Standard Precautions

Use Standard Precautions, or the equivalent, for the care of all patients. *Category IB*

A. Hand-washing
   (1) Wash hands after touching blood, body fluids, secretions, excretions, and contaminated items, whether or not gloves are worn. Wash hands immediately after gloves are removed, between patient contacts, and when otherwise indicated to avoid transfer of microorganisms to other patients or environments. It may be necessary to wash hands between tasks and procedures on the same patient to prevent cross-contamination of different body sites. *Category IB*
   (2) Use a plain (nonantimicrobial) soap for routine hand-washing. *Category IB*
   (3) Use an antimicrobial agent or a waterless antiseptic agent for specific circumstances (e.g, control of outbreaks or hyperendemic infections), as defined by the infection control program. *Category IB*

B. Gloves
   Wear gloves (clean, nonsterile gloves are adequate) when touching blood, body fluids, secretions, excretions, and contaminated items. Put on clean gloves just before touching mucous membranes and nonintact skin. Change gloves between tasks and procedures on the same patient after contact with material that may contain a high concentration of microorganisms. Remove gloves promptly after use, before touching noncontaminated items and environmental surfaces, and before going to another patient, and wash hands immediately to avoid transfer [of] microorganisms to other patients or environments. *Category IB*

C. Mask, Eye Protection, Face Shield
   Wear a mask and eye protection or a face shield to protect mucous membranes of the eyes, nose, and mouth during procedures and patient-care activities that are likely to generate splashes or sprays of blood, body fluids, secretions, and excretions. *Category IB*

D. Gown
   Wear a gown (a clean, nonsterile gown is adequate) to protect skin and to prevent soiling of clothing during procedures and patient-care activities that are likely to generate splashes or sprays of blood, body fluids, secretions, or excretions. Select a gown that is appropriate for the activity and amount of fluid likely to be encountered. Remove a soiled gown as promptly as possible, and wash hands to avoid transfer of microorganisms to other patients or environments. *Category IB*

E. Patient-Care Equipment
   Handle used patient-care equipment soiled with blood, body fluids, secretions, and excretions in a manner that prevents skin and mucous membrane exposures, contamination of clothing, and transfer of microorganisms to other patients and environments. Ensure that reusable equipment is not used for the care of another patient until it has been cleaned and processed appropriately. Ensure that single-use items are discarded properly. *Category IB*

F. Environmental Control
   Ensure that the hospital has adequate procedures for the routine care, cleaning, and disinfection of environmental surfaces, beds, bedrails, bedside equipment, and other frequently touched surfaces, and ensure that these procedures are being followed. *Category IB*

G. Linen
   Handle, transport, and process used linen soiled with blood, body fluids, secretions, and excretions in a manner that prevents skin and mucous membrane exposures and contamination of clothing, and that avoids transfer of microorganisms to other patients and environments. *Category IB*

H. Occupational Health and Bloodborne Pathogens
   (1) Take care to prevent injuries when using needles, scalpels, and other sharp instruments or devices; when handling sharp instruments after procedures; when cleaning used instruments; and when disposing of used needles. Never recap used needles, or otherwise manipulate them using both hands, or use any other technique that involves directing the point of a needle toward any part of the body; rather, use either a one-handed "scoop" technique or a mechanical device designed for holding the needle sheath. Do not remove used needles from disposable syringes by hand, and do not bend, break, or otherwise manipulate used needles by hand. Place used disposable syringes and needles, scalpel blades, and other sharp items in appropriate puncture-resistant containers, which are located as close as practical to the area in which the items were used, and place reusable syringes and needles in a puncture-resistant container for transport to the reprocessing area. *Category IB*
   (2) Use mouthpieces, resuscitation bags, or other ventilation devices as an alternative to mouth-to-mouth resuscitation methods in areas where the need for resuscitation is predictable. *Category IB*

I. Patient Placement
   Place a patient who contaminates the environment or who does not (or cannot be expected to) assist in maintaining appropriate hygiene or environmental control in a private room. If a private room is not available, consult with infection control professionals regarding patient placement or other alternatives. *Category IB*

From Garner JS, Hospital Infection Control Practices Advisory Committee. *Guideline for Isolation Precautions in Hospitals.* Public Health Service, US Dept. of Health and Human Services, Centers for Disease Control and Prevention, Atlanta, GA, 1996.

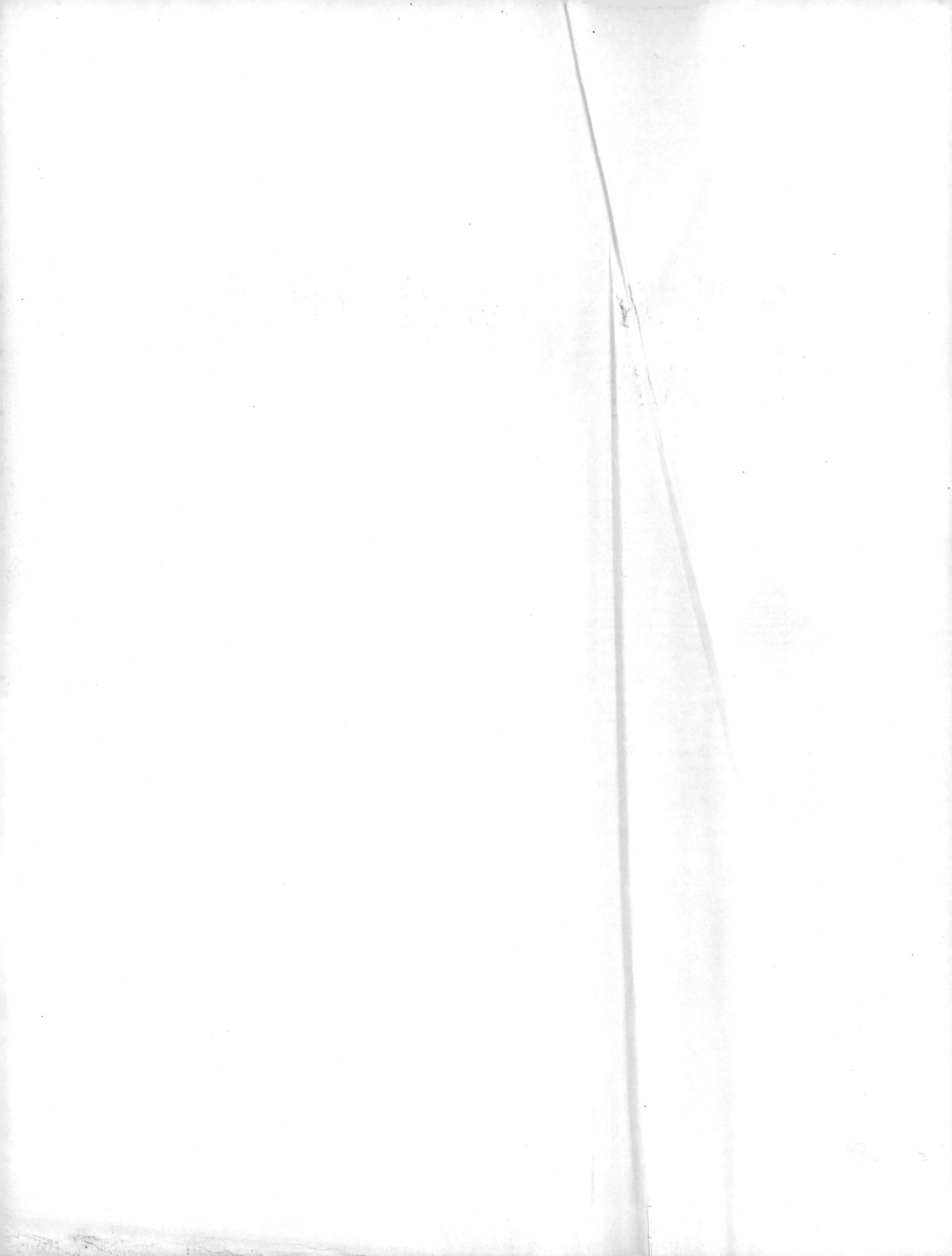

Medical-Surgical Nursing

Frances Donovan Monahan, Ph.D., R.N.

Professor and Director
Department of Nursing
Rockland Community College
State University of New York
Suffern, New York

Marianne Neighbors, Ed.D., R.N.

Professor
Eleanor Mann School of Nursing
College of Education
University of Arkansas
Fayetteville, Arkansas

Medical-Surgical Nursing

Foundations for Clinical Practice

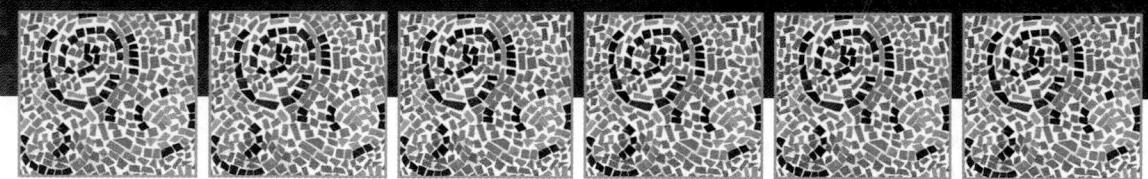

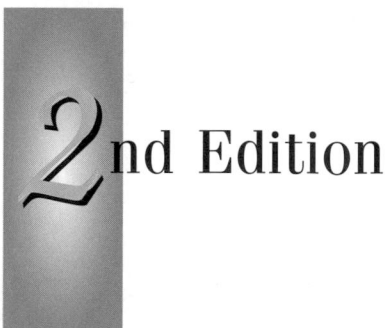

2nd Edition

W.B. SAUNDERS COMPANY
A Division of Harcourt Brace & Company
Philadelphia   London   Toronto   Montreal   Sydney   Tokyo

W.B. SAUNDERS COMPANY
A Division of Harcourt Brace & Company

The Curtis Center
Independence Square West
Philadelphia, Pennsylvania 19106

Library of Congress Cataloging-in-Publication Data

Monahan, Frances Donovan.
   Medical-surgical nursing/Frances Donovan Monahan, Marianne
Neighbors.—2nd ed.

      p.   cm.

   ISBN 0–7216–7006–7

   1. Nursing.   2. Surgical nursing.   I. Neighbors, Marianne.
II. Title.
   [DNLM: 1. Perioperative Nursing.   WY 162 M734m 1998]

RT41.M778   1998
610.73—dc21

DNLM/DLC   96-51069

NOTICE

Medical-Surgical Nursing is an ever-changing field. Standard safety precautions must be followed, but as new research and clinical experience broaden our knowledge, changes in treatment and drug therapy become necessary or appropriate. Readers are advised to check the product information currently provided by the manufacturer of each drug to be administered to verify the recommended dose, the method and duration of administration, and contraindications. It is the responsibility of the treating physician relying on experience and knowledge of the patient to determine dosages and the best treatment for the patient. Neither the Publisher nor the Editor assumes any responsibility for any injury and/or damage to persons or property.

THE PUBLISHER

MEDICAL-SURGICAL NURSING: FOUNDATIONS FOR CLINICAL PRACTICE   ISBN 0–7216–7006–7

Printed in the United States of America.

Last digit is the print number: 9   8   7   6   5   4   3   2   1

With all my love to my husband, William; to my son, Michael; to my daughter, Kerryane; and to the memory of my mother, Isabel Torpey Donovan.

—Fran

To my best friend and husband, Larry Butler. May you always be there for me as you were throughout this project.

—Marianne

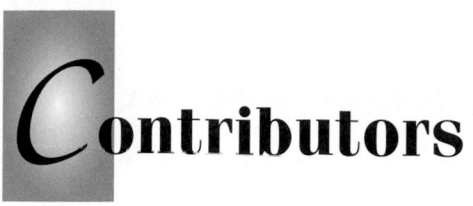ontributors

Fran Annand, BSN, MEd, RN, CAGS
Director of Nursing Education, Massachusetts Eye
   and Ear Infirmary, Boston, Massachusetts.
Knowledge Base for Patients with Eye Dysfunction

Francesca Armmer, PhD, RN
Assistant Professor, Chairperson, Department of
   Nursing, Bradley University, Peoria, Illinois.
Knowledge Base for Patients with Endocrine Dysfunction
*Nursing Care of Patients with Other Endocrine
Disorders*

Kathleen Barta, EdD, RN
Assistant Professor, Eleanor Mann School of
   Nursing, University of Arkansas, Fayetteville,
   Arkansas.
*Knowledge Base for Women with Reproductive
Dysfunction*
Nursing Care of Women with Reproductive Disorders
Research Abstracts

Ellen K. Boyda, MS, RN
Clinical Faculty–Graduate Program in Nursing,
   Widener University, Chester, Pennsylvania.
   Independent Pulmonary Clinical Nurse Specialist,
   Glen Mills, Pennsylvania.
*Knowledge Base for Patients with Fluid, Electrolyte, and
Acid-Base Imbalances*

Sally Brozenec, PhD
Assistant Professor, Rush University College of
   Nursing, Chicago, Illinois. Practitioner-Teacher,
   Rush Medical Center, Chicago, Illinois.
*Knowledge Base for Patients with Gastrointestinal
Dysfunction*
*Nursing Care of Patients with Disorders of the Upper
Gastrointestinal System*
*Nursing Care of Patients with Disorders of the Lower
Gastrointestinal System*
*Nursing Care of Patients with Disorders of the Accessory
Organs of Digestion*

Lori-Anne Cannata, BSN, RN
Staff Registered Nurse, The Laser and Skin Surgery
   Center of New York, New York, New York.
*Knowledge Base for Patients with Integumentary
Dysfunction*
Nursing Care of Patients with Integumentary Disorders

Ellen Clarke, MPH, RN, CIC
Infection Control Practitioner, Helen Hayes Hospital,
   West Haverstraw, New York.
*Nursing Care of Patients with Lower Respiratory
Disorders*

Zoela Clements, BSN, RNC, WHCNP
Women's Health Care Nurse Practitioner, Parkland
   Health and Hospital System, Dallas, Texas.
*Nursing Care of Patients with Sexually Transmitted
Diseases*

Barbara Cordell, PhD, RN
Associate Professor, Division of Nursing, Stephen F.
   Austin State University, Nacogdoches, Texas.
Knowledge Base for Patients with Immune Dysfunction
*Nursing Care of Patients with HIV/AIDS and Other
Immune Disorders*

Carol Covell, MS, RN
Vice President for Patient Services, Massachusetts
   Eye and Ear Infirmary, Boston, Massachusetts.
Knowledge Base for Patients with Eye Dysfunction

Patricia Cremins, MS, RNC
Assistant Professor, Division of Nursing, Laboure
   College, Boston, Massachusetts.
Knowledge Base for Patients with Hepatic Dysfunction
Nursing Care of Patients with Hepatic Disorders
Knowledge Base for Men with Reproductive Dysfunction
Nursing Care of Men with Reproductive Disorders

Dale A. Lange Crispell, MA, RN
Adjunct Professor, Rockland Community College,
   State University of New York, Suffern, New
   York.
*Nursing Care of Patients with Upper Respiratory
Disorders*

Audrey Reardon Delgrosso, MSN, RN, ET
Adjunct Professor of Nursing, Rockland Community
   College, State University of New York, Suffern,
   New York.
Nursing Care of Patients with Integumentary Disorders

Christine DeMarco, BSN, RN
Nurse Manager, Special Care and Respiratory Units,
   Helen Hayes Hospital, West Haverstraw, New
   York.

Nursing Care of Patients with Lower Respiratory Disorders

Patricia Dimick, BSN, RN
Nurse Manager, Burn Intensive Care, University of Washington Burn Center, Harborview Medical Center, Seattle, Washington.
Nursing Care of Patients with Burns

Sandra Eggenberger, MS, RN
Assistant Professor, School of Nursing, Mankato State University, Mankato, Minnesota.
Knowledge Base for Patients with Musculoskeletal Dysfunction
Nursing Care of Patients with Musculoskeletal Disorders

Sue-Ann Eitches, MA, RN
Associate Professor, Department of Nursing, Rockland Community College, State University of New York, Suffern, New York.
Clinical Thinking Features

Janice R. Ellis, PhD, RN
Professor and Director, Nursing Program, Shoreline Community College, Seattle, Washington.
Sociocultural Perspectives

Peggy Ellis, PhD, RN, CRNP
Assistant Professor, Acute Care Nurse Practitioner Program, School of Nursing, University of Alabama at Birmingham, Birmingham, Alabama.
Knowledge Base for Patients with Hematologic Dysfunction
Nursing Care of Patients with Hematologic Disorders

Karin Freas Gapper, MSN, RN
Assistant Professor, Queensborough Community College, Department of Nursing, Bayside, New York.
Nursing Care of Patients with Lower Respiratory Disorders

Rose Mary Gee, MSN, RN, CNS
Department of Nursing, Georgia Southern University, Statesboro, Georgia.
Research Abstracts

Pauline Laura Guay, MSN, RN
Associate Chairperson, Level I, Division of Nursing, Laboure College, Boston, Massachusetts.
Knowledge Base for Men with Reproductive Dysfunction
Nursing Care of Men with Reproductive Disorders

Kathleen Ann Hanrahan, BSN, RN
Staff Nurse–CORLN, Otolaryngology–Head and Neck Surgery Clinic, University of Iowa Hospitals and Clinics, Iowa City, Iowa.
Knowledge Base for Patients with Ear Dysfunction
Nursing Care of Patients with Ear Disorders

Barbara Fomenko Harrah, MSN, RN
Assistant Professor, Department of Nursing, Kent State University, East Liverpool Campus, East Liverpool, Ohio.
Knowledge Base for Patients with Cardiac Dysfunction
Nursing Care of Patients with Cardiac Disorders

Julie Hebenstreit, BSN, MA
Assistant Professor, School of Nursing, Mankato State University, Mankato, Minnesota.
Knowledge Base for Patients with Musculoskeletal Dysfunction
Nursing Care of Patients with Musculoskeletal Disorders

Melinda Henderson, EdD, RN
Assistant Professor, Department of Nursing, University of Central Oklahoma, Edmond, Oklahoma.
Knowledge Base for Patients with Urinary Dysfunction
Nursing Care of Patients with Urinary Disorders

Janet Jackson, MS, RN
Assistant Professor, Department of Nursing, Bradley University, Peoria, Illinois.
Knowledge Base for Patients with Neurologic Dysfunction
Nursing Care of Patients with Neurologic Disorders

Joyce Kee, MS, RN
Associate Professor Emeritus, College of Nursing, University of Delaware, Newark, Delaware.
Knowledge Base for Patients with Fluid, Electrolyte, and Acid-Base Imbalances

Nohra M. Leff, MSN, MPH, RN
Instructor, Department of Nursing, Rockland Community College, State University of New York, Suffern, New York. Clinical Instructor, Division of Nursing, New York University, New York, New York. Assistant Director of Nursing Staff Development, Beth Abraham Hospital, Bronx, New York.
Knowledge Base for Women with Reproductive Dysfunction
Nursing Care of Women with Reproductive Disorders

Dorothea Lever, MS, RN, CCRN
Instructor, Department of Nursing, Rockland Community College, State University of New York, Suffern, New York.
Nursing Care of Patients with Cardiac Disorders

Gay Lindsay, BSN, MSN
Emeritus Professor of Nursing and Assistant to the Vice Provost, Kent State University, Kent, Ohio.
Introduction to the Practice of Medical-Surgical Nursing

Jeanne Linhart, MSN, FNP
Assistant Professor, Department of Nursing, BLS Instructor, Rockland Community College, State University of New York, Suffern, New York.
Nursing Care of Patients with Cardiac Disorders
Knowledge Base for Women with Reproductive Dysfunction

Maryann Corrigan Magaldi, MSN, RN
Assistant Professor, Queensborough Community College School of Nursing, Bayside, New York.
Nursing Care of Patients with Lower Respiratory Disorders

Carol McAndrews, MA, RN
Clinical Instructor, Department of Nursing, North Harris County College, Houston, Texas. Staff-Resource Nurse, Northeast Medical Center Hospital, Humble, Texas.
Nursing Care of Patients with Upper Respiratory Disorders

Maureen McCracken, MA, RN, CCRN
Staff Nurse, Montefiore Medical Center, Bronx, New York.
Nursing Care of Patients with Cardiac Disorders

Phyllis McGrath, MS, RN
Vascular Clinical Nurse Specialist/Amputee Specialist, Veterans Administration Health Care System, Palo Alto, California.
Knowledge Base for Patients with Vascular Dysfunction
Nursing Care of Patients with Vascular Disorders

Carol Miller, MSN, RNC
Clinical Instructor, Frances Payne Bolton School of Nursing, Case Western Reserve University, Cleveland, Ohio. Clinical Specialist, Care and Counseling, Cleveland, Ohio.
Special Considerations for Nursing Care of Elderly Patients

Carolyn Milligan, BSN, RNC, WHCNP
Women's Health Care Nurse Practitioner, Parkland Health and Hospital System, Dallas, Texas.
Nursing Care of Patients with Sexually Transmitted Diseases

Josephine A. O'Callahan, MS, RN
Assistant Professor, Division of Nursing, Laboure College, Boston, Massachusetts.
Knowledge Base for Patients with Hepatic Dysfunction
Nursing Care of Patients with Hepatic Disorders

Lori O'Donnell, MSN, RN
Instructor, Department of Nursing, Saint Joseph's College, Standish, Maine. Staff Nurse, Cardiology Nursing Service, Maine Medical Center, Portland, Maine.
Knowledge Base for Patients with Cardiac Dysfunction
Nursing Care of Patients with Cardiac Disorders

Donna Peters, MA, RN
Instructor, Department of Nursing, Rockland Community College, State University of New York, Suffern, New York.
Nursing Care of Patients with Cardiac Disorders

Nancy Burns Reilly, MSN, RN, AOCN
Oncology Clinical Nurse Specialist, Thomas Jefferson University Hospital, Philadelphia, Pennsylvania.
Nursing Care of Patients with Breast Disorders

Ruth Rocheska, MSN, MA, RN
Assistant Professor, Department of Nursing,

Rockland Community College, State University of New York, Suffern, New York. Doctoral Candidate, Department of Nurse Education, Teachers College, Columbia University, New York, New York.
Knowledge Base for Patients with Cardiac Dysfunction
Nursing Care of Patients with Cardiac Disorders

Alison M. Rushing, MSN, RN, CCRN
Department of Nursing, Georgia Southern University, Statesboro, Georgia.
Research Abstracts

Angela Sammarco, PhD(C), RN
Instructor, Advanced Medical Surgical Nursing, St. Vincent's Medical Center of Richmond, School of Nursing, Staten Island, New York. Doctoral Candidate, Department of Nursing, Adelphi University, Garden City, New York.
Nursing Care of Patients with Breast Disorders

Theresa Schwarz, MPA, RN
Director of Nursing, Helen Hayes Hospital, West Haverstraw, New York.
Nursing Care of Patients with Lower Respiratory Disorders

Saundra L. Seidel, MNSc, APN CNOR, CNS, RN
Clinical Nurse Specialist, Perioperative, Veterans Administration Medical Center, Fayetteville, Arkansas.
Knowledge Base for Patients Undergoing Surgery

Catherine V. Smith, BSN, RN, CCRN
Nursing Education Associate, Cardiac Surgery, Robert Wood Johnson University Hospital, New Brunswick, New Jersey.
Nursing Care of Patients with Cardiac Disorders

Nan Smith-Blair, MSN, RN
Instructor, University of Arkansas, Mann School of Nursing, Fayetteville, Arkansas.
Knowledge Base for Patients in Shock

Joan Stackhouse, MSN, RN
Associate Professor, Retired, Department of Nursing, Rockland Community College, State University of New York, Suffern, New York.
Death, Dying, and Bereavement

Marilyn Stapleton, MS, RNC
Nurse Educator, Regents College, Albany, New York. Staff Nurse, Albany Medical Center Hospital, Albany, New York.
Knowledge Base for Patients with Respiratory Dysfunction

Marshelle Thobaben, MS, RNC, FNP, PHN
Professor, Department of Nursing, Humboldt State University, Arcata, California.
Medical-Surgical Nursing in Multiple Settings

Donna J. Gryetz Thomas, MSN, RN
Assistant Professor, Department of Nursing, Kent State University, East Liverpool Campus, East Liverpool, Ohio.
Knowledge Base for Patients with Cardiac Dysfunction
Nursing Care of Patients with Cardiac Disorders

Monica Toll, MSN, RNC
Assistant Professor of Nursing, Dominican College, Orangeburg, New York.
Nursing Care of Patients with Diabetes Mellitus

Barbara Ullman, BSN, RN, CRNO
Allied Health Professional Staff Member, Northern Dutchess Hospital, Rhinebeck, New York, and Columbia Memorial Hospital, Hudson, New York.
Knowledge Base for Patients with Eye Dysfunction
Nursing Care of Patients with Eye Disorders

Fran Walker, MSN, RN, AOCN
Nursing Care Coordinator, Bone Marrow Transplant Unit and Medical/Respiratory Intensive Care Unit, Thomas Jefferson University Hospital, Philadelphia, Pennsylvania.
Nursing Care of Patients with Oncologic Disorders

Pamela Becker Weilitz, MSN(R), RN, CS, ANP
Assistant Clinical Professor, Saint Louis University School of Nursing, St. Louis, Missouri. Director, Nursing Practice, BJC Health System, Barnes-Jewish Hospital, St. Louis, Missouri.
Nursing Care of Patients with Lower Respiratory Disorders

Judy Ellis White, MSN, RNC
Adjunct Faculty, Department of Nursing, Samford University, Birmingham, Alabama.
Nursing Care of Patients with Cardiac Disorders

Michelle Woodbeck, MSN, RN
Assistant Professor, Nursing, Hudson Valley Community College, Troy, New York.
Knowledge Base for Patients with Cardiac Dysfunction
Nursing Care of Patients with Cardiac Disorders

Elizabeth Wyskpisz, MS, RN
Cardiothoracic Nursing Director, Robert Wood Johnson University, New Brunswick, New Jersey.
Knowledge Base for Patients with Cardiac Dysfunction
Nursing Care of Patients with Cardiac Disorders

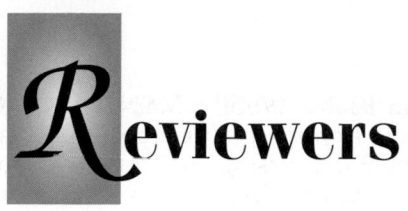

Reviewers

Sarah E. Angermuller, MSN, MEd, RN
Columbus State University
Columbus, Georgia

Susan Archbold, BSN, RN, CCRN
Mission Hospital Regional Medical Center
Mission Viejo, California

Donna Babao, MA, MSN, RN, PHN
Yuba College
Marysville, California

Marlene Beauregard, RN
Edmonton General Hospital
Edmonton, Alberta

Catherine F. Bennett, MSN, RNC
Lansing Community College
Lansing, Michigan

Elisa Bianchi-Smak, MS, RN
Charles E. Gregory School of Nursing
Perth Amboy, New Jersey

Wendy Blackburn, BScN, MAEd, RN, CNN
Parkwood Hospital
London, Ontario
St. Michael's Hospital
Toronto, Ontario

Betty Nash Blevins, MSN, RN, CS, CCRN
Bluefield State College
Bluefield, West Virginia

E. Ann Bokelman, MS, RN
Southside Regional Medical Center School of
    Nursing
Petersburg, Virginia

Cecilia Casey Boyer, MS, RN, CDE
The Ohio State University Medical Center
Columbus, Ohio

Clara W. Boyle, EdD, RN
Salem State College
Salem, Massachusetts

Lynne E. Bryant, MSN, RN, CCRN
Broward Community College
Davie, Florida

Carolyn Carlson, PhD, RN
Cedarville College
Cedarville, Ohio

Susan M. Chappell, MSN, RN, CDE
School of Nursing
University of Texas at Arlington
Arlington, Texas

Susan Coles, MSN, RN, OCN
Saint Thomas Hospital
Nashville, Tennessee

Claire B. Corbin, MS, RN
Carolinas College of Health Sciences
Charlotte, North Carolina

Vonna Roles Cranston, MS, RN
University of South Dakota
Vermillion, South Dakota

Maria Piccolo Cvach, MS, RN, CCRN, ACLS
Johns Hopkins Hospital
Baltimore, Maryland

Marla De Jong, MS, RN, Capt., CEN
United States Air Force Wilford Hall Medical Center
San Antonio, Texas

Charlie Jones Dickson, EdD, RN, FAAN
University of Alabama at Birmingham
Birmingham, Alabama

Julie Doyon, MScN, RN
University of Ottawa
Regional Geriatric Assessment Program
Ottawa, Ontario

Barbara Draude, MSN, RN
Middle Tennessee State University
Murfreesboro, Tennessee

Penny Dyess, MN, RN
Baton Rouge General Medical Center
Baton Rouge, Louisiana

Diane Ford, MS, RN, CCRN
Andrews University
Berrien Springs, Michigan

Cynthia Garrett, MSN, RNC
University of North Carolina Hospitals
Chapel Hill, North Carolina

Susan V. Gille, PhD, RN, CS
Missouri Western State College
St. Joseph, Missouri

Judy Goodhart, MSN, RN
Mesa State College
Grand Junction, Colorado

Renee Gould, MS, RN
University of Iowa Hospitals and Clinics
Iowa City, Iowa

Joan S. Grant, DSN, RN, CS
University of Alabama at Birmingham
Birmingham, Alabama

Connie L. Green, MSN, RN, CFNP, CCRN, CEN
Medical-Surgical Group
Beckley, West Virginia

Janis Richard Guilbeau, MSN, RN
University of Southwestern Louisiana
Lafayette, Louisiana

Karen Hammond, BSN, RN, CCRN
Washington College Hospital
Hagerstown, Maryland

Jean Heslin, MS, RN
Southside Regional Medical Center School of
    Nursing
Petersburg, Virginia

Wendy Hillman, MSN, RN
Kirtland Community College
Roscommon, Michigan

Betty Sue Hrouda, PhD, RN
Southside Regional Medical Center School of
    Nursing
Petersburg, Virginia

C. DaCosta Hunte, MSN, EdD, RN
Fayetteville State University
Fayetteville, North Carolina

Sandra Jesionek, MSN, RN, CARN, CCJS
Value Behavioral Health
Falls Church, Virginia

Anne G. Jones, MSN, RN
Mayo Foundation
Rochester, Minnesota

Janet B. Kasno, MSN, RNC
University of Detroit Mercy
Detroit, Michigan

Reita Keyes, PhD, RN
Mississippi College School of Nursing
Clinton, Mississippi

Helen Kissane, MA, RN
Rockland Community College
State University of New York
Suffern, New York

Jo Ann Kleier, MSN, EdDc, CURN, ARNP
Broward Community College
Ft. Lauderdale, Florida

Nancy Korchek, MSN, RN
Manatee Community College
Bradenton, Florida

Helene Krouse, PhD, RNC, ARNP
University of North Florida
Jacksonville, Florida

Janice Garrison Lanham, MSN, RN
Tri-County Technical College
Pendleton, South Carolina

Denise LeBlanc, BScN, RN
Humber College
Etobicoke, Ontario

Aggie Llewelyn, MS, RN, CS, CETN
Veterans Affairs Medical Center
Martinsburg, West Virginia

Pamela McKintuck, BA, RN
Humber College of Applied Technology
Etobicoke, Ontario

Mary E. Mancini, MSN, RN, CNA, FAAN
Parkland Memorial Hospital
Dallas, Texas

Linda Merse Markey, MSN, RN, CCRN
Baton Rouge General Medical Center School of
    Nursing
Baton Rouge, Louisiana

Sharon Melberg, MPA, RN
University of California Davis Medical Center
Sacramento, California

Rita Mertig, MS, RN, CCE
John Tyler Community College
Chester, Virginia

Dana Moore, MS, RN, CCRN
Johns Hopkins Hospital
Baltimore, Maryland

Sera Nicosia, BScN, MAEd, RN, MNI, CNN
McMaster University
Hamilton, Ontario

Nancy O'Quinn, MSN, MEd, RNC
Albany State College
Albany, Georgia

Patti O'Rourke, MA, RNC, CCRN
Craven Regional Medical Center
New Bern, North Carolina

AnneMarie Palatnik, MSN, RN, CS
Our Lady of Lourdes Medical Center
Camden, New Jersey

Kathleen M. Parsons, MS, RN, CS, CCRN
Physicians Memorial Hospital
La Plata, Maryland

Jane Pelosi-Kelly, MSN, RN, CS, ANP
Rush North Shore Medical Center
Skokie, Illinois

Phyllis Peterson, MN, RN, CNS
Our Lady of Holy Cross College
New Orleans, Louisiana

Jeanette Pletcher, MS, RN, CCRN
Alta Bates Medical Center
Berkley, California

Linda Reed, MSN, PhD, RN
University of Alabama at Birmingham
Birmingham, Alabama

Barbara Ryan, RN, CNS, APS
Ottawa Civic Hospital
University of Ottawa
Ottawa, Ontario

Angela Sammarco, MSN, RN
School of Nursing
St. Vincent's Medical Center of Richmond
Staten Island, New York

Mary Sampel, MSN, RN
Saint Louis University
Saint Louis, Missouri

Lorna Schumann, PhD, RN, CS, NPC, ARNP, CCRN
Intercollegiate Center for Nursing Education
Spokane, Washington

Almetta M. Shannon, MS, RNC
Modesto Junior College
Modesto, California

Lisa Anderson Shaw, MSN, MA, RNC
University of Illinois at Chicago
Chicago, Illinois

Sharon P. Shipton, MSN, PhD, RN
Youngstown University
Youngstown, Ohio

Mary Margaret Spica, MS, RN, CSE
Christ Hospital
Cincinnati, Ohio

Carol A. Stephenson, EdD, RNC
Harris College of Nursing
Texas Christian University
Fort Worth, Texas

Nancy Stotts, EdD, RN
University of California San Francisco
San Francisco, California

Katherine Sullivan, MA, RN
Rockland Community College
State University of New York
Suffern, New York

Kay Swiger, MN, RNC
York Technical College
Rock Hill, South Carolina

Maureen Tess, MS, RN, CCRN
Rush Presbyterian Hospital
St. Luke's Medical Center
Chicago, Illinois

Nancy Thornton, MSN, RN
British Columbia's Children's Hospital
Vancouver, British Columbia

Carroll Thorowsky, BScN, MSA, RN
Rehabilitation Hospital
Edmonton, Alberta

Tina Tiburzi, BSN, MBA, RN
Johns Hopkins Hospital
Baltimore, Maryland

Kuei-Shen Tu, MSN, RN
School of Nursing
University of Alabama at Birmingham
Birmingham, Alabama

Andrea Walton, MSN, RNC
Medical Center of Delaware
Wilmington, Delaware

Pamela Becker Weilitz, MSN, RN, CS
Barnes-Jewish Hospital
Saint Louis, Missouri

Ann White, MSN, MBA, RN, CNA
University of Southern Indiana
Evansville, Indiana

Patricia Sagan Wilkins, MSN, RN
University of Southern Mississippi
Long Beach, Mississippi

Emily Zabrocki, MSN, PhD, RN
Joliet Junior College
Joliet, Illinois

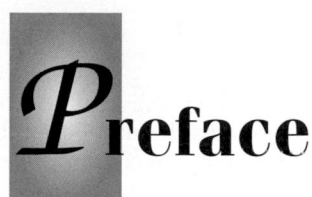

Preface

When we began to plan the second edition of *Nursing Care of Adults,* our goal was to produce a thoroughly new book that nevertheless retained the core strengths of the first edition:

- Clarity, readability, and logical organization
- A straightforward, no-nonsense, nursing process approach
- An abundance of practical pedagogical aids

The result of that planning is now before you: *Medical-Surgical Nursing: Foundations for Clinical Practice,* the second edition of *Nursing Care of Adults.*

We believe that *Medical-Surgical Nursing: Foundations for Clinical Practice,* like its predecessor, will facilitate learning by being clearly written, logical in sequence, and consistent in format and presentation, and by following a straightforward, familiar organizing framework. As in the first edition, we have employed a body systems approach, using the same headings and content sequence throughout the chapters, and consistently dividing units into Knowledge Base and Nursing Care chapters. This division of units clearly differentiates information that pertains to *all* patients with a problem in a particular body system from information that pertains to care of patients with a *specific* disorder in that system. Yet it leaves chapters sufficiently free-standing that they may be assigned in the order that best suits the curriculum of each particular nursing program.

The Knowledge Base chapters begin by succinctly reviewing the anatomy and physiology of the system. They then discuss the clinical manifestations common to different types of dysfunction in the system. Next, they cover assessment (patient history and physical examination) of the body system, diagnostic procedures, and medical and surgical interventions that are applicable to disorders of that system.

The Nursing Care chapters cover specific diseases, with a focus on their etiology and pathophysiology, clinical manifestations, diagnosis, and management. Cross references to the Knowledge Base chapters are provided as needed.

Because *Medical-Surgical Nursing: Foundations for Clinical Practice* is first and foremost a *nursing* text, both Knowledge Base and Nursing Care chapters focus on the contributions of *nursing* to patient care. We accomplish this goal by highlighting nursing care under the consistent headings "Nursing Process" (when the discussion warrants a full presentation of the nursing process) and "Nursing Process Guidelines" (when the discussion calls for only a brief presentation of nursing care) and by employing NANDA-approved nursing diagnoses throughout.

Yet any text that aims to help equip students for practice in the next millennium must recognize the collaborative nature of healthcare in today's world. It must also recognize that medical-surgical nursing care today is as likely to take place in the home or in a freestanding surgicenter as it is in a hospital. In special sections entitled "Settings, Providers, and Collaboration for Care," this text therefore underscores both the importance of collaboration in patient care and today's variety of care settings. Moreover, the text was rewritten from beginning to end with the aim of conveying the reality that care may take place in a variety of settings.

To further underscore today's changing patterns in healthcare delivery, this edition now includes a chapter entitled "Medical-Surgical Nursing in Multiple Settings" (Chapter 2). Throughout, the book also reflects the latest AHCPR clinical guidelines, includes early discharge and home care interventions, and provides tools for obtaining late-breaking information through the Internet. These tools are our new Internet Connections features and an extensive Resources listing (Appendix 3) at the end of the book.

Medical-Surgical Nursing: Foundations for Clinical Practice also fosters the development of the critical thinking skills that underlie safe, effective nursing practice. It does so through several means. First, it consistently presents nursing care divided into the five steps of the nursing process, with each nursing diagnosis clearly paired with related expected outcomes and nursing interventions. Second, it includes Nursing Care Guides—nursing care plans that demonstrate the relationship of assessment data, nursing diagnoses, outcomes, and interventions, with rationales. Third, it includes 13 Clinical Pathways, developed expressly for this book, to demonstrate the collaboration among the various healthcare disciplines and professionals. It also includes 22 Clinical Thinking features. These features are based on the concepts outlined in Dorothy del Bueno's clinical problems video series, which are used in the evaluation of new graduates, and Patricia Benner's *From Novice to Expert.* Written from the standpoint of an expert practitioner, these features bring to light the thinking processes underlying one nurse's clinical judgments and actions when confronted with clinical situations in which immediate, accurate nursing intervention made a critical difference. To help students take into account the impact of current sociocultural trends, we also commissioned Janice R. Ellis, PhD, RN, to write six Sociocultural Perspectives essays on such topics as the impact of the cost of healthcare on the elderly, how to overcome language barriers, and the impact of changes in family structure on healthcare. Also new to this edition are 25 Research Abstracts, which introduce readers to nursing research and how to incorporate its findings into practice. As a final tool to promote the development of critical thinking skills, each chapter concludes with a series of Chapter Review questions. These are not merely knowledge questions that evaluate reading comprehension point-by-point. Rather, they are challenging questions that prompt readers to dig back into the chapter to synthesize what they have read and apply it to practice.

Medical-Surgical Nursing: Foundations for Clinical Practice also focuses on health promotion and risk reduction for the adult health-care consumer. This focus is achieved primarily by means of the new Health Promotion & Risk Reduction Highlights that we have added to this edition. These 40 Highlights present information and strategies for students to use in planning patient education sessions and are found in the Patient History or Physical Examination section of each Knowledge Base chapter. They are also found in Nursing Care chapters when risk reduction strategies are applicable to the prevention of a specific disease.

The text continues to highlight the patient's role in self-care, and the patient's active role in making decisions about health management and treatment regimens. This is accomplished primarily through the expanded use of Patient Education Highlights (124 in this edition) and through the addition of the Health Promotion & Risk Reduction Highlights described above. Together, these informative Highlights equip students with a wide range of teaching strategies and resources to assist patients and families who are dealing with diseases and other health-care issues.

Also new to this edition is the use of full color throughout. For this edition we carefully reviewed all of the illustrations from the first edition. We compared them against the text to ensure that text and illustrations worked hand-in-hand to teach essential content. Where necessary, we revised and added color to illustrations. But we also commissioned hundreds of new illustrations and photographs, as well as photographs with overlays, a type of illustration not used so extensively in any other medical-surgical nursing text. We believe that the richness and visual clarity of these new and revised illustrations will help learners—especially those with a visual learning style—to attain a solid grasp of essential content.

Clear writing, logical organization, illustrations that unravel complex concepts, and sensitivity to current trends in health-care delivery—all are important in a medical-surgical nursing text, and all are reflected in this new edition. Yet what separates a good text from an outstanding one is its clinical content, and *Medical-Surgical Nursing: Foundations for Clinical Practice* has been updated and refocused throughout to provide the current, comprehensive clinical content that students need in today's world. In this edition we have therefore expanded, deepened, and updated our coverage of pain and pain management, cardiovascular disorders (including women's cardiovascular health), neurologic disorders, HIV/AIDS, and pressure ulcers. We have included an entirely new chapter on shock (Chapter 11). We have also included late-breaking information on such subjects as asthma management, thoracoscopic surgery, Heimlich valves, minimally invasive cardiac surgery, and necrotizing fasciitis ("flesh-eating disease").

Of course, no text stands alone. *Medical-Surgical Nursing: Foundations for Clinical Practice* therefore features a comprehensive ancillary package:

For the Student

- *Student Study Guide*
- *Pocket Companion*

For the Instructor

- *Instructor's Manual*
- *Transparencies*
- *Test Manual*
- *ExaMaster* computer test bank

In addition to these ancillaries, *Medical-Surgical Nursing: Foundations for Clinical Practice* is the first medical-surgical nursing text to feature a companion **home health manual.** Authored by Marianne Neighbors and Frances Donovan Monahan, and entitled *A Practical Guide to Medical-Surgical Nursing in the Home,* this pocket-sized book provides on-the-spot information that is essential to the practice of medical-surgical nursing in the home. It presents information on reimbursement, reportable diseases, home assessment, and documentation as well as common disorders, common therapeutic interventions, assessments and patient teaching guides for approximately 100 of the drugs most commonly prescribed for patients receiving care at home, and special diets in a format that is simple and easily accessible in the home-care setting. For more information about the home health manual or any other companion publications, please contact your W.B. Saunders Company sales representative or call W.B. Saunders Company Sales Support at 215-238-8406.

We wish you every success as you use *Medi-cal-Surgical Nursing: Foundations for Clinical Practice*, 2nd Edition. We are confident that it represents an ideal blend of clinical currency and comprehensiveness with the ease of use that is so important in nursing education today.

Frances Donovan Monahan
Marianne Neighbors

Acknowledgments

The support and encouragement of colleagues, of the students at Rockland Community College, and of family and friends have been invaluable during the preparation of *Medical-Surgical Nursing: Foundations for Clinical Practice*, 2nd Edition. I thank them all. Special thanks to Cynthia and John Donovan, my brother and sister-in-law, for their unqualified faith and love; to Mary Ellen Wyllie, MS, RN, my best friend, who is always there and willing to help; and to Liz Lonergan, Dawn Carolina, and Sophy Zayas, my office staff, who make days at work so pleasant that I have the energy to write in the evenings and on weekends. Special thanks also to Ramona Connelley, Health Science Librarian at York Hospital, York, Maine, for making the excellent resources at the York Hospital library available to me and for enthusiastically and willingly searching for needed information.

—*Frances Donovan Monahan*

I could not have persevered through this task if it were not for the loving support I received from my parents, Louis and Lillian Zadra; from my sister, Marji Schwickrath, who sent me daily e-mail notes of encouragement; and from my very special friends. I am so blessed to have such wonderful individuals in my life.

—*Marianne Neighbors*

Special thanks are also due to the many people at W.B. Saunders Company whose work has made this edition possible:

- Barbara Nelson Cullen, formerly Senior Editor, whose creativity, organization, and goal-directedness are inspiring and whose friendship is a treasure
- Lee Henderson, Senior Developmental Editor and quintessential gentleman, for his expert guidance and his unique attention to detail while maintaining a vision for the whole, and for his patience and understanding
- Catherine E. Harold, Developmental Editor, for her excellent queries and for providing the support that we needed to ensure that the book achieved a high level of quality
- Susan Hess Blaker, whose marvelous gift for art development and graphic design and whose commitment to finding and developing the perfect illustrations have resulted in a book of singular visual appeal and usefulness for teaching and learning
- Annette Ferran, Copy Editor, whose attention to detail and sensitivity to the special needs of textbook editing helped to ensure the accuracy, consistency, and readability of the second edition
- Linda R. Garber, Senior Production Manager, whose expertise in project management kept this edition on track from the beginning of production to the day of publication
- Ellen Zanolle, Senior Book Designer, whose talents are reflected in the cover of this edition and whose ability to overcome technical and design challenges were matched only by her amiability
- Peg Shaw, Senior Illustration Specialist, who carefully sized and managed the production of the book's illustrations
- Rachel Hubbs, Assistant Developmental Editor, and Marie Pelcin, then Editorial Assistant, who coordinated the peer reviews for the entire book and ably fielded countless editorial and administrative details
- Jean Rodenberger, Marketing Manager, whose creativity and marketing savvy ensured that this book got into the hands of the instructors and students for whom we created it.

Special thanks to Timothy J. Mullican, DVM, and the illustrators at Observatory Group, Inc: Emiko Koike, Jenny Robinson, Lisa Klancher, Quade Paul, Susan Young, Troy Hitch, and Scott Schneider. Their talent, mastery of digital illustration, hard work, patience, and commitment to this project have made a tremendous contribution toward our goal of developing a book that sets a new standard for clarity and visual presentation of complex information.

Contents in Brief

Unit I

Knowledge Base for Medical-Surgical Nursing   1

1
Introduction to the Practice of Medical-Surgical Nursing   3

2
Medical-Surgical Nursing in Multiple Settings   17

3
Death, Dying, and Bereavement   31

4
Special Considerations for Nursing Care of Elderly Patients   49

5
Knowledge Base for Patients with Fluid, Electrolyte, and Acid-Base Imbalances   75

6
Knowledge Base for Patients Undergoing Surgery   115

Unit II

Cardiovascular Dysfunction   161

7
Knowledge Base for Patients with Cardiac Dysfunction   163

8
Nursing Care of Patients with Cardiac Disorders   233

9
Knowledge Base for Patients with Vascular Dysfunction   323

10
Nursing Care of Patients with Vascular Disorders   351

11
Knowledge Base for Patients in Shock   401

Unit III

Hematologic Dysfunction   425

12
Knowledge Base for Patients with Hematologic Dysfunction   427

13
Nursing Care of Patients with Hematologic Disorders   467

Unit IV

Respiratory Dysfunction   521

14
Knowledge Base for Patients with Respiratory Dysfunction   523

15
Nursing Care of Patients with Upper
Respiratory Disorders   599

16
Nursing Care of Patients with Lower
Respiratory Disorders   639

Unit V

Neurologic Dysfunction   709

17
Knowledge Base for Patients with Neurologic
Dysfunction   711

18
Nursing Care of Patients with Neurologic
Disorders   767

Unit VI

Musculoskeletal Dysfunction   835

19
Knowledge Base for Patients with
Musculoskeletal Dysfunction   837

20
Nursing Care of Patients with Musculoskeletal
Disorders   887

Unit VII

Gastrointestinal Dysfunction   947

21
Knowledge Base for Patients with
Gastrointestinal Dysfunction   949

22
Nursing Care of Patients with Disorders of
the Upper Gastrointestinal System   1017

23
Nursing Care of Patients with Disorders of
the Lower Gastrointestinal System   1061

24
Nursing Care of Patients with Disorders of
the Accessory Organs of Digestion   1109

Unit VIII

Hepatic Dysfunction   1133

25
Knowledge Base for Patients with Hepatic
Dysfunction   1135

26
Nursing Care of Patients with Hepatic
Disorders   1169

Unit IX

Endocrine Dysfunction   1201

27
Knowledge Base for Patients with Endocrine
Dysfunction   1203

28
Nursing Care of Patients with Diabetes
Mellitus   1223

29
Nursing Care of Patients with Other
Endocrine Disorders   1265

Unit X

Urinary Dysfunction   1327

30
Knowledge Base for Patients with Urinary
Dysfunction   1329

31
Nursing Care of Patients with Urinary
Disorders   1371

Unit XI

Immune Dysfunction   1427

32
Knowledge Base for Patients with Immune Dysfunction   1429

33
Nursing Care of Patients with HIV/AIDS and Other Immune Disorders   1457

34
Nursing Care of Patients with Oncologic Disorders   1503

Unit XII

Integumentary Dysfunction   1565

35
Knowledge Base for Patients with Integumentary Dysfunction   1567

36
Nursing Care of Patients with Integumentary Disorders   1595

37
Nursing Care of Patients with Burns   1643

Unit XIII

Reproductive Dysfunction   1693

38
Knowledge Base for Men with Reproductive Dysfunction   1695

39
Nursing Care of Men with Reproductive Disorders   1727

40
Knowledge Base for Women with Reproductive Dysfunction   1765

41
Nursing Care of Women with Reproductive Disorders   1803

42
Nursing Care of Patients with Breast Disorders   1841

43
Nursing Care of Patients with Sexually Transmitted Diseases   1883

Unit XIV

Eye and Ear Dysfunction   1933

44
Knowledge Base for Patients with Eye Dysfunction   1935

45
Nursing Care of Patients with Eye Disorders   1963

46
Knowledge Base for Patients with Ear Dysfunction   1995

47
Nursing Care of Patients with Ear Disorders   2011

Appendix 1
Reference Values for Laboratory Tests   2023

Appendix 2
Common Abbreviations   2033

Appendix 3
Resources   2037

Index   2047

Contents in Detail

Unit I

Knowledge Base for Medical-Surgical Nursing   1

1

Introduction to the Practice of Medical-Surgical Nursing   3

Scope of Medical-Surgical Nursing Practice   3
Nature of Medical-Surgical Nursing Practice   3
Preparation for Medical-Surgical Nursing
    Practice   3
Certification   5
Trends in Medical-Surgical Nursing Practice   6
    Health-Care Reform   6
    Societal Changes   6
Standards of Practice   6
Clinical Practice Guidelines   7
The Nursing Process   8
    Assessment   8
    Nursing Diagnosis   8
    Planning   9
    Implementation   11
    Evaluation   11
Clinical Pathways   12
Culturally Competent Care   12
National Health Promotion and Disease Prevention
    Objectives   14

2

Medical-Surgical Nursing in Multiple Settings   17

The Shift to Nonhospital Settings   17
    Spiraling Health-Care Costs   18
    Demographic Changes   18
        Poverty   18
        Aging   18
        Domestic Violence   19

Homelessness   19
Human Immunodeficiency Virus Infection
    and Acquired Immunodeficiency
    Syndrome   19
Medicare Reimbursement and DRGs   20
The Advent of Managed Health Care   20
    Managed Care Organizations   20
    Health Maintenance Organizations   20
    Preferred Provider Organizations   20
    Case Management   21
Nonhospital Practice Settings   21
    Ambulatory Health-Care Settings   21
    Nurse-Managed Centers   22
    Outpatient and Ambulatory Surgical
        Facilities   22
    Adult Day Health Centers   22
    Home-Based Care   22
    Hospice Care Settings   23
    Community-Based, Long-Term-Care
        Services   23
    Rehabilitation in Long-Term-Care
        Facilities   23
    Public Health Departments   23
    Occupational Health Settings   23
    School-Based Settings   25
Nursing Practice Roles in Nonhospital
    Settings   26
    Supervisor of Unlicensed Assistive
        Personnel   26
    Discharge Planner   26
    Ambulatory Care Nurse   26
    Home Health Nurse, Visiting Nurse, Hospice
        Nurse   27
    Clinical Nurse Specialist, Nurse
        Practitioner   27
    Public Health Nurse   28
    Occupational Health Nurse   28
    School Nurse   28
    Provider of Telenursing Services   28
The Future of Medical-Surgical Nursing   29
    The NACNEP Study   29
    Pew Health Professions Commission
        Report   29

3
Death, Dying, and Bereavement   31

Death   31
   Personal Awareness of Death   31
Death as a Developmental Stage of Life   32
Dying   32
   Stages of Dying   32
      Denial   32
      Anger   32
      Bargaining   32
      Depression   32
      Acceptance   33
   Final Tasks Toward Achieving Acceptance of
   Death   33
      Developing Awareness of Impending
      Death   33
      Balancing Hope and Fear   33
      Relinquishing the Will to Live   33
      Letting Go of Autonomous Control   34
      Detaching from Former Experiences and
      Relationships   34
      Achieving Spiritual Preparation and
      Integration   34
   Nursing Process: The Dying Patient   34
Bereavement   36
   Stages of Bereavement   36
      Denial   36
      Anger   36
      Bargaining   37
      Depression   37
      Acceptance   37
   Stigmatized or Violent Death   37
   Sudden Death   38
   Nursing Process: The Patient Suffering
   Bereavement   38
Dysfunctional Grieving   39
   Nursing Process: The Patient with Dysfunctional
   Grieving   39
Spiritual Aspects of Death and Dying   40
Ethical and Legal Issues Related to Death and
   Dying   41
   The Changing Definition of Death   41
   Euthanasia   41
   Advance Directives   42
   Do Not Resuscitate Policies   43
   Organ Donations   45

4
Special Considerations for Nursing Care of Elderly Patients   49

Changes Associated with the Normal Aging
   Process   49
   Psychosocial Aspects   49
   Nursing Process Guidelines: Psychosocial Aspects
   of Aging   50
Body Composition   51
   Nursing Process Guidelines: Body Composition
   Changes   51
Nutritional Needs   51
   Nursing Process Guidelines: Nutritional Needs of
   Older Adults   52
Pharmacokinetics   52
   Nursing Process Guidelines:
   Pharmacokinetics   55
Integument   58
   Skin   58
      Nursing Process Guidelines: Skin
      Changes   58
   Hair and Nails   59
      Nursing Process Guidelines: Hair and Nail
      Changes   59
Thermoregulation   59
   Nursing Process Guidelines:
   Thermoregulation   59
Sensory Changes   60
   Vision   60
      Nursing Process Guidelines: Vision
      Changes   60
   Hearing   60
      Nursing Process Guidelines: Hearing
      Changes   60
   Taste and Smell   61
      Nursing Process Guidelines: Taste and
      Smell   61
   Tactile Sensation   61
      Nursing Process Guidelines: Tactile
      Sensation   61
Mental Processes   63
   Nursing Process Guidelines: Mental
   Processes   63
Sleep Patterns   63
   Nursing Process Guidelines: Sleep Patterns   64
Cardiovascular Function   64
   Nursing Process Guidelines: Cardiovascular
   Function   64
Respiratory Function   65
   Nursing Process Guidelines: Respiratory
   Function   65
Gastrointestinal Function   65
   Nursing Process Guidelines: Gastrointestinal
   Function   65
Urinary Function   66
   Nursing Process Guidelines: Urinary
   Function   66
Musculoskeletal Function   66
   Muscles   66
   Bones and Joints   67
      Nursing Process Guidelines: Musculoskeletal
      Function   67
Neurologic Function   67
   Nursing Process Guidelines: Neurologic
   Function   68

Reproductive Function   68
   Nursing Process Guidelines: Reproductive
   Function   68
Endocrine Function   68
   Nursing Process Guidelines: Endocrine
   Function   69
Assessment of the Elderly   69
   Patient History   69
Physical Examination   69

5
Knowledge Base for Patients with Fluid, Electrolyte, and Acid-Base Imbalances   75

Fluid Imbalances   75
   Extracellular Fluid Volume Deficit   75
      Nursing Process: Extracellular Fluid Volume
      Deficit   78
   Extracellular Fluid Volume Excess   79
      Nursing Process: Iso-Osmolar Extracellular Fluid
      Volume Excess   80
   Extracellular Third-Space Volume Shift   81
      Nursing Process Guidelines: Extracellular Third-
      Space Fluid Volume Shift   82
   Intracellular Fluid Volume Excess   82
      Nursing Process: Intracellular Fluid Volume
      Excess   83
Electrolyte Imbalances   84
   Potassium Imbalance   84
      Hypokalemia   84
         Nursing Process: Hypokalemia   86
      Hyperkalemia   89
         Nursing Process: Hyperkalemia   90
   Sodium Imbalance   91
      Hyponatremia   91
         Nursing Process: Hyponatremia   92
      Hypernatremia   93
         Nursing Process: Hypernatremia   94
   Calcium Imbalance   95
      Hypocalcemia   95
         Nursing Process: Hypocalcemia   96
      Hypercalcemia   97
         Nursing Process: Hypercalcemia   98
   Magnesium Imbalance   99
      Hypomagnesemia   99
         Nursing Process: Hypomagnesemia   100
      Hypermagnesemia   101
         Nursing Process: Hypermagnesemia   101
Acid-Base Imbalance   102
   Buffer System   103
   Respiratory Control of pH   103
   Renal Control of pH   103
   Metabolic Acidosis   104
      Nursing Process: Metabolic Acidosis   105
   Metabolic Alkalosis   106

   Nursing Process: Metabolic Alkalosis   107
   Respiratory Acidosis   108
      Nursing Process: Respiratory Acidosis   109
   Respiratory Alkalosis   111
      Nursing Process: Respiratory Alkalosis   111
The Elderly: Special Considerations   112

6
Knowledge Base for Patients Undergoing Surgery   115

Surgical Settings   115
Perioperative Nursing   116
   Legal Parameters   117
   Surgical Classifications   118
      Extent of Surgery   118
      Urgency of Surgery   118
      Surgical Approach   119
   Surgical Risk Factors   119
      Psychosocial Status   119
      Economic Influences   119
      Nutritional Status   120
      Fluid and Electrolyte Balance   121
      Immune Status   121
      Cardiovascular Status   121
      Respiratory Status   121
      Renal Status   122
      Hepatic Status   122
      Endocrine Status   122
      Neurologic Status   122
      Hematologic Status   122
      Therapeutic Drugs   122
      Substance Abuse   122
      Pregnancy   123
Preoperative Period   123
   Diagnostic Procedures   123
   Preoperative Management   124
      Food and Fluid Restrictions   124
      Elimination   124
      Skin Preparation   124
   Preanesthesia Management   127
   Nursing Process: The Preoperative Patient   128
Intraoperative Period   134
   Surgical Team   135
   Positioning   135
   Skin Preparation and Draping   135
   Anesthesia   136
      Regional Anesthesia   137
      General Anesthesia   137
   Nursing Process: The Intraoperative Patient   142
Postoperative Period   143
   Nursing Process: The Postanesthesia Patient   144
   Nursing Process: The Postsurgical Patient   150
Ambulatory Surgery   156

Nursing Process Guidelines: Ambulatory
    Surgery   156
The Elderly: Special Considerations   158
    Nursing Process Guidelines: Older Adults in
    Surgery   158

Unit II

Cardiovascular Dysfunction   161

7
Knowledge Base for Patients with Cardiac Dysfunction   163

Anatomy and Physiology   163
    The Heart   163
        Cardiac Chambers   165
        Cardiac Valves   167
    Coronary Arteries   167
    Coronary Veins   169
    The Cardiac Conduction System   169
        The Sinoatrial Node   169
        The Atrioventricular Node   169
        Ventricular Conduction   171
        Sequence of Impulse Conduction   171
    The Cardiac Cycle   171
    Mechanisms for Regulating Circulation   172
        Intrinsic Control   172
        Neural Control   173
        Humoral Control   173
Clinical Manifestations of Cardiac
    Dysfunction   174
    Dyspnea   174
        Nursing Process Guidelines: Dyspnea   174
    Chest Pain   175
        Nursing Process Guidelines: Chest Pain   175
    Syncope   176
        Nursing Process Guidelines: Syncope   176
    Palpitations   176
        Nursing Process Guidelines: Palpitations   176
    Edema   177
        Nursing Process Guidelines: Edema   177
    Altered Blood Pressure   177
    Altered Pulse   178
    Abnormal Heart Sounds   179
    Murmurs   181
    Pericardial Friction Rub   181
    Neck Vein Distention   181
    Altered Capillary Refill   181
    Cyanosis   181
    Pallor   182
    Fatigue   182
        Nursing Process Guidelines: Fatigue   182
    Clubbing   182
    Altered Renal Function   182

Nursing Process Guidelines: Altered Renal
    Function   183
Altered Gastrointestinal Function   184
    Nursing Process Guidelines: Altered
    Gastrointestinal Function   184
Altered Neurologic Function   185
Risk Factors for Cardiac Disease   185
    Uncontrollable Risk Factors   185
        Family History   185
        Age   185
        Sex   186
    Controllable Risk Factors   186
        Hyperlipidemia   186
        High Blood Pressure   186
        Diabetes Mellitus and Glucose
            Intolerance   186
        Obesity   186
        Cigarette Smoking   186
        Oral Contraceptive Use   187
        Sedentary Lifestyle   187
        Type A Personality   187
        Emotional Stress   187
        Multiple Role Expectations   187
Assessment of the Cardiovascular System   187
    Patient History   188
    Physical Examination   189
        Pulse   189
        Blood Pressure   190
        Heart   190
        Other Body Systems   192
Diagnostic Procedures   192
    X-Ray Studies   192
        Fluoroscopy   193
    Electrocardiography   193
        Signal-Averaged
            Electrocardiography   195
        Exercise Stress Testing   195
        Ambulatory Electrocardiographic
            Monitoring   197
    Electrophysiology Studies   197
    Radionuclide Imaging   197
    Technetium Pyrophosphate Scanning   198
    Thallium Scanning   198
    Gated Heart Studies   198
    Positron Emission Tomography   198
    Echocardiography   198
    Magnetic Resonance Imaging   199
    Electron Beam Computed Tomography   199
    Cardiac Catheterization   200
        Right-Sided Heart Catheterization   200
        Left-Sided Heart Catheterization   200
        Angiography   200
            Nursing Process Guidelines: Cardiac
            Catheterization   202
    Invasive Hemodynamic Monitoring   202
        Central Venous Pressure   202

Pulmonary Artery Pressure   202
Intra-Arterial Blood Pressure   206
Cardiac Output   207
Blood Studies   207
Complete Blood Count and
Differential   208
Electrolytes   208
Glucose   208
Blood Urea Nitrogen and Serum
Creatinine   208
Erythrocyte Sedimentation Rate   208
Prothrombin Time and Partial
Thromboplastin Time   208
Serum Lipids   209
Cardiac Enzymes   209
Cardiac Isoenzymes   209
Management   210
Nonsurgical Management   210
Reduction of Risk Factors   210
Pharmacologic Therapy   211
Surgical Management   217
Preoperative Preparation   219
Cardiopulmonary Bypass   220
Nursing Process: Cardiac Surgery   222
Cardiac Transplantation   227
Intra-Aortic Balloon
Counterpulsation   229
Ventricular Assistance   229
Cardiac Rehabilitation   229
The Elderly: Special Considerations   230

8
Nursing Care of Patients with Cardiac Disorders   233

Infections and Inflammations   233
Infective Endocarditis   233
Nursing Process: Infective Endocarditis   235
Rheumatic Heart Disease   236
Nursing Process Guidelines: Rheumatic Heart
Disease   237
Myocarditis   237
Nursing Process Guidelines: Myocarditis   238
Pericarditis   238
Acute Pericarditis   238
Chronic Constrictive Pericarditis   239
Nursing Process Guidelines: Pericarditis   239
Pericardial Effusion   239
Nursing Process Guidelines: Pericardial
Effusion   240
Cardiac Dysrhythmias   240
Sinus Dysrhythmias   240
Sinus Bradycardia   240
Sinus Tachycardia   241
Sinus Arrhythmia   242

Atrial Dysrhythmias   243
Premature Atrial Contraction   243
Paroxysmal Atrial Tachycardia   244
Atrial Flutter   245
Atrial Fibrillation   246
Junctional Dysrhythmias   247
Premature Junctional Contractions   247
Junctional Rhythm   247
Ventricular Dysrhythmias   248
Premature Ventricular Contractions   248
Ventricular Tachycardia   249
Ventricular Fibrillation   250
Atrioventricular Heart Blocks   251
First-Degree Atrioventricular Block   251
Second-Degree Atrioventricular Block,
Type I   251
Second-Degree Atrioventricular Block,
Type II   252
Third-Degree Atrioventricular Block   253
Nursing Process: Cardiac Dysrhythmias   255
Mechanical and Surgical Control of
Dysrhythmias   256
Artificial Pacemakers   256
Cardioversion   259
Cardiac Conduction Surgery   261
Cardiac Arrest   261
Nursing Process Guidelines: Cardiac Arrest   262
Heart Failure   264
Nursing Process: Heart Failure   276
Cardiogenic Pulmonary Edema   280
Nursing Process Guidelines: Cardiogenic Pulmonary
Edema   280
Coronary Artery Disease   280
Nursing Process Guidelines: Coronary Artery
Disease   284
Angina Pectoris   285
Myocardial Infarction   293
Nursing Process Guidelines: Myocardial
Infarction   298
Cardiomyopathies   303
Dilated Cardiomyopathy   303
Hypertrophic Cardiomyopathy   305
Restrictive Cardiomyopathy   306
Obliterative Cardiomyopathy   306
Nursing Process Guidelines: Nonsurgical Management
of Cardiomyopathy   306
Cardiac Valvular Disease   306
Aortic Valve Stenosis   307
Aortic Valve Regurgitation   308
Mitral Valve Stenosis   308
Mitral Valve Regurgitation   309
Mitral Valve Prolapse Syndrome   309
Nursing Process Guidelines: Nonsurgical Management
of Cardiac Valvular Disease   310
Valvular Surgery   310
Valvuloplasty   310

Commissurotomy   310
Chordoplasty   311
Leaflet Repair   311
Balloon Valvuloplasty   311
Valve Replacement Surgery   311
Nursing Process: Valve Repair or
Replacement   314
Cardiac Trauma   316
Nursing Process Guidelines: Cardiac Trauma   317
Cardiac Neoplasia   317
Nursing Process: Cardiac Neoplasia   318
The Elderly: Special Considerations   318

9
**Knowledge Base for Patients with
Vascular Dysfunction   323**

Anatomy and Physiology   323
Vascular Structures   323
Arteries and Arterioles   324
Capillaries   325
Veins and Venules   325
Factors That Affect Blood Flow   328
Structural Factors   328
Direct Control of Blood Flow   329
Lymphatic Vascular System   329
Clinical Manifestations of Vascular
Dysfunction   331
Pain   331
Intermittent Claudication   332
Rest Pain   332
Venous Insufficiency   332
Ischemic Neuropathy   332
Ulceration or Gangrene   333
Nursing Process: Pain   333
Changes in Skin Color, Temperature, and
Integrity   334
Trophic Changes   334
Color Changes   334
Temperature Changes   335
Ulceration   335
Gangrene   335
Nursing Process: Changes in Skin Color,
Temperature, and Integrity   335
Assessment of the Vascular System   337
Health History   337
Risk Factors   337
Physical Examination   337
Diagnostic Procedures   339
Management   342
Nonsurgical Management   342
Reduction of Risk Factors   342
Exercise   343
Medications   343
Angioplasty   343
Laser Thermal Angioplasty   344

Nursing Process Guidelines:
Angioplasty   344
Surgical Management   344
Grafts   344
Embolectomy   346
Endarterectomy   346
Amputation   346
Nursing Process: Peripheral Vascular
Surgery   346
The Elderly: Special Considerations   348

10
**Nursing Care of Patients with Vascular
Disorders   351**

Common Arterial Vascular Disorders   351
Thromboangiitis Obliterans (Buerger's
Disease)   351
Nursing Process: Thromboangiitis
Obliterans   352
Obstructive Disorders   354
Nursing Process: Arterial Vascular Obstructive
Disorders   354
Vasospastic Disorder (Raynaud's
Disease)   355
Nursing Process Guidelines: Vasospastic
Disorder (Raynaud's Disease)   356
Arterial Embolus and Thrombus   357
Nursing Process: Arterial Embolus or
Thrombus   357
Atherosclerosis   360
Nursing Process: Atherosclerosis   362
Chronic Arterial Occlusive Disease
(Arteriosclerosis Obliterans)   363
Nursing Process Guidelines: Chronic Arterial
Occlusive Disease   365
Aneurysms   365
Fusiform Aneurysm   366
Saccular Aneurysm   366
Dissecting Aneurysm   366
Abdominal Aortic Aneurysm   367
Thoracic Aortic Aneurysm   370
Peripheral Arterial Aneurysms   371
Nursing Process Guidelines:
Aneurysm   371
Hypertensive Vascular Disease   372
Nursing Process: Hypertension   376
Common Venous Vascular Disorders   384
Thrombophlebitis   384
Nursing Process: Thrombophlebitis   386
Chronic Venous Insufficiency   388
Varicose Veins   389
Nursing Process Guidelines: Varicose
Veins   390
Venous Stasis Ulcers   390
Nursing Process: Venous Stasis
Ulcers   392

Common Lymphatic Disorders   395
    Lymphangitis and Lymphadenitis   395
        Nursing Process Guidelines: Lymphangitis and
            Lymphadenitis   396
    Lymphedema   396
        Nursing Process Guidelines: Lymphedema   397
The Elderly: Special Considerations   397

11
Knowledge Base for Patients in
Shock   401

Principles for Understanding Shock   401
    Hemodynamic Principles   402
        Cardiac Output   402
        Heart Rate   402
        Preload   403
        Afterload   403
        Contractility   404
        Control of Peripheral Circulation   405
    Oxygen Transport Principles   405
Stages of Shock   406
    The Compensatory Stage   406
    The Progressive Stage   406
    The Refractory Stage   408
Types of Shock   408
    Hypovolemic Shock   408
    Cardiogenic Shock   411
    Distributive Shock   413
        Septic Shock   413
        Neurogenic Shock   416
        Anaphylactic Shock   417
    Nursing Process: Shock   418
The Elderly: Special Considerations   422

Unit III

Hematologic Dysfunction   425

12
Knowledge Base for Patients with
Hematologic Dysfunction   427

Anatomy and Physiology   427
    Blood   427
        Blood Components   428
        Blood Coagulation   429
        Anticoagulation   432
        Blood Grouping   432
    Blood-Forming Organs   433
        Lymph Nodes   433
        Bone Marrow   433
        Spleen   433
        Liver   433

Clinical Manifestations of Hematologic
    Dysfunction   433
    Fatigue, Weakness, Dyspnea, and Pallor   433
        Nursing Process: Fatigue and Dyspnea   434
    Hemorrhagic Tendencies   436
        Nursing Process: Hemorrhagic
            Tendencies   436
    Ulcerative Lesions   437
        Nursing Process: Ulcerative Lesions   437
    Bone and Joint Pain and Deformities   438
        Nursing Process: Bone and Joint Pain and
            Deformities   438
    Increased Susceptibility to Infection   438
        Nursing Process: Increased Susceptibility to
            Infection   438
    Jaundice, Pruritus, and Skin Problems   440
    Nutritional Deficiencies   440
        Nursing Process: Nutritional Deficiencies   440
    Gastrointestinal Symptoms   441
    Enlarged Organs   441
Assessment of the Hematologic System   442
Diagnostic Procedures   442
    Methods of Obtaining Blood   442
    Blood Tests   442
        Complete Blood Count   442
        White Blood Cell Count   442
        Differential   444
        Red Blood Cell Count   444
        Hematocrit   444
        Hemoglobin   444
        Red Blood Cell Indices   446
        Stained Red Cell Examination   446
        Platelet Count   446
    Coagulation Tests   447
        Platelet Aggregation   447
        Prothrombin Time   447
        Partial Thromboplastin Time and Activated
            Partial Thromboplastin Time   448
        Bleeding Time (Ivy Method)   448
        Coagulant Factor Assays   448
    Other Blood Component Tests   448
        Hemoglobin Electrophoresis   448
        Sickle-Cell Test   448
        Heinz Body Test   449
        Erythrocyte Fragility Test   449
        Erythrocyte Sedimentation Rate   449
        Reticulocyte Count   449
        Leukocyte Alkaline Phosphatase
            Stain   449
        Direct Coombs' Test   449
        Serum Iron   449
        Total Iron-Binding Capacity   450
        Serum Folic Acid   450
    Nursing Process Guidelines: Diagnostic Blood
        Tests   450
    Other Tests Specific to Hematologic
        Disorders   451

Schilling Test   451
Urobilinogen Test   451
Tests to Evaluate Blood-Forming Organs   451
Bone Marrow Aspiration and
Biopsy   451
Lymph Node Biopsy   451
Ultrasonography   451
Computed Tomography   452
Magnetic Resonance Imaging   452
Management   452
Nonsurgical Management   452
Bedrest and Exercise   452
Nutritional Support   452
Oxygen Therapy   452
Protective Isolation   452
Blood Transfusions   452
Nursing Process: Transfusion of Blood or
Blood Products   457
Surgical Management   462
Splenectomy   462
Nursing Process: Splenectomy   463
Other Surgical Procedures and Medical
Treatments   464
The Elderly: Special Considerations   464

Infections   512
Infectious Mononucleosis   512
Nursing Process Guidelines: Infectious
Mononucleosis   513
Bleeding Disorders   513
Purpuras   513
Nursing Process: Purpuras   514
Coagulation Disorders   515
Hemophilias   515
Nursing Process Guidelines:
Hemophilia   516
Acquired Hypoprothrombinemia   517
Nursing Process Guidelines: Acquired
Hypoprothrombinemia   517
Disseminated Intravascular
Coagulation   517
Nursing Process Guidelines: Disseminated
Intravascular Coagulation   517
The Elderly: Special Considerations   518

Unit IV

Respiratory Dysfunction   521

13
Nursing Care of Patients with Hematologic Disorders   467

Erythrocyte-Related Disorders   467
Anemias   467
Nursing Process: Anemia   468
Anemia from Blood Loss   470
Nursing Process: Anemia from Blood
Loss   471
Hypoproliferative Anemias   472
Hemolytic Anemias   482
Polycythemias   489
Polycythemia Vera   489
Nursing Process: Polycythemia Vera   490
Leukocyte-Related Disorders   491
Agranulocytosis   491
Nursing Process: Agranulocytosis   491
Neoplasia   493
Leukemias   493
Nursing Process: Leukemia   495
Hodgkin's Disease   503
Nursing Process: Hodgkin's Disease   505
Non-Hodgkin's Lymphomas   507
Nursing Process Guidelines: Non-Hodgkin's
Lymphoma   508
Multiple Myeloma   508
Nursing Process: Multiple Myeloma   512

14
Knowledge Base for Patients with Respiratory Dysfunction   523

Anatomy and Physiology   523
Thorax   523
Lungs   524
Conducting Airways   525
Upper Airways   525
Lower Airways   525
Respiratory Zone   526
Mechanics of Ventilation   527
Gas Exchange   528
Transport of Gases   528
Work of Breathing   528
Clinical Manifestations of Respiratory
Dysfunction   528
Local Manifestations   528
Cough   528
Excessive Nasal Secretions   529
Expectoration of Sputum   529
Pain   529
Dyspnea   529
Systemic Manifestations   529
Hypoxemia and Hypoxia   529
Hypercapnia   530
Hypocapnia   530

Respiratory Failure   530
Assessment of the Respiratory System   531
   Patient History   531
   Physical Examination   531
      Inspection   531
      Palpation   534
      Percussion   535
      Auscultation   536
Diagnostic Procedures   537
   Pulmonary Function Studies   537
   Blood Studies   539
      Arterial Blood Gases   539
      Pulse Oximetry   544
      Other Blood Studies   545
   Sputum Studies   545
      Collection of a Sputum Specimen   546
   Radiographic Studies   547
      Chest X-Rays   547
      Fluoroscopy   547
      Tomography   548
      Lung Scan   548
      Pulmonary Angiography   548
   Endoscopic Studies   548
      Bronchoscopy   548
         Nursing Process: Bronchoscopy   549
      Laryngoscopy   550
         Nursing Process Guidelines:
            Laryngoscopy   550
      Mediastinoscopy   550
   Thoracentesis   550
      Nursing Process: Thoracentesis   551
   Lung Biopsy   552
      Nursing Process Guidelines: Closed Lung
         Biopsy   552
Management   552
   Nonsurgical Management   552
      Respiratory Therapy   552
      Oxygen Therapy   556
      Mechanical Ventilation Therapy   567
         Nursing Process: Mechanical
            Ventilation   570
      Pharmacologic Therapy   574
      Chest Drainage   575
         Nursing Process: Chest Drainage   577
   Surgical Management   580
      Overview of Thoracic Surgery   580
      Patient Preparation for Thoracic
         Surgery   580
      Complications of Thoracic Surgery   581
      Pneumonectomy   581
         Nursing Process: Pneumonectomy   582
      Lobectomy   586
         Nursing Process: Lobectomy   587
      Thoracoscopic Surgery   587
         Nursing Process Guidelines: Thoracoscopic
            Surgery   587
The Elderly: Special Considerations   596

15
Nursing Care of Patients with Upper Respiratory Disorders   599

Infections and Inflammations   599
   Rhinitis   599
      Acute Viral Rhinitis   600
         Nursing Process Guidelines: Acute Viral
            Rhinitis   600
      Allergic Rhinitis   601
         Nursing Process Guidelines: Allergic
            Rhinitis   601
      Vasomotor Rhinitis   601
      Chronic Rhinitis   601
   Sinusitis   601
      Acute Sinusitis   602
         Nursing Process Guidelines: Acute
            Sinusitis   602
      Chronic Sinusitis   603
         Nursing Process: Chronic Sinusitis   603
   Pharyngitis   604
      Nursing Process: Pharyngitis   604
   Tonsillitis   606
      Nursing Process: Tonsillitis   606
   Peritonsillar Abscess   607
      Nursing Process: Peritonsillar Abscess   607
   Laryngitis   608
      Nursing Process: Laryngitis   609
Structural Disorders   610
   Epistaxis   610
      Nursing Process: Epistaxis   610
   Nasal Obstruction   611
      Nasal Polyps   611
      Hypertrophied Turbinates   611
      Deviated Nasal Septum   611
      Nursing Process: Nasal Surgery   612
Trauma   612
   Nasal Fracture   612
      Nursing Process Guidelines: Nasal
         Fracture   612
   Laryngeal Trauma   612
      Nursing Process Guidelines: Laryngeal
         Trauma   616
Neoplasia   616
   Cancer of the Larynx   616
      Laryngectomy   617
The Elderly: Special Considerations   632

16
Nursing Care of Patients with Lower Respiratory Disorders   639

Infections and Inflammations   639
   Acute Bronchitis   639
      Nursing Process: Acute Bronchitis   640
   Pneumonia   641
      Nursing Process: Pneumonia   644

Aspiration Pneumonia Syndrome   647
    Nursing Process Guidelines: Aspiration Pneumonia
        Syndrome   647
Lung Abscess   647
    Nursing Process: Lung Abscess   648
Influenza   648
    Nursing Process Guidelines: Influenza   649
Tuberculosis   650
    Nursing Process: Tuberculosis   655
Empyema   657
    Nursing Process Guidelines: Empyema   658
Pleuritis   658
    Nursing Process Guidelines: Pleuritis   659
Asthma   659
    Nursing Process: Asthma   664
Chronic Obstructive Pulmonary Disease   668
    Chronic Bronchitis   668
    Emphysema   669
    Nursing Process: Chronic Obstructive Pulmonary
        Disease   673
    Bronchiectasis   679
        Nursing Process Guidelines:
            Bronchiectasis   679
    Atelectasis   679
        Nursing Process Guidelines: Atelectasis   681
Disorders of the Pulmonary Circulation   681
    Pulmonary Embolism   681
        Nursing Process: Pulmonary Embolism   683
    Pulmonary Hypertension   685
        Nursing Process Guidelines: Pulmonary
            Hypertension   686
    Adult Respiratory Distress Syndrome   686
        Nursing Process: Adult Respiratory Distress
            Syndrome   687
Occupational Lung Diseases   688
    Silicosis   688
    Asbestosis   688
    Coal Workers' Pneumoconiosis   688
    Nursing Process: Occupational Lung Disease   689
Trauma   690
    Fractured Ribs   690
        Nursing Process: Fractured Ribs   690
    Flail Chest   691
        Nursing Process: Flail Chest   692
            Pneumothorax   692
            Hemothorax   694
                Nursing Process: Pneumothorax or
                    Hemothorax   694
    Pulmonary Contusion   695
        Nursing Process Guidelines: Pulmonary
            Contusion   695
    Subcutaneous Emphysema   695
Neoplasia   695
    Lung Cancer   695
        Nursing Process: Lung Cancer   697
    Tumors of the Mediastinum   698
        Nursing Process Guidelines: Mediastinal
            Tumor   698
The Elderly: Special Considerations   698

Unit V

Neurologic Dysfunction   709

17
Knowledge Base for Patients with
Neurologic Dysfunction   711

Anatomy and Physiology   711
    Cellular Structure   711
        Neurons   711
        Neuroglia   712
    Nerve Impulse Transmission   712
    Protective Coverings of the Brain and Spinal
        Cord   713
        Skull and Vertebral Column   713
        Meninges   714
    Blood Supply and Circulation   714
        Cerebral Circulation   714
        Spinal Circulation   716
    Blood-Brain Barrier   717
    Cerebrospinal Fluid and the Cerebral
        Ventricular System   718
    Central Nervous System   718
        Brain   718
        Spinal Cord   721
    Peripheral Nervous System   722
        Cranial Nerves   722
        Spinal Nerves   722
    Autonomic Nervous System   725
Clinical Manifestations of Neurologic
    Dysfunction   726
    Altered Levels of Consciousness   726
        Nursing Process: The Unconscious Patient   727
    Increased Intracranial Pressure   730
        Nursing Process: Increased Intracranial
            Pressure   733
    Speech and Language Dysfunction   738
        Nursing Process: Speech and Language
            Dysfunction   738
    Motor System Dysfunction   739
        Nursing Process: Motor System
            Dysfunction   740
    Sensory System Dysfunction   742
        Nursing Process: Sensory System
            Dysfunction   743
    Brain Death   745
Assessment of the Nervous System   745
    Patient History   745
    Physical Examination   745
        Mental Status   746
        Speech and Language Function   746
        Cranial Nerve Function   747
        Motor Function   747
        Sensory Function   747
        Reflex Function   748

Diagnostic Procedures   748
   Skull X-Ray Examinations   748
   Spine X-Ray Examinations   748
   Computed Tomography   749
   Positron Emission Tomography   749
   Magnetic Resonance Imaging   749
   Carotid Doppler Studies   749
   Cerebral Angiography   750
     Nursing Process Guidelines: Cerebral
      Angiography   752
   Myelography   752
     Nursing Process Guidelines: Myelography   753
   Lumbar Puncture   753
   Cisternal Puncture   754
   Electroencephalography   754
   Evoked Potential Studies   757
   Electromyography   757
   Nerve Conduction Studies   757
Management   757
   Intracranial Surgery   757
     Nursing Process: Intracranial Surgery   759
   Spinal Surgery   761
     Nursing Process: Spinal Surgery   762
The Elderly: Special Considerations   765
   Structural Changes Related to Aging   765
   Functional Changes Related to Aging   766
   Changes in the Special Senses Related to
     Aging   766

18
Nursing Care of Patients with Neurologic Disorders   767

Infections and Inflammations   767
   Meningitis   767
     Bacterial Meningitis   767
     Viral Meningitis   769
   Encephalitis   769
     Viral Encephalitis   769
   Brain Abscess   770
     Nursing Process: Meningitis, Encephalitis, or Brain
      Abscess   771
   Guillain-Barré Syndrome   773
     Nursing Process: Guillain-Barré Syndrome   774
Degenerative Disorders   775
   Amyotrophic Lateral Sclerosis   775
     Nursing Process: Amyotrophic Lateral
      Sclerosis   776
   Multiple Sclerosis   777
     Nursing Process: Multiple Sclerosis   780
   Myasthenia Gravis   782
     Nursing Process: Myasthenia Gravis   784
   Muscular Dystrophy (Limb-Girdle)   785
     Nursing Process: Limb-Girdle Muscular
      Dystrophy   786
   Parkinson's Disease   787

     Nursing Process: Parkinson's Disease   788
   Alzheimer's Disease   790
     Nursing Process: Alzheimer's Disease   791
   Disk Herniation   792
     Nursing Process: Disk Herniation   793
Functional Disorders   795
   Seizure Disorders   795
     Nursing Process: Seizure Disorders   798
   Headache   800
     Nursing Process: Headache   801
Structural Disorders   802
   Hydrocephalus   802
   Cerebrovascular Accident   804
     Nursing Process: Cerebrovascular
      Accident   808
   Subarachnoid Hemorrhage   814
     Nursing Process Guidelines: Subarachnoid
      Hemorrhage   816
Trauma   816
   Head Injury   816
     Scalp Injury   816
     Skull Fractures   817
     Brain Injury   818
     Complications of Head Injury:
      Hematomas   819
     Nursing Process: Head Injury   821
   Spinal Cord Injury   822
     Nursing Process: Spinal Cord Injury   825
   Peripheral Nerve Injury   827
     Nursing Process Guidelines: Peripheral Nerve
      Injury   828
   Cranial Nerve Disease   828
Neoplasia   828
   Brain Tumors   828
     Nursing Process Guidelines: Brain Tumors   831
The Elderly: Special Considerations   832
   Dementia and Delirium   832
   Cerebrovascular Accident   832
   Subdural Hematoma   832

Unit VI
Musculoskeletal Dysfunction   835

19
Knowledge Base for Patients with Musculoskeletal Dysfunction   837

Anatomy and Physiology   837
   Skeletal System   837
     Microscopic Anatomy   837
     Gross Anatomy   839
     Bone Repair   839
   Skeletal Muscular System   840

Skeletal Muscle   840
Ligaments and Tendons   842
Joints and Articulations   842
Cartilage   842
Clinical Manifestations of Musculoskeletal
  Dysfunction   843
  Mobility Impairment   843
    Nursing Process: Mobility Impairment   843
  Pain   846
    Nursing Process: Musculoskeletal Pain   846
Assessment of the Musculoskeletal System   847
  Patient History   847
  Physical Examination   848
Diagnostic Procedures   849
Management   849
  Nonsurgical Management   849
    Application of Heat and Cold   849
      Nursing Process: Application of Heat or
        Cold   852
    Cast Therapy   853
      Nursing Process: Cast Therapy   856
    Traction Therapy   858
      Nursing Process: Traction Therapy   862
  Surgical Management   863
    External Fixation Devices   863
      Nursing Process: External Fixation
        Devices   864
    Internal Fixation Devices   865
      Nursing Process: Internal Fixation
        Devices   866
    Total Joint Replacement   867
      Nursing Process: Total Joint
        Replacement   868
    Amputation   868
      Nursing Process: Amputation   873
  Assistive and Supportive Devices   878
    Ambulatory Aids   879
    Splints and Braces   881
    Nursing Process: Assistive and Supportive
      Devices   881
  External Prostheses   881
    Upper Extremity Prostheses   882
    Lower Extremity Prostheses   882
    Temporary Prostheses   883
  Self-Help Devices   884
The Elderly: Special Considerations   884

20
Nursing Care of Patients with
Musculoskeletal Disorders   887

Infections and Inflammations   887
  Osteomyelitis   887
    Acute Osteomyelitis   888
    Chronic Osteomyelitis   888
    Tuberculous Osteomyelitis   888
    Other Forms of Osteomyelitis   889
    Nursing Process: Osteomyelitis   889

Arthritis   890
  Rheumatoid Arthritis   890
    Nursing Process: Rheumatoid Arthritis   894
  Osteoarthritis   897
    Nursing Process Guidelines:
      Osteoarthritis   898
  Ankylosing Spondylitis   898
    Nursing Process Guidelines: Ankylosing
      Spondylitis   899
  Gout   899
    Nursing Process: Gout   900
  Lyme Disease   901
  Bursitis   902
  Tenosynovitis   902
Structural Disorders   902
  Osteomalacia   902
    Nursing Process: Osteomalacia   903
  Osteoporosis   904
    Nursing Process: Osteoporosis   906
  Paget's Disease   908
    Nursing Process Guidelines: Paget's
      Disease   908
  Disorders of the Wrist and Hand   909
    Carpal Tunnel Syndrome   909
    Dupuytren's Contracture   909
    Ganglion   909
    Nursing Process: Wrist and Hand
      Disorders   909
  Disorders of the Feet   910
    Hallux Valgus (Bunion)   910
    Plantar Digital Neuroma   910
    Hammer Toe   910
    Pes Planus   910
    Nursing Process: Foot Disorders   910
  Low Back Pain   911
    Nursing Process: Low Back Pain   912
Trauma   913
  Minor Musculoskeletal Injuries   913
    Contusions and Strains   913
    Sprains   913
    Meniscal Tears   914
  Major Musculoskeletal Injuries   915
    Subluxations and Dislocations   915
      Nursing Process: Subluxations and
        Dislocations   915
    Fractures   916
      Nursing Process: Fracture   919
    Fractures Common in Geriatric
      Patients   924
    Traumatic Amputations   930
      Nursing Process: Traumatic Amputation with
        Reattachment Surgery   930
Complications of Musculoskeletal
  Injuries   932
    Immediate Complications   932
    Delayed Complications   933
Neoplasia   935
  Benign Bone Tumors   935
    Nursing Process: Benign Bone Tumors   937
  Malignant Bone Tumors   938

Osteosarcoma   938
Ewing's Sarcoma   942
Nursing Process: Malignant Bone
Tumors   942
Metastatic Bone Tumors   943
The Elderly: Special Considerations   943

Unit VII

Gastrointestinal Dysfunction   947

21
Knowledge Base for Patients with Gastrointestinal Dysfunction   949

Anatomy and Physiology   949
Basic Structure and Function of the
Gastrointestinal Tract   949
Peritoneum   951
Mouth   951
Pharynx   951
Esophagus   951
Stomach   952
Small Intestine   955
Large Intestine   956
Liver   957
Gallbladder   957
Pancreas   957
Clinical Manifestations of Gastrointestinal
Dysfunction   958
Anorexia   958
Nursing Process: Anorexia   959
Nausea and Vomiting   959
Nursing Process: Nausea and Vomiting   960
Intestinal Gas   961
Constipation   961
Nursing Process: Constipation   961
Diarrhea   963
Nursing Process: Diarrhea   963
Pain   965
Bleeding   965
Nursing Process Guidelines: Bleeding   967
Assessment of the Gastrointestinal System   968
Patient History   968
Physical Examination   968
Assessment of the Gastrointestinal System   968
Patient History   968
Physical Examination   968
Diagnostic Procedures   969
Gastric Analysis   969
Nursing Process Guidelines: Gastric
Aspiration   970
Upper Gastrointestinal Series   970
Nursing Process Guidelines: Upper Gastrointestinal
Series   971

Barium Enema   971
Nursing Process Guidelines: Barium
Enema   971
Oral Cholecystogram   971
Nursing Process Guidelines: Oral
Cholecystogram   972
Cholangiogram   972
Endoscopy   973
Esophagogastroduodenoscopy   973
Nursing Process Guidelines:
Esophagogastroduodenoscopy   973
Colonoscopy   974
Nursing Process Guidelines:
Colonoscopy   975
Ultrasonography   975
Computed Tomography   976
Magnetic Resonance Imaging   976
Management   976
Gastrointestinal Intubation   976
Intubation for Decompression and
Drainage   976
Types of Tubes Used for Decompression
and Drainage   976
Intubation Procedure   978
Nursing Process: Intubation for Removal of
Gastric Contents   979
Removal of Gastrointestinal Tubes   980
Enteral and Parenteral Nutrition   980
Enteral Nutrition   980
Nursing Process: Enteral Feedings   984
Total Parenteral Nutrition   986
Nursing Process: Total Parenteral
Nutrition   988
Gastrointestinal Surgery   993
Abdominal Incisions   993
Gastrectomy   996
Nursing Process: Gastrectomy   997
Intestinal Resection   1000
Nursing Process: Anastomosed Intestinal
Resection   1002
Colostomy   1003
Nursing Process: Colostomy   1005
Ileostomy   1011
Nursing Process Guidelines:
Ileostomy   1013
The Elderly: Special Considerations   1015

22
Nursing Care of Patients with Disorders of the Upper Gastrointestinal System   1017

Infections and Inflammations   1017
Oral Infections   1017
Nursing Process: Oral Infection   1017
Esophagitis   1019
Nursing Process: Esophagitis   1020
Acute Gastritis   1023

Nursing Process: Acute Gastritis   1024
Chronic Gastritis   1025
Nursing Process Guidelines: Chronic
Gastritis   1025
Structural and Functional Disorders   1025
Peptic Ulcer Disease   1025
Nursing Process: Peptic Ulcer Disease   1032
Acute Stress Ulcers   1033
Nursing Process Guidelines: Stress
Ulcers   1033
Hiatus Hernia   1033
Nursing Process: Nonsurgical Treatment for Hiatus
Hernia   1043
Nursing Process Guidelines: Surgical Treatment for
Hiatus Hernia   1043
Achalasia   1044
Nursing Process: Achalasia   1045
Nursing Process Guidelines: Surgical Treatment for
Achalasia   1045
Trauma   1046
Fracture of the Mandible   1046
Nursing Process: Mandibular Fracture   1047
Neoplasia   1049
Oral Cancer   1049
Nursing Process: Oral Cancer   1050
Nursing Process Guidelines: Supportive Treatment
for Oral Cancer   1053
Cancer of the Esophagus   1053
Nursing Process: Surgery for Esophageal
Cancer   1055
Gastric Cancer   1058
Nursing Process Guidelines: Gastric
Cancer   1059
The Elderly: Special Considerations   1059

23
Nursing Care of Patients with Disorders of the Lower Gastrointestinal System   1061

Infections and Inflammations   1061
Peritonitis   1061
Nursing Process: Peritonitis   1062
Appendicitis   1063
Nursing Process: Appendectomy   1065
Inflammatory Bowel Disease   1066
Crohn's Disease   1066
Nursing Process: Crohn's Disease   1068
Ulcerative Colitis   1070
Nursing Process Guidelines: Ulcerative
Colitis   1071
Anorectal Abscess   1071
Nursing Process: Incision and Drainage of a Rectal
Abscess   1072
Functional Disorders   1074
Mechanical Obstruction   1074
Nursing Process: Mechanical Ileus   1075
Paralytic Ileus   1075

Nursing Process: Paralytic Ileus   1076
Malabsorption Syndrome   1077
Nursing Process Guidelines: Malabsorption
Syndrome   1078
Gluten-Induced Enteropathy   1078
Nursing Process: Gluten-Induced
Enteropathy   1079
Lactase Deficiency   1079
Nursing Process: Lactase Deficiency   1080
Structural Disorders   1081
Diverticular Disease   1081
Nursing Process: Diverticular Disease   1083
Intestinal Adhesions   1084
Nursing Process Guidelines: Intestinal
Adhesions   1084
Intestinal Hernias   1093
Nursing Process: Herniorrhaphy   1095
Hemorrhoids   1096
Nursing Process: Hemorrhoids   1097
Nursing Process: Post-Hemorrhoidectomy   1097
Neoplasia   1098
Polyps of the Colon   1098
Nursing Process Guidelines: Polyps of the
Colon   1100
Cancer of the Colon and Rectum   1100
The Elderly: Special Considerations   1106

24
Nursing Care of Patients with Disorders of the Accessory Organs of Digestion   1109

Infections and Inflammations   1109
Cholecystitis   1109
Acute Pancreatitis   1118
Nursing Process: Acute Pancreatitis   1118
Chronic Pancreatitis   1122
Nursing Process: Chronic Pancreatitis   1123
Structural Disorders   1124
Pancreatic Fistula   1124
Nursing Process: Pancreatic Fistula   1126
Neoplasia   1126
Cancer of the Pancreas   1126
The Elderly: Special Considerations   1131

Unit VIII
Hepatic Dysfunction   1133

25
Knowledge Base for Patients with Hepatic Dysfunction   1135

Anatomy and Physiology   1135
Carbohydrate Metabolism   1136
Lipid Metabolism   1137

Protein Metabolism   1137
Bile Production and Bilirubin
Conjugation   1137
Blood Filtration   1138
Detoxification   1138
Storage   1139
Clinical Manifestations of Hepatic
Dysfunction   1139
Jaundice   1139
Nursing Process: Jaundice   1140
Portal Hypertension and Ascites   1141
Nursing Process: Ascites   1145
Clotting Disorders   1149
Nursing Process: Risk for Bleeding   1149
Hepatic Encephalopathy   1149
Nursing Process: Hepatic
Encephalopathy   1150
Nutritional Deficiencies   1153
Nursing Process: Nutritional Deficiencies   1154
Assessment of Liver Status   1154
Patient History   1154
Physical Examination   1158
Diagnostic Procedures   1160
Blood Studies   1160
Liver Enzymes   1160
Bilirubin Levels   1163
Protein Studies   1163
Lipid Studies   1164
Alpha-Fetoprotein   1164
Prothrombin   1164
Urine and Fecal Studies   1164
Visualization Procedures   1164
Liver Biopsy   1164
Nursing Process: Diagnostic Studies of Hepatic
Function   1165
The Elderly: Special Considerations   1165

26
Nursing Care of Patients with Hepatic Disorders   1169

Infections and Inflammations   1169
Viral Hepatitis   1169
Nursing Process: Hepatitis   1176
Toxic and Drug-Induced Hepatitis   1177
Nursing Process Guidelines: Toxic
Hepatitis   1178
Liver Abscess   1179
Nursing Process Guidelines: Liver
Abscess   1179
Structural Disorders   1180
Cirrhosis   1180
Nursing Process Guidelines: Cirrhosis   1189
Nursing Process: Esophageal Varices   1189
Trauma   1193
Blunt and Penetrating Injuries   1193
Nursing Process Guidelines: Liver Trauma   1194

Neoplasia   1194
Benign Hepatic Tumors   1194
Malignant Hepatic Tumors   1195
Orthotopic Hepatic Transplant   1196
Selection Criteria for Recipients   1196
Selection Criteria for Donors   1196
Surgical Procedure   1196
Postoperative Complications   1196
Nursing Process Guidelines: Orthotopic Hepatic
Transplant   1197
The Elderly: Special Considerations   1198

Unit IX
Endocrine Dysfunction   1201

27
Knowledge Base for Patients with Endocrine Dysfunction   1203

Anatomy and Physiology   1203
Hormone Receptors   1203
Cell Membrane Receptors   1203
Intracellular Receptors   1204
Regulation of Hormone Secretion   1204
Thymus Gland   1204
Pineal Gland   1204
Hypothalamus   1208
Pituitary Gland   1209
Thyroid Gland   1210
Thyroxine and Triiodothyronine   1211
Calcitonin   1212
Parathyroid Glands   1212
Adrenal Glands   1213
Adrenal Cortex   1213
Adrenal Medulla   1215
Endocrine Dysfunction   1216
Primary Endocrine Gland Dysfunction   1216
Secondary Endocrine Gland
Dysfunction   1217
Inability to Use Hormone Produced   1217
Assessment of the Endocrine System   1217
Nursing Process Guidelines: Endocrine
Dysfunction   1217
The Elderly: Special Considerations   1218

28
Nursing Care of Patients with Diabetes Mellitus   1223

Hormonal Regulation of Blood Glucose
Levels   1223
Insulin   1223
Carbohydrate Metabolism   1223

Fat Metabolism   1224
Protein Metabolism   1224
Regulation of Insulin Secretion   1224
Counter-Regulatory Hormones   1224
Absence of Insulin   1224
Diabetes Mellitus   1225
Etiology and Pathophysiology   1225
Transcultural Considerations   1227
Classification of Diabetes Mellitus   1227
Type 1 Diabetes   1227
Type 2 Diabetes   1227
Gestational Diabetes   1228
Other Types of Glucose Intolerance   1228
Clinical Manifestations   1228
Diagnosis   1229
Fasting Blood Sugar   1229
Oral Glucose Tolerance Test   1229
Management   1231
Diet   1231
Exercise   1233
Insulin Therapy   1235
Oral Antidiabetic Agents   1239
Current Research in the Management of
Diabetes   1239
Management During Illness   1240
Management During Surgery   1241
Evaluation of Therapy   1241
Blood Glucose Monitoring   1241
Urine Testing for Glucose   1242
Urine Testing for Ketones   1243
Measurement of Glycosylated
Hemoglobin   1243
Acute Complications of Diabetes
Mellitus   1243
Diabetic Ketoacidosis   1243
Hyperglycemic Hyperosmolar Nonketotic
Syndrome   1249
Hypoglycemia   1250
Somogyi Phenomenon   1250
Dawn Phenomenon   1251
Long-Term Degenerative Changes of Diabetes
Mellitus   1251
Degenerative Vascular Changes   1251
Diabetic Retinopathy   1253
Diabetic Neuropathy   1253
Diabetic Nephropathy   1254
Nursing Process: Diabetes Mellitus   1255
The Elderly: Special Considerations   1261

29
Nursing Care of Patients with Other Endocrine Disorders   1265

Pituitary Disorders   1265

Anterior Pituitary Disorders   1265
Neoplasia   1265
Nursing Process: Pituitary
Neoplasms   1267
Hypersecretion of Somatotropin   1269
Nursing Process Guidelines:
Acromegaly   1274
Hypopituitarism   1274
Posterior Pituitary Disorders   1274
Diabetes Insipidus   1274
Nursing Process Guidelines: Diabetes
Insipidus   1275
Syndrome of Inappropriate Antidiuretic
Hormone   1277
Adrenal Disorders   1277
Adrenocortical Insufficiency: Addison's
Disease   1277
Nursing Process: Adrenocortical Insufficiency
(Addison's Disease)   1281
Adrenocortical Excess: Cushing's
Syndrome   1285
Nursing Process: Adrenocortical Excess (Cushing's
Syndrome)   1287
Primary Aldosteronism   1289
Nursing Process Guidelines: Primary
Aldosteronism   1291
Pheochromocytoma   1292
Nursing Process: Pheochromocytoma   1293
Thyroid Disorders   1295
Thyroiditis   1295
Acute Thyroiditis   1296
Subacute Granulomatous
Thyroiditis   1296
Silent (Painless) Thyroiditis   1296
Chronic Thyroiditis (Hashimoto's
Thyroiditis)   1296
Functional Disorders   1296
Hypothyroidism   1297
Nursing Process: Hypothyroidism   1301
Hyperthyroidism   1306
Nursing Process: Hyperthyroidism   1310
Thyroid Hormone Resistance   1314
Structural Disorders   1314
Simple Nontoxic Goiter   1314
Nodular Goiter   1315
Neoplasia   1315
Parathyroid Disorders   1316
Hypoparathyroidism   1316
Nursing Process: Hypoparathyroidism   1317
Hyperparathyroidism   1318
Nursing Process: Hyperparathyroidism   1321
The Elderly: Special Considerations   1322
Pituitary Disorders in Older
Adults   1322
Adrenal Disorders in Older Adults   1323
Thyroid Disorders in Older Adults   1323
Parathyroid Disorders in Older
Adults   1324

Unit X

Urinary Dysfunction   1327

30
Knowledge Base for Patients with Urinary Dysfunction   1329

Anatomy and Physiology   1329
    Kidneys   1329
        Formation and Excretion of Urine   1331
        Regulation of Fluid and Electrolyte
          Balance   1332
        Regulation of Acid-Base Balance   1333
        Stimulation of Red Blood Cell
          Production   1333
        Calcium Metabolism   1333
        Regulation of Blood Pressure   1333
    Ureters   1333
    Bladder   1334
    Urethra   1335
Clinical Manifestations of Urinary Tract
    Dysfunction   1335
    Dysfunctional Voiding   1335
        Frequency   1335
        Urgency   1335
        Dysuria   1335
        Nocturia   1335
        Nocturnal Enuresis   1335
        Hesitancy   1336
        Urinary Retention   1336
          Nursing Process: Urinary Retention   1336
    Incontinence   1336
      Nursing Process: Incontinence   1340
    Pain   1341
      Nursing Process: Urinary Tract Pain   1341
    Change in Urine Characteristics   1342
    Hematuria   1342
    Change in Urine Volume   1343
Assessment of the Urinary System   1343
    Health History   1343
    Physical Examination   1344
Diagnostic Procedures   1344
    Urine Studies   1344
        Urinalysis   1344
        Urine Culture   1344
        Urine Cytology   1345
        Twenty-Four-Hour Urine
          Collection   1345
    Blood Studies   1345
        Complete Blood Count   1345
        Blood Chemistry Studies   1345
        Serum Creatinine and Blood Urea
          Nitrogen   1345
      Nursing Process Guidelines: Blood
        Studies   1346

Radiologic Studies   1346
    Nursing Process: Excretory Urogram   1351
Cystoscopy   1352
    Nursing Process Guidelines: Cystoscopy   1353
Bladder Biopsy   1353
    Nursing Process: Bladder Biopsy   1356
Renal Biopsy   1357
    Nursing Process: Renal Biopsy   1357
Urodynamics   1358
    Nursing Process: Urodynamic Testing   1358
Management   1361
    Nonsurgical Management   1361
        Catheter Drainage   1361
        Medications   1363
        Self-Care Measures   1365
        Diet Therapy   1366
        Additional Treatment Options   1367
    Surgical Management   1367
The Elderly: Special Considerations   1368

31
Nursing Care of Patients with Urinary Disorders   1371

Infections and Inflammations   1371
    Cystitis   1371
      Nursing Process: Cystitis   1372
    Urethritis   1373
      Nursing Process Guidelines: Urethritis   1374
    Pyelonephritis   1374
      Nursing Process: Pyelonephritis   1374
    Perinephric Abscess   1375
      Nursing Process Guidelines: Perinephric
        Abscess   1375
    Glomerulonephritis   1376
      Nursing Process: Glomerulonephritis   1376
Obstruction   1377
    Urinary Calculi   1378
      Nursing Process Guidelines: Urinary
        Calculi   1380
    Upper Urinary Tract Obstruction   1380
        Ureteropelvic Junction Obstruction   1380
        Ureterovesical Junction
          Obstruction   1380
        Ureteral Stricture   1383
      Nursing Process: Upper Urinary Tract
        Obstruction   1384
    Lower Urinary Tract Obstruction   1385
        Urethral Stricture   1385
        Meatal Stenosis   1386
      Nursing Process: Lower Urinary Tract
        Obstruction   1387
Renal Failure   1388
    Acute Renal Failure   1388
      Nursing Process: Acute Renal Failure   1391
    Chronic Renal Failure   1394

Nursing Process: Chronic Renal Failure   1400
Dialysis   1400
  Peritoneal Dialysis   1401
    Nursing Process: Peritoneal Dialysis   1403
  Hemodialysis   1404
    Nursing Process: Hemodialysis   1406
Renal Transplantation   1408
  Nursing Process: Renal Transplantation   1410
Trauma   1411
  Renal Trauma   1411
    Nursing Process: Renal Trauma   1412
  Ureteral Trauma   1412
    Nursing Process: Ureteral Trauma   1413
  Bladder Trauma   1413
    Nursing Process: Bladder Trauma   1414
  Urethral Trauma   1414
    Nursing Process Guidelines: Urethral
    Trauma   1415
Neoplasia   1416
  Cancer of the Kidney   1416
    Nursing Process: Nephrectomy for Cancer of the
    Kidney   1417
  Cancer of the Renal Pelvis and Ureter   1418
    Nursing Process Guidelines: Cancer of the Renal
    Pelvis and Ureter   1419
  Cancer of the Bladder   1419
    Nursing Process: Papillary or Superficial Bladder
    Tumors   1422
    Nursing Process: Nonpapillary or Muscle-Invasive
    Bladder Cancer   1422
  Cancer of the Urethra   1424
    Nursing Process Guidelines: Urethral
    Cancer   1424
The Elderly: Special Considerations   1425

Unit XI

Immune Dysfunction   1427

32
Knowledge Base for Patients with Immune Dysfunction   1429

Anatomy and Physiology   1430
  Generative Lymphoid Organs   1430
    Thymus Gland   1430
    Bone Marrow   1430
  Peripheral Lymphoid Organs   1431
    Lymph Nodes   1431
    Spleen   1431
    Tonsils and Peyer's Patches   1432
    Liver   1432
  Cells of the Immune System   1432
    T Lymphocytes (T Cells)   1433
    B Lymphocytes (B Cells)   1434

The Immune Response   1434
  Nonspecific Immune Response   1435
  Specific Immune Response   1438
Types of Immunity   1441
  Natural Resistance   1441
  Acquired Immunity   1441
Assessment of the Immune System   1442
  Patient History   1442
  Physical Examination   1442
Diagnostic Procedures   1443
  Bone Marrow Aspiration and Biopsy   1443
    Nursing Process: Bone Marrow Aspiration and
    Biopsy   1444
  Laboratory Tests   1445
    Electrophoresis   1445
    Radioimmunoassay   1445
    Immunofluorescence   1445
    Agglutination   1445
    Complement Fixation Test   1445
    Genetic Testing   1446
    Allergy Tests   1446
      Nursing Process Guidelines: Allergy
      Testing   1447
Management   1447
  Immunizations   1447
  Immunosuppressive Therapy   1448
    Antigen-Specific
      Immunosuppression   1448
    Nonspecific Immunosuppression   1448
    Pharmacologic
      Immunosuppression   1448
    Radiation   1449
    Surgery   1449
      Nursing Process Guidelines:
      Immunosuppressive Therapy   1449
  Bone Marrow Transplantation   1449
    Types of Bone Marrow
      Transplantation   1449
    Nursing Process: Bone Marrow
    Transplantation   1451
The Elderly: Special Considerations   1455

33
Nursing Care of Patients with HIV/AIDS and Other Immune Disorders   1457

Immunodeficiency Disorders   1457
  Primary Immunodeficiencies   1457
  Secondary Immunodeficiencies   1458
  Nursing Process Guidelines:
  Immunodeficiency   1459
  Acquired Immunodeficiency Syndrome   1459
    Nursing Process Guidelines: Late Symptomatic and
    Advanced HIV Disease (AIDS)   1471
Hypersensitivity Disorders   1473
  Immediate Hypersensitivity Reactions
  (Type I)   1483

Allergy   1483
Cytotoxic Hypersensitivity Reactions
   (Type II)   1486
Immune Complex Hypersensitivity Reactions
   (Type III)   1486
   Serum Sickness   1487
      Nursing Process: Serum Sickness   1487
   Hypersensitivity Pneumonitides   1488
      Nursing Process: Hypersensitivity
         Pneumonitis   1488
Cell-Mediated Hypersensitivity Reactions
   (Type IV)   1489
   Skin Tests   1489
   Graft Rejection   1489
Autoimmune Disorders   1490
   Systemic Lupus Erythematosus   1490
      Nursing Process: Systemic Lupus
         Erythematosus   1492
   Scleroderma   1494
      Nursing Process Guidelines: Scleroderma   1495
   Autoimmune Hemolytic Anemia   1495
      Nursing Process Guidelines: Autoimmune
         Hemolytic Anemia   1496
   Chronic Fatigue Syndrome   1496
      Nursing Process: Chronic Fatigue
         Syndrome   1497
The Elderly: Special Considerations   1499
   Nursing Process Guidelines: Infection in the Elderly
      Patient   1500

34
Nursing Care of Patients with Oncologic Disorders   1503

Anatomy and Physiology   1503
Pathophysiology   1505
Incidence   1506
   Gender and Age   1506
   Race   1506
   Geography   1508
Etiology   1508
   Genetic Factors   1508
   Environmental Factors   1508
      Chemicals and Toxic Substances   1508
      Tobacco   1509
      Alcohol   1509
      Diet   1509
      Radiation   1510
   Viruses   1510
   Immunologic Defects   1510
   Psychosocial Factors   1510
Clinical Manifestations   1511
   Nursing Process: Cancer Prevention and
      Screening   1511
Diagnosis   1512

Staging   1513
Diagnostic Procedures   1513
   Blood Tests   1513
   Stool Tests   1513
   Cytologic Tests   1513
   Radiographic and Imaging Tests   1514
Nursing Process Guidelines: Diagnostic Tests for
   Cancer   1515
Nursing Process: Newly Diagnosed
   Cancer   1515
Cancer Management   1516
   Surgery   1516
      Preventive Surgery   1516
      Biopsy   1516
      Tumor Removal   1516
      Staging   1516
      Tumor Debulking   1516
      Hormonal Ablation   1516
      Surgical Palliation   1516
      Reconstruction and Rehabilitation   1517
   Nursing Process Guidelines: Cancer
      Surgery   1517
   Radiation   1517
      Therapeutic Uses of Radiation   1517
      Modes of Radiation Therapy   1518
      Safety Precautions   1519
      Side Effects of Radiation Therapy   1520
   Nursing Process: Radiation Therapy   1522
   Chemotherapy   1523
      Classification of Chemotherapeutic
         Agents   1524
      Combination Chemotherapy   1525
      Dosage   1525
      Treatment Schedules   1525
      Delivery of Chemotherapy   1527
      Safe Handling of Chemotherapeutic
         Agents   1528
      Side Effects of Chemotherapy   1528
   Nursing Process: Chemotherapy   1532
   Immunotherapy   1534
      Types of Immunotherapy   1544
      Side Effects   1544
   Unconventional Therapies   1544
      Nursing Process Guidelines: Unconventional
         Therapies   1545
Psychosocial Problems of the Patient Receiving
   Treatment for Cancer   1545
   Anxiety and Fear   1545
   Threats to Self-Concept   1545
   Altered Sexuality   1545
   Profound Loss and Helplessness   1545
   Isolation and Alienation   1545
   Family Stress   1546
   Nursing Process: Psychosocial Needs of Cancer
      Patients   1546
Cultural Considerations   1551
Complications   1551

Pain   1551
    Physiology of Pain   1551
    Pain Management   1552
        Nursing Process: Cancer Pain   1556
    Malnutrition   1558
        Cachexia   1559
        Nutritional Support   1559
        Nursing Process: Nutrition and Cancer   1559
    Home Care   1561
    Hospice Care   1561
The Elderly: Special Considerations   1561
    Nursing Process Guidelines: The Elderly Patient with
    Cancer   1562

Management   1579
    Nonsurgical Management   1579
        Pharmacologic Therapy   1579
        Topical Treatments   1582
        Radiation Therapy   1583
    Surgical Management   1584
        Dermatologic Surgical Procedures   1584
        Closure of Skin Wounds   1586
        Plastic Surgery Procedures   1590
            Nursing Process Guidelines: Rhytidoplasty or
            Liposuction   1591
The Elderly: Special Considerations   1591

Unit XII

Integumentary Dysfunction   1565

35
Knowledge Base for Patients with Integumentary Dysfunction   1567

Anatomy and Physiology   1567
    Epidermis   1567
    Dermis   1568
    Subcutaneous Fat   1568
    Glands   1569
    Hair   1569
    Nails   1569
Clinical Manifestations of Integumentary
    Dysfunction   1570
    Altered Skin Color   1570
    Altered Skin Turgor   1570
    Altered Skin Temperature   1570
    Altered Skin Sensation   1570
    Altered Skin Components: Lesions   1570
        Types of Lesions   1570
        Shapes of Lesions   1573
        Distribution of Lesions   1573
        Arrangement of Lesions   1573
        Evolution of Lesions   1573
        Scars   1573
        Atrophy   1573
Assessment of the Integumentary System   1574
    Patient History   1574
    Physical Examination   1575
Diagnostic Procedures   1575
    Cultures   1576
    Patch Test   1576
    Skin Biopsies   1577
        Types of Skin Biopsy   1577
        Procedures   1577
            Nursing Process Guidelines: Skin Biopsy   1578

36
Nursing Care of Patients with Integumentary Disorders   1595

Infections   1595
    Bacterial Infections   1595
        Nursing Process: Bacterial Skin Infection   1595
        Necrotizing Fasciitis   1599
            Nursing Process Guidelines: Necrotizing
            Fasciitis   1600
    Fungal Infections   1600
        Dermatophyte Infections   1600
            Nursing Process: Dermatophyte
            Infection   1601
        Nondermatophyte Infections   1601
    Viral Infections   1603
        Warts   1603
            Nursing Process Guidelines: Warts   1605
        Molluscum Contagiosum   1605
            Nursing Process Guidelines: Molluscum
            Contagiosum   1605
        Herpes Simplex   1605
            Nursing Process Guidelines: Herpes Simplex
            Virus Type 1 Oral Infection   1606
        Herpes Zoster   1606
            Nursing Process: Herpes Zoster   1606
Inflammations   1607
    Eczematous Dermatitis   1607
        Nonspecific Eczematous Dermatitis   1607
            Nursing Process: Eczema   1608
        Contact Dermatitis   1608
            Nursing Process: Contact Dermatitis   1610
        Seborrheic Dermatitis   1611
            Nursing Process Guidelines: Seborrheic
            Dermatitis   1611
        Stasis Dermatitis   1611
            Nursing Process Guidelines: Stasis
            Dermatitis   1612
    Drug Eruptions   1612
        Nursing Process Guidelines: Drug
        Eruption   1613
    Acne   1613
        Acne Vulgaris   1613

Nursing Process: Acne Vulgaris   1614
Acne Rosacea   1616
Nursing Process Guidelines: Acne
Rosacea   1616
Psoriasis   1616
Nursing Process: Psoriasis   1618
Structural Disorders   1619
Bullous Diseases   1619
Pemphigus Vulgaris   1619
Nursing Process Guidelines: Pemphigus
Vulgaris   1620
Bullous Pemphigoid   1620
Nursing Process Guidelines: Bullous
Pemphigoid   1621
Stings   1621
Nursing Process: Insect Sting   1621
Pressure Ulcers   1622
Nursing Process: Pressure Ulcers   1628
Neoplasia   1631
Benign Neoplasms   1634
Nursing Process: Benign Skin Neoplasm   1634
Malignant Neoplasms   1636
Basal Cell Epithelioma   1636
Squamous Cell Carcinoma   1637
Cutaneous Malignant Melanoma   1638
Nursing Process: Skin Cancer   1638
The Elderly: Special Considerations   1640

37
Nursing Care of Patients with Burns   1643

Assessment of the Burn Injury   1643
History of the Burn Injury   1644
Factors for Determining Burn Severity   1644
Burn Area   1645
Body Part Affected   1645
Burn Depth   1645
Burn Agent   1648
Age of the Patient   1648
Medical History   1648
Associated Injuries   1648
Criteria for Transport to a Burn Center   1648
Care of the Burn Injury   1649
Immediate Phase   1649
Stop the Burning Process   1649
Maintain a Patent Airway   1649
Treat Life-Threatening Injuries   1649
Maintain Peripheral Circulation   1655
Emergent Phase   1655
Respiratory Function   1655
Nursing Process: Altered Respiratory Function
After Burn Injury   1659
Hypovolemia and Electrolyte
Imbalance   1660
Nursing Process: Hypovolemia and Electrolyte
Imbalance After Major Burn Injury   1663

Circumferential Burns   1664
Nursing Process: Circumferential
Burns   1664
Acute Phase   1665
Fluid Mobilization and Electrolyte
Imbalance   1665
Nursing Process: Fluid Mobilization After a
Major Burn Injury   1669
Pain Management   1670
Nursing Process: Pain After a Burn
Injury   1670
Wound Care   1671
Nursing Process: Burn Wound Care   1675
Metabolic Needs   1678
Nursing Process: Increased Metabolic Needs
After Burn Injury   1679
Psychosocial Needs   1680
Nursing Process: Psychosocial Needs After
Burn Injury   1680
Rehabilitation Phase   1681
Contractures   1682
Hypertrophic Scarring   1682
Nursing Process: Rehabilitation After Burn
Injury   1682
Care of the Patient with a Chemical Burn
Injury   1684
Nursing Process Guidelines: Chemical Burn
Injury   1687
Care of the Patient with an Electrical Burn
Injury   1688
Nursing Process Guidelines: Electrical Burn
Injury   1689
Care of the Pregnant Patient After Burn
Injury   1690
The Elderly: Special Considerations   1690

Unit XIII

Reproductive Dysfunction   1693

38
Knowledge Base for Men with Reproductive Dysfunction   1695

Anatomy and Physiology   1695
External Genitalia   1695
Penis   1695
Scrotum   1696
Internal Genitalia   1696
Testes   1696
Epididymis   1697
Vas Deferens   1697
Seminal Vesicles   1697
Ejaculatory Ducts   1697

Prostate Gland   1697
Cowper's Glands   1697
Urethra   1697
Spermatic Cords   1697
Semen   1698
Male Sexual Response   1698
Clinical Manifestations of Male Reproductive
Dysfunction   1698
Sexual Dysfunction   1698
Pain   1699
Urinary Retention   1699
Assessment of the Male Reproductive
System   1700
Patient History   1700
Pelvic Examination   1700
Diagnostic Procedures   1703
Semen Analysis   1703
Laboratory Studies (Blood)   1704
Prostate-Specific Antigen   1704
Prostatic Acid Phosphatase   1704
Alkaline Phosphatase   1704
Alpha-Fetoprotein   1704
Human Chorionic Gonadotropin   1704
Testosterone   1704
Serum Follicle-Stimulating Hormone and
Serum Luteinizing Hormone   1704
Sequential Bacteriologic Localization
Cultures   1704
Visualization Techniques   1705
Urethrocystoscopy   1705
Ultrasonography   1705
Biopsies   1705
Prostate Biopsy   1705
Nursing Process Guidelines: Prostate
Biopsy   1705
Penile Biopsy   1706
Nursing Process Guidelines: Penile
Biopsy   1706
Management   1707
Surgical Management   1707
Vasectomy   1708
Nursing Process Guidelines: Vasectomy   1709
Prostatectomy   1709
Nursing Process: Simple Prostatectomy   1713
Penile Implants   1720
Nursing Process: Implantation of a Penile
Prosthesis   1722
The Elderly: Special Considerations   1724

**39
Nursing Care of Men with Reproductive
Disorders   1727**

Infections and Inflammations   1727
Balanoposthitis   1727
Nursing Process: Balanoposthitis   1728
Epididymitis   1728
Nursing Process: Epididymitis   1729
Orchitis   1731
Nursing Process: Orchitis   1732
Prostatitis   1733
Nursing Process: Prostatitis   1734
Structural Disorders   1735
Phimosis   1735
Nursing Process: Circumcision   1736
Paraphimosis   1737
Nursing Process: Paraphimosis   1738
Cryptorchidism   1739
Nursing Process Guidelines:
Orchiopexy   1739
Priapism   1740
Nursing Process: Priapism   1741
Hydrocele   1741
Nursing Process: Hydrocelectomy   1742
Varicocele   1743
Nursing Process Guidelines:
Varicocelectomy   1744
Neoplasia   1744
Cancer of the Penis   1744
Nursing Process: Penectomy   1747
Cancer of the Testis   1748
Benign Prostatic Hyperplasia   1752
Nursing Process Guidelines:
Prostatectomy   1754
Cancer of the Prostate   1754
Nursing Process Guidelines: Prostate
Cancer   1760
The Elderly: Special Considerations   1761

**40
Knowledge Base for Women with
Reproductive Dysfunction   1765**

Anatomy and Physiology   1765
External Genitalia   1765
Internal Genitalia   1766
Vagina   1766
Uterus   1766
Fallopian Tubes   1767
Ovaries   1767
Female Hormonal Cycle   1768
Proliferative Phase   1768
Secretory Phase   1768
Ischemic Phase   1769
Menstrual Phase   1769

Female Sexual Response   1769
Menopause   1769
  Physical Changes   1771
  Psychosocial Effects   1771
  Symptoms   1771
  Management   1772
  Nursing Process: Menopause   1773
Clinical Manifestations of Female Reproductive
  Dysfunction   1775
  Amenorrhea   1775
  Abnormal Uterine Bleeding   1775
  Leukorrhea   1776
  Dysmenorrhea   1776
    Primary Dysmenorrhea   1776
      Nursing Process: Primary
        Dysmenorrhea   1776
    Secondary Dysmenorrhea   1777
  Intermenstrual Pain   1777
Assessment of the Female Reproductive
  System   1777
  Patient History   1778
  Pelvic Examination   1778
    Patient Preparation   1778
    Examination Procedure   1779
Diagnostic Procedures   1781
  Papanicolaou Test   1781
  Schiller Test   1782
  Colposcopy   1782
  Cervical Biopsy   1783
    Punch Biopsy   1783
    Excision Biopsy   1783
    Cone Biopsy   1783
    Nursing Process Guidelines: Cervical
      Biopsy   1784
  Endometrial Cytology   1784
  Endometrial Biopsy   1785
  Hysteroscopy   1785
  Hysterosalpingography   1785
  Ultrasonography   1785
Management   1786
  Nonsurgical Management   1786
  Surgical Management   1786
    Preoperative Preparation   1786
    Complications of Gynecologic
      Surgery   1787
    Common Gynecologic Surgical
      Procedures   1787
The Elderly: Special Considerations   1800

41
Nursing Care of Women with Reproductive Disorders   1803

Infections and Inflammations   1803
  Vulvitis   1803

Nursing Process: Vulvitis   1804
Vaginitis   1804
  Nursing Process: Vaginitis   1806
Atrophic Vaginitis   1806
  Nursing Process Guidelines: Atrophic
    Vaginitis   1807
Toxic Shock Syndrome   1807
  Nursing Process Guidelines: Toxic Shock
    Syndrome   1808
Functional Disorders   1808
  Premenstrual Syndrome   1808
    Nursing Process: Premenstrual
      Syndrome   1810
  Endometriosis   1810
    Nursing Process Guidelines:
      Endometriosis   1814
Structural Disorders   1815
  Disorders Caused by Weakened Pelvic
    Supports   1815
  Retrodisplacement of the Uterus   1819
    Nursing Process Guidelines: Retrodisplacement of
      the Uterus   1820
  Genital Fistulas   1821
    Nursing Process Guidelines: Vaginal-Intestinal
      Fistula   1822
Neoplasia   1822
  Polyps   1822
    Cervical Polyps   1822
    Endometrial Polyps   1823
    Nursing Process Guidelines: Cervical or
      Endometrial Polyps   1823
  Leiomyomas   1823
    Nursing Process Guidelines: Leiomyomas   1824
  Benign Ovarian Tumors   1824
    Nursing Process Guidelines: Benign Ovarian
      Tumor   1825
  Malignant Neoplasms   1825
    Cancer of the Vulva   1825
    Cancer of the Cervix   1830
    Cancer of the Uterus   1836
      Nursing Process Guidelines: Uterine
        Cancer   1837
    Cancer of the Ovary   1837
      Nursing Process Guidelines: Ovarian
        Cancer   1838
The Elderly: Special Considerations   1838

42
Nursing Care of Patients with Breast Disorders   1841

Anatomy and Physiology   1841
  External Anatomy   1841
  Internal Anatomy   1841
  Physiology   1843
Assessment of the Breast   1843
  Patient History   1843

Physical Examination   1844
Breast Self-Examination   1846
Diagnostic Procedures   1848
Radiologic Examinations   1848
Mammography   1848
Xeromammography   1849
Thermography   1849
Diaphanography   1849
Ultrasonography   1849
Breast Biopsy   1849
Nursing Process: Breast Biopsy   1850
Infections and Inflammations   1852
Mastitis   1852
Nursing Process Guidelines: Mastitis   1852
Mammary Duct Ectasia   1853
Nursing Process Guidelines: Mammary Duct
Ectasia   1853
Structural Disorders   1853
Gynecomastia   1853
Nursing Process Guidelines:
Gynecomastia   1854
Neoplasia   1854
Benign Breast Disease   1854
Fibrocystic Breast Disease   1854
Nursing Process: Fibrocystic Breast
Disease   1855
Fibroadenoma   1856
Nursing Process Guidelines: Excision of a
Fibroadenoma   1856
Intraductal Papilloma   1856
Nursing Process Guidelines: Excision of an
Intraductal Papilloma   1857
Cancer of the Breast   1857
Plastic Surgery Procedures   1875
Breast Reconstruction   1875
Procedures   1876
Complications   1878
Nursing Process: Breast Reconstruction
Surgery   1878
Augmentation Mammoplasty   1879
Nursing Process Guidelines: Augmentation
Mammoplasty   1879
Reduction Mammoplasty   1879
Dermal Mastopexy   1880
Nursing Process Guidelines: Reduction
Mammoplasty or Dermal Mastopexy   1880
The Elderly: Special Considerations   1880

43
Nursing Care of Patients with Sexually
Transmitted Diseases   1883

Sexually Transmitted Vaginitis   1883
Vulvovaginal Candidiasis   1884
Trichomoniasis   1885
Gardnerella vaginalis Vaginitis   1886

Nursing Process: Vaginitis   1886
Genital Herpes   1889
Nursing Process: Genital Herpes   1904
Gonorrhea   1908
Nursing Process: Gonorrhea   1910
Syphilis   1914
Nursing Process: Syphilis   1917
Chlamydia trachomatis   1920
Nursing Process: Chlamydia trachomatis
Infection   1922
Nongonococcal Urethritis   1924
Nursing Process Guidelines: Nongonococcal
Urethritis   1925
Condylomata Acuminata   1926
Nursing Process Guidelines: Genital Warts   1928
Pediculosis Pubis   1928
Nursing Process: Pediculosis Pubis   1929
Scabies   1929
Nursing Process Guidelines: Scabies   1930

Unit XIV

Eye and Ear Dysfunction   1933

44
Knowledge Base for Patients with Eye Dysfunction   1935

Anatomy and Physiology   1935
Protective Structures of the Eye   1935
Muscles Controlling the Eye   1936
Eyeball Structure   1936
External Coat   1936
Middle Coat   1937
Inner Coat   1937
Inner Structure of the Globe   1937
Normal Vision and the Visual
Pathways   1938
Clinical Manifestations of Eye Dysfunction   1938
Blurred Vision   1938
Diplopia   1938
Photopsia   1939
Floaters   1939
Scotomata   1939
Photophobia   1939
Pain   1939
Loss of Vision   1939
Assessment of the Eye   1939
Patient History   1939
Physical Examination   1940
Visual Acuity   1940
Outer Eye Structures   1942
Extraocular Muscles   1943
Visual Fields   1943

Color Vision 1943
Ocular Fundus 1944
Diagnostic Procedures 1944
Measurement of Intraocular Pressure 1944
Slit-Lamp Examination 1945
Topical Fluorescein Staining 1945
Gonioscopy 1945
Fluorescein Angiography 1945
Ultrasonography 1945
Computed Tomography 1946
Magnetic Resonance Imaging 1946
Electroretinography 1946
Visual Evoked Potentials 1946
Management 1946
Pharmacologic Therapy 1946
Understanding Ophthalmic
Medications 1947
Administering Ophthalmic
Medications 1948
Surgical Interventions 1950
Ocular Surgery 1950
Nursing Process: Ocular Surgery 1951
Corneal Transplant 1954
Nursing Process Guidelines: Corneal
Transplant 1954
Enucleation 1955
Nursing Process Guidelines:
Enucleation 1956
Laser Therapy 1957
Nursing Process Guidelines: Laser Therapy
for an Eye Disorder 1958
Supportive Treatment for the Patient with Low
Vision 1958
Optical Aids 1958
Electronic Aids 1958
Nonoptical Accessory Aids 1959
The Elderly: Special Considerations 1961

45
Nursing Care of Patients with Eye Disorders 1963

Infections and Inflammations 1963
Conjunctivitis 1963
Nursing Process: Conjunctivitis 1964
Keratitis 1964
Nursing Process: Keratitis 1965
Other Infections and Inflammations 1967
Structural Disorders 1970
Refractive Errors 1970
Nursing Process Guidelines: Correction of
Refractive Error 1974
Entropion and Ectropion 1974
Nursing Process Guidelines: Entropion or
Ectropion 1975

Cataracts 1975
Nursing Process: Cataract Surgery 1977
Glaucoma 1978
Nursing Process: Glaucoma 1980
Nursing Process Guidelines: Laser Therapy for
Glaucoma 1982
Retinal Holes, Tears, and Detachments 1982
Nursing Process: Surgery for Retinal
Detachment 1984
Degenerative Disorders 1985
Macular Degeneration 1985
Nursing Process Guidelines: Macular
Degeneration 1986
Trauma 1987
Contusions, Abrasions, Lacerations, and
Penetrating Injuries 1987
Nursing Process: Ocular Trauma 1988
Chemical Burns 1989
Nursing Process Guidelines: Chemical Ocular
Burn 1991
Neoplasia 1991
The Elderly: Special Considerations 1991

46
Knowledge Base for Patients with Ear Dysfunction 1995

Anatomy and Physiology 1995
External Ear 1995
Middle Ear 1995
Inner Ear 1996
Process of Hearing 1997
Clinical Manifestations of Ear Dysfunction 1997
Hearing Loss 1997
Conductive Hearing Loss 1997
Sensorineural Hearing Loss 1997
Mixed Hearing Loss 1998
Severity of Hearing Loss 1998
Otalgia 1998
Otorrhea 1998
Tinnitus 1998
Vertigo 1998
Assessment of the Ear and Hearing 1999
Patient History 1999
Physical Examination 2000
Diagnostic Procedures 2001
Pneumatoscopy 2001
Tuning Fork Tests 2001
Audiometric Testing 2001
Vestibular Tests 2001
Management 2002
Pharmacologic Therapy 2003
Vestibular Rehabilitation 2003
Surgical Interventions 2003
Complications of Ear Surgery 2003

Common Surgical Procedures Performed on
the Ear   2003
The Elderly: Special Considerations   2009

47
Nursing Care of Patients with Ear Disorders   2011

Infections and Inflammations   2011
External Ear Infections   2011
Nursing Process Guidelines: External Ear
Infection   2012
Middle-Ear Infections   2012
Nursing Process Guidelines: Otitis Media or
Mastoiditis   2012
Labyrinthitis   2013
Nursing Process Guidelines: Labyrinthitis   2014
Structural Disorders   2014
Perforation of the Tympanic Membrane   2014
Nursing Process Guidelines: Perforated Tympanic
Membrane   2015
Otosclerosis   2015
Nursing Process Guidelines:
Stapedectomy   2016

Meniere's Disease   2016
Nursing Process: Meniere's Disease   2018
The Elderly: Special Considerations   2019
Presbycusis   2019
Nursing Process: Presbycusis   2019

Appendix 1

Reference Values for Laboratory Tests   2023

Appendix 2

Common Abbreviations   2033

Appendix 3

Resources   2037

Index   2047

Special Features

■■■■■▶ Clinical Pathways

Chapter

6 Endoscopy   116
8 Heart Failure   273
8 Coronary Artery Bypass Grafting   290
16 Pneumonia   644
17 Lumbar Laminectomy with Fusion   763
19 Amputation   875
20 Open Reduction and Internal Fixation of a Hip
    Fracture   926

Chapter

21 Colon Resection   1001
24 Open Cholecystectomy   1115
31 Acute Renal Failure   1392
39 Transurethral Resection of the Prostate   1755
40 Total Abdominal Hysterectomy   1796
42 Modified Radical Mastectomy or Lumpectomy
    with Axillary Node Dissection   1869

? Clinical Thinking

Chapter

8 Somnolence and Anxiety in a Patient on
   Digoxin Therapy   254
8 Dyspnea, Restlessness, and Anxiety in a Patient
   with a History of Myocardial Infarction   281
10 Sudden Abdominal Pain in a Patient with an
    Aortic Aneurysm   368
11 Flushing and Apprehension After Cardiac
    Catheterization   418
13 Fatigue, Weakness, and Dyspnea in a Patient
    Receiving a Blood Transfusion   483
14 Restlessness, Confusion, and Irritability in a
    Patient on Home Ventilator Support   572
15 Severe Dyspnea, Tachypnea, and Anxiety After
    Laryngectomy   624
16 Dyspnea, Chest Pain, and Anxiety After Pelvic
    Surgery   684
17 Headache After a Skiing Accident   735
18 Decreased Level of Consciousness in a 74-Year-
    Old Woman   810
20 Confusion, Tachycardia, and Tachypnea After a
    Fractured Hip   928

Chapter

21 Weakness, Headache, Thirst, and Nocturia
    in a Patient on Total Parenteral
    Nutrition   991
22 "Indigestion" After a Large Meal   1030
24 Abdominal Pain, Pallor, and Diaphoresis in a
    Man with Gallbladder Disease   1119
26 Coffee-Ground Vomitus in an Alcoholic
    Patient   1184
28 Palpitations, Diaphoresis, Pallor, and Anxiety
    in a Diabetic Patient   1260
29 Paresthesias After Thyroidectomy   1311
30 Anuria After Vascular Surgery   1337
34 Nausea, Chills, and Restlessness After
    Chemotherapy   1533
37 Hemorrhage After Severe Burn
    Injury   1666
38 Restlessness and Pain After Prosta-
    tectomy   1716
40 Abdominal Pain and Moist Dressings After
    Hysterectomy   1788

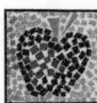

Health Promotion & Risk Reduction Highlights

Chapter

4 Maintaining Wellness in Older Adults   69
7 Cardiac Disease   189
8 Reducing Risk Factors for Patients with Coronary Artery Disease   285
9 Methods for Optimizing Peripheral Vascular Function and Reducing Risk Factors for Peripheral Vascular Disease   338
10 Self-Care for Prevention of Foot Problems in Vascular Disorders   355
12 Optimal Hematologic System Function   442
13 Sickle-Cell Anemia   485
14 Optimal Respiratory System Function   532
15 Laryngeal Cancer   617
16 Guidelines for Prevention of Hospital-Acquired Pneumonia   642
16 Preventing Tuberculosis Transmission in the Home-Care Setting   656
17 Optimal Neurologic System Function   746
18 Measures to Reduce Stress on the Lumbar Spine   794
18 Measures to Reduce the Risk of Cerebrovascular Accident   806
19 Optimal Musculoskeletal System Function   849
20 Preventing Lyme Disease   902
20 Osteoporosis   907
21 Optimal Gastrointestinal System Function   969
22 Self-Examination for Facial and Oral Cancer   1053
23 Strategies for Reducing the Risk of Colorectal Cancer   1100

Chapter

24 Primary Prevention of Gallstone Formation   1110
25 Guidelines for Maintaining a Healthy Liver   1159
27 Optimal Endocrine System Function   1219
30 Optimal Urinary System Function   1343
31 Self-Care for Prevention of Urinary Tract Infections   1372
31 Maintaining the Health of the Remaining Kidney   1418
32 Optimal Immune System Function   1443
32 Measures to Prevent Skin Damage After Bone Marrow Transplantation   1453
33 Infection Control Guidelines for Caregivers of People with HIV/AIDS   1472
33 Preventing Allergic Reactions   1486
33 Protecting Against Ultraviolet Light Rays   1494
34 Health Practices That May Reduce Cancer Risk   1512
35 Care of the Skin   1575
36 Preventing Recurrence of Dermatophyte Infections   1602
36 Instructions for Patients Allergic to Hymenoptera Stings   1622
36 Preventing and Detecting Skin Cancer   1636
38 Optimal Male Reproductive Function   1702
40 Optimal Female Reproductive Function   1779
44 Preventive Care of the Eyes   1941
46 Preventive Care of the Ears   2000

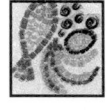

Nutrition Highlights

Chapter

4 Nutritional Needs of the Elderly   53
7 Potassium-Rich Foods   183
7 Foods High in Saturated and Unsaturated Fats   184
7 High-Sodium and Low-Sodium Foods   185
8 Dietary Guidelines for the Patient with Heart Failure   276
10 Diet Guidelines for Prevention of Atherosclerosis   363
10 Instructions for the Patient on a Low-Sodium Diet   382

Chapter

12 Requirements for Blood Cell Production   441
13 Special Considerations for Patients with Iron Deficiency Anemia   470
13 Food Sources for High-Protein, High-Vitamin Diets   472
14 Special Considerations for Patients with Endotracheal Tubes, Tracheostomy Tubes, or Mechanical Ventilation   563
15 Special Considerations for Patients with Pharyngitis and Tonsillitis   606
15 Discharge Instructions After Tonsillectomy   608

16 Common Nutritional Problems and Interventions for Patients with Pneumonia   646

16 Special Considerations for Patients with Chronic Obstructive Pulmonary Disease   678

20 High-Purine and Low-Purine Foods   901

20 Calcium Content of Some Common Foods   904

21 Special Considerations for Patients with a Colostomy   1009

21 Strategies for Reducing the Risk of Complications Following an Ileostomy   1014

22 Special Considerations for Patients with Hiatus Hernia   1044

23 Special Considerations for Patients with Crohn's Disease   1069

23 Special Considerations for Patients with Gluten-Induced Enteropathy   1080

23 Special Considerations for Patients with Lactase Deficiency   1081

23 Special Considerations for Patients with Diverticular Disease   1084

24 Special Considerations for the Patient with Cholecystitis   1111

24 Special Considerations for Patients with Pancreatitis   1122

25 Sample Daily Food Allowances for a 1000 mg Sodium-Restricted Diet   1143

25 Sample Daily Food Allowances for a 40 g Protein-Restricted Diet   1151

28 Meal-Planning Guidelines for Patients with Diabetes Mellitus   1233

30 Objectives of Diet Therapy for Patients with Chronic Renal Failure   1366

30 Calcium-Containing Foods   1367

31 Dietary Needs Related to Type of Calculus   1383

31 Dietary Restrictions in Acute and Chronic Renal Failure   1391

34 Special Considerations for Patients with Cancer   1560

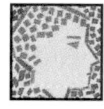

Patient Education Highlights

Chapter

4 Self-Administration of Medications for the Elderly   55

5 Use of Oral Potassium Supplements   88

6 Preoperative Patient Preparation and Teaching   129

6 Postoperative Patient Teaching   156

7 Discharge Instructions After Cardiac Catheterization   201

7 Special Instructions for Patients Taking Diuretics   218

8 Continuous Intravenous Antibiotic Therapy Administered at Home for Infective Endocarditis   235

8 Instructions for the Patient Recovering from Infective Endocarditis   236

8 Instructions for the Patient with an Implantable Cardioverter-Defibrillator   261

8 Discharge Instructions After Coronary Artery Bypass Grafting   291

8 Discharge Instructions After Myocardial Infarction   303

9 General Patient Instructions After Angioplasty   345

10 Discharge Instructions for the Patient with Buerger's Disease   353

Chapter

10 Relaxation Exercise for the Patient with Vascular Disease   354

10 Discharge Instructions for the Patient with Raynaud's Disease   356

10 Stepped Care Guidelines for the Patient with Hypertension   382

10 Behavior Modification Program for Improving Compliance with a Treatment Plan   383

10 Discharge Instructions for the Patient with Thrombophlebitis   388

10 Application of Antiembolic Stockings to Prevent Venous Stasis   389

11 Prevention of Anaphylaxis   422

12 Oral Hygiene   439

12 Prevention of Infection   440

12 Signs and Symptoms of Delayed Transfusion Reactions   462

13 Self-Care for a Bleeding Disorder   482

13 Methods to Prevent Infection in Leg Ulcers Related to Sickle-Cell Crisis   487

13 Prevention of Acute Attacks of Glucose-6-Phosphate Dehydrogenase Deficiency   488

13 Self-Care for Prevention of Leukemia Complications   504

14 Transtracheal Oxygen Therapy   558

14   Discharge Instructions After Pneumo-
      nectomy   585
15   Care for the Common Cold   600
15   Nonpharmacologic Treatments for
      Sinusitis   603
15   Discharge Instructions After Tonsil-
      lectomy   608
15   Discharge Instructions After Total
      Laryngectomy   631
16   Managing Acute Bronchitis   640
16   Recuperating from Pneumonia   646
16   Prevention and Treatment of Respiratory
      Irritation and Infection in Patients with
      Chronic Obstructive Pulmonary
      Disease   671
16   Managing Lung Cancer   699
18   Coping with Parkinson's Disease   789
18   Self-Care Related to Seizures   799
19   Discharge Instructions After Cast
      Application   857
19   Discharge Instructions After Application of an
      Internal Fixation Device   867
19   Care of the Skin and Prosthesis After an
      Amputation   878
20   Discharge Instructions for Patients with
      Osteoarthritis   898
21   Information for the Patient Having an
      Esophagogastroduodenoscopy   975
21   Self-Care After a Colonoscopy   976
21   Self-Care After an Ileostomy   1014
22   Use of Antacids   1043
22   Self-Management for Dysphagia   1046
22   Discharge Instructions After Intermaxillary
      Fixation   1049
22   Wound Care After Surgery for Oral
      Cancer   1052
23   Self-Care After Appendectomy   1066
23   Preventing Recurrence of Symptomatic
      Diverticulosis or Diverticulitis   1084
23   Self-Care After a Herniorrhaphy   1096
23   Self-Care After a Hemorrhoidectomy   1098
24   Discharge Instructions After Conventional
      Cholecystectomy with T-Tube Insertion   1117
25   Self-Management of Diuretic Therapy   1144
25   Self-Management of a LeVeen Shunt   1148
27   Self-Management of Endocrine
      Dysfunction   1219
28   Guidelines for Preparation and Injection of
      Insulin   1236
28   Guidelines for Taking Sulfonylureas   1240
28   Guidelines for Self-Monitoring of Blood
      Glucose   1242
28   Guidelines for Self-Care and Monitoring of
      Long-Term Degenerative Changes of Diabetes
      Mellitus   1252

29   Self-Management: Desmopressin Acetate
      Administration for Diabetes
      Insipidus   1276
29   Self-Management: Adrenocortical Insufficiency
      (Addison's Disease)   1284
30   Kegel Exercises   1365
30   Bladder Drills   1366
31   Self-Care for the Renal Transplant
      Patient   1410
32   Essentials of Self-Care After Bone Marrow
      Transplantation   1454
33   Tips to Relieve Nausea in People with
      AIDS   1473
33   Oral Care for the Patient with HIV
      Infection   1473
33   Symptoms That Require Immediate Medical
      Evaluation in the Patient with AIDS   1483
33   Managing Fatigue in Systemic Lupus
      Erythematosus   1493
34   Self-Care During External Radiation
      Therapy   1523
35   Self-Care After Skin Biopsy   1579
35   Self-Care After Dermatologic Cryo-
      surgery   1585
35   Self-Care After Dermatologic Carbon Dioxide
      Laser Surgery   1586
35   Self-Care of Grafts and Protection of
      New Skin   1590
35   Self-Care After Rhytidoplasty   1592
35   Self-Care After Liposuction   1592
36   Preventing the Spread of Bacterial Skin
      Infections   1599
36   Reducing Pruritus Caused by Psoriasis   1619
37   Discharge Instructions for Burn Care   1685
38   Testicular Self-Examination   1703
38   Discharge Instructions After
      Vasectomy   1710
38   Discharge Instructions After Prosta-
      tectomy   1720
38   Discharge Instructions After Penile Implant
      Surgery   1724
39   Preventing Recurrent Balanoposthitis   1729
39   Discharge Instructions After Circum-
      cision   1737
39   Discharge Instructions After
      Orchiopexy   1740
39   Discharge Instructions After Hydro-
      celectomy   1743
39   Using a Cunningham Clamp   1760
40   Basic Health Practices for the Postmenopausal
      Woman   1774
40   Discharge Instructions After Cervical
      Biopsy   1784
40   Discharge Instructions After Lapa-
      roscopy   1790

40 Self-Care After Gynecologic Laser Surgery   1791
40 Discharge Instructions After Dilatation and Curettage   1793
40 Discharge Instructions After Hysterectomy   1800
41 Preventing Vulvitis   1805
41 Vaginitis   1807
41 Preventing Toxic Shock Syndrome   1808
41 Relieving Premenstrual Syndrome   1809
41 Special Considerations for Patients with Premenstrual Syndrome   1812
41 Pelvic Floor Exercises   1817
41 Self-Care After Posterior Colporrhaphy   1819
41 Discharge Instructions After Radical Vulvectomy   1829
41 Discharge Instructions After Internal Radiation for Cancer of the Cervix   1835
42 Self-Care Measures for Relief of Discomfort Associated with Fibrocystic Breast Disease   1856
42 Hand and Arm Precautions After Modified Radical Mastectomy   1866
42 Postmastectomy Exercises   1867

42 Self-Care After Breast Reconstruction Surgery   1879
43 Sexually Transmitted Vaginal Infections   1901
43 Symptomatic Relief of Genital Herpes   1906
43 Preventing Transmission and Complications of Genital Herpes   1907
43 Treatment of Pediculosis Pubis   1929
44 Discharge Instructions After Eye Surgery   1953
44 Self-Care After Corneal Transplant   1955
44 Removal, Care, and Insertion of An Ocular Prosthesis   1956
45 Preventing the Spread of Conjunctivitis   1965
45 Preventing and Treating Blepharitis, Hordeolum, and Chalazion   1970
45 Removal, Cleaning, and Insertion of Contact Lenses   1972
46 Discharge Instructions After Tympanoplasty   2005
47 Preventing External Otitis   2012
47 Serous Otitis Media   2014
47 Discharge Instructions After Stapedectomy   2017

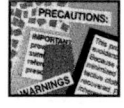

Pharmacology Highlights

Chapter

5 Potassium Supplements   87
7 Cardiac Glycosides   211
7 Nitrates   212
7 Alpha-Adrenergic Blocking Agents   213
7 Angiotensin-Converting Enzyme Inhibitors   214
7 Calcium Channel Blocking Agents   215
7 Anti-Arrhythmic Agents   216
7 Diuretics (Antihypertensives)   217
7 Antilipemics   218
8 Thrombolytic Agents   296
9 Lipid-Lowering Drugs (Hypolipidemics)   343
9 Anticoagulants   344
10 Beta-Adrenergic Blocking Agents   379
12 Plasma Substitutes   456
13 Epoetin Alfa   469
13 Hematinics   477
13 Filgrastim   492
13 Hemostatics   516
14 Decongestants   574
14 Antitussives   575
14 Bronchodilators   576

Chapter

17 Osmotic Diuretics   732
18 Cholinesterase Inhibitors (Anticholinesterase Agents)   783
18 Anticonvulsants   797
19 Skeletal Muscle Relaxants   846
20 Nonsteroidal Anti-Inflammatory Drugs (NSAIDs)   893
20 Uricosuric Drugs   900
20 Oral Calcium Supplements   903
20 Bone Resorption Inhibitors: Biphosphate-Alendronate Sodium   906
21 Laxatives   962
21 Nonspecific Antidiarrheal Agents   964
21 Antacids   967
22 Antacids   1021
22 Drugs That Decrease Gastric Acid Secretion   1022
24 Pancreatic Enzymes   1123
25 Bile Acid Sequestrants   1141
25 Neomycin Sulfate   1151
25 Lactulose   1152
26 Metronidazole (Flagyl)   1180

26 Cyclosporine   1197
29 Antidiuretic Hormones   1276
29 Adrenocorticosteroids   1285
29 Thyroid Hormone Preparations   1305
29 Thiomide Antithyroid Drugs   1309

33 Antihistamines   1484
40 Estrogens   1772
41 Progesterones   1814
44 Mydriatics   1947
44 Miotics   1948

Internet Connections

Chapter

 8 Cardiac Disorders   287
10 Vascular Disorders   361
13 Hematologic Disorders   506
15 Upper Respiratory Disorders   629
16 Lower Respiratory Disorders   665
18 Neurologic Disorders   779
20 Musculoskeletal Disorders   896
22 Upper Gastrointestinal System Disorders   1056
23 Lower Gastrointestinal System Disorders   1068
24 Disorders of the Accessory Organs of Digestion   1113
26 Hepatic Disorders   1176
28 Diabetes Mellitus   1258
29 Endocrine Disorders   1295

Chapter

31 Urinary Disorders   1425
33 HIV/AIDS and Other Immune Disorders   1498
34 Oncologic Disorders   1547
36 Integumentary Disorders   1639
37 Burn Injuries   1682
39 Disorders of the Male Reproductive System   1752
41 Disorders of the Female Reproductive System   1815
42 Breast Disorders   1864
43 Sexually Transmitted Diseases   1922
45 Eye Disorders   1986
47 Ear Disorders   2018

Nursing Care Guides

Chapter

 4 Promoting Compliance with Medication Regimen by Elderly Adults   56
 4 Geriatric Patients   70
 7 Patients Undergoing Cardiac Catheterization   203
 8 Patients Surviving a Cardiac Arrest   265
 9 Patients Undergoing Diagnostic Testing for Peripheral Vascular Dysfunction   341
10 Patients with Vasospastic Disorder (Raynaud's Disease)   358
10 Patients with Varicose Veins   391
12 Patients Receiving an Autologous Blood Transfusion   454
12 Patients with a Blood Transfusion Reaction   459
13 Patients with Acute Hemorrhagic Anemia   473
13 Patients with Chronic Lymphocytic Leukemia   497
13 Patients with Lymphomas   509
14 Patients Undergoing a Lobectomy   588

Chapter

15 Patients Undergoing Nasal Surgery   613
15 Patients Undergoing Conservation (Supraglottic) Laryngectomy   619
15 Postoperative Patients with a Radical Neck Dissection   634
16 Patients Undergoing Pneumonectomy for Cancer of the Lung   700
17 Patients Undergoing Lumbar Puncture   755
19 Patients Undergoing Total Joint Replacement   869
20 Patients Undergoing Surgery for a Fractured Femur   920
20 Patients Undergoing Surgery for Osteosarcoma   939
22 Patients Undergoing Subtotal Gastrectomy for Duodenal Ulcer Disease   1034
23 Patient Care After a Temporary Colostomy for Diverticular Disease   1085
25 Patients with Major Clinical Manifestations of Liver Dysfunction   1155

26 Patients with Cirrhosis   1190
28 Patients with Diabetes Mellitus   1244
29 Patient Care After Transsphenoidal
    Microsurgery for Excision of a Pituitary
    Adenoma   1270
29 Patients with Acute Adrenocortical
    Insufficiency: Addison's Crisis   1282
29 Patient Care After Adrenalectomy for Cushing's
    Syndrome   1290
29 Patients Learning Self-Management of
    Hypothyroidism   1303
29 Patients with Acute Hypoparathyroidism:
    Hypocalcemic Tetany   1319

30 Patients Undergoing Cystoscopy   1354
31 Patients with Renal Calculi   1381
31 Patients with Chronic Renal Failure   1395
33 Patients with Late Symptomatic and Advanced
    HIV Disease (AIDS)   1474
37 Patients with Thermal Burn Injuries   1650
42 Patients Having a Lumpectomy and
    Axillary Node Dissection for Cancer of the
    Breast   1870
43 Patients with Sexually Transmitted
    Diseases   1890

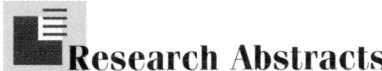

Research Abstracts

Chapter

 3 What Attitudes Do Nurses Hold Toward
    Euthanasia?   42
 5 What Role Do Electrolytes Play in Regulating
    Blood Pressure in Older Adults?   100
 6 Do Men and Women Cope Differently with
    Surgery?   120
 8 What Keeps People From Practicing Self-Care
    After a Myocardial Infarction?   299
 8 How Much Do Nurses Really Know About
    Recovery from Myocardial Infarctions?   301
10 Who Is at Risk for Development of Abdominal
    Aortic Aneurysms?   370
12 Does Aspirin Prevent Thrombotic Events in
    People with High Cholesterol?   432
14 Are Oximetry Probe Sheaths Effective?   545
14 What Care of Endotracheal Tube Cuffs Is
    Provided in Clinical Practice?   562
16 Are There Any Good Noninvasive Alternatives
    to Mechanical Ventilation in Chronic
    Obstructive Pulmonary Disease?   672
18 Does Cognitive Screening Help Prevent
    Disability in Young Patients with Mild Brain
    Injuries?   817
20 What Is It Like to Care for a Friend or
    Family Member Recovering from a Hip
    Fracture?   925
21 How Common Is Gastrointestinal Bleeding in
    ICU Patients with Strokes?   966

Chapter

26 What Hepatitis B Immunization Regimen
    Is Safe and Effective for Elderly
    Adults?   1175
28 How Effective Are Weight-Loss Strategies for
    People with Type II Diabetes?   1252
30 What Pads Work Best for Managing Urinary
    Incontinence in Women?   1339
33 What Factors Influence the Attitudes of Nurses
    Toward Patients with AIDS?   1470
34 What Approaches to Mouth Care Do Nurses
    Use for Patients Receiving Radiation Therapy to
    the Head and Neck?   1521
37 Can a 19th Century Dressing Promote Skin
    Graft Healing in the 1990s?   1676
39 Does Education Improve Prostate Cancer
    Awareness in African-American Men?   1756
40 How Can Nurses Develop Teaching Materials to
    Prepare Women for the Experience of
    Gynecologic Procedures?   1782
41 What Side Effects of Internal Radiation Therapy
    Are Most Common?   1833
42 How Can Nurses Best Help Women and Their
    Partners Facing a Breast Biopsy?   1850
43 What Factors Influence Condom Use in
    Divorced and Separated Women?   1924
44 What Do Patients Think of Outpatient Eye
    Surgery?   1950

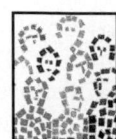 *S*ociocultural Perspectives

Chapter

4 The Elderly and the Cost of Chronic
      Illness   62
10 Planning Self-Care for the Homeless
      Person   394
16 Overcoming Language Barriers   666

Chapter

28 Cultural Competence in Nursing Care   1230
33 Access to Care   1462
43 The Impact of Changes in Family
      Structure on Health Care   1919

Unit I

Knowledge Base for Medical-Surgical Nursing

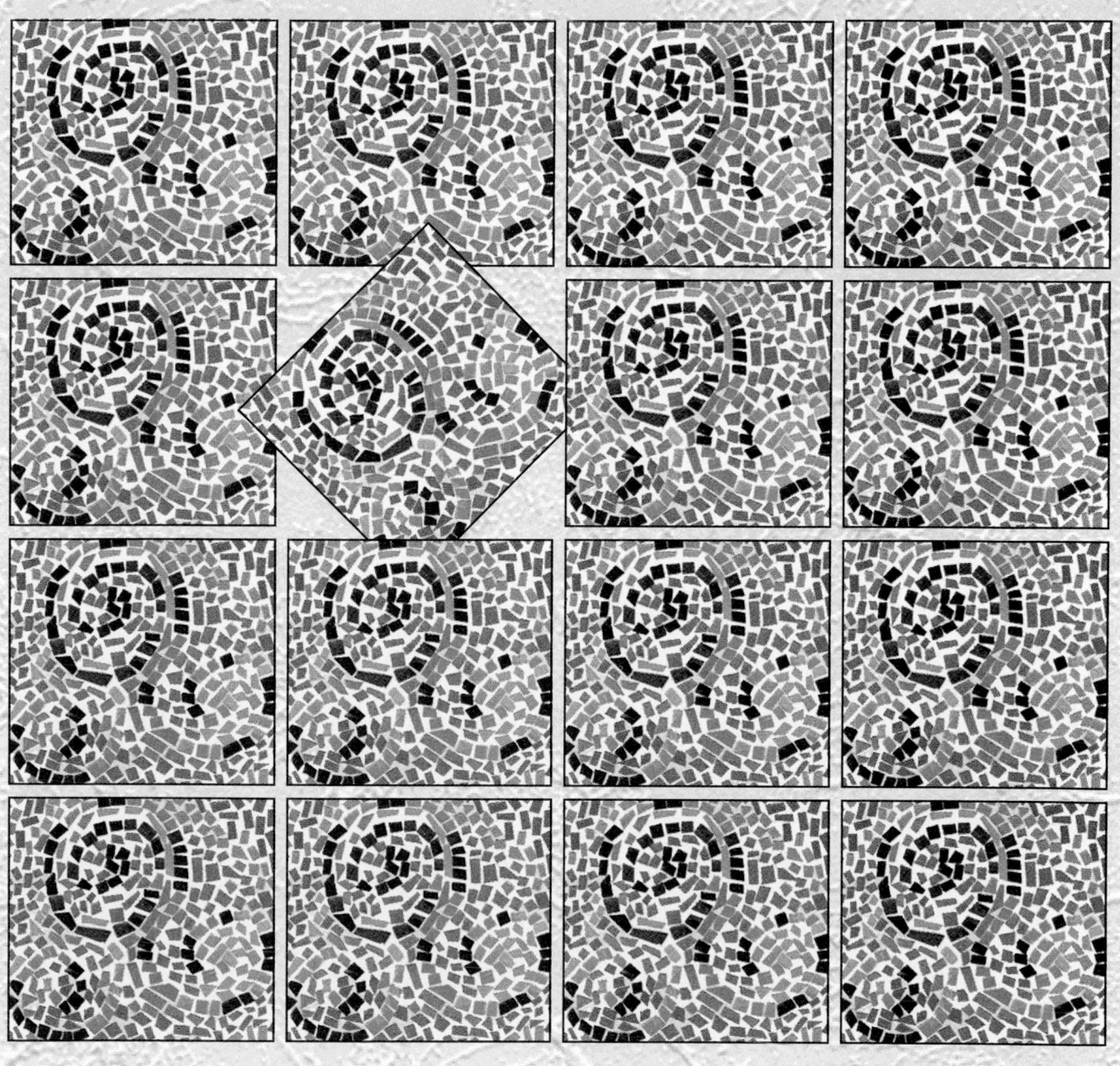

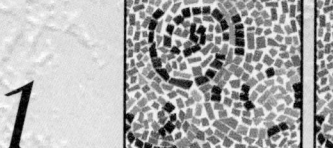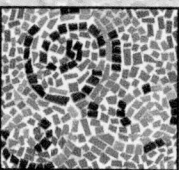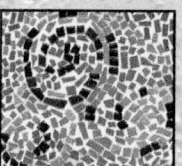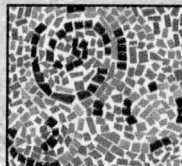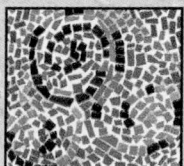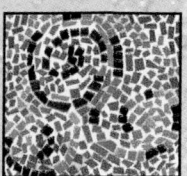

Introduction to the Practice of Medical-Surgical Nursing

Study Outcomes

After studying this chapter, you should be able to:

1. Describe the nature and scope of medical-surgical nursing practice.
2. List types of, and requirements for, certification in the area of medical-surgical nursing.
3. Identify major trends in the practice of medical-surgical nursing.
4. Define the standards of medical-surgical nursing practice.
5. Discuss the importance of Clinical Practice Guidelines in planning care for medical-surgical patients.
6. Explain the steps of the nursing process and their application to the practice of medical-surgical nursing.
7. Define clinical pathways and describe their use in medical-surgical nursing.
8. Describe the concept of culturally sensitive care.
9. Identify the national health promotion and disease prevention objectives that affect the nursing care of adults.

Scope of Medical-Surgical Nursing Practice

Medical-surgical nursing refers to the nursing care of adults with existing or predicted physiologic alteration, trauma, or disability (ANA, 1980). Within the broad range of medical-surgical nursing, there are specialized areas of practice. They include cardiovascular nursing, emergency nursing, gynecologic nursing, and infection-control nursing. Other specialties exist as well, and more are emerging as nursing expands and changes. Some medical-surgical nurses limit their practice to the care of patients with certain disorders. For example, medical-surgical nurses may limit their practice to the care of patients with respiratory diseases, diabetes, burns, eye disorders, ostomies, wounds, or other conditions. Medical-surgical nursing is practiced in a variety of settings. These include acute-care hospitals, urgent-care centers, health maintenance organizations, extended-care facilities, clinics, neighborhood health centers, schools, industrial settings, and patients' homes.

Nature of Medical-Surgical Nursing Practice

In the practice of medical-surgical nursing, all influences on health status are considered. Also considered are the related social and behavioral problems that arise as a result of the patient's physiologic condition. Practice is based on the nursing process, which encompasses patient assessment, nursing diagnosis, planning, implementation, and evaluation. Nursing care includes the following:

- Provision of comfort
- Promotion and maintenance of health
- Prevention, detection, and treatment of illness
- Restoration of function
- Assistance with a peaceful death

Through the nursing process, medical-surgical nursing care can be individualized to meet the unique needs of each patient. The nurse must be concerned not only with the physiologic component of the patient's response to a health disorder. She or he must also be concerned with psychologic, social, cultural, and spiritual components. Thus, the medical-surgical nurse must

- Understand principles and concepts from the basic biologic, physical, and social sciences
- Have a basic knowledge of the development, diagnosis, and treatment of disease
- Have a firm foundation in nursing theory, nursing skills, and use of the nursing process

Preparation for Medical-Surgical Nursing Practice

Medical-surgical nurses are prepared in a variety of ways and at different educational levels. Some are educated in hospital diploma schools, but most receive their education in colleges and universities. Generalist nurses are prepared at the associate or baccalaureate level. Advanced-practice nurses are educated at the master's or doctoral level. The role of the graduate of each level expands and changes as nursing adapts to meet society's needs.

Basic nursing study prepares the student to be a *generalist medical-surgical nurse*. The generalist has a broad base of knowledge and can function in a variety of settings. Generalist nurses may provide bedside care. More frequently, they assume responsibility for total patient care. This includes managing the work of others through assessing needs, delegating tasks, and maintaining accountability for the full range of nursing activities accomplished on behalf of

their patients. As with all medical-surgical nurses, generalist nurses monitor critical events. They make prompt judgment calls. They mobilize resources in a timely and efficient manner. And they ensure patient satisfaction. Whatever their work, generalist nurses structure their activities around the nursing process.

Medical-surgical nurse specialists are prepared through advanced study of medical-surgical nursing at the graduate level. Medical-surgical advanced-practice nurses may be either nurse practitioners or clinical nurse specialists.

Nurse practitioners engage in independent or collaborative nursing practice or both. They have advanced knowledge and skills that enable them to function as primary health-care providers who

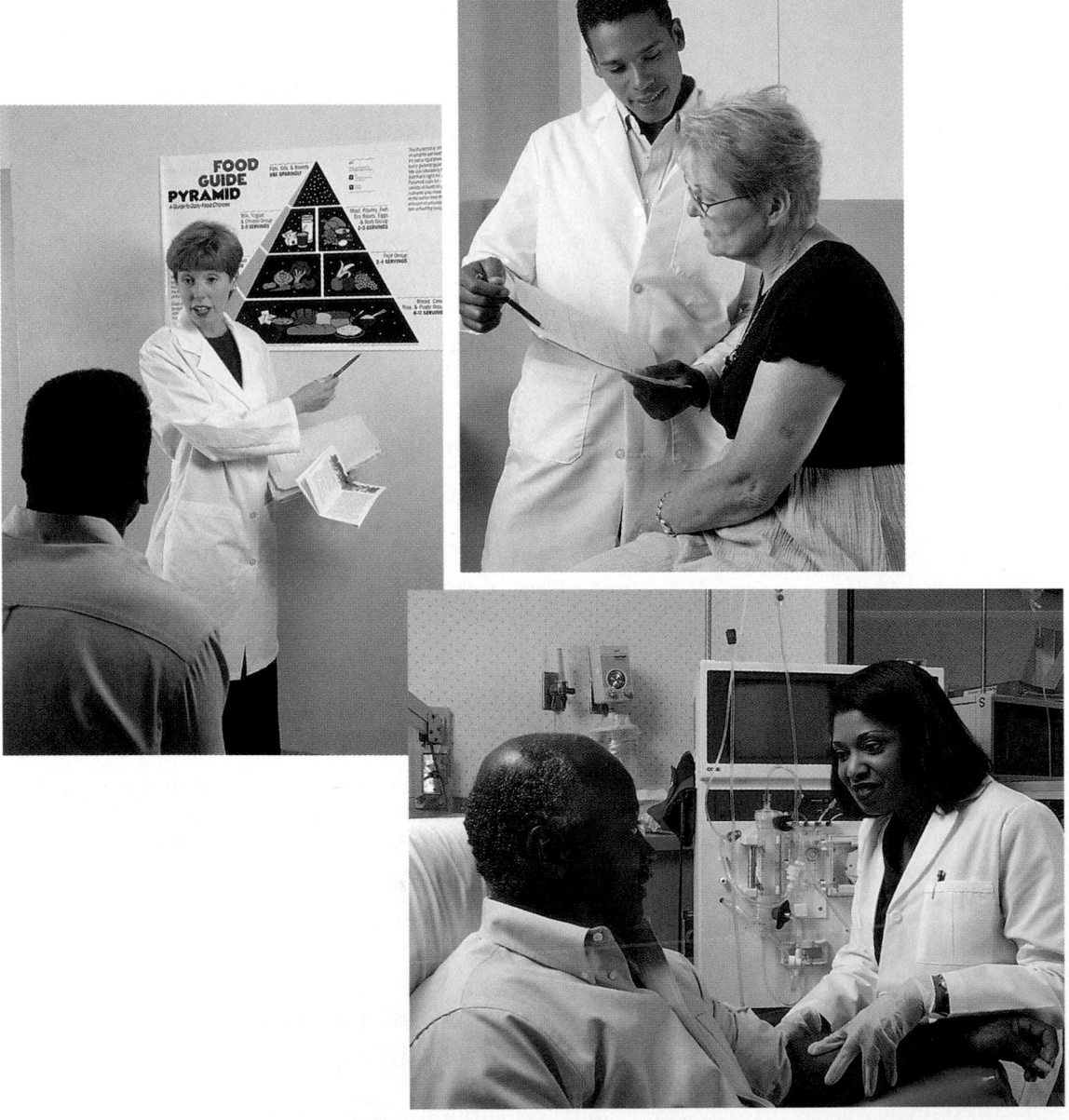

Figure 1–1

Because of their advanced knowledge and skills, nurse practitioners and clinical nurse specialists can provide comprehensive, specialized health care for a variety of clinical problems.

deliver comprehensive and continuous care (Fig. 1–1). Nurse practitioners conduct assessments of health status. Then, based on these assessments, they provide holistic health care. This includes health promotion, disease prevention, and management of acute and chronic health problems, with consultation and referral when appropriate. Nurse practitioners may be in private practice, in practice with a physician, or employed in a clinic or other ambulatory-care setting.

Clinical nurse specialists demonstrate an in-depth understanding of complex medical-surgical problems. They are prepared to provide and promote expert clinical care for a particular group of patients, such as those with diabetes, renal disease, or ostomy. Clinical nurse specialists use their in-depth knowledge of a specialty area to solve patient problems and to develop more effective approaches to patient care. They do this by

- Staying abreast of research and technologic developments affecting their area of practice

- Serving as consultants and role-models for other members of the health-care team
- Engaging in formal and informal teaching with coworkers, patients, and families
- Participating in the research process

Characteristics that define the unique roles of the clinical nurse specialist include accountability, change agency, collaboration, autonomy, leadership, and role-modeling.

*C*ertification

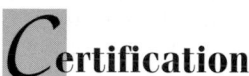

In addition to maintaining their academic credentials, medical-surgical nurses may elect to become certified. Although those who practice in specialized areas may seek certification from a variety of national specialty nursing organizations, the most widely used certification process in the United States

Table 1–1

Eligibility Requirements for Selected ANCC Certification Examinations	
Area of Practice	**Eligibility Requirements**
Medical-surgical nurse (generalist program)	Active Registered Nurse (RN) license in the United States or its territories.
	Have practiced as a licensed registered nurse a minimum of 4000 hours in medical-surgical nursing, 2000 of those hours within the past 2 years.
	Currently practice medical-surgical nursing an average of 8 hours per week.
	(Effective with the 1998 test administration, a baccalaureate or higher degree in nursing will be required.)
Clinical specialist in medical-surgical nursing	Active RN license in the United States or its territories.
	Master's degree with a major in nursing.
	Currently provide direct care to medical-surgical patients an average of at least 4 hours per week.
	At least 12 months of practice with an active RN license in the United States after completion of the master's degree.
	800 hours of post-master's practice giving direct patient care in the past 2 years, or full-time employment as a consultant, administrator, researcher, or educator for 2 of the past 3 years along with at least 400 hours of direct care to medical-surgical patients in the same time period.
Adult nurse practitioner	Active RN license in the United States or its territories.
	Master's degree with a major in nursing.
	Preparation as an adult nurse practitioner in an adult nurse or family nurse practitioner master's degree nursing program.
	or
	Preparation as an adult nurse practitioner in a formal postgraduate adult nurse practitioner or family nurse practitioner track or program in a school of nursing granting graduate credits.

Data from American Nurses Credentialing Center. Certification Catalog. Washington, DC, 1995.

is through the American Nurses' Association (ANA) and its Credentialing Center.

Nurses who meet the eligibility requirements (Table 1–1) can sit for a certification examination as a generalist medical-surgical nurse, clinical specialist in medical-surgical nursing, or adult nurse practitioner. The examination is based on nationally recognized standards of practice and is designed to have nurses demonstrate knowledge and functional expertise beyond that required for basic licensure. Upon passing the examination, the nurse is awarded certification for a period of 5 years. Recertification is obtained either by submitting evidence of required continuing education or by retesting.

Trends in Medical-Surgical Nursing Practice

No trend in medical-surgical nursing is more prevalent than the trend of constant change. The health-care industry in the United States is undergoing rapid and profound change. Some observers have characterized this period of change as a permanent "white water," or constant turbulence.

HEALTH-CARE REFORM

Among the many reasons for change, perhaps none is more powerful than a desire to reduce the cost of health care. To achieve cost containment, many sectors of the U.S. government and the public have called for health-care reform. Professional nurses have made major contributions to the reform movement by establishing an agenda for health-care change and by intensive political activity.

Because of the need for change, the goals, organizational arrangements, services, settings, and types of care that have been the norm in health-care delivery are all being reconfigured at a dramatic pace. Some of the many responses to the need for health-care reform have included

- Institutional downsizing and restructuring
- The development of managed-care programs, preferred-provider organizations, and health maintenance organizations
- The extension of services into the community
- The use of nonlicensed assistive personnel

This changing health-care environment is reshaping nursing practice and presenting unprecedented challenges for nurses.

Shortened hospital stays, increased acuity of inpatient care, and care provided on an outpatient basis are becoming common for many conditions seen in medical-surgical nursing. Thus, the nurse must identify and accomplish goals critical to the patient's well-being. She or he must support the patient's self-care abilities and collaborate with and supervise nonlicensed assistive personnel. And the nurse must recognize and encourage family responsibilities. All of this must occur within a shortened time frame. To respond appropriately to continued challenges, the nurse must work to provide care that is patient-based, that promotes the patient's optimal functional status and quality of life, and that is appropriate, satisfactory, and cost-effective.

SOCIETAL CHANGES

Adding to the rapid changes within the health-care system are the increasingly tumultuous changes in society. An epidemic of violence threatens the United States, and victims of gunshots, rape, and abuse are seen increasingly by the medical-surgical nurse. Caring for these victims requires understanding, compassion, and a recognition of the helplessness they may feel. In the United States, many state nurse licensure boards require nurses to receive continuing education on the subject of victim abuse. Supportive services from a variety of social agencies may need to be integrated into the plan of patient care.

Medical-surgical nursing practice is also influenced by other broad-based societal factors. Development of flexible patterns of education, coupled with greater access, is bringing into the profession a cadre of individuals with new and varied backgrounds and abilities. The women's movement is responsible for a new focus on women's health and is spawning changes in research, in access, and in care. Technologic developments are dramatically altering the diagnosis and management of disease, and computers are rapidly becoming an integral part of patient care management.

Standards of Practice

With the continual changes in U.S. society and its health-care delivery system, standards of practice are more important than ever. Standards are authoritative statements by which the nursing profession describes the responsibilities for which its practitioners are accountable (ANA, 1991). Regardless of level of preparation or certification, all practicing medical-surgical nurses in the United States are expected to meet the Standards of Clinical Nursing Practice developed by the ANA. The Standards of Clinical Nursing Practice consist of Standards of Care and Standards of Professional Performance. The Standards of Care are built around the steps of the nursing process and define a competent level of nursing care. The Standards of Professional Performance delineate a competent level of professional role behavior as it applies to quality of care, performance appraisal, education, collegiality, ethics, collaboration, research, and resource utilization. Each standard (Table 1–2) has accompanying measurement criteria that are considered key indicators of competent practice (ANA, 1991). Thus, the Standards of Practice address the nursing profession's responsibility

Table 1–2

American Nurses' Association Standards of Clinical Practice

STANDARDS OF CARE

Standard I. Assessment

The nurse collects client health data

Standard II. Diagnosis

The nurse analyzes the assessment data in determining diagnoses

Standard III. Outcome Identification

The nurse identifies expected outcomes individualized to the client

Standard IV. Planning

The nurse develops a plan of care that prescribes interventions to attain expected outcomes

Standard V. Implementation

The nurse implements the interventions identified in the plan of care

Standard VI. Evaluation

The nurse evaluates the client's progress toward attainment of outcomes

STANDARDS OF PROFESSIONAL PERFORMANCE

Standard I. Quality of Care

The nurse systematically evaluates the quality and effectiveness of nursing practice

Standard II. Performance Appraisal

The nurse evaluates his or her own nursing practice in relation to professional practice standards and relevant statutes and regulations

Standard III. Education

The nurse acquires and maintains current knowledge in nursing practice

Standard IV. Collegiality

The nurse contributes to the professional development of peers, colleagues, and others

Standard V. Ethics

The nurse's decisions and actions on behalf of clients are determined in an ethical manner

Standard VI. Collaboration

The nurse collaborates with the client, significant others, and health-care professionals in providing patient care

Standard VII. Research

The nurse uses research findings in practice

Standard VIII. Resource Utilization

The nurse considers factors related to safety, effectiveness, and cost in planning and delivering client care

From Standards of Clinical Nursing Practice, © 1991, American Nurses' Association, Washington, DC.

Clinical Practice Guidelines

Since 1992, U.S. nurses have had access to Clinical Practice Guidelines to assist them in determining what constitutes the best practices in dealing with specific health problems. These Guidelines have been developed through the support of the Agency for Health Care Policy and Research (AHCPR), an agency of the U.S. Public Health Service, Department of Health and Human Services.

Clinical Practice Guidelines are systematically developed statements designed to help practitioners and health-care consumers make decisions about appropriate care for specific health conditions. Guidelines reflect current scientific knowledge of practices and expert clinical judgment on the best ways to prevent, diagnose, treat, or manage diseases and disorders. They have been developed to discourage significant and unexplained practice variations that could potentially lead to inappropriate and ineffective treatment of patients and misused health-care dollars.

The AHCPR-supported Clinical Practice Guidelines are based on comprehensive reviews of the scientific literature and on evidence presented at open meetings. Where scientific or empirical evidence is lacking on a particular question, recommendations are based on the professional judgment of panel members and other experts in the field. Panels are composed of physicians, nurses, other health-care experts from academic and clinical environments, and consumer representatives.

The first AHCPR-sponsored Guideline, currently titled *Acute Pain Management in Adults: Operative Procedures*, was released in March 1992. Other Guidelines have been released and include the following that are of interest to the medical-surgical nurse:

- *Acute Low Back Problems in Adults*
- *Benign Prostatic Hyperplasia: Diagnosis and Treatment*
- *Cataract in Adults: Management of Functional Impairment*
- *Depression in Primary Care: Detection, Diagnosis, and Treatment*
- *Heart Failure: Management of Patients with Left Ventricular Systolic Dysfunction*
- *Management of Cancer Pain: Adults*
- *Managing Acute and Chronic Urinary Incontinence*
- *Post-Stroke Rehabilitation*
- *Pressure Ulcers in Adults: Prediction and Prevention*
- *Pressure Ulcer Treatment*
- *Quality Determinants of Mammography*
- *Unstable Angina: Diagnosis and Treatment*

to the public and provide a means of measuring the outcomes of care. It is through these Standards of Practice that nursing maintains professional autonomy and public confidence in its service.

Clinical Practice Guidelines for other diseases and concerns are under development. These Guidelines are available to nurses in desk reference form and in an abbreviated version that presents highlights for easy reference. Consumer versions in English and Spanish are available to enable the patient to be a partner in health-care decision-making. Guideline information is available by mail, by fax, and through online computer access.

The Nursing Process

Medical-surgical nurses must have a firm foundation in the use of the nursing process to provide effective, individualized nursing care for medical-surgical patients. Accordingly, a brief review of the nursing process follows.

The nursing process consists of five interrelated, interdependent, somewhat overlapping phases. They are assessment, nursing diagnosis, planning, implementation, and evaluation. These phases form a continuous cycle of thoughts and actions. Each phase relies on the accuracy of the previous phase.

ASSESSMENT

In the first phase of the nursing process, the nurse collects and organizes information about the patient to identify existing or potential health problems and factors that have an impact on them. Assessment is the most crucial phase of the nursing process, since the entire plan of care will be based on the information gathered. If this information is incorrect, identification of the problem will be incorrect, which leads to misguided interventions and inaccurate expected patient outcomes.

Data collection is an ongoing process that begins with the initial patient-nurse contact and continues until the patient is discharged from care. Data collection can be formal, as with a nursing history, or informal, as in conversation and observation during care.

Two basic types of data are collected: historical and current. Historical data include information about past events, such as previous illnesses, exposure to infections, and prior hospitalizations. Frequently, assessment of the patient's cultural background is included as well, to ensure culturally sensitive care. Current data derive from physical and laboratory findings and include such information as the presence of pain, an elevated temperature, and feelings of anxiety over a scheduled procedure.

The patient is the primary source of data because it is the patient who can most accurately describe symptoms; give a history; share perceptions, problems, and goals; and validate responses to treatment. All other sources of information are secondary.

Data are collected by interview, observation, physical examination, and chart review. Data collec-

tion varies with the condition and needs of the patient. If the patient has an urgent problem, such as severe pain or respiratory distress, data collection must be limited to evaluating the priority area and gathering additional information from secondary sources. Patient characteristics, such as intellectual development and communication ability, also influence data collection.

Once data are gathered, validated, and recorded, they can be organized and analyzed for patterns that suggest health problems.

The most common errors of assessment spring from inaccurate or incomplete data collection, inaccurate interpretation of data (usually the result of using only one clue to make an inference), and lack of clinical knowledge.

NURSING DIAGNOSIS

A nursing diagnosis is a clinical judgment about individual, family, or community responses to actual and potential health problems and life processes. Nursing diagnoses provide the basis for selecting nursing interventions and identifying outcomes. The nurse is accountable for the achievement of those outcomes (NANDA, 1994).

There are three types of nursing diagnoses: actual, risk, and wellness. An *actual* nursing diagnosis is one that describes human responses to health conditions or life processes that exist in an individual, family, or community (NANDA, 1994). An actual nursing diagnosis is supported by identifiable defining characteristics; that is, at least two signs or symptoms of the diagnosis are present.

A *risk* nursing diagnosis is one that applies to an individual, a family, or a community that has a greater risk of developing a problem than the risk others would face in the same or a similar situation. The diagnosis should be supported by risk factors that demonstrate this increased vulnerability (Carpenito, 1995).

A *wellness* diagnosis is a clinical judgment that an existing wellness response has the potential for enhancement to a higher state (NANDA, 1994).

A nursing diagnosis is a one-, two-, or three-part statement that follows from the analysis and interpretation of assessment data. The first part, the diagnostic label or category, represents a pattern of related cues. In actual and risk diagnoses, it identifies the alteration being experienced by the patient or for which the patient is at risk. It provides a clear idea of what needs to change and suggests expected patient outcomes. The second part, the related factors (or etiology), is joined to the diagnostic label by the words "related to" (or R/T) and expresses the reason for the alteration. It describes the physical, psychologic, sociocultural, spiritual, and environmental factors that relate to, or contribute to, the health problem. These related factors suggest the type of nursing interventions necessary to eliminate, reduce, or prevent the problem. The nursing diagnosis can be further specified by adding the phrase "secondary to." An example of a nursing diagnosis that includes these elements is "Altered nutrition: less than body requirements, related to anorexia secondary to chemotherapy."

With the exception of "Knowledge deficit" and "Rape-trauma syndrome," all actual and risk nursing diagnoses have an etiology. In cases in which the etiology cannot be identified, that should be noted by the words "related to unknown etiology." Wellness diagnoses also do not contain related factors but consist simply of the diagnostic label preceded by the phrase "Potential for enhanced" (Carpenito, 1995).

The third component, defining characteristics, specifies the signs and symptoms (identified during assessment) on which the nursing diagnosis rests. When present, the defining characteristics are joined to the related factor by the words "manifested by" (M/B).

Refer to Table 1–3 for the current list of nursing diagnostic categories accepted by the North American Nursing Diagnosis Association (NANDA).

PLANNING

The third phase of the nursing process is the planning phase. It consists of four steps: setting priorities, establishing expected patient outcomes, selecting nursing interventions (developing nursing orders), and documenting the plan of care.

Setting priorities serves to organize the delivery of nursing care so that more important problems are considered first. The problem that poses the greatest threat to the patient's well-being should be given the highest priority. Depending on the situation, this may be a problem directly affecting the patient's physical status, or it may be related to a knowledge deficit or a psychologic effect. Priorities in nonemergency situations may vary with the patient's perception of what is important.

Priorities can change day to day, shift to shift, and sometimes minute to minute. Thus, the delivery of nursing care must be flexible and geared toward the patient's current status. One problem need not necessarily be resolved before another is approached.

Expected outcomes are standards or measures used to evaluate the patient's progress. They are patient-oriented and derived from the nursing diagnosis. Each nursing diagnosis has one or more specific expected patient outcomes that define what the patient will do. Expected patient outcomes may relate to bodily appearance or function, relief or absence of specific symptoms, demonstration of knowledge or psychomotor skills, or psychosocial status. They are set in conjunction with the patient to help

ensure their achievement by encouraging patient participation.

Expected outcomes guide the nurse in selecting interventions and serve as criteria against which the interventions will be evaluated. According to Carpenito (1995), outcomes can represent resolution of a problem, evidence of progress toward resolution of a problem, progress toward improved health status, or continued maintenance of good health or function.

Expected patient outcomes can be short-term or long-term; the time frame established triggers their evaluation. Outcomes must be clearly defined, measurable, and observable. Each expected outcome should describe only one behavior and should be written as a positive statement. Each must be realistic concerning the patient's condition, abilities, and resources available.

The third step in the planning phase is selecting the nursing interventions—discrete nurse behaviors—that will best achieve the expected outcomes. This specific outline of nurse activities (nursing orders) is based on the etiology component of the nursing diagnosis and permits all nurses to provide comprehensive care. Interventions aim to reduce, eliminate, or prevent the cause or contributing factors. All nursing orders must be consistent with the therapeutic approaches of other health-care professionals involved in the patient's care. All must be individualized to the physical and psychologic needs of the individual patient. And all must be supported by rationales based on scientific principles. The plan of care is then documented in the patient's record (step four of the planning phase).

Recently, the Nursing Interventions Classification (NIC) has been under development to help unify and organize the nursing interventions database (McCloskey and Bulecheck, 1995). The NIC evolved after a number of other classification schemes, for the most part neither empirically derived nor validated, failed to provide a standardized comprehensive list of interventions that nurses could use to describe their treatments. The NIC is gaining acceptance among nurses because it seeks to determine relationships among interventions and to provide a taxonomy (a system of naming) that groups interventions by their similarities and differences.

The purpose of the classification is to list the direct-care treatments that nurses perform. Each nursing intervention contained in NIC has three parts:

- A label or name describing the concept
- The definition of the concept
- A set of defining activities or actions that a nurse must perform to implement the intervention concept

The development and use of NIC helps to advance nursing knowledge. And using a standardized language to document practice allows comparison

Table 1–3

NANDA-Approved Nursing Diagnoses

This list represents the NANDA-approved nursing diagnoses for clinical use and testing (1994).

Activity Intolerance
Activity Intolerance, Risk for
Adaptive Capacity: Intracranial, Decreased
Adjustment, Impaired
Airway Clearance, Ineffective
Anxiety
Aspiration, Risk for
Body Image Disturbance
Body Temperature, Risk for Altered
Breastfeeding, Effective
Breastfeeding, Ineffective
Breastfeeding, Interrupted
#Breathing Pattern, Ineffective
Caregiver Role Strain
Caregiver Role Strain, Risk for
Communication, Impaired Verbal
Community Coping, Ineffective
Community Coping, Potential for Enhanced
Confusion, Acute
Confusion, Chronic
Constipation
Constipation, Colonic
Constipation, Perceived
Decisional Conflict (Specify)
#Decreased Cardiac Output
Defensive Coping
Denial, Ineffective
Diarrhea
Disorganized Infant Behavior
Disorganized Infant Behavior, Risk for
Disuse Syndrome, Risk for
Diversional Activity Deficit
Dysfunctional Ventilatory Weaning Response (DVWR)
Dysreflexia
Energy Field Disturbance
Environmental Interpretation Syndrome, Impaired
#Family Coping: Compromised, Ineffective
#Family Coping: Disabling, Ineffective
Family Coping: Potential for Growth
Family Process: Alcoholism, Altered
Family Processes, Altered
Fatigue
Fear
#Fluid Volume Deficit
Fluid Volume Deficit, Risk for
#Fluid Volume Excess
Gas Exchange, Impaired
#Grieving, Anticipatory
#Grieving, Dysfunctional
Growth and Development, Altered
Health Maintenance, Altered
Health Seeking Behaviors (Specify)
Home Maintenance Management, Impaired
Hopelessness
Hyperthermia
Hypothermia
Incontinence, Bowel
Incontinence, Functional
Incontinence, Reflex
Incontinence, Stress

Incontinence, Total
Incontinence, Urge
#Individual Coping, Ineffective
Infant Feeding Pattern, Ineffective
Infection, Risk for
Injury, Risk for
#Knowledge Deficit (Specify)
Loneliness, Risk for
Management of Therapeutic Regimen: Community, Ineffective
Management of Therapeutic Regimen: Families, Ineffective
Management of Therapeutic Regimen: Individual, Effective
Management of Therapeutic Regimen (Individuals), Ineffective
Memory, Impaired
Noncompliance (Specify)
Nutrition: Less than Body Requirements, Altered
Nutrition: More than Body Requirements, Altered
Nutrition: Risk for More than Body Requirements, Altered
Oral Mucous Membrane, Altered
Organized Infant Behavior, Potential for Enhanced
#Pain
#Pain, Chronic
Parental Role Conflict
Parent/Infant/Child Attachment, Risk for Altered
Parenting, Altered
Parenting, Risk for Altered
Perioperative Positioning Injury, Risk for
Peripheral Neurovascular Dysfunction, Risk for
Personal Identity Disturbance
Physical Mobility, Impaired
Poisoning, Risk for
Post-Trauma Response
Powerlessness
Protection, Altered
Rape-Trauma Symdrome
Rape-Trauma Syndrome: Compound Reaction
Rape-Trauma Syndrome: Silent Reaction
Relocation Stress Syndrome
Role Performance, Altered
Self Care Deficit
    Bathing/Hygiene
    Dressing/Grooming
    Feeding
    Toileting
#Self Esteem, Chronic Low
#Self Esteem Disturbance
#Self Esteem, Situational Low
Self-Mutilation, Risk for
Sensory/Perceptual Alterations (Specify) (Visual, Auditory, Kinesthetic, Gustatory, Tactile, Olfactory)
Sexual Dysfunction
Sexuality Patterns, Altered
Skin Integrity, Impaired
Skin Integrity, Risk for Impaired
Sleep Pattern Disturbance
Social Interaction, Impaired
Social Isolation

Table 1–3 *continued*

NANDA-Approved Nursing Diagnoses

Spiritual Distress (Distress of the Human Spirit)
Spiritual Well-Being, Potential for Enhanced
Suffocation, Risk for
Sustain Spontaneous Ventilation, Inability to
Swallowing, Impaired
Thermoregulation, Ineffective
#Thought Processes, Altered
Tissue Integrity, Impaired

Tissue Perfusion, Altered (Specify Type) (Renal, Cerebral, Cardiopulmonary, Gastrointestinal, Peripheral)
Trauma, Risk for
Unilateral Neglect
Urinary Elimination, Altered
Urinary Retention
#Violence, Risk for: Self-Directed or Directed at Others

#Diagnoses revised by small work groups at the 1994 Biennial Conference on the Classification of Nursing Diagnoses; changes approved and added in 1996.

Copyright 1996, North American
Nursing Diagnosis Association.

and evaluation of the effectiveness of the nursing care delivered. For nurses and nursing, these advantages can be of particular importance in an era of rapid change in all aspects of health-care delivery.

IMPLEMENTATION

The fourth phase of the nursing process is the implementation phase. During this phase, actions are taken that enable the patient to achieve the expected outcomes identified in the planning phase.

The implementation phase begins with preparation for care. The nurse reviews the interventions to be carried out, estimates the time needed for their implementation, and selects the time for implementation based on the patient's needs and other nursing responsibilities. The nurse also evaluates the need for assistance from other personnel and, if necessary, arranges for that assistance before care begins. The nurse modifies the patient's immediate environment, if necessary, so that it supports efficient care and the goals of intervention. She or he makes the patient comfortable physically and psychologically. For example, the nurse positions the patient comfortably in bed and asks if a bedpan is needed before starting a lengthy procedure. The nurse also provides privacy, considers the patient's rights, and makes sure that the patient has given informed consent. When a patient does not consent to a procedure, the nurse respects the patient's right to refuse care.

Care may begin when preparation is complete. This may involve performing an action, assisting the patient with an action, supervising the family in performing an action, or teaching the patient and family.

The nurse maintains ongoing assessment during this phase of care. Such assessment provides the basis for any decision to initiate, continue, modify, or discontinue an intervention. It is also used in subsequent evaluation.

EVALUATION

The fifth phase of the nursing process involves making a judgement about the effectiveness of nursing care. Has this individual patient received the best possible plan of care? If not, how should the plan be modified?

Evaluation consists of two steps. First is the determination of whether the expected patient outcomes have been achieved. Second is a thorough reassessment of the entire plan to identify changes to further improve patient care.

To determine whether expected patient outcomes are achieved, the nurse compares the patient's status with the stated outcomes. Some of the data needed for this comparison may have been collected during the implementation of nursing interventions. Other data are collected at the time of evaluation by direct observation, examination, patient interview, pencil and paper tests, and feedback from other staff members. From this comparison, the nurse determines whether the expected outcomes have been met fully, partially, or not at all. The nurse documents the patient's progress or lack of progress and discusses the findings with the patient.

Then, based on all patient data, the nurse reassesses the entire plan of care. He or she changes, adds, or eliminates previous nursing diagnoses, expected patient outcomes, and nursing interventions as needed. If an expected outcome has been achieved, the nurse determines whether the problem has been resolved and the diagnosis can be eliminated, or whether the problem is ongoing and requires continued nursing intervention. For example, a patient with "Constipation related to immobility" may have achieved the expected outcome of one soft, formed bowel movement per day. But if the patient remains immobilized and nursing interventions cease, the problem would almost certainly recur. Thus, the most appropriate response would be to change the nursing diagnosis to "Risk for constipation related to immobility" and to continue the nursing intervention.

If the expected outcome is not achieved or only partly achieved, the nurse asks the following questions:

- Was the assessment complete and accurate?
- Was the nursing diagnosis correctly identified?
- Are the expected outcomes realistic for this patient?
- Are the nursing interventions appropriate?
- Have priorities changed?
- Have new nursing diagnoses arisen?

Depending on the answers to these questions, it may be necessary to reassess the patient, identify new nursing diagnoses, establish new expected outcomes, select new nursing interventions, set new priorities, or establish new dates for evaluation.

Clinical Pathways

The health-care industry has been challenged with the task of reducing the cost of health care while, at the same time, increasing the effectiveness of that care. To this end, everyone in a health-care organization must be concerned with the efficient and effective flow of patients through the system. The clinical pathway is a tool developed to help with this flow.

The clinical pathway (also called a critical path) is a guideline for patient care. It includes collaborative clinical practices aimed at delivering the most resource-efficient, clinically appropriate care within the shortest reasonable length of stay for a specific medical procedure or condition (Rudisill et al, 1994). It is a written document describing the optimal utilization, sequencing, and timing of interventions necessary to carry out a given procedure or treatment plan. Physicians, nurses, and other health-care personnel work together to execute a clinical pathway. The pathway is intended to clarify the overall plan. It is also intended to let everyone involved in the care of a patient, including the patient, know what to expect. A "good" clinical pathway minimizes the use of resources and, at the same time, maximizes the quality of care provided.

Agencies that develop clinical pathways typically do so for diagnoses that are high-volume, high-cost, and problematic. Examples of critical paths for selected conditions are incorporated throughout this text. In everyday practice, the nurse would use a clinical pathway as an adjunct to the plan of care, as a report mechanism, and as a treatment protocol. Staff members revise the patient's care based on differences between expected and actual outcomes. Variances from the standard are reported, documented, and reviewed to determine whether changes in practice are needed.

Culturally Competent Care

In 1986, the ANA called for nurses to include individual value systems and lifestyles in their plans for health care. The Association also urged the profession to meet the health- and nursing-care needs of a diverse and multicultural society (ANA, 1986). Nurses today recognize the need to know and understand people of different cultural backgrounds and to use this knowledge to guide nursing practice (Fig. 1–2). By learning to focus on the ways in which illness and health are expressions of a particular culture, and how culture influences patient expectations of nursing care, nurses can help their patients to move toward health and wellbeing.

Culture is a view of the world and a set of traditions used and transmitted from generation to generation. It includes the values, attitudes, roles, and behaviors acceptable to and expected by the cultural group. For nurses, the usefulness of culture as a concept is the direction it provides in understanding their own health values and behaviors as well as those of their patients.

The way in which a group of people explain life's events and offer solutions to life's mysteries is the group's world view. This, in turn, provides the guide for determining the values, beliefs, and practices of the group. Values are personal perceptions of what is good and useful. Norms or rules flow from values and form the roles by which human behavior is governed.

The dominant culture in the United States today is that of white, middle-class, Anglo-Saxon Protestants. This culture has had a profound influence on the values, beliefs, and practices held by many patients. However, there is also a rich mix of ethnic and cultural groups that cannot be ignored if the

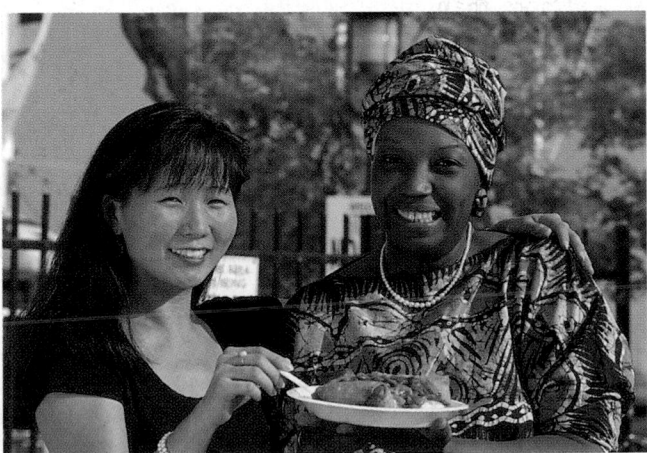

Figure 1–2

Many cultures coexist in today's population, making sensitivity to each patient's cultural background and beliefs a necessary facet of appropriate nursing care.

nurse is to individualize care (Andrews and Boyle, 1995). Other cultural groups that need health care include

- Hispanics (Mexicans, Puerto Ricans, Cubans, and others)
- Blacks (African-Americans, Haitians, persons from the Dominican Republic)
- Native Americans, and Asian/Pacific Islanders (Chinese, Japanese, Filipino, Korean, Vietnamese, Hawaiian, Guamian, Samoan, and Asian Indians)

The nurse must constantly distinguish the standards of the dominant white culture from those of the patient's cultural group.

A patient's thoughts about health, disease, illness, and appropriate treatment are usually culturally prescribed. For example, some ethnic groups believe that supernatural forces dominate in the world and that one's fate depends on the actions of a god or gods. In this magicoreligious paradigm, the person is at the mercy of these forces. Thus, religion can play a very important part in both treatment of disease and recovery of health.

Other paradigms that influence cultural beliefs are the scientific and the holistic. In the former, life is controlled by a series of physical and biochemical processes that can be studied and manipulated by humans. There is a cause-and-effect relationship in all phenomena, and life processes can be controlled by mechanical and other engineered interventions. The body can be reduced to its individual parts. Mind and body are separate. Disease is a breakdown of the human machine. The prevailing medical model of treatment, which we commonly see in our institutions, derives from this paradigm.

In the holistic health paradigm, nature is a dominant force and must be kept in balance or harmony. Humans are only one aspect of nature. Everything in the universe has a part to play in keeping the natural order. Health is a positive process that involves more than the absence of disease. Major socioeconomic problems such as poverty, discrimination, and suicide are as much illnesses as are pneumonia and diabetes. Many nurse theorists, beginning with Florence Nightingale, propose a holistic approach to health and the care of patients.

Common phenomena of concern to nurses occur in all cultures, but cultural symbols such as health, healing, illness, disease, and caring may have different meanings to people in different cultures. Therefore, the extent to which meanings are shared between patients and nurses may determine the effectiveness of the treatment approaches that are used.

Nurses are encouraged to use a cultural assessment for gathering relevant data about their patients. Leininger (1978) defines a cultural or culturologic nursing assessment as a systematic appraisal or examination of individuals, groups, and communities as to their cultural beliefs, values, and practices to determine explicit nursing needs and intervention practices within the cultural context of the people being evaluated. She suggests world view, language, cultural values, kinship, religion, politics, technology, education, and environment as areas that should be assessed.

Health-care agencies may include a cultural assessment as one of the tools for gathering data about patients. Of particular importance to the nurse's planning is a determination of the patient's beliefs about healing. Knowing the predominant health-care values of a particular culture may guide the nurse in relationships with the patient. However, assumptions can never take the place of a thorough and personal assessment.

The medical-surgical nurse can become more sensitive to the cultural norms and values of the patient by

Listening carefully
Being empathic
Recognizing the patient's self-interest and needs
Being flexible
Having a sense of timing
Using patient and family resources
Giving relevant information at the appropriate time

People search for meaning and purpose in their lives. Together with an individual's unique life experiences, such a search gives rise to spirituality. Religion, an integral part of culture, refers to an organized system of beliefs concerning the cause, nature, and purpose of the universe, and involves worship of a god or gods.

Religion plays an important role in patient beliefs about health and illness. Rituals, emotions, sets of beliefs, meanings, and standards of conduct are found in all religions. The ways in which different cultures emphasize each of these dimensions will affect the nurse providing care. Andrews and Hanson (Andrews and Boyle, 1995) suggest the following to guide the nurse:

- Determine what religious dimensions are important to the patient so that you and the patient can set mutual goals.
- Determine what the patient believes to be important.
- Validate the accuracy of information. Do not make assumptions.
- Be open to variations in patients' beliefs and practices and do not judge their religious values.
- Understand that ideal norms of conduct and actual behavior are not necessarily the same.

The goal of spiritual nursing care is to help patients find the god or truths that provide meaning in their lives during a time of illness. Be cautious never to impose beliefs and convictions on patients. A complex mosaic of religions exist around the world.

It is almost impossible for one nurse to understand the health-related beliefs and practices of very many of them. Fortunately, the patient, family, significant others, and spiritual counselor can provide guidance when the nurse is open to such direction. Recognizing the patient's needs and making an effort to include spirituality and religion in the plan of care is an appropriate goal for the medical-surgical nurse.

National Health Promotion and Disease Prevention Objectives

Healthy People 2000 is a publication of the Public Health Service of the U.S. Department of Health and Human Services. This report suggests a strategy for improving the health of the American people by the year 2000 by establishing objectives for health promotion and disease prevention (USDHHS, PHS, 1990). Included in the report are specific age-related objectives that address the populations normally cared for by medical-surgical nurses. For effective practice to occur, these objectives should form the basis of the nurse's educational approach to patients.

This report outlines three broad goals for the United States:

• Increase the span of healthy life for Americans
• Reduce health disparities among Americans
• Achieve access to preventive services for all Americans

Strategies related to health promotion, health protection, and preventive services are designed to achieve these goals.

The health profile of American adults is substantially determined by behavioral risk factors. The leading causes of death for adults ages 25 through 64 include cancer, heart disease, injuries, stroke, chronic lung disease, liver disease, HIV infection, and diabetes. Among persons 65 and older, heart disease, cancer, stroke, chronic obstructive pulmonary disease, pneumonia, and influenza are the leading causes of death. Many or all of these causes are associated with factors related to lifestyle.

To promote health and prevent disease, many adults would benefit from modifying their lifestyle behaviors. Because behavior changes are never easy, supportive social environments can be very important. Nurses can facilitate positive changes in the behaviors of patients through appropriate assessment and education. Table 1–4 lists the key risk reduction objectives found in the *Healthy People 2000* report. Recognizing and incorporating such factors as beliefs, practices, family networks, living situations, and economic circumstances can be very important to success.

The most important aspect of health promotion among older people is maintenance of health and functional independence. Even in later life, changing certain risk behaviors into healthy ones can improve health and reduce the likelihood of disability. Improvement in diet and nutrition, reduction in tobacco use, weight control, and increased physical

Table 1–4

Key Risk Reduction Objectives for Adults and Older Adults

OBJECTIVES FOR ADULTS

1. Reduce dietary fat intake to an average of 30% of calories or less and average saturated fat intake to an average of less than 10% of calories.
2. Increase complex carbohydrate and fiber-containing foods in the diets of adults to five or more daily servings for vegetables (including legumes) and fruits, and to six or more daily servings for grain products.
3. Reduce alcohol consumption to an annual average of no more than 2 gallons of ethanol per person.
4. Increase the effectiveness with which family-planning methods are used, as measured by a decrease to no more than 5% in the proportion of couples experiencing pregnancy despite the use of a contraceptive method.
5. Increase to at least 20% the proportion of people who seek help in coping with personal and emotional problems.
6. Increase to at least 50% the proportion of hypertensive people whose blood pressure is under control.
7. Reduce the mean serum cholesterol level among adults to no more than 200 mg/dL.
8. Reduce diabetes to an incidence of no more than 2.5 per 1000 people per year and a prevalence of no more than 25 per 1000 people per year.

OBJECTIVES FOR OLDER ADULTS

1. Increase to at least 30% the proportion of people ages 65 and over who engage regularly, preferably daily, in light to moderate physical activity lasting at least 30 minutes.
2. Reduce to no more than 22% the proportion of people ages 65 and over who engage in no leisure-time physical activity.
3. Increase to at least 80% the immunization levels for pneumococcal pneumonia and influenza among institutionalized chronically ill or older people.
4. Increase to at least 40% the proportion of adults ages 65 and over who have received, as a minimum within the appropriate interval, all of the screening and immunization services and at least one of the counseling services appropriate for their age and gender as recommended by the U.S. Preventive Services Task Force.

Derived from *Healthy People 2000*, U.S. Department of Health and Human Services, 1990.

activity can enhance the health of older people. Here, too, strong social support is important to risk reduction, and nurses can play a primary role in providing support.

Chapter Review

1. With what types of patients and in what settings do medical-surgical nurses practice?
2. How do the education and practice of a nurse practitioner differ from those of a clinical nurse specialist?
3. What criteria must a nurse meet to be certified as a generalist in medical-surgical nursing?
4. What effects have recent health-care reform initiatives had on the practice of medical-surgical nursing?
5. How do broad-based societal issues (other than health-care reform) affect the practice of the medical-surgical nurse?
6. Why are standards of practice for medical-surgical nursing important?
7. How do Clinical Practice Guidelines differ from standards of practice?
8. Why is the nursing process described as a continuous cycle of overlapping steps?
9. In what ways does a clinical pathway differ from other forms of patient-care planning?
10. What are some examples of how cultural competence can affect the outcomes of nursing care?

Bibliography

American Nurses' Association. Standards of medical-surgical nursing practice. Kansas City, MO: Author, 1980.

American Nurses' Association. Cultural diversity in the nursing curriculum: A guide for implementation. Kansas City, MO: Author, 1986.

American Nurses' Association. Standards of clinical nursing practice. Washington, DC: Author, 1991.

American Nurses Credentialing Center. Certification catalog. Washington, DC: Author, 1995.

Andrews M. Cultural perspectives on nursing in the 21st century. J Prof Nurs 1992; 8(1):7.

Andrews, MM, Boyle, JS. Transcultural concepts in nursing care. 2nd ed. Philadelphia: JB Lippincott, 1995.

Assembly of Advanced Practice Registered Nurses, Ohio Nurses Association. Resource manual for advanced practice registered nurses. Columbus, OH: Author, 1995.

Barnes R, Lawton L, Briggs D. Clinical benchmarking improves clinical paths: Experience with coronary artery bypass grafting. J Comm J Qual Improve 1994; 20(5):267.

Carpenito LJ. Nursing diagnosis application to clinical practice. 6th ed. Philadelphia: JB Lippincott, 1995.

Ellis J, Hartley C. Credentials for nursing practice. In Nursing in today's world: Challenges, issues and trends. 5th ed. Philadelphia: JB Lippincott, 1995, pp 109–135.

Fenton M. Education for the advanced practice of clinical nurse specialists. Oncol Nurs Forum 1992; 19(1)(Suppl):16.

Heacock D, Brobst R. A multidisciplinary approach to critical path development: A valuable CQI tool. J Nurs Care Qual 1994; 8(4):38.

Iyer P, Taptich B, Bernocchi-Losey D. Nursing process and nursing diagnosis. 3rd ed. Philadelphia: WB Saunders, 1995, pp 2–18, 84–111.

Leininger M. Transcultural nursing: Concepts, theories and practices. New York: John Wiley & Sons, 1978.

Leininger M. Transcultural nursing: An overview. Nurs Outlook 1984; 32(2):72.

McCloskey J, Bulechek G. Nursing interventions classification (NIC). 2nd ed. St Louis: Mosby-Year Book, 1996.

National Council of State Boards of Nursing. Position paper on the licensure of advanced nursing practice. Chicago, IL: NCSBN, Inc, 1992.

North American Nursing Diagnosis Association. Classification of nursing diagnoses: Proceedings of the tenth conference. Philadelphia: JB Lippincott Company, 1994.

North American Nursing Diagnosis Association. Nursing diagnoses: Definitions and classification, 1997–1998. Philadelphia: Author, 1997.

Rudisill P, Phillips M, Payne C. Clinical paths for cardiac surgery patients: A multidisciplinary approach to quality improvement outcomes. J Nurs Care Qual 1994; 8(3):27.

Snyder M, Mirr MP. Advanced practice nursing: A guide to professional development. New York: Springer Verlag, 1995.

Takacs P. Nursing roles in advanced practice. Ohio Nurses Review, June 1993.

Tuck I, Harris L. Teaching students transcultural concepts. Nurse Educator 1988; 13(3):36.

U.S. Department of Health and Human Services, Public Health Service. Healthy people 2000. Rockville, MD, Author, 1990.

U.S. Department of Health and Human Services, Public Health Service. AHCPR Fact Sheet. Rockville, MD: Agency for Health Care Policy and Research, 1993.

Woodyard L, Sheetz J. Critical pathway patient outcomes: The missing standard. J Nurs Care Qual 1993; 8(1):51.

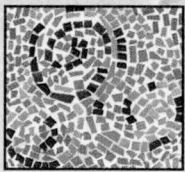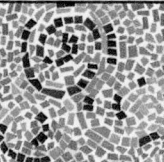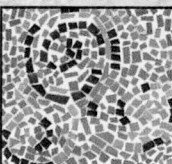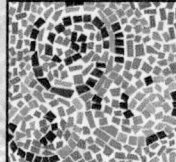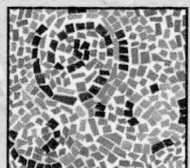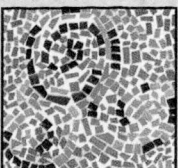

Medical-Surgical Nursing in Multiple Settings

Study Outcomes

After studying this chapter, you should be able to:

1. Discuss changes in health care and the society that have increased the need for medical-surgical nurses to practice in nonhospital settings.
2. Describe vulnerable populations in the United States and the unique health problems of those populations.
3. Define managed care and case management.
4. Identify nonhospital settings in which medical-surgical nurses work.
5. Identify the practice roles of medical-surgical nurses working in nonhospital settings.
6. Describe the discharge planning process.
7. Identify members of the multidisciplinary health-care team, their qualifications, and their responsibilities in patient care.
8. List the skilled nursing services performed by home health nurses, visiting nurses, and hospice nurses.
9. Describe future medical-surgical roles and responsibilities identified by the National Advisory Council on Nursing Education and Practice and by the Pew Health Professions Commission.

In the model of health-care delivery developed and practiced in the United States for much of the 20th century, the concept of medical-surgical nursing has been synonymous with acute-care hospital nursing. Indeed, in the past virtually all medical-surgical nurses worked for hospitals and provided inpatient care. Today, the majority of medical-surgical nurses still work in the hospital setting. But the tide of managed-health-care organizations and public policymakers is turning our traditional method of health-care delivery into a new model. Experts in both public and private sectors report that all but the most advanced medical services are shifting—and should shift—out of the hospital and into the community. As a consequence, many medical-surgical nursing functions are shifting into the community as well.

A myriad of reasons underlie this increasing shift out of the hospital and into diverse, community-based health-care settings. Spiraling health-care costs, sophisticated technologies, demographic changes, and political decisions have dramatically altered the provision of traditional inpatient services. As a result of these changes, hospital bed capacity exceeds the need in many communities and has prompted hospital mergers, closures, and alternative use of space. In response, we have seen an unprecedented increase in community-based health-care facilities and services. To staff these facilities and provide services, medical-surgical nursing roles and knowledge requirements have become increasingly diverse.

Indeed, today's medical-surgical nurse must handle much more than traditional nursing skills and procedures. Today's nurse must understand the entire health-care system, including mechanisms for distributing and reimbursing health-care services. Almost certainly, tomorrow's nurse will face an even greater need to work within an intensively managed and highly diversified health-care system.

This chapter outlines the major reasons for this shift out of the hospital and into the community. It also describes some of the most common nonhospital practice settings and the nursing roles they require.

The Shift to Nonhospital Settings

Several factors have contributed to the shift of patient care from the hospital to community-based clinics, long-term care facilities, schools, worksites, and the home. Among these are the increasing cost of health care, increasing numbers of poor and uninsured people, and significant population changes that have produced increased numbers of people with chronic illnesses or the inability to gain access to the health-care system in traditional ways. These population changes include a growing number of older adults, increasing numbers of homeless people and their families, and the epidemic of acquired immunodeficiency syndrome (AIDS).

SPIRALING HEALTH-CARE COSTS

In the United States, the cost of health care has risen faster and higher than in any of the world's other industrialized nations. There are many reasons for the escalating cost of health-care services. Historically, patients have received much of their care in the most expensive setting available: the hospital. And they have received much of their care from highly specialized—thus expensive—health-care professionals. To make matters worse, many health-care services have been overused, inefficiently used, wastefully used, sometimes fraudulently used by providers and patients whose goal was to provide the most and the best care possible for each person in need. Vigorous development of newer and better high-technology treatments whose success depends on highly trained professionals has helped some U.S. citizens receive the best medical care in the world. They have also created a demand for services. Few people want to miss an opportunity for better health or even continued life if a diagnostic or treatment procedure may improve the odds (Clark, 1996). However, for the nation at large, the result has been a staggering cost burden. So staggering, in fact, that government and public sectors have demanded a change.

National health-care expenditures are measured as a percentage the U.S. gross national product (GNP). The GNP is the total value of all goods and services produced in the U.S. economy in 1 year. In the mid-1990s, the U.S. allocated about 16% of GNP for health-care services. Experts projected that the percentage would reach 20% by the year 2000. In practical terms this means that out of every $100, $20 will be spent on health-care services. The more money spent on health care, the less is available for food, clothing, shelter, transportation, education, recreation, and other needs or interests (Stanhope & Lancaster, 1996).

Few patients can afford to pay for health-care costs out of their own pocket. To avoid financial devastation from a chronic or catastrophic illness or injury, patients rely on either government programs, such as Medicare and Medicaid, or employer-provided private insurance programs to pay for medical expenses. Even so, personal health-care costs have doubled every decade. By the year 2000, the average patient may spend more than $5,500 a year on insurance premiums, medications, and health care practitioners and services. In 1990, the yearly average was just $2,518 (Smith & Maurer, 1995)

Providing health care in community-based settings can reduce the cost of that care while still providing the patient with quality services. As insurance plans and other third-party payer services have honored claims for patient care delivered in nonhospital settings, the delivery of medical-surgical care is steadily moving to these arenas. Eventually, only patients who really need to be in the hospital will receive care there.

DEMOGRAPHIC CHANGES

Today, medical-surgical nurses must care for increasing numbers of poor patients, impaired elderly people, adult victims of domestic violence, homeless people, and people living with human immunodeficiency virus (HIV) infection or AIDS. Many of these patients are treated in the emergency department or outside the hospital setting.

Poverty

The U.S. Commerce Department's Census Bureau reported that 36.4 million people (13.8 percent of population) were living below the poverty level in 1995. The poverty rate of the native-born population was 13.0 percent, while the rate among foreign-born persons was 22.2 percent. About half the nation's poor were under the age of 18 years or over the age of 65. Medicaid was the most widespread type of health-care insurance among the poor, covering 46.4 percent of all poor people.

The Census Bureau also reported that nearly 40.6 million (15.4%) of the nation's population did not have health insurance (www.US Census Bureau, 1996). The relationship between poverty and health status has been well documented. There is a higher prevalence of chronic disease and disability among people who are poor than among the general population. Poor people often do not seek health care until they are in pain or acutely ill because they have neither health insurance nor money to pay for it. They are more often preoccupied with obtaining food and shelter than seeking preventive heath care.

Aging

Since 1900, the percentage of U.S. citizens 65 years of age and older has more than tripled, from 4.1% in 1900 to 12.8% in 1995. Moreover, the older population is itself getting older. In 1995, the 65- to 74-year-old age group (18.8 million) was eight times larger than in 1900, the 75- to 84-year-old age group (11.1 million) was 14 times larger and the 85 and older age group (3.6 million) was 29 times larger. By the year 2000, some 34.7 million people will be 65 years old or older. By 2030, more than 69.4 million people will be over the age of 65 (www.aoa.dhls.gov, 1996).

According to the U.S. Department of Health and Human Services, most older persons have at least one chronic medical condition and may have multiple chronic conditions. These conditions commonly include arthritis, hypertension, hearing impairment, cataracts, orthopedic problems, and heart disease.

In a recent study, about 6.1 million (23%) older people living in the community had health-related difficulties with one or more of the activities of daily living (ADLs). ADLs are basic personal care activities such as the ability to bathe, dress, eat, transfer from bed or chair, walk, get outside, and use the toilet without the assistance of others. Twenty-eight percent (7.6 million) had difficulty with one or more instrumental activities of daily living (IADLs). IADLs include the ability to prepare meals, shop, manage money, use the telephone, and do housework. The percentage of people having difficulty with ADLs or IADLs increased with age (www.aoa.dhhs.gov, 1996)

Elderly patients who have acute or chronic medical conditions or lack the capacity for self-care need a range of services to address their health-care, personal-care, and social needs. They need a continuum of long-term-care services that include both community-based services and institution-based services (Matteson et al, 1997). To complicate matters further, a significant number of older adults do not have adequate financial resources to meet the cost of those services. In total, about one-fifth (18%) of the older population was poor or near-poor in 1995.

Domestic Violence

An additional significant change in society is the increased prevalence of domestic violence. The U.S. Department of Justice estimates that 95% of assaults on spouses or ex-partners are committed by men against women. Nearly four million (7%) women in the United States who were married or living with someone as a couple were physically abused in 1995. Research studies have reported that more than 90% of women who were physically abused by their partners did not discuss these incidents with their physicians. This should come as no surprise, since U.S. institutions and society itself have not yet shown a willingness to offer consistent support to victims of violence. Nonetheless, although many victims of domestic violence do not require hospital care, most do require some form of health care.

Increasingly, agencies need established policies and procedures for identifying and treating women who are abused, including identifying when the nurse has a legal obligation to report domestic violence incidents to law enforcement agencies. Medical-surgical nurses need to remember that caring for these victims requires understanding, compassion, and a recognition of the helplessness they may feel. They need to be involved in designing an effective, coordinated, multidisciplinary response to the epidemic of domestic violence. Some state nurse-licensure boards are attempting to respond to the epidemic by requiring that nurses receive continuing education on family violence (www.igc.apc.org, 1996).

Homelessness

Homelessness is a major health and social problem in the United States. Two trends are largely responsible for the rise in homelessness: lack of affordable rental housing and increased poverty. Other factors that may contribute to homelessness include domestic violence, severe and persistent mental illness, addiction disorders, and underemployment or unemployment (www.ari.net).

Currently, women and children constitute the largest growing segment of the homeless population. Many health problems arise in this population, a result of poor nutrition, inadequate clothing, living in adverse weather conditions, being victims of violence, and being exposed to communicable diseases, such as tuberculosis, lice, scabies, and sexually transmitted diseases. Homeless persons typically have great difficulty gaining access to affordable health care, especially preventive care or early interventions.

Human Immunodeficiency Virus Infection and Acquired Immunodeficiency Syndrome

A major threat to the public health and a major concern to medical-surgical nurses is the epidemic cause by infection with HIV and the eventual development of AIDS. No one is immune from contracting the disease. The age-adjusted death rate from HIV infection was 15.4 deaths per 100,000 population in 1995. Through June 1996, the Centers for Disease Control and Prevention had received reports of 548,102 U.S. men, women, and children with AIDS. Some 343,000 had died. This epidemic has presented many new challenges to nursing practice, both inside and outside the hospital (www.cdc.gov, 1996).

The outbreak of AIDS has given rise to the concept of universal precautions (standard precautions) as a method of protecting nurses from contracting the disease while caring for patients infected with the virus. In every health-care setting, medical-surgical nurses who care for HIV-infected and AIDS patients require administrative support and information to maintain their own health. The number of reported cases of occupational transmission of HIV infection to nurses in the United States through December 1995 was 19. An additional 24 cases are considered possible occupational transmission (www.cdc.gov, 1996).

Those who care for HIV/AIDS patients need to wrestle with such ethical questions as, "Is the patient's right to privacy more important than the nurse's need to know the patient's diagnosis?" and, "Is mandatory testing for HIV infection in the best interest of patients and caregivers?" Education of patient, family, and the public about HIV and AIDS is an important aspect of the medical-surgical nurse's role in all health-care settings. The course of the epidemic will be determined by the effectiveness of health education programs in preventing new infections, prompt diagnosis of HIV infection, and the availability and effectiveness of new drug therapies.

These changes in populations that require a great deal of medical care have added to the spiraling costs of health care. Because access to health care is limited for some populations, such as many of the poor, the homeless, the aged, and those diagnosed with AIDS, medical-surgical nursing care delivered in the community allows for greater service to at-risk populations, at a lower cost. In addition, more people can be served at an overall lower cost to the health-care system.

MEDICARE REIMBURSEMENT AND DRGs

During the past decades, the U.S. health-care system has undergone significant public policy changes in an effort to control escalating costs and ensure accessibility. During the 1970s, the United States experienced a rapid increase in the cost of health care. It was predicted that costs would continue to spiral out of control because of the aging population and the growing cost of medical technology and personnel.

In an attempt to slow the escalating cost of care, Congress passed legislation in 1983 that provided hospitals with a prospective payment system (PPS) based on 467 diagnosis-related groups (DRGs). Medicare would reimburse hospitals a fixed, pre-established fee for each Medicare patient with a particular DRG, regardless of the services rendered or days of hospitalization. It allowed hospitals to make a profit by carefully monitoring the types of services provided and by discharging patients to their homes, residential facilities, or long-term care facilities at a much earlier stage of recovery and at a more acute level of illness. DRGs have resulted in hospitals downsizing, restructuring, and diversifying, and they have increased the need for noninstitutional health care services.

Patients are now discharged from the hospital earlier, sometimes with dressings still in place, with continuous needs for intravenous therapy, and without the level of discharge teaching that would have been completed in the hospital if the patient had stayed longer. This has significantly increased the demand for medical-surgical nurses to provide care and education to patients and families in such settings as the home, ambulatory care facilities, and long-term care settings (Dee-Kelly et al, 1994).

THE ADVENT OF MANAGED HEALTH CARE

Historically, the U.S. health-care system has been financed through health insurance systems that paid health-care providers on a fee-for-service basis and allowed patients relative freedom to select their health-care providers. As employers and other purchasers are increasingly taking steps to control health-care expenditures, managed care organizations (MCOs) are steadily gaining market share.

Managed Care Organizations

There is a broad and dynamic array of health plans that control health-care costs by regulating provision of care and using discounted fee schedules or capitated, prepaid fees for providers. Some MCOs contract with independent groups of health-care providers; others (called staff models) employ health-care providers.

As a group, MCOs are rapidly becoming a major payer or provider of health care for the beneficiaries of employer-funded and government-funded (Medicaid and Medicare) health-care programs. MCOs arrange for health care at predetermined or prepaid rates, specify which doctors and hospitals patients can use, and oversee physicians' treatment and referrals. These cost-reducing plans have become so popular so quickly that the majority of people with private insurance are currently enrolled in them. In fact, 7 of 10 U.S. workers were covered by some type of managed care plan in 1996 (Gray, 1996; Sederer & Bennett, 1996).

Health Maintenance Organizations

Health maintenance organizations (HMOs) are health plans that contract with medical groups to provide a full range of health services—including preventive and screening services—for their enrollees for a fixed, prepaid, per-member fee. Alternatively, some HMOs provide services themselves by employing health-care professionals directly. In either case, each member has a primary care physician (PCP) who functions as the plan's "gatekeeper" by directing the patient's medical care. For all but emergencies, the patient enters the health care system through the PCP and can receive covered care from a specialist only with the PCP's referral. For urgent problems that arise unexpectedly, many HMOs use free-standing urgent care centers rather than encouraging members to seek care in hospital emergency rooms (Fig. 2–1). Largely because of its cost-containment features and wide range of covered services, HMO enrollment has increased steadily. Some 51 million people were enrolled in HMOs in 1996 (www.wnet.org/mhc/info/index.html, 1996).

Preferred Provider Organizations

Preferred provider organizations (PPOs) are health plans that reduce costs by establishing a network of preferred providers, physicians, hospitals, and others who agree to provide comprehensive health services to subscribers while charging the PPO a discounted rate for those services. Compared with HMOs, PPOs typically offer members more latitude in choosing health-care providers. For example, a member can choose to see a specialist directly for covered care as long as that specialist appears on the plan's list of preferred providers. For members, the trade-off for this increased freedom usually is a

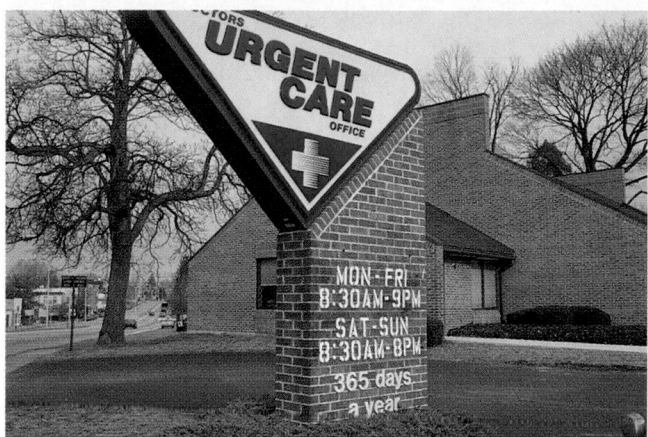

Figure 2–1

Urgent-care centers provide prompt care for patients with unforeseen urgent problems, thus avoiding the high cost of a visit to the emergency department.

higher out-of-pocket expense than is incurred with most HMOs. In 1996, about 50 million people were enrolled in PPOs (www.wnet.org/mhc/info/index.html, 1996).

Case Management

Case management is an essential component of managed care. The Case Management Society of America defines case management as a collaborative process designed to meet the health-care needs of patients by assessing, planning, coordinating, and monitoring their care. It evaluates patients' options and services to promote quality, cost-effective care.

Case managers (nurses, doctors, or social workers) affiliated with a health plan are responsible for coordinating the health care of the patients enrolled. They are the link between the patient, health and social service providers, the payer, and the community. They ensure the appropriate use of medical facilities and services and maintain cost effectiveness on a patient-by-patient basis.

Case management programs are operated by acute-care hospitals, public insurance (Medicaid, Medicare), private insurance (long-term care, liability, casualty, auto, accident, and health), managed care organizations (HMOs, PPOs), independent case management companies, and provider agencies and facilities (Smith, 1995).

Experts estimate that before 2010, 80 to 90% of insured patients will receive care through a managed system. The Pew Health Professions Commission predicts that by the end of the 20th century, the American health care system will be more managed, with better integration of services and financing; more accountable to those who purchase and use health services; and able to use fewer resources more effectively (www.futurehealth.ucsf.edu, 1997).

The managed care industry now includes large private insurance companies (such as Aetna, Travelers, and Cigna), Blue Cross and Blue Shield organizations, and consortia of hospitals, clinics, and community mental health centers (Sederer & Bennett, 1996). It is rapidly and dramatically shaping the delivery of health care and shifting it from the hospital to the community.

Nonhospital Practice Settings

With the advent of shortened hospital stays, advanced technology that allows more surgical interventions to be performed on an outpatient basis, and the increasing involvement of case management systems in the health-care industry, settings for delivery of medical-surgical interventions are expanding in the community. In fact, nonhospital practice settings are becoming the norm rather than the exception in providing health care to individuals, families, and communities. The type of care provided in these community settings may vary from general comprehensive care—such as that provided in nurse-managed centers—to highly specific treatments provided in outpatient surgery centers.

AMBULATORY HEALTH-CARE SETTINGS

Hospital- or community-based ambulatory care settings provide patients with primary health-care services. They do not offer inpatient services. They include hospitals, physician offices, community agencies, public health departments, medical clinics, ambulatory care centers, neighborhood health centers, free-standing urgent care centers, community outreach programs, and other types of services, such as cardiac rehabilitation. Ambulatory settings can provide a broad range of services and include medical care, diagnostic tests, surgery, administration of medications, physical therapy, kidney dialysis, counseling, and health education (Hunt & Zurek, 1997; Smith & Maurer, 1995). The types of patients served and services offered depend on the agency's mission.

Neighborhood health centers provide services for patients who live in geographically defined (urban or rural) areas. They may be free-standing buildings or mobile units. Mobile clinics are specially designed vans that provide ambulatory care services for patients in a variety of geographic locations (Fig. 2–2). Outreach programs offer health services to specific high-risk populations, such as children, migrant workers, Native Americans, or the elderly.

Free-standing urgent or emergency care centers are clinics that operate in shopping areas and malls and usually are open during regular business hours.

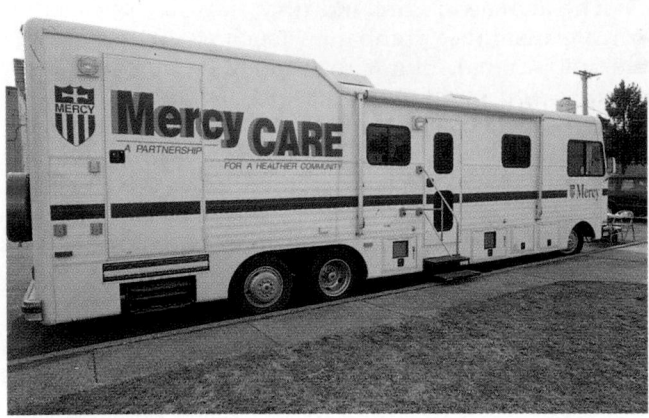

Figure 2–2
Mobile clinics can bring health-care services directly to patients' homes and gathering places.

They offer services without appointments for episodic illness or injury. Hospital-based or free-standing wellness centers offer activities and programs that promote health. Medical clinics offer care for acute and chronic health problems. Churches may hire parish nurses or use volunteers to offer screening, health education, information and referral services, counseling, and holistic care to parishioners (Hunt & Zurek, 1997; Smith & Maurer, 1995).

NURSE-MANAGED CENTERS

Nurse-managed centers are organizations where nurses control the practice and patient care and where education and research are paramount. They serve a variety of populations, such as the elderly, poor, rural, homeless, migrants, developmentally disabled, and handicapped. Colleges and universities were among the first to develop nurse-managed agencies to meet their students' health-care needs and to provide settings for nursing practice. Nurse practitioners are the primary care providers in the university nurse-managed agencies. Nursing care focuses on health promotion activities, such as physical assessments, health screenings, and health education classes. Services are reimbursed by private insurance, Medicare or Medicaid, and private pay (Clemen-Stone et al, 1995).

OUTPATIENT AND AMBULATORY SURGICAL FACILITIES

In outpatient and ambulatory surgical facilities (surgicenters) patients have scheduled operative procedures and are discharged on the same day. A variety of surgical procedures can be performed safely in these facilities, including herniorrhaphy, cataract extraction, plastic surgery, abdominal and thoracic

procedures using "video surgery," and many others. There has been a steady expansion of free-standing ambulatory surgical centers and the number of procedures performed. They have expanded because of improved surgical techniques, anesthetic agents, and practices and better operating facilities. The evolving technology will continue to make surgery easier on the patient and require less postoperative care and observation (Davis, 1993). Medical-surgical nurses working in surgical centers do patient preoperative care and teaching, postoperative care, self-care teaching for recovery at home, and postoperative follow-up at home.

ADULT DAY HEALTH CENTERS

Adult day health centers are congregate facilities for supervised care of frail, older patients during specified day hours. The patients return home in the evening. The purpose of the centers is to maintain or improve the functional abilities of impaired older patients by offering an array of structured health, social, recreational, and therapeutic activities. Medical-surgical nurses working at adult day health centers are responsible for patient assessments, administering medications and other treatments, designing and managing therapeutic regimens, and supervising nursing assistants and volunteers. They collaborate with a multidisciplinary team and families regarding the patient's condition and plans of care. The patients or families often pay for adult day health services with personal funds, because few health insurers pay for the service. In some states, public funds (Medicaid) cover these services for persons who meet eligibility criteria (Matteson et al, 1997).

HOME-BASED CARE

Home-based care provides health care to patients in residences that may be their own dwellings, apartments, relatives' homes, or homes for the aged, but not in a hospital or skilled nursing facility (SNF). Care is provided by a variety of agencies that are classified as official (public-funded by local or state government), nonprofit, proprietary chains (for-profit agencies operated by corporations), and hospital-based agencies. Most agencies provide comprehensive patient services, but some specialize in specific care, such as home infusion services. Between 1989 and 1995, the number of home health agencies increased by more than 50 percent. In 1995, Medicare expenditures for home care alone were $15 billion, up from $2 billion in 1988 (Clark, 1996; Marrelli, 1994).

Medicare patients and those covered by most other insurance plans must meet the following criteria to be eligible for home-based care.

- They must be homebound (leaving the house requires considerable and taxing effort).
- They must need part-time or intermittent skilled nursing care that is reasonable and necessary, physical therapy, or speech therapy.

Typically, patients have recently been discharged from a hospital with a new major diagnosis and a need for skilled health care. Medicare does not pay for custodial care. For many patients, home-based care can prevent lengthy or further hospitalization, or prevent admission to a nursing home (Marrelli, 1994).

Patients are provided health care and medical social services by a multidisciplinary team that includes registered nurses (RNs), physicians, home health aides, licensed practical or licensed vocational nurses (LPN/LVNs), medical social workers, and physical, speech, and occupational therapists. Table 2–1 describes the qualifications of the home health-care team and the services they provide patients. Medicare and Medicaid programs, private insurance, and patients themselves pay for the services. Each insurance program has its own requirements for reimbursement.

HOSPICE CARE SETTINGS

Hospice care is a palliative system of health services provided to terminally ill patients and their families. The care is provided in the patients' homes, in hospitals, in inpatient respite units, in long-term-care facilities, or in ambulatory care settings. Most patients have been diagnosed with cancer, end-stage cardiac disease, lung disease, renal disease, AIDS, end-stage Alzheimer's disease, amyotrophic lateral sclerosis, or another terminal debilitating degenerative disorder. They have elected not to continue with curative treatment. The focus of care is on improving the quality of the patient's life by controlling pain and other symptoms. Services are provided by a multidisciplinary team that includes physicians, RNs, LPN/LVNs, home health aides, social workers, dietitians, and speech, physical, and occupational therapists. In addition, clergy and volunteers are often important team members. (Gurfolina & Dumas, 1994; Rice, 1992).

Hospice home-care organizations are funded by Medicare, Medicaid, and private insurance. Hospice programs are frequently a component of home health services. Patient eligibility for hospice services varies depending on the funding source. Patients typically must have a life expectancy of 6 months or less according to their physician. They must not be undergoing or be contemplating active treatment for their disease. And they should have decided to forego resuscitative measures (such as cardiopulmonary resuscitation [CPR]). Families are eligible for bereavement benefits after the patients dies (Gurfolina & Dumas, 1994; Rice, 1992).

COMMUNITY-BASED, LONG-TERM-CARE SERVICES

Community-based, long-term-care services are provided to chronically ill or frail patients to sustain them in their residences at their highest level of functioning. Included are a broad spectrum of health and social services, including personal care, housekeeping, shopping services, respite care, senior companion, transportation, home-delivered meals, caregiver support groups, adult day care, home health, and hospice care.

REHABILITATION IN LONG-TERM-CARE FACILITIES

Rehabilitation services vary with the type of facility and payment (Medicare, Medicaid, or private pay). Some long-term-care facilities (LTCFs) provide primarily custodial care. Others are designed to provide rehabilitation for patients who have the potential to regain function. Services are provided by a professional multidisciplinary team. RNs assess patients in LTCFs during an acute or unstable phase of an illness, administer enteral or intravenous fluids and medications, do bowel and bladder training, and change sterile dressings. Patients not needing skilled nursing activities are not eligible for skilled nursing benefits under third-party reimbursement sources and are deemed to be in need of custodial care (Matteson et al, 1997).

PUBLIC HEALTH DEPARTMENTS

Public health departments have the responsibility for determining the health status and meeting the needs of communities. They provide community, mental health, personal, and environmental health services. They offer community-health programs aimed at controlling communicable diseases, mother-child health programs, nutrition education, and health education. They provide environmental health services, such as food hygiene, protection from hazardous substances, control of waste, occupational health, and control of air, noise, and water pollution. They receive government funding to provide services to groups and to individuals and families in clinics, schools, jails, and patients' homes (Swanson & Albrecht, 1993).

OCCUPATIONAL HEALTH SETTINGS

Occupational health focuses on the health and well-being of U.S. workers at the worksite. The federal Occupational Safety and Health Act of 1970 has had a major impact on the health and safety of employees. It protects employees against personal injury

Table 2–1

The Multidisciplinary Team: Member Qualifications and Responsibilities

Member	Qualifications	Responsibilities
Physician	Licensed by the State as a doctor of medicine (MD), osteopathy (DO), or podiatry (DPM)	Evaluate patient's medical status and provide medical care as needed Authorize patient's treatment plan Review patient's treatment plan as often as the patient's condition requires, but at least once every 62 days
Registered nurse (RN)	Licensed by the State as an RN	Use the nursing process to determine patient's needs and to establish the patient's care plans Provide skilled nursing services (see Table 2–2) Evaluate care delivered by the nursing team As case managers, determine the comprehensive needs of patients and families, make referrals to appropriate community resources, and coordinate care among the multiple agencies providing services
Physical therapist	Licensed by the State as a physical therapist. Completed a physical therapy curriculum approved by The American Physical Therapy Association (APTA), The Committee on Allied Health Education and Accreditation of the American Medical Association (AMA) or The Council on Medical Education of the AMA and the APTA	Work with patients who have functional impairments related to neuromuscular problems and help them conserve, restore, and improve neuromuscular functioning and increase their self-care capabilities Teach patients ambulating techniques and how to use assistive appliances Do prosthetic training, chest physiotherapy, electrotherapy, and muscle re-education and recommend the use of appropriate orthopedic and prosthetic devices
Occupational therapist	Completed an occupational therapy curriculum accredited jointly by the Council on Medical Education of the American Medical Association and the American Occupational Therapy Association	Work with patients who have difficulty carrying out activities of daily living Teach patients independent living/daily living skills, muscle re-education, perceptual motor training, fine motor coordination, neuro-development treatment, accessible sensory treatment, orthotics/splinting, and adaptive equipment fabrication and training Assess the patient's environment to identify safety hazards and barriers to self-care and recommend environmental modifications that could help the patient increase independence and prevent accidents
Dietitian (nutritionist)	Registered (or eligible) by the American Dietetic Association	Assess a patient's nutritional status Assist patients in meeting their basic nutritional needs Teach patients and families about therapeutic diets, how to plan economical nutritious meals, and food purchasing and preparation Often used as resource person by other members of the health-care team
Home health aide	Completed a State-sponsored or other training program that meets established requirements for home health aide training	Paraprofessionals trained to assist patients with personal care and light household tasks Required to report changes in the patient's condition and needs and complete appropriate records Must be supervised in patients' homes by RNS at least every 2 weeks if providing personal care If the patient needs only custodial care, supervisory visits must be made once every 62 days
Vocational/practical nurse	Licensed by the State as a vocational/practical nurse	Give skilled nursing care to patients under the supervision of RNs and physicians

Table 2–1

The Multidisciplinary Team: Member Qualifications and Responsibilities *(continued)*

Member	Qualifications	Responsibilities
Social worker	Completed a Masters degree from a school of social work accredited by the Council on Social Work Education and has gained 1 year of social work experience in a health-care setting	Conduct patient social and emotional assessments Work with patients who are experiencing significant psychosocial, financial, or environmental difficulties by providing short-term therapy and counseling for long-range planning Refer patients to community resources Help patients in attaining needed social and health-care services Help plan for institutional community placements, such as nursing-home or extended-care facility placement Resource person for other health-care team members who are dealing with difficult psychosocial, financial, or environmental problems
Speech pathologist (speech therapist)	Meets the educational and experience requirements for a Certificate of Clinical Competence in speech pathology or audiology from the American Speech-Language-Hearing Association	Assess patient's speech, language, and hearing abilities and identify barriers in the environment that inhibit effective communication Work with patients who have voice disorders, speech articulation disorders, dysphagia, and language disorder problems to help increase functional communication skills Initiate exercises to increase functional speaking skills, teach esophageal speech, and recommend the use of communication appliances, such as intraoral devices or hearing aids Teach caregivers how to effectively communicate with the patient

Information from California Association for Health Services at Home (CAHSAH). Side by side comparison of Title 22, Division 5, Chapter 6 and Medicare conditions of participation for home health agencies. Sacramento, CA: CAHSAH, 1995; Clemen-Stone S, Eigsti DG, McGuire SL. Comprehensive community health nursing. 4th ed. St. Louis: Mosby Year-Book, 1995; Marrelli TM. Handbook of home health standards and documentation guidelines for reimbursement. 2nd ed. St. Louis: Mosby Year-Book, 1994.

and illness resulting from hazardous working conditions. It encourages employers and employees to reduce hazards in the workplace by implementing new or improved safety and health programs. The Occupational Health and Safety Administration (OSHA) inspects workplaces for violations of existing health and safety standards and provides consulting services for management and for employer and employee training and education (Clemen-Stone et al, 1995).

Occupational health programs can reduce the costs associated with employee absenteeism, hospitalization, disability, and early death. There are several models for providing occupational health services. The ideal program is located at the work site. It is staffed by a multidisciplinary team that includes nurses, physicians, exercise physiologists, health educators, counselors, nutritionists, safety engineers, and industrial hygienists.

Occupational health programs range from worker safety and injury prevention to health promotion and emergency care. The leading work-related diseases and injuries are occupational lung dis-

eases, musculoskeletal injuries, occupational cancers, traumatic injuries and death, cardiovascular diseases, disorders of reproduction, neurotoxic disorders, noise-induced loss of hearing, dermatologic conditions, and psychologic disorders (Clemen-Stone et al, 1995).

SCHOOL-BASED SETTINGS

Health-care services provided in the school setting are governed by state and school district regulations and policies. They vary across the United States. Their purpose is to promote the optimal health of school-age children and adolescents so that they can reach their maximum potential for learning and participation in the educational process. School nurses collaborate with other school personnel to develop and implement a school health program. The multidisciplinary health team may include students, parents, teachers, homebound teachers, counselors, administrators, social workers, physicians, dentists, nutritionists, and youth service personnel.

School-based services provide health care for students and health education for students, parents, and school personnel. They also monitor and evaluate the environmental health and safety of students and school personnel. Common school health problems are substance abuse (alcohol and other drug use), pregnancy, sexually transmitted diseases, physical injuries, abuse and neglect, mental health problems, nutritional deficiencies, dental health problems, and physical ailments, such as dermatologic disorders and respiratory conditions. The school health program may include school-based clinics that provide physical health services, mental heath services, or both to school-age children (Igoe, 1994).

Nursing Practice Roles in Nonhospital Settings

Medical-surgical nurses who work in nonhospital practice settings provide care to patients with existing or predicted physiologic alteration, trauma, or disability. Their care is based on the nursing process and includes:

- Provision of comfort
- Promotion and maintenance of health
- Prevention, detection, and treatment of illness
- Restoration of function
- Assistance with a peaceful death

They work as members of multidisciplinary teams and are responsible for supervising unlicensed assistive personnel.

Medical-surgical nurses working in nonhospital practice settings usually take part in multidisciplinary health-care teams because no one discipline can address the array of needs experienced by many patients in the community. Nurses participate in team conferences, where they provide nursing assessments of patients, assist in establishing multidisciplinary patient care plans, and make referrals to other team members. They work as case managers and coordinate patient care with other health and social agencies to ensure continuity of care. The disciplines applied in each patient's care varies depending on the type of agency involved and the services needed by the patient (see Table 2–1).

SUPERVISOR OF UNLICENSED ASSISTIVE PERSONNEL

Managed care has increased the use of unlicensed assistive personnel in the delivery of health care. These are health-care providers who may be trained and certified but are not licensed to perform nursing tasks. They include certified nursing assistants, home health aides, and patient care technicians. RNs need to be knowledgeable about the unlicensed person's education and training and the agency's policies and procedures for supervision of unlicensed personnel (Barter, 1996; CAB of RN, 1994).

RNs supervise unlicensed assistive personnel in patients' homes and in ambulatory health-care facilities. To do so, they consider the competency of the particular unlicensed worker to perform the assigned tasks. This is especially challenging for RNs supervising unlicensed personnel who care for patients in their homes. RNs are responsible for assigning tasks to assist patients with ADLs (such as bathing, feeding, range-of-motion exercises, and transfers and ambulation) or IADLs (preparing meals, shopping, and doing housework). Medicare requires that RNs supervise unlicensed personnel in the patient's home at least every 2 weeks if they are providing personal care and at least every 62 days if the patient needs only custodial care. Other health insurance programs have similar supervisory requirements (Barter, 1996; CAHSAH, 1995).

DISCHARGE PLANNER

Recent changes in health-care delivery and reimbursement have increased the need for discharge planning in all health-care agencies to ensure that patients receive continuity of health care. Medical-surgical nurse discharge planners must efficiently coordinate continuity of care for patients who may move quickly from one health-care agency to another. They need to be knowledgeable about the community resources available for patients, including the services provided, their eligibility requirements, and their cost. These RNs act as service brokers for patients by obtaining formal and informal health-care resources to meet patients' unmet health needs. They work with the patients and other professionals to coordinate, plan, and arrange for patient transitions within an agency and between agencies (Clemen-Stone et al, 1995).

AMBULATORY CARE NURSE

Medical-surgical nurses employed in ambulatory care settings do interviews of patients in person and by telephone, perform patient assessments, do routine laboratory work, assist with examinations, administer injections and medications, change wound dressings, assist with surgery and other treatments, provide health education, and maintain records.

They function as triage nurses, clinic managers, supervisors of aides and LPN/LVNs, and discharge planners. They are employed in inpatient or outpatient hospital-owned or free-standing clinics, private group medical practices, clinics run by HMOs, public health clinics, industrial health service units, and school health clinics.

Table 2–2

Home-Health Skilled Nursing Services Covered by Medicare

Skilled observation and assessment of the patient's condition
Insertion and removal of a Foley catheter
Teaching patient or caregiver to care for indwelling catheter
Instilling medications into the patient's bladder
Skilled observation and care of surgical incision or suture line, irrigation of open post-surgical wounds, and application of medications and/or dressing changes
Irrigation, application of medication and/or dressing changes to decubitus, other skin ulcer, or lesion
Performing venipuncture for specific tests under physician's orders
Postoperative cataract care, including patient observation, dressing change, teaching, and so on
Bowel/bladder training for patients who have neurologic or muscular problems or other conditions in which the need for bowel or bladder training is clearly identified
Breathing exercises, postural drainage, chest percussion, conservation techniques, and so on
Administration of intramuscular and subcutaneous injections, including vitamin B_{12}
Preparation of insulin syringes for administration by the patient, caregiver, or nurse
Administration of intravenous fluids or medication or clysis
Teaching patient or caregiver about ostomy or ileal conduit care
Teaching the patient or caregiver to administer nasogastric feedings, and care of equipment and preparation of feedings
Reinsertion of nasogastric tube and changing the tube
Teaching the patient or caregiver to care for gastrostomy, care for equipment, and administer feedings
Teaching the patient or caregiver to administer parenteral nutrition, including teaching aseptic technique for dressing changes to catheter site
Teaching the patient or caregiver to care for a tracheotomy
Administration of tracheostomy care, including changing the tracheostomy tube and caring for equipment
Teaching patient or caregiver to administer inhalation therapy and care for equipment
Administration of inhalation treatment and care of equipment
Teaching patient or caregiver to administer an injection
All teaching of the diabetic patient (eg, diet, skin care, administration of insulin, urine testing)
Removal of an impaction and follow-up enema

Information from California Association for Health Services at Home (CAHSAH). Side by side comparison of Title 22, Division 5, Chapter 6 and Medicare conditions of participation for home health agencies. Sacramento, CA: CAHSAH, 1995; Health Care Financing Administration (HCFA): Medicare home health agency manual, HIM II: Coverage of services, 234.9. Washington, DC: U.S. Department of Health and Human Services, 1994. Marrelli TM. Handbook of home health standards and documentation guidelines for reimbursement. 2nd ed. St. Louis: Mosby Year-Book, 1994.

HOME HEALTH NURSE, VISITING NURSE, HOSPICE NURSE

Home health or visiting nurses visit patients who have acute and chronic health care problems in their home environments. They make the initial patient evaluation visits and develop comprehensive plans of care that address patients' physical, psychologic, and social environmental (safety) needs. They provide skilled nursing care to patients and families, as listed in Table 2–2. They serve as case managers and monitor the delivery of skilled and unskilled care provided to patients in their homes (Fig. 2–3). They are responsible for making intra-agency referrals to social workers and to speech, physical, and occupational therapists. They supervise and teach LPN/LVNs and home health aides. They document patient visits and report their findings to the patients' physicians and other members of the multidisciplinary team.

Hospice nurses visit patients who are terminally ill and their caregivers. Their care is focused on symptom relief, including pain management, comfort measures, education, and support during the dying process (Hunt & Zurek, 1997).

CLINICAL NURSE SPECIALIST, NURSE PRACTITIONER

Medical-surgical clinical nurse specialists are prepared through advanced study of medical-surgical nursing at the graduate level. They may be licensed as nurse practitioners or clinical nurse specialists. Nurse practitioners engage in independent or collaborative nursing practice. They have advanced knowledge and skills that enable them to function

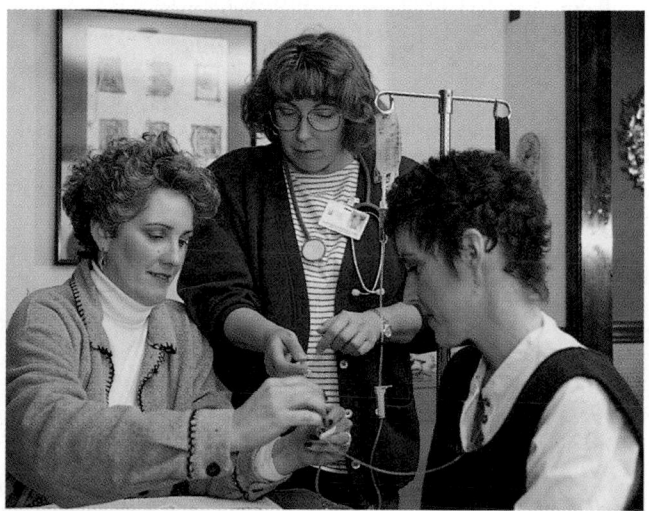

Figure 2–3

Home health care demands many skills, including provision of skilled nursing services and clear teaching of family members and other caregivers.

as primary health-care providers who deliver comprehensive and continuous care. They practice in a variety of settings, including private practice, physicians' offices, clinics, and other ambulatory settings. They specialize in adult health, gerontology, or other areas.

Clinical nurse specialists demonstrate an in-depth understanding of complex medical-surgical problems. They are prepared to provide expert clinical care for a particular group of patients, such as those with diabetes or renal disease. They use their advanced knowledge of a specialty area to solve patient problems and to develop more effective approaches to patient care. They serve as consultants and role models for other members of the health-care team. They engage in formal and informal teaching with coworkers, patients, and families, and participate in research activities and technologic developments affecting their area of practice.

PUBLIC HEALTH NURSE

Public health nurses (PHNs) are RNs who have completed a baccalaureate degree approved by the National League for Nursing (NLN) for PHN preparation or have completed post-RN study that includes content approved by the NLN for PHNs. The American Public Health Association (APHA) considers PHN a specialty in nursing practice that synthesizes the body of knowledge from the public health sciences and professional nursing theories for the purpose of improving the health of the entire community. Their practices have historically emphasized the control of communicable disease. Even though some communicable diseases have been eradicated, others—such as AIDS—still need public health nursing interventions to control, educate, investigate, and prevent.

PHNs participate in community assessment and planning projects to develop population-focused interventions to meet specific health objectives. Their work focuses on:

• Health promotion and health protection activities
• Teaching lifestyle adaptations to maintain health
• Detection, referral, and treatment for health problems

Their patients may be individual persons, a community, or a vulnerable population (such as the homeless). They work in patient homes, group or transitional housing for people with physical or mental disabilities, in occupational settings, schools, clinics, recreation centers, prisons, medical daycare centers, and wellness centers (Clark, 1996; Clemen-Stone et al, 1995; Spradley & Allender, 1996).

OCCUPATIONAL HEALTH NURSE

The American Association of Occupational Health Nurses (AAOHN) supports the baccalaureate degree in nursing as basic preparation for entry into occupational health nursing and recommends certification as an occupational health nurse (OHN). AAOHN defines occupational health nursing as the application of nursing principles in conserving the health of workers in all occupations. OHN roles have expanded in the last decade. They include wellness and lifestyle changes in addition to risk reduction associated with environmental dangers. OHN responsibilities include acting as a care provider, counselor, administrator, health educator, member of multidisciplinary team, and researcher. OHNs need to be knowledgeable about federal, state, and local regulations pertaining to occupational health, such as the Occupational Safety and Health Act, Workers' Compensation Acts, and Americans With Disabilities Act. The typical OHN is the only health-care provider in the agency where he or she is employed. Most OHNs work in medium-sized to large industrial sites, but they also work in many other settings, such as with environmental or occupational health consulting groups, worksite wellness consortia, and worker's compensation insurance carriers (Burgel, 1994; Smith & Maurer, 1995; Swanson & Albrecht, 1993).

SCHOOL NURSE

Most school nurses have a baccalaureate degree in nursing. In some states, they are required to become certified as a school nurse. Their primary responsibilities include the health and safety of school-age children and school personnel. Their roles include:

• Case manager
• Health screener (vision, hearing, scoliosis, for example)
• Provider of emergency care
• Provider of treatment for minor illnesses
• Care of students with special needs
• Health educator
• School health program developer
• Counselor
• Resource and consultant to parents and teachers regarding their health concerns about students

School nurses work in public and private preschools, elementary and secondary schools, and colleges and universities. School nurse practitioners work in school-based clinics as practitioners and perform physical examinations, education, and follow-up care (Hootman J, 1994; Stanhope M, Lancaster J, 1996).

PROVIDER OF TELENURSING SERVICES

An emerging role for medical-surgical nurses is the practice of telenursing. Technology allows the delivery of nursing care to patients in multiple, far-reaching locations. Nursing care can be provided using the telephone, facsimile, cellular phones, computers, teleconferencing, and video conferencing. Examples of nursing care include telephone triage, case managing, providing patient education, obtaining test results, and assisting physicians in the implementation of medical treatment protocols. Two-way interactive television is allowing electronic nursing calls via a two-way cable television line hookup to patients.

Technology-mediated nursing interventions will continue to emerge as equipment becomes more sophisticated and more patients and agencies have the technology available in their settings. Projects are underway to determine the efficacy of creating virtual hospitals and virtual clinics to provide assessment, diagnosis, and care electronically (National Council of State Boards of Nursing, 1996).

The Future of Medical-Surgical Nursing

As the health-care delivery system continues to change and evolve, so will the practice of medical-surgical nurses. The advancement and availability of health-care technology will have a significant influence on the nurse's role in the future. Several national studies are predicting the type of skills nurses will need in the next century.

THE NACNEP STUDY

The National Advisory Council on Nursing Education and Practice (NACNEP) recently reported that the focus of the health-care delivery system is changing the nature of practice of RNs. They found that the nation's previous emphasis on acute care and reliance on hospital-based patient care is shifting to focus on disease prevention and modification of patient lifestyles. This shift promotes maintenance of patients at home and the provision of treatment in ambulatory care settings (USDH&HS, 1996).

NACNEP identified the following future RN roles and responsibilities. RNs will manage patient care along a continuum that includes both community-based services (such as home health care) and institution-based services (such as board and care homes and nursing homes). They will work as peers in multidisciplinary teams and will need to integrate their clinical knowledge with knowledge of community resources. RNs will be focusing on primary care and health promotion. More nurses will manage patients with chronic conditions as the country's older population continues to expand (USDH&HS, 1996).

PEW HEALTH PROFESSIONS COMMISSION REPORT

The Pew Health Professions Commission identified the type of competencies that health care practitioners will need in the year 2005. They concluded that the key areas of practice will be to provide patients with primary care services, including preventive care, and to promote healthy lifestyles. Health-care professionals will be participating in coordinated, multidisciplinary care that involves patients and families in the decision-making process. They will be expanding and ensuring patient access to cost-effective and technologically appropriate care (Primomo, 1995).

As these studies indicate, the health-care environment is changing and presenting unprecedented challenges for medical-surgical nurses. Businesses and consumers have demanded a health-care system that is affordable, accessible, and of high quality. The aging population, changes in the leading causes of death and disability, an increasingly specialized health-care labor force, and increased health-care regulation has had major impact on the health care system. As a result of these changes, medical-surgical nursing roles have become multifaceted and practices have expanded to include community-based settings. Medical-surgical nurses will need to continue to be adaptive and responsive to the needs of society and the changes in health-care practice.

Chapter Review

1. What types of changes in the health-care system and society have increased the need for medical-surgical nurses to practice in nonhospital settings?
2. What are managed care and case management?
3. How have the roles of medical-surgical nurses changed recently?
4. Why is knowledge of the health-care needs of vulnerable populations important for medical-surgical nurses?
5. Compare and contrast the different roles of medical-surgical nurses working in nonhospital settings.
6. What is the discharge planning process?
7. Who takes part in the multidisciplinary health-care team?
8. What types of skilled care do the various team members give to patients?
9. In what types of nonhospital settings do medical-surgical nurses practice?
10. What are the future trends for medical-surgical nursing practice?

Bibliography

Barter M. Unlicensed assistive personnel and lay caregivers in the home. Home Care Provider 1996; 1(3):131.

Burgel BJ. Occupational health: Nursing in the workplace. Nurs Clin North Am 1994; 29(3):431.

California Association for Health Services at Home (CAHSAH). Side by side comparison of Title 22, Division 5, Chapter 6 and Medicare conditions of participation for home health agencies. Sacramento, CA: CAHSAH. August 4, 1995.

California Board of Registered Nursing (CAB of RN). Unlicensed assistive personnel. Sacramento, CA: State and Consumer Services Agency, 1994.

Clark MJ. Nursing in the community. Stamford, CT: Appleton & Lange, 1996.

Clemen-Stone S, Eigsti DG, McGuire SL. Comprehensive community health nursing. 4th ed. St. Louis: Mosby Year-Book, 1995.

Davis JE. Ambulatory surgery . . . How far can we go? Med Clin North Am 1993; 77(2):365.

Dee-Kelly PA, Heller S, Sibley M. Managed care: An opportunity for home care agencies. Nurs Clin North Am 1994; 29(3):471.

Gray J. Managed care 1996: A continuing revolution. Risk Manage 1996; 43(9):14.

Gurfolina V, Dumas L. Hospice nursing: The concept of palliative care. Nurs Clin North Am 1994; 29(3):533.

Health Care Financing Administration (HCFA). Medicare home health agency manual, HIM II: Coverage of services, 234.9. Rev. 272, Washington, D.C.: U.S. Department of Health and Human Services, 1994.

Hootman J. Nursing our most valuable natural resource: School age children. Nurs Forum 1994; 29(3):5.

Hunt R, Zurek EL. Introduction to community based nursing. Philadelphia: JB Lippincott, 1997.

Igoe JB. School nursing. Nurs Clin North Am 1994; 29(3):443.

Marrelli TM. Handbook of home health standards and documentation guidelines for reimbursement. 2nd ed. St. Louis: Mosby Year-Book, 1994.

Matteson MA, McConnell ES, Linton AD. Gerontological nursing concepts and practice. 2nd ed. Philadelphia: WB Saunders, 1997.

Miller CA. Nursing care of older adults: Theory and practice. 2nd ed. Philadelphia: JB Lippincott, 1995.

National Council of State Boards of Nursing. Issues: A newsletter of the National Council. 1996; 17(3).

Primomo J. Ensuring public health nursing in managed care: Partnerships for healthy communities. Public Health Nurs 1995; 12(2):69. [editorial]

Rice R. Home health nursing practice: Concepts and application. St. Louis: Mosby Year-Book, 1992.

Sederer LI, Bennett MJ. Managed mental health care in the United States: A status report. Admin Policy Mental Health 1996; 25(4):289.

Smith CL, Maurer FA. Community health nursing theory and practice. Philadelphia: WB Saunders, 1995.

Smith DS. Standard of practice for case management. J Case Manage 1995; 1(3):7.

Spradley BW, Allender JA. Community health nursing: Concepts and practice. 4th ed. Philadelphia: JB Lippincott, 1996.

Stanhope M, Lancaster J. Community health nursing: Process and practice for promoting health. 4th ed. St. Louis: Mosby Year-Book, 1996.

Swanson JM, Albrecht M. Community health nursing: Promoting the health of aggregates. Philadelphia: WB Saunders, 1993.

U.S. Department of Health & Human Services, Health Resources & Services Administration, (USDH&HS) Bureau of Health Professions, Division of Nursing. National advisory council on nurse education and practice report to the secretary of the Department of Health and Human Services on the basic registered nurse workforce. U.S. Government Printing Office 1996; publication no. 404–882/40043.

www.ari.net. The National Coalition for the Homeless (NCH) fact sheets on homelessness. Jan. 26, 1997. [website]

www.aoa.dhhs.gov. A profile of older Americans. Administration on Aging. 1996; Nov 29. [website]

www.cdc.gov. Income and poverty status of Americans improve, health insurance coverage stable, Census Bureau reports. U.S. Department of Commerce News. Economic & Statistics Administration, U.S. Census Bureau, 1996; Nov 27. [website]

www.futurehealth.ucsf.edu. Critical challenges: Revitalizing the health professions for the twenty-first century. The Pew Health Professions Commission Report 1997; Jan 26. [website]

www.igc.apc.org. The health care response to domestic violence. 1996; Nov 29. [website]

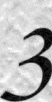 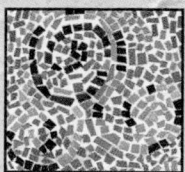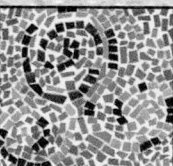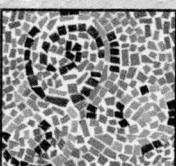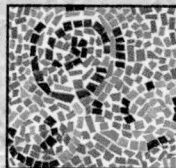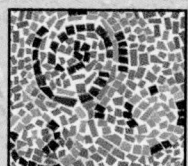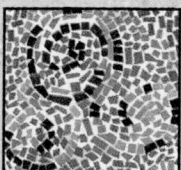

Death, Dying, and Bereavement

Study Outcomes

After studying this chapter, you should be able to:

1. Explain the stages of dying, including the final tasks toward achieving the acceptance of death.
2. Identify the stages of bereavement, as well as the risk factors and manifestations of dysfunctional grieving.
3. State basic beliefs of the major world religions that have implications for the care of dying patients.
4. Identify data essential to assessing the psychosocial status of dying patients, bereaved persons, and patients in spiritual distress.
5. State nursing diagnoses and related expected patient outcomes commonly applicable to dying patients, bereaved persons, and patients in spiritual distress.
6. Explain the basis for evaluation of nursing care provided to dying patients, bereaved persons, and patients in spiritual distress.

Nurses devote a great deal of time to caring for people who are either dying or grieving the death of a loved one. Consequently, nurses have both the opportunity and the responsibility to assist patients and their families through this difficult and painful time. To do so with skill and sensitivity requires clear, calm thinking about death and dying. To give bereaved and dying people the care they need, you must first understand your own thoughts about death. You must learn how to cope with the emotional stress that inevitably accompanies participation in the dying process. And you must find ways to share support with other colleagues who care for dying people.

This chapter presents a number of concepts that are important for nurses caring for people experiencing death, dying, bereavement, and spiritual distress. It provides an overview of how spiritual and religious beliefs can color the dying process and alter after-death practices. And it discusses some of the ethical issues—such as euthanasia and organ donation—that may arise for nurses and patients involved in death and dying.

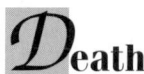eath

PERSONAL AWARENESS OF DEATH

Death is a natural part of life. Regardless of all our efforts to ignore, evade, or deny our death, it is inevitable for each one of us. But although death is a universal event, it is also a unique experience for each person.

Elisabeth Kübler-Ross called death the final stage of growth, and, as quoted in Beauchamp and Perlin (1978), said:

It is the denial of death that is partially responsible for people living empty, purposeless lives; for when you live as if you'll live forever, it becomes too easy to postpone the things you know you must do. You live your life in preparation for tomorrow or in remembrance of yesterday, and meanwhile, each today is lost. In contrast, when you fully understand that each day you awaken could be the last you have, you take the time that day to grow, to become more of who you really are, to reach out to other human beings.

When caring for dying persons, nurses expose themselves to an awareness of their own mortality as well as to their patients' grief and sadness. It is very important that nurses examine their philosophy about death and prepare themselves for those times when they are suddenly confronted by death in their professional and personal lives. A few questions follow regarding personal beliefs about death that nurses might examine and attempt to work through early in their career.

Do you equate death with termination, loss, and failure to survive? Do you see death as closure, conclusion, completion, fulfillment, and graduation? Is death actually a transition into richer, fuller existence, similar to the fetal transition from the security of the womb into this more complex, wondrous existence? Or is it the end of our existence? As health professionals, is the care of the dying basically a battle to be fought with death, the enemy? Can we be powerful, positive agents of healing even in death?

Everyone should develop his or her own philosophy and theology of death to care effectively and compassionately for the dying person.

Death as a Developmental Stage of Life

When John Quincy Adams was 80 years old he met on the streets of Boston an old friend who shook his trembling hand, and said, "Good morning, and how is John Quincy Adams today?" "Thank you," replied the former President, "John Quincy Adams is quite well, sir, but the house in which he lives at present is becoming dilapidated. It is tottering upon its foundations. Time and the seasons have nearly destroyed it. Its roof is pretty well worn out. Its walls are much shattered, and it trembles with every wind. The old tenement is becoming almost uninhabitable, and I think John Quincy Adams will have to move out of it soon; but he himself is quite well, sir, quite well."

Source unknown

Dying is the final developmental stage of life. With ever-lengthening life expectancies, the majority of deaths occur in the elderly between ages 70 and 80. Erik Erikson suggests that ego-integrity versus despair is the developmental task of old age. Death can be viewed as a meaningful conclusion to life if one feels satisfied with one's life as it is reviewed. Despair results from the realization that there is no more time to fulfill missed opportunities or correct mistakes or failures. Expectation of death is deeply resented.

Robert Peck identifies three developmental tasks for the elderly, all of which are preparation for death. The mourned loss of role in retirement is called *work preoccupation*. Many persons define their identity in terms of their work or role. In response to the question "Who are you?" they say, "I am a nurse," "I am a mother," "I was a policeman," or "I was a teacher." Successful adjustment and reinvestment in many roles and in being, rather than in doing, is called *ego differentiation* by Peck. The physical effects of aging bring diminished speed, strength, and sensory acuity along with various physical discomforts and annoying malfunctions, such as chronic constipation. The ability to continue to enjoy life rather than be dominated by these disabilities is called *body transcendence* versus *body preoccupation*. Calm acceptance and peaceful preparation for one's death as closure to one's life is called *ego transcendence*. Peck labels failure of this stage of development *ego preoccupation* and describes it as frequent, fearful, resentful thoughts about death.

Erikson and Peck both suggest that successful mastery of each developmental task is built on mastery of earlier developmental tasks. Therefore, it is no surprise that people usually face death the way they faced earlier life crises. We experience many small losses on an almost daily basis in life as we develop and adjust to the many changes required of us. Each loss is a small death. We learn that struggle and suffering along with pleasure and beauty are an integral part of life. As we struggle to cope and adjust to these small deaths, we prepare for our final death.

Dying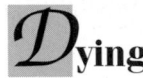

STAGES OF DYING

Much has been written and discussed about the five stages of grief and dying identified by Kübler-Ross. In her interviews with hundreds of dying persons, she witnessed them experiencing five emotional or subjective stages.

Denial

Denial is an initial normal reaction that helps push away the shock to allow us to cope with the reality bit by bit while the full impact settles into our consciousness. It has been characterized as the "No, not me" stage.

Anger

Anger typically follows denial. The rage can seem overwhelming. Fury is often displaced on healthcare professionals, who are accused of being incompetent and uncaring. Spiritual distress occurs when belief systems are challenged as one rages at God, asking "Why did you permit this to happen?" or "Why me?!"

Bargaining

Bargaining is the "Yes, me, but" stage, in which the person makes a promise, usually to God, to do a particular thing or to become a better person in exchange for longer time to live. Often the request is to be present at a special event like a wedding or a graduation or to be able to complete a specific project that is currently in process.

Depression

Depression occurs when the reality of the impending loss has registered. The enormity of what is happening is fully faced. This depression of mourning is normal, healthy behavior when one is dying. One grieves what has already been lost, such as health, attractiveness, independence, one's role in life. One also grieves future losses, such as separation from loved ones and from life itself. This is the resigned "Yes, me" stage.

Acceptance

Acceptance occurs when one has been allowed to work through the depression of mourning. Initially there are brief episodes of acceptance, which occur with greater and greater frequency. One has a sense of "Yes, me, and I am ready." The emotional tone of this stage fully realized is peaceful, calm acceptance. It is a quiet stage and is more positive than mere resignation. It occurs when one has been able to resolve the earlier stages to complete one's grief work. Acceptance, the final stage of dying, is not fully experienced by many persons. In some cases, the death is sudden and the dying person does not have time to complete the necessary tasks to achieve acceptance.

It is very important to note that the stages do not necessarily, or even usually, occur separately or in sequence as listed here. It is sometimes possible to identify indications of all five stages during one session when interviewing a dying patient. There are fluctuations in all emotions in humans on a daily, even an hourly, basis. Nor do all dying persons manifest all these stages. Any grief, regardless of the source of loss—whether life, object, person, or function—has been found to manifest these same five emotional stages.

Kübler-Ross made a significant contribution in the identification of these stages of dying and grief. She, more than any other individual, is responsible for bringing awareness and discussion of death issues out into the open. Some persons do not want to talk about their death, but many do. Their distress is compounded by loneliness and isolation when there is a conspiracy of silence by their loved ones and medical caregivers. Tolstoy described this very movingly in *The Death of Ivan Ilyich*:

What tormented Ivan Ilyich most was the deception, the lie, which for some reason all accepted, that he was not dying but was simply ill. . . . The deception tortured him. . . . This falsity around him and within him did more than anything else to poison his last days.

FINAL TASKS TOWARD ACHIEVING ACCEPTANCE OF DEATH

Tasks that must be completed for each of the subjective stages of denial, anger, bargaining, and depression to be resolved and the stage of acceptance reached are:

- Developing awareness of impending death
- Balancing hope and fear

- Relinquishing the will to live
- Letting go of autonomous control
- Detaching from former experiences and relationships
- Achieving spiritual preparation and integration

Some of these tasks may have been completed earlier in life by some patients. All of them blend together, overlap, and assume greater or lesser importance at different periods during the dying process. They commonly occur in more or less the following sequence.

Developing Awareness of Impending Death

Initially, this awareness may be only a suspicion, or it may be maintained for only brief periods as denial is worked through. Initial lack of awareness may relate to factors outside the patient's control, such as a pact of silence by family and caregivers. Persons whose life patterns have included a great deal of denial and avoidance and fear have difficulty working through denial and completing this task.

Balancing Hope and Fear

Fear is always a part of dying. Death itself is often less feared than a prolonged, suffering dying process. Fears include:

Pain
Uncertainty
Helplessness
Loss and deprivation
Isolation
Alienation
Abandonment
Disfigurement
Indignity
Judgment

Fear can be conquered only when hope is allowed to balance each fear whenever it emerges.

Nurses can do much to help provide hope. Patients must never be left without hope, because it is the antidote to fear. We need to listen as the patient's hope changes. An early expression might be "I hope there is nothing wrong," followed by "I hope there is a cure," then "I hope I am not a burden," then "I hope I will not have pain," and finally, "I hope I will die soon."

Relinquishing the Will to Live

Relinquishing the will to live is another final task necessary to arrive at acceptance of one's death. Reversal of the physical struggle for survival seems to be a conscious decision on the part of many patients near death, unless they are comatose or heavily sedated. Family and caregivers often notice the changes as withdrawal and diversion of energy away from the physical struggle. This fight for survival is so basic to life that a conflict and then a reversal of the will to live seems to take place before the actual acceptance of death is initiated. Often a patient manages to "hang on" and to continue the physical struggle to be alive for special family events like the birth of a grandchild, a homecoming, a graduation, or a wedding. Shortly thereafter, the patient relinquishes the struggle and dies peacefully. Sometimes loved ones need to be helped to give permission to the dying patient to cease a heroic fight to remain alive.

Letting Go of Autonomous Control

Letting go of autonomous control also occurs as the will to live is reversed. This is not the same loss of control experienced earlier in illness when one struggles to cope with the adjustment to debilitating illness. Rather, it is a positive "counter-control" in which one puts oneself peacefully into the hands of others for safe passage to death.

Detaching from Former Experiences and Relationships

Detachment from former experiences and relationships can cause loved ones misunderstanding and pain if they are not aware that this is a natural part of the final dying process. This liberating detachment enables peaceful preparation for impending death.

Achieving Spiritual Preparation and Integration

Spiritual preparation and integration are easiest for those who are devout or have actively practiced their faith and for those who believe in eternal life. Various patient surveys support what caregivers frequently observe, namely that persons with religious faith have an easier time achieving acceptance of their death.

Persons who are nonreligious should be supported in the review and integration of their life experiences and their search for meaning in life. This search is explained by Cicely Saunders, the founder of St. Christopher's Hospice near London, upon which many hospices have been modeled. Regardless of persons' beliefs, she often sees in them something that could be called "reaching out trustfully." "They come to remember things from the past, things that they have been too busy to listen to before, and as death approaches, they find that things begin to make sense. They bring a new attention to the old truths. This is something entirely different from plucking at straws, and is an extremely personal matter for each patient" (Doyle,

1972). Saunders feels that attending to individual spiritual needs is an important aspect of total care.

Dying is a very difficult process, full of fear and sadness. It requires great fortitude. Those who have completed these tasks report a sense of achievement and peace. They are observed to die with dignity, self-respect, and acceptance.

NURSING PROCESS
The Dying Patient

Assessment

To deliver quality nursing care to a person grieving about his or her impending death, the nurse needs information about the patient's prognosis and diagnosis and the expected clinical cause of death. Assess the patient's understanding of the illness, his or her desire or lack of desire to talk about dying, the subjective stages of the dying experience, and the communication patterns of patient and family. Review the patient's medical history, medical treatments, and past crises. Investigate the patient's religious and philosophic beliefs and practices as they relate to dying and death (Table 3–1). Assess resources available to help the patient and significant others deal with the crisis of death. Potential resources include family, friends, religious faith and advisors, financial resources, and personal coping patterns.

Nursing Diagnoses and Planning

Nursing diagnoses and related expected patient outcomes most commonly applicable to the dying patient include the following:

NDx: Anticipatory grieving related to impending death

Planning: Patient Outcomes
1. Patient demonstrates awareness of dying by talking about it, reviewing his or her life, putting affairs in order (such as drawing up a will), expressing farewells, giving keepsakes to significant others, and planning his or her funeral.
2. Patient identifies feelings of denial, anger, bargaining, depression, and acceptance as normal phases of dying, not as signs of weakness.
3. Patient demonstrates control of fear and expresses realistic and appropriate aspects of hope in the situation.
4. Patient communicates his or her decision to relinquish the will to live by ceasing the physical struggle to survive, by letting go of autonomous control, and by emotional detachment.
5. Patient prepares spiritually for death by examining beliefs and expressing a desire or lack of desire to have a religious leader visit for comfort, counseling, and religious rituals.
6. Patient expresses satisfaction with completion of his or her life's work.

Table 3–1

Beliefs and Practices of the Major World Religions Related to Death and Dying

Buddhism	Christianity	Hinduism	Judaism	Islam
BELIEFS AND PRACTICES REGARDING SUFFERING				
Pray for healing. May deny pain and refuse analgesics.	Suffering is God's will and should not be resisted.	Suffering is one's destiny for past lives' practices.	See no value in suffering. Encourage medical treatment.	Fatalistic. "Allah wills it."
DYING RITUALS				
Must stay alert and calm. Monk may chant last rites. Family is present.	Vary with subgroups. Anointing of the sick, Holy Communion, and Reconciliation (confession) important to Roman Catholics. Last rites by a priest are usually mandatory in Eastern Orthodox.	Must stay alert through death passage. Rituals performed by priests.	Family stays with patient.	Confession, seeking forgiveness.
PHYSICAL CARE AT DEATH				
Important for family to provide physical care.	Routine postmortem care given by nurses. Eastern Orthodox place hands in form of a cross.	Only family and close friends may touch the body.	Ritual cleansing by Burial Society. Shomrim stay with body (Orthodox).	Ritual washing by family. Body faced toward Mecca.
ORGAN DONATION AND TRANSPLANTATION				
Seldom oppose.	Generally allowed, but may vary by subgroup.	Problems: Caste beliefs, may need several hours for soul to pass.	Allowed with rabbinical permission. Some Orthodox oppose.	No body part is to be removed. Some liberals may permit it.
AUTOPSY				
Generally allowed.	Generally allowed, but may be opposed by some subgroups (such as Eastern Orthodox).	Generally allowed.	Opposed by Orthodox.	Opposed unless mandated by law.
CREMATION				
Usually preferred.	Generally allowed, but may be opposed by some subgroups (such as Eastern Orthodox.)	Generally allowed.	Opposed by Orthodox.	Generally not allowed.
REMOVAL OF LIFE SUPPORT				
Generally allowed.	Generally allowed, but may be opposed by some subgroups (such as Eastern Orthodox).	Generally allowed.	Do not believe in artificially prolonging life when no hope of recovery exists.	Life should be prolonged as long as possible.

Nursing Interventions and Evaluation

NDx: Anticipatory grieving

To aid the dying person in working through the stages of grief, to accept death and to die with dignity, provide the opportunity to talk about feelings. Stress that it is permissible, normal, and even healthy to grieve. Remember that there are many anticipated losses to be mourned, including:

Unfulfilled future plans and dreams
Roles that were enjoyed
Beloved family and friends
The beauty of the earth's environment
Former physical attractiveness
Abilities and health
Sense of a meaningful life
Hope of continued life on earth

Offer frequent, regular opportunities for the patient to talk out these feelings. Some patients may not wish to talk about their death. If so, respect this wish, but continue to gently provide occasional openers from time to time in case they change their mind. Some patients feel that they must act strong for their loved ones and should not burden them with their own suffering. They fear dragging the beloved downward by showing the extent of their own despair. Nurses and other helping persons can provide crucial opportunities for the patient to vent feelings through therapeutic communication techniques. Encourage the patient to accept visitors and other social contacts to reduce loneliness and isolation.

Display authentic respect for the person and consistent regard for his or her experience. To help counter bruised self-esteem, the sense of unreality, and the fear of breakdown, tell the patient that crying and other expressions of grief are not cowardly signs of weakness but healthy, normal aspects of the grief work. Tears can release feelings of helplessness in the face of tragedy. Keep advice to a minimum, but use nonverbal expressions of comfort to the maximum, since they carry the most potent messages.

Make every effort to combat hopelessness. Keep appointments and commitments with the patient faithfully and make only promises that can be fulfilled. Be open to communication, because everyone in this situation needs at least one person in whom to freely and honestly confide. Remember that pretense stifles hope. Do not pretend to be overly cheery, but be honest and genuine regarding your own feelings, without projecting them onto patients. Do not minimize or negate feelings, because this increases the patient's guilt and dependency. Provide positive experiences and a sense of accomplishment by dividing patient goals and tasks into short-term attainable units. Offer satisfying aesthetic experiences with music, nature, and art, to help inspire hope.

Keep hope alive when fear threatens, because hope is the antidote for fear and despair. Do not encourage hope that the death is not real. This is dishonest and inappropriate. Rather, by word and deed, assure the patient that he or she will be comfortable and well cared for and that the bereaved family will be helped. Provide opportunities to speak with peers who have worked through earlier stages of the process, if appropriate.

Sensitively offer opportunities to discuss life after death or the patient's religious beliefs. Offer to share experiences of prayer, because this commonly brings comfort and kindles the hope that a loving God is in control. Arrange visits by chaplains or other spiritual counselors of the patient's choice. Clergy visits can inspire a sense that God's blessing is being conveyed and can be deeply comforting. Do not proselytize. Convey respect for the patient's beliefs or lack of beliefs by learning and discussing the basic tenets of his or her religious or personal belief system.

Compare the patient's status with the expected outcomes. If the outcomes are not met, reassess the patient and revise the plan.

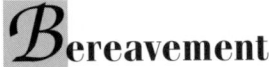ereavement

STAGES OF BEREAVEMENT

Denial

The first emotion felt by the bereaved after the death of a relative or friend is shock, even when the death is expected and invited. Denial is a useful buffer. Feelings of numbness, or of being in an unreal dream world, are experienced for several days or weeks. These feelings are followed by episodes of emotional pain and extremes of behavior in which a person becomes either hyperactive or almost inert. Various somatic complaints and mood swings arise. Physical symptoms include choking, sighing, shortness of breath, insomnia, and various gastrointestinal complaints, like anorexia and inability to taste the flavor of food. The bereaved person is preoccupied with thoughts of the deceased. Episodes of denial continue to resurface from time to time, right up to final acceptance of the death and resolution of the grief.

Anger

Throughout the mourning period, strong feelings of anger may arise suddenly in the bereaved. Typically, they gradually diminish in intensity over time. The person may feel rage at God for permitting the suffering, at health-care providers for failing to save the loved one, and at self for not being the one who died. Resentment may arise toward the loved one for the desertion, or toward others who are happy and not suffering a loss. Spiritual distress commonly occurs during this stage as beliefs are challenged by anger over the suffering.

Bargaining

Manifestations of bargaining in the bereaved surface throughout the process as "if only" thoughts and comments. These are attempts to negotiate, delay, and reduce the reality of the loss. They begin during the anticipatory grief period before death, with prayers like "Lord, if only you will spare her, I will be a good person and will serve you the rest of my life."

After death, there is a great deal of daydreaming about the deceased. Often the bereaved imagines the close presence of the deceased or suddenly seems to see him or her in a crowd of people. Magical thinking, like that of children, occurs frequently in thoughts like, "If only I pretend that he is here with me now, maybe it will happen." Restless searching for the beloved is a defense against recognition that the loss is final. Such seeking sometimes leads the bereaved to dabble in spiritualism and become fixated at this stage, unable to bring the grief work to resolution.

Depression

This is the most difficult stage of all and occurs as the permanence of death becomes real. It becomes very difficult for the bereaved to concentrate and to make decisions. Life seems out of control and seems to lose all meaning. A sense of hopelessness often pervades, as indicated by comments such as:

"It's no use."
"Why bother?"
"It will never work out now."
"Nothing can be done anyway."
"It's too late."
"Everything's going down the drain."
"It's all senseless."
"There's no hope."

Apathy, withdrawal, and passive acquiescence are noted. The bereaved lacks motivation and has little energy to invest in things and other people. Depression saps initiative, and the bereaved drifts along in seeming purposelessness. Guilt, remorse, and regret are common feelings and contribute to a decreased sense of self-worth. Withdrawal into isolation can occur, with frequent complaints of loneliness. Haunting and excessive fears about the security or health and safety of family and friends may be almost overwhelming. Complaints are usually irrational, and the bereaved may fear that he or she is having a mental breakdown. A few transient episodes might occur in which one hears the voice or senses the presence of the one who has died. This may either heighten the fear of losing one's sanity, or it may be very comforting to the bereaved.

Acceptance

Some months after the death, the bereaved typically begins to note a gradual reduction in the periods of depression with increased times of well-being. Confusion fades, and life begins to take on meaning again. The bereaved is finally able to experience real sources of comfort. Thoughts of the dead loved one find easier expression and are less and less idealized. The bad is remembered along with the good, and the bereaved feels an increasing calm acceptance. The old pain of loss is always there, especially on anniversaries and holidays, but the former fears, remorse, anger, and guilt diminish. Energy increases. The bereaved begins to reorder life. The grief work is over. Life starts to seem interesting and even to be fun again. Other people begin to capture the bereaved's attention, and gradually he or she begins to invest in new relationships.

Those who lose a loved one may engage in anticipatory grieving during the dying process. Experts believe that this anticipatory grieving may aid and shorten the grief process after the loved one dies. Even so, the final reality of death almost always comes as a shock.

Resolution of grief is vital for one's future mental and physical health. Dysfunctional grieving can cause crippling emotional problems. Death of a spouse rates highest on the scale of life stress events. A strong correlation exists between significant loss and subsequent deteriorating health, including cancer, of the survivors. Premature death of the bereaved often occurs.

Cathexis is a term used by Freud to refer to one's investment of emotional energy in a single idea or object. Mourning is the process of gradual decathecting or "letting go" of the dead loved one. Decathexis is an intense emotional process and cannot be rushed. Acceptance is attained when the earlier stages have been completed.

Tasks of mourning have been identified by Worden and expanded by Doka (Coolican et al, 1994). They include the following five tasks.

Task I: To accept the reality of the loss.
Task II: To work through the pain of grief.
Task III: To adjust to an environment in which the deceased is missing.
Task IV: To emotionally withdraw energy from the deceased and move on with life.
Task V: To rebuild faith and philosophical systems that were challenged by the loss.

STIGMATIZED OR VIOLENT DEATH

Stigmatized or violent deaths are particularly traumatic for the survivors. Humiliation and alienation are added to the anguish. Deaths caused by acquired immunodeficiency syndrome (AIDS), suicide, murder, or substance abuse are examples. Seldom does it help to tell the dying and their survivors that their guilt and shame are inappropriate and unwarranted. The isolating and alienating aspects of these deaths make it imperative that counseling be available to those who are closely involved. Many people need to talk out the grief over and over again. Keep in mind that if grief is buried, it festers and sooner or later erupts in an inappropriate manner. Health-care professionals must be sensitive to the dearth of opportunities available to survivors of stigmatized deaths to talk about their anguish. Nurses and other professionals must not become so preoccupied with physical care that they fail to address these tremendous psychosocial needs.

SUDDEN DEATH

Sudden, unexpected deaths and the deaths of persons who inspire ambivalent feelings also cause particular distress for survivors. In the former cases, survivors are denied opportunities for anticipatory grief and closure. Too many things are left unsaid and undone, and too many questions remain unanswered. In the latter, survivors feel relief that the difficult person is gone, possibly mixed with heavy guilt that complicates and compounds the grief process.

NURSING PROCESS
The Patient Suffering Bereavement

Assessment

Assess manifestations of each of the five stages of grief in the bereaved. Assess for signs of denial and for associated mood swings and physical symptoms. Observe for sighing or choking and note complaints of shortness of breath. Ask about insomnia and anorexia and other gastrointestinal complaints. Listen for expressions of anger or resentment toward God, health-care workers, the deceased, or survivors. Listen also for "if only" statements that indicate bargaining, and note daydreaming or magical thinking. Observe for signs of depression, such as apathy, withdrawal, and statements reflecting guilt or a sense that life is out of control or lacks meaning. Observe also for signs of acceptance, such as acknowledging the deceased person's weaknesses as well as strengths and expressing interest in resuming personal and social activities.

Nursing Diagnoses and Planning

Nursing diagnoses and related expected patient outcomes most commonly applicable to patients suffering bereavement include the following:

NDx: Grieving related to the recent death of a loved one

Planning: Patient Outcomes
1. Patient exhibits signs of shock for several days after the death and reaches out appropriately to others for comfort, support, and assistance.

2. Patient openly vents, projects, and displaces feelings of anger and guilt for several weeks after the death.
3. Patient gradually demonstrates acceptance of the death by talking freely and appropriately about it; expressing increasing themes of satisfaction and pleasure; demonstrating increased interest in new aspects of life; investing emotionally in new relationships; and showing renewed ability to solve problems and make major decisions.

Nursing Interventions and Evaluation

NDx: Grieving
To help the bereaved complete the grief work, allow the family to say farewell to the deceased by seeing and touching the body shortly after death. Physical contact helps to resolve the denial stage of grief. Survivors who have no opportunity to see their dead have difficulty progressing beyond denial. Keep in mind that some families assume total responsibility for care of the body based on religious beliefs. Provide strong support and protection of the bereaved during this traumatic, vulnerable period. Should the survivors develop physical complaints, assess them with honest concern and gentle reassurance.

Help the bereaved through the anger phase by demonstrating empathy, patience, and tolerance, especially when anger is directed at the health-care professionals. Explain that anger at the dead or rage at God is common and normal to help reduce guilt. Encourage contact with self-help organizations in the community, such as groups for widows and widowers or bereaved parents. Arrange contact with peers who can express feelings openly, to stimulate the bereaved to express his or her feelings and experiences freely. Provide frequent, regularly scheduled opportunities to vent, to sort out ambivalence, and to express resentments. Engage in frequent conversations with the bereaved about the deceased and their experiences together. Always be authentic and considerate to help promote the bereaved's self-esteem. Reinforce reality and reduce the nonproductive tendency to assign blame with gentle reminders to help correct misperceptions and misinterpretations regarding the cause of death. Be patient with constant negative expressions and attitudes and avoid the counterproductive tendency to advise the mourner to "Try to change your attitude and think more positively." Encourage participation in religious ceremonies and rituals, prayer, or counseling for spiritual support if consonant with the patient's beliefs. Be honest in communicating about anger, doubt, or disbelief, which commonly occur during this phase.

To intervene during this painful time, listen actively and patiently when the bereaved repeat accounts or thoughts over and over again about the death and the deceased. This enables the loss to become real and eventually accepted. Engage in frequent conversations with the bereaved, but keep in mind that the bereaved also need time by them-selves. Be alert to signs of excessive apathy and withdrawal.

Avoid suppressing the symptoms of grief with the use of tranquilizers and sedatives, which tend to mask reactions and delay the grief work. Be aware, however, that acute anxiety attacks or persistent in-somnia may need temporary drug therapy. Counsel the bereaved to avoid major changes and decisions during this time. Many bereaved people are too fragile to cope with added, unnecessary stress. They may make reactive decisions that they later regret. Encourage the bereaved to continue working unless the job is terribly stressful, since work can provide valuable structure, organization, and socialization during this chaotic period when life often seems out of control.

Make family and friends aware of the impor-tance of being patient with petty, irrational anxieties, fears, and phobias, and explain that strange feelings and compulsive behaviors bereaved people experi-ence are part of normal grieving. Encourage family and friends to take a positive approach with a griev-ing person rather than posing a question that is likely to be answered in the negative by a depressed person. For example, it is better to say, "We've made plans to have lunch together," rather than "Would you like to go?"

Try not to rush acceptance of the loss. It usually takes 6 months to a year, and sometimes up to 2 years. Feelings of acceptance occur gradually, with increased frequency and duration as the other phases are resolved. Assist the bereaved at this stage by continuing to encourage talk about the deceased but without a "halo" idealizing effect. Encourage the bereaved to remember the annoying, troublesome aspects of the relationship along with joyous, satis-factory aspects. Support the learning of new or re-discovered coping strategies. If the bereaved faces major decisions or life changes—such as selling a home, moving to another community, or moving in with a son or daughter—encourage the person to use the help of a neutral, objective, compassionate person in solving problems.

Compare the patient's status with the expected outcomes. If the outcomes are not met, reassess the patient and revise the plan.

Dysfunctional Grieving

Destructive, pathologic patterns of grief can some-times be predicted. Risk factors include a history of emotional problems with ineffective coping, and fre-quent conflict between the dying person and the survivors during their life together. Repression of feelings (manifested by an absence of expressed emotion) serves only to delay normal mourning. In-stead, the repressed emotions will probably arise to haunt the person at some unexpected time in the future.

The usual pattern is that dysfunctional grieving lasts beyond the normal 1- to 2-year period and becomes fixated at any of the stages leading up to acceptance or resolution. Acute grief continues well beyond the normal 6- to 8-week period. Months af-ter a death, the bereaved still manifests a dreamlike state of shock, as if the death had occurred the previous day. Psychosomatic symptoms result in se-rious illnesses or hypochondria or conversion hyste-ria. Severe anxiety reactions or an agitated de-pression can be easily triggered, and long-lasting phobias may develop. The bereaved may regress to childlike dependency for a prolonged period and be unable to carry responsibility. Severe egocentricity may alienate others. Prolonged self-deprecation and self-blame result from unresolved guilt. Sometimes there is continued rage at health-care professionals or God or deep resentment at feeling abandoned by the deceased. Idealization of the deceased is fre-quently and inappropriately expressed. Persistent re-fusal to discuss feelings regarding the death feeds dysfunctional patterns. Chronic hostility toward ev-eryone and everything may be openly expressed but is more apt to be manifested as passive-aggression or the super-sweetness of reaction-formation, which makes others uncomfortable because of the underly-ing hostility. Prolonged envy of others' happiness and security feeds this hostility and bitterness. Sui-cidal ideation is not uncommon. Self-destructive activities that induce pain and discomfort or are dangerous to health and well-being occur subcon-sciously. Deliberate suicide attempts may also occur and be successful.

NURSING PROCESS
The Patient with Dysfunctional Grieving
Assessment

Take a careful nursing history of past emotional problems. Try to accurately assess the quality of the relationship of the griever with the dead person, realizing the possibility of an increased need to maintain a halo effect, excessively glorifying the dead if the relationship was troubled. Learn the length of time since the death to determine whether grieving has exceeded the normal 1- to 2-year pe-riod. Listen for expressions of the various stages of normal grieving. Ask about situations that may have prevented the bereaved from freely expressing grief at the appropriate time. Assess the quality of life since the loss, including:

Sleeping pattern
Eating pattern
Social isolation or dependency
Emotional repression or lability
Psychosomatic manifestations

Assess the griever's ability to talk freely and honestly about the death and listen for themes of guilt or anger. It is especially important to ask about suicidal ideation and to consider the possibility of past or present suicide attempts.

Nursing Diagnoses and Planning

Nursing diagnoses and related expected patient outcomes most commonly applicable to patients with dysfunctional grieving include the following:

NDx: Dysfunctional grieving related to inability to express feelings as needed to complete the mourning process or ambivalent feelings resulting from chronic, unresolved conflict with the deceased

Planning: Patient Outcomes
1. Patient expresses awareness of the need to complete all phases of the grief work and a desire to emotionally accept the death.
2. Patient identifies some of the unresolved aspects of the grief process in his or her experience.
3. Patient openly and frequently expresses impacted or unresolved feelings of denial, anger, guilt, and despair and actively seeks constructive ways to complete the mourning.
4. Patient actively demonstrates efforts to change nonproductive behaviors and dysfunctional feelings by altering old patterns and adopting new ones.
5. Patient seeks and carries through on psychiatric consultations or psychotherapy as indicated.
6. Patient demonstrates healthy detachment from the deceased by talking freely of strengths and weaknesses of the relationship without pain and by reinvesting appropriately in new friendships or relationships.

Nursing Interventions and Evaluation

NDx: Dysfunctional grieving
Employ interventions for normal mourning to help an individual correct and resolve maladaptive responses to death and complete the grieving process. These are usually effective because dysfunctional grieving often results from the lack of such assistance at the time. Perhaps empathic listeners were unavailable to enable expression of the anger and despair. Perhaps the help of a caretaker was not there during the fragile, vulnerable period immediately after death. Sometimes the bereaved have had to be so brave and pretend to be so strong that they have suppressed or repressed their grief to the point that it has become impacted and later haunts them.

Give information and assist with referrals for counseling when basic interventions are not successful. Role play with an experienced counselor can help relieve such impacted pain so that the person can complete the grief process and resolve the emotional crisis. This can also help in reworking other unresolved feelings. Initiate an immediate referral for psychiatric consultation if the person displays evidence of deep depression with suicide potential, continuing hallucinations, or delusional thinking.

Compare the patient's status with the expected outcomes. If the outcomes are not met, reassess the patient and revise the plan.

Spiritual Aspects of Death and Dying

The spiritual nature is the very ground of one's being. Regardless of whether individuals adhere to an organized religion, all people have a spiritual nature. The self, or the soul, distinguishes humans from other animals. It transcends our body, our mind, our emotion, our relationships with other persons, and our relatedness to the environment.

A basic human drive that motivates all of us, consciously or not, is the desire to immortalize ourselves. We yearn to extend ourselves beyond the bounds of finitude, to be more than just an animal, more than just grass of the field that passes away. This is the basic human urge—to be unique, to matter, to count—not just for a little while or a few days, but for eternity. The terror of death is that the self will be extinct, our bodies will decay, our lives will be in vain, and we will be forgotten (Becker, 1973).

The comfort of most major religions is that God is at the very center of our existence and that the meaning and goal of human experience is to achieve perfect communion with God and to have eternal life.

Spiritual needs, when met, can be a powerful force in transcending illness and suffering. Spiritual distress can also be all-pervasive in its disruptive force. Recognition of patients' spirituality and attention to those needs demands high priority. Spiritual beliefs are so private and personal that nurses have typically avoided them. Fortunately, however, a growing number of nurses are coming to grips with the importance of this aspect of care and taking steps to learn about and deal with spiritual distress.

To meet the spiritual needs of patients, the nurse must know the core beliefs and practices of the patient's religion as they relate to death and dying. The nurse must respect the patient's beliefs and avoid imposing personal values and belief systems. Honest sharing of personal faith by the nurse may be helpful in small amounts, but only when done to help sustain the patient and never in an effort to change a patient or boost the nurse's ego.

The best way to learn about a patient's religious beliefs is to go to the primary source. Ask the patient: Are you a religious person? Would you like to tell me about your spiritual beliefs and how they affect your life? Spirituality is a very private matter for many, but most are willing and even eager to discuss these matters with an open-minded, nonjudgmental, sincerely interested listener. This is never more true than near the time of death. Bereaved family members usually need to be able to talk about life after death as well.

Another important reason for asking is that personal beliefs and practices may vary greatly from the person's stated religious affiliation. Most often, religious affiliation develops historically and culturally. It is derived from the early influences of family and community. Personal choice, commitment, and inspiration may follow later in life, but these things usually affect the degree of religious practice more than the choice of religious affiliation. Therefore, some personal beliefs and practices may not be totally consistent with one's religious "label." Avoid making assumptions or presuppositions.

*E*thical and Legal Issues Related to Death and Dying

THE CHANGING DEFINITION OF DEATH

Before the advent of modern medicine, doctors pronounced a person dead when breathing ceased, the heart stopped beating, and corneal reflexes were absent. Death usually resulted from infection and was not a prolonged process. Pneumonia became known as "an old man's friend."

Today, technologic developments such as mechanical ventilators, artificial feedings, and sophisticated medications make it possible to prolong life—even in a vegetative state—for an extended period of time. This ability, coupled with the growth of transplant surgery that requires viable organs (those that have not been deprived of oxygen and other nutrients as would occur with the cessation of breathing and heart beat), has resulted in a reconsideration of how to define death. It has also prompted creation of the concept of brain death. Brain death occurs when the vital centers in the brain stem cease to function and the heart and lungs operate only via a mechanical life-support system. Criteria for the definition of brain death were developed by a group at Harvard University Medical School and supported by The Hastings Center. These criteria have become widely accepted, especially in North America. They include the following:

- Unreceptivity and unresponsiveness. No response even to painful stimuli like strong pinching.
- No movements after observation by a physician for an hour continuously, and no breathing after 3 minutes off the respirator.
- No reflexes, including brain stem reflexes. Pupils are fixed and dilated.
- A flat electroencephalogram (EEG). This is considered of great confirmatory value if technically adequate.

- Absence of change in all these tests when repeated at least 24 hours later.
- Definite exclusion of hypothermia or central nervous system depression by drugs such as barbiturates.

Brain death is not the same as cortical or cerebral death. In cortical or cerebral death the patient is in a persistent vegetative state (PVS). All higher abilities mediated by the cerebral cortex are absent. However, the ability to maintain spontaneous respirations and heartbeat centered in the brain stem remains intact.

EUTHANASIA

The word *euthanasia* means "a good death." The prefix *eu* means good, or painless, and the root *thanasia* comes from the Greek word *thanatos,* meaning death. Active euthanasia is the commission of an act that directly and intentionally causes a person's life to end. Passive euthanasia is an act of omission. It involves letting a person die by withholding or withdrawing a therapy, such as artificial feedings or mechanical ventilation.

Active euthanasia is not legal in the United States. However, some people argue that active euthanasia on a voluntary basis or assisted suicide is more humane and has its place for patients suffering from incurable, intractable pain who want assistance in dying. Jack Kevorkian, MD, has openly challenged the United States legal system by participating in many assisted suicides. Some organizations, such as The Hemlock Society, support assisted suicides. Other people argue that, if assisted suicide is legalized, many patients will feel compelled to undergo it if they fear they are becoming a burden.

Passive euthanasia, although more universally acceptable, also presents many dilemmas and questions for nurses, patients, and family members. These include:

- When should life be prolonged and who should be resuscitated?
- Who should make the decision to begin extraordinary measures, such as a feeding tube or respirator, and who should discontinue them when the patient is unable to make the decision?
- When the family has various reasons for wishing an end to the ordeal, should they be forced to make the decision and bear the guilt of their decision?
- Should the decision rest with medical personnel, who may fear criticism for negligence or threat of malpractice suits if all possible measures to promote and prolong life are not used?
- Should such intimately personal and private matters of a profound nature become the domain of the courts and be impersonally decided legally for all of us?

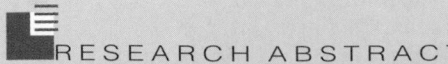

RESEARCH ABSTRACT

What Attitudes Do Nurses Hold Toward Euthanasia?

McInerny F, Siebold C. Nurses' definitions of and attitudes towards euthanasia. Journal of Advanced Nursing 1995; 22:171.

More and more, nurses face gray areas in caring for patients who are dying. How much and what type of intervention is needed with patients who are terminally ill? How should nurses talk with the families of dying patients? How should nurses care for dying patients who have no advance directives? How do professionals differentiate between active and passive euthanasia, or between a "good death" and assisted suicide?

These issues have become common topics of discussion since the 1991 publication of a book that described how dying patients could end their lives and since the beginning of widespread media coverage of Dr. Jack Kevorkian's assisted suicides. In the Netherlands, it is already legal for physicians to perform euthanasia. In the United States, the Supreme Court heard oral arguments on the legalization of assisted suicide in January of 1997, and it may be only a matter of time before assisted suicide becomes commonplace in the United States.

While teaching a class, McInerny and Siebold found that their students had difficulty in stating exactly what constituted euthanasia and in arriving at a consensus on a definition of euthanasia. The students agreed that withdrawal of aggressive therapy was sometimes appropriate and that maintaining the comfort of dying patients was always appropriate. On the other hand, ethical and moral conflicts erupted when the students tried to make a distinction between "killing" and "allowing to die." The debate within the group of nurses centered around ordinary and extraordinary treatment and "heroic measures."

Spurred on by this classroom discussion, the authors intensively interviewed 10 nurses from a variety of practice settings. From the results of their interviews, several themes and concerns arose. However, the researchers concluded that the stance taken by the nurses was an evolving one that depended heavily on context. The one consistent theme that emerged was that the stance emanated from a philosophy of caring for and comfort of the dying patient in an atmosphere that preserved human dignity.

Questions to Consider

1. What does the phrase "dying with dignity" mean to you?
2. Define "active" versus "passive" euthanasia.
3. How do *you* differentiate between euthanasia and withholding treatment or allowing death.
4. Give three to five reasons each for why you would support and why you would oppose euthanasia. What is your rationale for each reason?
5. Would you participate in legalized active euthanasia? Why or why not? Under what circumstances?

ADVANCE DIRECTIVES

All states recognize the right of individuals to make decisions about their medical treatments. The patient's right to refuse life-sustaining or life-prolonging medical intervention was the impetus for the Patient Self-Determination Act (PSDA) of 1990, passed as part of the Omnibus Budget Reconciliation Act of 1990. Although mandates about medical treatment choices (living wills) have been in existence for many years, it was not until the federal PSDA legislation that many health-care institutions and state laws began to recognize the wishes of an individual who is no longer able to articulate them.

There are two basic types of advance directives. A *living will* provides a way for the patient to specify which treatments to apply (or not apply) in the event that he or she is unable to choose. A *medical durable power of attorney* grants to a person of the patient's choosing the power to make decisions on the patient's behalf, should such decisions become necessary.

Many people think of a living will as little more than a do-not-resuscitate order. This is not correct. Rather, the patient chooses which treatments will be instituted, if any, and which will not be instituted should he or she not be capable of deciding. The person may state that "all life-sustaining measures are to be enacted", or that "only the following procedures, drugs, and treatments are to be used," or that "no treatment is to be initiated if I become permanently unconscious or terminally ill."

The medical durable power of attorney states the name of a proxy or surrogate, usually a relative or close friend, who is to make the medical treatment decisions for the patient when the patient is no longer able to make or express those decisions. Either of these directives applies only when the patient has been deemed by physicians to be incapable of making medical decisions. State laws vary as to how this decision is made.

The Patient Self-Determination Act requires that all agencies reimbursed for patient charges through Medicare and Medicaid must perform the following duties.

• Inform patients of their rights to make decisions concerning their medical care, including the right to receive or refuse medical treatments and the right to appoint another person (durable power of attorney) to make health-care decisions on his or her behalf.

- Inquire whether the patient has prepared a living will or written power of attorney.
- Provide written information to the patient at the time of admission concerning the right to submit or author an advance directive and the agency's policies about protection of that right.
- Document the treatment wishes of the patient and review these periodically with the patient.
- Have written policies about the use of advance directives in the institution according to state law.
- Organize an institutional ethics committee to initiate staff, patient, and community education programs on advance directives, and to advise staff and others about particular issues surrounding advance directives.

Institutions required to comply with the above mandates include hospitals, home health agencies, hospices, nursing homes, rehabilitation centers, subacute centers, and clinics.

Advance directives are legal documents. They are available in a variety of formats, either generic or state-specific. Figure 3–1 is an example of a living will for the state of Indiana. Figure 3–2 is an example of a health-care proxy, or durable power of attorney, form for Indiana. Some state-specific or generic forms may contain both types of advance directives on the same form. Preparation of an advance directive assures individuals, before a crisis occurs, that their wishes about medical treatments and life-sustaining or life-prolonging actions will be understood and followed.

DO NOT RESUSCITATE POLICIES

Cardiopulmonary resuscitation (CPR) is performed to revive a person who dies suddenly and unexpectedly. For terminally ill patients, it may serve no sound medical purpose and in fact may subvert the patient's wishes. When resuscitation is not in the patient's best interest, the attending physician may authorize a Do Not Resuscitate (DNR) order. All hospitals are required to have a DNR policy in effect to prevent the use of resuscitation when it is not in the best interest of the patient. DNR orders are

INSTRUCTIONS

INDIANA LIVING WILL DECLARATION

DECLARATION A
TO WITHHOLD OR WITHDRAW LIFE-PROLONGING PROCEDURES

PRINT THE DATE — Declaration made this ________ day of ________________.
(day) (month, year)

PRINT YOUR NAME — I, ______________________________,
(name)

being at least eighteen (18) years old and of sound mind, willfully and voluntarily make known my desires that my dying shall not be artificially prolonged under the circumstances set forth below, and I declare:

If at any time my attending physician certifies in writing that: (1) I have an incurable injury, disease, or illness; (2) my death will occur within a short time; and (3) the use of life prolonging procedures would serve only to artificially prolong the dying process, I direct that such procedures be withheld or withdrawn, and that I be permitted to die naturally with only the performance or provision of any medical procedure or medication necessary to provide me with comfort care or to alleviate pain, and, if I have so indicated below, the provision of artificially supplied nutrition and hydration. (Indicate your choice by initialling or making your mark before signing this declaration):

INITIAL THE STATEMENT THAT REFLECTS YOUR WISHES ABOUT ARTIFICIAL FEEDING

_____ I wish to receive artificially supplied nutrition and hydration, even if the effort to sustain life is futile or excessively burdensome to me.

_____ I do not wish to receive artificially supplied nutrition and hydration, if the effort to sustain life is futile or excessively burdensome to me.

_____ I intentionally make no decision concerning artificially supplied nutrition and hydration, leaving the decision to my health care representative appointed under Indiana Code 16-36-1-7 or my attorney in fact with health care powers under Indiana Code 30-5-5.

ADD PERSONAL INSTRUCTIONS (IF ANY) — Other directions:

INDIANA LIVING WILL DECLARATION — PAGE 2 OF 2

In the absence of my ability to give directions regarding the use of life prolonging procedures, it is my intention that this declaration be honored by my family and physician as the final expression of my legal right to refuse medical or surgical treatment and accept the consequences of the refusal.

SIGN THE DOCUMENT AND PRINT YOUR PLACE OF RESIDENCE

I understand the full import of this declaration.

Signed ______________________________

City, County, and State of Residence ______________________________

WITNESSING PROCEDURE

The declarant has been personally known to me, and I believe (him/her) to be of sound mind. I did not sign the declarant's signature above for or at the direction of the declarant. I am not a parent, spouse, or child of the declarant. I am not entitled to any part of the declarant's estate or directly financially responsible for the declarant's medical care. I am competent and at least eighteen (18) years of age.

WITNESSES MUST SIGN AND DATE THE DOCUMENT

Witness ______________________________

Date ________________

Witness ______________________________

Date ________________

Figure 3–1

Example of a living will form for Indiana. (Reprinted by permission of Choice in Dying, 200 Varick Street, New York, NY 10014; 212/366-5540.)

INSTRUCTIONS

INDIANA POWER OF ATTORNEY FOR HEALTH CARE DECISIONS AND APPOINTMENT OF HEALTH CARE REPRESENTATIVE

PRINT YOUR NAME AND ADDRESS

1) I, _____
(name)

of _____
(address)

PRINT THE NAME, ADDRESS AND TELEPHONE NUMBERS OF YOUR ATTORNEY-IN-FACT

hereby appoint _____
(name of attorney-in-fact)

_____
(address)

_____
(home telephone number)   _(work telephone number)_

as my attorney-in-fact to make health care decisions on my behalf whenever I am incapable of making my own health care decisions.

POWERS OF YOUR ATTORNEY-IN-FACT

I grant my attorney-in-fact the following powers in matters affecting my health care:

(1) to employ or contract with servants, companions, or health care providers involved in my health care;
(2) to admit or release me from a hospital or health care facility;
(3) to have access to my records, including medical records;
(4) to make anatomical gifts on my behalf;
(5) to request an autopsy; and
(6) to make plans for the disposition of my body.

© 1996
CHOICE IN DYING, INC.

---

2) In the event the person I appoint above is unable, unwilling or unavailable to act as my attorney-in-fact, I hereby appoint:

PRINT THE NAME, ADDRESS AND TELEPHONE NUMBERS OF YOUR ALTERNATE ATTORNEY-IN-FACT

_____
(name of successor attorney-in-fact)

of _____
(address)

_____
(home telephone number)   _(work telephone number)_

as my successor attorney-in-fact.

APPOINTMENT AND POWERS OF HEALTH CARE REPRESENTATIVE

Appointment of my Attorney-in-Fact as my Health Care Representative

In addition to the powers granted above, I appoint my attorney-in-fact as my health care representative to make decisions in my best interest concerning the consent, withdrawal or withholding of health care. I understand health care to include any medical care, treatment, service, or procedure to maintain, diagnose, treat, or provide for my physical or mental well-being. Health care also includes the providing of nutrition and hydration through intravenous, gastrostomy or nasogastric tubes.

If at any time, based on my previously expressed preferences and the diagnosis and prognosis, my health care representative is satisfied that certain health care is not or would not be beneficial, or that such health care is or would be excessively burdensome, then my health care representative may express my will that such health care be withheld or withdrawn and may consent on my behalf that any or all health care be discontinued or not instituted, even if death may result.

My health care representative must try to discuss this decision with me. However, if I am unable to communicate, my health care representative may make such a decision for me, after consultation with my physician or physicians and other relevant health care givers. To the extent appropriate, my health care representative may also discuss this decision with my family and others, to the extent they are available.

© 1996
CHOICE IN DYING, INC.

PRINT YOUR NAME AND THE DATE

I, _____, the principal, sign my name to this instrument this _____ day of _____ 19____, and do
(date)   _(month)_   _(year)_

hereby declare to the undersigned witness that I sign it willingly, and I execute it as my free and voluntary act for the purposes herein expressed, and that I am eighteen years of age or older, of sound mind, and under no constraint or undue influence.

SIGN THE DOCUMENT

_____
(principal)

A NOTARY PUBLIC MUST COMPLETE THIS SECTION OF YOUR DOCUMENT

Subscribed and acknowledged before me by _____,
the principal, this _____ day of _____, 19____.

_____
(notary public)

My Commission expires _____

(Drafted with the assistance of George G. Slater, J.D., Carmel, IN)

Courtesy of Choice In Dying, Inc.
200 Varick Street, New York, NY 10014 212-366-5540   6/96

© 1996
CHOICE IN DYING, INC.

Figure 3–2

Example of a health-care power of attorney (also called a health-care proxy) form for Indiana. (Reprinted by permission of Choice in Dying, 200 Varick Street, New York, NY 10014; 212/366-5540.)

often a part of advance directives. If an advance directive with a DNR order is not in place, the attending physician will address the issue when the patient's condition warrants it, as in these cases:

- When there is no medical benefit to treatment
- When the quality of life after resuscitation would be less desirable to the patient than death resulting from a cardiac arrest
- When the quality of life before resuscitation is such that the patient would prefer death resulting from a cardiac arrest
- When CPR would be futile

The possibility of a DNR order may also be raised with the physician by the patient, the family, or any member of the health-care team. In these discussions, every effort should be made to ensure that patients and their families understand the nature of CPR and are clear about the fact that a DNR order does not mean that the patient will not receive any treatment. A DNR order should not be written unless the patient approves the order. If the patient is not competent to approve the order, the next of kin, a legal representative, and adult family members should approve the order.

The order should be written on the appropriate form (Fig. 3–3) or in unabbreviated form on the physician's order sheet. Related information should be included in the patient's record. The latter includes supporting clinical information, documentation of any medical consults, and documentation of pertinent discussions with the patient, next of kin, other family members, and legal representatives. Once written, a DNR order should be reviewed regularly by all concerned individuals. The order may be rescinded at any time.

The DNR forms to be signed by the physician vary according to whether the patient is at home, in a hospital, or in a skilled nursing facility. Figure 3–3 is an example of a nonhospital DNR form.

ORGAN DONATIONS

The Uniform Anatomical Gift Act governs various aspects of donation, such as when, how, and who will decide that the donor's life has ceased. Organs must be removed within an hour after death. The patient's attending physician pronounces death but cannot participate in the organ removal process or

State of New York
Department of Health

Nonhospital Order Not to Resuscitate
(DNR Order)

Person's Name ____________________

Date of Birth ____/____/____

Do not resuscitate the person named above.

Physician's Signature ____________________
Print Name ____________________
License Number ____________________
Date ____/____/____

It is the responsibility of the physician to determine, at least every 90 days, whether this order continues to be appropriate, and to indicate this by a note in the person's medical chart. The issuance of a new form is **NOT** required, and under the law this order should be considered valid unless it is known that it has been revoked. This order remains valid and must be followed, even if it has not been reviewed within the 90 day period.

Figure 3–3
Example of a Do Not Resuscitate (DNR) order form for New York. (Courtesy of State of New York Department of Health.)

the transplantation. Because of a critical shortage of needed organs, some states have passed laws requiring "routine requests" for organs by hospital administrators or their designees if the patient's wishes are not known. Many times it is the nurse caring for the patient at the time of death who is designated to approach the family for a signed release that allows donation of organs. Many states now request that individuals record their decision in advance when applying for driver's licenses. Organ donor cards and information may be ordered from the United Network of Organ Sharing (see Appendix 1: Resources).

In cases of brain death, plans for organ donations are made before ventilators and other equipment are removed. The protocol encourages discretion and sensitivity to the survivors' suffering and respect for religious beliefs, as well as obvious non-suitability for organ and tissue donations. The American Nurses' Association encourages nurses to support organ procurement measures.

Chapter Review

1. How do you think a dying patient in the anger stage, the depression stage, the bargaining stage, and the acceptance stage would react to reassurance given by the nurse?
2. How do the stages and tasks of the dying patient compare with the stages and tasks of the person suffering bereavement?
3. What are some possible solutions to the problem of dysfunctional grieving?
4. In what ways does attending to spiritual needs affect the dying or the bereaved?
5. Why is it important to develop advance directives? Who should do so and when?
6. What are the meanings of the terms "durable power of attorney," "health-care proxy," and "living will"?
7. Why is it important to develop state-specific advance directives? Where can these forms be obtained?
8. How does emergency care for patients with DNR orders differ from that of other patients?
9. What arguments support the movement to legalize assisted suicides and what arguments oppose it?
10. What are possible reasons for the shortage of organs donated for transplantation?

Bibliography

Bailey S. Creativity and the close of life. In Corless B, Pillman M (eds). Dying, death and bereavement: Theoretical perspective and other ways of knowing. Boston: Jones and Bartlett, 1994, pp 327–335.

Barr P. DNR: A moral decision. Nebr Nurse 1994; 27(2):17.

Beauchamp TL, Perlin S. Ethical Issues in Death and Dying. Englewood Cliffs, NJ: Prentice-Hall, 1978.

Becker E. The denial of death. New York: The Free Press, Macmillan Publishing, 1973.

Bergevin PR, Bergevin RM. Discussing DNR issues. Am J Hosp Palliat Care 1995; 12(3):10.

Berrio M, Levesque M. CE credit advance directives: Most patients don't have one, do yours? Am J Nurs 1996; 96(8):24.

Callahan M, Kelly P. Final gifts: Understanding the special awareness, needs and communications of the dying. New York: Poseidon Press, 1992.

Choice in Dying. Dying at home. Choices 1996; 5(2).

Choice in Dying. Exploring the issue of physician assisted dying. Choices 1996; 5(3).

Choice in Dying. Medical treatments and your advance directives. Choices 1996; 5(2).

Coolican MB, Doka KJ, Stark J, Corr CA. Education about death, dying, and bereavement in nursing programs. Nurse Educator 1994; 19(6):35.

Corr CA, Doka KJ. Current models of death, dying, and bereavement. Crit Care Nurs Clin North Am 1994; 6(3):545.

Cox HB. The valley of the shadow. Point View 1990; 27(1):12.

DeSpelder LA, Strickland AL. The last dance: Encountering death and dying. 4th ed. Mountainview, CA: Mayfield Publishers, 1995.

Doyle N. The dying person and the family. Public Affairs Pamphlet. No. 485, New York: 1972, p 7.

Elsdon R. Spiritual pain in dying people: The nurse's role. Prof Nurse 1995; 10(10):641.

Erikson E. Childhood and society. 2nd ed. New York: Norton, 1963, pp 263–269.

Fade AE. Advance directives: Keeping up with changing legislation. Todays OR Nurse 1994; 16(4):23.

Fade AE. End-of-life decisions affect health care providers. Am Nurse 1994; 26(1):28.

Frankl V. Man's search for meaning. New York: Washington Square Press, 1963.

Golanowski M. Do not resuscitate: Informed consent in the operating room and postanesthesia care unit. J Post Anesth Nurs 1995; 10(1):9.

Henderson ML. Facilitating a "good death" in patients with end stage renal disease. Anna J 1995; 22(3):294.

Huber R. Relationship between right-to-die and satisfaction with life. Am J Hosp Palliat Care 1994; 11(5):13.

Johanson G. Physicians handbook of symptom relief in terminal care. 4th ed. Santa Rosa, CA: Sonoma County Academic Foundation for Excellence in Medicine, 1994.

Johnson B. Psychiatric mental health nursing. Adaptation and growth: 4th ed. Philadelphia: Lippincott-Raven, 1996.

Kauffman J. Awareness of immortality. Amityville, NY: Baywood Publishing Co, 1995.

Kingma R. Spotlight on revising death education. Nurse Educator 1994; 19(5):15.

Koenig H. Use of acute hospital services and mortality among religious and non-religious copers with medical illness. J Religious Gerontol 1995; 9(3):1.

Kübler-Ross E. On death and dying. New York: Macmillan Publishing, 1969.

Kübler-Ross E. Death: The final stage of growth. Englewood Cliffs, NJ: Prentice-Hall, 1975.

Lamm M. The Jewish way in death and mourning. New York: Jonathan David Publishers, 1969.

Lewis CS. A grief observed. New York: Harcourt Brace Jovanovich, 1958.

Mendyka BE. The dying patient in the intensive care unit: Assisting the family in crisis. AACN Clin Issues Crit Care Nurs 1993; 4(3):550.

Mitford J. The American way of death. Greenwich, CT: Fawcett Publications, 1963.

The Patient Self-Determination Act, Omnibus Reconciliation Act of 1990, Pub. L. No 101-508, Medicare 4206, Medicaid 4751.

Peck RC. Psychological developments in the second half of life. In Neugarten BL (ed). Middle-age and aging: A reader in social psychology. Chicago: University of Chicago Press, 1968, pp 88–92.

Perry J, Ryan A. A cross-cultural look at death, dying, and religion. Chicago: Nelson-Hall, 1995.

Schroeder-Sheker T. Music for the dying: A personal account of the new field of music-thanatology—history, theories, and clinical narratives. J Holist Nurs 1994; 12(1):83.

Shapiro P. Refusing treatment at home: A paramedic talks about nonhospital DNR orders. Choices 1995; 4(1):5.

Simpson SH. A study into the uses and effects of do-not-resuscitate orders in the intensive care units of two teaching hospitals. Intensive Crit Care Nurs 1994; 10(1):12.

Sloan A. Don't resuscitate, lose your job? RN 1996; 59(8):51.

Smith-Regojo P. Being with a patient who is dying. Holistic Nurs Pract 1995; 9(3):1.

Snyder R. Ethical decisions: Home healthcare providers and patients who choose to die. Home Healthc Nurse 1995; 13(5):75.

Tolstoy L. Death and the meaning of life. In A confession. New York: Thomas Crowell, 1899.

Tolstoy L. The death of Ivan Ilyich. New York: The New American Library, 1960, pp 137–138.

Ufema J. Death and dying. Nursing90 1990: 20:90.

Ufema J. Insights on death and dying. Nursing90 1990; 20:94.

Ufema J. Meeting the challenge of a dying patient [interview]. Nursing91 1991; 21:42.

Valko NG. The ethics of death: Selling euthanasia to nurses and doctors. Revolution 1995; 5(2):47.

Williams A. The last battle. Nurs Times 1995; 91(8):50.

Worden JW. Grief counseling and grief therapy: A handbook for the mental health practitioner. 2nd ed. New York: Springer Publishing Co; 1991.

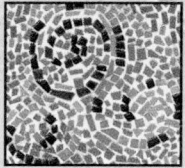
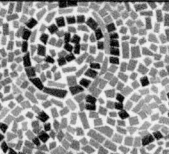
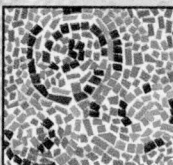
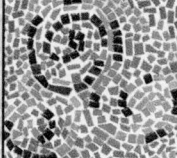
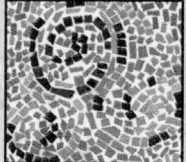
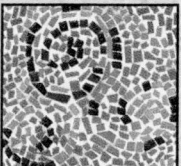

4

Special Considerations for Nursing Care of Elderly Patients

Study Outcomes

After studying this chapter, you should be able to:

1. Explain the physiologic, psychologic, and socioeconomic changes commonly associated with the normal aging process.
2. Describe normal assessment findings in the elderly.
3. Identify the nursing implications of altered function and pharmacokinetics in the elderly.
4. State nursing diagnoses and related expected patient outcomes commonly applicable to the elderly.
5. Describe nursing interventions, with their rationales, that promote wellness in the elderly.
6. Describe teaching strategies that promote learning in the elderly.
7. Explain the basis for evaluation of nursing care provided to the elderly.
8. Identify treatment and care settings for elderly patients and services related to community-based care.

United States Census Bureau projections indicate that by the year 2030, 23% of the population in the United States will be older than 65 years. Older adults, especially those older than 85 years, represent the fastest-growing segment of the population. Between 1960 and 1980, the population of those older than 84 increased by 141%. This spectacular growth in the number of older people is attributed to many factors. Chief among them are an increased health consciousness in the United States and a decline in mortality from chronic diseases, especially cardiovascular disorders. Despite common misconceptions, only 5% of the elderly are institutionalized.

The increased number of elderly people in the population has prompted the growth of research and specialized health fields in gerontology and geriatrics. *Gerontology* is the study of the process of aging and the needs of older people. It includes the physiologic, psychologic, and socioeconomic changes associated with aging. Gerontologists work to develop a body of knowledge to better meet the needs of older people. *Geriatrics* is a specialized health profession that addresses the physiology, pathology, diagnosis, and management of diseases in the elderly. Geriatric nurses specialize in the care of older peo-

ple in various settings, including homes, hospitals, and group arrangements.

Numerous changes are associated with the normal aging process. These changes occur at different points in the life span and are affected by such factors as

> Heredity
> Environment
> Age
> Daily activities
> Health habits
> Medical history
> Socioeconomic resources
> Psychosocial factors
> Support systems

Each person ages at a different rate, and each person adapts to the aging process individually. Although most changes associated with aging occur gradually, factors such as chronic or acute illnesses may accelerate changes. Also, life changes can have a major impact on the psychologic and physical status of the older person.

Understanding the changes associated with aging enables the nurse to accurately differentiate between normal and abnormal findings in assessing older adults. This chapter presents a brief overview of the normal changes of aging common in healthy older adults. It also outlines nursing actions that can help older people adapt to these changes. These actions seek to provide education, support, and services that enable older people to maintain optimal function and independence while also meeting their needs.

Changes Associated with the Normal Aging Process

PSYCHOSOCIAL ASPECTS

Most older adults must face the tremendous challenge of coping with difficult life changes. While many of the major life events of younger adulthood are familiar, positive, and purposefully chosen, the life events of older adulthood may be unknown, unwanted, unexpected, and associated with losses rather than gains. For example, major life events of younger adulthood may include establishing a career, moving away from the childhood family home, committing oneself to a partner, buying a house, and having children. In contrast, major life events of older adulthood may include retirement, widowhood, moving to a smaller home, losing significant relationships, and coping with illnesses and functional limitations.

Each major life event is likely to trigger related and significant coping challenges. For example, many older adults must cope with functional limitations, such as impairments in vision, hearing, mobility, memory, and cognition. Consequences of these limitations may include

Changes in lifestyle
Concerns about safety
An unpredictable future
Increased dependence on others
Loss of the ability to drive
Expenditures for assistance and medical care
Moving to a group or institutional setting

Emotional aspects of coping with functional limitations may involve feelings of fear, anger, inadequacy, poor self-esteem, and a loss of control over one's life.

Most older people cope well with major life events, particularly if they developed good coping skills throughout adulthood. However, older adults who face several major life events in close proximity typically have great difficulty in coping with the consequences. Factors that assist older adults in coping include financial assets, perceived control over life circumstances, and social supports, including a confidant relationship. Older adults who have not adjusted well in earlier adulthood are unlikely to cope well with the challenges of later adulthood. These people may experience depression, alcohol abuse, self-neglect, and serious threats to their self-esteem. It is important for the nurse to identify unhealthy coping responses so that interventions can be implemented. Table 4–1 lists some of the psychosocial adjustments of older adulthood and the healthy coping strategies that can be applied to these challenges.

Table 4–1

Coping Strategies for the Challenges of Older Adulthood

Psychosocial Adjustment	Coping Strategy
Retirement	Develop new skills.
	Use time for hobbies, volunteer activities, and personal pursuits.
Reduced income	Take advantage of discounts.
Declining physical health	Maintain good health practices (such as nutrition, exercise, rest).
Functional limitations	Adapt the environment to ensure optimal and safe functioning.
	Take advantage of assistive devices and equipment.
	Accept help when necessary.
Changes in cognitive skills	Take advantage of educational opportunities.
	Keep mentally stimulated.
	Avoid dwelling on things you cannot do and focus on abilities.
	Take advantage of increased potential for wisdom and creativity.
Death of spouse, friends, and family members	Allow yourself to grieve appropriately.
	Participate in group or individual counseling and support.
	Renew old relationships and establish new ones.
	Cherish happy memories.
	Realize new freedoms.
Relocation from family home	Look into various living arrangements.
	Appreciate the relief from responsibilities.
	Take advantage of new opportunities.
Other challenges to mental health	Maintain a sense of humor.
	Use stress-reduction techniques.
	Learn assertiveness skills.
	Participate in support groups.

Adapted from Miller CA. Nursing care of older adults: Theory and practice. 2nd ed. Philadelphia: JB Lippincott, 1995.

NURSING PROCESS GUIDELINES
Psychosocial Aspects of Aging

Identify major life events and other sources of stress that affect the older person. Assess the impact of major stressors by questioning the person directly and considering verbal and nonverbal cues as events are discussed. Pay particular attention to cues that indicate self-esteem during all interactions. Determine participation in social interactions and whether the person communicates with family, friends, or a confidant. Find out if there has been a change in patterns of social interaction. Ask whether the person has or has had a pet. Pets can be a valuable source of uninhibited love and emotional gratification for isolated people (Fig. 4–1). Compare this assessment information with data about lifelong patterns to detect changes in the person's quality of life.

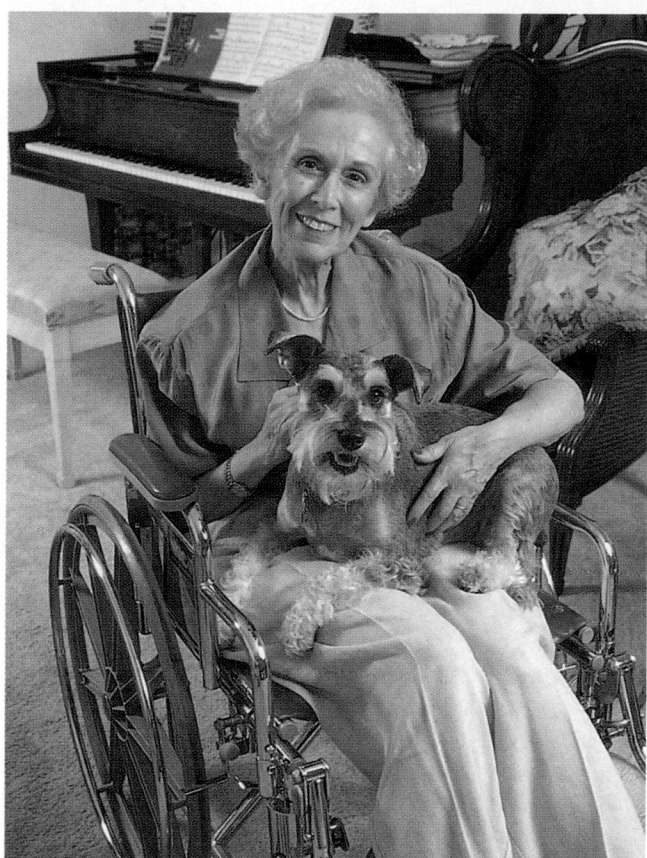

Figure 4–1

A relationship with a pet can provide mutual affection, purpose, and activity for an older adult.

Identify the older person's coping patterns and discuss coping mechanisms, such as those outlined in Table 4–1. Encourage verbalization about significant losses and provide opportunities for reminiscence. Allow the person to express feelings of grief and anger, and reassure the person that these are normal responses to loss. As grieving progresses, help the person focus first on short-term and then on long-term plans. Encourage socialization to help alleviate loneliness. If grief and anger remain unresolved or interfere with the person's ability to function, suggest that the person attend a support group or obtain group or individual therapy. If the person verbalizes suicidal ideation, obtain a prompt referral for psychiatric evaluation.

BODY COMPOSITION

As a person ages, changes occur in the distribution and functional capacity of the major body components. At about age 30, the number of functioning cells in most body organs begins to decrease. The cumulative effect of these gradual changes is that older adults experience a loss of functional reserve, which is the ability of organs to meet the body's

needs under conditions of stress or increased demand. Also beginning at about age 30, body fat gradually increases from 21 to 40% of body weight in men and from 35 to 53% in women. Lean tissue decreases until, by age 80, it has declined about 20%. Consistent with these age-related changes in body composition, total body water decreases by 10 to 15% between ages 20 and 80. Because adipose tissue contains little water, the increase in proportion of body fat to lean mass causes a decrease in the proportion of intercellular fluid and total body water to body weight. Distribution of body fat shifts, and fat deposits develop in and around muscle fibers and viscera. Subcutaneous body fat decreases. Many elderly persons, regardless of their body weight or build, develop a slightly protuberant abdomen and fat deposits on the hips.

NURSING PROCESS GUIDELINES
Body Composition Changes

Assess the older person's general size, weight, stature, and fat distribution. Ask about weakness, fatigue, and general response to stressful events. Determine whether the person has difficulty with physical activity, especially when performing more than the usual activities of daily living. Additional assessments related to body composition are found in the sections on thermoregulation and musculoskeletal function.

NUTRITIONAL NEEDS

Throughout the life cycle, nutritional and physical and emotional well-being are highly inter-related. In later adulthood, many factors can interfere with adequate nutrition and the enjoyment of food. Common factors that may contribute to nutritional problems include

- Limited financial resources
- Physical limitations
- Diminished smell and taste sensations
- Disorders, such as dementia and depression
- Dental problems, including loss of teeth, that may make it more difficult to enjoy food and obtain adequate nutrients
- Alcoholism, an often hidden problem that also may contribute to depression and mental changes
- Social and environmental circumstances, such as eating alone or in an institutional setting, may interfere with mealtime enjoyment.

Medications can interfere with food enjoyment and adequate nutrition in two ways. First, medications can interfere with food intake, digestion, and elimination through such common side effects as anorexia, dry mouth, diarrhea, or constipation. Second, medications can interfere with absorption of nutrients through food-drug interactions. For example, mineral oil can decrease absorption of vitamins A, D, E, and K. Aluminum-based antacids decrease absorption of fluoride and phosphorus. Malnutrition, dehydration, weight loss, and vitamin and mineral deficiencies are common problems associated with these and other factors that affect food ingestion and digestion in older adults.

Even healthy older adults who take no medications experience age-related changes that affect nutrition and digestion. The major change is a reduced need for calories. Thus, older adults need to consume higher-quality foods and beverages to achieve adequate nutrient intake with fewer calories. Another age-related change is a general slowing of the digestive tract. This process does not significantly affect digestion, nor does it directly cause constipation. It does, however, predispose older adults to constipation, especially in combination with risk factors for constipation, such as low intake of fiber and fluids.

The recommended dietary allowance (RDA) to meet the nutritional needs of healthy people suggests a 10% decrease in calorie intake for persons 51 to 75 years, and a 20 to 25% decrease for persons 76 years or older. Although there is no standard caloric requirement that fits all persons, the recommended average calorie intake for healthy people age 51 or older is 30 kcal/kg of body weight. Caloric requirements can be further adjusted to allow for activity level and advanced age. Current RDA standards indicate that the diet of all persons, including older adults, should contain 50 to 55% carbohydrate, 15% protein, and no more than 30% fat. Most of the carbohydrate calories should come from complex and high-fiber carbohydrates, such as grains. Less than 10% of the carbohydrate calories should come from simple carbohydrates, such as sugar. A person can reduce cholesterol by consuming soluble fiber, such as is found in oats and pectin, and polyunsaturated and monounsaturated fatty acids rather than saturated fats.

NURSING PROCESS GUIDELINES
Nutritional Needs of Older Adults

Assess the elderly person's general appearance, height, and weight to establish a baseline for future comparison. Ask whether this is the person's preferred weight. Find out about recent weight changes and ask if these changes were intended or unintended. Have the person describe a typical day's food preparation and intake. Include snacks, fluids, vitamin or mineral supplements, and alcohol. If the person takes a nutritional supplement, ask why. Ask whether the person avoids any foods because of difficulty chewing or digestive problems. Assess for such risk factors as depression, medications, and social circumstances that can interfere with the older adult's ability to obtain, enjoy, and digest food.

Teach the older person to choose varied foods from the basic food groups. Highlight 4–1 identifies nutritional guidelines for the elderly. Encourage consumption of complex carbohydrates, dietary fiber, polyunsaturated fats, caffeine-free beverages, and low-cholesterol protein sources. Suggest such food preparation methods as stewing or braising if chewing is difficult. Encourage the use of community resources, such as group meal programs and home-delivered meals. Eating at a community center offers the advantage of socialization (Fig. 4–2). If the person takes a vitamin or mineral supplement, suggest less costly generic brands and review how the preparation is to be taken. If loss, loneliness, or depression is affecting nutrition, consider a referral for mental health services. Consider the possibility of alcohol abuse in any malnourished older adult. If confirmed, make a referral to Alcoholics Anonymous or another appropriate resource.

PHARMACOKINETICS

Older adults make up 12% of the population in the United States but account for almost 50% of all drugs used. Many older adults take 10 or more prescription drugs, often prescribed by several different physicians. More than 70% of older adults use nonprescription drugs on a daily basis. Each additional drug taken increases the chance of interactions, altered effectiveness, and adverse reactions. In addition, older adults have altered pharmacokinetics because of normal age-related changes, diseases, and dietary deficiencies.

Normal physiologic changes of the aging process may alter drug absorption, metabolism, elimination, and effectiveness in a variety of ways. For example, glomerular filtration rate begins to decline in early adulthood and progresses at an annual rate of 1 to 2%. More than any other age-related change, diminished renal functioning has a profound impact on medication action. However, as with other aspects of pharmacokinetics, the specific chemical characteristics of each medication determine the degree to which age-related changes affect excretion. For example, medications excreted largely unchanged through the kidneys, such as amino glycoside antibiotics, will be more directly influenced by diminished renal functioning than those that are metabolized more extensively in the liver before excretion. Likewise, the effect of diminished renal functioning will be greater on medications with a narrow therapeutic index (such as digoxin) than on medications with a wide therapeutic index.

Changes in body composition also influence pharmacokinetics. Increased body fat and decreased total body water affect medications according to the degree to which those medications are fat- or water-soluble. Thus, drugs that are distributed primarily in body water or lean body mass may achieve higher serum concentrations in older adults, and their effects may be more intense. Similarly, highly fat-solu-

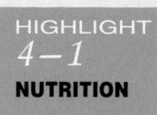
HIGHLIGHT
4–1
NUTRITION

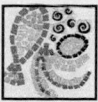

Nutritional Needs of the Elderly

Instruct the elderly individual in the following:
Plan a nutritionally sound diet by selecting a variety of familiar foods from the basic food groups.

Group	Servings	Examples of One Serving
Bread, Cereal, Rice, and Pasta	6–11	1 slice of bread $\frac{1}{2}$ muffin, bagel $\frac{1}{2}$ cup cooked cereal, pasta, rice, noodles 1 oz dry cereal
Vegetables	3–5	$\frac{1}{2}$ cup of most cooked or raw chopped vegetables 1 cup leafy raw vegetables $\frac{3}{4}$ cup vegetable juice
Fruit	2–4	$\frac{1}{2}$ cup of most fruits 1 small whole fruit 1 melon wedge $\frac{1}{2}$ banana or grapefruit $\frac{3}{4}$ cup fruit juice
Milk	2–3	1 cup low-fat or skim milk 1 cup low-fat yogurt $1\frac{1}{2}$ oz hard cheese 2 oz processed cheese
Meat, Poultry, Fish, Eggs, and Nuts	2–3	$2\frac{1}{2}$ to 3 oz cooked lean meat 3 to 4 oz cooked fish or poultry 1 cup cooked dry beans, peas 2 eggs (<3 eggs per week) 4–5 tbsp peanut butter

The minimum number of daily servings provides a caloric intake of approximately 1600 calories if low-fat, lean foods are selected. Add additional servings to achieve desired caloric intake.

Low-fat milk and milk products, canned fish with bones, and dark green leafy vegetables such as broccoli, collard greens, and kale are good sources of calcium.

Citrus fruit or juice, strawberries, cantaloupes, potatoes, tomatoes, and broccoli are good sources of vitamin C. Eat at least one serving daily.

Meat, fish, poultry, grains, legumes, and dark leafy vegetables are good sources of iron and B vitamins.

Dark green and yellow leafy vegetables, dark yellow fruits, liver, and fortified milk products are good sources of vitamin A. Eat at least three servings a week.

Whole-grain breads and cereals, brown rice, dried legumes, fresh fruits with skins, raw or minimally cooked vegetables, nuts, and seeds provide dietary fiber and help prevent constipation.

Apple juice, bananas, citrus fruits and juices, melons, prunes and prune juice, tomatoes and tomato juice, dried beans, white potatoes, sweet potatoes, beef, turkey, and most salt substitutes are good sources of potassium.

Food eaten in five or six small meals daily is generally tolerated and digested better by the elderly.

Chew food thoroughly before swallowing.

Eat soft, chopped, or puréed foods if chewing food well is difficult.

Drink six to eight glasses of fluid a day to help prevent constipation and maintain hydration.

Do not drink fluids within 1 hour before mealtime.

Use fats, oils, and sweets sparingly.

Avoid excessive salt and sodium intake.

Use nonsodium flavor enhancers and spices to season food.

Discuss ideal weight goal and dietary modifications with physician if appropriate.

Weigh weekly to monitor weight maintenance, loss, or gain.

Data from U.S. Department of Agriculture and U.S. Department of Health and Human Services.

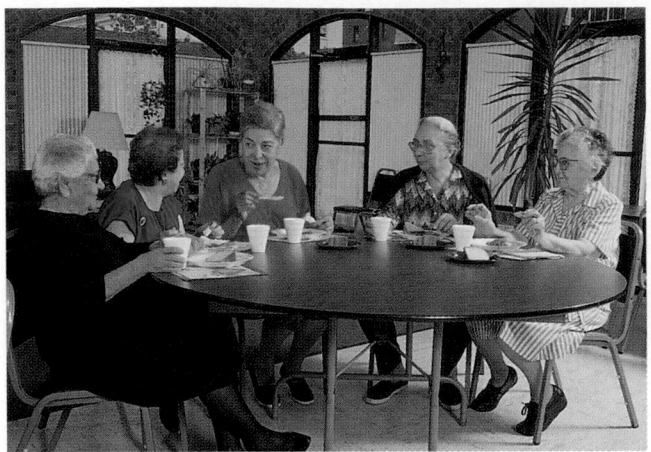

Figure 4–2

Eating in a community setting can help the older person maintain relationships in addition to providing nutritious meals.

ble medications, which are distributed and stored in fat tissue, may achieve lower serum concentrations and have a greater tendency to accumulate in adipose tissue. The end result is that fat-soluble medications may have a more prolonged duration of action, their overall effect may be erratic, and their short-term effects may be less intense.

Another age-related change that may affect pharmacokinetics is diminished serum albumin. As medications are distributed and metabolized in the body, some molecules are bound to serum albumin. The bound portion becomes inactive, while the unbound molecules remain active. The degree to which each medication binds with albumin varies. Some medications, such as warfarin, bind by as much as 99%. When serum albumin is lower than normal, or when two or more drugs compete for the binding sites, the risk of adverse effects and altered therapeutic effectiveness increases.

Compounding these problems, many older adults have an impaired ability to safely and correctly self-administer drugs. Sensory, cognitive, and musculo-

Table 4–2

Nursing Implications of the Altered Effects of Drugs in Geriatric Patients

Drug Classification	Nursing Implications Specific for Geriatric Patients
All drugs	Many side effects and signs of drug toxicity are common complaints that the elderly attribute to aging and therefore may ignore. Provide information about side effects and signs of toxicity in writing and emphasize the need to promptly report to the physician any occurrence lasting more than 24 hours.
Digitalis glycosides	Decreased renal excretion and increased cardiac sensitivity increase risk of toxicity. Antacids decrease absorption; do not administer within 1 hour of digitalis.
Diuretics	Adverse effects more frequent because of sensitivity to fluid loss. Higher risk for postural hypotension, hypokalemia, hyponatremia, muscle cramps, and thrombus formation
Anticoagulants	Increased drug activity from impaired plasma protein binding increases the risk of serious bleeding. This risk increases even more when the person takes other highly protein-bound drugs.
Antihypertensives	Postural hypotension common. Predisposition to bradycardia and respiratory and central nervous system side effects.
Antiarrhythmics	Elderly often treated with lower dose. Elderly more sensitive to central nervous system effects of drugs.
Calcium channel blockers	Higher risk of adverse reactions, especially orthostatic hypotension. Impaired renal and hepatic function prolong activity.
Anti-inflammatory agents	Risk of adverse reactions with indomethacin extremely high. Increased risk for peptic ulcer, aplastic anemia, and toxic reactions with phenylbutazone.
Oral hypoglycemic agents	Impaired hepatic and renal function impair excretion, prolong activity. Elderly especially vulnerable to hypoglycemia; early signs difficult to detect.
Antianxiety agents	Impaired hepatic and renal function impair excretion, prolong activity. Increased sensitivity to central nervous system effects.
Aminoglycosides	Monitor closely for nephrotoxicity and ototoxicity.
Narcotic analgesics	Increased sensitivity to central nervous system effects. Lower doses usually prescribed.

skeletal changes are common risk factors in older adults. Muscle weakness and stiff joints may reduce the older person's ability to open medicine containers. This, in turn, may tempt the person to either leave the medication open or pour it into another bottle. Visual impairment and decreased tactile sensitivity may cause the older person to misread labels or take incorrect doses. Depression and memory impairment may interfere with the older adult's ability and motivation to take medications correctly. Medication errors and noncompliance are also related to such factors as living alone, financial status, frequency of dosing, and complexity of the medication regimen. Lastly, when older adults experience adverse drug effects, these problems are likely to be overlooked, attributed falsely to the aging process, or treated with yet another medication.

NURSING PROCESS GUIDELINES
Pharmacokinetics

Assess the older person's knowledge of his or her medication schedule, the medications included in it, and their side effects. Ask about regular and periodic use of topical preparations, home remedies, dietary supplements, and nonprescription agents. Find out how many physicians and pharmacists the person is seeing. Determine whether each physician caring for the person is aware of all prescription and nonprescription preparations being taken. Ask if the older adult is following any special dietary or activity instructions because of medications. Ask what method the person uses to remember to take medications as prescribed and to remember that a dose was taken.

Always review medication information with the older person. Name the drug and state its purpose. Repetition reinforces learning. State how many pills or how much liquid must be taken. Administer oral medications with 6 to 8 ounces of water to facilitate swallowing and ensure their passage into the stomach. Have the person stand or sit upright to reduce the risk of choking or aspiration. It may be necessary to check the person's mouth to be sure pills have been swallowed.

Assess closely for adverse drug reactions. Mental confusion is a common early manifestation of drug toxicity. Recognize the possibility that any change in functioning or mental status could be drug-related. Anticipate that a drug may be given in smaller doses or less frequently to compensate for age-related changes. Use a body-weight formula to determine safe dosages for older adults who are frail. Consult with the physician to determine whether a medication can be administered once a day rather than in divided doses, since this may help improve compliance when the person is at home. Table 4-2 identifies specific geriatric nursing implications for classifications of drugs commonly prescribed for the elderly.

Teach the older person to take medications as prescribed and to bring a list of current medications to each doctor's visit. Recommend using one pharmacy to fill all prescriptions. Suggest asking the pharmacist to use easy-open containers and to type the label in all capitals to make it easier to read. Remind the person that the pharmacist is a good source of information about medications and their effects. Emphasize the need to notify the physician promptly about any changes in functioning or unusual sensations that develop while taking a medication. Refer to Highlight 4-2 for specific guidelines for teaching self-medication to older adults. Reinforce verbal instructions with clearly written instructions on cards. Nursing Care Guide 4-1 identifies some of the nursing interventions used to promote the older adult's compliance with a medication

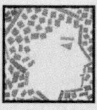

HIGHLIGHT 4-2

PATIENT EDUCATION   **Self-Administration of Medications for the Elderly**

Instruct the older person to take medications exactly as prescribed and provide clearly written instructions on the following:

Name, dose, frequency, expected effects, and untoward side effects of each medication.

How to take the medication.

How soon the expected effects should occur.

How to open the container and the availability of easy-open, non-childproof caps.

Whether medication is available in liquid or can be crushed and dissolved in fluid or mixed with food.

Methods to ensure accurate self-medication, such as a checkoff calendar or containers labeled with days of the week and medication times during the day.

Method of monitoring effects of medication.

Importance of reporting adverse reactions or absence of desired response to the physician so that the medication or dosage can be changed.

Dietary alterations; include foods or drugs to avoid.

Maintaining a list of current medications to take to each doctor's appointment.

Consulting physician before taking any over-the-counter preparation.

Whom to call for answers about prescribed and over-the-counter medications.

What to do if illness or other circumstances prevent taking medication.

Nursing Care Guide 4–1

Promoting Compliance with Medication Regimen by Elderly Adults

Assessment Findings: 81-year-old patient who has a history of congestive heart failure will be discharged on furosemide (Lasix) and digoxin (Lanoxin) following treatment for exacerbation of symptoms related to failure to follow prescribed medication regimen. When reviewing medications during hospitalization, patient repeatedly confuses medications, forgets when to take them, and cannot remember whether medication was taken.

Nursing Diagnosis: Ineffective management of therapeutic regimen (individuals) related to insufficient knowledge of medication regimen and inability to differentiate among medications or remember whether medication was taken as prescribed

Patient Outcomes	Nursing Interventions	Rationale
Patient verbalizes understanding of need to follow prescribed medication regimen before discharge.	Determine patient's readiness and ability to learn.	Teaching cannot be successful unless the patient is motivated and able to learn.
	Ask patient to identify reasons for current hospitalization. Reinforce with patient failure to take medications as prescribed as reason for hospitalization.	Determines level of knowledge and awareness of cause of hospitalization.
Patient correctly identifies a container of digoxin and a container of furosemide 100% of the time.	Assess patient's visual acuity and ability to read medication bottle labels.	Identifies possible cause of noncompliance.
	If patient is unable to read labels, ask the physician to write a note requesting that the patient's pharmacy mark the respective containers with a large "D" or "F" and type labels in all capitals.	Simplifies identification of correct medication. Capital letters are more easily read.
	Review identification method with patient daily.	Repetition reinforces learning.
Patient states the name, dose, frequency, expected actions, and untoward side effects of prescribed medications from memory or by reading printed cards.	Teach patient the name, dose, frequency, expected actions, and untoward side effects of prescribed medications.	Legally all persons must have this information to correctly and safely self-administer medication. Understanding increases compliance.
	Instruct patient to notify physician promptly if condition deteriorates or untoward side effects develop.	Medication or dosage may need to be altered.
	Reinforce verbal information with clearly printed cards.	Repetition reinforces learning.
	Ask patient to read each card.	To be sure lettering is large enough for patient to see.
Patient demonstrates ability to monitor effects of medications: a. accurately counts and records pulse	Teach patient how to count the radial or carotid pulse for a full minute and record.	Pulse rate indicates therapeutic effectiveness of digoxin.

(continued)

Nursing Care Guide 4–1
Promoting Compliance with Medication Regimen by Elderly Adults (continued)

Patient Outcomes	Nursing Interventions	Rationale
b. accurately weighs self and records weight	Teach patient to monitor and record body weight weekly.	Body weight indicates therapeutic effectiveness of furosemide.
	Have patient do return demonstration of ability to correctly monitor and record pulse and weight daily during remainder of hospitalization.	Evaluates learning and identifies need for further teaching and demonstration.
Patient states intent to notify physician if pulse is irregular, below 60 bpm, or above 110 bpm; if weight changes by more than 3 pounds in 1 week; or if ankle edema, nausea, vomiting, muscle weakness, cramps, or visual changes develop.	Instruct patient to notify physician promptly if untoward side effects of medications develop.	Pulse below 60 bpm or above 110 bpm and irregular pulse may indicate digoxin toxicity. Daily weight is the most accurate method of determining change in fluid balance. Each pound represents approximately 500 mL of fluid.
	Reinforce instructions and provide physician's telephone number on clearly printed card.	Repetition reinforces learning. The telephone number will be readily available if needed.
Patient states intent to avoid taking antacid within 1 hour of taking digoxin.	Advise patient that concurrent ingestion of antacids with digoxin inhibits absorption.	Patient must be aware of drug interactions to avoid altered therapeutic response.
Patient states intent to increase dietary intake of potassium-rich foods.	Instruct patient that potassium-rich foods such as bananas, oranges, peaches, and dates must be included in the diet daily to replace potassium lost during furosemide therapy.	Furosemide promotes potassium excretion.
Patient verbalizes intent and demonstrates ability to self-administer medications as prescribed.	Identify and reinforce patient's motivating factors to adhere to medication regimen.	Self-motivation increases learning and compliance.
	Provide method for monitoring self-administration of medication such as checkoff calendar or daily pill boxes.	Ensures therapeutic blood level of medications by preventing extra doses or omitted doses.
	Allow patient to learn at own rate.	Too much information too fast causes frustration and interferes with successful learning.
	Provide positive reinforcement.	Positive feedback increases motivation and reinforces learning.
	Have patient use monitoring method for remainder of hospitalization.	Develops familiarity with the method and reduces unexpected problems at home.

Evaluation: Compare the patient's status with the expected outcomes. If the outcomes are not met, reassess the patient and revise the plan.

regimen. Initiate a home-care referral for people who live alone and who appear unable to self-administer medications safely.

INTEGUMENT

Skin

Changes in an aging person's skin result from a combination of genetics, disease conditions, environmental factors, and normal effects of aging. Long-term exposure to the sun is the most significant environmental factor, and its effects accelerate the aging process. With age, cell division slows and replacement of damaged or dead skin cells declines. The epithelium thins, collagen fibers stiffen, elastin formation decreases, and the dermal-epidermal junction becomes flattened. As a consequence of these age-related changes, the skin becomes thinner, less pliable, and more likely to develop blisters in response to disease processes. Also, older skin has less resistance to shearing forces and is therefore more susceptible to bruises and shear-type injuries.

Decreased activity of the sebaceous and sweat glands causes the skin to be dry, rough, and flaky, especially on the extremities. Skin tags, which are small skin herniations composed of collagen and subcutaneous tissue, are common in elderly people. They can be removed if they bleed, cause pain, become inflamed, or undergo suspicious changes.

As subcutaneous adipose tissue is lost, the skin becomes wrinkled and, particularly on the arms and legs, loose and flabby. Loss of subcutaneous adipose tissue also makes the tendons, veins, and knuckles of the hands more prominent and exaggerates the bony prominence of the knees, scapulae, and trochanters. Without the cushioning effect of adipose tissue, the skin becomes more susceptible to physical trauma and pressure sores.

The melanocytes, or pigment cells of the skin, become larger but fewer in number. Pigment changes result from diminished melanocytes. The skin of white persons not exposed to the sun appears paler and more opaque. Skin with long-term sun exposure develops a blotchy appearance as areas of hyperpigmentation mix with areas of hypopigmentation. Flat brown macules of solar lentigines—commonly called senile lentigo, liver spots, or age spots—develop on sun-exposed areas of the arms, hands, and face. Solar lentigines are illustrated in Figure 4–3.

Western cultures place a high social value on personal appearance, especially the appearance of the parts of the body most visible to others, such as skin and hair. Thus, negative attitudes about and perceptions of old age may have a detrimental effect on the self-esteem of older adults who have visible age-related changes. It is important to recognize, challenge, and avoid conveying negative attitudes

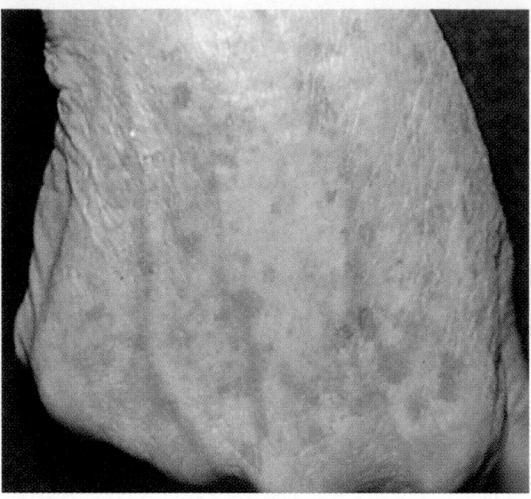

Figure 4–3

Solar lentigines, or liver spots, are characteristically seen on areas of sun-exposed skin in older adults. (From Lookingbill D, Marks J. Principles of dermatology. 2nd ed. Philadelphia: WB Saunders, 1993; p 89.)

about aging, including your own. If an older adult's self-esteem is affected by negative attitudes about his or her appearance, encourage the person to discuss changes in dress or grooming that could help minimize the changes in appearance and improve self-esteem.

NURSING PROCESS GUIDELINES
Skin Changes

Assess skin for alterations in color, turgor, dryness, texture, and overall condition, as described in detail in Chapter 35. Turgor is difficult to assess in the elderly because of wrinkling and dryness of the skin. However, skin that covers protected areas, such as the abdomen, may provide accurate information about hydration status. Observe for lesions and for signs of scratching, such as inflamed areas or linear scabs. Determine how long lesions have been present and whether their appearance has changed. Ask how long it usually takes for wounds to heal.

Teach the older adult that frequent applications of creams and lotions can help relieve dry skin. The chosen product should contain lanolin but little or no alcohol or perfume. Consider recommending that the person bathe less frequently and only with tepid water and superfatted soaps. When the person does bathe, suggest using soap only in the genital and axillary areas to minimize dryness. Application of emollients immediately after bathing may be beneficial. If the person uses bath oils, advise taking special precautions to avoid falls. In winter, a furnace humidifier, room humidifier, or pans of water placed near heat sources provide extra moisture in the air and diminish skin dryness. Encourage the person to limit sun exposure, to wear a wide-brimmed hat outdoors, and to apply sunscreen frequently. Recommend a sunscreen with a sun protection factor (SPF) of at least 15.

Hair and Nails

The hair of the scalp, trunk, pubis, axillae, and extremities gradually thins as a person ages, and the thickness of each hair shaft decreases. Hairs in the nostrils and ears thicken. Although the pattern of hair loss and onset of baldness are genetically determined, in general, scalp hair loss occurs primarily in the front and on the top of the head. The onset and pattern of gray hair, also genetically determined, occur as the function and number of melanocytes decrease. As estrogen production declines in women, facial hair may become more coarse and prominent.

An older person's nails grow more slowly than a younger person's, and they undergo cosmetic changes. As a person ages, the nails become dull, opaque, longitudinally striated, and yellow or gray in color. Under normal circumstances, age-related changes do not interfere with the protective function of the nails. However, because nails become fragile and brittle in older people, they are more likely to split. Also, if the nail has been injured, or if onychomycosis (a fungus infection of the nail) occurs, age-related changes will prolong the healing process.

NURSING PROCESS GUIDELINES
Hair and Nail Changes

Assess the hair and nails for alterations in color, texture, and distribution associated with the aging process. Assessment of the hair and nails is described in detail in Chapter 35. Ask whether the changes occurred gradually or rapidly. Rapid hair loss or a change in color, texture, or distribution may be related to a pathologic process. Note the presence of yellow-orange stains on the fingers and nails from smoking. Observe for evidence of poor hygiene and other clues to self-neglect that could be caused by conditions such as dementia or depression.

If an older adult is disturbed by loss and graying of the hair, discuss the availability of hair coloring products, hairpieces, and wigs. Encourage the person to examine negative attitudes that affect self-esteem. Facial hair can be bleached or removed by electrolysis. Long ear and nasal hairs can be trimmed. Fingernails should be rounded and smoothed with an emery board. To prevent ingrown toenails, teach the person to cut them straight across. If the person has impaired manual dexterity or vision, or if the person has a history of diabetes mellitus or peripheral vascular disorders, a podiatrist should cut the toenails.

THERMOREGULATION

Thermoregulation in older adults is altered by age-related changes that interfere with the ability to adapt effectively to environmental temperatures. Reduced sweat production decreases the body's ability to lose heat through evaporation, making the older person prone to heat stroke in hot weather. A reduction in insulating subcutaneous fat makes the older person more sensitive to cold environments as well. Other age-related changes that interfere with the ability to respond to cold temperatures include inefficient vasoconstriction, decreased cardiac output, decreased subcutaneous tissue, and delayed and diminished shivering. Many elderly persons feel chilled even in a warm room. The overall effect of these age-related changes is a dulled perception of cold and a concomitant lack of stimulus to initiate protective actions, such as adding more clothing or raising the environmental temperature. These changes increase the older person's susceptibility to hypothermia.

Another age-related change in thermoregulation is that even healthy older adults may have a lower normal body temperature and a diminished febrile response to illness. Risk factors that can further impair the thermoregulatory response of older adults include diseases, immobility, medication effects, and adverse environmental temperatures.

NURSING PROCESS GUIDELINES
Thermoregulation

Question the older person about tolerance to environmental temperature fluctuations. Ask about any history of hypothermia or heat-related illnesses. Determine the person's normal baseline body temperature so that any deviations can be detected. Assess the environment for risk factors for hypothermia or heat-related illnesses, such as inadequate heating or cooling. Assess for other risk factors, such as disease condition, medication effects, or diminished sweating during exercise.

Teach the older adult to avoid strenuous activity and to increase the intake of caffeine-free and alcohol-free beverages in extremely hot or cold weather. In hot weather, recommend a sun hat and light-weight clothing outdoors to protect from sun exposure while allowing air to circulate and cool the body. Insulating undergarments, multiple layers, hats, gloves, and scarves should be worn outdoors in cold temperatures to avoid chills. During cold weather, teach the person to maintain a constant room temperature as close to 24°C (75°F) as possible with a minimum temperature of 21°C (70°F). During hot weather, the person should maintain the room temperature below 29.5°C (85°F).

SENSORY CHANGES

Vision

Visual accommodation (the ability to focus on near and far objects) decreases with age as a result of weakening of the muscles that control the lens. Beginning in their forties, most people need reading glasses or bifocals to correct presbyopia (age-related decreased ability to focus on near objects) and to compensate for this loss in accommodation.

Cataracts are another common eye disorder in the elderly. Blurred vision, distortion of objects, and a gradual, progressive decrease in visual acuity result from altered protein metabolism in the crystalline lens and the lifetime effects of exposure to ultraviolet light. Color discrimination may deteriorate, and older adults may have difficulty discriminating between blues and greens. The lens may become discolored and develop scattered opacities that make the eye sensitive to glare. Degeneration may progress until the lens is completely opaque and rigid. The pupil, which is normally black, becomes gray, then milky white as the lens opacifies behind it. To restore vision, the opaque lens is removed in an elective surgical procedure described in Chapter 45.

Gradual fibrosis of the muscular iris causes the pupils to decrease in size. This diminishes the amount of light that enters the eye and inhibits the older person's ability to adapt to changes in light intensity. Bright, glare-free light is needed for the older person to be able to see well. As the blood supply to the oxygen-sensitive cells of the retina decreases, depth perception, peripheral vision, and night vision deteriorate. Loss of peripheral vision must be medically evaluated to rule out glaucoma, a common cause of preventable blindness. Glaucoma is discussed in Chapter 45. Decreased function of the lacrimal apparatus may cause dryness and itching of the eyes.

NURSING PROCESS GUIDELINES
Vision Changes

Assess the older person's vision for loss of acuity and accommodation as discussed in detail in Chapter 44. Ask where and how often the person receives eye care. Test visual fields and pupillary reaction to light. Ask about changes in depth perception, loss of color distinction, and difficulty seeing at night. Because visual deterioration occurs gradually, the person may not be aware that changes have occurred. Look for clues to visual changes, such as mis-

matched clothing, groping for objects, recent automobile accidents, or bruises on arms or legs caused by bumping into surrounding objects.

Recommend that the older person have an annual eye examination and glaucoma screening. Demonstrate how to turn the head to compensate for loss of peripheral vision to prevent accidents. Suggest the use of railings, adequate lighting, and removal of environmental hazards such as loose floor coverings to avoid falls. Use of wetting drops or artificial tears may help relieve ocular dryness. Advise the older person to allow additional time for the eyes to adjust to changes in light intensity. Also discuss the need to limit driving to daylight hours if night vision is impaired. A referral to a local sight center may be helpful in obtaining aids for improving visual performance. If vision is impaired to the point of making food preparation tasks dangerous, referral to social services, home-care agencies, home-delivered meal services, or a group meal program may be appropriate. Use good color contrast, such as red print on a yellow background, in teaching aids.

Hearing

The ability to hear high-frequency sounds begins to deteriorate in childhood and usually becomes noticeable by late middle age. As the person continues to age, the ability to hear high-pitched sounds continues to decrease. This problem is worsened by background noise. These changes are caused by

- increased rigidity of the small bones of the middle ear
- degeneration of hair cells in the organ of Corti
- atrophy of cochlear capillaries
- reduced sound transmission through a thickened tympanic membrane

Sudden loss of hearing is not normal at any age and requires investigation by a physician to identify factors such as impacted wax, physiologic disorders, or adverse medication effects.

NURSING PROCESS GUIDELINES
Hearing Changes

Assess the older person's ears and hearing, as discussed in detail in Chapter 46. Ask whether any hearing loss has been noted. Observe for nonverbal cues of impaired hearing, such as leaning forward or turning one ear toward the speaker, cupping a hand behind the ear, or frequent misunderstanding of questions. If the person wears a hearing aid, examine the auditory canal for signs of irritation (Fig. 4–4).

Encourage older adults to have their hearing evaluated periodically for early detection and correction of hearing problems. Find out if the person has

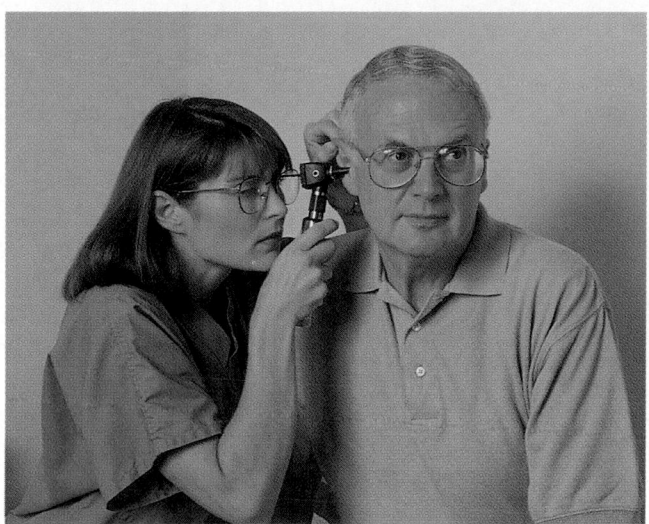

Figure 4-4
Although hearing ability normally declines with age, abrupt loss of hearing is not normal and requires prompt examination to determine its cause.

ever had a hearing evaluation and, if appropriate, ask whether the person has considered buying a hearing aid. Discuss the availability of hearing aids and adaptive devices that modify telephone transmission for the hearing impaired. Encourage the person to find out about assistive hearing devices, such as closed-captioned television, that might improve communication and quality of life.

Teach methods of improving communication for hearing-impaired people. Encourage the person to ask others to face him or her when speaking and to speak clearly in a normal voice. Also, the hearing-impaired person can ask people to avoid shouting because this produces distorted, high-pitched sounds that are more difficult to understand. Identify and implement ways of eliminating or reducing background noise.

Taste and Smell

The ability to taste depends primarily on receptor cells in the taste buds, which are located on the tongue, palate, and tonsils. Unlike other neural cells, taste cells have the ability to regenerate and are replaced every few days. Although many early studies identified age-related declines in taste sensation, more recent studies conclude that taste, particularly the sweetness of sugar, is well preserved in older adults despite a decline in the number of taste buds. Many older adults experience decreased saliva flow, but this typically stems from medication and disease effects rather than age-related changes.

The ability to smell depends on the perception of odorants by sensory cells in the olfactory mucosa and on central nervous system processing of that information. Olfactory ability begins to decline after about age 30 and declines to a greater extent than

the sense of taste. Because the perception of food flavor is highly associated with olfactory stimulation, age-related declines in the sense of smell interfere with the older person's ability to discern flavors or identify foods in the mouth.

NURSING PROCESS GUIDELINES
Taste and Smell

Ask whether the older person has noticed any decrease in the ability to smell or taste food or to smell other odors. Examine the lips and mouth for excessive dryness. Assess for medications or disease processes that may cause dry mouth. Ask what seasonings the person uses on food, with particular attention to seasonings containing sodium or monosodium glutamate. Assess for environmental hazards that might cause problems because of the person's diminished ability to smell.

Teach the older person that the taste of food can be improved by increasing the use of non-sodium flavor enhancers and spices. Sucking hard candy and performing frequent oral hygiene with a soft-bristled toothbrush may increase saliva production, relieve dry mouth, and help prevent gum disease. Encourage the proper use of smoke and gas detectors because the older person may be unable to smell smoke.

Tactile Sensation

The older person experiences diminished sensitivity to touch, temperature, pressure, and pain as a result of decreased capillary circulation and the loss of nerve fibers. Older people may not perceive or complain of pain because of increased pain tolerance. Also, they are more susceptible to scald burns because of decreased tactile sensitivity.

NURSING PROCESS GUIDELINES
Tactile Sensation

Assess for decreased tactile sensitivity and altered pain sensitivity. Examine the hands, feet, and bony prominences for evidence of burns, injuries, pressure areas, or signs of healed injuries. Observe the person's nonverbal behavior to determine response to touch.

Teach the older person to always use potholders to prevent burns when cooking. Demonstrate how to examine the feet and other injury-prone areas to detect wounds and how to test water temperature with the inside of the elbow or a thermometer before washing or bathing to avoid accidental burns. Suggest that the person lower the thermostat on the hot water heater as a safety measure.

Tactile stimulation is important to many older people, especially as vision and hearing diminish. For many people, a gentle touch on the hand, arm,

SOCIOCULTURAL PERSPECTIVES

The Elderly and the Cost of Chronic Illness

by Janice R. Ellis, PhD, RN

As people approach retirement, financial advisers, banks, insurance companies, and pension plan administrators all urge them to plan for adequate retirement income. The list of expenses that the elderly are usually advised to consider when planning for retirement includes food, clothing, housing, transportation, travel, and even gifts. In the United States, many advisers go so far as to suggest planning to pay insurance premiums for a Medicare supplement. *Rarely*, however, are elderly people encouraged to consider the costs of maintaining health in the face of a chronic illness. Yet statistics tell us that 40% of the elderly not living in institutions have chronic conditions that impose limitations on their lives. The most common of these are arthritis, hypertension, and heart disease. Diabetes, hypothyroidism, and chronic respiratory disease lead to still more illness, and risk of disability.

Inflation has affected all of life, but its impact has been much greater in health care than in any other sector of the economy. Prescription drugs have skyrocketed in price. In the United States, a health insurance policy to supplement Medicare is very costly.

People with chronic illness usually require medications on a consistent basis. This need for medication may put a significant strain on financial resources. For example, one elderly woman with a need for thyroid replacement hormone, an anti-inflammatory drug for her arthritis, and medication to lower her cholesterol level found herself looking at the prospect of spending $160 each month for medications. A 69-year-old man found that after his heart attack, his monthly medication bill for a long list of cardiac, blood pressure, and cholesterol-lowering agents amounted to $240.

As you read about the high cost of medications for the elderly, you might find yourself saying—as many people do—"Well, sure, the medications are expensive, but Medicare covers all that." Like many people who haven't reached retirement age, you might be shocked to learn that Medicare does *not* cover the cost of outpatient prescriptions, and many insurance plans for the elderly do not either.

Often, people on low incomes must therefore choose between filling prescriptions and paying for other basic necessities of life such as housing, groceries, and utilities. For example, in the United States, an elderly woman may have a total retirement income of $650 per month. Depending on the area of the country, rent may take 50 to 60% of this income unless the woman has subsidized housing.

Heating bills in the winter may be $150 a month (although this cost may be spread evenly in payments due throughout the year to facilitate budgeting). Healthy eating patterns demand that the woman be able to purchase appropriate groceries, including fresh fruits and vegetables. As you begin to consider these and other aspects of the budget, it is easy to see how quickly the money runs out. How much of the $650 is left over for the cost of medications when the woman must first spend $350 for rent, $150 for heat, and $120 for food each month? The older the person, the more critical these problems become because the number of chronic conditions increases with age, while inflation erodes the value of retirement income over time. For a person 85 years of age, the retirement income that seemed adequate at retirement 20 years ago may be completely inadequate to meet the demands of today.

Further complicating the situation is the reluctance of many elderly people to ask for help. Older adults usually value self-reliance and independence. They take pride in having survived a world war and a major economic depression. A great fear of many elderly people is that they will become dependent on others. Therefore, when confronted with economic problems, they return to the old Depression adage, "Make do, or do without!" Unfortunately, health-care professionals may completely overlook this philosophy and simply express annoyance at the lack of "compliance" that they identify in their elderly patients.

As you look at the older adults who come to you for care, what do you see? Do you see a neatly dressed, cooperative, agreeable person? Does it occur to you that neat clothes may cover an empty wallet? That an agreeable demeanor may mask concerns and problems? Do you have any idea of the cost of the recommended treatments, the prescribed medications, or the dietary supplements that are part of the patient's health maintenance plan?

Increasingly, nurses must reach out and take on the role of patient advocate in the health-care system. Assessment must include attention to all of the many factors that might affect an elderly person's ability to carry out the recommended health-care regimen. A simple interaction beginning, "I see that you'll be taking many medications now. Sometimes people find the cost of so many medications a real concern. Has this been a concern for you?" will provide the opportunity to explore problems from the patient's perspective.

(continued)

SOCIOCULTURAL PERSPECTIVES
The Elderly and the Cost of Chronic Illness
(continued)

The next consideration is to ask yourself, "What do I do with this information when I have it?" To be effective, you will need to understand the resources available to patients in your setting. Drugs ordered in their generic forms may provide significant cost savings, but not all brand-name drugs are available in generic forms, and generic forms may not be as effective as brand-name drugs. It may be that you can facilitate a conversation between the physician and the pharmacist to select a more cost-effective drug regimen. A social worker or specialized nurse discharge planner may be available in a hospital to work with the patient in finding resources to assist with the cost of medications. Your role may be to refer the patient to this professional. As a nurse in a long-term-care facility, you may need to make the contacts and begin procedures to facilitate some type of assistance. In the ambulatory care setting, you may need to explore community resources and help the patient to contact them. Sometimes it is the nurse who acts for the patient to persuade an insurance company or managed-care organization that an initial, costly treatment may save the organization money in the long run. For example, you may need to persuade an insurance company that if the company doesn't pay for a patient's outpatient drug treatment, it may have to pay for the patient's resulting hospitalization. Effective advocacy for patients takes many forms, but it always takes commitment from you, the nurse.

or shoulder during conversations conveys a sense of caring and acceptance. However, keep in mind that some people feel uncomfortable being touched, and that it is normal for touch to be welcome on some occasions and rejected on others.

MENTAL PROCESSES

Very few changes in cognition are attributable to age-related factors alone. In healthy, mentally stimulated older adults, deficits are minor and nonprogressive. They are most noticeable in conditions of stress. The phrases *benign senescent forgetfulness* or *age-associated memory impairment* have been used in reference to age-related changes in mental processes. These changes in mental processes include a modest decline in short-term memory and a slight and gradual decline in some cognitive skills, such as abstraction, calculation, word fluency, verbal comprehension, spatial orientation, and inductive reasoning. Older adults are as capable of learning new things as younger people, but their speed of processing information is slower.

Examples of mental changes that are not part of the normal aging process include confusion, depression, disorientation, inappropriate behavior, and inability to concentrate or follow directions. Any major declines in mental processes typically result from

• Diseases, such as dementia and metabolic disorders
• Stress, such as that caused by relocation
• Chemical effects, such as from alcohol
• Medication effects
• Vision or hearing impairments

NURSING PROCESS GUIDELINES
Mental Processes

An older person with major changes in mental functioning should undergo a comprehensive assessment. Do not attribute these changes to irreversible or untreatable age-related causes. Use the guidelines in Chapter 17 to assess for alterations in mental processes. Be sure to allow enough time for older people to respond to questions. Compensate for hearing or vision limitations during all interactions. Assess for factors that might cause or contribute to altered mental processes, such as medication effects, disease processes, an unfamiliar environment, fluid and electrolyte imbalance, and psychosocial stressors.

Encourage the use of memory training techniques and "memory aids," such as calendars and appointment schedules, to compensate for memory problems. Suggest activities, such as volunteering, that are meaningful and mentally stimulating. Allow for step-by-step processing of new information and reinforce verbal instructions with easy-to-read written materials. If mental changes do result from an irreversible condition, suggest that the older adult and family contact the Alzheimer's Association for educational information and support services.

SLEEP PATTERNS

The normal sleep pattern consists of cycles of the four stages of non–rapid eye movement (non-REM) sleep, followed by REM sleep. Each stage of non-REM sleep is progressively deeper and represents a different stage of relaxation. REM sleep, the period when most dreams occur, is a relatively active state characterized by muscle twitching, rapid eye movement, and fluctuations in vital functions. Older adults commonly experience changes in their sleep patterns. It may take longer to fall asleep. They may awaken more frequently. They may spend a longer time in bed but sleep for the same or a shorter amount of time than when they were younger. Also, because they tend to awaken frequently and spend less time in the deep stages of sleep, they may feel that the quality of their sleep is unsatisfactory.

Factors that may interfere with the sleep patterns of older adults include

- Sleep apnea
- Periodic leg movements while sleeping
- Adverse medication effects
- Physical pain, illness, or discomfort
- Environmental factors, especially in institutional settings
- Psychosocial disturbances such as anxiety, dementia, or depression

Hypnotic medications interfere with REM and deep sleep stages and they tend to cause paradoxical effects such as nightmares and agitation, particularly in older adults. Although hypnotics may be effective initially or for a short time, they are not effective for consistent or long-term use.

One or two short naps during the day help maintain energy levels in older adults and, if integrated into a regular sleep-wake pattern, will not interfere with night-time sleep. However, frequent or long naps taken at irregular intervals are usually prompted by boredom and may interfere with night-time sleep.

NURSING PROCESS GUIDELINES
Sleep Patterns

Assess the older person's sleep-wake pattern for alterations and ask when the person usually retires and awakens. If the person wakes during the night, ask about frequency and about any difficulty returning to sleep. Ask whether the person feels rested upon awakening. Determine any napping pattern and reasons for taking naps. Ask about pre-bedtime activities and identify factors that affect sleeping patterns. Ask about medications or nonpharmaceutical methods of facilitating sleep.

Teach the older person about age-related changes in sleep and emphasize the importance of feeling rested. If the person naps, explain the importance of a regular pattern of short naps. Encourage participation in meaningful activities if boredom or inactivity affects sleep patterns. Tell the older adult that daytime exercise typically improves night-time sleeping. Also explain that warm milk, meditation, soft music, or a light carbohydrate snack at bedtime enhances the production of serotonin, a chemical in the brain that helps to induce sleep. Urge the older person to

avoid alcohol, caffeine, protein snacks, and strenuous exercise for at least 2 hours before bedtime because they decrease serotonin production and may make it difficult to fall asleep. Cigarette smoking should also be avoided before bedtime because nicotine is a stimulant. Teach about the adverse effects of hypnotic medications and explore nonpharmaceutical interventions for addressing sleep disturbances.

CARDIOVASCULAR FUNCTION

In the normal aging process, cardiac output gradually decreases by 30 to 40% as a result of fibrosis, hypertrophy, and fat infiltration of the heart muscle and valves. The ability of the cardiovascular system to respond to fluctuations in body needs diminishes. It also takes longer for the heart to return to a normal rate after stress. Slowed response of the autonomic nervous system to changes in physical position may cause episodes of orthostatic hypotension. Thickening and fibrosis of the venous walls may lead to varicosities and dependent edema. Fibrosis and calcification of the arterial walls may lead to hypertension, atherosclerosis, arterial insufficiency, a wide pulse pressure, and weak peripheral pulses. Hypertension is defined as a systolic pressure of more than 140 mm Hg and a diastolic pressure of more than 90 mm Hg based on the average of two or more readings on at least two occasions. The 1992 report of the Joint National Committee on Detection, Evaluation, and Treatment of High Blood Pressure recommended that the same criteria be applied to all adults, regardless of age, because any degree of high blood pressure is a risk factor for cardiovascular disease.

NURSING PROCESS GUIDELINES
Cardiovascular Function

Assess for alterations in cardiovascular function, as discussed in detail in Chapters 7 and 9. Obtain blood pressure readings with the patient in lying, sitting, and standing positions to assess for orthostatic hypotension. Ask about symptoms of hypotension, such as lightheadedness, especially on rising from a sitting or lying position. If the person has symptomatic or asymptomatic orthostatic hypotension, assess for medications that may affect the blood pressure, such as anticholinergics or cardiovascular agents. Ask whether the person experiences any unusual fatigue, difficulty breathing, or tightness of the chest. Anticipate that the hands and feet may be cool to the touch and peripheral pulses difficult to palpate. Assess for dependent edema and varicosities. Ask about the kind and amount of exercise the person engages in as part of the daily routine.

Teach the older person to change positions slowly and to rest when tired or short of breath. If the person has varicosities or dependent edema or if orthostatic hypotension develops, encourage the use of elastic stockings and elevation of the feet. Socks worn to bed at night help relieve the discomfort of cold feet caused by decreased peripheral circulation.

Encourage participation in a medically approved exercise program to maintain and improve cardiovascular status. Walking is excellent exercise, promotes respiratory and cardiovascular fitness, helps maintain proper weight, and provides opportunity for socialization. Many shopping malls open before their regularly scheduled business hours to accommodate older walkers.

RESPIRATORY FUNCTION

Several changes in the normal aging process result in diminished respiratory capacity. Atrophy of the respiratory muscles, combined with kyphosis and an increase in the anteroposterior diameter of the chest, produces a "barrel chest" appearance in many older people and interferes with chest movement and gas exchange. Loss of elasticity of the respiratory muscles and lungs reduces vital capacity and increases residual volume. Thickening of the walls of the alveolar sacs and capillaries further impairs oxygen–carbon dioxide exchange. The older person may be less able to adjust to increased oxygen requirements. As the respiratory passages lose muscle tone, mucus secretion and ciliary movement diminish.

If the older person does not smoke or have a respiratory illness, these changes typically cause no significant respiratory problems during daily activities. However, under conditions of physical stress, older adults are likely to become dyspneic and fatigued because they have less efficient gas exchange. Other consequences of age-related changes in respiratory functioning include a slowed and less effective cough reflex and increased susceptibility to lower respiratory infections, such as pneumonia and influenza. Also, older adults are more prone to tuberculosis. This disease is increasingly common among nursing home populations.

NURSING PROCESS GUIDELINES
Respiratory Function

Assess for alterations in respiratory function, as discussed in detail in Chapter 14. Ask whether the person has modified any activities to compensate for respiratory problems. Obtain a smoking history and history of immunizations for influenza and pneumonia. If the person smokes, ask about any attempts to quit smoking. Find out whether the person would be willing to consider quitting. Determine what effects weather and changes in air quality have on respiratory function. Ask whether the person humidifies indoor air during the winter.

To help reduce the risk of respiratory problems, teach the older adult to use diaphragmatic breathing

and to use abdominal muscles for deep breathing. Encourage daily exercise, such as walking. Recommend seeing a physician about shortness of breath, respiratory infection that lasts more than 3 days, and inability to retain fluids for more than 24 hours. For older adults who have trouble getting to the doctor's office, suggest the use of a transportation service (Fig. 4–5). Annual influenza and once-in-a-lifetime pneumonia vaccines are recommended for all persons older than 65 years. Discourage smoking in persons of all ages. Encourage older adults to explore options that could help them quit smoking.

GASTROINTESTINAL FUNCTION

Tooth loss, decreased saliva production, and poor oral or dental condition are common causes of difficulty with chewing and enjoying food. A slight loss of muscle tone throughout the gastrointestinal tract may cause some difficulty swallowing and may slow the transit of food. Although slowed food transit may predispose the older adult to constipation, it does not cause constipation in the absence of other factors. Factors that commonly contribute to constipation include inactivity, adverse medication effects, and limited fluid and fiber intake. Diarrhea may develop from food intolerance, fecal impaction, and adverse medication effects. At about age 50, liver size, blood flow, enzyme activity, and synthesis of plasma proteins begin to decrease. Fat intolerance may develop as a result of increased viscosity of the bile and diminished elasticity of the gallbladder.

NURSING PROCESS GUIDELINES
Gastrointestinal Function

Assess for alterations in gastrointestinal function as discussed in detail in Chapter 21. Ask about daily

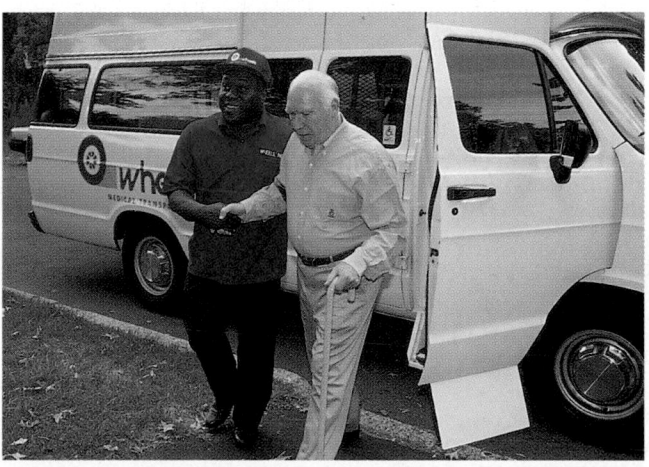

Figure 4–5

Use of a transportation service can help the older adult travel safely to the physician's office and other medical appointments. In some communities, transportation may be provided at no charge.

fluid and fiber intake. Examine the mouth to assess hydration and dental conditions. Look for inflamed or irritated areas that suggest poor denture fit. Ask how foods are prepared and whether the person avoids any foods because of decreased tolerance or difficulty chewing or swallowing. Determine bowel pattern and obtain a description of the stool, as well as complaints of constipation, diarrhea, or hard or loose stools.

Recommend a semiannual dental cleaning and examination, especially if the person wears dentures. Teach the older person to chew food thoroughly before swallowing and to modify the diet if chewing food is difficult. Suggest eating five or six small meals daily that include a variety of foods from the basic food groups. This plan is nutritionally sound and well tolerated by most older people.

Discuss normal bowel movement patterns and explain that normal patterns vary from several movements a day to one every 3 or 4 days. Teach that increased fluids and fiber and regular exercise are useful in preventing constipation and that laxatives often exacerbate bowel problems.

URINARY FUNCTION

Age-related kidney changes include decreased blood flow and a decreased number of functioning nephrons. These changes result in a diminished glomerular filtration rate and delayed excretion of water-soluble medications. Age-related changes of the renal tubules cause nocturia and decreased efficiency of homeostatic mechanisms. In the urinary musculature, the bladder muscles hypertrophy, the pelvic floor muscles relax, and smooth muscle tissue is replaced with connective tissue. Diminished bladder capacity and decreased perception of sensory impulses are normal age-related changes that also affect urinary function. Bladder emptying is incomplete, causing chronic residual urine.

As a result of these changes, older adults may experience urinary urgency, frequency, and dribbling. Chronic residual urine predisposes older adults to urinary tract infections. Between 15 and 30% of noninstitutionalized older Americans suffer from some reduction in urinary control. This problem causes embarrassment, loss of self-esteem, and withdrawal from activities outside the home. Local or systemic disorders that are common in older adults—such as vaginitis, prostate enlargement, impacted bowels, or neurologic diseases—can further interfere with urinary function and control.

NURSING PROCESS GUIDELINES
Urinary Function

Assess for alterations in urinary pattern associated with the aging process. Assessment of urinary func-

tion is discussed in detail in Chapter 30. Determine urinary pattern and any factors that influence urinary function, such as fluid intake. Ask men to describe the urine stream and whether starting urination is difficult. Find out when the last prostate examination occurred. Ask women about vaginal irritation or infections and about any history of surgery for pelvic, bladder, or uterine disorders.

Inquire about urinary frequency, urgency, dribbling, and stress incontinence, and be aware of reluctance on the part of the older person to volunteer information that might be perceived as embarrassing. Ask whether treatment has been sought to correct any problems. Many older adults do not seek treatment because they are embarrassed, do not know treatment is available, or think some loss of urinary control is a normal part of aging. Teach the older person that urinary incontinence is not a necessary part of aging and that interventions are available to address incontinence. Emphasize the importance of adequate fluid intake to maintain continence and urinary function. Encourage older adults to drink eight to 10 glasses of noncaffeinated beverages during the day but to avoid fluids for 3 to 4 hours before bedtime. Encourage pelvic exercises to improve the tone of the pelvic muscles and the urethral sphincter. This helps reduce dribbling and stress incontinence in both men and women.

A person can strengthen the pelvic muscles by tightening them for a count of 10 and then relaxing. This exercise should be performed at least three or four times a day. Also teach the person to void, wait a moment, and then attempt to void again to promote complete emptying of the bladder. Referral to a specialized incontinence clinic may be appropriate if these measures prove ineffective. Discuss the many commercial products available to prevent embarrassment if incontinence cannot be treated.

MUSCULOSKELETAL FUNCTION

Muscles

Beginning at about age 40, muscle strength declines gradually, resulting in an overall decrease of 30 to 50% by age 80. Diminished muscle strength stems primarily from an age-related loss of muscle mass. In addition, a person's current level of activity and lifelong patterns of exercise can influence muscle strength at any age. Muscle endurance and coordination diminish as a result of age-related changes in the muscles and central nervous system. As a consequence of these changes, older adults experience muscle fatigue after a shorter duration of exercise. Movement slows and agility diminishes because of a reduced sensitivity to neural stimulation and a slowed reaction time. Tendons shrink and become sclerotic, further slowing muscle movement.

Bones and Joints

Years of use cause gradual thinning and erosion of joint cartilage. The synovial membrane and synovial fluid thicken, causing stiffness, crepitation, and reduced joint lubrication. Ligaments become calcified and lose elasticity. Joint function begins to decline in the twenties and diminishes gradually throughout one's lifetime. The outcome of these degenerative changes is decreased flexion of the lower back and diminished range of motion in the ankles, knees, hips, and upper arms. The overall impact of diminished joint functioning is that older people are slower in their ability to respond to environmental stimuli and to perform some activities of daily living.

Increased resorption of bone matrix and minerals causes bone density to decrease with age. This loss of bone mass is called osteoporosis. As calcium is resorbed from the bones, they become increasingly porous, brittle, and more susceptible to fracture, even without severe trauma. Although it occurs in all aging people, osteoporosis is most severe in postmenopausal women who do not take estrogen replacement therapy or other medications to prevent osteoporosis. Other factors that increase the risk and severity of osteoporosis include white race, genetic predisposition, low calcium intake, and long-term use of corticosteroids.

In the vertebral column, thinning of the intervertebral cartilaginous disks and collapse of the porous vertebral bodies result in kyphosis (dowager's hump). As illustrated in Figure 4–6, kyphosis increases the anteroposterior diameter of the chest and decreases trunk height. This latter effect is primarily responsible for the decrease in height that occurs in the older person.

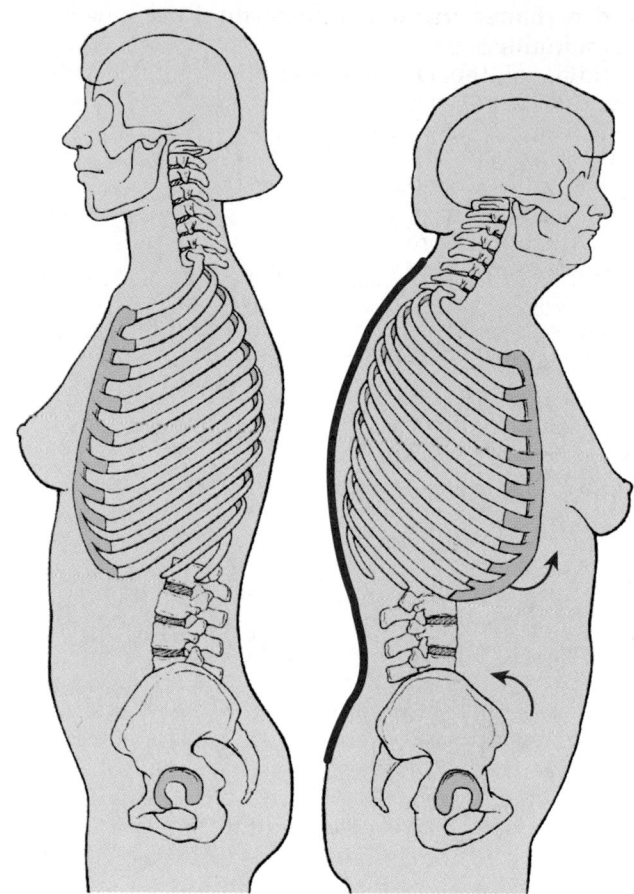

Figure 4–6

Height and posture change as a person ages. Deterioration of vertebrae and intervertebral disks results in loss of height, kyphosis of the thoracic spine, straightening of the lumbar curve, slight posterior rotation of the hips, and an increase in anteroposterior diameter of the thorax.

NURSING PROCESS GUIDELINES
Musculoskeletal Function

Assess for alterations in musculoskeletal function and for the risk of osteoporosis and falls. Assessment of musculoskeletal function is discussed in detail in Chapter 19. Note the older person's mobility pattern and stability to identify any safety risks. Assess the environment for safety hazards. Ask whether the person participates in daily physical activity or in a daily exercise program. Ask about limitations in performing daily activities. Examine joints for swelling, deformity, crepitation, or decreased function. When assessing range of motion, move the person's limbs gently to avoid pain or discomfort. Determine whether the person eats calcium-rich foods or takes calcium supplements.

Teach the older person to use assistive devices, such as canes and walkers, for safety as needed. Encourage walking and other forms of weight-bearing exercise. Advise women approaching or in menopause to ask their physicians about advantages and disadvantages of estrogen replacement therapy to slow bone demineralization. Encourage a daily intake of 400 IU of vitamin D and 1500 mg of calcium for older men and postmenopausal women.

NEUROLOGIC FUNCTION

The number of nerve cells throughout the central nervous system decreases with age. Because neurons cannot reproduce, this loss is irreversible. Although loss of neurons is a definite part of the aging process, the implications of this age-related change are not clear. For example, a computed tomographic evaluation may show atrophy of brain cells, but the person may show no decline in cognitive ability. Healthy older adults show little or no neurologic dysfunction other than a slower response time. Diminished sensory abilities is another central nervous system change that may affect neurologic function in older adults.

Some of the changes identified in older brains include

- Loss of neurons
- Diminished blood flow
- Accumulation of lipofuscin
- Reduction of brain weight
- Decline in synaptic function
- Changes in neurotransmitter activity
- Decreased utilization of glucose and oxygen
- Presence of senile plaques and neurofibrillary tangles

NURSING PROCESS GUIDELINES
Neurologic Function

Assess for alterations in neurologic function, as discussed in detail in Chapter 17. Inquire about falls, dizziness, lightheadedness, numbness or tingling, altered speech or behavior patterns, and loss of consciousness. These manifestations may indicate an impairment that requires evaluation by a physician.

Reassure the older person that it is normal to require more time to perform daily activities because reactions may be slower. Special care must be taken to avoid touching surfaces that may be hot or cold, since pain sensitivity may be impaired. In addition, care must be taken to avoid falls because of the combination of slowed response time and common disorders such as arthritis, which may increase the risk of falls.

REPRODUCTIVE FUNCTION

Both men and women experience reduced sex hormone secretion as they grow older. Pubic hair thins, reproductive organs atrophy, and secretions diminish. In women, the breasts become less firm and more pendulous and the nipples become smaller, flatter, and less responsive. Decreased estrogen levels cause the vaginal mucosa to become pale, thin, and dry. Painful intercourse (dyspareunia) may result from slow arousal and decreased vaginal lubrication. In men, sperm production decreases. Men may experience slower erection and weaker ejaculation. Longer stimulation is required before ejaculation.

These age-related changes result in the loss of reproductive ability in women and a diminished reproductive ability in men. These changes alone do not, however, interfere with the ability of older adults to maintain satisfying sexual activities and relationships. The factors that most often interfere with sexual relationships are medical conditions, functional limitations, social circumstances, and adverse medication effects.

NURSING PROCESS GUIDELINES
Reproductive Function

Assess for alterations in reproductive function associated with the aging process. Assessment of male reproductive function is discussed in detail in Chapter 38, female reproductive function in Chapter 40. Anticipate that many people will be reluctant to volunteer information about sexuality and reproductive function because of the intimate nature of this subject. Maintain eye contact while asking tactful, direct questions to help put each person at ease and facilitate collection of accurate information.

Be cautious not to convey negative attitudes about sexuality and older adults. Also, be aware of the possibility that older adults, like younger adults, may have nontraditional sexual relationships. If appropriate, ask nonjudgmental questions to assess sexual activity that may include gay, lesbian, or unmarried relationships.

Use a matter-of-fact approach and discuss sexual desire and activity as normal and healthy aspects of daily life that do not necessarily cease or diminish in older adulthood. If appropriate, explain that older people remain fully capable of enjoying orgasm, but their response to sexual stimulation may be slower, less intense, and of shorter duration. Increasing the amount and diversity of sexual stimulation and experimenting with different positions can compensate for these changes and increase sexual enjoyment. It may also be appropriate to discuss delayed ejaculation as an opportunity to increase satisfaction of both partners. A water-soluble lubricant relieves painful intercourse caused by diminished vaginal secretions.

Teach older women to perform monthly breast self-examination as described in Chapter 42 and to obtain an annual gynecologic examination. Teach older men to perform monthly breast and testicular self-examination (Chapter 38) and to have an annual prostate examination.

ENDOCRINE FUNCTION

Because the endocrine system has a large functional reserve, changes associated with the aging process often have minimal physiologic effect. Pituitary and adrenal function is unchanged. Thyroid disorders are more common with increased age, and manifestations of thyroid disorders may be more subtle in older adults. Researchers are trying to determine whether age-related changes in thyroid calcitonin secretion and parathyroid function may be linked to osteoporosis in the elderly (see Chapter 29).

Glucose intolerance is another condition more common in older adulthood. The exact cause is unclear, but it may be related to delayed insulin response to glucose ingestion or increased insulin resistance. Non-insulin-dependent diabetes mellitus occurs frequently in older adults.

NURSING PROCESS GUIDELINES
Endocrine Function

Assess for signs of endocrine dysfunction as described in Chapter 27. Ask the person about activity restrictions caused by fatigue. Review the nutritional patterns of the older person. Check for foods that provide adequate calcium. Observe for early signs of non-insulin-dependent diabetes as discussed in Chapter 28.

$\mathcal{A}$ssessment of the Elderly

In assessing older people, remember that each person ages at a different rate and adapts to the aging process differently. Because it takes an older person longer to process and respond to questions, allow at least 30 minutes for the health interview. If the person uses a hearing aid or glasses, be sure they are worn. Determine whether the person has brought all currently used medications, or a list of them, to the appointment. Provide bright, glare-free lighting in a comfortably warm environment. Complete an assessment of mental processes and neuromuscular coordination early in the examination to avoid inaccurate results caused by fatigue. Also be sure to assess the person's health promotion behaviors and health risks. Encourage the older adult to reduce risks by participating in positive health behaviors as described in Highlight 4–3.

HIGHLIGHT
4–3
HEALTH PROMOTION & RISK REDUCTION

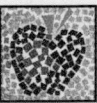

Maintaining Wellness in Older Adults

To maintain health and wellbeing, give older adults the following advice:

- Visit a physician yearly for a thorough examination and laboratory studies.
- Perform self-examinations (such as breast, testicular, and skin) monthly.
- Report any unusual signs and symptoms to the physician.
- Maintain good nutritional habits.
- Rest as needed throughout the day.
- Try to get at least 6 hours of sleep nightly.
- Participate in planned physical activity at least three or four times weekly (walking, moderate weight lifting, swimming, etc).
- Stay involved in social activities.

PATIENT HISTORY

Sit face-to-face, identify yourself, and state your questions one at a time in a clear voice. Allow time for the person to answer. If an answer seems inappropriate, do not assume impaired mental processes. The person may have misunderstood the question or not heard it clearly. Clarify the answer or restate the question.

Many older adults have a high tolerance for pain and may dismiss many symptoms as being signs of old age. Make sure to ask specific questions to help obtain accurate information. For example, instead of asking about the presence of skin problems, ask specifically about itching, burning, dryness, and skin lesions. Ask additional specific questions about physical assessment findings as they are identified to clarify information collected in the history.

Conclude the interview by asking the person to describe a typical day. This provides an opportunity to assess the person's ability to perform self-care activities and activities outside the home. Family members or friends can help clarify information and provide missing information or can be used as an additional source if the person has difficulty communicating or if the information is not accurate.

PHYSICAL EXAMINATION

Physical assessment of the normal changes associated with the aging process has been identified in each of the preceding sections. Maintain a warm environment and avoid unnecessary or prolonged exposure during physical examination to prevent excessive heat loss. Explain each procedure as you perform it. Provide assistance during position changes and maintain safety measures to prevent injury. Palpate and percuss gently to avoid trauma to fragile skin. Move joints carefully to avoid discomfort.

Recognize that assessment of older adults is a complex and challenging process. Not only are the manifestations of illness less predictable, but the causes are more variable and the consequences more far-reaching. For example, older adults are much more likely than their younger counterparts to experience mental changes, rather than physical complaints, in response to medications and physiologic disturbances. Symptoms of illness, even acute illness, in older adults tend to be more subtle and less predictable. Also, older adults with infections may have little or no temperature elevation. Further, by the time illnesses in older adults are noted and attended to, the physiologic disturbances may be in an advanced stage, and additional complications may have developed. Selected nursing diagnoses with patient outcomes and nursing interventions frequently applicable in the care of geriatric patients are identified in Nursing Care Guide 4–2.

Nursing Care Guide 4–2
Geriatric Patients

Assessment Findings: Geriatric patient complaining of discomfort in right hip and back upon awakening. Examination reveals mild kyphosis and redness over thoracic spine, right scapula, right trochanter, and sacrum. Skin is dry and intact. Patient states difficulty repositioning in bed.

Nursing Diagnosis: Risk for impaired skin integrity related to prolonged pressure over bony prominences and limited independent mobility in bed

Patient Outcomes	Nursing Interventions	Rationale
Patient identifies lying or sitting in one position for extended periods of time as cause of discomfort and reddened skin.	Inform patient that immobility increases pressure over bony prominences and impairs circulation. Identify impaired circulation as cause of redness, discomfort, and potential skin breakdown.	A simple explanation directly relating the patient's immobility to the skin alterations increases understanding of the need to change positions more frequently.
Patient shifts weight every hour while sitting.	Instruct patient to sit in arm chair with padded seat when possible. Provide egg-crate chair pad.	Use of padded seat and egg-crate cushion reduces pressure over bony prominences and reduces impairment of capillary blood flow.
	Demonstrate how to use chair arms to shift weight, and have patient do return demonstration.	Increases the frequency of position changes by encouraging independence.
Patient verbalizes understanding of need to be repositioned every 2 hours while in bed.	Apply egg-crate mattress or other weight-distributing product to bed.	Reduces pressure over bony prominences and reduces impairment of capillary blood flow.
	Assist patient with repositioning every 2 hours while in bed.	Position changes relieve pressure and allow return of capillary blood flow.
	Consider use of overhead trapeze.	Enables patient to assist with position changes or to move independently.
Patient maintains skin that is clean, dry, and intact.	Examine skin daily to detect potential areas of skin breakdown.	To evaluate effectiveness of care.
	Instruct patient to use nondrying products for bathing and skin care. Gently apply lanolin-based lotions to skin and bony prominences. Encourage intake of six to eight glasses of fluid daily. Keep linens clean, dry, and wrinkle-free.	Adequate hydration and clean, dry, supple skin that is free of irritants reduce the risk of altered skin integrity.

Evaluation: Compare the patient's status with the expected outcomes. If the outcomes are not met, reassess the patient and revise the plan.

(continued)

Nursing Care Guide 4–2
Geriatric Patients (continued)

Assessment Findings:	Geriatric female who has recently recovered from a fractured wrist suffered in a fall during a dizzy spell while going to the bathroom at night. Patient identifies occasional lightheadedness when standing from sitting or lying position and difficulty seeing at night. Examination reveals decreased visual acuity, steady gait, mild kyphosis.
Nursing Diagnosis:	Risk for trauma related to lack of knowledge of safety precautions needed secondary to orthostatic hypotension, impaired vision, and osteoporosis

Patient Outcomes	Nursing Interventions	Rationale
Patient states intent to use night-lights in bedroom, bathroom, and hall.	Inform patient of the visual changes that accompany aging.	To relieve anxiety.
	Advise patient to use bright, glare-free lighting at home. Recommend use of night-lights and bedside lamps to lessen danger of falls.	Adequate lighting reduces the risk of falls.
	Suggest that patient keep eyeglasses at bedside and put them on before getting out of bed at night or in the morning.	Poor vision increases the risk of injury.
	Advise patient to allow extra time for eyes to adjust to changes in light intensity.	Adjustment to changes in light is slower in the elderly, and vision is poor until eyes adjust.
Patient demonstrates rising slowly from a sitting position and sitting on the side of the bed before standing.	Explain to patient circulatory changes that accompany the aging process and may cause episodes of orthostatic hypotension.	Understanding increases compliance with safety measures.
	Explain rationale of increased safety with slow position changes. Teach patient to rise slowly from a sitting position and to sit at the edge of the bed for a minute or two before standing.	Changing position slowly allows the peripheral vascular system to adjust to fluctuations in blood pressure and prevents orthostatic hypotension.
	Have patient do return demonstration and continue practice during rest of hospital stay.	Return demonstration allows evaluation of learning.
Patient identifies foods high in calcium that she will include in her diet daily.	Teach patient changes in bone structure that accompany the aging process and the possible benefits of increased calcium intake.	Understanding increases compliance.
	Help patient identify her preferences from a list of high-calcium foods.	Preferred foods are more likely to be eaten.
	Clearly print these foods on a card, with serving size and percentage of daily calcium requirement.	Provides an easily read, handy reference.
	Review menu selections during remainder of hospitalization to reinforce selection of good calcium sources.	Positive feedback increases motivation. Repetition increases learning.

(continued)

Nursing Care Guide 4–2
Geriatric Patients (continued)

Evaluation:	Compare the patient's status with the expected outcomes. If the outcomes are not met, reassess the patient and revise the plan.
Assessment Findings:	Ambulatory geriatric patient identifies irregular bowel pattern during interview: soft, formed stools with periods of infrequent hard stools, treated with laxatives. Last bowel movement was soft, formed, 2 days ago. Examination reveals abdomen soft on palpation, active bowel sounds on auscultation. Passing flatus. Drinks approximately two cups of coffee and two glasses of beverage daily.
Nursing Diagnosis:	Risk for colonic constipation related to inadequate fluid intake and laxative abuse

Patient Outcomes	Nursing Interventions	Rationale
Patient identifies nonlaxative measures to prevent constipation.	Teach patient that constipation is a long-term effect of laxative use caused by decreased intestinal muscle tone.	Understanding the undesirable effects of laxatives may encourage reduced use.
	Teach patient that regular exercise, adequate fluids, and high-fiber diet help prevent constipation.	Exercise stimulates peristalsis, fluids soften stool, and fiber increases bulk to promote regular passage of soft, formed stool.
Patient drinks at least eight glasses of fluid daily.	Identify beverage preferences. Teach patient that any beverage counts toward fluid total.	Preferred fluids are more readily consumed.
	Suggest keeping track of intake by marking off numbers 1–8 written on a card each morning.	Accurate recording provides feedback and promotes consumption of desired amount.
Patient chooses high-fiber foods from daily menu selections and states intent to eat high-fiber foods daily at home.	Help patient identify preferences from a list of high-fiber foods.	Preferred foods are more likely to be eaten.
	Clearly print these foods on a card.	Provides an easily read, handy reference.
	Review menu selections during remainder of hospitalization to reinforce selection of good fiber sources.	Positive feedback increases motivation. Repetition increases learning.

(continued)

Nursing Care Guide 4–2
Geriatric Patients (continued)

Patient Outcomes	Nursing Interventions	Rationale
Patient has a soft bowel movement within 48 hours and at least one every 3 days thereafter.	Encourage patient to ambulate freely about unit unless contraindicated.	Walking improves abdominal muscle tone and increases peristalsis.
	Identify time of day patient normally defecates. Recommend that a regular time for defecation be part of daily routine.	Identifies patient's regular pattern of elimination and aids in reestablishing regular pattern.
	Advise that urge to defecate often occurs an hour or so after meals. Teach patient to respond to urge to defecate promptly.	Eating stimulates the colorectal reflex to defecate. Failure to respond to urge to defecate suppresses it.
	Provide prune juice or warm beverage 30 minutes before normal defecation time.	Helps stimulate defecation.
	Advise not to hold breath or strain during bowel movement.	Stimulates the vagus nerve and slows the heart rate.

Evaluation:	Compare the patient's status with the expected outcomes. If the outcomes are not met, reassess the patient and revise the plan.

Assessment Findings:	Geriatric male patient recovering from fractured hip. Ambulates well with walker but tires easily and cannot climb stairs. Previously lived independently but will temporarily live with son after discharge. Patient verbalizes frustration over loss of independence, is no longer participating in decision-making, and verbalizes doubts about ability to ever return home.
Nursing Diagnosis:	Powerlessness related to loss of independence, decreased stamina, limited mobility, and potential loss of home and possessions

Patient Outcomes	Nursing Interventions	Rationale
Patient identifies previous coping mechanisms.	Encourage patient to reminisce about previous successes in solving problems and overcoming obstacles.	Helps patient identify previous coping mechanisms to assist in transferring them to current situation.
	Acknowledge past accomplishments and praise progress since injury.	Positive feedback promotes self-esteem and motivation.
Patient makes decisions in areas over which he has control.	Help patient identify areas over which he has control.	Promotes independence and a sense of control.
	Provide positive reinforcement when patient participates in decision-making process.	Positive feedback increases participation.

(continued)

Nursing Care Guide 4–2
Geriatric Patients (continued)

Patient Outcomes	Nursing Interventions	Rationale
Patient expresses sense of control over events and anticipates future return to own home.	Recognize when patient is seeking information and provide rationale for actions. Encourage patient to verbalize feelings about current status and potential discharge.	Accurate information increases knowledge and understanding and reduces anxiety.
	Schedule health team conference with patient and family to assist patient in formulating realistic goals.	Realistic goals and expectations increase motivation and reduce frustration.
Evaluation:	Compare the patient's status with the expected outcomes. If the outcomes are not met, reassess the patient and revise the plan.	

Chapter Review

1. Describe strategies older adults might use to cope effectively with the psychosocial challenges common in later adulthood.
2. What adverse medication effects are more likely to occur in older adults, in contrast to younger adults?
3. Identify five health-education tips that can be taught to older adults to assist them in adjusting to age-related vision changes.
4. Name five factors that should be assessed as potential underlying causes of mental changes in older adults.
5. What would you teach about age-related changes in sleep patterns and ways of coping with these changes?
6. What is unique about assessing blood pressure in older adults?
7. What would you teach an older adult about constipation?
8. What would you teach an older person about incontinence?
9. What would you teach an older adult about prevention of falls and fractures?
10. Describe the approach you would use for an assessment of sexual functioning in older adults.

Bibliography

Abrams WB, Beers MH, Berkow R (eds). The Merck manual of geriatrics. 2nd ed. Whitehouse Station, NJ: Merck Research Laboratories, 1995.

Brocklehurst JC. Textbook of geriatric medicine and gerontology. New York: Churchill-Livingstone, 1992.

Carpenito LJ. Nursing diagnosis: Application to clinical practice. 6th ed. Philadelphia: JB Lippincott, 1995.

Chalkins E, Ford AB, Katz PR (eds). The practice of geriatrics. Philadelphia: WB Saunders, 1992.

The fifth report of the Joint National Committee on Detection, Evaluation, and Treatment of High Blood Pressure (JNC V). Arch Intern Med 1993; 153:154.

Miller CA. Nursing care of older adults: Theory and practice. 2nd ed. Philadelphia: JB Lippincott, 1995.

National Academy of Sciences/National Research Council. Recommended dietary allowances. 10th ed. Washington, DC: National Academy Press, 1989.

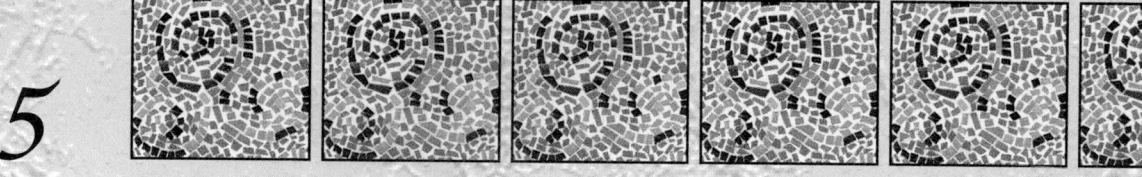

5

Knowledge Base for Patients with Fluid, Electrolyte, and Acid-Base Imbalances

Study Outcomes

After studying this chapter, you should be able to:

1. Explain normal fluid, electrolyte, and acid-base balance physiology, including normal laboratory test values.
2. Define the major fluid, electrolyte, and acid-base imbalances.
3. Describe each of the major fluid, electrolyte, and acid-base imbalances, including the cause, pathophysiology, clinical manifestations, related diagnostic tests, and medical management.
4. Identify information and physical examination data essential to the assessment of fluid, electrolyte, and acid-base status.
5. State nursing diagnoses and related expected patient outcomes commonly applicable to patients with fluid, electrolyte, or acid-base imbalance.
6. Describe nursing interventions, with their rationales, commonly applicable to patients with fluid, electrolyte, or acid-base imbalance.
7. Explain the basis for evaluation of nursing care provided to patients with fluid, electrolyte, or acid-base imbalance.
8. Identify special considerations for the elderly patient with fluid, electrolyte, or acid-base imbalance.

Fluid, electrolyte, and acid-base imbalances accompany a wide variety of health problems. They may be a life-threatening result of acute traumas, such as burns. They may result from chronic illness, such as chronic obstructive pulmonary disease, diabetic ketoacidosis, and liver, renal, and gastrointestinal (GI) disorders. They may even result from the vomiting and diarrhea that occur during relatively minor illnesses, such as the flu.

Patients with fluid, electrolyte, and acid-base imbalances are treated in varied settings. These include the home, clinics, and chronic- and acute-care institutions. Regardless of setting, assessments and interventions needed to manage these imbalances are an ongoing nursing responsibility.

Fluid Imbalances

In the adult, water accounts for approximately 60% of body weight. It is distributed between two major fluid compartments: intracellular and extracellular (Fig. 5–1). Intracellular fluid (ICF) is the fluid within cells. Extracellular fluid (ECF) is the fluid between cells and within blood vessels. Fluid between cells is called interstitial fluid. Fluid within blood vessels is called intravascular fluid. Also included in the ECF category are cerebrospinal, synovial, pleural, abdominal, GI, and lymphatic fluids. Body fluids shift between these compartments to maintain fluid balance.

EXTRACELLULAR FLUID VOLUME DEFICIT

Extracellular fluid volume deficit, also called hypovolemia, is a loss of fluid from the interstitial and intravascular spaces. The loss of fluid can be accompanied by a loss of electrolytes, particularly sodium. Sodium is a major extracellular electrolyte whose primary function is to regulate body fluid. Water loss can also occur without sodium loss. When water and sodium decline in equal amounts, the fluid loss is referred to as an iso-osmolar (isotonic) fluid volume deficit. When water loss exceeds sodium loss, the fluid deficit is referred to as a hyperosmolar (hypertonic) fluid volume deficit.

The concentration of solutes in body fluid is described as *osmolarity* or *osmolality*. These terms are used interchangeably. Osmolarity is the osmotic pull exerted by all particles (solutes) per unit of solution, expressed as osmols or milliosmols per liter of solution. Osmolality is the osmotic pull exerted by all particles (solutes) per unit of water, expressed as osmols or milliosmols per kilogram of water. If there are more particles (sodium, glucose, urea, pro-

Osmotic pull- fluid lost from intravascular spaces but the electrolytes remain the same.

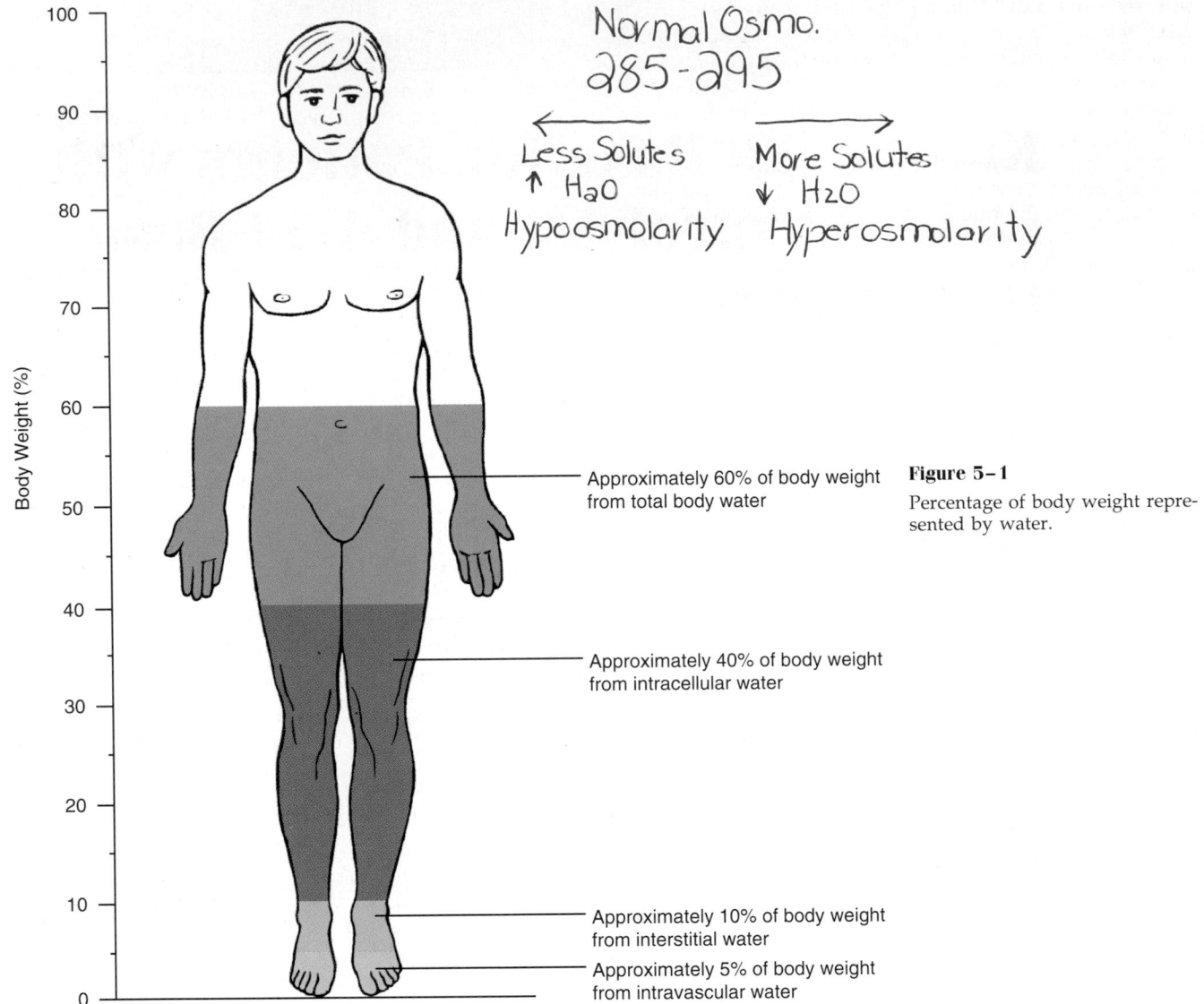

Normal Osmo.
285-295

← Less Solutes
↑ H₂O
Hypoosmolarity

More Solutes →
↓ H₂O
Hyperosmolarity

Approximately 60% of body weight from total body water

Approximately 40% of body weight from intracellular water

Approximately 10% of body weight from interstitial water

Approximately 5% of body weight from intravascular water

Figure 5–1

Percentage of body weight represented by water.

tein) than water, a hyperosmolar fluid results. If particles and water are of equal proportion, an iso-osmolar fluid results. Hypo-osmolar (hypotonic) fluid has fewer particles than water.

Normal serum osmolality is 285 to 295 mOsm/kg water or 285 to 295 mmol/kg water. If the serum osmolality is less than 285 mOsm/kg water, it is hypo-osmolar (fewer particles and more water); and if the serum osmolality is more than 295 mOsm/kg water, it is hyperosmolar (more particles and less water).

Etiology and Pathophysiology

Hyperosmolar fluid volume deficit occurs when the loss of water exceeds the loss of sodium. Another term for this type of fluid volume deficit is *dehydration*. Causes of hyperosmolar fluid volume deficit include severe diarrhea, inadequate water intake, diabetic acidosis, renal disease, and sweating. Hyper-

osmolar fluid volume deficit may also occur when intake of salt and other solutes rises without an increase in water intake.

Iso-osmolar fluid volume deficit occurs when water, electrolytes, and other solutes are lost in equal proportion from the ECF space. Profuse diaphoresis, vomiting, diarrhea, GI suction, fistulas, draining abscesses, fever, burns, and hemorrhage can result in iso-osmolar fluid loss. Other causes include diuretic therapy and maintenance on a "nothing by mouth" (NPO) order for a prolonged period of time. Iso-osmolar fluid volume loss is not classified as dehydration, although it is frequently referred to as such.

With hyperosmolar dehydration, the osmotic pressure of the ECF is increased, and, as a result, fluid moves quickly out of the ICF into the ECF. This shift maintains relatively normal vascular volume, so symptoms of hypovolemic shock do not occur. However, the shift causes cellular dehydration (cellular fluid deficit) and imbalance of electrolytes such as potassium and calcium, which results in unstable excitable cellular membranes.

With iso-osmolar fluid loss, ECF osmolality is unchanged; therefore, fluid does not shift from the ICF to ECF, and a decrease in circulatory volume occurs. Compensatory mechanisms begin to function as soon as a decrease in volume occurs, and they are successful in maintaining the perfusion of vital organs until one-fourth to one-third of the circulating volume is lost. At this point, symptoms of severe hypovolemic shock occur.

Clinical Manifestations

Whether as a result of water loss in excess of loss of solutes, or water and solute loss in approximately the same proportions, extracellular fluid volume deficit can be mild, moderate, or severe. Signs and symptoms vary with the degree of fluid loss, as shown in Table 5–1.

Thirst is a common symptom that occurs with mild, moderate, and severe fluid deficit. Both lack of fluid intake and fluid loss lead to thirst in most clinical situations. Water intake may correct the fluid deficit before it becomes severe; however, in an elderly person, the thirst mechanism in the medulla may not alert the person to drink fluids. Also, fluids may not be easily accessible to the person. Thus, a mild type of fluid deficit can lead to moderate fluid deficit.

When fluid loss becomes moderate or severe, shocklike symptoms arise. These include tachycardia, a moderate to severe decrease in blood pressure, and increased respiration. Evidence of decreased intravascular fluid volume may arise when the person shifts from a sitting to a standing posi-

tion. Watch for a drop in systolic blood pressure of 20 mm Hg and an increase in pulse rate of 10 beats per minute at 1 minute after the position change (Gettrust & Brabec, 1992). Weight loss also occurs with moderate and severe fluid deficit. A 1 kg (2.2 lb) change in body weight corresponds to a 1 L net change in fluid balance.

Diagnosis

Normal 1.005 to 1.030 — Specific gravity will be ↑

Laboratory tests, such as a general chemistry profile, can reveal the type of fluid deficit. A serum osmolality greater than 295 mOsm/kg and a serum sodium level greater than 156 mEq/L usually indicate hyperosmolar fluid volume deficit. Other laboratory indicators of fluid volume deficit include levels of blood urea nitrogen (BUN) greater than 30 mg/dL, hemoglobin greater than 18 g/dL, and hematocrit greater than 55%.

Poor skin turgor, cracked gums and tongue, oliguria, decreased central venous pressure, and decreased pulmonary capillary wedge pressure (less than 6 mm Hg) are additional diagnostic indicators of fluid deficit. Narrowing of pulse pressure (difference between systolic and diastolic pressures) may also suggest fluid loss.

Management

Medical management of fluid volume deficit depends on the severity and type of fluid deficit. If the patient has mild extracellular fluid volume deficit, oral fluid intake can be increased as long as the patient is conscious, not nauseated, and can drink. A patient with hyperosmolar fluid volume deficit will need intravenous fluids, such as 5% dextrose in water (D_5W) or 0.2% dextrose in saline. For moderate or severe extracellular fluid volume deficit, intrave-

Table 5–1

Clinical Manifestations of Body Fluid Volume Deficit

Mild ECFVD	Moderate ECFVD	Severe ECFVD
2% weight loss	5% weight loss	8% weight loss
1–2 L water loss	3–5 L water loss	5–10 L water loss
Thirst	Marked thirst	Marked thirst
Apprehension	Restlessness	Lethargic or irritable, delirium or disorientation
	Flushed skin	Cold, clammy skin
	Dry mucous membranes	Dry mucous membranes
	Poor skin turgor	Poor skin turgor
	Hand veins slow in filling with hand lowered	Hand veins slow in filling with hand lowered
	Increased pulse rate	Tachycardia
	Increased respiration	Increased respiration
	Systolic BP drops 10–15 mm Hg in standing position	Systolic BP <70 mm Hg
	Urine volume decreased, concentrated urine	Urine volume <25 mL/h
	Increased BUN, Hgb	Increased BUN, Hgb

ECFVD, extracellular fluid volume deficit; BP, blood pressure; BUN, blood urea nitrogen; Hgb, hemoglobin.

nous fluids such as dextrose in 0.45% or 0.9% saline might be prescribed. Lactated Ringer's solution may also be used, provided that the patient does not have liver disease or lactic acidosis. Blood replacement may be necessary if the patient's extracellular fluid volume deficit results from hemorrhage of more than 1 L of blood. Balanced salt solutions, such as normal saline and lactated Ringer's solution, may be used to replace blood and fluid losses of less than 1 L.

Medical management is also directed at correcting the underlying causes of the fluid volume deficit to decrease or prevent further fluid loss. For example, if the cause is diarrhea, antidiarrheal agents and dietary restrictions are usually ordered.

NURSING PROCESS
Extracellular Fluid Volume Deficit

Assessment

Obtain a patient history to identify factors that place the patient at risk for extracellular fluid volume deficit. Question the patient about any history of renal disease, diabetes mellitus or insipidus, liver disease, burns, or large draining wounds. Also ask about recent surgery, episodes of excessive sweating, salivating, vomiting, diarrhea, fever, or periods of restricted fluid intake. Question also about the use of diuretics, noting brand name, frequency of use, and dose. Determine whether any physical limitations exist that would prevent adequate fluid intake, such as limited mobility or difficulty swallowing. Obtain a list of fluids (type and amount) ingested in the previous 24 hours and ask whether it represents typical fluid intake. Also question the patient about frequency and amount of urination.

Assess the skin for turgor. Pinched skin on the arm that remains pinched or returns slowly to normal typically indicates poor turgor. Note skin color and temperature. Observe for dry mucous membranes and dry, cracked lips or tongue.

Assess mental status. Observe for apprehension, restlessness, irritability, lethargy, or confusion.

Check pulse rate, respirations, and blood pressure. Remember that as fluid volume deficit occurs, the heart compensates for the fluid loss by increasing its rate. If fluid volume continues to decline, systolic blood pressure begins to fall. Check blood pressure while the patient is sitting and again while the patient is standing. A drop in systolic or diastolic blood pressure of 10 to 15 mm Hg or an increase of 10 to 20 beats per minute (bpm) in heart rate could indicate moderate fluid volume loss.

Assess hand and neck vein filling. Decreased filling of hand veins when the hand is below heart level and of the jugular vein when the patient is in a low Fowler's position (head elevated 30–45 degrees) suggests fluid volume deficit.

Measure urinary output and note urine color. With extracellular fluid volume deficit, urine may be dark yellow. Increased urine output as a result of osmotic diuresis from hyperosmolar fluid (diabetic ketoacidosis) suggests fluid volume loss. Keep in mind that decreased urine output may be due to a lack of fluid intake. Review laboratory reports for increased BUN or hemoglobin levels.

Nursing Diagnoses and Planning

Nursing diagnoses and related expected patient outcomes commonly applicable to patients with extracellular fluid volume deficit include the following:

NDx: Fluid volume deficit related to insufficient intake, vomiting, diarrhea, or diaphoresis (specify for individual patient)

Planning: Patient Outcomes
1. Skin is warm and dry with normal turgor.
2. Capillary refill is within normal limits.
3. Vital signs are within patient's baseline range.
4. Urinary output is 30 to 50 mL/hour or more, or 1500 mL/day.

NDx: Altered oral mucous membrane related to dehydration

Planning: Patient Outcomes
1. Oral mucous membrane is moist and pink.
2. Lips are supple, moist, and free of cracks.
3. Patient denies dryness of the mouth.

Nursing Interventions and Evaluation

NDx: Fluid volume deficit
Monitor vital signs and compare with the patient's baseline vital signs. Report any marked differences from baseline. Check blood pressure with the patient in lying, sitting, and standing positions. Report if the standing (postural) systolic blood pressure falls 20 mm Hg and is accompanied by a pulse rate increase of 10 bpm at 1 minute after the position change.

Provide oral fluid intake to replace mild fluid volume loss. Increase oral intake by offering a variety of fluids at frequent intervals between meals. Offer small amounts at one time if the patient has difficulty drinking or is reluctant to drink. Offer both hot and cold fluids unless otherwise contraindicated and provide assistance as needed. Administer intravenous fluids as ordered for moderate and severe fluid losses.

Monitor skin turgor and mucous membranes for changes, improvement, or deterioration. Also monitor hand and neck veins. Flattened veins may indicate lack of improvement in fluid status.

Track urinary output and report the results. Report immediately if urinary output increases or decreases by 30 mL/hour or more.

Check body weight at the same time every morning, after the patient has voided and before he or she has eaten. Loss of 1 kg (2.2 lb) of weight equals 1 L (1000 mL) of fluid loss. For example, if the patient dropped 3.4 kg (7.5 lb), the fluid loss would be approximately 3 L, indicating a moderate fluid volume deficit.

NDx: Altered oral mucous membrane
Assist the patient with oral hygiene, including toothbrushing and mouth-rinsing, after meals. Avoid agents with a drying effect on mucous membranes, such as commercial mouthwash or lemon and glycerin. Use a solution of equal parts hydrogen peroxide and water to remove debris and deodorize the mouth or use a solution composed of a half teaspoon of sodium bicarbonate and a pint of warm water to cleanse and soothe the mouth. Apply a water-soluble lubricant to the lips to keep them supple and prevent cracking.

Compare the patient's status with the expected outcomes. If the outcomes are not met, reassess the patient and revise the plan.

EXTRACELLULAR FLUID VOLUME EXCESS

Extracellular fluid volume excess is a condition of increased fluid in the vascular system and interstitial spaces. When sodium and water are retained in the same proportion, the excess is referred to as iso-osmolar (isotonic) fluid volume excess. As a result of hemodilution, the serum sodium level may be within normal range even though the actual sodium level is increased. Because sodium promotes water retention, both would be increased.

Etiology and Pathophysiology
Causes of iso-osmolar fluid volume excess include heart failure, chronic renal disease, cirrhosis, and increased ingestion of sodium-laden products, such as packaged foods, salt, and foods with a high sodium content.

Iso-osmolar fluid volume excess is also called *hypervolemia* or *fluid overload*. Normally, fluid shifts freely between the intravascular and interstitial spaces to maintain fluid balance in the ECF compartment. This exchange results from fluid pressure (hydrostatic pressure) and colloid osmotic (oncotic) pressure in the intravascular and interstitial spaces. Fluid pressure (force exerted by intravascular fluid against the walls of the blood vessels) acts to push fluid into the tissue spaces. Oncotic pressure (colloid osmotic pressure caused by albumin and other proteins) holds fluid in the vessels. In fluid overload, the fluid pressure is greater than the oncotic pressure in the vessels. Fluid is pushed into the tissue spaces, and peripheral edema results. As fluid pressure increases, fluid also moves across the alveolo-capillary membrane of the lungs, causing pulmonary edema.

In heart failure, when the heart fails to maintain adequate blood flow throughout the circulatory system, the buildup of intravascular fluid pressure causes fluid shifts into the interstitial spaces. Thus, left-sided heart failure can cause pulmonary edema as a result of fluid shifts into the alveolar spaces. Right-sided heart failure leads to systemic and pe-

ripheral edema. Renal disease can cause a decrease in sodium and water excretion, with resultant fluid overload. With cirrhosis of the liver, serum protein and albumin levels are decreased; therefore, the oncotic pressure is decreased in vascular fluids, causing fluid to move into tissue spaces. With malnutrition, as with cirrhosis, the serum protein level is decreased, and low oncotic pressure causes fluid to leave the vessels and shift into the tissue spaces, causing edema.

Clinical Manifestations
Weight gain, puffy eyelids, and pitting edema in the extremities occur as a result of excess fluid volume. Pulse is rapid, full, and bounding. Blood pressure is elevated, and pulse pressure is decreased. Hand and neck veins are engorged. Hemorrhoids, if present, enlarge. The liver enlarges. Ascites develops as the condition worsens. As fluid shifts into the alveolar spaces, the patient will develop rapid and shallow respirations, dyspnea, moist crackles, and an irritable cough.

Diagnosis
Iso-osmolar extracellular fluid volume excess is diagnosed from the following data:

- The patient's history
- Presenting symptoms such as dyspnea, orthopnea, shortness of breath, edema, weight gain, increased central venous pressure or pulmonary capillary wedge pressure, and distended neck veins
- Serum osmolality of less than 285 mOsm/kg
- Possibly decreased serum protein and albumin levels
- Decreased hematocrit and BUN levels because of diluting effect.

Management
The three "Ds" (diuretics, digitalis, and diet) are frequently prescribed for iso-osmolar extracellular fluid volume excess. Diuretics promote excretion of sodium and water. The potassium-wasting diuretics, which excrete sodium and potassium, are more potent than the potassium-sparing diuretics, which excrete sodium but not potassium. Potassium-wasting diuretics include the thiazide diuretics, such as hydrochlorothiazide (HydroDIURIL), and the loop or high-ceiling diuretics, such as furosemide (Lasix). As water and sodium are lost in urine, blood volume decreases. Furosemide has the added ability to increase venous vasodilation, which increases venous capacitance to decrease the volume returned to the heart. This is especially useful in heart failure.

Digoxin, a digitalis preparation, is ordered to decrease the heart rate and increase the force of myocardial contraction. Because hypokalemia can precipitate digitalis toxicity, potassium-rich foods or a potassium supplement may be suggested for patients also taking thiazide or loop diuretics. Examples of potassium-rich foods include green leafy vegetables, carrots, sweet potatoes, bananas, cantaloupe, apricots, and watermelon.

A diet low in sodium decreases fluid volume because less sodium is available for water retention. In individuals with low serum albumin caused by malnutrition, dietary protein is increased to enable the liver to manufacture albumin. Because albumin is the major determinant of oncotic pressure in the vascular space, increasing albumin increases the oncotic pressure. As a result, fluid moves out of the tissues into the blood vessels, and edema is decreased.

NURSING PROCESS
Iso-Osmolar Extracellular Fluid Volume Excess

Assessment

Obtain a patient history to identify risk factors for iso-osmolar extracellular fluid volume excess. Ask about any history of cardiac disease, renal disease, or cirrhosis. Question the patient about recent weight gain. Determine whether the patient takes any medications. Obtain a diet history to evaluate sodium and fluid intake.

Assess vital signs. Take blood pressure, keeping in mind that the pulse pressure narrows as compensatory mechanisms reach their limit. Check the pulse. Expect it to be rapid, bounding, and full, with peripheral pulses difficult to obliterate in the presence of iso-osmolar extracellular fluid volume excess.

Assess respirations. Note rate and depth. Auscultate breath sounds. Note location of crackles in the chest and whether breathing is difficult. Ask about shortness of breath, particularly orthopnea. Observe for a constant irritated cough, because this is an early sign of fluid overload.

Check lower extremities for pitting edema in the morning before the patient rises. Edema present in the morning is not dependent edema (edema caused by gravity), but may result from a cardiac or renal disorder. If the patient is bedridden, check the sacral

area for edema. Weigh the patient daily. Keep in mind that 1 L of fluid retained causes a 1 kg (2.2 lb) weight gain.

Check hand veins for engorgement. Place the hand below the patient's heart level until the veins are full. Then raise the hand above heart level and note the time needed for veins to flatten. Normally, they should flatten in 10 to 20 seconds. If they stay engorged after 30 seconds, overhydration or fluid overload is most likely present. Also check for neck vein distention, because it also occurs with fluid overload. Assess for liver enlargement, ascites, and enlarged hemorrhoids.

Nursing Diagnoses and Planning

Nursing diagnoses and related expected patient outcomes commonly applicable to patients with extracellular fluid volume excess include the following:

NDx: Fluid volume excess related to excessive fluid/sodium intake or fluid retention (specify for individual patient)

Planning: Patient Outcomes
1. Vital signs are within patient's baseline range.
2. Chest sounds are clear.
3. Extremities are free of edema.

NDx: Risk for impaired skin integrity related to peripheral edema

Planning: Patient Outcomes
1. Skin is warm.
2. Cyanosis is absent.
3. Skin is intact.

Nursing Interventions and Evaluation

NDx: Fluid volume excess
Monitor vital signs and chest sounds. Report elevated blood pressure and a bounding pulse. Be alert for shortness of breath, particularly orthopnea.

Check for pitting edema each morning in the patient's extremities (Fig. 5–2). Press one or two fingers on the edematous area over a bony prominence. If the indentation remains for 15 seconds or

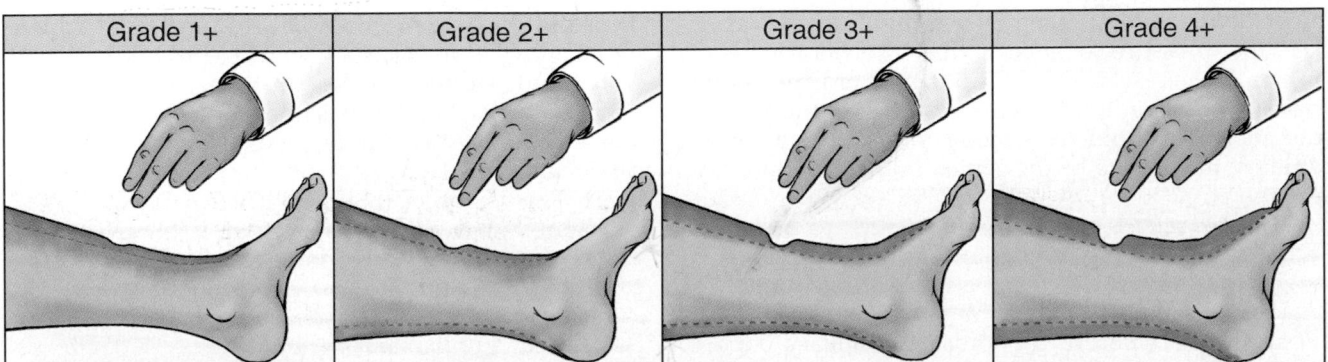

| Grade 1+ | Grade 2+ | Grade 3+ | Grade 4+ |

Figure 5–2
Assessment of pitting edema.

*Patient has FVE

more, record the degree of pitting edema according to the depth of the indentation, as shown:

- 1+ for a 2 mm indentation
- 2+ for a 4 mm indentation
- 3+ for a 6 mm indentation
- 4+ for an 8 mm indentation

Also check the patient's weight each morning. A gain of 1 kg (2.2 lb) equals 1 L of body fluid. Usually edema does not occur unless the patient has 3 L or more of excess fluid.

Administer diuretics as ordered and monitor intake and output. Also monitor for electrolyte and acid-base imbalances during diuretic therapy. Restrict fluid and sodium in the diet according to physician's order. Encourage the patient to drink small amounts of the total fluid allowed at intervals throughout the day to avoid long periods when fluids cannot be taken. In preparation for self-care, teach the patient or significant other about sources of sodium in the diet. Provide a list of sodium-rich foods and condiments to be avoided. Stress that salt (sodium chloride) is only one source of sodium. Foods containing other sodium compounds, such as monosodium glutamate, must also be limited. Encourage the patient to read food labels.

NDx: Risk for impaired skin integrity
Keep the edematous skin areas that are at risk for breakdown clean. Apply an emollient to prevent dryness and flaking. Before getting the patient out of bed, apply antiembolic stockings to minimize pooling of fluid in the legs and feet as a result of gravity. Assist with repositioning at least every 2 hours as needed to prevent pressure, which will further impair circulation. It is critical to prevent skin breakdown, because edema slows oxygen transport to the cells and thus impairs healing.

Compare the patient's status with the expected outcomes. If the outcomes are not met, reassess the patient and revise the plan.

EXTRACELLULAR THIRD-SPACE VOLUME SHIFT

Fluid shifts constantly in the ECF compartment between the intravascular and interstitial spaces to maintain fluid balance. When an abnormal amount of fluid shifts into the interstitial space and remains there, it is called third-space fluid. Third-space fluid is physiologically useless because it does not circulate to provide nutrients to cells.

Etiology and Pathophysiology
Common causes of fluid shift from intravascular to interstitial spaces include:

1. Severe inflammation and tissue damage from burns, abdominal surgery, crushing injury, or severe infection.
2. Increased hydrostatic fluid pressure resulting from heart failure, renal disease, or corticosteroid therapy.
3. Decreased colloid (oncotic) pressure from protein deficit caused by cirrhosis of the liver, malnutrition, or renal disease.

When tissue is injured, increased capillary permeability allows fluid, protein, and other solutes to shift into the interstitial spaces. In cirrhosis, serum albumin levels are typically decreased because of poor dietary practice. This results in a decreased plasma oncotic pressure, so fluid shifts from the blood vessels to the peritoneal cavity and to the interstitial spaces in the extremities. Ascites and peripheral edema result. Heart failure can precipitate fluid and sodium overload. This, in turn, increases hydrostatic fluid pressure and pushes fluid into the interstitial spaces of the extremities (peripheral edema) and into the lung tissues (pulmonary edema).

Two phases of fluid shift to the third space usually occur as a result of tissue injury, such as burns or abdominal surgery. The first phase is from the intravascular space to the interstitial space. The second phase is from the interstitial space back to the intravascular space. In the first phase, fluid volume deficit (hypovolemia) results, which may lead to shock. In the second phase, fluid volume excess occurs if the kidneys are unable to excrete excess fluid. Table 5–2 presents the two phases of fluid volume shift.

Clinical Manifestations
In fluid shifts resulting from tissue injury, it usually takes 24 to 48 hours for the fluid to leave the blood vessels and accumulate in the interstitial spaces at

Table 5–2

Phase	Fluid Shift	Time	Cause
Fluid Volume Shift			
I	Intravascular (vessel) to interstitial (tissue) spaces	24–48 h (1–2 d)	Major: Burns, abdominal surgery, intestinal obstruction, crushing wounds, severe infection Minor: Blister, sprain
II	Interstitial to intravascular spaces	72–120 h (3–5 d)	

the injured site. Edema may or may not be visible. Vital signs may indicate hypovolemia, with shock-like symptoms of tachycardia, a decrease in systolic pressure, and tachypnea.

Three to 5 days after an injury caused by burns, surgery, or tissue destruction, the fluid shifts from the injured site to the blood vessels. If the kidneys cannot excrete this extra fluid from the vascular compartment, hypervolemia results. Clinical manifestations of hypervolemia include dyspnea, chest crackles, engorgement of the jugular vein, and increased central venous pressure.

In cirrhosis, heart failure, or renal disease, pitting edema occurs because of a decreased oncotic pressure and an increased fluid (hydrostatic) pressure. Edema in the extremities occurs when there is an accumulation of approximately 3 L of fluid. Plus one (+1) edema indicates a mild case, whereas +4 edema indicates a large amount of fluid accumulation (severe peripheral edema).

Diagnosis

Serum albumin and electrolytes are among the laboratory tests used for diagnosing ECF shift. A decreased serum albumin level causes decreased oncotic pressure and fluid accumulation in the extremities. A decrease in urinary output may indicate a fluid shift to the tissue spaces, and an increase in urinary output can indicate fluid shift back to the intravascular space.

Clinical findings confirm the fluid imbalance. Pitting edema indicates fluid shift to the interstitial spaces of the extremities. Crackles, dyspnea, and vein engorgement signal hypervolemia involving the lung tissues.

Management

Albumin IV fluid ~~volume~~ is given for fluid volume excess

Medical management begins with determination of the cause of the fluid shift. Hypovolemia resulting from tissue injury such as burns requires large amounts of intravenous fluid replacement. The amount of fluid infusion may be three times greater than the urinary output. The type of intravenous fluid replacement used is iso-osmolar solution. During the second phase, in which fluid shifts back into the circulation, urinary output may be three times greater than the fluid intake. Fluid intake is restricted.

Diuretics may be used for peripheral and pulmonary edema. Electrolyte replacement is determined by the serum electrolyte results. A diet rich in protein and low in sodium may increase the serum protein level, thus increasing the oncotic pressure, which pulls fluid back from the third space.

NURSING PROCESS GUIDELINES
Extracellular Third-Space Fluid Volume Shift

Assessment, nursing diagnoses, expected patient outcomes, nursing interventions, and evaluation for patients with an extracellular third-space fluid volume shift are a combination of those described previously for patients with extracellular fluid volume deficit or extracellular fluid volume excess (depending on the stage of the fluid shift) and those that derive from the specific disorder underlying the fluid shift.

INTRACELLULAR FLUID VOLUME EXCESS

Intracellular fluid volume excess is not as common a fluid imbalance as extracellular fluid volume deficit or extracellular fluid volume excess. Intracellular fluid volume excess results from hypo-osmolar fluid in the intravascular system, which can be due to either excess water or decreased solutes. The hypo-osmolar fluid moves to the cells that contain iso-osmolar fluid to maintain fluid balance. The fluid moves by osmosis, from an area of lesser solute concentration to one of greater solute concentration. Intracellular fluid volume excess caused by hypo-osmolar (hypotonic) fluid is also called water intoxication. Water intoxication is not the same as edema. Edema is the accumulation of water and sodium in the interstitial spaces. Water intoxication is an accumulation of water in the cells (Fig. 5–3). Individuals at greatest risk for water intoxication are the elderly, the malnourished, and the debilitated.

Etiology and Pathophysiology

Conditions that cause intracellular fluid volume excess, or water intoxication, include:

- Excessive intake of water
- Solute (electrolytes, protein) deficit *secondary to malnutrition*
- Increased secretion of antidiuretic hormone (ADH)
- Inability of the kidneys to excrete excess water

Specific causes of each of these conditions are presented in Table 5–3.

Intracellular fluid volume excess causes cellular edema and electrolyte dilution. In the brain, this edema causes increased intracranial pressure and can either depress or stimulate various nerve centers.

Clinical Manifestations

Increased fluid in the cerebral cells (cerebral edema) causes headache and behavioral changes, such as incoordination, apprehension, irritability, and changes in level of consciousness, including lethargy, disorientation, and confusion. Anorexia, nausea, projectile vomiting, blurred vision, and papilledema may also occur. Changes in vital signs also develop, including increased blood pressure, decreased pulse rate, and increased or decreased respirations. Acute weight gain is evident. Convulsions are common in severe intracellular fluid volume excess.

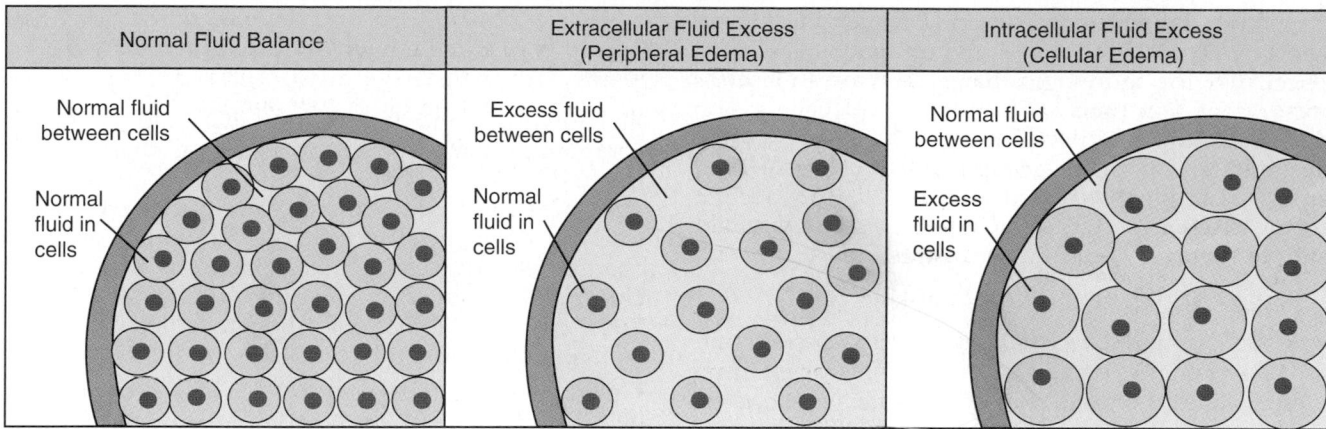

Figure 5–3

Schematic view of extracellular and intracellular fluid volume excess.

Diagnosis

The diagnosis of intracellular fluid volume excess is based on patient history, clinical findings, and laboratory values. Serum osmolality of less than 285 mOsm/kg suggests the possibility of intracellular fluid volume excess, but no one laboratory test is diagnostic.

Management

Medical management begins with water restriction. For severe intracellular fluid volume excess, diuretics and hypertonic saline solutions may be prescribed.

Table 5–3

Causes of Intracellular Fluid Volume Excess

Condition	Causes
Excess water	Excessive intake of water or ice chips
	Psychogenic polydipsia
	Continuous use of intravenous D_5W
	Brain injury or tumor with increased ADH production
Solute deficit	Diet low in electrolytes and protein
	Multiple tap-water enemas
	Irrigation of nasogastric tube with water and not normal saline
Impaired excretion	Kidney dysfunction
	Heart failure
	SIADH, which may result from stress, surgery, drugs (narcotics, anesthesia), pain, and tumors (brain, lung)

ADH, antidiuretic hormone; D_5W, 5% dextrose in water; SIADH, syndrome of inappropriate antidiuretic hormone.

Intracellular fluid volume excess can result from the syndrome of inappropriate antidiuretic hormone. In this syndrome, excessive ADH from the posterior pituitary promotes increased water resorption in the renal tubules. Syndrome of inappropriate antidiuretic hormone can be caused by surgery, head trauma, anesthesia, narcotic use, or continuous parenteral administration of D_5W. If a patient's excess fluid results from syndrome of inappropriate antidiuretic hormone, treatment involves changing the intravenous solution to dextrose in normal saline (0.9%), dextrose in one-half normal saline (0.45%), or lactated Ringer's solution.

Prevention should be the main medical management for intracellular fluid volume excess. Continuous parenteral administration of D_5W and excess oral water intake dilute the vascular fluid, causing intracellular fluid volume excess. This can be avoided by making certain that intravenous solutions and oral fluid intake contain solutes such as sodium chloride and other electrolytes.

NURSING PROCESS
Intracellular Fluid Volume Excess

Assessment

Assess for factors that place the patient at risk for intracellular fluid volume excess. Note the patient's age and explore any history of chronic or debilitating disease. Inquire specifically about any history of renal disease and ask about current urinary output (frequency and amount). Explore recent medical problems or treatments, such as surgery, head trauma, intravenous therapy, and enemas. Assess the patient's recent fluid intake. Determine the volume and type of both oral and intravenous fluids. Note the intake of hypo-osmolar fluids, such as water, ice chips, and D_5W relative to the intake of iso-osmolar or hyperosmolar fluids.

Assess vital signs and compare them with baseline values. Observe for an increase in blood pressure; slow, bounding pulse; and an increased respiratory rate, which are signs of cerebral edema. Check also for neurologic changes. Observe alertness and orientation and ask about headache, vision changes, and projectile vomiting.

Check the patient's weight, because intracellular fluid volume excess usually involves acute weight gain. Assess for peripheral edema, which is slight with intracellular fluid volume excess.

Nursing Diagnoses and Planning

Nursing diagnoses and related expected patient outcomes commonly applicable to patients with intracellular fluid volume excess or water intoxication include the following:

NDx: Fluid volume excess: water intoxication related to excess water intake, decrease in solutes, oversecretion of ADH, or renal dysfunction secondary to intracellular fluid volume excess

Planning: Patient Outcomes
1. Serum osmolality returns to between 285 and 295 mOsm/kg.
2. Vital signs return to patient's baseline level.
3. Neurologic signs of brain-cell edema are absent.

NDx: Risk for injury related to incoordination, confusion, and convulsion

Planning: Patient Outcomes
1. Patient complies with safety measures.
2. Patient remains free of injury.

Nursing Interventions and Evaluation

NDx: Fluid volume excess
Monitor fluid replacement. Keep in mind that if intravenous D_5W is given continuously and oral intake is only water and ice chips, intracellular fluid volume excess is likely to occur. Dextrose is metabolized quickly, leaving only water, which is a hypoosmolar fluid. Ensure that several of the intravenous solutions contain saline (0.45% or 0.9%). When clear liquids are ordered, give broth because it contains solutes that increase the serum osmolality.

Monitor urinary output. As output increases, intracellular fluid volume excess should decrease.

NDx: Risk for injury
Protect the patient from falls or other injury that may result from incoordination or confusion. Keep the bedside rails up. Provide assistance and supervision if the patient is out of bed. Keep personal items and the call bell within reach. If the patient is confused, reorient with each interaction.

 To decrease central nervous system (CNS) stimulation and the risk of seizures, maintain a quiet environment. Eliminate sources of loud noise and avoid sudden stimuli. Institute seizure precautions to protect the patient from injury should a seizure occur.

Compare the patient's status with the expected outcomes. If the outcomes are not met, reassess the patient and revise the plan.

*E*lectrolyte Imbalances

Electrolytes, found in ECF and ICF (Fig. 5–4), are compounds that produce an electrical charge when in fluid. These compounds break up into particles known as ions, which carry either a positive charge (cation) or a negative charge (anion). Positively charged electrolytes include potassium, sodium, calcium, and magnesium. Negatively charged electrolytes include chloride, bicarbonate, phosphate, and sulfate. Potassium and phosphate are the electrolytes most plentiful in the cells (ICF). Sodium, chloride, and bicarbonate are the electrolytes most plentiful in the ECF.

Cations are discussed in relation to deficits and excesses. Names for these deficits and excesses are

> Hypokalemia and hyperkalemia (potassium deficit and excess)
> Hyponatremia and hypernatremia (sodium deficit and excess)
> Hypocalcemia and hypercalcemia (calcium deficit and excess)
> Hypomagnesemia and hypermagnesemia (magnesium deficit and excess)

POTASSIUM IMBALANCE

Potassium, the predominant intracellular cation, is essential for the transmission and conduction of nerve impulses and for contraction of skeletal, smooth, and cardiac muscle. Potassium is absorbed through the GI tract. About 80 to 90% is excreted by the kidneys. Potassium is not stored in the body, so 40 to 60 mEq must be ingested daily. Foods rich in potassium include vegetables, fruits, dry fruits, nuts, and meats. Increased sodium intake promotes potassium loss.

Potassium moves continually between the ICF and the ECF under control of the sodium-potassium pump. Normal potassium level in the cells (ICF) is 150 mEq/L, whereas the serum potassium level (ECF) is 3.5 to 5.3 mEq/L, or 3.5 to 5.3 mmol/L. Body potassium levels can be obtained only from intravascular (serum) fluid, so actual intracellular potassium levels are unknown. A serum potassium level less than 3.5 mEq/L is called *hypokalemia*, and a serum potassium level greater than 5.3 mEq/L is called *hyperkalemia*.

Hypokalemia

Etiology and Pathophysiology
Decreased serum potassium is a common disorder that can result from an abnormal loss of potassium from the body, movement of excessive amounts of potassium into the cells, or rarely, inadequate intake. The major source of abnormal loss of potas-

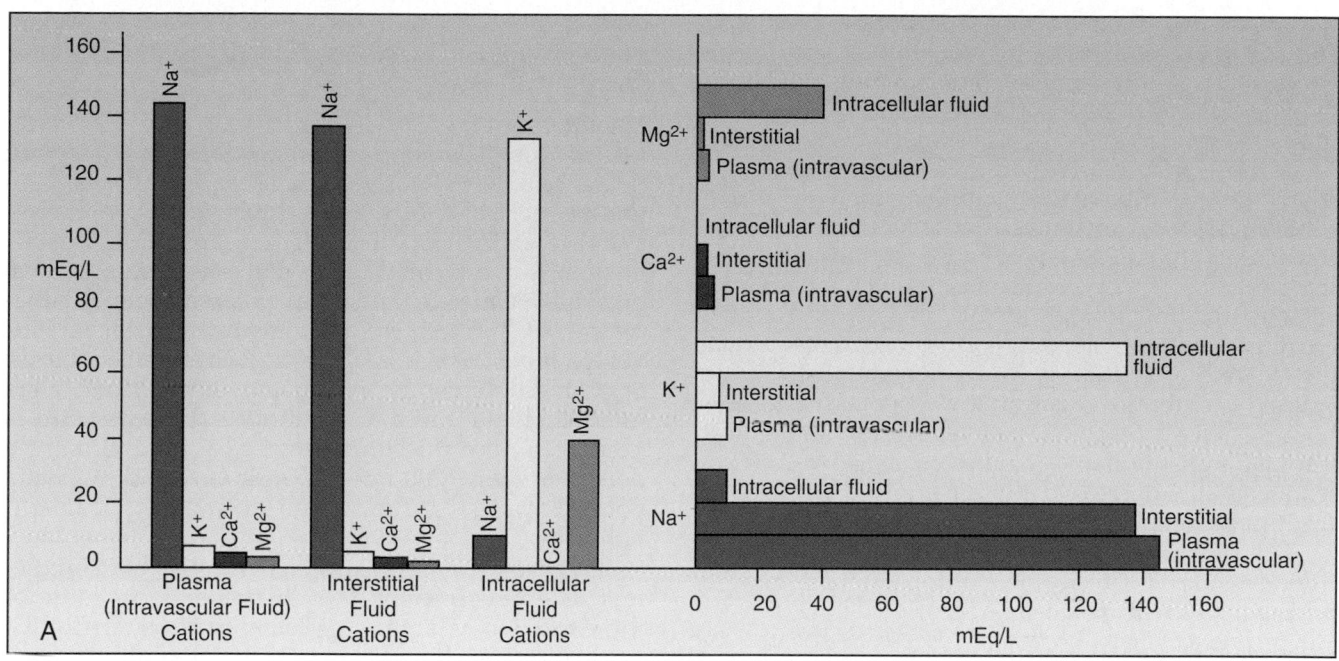

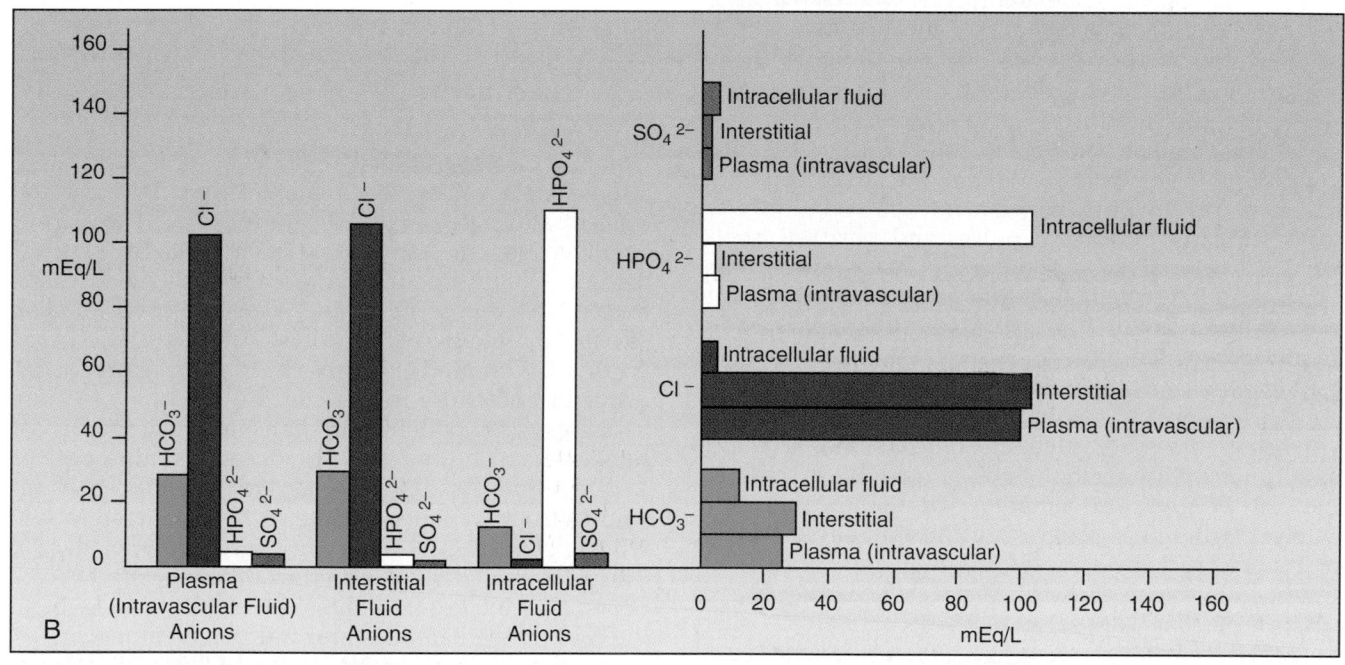

Figure 5–4

Distribution of the major cations sodium (Na^+), potassium (K^+), calcium (Ca^{2+}), and magnesium (Mg^{2+}) *(A)* and the major anions bicarbonate (HCO_3^-), chloride (Cl^-), phosphate (HPO_4^{2-}), and sulfate (SO_4^{2-}) *(B)* in body fluid compartments.

sium from the body is the GI tract. Because there are large amounts of potassium in the tract, vomiting, diarrhea (including that from abuse of laxatives), GI suction, and drainage from a fistula or an ostomy all result in loss of potassium. Hypokalemia resulting from the movement of large amounts of potassium from the ECF into the ICF occurs secondary to metabolic alkalosis. Hypokalemia is worsened if metabolic alkalosis develops, because the condition increases renal potassium excretion. Other causes of abnormal potassium loss include:

- Increased aldosterone secretion (aldosterone promotes sodium retention and potassium excretion)
- Use of steroids
- Use of potassium-wasting diuretics such as the thiazides, ethacrynic acid, furosemide, and acetazolamide

Hypokalemia may also result from excessive insulin in the blood (hyperinsulinism), as seen in patients receiving hyperalimentation therapy. Hypokalemia resulting from insufficient intake of potassium may arise in patients on NPO status for several days or in those who receive large volumes of parenteral fluids without a potassium supplement.

Decreased serum potassium levels relative to intracellular potassium levels cause an increased resting potential in nerve and muscle fiber membranes, causing the membranes to be less readily excited. Further, when depolarization does occur, a return to the resting potential is slowed because of a decreased membrane permeability to potassium. Thus, both decreased responsiveness to stimuli and slowed impulse transmission—manifested as slowed neural response and decreased muscle contractility—result from hypokalemia.

The severity of the pathophysiologic effects of hypokalemia is directly proportional to the rapidity with which the hypokalemia occurs.

Clinical Manifestations

Clinical manifestations of hypokalemia involve most body systems. Effects on the respiratory and cardiovascular systems are those most likely to be fatal. In the respiratory system, the depressive effect of hypokalemia on excitable neuromuscular membranes can cause weak, shallow breathing with inadequate ventilation. In the cardiovascular system, hypokalemia affects ventricular contractility. A serum potassium level below 3.0 mEq/L decreases the strength of myocardial contraction, resulting in weak, thready peripheral pulses and postural hypotension. Ventricular dysrhythmias may also occur. Electrocardiographic (ECG) changes associated with hypokalemia include a depressed and prolonged ST segment and a depressed or inverted T wave. Cardiac arrest can occur with severe hypokalemia.

Depression of membrane excitability in the nervous system results in changes in mental status and tactile perception. Initial signs of anxiety or irritability can progress to lethargy, confusion, and even coma. During this progression, peripheral sensation of touch, pain, heat, and cold may be diminished. Changes in tissue excitability also affect skeletal and smooth muscle. Skeletal muscles become weak, deep tendon hyporeflexia develops and, in severe cases, flaccid paralysis occurs. Hypokalemia similarly decreases the contractility of smooth muscle. This leads to decreased peristalsis in the GI tract. Bowel sounds are hypoactive, and nausea, vomiting, constipation, abdominal distention, and even paralytic ileus may occur.

Renal manifestations of hypokalemia include polyuria, with decreased specific gravity secondary to the decreased ability of the kidney to concentrate urine.

Diagnosis

The diagnosis of hypokalemia is based on the patient history and laboratory and clinical findings. A serum potassium level lower than 3.5 mEq/L indicates hypokalemia. It does not indicate, however, whether there is a real deficit of potassium or a shift from ECF to ICF.

Management

Medical management is designed to return serum potassium to its normal range and to correct the underlying cause of the hypokalemia to prevent recurrence. Treatment instituted to return serum potassium to the normal range varies with the severity of hypokalemia. If the serum potassium level is between 3.0 and 3.5 mEq/L, treatment typically involves foods rich in potassium accompanied by an oral or intravenous potassium supplement. One hundred to 200 mEq/L of intravenous potassium is needed to raise the serum level by 1 mEq/L. Larger deficits require 200 to 400 mEq/L of intravenous potassium to raise the serum level 1 mEq/L (Highlight 5–1).

Hypokalemia is accompanied by hypomagnesemia in approximately 4 of 10 patients. In most of these cases, potassium supplements prove ineffective in treating the hypokalemia until after the magnesium deficit is corrected.

NURSING PROCESS
Hypokalemia

Assessment

Obtain a patient history to identify risk factors for hypokalemia. Note the patient's age, because the concentrating power of the kidney decreases with age. Question the patient about any history of renal disease. Obtain detailed information on medications taken, both prescribed and over-the-counter. Ask specifically about the use of steroids, diuretics, and laxatives. Obtain a dietary history to assess adequacy of potassium intake.

Assess the patient for signs and symptoms of hypokalemia, noting time of onset and duration of each episode. Assess for respiratory insufficiency resulting from weakness of the muscles of respiration, which can cause death in severe hypokalemia. Check the rate, depth, and effort of respiration every 2 hours. Auscultate for diminished breath sounds. Note the color of the nail beds and mucous membranes.

Assess cardiovascular status. Check peripheral pulses for strength and regularity. With hypokalemia, the pulse is usually weak and thready with a variable rate, depending on the dysrhythmia produced. Review ECG findings. Measure blood pressure with the patient lying, sitting, and standing to check for postural hypotension.

Assess mental status. Obtain baseline information on usual mental status, mood, and personality from a family member or significant other. Assess for tactile sensation (ie, perception of touch, pain, heat, and cold).

Assess for skeletal muscle weakness. Observe the patient's ability to move, stand, ambulate, and perform activities of daily living. Check lifts and grips.

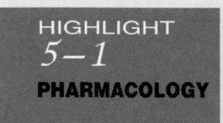 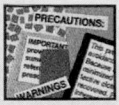

HIGHLIGHT
5–1
PHARMACOLOGY

Potassium Supplements

Definition:

Potassium preparations for oral or intravenous administration, designed to increase the amount of potassium, the principal intracellular cation, in the body. Most are in the form of potassium chloride.

Action:

Potassium is essential for nerve impulse transmission and muscular contraction, tissue growth and repair, and maintenance of acid-base balance.

Uses:

Oral supplements: prevention and treatment of mild hypokalemia.

Intravenous supplements: treatment of moderate to severe hypokalemia.

Side Effects:

Nausea, vomiting, abdominal discomfort, diarrhea, ulceration, and gastrointestinal (GI) bleeding, skin rash, and hyperkalemia, which is characterized by paresthesias, muscle weakness progressing to flaccid paralysis, confusion, hypotension, and cardiac dysrhythmias. Intravenous preparations can cause chemical phlebitis and, if extravasated, tissue irritation and necrosis.

Interactions:

Severe hyperkalemia can occur when potassium supplements are used concurrently with potassium-sparing diuretics or with salt substitutes containing potassium salts.

Increases in serum potassium decrease both effectiveness and toxicity of digitalis.

Anticholinergic agents increase the risk of GI ulceration resulting from oral potassium supplements because they decrease GI motility and gastric emptying.

Nursing Implications:

Check for patient history of renal dysfunction, which would increase risk of hyperkalemia.

Never administer parenteral potassium intramuscularly or subcutaneously.

Always dilute intravenous preparation. Never give as a bolus.

Give slowly because rapid administration can cause severe hyperkalemia with cardiac dysrhythmias and cardiac arrest.

Always use a controller or pump for administration.

Do not mix intravenous potassium in solutions containing calcium or magnesium because precipitation results.

Protect against extravasation because severe irritation and necrosis result.

Monitor for chemical phlebitis at the site of administration because potassium is highly irritating.

Monitor electrolyte levels, electrocardiogram, and urinary output.

Stop potassium infusion if urinary output drops to less than 20 mL/h for 2 consecutive hours.

Instruct patients on the correct use of oral potassium supplements as presented in Highlight 5–2.

Geriatric Considerations:

Elderly are at increased risk for hyperkalemia secondary to potassium replacement because of lower lean body mass and total body potassium. Decreased renal function that occurs with age can increase the amount of retained potassium. Elderly are at increased risk for ulcerative GI lesions.

Assess GI function. Ask about nausea, vomiting, and constipation. Auscultate bowel sounds in all quadrants and check for abdominal distention by measuring abdominal girth. Assess renal function. Measure urinary output and check specific gravity. Note color and volume of urine.

Nursing Diagnoses and Planning

Nursing diagnoses and related expected patient outcomes commonly applicable to patients with varying degrees of hypokalemia include the following:

NDx: Risk for decreased cardiac output related to weak or dysrhythmic myocardial contraction

Planning: Patient Outcomes
1. Vital signs remain within the patient's normal range.
2. ECG readings indicate a normal sinus rhythm free of ventricular dysrhythmias.

NDx: Risk for injury related to muscle weakness and changes in mental status

Planning: Patient Outcomes
1. Patient complies with safety precautions.
2. Patient uses assistance as needed.
3. Patient remains free of injury.

NDx: Constipation related to decreased peristalsis

Planning: Patient Outcomes
1. Patient passes soft, formed stool at regular intervals.
2. Defecation occurs without undue straining.
3. Defecation occurs without pain.

NDx: Risk for altered health maintenance related to lack of knowledge of measures to prevent hypokalemia

Planning: Patient Outcomes
1. Patient defines hypokalemia.
2. Patient lists good dietary sources of potassium.
3. Patient describes factors that can lead to hypokalemia.

Nursing Interventions and Evaluation

NDx: Risk for decreased cardiac output
Monitor cardiovascular status. Measure blood pressure when the patient is lying, sitting, and standing, because postural hypotension develops before a generalized hypotensive state. Report ECG changes that indicate hypokalemia, such as prolonged, depressed ST segments and flat or inverted T waves. Be alert for severe bradycardia and the development of heart block, especially in patients taking digitalis, because low serum potassium levels potentiate digitalis toxicity. Monitor serum potassium levels and administer supplemental potassium.

NDx: Risk for injury
Protect the patient from accidental falls caused by muscle weakness or confusion. Keep the side rails up when the patient is in bed. Provide assistance and supervision when the patient is out of bed. Ensure that personal items are easily accessible to limit the need for reaching or for getting out of the bed or chair. Also keep the call bell within reach. Assist with self-care as necessary. If the patient is experiencing changes in mental status, reorient to time and place with each interaction. Also restate who you are, what you are going to do, and what is expected of the patient.

NDx: Constipation
Explain the role of low serum potassium level in causing constipation. Reassure the patient that as the serum potassium level returns to normal, bowel function will as well. Within the limits of any dietary restrictions, ensure that the patient consumes a high-fiber diet and 2500 mL of fluid daily. When possible, have the patient use a toilet or commode rather than a bedpan. Provide privacy.

Encourage physical activity, whether it be bed exercises or ambulation, to promote bowel function. According to physician's order, assist evacuation by using stool softeners or drugs that stimulate GI activity, such as metoclopramide hydrochloride (Reglan).

NDx: Risk for altered health maintenance
Explain to the patient what hypokalemia is and how it can be prevented. Provide the patient with a list of foods high in potassium (bananas, oranges, cantaloupe, dates, raisins, avocado, apricots, dried fruits, leafy green vegetables, broccoli, carrots, potatoes, beans, meats, nuts, coffee, cocoa, and cola beverages).

Stress the importance of including potassium-containing foods in the daily diet, especially if the patient takes drugs such as potassium-wasting diuretics, cortisone, laxatives, or lithium carbonate. Explain that boiling foods depletes potassium; suggest steaming or broiling as alternative preparation techniques. If the patient uses a salt substitute, explain that some contain potassium salts and, therefore, may provide all the extra dietary potassium needed. If oral potassium supplements are ordered, instruct the patient in correct administration, as presented in Highlight 5–2. If the patient is very weak, lethargic,

---

HIGHLIGHT 5–2

PATIENT EDUCATION

Use of Oral Potassium Supplements

Instruct the patient in the following:

Dissolve liquid, powder, or effervescent tablets in 4 to 8 oz of cold fruit juice or water.

Measure liquids in drops to avoid overdose.

Wait until effervescent preparations have stopped fizzing before drinking.

Avoid chewing or breaking tablets unless they are specifically designated as "chewable."

Avoid dissolving tablets in the mouth because ulcerations can occur.

Expect a strong, salty taste.

Sip dissolved preparations over 5- to 10-minute period.

Take in divided doses over the day as directed to help maintain extracellular fluid levels.

Take with meals to decrease gastrointestinal distress.

Return for scheduled visits and to have serum potassium levels measured.

Report muscle weakness, numbness, tingling, or pulse changes.

Observe for and report tarry or bloody stools.

or confused, instruct a family member or significant other in correct administration. Teach the correct use of laxatives and diuretics and stress the importance of having blood drawn as scheduled to check serum potassium levels. Tell the patient to report signs of hypokalemia, including the following:

> Slow or irregular heartbeat
> Muscle cramps
> Numbness or tingling in the hands or the feet
> Weakness
> Difficulty concentrating
> Forgetfulness or confusion
> Constipation
> Abdominal distention
> Nausea

Additional Interventions

Chop or purée foods and assist the patient with eating if muscles are weak. Give small, frequent meals. If a GI tube is in place, irrigate the tube with normal saline to avoid electrolyte loss. Measure and record intake and output. Record and report signs and symptoms of progressive hypokalemia. Remember that immediate medical intervention is needed if the serum potassium level drops below 3.0 mEq/L.

Compare the patient's status with the expected outcomes. If the outcomes are not met, reassess the patient and revise the plan.

Hyperkalemia

Etiology and Pathophysiology

Hyperkalemia occurs less often than hypokalemia and rarely in persons with normal renal function. This is because potassium is not stored in the body but is continuously excreted by the kidneys. When hyperkalemia does occur, it may result from impaired potassium excretion, movement of potassium from ICF to ECF, or excessive intake of potassium.

Impaired excretion can occur under the following conditions:

- In kidney failure with oliguria
- From hypoaldosteronism secondary to adrenalectomy, adrenal insufficiency, or Addison's disease
- As an effect of potassium-sparing diuretics, such as spironolactone (Aldactone) and amiloride (Midamor)

Movement from ICF to ECF occurs secondary to starvation, surgery, burns, and crushing tissue injuries. It also occurs secondary to metabolic acidosis, because, in the acidotic state, hydrogen ions are taken into the cells and potassium is released.

Hyperkalemia resulting from excessive intake can develop from overuse of potassium supplements or salt substitutes, rapid administration of intravenous potassium, or transfusion of cell-damaged blood. Cell damage can result from blood storage for longer than 48 hours or from physical disruption of cells caused by improper handling or administration through a small access device.

Increased serum potassium levels relative to the ICF level decrease the resting membrane potential, resulting in increased membrane excitability. However, repolarization is slow. Thus, the additional time taken for return to resting membrane potential limits the speed of, and eventually prevents, response to stimuli. Of all excitable membranes, cardiac muscle is the most sensitive to hyperkalemia. As with hypokalemia, the severity of pathophysiologic change varies directly with the speed of onset of the increased serum potassium level.

Clinical Manifestations

The cardiovascular system is most seriously affected by hyperkalemia. Hypotension and bradycardia occur, sometimes preceded by tachycardia and ectopic beats. As hyperkalemia worsens, ECG changes develop, including a tall, peaked T wave, a prolonged PR interval, and a wide QRS complex. The patient risks ventricular fibrillation and cardiac arrest as the serum potassium level approaches 7 mEq/L.

Neurologic symptoms associated with mild hyperkalemia are due to membrane hyperexcitability and include muscle twitching, cramps, and paresthesias. As hyperkalemia persists or worsens, neural responses to stimuli are slowed or blocked because of prolonged membrane repolarization time. Weakness begins in the hands and feet and moves medially, progressing to flaccid paralysis in the muscles of the upper and lower extremities.

GI effects of hyperkalemia relate to increased motility. Bowel sounds are hyperactive, and nausea, abdominal cramping, and diarrhea occur.

Diagnosis

The diagnosis of hyperkalemia is confirmed by a serum potassium level higher than 5.3 mEq/L.

Management

Treatment of hyperkalemia varies with its severity. With a slight elevation of serum potassium level, 5.3 to 5.6 mEq/L, potassium intake is restricted. A low-potassium diet is instituted, and all potassium supplements, parenteral solutions containing potassium, and drugs containing potassium, such as potassium penicillin, are eliminated. Blood transfusions are avoided whenever possible. If a transfusion is required, only blood stored for fewer than 48 hours is used.

For severe hyperkalemia, sodium polystyrene (Kayexalate) is administered to increase potassium excretion. This drug is a cation-exchange resin. It is nondigestible and releases sodium and absorbs potassium in the GI tract before being excreted in the feces. It may be administered orally or rectally. Because time is required for the desired effect to occur, dialysis or ultrafiltration may be used to rid the body of the excess potassium in cases in which the level is critically high.

Measures designed to lower serum potassium level by promoting the movement of potassium from the ECF to the ICF can also be used. Glucose

(10–50%) with insulin can be given, because potassium moves with glucose and insulin into the cells. If acidosis is present, sodium bicarbonate can also be given to elevate the pH and further promote the movement of potassium into the cells. Calcium gluconate (10%) can be used to decrease the irritability of the myocardium.

NURSING PROCESS
Hyperkalemia

Assessment

Obtain a patient history to identify risk factors for hyperkalemia. Ask about any history of renal or adrenal disorders and explore any recent medical or surgical problems and their treatment. If the patient denies any history of renal disease, ask specific questions about urinary output (frequency, amount, and appearance of urine). Question the patient about the use of prescribed and over-the-counter medications. Ask specifically about potassium-sparing diuretics. Review the patient's diet. Explore the intake of potassium-rich foods and use of salt substitutes containing potassium salts.

Assess the patient for signs and symptoms of hyperkalemia, noting time of onset and duration of each episode. Begin with cardiovascular status. Check pulse and blood pressure and question the patient about palpitations and skipped beats. Review ECG results. Assess neuromuscular status. Ask about and observe for muscle twitching, cramping, and paresthesias. Assess for muscle weakness in the extremities. Check lifts and grips. Auscultate for hyperactive bowel sounds and ask about cramping and diarrhea.

Nursing Diagnoses and Planning

Nursing diagnoses and related expected patient outcomes commonly applicable to patients with hyperkalemia include the following:

NDx: Risk for decreased cardiac output related to dysrhythmia secondary to the effect of hyperkalemia on the myocardium

Planning: Patient Outcomes
1. Vital signs remain within the patient's normal range.
2. ECG readings indicate a normal sinus rhythm.

NDx: Diarrhea related to increased peristalsis

Planning: Patient Outcomes
1. Stool is formed.
2. Frequency of defecation is consistent with patient's normal pattern.
3. Perianal skin remains free of irritation.

NDx: Altered health maintenance related to lack of knowledge of potassium restriction

Planning: Patient Outcomes
1. Patient describes need to restrict potassium.
2. Patient identifies sources of potassium.
3. Patient describes plan for avoiding excessive potassium.

Nursing Interventions and Evaluation

Eliminate all external sources of potassium. According to physician's orders, discontinue parenteral infusions containing potassium, oral potassium supplements, and medications containing potassium. Also place the patient on a potassium-restricted diet. If the patient must have a blood transfusion, check that the blood has been stored for no longer than 48 hours. Monitor urinary output to check renal function. Output should be at least 25 mL/hour or 600 mL/day.

NDx: Risk for decreased cardiac output
Monitor cardiovascular status. Be alert for hypotension, tachycardia or bradycardia, and ECG changes such as QRS spread and peaked T waves that occur as the serum potassium level drops. Monitor serum potassium levels and report those greater than 5.3 mEq/L. Remember that levels greater than 7.0 mEq/L can cause ventricular fibrillation and cardiac arrest.

NDx: Diarrhea
Record the time, amount, and characteristics of stool passed. Administer medications prescribed to decrease intestinal motility. Provide a diet low in fiber residue and milk products to avoid stimulating peristalsis. Record intake and output. Increase fluids as necessary to maintain normal urine specific gravity. Provide fluids such as water and flat ginger ale, which are low in potassium and do not further stimulate peristalsis. Do not serve very hot or very cold liquids.

NDx: Altered health maintenance
Explain the risk of hyperkalemia to patients with renal dysfunction and to those taking potassium-sparing diuretics (spironolactone and amiloride). Stress the importance of adhering to a potassium-restricted diet. Provide patients with both a list of high-potassium foods to be avoided and a list of low-potassium foods, which may be ingested at will. Such low-potassium foods include cranberry juice, cranberry sauce, ginger ale, root beer, sugar, honey, jelly, beans, gumdrops, butter, and margarine. Caution patients that many salt substitutes contain potassium salts. These should be used sparingly, if at all.

If the episode of hyperkalemia is related to incorrect use of diuretics or potassium supplements, review the correct administration procedure and stress its importance.

Compare the patient's status with the expected outcomes. If the outcomes are not met, reassess the patient and revise the plan.

SODIUM IMBALANCE

Sodium, the predominant extracellular cation, is essential for the conduction and transmission of nerve impulses, contraction of muscles, regulation of body fluid volumes, and regulation of the distribution and concentration of other electrolytes. The sodium-potassium pump keeps the concentration of sodium low in the ICF and high in the ECF.

Sodium, like potassium, is plentiful in the GI tract. The daily sodium requirement is 2 to 4 g. Most Americans consume 5 to 15 g per day (1 tsp of salt contains 2.3 g of sodium). Sodium levels in the body are regulated by the kidney, which can excrete excess sodium or conserve sodium under the influence of aldosterone. When sodium levels decrease, serum osmolality decreases, and secretion of ADH by the posterior pituitary is inhibited. The subsequent decrease in ADH increases excretion of water by the kidney. This results in less dilution of the sodium in the body fluids and therefore increases its concentration.

Decreases in sodium concentration are also picked up by sensors in the renal afferent arteriole. When this occurs, a series of reactions is initiated through the renin-angiotensin mechanism, resulting in increased secretion of aldosterone. This increases renal reabsorption of both sodium and water. The normal serum sodium level is 136 to 145 mEq/L or 136 to 145 mmol/L. A serum sodium level less than 136 mEq/L is called *hyponatremia*, and a serum sodium level higher than 145 mEq/L is called *hypernatremia*.

Hyponatremia

Etiology and Pathophysiology

Decreased serum sodium can result from dilution caused by excessive gain of water or excessive loss of sodium. Hyponatremia from dilution is associated with an increase in ECF volume. Causes of this dilution-induced hyponatremia include the following:

- Cardiac, renal, or hepatic failure
- Excessive irrigation of body cavities with water or other hypotonic fluids
- Near-drowning in fresh water

Excessive loss of sodium can occur in the presence of either normal or decreased ECF volume. Causes of hyponatremia with a normal ECF volume include:

- Diaphoresis with water but not electrolyte replacement
- Hyperglycemia
- Long-term use of drugs such as morphine sulfate or vincristine
- Syndrome of inappropriate antidiuretic hormone

In the syndrome of inappropriate antidiuretic hormone, excessive amounts of ADH are released from the posterior pituitary gland, which promotes increased water reabsorption in the renal tubules. The reabsorbed water dilutes the sodium concentration and causes hyponatremia. The syndrome of inappropriate antidiuretic hormone is seen in patients with head injuries and cerebrovascular accidents and for 1 or 2 days after surgery.

Hyponatremia with decreased ECF volume occurs secondary to hemorrhage, excessive wound drainage, vomiting, diarrhea, adrenal insufficiency, and use of diuretics.

The pathophysiologic effects of hyponatremia are most pronounced on excitable membranes because the movement of sodium from the ECF across the membrane to the ICF is a primary trigger of depolarization. The most common effect of hyponatremia on excitable membranes is to depress them, making them less responsive to stimuli. The excitable membranes most sensitive to hyponatremia are those in the CNS, the neuromuscular tissues, and the smooth muscle of the GI system. Tissues such as cardiac muscle that autoinitiate depolarization are basically unaffected by a decrease in serum sodium.

In some cases, CNS hyperexcitability occurs instead of or in conjunction with depression. This happens if fluid shifts into the nerve cells secondary to decreased ECF osmolality and osmotic pressure caused by the decreased sodium. This swelling of the brain can cause increased intracranial pressure, which depresses some nerve centers and stimulates others.

Clinical Manifestations

The severity of the clinical manifestations of hyponatremia varies with the speed of onset and the extent of the sodium decrease. Of these two factors, however, speed is more critical, and a patient with mild to moderate rapid-onset hyponatremia has clinical manifestations of greater severity than a patient with more severe hyponatremia of gradual onset.

The most common CNS manifestations of hyponatremia include headache, decreased attention span, drowsiness, and confusion. Less commonly, signs of hyperexcitability occur, such as apprehension, agitation, and seizures. Neurologic symptoms usually arise when serum sodium drops to 125 mEq/L or less.

Neuromuscular symptoms include generalized muscle weakness with decreased muscle tone and deep tendon hyporeflexia. Motility of the GI smooth muscle is increased, resulting in nausea, abdominal cramping, and frequent, explosive passage of watery stool.

When hyponatremia accompanies a fluid volume change, cardiovascular symptoms also occur. If hypovolemia coexists, the pulse is rapid, weak, and thready. Peripheral pulses are easily obliterated. An orthostatic progression to generalized hypotension develops. If hypervolemia coexists, pulses are full and strong and blood pressure is normal or elevated.

Urine specific gravity in hyponatremia is less than 1.003. Other renal manifestations vary with ECF volume and underlying disease. In the syndrome of inappropriate antidiuretic hormone, urinary output is decreased, accompanied by weight gain without peripheral edema.

Diagnosis

History of the health problem, laboratory findings (serum sodium level and serum osmolality), and clinical findings are used to diagnose a sodium imbalance.

The osmolality of the plasma or serum is determined mainly by the concentration of sodium. When serum sodium level is decreased, the plasma/serum osmolality is also decreased. Normal serum osmolality is 285 to 295 mOsm/kg. Serum osmolality of less than 285 mOsm/kg indicates hypo-osmolality, fluid volume excess, or hyponatremia.

Management

Oral sodium replacement is usually prescribed for mild hyponatremia resulting from excessive loss of sodium. For moderate hyponatremia, 125 mEq/L, intravenous solutions of normal saline (0.9% sodium chloride) or lactated Ringer's solution may be ordered. With severe hyponatremia, 115 mEq/L, concentrated saline solution (3% sodium chloride) is generally indicated.

If the hyponatremia is due to dilution secondary to fluid volume excess, sodium may not need to be replaced. In such cases, sodium-conserving water-excreting diuretics such as the osmotic diuretics, water restriction, and the treatment of the underlying disorder may return the serum sodium level to normal.

In the treatment of hyponatremia caused by the syndrome of inappropriate antidiuretic hormone, ADH receptor blockers or ADH antagonists may be used.

NURSING PROCESS
Hyponatremia

Assessment

Obtain a patient history to identify risk factors for hyponatremia. Note the patient's age. Question the patient about any history of renal, cardiac, or hepatic disorders. Ask about any recent episodes of vomiting, diarrhea, or fever. Ascertain what prescribed or over-the-counter medications the patient uses. Inquire specifically about diuretics, morphine, and chemotherapeutic agents.

Explore the patient's usual diet. Determine whether the patient purposefully limits salt and, if so, how. For example, determine whether the patient avoids using table salt, avoids cooking with salt, limits high-salt foods, or uses a salt substitute. Question the patient about recent activities, especially strenuous activities in a hot, humid environment in which marked diaphoresis can be expected.

Assess the patient for signs and symptoms of hyponatremia, noting time of onset of each episode. Assess neuromuscular status. Obtain baseline information on the patient's usual mental status from a family member or significant other, and ask whether any changes have been noted. Assess the patient's current orientation and alertness. Ask about headaches, drowsiness, and lethargy. Check lifts and grips to assess muscle tone. Check patellar and Achilles tendon reflexes. Auscultate for hyperactive bowel sounds and ask about nausea, cramping, and diarrhea. Question the patient about the frequency and amount of urination. Observe the color of urine and measure its specific gravity. Assess cardiovascular status. Check apical rate, blood pressure, peripheral pulses, and venous filling capacity. Observe for edema.

Nursing Diagnoses and Planning

Nursing diagnoses and related expected patient outcomes commonly applicable to patients with varying degrees of hyponatremia include the following:

NDx: Diarrhea related to increased GI motility

Planning: Patient Outcomes
1. Stool is formed.
2. Frequency of defecation is consistent with patient's normal pattern.
3. Perianal area remains free of irritation.

NDx: Risk for injury related to potential altered thought processes and muscle weakness

Planning: Patient Outcomes
1. Patient complies with safety precautions.
2. Patient remains free of injury.

NDx: Pain (headache) related to increased intracranial pressure secondary to intracellular edema

Planning: Patient Outcomes
1. Patient complies with position restrictions.
2. Patient reports relief of headache.

NDx: Risk for altered health maintenance related to lack of knowledge of dietary sodium and water requirements

Planning: Patient Outcomes
1. Patient describes need for increased dietary sodium.
2. Patient identifies foods high in sodium.
3. Patient affirms plan to ingest needed daily sodium.

Nursing Interventions and Evaluation

Administer saline infusions per physician's order. Use a controller or pump to control the rate because too rapid administration can cause serious problems as a result of overresponse of excitable membranes. In general, the rate of replacement of sodium should parallel the rate of loss.

Monitor the patient for signs and symptoms of fluid volume excess when the patient is receiving saline solutions, especially concentrated saline solutions.

Administer diuretics as ordered. Record intake and output and monitor the patient closely for signs and symptoms of excessive loss of fluid or potassium. Also monitor for signs and symptoms of too rapid or excessive sodium increase.

NDx: Diarrhea

Explain to the patient or significant other that diarrhea will be relieved as sodium is replaced. Assist the patient onto the bedpan or to the bathroom promptly. Protect the perianal skin by gentle washing with mild soap and warm water. Apply a skin-barrier ointment. If perianal irritation develops despite precautions, apply witch hazel compresses or topical anesthetic ointment. Record the time, amount, and characteristics of stool passed.

NDx: Risk for injury

Protect the patient from injury that may result from muscle weakness or confusion. Keep the side rails up when the patient is in bed. Provide assistance and supervision when the patient is out of bed. Keep the call bell within reach. Also keep personal items within reach to limit the need for reaching or getting out of the bed or chair. Provide a quiet environment free of unnecessary stimuli, because the patient with hyponatremia is abnormally sensitive to sensory input. Remove the telephone and eliminate loud noise from the television, radio, and the like. Reorient the patient to time and place with each interaction if needed.

NDx: Pain

Administer analgesics for headache as ordered. Keep in mind that morphine aggravates the syndrome of inappropriate antidiuretic hormone and should be avoided if this is the cause of the hyponatremia. Keep the head of the bed elevated to promote venous return from the brain. Also instruct the patient to avoid bending over, because it increases intracranial pressure.

NDx: Risk for altered health maintenance

The patient who is losing abnormal amounts of sodium but on a regular diet should be instructed to ingest daily fluids and foods high in sodium. Provide a list of dietary sources of sodium, including condiments. Suggest nutritious, sodium-rich snacks that are easy to prepare and ingest, such as tomato juice, saltine crackers, and beef bouillon. Advise the patient against drinking plain water.

If fluids are also restricted, explain why. Encourage the patient to plan a spaced pattern of fluid intake over each 24-hour period to avoid ingesting the entire amount of fluids permitted early in the day, thus leaving a period of thirst. Teach patients to monitor intake and output.

Compare the patient's status with the expected outcomes. If the outcomes are not met, reassess the patient and revise the plan.

Hypernatremia

Etiology and Pathophysiology

Hypernatremia develops as a result of either excessive sodium in the body or concentration of normal amounts of sodium because of the loss of water. Excessive sodium in the body can be due to excessive intake or to decreased renal excretion. Sources of excessive intake include sodium chloride in foods, sodium bicarbonate preparations, and sodium-containing parenteral fluids. Causes of decreased renal excretion include renal insufficiency, hyperaldosteronism, Cushing's disease, and the use of cortical steroids. Hypernatremia from concentration of sodium resulting from the loss of water can be caused by decreased fluid intake or increased water loss. Causes of increased water loss include excessive diaphoresis, hyperventilation, pyrexia, diarrhea, and osmotic diuresis.

An increase in serum sodium results in a greater concentration gradient for sodium between the ECF and the ICF. This means that sodium passes more easily across excitable membranes and thus initiates depolarization more quickly and in response to less intense stimuli (the excitable membranes become irritable). As hypernatremia worsens, however, the opposite effect sets in. Water moves out of the cells into the ECF in an attempt to dilute the sodium concentration, and this leaves the cells dehydrated and excitable membranes nonresponsive to stimuli. The excitable membranes most sensitive to these changes are those of the brain, skeletal muscle, cardiac muscle, and smooth muscle.

Clinical Manifestations

Symptoms of hypernatremia depend on the severity and speed of the sodium increase and the presence or absence of a coexisting volume imbalance. Mental status changes that occur with hypernatremia in the presence of normal or decreased fluid volumes include shortened attention span, lack of concentration, hypersensitivity to sensory stimuli, agitation, confusion, and even convulsions.

When hypernatremia accompanies increased fluid volume, mental activity is depressed, and lethargy, drowsiness, stupor, and coma can occur. Changes in skeletal muscles proceed from twitching and spasms with mild levels of hypernatremia to weakness with hyporeflexia and even rigid paralysis as the hypernatremia worsens.

The effect of hypernatremia on cardiac muscle is generally depressive, manifested by decreased contractility and decreased cardiac output. Pulse and blood pressure vary with fluid volume changes as described for hyponatremia. Changes in the skin that occur with hypernatremia also vary with fluid volume status. When ECF volume is decreased, the skin is pale and has poor turgor. With increased ECF volume, color ranges from pale to flushed and turgor is increased. The skin does not pinch up and pressure leaves depressions that are very slow to disappear. In all cases, the skin is dry and flaky.

Renal changes also occur as a result of hypernatremia. Urinary output is decreased, and the urine is concentrated (specific gravity greater than 1.030) and is marked by a strong odor.

Diagnosis

History, clinical findings, serum sodium, and serum osmolality all contribute to the diagnosis of hypernatremia. Serum sodium levels higher than 145 mEq/L indicate hypernatremia. A serum osmolality higher than 295 mOsm/kg indicates hyperosmolality, fluid volume deficit, and hypernatremia.

Management

Management of hypernatremia depends on its severity as well as the underlying cause. Dietary restriction of sodium, often in conjunction with water restriction, can prevent hypernatremia when renal excretion of sodium is impaired and can prevent existing hypernatremia from worsening. It cannot rapidly lower serum sodium levels. Loop diuretics (furosemide and ethacrynic acid), which are sodium-excreting, are used to increase renal excretion of sodium and therefore lower serum levels if renal function allows. If hypernatremia results from fluid loss, parenteral administration of glucose and water can restore volume, thus diluting sodium concentration and returning serum sodium to a normal range.

NURSING PROCESS
Hypernatremia

Assessment

Obtain a patient history to identify risk factors for hypernatremia. Question the patient about any history of renal disease, adrenal disease, or recent episodes of fever, vomiting, diarrhea, or diaphoresis. Assess for factors that might indicate difficulty maintaining oral fluid intake. Note the patient's age and mental and mobility status. Ascertain what prescribed or over-the-counter medications the patient takes. Specifically, explore the use of osmotic diuretics as well as drugs that contain sodium, such as cortisone preparations, certain antibiotics, cough syrups, and cold medications. Also explore the patient's dietary intake of sodium. Identify usual intake of high-sodium foods, including processed and canned foods, fluids, and condiments. Establish fluid intake for the past 24 hours, noting both the type and the amount of ingested fluids. Also establish the frequency and amount of urinary output.

Assess the patient for signs and symptoms of hypernatremia, noting the time of onset of each episode. Assess neuromuscular status. Ask about the presence of insomnia, irritability, agitation, muscle twitches, or convulsions. Observe for signs of confusion or inability to maintain attention. Assess for signs of late or severe hypernatremia and hyperkalemia. Check for hypoactive, deep tendon reflexes.

Check lifts and grips to assess muscle weakness. Observe for lethargy.

Assess cardiovascular status. Measure blood pressure and heart rate. Check the quality of peripheral pulses. Observe the neck veins for distention. Observe for dry, flaky skin, and inspect the oral mucous membranes for dryness. Check skin turgor and note skin color. Measure urinary output, and note the color and odor of the urine.

Review serum sodium and osmolality values. Remember that doubling the serum sodium level gives an estimate of the serum osmolality value.

Nursing Diagnoses and Planning

Nursing diagnoses and related expected patient outcomes commonly applicable to patients with varying degrees of hypernatremia include the following:

NDx: Risk for injury related to altered sensorium

Planning: Patient Outcomes
1. Patient complies with safety measures
2. Patient remains free of injury.

NDx: Altered nutrition: more than body requirements related to excessive sodium intake

Planning: Patient Outcomes
1. Patient states reason for sodium-restricted diet.
2. Patient identifies sources of dietary sodium to be avoided.
3. Patient selects and plans low-sodium meals and snacks.

Nursing Interventions and Evaluation

NDx: Risk for injury
Protect the patient from injury that may be caused by muscle weakness, confusion, or convulsions. Keep the side rails up, the bed low, and the call bell within reach. Provide assistance with moving and self-care activities. If the patient is confused, reorient at each interaction. To decrease CNS stimulation and the risk of seizures, maintain a calm, quiet environment. Eliminate bright lights, loud noises, and sudden movement. Pad the side rails to guard against injury if a seizure occurs.

NDx: Altered nutrition: more than body requirements
Explain the role of dietary sodium in hypernatremia. Stress the importance of adhering to a sodium-restricted diet. Discuss sources of ingested sodium with the patient, and provide a list of high-sodium foods to be avoided. These include canned foods, lunch meats, ham, pork, pickles, potato chips, and pretzels. Caution the patient to avoid using salt when cooking or eating.

Compare the patient's status with the expected outcomes. If the outcomes are not met, reassess the patient and revise the plan.

CALCIUM IMBALANCE

Calcium is an extracellular and intracellular electrolyte with many functions. It is essential for the following:

1. Transmission of nerve impulses and contraction of the skeletal, smooth, and cardiac muscles
2. Maintenance of cellular permeability
3. Formation of teeth and bones
4. Coagulation of blood

Approximately 55% of serum calcium is bound to albumin, and 45% is free ionized calcium. The free calcium is physiologically active and affected by pH. During acidosis (decreased pH), more calcium is ionized even if the serum calcium level is decreased. During alkalosis (increased pH), there is a decrease in free ionized calcium.

Normally, the total serum calcium level is 4.5 to 5.5 mEq/L or 9 to 11 mg/dL. The ionized calcium level is 2.2 to 2.5 mEq/L or 4.25 to 5.25 mg/dL. The serum calcium result given in laboratory reports is the combined ionized and nonionized calcium. A decreased serum calcium level, less than 4.5 mEq/L or 9 mg/dL, is called *hypocalcemia*, and an increased serum calcium level, more than 5.5 mEq/L or 11 mg/dL, is called *hypercalcemia*.

Vitamin D promotes calcium absorption from the GI tract, and phosphorus inhibits calcium absorption. The physiologic relationship of calcium and phosphorus is inverse. Both calcium and phosphorus are stored in bone and excreted by the kidneys. When the serum calcium level is increased, the serum phosphorus level is decreased. Parathyroid hormone (PTH) maintains the serum calcium level; however, PTH and vitamin D promote calcium movement from the bone to the vascular fluid, causing an increase in the serum calcium level. Phosphorus and calcitonin (from the thyroid gland) promote calcium return to the bone, causing a decrease in serum calcium level.

Hypocalcemia

Etiology and Pathophysiology

Calcium deficit, or hypocalcemia, usually occurs from decreased absorption of calcium from the GI tract, decreased release of calcium from the bone, increased calcium binding to albumin (less free calcium), or increased loss of calcium by urine excretion. With renal failure, the serum calcium level is decreased and the serum phosphorus level is increased.

Decreased absorption from the GI tract can result from inadequate intake of calcium or vitamin D, lactase deficiency, Crohn's disease, or other malabsorption disorders. A decrease in the release of calcium from bone may result from lack of PTH. This can occur as a result of a loss of parathyroid tissue secondary to thyroidectomy or radiation. It can also be the result of neck injury. An increase in protein-bound calcium, and therefore a decrease in the ionized fraction of calcium, can be the result of hyperproteinemia, alkalosis, calcium chelates or binders such as citrate (found in blood transfusions), and acute pancreatitis. Because citrate is a chelating agent that binds ionized calcium, temporary hypocalcemia may occur as a result of massive administration of citrated blood. Drugs that can decrease serum calcium levels include the following:

Glucocorticoids
Heparin
Loop diuretics such as furosemide
Glucagon
Mithramycin
Sodium nitroprusside
Theophylline

Infusion of phosphate and sulfate salts can decrease calcium. Calcium can also be lost through diarrhea, steatorrhea, and wound drainage.

There is a correlation between calcium and magnesium. Usually with a magnesium deficit, there is a calcium deficit. Hypomagnesemia (serum magnesium deficit) can cause a decrease in PTH secretion. A PTH deficiency affects the bone, thus causing hypocalcemia. Also, magnesium deficit can cause a decrease in vitamin D metabolites, which impairs calcium absorption from the intestine.

Calcium normally acts as a sedative on nervous tissue. Consequently, hypocalcemia leads to nervous irritability. Decreased serum calcium levels increase permeability of excitable membranes to sodium. As a result, the membrane is more readily depolarized and an action potential is easily generated. Tissues most affected by hypocalcemia are peripheral nerves, skeletal muscles, and GI smooth muscle (whose actions are stimulated) and cardiac muscle (whose contractions are depressed). Prolonged hypocalcemia leads to osteoporosis. A marked or prolonged decrease in serum calcium can interfere with the conversion of prothrombin to thrombin and thus impair clotting.

Clinical Manifestations

The most common clinical manifestation of hypocalcemia (decreased ionized calcium) is tetany. This is a condition resulting from the excitability of peripheral nerves and muscles characterized by tingling and numbness of the extremities, muscle twitching, cramps, carpopedal spasm, laryngeal spasm, and convulsions. Typically, the onset of tetany is heralded by paresthesias (numbness and tingling) of the hands and feet. As the condition progresses, carpopedal spasm, twitching of the mouth, and sustained contraction of individual muscle groups can lead to convulsions, respiratory paralysis, and death. Tetany does not occur with metabolic acidosis, even when the serum calcium level is decreased, because more albumin-bound calcium is freed as the pH is decreased. It is when the acidotic state is corrected and calcium rebinds with protein that tetany symptoms might occur.

Other clinical manifestations of hypocalcemia include diarrhea resulting from increased intestinal motility, restlessness, and lack of concentration. Marked hypocalcemia may also result in a weak, slightly more rapid heartbeat.

Diagnosis

The diagnosis of hypocalcemia is based on history, laboratory results, and clinical findings. A serum calcium level less than 4.5 mEq/L and 9 mg/dL indicates hypocalcemia.

Tetany resulting from a decrease in free ionized calcium can be confirmed by a positive Chvostek's test and positive Trousseau's test (Fig. 5–5). Chvostek's test involves tapping the patient's face over the facial nerve (2 cm anterior to the ear lobe). If the facial muscle twitches, the test is positive. Trousseau's test involves inflating a blood pressure cuff on the upper arm to slightly above the systolic presence to constrict circulation. If carpal spasm (palmar flexion) of the hand occurs after 1 to 5 minutes, the test is positive.

Management

Acute hypocalcemia requires immediate medical intervention. Calcium gluconate or calcium chloride is given intravenously to correct it. Calcium chloride provides more ionized calcium than calcium gluconate. However, it is more irritating to the subcutaneous tissue. Also, if calcium chloride infiltrates, sloughing of the tissue results. If 10% calcium gluconate (10–20 mL) is prescribed, the solution should be given slowly, 2 mL/min. For a severe calcium deficit, intravenous 10% calcium gluconate (100 mL) can be administered in a liter of D_5W over 4 hours.

In cases of mild hypocalcemia, oral calcium supplements (calcium carbonate, calcium gluconate, or calcium lactate) are prescribed. Calcium carbonate may cause GI upset due to carbon dioxide forma-

tion. For best absorption, these supplements are taken $\frac{1}{2}$ hour before meals.

Aluminum hydroxide is sometimes used to treat hypocalcemia because it decreases serum phosphorus, which in turn increases serum calcium. Magnesium preparations are also used because an increase in serum magnesium may result in an increase in serum calcium. Vitamin D may be prescribed in an effort to increase the absorption of calcium from the GI tract.

NURSING PROCESS
Hypocalcemia

Assessment

Question the patient about any history of health problems that can cause hypocalcemia. Ask about hypoparathyroidism, previous thyroidectomy, radiation, or injury to the neck. Question the patient about any chronic diarrhea, and check for overuse of laxatives or antacids. Obtain a dietary history to assess intake of calcium and vitamin D. Question the patient about usual intake of dairy products, legumes, and other foods rich in calcium and vitamin D. Also question the patient about the use of calcium and vitamin D supplements. Determine the patient's activity level and the usual amount of exposure of the skin to sunlight.

Assess for signs and symptoms of hypocalcemia such as the following:

Numbness and tingling in the hands or feet
Carpopedal spasm
Twitching of the mouth
Laryngeal spasm
Abdominal cramping
Hyperactive bowel sounds
Diarrhea
Rapid, weak pulse
Bleeding tendencies

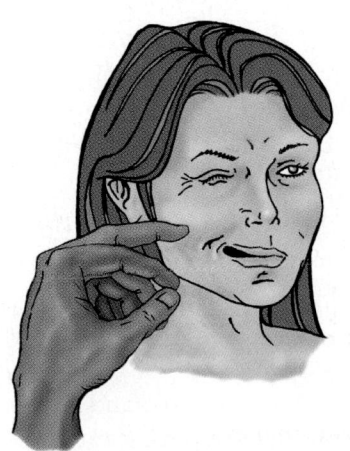

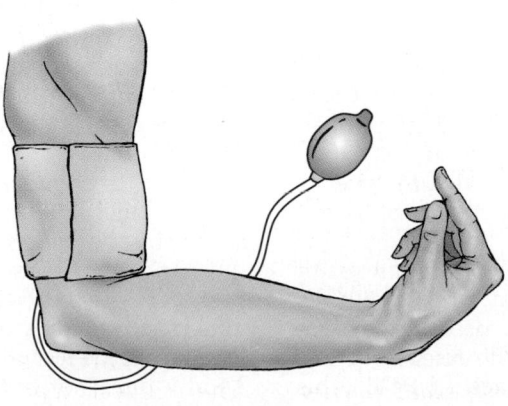

A   B

Figure 5–5

Manifestations of hypocalcemia. *A,* Positive Chvostek's sign. A tap on the facial nerve anterior to the ear lobe below the zygomatic process causes muscles supplied by the facial nerve to spasm. *B,* Positive Trousseau's sign. Carpal spasm occurs when compression of the upper arm causes ischemia to the distal nerves.

Check for positive Chvostek's and Trousseau's signs. Review serum calcium levels.

Nursing Diagnoses and Planning

Nursing diagnoses and related expected patient outcomes commonly applicable to patients with **acute** hypocalcemia include the following:

NDx: Risk for injury related to tetany secondary to hypocalcemia

Planning: Patient Outcomes
1. Serum calcium level returns to normal range.
2. Signs of skeletal muscle hyperexcitability are absent.

Nursing diagnoses and related expected patient outcomes commonly applicable to patients with **chronic** hypocalcemia include the following:

NDx: Altered nutrition: less than body requirements related to inadequate intake of calcium or vitamin D

Planning: Patient Outcomes
1. Patient reports adequate dietary intake of calcium.
2. Signs and symptoms of calcium deficit are absent.
3. Serum calcium is within normal range.

Nursing Interventions and Evaluation

NDx: Risk for injury
Administer intravenous calcium replacement as prescribed. Mix calcium for intravenous administration in D_5W instead of saline solution, because sodium promotes calcium loss. Do not add calcium to solutions containing bicarbonate because rapid precipitation will occur. Administer intravenous calcium solutions slowly whenever the patient's condition permits. During administration, monitor for positive Chvostek's and Trousseau's signs every 15 minutes and check serum calcium levels hourly. Monitor the infusion site for infiltration every 15 minutes, and monitor the ECG continuously if possible. Keep in mind that with hypocalcemia, the ST segments and the QT intervals are prolonged.

Because any stimulation of the neuromuscular condition can worsen the tetanic condition, control environmental stimuli. If Chvostek's and Trousseau's signs are positive, maintain the patient on complete bedrest in a quiet, darkened room. Avoid unnecessarily touching the patient and protect against loud noises, bright lights, and sudden position changes. Avoid accidentally bumping the patient's bed, turn off the telephone ringer, eliminate access to television, and limit visitors. Maintain seizure precautions. Keep the side rails up and padded and keep the bed in its lowest position. Have oxygen, suction, ventilation (Ambu) bag, and tracheostomy tray readily available at the patient's bedside.

NDx: Altered nutrition: less than body requirements
Suggest that the patient consume foods high in calcium, such as milk, milk products, and protein. Pro-tein enhances calcium absorption. Administer oral calcium supplements before or after meals.

Monitor pulse regularly if the patient is receiving a digitalis preparation in addition to calcium supplements. Calcium excess enhances the action of digitalis and can cause digitalis toxicity, which is characterized by nausea, vomiting, anorexia, bradycardia, cardiac dysrhythmias, and visual changes.

Additional Interventions
Instruct the patient to avoid overuse of antacids and to avoid chronic laxative use. Chronic use of laxatives decreases calcium absorption from the GI tract. Suggest fruits, foods rich in fiber, plenty of fluids, and exercise for improving bowel elimination. Excessive use of certain antacids can cause alkalosis, decreasing calcium ionization. In addition, many antacids contain magnesium, which can lower the serum calcium level. Many laxatives contain phosphates (phosphorus), which have an opposing effect on calcium, causing calcium loss.

Compare the patient's status with the expected outcomes. If the outcomes are not met, reassess the patient and revise the plan.

Hypercalcemia

Etiology and Pathophysiology
Calcium excess, or hypercalcemia, can result from increased absorption, decreased excretion, or increased resorption of calcium from bone. Increased absorption can occur secondary to excessive oral intake of either calcium or vitamin D. Decreased excretion can be due to renal failure or the use of thiazide diuretics (hydrochlorothiazide [Hydro-DIURIL]). Increased resorption from bone can be caused by prolonged immobilization, bone-destroying cancer, hyperparathyroidism, and use of glucocorticoids. Fractures also release calcium into the vascular fluid, thus increasing the serum calcium level.

Increased levels of calcium in ECF (hypercalcemia) decrease the permeability of excitable membranes to sodium. This means that the membranes are less easily depolarized, and action potentials are less easily generated. Depression or decreased irritability of the excitable membrane is the result. Excitable membranes most sensitive to this effect of hypercalcemia are found in cardiac muscle, skeletal muscle, smooth muscle of the GI tract, and peripheral and CNS tissue.

Hypercalcemia also affects many enzyme systems within the body, including those involved in blood clotting. The effect of hypercalcemia on the latter is to decrease clotting time, thus predisposing to excessive clot formation, particularly in areas of slow blood flow.

Clinical Manifestations
The clinical manifestations of hypercalcemia are most pronounced in systems containing excitable membranes easily depressed by the increase in cal-

cium. The severity of the clinical manifestations is generally a function of both the amount of calcium increase and the speed with which it occurs. The greater the increase and the faster it develops, the more severe the symptoms. Rapid onset of mild hypercalcemia may present with more serious clinical manifestations than the gradual onset of a more marked hypercalcemia.

Clinical manifestations of hypercalcemia related to the GI tract include decreased peristalsis, anorexia, nausea, constipation, abdominal distention, and decreased bowel sounds. Effects of hypercalcemia on neuromuscular function include:

Weak, flabby muscles
Diminished or absent deep tendon reflexes
Lack of coordination
Slurred speech
Lethargy
Memory lapses
Depression
Confusion, psychotic behavior, or coma in severe cases

In the heart, effects on both muscle function and electrical conduction occur. These result in:

Tachycardia
Elevated blood pressure
Full, bounding peripheral pulses
A shortened QT interval and prolonged PR interval on ECG

With severe hypercalcemia, ventricular dysrhythmia, bradycardia, and even cardiac standstill can occur. Hypercalcemia also affects renal function. The increased extracellular calcium results in polyuria, which in turn can lead to dehydration. Renal calculi (kidney stones) characterized by flank pain can also develop as a result of the precipitation of excess calcium.

Hypercalcemic crisis occurs when serum calcium levels reach 16 to 17 mg/dL. Clinical manifestations include severe thirst, polyuria, altered levels of consciousness (confusion to coma), nausea, vomiting, and severe abdominal pain. Correction of hypercalcemic crisis is a medical emergency.

Diagnosis

The diagnosis of hypercalcemia is suggested by history and clinical findings. Diagnosis is confirmed by a serum calcium level higher than 5.5 mEq/L and 11 mg/dL.

Management

Medical management of hypercalcemia aims to promote calcium excretion while limiting sources of external calcium. No intravenous fluids containing calcium (eg, calcium gluconate) are administered. All thiazide diuretics, antacids containing calcium, calcium supplements, and vitamin supplements are discontinued. To promote calcium excretion, intravenous isotonic saline may be given both to dilute the ECF and to provide sodium, which inhibits the tu-

bular resorption of calcium. Loop diuretics such as furosemide (Lasix), which enhance calcium excretion, can be given. Calcium binders or chelates, such as the cytotoxic antibiotic mithramycin (plicamycin), can be given as well. Drugs that inhibit calcium resorption from bone can also be administered, such as calcitonin (Calcimar) and prostaglandin inhibitors (aspirin and nonsteroidal anti-inflammatory drugs). In acute cases of hypercalcemia, dialysis can be performed to quickly lower the serum calcium level.

NURSING PROCESS
Hypercalcemia

Assessment

Question the patient about any history of health problems associated with hypercalcemia, such as cancer, hyperparathyroidism, immobility, hyperthyroidism, and renal failure. Ask about the patient's use of medications that could affect calcium levels, such as glucocorticoids, thiazide diuretics, calcium or vitamin D supplements, and antacids. Explore the usual daily intake of milk and other dairy products.

Assess for signs and symptoms of hypercalcemia. Review serum calcium levels. Ask the patient about anorexia, nausea, and constipation. Assess for abdominal distention and listen to bowel sounds. Assess muscle tone, strength, and deep tendon reflexes. Observe for coordination and check orientation. Question a family member or significant other about the patient's usual level of alertness, interest, and activity to establish a basis for assessment of mental status changes.

Assess cardiac status. Observe for changes in heart rate and rhythm and review ECG strips for changes in the QT interval. Measure urinary output and question the patient about symptoms of renal calculi. Assess for factors leading to slow or impaired blood flow, because the patient with hyperglycemia is prone to blood clots. Note the time of onset of all reported symptoms.

Nursing Diagnoses and Planning

Nursing diagnoses and related expected patient outcomes commonly applicable to patients with hypercalcemia include the following:

NDx: Constipation related to decreased intestinal motility

Planning: Patient Outcomes
1. Patient defecates at regular intervals.
2. Stool is soft and moist.
3. Patient defecates without straining.

NDx: Risk for injury related to muscle weakness, incoordination, memory lapses, and confusion

Planning: Patient Outcomes
1. Patient complies with safety precautions.
2. Patient remains free of injury.

Nursing Interventions and Evaluation

Discontinue all calcium-containing parenteral fluids and oral medications per physician's order. Administer diuretics that enhance calcium excretion or drugs that inhibit calcium resorption from bone as ordered. Promote active and passive exercises for the bedridden patient to decrease calcium loss from the bone. Instruct the patient to avoid foods high in calcium and to increase fluid intake to dilute calcium in the serum and decrease the risk of urinary calculi.

NDx: Constipation

Explain the role of elevated serum calcium in causing constipation. Reassure the patient that, as serum calcium returns to normal, bowel function will as well. Within the limits of any dietary restrictions, encourage a high-fiber diet and the consumption of 2500 mL of fluid or more daily. When possible, have the patient use a toilet or commode rather than a bedpan. Always provide privacy.

Encourage physical activity, whether it be bed exercises or ambulation, to promote bowel function. Administer drugs to stimulate GI activity as ordered.

NDx: Risk for injury

Institute measures to protect the patient from falls or other injuries that may result from muscle weakness, incoordination, or changes in mental status. Keep the side rails of the bed up and the call bell within easy reach. Provide assistance and supervision when the patient is out of bed. Keep personal or other items the patient may want within reach to discourage leaning over the side rails and attempting to get up without assistance. If the patient is confused, reorient at each interaction.

Compare the patient's status with the expected outcomes. If the outcomes are not met, reassess the patient and revise the plan.

MAGNESIUM IMBALANCE

Magnesium is the second most plentiful intracellular cation. Like other cations, magnesium promotes the transmission and conduction of nerve impulses and the contraction of skeletal, smooth, and cardiac muscle. Additional functions of magnesium include:

- Activating enzymes for carbohydrate and protein metabolism
- Influencing utilization of potassium, calcium, and protein
- Exerting a sedative action on the CNS
- Directly affecting peripheral arteries by producing vasodilation

More than 50% of the magnesium in an adult's body is in bone. Vitamin D and its metabolites enhance intestinal absorption of magnesium but to a lesser degree than calcium absorption.

The normal serum magnesium level is 1.5 to 2.5 mEq/L or 1.8 to 3.0 mg/dL. One-third of the serum magnesium is bound to protein, and the remaining two-thirds is free ionized circulating magnesium (physiologically active magnesium). Therefore the serum magnesium level must be evaluated along with serum albumin levels. A serum magnesium level less than 1.5 mEq/L or 1.8 mg/dL is called *hypomagnesemia* (magnesium deficit). A serum magnesium level more than 2.5 mEq/L or 3.0 mg/dL is known as *hypermagnesemia* (magnesium excess). Magnesium is absorbed primarily from the distal small intestine and is excreted by the kidneys. A decreased serum calcium level promotes magnesium absorption, while the kidneys conserve magnesium when intake magnesium is decreased.

The minimum daily adult requirement for magnesium is an average of 250 mg (200–300 mg); for an infant, it is 150 mg. Foods rich in magnesium include green vegetables, dairy products, chocolate, seafood, whole grains, beans, and nuts.

Hypomagnesemia

Etiology and Pathophysiology

Hypomagnesemia can result from decreased absorption of dietary magnesium or from an increase in the amount of magnesium excreted by the kidneys. Causes of decreased absorption include:

Inadequate intake
Chronic alcoholism with or without cirrhosis
Prolonged gastric suction
Severe diarrhea
Prolonged intravenous or hyperalimentation therapy without magnesium replacement
Loss of absorbing surface resulting from distal small-bowel resection or destruction of the distal mucosa, as in ileitis
Excessive phosphorus in the GI tract

Hypomagnesemia resulting from an increase in renal excretion of magnesium can be due to the effect of drugs such as thiazide and loop diuretics, osmotic diuretics, aminoglycosides, amphotericin B, and some antineoplastic agents such as cisplatin. It can also occur with diabetic ketoacidosis because of diuresis resulting from concentrated blood glucose, hypoparathyroidism, and primary aldosteronism.

With moderate to severe magnesium deficit, symptomatic hypocalcemia can occur. Hypomagnesemia can occur with hypercalcemia due to hyperparathyroidism or malignant tumors that have metastasized to the bone, releasing calcium.

Decreased magnesium in the ECF results in an increased release of acetylcholine from the presynaptic membrane. This increases impulse transmission from nerve to nerve or nerve to muscle and thus increases neuromuscular irritability.

Clinical Manifestations

Neuromuscular clinical manifestations of hypomagnesemia and related changes in calcium and potas-

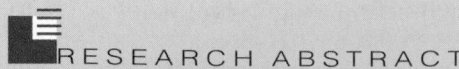

RESEARCH ABSTRACT

What Role Do Electrolytes Play in Regulating Blood Pressure in Older Adults?

Geleijnse JM, Witteman JCM, den Breeijen JH, et al. Dietary electrolyte intake and blood pressure in older subjects: The Rotterdam study. J Hypertension 1996; 14(6):737.

It is an established fact that diet plays an important part in the management of blood pressure problems. The researchers in this study wanted to focus on the role that certain electrolytes (potassium, magnesium, and calcium) play in regulating blood pressure in older adults.

The subjects were a large group of older adults (>55 years) who lived in the suburb of a large city. For a 1-year period, Geleijnse and colleagues assessed the subjects for medical history, use of cardiovascular medications, and foods consumed. The researchers also periodically recorded the blood pressure measurements of the subjects.

The researchers found a strong correlation between increased levels of potassium and magnesium and decreases in both systolic and diastolic blood pressure in the older adults studied. There was also a similar lowering of diastolic blood pressure in pa-

tients already diagnosed with hypertension who increased their intake of calcium.

The overall recommendation of the researchers was that older adults should increase their intake of foods high in potassium and magnesium as part of a healthy diet to help lower blood pressure.

Questions to Consider

1. What are the dietary recommendations supported by the Joint National Committee for the detection, evaluation, and treatment of hypertension?
2. What is the clinical picture of a patient with elevated levels of calcium, magnesium, or potassium? Depressed levels? What observations and interventions are appropriate?
3. Plan a 2-day diet for a patient who needs to increase intake of calcium, magnesium, or potassium, or a combination of these.

sium levels include hyperactive reflexes, tremors, muscle spasms, positive Chvostek's and Trousseau's signs, tetany, generalized tonic-clonic seizures, and, in some cases, depression, agitation or confusion. Hypomagnesemia is also associated with hypertension and cardiac dysrhythmias, such as premature ventricular contractions and ventricular fibrillation. ECG changes are similar to those found with hypokalemia. The T wave is flat or inverted, the ST segment is depressed, and the QRS complex is widened. Hypomagnesemia also enhances the action of digitalis, which can lead to digitalis toxicity.

Diagnosis

Hypomagnesemia often goes unrecognized because serum magnesium tests are rarely ordered. In addition, symptoms usually do not occur until the serum level drops to 1.0 mEq/L or 1.2 mg/dL or lower. ECG changes suggest hypomagnesemia when combined with other findings.

A urine magnesium tolerance test is an accurate method to determine magnesium imbalance. If there is a greater than 25% retention of IV magnesium load present in 24 hours, this could indicate a probable magnesium deficit. A greater than 50% retention of IV magnesium load in 24 hours can indicate hypomagnesemia.

Management

Mild hypomagnesemia can be corrected by a diet high in magnesium-containing foods, such as green vegetables, nuts, legumes, chocolate, bananas, oranges, and grapefruit. Supplementary oral magne-

sium sulfate is also available. For moderate magnesium deficit, 1 to 2 g of intramuscular 50% magnesium sulfate solution may be prescribed every 8 hours. Oral or intramuscular magnesium salts should be given in divided doses to prevent diarrhea. If the deficiency is severe, intravenous magnesium salts are diluted in 100 mL or more of intravenous fluid.

It may take 3 to 4 days before a magnesium deficit is corrected. Magnesium can restore calcium levels in patients with hypocalcemic hypomagnesemic imbalance. Magnesium therapy can increase parathyroid hormone secretion, which normalizes serum calcium levels.

NURSING PROCESS
Hypomagnesemia

Assessment

Assess the patient for risk factors for hypomagnesemia. Be certain to check dietary intake of magnesium. If the patient has been receiving prolonged intravenous or hyperalimentation therapy, determine whether magnesium supplements have been provided. Also assess for symptoms of hypomagnesemia, such as muscle tumors, twitching, spasms, hyper-reflexia, and cardiac dysrhythmias. Check the ECG for flat or inverted T waves and widened QRS complexes, which are associated with both hypomagnesemia and hypokalemia.

Nursing Diagnoses and Planning

Nursing diagnoses and related expected patient outcomes commonly applicable to patients with hypomagnesemia include the following:

NDx: Risk for injury related to neuromuscular excitability

Planning: Patient Outcomes
1. Patient remains free of injury.

NDx: Altered nutrition: less than body requirements related to intake of magnesium

Planning: Patient Outcomes
1. Patient describes the importance of adequate dietary magnesium for health.
2. Patient identifies foods rich in magnesium.
3. Patient states the intent to incorporate recommended amounts of these foods into the daily diet.

Nursing Interventions and Evaluation

NDx: Risk for injury
If the patient is confused, institute safety precautions as for the patient with hypernatremia. Institute seizure precautions if the magnesium deficit is marked.

NDx: Altered nutrition: less than body requirements
Administer oral or intravenous magnesium sulfate as ordered. If the oral drug is given, monitor the patient for diarrhea, a common side effect that may exacerbate a magnesium deficit. If the intravenous drug is ordered, administer it slowly to prevent a hot or flushed feeling. Monitor vital signs.

Explain to the patient the need for magnesium in the daily diet. Identify foods that are rich in magnesium, such as meat, green vegetables, seafood, whole grains, and nuts. Provide the patient with a list of these foods, and assist in planning how to incorporate adequate amounts of them into the daily diet.

Additional Interventions
Because the patient with a magnesium deficit is at risk for dysphagia, use water to check the patient's ability to swallow before giving other oral fluids, medications, or foods. If the patient is taking digitalis, assess for symptoms of toxicity (bradycardia, nausea, vomiting, and visual disturbances), because hypomagnesemia enhances the action of digitalis.

Compare the patient's status with the expected outcomes. If the outcomes are not met, reassess the patient and revise the plan.

Hypermagnesemia

Etiology and Pathophysiology
Hypermagnesemia results most often from renal insufficiency. It can also occur as a result of severe dehydration, untreated diabetic ketoacidosis, and excessive use of magnesium-containing laxatives (magnesium sulfate, milk of magnesia, and citrate solutions) or antacids (Maalox, Mylanta, Di-Gel, Aludrox).

Increased serum magnesium inhibits the release of acetylcholine at the neuromuscular junction and depresses the excitability of nerve fibers.

Clinical Manifestations
Mild hypermagnesemia is characterized by vasodilatation with flushing and sweating and resultant hypotension. Bradycardia and ECG changes consisting of a peaked T wave, prolonged PR intervals, and broad QRS complex also develop.

Other symptoms that develop as the magnesium level continues to increase include drowsiness, lethargy, muscle weakness, loss of deep tendon reflexes, and paralysis. Respiratory depression, coma, and cardiac standstill can ultimately occur.

Diagnosis
A serum magnesium level higher than 2.5 mEq/L or 3.0 mg/dL is diagnostic of hypermagnesemia. In the absence of serum levels, characteristic ECG changes suggest the diagnosis when combined with other findings.

Management
When possible, medical management of hypermagnesemia aims to correct the underlying cause, thereby decreasing serum magnesium and preventing further increases. When renal failure is the underlying problem, dialysis may be necessary to return serum magnesium to normal levels. In acute situations, intravenous calcium, which is an antagonist to magnesium, may be given to control symptoms. Excess parenteral magnesium infusion can be reversed with administration of intravenous calcium salt.

NURSING PROCESS
Hypermagnesemia

Assessment

Assess the patient for risk factors of hypermagnesemia. Check for a history of renal insufficiency or failure and for chronic use of laxatives or antacids containing magnesium salts. Also assess for symptoms of hypermagnesemia, such as a change in level of consciousness, hyporeflexia, shallow respirations, bradycardia, and hypotension.

Nursing Diagnoses and Planning

Nursing diagnoses and related expected patient outcomes commonly applicable to patients with hypermagnesemia include the following:

NDx: Altered nutrition: more than body requirements related to intake of magnesium

Planning: Patient Outcomes

1. Patient describes need to limit dietary magnesium.
2. Patient identifies foods rich in magnesium to be restricted.
3. Patient states an intent to restrict dietary magnesium as recommended.

Nursing Interventions and Evaluation

Discontinue administration of magnesium-containing drugs and parenteral fluids per physician's order. Monitor urinary output, because output of more than 750 mL daily is necessary to allow for excretion of magnesium. If not contraindicated, increase fluid intake to dilute serum magnesium and increase urinary output. Administer loop diuretics as prescribed to increase renal excretion of magnesium further.

NDx: Altered nutrition: more than body requirements

Explain the need to restrict intake of magnesium. Instruct the patient to limit intake of magnesium-rich foods such as meat, seafood, nuts, green vegetables, and whole grains. Assist the patient in planning and selecting meals low in magnesium. Refer to the dietitian if needed. Also instruct the patient to avoid over-the-counter drugs that contain large amounts of magnesium, especially laxatives and antacids. Show the patient how to read drug labels to ascertain magnesium content.

Compare the patient's status with the expected outcomes. If the outcomes are not met, reassess the patient and revise the plan.

$\mathcal{A}$cid-Base Imbalance

Hydrogen ions (H^+) are vital to life and health. Although hydrogen ions exist in far lower concentrations in body fluids than other ions (such as chloride and potassium), they play a major role in regulating biochemical and metabolic activities necessary for proper cellular function.

The H^+ concentration determines the acidity or alkalinity of a solution. The greater the H^+ concentration, the more acidic the solution. The lower the H^+ concentration, the more alkaline the solution.

pH is the symbol used to indicate the H^+ concentration in a solution, or the acidity or alkalinity of that solution. Neutral pH is 7.0. The higher the pH, the lower the H^+ concentration in the solution and vice versa. The normal pH range of arterial blood is 7.35 to 7.45. A blood pH below 7.35 indicates acidosis (a high H^+ concentration). A pH above 7.45 indicates alkalosis (a low H^+ concentration). pH limits that are compatible with life are 6.9 to 7.9 (Fig. 5–6).

Hydrogen circulates through body fluids in two forms: the volatile H^+ of carbonic acid (H_2CO_3) and the nonvolatile hydrogen ions of metabolic acids. Volatile acids are eliminated as CO_2 is exhaled by the lungs. Nonvolatile hydrogen ions are derived from acids such as sulfuric, pyruvic, phosphoric, and lactic acids. Nonvolatile hydrogen ions are eliminated by the kidneys.

Maintaining a proper H^+ concentration and normal pH is the key to acid-base balance. This balance between acids and bases in the blood is best ex-

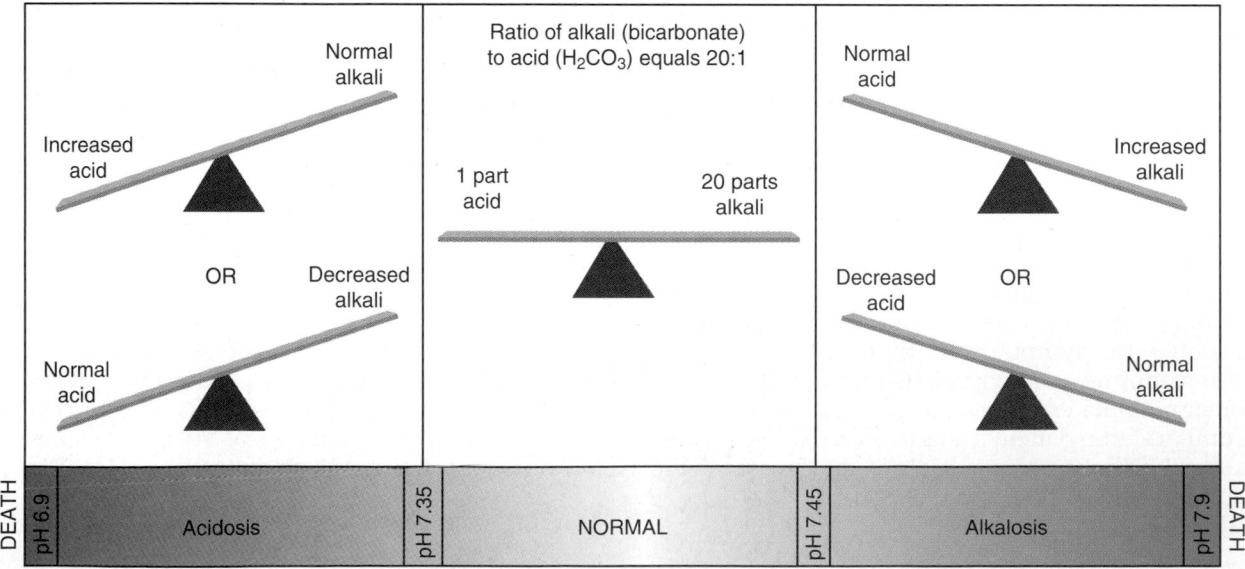

Figure 5–6

Limits of pH and bicarbonate–carbonic acid balance. The relationship of 20 parts bicarbonate to 1 part carbonic acid maintains H^+ and pH within normal limits. An increase in acid or a decrease in alkali causes acidosis; a decrease in acid or increase in alkali causes alkalosis.

pressed by the relationship between the bicarbonate ion (HCO_3^-) and H_2CO_3. This relationship is represented as follows:

$$pH = pk \times \log \frac{HCO_3^-}{H_2CO_3}$$

The ratio of bicarbonate to carbonic acid is 20:1 (see Fig. 5–6). The body strives to maintain this ratio at all times. This is done by retaining or blowing off CO_2 by the lungs or by retaining or excreting HCO_3^- by the kidneys. The relationship is expressed in Figure 5–7.

The body has three main defense systems that regulate H^+ concentration and, therefore, acid-base balance. They are the chemical buffer systems, the respiratory system, and the kidneys (Table 5–4).

BUFFER SYSTEM

A buffer is a substance that can act as a chemical sponge by either releasing or soaking up H^+. This is an immediate process that functions to keep the pH at 7.40. This system works by adding a buffered solution to a strong acid (or base), which results in a weak acid (or base) and a salt. A weak acid (or base) does not ionize in solution as much as a strong acid (or base), so there is less free H^+ to alter the pH. The pH of the solution then remains within the normal range.

Buffer systems exist in both the intracellular and extracellular fluid compartments. The main buffer systems are the bicarbonate–carbonic acid system, the protein (or hemoglobin) system, and the phosphate system. The bicarbonate–carbonic acid system is the one that is monitored clinically. If this buffer system is stable, the others are also stable. Within the body fluids, HCO_3^- and H_2CO_3 operate together, buffering and protecting the body from large amounts of acid. H_2CO_3 is a weak acid. Sodium HCO_3 ($NaHCO_3$) is its salt, which ionizes into Na^+ and HCO_3^-. Again, it is not absolute values that regulate acid-base balance but the ratio of HCO_3^- to

H_2CO_3 (a 20:1 ratio) that is crucial to H^+ balance. When the ratio is altered, a pH imbalance exists, as described in Figure 5–6.

The phosphate buffer system is almost identical to the bicarbonate–carbonic acid buffer system. The major components of this system are dihydrogen phosphate ion ($H_2PO_4^-$ and the hydrogen phosphate ion (HPO_4). Because phosphate is excreted in the urine, this system is helpful in buffering fluids in the renal tubules.

The protein buffer system is active in the plasma and in the cells. Protein hemoglobin in red blood cells provides much of the chemical buffering power of body fluids. Proteins are important buffers because they are found throughout the body.

RESPIRATORY CONTROL OF pH

Respiratory control of H^+ levels in the body occurs by varying the rate of CO_2 removal in the lungs. The respiratory control center in the medulla of the brain responds to changes in CO_2 and H^+ in the body. A rise in the partial pressure of arterial CO_2 ($PaCO_2$) is a strong stimulus for breathing. In the presence of a low pH (acidosis), the respiratory rate and depth are increased, causing a greater removal of CO_2, which reduces the amount of acid in solution, thereby raising the pH. Conversely, when the pH is high (alkalosis), the respiratory rate is decreased, causing CO_2 to be retained, which raises the amount of acid in solution and lowers the pH. This response occurs within minutes to maintain acid-base balance within the body.

RENAL CONTROL OF pH

Renal control of H^+ is accomplished by regulating bicarbonate via the bicarbonate–carbonic acid buffer system and eliminating nonvolatile H^+. This response takes hours to days. But the renal system is powerful and complete in its acid-base regulation. To correct H^+ imbalance, the kidneys alter the rate

Figure 5–7

The lungs help control acid-base balance by blowing off or retaining CO_2. The kidneys help regulate acid-base balance by excreting or retaining HCO_3^-.

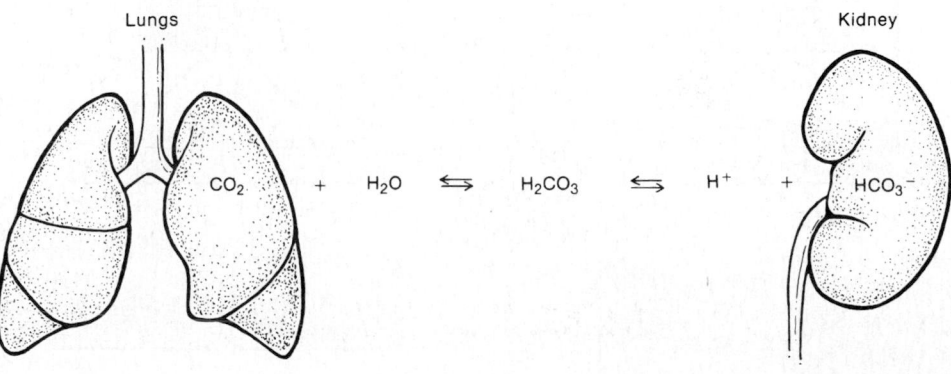

Table 5–4

Body Defenses that Regulate H⁺ Concentration

Mechanism	Action Time	Effect
Chemical buffers	Immediate	Combine with acids or bases to buffer them and prevent marked changes in pH
Respiratory system	Minutes	Controls carbon dioxide concentration by changing rate and depth of respirations
Renal system	Hours to days	Controls HCO_3^- by reabsorption of HCO_3^-; excretion of H^+ in urine; and production of NH_3

H^+, hydrogen ion; HCO_3^-, bicarbonate ion; NH_3, ammonia.

of excretion of metabolic acids by three major processes: reabsorption of HCO_3^-, secretion of H^+ by the proximal and distal tubules, and production of ammonia (NH_3).

Maintenance of acid-base balance depends on the healthy functioning of the kidneys, lungs, and buffer systems. These systems normally respond swiftly and efficiently to changes in H^+ concentration. However, when there is an excessive amount of acid or HCO_3^- in the body fluids, or in the presence of certain diseases, H^+ regulation fails and imbalances result. There are two major types of imbalances: acidosis and alkalosis. There are two types of acidosis (respiratory and metabolic) and two types of alkalosis (respiratory and metabolic). Figure 5–8 summarizes the four types of imbalances. Table 5–5 lists the laboratory significance for the four imbalances.

METABOLIC ACIDOSIS

Etiology and Pathophysiology

Metabolic acidosis is characterized by a pH below 7.35 (decreased pH and increased H^+ concentration) and a bicarbonate concentration below 22 mEq/L (decreased HCO_3^-). The general cause of metabolic acidosis is either an abnormal loss of $NaHCO_3$, which decreases the HCO_3^- in the HCO_3^-/H_2CO_3 ratio and thus the pH, or an excess of nonvolatile acid, which is more acid than the kidneys are able to handle. Table 5–6 lists some causes of metabolic acidosis.

Clinical Manifestations

As in all acidotic states, a decreased pH produces CNS depression, which may include apathy, headache, disorientation, weakness, stupor, and coma. The skin is typically warm and flushed because skin vessels become less responsive to sympathetic nervous system vasoconstrictor input. Skin is commonly dry and skin turgor poor when fluid deficit accompanies acidosis. The hyperventilation of Kussmaul's respirations occurs as a compensatory attempt to blow off CO_2, thereby correcting the acidosis. Hyperkalemia may occur from the movement of potassium out of the cells as hydrogen ions move in, and from retention of potassium by the kidneys. In addition, when the pH falls below 7.0, cardiac dysrhythmias develop, and heart rate and cardiac output decrease.

Diagnosis

Arterial blood gas measurements are essential in diagnosing all acid-base disturbances. In metabolic aci-

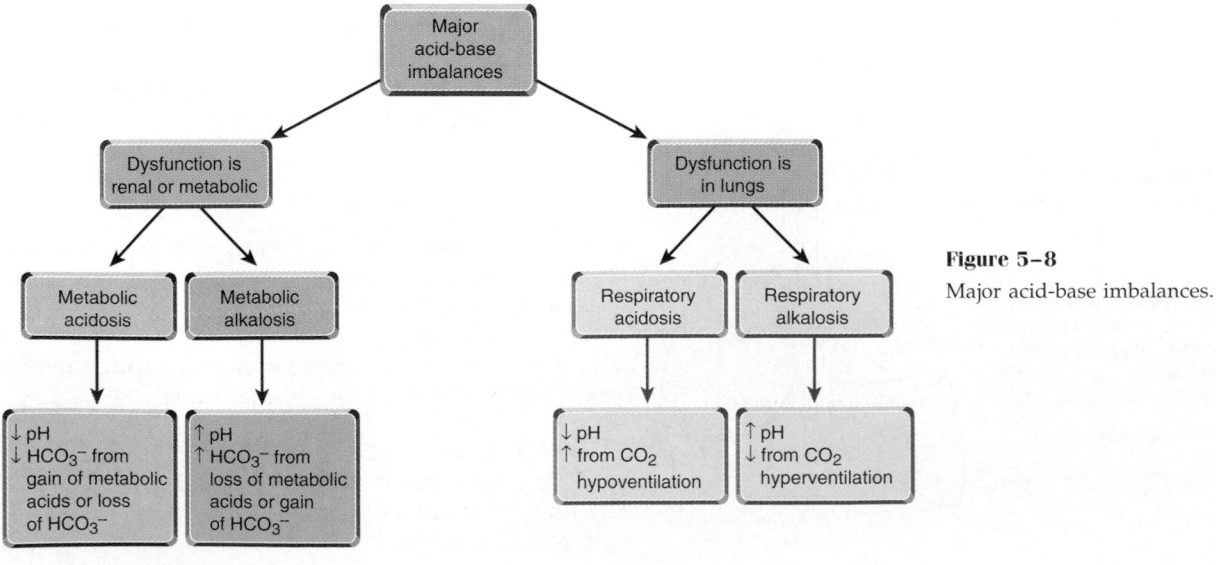

Figure 5–8

Major acid-base imbalances.

Table 5–5

Laboratory Values for Acid-Base Disturbances

Imbalance	pH	Paco$_2$	HCO$_3$
Metabolic acidosis			
Uncompensated	↓	Normal	↓
Partially compensated	↓ or normal	↓	↓
Metabolic alkalosis			
Uncompensated	↑	Normal	↑
Partially compensated	↑ or normal	↑	↑
Respiratory acidosis			
Uncompensated	↓	↑	Normal
Partially compensated	↓ or normal	↑	↑
Respiratory alkalosis			
Uncompensated	↑	↓	Normal
Partially compensated	↑ or normal	↓	↓

HCO$_3^-$, bicarbonate ion; PaCO$_2$, partial pressure of arterial carbon dioxide; ↓, decreased; ↑, increased.

dosis, there is a low arterial blood gas pH (<7.35) and a low blood gas bicarbonate level (<22 mEq/L). High serum potassium (hyperkalemia) may also occur as potassium leaves the cell. Compensatory hyperventilation decreases blood gas CO_2 levels (<40 mm Hg). Diagnosis is made by correlating the arterial blood gas findings to other known abnormal conditions.

Management

Management of metabolic acidosis is directed toward treating the underlying cause and correcting the electrolyte imbalance. Through supportive intervention, renal and respiratory systems can help correct and compensate for the imbalance. If the acidosis is severe enough, intravenous sodium bicarbonate is given. When acidosis is caused by renal failure, renal dialysis is necessary. If osmotic diuresis occurs, fluid replacement, along with careful monitoring of intake and output, is necessary.

NURSING PROCESS
Metabolic Acidosis

Assessment

Obtain and review the arterial blood gas results. Remember that metabolic acidosis may exist in the

Table 5–6

Causes of Metabolic Acidosis

Diabetic ketoacidosis	Hypothyroidism
Lactic acidosis	Trauma
Starvation	Salicylate poisoning
Renal failure	Diarrhea
High fever	Alcoholic ketoacidosis

presence or absence of clinical manifestations or assessment findings. Review the patient's medical problems, because they can suggest the possible cause of metabolic acidosis. Ask specifically about renal problems, diabetes mellitus, and persistent diarrhea. Also ask about the use of prescribed and over-the-counter medications. Note those medications that may affect acid, base, fluid, and electrolyte balance.

Assess for apathy, decreased alertness, disorientation, weakness, stupor, and coma, which can occur in acidosis as a result of CNS depression. If necessary, obtain or confirm this information with a family member or significant other. Acidosis, if severe enough, also affects cardiac muscle function, so assess for cardiac dysrhythmias, low heart rate, and low cardiac output. Assess fluid status to determine whether a volume deficit exists. Obtain a detailed dietary history. Review serum electrolytes for abnormal findings that may cause or result from metabolic acidosis. Observe for Kussmaul's respirations, which are present if the patient is having a compensatory reaction by the lung. Keep in mind that skin and mucous membranes are pink, warm, and dry as a result of the increased gas exchange and vasodilatation.

Nursing Diagnoses and Planning

Nursing diagnoses and related expected patient outcomes commonly applicable to patients with metabolic acidosis include the following:

NDx: Risk for ineffective breathing pattern related to compensatory changes in lung function

Planning: Patient Outcomes
1. Respiratory rate remains within normal limits.
2. Patient verbalizes that breathing is easy and not labored or hard.

NDx: Risk for fluid volume deficit related to vomiting and diarrhea

Planning: Patient Outcomes

1. Intake and output record demonstrates adequate fluid intake.
2. Intake and output record indicates that intake approximates output.
3. Vomiting and diarrhea are absent.

NDx: Risk for decreased cardiac output related to hyperkalemia and altered cardiac muscle function from low pH levels

Planning: Patient Outcomes

1. Patient is in normal sinus rhythm.
2. Cardiac output is within normal limits.
3. Serum potassium is within normal limits.

NDx: Risk for altered thought processes related to CNS depression

Planning: Patient Outcomes

1. Patient is alert.
2. Patient is coherent.
3. Patient responds appropriately to questions and commands.

NDx: Risk for injury related to disorientation, weakness, or stupor

Planning: Patient Outcomes

1. Patient remains free of injury.

Nursing Interventions and Evaluation

NDx: Risk for ineffective breathing pattern

Maintain good pulmonary function to facilitate compensatory excretion of CO_2. Encourage airway clearance through deep breathing, coughing, and incentive spirometry. Monitor work of breathing and be alert for signs of respiratory muscle fatigue. Facilitate rest, which is essential for sufficient energy to maintain a higher level of ventilation. Remember that as the primary disorder is treated, the level of ventilation will return to normal.

NDx: Risk for fluid volume deficit

Monitor and record accurate fluid intake and output. Weigh the patient daily at the same time with the same scale and the same clothing. Be alert for signs of dehydration and hypovolemia such as decreased blood pressure, increased heart rate, dry tongue, flattened neck veins, and poor skin turgor. Administer fluid replacement as ordered. Provide mouth care at least every 4 hours. Apply petroleum jelly or other moisturizer to lips. If vomiting occurs, support the patient. Document the amount and provide a description of vomitus. If diarrhea occurs, provide adequate skin care and provide bedpan or commode (if needed) for easy access. Document the amount, color, consistency, and frequency of diarrhea.

NDx: Risk for decreased cardiac output

Place the patient on a cardiac monitor if severe acidosis is present. Monitor heart rate closely and be alert for dysrhythmias. Measure the cardiac output if ordered. Measure arterial blood pressure regularly. Review relevant laboratory data including potassium, magnesium, and chloride. Monitor level of consciousness and urinary output. Reassure and comfort the patient to alleviate anxiety that may arise from cardiac symptoms.

NDx: Risk for altered thought processes

For the patient with metabolic acidosis, intervention directed toward returning the pH to normal also corrects the change in thought process. Implement the medical plan designed to correct the pH. If dialysis is necessary, provide appropriate nursing care.

If the patient has diabetic ketoacidosis, administer insulin as ordered by the physician. Administer replacement fluids, bicarbonate, and other medical treatments per physician orders. Monitor the patient's mental status throughout care to detect improvement. Orient the patient to time and place and restate who you are and what you are doing at each interaction. When feasible and appropriate, encourage the patient to wear his or her eyeglasses or hearing aid.

NDx: Risk for injury

Keep side rails raised and maintain the bed in a low position. Keep the call bell within easy reach. Assist the patient in meeting physical needs until he or she is capable of self-care. Closely observe and assist the patient when out of bed. Keep the environment adequately lit for safety.

Compare the patient's status with the expected outcomes. If the outcomes are not met, reassess the patient and revise the plan.

METABOLIC ALKALOSIS

Etiology and Pathophysiology

Metabolic alkalosis is characterized by a pH higher than 7.45 (increased pH and decreased H^+) and a bicarbonate concentration greater than 28 mEq/L (increased HCO_3^-). It is produced when there is an excess amount of bicarbonate or a loss of H^+. This disturbance does not occur often. When it does, the most common cause is vomiting or prolonged nasogastric suctioning that results in a loss of hydrochloric acid with gastric contents. Other causes include those associated with the loss of potassium, such as drainage from an intestinal fistula, diarrhea, and the use of potassium-wasting diuretics (thiazides, furosemides, and ethacrynic acid). Others are associated with excessive adrenocorticoid hormones, as in hyperaldosteronism and Cushing's disease. Hypokalemia produces metabolic alkalosis by the conservation of potassium in the kidneys, creating increased excretion of H^+ and by cellular potassium moving out of the cells into the ECF in an attempt to achieve a near-normal serum level. Other causes of metabolic alkalosis include excessive alkali ingestion (such as antacids and baking soda) to alleviate acid

Table 5–7

Causes of Metabolic Alkalosis

Vomiting	Hypokalemia
Nasogastric suctioning	Hyperaldosteronism
Intestinal fistulas	Cushing's disease
Diuretic therapy (thiazides,	Alkali ingestion
furosemides, and etha-	Sodium bicarbonate
crynic acid)	administration

indigestion or ulcer symptoms and administration of intravenous sodium bicarbonate during cardiopulmonary resuscitation. Table 5–7 lists the causes of metabolic alkalosis.

Clinical Manifestations

In metabolic alkalosis, as in all alkalotic conditions, an elevated pH results in CNS excitation, which produces such neurologic symptoms as belligerence, irritability, mental confusion, tingling of the fingers and toes, dizziness, hyperactive reflexes, tetany, and convulsions. These neurologic findings usually occur only with acute and severe metabolic alkalosis.

Metabolic alkalosis also leads to compensatory hypoventilation (which results in retention of CO_2 by not blowing it off, thereby increasing the carbonic acid and H^+ concentration). This is manifested by shallow, slow respirations with decreased thoracic movements that are limited by the body's need for oxygen. In some cases, hypokalemia, hypochloremia, or fluid volume deficit may also occur.

Diagnosis

The diagnosis of metabolic alkalosis is based on arterial blood gas evaluation showing a pH higher than 7.45 and an HCO_3^- level higher than 28 mEq/ L. Hypokalemia may occur when the body attempts to conserve H^+, thereby excreting potassium, or when potassium-wasting diuretics are given. Hypochloremia exists in the presence of metabolic alkalosis when Cl^- is lost in the gastric contents through vomiting or nasogastric suction. Compensation by the lungs is apparent when the $PaCO_2$ increases. Hypoventilation may be more pronounced in the unconscious and debilitated patient, and hypoxemia may occur as a result of the hypoventilation. Diagnosis is made by correlating the arterial blood gas findings to the underlying cause or medical condition.

Management

The treatment of metabolic alkalosis is directed at correcting the underlying cause or condition. Nasogastric suction should be avoided and vomiting controlled when possible. Administration of alkali is discontinued, as is administration of diuretics when those therapies contribute to the metabolic alkalosis. Fluid-volume deficit as well as chloride depletion is usually corrected with lactated Ringer's solution (which contains chloride) or normal saline. In severe

cases, ammonium chloride or hydrochloric acid may be administered intravenously to replace the H^+ and chloride loss. To correct a potassium loss, potassium chloride is administered. Diamox, a carbonic anhydrase inhibitor, is a diuretic that relieves alkalosis by increasing the excretion of bicarbonate by the kidneys.

NURSING PROCESS
Metabolic Alkalosis

Assessment

Because the patient with metabolic alkalosis has few symptoms, it is essential to anticipate and assess for the conditions that cause metabolic alkalosis. Review results of laboratory tests for depletion of chloride and potassium.

Check arterial blood gas results for elevated pH and HCO_3^- values. Assess fluid intake and output for volume deficit. Measure the amount of nasogastric drainage or vomiting when applicable. Assess the patient's neurologic status. Look for symptoms of alkalosis, such as dizziness, irritability, numbness in fingers and toes, mental confusion, tetany, and convulsions. If the patient has a history of ulcers or acid indigestion, ask about the amount of antacids or baking soda ingested. Assess the patient's respiratory status for decreased rate and depth of ventilation.

Nursing Diagnoses and Planning

Nursing diagnoses and related expected patient outcomes commonly applicable to patients with metabolic alkalosis include the following:

NDx: Risk for ineffective breathing pattern related to the compensatory mechanism of decreased rate and depth of ventilation

Planning: Patient Outcomes
1. Ventilation is of normal rate and depth.
2. Oxygen levels/saturation are within normal limits.

NDx: Risk for fluid volume deficit related to vomiting or nasogastric suction and potassium or chloride loss

Planning: Patient Outcomes
1. Vomiting has ceased.
2. Nasogastric suction is discontinued.
3. Fluid intake is greater than output.
4. Potassium and chloride values are within normal limits.

NDx: Risk for altered thought processes related to increased excitability of the nervous system secondary to increased pH and bicarbonate level, resulting in irritability, dizziness, and mental confusion

Planning: Patient Outcomes
1. Patient is alert and responsive.
2. Patient is cooperative.

3. Patient follows directions.
4. Patient denies dizziness.

NDx: Risk for injury related to belligerence, mental confusion, dizziness, tetany, and convulsions secondary to CNS excitement

Planning: Patient Outcomes
1. Patient complies with safety precautions.
2. Patient remains free of injury.

Nursing Interventions and Evaluation

NDx: Risk for ineffective breathing pattern
Encourage deep breathing, coughing, and the use of incentive spirometry to keep the airways clear and prevent atelectasis. Support the patient in a semi-Fowler's position if necessary to aid chest expansion and ease breathing. Administer oxygen therapy as ordered by the doctor if hypoxemia is present. Monitor oxygen saturation and the rate and rhythm of respirations. Explain the reason for the change in breathing pattern and reassure the patient that breathing will return to normal once the cause of the alkalosis is treated.

NDx: Risk for fluid volume deficit
For the person with metabolic alkalosis resulting from prolonged vomiting or nasogastric suctioning, record and report the amount of emesis or drainage if excessive. Use isotonic saline to irrigate nasogastric tubes since water can cause electrolyte washout. Encourage fluid intake as ordered. Monitor laboratory values for alterations in potassium or chloride. If potassium or chloride replacement is ordered, give oral or intravenous medication as prescribed. Administer intravenous fluids carefully and in appropriate time intervals as ordered by the physician. Weigh the patient daily, at same time and with the same scale and clothing.

NDx: Risk for altered thought processes
Be aware that a change in the patient's mood or personality to one of irritability or belligerence may result from chemical excitability of the CNS from alkalosis. Treat the patient with understanding and support until the underlying cause is treated and the mental confusion subsides. By appropriate conversation, keep the patient oriented to time and place and to what is going on. Encourage a family member or significant other to stay with the patient to decrease anxiety. Protect the patient from harm by keeping the bedside rails up while in bed and assist with ambulation when needed.

NDx: Risk for injury
Because a patient with severe metabolic alkalosis may become confused or dizzy and has the potential to develop convulsions, institute precautions for the patient's protection. Keep side rails up when the patient is in bed. Stay with the patient or assist with ambulation if the alkalosis is severe. Explain the importance of safety precautions to the patient and enlist cooperation while the alkalosis is present.

Compare the patient's status with the expected outcomes. If the outcomes are not met, reassess the patient and revise the plan.

RESPIRATORY ACIDOSIS

Etiology and Pathophysiology
Respiratory acidosis is characterized by a pH less than 7.35 and a $PaCO_2$ higher than 45 mm Hg. Any condition that decreases the level of pulmonary ventilation increases the concentration of CO_2, which increases carbonic acid and H^+ concentration. In addition to an elevated $PaCO_2$, which causes hypoventilation, hypoxemia (partial pressure of arterial oxygen, or PaO_2) usually exists. Respiratory acidosis may be either acute or chronic.

The causes of respiratory acidosis include any condition that impairs gas exchange. Acute respiratory acidosis can result from impaired function of the medullary center, from chest injury, from weakness of the respiratory muscles, or from airway obstruction. Chronic respiratory acidosis is most commonly caused by chronic obstructive pulmonary disease. Table 5–8 lists specific causes of acute and chronic respiratory acidosis.

Because renal compensation (retention of bicarbonate) takes hours to days to stabilize the pH, the pH can drop severely in patients with acute respiratory acidosis. Respiratory acidosis is often accompanied by hypoxemia. In fact, signs of hypoxemia often develop before those of respiratory acidosis because CO_2 diffuses 20 times faster than oxygen (O_2) across the alveolar-capillary membrane. When CO_2 accumulates in the blood, ventilation increases and eliminates a portion of the CO_2, but the O_2 uptake moves more slowly.

Acute respiratory acidosis can occur in patients with chronic lung disease who have chronically elevated $PaCO_2$ levels. This is often called CO_2 narcosis.

Table 5–8

Causes of Respiratory Acidosis	
Acute	**Chronic**
Drug overdose	Chronic obstructive
Head injury	pulmonary disease
Oversedation	Emphysema
Postanesthesia	Chronic bronchitis
Chest injuries	Asthma
Paralysis of the respi-	Bronchiectasis
ratory muscles (as in	Kyphoscoliosis
Guillain-Barré syn-	Extreme obesity
drome)	
Pneumonia	
Pulmonary edema	
Respiratory distress	
syndrome	

In this situation, the medullary respiratory center has become insensitive to elevated levels of CO_2 and no longer responds to increases in $PaCO_2$. Rather, the oxygen level in the blood now becomes the major stimulus for breathing. If oxygen is administered at a level that suppresses this stimulus, the rate and depth of respiration decrease, $PaCO_2$ rises, and respiratory distress ensues.

Clinical Manifestations

The signs and symptoms of respiratory acidosis vary depending on whether the condition is acute or chronic. Because respiratory acidosis is often accompanied by hypoxemia, manifestations are often intermixed. Acute onset of hypercapnia (increased $PaCO_2$) can cause an increased pulse, respiration, and blood pressure; mental cloudiness; and a feeling of fullness in the head. An increased $PaCO_2$ can cause cerebral vasodilatation and increased cerebral blood flow. If the condition is severe and prolonged, it can cause such signs and symptoms as papilledema, dull headache, blurred vision, behavioral changes (such as depression, paranoia, and hallucinations), weakness, paralysis, stupor, and coma. In less severe cases, warm, flushed skin, weakness, and tachycardia may be present. Ventricular fibrillation may be the first sign of respiratory acidosis in anesthetized patients.

Diagnosis

The diagnosis of respiratory acidosis is based on arterial blood gases with a pH less than 7.35 and a $PaCO_2$ level higher than 45 mm Hg. When compensation (the kidney's retention of bicarbonate) has occurred, the pH may return to the lower limits of normal.

The patient's underlying pulmonary dysfunction or medical condition often suggests the possibility of respiratory acidosis. Hypoventilation and hypoxemia strongly suggest respiratory acidosis as well. The diagnosis is made by correlating the arterial blood gas findings to the underlying cause or medical condition.

Management

Management of respiratory acidosis is directed at treating the underlying condition and restoring effective alveolar ventilation. This is accomplished by using respiratory care techniques such as:

- Bronchodilators to help reduce bronchospasm
- Postural drainage and percussion to loosen and raise thickened mucus
- Suctioning to rid the airway of secretions
- Humidity to loosen secretions
- Antibiotics for respiratory infections

Low-flow oxygen (1–3 L/minute) is given to the hypoxemic patient who has a chronically high $PaCO_2$ value. In severe cases, mechanical ventilation may be necessary to correct the hypoxemia or the acidosis and hypercapnia adequately. In such cases, the elevated $PaCO_2$ must be brought down slowly. If the acidosis is severe enough, intravenous sodium bicarbonate may be administered to bring the pH to within a safe range quickly. Close monitoring and frequent arterial blood gas measurements are necessary in this case to avoid severe alkalosis from overcompensation.

NURSING PROCESS
Respiratory Acidosis

Assessment

Assessment of the patient with respiratory acidosis reveals mainly cardiopulmonary findings, since hypercapnia causes release of epinephrine and norepinephrine, which increase heart rate and cardiac output. Question the patient about and observe for dyspnea on exertion. This is often the patient's prominent symptom. Also assess for indications of cerebral vasodilatation caused by hypercapnia. These include blurred vision, headache, papilledema, behavioral changes such as depression and paranoia, hallucinations, weakness, paralysis, stupor, and coma. Be aware that a patient's moodiness, belligerence, anxiety, irritability, or paranoia may result from chemical changes in the blood, such as hypercapnia and hypoxemia. Review and relate the arterial blood gas values to the patient's medical problems.

Auscultate lung sounds for crackles, wheezes, and decreased breath sounds, which suggest impaired gas exchange or airway clearance. Check vital signs regularly for tachycardia, tachypnea, and elevated blood pressure. Monitor for cardiac dysrhythmias. Examine the skin condition to determine whether the skin is warm and flushed.

Nursing Diagnoses and Planning

Nursing diagnoses and related expected patient outcomes commonly applicable to patients with respiratory acidosis include the following:

NDx: Impaired gas exchange related to inadequate ventilation

Planning: Patient Outcomes
1. pH, PaO_2, and $PaCO_2$ are within the patient's normal limits.
2. Respiratory rate is within the patient's normal limits.
3. Heart rate returns to within patient's normal limits.
4. Patient is alert and oriented without being agitated.
5. Color of skin and mucous membranes is normal for the patient.

NDx: Ineffective airway clearance related to inadequate ventilation and lung condition

Planning: Patient Outcomes
1. Crackles and wheezes are absent.
2. Patient coughs and raises secretions effectively.

3. Patient describes the need to increase fluids to keep secretions loose.
4. Vital signs are within patient's normal limits.

NDx: Ineffective breathing pattern related to inadequate ventilation and underlying lung condition

Planning: Patient Outcomes
1. Respiratory rate, depth, and rhythm return to within patient's normal limits.
2. Patient demonstrates effective diaphragmatic breathing pattern.
3. Adventitious breath sounds return to within patient's normal limits.
4. Patient demonstrates correct use of prescribed respiratory drugs and equipment.

NDx: Decreased cardiac output related to poor gas exchange of O_2 and CO_2

Planning: Patient Outcomes
1. Heart rate is within patient's normal limits.
2. Serious dysrhythmias are absent.
3. Blood pressure is within patient's normal limits.

NDx: Activity intolerance related to dyspnea on exertion and ineffective breathing patterns

Planning: Patient Outcomes
1. Patient verbalizes need to pace activity.
2. Activity level returns to patient's normal level.
3. Patient verbalizes plan to engage in regular exercise.
4. Patient describes need for effective breathing with activity.

NDx: Anxiety related to dyspnea

Planning: Patient Outcomes
1. Patient discusses fear of breathlessness.
2. Patient demonstrates effective breathing pattern.
3. Patient verbalizes ability to deal with anxiety level.

Nursing Interventions and Evaluation

NDx: Impaired gas exchange
When hypoventilation is present, interventions to improve the level of ventilation also improve the respiratory acidosis. Perform bronchial hygiene measures, such as nebulizer treatments, postural drainage, and percussion, as ordered.

Coordinate the patient's plan of care to ensure that all aspects of care are implemented. If oxygen therapy is ordered for hypoxemia, frequently assess proper function of the oxygen administration equipment and patient compliance. Administer antibiotics to treat respiratory infection and bronchodilators to open the airways as prescribed. Monitor white blood cell count, temperature, work of breathing, and lung sounds to evaluate the effectiveness of these medications. If chronic lung disease is present, teach the patient to use an effective breathing pattern, such as pursed lip or diaphragmatic breathing.

If the level of ventilation is very poor and the respiratory acidosis suggests respiratory failure, maintain mechanical ventilation as ordered. In this event, assess the patient's respiratory status and function of the ventilator closely. Throughout care, monitor the patient for changes in gas-exchange status.

NDx: Ineffective airway clearance
With many pulmonary disorders, increased secretions develop as a result of the primary lung problem or a secondary lung infection. Implement measures to loosen and raise secretions, such as effective coughing, increased fluids, and postural drainage. Teach the patient effective breathing and coughing techniques as well as the need to drink six to eight glasses of liquid a day. Administer medication to loosen secretions or antibiotics to treat an infection as prescribed. If the patient cannot cough up secretions, suction as necessary. Observe and document color, consistency, amount, and odor of sputum.

NDx: Ineffective breathing pattern
Implement nursing interventions as described for impaired gas exchange and ineffective airway clearance. As the patient's method of breathing, clearing of secretions, and stabilization of oxygenation all improve, gas exchange and breathing pattern also improve. If the patient has a chronic breathing problem, instruct in breathing techniques, methods to maintain a patent airway, and use of medication to improve ventilation.

NDx: Decreased cardiac output
Hypoxemia affects cardiac status, causing an increased heart rate, dysrhythmias, and changes in blood pressure. Closely monitor heart rate and cardiac rhythm during the unstable phase of hypoventilation. Administer cardiac medication as ordered and monitor effectiveness. Maintain an accurate record of intake and output.

NDx: Activity intolerance
When dyspnea occurs as a result of an ineffective breathing pattern and poor gas exchange, the patient's activity level is affected. Provide assistance as needed with bathing, shaving, getting out of bed, and eating. Take care to pace activities, and plan care so that severe dyspnea does not occur. Teach the patient the importance of self-pacing activities so that the respiratory condition is not aggravated. If the patient has a chronic lung condition, teach the importance of regular, planned exercise as well as how to coordinate breathing with exercise. Encourage attendance at a pulmonary rehabilitation program.

NDx: Anxiety
Dyspnea, whether acute or chronic, causes anxiety. Explain to the patient, in simple terms, what is happening. Also explain the plan of care. Part of the anxiety may be due to impaired gas exchange, so interventions previously mentioned to correct hypoxemia and hypoventilation will reduce the anxiety. If the patient has a chronic lung condition, teach

proper breathing techniques and methods to control breathlessness.

Compare the patient's status with the expected outcomes. If the outcomes are not met, reassess the patient and revise the plan.

RESPIRATORY ALKALOSIS

Etiology and Pathophysiology

Respiratory alkalosis is characterized by a pH greater than 7.45 and a $PaCO_2$ less than 35 mm Hg. Respiratory alkalosis results from hyperventilation, which is the excessive exhaling of CO_2. This causes a decrease in $PaCO_2$, which causes a decrease in carbonic acid and consequently a rise in pH. Hyperventilation means that the respiratory rate and depth are greater than needed to maintain a normal $PaCO_2$ and should not be confused with the hyperpnea of exercise. Respiratory alkalosis can also occur from overstimulation of the respiratory center in the brain. Table 5–9 lists some of the causes of hyperventilation and overstimulation of the respiratory center that contribute to development of respiratory alkalosis.

Renal compensation exists when the HCO_3^- decreases until it restores the 20:1 ratio of HCO_3^- to H_2CO_3. The kidney is slow in the reabsorption of HCO_3^- and the decrease of H^+ secretion as well as the decrease in NH_3 production. If respiratory alkalosis is self-limited, renal compensation will not have time to develop.

Clinical Manifestations

The major characteristics of respiratory alkalosis are those associated with hyperexcitability of the nervous system and decreased cerebral blood flow. They include an inability to concentrate, lightheadedness, numbness and tingling of the fingers and toes, hyper-reflexia, and positive Chvostek's and Trousseau's signs. There may also be associated sweating, palpitations, panic, and air hunger. If respiratory alkalosis becomes severe, tetany and convulsions may occur. Cardiac dysrhythmias and ST-T wave changes develop, caused by a decreased serum potassium level.

Diagnosis

Diagnosis of respiratory alkalosis is made by analyzing the arterial blood gases. Respiratory alkalosis is present when the pH is greater than 7.45 and the $PaCO_2$ is less than 35 mm Hg. If the situation is compensated, the kidneys lower the bicarbonate level to lower the pH to normal. The kidneys cannot do this quickly, however.

Management

Management of respiratory alkalosis is directed toward treatment of the underlying cause. People who are hyperventilating can inhale their own exhaled CO_2 from a paper bag, thus lowering the $PaCO_2$ and increasing H_2CO_3 in their blood. This is especially useful when anxiety or pain is the cause of the respiratory alkalosis. If the patient is on a mechanical ventilator and the $PaCO_2$ is less than 35 mm Hg, it is likely that the level of ventilation is too great. If so, the respiratory rate of the machine should be decreased. If the alkalosis is severe and tetany is present, calcium gluconate is given intravenously. Renal function is maintained to allow for adequate compensation of the disturbance.

NURSING PROCESS
Respiratory Alkalosis

Assessment

Obtain a patient history. Determine when the onset of symptoms occurred and identify a precipitating event if possible. Ask about prior similar episodes. Assess current respiratory status, observing for such signs of pulmonary disorders as pneumonia or pulmonary edema. Ask about lightheadedness and numbness or tingling of the fingers and toes. Examine the patient for hyper-reflexia, Chvostek's and Trousseau's signs, muscle twitching, tetany, or seizure activity.

Review arterial blood gas results to identify respiratory alkalosis. Check the patient's temperature routinely because fever may cause hyperventilation. Assess the patient for anxiety. Observe for associated symptoms, such as sweating, palpitations, panic, air hunger, and dyspnea. If the patient is on a ventilator, perform routine ventilator checks to identify inappropriate settings that may cause hyperventilation.

Nursing Diagnoses and Planning

Nursing diagnoses and related expected patient outcomes commonly applicable to patients with respiratory alkalosis include the following:

NDx: Ineffective breathing pattern related to hyperventilation or an incorrectly adjusted respiratory rate on mechanical ventilator

Table 5–9

Causes of Respiratory Alkalosis	
Hyperventilation	**Overstimulation of the Respiratory Center**
Anxiety	Fever
Pain	Gram-negative sepsis
Hypoxemia	CNS disease (meningitis, encephalitis, brain tumor)
Overventilation with mechanical ventilator	Early salicylate poisoning
	Hyperthyroidism

CNS, central nervous system.

Planning: Patient Outcomes
1. Breathing pattern is effective, with pH and $PaCO_2$ within normal limits.

NDx: Anxiety related to the symptoms of respiratory alkalosis and the precipitating event

Planning: Patient Outcomes
1. Hyperventilation is absent.
2. Patient states anxiety has decreased.
3. Patient expresses confidence in ability to cope.

NDx: Risk for injury related to nervous system hyperexcitability

Planning: Patient Outcomes
1. Patient complies with safety precautions.
2. Patient remains free of injury.

Nursing Interventions and Evaluation

NDx: Ineffective breathing pattern
Demonstrate the slow, relaxed breathing pattern necessary to help reduce symptoms caused by hyperventilation and alkalosis (panic, dizziness, tingling, hyper-reflexia, and lightheadedness). Encourage slow, even breaths. When indicated, help the patient blow into a paper bag to reinhale CO_2 and arrest the hyperventilation.

NDx: Anxiety
Listen to the patient who is emotionally upset. Encourage expression of feelings and help the patient work through anxiety. Administer sedation as ordered if the patient is extremely anxious. Monitor its effectiveness.

NDx: Risk for injury
If the patient is in danger of developing the serious consequences of alkalosis, institute precautions to ensure safety. Keep side rails up while the patient is in bed. Assist with moving and walking if dizziness or lightheadedness is present. Routinely monitor for mental alertness throughout the course of the patient's stay in the hospital. Be alert for hyper-reflexia, tetany, and seizure activity.

Compare the patient's status with the expected outcomes. If the outcomes are not met, reassess the patient and revise the plan.

The Elderly: Special Considerations

Older people are at greater risk for fluid imbalance than younger people, with dehydration (hyperosmolar extracellular fluid volume deficit) being the most common imbalance. There are numerous reasons for this tendency. First, with advancing age, lean body mass is replaced with fat tissue. This results in a decrease in total body fluid because fat tissue has a lower volume of ICF. Second, the kidney's ability to concentrate urine decreases with advancing age. This results from decreased sensitivity of the renal tubules to ADH, with progressive loss of renal mass and a decrease in renal perfusion. By 80 years of age, renal mass has decreased by approximately 30% and renal perfusion by 50%.

The third factor predisposing the elderly to dehydration is insufficient intake. Age-related changes diminish the thirst sensation, which in turn may lead to decreased fluid intake. Other factors that might cause or contribute to insufficient fluid intake include functional limitations or environmental factors, such as impaired mobility or an institutional setting, which limit access to fluids. Also, older adults may intentionally restrict their fluid intake based on the mistaken belief that this will control incontinence.

A fourth predisposing factor is the presence of a health problem, such as vomiting or diarrhea, that increases the need for fluids because of excessive loss. A final factor that can lead to dehydration and hyperosmolality is the excessive use of salt without an associated increase in water intake, which may be associated with diminished taste perception.

Identifying signs of dehydration is more difficult in older than in younger adults. For example, the skin turgor of older adults may be poor because of disease conditions and the age-related loss of skin elasticity. Similarly, oral mucous membranes may be dry from decreased saliva production associated with disease conditions and adverse medication effects. Therefore, poor skin turgor and dry mucous membranes are not necessarily accurate indicators of dehydration in the elderly. A more accurate indicator may be altered cognitive function, such as the development of mild confusion or disorientation. Other signs of dehydration include constipation, concentrated urine, and orthostatic hypotension.

Dehydration is a particularly dangerous problem to the person with a respiratory infection. It contributes to the development of very thick and tenacious sputum, which is difficult to expectorate. This can both prolong the existing infection and contribute to reinfection.

Just as there is impaired ability to concentrate urine and conserve water on the part of the aged kidney, there is also an impaired ability to dilute urine. Excretion of excess water by the aged kidney is slow. Give intravenous solutions containing sodium to the elderly with caution because their use can lead to hypervolemia and precipitate heart failure.

Older adults are also at increased risk for electrolyte imbalance. As with fluid imbalances, this increased risk is related to a loss of adaptive capacity. For example, it takes the aged kidney half again as long as the younger kidney to decrease the amount of sodium excreted in the urine in response to a decreased sodium intake. Because the aged kidney is less sensitive to the effects of aldosterone, the elderly are at risk for hyperkalemia, especially if they have GI bleeding or are receiving intravenous potassium. Also, any condition or medication that stimulates ADH secretion, such as pneumonia or chlorpropamide, is likely to cause water intoxication and hyponatremia in older adults because of their diminished ability to compensate for excessive levels of ADH.

Chapter Review

1. What clinical manifestations should the nurse assess for to determine whether extracellular fluid volume deficit is moderate or severe?

2. Why should the nurse assess the types and osmolality of intravenous fluids a patient receives?

3. In what ways can the nurse determine whether a patient is hypokalemic?

4. What nursing responsibilities are related to the administration of potassium preparations, orally and intravenously?

5. How is the care of a patient with hypokalemia similar to that of a patient with hypomagnesemia?

6. How can the effectiveness of calcium replacement be evaluated when caring for a patient with hypocalcemia?

7. How is the care of a patient with respiratory acidosis different from that of a patient with respiratory alkalosis?

8. What would happen to the acid-base balance of a patient with severe vomiting if it were not controlled or stopped?

9. How can the effectiveness of treatment be evaluated when caring for a patient with respiratory acidosis who is on mechanical ventilation?

10. What laboratory values are considered when assessing a patient with a metabolic acid-base disturbance?

Bibliography

Abraham WT, Schrier RW. Body fluid volume regulation in health and disease. Adv Int Med Vol 1994; 39:23.

Andrews BT. Fluid and electrolyte disorders in neurosurgical intensive care. Neurosurg Clin North Am 1994; 5(4):707.

Berne RM, Levy MN. Physiology. 3rd ed. St Louis: Mosby Year-Book, 1993.

Brenner M, Williver J. Pulmonary and acid-base assessment. Nurs Clin North Am, 1990; 25(4):761.

Brensilver JM, Goldberger E. A primer of water, electrolyte acid-base syndromes. 8th ed, Philadelphia: FA Davis, 1996.

Brown RG. Disorders of water and sodium balance. Postgrad Med 1993; 93(4):227.

Carlin K, Carlin S. Acid/base may be more variable than previously thought (Review). Med Hypotheses 1993; 41(1):42.

Carpenito LJ. Nursing diagnosis: Application to clinical practice. 6th ed. Philadelphia: JB Lippincott, 1995.

Carroll HJ, Oh MS. Water, electrolyte and acid-base metabolism. 2nd ed. Philadelphia: JB Lippincott, 1989.

Chernow B, Bamberger S, Stoiko M, et al. Hypomagnesemia in patients in postoperative intensive care. Chest 1989; 95(2):391.

Clark BA, Brown RS. Potassium homeostasis and hyperkalemic syndromes. Endocrin Metab Clin North Am 1995; 24(3):573.

Cody RJ, Pickworth KK. Approaches to diuretic therapy and electrolyte imbalance in congestive heart failure. Cardiol Clin 1994; 12(1):37.

D'Addesio J. Metabolic and respiratory acidosis. Top Emerg Med 1992; 14(1):51.

Dafnis EK, Laski ME. Fluid and electrolyte abnormalities in the oncology patient. Semin Nephrol 1993; 13(3):281.

DuBose TD. Acid-base emergencies. Patient Care 1992; 26(3):214.

Faber MD, Kupin WL, Heilig CW, Narins RG. Common fluid-electrolyte and acid-base problems in the intensive care unit: Selected issues. Semin Nephrol 1994; 14(1):8.

Fencel V, Leith DE. Stewart's quantitative acid-base chemistry: Application in biology and medicine (Review). Resp Physiol 1993;91(1):1.

Gershan JA, Freeman CM, Ross MC, et al. Fluid volume deficit: Validating the indicators. Heart Lung 1990; 19(2):152.

Gettrust KV, Brabec PD. Nursing diagnoses. Albany, NY: Delmar, 1992.

Guyton AC. Textbook of medical physiology. 9th ed. Philadelphia: WB Saunders, 1996.

Ham RJ, Sloane PD. Primary care geriatrics. 2nd ed. St. Louis: Mosby Year-Book, 1991.

Heitkemper MM, Bond E. Fluid and electrolytes: Assessment and interventions. J Enterostomal Ther 1988; 15(1):18.

Held JL. Correcting fluid and electrolyte imbalances. Nursing 1995; 25(4):71.

Horne M, Heitz U, Swearingen P. Fluid, electrolyte and acid-base balance: A case study approach. St Louis: Mosby Year-Book, 1991.

Jennings DB. The physiochemistry of [H+] and respiratory control: Roles of PCO₂, strong ions, and their hormonal regulators. (Review) Can J Physiol Pharm 1994; 72(12):1499.

Kee JL. Laboratory and diagnostic tests with nursing implications. 4th ed. Norwalk, CT: Appleton & Lange, 1995.

Kee JL, Paulanka BJ. Fluids and electrolytes with clinical applications. 5th ed. New York: Delmar, 1994.

Kositzke JA. A question of balance: Dehydration in the elderly. J Gerontol Nurs 1990; 16(5):4.

Kowalchuk JM, Scheuermann BW. Acid-base regulation: A comparison of quantitative methods. Can J Physiol Pharm, 1994; 72(7):818.

Leier, CV, DelCas L, Metra M. Clinical relevance and management of the major electrolyte abnormalities in CHF: Hyponatremia, hypokalemia, and hypomagnesemia. Am Heart J 1994; 28(3):564.

McCance KL, Huether SE. Pathophysiology: The biologic basis for disease in adults and children. 2nd ed. St Louis: Mosby Year-Book, 1994.

Metheny NM. Fluid and electrolyte balance. 3rd ed. Philadelphia: JB Lippincott, 1996.

Nadler JL, Rude RK. Disorders of magnesium metabolism. Endocrin Metab Clin North Am 1995; 24(3):623.

Paulson WD, Gadallah MF. Diagnosis of mixed acid-base disorders in diabetic ketoacidosis. Am J Med Sci 1993; 306(5):295.

Porth CM. Pathophysiology. 4th ed. Philadelphia: JB Lippincott, 1995.

Seshadri V, Meyer-Tettambel OM. Electrolyte and drug management in nutritional support. Crit Care Nurs Clin North Am 1993; 5(1):31.

Sica DA. Renal disease, electrolyte abnormalities, and acid-base imbalance in the elderly. Clin Geriatr Med 1994; 10(1):197.

Terry J. The major electrolytes: Sodium potassium and chloride. J Intraven Nurs 1994; 17(5):240.

6

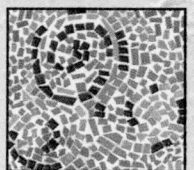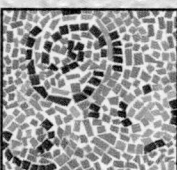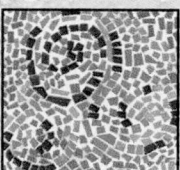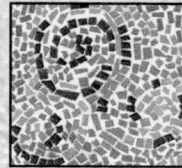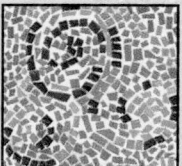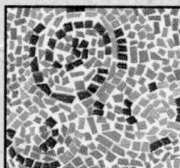

Knowledge Base for Patients Undergoing Surgery

Study Outcomes

After studying this chapter, you should be able to:

1. Describe the nature and scope of perioperative nursing practice.
2. Define the standards of perioperative nursing practice.
3. Identify the legal parameters associated with the care of patients undergoing surgery.
4. Describe common preoperative diagnostic procedures and preoperative management of patients undergoing surgery.
5. Identify information and physical examination data essential to the assessment of preoperative, intraoperative, and postoperative patients.
6. State nursing diagnoses and related patient outcomes commonly applicable to patients undergoing surgery.
7. Describe nursing interventions, with their rationales, commonly applicable to patients undergoing surgery.
8. Explain the basis for evaluation of nursing care provided to patients undergoing surgery.
9. Identify special considerations for the patient undergoing ambulatory surgery.
10. Identify special considerations for the elderly patient undergoing surgery.
11. Identify alternative settings for perioperative nursing care.

Surgery is any procedure performed on the human body that uses instruments to alter tissue or organ integrity. The purpose of a surgical procedure may be diagnostic, as in excision of tissue for biopsy. It may be corrective, as in repair of a defective heart valve. It may be reconstructive, as in skin grafting after a burn injury. Or it may be palliative, as in debulking an inoperable tumor to relieve pain or temporarily restore function.

Nursing care of the patient undergoing surgery requires clinical expertise based on a sound understanding of anatomy and physiology, the planned surgical procedure, and the effects of surgery on the body's homeostatic mechanisms. The patient and loved ones depend on the nurse's knowledge, understanding, compassion, and technical expertise to allay their concerns, demystify the surgical experience, and help the patient through a smooth, successful surgery and recovery. The nurse's roles as educator and patient advocate remain a primary focus throughout the perioperative period. This chapter presents physiologic and psychologic factors that affect the patient undergoing surgery and outlines perioperative nursing activities that promote a successful surgical experience.

Surgical Settings

Not so long ago, patients who needed surgery were almost always admitted to a hospital. However, as insurance reimbursement practices have evolved, so too have the settings in which surgical procedures take place. To streamline care and reduce costs, an increasing number of surgical procedures that once would have required hospitalization now take place in ambulatory or short-stay settings.

Ambulatory surgical centers are designed for outpatient care. In 1995, roughly 70% of surgical procedures took place in an outpatient setting. These procedures include endoscopy, obstetrics, urology, orthopedics, plastics, and special procedures. Advances in anesthesia and state of the art technology allow physicians to perform operations with fewer complications and side effects. The patient leaves shortly after recovering from anesthesia.

Short-stay surgical centers can accommodate patients overnight, or for two to three days if necessary. These centers are used for patients who need somewhat more complex surgery, who have no one to assist with postsurgical care at home, or who have other medical problems that require supervision and assistance from health professionals in a structured setting.

Ambulatory and short-stay settings may be hospital-based or privately owned free-standing centers. On average, a procedure performed in one of these settings costs some 30 to 50% less than a comparable

■■■■■■▶

■ Clinical Pathway for Endoscopy

Patient Name _____   Date _____

DRG# _____   Expected LOS <u><23 hours</u>

	Preprocedure	Preoperative	Intraoperative	Postoperative Phase I PACU	Postoperative Phase II PACU	Discharge	Postoperative Home Day I
Medication	Review medical history	Start IV	Administer midazolam, meperidine, promethazine	Administer naloxone, flumazenil prn	Antiemetic, PO pain med prn	Start on new Rx, omeprazole	Continue medications
Diagnostic tests	History & physical, chest x-ray, ECG, blood work	Review tests, report abnormalities	Endoscopy procedure	None, unless procedure complications	None or if complications, plan for follow-up exam	None or schedule follow-up exam & procedure	None
Diet	Regular	NPO	NPO	NPO	Clear liquids & progress	Regular	Regular
Activity	Not restricted	Ambulate, turn, cough, and deep-breathe	Sedated, little movement	Turn, cough, and deep-breathe, leg exercises	Increase activity to ambulation	Normal ambulation with rest periods	Not restricted
Treatments/ nursing action	Assessment of needs	Vital signs, assess further education needs, check list	Monitor vital signs, level of consciousness parameters, O$_2$ saturation, and cardiac status	Monitor vital signs, level of consciousness parameters, O$_2$ saturation, and cardiac status	Continue to monitor as before and assess further needs, start exercises	Prepare for discharge with education for continued care needs	Follow-up evaluation via phone call (or home visit in special needs cases)
Teaching/ discharge planning	Phone call to remind patient about scheduled surgery, answer questions, tell patient to bring a driver to escort the patient home	Patient education about procedure and follow-up care	Transport to PACU	Discharge when Aldrete criteria I met	Discharge when Aldrete criteria II met	Postoperative instructions reviewed	Postoperative phone call for follow-up (or home visit in special needs cases)

procedure performed in a hospital. Although the cost-savings is necessary and the short stay is less disruptive to patients' increasingly hectic lives, this trend toward earlier discharge means that patients tend to go home sicker than ever. Since nurses in the outpatient surgical setting have a shorter length of time to care for patients, a greater emphasis must be placed on patient responsibility and health teaching.

Certainly, many procedures still require traditional inpatient hospitalization. But even here, length of stay is decreasing and illness at discharge is increasing. Patients planning to stay in the hospital may arrive the day of surgery, which makes routine preoperative care more hurried. Some patients stay 23 hours and leave the hospital as soon as they are fully awake from anesthesia and considered stable enough for discharge. Shown above is a sample clinical pathway for such a patient. Other hospitalized surgery patients are acutely ill and may require

emergency care. As more procedures take place in outpatient settings, the level of acuteness of inpatient care will continue to increase.

𝒫erioperative Nursing

Perioperative nursing is the term used to describe nursing care of the patient who requires surgical intervention. Perioperative nursing is divided into three phases: preoperative, intraoperative, and postoperative. The Association of Operating Room Nurses (AORN) has established standards and recommended practices for perioperative nursing. These standards, which are represented by the examples of nursing activities listed in Table 6–1, help define the scope of nursing practice during the perioperative period.

Table 6-1

Examples of Nursing Activities in Perioperative Nursing Practice

Preoperative Phase	Intraoperative Phase	Postoperative Phase

PREOPERATIVE ASSESSMENT
Home/clinic
1. Initiates first preoperative assessment
2. Plans teaching methods appropriate to patient's needs
3. Involves family in interview
Surgical unit
1. Completes preoperative assessment
2. Coordinates patient teaching with other nursing staff
3. Explains phases in perioperative period and expectations
4. Develops a plan of care
Surgical suite
1. Assesses patient's level of consciousness
2. Reviews chart
3. Identifies patient
4. Verifies surgical site
 	
PLANNING
1. Determines a plan of care based on individualized assessment
 	
PSYCHOLOGIC SUPPORT
1. Tells patient what is happening
2. Determines psychologic status
3. Gives prior warning of noxious stimuli
4. Communicates patient's emotional status to other appropriate members of the health-care team
	MAINTENANCE OF SAFETY
	1. Verifies that the sponge, needle, and instrument counts are correct
	2. Positions the patient
	  a. Functional alignment
	  b. Exposure of surgical site
	  c. Maintenance of position throughout procedure
	3. Applies grounding device to patient
	4. Provides physical support
	
	PHYSIOLOGIC MONITORING
	1. Calculates effects on patient of excessive fluid loss
	2. Distinguishes normal from abnormal cardiopulmonary data
	3. Reports changes in patient's pulse, respirations, temperature, and blood pressure
	
	PSYCHOLOGIC MONITORING
	(prior to induction and if patient is conscious)
	1. Provides emotional support to patient
	2. Stands near/touches patient during procedures/induction
	3. Continues to assess patient's emotional status
	4. Communicates patient's emotional status to other appropriate members of the health-care team
	
	NURSING MANAGEMENT
	1. Provides physical safety for the patient
	2. Maintains aseptic, controlled environment
	3. Effectively manages human resources
		COMMUNICATION OF INTRAOPERATIVE INFORMATION
		1. Gives patient's name
		2. States type of surgery performed
		3. Provides contributing intraoperative factors; ie, drain, catheters
		4. States physical limitations
		5. States impairments resulting from surgery
		6. Reports patient's preoperative level of consciousness
		7. Communicates necessary equipment needs
		
		POSTOPERATIVE EVALUATION
		Recovery area
		1. Determines patient's immediate response to surgical intervention
		Surgical unit
		1. Evaluates effectiveness of nursing care in the operating room
		2. Determines patient's level of satisfaction with care given during perioperative period
		3. Evaluates products used on patient in the operating room
		4. Determines patient's psychologic status
		5. Assists with discharge planning
		Home/clinic
		1. Seeks patient's perception of surgery in terms of the effects of anesthetic agents, impact on body image, distortion, immobilization
		2. Determines family's perceptions of surgery

LEGAL PARAMETERS

Written permission must be obtained from the patient before performing

- Any surgical procedure
- Any procedure during which anesthesia is administered

- Any procedure in which the physician plans to enter a body cavity
- Any procedure that carries a high risk
- Diagnostic tests that have potentially sensitive outcomes, such as human immunodeficiency virus (HIV) antibody testing

This written permission is called the patient's

informed consent. Informed consent protects the patient's right to make an informed decision about medical treatment and protects the health-care facility and staff from legal action should the patient or significant other claim the procedure was performed without the patient's permission or knowledge.

Competent adults 18 years of age and older must consent to their treatment. Minors may consent to treatment if they are

- Emancipated, that is, living without parents or guardians and managing their own financial affairs
- On active duty with the United States armed forces
- Pregnant
- Married, whether or not the marriage has been dissolved

Otherwise, a parent or legal guardian must give consent for surgery involving a minor. A parent or legal guardian must also give consent for surgery involving an incompetent adult. An adult is considered incompetent if he or she is unconscious or mentally unable to understand the procedure or make a reasoned decision.

The key to informed consent is that it must indeed be "informed." The patient, parent, or legal guardian must be informed by the physician about the nature, risks, desired results, and possible complications associated with the planned procedure. The physician must also explain any alternative treatment available. The explanation must be given in terminology and a language understood by the person signing the consent and must include information that any reasonably prudent person would need in order to make an intelligent decision about the proposed procedure or treatment. Consent must be given voluntarily and without coercion. It cannot be obtained from a person under the influence of a potentially mind-altering substance.

In an emergency situation, the physician is permitted to proceed with treatment or surgery based on implied consent, when it is believed that the patient would have given permission if competent, able to understand the situation, and able to do so. In a nonemergency situation, when the patient's health is at risk but consent is either not obtainable or refused, the hospital may obtain a court order for treatment such as blood transfusions or necessary surgery.

Each agency has a form that must be signed, dated, and witnessed indicating informed consent. It specifies the patient, the surgery or procedure, and the physician performing the surgery or procedure. The agency defines in its procedure policies the role of the nurse in obtaining consent forms and in witnessing such forms. As a witness, the nurse verifies that the patient has signed the form voluntarily and understands the procedure to which he or she is consenting. The physician is responsible for explaining both the benefits and the risks to the patient before the patient gives a valid informed consent. If a patient indicates lack of understanding, confusion, or ambivalence regarding the consent, the nurse should notify the physician immediately and wait until the patient's issues have been resolved before obtaining consent.

Finally, remember that a patient can revoke consent at any time before the procedure. Document the patient's unwillingness to proceed with the procedure and notify the physician immediately.

SURGICAL CLASSIFICATIONS

Surgical procedures are classified in many different ways. The most common classifications are based on the extent of surgery, the urgency of surgery, and the surgical approach used.

Extent of Surgery

Procedures are described as major or minor on the basis of risk involved and extent of surgery. Minor surgical procedures involve a limited body area and a short period of time to complete the procedure. They constitute minimal risk to the patient. An example is the removal of a benign skin lesion that could be performed in a hospital ambulatory setting or in a physician's office.

Major surgical procedures involve an extended body area or a longer period of surgical time. They present an increased risk to the patient. These procedures are performed in an operating room and require a surgical team. Examples of major surgery are an abdominal bowel resection (opening into the abdominal cavity to excise a portion of the bowel) or a craniotomy (an opening into the skull to operate on a portion of the brain).

Urgency of Surgery

Another method of classifying surgical procedures is based on the degree of urgency surrounding the procedure.

Emergency surgery must be performed immediately to save the patient's life, to maintain organ or limb function, to remove a damaged organ or limb that endangers the patient's life, or to stop a hemorrhage. A gunshot or stab wound lacerating a large blood vessel would require emergency surgery.

Urgent surgery must be performed within 24 to 48 hours, and includes such procedures as removal of kidney or ureteral calculi.

Required surgery must be performed, but can be scheduled a few weeks or months ahead of time. Examples include cataract removal and tonsillectomy.

Elective surgery involves a condition for which surgery is recommended, but if the procedure was delayed or not done there would be no adverse effects. A vaginal repair and a scar removal are examples of elective surgical procedures. To ensure the necessity of elective surgical procedures, many insurance companies require the opinion of a second surgeon.

Optional surgery is performed on the basis of the patient's personal choice. Cosmetic surgery in most instances is optional.

Surgical Approach

The surgical approach and location of the surgical incision are influenced by many factors, including

> The patient's diagnosis
> Expected pathology
> Provision for maximum exposure of the operative area
> Ease of increasing the size of the incision if necessary
> Ease of closure
> Minimum postoperative discomfort
> Maximum provision for wound healing and aesthetic effect.

Examples of surgical procedures classified by approach include vaginal hysterectomy (removal of the uterus through the vagina), abdominal hysterectomy (removal of the uterus through an abdominal incision), transurethral prostatectomy (removal of the prostate gland through the urethra), and perineal prostatectomy (removal of the prostate gland through a perineal incision).

Some surgery can also be performed through straight or flexible fiberoptic/endoscopic tubes inserted into the body through external orifices or small surgical incisions. These tubes allow instruments for cutting, applying clips, electrical cauterization, and laser light to be guided into the body and manipulated by the surgeon, who visualizes the procedure either through an optical scope inside the tube or on a visual display monitor attached to a camera on the end of the tube. Surgery of the gastrointestinal tract, the urinary tract, the respiratory tract, the circulatory system, and the reproductive organs can be performed through fiberoptic/endoscopic tubes.

Other surgical techniques include application of chemical agents to superficial skin lesions to damage the tissue and cause it to die and slough off. Electric current can be applied to a lesion to cauterize it or its vascular supply and its base of attachment to underlying structures. The lesion is then manually removed or allowed to die and slough off. Laser light can be used to vaporize lesions or cauterize blood vessels supplying a lesion. Surgical approaches and the nursing care specific to each are discussed in detail in the appropriate chapters throughout the text.

SURGICAL RISK FACTORS

Every surgical procedure involves risk. The amount of risk depends on the patient's overall physical and mental health status, the presence of factors known to increase surgical risk, the nature and extent of the disease being treated, and the location and extent of the planned procedure. To determine surgical risk, the surgeon evaluates the patient's history, physical examination, and diagnostic evaluation. The surgeon also assesses the patient's condition and any other physical attributes that might alter the surgical outcome or affect the patient's ability to tolerate the procedure. If the risks of surgery appear to be greater than its potential benefits, surgery may be delayed until the patient is in better condition, or it may be canceled altogether.

Psychosocial Status

Regardless of the extent or urgency of the surgical procedure, it is a stressful event and has an emotional impact on the patient as well as a physical impact. Most patients have many fears about surgery. They fear the unknown, an altered body image, a change in lifestyle, separation from loved ones, cancer, pain, death, and more. At the same time, a patient may feel relief at reaching a diagnosis and deciding on a treatment, even if the treatment is surgery. For many patients, fear and relief exist together.

Stress can elicit a physical as well as an emotional response, depending on the degree of stress experienced. Age, physical condition, and past experience with stressful situations (including surgery) affect the patient's response. A patient under stress may be overly anxious or appear deceptively calm and relaxed. The person may have difficulty concentrating and be easily distracted, or may focus exclusively on one detail. The patient may become withdrawn, agitated, angry, hostile, or demanding. Stimulation of the sympathetic nervous system and neuroendocrine response to stress are manifested by decreased urinary output, increased heart rate and cardiac output, increased blood pressure, and increased physical activity, such as pacing.

During the preoperative period, the patient requires psychologic and emotional support. The nurse can give support by explaining the surgical procedure in easily understood language. Diagrams and pictures usually help in explaining the surgical procedure. Preoperative teaching, tailored to the patient's cultural and educational background, provides psychologic and emotional support and will probably help to alleviate anxiety.

Economic Influences

The financial implications of surgery depend on the type and extent of the procedure, as well as on the patient's course of recovery. Extensive surgery requires a longer recuperation than a minor surgical procedure. The impact of the hospitalization, surgery, and recovery may add to the patient's stress and alter postsurgical lifestyle and independence.

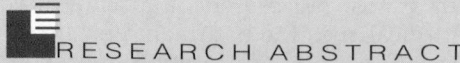

RESEARCH ABSTRACT

Do Men and Women Cope Differently with Surgery?

Crumlish CM. Coping and emotion in women undergoing cardiac surgery: A preliminary study.
MEDSURG Nursing 1993; 2(4):283.

For several years, there has been growing concern over the practice of extrapolating the results of research conducted using male subjects to populations of women.

In this article, Crumlish points out that although one in seven women between the ages of 45 and 64 has some form of heart disease, they are protected from the disease to some degree before menopause and usually do not develop significant cardiac problems until about age 65. When significant cardiac problems do develop, the presenting symptoms are often very different from those with which men with the same problems present. Additionally, for patients undergoing cardiac surgery, the expected coping responses in the immediate preoperative and postoperative periods are postulated primarily based on experience with male patients. There is therefore little information about how female patients undergoing cardiac surgery cope in these same periods.

Crumlish sought to examine how a pooled sample of women coped with the experience of cardiac surgery preoperatively and postoperatively and to examine their emotional reactions to the surgical experience in those periods. Crumlish wanted to answer the following questions:

- Does coping change in women from the preoperative to the postoperative period?
- What is the relationship between coping and emotion preoperatively in women?
- What is the relationship between coping and emotion postoperatively in women?

To answer these questions, Crumlish used Lazarus and Folkman's stress and coping theory as the basis for the study. According to Lazarus and Folkman, psychologic stress is mediated by cognitive appraisal, which determines the meaning of an event that stimulates an emotional response. Coping is defined as how the person manages the stressor and the accompanying emotion. According to Lazarus and Folkman, coping changes over time as the appraisal of a situation changes. The relationship between emotion and coping is seen as bidirectional. That is, each affects the other.

Crumlish found that while the strategies used by men and women were similar, women's thoughts and behaviors remained stable and consistent during the preoperative and postoperative periods. Crumlish found that neither gender perceived cardiac surgery as a highly distressing experience, because by the time of surgery most patients were well-prepared, educated, and knowledgeable about cardiac surgery. Crumlish also found that even if the patients perceived the surgery as stressful, most of them were well prepared to handle the experience and their emotions.

Questions to Consider

1. Why should there be such concern about the extrapolation of research data compiled on a primarily male population to the general population?
2. What agencies are now requiring or encouraging replication of research formerly conducted on males using a female population?
3. What percentage of research performed in any area uses a mixed group of both males and females?
4. What type of research should be carried out using only one gender as the target group?
5. Why is it important to incorporate stress and coping theory into the care of the perioperative patient?

At the very least, surgery may take time away from responsibilities at work and at home. The patient may lose income, possibly the job itself, while unable to work. Surgery may render the person unable to continue in a former occupation, further altering income and socioeconomic status. Many individuals have no insurance to cover health-care costs. Others may undergo treatments not covered by insurance. Referral to resources for financial assistance, often coordinated by the agency's social workers, helps the patient cope with the economic impact of surgery. And by increasing the patient's sense of control over the situation, it can reduce stress.

Nutritional Status

Malnutrition, including obesity, increases the risk of surgery. Nutritional deficits can lead to poor wound healing, inadequate hemostasis, and postoperative infection. These deficits are found primarily in elderly patients or those with chronic illnesses, cancer, or intestinal disease. They are also common among the homeless and abusers of alcohol and drugs. Malnourished patients may require oral supplements, enteral feedings, or parenteral hyperalimentation therapy before and after surgery.

Obesity increases surgical risk because of a

higher incidence of postoperative wound complications and concomitant disease. Poor wound healing and infection are common in obese patients because fat tissue has a poor blood supply, which reduces the amount of nutrients and antibodies that can reach the operative area. Pulmonary complications are also more likely in the obese because

1. Ventilatory expansion may be compromised by abdominal fat.
2. Obese patients have more difficulty moving, coughing, and deep-breathing after surgery.
3. Postanesthetic recovery is prolonged because fat cells retain anesthetic agents longer than other cells.

To decrease risks, a nutritionally sound weight-loss program may be undertaken before elective surgery.

Fluid and Electrolyte Balance

Fluid and electrolyte disturbances increase surgical risk by altering the body's ability to adjust to and recover from the stress and trauma of surgery. These imbalances are more common in the elderly because the aging process reduces renal function, decreases cardiovascular and respiratory function, alters hormonal regulatory functions, and decreases total body fluids.

Excess fluid increases the risk of cardiovascular and respiratory complications. Such excess may be caused by acute or chronic cardiac disorders, renal disorders, liver disorders, overadministration of parenteral fluids, and hypernatremia. Fluid volume deficit increases the risk of altered tissue perfusion, cardiovascular complications, and hypovolemic shock. The deficit may be caused by inadequate fluid intake or by fluid loss from vomiting, diarrhea, or hemorrhage. Additional fluids are lost during surgery from evaporation and blood loss. Blood loss is always measured or estimated during the surgical procedure.

Electrolyte imbalances may develop in many acute and chronic conditions. They most commonly result from altered electrolyte intake or absorption, altered electrolyte excretion, or electrolyte shift between the cells and extracellular fluid. A loss or gain of sodium is usually associated with a loss or gain of water. Electrolyte imbalance places the patient at risk for fluid imbalance, acid-base imbalance, and disturbances in neuromuscular impulse transmission and response. In nonemergency situations, fluid and electrolyte imbalances are corrected before surgery. Fluid and electrolyte imbalances are discussed in detail in Chapter 5.

Immune Status

An infection anywhere in the body can affect the outcome of a surgical procedure. The body's defenses are involved in fighting the infection; there-fore, the ability to withstand the stress of surgery is compromised. For this reason, elective surgery may be postponed if any signs or symptoms of infection are present, such as an elevated temperature, skin lesions, sore throat, coughing, or sneezing. For a patient with an immunodeficiency disorder, the risk of postoperative complications and even death is greatly increased.

A strong personal or family history of allergic disorders might indicate a hypersensitivity to drugs. The surgeon and anesthesiologist will consider this possibility carefully because drug allergies, sensitivities, and incompatibilities—as well as adverse drug reactions—may be fatal. Chapters 32 and 33 discuss the immune system and its disorders in detail.

Cardiovascular Status

Concurrent cardiac disease increases the risk of surgery because it alters or exaggerates myocardial responses to anesthetic agents, electrolyte imbalance, and catecholamine release stimulated by the stress and trauma of the procedure. Previous cardiovascular disorders compromise the patient's ability to adjust to alterations in fluid balance and tissue perfusion and to recover from the effects of blood loss and shock. Recent or unstable anginal pain, signs of a recent myocardial infarction, cardiac dysrhythmia, valvular heart disease, and cardiac failure should be evaluated, treated, or controlled before surgery. An electrocardiogram is often done for adults who will undergo surgery. If not an emergency or urgent procedure, surgery may be postponed for 6 months after a myocardial infarction. Cardiac function and disorders are discussed in detail in Chapters 7 and 8.

Peripheral vascular disease and hypertension increase the risk of clot and emboli formation postoperatively. The patient should be evaluated and, if necessary, treated to control the problem and reduce surgical risk. The vascular system and its disorders are discussed in detail in Chapters 9 and 10.

Respiratory Status

Upper and lower respiratory tract infections contra-indicate required and elective surgery because of the increased risk of airway obstruction and postoperative atelectasis. Chronic obstructive pulmonary disease, bronchial asthma, and restrictive lung disease increase the number and severity of postoperative complications because they hamper exchange of respiratory gases. During the history and physical examination, the finding of a pulmonary disease or the possibility of one may suggest the need for further evaluation and pulmonary function tests. Suspicious findings include exertional dyspnea, exercise intolerance, cough, production of sputum, or history of smoking. Before surgery, the anesthesiologist will conduct an extensive examination focused on the patient's respiratory system. A chest x-ray may be ordered to rule out active pulmonary disease. Respiratory functions and disorders are discussed in detail in Chapters 14, 15, and 16.

Renal Status

Impaired renal function places the patient at risk for fluid and electrolyte imbalances that result from altered excretion of catabolic waste products and fluid retention. Renal function is evaluated through a complete urinalysis and measurement of serum creatinine, albumin, and blood urea nitrogen. Dialysis patients will need to receive a dialysis treatment the day before surgery and as soon as possible afterward to reduce accumulation of toxic metabolites.

Many medications commonly used during the perioperative period are toxic to the kidney, and dosages are modified in patients with renal disease. These include:

Antibiotics
Antituberculosis agents
Anti-inflammatory agents
Hypoglycemic agents
Analgesics
Anesthetics
Hypnotics
Antineoplastic drugs

Renal function and urinary tract disorders are discussed in detail in Chapters 30 and 31.

Hepatic Status

Liver disease is associated with increased surgical risk because adequate liver function is necessary for biotransformation and detoxification of drugs and anesthetic agents and for production of clotting factors. Further hepatic studies are indicated if the history and physical examination reveal the possibility of liver disease, chronic malnutrition, alcoholism, or drug abuse. Hepatic function and disorders are discussed in detail in Chapters 25 and 26.

Endocrine Status

Endocrine abnormalities must be recognized and treated preoperatively to prevent acute hormone imbalances triggered by stress or anesthetic agents. Diabetes mellitus and chronic thyroid, adrenal, or other endocrine disorders increase the patient's risk for infections, impaired wound healing, and cardiovascular complications. Endocrine disorders require evaluation, treatment, and control before elective surgery to minimize perioperative risk. Endocrine gland functions and disorders are discussed in detail in Chapters 27, 28, and 29.

Neurologic Status

Neurologic disorders increase the risk for impaired respiratory function and altered response to anesthetic and analgesic agents. Anesthesia and the stress of surgery may exacerbate a chronic neurologic disorder such as epilepsy, multiple sclerosis, or myasthenia gravis, increasing the risk for injury and poor wound healing. Chronic neurologic conditions should be stabilized before elective surgery. A preoperative neurologic examination for all surgical candidates provides baseline data for postoperative reference and evaluation. Neurologic function and disorders are discussed in detail in Chapters 17 and 18.

Hematologic Status

In general, moderate anemia does not increase the hazards of surgery, although it may prolong the recovery period. Ideally, moderate anemia and deficiencies of iron, folic acid, and vitamin B_{12} should be corrected before elective surgery. Elective surgery is usually postponed for severe anemia. Anticoagulants usually are discontinued before surgery to prevent delayed clotting. Sickle-cell disease usually is accompanied by chronic anemia and increased risk of thrombosis formation because the stress of surgery causes sickling of the red blood cells. Before surgery, hydration is increased and blood transfusions may be administered to increase the hemoglobin to normal levels. The hematologic system and its disorders are discussed in detail in Chapters 12 and 13.

Therapeutic Drugs

Many prescription and nonprescription medications can alter a person's response to surgery or anesthetic agents. Antihypertensives, antiarrhythmics, antibiotics, and anticonvulsants can interact adversely with anesthetic agents. Corticosteroids typically diminish the patient's ability to withstand the stress of surgery. Aspirin and other anticoagulants increase the chance of hemorrhage. Diuretics increase the risk for postoperative electrolyte imbalance. For these reasons, all medications that the patient takes routinely are evaluated before surgery. They may be discontinued or dosages adjusted as needed.

Substance Abuse

Patients who abuse such substances as alcohol, caffeine, nicotine, and drugs are at increased surgical risk. The surgical team needs to be aware of the patient's use of these substances before surgery because they may affect the patient's response to medication and ability to recover from the surgery.

ALCOHOL

Alcohol is a central nervous system depressant that can interact with medications given during the perioperative period and result in unexpected and often dangerous reactions. Patients tend to understate their alcohol consumption and deny symptoms that might be associated with alcoholism. Withdrawal from alcohol can lead to delirium tremens and unexpected gastrointestinal bleeding. In some instances, the surgeon, anesthesiologist, and nurse are unaware of the substance abuse and discover it because of the withdrawal effects that begin during the postoperative period.

Chronic alcoholism leads to malnutrition and clotting disorders. Cirrhosis of the liver leads to a reduction of the clotting factors II (prothrombin), V, VII, and X. Platelets may be severely reduced in acute alcoholism and may cause bleeding problems. Bleeding from the gastrointestinal tract is usually caused by esophageal varices, gastritis, or hemorrhoids. Bleeding further compromises the patient's condition and increases the risk of complications. Liver disorders related to alcohol abuse are discussed in Chapter 26.

OTHER SUBSTANCES

Smoking and pulmonary disease greatly increase the surgical patient's risk. Smoking irritates the respiratory passages, destroys cilia, and decreases vital capacity. The person is less able to cough effectively to clear pulmonary secretions and faces increased risk for pulmonary tract infections, atelectasis, and impaired clearance of inhaled anesthetic agents. Smokers should be encouraged to stop smoking altogether, or at least for 24 hours before anesthesia. After surgery, heavy smokers may become restless or agitated from nicotine withdrawal. They may ignore activity restrictions in order to smoke. And they may create a fire hazard by smoking while confined to bed.

Although most patients are well aware of their coffee-drinking habits, they may not realize that other beverages contain caffeine, such as colas. Caffeine withdrawal can lead to headache, jitters, tremors, insomnia, or agitation.

Patients may also use illicit drugs or even abuse over-the-counter drugs. Specific responses to drug withdrawal depend on the substance abused by the patient.

Pregnancy

The need for surgery arises in the pregnant woman just as often as in the nonpregnant woman of the same age. When it does, fetal risk must be considered. Maternal surgery raises the risk of morbidity and mortality in the fetus. The risk of preterm delivery also increases in women who undergo surgery. Only emergency and urgent operations are performed during pregnancy. Elective operations are postponed until the postpartum period. In addition, radiologic examinations of the lower abdomen and pelvis are avoided, if possible, especially during the first 6 weeks of pregnancy.

The more common disease entities that require surgical intervention during pregnancy include appendicitis, hiatal hernia, and cholecystitis. Less frequently, intestinal obstruction, breast cancer, and ovarian tumor may require surgery during pregnancy. To reduce surgical risk, general considerations for the pregnant surgical patient for specific affected systems are as follows:

1. Maintain left lateral tilt in second and third trimester to help with cardiovascular status and enhance urinary output.
2. Monitor fetal heart rate continuously.
3. Do not expect cool, clammy skin to develop in shock.
4. Administer supplemental oxygen to maintain pulse oximeter reading of 94% or greater.
5. Insert a nasogastric tube to prevent aspiration.
6. Avoid urinary catheterization to prevent urinary tract infections.

Preoperative Period

The preoperative period begins with the recommendation for surgery and ends with the patient's entrance into the operative suite. During the preoperative period, diagnostic studies are completed, preoperative teaching is initiated, disorders are stabilized, and the consent for treatment is obtained. The preoperative period can be very short, as with emergency surgery, or extended in length, as with elective or optional surgery.

DIAGNOSTIC PROCEDURES

Depending on the surgical procedure planned and the age and condition of the patient, a variety of diagnostic procedures may be completed before surgery. The purposes of these procedures are as follows:

- Establish baseline values for intraoperative and postoperative comparison.
- Screen for diseases or conditions that may affect the surgical result (such as infectious processes).
- Identify diseases that may contraindicate elective surgery or require treatment before surgery (such as diabetes mellitus or respiratory disorders). If elective surgery is being contemplated, surgery could be delayed by low blood counts, infection, or fluid and electrolyte imbalance.
- Initially diagnose or further evaluate conditions that require surgery (such as appendicitis or a fracture).
- Evaluate the extent and nature of pre-existing medical conditions (such as heart and renal disease).

Diagnostic examinations depend on the planned surgical procedure and the condition of the patient. A complete blood count, serum electrolytes and chemistries, and urinalysis are the most common preoperative diagnostic procedures. Completion of blood coagulation studies, radiologic studies of the chest, and an electrocardiogram depend on the patient's age, condition, diagnosis, and medical history, as well as agency policy and physician preference.

Additional diagnostic studies may be required to clarify results of these examinations or to further aid the surgeon in determining the patient's diagnosis or the extent of the area involved in the planned surgery. Radiologic studies of specific body parts or organs, computed tomography, magnetic resonance imaging, ultrasonography, and nuclear medicine studies are examples of these types of diagnostic procedures. Table 6–2 describes common preoperative diagnostic studies and their nursing implications.

PREOPERATIVE MANAGEMENT

Patients who have an extensive medical history or who have been treated medically before surgical intervention are examined by their primary care physician before surgery and their progress followed throughout recovery to ensure consistent, ongoing management of concurrent medical conditions. The surgeon, during a final preoperative examination and evaluation, reviews diagnostic findings with the patient as well as the anticipated plan for surgery, answers questions to clarify areas of concern, and writes specific orders for preoperative restrictions and final preparation of the patient for surgery.

Food and Fluid Restrictions

Dietary modifications depend on the scheduled time of surgery, the type of anesthesia to be used, and the surgical procedure. Solid food intake is restricted for a minimum of 7 hours preoperatively, and fluids for at least 4 hours, to prevent regurgitation or vomiting, which could result in airway obstruction, aspiration pneumonia, or atelectasis.

If surgery is scheduled for the morning, the patient usually receives a light meal the evening before and then nothing by mouth (NPO) after midnight. If surgery is scheduled for the afternoon and does not involve the gastrointestinal tract, the patient may receive a soft or liquid meal for breakfast, then be on NPO status. Intravenous fluids may be started the day or night before surgery to prevent dehydration in the elderly and other patients at risk for dehydration during fluid restriction.

It is particularly important that outpatients or ambulatory patients understand the importance of food and fluid restrictions. The nursing staff needs to fully assess NPO time status, since the patient arrives the day of surgery and has not been monitored. In preoperative teaching, stress that elective surgery may be canceled if food or fluids are taken.

Frequently, outpatient surgeries are scheduled in the morning to accommodate this inconvenience.

Elimination

All patients are instructed to void and defecate before administration of preoperative medications. Preoperative laxatives and cleansing enemas are not routinely ordered, except for bowel or gastrointestinal surgery. In those situations, multiple cleansing enemas as well as cathartics might be ordered to reduce microorganisms in the operative area and the risk of contamination of the abdomen with stool. Gastric or intestinal suction tubes to remove gastrointestinal contents and to prevent aspiration and abdominal distention may be inserted preoperatively or in the operating room.

For abdominal surgery or surgery of the genitourinary or reproductive tract, an indwelling urinary catheter is commonly inserted to lessen the risk of accidental bladder injury by maintaining bladder decompression. It may be inserted preoperatively or in the operating room.

Skin Preparation

The purpose of skin preparation is to reduce the risk of postoperative wound infection by minimizing the number of microorganisms on the skin. In most instances, it is begun at home or on the unit and is completed in the operating room. If possible, the patient bathes or showers the evening before or the morning of surgery. Outpatients or ambulatory patients may be instructed to wash or scrub the surgical site with a particular antimicrobial solution at home before the procedure.

Hair removal at and surrounding the operative site may be requested before an operative procedure. Some institutions remove hair only if it interferes with the surgical procedure (craniotomy, for example) because of the risk of nicks, cuts, rash, and infection. Hair is removed just before surgery. Research studies have shown a direct correlation between length of prep time and infection rates; that is, the closer the preoperative preparation is to the actual surgery (incision time), the less the risk of infection. Depending on agency policy and surgeon preference, hair can be removed with an electric clipper, a depilatory, or a sharp, disposable razor. An antimicrobial agent is used to cleanse the area. The anatomical area to be prepared, the type of solution, and the length of scrub time after hair removal varies with each surgery and with agency policy.

If a rash is present or develops after skin preparation, or if skin integrity is broken during hair removal, the surgeon should be notified immediately. Altered skin integrity increases the risk of infection and may necessitate a delay in surgery. Document skin preparation in the patient record.

Table 6-2

Common Preoperative Diagnostic Studies

Study	Purpose and Procedure	Nursing Implications
BLOOD STUDIES		
Complete blood count (CBC)	Examination of venous blood sample to evaluate Hgb concentration, Hct, RBC, and WBC. White cell differential identifies percentages of each type of leukocyte.	No special preparation needed. There is slight discomfort during needle insertion. The arm is elevated without bending the elbow, and pressure applied until bleeding stops.
Platelet count and coagulation studies	Evaluation of venous blood sample for platelet level and PT, PTT. Used to evaluate homeostatic function and identify patients at risk for prolonged bleeding or coagulation abnormalities during and after surgery.	Same as CBC. Assess skin and mucous membranes for petechiae and ecchymoses. Ask about bleeding from gums or rectum to identify patients at risk.
Serum test profile (SMA 12)	Automated electronic system examines venous serum sample for multiple diagnostic studies. 12 determinations include glucose, cholesterol, albumin, and total protein (nutrition status); bilirubin level (liver function); BUN and uric acid levels (renal function); AST (tissue injury); alkaline phosphatase (bone-tissue injury); and calcium and phosphate levels (parathyroid function).	Instruct the patient to maintain NPO status except for water for 4 hours before test. Venous blood sample per CBC.
Serum electrolytes	Sodium, potassium, chloride, calcium are measured; magnesium may be included.	No special preparation. Venous blood sample per CBC. Report abnormal electrolyte values to physician immediately.
RENAL FUNCTION STUDIES		
Urinalysis	Screening test for urinary tract and renal disease as well as some metabolic and systemic disorders.	No special preparation. Send random sample of at least 15 mL of fresh urine for analysis immediately or refrigerate. First morning urine preferred. Collect specimen in clean, dry container. Indicate current medications on laboratory requisition.
CARDIAC FUNCTION STUDIES		
Electrocardiogram (ECG)	Evaluate cardiac status, provide baseline data. Electrodes are placed on the four extremities and the chest.	Test involves no special preparation or discomfort. Male patients may need some chest hair shaved to permit proper adhesion of leads.
RADIOLOGIC STUDIES		
Radiography (x-ray examination)	Shadow image of the contour and density of a part of the body produced by roentgen rays. Used to visualize size, position, foreign objects, or injury.	Patient preparation depends on examination. Determine date of LMP: radiographic studies are avoided during pregnancy, especially in first trimester. Jewelry in the area to be examined must be removed.

Table continued on following page

Table 6–2

Common Preoperative Diagnostic Studies *(continued)*

Study	Purpose and Procedure	Nursing Implications
Chest roentgenogram (chest x-ray examination)	Assess pulmonary status and determine location and size of pulmonary lesions.	Patient preparation depends on view. Instruct patient to hold breath on inhalation while the films are taken.
Computed tomography (CAT scan or CT scan)	An x-ray system that produces detailed cross-section images of body tissues and organs not clearly seen with regular x-ray films. Contrast agent may be injected to improve visualization. Used to detect organ dysfunction and to determine size and volume of tumor.	Patient preparation depends on area examined. If contrast agent is used, NPO for 3 hours before examination; oral medications may be taken with sip of water. Determine whether patient is claustrophobic and explain that he or she will be positioned flat on narrow table that slides into center of a donut-shaped scanner, that the table moves every few seconds, and that the examination may take 15–60 minutes, depending on the body part being examined.
MAGNETIC RESONANCE IMAGING (MRI)		
	Uses a strong magnetic field and radiowaves to produce precise images of the body's internal organs and tissues. Contrast agent may be injected to improve visualization. Used to detect organ and tissue dysfunction not visible by x-ray film or CT scan.	All metal objects and jewelry must be removed. All items with metal clips and parts, including hearing aids, must be removed. Patients with pacemakers, neurostimulators, or any type of metal implants, clips, prostheses, or metal shrapnel or fragments cannot have MRI scans because of strong magnetic fields created. Determine date of LMP: Study not recommended during pregnancy. Keep patient NPO for 3 hours before scan if contrast agent will be used; oral medications may be taken with sips of water. Determine whether patient is claustrophobic and explain that he or she will be positioned flat on a narrow table that slides into the center of a donut-shaped magnet, and that examination may take 15–90 minutes, depending on the body part being examined.
ULTRASONOGRAPHIC IMAGING		
Ultrasonography (ultrasound examination)	Produces image of deep body structures by measuring and recording reflection of pulsed or continuous high-frequency sound waves. Used to visualize organs.	Patient preparation depends on body organ being examined. Electrode jelly applied over body surface to facilitate movement of transmitter/receiver.

Table 6-2

Common Preoperative Diagnostic Studies *(continued)*

Study	Purpose and Procedure	Nursing Implications
NUCLEAR MEDICINE STUDIES	Patient receives radioactive compound that circulates through body. Gamma rays given off by compound are detected in tissues and organs by gamma scanners and imagers and in blood and urine by gamma counters. Used to evaluate organ function and extent of certain diseases.	Patient preparation and participation depend on study. Reassure patient that radioactive dose is very low; agents lose most of their activity in hours or days and are usually quickly eliminated from the body. Refer to facility procedure manual for specific precautions. Determine date of LMP: study not done during pregnancy.

AST, aspartate aminotransferase (formerly SGOT); BUN, blood urea nitrogen; Hct, hematocrit; Hgb, hemoglobin; LMP, last menstrual period; NPO, nothing by mouth; PT, prothrombin time; PTT, partial thromboplastin time; RBC, red blood cells; WBC, white blood cells.

PREANESTHESIA MANAGEMENT

Patients scheduled for surgery are assessed by the anesthesiologist either the day before or the day of surgery. The anesthesiologist reviews the medical history and current diagnostic findings and obtains a history of anesthetic experiences, current and past medication use, drug reactions, and allergies. Ambulatory surgery patients are classified according to the following categories:

Physical status I
Healthy patient with no systemic disease
Physical status II
Mild systemic disease without functional limitations; Examples: moderate obesity, old MI, mild hypertension
Physical status III
Severe systemic disease associated with definite functional limitations; Examples: persisting angina, morbid obesity, moderate to severe pulmonary insufficiency
Physical status IV
Not a candidate for ambulatory surgery; severe systemic disease that is a constant threat to life; Examples: advanced pulmonary, renal, hepatic insufficiency
Physical status V
Not a candidate for ambulatory surgery; moribund patient who is not expected to survive without the operation; Example: ruptured abdominal aneurysm with shock
Physical status VI
Not a candidate for ambulatory surgery; a declared brain-dead patient whose organs are being removed for donor
Physical status E (emergency)

Used to denote a presumed poorer physical status of a patient in any of these categories who is operated on as an emergency.

A physical examination emphasizing the head, neck, chest, back, and arms is completed to identify potential intravenous sites and difficulties with intubation and airway management. Anesthesia and operating room procedures are explained. The anesthesiologist writes orders for preanesthesia medication and determines the type of anesthesia to be administered.

The goals of preoperative medication are to

- Reduce anxiety, fear, and stress
- Lower the incidence of nausea and vomiting
- Decrease discomfort and pain
- Reduce secretions and potential for aspiration and laryngospasm

Antibiotic medications may be given prophylactically to decrease the risk of infection. Medications are given to control diabetes, hypertension, seizures, or steroid replacement, although they may be held or modified when given preoperatively. They're given with a small sip of water. The choice of preoperative medications depends on specific patient needs. The preanesthetic medication regimen usually consists of medications given about an hour before surgery, consisting of a variety of narcotics, benzodiazepines, antiemetics, antihistamines, and anticholinergics.

Narcotic analgesics (such as morphine and meperidine) minimize the perception of pain and supplement the action of general anesthesia. However, narcotics depress the respiratory and cardiovascular systems and decrease gastric motility, which may predispose the patient to nausea and vomiting. The narcotic antagonist naloxone hydrochloride rapidly reverses respiratory depression and should be readily available.

Benzodiazepines (such as diazepam and midazolam) provide sedation with mild circulatory depression but rarely cause postoperative nausea or vomiting. They also reduce anxiety and apprehension. The respiratory system may be severely depressed. The benzodiazepine antagonist flumazenil rapidly reverses respiratory depression and should be readily available.

Antiemetics (such as droperidol, metoclopramide, and ondansetron) potentiate sedative effects from other medications. The circulatory system may be compromised by hypertension or hypotension.

Antihistamines (such as promethazine and hydroxyzine pamoate) provide sedation. They potentiate the action of other medications; therefore, a decreased dose of analgesic can be administered with the same effect.

Anticholinergics (such as atropine, Robinul, and scopolamine) reduce oral, respiratory, and gastric secretions to facilitate intubation and also prevent reflex bradycardia caused by surgical manipulation.

NURSING PROCESS
The Preoperative Patient
Assessment

Assessment of the surgical patient begins with the first encounter, whether in the physician's office, the clinic, or the emergency room, or on admission to the hospital. Determine the patient's understanding of the current diagnosis, diagnostic procedures, planned surgery, expected outcome of surgery, sequence of recovery, and impact of surgery and recovery on lifestyle to identify areas of concern and teaching needs. Assess the patient's ability to understand and cooperate with diagnostic procedures.

A thorough medical history and physical examination are essential to a successful surgical outcome. Each agency has a patient history form to guide data collection and to facilitate documentation. Common symptoms that require special emphasis during data collection include pain, vomiting, change in bowel habits, hematemesis, passage of blood through the rectum, and trauma. The physician obtains information about the present illness, family history (such as a family member's trouble with anesthesia), and the patient's history and emotional background. Allergies are verified. Range of motion and mobility is assessed to prevent positioning problems during surgery.

Review the medical history and therapeutic drug use and assess physical status to identify factors that increase surgical risk or the risk of postoperative complications. Specifically ask about current and past alcohol consumption, drug use, smoking habits, and allergies.

Ask female patients whether they might be pregnant and determine the date of the last menstrual period. Determine how the patient copes with stress and identify family members or significant others who provide emotional support and encouragement.

Cultural influences vary, and an individual's family can be an important support system during the perioperative phase. Be aware of religious beliefs that may interfere with routine practices, such as a Catholic patient requesting to wear religious jewelry (medal or rosary), or a Jehovah's Witness patient refusing blood products. Attempt to include family members or significant others in the discussion when possible. Offer spiritual support through consultation with available pastoral care providers.

Nursing Diagnoses and Planning

Nursing diagnoses and related expected patient outcomes commonly applicable to preoperative patients include the following:

NDx: Anxiety related to hospitalization, surgery, outcome of surgery, and impact on lifestyle

Planning: Patient Outcomes
1. Patient asks questions and verbalizes concerns.
2. Patient states that feelings of apprehension have decreased.

NDx: Knowledge deficit: diagnosis, diagnostic procedures, planned surgery, expected outcome of surgery, admission procedures

Planning: Patient Outcomes
1. Patient states diagnosis and verbalizes an understanding of the diagnosis.
2. Patient verbalizes understanding of diagnostic procedures and cooperates in their timely completion.
3. Patient identifies planned surgery and states the reason it was chosen as treatment.
4. Patient verbalizes realistic expectations of surgery.
5. Patient arrives at the hospital or ambulatory surgery unit and is admitted as scheduled.

NDx: Risk for altered health maintenance related to insufficient knowledge of postoperative activities and exercises to promote respiratory and circulatory function

Planning: Patient Outcomes
1. Patient verbalizes understanding of the benefits of each exercise.
2. Patient demonstrates each exercise.
3. Patient states intention to perform each exercise hourly as instructed.

NDx: Knowledge deficit: preoperative preparations and postoperative routines

Planning: Patient Outcomes

1. Patient verbalizes understanding of preoperative preparations and postoperative routines.
2. Patient participates in preoperative preparations and postoperative routines.

Nursing Interventions and Evaluation

The primary goal of preoperative nursing care is to ensure that the patient is prepared physically and mentally for surgery to the fullest extent possible given the specific circumstances. Preoperative teaching is a major focus of patient preparation and preoperative nursing care. It facilitates recovery and decreases the length of hospital stay. Studies have documented that patients who receive preoperative teaching have a smoother induction into anesthesia, fewer postoperative complications, more rapid recovery, less anxiety, and a better feeling about themselves than patients who do not receive preoperative instruction. Highlight 6–1 summarizes important points to include in the patient's preoperative preparation.

HIGHLIGHT 6–1 **PATIENT EDUCATION**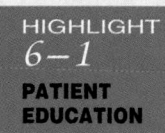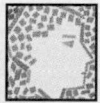

Preoperative Patient Preparation and Teaching

Instruct the patient on the following topics. Provide written instructions when possible.

Before Admission

Review the physician's explanation of scheduled surgical procedure, anticipated location of incision, possibility of surgical drains, anticipated surgical outcome, and typical recovery. Clarify information, answer questions, and identify teaching goals.

Outline the anticipated sequence of events from preadmission diagnostic procedures through admission, preoperative preparation, intraoperative procedures, and postoperative care.

List the diagnostic procedures to be completed before admission and their scheduled date, time, location, patient preparation, and participation.

Note the date and time of admission and location of the hospital and admitting office.

Explain food and fluid restrictions and skin preparation to be performed at home if surgery is scheduled the day of admission.

Instruct about personal items to leave at home for safekeeping and which documents and items should be brought to the hospital.

Specify what to wear and who must accompany the patient if ambulatory or same-day surgery is scheduled.

Before Surgery

Review diagnostic procedures, patient preparation, and participation.

Review (again) the physician's explanation of scheduled surgical procedure, anticipated location of incision, possibility of surgical drains, anticipated surgical outcome, and typical recovery. Clarify information, answer questions, and identify teaching goals.

Check the informed consent form to make sure that signatures have been obtained. Evaluate the patient's wishes for advance directives for treatment and organ donation.

Note the time at which surgery has been scheduled.

Remind the patient to increase fluid intake the day and evening before surgery.

Also remind the patient about food and fluid restrictions and when they take effect.

Review preoperative skin preparation and bowel and bladder preparation.

Instruct the patient to remove jewelry, nail polish, dental appliances, contact lenses, and prostheses, and to ensure their safekeeping during surgery.

Explain the appropriate preoperative procedures, including changing into the hospital gown, removing underwear, emptying bowel and bladder before premedication, preoperative medications, parenteral fluids, transport to the operating room or preanesthesia holding area.

Describe the surgical procedure, including positioning on the operating table, skin preparation, expected sensations, the environment, induction of anesthesia and its expected sensations.

Tell the patient about postanesthesia care unit procedures, expected sensations, transport to the postsurgical unit.

Review postoperative positioning, movement, respiratory exercises, circulatory exercises, splinting techniques, pain management, and early ambulation.

NDx: Anxiety

Provide ample opportunity for the patient and significant others to express thoughts and concerns about diagnosis, planned treatment, hospitalization, and their possible impact on current lifestyle and financial situation. Encourage questions to demonstrate interest and concern. Answer honestly in terms the patient can understand. Do not offer false reassurance. Reinforce the physician's explanations of the planned surgery and its expected outcome to help increase the patient's understanding. Refer questions you cannot answer to an appropriate resource. Offer a referral to social service or clergy if needed.

NDx: Knowledge deficit: diagnosis, diagnostic procedures, hospitalization procedures, planned surgery, expected outcome of surgery, admission procedures

Depending on the patient's diagnosis, condition, and urgency of the planned surgery, diagnostic procedures may be completed before or after hospitalization. Explain the diagnostic procedures, their purpose, patient preparation and participation, and expected sensations during each procedure. When possible, provide written as well as verbal instructions. Answer questions and provide necessary assistance to ensure timely and accurate completion of diagnostic evaluation.

Once diagnosis is confirmed and surgery is planned, answer questions and reinforce the physician's explanations of the diagnosis, planned surgery, and its expected outcome to correct misconceptions and reduce anxiety. Encourage the patient to telephone if he or she has any further questions. New questions frequently come to mind after the patient has had time to think about the planned surgery.

Review hospital admission procedures and how and when the patient will be advised of the date of surgery and admission date and time. Remind the patient to bring all hospitalization and medical insurance information to the admitting office.

NDx: Risk for altered health maintenance

Teach and reinforce postoperative activities that promote respiratory and circulatory function and help prevent postoperative complications. Explain the benefit of each activity or exercise. Tell the patient that he or she will be encouraged and assisted to perform exercises hourly on the day of surgery and the first postoperative day. Frequency thereafter depends on the patient's condition, risk factors, and ability to ambulate. Place the patient in a semi-Fowler's to high Fowler's position to promote maximum lung expansion during respiratory exercises. Document teaching, return demonstration, and independent performance of exercises in the patient record. Many agencies use a checklist for each teaching topic and for documenting demonstration of learning by the patient.

DEEP-BREATHING EXERCISES. Teach the patient the following: Breath deeply using the diaphragm, as illustrated in Figure 6–1. Exhale completely and then place a fist high up on the abdomen, just below the breast bone, and inhale gently and deeply through the nose, making the fist move outward without making the shoulders rise. Hold the breath 3 seconds and then exhale slowly and gently through pursed lips, as if whistling. Repeat the cycle three to five times. Tell the patient to perform this exercise each hour after surgery. This exercise dilates the respiratory passages and alveoli, increases gas exchange, helps prevent atelectasis, and enables the patient to get more air into the lungs with less effort.

COUGHING EXERCISES. Teach the patient the following: Sit upright and lean slightly forward, or bend the knees while seated in a high Fowler's position in bed, and breathe in and out deeply, using the diaphragm as just described. Repeat the procedure. Take a third deep breath and then, with the mouth open, give three short, shallow coughs with short breaths in between. Keeping the mouth open, inhale quickly and immediately cough forcibly once or twice from below the diaphragm where the fist is pressed, using the abdominal muscles. Inhale deeply to reinflate collapsed alveoli. If abdominal surgery is scheduled, teach the patient to splint the incision with both hands and interlaced fingers or a folded blanket or sheet to decrease discomfort when coughing, as illustrated in Figure 6–2. This exercise mobilizes secretions to clear the lungs of mucus.

INCENTIVE SPIROMETER. This device motivates the patient to get more air into the lungs. The exact apparatus varies with each institution. One example is shown in Figure 6–3. All devices measure the amount of inhaled air and display the amount clearly to the patient. Teach the patient to place the mouthpiece between the lips and take slow, deep

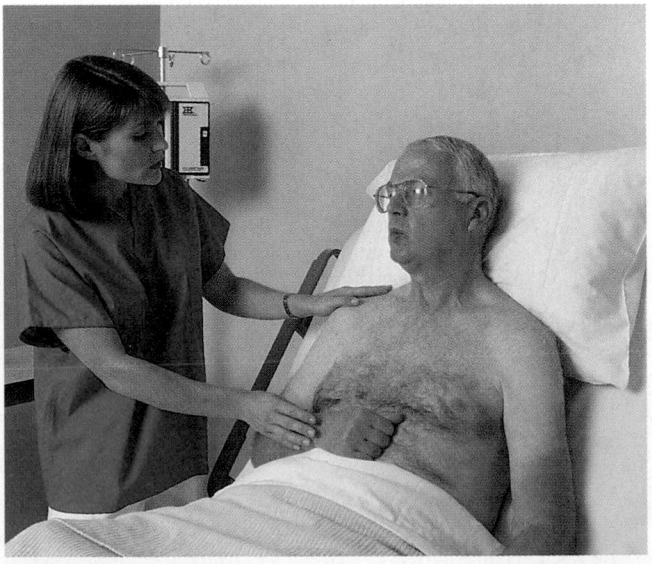

Figure 6–1

Deep-breathing exercises.

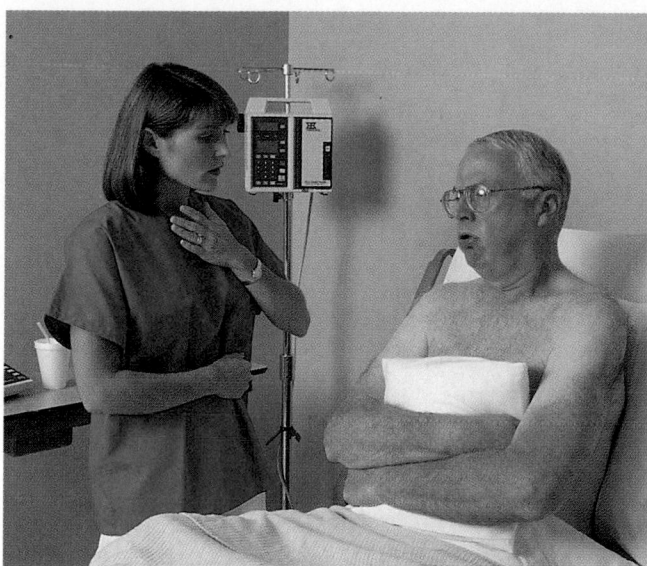

Figure 6-2

Splinting an abdominal incision.

breaths through the mouth, moving the spirometer indicator. Repeat 5 to 10 times. Tell the patient to perform this exercise every hour after surgery. Encourage the patient to use the spirometer before surgery to increase vital capacity and to promote alveolar inflation. Mark the preoperative inspiratory level to provide a postoperative comparison.

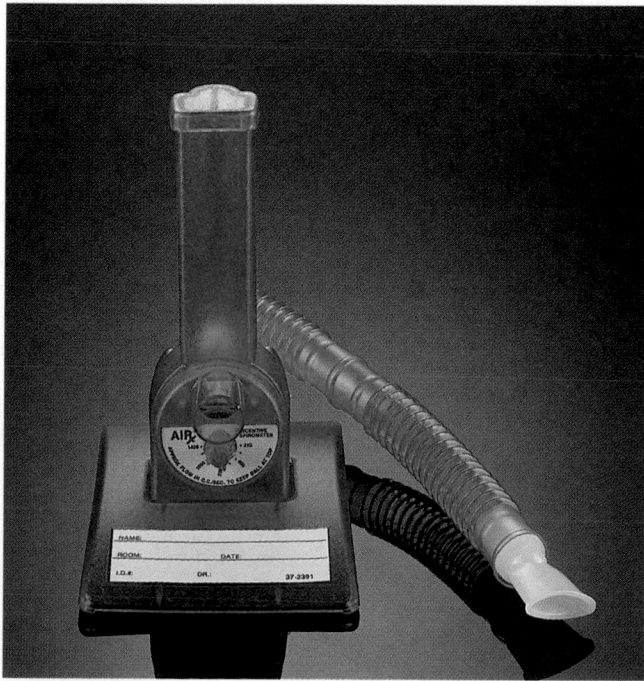

Figure 6-3

Incentive spirometer. (Courtesy of Baxter Healthcare Corporation, Round Lake, IL.)

TURNING AND POSITIONING. Teach the patient to use the side rails to turn and change position at least every 2 hours. If the patient cannot move independently, assist in changing position at least every 2 hours. Active movement stimulates circulation, promotes venous return, and prevents thrombus formation by minimizing venous stasis. Repositioning promotes comfort, helps maintain skin integrity, and mobilizes respiratory secretions. Early ambulation is the best postoperative activity to regain health maintenance.

LEG EXERCISES. These strengthen the muscles and improve blood circulation in the feet and legs. As illustrated in Figure 6-4, teach the patient the following: Flex the foot toward the head, stretching the toes upward, and then point the feet toward the bottom of the bed, curling the toes downward. Trace circles with the feet by rotating the ankle in a circle in one direction and then in the opposite direction. Flex the leg by bending the knee, sliding the foot along the mattress as far back as possible, lift the foot, and then stretch the leg out completely. Exercise the quadriceps by tightening the buttocks for a count of 10 and releasing. Tell the patient to repeat each exercise 5 to 10 times every hour after surgery.

NDx: Knowledge deficit: preoperative preparations and postoperative routines

Ideally, preoperative teaching begins at the point that surgery is recommended. In elective surgery, the nurse in the surgeon's office usually begins the instruction. Information presented to the patient before admission to the hospital (especially written information) is often retained better than information presented the day or evening before surgery. Concrete, factual information on the upcoming sequence of events will help decrease patient anxiety, clarify information, and increase patient understanding and participation in these events. Teaching is continued during preadmission diagnostic procedures and on admission to the hospital. Group instruction, closed-circuit television, videotapes, and slide presentations can be used as teaching aids to supplement individual instruction.

In-hospital preoperative teaching is designed to decrease anxiety by familiarizing the patient and significant others with the environment and routine procedures associated with surgical care. It also promotes cooperation and participation in postoperative care necessary for a smooth recovery free from complications. Explain the consent form, examinations, and tests performed at admission, preoperative preparation, and the preanesthesia assessment by the anesthesiologist.

Review the sequence of events as the patient goes from the surgical unit to the preoperative holding area, the operating room, the postanesthesia care unit (PACU or recovery room), and finally back to the surgical unit. Describe the holding area, the PACU, and the routines. Include the fact that male

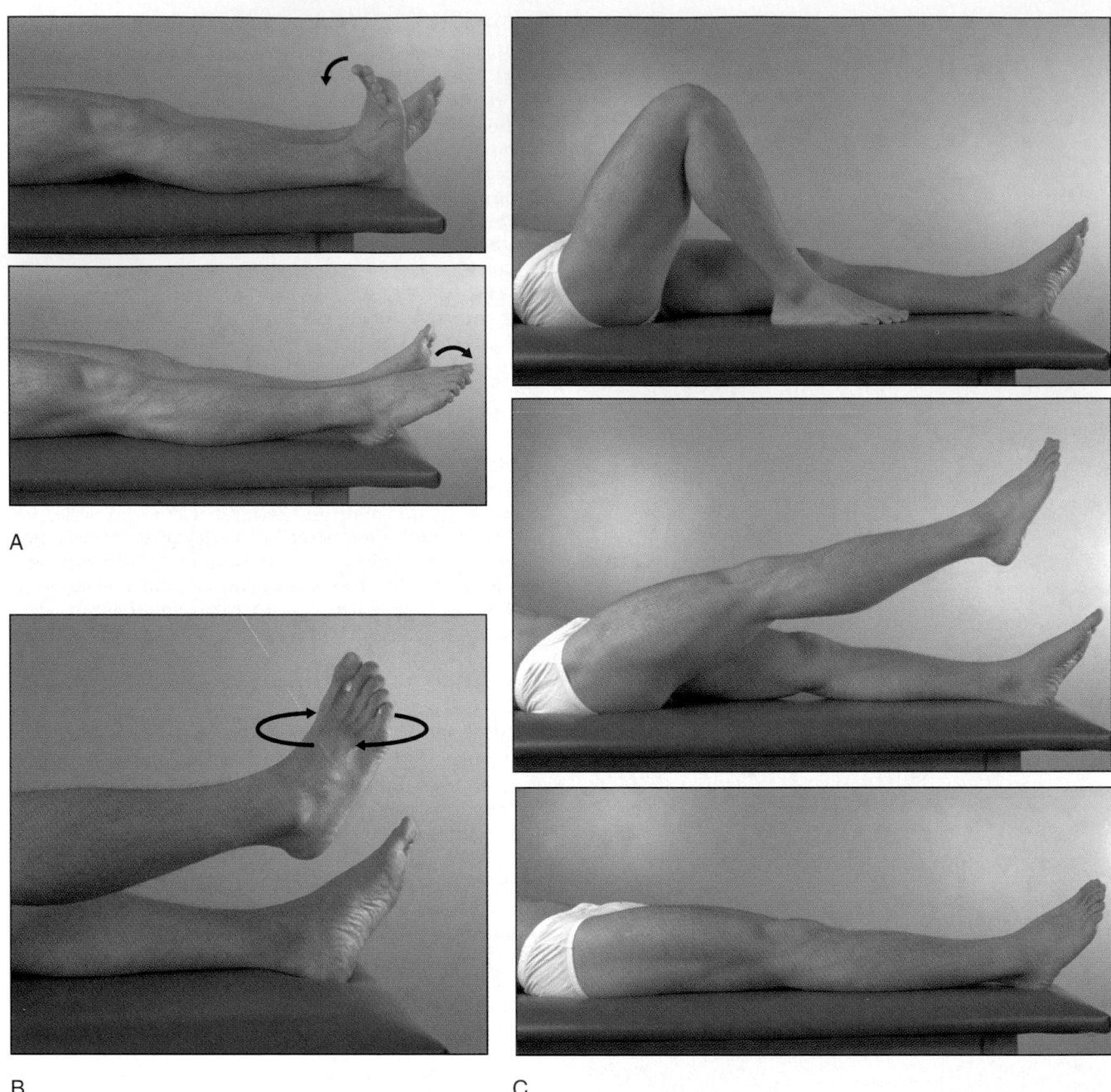

Figure 6–4

Exercises to strengthen muscles and improve circulation in the feet and legs. *A,* Flex and extend the feet. *B,* Make circles with the feet. *C,* Bend the knee, raise the foot and extend the leg, then relax.

and female patients and, in some cases, children are cared for in the unit immediately after surgery.

If the patient is scheduled to go to an intensive care unit rather than return to the surgical unit, be sure the change and its rationale are clearly understood by the patient and significant others to avoid unnecessary anxiety after surgery. Advise the patient to expect pain as the anesthesia wears off but provide reassurance that medication will be given to relieve the discomfort. Stress that the patient should

not hesitate to ask for medication because pain relief reduces anxiety and facilitates coughing, deep breathing, easier movement, and early ambulation. These activities prevent complications of immobility and promote respiratory and circulatory function.

Advise the family and significant others of the scheduled time for surgery, and inform them that the patient will be taken to the PACU before returning to the nursing unit. Assure them that the surgeon will speak to them as soon as possible after surgery. Explain where they wait during surgery and how to find out when the operation is over, when the patient returns to the unit, and when they can see the patient. Be sure they know where the patient will go after he or she leaves the PACU.

Additional Interventions

If not contraindicated, encourage increased fluid intake between diagnostic procedures and on the day and evening before surgery to promote hydration and reduce discomfort during food and fluid restrictions. Explain and implement preoperative food and fluid restrictions to reduce the risk of aspiration during or after surgery. Advise the patient at what time bedside food and fluids will be removed, and reinforce instructions not to eat or drink afterward. Notify oncoming staff and document the NPO status in the chart and on the patient care plan. Follow agency policies to alert other staff and departments of NPO status.

Before surgery, review the chart to confirm that the consent for surgery, preoperative diagnostic procedures, and health-team evaluations and consultations are complete and documented. Encourage and respond to last-minute questions to allay anxiety. Review the planned time of surgery and what preparations to expect.

Review skin-preparation procedures and provide the ambulatory patient with supplies for showering or bathing and with a clean hospital gown. Assist nonambulatory patients in bathing and changing clothes in bed. If surgery is scheduled for the afternoon, bathing may be performed in the morning. Remove hair in the operative site according to agency policy and procedures as close to time of surgery as possible. Enemas to cleanse the bowel are usually administered the evening before surgery but may be repeated in the morning.

If the patient is in the hospital the night before surgery, offer physical comfort measures, such as a back rub or warm, noncaffeinated beverage, and provide a quiet atmosphere to increase comfort, help reduce anxiety, and promote sleep. Offer a sedative if one is ordered by the surgeon or anesthesiologist.

Before readying the patient for surgery, assess vital signs (including oxygen saturation) to determine current hemodynamic status and provide baseline values to compare with measurements obtained during and after surgery. If the temperature is elevated or another abnormal value is present, report it immediately to the anesthesiologist or the surgeon because the surgery may have to be delayed.

Instruct the patient to cleanse the mouth and teeth without swallowing water, remove all undergarments, and put on a clean hospital gown. Provide assistance as needed. If time allows, the patient may wish to bathe or shower. Remove facial makeup and nail polish and artificial nails on at least one finger of each hand so peripheral perfusion can be accurately evaluated by the anesthesiologist

during the operation. Remove all jewelry, dentures, prostheses, and wigs to prevent injury, loss, or damage. These valuables should either be sent home or labeled and placed in the hospital safe.

Ask the patient to urinate and defecate just before leaving the unit or receiving the preoperative medications. Double-check that the operative consent form is signed before administering preoperative narcotic medications. A consent signed after administration of narcotic medication is invalid. If the patient has received premedication, raise the side rails, place the call bell within reach, and, to prevent falls caused by dizziness from the medications, tell the patient not to get out of bed. Reinforce that the medication promotes relaxation but does not necessarily induce sleep. A quiet, darkened room enhances the effect of preoperative medication. To evaluate response and detect adverse effects from the medications assess the patient 15 minutes and 30 minutes after he or she has received premedication.

Document preoperative preparations and premedication in the patient record. In most agencies, a preoperative checklist on the front of the chart is started before the patient is transported to the preoperative holding area. Although the form varies with the institution, Figure 6–5 illustrates possible contents, flowing from the preoperative area to the holding area.

Transport the surgical patient to the holding area on a stretcher, with the side rails elevated and safety belt in place. The surgical floor nurse confirms the patient's identity with the holding room and operating room nurses. The holding area allows for planning that is efficient and moves at a fast pace without patients feeling rushed. One of the main goals of the holding area is to reduce patient anxiety and provide emotional support. The holding area nurse reviews the chart and completes the preoperative checklist and reports on:

Vital signs
Allergies
General condition
Surgical risk factors
Alterations in mobility or neurologic function
Parenteral infusions
Preoperative preparations
Medications to ensure continuity of care

Advise the surgical nurse if the patient is wearing a prosthesis or if family members are present. Frequently, procedures such as insertion of lines (arterial or central venous), insertion of epidural catheters, and administration of spinal or local anesthesia are performed in the holding area. Occasionally family members will be allowed into the preoperative holding area.

Compare the patient's status with the expected outcomes. If the outcomes are not met, reassess the patient and revise the plan.

Surgical procedure(s): _____   Date: _____

_____

Allergies: _____   NPO since: _____

Vital signs at (time) _____: Temp: _____   P: _____   R: _____   B/P: _____

Ht: _____   Wt: _____   Age: _____   Tobacco Use: ❑ No   ❑ Smokes   ❑ Smokeless

PREOPERATIVE CHECKLIST (if no, explain)

	PREOP Y	N	N/A	HOLD. RM		PREOP Y	N	N/A	HOLD. RM
Operative area prepped	❑	❑	❑	❑	EKG _____	❑	❑	❑	❑
Type _____					Dr. _____ notified	❑	❑	❑	❑
ID Band	❑	❑		❑	of any abnormal results				
Verbal ID	❑	❑		❑	H&P dictated/on chart	❑	❑		❑
Dentures/partial plate removed	❑	❑	❑	❑	MAR on chart	❑	❑	❑	❑
disposition _____					Pre-med given	❑	❑	❑	❑
Glasses/contacts removed	❑	❑	❑	❑	Side rails up after pre-med	❑	❑	❑	❑
disposition _____									

PREOP EDUCATION: PATIENT FAMILY NA

	PREOP Y	N	N/A	HOLD. RM
Hearing aid(s) removed: (circle R L)	❑	❑	❑	❑
disposition _____				
Prosthesis type _____	❑	❑	❑	❑
disposition _____				
Jewelry, hairpins, barrettes removed	❑	❑	❑	❑
Surgical cap on	❑	❑		❑
Nail polish removed	❑	❑	❑	❑
Hospital gown on	❑	❑		❑
Undergarments removed	❑	❑		❑
TED hose on	❑	❑	❑	❑
Voided time _____ amt _____	❑	❑	❑	❑
❑ Foley				
Operative permit	❑	❑		❑
Sterilization permit	❑	❑	❑	❑
Blood consent	❑	❑	❑	❑
Father's permit (c-section)	❑	❑	❑	❑
Anti-thrombic pump/calf size _____	❑	❑	❑	❑
CBC _____	❑	❑	❑	❑
U.A. _____	❑	❑	❑	❑
Lytes _____	❑	❑	❑	❑
Other Lab _____	❑	❑	❑	❑
T + C/S with blood band _____	❑	❑	❑	❑
CXR _____	❑	❑	❑	❑

	PATIENT	FAMILY	NA
NPO	❑	❑	
Preps	❑	❑	❑
Preop medication	❑	❑	❑
Transport by stretcher	❑	❑	
Estimated OR & RR time	❑	❑	
Waiting room location	❑	❑	
Postop vital signs	❑	❑	
Postop pain/nausea	❑	❑	
PCA pump	❑	❑	❑
IV, drains, dressings, catheter	❑	❑	❑
TCDB, leg exercises	❑	❑	❑
Respiratory treatments	❑	❑	❑
Postop diet, I/O	❑	❑	
Postop activity	❑	❑	
TED hose/anti-thrombic pump	❑	❑	❑

Literature given _____

Videos seen _____

Response to teaching: ❑ Expressed understanding
❑ Distracted   ❑ Unable to teach pt./family because:

_____

Nurse signature (only if other than pre-op nurse):

To surgery at _____ / _____
(time)   (date)

Nurse Signature: _____

Northwest Medical Center
INPATIENT PERIOPERATIVE
ASSESSMENT FORM, page one
NS 4-35a 12/93

PATIENT LABEL

Figure 6–5

Example of a preoperative checklist. (Courtesy of Northwest Medical Center, Springdale, AR.)

Intraoperative Period

The intraoperative period is the time during which the patient is transported to the operating room, receives anesthesia, undergoes surgical intervention, and is transferred to the PACU. The patient is sedated and anesthetized during the intraoperative period and is, therefore, unable to prevent injury or make needs known. The nurse, as part of the surgical team, is the patient's advocate. The nurse monitors patient safety, maintains asepsis, and initiates activities that facilitate completion of the surgical procedure with minimal anesthesia time and patient trauma. Nursing interventions reduce the risk of intraoperative complications and promote optimum recovery.

SURGICAL TEAM

The surgical team is composed of a group of specialized individuals working together for the welfare and safety of the patient. It includes the surgeon, assistants to the surgeon, anesthesiologist, scrub assistant, and circulating nurse.

The surgeon is the physician whose primary responsibility is to perform the operative procedure. The surgeon may assist with positioning, preparing, and draping the patient or may delegate these duties to the first assistant or to a perioperative nurse.

The assistant to the surgeon may be another surgeon, resident, intern, physician's assistant, or registered nurse (RN) first assistant. The assistant's responsibilities include:

- Preparation of the operative site
- Exposure of the operative field with retractors
- Sponging and suctioning blood and fluid that might obscure visualization of the operative field
- Tissue handling
- Suturing
- Providing hemostasis

Preparation for the RN first assistant program includes a minimum of 2 years of recent perioperative nursing experience with competencies in scrubbing, circulating or assisting roles, and certification as a certified nurse in the operating room (CNOR). The structured RN first assistant program is equivalent to 1 year of post–basic nursing study and consists of curricula that address specific nursing concepts and behaviors to provide care to patients experiencing surgical intervention.

The anesthesiologist is a physician who specializes in the administration of anesthesia to relieve pain and relax muscles. A certified registered nurse anesthetist (CRNA) is specially trained in the administration of anesthesia at the nursing advance practice level. The person who administers anesthesia is also responsible for airway insertion and for maintaining a patent airway and adequate exchange of respiratory gases. He or she monitors fluid and blood loss, provides intravenous fluid replacement, and monitors respiratory and cardiac function.

The scrub assistant may be a nurse or a surgical technician. The scrub assistant is responsible for maintaining a sterile environment and preparing sterile instruments and supplies that will be needed during surgery. The scrub assistant and circulating nurse count the instruments, needles, and sponges before the surgery and again before closure of the wound to ensure that all instruments have been removed from the patient. The scrub assistant prepares and hands surgical instruments to the surgeon and assistant, advises the circulating nurse when additional supplies are needed, and ensures that all team members adhere to the principles of surgical asepsis.

The circulating nurse is an RN who manages and coordinates activities in the operating room, brings needed supplies and medications, and removes used or contaminated items. The circulating nurse implements the nursing care plan, provides emotional support before anesthesia and during emergence from anesthesia, assists the anesthesiologist with induction, monitors patient safety and positioning, monitors the patient's fluid losses and general condition, and documents assessments and interventions throughout the surgical procedure. At the close of surgery, the circulating nurse supervises, confirms, and records the final sponge and instrument count with the scrub assistant and then accompanies the anesthesiologist and patient to the PACU and reports to the PACU nurse.

POSITIONING

Position for surgery is determined by the site of the operation, type of anesthesia, maintenance of respiratory and cardiac function, age and size of the patient, and pre-existing physical limitations or disease conditions. Regardless of the selected position, basic principles must be observed to maintain the patient's dignity and safety and to prevent neuromuscular and peripheral vascular complications. Such complications can arise despite depression of normal responses to pain and pressure by preoperative medications and anesthesia. These principles are as follows:

- Expose only the operative area.
- Use a safety belt.
- Maintain normal body alignment.
- Pad all equipment used for positioning.
- Do not cross the legs.
- Do not allow extremities to rest on body surfaces or to hang off the table.

Positioning injuries may be temporary or permanent and include nerve damage (ulnar, radial, peroneal, tibial), brachial plexus injury, foot drop, and finger or toe injuries.

Common surgical positions are illustrated in Figure 6–6. These include supine or dorsal recumbent, Trendelenburg, reverse Trendelenburg, modified Fowler's, lithotomy, prone, jackknife, and lateral. The lateral position may be either level or jackknife, depending on the surgery planned.

SKIN PREPARATION AND DRAPING

The purpose of skin preparation is to minimize the number of microorganisms. Skin preparation continues in the operating room and, in most instances,

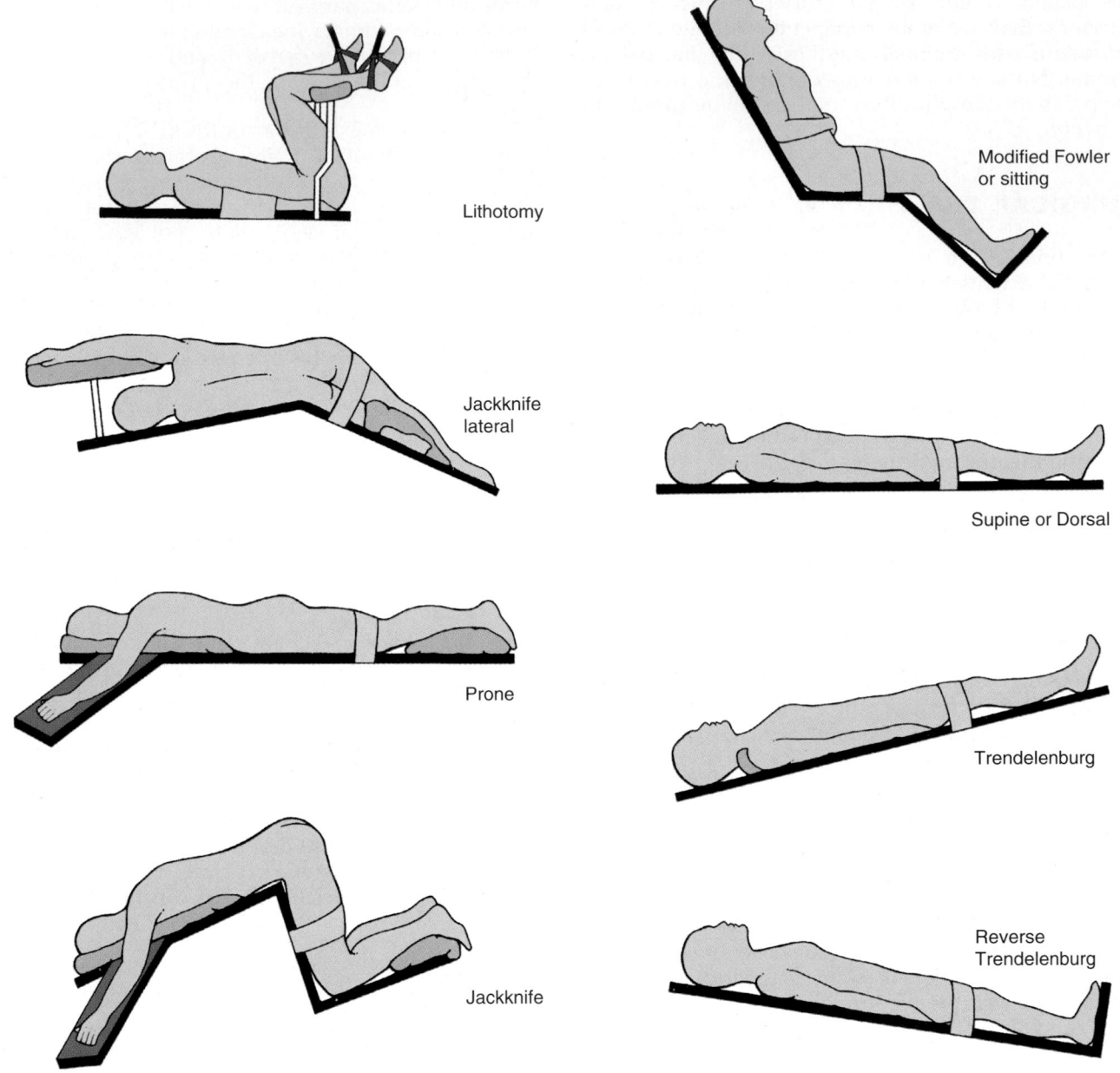

Figure 6-6
Common surgical positions.

includes scrubbing the operative area with an antimicrobial solution and applying an antiseptic agent. The circulating nurse must diligently assess the skin and document so that comparisons can be done postoperatively. Occasionally, pressure ulcers begin in the operating room.

On completion of the surgical scrub, a sterile operating field is created by covering the body with sterile drapes that leave a minimum area of skin exposed around the operative site. Surgical drapes maintain a barrier between nonsterile and sterile areas. They are made of disposable or reusable materials that are safe for use in the operating room. In addition to surgical drapes, a sterile, transparent, impermeable adhesive drape may be applied to the skin over the surgical area. This adhesive drape forms a seal over the operative site and minimizes the risk of skin bacteria coming in contact with the surgical wound. The surgical incision is made directly through the adhesive drape.

ANESTHESIA

Administration of anesthetic agents produces a partial or complete loss of pain sensation (with or without loss of consciousness), muscle relaxation, and loss of reflexes. The two major types of anesthesia are regional and general.

Regional Anesthesia

Regional anesthesia includes local, nerve block, epidural, and spinal. The anesthetic agent is deposited either directly into the area to be anesthetized or along a nerve or nerve pathway to the central nervous system that transmits the pain stimulus to the brain. It temporarily blocks transmission of pain and sensory impulses from a specific part of the body. Motor function may or may not be affected. The size of the anesthetized field depends on the site of application, the amount of anesthetic used, and the specific effects of the anesthetic agent.

Regional anesthesia can be used for most surgical procedures and is particularly suitable for the following operations:

Cosmetic procedures
Biopsies
Excisions of moles and cysts
Hernia repairs
Cesarean sections
Some abdominal and pelvic procedures
Many eye, ear, nose, and throat procedures
Endoscopic examination of the respiratory, urinary, and gastrointestinal tracts

The most commonly used regional anesthetic agents include cocaine, lidocaine hydrochloride (Xylocaine), tetracaine hydrochloride (Pontocaine), mepivacaine hydrochloride (Carbocaine), procaine hydrochloride (Novocain), and chloroprocaine hydrochloride (Nesacaine). Table 6–3 presents the types of regional anesthesia, their uses, and nursing implications.

Complications from regional anesthesia are rare. However, local and systemic hypersensitivity or idiosyncratic reactions can occur. Complications of spinal anesthesia resulting from prolonged depression of the central nervous system include hypoxia, irregular respirations, respiratory depression, drowsiness, and convulsions. Temporary paralysis of the respiratory muscles requires intubation and mechanical ventilation. Adverse cardiovascular reactions caused by interruption of sympathetic nerve pathways and loss of vasomotor tone are manifested by hypotension, bradycardia, and thready pulse. Bladder control is the last function to return after spinal anesthesia.

Headache after spinal anesthesia is thought to result from leakage of cerebrospinal fluid through the hole in the dura. It typically occurs up to 48 hours after spinal placement when the patient assumes an upright position but is unrelated to how soon the patient ambulates. With adequate hydration, it usually resolves spontaneously in 1 to 3 days. Occasionally a blood patch is performed to help seal the fluid leak.

General Anesthesia

General anesthesia is produced either by injection of an anesthetic agent into a vein or by inhalation and absorption of the agent into the blood from the alveoli. These anesthetic agents are carried to all body tissues via the circulatory system. In the brain, the anesthetic agent interrupts nerve-cell activity. Central nervous system alterations begin at the cortex and work down the brain stem. As the patient loses consciousness, sensory messages are no longer processed by the brain and motor responses are no longer issued to body parts. Behavioral changes and loss of social inhibitions occur first, followed by loss of memory, consciousness, voluntary muscle control, response to pain, body temperature control, muscle and vascular tone, protective reflexes and, finally, respiratory and circulatory control.

STAGES OF GENERAL ANESTHESIA

Administration of general anesthesia produces four characteristic stages.

Stage 1: Relaxation
This is the period of induction. The patient is drowsy and dizzy and appears inebriated. Hearing is exaggerated; pain sensation is decreased.

Stage 2: Excitement
This stage is characterized by irregular breathing, increased muscle tone, and involuntary motor movements of all extremities. Movement, touch, or noise may trigger vomiting, breathholding, and thrashing about. Avoid stimulation, be sure safety straps are properly applied, and be prepared to assist with patient restraint.

Stage 3: Surgical Anesthesia
This period is characterized by quiet regular breathing, a relaxed jaw, constricted pupils that respond to light, loss of auditory and pain sensation, absence of eyelid reflex, and decreased muscle tone.

Plane 1. Muscle tone decreases. Eyelid, gag, cough, and swallow reflexes are lost. Type of surgery: craniotomy, mastectomy, reduction of small-bone fractures.

Plane 2. Muscle tone further decreases. Pause between respirations increases. There is a slight increase in pupil size. Type of surgery: amputation, large-bone surgery, thoracic.

Plane 3. Muscle tone markedly decreases. Pupils are more dilated. Type of surgery: upper abdominal, hernioplasties, rectal procedures, cesarean section.

Plane 4. Anesthesia should not reach this level. Pupils are widely dilated and do not react to light. Intercostal muscles are paralyzed. Diaphragm maintains respirations. Blood pressure and pulse decrease.

Table 6-3

Types of Regional Anesthesia

Type	Administration	Use	Possible Complications	Nursing Implications
Topical	Spray, gargle, or application of packs soaked with anesthetic agent to surface area to be anesthetized	Anesthesia of respiratory passage to facilitate intubation; diagnostic procedures of larynx, bronchus, vagina, rectum, or urinary bladder	Cardiovascular collapse when applied to respiratory tract	Monitor vital signs frequently
Local infiltration	Injection of agent into subcutaneous tissue with needle and syringe	Minor operations of short duration; before administration of spinal anesthesia	Myocardial and circulatory depression, toxicity, drowsiness, disorientation, twitching	Monitor vital signs frequently
Nerve block	Injection of agent into and around nerve or group of nerves supplying a specific region	Common nerve blocks: digital, radial, ulnar, intercostal, sciatic, femoral, brachial plexus, cervical plexus Also used to identify cause of pain, to increase circulation in some vascular diseases, and for relief of chronic pain	Nerve damage	Monitor neuromuscular function
Caudal and epidural blocks	Injection of agent into epidural space through sacral hiatus (caudal) or into epidural space between vertebrae (epidural)	Anorectal, vaginal, and perineal procedures	Nerve damage	Monitor vital signs frequently
Spinal anesthesia	Injection of agent into subarachnoid space (most frequently the interspace between third and fourth lumbar vertebrae); to achieve level of anesthesia, patient's head is immediately lowered after injection of anesthetic agent until desired height of anesthesia is realized; after 15–20 min, level is set and cannot be altered by positional changes		Hypotension, spinal headache (up to 48 hours) postoperatively caused by dura mater not sealing off after removal of needle and resultant leakage of cerebrospinal fluid (CSF) into epidural space and decreased CSF pressure; nausea and vomiting; respiratory paralysis; paresthesia or paralysis of legs	Maintain client flat in bed for 12–24 hours as ordered Monitor vital signs frequently Monitor neuromuscular function
Low spinal (saddle block)	Involves sacral nerves (S-1 to S-5)	Perineal and anal region procedures		
Midspinal	Thoracic nerves (T-10)	Procedures below umbilicus		
High spinal	Thoracic nerves (T-4)	Procedures below nipple line		

Stage 4: Danger

The patient is near death with fixed, dilated pupils. Respirations are absent and pulse is rapid and thready. All reflex activity is absent. Vital organs are compromised during this stage, and respiratory failure and cardiac arrest can occur if the patient is not returned to the appropriate surgical anesthesia plane.

INHALATION ANESTHESIA

Anesthetic agents that are inhaled are either in gaseous form (nitrous oxide) or liquid form that can easily be vaporized (halothane, enflurane) and then inhaled. Table 6–4 lists the most common inhalation agents and their nursing implications. All these agents produce rapid induction. The principal advantage of inhalation anesthetics is the ability to control the depth of anesthesia by controlling the rate at which the agent enters and exits the lungs. Another advantage is that the rate of recovery from inhaled anesthesia with adequate alveolar ventilation is quite predictable.

Inhalation anesthetics are administered by a mask placed over the nose and mouth or by endotracheal tube. Use of an endotracheal tube allows anesthetic gases and oxygen to flow directly into the tracheobronchial tree, as illustrated in Figure 6–7. The anesthesia provider inserts the endotracheal tube after the patient is anesthetized sufficiently by intravenous or mask inhalation anesthesia to be unaware of the procedure. Postoperatively, many patients who have been intubated complain of a sore throat caused by irritation.

Inhalation anesthetics are primarily eliminated from the body through the respiratory system. Unless surgery lasts more than a few hours, the inhalation agent is almost completely excreted by the time the patient returns to the postoperative surgical unit.

Table 6–4

Inhalation Anesthetic Agents

Agent	Use	Potential Implications	Nursing Implications	Comments
Nitrous oxide	Short procedures	Hypertension, tachycardia	Monitor vital signs frequently	Used in combination with other agents because of minimal anesthetic potency
Halothane (Fluothane)	Not recommended for individuals who might require multiple surgeries (hepatotoxicity may result)	Cardiovascular depression Hypothalamus depression, shivering immediately postoperatively	Monitor vital signs frequently Maintain warm environment; provide warmed blankets	Provides smooth induction and rapid emergence with minimal excitement
		Liver damage in some individuals	Liver function screening before and after surgery	
Enflurane (Ethrane)	Intra-abdominal surgical procedures	With increased depth of anesthesia, ventilation decreases and blood pressure is lowered	Monitor vital signs frequently	Provides abdominal muscle relaxation; rapid and smooth induction
		Liver damage	Liver function screening before and after surgery	Associated with seizures and renal failure
Desflurane (Suprane)	Ambulatory surgery setting	No lingering analgesia; patient immediately wakens and is aware of pain	Monitor vital signs; assess and manage pain postoperatively	Fast onset and offset of CNS effects
		May cause laryngospasm		Requires specially designed electrically warmed vaporizer
Isoflurane (Forane)	Appears to be most ideal inhalation agent	Mild respiratory depression	Monitor vital signs frequently	Cardiac output and myocardial contractility well maintained
				Agent of choice for diminished renal or liver function

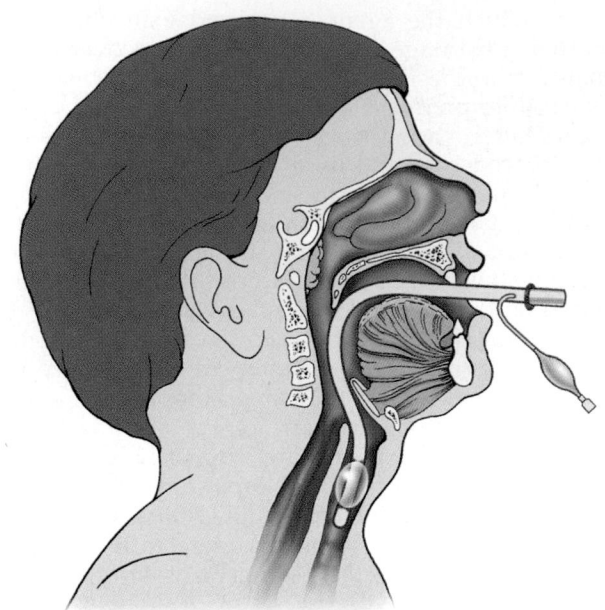

Figure 6–7
Endotracheal tube in position for ventilation.

INTRAVENOUS ANESTHESIA

General anesthesia can also be produced by intravenous administration of one or more central nervous system depressants, narcotic analgesics, and neuromuscular blocking agents. They may be administered alone or in combination with an inhalation agent. Intravenous anesthetics cause a rapid onset of unconsciousness and are often used to initiate anesthesia. Their disadvantage is that they must be metabolized by the liver before they are excreted by the kidneys. Therefore, they are not rapidly removed from the body, and their action cannot be stopped once they are injected. Reversal agents may be required to overpower the effects. Table 6–5 lists the most common intravenous anesthetic agents.

COMPLICATIONS OF GENERAL ANESTHESIA

The most common complications of general anesthesia include hypothermia, hypotension, hypoxia from inadequate ventilation or oxygen administration, and unexpected individual variations in response. Complications are most likely to occur at the time of induction or emergence. Transient decreased urinary output after general anesthesia is common. It is caused by reduced renal perfusion during surgery and release of antidiuretic hormone in response to the stress of surgery. Slow return of bladder tone may cause transient postoperative urinary retention.

Hypothermia

The operating room is a cool, air-conditioned environment. Evaporation of skin-preparation solutions and exposure of internal organs and blood vessels in air-conditioned operating rooms cause excessive loss of body heat and a decrease in body temperature during surgery. More than 90% of patients undergoing surgery experience some degree of postoperative hypothermia (body temperature below 36.6°C [97.8°F]).

Hypothermia is reduced by minimizing exposure of nonsurgical body parts, minimizing exposure time between skin preparation and application of surgical drapes, use of a head covering and blankets, specialized warming equipment, and administration of warmed intravenous fluids and anesthetic agents during surgery. In some instances, hypothermia is induced to lower cellular metabolism and thereby reduce oxygen requirements. Shivering is an attempt by the body to raise core temperature, but it increases oxygen consumption and energy expenditure and could compromise myocardial and peripheral tissue perfusion. Shivering that occurs on emergence from anesthesia is a side effect of inhalation anesthetic agents.

Respiratory Complications

Hypoxia is a major concern during general anesthesia. Aspiration of secretions or vomitus can occur with loss of pharyngeal and cough reflexes. Gaseous exchange is affected by inhaled anesthetic agents that alter pulmonary ventilation percentages of oxygen and carbon dioxide. Along with preanesthetic medications, they can cause respiratory depression. Neuromuscular relaxants weaken or paralyze respiratory muscles. Lung expansion may be further compromised by the patient's position on the operating table. Anesthesia-induced vasodilation reduces cardiac output and pulmonary tissue perfusion.

The anesthesia provider is responsible for maintaining a patent airway. Perfusion of the patient's skin, conjunctivae, mucous membranes, and fingers are monitored by the anesthesia provider and circulating nurse. A pulse oximeter applied to a finger, toe, or ear lobe constantly monitors blood-oxygen saturation.

Peripheral Vascular Complications

Effective peripheral perfusion requires adequate blood volume as well as sufficient stroke volume and heart rate to maintain cardiac output. Anesthetic agents decrease the heart rate or the force of contractions and cause vasodilation and pooling of blood, which reduces venous return to the heart. These actions combine to reduce cardiac output and are manifested by a rapid drop in blood pressure during induction and hypotension during anesthesia. Adequate fluid and blood replacement helps to minimize hypotension.

Reduced peripheral perfusion increases the risk of compromised blood flow, tissue ischemia, and nerve damage caused by direct pressure, hyperextension, flexion, or twisting of body parts. In many surgical positions, body weight is supported over bony prominences, increasing the risk of pressure ulcers. Impaired peripheral perfusion and nerve and

Table 6-5

Intravenous Anesthetic Agents

Agent	Use	Potential Complications	Nursing Implications	Comments
BARBITURATES				
Thiopental sodium (Pentothal) and general characteristics	To induce surgical anesthesia	Large doses can cause respiratory and cardiac depression	Make mechanical ventilator available to control or assist ventilation Monitor vital signs frequently	Onset of action is 30 seconds and duration is ultra-short
Propofol	Used as induction agent; rapid and alert emergence	Hypotension if injected rapidly; high incidence of pain on injection	Rapid emergence may hasten pain awareness Administer analgesics during or after surgery	
NARCOTICS				
General characteristics	Used as adjunct to anesthesia to improve analgesia	Cardiac and respiratory depression	Monitor vital signs frequently Have naloxone (Narcan) or nalbuphine (Nubain) available.	Given in small, repeated doses to provide more intense analgesia
Fentanyl citrate (Sublimaze)	Used as analgesic/anesthetic induction agent	Bradycardia; miosis; nausea and vomiting; hypotension; respiratory depression	Observe for respiratory depression Monitor vital signs Have naloxone readily available	Synthetic narcotic with potency 100 times greater than morphine; administered intravenously or intramuscularly
NEUROMUSCULAR BLOCKERS				
General characteristics	Provide profound muscle relaxation without deep levels of anesthesia	Profound respiratory depression	Must monitor respirations carefully for at least 1 hour after effects of drug appear to have worn off Monitor ability to lift and hold head up for 10 seconds Monitor for firm handgrip Must be provided with artificial ventilation	
Tubocurarine chloride	Short-acting, nondepolarizing agent	Hypotension, bronchospasm		Produces muscle relaxation in 3-5 minutes; duration is 20-60 minutes
Pancuronium bromide (Pavulon)	Long-acting	Hypertension, tachycardia		More long-acting than curare
Succinylcholine chloride (Anectine)	Depolarizing blocking agent; frequently used for intubation			Rapid-acting; duration 3-5 minutes

tissue damage are prevented by avoiding extreme surgical positions, by anatomical positioning of uninvolved body parts, and by padding potential pressure areas and instruments used in positioning.

Bodily Injury

General anesthesia interferes with the body's protective mechanisms for maintaining homeostasis. The patient is unconscious, and pain sensation and reflexes are abolished as the central nervous system is depressed by anesthetic agents. The patient must be protected from injury caused by trauma, thermal and electrical burns, impaired peripheral circulation, pressure damage to the skin or nerves, corneal abrasions, and joint injuries or nerve palsies caused by unnatural positions. Lip, tongue, tooth, and vocal cord injuries can be caused by intubation. The circulating nurse is responsible for patient safety.

Malignant Hyperthermia

Malignant hyperthermia is a rare but potentially fatal complication of surgery. The incidence of malignant hyperthermia in North America is about 1 of 100,000 cases of adults receiving anesthesia. It is a hypermetabolic state of the skeletal muscles caused by a defect in the muscle-cell membrane manifested by excess calcium release and heat production. This hypermetabolic crisis is most commonly triggered by administration of succinylcholine and halothane anesthetic agents. It can also be induced by other anesthetic agents, stress, muscle trauma, infection, and strenuous exercise.

Malignant hyperthermia is characterized by a rapid rise in body temperature of up to 1°C (1.8°F) every 5 minutes. Temperatures as high as 46°C (114.8°F) have been recorded. Primary signs include tachycardia, tachypnea, fever, generalized rigidity, respiratory and metabolic acidosis, hypercarbia, and increasing end-tidal carbon dioxide (ET CO_2), which is the most sensitive of the signs. The patient's skin first has a flushed, rosy color from dilated peripheral vessels and then a mottled, cyanotic appearance caused by hypoxia.

Surgery and anesthesia are stopped immediately, if possible. Otherwise the anesthetics are changed to nontriggering agents. Intravenous dantrolene sodium, a skeletal muscle relaxant, is administered. The patient is hyperventilated with 100% oxygen. Cooling blankets and ice packs are used to reduce body temperature. Refrigerated IV normal saline is administered and a nasogastric tube inserted for stomach irrigation. Cardiac dysrhythmias and acidosis are corrected. A high urine output should be maintained by administering IV fluids, furosemide, and mannitol.

Malignant hyperthermia is a genetically transmitted autosomal dominant trait more common in male children and adolescents. It is associated with inherited skeletal muscle disorders and dystrophies, although most individuals are not aware a disorder exists. Inheritance also has been suggested to be multifactorial and multigenetic. Individuals with scoliosis, a large bulky muscular build, a family history of malignant hyperthermia or skeletal muscle disorders, or a history of muscle or joint injuries preceded by minimal trauma are at risk for malignant hyperthermia. If a patient has an equivocal malignant hyperthermia episode or is a first-degree blood relative of a newly diagnosed patient, a referral may be made to a regional medical testing center for a skeletal muscle biopsy. Currently, this is the only definitive diagnostic test and is available only at specific centers.

For these patients, regional or local anesthesia is preferred for surgery. If this is not possible, then triggering agents such as halothane, enflurane, isoflurane, desflurane, and succinylcholine should not be used. Body temperature is monitored continually by a probe if general anesthesia is used. Dantrolene sodium is administered as prophylaxis to individuals with a known history of malignant hyperthermia if general anesthesia is required. A careful and complete patient and family assessment that includes questions about previous anesthesia should be conducted along with a physical examination to alert for connective tissue abnormalities that suggest potential malignant hyperthermia.

NURSING PROCESS
The Intraoperative Patient

Assessment

In some instances, assessment of the intraoperative patient begins with a preanesthesia visit by the operating room nurse. However, the patient's admission to the operating suite may be the initial contact.

Greet the patient and identify yourself. Confirm the patient's identity with the holding room nurse by checking the identification band and chart, and ask the patient's name. Review the chart, consent, advance directive for treatment, allergies, general condition, surgical risk factors, location and types of permanent prostheses, alterations in mobility or neurologic function, special needs, preoperative checklist, and preoperative vital signs to ensure continuity of care and compliance with legal requirements. Confirm food and fluid restrictions, parenteral infusions, preoperative preparations, removal of prostheses and jewelry, and whether preoperative medications were administered. Assess the patient's emotional state and general condition, vital signs, and response to preanesthetic medications.

Nursing Diagnoses and Planning

Nursing diagnoses and related expected patient outcomes commonly applicable to intraoperative patients include the following:

NDx: Risk for injury related to loss of independent defense mechanisms secondary to anesthesia

Planning: Patient Outcomes
1. Patient remains free from injury.

NDx: Risk for infection related to contamination of wound during surgical procedure

Planning: Patient Outcomes
1. Patient remains free from infection the first 48 hours after surgery as evidenced by absence of the following:
   a. Fever
   b. Purulent or malodorous wound drainage
   c. Increasing redness or edema around the incision

Nursing Interventions and Evaluation

The primary goals of intraoperative nursing care are to ensure patient safety, maintain asepsis, prevent intraoperative complications, and promote optimal recovery. The circulating nurse coordinates the activities of all individuals who enter the operating room and documents nursing care provided during the intraoperative period in the patient's chart. A special surgical record form is completed for perioperative documentation.

NDx: Risk for injury

Throughout the intraoperative period, the circulating nurse functions as patient advocate to prevent injury. Because the patient has received premedication and might be drowsy or disoriented, maintain safety measures and remain with the patient, if possible, before transfer to the operating table. An agitated or confused patient cannot be left alone. Speak in a calm, reassuring voice, explaining procedures and anticipated sensations to reduce anxiety.

Confirm patient identity, diagnosis, and planned surgery with the scrub assistant and anesthesiologist on transfer to the operating room and with the surgeon before surgery. Assist with patient transfer to and from the operating table, and with positioning for surgery. Avoid extreme positions when possible to prevent injury from hyperextension of joints and muscles that are atonic from anesthesia. Maintain functional anatomical position of uninvolved body parts to prevent injury to nerves, vessels, and muscles. Pad all equipment that could compromise peripheral circulation. Determine the presence of peripheral pulses and assess skin color and temperature after positioning and throughout surgery. Attach safety straps to prevent falls and injury from uncontrolled movement during induction and recovery from anesthesia. Assist with draping to ensure maximum access to the surgical site and access for the anesthesiologist while maintaining the patient's dignity. Minimize exposure of uninvolved body parts to reduce heat loss.

Confirm and document instrument, needle, and sponge count before surgery begins and before wound closure. Ensure that electrical grounding pads are properly applied away from pressure points but as close to the operative site as possible to prevent electrical injury. Monitor fluid loss and replacement, body temperature, and cardiovascular status to prevent hemodynamic disequilibrium.

NDx: Risk for infection

The circulating nurse is responsible for maintaining surgical asepsis. Assist with surgical skin scrub and draping to minimize risk of wound contamination. Assist surgeon and scrub assistant in putting on sterile gloves and gowns. Monitor sterile fields and supplies and provide additional supplies as needed. Remove specimens and used or contaminated supplies from the operating area. Assist in applying dressings to protect the wound. Document skin preparation, wound drains, and irrigation devices and dressings.

Compare the patient's status with the expected outcomes. If the outcomes are not met, reassess the patient and revise the plan.

$\mathcal{P}$ostoperative Period

The postoperative period begins when the patient is transferred to either the PACU or the surgical floor. Postanesthesia care, phase I, begins with admission to PACU and ends with safe discharge to phase II. Phase II begins with transfer to the surgical floor or ambulatory section and ends with discharge home.

The surgical team transfers the patient from the operating room table to a stretcher by lifting or using a roller. Apply safety straps and raise the side rails to prevent injury. Protect the incision and any drainage tubes, intravenous tubing, and airway to prevent trauma and dislodgement. The anesthesia provider and circulating nurse accompany the patient to the PACU, confirm the patient's identity with the PACU nurse, give a report, and review postoperative orders. The report includes:

Name
Age
Language spoken
Allergies
Type and extent of the surgical procedure
Preoperative and intraoperative vital signs
Position during surgery
Type of anesthetic agent used
Estimated blood loss
Drugs and intravenous solutions administered
Complications
Location and type of catheters, drains, or packs
Altered sensory or motor functions
Intraoperative events that might affect the postoperative course

The PACU is an area, usually adjacent to the operating room, staffed by nurses and personnel specially trained to assess and care for surgical patients who have received general or regional anesthesia. To meet the patient's needs during recovery and to respond to emergencies, the PACU is equipped with oxygen and suction outlets; bedside cardiac monitors; pulse oximeters; an emergency cart with defibrillator, endotracheal equipment, and emergency drugs; supplies for drawing arterial and venous blood samples; chest tube equipment; ventilators; cutdown infusion equipment; blanket warmer; various medications; and intravenous solutions and supplies.

The patient remains in the unit until the effects of anesthesia have worn off. Criteria for discharge from the PACU include the following:

• The patient is sufficiently awake or easily aroused to respond to simple questions.

- Vital signs are stable with patent airway and spontaneous respirations.
- The gag reflex is present.
- Peripheral pulses distal to the operative site are present.
- Pain is minimal.
- Postoperative complications are resolved or under control.

A numeric scoring system, such as Aldrete, can be used on admission and discharge to measure parameters. These include activity, respiration, circulation, consciousness, and oxygen saturation as presented in Table 6–6. The scale may use color instead of SaO_2.

If regional anesthesia was administered, the patient must have return of motor function and partial sensory return to all anesthetized parts. The patient is discharged from the PACU by the anesthesiologist. If the surgery was major, if concurrent illnesses may complicate recovery, or if the operative or anes-

thetic course was complicated, the patient might be transferred to an intensive care unit.

NURSING PROCESS
The Postanesthesia Patient
Assessment

On admission to the PACU, confirm the patient's identity. Listen to breath sounds and assess blood pressure, pulse quality and rhythm, oxygen saturation percentage, and respiratory status immediately on arrival. Review the postoperative report and orders with the anesthesiologist and circulating nurse. Complete a head-to-toe assessment, including blood pressure, apical pulse, temperature, respiratory status and breath sounds, skin color, condition and temperature, level of consciousness, and response to commands. Determine the rate of flow of parenteral infusions and the solution being infused and compare with the doctor's orders. Assess the infusion site for signs of infiltration or inflammation. Examine dressings to ensure placement and adherence and note drainage. Check beneath the patient for wound drainage or bleeding or skin compromise. Determine the placement of drains or irrigating devices, connect drains to appropriate receptacles and irrigating devices to solutions, and ensure proper function. Note the amount and characteristics of all drainage. Examine bony prominences and pressure areas for redness or unusual pallor and for signs of altered perfusion caused by pressure from the operating table or equipment used for positioning during surgery.

Nursing Diagnoses and Planning

Nursing diagnoses and related expected patient outcomes commonly applicable to patients in a PACU include the following:

NDx: Risk for ineffective airway clearance related to tracheobronchial obstruction by tongue or secretions, depressed cough and gag reflexes, impaired swallowing, possible regurgitation, or vomiting secondary to general anesthesia

Planning: Patient Outcomes
1. Patient maintains clear, open airway as evidenced by normal breath sounds.

NDx: Risk for ineffective breathing pattern related to hypoventilation secondary to the effects of general anesthesia, pain, and positioning

Planning: Patient Outcomes
1. Patient maintains spontaneous, unlabored respirations of more than 10/minute and fewer than 30/minute.
2. Patient remains free of dyspnea and cyanosis.

NDx: Risk for altered systemic tissue perfusion related to hypovolemia, peripheral vasodilation and blood pooling, hypothermia

Table 6–6

Aldrete's Modified Phase I Postanesthetic Recovery Score

Patient Sign	Criterion	Score
Activity	Able to move 4 extremities*	2
	Able to move 2 extremities*	1
	Able to move 0 extremities*	0
Respiration	Able to deep-breathe and cough	2
	Dyspnea or limited breathing	1
	Apneic, obstructed airway	0
Circulation	BP ±20% of preanesthesia value	2
	BP ±20–49% of preanesthesia value	1
	BP ±50% of preanesthesia value	0
Consciousness	Fully awake	2
	Arousable (by name)	1
	Nonresponsive	0
Oxygen saturation	SpO_2 >92% on room air	2
	Requires supplemental O_2 to maintain SpO_2 > 90%	1
	SpO_2 <90% even with O_2 supplement	0

*Voluntarily or on command.
BP, blood pressure; SpO_2, oxyhemoglobin saturation determination via pulse oximetry.
From Aldrete JA: Discharge criteria. In Thomson D, Frost E (eds). Baillière's Clinical Anaesthesiology: Postanaesthesia Care. London, Baillière-Tindall, 1994, pp 763–773.

Planning: Patient Outcomes
1. Patient maintains adequate tissue perfusion as evidenced by the following:
   a. Pulse greater than 60 beats per minute (bpm) but less than 100 bpm, with regular rhythm
   b. Blood pressure stable, more than 90 mm Hg systolic
   c. Capillary refill less than 3 seconds
   d. Urine output greater than 30 mL/hour
   e. Easily aroused and oriented

NDx: **Risk for injury** related to restlessness during recovery from anesthesia and diminished awareness of, and responses to, internal and external stimuli

Planning: Patient Outcomes
1. Patient remains free of injury.

Nursing Interventions and Evaluation

The goals of nursing care in a PACU are to support hemodynamic stabilization after anesthesia and surgery, promote recovery from anesthesia, promote physical comfort and wound healing, and prevent injury and postoperative complications. Table 6–7 describes common postoperative complications and their management.

Patient status is monitored and documented on admission, every 5 to 10 minutes for the first hour, and then every 15 minutes until stable. A special PACU documentation form is used during the immediate postoperative period.

NDx: Risk for ineffective airway clearance
Nursing priorities for the postoperative patient include maintaining a patent airway and adequate respiratory exchange. On admission to the PACU, the patient's reflexes, including the pharyngeal cough and gag reflex, may be absent because of the effects of general anesthesia. Many patients feel nauseated and retch within the first 5 or 10 minutes after waking from anesthesia. Airway obstruction most commonly occurs as a result of the tongue, which is relaxed from anesthesia, falling back against the pharynx or from secretions or gastric fluids collecting in the oropharynx. Keep the bed flat. Unless contraindicated, position the patient to the side to allow secretions to drain until the patient is conscious and swallowing. Monitor breath sounds to detect airway obstruction. Noisy respirations, snoring, wheezes, and gurgling indicate partial airway obstruction. Suction to remove vomitus or mucus that may be obstructing the airway. An oropharyngeal airway to prevent obstruction by the tongue is often in place on transfer to the PACU. The patient usually pushes the airway out on regaining consciousness. If the tongue obstructs the airway because no oropharyngeal airway is in place, and a side-lying position is contraindicated, tilt the head back slightly and thrust the jaw forward by lifting at the angle of the jaw or lift the jaw under the chin to move the tongue forward and reopen the airway.

NDx: Risk for ineffective breathing pattern
Monitor the quality and rate of respirations at least every 5 or 10 minutes until breathing is regular and unlabored, then every 15 minutes until the patient is discharged from the PACU. Administer continuous humidified oxygen and encourage deep breathing and coughing every 5 to 15 minutes to promote gaseous exchange and removal of inhaled anesthetic agents. Reposition the patient side to side every 15 minutes to promote lung expansion and prevent atelectasis. Administer analgesics to promote pain relief and participation in respiratory exercises. Because of the potential side effect of respiratory depression, narcotic analgesics are commonly administered in reduced dosages in the PACU.

Attach a pulse oximeter to a finger, a toe, or an ear lobe to monitor arterial oxygen saturation. Note the color of the skin, lips, mucous membranes, and nail beds to detect cyanosis caused by hypoxia. If an endotracheal tube is in place, maintain patency and mechanical ventilation or oxygen administration as prescribed. Monitor the patient's ability to follow commands and to lift the head or a limb and hold it steady for 5 seconds. Check that the patient can maintain spontaneous respirations of more than 10 per minute and fewer than 30 per minute with pulse oximeter readings of greater than 95%. These are criteria for extubation by the anesthesiologist. Usually, arterial blood gas levels confirm adequate oxygenation before extubation.

NDx: Risk for altered systemic tissue perfusion
Hypoxemia and respiratory acidosis are common causes of cardiac dysrhythmias in the immediate postoperative period. Use a cardiac monitor to monitor heart rate and rhythm continuously. Monitor vital signs, heart sounds, the quality and rate of peripheral pulses, and capillary refill every 5 to 15 minutes until stable and then every 30 minutes. Compare with preoperative and intraoperative assessments to detect changes in cardiac output and cardiovascular function. Monitor temperature and urine output every hour. Immediately report a rapid, thready pulse and a drop in blood pressure. These changes may indicate shock. Other clinical manifestations of shock include the following:

Rapid, shallow respirations
Restlessness or slowed responses
Pallor
Cold, moist skin
Cyanosis
Decreased urine output
Decreased temperature

Possible causes of shock include untoward reaction to the anesthetic or other medications, fluid or blood loss, and bacterial infection.

Administer intravenous infusions to replace intraoperative fluid losses. Monitor the type of solution, flow rate, and infusion site to prevent fluid

Table 6-7

Common Postoperative Complications

Complication	Causes	Major Clinical Manifestations	Treatment	Preventive Nursing Interventions
Atelectasis (collapse of alveoli with retained mucous secretions)	Obstruction of airway by secretions; closure of bronchioles because of shallow breathing or failure to periodically hyperventilate lungs	Fever, tachypnea, tachycardia; decreased breath sounds, scattered crackles	Chest percussion, coughing, suctioning; bronchodilators and mucolytics via nebulizer	Early ambulation, turning, coughing and deep breathing, incentive spirometry
Aspiration	Depression of gastroesophageal and pharyngoesophageal sphincter reflexes resulting from drugs and irritation from endotracheal or nasogastric tubes; food in stomach when given general anesthesia; improper positioning of the patient	Signs of airway obstruction, atelectasis, pulmonary abscess, pneumonitis, pneumonia, or shock	Establish a patent airway by endotracheal suctioning or bronchoscopy	Avoid general anesthesia for patients who have recently eaten; position patient correctly before intubation; use pressure cuffs when prolonged intubation is required; use cricoid pressure prior to induction in emergency cases
Pneumonia	Atelectasis, aspiration, copious secretions as found in a heavy smoker or patient with chronic obstructive lung disease	Fever, tachypnea, increased secretions, crackles, rhonchi	Antibiotics on basis of sputum culture and sensitivity, chest physiotherapy	Coughing and deep breathing, frequent position changes, early ambulation
Thrombophlebitis	Venous stasis caused by prolonged immobilization or pressure on vein walls from leg straps in the operating room, leg holders for lithotomy position	Redness, heat, pain, swelling in calf	Anticoagulation, bedrest, moist heat on affected area	Antiembolic stockings or pumps, postoperative leg exercises, early ambulation
Pulmonary embolism	Formed from venous thrombus; usually originating in legs, pelvis, or right side of heart, then traveling to and being trapped in pulmonary circulation	Sudden severe chest pain or tightness, tachycardia, hypotension, pallor or cyanosis, restlessness, anxiety	Oxygen administration, Fowler's position, anticoagulant therapy, analgesics	Passive and active range-of-motion exercises to legs, antiembolic stockings, low-dose heparin administration if predisposing factors present, early ambulation
Shock	Two most common causes: hemorrhage and sepsis	Decreased blood pressure; elevated pulse; cold, clammy skin; decreased urinary output	If hemorrhage, ligate bleeder and give blood; if septic, antibiotics on basis of blood culture sensitivity	

Table 6–7

Common Postoperative Complications (continued)

Complication	Causes	Major Clinical Manifestations	Treatment	Preventive Nursing Interventions
Wound infection	Break in aseptic technique or a dirty wound; predisposing factors: inadequate preoperative screening and preparation, coexistent conditions such as diabetes mellitus or uremia, obesity, malnutrition, corticosteroid therapy	Fever; foul-smelling, greenish-white drainage from wound; persistent edema, redness	Antibiotics on basis of culture and sensitivity of wound	Strict aseptic technique in operating room and during postoperative dressing changes
Wound dehiscence (opening of the wound) and wound evisceration (protrusion of viscera through opening)	Inadequate surgical closure; increased intra-abdominal pressure from coughing, vomiting, or straining at stool; poor wound healing caused by malnutrition, poor circulation, old age, or preoperative radiation	Discharge of serosanguineous drainage from the wound; sensation that "something gave or let go"	Lay patient down, cover wound with sterile saline-soaked gauze or towels; return to operating room for repair, monitor for shock	Splint wound when patient coughs, medicate for nausea and vomiting; highest risk during 5th to 8th postoperative days, so teach patient signs and symptoms as they may already be discharged
Delayed wound healing	Inadequate supplies of protein, vitamin C, and trace minerals ferrous iron and zinc manganese; inadequate oxygen supply; administration of steroids; wound infections; additional injuries	Edges of wound are not approximated; granulation is not evident	High-protein, high-vitamin, high-calorie diet; splint and support wound during activity	Provide adequate dietary intake; maintain aseptic technique; promote rest for adequate healing
Wound infection with abscess	Poorly nourished individual; surgical contamination; wound drains create entrance site for bacteria; deep wounds more prone to abscess	Temperature elevation; inflammation and edema around wound; malaise; persistent pain	High-protein, high-vitamin, high-calorie diet; antibiotics on basis of wound culture and sensitivity; aseptic technique with dressing changes; abscess treated with incision and drainage	Aseptic technique throughout perioperative period; improve nutritional status preoperatively
Hematoma (collection of blood and clots in wound)	Imperfect hemostasis, use of anticoagulants, coagulation disorders, active bleeding	Elevation and discoloration of wound edges	If small, may reabsorb; otherwise surgical evacuation	
Seroma (collection of fluid other than blood or pus in the wound)	Inadequate drainage from incisional area	Elevation of wound edges	Needle aspiration or surgical drainage	

Table continued on following page

Table 6–7

Common Postoperative Complications (continued)

Complication	Causes	Major Clinical Manifestations	Treatment	Preventive Nursing Interventions
Adhesions after abdominal surgery (fibrous bands between abdominal wall and viscera or between viscera)	Unknown; represents overhealing of tissue and is more extensive if inflammatory process is present	Bowel obstruction, pain	Surgery for lysis of adhesions	Aseptic technique in operating room; aseptic dressing changes
Paralytic ileus	Anesthetic agents, manipulation of the bowel, wound infection, electrolyte imbalance	Absent bowel sounds, no passage of flatus or feces, abdominal distention	Nasogastric suction, IV fluids, rectal tube, ambulate	Early ambulation, abdominal tightening exercises, keep NPO if inactive bowel sounds
Bowel obstruction	Intestinal adhesions	Similar to paralytic ileus although BM may occur before obstruction	Bowel decompression with a Miller-Abbott tube, surgical correction	
Urinary retention	Lack of urge to void because of anesthetics, narcotic, or anticholinergic drugs; surgery of pelvic or perineal area resulting in edema in area of bladder	Little or no output or frequent small amounts; palpably distended bladder, restlessness, discomfort	Measures to promote voiding (privacy, run water, sit patient up); catheterization if above methods fail	Adequate hydration; early ambulation
Urinary tract infection	Urinary retention, catheterization, contamination of urinary tract	Mild fever, dysuria, hematuria, malaise	Adequate hydration, maintenance of good bladder drainage, antibiotics on basis of urine culture and sensitivity	Encourage fluid intake, early ambulation; avoid catheterization or remove within 2 days
Gastric erosion and stress ulcer	Intense physical or emotional stress resulting in increased secretion of adrenocorticotropic hormone from pituitary and cortisol from adrenal cortex	Bleeding often first symptom, epigastric pain	Antacids; small, frequent meals; emotional support	Identification of patients at risk: gram-negative sepsis, acute renal failure, central nervous system lesions, severe injuries
Temperature elevation	Infection dehydration, response to stress and trauma, prolonged hypotension, transfusion reaction, respiratory congestion, thrombophlebitis	Temperature elevated above 37.5°C (99.5°F); elevated pulse and respiratory rates; diaphoresis; lethargy	Antipyretics; cooling sponge baths; increasing fluids	Dependent on cause
Parotitis (inflammation of parotid glands)	Poor oral hygiene, malnutrition	Mild fever, edema anterior to the ear lobe, discomfort	Antibiotics; incision and drainage	Frequent oral hygiene, adequate fluid intake

Table 6-7

Common Postoperative Complications (continued)

Complication	Causes	Major Clinical Manifestations	Treatment	Preventive Nursing Interventions
Hiccups (singultus)	Idiopathic; irritation of phrenic nerve	Periodic release of air through glottis, emanating noise; abdominal distention	Breathe in and out of paper bag for 5-minute intervals; administration of 5% carbon dioxide in oxygen mix for a few minutes	None
Sore throat	Intubation; presence of oral or nasopharyngeal airways, nasogastric tubes; dry, irritating nature of inhalants	Pain in throat	Mouthwash; ice chips; throat lozenges; warm beverages if allowed oral fluids	None

overload or infiltration. Auscultation of crackles with breath sounds indicates fluid overload. If the patient has lost an excessive amount of blood during surgery, a transfusion may be administered. Ensure blood compatibility according to agency policies, regulate infusion flow rate to complete transfusion within 4 hours, and monitor for signs of a transfusion reaction. Chapter 12 discusses administration of blood products in detail.

Examine dressings and check the patient every 15 to 30 minutes for bleeding or drainage. Report rapid saturation of the dressing or frank bleeding to the surgeon immediately. Circle a small amount of drainage on the dressing and record the time and date on the dressing so the amount of subsequent drainage in a given period of time can be monitored. The operative dressing can usually be reinforced as necessary, but do not remove the original dressing without the surgeon's order. Check placement of drains or irrigating devices, gastrointestinal tubes, indwelling urinary catheters, and monitoring devices every 5 to 10 minutes to ensure proper function. Note the color, odor, amount, and consistency of all drainage.

Reposition the patient every 10 to 15 minutes to prevent venous stasis and to promote return of vasculomotor function. Examine bony prominences each time the patient is repositioned for early detection and prevention of pressure areas. Gently massage bony prominences and pressure areas to promote capillary circulation. The risk of rapid development of pressure areas remains high until full vasculomotor function returns. Provide blankets to promote warming and to prevent vasoconstriction associated with shivering. To prevent venous impairment, apply antiembolic stockings or pumps, if

not already in use, and remind the patient not to cross the legs or ankles. Do not massage the calves or legs; massage can cause dislodgement of a thrombus. As the patient becomes more alert, encourage independent movement of feet and legs and position changes per preoperative teaching to promote circulation and vascular tone.

NDx: Risk for injury
Keep the side rails of the stretcher raised and the wheels locked. Monitor level of consciousness frequently. Stimulate verbal interaction and reorient the patient to surroundings each time vital signs are assessed. Speak in a calm, reassuring manner and explain all procedures to reduce anxiety. The first responses that the patient will make are reflex motor responses. These are followed by spontaneous movements or movement in response to a command. The patient will at first be drowsy, then more alert, talkative, and oriented to time and place. Some patients become temporarily combative or disoriented. Determine the cause of agitation or restlessness. Although it is a common response to recovery from anesthesia, it may also be caused by pain, hypoxia, cardiac ischemia, hemorrhage, urinary retention, lying too long in one position, and impaired circulation or limb constriction caused by bandages or casts. If restlessness or agitation persists despite interventions, the patient may need to be restrained to prevent injury. Restraints are always a last resort because restriction of movement increases the risk of circulatory impairment and may aggravate the patient's emotional status.

Compare the patient's status with the expected outcomes. If the outcomes are not met, reassess the patient and revise the plan.

NURSING PROCESS
The Postsurgical Patient

The postsurgical unit is notified when the patient has met the Aldrete discharge criteria and is ready to be released. A score of 8 or above is needed for discharge unless the patient's preoperative score was lower than 8. In that case, an individual assessment and decision are made as to whether the patient is ready to be discharged from the PACU. The PACU nurse accompanies the patient to the unit, gives a report to the receiving nurse, and reviews postoperative medical orders. The report includes the same items included on entry to the PACU, plus a summary of the patient's stay in the PACU and any special instructions. The patient is transferred to the bed in the postsurgical unit. Family members or significant others are notified of the patient's return and told when they may visit.

Assessment

On transfer from the PACU, confirm the patient's identity and assist with transfer into bed. Listen to breath sounds and assess blood pressure, pulse quality and rhythm, and respiratory status immediately on arrival. Receive the report and review postoperative orders with the PACU nurse. Complete a head-to-toe assessment, including:

> Blood pressure
> Apical pulse
> Temperature
> Respiratory status
> Skin color, condition, and temperature
> Level of consciousness
> Response to commands
> Independent movement

Examine dressings to ensure placement and adherence and note drainage. Check beneath the patient for wound drainage or bleeding and skin breakdown. Determine placement of drains or tubes, connect to appropriate receptacles, and ensure proper function. Note the amount and characteristics of all drainage. Determine the rate of flow of parenteral infusions and the solution being infused and compare with the physician's orders. Assess the infusion site for signs of infiltration or inflammation.

Nursing Diagnoses and Planning

Nursing diagnoses and related expected patient outcomes commonly applicable to postsurgical patients include the following:

NDx: Risk for ineffective breathing pattern related to tracheobronchial obstruction by secretions or hypoventilation secondary to the effects of general anesthesia, postoperative analgesics, pain, and positioning

Planning: Patient Outcomes
1. Patient maintains patent airway as evidenced by normal breath sounds.

2. Patient maintains spontaneous, unlabored respirations of more than 10/minute and fewer than 30/minute.
3. Patient remains free of dyspnea and cyanosis.

NDx: Risk for fluid volume deficit related to NPO status and inadequate replacement of fluid loss in surgery, or from gastrointestinal tract and/or wound drainage

Planning: Patient Outcomes
1. Patient maintains adequate hydration as evidenced by the following:
   a. Pulse greater than 60 bpm but less than 100 bpm, with regular rhythm
   b. Blood pressure stable, more than 90 mm Hg systolic or within 10% of preoperative baseline
   c. Capillary refill less than 3 seconds
   d. Urine output more than 30 mL/hour
   e. Easily aroused and oriented
   f. Moist mucous membranes
   g. Skin supple with good turgor

NDx: Pain related to surgical incision, manipulation of internal structures during surgical procedure

Planning: Patient Outcomes
1. Patient verbalizes relief of pain to tolerable levels.

NDx: Risk for injury related to diminished awareness of, and response to, internal and external stimuli secondary to postoperative analgesics

Planning: Patient Outcomes
1. Patient remains free of injury.

NDx: Risk for infection related to presence of surgical incision and wound drains

Planning: Patient Outcomes
1. Patient remains free from infection as evidenced by absence of the following:
   a. Fever
   b. Purulent or malodorous wound drainage
   c. Increasing redness or edema around the incision

NDx: Impaired physical mobility related to pain, surgical procedure, and side effects of narcotic analgesics

Planning: Patient Outcomes
1. Patient resumes independent ambulation and physical care activities within physical limitations by the second postoperative day.

NDx: Risk for altered urinary elimination related to decreased bladder tone secondary to effects of general or spinal anesthesia

Planning: Patient Outcomes
1. Patient voids within 8 hours of surgery.

NDx: Risk for altered nutrition: less than body requirements, related to nausea or absence of peristalsis secondary to general anesthesia

Planning: Patient Outcomes
1. Patient has return of peristalsis as evidenced by presence of bowel sounds by the third postoperative day.
2. Patient ingests and retains 75% of prescribed diet within 24 hours of return of peristalsis.

NDx: Risk for body image disturbance related to surgical procedure, surgical incision, presence of wound drains, loss of independence

Planning: Patient Outcomes
1. Patient verbalizes acceptance of permanent changes in appearance and physical status.
2. Patient assumes as much independence as possible.
3. Patient makes positive statements about self.

NDx: Risk for altered health maintenance related to insufficient knowledge of postoperative self-management after discharge

Planning: Patient Outcomes
1. Patient verbalizes understanding of wound-care procedures and postoperative instructions.
2. Patient demonstrates correct technique in wound care, if appropriate.

Nursing Interventions and Evaluation

The goals of nursing care of the postsurgical patient are to promote physical comfort and wound healing, to prevent injury and postoperative complications, and to prepare the patient for discharge. The risk of altered tissue perfusion as a result of postoperative hemorrhage is highest in the first 48 hours postoperatively. Expected outcomes and nursing interventions for this nursing diagnosis continue as previously discussed in PACU care.

Cardiovascular and respiratory status, level of consciousness, and the condition of all infusions, wounds, drains, and dressings must be monitored and documented at least every 15 minutes for the first hour, every 30 minutes for the next hour, every hour for 4 hours, and every 4 hours for at least 24 hours after transfer to the postsurgical unit. Status is monitored more frequently if the patient's condition warrants it.

As the patient progresses through the postoperative period, some assessments, such as frequent determination of level of consciousness or vital signs, may no longer be necessary, whereas other assessments, such as auscultation of bowel sounds, ability to perform self-care procedures, and understanding of discharge instructions, become more significant.

NDx: Risk for ineffective breathing pattern
Turn the patient every hour until fully conscious, and then every 2 hours, to prevent aspiration and stasis of secretions. Auscultate breath sounds and monitor rate and depth of respirations to detect accumulation of secretions or reduced ventilation. Manifestations of compromised respiratory status include rapid, thready pulse; restlessness; apprehen-

sion; rapid, shallow breathing; confusion; and cyanosis. Arouse the patient every time status is monitored and encourage deep breathing and coughing to expel residual anesthetic agents and to promote gas exchange and respiratory function. As the patient becomes more alert, elevate the head of the bed to promote chest expansion and diaphragmatic excursion. Encourage the patient to perform respiratory exercises and to use the incentive spirometer every hour the day of surgery, then at least every 2 hours as taught preoperatively to mobilize secretions and to prevent atelectasis. Administer prescribed analgesics, and assist the patient in sitting upright and in splinting abdominal incisions when coughing and deep breathing to reduce incisional pain. Monitor respiratory rate and depth before analgesic administration to avoid respiratory depression from narcotic agents.

Early ambulation and mobility are major factors in preventing postoperative respiratory complications. Assist the patient in getting out of bed to a chair and in ambulating short distances within 24 hours after surgery to minimize the risk of respiratory complications.

NDx: Risk for fluid volume deficit
Adequate circulating fluid volume is necessary for tissue oxygenation and repair, and to reduce the risk of postoperative circulatory complications such as thrombophlebitis. Monitor heart rate and quality of pulse, blood pressure, level of consciousness, capillary refill, and urine output to detect changes in cardiovascular function and fluid balance. Inspect mucous membranes and skin turgor to detect dryness. Other manifestations of fluid volume deficit include increased heart rate, a drop in blood pressure, decrease in level of consciousness, slow capillary refill, decreased urine output, and dry mucous membranes. Monitor and maintain intravenous infusions to replace intraoperative and postoperative fluid losses as discussed for altered tissue perfusion in PACU care. Document all fluid intake and output, including wound drainage, catheters, urine, emesis, gastrointestinal tubes, and liquid stool, to monitor fluid balance. When oral intake is resumed, encourage up to 3000 mL daily, unless contraindicated, to promote and maintain good hydration.

Promotion of good blood flow is also supported by measures that prevent venous stasis. Apply antiembolic stockings or pumps, or both, if ordered by the physician. Encourage the patient to perform leg exercises at least every hour while awake. Assist with early ambulation. To promote venous return, elevate the patient's legs when he or she is sitting in a chair. Do not raise the bed's knee support unless the foot of the bed is also elevated. To avoid putting pressure on the popliteal space, do not place anything under the knees. To prevent impaired venous flow, teach the patient to avoid crossing the legs or ankles.

NDx: Pain

Remind the patient that postoperative pain is expected. Offer and administer prescribed analgesics to provide relief. Explain that analgesics should reduce pain to a tolerable level but not necessarily eliminate it altogether. Do not assume that all pain after surgery is related to the surgical procedure. Determine the location, type, and characteristics of pain to rule out other causes. Ask the patient to rate the pain on a scale of 1 (minimal) to 10 (excruciating) to quantify the severity of pain. Administer the analgesic and document the patient's stated or apparent (the patient is asleep, for example) degree of pain relief. Use other comfort measures, such as distraction, imagery, a quiet environment, position changes, and back massage to enhance the effect of analgesics. Advise the surgeon if pain is not relieved.

Adequate analgesia promotes not only patient comfort but also independent movement and position changes and early ambulation and improves patient participation in exercises to promote respiratory and circulatory function. Pain relief reduces anxiety and fear of movement and promotes recovery. Most institutions have a pain management program with protocols. The Agency for Health Care Policy and Research has developed Acute Pain Management Clinical Practice Guidelines.

Patient-controlled analgesia (PCA) (Fig. 6–8) allows the patient to control the amount and frequency of self-administered narcotic analgesic within set limits. Intravenous morphine sulfate (Duramorph) is the most commonly used drug. The patient usually receives a loading dose of narcotic, and then the PCA pump delivers an additional bolus dose when the patient pushes a button. The PCA pump can also deliver a set basal dose independent of the patient's control. For safety, the PCA pump has a set lock-out time to maintain a minimum interval between bolus doses and a maximum number of bolus doses per hour. The patient must be able to operate the PCA control button and understand the instructions. PCA promotes patient independence through optimal pain relief and minimizes the patient's fear of severe pain by avoiding peaks and troughs of serum drug levels.

Document the programming mode each shift or when the program is altered. Monitor and document respiratory rate, blood pressure, pulse, level of consciousness, pain relief, and infusion site every hour for 4 hours when PCA is initiated and at least every 4 hours throughout PCA therapy. Notify the physician if respirations are less than 10 per minute and prepare for administration of a narcotic antagonist, such as naloxone hydrochloride (Narcan). The antagonist must be available on the postsurgical unit throughout PCA therapy.

Narcotic analgesics, usually morphine, may also be administered via catheter into the epidural or subarachnoid space. Postoperative use is usually

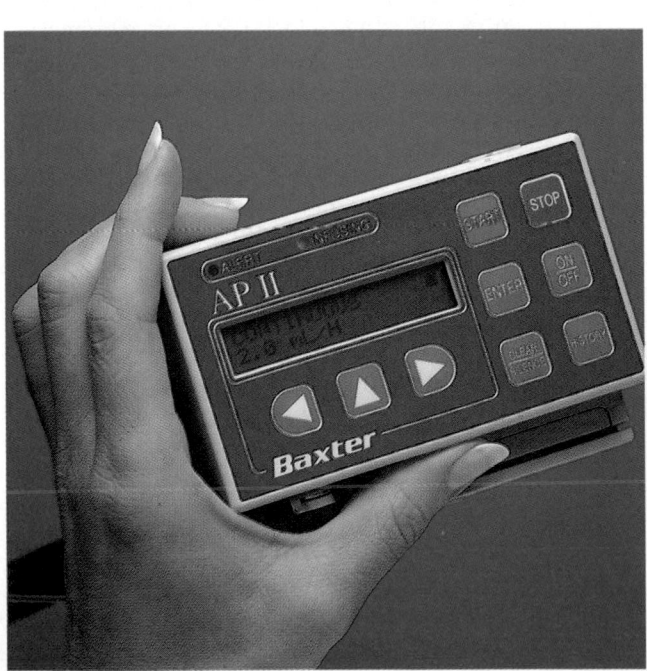
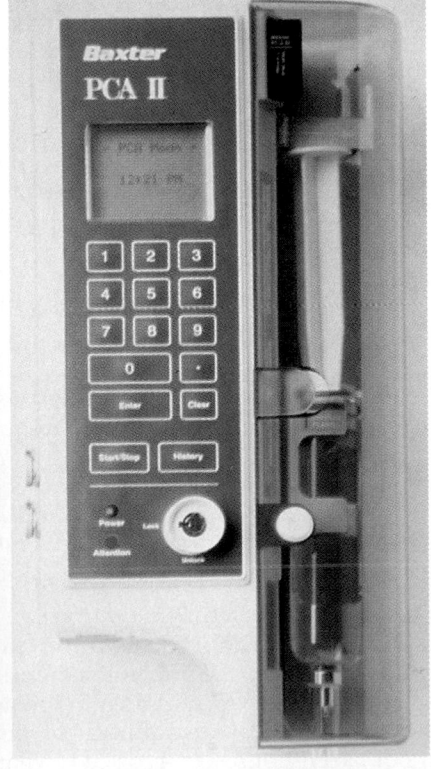

Figure 6–8

Examples of patient-controlled analgesic infusion pumps. (Courtesy of Baxter Healthcare Corporation, Round Lake, IL.)

limited to 48 to 72 hours to reduce the risk of central nervous system infection. The physician or anesthesiologist administers a loading dose of narcotic and may administer additional bolus doses at 12- to 36-hour intervals, depending on patient comfort. Respiratory depression, sedation, nausea and vomiting, urinary retention, and pruritus are possible side effects. A pulse oximeter or apnea monitor is used to continuously monitor oxygenation and respiratory function. Monitor for side effects of the analgesic, and document monitor readings, respiratory rate, level of consciousness, and pain relief every hour or per agency policy to detect respiratory depression. Notify the physician if respirations are less than 10 per minute and have naloxone available for rapid treatment.

Continue to monitor the patient for residual respiratory depression for 24 hours after the last dose of narcotic. Be sure the catheter is securely taped and protected by a dressing to prevent dislodgement. Examine the catheter insertion site every 4 hours for redness, swelling, and discomfort to detect early signs of irritation or infection.

NDx: Risk for injury

Anesthesia and postoperative analgesics can alter patient awareness of the environment, reduce protective reflexes, cause confusion and disorientation, and increase the risk of injury. Keep side rails elevated until the patient is fully alert, oriented, and recovered from anesthesia. Encourage the patient to use the call bell and to ask for assistance when getting out of bed. To prevent injury, assist the patient in getting out of bed and ambulating until his or her gait is steady. Demonstrate how to get in and out of bed safely and how to manage infusion lines and poles, drains, and catheters.

NDx: Risk for infection

Wash hands before and after patient contact and use aseptic technique in all wound care to prevent contamination. Examine dressings for excess drainage and change saturated dressings to prevent contamination of the wound by capillary action. Soiled, warm, moist dressings provide an excellent environment for the growth of pathogens. Ensure proper function of wound drains to promote tissue approximation and healing. Examine wounds for early signs of infection or delayed healing. Wound edges should be approximated, or touch, when healing by primary intention. Granulation tissue should be present in wounds healing by secondary intention. Figure 6–9 illustrates the wound healing process. Inflammation, edema, and bloody or serosanguineous drainage are normal the first 3 days postoperatively. Redness and edema should gradually subside, and the drainage should cease as healing progresses. Increasing inflammation or edema, purulent drainage, foul odor, persistent pain, delayed healing, and fever are signs of wound infection.

Wound healing may also be delayed by dehiscence (partial or complete separation of the wound edges) and evisceration (protrusion of internal organs through a dehisced wound). Infection, fluid accumulation in the wound, obesity, malnutrition, fragile skin in elderly patients, cancer, and excessive coughing increase the risk of dehiscence and evisceration. Immediately examine any wound if a sudden increase in drainage or bleeding occurs or if the patient reports a sensation that something "popped" or "gave way." Notify the surgeon immediately if wound disruption has occurred and instruct the patient to avoid coughing or moving. Position the patient to prevent further stress on the wound. Wound dehiscence may or may not require surgical repair. Evisceration requires emergency surgery to prevent impaired perfusion and possible gangrene of protruding organs. Cover protruding internal organs with sterile gauze moistened with sterile saline to prevent drying. Place the patient on NPO status and initiate preparations for surgery as ordered by the surgeon. Prophylactic antibiotics are usually administered to minimize the risk of peritonitis. Explain all procedures and provide emotional support to reduce patient anxiety.

Most patients are discharged from the hospital before wounds are completely healed. Advise the patient to wear loose-fitting clothes to avoid irritating the incision. Describe the expected appearance of the wound as it heals and the signs of infection to promote early detection of altered healing. Teach the patient to wash hands before and after wound care. Determine whether the patient can bathe or shower. Teach the patient how to remove and apply the dressing without contaminating the wound and how to cleanse the wound. Provide written instructions to reinforce teaching. Observe return demonstration to evaluate learning. If the wound is large or requires irrigation or if the dressing is complicated, a home-care referral may be appropriate. If sutures or staples are in place, confirm with the patient when to return to the surgeon for their removal.

NDx: Impaired physical mobility

Physical mobility promotes positive self-esteem and is essential to the optimal function of all body systems. The stress of surgery and limitation of nutritional intake can leave the patient weak and unsteady. Encourage and assist the patient to turn, change position, and perform leg exercises to begin physical activity immediately after surgery. Assist the patient out of bed as soon as possible after surgery to promote respiratory and circulatory function. Most patients should be able to sit in a chair the evening of surgery and ambulate short distances by the end of the first postoperative day. Monitor activity tolerance by changes in pulse rate. A rise or drop of more than 10 bpm indicates poor tolerance and the patient should return to bed. Gradually increase activity based on the patient's response. Encourage the patient to sit or stand upright when out

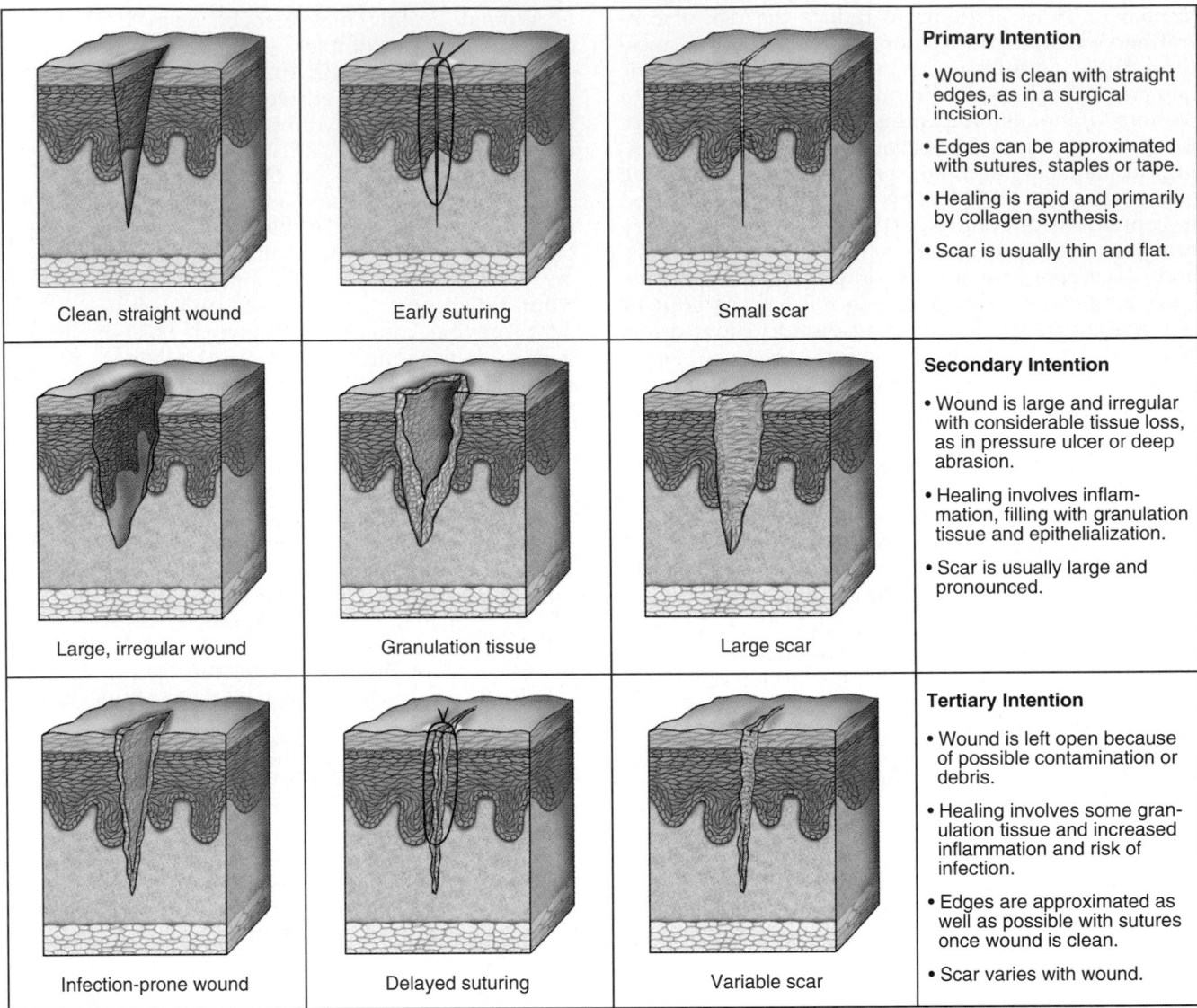

Primary Intention
- Wound is clean with straight edges, as in a surgical incision.
- Edges can be approximated with sutures, staples or tape.
- Healing is rapid and primarily by collagen synthesis.
- Scar is usually thin and flat.

Clean, straight wound   Early suturing   Small scar

Secondary Intention
- Wound is large and irregular with considerable tissue loss, as in pressure ulcer or deep abrasion.
- Healing involves inflammation, filling with granulation tissue and epithelialization.
- Scar is usually large and pronounced.

Large, irregular wound   Granulation tissue   Large scar

Tertiary Intention
- Wound is left open because of possible contamination or debris.
- Healing involves some granulation tissue and increased inflammation and risk of infection.
- Edges are approximated as well as possible with sutures once wound is clean.
- Scar varies with wound.

Infection-prone wound   Delayed suturing   Variable scar

Figure 6–9
Types of wound healing.

of bed to prevent pressure on internal organs from poor posture. Adequate pain relief encourages patient willingness to ambulate.

NDx: Risk for altered urinary elimination

The urge to void may be reduced postoperatively because of reduced bladder tone from the effects of general anesthesia. Bladder distention and urinary retention are possible up to 24 hours after spinal anesthesia as a result of blocked bladder innervation. More men than women suffer from urinary retention postoperatively. Review intraoperative, PACU, and postoperative intake and output records and compare fluid loss and intake to determine whether failure to void may be due to inadequate fluid replacement. If hydration is adequate, the patient should void within 6 or 8 hours after

surgery. Ask if the patient feels discomfort or an urge to void. Palpate the abdomen to detect a distended bladder. Offer a bedpan or urinal, assist a male patient to stand to void or assist a female patient to a bedside commode, and provide privacy to facilitate relaxation and voiding. Run water or place the patient's hand in a basin of warm water to stimulate voiding. Encourage voiding before administration of analgesic medications, which may promote further muscle relaxation or have a sedating or antimicturition effect on the patient.

If the patient cannot void and the bladder is distended, straight catheterization may be necessary. Acute postoperative urinary retention usually resolves spontaneously within 48 hours. Straight catheterization is repeated every 6 to 8 hours as necessary during this period to prevent bladder distention. An indwelling catheter may delay return of bladder tone and is not recommended.

NDx: Risk for altered nutrition: less than body requirements

General anesthesia causes temporary loss of gastrointestinal muscle tone and interruption of peristaltic function. Patients who had surgery that did not involve gastrointestinal organs can often begin taking oral fluids as soon as they are fully awake and free of nausea. Manipulation of gastrointestinal organs delays the return of peristalsis. To prevent vomiting and abdominal distention, patients who had surgery that involved manipulation of the gastrointestinal tract are allowed nothing by mouth until gastrointestinal function returns.

Gastrointestinal function should resume by the third postoperative day and may resume within hours. Auscultate bowel sounds in all four quadrants to detect return of peristalsis. Listen for 2 minutes at a point midway between the umbilicus and the anterior iliac crest before documenting absence of bowel sounds. Determine whether the patient has passed flatus or is experiencing gas pains. Patients swallow air while on NPO status. The air accumulates in the stomach while peristalsis is absent and may cause abdominal distention. As peristalsis returns, the air moves slowly along the intestinal tract and gas pains are common. The passage of flatus and then a bowel movement usually follow. Encourage ambulation to promote peristalsis and relief of gas pains.

Paralytic ileus is the absence of peristalsis beyond the third day after surgery. Abdominal distention, nausea, and a feeling of fullness may also be present. The patient is allowed nothing by mouth, and a nasogastric tube may be inserted to decompress the stomach until peristalsis returns.

The patient is maintained on intravenous dextrose and electrolyte solutions until oral intake is adequate to prevent dehydration and electrolyte imbalance. Begin oral intake with clear fluids in small amounts to avoid distention and vomiting once bowel sounds indicate return of gastrointestinal function. Progress the diet as tolerated to full fluids, then a soft diet, and finally a regular diet or one prescribed by the physician. Monitor for nausea or vomiting. Administer antiemetics at the onset of nausea to prevent vomiting and withhold solid food for several hours. Document dietary tolerance. Encourage a diet high in vitamins and protein to promote wound healing.

NDx: Risk for body image disturbance

The body image of a surgical patient may be threatened by the appearance of the wound, dressings, drainage, dependence on others for self-care activities, impaired mobility, changes in body function, and loss of body parts. Encourage the patient to look at the surgical site to ensure realistic knowledge of its appearance and the extent of surgery. Encourage as much independence as possible in hygiene and grooming but provide necessary assistance to prevent fatigue.

Assist the patient in getting out of bed and ambulating to promote return to independence. Encourage the patient to wear his or her own clothing when feasible and to use light cosmetics if usually worn to foster a positive self-image. Keep the bedside unit neat and orderly and provide privacy for all treatments and dressing changes to promote a sense of self-worth. To promote a sense of control, allow the patient to make decisions about care, clothing, and activities whenever possible. Provide opportunities for the patient and family members or significant others to discuss feelings, fears, or concerns about appearance, self-care, and activities after discharge. Provide information on community support services if appropriate.

NDx: Risk for altered health maintenance

Patients who have an uncomplicated postoperative course are often discharged before complete wound healing. Early discharge minimizes exposure to nosocomial (hospital-based) infections, promotes recovery, and helps to minimize hospital costs. Provide all discharge information in writing to reinforce instructions, minimize errors, and reduce anxiety. Highlight 6–2 summarizes topics to include in discharge teaching.

If dressings are still in place, determine the patient's ability to change them and care for the wound. Teach the patient and a caregiver how to remove and dispose of the old dressing, how to examine the wound for healing and infection, what changes in the wound or patient's condition should be reported to the physician immediately, how to care for and prevent dislodgement of drains, and how to cleanse the wound and apply a fresh dressing. Observe the patient's wound-care technique. Help the patient determine where to purchase wound-care supplies. A visiting nurse or home care referral may be necessary if the patient or caregiver cannot care for the wound.

Review activity restrictions to prevent injury to the operative site that may delay healing. Stress the need for planned rest periods to avoid fatigue and promote recovery. Specify when the patient can expect to resume household chores, lifting, work, driving, sexual intercourse, and leisure activities. Review prescribed medications, administration schedule, expected action, and possible side effects to prevent self-medication errors that may complicate recovery. Review dietary modifications or restrictions and the effect of proper nutrition on recovery. Protein and vitamins B and C promote tissue repair and wound healing. Reinforce the need for follow-up care and identify when the patient should return to the physician, hospital, or clinic for evaluation of the recovery progress.

Compare the patient's status with the expected outcome. If the outcomes are not met, reassess the patient and revise the plan.

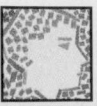

HIGHLIGHT 6–2
PATIENT EDUCATION
Postoperative Patient Teaching

Instruct the patient on the following topics. Provide written instructions when possible.

Tell the patient to follow the physician's instructions for cleansing and dressing the wound. Demonstrate and explain aseptic technique if it is required for wound care. Observe the patient performing wound care.

Urge the patient to allow for additional rest during the recovery period and to resume previous activities of daily living gradually according to the physician's instructions. Specify a schedule if possible.

Instruct the patient to take medications as prescribed and to take *all* doses of any antibiotic.

Teach the patient to modify or restrict the diet as specified by the physician. Provide a written diet plan.

Tell the patient to return for a follow-up appointment and specify the date.

Tell the patient what to do if problems arise. Give the patient a phone number to call in case his or her condition worsens.

Ambulatory Surgery

Ambulatory surgical procedures are usually elective procedures of short duration (less than 90 minutes) that present minimal risk for perioperative complications, do not require an overnight stay, and are associated with minimal postoperative nausea, vomiting, and pain. Examples of surgical procedures that can be performed in an ambulatory unit are listed in Table 6–8. Regional or general anesthesia can be used if the facility has a PACU.

Patients who are candidates for this form of surgery are screened to ensure general good health. Preoperative diagnostic procedures are completed before the day of surgery. Any chronic health problems must be well controlled and present minimal risk for perioperative complications. The patient must be capable of understanding and following preoperative and postoperative instructions. Depending on the surgery, it may also be necessary for someone to be available to assist with self-care in the immediate postoperative period.

NURSING PROCESS GUIDELINES
Ambulatory Surgery

Nursing care of the patient in ambulatory surgery includes all of the aspects of care of the patient undergoing in-hospital surgery already discussed, except for the extended recovery period on a post-surgical unit. The goals of nursing care of a patient in an ambulatory surgical unit are to

Provide safe, well-organized, cost-effective care
Promote patient participation through education
Minimize patient anxiety
Promote rapid recovery
Reduce the risk of postoperative complications

PREOPERATIVE PERIOD

In most instances, the office nurse initiates nursing care of the ambulatory surgical patient. Collect data to develop an individualized plan of care. Initiate preoperative teaching and provide information booklets or written instructions to reinforce verbal instructions. Describe and discuss the preoperative preparations and intraoperative and postoperative

Table 6–8

Examples of Ambulatory Surgery Procedures

Specialty	Ambulatory Surgery Procedures
General surgery	Hernia repair; hemorrhoidectomy; laparoscopic cholecystectomy; laser procedures; excision and biopsy of small masses, lesions, cysts, tumors
Ear, nose, and throat	Tonsillectomy, adenoidectomy, myringotomy, nasal polypectomy, oral surgery
Gynecology	Laparoscopy; tubal ligation; dilation and curettage; abortion; cervical laparoscopy, biopsy, and conization
Urology	Cystoscopy, vasectomy, circumcision
Ophthalmology	Cataract excision and lens implant, laser surgery
Orthopedics	Arthroscopy, fracture reduction, tendon repair, carpal tunnel surgery, bunionectomy
Neurology	Hand surgery, ganglionectomy, nerve repair
Plastic surgery	Face lift, rhinoplasty, eyelid surgery, breast augmentation

course to reinforce the surgeon's explanation and increase understanding of perioperative routines. Encourage questions and correct any misconceptions to reduce anxiety and to promote realistic expectations. Instruct the patient to make arrangements for transportation home after the procedure, since driving will be prohibited. Review discharge instructions and home care to promote uncomplicated recovery. Advise the patient of the need for preadmission diagnostic evaluation and how he or she will be notified of the date and time to report for the tests. Review the date and time to report to the facility for surgery.

On the day of surgery, review the preadmission documents and assess the patient's physical and psychologic status to ensure readiness for surgery. Obtain baseline vital signs and complete the preoperative checklist. Review the anticipated sequence of events and answer questions to reduce anxiety. Accompany the patient to the dressing area and give instructions on how to secure personal possessions and where to go after changing.

POSTOPERATIVE PERIOD

The recovery period is divided into two phases. Phase I involves those patients who have received general anesthesia, or local or regional anesthesia with sedation. Nursing care for these patients parallels that for PACU inpatients.

Patients in phase II have received only local or regional anesthesia without sedation or have progressed from phase I and are now conscious. Monitor vital signs every 30 minutes to detect changes in hemodynamic status and vital functions. To promote recovery from anesthesia, transfer the patient to a reclining chair and encourage him or her to awaken, cough and deep-breathe, move about, and get ready to ambulate. Monitor closely for disorientation and maintain safety measures to prevent injury. Gradually adjust the recliner to the sitting position as the patient recovers. Offer oral fluids as tolerated. Administer oral analgesics for pain control.

DISCHARGE

Review the discharge instructions received before surgery to ensure understanding. Criteria for discharge from the ambulatory surgery unit include stable vital signs; presence of swallow, cough, and gag reflexes; ability to ambulate; minimal nausea, vomiting, and dizziness; no respiratory distress; ability to void; and alertness and orientation. The Phase II Aldrete Postanesthesia Recovery Score is often used for discharge criteria, as presented in Table 6–9. Determine how the patient is returning home. In most instances, a follow-up telephone call is made during the 24-hour period after discharge to review home-care instructions, answer questions, detect any problems or complications, and reconfirm the first follow-up appointment.

Table 6–9

Ambulatory Patient Discharge
ALDRETE'S PHASE II POSTANESTHETIC RECOVERY SCORE

Patient Sign	Criterion	Score
Activity	Able to move 4 extremities*	2
	Able to move 2 extremities*	1
	Able to move 0 extremities*	0
Respiration	Able to deep-breathe and cough	2
	Dyspnea, limited breathing, or tachypnea	1
	Apneic or on mechanical ventilator	0
Circulation	BP ±20% of preanesthesia level	2
	BP ±20–49% of preanesthesia level	1
	BP ±50% of preanesthesia level	0
Consciousness	Fully awake	2
	Arousable on calling	1
	Not responding	0
Oxygen saturation	SpO_2 >92% on room air	2
	Requires supplemental O_2 to maintain SpO_2 >90%	1
	SpO_2 <90% even with O_2 supplement	0
Dressing	Dry and clean	2
	Wet but stationary or marked	1
	Growing area of wetness	0
Pain	Pain-free	2
	Mild pain handled by oral meds	1
	Severe pain requiring IV or IM meds	0
Ambulation	Can stand up and walk straight†	2
	Vertigo when erect	1
	Dizziness when supine	0
Fasting-feeding	Able to drink fluids	2
	Nauseated	1
	Nauseated and vomiting	0
Urine output	Has voided	2
	Unable to void but comfortable	1
	Unable to void and uncomfortable	0

BP, blood pressure; IV, intravenous; IM, intramuscular; SpO_2, oxyhemoglobin saturation determination via pulse oximetry.

* Voluntarily or on command.

† May be substituted by Romberg's test, or picking up 12 clips in one hand.

NOTE: The total possible score is 20. A score of 18 or more is required before patient discharge.

From Aldrete JA: Discharge criteria. In Thomson D, Frost E (eds). Baillière's Clinical Anaesthesiology: Postanaesthesia Care. London: Baillière-Tindall, 1994, pp 763–773.

Although patient education is usually done before surgery, continued education just before discharge is necessary for the patient and other caregivers since the patient will not be observed by a professional nurse in most cases. Referrals to health professionals, such as a home health nurse or physical therapist, may be needed. Tell the patient to expect a phone call within 24 hours to check if any problems have arisen or to answer questions. Give the patient written instructions as well as verbal to reinforce the information and for reference at home for the patient and other caregivers.

The Elderly: Special Considerations

Surgical mortality and morbidity of frail or functionally impaired geriatric patients are higher than for the rest of the adult population. The physiologic changes of aging (discussed in Chapter 4) and concurrent health problems (such as diabetes, cardiovascular disease, altered mental status, and impaired renal or hepatic function) can compromise physiologic response to surgery and can slow recovery. Except in emergency situations, concurrent health problems usually are corrected or brought under control before elective surgery.

In general, the older adult has less tolerance for the stresses of surgery and less physiologic reserves to aid in recuperation. Bedridden and less active patients have a higher risk than those who are active. The risks of surgery increase with advanced age, the duration of anesthesia, the number and severity of coexisting health problems, and the extent of physiologic disturbance associated with the surgery.

The incidence of postoperative and life-threatening complications is three times higher in patients 75 years of age and older compared with those 65 to 74 years of age. However, because each person's physical and psychologic response to the aging process is different, chronologic age is not necessarily the primary determinant of surgical risk.

Many times it is ethically difficult to determine the benefit of and necessity for surgical intervention. When weighing surgical risk against potential benefits, it is important that the surgeon, older adult, and significant others explore the consequences of the proposed elective surgery on both survival rate and quality of life.

NURSING PROCESS GUIDELINES
Older Adults in Surgery

The increasing numbers of older patients undergoing surgery present a challenge in perioperative nursing care. The goals of nursing care are the same as for a younger patient, with emphasis on recovery of functional abilities. The nurse must understand the impact of age-related changes, disease processes, and medication side effects on the person's response to surgery. Then the nurse must develop a comprehensive care plan to minimize surgical risks and postoperative complications. Early activity is essential after surgery to prevent complications and long-term disability from immobility and bedrest.

PREOPERATIVE PERIOD

Obtain a complete health history to identify potential surgical risks. Allow adequate time for the interview so the patient will not feel rushed. Identify drug allergies, previous response to surgical anesthetics, and use of over-the-counter and prescribed medications. Document all prosthetic and assistive devices used. Tell the patient how and where they will be secured. Be alert to nonverbal cues and ask specific questions, such as "Have you recently experienced . . ." to elicit information the patient may omit. Older people may omit information because they do not consider it important, they consider it a normal part of aging, they fear a serious illness will be diagnosed, or they are afraid of losing their independence or autonomy. Severely depressed older people are considered at high risk from surgery because psychologic response and motivation may be impaired. Mental function, economic resources, functional status, coexisting health problems, social support system, ability to perform activities of daily living, and previous experience coping with illness and stress have an impact on the person's recovery from surgery.

The physical examination includes assessment of fluid balance, cardiovascular status, pulmonary function, and hepatic and renal function. Diagnostic studies further evaluate physical status, concurrent health problems, and potential risk factors. Studies that require food and fluid restrictions are scheduled as early in the day as possible to avoid dehydration and other physiologic disturbances. Review with the patient the required oral intake restrictions for diagnostic procedures. Often fluids are permitted, whereas solid foods are restricted. Intravenous infusions may be necessary to maintain hydration during fluid restrictions for multiple diagnostic procedures and before surgery.

Problems such as dehydration, malnutrition, and constipation are corrected before surgery by fluid intake, dietary support, and stool softeners or enemas. If enemas are required, assess the patient between irrigations for fatigue, excess fluid loss, bradycardia, or cardiac dysrhythmias.

Assess and document range of motion and condition of teeth and skin. Stiff neck or loose teeth may interfere with intubation. Fragile skin, stiff joints, and loss of subcutaneous tissue over bony prominences require additional padding and special precautions during intraoperative positioning. Encourage ambulation, frequent position changes, and joint exercises to maintain mobility and muscle tone. Maintain a safe, uncluttered, and well-lighted environment to prevent injury.

Allow extra time for preoperative teaching and reinforce instructions frequently. Preoperative medication doses may need adjustment to prevent mental changes and suppression of vital functions associated with adverse effects. Elevate side rails to prevent injury and monitor the patient closely after administration of preoperative medication to detect untoward reactions.

INTRAOPERATIVE PERIOD

Operating time will be minimized to reduce exposure to anesthetic agents. Older patients may require lower doses of anesthetic agents and are at higher risk for toxicity and untoward reactions from their immediate and cumulative effects. When possible, regional or local anesthesia is used. Monitor for hypotension with all anesthetics.

Older patients have a higher risk for hypothermia because of their lower basal metabolism and loss of subcutaneous fat. Minimize exposure and use a head covering, blankets, and warmed intravenous and irrigating solutions to prevent hypothermia. Decreased joint mobility, impaired peripheral circulation, loss of subcutaneous fat, prolonged immobilization, and hard operating tables increase the risk of tissue ischemia. Risk increases with the length of time the operation requires. Handle body parts gently, use care in positioning, provide extra padding of pressure areas, and monitor peripheral circulation frequently.

POSTOPERATIVE PERIOD

Immediate postoperative care of the older patient is similar to the care for a younger patient. However, recovery is slower. Closely monitor renal, respiratory, and cardiovascular function to ensure early detection and treatment of complications. Ability to compensate for fluctuations in blood pressure and fluid volume status is impaired by reduced cardiac output, impaired peripheral circulation, and diminished vasomotor response. Impaired peripheral circulation increases the risk for pressure sores and thrombus formation.

Change the patient's position slowly, to prevent rapid fluctuations in blood pressure. Change it frequently to prevent tissue ischemia and circulatory stasis. Encourage early ambulation, exercises, and movement of limbs in bed to promote circulation and improve muscle tone. Antiembolic stockings and low-dose prophylactic heparin reduce the risk of deep vein thrombosis. Monitor for signs of fluid overload, and regulate intravenous infusions to prevent congestive heart failure caused by diminished cardiac efficiency. Monitor urine output to detect fluid volume deficit or inadequate renal perfusion.

A decrease in lean body mass and a relative increase in body fat content delay excretion of fat-soluble anesthetic agents. Monitor for restlessness, mental changes, and other signs of cerebral hypoxia.

The elderly are at increased risk of atelectasis and pneumonia because of decreased ciliary action, loss of lung elasticity, reduced vital capacity, and weakened respiratory muscles. Encourage deep breaths and coughing to stimulate respiratory function, to mobilize secretions, and to promote excretion of inhaled anesthetic agents. Low concentrations of humidified oxygen reduce the risk of hypoxia. Older patients are also at high risk of aspirating gastric contents because of a diminished cough reflex. Withhold solid food intake until bowel sounds return, position the patient upright before oral intake, and maintain a semi-Fowler's position immediately after intake to prevent aspiration.

Postoperative confusion after general anesthesia or heavy sedation with regional anesthesia is common and sometimes lasts several days. It occurs more frequently in elderly patients who have experienced hypothermia, cerebral hypoxia, or excess blood loss. Assess the patient for manifestations of pain, hypoxia, cerebrovascular accident, and adverse medication effects. Observe for any changes in mental status. Keep in mind that older adults may have a dulled response to pain. Administer analgesics to promote comfort but monitor closely for mental changes and other signs of adverse effects, which occur more frequently in the elderly. Evaluate whether non-narcotic analgesics can be used rather than narcotic analgesics. Speak in short phrases to reorient and communicate with the patient. Be sure that hearing aids, if worn, are inserted properly and turned on. Maintain safety measures to prevent injury but avoid restraints. They typically increase disorientation and anxiety.

Wounds heal more slowly in the elderly, and risk of infection is greater because of impaired immune response. Use strict aseptic technique in wound care to avoid contamination. Remove tape gently by pulling toward the wound to avoid tension on the edges of the wound. Apply countertraction while removing the tape to prevent tearing fragile skin. If the patient is likely to disturb the dressing, protect it with fluffed gauze or a gauze wrap.

Discharge planning requires collaboration among the patient, family, nurses, physicians, and home-care or discharge-planning staff. Placement in an extended-care or rehabilitation facility may be necessary before discharge home. Discharge teaching begins as soon as possible and should include family members and caregivers. Reinforce instructions with large-lettered information. A follow-up telephone call after discharge to answer questions and reinforce instructions may help reduce anxiety and prevent errors.

Chapter Review

1. Upon admission to the hospital, how is the care of a surgical patient different from that of a medical patient?
2. What evidence supports the therapeutic effect of preoperative teaching as part of the nursing care plan for a surgical patient?
3. What would happen to a patient with malignant hyperthermia if it developed during the course of surgery?
4. What are the advantages and disadvantages of the types of pain management programs for a postoperative patient?
5. What is the meaning of exercises or movement when seen in the postoperative patient?
6. How is the care of an ambulatory surgery patient different from that of a hospitalized surgery patient?
7. How can anxiety best be assessed before surgery?
8. What implementations might be different on a teaching plan for the hospitalized surgical patient as compared with one for the ambulatory surgical patient?
9. What are possible solutions to the problem of hypothermia in the surgical patient?
10. Compare the differences in the nursing care plan for an older adult and that for a young adult having the same surgery.

Bibliography

Aldrete JA. Discharge criteria. In Thomson D, Frost E (eds). Baillières Clinical Anaesthesiology: Postanaesthesia Care. London: Baillière-Tindall, 1994, pp 763–773.

Association of Operating Room Nurses, Inc. Recommended practices for positioning the patient in the perioperative setting. AORN J 1995; 61(2):414.

Association of Operating Room Nurses, Inc. Standards and recommended practices. Denver, CO: AORN Inc, 1996.

Ball KA. Lasers: The perioperative challenge. St. Louis: CV Mosby, 1995.

Beck CF. Malignant hyperthermia: Are you prepared? AORN J 1994; 59(2):367.

Benjamin RB. Atlas of outpatient and office surgery. Baltimore: Williams & Wilkins, 1994.

Burden N. Ambulatory surgical nursing. Philadelphia: WB Saunders, 1993.

Dennison D. Thermal regulation of patients during the perioperative period. AORN J 1995; 61(3):827.

Donnelly AJ. Malignant hyperthermia: Epidemiology, pathophysiology, treatment. AORN J 1994; 59(2):393.

Eliopoulos C. Gerontological nursing. 3rd ed. Philadelphia: JB Lippincott, 1993.

Gaberson KB. The effect of humorous and musical distraction on preoperative anxiety. AORN J 1995; 62(5):784.

Kendrick JM, Powers PH. Perioperative care of the pregnant surgical patient. AORN J 1994; 60(2):205.

Litwack K. Core curriculum for postanesthesia nursing practice. 3rd ed. Philadelphia: WB Saunders, 1995.

Martin JH, Larsen PD. Dehydration in the elderly surgical patient. AORN J 1994; 60(4):666.

Meeker MH, Rothrock JC. Alexander's care of the patient in surgery. 10th ed. St. Louis: CV Mosby, 1995.

North American Nursing Diagnosis Association. NANDA Nursing diagnoses: Definitions and classifications. St. Louis: North American Nursing Diagnosis Association, 1994.

Null S, Richter D, Kovac J. Development of a perioperative nursing diagnosis flow sheet. AORN J 1995; 61(3):547.

Phippen ML, Wells MM. Perioperative nursing practice. Philadelphia: WB Saunders, 1994.

Pica-Furey W. Ambulatory surgery-hospital based versus freestanding: A comparative study of patient satisfaction. AORN J 1993; 57(5):1119.

Stein RH. The perioperative nurse's role in anesthesia management. AORN J 1995; 62(5):794.

Way LW. Current surgical diagnosis and treatment. 10th ed. Norwalk, CT: Appleton & Lange, 1994.

Unit II

Cardiovascular Dysfunction

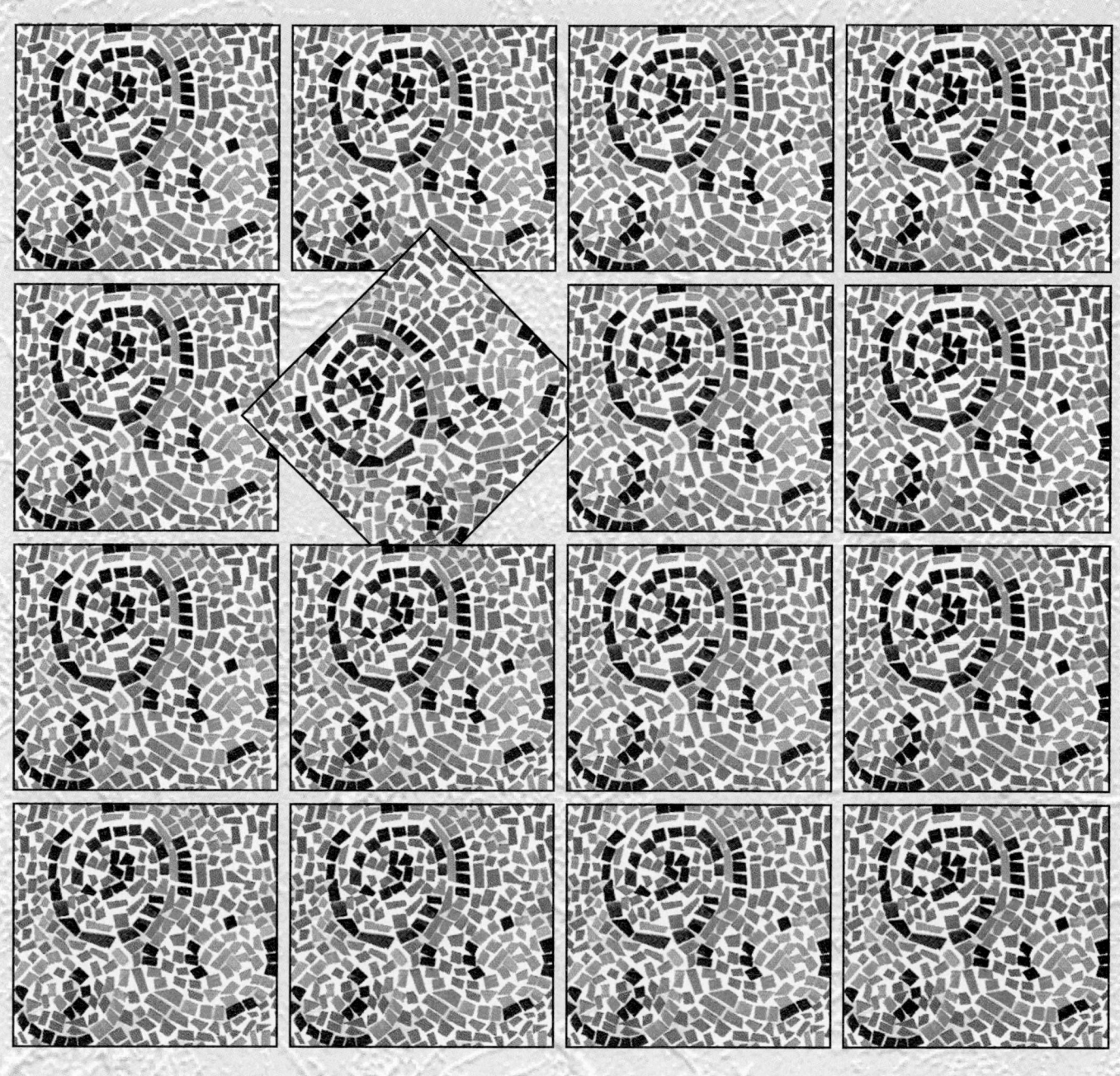

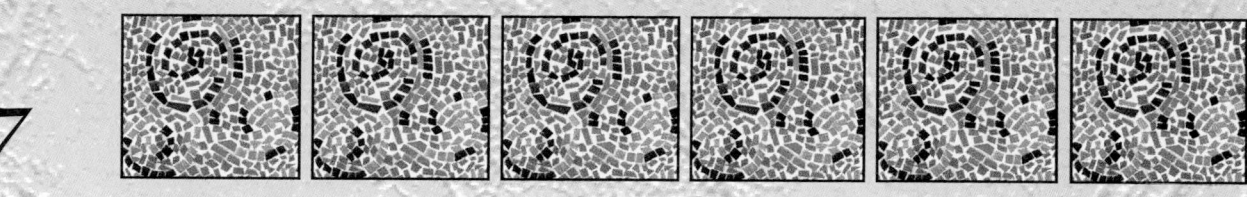

Knowledge Base for Patients with Cardiac Dysfunction

Study Outcomes

After studying this chapter, you should be able to:

1. Explain the normal anatomy and physiology of the heart.
2. Describe common clinical manifestations of cardiac dysfunction.
3. Identify information and physical examination data essential to the assessment of cardiac status.
4. Describe basic diagnostic tests and treatment modalities used in the collaborative management of patients with cardiac disorders.
5. Describe basic surgical procedures used in the treatment of patients with cardiac disorders.
6. Identify data essential to the assessment of patients undergoing surgical treatment of cardiac disorders.
7. State nursing diagnoses and related expected patient outcomes commonly applicable to patients undergoing surgical treatment of cardiac disorders.
8. Describe nursing interventions, with their rationales, commonly applicable to patients undergoing surgical treatment of cardiac disorders.
9. Explain the basis for evaluation of nursing care provided to patients undergoing surgical treatment of cardiac disorders.
10. Identify alternative treatment and care settings for patients with cardiac dysfunction and the services related to community-based care.
11. Identify special considerations for the elderly patient with altered cardiac function.

Human life cannot exist without a functioning heart. The heart is unique in many ways when compared with other organs of the body. The heart's function is purely mechanical. It is simply a pump. It does not secrete, excrete, or produce any substances. It does not filter blood or exchange oxygen. The heart functions to propel blood through a vast network of vessels to all body tissues. The heart's delivery system requires it to beat steadily—averaging more than 60 times per minute, 3600 times per hour, 86,400 times per day—throughout the lifespan. The heart is a highly durable organ, able to accomplish this task without tiring or stopping to rest for many decades in the healthy person. The heart compen-

sates quickly to accommodate a variety of insults and typically fails only in later stages of disease processes.

Anatomy and Physiology

THE HEART

The heart is a hollow muscular pump comprising four chambers and four valves (Fig. 7–1). Its function is characterized by a rhythmic pattern of relaxation (diastole), during which blood fills the chambers, and contraction (systole), during which blood is ejected from the chambers.

By pumping rhythmically, the heart circulates blood through the body's vast network of blood vessels. The right side of the heart pumps deoxygenated venous blood returning from the systemic circulation to the lungs, where it is reoxygenated. The left side of the heart pumps freshly oxygenated blood returning from the pulmonary vascular bed throughout the body. This blood provides oxygen and other essential nutrients to the body's tissues and removes carbon dioxide and other metabolic wastes.

The normal adult heart varies in size based on such factors as sex, weight, and amount of exercise. Typically, it is about the size of a fist. In the average adult, the heart contracts between 60 and 100 times per minute, for a total output of about 5 L per minute.

The heart lies diagonally in the chest, behind and slightly to the left of the sternum, in an area called the mediastinum. The top of the heart is usually level with the third rib and is referred to as the base of the heart. The bottom of the heart, which extends to a point on the midclavicular line just below the left nipple, is called the apex (Fig. 7–2).

Surrounding the heart is the pericardium, a fibrous sac that consists of two layers: the inner layer (visceral pericardium) and the outer layer (parietal pericardium). Between these layers is the pericardial

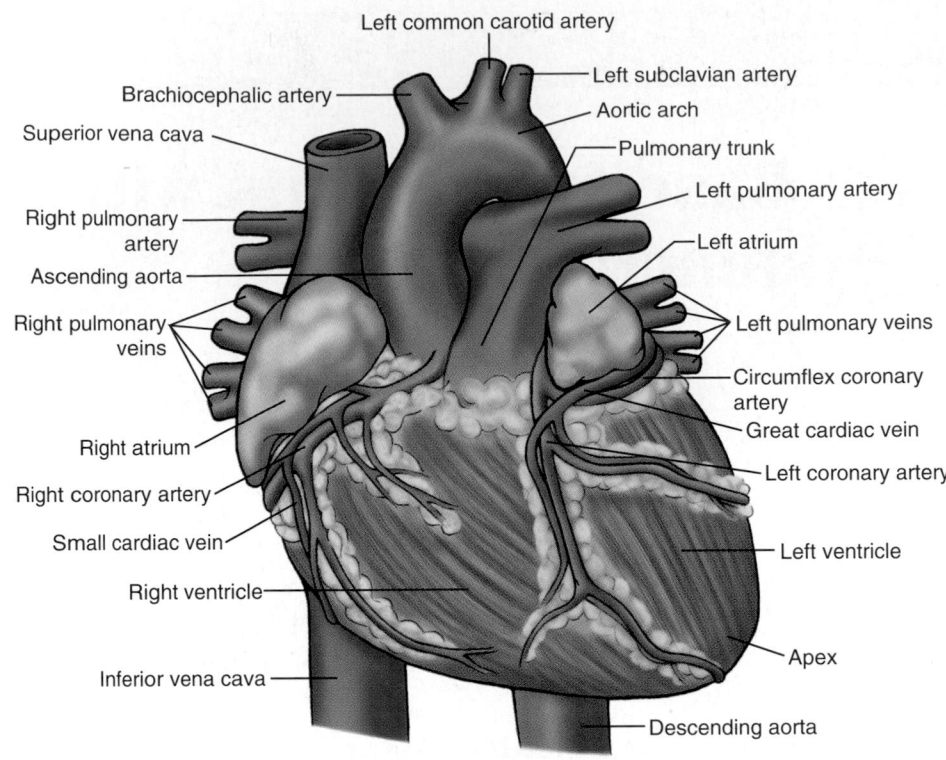

Left common carotid artery

Brachiocephalic artery

Superior vena cava

Right pulmonary artery

Ascending aorta

Right pulmonary veins

Right atrium

Right coronary artery

Small cardiac vein

Right ventricle

Inferior vena cava

Left subclavian artery

Aortic arch

Pulmonary trunk

Left pulmonary artery

Left atrium

Left pulmonary veins

Circumflex coronary artery

Great cardiac vein

Left coronary artery

Left ventricle

Apex

Descending aorta

Figure 7–1
Structures of the heart.

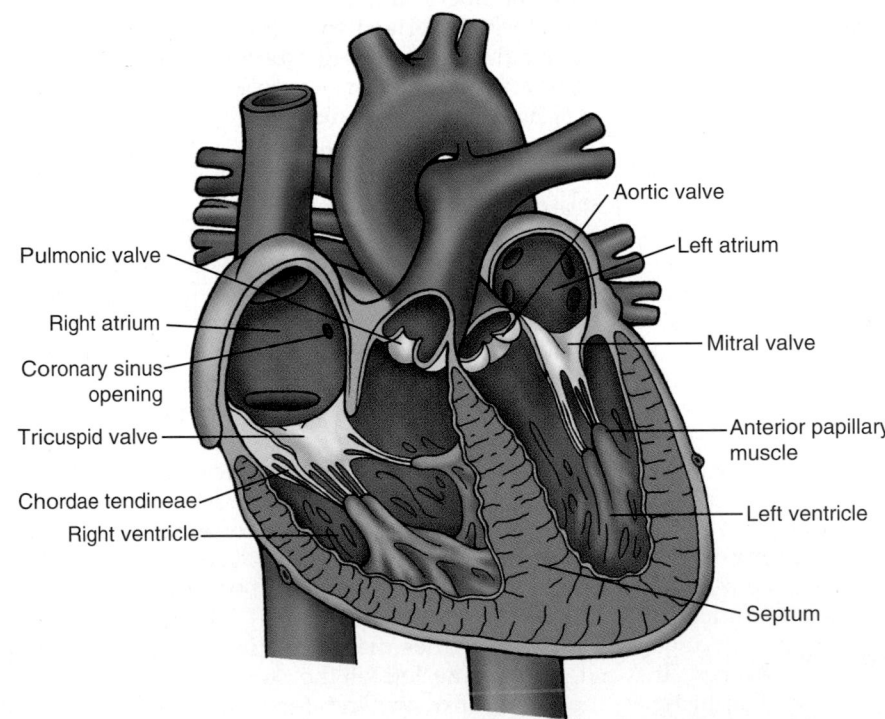

Pulmonic valve

Right atrium

Coronary sinus opening

Tricuspid valve

Chordae tendineae

Right ventricle

Aortic valve

Left atrium

Mitral valve

Anterior papillary muscle

Left ventricle

Septum

space, which is filled with 10 to 30 mL of clear lubricating fluid. This pericardial fluid reduces friction against the heart muscle and allows the pumping heart to move freely. The pericardium forms a barrier that protects the heart from infections of the lung and mediastinum, and from external trauma to the chest wall.

The heart is composed of three layers of cardiac tissue: epicardium, myocardium, and endocardium. The epicardium is synonymous with the visceral

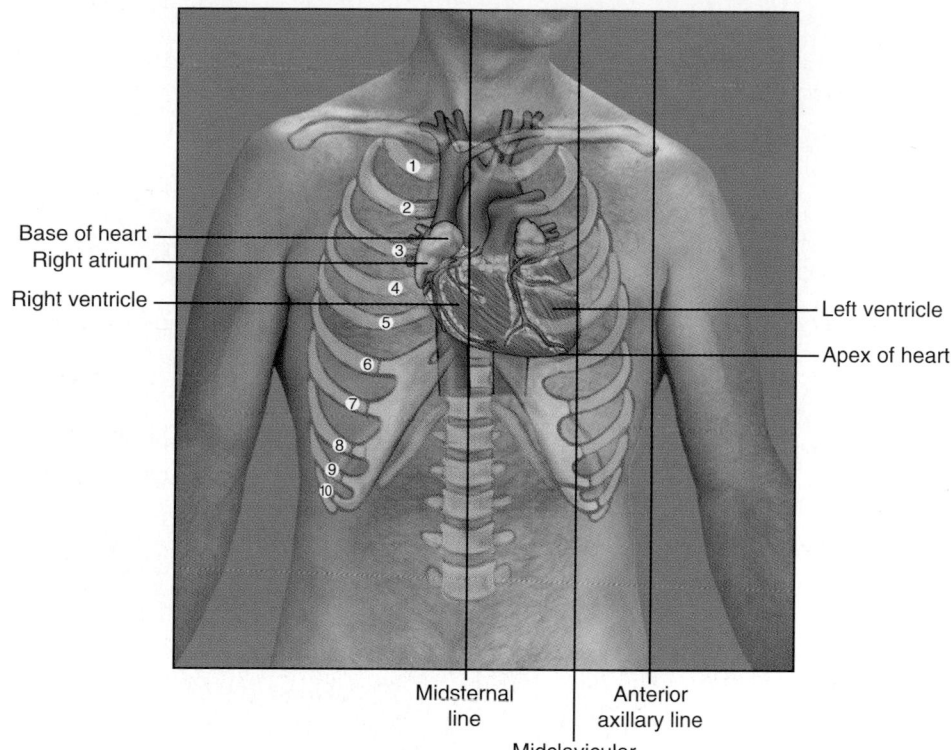

Figure 7–2

Anatomical position of the heart within the chest.

Base of heart
Right atrium
Right ventricle
Left ventricle
Apex of heart

Midsternal line
Anterior axillary line
Midclavicular line

pericardium. It is the outermost layer and covers the surface of the heart and the great vessels. The myocardium, or middle layer, is composed of involuntary striated muscle arranged as an interconnected mass. It provides the coordinated, contractile force needed to pump blood through the circulatory system. The endocardium is the innermost layer. This layer is a thin, delicate sheath of tissue lining the inside of the cardiac chambers and covering the surface of the cardiac valves. The endocardium is in direct contact with blood as it moves through the heart.

Cardiac Chambers

The heart is divided into right and left sides by a midline muscular wall called the cardiac septum. Each side contains two chambers: an upper receiving chamber called the atrium and a lower pumping chamber called the ventricle. The right atrium collects venous blood returning to the heart from the following vessels:

- The superior vena cava, which drains blood from the upper body
- The inferior vena cava, which drains blood from the lower body
- The coronary sinus, which drains blood from the coronary circulation
- The multiple thebesian veins, which drain blood from the atrial wall itself

The right atrium contains this blood during right ventricular systole (right ventricular contraction).

When the right ventricle relaxes (right ventricular diastole), about 80% of this blood flows out of the atrium and into the ventricle by gravity. The remaining 20% is propelled into the ventricle by contraction of the atrium (atrial systole). This is the so-called "atrial kick" that distends the ventricle, thereby readying it for its pumping action. The right ventricle then contracts and ejects blood into the pulmonary artery. From here, the blood enters the pulmonary vascular bed where carbon dioxide is exchanged for oxygen.

The left atrium collects freshly oxygenated blood returning from the lungs via the pulmonary veins. As in the right side of the heart, blood is stored in the atrium during left ventricular systole. During ventricular diastole, blood flows into the ventricle, first by gravity and then as a result of atrial systole. The left ventricle pumps blood into the aorta and the systemic circulation (Fig. 7–3). The right ventricle is the most anterior chamber of the heart and lies just beneath the sternum. The left atrium is the most posterior chamber of the heart. The left ventricle lies laterally on the left side.

The division between the atria and the ventricles is indicated on the exterior heart by the atrioventricular groove, and the division between the right and left ventricles is indicated by the interventricular groove. These two anatomical grooves meet on the posterior surface of the heart at a point known as the crux.

The thickness of the muscular wall of the cardiac chambers differs according to the force needed to

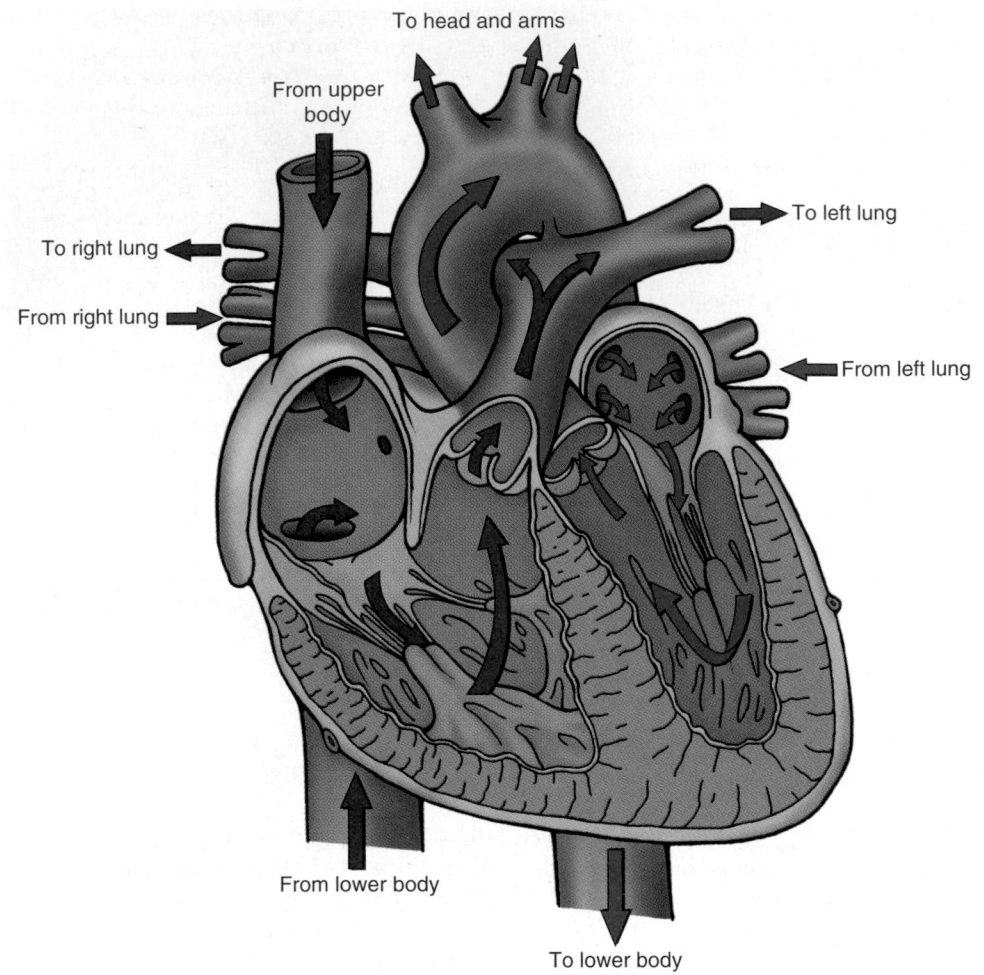

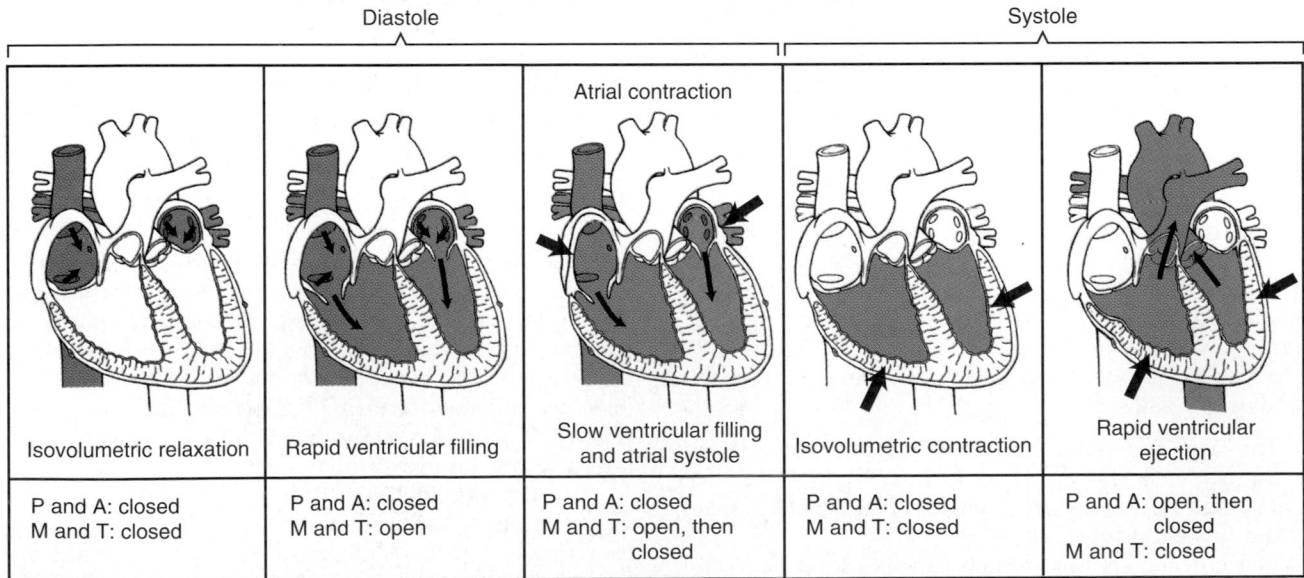

Figure 7–3

Blood flows in a forward motion through the chambers of the heart, with the valves opening and closing in a coordinated manner. A, atrial valve; M, mitral valve; P, pulmonary valve; T, tricuspid valve.

pump blood out of them. The atria have the thinnest walls because they pump small amounts of blood and only as far as the adjoining ventricle. Pressure generated in the right atrium is about 2 to 7 mm Hg; in the left atrium, it is about 5 to 10 mm Hg. The left ventricle has the thickest wall because it must generate pressures of 120 mm Hg to pump blood into the high-pressure arterial circulation. The thickness of the right ventricle wall is greater than that of the atria, but less than that of the left ventricle. It must generate pressures of about 20 mm Hg to pump blood into the pulmonary system.

Cardiac Valves

The cardiac valves maintain forward blood flow through the heart by opening and closing in response to changes in volume and pressure in the cardiac chambers (Fig. 7–4). Of the four cardiac valves, two are atrioventricular valves and two are semilunar valves.

As the name suggests, the atrioventricular valves lie between the atria and the ventricles. These valves are composed of several parts, including a fibrous supporting ring called the annulus and fibrous leaflets, or cusps, that open and close. The atrioventricular valves are open during ventricular diastole, allowing blood to enter the ventricle. These valves then close as pressure rises in the ventricle, thus preventing backflow (regurgitation) of blood during ventricular systole. The valve between the right atrium and the right ventricle is called the tricuspid valve because it has three cusps. The valve between the left atrium and the left ventricle is called the bicuspid valve because it contains two cusps. This valve is also referred to as the mitral valve. Fibrous bands called the chordae tendineae connect the free edges of the atrioventricular valve cusps to the papillary muscles, which are muscle bundles on the

walls of the ventricles. During ventricular systole, the papillary muscles contract, pulling the chordae tendineae taut and preventing the valve cusps from prolapsing into the atrium and allowing regurgitation of blood (Fig. 7–5).

The two semilunar (half-moon shaped) valves in the heart are the aortic and the pulmonic. The aortic valve lies between the left ventricle and the aorta; the pulmonic valve lies between the right ventricle and the pulmonary artery. These valves consist of an annulus, three cup-like cusps, and a small recess or outpocketing above each cusp. This recess is called the sinus of Valsalva in the aortic valve. During ventricular systole, the cusps of the aortic and pulmonic valves float upward and toward the side walls of the aorta and pulmonary artery, respectively, creating a wide opening through which blood is ejected into the artery from the ventricle. During ventricular diastole, backward pressure from the blood-filled artery causes the cusps to descend until the edges meet, thereby preventing regurgitation of blood through the valve.

CORONARY ARTERIES

The coronary arterial system delivers oxygen- and nutrient-rich blood to the cells of the myocardium. This system begins with the right and left coronary arteries and ends in an extensive capillary system. The coronary arteries branch from the aorta just above the aortic valve and traverse the epicardial surface of the heart embedded in a layer of protective fat. Multiple smaller arteries branch from the coronary arteries and penetrate the myocardium (Fig. 7–6). The terminal portions of these arteries form a plexus of small vessels just inside the lining of the cardiac chambers and supply blood to the papillary muscles. The coronary arterial system also

Figure 7–4

Cardiac valves during diastole and systole. Note that the mitral and tricuspid (atrioventricular) valves are open during diastole and closed during systole. The aortic and pulmonic (semilunar) valves are closed during diastole and open during systole.

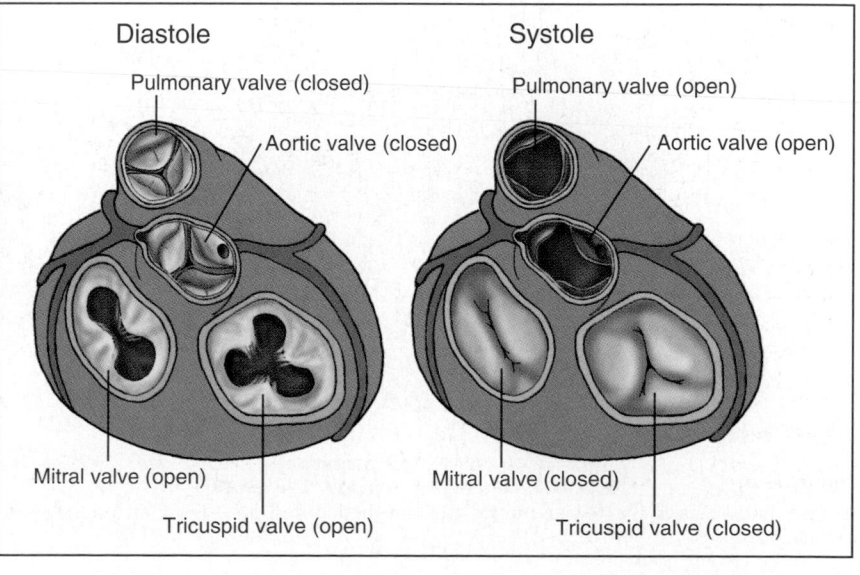

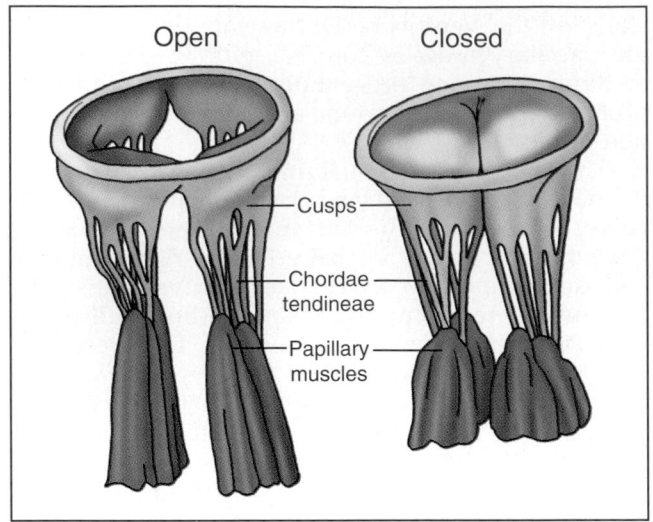

Figure 7–5

Position of papillary muscles, chordae tendineae, and cusps when the mitral valve is open and when it is closed.

includes collateral vessels that connect the various branches of the coronary arteries and serve as a backup system for delivery of oxygenated blood to the myocardium in the event that one of the main vessels is damaged.

The precise pattern of branching between the coronary arteries and the capillary bed varies from person to person. However, basic similarities exist,

and thus a typical pattern can be described as follows. After exiting from the anterior surface of the aorta, the right coronary artery (RCA) passes diagonally toward the right side of the heart and travels in the atrioventricular groove that circles the heart between the atria and ventricles. A branch of the RCA descends along the lateral margin of the heart to the apex, supplying blood to both the anterior and posterior surfaces of the right ventricle. The RCA itself continues high across the posterior surface of the right ventricle. A small branch goes to the atrioventricular node. In persons with a "right dominant" heart (an estimated four-fifths of the population), the RCA turns at the crux and descends in the interventricular groove as the posterior descending branch of the artery and terminates in the left ventricular wall. The RCA supplies blood to the following areas:

- The anterior portions of the right and left ventricles
- The posterior portion of the right ventricle
- The sinoatrial and atrioventricular nodes
- When it forms the posterior descending branch, the posterior portion of the interventricular septum and the posterior papillary muscle

After exiting from the posterior surface of the aorta, the left coronary artery passes behind the pulmonary artery, extends small branches to the left atrium, and then separates into two major divisions: the left anterior descending artery and the circum-

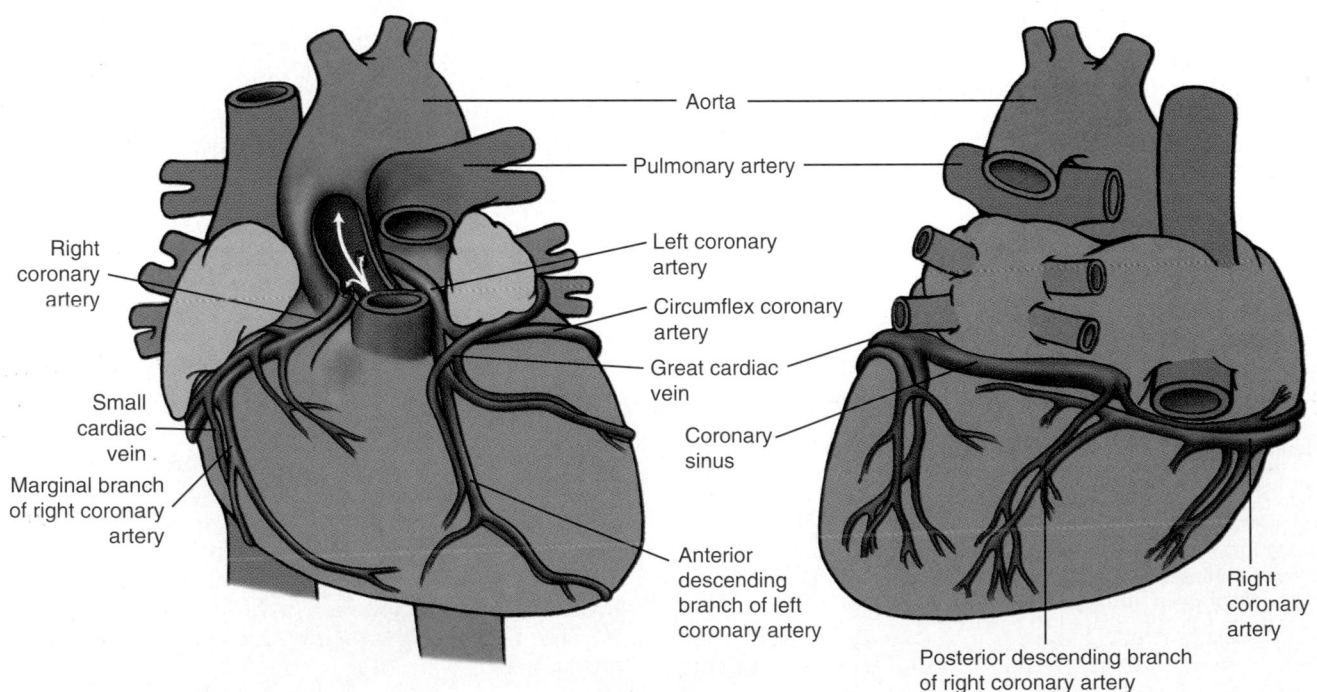

Figure 7–6

Arteries and veins of the heart (anterior view on the left and posterior view on the right). Note that the major cardiac veins parallel the coronary arteries.

flex artery. The left anterior descending artery descends on the anterior surface of the heart in the interventricular groove. Branches off of the left anterior descending supply the anterior portion of the interventricular septum and the anterior surface of the left ventricle. A large diagonal branch supplies the lateral margin of the left ventricle. The circumflex artery passes around the left atrium and flows from right to left, high across the posterior surface of the heart in the atrioventricular groove. It supplies the left atrium and lateral wall of the left ventricle with blood. The major branch of the circumflex artery is the obtuse marginal branch, which supplies much of the posterior surface of the left ventricle. In the approximately one-fifth of the population with "left dominant" hearts, the left coronary also provides the posterior descending branch that terminates in the left ventricular wall.

Blood flow through the coronary arteries differs from the flow in other arteries in that it occurs primarily during diastole rather than systole. The reason for this is that ventricular contraction increases tension in the ventricular wall and thereby increases resistance to blood flow through the ventricular arteries. When the ventricular wall is relaxed, vascular resistance is decreased and blood flow is relatively unimpeded.

CORONARY VEINS

The venous drainage system of the heart closely parallels the arterial inflow (see Fig. 7–6). Coronary veins run alongside each of the major coronary arteries. All of the coronary veins flow into the coronary sinus, which is the large vein that passes from left to right, high across the posterior cardiac surface. This coronary sinus ends in the right atrium at the coronary sinus ostium between the tricuspid valve and the opening of the inferior vena cava.

THE CARDIAC CONDUCTION SYSTEM

Cardiac tissue is capable of automatic, spontaneous depolarization. This means that any muscle cell within the heart can initiate its own rhythmic action potentials without any nervous intervention or other stimulation. Rhythmic waves of contraction normally occur repeatedly to activate the pumping mechanism of the heart. The contractile characteristics of cardiac muscle reside in the biochemical properties of substances found in the tissue itself. Changes in these chemicals induce changes in cardiac rhythm and rate.

Cardiac muscle cells are polarized cells. They carry an electrical charge. This charge (or resting potential) results from the relative distribution of sodium and potassium on either side of the cell membrane. The cell membrane is permeable to both sodium and potassium ions, but in the resting state,

the cell membrane has a positive charge on the outside of the membrane because the sodium-potassium pump functions to keep a large number of positively charged sodium ions outside of the cell.

When a cardiac muscle cell is stimulated, whether by its own automaticity, by another cell, or by an external source, an action potential develops. Depolarization, which is a reversal of the resting membrane potential, is the first phase of the action potential. During depolarization, the cell membrane's permeability to sodium increases and sodium pours into the cell via the fast channels while potassium exits. Slow calcium-sodium channels also open up at this time, allowing calcium into the cell. The cell membrane now has a positive charge on the inside of the membrane and a negative charge on the outside of the membrane. This movement of ions creates an electric current and ultimately generates an impulse that spreads to adjacent cells (Fig. 7–7). Following depolarization, the myocardial cell contracts.

The second phase of the action potential is repolarization. During repolarization, the cell membrane's permeability to sodium decreases. Sodium leaves the cell and potassium enters the cell. With repolarization, the myocardial cell returns to its relaxed state and enters a refractory period. The first part of this period is the absolute refractory period, during which the myocardial cell cannot respond to any stimulus. This is followed by the relative refractory period, during which the myocardial cell can respond to a stimulus of sufficient strength. The refractory state protects the heart from prolonged contraction, which would halt blood flow and cause death.

After the refractory period, a brief supernormal period occurs as the cell regains a resting potential. During this interval, the myocardial cell is very sensitive and will respond to even a mild stimulus. The electrochemical changes that occur in myocardial cells can be detected on the surface of the body and recorded. The resultant recording is the electrocardiogram (ECG, formerly called EKG).

The Sinoatrial Node

Normal cardiac conduction begins at the sinoatrial node. This node is called the pacemaker of the heart because it has the fastest innate rate of spontaneous depolarization. Its innate rate is 60 to 100 beats per minute. Thus, in an adult, a heart rate of 60 to 100 beats per minute is considered normal. The sinoatrial node lies close to the epicardial surface of the right atrium above the tricuspid valve near the entrance of the superior vena cava (Fig. 7–8). It is supplied with blood by a small atrial branch of the RCA.

The Atrioventricular Node

The impulse generated at the sinoatrial node is transmitted to the atrioventricular node through in-

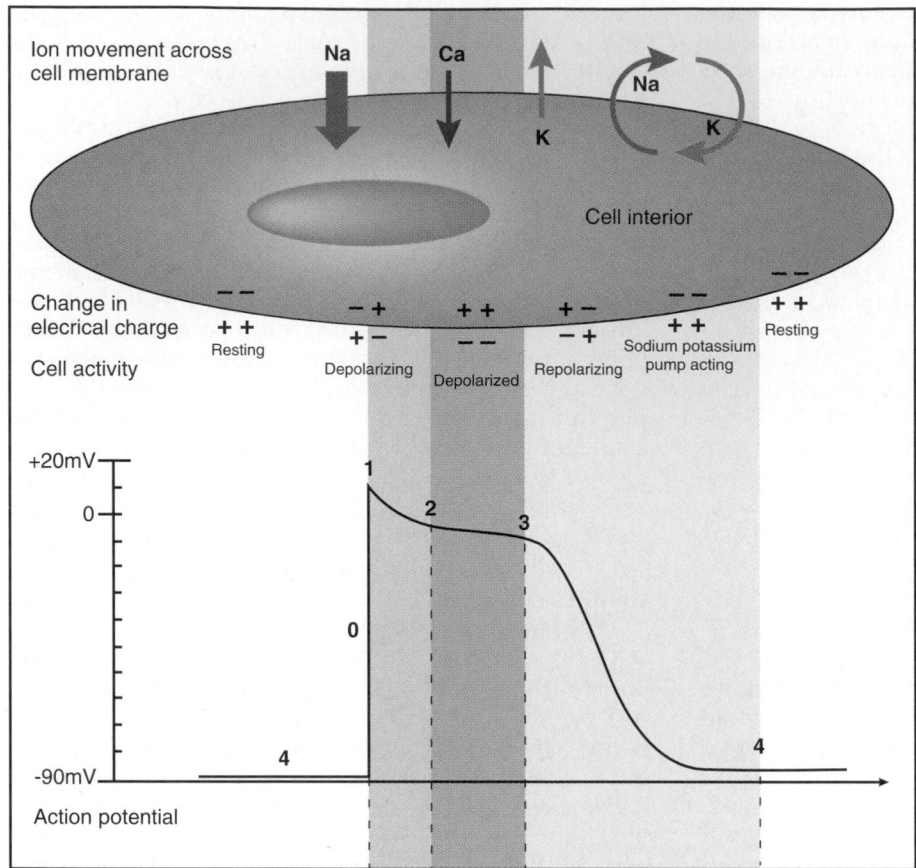

Figure 7–7

Phases of the action potential of a cardiac cell. In the resting phase (4), the cell membrane is polarized. The cell's interior has a net negative charge and the membrane is more permeable to potassium ions than to sodium. When the cell is stimulated and begins to depolarize (0), sodium ions enter the cell, potassium leaves the cell, calcium channels open, and sodium channels close. In its depolarized phase (1), the cell's interior has a net positive charge. In the plateau phase (2), calcium and other positive ions enter the cell and potassium permeability declines, lengthening the action potential. Then (3), calcium channels close and sodium is pulled from the cell by the sodium-potassium pump. The cell's interior then returns to its polarized, negatively charged state (4).

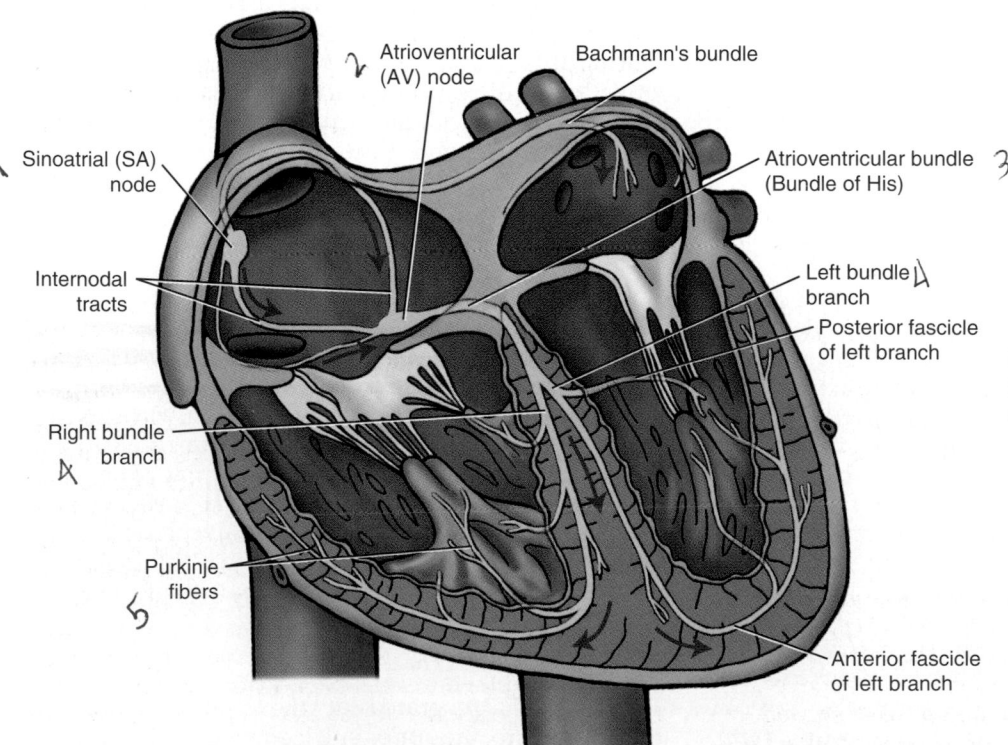

Figure 7–8

Sequence of impulse conduction over the myocardium.

ternodal tracts in the atrial muscle. The atrioventricular node is also called the atrioventricular junction or the junctional pacemaker of the heart. Its innate rate is 40 to 60 beats per minute. It is the secondary pacemaker and takes over if the sinoatrial node fails because of damage or disease. Because the atrioventricular node fires at a slower rate than the sinoatrial node, a patient with a failed sinoatrial node will have a slower-than-normal heart rate that reflects the atrioventricular node's innate rate.

The atrioventricular node is seated on the right atrial wall close to the tricuspid valve and the ostium of the coronary sinus. The atrioventricular node receives its signals from the atrium and, after a delay of about 0.04 second, sends the impulses toward the ventricles. This normal delay is important because it postpones activation of the ventricles long enough for the atria to eject their blood through the atrioventricular valves into the ventricles.

Ventricular Conduction

The impulse is transmitted to the ventricles via the bundle of His located at the junction of the atrial and ventricular septa beneath the noncoronary cusp of the aortic valve. As the bundle of His reaches the upper portion of the interventricular septum, it divides into a right bundle branch and a left bundle branch. These branches then descend in the interventricular septum and terminate in the Purkinje fibers, which carry the impulse to all the ventricular musculature. The right bundle branch spreads out over the right ventricle. The left bundle branch divides into anterior and posterior branches as it exits the septum, supplying electrical conduction to the large left ventricle. Impulses are further spread cell to cell outside the conduction system. This spread is facilitated by the intercalated disks, which are thickened portions of the sarcolemma (surface membrane around each cell) that connect myocardial cells end-to-end. These intercalated disks act as low resistance pathways for impulse transmission.

The ventricles are capable of initiating their own action potentials and may do so if both the sinoatrial and atrioventricular nodes are incapable of providing pacemaking for the heart. The innate rate of the ventricles is about 20 to 40 beats per minute, a heart rate that is not very compatible with an active life. Therefore, patients whose ventricles perform the pacing function typically receive an artificial pacemaker.

Sequence of Impulse Conduction

In the normal heart, the sinoatrial node generates an impulse that initiates depolarization. Depolarization spreads over the right atrium, to the left atrium, on to the junctional region, and then to the atrioventricular node. Here, a delay of about 0.04 second occurs. The impulse-initiating depolarization then proceeds down the bundle of His, through the bundle branches to the cardiac septum, and continues down the bundle branches to the Purkinje fibers in the walls of the ventricles. From the Purkinje fibers, depolarization spreads through the ventricular myocardium from its apex to its base. In all areas of the myocardium, depolarization occurs first in the endocardium and moves outward to the epicardium. Repolarization occurs in the same sequence in the atria but in reverse sequence (epicardium to endocardium) in the ventricles.

THE CARDIAC CYCLE

The cardiac cycle is the period from the beginning of one heart beat to the beginning of the next beat. It consists of two phases: systole and diastole. Diastole is the period during which both atria and then both ventricles fill with blood. Systole is the period during which both atria and then both ventricles contract and propel the blood forward.

Diastole begins when the aortic and pulmonic valves close to prevent backflow of blood from the aorta and pulmonary arteries into the ventricles. The myocardium relaxes and ventricular pressure begins to decrease. Initially, the ventricular pressure, although decreasing, is still higher than the pressure in the atria so the atrioventricular valves remain closed and a large amount of blood collects in the atria. When the falling ventricular pressure drops below the atrial pressure, the atrioventricular valves open and the blood that has collected in the atria begins to flow rapidly into the ventricles because of the difference in pressure. As the volume of blood in the ventricles increases, ventricular pressure rises and filling slows. At this point, atrial systole occurs. This provides the "atrial kick" or the pumping of about 20% of the blood remaining in the atria into the ventricles, after which the atrioventricular valves close.

Ventricular systole ensues. Tension in the myocardium begins to rise. The aortic and pulmonic valves are still closed because pressure in the large arteries (aorta and pulmonary) is greater than that in the ventricles because of the blood that was pumped into them with the previous systole. As systole continues, intraventricular pressure continues to rise and pressure in the large arteries falls as blood within them moves toward the capillary beds. When intraventricular pressure exceeds pressure in the large arteries, the aortic and pulmonic valves open and blood is propelled rapidly into the pulmonary and systemic circulations. Following this rapid ejection of blood, the ventricles stay contracted but the outflow of blood slows. Systole then ends abruptly: the ventricles relax and intraventricular pressure falls below pressure in the large arteries. As a result, blood surges backward toward the ventricles and closes the aortic and pulmonic valves for the start of the next diastole.

MECHANISMS FOR REGULATING CIRCULATION

Three types of regulatory mechanisms maintain blood circulation in the body: intrinsic control, neural control, and humoral control. The three mechanisms of circulatory control work together to provide maximum delivery of blood containing oxygen and nutrients to all tissues of the body.

Intrinsic Control

Intrinsic circulatory control refers to the natural ability of the cardiovascular system to regulate cardiac output. Cardiac output is the volume of blood ejected from the ventricles into the circulation in 1 minute. Expressed as an equation, cardiac output equals stroke volume (the amount of blood ejected from the ventricles with each beat) times heart rate (the number of beats per minute). A sufficient cardiac output provides adequate perfusion and oxygenation to all the tissues of the body. Normally, cardiac output ranges from 4 to 8 L per minute.

Cardiac output varies with the body's size and metabolic needs. Such factors as stress, illness, and exercise can increase cardiac output as much as four times the normal resting volume. These variations result from changes in either heart rate or stroke volume, which directly affect cardiac output. Factors influencing stroke volume, which averages 70 mL, include contractility, preload, and afterload (Fig. 7–9).

Contractility refers to the ability of muscle fibers to shorten during contraction. This ability depends on actin-myosin complexes within the muscle. Contractility determines the strength of muscle contraction and can be affected by a variety of factors. These factors include myocardial oxygen consumption, coronary artery disease, primary cardiac muscle disease, calcium or potassium imbalances, and autonomic nervous system stimulation. An increase in contractility improves stroke volume and cardiac output. A decrease in contractility diminishes stroke volume and subsequently cardiac output.

Preload, another factor determining stroke volume, refers to the volume of blood within each ventricle at the end of diastole. This volume is responsible for stretching the ventricular muscle fibers during diastole and determines the force of contraction in accord with Frank-Starling's Law. This law states that, within limits, the force of cardiac muscle contraction is directly related to the amount of stretch placed on the muscle fibers. Therefore, the larger the volume of blood that fills the ventricles in diastole, the greater the muscle fiber stretches in diastole. This greater muscle stretch creates a stronger contraction in systole and thereby increases stroke volume and cardiac output. The exception to this law is the failing heart, in which the muscles are overstretched. In overstretched muscles the actin and myosin complexes of the muscle fibers are disengaged and cannot increase the force of contraction. Preload is affected by venous return from the systemic and pulmonary circulations. As a result, changes in the amount of venous return to the heart directly affect the strength of cardiac muscle contraction, stroke volume, and ultimately cardiac output.

Afterload, a third determinant of stroke volume, refers to the tension that develops in the ventricular wall during systole. This tension reflects the force needed to eject blood from the ventricles. It is affected by the volume of blood that must be moved with each systolic ejection, and by the resistance to blood flow (systemic vascular resistance). This systemic vascular resistance is determined by the diameter of the vessels in the arterial circulation.

Left ventricular afterload is the amount of resistance that the myocardial contraction must overcome to open the aortic valve and eject blood into the arterial circulation. Right ventricular afterload is normally lower than the left because of the low vascular resistance in the pulmonary circulation. Left ventricular afterload increases as systemic blood pressure increases. Right ventricular afterload increases as pressure in the pulmonary vessels increases.

Afterload is also affected by the size of the heart.

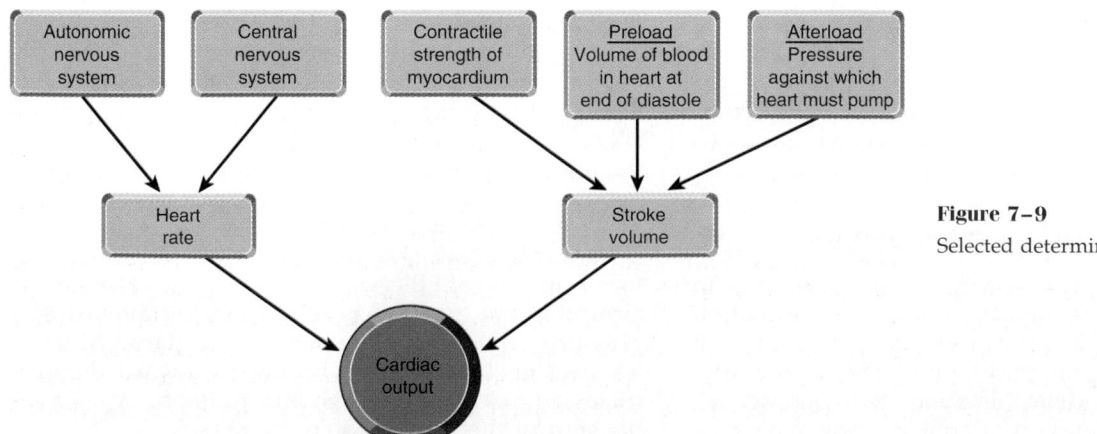

Figure 7–9

Selected determinants of cardiac output.

Dilatation of the ventricles increases the volume of blood to be moved and therefore increases the afterload. The higher the afterload, the harder the ventricles must work. As the work demand of afterload approaches the work capacity of the ventricles, blood flow is impeded and stroke volume and cardiac output decrease.

The second part of the cardiac output equation is heart rate (cardiac output = stroke volume × heart rate). Changes in heart rate alter the frequency with which blood is pumped from the heart. All other factors being equal, within the normal range of 60 to 100 beats per minute, an increase in heart rate means an increase in the amount of blood ejected. Tachycardias (rates over 100) however, result in a reduced ventricular filling time during diastole. Decreased stroke volume and cardiac output may result. Conversely, bradycardias (rates below 60) allow for longer diastolic filling time and a subsequent increase in ventricular volume before systole. Therefore, stroke volume has the potential to be enhanced.

Neural Control

The neural control of circulation is a combination of sympathetic, parasympathetic, and reflex nerve functions. The cardiovascular control center in the medulla has fibers that synapse with the parasympathetic and sympathetic nervous system to regulate circulation. Sympathetic nerves, which permeate atrial and ventricular tissue, leave the spinal column through the cervical and thoracic vertebrae. Other sympathetic nerve fibers travel to all body tissues and organs, ending in peripheral sympathetic nerves.

At the ends of the sympathetic nerve fibers are postganglionic neurons and preganglionic neurons. The postganglionic neurons secrete norepinephrine, which stimulates vasoconstriction of vessels in tissues and organs. The preganglionic neurons secrete acetylcholine, which stimulates vasodilation of the same vessels. With stimulation of the sympathetic fibers, powerful vasodilation occurs in skeletal muscle, cardiac muscle, and the brain. These sympathetic effects underlie the "fight or flight" response. In order to fight or flee, the person needs an increased amount of blood circulated to the heart, brain, and skeletal muscles for quick thinking and quick action. To obtain an increased blood flow, vasoconstriction shunts blood from the kidneys (which reduces urine output), from the gut (which decreases digestion), from the spleen, and from the skin (which causes chills), to the core of the body (the heart and brain) and to the skeletal muscles as needed. These changes, which constitute the usual response to any stressful event, require a concomitant increase in heart rate and blood pressure. Direct stimulation of the heart by an increase in circulating epinephrine from the adrenal medulla further supports these increases.

At the end of the stressful situation, the parasympathetic nervous system buffers the sympathetic nervous system. Parasympathetic stimulation via the vagus nerve predominates in the normal resting heart. Like the sympathetic nervous system, the parasympathetic nervous system contains both postganglionic and preganglionic neurons. However, acetylcholine is secreted at both its preganglionic and postganglionic endings. Because acetylcholine stimulates vasodilation, this is the only effect the parasympathetic nervous system exerts on the vessels. Thus, blood flow is increased to the kidneys, gut, spleen, and skin, leveling off the increased blood flow in the skeletal muscle, cardiac muscle, and brain. These areas are not vasoconstricted because they need high blood flow to maintain normal functions. Parasympathetic stimulation decreases heart rate and blood pressure.

Located in the walls of the large arteries, such as the internal carotid arteries and the aortic arch, are sensory nerve endings called baroreceptors. They are stimulated when pressure from increased blood flow causes the vessel to stretch. Stimulation of baroreceptors inhibits the vasomotor center in the brain (decreased sympathetic stimulation) and excites the vagal center (increased parasympathetic stimulation). The result is decreased blood pressure and heart rate. An increase in blood pressure of 0 to 50 mm Hg usually does not result in significant stimulation of the baroreceptors. An increase of 50 to 200 mm Hg stimulates a maximum response. An increase in blood pressure of more than 200 mm Hg stretches the receptors to a point at which they can no longer respond. A rising pressure stimulates more of a response than a stationary or falling pressure.

Humoral Control

Humoral control of circulation is accomplished by release of hormones from various organs. Epinephrine and norepinephrine are released from the adrenal medulla. Epinephrine and norepinephrine are vasoconstricting substances that increase blood pressure and heart rate and can divert blood from peripheral areas of the body to the core when needed.

Another potent vasoconstrictor is angiotensin II. The kidney secretes renin, which causes angiotensinogen to convert to angiotensin I. An enzyme in the lungs converts angiotensin I to angiotensin II. While angiotensin II increases blood pressure and heart rate, it also stimulates the secretion of aldosterone by the adrenal cortex, which aids in fluid control by retaining sodium and water in the vascular system when the body needs to conserve fluid.

Atrial natriuretic factor is a hormone secreted by atrial tissue in response to abnormal stretch and the related increase in blood pressure. The hormone promotes the excretion of sodium and water, decreasing blood volume and blood pressure. It also is a vasodilator and thus further decreases the heart's workload.

Clinical Manifestations of Cardiac Dysfunction

All body systems are affected by cardiac changes because all systems depend on the heart to supply oxygenated blood and nutrients to the tissues. There are, however, five classic signs and symptoms of heart disease. These are dyspnea, chest pain, syncope, palpitations, and edema. Other signs and symptoms associated with heart disease include altered blood pressure and pulse, abnormal heart sounds and murmurs, neck vein distention, delayed capillary refill, cyanosis, pallor, fatigue, clubbing, and alterations in the renal, gastrointestinal, and neurologic systems. These symptoms usually are not specific and seldom present as the most prominent indication of cardiac dysfunction.

DYSPNEA

Dyspnea is a general term used to describe difficulty breathing. It is commonly associated with heart disease but may be a symptom of many other diseases, even acute anxiety. Dyspnea can be either inspiratory or expiratory in nature. Inspiratory dyspnea occurs primarily when airflow is obstructed in the larger airways, such as the trachea or large bronchi. Usually, it is associated with heart failure. Expiratory dyspnea prolongs the expiratory phase of breathing. Usually, it is associated with such pulmonary conditions as asthma and emphysema.

Dyspnea occurs in many forms, including:

- Dyspnea on exertion
- Positional dyspnea
- Paroxysmal nocturnal dyspnea
- Orthopnea

Dyspnea on exertion is shortness of breath caused by physical exertion and relieved by rest. It is a common early symptom of heart failure. As the left ventricle begins to fail, blood begins to back up into the left atrium and, from there, into the lungs. The alveoli swell with fluid, and gas exchange becomes impaired. This limits the heart's ability to meet the increased demand for oxygenated blood that occurs with exertion. Thus, the person experiences shortness of breath. As heart failure progresses, the amount of exertion needed to induce dyspnea decreases.

Positional dyspnea is shortness of breath that develops when a person turns from a supine to a side-lying position. Most affected patients become short of breath when turning onto the left side. Usually, positional dyspnea indicates advanced failure of the left ventricle. In inactive people, however, it may be the first symptom of heart failure.

Paroxysmal nocturnal dyspnea is a form of shortness of breath that occurs suddenly, at night. It is a very specific sign of heart failure. A few hours after going to sleep as usual, the patient is awakened by an intense feeling of suffocation, possibly accompanied by wheezing or sweating. It occurs because the supine position allows fluid pooled in previously dependent areas to be resorbed into the circulation. As a result, venous return increases, the left ventricle becomes overloaded, and fluid backs up into the lungs. Change of position from supine to upright, as in sitting up or going to the window for air, allows gravity to redistribute fluid away from the lungs back to the legs and feet. This relieves the distress and the patient can return to sleep, usually for the rest of the night.

Orthopnea is shortness of breath that develops any time the patient lies flat. It resolves less than 5 minutes after the patient sits up. This manifestation often occurs in patients with heart failure. Gravitational forces that pull fluid to the lower extremities while the patient is sitting no longer operate when the patient is in the supine position. Thus, fluid is mobilized and redistributed to an already compromised pulmonary circulation. Pulmonary venous and capillary pressures increase, resulting in pulmonary congestion. As heart failure progresses, patients must prop themselves up on an increasing number of pillows to sleep. In its most severe form, orthopneic patients must sleep upright in a chair. Asking how many pillows a patient sleeps on can be helpful in assessing orthopnea, but be sure to differentiate between the person who simply prefers sleeping with several pillows and the person who must sleep with several pillows to breathe.

Orthopnea sometimes is accompanied by a dry, nonproductive cough called a cardiac cough. This cough usually occurs at night and results from an accumulation of fluid in the lungs. It is precipitated by lying down or exercising and is relieved by sitting up.

NURSING PROCESS GUIDELINES
Dyspnea

For the patient with dyspnea, obtain a pulse oximetry reading if possible. Count the respiratory rate and observe for the use of accessory muscles of breathing. Count the pulse, noting rate and rhythm. Check the blood pressure and compare the results to the patient's baseline values. Assess breath sounds, listening for inspiratory and expiratory adventitious sounds. Auscultate heart sounds, assessing for abnormalities. Note any concomitant symptoms such as fatigue, cough, sputum production, or cyanosis. Check capillary refill. Question the patient as to precipitating activities. Note what position or activities seem to relieve symptoms. Monitor arterial blood gas values if available.

Elevate the head of the bed to relieve dyspnea. Encourage the patient to rest with the feet lowered. Maintain a calm quiet environment and stay with the patient, providing reassurance as appropriate. Administer oxygen as ordered. Based on assessment data, help the patient alter the activity level as needed.

CHEST PAIN

Chest pain is considered a classic symptom of cardiac disease. However, not all cardiac disease presents with chest pain and not all chest pain results from cardiac disease. Chest pain of cardiac origin is most often caused by myocardial ischemia, a condition in which the oxygen supply is inadequate to meet the metabolic needs of cardiac muscle. If the ischemia is temporary and does not result in the death of myocardial tissue, it is called angina pectoris. If the ischemia is sufficiently severe or prolonged to kill myocardial cells, a myocardial infarction (heart attack) has occurred.

The pain of angina pectoris typically is substernal or retrosternal, spreads across the chest, and radiates to the left shoulder and down the left arm. It may also radiate to the back or to the jaw. The pain of angina typically lasts 3 to 5 minutes, but it may last close to 15 minutes. The pain may be precipitated by exertion, emotional stress, exposure to cold, or eating. Some patients experience anginal pain at rest. Usually it can be relieved by rest and sublingual nitroglycerin.

Chest pain associated with a myocardial infarction typically is a severe substernal or precordial sensation of crushing or squeezing felt throughout the chest. It may radiate to the shoulder, neck, arm, and to the fourth and fifth fingers of the left hand. It also may radiate to the back, teeth, jaw, or to the right shoulder and arm. It occurs without a specific precipitating factor, is steady, and lasts longer than 15 minutes, even during rest. This pain typically is not relieved by sublingual nitroglycerin. In addition to the pain, the person may experience dyspnea, diaphoresis, nausea, vomiting, syncope, and palpitations.

A third cardiac cause of chest pain is pericarditis (inflammation of the pericardium). Chest pain from pericarditis is intermittent, severe, sharp pain of sudden onset, felt under or to the left of the sternum. The pain worsens on inspiration, swallowing, coughing, or turning the upper body. It may be referred to the epigastrium, back, neck, or arms. This pain may be relieved by sitting up and leaning forward.

Noncardiac causes of severe chest pain include:

- Dissecting aortic aneurysm
- Pulmonary disorders, such as pulmonary embolism and pleuritis
- Esophageal disorders, such as esophagitis and esophageal spasm
- Anxiety

Pulmonary pain differs from cardiac pain in that it typically is referred to the costal margins or upper abdomen and is associated with inspiration. Many patients can point to one area on the chest with pulmonic pain. Esophageal pain is substernal and spreads over the chest to the shoulders. Chest pain caused by anxiety extends over the left chest and does not radiate. It typically lasts 2 to 3 minutes and may be accompanied by a tingling sensation of the hands and mouth. A detailed history and physical examination helps to distinguish one cause of chest pain from another. Until another cause is definitively established, chest pain in any patient—even one without known coronary artery disease—is assumed to result from myocardial ischemia.

NURSING PROCESS GUIDELINES
Chest Pain

When assessing a patient with chest pain, adjust your approach to the condition at hand. If the patient is in acute distress, focus on obtaining information most critical in determining the need for immediate intervention. Obtain vital signs and basic information related to the chest pain (type, location, intensity, onset), associated symptoms (dyspnea, palpitations, diaphoresis, nausea), medications, and allergies. When determining the location of chest pain, ask the patient to point to where the pain is and also ask where it radiates.

Interventions for the patient with chest pain of assumed cardiac origin include those identified in Table 7–1.

Table 7–1

Interventions for the Patient with Chest Pain of Assumed Cardiac Origin

Start oxygen using a nasal cannula at 2–4 L/min.
Provide a quiet, nonstressful environment.
Help the patient assume a comfortable upright position.
Start an intravenous line.
Attach the patient to a cardiac monitor and obtain a full 12-lead electrocardiogram.
Administer nitroglycerin, pain medication, or both, as ordered.
Monitor vital signs frequently. Keep the blood pressure cuff in place.
Stay with the patient. Most are frightened and fearful.
Help reduce anxiety by explaining all procedures and medications and allowing family or a significant other to remain with the patient.
Assess response to medication by asking the patient to rate the pain on a scale of 0 to 10 or 0 to 5, 5 minutes after administering nitroglycerin and 15 to 30 minutes after administration of other medications.
Warn the patient about nitroglycerin's common side effects, including headache, flushing, and dizziness.
Identify precipitating factors and eliminate them.

SYNCOPE

Syncope (fainting) is a transient loss of consciousness caused by cerebral hypoxia. The precipitating factor is a drop in arterial blood pressure to less than 50 mm Hg, which results in a temporary reduction of blood supply to the brain. Syncope may have a sudden onset and last only a short period of time. Usually, it is preceded by lightheadedness, dizziness, pallor, and diaphoresis. Syncope may be cardiac or noncardiac in origin. Cardiac causes include sick sinus syndrome, valvular heart disease, brady and tachy dysrhythmias, and pacemaker failure. Noncardiac causes include seizure disorders, hypoglycemia, orthostatic hypotension, hyperventilation, or emotional disturbance. In most cases of syncope, the cause is not a cardiac problem. However, it may provide an early clue to a cardiac disorder and treatment may prevent a future cardiac emergency.

Specific types of cardiac syncope include effort, Stokes-Adams syndrome, pacemaker, and hypersensitive carotid sinus. Effort syncope occurs shortly after exertion. The patient collapses and usually recovers spontaneously after several moments. It is caused by aortic stenosis or subaortic stenosis, which is a narrowing of the aortic valve or the area just below the valve. Both of these conditions reduce the amount of blood flow through the stenosed areas, leading to decreased cerebral and coronary perfusion. When the person begins to exercise, the body's demands for oxygen increase beyond what the heart can pump through the narrowed vessel and fainting results.

Stokes-Adams syndrome refers to syncope caused by heart block or other rhythm disturbances. The person has a sudden and unexpected loss of consciousness associated with an absence of pulse and ashen color. Breathing may also stop. If the heart does not begin to beat within 15 to 30 seconds, cyanosis may develop, along with twitching of the face and upper extremities. The pupils may become fixed. Attacks usually last only a few seconds and therefore may be mistaken for absence seizures. If the patient fails to recover after a few seconds, there is a danger of complete cardiopulmonary arrest and death.

Pacemaker syncope is caused by the malfunction or failure of an artificial pacemaker. This type of syncope means that the pacemaker should be checked or replaced, even if the patient recovers immediately.

Hypersensitive carotid sinus syncope is a type of vagal syncope that occurs most often in older men with atherosclerotic carotid arteries. Fainting is precipitated by sudden turning of the head, shaving the neck, buttoning a tight collar, or another activity during which the patient inadvertently applies pressure to the carotid artery sinus just below the angle of the jaw. This pressure results in a reflex vagal inhibition of the heart, leading to a sudden, severe slowing of the heart rate, a heart block, or even cardiac arrest.

Because of the risk of vagal syncope, only one carotid is examined at a time. Diagnostic carotid massage is never done on both sides at the same time and is always performed in a controlled setting where a monitor and cardiac resuscitative drugs and equipment are available.

Management of syncope depends on its cause or causes. Management options for the various types of cardiac syncope include drug therapy, corrective surgery, and insertion of a pacemaker.

NURSING PROCESS GUIDELINES
Syncope

When assessing the syncopal patient, first ascertain that the patient is breathing spontaneously and that a pulse is palpable. Next check the pupillary response to light. Loosen any constricting clothing and protect the patient from harm if necessary. Stay with the patient. Note the duration of the attack as well as the patient's color, and vital signs.

PALPITATIONS

Palpitation refers to the discomforting, often anxiety-producing, sensation or awareness of a rapid "racing" heartbeat or of a pounding or skipped heartbeat. Onset and termination of this sensation may be sudden. Physiologic palpitations occur during or after strenuous exercise. Nonphysiologic or pathologic palpitations of cardiac origin most often result from premature beats or some other rhythm disturbance. These include rhythm disturbances that can be induced by cardiac medications when taken in excess. A prime example of this type of medication is digitalis, where the therapeutic level is differentiated from the toxic level by only a narrow range. Pathologic palpitations also may be caused by noncardiac factors, such as large amounts of caffeine or nicotine, heavy meals, lack of sleep, or stress. Palpitations that occur with mild exercise can indicate heart failure, anemia, or hyperthyroidism.

NURSING PROCESS GUIDELINES
Palpitations

Obtain vital signs. Assess pulse carefully; if possible place the patient on a cardiac monitor. Note and document associated symptoms, such as chest pain, dyspnea, lightheadedness, dizziness, syncope, or diaphoresis. Ask questions about precipitating events and obtain a thorough medication history. Stay with the patient to reduce anxiety. Encourage the patient to rest, and administer oxygen when necessary.

If the cause of the palpitations is found to be

related to caffeine or nicotine, discuss with the patient ways to decrease their use. Explore the sources and patterns of caffeine intake and suggest substitute liquids or activities. Provide information on methods of smoking cessation. If palpitations are stress related, help the patient recognize sources of stress and identify ways to manage it.

EDEMA

Edema is an abnormal accumulation of serous fluid in the soft tissues. It occurs when the normal balance between hydrostatic and osmotic pressure is disturbed and excess fluid is released through the capillary walls into the subcutaneous tissues. It can be caused by inadequate venous return to the heart because of venous obstruction from external pressure on the veins, incompetent valves, and/or the effects of gravity. Edema from these causes is nonpitting and disappears when pressure is removed from the veins or the body part is elevated.

Edema is called "pitting" when the skin in the edematous area maintains an indentation for 5 to 30 seconds after being pressed with a finger. It is best palpated over a bony prominence. The degree of pitting is described in terms of depth according to the rating system described in Chapter 5. Pitting edema does not disappear when the body part is elevated. It indicates such pathology as fluid overload or heart failure.

Depending on its cause, edema can be localized or generalized. In the ambulatory cardiac patient, edema is usually bilateral and dependent. It appears in the hands, feet, and ankles from the effect of gravity. The more proximally the edema extends, the more severe the condition. In the bedridden patient, edema occurs in the sacral area and posterior thighs. Four to seven liters of fluid, causing a weight gain of 4.5 to 6.8 kg (10–15 lbs), can accumulate in the tissues before obvious edema occurs.

Edema is treated by limiting fluid intake and eliminating excess fluid that has accumulated within the tissues. Typically, the patient is allowed 800 to 1500 mL of fluid per day and follows a low-sodium diet and diuretic therapy.

NURSING PROCESS GUIDELINES
Edema

For all patients with edema, regardless of cause, the focus of nursing care is monitoring fluid and electrolyte balance and educating the patient or caregiver in how to maintain this balance. Maintain accurate intake and output records. Obtain daily weights at the same time each day, on the same scale, and with the same amount of clothing. Monitor for signs of electrolyte imbalance. Because the accumulation of extra fluid in the tissues disrupts the normal transport of nutrients to the cells, skin breakdown occurs easily. Therefore, observe the skin frequently for any sign of redness or irritation.

Clean the skin gently. Avoid soaps and other drying agents. Pat the skin dry and apply lotion to prevent dryness. Reposition bedridden patients every 2 hours. Unless contraindicated, elevate affected extremities to promote drainage of fluid. Assess the patient's understanding of diet, medications, diagnosis, and activity. Provide information about low-sodium diets and consult a dietitian as needed. If possible, discuss dietary restrictions with the person who will do the cooking and shopping. Teach the patient or other involved person to read labels for sodium content and to avoid canned and "fast" foods, which have a high sodium content. Encourage experimentation with other spices—such as basil, lemon, and tarragon—rather than sodium.

ALTERED BLOOD PRESSURE

Blood pressure is the force exerted by the blood against the arterial walls. Systolic pressure is the maximum force exerted on the arterial walls during left ventricular contraction (systole). Diastolic pressure is the force exerted on the arterial walls when the heart is in its relaxed phase (diastole). Pulse pressure is the difference between systolic and diastolic pressures. Normally, blood pressure in the aorta and large arteries (such as the brachial) ranges from 90 to 140 mm Hg for the systolic pressure and 60 to 90 mm Hg for the diastolic pressure. Pulse pressure is normally 30 to 40 mm Hg.

Blood pressure is determined by several factors, including cardiac output, arterial wall distensibility, peripheral vascular resistance, and total blood volume. Systolic blood pressure is determined mainly by stroke volume, and diastolic pressure by the condition of the arteries. A change in any one of these factors can result in changes in blood pressure. For example, the decreased elasticity of vessel walls that accompanies the aging process lowers the diastolic blood pressure and increases the systolic blood pressure. Because many physical and psychologic factors influence blood pressure, the healthy person's blood pressure fluctuates to some degree from moment to moment. Thus, an isolated blood pressure measurement has little significance unless compared to the patient's baseline blood pressure.

The two most common abnormalities of blood pressure are hypertension and hypotension. Hypertension is defined as a persistent elevation of systolic pressure above 140 mm Hg, or a persistent elevation of diastolic pressure above 90 mm Hg. Systolic hypertension refers to an elevation of only systolic pressure, with a consequent widening of the pulse pressure. It occurs with atherosclerosis and thyrotoxicosis. Elevated diastolic pressure is always accompanied by elevated systolic pressure. It typically has no specific identifiable cause.

Hypotension is defined as a persistent blood pressure of less than 90/60 mm Hg. It can result from decreased cardiac output or decreased peripheral vascular resistance. Hypotension that results from decreased cardiac output occurs with:

Myocardial infarction
Myocarditis
Addison's disease
Hypovolemia resulting from hemorrhage
Vomiting
Diarrhea
Dehydration

Hypotension that results from decreased peripheral vascular resistance occurs with pneumonia, septicemia, and drug overdose. Signs and symptoms associated with hypotension include:

Increased pulse rate
Diaphoresis
Confusion
Restlessness
Cool, clammy skin
Decreased urinary output

A specific type of hypotension is orthostatic or postural hypotension. This is a transient drop in blood pressure in response to a change in body position in relationship to gravity. Typically, the patient experiences dizziness, lightheadedness, or actual syncope when quickly standing up or moving from a supine to an upright position. Common factors underlying this response in the cardiac patient are hypovolemia, impaired vasoconstriction, and/or impaired autonomic nervous system function.

Normally, blood pressure rises almost instantly to maintain blood flow to the brain against the altered gravitational force caused by a change in position. This compensation results from increased heart rate and peripheral vasoconstriction. In the presence of extracellular fluid volume depletion, these compensatory mechanisms are inadequate and blood pressure drops on position change despite them. With impaired vasoconstriction, heart rate increases but cannot overcome the effect of gravity in the absence of normal vasoconstriction. With autonomic nervous system impairment, the heart rate cannot increase and peripheral vasoconstriction is decreased or absent, thus eliminating both normal compensatory mechanisms.

ALTERED PULSE

Pulse is the fluid wave of blood that travels through the arterial system as a result of ventricular systole. Palpating pulses to determine their rate, rhythm, amplitude, and symmetry provides information about cardiac function and peripheral circulation. Palpation of the carotid pulse provides the most accurate information about cardiac function because it best correlates with central aortic pressure. Therefore it is the best artery to use when assessing the characteristics of the arterial pulse. The carotid pulse is also easily accessible and thus well suited for use in emergency situations. Palpation of peripheral pulses provides information about both cardiac function and peripheral circulation.

The normal pulse rate for a resting adult is between 60 and 100 beats per minute. Pulse rate is lower in the conditioned athlete and tends to increase slightly with aging. Tachycardia is an abnormally rapid pulse rate, above 100 beats per minute. Bradycardia, an abnormally slow pulse rate, is less than 60 beats per minute.

The normal pulse has a regular rhythm, that is, the interval between pulse beats is equal. An exception to this is a regularly irregular rhythm, in which the pulse speeds up with inspiration and slows down with expiration. This is called sinus dysrhythmia and is common in children and young adults. The irregularity disappears if the patient holds his or her breath.

Other rhythm abnormalities are caused by disturbances in the heart's conduction system. The most common of these irregularly irregular pulse rates is atrial fibrillation. In this condition, there is an extremely rapid rate (350–600 per minute) of impulses discharged from the atria. Since the atrioventricular junction is only able to respond to some of them, an irregular ventricular rate of 40 to 170 results. Although this dysrhythmia can occur transiently in healthy, young persons, it is almost always associated with underlying heart disease.

The amplitude or force of the pulse reflects pulse pressure, which is determined by the strength of contraction of the left ventricle and the peripheral vascular resistance. The amplitude of the pulse is described according to the following scale.

0   absent
1+ weak, thready (hypokinetic)
2+ normal
3+ bounding, full (hyperkinetic)

A weak pulse indicates a narrowed pulse pressure secondary to weak left ventricular contraction, with low cardiac output and increased peripheral vascular resistance (Fig. 7–10). It may indicate impaired circulation, left ventricular failure, mitral or aortic stenosis, or hypovolemia. It also can be a normal variation. This is particularly true of the popliteal, brachial, and posterior tibial arteries, which are more deeply buried in surrounding tissue in some individuals than in others. A weak pulse typically is not significant as long as a more distal pulse is palpable. If the more distal pulse is decreased or absent, other measures of circulatory status must be assessed, such as color, temperature, capillary refill, movement, and hair growth.

A bounding pulse indicates a widened pulse pressure that results from strong left ventricular contraction with an increase in stroke volume and a decrease in peripheral vascular resistance. A bound-

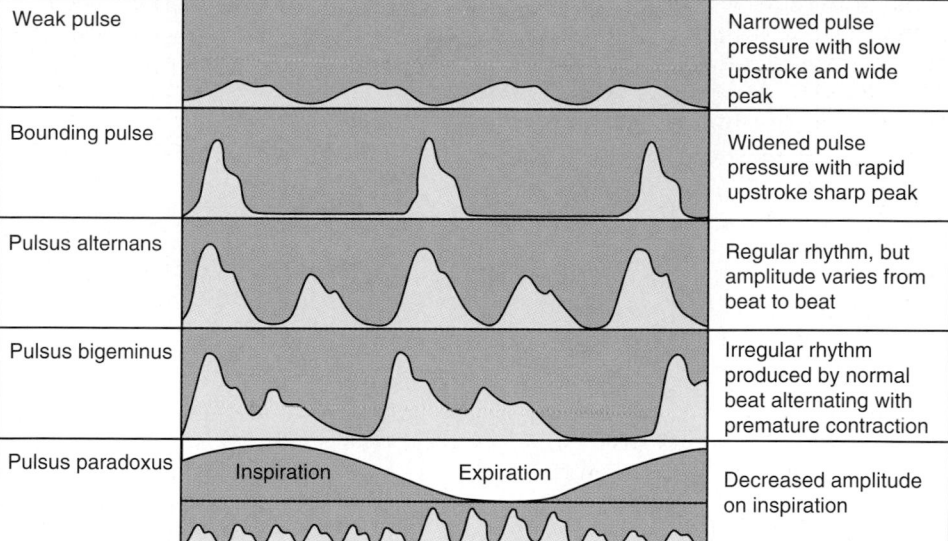

Figure 7–10

Schematic representation of abnormal pulses.

Weak pulse		Narrowed pulse pressure with slow upstroke and wide peak
Bounding pulse		Widened pulse pressure with rapid upstroke sharp peak
Pulsus alternans		Regular rhythm, but amplitude varies from beat to beat
Pulsus bigeminus		Irregular rhythm produced by normal beat alternating with premature contraction
Pulsus paradoxus	Inspiration Expiration	Decreased amplitude on inspiration

ing pulse occurs with exercise, fever, anemia, and hyperthyroidism.

If a pulse varies in amplitude from beat to beat, it is called pulsus alternans. The cause of this abnormality is variation in the force of left ventricular contraction. For pulsus alternans to be detected, the pulse must be regular. When pronounced, the alternation from a strong beat to a weak beat can be felt on palpation. Less pronounced cases can be identified only during auscultation of blood pressure. Pulsus alternans is associated with left ventricular failure.

A bigeminal pulse is also characterized by change in amplitude from beat to beat. However, the rhythm of a bigeminal pulse is irregular and is produced by a normal beat alternating with a premature contraction.

Pulsus paradoxus is an abnormal pulse in which there is a greater-than-normal change in amplitude of the arterial pulse with inspiration. It results from a combination of low left ventricular stroke volume and intrathoracic pressure. It can occur with constrictive pericarditis, cardiac tamponade, and some cases of chronic obstructive lung disease.

ABNORMAL HEART SOUNDS

Heart sounds are produced by the closing of the heart valves and thus are directly correlated with events of the cardiac cycle (Fig. 7–11). As the valves close, they create turbulence in the blood flow, which sets up vibrations. These vibrations are transmitted to the chest wall and can be heard with a stethoscope.

Normal heart sounds are labeled S_1 and S_2. The first heart sound, S_1, is produced by the nearly simultaneous closure of the mitral and tricuspid valves. The mitral valve produces most of the first heart sound, so S_1 is best heard in the mitral (apical)

area, which is on the left side, fifth intercostal space at the midclavicular line (Fig. 7–12). The first heart sound is about 0.10 seconds long and corresponds with the beat of the carotid pulse. It marks the start of ventricular systole. Splitting of S_1 (hearing the sounds of the mitral and tricuspid valves closing individually rather than as one sound) may occur with right bundle branch block, mitral stenosis, or dysfunction of the tricuspid valve.

The second heart sound, S_2, is shorter and higher pitched than S_1. It is produced by the nearly simultaneous closure of the aortic and pulmonic valves. As the aortic and pulmonic valves close, the mitral and tricuspid valves open, atrial contraction occurs, and blood flows into the ventricles from the atria during diastole. The aortic valve produces the major portion of the second heart sound, so S_2 is heard loudest in the aortic area. This is at the base of the heart on the right side, second intercostal space. Splitting of S_2 occurs normally on inspiration from pressure changes within the chest that delay closure of the pulmonic valve. This is called physiologic splitting. When S_2 is split on both inspiration and expiration it is a pathologic "fixed split." A fixed split can occur with right bundle branch block, pulmonary hypertension, and right ventricular failure secondary to a septal defect.

The third heart sound, S_3, is a faint, high-pitched sound. It is normal in children and may be heard until the age of 25 or 30 years. If S_3 can be heard after the patient reaches age 30, it is called a ventricular diastolic gallop and is considered pathologic. It is produced by rapid, passive filling of a partially filled ventricle during early diastole when the mitral and tricuspid valves are open. A pathologic S_3 can be associated with constrictive pericarditis, left-to-right shunts, and mitral regurgitation, but is most commonly found in ventricular failure. In right or left ventricular failure, the ventricle cannot initiate a contraction adequate to eject the blood it receives,

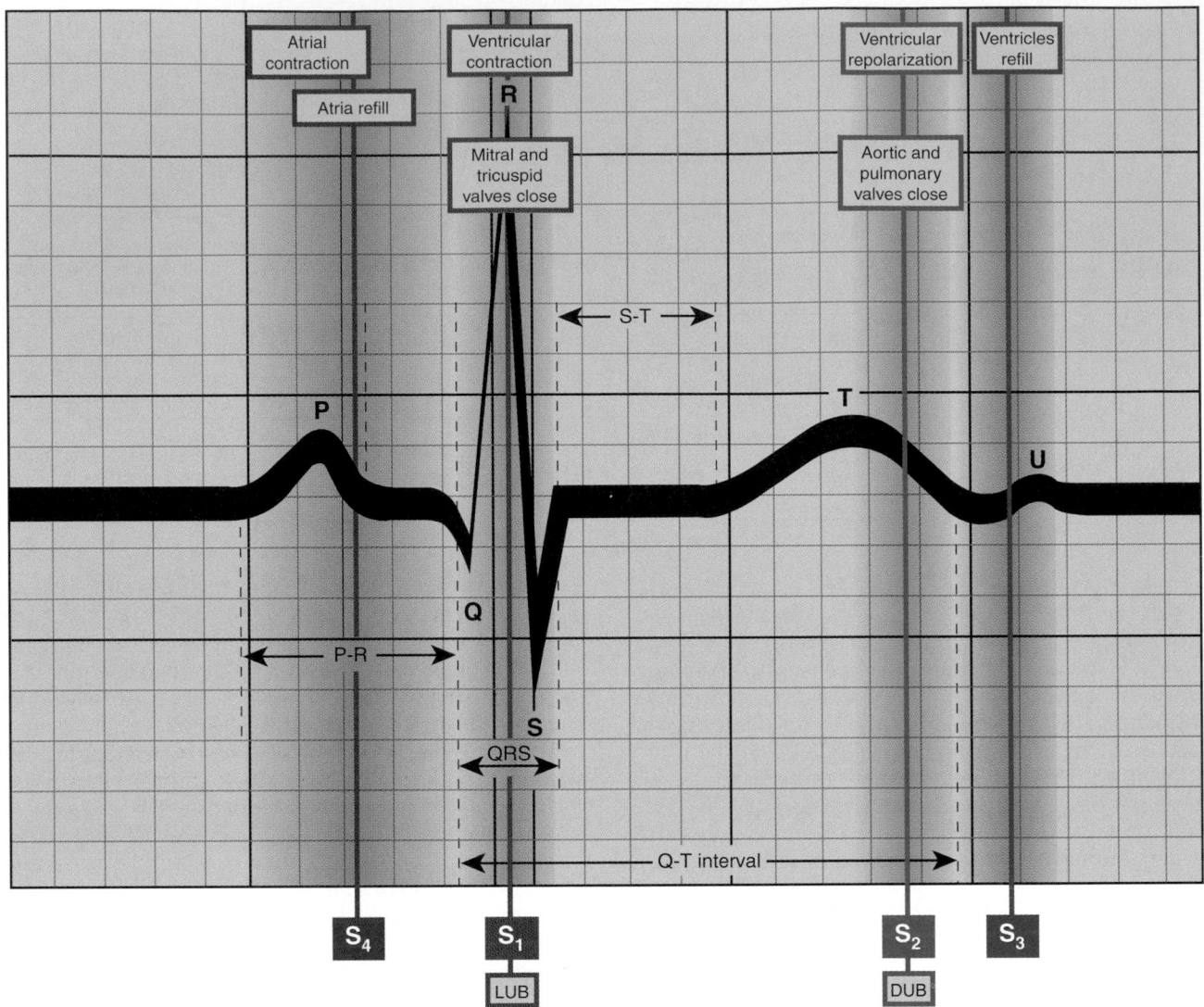

Figure 7–11

Relationship between the cardiac cycle and the heart sounds.

resulting in a partially filled chamber during diastole. As blood flows into the partially filled ventricle during early diastole, turbulent flow is produced and is heard as a low-pitched thud. A left ventricular S_3 is best heard on the left side at the apex of the heart. A right ventricular S_3 is best heard in the right ventricular area near the left sternal border. The timing sequence of S_1, S_2, and S_3 can be compared with the timing of the syllables in the word *Kentucky*. S_3 closely follows S_2 with a normal separation of S_1 and S_2.

An abnormal fourth heart sound, S_4 or atrial diastolic gallop, is produced by high-velocity blood flow during atrial contraction as the blood enters a noncompliant ventricle, causing turbulent flow. An S_4 is almost always pathologic in adults and may be caused by cardiomyopathy, aortic and pulmonic stenosis, pulmonary hypertension, systemic hypertension, myocardial infarction, heart block, or coronary artery disease. A left atrial S_4 is best heard in the

mitral (apical) area, whereas a right atrial S_4 is best heard in the right ventricular area close to the left sternal border. The timing of S_1, S_2, and S_4 can be compared with the timing of the syllables in the word *Tennessee*. The S_4 is a lower pitch than S_1 and closely precedes S_1 when S_1 and S_2 have a normal separation.

When all four heart sounds are present, the condition is called a quadruple rhythm. If the heart rate is abnormally fast, the sounds may fuse together so that four distinct sounds cannot be heard. This may be called a summation gallop.

An opening snap is an abnormal sound that occurs early in diastole. It is sharp, of higher pitch than S_3, and does not vary with inspiration or expiration. It is caused by the opening of a stiff or stenotic mitral valve.

An ejection click is a high-frequency sound produced by rapid ejection of blood through a normal valve or by the opening of an abnormal semilunar

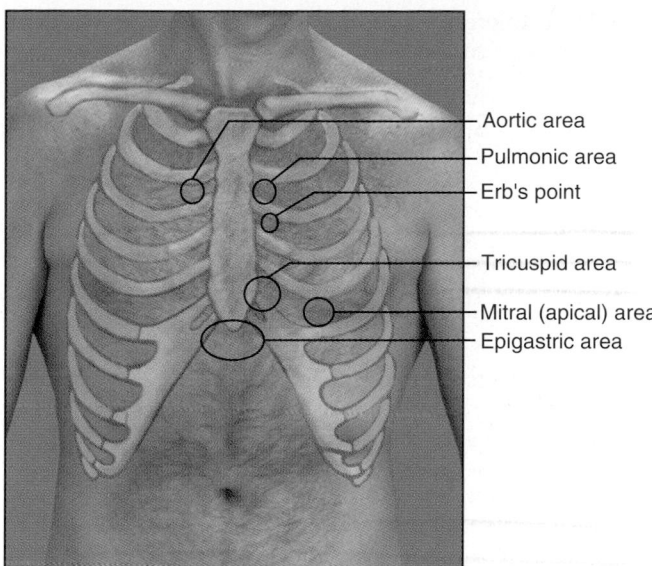

Figure 7-12
Major anatomical landmark areas on the anterior chest.

Labels on figure:
- Aortic area
- Pulmonic area
- Erb's point
- Tricuspid area
- Mitral (apical) area
- Epigastric area

(aortic or pulmonic) valve. An ejection click is heard just after the first heart sound. A midsystolic click results from the prolapse of a leaflet of the mitral valve. It is a high-pitched, snapping sound heard over the mitral or apical area.

MURMURS

A murmur is an abnormal swishing, whooshing, or blowing sound that may occur either in systole or diastole. It is a vibration caused by turbulent blood flow. Conditions that can cause a cardiac murmur include:

- An increased rate of blood flow through a normal structure
- Normal blood flow through a narrowed structure
- Backflow of blood through an incompetent valve, septal defect, or patent ductus arteriosus
- Normal blood flow into a dilated or enlarged structure

Systolic murmurs are the most common. Most are insignificant "functional" murmurs heard in pediatric and geriatric patients. Pathologic systolic murmurs may be caused by aortic or pulmonic stenosis, tricuspid or mitral regurgitation, and ventricular septal defects.

Diastolic murmurs occur during ventricular diastole. A diastolic murmur almost always signifies heart disease. Two common causes of diastolic murmurs are mitral stenosis and aortic regurgitation. Other causes are tricuspid stenosis and aortic regurgitation.

Murmurs are described not only as systolic or diastolic to indicate their place in the cardiac cycle,

but also by their intensity, quality, pitch, location, and direction of radiation.

PERICARDIAL FRICTION RUB

A pericardial friction rub is a scratching, grating sound that seems very close to the ear of the examiner. This sound occurs when the parietal and visceral layers of the pericardium rub against each other as a result of inflammation. Hence, this sound indicates pericardial inflammation. It is a highly transient sound, sometimes occurring for no more than a few hours, especially after a myocardial infarction. This sound is best heard at the third intercostal space to the left of the sternum. It is associated with pain.

NECK VEIN DISTENTION

Jugular venous distention warns of elevated pressure within the venous system. As pressure in the right atrium increases, the elevated pressure backs up into the jugular vein and the jugular vein becomes more distended and prominent. Jugular veins are normally distended and visible in the supine position, but should collapse and disappear as the patient is elevated 30 to 45 degrees above recumbent position. Venous engorgement is most commonly observed in patients with heart failure, but it can result from any condition that obstructs blood return to the heart.

ALTERED CAPILLARY REFILL

Capillary refill time provides an estimate of the rate of peripheral blood flow. After light pressure is applied to the nailbed to create pallor, color normally returns in less than 3 seconds and appears to return from the periphery as well as from within the pallid area. With cyanosis, color returns more slowly, and from the periphery toward the center. Capillary refill time is prolonged when the rate of peripheral blood flow is slow, as occurs in heart failure.

CYANOSIS

Cyanosis is a slightly blue-gray discoloration of the skin and mucous membranes caused by abnormal amounts of reduced hemoglobin or other hemoglobin compounds in the capillary blood. It can result from cardiovascular diseases, pulmonary diseases, hemoglobin abnormalities, or cold.

There are two types of cyanosis: central and peripheral. Central cyanosis results from insufficient amounts of oxygen (low oxygen saturation) in a normal volume of circulating blood. It is more serious than peripheral cyanosis and manifests itself on the lips, buccal mucosa, and underside of the tongue. Peripheral cyanosis may or may not be co-existent. The presence of central cyanosis indicates serious cardiac or pulmonary disease.

Peripheral cyanosis appears on the earlobes, tip of the nose, and the extremities. It does not appear in the mouth. In dark-skinned individuals, cyanosis, which appears as a pale gray ashen color or a yellow-brown color, depending on basic skin tone, can be difficult to detect. Thus, less highly pigmented areas of the body such as the nailbeds, lips, palpebral conjunctiva, palms, and soles of the feet should be inspected. In peripheral cyanosis, oxygen levels in the blood are normal but blood flow to the area of cyanosis is inadequate. Because of the reduced blood flow to the extremities, there is more time available for the tissues to remove oxygen from hemoglobin. This can occur normally due to the vasoconstriction that results from a cold room or from anxiety.

Cyanosis is a late and unreliable manifestation of oxygen deprivation. It does not appear until there are at least 5 g of deoxygenated blood in the vascular tree. Thus, persons with anemia rarely become cyanotic, regardless of the degree of oxygen deprivation, because of the limited amount of hemoglobin in their circulation.

Cyanosis, like all other color changes, must be assessed in natural daylight or under a lamp designed to simulate sunlight. A flashlight or overbed light is not adequate.

PALLOR

Pallor is a decrease in skin color. It occurs when there is a decrease in the amount of hemoglobin in the blood or a decrease in blood flow to the superficial vessels. Anemia, acute blood loss, and cardiovascular disorders that impair peripheral circulation can cause pallor. Like cyanosis, pallor is most readily seen in the face, mouth, conjunctiva, and nailbeds of light-skinned persons. In dark-skinned persons, pallor is best seen in the buccal mucosa and palpebral conjunctiva.

FATIGUE

Fatigue is not specific to cardiac disease but is a common manifestation. Normally, cardiac output increases during activity as a result of an increased heart rate and stroke volume. If this compensatory increase in cardiac output is inadequate because of cardiac disease, then fatigue occurs as a direct effect of an inadequate oxygen supply to the body's tissues. Thus, patients with chronic decreased cardiac output have difficulty performing activities of daily living, such as walking, bathing, dressing, cooking and eating, and doing household chores that involve the use of large muscles. This type of fatigue typically worsens over time, manifesting as progressive

activity intolerance accompanied by other signs and symptoms of cardiac failure.

NURSING PROCESS GUIDELINES
Fatigue

Nursing care of the cardiac patient with fatigue is directed toward decreasing the cardiac workload by providing comfort and promoting rest. Encourage the patient to reduce the demand on the heart by practicing energy-saving techniques, such as placing frequently used items within easy reach, and sitting rather than standing to perform such chores as food preparation. Help the patient develop a plan of activity that includes frequent rest and relaxation times throughout the day.

Specifically encourage rest periods before and after meals because good nutrition is essential to maintaining and increasing the patient's energy level. If necessary, suggest frequent, small meals to avoid fatigue while eating, or arrange for the patient to be fed to prevent cardiac strain and nutritional deficiency.

Encourage the patient to slowly build up a tolerance for increased activity. Instruct the patient to do this by monitoring vital signs before an activity, immediately after an activity, and then again after a 3-minute rest period. If the pulse fails to return to its resting rate, if respiratory rate remains elevated, or if other signs of anoxia (such as confusion or lightheadedness) are present after 3 to 4 minutes, reduce the duration of the activity. Also instruct the patient to discontinue activity and notify the healthcare provider about dyspnea, increased pulse rate, palpitations, or chest pains. Refer the patient to an exercise therapist or a cardiac rehabilitation program if needed.

CLUBBING

Clubbing is an abnormality of the nailbase in which the angle between the nail and the nailbase exceeds 180 degrees. With clubbing, the base of the nail becomes swollen, soft, and spongy, and the fingertips enlarge and look like clubs (see Chap. 14).

Clubbing develops in stages and occurs with pulmonary disease as well as cardiovascular disease. Since it tends to be associated with conditions of hypoxia and ischemia, it is thought to result from a diminished oxygen supply to the tissues.

ALTERED RENAL FUNCTION

A number of cardiac conditions decrease cardiac output. With a decreased cardiac output, there is decreased perfusion of the kidneys via the renal arteries. Activation of the renin-angiotensin-aldosterone system is a response to decreased renal blood flow. The result is increased blood pressure and retention of sodium and water. If further decreases in cardiac output develop—as may occur with cardiogenic shock, oliguria, and anuria—acute tubular necrosis may develop (see Chap. 31).

With prolonged renal vasoconstriction, the kidneys lose their ability to filter, excrete, and reabsorb necessary particles. Urinary output falls to 20 to 30 mL/hour or less. Blood urea nitrogen (BUN) and serum creatinine undergo a disproportionate rise. Urinary sodium concentration is high because the kidneys are unable to reabsorb sodium. As the kidneys lose their ability to concentrate urine, urine osmolarity drops and urine specific gravity decreases. Metabolic wastes plus metabolic byproducts of drugs given to the patient are recirculated because the kidneys cannot filter them from the blood. Thus, drug toxicity symptoms may be seen in patients with renal alterations from cardiac malfunction.

NURSING PROCESS GUIDELINES
Altered Renal Function

Assess and record the patient's vital signs, intake, and output. Note the color and consistency of urine. Observe for signs of fluid overload, such as oliguria, edema, crackles, wheezes, increased blood pressure, and weight gain. Notify the physician if urinary output falls below 30 mL per hour. Monitor hematocrit, BUN, creatinine, electrolyte levels, and other laboratory data related to renal function. Check for disorientation, confusion, sensory loss, and other cerebral signs indicating high levels of toxic wastes. Assess for signs of drug toxicity.

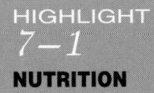 **HIGHLIGHT**
7–1
NUTRITION

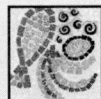

Potassium-Rich Foods

Fruits	Vegetables*	Seafood	Meats†	Dairy Products
Apple juice	Beans, dried	Scallops	Beef	Powdered milk
Bananas	Green beans	Clams	Ham	Whole milk
Cantaloupe	Broccoli	Cod	Pork	Skim milk
Honeydew	Artichokes	Flounder	Veal	Ice cream
Grapefruit	Asparagus	Haddock	Liver	
Nectarine	Greens	Lobster	Chicken	
Oranges	Carrots	Sardines	Goose	
Orange juice	Cabbage	Tuna		
Peaches	Cauliflower			
Plums	Chard			
Raisins	Cucumber			
Avocado	Potatoes			
Rhubarb	Peanuts			
	Peas			
	Green pepper			
	Pumpkin			
	Spinach			
	Squash			
	Tomatoes			
	Tomato juice			

*Fresh or frozen vegetables are higher in potassium than canned.
†Meats in general are not as high in potassium as fruits or vegetables.

ALTERED GASTROINTESTINAL FUNCTION

Hepatomegaly occurs with impaired venous return to the heart secondary to right-sided heart failure. This causes abdominal pressure, pain, tenderness, a feeling of fullness, anorexia, and, in some cases, nausea and vomiting.

Severe vasoconstriction causes detrimental changes in the pancreas. As the pancreatic cells become ischemic and necrotic, they release amylase and lipase into the circulating blood. Measuring serum amylase and lipase gives an indication of the severity of the pancreatic injury. Pancreatic injury leads to pancreatitis, pancreatic hemorrhage, and peritonitis, which may be life-threatening.

NURSING PROCESS GUIDELINES
Altered Gastrointestinal Function

Assess the patient for gastric discomfort and abdominal distention. Auscultate bowel sounds and ascertain bowel habits. Note any diarrhea. Ask the patient about nutritional habits and ability to eat. Ask about episodes of nausea, vomiting, anorexia, and weight loss. Observe for signs of hypovolemia and malnutrition, such as poor skin turgor, dry skin, weakness, brittle nails and hair, mucous membrane ulcerations, and depression. Check intake, noting the foods and fluids consumed and whether a particular food stimulates the distress. Determine whether the patient is too fatigued to eat or whether eating causes respiratory distress, making it more difficult for the patient to consume the entire meal. Check the amount usually served at mealtime and the type of foods the patient prefers.

Help the patient maintain adequate nutrition by providing attractive meals in a pleasant atmosphere. Serve foods the patient prefers when possible. Encourage the patient to eat foods high in potassium and fiber, low in saturated fat, and low in sodium (Highlights 7–1, 7–2, and 7–3). Provide six to eight small meals daily to prevent distention and reduce fatigue.

Instruct the patient to avoid foods that are gas-forming because they distend the abdomen, which may decrease appetite and interfere with respiratory efforts. Avoid hot, spicy foods and acidic fluids to

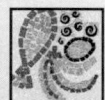

**HIGHLIGHT
7–2
NUTRITION**

Foods High in Saturated and Unsaturated Fats

Saturated Fat	Unsaturated Fat
Bacon	Chicken breast
Butter	Corn oil
Cheese	Dressings made with the oils on this list
Coconut oil	Fish (freshwater)
Eggs	Imitation foods (bacon, cheese)
Gravies	Plant foods (such as olives, peanut butter, pumpkin seeds)
Ice cream	Polyunsaturated margarine
Lard	Safflower oil
Milk	Soybean oil
Most meats	Sunflower oil
Nondairy creamer	
Palm oil	
Poultry skin	
Salad dressings containing other than low-fat oils	
Sauces	
Whipped dairy dessert toppings	

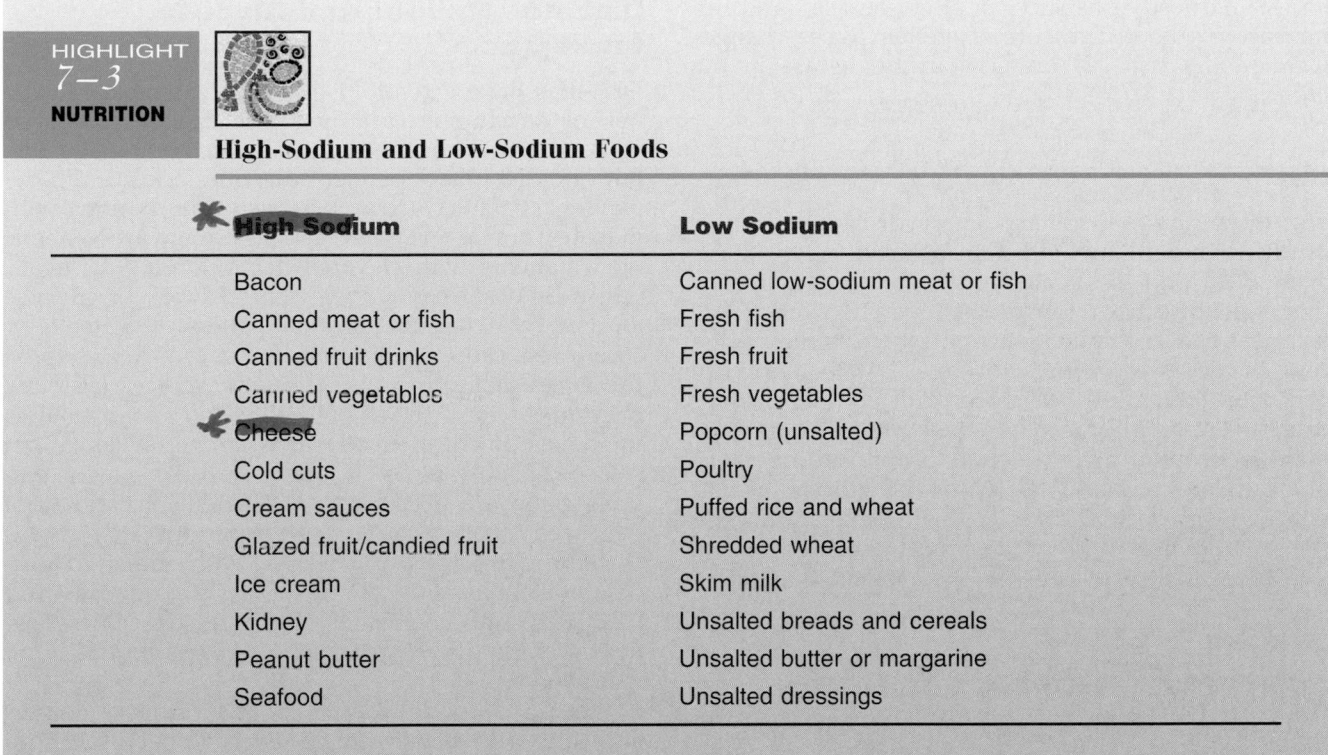

(See Chaps. 21 through 24 for the care of patients with gastrointestinal dysfunction.)

decrease gastrointestinal irritation. Encourage increased fluid intake, unless contraindicated, to prevent constipation and promote adequate hydration.

Review the cause, symptoms, and nutritional implications of the gastrointestinal problems with the patient and family. Allow time for questions and verbalization of concerns and misunderstandings. (See Chaps. 21 through 24 for the care of patients with gastrointestinal dysfunction.)

ALTERED NEUROLOGIC FUNCTION

The level of consciousness is assessed frequently in patients with cardiac dysfunction because it may change quickly. With cardiac failure and its concomitant decrease in circulating oxygen, the brain may not receive the necessary amount of oxygen for normal functioning. This oxygen deficit alters the level of consciousness. Restlessness is usually the first sign of decreased circulation of oxygen to the brain. Periods of disorientation and confusion are common. Any change in the patient's neurologic status should be assessed, and safety must be maintained.

Risk Factors for Cardiac Disease

Coronary artery disease is the most common acquired cardiac disease. It is associated with a num-

ber of risk factors, many of which can be influenced by lifestyle and personal choices.

UNCONTROLLABLE RISK FACTORS

Not all risk factors for cardiac disease can be influenced or controlled by the affected person. These uncontrollable risk factors include family history, age, and sex.

Family History

The risk of developing cardiac disease (atherosclerosis) is increased in a person whose parent or other close blood relative has been diagnosed with angina or myocardial infarction. The magnitude of familial risk depends on the sex of the relative and the age of onset of coronary artery disease in the person at risk. Greatest risk exists when there is a family history of a female with a premenopausal cardiac event. Also at increased risk are members of African-American families, owing to the increased incidence of hypertension in this group.

Age

Along with the normal aging process comes an increase in arterial deposition of cholesterol, an accumulation of calcium deposits in the coronary arteries, reduced elasticity of the vessels, and an increase in blood pressure. Together, these changes increase the risk of coronary artery disease in the older patient.

Sex

The incidence of coronary artery disease is significantly higher in men than in women between the ages of 35 and 44, probably because of the protective effect of estrogen in premenopausal women. After menopause, the incidence of coronary artery disease increases in women; by age 75, the morbidity and mortality rates associated with coronary artery disease are approximately equal in males and females. Coronary artery disease is the leading cause of death and disability in women over age 40 and one of every two women will die of heart disease (Jensen & King, 1997). Men are at the highest risk for coronary disease between the ages of 40 and 55.

CONTROLLABLE RISK FACTORS

Many risk factors for cardiac disease can be influenced by a person's lifestyle choices. These controllable risk factors play a very important role in planning long-term care for the patient with identified heart disease.

Hyperlipidemia

Several lipids (cholesterol lipoproteins) circulate in the blood, including:

High-density lipoproteins (HDL)
Low-density lipoproteins (LDL)
Very-low-density lipoproteins (VLDL)

When lipids are elevated in the serum, there is a higher risk that they will collect in the coronary arteries (as well as other arteries of the body) and, over a period of time, clog the arterial lumen, resulting in decreased blood flow to myocardial tissue, ischemia, and angina. Increased levels of HDL exhibit a protective effect against coronary artery disease. Consequently, a diet low in animal fats (saturated fats), high in fiber, and calorically balanced to maintain appropriate body weight can decrease the risk of coronary artery disease.

High Blood Pressure

Blood pressure fluctuates normally in all persons, but a sustained high blood pressure over a period of years leads to atherosclerosis. Atherosclerosis probably results from the mechanical damage of arterial linings that accompanies elevated pressure.

Diabetes Mellitus and Glucose Intolerance

Diabetics have a twofold to fourfold increase in the risk of developing cardiovascular disease compared with people who have normal glucose metabolism. Both non-insulin-dependent diabetics and insulin-dependent diabetics are at increased risk. Women with diabetes are at even greater risk than are diabetic men. Patients with elevated hemoglobin A_1C levels, which indicate poor long-term control of glucose levels, are at higher risk than others. Elevated glucose levels cause sorbitol and other substances to be produced in high levels. These substances alter cell membranes, and these alterations may contribute to the development of cardiovascular disease, as do decreased insulin levels. In addition, people with diabetes often are obese, have hypertension, and have increased cholesterol and triglyceride levels. It is therefore important for people with impaired glucose metabolism to use measures to monitor and maintain good control of blood glucose. These patients should also institute measures to control other risk factors.

Persons, especially women, with glucose intolerance (not just diabetes mellitus) have been found to have a greater prevalence of coronary atherosclerosis. These patients typically are obese and have increased cholesterol and triglyceride levels as well as hypertension. It is important for persons with impaired glucose tolerance to keep blood glucose levels under control in addition to modifying the other controllable risk factors listed here.

Obesity

The obese patient has an increase in cholesterol synthesis and usually a decrease in HDL, possibly caused by inactivity. Obesity appears to be a major determinant of glucose intolerance and of adult-onset diabetes mellitus. Obesity probably contributes to the development of coronary artery disease through its association with the other risk factors of hypertension, hyperlipidemia, and diabetes mellitus.

Cigarette Smoking

All by itself, cigarette smoking increases the risk of coronary artery disease 2.5 times in persons who smoke two or more packs daily. This increased risk is reversible through smoking cessation. Therefore, it is reasonable to suspect that smoking triggers cardiovascular events rather than being primarily atherogenic in nature or that atherogenesis may depend on the continuation of smoking. Mechanisms that have been suggested to explain the increased risk in smokers include the following:

- Vasoconstriction secondary to nicotine inhalation
- Neutralization of heparin, which promotes thrombus formation
- Platelet aggregation and the release of products during aggregation that may lead to vasospasm
- Increases in catecholamines, which lead to increases in heart rate and blood pressure
- Dysrhythmias, which diminish cardiac output and may precipitate fatal rhythms in vulnerable persons
- Decreased vital capacity in the lungs
- Increased carbon monoxide intake, which reduces the oxygen-carrying capacity of the blood, thus reducing the duration of smokers' exercise tolerance

In addition, smoking is associated with an increase in LDLs and a decrease in HDLs, which is in itself a risk factor for coronary artery disease. Exposure to second-hand smoke is also a significant risk factor. A 10-year study of more than 32,000 nonsmoking women showed that risk of heart disease was almost doubled among those with regular exposure to second-hand smoke at home or at work (Kawachi, 1997).

Oral Contraceptive Use

It is not known how oral contraceptives contribute to coronary artery disease. Serum lipids, specifically triglyceride, cholesterol, LDL, and VLDL levels, are elevated by oral contraceptives. Abnormalities of clotting factors and platelet functions have also been noted with the use of oral contraceptives. Users of oral contraceptives have elevated mean blood pressures, with systolic increases rather than diastolic increases. The risk from cigarette smoking acts synergistically with the risk from oral contraceptives to increase the risk of coronary artery disease in women at least fivefold.

Sedentary Lifestyle

Physical exercise raises HDL cholesterol, which protects against coronary artery disease. Exercise has also been shown to reduce resting heart rates, control obesity, and increase the vital capacity of the lungs, thus promoting oxygenation. Physical activity also helps dispel some of the effects of emotional stress on the cardiovascular system. It has been shown that a sedentary lifestyle, independent of other factors, increases risk of coronary artery disease.

Type A Personality

The Type A behavior pattern, characterized by an increased sense of time urgency, a profound eagerness to compete, and a drive for recognition, has been identified by some studies as a potential partially modifiable risk factor for heart disease. It is hypothesized that these behaviors can lead to profound stress, a higher serum cholesterol level, increased amounts of circulating norepinephrine and adrenocorticotropic hormone, elevated serum triglyceride levels, and increased sludging of red blood cells, particularly during episodes of hypertriglyceridemia—all risk factors for developing coronary artery disease. Studies have produced conflicting results as to whether personality type alone increases the risk for heart disease.

Emotional Stress

The physiologic concomitants of anxiety and other forms of emotional stress can increase the risk of heart disease. Sources of stress in everyday life are many, although what is stressful for one person may differ from what is stressful for another. Potential sources of stress include sociocultural mobility (major changes in residence, occupation, and cultural situations), socioeconomic pressures, life changes (marriage, divorce, major illnesses, and death of family or friends) and personal factors (life dissatisfaction, sleep disturbances, and depression). Recognizing personal stressors and learning to cope with life's changes are necessary components of good cardiac health.

Multiple Role Expectations

Multiple role expectations are considered a probable risk factor for cardiac disease in women (Jensen, 1997). It is suggested that the multiple role expectations of primary caretaker of nuclear and extended families and of member of the workforce increase the risk of heart disease because the time demands of these roles interfere with regular exercise and other healthy lifestyle choices. The multiple role expectations, which may be conflicting at times, may also increase the risk by inducing emotional stress and its associated physiologic responses.

Assessment of the Cardiovascular System

Despite the wide array of highly technologic tests available today, the health history and physical examination, along with an ECG and chest x-ray, are the essential elements of high-quality, cost-effective assessment of cardiac status. A major focus of both the history and the physical examination is the detection and evaluation of the risk factors for cardiac disease and the classic cardiac symptoms of chest pain, palpitations, syncope, dyspnea, and edema. These symptoms are classic because one or more of them can result from any of the three types of pathophysiology (rhythm abnormality, myocardial ischemia, and ineffective pumping) that underlie most common forms of heart disease. The history and physical examination must be comprehensive because cardiac disturbances affect almost all body systems and symptoms typically do not appear until compensatory mechanisms fail or a complication occurs.

PATIENT HISTORY

From the moment you meet the patient, work to establish a sense of trust. Trust is essential to obtaining the detailed, comprehensive history needed to provide an accurate assessment of cardiac status. Help to establish trust by:

- Introducing yourself by name and role
- Calling the patient by name
- Exhibiting respect for the patient
- Listening to the patient attentively
- Avoiding any indication of a need to rush
- Indicating that you welcome the patient as a partner in his or her health care

Begin the history by asking about the problem that prompted the patient to seek health care. This conveys a sense of concern and acceptance and aids in establishing a sense of trust. Use open-ended questions to determine the onset of the problem and the patient's perception of it. Throughout the history, allow the patient to describe symptoms in his or her own words to minimize the risk of misinterpretation. During the history-taking process, observe the patient for signs of distress, such as dyspnea, coughing, or breathlessness. Since cardiac symptoms frequently are absent at rest and appear only with a critical level of activity, make sure to assess activity tolerance.

Review the patient's health history. Elicit information about the type, frequency, and treatment of illnesses. Pay particular attention to any history of cardiovascular disease, such as a congenital defect, murmur, dysrhythmia, coronary artery disease, heart failure, angina, myocardial infarction, hypertension, or cerebrovascular accident. Also ask about any history of diabetes mellitus, hyperlipidemia, or thyroid disease, which are known to increase the risk for cardiac disease. Note the date and results of the last blood pressure check, cholesterol test, and ECG or other cardiac function test.

Review the family history. Ask whether any family members have cardiovascular disease, diabetes mellitus, or thyroid disease. If the history is positive, note the relationship to the patient, the specific problem, age of onset, and course of the disease.

Explore lifestyle factors that could put the patient at increased risk for cardiac disease. Determine if the patient smokes (or used to smoke) cigarettes or uses other tobacco products. If yes, note how many packs per day, and for how long. If the patient no longer smokes, also note the quitting date. Does the patient take oral contraceptives? What type and for how long have they been taken? Explore the amount of stress the patient is experiencing in daily life and determine if the patient has a sedentary lifestyle. Review the patient's dietary habits.

Next, direct the interview toward specific clinical manifestations of cardiac disease: chest pain, palpitations, dyspnea, syncope, cough, fatigue, and edema. If the patient complains of chest pain, assess it using the "PQRST" format:

Provocative/palliative
Quality
Region
Severity
Timing

Explore what provoked the pain, for example exertion, rest, eating, position changes, emotions, weather changes. If associated with activity, determine what type, how much, and whether or not the amount of activity required to provoke the pain has changed over time. Determine what the patient does to improve or alleviate the pain. Ask about effect of such factors as rest, nitroglycerin, position change, warmth, and stress reduction. Ask the patient to describe the quality of the pain. Keep in mind that patients often perceive pain of cardiac origin as discomfort, pressure, tightness, a feeling of being in a vise or being crushed, or like something heavy sitting on the chest. Some patients simply describe the feeling by showing a clenched fist. Ask the patient to describe or point to the location of the pain. Note whether it is localized or diffuse. Determine if it radiates to the neck, jaw, back, shoulders, or down the arms. Finally, determine its severity. Would the patient describe it as mild, moderate, or severe? Ask the patient to rate the pain on a scale of 0 to 10 or 0 to 5 where 0 is no pain and 10 or 5 is the worst pain imaginable.

Ask if the patient experiences palpitations. If yes, ask the patient to describe them (skipping beats, racing, trembling?). Do any other symptoms accompany the palpitations, such as shortness of breath, chest pain, lightheadedness, or diaphoresis? How often and when do these symptoms occur? What, if anything, does the patient do in response to them?

Question the patient about dyspnea. If it occurs, is it constant or intermittent? If intermittent, does it occur without warning? Does it occur at rest or on exertion? If the latter, determine the type of activity that induces dyspnea and whether it has changed over time. Ask if dyspnea occurs at night, how many pillows the patient sleeps on, and whether the patient awakens because of the dyspnea. Determine if dyspnea is accompanied by other symptoms, such as cough, fever, chest pain, or diaphoresis.

Ask whether the patient coughs. If so, is it constant, intermittent, or occasional? What time of day does it occur and are there specific activities that induce it? Is it productive or nonproductive? If productive, ascertain the quantity, color, consistency, and odor of the expectorate. Determine what the patient does to control the cough and how effective it is.

Ask about fatigue. Determine if it is sudden or gradual in onset, if it is increasing, and if it is related to time of day. Also be as specific as possible in describing what level of activity is associated with fatigue.

Question about edema of the legs and feet. Ask what areas of the extremities are swollen, how often, and at what time of day (at night, in the morning, after standing?). Is the edema unilateral or bilateral and is there any associated pain? If the patient denies edema, ask about feelings of shoes being too tight or if indentations from socks have been noticed since significant amounts of edema fluid can accumulate in the tissues before swelling is obvious. Determine whether the patient gets weighed daily, whether any weight gain or loss has occurred, and over what interval of time. Ask if the patient is experiencing nocturia. Does the patient get up at night with an urgent need to urinate? How many times per night?

Assess the patient's understanding of and compliance with risk reduction and health maintenance information related to preventing heart disease (Highlight 7–4).

PHYSICAL EXAMINATION

Physical assessment follows the cardiac health history. The four components of physical assessment (inspection, palpation, percussion, and auscultation) are used to gather data about cardiac function. The physical assessment is completed in a systematic, structured manner. Typically, assessment begins with general observation of the patient, followed by evaluation of pulse and blood pressure, progressing to the heart and the other body systems. Observation of the patient gives immediate, useful information about the current cardiac status. The patient who is fatigued may look unkempt, pale, and haggard. Dyspnea may be obvious, with an increased respiratory rate and difficulty answering questions during the assessment. Pallor may be evident if the patient has increased systemic vascular resistance or anemia. Peripheral cyanosis, the result of decreased circulation, may be noted in the fingernail or toenail beds.

Pulse

To obtain information about both cardiac function and the circulation, palpate peripheral pulses. Note their rate, rhythm, and amplitude. To obtain the rate, count the number of beats palpated in a 60-second interval. Count for the full 60 seconds the first time the pulse is taken and whenever you detect any irregularity of rhythm or rate outside of the normal 60 to 100 bpm range. Otherwise, count for 30 seconds and multiply by 2.

Note the rhythm of the pulse. Normally, it is regular, with an equal interval of time between each

---

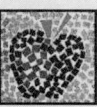

HIGHLIGHT 7–4

HEALTH PROMOTION & RISK REDUCTION   **Cardiac Disease**

To decrease the risk of cardiac disease and promote cardiac health, instruct the patient to:

Stop smoking

Eat a diet low in saturated fats and cholesterol

Avoid excessive use of alcohol

Be physically active:
  Start with a 5-minute walk every day
  Take a friend for company and motivation
  Increase to two 5-minute walks per day
  Increase to a 15-minute walk
  Continue to increase to the optimal 30- to 60-minute walks three to four times per week
  Maintain weight at recommended levels for age, sex, and bone size
  Have periodic checks of blood pressure*
  Control hypertension if diagnosed
  Have periodic measurements of serum cholesterol between ages 35 and 65 (for men) or between ages 45 and 65 (for women)*
  Discuss with your physician the need for a periodic electrocardiogram or prophylactic aspirin if at high risk for heart disease (male over age 40 with a family history of heart disease, a history of smoking, high blood pressure, diabetes, or elevated cholesterol)

---

*Recommendations from US Preventative Services Task Force (USPSTF) Guide to Clinical Preventative Services. 2nd ed. Baltimore: Williams & Wilkins, 1996.

---

beat. If the rhythm is irregular, note if it is regularly irregular or irregularly irregular. In cases in which a regularly irregular rhythm exists, ask the patient to hold his or her breath and note if the irregularity disappears. If it does not disappear, obtain an apical-radial pulse to determine if a pulse deficit exists. A pulse deficit exists when the apical rate exceeds the radial rate.

Except for the carotids, check for symmetry of pulses by palpating the same pulse on both sides of the body at the same time (Fig. 7–13). Proceed in a systematic fashion following a cephalocaudal direction. Corresponding pulses should be equal in quality.

As you palpate the peripheral pulses, note the temperature and moistness or dryness of the skin. Observe the extremities for edema and, if present, note the degree and check for pitting.

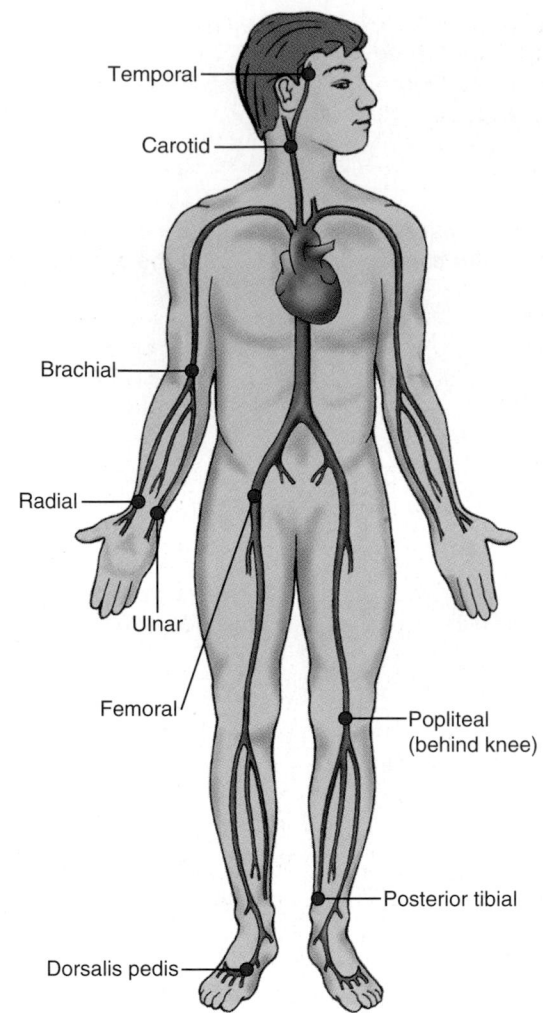

Figure 7–13
Sites for palpating peripheral pulses.

Blood Pressure

To be meaningful, blood pressure readings must be accurate. Inaccurate readings often result from incorrect technique. Common errors in technique that result in falsely high pressures include the following:

- Use of a cuff that is too small. The cuff should be 20 to 25% wider than the circumference of the patient's arm. This is especially important when taking blood pressure on an obese person or on a thigh.
- Poor timing. Blood pressure should not be taken after eating a meal, during or after exercise, during an emotional upset, or just before or after defecating or urinating.
- Incorrect position of the brachial artery. The brachial artery should be at heart level. If it is positioned below the heart, a falsely high blood pressure reading results.
- Poor cuff fit. The cuff should fit snugly and securely around the upper arm.

- Improper speed of deflation. When the cuff is deflated too slowly, venous congestion in the extremity results in a falsely high reading.

Common errors in technique that result in falsely low blood pressure measurements include:

- Use of a cuff that is too wide.
- Positioning the brachial artery above the level of the heart.
- Inaudible sounds from positioning the stethoscope incorrectly (not over the brachial artery) or from venous engorgement in the arm after repeated cuff inflations. To eliminate engorgement, remove the cuff and elevate the arm over the head for 1 to 2 minutes. Then reapply the cuff and try again.
- Failure to recognize the auscultatory gap. Some patients, especially hypertensive patients, have a silent period of about 10 to 15 mm Hg partway between the systolic and diastolic pressures. Failure to recognize this gap results in a falsely low systolic pressure or an overestimation of diastolic pressure.

For the initial assessment of blood pressure in the cardiac patient, take measurements in both arms. Normally, pressure may differ by 5 to 10 mm Hg between the two arms. Differences of more than 10 mm Hg may indicate aortic stenosis, arterial compression, or obstruction of blood flow in the arm with the lower pressure. Take future readings from the arm with the higher reading.

If the patient's history warrants it, assess for postural changes in blood pressure. Have the patient lie as flat as possible for 10 minutes. Take pulse and blood pressure at the end of this interval with the patient still in the flat position. Without removing the blood pressure cuff, have the patient assume a sitting position on the side of the bed with feet dangling over the side. Wait at least 1 minute, but not more than 3 minutes, check that the cuff remains correctly in place, and repeat pulse and blood pressure measurements. Then, obtain measurements 1 to 3 minutes after the patient assumes a standing position. Throughout the procedure, observe the patient for signs of distress, dizziness, or syncope. Protect the patient from possible injury if you note any of these problems. Record pulses and blood pressures, indicating the position in which each was taken. Also record the type and timing of any symptoms the patient experienced during the procedure.

Heart

To assess the heart, ask the patient to undress to the waist and to assume either a supine or upright sitting position. Begin the examination by inspecting and palpating the six major anatomical landmark areas of the anterior chest (see Fig. 7–12). These include

The aortic area, located at the right second intercostal space

The pulmonic area, at the left second intercostal space

Erb's point, at the left third intercostal space

The tricuspid area, at the sternum at the level of the fifth intercostal space

The apical area, at the left fifth intercostal space

The epigastric area just below the tip of the sternum

Inspect each of these areas from the side and in good light for pulsations. Next use the ball of your hand and your finger pads placed lightly on the chest to palpate each of these areas for pulsations, heaves (forceful pulsations which bound against the hand), or thrills (palpable vibrations). If you feel any pulsations, determine whether they occur with systole or diastole by simultaneously palpating the carotid artery or auscultating the apical pulse.

With the patient in a flat or slightly elevated supine position, palpate the apical impulse, which is usually the point of maximum impulse. It is a faint heaving of the chest wall resulting from the forward thrust of the ventricles during systole. Press lightly with finger pads over the left fifth intercostal space at the midclavicular line. Feel for a tapping sensation, which normally occurs in an area 1 to 2 cm in diameter and is confined to one intercostal space.

Next palpate the carotid pulse. Find this pulse by asking the patient to tilt the chin up, then place your index and middle finger on the Adam's apple and let them slide off to the side onto the carotid pulse area. Alternatively, ask the patient to turn the head away from the side being palpated to relax the sternocleidomastoid muscle and then proceed as above.

This lower portion of the artery is palpated to avoid pressure on the carotid sinus, which can precipitate bradycardia and a drop in blood pressure. Palpate the right and left carotids separately to avoid inducing cerebral ischemia. Note rate, rhythm, and amplitude.

Next, use the diaphragm of the stethoscope to auscultate in the apical (mitral) area of the heart. Count the apical pulse. Do this by counting the first (S_1) and second (S_2) heart sounds, *lub-dub* in combination as one beat, for 1 full minute. Assess the cardiac rhythm. Listen to several cycles, noting the lengths of the systolic pauses between S_1 and S_2 and the longer diastolic pauses between S_2 and S_1. If the length of the systolic and diastolic pauses are consistent in all cycles, the rhythm is regular. If there is variation in the length of the pauses, or sudden increases or decreases in heart rate, over a number of cycles, the rhythm is irregular. If an irregular rhythm is present, proceed to check for a pulse deficit. Do this by simultaneously counting the apical and radial pulses.

Heart sounds are most clearly heard with a stethoscope in a quiet environment. The diaphragm is best used to hear high-pitched sounds, such as S_1, S_2, and friction rubs. The bell of the stethoscope is best used to listen for low-pitched sounds, such as S_3, S_4, and diastolic murmurs. Place the bell lightly on the patient's chest with just enough pressure to produce an air seal with its full rim. (Firm pressure seals the bell and it then conducts sounds like a diaphragm).

When auscultating, first use the diaphragm and then the bell to auscultate the heart over the six anatomical landmark areas, noting rate and rhythm of the heart beat at each. Since the sounds produced by closing cardiac valves can be heard all over the precordium, auscultate by edging the stethoscope over the base of the heart and down to the apex in a Z type pattern to evaluate more surface area over the heart. Apply firm pressure when using the diaphragm and light pressure when using the bell.

Evaluate the heart sounds. Begin by identifying the first heart sound (the *lub*), which occurs at the same time as the carotid pulse and is followed by a short pause or systole. This sound is heard best over the apex and is normally louder than the second sound at the apex, the tricuspid, and Erb's point. Next, identify the second heart sound (the *dub*), which is heard best in the aortic area and is louder than S_1 at the aortic and pulmonic areas. Listen to these sounds carefully and note if they are normal, accentuated, or split. Identify systole and diastole. Remember that systole is the pause between S_1 and S_2 and is a shorter pause than diastole, which is the pause between S_2 and S_1. Normally these are silent pauses. During auscultation, also listen for extra heart sounds, systolic clicks, prosthetic valve sounds, or an S_3 (following S_2) or S_4 (preceding S_1). Note the location, timing, and characteristics of any extra sounds, and whether they occur in diastole or in early, mid, or late systole.

Also listen for heart murmurs, which are heard as swooshing or blowing sounds in areas of turbulent blood flow in the heart or great vessels. Evaluate any murmur detected according to its intensity, pattern, quality, location, radiation, and patient position. Grade murmur intensity using the following scale:

Grade I	Barely audible
Grade II	Audible but faint
Grade III	Moderately loud
Grade IV	Loud and associated with a thrill
Grade V	Loud and heard with the corner of the stethoscope lifted off the chest wall
Grade VI	Loudest and heard easily without a stethoscope, or with a stethoscope held an inch above the chest wall

Describe the pattern in terms of variation in intensity and timing within the cardiac cycle.

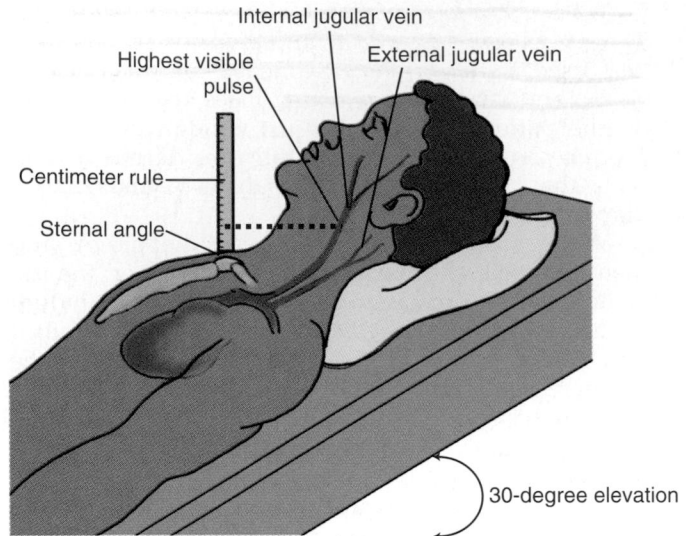

Internal jugular vein

Highest visible pulse

External jugular vein

Centimeter rule

Sternal angle

30-degree elevation

Figure 7–14

To assess jugular venous distention, place the patient in a supine position and raise the head of the bed about 30 degrees. Use tangential lighting to locate the highest point of pulsation in the internal jugular vein. While holding a straight-edge horizontally from the pulsation over the sternum, hold a centimeter rule vertically from the sternal angle (the notch at the top of the sternum). The jugular venous pressure is the height in centimeters where the horizontal and vertical edges cross. It normally does not exceed 3 or 4 cm.

Finally, check for neck vein distention. Elevate the head of the bed 30 degrees and use tangential lighting to illuminate the neck. Observe for the highest point along the vein where jugular vein pulsations are visible. Record the vertical distance above the sternal angle as "centimeters above" sternal angle (Fig. 7–14).

Other Body Systems

Examine other body systems specifically for changes associated with cardiac disease. Auscultate lung sounds by moving the diaphragm of the stethoscope across all lobes of the lungs anteriorly and posteriorly. Listen for crackles, which occur as air passes through alveoli containing fluid. Crackles may result from any cardiac disorder that impedes blood flow through the left heart, thus causing congestion in the pulmonary vascular bed and escape of fluid into the alveolar spaces.

Percuss the chest. Listen for the dull percussion note revealing areas of lung consolidation. This dullness results from fluid-filled spaces rather than the normal hollow sound produced by air-filled alveoli.

Percuss and palpate the abdomen. A dull sound rather than the normal tympanic sound over the liver can indicate engorgement secondary to right-heart failure and backup of blood in the portal venous system. Similarly, since the liver is not normally palpable, a palpable liver at the lower edge of the right rib cage can indicate engorgement from right-sided heart failure. Keep in mind that an engorged liver may be painful when palpated.

Observe for skin color changes: cyanosis, pallor, or jaundice. Assess for these color changes using natural or simulated sunlight. Areas to assess are nailbeds, lips, conjunctiva, hard palate, palms of the hands, and soles of the feet, where skin pigmentation is minimal and capillary beds are superficial. Keep in mind that in dark-skinned individuals, cyanosis appears as a light gray, ashen tone or a brownish yellow tone, depending on whether black or brown pigment predominates in the skin.

Diagnostic Procedures

A variety of diagnostic procedures is used to confirm suspected cardiac diagnoses. Explanations and expectations of the tests should be given to the patient and family for each procedure. Some diagnostic procedures for determining cardiac dysfunction are noninvasive, while others are invasive. Most invasive studies require informed consent forms to be signed before the study.

X-RAY STUDIES

The most common x-ray examination ordered for cardiac patients is the routine chest x-ray. The chest x-ray is used to visualize the silhouette of the heart, to determine the size of the heart, and to detect pulmonary congestion and pleural and pericardial effusions. The size of the heart is studied because an enlarged heart usually signifies impaired cardiac function. In assessing heart size, evaluation of previous chest x-rays is important because heart enlargement occurs over a period of time.

Areas of fluid in the normally air-filled lungs appear as dense or cloudy areas on a chest x-ray. Pulmonary congestion appears as a cloudiness or distension of the pulmonary vasculature even before crackles can be auscultated on physical examination. Pulmonary edema causes fluffy densities around the root of the lung, while pleural effusions obscure the sharp costophrenic angles.

Calcifications within the heart and coronary arteries can also be seen on chest x-ray. These commonly occur from aging or an infectious process.

Chest x-rays are also used to verify placement of

invasive catheters. A chest x-ray is taken after insertion of central venous catheters, pulmonary flotation catheters, and temporary pacemakers.

Chest x-rays are best taken with the patient in an erect position and during deep inspiration. All metal (such as jewelry) must be removed from the patient's chest. For a posteroanterior film, the x-ray plate is placed in front of the patient's chest. For an anteroposterior film, it is placed in back of the patient's chest. The cardiac silhouette appears different in each of these views as well as on chest x-rays taken in the supine position.

A chest x-ray may be taken in the x-ray department, which gives the best contrast films for diagnostic purposes, or in the patient's room with a portable x-ray machine if the patient cannot be moved. In portable chest films, the heart and great vessels assume a different size and configuration because of the placement of the chest plate at a shorter distance from the machine (about 4 feet versus 6 feet in the x-ray department). A portable chest film should not be directly compared with an x-ray department film because of these changes.

Fluoroscopy

Fluoroscopy allows visualization and analysis of the heart and lungs in motion, with the heart beating and the lungs inflating and deflating. It also allows visualization of invasive catheters with radiopaque tips as they are moved through the blood vessels. Thus, fluoroscopy is used during insertion of temporary pacemakers, pulmonary flotation catheters, and during such procedures as cardiac catheterization. During fluoroscopy, the x-ray machine is positioned directly above the chest as the patient lies in the supine position. The room is darkened and intrathoracic movements are viewed on a luminescent x-ray film screen or monitor.

ELECTROCARDIOGRAPHY

An ECG is a graphic recording of the heart's electrical activity. It provides information about cardiac rate, rhythm, and conduction. It can also determine atrial and ventricular enlargement and drug effects. Since ischemic or infarcted tissue does not conduct electrical activity normally, an ECG can be used to pinpoint the location and size of a myocardial infarction. In some cases, ECG changes only occur when the patient is having cardiac symptoms, and a normal ECG tracing is obtained at all other times.

An ECG is a noninvasive test easily performed at the bedside. Four electrodes are placed on the limbs and six are placed on the chest (precordium) to record the electrical current produced by the heart from 12 different angles, or leads. Hence the name 12-lead ECG. The heart's electrical activity can be recorded in this way because the body and its fluid are good conductors of electrical current. When the sinoatrial node initiates an impulse and the myocardial cells begin to depolarize and spread the electrical stimulus through the conduction system to the rest of the myocardium, the current is also conducted to the body's surface and the electrodes. The wave patterns generated by these impulses are recorded on the ECG machine to which the electrodes are attached and a graphic printout of myocardial activity from the 12 angles of the heart is produced. As the wave patterns are recorded on the ECG, they are labeled P, Q, R, S, and T (Fig. 7–15).

As atrial excitation begins in the sinoatrial node and spreads through the right and left atria, atrial depolarization is initiated. Atrial depolarization is represented on the ECG as a P wave. In normal rhythm, the P wave is the first wave seen in the cardiac cycle. The upstroke of the P wave represents the beginning of atrial depolarization, and the return of the P wave to baseline marks the completion of atrial depolarization. Thus, the width of the P wave represents the time necessary for the atrial activation process.

After atrial depolarization, an absence of electrical activity is noted on the ECG for a brief period, representing passage of the impulse from the atria through the atrioventricular node and the bundle of His to the ventricular myocardium. This flat, or isoelectric, line represents the early phase of atrial repolarization. The passage of time is labeled as the PR interval and is measured from the beginning of the P wave to the beginning of the QRS complex.

Ventricular depolarization is represented on the ECG by the waveform labeled QRS. The Q wave is always the first downward or negative deflection, and the R wave is always the first upward or positive deflection. If there is a second negative deflection after the R wave, it is labeled an S wave. In certain leads of the ECG, a Q wave may not be obvious. Even if a Q wave is not obvious, the ventricular depolarization wave is still called the QRS complex. The QRS waveform represents ventricular depolarization. It is during this period of time that actual atrial repolarization occurs. It is important to remember that electrical depolarization occurs before cardiac muscle contraction and that electrical repolarization follows cardiac muscle contraction.

After ventricular activation, ventricular repolarization begins. The ST segment is a flat (isoelectric) line between the S wave and the T wave, and it represents the early phases of ventricular muscle recovery. The T wave represents the actual recovery, or repolarization, of the ventricular muscle. Occasionally, an additional waveform, a U wave, can be observed after the T wave. The origin of the U wave is not well understood, but it is considered a significant finding in hypokalemic states.

The ECG recording paper runs at a uniform speed of 25 mm/second to facilitate time measurement of the various electrical events. ECG paper is subdivided horizontally and vertically with 1 mm and 5 mm boldfaced, spaced lines (Fig. 7–16). The

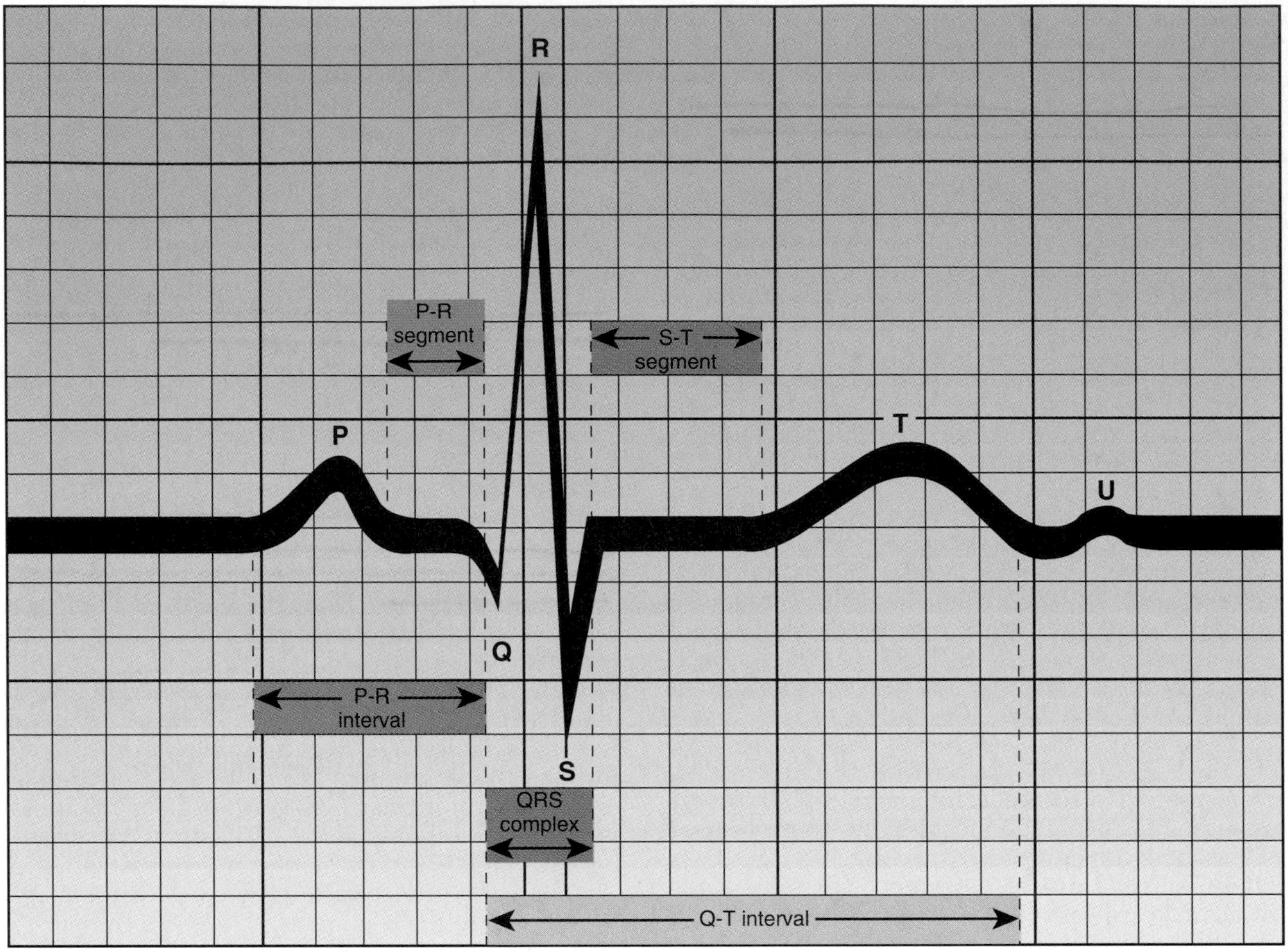

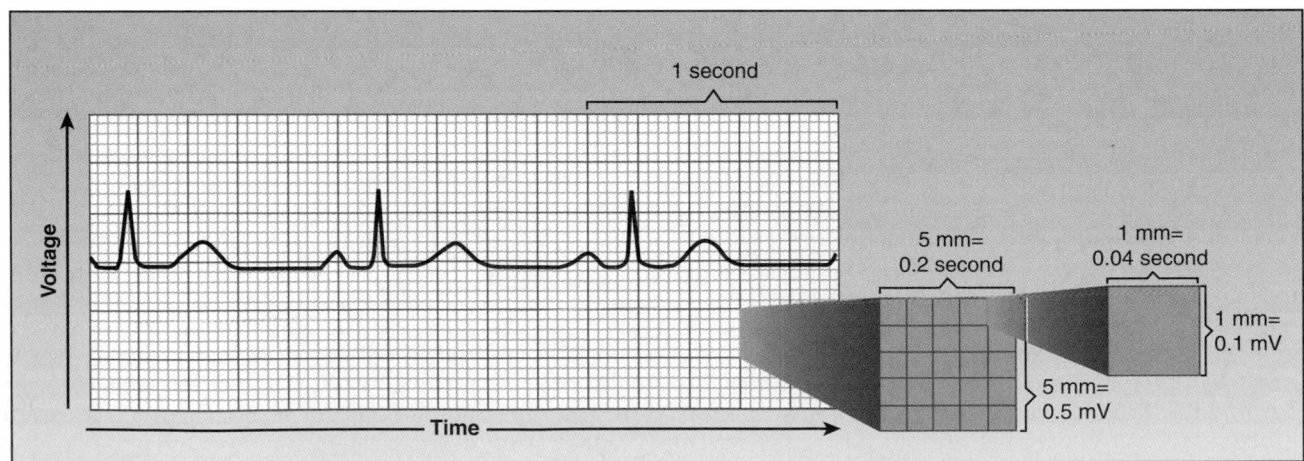

Figure 7–15

Normal electrocardiogram (ECG) complex. The complex is superimposed on the standard electrocardiographic paper at customary amplitude (1 mm = 0.1 mV) and paper speed (25 mm per second).

Figure 7–16

One small ECG square (1 mm) equals 0.04 seconds of time and 0.1 mV. One large ECG square (5 mm) equals 0.20 seconds and 0.5 mV. Five large ECG squares equal 1 full second.

horizontal lines represent time intervals, and the space between two 1 mm lines, or the space in one small square, represents 0.04 second. Thus, two small squares represent 0.08 second, three small squares represent 0.12 second, and so forth. The space across five small squares or one large square represents 0.20 second. The space across five large squares represents 1 second.

For convenience, ECG recording paper displays a marker every 3 seconds. There are 15 large (5 mm) squares per 3-second marker. Fifteen large squares, the distance between two markers, represent 3.0 seconds. Two of these distances is equal to 6.0 seconds; thus, the number of QRS complexes in a 6-second period can be counted. This is multiplied by 10 to obtain an approximate heart rate per minute (Fig. 7–17).

Normal conduction time from the atria, through the atrioventricular node, and to the ventricular myocardium is between 0.12 and 0.20 second and is represented by the PR interval. The PR interval is measured from the beginning of the P wave to the beginning of the QRS complex, not including the Q wave. A deviation from this "normal" PR interval represents pathology that either accelerates or delays conduction of the impulse.

Normal ventricular depolarization time should last less than 0.10 second and is represented by the QRS interval. The QRS interval is measured from the beginning of the Q wave to the point at which the S wave ends or reaches baseline. This is referred to as the ST segment.

The physiologic pacemaker of the heart is the sinoatrial node because of its high rate of automaticity. The rhythm generated by the sinoatrial node is known as the sinus rhythm. It is characteristically regular. To determine regularity, the distance between two R waves is measured and that distance is then compared with other R-R intervals. Normal sinus P waves have smooth contours and appear uniform across the monitor tracing. The P wave precedes each QRS complex. The QRS complexes are uniform in appearance and follow each P wave by the same distance. Each rhythm that is interpreted is done so in comparison with its deviation from a sinus rhythm; therefore, the normal sinus rhythm characteristics should be known by all practitioners responsible for interpreting ECG rhythms. Basic guidelines for interpreting ECG rhythms are helpful and can be used to interpret all types of rhythms. Basic guidelines are provided in Table 7–2.

To aid in ECG interpretation, note any medications or treatments received by the patient that have potential cardiac effects. Also note any cardiac symptoms or changes in vital signs at the time the ECG is done.

Signal-Averaged Electrocardiography

Signal-averaged electrocardiography involves placing six electrodes on the anterior and posterior chest and obtaining a 15- to 30-minute recording. The electrical current is amplified about 1000 times and the equipment filters and screens artifacts. The result is one QRS complex that is the average of many. Since the current is amplified many times, signal-averaged electrocardiography can detect signals of a frequency too low to appear on a regular ECG, but which predispose some patients to ventricular tachycardia and sudden cardiac death.

Exercise Stress Testing

The exercise stress test evaluates the heart's response to an increased workload. It is a noninvasive test that involves recording of an ECG during exercise (stress). Exercise increases the myocardial need for oxygen and, in response, increases the rate, force of contraction, and stroke volume of the left ventricle. Thus, a person who has a normal ECG under resting conditions may develop significant abnormalities and require therapy when increased demand is placed on the heart.

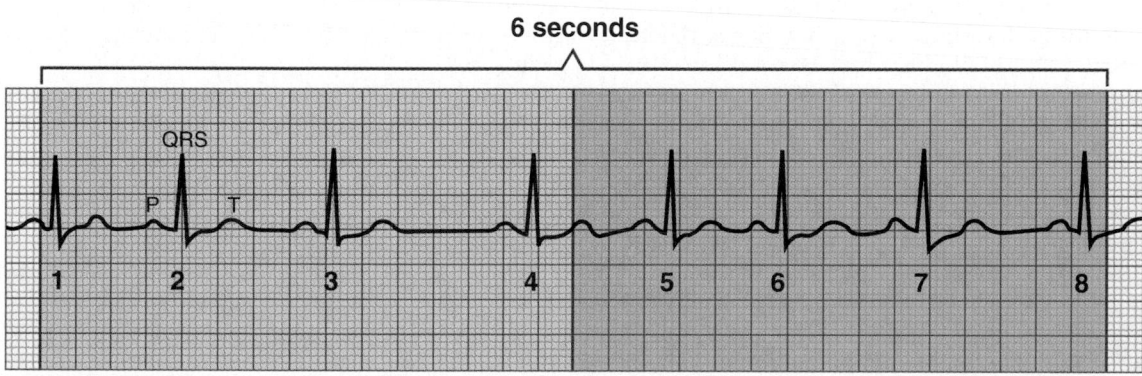

6 seconds

Figure 7–17

Counting QRS complexes on an ECG strip is a quick and relatively accurate way to determine heart rate. Simply count the number of QRS complexes that appear during a 6-second interval and multiply by 10. In the example shown here, the patient's heart rate is about 80.

Table 7–2

Guidelines for Interpreting Electrocardiographic Rhythms

Assessment Step	Description
Check rhythm regularity	To determine regularity, measure the distance between two R waves (R-R interval), and compare that distance with other R-R intervals. If the rhythm is not regular, identification of what causes the irregularity is required.
Check the heart rate	If the rhythm is regular, the rate can be estimated by counting the number of QRS complexes in 6.0 seconds and multiplying that number by 10. If the rhythm is irregular, the actual rate must be calculated over an entire minute.
Check the relationship between the atria and the ventricles	Look for P waves in front of every QRS complex. Look for uniform P waves. Determine whether the P waves are of equal distance from every QRS complex. If P waves are absent, are not uniform, or have a varying PR interval, the abnormalities must be explained.
Check the QRS complexes	QRS complexes should all look the same. The QRS interval should be normal. Variation in the QRS complexes in the tracing must be explained. The reason for the extra complexes or missing complexes should be determined. Assessing and describing abnormalities helps the practitioner determine possible pathology, its location, and the possibilities for treatment.

Remember: Women have more rapid resting heart rates than men, shorter PR and QRS intervals, and smaller-amplitude R, S, and T waves across the pericardium (Jensen & King, 1997).

Because the stress test evaluates the compensatory ability of the myocardium, exercise stress testing is used to:

- Detect latent coronary artery disease
- Provide sequential evaluations of the exercise response in patients who have known coronary artery disease or a history of myocardial infarction
- Evaluate the effects of medical or surgical treatment
- Monitor the effects of cardiac rehabilitation programs

An exercise stress test is performed on a bicycle or treadmill, the speed and incline of which can be adjusted to incrementally increase workload. Before the test, a baseline resting ECG is taken, and resting blood pressure is determined. During the entire test, the electrical pattern of the heart is monitored, frequent blood pressure readings are obtained, and activity intolerances are assessed. The test is continued until the patient reaches his or her maximal heart rate, previously determined by age, or until there is an indication to stop the test. Absolute indications to stop the test include hypotension, three consecutive premature ventricular contractions, ST depression of 1 mm or more, physical exhaustion, severe angina, and a staggering gait. ECG monitoring is continued for 5 to 10 minutes after the exercise while the patient's heart rate and blood pressure responses return to normal.

In a graded exercise stress test workload is carried out in stages. Each stage is 3 minutes in dura-

tion. Monitoring is as just described, with blood pressure readings obtained as each workload segment ends.

A positive stress test is one that shows a 2 mm depression in ST segment at any heart rate. An absence of a 2 mm ST depression at the desired heart rate constitutes a negative stress test. A high correlation exists between significant obstructive coronary artery disease and a positive stress test. Factors that can produce a falsely positive test include digitalis, hypertension, and electrolyte abnormalities. Other possible causes of false positive results in women are women's normally lower hematocrits, blood volumes, and oxygen carrying capacities; their normally higher stroke volumes, at-rest ejection fractions, and lower left ventricular pressures and volumes; and their gender-specific ECG characteristics (Jensen & King, 1997).

Complications of stress testing are cardiac dysrhythmias, which may lead to cardiac arrest and myocardial infarction. Because of this, emergency resuscitation equipment must be kept readily available and cardiac monitoring may be continued for several hours.

Before stress testing, the patient is instructed to not smoke and to avoid caffeine for 2 hours. The patient may be instructed to withhold cardiac drugs as well, because they could influence the outcome of test results. The patient should be advised to wear walking shoes and comfortable clothing.

Exercise stress testing is contraindicated for any patient suspected of having a recent myocardial infarction. It also is not performed on patients with recent episodes of angina or chest pain associated with shortness of breath, diaphoresis, nausea, or vomiting. Mini stress tests may be done before discharge for patients who have had a myocardial infarction to assess ability to resume activities of daily living. In cases in which the patient cannot exercise because of physical limitations or positive cardiac history, the heart may be stressed with medications such as dipyridamole (Persantine), dobutamine, or adenosine. Complete stress testing is usually done 4 to 6 weeks after a myocardial infarction or cardiac surgery to establish an exercise routine.

Ambulatory Electrocardiographic Monitoring

Ambulatory electrocardiographic monitoring allows continuous recording of myocardial activity while the patient performs normal daily activities. This provides significantly more data than a conventional ECG, which records only 45 seconds of myocardial activity and therefore does not demonstrate the effects of normal physical and psychologic stresses at home and at work.

Ambulatory monitoring is used to evaluate patients who have experienced intermittent dysrhythmias, dizziness, syncope, angina, and palpitations. It can also be used to evaluate the function of a permanent pacemaker and the patient's response to medications. Ambulatory monitoring is usually conducted for 24 hours, although it may be continued for a longer period.

The monitor commonly used is called the Holter monitor. It consists of a recording box (like a cassette tape recorder) attached to the patient via electrodes placed on the chest. The patient wears the electrodes and recorder for the total recording time. Simultaneously, the patient keeps a diary of daily activities and symptoms experienced and notes the time of each. Most Holter monitors have a recording clock so variations in ECG can be compared with activities in the diary by using the times recorded. The patient can mark events by pushing a button on the recorder when experiencing such symptoms as chest pain, dizziness, or palpitations. If the symptoms are caused by a change in cardiac rhythm, this type of ambulatory ECG recording helps diagnose the problem and provides guidelines to planning care for the patient.

At the end of the recording period, the patient returns the monitor to the physician, clinic, or hospital, and the tape is scanned by special equipment that can evaluate a 24-hour period in just a few minutes. ECG abnormalities are identified by the scanner and recorded at normal ECG paper speed for careful consideration and diagnosis by the physician.

Before ambulatory monitoring, the skin areas where electrodes will be attached must be thoroughly cleansed and dried. Areas of heavy hair growth should be shaved because the electrodes must make good skin contact for 24 or more hours.

Ambulatory monitoring is also done in hospitals via telemetry units. Patients who have had an acute cardiac event or dysrhythmia, or who have been started on cardiac medications that may affect heart rhythm, wear electrodes connected to a battery powered unit. The ECG is viewed on a monitor at a nurse's station in a critical care or telemetry unit. The patient's cardiac rhythm is monitored during activities of daily living. If dysrhythmias occur during eating, bathing, walking, or other activities, they can be treated before the patient is discharged.

ELECTROPHYSIOLOGY STUDIES

Electrophysiologic studies or programmed electrical stimulation is used to evaluate conduction abnormalities in patients with dysrhythmias that do not respond to conventional therapies. In a laboratory similar to a cardiac catheterization laboratory, the patient undergoes a percutaneous puncture of a vein and a multipolar electrode catheter is advanced into the heart. The heart is then stimulated by these electrodes to induce the dysrhythmia. Tracings are recorded and analyzed by a computer to identify the site of the ectopic focus and abnormal pathways of the patient's dysrhythmia. Medications can be administered or abnormal pathways eliminated by treatment with high-frequency waves.

In preparation for the test, antiarrhythmic medications are discontinued, the patient remains on nothing-by-mouth status (NPO) for 4 to 6 hours, and the fact that palpitations may develop during the test is explained. Following the examination, the puncture site is covered with a pressure dressing; the patient is kept on bedrest for 6 to 12 hours; and the affected extremity is maintained in a straight position. The patient is assessed frequently for bleeding or hematoma formation at the puncture site. Pulses distal to the site are monitored frequently. Potential complications of this test include thromboembolism, infection, and perforation of the myocardium, which could result in pericardial effusion or cardiac tamponade.

RADIONUCLIDE IMAGING

Radionuclide imaging uses radioactive isotopes that have an affinity for specific types of tissue. The selected radioactive agent is injected into a peripheral vein and the patient is placed beneath a gamma scintillation camera. This camera detects gamma radiation and produces images recorded on magnetic disc or tape that show areas where the radioactive agent was or was not absorbed by the tissue. Complications of radioactive imaging are rare.

TECHNETIUM PYROPHOSPHATE SCANNING

Technetium stannous pyrophosphate scanning is used to confirm the diagnosis of myocardial infarction when ECG and enzyme studies are inconclusive. In this scan, the radioactive isotope technetium-99 pyrophosphate, which has a particular affinity for areas of acute myocardial necrosis, is injected into the patient's blood stream. This radioisotope circulates to the heart, where it combines with calcium, permeating damaged myocardial tissue. These damaged areas then show up as "hot spots" on the scan produced by the scintillation camera. Hot spots that appear within 12 hours after the onset of infarction indicate infarct size. Because hot spots disappear within a week, old areas of infarction cannot be detected. In addition to an acute infarction, hot spots can appear because of ventricular aneurysm, cardiac tumor, or cardiac trauma.

THALLIUM SCANNING

In contrast to hot-spot imaging, use of the radioactive isotope thallium-201 results in images referred to as "cold spots." Thallium-201 concentrates in healthy myocardial cells, provided that an adequate coronary blood flow to these cells is available. Cold spots, or areas free of thallium-201, appear anywhere tissue perfusion is decreased. Thus, old and new areas of infarction are detectable, as well as areas of ischemia. An acute myocardial insult can be demonstrated within hours of its onset, even before elevated enzyme levels or ECG changes. This test may also be done in conjunction with exercise to detect reversible perfusion defects. For patients unable to exercise, drugs (such as dipyridamole) that mimic the effect of exercise by dilating nonstenotic arteries may be administered.

GATED HEART STUDIES

Gated heart studies use radioactive tracers to determine the location and size of an infarct and to evaluate ventricular function by assessing the motion of the myocardial wall. In these studies, the scintillation camera takes a series of images of the heart in action. These images are then played as a motion picture. One study of this type is the MUGA (multiple-gated acquisition) scan. The MUGA scan employs the radioisotope technetium-99m and is triggered by the patient's ECG. It visualizes the cardiac wall in motion, providing an outline of the heart through the cardiac cycle. Areas of dyskinesia or akinesia can be visualized and the left ventricular ejection fraction calculated via computer.

When used in conjunction with stress tests, gated heart studies help determine the severity of coronary artery disease. They also allow detection of right ventricular infarction, which is not detectable by the standard ECG.

POSITRON EMISSION TOMOGRAPHY

Positron emission tomography distinguishes between ischemic tissue and necrotic nonviable tissue. This information is useful in selecting patients who are candidates for revascularization surgery. Following injection of a radionuclide, positrons concentrate in the myocardium, which outlines perfusion of the organ. A second injection is administered that monitors glucose uptake by cells in the myocardium, indicating the viability of the cells.

ECHOCARDIOGRAPHY

Echocardiography is a noninvasive, painless procedure that uses high-frequency sound waves to provide information about ejection fraction, ventricular volumes, cardiac wall motion, valve structure and competency, and thrombi. In this procedure, high-frequency sound waves are emitted from a transducer that is placed on the patient's anterior chest wall. Because the frequencies of the sound waves used are above the audible range, they are called ultrasound waves. As the ultrasound waves pass through the chest wall, they encounter the cardiac wall or other tissue and bounce, or echo, back to the transducer. The echoes are then recorded. The recording depicts the depth of a cardiac structure (wall, chamber, septum, valve) by converting to distance the time taken by the echo to travel to the reflecting surface and return to the transducer (Fig. 7–18). By changing the position of the transducer, a structure can be viewed from different angles. Simultaneously, the patient is monitored on an ECG lead to relate the echoes to the cardiac cycle.

This procedure involves no risk to the patient and can be performed in the physician's office, in the cardiopulmonary department, or at the bedside. An echocardiogram takes about 20 to 30 minutes to perform.

Transesophageal echocardiography is an invasive form of echocardiography that gives superior images, especially of the posterior cardiac wall. A transducer attached to a flexible endoscope is introduced through the oropharynx into the esophagus, after which an echocardiogram is taken. The patient must be NPO for about 6 hours before the test. The patient may be sedated and given local anesthesia to block the gag reflex. Suction and resuscitation equipment must be available during the procedure, and

Figure 7–18

Two-dimensional echocardiographic images of the heart. The schematic (*A*) shows the position of the heart in the echocardiograms. AMVL, anterior mitral valve leaflet; ATVL, anterior tricuspid valve leaflet; DA, descending aorta; LA, left atrium; LV, left ventricle; MB, moderator band; PMVL, posterior mitral valve leaflet; RA, right atrium; RSPV, right superior pulmonary vein; RV, right ventricle; STVL, septal tricuspid valve leaflet; VAS, ventriculoatrial septum. (From Otto CM, Pearlman AS. Textbook of clinical echocardiography. Philadelphia: WB Saunders, 1995; p. 42.)

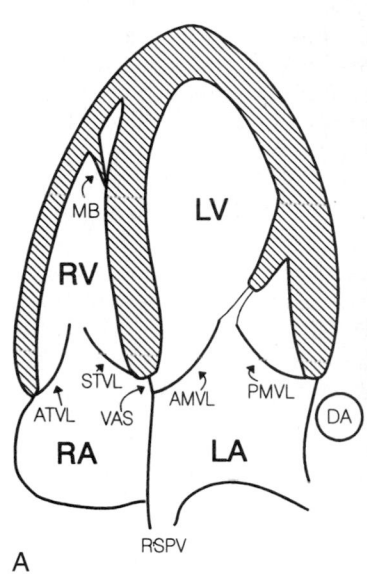

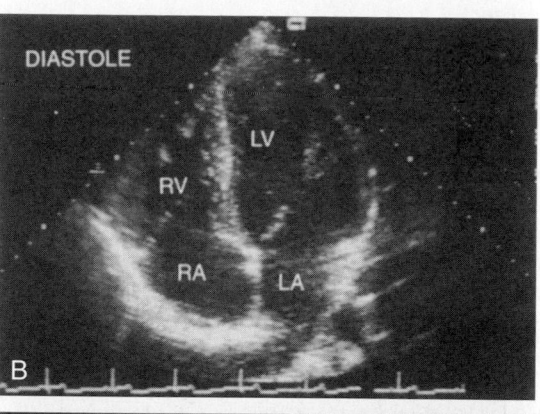

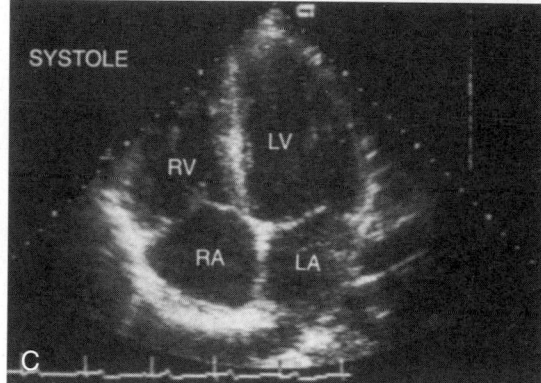

the patient must remain NPO until the gag reflex returns.

Stress (exercise and pharmacologic) echocardiography is also commonly done, and studies have shown this to be a particularly reliable test of cardiac function in women.

MAGNETIC RESONANCE IMAGING

Magnetic resonance imaging (MRI) is currently being studied as a noninvasive method of diagnosing coronary artery disease without the discomfort, trauma, and risk of coronary angiography. MRI produces a three-dimensional picture of the heart and coronary arteries. Difficulties with the technique include blurred images, inability to image small vessels, and inability to detect small blockages in large vessels.

Blurring of images is a result of movement, both of the heart beating and of the heart moving up and down as the diaphragm moves with inspiration and expiration. To overcome these movement problems, the patient's ECG is monitored during the procedure, and ECG signals are used to time image production during still portions of the cardiac cycle.

This timing is called ECG gating. During still portions of the cardiac cycle, the patient is asked to hold his or her breath. With ECG gating, large arteries where atherosclerotic plaques frequently occur can be seen. Even with this technique, however, diagnosis of cardiac disease with MRI is not precise, and false-positive and false-negative results do occur. Work is under way to develop intravenous contrast agents to enhance MRI images, as well to improve other aspects of MRI technology.

As with MRI of any structure, MRI of the coronary arteries is contraindicated for patients with implants or other devices, such as pacemakers, that contain magnetic material. During MRI, these devices could become dislodged by the powerful magnetic field generated by the MRI equipment.

ELECTRON BEAM COMPUTED TOMOGRAPHY

Electron beam computed tomography (EBCT), also called ultrafast CT, is a noninvasive test currently under study. It is designed to produce images of the coronary arteries by taking pictures so rapidly that blurring caused by the motion of the heart is minimized. EBCT does not produce a clear image of the arteries, but it does allow calcium deposits, which are part of most atherosclerotic plaques, to be seen and counted as a "calcium score." This score is currently the focus of research to determine whether it can be used as an indicator of coronary artery disease in asymptomatic patients. If it can, patients could avoid having to undergo invasive coronary angiography for diagnosis. Interpreting the calcium score is difficult because calcium deposits are common and do not always indicate severe arterial narrowing.

CARDIAC CATHETERIZATION

Cardiac catheterization is an invasive procedure that can provide information about the anatomical, hemodynamic, and functional status of the right heart, the left heart, and the coronary arteries. It is used to diagnose congenital heart disease, valvular disease, and myocardial disease. It is also done to assess the need for surgery, to evaluate cardiac function after medical or surgical treatment, and as a means by which other diagnostic or therapeutic procedures are performed. An example of the latter is cardiac catheterization during the acute phase of a myocardial infarction as a means of injecting a thrombolytic agent directly into the coronary arteries to reduce the infarction by dissipating the clot and promoting reperfusion of the ischemic area.

Cardiac catheterization is performed in a special laboratory. It takes anywhere from 1 to 3 hours and requires a signed consent. The patient is awake but mildly sedated for relaxation during the procedure. It is basically painless, although some pressure may be felt as the catheter is introduced into the vascular system. Because women have smaller hearts and coronary arteries, cardiac catheterization (as well as other procedures which require cannulation) is more difficult to perform on women.

To change pressures in the chest cavity and aid circulation as it is viewed on the oscilloscope, the patient is frequently instructed by the physician to cough or change breathing patterns. In addition, the table to which the patient is strapped may be tilted to view different angles of the heart during the catheterization.

Throughout testing, a heparinized solution may be infused through the catheterized artery to prevent clotting. The ECG is continuously monitored to detect dysrhythmias caused by the catheter touching the myocardium or occurring secondary to ischemia. An intravenous line is maintained throughout the procedure at a keep-open rate in case medications need to be rapidly administered.

Right-Sided Heart Catheterization

Right-heart catheterization evaluates the function of the tricuspid and pulmonic valves and the right

ventricle, and allows diagnosis of cardiac shunts and pulmonary hypertension. For right-heart catheterization, a small plastic catheter is inserted through a cut-down into a large peripheral vein (femoral or antecubital). It is advanced under fluoroscopic control through the venous system into the vena cava and into the right atrium. The catheter is manipulated through the tricuspid valve into the right ventricle, through the pulmonic valve, and into the main pulmonary artery. From there, it is advanced into the smaller branches of the pulmonary vessels until it becomes wedged in a very small peripheral branch. As the catheter is advanced, right atrial, right ventricular, pulmonary artery, and pulmonary artery wedge pressures are recorded. Cardiac output can be calculated using the thermodilution technique and blood samples can be drawn for analyses, such as oxygen and carbon dioxide content.

When the catheter is wedged in a peripheral pulmonary artery branch, the pressure reflected is the pulmonary wedge pressure, or pulmonary capillary wedge pressure. The wedged catheter obstructs pulmonary artery blood flow in that small vessel and senses the pressure transmitted by the pulmonary veins and the left atrium, thus reflecting indirectly the pulmonary venous or left atrial pressures.

Left-Sided Heart Catheterization

Left-heart catheterization evaluates the function of the mitral and aortic valves and the left ventricle. To do this, a catheter is passed into the left side of the heart by inserting it, via a cut-down, into a large peripheral artery (femoral or brachial) and advancing it, under fluoroscopy, through the aorta and the aortic valve into the left ventricle, through the mitral valve, and into the left atrium. At times, the catheter cannot be advanced into the left atrium because of the action and pressures of blood flowing through the mitral valve. Therefore, access to the left atrium is gained by trans-septal puncture. In this procedure, the right-sided heart catheter, with a catheter-sheathed needle on its end, is advanced through the interatrial septum from the right atrium to the left atrium. In patients who have had an aortic valve replacement or who have a stenotic aortic valve, percutaneous puncture through the chest wall for access to the left ventricle may be required. As in right-sided heart catheterization, pressure measurements are taken, blood samples drawn, and cardiac output determined as a measure of hemodynamic function.

Angiography

Cardiac angiography (called *arteriography* when the vessels to be studied are arteries) is a procedure in which a radiopaque contrast dye is injected into the heart and its blood vessels. Films called cineangiograms are then taken in rapid sequence to record the flow of the contrast media. This allows the myocardium's performance to be observed throughout several cardiac cycles and the coronary circulation to be visualized. The recordings can be studied at various speeds for detailed diagnosis of coronary artery and cardiac chamber problems.

Right-heart angiography is done to detect congenital anomalies, identify valve problems, and evaluate the motion of the right myocardial wall. A contrast medium is injected into the inferior or superior vena cava, right ventricle, and pulmonary artery. A contrast medium is injected into the left ventricle to allow assessment of the mitral and aortic valves as well as of left ventricular performance. Less efficient myocardial contraction, which occurs following a myocardial infarction or in the presence of a ventricular aneurysm, can be detected by observing ventricular size during the diastolic and systolic phases of the cardiac cycle.

Coronary angiography can demonstrate occlusion, narrowing, or congenital defect of the coronary arteries and allows visualization of collateral circulation (Fig. 7–19). For coronary arteriography, the catheter is advanced into the openings of the coronary arteries located just superior to the aortic valves. A small amount of contrast medium is then injected into each artery and angiographic films are taken. This procedure is commonly done to assess the need for coronary artery bypass grafting or angioplasty.

Patient Preparation

Since the contrast media used are largely composed of iodide salts, patients must be assessed for allergy to iodine or shellfish. Those who are allergic are treated prophylactically with prednisone or antihis-

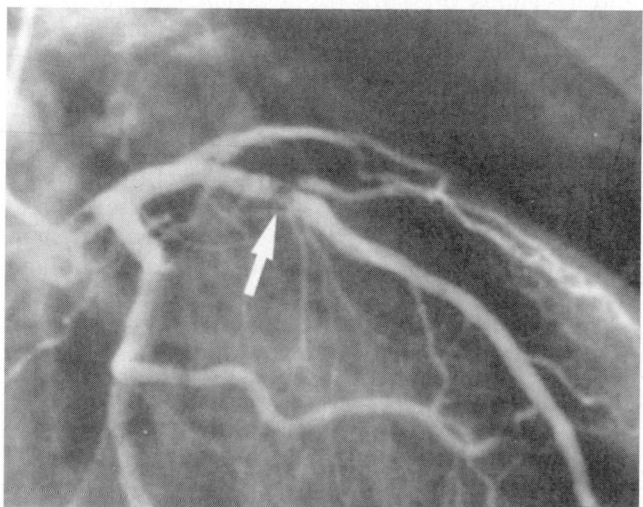

Figure 7–19

Coronary arteriogram showing a coronary artery thrombus (arrow) in a patient with unstable angina. (From Braunwald E. Heart disease: A textbook of cardiovascular medicine. 5th ed. Philadelphia: WB Saunders, 1997; p. 1333.)

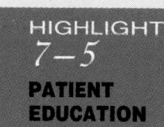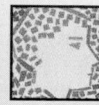
Discharge Instructions After Cardiac Catheterization

On discharge, instruct the patient who has had cardiac catheterization to:

Watch for bleeding or swelling at dressing sites (puncture sites).

Apply direct pressure over the dressing and notify the physician if bleeding occurs.

Observe for signs of circulatory impairment to the extremities, such as discoloration, numbness, tingling, and lack of warmth.

Report any of these untoward signs to the physician.

Expect some pain at puncture sites. Take an analgesic as ordered.

Increase fluid intake for 24 hours, unless contraindicated, to help clear the contrast medium.

tamines before testing. Contraindications to cardiac catheterization include ventricular irritability, hypertension, fever, anemia, digitalis toxicity, and electrolyte imbalances. During the catheterization, the patient is told to expect a warm, tingling sensation when the dye is injected. If the patient experiences chest pain, appropriate analgesics or nitrates are administered.

Postprocedure Care

After catheterization, the patient is assessed for pain, stability of vital signs, bleeding, edema, and temperature change. Pulses distal to the catheter insertion site are palpated and compared with the opposite side. Changes in peripheral pulses, such as a weak and thready pulse, are reported immediately because they indicate compromised circulation.

Arterial puncture sites are bandaged with pressure dressings. The site is monitored for bleeding and hematoma formation and pulses distal to the site are palpated every 15 minutes to 1 hour, as ordered. The patient is on bedrest with the extremity extended for 8 to 10 hours after the procedure to ensure stability of vital signs and absence of bleeding. Before discharge, the patient is given instructions for self-management at home (Highlight 7–5).

Complications of cardiac catheterization include allergic reactions to the contrast agent, bleeding at the catheter site, perforation of the heart or a blood vessel, dysrhythmias, pulmonary embolism, myocardial infarction, cerebral vascular accident, heart failure, and infection. The mortality rate associated with cardiac catheterization is extremely low and correlates with the severity of existing cardiac disease.

NURSING PROCESS GUIDELINES
Cardiac Catheterization

Refer to Nursing Care Guide 7–1 for assessments, nursing diagnoses, expected outcomes, nursing interventions and evaluation for patients undergoing cardiac catheterization.

INVASIVE HEMODYNAMIC MONITORING

Invasive hemodynamic monitoring is used to monitor cardiovascular function and blood volume. The monitoring is done by means of catheters placed in the vascular system. Hemodynamic monitoring is indicated for critically ill patients with severe heart failure or other major cardiovascular disorder.

Three specific types of invasive hemodynamic monitoring are central venous pressure monitoring, pulmonary artery pressure monitoring, and intra-arterial blood pressure monitoring.

Central Venous Pressure

Central venous pressure is the pressure in the right atrium and in the great veins as they enter the right atrium. Central venous pressure is determined primarily by the volume of blood entering the great veins, the pumping action of the right heart, and the degree of vasoconstriction in the vascular system. Hence, central venous pressure is an indicator of circulating blood volume and right-heart pumping effectiveness. A high central venous pressure reading may indicate hypervolemia or poor myocardial contraction and right-heart pump failure. A low central venous pressure is consistent with hypovolemia. Of equal or greater importance than a single central venous pressure reading is the direction of change indicated by a series of readings. For example, a change of 6 mm H_2O in 30 minutes is significant even though numerically the central venous pressure may be within the normal range of 5 to 15 mm H_2O. When assessing patient status, it must be remembered that significant changes in hemodynamic state can occur before the central venous pressure changes. Measurement of central venous pressure is primarily used to guide fluid replacement in seriously ill patients.

Central venous pressure is measured by means of a catheter inserted into a large vein (the external jugular vein in the neck, the subclavian vein in the upper chest, the antecubital vein in the arm, or the femoral vein in the leg) and advanced through the vena cava until it reaches the right atrium. The free end of this catheter is most often attached to a pressure transducer, which allows for continuous monitoring, although occasionally it is attached to a water monitor, which allows for intermittent monitoring. Central venous pressure is measured in millimeters of mercury (mm Hg) when a transducer is used and in centimeters of water (cm H_2O) when a water manometer is used. Normal limits are generally accepted as 1 to 6 mm Hg and 2 to 8 cm H_2O, respectively, although what constitutes normal continues to be debated.

Two major complications associated with this procedure are infection and embolism. To prevent infection, the catheter insertion site is covered with a dry sterile or transparent dressing. This dressing, along with the line set-up, is changed at regular intervals set by agency protocol. CDC recommendations (1995) regarding dressing and tubing changes are to (1) leave dressings in place until the catheter is removed or changed or until the dressing becomes damp, loosened, or soiled, and (2) change intravenous tubing, including "piggy back tubing" no more frequently than at 72-hour intervals.

Pulmonary Artery Pressure

Since cardiac patients do not usually have sudden changes in blood volume except in response to aggressive diuresis, central venous pressure measurements are of limited value in managing their care. Much more useful are pulmonary artery pressure measurements that reflect left ventricular function and thus effectively monitor a left-failing heart. These measurements are obtained by means of a pulmonary artery catheter, which is a multilumen, balloon-tipped catheter inserted into the right side of the heart via the venous system (brachial, subclavian, jugular, or femoral veins). One lumen of the catheter remains in the right atrium and provides central venous pressure (right atrial pressure) readings and an avenue for fluid administration.

When in the right atrium, the balloon on one port is inflated with air, and the catheter advances with the flow of blood through the tricuspid valve and into the right ventricle. From the right ventricle, the catheter is advanced through the pulmonic valve into the pulmonary artery. Pulmonary artery pressure can then be measured and the catheter left in place. When needed, the balloon is inflated again and the catheter is carried into a distal branch of the pulmonary artery until it stops or is wedged into place by the inflated balloon in a small vessel (Fig. 7–20). A pressure reading is taken at this point: it is known as pulmonary artery wedge pressure, pulmonary capillary wedge pressure, or pulmonary artery occluded pressure. Normal pulmonary artery pressure is 10 to 25 mm Hg, with a mean pressure of 10 to 20 mm Hg. Normal pulmonary wedge pressure is 5 to 12 mm Hg.

Pulmonary artery pressure is monitored continuously on an oscilloscope, and pulmonary wedge pressures are obtained as needed. The balloon is

Nursing Care Guide 7-1
Patients Undergoing Cardiac Catheterization

Precatheterization

Assessment Findings: Patient presents with signs of restlessness, nervousness, and increased respiratory and heart rate, asks questions about procedures, clenches hands, and cries.

Nursing Diagnosis: Anxiety related to fear of procedure, diagnosis, and future medical/surgical management

Patient Outcomes	Nursing Interventions	Rationale
Patient is less anxious, as evidenced by lack of restlessness, crying, or nervousness.	Explain the procedure to the patient and family. Allow time for questions and concerns.	An understanding of the procedure may alleviate the stress induced from the unknown or misunderstandings.
Patient's vital signs are within normal limits for the patient.	Teach relaxation techniques. Allow time for rest; provide a quiet, comfortable atmosphere.	Practicing relaxation techniques alleviates tension, as indicated by normal vital signs.
Patient states relief of anxiety.	Help the patient find coping strategies that help alleviate the stress and anxiety.	Appropriate coping strategies may reduce levels of anxiety.

Evaluation: Compare the patient's status with the expected patient outcomes. If the outcomes are not met, reassess the patient and revise the plan.

Assessment Findings: Patient asks questions about procedure, seems uninformed about preprocedure and postprocedure care and treatments; patient and family voice concerns about risks and necessity for the procedure.

Nursing Diagnosis: Risk for altered health maintenance related to lack of knowledge about the nature of procedure and postprocedure care

Patient Outcomes	Nursing Interventions	Rationale
Patient reports accurate information about the procedure, the necessity for it, and the expectations after procedure.	Be sure the physician has discussed the procedure, risks, complications, and expectations with the patient.	Checking the information the patient has received reinforces understanding.
	Allow the patient to ask questions and try to expand on the understanding about the procedure for the patient and family.	Allowing time for questions gives the patient a chance to be fully knowledgeable about the procedure.
	Have the patient state the information received from the physician so any misconceptions can be eliminated.	Asking the patient to repeat the information allows for correction of misinformation.

(continued)

Nursing Care Guide 7-1
Patients Undergoing Cardiac Catheterization (continued)

Patient Outcomes	Nursing Interventions	Rationale
Patient and family state they have an understanding of the procedure, the risks, and the postprocedure care needed.	Explain the postprocedure care needed to both the patient and the family, and tell the patient it will be repeated before discharge (see Highlight 7–5).	Giving information to both patient and family provides support and reinforcement for the patient, especially after discharge. It also alleviates some of the anxiety for the family.

Evaluation: Compare the patient's status with the expected patient outcomes. If the outcomes are not met, reassess the patient and revise the plan.

Postcatheterization

Assessment Findings: Patient has had an arterial puncture.

Nursing Diagnosis: Risk for decreased cardiac output related to bleeding secondary to arterial puncture

Patient Outcomes	Nursing Interventions	Rationale
Patient's vital signs are stable.	Monitor vital signs, usually every 15 minutes for first 2 to 3 hours.	Tachycardia, tachypnea, and hypotension are signs of bleeding.
Signs of bleeding are absent.	Inspect the site and palpate peripheral pulses distal to puncture site. Observe for bleeding and hematoma. A sand bag may be applied for 2 to 4 hours postprocedure.	Bleeding may be evident on dressings and a clot may disrupt distal circulation.
	Maintain bedrest with the extremity in a straight position.	Flexion may disrupt hemostasis.

Evaluation: Compare the patient's status with the expected patient outcomes. If the outcomes are not met, reassess the patient and revise the plan.

Assessment Findings: Patient has recently undergone cardiac catheterization and angiography.

Nursing Diagnosis: Risk for fluid volume deficit related to extreme diuresis from effects of contrast dye

Patient Outcomes	Nursing Interventions	Rationale
Patient remains well hydrated.	Encourage increased fluid intake to match the output.	Increased intake of fluids replaces losses.
Vital signs are within normal limits for the patient.	Observe for signs of hypovolemia such as poor skin turgor, dry, cracked lips, and vital sign changes.	Vital sign changes and dry skin and mucous membranes may reflect dehydration.
Patient's output is adequate but not excessive.	Check the patient's output frequently. Compare fluid intake and output amounts.	Balance between intake and output is indicative of fluid balance.

(continued)

Nursing Care Guide 7–1
Patients Undergoing Cardiac Catheterization (continued)

Evaluation:	Compare the patient's status with the expected patient outcomes. If the outcomes are not met, reassess the patient and revise the plan.
Assessment Findings:	Patient complains of confusion, disorientation, paresthesia, weakness, or syncope.
Nursing Diagnosis:	Altered cerebral tissue perfusion related to potential complication of blood clot or plaque being dislodged during procedure and traveling to the brain

Patient Outcomes	Nursing Interventions	Rationale
Patient remains alert and oriented.	Watch for signs of confusion, dizziness, altered level of consciousness, and lethargy. Notify the physician if these signs are evident.	Although a clot or plaque embolus may not be preventable, observe for early signs of decreased cerebral tissue perfusion so early intervention can occur.
Patient experiences no further complications from the results of the procedure.	Assist the patient in getting out of bed when able if patient is dizzy or confused or if blood pressure is low.	Because the patient may have some weakness and orthostatic hypotension, assistance is needed to prevent injury.

Evaluation:	Compare the patient's status with the expected patient outcomes. If the outcomes are not met, reassess the patient and revise the plan.
Assessment Findings:	Patient asks questions about necessary home care and other discharge instructions.
Nursing Diagnosis:	Risk for altered health maintenance related to lack of knowledge about self-management after discharge

Patient Outcomes	Nursing Interventions	Rationale
Patient states accurate information about discharge care. Patient states when to report to the physician for follow-up.	Give the patient written instruction for self-care after discharge as listed in Highlight 7–5.	Written instructions reinforce verbal information and allow for review after discharge.
	Have patient repeat information. Allow time for questions and concerns, and correct misunderstandings. Explain in terminology the patient can understand and ask for the patient's perception of what was said.	Having patient repeat information and providing time for questions allow further patient education and correction of misunderstandings.
Patient and family report an understanding of the instructions given.	Include the family in the discharge instruction session. Allow time for questions.	Including the family gives additional support to the patient, especially if the patient cannot provide the self-care necessary on discharge.

Evaluation:	Compare the patient's status with the expected patient outcomes. If the outcomes are not met, reassess the patient and revise the plan.

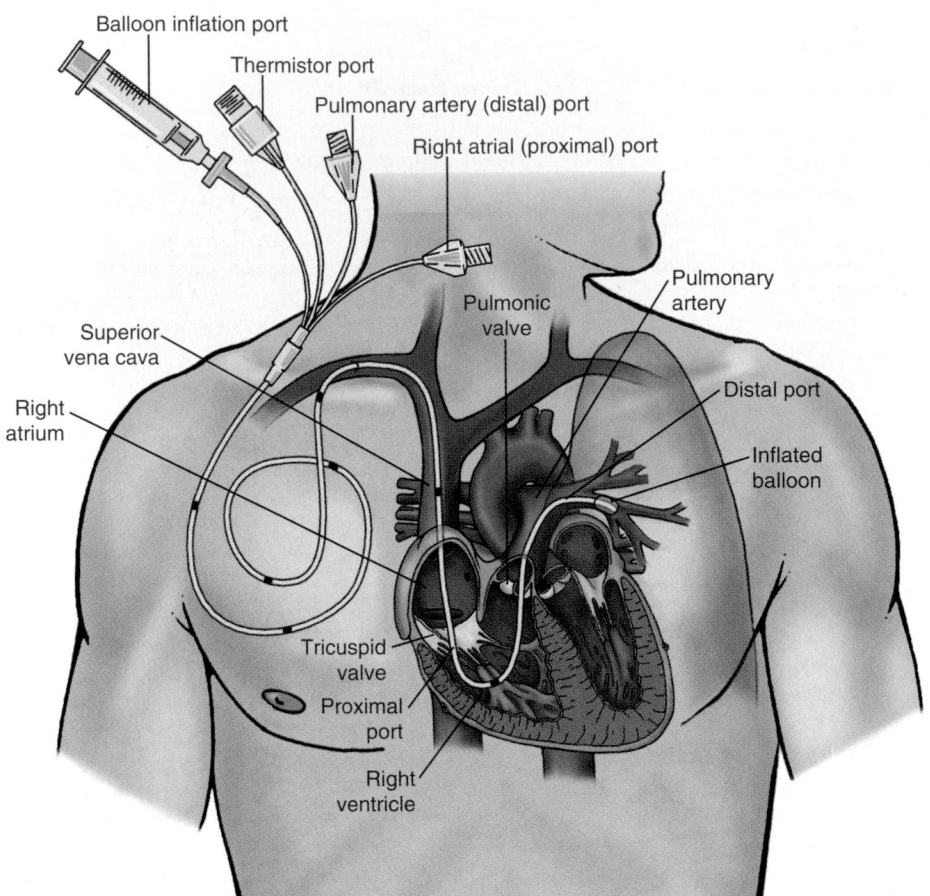

Balloon inflation port
Thermistor port
Pulmonary artery (distal) port
Right atrial (proximal) port

Superior vena cava
Right atrium

Pulmonic valve

Pulmonary artery

Distal port

Inflated balloon

Tricuspid valve
Proximal port
Right ventricle

Figure 7–20

The pulmonary artery catheter enters the heart via the superior vena cava and travels through the right atrium, tricuspid valve, right ventricle, pulmonic valve, and pulmonary artery and into a distal branch of the pulmonary artery, where the inflated balloon wedges in the vessel.

inflated with the amount of air needed to change the pulmonary artery pressure curve into a pulmonary wedge pressure curve. Usually 0.6 to 0.8 mL of air is sufficient to inflate the balloon to a wedge position. Air is never forced into the balloon, because it may break and injure the pulmonary artery tissue. When the pulmonary wedge pressure has been obtained, the balloon is deflated. The balloon is not left inflated because, during inflation, no blood is able to pass by the balloon to the pulmonary artery branch that contains the catheter. Patients who require pulmonary artery pressure monitoring are critically ill and should be cared for in a critical-care setting.

Although the pulmonary artery catheter is placed in the right side of the heart, it gives information about the function of the left side of the heart as well. This is because, when the balloon is inflated, blood cannot flow from the right side of the heart toward the lungs in that branch of the pulmonary artery. Consequently, the opening in the tip of the catheter distal to the balloon can measure back pressure from the pulmonary veins. This pressure reflects the left side of the heart. During ventricular diastole, when the mitral valve is open, the pressure in the left ventricle is reflected in the left atrium, which in turn is reflected in the pulmonary veins

and against the tip of the pulmonary artery catheter with the balloon inflated. Pulmonary capillary wedge pressure is a good indication of left ventricular end-diastolic pressure. Furthermore, pulmonary capillary wedge pressure correlates very closely with pulmonary artery diastolic pressure (Fig. 7–21).

Intra-Arterial Blood Pressure

Intra-arterial blood pressure measurement, most often used in critical-care units and cardiac telemetry units, provides continuous, direct blood pressure readings. It is used to accurately titrate vasoactive drugs such as TNG and dopamine whether given orally or intravenously.

Measurements of intra-arterial blood pressure are obtained by means of a catheter introduced percutaneously into an artery. This catheter is attached to a transducing system that converts pressure generated by the pulse wave into electrical impulses and produces a display of intra-arterial systolic, diastolic, and mean arterial pressure readings.

The catheter is commonly inserted in the radial artery but others—such as the femoral, brachial or axillary—may also be used. Before insertion, collateral circulation feeding the area distal to the insertion site must be checked to ascertain that it is

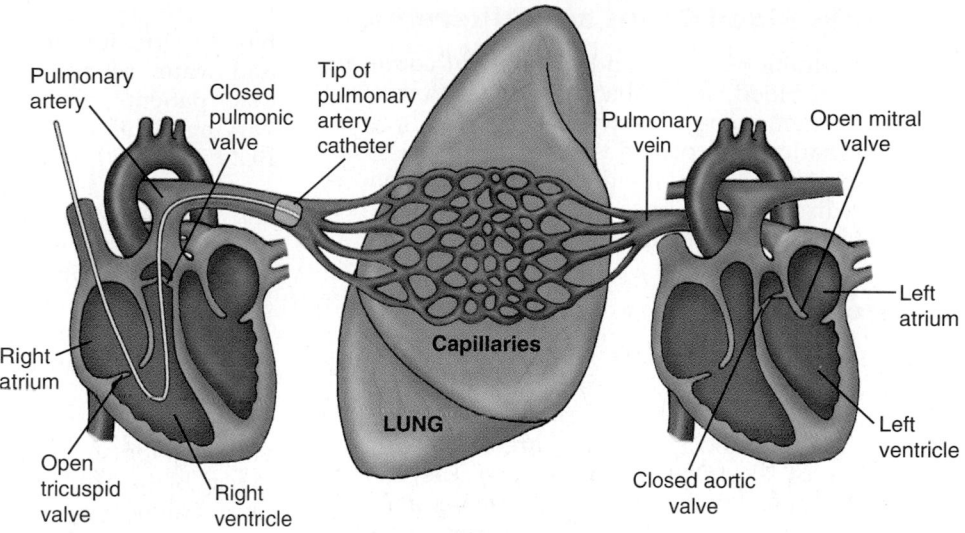

Figure 7–21

With the balloon inflated, blood can no longer flow from the right side of the heart to the pulmonary vasculature. Consequently, the port distal to the catheter balloon can measure back pressure from the pulmonary veins, yielding a reliable measurement of left ventricular end-diastolic pressure during diastole.

adequate to provide the area with oxygenated blood if the intra-arterial catheter became obstructed. Obstruction of the catheter in the absence of adequate collateral circulation would result in ischemia and infarction of distal tissues. Collateral circulation can be checked by means of an ultrasonic Doppler test or, for the radial and ulnar arteries, with an Allen test.

Once the catheter is in place, patency is maintained via a heparinized normal saline arterial flush system. Extreme care must be taken to ensure that the catheter does not become disconnected from the system because arterial bleeding would result and exsanguination could occur. As a precaution, the extremity containing the insertion site is kept uncovered so that any bleeding can be easily seen. Color, temperature, and pulses distal to the insertion site are assessed every 2 hours to check for any developing circulatory problems. To prevent infection, antibiotic ointment and a dry sterile dressing are applied to the insertion site per agency protocol.

Cardiac Output

Cardiac output refers to the volume of blood ejected from the ventricles each minute. It can be determined at the bedside and in the cardiac catheterization laboratory by several different methods. It is measured in liters of blood per minute and varies with the metabolic needs of the body and with body size. In an average-size adult at rest, cardiac output is about 6 L/minute. In disease states, cardiac output is usually less than normal and may be so low that the body's tissues receive inadequate blood supply, especially in times of stress.

Cardiac output measurements can be obtained at the bedside with a four-lumen pulmonary artery catheter (thermodilution catheter). The catheter contains lumens for measuring central venous pressure,

pulmonary artery pressure, and pulmonary wedge pressure, plus a lumen containing a thermistor for measurement of blood temperature in the heart. A bolus of 10 mL of cold or room-temperature (cooler than body temperature) intravenous fluid is injected into the external port of the central venous pressure portion of the catheter. As the fluid exits into the right atrium, it cools the blood in the right atrium. This volume of cooled blood moves into the right ventricle and then into the pulmonary artery. In the pulmonary artery, the thermistor senses the temperature change as the cooled blood passes over it. The pulmonary artery temperature monitoring port (containing the thermistor) records a decrease in temperature followed by a gradual return to the patient's body temperature as the cold solution is "washed out." The resulting temperature-time curve is analyzed by a computer and cardiac output is thereby calculated.

Once cardiac output is known, systemic vascular resistance can be calculated, giving an indication of afterload. As afterload increases, the work of the heart increases, myocardial oxygen consumption increases, and stroke volume falls. Based on this data, medications can be administered to reduce or elevate afterload as necessary.

BLOOD STUDIES

The usual blood studies for cardiac disorders include complete blood count, electrolytes, cholesterol, lipids, and enzymes. If specific enzymes are elevated in the blood, further delineation is accomplished by determining isoenzymes. Additional blood studies may be ordered for patients with complicating problems, such as diabetes. If a patient has a family history of other diseases, further blood studies may also be ordered.

Complete Blood Count and Differential

The complete blood count and differential count are a series of blood tests that provide information about the hematologic system and other organs. This information also provides clues to cardiac problems, especially those related to oxygenation. A complete discussion of these tests and possible abnormalities is found in Chapter 15.

Electrolytes

Serum electrolytes important to the management of the cardiac patient include sodium (Na^+), potassium (K^+), chloride (Cl^-), calcium (Ca^{2+}), and magnesium (Mg^{2+}). Sodium and potassium are necessary for conduction of electrical impulses over the cardiac muscle. An elevated serum potassium level acts as a myocardial depressant. A decreased serum potassium level acts to increase the excitability of the myocardium and places the patient receiving digitalis therapy at increased risk for digitalis toxicity. Both increased and decreased potassium levels predispose the patient to lethal dysrhythmias, such as ventricular tachycardia and asystole. Normal levels for sodium range from 136 to 145 mEq/L while normal potassium levels are 3.5 to 5.0 mEq/L.

Chloride maintains electrical neutrality as a salt with sodium and serves as a buffer in acid-base balance. The normal level for chloride is 98 to 106 mEq/L.

Hypercalcemia enhances the inotropic or contractile effect of the myocardium. In contrast, hypocalcemia acts as a depressant of myocardial contractility. Low magnesium levels increase the effect of hypercalcemia, while high magnesium levels reverse the effect of hypocalcemia. The normal serum levels for calcium and magnesium are 4.5 to 5.5 mEq/L and 1.5 to 2.5 mEq/L, respectively.

Although not an electrolyte, carbon dioxide in the blood also affects the normal conduction system of the heart through its effect on acid-base balance. The normal level for carbon dioxide is 22 to 30 mEq/L. Acid-base imbalances may produce cardiac dysrhythmias that can be noted on the ECG.

Glucose

Epinephrine, which is secreted in response to stress, elevates the blood glucose level. Thus, patients experiencing a myocardial infarction may have hyperglycemia on admission even in the absence of diabetes mellitus.

Blood Urea Nitrogen and Serum Creatinine

Kidney function is assessed by evaluating BUN and serum creatinine. Urea is formed in the liver as an endproduct of protein catabolism and is excreted entirely by the kidney. Therefore, BUN is related to the excretory function of the kidney. Diminished blood perfusion to the kidneys can elevate BUN, and water retention can decrease BUN. Thus, cardiac patients with changing hemodynamics have varying BUN levels from day to day. The normal BUN is 8 to 20 mg/dL.

Creatinine is excreted entirely by the kidneys and is directly proportional to renal excretory function. Creatinine is a catabolic product of creatine, which is used in skeletal muscle contraction. The daily production of creatine, and subsequently creatinine, depends on muscle mass, which fluctuates very little. The normal serum creatinine level is 0.6 to 1.3 mg/dL.

BUN is affected by dehydration, malnutrition, and hepatic function, whereas creatinine is not. When BUN rises out of proportion to the creatinine level, dehydration, gastrointestinal bleeding, and malnutrition are suspected. When both BUN and creatinine levels rise, the patient is assessed for kidney disease or failure. Low protein intake, overhydration, or severe liver failure will reduce the BUN level but not the creatinine level.

Erythrocyte Sedimentation Rate

The erythrocyte sedimentation rate is a nonspecific test used to detect inflammatory response, infection, or necrotic processes. The erythrocyte sedimentation rate is not diagnostic for any specific disorder or disease, but it is useful in the detection of inflammatory disease not otherwise suspected or to confirm a suspected disease, such as endocarditis, rheumatic fever, or pericarditis.

Prothrombin Time and Partial Thromboplastin Time

The prothrombin time is used to evaluate the adequacy of the extrinsic clotting system. The partial thromboplastin time is used to assess the intrinsic clotting system. Both of these tests are discussed in detail in Chapter 12. These tests are useful for monitoring the patient on anticoagulant therapy. Heparin, an anticoagulant, is commonly given during cardiac and vascular surgery and is also used for thromboembolic episodes, such as pulmonary embolism, arterial embolism, and thrombophlebitis. The partial thromboplastin time should be 1.5 to 2.5 times normal in these patients. Warfarin (Coumadin) is often used for long-term oral anticoagulation in cardiac patients such as those with chronic atrial fibrillation, or those with prosthetic heart valve or intracoronary stent. Because of variations in reagents used in the laboratory, prothrombin times on which this therapy is based are usually reported as two numbers: a patient value and a control value. Depending on the patient's condition, therapeutic anticoagulation is usually considered 1.5 to 2.5 times the control. Alternatively, prothrombin time may be reported as an international normalized ratio (INR) value. This eliminates individual laboratory variations in reporting prothrombin times through comparison to a standard reagent and calculation from a standard nomogram. Therapeutic INR value ranges from 2.0 to 3.0. However, certain cardiac patients, such as those with intracoronary stents and recurrent systemic emboli, may be maintained with an INR value of 3.0 to 4.5.

Serum Lipids

A serum lipid study usually includes total blood lipids, cholesterol, triglycerides, phospholipids, and cholesterol lipoproteins. Lipids—such as cholesterol, triglycerides, and phospholipids—are transported in the blood by combining with proteins. This is why they are called *lipoproteins*.

Lipoproteins can be separated by electrophoresis and fractionated into HDL, LDL, and VLDL. HDL is inversely associated with coronary artery disease; that is, patients with increased HDL levels are less likely to develop coronary artery disease and may have a protective effect against this disease. LDL is about 50% cholesterol and has the highest positive association with coronary artery disease. VLDL is composed of triglycerides synthesized by the liver and is probably associated with coronary artery disease. The patient must fast for 12 hours before these blood studies and should eat a low-fat meal and avoid alcoholic beverages (which are high in triglycerides) the night before testing.

Cardiac Enzymes

Enzymes are protein catalysts of biochemical reactions in cells. When cell membranes are damaged or broken, as occurs when cardiac cells are damaged by a myocardial infarction, enzymes inside the cells are released through the damaged membranes into the circulating blood. Three enzymes are released when cardiac tissue is damaged: lactate dehydrogenase (LDH), serum aspartate aminotransferase (AST) (formerly measured as serum glutamic oxaloacetic transaminase), and creatine kinase (CK), or creatine phosphokinase.

CK is the first enzyme that becomes elevated after any cardiac damage. Its level rises within 3 to 6 hours of the onset of ischemia, peaks in 10 to 30 hours, and returns to the normal range within 3 to 4 days (Fig. 7–22). In addition to being found in cardiac muscle, CK is also found in skeletal muscle and brain tissue and is released in response to damage to these organs. Patients who are suspected of having an acute cardiac disease should not be given any intramuscular injections because injury to skeletal muscle may elevate the CK level and mask an increase that is actually due to cardiac damage.

AST is also found outside of cardiac tissue, so not all institutions test AST levels to rule out a myocardial infarction. When it is performed, the AST level rises within 6 hours after cardiac damage, peaks in 12 to 14 hours, and returns to the normal range in 4 days. It is found in cardiac muscle, skeletal muscle, and liver, pancreas, and kidney tissue.

The LDH level rises within 24 to 48 hours after cardiac damage, peaks in 72 to 144 hours, and returns to the normal range within 14 days. Besides being found in cardiac muscle, LDH is found in red blood cells, skeletal muscle, and brain, liver, kidney, lung, and skin tissue.

Levels of cardiac enzymes can signal an impending threat to a patient's life. The longer an enzyme remains at peak level, the more tissue damage is likely to have occurred and the poorer the prognosis. Patients who demonstrate high peak levels immediately after an acute myocardial infarction tend to develop more hemodynamic problems and are more prone to complications. When a patient's enzyme levels peak, begin to return to normal, and then begin to rise again, an extension of tissue damage may have occurred.

Cardiac Isoenzymes

CK can be fractionated into three subunits, or isoenzymes: MM, BB, and MB. These isoenzymes, each of which has a slightly different molecular structure, help to show whether the CK came from the heart muscle (MB), from skeletal muscle (MM), or from the brain (BB). The isoenzyme MB provides a unique marker for damaged myocardial cells. The

Figure 7–22

Levels of cardiac enzymes and isoenzymes following acute myocardial infarction. AST, aspartate aminotransferase; CK, creatine kinase; LDH, lactate dehydrogenase.

Enzyme/Isoenzyme	Onset of Elevation	Peak Elevation	Return to Normal Range
CK	3 to 6 hours	10 to 30 hours	3 to 4 days
AST	6 hours	12 to 14 hours	4 days
LDH	24 to 48 hours	72 to 144 hours (3 to 6 days)	14 days
CK-MB	4 to 8 hours	12 to 24 hours	3 days
CK-MB$_2$: CK-MB$_1$ ratio	2 to 8 hours	———	12 to 24 hours

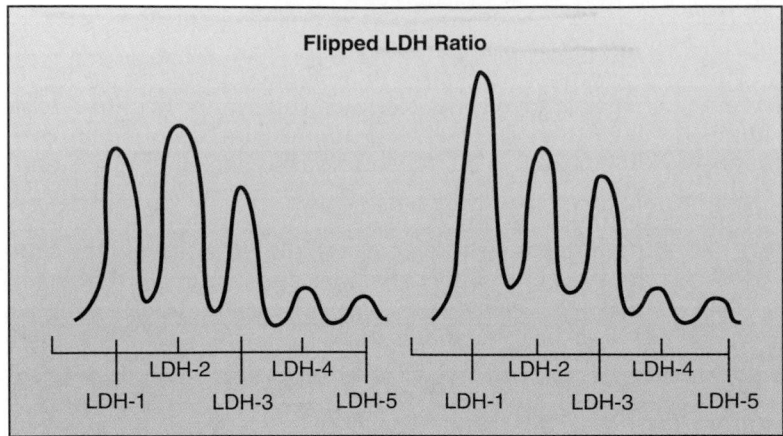

Figure 7–23
In a flipped lactate dehydrogenase (LDH) ratio, the amount of LDH-1 is greater than the amount of LDH-2, suggesting a myocardial infarction. (From Owen A. Tracking the rise and fall of cardiac enzymes. Nursing 1995;25(5):37.)

CK-MB level does not rise with chest pain unless a myocardial infarction occurs. For this reason, it is a more valuable test for evidence of myocardial infarction than measurement of the total CK. After a myocardial infarction, the CK-MB level rises within 4 to 8 hours, peaks in 12 to 24 hours, and returns to the normal range within 3 days. The CK-BB isoenzyme is found primarily in the brain and lungs and will be elevated when these organs are damaged. The CK-MM isoenzyme is found primarily in skeletal muscle and increases with muscle damage.

CK-MB can be further broken down into to isoforms or subforms of the enzyme. Normally, CK-MB_1 and CK-MB_2 are present in the blood in equal amounts. Following a myocardial infarction, however, the ratio of MB_2 to MB_1 is $1:5$ or greater. This rise may be seen within 2 hours of an infarct and is positive in almost all myocardial infarction patients within 8 hours. The ratio change may last only 12 hours, so patients who seek care more than 12 to 24 hours after an infarct may not show this enzyme change.

There are five LDH isoenzymes, LDH-1 to LDH-5, which may be separated by electrophoresis. LDH-1 is primarily found in the heart and red blood cells. Normally LDH-2 is greater than LDH-1, but, in cardiac cellular damage, LDH-1 becomes greater than LDH-2. This is called a "flipped LDH." An LDH flip is diagnostic of an acute myocardial infarction (Fig. 7–23).

*M*anagement

NONSURGICAL MANAGEMENT

Once the risk factors for cardiac dysfunction have been identified, the goal of nonsurgical management is reduction of risk for myocardial disease. Some

risk factors, such as heredity, cannot be altered, but many others can be modified or eliminated, thus changing the risk for future cardiac problems.

Reduction of Risk Factors

Hyperlipidemia is reduced by adhering to a diet low in animal fats and other saturated fats, but high in fiber. Caloric intake is regulated to achieve the target body weight and a normal glucose level. Because obesity is also a risk factor for cardiac disease, weight reduction is a goal to be achieved. For these people, this may mean a reduction in caloric intake to lose weight.

Associated disease processes need to be controlled. Hypertension and diabetes mellitus are treated with a combination of diet changes, exercise, and drug therapy. The goal is to keep blood pressure and the glucose level stable and within normal limits.

Cessation is the only way to combat the risk that smoking plays in cardiac disease. Management in smoking cessation may include referral to education and support classes for smokers or nicotine-replacement drug therapy.

Physical exercise is recommended as a component of every person's daily life. The specific exercise prescription is modified for each patient based on history, ability, and other interfering disorders or limitations.

People with Type A personality patterns are confronted with behaviors that may aggravate stress levels, such as time urgency, competitiveness, compulsive work schedules, and interrupted sleep patterns. A frank explanation of the risk of cardiac disease from these continued behaviors is usually necessary. Referral to stress-management seminars or relaxation sessions may be indicated. Professional assistance from a psychiatrist, psychologist, or counselor may also be beneficial.

Women taking oral contraceptives are periodically tested for serum lipid, triglyceride, and cholesterol levels. Baseline levels are determined before initiating contraceptive therapy. Any significant elevation in the values after initiating use is evaluated. Other birth-control measures may be recommended if the values indicate an increased risk of cardiac disease. Blood pressure measurements are taken along with the serum testing because an elevation in blood pressure may accompany oral contraceptive use. Cigarette smoking is highly discouraged because smoking and oral contraceptive use together increase the risk of coronary artery disease at least fivefold.

Pharmacologic Therapy

A multitude of pharmacologic agents are available for treating cardiovascular disease. Most of these drugs can be categorized into six groups that are used to treat cardiac failure, angina pectoris, blood pressure variations, and dysrhythmias. The six groups are cardiac glycosides, vasodilators, catecholamines, beta blockers, anti-arrhythmics, and diuretics. The drugs in each category have many similar characteristics, but individual drugs in each group also have some unique properties, side effects, routes of administration, and nursing implications.

CARDIAC GLYCOSIDES

Cardiac glycosides are used to treat patients with heart failure. They strengthen cardiac muscle contractions, which increases stroke volume and cardiac output. As cardiac output increases, more blood flows to the kidneys and urine output increases. Blood volume decreases as urine output increases, thus reducing preload and easing the work of the heart (Highlight 7–6).

Cardiac glycosides also slow the transmission of electrical impulses across the atrioventricular node and through the bundle of His. An increase in diastolic filling time may improve cardiac output in patients with rapid heart rates. Also, patients who have supraventricular dysrhythmias (coming from above ventricular tissue) may benefit from drug therapy that slows the heart rate, thus increasing cardiac filling time and cardiac output.

The most commonly used cardiac glycoside is digoxin (Lanoxin). The side effects of the drugs in this category are similar for the different preparations. They include anorexia, nausea, vomiting, weakness, heart block, and visual disturbances, such as seeing halos around lights and greenish-yellow hues. Since dysrhythmias may occur, the apical pulse should be counted for one minute and should

---

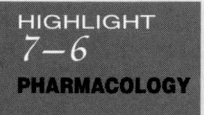 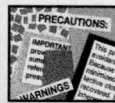

HIGHLIGHT 7–6 PHARMACOLOGY

Cardiac Glycosides

Definition:

Group of drugs derived from natural sources containing a glycoside, a steroid, and a lactone.

Action:

Strengthen contraction of cardiac muscle, thereby increasing stroke volume and cardiac output. Reduce preload and slow transmission of electrical impulses across atrioventricular node and bundle of His.

Uses:

Treatment of heart failure.

Side Effects:

Anorexia, nausea, vomiting, headache, visual disturbances, weakness, restlessness, confusion, and cardiac dysrhythmias

Interactions:

May interact with such drugs as antacids and antidiarrheal agents.

Nursing Implications:

Check heart rate before administering; if less than 60 bpm or more than 110 bpm, check with physician.

Some glycosides are best absorbed in liquid form.

Give tablets with food to decrease gastric irritation.

Protect intravenous solution from light.

Observe for side effects and toxicity.

Monitor cardiac status, checking for bigeminy or other dysrhythmias.

Check laboratory data for potassium level (should be at least 4.0).

Monitor digoxin levels.

Encourage patient to eat potassium-rich foods.

Instruct patient about medication, side effects, and importance of checking pulse.

be between 60 and 110 before digoxin is administered. Loading doses may sometimes be given to digitalize the patient. Serum digoxin levels (normally 0.5–2.0 ng/mL) should be monitored when the patient begins digoxin therapy, when dosages are changed, or if any signs of toxicity or ineffectiveness occur. Serum digoxin levels should be drawn 4 to 6 hours after intravenous administration and 6 to 8 hours after an oral dose.

Hypokalemia, hypomagnesemia, and hypercalcemia make a patient hypersensitive to digoxin; thus, toxicity may result with low serum levels of digoxin. Patients taking nifedipine, verapamil, or quinidine may have high serum digoxin levels, thus indicating that their doses of digoxin need to be lowered while they are concurrently taking these drugs.

Symptoms of toxicity are the more severe side effects of digoxin. Toxicity is usually treated by discontinuing the drug or giving a lower dose. The physician is notified of toxicity symptoms so orders to treat the problem may be obtained. If dysrhythmias are severe, they are treated with the appropriate antiarrhythmic drug therapy or a pacemaker if indicated.

VASODILATORS

Vasodilators act on the smooth muscle walls of blood vessels to widen the vascular lumen, thus decreasing resistance to blood flow and increasing flow through the vessels. Some vasodilators act primarily on the walls of veins, some on the walls of arteries, and some on both. Those that act primarily on veins are used to prevent angina and to treat acute anginal attacks. Common drugs that act on veins are nitroglycerin, isosorbide dinitrate (Isordil), and other nitrates (Highlight 7–7).

Vasodilators dilate veins and venules so that more blood collects in these vessels rather than returning to the heart, decreasing venous return to the heart. Blood is said to "pool" in these peripheral vessels. Pooling of blood away from the heart reduces preload, allowing the heart to expend less oxygen to empty its chambers. Chest pain resulting from decreased oxygen flow to the heart muscle is

---

HIGHLIGHT 7–7
PHARMACOLOGY

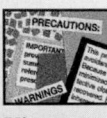

Nitrates

Definition:

Group of drugs used for symptomatic relief or prevention of chest pain.

Action:

Reduce oxygen consumption by coronary vessels, relieving ischemia; relax coronary smooth muscle, producing vasodilation; and increase coronary blood flow.

Uses:

Treatment of angina pectoris; provide relief of cardiac ischemia, thus relieving angina.

Side Effects:

Headache, flushing of face, nausea, vomiting, dizziness, hypotension, and confusion.

Interactions:

May enhance effects of alcohol, and alcohol in turn may increase the effects of the antianginal agents.

Nursing Implications:

Give at first symptom of an anginal attack and prior to activities that cause pain or place at the bedside after teaching the patient when to self-administer.

Watch for signs of hypotension, check blood pressure.

Instruct patients taking nitrates to:

Store tablets in a tightly closed container protected from light.

Discard any tablets older than 6 months.

Avoid drinking alcohol while taking the medication.

Take oral tablets on an empty stomach and swallow whole; place sublingual tablets under the tongue.

Apply topical medication to non-hairy areas of the body, rotate sites, and remove all of old dose before applying new medication.

Lie down or sit in a chair when taking the medication. Stay in that position for 5 to 10 minutes because of potential weakness or dizziness.

Repeat dose of sublingual medication (if pain is not relieved immediately) every 5 minutes for up to three doses.

Notify the physician if pain persists.

Record episodes of pain and number of doses of medication taken and report to the physician.

Watch for side effects, such as headache, weakness, confusion, dizziness, nausea, and vomiting.

less likely to occur when preload is reduced. Nitrates may also dilate coronary arteries, thus improving collateral circulation to the heart tissues. Myocardial ischemia is further reduced when this occurs. Nitrates also alleviate the symptoms of heart failure because of a reduction of preload.

Nitrates can be administered by various routes. These drugs may be administered intravenously in acute situations and are titrated according to the patient's clinical manifestations. They are easy to administer in sublingual form. A nitroglycerin tablet may be placed under the patient's tongue just before he or she engages in activities known to provoke angina (exercising, going out into cold weather, eating a heavy meal, sexual intercourse, or dealing with an emotionally stressful situation).

When angina occurs, the patient is taught to place a nitroglycerin tablet under the tongue every 3 to 5 minutes until three tablets have been used. If relief is not obtained with three sublingual nitroglycerin tablets, the patient needs to seek immediate medical assistance because a heart attack may be occurring and further use of nitroglycerin tablets will delay needed care.

Oral and transdermal nitrates give longer-lasting protection against angina, although they take effect more slowly than sublingual nitrates. Some transdermal patches last up to 24 hours; thus, the patient has to apply a new patch only once each day. Skin irritation may occur with transdermal patches. It is important to rotate application sites and to cleanse the skin carefully after removing a patch. Since nitrates are vasodilators, they may cause hypotension and headache.

Arterial dilators relax the walls of arteries and make it easier for the heart to expel blood from the left ventricle into the arterial circulation (afterload). Cardiac output increases when the heart does not have to pump against a highly resistant system. The most common arterial dilators are diazoxide (Hyperstat), hydralazine (Apresoline), and minoxidil (Loniten). Arterial dilators also lower blood pressure in patients with arterial hypertension.

Mixed vasodilators widen the lumens of arteries and veins. With arterial relaxation, afterload is reduced, making it easier for the left ventricle to eject blood. With venous relaxation, preload is reduced. Drugs that contain both arterial and venous dilating properties include nitroprusside (Nipride) and prazosin (Minipress). Both of these drugs directly relax vascular smooth muscle, and prazosin also blocks sympathetic alpha$_1$-receptors, interfering with nerve impulses that cause vascular smooth muscles to contract (Highlight 7–8).

Captopril (Capoten), enalapril (Vasotec), lisinopril (Prinivil), and other angiotensin converting enzyme inhibitors block the conversion of angiotensin I to angiotensin II, the most powerful vasoconstrictor produced by the body. This lowers peripheral resistance and results in a decreased afterload. Because these drugs decrease pressure in the pulmo-

---

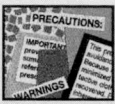

HIGHLIGHT
7–8
PHARMACOLOGY

Alpha-Adrenergic Blocking Agents

Definition:

Group of drugs, such as prazosin, used to dilate arteries and veins.

Action:

Relaxes arterial smooth muscle, decreasing preload and afterload.

Uses:

Treatment of hypertension and heart failure.

Side Effects:

Drowsiness, weakness, postural hypotension, palpitations.

Interactions:

Many different agents; sequelae include profound hypotension, vascular collapse, cardiac dysrhythmias, hypertensive crisis, and cerebrovascular accident.

Nursing Implications:

Monitor blood pressure.

Instruct patient to avoid postural hypotension by rising from bed slowly, sitting for a few minutes before rising.

Check for dizziness or headache.

---

nary capillaries and increase cardiac output, they are a mainstay of therapy for heart failure. Post–myocardial infarction patients who take angiotensin-converting enzyme inhibitors live longer and are less likely to develop heart failure. By inhibiting angiotensin II production, these drugs also indirectly reduces production of aldosterone. As a result, the body excretes more sodium and water, thus reducing blood volume and causing a decrease in blood pressure (Highlight 7–9).

Calcium channel blocking agents slow the movement of calcium into the coronary and systemic arteries and dilate these vessels, thus increasing circulation to the myocardium, decreasing heart rate and afterload. They may also retard the deposition of calcium in plaque that has accumulated on vessel walls and decrease the likelihood of a second myocardial infarction (Highlight 7–10). Common cal-

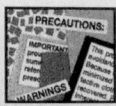

HIGHLIGHT
7–9
PHARMACOLOGY

Angiotensin-Converting Enzyme Inhibitors

Definition:

Class of drugs that dilate blood vessels and decrease fluid volume

Action:

Inhibit conversion of angiotensin I to the patent vasoconstrictor angiotensin II resulting in vasodilation. They also inhibit the release of aldosterone, promoting sodium and water excretion.

Uses:

Treatment of hypertension and heart failure; protect against cardiac events following myocardial infarction.

Side Effects:

Hypotension, especially with first dose, persistent dry cough, renal failure, neutropenia.

Nursing Implications:

Monitor complete blood count results.

Instruct the patient to:

Take before meals.
Change positions slowly.
Avoid use of over-the-counter cough and cold medicines.
Report fever, sore throat, or other signs of infection.

cium blocking agents include nifedipine (Procardia), nicardipine (Cardene), diltiazem (Cardizem), and verapamil (Calan).

CATECHOLAMINES

Catecholamines are most often used in cardiac emergencies because of their positive inotropic and vasopressor action. They increase cardiac output, blood pressure, and systemic vascular resistance.

Dopamine is a naturally occurring catecholamine, a precursor of norepinephrine. At low doses it dilates renal arteries and increases urine output. At moderate doses dopamine stimulates beta$_1$ receptors in the heart to increase myocardial contractility, thereby increasing stroke volume and raising blood

pressure. At high doses, it stimulates sympathetic alpha$_1$-receptors in the smooth-muscle walls of arterioles to cause vasoconstriction. This increases arterial blood pressure. This combination of effects helps prevent a patient from going into shock. Before initiating dopamine therapy, any pre-existing hypovolemia should be corrected so there is enough vascular volume to contribute to an increase in cardiac output. Unfortunately, the vasoconstrictive effects of high-dose therapy may actually promote decreased tissue perfusion and the elevation in heart rate may promote myocardial ischemia.

Dobutamine is a synthetic catecholamine that is primarily a myocardial beta$_1$ receptor stimulator. Dobutamine increases the force of contraction by as much as 30 to 70%. Its peripheral vascular effects are minimal even in high doses. It increases stroke volume and cardiac output without as much increase in cardiac rate as produced by dopamine. Thus, it uses less cardiac energy and tends to produce fewer dysrhythmias.

Dobutamine may be used with the balanced vasodilator nitroprusside to sharply decrease preload and circulating blood volume in patients with severe refractory heart failure (intractable heart failure). It can also be used with dopamine because dopamine improves renal blood flow while dobutamine increases cardiac output.

Patients receiving catecholamine therapy should be in a critical care area with continuous ECG monitoring and invasive hemodynamic monitoring. Small dosage changes in catecholamines may mean life-threatening changes in blood pressure and cardiac rate. Such patients need close nursing observation and intervention as indicated by changes in their status.

BETA BLOCKERS

Beta-adrenergic blocking agents find widespread use in the cardiac patient. These drugs compete with epinephrine at the beta-adrenergic receptor sites to decrease heart rate, blood pressure, and cardiac output. They also act on β_2 sites in the kidney to inhibit the renin-angiotensin-aldosterone system. Some of the agents are considered nonselective drugs in that they work on both cardiac (β_1-receptors) and noncardiac (β_2-receptors). Examples of these agents are nadolol (Corgard) and propranolol (Inderal). Because of their nonselective activity, they are more likely to cause side effects such as bronchospasm than are the selective agents. The selective agents, such as atenolol (Tenormin) and metoprolol (Lopressor) have a more limited action on the cardiac (β_1) receptors.

Because these agents block receptor sites in the conduction system in the heart, they slow atrioventricular conductivity and are useful anti-arrhythmic agents. By slowing the heart rate and decreasing the force of myocardial contractility, these drugs de-

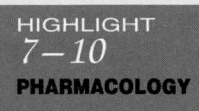 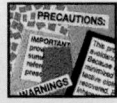

HIGHLIGHT
7–10
PHARMACOLOGY

Calcium Channel Blocking Agents

Definition:

Group of drugs, such as nifedipine, verapamil, and nicardipine, that cause arterial dilatation.

Action:

Inhibit movement of extracellular calcium into cardiac muscle, thus slowing conduction and reducing cardiac workload; they dilate coronary arteries and prevent coronary spasms.

Uses:

Management of anginal episodes; control of ventricular rate in atrial fibrillation and flutter and supraventricular dysrhythmias; and control of hypertension.

Side Effects:

Headache, dizziness, weakness, confusion, edema, and constipation.

Interactions:

May be less effective if taken with calcium tablets; may be enhanced by cimetidine (Tagamet); may be enhanced by the addition of beta blockers; may cause increased serum digoxin levels; and may cause decreased blood pressure if taken with beta blockers.

Nursing Implications:

Monitor blood pressure for hypotension.

Monitor the electrocardiogram for bradycardia and dysrhythmias.

Observe for side effects.

Assess for symptoms of heart failure such as edema, cough, changes in vital signs, and decreased circulation.

Check laboratory data, especially liver function studies, because some enzymes may be increased.

---

crease the oxygen requirements of the myocardium. This decreased need of the cardiac muscle for oxygen is useful in preventing anginal attacks. Patients receiving these drugs often report increased exercise tolerance and fewer episodes of angina. However, the decreased force of myocardial contraction leads to a decreased cardiac output, so these drugs should be used cautiously in a patient with heart failure. Beta blockers may also limit infarct size following a myocardial infarction.

ANTI-ARRHYTHMICS

Anti-arrhythmic drugs suppress cardiac automaticity, thus altering the rate of conduction, the refractory period, or the shift in impulse. There are many different classes of drugs in the anti-arrhythmic category. The drug prescribed is chosen on the basis of the patient's history, concomitant problems, specific drug effect, and tolerability (Highlight 7–11).

Lidocaine hydrochloride (Xylocaine) exerts antiarrhythmic action by suppressing automaticity in the His-Purkinje system and by elevating the electrical stimulation threshold of the ventricles during diastole. It decreases the irritability of the ventricles and controls ventricular tachycardia, ventricular fibrillation, and premature ventricular contractions. It is given by an intravenous bolus, followed by an intravenous drip titrated to control the undesired dysrhythmia. Procainamide hydrochloride (Pronestyl) is given intravenously to patients who do not respond to lidocaine, and it can be given orally for long-term management of ventricular dysrhythmias. Tocainide (Tonocard) may be considered an oral equivalent of lidocaine. All of these drugs have multiple side effects, especially CNS disturbances such as dizziness, drowsiness, and confusion. They can also actually worsen dysrhythmias and cause hypotension.

Verapamil (Calan) and diltiazem (Cardizem), which slow the inflow of calcium needed for conduction, are useful in supraventricular tachycardia because they increase the relative refractory period in the atrioventricular node. They also slow the ventricular response to atrial flutter and fibrillation by slowing conduction in the atrioventricular node. Thus, patients who have fast heart rates because of atrial flutter or fibrillation, with a resultant decrease in cardiac output, can improve with administration of intravenous or oral verapamil or diltiazem. Beta-adrenergic blocking agents, such as sotalol (Betapace) and metaprolol (Lopressor) slow atrioventricular conductivity and are often used to decrease abnormally rapid heart rates.

Adenosine (Adenocard), which slows conduction in the atrioventricular node, may be given by intravenous bolus to convert supraventricular tachycar-

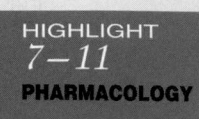 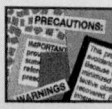

HIGHLIGHT
7–11
PHARMACOLOGY

Anti-Arrhythmic Agents

Definition:

Group of drugs that suppress cardiac automaticity. They may be subdivided into four categories on the basis of other electrophysiologic effects of the drugs.

Action:

Alter rate of conduction and refractory period or correct shift in impulse origin or automaticity of cardiac tissue.

Uses:

Treatment of rhythm disturbances.

Side Effects:

Anorexia, nausea, vomiting, dry mouth, blurred vision, cardiac dysrhythmias, urinary retention, drowsiness, tremors, paresthesia.

Interactions:

Some anti-arrhythmic agents may prolong bleeding times, potentiate actions of other drugs (such as anti-hypertensives and diuretics), react with other drugs to cause dysrhythmias, and enhance the action of curariform drugs and antibiotics.

Nursing Implications:

Give with meals to prevent gastrointestinal distress unless specifically directed to give on an empty stomach.

Check laboratory studies for liver function and bleeding times.

Observe for side effects as listed above.

Monitor electrocardiographic reading and blood pressure.

Check output; watch for signs of renal insufficiency or urinary retention.

Observe for signs of bleeding.

Instruct patient about medications and side effects.

Teach patient to monitor heart rate and blood pressure and to report palpitations, dizziness, or tremors.

---

dia without the side effect of hypotension, which may occur with verapamil. Adenosine's half-life is 10 to 15 seconds; thus, possible side effects of chest pain, dyspnea, or transient dysrhythmias disappear very rapidly. All of the anti-arrhythmic drugs can have a proarrhythmic effect, that is, they can induce a new dysrhythmia when one is already present.

Atropine sulfate stimulates sinus node automaticity and atrioventricular node conduction. It is used to treat sinus bradycardia because of its ability to speed conduction and increase heart rate. Atropine is given as an intravenous bolus.

DIURETICS

Diuretics are used commonly in the treatment of cardiac disease because cardiac failure causes retention of fluid (Highlight 7–12). Excess fluid may collect in the pulmonary system and lead to pulmonary edema. Peripheral edema may also result from cardiac failure. An increase in preload makes it difficult for the heart to pump effectively. Furosemide (Lasix) is a potent, rapid-acting diuretic used to decrease total body fluid. It inhibits reabsorption of sodium and chloride in the ascending loop of Henle in the kidneys. The onset of diuresis after an intravenous dose of furosemide is about 10 minutes, with a total diuretic effect that lasts about 6 hours. Furosemide may also be given orally. Less potent diuretics, such as hydrochlorothiazide (Hydrodiurl), spironolactone (Aldactone), and others, may be used to treat chronic cardiac failure and are usually given orally (Highlight 7–13). Diuretics also have an antihypertensive effect from the reduction in circulating volume.

ANTILIPEMICS

Patients who have elevated serum cholesterol levels (greater than 200 mg/dL) have a greater risk for coronary artery disease or myocardial infarction. The long-range health status of patients prone to hyperlipidemia can be positively affected through the use of antilipemic agents in conjunction with diet therapy and other nonpharmacologic agents.

Drugs in this classification exert two actions. They increase lipoprotein removal and restrict lipoprotein production. Most commonly used are lova-

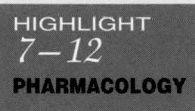
HIGHLIGHT
7–12
PHARMACOLOGY

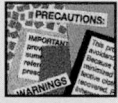

Diuretics (Antihypertensives)

Definition:

Group of drugs affecting sodium and water excretion. Some cause potassium depletion; others are potassium sparing.

Action:

Varies with type of diuretic; generally, they inhibit sodium and chloride absorption, thus promoting their excretion along with excess fluid.

Uses:

Treatment of high blood pressure and hypervolemia as well as pulmonary edema, peripheral edema, and heart failure.

Side Effects:

Hypokalemia, cardiac dysrhythmias, postural hypotension, weakness, dizziness, dehydration, nausea, vomiting, headache, and confusion.

Interactions:

May cause digitalis toxicity because of hypokalemic state; may potentiate effects of alcohol; may react with probenecid; and may enhance effects of other antihypertensive drugs.

Nursing Implications:

Give early in day to prevent nocturia.

Monitor intake and output.

Check laboratory data and electrolytes, especially potassium level.

Observe for signs of hypokalemia. (If patient is taking a potassium supplement, also observe for hyperkalemia.)

Monitor weight and blood pressure.

Check for symptoms of digitalis toxicity.

Provide potassium-rich foods (if patient is taking a non–potassium-sparing diuretic). Instruct patient about medication, side effects, and possible hypotensive episodes.

---

statin (Mevacor) and simvastatin (Zocor), which are enzymes that inhibit cholesterol synthesis. They are well tolerated except for rare mild headaches or gastrointestinal symptoms. Also used is gemfibrozil (Lopid), which decreases triglycerides and very low density lipids. All these drugs should be used cautiously in patients with liver disease (Highlight 7–14).

THROMBOLYTICS

The lysing or dissolving of clots within the coronary arteries may prevent myocardial damage from prolonged ischemia. If a clot can be lysed and blood flow restored through the coronary artery to the myocardium, ischemia will be reversed. There is about a 6 hour window in which thrombolytic therapy will be effective; after this period of time, irreversible tissue death will have occurred.

Thrombolytics convert plasmin into plasminogen, which breaks down clots. Streptokinase (Streptase) is a nonenzymatic enzyme excreted by group C beta-hemolytic streptococci. It generates the proteolytic enzyme plasmin, which lyses clots (Fig. 7–24). Alteplase recombinant (Activase) is a form of tissue

plasminogen activator, a naturally occurring protein that plays a major role in dissolving clots.

Thrombolytic therapy is contraindicated in patients with

- Active internal bleeding
- A history of cerebral vascular accident
- Recent surgery or trauma (usually within the last 2 months)
- Intracranial neoplasm
- Arteriovenous malformation or aneurysm
- Severe, uncontrolled hypertension
- Any bleeding disorder

Patients with any other condition in which bleeding would constitute significant risk or a management problem are also not candidates for thrombolytic therapy.

SURGICAL MANAGEMENT

The goal of cardiac surgery is to better the quality and length of life by restoring or improving the functional capacity of the heart. Cardiac surgery is used to treat many acquired and congenital heart

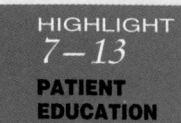 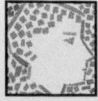

HIGHLIGHT 7–13
PATIENT EDUCATION
Special Instructions for Patients Taking Diuretics

Instruct the patient taking diuretic medications to:

Expect the amount of urine and the frequency of voiding to increase.

Avoid restricting normal fluid intake, unless specifically ordered, because of the increased output.

Take medication early in the morning to prevent nocturia. If ordered twice a day, take early in the morning and early in the evening.

Eat meals that include potassium-rich foods.

Observe for signs of hypokalemia such as fatigue, anorexia, vomiting, paresthesia, and palpitations.

Observe for signs of hyperkalemia (if also taking a potassium supplement) such as muscle weakness, nausea, respiratory distress, and diarrhea.

Observe for signs of hypovolemia such as dry skin, hypotension, weakness, dizziness, and excessive thirst.

Report any of the above untoward signs to the physician.

Be safety conscious and change positions slowly; hypotension may occur, causing weakness, dizziness, and syncope.

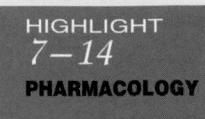 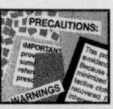

HIGHLIGHT 7–14
PHARMACOLOGY
Antilipemics

Definition:
One of several different types of drugs given to decrease cholesterol or triglyceride levels.

Action:
Varies with drug. Some decrease synthesis of cholesterol and triglycerides; other promote excretion of these.

Side Effects:
Constipation, nausea, bloating, abdominal pain, diarrhea, flatulence, bleeding, tenderness, and cataract development.

Nursing Implications:
Assess liver function tests.

Monitor prothrombin times.

Monitor serum cholesterol and triglyceride levels.

Administer with meals to decrease gastrointestinal distress.

Instruct patient to schedule eye examinations regularly.

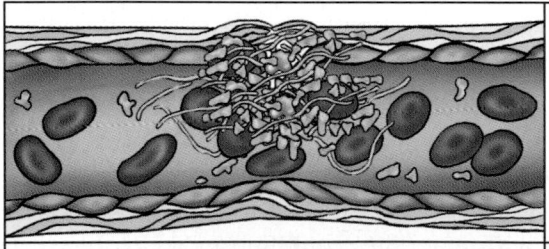
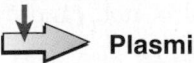
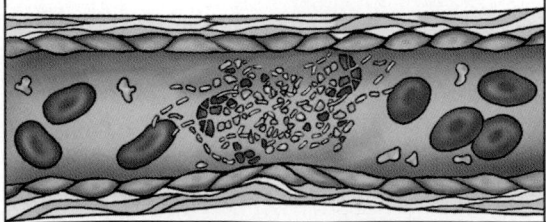

- Fibrin threads tangle with platelets and trap red blood cells, forming a clot

Thrombolytic therapy

Plasminogen ⟹ **Plasmin**

- Thrombolytic drug accelerates conversion of activated plasminogen to plasmin

- Plasmin breaks the clot into fibrin split products, helping to dissolve it

Figure 7–24

Thrombolytic medications convert plasminogen present in clots into plasmin. Plasmin then breaks down fibrin threads, dissolving the clot.

disorders. It can be used to repair septal defects (congenital and those that develop after a myocardial infarction). It can be used to reconstruct or replace valves narrowed or deformed by infection, age-related degeneration, or other pathologic processes. It can be used to revascularize the myocardium at risk for ischemic damage from coronary artery disease. It can be used to remove areas of diseased tissue, such as ventricular aneurysms or hypertrophic myocardium. And it can be used to repair damage caused by traumatic injury. In some cases, surgery must be immediate and is the only option. In other cases, surgery is performed when the response to medical management is no longer satisfactory. Common cardiac surgical procedures are summarized in Table 7–3.

Most cardiac surgery is performed by splitting the sternum and retracting the ribs to expose the heart and using cardiopulmonary bypass and cold cardioplegia to create a blood-free, still operating field. Because this approach is very traumatic and painful to the patient and requires an extensive recovery period, new techniques of minimally invasive cardiac surgery are rapidly evolving. These minimally invasive techniques are performed through a small left thoracotomy incision and sometimes a second small incision on the left anterior chest and may or may not use cardiopulmonary bypass and cardioplegia.

Preoperative Preparation

The preoperative interval may vary from a few hours to several months or even years depending on the patient's state of health and the underlying cardiac pathology. Some conditions—such as a ruptured ventricular aneurysm or blunt trauma—may require immediate surgical intervention. Other conditions, such as heart failure and valvular disease, may evolve over years. In either case, it is always desirable to stabilize the patient and optimize cardiac status before surgery. This means that dysrhythmias should be under control, heart failure treated, and anginal pain relieved. Also, such coexisting diseases as diabetes and hypertension should be well managed and stable.

Extensive studies are usually performed before surgery to confirm the diagnosis and validate the surgical plan. These include echocardiograms, stress testing, and nuclear scanning. In addition, most patients undergo cardiac catheterization to check for structural abnormalities and assess left ventricular function. Arteriography may also be performed during catheterization to observe how well the coronary arteries perfuse the myocardium. For patients with pulmonary disease or a history of smoking, pulmonary function studies are required.

In an attempt to improve respiratory status, patients who smoke are encouraged to stop or at least reduce their habit before surgery. Doing so helps to decrease the amount of bronchial secretions and re-

Table 7–3

Common Cardiac Surgical Procedures

Surgical Procedure	Description
Pericardiectomy	Removal of the pericardium through a median sternotomy
Pericardiostomy	Surgical incision into the pericardial sac with insertion of a drainage tube
Pericardial fenestration	Surgical creation of a window (opening) in the pericardium to allow for continuous drainage of pericardial fluid
Coronary artery bypass grafting (CABG)	Use of an artery or vein from another part of the body as a conduit to bring oxygenated blood to the myocardium around an obstructed artery
Minimally invasive coronary artery bypass (MICAB)	Coronary artery bypass grafting through a small "keyhole" incision through the chest wall, with or without cardiopulmonary bypass, sometimes with thorascopic guidance
Dynamic cardiomyoplasty	A procedure in which the latissimus dorsi muscle is wrapped around the ventricle to improve contractile force and cardiac output
Myotomy/myectomy	Incision into or removal of a section of hypertrophied myocardium to relieve obstruction and increase cardiac output
Valvuloplasty	Repair of a cardiac valve
Commissurotomy	A type of valvuloplasty in which fused valve leaflets are separated to relieve valve stenosis. In a closed commissurotomy, the surgeon's finger or a dilator is inserted into the valve through a small incision in the heart. In an open commissurotomy, cardiopulmonary bypass is used, and the valve is visualized for repair.
Annuloplasty	Repair of a narrowed or dilated annulus (the ring that supports a cardiac valve)
Chordoplasty	Repair of the chordae tendineae, usually of the mitral valve
Leaflet repair	Repair of a cardiac valve leaflet by means of a pericardial patch to close a hole in the leaflet, removal of excess leaflet tissue by excision or plication, or changing the length of the leaflet by chordoplasty
Valve replacement	Replacement of a diseased cardiac valve with a mechanical or biologic valve

duces the postoperative risk of complications, such as atelectasis and pneumonia.

Patients are also typed and cross-matched for blood transfusion. If surgery is not an emergency procedure, they may elect to participate in a predeposit transfusion. This type of transfusion involves removing whole blood, storing it, and transfusing it back to the donor at a later time. Under these circumstances, the problems of incompatibility, allergic reaction, and disease transmission are avoided.

In many cases, it is necessary to modify the patient's medication regimen before surgery to prevent adverse reactions. Except for patients with atrial fibrillation, digoxin (Lanoxin) is usually discontinued 24 to 36 hours before surgery because toxicity is common in the early postoperative period. Propranolol (Inderal) is commonly tapered 24 hours to 2 weeks before surgery provided the patient tolerates the weaning process and has no anginal or hypertensive episodes. For those who do not tolerate weaning, positive inotropic agents or glucagon may be given postoperatively to counteract propranolol's effects.

Unless the patient has decompensated heart failure, diuretics are typically discontinued 24 to 48 hours before surgery to help reduce potassium loss and hypovolemia. Diabetic patients receiving long-acting insulins are switched to regular insulin coverage on the day before surgery and remain on a sliding scale into the postoperative period. Other drugs that may need modification include corticosteroids, anticoagulants, antihypertensives, and phenothiazines.

Many patients are admitted to the hospital on the day of surgery and are prepped in a holding area. Baseline information obtained at this time includes a chest x-ray, ECG, complete blood count, urinalysis, serum chemistry levels, and cardiac enzymes. Body weight is obtained to guide fluid management during the postoperative period. Vital signs are documented and any elevation in temperature reported to the surgeon because it may cause the surgery to be postponed.

Preoperative preparation for cardiac surgery has psychologic as well as physiologic components and underscores the importance of a multidisciplinary approach if the goal of safe, effective quality patient care is to be met. A psychosocial assessment should focus on the patient's anxiety level, established patterns of handling stress, understanding of the operative experience and available support system. To decrease the risk of infection, a preoperative dose of antibiotic is given within 1 to 2 hours of incision. Patients are also instructed to shower several times the morning before surgery using a bacteriostatic soap, such as one containing povidone-iodine or hexachlorophene. For further detail on basic aspects of preoperative preparation, see Chapter 6.

The operative mortality of patients undergoing cardiac surgery has been reduced because of improved preoperative stabilization, adjustment of hemodynamic parameters during surgery, suitable postoperative management, and blood conservation. However, the most significant improvement is related to the use of cardiopulmonary bypass machines and cold chemical cardioplegic solutions and the development of minimally invasive cardiac surgery techniques.

Cardiopulmonary Bypass

Cardiopulmonary bypass allows the heart to be still and empty during surgery. It is accomplished through the use of a cardiopulmonary bypass machine. This machine, also called a heart-lung machine, is used to oxygenate the blood, remove carbon dioxide, and provide peripheral blood flow to meet the body's metabolic needs.

Cardiopulmonary bypass uses a cannula placed in a vein to direct blood flow from the heart to the bypass machine, and a cannula placed in an artery to return it to the patient. The specific sites for vessel cannulation are determined by the type of surgery performed. Venous cannulas are usually placed in the vena cava or the right atrium. Arterial cannulas can be placed in the femoral artery, the iliac artery, or the ascending aorta. Blood exiting the venous cannula enters the venous reservoir. The venous reservoir is connected to the oxygenator, where blood is oxygenated and carbon dioxide removed. Oxygenated blood then enters a heat exchanger, where it is cooled to lower the patient's core body temperature and reduce the metabolic rate and the oxygen demands of tissues (Fig. 7-25).

ESTABLISHING BYPASS

Before the patient is placed on cardiopulmonary bypass, the machine is primed with a balanced electrolyte solution; blood is not used. This causes hemodilution, which is advantageous because it reduces the need for blood and counteracts the increased blood viscosity that occurs during hypothermia, thus reducing the risk of microemboli. The disadvantage to the primer solution is that it tends to dilute the patient's blood volume, and measures must be taken to keep the hematocrit at a minimum of 25%. To further prevent blood from clotting in the extracorporeal circuit, the patient is anticoagulated with high doses of heparin, given initially as a bolus and then at frequent intervals during the procedure.

Once cardiopulmonary bypass is established and systemic hypothermia is achieved, the aorta is cross-clamped, and a cold hyperkalemic cardioplegic solution is used to arrest the heart and cool and perfuse the coronary arteries. As a result of hypothermia and chemically induced arrest, metabolic demands of the heart are lowered; the operative field is quiet and bloodless; the amount of cellular damage that occurs during surgery is limited; and the incidence of perioperative infarction is reduced.

Because cardiopulmonary bypass alters capillary

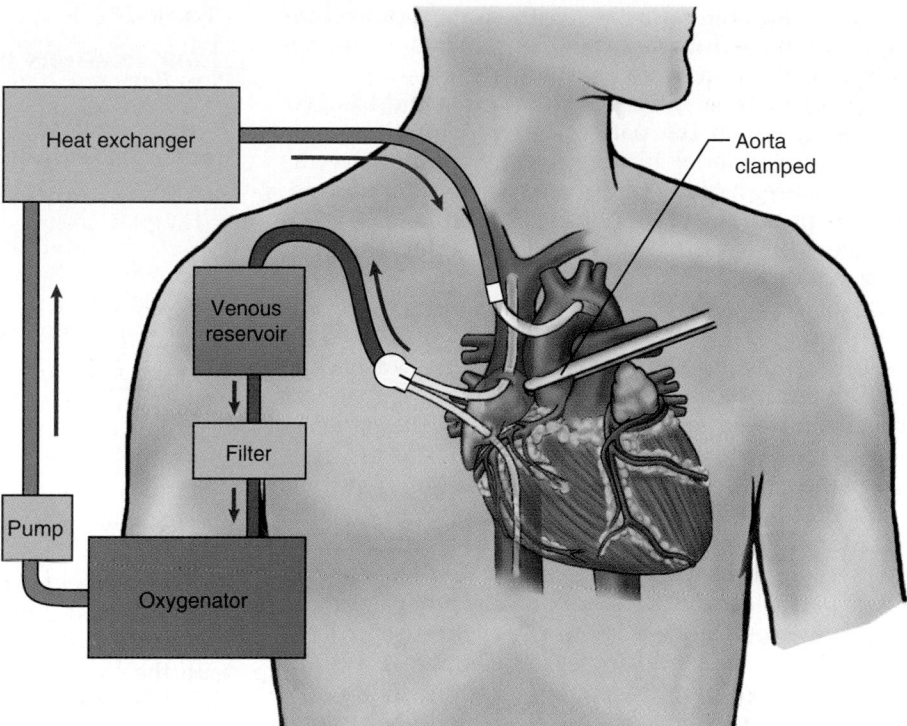

Figure 7–25

Major components of a cardiopulmonary bypass machine. Blood leaves the right atrium or superior vena cava and goes to a venous reservoir. From there, it moves through a filter and to the oxygenator, which adds oxygen and removes carbon dioxide. A pump moves the blood to the heat exchanger, which cools it during surgery and rewarms it afterward. The blood then returns to the body just above the patient's clamped aorta.

permeability, fluid shift from the intravascular to the interstitial space is common. To limit this shift and the concomitant visceral edema, fluid replacement is kept to a minimum (Riddle, 1996).

DISCONTINUING BYPASS

Before removing the patient from bypass, anesthetics are discontinued, the patient is ventilated with 100% oxygen and suctioned, and the blood is rewarmed to raise the patient's body temperature. The heart is restarted by defibrillation. Bypass perfusion is discontinued slowly. The cannulas are not removed until satisfactory arterial pressure and cardiac function are achieved. If the patient cannot maintain adequate cardiac output during the weaning process, positive inotropic agents or intra-aortic balloon counterpulsation may be instituted. A pulmonary artery catheter and arterial line may be placed to facilitate postoperative hemodynamic monitoring.

In some patients, epicardial pacing wires are placed on the right atrial and ventricular wall and threaded out through the chest surface in case the patient requires temporary pacing in the postoperative period. Chest tubes are inserted to drain blood, air, and fluid from the chest. Protamine sulfate is given to neutralize the effects of heparinization.

POSTOPERATIVE COURSE

Upon completion of surgery, most patients are transferred directly to a critical care unit for up to

24 hours, although with the increasing use of lighter anesthesia induced by rapidly acting agents and extubation in the operating room, some patients do not go to a critical care unit. Those who do are usually admitted by a team of nurses who immediately connect suction equipment and monitoring devices so that a patent airway can be maintained and hemodynamic parameters continuously assessed. Most patients have an intra-arterial line, a pulmonary artery catheter, and a central venous pressure line in place. Since atrial or ventricular dysrhythmias are the most common complications after heart surgery, all have continuous ECG and blood pressure monitoring, and an indwelling urinary catheter. If the patient has not been extubated, placement of the endotracheal tube is checked by auscultation and then is attached to a ventilator. Immediately following connection and calibration of the equipment, the patient's respiratory, cardiac, and neurologic status is assessed to determine the level of anesthesia as well as ventilation and perfusion status. Specimens for baseline laboratory data are then collected, including arterial blood gases, serum electrolytes, complete blood count, clotting profile, and cardiac enzymes.

On admission to the critical care unit, patients generally manifest a mild hypothermia because of a 2° to 5°C (3.6°–9°F) drop in core body temperature that occurs 60 to 90 minutes after separation from cardiopulmonary bypass. Weaning and extubation occur as soon as the patient completely recovers from anesthesia. Early extubation (within 6 hours) is becoming standard practice, with some rapid recovery programs extubating low-risk patients in the operating room as indicated earlier.

The heart is monitored continuously and baseline data obtained on the patient's cardiovascular status by checking arterial blood pressure, pulmonary artery pressure, heart sounds, cardiac rhythm, and peripheral pulses. Cardiac output is maximized by adjustments in cardiac rate, preload, afterload, and contractility. In most patients, reduced preload is the cause of low postoperative cardiac output. To enhance preload, volume usually is administered in the form of colloid or packed red cells. Vasoactive and/or inotropic medications or volume expanders are administered as needed to maintain the patient's blood pressure and cardiac output. Blood pressure is maintained in the 90 to 150 mm Hg range. If systolic blood pressure is less than 90 mm Hg, the patient is considered hypotensive because saphenous vein grafts can collapse at this pressure and tissue and organ perfusion can be inadequate. Hypertension is also dangerous because it can cause rupture or leakage at suture lines and increase bleeding. A systolic blood pressure of 150 mm Hg or more is usually considered hypertensive and is treated. Nitroprusside or nitroglycerine, vasodilators, can be titrated to bring blood pressure into an acceptable range. Blood products are also given as needed to stabilize the hematocrit.

Most often, patients are turned side to side and, when vital signs are stable, the head of the bed is elevated 30 degrees. Patients free of complications can be up in a chair and beginning to ambulate immediately after extubation (Riddle, 1996). Activity is then progressively resumed. Most tubes and lines are removed in 72 hours, although additional ECG monitoring may be necessary for some patients. In line with the current movement away from overuse of antibiotics, if they are given postoperatively, it is generally only until the chest tubes are removed. For patients with a prosthetic valve replacement, anticoagulants are begun 72 hours after surgery. In preparation for discharge, referrals are made to appropriate community resources. Home regimens and medications are discussed, and the patient or family is given written instructions on wound care, diet, and activity levels.

COMPLICATIONS

There are many potential complications of cardiac surgery. These complications arise from preoperative cardiac risk factors, the cardiac disease that necessitated the surgery, and the opening of the chest (Table 7–4). All patients who have a thoracotomy are at risk for complications, as discussed in Chapter 14. Another source of potential complications is the cardiopulmonary bypass procedure. Time on the bypass machine is closely monitored and kept to a minimum because, the longer a patient is on it, the more complications are likely to develop. Both the

Table 7–4

Complications of Cardiac Surgery

Common Complications	Less Common Complications
Acute myocardial infarction	Renal failure
Vein graft closure	Stress ulcer
Dysrhythmias	Respiratory failure
Pneumonia	Cardiac tamponade
Pericarditis	Cardiogenic shock
Embolism/cerebrovascular accident	Gastrointestinal bleeding
Atelectasis	Infection
Pneumothorax	Paralytic ileus
Hemothorax	

formed elements (red blood cells, white blood cells, and platelets) and the unformed elements (plasma proteins) of blood are traumatized by direct contact with the surfaces of the pump, its mechanical action, and the resulting turbulent flow. This damage is typically tolerated well by most patients. However, a small number—particularly those whose pump times extend beyond 3 hours—do not tolerate it well. Postoperatively, these patients may be prone to develop blood dyscrasias, pulmonary edema, and transient neurologic alterations. Table 7–5 lists these and other pathophysiologic effects of cardiopulmonary bypass and their causes.

Patients are also at risk for many fluid and electrolyte imbalances, especially if cardiopulmonary bypass was used. Thus, intake, output, and electrolyte values must be closely monitored and daily weights obtained and compared to the preoperative baseline weight.

NURSING PROCESS
Cardiac Surgery

PREOPERATIVE NURSING CARE

Assessment

Review the patient's history, personal risk factor profile, and diagnostic findings as a basis for assessing current status and projecting postoperative needs and possible complications. Determine the patient's functional status by asking about the patient's activities and whether they are associated with dyspnea, palpitations, or angina.

Obtain a list of medications the patient takes and note the time and dose last taken. This is particularly important for medications (such as digoxin and anticoagulants) that may be discontinued in preparation for surgery. Determine nutritional intake and whether the patient has any dietary restrictions.

Perform a baseline physical assessment with particular focus on the cardiopulmonary systems. Aus-

Table 7–5

Pathophysiologic Effects of Cardiopulmonary Bypass

Pathophysiologic Effects	Possible Causes
Intravascular fluid deficit (hypotension)	Third spacing
	Postoperative diuresis
	Vasodilation due to drugs and rewarming
Third spacing (weight gain, edema)	Decreased plasma protein concentration
	Increased capillary permeability
Decreased cardiac output	Hypothermia
	Increased systemic vascular resistance
	Pre-existing heart disease
Increased bleeding	Systemic heparinization
	Mechanical trauma to platelets
	Depressed release of clotting factors from liver due to hypothermia
Hemolysis and hemoglobinuria	Red blood cells damaged in pump circuit
Hyperglycemia	Decreased insulin release
	Glycogenolysis
Neurologic dysfunction	Inadequate cerebral perfusion
	Microemboli
Hypertension	Catecholamine release and vasoconstriction due to hypothermia

cultate the heart in all six areas to check for extra heart sounds, gallops, rubs, or murmurs. Take vital signs. Obtain apical and radial pulses and bilateral blood pressure readings. Assess and record all peripheral pulses, comparing the quality of each bilaterally. Auscultate each carotid artery from the base of the neck to the corner of the jaw. Listen for bruits, which usually indicate arterial stenosis at or proximal to the site of auscultation. Observe the neck for jugular venous distention. Check for edema and, if present, note its location, amount, and relationship to time of day and activity. Determine whether it is pitting or non-pitting.

Ask the patient about any history of smoking and calculate the number of pack years. (For example, 2 packs a day for 10 years equals 20 pack years.) Assess the rate, depth, and work of respiration. Auscultate the patient's lungs and document adventitious sounds, crackles, or wheezes. Check baseline oxygen saturation on room air.

Assess and document neurologic status, including any history of episodes of confusion. This is critical to interpretation of postoperative assessment findings since cardiopulmonary bypass, a low-flow state during surgery, and postcardiotomy syndrome can cause postoperative confusion.

Assess the patient's and the family's understanding of the underlying cardiac disease, the need for surgery, the operative procedure to be done and its expected outcomes. Determine the nature of past hospitalization experiences and the patient's expectations of the current one. Observe for signs of anxiety, such as nervousness, hyperventilation, and inability to focus or follow directions. Determine how the patient usually copes with anxiety and what support systems are available. Be sure to consider information documented by members of the multidisciplinary team, such as the psychologist, social worker, and spiritual advisor.

Nursing Diagnoses and Planning

Nursing diagnoses and related expected patient outcomes commonly applicable to patients in the preoperative stage of cardiac surgery include the following:

NDx: Anxiety related to the life-threatening nature of the surgery and the perioperative experience

Planning: Patient Outcomes
1. Patient and family accurately describe the nature of the cardiac disease, the need for surgery, the planned surgical procedure and its outcomes, the postoperative environment, and postoperative routines.
2. Patient uses anxiety-reduction techniques.
3. Signs of anxiety (such as nervous mannerisms, hyperventilation, and inability to focus or follow directions) are absent.

NDx: Risk for altered health maintenance related to insufficient knowledge of postoperative pulmonary hygiene and pain control

Planning: Patient Outcomes
1. Patient demonstrates coughing, deep-breathing, use of assistive breathing devices, and wound splinting.
2. Patient explains the importance of postoperative pulmonary hygiene.
3. Patient explains use of patient-controlled analgesia.

Nursing Interventions and Evaluation

NDx: Anxiety
Because the heart is essential to life, expect a high level of anxiety in both the patient and the family over the impending surgery. Assisting the patient to control anxiety is critical because of the detrimental physiologic effects that stress exerts on the body and its potential for contributing to the development of perioperative complications. Lowering the family's

anxiety level is important as well, because it allows them to better support the patient.

In assisting the patient and family to control anxiety, use a calm, caring approach. Reassure them that anxiety is normal and encourage them to ask questions and discuss their concerns about the disease, the life-threatening nature of the surgery, and fears of death. Provide physical comfort measures for the patient and family. Teach relaxation techniques and collaborate with other members of the multidisciplinary team to support the patient in using effective coping strategies.

Because fear of the unknown is a major determinant of anxiety, a key aspect of anxiety control is familiarizing the patient and the family with the care environment, perioperative procedures, and expected postoperative course (Table 7–6). Thus, providing a tour of the postoperative unit may be beneficial to the patient and family. Meeting and speaking with a patient who has successfully recov-

ered from cardiac surgery may also help to inspire confidence and lessen anxiety.

In presenting information to anxious patients and families, take care not to overwhelm them. Present information in simple terms and manageable segments, repeating as necessary. Tailor the information to their specific needs. Keep in mind that highly anxious people commonly have misconceptions about the disease, the surgical procedure, or the outcomes. Be sure to allow time for questions. Reinforce information as necessary because patients and their families have limited knowledge retention in the high-stress period before surgery.

NDx: Risk for altered health maintenance
Instruct the patient in coughing, deep-breathing, use of an incentive spirometer or other assistive breathing device, and splinting the incision (see Chap. 6). Obtain a return demonstration. Explain the importance of pulmonary hygiene in avoiding post-

Table 7–6

Preoperative Teaching Plan: Cardiac Surgery

Teaching Areas	Topics to Include
Tour the critical care unit	Introduce the staff Tour the patient room and family waiting area Explain noises, lights, and alarms Explain visiting hours, approximate length of surgery, length of stay in unit, what items patient may bring to unit

Explain the equipment, tubes, and lines	Cardiac monitor
	Arterial line
	Pulmonary artery catheter
	Intravenous lines and infusion pumps
	Endotracheal tube and ventilator
	    Suctioning
	    Inability to talk and how to communicate
	    When extubation can be anticipated
	Foley catheter
	Chest tubes
	Pacing wires
	Nasogastric tube

Describe the incision and dressings	
Discuss the patient's immediate post-operative appearance	Skin color change from use of povidone-iodine solution in operating room Skin will be pale and cool to touch due to hypothermia Generalized swelling of neck, face, and hands from third spacing of fluid
Explain the process of awakening from anesthesia	Patient goes directly to critical care unit and does not go to the surgical recovery room Sensations patient will experience, may be aware of, or able to hear but unable to respond
Discuss discomfort from incision, chest tubes, and endotracheal tube	Amount of discomfort to be expected Relief measures provided
Explain and demonstrate postoperative respiratory care measures	Turning Effective coughing and deep-breathing Use of pillow to splint incision Incentive spirometry Have patient practice these techniques preoperatively
Describe progression of postoperative activity	Sitting Dangling Ambulation

operative complications. Allay fears of pain associated with turning, coughing, and deep breathing by reassuring the patient that adequate analgesia will be available at all times.

Describe the plan for progressive activity: up in chair and ambulating on the first postoperative day and ambulating in the hall on day 2. Explain the role progressive activity plays in mobilizing secretions, improving oxygenation, and preventing atelectasis.

If patient-controlled analgesia will be used postoperatively, teach the patient about its use. Stress the importance of taking pain medications at regular intervals.

Additional Interventions

Anticipate discharge concerns and begin discharge planning.

Compare the patient's status with the expected outcomes. If the outcomes are not met, reassess the patient and revise the plan.

POSTOPERATIVE NURSING CARE

Assessment

Assess respiratory status. Check the integrity of the endotracheal tube and ventilator. Auscultate breath sounds to assure bilateral aeration of the lungs and to check for secretions and pneumothorax. Monitor SAO_2 (percentage of oxygen carried in hemoglobin in arterial blood). Obtain a chest x-ray and arterial blood gases within the first 30 minutes of admission to the critical care unit. Observe amount, color, and consistency of secretions. When the patient has been extubated, monitor rate, depth, and quality of respirations.

Assess cardiovascular function. Monitor and document blood pressure and heart rate every 15 minutes until stable and then every hour. Auscultate heart sounds. Measure central venous pressure, pulmonary artery pressure, pulmonary capillary wedge pressure, and cardiac output every 2 to 4 hours and as warranted by changes in the patient's condition. Check the rate, rhythm, and volume of radial pulses and compare bilaterally. Assess for a pulse deficit by counting apical and radial pulses simultaneously. Palpate dorsalis pedis or posterior tibial pulses for strength and equality.

Check skin temperature, color, and capillary refill. Note cool, pale skin; central or peripheral cyanosis; and delayed capillary refill because they can indicate poor perfusion, inadequate oxygenation, or the onset of cardiogenic shock.

Assess ECG pattern, which is monitored continuously for changes from the patient's preoperative baseline. Be alert to the development of dysrhythmias, which commonly occur in the initial preoperative period from such factors as trauma to the myocardium, cardiopulmonary bypass, anesthesia, and variations in serum potassium.

Monitor serum electrolyte levels, especially potassium and calcium, because increased or decreased electrolyte levels may exacerbate dysrhythmias or impede their treatment.

Check the patient's temperature upon admission to the unit and every 1 to 2 hours thereafter. Use a tympanic membrane probe because rectal temperatures do not correlate with core temperature measurements until 8 hours postoperatively. Expect the temperature to be in the 35° to 36°C (95°–97°F) range because, although the patient is rewarmed before separation from the bypass machine, a drop of 2° to 5°C (3.6°–9°F) typically occurs 60 to 90 minutes after separation.

Assess the patient's neurologic status on admission to the critical care unit, then hourly and whenever a change is noticed until the patient is fully recovered from anesthesia. Check the following:

- Level of consciousness
- Pupil size and reaction
- Orientation to time, place, and person
- Ability to follow commands
- Sensation, strength, and movement of the extremities

Neurologic assessment is done to monitor the patient's awakening from anesthesia, which typically occurs over a period of 1 to 2 hours following admission to the critical care unit. It is an indicator of the patient's ventilation and perfusion status and allows for early detection of neurologic complications, such as cerebral embolism or neurologic damage from low cerebral perfusion during bypass. Patients at greatest risk for neurologic complications are those with prolonged cardiovascular bypass time, pre-existing carotid or cerebrovascular disease, and valve disease, especially with atrial fibrillation. The risk of neurologic complications also increases with age.

Check the dressing over the chest wound for signs of excessive bleeding. Also assess the character and amount of chest tube drainage every 15 to 30 minutes immediately postoperatively, then every hour for 16 hours. Normally, chest drainage is dark red, thin, serosanguineous, and does not clot because it is defibrinated. Chest drainage normally does not exceed 100 mL per hour after the first 2 postoperative hours for a 24-hour total averaging 500 mL. Persistent mediastinal bleeding, in excess of 500 mL in 1 hour or 400 mL/hr for 2 consecutive hours, is an indication for re-exploration of the surgical site. Assess function of the chest drainage system as discussed in Chapter 14.

Assess postoperative pain. Ask the patient to rate the pain on a scale of 0 to 10 or 0 to 5, with 0 being no pain. Also ask about the character, location, and duration of the pain. Observe for signs of pain, such as moaning, a tense posture, and reluctance to move. To judge their effectiveness, compare pain assessments before and after administration of analgesic medications and use of other comfort measures.

Check the patency and integrity of the indwelling urinary catheter drainage system. Measure and record the amount and color of urine output every hour. Hourly urine volume should be at least 20 to 30 mL. Volume in the 100 to 200 mL range is not uncommon because of postoperative diuresis secondary to the hemodilution that occurs during cardiopulmonary bypass. Observe for hematuria and monitor BUN and serum creatinine levels. Notify the physician if BUN is elevated because, when associated with oliguria, it indicates acute tubular necrosis that can be caused by low perfusion of the kidney during surgery. Renal insufficiency can also occur from buildup of products of red blood cell destruction during bypass.

Assess hydration status, looking for signs of dehydration or fluid overload. Check skin turgor and the condition of mucous membranes. Measure intake and output. Track the number of dressing changes and estimate the amount of drainage on each discarded dressing. Check for edema and obtain daily weights. Assess gastrointestinal function as for any postoperative patient. Keep in mind that a decreased appetite and nausea are not unusual and may occur secondary to perioperative hypotension and hypoperfusion, hypothermia, anxiety, and stress, or as a side effect of many cardiac medications. Assess the patient's sleep pattern and need for sleep aids. Observe for signs of sleep deprivation, such as marked fatigue, nausea, headache, inability to concentrate, irritability, or emotional lability. See Table 7–7 for the interpretation of selected assessment findings in postoperative cardiac surgery patients.

Nursing Diagnoses and Planning

Nursing diagnoses and related expected patient outcomes commonly applicable to patients who have had cardiac surgery include the following:

NDx: Impaired gas exchange related to anesthesia, poor chest expansion and retained secretions

Planning: Patient Outcomes
 1. Airway is patent.
 2. Lung sounds are clear.
 3. Arterial blood gases are within normal limits.

NDx: Hypothermia related to separation from cardiopulmonary bypass

Planning: Patient Outcomes
 1. Temperature returns to 37°C (98.6°F) without shivering or rapid vasodilation.
 2. Temperature is maintained at 37°C (98.6°F) or above.

NDx: Pain related to surgical trauma

Planning: Patient Outcomes
 1. Patient states that pain is relieved or controlled.
 2. Patient appears comfortable.
 3. Patient is able to rest.

NDx: Sleep pattern disturbance related to pain, anxiety, and environmental distraction

Planning: Patient Outcomes
 1. Patient reports adequate rest.
 2. Signs of sleep deprivation are absent.

Table 7–7

Interpretation of Selected Assessment Findings After Cardiac Surgery

Assessment Finding	Interpretation
Failure to regain consciousness for more than 2 hours postoperatively	Unusually deep anesthesia
	Possible air, calcium, fat, or thrombotic emboli to brain
Slow return to consciousness and less than fully alert 24 to 48 hours postoperatively	Poor cerebral perfusion or microemboli to brain during cardiopulmonary bypass
Dilated pupils	Hypercalcemia
	Medications, such as atropine
Constricted pupils	Dopamine
Disorientation	Hypoxia, brain embolism, sensory overload, fatigue
Sugar and acetone in the urine	Benign effect of cardiopulmonary bypass
Increased urine specific gravity	Oliguria or presence of red blood cells from cardiopulmonary bypass
Absence of chest tube drainage in initial hours after surgery	Clotting of the tube within the mediastinum. This can lead to cardiac tamponade from compression of the heart by blood or clots caught between the heart and the chest wall.
	Other indications of tamponade are increased incisional bleeding, fall in blood pressure, rise in central venous and pulmonary artery pressures, decreased urinary output, and restlessness.

NDx: Risk for ineffective management of therapeutic regimen (individuals) related to lack of knowledge or motivation

Planning: Patient Outcomes
1. Patient and family explain discharge instructions.
2. Patient and family describe importance of complying with discharge instructions.
3. Patient and family verbalize intent to comply with discharge instructions.

Nursing Interventions and Evaluation

NDx: Impaired gas exchange
Maintain a patent airway while the patient is intubated. Preoxygenate and suction as often as needed to clear secretions. Turn the patient every 2 hours to help loosen and prevent pooling of secretions. After extubation, administer oxygen to maintain oxygen saturation levels. Encourage the patient to splint the incision, cough, and deep-breathe every hour initially and then every 2 hours when awake. Also encourage use of an incentive spirometer every 2 hours. To promote the effectiveness of these measures, reinforce preoperative teaching on coughing and deep breathing techniques and use of the incentive spirometer. If a change occurs in secretions, obtain a specimen for culture.

NDx: Hypothermia
Because hypothermia causes peripheral vasoconstriction and a shift to the left on the oxyhemoglobin dissociation curve (where less oxygen is released from the hemoglobin to the tissues), warming the patient is important to good tissue perfusion and oxygenation. Institute warming measures for patients whose core body temperature is below 37°C (98.6°F). These measures may include:

- Raising the room temperature
- Covering the patient with warmed blankets, perfusion blankets, fluid-filled thermal blankets, or other mechanical heating blanket
- Covering the top and back of the patients head with blankets or plastic

In some cases nitroprusside may be ordered to induce vasodilation. Slow rewarming is also necessary to prevent shivering, which increases metabolic rate, oxygen consumption, carbon dioxide production, and myocardial workload. It also can precipitate dysrhythmias.

NDx: Pain
Medicate the patient to relieve pain. Typically, this means giving narcotic analgesics every 3 hours during the first 24 hours and then as needed. If patient-controlled analgesia is used, encourage the patient to use it as needed. Explain that pain increases the need for oxygen and the work of the heart. Therefore, relieving pain is desirable and promotes recovery. Support the effects of analgesics with other comfort measures, such as splinting the incision during coughing or moving, careful positioning, attention to oral and body hygiene, back rubs, and other relaxation measures. Minimize factors that enhance pain perception, such as fatigue and anxiety. Instruct the patient to report if pain relief is not achieved. Confer with the physician or clinical specialist on pain management and evaluate the need for a change in pain medication and use of nonpharmacologic interventions.

NDx: Sleep pattern disturbance
Encourage sleep through such relaxation measures as back rubs and soft music. Avoid loud noises and overhead lights during nighttime sleep. Provide a quiet and peaceful environment and minimize interruptions. Plan activities to allow time for sleep and rest. Avoid unnecessary procedures during sleep period, and limit visiting during rest periods. Confer with the physician about revising the patient's medication regimen when it interferes with the sleep pattern.

NDx: Risk for ineffective management of therapeutic regimen (individuals)
Instruct the patient and family in care needed after discharge. Include information on medications, wound care, diet, activity, symptoms to report, and follow-up examinations.

Additional Interventions
Postoperatively, patients face an increased risk of fluid overload from hemodilution (from bypass) and increased vasopressin and aldosterone levels. If it occurs, administer mannitol, furosemide (Lasix), or other diuretics, and restrict fluids as ordered. Double concentrate intravenous drug drips when possible to decrease the volume infused to the patient. Monitor electrolytes, especially potassium and sodium. Report abnormalities and be prepared to replace as necessary.

If temporary pacing is used postoperatively, provide care as described in Chapter 8. If prolonged, severe acute tubular necrosis develops secondary to bypass and hemodialysis is instituted, provide care as described in Chapter 31.

Compare the patient's status with the expected patient outcomes. If the outcomes are not met, reassess the patient and revise the plan.

Cardiac Transplantation

The first successful human to human heart transplant was performed in 1967. However, because of a poor long-term survival rate, cardiac transplantation remained primarily an experimental procedure until the development of cyclosporine in 1983. Today, the 1-year survival rate is 80 to 90% and the 5-year survival rate is 60 to 70%.

Candidates for a heart transplant have end-stage heart disease, no other medical or surgical options, and a poor prognosis for survival greater than 6 months. Cardiomyopathy, ischemic heart disease, congenital heart disease, valvular disease, and rejection of previously transplanted hearts are the most common indications for transplantation.

The potential recipient is screened by a multidisciplinary team before becoming a candidate. Age, pulmonary status, chronic health conditions, infections, history of other transplants, and current health status are all taken into consideration. Candidates must also demonstrate emotional and psychosocial stability and a willingness to comply with lifelong immunosuppressive drug therapy. Exclusion because of age is based on the person's physiologic rather than chronologic age. Many centers now consider insulin-dependent diabetic patients as long as they are free of diabetic retinopathy, neuropathy, nephropathy, and vascular disease.

When a donor heart becomes available, a list of potential recipients is generated based on ABO blood group compatibility, size of the donor heart, and the geographic distance between the donor and potential recipient. To minimize tissue damage, the maximum time the donor heart can be ischemic is 4 to 5 hours. Therefore, distance for transport is limited to a flying radius of about 3 hours.

The recipient is prepared for surgery using a sternotomy incision. Then, either an orthotopic or a heterotopic procedure is performed. The orthotopic technique is the most common (Fig. 7–26). In this procedure, a portion of the recipient's atria, usually the posterior wall, is left in place. The rest of the heart is removed. The donor heart is then trimmed to match the recipient's and implanted by suturing the donor atria to the residual tissue of the recipient's heart. The pulmonary artery and aorta are then anastomosed.

A second method, the heterotopic or piggyback procedure, is less common. Using this approach, the recipient's heart is left in place and the donor heart is placed next to it in the right chest. The two hearts are then connected by anastomoses between the left and right atria, aortas, and pulmonary arteries, using synthetic graft. This allows blood to flow through both hearts and the two functional hearts work together to provide one cardiac output.

Postoperatively, heart transplant recipients receive immunosuppressive drugs for the rest of their lives to minimize the possibility of rejection. Cyclosporine, the drug of choice, is used to prevent rather

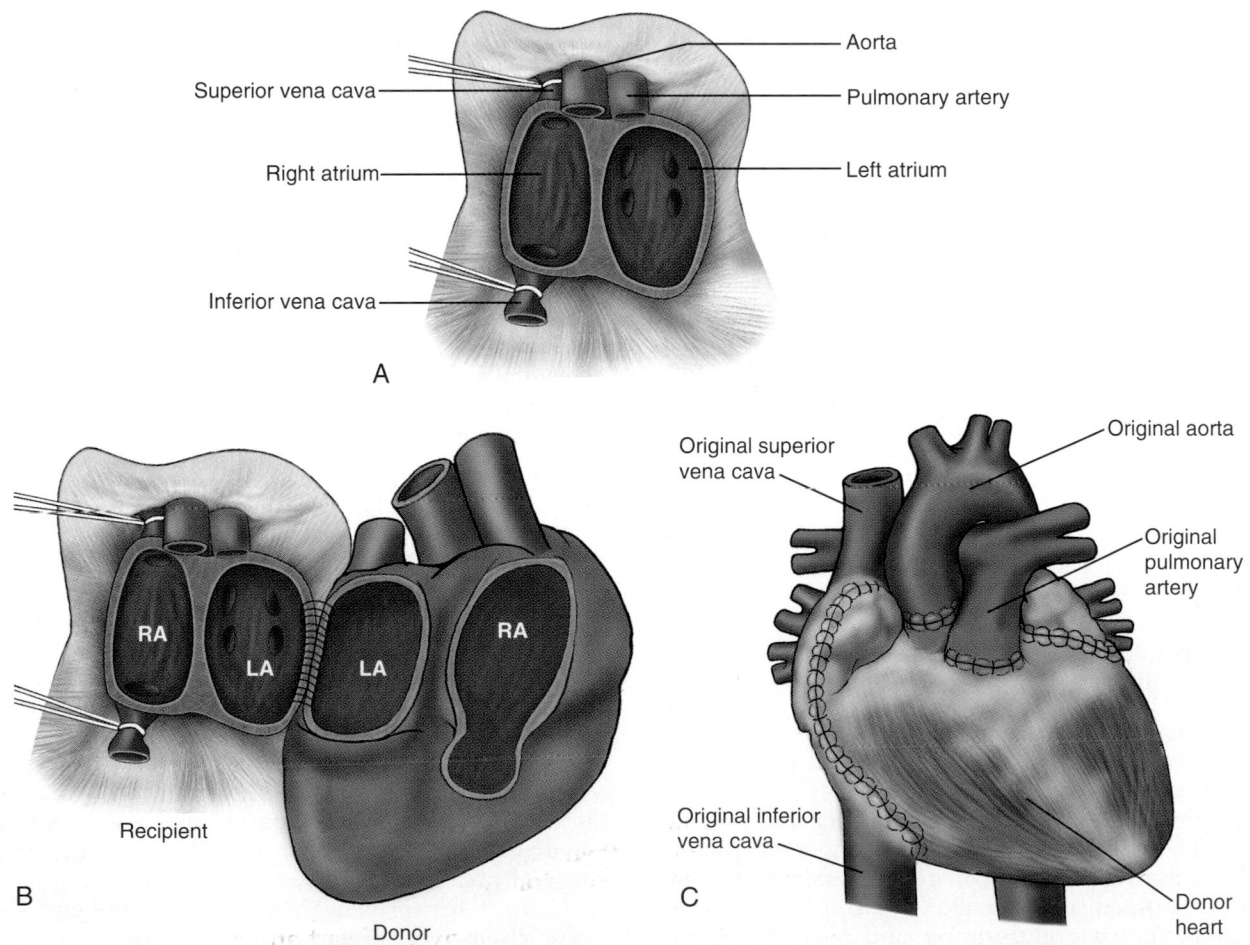

Figure 7–26

Orthotopic technique of heart transplantation. *A,* Patient's heart is removed except for a portion of the posterior atrial walls. *B,* Atria of the donor heart, trimmed to match, are sutured to the remaining portion of the patient's atria. *C,* The great vessels are anastomosed.

than reverse acute rejection. It does, however, decrease the body's ability to resist infections. A delicate balance must be achieved between suppressing rejection and avoiding infection. Heart transplant also places the patient at risk for accelerated arteriosclerotic heart disease, hypertension and hypotension, respiratory and gastrointestinal disturbances, renal failure, and psychosocial responses to the stresses imposed by organ transplantation.

Other complications relate to the fact that the transplanted heart is a denervated heart. That is, it does not have central nervous system connections to the recipient's body. As a result, it is unaffected by the recipient's sympathetic and parasympathetic nervous system. Because vagal influence is lost, the resting heart rate is higher than normal, usually between 90 and 110 beats per minute, and it does not vary with the patient's respirations. Similarly, atropine (which blocks vagal stimulation) is ineffective in treating bradydysrhythmias in the transplanted heart because there is no parasympathetic innervation. With exercise, heart rate and cardiac output increase gradually over 3 to 5 minutes and remain elevated for a longer period of time after exercise. Therefore, patients must gradually increase and decrease demands on heart rate by means of extended warm-up and cool-down periods.

Intra-Aortic Balloon Counterpulsation

Intra-aortic balloon counterpulsation is a method of mechanically supporting circulation with a device called an intra-aortic balloon pump. It is used to support cardiac output and thereby prevent or treat cardiogenic shock in patients who have had cardiac surgery or a massive myocardial infarction.

The balloon is positioned in the thoracic aorta after being passed through the femoral artery via a cutdown or percutaneous insertion. The balloon is positioned distal to the left subclavian artery as it branches off the aortic arch and proximal to the renal arteries as they branch off the descending aorta.

The balloon is inflated during diastole, when the aortic valve is closed, forcing blood from the aorta in two directions: into the coronary arteries and into the arteries of the general systemic circulation. This increases the amount of oxygen delivered to the myocardium and enables the heart to increase its contractile strength. Perfusion of blood and oxygen to the brain, kidneys, and tissues also increases. Myocardial function, cardiac output, and renal function improve.

Deflation of the balloon occurs just before and during the beginning of systole. Because most of the blood has been pushed out of the aorta by the inflated balloon during diastole, the heart pumps against low peripheral vascular resistance, which reduces the workload of the left ventricle.

Patients who require intra-aortic balloon counterpulsation are critically ill, so nursing care is focused on life-sustaining interventions. These patients are monitored and cared for in critical care units.

Ventricular Assistance

Ventricular assistance is commonly required by the patient with a failing heart. A ventricular assist device (VAD) is a mechanical pump used to maintain life until another procedure can be implemented, a transplant can be performed, or the heart can recover and support itself. A VAD is used most frequently in patients with severe cardiomyopathy, myocarditis, endocarditis, myocardial infarction, or a rejected heart transplant. The VAD can support the right ventricle, the left ventricle, or both. Usually, it is the left ventricle that needs assistance.

When the VAD is attached to the heart surgically, blood can be shunted from the inadequate ventricle to a battery-powered pump. The pump does not replace the work of the ventricle, but rather enhances it. The pump and battery may be implanted in the patient's chest, or they may be attached externally with tubes extending to the heart.

Complications are common in patients with VADs. Thrombi are the most common complication. This leads to pulmonary emboli, cerebral clots, and peripheral thrombophlebitis. Clots tend to develop even with heparin therapy.

A VAD is usually considered to be only a temporary therapy to sustain life for a patient with serious cardiac dysfunction. Many patients receiving ventricular assistance are awaiting heart transplantation. However, patients with severe cardiac disease who are not candidates for transplantation may have a permanent VAD implanted in the chest. This is still considered palliative treatment.

CARDIAC REHABILITATION

Cardiac rehabilitation is a medically supervised, individualized program of care designed to return the patient with heart disease to normal living and to decrease the risk of further cardiac damage. To accomplish these goals, cardiac rehabilitation programs focus on promoting psychologic and social—as well as physical—wellbeing. They accomplish this goal through medical evaluation, prescribed exercise, modification of cardiac risk factors, patient education, and counseling. Health-care providers involved in the delivery of these services include physicians, registered nurses, physical therapists, nutritionists, psychologists, social workers, occupational therapists, and vocational counselors. Cardiac rehabilitation is most often prescribed for patients who

Have survived a heart attack.
Have had coronary artery bypass surgery or balloon angioplasty to increase blood flow to the myocardium.

Have had a heart transplant.

Have angina or stable heart failure.

For hospitalized patients, cardiac rehabilitation begins with admission and continues throughout hospitalization and during recovery at home. Ultimately, cardiac rehabilitation is a lifelong program. In fact, cardiac rehabilitation is no longer just for hospitalized patients. Programs are becoming available for a wide range of patients in a variety of settings, such as clinics, community centers, and patients' homes. Among the last are programs that feature telephone monitoring of the patient and the patient's ECG, and group discussion via conference calls facilitated by a registered nurse.

❖ Settings, Providers, and Collaboration for Care

Screening for heart disease occurs in a variety of settings. Blood pressure clinics are held in workplaces, schools, churches, shopping malls, and pharmacies. Cholesterol screening is also done in workplaces and at health fairs held throughout the community. Screening for heart disease is also a part of regular health check-ups in physician offices and clinics.

Diagnostic studies are primarily done in outpatient settings. These include both invasive tests, such as transesophageal echocardiography, and noninvasive tests, such as stress testing. Some procedures, such as electrophysiology studies and cardiac catheterization, may require admission to an observation unit for several hours following the procedure.

Care settings for patients diagnosed with heart disease vary according to the acuity of the problem and the type of care required. Patients who have experienced open heart surgery, an acute myocardial infarction, acute heart failure, or other major cardiac event are initially cared for in a critical care unit, When the patient's condition begins to stabilize, care may be provided on a telemetry unit to allow continuous monitoring of cardiac status or on a general medical-surgical unit. In some cases, care may continue in a rehabilitation setting, either inpatient or outpatient, to increase the patient's functional ability and overall level of wellness.

The diversity of health-care professionals essential to comprehensive care of the cardiac patient is as great as the diversity of settings in which care is provided. These health-care providers may include the cardiologist, the invasive cardiologist, the cardiothoracic surgeon, the respiratory therapist, the dietitian, the exercise physiologist, and nurses across all settings. Because of the life-threatening and anxiety-producing nature of many cardiac disorders, spiritual advisors, mental-health practitioners, and representatives of support groups may also be involved with care. Social service personnel play a role in obtaining financial support needed to ensure that medication and equipment can be purchased and that transportation is available for follow-up care. Many patients require a home health nurse for continued assessment of cardiac status and for health teaching and monitoring of medications and diet.

The Elderly: Special Considerations

Physiologic changes in the cardiovascular system present in a variety of ways in the older person. Throughout the adult years, the heart muscle loses its efficiency and contractile strength, resulting in reduced cardiac output. Adjustment to this change is made by pacing activities. For example, the patient may drive rather than walk long distances, or take an elevator rather than walk up several flights of stairs.

Elevated pulse rates in the elderly may not be as high as in younger persons, but tachycardia experienced with activity or stress in the elderly lasts for a longer period of time. Stroke volume may increase as the heart tries to increase cardiac output in stressful situations, resulting in elevated blood pressure and a bounding pulse.

The increased rigidity of vessel walls and narrowing of lumens that occur with aging necessitate increased force from the heart to pump blood through the vessels. Thus, systolic and diastolic blood pressures rise. Heart valves become thick and rigid from sclerosis and fibrosis, compounding the need for increased force to deliver adequate blood and oxygen to the body's tissues. There is controversy among physicians about treating elevated blood pressures in the elderly because some elevation is necessary to compensate for changes associated with the aging process.

The elderly may be spared the lethal complications associated with myocardial infarction because, over the years, they develop collateral circulation of the myocardium. Instead, they may develop compromised tissue perfusion because of increased peripheral vascular resistance resulting from the arteriosclerosis of the peripheral vessels. Just as the heart ages, so do the other organ systems of the body. With acute cardiac disease, the elderly often acquire associated problems, such as renal failure from decreased cardiac output in heart failure, respiratory failure from fluid accumulation in heart failure, and disorientation, syncope, or coma resulting from inadequate circulation to the brain.

Medication therapy is a specific concern in the elderly. Older adults take medications frequently, both prescription and over-the-counter. Some of their health problems may result from adverse reactions to medications. Many older adults take more than one medication, so possible drug interactions must be monitored. Decreased blood flow to the liver diminishes hepatic drug metabolism, and decreased blood flow to the kidneys decreases drug elimination. Thus, the common adult dosages of many cardiac medications must be reduced for the elderly. Their responses to medications should be monitored and dosages altered according to individual response. Laboratory tests that measure drug levels in the blood may be needed to adjust specific medications. Signs of toxicity for any medication must be assessed, documented, and reported when caring for elderly patients.

Anginal pain in the elderly is more diffuse and less severe than in younger patients. It may be regarded as not bothersome and therefore may not be reported until cardiac damage has resulted. Dyspnea, rather than pain, may be the most prominent symptom of acute myocardial infarction in an older adult.

Peripheral edema may result from nutritional deficiency rather than ventricular dysfunction. A low serum albumin level associated with edema in all soft tissue areas indicates inadequate nutrition in the elderly.

There are age-related changes in all systems of the body. These changes mandate that nursing assessment, planning, implementation, and evaluation be examined in relationship to the aging process. Cardiac problems in the elderly should be evaluated for each individual and a plan of care developed accordingly. The goal of nursing care is to help the aging patient remain a functioning, contributing member of society.

Chapter Review

1. How does an increase in afterload affect cardiac output?
2. What electrical events in the heart cause the P wave, the QRS complex, and the T wave?
3. What is the physiologic basis for decreased activity tolerance in patients with heart disease?
4. What factors encourage and discourage patient compliance with cardiac disease risk-reduction measures?
5. How does the diagnostic information provided by a standard ECG differ from that provided by an exercise stress test?
6. What are the similarities and differences between echocardiography and thallium scanning?
7. Why is it important to deflate the balloon on a pulmonary artery catheter immediately after a pulmonary capillary wedge pressure reading is taken?
8. Why are patients with heart disease at risk for fluid and electrolyte problems?
9. What are the advantages and disadvantages of cardiopulmonary bypass?
10. How is the postoperative cardiac surgery patient guarded against potentially lethal atrial and ventricular dysrhythmias?

Bibliography

Armstrong PJH. Your guide to continuing cardiac care. Medford, OR: Rogue Valley Medical Center, 1995.

Barkman A, Lunse CP. The effect of early ambulation on patient comfort and delayed bleeding after cardiac angiogram: A pilot study. Heart and Lung 1994; 23(2):112.

Bertrand M. The prevention of cardiovascular events: An new challenge for calcium channel blockers. In The prevention of cardiovascular events: A new challenge for calcium channel blockers (satellite symposium to the XVIIth congress of the Europena Society of Cardiology). Auckland, NZ: Adis International, 1996.

Carpenito LJ. Handbook of nursing diagnosis. 6th ed. Philadelphia: JB Lippincott, 1995.

Copstead LC. Perspectives on pathophysiology. Philadelphia: WB Saunders, 1995.

Cornock MA. Psychological approaches to cardiac pain. Nurs Stand 1996; 11(12):34.

Cusimano RJ, Dale L, Butany JW. Minimally invasive cardiac surgery for removal of the greater saphenous vein. Can J Surg 1996; 39(5):386.

Das BN, Banka VS. Coronary artery disease in women: How it is and isn't unique. Postgrad Med 1992; 91(4):197.

Das DK, Engelman RM, Cherian KM. Myocardial preservation, preconditioning, and adaptation. Ann N Y Acad Sci 1996; 793:1.

Davidson CJ, Crawford MH. Intravascular imaging and Doppler. Philadelphia: WB Saunders, 1997.

Davies MK, Giles TD. ACE inhibitors in heart failure: Advancing clinical practice. In Mechanisms and management (satellite symposium to the 3rd International Congress on Heart Failure, Geneva, May 21–25, 1995). Basel: S. Karger, 1996.

Department of Health and Human Services, Centers for Disease Control and Prevention. Intravascular device-related infections prevention. Federal Register, Part II, Sept 27, 1995.

DiNardo JA. Anesthesia for cardiac surgery. 2nd ed. Stamford, CT: Appleton & Lange, 1998.

Donlevy JA, Pietruch BL. The connection delivery model: Care across the continuum. Nurse Manage 1996; 27(5):34.

Doty DB. Cardiac surgery: Operative technique. St. Louis: Mosby, 1997.

Earp JK, Shah HS. Cardiac surgery. AACN Clin Issues Adv Pract Acute Crit Care 1997; 8(1):1.

Edmunds LH. Cardiac surgery in the adult. New York: McGraw-Hill, 1997.

Edwards D, Hess L: Aggressive weaning in cardiac surgical patients. Dimens Crit Care Nurs 1996; 15(4):181.

Ellis MF. Low cardiac output following cardiac surgery: Critical thinking steps. Dimens Crit Care Nurs 1997; 16(1):48.

Elkayam U. A symposium—Nitrates in congestive heart failure: New mechanisms and rationale for use. Am J Cardiol 1996; 77(13):1.

Fowler JP. How to respond rapidly when chest pain strikes your patient. Nursing 96 1996; 26(4):42.

Froelicher VF, Quaglietti S. Handbook of ambulatory cardiology. Boston: Lippincott-Raven, 1997.

Glaxo Wellcome, Inc. Pre-operative cardiac risk assessment: Working towards a consensus (videocassette). Salt Lake City: University Hospital, 1997.

Glennen S, Metcalfe H. Cardiology: Minimally invasive cardiac surgery (MICS). Nurs Stand 1996;11(5):54.

Grech ED, Ramsdale DR. Practical interventional cardiology. St. Louis: Mosby, 1997.

Holmes DR, Serruys PW. Current review of interventional cardiology. 3rd ed. Philadelphia: Current Medicine, 1997.

Intili H. Overlooked drug effect: Cardiovascular drugs and older patients. Am J Nurs 1995; 95(12):17.

Jarvis C. Physical examination and health assessment. 2nd ed. Philadelphia: WB Saunders, 1996.

Jensen L, King KM. Women and heart disease: The issues. Crit Care Nurse, 1997; 17(2):45.

Kawachi I, Colditz GA, Speizer FE, et al. A prospective study of passive smoking and coronary heart disease. Circulation 1997; 95(10):2374.

Kee JL. Laboratory and diagnostic test with nursing implications. 4th ed. Norwalk, CT: Appleton & Lange, 1995.

Kenny RA. Syncope in the older patient: Causes, investigations and consequences of syncope and falls. London: Chapman & Hall, 1996.

Keresztes PA, Kuruzar L. Very early extubation: Extubating in the OR following coronary artery bypass. Dimens Crit Care Nurs 1996; 15(4):198.

Khonsari S, Sintek C. Cardiac surgery: Safeguards and pitfalls in operative technique. 2nd ed. Philadelphia: Lippincott-Raven, 1997.

Krieger KH, Isom OW. Blood conservation and transfusion in cardiac surgery. New York: Springer, 1997.

Landreneau RJ, Mack MJ, Magovern JA, et al. "Keyhole" coronary artery bypass surgery. Ann Surg 1996; 224(4):453.

Lau KW, Ding ZP, Gao W, et al. Percutaneous balloon mitral valvuloplasty in patients with mitral restenosis after previous surgical commissurotomy: A matched comparative study. Eur Heart J 1996; 26(11):42.

Lazzara D, Sellergren C. Chest pain emergencies: Making the right call when the pressure is on. Nursing 96 1996; 26(11):42.

Leier CV. Positive inotropic therapy: An update and new agents. St. Louis: Mosby, 1996.

Lytle BW. Minimally invasive cardiac surgery (editorial, comment). J Thorac Cardiovasc Surg 1996; 111(3):554.

MacKenzie GS, Heinle SK. Echocardiography and Doppler assessment of prosthetic heart valves with transesophageal echocardiography. Crit Care Clin 1996; 12(2):383.

Metcalfe H, Cox W. Cardiology: Cardiomyoplasty. Nurs Stand 1996; 11(5):49.

Moreira LF, Bocchi EA, Stolf NA, et al. Dynamic cardiomyoplasty in the treatment of dilated cardiomyopathy: Current results and perspectives. J Card Surg 1996; 11(3):207.

Moss AJ, Stern S. Noninvasive electrocardiology: Clinical aspects of Holter monitoring. London: WB Saunders, 1996.

Nagueh SF, Zoghbi WA. Stress echocardiography for the assessment of myocardial ischemia and viability. St. Louis: Mosby, 1996.

Nightingale K. Minimal invasive cardiac surgery. Br J Theatre Nurs 1996; 6(7):41.

Peterson KL, Nicod P. Cardiac catheterization: Methods, diagnosis, and therapy. Philadelphia: WB Saunders, 1997.

Pinnell N. Nursing pharmacology. Philadelphia: WB Saunders, 1996.

Pratt CM. Calcium antagonists: Class distinctions, current controversies, and future trends. Am J Cardiol 19XX; 79(9A):1.

Rahimtoola SH. The use of digitalis in heart failure. St. Louis: Mosby, 1996.

Redecker NS, Sadowski AV. Update of cardiovascular drugs and elders. Am J Nurs 1995; 95(9):34.

Riddle MM, Dunstan JL, Castanis JL. A rapid recovery program for cardiac surgery patients. Am J Crit Care 1996; 5(2):152.

Salerno TA. Warm heart surgery. London: Edward Arnold, 1995.

Salisbury C. Rehabilitation after myocardial infarction: The role of the community nurse. Nurs Stand 1996; 10(23):49.

Shannon MT, Wilson BA, Stang CL. Govoni & Hayes drugs and nursing implications. 8th ed. Norwalk, CT: Appleton & Lange, 1995.

Shyu KG, Lin JL, Chen JJ, Chang J. Use of cardiac troponin t, creatine kinase and its isoform to monitor myocardial injury during radiofrequency ablation for supraventricular tachycardia. Cardiology 1996; 87(5):392.

Smalling RW. A symposium—Controveries in thrombolytic therapy. Am J Cardiol 1996; 78(12A):1.

Smith DF, Bumann R. Assessing and treating decreased cardiac output. MEDSURG Nurs 1993; 2(5):351.

Stamatis SJ, Spadoni SM. Getting to the heart of IABP therapy. RN 1997; 60(1):38.

St. John Sutton MG, Oldershaw PJ, Kotler MN (eds). Textbook of echocardiography and Doppler in adults and children. 2nd ed. Cambridge, MA: Blackwell Scientific Publications, 1996.

Taylor SH. Beta-blockers in heart failure: Myths and realities (satellite symposium to the XIIth World Congress of Cardiology and the XVth Congress of the European Society of Cardiology, Berling, Sept 13, 1994). London: WB Saunders, 1996.

US Preventive Services Task Force (USPSTF) Guide to Clinical Preventive Services. 2nd ed. Baltimore: Williams & Wilkins, 1996.

Vaca KJ, Lohamnn DP, Moskoff ME. Cardiac surgery in the octogenarian: Nursing implications. Heart Lung 1994; 23(5):413.

Williams JP. Postoperative management of the cardiac surgical patient. New York: Churchill-Livingstone, 1996.

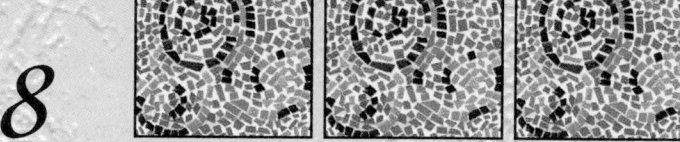
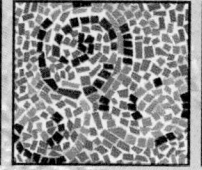
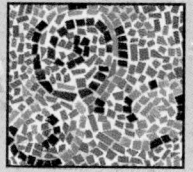
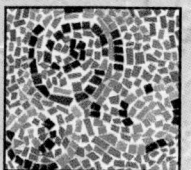

8

Nursing Care of Patients with Cardiac Disorders

Study Outcomes

After studying this chapter, you should be able to:

1. Describe the etiology, pathophysiology, clinical manifestations, diagnostic procedures, and collaborative management of common cardiac disorders.
2. Identify pharmacologic agents commonly used to treat cardiac disorders.
3. Describe health teaching appropriate for the patient at risk for coronary artery disease.
4. Identify information and physical examination data essential to the assessment of patients with common cardiac disorders.
5. State nursing diagnoses and related expected patient outcomes commonly applicable to patients with cardiac disorders.
6. Describe nursing interventions, with their rationales, commonly applicable to patients with cardiac disorders.
7. Explain the basis for evaluation of nursing care provided to patients with common cardiac disorders.
8. Identify alternative treatment and care settings for patients with cardiac disorders and the services related to community-based care.
9. Identify special considerations for the elderly patient with a cardiac disorder.

Cardiac disorders range from coronary artery disease to disorders of the cardiac valves to cardiac tumors and trauma. Regardless of the specific cardiac problem, however, cardiac disorders have a number of features—such as treatments, clinical manifestations, and complications—in common. Because the heart is responsible for delivering oxygen and nutrients via the blood to all parts of the body, the impact of cardiac disorders on other body systems is an important consideration. For all cardiac disorders, the primary goal of medical, surgical, and nursing management is to restore the patient to optimal cardiac function with minimal restrictions in daily activities.

The current trend toward early discharge and toward management of patients at home also extends to patients with cardiac problems. Therefore, careful early planning is an essential aspect of car-

diac care. Thorough assessment of the patient's home environment, and of the support systems that the patient has in place, is critical to ensure optimal restoration of function. Early planning also helps ensure that essential services are in place for the patient. Detailed teaching of the patient and family members is more crucial than ever in this era of early hospital discharges.

*I*nfections and Inflammations

INFECTIVE ENDOCARDITIS

Infective endocarditis is a microbial infection of the endothelial surface of the heart. This infection may involve a cardiac valve or an area of cardiac wall. Infective endocarditis can occur in an acute or a subacute form and is classified according to the causative organism.

Etiology and Pathophysiology

Infective endocarditis most often is caused by bacteria but may also be caused by fungi, rickettsiae, or chlamydiae.

Persons with rheumatic or degenerative disease of the cardiac valves, those with prosthetic valves, and those with a congenital cardiac anomaly are at increased risk for endocarditis. In this group, normal body flora become common causative organisms. These normal flora include the following:

- *Streptococcus viridans*, which inhabits the oral cavity
- Enterococci from the bowel, the female genitourinary system, and the urinary tract of men with prostatic obstruction.

Bacteria from the oropharynx may enter the blood stream during surgical or dental procedures (including cleaning), or from vigorous chewing or use of an oral irrigating jet in patients with gum disease. Bacteria from the bowel or genitourinary system may enter the blood stream during gastrointestinal or genitourinary surgical procedures or instrumentation, including catheter insertion and pelvic examination. When these bacteria enter the blood stream, they may result in subacute bacterial endocarditis, which is characterized by gradual onset and a clinical course of longer than 6 weeks.

Subacute infection in persons with pre-existing cardiac lesions is also caused by gram-negative coccobacilli referred to as the HACEK organisms. They include:

> Haemophilus aphrophilus and other Haemophilus species
> Actinobacillus actinomycetemcomitans
> Cardiobacterium hominis
> Eikenella corrodens
> Kingella kingae

More virulent and invasive organisms can attack the endothelium of normal valves and heart walls, causing rapid tissue destruction and sites of suppuration. This acute bacterial endocarditis has a rapid onset and, if untreated, can lead to death in a matter of days or weeks. The most frequent cause of native valve bacterial endocarditis is Staphylococcus aureus, which occurs as a nosocomial acquired infection and is also common among intravenous drug abusers who use unsterile needles or drugs. Other frequent causes of native valve bacterial endocarditis among intravenous drug abusers are the gram-negative bacilli Pseudomonas aeruginosa, P. cepacia, and Serratia marcescens. Fungal endocarditis occurs in intravenous drug abusers as well as in persons with prosthetic valves, long-term central venous catheters, and those on steroids or immunosuppressive medications.

Valve disorders and congenital anomalies predispose to infective endocarditis because blood is driven from an area of high pressure on one side of the defect to an area of low pressure on the other. This promotes platelet adhesion and formation of a fibrin clot to which microorganisms traveling in the blood stream can adhere. The resultant mass is called a *vegetation*. These vegetative growths can scar and perforate the valve leaflets, rupture the chordae tendinae, or erode into the septum or myocardium. Vegetations may also break free and embolize to the skin, kidneys, or lungs, causing petechiae, renal injury, or pulmonary infarcts.

Clinical Manifestations

Patients with acute bacterial endocarditis become ill suddenly, have a high fever, and exhibit symptoms of septicemia, valvular insufficiency, and heart failure. Patients with subacute bacterial endocarditis become ill gradually. They complain of flu-like symptoms of headache, general malaise, anorexia, weakness, fatigue, muscle aches, joint pain, low back pain, and sweats. They have weight loss and anemia. A low-grade fever is also typical, although it may be absent in the elderly and in patients taking corticosteroids or anti-infective agents.

Linear splinter hemorrhages appear in the nail-bed, and petechiae develop on the conjunctivae, the oropharynx, and the skin, particularly that of the lower extremities. Splenomegaly and heart murmurs develop and may change over time as valve damage occurs. If undiagnosed or untreated for an extended length of time, clubbing and Osler's nodes (tender, purplish nodules in the subcutaneous tissue of the finger pads) may also be seen.

In some patients, initial symptoms result from systemic embolization. They may include dyspnea, palpitations, symptoms of cerebrovascular accident (such as headache and transient ischemic attack), myocardial infarction, recurrent pneumonia, pulmonary abscess, or renal failure.

Diagnosis

The diagnosis of bacterial endocarditis is based on positive blood cultures, usually a series of cultures to ensure adequate sampling. These cultures are best obtained over a 3- to 4-day period while the patient is running a fever. An echocardiogram may demonstrate the presence of vegetations on the valves. Cardiac catheterization may be performed to evaluate valve function.

Management

Basic management consists of continuous intravenous antibiotic therapy administered at home for 4 to 6 weeks to eliminate the infecting organisms from the vegetative growths (Highlight 8–1). Bacteriocidal serum levels of the antibiotic are monitored. If the serum does not demonstrate bacteriocidal activity, the dose is increased or a different drug is given. Amphotericin B is the agent of choice for fungal endocarditis. Blood cultures are also done to monitor the course of treatment.

If bacteria have produced widespread valve destruction, the patient may need valve replacement and surgical débridement of infected perivalvular tissue. Valve replacement is also performed in patients who have experienced more than one serious systemic embolic episode. Valve-replacement surgery cannot be done until all traces of bacterial infection are eliminated, because sutures into bacteria-invaded tissue will not hold and the prosthetic valve will ultimately disengage.

Prevention is a key aspect of management. Prophylactic antibiotic therapy is recommended for patients with most congenital heart diseases, rheumatic or other acquired valvular disease, hypertrophic cardiomyopathy, mitral valve prolapse or insufficiency, prosthetic heart valves, and a history of infective endocarditis. Because of the risk of bacteria lodging in the heart, these patients should receive prophylactic antibiotics for any procedures associated with transient bacteremia, including the following:

- Oral procedures likely to cause bleeding
- Upper respiratory tract surgery
- Procedures that employ a rigid scope (such as bronchoscopy) and balloon dilatation of the esophagus, which disrupt the respiratory or gastrointestinal mucosa

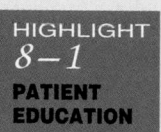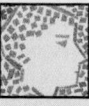

HIGHLIGHT
8–1

PATIENT EDUCATION

Continuous Intravenous Antibiotic Therapy Administered at Home for Infective Endocarditis

Include the following topics in patient teaching for home parenteral antibiotics:

Site care (may be peripheral, a peripherally inserted central line, or a central line)

- Reinforce the need for strict asepsis.
- Demonstrate dressing changes for the site, and have the patient or a family member give a return demonstration.
- Instruct the patient to report redness, swelling, tenderness, or drainage.
- Tell the patient to check temperature if unusual symptoms develop.

Flushing routine

- Review strict asepsis.
- Provide a telephone number for the patient or family to call in case of difficulty with the flushing routine.

Medication administration

- Teach about the pump, tubing, needles, and any other pertinent parts of the system.
- Reinforce the importance of administering antibiotics on time.
- Check to be sure that medication delivery and pick-up services are in place.

- Surgery or instrumentation of the genitourinary tract, and surgery involving infected tissue

❖ Settings, Providers, and Collaboration for Care

Patients with infective endocarditis typically are managed at home, with home health nurses monitoring the long-term intravenous administration of antibiotics and compliance with activity restrictions and other aspects of the plan of care. The home health nurse also assesses the patient's response to therapy and contacts the physician if symptoms of complications arise, such as embolization or heart failure. Assistance from a home health aide may be required if the patient lives alone or with someone unable to maintain the household. Hospitalization is required if the patient develops complications or needs valve replacement surgery.

NURSING PROCESS
Infective Endocarditis

Assessment

Review the patient's history, present signs and symptoms, and diagnostic test results. Determine if the patient has a history of strep throat, scarlet fever, rheumatic fever, congenital heart disease, cardiac surgery, or IV drug use. Assess the patient's vital signs. Ask about headache, malaise, fatigue, weakness, dyspnea, palpitations, and fainting spells. Inquire about anorexia, weight loss, muscle aches, back pain, joint pain, chest pain, or night sweats. Auscultate heart sounds to determine whether any abnormal sounds are present, such as an S_3 or S_4, friction rubs, or murmurs. Check breath sounds for crackles and observe for cough, dyspnea, and use of accessory muscles that could indicate left-sided heart failure. Observe for edema and neck vein distention that could indicate right-sided heart failure. Examine the patient for petechiae in the conjunctiva, mouth, and skin.

Nursing Diagnoses and Planning

Nursing diagnoses and related expected patient outcomes commonly applicable to patients with infective endocarditis include the following:

NDx: Pain (muscle aches, back, joint, or chest) related to systemic infection and inflammation of the myocardium and pericardium

Planning: Patient Outcomes
1. Patient rates pain as less than 3 on a scale of 0 to 10.
2. Patient uses relaxation skills and diversional activities to decrease awareness of pain.

NDx: Activity intolerance related to fatigue

Planning: Patient Outcomes
1. Patient rates fatigue as less than 4 on a scale of 0 to 10 during or after activity.
2. Patient tolerates increasing levels of activity, as indicated by systolic blood pressure less than 10 over baseline, pulse rate less than 20 over baseline during activity, and freedom from chest pain, dyspnea, and lightheadedness.
3. Patient describes a realistic and appropriate plan of activity to follow after discharge.

NDx: Risk for altered health maintenance related to insufficient knowledge about the need for long-term therapy, follow-up, and ways to prevent recurrence or complications

Planning: Patient Outcomes
1. Patient describes the treatment program, possible complications, and prevention plan.
2. Patient verbalizes ability and willingness to comply with the plan of treatment and prevention.

Nursing Interventions and Evaluations

NDx: Pain
Investigate all complaints of chest pain and joint

pain. Use a pain scale of 0 to 10 or 0 to 5 (on which 0 equals no pain) for objective measurement. Document the onset of pain and factors that aggravate and relieve the pain. Maintain a quiet environment and provide comfort measures as needed. They may include positioning, back rubs, application of heat or cold, and emotional support. Teach relaxation exercises to help the patient control pain. Give prescribed medications, such as nonsteroidal anti-inflammatories (NSAIDs), for pain as necessary. Evaluate the patient's response to all pain-control measures and maintain ongoing collaboration with the health-care team to implement an effective plan to control pain and provide rest.

NDx: Activity intolerance

Arrange for uninterrupted sleep periods to reduce fatigue. Plan care to limit interruptions and schedule visitors, as needed, so the patient can have uninterrupted periods of rest. Have the patient perform range-of-motion exercises as tolerated during the day to maintain and increase strength and endurance. If active range-of-motion exercises are not possible, provide passive range-of-motion at least twice daily. Allow at least 30 minutes of rest between all activities and provide assistance with activities as necessary. Provide six small meals during the day to conserve the patient's strength and energy. In cases of severe activity intolerance, judge the patient's tolerance by observing for dyspnea and by checking blood pressure and heart rate before, during, and after activity. Stress the importance of not becoming over-fatigued and of resting immediately if chest pain, lightheadedness, or difficulty breathing occurs.

NDx: Risk for altered health maintenance

Explain the effects of inflammation on the heart and other affected tissues. Educate the patient and family about signs and symptoms of recurrence, symptoms to report, and actions to take that will reduce the possibility of future recurrence. Discuss the use of antibiotics, the time period for their use, and procedures that require prophylaxis throughout the patient's remaining life (Highlight 8–2).

Compare the patient's status with the expected outcomes. If the outcomes are not met, reassess the patient and revise the plan.

RHEUMATIC HEART DISEASE

Rheumatic fever is a systemic inflammatory disorder that follows pharyngeal infection with Group A *Streptococcus* in about 1 in 10 affected people. Rheumatic heart disease refers to the effects of rheumatic fever on the heart during the acute stage of the disease as well as to its long-term cardiac sequelae. Rheumatic fever, and hence rheumatic heart disease, can be prevented by treating the Group A streptococcal infections.

The incidence of rheumatic fever in the United States, as in all developed countries, has decreased markedly since World War II; however, pockets and

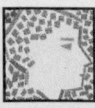

HIGHLIGHT 8–2

PATIENT EDUCATION

Instructions for the Patient Recovering from Infective Endocarditis

Instruct the patient with infective endocarditis to:

- Take the prescribed antibiotics exactly as ordered for the full length of time specified. Stress that although symptoms may disappear, it is imperative that they be taken as ordered to clear the infection completely and to prevent other infections from developing during recuperation.
- Report chest pain, dyspnea, and recurrence or worsening of other symptoms to the health-care provider.
- Avoid close contact with individuals with infections, colds, or influenza.
- Practice good dental hygiene: use a soft-bristled tooth brush and floss regularly.
- Practice good skin care: Do not pick scabs or pimples; do not cut cuticles too short; avoid body piercing and tattoos.
- Prevent constipation since difficult passage of dry stool may traumatize rectal tissues.
- Avoid sexual activities such as anal intercourse that may traumatize delicate tissues.
- Avoid illicit injectable drugs.
- See a dentist regularly and inform him or her of history since any procedure that causes bleeding gums may require antibiotic prophylaxis.
- Inform physician of history before any gynecologic, genitourinary, or gastrointestinal instrumentation.

outbreaks of the disease still persist. Social factors that predispose to rheumatic fever include overcrowding (with its increased incidence of pharyngeal streptococcal infection) and low socioeconomic status (associated with poor access to medical care and the antibiotics needed to treat pharyngeal streptococcal infection). Rheumatic heart disease in the form of chronic valvular disease remains prevalent among adults who had rheumatic fever as children or adolescents.

Etiology and Pathophysiology

Focal inflammatory lesions called Aschoff's nodules are characteristic of rheumatic fever. These lesions, which have a central area of necrotic connective tissue surrounded by inflammatory cells, develop around small blood vessels and throughout the heart. As they regress with time, areas of fibrosis remain. In the heart, these lesions can result in pericarditis, myocarditis (which is associated with decreased contractile strength of the heart), and endocarditis. Rheumatic pericarditis and myocarditis typically resolve without consequence. Rheumatic endocarditis, on the other hand, can damage the cardiac valves that develop fibrotic scarring, which thickens, retracts, and fuses the leaflets. This process leaves the valve narrowed (stenotic) and commonly incompetent. An incompetent valve cannot close completely, thus allowing blood to regurgitate or flow backward through the valve. The mitral valve is affected most commonly, followed by the aortic valve, and then the tricuspid.

Clinical Manifestations

Rheumatic fever has four distinct clinical stages. The clinical manifestations of rheumatic fever and rheumatic heart disease vary with the stage at which the disease is detected. The first stage is that of acute streptococcal pharyngeal infection. This stage lasts about a week and is characterized by fever, chills, acute onset sore throat with diffuse erythema and exudate on the oropharynx, and lymphadenopathy. This is followed by a latent period of a few days to 3 weeks, during which time the patient looks and feels well.

Stage III then ensues and may last from a few weeks to more than a year. It is during stage III that the acute manifestations of rheumatic fever appear. They include:

- Carditis
- Acute migratory polyarthritis, which usually causes severe pain and swelling of the large joints of the lower extremities
- Chorea (involuntary motor movements)
- Rash and subcutaneous nodules over tendons and bony surfaces

The fourth clinical stage is known by chronic sequelae, such as valvular deformity. Rheumatic fever does not always result in the chronic sequelae of rheumatic heart disease. In some patients, valvular damage heals spontaneously after the acute stage of the disease. In others, valvular damage worsens over time and symptoms of heart failure develop when the myocardium can no longer overcome the effects of valvular stenosis and regurgitation. Refer to the discussion of valvular disease and heart failure in this chapter for signs and symptoms specific to these disorders. Rheumatic fever is rare in adults and tends to be mild. It has more significant effects on the joints than on the heart. For this reason, rheumatic fever in adults is sometimes called *poststreptococcal arthritis*.

Diagnosis

There is no definitive test for rheumatic fever. The diagnosis is based on a combination of clinical and laboratory findings. These include a history of throat cultures positive for *Streptococcus,* a rising antistreptolysin O titer (which indicates antibody production), an elevated erythrocyte sedimentation rate (ESR), the appearance of C-reactive protein in the serum, leukocytosis in the presence of fever, polyarthritis, and symptoms of carditis. Some cases of rheumatic fever are relatively asymptomatic and remain undiagnosed until a health-care provider hears a heart murmur and an echocardiogram reveals valvular abnormalities. Upon careful review of the patient's history in these cases, a childhood episode of "growing pains" typically appears.

Management

There is no cure for rheumatic fever, so the goal of treatment is to prevent or control it to avoid recurrence. An initial attack of rheumatic fever can be prevented by prompt treatment of streptococcal pharyngitis with 1.2 million units of long-acting benzathine penicillin intramuscularly or 400,000 to 600,000 units orally every 4 hours for 10 days. If rheumatic fever has developed, salicylates are given to reduce joint inflammation, thereby relieving pain and swelling. Corticosteroids also may be used to help reduce inflammation and scarring of cardiac tissue, although their effectiveness for this purpose is still debated. For patients with severe cardiac involvement, physical activity is restricted for 6 weeks or more during the acute stage.

Since patients who have one attack of rheumatic fever are highly likely to have another, prophylaxis with 1.2 million units of long-acting benzathine penicillin IM every 28 days or 200,000 units orally twice a day continuously is begun as soon as the initial disease is treated. Prophylaxis is continued for at least 5 years. Once discontinued, it is resumed before any surgical, invasive diagnostic, or dental procedure.

For patients with long-term rheumatic heart disease, management is as described for cardiac valvular disease and may involve valve replacement or repair.

NURSING PROCESS GUIDELINES
Rheumatic Heart Disease

Nursing care of patients during the acute phase of rheumatic heart disease is similar to that for patients with endocarditis, with additional considerations related to the discomfort and activity limitation imposed by significant joint involvement.

MYOCARDITIS

Myocarditis is an inflammation of the heart muscle. It may be acute or chronic.

Etiology and Pathophysiology

Myocarditis occurs as both a primary and a secondary disorder. The cause of primary myocarditis is unknown. The cause of secondary myocarditis may be either infectious or noninfectious. Infectious causes include bacteria, rickettsiae, fungi, and such viruses as the picornavirus, coxsackievirus B and A, and echovirus. Noninfectious causes include drug hypersensitivity reactions, autoimmune reactions (as in systemic lupus erythematosus and rheumatic fever), and toxic reactions. Myocarditis usually develops secondary to acute endocarditis, pericarditis, or systemic infection. It also occurs in patients on immunosuppressive therapy and is associated with acquired immunodeficiency syndrome.

Clinical Manifestations

With acute viral myocarditis, patients have flu-like symptoms, including fatigue, fever, lymphadenopathy, pharyngitis, myalgias, and gastrointestinal problems. Cardiac signs and symptoms include pericardial pain, a friction rub, distant heart sounds, systolic murmur, pulsus alternans (a regular alteration between weak and strong beats), syncope, symptoms of heart failure, and pericardial effusion. In addition, hepatitis, encephalitis, nephritis, and orchitis may occur.

Diagnosis

Diagnosis is based on history and physical examination. Nonspecific laboratory findings include mild to moderate leukocytosis with atypical lymphocytes, elevated ESR, and elevated enzymes, such as lactic dehydrogenase, creatinine kinase, and transaminase. Chest x-ray may reveal an enlarged heart. Electrocardiographic changes include ST elevation or T wave flattening, appearance of Q waves, and a prolonged QT interval. These abnormal findings may return to normal after recovery or may persist for several years. Diagnosis can only be confirmed by an endomyocardial biopsy within the first 6 weeks of acute illness, during the time when lymphocytic infiltration and myopathic damage are present.

Management

Treatment is aimed at the underlying cause of the myocarditis, if it is known. Antimicrobial therapy is used to eradicate infection in cases in which an infecting organism has been identified. In noninfectious cases, immunosuppressive agents may be used to decrease the inflammatory response. In all instances, the patient is maintained on bedrest to reduce cardiac workload and the risk of myocardial damage. To decrease the risk of venous thrombosis and embolism, antiembolism stockings are applied and active and passive range-of-motion exercises are performed. Daily aspirin or anticoagulant therapy may be instituted. If heart failure occurs, standard pharmacologic and other supportive therapy for that disorder is instituted. If dysrhythmias develop, treatment includes continuous cardiac monitoring and anti-arrhythmic therapy.

Complications

Complications of myocarditis include damage to the heart muscle that results in cardiac enlargement and mural and venous thrombi. Pericardial effusion and tamponade may also occur.

❖ **Settings, Providers, and Collaboration for Care**

Patients with myocarditis are treated at home unless dysrhythmias or complications that require telemetry or other monitoring develop. A home health nurse monitors the patient's condition, administration of antibiotic therapy (if the disease has a bacterial origin), and compliance with instructions to remain on bedrest to decrease cardiac workload. Depending on the availability of support from significant others, the patient also may need assistance with meals, household maintenance, and self-care.

NURSING PROCESS GUIDELINES
Myocarditis

Nursing care of patients with myocarditis is essentially the same as for patients with endocarditis, with the following considerations. Patients with myocarditis are prone to digitalis toxicity and must be monitored closely for signs of toxicity if this drug is used to improve cardiac function. Further, patients must be instructed to increase activity gradually, and to avoid alcohol and competitive sports because of the risk of further myocardial damage.

PERICARDITIS

Pericarditis is an inflammation of the membrane that surrounds that heart. It may be acute or chronic.

Acute Pericarditis
Etiology and Pathophysiology

Acute pericarditis occurs as both a primary and a secondary disorder. Primary pericarditis is assumed to be viral in origin. Secondary pericarditis can result from rheumatic disease, radiation therapy, or a transmural infarct. Both types tend to follow a short, uncomplicated course. Rarely, acute pericarditis may become recurrent, probably from a hypersensitivity reaction, or may progress to chronic constrictive pericarditis.

Clinical Manifestations

A major clinical manifestation of acute pericarditis is sudden, severe, constant pain over the anterior chest that worsens on inspiration and typically lasts up to 48 hours. The pain may radiate to the back or neck, over the left shoulder, or down the left arm. Usually, it is accompanied by sinus tachycardia and a low-grade fever. Patients with acute pericarditis may also complain of weakness, malaise, irritability, and dysphagia.

On auscultation, a pericardial friction rub is audible in most patients. It sounds like two pieces of leather being rubbed together or like a squeaky shoe. The friction rub may be transient throughout the inflammatory period of 7 to 10 days. Leukocytosis and an elevated ESR are present.

Diagnosis

Diagnosis of acute pericarditis is based on the history, physical examination findings, and electrocardiographic changes. The latter include elevation of the ST segment in some leads and depression of the P-R segment. As the infection resolves, electrocardiographic waveforms return to normal. Echocardiography may demonstrate nonspecific pericardial thickening in cases of constrictive pericarditis. However, this disorder is best diagnosed by computed tomography (CT) scan.

Management

Since the cause of acute pericarditis is usually unknown, relief of symptoms is the goal of treatment. Rest is encouraged. Oral analgesics, such as codeine, are given for pain. Salicylates or NSAIDs are given to reduce inflammation. If symptoms are not relieved by these conservative measures, corticosteroids may be given. They are tapered gradually to zero over 2 to 4 weeks as soon as symptoms resolve.

If bacterial or fungal infection causes pericarditis, antimicrobial therapy begins as soon as the infectious organism is identified.

Chronic Constrictive Pericarditis

Chronic constrictive pericarditis is characterized by a thickened fibrous pericardium that restricts the movement of the heart and hence interferes with its ability to pump. It can result from trauma, neoplastic disease, or, rarely, the progression of acute pericarditis. Symptoms of chronic constrictive pericarditis result from impaired cardiac pumping and include dyspnea on exertion, fatigue, anorexia, weight loss, edema, and distended neck veins.

Treatment is designed to improve the heart's pumping action, usually with digitalis, diuretics, and a low-sodium diet. If medical management is not effective, the patient may undergo a pericardiectomy, during which the pericardium is opened through a median sternotomy approach.

NURSING PROCESS GUIDELINES
Pericarditis

Closely monitor the patient for signs and symptoms of cardiac tamponade and heart failure. Give analgesics for pain and help the patient find a position of comfort. Often this means sitting up supported with pillows, or leaning forward on an overbed table or other support. Since the pain tends to worsen with turning, twisting, and coughing, these activities should be avoided as much as possible. Teach the patient and family about prescribed medications and explain the expected course of the disease. If a pericardiectomy is performed for chronic constrictive pericarditis, provide care as described in Chapter 7 for the patient undergoing heart surgery.

PERICARDIAL EFFUSION

Pericardial effusion is an abnormal accumulation of fluid in the pericardial cavity.

Etiology and Pathophysiology

Virtually all pericardial disorders can cause fluid to accumulate in the pericardial space, but the type of fluid varies with the specific disease process involved (Table 8–1). Pericardial effusions may develop rapidly or slowly over a period of days or weeks. Effusion that develops rapidly, even if it involves a relatively small amount of fluid over the usual 30 to 50 mL in the pericardial space, can cause cardiac tamponade, which is a medical emergency because the heart loses its ability to pump and, as a result, cardiac output falls dramatically.

After cardiac surgery, localized cardiac tamponade may occur. In this type, one or more of the cardiac chambers is selectively compressed and symptoms vary accordingly.

Clinical Manifestations

Pericardial effusions do not always cause significant clinical manifestations. If the effusion occurs gradually and the pericardium stretches to accommodate it, the patient may be asymptomatic or complain of only a vague pain in the chest or a feeling of fullness. Distant heart sounds may be present. If cardiac tamponade occurs, symptoms depend on its severity and mimic those of right-sided heart failure. Central venous pressure is elevated, as evidenced by jugular venous distention with the head of the bed elevated, edema, hepatomegaly, tachycardia, pulsus paradoxus (greater than 10 mm Hg drop in arterial pressure during inspiration), and narrowed pulse pressure.

Diagnosis

Pericardial effusion is most accurately detected by echocardiography, which can demonstrate an effusion as small as 20 mL. MRI and CT can also demonstrate pericardial effusion and pericardial thickening.

Table 8–1

Types and Causes of Pericardial Effusion	
Type of Fluid	**Possible Causes**
Transudate	Heart failure
	Overhydration
	Hypoproteinemia
Exudate	Pericardial injury
Serosanguineous	Tuberculosis
	Neoplastic disease
	Uremia
	Radiation
	Idiopathic
	Acute myocardial infarction with cardiac rupture
	Perforation of the heart
	Coagulation defect

Clinical evaluation is the basic method of diagnosing cardiac tamponade.

Management

Treatment is aimed at eliminating the underlying cause of the effusion. Thus, conventional treatment of heart failure, pericarditis, or any other precipitating disorder begins promptly. If mild cardiac tamponade is present, it is treated with diuretics while the underlying problem is corrected.

In cases of severe tamponade, intravenous fluids are used to combat shock temporarily until the fluid causing the tamponade can be removed. Pericardial fluid can be removed by:

- Pericardiocentesis—aspiration via a needle inserted through the chest wall into the pericardial sac
- Pericardiostomy—surgical incision into the pericardial sac with tube drainage
- Pericardial fenestration—creation of a pericardial window to allow for continuous drainage of pericardial fluid through the lymphatic system and into the pericardial cavity

If the patient's central venous pressure is elevated, it is measured before and after the procedure to determine if the tamponade has been removed. Effusion fluid is sent for laboratory analysis to aid in determining the nature of the underlying disorder. Pericardiectomy may also be done. This procedure promotes formation of adhesions that obliterate the pericardial space and prevent future effusions.

NURSING PROCESS GUIDELINES
Pericardial Effusion

When caring for patients with disorders known to be associated with pericardial effusion, assess regularly and carefully for signs or symptoms of effusion. This is critical because early detection is essential to the prevention of cardiac tamponade, which carries the risk of sudden death. Once effusion is diagnosed, monitor for signs and symptoms of compromised cardiac output from tamponade. Observe for jugular venous distension, dyspnea, edema, and changes in vital signs, including pulsus paradoxus.

If a pericardiocentesis is done, maintain electrocardiographic and hemodynamic monitoring throughout and have resuscitation equipment available nearby. Check the drainage for blood during the procedure because the presence of blood that clots indicates inadvertent puncture of a cardiac structure. After the procedure, monitor heart sounds, blood pressure, and venous pressure to detect a recurrence of tamponade.

Cardiac Dysrhythmias

Cardiac dysrhythmias are abnormalities in the rate or rhythm, or both, of the heartbeat. The diagnosis of dysrhythmias is made on the basis of patient history, physical assessment, and diagnostic studies. The history and physical examination identify the presence of a symptomatic dysrhythmia and the degree to which it is affecting the patient. Diagnostic studies, especially electrocardiography, are done to confirm the presence of a dysrhythmia and to identify its type, severity, and cause (Fig. 8–1).

Dysrhythmias are named according to the site of origin and type of abnormality.

SINUS DYSRHYTHMIAS

Sinus dysrhythmias originate in the sinoatrial node. They are the most common type of dysrhythmias, often occurring in young adults and the elderly. A sinus dysrhythmia is said to exist if the P-P intervals vary by more than 0.16. Variation of less than 0.16 is considered normal because of the fluctuation of sympathetic and parasympathetic stimulation.

Sinus Bradycardia

Sinus bradycardia is a heart rate of less than 60 beats per minute arising from the sinoatrial node (Fig. 8–2). It can be a normal finding in highly trained athletes and other healthy adults, particularly during sleep.

Etiology and Pathophysiology

Pathologic causes of this dysrhythmia include inferior wall myocardial infarction, increased intracranial pressure, Addison's disease, myxedema, hypothermia, and anorexia nervosa. It can be caused by such drugs as digitalis and beta blockers (propranolol, nadolol), which can reduce the automaticity of the sinoatrial node, thus producing a slower heart rate. Sinus bradycardia can also be induced by vagal stimulation from severe pain, fear, vomiting, and bearing down during defecation. In many people, carotid sinus stimulation also results in bradycardia.

Clinical Manifestations

Most often, sinus bradycardia is asymptomatic. However, because cardiac output is determined by both heart rate and stroke volume, bradycardia has the potential to decrease cardiac output. If cardiac output falls, the patient may develop dizziness, angina, disorientation, hypotension, syncope, and even heart failure.

Management

Treatment of sinus bradycardia is warranted only for symptomatic patients and is aimed at increasing the heart rate. The simplest form of treatment is

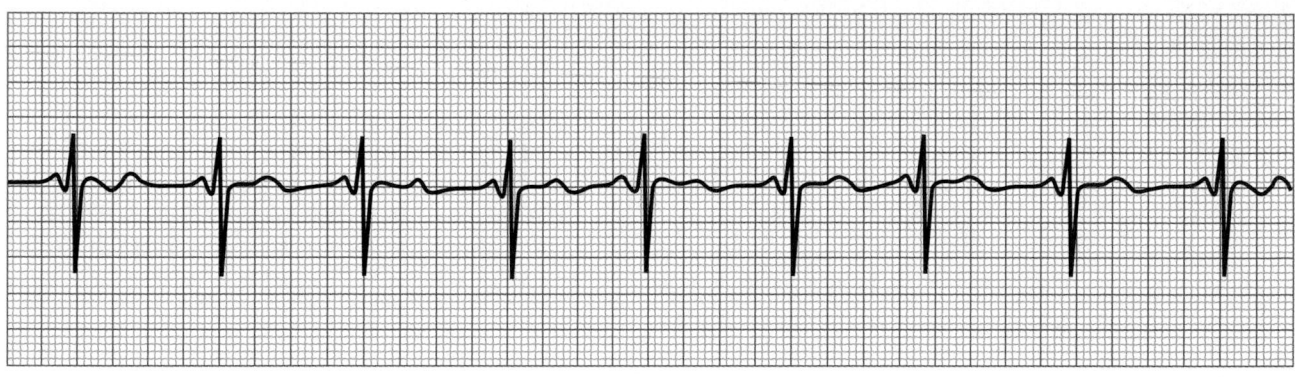

Classic Characteristics:

Pacemaker site:	Sinoatrial node
Rhythm:	Regular
Rate:	60–100 beats per minute
P waves:	Normal
QRS complex:	Normal
Intervals:	Normal
Ectopic beats:	Escape beats may be present.

Figure 8–1

Normal sinus rhythm.

removal of the causative factor. For example, if the cause is hypothermia, the patient is warmed. If the cause is drug toxicity, the drug is withheld. If the cause is vagal stimulation, factors causing vagal stimulation are controlled. If the problem cannot be managed in this way, atropine or, more rarely, isoproterenol may be administered intravenously to raise the heart rate. In refractory cases, a temporary or permanent pacemaker may be used to reverse the bradycardia and control symptoms.

Sinus Tachycardia

Sinus tachycardia is a heart rate of between 100 and 160 beats per minute arising from the sinus node (Fig. 8–3).

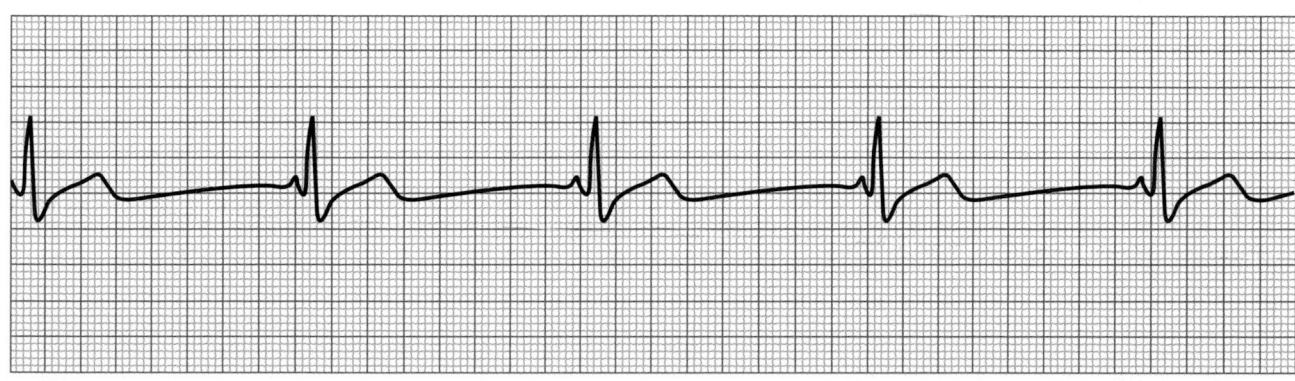

Classic Characteristics:

Pacemaker site:	Sinoatrial node
Rhythm:	Regular
Rate:	Fewer than 60 beats per minute
P waves:	Normal
QRS complex:	Normal
Intervals:	Normal
Ectopic beats:	Escape beats may be present.

Figure 8–2

Sinus bradycardia.

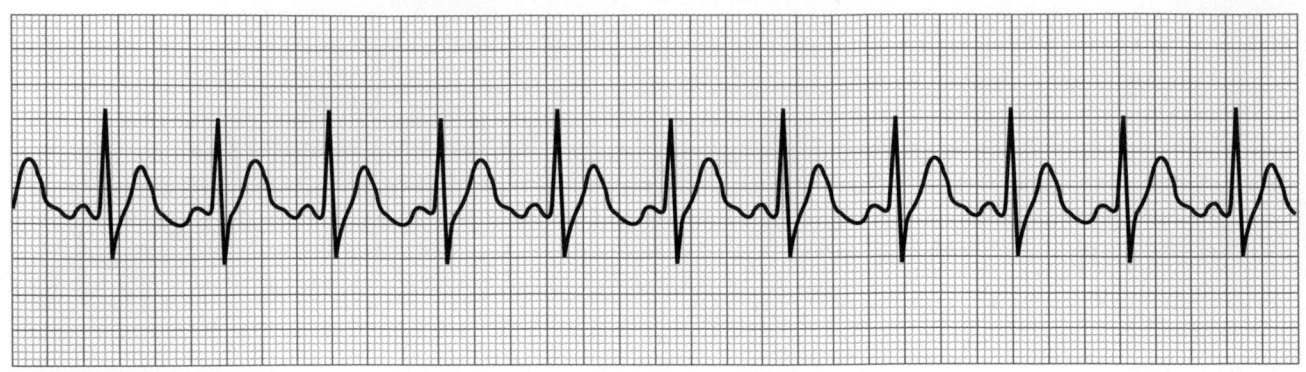

Classic Characteristics:

Pacemaker site: Sinoatrial node
Rhythm: Regular
Rate: More than 100 beats per minute
P waves: Normal but in rapid rhythms may be more peaked or lost in the T wave.
QRS complex: Normal
Intervals: P-R and Q-T intervals may shorten as the rate increases.

Figure 8-3

Sinus tachycardia.

Etiology and Pathophysiology

Sinus tachycardia is a normal response to sympathetic nervous system stimulation and to any condition that produces an increase in metabolic rate. Thus it occurs in healthy individuals as a result of excitement, fear, anxiety, and physical exertion. It is associated with the ingestion of alcohol and caffeine, with the use of nicotine, and with use of atropine and catecholamines such as epinephrine, isoproterenol, dopamine, and dobutamine. Sinus tachycardia accompanies pathologic processes, such as fever and thyrotoxicosis, that raise metabolic rate. It also occurs as a short-term compensatory mechanism to maintain circulation of oxygenated blood to body tissues in the presence of pathology such as myocardial ischemia and infarction, pulmonary embolism, heart failure, anemia, hypoxemia, and hypovolemia.

Clinical Manifestations

Sinus tachycardia produces a regular pulse rate between 100 and 160 beats per minute that may or may not be accompanied by a subjective feeling of palpitations. Most often, there are no symptoms. However because the workload (and hence the oxygen requirements) of the myocardium increases, and ventricular filling time (and hence the amount of oxygenated blood available to be pumped) decreases as the heart pumps faster, the patient with pre-existing heart disease is at risk for a drop in cardiac output and ultimately for cardiac failure. These patients may experience light-headedness, angina, disorientation, and syncope.

Management

Patients with sinus tachycardia are treated if it is causing symptoms, such as disorientation, confusion, or chest pain. The goal of management is correction or elimination of the underlying cause. Such drugs as beta-adrenergic blocking agents, calcium channel blockers, digoxin, and adenosine may be used to control the dysrhythmia while the underlying cause is being corrected.

Sinus Arrhythmia

Sinus arrhythmia is a normal variation in rhythm related to respiration (Fig. 8-4).

Etiology and Pathophysiology

With a sinus arrhythmia, the heart rate commonly is within the normal limits of 60 to 100 beats per minute, but it increases with inspiration and decreases with expiration. This slight variation in rhythm results from slowing of the automaticity of the sinoatrial node from changes in vagal tone secondary to changes in intrathoracic pressure during the cycles of respiration. Sinus arrhythmia is seen in children, the elderly, and athletes. This arrhythmia occurs rarely in other adults but can be observed in patients with heart disease who receive morphine therapy or who have digitalis toxicity.

Clinical Manifestations

Sinus arrhythmia is asymptomatic. If there is an underlying cause, clinical manifestations of the underlying cause may be present.

Management

Sinus arrhythmia is of no clinical significance, and no treatment is necessary. If the underlying cause is identified, treatment is initiated. Atropine may be indicated if the heart rate is too slow and the patient is symptomatic.

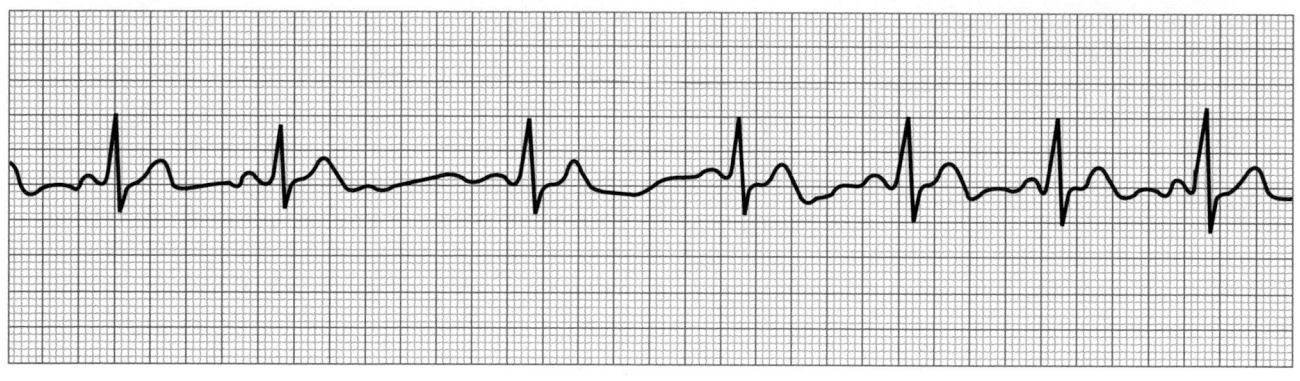

Classic Characteristics:

Pacemaker site:	Sinoatrial node
Rhythm:	Irregular
Rate:	60–100 beats per minute
P waves:	Normal
QRS complex:	Normal
Intervals:	R-R intervals are irregular.

Figure 8–4

Sinus arrhythmia.

ATRIAL DYSRHYTHMIAS

Atrial dysrhythmias result when the focus of impulse generation arises outside the sinoatrial node in the atrial tissue. The atrial tissue or ectopic focus acts as the heart's pacemaker for one or more beats. Because the origin of the impulse is in atrial tissue, the P waves differ in configuration from those that originate in the sinoatrial node. There are several atrial dysrhythmias. The most common include premature atrial contraction, paroxysmal atrial tachycardia, atrial flutter, and atrial fibrillation.

Premature Atrial Contraction

Premature atrial contraction is an ectopic beat that originates in an atrial site other than the sinoatrial node and occurs earlier than the next expected beat (Fig. 8–5).

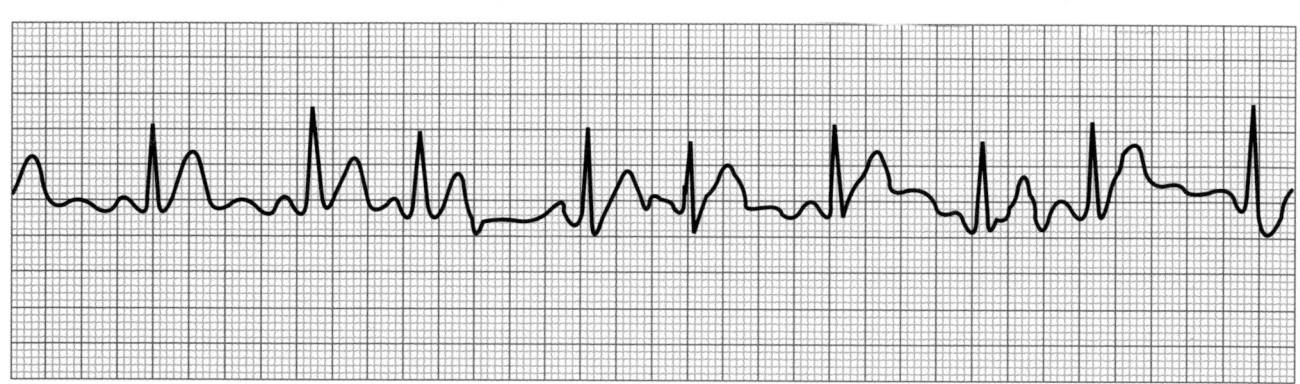

Classic Characteristics:

Pacemaker site:	Atrial tissue (single or multiple foci)
Rhythm:	Irregular because of premature beat
Rate:	Usually 60–100 beats per minute
P waves:	P wave of the ectopic beat is usually abnormal, often pointed or hidden in the previous T wave.
QRS complex:	Normal
Intervals:	P-R and R-R intervals are irregular.

Figure 8–5

Premature atrial contraction.

Etiology and Pathophysiology

Premature atrial contractions can occur in healthy individuals as a result of excessive use of caffeine, alcohol, or tobacco products as well as from stress and fatigue.

Premature atrial contractions may originate in one ectopic site or multiple sites, usually from enhanced automaticity or a re-entry phenomenon. Because impulse conduction is delayed long enough for myocardial cells to repolarize, the impulse re-enters the same tissue over and over again, resulting in many depolarizations. Premature atrial contractions are not in themselves a threat to the patient. They are of concern, however, in that they may indicate a more serious underlying problem, such as myocardial infarction, heart failure, pericarditis, valvular disorder, hypoxemia, digitalis toxicity, hypokalemia, hypomagnesemia, or metabolic alkalosis.

Clinical Manifestations

Few clinical manifestations occur with premature atrial contractions. If they occur frequently, the patient may complain of palpitations or a fluttering sensation.

Management

In most cases, patients experiencing premature atrial contractions do not require treatment. When it is necessary, treatment is based on the cause of the premature atrial contractions. If the cause is stress or excessive use of caffeine, alcohol, or tobacco, treatment involves elimination of the precipitating factor. To this end, the patient is provided with the needed education or counseling. If pharmacologic management is required, drugs such as quinidine sulfate, procainamide, digitalis (if not the cause), or disopyramide may be prescribed.

Paroxysmal Atrial Tachycardia

Paroxysmal atrial tachycardia is a very rapid, regular heart rate that occurs and stops suddenly (Fig. 8–6). The heart rate is 150 to 250 beats per minute.

Etiology and Pathophysiology

Paroxysmal atrial tachycardia, also called paroxysmal supraventricular tachycardia, may occur in the healthy person and is usually preceded by frequent premature atrial contractions, one of which precipitates the paroxysmal atrial tachycardia. This dysrhythmia involves a very rapidly firing ectopic focus involving enhanced automaticity of the atrial tissue. The conduction of the ectopic impulse occurs through a re-entry loop in and around the atrioventricular node.

Paroxysmal atrial tachycardia may be caused by sympathetic nervous system stimulation or hypermetabolic states, as seen with hyperpyrexia and hyperthyroidism. Patients with ischemic heart disease, rheumatic heart disease, and myocarditis are also at risk of developing paroxysmal atrial tachycardia.

Clinical Manifestations

The patient with paroxysmal atrial tachycardia may experience symptoms of decreased cardiac output. The rapid heart rate causes inadequate ventricular filling, resulting in reduced cardiac output with decreased perfusion to the brain and other vital organs. In addition, the rapid heart rate increases the heart's workload, thus creating a greater myocardial oxygen demand, which can lead to myocardial ischemia. The patient may complain of palpitations and a rapid (racing) heartbeat as well as dizziness, dyspnea, angina, diaphoresis, and fatigue.

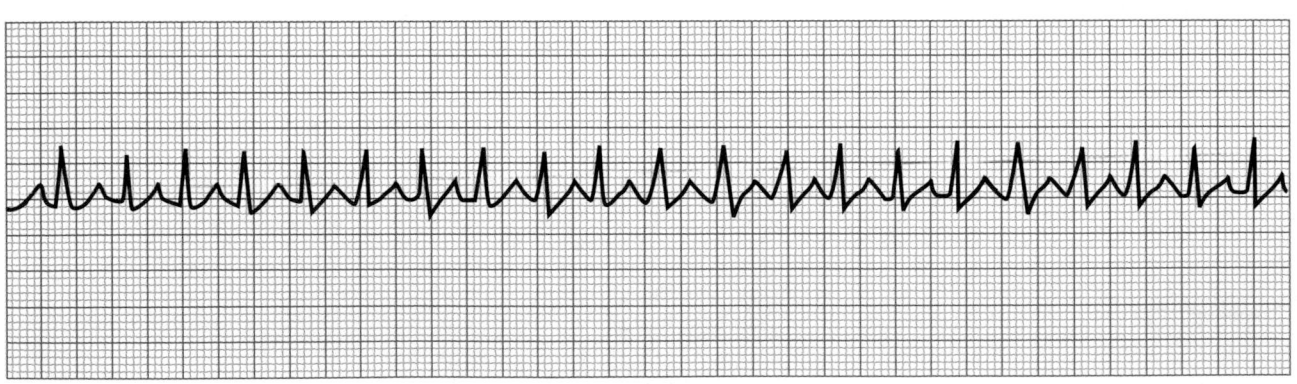

Classic Characteristics:

Pacemaker site:	Atrial tissue
Rhythm:	Regular
Rate:	150–250 beats per minute
P waves:	Usually hidden in previous T wave
QRS complex:	Normal
Intervals:	P-R intervals not measurable. The R-R interval is regular.

Figure 8–6

Paroxysmal atrial tachycardia.

Management

The management of paroxysmal atrial tachycardia depends on the patient's tolerance of the dysrhythmia. If the patient is hemodynamically stable, treatment may involve stimulating the vagus nerve by means of Valsalva's maneuver (the patient is directed to strain as if to defecate) or carotid sinus pressure (applied to one side only for not longer than 8 seconds) to slow impulse formation. If vagal stimulation fails, a 6 mg intravenous bolus of adenosine is administered rapidly over 1 to 2 seconds, followed by a 20 mL saline flush. If adenosine is administered too slowly, the conversion efficacy is decreased. If the initial dose of adenosine fails after 2 minutes, a 12 mg IV bolus is administered, again followed by a 20 mL saline flush. Patients who fail to respond to adenosine can be treated with verapamil, propranolol, or digitalis. If the patient remains unresponsive to drug therapy or is hemodynamically unstable, synchronized cardioversion is used.

Atrial Flutter

Atrial flutter is an atrial dysrhythmia that occurs when an atrial ectopic pacemaker discharges impulses at a rate of 250 to 400 beats per minute (Fig. 8–7). Atrial flutter is a less common dysrhythmia than atrial fibrillation.

Etiology and Pathophysiology

Atrial flutter is not usually identified in people with normal hearts. It occurs in relation to a variety of heart diseases, such as rheumatic, coronary, or hypertensive heart disease. It is also seen in patients with cardiomyopathy, hypoxia, heart failure, pericarditis, myocarditis, hyperthyroidism, pulmonary disease, and pulmonary emboli.

Atrial flutter is triggered by re-entry conduction. The atrial muscles respond to these rapid impulses, producing waves called flutter (F) waves. The flutter waves produce a V-shaped waveform, giving an appearance of a sawtooth. These sawtooth waves affect the baseline. Therefore, there is no isoelectric line between the F waves. T waves are often obscured by the flutter waves.

The atrioventricular node is bombarded with the rapid atrial rate but only allows some of the impulses to reach the ventricles. The other impulses are not conducted. The atrioventricular node may allow every other impulse through the atrioventricular junction, producing a 2:1 atrioventricular conduction ratio. In other words, for every two flutter waves, one is followed by the QRS complex. If the ratio remains constant, the ventricular rhythm is regular. If the conduction varies (2:1 to 4:1), the ventricular rate is irregular.

Clinical Manifestations

Patients with atrial flutter may be asymptomatic or complain of palpitations or a fluttering feeling in the chest or throat. Atrial flutter with a rapid ventricular response produces manifestations of a lowered cardiac output, as in other rapid atrial dysrhythmias. The patient may become hypotensive and develop cool, clammy skin.

Management

Digitalis, beta blockers, and calcium channel blockers are used to slow impulse conduction through the atrioventricular node. In situations in which the atrioventricular conduction rate is 1:1, immediate syn-

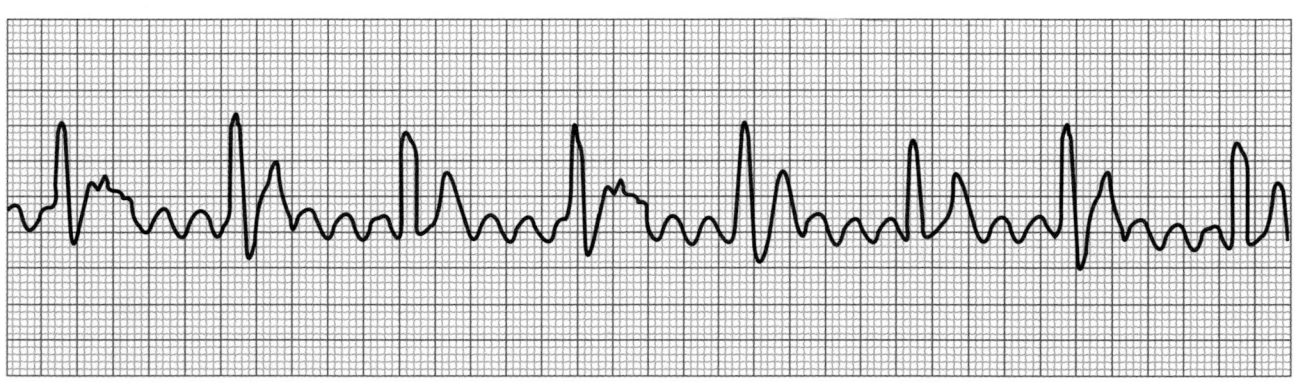

Classic Characteristics:

Pacemaker site:	Ectopic focus in atrial tissue
Rhythm:	Usually regular, but may be irregular
Rate:	Atrial rate is 250–400; ventricular rate depends on the atrioventricular conduction ratio.
P waves:	Flutter (F) waves are present, producing a sawtooth appearance.
QRS complex:	Normal
Intervals:	P-R interval not measurable. The R-R interval can be regular or irregular.

Figure 8–7

Atrial flutter.

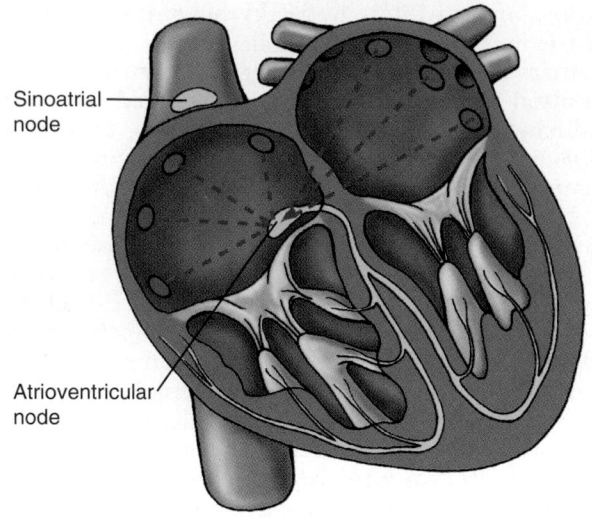

Figure 8-8

In atrial fibrillation, atrial cells other than those of the sinoatrial node discharge at a rapid, erratic rate.

chronized cardioversion is done. Atrial overdrive pacing may also be considered if time and the patient's condition permit.

Atrial Fibrillation

Atrial fibrillation is a dysrhythmia in which there are chaotic (several) ectopic atrial foci causing the atria to quiver rather than contract (Figs. 8-8 and 8-9). The atrial rate is greater than 400 beats per minute.

Etiology and Pathophysiology

Atrial fibrillation can occur in healthy people as well as in those with a variety of cardiac diseases. In healthy people, this dysrhythmia may last for a few hours to several days and is usually associated with stress or excessive alcohol consumption. Chronic atrial fibrillation is seen in patients with heart failure, mitral valve disease, rheumatic heart disease, hypertension, and hyperthyroidism.

The pathophysiology underlying atrial fibrillation is believed to be an atrial re-entry mechanism. The atrioventricular node is bombarded with multiple impulses from the atria but allows only a few impulses through to the ventricle. Because of the refractory time in the atrioventricular node, the ventricular response is grossly irregular and the ventricular rate depends on the number of impulses conducted through the atrioventricular node. When the ventricular rate is under 100, it is called *controlled atrial fibrillation*. Ventricular rates over 100 are called *uncontrolled atrial fibrillation*.

Impulses caused by the quivering atria produce irregular electrocardiographic deflections of various shapes and sizes. The waves are called flutter waves, fibrillary waves, or F waves. As in atrial flutter, these fibrillary waves affect the ECG baseline. Atrial flutter waves are sometimes mixed with atrial fibrillation waves and this mixed rhythm is called atrial fib-flutter.

Clinical Manifestations

The signs, symptoms, and significance of atrial fibrillation are related to the rate of the ventricular response. With rapid ventricular response, the patient experiences manifestations of decreased cardiac output. Because the atria do not contract as a whole, the atrial kick is lost. The cardiac output decreases

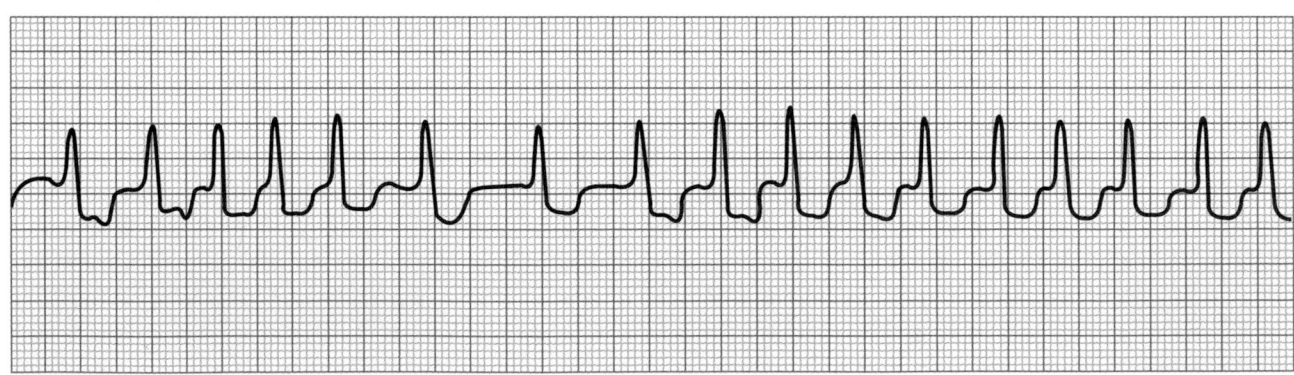

Classic Characteristics:

Pacemaker site:	Many ectopic foci in atrial tissue
Rhythm:	Irregular
Rate:	Atrial rate greater than 400 beats per minute.
P waves:	F waves are seen and are chaotic.
QRS complex:	Normal
Intervals:	No P waves are seen. The R-R interval is irregular.

Figure 8-9

Atrial fibrillation.

15% to 30%, placing the patient at risk for heart failure and myocardial ischemia. Blood pools in the atria, placing the patient at high risk for thrombus formation and embolization to the brain and other organs.

Management

Management of atrial fibrillation involves controlling the ventricular rate, anticoagulation therapy to prevent thrombus formation, and conversion of the dysrhythmia to a sinus rhythm. Patients who tolerate atrial fibrillation are treated with digitalis, beta blockers, or calcium channel blockers, all of which delay conduction through the atrioventricular node, thus slowing the heart rate. If the patient is hemodynamically unstable (experiencing hypotension, syncope, dyspnea), synchronized cardioversion is the treatment of choice. Cardioversion is also attempted for those patients who need the atrial kick to improve cardiac output and who were not converted to sinus rhythm by pharmacologic treatment. Patients are placed on anticoagulant therapy prior to cardioversion to prevent thrombus formation and cerebral embolism. Patients experiencing chronic atrial fibrillation may never be converted to sinus rhythm, and management is directed toward controlling the ventricular rate and preventing embolization to distant organs. Aspirin, one tablet daily, is recommended by the AMA for embolism prophylaxis in these patients.

JUNCTIONAL DYSRHYTHMIAS

Premature Junctional Contractions

Premature junctional contractions are beats that occur early in the cycle and originate in an ectopic site in the atrioventricular node. They are often referred to as junctional beats.

Premature junctional contractions are caused by enhanced automaticity of the junctional tissue related to ischemia. Other conditions that may cause premature junctional contractions include stress, excessive caffeine or alcohol intake, heart failure, pericarditis, valvular disease, hyperthyroidism, electrolyte imbalance, and digitalis toxicity.

Occasionally, junctional beats occur late instead of prematurely, and these beats are called junctional escape beats. These escape beats are a safety mechanism and should never be treated.

Junctional Rhythm

Junctional rhythm originates in or around the atrioventricular node. It is a continuous rhythm with a rate of 40 to 60 beats per minute. This rhythm is often referred to as *junctional escape rhythm* (Fig. 8–10).

Etiology and Pathophysiology

Junctional rhythm only occurs when the dominant pacemaker of the heart fails to function. The pacing rate of the sinoatrial node becomes less than the pacing rate of the atrioventricular node. Another cause of junctional rhythm is failure of electrical impulses from the sinoatrial node to reach the atrioventricular node.

With this rhythm, there is retrograde or backward stimulation of the atria. Consequently, the atria do not contract simultaneously with the ventricles and the atrial kick is lost, reducing cardiac output. This retrograde stimulation of the atria also produces a characteristic P wave, which is either a negative deflection before or after the QRS complex or no P wave at all. Junctional rhythm may be

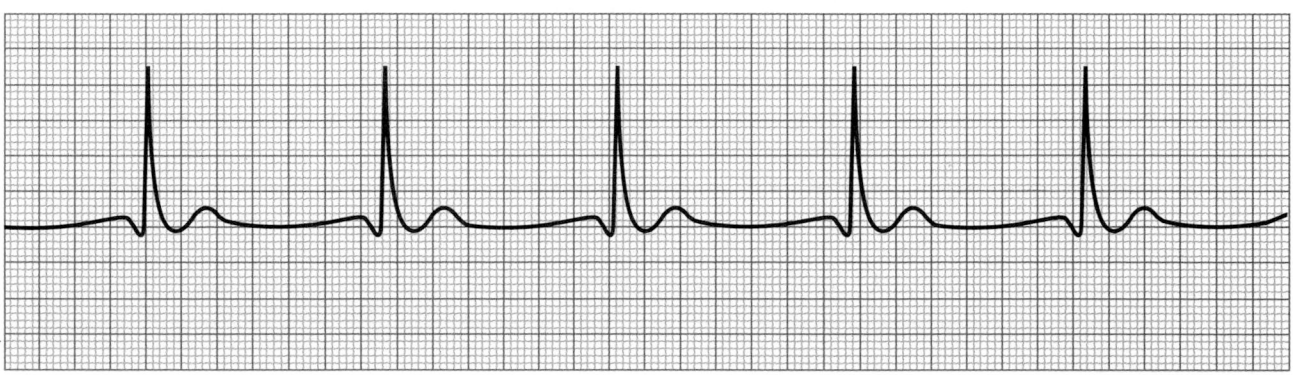

Classic Characteristics:

Pacemaker site:	Atrioventricular node
Rhythm:	Regular
Rate:	40–60 beats per minute
P waves:	May or may not be present. May be inverted and found before, in, or after the QRS.
QRS complex:	Usually normal
Intervals:	P-R interval shorter than normal. The R-R interval is normal.

Figure 8–10

Junctional rhythm.

caused by certain drugs (digitalis, beta blockers, and calcium channel blockers), or damage to the atrioventricular node secondary to acute myocardial infarction or ischemia. Other causes are electrolyte disturbances, heart failure, valvular heart disease, cardiomyopathy, and myocarditis.

Clinical Manifestations
The clinical signs and symptoms are similar to other bradydysrhythmias and include manifestations of decreased cardiac output.

Management
The major goal of pharmacologic management is to increase the heart rate. The drug of choice is atropine. A temporary pacemaker may be inserted to support the ventricular rate. Treatment is geared to identifying and managing the underlying cause.

VENTRICULAR DYSRHYTHMIAS

Ventricular dysrhythmias have their origin in the ventricles below the branching portion of the bundle of His. These dysrhythmias include premature ventricular contraction, ventricular tachycardia, ventricular fibrillation, and ventricular standstill. Ventricular dysrhythmias usually result from drug toxicity (digoxin, amiodarone, cocaine), hypoxia, hypothermia, or unrecognized electrolyte imbalances. The patient with coexisting coronary disease is prone to ventricular dysrhythmias.

Premature Ventricular Contractions

A premature ventricular contraction is an ectopic beat that originates in the ventricles below the bun-

dle of His. The premature ventricular contraction occurs earlier than the normally expected beat and is commonly followed by a compensatory pause (Fig. 8–11). A compensatory pause is the measurement between the R wave preceding the premature ventricular contraction and the R wave following the premature ventricular contraction and is equal to two R-R intervals of the underlying regular rhythm. Premature ventricular contractions result from either enhanced automaticity or the re-entry phenomenon.

Etiology and Pathophysiology
Premature ventricular contractions are associated with stimulants such as caffeine, alcohol, aminophylline, epinephrine, isoproterenol, and digoxin. Associated disease entities include acute myocardial infarction, mitral valve prolapse, heart failure, and coronary artery disease. Premature ventricular contractions may be unifocal (arising from the same ectopic focus) or multifocal (arising from several different ventricular sites).

When the premature ventricular contraction occurs with every other beat, it is called *ventricular bigeminy*. When every third beat is a premature ventricular contraction, it is called ventricular trigeminy. Two consecutive premature ventricular contractions are called couplets. Three consecutive premature ventricular contractions are called triplets. When three or more premature ventricular contractions occur together, the patient has ventricular tachycardia. When a premature ventricular contraction falls on the T wave of the preceding beat, the R-on-T phenomenon occurs and is a more ominous sign because ventricular tachycardia or ventricular fibrillation may occur.

Clinical Manifestations
Most patients with premature ventricular contrac-

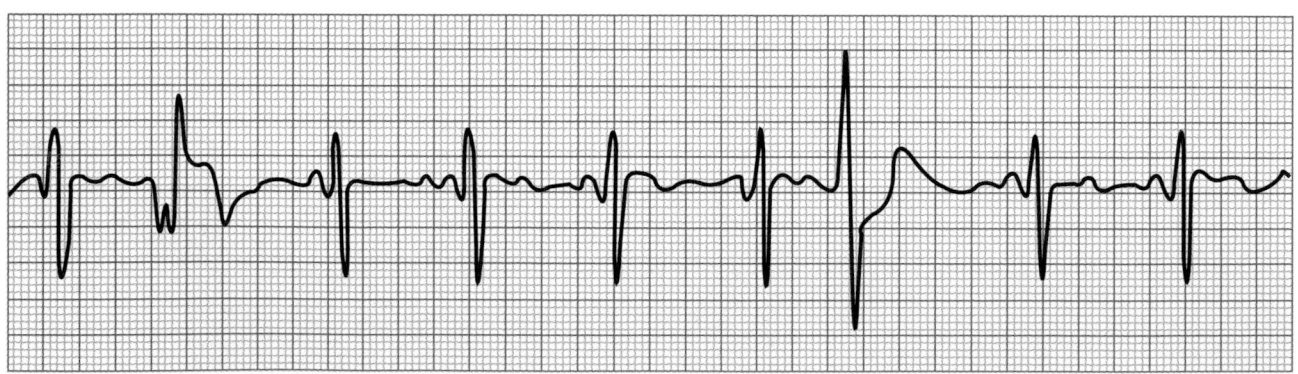

Classic Characteristics:

Pacemaker site:	Ventricular tissue (single or multiple foci)
Rhythm:	Irregular
Rate:	Normal, 60–100 beats per minute
P waves:	Will not be present because impulses originate in the ventricles.
QRS complex:	Usually wide and bizarre. Usually no longer than 0.10 second. May have the same focus in the ventricles or may have a variety of configurations if occurring from multiple foci in the ventricles.
Intervals:	P-R intervals are absent in PVCs.

Figure 8–11

Premature ventricular contractions.

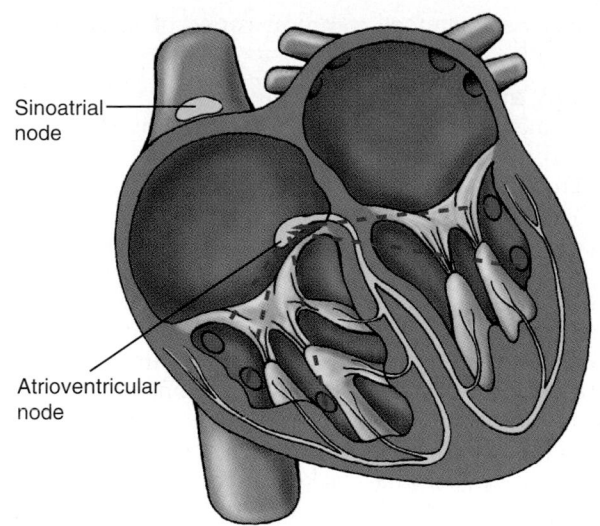

Figure 8-12

In ventricular tachycardia, ventricular cells discharge at a rapid, erratic rate.

tions are asymptomatic, although some complain of palpitations and skipped beats. A longer-than-normal pause immediately after the premature beat can be identified when the radial pulse is checked or the heart auscultated. If premature ventricular contractions are frequent, signs of decreased cardiac output may occur.

Management

Treatment for premature ventricular contractions is indicated when six or more occur per minute, when ventricular couplets or triplets appear, or when multifocal premature ventricular contractions or R-on-T

phenomena occur. If treatment is not initiated, ventricular tachycardia or ventricular fibrillation may ensue. Lidocaine is the drug of choice for treatment of premature ventricular contractions. An initial IV bolus of 1 to 1.5 mg/kg followed by a second bolus if needed in 5 minutes of one-half to one-third the initial dose and a continuous lidocaine infusion of 2 to 4 mg per minute is administered. Procainamide is the second drug of choice if lidocaine is ineffective.

Ventricular Tachycardia

Ventricular tachycardia is a dysrhythmia originating in an ectopic focus in the ventricles. The rate of ventricle discharge is 100 to 250 impulses per minute (Figs. 8-12 and 8-13).

Etiology and Pathophysiology

Ventricular tachycardia occurs when more than three premature ventricular contractions occur in succession with a heart rate of more than 100 per minute. It is associated with enhanced automaticity and re-entry phenomenon. This increased myocardial irritability is usually associated with coronary artery disease, acute myocardial infarction, electrolyte imbalances, or cardiomyopathy or may be the antecedent to ventricular fibrillation.

The QRS complexes associated with ventricular tachycardia are wide, distorted, and bizarre. They are often notched, with a duration greater than 0.12 second. The rhythm is usually regular but at times may be slightly irregular.

Clinical Manifestations

Ventricular tachycardia may cause the patient to complain of palpitations, dizziness, chest pain, and shortness of breath. Signs and symptoms of de-

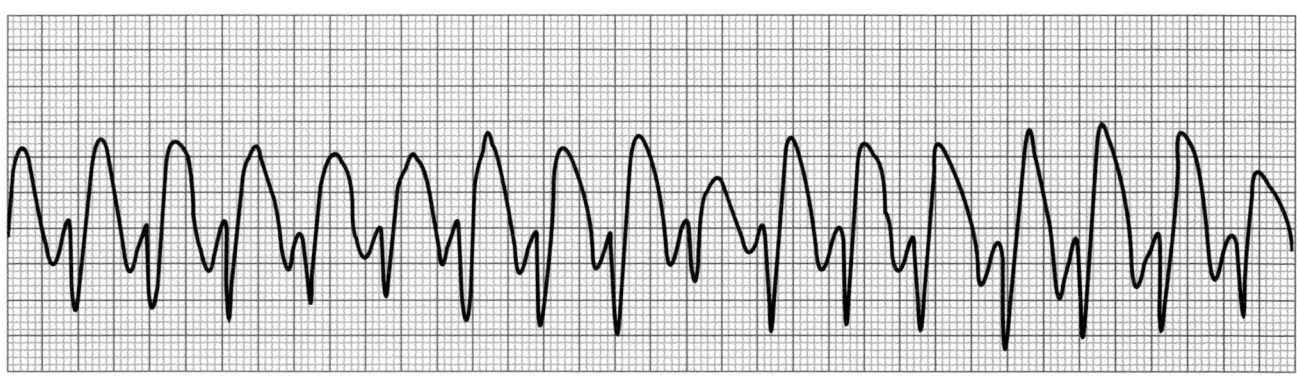

Classic Characteristics:

Pacemaker site: Ventricular (single or multiple foci)
Rhythm: Atrial cannot be determined. Ventricular is typically regular but may be slightly irregular.
Rate: Ventricular rate 100-250 beats per minute
P waves: Usually buried in the QRS complex. Retrograde P waves may be present.
QRS complex: Wide, bizarre, and independent of P waves. May have the same configuration as PVCs.
Intervals: Cannot be determined.

Figure 8-13

Ventricular tachycardia.

creased cardiac output are present. If ventricular tachycardia is rapid or sustained, loss of consciousness may occur.

Management

Treatment depends on the severity of the situation. If ventricular tachycardia occurs at a rate below 100 beats per minute and the patient is hemodynamically stable, no treatment is necessary. If hemodynamic status is stable but this dysrhythmia occurs with higher heart rates, treatment involves administration of a lidocaine bolus of 1 to 1.5 mg/kg per minute, not to exceed 200 to 300 mg in 1 hour. If this controls the tachycardia, a continuous lidocaine infusion of 1 to 4 mg per minute is started.

In the event of lidocaine ineffectiveness, procainamide may be started. It is given in an infusion of 20 mg per minute until the dysrhythmia is suppressed, hypotension occurs, the QRS complex is widened by 50% of its original width, or a total of 17 mg/kg of the drug has been injected.

Bretylium is a third drug of choice for treating ventricular tachycardia. A 5 mg/kg dose is given IV over several minutes. If the dysrhythmia is unresolved, it is then increased to 10 mg/kg at 15- to 30-minute intervals. The maximum dose of bretylium is 30 mg/kg. A continuous infusion (1 to 2 mg/kg) may be initiated. For the patient with hemodynamic compromise, immediate synchronized cardioversion is the treatment.

Ventricular Fibrillation

Ventricular fibrillation is a rapid, ineffective, and disorganized depolarization of the ventricles (Fig. 8–14). It is the most common cause of sudden cardiac death.

Etiology and Pathophysiology

Ventricular fibrillation is characterized by disorganization of electrical impulses, conduction, and ventricular contraction. It is the result of multiple ectopic foci in the ventricles.

As in atrial fibrillation, the ventricles quiver and do not contract simultaneously. The electrocardiographic waveforms appear irregular and chaotic, reflecting no coordinated ventricular activity. The severe derangement of ventricular fibrillation is characterized by irregular undulations of varying contour and amplitude. Ventricular fibrillation occurs with coronary artery disease, acute myocardial infarction, myocardial ischemia, and cardiomyopathy. Procedures such as cardiac catheterization or cardiac pacing may induce ventricular fibrillation via irritation of the ventricles from the catheter. It may also occur with thrombolytic therapy, coronary reperfusion, accidental electrical shock, hyperkalemia, and hypoxia. Ventricular fibrillation is life-threatening because cardiac output stops and death follows immediately.

Clinical Manifestations

The patient with ventricular fibrillation presents with a loss of consciousness and absent pulse, heart sounds, and blood pressure. The patient has dilated pupils, rapid development of cyanosis, and possible seizures.

Management

Immediate initiation of cardiopulmonary resuscitation (CPR) and defibrillation following advanced

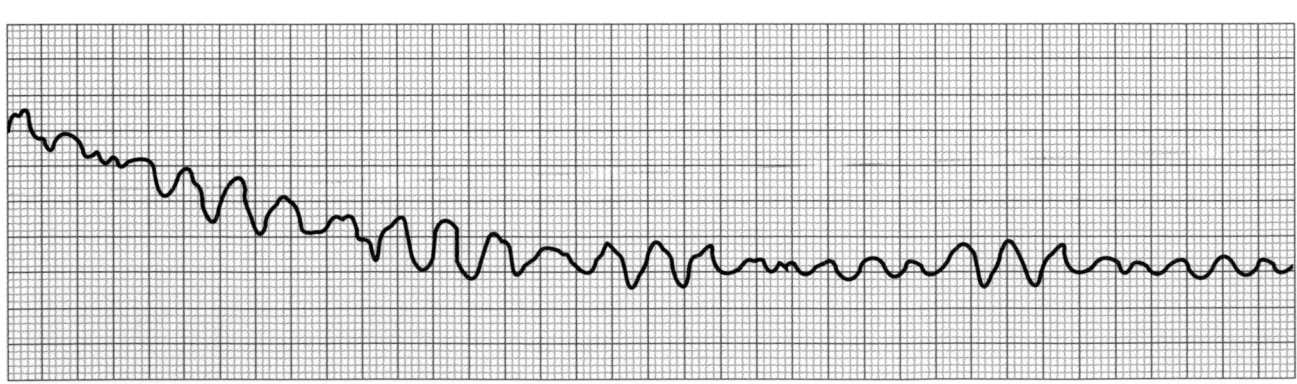

Classic Characteristics:

Pacemaker site:	Ventricular tissue (multiple foci)
Rhythm:	Irregular, uncoordinated, without specific pattern
Rate:	Rapid, uncoordinated, cannot be determined
P waves:	None
QRS complex:	Rapid, irregular, not discernible
Intervals:	Not discernible

Figure 8–14

Ventricular fibrillation.

cardiac life support measures and drug therapy is necessary (see Cardiac Arrest, later in this chapter).

ATRIOVENTRICULAR HEART BLOCKS

Heart block is a term used to describe disturbances in the atrioventricular conduction system. The atrioventricular node normally acts as a bridge between the atria and ventricles. When an atrioventricular block exists, there is an abnormal delay in conduction across this bridge. Atrioventricular blocks are classified into first-degree, second-degree (type I and type II), and third-degree. The site of the block and severity of the conduction disturbances serve as the basis for classification.

First-Degree Atrioventricular Block

First-degree atrioventricular block is a block in which every impulse from the sinoatrial node is conducted to the ventricles, but a delay occurs at the atrioventricular node (Fig. 8–15).

Etiology and Pathophysiology
In first-degree atrioventricular block, the sinus impulse is conducted normally through the atrioventricular node but is delayed longer than the normal 0.20 second before being conducted to the ventricles. This delay in the atrioventricular node results in a prolonged P-R interval. The rhythm is regular, while the QRS is narrowed. First-degree atrioventricular block is associated with organic heart diseases, such as rheumatic fever, chronic ischemic heart disease, myocardial infarction, hyperthyroidism, vagal stimulation, or drugs such as digitalis, beta-blockers, and calcium channel blockers.

Clinical Manifestations
Patients with first-degree atrioventricular block may have a soft S_1. They may also have asymptomatic bradycardia or be otherwise asymptomatic.

Management
If an underlying cause exists, treatment is aimed at resolving the source. Normally, first-degree atrioventricular block does not require treatment. Close monitoring of these patients is important, however, because this type of heart block may lead to more serious forms of heart block.

Second-Degree Atrioventricular Block, Type I

Second-degree atrioventricular block, type I, also known as Mobitz I or Wenckebach block, is characterized by failure of some of the sinoatrial impulses to be conducted to the ventricles (Fig. 8–16).

Etiology and Pathophysiology
Second-degree atrioventricular block usually results from myocardial ischemia in an acute inferior-wall myocardial infarction. Other contributing causes include digitalis toxicity, acute rheumatic fever, electrolyte imbalance, vagal stimulation, or quinidine or procainamide therapy.

Clinical Manifestations
The S_1 tends to become progressively softer with intermittent pauses. Otherwise, the patient with second-degree atrioventricular block, type I, is usually asymptomatic. If the ventricular rate is slow, hypotension and syncope can occur.

Management
Although no treatment is necessary for most pa-

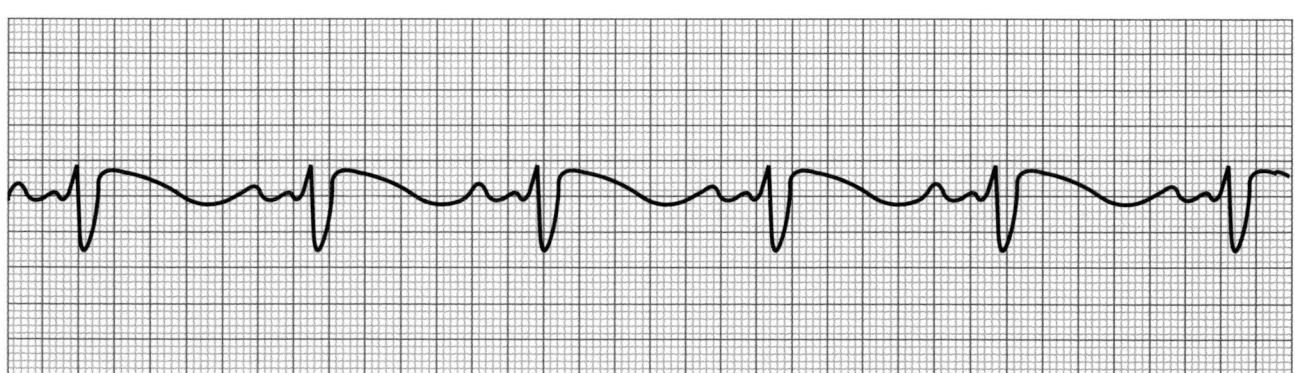

Classic Characteristics:

Pacemaker site:	Sinoatrial node
Rhythm:	Regular
Rate:	60–100 beats per minute
P waves:	Normal
QRS complex:	Normal
Intervals:	P-R interval greater than 0.20 second

Figure 8–15

First-degree atrioventricular block.

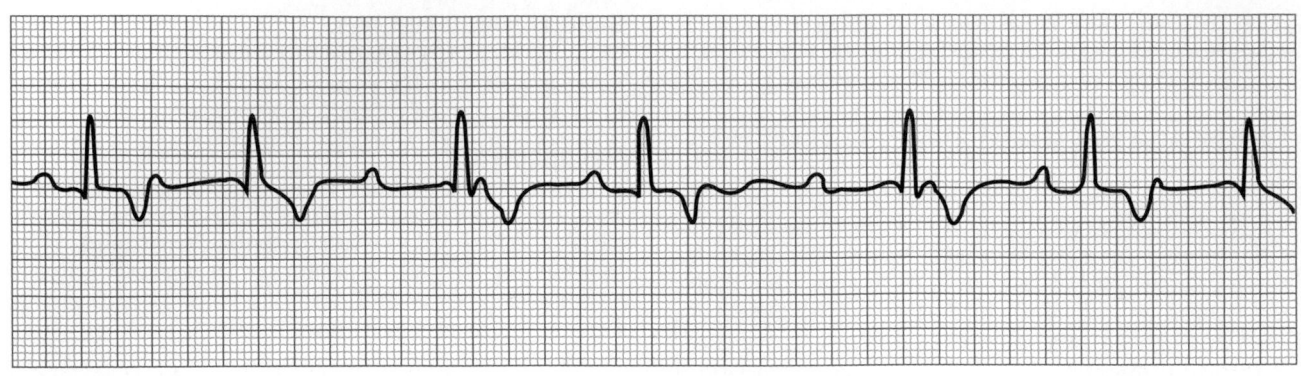

Classic Characteristics:

Pacemaker site:	Sinoatrial node
Rhythm:	Slow: Atrial regular; ventricular irregular
Rate:	Reduced: 30–55 beats per minute
P waves:	Normal: 2–4 for each QRS complex
QRS complex:	Normal, but dropped periodically
Intervals:	P-R interval lengthens with each cycle until a beat is dropped; then the cycle repeats.

Figure 8–16

Second-degree atrioventricular block, type I, also called Mobitz type I or Wenckebach.

tients, the underlying cause is treated when necessary. Atropine, a temporary pacemaker, or both may be used if the patient is symptomatic.

Second-Degree Atrioventricular Block, Type II

Second-degree type II atrioventricular block, also called Mobitz II, is characterized by the failure of some sinus impulses to be conducted to the ventricles. In atrioventricular second-degree type II block, every second, third, or fourth sinus impulse is blocked and not conducted to the ventricles but there is a constant PR interval (Fig. 8–17).

Etiology and Pathophysiology

Type II block is associated with acute anterior wall or anteroseptal wall myocardial infarction, rheumatic and other silent heart diseases, or digitalis toxicity. Type II block occurs lower in the A-V node than type I block.

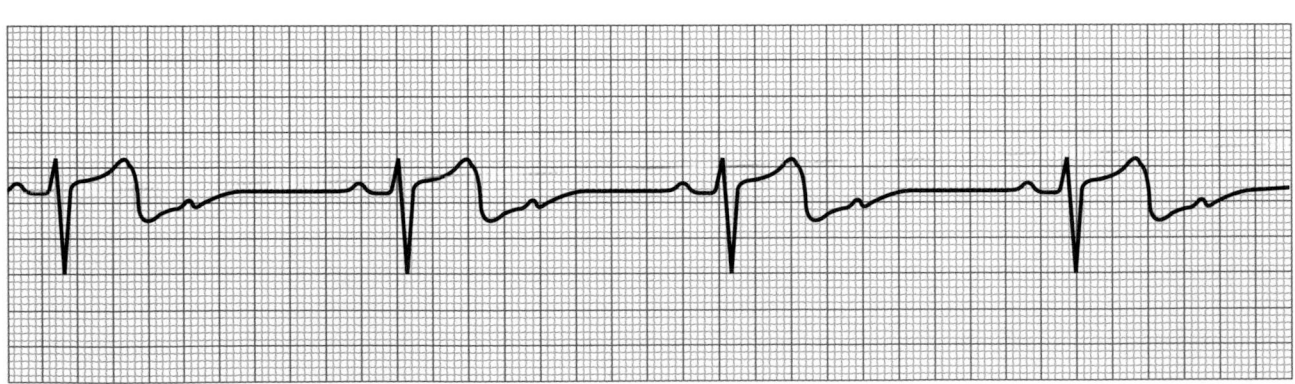

Classic Characteristics:

Pacemaker site:	Sinoatrial node
Rhythm:	Atrial regular, ventricular irregular
Rate:	Atrial normal; ventricular normal, but may be slower than atrial rate
P waves:	Normal or prolonged
QRS complex:	Widens to more than 0.12 second
Intervals:	Normal

Figure 8–17

Second-degree atrioventricular block, type II, also called Mobitz type II.

Clinical Manifestations

The patient with type II second-degree block has a more serious condition than the person with type I second-degree block. Second-degree type II block is more unpredictable and can progress to third-degree (complete) heart block. The patient may be hypotensive, have bradycardia, and exhibit symptoms of decreased cardiac output.

Management

Treatment for type II second-degree heart block is necessary for the symptomatic patient. In the event of an acute myocardial infarction, a pacemaker is inserted to prevent development of third-degree atrioventricular block or asystole. To maintain cardiac output until a pacemaker can be inserted, a transcutaneous external pacemaker may be used or, as a last resort in an emergency situation, isoproterenol may be administered.

Third-Degree Atrioventricular Block

Etiology and Pathophysiology

Third-degree atrioventricular heart block, also known as complete heart block, occurs when all atrial impulses are blocked at the atrioventricular node. The atria are stimulated and contract independently of the ventricles. The ventricles are stimulated by a secondary (escape) ventricular pacemaker (Fig. 8–18). This block may occur at the level of the atrioventricular node, within the bundle of His, or in the Purkinje system. Complete heart block can be transient or permanent. Common causes include:

- Inferior and anterior wall myocardial infarction

- Drug toxicity from digitalis, beta-blockers, or calcium channel blockers
- Vagal stimulation
- Congenital abnormalities
- Post-surgical complication of mitral valve replacement

Regardless of cause, complete heart block is a serious and potential life-threatening dysrhythmia that can lead to ventricular standstill.

Clinical Manifestations

The patient with third-degree heart block may experience fatigue, hypotension, syncope, heart failure, or other signs of inadequate cardiac output. If the heart block is congenital or caused by digitalis toxicity, the patient is asymptomatic. Symptoms vary depending on the stability of the escape rhythm and the patient's response to the decreases in ventricular rate.

Management

Atropine may be effective on narrow-complex third-degree atrioventricular block, but has little or no effect on wide-complex third-degree atrioventricular block. Pacemaker insertion is required when cardiac output is inadequate.

❖ SETTINGS, PROVIDERS, AND COLLABORATION FOR CARE

The patient with a new onset of dysrhythmias may be treated in a critical care setting or in an acute care setting with telemetry monitoring. Discharge planning may include arranging visits from a home

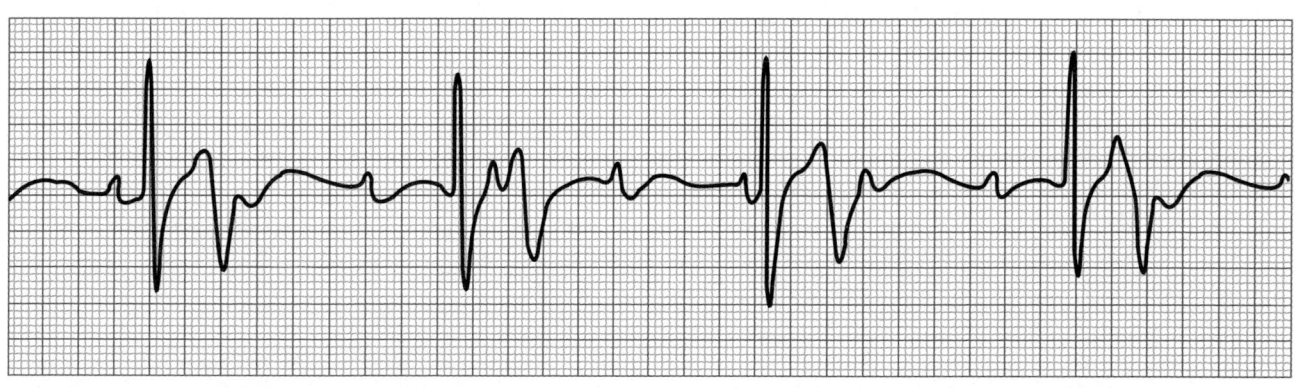

Classic Characteristics:

Pacemaker site:	Atrial rate impulses are from the sinoatrial node. The ventricular pacer is an escape pacemaker in the atrioventricular node or ventricle.
Rhythm:	Regular but slow
Rate:	Atrial 60–100; ventricular 40–60 if originating in the junction, 20–40 if originating in the ventricle
P waves:	Normal
QRS complex:	Normal if blocked at the level of the atrioventricular node or the bundle of His, wide if blocked at the level of the bundle branches
Intervals:	Vary greatly

Figure 8–18

Third-degree atrioventricular block.

CLINICAL ? THINKING

SOMNOLENCE AND ANXIETY IN A PATIENT ON DIGOXIN THERAPY

At 11 AM, I entered the room of a 67-year-old female patient who had undergone extensive oral surgery, to review her discharge instructions. She was seated in the armchair and I noted that her breakfast tray was untouched. She stated that she felt too tired to eat and was dreading the trip home. She appeared to be slightly anxious but in no acute distress. Her medical history included aortic valve stenosis, which was currently being treated with digoxin and an angiotensin-converting enzyme (ACE) inhibitor (Capoten). Her postoperative course had been unremarkable, with the exception of the development of nausea, vomiting, and diarrhea secondary to the prophylactic antibiotics prescribed prior to and following surgery.

Because the patient was taking digoxin, I knew I had to be extremely vigilant for the signs and symptoms of digitalis toxicity. I helped the patient back to bed and assessed her further. Her vital signs revealed a regular apical heart rate of 68 bpm (just slightly lower than her usual range of 72–76 bpm), a respiratory rate of 20 per minute, a temperature of 36.3°C (97.4°F), and a blood pressure of 122/76 mm Hg. Her skin was dry and pink, and there was no evidence of decreased peripheral perfusion. Anterior and posterior breath sounds were clear on auscultation. She denied any visual disturbances, light-headedness, chest discomfort, or shortness of breath.

Despite her cardiovascular stability and the possibility that the fatigue and anorexia might simply be related to her surgical recovery, I sensed that something was wrong and decided to investigate further. The patient was not scheduled for another dose of digoxin until that evening.

I attached a cardiac monitor and ran a rhythm strip. Analysis of the electrocardiographic strip revealed a heart rate of 66 bpm, a P-R interval of 0.24 seconds, and a flat T wave. Both the atrial and ventricular rates were regular, and the configuration of the P wave and QRS complex were normal. Each P wave was followed by a QRS complex. These findings are indicative of a first-degree atrioventricular heart block and led me to believe that the patient had developed digitalis toxicity. Although the heart rate was above 60 bpm and remained regular, the combination of the patient's noncardiac symptoms (fatigue and anorexia) along with the cardiac clinical manifestations (an increased P-R interval greater than 0.20 seconds and a flat T wave) supported my suspicion of digitalis toxicity.

Knowing that the toxic effects of digoxin on the heart could progress to a second- or third-degree heart block and be life threatening, I implemented the following nursing actions:

1. I notified the physician.
2. I checked the latest serum digoxin level.
3. I checked the latest serum potassium and serum magnesium levels.
4. I checked the patient's blood urea nitrogen (BUN) and creatinine levels as well as the liver function tests (aspartate transaminase and alanine transaminase).
5. I continued to monitor the heart rate and rhythm as well as the patient's respiratory and neurologic status.
6. I documented my findings and actions.

The physician ordered a 12-lead electrocardiogram (ECG), continuous cardiac monitoring, and a serum digoxin, potassium, and magnesium level assessment. The results of the diagnostic tests revealed a normal serum digoxin level and lower than normal levels of potassium and magnesium. The 12-lead ECG confirmed my suspicion of first-degree heart block.

The patient remained in the hospital for observation and further treatment. The physician ordered the evening dose of digoxin to be held and prescribed supplemental potassium, which I administered. By the following morning, the atrioventricular block had resolved, her ECG returned to normal, and the digoxin was resumed.

The recognition of early clues to digitalis toxicity, along with the additional observations, clinical decisions, and appropriate interventions, ensured a positive outcome for this patient.

Think Critically

What possible sequela might have developed if the early signs and symptoms had gone unheeded by the nurse and the patient had been discharged as scheduled?

What knowledge must the nurse ensure the patient has to minimize the risk of a future episode of digitalis toxicity developing at home?

Why were prophylactic antibiotics ordered for this patient? What role did they play in the development of digitalis toxicity?

What medical interventions should the nurse have anticipated if the patient's condition had deteriorated to a complete (third-degree) heart block? What if the serum digoxin levels had been alarmingly high? How does digitalis toxicity develop when serum digoxin levels are normal?

Why did the nurse check the patient's BUN, creatinine, and liver function tests?

health care nurse for ongoing assessment for signs of worsening condition in the home setting. Compliance with pharmacologic management is crucial to the wellbeing of the patient, and the home care nurse is invaluable in giving instruction and in monitoring patient compliance.

NURSING PROCESS
Cardiac Dysrhythmias

Assessment

Assess the effect of the dysrhythmia on cardiac output by checking the patient's level of consciousness and blood pressure. Review the patient's medical history and diagnostic test results for the type of dysrhythmia present. Monitor the electrocardiogram (ECG) and telemetry patterns. Check the vital signs and watch for changes with activity. Monitor for hypotension, which may indicate decreased cardiac output.

Check for mental status changes from decreased cardiac output, including disorientation, confusion, memory loss, or loss of consciousness. Decreased cerebral perfusion can also lead to behavior changes, such as combativeness, lethargy, and hallucinations. Auscultate the chest for abnormal heart sounds. Auscultate the lungs for crackles, which indicate left-sided heart failure. Assess for signs of right-sided heart failure, such as edema, jugular vein distension, and an engorged, painful liver. Assess for nausea and vomiting, which may be signs of vagal nerve stimulation. Assess for fatigue and generalized weakness that cannot be attributed to any specific change in living pattern. Ask about a history of cardiac dysrhythmia or other disease.

Nursing Diagnoses and Planning

Nursing diagnoses and related expected patient outcomes commonly applicable to patients with dysrhythmias include the following:

NDx: Decreased cardiac output related to altered electrical conduction

Planning: Patient Outcomes
1. Cardiac output is adequate as evidenced by systolic blood pressure between 90 and 140, diastolic blood pressure between 50 and 90, and heart rate between 60 and 100.
2. Patient avoids activities that increase the heart rate by more than 20 over baseline.
3. Frequency of dysrhythmias causing decreased cardiac output is reduced.

NDx: Anxiety related to presence of a potentially life-threatening dysrhythmia and the treatment regimen necessary

Planning: Patient Outcomes
1. Patient reports reduced anxiety and fear related to the dysrhythmia.
2. Patient appears relaxed and is resting and sleeping well.

3. Outward signs of anxiety are absent, such as nervousness, clenching of hands, withdrawal, hyperventilation, or twitching.

NDx: Risk for altered health maintenance related to lack of information about electrical conduction of the heart, nature of dysrhythmias (specify the particular dysrhythmia), and the drug intervention or other therapies required

Planning: Patient Outcomes
1. Patient verbalizes accurate information about the electrical conduction of the heart and the nature of the dysrhythmia present.
2. Patient lists the medications prescribed, giving the dose, side effects, and expected therapeutic results.
3. Patient accurately checks and records heart rate.

Nursing Interventions and Evaluation

NDx: Decreased cardiac output
Use telemetry monitoring whenever possible, especially if the patient experiences dysrhythmias or is taking anti-arrhythmic drugs. Auscultate the apical pulse, noting the rate and rhythm. Review the results of laboratory studies, especially potassium level, and hemodynamic monitoring.

Monitor the patient's vital signs both at rest and during activity, and document the data. Encourage the patient to take frequent rest periods throughout the day to prevent fatigue and strain on the myocardium. Note any dyspneic episodes and precipitating factors. Ask whether the patient is getting enough rest and sleep, and prevent disturbances.

Check the patient's intake and output, observing for adequacy and balance. Keep the patient's legs in a nondependent position while sitting. Provide support for the extremities while sitting or lying in bed. Pad bony prominences to prevent breakdown from pressure and poor circulation.

Teach the patient relaxation techniques and range-of-motion exercises to increase circulation while lying in bed. Keep the patient warm and comfortable. Prevent constriction of circulation from tight-fitting clothing or bed linen.

NDx: Anxiety
Help the patient find effective relaxation methods. Teach relaxation techniques that the patient can practice throughout the day. Allow the patient and family time to be alone. Give explanations that the patient can understand, and allow for patient input in the daily care plan. Teach the patient about the disease and medications used to control the effects of the disorder.

Answer the patient's questions in a professional, informative manner. Help the patient find coping strategies that relieve stress and anxiety. Ask for assistance from clergy or counseling staff if necessary.

NDx: Risk for altered health maintenance
Plan education sessions with the patient when he or she is rested and relaxed. Provide time for questions

and concerns to be voiced. Include the family in the teaching. Review normal cardiac function and electrical conduction with the patient using terminology the patient can understand. Explain specific changes in rhythm in relation to the normal patterns. Identify symptoms of the dysrhythmia, such as fatigue, edema, anorexia, and changes in mentation.

Instruct the patient about prescribed medications, their side effects, dosages, frequency, and when to seek medical intervention if untoward symptoms are present. Provide written instructions about the medications. Tell the patient to keep a record of pulse rates, untoward symptoms, and medication administration for the physician's information at the next visit.

Compare the patient's status with the expected outcomes. If the expected outcomes are not met, reassess the patient and revise the plan.

MECHANICAL AND SURGICAL CONTROL OF DYSRHYTHMIAS

Two mechanical treatment options are available for patients with cardiac dysrhythmias: pacemakers and cardioversion.

Artificial Pacemakers

An artificial pacemaker is a device that initiates and maintains heartbeats. It is used to control heart rate and prevent dangerous dysrhythmias when the heart's natural pacemakers cannot do so because of a disorder of the conduction system. Artificial pacemakers come in temporary and permanent single-chambered or dual-chambered models. One type of temporary pacemaker is external (transcutaneous), or noninvasive. All other temporary or permanent pacemakers are internal, or invasive.

INTERNAL PACING

Internal, or invasive, pacemakers consist of a pulse generator and a pacing wire or wires. The pulse generator produces an electrical impulse that stimulates the myocardium to depolarize, thereby initiating a heartbeat. The pacing wire carries the electrical impulse from the generator to the myocardium. Single-chambered pacemakers have one pacing wire positioned in the chamber to be paced, usually the right ventricle. Dual-chambered pacemakers have two lead wires, one in the right ventricle and one in the right atrium. By depolarizing the atrium, the dual-chambered pacemaker preserves the atrial kick. A programmed interval between stimulation of the atrium and the ventricle ensures that ventricular contraction will follow atrial contraction. These atrioventricular pacemakers, which simulate normal cardiac function, are sometimes referred to as *physiologic pacemakers*.

Because of the variety of terms used to describe pacemakers and their function, a *universal pacemaker code* has been developed to standardize language and facilitate clear communication. The code consists of five positions, of which the first three are most commonly used and are presented here. Position 1 refers to the chamber(s) being paced. Position 2 refers to the chamber(s) being sensed. Position 3 refers to the mode of response. Letter options for positions 1 and 2 are

A for atrium
V for ventricle
D for dual (both atrium and ventricle)
0 for none

Letter options for position 3 are

I for inhibited (when the pacemaker senses an intrinsic beat, it does not deliver an impulse)
T for triggered (when the pacemaker senses an intrinsic beat, it does deliver an impulse)
D for atrial inhibited and ventricular triggered (when the pacemaker senses an intrinsic beat arising in the atrium, it does not deliver an impulse; but when it senses a beat arising in the ventricle, it does deliver an impulse)
0 for no response mode (fixed rate, asynchronous impulses delivered)

Use of this system can be illustrated with the following example, which shows how to interpret the universal pacemaker code DVI:

Code = DVI		
Position 1 =	D = Dual:	Both the atrium and the ventricle are being paced
Position 2 =	V = Ventricle:	The ventricle is being sensed
Position 3 =	I = Inhibited:	When the pacemaker senses an intrinsic heartbeat, it does not deliver an impulse

Most pulse generators are powered by lithium batteries, which last up to 10 years. Others are nuclear powered and last 20 or more years. Controls on the pulse generator allow energy output, heart rate, and mode of pacing to be determined according to the needs of the individual patient.

Energy output is the intensity of the electrical impulse delivered to the myocardium, measured in milliamperes (mA). It is set by the physician at the lowest level needed to produce depolarization, typically 1.5 mA.

Heart rate is usually set at 70 to 80 beats per minute. It is set higher if the pacemaker is being used to suppress dysrhythmias.

The mode of pacing may be demand (synchronous, noncompetitive), fixed (asynchronous, competitive), or rate-responsive. In the demand mode, heartbeats triggered naturally by the heart are sensed by an electrode at the tip of the pacing wire and a stimulus from the artificial pacemaker is delivered to the myocardium only when the natural heart rate falls below the level preset on the impulse generator. Thus the pacemaker is synchronized with the heart and does not compete with it.

In the fixed mode, the artificial pacemaker stimulates the heart at the preset number of times per minute regardless of the beats generated by the pacemakers of the heart itself. In this mode, the pacemaker is not synchronized with the heart and is in competition with it. The use of the fixed mode is usually limited to situations in which the heart is basically asystolic, as after open heart surgery. It is not used when the natural pacemakers of the heart are initiating a significant number of beats because of the danger of a pacemaker impulse reaching the myocardium during the vulnerable period of repolarization and causing ventricular fibrillation.

A rate responsive mode is one in which the rate of pacing changes in response to body demands. This newer type of dual-chambered pacemaker senses some physiologic variable, such as oxygen saturation or an acid-base parameter, and alters the pacing rate accordingly in patients with sinus or atrial impairment.

Internal Permanent Pacing

Permanent pacemakers are surgically implanted in the patient. They are used to treat irreversible or recurrent conditions, such as complete heart block and sick sinus syndrome. The pulse generator is placed in a surgically created space in the subcutaneous tissue either below the right or left clavicle or in the upper left abdomen. If the pulse generator is below the clavicle, the free end of the pacing wire or wires attached to it is fed through the cephalic or subclavian vein into the endocardium of the right side of the heart. If the pulse generator is placed in the abdomen, the pacing wire is sutured to the epicardium through a thoracotomy incision (Fig. 8–19).

Following implantation of a pacemaker, periodic checks of its function are necessary. As part of these follow-ups, which are done in a pacemaker clinic or other specialized facility, an electrocardiographic rhythm strip is obtained and the pulse generator tested for signs of battery depletion and other signs of impending system failure. If necessary, the pulse generator settings can be reprogrammed by placing the head of the reprogramming device on the patient's skin over the pulse generator. Intermittent, less detailed checks on pacemaker function can be made via the telephone. For this type of check, electrodes from a transmitting unit are attached to the patient's wrists and the telephone receiver is placed in the transmitting unit. Sound signals go out over the telephone lines to the receiving unit in a physician's office or clinic, where they are converted into an electrocardiographic rhythm strip and other information on the pacemaker.

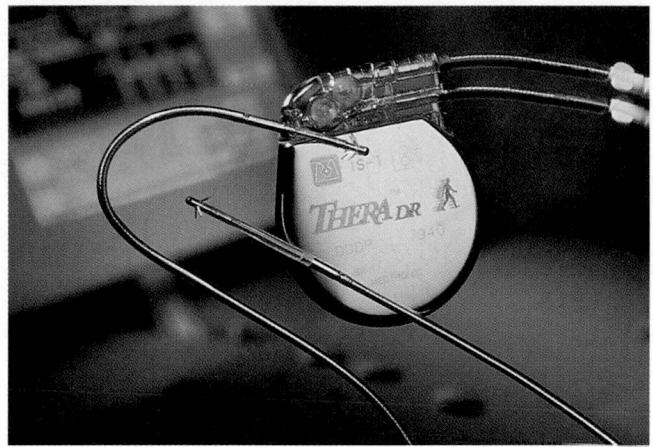

Figure 8–19

A permanent pacemaker (pulse generator) that can be implanted in subcutaneous tissue below the patient's clavicle or in the abdomen. The pacing wires are then threaded to the patient's heart. (Courtesy of Medtronic, Inc, Minneapolis, MN.)

When battery power is lost, the battery is either changed or, in some pacemaker models, recharged in place. Since the battery cells are sealed in the pulse generator, a battery change is actually a pulse generator change. This change is a simple surgical procedure. Under local anesthesia, the subcutaneous implantation site is opened at the site of the original incision and the old pulse generator is disconnected from the pacing wires and removed. The new pulse generator is then inserted.

Complications of permanent pacing include wound infection, sepsis, ectopic beats from irritation of the myocardium by the pacing wire, and development of dysrhythmias from dislodgment of the pacing wire and resultant stimulation of various areas of the myocardium. Loss of capture (depolarization does not occur in response to the impulse delivered to the myocardium) can occur from low current or an increase in the stimulation threshold of the myocardium as a result of ischemia, drug therapy, or metabolic changes. Pacemaker failure can also result from pacing wire dislodgment, loss of system integrity (wire breaks, impulse generator malfunction), or loss of battery power.

NURSING PROCESS GUIDELINES
Internal Permanent Pacing

Immediately following insertion of a pacemaker, monitor the electrocardiographic rhythm to determine if the pacemaker is functioning correctly. A sharp spike immediately preceding a QRS complex indicates a paced beat (Fig. 8–20). Document the type, model, date and time of insertion, and location of the pacemaker as well as its settings in the patient record. Monitor vital signs for stability. Report

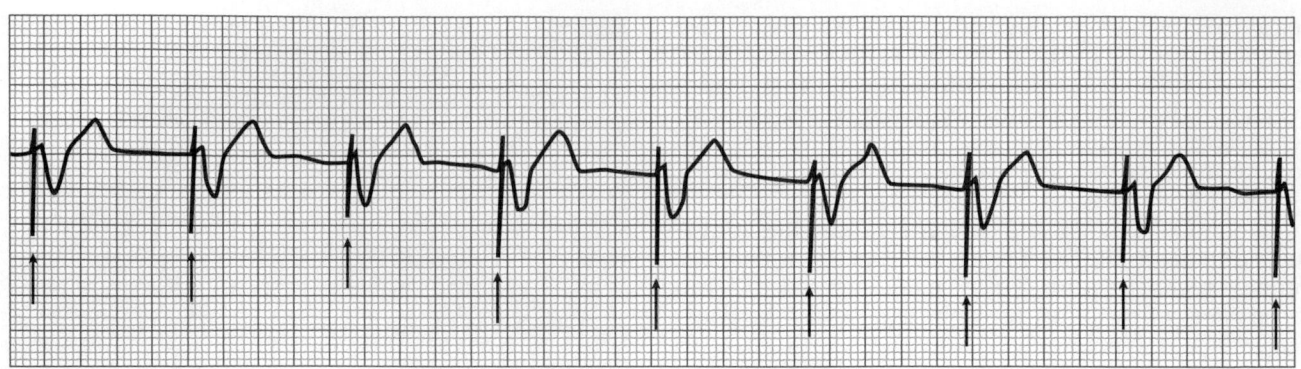

Figure 8–20
Sharp spikes (arrows) just preceding the QRS complexes indicate the action of a ventricular fixed-rate demand pacemaker. These spikes are known as "pacemaker artifact."

the development of any new dysrhythmia or the increasing frequency of an existing one. Maintain an open intravenous line in case anti-arrhythmic or other drugs are needed. Limit the patient's activity for the first 24 hours to decrease the risk of dislodging the pacing wire.

Observe the dressing over the implantation site for drainage. When the dressing is removed, assess the site itself. The wound should be approximated and free of drainage, swelling, or marked erythema. Instruct the patient on care of the wound and the need to report any signs of infection (increased redness, heat, swelling, pain, drainage, odor, or fever) to the health-care provider. Suggest that loose clothing be worn over the implantation site for comfort. Explain that activity should be increased gradually in accordance with the physician's directions and that trauma to the implantation site should be avoided.

In the past, it was necessary to explain the need to avoid proximity to magnetic fields and microwave ovens because of the risk of current being carried over the pacing wires to the heart and precipitating a dysrhythmia. With newer pacemakers, this is not a problem, but electromagnetic interference from welding areas or large motors can occur. Thus, this equipment must be grounded and persons with a pacemaker using the equipment need to wear insulated gloves. Explain this to the patient and instruct him or her to avoid leaning over large motors. Also, instruct the patient to self-identify as a pacemaker user at airport and other similar security systems so that a hand-held metal detector will be used. Teach the patient and a significant other to take a pulse. Instruct the patient to count the pulse for a full minute every day at about the same time and to report any sudden slowing or increase in rate. Stress the importance of returning for follow-up checks on the pacemaker's function. Make certain the patient understands that transtelephone checks cannot totally replace in-person checks on the pacemaker.

Encourage the patient to carry an identification card or emergency alert tag identifying the type, model, and manufacturer of the pacemaker, settings, date of insertion, and name of physician and hospital.

Internal Temporary Pacing

Internal temporary pacing is used as adjunctive therapy in patients with a short-term, reversible problem of the conduction system such as following open-heart surgery or a myocardial infarct. It may be transvenous or epicardial. In transvenous pacing, the pacing wires, which are in a sterile catheter with an electrode tip, are threaded under fluoroscopy, through a vein (antecubital, brachial, jugular, subclavian, or femoral) to the right ventricle. There, the electrode tip comes into contact with the endocardium. If the atrial kick is needed, a double-chambered pacemaker is used with one catheter tip placed in the atrium and one in the ventricle.

Epicardial pacing is used after open-heart surgery. As the name indicates, the pacing wires are placed on the outer surface of the heart, usually two on the atrium and two on the ventricle, and exit through the chest wall to attach to a pulse generator. The pulse generator used for temporary pacing is larger than an implantable one for permanent pacing but can be attached to the arm or leg or placed in a specially constructed pacemaker pocket of a hospital gown.

During insertion of a pacemaker, there is a risk of ventricular dysrhythmia, and for this reason a defibrillator should be at hand during the procedure. Cardiac perforation is also a potential complication but occurs very rarely. Complications following insertion are similar to those associated with permanent pacing. In addition there is risk of infection or hematoma at the venous insertion site, increased risk of dislodging the pacing wires, and risk of dysrhythmias due to a small electric charge passing along the pacing wires from improperly grounded electrical equipment or from magnetic fields.

NURSING PROCESS GUIDELINES
Internal Temporary Pacing

Following insertion of a internal temporary pacemaker, monitor the electrocardiographic rhythm to determine pacemaker function. Check that pacer spikes appear and that they are followed by a QRS complex. Assess vital signs regularly and notify the physician if the heart rate falls below the preset level. Assess the patient for dizziness, weakness, and syncope, which could indicate decreased cardiac output due to pacemaker malfunction. Check the pacing wire insertion site for signs of hematoma or infection. Immobilize the extremity through which the pacing wires are inserted, limit the patient's movement as necessary, and keep the pulse generator secured to the patient to avoid accidental displacement of the pacing wires. Take precautions to ensure that no ungrounded electrical current is conducted through the pacing wire, as this could lead to ventricular fibrillation. Ground all electrical equipment in the patient's room with a three-prong plug. Remove equipment with frayed or broken wires. Make certain the ends of the pacing wires are insulated (eg, covered with rubber gloves or taped to the chest) when not attached to a pulse generator. Protect the patient from exposure to magnetic fields.

EXTERNAL TEMPORARY PACING

External temporary pacing is used chiefly as a stop-gap measure in emergency situations in which a patient is asystolic or in extreme bradycardia. It is a means to maintain the pumping action of the heart and hence the circulation of oxygenated blood until the patient's intrinsic rate returns to normal or invasive pacing can be instituted. It is sometimes used as a prophylactic measure during invasive procedures or during transport of patients at risk for bradydysrhythmias.

An external temporary pacemaker consists of a pulse generator and two large patch electrodes, an anterior and a posterior, connected to it by wire leads. The posterior electrode is placed between the spinal column and the left scapula on the patient's back so it is behind the heart. The anterior electrode is placed on the patient's chest over the apex of the heart (Fig. 8–21). Since the electrode cannot be placed over the female breast and must be above the diaphragm, in female patients the breast must be displaced upward before its placement. This system provides transcutaneous electrical stimulation to initiate ventricular depolarization when the patient's intrinsic heart rate drops lower than the preset rate on the generator. Impulses of 60 mA or more are generally needed for depolarization to occur. Because this current is so high, the external temporary pacemaker comes equipped with a filter that attaches to the bedside monitor to prevent distortion of the electrocardiographic signal on the monitor.

External pacing is uncomfortable. The electrical impulse flows through the skin and muscle under

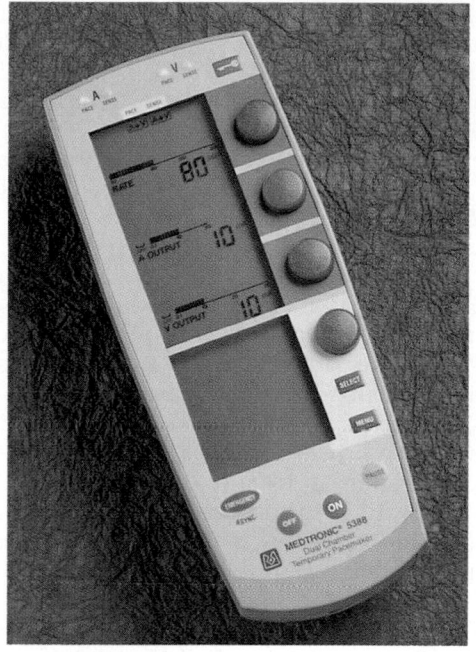

Figure 8–21

An external temporary pacemaker. (Courtesy of Medtronic, Inc, Minneapolis, MN.)

the patch, causing muscle twitching, skin irritation, and diaphoresis. To minimize discomfort, the areas under the electrodes are never shaved, rubbed, or treated with alcohol or other potentially irritating agents, and the energy output is set at the lowest effective level. Before electrode placement, the skin is washed with soap and water both to cleanse the area and to promote good contact between the electrode and the skin.

NURSING PROCESS GUIDELINES
External Temporary Pacing

Check that ventricular contraction is occurring with each pacing stimulus by palpating for a right carotid or right radial pulse and obtaining a blood pressure on the right arm. Pulses and blood pressure are not taken on the left side of the body because they may be altered by the effects of the electrical stimulus. Give prescribed analgesics or sedatives for comfort. Maintain the electrodes in good contact with the skin and observe the ECG to ascertain that each pacing spike is followed by a QRS complex. Pacing spikes not followed by a QRS complex indicate that the electrodes are not in good contact with the skin or the milliamperage of the impulse is too low to depolarize the ventricle.

Cardioversion

Cardioversion is a procedure in which an electrical impulse is delivered to the heart during ventricular depolarization. Its purpose is to change a hemodynamically unstable cardiac dysrhythmia such as atrial fibrillation or atrial flutter into a normal sinus rhythm or at least a more stable rhythm. Voltage of between 25 and 400 watt-seconds is delivered one or more times by a machine called a defibrillator. This is done to completely depolarize the cardiac fibers, thus terminating the existing dysrhythmia and allowing the sinoatrial node to re-establish control. To prevent the electrical current from reaching the cardiac fibers during the vulnerable period (T wave), thereby triggering ventricular tachycardia or fibrillation, the defibrillator is synchronized with a cardiac monitor. The synchronizer is programmed to sense QRS waves, ensuring that the electrical discharge from the defibrillator occurs during this period. Cardioversion is not possible in ventricular fibrillation, since there is no discernible QRS wave.

Cardioversion is usually an elective procedure and is performed under conscious sedation with intravenous diazepam (Valium) or midazolam (Versed). In preparation for the procedure, oral antiarrhythmics may be given. Digoxin, however, is generally withheld for 24 to 72 hours and oral food and fluids withheld for 8. Patients with atrial fibrillation usually are given anticoagulation therapy with coumadin before cardioversion to prevent cerebral embolization. The patient's airway, vital signs, ECG, and level of consciousness are carefully monitored during and after the procedure. Expected outcomes of the procedure include a sinus rhythm, strong peripheral pulses, and stable blood pressure.

DEFIBRILLATION

Defibrillation is unsynchronized cardioversion. Delivery of the electrical impulse is not programmed to occur during the QRS interval. It is used in emergency situations when there is no discernible cardiac rhythm. The voltage used is generally 200 to 360 watt-seconds, higher than that used in cardioversion because the aim is to depolarize all myocardial cells simultaneously. Defibrillator paddles or, on newer models, large self-adhesive patches containing electrodes (for pacing or cardioversion as well as defibrillation, depending on how the machine is set) are placed at the right third intercostal space just lateral to the sternum and at the left fifth intercostal space at the midaxillary line to create an effective arc. A conducting agent, such as electrode paste or saline pad, is used beneath each paddle to promote good conductance and to protect the skin from burning. In addition, 20 to 25 pounds of pressure is exerted on each paddle to create good skin contact. When it is determined that no one is touching the bed or the patient, buttons on both paddles are depressed simultaneously to deliver the electrical discharge.

IMPLANTABLE CARDIOVERTER-DEFIBRILLATOR

An automatic implantable cardioverter-defibrillator is a device that senses a dysrhythmia and, in 10 to 20 seconds, delivers an electric shock to the myocardium, thus automatically cardioverting the heart.

The technology of this device is rapidly evolving. Until recently, the device weighed about 225 g ($\frac{1}{2}$ lb) and the generator was implanted into the abdominal cavity. New advances in the development of implantable cardioverter-defibrillators have made a wide variety of devices available. Many are capable of dual chamber sensing and pacing as well as cardioversion and defibrillation. There are devices in use, however, that have anti-tachycardia pacing properties but do not defibrillate. Most patients today have a single lead inserted onto the epicardial surface of the right ventricle. This unipolar lead is inserted transvenously under local anesthesia. The generator is then inserted into the subcutaneous tissue of the subpectoral region of the chest, similar to a pacemaker. In the past, the leads were inserted through a median sternotomy, left subcostal, left subxiphoid, or left thoracotomy incision, and this technique is still used in patients in whom transvenous insertion is not possible. This system can detect and respond to ventricular fibrillation and ventricular tachycardia because the generator is set to a specific cut-off rate and, when the sensing leads detect a heart rate that exceeds the set rate, an electric shock is delivered to the myocardium. In the event that the shock is unsuccessful in converting the heart to a more stable rhythm, up to five additional shocks can be delivered.

Implantable cardioverter-defibrillators are used for:

- People who have survived an episode of sudden cardiac death from ventricular tachycardia or ventricular fibrillation in the absence of a myocardial infarct
- Those with repeated episodes of ventricular tachycardia or ventricular fibrillation not responsive to treatment with anti-arrhythmic drugs alone
- Patients who have survived a myocardial infarction and are asymptomatic except for ECG-documented erratic heart rhythms.

Implantable cardioverter-defibrillators do not eliminate the need for antiarrhythmic agents but are used in conjunction with them. Since the patient may feel the electric shock when the implantable cardioverter-defibrillator discharges, the patient should be informed of this and also instructed to contact his or her health-care provider for follow-up after the device discharges.

NURSING PROCESS GUIDELINES
Implantable Cardioverter-Defibrillator

The postoperative care associated with implantation of an implantable cardioverter-defibrillator is similar to the care of the patient who has had a pacemaker insertion, with the additional instruction to avoid driving a car for at least 6 months. Instruct the patient in self-care related to the implantable cardioverter-defibrillator as presented in Highlight 8–3. If

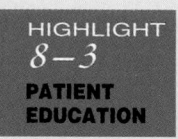 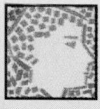

HIGHLIGHT
8–3

PATIENT EDUCATION

Instructions for the Patient with an Implantable Cardioverter-Defibrillator

Instruct the patient to:

- Check the incision daily until it heals for signs of infection: redness, swelling, heat, and drainage.
- Avoid tight clothing or rough fabrics, which can cause irritation directly over the incision.
- Avoid trauma to the area of implantation.
- Engage only in activities identified as safe by the physician. Avoid exposure to magnetic fields, such as at the airport, the library, and other security checkpoints, and magnetic resonance imaging machines. Do not drive a car.
- Alert family, friends, and most importantly, sexual partners, to the fact that if they are touching you when the ICD discharges, they may feel the shock and, with some models, hear a sound.
- Call for help if dizziness develops.
- Maintain a record of the times the ICD discharges, symptoms noted, and activities that preceded the discharge to provide a guide to adjusting the medical treatment plan.
- Return for follow-up appointments to check the functioning of the system.

fibrillation occurs postoperatively, while the patient is still hospitalized, respond by bringing a crash cart with a defibrillator to the bedside in case the newly implanted cardioverter-defibrillator does not work.

Cardiac Conduction Surgery

Surgery on the conduction system of the heart is done to treat atrial and ventricular tachycardias that cannot be successfully controlled by anti-arrhythmic medications or by pacing. There are a variety of techniques in use. Endocardial isolation is designed to prevent the dysrhythmia from affecting the entire heart. This is accomplished by incising the endocardium around the source of the dysrhythmia, reapproximating the edges of the incision with sutures, and allowing scar tissue to form. The resultant ring of scar tissue prevents the spread of the dysrhythmia.

Other types of conduction surgery are designed to eliminate the source of the dysrhythmia. In endocardial resection, this is done by dissecting away the endocardium at the origin of the dysrhythmia. In ablation procedures, cold (cryoablation), electrical shocks (electrical ablation), or high frequency sound waves (radiofrequency ablation) are used to create damage and scarring thus destroying the site of origin.

Cardiac Arrest

Etiology and Pathophysiology

Cardiac arrest is defined as the cessation of effective cardiac output due to the absence of mechanical cardiac activity. When cardiac arrest occurs, the patient is only minutes away from irreversible biologic death unless the condition is recognized and CPR is begun immediately.

Cardiac arrest may be secondary to respiratory arrest, or it may immediately precede a respiratory arrest because the failure of one of these systems causes rapid failure in the other. The most frequent cause of cardiac arrest is coronary heart disease in which atherosclerosis leads to a decrease in the supply of oxygenated blood to the cardiac muscle. Cardiac arrest may also follow a number of other medication conditions and emergency situations, such as cerebrovascular accidents, seizures, trauma, drugs, electrocution, or hemorrhagic, anaphylactic, or septic shock.

Clinical Manifestations

Unresponsiveness and the inability to arouse the patient may be the first indication of cardiac arrest in the unmonitored patient. The absence of a palpable pulse in a major artery such as the carotid or femoral artery indicates that cardiac arrest has occurred. When cardiac output ceases, the skin becomes cool and cyanotic. Hypoxemia, followed by acidemia, occurs rapidly when circulation stops or slows.

Diagnosis

When cardiac arrest occurs, the cardiac monitor may display asystole, which indicates the complete cessation of myocardial electrical activity. Other dysrhythmias that may be noted at the time of cardiac arrest include ventricular fibrillation and ventricular tachycardia. Ventricular fibrillation is chaotic electrical activity that causes asynchronous, fluttering contractions in the ventricles. Ventricular tachycardia usually deteriorates quickly into ventricular fibrillation. In these dysrhythmias, cardiac output drops toward zero and thus the heart is unable to supply enough oxygenated blood to the body to maintain cellular life.

Management

There are two components to management in cases of sudden cardiac arrest. The first is basic life support, and the second is advanced cardiac life support. Baxic life support includes recognition of cardiac arrest, accessing advanced medical support, and implementation of cardiopulmonary resuscitation. CPR involves external cardiac massage to create manual heart compression, and artificial respiration by means of mouth-to-mouth or mouth-to-face mask breathing, to sustain circulation and ventilation during cardiac arrest. Since it requires no special equipment, basic life support can be administered by trained persons in the community as well as trained health-care personnel.

When cardiac arrest occurs in the hospitalized patient, resuscitation efforts begin with the initiation of code procedures. Most hospitals use an emergency notification system to summon members of a resuscitation team and a crash cart (also called a *code cart*) that contains resuscitation equipment, drugs, and intravenous solutions (Table 8–2) to the patient's bedside. Although exceptions have occurred, in the vast majority of cases, resuscitation must begin within 4 to 6 minutes of the arrest to be successful. Therefore, CPR should be begun by the first person on the scene. The physician may take over CPR or may choose to monitor the patient's status and supervise the resuscitation activities.

Advanced cardiac life support is performed by physicians, nurses, and paramedics trained in the techniques, which include:

- CPR to sustain tissue oxygenation
- Endotracheal intubation to obtain a patent airway and provide supplemental oxygen
- Intravenous drugs to correct acidosis, maintain blood pressure, and stimulate normal cardiac rhythm (Table 8–3)
- Defibrillation to terminate ventricular fibrillation by means of an electrical counter-shock to the myocardial cells

Studies have shown that defibrillation is the most successful way to convert ventricular fibrillation to a perfusing rhythm and that early defibrillation is a key to improving survival rates in sudden cardiac death (AHA, 1994). As a result, communities are now training emergency medical technicians and volunteers to defibrillate in the field by means of automated external defibrillators. These computerized devices read the cardiac rhythm and determine the need for defibrillation. In the hospital, the need for defibrillation is determined by the physician or other qualified personnel and is ordered according to standard defibrillation protocols.

NURSING PROCESS GUIDELINES
Cardiac Arrest

Be prepared to perform CPR when needed. Review and practice on a regular basis the psychomotor skills necessary to perform CPR correctly and with the least possible risk to the patient. Include practice using manual resuscitators with a bag-valve-mask device and other barrier masks, as these are used in clinical settings.

When administering CPR, perform steps in the

Table 8–2

Supplies Commonly Found on a Crash Cart

Arterial blood gas kit
Alcohol wipes
Angiocatheters (assorter)
Cardiac arrest board
Central venous catheters
Chest tubes (assorted)
Defibrillator
Defibrillator pads
Dressing materials
Electrocardiographic electrodes
Endotracheal tubes
Foley catheters and drainage bags
Irrigation tray
Intravenous fluids (assorted)
Intravenous tubing
Laryngoscope
Manual resuscitator bag with face mask
Medications
   Adenosine (Adenocard)
   Atropine sulfate
   Digoxin (Lanoxin)
   Dopamine hydrochloride (Intropin)
   Epinephrine
   Furosemide (Lasix)
   Heparin
   Hydrocortisone sodium succinate (Solu-Cortef)
   Isoproterenol hydrochloride
   Lidocaine hydrochloride
   Magnesium sulfate
   Methylprednisolone sodium succinate (Solu-Medrol)
   Naloxone hydrochloride (Narcan)
   Nitroglycerin (glyceryl trinitrate)
   Norepinephrine bitartrate (Levophed)
   Phentolamine mesylate (Regitine)
   Procainamide hydrochloride (Pronestyl)
   Propranolol hydrochloride (Inderal)
   Sodium bicarbonate
   Verapamil hydrochloride
Nasogastric tubes
Needle discard box
Oral and nasal airways
Portable oxygen
Protective coverings (gowns, gloves, goggles, masks)
Tape
Tourniquets
Tracheostomy tray
Tracheostomy tubes
Wrist and vest restraints
Emergency carts are checked daily to be sure that all equipment is functioning and in place, and that drugs and intravenous solutions stored on the cart have not expired.

order shown in Table 8–4. Begin each step with assessment and base interventions on the assessment findings. To aid in recalling the correct sequence of assessments and interventions, remember the American Heart Association's "ABCs of CPR": airway, breathing, and circulation.

Table 8–3

Drugs Used for Cardiac Arrest

Drug	Purpose	Dose	Comments
Epinephrine	Vasoconstrictor Improves blood flow to heart and brain during resuscitation	1.0 mg IV If ventricular fibrillation or asystole persists, repeat at 3- to 5-minute intervals (designated as standard-dose epinephrine or SDE)	If IV route not available, drug may be administered endotracheally. Dosage may be adjusted upward to maintain effectiveness. Consideration now being given to higher doses (called HDE) after two unsuccessful attempts at SDE.
Lidocaine	Antifibrillatory Used to treat ventricular fibrillation that does not respond to epinephrine	1.5 mg/kg of body weight Repeat once in 3 to 5 minutes	A continuous IV infusion of lidocaine may be started after the two doses have been given. The rate is usually 2 mg per minute.
Bretylium	Antifibrillatory Used if treatment with lidocaine is unsuccessful	5 mg/kg of body weight followed by defibrillation. Increase to 10 mg/kg and repeat every 5 minutes to maximum dose of 35 mg/kg	May take as long as 5 minutes before heart responds. Perform CPR for at least this long. Bretylium is not a first-line drug and may cause severe hypotension.
Atropine	Used to treat symptomatic bradycardia.	0.5 to 1 mg IV push. Repeat every 3 to 5 minutes.	Use cautiously with myocardial infarction. Do not give less than 0.5 mg per dose because doing so may cause a paradoxical slowing of the heart.
Adenosine	Slows conduction through the atrioventricular node Used in paroxysmal supraventricular tachycardia or wide-complex tachycardia of unknown origin	6 mg rapidly by IV push If no response in 1 to 2 minutes, give 12 mg by IV push Repeat 12 mg dose in 1 to 2 minutes if necessary	Must be given rapidly because half-life is 5 seconds. A brief period of asystole is common after administration.
Dopamine	Used to treat shock and correct hemodynamic imbalances Improves perfusion to vital organs, increases cardiac output, and corrects hypotension	Titrated dosage starting with 2 to 5 μg/kg/minute IV up to 50 μg/kg/minute	Not a substitute for fluid volume replacement. Extravasation may cause tissue sloughing and necrosis.
Magnesium sulfate	An element necessary for many cellular reactions Used to treat hypomagnesemia	1 to 2 grams diluted in 10 ml of D_5W given IV push over 1 to 2 minutes	Rapid administration may cause flushing, sweating, and hypotension.

CPR, cardiopulmonary resuscitation; IV, intravenous.

Once initiated, continue uninterrupted cardiopulmonary resuscitation until the return of a spontaneous cardiac rhythm or the physician orders it stopped. The exception to this is the brief period when CPR is interrupted for the patient to be intubated, defibrillated, or both. While CPR is being done, other personnel will be starting intravenous lines, connecting cardiac monitors, and administering medications according to the physician's orders.

Once the cardiac rhythm is re-established, the patient will be transferred to a critical care unit for monitoring and further treatment.

Patients who experience a cardiac arrest have special concerns and needs following a successful resuscitation. Nursing Care Guide 8–1 addresses some of the needs of patient surviving a cardiac arrest.

Family members of the patient also have needs and concerns beginning with the resuscitation effort and continuing through the patient's recovery or death. Families who are present when the patient goes into arrest need emotional support while they await the outcome of the resuscitation effort. Some facilities allow the family to remain in the room to witness the resuscitation while other facilities request the family wait in a separate room. In either

Table 8–4

Basic Steps in Cardiopulmonary Resuscitation

Step	Assessment	Intervention	Rationale
A: Airway	Determine the patient's responsiveness. Grasp the patient's shoulder and shake gently while calling the patient's name. (Never shake if you suspect a neck injury.)	If unresponsive, call for help from other hospital personnel by instituting code procedures. Open the patient's airway using the chin lift or jaw thrust maneuver. (Use the jaw thrust if you suspect a neck injury.) Remember that the tongue is the most common cause of airway obstruction in an unconscious adult.	It is difficult for one person to carry out successful CPR because of its physical and emotional demands. Expert medical assistance will be needed to initiate advanced cardiac life support procedures as indicated by the patient's condition.
B: Breathing	Determine breathing. Look for chest movement, listen for air moving in and out of the patient's nose and mouth, and feel for the patient's breath on your cheek.	If the patient is not breathing, give two rescue breaths. Use a barrier mask to prevent exchange of body fluids between patient and nurse. Supply supplemental oxygen by connecting the resuscitation bag to the oxygen flow meter.	Ventilation prevents and corrects acidosis associated with hypercapnia secondary to anaerobic metabolism.
C: Circulation	Check for circulation. Using the first and second finger of the hand closest to the chest, feel for the carotid pulse. Assessment should take 5 to 10 seconds and should not be hurried.	If there is no pulse, begin cardiac compressions at the rate of 15 compressions to two respirations. If two rescuers are present, the ratio is five compressions to one respiration. Compressions should be 1.5 to 2 inches deep and over the lower half of the sternum. If the patient is in bed, use a cardiac arrest board to create a hard surface. Complications may include pneumothorax, fractured ribs and sternum, laceration of the liver and spleen, and fat emboli.	External cardiac massage changes intrathoracic pressure, closing the mitral and tricuspid valves and forcing blood into the pulmonary artery and aorta.

Based on information in *Textbook of Basic Life Support for Healthcare Providers.* Copyright © 1994, American Heart Association.

situation, assign a support person to the visitors to inform them of what is being done and why. This support person should be present when any information is being shared with the family to help clarify, if necessary, what the family is told.

Family members generally want to see their loved one as soon as possible after the resuscitation effort regardless of the outcome. The nurse should be present to continue the emotional support during these visits. Prior to the family entering the patient's room, equipment and medical apparatus they will see should be explained to them. Remember that the family may be hesitant to talk to or touch the patient without "permission" from the nurse.

The nurse who assumes the support role often has a more difficult role than the nurse actively involved in the resuscitation effort. Good communication skills and the use of clear and explicit language as well as appropriate silence are necessary to help the family cope with the situation.

Heart Failure

Some three to four million Americans suffer from heart failure. It is the most common discharge diagnosis for patients over age 65. As the present popu-

Nursing Care Guide 8–1
Patients Surviving a Cardiac Arrest

Assessment Findings: Patient is nervous, restless, and tense; withdraws from others; expresses feelings of fear, helplessness, and concern about the future.

Nursing Diagnosis: Anxiety related to fear of cardiac disease, uncertainties about the future, and the possibility of death

Patient Outcomes	Nursing Interventions	Rationale
Patient appears relaxed with no visible signs of anxiety such as nervousness, restlessness, or clenching of the hands.	Allow time for discussion of the patient's concerns and fears without expressing opinions about the patient's status.	Accepting but not encouraging denial of the patient's condition or seriousness of the illness leaves the atmosphere open for free expressions of feelings.
	Invite questions about the patient's condition, and share the information with the family.	Including significant others will encourage their continued support.
	Provide rest periods and time for privacy.	These are measures that can improve cardiac output.
Patient reports feeling less anxious, verbalizes methods for coping with illness, joins in conversations, and participates in care regimen.	Help the patient find effective coping strategies to manage the lifestyle changes that may be necessary.	Using coping techniques helps alleviate stress.
	Teach relaxation techniques.	Relaxation techniques assist in anxiety reduction and allow for rest.
	Acknowledge that feelings of fear are normal and expected after such a traumatic event.	Acknowledgment of feelings provides understanding and support.
	Encourage participation in the daily care regimen.	Encouraging patient participation in the care acknowledges the patient's worth and the expectation of return to normal activities.

Evaluation: Compare the patient's status with the expected patient outcomes. If the outcomes are not met, reassess the patient and revise the plan.

Assessment Findings: Patient presents altered hemodynamics, decreased output, poor peripheral circulation, and cyanosis.

Nursing Diagnosis: Decreased cardiac output related to electrical and mechanical malfunction

Patient Outcomes	Nursing Interventions	Rationale
Patient exhibits a cardiac rhythm that is stable to support an adequate cardiac output and demonstrates a decrease in dysrhythmias as seen by the hemodynamic monitoring.	Promptly treat life-threatening dysrhythmias with DC shock and medications.	Immediate intervention may prevent arrest.
	Monitor the heart rate and rhythm continuously. Assess for dysrhythmias and accompanying symptoms. Prepare for defibrillation, pacemaker insertion, or ICD if the patient has a life-threatening cardiac rhythm.	Careful monitoring provides for early interventions if problems arise.

(continued)

Nursing Care Guide 8–1
Patients Surviving a Cardiac Arrest (continued)

Patient Outcomes	Nursing Interventions	Rationale
	Assist the patient in turning and performing other self-care activities. Perform passive range-of-motion exercises as tolerated.	Implementing these actions will reduce cardiac workload and promote rest.
	Administer oxygen, and raise the head of the bed for maximum chest expansion.	Reduces cardiac workload by enhancing oxygenation of the blood. Elevated position also decreases venous return to the heart.
	Allow the patient frequent rest periods during delivery of nursing care.	Rest during activities decreases demand on the heart and reduces cardiac workload.
	Use a bedside commode.	Decreases straining and the Valsalva maneuver.
	Reduce disturbances. Plan care to allow uninterrupted periods of rest.	Reducing external stimuli allows for rest and reduces cardiac strain.
Patient's vital signs are within normal ranges for the patient.	Assess vital signs frequently, noting any changes.	Vital signs within normal ranges may indicate patient stability.
	Evaluate mentation and urinary output.	Mental alertness and adequate urinary output indicate adequate cardiac output and perfusion of vital organs.
	Notify physician according to protocol.	Protocol ensures patient safety.

Evaluation: Compare the patient's status with the expected patient outcomes. If the outcomes are not met, reassess the patient and revise the plan.

Assessment Findings: Patient complains of pressure, heaviness, or pain in the chest and states pain is radiating into the neck and arm.

Nursing Diagnosis: Pain (chest) related to myocardial ischemia secondary to coronary artery occlusion

Patient Outcomes	Nursing Interventions	Rationale
Patient rates pain as less than 3 on a scale of 0 to 10. Patient rests and sleeps well.	Give prescribed pharmacologic agents for anginal pain, and repeat as ordered.	Antianginal agents are vasodilators that increase myocardial perfusion and can quickly reduce the anginal episode or prevent another attack.
	Teach relaxation techniques and position the patient for comfort.	Relaxation and comfort measures may help reduce the pain or make it more tolerable for the patient.
	Obtain 12-lead ECG.	Documents location of pathologic changes and guides treatment.

(continued)

Patients Surviving a Cardiac Arrest (continued)

Patient Outcomes	Nursing Interventions	Rationale
Patient describes relaxation methods and coping strategies to assist in the control or prevention of anginal episodes.	Support the patient in the use of coping methods that help patient to relax and relieve or prevent episodes of pain. Place articles within reach. Help prevent anginal episodes by teaching the patient to use energy-saving activities.	Reduction of anxiety decreases sympathetic nervous system stimulation and hence myocardial workload and assists the patient to rest. Energy-saving practices reduce the workload of the myocardium.

Evaluation: Compare the patient's status with the expected patient outcomes. If the outcomes are not met, reassess the patient and revise the plan.

Assessment Findings: Patient is dyspneic, tachypneic, and cyanotic; blood pressure is elevated, and tachycardia is present; some confusion, dizziness, and a headache are present; urine output is decreased; gastric distress and distention are evident; peripheral pulses are diminished; toes are pale and cool.

Nursing Diagnosis: Altered cardiopulmonary, cerebral, renal, peripheral, and gastrointestinal tissue perfusion related to decreased cardiac output secondary to decreased effectiveness of ventricular pumping.

Patient Outcomes	Nursing Interventions	Rationale
Patient demonstrates appropriate functioning of all body systems as seen on hemodynamic monitoring, and by freedom from gastrointestinal or neurologic symptoms; and adequate output.	Monitor and assess the adequacy of cardiac function, respiratory status, urine output, mentation, gastrointestinal functioning, and peripheral circulation. Provide frequent, small, nonirritating meals. Complete range-of-motion exercises, and reposition the patient frequently.	Decreased cardiac output may affect all body systems. Careful monitoring for changes and the promotion of activities that improve circulation are important to the patient's progress. Early intervention may reduce the effects of the disorder. Large meals require an increase in blood supply to the gastrointestinal tract for digestion to take place. Such foods as caffeine, tea, chocolate are myocardial stimulants and increase oxygen consumption. Stimulates circulation and decreases the risk of pressure sores and maintains joint motion.

(continued)

Nursing Care Guide 8–1
Patients Surviving a Cardiac Arrest (continued)

Patient Outcomes	Nursing Interventions	Rationale
	Have the patient take frequent deep breaths with good chest expansion.	Increases O_2 intake and reduces cardiac workload.
	Keep the patient in a high Fowler's position, and administer oxygen by nasal cannula, mask, or intubation.	
Patient is warm, with good skin color, palpable peripheral pulses, and no signs of tissue ischemia.	Check for skin breakdown caused by decreased circulation to the extremities.	Maintenance of skin integrity is important. Decreased circulatory status predisposes the patient to skin breakdown and infections.
	Keep the patient warm.	Keeping patient warm prevents cold stress.
	Remove constricting clothing.	Removing constricting clothing facilitates ventilation and circulation; decreases risk of thromboembolism.
	Give prescribed medications to increase circulation and monitor for therapeutic and non-therapeutic effects.	Monitoring allows need for change in drug or dosage to be identified.
	Do not allow patient to smoke.	Smoking causes vasoconstriction.
	Teach the patient to use relaxation methods.	Relaxation will reduce stress, thus reducing cardiac workload.
Evaluation:	Compare the patient's status with the expected patient outcomes. If the outcomes are not met, reassess the patient and revise the plan.	

lation ages, heart failure is predicted to become an increasingly prevalent cause of hospitalization. Heart failure has a significantly high mortality rate, with many patients dying within the first few years of diagnosis. Early diagnosis and interventions can lower the mortality rate, reduce subsequent hospitalizations, and improve the quality of life for these patients.

Heart failure is not a disease; it is a syndrome caused by a variety of disease processes. Heart failure can be defined as a physiologic state in which the heart fails to pump enough blood to meet the metabolic demands of the body during activity and when at rest. This broad definition encompasses two distinct categories of heart failure: high-output failure and low-output failure. High-output failure occurs in the absence of cardiac disease. Cardiac output is normal or above normal in this type of heart failure, but the metabolic demands of the body are so high that the amount of oxygenated blood

pumped to the tissues is inadequate to meet the need. Causes of high-output failure include sepsis, hyperthyroidism, Paget's disease, and anemia. In low-output failure, the heart fails as a pump. Cardiac output is diminished and does not meet even normal metabolic demands. Low-output failure is caused by conditions such as arteriosclerosis, hypertension, myocardial infarction, and valvular disorders. Low-output failure is more common and is the primary focus of this discussion. Fig. 8–22 shows the compensatory mechanisms in heart failure.

Etiology and Pathophysiology
There are four basic factors that can cause the heart to fail as a pump:

- An increase in volume of blood to be pumped
- An increase in resistance against which the blood must be pumped
- A decrease in the heart's contractility
- A decrease in filling of the cardiac chambers

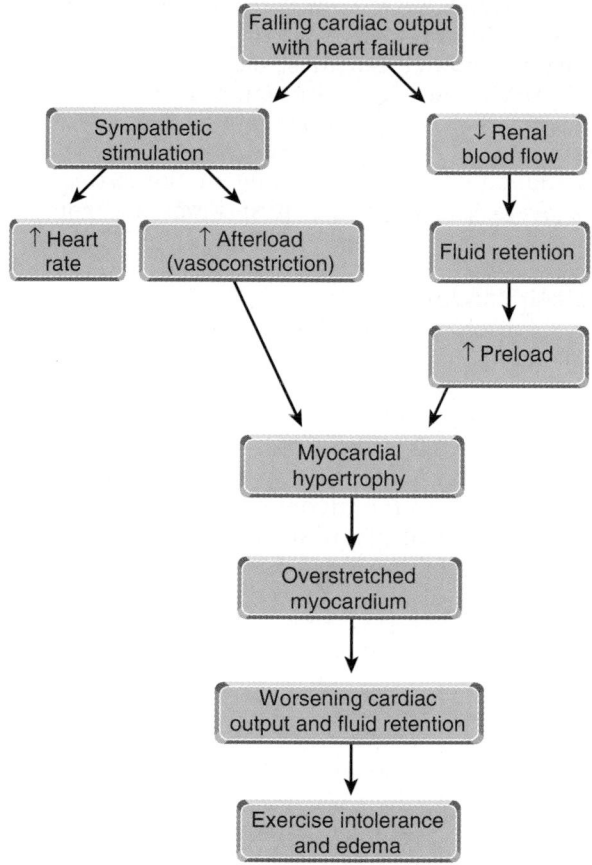

Figure 8–22

Schematic representation of compensatory mechanisms in heart failure.

Causes of an increased volume of blood to be pumped (increased preload) include mitral regurgitation, aortic regurgitation, and left to right shunts through atrial or ventricular septal defects. Causes of increased resistance against which blood must be pumped (increased afterload) include systemic hypertension and aortic stenosis. Decreased contractility results from damage to the myocardium and thus can be caused by myocardial infarction, myocarditis, or cardiomyopathy. Decreased filling occurs if the ventricle is constricted or unable to relax, such as in cardiac tamponade or pericarditis.

Heart failure is termed *systolic*, or forward, failure when the contraction of the ventricle is not strong enough to empty itself by ejecting an adequate volume of blood into the circulation. Systolic failure results in diminished tissue perfusion so symptoms of specific organ or system dysfunction present.

Heart failure is termed *diastolic*, or backward, failure when the ventricles fail to adequately relax and are unable to fill properly. This leads to an accumulation of blood and increased pressure in the atrium and the pulmonary or systemic venous system.

When the heart begins to fail, the compensatory mechanisms that allow the healthy heart to adjust to normal variations in workload and metabolic demand immediately come into play. These mechanisms maintain cardiac output temporarily despite the failing function of the heart. However, as the failure worsens, these mechanisms become unable to sustain the cardiac output and ultimately end up contributing to the failure.

One of the most important of these compensatory mechanisms is the Frank-Starling mechanism in which the tension in a muscle as it contracts increases as the length of the muscle at rest increases. In the heart, this means that increased stretch of the ventricle during diastole results in a stronger systolic contraction. Since stretch increases as the volume of blood in the ventricle increases, an increase in end-diastolic volume results in an increased force of contraction, increased stroke volume, and hence increased cardiac output.

But, stretch can only increase tension in the contracting muscle to a certain degree. Once this limit is reached, no further increase in stroke volume due to the Frank-Starling mechanism can occur.

A second compensatory mechanism is an increase in heart rate. As cardiac output decreases, arterial pressure decreases and the baroreceptors are stimulated. This in turn stimulates the sympathetic nervous system and norepinephrine is released. Norepinephrine raises heart rate by stimulation of the cardiac β-receptors. Since heart rate, along with stroke volume, determines cardiac output, an increase in heart rate supports an increase in cardiac output up to the point that diastole becomes so brief that the ventricle cannot fill adequately and cardiac output drops.

With chronic overloading of the heart, two other compensatory mechanisms develop. The first is ventricular hypertrophy. This is an increase in thickness of the muscle fibers, which in turn thickens the ventricular wall and results in a more effective contraction. Hypertrophy results from chronic pressure overload, as occurs with stenosis of the aortic valve or systemic hypertension. Initially the thickening of the heart muscle results in a more forceful contraction and improves cardiac output. However, as hypertrophy progresses, the muscle works at a lower inotropic state and contraction becomes less effective. In addition, when the myocardial mass expands beyond the point at which the coronary circulation is capable of meeting its need for oxygen, myocardial hypoxia occurs. This further impairs the effectiveness of pumping.

Ventricular dilatation is an enlargement of the ventricular chamber. It results from chronic overstretching of the ventricular muscle fibers by excessive volumes of blood.

In addition to these cardiac compensatory mechanisms, peripheral mechanisms also come into operation in an attempt to maintain cardiac output. The norepinephrine secreted in response to baroreceptor stimulation causes vasoconstriction in addition to increasing the heart rate. Venous vasoconstriction results in decreased pooling of venous blood in the periphery due to a contraction of venous space. This in turn increases venous return to the heart. Arteriolar constriction maintains blood pressure despite a decrease in cardiac output. It also shunts blood away from the kidneys, gastrointestinal system, skin, and skeletal muscle to the heart and brain in order to maintain adequate perfusion of these vital organs that have high metabolic rates.

In response to this decreased blood flow to the kidneys, the renin-angiotensin system is activated. Activation of this system causes further vasoconstriction as well as secretion of aldosterone and antidiuretic hormone. Aldosterone promotes water retention as a result of increased sodium resorption in the renal tubules, and antidiuretic hormone inhibits water excretion in the distal tubules. These peripheral mechanisms effectively maintain cardiac output in the face of hypovolemia. However, with a failing myocardium, they can cause a decrease in cardiac output as a result of the extra workload placed on the heart. Atrial natriuretic peptide, a hormone stored in atrial muscle, protects the failing heart against these effects to some extent. Atrial natriuretic peptide, which is released in response to atrial stretching, promotes the excretion of sodium and water. It suppresses the secretion of aldosterone and antidiuretic hormone, lowers serum renin and norepinephrine levels, and directly relaxes peripheral blood vessels. With long-term atrial distention, stores of atrial natriuretic peptide are depleted and its balancing effect on the peripheral compensatory mechanisms is lost.

Once these cardiac and peripheral mechanisms no longer effectively compensate for the failing heart, symptoms of decompensation ensue.

Because the heart consists of two separate pumping systems, failure may affect one or both sides. Typically, failure of one side progresses to failure of both sides. Most often failure occurs first in the left side of the heart because of its heavy workload and high oxygen requirement. With left-sided heart failure, the left ventricle does not empty completely because of ineffective contraction. This results in reduced cardiac output and an accumulation of blood in the heart. The effect of reduced cardiac output is poor tissue perfusion, so changes in the function of organs and systems occur. Accumulation of blood in the heart results in an increase in atrial and ventricular end-diastolic pressure and poor filling, causing blood to back up in the pulmonary veins. This congestion raises pressure in the pulmonary vessels and causes fluid to move out of the vessels and into the interstitial spaces. Fluid in the tissues of the lung is called pulmonary edema and constitutes a life-threatening complication of left-sided heart failure (see the next section on pulmonary edema).

Right-sided heart failure can develop as a result of primary pulmonary hypertension or a right-side myocardial infarct, but most often it develops as the result of the work of pumping against increased pulmonary pressure secondary to left-sided heart failure. As the right ventricle fails, blood backs up into the right atrium and then in the systemic venous system. Congestion of abdominal organs and peripheral edema results.

Clinical Manifestations

Heart failure can be either acute or chronic. Acute heart failure has an abrupt onset, often without warning. It may present as pulmonary edema—an acute life-threatening situation in which the alveoli of the lungs fill with fluids—syncope, shock, or sudden death. Acute heart failure can result from severe damage to the myometrium of the left ventricle as with a myocardial infarction. Conversely, chronic heart failure develops gradually over time. Symptoms of chronic failure are less severe and the patient often presents in less acute distress because compensatory mechanisms develop over time.

Left-Sided Heart Failure

Dyspnea in its many forms is one of the earliest symptoms of left-sided heart failure. It occurs because edema in the interstitial tissues of the lungs makes the lungs stiffer, thereby increasing the work of breathing (Fig. 8–23). Dyspnea occurs initially on exertion but as the heart progressively fails it occurs at rest. Orthopnea and paroxysmal nocturnal dyspnea are also characteristic of left-sided heart failure. Orthopnea, or dyspnea that occurs on lying down flat, is relieved by sitting up. Patients with this condition typically sleep with the head and thorax elevated. Paroxysmal nocturnal dyspnea is a sudden intense feeling of suffocation or shortness of breath that awakens the patient a few hours after lying down and going to sleep. It is relieved by sitting up, opening a window, or walking around. Both orthopnea and paroxysmal nocturnal dyspnea occur because the supine position allows fluid that has previously collected in dependent areas to return to the general circulation, thus overloading the failing left ventricle and causing a back-up of fluid in the lungs. Sitting up or standing relieves the distress, because venous return is decreased by the effect of gravity so that the volume of blood to be pumped by the heart is reduced.

In some patients, orthopnea manifests as a dry, nonproductive, hacking cough rather than as difficulty breathing. Like classic orthopnea, this cough develops in the supine position and is relieved by sitting up.

The major sign of left-sided heart failure found on physical examination is the presence of moist crackles on auscultation. In early left-sided failure, these crackles may be limited to the lung bases, but as failure worsens, they are heard over a progressively greater area of the lung fields. Other signs of

Decreased cardiac output:

Tachycardia
Fatigue
Dizziness
Decreased urination
Angina
Restlessness

Enlarged left atrium

Pulmonary congestion:

Cough, especially at night
Dyspnea
Tachypnea
Crackles
Frothy, pinkish sputum

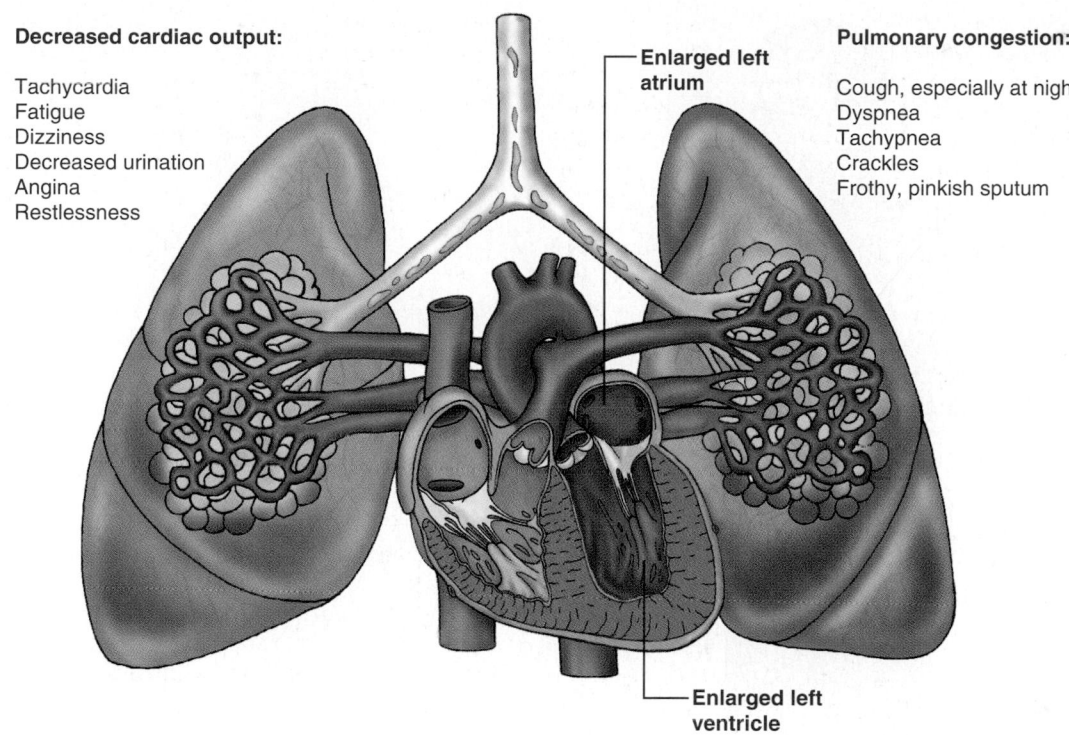

Enlarged left ventricle

Figure 8–23

Left-sided heart failure.

left-sided heart failure are tachypnea, wheezing, an S₃ gallop, and paradoxical splitting of the second heart sound.

Right-Sided Heart Failure
Symptoms of right-sided heart failure result from a back-up of blood in the systemic venous system (Fig. 8–24). Early signs of this venous congestion are distended neck veins (jugular venous distention) and peripheral edema. Retention of sodium and water secondary to elevated aldosterone levels contributes to dependent pitting edema. It increases gradually as right-sided heart failure worsens, appearing first in the feet and ankles and progressing to involve the upper leg and then the external genitalia and lower trunk. The exception is in bedridden patients in whom edema first appears in the sacral area.

Venous congestion can also affect organs. The first organ to be affected is usually the liver. Hepatomegaly (enlargement of the liver) occurs due to congestion of the hepatic veins. This congestion causes the liver to distend and stretch its capsule, producing right upper quadrant pain or tenderness. With chronic congestion and hypoxia, liver cells eventually become fibrosed and necrotic. As this occurs, liver function tests, such as alkaline phosphatase, aspartate transaminase, and alanine transaminase, become abnormal and prothrombin time may be prolonged. In rare cases, jaundice, ascites, and frank liver failure may ensue. Occasionally, the spleen and splanchnic vessels also become congested. With the latter condition, anorexia, nausea, diarrhea, and malabsorption are common because of the congestion of the gastrointestinal tract.

Low Cardiac Output Syndrome
Patients with either left- or right-sided heart failure often exhibit the signs and symptoms of low cardiac output syndrome. These include fatigue resulting from tissue hypoxia and inadequate removal of toxic wastes; cachexia secondary to loss of lean muscle mass; and lethargy, light-headedness and confusion due to decreased cerebral blood flow. An increase in blood urea nitrogen relative to serum creatinine indicates a decrease in renal perfusion, and, in severe cases, oliguria and renal failure may occur.

Diagnosis
Diagnosis of heart failure is not based on a single diagnostic measure or test. Diagnosis of heart failure begins with the patient's history, physical examination, and clinical manifestations and is followed by a variety of invasive and noninvasive tests done to support the diagnosis, identify the underlying cause, and determine the severity of the heart failure.

These tests include chest x-rays, electrocardiograms, echocardiograms, radionuclide studies (thallium or technetium scans), multigated angiographic scans, and basic laboratory studies (arterial blood gases, serum electrolytes, complete blood count), and tests of hepatic and renal function. On an upright chest x-ray, distention of the pulmonary veins

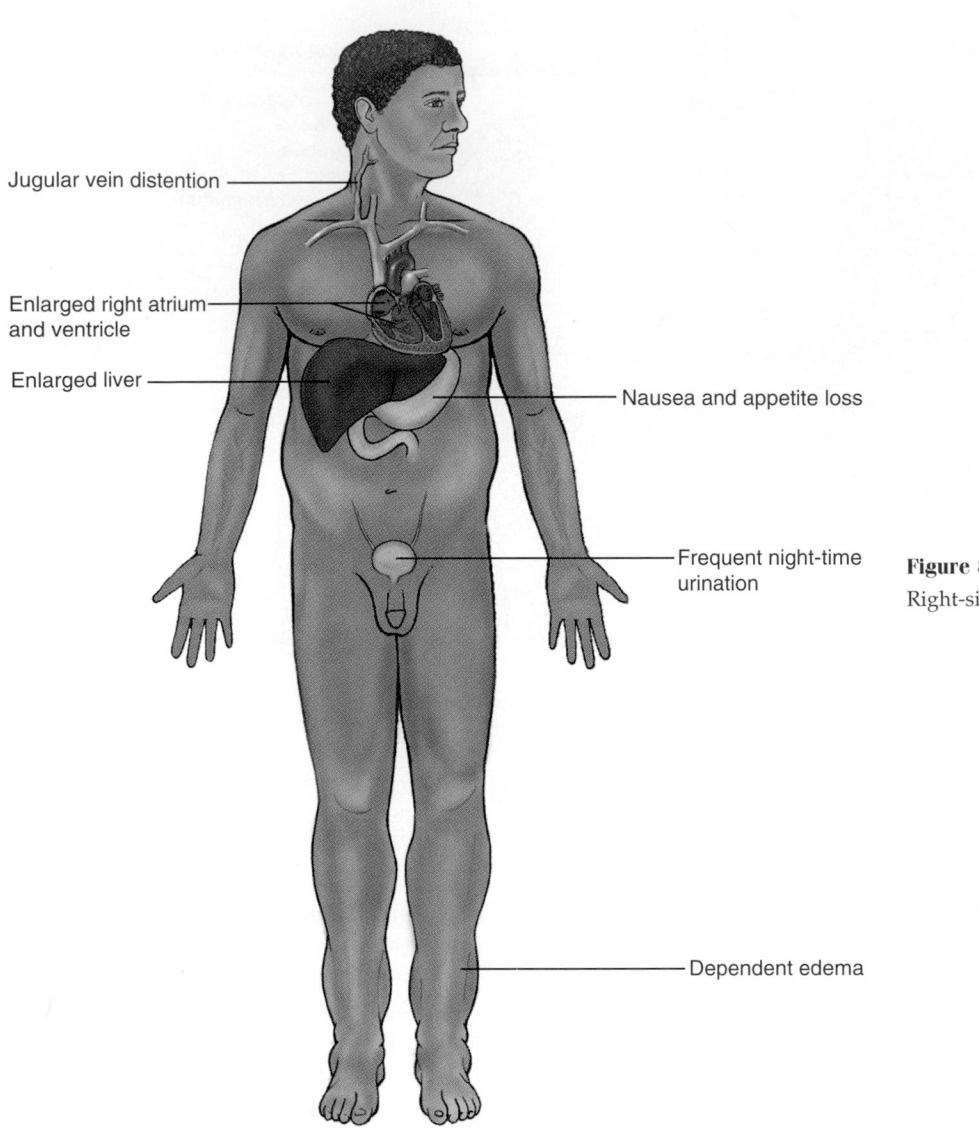

Jugular vein distention

Enlarged right atrium and ventricle

Enlarged liver

Nausea and appetite loss

Frequent night-time urination

Dependent edema

Figure 8–24
Right-sided heart failure.

of the upper lobe is the earliest sign of pulmonary congestion. As congestion progresses and interstitial fluid builds up around the blood vessels, the film takes on a hazy appearance. As edema develops in the alveoli, densities appear in the lung fields. An enlarged cardiac silhouette indicative of cardiac hypertrophy and dilatation can also be seen on x-ray. Electrocardiographic tracings can also demonstrate cardiac hypertrophy as well as dysrhythmias or myocardial damage. Echocardiography can document valvular changes and chamber enlargement as well as hypertrophy.

Hemodynamic monitoring, using pulmonary arterial catheters, can be used to measure cardiac pressures. Pulmonary artery pressure and pulmonary artery wedge pressure measure the left ventricular pressure in patients with left-sided failure. Central venous pressure measurements monitor right ventricular pressure in patients with right-sided failure (see Chap. 7).

Management
Management of heart failure is first aimed at correction of the underlying cause. Thus dysrhythmias or heart blocks should be controlled with drug therapy or a pacemaker, systemic hypertension should be treated, and surgical correction of cardiac deformities should be considered. Heart failure not corrected by measures such as these is managed primarily by pharmacologic therapy, dietary therapy, and rest.

Pharmacologic Therapy
Since heart failure is a complex syndrome, a combination of drugs is typically required for effective management. The specific types of drugs utilized depend on the clinical manifestations but most often include inotropic agents, angiotensin-converting enzyme (ACE) inhibitors, diuretics, and vasodilators.

INOTROPIC AGENTS. Inotropic drug therapy maximizes cardiac function by increasing myocardial

■■■■■■▶
■ **Clinical Pathway for Heart Failure**
■

Patient Name _____ Date _____

DRG# _____ Expected LOS _____

	Day 1 (Critical Care Unit)	Day 2 (Critical Care Unit)	Day 3 (Critical Care Unit/ Telemetry Unit)	Day 4 (Telemetry Unit)	Day 5 (Telemetry Unit/ Medical-Surgical Unit)
Medication	• ACE inhibitors • Digitize patient (inotropics IV) • Diuretics IV • Vasodilators to reduce preload, afterload • Nitroglycerin IV	• Continue meds • Switch to topical nitroglycerin • Add stool softener	• Continue ACE inhibitors PO • Give digoxin, diuretics, stool softener PO • Continue topical nitroglycerin	• Continue orally	• Continue orally
Diagnostic Tests	• ECG • ABGs • Electrolytes • BUN • Serum enzymes • Digoxin level	• ECG • Enzymes • Electrolytes • Echocardiogram	• Enzymes • Electrolytes • Digoxin level • Cardiac catheterization if needed	• Potassium levels • Pulse oximetry on room air • EPS if needed	• Digoxin level
Diet	• Clear liquid • Fluid restriction • Low sodium	• Full liquid • Fluid restriction	• Soft • Low sodium • Low fat • Assist as needed • Fluid restriction	• Restricted sodium and fat • Normal fluids	• Restricted sodium and fat • Normal fluids
Activity	• Bedrest • Elevate HOB 30 to 60 degrees • Commode if needed for BM • Provide hygiene • Leg extension and dorsiflexion	• Bedside chair × 1–2 • Commode • Elevate HOB when in bed • Assist with ADLs • Leg exercises, ROM	• Ambulate short distance × 2–3 • OOB for meals • Bedrest after cardiac catheterization per unit protocol • Assist with ADLs	• Ambulate × 5–6	• As tolerated
Treatments/ Nursing Actions	• Baseline bed weight • O₂ to keep SO₂ above 94% • Hemodynamic monitoring (CVP, PA, PWP) • Cardiac monitor • Central line • Vital signs q 1h • Breath sounds, pulmonary hygiene, skin assessment • I & O	• Weight • O₂ to keep SO₂ above 94% • Discontinue hemodynamic monitor • Cardiac monitor • IV at keep-vein-open rate • Vital signs q 2h • Breath sounds, pulmonary hygiene, skin assessment	• Weight • Discontinue O₂ if SO₂ is above 94% • Telemetry • Continue venous access device • Vital signs q 4h • Breath sounds, pulmonary hygiene, skin assessment	• Weight • Telemetry • Discontinue venous access device • Vital signs q 4h • Continue pulmonary hygiene	• Weight • Discontinue telemetry
Teaching/ Discharge Planning	• Deep-breathing and leg exercises • Assess family support	• ROM • Skin care • Social service consult	• Visiting nurse consult • Dietary consult • Teach to take pulse • Teach about heart failure (what it is and how it is managed)	• Cardiac rehab consult • Verify that home services are in place • Written and oral teaching about each medication • Review diet • Teach symptoms that require MD consult	• Review meds • Review diet • Review activity • Teach patient to obtain weight daily or 2 to 3 times weekly

contractility and, therefore, stroke volume and cardiac output. This ability of the heart muscle to improve contractility is called a positive inotropic action. This action decreases preload (filling pressure), relieves venous congestion, and decreases end-diastolic pressure, with the net result of alleviating the signs and symptoms of heart failure.

DIGITALIS. Digitalis increases stroke volume and cardiac output in patients with systolic heart failure. It does this by increasing the contractility of the myocardium (positive inotropic effect) through inhibition of the enzyme Na^+,K^+-ATPase. This enzyme governs the transport of sodium and potassium across the cell membrane. As a result of this inhibition, potassium moves out of the cell and sodium and calcium enter. The resultant increase in intracellular calcium facilitates the interaction of the contractile elements of the myofibrils thereby increasing the force of contraction. As cardiac output increases, arterial blood pressure rises and suppresses the baroreceptor reflexes, decreasing sympathetic stimulation of the cardiovascular system. As a result of this decreased sympathetic stimulation, the heart rate slows. This allows for more complete emptying of the ventricle. Also, arteriolar tone is decreased, thus reducing afterload. Finally, venous tone is decreased, thus reducing preload.

Increased cardiac output also improves renal blood flow. This increases production of urine, which lowers blood volume and reduces peripheral edema and pulmonary congestion.

Improved renal perfusion also inhibits the release of renin, which decreases aldosterone secretion and water retention. It also decreases the production of angiotensin II, thereby decreasing vasoconstriction. As a result of these actions, symptoms of heart failure are reversed and activity tolerance is increased.

Treatment with digitalis is begun with a loading (digitalizing) dose when rapid onset of action is desired. Once therapeutic blood levels have been achieved, a maintenance dose is prescribed for digoxin, the most commonly used digitalis preparation. The average digitalizing dose is 1.0 to 1.5 mg given orally in divided doses over 24 hours, or 0.75 to 1.0 mg given intravenously. The usual maintenance dose of digoxin required to maintain blood levels in the therapeutic range of 0.5 to 2.0 ng/mL is 0.125 to 2.00 mg per day.

Digitalis has a narrow therapeutic range and a wide variety of factors can lead to toxicity. These include impaired renal function (because digitalis is excreted by the kidney), hypokalemia, hypomagnesemia, hypercalcemia, hypoxemia, and acidosis. Recent myocardial infarction and use of quinidine or procainamide can also induce digitalis toxicity.

Extracardiac signs of digitalis toxicity include anorexia, nausea, vomiting, diarrhea, and, less frequently, visual disturbances such as seeing objects colored green or yellow or surrounded by halos of these colors. The most serious toxic effects are cardiac dysrhythmias, which often occur in the absence of other toxic symptoms. The most common dysrhythmias include premature beats, atrial fibrillation, and first-degree heart block.

Treatment of toxicity consists of withholding the digitalis preparation, correcting the precipitating cause if possible, and providing supportive treatment. In the case of life-threatening dysrhythmias, treatment may involve temporary pacing. Digoxin immune Fab (Digibind), which binds digoxin and is excreted in the urine, is sometimes used to reverse severe toxicity. The role of digitalis in the long-term management of patients with heart failure is controversial because patients with heart failure receiving digitalis have been shown to have a shorter life span than those not on digitalis. It is suggested that this effect occurs because, over time, digitalis depletes energy stores in the myocardium by increasing the force of contraction. Studies are ongoing to determine which patients benefit from digitalis therapy (Wright, 1995).

PHOSPHODIESTERASE INHIBITORS. Phosphodiesterase inhibitors have two effects that are beneficial in the treatment of heart failure. First, they increase myocardial contractility through a positive inotropic effect on the heart. Second, they reduce afterload by producing vasodilation. As a result of these effects, cardiac output is improved. Phosphodiesterase inhibitors are also useful because they can be given to digitalized patients for an apparently additive inotropic effect without a significant increase in the risk of dysrhythmia.

The phosphodiesterase inhibitor amrinone lactate (Inocor) is most often used for short-term (24 hours or less) management of severe heart failure in patients unresponsive to other drug therapy. It is given intravenously mixed with normal or half-normal saline (never dextrose), and invasive hemodynamic monitoring is essential to establish the dose needed to obtain the desired response. Because adverse effects include hepatotoxicity and thrombocytopenia, although mainly with long-term use, liver and blood tests prior to and during therapy are desirable.

Milrinone (Primacor) is another phosphodiesterase inhibitor that is administered intravenously and used as short-term therapy for patients in heart failure. These agents are contraindicated for patients with acute myocardial infarction or severe aortic or pulmonic valve disease. They are used with caution in the elderly, pregnant women, renal or hepatic failure patients, and those who present with hypokalemia. Side effects, which are few with short-term use, include nausea, vomiting, anorexia, and abdominal cramps.

BETA-ADRENERGIC AGONISTS. Beta-adrenergic agonists increase cardiac output by stimulating the β-receptors on the heart, thereby increasing the force of myocardial contraction. Two beta-adrenergic agonists widely used in the treatment of heart failure are dopamine (Intropin) and dobutamine (Dobutrex). Both have strong positive inotropic effects on the heart, but dopamine at moderate dosages also causes dilatation of renal, mesenteric, cerebral, and coronary vasculature. Overall, this vasodilation decreases ventricular afterload and in addition, the increase in renal blood flow promotes diuresis. At higher doses, dopamine can stimulate α-receptors and cause vasoconstriction. This increases cardiac workload by increasing afterload and reduces perfusion to the kidneys and other areas.

ANGIOTENSIN-CONVERTING ENZYME INHIBITORS. ACE inhibitors are widely used to treat heart failure. When used early, they have been shown not only to reduce symptoms but also to slow the progression of pathologic changes in the myocardium (Elkayam, 1997).

ACE inhibitors interfere with the conversion of angiotensin I to angiotensin II in the renin-angiotensin system. Angiotensin II increases cardiac workload because it is a potent vasoconstrictor (increases afterload) and also stimulates the release of aldosterone. This causes the kidney to retain salt and water (increases preload). By blocking the production of angiotensin II, the ACE inhibitors block its effects. Thus ACE inhibitors support vasodilation and decrease resorption of sodium. They improve cardiac output by increasing stroke volume, lower blood pressure, improve renal blood flow, and reduce cardiac workload. Common ACE inhibitors include captopril (Capoten), benazepril hydrochloride (Lotensin), and enalapril maleate (Vasotec). Side effects of the ACE inhibitors include hypotension, cough, skin rash, angioedema, and neutropenia.

DIURETICS. Diuretics are used in the treatment of heart failure because they increase urine production, thereby reducing the volume and pressure of blood to be pumped by the heart. These effects provide prompt relief of symptoms since most symptoms result from increased volume in the pulmonary or systemic circulation.

Major types of diuretics are loop or high-ceiling diuretics, thiazide diuretics, and potassium-sparing diuretics. Loop diuretics such as furosemide (Lasix), bumetanide (Bumex), and ethacrynic acid (Edecrin) are used to treat severe heart failure. These diuretics reduce preload by preventing the reabsorption of sodium and chloride in the descending loop of Henle, thereby increasing fluid excretion. Loop diuretics are the most potent diuretics and have the greatest potential for undesired clinical responses. The major undesired response is extracellular fluid volume deficit. Hypokalemia can also develop rapidly, so potassium supplements are commonly used in conjunction with these diuretics.

Thiazide diuretics are generally used for mild to moderate heart failure. This group, of which hydrochlorothiazide (Hydrodiuril, HCTZ) is the most commonly used, inhibits the reabsorption of sodium and chloride in the proximal and distal convoluted tubules. As with the loop diuretics, hypokalemia, which can cause ventricular ectopic activity, is a risk. Potassium levels must be checked at regular intervals, and oral potassium supplements in the form of potassium chloride may be prescribed.

The potassium-sparing diuretics, such as spironolactone (Aldactone), amiloride (Midamor), and triamterene (Dyrenium), are relatively weak diuretics that do not all work by the same mechanisms. These diuretics may be used in combination with other types to counteract potassium loss and enhance diuresis.

VASODILATORS. Venous vasodilators are important in the short-term management of heart failure. They are given to reverse the vasoconstriction that occurs as a compensatory mechanism in response to reduced cardiac output.

Vasodilators, such as the nitrates, that primarily affect the veins cause blood to pool in the periphery, thereby decreasing venous return to the heart (preload) and cardiac output. These drugs can decrease pulmonary congestion without affecting systemic blood pressure.

Vasodilators, such as hydralazine hydrochloride (Apresoline), that primarily affect arterioles reduce systemic vascular resistance (afterload) and increase cardiac output.

Vasodilators such as nitroprusside (Nipride) and prazosin hydrochloride (Minipress) affect both venous and arterial dilation. These drugs reduce both preload and afterload.

Dietary Management

The goal of dietary management is to reduce sodium and water retention, thereby improving cardiac status (Highlight 8–4). Often the patient is placed initially on a 2 to 4 g sodium restriction diet with further sodium restriction prescribed as the severity of the heart failure increases. A severely sodium-restricted diet is rare because it is unpalatable, costly, and usually results in patient noncompliance.

In cases of severe heart failure, fluid intake by all routes may be restricted to 1000 mL or less per 24 hours. Otherwise, fluids are not generally restricted.

Rest

Bedrest mobilizes fluid from the periphery into the systemic circulation and thereby increases venous return. The increased venous return stretches the myocardial muscle fibers and increases contractility (by the Frank-Starling mechanism), thereby increasing cardiac output. The increased cardiac output improves renal perfusion and promotes diuresis. Bedrest also reduces metabolic activity and therefore the demand for blood flow and cardiac workload. Planned rest periods throughout the day are therapeutic for patients with chronic heart failure.

Prophylactic anticoagulant therapy is used for patients on prolonged bedrest because of the risk of thromboembolism.

Surgical Management

Surgery may be considered for patients in end-stage cardiac disease or refractory heart failure. Correction of the underlying cause of heart failure is attempted

HIGHLIGHT 8-4

NUTRITION

Dietary Guidelines for the Patient with Heart Failure

Instruct the patient with heart failure to follow these dietary guidelines:

- Follow a sodium-restricted diet to help the body get rid of excess fluid. This diet may vary, from the restriction of the addition of table salt to eating foods that contain no sodium. The amount of sodium ingested daily should be based on the severity of the disease and the amount of edema present. The exact amount of sodium allowed is prescribed by the physician. Remember the taste for salt gradually decreases.
- Learn to use other seasonings that enhance food flavor but contribute no sodium to the diet such as lemon juice, vinegar, and herbs.
- Learn to read labels carefully for sodium content. Be aware that baking soda, baking powder, and monosodium glutamate are sources of sodium in foods. Also be aware that toothpastes and over-the-counter drugs such as cough medications and antacids may contain sodium.
- Avoid foods naturally high in sodium, presalted, or preserved with salt. Be especially careful about canned, frozen, and prepared foods.
- Check with physician before using salt substitutes, since they may contain potassium.
- Eat frequent small meals to prevent gastric distention, fatigue, and cardiac or respiratory distress from increased workload on the heart.
- Limit caloric intake to maintain weight or reduce weight if obese.

if the cause is a valvular disorder (see Valvular Surgery) or coronary atherosclerosis (see Coronary Artery Bypass Grafting). In cases of acute myocardial infarction, patients may be placed on a mechanical assist device to improve coronary perfusion until the heart recovers. If no corrective option is available, patients may be considered for a heart transplant (see Chap. 7) or a procedure called dynamic cardiomyoplasty. In dynamic cardiomyoplasty, the patient's latissimus dorsi muscle (skeletal muscle) is wrapped around the ventricle of the patient's heart to improve contractile force and cardiac output. The skeletal muscle is stimulated to contract in synchrony with the myocardium by a cardiomyostimulator implanted in the subcutaneous tissue of the

upper abdomen. A sensing electrode from this device is placed on the epicardium and its two pacing electrodes are placed on the skeletal muscle. Stimulation is begun about 2 weeks postoperatively to allow time for adhesions to form between the skeletal muscle and the heart and for good circulation to be established.

❖ Settings, Providers, and Collaboration for Care

Compliance with the therapeutic plan is essential for the control of heart failure. Because the plan involves not only a medication regimen and need for regular laboratory studies and follow-up examinations but also a dietary regimen, activity limitations, and other lifestyle changes, collaboration among a variety of health-care professionals, the patient, and the family is needed for compliance to occur. In addition to the physician and the acute care nurses, health-care professionals likely to be involved in the care of patients with heart failure are

- The dietitian, who provides information on appropriate menu planning, food selection, and food preparation
- The physical therapist, who guides a graded exercise program
- The discharge planner, who evaluates the home environment in relation to the patient's activity restrictions
- The home care nurse, who assesses for compliance with the treatment plan and monitors cardiac status

A home health or personal care aide may also be needed to provide assistance to patients with significant activity limitation.

Because heart failure can be exacerbated by many factors, including another illness and emotional stress, patients with heart failure, though treated primarily as outpatients, frequently have a number of hospitalizations. Thus collaboration for effective treatment must occur across as well as within settings.

NURSING PROCESS
Heart Failure

Assessment

Review the patient's history. Check for any personal or family history of heart disease. Note type of disease, date of diagnosis, treatment, and treatment outcomes. Identify lifestyle factors known to be associated with or to have an impact on heart disease. Examples of the latter include smoking and use of caffeine-containing food products. Both nicotine and caffeine increase heart rate, which in turn increases the cardiac workload and the need of the myocardium for oxygen. Determine any history of the signs and symptoms of left- and right-sided heart failure. Question the patient about dyspnea. Quantify the degree of dyspnea by asking how many stairs can be climbed or the distance that can be walked before dyspnea occurs. Have the patient rate the severity of dyspnea on a scale of 0 to 10 or 0 to 5. Ask when dyspnea was first noticed and whether it has worsened.

Explore any history of orthopnea. This can be approached by asking how many pillows the patient sleeps on, but care must be taken to ask why extra pillows are used, to differentiate orthopnea from preference. Also question about episodes of paroxysmal nocturnal dyspnea or the presence of "cardiac cough."

Ask the patient about edema, including the following:

- Areas involved, eg, feet and ankles
- Degree, eg, half again normal size or too swollen to fit into shoes
- Relationship to activity or time of day, eg, occurs only after sitting for an extended time, occurs at end of day but gone on arising in the morning

If noticeable edema is denied, asking a question such as, "Do your shoes ever get tight in the evening?" can help identify mild, transient dependent edema.

Question about any upper right abdominal pain or tenderness. These symptoms could be indicative of venous congestion of the liver. Also ask about anorexia, nausea, or diarrhea, which can be indicative of splanchnic congestion.

Since low cardiac output syndrome is often seen with either left- or right-sided heart failure, assess sleep and rest pattern, strength and endurance, and ability to complete activities of daily living. Ask about activity tolerance. Determine what activities are engaged in and for how long before fatigue sets in. Further determine if and how this pattern of activity and fatigue has changed and over what period of time. Check for symptoms of decreased cerebral blood flow such as lethargy, light-headedness, syncope, memory loss, confusion, combativeness, and hallucinations.

If the patient has previously been diagnosed with heart failure, ascertain the time of diagnosis, the presenting symptoms, and the treatment instituted both immediately and over the long-term. Note any current medication or dietary regimen and determine the patient's compliance with it.

Assess the patient's current status. Take vital signs. Remember that in early stages of heart failure, blood pressure may be normal or elevated due to compensatory vasoconstriction, whereas later, as compensatory mechanisms fail, blood pressure is low. Check the rate, rhythm, and quality of the pulse, keeping in mind that tachycardia is common in heart failure because heart rate increases in an attempt to maintain an adequate cardiac output. Be alert for dysrhythmias, which can result from decreased perfusion of the myocardium secondary to a reduction in cardiac output. Assess the strength of the patient's peripheral pulses, which may be bilaterally diminished secondary to decreased cardiac output and reduced tissue perfusion. Diminished peripheral pulses may be accompanied by bounding central pulses with visible jugular, carotid, or abdominal pulsations. Note the rate, rhythm, and depth of respirations and any use of accessory muscles. Auscultate heart sounds. Listen for a diminished S_1 and S_2 as well as for an S_3 or gallop rhythm, which is an early sign of heart failure. Auscultate lung sounds. Expect moist crackles in the lung bases in the early stages of left ventricular failure. The greater the area over which crackles or wheezes are heard, the greater the severity of the failure. Observe for signs of air hunger and for cough, which may be productive or dry and hacking.

Check capillary refill in the nailbeds. Slow capillary refill occurs with decreased peripheral perfusion and therefore is common in heart failure. Assess skin for signs of decreased perfusion. Look for pallor, cyanosis, duskiness, or an ashen appearance. Check for cool temperature, moistness, and any breaks in integrity.

Observe for jugular venous distention and for peripheral edema characteristic of right-sided heart failure. Check for edema of the lower extremities (edema of the sacrum in bedridden patients) and note if it is pitting or nonpitting. Classify it as 1+ to 4+ according to its depth (see Chap. 5). Weigh the patient and document any weight gain and the time period over which it has occurred. Since 500 mL (1 pint) of retained fluid weighs approximately 2.2 kg (1 lb), changes in weight can be used to monitor the effectiveness of diuretic therapy.

Palpate for enlargement of the liver and right upper abdominal tenderness and pain.

Assess the patient's overall level of stress and anxiety, since sympathetic nervous stimulation increases the workload of the heart.

Nursing Diagnoses and Planning

Nursing diagnoses and related expected patient outcomes commonly applicable to patients with heart failure include the following:

NDx: Decreased cardiac output related to altered myocardial contractility, increased preload and/or increased afterload, and alterations in rate, rhythm, or electrical conduction.

Planning: Patient Outcomes
1. Vital signs are within acceptable ranges for the patient.
2. Patient maintains an adequate cardiac output as demonstrated by hemodynamic monitoring.
3. Dysrhythmias are absent or controlled.
4. Patient participates in activities consistent with abilities.
5. Patient is free of dyspnea.

NDx: Risk for ineffective breathing pattern related to pulmonary edema secondary to heart failure.

Planning: Patient Outcomes
1. Vital signs are within normal ranges for the patient.
2. Patient is free of dyspnea, tachypnea, or cough.
3. Breath sounds are clear to auscultation.
4. Patient completes activities of daily living without shortness of breath.

NDx: Activity intolerance related to generalized weakness or an imbalance between oxygen supply and oxygen demand.

Planning: Patient Outcomes
1. Patient increases participation in activities without intolerable dyspnea or fatigue.
2. Patient seeks assistance as needed.
3. Patient demonstrates energy-saving activities.
4. Patient sets a daily schedule that allows for intermittent periods of rest.
5. Patient describes the need for and importance of oxygen, medications, and supportive equipment to increase tolerance for activity.

NDx: Fluid volume excess related to retention of sodium and water secondary to the stimulation of the renin-angiotensin-aldosterone system in response to inadequate cardiac output

Planning: Patient Outcomes
1. Patient maintains a balanced intake and output.
2. Breath sounds are clear.
3. Shortness of breath is absent.
4. Hemodynamic parameters are within normal limits.
5. Peripheral edema is absent.
6. Patient is free of daily weight gain attributable to fluid retention.
7. Patient explains dietary and fluid restrictions.

NDx: Knowledge deficit: disease process, complications, and self-care after discharge.

Planning: Patient Outcomes
1. Patient describes heart failure.
2. Patient explains medication, dietary, and activity regimen and the need for follow-up care.

Nursing Interventions and Evaluation

NDx: Decreased cardiac output
Monitor for indications of further drop in cardiac output: increasing tachycardia, increased and then decreased blood pressure, diminished peripheral pulses, cold, clammy skin, and pallor or cyanosis. Measure intake and output to monitor for oliguria. Report and document signs of worsening status. Also monitor temperature and report any elevation because as temperature increases, metabolic rate and the need for oxygen increases, thus placing a greater workload on the heart.

Administer prescribed medications and monitor for the expected therapeutic response and for toxic effects. If a digitalis preparation is ordered, be certain to check the cardiac monitor pattern or the apical pulse for a full minute prior to administration. Withhold the drug and notify the physician if the pulse is less than 60 or more than 100 beats per minute. Monitor serum levels of digitalis (therapeutic range is 0.5 to 2.0 ng/mL) and serum potassium levels. Monitor for signs of digitalis toxicity: anorexia, nausea, vomiting, diarrhea, visual disturbances, and dysrhythmias. Notify the physician if any of these signs occur.

Since decreased cardiac output results in decreased perfusion of body tissues with oxygenated blood, provide care designed to lower the need for oxygen to decrease the risk of tissue damage from inadequate perfusion and hypoxia.

Begin by encouraging physical and psychologic rest. The latter is important because psychologic stress activates the sympathetic nervous system, thereby increasing the workload of the heart.

Provide a calm, quiet environment. While the patient is on bedrest, elevate the head of the bed to ease the work of breathing. Reposition frequently for comfort and to prevent pooling of blood in dependent areas. Place needed items within reach of the patient to limit the effort required and decrease the frustration associated with limitations on activity and independence.

Because the Valsalva maneuver—bearing down while holding the breath—causes a sudden increase in preload, instruct the patient not to strain at stool. When permitted for patients on bedrest, use a bedside commode rather than a bed pan to facilitate defecation. Monitor number and consistency of bowel movements and ask patients to report any difficulty passing stool. Administer prescribed stool softeners or laxatives if needed. In preparation for discharge, instruct patients to prevent constipation and the need to strain by eating a diet high in fiber, drinking at least six glasses of fluid per day (unless on a fluid restriction), and obeying the urge to defecate. Also instruct patients to avoid isometric exercise and heavy lifting, as these activities can also involve the Valsalva maneuver.

Advise patients to avoid the use of nicotine- and caffeine-containing products because they stimulate the heart, causing tachycardia and increasing the workload and the need for oxygen.

NDx: Risk for ineffective breathing pattern
Because congestion in the lungs impedes the diffusion of oxygen across the alveolar membrane and into the blood stream, it is important to promote effective breathing to bring a maximum of oxygen to the alveolar membrane, thereby enhancing diffusion into the blood stream. Monitor breath sounds and respiratory rate, rhythm, and depth every 1 to 4 hours. Facilitate respiration through positioning. Have the patient assume a semi-Fowler's or high Fowler's position while in bed to combat orthopnea and to aid chest expansion. Further support good chest expansion by placing a pillow lengthwise behind the head, shoulders, and back, by supporting the forearms away from the chest on pillows or an over-the-bed table, and by using a foot board to prevent the patient from slipping down in bed,

which compresses the chest. If the patient is sitting in a chair, elevate the feet to prevent pooling of fluid and support maximum chest expansion as described. Coach the patient in coughing and deep-breathing every 2 hours to expand the alveoli to improve oxygenation.

Administer supplemental oxygen as prescribed. A common dosage is 2 to 4 L/min by nasal cannula. Obtain baseline oxygen saturation before initiating oxygen therapy. Monitor oxygen saturation throughout therapy via pulse oximetry or arterial blood gases or both.

NDx: Activity intolerance

Patients' ability to tolerate activity varies with the degree of heart failure. With severe heart failure, there is little or no cardiac reserve and even slight increases in oxygen demand cannot be met by the failing heart. Therefore, bedrest and assistance with activities of daily living such as bathing and eating may be needed. As symptoms regress, have the patient increase activity gradually. Progress from passive and active range-of-motion exercises performed while on bedrest to maintain muscle tone, strength, joint mobility, and circulation, to sitting up in a chair, to short walks, and then to increasingly longer walks. Judge how well activity is tolerated by observing the patient for fatigue and dyspnea and taking vital signs before and after activity. Indications of activity intolerance include a change in blood pressure of greater than 20 mm Hg, a sustained increase in heart rate of 20 beats per minute, and the occurrence of dyspnea, chest pain, palpitations, dizziness, or excessive fatigue. If these occur, discontinue the activity and have the patient rest.

Organize care to provide for needed rest. Space care activities so that the patient is not too overtaxed at any one time but so that uninterrupted periods of rest are possible. Since good nutrition is necessary to increase energy level, encourage eating by offering four to six small meals per day, as this is less tiring for the patient. Small meals also prevent gastric overdistention and help prevent dyspnea while eating. Schedule rest periods after meals.

Explain to the patient the importance of frequent rest periods even when symptoms are stabilized. Stress the need to avoid sudden movements because they cause decreased blood flow to the brain and increase strain on the heart. Teach the patient energy-saving strategies, of which one of the most important is to perform normal activities more slowly than usual to decrease cardiac workload.

NDx: Fluid volume excess

Fluid volume excess develops as a result of normal compensatory mechanisms, which increase the retention of sodium and water in an effort to maintain cardiac output. The resultant increase in fluid volume increases the workload of the heart and further contributes to its failure. Because of this fact, monitoring fluid status of the patient with heart failure is critical. Track hemodynamic parameters. Weigh the patient daily at the same time, in the same clothes, and on the same scale. Record intake and output. Report urinary output of less than 30 mL/h to the physician. Monitor for jugular venous distention, peripheral edema, and signs of acute pulmonary edema.

Provide a sodium-restricted diet as prescribed. Explain the relation of sodium to fluid retention, and stress the importance of sodium restriction in the control of heart failure. Teach the patient about sources of sodium in the diet and provide a list of sodium-rich foods and condiments to be avoided. Provide sample meal plans and guidelines for compliance with the prescribed diet.

If fluids are restricted, encourage the patient to drink small amounts of the total fluid allowance at intervals throughout the day to avoid long periods when fluids cannot be taken. Allow the patient to select the type of fluid within the prescribed dietary guidelines. Provide frequent mouth care and offer hard candy or lozenges if allowed.

NDx: Knowledge deficit: disease process, complications, and self-care after discharge

Explain the cause, effects, and clinical course of heart failure to the patient and the family. Stress the importance of rest in decreasing the workload of the heart. Allow time for questions and for verbalization of concerns and fears. Provide appropriate literature about heart failure for the patient and family to review. Refer the patient to cardiac support groups if available and recommend the American Heart Association as a good source of information with pamphlets and videos on living with heart disease. Teach the patient the signs and symptoms of heart failure, such as fatigue, dyspnea, and weight gain, which should be reported to the physician. Have the patient keep a daily weight record.

Instruct the patient in dietary changes and any fluid restrictions prescribed to reduce symptoms or prevent recurrence of the heart failure. Explain the need for reduction in the use of nicotine and caffeine products, which increase the workload of the heart. Initiate counseling with a dietitian to assist with meal planning if needed.

Explain the prescribed medication regimen to the patient and family. Include name, use, dose, frequency, and potential side effects of all medications the patient is to take. Stress the importance of taking correct dosages at correct times and design, with the patient, a schedule and reminder system that fits his or her lifestyle. Explain the need to contact the physician prior to taking any over-the-counter drugs, since these may interact with the prescribed medication. Provide information and instructions about all medications in writing so the patient can refer to them as needed.

Additional Interventions

For patients on bedrest, be aware of their risk for skin breakdown due to poor tissue perfusion and pressure. Inspect the skin at least once every 8 hours. Pay special attention to edematous areas and areas over bony prominences. Keep skin clean and dry. Apply an emollient to prevent drying and cracking.

Use protective devices to relieve pressure from tissues over bony prominences. Reposition the patient (or teach the patient to reposition self) every half hour to stimulate circulation and relieve pressure. For further information on the prevention and management of pressure ulcers, refer to Chapter 36.

Compare the patient's status with the expected outcomes. If the outcomes are not met, reassess the patient and revise the plan.

Cardiogenic Pulmonary Edema

Etiology and Pathophysiology

Cardiogenic or hydrostatic pulmonary edema is a diffuse extravascular accumulation of fluid in the tissues and airspaces of the lungs due to increased pressure in the pulmonary capillaries. Normally fluid that crosses the capillary membrane and enters the lung is removed by the pulmonary lymphatic system. However, with failure of the left ventricle, blood backs up into the pulmonary vascular system, capillary pressure increases, and fluid crosses the capillary membrane in amounts greater than the lymphatics can drain. The result is that fluid builds up first in the interstitial tissues around the airways, then around the alveoli, and finally in the alveoli.

Clinical Manifestations

Classic symptoms of cardiogenic pulmonary edema are extreme breathlessness (air hunger), a sense of impending doom, tachypnea, tachycardia, hypertension, and diaphoresis. Dyspnea is prominent, as is the use of accessory muscles of respiration. Peripheral cyanosis due to vasoconstriction is common. Pink frothy sputum may be expectorated. On auscultation of the lungs, wheezes are heard initially, progressing to diffuse crackles.

Diagnosis

Diagnosis of cardiogenic pulmonary edema is based on physical examination and characteristic findings on chest x-ray. Cardiogenic pulmonary edema can be differentiated from noncardiogenic pulmonary edema (that caused by increased capillary permeability, as in adult respiratory distress syndrome) by determination of pulmonary artery wedge pressure. A wedge pressure of 22 to 24 mm Hg is indicative of cardiogenic pulmonary edema.

Management

Supplemental oxygen is immediately given to relieve hypoxemia, and then measures are instituted to improve the function of the left side of the heart. Morphine, loop diuretics, and nitroglycerin are given IV to reduce preload and vasodilators are given to reduce afterload. In some cases, mechanical ventilation is required.

NURSING PROCESS GUIDELINES
Cardiogenic Pulmonary Edema

If signs of acute pulmonary edema develop, immediately notify the physician because this is a life-threatening situation that requires immediate intervention. Sit the patient upright with legs dangling to trap blood in the lower extremities, thereby decreasing venous return and reducing the workload of the heart. This in turn decreases pulmonary congestion and facilitates gas exchange. Suction if needed to keep the airway patent and administer oxygen, keeping the oxygen partial pressure (PO_2) at greater than 60 mm Hg. Auscultate lung and heart sounds and monitor the ECG for dysrhythmias. Record intake and output. Provide emotional support to the patient through the use of calming words and touch. Also support the family. Keep them informed and allow time for them to ask questions and express concerns.

Coronary Artery Disease

Of all forms of heart disease, coronary artery disease (CAD) is the most common. It is the leading killer of Americans today. Most diagnosed cases of CAD are the result of a lifetime of gradual buildup of atherosclerotic plaque that narrows the coronary arteries and restricts blood flow (Fig. 8–25). Despite widespread public education regarding reduction of risk factors and modification of lifestyle (see Chap. 7), CAD remains one of the biggest public health problems in America. It is estimated that 1.5 million people in America with CAD will have suffered an acute myocardial infarction in 1996. About 500,000 of these will die (American Heart Association, 1996).

CAD affects both men and women and is the leading cause of death in both sexes. In recent years, awareness of the incidence of CAD in women has increased, and a new body of literature is emerging regarding the uniqueness of CAD in women. It is now known that women are often diagnosed with CAD later in life than men. Also, women who experience acute myocardial infarction have higher mortality rates in the first few weeks and in the year after the heart attack than men. Finally, women often have more numerous coexisting disease states when diagnosed with CAD (Beery, 1995). It is further known that one of the primary reasons that women develop heart disease at an older age than men is that estrogen protects younger women against damage to the heart and against high serum lipid levels. Menopause is accompanied by an increase in low-density lipoproteins, or LDL cholesterol ("bad cholesterol"), and a decrease in high-density lipoproteins, or HDL cholesterol ("good

CLINICAL ? THINKING

DYSPNEA, RESTLESSNESS, AND ANXIETY IN A PATIENT WITH A HISTORY OF MYOCARDIAL INFARCTION

A 68-year-old man was admitted to the medical unit with complaints of increasing fatigue and weakness, shortness of breath with activity, swelling of the ankles, tightening shoes, a decreased appetite, and a weight gain of 2 kg (4.5 lbs) over the previous 3 days. The patient's medical history included coronary artery disease, hypertension, and an acute myocardial infarction that had occurred 4 months earlier.

The patient was alert and oriented. He had an irregular pulse rate of 96 beats per minute, a respiratory rate of 22 per minute, and blood pressure of 138/92 mm Hg. The physician suspected heart failure and initiated therapy with a mild diuretic and an angiotensin converting enzyme inhibitor.

When I arrived at the patient's bedside during my 3 AM rounds, I found an acute change in the patient's status. He was lying flat, had a persistent dry cough, and said, "I just woke up and I don't feel right. I'm having trouble breathing." The patient was visibly short of breath, restless, and extremely anxious.

I recognized that dyspnea, cough, restlessness, and anxiety might be associated with a number of medical conditions, including pneumonia, iatrogenic fluid overload, noncardiogenic pulmonary edema (adult respiratory distress syndrome), acute myocardial infarction, pulmonary embolism, and cardiac tamponade. However, the presence of paroxysmal nocturnal dyspnea in conjunction with the patient's medical history and admitting medical diagnosis led me to believe that the patient's condition had deteriorated, resulting in acute pulmonary edema secondary to left ventricular failure.

Because acute pulmonary edema is a medical emergency that can rapidly become fatal, I placed the patient in semi-Fowler's position to facilitate breathing and quickly assessed him for associated clinical manifestations. My focused assessment revealed tachycardia (his pulse rate had increased to 134 bpm and was thready and irregular), tachypnea (respirations had increased to 32 per minute and were shallow), a normal temperature, and a blood pressure that had fallen to 112/78 mm Hg. I noted that the patient was using accessory muscles of respiration to breathe, his skin was pale, cool, and clammy, and his capillary refill was sluggish. Auscultation revealed crackles at the base of both lungs. I heard an S₃ heart sound despite his noisy breathing. The patient denied having chest pain.

These nursing assessments further strengthened my suspicion of cardiogenic pulmonary edema. In addition, the absence of fever and chest discomfort, and the lack of evidence pointing to direct or indirect lung trauma during the previous 48 to 72 hours helped me eliminate some of the other possible conditions.

Knowing that acute pulmonary edema is a life-threatening condition that requires immediate intervention, I implemented the following actions:

1. I placed the patient in high-Fowler's position with his legs dangling in a dependent position to promote lung expansion and reduce venous return (preload).
2. I notified the physician.
3. I administered oxygen and established an intravenous line for administering medications, per hospital protocol.
4. I requested that another staff member bring the crash cart to the bedside in case the patient required intubation. I remained with the patient.
5. I provided emotional support to the patient and gave clear, accurate explanations of all procedures.

The physician arrived and ordered a stat portable chest x-ray, 12-lead electrocardiogram, arterial blood gas (ABG) analysis, complete blood count, and serum electrolytes. He also ordered the following medications, which I administered: morphine sulphate, furosemide, digoxin, and aminophyllin.

I also took the following additional nursing actions:

1. I inserted an indwelling urinary catheter as per medical order.
2. I monitored fluid intake and output and electrolyte levels.
3. I encouraged the patient to cough and monitored for the presence of pink frothy sputum (an indication of worsening condition).
4. I monitored ABGs and applied a pulse oximeter to monitor oxygen saturation levels.
5. I monitored the patient's response to the medications.
6. I continued to monitor the patient's respiratory, cardiovascular, and mental status.
7. I documented my findings and actions.

The patient's chest x-ray revealed pulmonary congestion, and his ABGs reflected hypoxemia. These results verified my clinical suspicion of acute cardiogenic pulmonary edema. Within 6 hours of my response to the patient's emergency situation,

(continued)

CLINICAL ❓THINKING

(continued)

the acute phase of pulmonary edema was resolved. Baseline vital signs were restored, breath sounds were clear, ABGs were within normal limits, and he appeared calm and said that he could breathe again.

The patient was spared the possibility of endotracheal intubation, mechanical ventilation, hemodynamic monitoring, and transfer to a critical care unit. His life was saved because of the rapid identification and prompt, effective treatment of this complication of heart failure.

Think Critically

Why did the nurse position the patient as described?

How might the nurse have positioned the patient if he had been hypotensive?

Which medication orders would the nurse have questioned if the patient had been hypotensive?

How would the nurse's actions have differed if the medical diagnosis had been noncardiogenic pulmonary edema (adult respiratory distress syndrome)?

What action would the nurse have taken if she was caring for the patient in the home?

How might the administration of digoxin, furosemide, and aminophylline result in dysrhythmias?

For which additional cardiac problems must the nurse monitor the patient while he is receiving diuretic therapy (which depletes serum electrolytes)?

Which additional nursing assessments are required after administering morphine sulphate?

What would you expect the ABGs to reveal at the point the nurse discovered the patient?

What would you expect the ABGs to reveal if the patient's condition continued to deteriorate? Why?

What was the rationale for inserting the indwelling urinary catheter?

Although infrequently used, how would the application of rotating tourniquets have benefited the patient if they were necessary?

Which topics should the nurse include in discharge teaching to prevent future hospital admissions for heart failure?

Which additional medical treatments might the nurse anticipate if further diagnostic tests revealed progressing coronary artery disease?

Was the insertion of an IV line the best action? What alternative action might the nurse have taken? Why?

---

cholesterol"). After menopause women have the same incidence of CAD as men (Douglas & Ginsburg, 1996).

CAD is a largely preventable disease. Primary prevention of CAD begins early in life with the adoption of healthful lifestyle habits. Secondary prevention of CAD occurs after the diagnosis of the disease and focuses on risk factor reduction and lifestyle changes such as smoking cessation and participation in a regular exercise program, designed to prevent the progression of atherosclerotic plaque formation in the coronary arteries.

Etiology and Pathophysiology

The coronary artery, like other arteries, has three layers. The outermost supporting layer is the adventitia. The thick middle layer composed of smooth muscle is the media. The innermost layer is the in-

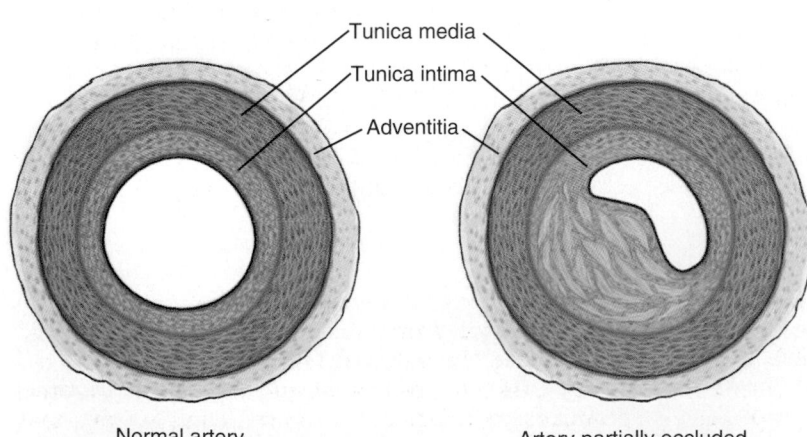

Normal artery

Artery partially occluded by atherosclerotic plaque

Fiigure 8–25

In coronary artery disease, atherosclerotic plaque narrows the coronary arteries and restricts blood flow.

tima. The intima is composed of a thin, fibrous lining and a very delicate sheet of cells called the endothelium. The endothelium lines the lumen of the vessel and secretes chemical mediators that regulate vascular activity and integrity.

Injury to the endothelium with disruption of this regulatory activity is believed to initiate atherosclerotic plaque formation (Feister, 1996). Factors that have been associated with endothelial injury include increased intra-arterial blood pressure, elevated levels of serum lipids, turbulent patterns of blood flow with shearing forces, catecholamines, and irritants from cigarette smoke. Inflammation of the vascular wall as an important factor in the development of atherosclerosis is supported by findings of the Physician's Health Study (New England Journal of Medicine, 1997), which showed that the serum level of C-reactive protein, an indicator of chronic inflammation, was significantly higher in men who suffered a myocardial infarction or a stroke than in those who did not.

Atherosclerotic plaques form gradually over a period of years and can be described in terms of three distinct stages: early, advanced, and acute disruptive. In the early stage, the lesion appears as a fatty streak. There is no significant narrowing of the vessel, and the patient is free of symptoms. The advanced stage is characterized by complex plaques that narrow the artery and can result in angina. The third stage involves acute disruptive changes in the plaque that cause sudden occlusion of the artery with unstable angina, myocardial infarction, or even sudden death as the result.

The early plaque or fatty streak is composed of lipid-laden cells in the intima. In accord with the response-to-injury hypothesis of plaque development, adhesive molecules, which are released in increased numbers by damaged endothelium, cause monocytes circulating in the blood to adhere to the endothelium at the site of damage. These monocytes then pass between the endothelial cells and enter the intima where they take up lipid and become macrophages. Subsequently, with additional uptake of lipid, they become foam cells. The fatty streak produces a roughened irregular endothelial surface that attracts additional monocytes and also causes platelets to aggregate. Under the influence of platelet-derived growth factor released by the activated platelets, smooth muscle cells from the media migrate into the intima and proliferate there. These cells, like the monocytes, also take up lipid and become foam cells.

As plaque development advances, foam cells continue to take up lipid, and collagen, elastic fibers, and ground substance begin to be deposited in the lumen of the artery. This significantly increases the bulk of the plaque and begins to narrow the arterial lumen. A fibrotic reaction, which is most marked on the aspect of the plaque facing the arterial lumen, occurs and seals the lesions with a fibrous cap. As the lesion continues to progress, fissures or tears in plaques cause small hemorrhages and the resulting thrombus is commonly incorporated into the existing plaque by the vascular repair process. This further enlarges the plaque, which in its most complex form can exhibit areas of lipid, fibrosis, calcification, and hemorrhage.

Plaques continue to enlarge as local chemical mediators continue to stimulate proliferation of smooth muscle and these processes repeat themselves.

Acute disruption of a plaque can take three basic forms:

• Coronary artery thrombosis
• Hemorrhage into a plaque that dramatically and suddenly increases in size
• Rupture of a plaque, with extrusion of its contents into the coronary artery

Plaques most likely to rupture are softer, less formed lesions containing lipid material as opposed to firm lesions with a well-defined fibrous cap.

Plaques may be crescent-shaped and eccentric or concentric. Eccentric plaques develop in an asymmetric region of the arterial wall. Concentric plaques involve the entire circumference of the artery. Once the disease has developed, the progression of CAD is individual. Often it is a slow, gradual process of progressive narrowing of the arterial lumen and some patients can have lesions that remain stable for many years. In some cases, new blood vessels grow around the artery to compensate for the reduced blood supply. The development of this collateral circulation is an adaptive mechanism and serves to protect the myocardium in the event of total obstruction.

Clinical Manifestations

The clinical manifestations of CAD are dependent on the severity of the disease. In the early stages of coronary artery disease, the patient is asymptomatic but is positive for a number of CAD risk factors. These risk factors, as discussed in Chapter 7, include family history of heart disease, hyperlipidemia, cigarette smoking, obesity, physical inactivity, aggressive, time-oriented personality, hypertension, diabetes, and use of oral contraceptives and premature menopause. As plaque formation progresses and the lumen of the artery is narrowed, angina (chest pain associated with temporary ischemia of myocardial tissue) occurs. With acute disruption of a plaque and complete, prolonged obstruction to blood flow, myocardial infarction occurs. (Refer to subsequent sections for detailed discussion of angina and myocardial infarction.)

Diagnosis

The presence of CAD in asymptomatic individuals is usually inferred from the patient's history and risk factor profile. In patients with a strong family history of CAD, a positive stress test result, or other significant risk factors, coronary angiography may be performed to confirm the diagnosis and verify the extent of the disease.

Management

Management of asymptomatic CAD is focused on primary prevention of cardiac events. This is accomplished through extensive and ongoing patient education to promote lifestyle modifications designed to reduce or eliminate cardiac risk factors.

Risk factor interventions such as smoking cessation, weight reduction, decreasing blood lipid levels, and regular exercise, extend overall survival from CAD, improve quality of life, decrease the need for interventions like balloon angioplasty and bypass surgery, and reduce the incidence of another heart attack (Smith et al, 1995).

For patients with elevated cholesterol levels (LDL cholesterol levels over 190 mg/dL or over 160 mg/dL with two other risk factors) not responsive to dietary control, antilipidemia and cholesterol-lowering drugs may be prescribed in addition to, not as a substitute for, diet therapy.

Drug therapy may consist of cholesterol-synthesis inhibitors such as lovastatin (Mevacor), pravastatin (Pravachol), or simvastatin (Zocor); fibric acid derivatives such as clofibrate (Abitrate), or gemfibrozil (Lopid), which decrease triglyceride levels by increasing lipoprotein lipase activity; bile acid–binding resins such as colestipol (Colestid); or agents such as nicotinic acid (Niacor) or probucol. Lowering blood cholesterol dramatically decreases the risk of subsequent cardiac events (Sachs et al, 1996; Treasure et al, 1996) and these medications have been demonstrated to be highly effective for both primary and secondary prevention of heart disease.

Other drug therapy used in the treatment of CAD includes prophylactic low-dose aspirin therapy (81 mg every day), estrogen replacement for postmenopausal women, and niacin or nicotinic acid. Initial studies indicate that clopidogrel, which inhibits platelet activity and therefore blood clotting, may be more effective than aspirin in preventing myocardial infarction and stroke in people with atherosclerosis. Other initial studies suggest that red grape juice has a similar effect. In people with significant inflammation, as indicated by serum C-reactive protein levels, it appears that the anti-inflammatory effect of aspirin contributes to its effectiveness in preventing myocardial infarction.

Coronary artery bypass grafting or balloon dilatation may be performed prophylactically in patients with significant disease documented by angiography.

❖ Settings, Providers, and Collaboration for Care

The patient with coronary artery disease is usually treated in the outpatient setting unless invasive treatment becomes necessary. The nurse in the primary care setting provides instructions about medication, dietary modifications, and lifestyle changes that may be needed to slow the progression of the disease. On subsequent visits with the patient, the nurse will review progress toward these goals. Consultation with a nutritionist and exercise physiologist may be needed to help the patient modify long-term patterns of living. It may be necessary for the home health nurse to become involved to assess compliance with therapy and to stress the importance of follow-up care.

NURSING PROCESS GUIDELINES
Coronary Artery Disease

The goal of nursing care is to help the patient lower his or her risk factor profile (Highlight 8–5). Achievement of this goal requires intensive patient education and development of a plan for implementing lifestyle changes that is realistic, tailored to the individual patient's needs, and able to be implemented.

Explain the cause, effects, and clinical course of coronary atherosclerosis. Stress the patient's role in preventing progression of the disease by reducing modifiable risk factors. Provide literature at an appropriate literacy level for the patient to review. Encourage discussion and allow time for patient questions.

Explain the importance of a diet low in fat and cholesterol in preventing progression of the disease. Recognize that patients often have a great deal of difficulty adapting to such a diet because of dietary likes and dislikes developed over many years of eating a traditional American diet, which is rich in saturated fats. Teach the patient about the food pyramid and healthy substitutes (fruits, vegetables, grains) for meat and other fatty foods. Show how to read food labels for fat content and serving sizes. Provide literature on healthy approaches to diet and recipe modification. Discuss methods of preparing and cooking foods that lower fat content, and refer the patient to a cookbook containing low-fat recipes. To increase the likelihood of compliance with recommended dietary changes, encourage the patient to take a moderate approach that allows for occasional small amounts of favorite foods. Reinforce that dietary modifications represent lifelong changes, not temporary treatment measures. Initiate counseling with a dietitian if assistance with meal planning is needed or if the patient is obese or has another condition such as diabetes that must be considered when planning diet.

Discuss the importance of regular exercise in the prevention and control of heart disease. Explain that regular exercise strengthens and conditions heart muscles in the same manner it improves and strengthens other muscles in the body. Explore the patient's usual level of activity and discuss ways in which exercise can be incorporated into the daily routine. Suggest walking as a good form of exercise (see Highlight 7–4 in Chapter 7). Current recommendations include using the "talk test" to gauge

HIGHLIGHT
8–5

HEALTH PROMOTION
& RISK REDUCTION

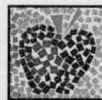

Reducing Risk Factors for Patients with Coronary Artery Disease

Instruct the patient with coronary artery disease from atherosclerosis to modify lifestyle and to lower risk by:

Reducing serum lipid levels. The blood cholesterol level directly relates to the development of atherosclerosis. Increased cholesterol levels can be modified by following a low-fat, low-cholesterol diet and exercising daily.

Reducing high blood pressure or preventing high blood pressure. The risk for atherosclerosis may double with high blood pressure. It can be lowered by reducing weight, reducing stress levels, and participating in a regular exercise program.

Ceasing smoking. Because nicotine is a vasoconstrictor, blood flow through arteries is decreased in smokers.

Keeping diabetes mellitus under control. If the patient is diabetic, risk for atherosclerosis is increased because of the high levels of blood lipids, but it may be less severe if the diabetes is well controlled.

Reducing weight. The patient who is obese is at high risk for atherosclerosis. This can be corrected by following a weight-reduction plan and an exercise plan.

Changing from a high-fat diet to a low-fat diet. A diet that is high in fat contributes to elevated blood lipid levels, which is a major risk factor for atherosclerosis. Following a low-fat (low saturated fat) diet helps prevent atherosclerosis, contributes to weight loss, and decreases the workload on the myocardium.

appropriate exercise level. That is, the person should exercise to the point of being slightly breathless, but should be able to talk without difficulty. This level of exercise should be performed for 30 minutes most days of the week.

If the patient smokes, discuss the need to stop. Explain the role of nicotine in causing endothelial injury and CAD. Also explain that smoking causes constriction of coronary arteries, thus worsening narrowing that may already be present. Refer the patient to a smoking cessation program after exploring the type of program that best fits the patient in terms of location, cost, and approach.

Discuss the relationship between stress and CAD. Encourage the patient to analyze sources of stress in his or her life and to identify ways in which they can be minimized or eliminated. Explore with the patient strategies for coping with unavoidable stress. Teach basic relaxation techniques such as deep-breathing, progressive muscle relaxation, and visualization.

Emphasize the importance of early diagnosis and good control of hypertension and diabetes. Stress the need for regular health examinations and follow-up care as needed.

Angina Pectoris

Etiology and Pathophysiology

Angina pectoris is an acute pain in the chest caused by myocardial ischemia. It is not a disease in itself but is a symptom of an imbalance between the need of the myocardium for oxygen and its supply. Angina occurs when the supply of oxygen reaching the myocardium is inadequate to meet its need. By far the most common cause of angina is coronary artery disease in which atherosclerotic plaques narrow the coronary arteries and impair their ability to dilate (see Coronary Artery Disease for a detailed description of the pathophysiology), thus diminishing the flow of oxygenated blood to the myocardium. This is usually compounded by increased metabolic demands associated with exercise or activity. Other conditions that can induce angina because they decrease the supply or increase the demand for oxygenated blood to the myocardium include

- Thromboembolism
- Aortic stenosis, which increases the workload of the left ventricle and can ultimately decrease cardiac output
- Pulmonary stenosis, which increases the workload of the right ventricle and eventually leads to decreased blood flow through the pulmonary vascular bed and therefore limits oxygenation of the blood
- Coronary artery spasm
- Small vessel disease associated with inflammatory and connective tissue disorders such as rheumatoid arthritis, radiation injury, and lupus erythematosus

Thyrotoxicosis, cocaine abuse, heavy exercise, and emotional stress are examples of extracardiac factors that increase the need of the myocardium for oxygen by virtue of increasing its workload.

As oxygen supply to the myocardium falls short of its need, myocardial cells change from aerobic to anaerobic metabolism. This causes lactic acid to accumulate and alters cell membrane permeability, allowing the release of chemical mediators that stimulate nerve fibers on the myocardium and cause pain.

Clinical Manifestations

Angina pain may occur in the left anterior chest, jaw, neck, arms, or in the back epigastric or scapular areas. Sometimes it radiates down the right arm and may be oppressive or sharp, localized, or radiating. Although most patients describe the sensation as pain, some describe it as indigestion, heartburn, heaviness, a dull ache, or even shortness of breath. The precise type, intensity, and location of pain can vary significantly from person to person but tends to be the same each time it recurs in a given patient. The most common type of angina is stable angina. Stable angina is induced by exercise and relieved by rest or nitroglycerine tablets. It can also be precipitated by a large meal, exposure to cold, emotional stress, or any other factor that increases the workload of the heart. It is generally the first symptom of coronary artery disease that the patient experiences.

A second type of angina is unstable angina, which occurs at lower and lower levels of activity or at rest. This angina is far less predictable and is often a precursor of myocardial infarction. The pain of unstable angina tends to occur with increasing frequency and becomes increasingly prolonged and severe. It represents progressive obstruction of a coronary artery and development of an unstable plaque.

Variant, or Prinzmetal's, angina is a third type of angina. This is prolonged, severe pain that tends to occur at the same time each day, often in the morning. It occurs in the absence of identified precipitating factors and is often caused by coronary artery spasm, as opposed to a blockage in the vessel. It is usually quickly relieved by nitrates or calcium channel blockers.

Diagnosis

The diagnosis of angina pectoris is suggested by a characteristic pattern of chest pain relieved by rest and nitroglycerin, risk factor profile, and auscultation of a transient S_4 gallop or paradoxical splitting of the second heart sound during episodes of pain. The diagnosis can be confirmed by finding a transient ST segment depression on an ECG taken during pain. Unlike other types of angina, variant angina is characterized by ST segment elevation and this must be documented on ECG during pain for the diagnosis to be made. In all types of angina, the ECG may be normal when pain is absent.

Exercise stress testing may be done as part of the diagnostic work-up particularly in patients whose resting electrocardiographic results are normal. This test uses controlled exercise, done with a cardiac monitor in place, to increase the metabolic rate and hence the demand on the heart. If the coronary arteries are partially occluded, the patient may develop anginal pain as the heart rate and the myocardium's need for oxygen increases and waveform changes (such as depression of the ST segment) diagnostic of angina appear on the electrocardiographic strip. If the patient is unable to exercise on a treadmill, a pharmacologic agent such as dobutamine may be given to increase heart rate and cardiac workload.

For further specificity in the diagnosing of CAD, nuclear imaging using thallium or technetium may be done. Coronary angiography may be used to determine the precise location and extent of the disease and to evaluate the patient's suitability for coronary angioplasty or bypass surgery.

Management

Management of acute angina is designed both to reduce myocardial oxygen demand and to increase the supply of oxygen-rich blood to the myocardium. Relief of pain is essential to this goal because pain not only signals myocardial ischemia but increases the heart's oxygen consumption, thereby worsening the ischemia.

Pharmacologic Therapy

Initial treatment consists of drug therapy. Nitrates, beta blockers, and calcium channel blockers are the most commonly used drugs in the treatment of angina.

Sublingual nitroglycerin is the mainstay of pharmacologic management of acute angina. Absorbed into the systemic circulation in 1 to 2 minutes, nitroglycerin dilates coronary veins and arteries. It also dilates systemic vessels, decreasing preload and afterload. Nitroglycerin may also be used in a buccal spray, metered dose form to treat acute angina. For a sustained vasodilator effect, and hence prevention of attacks of angina, long-acting forms of nitroglycerin such as oral tablets, ointments, and transdermal patches are used. To decrease tolerance to nitroglycerin, which develops in almost all patients, doses of long-acting forms are scheduled so the patient is nitrate free for 8 to 10 hours out of 24. Typically, the nitrate-free period is scheduled for sleep time when angina is least likely to occur.

If anginal pain is prolonged and unresponsive to nitroglycerin, it may herald an increasingly unstable coronary artery lesion that may progress to total arterial occlusion and myocardial infarction.

Beta-adrenergic blocking agents are also important in the management of angina. These agents decrease sympathetic stimulation of the cardiac muscle, smooth muscle of the bronchi, and smooth muscle of the vasculature. The primary therapeutic effect of beta blockade is a decreased heart rate and lowered blood pressure. Beta blockers are negative inotropes, meaning they decrease myocardial contractility, thereby diminishing the myocardial oxygen requirements and workload of the heart. By slowing the rate, the diastolic period is lengthened. Since diastole is the time when the myocardium is perfused by the coronary arteries, lengthening diastole provides a longer period of time for delivery of fresh, oxygen-rich blood to the heart muscle, thus perfusion of the myocardium is increased and the risk of angina is decreased.

Calcium channel blockers may also be used in

the management of angina with a select group of patients. The calcium channel blockers cause coronary artery dilatation and also lessen workload on the heart by a negative inotropic action. These agents have been demonstrated to be particularly effective with patients who experience coronary vasospasm as the underlying etiology of their angina.

Because the process of atherosclerosis, which is the cause of angina in the vast majority of cases, is dynamic, the progression of plaques should be slowed by intensive interventions to lower blood cholesterol (Smith et al, 1996). Based on this premise, the effectiveness of anti-lipid drugs in the reduction of angina symptoms and regression of existing coronary disease is under study and initial results have been promising. Thus, patients with elevated blood cholesterol levels should be closely monitored after a low-fat diet is started and if no significant improvement occurs, an antilipemic agent may be prescribed.

When drug therapy is not effective, invasive procedures designed to open or bypass the obstructed artery may be used to re-establish adequate blood flow to the myocardium. Risk factor reduction is an integral part of all management protocols and is essential to long-term control of angina.

❖ **Settings, Providers, and Collaboration for Care**

Although some patients with angina are diagnosed on an outpatient bases, others may enter the healthcare system via the emergency department if acute chest pain is the presenting symptom. Once the patient is stabilized and other acute processes are ruled out, patients with angina are usually treated on an outpatient basis. A nutritionist and a physical therapist may be consulted to help the patient modify the lifestyle. The home care nurse or the nurse in the primary care setting must work closely with the patient and the family to assess compliance with therapy. The nurse in this setting also assesses the patient with each contact for any signs of deterioration of the patient's condition.

NURSING PROCESS
Pharmacologic Management of Angina Pectoris

Assessment

A thorough history of pain and a comprehensive risk factor assessment are essential to the care of patients with angina. Assess for signs and symptoms of pain, noting the onset, intensity, duration, radiation, and location. Use an objective measure such as a pain scale to help quantify the pain. Determine when the pain is present, if it occurs only during exercise or while at rest. Ask if the patient has ever been awakened with chest discomfort. Look for signs of pain such as grimacing, clenching

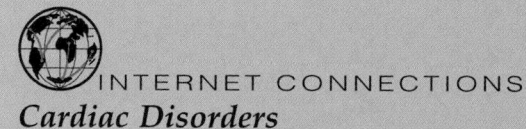

of hands, moaning, or guarding. Often the patient experiencing anginal pain will place a clenched fish against his chest. Patients also tend to remain very still or may appear apprehensive. Question the patient as to what makes the pain better and worse.

Assess vital signs. Obtain an apical pulse and listen to heart sounds in all six cardiac areas. Use both the diaphragm and bell to pick up high- and low-pitched heart sounds, gallops, friction rubs, or murmurs. Document type and location of any abnormal heart sounds heard. Check blood pressure in both arms and document discrepancies. Palpate all the peripheral pulses and compare bilaterally for quality. Listen for adventitious lung sounds and observe for jugular venous distention and peripheral edema. Auscultate for bruits over the carotid arteries. Check laboratory values including cholesterol levels, triglycerides, and cardiac isoenzymes.

Assess the patient's activity level and tolerance. Determine the patient's usual activities and what, if any, assistance is required for activities of daily living. Inquire about symptoms such as shortness of breath, anorexia, and fatigue.

Assess the patient's knowledge of the disorder and its treatment. Determine his or her understanding of the relationship of risk factors to cardiac disease. Assess the patient's emotional response to the disorder and his or her ability to cope with the fact of the disease and its manifestations.

Nursing Diagnoses and Planning

Nursing diagnoses and related expected patient outcomes commonly applicable to patients with angina include the following:

NDx: Pain related to imbalance between myocardial oxygen supply and oxygen need secondary to atherosclerosis and progressive coronary artery obstruction

Planning: Patient Outcomes
1. Patient states pain is relieved.
2. Patient describes ways to prevent anginal episodes.
3. Patient states what to do when angina occurs.
4. Patient reports a decrease in the frequency, duration, and severity of the anginal episodes.

NDx: Activity intolerance related to insufficient myocardial blood flow to meet the myocardial need for oxygen

Planning: Patient Outcomes
1. Patient identifies activities that aggravate pain and fatigue.
2. Patient sets a daily schedule that allows for intermittent periods of rest.
3. Patient demonstrates energy-saving activities.
4. Patient seeks assistance when needed.
5. Patient is able to perform activities of daily living without fatigue, dyspnea, or chest pain.

NDx: Risk for altered health maintenance related to insufficient knowledge related to disease state, risk factor reduction, and management of clinical manifestations of the disease

Planning: Patient Outcomes
1. Patient describes the disease process and the risk factors.
2. Patient describes lifestyle changes needed to prevent progression of the disease.
3. Patient explains prescribed medications in terms of name, use, dose, route, and potential side effects.

Nursing Interventions and Evaluation

NDx: Pain
If sublingual nitroglycerin is prescribed for anginal pain, keep it at the bedside of the hospitalized patient if agency protocol allows. Instruct the patient to take it at the onset of pain and then notify the nurse so that status can be assessed and documented. If intravenous narcotic analgesics are ordered, titrate to the patient's pain and closely monitor the patient's respiratory status. Note the time, duration, characteristics, and severity of the pain as well as the patient's response to the episode. Determine if the pain radiates into the jaw, neck, shoulder, inner aspect of the arm, or hand and observe for associated signs and symptoms such as dyspnea, hypotension, nausea and vomiting, dizziness, palpitations, or diaphoresis. Place the patient in a comfortable position, elevate the head of the bed, and administer oxygen by nasal cannula with 4 to 6 L/min unless contraindicated by chronic pulmonary disease. Monitor vital signs and respiratory status every 5 minutes during the anginal episode. Initiate cardiac monitoring during episodes of chest pain if it is not already in progress and obtain a twelve-lead ECG to be compared to the patient's baseline ECG. Assess heart rate and rhythm and observe for ST changes characteristic of ischemia.

Allay anxiety. Exhibit a calm, reassuring manner and stay with the patient during the episode of angina. Chest pain is anxiety-provoking to most patients regardless of how many times they have experienced it, and anxiety can worsen angina because it increases heart rate and thereby increases the myocardial need for oxygen.

Teach all patients about the medications prescribed for angina: name, dose, route, frequency, expected action, and proper handling and storage. Teach the patients to carry nitroglycerin with them at all times in a light-proof container to prevent breakdown of the medication and to check the expiration date on the bottle and replace with a new bottle before that date. In case of chest pain, tell them to stop activity, sit or lie down and place a nitroglycerin tablet under the tongue. (Nitroglycerin often causes light-headedness so sitting or lying down is important.) Tell the patient to put one tablet under the tongue every 5 minutes for a total of three tablets. Make certain patients understand the difference between rapid-acting nitroglycerin to be taken when anginal pain occurs and long-acting nitrates, beta blockers, and calcium channel blockers designed to prevent pain, not to relieve it. Instruct patients to go to a hospital emergency department or to call 911 if chest pain is not relieved by three nitroglycerin sublingual tablets taken over 15 to 20 minutes.

Remember that all patients experiencing chest pain are considered at risk of myocardial infarction until it is ruled out. Therefore, consider the patient complaining of chest pain a priority and institute interventions rapidly.

NDx: Activity intolerance
Instruct the patient to cope with the activity intolerance related to angina in the following ways:

- Avoid unnecessary activities that require overexertion.
- Take prophylactic nitroglycerin prior to engaging

in activities likely to induce angina, such as stair climbing or sexual intercourse.

- Space activities to avoid precipitating angina due to increased cardiac workload.
- Practice energy-saving techniques.
- Rest between activities.
- Participate in a program of gradually increasing exercise.
- Avoid sudden temperature changes, especially prolonged exposure to cold.

NDx: Risk for altered health maintenance
Instruct the patient in the reduction of risk factors for CAD as discussed in Chapter 7 and under Nursing Process Guidelines: Coronary Artery Disease.

If the patient is discharged on cardiac medications, teach about the therapeutic effects, dosage, time, frequency, and side effects. Reinforce the importance of taking the medication as directed and reporting any adverse effects. Teach patients never to suddenly stop cardiac medications without consulting their physician. Also teach patients about the dangers of polypharmacy and drug interactions. Communicate, without inducing fear, that cardiac medications are powerful drugs with potentially serious consequences when taken incorrectly or mixed with other drugs. If the patient is discharged on lipid-lowering drugs, stress that these medications are not a substitute for following a low-fat diet.

Refer patients who are newly diagnosed with CAD to a cardiac rehabilitation program. Cardiac rehabilitation programs, which can be defined as secondary prevention of CAD, allow patients to begin an exercise regimen in a closely monitored situation. They also provide the education and guidance that persons with CAD need to regain control over their lives and their disease.

Compare the patient's status with the expected outcomes. If the outcomes are not met, reassess the patient and revise the plan.

Coronary Artery Bypass Grafting
Myocardial revascularization, or coronary artery bypass grafting (CABG), is the primary surgical treatment for coronary artery disease. The goal of the procedure is to improve blood supply to an often chronically ischemic heart, thereby alleviating symptoms and prolonging survival.

Candidates for CABG are patients who have chronic angina with pain that is unmanageable with maximum medical therapy, particularly those with left main stem stenosis or severe "three-vessel disease" (several diseased arteries), or both. CABG is also done on patients with acute unstable angina not amenable to percutaneous transluminal coronary angioplasty and those with acute myocardial infarction and severe vessel disease.

In CABG, a conduit of the patient's own tissue such as the saphenous vein, internal mammary artery, gastroepiploic artery, or radial artery is used to bring blood from the aorta to the coronary artery distal to the obstruction (Fig. 8–26). Thus blood flow to the myocardium is re-established by bypassing the obstruction. When the saphenous vein is used for the graft, a segment is harvested from the lower leg or thigh through either an open or an endoscopic approach. It is then grafted into place in a reversed position to avoid interruption of blood flow by the venous valves. When either the right or left internal mammary artery is used, it is dissected off the chest wall already attached to the subclavian artery and is grafted to the coronary artery below the obstruction. Use of the internal mammary artery has become the procedure of choice because studies have shown that 40 to 50% of saphenous vein grafts close within 10 years, whereas 90% of internal mammary artery grafts remain patent 10 years after surgery. Use of the radial artery is a newer technique but carries the risk of paralysis of the hand on the affected side. Multiple arteries are usually diseased and one to five bypasses are done to improve blood supply to the myocardium.

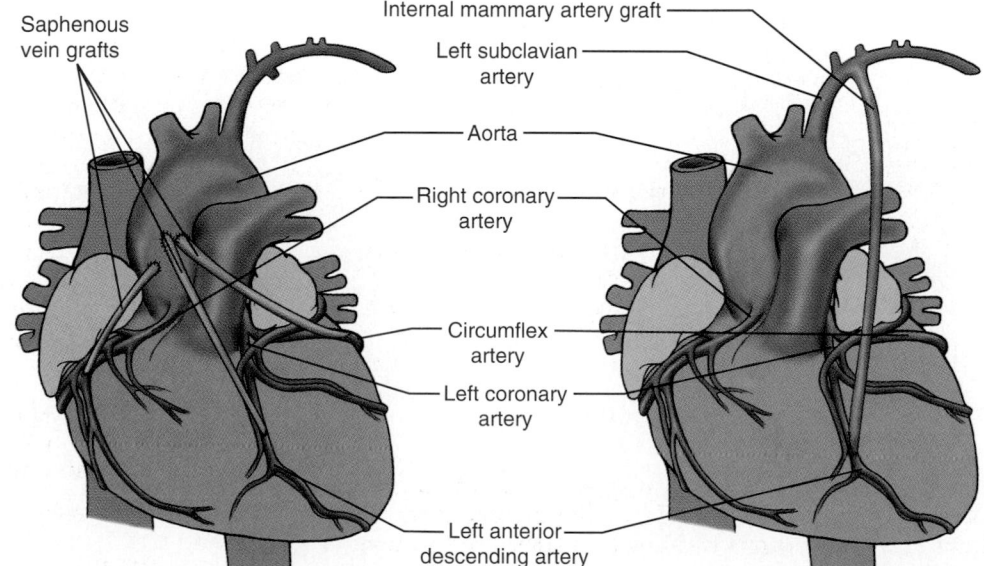

Figure 8–26

Coronary artery bypass grafting.

■■■■■■■▶

■ Clinical Pathway for Coronary Artery Bypass Grafting

Patient Name _____   Date _____

DRG# _____   Expected LOS _____

	Day 2 (PO #1)	Day 3 (PO #2)	Day 4 (PO #3)	Day 5 (PO #4)	Day 6 (PO #5)
Medication	IV PCA pain med; change to PO Antiemetics Anxiolytic, sleeping med Stool softener SC heparin Aspirin IV nitro; change to nitropaste	PO pain med Antiemetics Anxiolytic, sleeping med Stool softener SC heparin Aspirin Nitropaste	PO pain med Antiemetics Anxiolytic, sleeping med Laxative if no BM SC heparin Aspirin Nitropaste	PO pain med Sleeping med Stool softener SC heparin Aspirin Nitropaste	PO pain med Sleeping med Stool softener SC heparin Aspirin Nitropaste Consider antilipemic post-discharge
Diagnostic Tests	Telemetry monitor ECG CBC, electrolytes, BUN, Cr	Telemetry monitor ECG H&H, K^+	Telemetry monitor Pulse oximetry	D/C telemetry if rhythm stable Pulse oximetry H&H, K^+	
Diet	Advance from clear to AHA diet*	AHA diet	AHA diet	AHA diet	AHA diet
Activity	Phase I cardiac rehab, step 1 Dangle and progress to cardiac chair OOB to chair 20 min bid Partial self-care	Phase I cardiac rehab, step 2 OOB to chair; ambulate in room Partial self-care	Phase I cardiac rehab, step 3 Ambulate in hall Self-care	Phase I cardiac rehab, step 4 Shower Ambulate 10 min 3x/day	Phase I cardiac rehab, step 5 Shower Ambulate 20 min 3x/day
Treatments/ Nursing Actions	Vitals q4h if stable Strict I&O, daily weight Epicardial wire care O_2 titrated to sats > 92% Chest PT q4h Incentive spirometry q1h D/C chest tubes if drainage < 10 mL/hr IV infusing at 50 mL/hr until POs Sternal wound care, dressing; SVG site care, dressing TEDs stockings Heparin lock IV	Vitals q4h I&O, weight Epicardial wire care O_2 with sat checks Chest PT q4h Incentive spirometry q1h D/C Foley Incision care TEDs stockings Heparin lock care	Vitals q4h I&O, weight Epicardial wire care D/C O_2 Chest PT q4h Incentive spirometry q1h Incision care TEDs stockings Heparin lock care	Vitals q8h if stable Weight Epicardial wire care D/C chest PT if lungs clear Incentive spirometry q2–4h Incision care TEDS stockings Heparin lock care	Vitals q8h Weight D/C epicardial wires Incentive spirometry q4h Incision care Remove staples, sutures TEDS stockings D/C heparin lock
Teaching/ Discharge Planning		Begin classes: • Diet class/lipid education • Activity class • Going Home class • Support group • Risk factor reduction class		Reinforce classroom materials Initiate appropriate referrals	Medication teaching Wound care teaching Follow-up teaching Phase II referral Reinforcement of all teaching "Survival skills"

---

* "A Healthy Approach" diet with restriction of 30 g of fat per day.
Adapted from the post–open heart protocol of the Maine Medical Center, Portland, Maine, 1996.

CABG is most often done through a median sternotomy incision with cardiopulmonary bypass. A variation on this conventional CABG procedure is the minimally invasive coronary artery bypass (MICAB) or "keyhole" approach, in which the chest is entered through a mini-thoracotomy incision of about 6 cm in length at the level of the fourth intercostal space under the breast. This procedure, which is done "off-bypass" (without cardiopulmonary bypass), provided that myocardial function remains effective when the coronary artery is occluded in preparation for the anastomosis of the bypass graft, has many advantages. These include less postoperative pain, better postoperative arm movement on the affected side, faster resumption of activity, discharge after 3 days, and absence of a long mid-chest scar. In addition, the risk of postoperative neural, renal, and pulmonary complications is decreased. As a result, MICAB can be done in patients with coexisting medical problems that would prohibit the use of conventional CABG. Because "off-bypass" MICAB is done on the beating heart, an infusion of osmolar or other pharmacologic agent is given to decrease the heart rate and strength of contraction, thereby making the surgical procedure easier.

MICAB that can be done directly (sometimes referred to as MIDCAB) or with thorascopic guidance is best suited to one-artery disease involving the left anterior descending and right coronary arteries. The use of a second incision under the clavicle and arm and leg vessels extends the application of MICAB to multivessel disease.

NURSING PROCESS GUIDELINES
Coronary Artery Bypass Grafting

The care of the patient undergoing a traditional coronary artery bypass graft is essentially the same as for any patient undergoing cardiac surgery with cardiopulmonary bypass, with the following considerations. (Refer to Chapter 7 for a detailed discussion of the preoperative, intraoperative, and postoperative care of the patient having cardiac surgery.) When assessing the patient with CABG, keep in mind that both hypotension and hypertension have the potential to cause injury to the new grafts and compromise blood flow to the myocardium. Also remember that, depending on the source of the graft, a second incision may be present. This second incision must also be checked for drainage and signs of infection. Be certain also to assess for chest pain unrelated to the incision, noting the quality of the pain and any similarities to angina. In patients with a graft involving the radial artery, check color, temperature, and motion of the hand on the affected side when the patient awakens from anesthesia. In preparation for discharge, instruct the patient in self-care as presented in Highlight 8–6. Teach about prescribed medications. Expect some patients to be surprised at the few medications to be taken com-

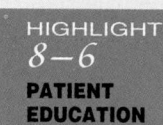 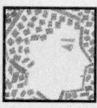

HIGHLIGHT
8–6

PATIENT EDUCATION

Discharge Instructions After Coronary Artery Bypass Grafting

On discharge, instruct the patient who has undergone CABG to:

- Take medications as ordered.
- Keep nitroglycerin available at all times.
- Do not sit for more than 45 minutes at a time without getting up and walking a few feet.
- Exercise twice a day, preferably by walking. Increase distance gradually. In inclement weather, consider walking indoors, perhaps at a shopping mall.
- Expect fatigue for 4 to 6 weeks.
- Rest at frequent intervals.
- Sleep 6 to 10 hours a night.
- Perform light housework such as dusting if desired.
- Do not perform heavy housework such as mopping floors or vacuuming and do not lift more than 10 pounds for the 6 weeks it takes for the sternum to heal.
- Inspect chest and leg incisions (if present) daily and report redness, increasing tenderness or drainage. Gently cleanse as prescribed.
- Take temperature twice a day and report fever.
- Call surgeon if unusual symptoms such as chest pain, cough, or shortness of breath develop.
- Eat a well-balanced, heart-healthy diet. Limit total fat intake, being especially careful about saturated fats. Limit salt in diet.
- Eat frequent small meals to prevent gastric distress and fatigue.
- Prevent straining with bowel movements by using a stool softener, drinking fluids, and including fiber in the diet unless otherwise contraindicated.
- Avoid smoking.
- Control blood sugar carefully, if diabetic, to promote wound healing.

pared to the number taken preoperatively. To aid the patient in complying with the low-fat, low-sodium, heart-healthy diet requirement, provide lists of foods to be avoided for reference when meal planning. Involve the dietitian in teaching if complicated problems coexist, such as malnutrition, diabetes, or hypercholesterolemia.

If the patient smokes, refer to a smoking cessation program. Explain how smoking impairs wound healing and increases the risk of damage to the new grafts by direct trauma and depletion of oxygen.

Refer the patient to a Phase II cardiac rehabilitation program to assist both the patient and his family in dealing with the diagnosis of CAD and CABG, and in maintaining a healthy and active lifestyle.

Above all, stress that CABG surgery is not a cure for CAD. CAD is a chronic disease, and lifestyle modifications and medical management will be needed throughout life.

Percutaneous Transluminal Coronary Angioplasty
Percutaneous transluminal coronary angioplasty (PTCA) compresses plaque and stretches the walls of the coronary vessels (Fig. 8–27), resulting in improved myocardial perfusion. PTCA is done in the cardiac catheterization laboratory. First, stenosis of a coronary artery is confirmed by a coronary arteriogram, then a coronary artery guide wire is passed into the aorta (as in cardiac catheterization) and positioned in the orifice of the stenosed coronary artery to be dilated. A special double-lumen catheter with a nonelastic dilating balloon and a soft wire tip is advanced through the guide wire into the coronary artery and positioned so the catheter tip is

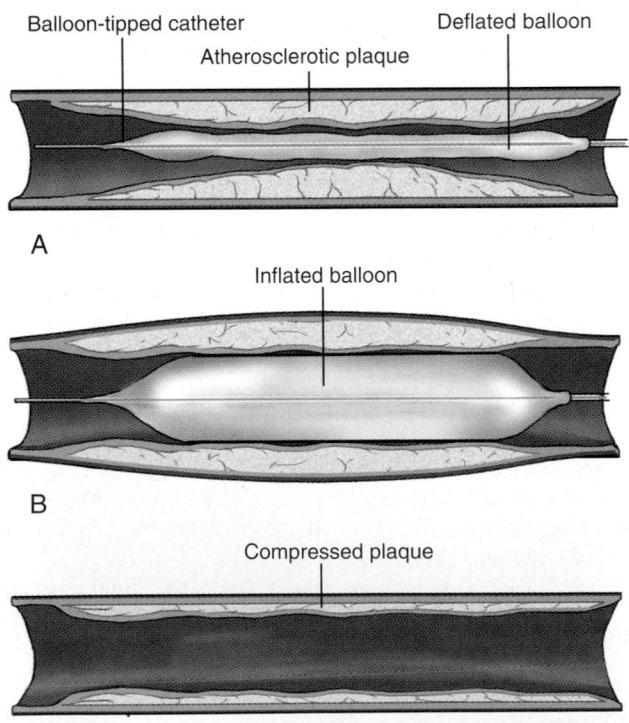

A

B

C

Figure 8–27
Percutaneous transluminal coronary angioplasty. *A,* The deflated balloon is advanced to the area of plaque buildup. *B,* The balloon is inflated, compressing the plaque against the artery walls. *C,* The balloon is deflated and withdrawn, leaving the plaque compressed and the artery lumen enlarged.

beyond the atherosclerotic obstruction and the dilating balloon is within the stenotic area. The dilating balloon is inflated for 3 to 4 seconds and then deflated. The coronary arteriogram is repeated to document the effect of the forceful dilatation on the obstructing lesion. It is believed that the balloon causes compression of the soft atheromatous material of the stenotic lesion, a "flattening out" of the obstruction, which opens the lumen to permit increased blood flow.

Complications of PTCA include those of routine cardiac catheterization plus possible dissection of the coronary artery, blockage of a branch artery in the area where plaque is compressed, and acute myocardial infarction. Cardiac surgery facilities should be available to a patient undergoing PTCA. Immediate surgery may be indicated when complications of dissection, rupture, or bleeding of coronary arteries occur, as well as when PTCA is unable to open the lesion and the patient is at risk for myocardial infarction. Vasospasm of coronary arteries may also develop during PTCA. Signs and symptoms are similar to those of a developing myocardial infarction. Vasospasm may be self-limiting or may respond to pharmacologic therapy with drugs such as the calcium channel blocking agents.

Since restenosis of vessels may develop in as many as 40% of patients within 6 months following PTCA, some patients may undergo directional coronary atherectomy at the time of the procedure. This technique widens the vessel lumen by using special cutting blades on the catheter to excise and remove or pulverize plaque.

When balloon angioplasty is unsuccessful because of the presence of hard, calcified lesions or distal lesions, coronary endoscopic laser therapy may be performed.

NURSING PROCESS GUIDELINES
Percutanous Transluminal Coronary Angioplasty

Both during and after the procedure, assess the patient for complications and monitor hemodynamic status. Maintain telemetry monitoring and observe for signs of cardiac rhythm changes. Monitor for bleeding at the puncture site. Since reocclusion of a vessel can occur, also monitor for chest pain and track enzyme levels. Measure intake and output while the patient is receiving intravenous fluid therapy.

Coronary Stenting
Coronary stents are tiny slotted or meshed tubes that are implanted within the coronary vessels to prevent restenosis after PTCA by providing structural support to the vessels and holding plaque firmly against the vessel walls (Fig. 8–28). Much like an angioplasty, a catheter is threaded into the area of the lesion and a stent is deployed. Over time, endothelial cells grow along the inner surface

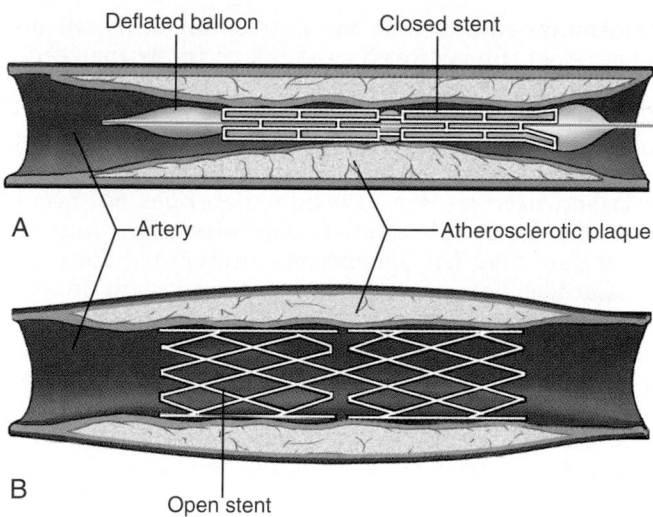

Figure 8–28

Placement of a stent in a coronary artery. *A,* The stent is advanced to the area of plaque buildup on a deflated balloon. *B,* The balloon is opened, expanding the stent and compressing the plaque against the artery walls. The balloon is then deflated and withdrawn.

of the stent, producing a smooth lining. Nonetheless, clots can easily form on stents and long-term, high-level anticoagulation is needed.

Laser Angioplasty

In a laser angioplasty, pulsed laser energy is used to vaporize plaque that is obstructing blood flow in a coronary artery. Laser angioplasty is performed in the cardiac catheterization laboratory and post-procedure care is similar to care after cardiac catheterization.

❖ Settings, Providers, and Collaboration for Care

Although some cases of angina are diagnosed on an outpatient basis, many patients enter the health-care system via the emergency department if acute chest pain is the presenting symptom. Once the patient's condition is stabilized and other acute problems are ruled out, the patient is usually treated on an outpatient basis. A nutritionist and a physical therapist may be consulted to help the patient modify his or her lifestyle. A home care nurse or a nurse in a primary care setting must work closely with the patient and family to assess compliance with therapy. The nurse in this setting also assesses the patient with each contact for any signs of deterioration of the patient's condition.

*M*yocardial Infarction

Etiology and Pathophysiology

Myocardial infarction is death of myocardial tissue as a result of insufficient oxygen. Factors that can cause myocardial oxygen insufficiency fall into two categories: those that decrease the flow of oxygenated blood to the myocardial tissues and those that increase the myocardial need for oxygen beyond what the circulation can supply. Factors in the first category include occlusion of a coronary artery by a thrombus, coronary artery spasm, embolus lodging in the coronary artery, and a sudden, dramatic drop in blood pressure during anesthesia. Factors in the second category, those that increase need for oxygen, include acute stress as in heavy exertion, an abrupt increase in blood pressure, excessive catecholamine levels, and cocaine abuse.

Of all these potential causes of myocardial infarction, by far the most common is the sudden total occlusion of a major coronary artery by a thrombosis. Thrombosis almost always occurs as the result of an acute change in an atherosclerotic plaque already present in the coronary artery. Types of acute change that can initiate thrombosis include hemorrhage within the plaque, fissuring of the plaque, or actual rupture of the plaque. Plaques that are the most likely to undergo acute change are those that are soft and filled with fatty deposits. Older, more fibrotic plaques are more stable. In response to these acute changes, vasoactive substances are released and platelets aggregate at the site. Ultimately a thrombus forms, which obstructs the artery (Fuster, 1995). If the area of myocardium perfused by the obstructed artery has collateral circulation from other nearby vessels, this may compensate for the blocked vessel, and myocardial infarction may be averted. However, if there is no collateral blood flow, the area of myocardium normally supplied by the obstructed vessel becomes ischemic. Initially, this is a reversible process. However, necrosis of the cardiac muscle begins 20 to 30 minutes after total occlusion and spreads out in a wave over the next 3 to 6 hours. Necrosis cannot be reversed, but the size of the necrotic area may be limited by restoration of oxygen to the affected tissue during this 3- to 6-hour period. Following infarction, over 3 to 6 weeks, scar tissue gradually forms over the necrotic area. The cells in the infarct-related zone thin, the ventricular chamber dilates, and the surrounding muscle hypertrophies to compensate. Eventually, connective tissue enters the area so the scar becomes interspersed with muscle fibers. The entire process is called ventricular remodeling.

Depending on their location in the heart, myocardial infarctions are described as anterior wall, inferior with extension to the posterior wall or right ventricular wall, or lateral wall infarcts. Location is determined by which artery is obstructed, and location in turn determines the effect on cardiac function. Thrombosis of the left anterior descending branch of the left coronary artery results in an anterior myocardial infarction affecting the left ventricle and can result in cardiogenic shock. Thrombosis of the right coronary artery causes an inferior myocardial infarction affecting the sinoatrial node, atrioventricular node, and proximal bundle of His, thus predisposing to conduction disturbances. Thrombosis of the left circumflex artery causes a lateral wall infarct with effects similar to those of an anterior infarct.

Most myocardial infarcts occur in the left ventricle, as this is the largest area of heart muscle and has the greatest workload and the greatest oxygen requirement.

Clinical Manifestations

The most prominent symptom of myocardial infarction is sudden, acute chest pain. The pain, which is described as crushing, heavy, viselike, constricting, or "like an elephant sitting on my chest," persists and increases in severity. Pain is most often felt in the lower substernal area and may radiate to the neck, jaw, back, shoulder, or left arm. Although this is the typical picture of the pain of myocardial infarction, there is individual variation. Women, for example, do not always present with the same classic crushing chest pain that men do, and so-called "silent" myocardial infarctions (infarcts) are not uncommon in the elderly and in diabetics with neuropathy. The pain associated with a myocardial infarction differs from angina in that it is prolonged and unrelieved by rest or nitroglycerin.

In addition to pain, patients are frequently pale, diaphoretic, short of breath, and dizzy or lightheaded. A feeling of impending doom is common. Vagal stimulation, which is most pronounced when the right coronary artery is involved, can result in nausea and vomiting. This sometimes causes patients to interpret the problem as indigestion or heartburn and to self-treat with antacids rather than seeking immediate medical attention. Symptoms of full-fledged cardiogenic shock ensue if the ventricle becomes so ischemic that it is unable to pump sufficiently to maintain cardiac output.

Diagnosis

The diagnosis of myocardial infarction is made on the basis of symptoms, history, electrocardiographic changes, and cardiac isoenzyme elevations. The description of the pain and its onset suggest the diagnosis in most cases. A history of coronary artery disease or risk factors for it such as obesity, smoking, familial history of cardiac disease, diabetes, hypertension, and a high-stress lifestyle support the clinical impression.

Electrocardiograms show serial changes in response to myocardial infarction because ischemic and necrotic cells do not respond normally to electrical stimulation. In the majority of cases, appearance of Q waves, ST segment elevation or depression, and T wave abnormalities accompany transmural myocardial infarction (infarction involving all the layers of the myocardium). In the remaining cases, the so-called non-Q wave infarction, only changes in the ST segment and the T waves occur. Previously, the absence of Q waves was considered indicative of a subendocardial (infarction involving the inner muscle beneath the endocardium) rather than a transmural infarct, but the correlation does not always exist. Since wave changes occur in the leads that overlie the area of tissue damage, the size and location of the infarct can also be determined. Electrocardiographic tracings also detect dysrhythmias, which may occur as the result of myocardial ischemia and necrosis. Because infarction does not occur instantaneously, the initial ECG after the onset of chest pain may not demonstrate myocardial damage.

Cardiac enzyme studies most important in the diagnosis of myocardial infarction are creatine kinase and lactate dehydrogenase. Creatine kinase is found in skeletal muscle, cardiac muscle, and the brain and is released when these tissues are injured. The isoenzymes of creatine kinase specific to each of these tissues are CK-MM (skeletal muscles), CK-MB (cardiac muscle), and CK-BB (brain). With a myocardial infarction, the total level of creatine kinase begins to rise within 3 hours after the onset of pain, peaks about 12 hours later, and then declines to normal in the next 12 to 24 hours. By itself, an increase in creatine kinase is not diagnostic of myocardial infarction; however, an increase in CK-MB only occurs with damage to cardiac tissue. CK-MB levels consistent with a myocardial infarction are a peak level of more than twice the normal limit or a peak of over 13 IU/L with a 50% rise having occurred in the 4 to 12 hours after the onset of pain. CK-MB is the most specific indicator of myocardial infarction. The peak levels of CK and CK-MB correlate positively with the size of the infarct and thus serve as predictors of prognosis and likelihood of complications.

Lactate dehydrogenase levels rise after creatine kinase levels and remain elevated for a week or more after myocardial infarction. Though not as reliable as creatine kinase levels in reflecting cardiac tissue damage, they can be of use when evaluating patients seen more than 24 hours after the onset of chest pain.

Another, more recently developed test for the diagnosis of myocardial infarction measures the serum levels of troponin. Troponin, which can be measured in the form of troponin I and troponin T, is a protein released by damaged myocardial cells. It begins to appear in 6 hours, even after mild heart attacks that might not cause creatine kinase to rise above its upper normal limit. Troponin T may be present for up to 14 days following a myocardial infarction, and high levels of Troponin I may be present for 7 days.

Laboratory findings indicative of tissue necrosis or inflammation, though not specific to cardiac tissue, also support the diagnosis of myocardial infarction. These findings include leukocytosis of up to 15,000/mm that begins within a few hours of the onset of pain and lasts for 3 days to a week. The ESR also rises during the first weeks after myocardial infarction and remains high for several weeks.

Echocardiography and nuclear scans may also be used in the diagnosis of areas of ischemia and infarct (see Chap. 7 for a discussion of these tests).

Management

Early treatment following a myocardial infarction is important to prevent the development of life-threatening complications. Serious dysrhythmias and cardiac arrest can occur at the time of infarct and are the leading cause of death before hospitalization. Up to 95% of myocardial infarction patients experience irregularities in heart rhythm at some point in the postinfarction period. If the contractility of the ventricles is impaired from damaged heart muscle, heart failure and pulmonary edema can ensue. If a large amount of the left ventricle is damaged, cardiac output is inadequate to maintain blood pressure, and tissue perfusion and cardiogenic shock develops, with serious sequelae. Pericarditis is a complication that can develop, particularly following a transmural myocardial infarction. As ventricular remodeling occurs, the ventricular wall can thin, leading to ventricular aneurysm and, in some instances, to rupture of the ventricle and death. Early entry into the emergency medical system and admission to an acute care facility improve the chances of survival for the patient with a myocardial infarction.

The major treatment goal for the patient with a myocardial infarction is to prevent or limit damage to the myocardium. To accomplish this goal, a balance between the supply of oxygen to the myocardial tissue and its need for oxygen must be restored. Thus treatment measures consist of those designed to increase the flow of oxygenated blood to all areas of the myocardium and those designed to decrease the workload of the myocardium and therefore its need for oxygen.

Immediate management of the patient with a possible myocardial infarction includes a 12-lead ECG; cardiac monitoring; oxygen therapy for 2 to 3 hours in cases of uncomplicated myocardial infarction, because longer therapy can lead to systemic vasoconstriction and problems for patients with COPD (Cerrato, 1997); administration of intravenous fluids; and blood studies. The severe pain associated with myocardial infarction is treated with morphine sulfate or meperidine unless thrombolytic or beta-adrenergic blocking agents are to be used. In that case, sublingual nitroglycerin, repeated twice at 5-minute intervals, is given, provided that systolic arterial pressure is not less than 90 mm Hg and heart rate is not less than 50 or more than 100. If pain is not relieved, nitroglycerin is given IV and titrated relative to blood pressure and pain relief.

Since research has demonstrated a dramatic decrease in mortality with early restoration of blood flow to the infarcted area, once the diagnosis of myocardial infarction is made, the first priority is to limit damage by opening the artery. Thrombolytic agents are given intravenously when patients present to the hospital within 6 hours of the onset of symptoms. These agents dissolve the existing clot and restore blood flow to the ischemic zone. They are most effective when the infarct is large and

when given within the first 3 hours after the onset of symptoms. The thrombolytics most commonly utilized include tissue plasminogen activator (t-PA), which is a naturally occurring enzyme, and streptokinase. A third thrombolytic with the advantage of being given as a single intravenous injection is anistreplase (APSAC [anisoylated plasminogen streptokinase activator complex]). A major risk associated with these drugs is bleeding, including cerebral hemorrhage, so a careful history must be obtained from any potential candidate to determine whether any contraindications to thrombolytic therapy exist (Highlight 8–7). Other risks associated with thrombolytic therapy include

- "Stunned myocardium," which is a condition of prolonged contractile dysfunction following reperfusion
- Reperfusion injury to cells, which can manifest in a variety of ways, including further myocardial necrosis or reperfusion dysrhythmias

Since reocclusion can occur following thrombolytic therapy, heparin is often given for 24 hours thereafter.

Other options for opening the infarct-related artery are emergency PTCA and CABG surgery. Because these procedures require specialized facilities, such as catheterization laboratories and operating rooms, as well as the necessary personnel, thrombolytic therapy is generally the preferred treatment. The American Heart Association/American College of Cardiology Guidelines (1996) recommend thrombolytic therapy or PTCA only in cases in which an ST elevation is evident on ECG.

Also important in the medical treatment of myocardial infarction is the use of aspirin (162–325 mg) immediately when myocardial infarction is being considered as a diagnosis. Aspirin is routinely stocked on ambulances and given to patients with a high index of suspicion for myocardial infarction. Aspirin is believed to decrease the inflammatory response in the endothelium and the aggregation of platelets at the site of injury. Prior to the administration of aspirin the patient must be carefully questioned as to a history of allergy to the drug or bleeding problems.

The patient with an acute myocardial infarction should be admitted to a coronary care or telemetry unit for close cardiac monitoring and intensive care, which includes complete rest, analgesia, oxygen, and early detection and treatment of dysrhythmias. For uncomplicated cases in patients without ischemia-related chest discomfort, bedrest and use of a bedside commode are maintained for the first 12 hours. After this time, the patient is encouraged to use the toilet, take short walks, and bathe with assistance. Indications for prolonged bedrest are the development of unstable vital signs, dysrhythmias, cardiogenic shock, or recurrent chest pain that may indicate extension or expansion of the infarct-related zone.

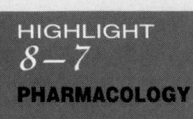 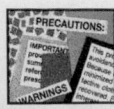

Thrombolytic Agents

Definition:

Enzymes such as alteplase, t-PA, streptokinase, and urokinase

Action:

Convert plasminogen to plasmin, which breaks up fibrin clots.

Uses:

Lysis of thrombi after an acute myocardial infarction or for pulmonary emboli, thereby limiting the size of the infarct.

Side Effects:

Excessive bleeding and bruising, bleeding at puncture sites, internal hemorrhage, fever, or headache. As myocardium reperfuses, it can also become irritable, predisposing the patient to dysrhythmias.

Interactions:

Risk of bleeding is increased if used in combination with anticoagulants.

Contraindications:

Bleeding disorders or recent cerebrovascular accident, intracranial or intraspinal surgery, or neoplasm.

Nursing Implications:

• Monitor for signs of reperfusion, eg, relief of chest pain, reperfusion dysrhythmias (premature ventricular contractions or short runs of ventricular tachycardia), return of the ST segment to baseline, and early elevation of creatine kinase.
• Check vital signs.
• Evaluate hematocrit levels.
• Monitor for signs of intracerebral bleeding: altered levels of consciousness, headache, weakness, paralysis, unilateral change in pupil size.
• Monitor the electrocardiogram for dysrhythmias, taking appropriate action as necessary.
• Observe for bleeding every 15 minutes for 8 hours and then every hour for 8 hours, especially at puncture sites. Be alert for hematomas, bruising, or petechiae.
• Avoid needle sticks if possible; when unavoidable, hold pressure on the site for 5 minutes. Three venous lines should be in place before thrombolytic therapy is given. Blood specimens should be obtained through one of them.
• Protect the patient from accidental bruising or other injury that may cause bleeding.
• Avoid over-manipulation of the patient.
• Observe for new back or leg pain, which may indicate retroperitoneal bleeding.
• Teach the patient signs of bleeding to be alert for: tea-colored urine, nose bleeds, bleeding gums, black stool, and abdominal pain.
• Teach the patient how to prevent bleeding episodes, eg, brush teeth gently with a very soft toothbrush, shave with an electric razor.
• Direct the patient to report any signs of bleeding that occur.

Sufficient analgesia is administered to control the severe chest pain as well as the accompanying anxiety, since pain and stress increase myocardial oxygen requirements. Morphine sulfate is the analgesic of choice unless thrombolytic or beta-adrenergic blocking agents are to be used because it also dilates the peripheral vasculature and lessens cardiac workload. Morphine also induces a state of well-being or euphoria, which serves to diminish the patient's anxiety. Small intravenous doses of 2 mg are titrated to pain relief. The intravenous route is used rather than the intramuscular because IM administration damages the muscles, thereby falsely elevating the creatinine kinase levels. The IV route also allows for rapid absorption of the medication. Other medications such as hydroxyzine (Vistaril) or promethazine (Phenergan) may be used concomitantly because of their antiemetic properties and the potentiating effects they have on narcotics. Less narcotic is needed when given in conjunction with these medications.

Oxygen is administered at a flow rate of 2 to 4 L per minute by nasal cannula. If the patient has evidence of chronic obstructive lung disease with carbon dioxide retention, the oxygen flow rate is adjusted downward to 2 L/min. Oxygen helps to relieve ischemia of the myocardium by raising the blood oxygen level.

Cardiac monitoring with serial ECGs is essential to assess the electrical activity of the heart. Ischemia and necrosis of the cardiac muscle cause alteration of electrical conduction through the muscle because dead tissue cannot conduct electricity—it is inert and unable to depolarize. Ischemic cells may become excessively irritable and initiate impulses outside the normal conduction pathways. This disruption may produce ectopic beats—beats that come from an area other than the sinoatrial node. These beats often originate in the ventricles and come prematurely in the conduction cycle, hence they are called premature ventricular contractions. In the presence of myocardial infarction, premature ventricular contractions may herald impending ventricular tachycardia or fibrillation. Dysrhythmias are the leading cause of death in patients with myocardial infarction, and one of the primary reasons why patients are placed in coronary care units during the acute phase of their myocardial infarction is to allow life-threatening dysrhythmias to be promptly recognized and treated. Drugs commonly used to treat ventricular dysrhythmias are procainamide, bretylium, and amiodarone. The use of lidocaine, once used prophylactically to decrease the risk of dysrhythmias in the care of the patient with acute myocardial infarction, has become much less common. Current recommendations are to use lidocaine sparingly and only for frequent ectopy, beats originating from different focal points indicating irritability, or for life-threatening ventricular rhythms. Although lidocaine is an anesthetic and has many toxic side effects, it is still a first-line drug when malignant dysrhythmias develop. Its use should be short-term, and careful monitoring for symptoms of toxicity such as seizure activity and depressed mental status is essential.

If thrombolytic agents are used, reperfusion dysrhythmias are common and may signal arterial opening. Ventricular tachycardia and fibrillation occur frequently, so close monitoring and immediate treatment are necessary. Although alarming, these reperfusion rhythms may simply indicate that the artery is open. Another indicator of restored blood flow is the patient's report of decreased or completely relieved chest pain.

Vessels that have been successfully opened with thrombolysis or emergency PTCA are susceptible to reocclusion; therefore, anticoagulant therapy is instituted. The use of heparin after thrombolysis prevents the formation of new clots and keeps the blood flow smooth across the irritated and injured vascular wall.

The patient's partial thromboplastin time (PTT) is monitored every few hours after thrombolysis is given and per hospital policy while he or she is maintained on heparin. Generally, the PTT is maintained at one and a half times the normal control value. Aspirin, which prevents platelet aggregation and reduces inflammation, thus reducing the risk of another myocardial infarction by up to 50%, is given daily.

Nitrates are used in the management of acute myocardial infarction to dilate coronary arteries and improve blood flow, thus reducing pain. Intravenous nitroglycerin infusion carefully titrated to pain control and blood pressure provides a continuous therapeutic effect. Titration to blood pressure is critical because nitroglycerin is such a potent vasodilator that it can cause severe hypotension.

Beta blockers are now standard for the treatment of acute myocardial infarction because they decrease the heart rate, decrease the workload of the heart, and in some patients prevent heart failure after a myocardial infarction. Cardioselective beta-blockers, such as atenolol (Tenormin) and metoprolol (Lopressor), are the drugs of choice. Because these medications are cardioselective, they have less effect on the β-receptors located in the bronchioles, thus less risk of inducing bronchospasm. Beta blockers are initially given intravenously, then orally. Most patients are discharged on a beta blocker after acute myocardial infarction unless there is a strong contraindication to its use (Smith, 1997).

Many patients with acute myocardial infarction are also started on ACE inhibitors such as enalapril (Vasotec), lisinopril (Prinivil), or captopril (Capoten). ACE inhibitors prevent heart failure in a select group of patients after myocardial infarction by decreasing afterload or lessening the workload of the heart by decreasing the systemic blood pressure. These drugs influence ventricular remodeling and also have contributed significantly to decreasing mortality rates. Calcium channel blockers are not recommended.

Patients are maintained on a clear liquid diet for about 24 hours depending on their condition and response to treatment. Clear liquids are advanced to bland, solid food according to patient toleration and desire, with meals ideally given frequently in small portions. There is no longer any restriction on hot or cold foods, as research does not support that they will precipitate an angina attack. Decaffeinated coffee or tea is recommended because caffeine is a potent cardiac stimulant that raises heart rate and blood pressure.

On transfer out of the critical care unit, patients are maintained on telemetry and watched for changes in cardiac rate or rhythm as activity progresses. Initially, patients ambulate with assistance at least twice a day, beginning with 5-minute walks. Walking is gradually increased to 30 minutes twice a day, after which stair-climbing is begun. When 30-minute unassisted walks and stair-climbing are tolerated, patients are usually able to perform most activities of daily living.

Tolerance to this progressive exercise program is evaluated by pulse rate and rate of perceived exertion. A resting pulse rate is obtained prior to exercise. The exercise is considered to be well-tolerated if the pulse rate does not increase by more than 20 beats per minute. Rate of perceived exertion is a measure of the patient's subjective sense of how much exertion is required to perform an activity. The scale ranges from No Exertion, with a score of

0, to Very Light Exertion, with a score of 7, to Very Hard Exertion, with a score of 19. A rate of perceived exertion score less than 14 is considered to indicate tolerance. Prior to walking and stair-climbing, a baseline blood pressure is also obtained and the patient is asked to perform a series of flexibility exercises.

Prior to discharge, a submaximal exercise stress test is generally performed to evaluate the patient's status. A submaximal exercise stress test is a stress test that ends when the patient's pulse rate increases to a preselected level, when the rate of perceived exertion score reaches a preselected level, or when symptoms occur.

Following discharge, patients are sometimes instructed to gauge their activity based on pulse rate and rate of perceived exertion. In other cases, patients may be instructed to engage in only those activities that fall within a certain MET (metabolic equivalent) range. METs are measures of cardiovascular workload and oxygen consumption associated with various activities. One MET is the amount of oxygen used when sitting at rest. Two METs are twice that amount. Three METS are three times that amount, and so on. The MET scale categorizes activities as follows:

Very light	Less than 3 METs
Light	3 to 5 METs
Moderate	5 to 7 METs
Heavy	7 to 9 METs
Very heavy	More than 9 METs

Examples of very light activities include washing, shaving, dressing, cooking, driving a car, walking 2 miles per hour, using a stationary bicycle at low resistance, and playing golf with a cart. Light activities include carrying 15 to 30 pounds, raking leaves, using a power lawn mower, dancing, playing doubles tennis, walking 3 to 4 miles per hour, and bicycling on level ground. Moderate activities include slow stair-climbing, carrying 30 to 60 pounds, walking 4 to 5 miles per hour, swimming using the breaststroke, skating, and playing singles tennis. Heavy activities include carrying 60 to 90 pounds, climbing stairs at a moderate pace, jogging, swimming using the crawl stroke, and bicycling at 12 miles per hour. Very heavy activities include carrying more than 90 lb, carrying loads up stairs, bicycling up steep hills, and running at 6 miles per hour or more (Haskell, 1984).

❖ **Settings, Providers, and Collaboration for Care**

Care of the patient with a myocardial infarction generally begins with the arrival of ambulance personnel, emergency medical technicians, or paramedics at the patient's location. In some cases however, the patient may present at a hospital emergency department, clinic, or physician's office and treatment be-

gins there. Subsequent to immediate care, the patient is admitted to a coronary or critical care unit for monitoring and treatment. Once the patient's condition is hemodynamically stable, he or she may be transferred to a telemetry unit for further monitoring or to a general medical floor. Discharge home with follow-up outpatient care usually occurs within 5 days in uncomplicated cases. Because a myocardial infarction requires pharmacologic and dietary treatment, lifestyle changes, and psychologic adjustment to a potentially lethal disorder, a wide variety of health-care professionals is essential to comprehensive, effective care. These include all the members of the cardiac rehabilitation team: the primary care physician, cardiologist, cardiac care nurses, physical therapist, nutritionist, psychologist, and social worker. Home care nurses and physicians responsible for handling coexistent problems such as diabetes or a rheumatic disease, family members, and support group representatives also play a critical role. Good communication among care givers and across settings is a key element to successful care.

NURSING PROCESS
Myocardial Infarction

Assessment

Determine the patient's level of consciousness and hemodynamic stability, as these findings guide subsequent assessment. Obtain a targeted history since the patient with acute myocardial infarction has the potential for life-threatening complications in the initial phases of the disease.

Assess for signs and symptoms of severe and unrelenting pain, noting the onset, duration, radiation, and location. Determine if anything (such as nitroglycerin or rest) relieves the pain. Look for nonverbal signs of pain such as restlessness, grimacing, clenching of fists, moaning, or crying. Check if patient has associated symptoms with the pain, such as profuse diaphoresis or vomiting.

Assess for any skin changes, such as cyanosis or pale, clammy, mottled skin indicating shock. Ask the patient about numbness, tingling, or paresthesias of the extremities. Continually observe the cardiac monitor for dysrhythmias or ischemic changes such as ST segment elevation to T wave changes. Monitor the vital signs, including an apical pulse and heart sounds in all six cardiac areas. Use both the diaphragm and bell to pick up high- and low-pitched heart sounds, gallops, rubs, or murmurs. Document where the abnormal heart sounds are heard. Check the blood pressure at frequent intervals and observe for hypotension. Palpate all the peripheral pulses, noting strength and equality on both sides of the body.

Listen to the lung sounds for crackles and check for jugular venous distention. Observe for produc-

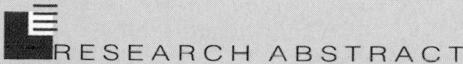

RESEARCH ABSTRACT

What Keeps People From Practicing Self-Care After a Myocardial Infarction?

Beach EK, Smith A, Luthringer L, et al. Self-care limitations of persons after acute myocardial infarction. Appl Nurs Res 1996; 9(1):24.

After a myocardial infarction (MI), a patient has much to learn about the lifestyle changes that he or she will need to make in order to return to optimal function. At the same time as the patient is beginning to cope with the physical changes that result from the MI, he or she must also make emotional and psychologic adjustments, which can make recovery from MI a complicated process. Traditionally, nurses have relied heavily on cardiac rehabilitation programs to teach patients about the lifestyle changes that will be needed. But is this trust in cardiac rehabilitation programs well placed? According to Beach and colleagues, it may not be.

Beach and colleagues discovered that the complex adjustments that patients need to make after MIs are *not* achieved by a significant number of people, despite extensive "education." This finding suggested to the researchers that education was not always the key. The authors suggested that in addition to providing education, nurses should be looking at factors that affect the *willingness* of patients to participate in their own recovery, and at how compliance or lack of it affects long-term outcomes.

Because the current health-care climate focuses more and more on the participation of patients and families in care, the researchers used Orem's self-care model to study a group of patients who had experienced their first MI. The researchers posed the question, "What are the limitations that keep people from practicing self-care after an MI?"

Orem defines self-care as the "actions people develop to take care of themselves." She defines self-care agency as the "ability of persons to meet their requirements for actions to regulate their own functioning and development." Those factors that restrict people from taking the actions necessary to regain health and well-being she dubs "limitations." Orem has suggested that nurses use her list of limitations to assess readiness for learning and change. The researchers, using this framework, sampled a group of patients who had experienced their first MI. The researchers sought to discover the limitations that may have adversely affected the patients' learning of or participation in needed lifestyle changes and their adaptation or incorporation of these changes into everyday life.

Beach and colleagues found that the categories of limitations outlined by Orem *did* apply to these patients. The categories were as follows:

Limitations of knowing
Limitations for making judgments and decisions
Limitations for engaging in result-achieving courses of action

The research team carried out extensive interviews with their target group. After analyzing the data, the researchers found that three of the most frequently cited limitations were:

- Patterns of personal or family living that interfered with self-care (ie, work; and the dependence of a spouse, children, or parents on the patient for care)
- Intense emotional states or sudden, strong likes, dislikes, or concerns (ie, emotional stress, anxiety, or depression)
- Alterations (not in accord with reality) in the perceptions, meanings, and appraisals of situations (ie, the use of denial as a coping mechanism, especially to the point that it interferes with compliance)

Based on their findings, Beach and colleagues strongly recommend the use of some type of appraisal tool for patients who have suffered MIs to examine factors that may affect self-care.

Questions to Consider

1. What type of rehabilitation/education program is available for post-MI patients at your facility?
2. Why is it important for patients to participate in all aspects of rehabilitation after an MI?
3. If you were to follow a group of patients recovering from uncomplicated MI, what do you think you would find?
4. If you could design your own post-MI rehabilitation program, what would it look like?
5. Other than the factors identified in this study, what are some other factors that you think might interfere with compliance with a rehabilitation program for patients recovering from MI? Why did you include these particular factors?

tion of pink, frothy sputum indicative of pulmonary edema.

Nursing Diagnoses and Planning

Nursing diagnoses and related patient outcomes commonly applicable to patients with a myocardial infarction include the following:

NDx: Pain related to tissue ischemia secondary to complete coronary artery occlusion

Planning: Patient Outcomes
1. Patient states chest pain is relieved or controlled.
2. Nonverbal signs of pain are absent.
3. Patient rests quietly.

NDx: Anxiety related to sympathetic nervous stimulation, severe pain, and fear of death due to myocardial infarction

Planning: Patient Outcomes
1. Patient verbalizes feelings and concerns.
2. Patient verbalizes acceptance of the diagnosis of myocardial infarction.
3. Patient describes anxiety as decreasing and under control.
4. Behavioral signs of anxiety are absent.

NDx: Altered myocardial tissue perfusion related to obstruction of a coronary artery

Planning: Patient Outcomes
1. Patient complies with activity restrictions designed to decrease cardiac workload.
2. Patient rests quietly, free of signs of anxiety or agitation.
3. Patient tolerates gradual increases in activity without pain or dyspnea.

NDx: Risk for decreased cardiac output related to loss of mechanical pumping ability, changes in cardiac rate, rhythm, or electrical conduction secondary to tissue ischemia

Planning: Patient Outcomes
1. Patient remains hemodynamically stable, free of signs of shock as indicated by heart rate less than 100 and regular, systolic blood pressure between 90 and 140, diastolic blood pressure between 50 and 90, an alert and oriented mental status, warm, pink skin, urine output of at least 30 mL/hour, and oxygen saturation about 95%.
2. Patient remains free of chest pain.
3. Patient demonstrates a stable cardiac rhythm on the monitor.
4. Patient activity tolerance increases daily.

NDx: Risk for altered health maintenance related to insufficient knowledge about the nature of myocardial infarction and CAD, treatment, expected outcomes, and need for significant lifestyle changes

Planning: Patient Outcomes
1. Patient verbalizes understanding of heart disease, present condition, and symptoms that require immediate attention.

2. Patient describes personal risk factors and the need for lifestyle changes such as low-fat diet, exercise, and cessation of smoking to prevent progression of CAD.
3. Patient states the name and purpose of prescribed medications, their dose, time, and side effects.
4. Patient explains the need for involvement in a cardiac rehabilitation program.

Nursing Interventions and Evaluation

NDx: Pain
Instruct the patient to report onset of chest pain immediately. Document both the characteristics of chest pain as described by the patient and the concurrent wave changes seen on the cardiac monitor. Note nonverbal cues indicating pain as well as hemodynamic changes during pain. Monitor heart rate, respiratory rate, and blood pressure at regular, frequent intervals as well as whenever pain changes character and prior to the administration of pain medication. Also obtain a 12-lead ECG whenever the pain changes in nature or if the monitor shows a dysrhythmia. Compare to baseline. Perform a complete cardiovascular assessment every 4 hours.

Administer analgesics as ordered to achieve pain control.

NDx: Anxiety
Acknowledge the patient's anxiety and the perception of the threat of the situation. Encourage expression of feelings of anger, fear, and grief. Support the patient's coping mechanisms, which may initially include denial of the situation. In a calm and non-threatening manner, gradually reinforce the idea that a myocardial infarction has occurred.

Administer sedative medications as ordered and monitor the patient's response to them. Explain the necessity of remaining quiet and relaxed to allow the myocardium to begin healing.

Orient the patient to the coronary care unit and routine procedures, and explain all activities in the patient's room. Allow the family to visit the patient at short intervals during the acute phase. Encourage questions and provide updated information at frequent intervals, keeping both the patient and family apprised of changes in the patient's status or treatment plans. Involve social services or clergy if appropriate to assist the family to cope with the situation. Answer all questions with simple, factual responses and provide consistent reinforcement, as anxiety impairs the ability to retain information.

Support grieving behavior and let the patient know this is a normal and appropriate response. Encourage increasing independence, self-care, and decision-making as the patient's hemodynamic status improves.

NDx: Altered myocardial tissue perfusion
Provide physical and emotional rest because stress activates the sympathetic nervous system, induces

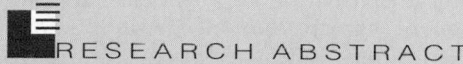

RESEARCH ABSTRACT

How Much Do Nurses Really Know About Recovery from Myocardial Infarction?

Newens AJ, McColl E, Bond S, Priest JF. Patients' and nurses' knowledge of cardiac-related symptoms and cardiac misconceptions. Heart Lung 1996; 25(3):190.

One primary nursing intervention is educating patients and families to enable them to provide safe self-care at home. These patients trust that nurses will provide information that is sufficiently reliable and timely to prevent complications. In order to provide that information, however, nurses must have current, accurate information. Nowhere is this more important than in the area of cardiac rehabilitation.

To ascertain the accuracy of nursing knowledge in cardiac rehabilitation, Newens and colleagues studied the relationship between what symptoms patients recovering from myocardial infarctions (MIs) *actually* experienced and what their nurses *predicted* they would experience.

The results of this study were interesting. When the researchers compared the *estimated* incidence of common post-MI symptoms against the incidence actually *reported* by patients, they found a significant gap. The researchers also found that the nurses had a significant lack of understanding of post-MI symptoms, and that they were ill-equipped to correct misconceptions verbalized by post-MI patients.

These findings are important because nurses are perceived to be a critical source of accurate information about recovery from MIs. The researchers point out that although nurses cannot always predict the exact symptoms that a particular patient will experience, nurses must nevertheless have an accurate knowledge of the most common symptoms to reassure patients that many of these experiences are not uncommon during recovery.

The research team also discovered that although most nurses were informed about the risks of smoking, they did not have an accurate understanding of the impact of the length of time that a person smoked. Additionally, the researchers found that nurses were not well informed about the risks of heavy physical work, excessive alcohol consumption, and the consumption of certain types of foods after MI.

The researchers also found deficiencies and inconsistencies in the provision of information to patients. They found that in many instances, nurses thought another health-care professional should provide certain information. The result? The patient was given information that was incomplete or difficult to apply.

The investigative team also discovered little association between specialization in cardiac or intensive care and the knowledge of the nurses studied. They speculated that this may be due to an emphasis on skills or symptoms, to the exclusion of information on patient education or rehabilitation. They also found that the nurses gave low priority to patient education.

The outcome of this study has important implications both for nurses caring for cardiac patients and for educators. As the emphasis on early discharge continues and more and more care is provided by patients and family, information provided by nurses *must* be accurate. Patients must know what to expect in their recovery, as well as what to report to their physicians. They must have accurate education about risk factors and the lifestyle modifications that must be made to prevent or minimize recurrence. In this era of cost containment, nurses at the bedside may not have the luxury of calling on a specialist to provide accurate home care information. The information that all of us provide must therefore be timely, accurate, and understandable if patients are to have the best possible chances for a full recovery and good quality of life.

Questions to Consider

1. What information do accrediting agencies require to be given to patients?
2. What might happen if a patient is given inaccurate or incomplete discharge information?
3. What symptoms might a patient experience in the immediate post-MI recovery period? Why might these symptoms occur?
4. What information is given to patients about MI recovery at your clinical facility?
5. How much time do nurses in your clinical facility give to answering patient questions about home care? Do the nurses just hand out books, pamphlets, and show videos, or do they also teach and answer questions? Is there a mechanism in place to address questions or concerns that patients have during their recovery? How does it operate?

the "fight or flight" response, and increases myocardial oxygen consumption. Remain at the bedside and be calm and confident in your approach to care. Provide a quiet, restful environment and basic comfort measures to enhance the effectiveness of the pain medications. If ordered, administer sedatives to keep the patient relaxed. Assist the patient to relax by using guided imagery or visualization techniques. Teach alternative methods of relaxation such as music or massage to alleviate pain and anxiety. Allow the family to participate in the patient's care if they request.

Keep the patient on bedrest with use of a bedside commode for the first 12 hours, then progress to use of the toilet, short walks, and bathing. If no untoward effects occur, gradually progress the patient's activity and plan care around scheduled, uninterrupted periods of rest. Initially, if necessary, provide total care such as washing and feeding the patient to decrease myocardial oxygen consumption and risk of injury from bleeding after thrombolysis or anticoagulation therapy.

Administer oxygen by nasal cannula to increase the myocardial oxygen supply. Place a humidification device on the oxygen set-up to prevent drying of the mucous membranes and prevent cracking and bleeding. Auscultate lung fields every 4 hours and with any change in the patient's condition. Assess for dyspnea at rest and with activities and assist the patient with care as needed.

Administer stool softeners and prevent constipation, which can cause gastric discomfort. Instruct the patient not to strain at stool since this can induce a vagal response and increase the workload of the heart, precipitating angina or dysrhythmia.

NDx: Risk for decreased cardiac output

Monitor vital signs continuously. Document and report immediately any changes. Monitor for life-threatening dysrhythmias and keep a code cart and defibrillator available near the bedside. Familiarize yourself with all emergency procedures and protocols and implement them promptly should a life-threatening dysrhythmia occur. Remain vigilant at the bedside during the first few hours of the event, since fatal complications can develop rapidly in a patient with an acute myocardial infarction.

Monitor for symptoms of cardiogenic shock, including tachycardia, hypotension, decreased urine output, impaired mental status, and cool, clammy skin. Insert a Foley catheter and record urine output at least hourly, noting the amount and character. Maintain at least two patent intravenous lines for emergency medications and fluids. Track laboratory values such as hematocrit and hemoglobin if the patient has received thrombolytic therapy. Watch for any signs of external bleeding especially from puncture sites. Check all stool specimens and emesis for occult blood.

Give supplemental oxygen, 2 to 4 L by nasal cannula. If the patient has a history of chronic obstructive lung disease, adjust the flow rate downward to prevent suppression of the hypoxic drive for respiration. Place the patient in semi-Fowler's position to allow maximum lung expansion and promote comfort. Auscultate lung fields at least every 4 hours to check for crackles indicative of heart failure. Monitor oxygen saturation values and arterial blood gases.

Allow the patient frequent and uninterrupted periods of rest. Place necessary items within reach to save energy from excessive movement. Limit visitors if they appear to be fatiguing the patient. Provide a quiet environment that promotes rest with a minimum of noise and stimuli. Dim the lights and restrict extraneous personnel from entering the room. As the patient stabilizes, begin a program of gradually increasing exercise as described previously under Management.

NDx: Risk for altered health maintenance

Begin patient education when the patient is hemodynamically stable. Be sensitive to cues indicating that the patient has questions or concerns about the disease and schedule teaching sessions accordingly. Explain the cause, effects, and clinical course of CAD and myocardial infarction to the patient. Allow time for questions from the patient and family. Provide written materials at educationally appropriate levels. Evaluate discharge concerns of the patient and family and initiate continuing care referrals as necessary (Highlight 8–8).

Provide the patient and family with "survival information." Review the signs and symptoms of acute myocardial infarction, so that if another occurs there will be early recognition. Stress the importance of calling 911 or going to the hospital emergency department immediately after three sublingual nitroglycerin tablets have failed to relieve the pain. Teach the concept that "time is muscle" when discussing myocardial infarction. Be sure the patient understands the use and function of nitroglycerin, its storage, the need to keep it with him or her at all times, and the need to replenish the supply at 6-month intervals.

Explain that fatigue and decreased endurance are part of the course of myocardial infarction and that strength will gradually improve. Instruct the patient to ask for help with activities of daily living. Ensure that there is someone who will be able to assist the patient at discharge. Stress the importance of not overdoing activity and taking time to rest at frequent intervals. Teach the patient to monitor his or her own pulse rate before and during activity and to use the rate of perceived exertion scale. Instruct the patient to stop activities if an increase in pulse rate of more than 20 beats per minute occurs or if the rate of perceived exertion scale is 14 or higher. If required by the plan of treatment, teach the patient about METs and provide a chart of activities (and the METs that they require) tailored to the patient's lifestyle. Make certain that the patient understands

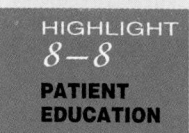 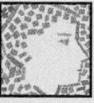

HIGHLIGHT 8–8 PATIENT EDUCATION

Discharge Instructions After Myocardial Infarction

Instruct the patient being discharged after a myocardial infarction to:

- Modify activities of daily living. Avoid overexertion, tiring activities, or any activity that induces fatigue or chest pain. Add a few new activities daily as tolerated without dyspnea, fatigue, or other untoward signs.
- Participate in a cardiac rehabilitation program. Begin an exercise regimen that is designed specifically for the individual's ability and limitations. Build strength and endurance slowly but steadily. If symptoms reappear with the exercise, revert to the previous exercise level, and then repeat the gradual increase.
- Resume sexual activity when permitted by the physician, usually when two flights of stairs can be climbed without symptoms. Initially, assume a relaxed position. Avoid sexual activity after heavy meals or alcohol intake. Take nitrates as directed prior to sexual activity to prevent angina.
- Avoid extreme temperature changes, close contact with individuals who are ill, large crowds, and other situations that present a high risk for acquiring an infection.
- Follow the prescribed diet therapy plan. Reduce caloric intake if overweight, and eat low-fat, low-sodium, well-balanced, frequent, small meals.
- Rest and relax frequently throughout the day to decrease stress and decrease the workload on the myocardium during the healing process.
- Stop smoking and avoid settings where others are smoking.
- Adhere to the prescribed medication regimen carefully.

what level of METs is permitted. Stress the importance of taking time off from work until the physician approves return. This is important because many people with acute myocardial infarction are highly motivated, hard-working individuals with a high-stress lifestyle, the so-called type A personality, and they need much reinforcement to slow down and take time for relaxation. Teach about the effect of stress on the body and heart muscle to reinforce the need for relaxation.

Instruct the patient about dietary modifications needed to prevent progression of atherosclerotic plaques. Provide written information and recipes and initiate a dietary consultation if complex issues are present, such as elevated blood cholesterol and triglycerides or diabetes. Teach modification of recipes and limitation of saturated fats and a healthy, balanced approach to diet. Reinforce the positive effects of graded exercise on cardiovascular health and stress the importance of long-term participation in a cardiac rehabilitation program. Make certain that the patient understands that, in order to be effective, exercise should be performed most days of the week (five times) and should include 20 to 40 minutes of aerobic exercise, sufficient to induce slight shortness of breath without interfering with the ability to easily talk.

Compare the patient's status with the expected outcomes. If the outcomes are not met, reassess the patient and revise the plan.

Cardiomyopathies

The cardiomyopathies are a diverse group of diseases characterized by structural changes involving the heart muscle and associated changes in hemodynamics. The four basic types of cardiomyopathy based on the type of structural change and hemodynamic profile are *dilated*, *hypertrophic*, *restrictive*, and *obliterative* (Fig. 8–29). Cardiomyopathies are further described in terms of etiology. In many cases, the cause is unknown and they are labeled *idiopathic*. In other cases, the cause can be identified as

- An infectious disorder
- Toxicity to alcohol, cocaine, other drugs such as anticancer or antiviral agents, or other toxins
- A systemic disorder such as a neuromuscular disease, a collagen-vascular disease, sarcoid, or endocrine disease
- An infiltrative disorder
- A nutritional disorder
- An ischemic disorder

DILATED CARDIOMYOPATHY

Etiology and Pathophysiology

Dilated cardiomyopathy is associated with excessive alcohol intake on a regular basis over an extended period, the use of cocaine, and treatment with cancer chemotherapeutic drugs such as doxorubicin and daunorubicin, which are anthracycline agents. The incidence of dilated cardiomyopathy caused by these chemotherapeutic drugs increases as the total cumulative dose increases and is most likely to occur in patients over the age of 70, those with pre-existing cardiac disease, and those treated with mediastinal radiation as well as chemotherapeutic agents.

Dilated cardiomyopathy is also associated with CAD. Ischemia is considered a possible contributing

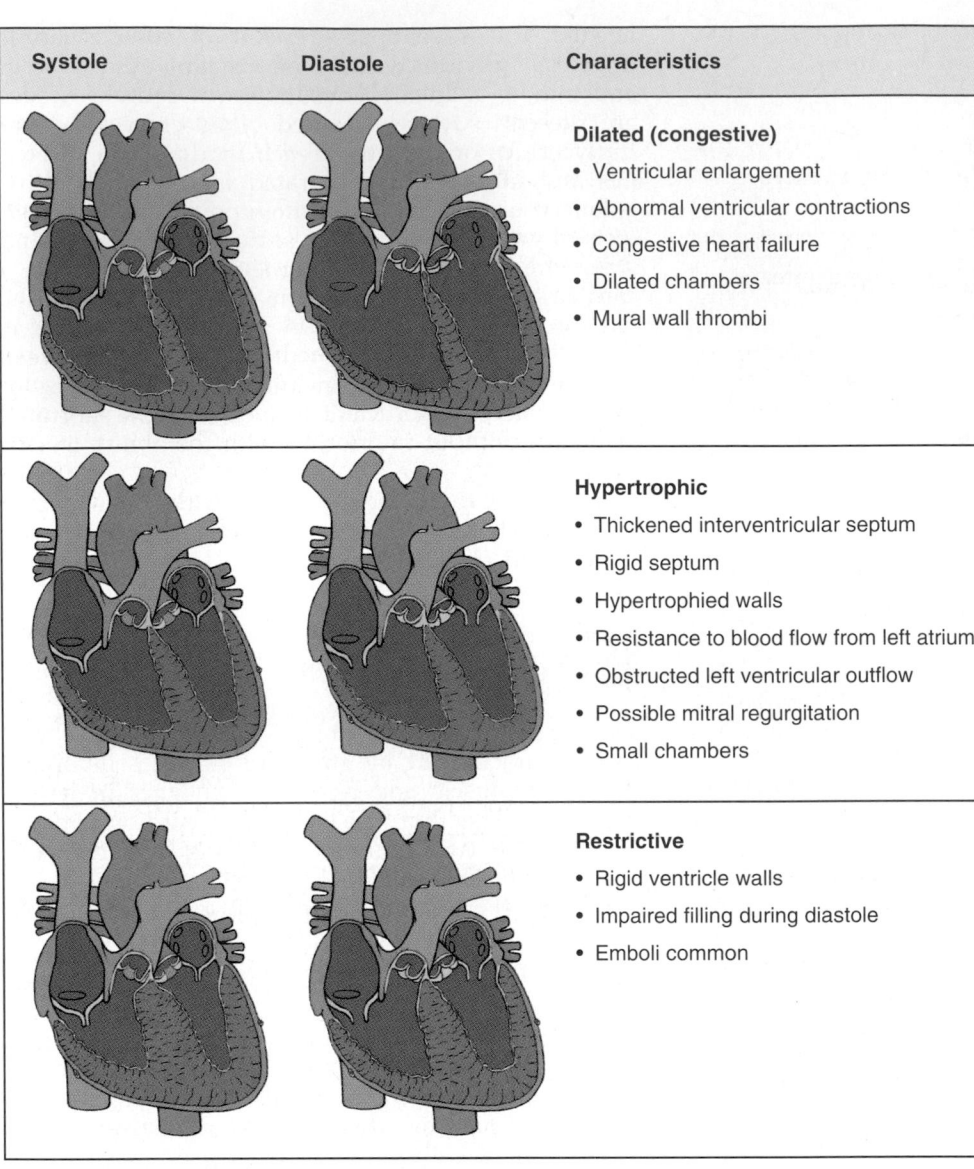

Systole	Diastole	Characteristics
		Dilated (congestive) • Ventricular enlargement • Abnormal ventricular contractions • Congestive heart failure • Dilated chambers • Mural wall thrombi
		Hypertrophic • Thickened interventricular septum • Rigid septum • Hypertrophied walls • Resistance to blood flow from left atrium • Obstructed left ventricular outflow • Possible mitral regurgitation • Small chambers
		Restrictive • Rigid ventricle walls • Impaired filling during diastole • Emboli common

Figure 8–29

Characteristics of the three types of cardiomyopathy most common in the United States. (Obliterative cardiomyopathy is very rare.)

factor, but direct evidence of the relationship is lacking. It is known, however, that multiple large myocardial infarcts cause symptoms of cardiomyopathy, as does obliterative disease of the small coronary arteries.

Autoimmune processes and long-term effects of infection with viruses such as the coxsackie B virus are also considered to be etiologic factors in some cases of dilated cardiomyopathy.

With dilated cardiomyopathy, the contractility of the myocardium is decreased. This decreased contractility usually involves both ventricles and results in impaired pumping. Chamber size and ventricular filling pressure are increased. Cardiac output and stroke volume are decreased. The ejection fraction is reduced, and functional regurgitation through the mitral or tricuspid valves may occur. In the occasional case in which the pathologic changes occur primarily in the right ventricle, the condition is referred to as right ventricular dysplasia.

Clinical Manifestations

Clinical manifestations of dilated cardiomyopathy range from asymptomatic cardiac enlargement to symptoms of heart failure. The most common symptoms experienced by patients are dyspnea and fatigue. Other symptoms include

- Pulmonary congestion that rarely progresses to pulmonary edema
- Palpitations due to ectopic beats or dysrhythmias
- Syncope secondary to dysrhythmias
- Chest pain

Systemic or pulmonary emboli may also occur. Physical findings in addition to an enlarged heart include a displaced, heaving cardiac impulse, an S_4 gallop, and an S_3 gallop. Functional murmurs may also be present.

In some patients, spontaneous improvement in ventricular function occurs. In others, the condition progresses quickly into heart failure; and in still others, sudden death occurs secondary to a dysrhythmia. The average survival time is 5 years.

Diagnosis

Diagnosis of dilated cardiomyopathy is based on the following:

- History
- Characteristic findings on physical examination
- Chest films that show massive cardiac enlargement involving all chambers
- An abnormal ECG
- An echocardiogram that documents cardiac enlargement and decreased ventricular contractility

On radioisotope imaging, dilatation of the ventricles and decreased contractility are also seen.

Management

The overall goal of management is to prolong life and maintain its quality. Further cardiac enlargement must be prevented and ability to function improved. Thus, if the cause of the cardiomyopathy is known, management focuses first on its treatment. Lifestyle adjustments to ensure adequate rest and avoidance of smoking and alcohol use are promoted. Heart failure is treated with a restricted sodium diet, cardiac glycosides, diuretics, and vasodilators. Of the latter, the preferable initial therapy in symptomatic patients is with vasodilators rather than with an ACE inhibitor. Vasodilation is desirable because venous dilatation decreases preload, whereas arterial dilatation decreases afterload. Anticoagulant therapy such as warfarin therapy is given to patients with significant impairment of left ventricular function because of the risk of pulmonary and systemic emboli. If active myocarditis exists, immunosuppressive therapy with prednisone and azathioprine is indicated for 3 to 6 months. For patients not responsive to medical therapy, surgical measures may be utilized. If severe dilated cardiomyopathy coexists with coronary arteriosclerosis, coronary bypass surgery may be performed to try to improve ventricular function. In cases of advanced heart failure and poor prognosis, cardiac transplantation may be done. For these patients, a mechanical heart or a left ventricular assist device may be used until a donor organ is obtained. A new procedure that may be appropriate for some patients is a dynamic cardiomyoplasty. In this procedure, the left or right latissimus dorsi muscle is mobilized and wrapped around the ventricles. It is then electronically stimulated to condition it to function as myocardium.

HYPERTROPHIC CARDIOMYOPATHY

Etiology and Pathophysiology

Hypertrophic cardiomyopathy is an autosomal dominant inherited disorder in more than half of the affected patients. Of the remaining cases, some occur following a viral infection and some occur spontaneously and are considered to be idiopathic. Pathophysiologically, the disorder manifests as unexplained hypertrophy of the myocardium. This hypertrophy can occur in many areas of the heart. Most often the interventricular septum is more thickened than the outer ventricular wall, and the left ventricular papillary muscles are hypertrophied. This hypertrophy may result in mitral insufficiency due to restricted movement of the septal leaflet of the mitral valve. It may also cause a fixed or labile obstruction to the left ventricular outflow because the opening of the valve leaflets is blocked by the enlarged septum. Hemodynamically, this hypertrophy of the ventricle reduces its compliance, but systolic function is maintained at least initially. The heart is hypercontractile and the ejection fraction is increased.

Clinical Manifestations

Clinical manifestations of hypertrophic cardiomyopathy include angina, palpitations, and syncope. Dyspnea, fatigue, fluid retention, and other signs and symptoms of heart failure also occur. In many patients, an abnormal cardiac impulse is noted on palpation, and an S_4, often accompanied by an S_3, is noted on auscultation. Murmurs due to left ventricular outflow obstruction or mitral regurgitation may also be present. Hypertrophic cardiomyopathy predisposes to dysrhythmias. Paroxysmal or established atrial fibrillation and premature ventricular beats are the most common. Systemic emboli are a common complication of atrial fibrillation in hypertrophic cardiomyopathy. Sudden death is not uncommon with this disease, especially in young patients. Death is often due to a lethal dysrhythmia but can also occur secondary to a sudden outflow obstruction. In older patients, this hypertrophy and related symptoms tend to remain stable or progress very slowly.

Diagnosis

The diagnosis of hypertrophic cardiomyopathy is suggested by history, findings on physical examination, chest films showing cardiac enlargement particularly of the left side of the heart, and characteristic changes on the ECG. With marked septal hypertrophy, abnormal Q waves similar to those seen with a myocardial infarct may appear. In many patients, electrocardiographic changes occur before any other signs or symptoms of the disease. The diagnosis can usually be confirmed by an echocardiogram and cardiac catheterization. The echocardiogram allows the thickness of the septum and the ventricular wall to be measured and compared and also allows detection of outflow obstruction through calculation of the pressure gradient across the ventricular outflow tract. On cardiac catheterization, an elevated left ventricular end-diastolic pressure is usually found. Thickened papillary muscles, a small hyperdynamic left ventricle, and mitral regurgitation are seen on angiography.

Management

Management of patients with hypertrophic cardiomyopathy is variable. Generally, treatment of symptomatic patients with hypertrophic cardiomyopathy with or without obstruction begins with drug therapy. Beta-adrenergic blocking agents (atenolol, metoprolol) may be used to help prevent dysrhythmias, relieve angina, syncope, and dyspnea, and improve exercise tolerance. Alternatively, the calcium channel blocking agents diltiazem and verapamil may be used. These drugs reduce myocardial oxygen consumption, relieve obstruction, and may improve diastolic compliance. Because of their hypotensive and negative inotropic effects, they must be used with caution in patients with severe heart failure and outflow obstruction. Nitroglycerin and related drugs are contraindicated. Digitalis glycosides, which can worsen obstruction, must be used with caution. Diuretics must also be used with caution, since patients with hypertrophic cardiomyopathy are very sensitive to depletion of intravascular volume. Sequential atrioventricular pacing may be tried in patients with obstruction whose symptoms do not respond to drug therapy. If this is not successful, and the obstruction is fixed, surgery in the form of a myotomy (incision into the myocardium) or myectomy (removal of a section of hypertrophied myocardium), or both, may be performed to relieve the obstruction. This surgery is done by means of a transaortic approach and requires the use of cardiopulmonary bypass. Young patients and those with a family history of sudden cardiac death should be screened for potentially fatal dysrhythmias by a 24-hour ambulatory cardiac monitor. Maintenance of a sinus rhythm is a priority but not always possible, and repeated cardioversion may be used for some patients.

RESTRICTIVE CARDIOMYOPATHY

Etiology and Pathophysiology

Restrictive cardiomyopathy is commonly due to infiltrative disease such as amyloidosis or hemochromatosis. It may also be idiopathic. In some patients, it may be associated with diabetes. With restrictive cardiomyopathy, the heart muscle is rigid and noncompliant. As a result, ventricular filling is impaired, particularly in the left side of the heart, and filling pressure is elevated. Cardiac output, stroke volume, and ejection fraction may be normal or decreased. Chamber size may be normal or increased.

Clinical Manifestations

Right-sided heart failure with edema, ascites, and hepatomegaly is the most common clinical manifestation of restrictive cardiomyopathy. Systemic venous pressure is elevated and it rises rather than falls on inspiration. Cardiac enlargement, an early diastolic third sound, low-voltage ECG, and dysrhythmias are also common.

Diagnosis

Diagnosis is based on history, physical examination, chest films, electrocardiographic tracings, echocardiograms, and cardiac catheterization. Definitive diagnosis can be made based on percutaneous myocardial biopsy.

Management

There is no known treatment for the majority of restrictive cardiomyopathies. Death occurs because of a dysrhythmia or heart failure.

OBLITERATIVE CARDIOMYOPATHY

Obliterative cardiomyopathy is very rare in the United States. Those cases that occur are due to hypereosinophilic syndrome, a highly fatal disease characterized by huge numbers of degranulated eosinophils and multiple organ involvement. In the heart, thickened endocardium or mural thrombi act as space-occupying lesions and cause a decrease in chamber size and diastolic compliance. Ventricular filling pressure is usually increased. Cardiac output, stroke volume, and the ejection fraction may be normal or decreased. Rapidly progressive heart failure, systemic embolism, dysrhythmias, and conduction disturbances occur.

NURSING PROCESS GUIDELINES
Nonsurgical Management of Cardiomyopathy

Because the cardiomyopathies result in heart failure, assessments, nursing diagnoses, expected outcomes, interventions, and evaluation are the same as those previously discussed under the care of the patient with heart failure. In addition to these measures, be certain to explain to the patient with hypertrophic cardiomyopathy the need for prophylactic antibiotics prior to having dental work or a surgical procedure to decrease the risk of infective endocarditis. Instruct the patient to inform his or her dentist or other health-care provider about this need. Also, reinforce to these patients the advisability of avoiding competitive sports because of the risk of sudden cardiac death.

For the patient undergoing a dynamic cardiomyoplasty for dilated cardiomyopathy, provide perioperative care as described in Chapter 7 under Cardiac Surgery.

*C*ardiac Valvular Disease

Cardiac valvular abnormalities are classified as pure stenosis, pure regurgitation, or mixed, with both stenosis and regurgitation. *Stenosis* is the term used to describe the condition in which the valve opening is narrowed, so that the valve does not open com-

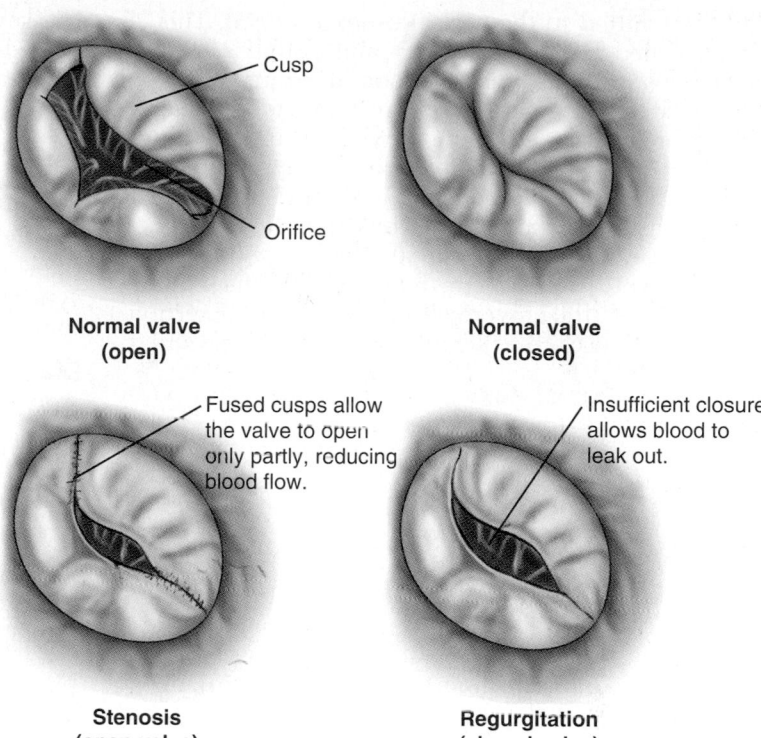

Figure 8–30
Valvular stenosis and regurgitation.

pletely (Fig. 8–30). This causes an obstruction to forward blood flow. *Regurgitation* (also called insufficiency) is the term used to describe the condition in which the valve does not close completely, thus allowing blood to flow backward, or regurgitate, through the valve's orifice (see Fig. 8–30). When both stenosis and regurgitation are present, it is termed a mixed lesion. Valvular disease can be further classified as rheumatic heart disease, nonrheumatic heart disease, and disease associated with other factors or systemic disorders such as radiation therapy, rheumatoid arthritis, and systemic lupus erythematosus. Typically, rheumatic heart disease and valvular disease caused by other systemic disorders involve more than one valve and present as a mixture of stenosis and regurgitation. Lesions affecting a single valve, on the other hand, tend to be congenital or degenerative in origin.

Cardiac valve disease is a common form of heart disease in individuals of all ages. It may cause disability ranging from slight to severe, depending on the amount of involvement and the rapidity with which the changes occurred. Although rheumatic fever has decreased in incidence and severity in developed nations, it is still an important cause of valvular disease in adults.

AORTIC VALVE STENOSIS

Etiology and Pathophysiology
Stenosis of the aortic valve can be caused by rheu-

matic heart disease. However, when it occurs in the absence of other valvular lesions, it is usually nonrheumatic in origin. In individuals under the age of 60, aortic stenosis is most often due to progressive calcification and stenosis of a congenitally abnormal valve. In patients over the age of 60, degenerative thickening and calcification of leaflets in an originally normal valve are the usual causes. In the latter cases, similar changes also tend to be found in the coronary arteries.

Valvular stenosis obstructs blood flow and usually causes increased pressure in the cardiac chamber upstream from the obstruction, that is, the area through which the blood flows immediately before it encounters the obstruction. Thus with aortic stenosis, left ventricular systolic pressure is abnormally increased and higher than aortic systolic pressure. The amount of the increase varies with the degree of stenosis and may be as much as four or five times normal. The effect of this increased pressure in the ventricle is concentric hypertrophy (a thickened ventricular wall with a normal-sized chamber), which develops as a compensatory mechanism to allow the heart to effectively pump blood against the increased pressure. This can ultimately lead to increased left ventricular diastolic pressure, dilatation of the ventricle, and cardiac failure.

Clinical Manifestations
The primary clinical manifestation of aortic stenosis is a loud, harsh, crescendo-decrescendo, systolic ejection murmur heard over the right second interspace

and transmitted to the neck (Resnekov, 1993). This is accompanied by an absent or faint sound of aortic valve closure. The characteristic murmur may be less distinct in the elderly and in patients with heart failure or obstructive pulmonary disease. Pulses are faint and pulse pressure is narrowed. Symptoms experienced by patients with aortic stenosis are caused by the onset of heart failure and consist of fatigue, dyspnea, and possibly syncope. Angina pectoris and even myocardial infarction may occur if inadequate perfusion of the myocardium develops. Exertion usually increases the symptoms of left ventricular failure.

Diagnosis

A diagnosis of aortic stenosis is suggested by its characteristic murmur and change in the sound of closure of the aortic valve. Electrocardiographic changes consistent with left ventricular hypertrophy occur. Echocardiography demonstrates a thickened ventricular wall, thickening and calcification of the valve, and decreased movement of the valve leaflets. The pressure difference on each side of the valve (in the ventricle and in the aorta), which is an indicator of the severity of the disease, can be determined by Doppler ultrasonography.

Management

Valve replacement is the treatment of choice for patients with aortic stenosis who are experiencing symptoms of angina, syncope, dyspnea on exertion, or left ventricular failure. Valve replacement is done even when symptoms are mild because of the risk of sudden death or progression to irreversible heart failure. For persons who are not good candidates for surgery because of pulmonary, renal, or coronary artery disease, percutaneous aortic balloon valvuloplasty may be done. Surgery is not indicated for asymptomatic patients because sudden death is not considered a risk for this group.

AORTIC VALVE REGURGITATION

Etiology and Pathophysiology

Pure aortic regurgitation (insufficiency) occurring in the absence of other valvular lesions is also usually nonrheumatic in origin. This is especially true when it develops in middle-aged or older adults. Its most common cause is dilatation of the ascending aorta, which is often an idiopathic disorder. Aortic valve regurgitation may also be due to valve perforation from infective endocarditis or a congenital anomaly.

With valvular regurgitation, each time a volume of blood is pumped from one chamber to another through a valve, some of it leaks back into the chamber from which it came. In the case of aortic regurgitation, blood leaks from the aorta back into the left ventricle. To compensate for this volume overload, the stroke output is increased, thus overworking the ventricle, which dilates to accommodate the additional blood volume at normal diastolic

pressure. Eventually, however, pumping effectiveness decreases, diastolic pressure increases, and the left ventricle fails.

Clinical Manifestations

Aortic regurgitation is characterized by soft blowing diastolic and systolic murmurs heard on auscultation over the aortic area (second intercostal space) to the right of the sternum. Diastolic blood pressure is often low. Dyspnea on exertion, orthopnea, fatigue, syncope, and angina pectoris are common symptoms.

Diagnosis

Aortic regurgitation is suggested by the characteristic diastolic murmur. It can also be detected through color Doppler imaging and echocardiography. The severity of the problem is indicated by the loudness of the murmur and by signs of left ventricle enlargement on chest x-ray and ECG. Cardiac catheterization with angiography, which allows the regurgitation to be visualized, is the most definitive method of diagnosis.

Management

Valve replacement is the treatment of choice for patients with aortic regurgitation. It is done immediately if severe aortic regurgitation develops during an episode of infective carditis. In other cases, optimal timing of the surgery is debatable, since on the one hand many patients remain asymptomatic for years and there is low risk of sudden death, and on the other, once heart failure develops valve replacement may not reverse it. Thus individual decisions are made based on symptoms and heart size. Some cardiologists believe that surgery is indicated for all patients with left ventricular hypertrophy even in the absence of other symptoms.

MITRAL VALVE STENOSIS

Etiology and Pathophysiology

Rare cases of mitral valve stenosis occur as congenital valve defects; all other cases are presumed to be sequelae of rheumatic fever even in the absence of a known history of the disease. Rheumatic disease causes scarring of the valve tissue, which results in the valve leaflets being thickened, retracted, and fused. These structural changes produce stenosis, which is often accompanied by some regurgitation. The narrowed mitral valve results in poor left atrial emptying and increased left atrial pressure. This causes the left atrium to hypertrophy but does not significantly impact cardiac function. Subsequently, the left atrium dilates, contractility decreases, and pulmonary venous congestion develops, since no valve protects the pulmonary veins from backward blood flow from the atrium. Eventually, right ventricular failure ensues.

Clinical Manifestations

The primary clinical manifestation of mitral valve

stenosis is an opening snap and a low rumbling diastolic murmur heard on auscultation over the mitral area (midclavicular line at the fifth intercostal space). Symptoms, which often gradually worsen due to low cardiac output, include fatigue, weakness, ascites, hepatomegaly, chest pain, and dyspnea on exertion. Hemoptysis, cough, and recurrent respiratory infections may also occur. Atrial fibrillation is a common occurrence due to left atrial hypertrophy.

Diagnosis
Diagnosis of mitral valve stenosis is suggested by auscultation of the characteristic opening snap and rumbling diastolic murmur as well as by evidence of atrial enlargement and pulmonary venous congestion seen on chest x-ray. Echocardiography shows abnormal movement of the valve leaflets and failure of the valve to close during diastole. Doppler ultrasonography can measure the pressure difference across the valve. Cardiac catheterization, however, provides the best information on the degree of stenosis.

Management
Antibiotics are given to protect against infective endocarditis when surgical or invasive diagnostic or dental procedures are done.

Symptoms of heart failure are treated with diuretics, digoxin, vasodilators, a no-added-salt diet, and activity limitations. Dysrhythmias that occur are treated with appropriate anti-arrhythmics. Surgery in the form of valve replacement or commissurotomy is performed when there is a significant degree of disability due to dyspnea and fluid retention. Systemic embolization is also a reason for surgery but not for prosthetic valve replacement, which creates its own risk of systemic embolization. For patients unable to tolerate surgery, percutaneous transluminal (balloon) valvuloplasty may be done.

MITRAL VALVE REGURGITATION

Etiology and Pathophysiology
Mitral valve regurgitation can be rheumatic in origin or can occur because of a floppy, prolapsed valve or secondary to CAD. A valve becomes floppy and prolapsed when there is a loss of fibrous and elastic tissue in the leaflets or chordae tendineae. The cause of this loss is unknown. However, the process, which is termed *myxomatous degeneration*, is also characterized by an increase in the mucopolysaccharide component of the involved tissues. Coronary artery disease can result in mitral regurgitation due to damage to the papillary muscle. Dysfunction of the papillary muscle can be caused by ischemia. Actual rupture of the papillary muscle can occur secondary to an acute myocardial infarction or as a late complication of a healed infarct.

Mitral valve regurgitation permits a backflow of blood into the left atrium, causing atrial stretching

and thinning. Pulmonary congestion and right-sided heart failure develop. Eventually, the left ventricle hypertrophies and left-sided heart failure develops.

Clinical Manifestations
A blowing, high-pitched systolic murmur heard at the apex of the heart on auscultation is a primary clinical manifestation of mitral valve regurgitation. Common manifestations are fatigue, weakness, dyspnea, and atrial fibrillation.

Diagnosis
Diagnosis is based on clinical findings, chest x-ray, color Doppler ultrasonographic studies, and echocardiography.

Management
Treatment of mitral valve regurgitation varies with the type and severity of symptoms and with the cause of the regurgitation. Surgery is most successful in relieving symptoms due to left ventricular volume overload or to increased left atrial pressure secondary to rheumatic heart disease, ruptured chordae or papillary muscles, or floppy valve syndrome.

MITRAL VALVE PROLAPSE SYNDROME

Etiology and Pathophysiology
Mitral valve prolapse develops when the leaflets of the valve balloon backwards into the left atrium during systole. This can result in incomplete closure of the valve with regurgitation of blood from the left ventricle to the left atrium. Mitral valve prolapse is prevalent in young women.

Clinical Manifestations
Mitral valve prolapse can be asymptomatic or lead to sudden death. If symptoms appear, they are often not typical cardiac symptoms. Anxiety, panic attacks, hyperventilation, light-headedness, and depression are common complaints. Symptoms similar to those of mitral valve regurgitation may appear: fatigue, weakness, dyspnea, and palpitations. Atypical chest pain may be present. For most patients with mitral valve prolapse, the psychologic effects of the diagnosis are more disabling than the disease itself, although the individual is at risk for developing dysrhythmias, infective endocarditis, and stroke. On auscultation of the heart, an extra sound—a mitral "click"—may be heard. As the valve becomes progressively incompetent, this click may evolve into a murmur, and signs of heart failure may develop.

Diagnosis
Mitral valve prolapse can be detected by echocardiography. It can also be demonstrated by angiocardiography.

Management
Significant dysrhythmias are treated with anti-arrhythmic agents, and heart failure is treated with

diuretics, digoxin, vasodilators, and a no-salt-added diet. Prophylactic antibiotic therapy is given prior to dental work and surgical procedures because valvular pathology predisposes to infective endocarditis. Mitral valve replacement may be necessary if progression to severe mitral regurgitation occurs.

NURSING PROCESS GUIDELINES
Nonsurgical Management of Cardiac Valvular Disease

Because heart failure is common in patients with valvular disease, their care is similar to that of patients with heart failure from any other cause.

Explain to the patient the cause, effects, and clinical course of the specific cardiac valvular disease and the resulting complications. Review with the patient signs of worsening disease and heart failure and when to call the physician.

Stress the risk of endocarditis and the need for prophylactic antibiotics prior to dental, gynecological, genitourinary, and gastrointestinal procedures.

VALVULAR SURGERY

Valvuloplasty

Valvuloplasty is a valve repair. The major advantages of valve repair over valve replacement are as follows:

- Repaired valves remain functional for a longer time than do replacement valves.
- Repaired valves do not necessitate the use of continuous anticoagulation therapy.
- Some repairs do not require general anesthesia or cardiopulmonary bypass.

Specific types of valvuloplasty are commissurotomy (open and closed), annuloplasty (Fig. 8–31), leaflet repair, chordoplasty, and balloon valvuloplasty. The type of valvuloplasty performed depends on the type and extent of valvular pathology. Mitral valve repair is most common and many advances have been made in surgical techniques. Tricuspid valve repair is generally preferred over replacement because of better results. Conversely, aortic valve replacement is more common than repair because of technical difficulty, although aortic valvuloplasty is done to treat aortic stenosis in adults for whom the risk of operation or anticoagulant use is great. Pulmonary valve surgery is rare because it is a technically difficult procedure that does not necessarily produce good results.

Commissurotomy

Commissurotomy is a repair procedure in which valve leaflets that have fused together, resulting in a narrowed valve opening and sometimes incomplete valve closure, are separated. Open commissurotomy, which is done via a median sternotomy or thoracotomy incision, uses cardiopulmonary bypass to allow visualization of the valve. With this technique, the

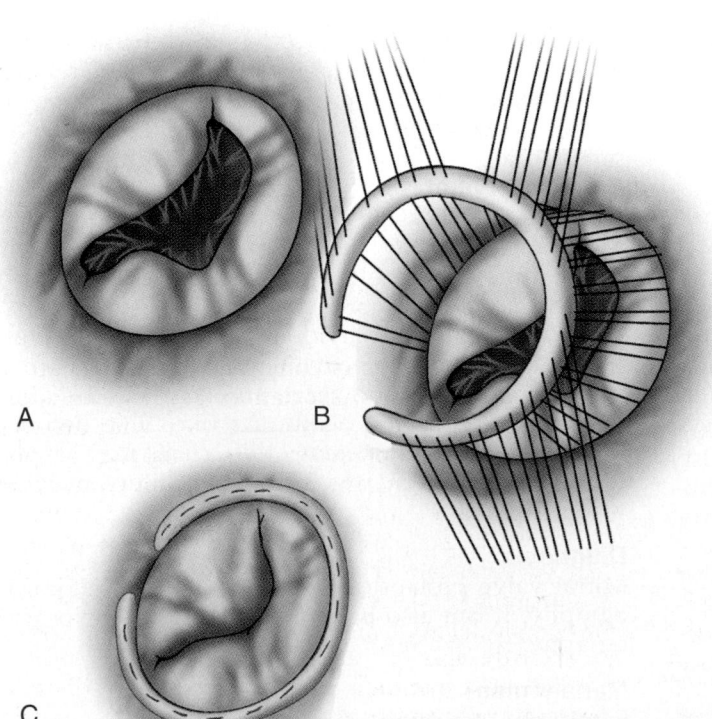

Figure 8–31
Annuloplasty.

commissure can be incised in a controlled fashion and other reconstructive efforts such as débridement of calcium, separation of fused chordae, removal of atrial thrombi, and plication or annuloplasty for mild regurgitation can be performed if needed.

In a closed commissurotomy, a small opening is made in the heart and a dilator or the surgeon's finger is inserted to break apart the valve leaflets. Because the valve is not actually seen, closed commissurotomy is suitable only for cases uncomplicated by calcifications, regurgitation, atrial thrombi, or significant fusion or shortening of the chordae.

Commissurotomy is considered a palliative as opposed to a curative procedure and is done to delay the need for an artificial valve.

Chordoplasty

Chordoplasty is a repair of the chordae tendineae, usually of the mitral as opposed to the tricuspid valve. It is typically done to shorten chordae that have become elongated and are allowing the leaflets to prolapse into the left atrium during systole, resulting in mitral incompetence. An alternative procedure leaves the existing chordae in place but uses an artificial graft to correct the valve prolapse. Chordoplasty may also involve reattachment of torn chordae to the valve leaflets or elongation of chordae that have shortened. A risk of chordoplasty is that the sutures used to shorten the chordae or attach the graft may injure or tear the leaflet. This can interfere with the repair and require a valve replacement.

Leaflet Repair

Leaflet repair is done when damage to the leaflet from rheumatic fever, valve prolapse, idiopathic causes, or chordal rupture causes regurgitation. Leaflet repair may involve use of a pericardial patch to close a hole in the leaflet, removal of excess leaflet tissue by means of leaflet resection or plication, or elongating a shortened leaflet by chordoplasty.

Balloon Valvuloplasty

Balloon valvuloplasty is a procedure that uses an inflated balloon-tipped catheter to increase the surface area of a valve. It is performed under local anesthesia in the cardiac catheterization laboratory and is used to treat both mitral and aortic valve stenosis.

MITRAL VALVULOPLASTY

In mitral valvuloplasty, a one- or two-balloon dilatation catheter is inserted percutaneously in the patient's right femoral artery. It is progressed into the right atrium, through the atrial septum into the left atrium, and across the valve. A sheath is placed through the mitral and aortic valves and then a guide wire is inserted through the sheath and placed externally to the patient. The sheath is withdrawn into the left atrium, and the balloon catheters are inserted from the femoral arteries over the guide wires. The balloons are inflated with a mixture of contrast medium and saline. Inflations are repeated until the balloon expands fully at the level of the mitral valve. Balloons of different sizes may be used. Variation in size decreases the potential for the creation of an atrial septal defect. Other complications include embolism and bleeding from the catheter site. Some mitral regurgitation always occurs. Four to 8% of patients undergoing this procedure experience a cerebral vascular accident due to dislodgment of thrombi or calcium. To reduce this risk, patients are usually placed on warfarin (Coumadin) therapy for 4 to 6 weeks before the procedure. Use of mitral valvuloplasty has proved to increase cardiac output, increase mitral valve surface area, and decrease mitral gradients.

AORTIC VALVULOPLASTY

The aortic procedure can be performed by either a femoral or brachial artery approach and is similar to that for mitral valvuloplasty. Aortic valvuloplasty results in improved ejection fraction, lower aortic gradients, and increased aortic valve area. This procedure is usually reserved for patients at high risk for a surgical procedure or for patients urgently needing noncardiac surgical procedures, the elderly, and patients with severe left ventricular dysfunction. It is also used to delay the need for valve replacement.

Valve Replacement Surgery

Cardiac valve replacement is a common surgical procedure. The decision to perform valve replacement surgery is dependent upon many factors. These factors include

- The cardiac valve involved
- The underlying disorder (stenosis or regurgitation)
- The degree of myocardial dysfunction
- The patient's symptoms and the degree of associated disability

Cardiac disability is commonly judged based on the New York Heart Association (NYHA) Functional Classification system (Table 8–5). As with any type of surgery, the operative risks must be weighed against the long-term benefits of the procedure. Presently, the operative mortality for a single valve replacement is approximately 4 to 8%, and the 5-year survival rate is approximately 75 to 80%. These are acceptable statistics considering the poor prognosis associated with medical treatment of severe valvular disease.

The most common adult cardiac valve disorders that may progress to the point of requiring surgical replacement of the valve are aortic valve regurgita-

Table 8–5

New York Heart Association Functional Classification System

Class	Description
I	Ordinary physical activity does not cause undue fatigue, palpitation, dyspnea, or angina.
II	Ordinary physical activity causes undue fatigue, palpitation, dyspnea, or angina.
III	Less than ordinary physical activity causes undue fatigue, palpitation, dyspnea, or angina.
IV	Fatigue, palpitation, dyspnea, or angina occurs at rest.

tion, aortic valve stenosis, mitral valve regurgitation, and mitral valve stenosis.

PROSTHETIC HEART VALVES

Prosthetic heart valves are broadly classified into two main categories: mechanical and biologic (or tissue) valves. Both types of valves are associated with different valve-related complications, and the clinical

Table 8–6

Advantages and Disadvantages of Valve Types

Valve Type	Advantages	Disadvantages
MECHANICAL VALVES		
Caged ball	Excellent durability	Thrombogenic Turbulent flow Hemolysis Loud and large
Tilting disc	Excellent durability Good performance Less hemolysis	Thrombogenic Embolization
Bileaflet	Large, unobstructed orifice Decreased turbulence Excellent durability Excellent performance	Thrombogenic
BIOLOGIC (TISSUE) VALVES		
Xenografts	Minimally thrombogenic	Less durable Structure/size
Homografts (allografts)	Durable Nonthrombogenic	Technically difficult to implant Require donors Preservation
Autografts	Durable Nonthrombogenic	Prolonged surgery time

superiority of one type over the other has not been established (Table 8–6).

Mechanical Valves

The three types of mechanical valves in use are: caged-ball valve, tilting-disc valve, and bileaflet valve (Fig. 8–32). All three have excellent durability but all are thrombogenic and therefore require that the patient receive lifelong anticoagulation therapy.

Caged-Ball Valve

The caged-ball valve consists of a metal orifice and a cage that houses a silicone rubber ball. The major problems associated with this type of valve are

Turbulent blood flow, which contributes to hemolysis of red blood cells
A tendency to promote thrombosis
The audible sound of the valve, which is disturbing to many patients

Caged-ball valves are rarely used today but may be encountered in patients who have had a past valve replacement.

Tilting-Disc Valve

Tilting-disc valves use a disc that tilts within a valve ring. When the valve is closed, the disc rests flat within the valve ring. When the valve opens, the disc tilts within the ring, causing minimal obstruction to blood flow. The advantages of the tilting-disc valve over the caged-ball valve are less turbulent flow, less hemolysis of red blood cells, and improved hemodynamic performance. The tendency to develop blood clots remains a problem, so patients do require lifelong anticoagulation. Also, structural failure of the tilting-disc valves is a rare but catastrophic complication. Survival after such a complication depends on rapid recognition and emergency surgery to replace the valve.

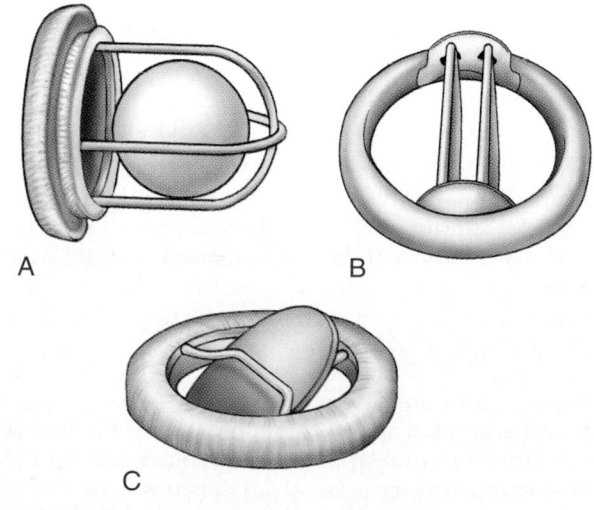

Figure 8–32

Types of mechanical valves. *A,* Caged-ball valve. *B,* Bileaflet valve. *C,* Tilting-disk valve.

Bileaflet Valve

The bileaflet mechanical valves are the most recently developed and have greatly improved hemodynamic performance. In this type of valve, the leaflets move apart as they open to create a central orifice for blood flow. This central orifice allows unobstructed blood flow and eliminates turbulence. The bileaflet valve has proven durability, excellent hemodynamic function, an insignificant amount of hemolysis, and a low rate of thromboembolism. The St. Jude bileaflet prosthesis is the most widely implanted type of mechanical valve.

Biologic Tissue Valves

Biologic tissue valves are characterized by a low incidence of thromboembolism and valve thrombosis. Thus, they possess a major advantage over mechanical valves, particularly for patients in whom anticoagulation is contraindicated. The disadvantages to biologic tissue valves is that progressive deterioration and leaflet calcification may occur as early as 5 to 7 years postoperatively.

Biologic and bioprosthetic valves are classified according to their biologic source. The three types of biologic valves currently available are xenografts, homografts, and autografts.

Xenografts

Xenografts are the most extensively used biologic valves. Xenograft valves are derived from animal sources, especially pigs and cows, because of the similarity of their physical characteristics to those of human valves. Bioprosthetic cardiac valve substitutes include the porcine aortic valve mounted on a stent (Fig. 8–33) and the bovine pericardial valve also mounted on a stent.

Homografts

Aortic valve homografts, also known as allografts, are human heart valves obtained from cadavers. The homograft procedure is technically difficult because the valve is not mounted on a stent. However, its results are excellent in terms of the flow across the valve orifice and the patient survival rate, which surpasses that of grafting procedures using other bioprostheses. However, use of this type of valve is limited by availability. Too few donors have been obtained to supply all patients requiring valve replacement.

Autografts

The closest to ideal valve replacement is the use of the native pulmonic valve to replace a diseased aortic valve. In this procedure, the aortic valve is replaced with the patient's native pulmonic valve, and a homograft is used to replace the pulmonic valve. Autografts, although they require a prolonged operation, are durable, unlikely to produce blood clots, and less prone to degeneration than xenografts. This type of valve replacement is particularly suitable for children and young adults because of the excellent long-term outcome and the lack of need for anticoagulation.

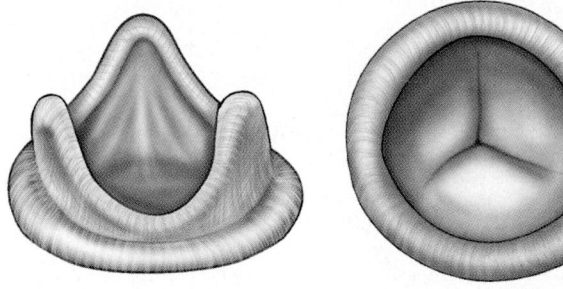

Figure 8–33
Porcine aortic valve.

SELECTION OF A PROSTHETIC VALVE

Selection of a prosthetic valve is based on the patient's specific needs in relationship to the characteristics of the various valve substitutes. Generally speaking, where there are problems with anticoagulation, such as with the elderly or women of childbearing age, patients with a history of bleeding, or patients unlikely to follow an anticoagulation regimen, biologic valves are favored. When longevity and functional capacity are major concerns, a mechanical valve is indicated.

VALVE REPLACEMENT PROCEDURE

The heart is accessed through a midsternotomy incision for most valve replacement procedures. Cardiopulmonary bypass is established and the diseased valve is excised. The remaining orifice into which the new valve will be placed is then sized by placing a temporary sizer prosthesis. Sutures are placed around the annulus and into the skirt of the replacement valve. The new valve is then lowered into place and the sutures tied (Fig. 8–34).

❖ SETTINGS, PROVIDERS, AND COLLABORATION FOR CARE

Patients with stable valvular disease are treated at home with regular assessments in a primary care setting. Patients who have undergone surgery for valvuloplasty and valve replacement need ongoing care similar to that given to a patient who has undergone cardiac surgery. A discharge planning nurse may need to assess the patient's home environment to determine the patient's ability to recuperate in the home. Some patients with complicated needs or inadequate home support may need a referral to a subacute facility or a facility with a cardiac rehabilitation program in place to complete postoperative recovery prior to returning home. Patients who are discharged from the hospital directly home may need the assistance of the home health nurse for evaluation of wound status and cardiac functioning. Depending on the level of functioning

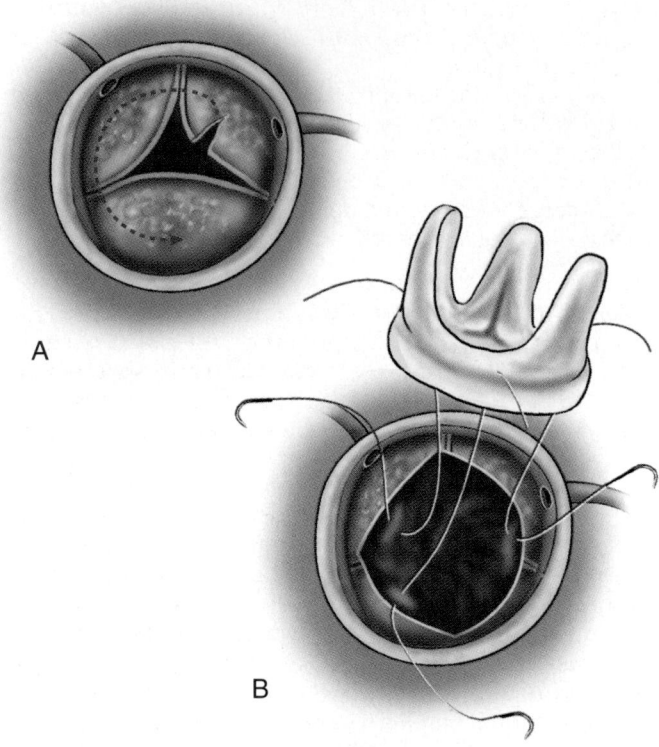

Figure 8–34

Valve replacement procedure. *A*, Excision of the diseased valve. *B*, Suturing the prosthetic valve in place.

of the patient and available family support, the patient may need the assistance of a home health aide. Patients may need referral to a dietitian or to a physical therapist for development of an exercise plan.

NURSING PROCESS
Valve Repair or Replacement

PREOPERATIVE NURSING CARE

Preoperative nursing care for patients undergoing a valve repair or replacement is as described under cardiac surgery in Chapter 7.

POSTOPERATIVE NURSING CARE

Assessment

Review the patient's history prior to surgery. Obtain information about the type of surgical procedure performed and the cardiac valve involved. In the case of valve replacement surgery, identify the type of prosthetic valve used for the replacement. Obtain baseline vital signs, including arterial blood pressure, pulmonary artery pressures, pulmonary capillary wedge pressure, and cardiac output. In the immediate postoperative period, these hemodynamic parameters are routinely monitored every hour. This is critically important because new valves cause sud-

den changes in pressures within a heart that had adapted over a long period to the pressure of pathology. Once the patient is stabilized, usually after 12 to 24 hours, measure vital signs every 4 hours. Obtain and record the patient's body temperature. In the immediate postoperative period, the patient may be hypothermic. This contributes to hemodynamic instability. Later in the postoperative period, an elevated body temperature may signal pulmonary complications or other infection. Any type of infection in a patient with a prosthetic cardiac valve is extremely serious, as the prosthetic valve may become seeded with bacteria and lead to endocarditis. Monitor ECG for dysrhythmias and heart blocks. Either one of these complications may occur as a result of cardiac manipulation, edema at the surgical site, or sutures interrupting the conduction system. Auscultate heart tones, noting rate, rhythm, extra heart sounds, and the presence of any murmurs. Monitor chest tube drainage every hour initially and then every 4 hours after 24 hours. Assess the patient for signs of bleeding (excessive chest tube drainage) or cardiac tamponade (hypotension, elevated central venous pressure, decreased cardiac output, decreased urine output). Auscultate the lung sounds for crackles or wheezes, which may indicate heart failure. When the patient awakens from anesthesia, immediately perform a complete neurologic evaluation, as the incidence of cerebral vascular accident is higher with valvular surgery because of the increased risk of emboli from the diseased valve. Carefully monitor intake and output to assess for alterations in fluid volume status. Once anticoagulation is initiated (if indicated), monitor prothrombin time daily. Assess the patient for signs of bleeding related to anticoagulation therapy. Refer to Chapter 7 for additional assessment guidelines that apply to all patients undergoing cardiac surgery.

Nursing Diagnoses and Planning

Nursing diagnoses and related patient outcomes commonly applicable to patients who have had cardiac valve surgery include the following:

NDx: Risk for decreased cardiac output related to dysrhythmias, hypovolemia, or persistent right- or left-sided heart failure

Planning: Patient Outcomes
1. Patient demonstrates adequate cardiac output as evidenced by systolic blood pressure between 90 and 140, diastolic blood pressure between 50 and 90, heart rate between 60 and 100, and urine output (greater than 30 mL/h) and alert and oriented demeanor.
2. Patient has a normal sinus rhythm without ectopy.
3. Patient demonstrates signs of adequate fluid and electrolyte balance including moist mucous membranes, good skin turgor (<3 sec), and urine output of greater than 30 mL/h.
4. Patient is free of signs and symptoms of persist-

ent right- or left-sided heart failure (jugular venous distension, edema, hepatomegaly, dyspnea, crackles, wheezes).

NDx: Risk for infection related to multiple invasive lines, surgical incision, and future valve protection needs

Planning: Patient Outcomes
1. Patient is afebrile.
2. White blood cell count is less than 10,000.
3. Patient's incision is clean, dry, and approximated.
4. Patient verbalizes the need for prophylactic antibiotics before undergoing any invasive procedures in the future.

NDx: Risk for altered health maintenance related to lack of knowledge regarding self-care after cardiac valve surgery

Planning: Patient Outcomes
1. Patient verbalizes understanding of the surgical procedure performed.
2. Patient states the type of prosthetic valve used if applicable.
3. Patient reports accurate information about postoperative treatments, including activity restrictions, dietary guidelines, drug therapy, and incision care.
4. Patient demonstrates understanding of anticoagulation therapy, risks associated with the therapy, lifestyle modifications, and blood work regimen.
5. Patient verbalizes signs and symptoms that would prompt him or her to notify the physician (signs and symptoms of bleeding, infection, or valve dysfunction).
6. Patient demonstrates understanding of the treatment plan and follow-up care.

Nursing Interventions and Evaluation

NDx: Risk for decreased cardiac output
Monitor vital signs, hemodynamic parameters, ECG, and intake and output as ordered. Notify the physician of any alterations, including hypotension, dysrhythmias, or low urine output (<30 mL/h). Maintain the patient on a cardiac monitor or telemetry as ordered. Most patients remain on a monitor for several days following cardiac valve surgery. This is because atrial or ventricular dysrhythmias and other conduction disturbances, may occur, depending on which cardiac valve is repaired or replaced, and also on the underlying disorder. In the event of postoperative bradycardias or heart blocks, temporary pacing via epicardial pacing wires (wires that are surgically implanted during surgery) may be initiated. If indicated, initiate and maintain a temporary pacemaker as prescribed. Administer fluids intravenously or by mouth as ordered. Note any fluid restrictions and maintain such restrictions by notifying ancillary staff members and the patient. Weigh the patient daily to detect any excess fluid gain or

loss. Administer prescribed medications, including digitalis preparations, anti-arrhythmics, diuretics, or vasoactive agents.

If the patient exhibits signs of right- or left-sided heart failure, institute measures directed at relief of symptoms and promotion of comfort. Elevate the head of the bed to promote lung expansion. Administer oxygen as needed and as ordered. Administer medications as ordered.

NDx: Risk for infection
Monitor invasive line sites and incision daily for signs of infection. Change invasive line dressings according to institutional protocol using strict aseptic technique. Report any signs of inflammation or infection to the physician immediately. Provide care of the Foley catheter according to institutional policy and discontinue the use of the catheter as early as possible following a physician's order. Change intravenous catheter sites according to protocol. Maintain aseptic technique when handling intravenous catheters and tubing. Prevent contamination of intravenous ports, which may lead to bacteremia and subsequent prosthetic valve infection. Clean the incision daily with a clean, dry cloth. Incisions are routinely cleaned with soap and water, but normal saline or an iodine solution may be used. Prior to discharge, teach the patient to wash the incision daily with soap and water, and then to dry it with a clean towel. Unless the incision is draining or open, it is usually left exposed to air. If drainage is present, a dry sterile dressing may be applied.

NDx: Risk for altered health maintenance
Explain the exact procedure that was performed to the patient. Provide the patient with literature on the subject when available. Explain to the patient which type of prosthetic valve was used, in what position it was placed (aortic, mitral, etc), and the implications associated with the type of prosthesis that was implanted. Most prosthetic valves come with a patient identification card that the patient should be instructed to keep with him or her at all times.

Review with the patient the postoperative instructions, including progressive activity guidelines, any dietary restrictions, medication regimens, and incision care. Activity following cardiac valve surgery is progressive and is guided by the patient's tolerance. Most patients are out of bed to the chair within 24 hours after surgery. Ambulation outside of the patient's room is usually begun on postoperative day 2 after the chest tubes are removed. Patients who were generally debilitated prior to the surgery may not progress as quickly and may require physical therapy to rebuild their strength. In either case, encourage frequent rest periods to prevent fatigue.

Patients do not necessarily require any dietary restrictions following cardiac valve surgery. If the patient was on a special diet preoperatively for another medical problem (ie, diabetes), then the previous diet should be resumed. Most patients begin a clear liquid diet within several hours after the endotracheal tube is removed in the intensive care unit. If tolerated, the diet is then progressed through full liquids to regular consistency over the next 24 hours. Although the appetite may be poor initially after surgery, encourage the patient to eat to promote healing and prevent complications. Consult the dietitian as needed for problems with intake. If the patient exhibits signs of fluid overload or heart failure, he or she may be placed on a sodium- or fluid-restricted diet. In such instances, review with the patient the rationale for the restrictions and assist the patient in selecting items that are consistent with the prescribed restrictions. In the event that the patient has received a mechanical valve and will require anticoagulation, provide special dietary counseling. This is needed to ensure that the patient will avoid excess intake of foods (such as green leafy vegetables) that are high in vitamin K. Such vitamin K-rich foods would counteract the anticoagulant effects of sodium warfarin.

Prior to discharge, review with the patient all medications that will be prescribed upon discharge. Examples of typical postoperative medications include iron preparations to correct perioperative anemia, digitalis preparations to control dysrhythmias or to improve cardiac output, and diuretics to prevent fluid overload. Discuss each of the medications in detail, including indications, actions, side effects, and dosages. Provide literature whenever possible. Assist the patient to develop a schedule for safe and proper self-administration of medications.

Review with the patient proper incision care as detailed earlier. Have the patient provide a return demonstration so that you can assess understanding and identify areas for improvement. Teach the patient signs and symptoms of wound infection and instruct the patient to notify the physician should any of these signs occur.

Depending on the type of valve surgery performed and on past medical history, the patient may also have short- or long-term anticoagulation therapy prescribed postoperatively. Anticoagulant therapy, specifically sodium warfarin, is indicated for patients who receive a mechanical valve prosthesis, suffer from chronic atrial fibrillation, or have a history of prior embolization. Prior to discharge, the patient and the family must demonstrate a complete understanding of the anticoagulation regimen. Teach the patient about the effects of the medication, the importance of regularly scheduled blood work to assess prothrombin time, the signs and symptoms of excessive blood thinning, and lifestyle changes associated with anticoagulation. Instruct the patient to avoid activities that place him or her at high risk for injury or bleeding. These include simple activities of daily living such as shaving with a nonelectric razor or other activities such as aggressive sports. Teach the patient about over-the-counter medications that

can potentiate the effects of warfarin and contribute to excessive anticoagulation. Examples of such medications include aspirin and nonsteroidal anti-inflammatory agents such as ibuprofen (Motrin).

Discuss with the patient the expected postoperative concerns such as fatigue, poor appetite, and feelings of sadness. Stress that these are normal concerns and offer suggestions for coping, such as frequent rest periods, small frequent meals, and participation in leisurely activities that are satisfying to the patient. Reinforce that if any symptom is persistent or troublesome, it should be reported to the physician. Instruct the patient to promptly report to the physician any of the signs and symptoms of heart failure such as dyspnea, orthopnea, chest pain, or excessive leg swelling, since an acute onset of such symptoms following cardiac valve surgery may signal valve dysfunction and needs to be addressed immediately. Also, teach the patient the signs of wound infection, respiratory system infection, and urinary tract infection and instruct him or her to notify the physician immediately if any of these signs develop. Instruct the patient to notify the physician if a fever develops, even in the absence of signs of infection. If the patient has a prosthetic valve in place, emphasize the importance of prophylactic antibiotics prior to any invasive procedures in the future. This is particularly important if the patient is to have dental work or gastrointestinal procedures performed. If the patient is to have a procedure done and is not sure whether or not antibiotics are indicated, he or she should check with the physician prior to the procedure. Also, if the patient is receiving anticoagulant therapy, the physician should be notified for any signs of excessive blood thinning such as blood in the urine or stool, or bleeding gums.

Prior to discharge, assess the patient's complete understanding of the discharge instructions, medical regimen, and potential complications. Allow time for the patient and the family to ask questions. Provide written materials whenever possible for future reference. Discuss follow-up care and emphasize the importance of completing blood work or any diagnostic studies that may be ordered to assess the outcome of the surgery. Provide the patient with the names and phone numbers of all available resources.

Compare the patient's status with the expected outcomes. If the outcomes are not met, reassess the patient and revise the plan.

Cardiac Trauma

Etiology and Pathophysiology

Cardiac trauma is usually divided into two categories: penetrating trauma and blunt trauma. Stab wounds may result in puncture of any chamber of the heart, valvular laceration, coronary artery transection, or lacerations to the great vessels of the heart. Rapid exsanguination may ensue, or the patient may present with signs of acute cardiac tamponade. Only about one-half of the patients receiving stab wounds to the heart survive long enough to obtain medical treatment. Of those that do, survival potential is greatest if the patient is transported to a trauma center with the capability of immediate open-heart surgery. Gunshot wounds to the heart are even more severe because they are usually through the entire heart. The survival rate is only 10% to 15%. The chambers of the heart that are damaged and the amount of blood lost determine the chance of survival of most cardiac trauma patients.

Crushing injuries to the heart from automobile accidents or other blunt trauma incidents usually cause damage to the cardiac walls, septum, valves, and great vessels. The damage inflicted may range from minor to being incompatible with life. If a large myocardial contusion occurs, potential complications are the same as following a myocardial infarction.

Clinical Manifestations

Massive blood loss is common in traumatic injuries to the myocardium. Trauma to the chest injures not only the heart but also the large vessels, the lungs, and possibly the liver. These multiple-organ injuries compound the blood loss from the injury. Hypotension and shock result from massive hemorrhage. The trauma may also cause bleeding into the pericardial sac causing cardiac tamponade, with resultant poor cardiac filling. Clinical manifestations of cardiac tamponade are termed Beck's triad. They consist of jugular neck vein distention, muffled heart sounds, and pulsus paradoxus (a drop in systolic pressure greater than 10 mm Hg during inspiration).

Blunt trauma may result in potentially life-threatening dysrhythmias.

Diagnosis

The diagnosis is made on the basis of assessment of the trauma site, symptoms, and diagnostic tests. Immediate assessment is made to determine life-threatening symptoms. Vital signs and the overall clinical condition are used to determine the amount of damage present. Electrocardiographic changes may mimic those of myocardial injury, ischemia, or infarction. An echocardiogram may be done to aid in identifying the trauma. Immediate thoracotomy with possible open-heart surgery is often necessary to reveal the specific damage.

Management

Patients with penetrating cardiac trauma who survive long enough to reach a major trauma center usually must undergo corrective surgery. If a patient arrives with an object protruding from the chest, the object should be left in place until the patient reaches the operating room because the object may act as a dam, preventing exsanguination. The initial surgery may be only the life-saving intervention, and several other reconstructive surgeries may need to follow. The prognosis for such injuries is usually grave.

The patient with blunt cardiac trauma is observed for symptoms related to the injury. Complications such as dysrhythmias and pericarditis may be treated with medications. Pericardiocentesis (aspiration of fluid from the pericardial sac) is necessary for cardiac tamponade. The patient may require open-heart surgery if tearing or rupture of cardiac structures is suspected.

NURSING PROCESS GUIDELINES
Cardiac Trauma

Nursing management of the patient with cardiac trauma varies with the type of trauma the patient experienced and the medical intervention necessary to correct the effects of the trauma. Because of the typical effects of most cardiac trauma, the assessment, nursing diagnoses, expected patient outcomes, nursing interventions, and evaluation for patients with cardiac trauma are similar to those described previously for patients with cardiac valvular disease. If the patient undergoes surgery for correction of the damage from the trauma, the nursing care may change. (See Chap. 7 for care of the patient undergoing cardiac surgery.)

Cardiac Neoplasia

Etiology and Pathophysiology

Tumors within the heart are rare and are usually not malignant. The rare tumor that is malignant may be either a primary-site tumor or a metastatic tumor. The metastatic tumors implanting on the heart are usually from primary cancers of the breast, bronchus, or lymph nodes or from malignant melanoma.

Clinical Manifestations

Benign cardiac tumors often project into the chambers of the heart, providing a place for thrombi to develop, so the patient may exhibit symptoms of embolism to the brain or other organs. Any cardiac tumor can cause pericardial effusion and constriction of the heart and may even grow into the heart muscle, impairing contractility or obstructing blood flow. By the time symptoms of a malignant tumor occur, the tumor is usually large and has thoroughly invaded the surrounding tissue.

Diagnosis

The diagnosis of a cardiac tumor is made on the basis of symptoms, x-ray films, and other diagnostic tests. The patient usually presents with symptoms of fatigue, dyspnea, heart failure, or pain. Pericardial effusion may be present. Chest x-rays and cardiac catheterization are done to reveal the presence of a tumor and the involved structures.

Management

Surgical intervention may be indicated for cardiac tumors that obstruct major vessels or valves. Cardiopulmonary bypass is necessary for cardiac tumor excision, except when the tumor is only in the epicardial area. If the tumor is not causing a major obstruction, treatment focuses on the presenting symptoms. Fluid accumulation is reduced with diuretic therapy. Other cardiac drugs specific to the dysrhythmias present are ordered.

NURSING PROCESS
Cardiac Neoplasia

Assessment

Before the physical assessment of the patient, review the medical notes and the diagnostic studies completed to determine the structures involved. Assess for interferences with all systems, because impaired blood flow through the cardiac chambers or valves affects the lungs, kidneys, liver, digestive tract, and neurologic function. Look for signs of respiratory difficulty such as dyspnea, tachypnea, wheezes, or cyanosis. Monitor the vital signs for indications of pericardial effusion. Observe for changes in intake and output, edema, digestive problems, and either constipation or diarrhea. Ask the patient whether there have been episodes indicating neurologic dysfunction such as confusion, dizziness, or memory lapses. The symptoms are usually progressive, and the patient may not have sought medical treatment until the symptoms were no longer tolerable.

Nursing Diagnoses and Planning

Nursing diagnoses and related expected patient outcomes commonly applicable to patients with cardiac tumors vary with the type and the location of the tumor. The nursing diagnoses, patient outcomes, and nursing interventions previously discussed under Cardiomyopathy are applicable to the patient with a cardiac tumor. In addition, the following nursing diagnosis, patient outcomes, and nursing interventions apply:

NDx: Fear related to the negative diagnosis of cardiac tumor and perceived threat of death

Planning: Patient Outcomes
1. Patient acknowledges and discusses fears and concerns.
2. Patient reports that anxiety and fear are reduced to a manageable level.

3. Patient demonstrates appropriate coping behaviors relative to the diagnosis and possible outcomes of the condition.

Nursing Interventions and Evaluation
NDx: Fear

Acknowledge the reality of the patient's fears and concerns, and encourage expression of feelings. Accept but do not reinforce the patient's behaviors of denial. Involve the patient and family in discussions, planning, and education sessions for short-term and long-term therapy. Provide information in a professional, empathetic manner, and allow time for questions and concerns. Use the services of professional counselors or clergy if appropriate. Help the patient to identify coping strategies and to use them effectively.

Compare the patient's status with the expected outcomes. If the outcomes are not met, reassess the patient and revise the plan.

The Elderly: Special Considerations

Because of the aging of the cardiovascular system, complications can occur in the older adult. There is less elasticity of the aorta and arteries. The valves become thick and rigid as a result of fibrosis and sclerosis. Also, the heart muscle contains increased collagen and scar tissue. Cardiac output is reduced about 1% each year beginning at approximately 25 years of age. Maximum coronary blood flow at age 60 is estimated to be 35% less than that of younger persons. Systolic blood pressure rises to compensate for the inelasticity and increased resistance of peripheral vessels.

Pain described by the elderly person may be atypical for cardiac disease as a result of altered pain sensation related to aging. Because of other organ dysfunction associated with aging, cardiac pain may be interpreted by the individual as respiratory, gastric, or musculoskeletal.

Edema associated with heart failure or other cardiac problems may lead to skin breakdown in older individuals who have fragile skin. Protective padding for pressure points and gentle changes of position are important nursing measures to prevent problems. Intravenous fluids are monitored carefully in the elderly because excessive fluid infusion results in hypervolemia and may lead to heart failure in the older adult.

Temperature elevations increase metabolism, thereby increasing the body's requirements for oxygen as the heart muscle works harder. For every degree of temperature elevation, the heart rate increases approximately 10 beats per minute. Older hearts cannot tolerate this type of stress very well. Therefore, temperature elevations need to be treated promptly to decrease the stress on the heart muscle.

Anorexia that accompanies some forms of cardiac disease may lead to decreased nutritional status in the older adult. Several small meals throughout the day help to compensate for a poor appetite and reduce the workload on the heart as it supplies blood to the digestive system.

A healthy cardiac lifestyle that begins in childhood can prevent many of the cardiac problems that occur in later life. Individuals who do not begin the habit of cigarette smoking, who develop lifelong exercise programs, who eat low-fat, low-cholesterol foods, and who learn to manage life's stressors in a healthy manner are less likely to experience the common cardiac disorders in their elderly years. Prevention is the best treatment for potential cardiac disorders, even with the older adult. Education programs for the elderly focusing on exercise (designed for their age and ability), appropriate nutrition and meal planning, and information about other lifestyle changes can contribute to decreasing severe cardiac disease in the older adult or assist them in managing the effects of the disorder.

Chapter Review

1. What is the meaning of a new heart murmur in a patient with pericarditis?
2. What is the meaning of a paradoxical pulse in a patient with pericarditis?
3. What are the therapeutic effects of magnesium sulfate, digoxin, captopril, prazosin, dobutamine, and furosemide when given to a patient in heart failure? By what mechanisms do they exert these therapeutic effects?
4. How are central venous pressure, renal artery pressure, pulmonary artery pressure, pulmonary artery wedge pressure, and cardiac output affected by the development of pulmonary edema?
5. How do sinus bradycardia, sinus tachycardia, atrial fibrillation, ventricular tachycardia, and ventricular fibrillation cause a decrease in cardiac output?
6. What other assessment data should be collected when redness is noted at the site of pacemaker insertion 3 days after the operative procedure?
7. How does thrombolytic therapy affect recovery after a myocardial infarction?
8. How is the care of a patient with cardiomyopathy similar to that of a patient with heart failure?
9. What is the meaning of a sudden onset of dyspnea, orthopnea, crackles, and wheezes in a patient recovering from a myocardial infarction?
10. What signs and symptoms are indicative of cardiac tamponade in a patient with cardiac trauma?

Bibliography

Ahrens SGL. Managing heart failure: A blueprint for success. Nurs 95 1995; 25(12):27.

American College of Cardiology. Guidelines for the management of patients with acute myocardial infarction: Report of the American College of Cardiology/American Heart Association Task Force on Practice Guidelines (Committee on Management of Acute Myocardial Infarction). Bethesda, MD: American College of Cardiology and the American Heart Association, 1996.

American Heart Association. Heart and stroke facts. Dallas: Author, 1996.

Aragon D, Martin M. What you should know about thrombolytic therapy for acute MI. Am J Nurs 1993; 93(9):24.

Armstrong PJH. Your guide to continuing cardiac care. Medford, OR: Rogue Valley Medical Center, 1995.

Asensio JA, Demetriades D, Berne TV. Complex and challenging problems in trauma surgery. Surg Clin North Am 1996; 76(4):645.

Bahr R, Giurfa L. Early heart-attack care: The critical paradigm shift toward prevention [interview by Michael Villaire]. Crit Care Nurse 1996; (1):78.

Bashford CW. When a patient survives sudden cardiac death. RN 1994; 57(4):34.

Beery TA. Gender bias in the diagnosis and treatment of coronary artery disease. Heart Lung 1995; 24(6):427.

Bernat JJ: Smoothing the CABG patient's road to recovery. Am J Nurs 1997; 97(2):23.

Bertrand M. The prevention of cardiovascular events: A new challenge for calcium channel blockers. In The Prevention of Cardiovascular Events: A New Challenge for Calcium Channel Blockers (proceedings of a satellite symposium to the XVIIth Congress of the European Society of Cardiology, Amsterdam, August 23, 1995). Auckland, NZ: Adis International, 1996.

Bharati S, Lev M. Pathologic changes of the conduction system with aging. Cardiology in the Elderly 1994; 2(2):152.

Blaker GJ. Close up on atrial natriuretic factor. Nurs 94 1994; 24(12):61.

Boltz MA. Nurse's guide to identifying cardiac rhythms. Nurs 94 1994; 24(4):54.

Boncheck LI. The basis for selecting a valve prosthesis. In McGoon DC (ed). Cardiac surgery. Philadelphia: FA Davis, 1982.

Bosley CL. Assessing cardiac output: Don't stop at the heart. Nurs 95 1995; 25(9):43.

Brown C, Clark L, Williams L, et al. Coronary restenosis. J Am Acad Nurse Pract 1996; 8(6):283.

Brown KK. Boosting the failing heart with inotropic drugs. Nurs 93 1993; 23(4):34.

Calafiore AM, Angelini GD, Bergsland J, Salerno TA. Minimally invasive coronary artery bypass grafting. Ann Thoraci Surg 1996; 62(5):1545.

Carpenito LJ. Nursing diagnosis: Application to clinical practice. 6th ed. Philadelphia: JB Lippincott, 1995.

Cash LA. Heart failure from diastolic dysfunction. Dimens Crit Care Nurs 1996; 15(4):170.

Casimir-Ahn H, Rutberg H, et al. Recent advances in treatment of severe cardiac failure (international symposium, Linkoping Heart Center, Sweden, March 3–4, 1994). Ann Thorac Surg 1995; 59(2)Suppl:1.

Catania U-M. Monitoring Coumadin therapy. RN 1994; 57(2):29.

Cerrato PL. New acute MI guidelines. RN 1997; 60(1):25.

Cerrato PL. New parameters for cholesterol screening. RN 1994; 57(11):37.

Child JS. Diagnosis and management of infective endocarditis. Cardiol Clin 1996; 14(3):327.

Cochrane BL. Acute myocardial infarction in women. Crit Care Nurs Clin North Am 1996; 4(2):279.

Cohen JD. Current concepts in the management of hypercholesterolemia with an update on fluvastatin. Am J Cardiol 1996; 78(6A):1.

Collins MA. When your patient has an implantable cardioverter defibrillator. Am J Nursing 1994; 94(3):34.

Collins R, Peto R, Baigent C, Sleight P. Aspirin, heparin, and fibrinolytic therapy in suspected acute myocardial infarction. N Engl J Med 1997; 336(12):847.

Cotran RS, Kumar V, Robbins SL. Robbins pathologic basis of disease. 5th ed. Philadelphia: WB Saunders, 1994.

Cronin LA. Beat the clock: Saving the heart with thrombolytic drugs. Nurs 93 1993; 23(8):34.

Dahlen R, Roberts SL. Acute congestive heart failure: Preventing complications. Dimens Crit Care Nurs 1996; 15(5):226.

Dajani AS, Taubert KA, Wilson W, et al. Prevention of bacterial endocarditis: Recommendations by the American Heart Association. JAMA 1997; 277(22):1794.

Davies MK, Giles TD. ACE inhibitors in heart failure: Advancing clinical practice. In Mechanisms and Management (proceedings of a satellite symposium of the 3rd International Congress on Heart Failure, Geneva, Switzerland, May 21–25, 1995). Basel: S. Karger, 1996.

Dennison RD. Making sense of hemodynamic monitoring. Am J Nurs 1994; 94(9):24.

DeVane GG. Valvular heart disease: A review for nurse anesthetists. CRNA 1996; 7(1):14.

DiMarco JP. Atrial fibrillation. Philadelphia: WB Saunders, 1996.

Donlevy JA, Pietruch BL. The connection delivery model: Care across the continuum. Nurse Manage 1996; 27(5):34.

Doty DB. Cardiac surgery: Operative technique. St Louis: Mosby, 1997.

Dougals PS, Ginsburg GS. The evaluation of chest pain in women. N Engl J Med 1996; 34(20):137.

Dunn D, Corrubia N. Patient teaching: Cardioversion. RN 1993; 56(1):45.

Edmunds LH. Cardiac surgery in the adult. New York: McGraw-Hill, 1997.

Elder AN. Sinus tachycardia: Lowering a high heart rate. Nurs 94 1994; 24(12):63.

Elkayam U. Congestive heart failure. In Rakel RE (ed). Conn's current therapy. Philadelphia: WB Saunders, 1997, pp 288–294.

Elkayam U. Nitrates in congestive heart failure: New mechanisms and rationale for use (symposium). Am J Cardiol 1996; 77(13):1.

Fair JM, Berra K. Endothelial function and coronary risk reduction: Mechanisms and influences of nitric oxide. Cardiovasc Nurs 1996; 32(3):17.

Finkelmeier BA. Cardiothoracic surgical nursing. Philadelphia: JB Lippincott, 1995.

Fitzgerald CA. Current perspectives on prosthetic heart valves and valve repair. AACN Clin Issues 1993; 4(2):228.

Fowler JP. When CHF turns deadly. Nurs 95 1995; 25(1):54.

Froelicher VF, Quaglietti S. Handbook of ambulatory cardiology. Boston: Lippincott-Raven, 1997.

Fuster V. Elucidation of the role of plaque instability and rupture in acute coronary event. Am J Cardiol 1995; 76:24C.

Fuster V, Gotto AM, Libby P, et al. Task force I. Pathogenesis of coronary disease: The biologic role of risk factors. J Am Coll Cardiol 1996; 27(5):964.

Gersh BJ, Rahimtoola SH. Acute myocardial infarction. 2nd ed. New York: Chapman & Hall, 1997.

Glennen S, Metcalfe H. Cardiology: Minimally invasive cardiac surgery (MICS). Nurs Stand 1996; 11(5):54.

Grech ED, Ramsdale DR. Practical interventional cardiology. St Louis: Mosby, 1997.

Hayes DL, Wang PJ, Reynolds DW, et al. Interference with cardiac procedures by cellular telephone. N Engl J Med 1997; 336(21):1473.

Hicks SL. Standing guard against silent ischemia and infarction. Nurs 94 1994; 24(1):34.

Holcomb SS. Atherectomy: A different way to unblock coronary arteries. Nurs 93 1993; 23(2):45.

Holmes DR, Serruys PW. Current review of interventional cardiology. 3rd ed. Philadelphia: Current Medicine, 1997.

Hudak CM, Gallo BM. Critical care nursing: A holistic approach. 6th ed. Philadelphia: JB Lippincott, 1994.

Jensen L, King KM: Women and heart disease: The issues. Crit Care Nurse 1997; 17(2): 45.

Jordaens L. The implantable defibrillator: From concept to clinical reality. Basel: S. Karger, 1996.

Kayser SR. Therapeutic advances in management of heart failure and acute myocardial infarction. Prog Cardiovasc Nurs 1993; 8(2):29.

Kayser SR. Management of chronic congestive heart failure: Part 1—General introduction to treatment. Prog Cardiovasc Nurs 1994; 9(1):39.

Kegel LM. Case management, critical pathways, and myocardial infarction. Crit Care Nurs 1996; 16(2):97.

Keresztes PA, Kuruzar L: Very early extubation: Extubating in the OR following coronary artery bypass. Dimens Crit Care Nurs 1996; 15(4):198.

Khonsari S, Sintek C. Cardiac surgery: Safeguards and pitfalls in operative technique. 2nd ed. Philadelphia: Lippincott-Raven, 1997.

Kirklin JW, Barratt-Boyes BC. Cardiac surgery. 2nd ed. New York: Churchill-Livingstone, 1993.

Koneru CL. Staff education: A quick in-service program on the new cardiac serum enzyme markers. J Emerg Nurs 1996; 22(3):246.

Kontos CD, Hess ML. Today's approach to managing severe myocarditis. J Crit Illness 1994; 9(2):152.

Kuc J. When heparin causes clots. RN 1993; 56(3):34.

Landreneau RJ, Mack MJ, Magovern JA, et al. "Keyhole" coronary artery bypass surgery. Ann Surg 1996; 224 (4):453.

Lau KW, Ding ZP, Gao W, et al. Percutaneous balloon mitral valvuloplasty in patients with mitral restenosis after previous surgical commissurotomy: A matched comparative study. Eur Heart J 1996; 17(9):1367.

Leier CV. Positive inotropic therapy: An update and new agents. St Louis: Mosby, 1996.

Luquire R, Houston S. Cardiomyopathy: How to buy time. RN 1993; 53(5):29.

MacKenzie GS, Heinle SK. Echocardiography and Doppler assessment of prosthetic heart valves with transesophageal echocardiography. Crit Care Clin 1996; 12(2):383.

Mailhot C: Mini-coronary artery bypass grafting. Nurs Manage 1996; 27(6):56.

Maye J, Marshall NE. Penetrating mine injury to the heart with a pericardial tamponade. CRNA 1996; 7(1):25.

McCafferty M, Welsh C. Teaching tools for heart failure. J Emerg Nurs 1996; 22(5):451.

McCance KL, Huether SE. Pathophysiology: The biologic basis for disease in adults and children. 2nd ed. St. Louis: Mosby-Year Book, 1994.

Meissner JE, Gever LN. Reducing the risks of digitalis toxicity. Nurs 93 1993; 23(7):47.

Merva J. A closer look at the heart: SAECG. RN 1993; 53(5):50.

Miller S: Congestive heart failure: Clinical assessment and pharmacologic management. ADVANCE Nurse Pract 1997; 5(6): 16.

Moreira LF, Bocchi EA, Stolf NA, et al. Dynamic cardiomyoplasty in the treatment of dilated cardiomyopathy: Current results and perspectives. J Card Surg 1996; 11(3):207.

Morton PG. Using the 12-lead ECG to detect ischemia, injury, and infarction. Crit Care Nurse 1996; 16(2):85.

Moser DK. Maximizing therapy in advanced heart failure patients. J Cardiovasc Nurs 1996; 10(2):29.

Nagueh SF, Zoghbi WA. Stress echocardiography for the assessment of myocardial ischemia and viability. St Louis: Mosby, 1996.

Nightingale K: Minimal invasive cardiac surgery. Br J Theatre Nurs 1996; 6(7):41.

O'Donnel L. Complications of MI: Beyond the acute stage. Am J Nurs 1996; 96(9):25.

Olbrych DD. Interpreting CPK and LDH results. Nurs 93 1993; 23(1):49.

Ondrusek RS. Spotting an MI before it's an MI. RN 1996; 59(4):26.

Owen A. Tracking the rise and fall of cardiac enzymes. Nurs 95 1995; 25(5):35.

Page JG, Hubble MW. Recognizing infective endocarditis: Case study of a 28-year-old. J Emerg Nurs 1996; 22(1):24.

Paul S. The pathophysiologic process of ventricular remodeling: From infarct to failure. Crit Care Nurs Q 1995; 18(1):7.

Petrosky-Pacini AJ. The automatic implantable cardioverter defibrillator in home care. Home Healthc Nurse 1996; 14(4):238.

Place B. Critical care: Inotrope therapy. Nurs Times 1996; 92(35): 55.

Porterfield LM. The cutting edge in arrhythmias. Crit Care Nurse 1993; (Suppl) June:8.

Potts A, Elliot D. Radiofrequency ablation: A review of its application and nursing considerations. Aust Crit Care 1996; 9(1):4.

Pratt CM. Calcium antagonists: Class distinctions, current controversies, and future trends. Am J Cardiol 78(9A):1.

Rahimtoola SH. The use of digitalis in heart failure. St Louis: Mosby, 1996.

Raimer F, Thomas M. Clot stoppers: Using anticoagulants safely and effectively. Nurs 95 1995; 25(3):34.

Reeder GS, Gersh BJ. Modern management of acute myocardial infarction. St Louis: Mosby-Year Book, 1996.

Ribeiro PA. Unstable angina: New insights in pathophysiologic characteristics, prognosis, and management strategies. St Louis: Mosby, 1996.

Riddle MM, Dunstan JL, Castanis JL: A rapid recovery program for cardiac surgery patients. Am J Crit Care 1996; 5(2):152.

Ridker PM, Cushman M, Stampfer M-J, Tracy RP, Hennekens CH. Inflammation, aspirin, and the risk of cardiovascular disease in apparently healthy men. N Engl J Med 1997; 336(14): 973.

Riley MC: Elective cardioversion: Who, when and how. RN 1997; 60(5):27.

Sabiston DC, Spencer FC. Surgery of the chest. 6th ed. Philadelphia: WB Saunders, 1996.

Sacks FM, Pfeffer MA, Moye LA, et al. The effect of pravastatin on coronary events after myocardial infarction in patients with average cholesterol levels. N Engl J Med 1996; 335(14): 1001.

Salisbury C. Rehabilitation after myocardial infarction: The role of the community nurse. Nurs Stand 1996; 10(23):49.

Salter DR. Acquired valvular heart disease. In Levine BA, Copeland EM, Howard RJ, et al (eds). Current practice of surgery. Vol 2: Cardiac surgery. New York: Churchill-Livingstone, 1994.

Schwabauer NJ. Retarding progression of heart failure: Nursing actions. Dimens Crit Care Nurs 1996; 15(6):307.

Schwartz DS, Ribakove GH, Grossi EA, et al. Minimally invasive cardiopulmonary bypass with cardioplegic arrest: A closed chest technique with equivalent myocardial protection. J Thorac Cardiovasc Surg 1996; 111(3)556.

Shyu KG, Lin JL, Chen JJ, Chang H. Use of cardiac troponin T, creatine kinase and its isoform to monitor myocardial injury during radiofrequency ablation for supraventricular tachycardia. Cardiology 1996; 87(5):392.

Sigwart U. Endoluminal stenting. London: WB Saunders, 1996.

Singh P. Managing congestive heart failure in the home. Home Healthc Nurse 1995; 13(2):11.

Smalling RW. Controversies in thrombolytic therapy (symposium). Am J Cardiol 1996; 78(12A):1.

Smith SC Jr, Blair SN, Criqui MH, et al. Preventing heart attack and death in patients with coronary disease. Endorsed by the board of trustees of the American College of Cardiology. Cardiovasc Nurs 1996; 32(4):26.

Smith SL. Acute myocardial infarction. In Rakel RE (ed). Conn's current therapy. Philadelphia: WB Saunders, 1997; pp 324–330.

Snowberger P. Second-degree atrioventricular block. RN 1993; 56(2):43.

Snowberger P. Third-degree heart block. RN 1993; 56(6):52.

Solomon J. Hypertension: New guidelines, new roles. RN 1993; 56(12):54.

Solomon J. Hypertension: New drug therapies. RN 1994; 57(1):26.

Spirito P, Seidman CE, McKenna WJ, Maron BJ. Medical progress: The management of hypertrophic cardiomyopathy. N Engl J Med 1997; 336(11):775.

Stahl L. How to manage common arrhythmias in medical patients. Am J Nurs 1995; 95(3):36.

Steinke E, Patterson-Midgley P. Sexual counseling following acute myocardial infarction. Clin Nurs Res 1996; 5(4):462.

Symanski JD, Nishimura RA. The use of pacemakers in the treatment of cardiomyopathies. St Louis: Mosby, 1996.

Taylor SH. Beta-blockers in heart failure: Myths and realities. (Proceedings of a satellite symposium of the XIIth World Congress of Cardiology and XVIth Congress of the European Society of Cardiology, 13 September 1994, Berlin, Germany.) London: WB Saunders, 1996.

Timmis AD, Brecker S. Cardiology. London: Mosby-Wolfe, 1997.

Treasure CB, Klein JL, Weintraub WS, et al. Beneficial effects of cholesterol lowering therapy on the coronary endothelium in patients with coronary artery disease. N Engl J Med 1996; 332(8):481.

Vitello-Cicciu J, Lapsley DP. Valvular heart disease. In Kinney MR, Packa DR, Dunbar SB (eds). AACN's clinical reference for critical care nursing. 3rd ed. St. Louis: Mosby-Year Book, 1993.

Waldo AL. Acute débridement of atrial fibrillation and flutter: Ibutilide in perspective. Am J Cardiol 1996; 78(8A):1.

Weeks SM. Caring for patients with heart failure. Nurs 96 1996; 26(3):52.

Weland AP, Walter WE. Physiologic principles and clinical sequelae of cardiopulmonary bypass. Heart Lung 1986; 15(1):34.

Williams JP. Postoperative management of the cardiac surgical patient. New York: Churchill-Livingstone, 1996.

Woodhouse KW, Pascual J. Hypertension in elderly people. London: Martin Dunitz, 1996.

Wright JM. Pharmacologic management of congestive heart failure. Crit Care Nurs Quarterly 1995; 18(1):32.

Wu KT, Baker-Carpenter K. ST-T segment changes in a patient with ECG evidence that suggests stenosis of the proximal left anterior descending artery. Crit Care Nurse 1996; 16(6):56.

Yacone-Morton LA. Inotropic drugs and nitrates. RN 1995; 58(3): 22.

Yager M. Right ventricular infarction in the emergency department: A review of pathophysiology, assessment, diagnosis, treatment, and nursing care. J Emerg Nurs 1996; 22(4):288.

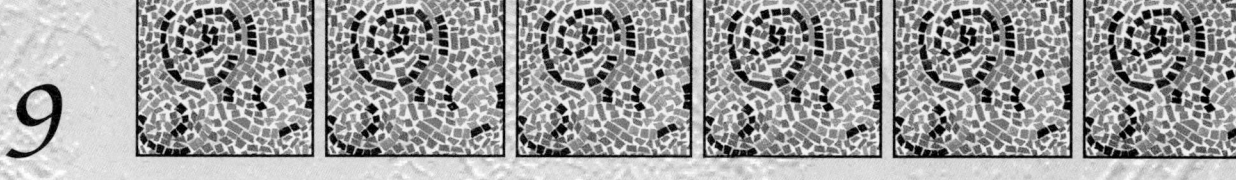

9

Knowledge Base for Patients with Vascular Dysfunction

Study Outcomes

After studying this chapter, you should be able to:

1. Explain the normal anatomy and physiology of the vascular system.
2. Identify the important risk factors for vascular disorders.
3. Describe common clinical manifestations of vascular dysfunction.
4. Identify information and physical examination data essential to the assessment of vascular status.
5. Compare and contrast the diagnostic studies used to identify vascular problems.
6. Describe medical management and surgical procedures commonly used in the treatment of patients with vascular disorders.
7. Describe the healing stages of leg ulcers.
8. Identify data essential to the assessment of patients undergoing treatment of vascular disorders.
9. State nursing diagnoses and related expected patient outcomes commonly applicable to patients undergoing treatment of vascular disorders.
10. Describe nursing interventions, with their rationales, commonly applicable to patients undergoing treatment of vascular disorders.
11. Explain the basis for evaluation of nursing care provided to patients undergoing treatment of vascular disorders.
12. Identify special considerations for the elderly patient with altered vascular function.
13. Identify alternative treatment and care settings for patients with vascular dysfunction and the services related to community-based care.

The peripheral vascular system is responsible for circulating blood from the right side of the heart to the lungs, returning it to the left side of the heart, carrying it throughout the body, and bringing it back to the right side of the heart again (Fig. 9–1). These transportation vessels are called the systemic circulatory system. Arteries, veins, and capillaries are the major components of systemic circulation. In addition to blood vessels, the lymphatic system is also closely related to circulatory function. This chapter presents an overview of the peripheral vascular system, the lymphatic system, vascular dysfunction, and how the nursing process applies to patients with vascular dysfunction.

Remember that patients with vascular dysfunction are commonly older adults with chronic circulatory problems. In addition to the acute care setting, these patients may be monitored, treated, and cared for in outpatient facilities, private clinics, and at home. Consultation and assistance from several health-care professionals may be necessary to preserve quality of life for the patient with peripheral vascular dysfunction.

*A*natomy and Physiology

VASCULAR STRUCTURES

The vascular structures found in the transport loop of the systemic circulation have many structural similarities. Except for the capillaries, blood vessels are composed of three distinct layers (Fig. 9–2). The tunica adventitia, or externa, is the outermost layer. It is composed of fibrous and connective tissue that provide support to the vascular structure. The tunica media, or middle layer, is predominantly smooth muscle. This smooth muscle layer is the one most responsive to the neural and chemical input that regulates blood-vessel diameter. The tunica intima, the innermost layer, is composed of connective tissue and a smooth endothelial inner surface to facilitate the flow of blood. This slippery surface prevents blood from clotting. Blood vessels vary in density

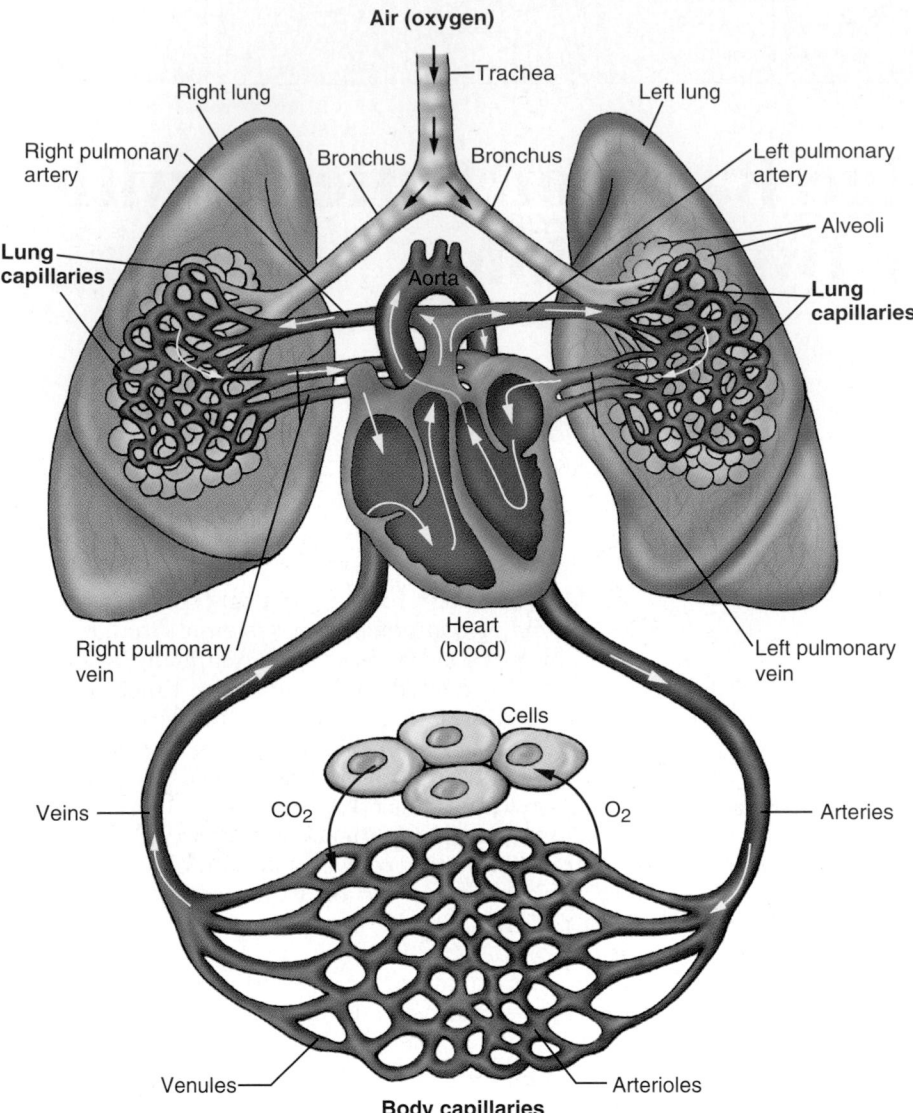

Figure 9–1

Systemic circulation. Blood from the body capillaries returns to the right atrium of the heart via the venules and veins. It then flows to the lungs, where it loses carbon dioxide and gains oxygen. It then flows to the left atrium, into the ventricle, and out of the heart through the aorta. It travels by arteries and arterioles until it reaches the capillaries, where it oxygenates the tissues and removes carbon dioxide and metabolic waste products.

and size to accommodate their function and anatomical position in the vascular system (Fig. 9–3).

Arteries and Arterioles

The arterial tree of vessels begins the transport of oxygenated blood in the aorta and culminates in the arterioles. The large arteries are thick-walled and quite elastic. They stretch in response to cardiac systole and recoil during diastole. This structural characteristic propels blood forward rapidly with much greater pressure than in the venous system.

The arterioles are just a few millimicrons in length, have diameters of 8 to 50 μ, and are composed predominantly of smooth muscle. They branch many times to supply as many as 100 capillaries. The contraction or relaxation of this smooth muscle changes the diameter of the vessel, thus influencing peripheral vascular resistance. Arterioles are high-resistance vessels innervated by sympathetic fibers of the autonomic nervous system. Sympathetic stimulation results in vasoconstriction. Decreased sympathetic activity results in vasodilation; thus, arterioles have a major influence on blood pressure and blood distribution to the capillaries. Precapillary sphincters located at the termination of some arterioles act as control valves through which blood is released into the capillaries.

Arterioles may also connect directly with capillaries or first connect with precapillaries (metarterioles). These structures serve as either thoroughfare channels or pipelines to supply the capillary network. Blood flows through the arterial system rapidly. Some 20% of the total circulating volume exists within the high-pressure arterial component at any one time.

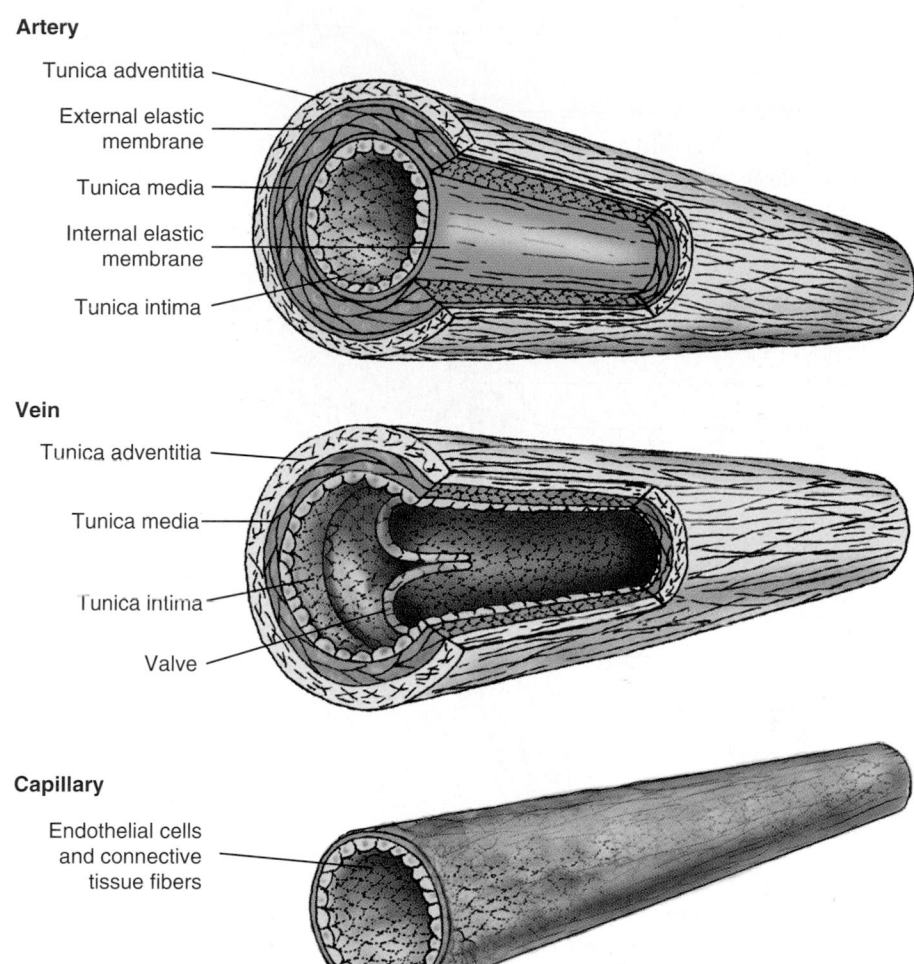

Artery
- Tunica adventitia
- External elastic membrane
- Tunica media
- Internal elastic membrane
- Tunica intima

Vein
- Tunica adventitia
- Tunica media
- Tunica intima
- Valve

Capillary
- Endothelial cells and connective tissue fibers

Figure 9–2

Microscopic view showing the anatomical structures of an artery, a vein, and a capillary.

Capillaries

Blood flowing through the capillary system delivers nutrition and removes the waste products of circulation. There are approximately 10 billion capillaries in the peripheral vascular network. The number of capillaries in a particular body tissue depends on its metabolic needs. For example, muscles contain abundant capillaries. They comprise more than 40% of total body tissue and, at rest, they receive 20% of blood flow. During exercise, however, they receive up to 85% of blood flow.

Capillaries are microscopic and composed of a single-thickness layer of endothelial tissue. Red blood cells must move through the small capillary lumen in single file. There are no smooth muscle fibers in capillaries. Lumen size is controlled passively through alterations in precapillary or postcapillary resistance. Capillaries contain small pores that make the capillary bed extremely permeable to the exchange of gases, nutrients, and metabolic wastes between blood and tissue cells. Fluid volume transfer between plasma and interstitial fluid occurs in the capillary system. The capillaries contain 5% of the total circulating blood volume. Arterioles, capillaries, and venules as a unit are referred to as the microcirculation (Fig. 9–4).

Arteriovenous anastomoses occur in some capillary beds. In these structures, blood passes directly from arteriole to venule. They are believed to be local thermoregulation centers between the body and the external environment.

Veins and Venules

The venules connect with capillaries and veins and begin the chain of vessels that return blood to the right atrium of the heart. Venules are thin-walled transit tubules. White blood cells can enter or exit the circulatory system through the venule.

Veins have a thinner tunica media than arteries do, so their walls are extremely distensible and collapsible. They can hold large volumes of blood: up to 75% of total volume. Their characteristic ability to stretch and act as a reservoir earns the venous system the name *capacitance vessels*.

The venous system is a low-pressure unidirec-

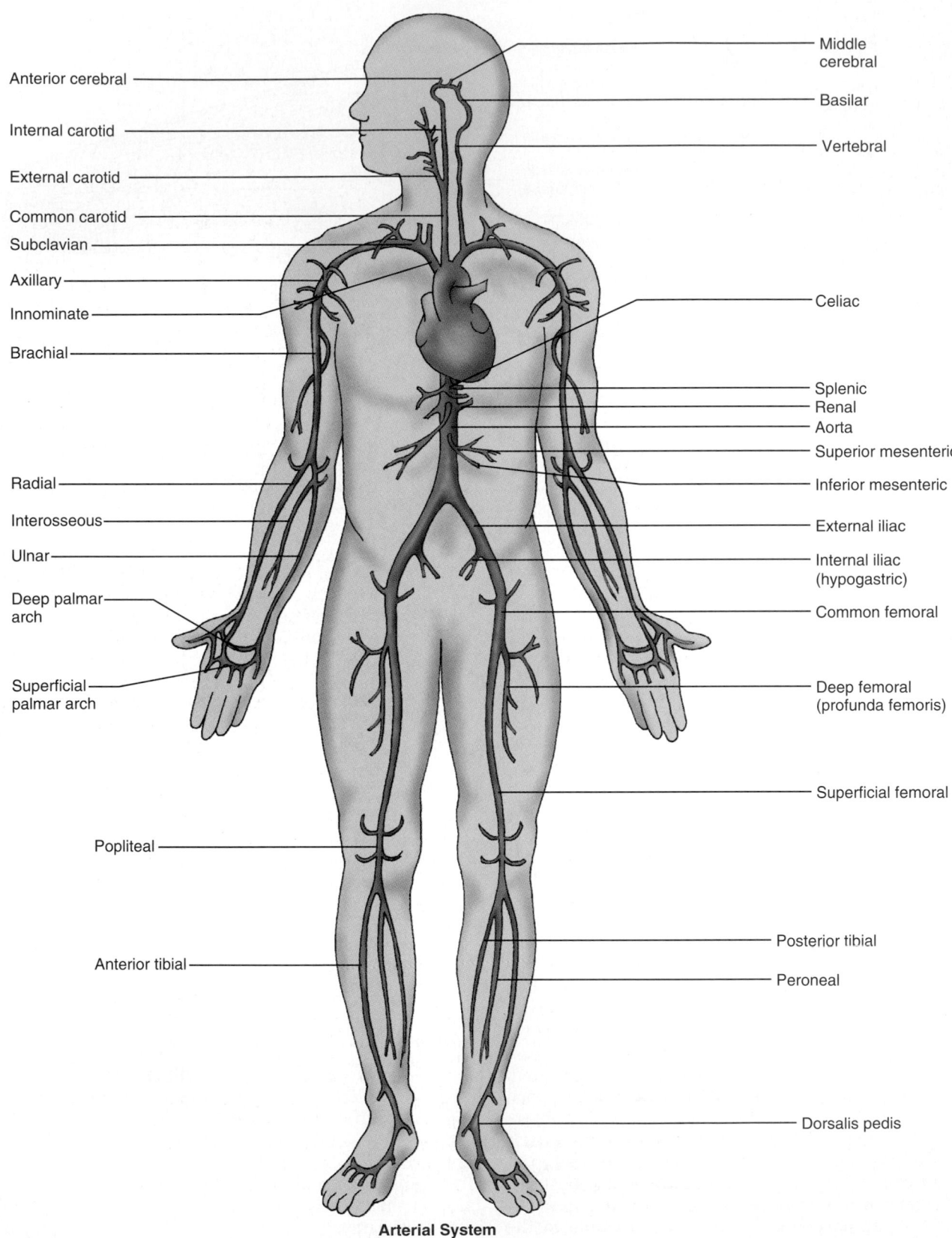

Anterior cerebral

Internal carotid

External carotid

Common carotid

Subclavian

Axillary

Innominate

Brachial

Radial

Interosseous

Ulnar

Deep palmar arch

Superficial palmar arch

Popliteal

Anterior tibial

Middle cerebral

Basilar

Vertebral

Celiac

Splenic

Renal

Aorta

Superior mesenteric

Inferior mesenteric

External iliac

Internal iliac (hypogastric)

Common femoral

Deep femoral (profunda femoris)

Superficial femoral

Posterior tibial

Peroneal

Dorsalis pedis

Arterial System

Figure 9–3

Vessels of the arterial system.

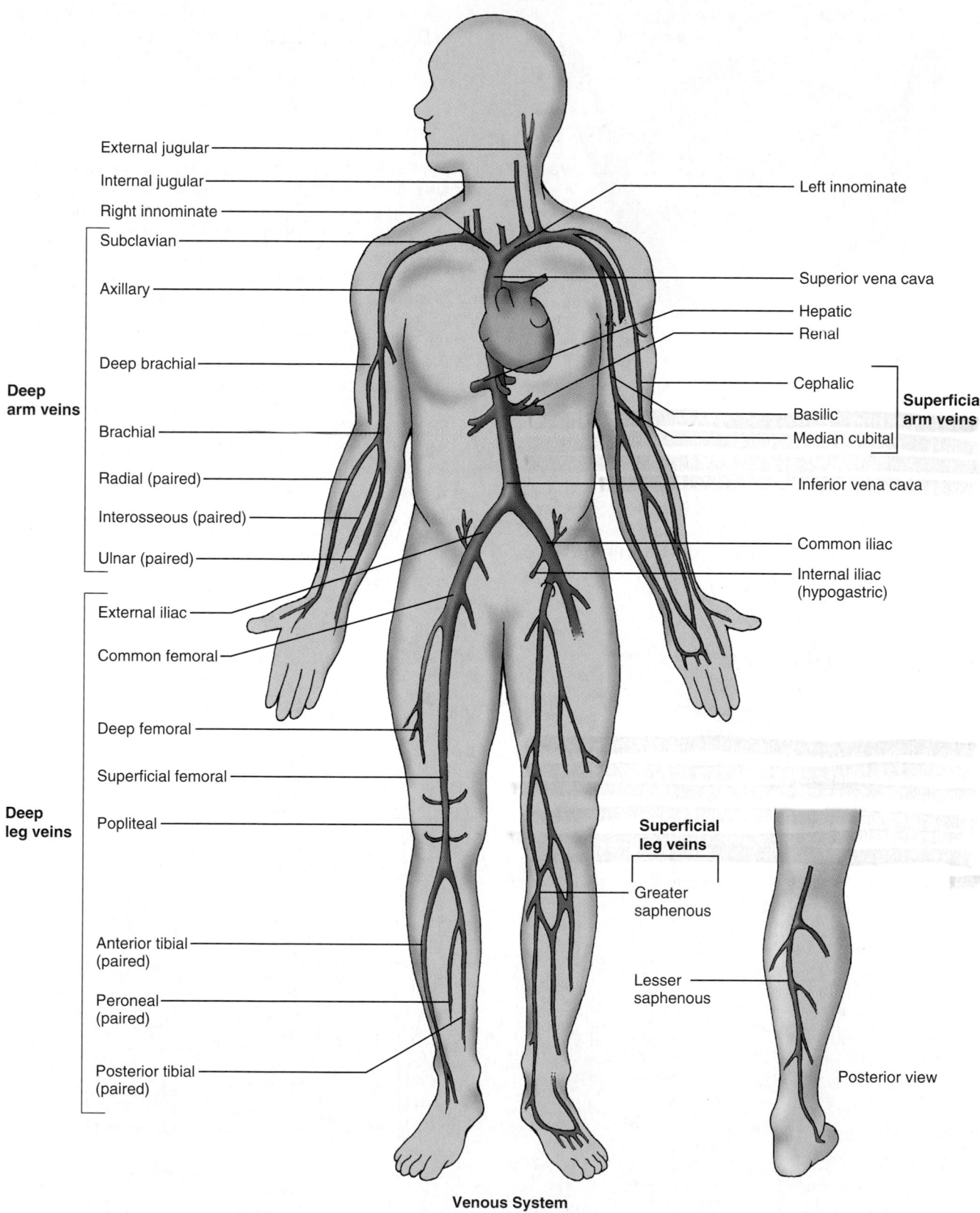

Figure 9–3 *Continued*
Vessels of the venous system.

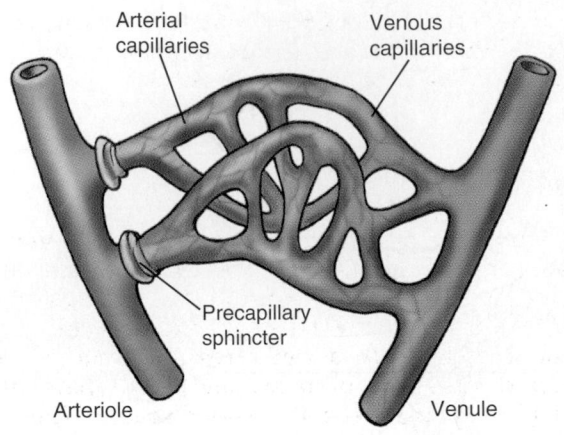

Figure 9-4

Arterioles, venules, and capillaries make up the microcirculation.

tional conduit. It relies on the muscular pumping action of the skeletal muscle contraction and changes in thoracic, intra-abdominal, and right atrial pressure to move blood back to the heart. The peripheral veins, especially those of the lower extremities, are equipped with one-way valves or endothelial flaps that maintain forward flow and prevent retrograde movement (Fig. 9-5). Large central veins do not have these valves.

FACTORS THAT AFFECT BLOOD FLOW

Structural Factors

Blood flow is governed by the difference in pressure gradients within the circulatory system. Fluid always flows from an area of higher pressure to an area of lower pressure. The high-pressure gradient begins in the high-pressure arterial tree and ends with the low-pressure gradient in the venous system. The pressure gradient ranges from an average mean arterial pressure of 100 mm Hg to a venous pressure in the vena cava of 4 to 0 mm Hg.

The rate of blood flow through the circulatory system is regulated by a number of factors. Some mechanisms impede or cause resistance to the flow. Structural factors include the diameter of the vessel, the elastic recoil ability of the vessel wall, and the viscosity of the blood itself. These three contribute to hemodynamic or peripheral vascular resistance.

DIAMETER OF THE VESSEL

The velocity of the flow of any liquid is inversely proportional to the cross-sectional areas of the lumen or opening through which the fluid must flow. In the vascular system, the differences in the lumens of the arteries, capillaries, and veins exert an influence on the rate of flow. Arterioles, the smallest and most distant branches of the arterial tree, alter their diameter in response to the metabolic needs of the

tissues and various chemical and hormonal stimulation. These vessels are often called resistance vessels because of the effect of their changing lumen size on blood flow to the capillaries and on blood pressure.

ELASTIC RECOIL

Arteries have thick, muscular walls and thus have a considerable amount of recoil ability. This recoil moves blood quickly to the capillary networks under high pressure. Capillaries alter diameter negligibly and have little recoil ability with their single-cell-layer thickness. Veins, with their less muscular walls and a great capacity for distending and collapsing, provide no resistance to blood flow if valves are competent.

Blood moves through healthy vessels smoothly because of streamlined or laminar flow. In this type of flow, the blood components are layered. Plasma is in closest proximity to the vessel wall, and erythrocytes, platelets, and cellular components move through the center of the vessel. Narrowing of the vessel lumen at anatomic bifurcations, or by atherosclerosis or other structural changes in vessel integrity, can cause turbulence or eddy currents of blood flow. These areas of turbulent flow may produce a murmur, or bruit, that can be auscultated with a stethoscope.

VISCOSITY OF BLOOD

The last basic controller of the rate of blood flow is the viscosity of blood itself. This factor is usually of little consequence with normal concentrations of red

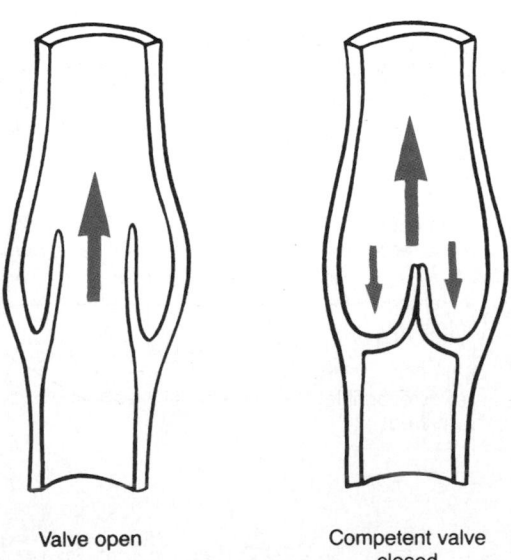

Valve open   Competent valve closed

Figure 9-5

A normal venous valve in open and closed positions. Colored arrows signify the forward flow of blood (toward the heart). A competent venous valve in the closed position prevents retrograde blood flow, signified by the black arrows. Thus, venous valves help maintain the movement of blood back to the heart.

blood cells. However, if viscosity increases (indicated by an increasing hematocrit of 55% or higher) the "thicker" blood flows more slowly. This viscous blood will have a greater tendency to clot and contribute to impeded flow. See Chapter 12 for a detailed discussion of hematocrit.

Direct Control of Blood Flow

There are three mechanisms that influence blood flow by direct effects on the vessels: Local control, neural control, and humoral control.

LOCAL CONTROL

Local control of blood flow in all body tissues is governed by each tissue's need for nutrition and perfusion. The tissues regulate flow independently of the autonomic nervous system through a mechanism of metabolic autoregulation. Although this mechanism is not fully understood, it appears to be regulated by a lack of oxygen or accumulation of tissue metabolites. When oxygen and the level of other cellular nutrients decrease or metabolites increase, arterioles and metarterioles dilate to increase blood flow. During exercise, muscles demand an increased flow and arterioles dilate. At rest, arterioles constrict and blood flow moves to other parts of the body. Local autoregulation has a major influence on vasoconstriction or vasodilation—and thus on blood flow—by varying lumen size.

NEURAL CONTROL

Neural control of blood flow is mediated by the sympathetic branch of the autonomic nervous system. The sympathetic pathway begins in the vasomotor center located in the lower pons and medulla. The vasomotor center also receives input from the hypothalamus. All blood vessels except capillaries are supplied with sympathetic nerve fibers. Sympathetic input impacts the blood vessels, producing selective vasoconstriction in 1 to 30 seconds. The sympathetic nerve fibers secrete norepinephrine, a potent vasoconstricting neurotransmitter. The effect of this vasoconstriction in the arterioles is increased arterial blood pressure. In veins, norepinephrine causes venoconstriction, which increases venous return to the heart.

HUMORAL CONTROL

Various substances released into or circulating in the blood can influence blood flow. Hormones are released from the adrenal medulla in response to acute stress as part of the "fight or flight" response. The hormones epinephrine and norepinephrine (catecholamines) act directly on the smooth muscle of blood vessels to cause vasoconstriction and some selective vasodilation. Other substances found in circulation that influence lumen diameter, and thus blood flow, are listed in Table 9–1.

LYMPHATIC VASCULAR SYSTEM

The lymphatic system consists of lymph capillaries, vessels, ducts, nodes, and the lymph that flows through its channels to return to the venous system. Figure 9–6 illustrates the lymphatic network. Lymphatic vessels serve as an accessory route for the transport of fluid, proteins, and large particulate matter away from the interstitial spaces. They remove excess interstitial fluid or plasma that the venous capillaries are unable to reabsorb (Fig. 9–7). The lymphatic system plays an important role in immunity and prevention of edema in body tissues.

The lymphatic capillaries are thin-walled, endothelially lined, and slightly larger than systemic circulatory capillaries. They have varying diameters. Lymphatic capillaries have wider spaces between endothelial cells than venous capillaries do, making them more permeable by large protein molecules and colloids. Lymphatic capillaries are found at the venous end of the body tissues, except in the central

Table 9–1

Substances that Affect Blood Flow	
VASOCONSTRICTORS	
Angiotensin	The most potent vasoconstrictor known. Formed after activation of the renin-angiotensin system of the kidney. Released in response to decreased arterial pressure or decreased sodium.
Cold	Direct application causes local vasoconstriction.
Serotonin	Particularly potent in cutaneous arterioles. It is found in platelets, gastrointestinal mucosa, and cancerous tumors.
Trauma	Arterial injury causes local reaction.
VASODILATORS	
Bradykinin	Vasoactive polypeptide found in plasma. It also increases capillary permeability.
Heat	Direct application causes local reaction.
Histamine	Released from injured body cells and affects arterioles. It also increases the porosity of capillaries, causing them to leak fluid and plasma proteins into tissues.
Muscle metabolites	Lactic acid is the most common muscle metabolite.

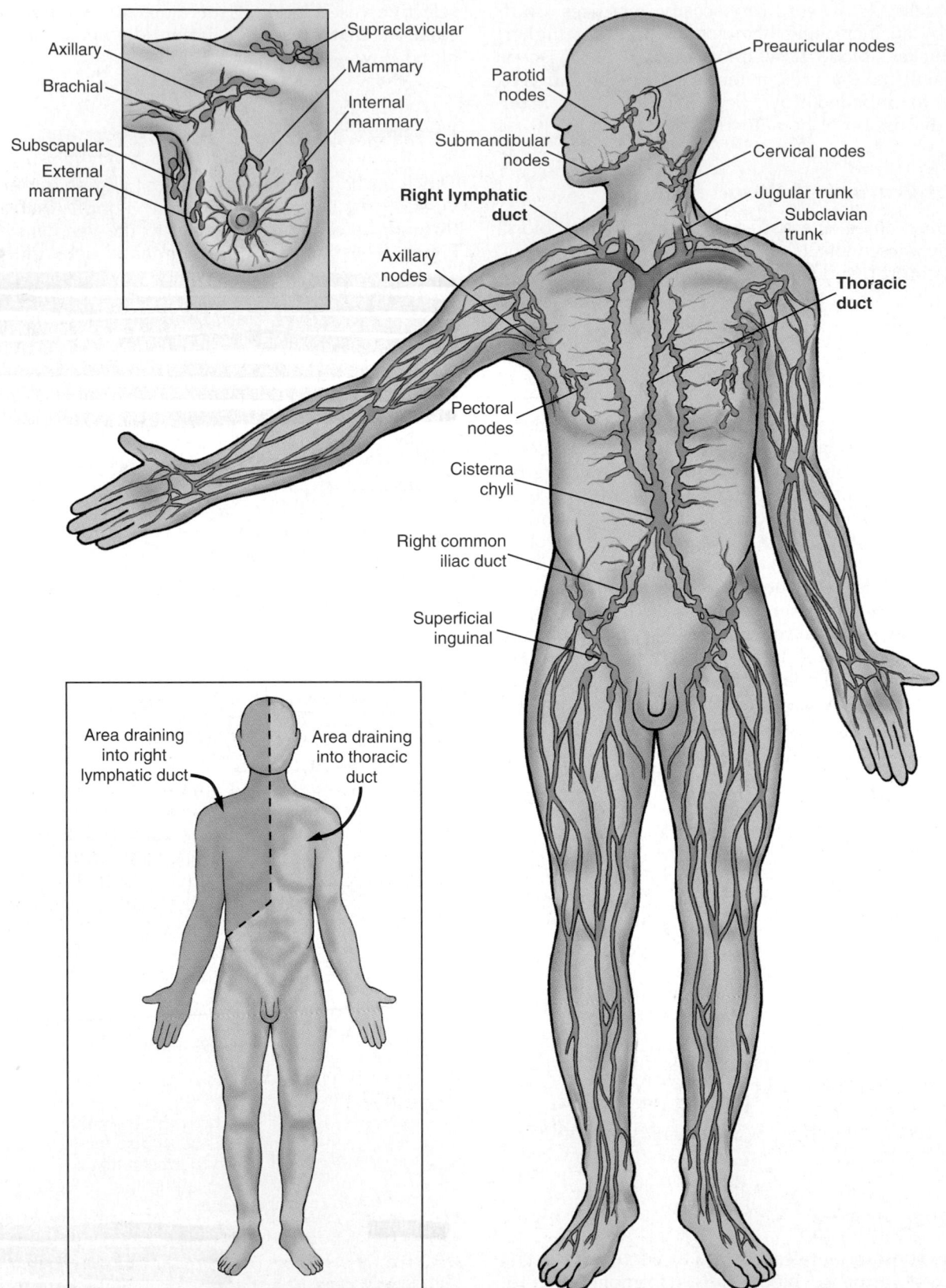

Figure 9–6
The lymphatic system.

Arterial end

Blood capillary

Venous end

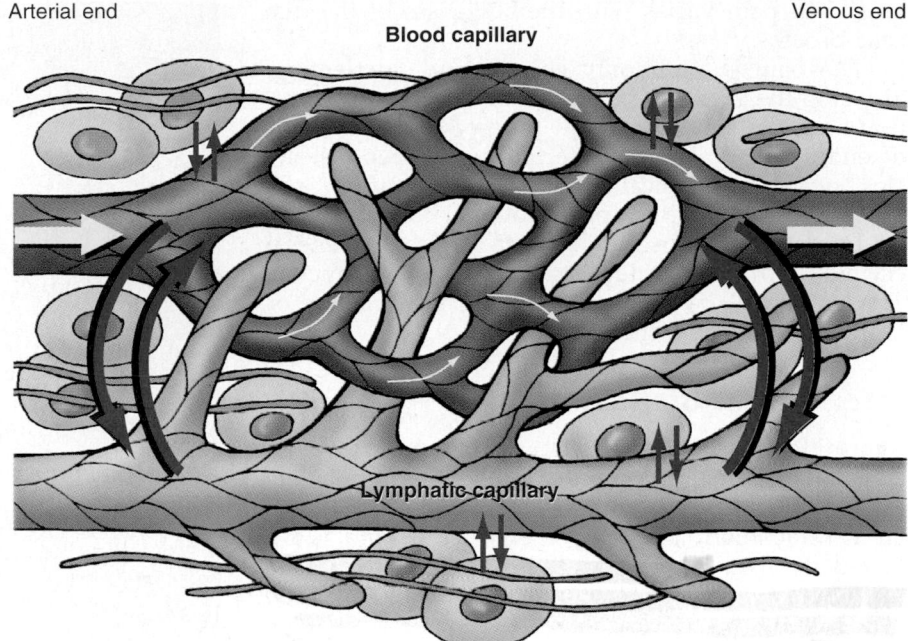

Lymphatic capillary

Figure 9–7

The lymphatic system is integrally related to the systemic vascular system. Excess fluid and plasma diffuse between the capillaries, interstitial spaces, and lymphatic vessels. Because lymphatic capillaries have larger spaces between endothelial cells, they can remove excess interstitial fluid or plasma that venous capillaries cannot reabsorb.

nervous system and in such nonvascular structures as cartilage.

Lymphatic capillaries and vessels have one-way valves, as does the venous system, but they are more numerous in the lymphatics. At the capillary level, the valvular structure originates between the spaces of the endothelial cell wall. These valve flaps are attached to filaments that pull inward, allowing excess interstitial fluid to enter the capillary but preventing backflow.

Lymphatic capillaries increase in diameter to form lymphatic vessels. The lymphatic network propels lymph forward to enter the venous circulation. Lymph empties into two major ducts: the thoracic duct and the right lymphatic duct. The thoracic duct receives lymph from most of the body. The right lymphatic duct empties the right side of the head, neck, arm, and thorax directly into the venous system at the junction of the subclavian and internal jugular veins.

Lymph nodes are small, ovoid masses of lymphatic tissue located along the circuit of lymphatic channels. The internal structure of the node is spongy, enabling it to serve as a filter for bacteria. Granulocytes, macrophages, and lymphocytes are able to pass into the lymph nodes and return to systemic circulation via the lymphatic network.

Lymph has many similarities to plasma. It is pale yellow to milky white in color, depending on the concentration of molecules of digested fats. The fluid also contains lymphocytes, granulocytes, enzymes, hormones, antibodies, and excess interstitial fluid. Because it is deficient in fibrinogen, erythrocytes, and platelets, it coagulates very slowly. Lymph movement is generated by contraction of the lym-

phatic walls and compression of tissues through skeletal muscle activity.

*C*linical Manifestations of Vascular Dysfunction

Vascular dysfunction produces clinical manifestations because impaired blood flow deprives tissues of adequate oxygen and nutrients and fails to adequately remove metabolic waste products. As a result, the person with impaired blood flow typically experiences pain and tissue changes in areas of poor perfusion. Complete obstruction of blood flow results in rapid tissue death. The progression of symptoms depends on several variables, including:

- Origin (arterial or venous)
- Duration and onset (acute or chronic)
- Obstruction (partial or complete)
- Availability of collateral or alternate vessels to perfuse the area

PAIN

For many people, pain is an omnipresent effect of vascular dysfunction. When blood flow is obstructed, tissue oxygenation decreases and metabolic waste products accumulate. The tissue becomes hypoxic or ischemic. Although the exact mechanism is unknown, pain probably results from a metabolic factor released from the ischemic tissues. This factor irritates peripheral sensory nerve endings. The intensity of pain varies with the acuteness of the disease process.

The pain is commonly chronic and unrelenting, affecting the person's quality of life. In fact, its duration and intensity may push the person to the limit of endurance. Pain may interfere with sleep-rest cycles, appetite, physical activity, concentration, and interpersonal relationships. Emotional stress brought on by constant pain manifests in irritability, anger, crying, withdrawal, depression, and even suicide. The pain may be resolved only by nerve block or amputation of the ischemic area.

Intermittent Claudication

Intermittent claudication is a severe aching or cramp-like pain most frequently experienced in the calf muscles. It is precipitated by walking or muscular contractions of the lower extremities and is relieved by rest. The pain of claudication can be re-elicited by walking the same distance that caused pain to begin the first time. The pain is usually bilateral.

Claudication pain is associated with arterial insufficiency caused by atheromatous plaque, which obstructs blood flow to the extremities. The femoral artery is usually the occlusive site for calf claudication. Occlusions of the aortic and iliac arteries cause claudication pain in the hip or thigh. Figure 9–8 illustrates sites of obstruction and corresponding levels of claudication.

The circulatory needs of muscles for oxygen and metabolite waste removal increase with exercise. The mechanically impaired arteries are not able to dilate to increase blood flow through the obstruction. The pain of intermittent claudication appears to be related, in order of occurrence, to the following:

1. Tissue ischemia
2. Metabolite accumulation in tissue
3. Painful muscle spasm

Rest Pain

Rest pain is a sign of acute arterial insufficiency and is associated with severe ischemia. It typically precedes gangrene. Affected people describe rest pain as a severe aching, throbbing, gnawing, or burning pain, usually in the forefoot. The discomfort is often more severe at night and may last for interminable hours. The pain of arterial insufficiency is aggravated by elevating the affected part. It may be relieved by placing the part below heart level.

Many patients may be able to rest only by sitting in a chair or by dangling the affected extremity from the bed. People often rub and cradle an ischemic leg in their lap to try to alleviate the pain.

Venous Insufficiency

Venous dilatation, congestion, edema, and stasis from incompetent valves produce a heaviness or

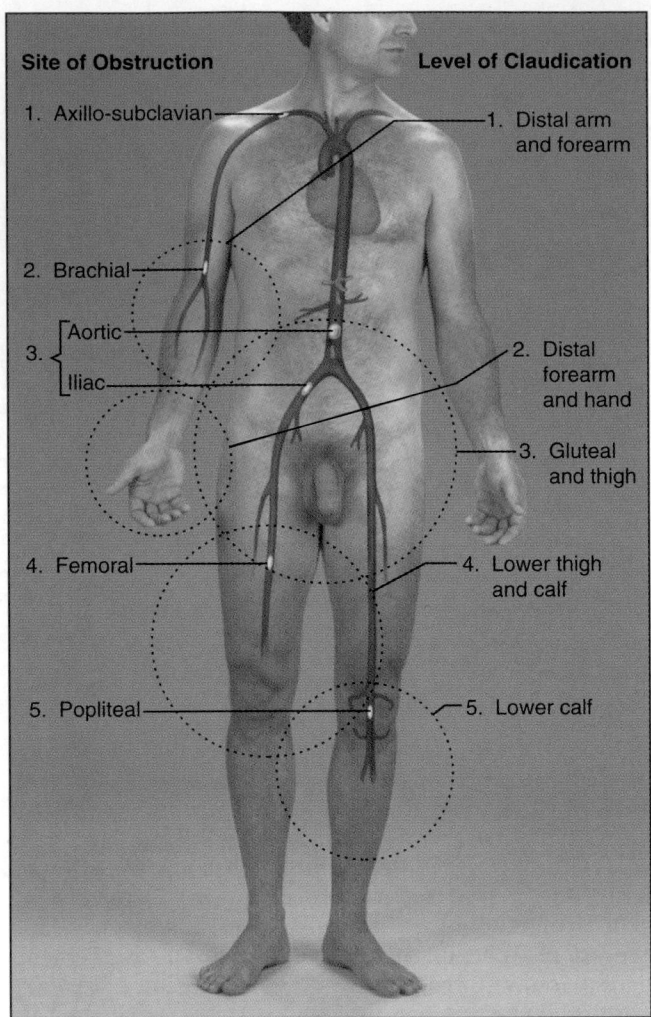

Figure 9–8
Arterial obstructions and their corresponding areas of claudication.

dull, aching pain in the affected extremity. Some people experience leg cramps, especially at rest. Elevation of the congested extremity facilitates venous return of excess blood volume and often relieves the pain.

Stasis of deoxygenated blood unable to remove the toxic byproducts of cellular metabolism causes tissue deterioration and the development of stasis ulcers. These ulcerations produce localized pain in the area of deterioration.

Ischemic Neuropathy

This type of pain manifests late in the course of acute arterial insufficiency and is described as a shock-like sensation in the leg and foot. Paresthesias often accompany progressive ischemia. The pain is believed to be associated with irritation of the peripheral sensory nerves by the effects of chronic ischemia.

Ulceration or Gangrene

The pain of arterial ulcerations or gangrene is described as aching, sharp, stabbing, and unrelenting. It is so intense that rest and sleep are greatly impaired. This type of severe rest pain is the result of acute or progressively chronic ischemia and is frequently the precursor to amputation. Venous stasis ulcerations are less painful than ischemic arterial ulcers.

NURSING PROCESS
Pain

Assessment

Obtain a patient history and description of the pain. Identify the location, intensity, and quality. Have the patient rate the intensity of pain on a scale of 0 to 10. Include the present pain level, the most severe level, and the least severe level experienced on this scale. Use the patient's own words to describe the quality of the pain. Ask about the onset, duration, and any variations or rhythms to the occurrence of pain.

Determine precipitating factors, such as exercise or exposure to cold. Evaluate activity and exercise tolerance, such as distances walked when pain occurs, to establish a baseline. Each individual with claudication experiences pain with walking. The individual has a unique and consistent distance at which he or she experiences the pain. By obtaining this history or activity baseline, you can begin planning a slowly progressive exercise regimen. Inquire about measures that have helped alleviate the patient's pain, such as rest or position changes.

Ask about the effects of pain on sleep-rest patterns, appetite, physical activity, and relationships with others. Evaluate the patient's ability to cope with the pain and the effects on emotional stability.

Assess the patient's level of knowledge about what is causing the pain, and instruct accordingly. Evaluate the effectiveness of pain-management measures.

Nursing Diagnoses and Planning

Nursing diagnoses and related expected patient outcomes commonly applicable to patients with peripheral vascular pain include the following:

NDx: Pain related to altered tissue perfusion

Planning: Patient Outcomes
1. Patient verbalizes a decrease in the level of pain.
2. Patient follows a regimen of exercise and rest.
3. Patient participates in relaxation techniques to help manage pain.

Nursing Interventions and Evaluation

NDx: Pain
Because impaired circulation is the cause of the pain, measures that improve blood flow can help alleviate or lessen the discomfort. Tell the patient to begin a slow, progressive, moderate exercise program of walking short distances several times a day, followed by rest periods. This is helpful for many patients with intermittent claudication. Note the distance or amount of muscular activity the patient can tolerate before pain occurs. Exercise promotes not only blood flow and removal of metabolites that cause muscle spasm, but also the development of collateral circulation channels that bypass blocked areas. Walking assists the venous pump because muscle contractions help return blood to the heart. It is helpful in people with venous insufficiency if followed by a period of elevation.

Position the patient for pain relief. If the person has arterial insufficiency, do not elevate the extremities because doing so usually increases pain and further impairs circulation. Instead, place the extremities in a dependent position to the torso. This works with the force of gravity and assists circulatory perfusion.

If the person has a venous disorder, elevate the extremities. Doing so helps relieve venous engorgement, edema, and pain. Instruct the patient to elevate the extremities several times throughout the day. Tell the patient to avoid standing for prolonged times in one position. If the person must stand, suggest shifting the weight from one foot to the other. Encourage flexion and dorsiflexion of the ankles when at rest. These muscular contractions assist the venous muscular pumping action.

Pharmaceutical and non-pharmaceutical treatments may also help alleviate pain. Use the clinical practice guidelines developed by the Agency for Health Care Policy and Research to help the patient relieve pain. Teach the patient to combine several methods for best pain relief.

Administer prescribed analgesics, tranquilizers, vasodilators, and sleep medications, and evaluate their effectiveness. These medications may relieve or lessen the severity of pain and make it possible for the patient to participate more actively in exercise that improves circulation. Encourage adequate rest and sleep to maintain psychologic integrity.

Teach relaxation exercises, such as deep abdominal breathing with a focal point, guided imagery, and autogenic training. These produce a sense of control over pain and decrease feelings of powerlessness. Also, physiologic production of the relaxation response decreases sympathetic vasoconstriction in peripheral vessels. Peripheral vessels dilate and increase cutaneous temperature during the relaxation response.

Sit down at the bedside and practice relaxation exercises with the patient. These exercises are most successful when the nurse is actively involved rather than just providing a relaxation tape or written instructions. Once the patient has learned the technique, reinforce it with additional material. Provide back and neck massage to promote relaxation and circulation. Massage the calves of the legs unless the patient is on bedrest or limited mobility or recently had surgery. Massaging the calves at these times could release a thrombus, causing embolization.

Compare the patient's status with the expected outcomes. If the outcomes are not met, reassess the patient and revise the plan.

CHANGES IN SKIN COLOR, TEMPERATURE, AND INTEGRITY

The clinical manifestations vary with arterial or venous dysfunction. Table 9–2 compares and summarizes changes in skin, color, temperature, and integrity.

Trophic Changes

Trophic changes are the result of a prolonged lack of cellular nutrition and ischemia. The growth of nails, hair, and skin are affected. Skin becomes thin,

shiny, and frail. Hair growth becomes scanty to absent. Nails become thickened, yellowish, flaky, and fungal.

Color Changes

Cyanosis, or bluish discoloration, develops in tissues that contain blood deficient in oxygenated hemoglobin. Many people with venous insufficiency acquire positional cyanosis when the legs are in a dependent plane. Mottling, or cyanotic discoloration, of the toes or foot occurs in end-stage arterial obstruction and precedes ischemic gangrene. The extremity assumes a normal color when not dependent.

Pallor results from a deficient blood supply. When blood flows normally, tissue manifests a pink or rosy hue. Extremities with advanced arterial disease become extremely pale (in light-skinned individuals) and cadaveric gray (in dark-skinned individuals) when elevated above heart level.

Rubor (redness) in chronic arterial insufficiency

Table 9–2

Clinical Manifestations of Changes in Skin Temperature, Color, and Integrity with Arterial and Venous Insufficiency

Assessment	Arterial	Venous
Extremity characteristics	Extremities typically exhibit muscular atrophy and decreased hair growth. Skin is dry, smooth, shiny in appearance. Toenails are thickened and discolored.	Brownish pigmentation on anterior surface of lower leg and ankle. Skin is thickened and rough. Dermatitis.
Skin color	Ghostly white or cadaveric gray pallor when elevated. Rebound rubor when placed in dependent position. Blotchy cyanosis as severe ischemia progresses.	Feet and lower leg become cyanotic with prolonged dependent position. Normal coloration to rosy when not dependent, pale when elevated.
Skin temperature	Poikilothermy (decreased temperature). Cool feet. Extremity becomes cold below the level of occlusion with acute blockage.	Warm. Cooler with presence of tissue edema.
Edema	Not characteristically present.	Persistent chronic swelling, especially in prolonged dependent position. Elevation decreases venous dilatation and swelling.
Pathologic ulcerations	Caused by prolonged small artery and arteriole constriction. Acutely painful. Pale grayish base. Located on heel, lateral malleolus of ankle, toes, top of the foot.	Caused by venous stasis or pooling of blood. Chronic slow healing. Moderately painful. Pink base. Found on medial malleolus of ankle.
Gangrene	Dry gangrene starting with the toes. Dry, hard, black, shriveled appearance. Toes may autoamputate. Pregangrenous areas appear dark purple and do not change color with pressure.	Not present.
Paresthesia	Tingling, numb, or prickly sensation with progressive ischemia.	Not present.

Artery → red   Venous → blue when dependant skin will be

is the result of a permanent dilatation of the arterioles caused by damage to the vascular smooth muscle layer. Arterioles lose their basic vasomotor tone and responsiveness. They become dilated with blood. Muscle metabolite accumulation of lactic acid also has a vasodilating effect that produces rubor.

Rubor may also be produced as a rebound response to placing the arterially affected extremity in an elevated position (where it becomes pale) and then lowering it below the heart (where it becomes ruddy). Pallor followed by rubor is a sign of severe arterial disease.

Rubor localized in the hands and feet is characteristic of arterial spasms or occlusions. Exposure to cold temperatures often precipitates spasms in individuals with arterial vessel dysfunction.

Brownish pigmentation commonly appears on the anterior surface of the lower leg in venous insufficiency. This coloration results when hemosiderin deposits are left behind from chronic stasis and poor cellular nutrition and waste removal.

Temperature Changes

Skin temperature reflects the adequacy of blood circulation. A cool extremity denotes deficient blood supply. A rapid change to coldness signifies an acute occlusion. Emergency measures must be taken to salvage the limb.

Ulceration

In arterial disorders, ulcerations are caused by chronic occlusion of arterioles and small arteries. In venous insufficiency, the precipitating factor is venous stasis and the accumulation of deoxygenated blood. Tissues receive inadequate nutrition, making them vulnerable to bacterial growth and tissue breakdown or ulceration.

Gangrene

Gangrene is characterized by black devitalized tissue, the net result of tissue death from severe ischemia. Gangrene is usually confined to one extremity.

NURSING PROCESS
Changes in Skin Color, Temperature, and Integrity

Assessment

Review the patient's medical history to determine how long symptoms have been present. Perform a physical examination of the affected extremity for evidence of peripheral vascular dysfunction. See Table 9–2 for a summary of assessment parameters for skin integrity in vascular disorders. Thoroughly examine all extremities for changes in skin color, temperature, or presence of ulcerations or gangrene.

Palpate the distal pulses bilaterally and note their presence, absence, and quality. Move up the extremity if the distal pulses are absent (Fig. 9–9). Use Doppler ultrasonography if pulses are not palpable (Fig. 9–10). Assessment of pulses helps estimate the degree of vascular dysfunction. Pulses are present with venous disorders but are usually diminished or absent in arterial insufficiency. Check capillary refill in extremities. Refill in less than 3 seconds indicates adequate perfusion.

Observe skin color or temperature changes while the extremity is elevated or dependent to the heart. Ask the patient about skin-color changes with exposure to cold temperatures. Also ask whether the patient perceives coolness or warmth in the part. Examine toenails and skin for changes in thickness, pigmentation, or coloration. Check for edema, ulceration, gangrene, or paresthesia.

If ulceration or gangrene is present, carefully document the location, color, shape, and qualities of healing or granulation. Measure the area precisely for baseline data for future comparison. Ask how the patient cares for an ulceration. Assess learning needs for wound care. Gangrene is end-stage ischemia, and amputation is probable. Provide support in the grieving process for limb loss.

Nursing Diagnoses and Planning

Nursing diagnoses and related expected patient outcomes commonly applicable to patients with changes in skin color, temperature, and integrity include the following:

NDx: Altered peripheral tissue perfusion related to compromised blood flow

Planning: Patient Outcomes
1. Patient exhibits improved blood supply to the affected extremity as evidenced by improvement in color, temperature, and integrity.
2. Patient participates in exercises and positioning that facilitate blood flow.

NDx: Risk for impaired skin integrity related to impaired circulation

Planning: Patient Outcomes
1. Patient maintains or re-establishes skin integrity with no signs of tissue damage.
2. Patient demonstrates daily protective measures in skin care and activities.

Nursing Interventions and Evaluation

NDx: Altered peripheral tissue perfusion
Determine whether altered tissue perfusion is the result of arterial or venous insufficiency, or both. Position the patient appropriately. In venous insufficiency, feet should be elevated to promote venous return. In arterial insufficiency, feet should be dependent to the heart or on a straight plane to foster gravitational flow to the extremity. Tell the patient to avoid crossing the legs, wearing constrictive shoes

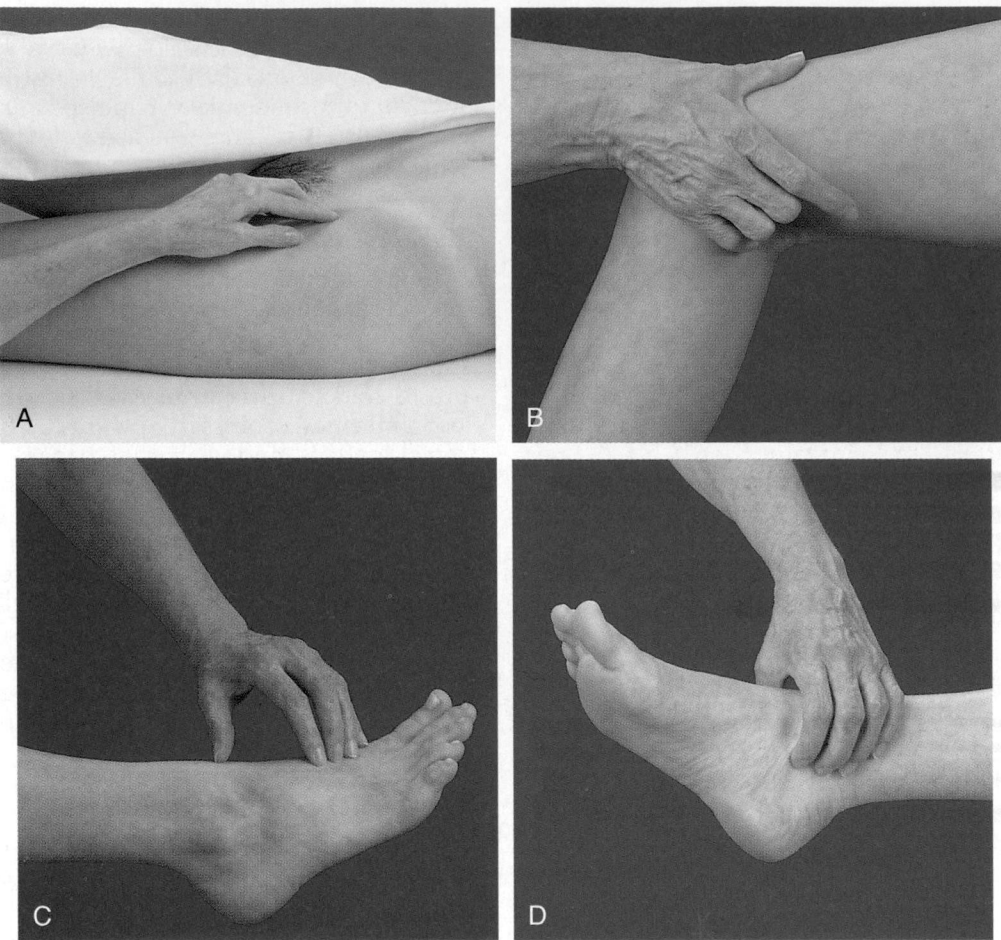

Figure 9–9

Palpating distal pulses. *A*, Femoral. *B*, Popliteal. *C*, Dorsalis pedis. *D*, Posterior tibial.

or clothing, or using the knee gatch on hospital beds because these impede blood flow.

Encourage moderate muscular activity, such as graded extremity exercise or walking short distances several times a day. Muscular contraction promotes development of collateral circulation and increases blood flow. Collateral channels for blood flow may decrease the speed at which symptoms of arterial or venous insufficiency develop.

NDx: Risk for impaired skin integrity
Continue daily assessment of skin for changes in color, temperature, and integrity (see Table 9–2). Document any changes seen.

Urge the patient and family to perform daily skin and foot care and to observe the skin and feet closely when they do. Teach the patient to keep the skin clean, warm, and dry by washing with warm water and mild soap and blotting dry gently and thoroughly. This will decrease bacterial count on the skin and help improve blood flow. Tell the patient to apply a lanolin-based lotion after cleansing. Lotion keeps the skin soft and prevents cracks or fis-

sures that could be a portal to infection. Before cutting toenails, tell the patient to soften them by soaking them in warm water for 10 minutes. Then cut straight across to prevent ingrowth. Recommend consultation with a podiatrist if the patient has extremely thick nails.

Instruct the patient to report promptly to the physician any cuts, abrasions, or lesions that do not show evidence of healing after 2 or 3 days. Explain the need to seek medical attention immediately for abrupt onset of pain, discoloration, and temperature change.

Use a bed cradle, if needed, to protect the affected extremity from injury caused by pressure from linens. Teach the patient to avoid direct heat from heating devices and to use nonconstricting footlets or socks to keep the feet warm. Maintain an environmental temperature of 21 to 23.5°C (70–74°F).

Assess risk factors and stress the importance of controlling them. Discourage smoking because nicotine is a powerful vasoconstrictor. Discuss strategies to reduce stress, which will reduce the release of norepinephrine and epinephrine. These catechol-

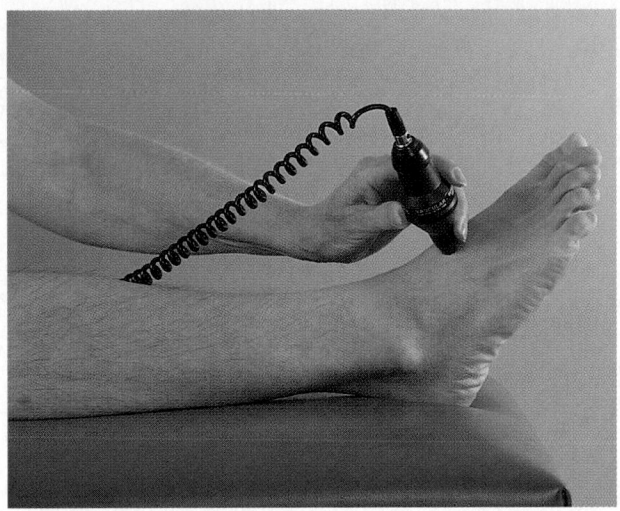

Figure 9-10
Doppler transducer placed on the dorsalis pedis pulse for audible recording.

amines cause vasoconstriction, especially in peripheral tissues.

Manage ulcerations per physician's protocol. Carefully document progression of wound healing.

Compare the patient's status with the expected outcomes. If the outcomes are not met, reassess the patient and revise the plan.

Assessment of the Vascular System

The health history, along with identification of risk factors for vascular disease, is the most important part of diagnosing a peripheral vascular problem. A physical assessment follows the history so that specific problems can be identified and a plan for care established.

HEALTH HISTORY

The health history is an organized method of eliciting comprehensive, pertinent information from a patient regarding past and present health in relation to the peripheral vascular status. This information allows you to formulate a database for problem identification. The health history serves to direct attention toward specific body systems during the physical examination and allows observation of the patient during responses to the questions. Time must be allowed during the health history to establish a relationship of trust with the patient by listening attentively and with concern and by allowing the patient to assume an active, integral role in his or her health care.

Collect the appropriate data using understand-

able terminology and allow the patient to respond fully and voice concerns. Ask the patient about the history of the present illness or disorder. Inquire about the patient's chief complaint and obtain a detailed description of it. If pain is the most significant problem, ask for the location, intensity, duration, precipitating factors, and relief methods. For example, the patient may indicate that pain occurs in the calves but only after walking short distances and it stops after resting for a few moments. Ask whether this happens every time the patient walks or just at specific times. Find out how severe the pain becomes and if it is always relieved by rest.

Ask the patient about past medical problems, medications, and surgeries. Also ask about the family history of illness. Determine the patient's usual activities of daily living and whether the present condition interferes with the normal daily routine. Complete a brief review of systems, determining whether dysfunctions in any other system are affecting peripheral vascular status. Carefully document the information obtained.

Assess the patient's understanding and compliance with health promotion and risk reduction measures related to the peripheral vascular system (Highlight 9-1).

RISK FACTORS

The risk factors for peripheral vascular disease are essentially the same as those for coronary artery disease (see Chapter 7). Review them with the patient to assess the patient's risk level. Determine the patient's understanding of the risk factors and the importance of reducing risk for vascular disease when possible. Some risk factors, such as age and sex, cannot be modified. Men over age 50 have a higher incidence of peripheral vascular disease than women of the same age. Elderly male diabetic smokers have the highest incidence.

Elevated cholesterol levels are associated with atherosclerosis and resultant peripheral vascular problems. Current recommended blood cholesterol levels are as follows:

- Desirable: Less than 200 mg/dL
- Borderline to high risk: 200 to 239 mg/dL
- High risk: 240 mg/dL or more

Most cholesterol is contained in low-density lipoproteins. High-density lipoproteins remove cholesterol from the blood and return it to the liver. Table 9-3 summarizes modifiable risk factors for peripheral dysfunction.

PHYSICAL EXAMINATION

Complete a general inspection, focusing on the overall appearance of the patient and the extremities. In particular, note skin color, temperature, and integrity. Note obvious venous insufficiency, which may

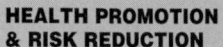 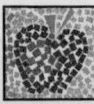

Methods for Optimizing Peripheral Vascular Function and Reducing Risk Factors for Peripheral Vascular Disease

- Begin an exercise program, walking to the limits of pain. Rest, and then continue to walk. Set a goal of 1 mile a day.
- If a smoker, join a smoking cessation program. Rejoin if you have tried unsuccessfully to stop in the past.
- Modify the diet to reduce fat consumption and cholesterol intake.
- If overweight, begin a reasonable weight reduction program that includes calorie reduction and moderate exercise.
- Have blood pressure checked routinely.
- Make lifestyle adjustments and behavioral changes (such as reducing stress) as needed to improve overall health.
- Visit a physician yearly for evaluation, including laboratory assessments focused on the cardiovascular system.

be evident by tortuous veins, peripheral edema, and brown pigmentation. Poor color, a cool skin temperature, or the presence of edema or lesions indicate potential peripheral vascular disease. Check the nail beds for color and clubbing. Hair on the extremity may be diminished or absent. Skin may be thin, fragile, and shiny, which indicates poor circulation to the area. Note any areas of localized redness or cyanosis.

Assessment of the pulses is a first-line diagnostic test. This assessment is ongoing after many invasive diagnostic procedures, vascular surgery, and daily nursing care of the patient with peripheral vascular disease. Evaluation of the pulses is an essential and reliable indicator of the progression or severity of peripheral arterial insufficiency or arterial occlusive disease.

Compare both extremities at one time and evaluate pulses for their presence or absence. Note the amplitude, equality, rate, and rhythm of the pulse. Pulse amplitude is rated on a scale of 0 to 4.

0   not present
1   weakly present
2   slightly diminished
3   normal
4   full and bounding

Begin with the most distal pulses and proceed upward. If an occlusion exists, pulses below it will be affected. Begin assessing pulses in this order: dorsalis pedis, posterior tibial, popliteal, and femoral (see Fig. 9–9). Congenital absence of either the dorsalis pedis or posterior tibial can occur, but

Table 9–3

Modifiable Risk Factors	
Elevated lipid levels	Directly associated with atheromatous plaque buildup.
	Diet and exercise can lower LDL levels.
Obesity	Raises blood lipid levels, increasing deposition of atheromatous plaque.
	Greater tissue needs for circulation.
	Associated with decreased physical mobility and activity, which raises LDL levels.
Sedentary lifestyle	Increased LDL.
	Exercise promotes utilization of lipids and raises level of beneficial HDL.
Stress	Blood coagulates more easily.
	Vasoconstriction of peripheral vessels.
	Related to an increase in LDL.
	Decreases immune response.
Cigarette smoking	Direct stimulation of the sympathetic nervous system.
	Peripheral vasoconstriction is immediate and lasts up to 1 hour.
	Even one cigarette affects platelets, making them more "sticky," and increases platelet aggregation.
	Carbon monoxide damages red blood cells' ability to carry oxygen to nourish tissues.
	Increased chance of blood clot formation.
Elevated lipid levels	Directly associated with atheromatous plaque buildup.
	Diet and exercise can lower LDL levels.
Hypertension	Arterial walls damaged from elevated blood pressure become thickened and demand more oxygenation.
Diabetes	Associated with high incidence and accelerated rate of peripheral vascular disease, especially in distal vessels.
	Damage to microcirculation.
	Poor wound healing from tissue malnourishment.

HDL, high-density lipoproteins ("good cholesterol"); LDL, low-density lipoproteins ("bad cholesterol").

this defect does not affect both of these distal pulses in any one individual. Use Doppler ultrasonography (see Fig. 9–10) on sites of absent pulses because it can detect blood flow that is not palpable. Auscultate with a stethoscope for bruits, especially over the popliteal, femoral, and abdominal areas.

Assess arterial flow by having the patient lie flat with the arms (or legs) raised above heart level. Have the patient wave the extremities for a few moments. Then have the patient sit upright. The extremity appears slightly pale at first, but color should return within 10 seconds. Delayed pallor or mottling indicates arterial insufficiency. Compare the extremities bilaterally and document all findings.

Diagnostic Procedures

Numerous diagnostic studies are used for peripheral vascular dysfunction. They are classified as noninva-

Table 9–4

Common Arterial Diagnostic Studies

Study	Purpose	Procedure
NONINVASIVE		
Doppler ultrasonography	Detection of disrupted flow in arteries or veins caused by stenosis, occlusion, thrombus. Used when pulses are not palpable. Sound frequencies produced relate to blow flood and velocity.	Conductive jelly applied to skin. Doppler flowmeter detects flow through vessels and magnifies sound. Differences in pitch noted. Doppler ultrasonogram used with a blood pressure cuff to obtain thigh, calf, ankle pressures.
Doppler treadmill	Measurement of ankle pressures with exercise to test for intermittent claudication.	Patient walks on a treadmill after Doppler study until claudication pain develops. Doppler ultrasonogram again records extremity pressures.
Cold stimulation test	Determination of temperature changes in fingers. Used to diagnose Raynaud's phenomenon.	Thermistors are attached to fingers, and baseline temperature obtained. Fingers are submerged in ice water for 20 seconds. Temperature measured every 5 minutes until pretest temperature established.
INVASIVE		
Angiogram (arteriogram, arterial angiography, or arteriography)	Visualize arteries and assess blood flow. Detect obstruction, narrowing or aneurysm, collateral circulation.	Iodine-based contrast medium injected into artery. X-ray films taken. Test takes 1 to 2 hours.
Digital subtraction angiography	Visualize arteries and assess blood flow. Detect obstruction, narrowing, aneurysm, collateral circulation.	Computer-based techniques make vessel-specific images of arteries. Fluoroscopic image intensifier displays vessel. Data fed to computer. Images not required are subtracted to provide detailed image of desired area of study.
Lumbar sympathetic block	Determine feasibility of sympathectomy to provide increased flow in extremity by blocking vasoconstriction input from sympathetic nervous system.	Procaine hydrochloride, a local anesthetic, is injected to block sympathetic nerves at the 2nd to 3rd lumbar vertebra. Patient observed for warming of the extremity or decrease in pain.

sive or invasive. Tables 9–4 and 9–5 summarize arterial and venous diagnostic testing, respectively.

Explain to the patient the purpose and procedures involved in the diagnostic examination to alleviate anxiety and elicit cooperation. Provide time for the patient to ask questions (Nursing Care Guide 9–1). All invasive diagnostic procedures require a signed informed consent. Table 9–6 summarizes nursing actions for patients undergoing invasive venography or arteriography.

Table 9–5

Common Venous Diagnostic Studies

Study	Purpose	Procedure
NONINVASIVE		
Impedance plethysmography	Evaluate patency of iliac or femoral veins. Gain information on changes in venous volume after impedance. Measure electrical resistance in veins related to blood volume.	Electrodes wrapped around calf. Pressure cuff inflated on thigh to impede venous flow. Cuff deflated rapidly and venous flow measured. Normally, impedance increases venous volume; if volume remains the same, test is positive for blockage caused by clot along with presence of Homans' sign or other symptoms of DVT.
Perthes' test	Evaluate the competence of valves in saphenous vein, varicose veins, or DVT.	Tourniquet applied around thigh or knee. Patient asked to walk. Previously distended veins collapse if valves are competent. Veins remain distended if obstruction or incompetent valves.
Doppler ultrasonogram	Detect auditory signs of blood flow. Sound waves bounced off RBCs in vein or artery can detect incompetent valves. Sounds of retrograde flow can be discriminated.	Conductive jelly applied to skin. Doppler flowmeter detects flow through vessels and magnifies sound. Differences in pitch noted. Doppler ultrasonogram used with a BP cuff to obtain thigh, calf, ankle pressures.
INVASIVE		
Angiogram (venogram or venography)	Visually examine veins and valves. Definitive examination to visualize clots.	Contrast medium (50 mL) injected into veins. Procedure is dangerous and contraindicated in patients with suspected or acute phlebitis. Examination can precipitate thrombophlebitis.
Digital subtraction venography	Visualize veins and assess blood flow.	Computer-based techniques make vessel-specific images of veins.
Radionuclide venography	Detect early thrombi in leg veins. Useful in patients too ill for venogram. Not useful for thrombus in pelvis or femoral area.	Radioactive fibrinogen-125 is injected. If thrombi are present, iodine isotope will combine with existing clot. Clot then can be detected with scintillator scan counter. Scan done 12 and 24 hours after injection.

BP, blood pressure; DVT, deep venous thrombosis; RBCs, red blood cells.

Nursing Care Guide 9–1

Patients Undergoing Diagnostic Testing for Peripheral Vascular Dysfunction

Assessment Findings: Patient presents with signs of restlessness, nervousness, increased respiratory and heart rate; asks questions about procedures; and clenches hands and cries.

Nursing Diagnosis: Anxiety related to fear of procedure, diagnosis, and future medical/surgical management

Patient Outcomes	Nursing Interventions	Rationale
Patient practices relaxation techniques for relief of tension and anxiety.	Teach relaxation techniques. Help the patient find coping strategies that help alleviate the stress and anxiety.	Implementation of relaxation exercises reduces stress and anxiety.
Patient appears less anxious, as evidenced by smiling; lack of restlessness, crying, or nervousness; and vital signs within normal limits.	Explain the diagnostic procedure to the patient and family. Allow time for questions and concerns. Check vital signs.	An understanding of the procedure may alleviate some of the fear and anxiety. Vital signs within normal limits may indicate relief of anxiety.

Evaluation: Compare the patient's status with the expected outcomes. If the outcomes are not met, reassess the patient and revise the plan.

Assessment Findings: Patient and family ask questions about the diagnostic procedure and seem uninformed about preprocedure and postprocedure care. Patient and family voice concerns about risks and necessity for the procedure, especially if an invasive test is to be done.

Nursing Diagnosis: Knowledge deficit: nature of the diagnostic procedure and postprocedure care

Patient Outcomes	Nursing Interventions	Rationale
Patient and family state they have an understanding of the diagnostic procedure, the risks, and the postprocedure care needed, if applicable.	Be certain the physician has discussed the procedure, risks, complications, and expectations with the patient.	An understanding of the procedure is important to increase patient compliance and reduce fears about the diagnostic testing.
	Give the patient and family literature about the procedure if available. Allow the patient to ask questions, and try to expand the patient's and family's understanding of the procedure.	Including the family in the sessions reinforces the information provided. Misinformation can be corrected during the question session.
Patient reports accurate information about the diagnostic procedure, the potential risks, and the necessity for the procedure.	Have the patient restate the information received.	Reiterating the information allows an assessment of the patient's understanding.
	Explain the postprocedure care needed.	
	Tell the patient to notify the physician if any untoward symptoms occur after discharge.	Follow-up care is necessary to prevent complications.

Evaluation Compare the patient's status with the expected outcomes. If the outcomes are not met, reassess the patient and revise the plan.

Table 9–6

Nursing Actions for Invasive Contrast Media Studies: Arteriography and Venography

Action	Rationale
BEFORE PROCEDURE	
1. Check extremities to obtain baseline data: Pulse Color Sensation Temperature Movement Vital signs	Baseline data are used for postprocedure comparison. Changes in neurovascular parameters after procedure indicate increased occlusion and limb-threatening ischemia.
2. Assess patient for allergy to iodine or seafood.	Iodine is used in contrast medium injected during the procedure. Allergic reaction and anaphylactic shock could occur.
3. Clarify purpose and patient involvement during procedure and explain that contrast medium causes feeling of warmth or burning during injection.	Clarification alleviates anxiety and ensures patient cooperation.
4. Obtain informed consent.	These are invasive procedures that require legal documentation of the patient's informed consent.
DURING AND AFTER PROCEDURE	
1. Observe for signs and symptoms of allergic reaction: Dyspnea Flushing or hives Nausea or vomiting Tachycardia or hypotension Numbness in extremity	Allergic reactions may occur during or even a few hours after the procedure.
2. Monitor and compare baseline vital signs, extremity pulses, and neurovascular integrity, per recovery protocol, beginning every 15 minutes and then hourly for up to 4 hours.	Changes in vital signs may indicate complications.
3. Check extremity for the following: Pulses Pallor Cyanosis Decreased temperature Numbness or paralysis	Bleeding and neurovascular compromise can be life- or limb-threatening.
4. Maintain patient on bedrest with extremity extended for 4 to 6 hours after procedure.	Rest helps reduce bleeding.
5. Check injection site dressing for bleeding or hematoma with each vital sign and neurovascular assessment.	Bleeding may indicate serious complications.
6. Encourage oral fluids.	Consumption of oral fluids enhances excretion of contrast media.

Management

The overall objective in managing patients with peripheral vascular dysfunction is to increase blood flow to the ischemic tissues. The approaches taken depend on the acuteness of the disease process. Specific management is discussed with each disorder in Chapter 10. This chapter includes some general approaches to management.

NONSURGICAL MANAGEMENT

Conservative approaches to management include reduction of risk factors, exercise, and medication.

Nonsurgical procedures such as angioplasty and laser thermal angioplasty are common nonsurgical techniques used for some patients to improve peripheral circulation.

Reduction of Risk Factors

A reduction in modifiable risk factors is accomplished through diet, exercise, and other lifestyle adjustments. For patients with high cholesterol levels and atherosclerosis, drug therapy may be instituted. Cigarette smoking is discouraged. Education is provided to assist the patient in changing behaviors. Routine medical evaluation with laboratory assessments is prescribed (see Highlight 9–1).

Exercise

A slow, progressive exercise program can be effective for patients with intermittent claudication if they have no contraindication or performance deficit, such as severe respiratory, cardiac, or musculoskeletal dysfunction. Exercise is also beneficial in reducing some modifiable risk factors. The patient may be referred to an exercise therapist for a prescribed regimen of physical activity.

Medications

A combination of drugs may be used in arterial peripheral vascular disease, but their efficacy in improving circulation is questionable because atherosclerosis—the basic problem—is irreversible. At best, they may provide some relief of symptoms or prevent further arterial plaque accumulation. These medications include vasodilators, hypolipemics, anticoagulants, defibrination agents, and antiplatelet therapy (Highlights 9–2 and 9–3). Drug therapy may improve blood flow at rest but has a negligible effect on the increased tissue oxygenation needs with activity. Table 9–7 summarizes some representative drugs used.

Pain management is a challenge. Pain relief may not be fully accomplished until measures are taken to remove the source of pain: the obstructed blood flow. Narcotic and non-narcotic analgesics are used to control the pain of advanced ischemia. The patient commonly requires increasing doses as the disease progresses. It is important to keep the analgesic level stable. Instruct the patient to ask for medication before the pain becomes intolerable. Patient-controlled analgesia is usually used. It has the added benefit of increasing the patient's sense of control and decreasing powerlessness in coping with the pain.

Sustained-action morphine sulfate (MS Contin) is a 12-hour sustained-release tablet that may provide relief. Sympathetic nerve blocks are occasionally used when other analgesics have failed.

Angioplasty

Peripheral angioplasty is a nonsurgical but invasive procedure. Percutaneous transluminal angioplasty involves insertion of an inflatable balloon-tipped catheter into an identified area of arterial blockage. The balloon is inflated, compressing atherosclerotic plaque and thereby enlarging and smoothing the lumen of the affected vessel and increasing blood flow. Blockages in the iliac and femoral arteries have had the greatest success with percutaneous transluminal angioplasty. The procedure can be repeated if the vessel reoccludes. Reocclusion of the artery may be immediate. Thirty percent of vessels reocclude during the first 6 months. Many arteries remain patent from 1 to 5 years. The procedure is of benefit

for patients who are poor surgical risks, because local anesthesia is used. Successful angioplasty restores pulses, improves extremity tissue integrity, and abates or lessens claudication pain.

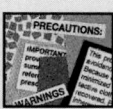

HIGHLIGHT
9–2
PHARMACOLOGY

Lipid-Lowering Drugs (Hypolipemics)

Definition:

Lipid-lowering drugs used in patients with levels of hyperlipoproteinemia that are associated with an increased risk of atherosclerosis and its complications.

Action:

The prototype drug, cholestyramine (Questran), lowers cholesterol by binding with bile acids in the intestine, changing cholesterol into an insoluble complex that is eliminated in feces. Lovastatin (Mevacor) blocks the enzyme necessary for the synthesis of cholesterol in the liver.

Use:

As adjunct therapy when diet, exercise, weight reduction, and other nonpharmacologic methods of risk-factor control have failed to reduce blood lipid levels.

Side Effects:

May interfere with or enhance oral absorption of anticoagulants. The bile-sequestering resins may interfere with absorption of vitamin K and thus reduce prothrombin. They can produce flatulence, constipation, liver function abnormalities, diarrhea, abdominal pain, or heartburn. They interfere with absorption of digitalis, folic acid, and corticosteroids.

Interactions:

Bile acid sequestrants and vitamins A, D, E, and K (may bind with the vitamins).

Nursing Implications:

Establish baseline lipid levels before therapy is begun and periodically during therapy. Administer routine medications before meals or 4 hours after. Monitor for bleeding tendencies. Assess for constipation, especially in the elderly. Report gastrointestinal symptoms that persist. Lipid-lowering drugs are contraindicated in pregnancy.

HIGHLIGHT
9–3
PHARMACOLOGY
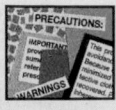
Anticoagulants

Definition:

Drugs that affect the ability of blood to form fibrin clots. Anticoagulants include heparin, warfarin sodium, and dicumarol.

Action:

Inhibit various stages of the blood-clotting cycle depending on the specific anticoagulant.

Uses:

Treatment of deep vein thrombosis, pulmonary emboli, myocardial infarction, and rheumatic heart disease. Also prevention of clot formation.

Side Effects:

Excessive anticoagulation, causing petechiae, bruising, hematomas, ecchymoses, and hemorrhage.

Interactions:

May interact with other protein-bound drugs, such as salicylates. Metabolism of anticoagulants may also be enhanced by drugs that increase liver enzyme production.

Nursing Implications:

Check coagulation studies before giving each dose of anticoagulant and intermittently throughout the patient's hospital stay. Check frequently for signs of bleeding, such as petechiae and ecchymoses. Teach the patient to practice safety measures to prevent cuts and scratches because they may bleed excessively.

Geriatric Considerations:

Bruising, especially on the hands, arms, and legs, and bleeding of mucous membranes may be more prominent. Special safety and care measures are needed to prevent injury and bleeding episodes because capillaries are more fragile in the older adult.

Complications of angioplasty include stenosis, thrombi formation, embolism, and bleeding. Heparin typically is given for 3 days after the procedure. The patient is prescribed home-maintenance antiplatelet therapy with aspirin.

Laser Thermal Angioplasty

Laser thermal angioplasty can be performed in conjunction with percutaneous transluminal angioplasty. The laser-tipped fiberoptic catheter heats to approximately 400°C, vaporizes the atherosclerotic plaque, and opens a channel for blood flow. This procedure is believed to produce a smoother vessel lumen and a decreased frequency of reocclusion.

NURSING PROCESS GUIDELINES
Angioplasty

Nursing care for the patient undergoing angioplasty is essentially the same as with arteriography (see Table 9–6). Preprocedure, instruct the patient to eat nothing by mouth (NPO) for 8 hours before the procedure. The groin area is prepared with a surgical scrub. The physician may order the area shaved before the scrub.

After the procedure, the patient will be on bed rest, with the affected extremity maintained in straight alignment for 6 to 8 hours. Monitor laboratory values for prolonged clotting times because the patient is commonly heparinized during and after the procedure. Blood coagulation studies include prothrombin time, international normalized ratio (INR), partial thromboplastin time, and activated clotting time. Activated clotting time can be done at the bedside. Desirable levels for these laboratory tests to maintain vessel patency is two times the control level. (See Chap. 12 for explanation of these diagnostic tests.)

Assess for bleeding or hematoma formation at the angioplasty insertion site. Palpate the tissues around the site for distention from hematoma. Measure abdominal girth every 4 hours for patients with iliac artery angioplasty. They are more likely to manifest retroperitoneal bleeding. Monitor for signs of shock from retroperitoneal hemorrhage. Highlight 9–4 contains general instructions for the patient after angioplasty.

SURGICAL MANAGEMENT

Management by surgical intervention is necessary when ischemic pain interferes with activity and threatens tissue loss. Many surgical procedures can restore circulation and thus decrease pain and improve tissue integrity. These procedures may help to improve the patient's quality of life.

Grafts

A bypass graft leaves the diseased area intact but bypasses it with a graft, either the patient's saphenous vein or a synthetic material. The saphenous vein is the preferred grafting material, but many patients have concomitant coronary artery disease and the saphenous vein may have already been

Table 9–7

Medications Used in Peripheral Vascular Disease

Classification	Drug	Effects
Vasodilator	Isoxuprine hydrochloride (Vasodilan)	Acts directly on vascular smooth muscles. High doses also inhibit platelet aggregation and decrease blood viscosity.
Antiplatelet or defibrination agent	Pentoxifylline (Trental)	Makes RBCs more flexible, thereby facilitating movement through the capillary. Decreases platelet and RBC aggregation and decreases blood viscosity.
Antiplatelet	Aspirin	Powerfully inhibits platelet aggregation. Effects may persist 3 to 8 days.
Antiplatelet and vasodilator	Dipyridamole (Persantine)	Vasodilation effects are only slight in peripheral arteries. Drug inhibits platelet aggregation. It is usually prescribed with aspirin.
Anticoagulant	Heparin	Prevention of clot (thrombosis) formation by blocking several factors essential to normal blood clotting. It is used prophylactically or in acute disease states.

used or may be needed for a future coronary artery bypass graft. In this case, an arm vein may be used. Before grafting, arteriography is performed to look at the blood flow in vessels below the obstruction and to find the best location for the graft. Bypass grafting is preferred over excision and replacement grafting because collateral circulation is maintained. The success rate of grafting is better in larger vessels. The successful re-establishment of blood flow is evidenced by return of pulses, warming of the extremity, and decreased ischemic pain.

A patch graft removes the diseased part of the artery and replaces it with a "patch" from the patient's vein, usually the saphenous vein. This method is preferred over a synthetic graft made of Dacron or Teflon because thrombosis is less likely to occur. A vein patch may also be used to widen an artery.

PATIENT PREPARATION

Inform the patient about nursing procedures that will be implemented before surgery and about the usual postoperative course. Begin physical preparation after the patient gives informed consent. Prepare the surgical site per protocol. Administer prophylactic antibiotics if they are ordered.

POSTOPERATIVE COURSE

If the surgically revascularized vessel remains patent, the postoperative course is usually uneventful. The patient will be ambulating on the first postoperative day. Anticoagulation therapy is typically instituted using heparin or low-molecular-weight dextran to prevent thrombus formation. Postoperative noninvasive arterial studies give baseline information for future management. The graft should be

---

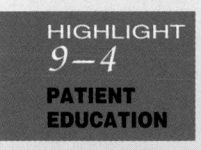 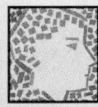

HIGHLIGHT
9–4
PATIENT
EDUCATION

General Patient Instructions After Angioplasty

Instruct the patient to:

- Remain on bedrest with extremity extended for 4 to 6 hours after procedure.
- If discharge is the same day, plan for a driver other than yourself.
- Observe for active bleeding or bruising at the puncture site.
- Check the extremities for pallor, coldness, discoloration, numbness, or tingling.
- Drink an increased amount of fluid, unless otherwise contraindicated, to assist the excretion of the contrast media.
- Check for temperature elevation because it may indicate an infection.
- Check the puncture site for drainage (other than bleeding) or swelling because it may indicate localized infection.
- Notify the physician if any of the symptoms listed above occur.

followed with noninvasive studies every 3 months for the first year, every 6 months for the second year, and yearly thereafter, or as needed if claudication symptoms return.

COMPLICATIONS

The most common postoperative complication is graft occlusion. It usually occurs in the first 24 hours. Other complications include bleeding, infection, and delayed wound healing resulting from the effects of prolonged tissue ischemia.

Embolectomy

An embolectomy is the surgical removal of a clot (thrombus) from the vessel. This procedure is performed when a major vessel is acutely occluded, thus impeding blood flow to a large area of tissue. Ischemia is severe. Distal extremities become cyanotic and mottled. Often, this surgery is an emergency. It is most successful when performed within 10 hours after the clot has formed. Anticoagulant therapy is used postoperatively to prevent further thrombus formation (see Highlight 9–3).

Endarterectomy

Endarterectomy is the surgical removal of fatty plaques from the inner (tunica intima) and middle (tunica media) layers of vessel walls. The artery is incised, cleaned out, and then sutured closed. An endarterectomy is most successful with localized atheromatous plaque. This procedure is contraindicated in patients with aneurysmal changes, total occlusion of the aortic branch to renal arteries, or a major aortic occlusion that extends into the iliac and femoral arteries.

Amputation

Surgical removal of part or all of an extremity may be the only therapeutic option when tissues are hopelessly ischemic, painful, and gangrenous. It is often the culmination of months of ischemic rest pain and progressive tissue degeneration. Approximately 85% of all surgical amputations result from severe peripheral vascular circulatory impairment. Elderly people with arterial disease constitute the largest amputation population group. Of this group, diabetic elderly male smokers have the highest amputation rate. Even though the surgical procedure provides relief from the ischemic pain, it greatly disrupts the independence and coping ability of an elderly person.

The level of amputation is dictated by peripheral vascular diagnostic studies. In arterial obstructive gangrene, these studies demonstrate the location where circulation is adequate to provide optimal tissue healing after the surgery.

The length of time needed for the patient to resume functional upright ambulation depends on how well the stump heals, adequacy of circulation in the remaining leg, the patient's overall health, and personal motivation. Ambulation with a prosthesis requires a tremendous expenditure of energy and coordination. It may not be a viable option for a person with a peripheral vascular disease–induced amputation. The optimal goal may be the patient's eventual acceptance of wheelchair independence.

Loss of an extremity is always a devastating event. In fact, the grieving process may start even before the amputation occurs. Support the patient throughout the process to help hasten acceptance of a changed body image.

Many arterial disease–induced amputations could be prevented by meticulous foot care and prevention of cuts and abrasions of the extremities. The foot is quite vulnerable, being the most distal to the area of ischemic flow. Wound healing is impaired because of the poor tissue nutrition. Dry, gangrenous toe tips with no evidence of infection or cellulitis may be allowed to autoamputate. This is a nonsurgical spontaneous separation of the devitalized tissue.

NURSING PROCESS
Peripheral Vascular Surgery

PREOPERATIVE NURSING CARE

Assessment

Obtain a history and perform a complete physical assessment to evaluate the health status of all body systems. Determine risk factors presented by nutritional deficits, lifestyle, and involvement of cardiac, respiratory, or endocrine systems that could complicate surgery.

Nursing Diagnoses and Planning

Nursing diagnoses and related expected patient outcomes commonly applicable to patients scheduled for peripheral vascular surgery include the following:

NDx: Knowledge deficit: surgical procedure and postoperative course

Planning: Patient Outcomes
1. Patient states accurate information about the surgical procedure and expected results.
2. Patient describes the typical postoperative course.

Nursing Interventions and Evaluation

NDx: Knowledge deficit: surgical procedure and postoperative course

Assess the patient's understanding of the surgical procedure, its risks, the usual postoperative course, and self-care responsibilities after discharge. Explain all facets of the procedure, the recovery period, and the postoperative care required. Tell the patient about medications, activity progression, and routine postoperative deep-breathing exercises. Provide time for the patient and family to ask questions and verbalize concerns.

Compare the patient's status with the expected outcomes. If the outcomes are not met, reassess the patient and revise the plan.

POSTOPERATIVE NURSING CARE

Assessment

Assess the dressing for bleeding and the patient's vital signs, level of consciousness, respiratory pattern, skin temperature, and skin color. Check the integrity of the intravenous site. Evaluate the patient's level of pain.

Complete a critical assessment of pulses and other parameters of neurovascular compromise that indicate thrombosis or reocclusion. Monitor results of blood coagulation studies for abnormal bleeding times.

Nursing Diagnoses and Planning

Nursing diagnoses and related expected patient outcomes commonly applicable to patients undergoing peripheral vascular surgery include the following:

NDx: Altered peripheral tissue perfusion related to thrombus formation or reocclusion induced by existing vascular dysfunction or excessive bleeding

Planning: Patient Outcomes
1. Patient exhibits palpable pulses and adequate temperature, sensation, and color in extremities.
2. Quality of pulse and/or Doppler signal remains the same or improves, but does not diminish.
3. Excessive bleeding is absent.
4. Patient experiences no ischemic pain.
5. Patient's laboratory coagulation studies are within safe range.

NDx: Risk for infection related to surgical incision, location, length, and presurgical tissue integrity

Planning: Patient Outcomes
1. Patient demonstrates a dry, nondraining wound with no evidence of erythema or swelling.
2. Patient is free from signs of infection (afebrile, normal white blood cell count).

NDx: Pain related to incision or acute postsurgical thrombus occlusion

Planning: Patient Outcomes
1. Patient states pain is relieved.

2. Patient is able to mobilize freely without extreme discomfort.
3. Patient is able to participate in self-care.

NDx: Altered health maintenance related to lack of knowledge of self-care after discharge

Planning: Patient Outcomes
1. Patient relates accurate information about wound care, medications, potential complications, and the need to seek medical attention if these occur.
2. Patient palpates pulses and inspects incision and skin daily for changes in color, temperature, and integrity.
3. Patient is able to increase activity as prescribed.
4. Patient states the need for follow-up care.

Nursing Interventions and Evaluation

NDx: Altered peripheral tissue perfusion
Monitor neurocirculatory status for signs of reocclusion. Ask the patient to report changes in color or sensation. Assess pulses, mark location of distal pulses, and use Doppler ultrasonography for nonpalpable pulses. Check color, sensation, temperature, and motor ability in the affected extremities. Document the changes. Notify the physician of abnormalities because sudden changes may indicate acute occlusion, which requires emergency medical intervention.

Ask the patient to wiggle the toes and to perform dorsiflexion and flexion of the plantar area of the foot. Note any complaints of pain in the extremity at rest or excessive pain with movement. Check for paresthesia. Measure the girth of the extremity and check for swelling. Document findings for a postoperative baseline. Some swelling is expected as the result of surgical tissue trauma and as a rebound effect of tissues becoming revascularized after a period of ischemic flow. Edema can also be caused by hemorrhage into the tissues from a leaking graft. Excessive accumulation of fluid in the muscle compartment can compromise tissue perfusion and cause nerve compression, resulting in compartment syndrome (increased pressure within a fascial muscle compartment). Classic signs of compartment syndrome include excessive pain at rest that increases with movement, and paresthesias. Notify the physician immediately. The patient may require an emergency fasciotomy.

Keep the extremity in straight alignment per physician's protocol, usually for 24 hours after major grafting. Position the patient off the graft site or drains. Avoid extreme flexion of the extremity. These interventions prevent trauma to the graft and promote optimal circulation.

Monitor vital signs for evidence of shock. Elevated blood pressure can place too much stress on the graft and cause rupture and hemorrhage. Diminished blood pressure can cause low flow states, stasis, and occlusion.

NDx: Risk for infection

Use strict aseptic technique when changing dressings or handling intravenous equipment. Monitor temperature and white blood cell count. Inspect the incision for warmth, erythema, swelling, unusual drainage, and wound approximation.

Observe and prevent skin breakdown with position changes and early mobilization. Have the patient cough and deep-breathe every 2 hours to prevent respiratory infection.

NDx: Pain

Manage operative pain with prescribed analgesics and note how the patient responds. Encourage the patient to verbalize discomfort before pain becomes intolerable; patient-controlled analgesia is often used. Incisional pain is usually the greatest during the first 4 postoperative days. Revascularization pain is sometimes experienced as a throbbing sensation. The return of ischemic pain indicates reocclusion. Notify the physician immediately.

NDx: Altered health maintenance

Teach the patient how to care for the surgical incision and how to complete an aseptic dressing change. Explain the signs and symptoms of complications and when to seek medical intervention. Inform the patient of activity restrictions, such as avoiding long periods of sitting, leg crossing, extreme flexion, and heavy lifting. Reinforce teaching of the prescribed progression of ambulation. Teach how to perform pulse checks and assess extremities. Reinforce teaching on the importance of daily foot care and the reduction of risk factors for peripheral vascular dysfunction.

Compare the patient's status with the expected outcomes. If the outcomes are not met, reassess the patient and revise the plan.

❖ Settings, Providers, and Collaboration for Care

Patients with peripheral vascular dysfunction are commonly diagnosed in outpatient clinics and treated in the home. Frail elderly patients may be treated in intermediate care facilities or nursing homes. Patients with severe peripheral perfusion problems or with other complicating diseases, such as diabetes, may be hospitalized during the acute phase of treatment.

It takes a collaborative effort by several health professionals to establish a therapeutic regimen that allows the patient to manage the pain and skin integrity problems created by peripheral vascular dysfunction. The nurse works with the physician and patient to establish pain control methods that meet the patient's needs. Patients treated in the home may need referral to a home health agency. The nurse instructs the patient and family members about the prescribed regimen and monitors the patient's progress. Intermittent evaluation of the patient's success at pain management and skin care is necessary so that changes can be made as needed.

A podiatrist can be helpful in providing proper foot care, especially in diabetic patients or those with severe circulatory impairment. A referral can be made to an exercise therapist for a prescriptive plan of physical activity based on the patient's particular needs and abilities.

The Elderly: Special Considerations

Peripheral vascular disease is a common disorder of later adulthood. The elderly comprise the largest peripheral vascular disease population group. Older men who smoke have the highest incidence of dysfunction of the vascular system. Diabetes, which is also increasing in the elderly population, increases the incidence of atherosclerosis, severe perfusion problems in the extremities, and risk for amputation.

Changes in blood vessel integrity occur with aging even without disease. The aorta becomes thicker and less elastic, which places additional strain on the left ventricle of the heart to pump blood into the systemic circulation. The outer arterial layers develop increased connective tissue. Smooth muscle fibers in the middle layer become less responsive to hormonal influence and vasoconstrictor input from the sympathetic nervous system. Calcium deposition in the medial layer makes the vessel stiffer and less distensible. These age-related changes increase the probability of disease.

With increased age, veins lose elasticity and vessel walls become weakened. Varicosities, or abnormal dilation of the veins, can result from distention of these weakened vessels. Decreased muscular activity impedes venous return. Venous stasis caused by surgery and immobility is associated with a high incidence of venous thrombus formation, embolization, and death.

Capillaries are also altered by the aging process. The single-layer endothelial cells rest on a collagen-like material called the basement membrane. This membrane thickens with age, hampering cellular nutrition and removal of waste products. A chronic lack of cellular nutrition increases the risk for infection and poor wound healing.

Older people with peripheral vascular disease may have difficulty coping with its chronic pain, mobility limitations, and disruptions in skin integrity. Intermittent claudication can be a particularly ominous condition in the older adult. It is usually treated with conservative management, but may take special nursing intervention to assist the patient in managing the pain cycles. Nursing measures that help the patient understand the disease process and identify preventive factors and interventions may facilitate a healthy coping response.

Chapter Review

1. What factors affect blood flow in the vascular system?
2. How do physiologic changes in vascular dysfunction cause the clinical manifestations of pain and poor tissue perfusion and integrity?
3. What teaching strategies should be employed to help the patient with vascular dysfunction reduce the various types of pain that may occur?
4. What should the nurse assess for in the patient with vascular dysfunction?
5. Which diagnostic studies are commonly ordered for the patient with suspected vascular dysfunction?
6. What nursing care should be implemented for the patient undergoing diagnostic testing for vascular dysfunction?
7. How can the nurse evaluate the effectiveness of medications ordered to reduce the manifestations of vascular dysfunction?
8. What are some risk reduction strategies that the patient can use to help prevent vascular dysfunction?
9. Why is the patient with vascular dysfunction on anticoagulant therapy postoperatively?
10. What special nursing considerations should be employed when caring for an elderly patient with vascular dysfunction?

Bibliography

Agency for Health Care Policy and Research. Acute pain management: Operative or medical procedures and trauma. U.S. Department of Health and Human Services. AHCPR 92-0032, 1992.

Allen SL. Perioperative nursing interventions for intravascular stent placements. AORN Journal 1995; 61(4):689.

Allsup DJ. Use of the intermittent pneumatic compression device in venous ulcer disease. J Vasc Nurs 1994; 12(4):106.

Bloomfield R, Pearce K, Cross H. Hypertension: Choosing therapy when coexisting disease confounds the choice. Consultant 1993; 33(7):69.

Borriello SL, Siegel SC, Fishman RF. Directional coronary atherectomy: A new treatment for coronary artery disease. Heart Lung 1994; 23(3):199.

Czyrny JJ, Merrill A. Rehabilitation of amputees with end-stage renal disease: Functional outcome and cost. Am J Phys Med Rehabil 1994; 73(5):353.

Dimengo J. Commentary on tissue renin-angiotensin system in myocardial hypertrophy and failure. AACN Nurs Scan Crit Care 1993; 3(6):4. [Original article by Dzau appears in Arch Intern Med 1993; 153(8):937.]

Edwards LH. Commentary on homelessness as a determinant of health. Nurs Scan Admin. 1993; 8(3):20. [Original article by Jackson appears in MCN 1982; 9(3):185]

Flett R, Harcourt B, Alpass F. Psychosocial aspects of chronic lower leg ulceration in the elderly. West J Nurs Res 1994; 16(2):183.

Galindo-Ciocon D. Nursing care of the elders with leg edema. J Gerontol Nurs 1995; 21(7):7.

Galloway S, Bubela N, McKibbon A, et al. Symptom distress, anxiety, depression, and discharge information needs after peripheral arterial bypass. J Vasc Nurs 1995; 13(2):35.

Gardner AW, Skinner JS, Bryant CX, Smith LK. Stair climbing elicits a lower cardiovascular demand than walking in claudication patients. J Cardiopulm Rehabil 1995; 15(2):134.

Grace ML, Crosby FE, Ventura MR. Nutritional education for patients with peripheral vascular disease. J Health Educ 1994; 25(3):142.

Harley JR. Preventing diabetic foot disease. Nurse Pract 1993; 18(10):37.

Hatswell EM. Abdominal aortic aneurysm surgery: An overview and discussion of immediate perioperative complications. Part I. Heart Lung 1994; 23(3):228.

Hebdon B, Letourneau JG. Duplex sonography of extremity arteries and veins. Part 2. Appl Radiol 1994; 23(4):39.

Henderson LJ, Kirkland JS. Angioplasty with stent placement in peripheral arterial occlusive disease. AORN J 1995; 61(4):669.

Hiash J, Oalen JE, Deykind D, Poller L, Bussey H. Oral anticoagulants. Mechanisms of action, clinical effectiveness and optimal therapeutic range. Chest 1995; 108(4):2315.

Johnson M. Interactional aspects of self-efficacy and control in older people with leg ulcers. J Gerontol Nurs 1995; 21(4):20.

Kashyap A, Deshmukh N. Abdominal aortic aneurysms in females: A comparative analysis. J Womens Health 1994; 3(4):291.

Lacey KO, Meier GH, Krumholz HM, Gusberg RJ. Outcomes after major vascular surgery: The patient's perspective. J Vasc Nurs 1995; 13(1):8.

Lovell MB, Cameron D, Harris KA, et al. Peripheral aneurysms. J Vasc Nurs 1994; 12(2):44.

MacLean N, Fick GH. The effect of semirigid dressings on below-knee amputations. Phys Ther 1994; 74(7):668.

Maklebust J, Magnan MA. Risk factors associated with having a pressure ulcer: A secondary data analysis. Adv Wound Care 1994; 7(6):25.

Margolis S. Point/counterpoint. Chelation therapy is ineffective for the treatment of peripheral vascular disease. Alternative Ther Health Med 1995; 1(2):53.

McAbee R. Primary prevention of hypertension: A challenge for occupational health nurses. AAOHN J 1995; 43(6):306.

Orsted H. Physiology of venous leg ulceration. CAET J 1994; 13(3):6.

Phillips NA, Mate-Kole CC, Kirby RL. Neuropsychological function in peripheral vascular disease amputee patients. Arch Phys Med Rehabil 1993; 74(12):1309.

Plummer ES, Albert SG. Foot care assessment in patients with diabetes: A screening algorithm for patient education and referral. Diabetes Educ 1995; 21(1):47.

Podmore J. Leg ulcers: Weighing up the evidence. Nurs Stand 1994; 8(38):25.

Provan JL. Peripheral vascular disease: What's urgent, what's not. Med North Am 1993; 16(10):772.

Robertson C. Diabetes 2000: Chronic complications. RN 1995; 58(9):34.

Sabatino KA, Dougher MJ, Kee JC. Research: Conception to completion. J Vasc Nurs 1993; 11(4):111.

Sepka RS. Transcutaneous PO$_2$ measurement in peripheral vascular disease. Physician Assist 1993; 17(5):86.

Tosone NC, Marcley DM, Thielen JB, Vyhlidal SK. Discharge teaching for the directional coronary atherectomy patient. DCCN 1994; 13(4):208.

Waite LG. Commentary on cardiogenic shock complicating acute myocardial infarction in patients without heart failure on admission: Incidence, risk factors and outcome. AACN Nursing Scan Crit Care 1993; 3(5):23. [Original article by Leor et al appears in Am J Med 1993; 94(3):265.]

Waite LG. Commentary on circadian variations and possible external triggers of onset of myocardial infarction. AACN Nurs Scan Crit Care 1993; 3(5):22. [Original article by Behar et al appears in Am J Med 1993; 94(4):395.]

Wymelenberg S. Hit the road, Jack: Peripheral vascular disease. Harv Health Lett 1993; 18(10):4.

teacher and nursing homes, continue

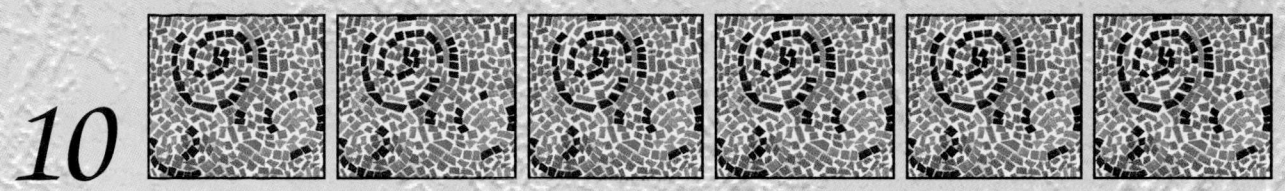

10

Nursing Care of Patients with Vascular Disorders

Study Outcomes

After studying this chapter, you should be able to:

1. Describe the etiology, pathophysiology, clinical manifestations, diagnostic procedures, and management of common vascular disorders.
2. Compare the common pharmacotherapeutic agents used to treat vascular disorders.
3. Identify information and physical examination data essential to the assessment of patients with common vascular disorders.
4. State nursing diagnoses and related expected patient outcomes commonly applicable to patients with vascular disorders.
5. Describe nursing interventions, with their rationales, commonly applicable to patients with vascular disorders.
6. Explain the basis for evaluation of nursing care provided to patients with common vascular disorders.
7. Identify alternative treatment and care settings for patients with vascular disorders, and the services related to community-based care.
8. Identify special considerations for the elderly patient with a vascular disorder.

Vascular disorders encompass all the diseases of the blood vessels and lymphatic vessels. The most common vessel disorders are obstructive, such as atherosclerosis and arteriosclerosis. Although many vessel changes occur naturally as a result of aging, lifestyle is a significant contributing factor to the incidence of occlusive vascular diseases. Disorders of the vascular system may cause pain, decrease mobility, interfere with peripheral circulation, and exacerbate other disease processes.

Many diseases of the vascular system are chronic and debilitating. This presents specific implications for nursing care. Because the elderly, in particular, are prone to vascular disorders, long-term care planning, home-care instructions, and follow-up care are all important facets of nursing intervention. Treatment settings for vascular disorders are as likely to be in outpatient clinics as in an acute-care setting.

Since many older adults reside in residential care facilities and nursing homes, continued care of vascular disorders may occur in these facilities. Referrals to other agencies outside the hospital for continuity of care may be necessary for the patient with a vascular disorder because of the chronic nature of the disease.

Common Arterial Vascular Disorders

The collective group of common arterial vascular disorders includes inflammatory conditions such as Buerger's disease and inflammations of the aorta; functional and structural problems that are obstructive in nature, such as Raynaud's disease or atherosclerosis and arteriosclerosis; and other structural abnormalities, such as aneurysms.

THROMBOANGIITIS OBLITERANS (BUERGER'S DISEASE)

Etiology and Pathophysiology

Thromboangiitis obliterans is a chronic inflammatory process involving medium-size blood vessels. Although the disease affects both arteries and veins, arteries are more commonly and more severely affected. In fact, the disease commonly leads to arterial occlusion. It most often affects male smokers between ages 20 and 45. The greatest incidence occurs among Jewish and Asian populations. Although the exact cause is unknown, it is thought to be a reaction to excessive use of nicotine over a long period of time. The incidence of the disease has decreased in recent years.

The arteries of the lower extremities are most often involved. Early stages are characterized by acute inflammation, followed by remission lasting weeks to years. Large arteries and veins are rarely involved until late in the disease process. Then, abscesses develop in specific areas. The arteries contract and finally occlude in the region of the destruction. Cellular proliferation of the intima predisposes to thrombi development in the vessels, contributing to the occlusion and causing intense pain. Spasms may also occur in the vessels, further decreasing the blood flow and causing increased ischemia.

Clinical Manifestations

Peripheral vascular ischemia results in cold extremities. The distal portions of the hands and feet are extremely pale. In later stages of the disease, rubor may occur when the extremity is in a dependent position. Pain is one of the most common and most severe manifestations of thromboangiitis obliterans. In early stages, it may affect only the palm of the hand and the arch of the foot. As the disease progresses, however, the pain may become excruciating. Rest pain, numbness, burning, and impaired sensation result from ischemic neuropathy.

Pulses of the dorsalis pedis, posterior tibial, ulnar, and radial arteries are weak or absent from decreased peripheral blood supply. The extremities may become edematous in advanced stages. Nail ulcers and gangrene may result from infections and tissue necrosis.

Diagnosis

The diagnosis is based on history, physical assessment, and laboratory studies. Arteriography of the extremities, oscillometry, skin temperature studies, and x-rays may also be used to determine the diagnosis. The peripheral pulses are checked with a Doppler ultrasonogram.

Management

Smoking is prohibited because nicotine produces vasoconstriction and exacerbates the disease. Pharmacologic intervention includes analgesics for pain control and vasodilators to increase blood flow to the extremities. Buerger-Allen exercises are prescribed to promote vasodilation (Highlight 10–1). Usually, this disease is treated palliatively, with interventions focusing on the clinical manifestations of the disorder.

Peripheral angioplasty is a nonsurgical procedure for treating chronic arterial occlusive disease. It may be beneficial for patients who are poor surgical risks, and for those who are not obtaining relief through palliative treatment.

Although a sympathectomy may be done to promote vasodilation, enhance circulation to the skin, and relieve rest pain, it is now used only in rare cases. It is a palliative surgery involving excision of the second and third lumbar sympathetic ganglia. It blocks vasoconstricting input, thus reducing pain and improving peripheral circulation.

Amputation of the fingers and toes or a below-the-knee amputation may be necessary if the patient has gangrene or uncontrolled pain.

❖ Settings, Providers, and Collaboration for Care

Since patients with thromboangiitis obliterans are more commonly seen in outpatient clinics for diagnosis and management of the disorder, continuity of care may be difficult to maintain. Usually, the nurse instructs the patient in the appropriate care regimen after consulting with the physician. If the patient has severe peripheral vascular ischemia, ulcerations on the extremities, or other complicating disorders, follow-up care in the home is necessary.

In the long-term care facility or in the home setting, the nurse may continue the exercise instructions to the patient (and family). The nurse should observe the patient during the Buerger-Allen exercise routine to make sure it is being done correctly. The nurse also assesses the patient's extremities, checking pulses, skin integrity and color, and areas of pain. If the patient has ulcerations, the nurse will dress them. If applicable, the nurse may also review the patient's progress to stop smoking. The patient will also need ongoing monitoring.

Since the patient's arterial circulation may be severely compromised, foot care can present problems. A podiatrist visit may be necessary to assist the patient in maintaining healthy feet. The podiatrist may trim the toe nails, treat ulcerations, and assist the patient with pain control strategies.

NURSING PROCESS
Thromboangiitis Obliterans

Assessment

Review the patient's history and diagnostic findings. Perform a physical assessment, focusing on circulation in the extremities. Palpate distal pulses bilaterally. Note the presence, rate, regularity, and intensity of each. Assess the extremities for color, temperature, and sensation. Assess for the presence of pain, noting the location, intensity, precipitating factors, duration, frequency, radiation, and relief methods. Check for edema, lesions, or gangrene of the extremities. Note whether the patient is taking any medications or smokes cigarettes.

Nursing Diagnoses and Planning

Nursing diagnoses and related expected patient outcomes commonly applicable to patients with thromboangiitis obliterans include the following:

NDx: Pain related to inflammation and ischemia secondary to the disease state

Planning: Patient Outcomes

1. Patient reports an absence or reduction of pain.
2. Signs of pain, such as grimacing, clenching hands, or guarding, are absent.
3. Patient states methods of relaxation to reduce pain and coping strategies to deal with pain.

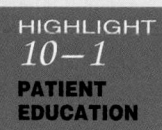 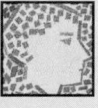

HIGHLIGHT
10–1
PATIENT EDUCATION

Discharge Instructions for the Patient with Buerger's Disease

Teach the patient with Buerger's disease to perform Buerger-Allen exercises to improve circulation to the legs and feet:
As shown in *A*, elevate and support the legs at a 45- to 90-degree angle, or until the skin blanches, for 2 to 3 minutes. Then, as shown in *B*, sit with feet in a dependent position so the skin turns red. Support the legs in this position for 5 to 10 minutes. Then flex, extend, pronate, and supinate each foot three times. Finally, lie flat in a supine position for 10 minutes.

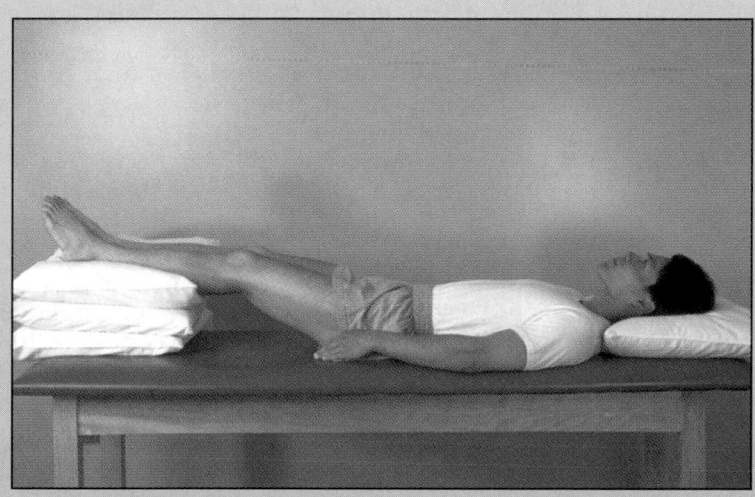

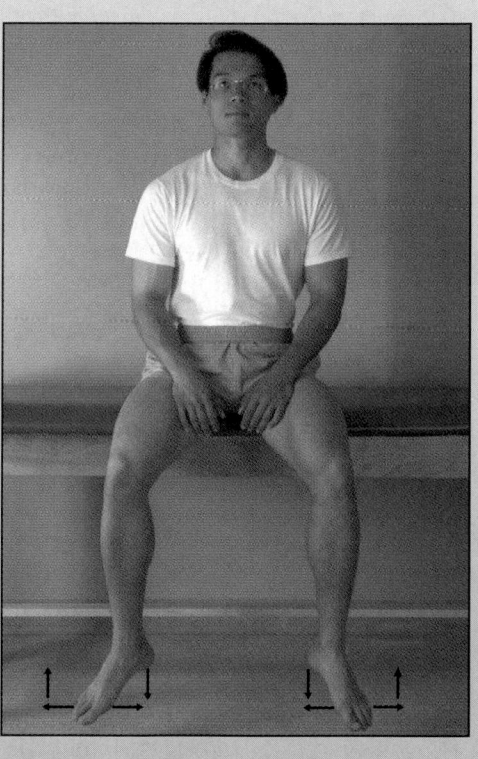

A   B

4. Patient describes and practices exercises to increase circulation and prevent ischemic pain (see Highlight 10–1).
5. Patient displays behaviors that may reduce painful effects of the disease, such as trying to quit smoking.

NDx: Knowledge deficit: nature of disease, factors contributing to manifestations of disease, and preventive measures

Planning: Patient Outcomes
1. Patient states accurate information about the disease process and the manifestation of the disorder.
2. Patient relates measures to decrease the effects of the disease.
3. Patient complies with behavioral changes necessary to reduce manifestations of the disease.

Nursing Interventions and Evaluation

NDx: Pain
Tell the patient to stop smoking. Smoking causes vasoconstriction while also increasing the demand for blood and oxygen to tissues. This combination increases ischemia and, thus, increases pain.

Use diversional activities to decrease the patient's awareness of pain. Determine coping strategies that help the patient deal with the pain, especially when severe. Administer pain medication as prescribed. Teach the patient about the effects of the medication, frequency of use, and potential side effects. Help the patient relieve the pain of increased vasoconstriction by decreasing stress and tension through relaxation methods (Highlight 10–2). Allow for periods of rest during episodes of intense pain.

Teach the patient Buerger-Allen exercises to in-

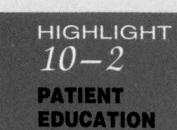 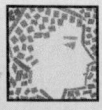

HIGHLIGHT 10-2 PATIENT EDUCATION

Relaxation Exercises for the Patient with Vascular Disease

Instruct the patient to:

Sit or lie in a comfortable position with loose clothing in a quiet, dark room.

Close the eyes and breathe slowly and naturally.

Starting at the head, tighten and relax each muscle, ending with the feet.

Continue to breathe slowly and deeply.

Repeat the words *relax, peace,* and so on each time exhalation occurs.

Disregard all outside thoughts and concerns.

Focus on each muscle being relaxed more and more with each exhalation.

Tell the patient this exercise should take only about 10 minutes or so to complete. Visualizing a favorite quiet place (the beach, woods, mountain, and so on) may be helpful to relax the mind and muscles.

crease circulation to the extremities to reduce the ischemia. Encourage continued participation in the exercise regimen (see Highlight 10–1).

Be sure the patient avoids wearing constricting clothing because it interferes with circulation in the extremities. Tell the patient to wear warm clothing and to protect the extremities against extreme heat or cold.

NDx: Knowledge deficit: nature of disease, factors contributing to manifestations of disease, and preventive measures
Explain the disease process to the patient in understandable terms. Allow time for questions and concerns. Give the patient and family appropriate literature about the disease. Tell them about the manifestations of the disorder and preventive measures to protect the patient from complications, such as keeping warm, exercising to increase circulation, preventing stress (which aggravates the condition), and avoiding injury to the extremities.

Compare the patient's status with the expected outcomes. If the outcomes are not met, reassess the patient and revise the plan.

OBSTRUCTIVE DISORDERS

Obstructive vascular disorders are most common among older adults. Several of the diseases, including atherosclerosis, are insidious in their develop-

ment and heavily influenced by lifestyle. Because many of these disorders have similar characteristics and effects, there are several common areas of nursing care applicable to patients with obstructive arterial vascular disorders.

NURSING PROCESS
Obstructive Arterial Vascular Disorders

Assessment

Review the history and diagnostic studies results for the patient. Complete a physical assessment. Check the patient for circulatory impairment, especially in the periphery. Palpate all distal pulses and compare them bilaterally. Auscultate for bruits in the major arteries. Note temperature, color, and sensation in the extremities. Look for signs of poor capillary refill, which indicates decreased circulation.

Ask the patient about pain in the extremities. Obtain a description of the pain, including onset, duration, precipitating factors, and relief measures.

Check for signs of injury caused by falls, burns, or cuts. Ask the patient about the amount of sensation in the extremities. Check for numbness, tingling, and equal feeling bilaterally.

Observe for breaks in the skin. Look for tears, ulcerations, necrotic spots, or gangrene. Note any drainage from lesions.

Nursing Diagnoses and Planning

Nursing diagnoses and related expected patient outcomes commonly applicable to patients with obstructive arterial vascular disorders include the following:

NDx: Altered peripheral tissue perfusion related to the disease state, causing arterial occlusion and decreased circulation to the extremities

Planning: Patient Outcomes
1. Patient demonstrates increased perfusion as noted by skin that is warm and dry, strong pulses, and absence of edema and cyanosis in the extremities.
2. Vital signs are within normal ranges for the patient.
3. Patient demonstrates changes in behaviors that promote improved circulation such as mild exercise, cessation of smoking, and relaxation techniques.

NDx: Risk for injury related to decreased sensation in the extremities secondary to arterial occlusion, causing hypoxia

Planning: Patient Outcomes
1. Patient states need for assistance when out of bed and ambulating to prevent injury.
2. Patient states preventive measures such as requesting assistance when needed and following foot-care guidelines as described in Highlight 10–3.

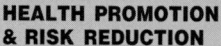
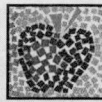

HIGHLIGHT 10–3
HEALTH PROMOTION & RISK REDUCTION

Self-Care for Prevention of Foot Problems in Vascular Disorders

Instruct the patient with vascular problems to institute the following foot-care measures to prevent complications:

Wear soft, comfortable shoes that are not too tight and that do not have any pressure areas.

Cleanse feet frequently. Be sure to dry them well, especially between the toes.

Apply skin moisturizer if feet are excessively dry or cracked.

Put on clean antiembolic stockings or socks daily.

Massage the feet frequently to promote circulation.

Keep toenails trimmed short. When trimming, be extremely careful not to cut the skin and not to cut the nails too short, which might cause bleeding.

Check the feet daily for discoloration, edema, bleeding, blisters, or any other lesions.

Consult a physician if any of these symptoms become apparent.

3. Patient conforms to the safety measures.
4. Patient remains free from injury.

NDx: Impaired skin integrity (in the extremities) related to inadequate oxygen and nutrients secondary to decreased circulation

Planning: Patient Outcomes
1. Patient's skin remains intact without evidence of shearing, infection, ulcerations, or gangrene.
2. Patient states appropriate skin-care measures to prevent impairment of skin integrity.

Nursing Interventions and Evaluation

NDx: Altered peripheral tissue perfusion
Help the patient conserve oxygen needs by encouraging rest and limiting activities. Elevate the head of the bed to aid in lung expansion. Initiate oxygen therapy if needed. Assist patient with activities of daily living, if needed, to conserve energy.

Keep the patient in a comfortable position and reposition frequently to release pressure. Use range-of-motion exercises to stimulate circulation. Monitor vital signs and laboratory studies to assess for changes and improvements in status. Encourage ambulation as tolerated, but provide for frequent rest periods to decrease cardiac workload. Discourage

smoking to avoid vasoconstriction. Discuss strategies to reduce stress, which could cause increased blood pressure. Remove constricting clothing, and keep heavy bed linen from constricting peripheral circulation.

Give prescribed medications to promote increased circulation. Discuss risk factors and preventive health-care measures with the patient. Explain lifestyle changes that will promote circulation and decrease risk of further arterial occlusion.

NDx: Risk for injury
Teach the patient to ask for assistance when getting out of bed or ambulating. Keep the bed rails raised and the patient's call light within reach. Explain the effects of decreased circulation to the extremities and describe safety measures to prevent injury.

Instruct the patient to use care when bathing the extremities. With decreased sensation, it is easy to burn the feet or legs by using water that is too hot. Give the patient and family a list of foot-care measures (see Highlight 10–3). Teach the patient to use special care when trimming toenails.

NDx: Impaired skin integrity
Handle the patient's legs and feet with care, especially if the skin is not intact. Use aseptic technique when bathing or dressing areas where the skin is broken to prevent infection. Keep linen off the extremities with the use of a bed cradle. Have the patient avoid wearing constricting clothing. Keep the extremities warm and dry at all times.

Check peripheral circulation frequently. Observe for early signs of problems developing as a result of decreased circulation, such as pressure spots, absent pulses, coldness, and discoloration. Report any untoward signs. Have the patient change position frequently to stimulate circulation and prevent pressure ulcers. Use heel pads to prevent skin breakdown if the patient is in bed for long periods of time.

To promote healing and minimize tissue damage, teach the patient to eat a diet high in protein and vitamins. Encourage foods low in cholesterol and triglycerides to decrease the formation of atherosclerotic plaques.

Compare the patient's status with the expected outcomes. If the outcomes are not met, reassess the patient and revise the plan.

Vasospastic Disorder (Raynaud's Disease)

Etiology and Pathophysiology
Vasospastic disorder, also called Raynaud's disease, has an unknown cause. The incidence of this disorder is higher in people who have immunologic disorders. The disease is more common in women and usually begins between ages 20 and 30. It is often associated with other diseases but is not precipitated by any one condition. The onset is insidious, with initial episodes occurring in the winter months. Characteristic vasospastic episodes usually affect the

fingers, lasting from a few minutes to hours, and may occur several times daily or not for weeks at a time. Episodes are frequently precipitated by a chilly or damp environment.

Raynaud's disease is characterized by paroxysmal, bilateral digital ischemia induced by cold or emotional stress. The vasospastic episodes may end spontaneously or be relieved by a warm environment or by placing the fingers in warm water. The ischemia stems from constriction of the digital and plantar arteries, which over-react to vasospastic stimuli. As the disease progresses, the intima of the arteries becomes thick and the muscular layers hypertrophy. Thrombosis of small arteries and gangrene of the digit tips may result.

Raynaud's phenomenon is a condition with the same symptoms of Raynaud's disease that may occur in conjunction with other diseases or conditions. It may result from collagen disorders such as scleroderma, arterial disorders causing occlusion such as Buerger's disease, drug or chemical exposures, or neuropathy such as carpal tunnel syndrome. Raynaud's phenomenon is a temporary disorder without the pathology of Raynaud's disease.

Clinical Manifestations

Vasospastic disease, or Raynaud's disease, is characterized by intermittent episodes of vasospasms in the fingers, causing pallor and cyanosis. It rarely occurs in the thumbs or toes and may be confined to two or three digits of the hand. Although it is usually bilateral and symmetric, more digits of one hand may be affected than of the other hand. Initially, one or two digits may be symptomatic, but eventually all fingers extending to the distal palm area become affected.

During a vasospastic episode, the digits become pale, cold, and cyanotic from vasoconstriction of the small cutaneous vessels. Pulses are usually still palpable. As the vasospasm ends, the fingers become bright red (rubor), starting at the base, from the increased blood flow and blood volume. Throbbing pain and a burning sensation accompany the return of circulation.

Numbness, edema, and decreased sensations may develop as the disease progresses through repeated ischemic episodes. Trophic changes occur, such as:

Atrophy of the fingers
Smooth, shiny, stretched skin
Slow-growing, ridged nails
Infections
Blisters
Small, painful gangrenous areas on the tips of the digits

These changes may occur 1 to 4 years after the onset of the disorder because of obstruction of the digital blood vessels.

Diagnosis

The diagnosis is based on history, physical assessment, patient description of vasospastic episodes, ar-

teriography, and plethysmography. When symptoms are unilateral, nerve conduction tests may be done to rule out carpal tunnel syndrome. Doppler ultrasonography is used to detect digital pulses. Although Raynaud's disease is not a fatal disorder, it may cause deformity or disability in severe cases.

Management

Management of Raynaud's disease includes avoiding precipitating factors, especially by protecting the hands from exposure to a cold and damp environment. Sedatives or tranquilizers may be prescribed to help relieve symptoms by relaxing the patient. Large doses of vasodilators are prescribed in some cases to increase blood flow to the distal areas, but they are frequently of limited value. Reserpine may be injected directly into veins in the hands to promote vasodilation and to produce symptomatic relief for up to 2 weeks. Because this is a very temporary treatment, it is not commonly used. A sympathectomy can be performed to help alleviate the symptoms. In most cases, the disease is treated conservatively through prevention methods. Highlight 10–4 provides discharge instructions for the patient with Raynaud's disease.

NURSING PROCESS GUIDELINES
Vasospastic Disorder (Raynaud's Disease)

Assessment, nursing diagnoses, expected patient outcomes, nursing interventions, and evaluation for patients with vasospastic disorder (Raynaud's dis-

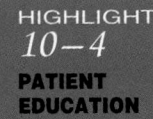 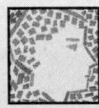

HIGHLIGHT
10–4
PATIENT EDUCATION
Discharge Instructions for the Patient with Raynaud's Disease

On discharge, instruct the patient with Raynaud's disease to observe the following preventive and safety measures:

Avoid exposure to chilly, damp, or cold temperatures.

Wear protective clothing, such as gloves and heavy socks, when out in cold or damp weather.

Use relaxation exercises to decrease stress levels.

Try to get plenty of rest and sleep every day.

Stop smoking.

Stop activity during an episode of vasospasm to protect the area until sensations return.

ease) are similar to those described previously for patients with thromboangiitis obliterans and obstructive arterial vascular disorders (Nursing Care Guide 10–1).

Arterial Embolus And Thrombus

Etiology and Pathophysiology
An arterial embolism is characterized by fragments of atheromatous material or thrombi (the embolus) that enter the arterial system and obstruct a vessel. The embolus is carried by the blood flow to the site where it lodges.

A thrombus may also block an artery at the site where it develops rather than traveling to another site. It usually develops in an artery damaged by atherosclerosis or inflammation. Arteriosclerotic heart disease accounts for about two-thirds of cases of thrombus formation. Rheumatic heart disease accounts for about one-fourth of cases. Other cardiac and vascular disorders, such as fibrillation and aneurysms, are also associated with the development of thrombi. Symptoms do not usually appear until the vessel is occluded.

A thrombus may develop at the point where blood flow is restricted in the vessel from a lesion, fatty plaques, inflammation, or any other obstruction. The term *thrombosis* refers to the process of the development of a thrombus. Any disease, drug, or process that slows circulation, especially in the peripheral circulatory system, may place the patient at risk for thrombus formation. A piece of a fatty plaque or a thrombus that breaks loose and travels to another location in the circulatory system and obstructs a vessel is called an *embolus*. The blockage is called an *embolism*.

Clinical Manifestations
When an embolus lodges in a vessel or when a thrombus develops in a vessel in the extremities, pain occurs distal to the site of occlusion. The pain may be either gradual or sudden, depending on the blockage. Numbness, tingling, and a cold sensation may precede the pain. The pain is described as a burning or aching discomfort in most patients. Exercise aggravates the discomfort in the extremity. Tenderness directly over the site of the blockage may be present. Muscle weakness or paralysis of the affected part can also occur.

Mottling, rigidity, collapsed veins, and impaired reflexes are present. The extremity may display pale to blotchy discoloration. Arterial pulses are absent distal to the occlusion if the blockage is in a large artery.

Diagnosis
The diagnosis is based on physical assessment, with confirmation from diagnostic studies. An angiogram is used to determine the presence of ulcerative atherosclerotic lesions or abnormalities of blood flow caused by the arterial obstruction. Doppler ultrasonography may be used to locate the obstruction.

Management
The goal of medical care is to improve blood flow through the affected vessel. Heparin is administered to prevent further clot formation. The patient is placed on long-term anticoagulant therapy once the acute phase has passed and is monitored for effects of the therapy. Thrombolytic therapy may be used to dissolve the clot and restore circulation. Procaine or lidocaine (Xylocaine) may be injected into the subarachnoid space of the spinal column as a lumbar sympathetic block to relieve constriction and spasms of the affected vessel. Vasodilators may be prescribed as adjunct therapy. Analgesics are given for pain relief.

If the embolus or thrombus is completely occluding a major vessel so that circulation is severely compromised or interrupted in the extremity, surgical intervention is required. A thromboendarterectomy or an arterial graft may be done. (Refer to Chapter 9 for a discussion of endarterectomy and grafts.)

The prognosis depends on the location and extent of the blockage, age of the patient, and other complicating conditions. Early treatment is essential for a good prognosis. Removing or treating the underlying cause is important. The recurrence of thrombi and emboli is common, particularly if the cause is atherosclerotic disease.

NURSING PROCESS
Arterial Embolus or Thrombus

Assessment

Review the patient's history and diagnostic studies. Assess the patient for changes in sensation, color, temperature, strength, and endurance. Palpate for pulses in the affected area. Note any pain and determine its onset, duration, intensity, radiation, and location.

Check the patient's understanding of the disorder, the treatment, and expected outcomes of the treatment, especially if surgery is indicated. Observe for signs of anxiety, such as increased blood pressure and heart rate, nervousness, withdrawal, twitching, and continual questions related to the medical intervention. If the condition is a highly acute, complete occlusion of a major vessel, the patient may fear surgery, the risk of death, or loss of a limb.

Nursing Diagnoses and Planning

Nursing diagnoses and related expected patient outcomes commonly applicable to patients with an arterial embolus or thrombus include those discussed under obstructive arterial vascular disorders as well as those discussed here. (Also refer to Chapter 9 for application of the nursing process to the patient undergoing peripheral vascular surgery.)

NDx: Anxiety related to the disease state, treatment, and possible surgical intervention

Nursing Care Guide 10-1
Patients with Vasospastic Disorder (Raynaud's Disease)

Assessment Findings: Patient experiences numbness in digits of hands progressing to pain; fingers are blanched; radial pulses are present.

Nursing Diagnosis: Altered peripheral tissue perfusion related to obstructed circulation secondary to vasospasms

Patient Outcomes	Nursing Interventions	Rationale
Patient exhibits improved blood supply to ischemic areas as seen by warm, pink digits.	Provide warmth, especially for the extremities, and prevent drafts.	Providing warmth to the extremities may prevent some problems resulting from the circulatory deficiency.
	Assess pulses. Assess the skin temperature, color, and texture frequently. Document any changes.	Observation for problems leads to early intervention and prevention of complications.
Patient identifies activities to improve circulation and prevent vasospastic episodes.	Teach the patient to wear warm clothing, protect the digits from exposure, and avoid damp, chilly environments. Instruct about the effects of smoking and encourage the patient in the cessation of smoking.	Some vasospastic episodes may be prevented by removing the precipitating factors such as sudden chilling or smoking.
	Have the patient reiterate the information provided.	Having the patient repeat the information allows for correction of misunderstandings and reinforcement of the information.
Patient ceases smoking.	Talk to the attending physician about smoking cessation programs. Make a referral to a smoking cessation program.	There are a variety of programs for assisting patients in quitting smoking, such as nicotine patch programs and behavioral modification programs.

Evaluation: Compare the patient's status with the expected outcomes. If the outcomes are not met, reassess the patient and revise the plan.

Assessment Findings: Patient reports pain in digits after vasospastic episode; at times, the pain is extreme.

Nursing Diagnosis: Pain related to aftereffects of vasospasms in digits.

Patient Outcomes	Nursing Interventions	Rationale
Patient reports absence of pain or that pain is reduced to tolerable level.	Give analgesics as prescribed.	Analgesics reduce the pain sensations.
	Allow patient to rest and relax frequently. Keep the patient free from chilling.	Prevention of vasospasms reduces the number of pain episodes the patient experiences.

(continued)

Nursing Care Guide 10–1
Patients with Vasospastic Disorder (Raynaud's Disease) *(continued)*

Patient Outcomes	Nursing Interventions	Rationale
Patient states methods to deal with pain and measures to prevent vasospasms from occurring.	Teach relaxation exercises, as described in Highlight 10–2. Help the patient find coping methods to deal with the pain after the vasospasms.	Relaxation techniques may reduce some of the pain or help the patient tolerate it better.
	Instruct the patient on how to avoid the vasospasms as described in Highlight 10–4.	Prevention of the vasospasms or a reduction in the occurrence reduces the painful episodes after spasm.

Evaluation: Compare the patient's status with the expected outcomes. If the outcomes are not met, reassess the patient and revise the plan.

Assessment Findings: Patient presents cold, numb, and pale digits; there is potential for lesions or gangrene.

Nursing Diagnosis: Impaired skin integrity related to decreased circulation to the digits secondary to disease process.

Patient Outcomes	Nursing Interventions	Rationale
Patient's skin on digits remains intact, warm, pink, and smooth without signs of breakdown or gangrene.	Instruct the patient to observe for early signs of breakdown and seek medical assistance if symptoms appear.	Early recognition and intervention may prevent severe complications.
	Tell the patient how to protect the digits from the vasospastic episodes.	Prevention of vasospastic episodes reduces the risk of complications
	Explain the necessity of keeping the hands warm and covered in cold weather. Instruct on skin care if any breakdown is apparent such as keeping skin clean, using aseptic dressing, if needed, and moisturizing the dry areas to prevent cracks.	Patient education is important because the patient needs to observe for signs of skin problems and to properly care for the skin after discharge.

Evaluation: Compare the patient's status with the expected outcomes. If the outcomes are not met, reassess the patient and revise the plan.

Assessment Findings: Patient asks questions about care of hands and prevention of vasospasms; seems anxious about managing effects of disease; is unsure about future effects of disease.

Nursing Diagnosis: Knowledge deficit: nature of disease and preventive care

(continued)

Nursing Care Guide 10–1
Patients with Vasospastic Disorder (Raynaud's Disease) *(continued)*

Patient Outcomes	Nursing Interventions	Rationale
Patient states accurate information about the disease process and the preventive measures, as listed in Highlight 10–4.	Explain the disease process to the patient in understandable terms. Give the patient appropriate literature about the disease. Explain the preventive measures, as listed in Highlight 10–4. Allow time for questions, concerns, and repeated explanations. Have the patient repeat the information provided.	An understanding of the disease process and the preventive behaviors may increase patient compliance with the medical regimen and prevent complications of the disease process. Planning time for questions and having the patient repeat the information allow for correction of any misunderstandings.
Evaluation:	Compare the patient's status with the expected outcomes. If the outcomes are not met, reassess the patient and revise the plan.	

Planning: Patient Outcomes

1. Patient states accurate information about the disease, its effect on the extremities, potential treatment, and expected outcomes.
2. Patient exhibits signs of decreased anxiety, such as normal vital signs, a cheerful and relaxed posture, and lack of nervousness or twitching.
3. Patient reports feeling less anxious.

Nursing Interventions and Evaluation

NDx: Anxiety

Explain the disease process, typical interventions, and expected outcomes to the patient. If the situation requires surgery, explain its necessity and all preoperative preparations as they are instituted. Allow the patient time to adjust to the information and to voice concerns. Encourage questions and give explanations in terms the patient can understand. Include the family in the discussions when appropriate.

Encourage rest and teach relaxation techniques to reduce anxiety (see Highlight 10–2). Provide uninterrupted rest periods throughout the day. Seek assistance from clergy or other professionals as needed.

Compare the patient's status with the expected outcomes. If the outcomes are not met, reassess the patient and revise the plan.

Atherosclerosis

Etiology and Pathophysiology

Atherosclerosis is the most common arterial occlusive disorder. Its exact cause is unknown; however, the fatty tissue found in the disease may be the continuation of a fatty streak that is present at birth in the vessels. Any artery may be involved, but the aorta, iliac arteries, carotid arteries, and coronary arteries are the most commonly affected. In the aorta, the abdominal section is affected more often than the ascending section. In the lower extremities, it occurs more frequently in the femoral arteries than other smaller arteries.

Atherosclerosis is primarily recognized in adults age 20 or older and is most commonly found in the older adult. It is the major cause of death in the individual older than 65 years. Risk factors associated with atherosclerosis include increased cholesterol (particularly low-density lipoproteins), cigarette smoking, hypertension, diabetes, and a familial history of heart disease.

In atherosclerosis, the arterial wall becomes calcified from fatty plaques. The plaques are white fibrous tissue and yellowish fatty deposits of cells, lipids, carbohydrates, and calcium in the intima of the vessel. Thrombosis develops, causing obstruction.

Calcium deposits in the vessel wall prevent dilatation and contraction. The lumen of the artery becomes narrowed and weak and loses its flexibility. As the intima thickens with age, vessels become more rigid, resulting in a rise in peripheral resistance and increased cardiac workload. An aneurysm may develop, obstructing or occluding the vessel and leading to fibrosis of tissues and organs from lack of blood supply. Calcification, necrosis, and rupture of the vessel may also occur.

Clinical Manifestations

Clinical manifestations of atherosclerosis depend on the location and extent of arterial occlusion. Ische-

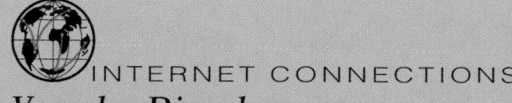

INTERNET CONNECTIONS
Vascular Disorders

Atherosclerosis
Arteriosclerosis
http://web.bu.edu/COHIS/cardvasc/vessel/artery/
arterio.htm
A patient information resource featuring an extensive list of frequently asked questions about atherosclerosis and arteriosclerosis. This site also includes such topics as aneurysm, stroke, vasculitis, and hypertension.

Hypertension
Hypertension, Dialysis, and Clinical Nephrology:
Renal Diseases Electronic Journal
http://www.medtext.com/hdcn.shtml
Designed for physicians, this site provides answers to frequently asked questions, summaries of new information and presentations, and links to related sites.

National Institute on Aging Age Page:
High Blood Pressure: A Common but Controllable
Disorder
http://www.aoa.dhhs.gov/aoa/pages/agepages/
hibldpr.html
A patient-oriented resource that answers frequently asked questions about hypertension in straightforward language. In addition, this site includes a high blood pressure checklist for patients and directs patients to national information resources.

High Blood Pressure: American Heart Association
Heart and Stroke Guide
http://www.amhrt.org/hs96/hbp.html
An excellent resource providing basic patient-oriented information about high blood pressure in clear, easy-to-understand language. This site also links patients to further information related to hypertension, other cardiovascular disorders, and stroke, all found within the Heart and Stroke Guide.

---

mia occurs in the lower extremities if the atherosclerotic area is in the abdominal aorta or iliac or femoral arteries. Manifestations of the ischemia include impotence in the male, decreased or absent pulses, cold feet, gangrene of the toes or feet, intermittent claudication, and aneurysms.

If the blockage is in the carotid arteries, manifestations may be numbness, tingling, or weakness on the side of the body contralateral to the involved carotid artery, transient ischemic attacks, dizziness, confusion, and cerebrovascular accidents. They may also include amaurosis fugax (temporary loss of vision) involving the ipsilateral eye of the involved carotid. Atherosclerotic plaques in the coronary arteries usually cause angina pectoris and myocardial infarction. Hypertension may be caused by occlusion in the renal arteries.

Diagnosis
The diagnosis of atherosclerosis is based on history, physical assessment, and diagnostic studies. Present symptoms, palpation of peripheral pulses, and skin temperature studies are also used for determining the diagnosis. A treadmill exercise test and Doppler ultrasonogram demonstrate the quality of peripheral blood flow and the presence of intermittent claudication. Angiography, tomography, and magnetic resonance imaging evaluate blood flow and the severity of the obstruction or narrowing of the arteries.

Laboratory studies of levels of cholesterol, low-density lipoproteins, and high-density lipoproteins may add support to the diagnosis. High cholesterol levels, with a high level of low-density lipoproteins and low level of high-density lipoproteins, are common in atherosclerosis.

Management
The management of atherosclerosis depends on the location and severity of the disorder. It may consist of palliative treatment, supportive care, or pharmacologic intervention. The patient must be educated about lifestyle changes, such as diet modifications, cessation of smoking, and initiation of a mild exercise regimen. A low-cholesterol, low-fat diet is encouraged. The patient may be referred to a smoking cessation program. Exercise increases circulation to the periphery, so a regular exercise program will be prescribed on the basis of the patient's ability and other influencing factors. Antiplatelet therapy may be prescribed for carotid arterial occlusion.

Interventional radiologic procedures such as angioplasty may enhance blood flow to the affected areas. Surgical intervention may be necessary to enhance blood flow to the affected areas. Endarterectomy and bypass grafts are the most common surgeries performed for atherosclerotic disorders. Refer to Chapter 9 for a discussion of the surgeries for vascular disorders.

NURSING PROCESS
Atherosclerosis

Assessment

Assess for pain, noting the onset, intensity, duration, radiation, and location. Determine whether the pain is present only during exercise or also at rest. Look for signs of pain, such as grimacing, clenching of hands, moaning, or guarding when the patient is moving in bed, ambulating, or resting after ambulation.

Assess for any skin changes. Ask the patient about numbness, tingling, or paresthesia of the extremities. Check the temperature and color of extremities, when the extremity is elevated and dependent. Observe the condition of the feet. Palpate for pulses and compare bilaterally. Look for signs of skin breakdown. Auscultate for bruits over stenotic arteries. Monitor serum cholesterol levels and other laboratory data.

Check the patient's physical mobility. Ask about assistance needed to perform activities of daily living. Determine the patient's flexibility, range of motion, and strength in the extremities.

Assess the patient's level of knowledge about the disorder and treatment. Ask about lifestyle and associated risk factors. Assess the level of adaptation to the disorder and ability to manage the disease process and its manifestations.

Nursing Diagnoses and Planning

Nursing diagnoses and related expected patient outcomes commonly applicable to patients with atherosclerosis include those discussed under obstructive arterial vascular disorders as well as the following.

NDx: Pain related to ischemic tissues secondary to decreased circulation from disease process

Planning: Patient Outcomes
1. Patient reports an absence or reduction in pain when ambulating or at rest.
2. Nonverbal signs of pain, such as grimacing, clenching hands, or guarding, are absent.
3. Patient states methods of relaxation to reduce pain and coping strategies to deal with the pain.

NDx: Impaired physical mobility related to pain and decreased strength and sensation secondary to disease state

Planning: Patient Outcomes
1. Patient reports increased mobility, strength, and endurance.
2. Patient is able to perform activities of daily living.

NDx: Knowledge deficit: nature of the disease, nutritional needs, treatments, and measures to reduce risk

Planning: Patient Outcomes
1. Patient describes cause, effects, and risk factors associated with atherosclerosis.

2. Patient lists symptoms and treatments for the complications of the disorder.
3. Patient relates the nutritional therapy for lowering cholesterol levels.
4. Patient states the self-care needed to prevent risk or complications of atherosclerosis.

NDx: Self esteem disturbance related to chronic illness, changes in lifestyle to manage disease and reduce risk factors, and inability to perform activities of daily living

Planning: Patient Outcomes
1. Patient states methods to cope with illness.
2. Patient denies feelings of inadequacy, helplessness, or dependency.
3. Patient appears positive, friendly, and cheerful and actively participates in plans for discharge and patient education sessions.
4. Patient takes responsibility for self-care.

Nursing Interventions and Evaluation

NDx: Pain
Counsel the patient to stop smoking. It causes vasoconstriction while also increasing demand for blood and oxygen to tissues. This combination increases ischemia and thus pain. Use diversional activities to decrease the patient's awareness of pain. Determine coping strategies that help the patient deal with the pain, especially when it is severe. Be sure the patient avoids wearing constricting clothing, which interferes with circulation in the extremities.

Administer pain medication as prescribed. Teach the patient about the effects of the medication, frequency of use, and potential side effects. Help the patient decrease stress and tension through the use of relaxation methods to relieve the pain caused by increased vasoconstriction. Allow for periods of rest during episodes of intermittent claudication.

NDx: Impaired physical mobility
Assist the patient when getting out of bed and ambulating. Use durable medical equipment accessories, when appropriate, to assist the patient in maintaining mobility. Teach the patient to perform range-of-motion exercises to increase circulation and to maintain or improve strength and endurance.

Prepare a daily exercise schedule for the patient, increasing the level as tolerable. Tell the patient to walk slowly and avoid stairs or inclines at first, if necessary, and to stop for a few minutes when pain occurs. Encourage the patient to persist in the exercise regimen, even if it must be moderated during times of pain or lack of endurance. Praise the patient on progress made.

NDx: Knowledge deficit: nature of the disease, nutritional needs, treatments, and measures to reduce risk
Explain the cause, effects, and clinical course of atherosclerosis to the patient. Allow opportunities for

the patient to ask questions at any time. Provide appropriate literature about atherosclerosis for the patient and family to review. Allow the patient to verbalize concerns and fears. Evaluate the discharge needs of the patient and family.

Alert the patient to signs and symptoms of atherosclerosis and complications, such as impaired mobility, skin breakdown, and infection or gangrene of the extremities. Teach the patient to use safety measures or to ask for assistance when out of bed or when ambulating.

Instruct the patient about dietary modifications needed to reduce risk or prevent complications of the disorder. Explain the need for decreases in dietary fats and cholesterol to prevent the effects of the disease and increases in protein and vitamins to promote good health and healing (Highlight 10–5). Initiate counseling with a dietitian to assist with meal planning if needed.

Teach the patient how to achieve comfort by frequent repositioning and padding of bony prominences. Show family members how to massage the patient with lotion to promote circulation and prevent skin breakdown. Tell the patient to avoid using heating pads because thermoreceptors in the tissue may be dulled from oxygen deprivation. Explain the

use of a bed cradle to prevent pressure on joints and sensitive areas.

Teach the patient dosage, route, time, frequency, side effects, and toxic effects of any medication prescribed. Explain the diagnostic studies completed and the need for any follow-up studies after discharge. Include the family in the teaching sessions, when appropriate.

NDx: Self esteem disturbance

Teach the patient self-care measures, encouraging participation and decision-making by the patient. Explain how changes in lifestyle can benefit the patient and significant others. Allow time for expression of concerns, questions, and clarification of misunderstandings. Praise the patient for knowledge gained about the disorder, for attempts at lifestyle change, and for participation in self-care.

Seek assistance from clergy, family members, or other professionals when appropriate. Make referrals for the patient on discharge as needed.

Compare the patient's status with the expected outcomes. If the outcomes are not met, reassess the patient and revise the plan.

Chronic Arterial Occlusive Disease (Arteriosclerosis Obliterans)

Etiology and Pathophysiology

The cause of chronic arterial occlusive disease is usually atherosclerosis, resulting in gradual blockage of the large vessels. It may also be caused by thrombosis or chronic inflammation. Chronic arterial occlusive disease is most common in men older than 50 years and primarily affects the vessels of the lower extremities. Diabetes mellitus is frequently a precursor to the disorder because of the prevalence of hyperlipidemia in the disease. Chronic arterial occlusive disease affects the distal part of the aorta and the iliac, femoral, and popliteal arteries.

Arteriosclerosis of smaller arterial vessels is considered to be part of the aging process. This may cause a hypertensive state in the patient if it is severe in the renal arterioles.

Fatty plaques or atheromas gradually occlude the involved artery, causing the symptoms of the disease. Occlusions of the aorta and iliac arteries usually occur proximal to the bifurcation of the common iliac arteries or distal to the aortic bifurcation. Complete occlusion may also be present. Occlusion of the femoral and popliteal arteries usually begins distal to the femoral artery and spreads into the popliteal artery. The superficial femoral artery is the most commonly affected area.

Clinical Manifestations

The clinical manifestations of chronic arterial occlusive disease result from ischemia distal to the occluded blood flow. Occlusion of the aorta and iliac artery may produce male impotence and intermittent claudication in the lower back, buttocks, thighs,

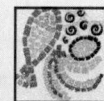

HIGHLIGHT
10–5
NUTRITION

Diet Guidelines for Prevention of Atherosclerosis

- Eat only the number of calories necessary to maintain an ideal weight, or reduce intake of calories to achieve target weight.
- Decrease fat intake to 30 to 35% of total calories.
- Decrease intake of saturated fat.
- Decrease intake of cholesterol to 300 mg/day.
- Decrease sodium to 130 mg/day.
- Maintain protein intake at 12 to 15% of total calories.
- Increase carbohydrate intake to 50 to 55% of total calories.
- Eat no more than three egg yolks per week.
- Use more poultry meats (white meat, skinless).
- Use skim milk dairy products.
- Remove visible fat from meat, use more polyunsaturated fats, and add no salt to cooking.
- Eat more fresh fruits and vegetables.

Data from American Heart Association. The American Heart Association diet: An eating plan for healthy Americans. Dallas, TX: American Heart Association, 1991.

and calf muscles. Occlusion in the femoral and pop-liteal arteries produces intermittent claudication in the calf muscles and feet. Pain increases with exercise.

Rest pain usually results from ischemia of the distal tissues and nerves. It worsens at night when cardiac output decreases. Elevation of the affected extremity aggravates the condition.

Dependent rubor results from the inadequate blood supply, causing anoxia and paralysis of the capillaries. Dependent rubor indicates moderate to severe arterial occlusive disease. With the extremity in a dependent position, the amount of color change relates directly to the severity of the disease. Pallor occurs when the extremity is elevated.

As a result of the decreased arterial blood flow, the lower leg and foot lose hair, decrease muscula-ture, and develop thin, dry, shiny skin. If the foot is elevated, it blanches immediately. When the foot is lowered, venous filling is delayed. The foot is usu-ally cold and often numb. The toenails may be hy-pertrophied. Ulcerative lesions appear on the ex-tremities because of a lack of oxygen and nutrients from diminished circulation. The extremities usually become very painful from the lesions. The develop-ment of secondary infection, which aggravates and spreads the ulcerations, is common. Gangrene de-velops from bruising, shearing, and trauma to the tissue.

The extremities may become edematous, espe-cially if the patient keeps them in a dependent posi-tion for long periods of time. Edema may range from mild to the severe, pitting type. The edema is the result of position and obstruction in the vessel.

Popliteal and pedal pulses are usually absent. Pulsation in the abdominal aorta may be present. Bruits are audible with a stethoscope over the ste-notic arteries. If pulses are palpable, they tend to be obscured with exercise if an artery is obstructed.

Diagnosis

The diagnosis of chronic arterial occlusive disease is based on history, present symptoms, physical assess-ment, and diagnostic studies. Coronary arteriogra-phy may be conducted if heart disease is also present. Ultrasonography, oscillometry, plethysmog-raphy, and a Doppler ultrasonogram can be used to determine the degree of stenosis or the presence of occlusion.

Management

The goal of treatment is to restore blood flow through the narrow or occluded artery and to relieve the patient's symptoms. Conservative treatment in-cludes reduction of risk factors to slow disease pro-gression and improve blood flow. Management also includes pharmacologic therapy, such as vasodila-tors and anticoagulants, to enhance circulation.

Surgical intervention may be required to bypass the occluded artery. An aortofemoral graft or an aortoiliac graft may be necessary to bypass the

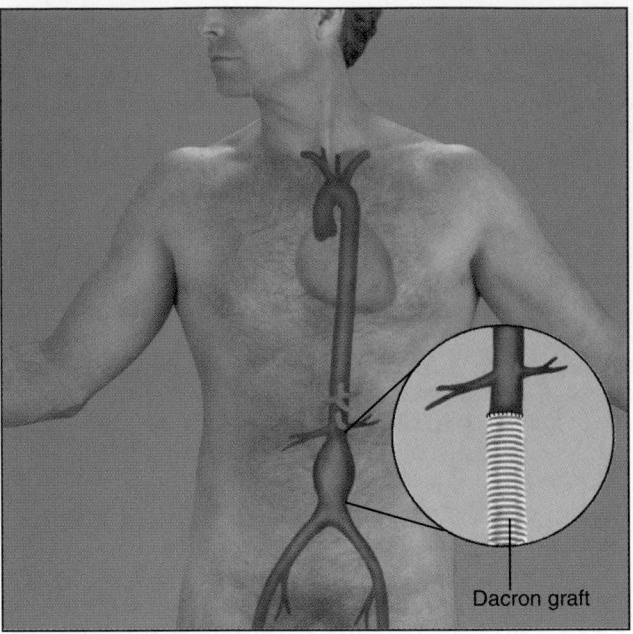

Figure 10–1

Bifurcated synthetic aortoiliac graft inserted after surgical excision of aortoiliac aneurysm. The graft permits arterial blood flow to the lower extremities.

blockage. An aortoiliac graft is illustrated in Figure 10–1. A graft from the axillary artery to the femoral artery (Fig. 10–2) may be required for a patient unable to tolerate abdominal surgery. A femoropop-

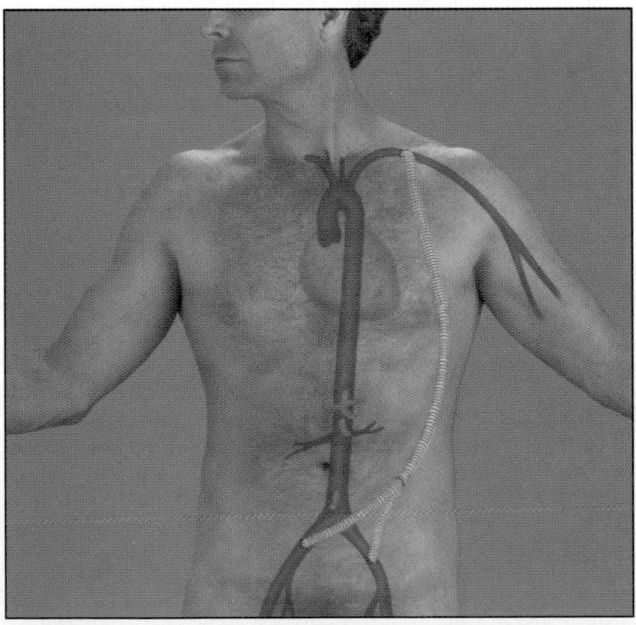

Figure 10–2

An axillobifemoral bypass graft. The axillary artery is connected to the femoral artery, with a branch graft connecting to the other femoral artery.

liteal bypass graft or a longer graft extending to the tibioperoneal trunk or ankle may be performed (Fig. 10–3). The patient's saphenous vein is the preferred material for the bypass graft for distal reconstruction to prevent complications of thrombosis and sepsis. (Refer to Chapter 9 for a discussion of bypass grafts.)

A thromboendarterectomy can be performed for occlusions in the common iliac and femoral arteries. For patients unable to tolerate surgery, a sympathectomy may be performed to dilate the arteries permanently, allowing increased blood supply to the lower legs and feet. Amputation may be necessary if the artery is completely occluded, especially if gangrene is present.

NURSING PROCESS GUIDELINES
Chronic Arterial Occlusive Disease

Assessment, nursing diagnoses, expected patient outcomes, nursing interventions, and evaluation for patients with chronic arterial occlusive disease are similar to those described previously for patients with atherosclerosis and obstructive arterial vascular disorders.

❖ Settings, Providers, and Collaboration for Care

Patients with obstructive arterial vascular disorders, although frequently diagnosed in the hospital set-ting, are usually managed in the home setting with visits to the physician's office for follow-up care. Many of these patients are older adults who live in residential care settings or nursing homes. The chronic nature of obstructive arterial diseases requires ongoing assessment and treatment.

Patients who have had surgery for the disease, such as an endarterectomy or a bypass graft, need continuity of care after being discharged. The home health nurse (or nurse in the residential care facility or nursing home) can assess the site for healing or early signs of complications and collaborate with the physician about further treatment. The nurse can also instruct the patient and family about dressing changes, signs and symptoms of problems, and the medications prescribed.

A nutritionist can assist with dietary instructions as needed. An exercise therapist can evaluate the patient and prescribe physical activities to help alleviate the symptoms of occlusive arterial vascular disease. The exercise plan is tailored to the patient's age, ability, symptoms, and other disease factors. The physician, exercise therapist, nutritionist, and nurse work together to plan a diet and activities for the patient to lose weight or maintain ideal weight while reducing risk factors for arterial disease. The nurse monitors the patient's progress in this area.

ANEURYSMS

An aneurysm is an outpouching of a vessel wall or sac caused by the dilatation or expansion of a partic-

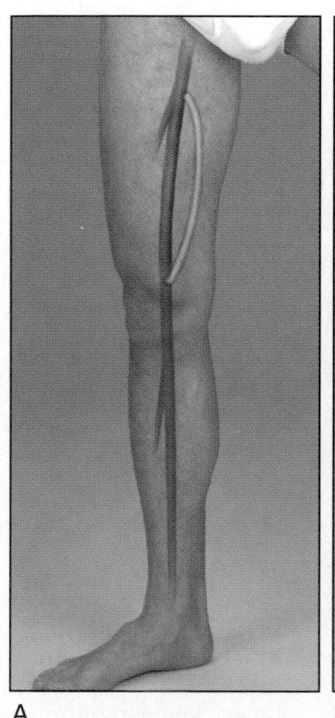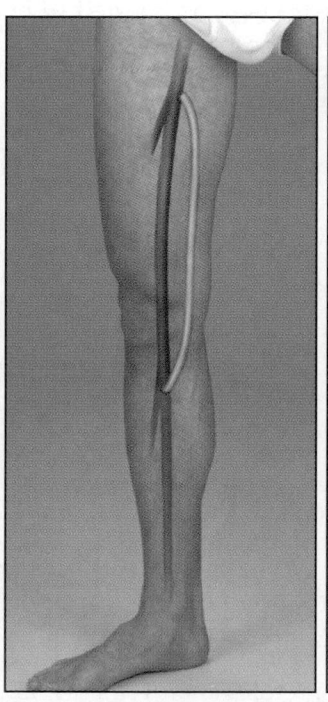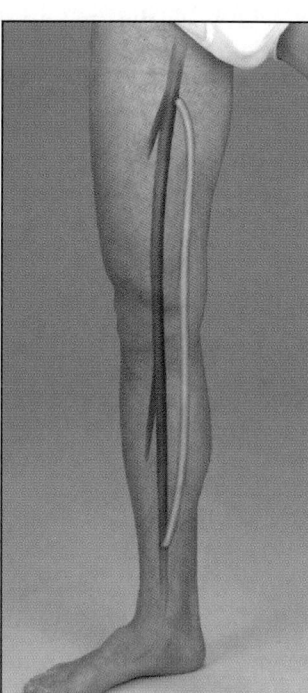

Figure 10–3

A, A femoropopliteal bypass graft. *B,* A graft extending to the tibioperoneal trunk. *C,* A long graft extending to the ankle.

A   B   C

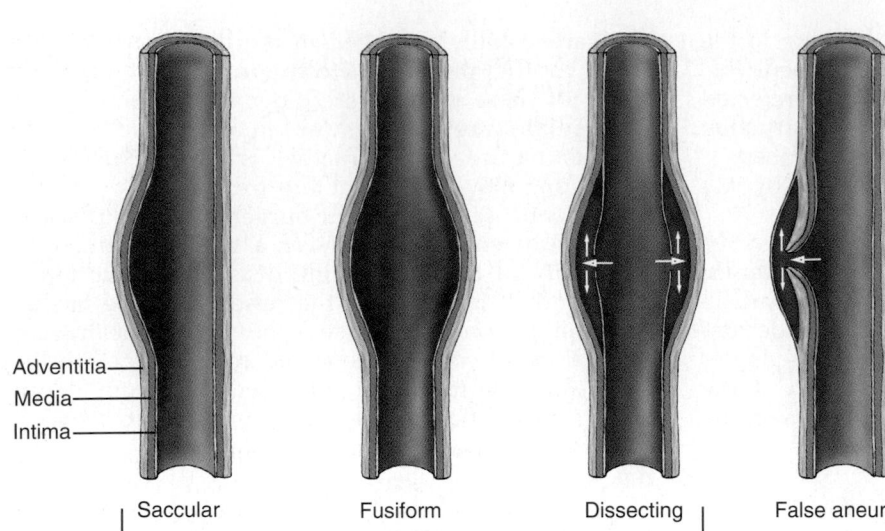

Adventitia
Media
Intima

Saccular   Fusiform   Dissecting   False aneurysm

True aneurysms

Figure 10–4

Classification of aneurysms. True aneurysms include the saccular, fusiform, and dissecting types. A false aneurysm occurs from a rupture in the vessel wall, which allows blood to leak into an outpouching of tissue.

ular site on the vessel. It usually results from atherosclerosis but may also be caused by hypertension, infection, inflammation, congenital abnormalities of vessel walls, or trauma that weakens vessel walls.

Aneurysms usually develop in people older than age 60 and are more likely to occur in men than in women. Aneurysms are found more frequently in the aorta than in other vessels, but they can occur in any artery. They are classified by their location, cause, and shape. They may also be referred to by the blood vessel involved, such as in aortic, splenic, or femoral aneurysm. Or they may be referred to by the part of the vessel involved, such as in ascending aortic and descending aortic aneurysms.

True aneurysms include the fusiform, saccular, and dissecting types (Fig. 10–4). In these types, the outpouching or sac involves all three layers of the artery wall. A false aneurysm usually results from trauma that damages the vessel, allowing blood to form a channel within the vessel wall. A false aneurysm is more likely to rupture and leak into the surrounding tissues.

Although the underlying pathologic process resulting in an aneurysm is usually atherosclerosis, other pathologic processes may also be responsible for arterial changes resulting in a weakened vessel wall. Over the years, increased vascular pressures and stretching of the layers of the damaged vessel can result in the outpouching. The aneurysm gradually increases in size and may rupture. This is an emergency and requires immediate surgical intervention. A ruptured cerebral aneurysm produces one type of cerebrovascular accident. A ruptured aortic aneurysm will result in death in a few minutes.

A small aneurysm may be present for years before diagnosis because it may cause few symptoms,

if any. Many large popliteal, femoral, and abdominal aneurysms are palpable and found during a routine physical examination or chest x-ray. These are usually asymptomatic as well.

Fusiform Aneurysm

A fusiform or spindle-shaped aneurysm is the most common type of aneurysm diagnosed. The entire circumference of the vessel is dilated by the aneurysm. A fusiform aneurysm occurs most commonly in the abdominal aorta and iliac arteries and is usually caused by atherosclerosis.

Saccular Aneurysm

A saccular aneurysm is an outpouching or saclike aneurysm of the artery that involves only a part of the vessel wall. The primary cause of a saccular aneurysm is trauma to the site and thinning and stretching of the medial layer of the vessel. Saccular aneurysms occur most commonly in the abdominal aorta and popliteal and femoral arteries. Aneurysms occurring in the transverse and descending thoracic aorta are also frequently saccular. A saccular aneurysm in the circle of Willis in the brain (berry aneurysm) results from a congenital anomaly.

Dissecting Aneurysm

A dissecting aneurysm occurs when blood penetrates the intimal layer of the aortic wall and separates the layers of the arterial wall, forming a hematoma. The intima and medial layers are torn in most cases, and the hematoma extends to the adventitial layer. The separation may extend in either direction.

The separation may obstruct an artery branching from the aorta, or the hematoma may rupture, causing a life-threatening situation.

If the dissecting aneurysm is in the ascending aorta, it is called a type A dissecting aneurysm. If the aneurysm is in the descending aorta, it is called a type B dissecting aneurysm. Dissecting aneurysms occur more frequently in men than in women and are usually located in the thoracic arch of the aorta. Predisposing factors include hypertension and left ventricular hypertrophy. Surgical intervention is the usual treatment for a dissecting aneurysm.

Abdominal Aortic Aneurysm

Etiology and Pathophysiology
Usually, abdominal aortic aneurysms develop in the abdominal aorta below the renal arteries. They may also extend to the iliac arteries. Atherosclerosis is the most common predisposing factor for an abdominal aortic aneurysm. Other causes include infection, trauma, or congenital abnormalities. The medial layer of the vessel wall is weakened, affecting the elastin and collagen, and the adventitia layer becomes inflamed.

An abdominal aortic aneurysm is usually of the fusiform type and contains ulcerated plaques, mural thrombi (clots attached to the wall of the vessel or heart), and necrotic material. The aneurysm may vary in size. The normal abdominal aorta is 2.5 cm in diameter. Anything greater than 3 cm is considered aneurysmal. Undetected silent abdominal aortic aneurysms are occasionally found as large as 10 cm, 12 cm, or even 15 cm. The incidence of abdominal aortic aneurysms has risen in recent years, primarily because of increased longevity and increased incidence of atherosclerotic problems. It is more common in people over age 60 with a history of cardiovascular disease, including myocardial infarction, hypertension, angina pectoris, and congestive heart failure.

Clinical Manifestations
Typically, abdominal aortic aneurysms are asymptomatic. However, complications are just as likely to occur in an asymptomatic patient as in a symptomatic patient. Abdominal pain from pressure on the somatic sensory nerve is an occasional manifestation. The pain ranges from mild to severe and may be localized in the lumbar, midabdominal, or pelvic area. It may also radiate to the lower extremities. Low back pain may indicate impending rupture.

The patient may feel a throb or pulsation in the abdomen, especially when supine. This pulsation may also be auscultated as a bruit over the abdomen. Large aneurysms can easily be palpated in thin individuals and may cause some abdominal distention. Tenderness with palpation may be present directly over the aneurysm. Extremities may be pale, cold, or mottled and pulses absent if the aneurysm dissects, enlarges, or ruptures, interrupting blood flow to the periphery.

Because approximately half the patients with an abdominal aortic aneurysm have hypertension, systolic readings in the thigh (which are normally higher than in the arm) may be decreased as a result of arterial occlusion of the femoral artery. Occlusion of arteries related to abdominal aneurysms is illustrated in Figure 10–5.

Diagnosis
The diagnosis is based on physical assessment and diagnostic test results. Most large abdominal aortic aneurysms are discovered by palpation during a physical examination. Small aneurysms are not usually palpable, especially if the patient is obese. Even large abdominal aortic aneurysms may not be detected on physical examination if they are beneath many layers of adipose tissue. Some are found on routine chest x-rays, but ultrasonography and com-

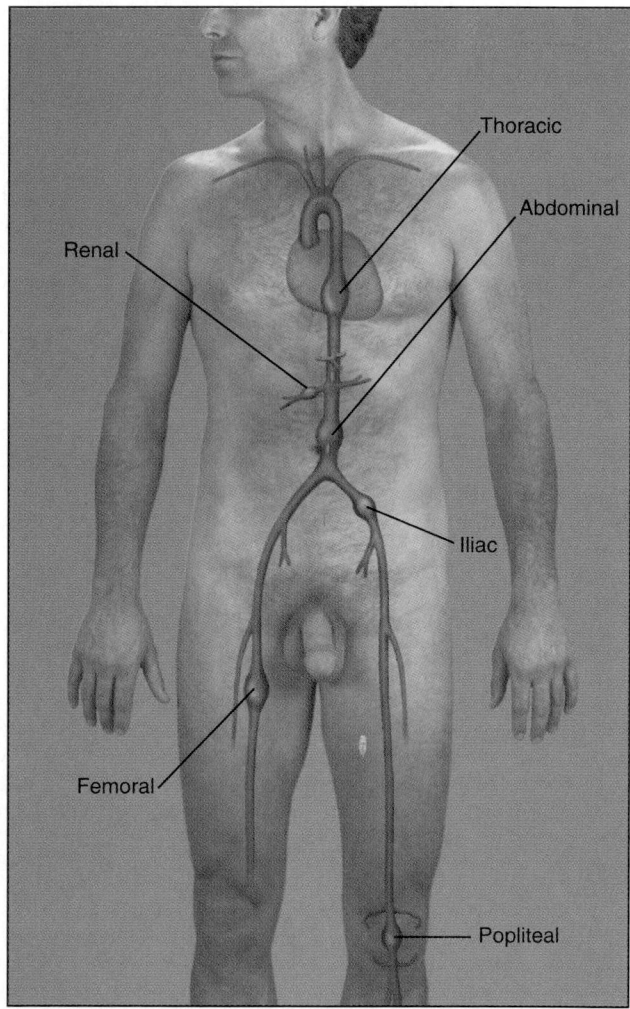

Figure 10–5
The relative location of arterial occlusion and arterial aneurysms.

SUDDEN ABDOMINAL PAIN IN A PATIENT WITH AN AORTIC ANEURYSM

A 78-year-old male patient turned on his call light and screamed in pain as I reached his room. The patient was admitted with a medical diagnosis of abdominal aortic aneurysm (AAA) which had been treated medically with antihypertensive medication and a sodium-restricted diet for the previous year. Recent complaints of difficulty walking, cramping at night, and claudication of the legs resulted in this hospital admission for further evaluation of his condition. His medical history included long-standing atherosclerotic cardiovascular disease, hypertension (HTN), and Type II diabetes mellitus. The patient stopped smoking 15 years previously; before that, he smoked at least a pack a day for more than 40 years.

As I approached his bed, I could see that the patient was extremely apprehensive and was attempting to sit up. He was pale, sweating profusely, and reported that the pain had started suddenly, was located in the epigastric area, and went clear through to his back. He felt nauseous and verbalized an impending sense of doom.

I immediately recognized that an acute change in the patient's condition had occurred, and because the required interventions vary, I quickly considered the possible causes. The patient's pain, anxiety, pallor, and diaphoresis might have resulted from gastrointestinal disorders such as indigestion, esophagitis, or peptic ulcer; or from cardiovascular disorders such as acute myocardial infarction, pulmonary embolism, pericardial tamponade, pericarditis, dissecting aortic aneurysm, threatened aortic rupture, or an already leaking or ruptured aortic aneurysm. His medical history certainly supported the likelihood of a cardiovascular

condition, but further assessment was required to sort out the symptoms of a potentially-life threatening condition from a less serious one.

Because the patient's condition was potentially fatal, I focused my assessment on his airway, breathing, and circulation first. His airway was clear, his respirations were rapid (32 per minute), shallow and unlabored, and his breath sounds were clear. His apical rate was tachycardic (126 bpm) and regular, and no abnormal heart sounds were auscultated. The patient was hypotensive (92/62 mm Hg), his skin was cool and clammy, and a prolonged capillary refill time was noted.

These findings are typical clinical manifestations of a decreased circulating volume secondary to bleeding and hemorrhage, but might also accompany an acute myocardial infarction and cardiogenic shock. Brief questioning regarding the patient's pain revealed that it remained constant and boring, rated a 9 on a scale of 1 to 10, and radiated to the groin. The location, nature, and severity of the pain, along with its unrelatedness to respirations, position, movement or meals, helped me to eliminate some potential conditions. I quickly palpated the patient's peripheral pulses and found them to be stronger in the upper extremities and diminished in the legs. This information, in addition to the above findings, led me to suspect that the patient was suffering from a leaking or ruptured abdominal aortic aneurysm.

The patient complained of thirst and was becoming confused. Gentle palpation of his abdomen revealed a large pulsating mass, while inspection revealed abdominal distention and slight ecchymosis in the perumbilical area.

The patient's medical history, signs and symptoms of shock, and decreasing level of consciousness coupled with the pulsating abdominal mass,

(continued)

puted tomographic scanning are the most accurate tests used for diagnosis. These diagnostic tools are used to detect the size and exact location of the aneurysm. Abdominal aortic angiography (aortogram) is used to evaluate the neck of the aneurysm, extension into the iliac arteries, the location and condition of the renal, celiac, splenic, and superior and inferior mesenteric arteries prior to surgical resection of the abdominal aortic aneurysm.

Management

Surgical resection is the treatment of choice for most abdominal aortic aneurysms. If the patient is a poor

surgical risk, in extremely poor health, or has a history of cardiac dysfunction, the surgery may be delayed. If the aneurysm is very small, the prognosis may still be good without surgery. The aneurysm should be screened every 6 months with ultrasonography to follow the progression of enlargement.

Patients undergoing elective surgery for resection of an abdominal aortic aneurysm have a good prognosis, but some complications may occur. Complications include emboli in the peripheral arteries, renal failure from decreased cardiac output, and myocardial infarction from previous coronary artery dis-

CLINICAL ? THINKING

(continued)

ecchymotic area, and increasing abdominal girth increased the likelihood of rupture and further supported my suspicion.

Knowing that a ruptured aortic aneurysm is a rapidly life-threatening condition with a very high risk of death resulting from hemorrhage and exsanguination, I recognized that there was little time to spare and immediately implemented the following actions:

1. I remained with patient and called for help.
2. I asked the other staff nurse to notify the physician of my findings STAT and to bring the crash cart to the bedside.
3. I placed the patient in a supine position with legs elevated.
4. I initiated an IV line and administered oxygen as per hospital protocol.
5. I provided the patient with brief explanations of procedures, and offered realistic reassurance.
6. I continued to monitor the patient's vital signs and mental status.
7. I documented my findings and actions.

The physician arrived and ordered a STAT portable abdominal x-ray and blood specimens for CBC, blood type, and cross match. My suspicion was confirmed by the x-ray, a decreased RBC count, and the physician's evaluation of the patient's clinical picture.

The patient was prepared for emergency surgery and underwent a 6-hour resection and repair of his ruptured abdominal aortic aneurysm. He arrived in the surgical intensive care unit in critical but stable condition. Although he faced numerous potential postoperative complications during recovery, careful assessment and quick response to this crisis helped prevent the patient's immediate death and increased his chance for long-term survival.

Think Critically

Why did the nurse remain with the patient at all times?

Was placing the patient flat in bed with legs elevated the best action? What was the rationale behind this action?

Should oxygen have been administered? What was the rationale for this nursing action when respiratory distress is not evident?

What additional nursing actions would have been implemented if the patient's systolic pressure had been less than 80 mm Hg? What medications would the nurse have anticipated for administration?

What additional emergency measures would have been implemented if this patient was discovered at home?

Before going to surgery the patient said to the nurse, "I know I'll never survive this operation." What would have been the best response by the nurse? What constitutes "realistic" reassurance?

What preparation for surgery can the nurse realistically plan for in the limited period of time permitted?

What priority nursing assessments will the nurse make following surgery? What postoperative complications should the nurse be particularly alert for?

What similarities and differences would the nurse have noted if the patient's medical diagnosis was ruptured thoracic aneurysm?

---

ease. Patients at risk for myocardial infarction may need to have a coronary artery bypass graft completed before undergoing surgery for the aneurysm.

Additional complications may develop before surgery if a large aneurysm presses on adjacent structures. Pressure on the duodenum can result in blockage of the intestine or bleeding from ulcerations caused by inadequate blood flow to the organ.

For patients whose aneurysms are untreated, rupture and hemorrhage is the most common cause of death. The larger the aneurysm, the more likely it is to rupture. The presence or absence of symptoms has no effect on the likelihood of rupture or development of other complications. Less than 30% of abdominal aortic aneurysms rupture. A size greater than 5 cm or one rapidly increasing at a rate greater than 1 cm per year is a poor prognosis and is a greater risk of rupture. The risk of rupture increases exponentially after 5 cm. That is why surgical repair is typically undertaken when the aneurysm reaches 5 cm. Before then, the size of the aneurysm is followed by ultrasonography every 6 months.

Symptoms of a ruptured aneurysm include sudden back or abdominal pain, decreased blood pressure, increased pulse rate, and ecchymoses in the lower back area. Although laboratory findings

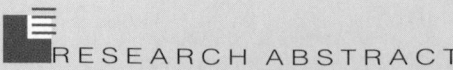
RESEARCH ABSTRACT

Who Is at Risk for Development of Abdominal Aortic Aneurysms?

Alcorn H, Wolfson S, Sutton-Tyrrell K, Kuller L, O'Leary D. Risk factors for abdominal aortic aneurysms in older adults enrolled in the cardiovascular health study. Arterioscler Thromb Vasc Biol 1996; 16(8):963.

Abdominal aortic aneurysms cause few symptoms until they enlarge or begin to dissect. Alcorn and colleagues therefore sought to develop a profile of people at risk for development of abdominal aortic aneurysms, so that high-risk patients could be screened and treated early in the course of their disease. The study was part of the long-term Cardiovascular Health Study and was based on four sources of data:

Routine mortality statistics
Autopsy studies
Clinical and epidemiologic studies
Population screening

The researchers found that the factors that presented the highest risk for development of abdominal aortic aneurysms were male sex, increasing age, smoking, tall stature, and obesity. Interestingly, the study did *not* find a correlation between elevated blood pressure and risk for development of abdominal aortic aneurysms. People who had been treated for hypertension *were* at risk for expansion of a pre-existing abdominal aortic aneurysm, but the mere presence of hypertension was not a risk factor in itself. The prevalence of abdominal aortic aneurysms was also higher among people with a history of atherosclerotic disease, especially those with a history of angina. The researchers also found a familial clustering of abdominal aortic aneurysms, suggesting genetic and environmental components.

The results of blood studies that correlated highly with abdominal aortic aneurysms were increased cholesterol and low-density lipoprotein levels, and decreased high-density lipoprotein levels. Increased creatinine levels were also associated with abdominal aortic aneurysms.

Nurses do not easily give up sacred cows, but the use of abdominal palpation in screening for abdominal aortic aneurysms may need to be abandoned. One finding of this study was that abdominal palpation was an inaccurate means of detecting the presence of abdominal aortic aneurysms. According to Alcorn and colleagues, a better means of diagnosing abdominal aortic aneurysms would be to determine on an ultrasonogram the ratio of infrarenal diameter to suprarenal diameter.

The researchers also found that the prevalence of abdominal aortic aneurysms appears to be increasing, as is the rate of growth of abdominal aortic aneurysms less than 5 cm in diameter.

Questions to Consider

1. Why is it important to educate the public about the risk factors for abdominal aortic aneurysm?
2. Is screening for abdominal aortic aneurysms feasible? Why or why not?
3. Are all of the risk factors that were identified in this study covered on a routine admission form in your clinical facility? What factors might your form miss? What questions would you need to ask to compensate for that omission?

would show a decreased red blood cell count and hemoglobin related to the hemorrhage, this is not the time to send the patient to the laboratory for a blood test. Call a surgeon immediately. This is a true surgical emergency. Even with immediate surgery, the prognosis can be very poor after rupture, especially if the patient is over age 65 years or has a history of other disorders. Spinal paralysis, resulting in paraplegia, is one potential complication. Death is another.

Thoracic Aortic Aneurysm

Etiology and Pathophysiology

Atherosclerosis is the primary cause of thoracic aortic aneurysms. They occur most often in men between the ages of 40 and 70 years. Thoracic aneurysms are frequently the dissecting type, but they may also be fusiform or saccular.

Clinical Manifestations

Thoracic aortic aneurysms are usually asymptomatic. Patients with symptoms may experience constant pain in the chest or upper back, neck, and shoulders. The pain may be more prominent when the patient is supine. Dyspnea may result from pressure of the aneurysm against the trachea, bronchi, or lungs. A brassy cough, stridor, hoarseness, and weak voice are caused by pressure on the trachea and laryngeal nerve. Dysphagia occurs from pressure on the esophagus. Pressure on the cervical sympathetic nerve chain causes unequal dilatation of the pupils. The aneurysm may compress large veins in the chest, causing edema, cyanosis, and dilated superficial veins of the neck, chest, and upper extremities. Distention of neck veins occurs from pressure on the superior vena cava.

Diagnosis

A thoracic aortic aneurysm is diagnosed by physical assessment, history (if symptomatic), chest x-ray, aortography, and computed tomographic scan. These tests help determine the exact location of the aneurysm and which surrounding vessels are involved.

Management

Antihypertensive medications are given to keep systolic pressure below 120 mm Hg, thus reducing pressure in the aorta. Other medications, such as propranolol, may be prescribed to reduce cardiac contractions and decrease the pulsating flow of blood.

Surgical resection of the aneurysm with a synthetic vascular graft is the treatment of choice (see Chapter 9 for a discussion of grafts). With surgery, prognosis is very good. However, the prognosis worsens if the patient is over age 50, has a history of hypertension, or if the aneurysm is extremely large. Death from rupture of the aneurysm occurs in approximately one-third of patients. A small asymptomatic aneurysm may not be treated unless it enlarges.

Peripheral Arterial Aneurysms

Etiology and Pathophysiology

Most peripheral aneurysms occur in men between ages 50 and 80. Aneurysms of the peripheral vessels usually result from atherosclerosis. Other causes include trauma, infection, stress, and shear factors of blood flow. Peripheral aneurysms are often bilateral and multiple. Symptoms are absent in about half the patients.

Peripheral aneurysms occur more often in the lower extremities than in the upper extremities. Two-thirds of all peripheral arterial aneurysms occur in the popliteal artery, and about one-third occur in the femoral artery. Femoral aneurysms appear as a pulsating mass along the femoral artery. Popliteal aneurysms are located in the popliteal fossa and also appear as a pulsating mass. The aneurysm is usually elongated and fusiform (Fig. 10–6). Flexion of the knee may predispose the popliteal artery to dilatation.

Clinical Manifestations

Clinical manifestations of peripheral arterial aneurysms include intermittent claudication from arterial insufficiency in the lower legs and feet. Rest pain or gangrene may occur from thrombosis or embolism. The risk is embolization of the mural clot down the limb, occluding smaller distal vessels. Multiple small emboli may appear as black dots on the plantar surface of a toe or toes or as blue toe syndrome. The aneurysmal source of the emboli needs to be located and surgical repair considered to prevent limb loss.

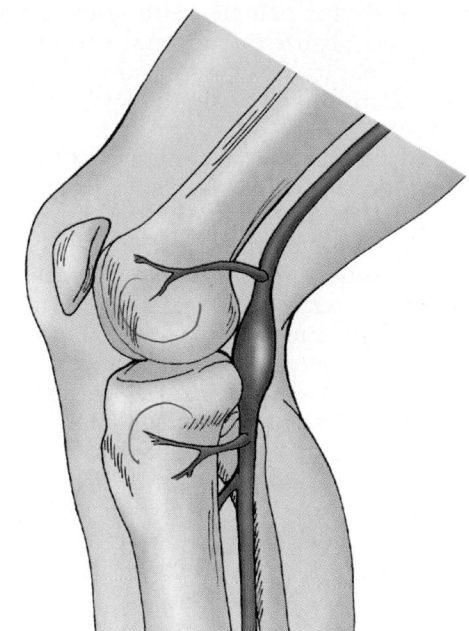

Figure 10–6
Fusiform aneurysm of the popliteal artery.

Tenderness, pain, edema, coldness, and numbness in the lower extremities are caused by pressure on the nerves, veins, and arteries.

Diagnosis

The diagnosis is based on the symptoms present, physical assessment, and diagnostic studies, such as angiography and ultrasonography.

Management

Surgical resection of the aneurysm with a saphenous vein graft is the treatment of choice. Occasionally, a prosthetic graft is used, but it does not have the longevity of autogenous material. Prognosis is excellent after surgery if the patient takes steps to reduce the risk factors associated with atherosclerosis. The most common postoperative complication is bleeding. (Refer to Chapter 9 for a discussion of grafts.)

Without surgery, complications develop within 8 years in most patients. Thrombosis may result in ischemia and possible loss of the extremity. The aneurysm may cause pressure on surrounding veins and nerves, causing occlusion and pain. Other complications include rupture, which is rare, or infection and gangrene from interruption of the circulation.

NURSING PROCESS GUIDELINES
Aneurysm

The assessment, nursing diagnoses, expected patient outcomes, nursing interventions, and evaluation for patients with an aneurysm are similar to those described previously for patients with arterial embolus or thrombus and obstructive arterial vascular disorders. Refer to Chapter 9 for application of the nursing process to the patient undergoing peripheral vascular surgery.

The following additional assessments apply to the care of patients with aneurysm. Assess cardiopulmonary and renal status by observing hemodynamic monitoring, laboratory tests, and output. Check for tenderness and distention of the abdomen. Auscultate arteries for bruits. Do not use deep palpation if a dissecting aneurysm is suspected. Assess all pulses to detect occlusion of arteries. Observe the color and temperature of the extremities. Look for venous distention and edema. Check for pain in the back, neck, shoulders, or extremities. Observe for ecchymoses on the lower back.

Assess changes in respiratory status. Observe for fever and leukocytosis, which indicate pulmonary complications. Auscultate for wheezes and crackles, indicating pulmonary congestion from increased hydrostatic pressure in the pulmonary vascular system. Respiratory distress may indicate impending shock from hemorrhage after rupture of the aneurysm. Observe for other changes that could indicate a ruptured aneurysm, such as sudden, intense pain and vital sign changes.

The following additional interventions apply to the care of patients with aneurysm. If the patient is at high risk, surgery may be delayed or not recommended. Explain the effects of the disorder to the patient and family. Teach the signs of rupture and tell the patient to seek immediate medical assistance if any of the signs become apparent. Explain the lifestyle restrictions prescribed by the physician. Allow the patient and family time to ask questions and to voice fears and concerns about the patient's future. Make appropriate referrals for home-care assistance as needed.

❖ Settings, Providers, and Collaboration for Care

Most patients with aneurysms are hospitalized for diagnosis and treatment. After surgery, the patient may be discharged with dressings still in place. The nurse teaches the patient about dressing changes, signs of complications, when to call the physician, and the medication regimen to be followed at home. If the patient is alone or has other debilitating disorders, a home health nurse may assist with the dressing changes after discharge. The nurse also observes for signs of healing or complications and communicates these findings to the physician. The patient will have follow-up appointments at the physician's office.

ℋypertensive Vascular Disease

Hypertensive vascular disease is defined as a persistent systolic blood pressure greater than 140 mm Hg and a persistent diastolic blood pressure greater than 90 mm Hg. A persistent systolic blood pressure greater than 140 mm Hg with a diastolic pressure less than 90 mm Hg is termed *systolic hypertension*. In 1992, federal health officials released a new system for classifying blood pressure, dividing levels of hypertension into four stages (Table 10–1).

Hypertensive vascular disease is the most common cardiovascular disorder in the United States. It is estimated that at least 20% of the adult population may be affected. In the elderly, the numbers are significantly higher. Approximately 65% of African-American elderly and 40 to 50% of white elderly are hypertensive. Because people with hypertension are commonly free of symptoms until complications de-

Table 10–1

Classification of Blood Pressure for Patients Age 18 and Older

Average Diastolic Blood Pressure (mm Hg)	Average Systolic Blood Pressure (mm Hg)						
	Less Than 120	120–129	130–139	140–159	160–179	180–209	210 or Over
Less than 80	Optimal*	Normal	High normal	1	2	3	4
80–84	Normal	Normal	High normal	1	2	3	4
85–89	High normal	High normal	High normal	1	2	3	4
90–99	1	1	1	1	2	3	4
100–109	2	2	2	2	2	3	4
110–119	3	3	3	3	3	3	4
120 or over	4	4	4	4	4	4	4

*Unusually low readings should be evaluated for clinical significance.

Adapted from National Heart, Lung, and Blood Institute, National Institutes of Health. National high blood pressure education program. Washington, DC: U.S. Government Printing Office, 1992.

Table 10–2

Risk Factors Associated with Hypertension

Risk Factors	Rationale
Age	Loss of arterial elasticity
Sex	Higher blood pressure in males over age 40
Race	Blood pressure higher in African-Americans; possibly due to high-fat dietary intake, genetics, high-stress lifestyle
Obesity	Extra weight increases cardiac workload and strains vessels
Smoking	Nicotine constricts vessels
Caffeine	Vasoconstriction
Sodium	Water retention causes volume expansion
Stress	Vasoconstriction

velop, only about half of those with hypertension are diagnosed. Of those diagnosed, only about half comply with their prescribed treatment plan.

The incidence of hypertension in the United States is higher among men than women and is highest in the African-American population. In addition to a higher incidence of hypertension, this population also tends to have more severe disease and a higher incidence of mortality associated with the disease.

Hypertension is classified as either primary (essential) hypertension or secondary hypertension. About 90% of all individuals who have hypertension have primary hypertension. The onset is usually between ages 25 and 55. Primary hypertension is further categorized as benign, which has a slow onset and is initially asymptomatic, or malignant, which is a rare form characterized by sudden onset, rapid development of symptoms, and accelerated progression of the disease.

Secondary hypertension is characterized by an underlying known cause that impairs peripheral blood flow, alters cardiac output, or increases blood viscosity. Secondary hypertension may also be associated with endocrine gland disorders and side effects of some medications. When the underlying cause is treated, the hypertension resolves. Ten per-

cent of all individuals with hypertension have secondary hypertension.

Etiology and Pathophysiology

Primary hypertension has no known cause; however, a variety of factors contribute to its occurrence. These factors, which are identified in Table 10–2, include heredity, age, and lifestyle patterns. A diet high in fat and sodium also increases the risk of hypertension. There is a direct relationship between the incidence of hypertension and atherosclerosis. Hypertension is a risk factor in the development of atherosclerosis, and atherosclerosis, with its associated impairment of arterial blood flow, contributes to the development of hypertension.

Peripheral vascular resistance and cardiac output directly affect blood pressure. Resistance is determined by the diameter of the blood vessels and blood viscosity. Primary benign hypertension is characterized by narrowed arteries, which increase peripheral resistance. In many instances, it is unclear whether increased peripheral resistance precedes or results from increased blood pressure.

In some individuals with primary hypertension, a pathologic response to stress causes excessive stimulation of the sympathetic nervous system. Increased sympathetic nervous system stimulation produces peripheral vasoconstriction and increased heart rate, which results in increased blood pressure.

In some cases of hypertension, excess quantities of renin are secreted by the kidneys. Excess renin may be secreted in response to sympathetic nervous system stimulation or in the absence of any stimulating factors. Renin converts angiotensinogen into angiotensin I, which is subsequently converted by an enzyme to angiotensin II. Angiotensin II causes arteriole constriction and stimulates the adrenal cortex to increase the secretion of aldosterone. Aldosterone promotes sodium and water retention, which increases extracellular fluid volume. The combination of excess peripheral vasoconstriction and an increase in the blood volume results in pathologic elevation in blood pressure (Fig. 10–7).

In the early stages of primary benign hypertension, changes in the blood vessels and organs are not apparent. However, as the disorder progresses, changes can be detected in blood vessels and the major target organs, such as the heart, kidneys, brain, and eyes.

Under constant stress from abnormally high

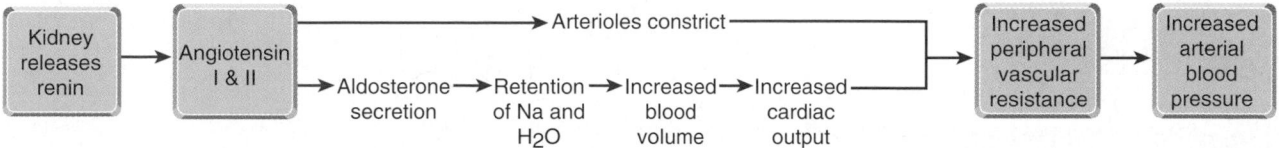

Figure 10–7

Effect of the release of renin-angiotensin on blood pressure.

pressure, the intima of the arteries is damaged, resulting in edema, fibrin accumulation, and clot formation. Arterial walls weaken, and the vessels become sclerosed and tortuous. As the lumens narrow, blood flow to the major target organs and peripheral tissues decreases. Because the blood supply to organs and peripheral tissues is impaired, ischemia, atrophy, fibrosis, and loss of function occur. Damaged vessels may eventually become occluded or may hemorrhage as a result of weakened vascular walls.

Cardiovascular disorders associated with hypertension result from the heart's attempt to overcome increased peripheral resistance. When the blood vessels constrict, the heart pumps harder, resulting in cardiac hypertrophy, especially of the left ventricle. This, in turn, may lead to left ventricular failure, progressing to right ventricular failure and con-

gestive heart failure. Venous congestion occurs throughout the entire vascular system. Figure 10–8 illustrates the events in hypertensive vascular disease that lead to target organ destruction.

Decreased arterial blood flow to the kidneys may cause ischemia and necrosis of renal nephrons and may lead to renal failure. Weakened arteriosclerotic vessels under prolonged above-normal pressure may rupture or develop aneurysms. Cerebral aneurysms may result in cerebral hemorrhage, transient ischemic attacks, cerebral infarctions, or cerebrovascular accidents. Arteriosclerosis, ischemia, and hemorrhage of retinal vessels may result in visual disturbances and blindness. Arterial atherosclerosis with reduced blood flow to the lower extremities results in arterial peripheral vascular disease, ischemia, and intermittent claudication. The incidence of these long-term degenerative changes associated with hy-

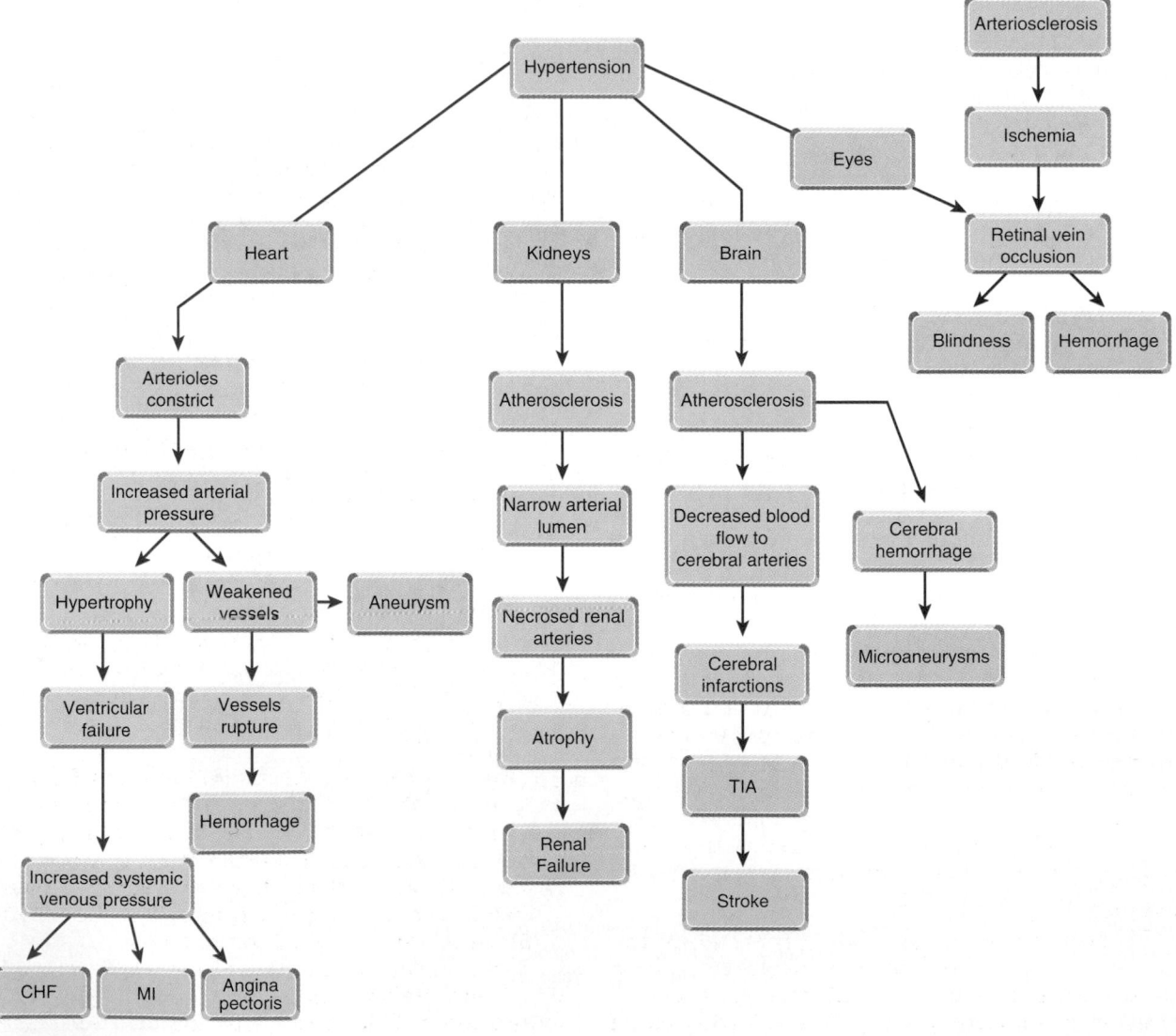

Figure 10–8

How hypertension affects major target organs. CHF, congestive heart failure; MI, myocardial infarction; TIA, transient ischemic attack.

pertension is greatly reduced if the condition is adequately controlled.

The pathologic deterioration associated with malignant hypertension is more severe and may progress more rapidly than in benign hypertension. In malignant hypertension, blood pressure rises suddenly, possibly as high as 200/140 mm Hg. It occurs most commonly in people between ages 40 and 50.

More than half the people with malignant hypertension have an underlying chronic kidney disease. Hyperplasia of the intima of the arteries in the kidneys leads to nephron ischemia and atrophy. As the arterial lumen becomes permanently narrowed, renal failure results. Cardiovascular disorders such as left ventricular failure, congestive heart failure, arteriosclerosis, and myocardial infarctions develop rapidly. The high sustained blood pressure causes papilledema, hemorrhage, and exudates in the retinas. Without treatment, the mortality rate is about 80% within 1 year and almost total within 2 years.

Clinical Manifestations

An absence of symptoms in the initial stages is typical of benign hypertension. This is one reason that rates of early diagnosis and compliance to treatment regimens are so low. Initially the patient feels well even without treatment.

Ophthalmoscopic examination of the retina shows:

- Hemorrhages
- Crossing over, narrowing, and nicking of the retinal arteries
- Tortuous vessels
- Patchy white areas with indefinite edges (cotton wool exudates)
- Papilledema with blurring of the disk margins

Cerebrovascular manifestations include epistaxis, vertigo, lightheadedness, tinnitus, occipital headaches in the early morning, and blurred vision. Decreased sensations and hemiplegia may indicate a transient ischemic attack or stroke. Personality changes, nausea, and vomiting result from reflex spasms of cerebral vessels associated with extremely high blood pressure readings.

Cardiac changes include palpitations, fatigue, paroxysmal nocturnal dyspnea, angina pectoris, and left ventricular hypertrophy, which result from the increased workload on the heart and tissue ischemia from impaired blood supply.

Renal involvement results in nocturia, hematuria, and increased blood urea nitrogen and creatinine levels. Skin changes, such as discoloration and edema, may indicate vessel inflammation.

Diagnosis

The diagnosis is based on history, physical assessment, and blood pressure measurements. Blood pressure measurements are obtained over a period of a few days to several weeks. The recorded blood pressure at each measurement is the average of three readings taken at least 2 minutes apart. On the first measurement, the patient's pressure is obtained in both arms while he or she is lying, sitting, and standing.

A chest x-ray and ECG are done to determine cardiac changes, and a urinalysis is completed to detect protein. Complete blood count, fasting blood sugar, blood urea nitrogen, serum creatinine, and urine specific gravity help determine the extent of renal damage.

Renal function studies, renal angiography, intravenous urograms, and tomography are used to detect secondary causes. Urine is tested for excessive serum catecholamines. Studies are conducted to evaluate plasma renin, angiotensin, and aldosterone. A serum potassium level is determined because hypokalemia may indicate primary aldosteronism. Thyroid studies are conducted because hyperthyroidism can cause excessively high blood pressure and heart rate, leading to vasoconstriction and hypertension. High serum cholesterol and triglyceride levels may predispose to the development of atheromatous plaques.

Management

The management goal for primary hypertension is to reduce blood pressure. For a patient whose diastolic blood pressure is less than 100 mm Hg, the treatment of choice involves minimizing risk factors by adopting a diet low in cholesterol and sodium, losing weight if necessary, performing relaxation exercises, and following a regular regimen of moderate exercise. If diastolic pressure is consistently greater than 105 mm Hg, drug therapy may be indicated. Table 10–3 outlines actions recommended by the National Institutes of Health. The goal in drug therapy is to use the least amount of medication with the most effectiveness and the least side effects.

The drugs of choice for hypertension vary with physician preference, patient history, concurrent medications, and tolerance. Commonly prescribed antihypertensive drugs are listed in Table 10–4. Diuretics may be used to suppress renal tubular reabsorption of sodium. Sympathetic blocking agents or beta blockers and vasodilators may be added. The medications are given to relax smooth-muscle walls, decrease cardiac output, block or interfere with sympathetic impulses, decrease release of renin, and decrease peripheral resistance and arterial constriction (Highlight 10–6).

Noncompliance to treatment regimens for hypertension is extremely common. It is estimated that only about one-ninth of all patients with hypertension are being treated adequately. Of newly diagnosed patients, about half discontinue therapy within 1 year of treatment. Almost three-fourths discontinue therapy within 5 years.

Many theories have been proposed to explain why noncompliance is so high among patients with hypertension. One reason may be that the disorder is usually asymptomatic in its early stages. Another may be that treatment requires lifestyle changes and,

Table 10-3

Recommended Actions for Patients with High Systolic or High Diastolic Readings

RECOMMENDED ACTION FOR PERSONS WITH HIGH SYSTOLIC READINGS

Systolic Readings with Diastolic ≤90 mmHg	Recommended Action
≥200	Immediate evaluation and treatment no later than 2 weeks
140–199	Re-evaluate within 1–2 months
<140	Re-evaluate in 2 years

RECOMMENDED ACTION FOR PERSONS WITH HIGH DIASTOLIC READINGS

Diastolic Readings	Recommended Action
≥115	Immediate evaluation and treatment
105–114	Evaluation/treatment no later than 2 weeks
90–104	Re-evaluate within 1–2 months
<90	Re-evaluate in 1 year

Adapted from The Joint National Committee on Detection, Evaluation and Treatment of High Blood Pressure. The Fourth Report of the Joint National Committee on Detection, Evaluation and Treatment of High Blood Pressure (JNC IV). Bethesda, MD: National Institutes of Health, 1988.

in some cases, medications. The patient may feel well without treatment and may even feel ill when taking medication because of the side effects. It is difficult to motivate patients to adhere to a treatment regimen when benefits are not easily apparent. Other factors associated with noncompliance include long waiting times at clinics or physician's offices, treatment and medication costs, and poor follow-up care.

With asymptomatic diseases like hypertension, patients have a 50% appointment failure rate and at least a 60% noncompliance rate with medications. It is estimated that one-third of patients almost always take the prescribed medications, one-third take the prescribed medication sometimes, and one-third never take the prescribed medication. It is difficult to predict which patients will be noncompliant with the prescribed treatment regimen. Evidence suggests that increased patient education about the disease and treatment modalities may enhance compliance.

Complications

Excessively high blood pressure that requires immediate treatment is termed *hypertensive crisis*. Less than 5% of patients with primary hypertension progress to hypertensive crisis. During a crisis, the diastolic pressure may be as high as 130 mm Hg. Retinal hemorrhages, exudates, and papilledema are usually present. The patient may be restless and confused and experience blurred vision, headache, nausea, and vomiting. A cerebrovascular accident, renal failure, or cardiac failure may occur within days. A hypertensive crisis is a medical emergency. The patient is admitted to an intensive care unit for close monitoring of blood pressure and target organ damage. Quick-acting parenteral medications—such as the vasodilators, sympathetic inhibitors, and diuretics identified in Table 10–5—are administered to lower the blood pressure rapidly.

❖ Settings, Providers, and Collaboration for Care

Patients with hypertensive vascular disease are usually managed as outpatients with frequent visits to the physician's office for continued evaluation and review of the treatment plan. The nurse, in collaboration with the physician, informs the patient about the disease and the treatment regimen. The patient is given detailed instructions about the diet, exercise, and medication plan. Complications of the disease and results of lack of compliance are explained to the patient. The nurse teaches the patient to monitor blood pressure and to keep a record of the results. The nurse emphasizes the lifestyle changes the patient can make to reduce the modifiable risks of the disorder.

If the patient has other complications of the disease, cannot comply with the treatment regimen, or lacks assistance from family members, a referral to a home health agency is recommended. The home health nurse assesses the patient's status, checks on compliance with the treatment plan, and refers the patient to the physician's office as needed.

An exercise therapist may assist the patient to devise a moderate physical activity plan. A nutritionist can teach the patient and family meal-planning strategies to reduce weight and risk factors. Sample menus can help direct the meal-planning process and simplify it for the patient or family members.

NURSING PROCESS
Hypertension

Assessment

Review the patient's history and diagnostic studies and complete a physical assessment. Assess blood pressure while the patient is lying, sitting, and standing. Take the measurements in both arms and legs to determine baseline data and note any differences bilaterally. Before taking the blood pressure, have the patient rest quietly for at least 5 minutes. Compare the readings with previous data. Measurements may be affected by the time of day, the pa-

Table 10–4

Oral Antihypertensive Medications

Medication	Action	Contraindications	Side Effects
THIAZIDE DIURETICS			
Bendroflumethiazide (Naturetin)	Renal excretion of Na$^+$, water, K$^+$; initial decrease in blood volume and cardiac output	Renal failure	↑ BUN
Benzthiazide (Exna)		Hepatic disease	↑ Uric acid
Chlorothiazide (Diuril)		Lactation/pregnancy	↑ Blood glucose
Chlorthalidone (Hygroton)		Hypokalemia	↑ Calcium
Hydrochlorothiazide (Esidrix, HydroDIURIL, Oretic)		Gout	↓ Potassium
		Diabetes	Restlessness
Hydroflumethiazide (Saluron)		Peripheral vascular disease	Lethargy, weakness, vertigo, thirst, dry mouth
Indapamide (Lozol)			GI disturbances
Metolazone (Zaroxolyn, Diulo)			Muscle cramps
Methyclothiazide (Ethon, Enduron)			Hypotension, tachycardia
			Polyuria
Polythiazide (Renese)			Leukopenia
Trichlormethiazide (Metahydrin, Naqua)			Agranulocytosis
Quinethazone			
LOOP DIURETICS			
Furosemide (Lasix)	Same as thiazides	Same as thiazides	Similar to thiazides
Ethacrynic acid (Edecrin)			Hypocalcemia
Bumetanide (Bumex)			Hypovolemia
			Dehydration
			Gynecomastia
			Photosensitivity
POTASSIUM SPARING (NONTHIAZIDES)			
Spironolactone (Aldactone)	Renal excretion of Na$^+$ and water; retention of K$^+$	Renal failure	↑ BUN
		Hyperkalemia	Hyperkalemia
		Diabetes	Hyponatremia
		Calcium channel blocking agents	Gynecomastia
			Hirsutism
			Irregular menses
			Rash
			Lethargy, ataxia
			Confusion
Triamterene (Dyrenium)			Hyperkalemia, hyperchloremic acidosis, diarrhea, nausea, vomiting, rash, photosensitivity, blood dyscrasias
Amiloride (Midamor)			
Spironolactone with HCTZ (Aldactazide, Dyazide)	Blocks reabsorption of Na$^+$		Vertigo, headache, dry mouth, GI disturbances
ADRENERGIC INHIBITORS			
Beta Blockers			
Acebutolol (Sectral)	Decreases cardiac output, sympathetic stimulation, and renin secretion	Bronchial asthma	Lethargy, fatigue, depression, vertigo, insomnia, headache
Atenolol (Tenormin)		Rhinitis	
Metoprolol (Lopressor)		Cardiomegaly	
Nadolol (Corgard)		CHF	Bronchospasm
Pindolol (Visken)		Peripheral vascular disease	Dyspnea
Propranolol (Inderal)			Bradycardia, palpitations, orthostatic hypotension
Timolol (Blocadren)		Bradycardia	Raynaud's phenomenon
		Diabetes, hypoglycemia	GI disturbances, nausea, vomiting, diarrhea, fluid retention
		MAO inhibitors	
		Bronchodilators	
		Liver disease	Hypoglycemia
		Pheochromocytoma	Thrombocytopenia
		Pregnancy, lactation	Rash, fever, nasal stuffiness
			Impotence

Table continued on following page

Table 10–4

Oral Antihypertensive Medications *(continued)*

Medication	Action	Contraindications	Side Effects
Alpha Inhibitors			
Prazosin (Minipress)	Decreases peripheral vascular resistance, vasodilation		
Beta/Alpha Combined			
Labetalol (Normodyne, Trandate)	Same as prazosin		
Central Inhibitors			
Clonidine (Catapres)	Initially decreases cardiac output; decreases peripheral vascular resistance and heart rate	Hepatic disease Pregnancy Tricyclic antidepressants Mental depression	Orthostatic hypotension, vertigo, sedation, rash, constipation, dry mouth, headache, fatigue, anorexia, bradycardia, fluid retention, insomnia, nightmares
Guanabenz (Wytensin)			Drowsiness, dry mouth, fluid retention, rash, postural hypotension, loss of libido, dark or blue urine
			Same as clonidine
Methyldopa (Aldomet)			Fever, anemia, impotence
Peripheral Inhibitors			
Guanadrel (Hylorel) Guanethidine (Ismelin) Reserpine (Serpasil, Serpalan, Reserfia)	Relaxes smooth muscle, decreases peripheral vascular resistance, heart rate, and blood pressure when upright	CHF, pheochromocytoma, peptic ulcer, surgery, ulcerative colitis, bronchial asthma, tricyclic antidepressants, MAO inhibitors, orthostatic hypotension, severe coronary artery or cerebrovascular disease, mental depression	Orthostatic hypotension, bradycardia, diarrhea, edema, impotence, decreased libido, depression, nasal congestion, increased appetite, weight gain, gastric hyperacidity, salt and water retention, drowsiness, bizarre dreams
VASODILATORS			
Diazoxide (Hyperstat) Hydralazine (Apresoline) Minoxidil (Loniten) Sodium nitroprusside (Nipride)	Relaxation of arteriolar smooth muscle resulting in vasodilation; initial decrease in cardiac output; decreased peripheral vascular resistance	Coronary artery disease CHF Lupus erythematosus Cerebrovascular disease Migraine	Headache, vertigo, fever, flushing, tachycardia, palpitations, nausea, anorexia, diarrhea, dyspnea, rash, angina, fluid retention, muscle aches, tremors, cramps, lupus-like syndrome with long-term usage
CALCIUM CHANNEL BLOCKING AGENTS			
Diltiazem (Cardizem) Nifedipine (Procardia) Verapamil (Calan, Isoptin)	Inhibits calcium into smooth muscle cells; arteriolar vasodilation, decreases peripheral vascular resistance; increases cardiac output, with the exception of verapamil.	CHF Heart block Beta blocking agents	Headache, vertigo, weakness, palpitations, tachycardia, dysrhythmia, flushing, rash, hypotension, peripheral edema, nausea, constipation, diarrhea, fluid retention, bradycardia, muscle aches, tremors, cramps

Table continued on following page

Table 10–4

Oral Antihypertensive Medications *(continued)*

Medication	Action	Contraindications	Side Effects
ANGIOTENSIN-CONVERTING ENZYME INHIBITORS			
Captopril (Capoten) Enalapril (Vasotec)	Decreases peripheral vascular resistance	Renal insufficiency Renal artery stenosis	Hypotension Hyperkalemia Granulocytopenia, hemolytic anemia, proteinuria, stomatitis, loss of taste, tongue ulcers, fever, rash

BUN, blood urea nitrogen; CHF, congestive heart failure; GI, gastrointestinal; HCTZ, hydrochlorothiazide; K$^+$, potassium ion; MAO, monoamine oxidase; Na$^+$, sodium ion.

tient's emotional status, pain, smoking, eating, talking, coldness, bladder distention, or drugs. Blood pressure readings are often higher at midmorning and noon.

Palpate the apical pulse at the midclavicular line in the fifth intercostal space and the peripheral pulses to determine the rate, rhythm, and amplitude. Palpate extremities for edema. Auscultate for dysrhythmias, tachycardia, or abnormal breath sounds, which may indicate cardiac involvement.

Ask about episodes of angina and obtain a description of the pain as to intensity, precipitating factors, duration, radiation, and relief methods. Examine the neck for enlarged thyroid or vein disten-

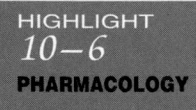 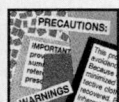

HIGHLIGHT
10–6
PHARMACOLOGY

Beta-Adrenergic Blocking Agents

Definition:

Drugs that block receptor sites affected by catecholamines.

Action:

Exhibit effective blocking at specific receptor sites, resulting in decreased heart rate, slowed conduction, decreased plasma renin, and decreased force of myocardial contraction.

Uses:

To reduce hypertension, dysrhythmias, aortic stenosis, and other noncardiovascular effects.

Side Effects:

May be selective depending on the particular drug; they include drowsiness, malaise, nausea, tingling, paresthesia, dizziness, and decreased heart rate.

Interactions:

May interact with cardiac depressants. May be inactive when used in conjunction with sympathomimetic drugs. May antagonize the bronchodilating effect of theophylline. May increase problems with orthostatic hypotension. May enhance neuromuscular blocking agents.

Nursing Implications:

Watch for signs of drug interactions as listed above.

Monitor vital signs while patient is on medications; especially observe for bradycardia and measure blood pressure frequently to monitor the effect of the drug if given for hypertension.

Tell the patient being discharged on medication to return, as ordered, for follow-up laboratory studies to check kidney, liver, cardiac, and respiratory function.

Give the medication before meals except when otherwise indicated, because most beta blockers should be taken before meals.

Geriatric Considerations:

Caution the elderly patient to change positions slowly because the drug may cause orthostatic hypotension. This could be a safety concern for older adults, especially those with physical mobility impairment. Tell the patient the drug may cause increased sensitivity to cold, which is a common problem in the elderly.

Table 10–5

Parenteral Medications Used in Treating Hypertensive Crisis

Medication	Action	Indications	Nursing Considerations
DIURETICS			
Furosemide (Lasix)	Inhibits reabsorption of Na+ and chloride by the renal tubule; large amounts of Na+ and chloride are excreted; smaller amounts of K+ and bicarbonate ion are excreted	Malignant hypertension Hypertensive encephalopathy CHF Intracranial hemorrhage Pulmonary edema Lymphedema	Never use with ethacrynic acid; assess for electrolyte losses (ie, chest pain, calf and pelvic pain); do not give with whole blood or its derivatives; assess for vestibular disturbance with renal impairment; assess for vascular thrombosis and embolism, especially in elderly
Ethacrynic acid (Edecrin)	Same as for Lasix	Same as for Lasix	Same as for Lasix; pain and irritation at injection site when given IM and SC
VASODILATORS			
Sodium nitroprusside (Nipride)	Vasodilation of peripheral arterioles	Hypertensive encephalopathy Malignant hypertension CHF, pheochromocytoma Intracranial hemorrhage	Monitor BP closely; check for excessive hypotensive effect
Diazoxide (Hyperstat)	Vasodilation of peripheral arterioles	Hypertensive encephalopathy Intracranial hemorrhage Malignant hypertension	Potent diuretic; assess BP before each bolus dose; inject rapidly within 30 sec into peripheral vein; keep patient flat 30 min after injecting
Hydralazine (Apresoline)	Vasodilating effect on vascular smooth muscle and CNS effects (reflex action)	Malignant hypertension Eclampsia	Assessing BP within 5 min after injecting; may cause headaches, palpitations, arrhythmias; weigh daily; observe for edema, I & O
SYMPATHETIC INHIBITORS			
Methyldopa (Aldomet)	Depresses sympathetic nervous system, relaxes smooth muscle	Malignant hypertension Intracranial hemorrhage	Weigh daily; observe for edema, I & O; usually used with other antihypertensive drugs
Reserpine (Serpasil)	Same as Aldomet	Malignant hypertension	Same as above
GANGLIONIC BLOCKER			
Trimethaphan (Arfonad)	Dilates blood vessels, increases heart rate and cardiac output	Malignant hypertension Hypertensive encephalopathy Pulmonary edema Dissecting aortic aneurysm Ischemic heart disease	Instruct patient with history of angina that it may precipitate an attack; monitor BP closely; assess for peripheral vascular collapse (ie, hypotension; rapid pulse; cold, clammy skin; cyanosis)

BP, blood pressure; CHF, congestive heart failure; CNS, central nervous system; IM, intramuscularly; I & O, input and output; K+, potassium ion; Na+, sodium ion; SC, subcutaneously.

tion. Observe for decreased urinary output, or increased output if the patient is on diuretic therapy. Palpate the abdomen for masses and bruits that indicate aneurysms or stenosis of the abdominal aorta or renal arteries.

Assess neurologic status to detect changes associated with altered cerebral perfusion, cerebrovascular accident, or hemorrhage. Assess for pallor, diaphoresis, and vertigo when the patient rises from a supine position, which may indicate orthostatic hypotension.

Assess for skin and retinal changes that indicate progressive hypertension. Obtain height and weight measurements to determine obesity. Review the patient's dietary pattern; check calorie levels and the amount of fat, cholesterol, and sodium regularly consumed. Determine food preferences and financial influences on food choices.

Assess the patient's level of knowledge, stressors, and risk factors, such as smoking, obesity, and lack of exercise. Determine whether the patient is taking birth-control pills, diet pills, cold medications, amphetamines, or alcohol, which may be associated with hypertension. Check the family history for hypertension, other cardiovascular diseases, and diabetes.

Nursing Diagnoses and Planning

Nursing diagnoses and related expected patient outcomes commonly applicable to patients with hypertension include the following:

NDx: Decreased cardiac output related to increased workload of the heart and vasoconstriction

Planning: Patient Outcomes
1. Vital signs are within normal ranges for the patient.
2. Patient has a balanced intake and output and is free of peripheral and central edema.
3. Patient's skin is warm, color is appropriate, no cyanosis is present, and peripheral pulses are palpable.
4. Patient maintains an adequate cardiac output as seen by the hemodynamic monitoring.

NDx: Altered nutrition: more than body requirements, related to lifestyle, resulting in obesity, atherosclerosis, and hypertension

Planning: Patient Outcomes
1. Patient states accurate information about an appropriate diet plan for weight loss, including low-fat, low-cholesterol, and low-sodium foods.
2. Patient chooses food as allowed on the diet plan.
3. Patient's weight decreases.

NDx: Self esteem disturbance related to hypertensive disease state, changes in lifestyle to manage disease and reduce risk factors, or inability to comply with the treatment plan

Planning: Patient Outcomes
1. Patient states methods to cope with illness.
2. Patient denies feelings of inadequacy, helplessness, or dependency.
3. Patient appears positive, friendly, and cheerful and actively participates in plans for discharge and patient education sessions.
4. Patient takes responsibility for self-care and complies with treatment plan.

NDx: Knowledge deficit: nature of the disease, nutritional needs, treatments, and measures to reduce risk

Planning: Patient Outcomes
1. Patient describes cause, effects, and risk factors associated with hypertension.
2. Patient lists symptoms and treatments for the complications of the disorder.
3. Patient relates the nutritional therapy for lowering cholesterol levels and consumes low-fat, low-sodium meals.
4. Patient states the self-care needed to prevent risk or complications of hypertension.

NDx: Noncompliance to treatment regimen related to asymptomatic disorder, side effects of medications, financial problems, inability to make lifestyle adjustments, or lack of education about disease state

Planning: Patient Outcomes
1. Patient relates accurate information about the disease and the importance of following the prescribed treatment plan.
2. Patient states the potential consequences or risks of not following the prescribed treatment plan.
3. Patient demonstrates compliance with the plan.
4. Patient's vital signs stay within normal ranges for the patient.

Nursing Interventions and Evaluation

NDx: Decreased cardiac output
Monitor vital signs while the patient is lying, sitting, and standing. Encourage the patient to rest frequently throughout the day to prevent fatigue and strain on the myocardium. Instruct the patient to stop activity if it initiates episodes of chest pain, aggravates chest discomfort, or causes headache, confusion, or dizziness, indicating possible neurologic problems.

Use telemetry monitoring whenever possible, especially if the patient experiences dysrhythmias or if the patient is taking antidysrhythmic drugs. Review the results of laboratory studies and hemodynamic monitoring.

Check the patient's intake and output, observing for adequacy and balance. Keep the patient's legs in a nondependent position while he or she is sitting, to prevent edema. Provide support for the extremities while the patient is sitting or lying in bed.

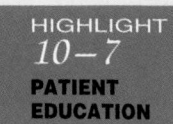
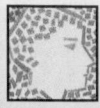

HIGHLIGHT
10–7
PATIENT EDUCATION

Stepped Care Guidelines for the Patient with Hypertension

The Joint National Committee on Detection, Evaluation, and Treatment of High Blood Pressure recommends the following guidelines for hypertensive patients:

Upon discharge, instruct the patient to:

Set a plan for lifestyle changes to reduce weight.

Stop smoking.

Reduce the dietary intake of salt.

Consume no more than 2 oz of hard liquor, 8 oz of wine, or 24 oz of beer per day.

Adapted from the National Committee on Detection, Evaluation, and Treatment of High Blood Pressure. 1988 report. Bethesda, MD: National Institutes of Health, 1988.

Teach the patient relaxation techniques and range-of-motion procedures to increase circulation while he or she is lying in bed. Keep the patient warm and comfortable. Prevent constriction of circulation from tight-fitting clothing or bed linen.

NDx: Altered nutrition: more than body requirements
Teach the patient about dietary modifications needed to reduce weight. Give the patient literature explaining the caloric content of foods and the fat, cholesterol, and sodium content. Plan a dietary regimen for the patient, including foods of choice when possible, and give sample menus to the patient and family to follow at home. Seek dietary counseling with the dietitian as needed.

Devise an exercise regimen for the patient that will help burn calories and increase circulation as well as make the heart more efficient and lower the blood pressure. Encourage the family to participate with the patient in the exercise program.

NDx: Self esteem disturbance
Teach the patient self-care measures and encourage participation and decision-making. Explain how changes in lifestyle can benefit the patient by reducing blood pressure and the risk of other disorders. Allow time for expression of concerns, questions, and clarification of misunderstandings. Praise the patient for knowledge gained about the disorder, for

---

HIGHLIGHT
10–8
NUTRITION

Instructions for the Patient on a Low-Sodium Diet

Some Common Foods to Avoid on a Low-Sodium Diet

- Presalted canned foods, meats, and snacks
- Foods preserved by sodium addition
- Soups, bouillon, and gravies
- Condiments and sauces
- Cheese, butter, and cheese spreads
- Seasonings prepared with salt such as garlic salt and onion salt
- Frozen fish, pizza, and sausage products

Herbs and Spices to Substitute for Salt

Allspice	Ground meats, stews, tomatoes, peaches
Almond extract	Pudding, fruits
Basil	Fish, lamb, ground meats, stews, salads, soups, sauces
Bay leaves	Meats, stews, poultry, soups, tomatoes
Caraway seeds	Meats, stews, soups, salads, breads, cabbage, noodles
Chives	Salads, sauces, soups, meat dishes, vegetables
Cinnamon	Fruits, breads, pie crust, desserts
Curry powder, cumin	Lamb, chicken, fish, tomatoes, soup
Dill	Fish, soups, salads
Onion powder	Meats, vegetables, salads
Paprika, parsley	Meats, eggs, fish, soups, salads, vegetables, potatoes
Peppermint	Puddings, fruits, desserts
Rosemary	Chicken, veal, beef, pork, sauces, potatoes, peas
Sage	Meats, stews, biscuits, beans
Savory	Salads, ground meats, soups, beans, squash, peas
Thyme	Veal, pork, sauces, onions, peas, tomatoes
Turmeric	Meats, fish, rice

attempts at lifestyle change, and for participation in self-care.

Seek assistance from clergy, family members, or other professionals when appropriate. Make referrals for the patient on discharge as needed.

NDx: Knowledge deficit: nature of the disease, nutritional needs, treatments, and measures to reduce risk

Explain the cause, effects, and clinical course of hypertension to the patient. Provide opportunities for the patient to ask questions at any time. Provide appropriate literature about hypertension for the patient and family to review. Allow the patient to verbalize concerns and fears. Evaluate discharge needs of the patient and family (Highlight 10–7). Teach the patient or family how to take a blood pressure reading.

Alert the patient to signs and symptoms of uncontrolled hypertension and the complications such as impaired renal function, hemorrhage, and neurologic disturbances.

Instruct the patient about dietary modifications needed to reduce risk, reduce weight, or prevent complications of the disorder. Explain the need for decreases in dietary fats and cholesterol to prevent the effects of the disease and increases in protein and vitamins to promote good health and healing (see Highlight 10–5). Also instruct the patient to follow a reduced-sodium diet (Highlight 10–8). Devise a diet plan for weight reduction as needed and appropriate for the patient. Initiate counseling with a dietitian to assist with meal planning if needed.

Teach the patient dosage, route, time, frequency, side effects, and toxic effects of any medication prescribed. Explain the diagnostic studies completed and the need for any follow-up studies after discharge. Include the family in any of the teaching sessions when applicable.

NDx: Noncompliance to treatment regimen

Encourage the patient to comply with the prescribed treatment plan by explaining the consequences and risks of noncompliance and the benefits of compliance. Refer the patient to a support group if applicable. Seek assistance from social services for financial counseling and support. Encourage the family to become involved with the treatment regimen, especially the lifestyle changes. Have a family member check the patient's blood pressure and weight

---

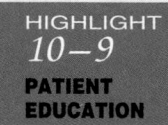 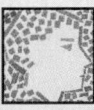

HIGHLIGHT 10–9

PATIENT EDUCATION

Behavior Modification Program for Improving Compliance with a Treatment Plan

Using a behavior modification program can assist in improving the patient's compliance with a treatment program. Set up the program with the patient as follows:

Identify the behavior to be changed with the patient's approval.

Write the behavior that is to be changed in the form of a goal-oriented contract (see example below).

Identify a reward for the patient if the behavior is achieved.

Be sure the contract is realistic, measurable, positively stated, dated, and timed with a deadline.

Have both the nurse and the patient sign the contract and give each party a copy.

Be sure that follow-up occurs on the stated date. Renegotiation may be done if necessary.

I, _____ , will _____
       (Patient Name)   (Behavior to be changed)

by _____ for _____
      (Deadline)   (Reward)

_____
Patient's Signature

_____
Nurse's Signature

weekly, if needed. Praise the patient for compliance with the regimen. Institute a behavior-modification program using a contract signed by the patient and the nurse to improve compliance (Highlight 10–9).

Compare the patient's status with the expected outcomes. If the outcomes are not met, reassess the patient and revise the plan.

Common Venous Vascular Disorders

The collective group of venous vascular disorders includes those that are inflammatory in nature, such as thrombophlebitis, and those that result from other vascular problems, such as varicose veins.

THROMBOPHLEBITIS

Etiology and Pathophysiology

Thrombophlebitis, or venous thrombosis, is the development of a clot in the vein with inflammation of the vessel walls. If inflammation is not present but a clot is, the condition is referred to as phlebothrombosis. The clot, or thrombus, causes partial or complete occlusion of the vein. The primary cause of venous thrombosis is venous stasis. Immobilization and surgical procedures predispose patients to venous stasis. Bedrest reduces blood flow in the legs by half. Injury to the vessel wall and increased blood coagulation when anticoagulants are suddenly withdrawn may also cause a thrombus to form. The estrogen oral contraceptives affect the clotting mechanism of the blood by increasing platelet adhesiveness, increasing the risk of clot formation. Some blood dyscrasias and dehydration may increase the

risk by increasing the concentration of platelets and the blood viscosity (Table 10–6).

It is estimated that about one-third of patients over age 40 and having major surgery acquire small thrombi in the deep calf veins within 24 hours postoperatively. Patients with cerebrovascular accidents or hip fractures have a 50% or greater chance of acquiring thrombi as a result of immobilization from prescribed extended bedrest.

Phlebitis is the inflammation of a vein without thrombosis. It occurs most commonly in the lower extremities. Phlebitis in deep veins is more common than in superficial veins. It occurs in women more often than men, and the occurrence increases with age.

The thrombus or clot formation process (thrombosis) begins with an aggregation of platelets on the vein wall. Platelets may be released in the blood in the presence of viruses, bacteria, endotoxins, some diseases, and trauma to the vein wall. The platelets adhere to the vessel wall within 7 to 10 days, forming deposits of fibrin, white blood cells, and red blood cells. As the thrombus develops, it causes further scarring and damage to the vessel. A free-floating tail grows on the thrombus and may break off, particularly if from a deep vein thrombus. This piece of the thrombus may travel to other parts of the body, such as the lungs, causing an embolus. Thrombi from superficial veins rarely dislodge.

Thrombi tend to develop from the outer edges toward the center. They may occlude the vessel completely or only partially. If a thrombus develops in superficial veins, collateral circulation usually compensates for the blockage. If the thrombus develops in larger veins, collateral circulation may not be sufficient to provide the affected extremity with enough blood flow. Then, symptoms will appear.

Clinical Manifestations

Many patients with thrombophlebitis present no symptoms, especially if the inflammation is in superficial veins. When symptoms do develop, they tend to appear suddenly and last 1 to 2 weeks after the onset of the inflammation. Clinical manifestations vary with the amount of involvement and vein affected.

Deep venous thrombophlebitis causes severe pain, fever, chills, edema, and cyanosis along the affected vein. It typically produces complications of venous insufficiency and varicosities. Homans' sign, calf pain with dorsiflexion of the foot, may be present in deep venous thrombophlebitis, but it is not diagnostic of the condition.

Superficial thrombophlebitis may cause minor pain, edema, rubor, warmth, and topical tenderness along the affected vein. Needle trauma to superficial veins may cause septic phlebitis, resulting in red, warm, tender inflamed areas. The veins feel hard and thready when palpated. Fever and leukocytosis may also occur.

Table 10–6

Risk Factors Associated with Thrombophlebitis

Obesity
Pregnancy (through 10 days after delivery)
Oral contraceptives
Intravenous therapy
Smoking
Bedrest, immobilization
Prolonged sitting or standing
Hypercoagulability of blood (malignant neoplasms)
Blood dyscrasias
Infections (pneumonia)
Trauma (accidents, fractures)
Surgery (postoperative venous stasis)
Dehydration

Diagnosis

The diagnosis is based on history, physical assessment, and diagnostic studies. Phlebography (a graphic study of the structure and function of the veins) is used to detect the location and degree of attachment of the thrombus and to confirm the diagnosis of thrombophlebitis. Plethysmography measures changes in blood volume and shows decreased circulation distal to the thrombus. (See Chapter 9 for a description of the study.) A radioactive fibrinogen uptake test determines the presence of small thrombi in the calf. Angiography, venography, and Doppler venous flow studies may detect further damage to the vessels.

Management

The goal of therapy is to control thrombosis, relieve symptoms, prevent complications, and prevent recurrence of the disorder. The primary treatment is bedrest with elevation of the affected extremity, application of warm compresses, analgesics for pain, and anticoagulant therapy. The dosage, action, side effects, and contraindications for anticoagulant therapy are presented in Table 10–7.

Heparin is the drug of choice for initial anticoagulation and short-term therapy, although it can be used for long-term therapy as well. Heparin is administered by intravenous or subcutaneous routes. The injection site is monitored to ensure that the locations are rotated. While the patient is on heparin therapy, minor trauma, injections, use of razor blades, and aspirin use are avoided to prevent bleeding.

Baseline coagulation studies—such as clotting time, prothrombin time, International Normalized Ratio partial thromboplastin time, and platelet count—are evaluated before the initiation of therapy and throughout administration of the anticoagulants. Heparin doses are determined by maintaining the coagulation time within a preset therapeutic range, usually 1.5 to 2.5 times the control. (Refer to Chapter 12 for a discussion of coagulation times.)

Oral anticoagulants are used for long-term therapy. Coumarin derivatives prevent synthesis of clotting factors and may be administered for several months after discharge to prevent recurrence of the thrombosis. Coagulation studies may be monitored at 1-week to 4-week intervals on an outpatient basis, depending on the case.

Bleeding complications can occur from the anticoagulant therapy. Bleeding usually develops after the first 3 days of therapy. If the venous occlusion is

Table 10–7

Anticoagulants

Medication	Action	Contraindications	Side Effects
Heparin sodium (parenteral)	Delays clotting time, prevents thrombus formation; does not resolve clot; used first 7–14 days of thrombus development Administration: IV bolus 100 units/kg initially, then 1000–1500 U/h infused in D_5; SC 15–20,000 U every 12 h if veins cannot be used Dosage: determined by hematocrit and coagulation tests (PTT)	Hypertension CHF Uremia Duodenal ulcer GI bleeding Recent trauma or surgery Blood dyscrasias Aneurysms Alcoholism Renal and liver diseases Pregnancy Women older than 60 years	Alopecia, flushing, bleeding, hematuria, ecchymosis, bleeding gums, thrombocytopenia, GI bleeding, osteoporosis, epistaxis, rashes Caution: If heparin is given SC, do not stretch skin or rub injection site to prevent hematomas. Use smaller doses in elderly.
Coumarin (oral) Dicumarol (bishydroxycoumarin) Warfarin sodium (Coumadin)	Inhibits synthesis of clotting factors II, VII, IX, X On first day of heparin, start 5 mg/d coumadin and adjust as needed daily. (Because of shorter stay in hospital, coumadin is started sooner without a loading dose.) The dosage is determined by INR (average, 2.5–7.5 mg; range, 1–15 mg/d). Dosage: determined by prothrombin time and INR	Same as for heparin	Avoid drugs that may enhance or inhibit effects (see Table 10–8).

CHF, congestive heart failure; D_5, dextrose 5%; GI, gastrointestinal; INR, International Normalized Ratio; IV, intravenous; PPT, partial prothrombin time; SC, subcutaneously.

severe enough to cause total obstruction of blood flow, ischemia of the extremity and gangrene may result. Approximately half of the patients with deep venous thrombosis acquire chronic venous insufficiency or stasis dermatitis within 5 years. Venous stasis ulcers develop in about 20% of the patients with chronic venous insufficiency. Varicose veins may develop secondary to deep thrombophlebitis as a result of incompetent valves.

Pulmonary embolism may result if parts of the thrombus break loose and travel through the right side of the heart into the pulmonary artery. The pulmonary blood flow is obstructed, resulting in pulmonary infarction from ischemia and necrosis. Venous pressure in the pulmonary artery is increased. A pulmonary embolism is characterized by an abrupt onset of dyspnea, chest pain, cough, hemoptysis, fever, restlessness, petechiae, and shock.

Thrombolytic agents such as alteplase, anistreplase, streptokinase, and urokinase may be used to dissolve fresh clots, but they are more frequently used for major arterial blockages rather than venous blockages. Complications of thrombolytic therapy include bleeding and anaphylaxis.

A femoral vein thrombectomy may be performed in the presence of massive venous occlusion. Vein ligation or interruption of the inferior vena cava may be performed to prevent pulmonary embolism. This is accomplished by implanting a filter in the inferior vena cava to preserve blood flow while preventing clots from moving to the lungs. Prognosis improves after 2 to 3 weeks if the patient remains free from pulmonary embolism. (Refer to Chapter 9 for the discussion on peripheral vascular surgery.)

NURSING PROCESS
Thrombophlebitis

Assessment

Review the patient's history and diagnostic study results. Palpate and compare the lower extremities for edema, discoloration, and tenderness. Measure the circumference of the limbs. Ask about pain in the extremities, noting the intensity, location, and duration. Assess skin temperature of both limbs. Check for the presence of Homans' sign.

Review the laboratory studies, especially hematocrit and coagulation time, if the patient is on heparin therapy. Ask whether the patient is taking any drugs that may potentiate or inhibit the anticoagulant (Table 10–8). Check the urine for blood and assess the stool for occult blood. Observe for ecchymoses, petechiae, epistaxis, or bleeding from the gums.

Check the patient's activity level. If the patient is on bedrest, observe for complications of immobility, such as skin breakdown, infection, and pressure areas. Observe for signs of pulmonary embolism, in-

Table 10–8

Drugs that Affect Anticoagulants	
Drugs that Potentiate Oral Anticoagulants	**Drugs that Inhibit Oral Anticoagulants**
Anabolic steroids	Griseofulvin
Aspirin	Barbiturates
Phenylbutazone (Butazolidin)	Cholestyramine
Chloral hydrate	Corticosteroids
Chloramphenicol	Glutethimide (Doriglute)
Neomycin	Oral contraceptives
Glucagon	Ethchlorvynol (Placidyl)
Quinidine	Tranquilizers

cluding sudden chest pain, dyspnea, restlessness, diaphoresis, and cyanosis. Auscultate breath sounds to check for wheezes or crackles indicative of respiratory distress from infection or embolus.

Assess the patient's level of understanding about the disorder and the complications. Note the patient's history and risk assessment.

Nursing Diagnoses and Planning

Nursing diagnoses and related expected patient outcomes commonly applicable to patients with thrombophlebitis include the following:

NDx: Pain in extremities related to venous inflammation

Planning: Patient Outcomes
1. Patient reports absence of pain or decrease in pain to a tolerable level.
2. Patient states comfort measures to help relieve pain, such as positioning and relaxation techniques.
3. Patient does not present nonverbal signs of pain, such as grimacing, withdrawal, nervousness, and clenching of hands.

NDx: Altered peripheral tissue perfusion related to impaired venous flow from thrombus formation

Planning: Patient Outcomes
1. Patient demonstrates increased perfusion by skin that is warm and dry, with absence of edema, and absence of cyanosis in the extremities.
2. Vital signs are within normal ranges for the patient.

NDx: Impaired physical mobility related to extended bedrest and pain secondary to disease state

Planning: Patient Outcomes
1. Patient reports increased mobility, strength, and endurance.
2. Patient is able to perform activities of daily living.

NDx: Impaired skin integrity (in the extremities) related to immobility

Planning: Patient Outcomes
1. Patient's skin remains intact without evidence of shearing, infection, ulcerations, or gangrene.
2. Patient states appropriate skin-care measures to prevent impairment of skin integrity.

NDx: Knowledge deficit: nature of the disease, complications of bedrest, treatments, and measures to reduce risk

Planning: Patient Outcomes
1. Patient describes cause, effects, and risk factors associated with thrombophlebitis.
2. Patient lists symptoms and treatments for the complications of the disorder.
3. Patient states the self-care needed to prevent risk or complications of thrombophlebitis.

Nursing Interventions and Evaluation

NDx: Pain
Refer to Clinical Practice Guidelines from the Agency for Health Care Policy and Research for suggestions to assist patients in alleviating pain. Counsel the patient to stop smoking. Smoking causes vasoconstriction and increases demand for blood and oxygen to tissues. This combination increases ischemia and thus pain. Use diversional activities to decrease the patient's awareness of pain. Determine coping strategies that help the patient deal with the pain, especially when it is severe.

Administer pain medication as prescribed. Teach the patient about the effects of the medication, frequency of use, and potential side effects. Help the patient relieve pain by using relaxation methods that decrease stress and tension (see Highlight 10–2). Allow for periods of rest during episodes of intense pain. Apply warm, moist compresses to the extremities to decrease edema, relieve spasms, and promote comfort.

Be sure the patient avoids constricting clothing, which interferes with circulation in the extremities and may exacerbate the complications of the disorder. Avoid placing a pillow behind the knees because it can be constricting. Tell the patient to wear warm clothing and to protect the extremities from extreme heat or cold exposure.

NDx: Altered peripheral tissue perfusion
Help the patient conserve oxygen needs by encouraging rest and limiting activities. Elevate the head of the bed to aid in lung expansion. Initiate oxygen therapy if needed. Assist the patient with activities of daily living, if needed, to conserve energy.

Keep the patient in a comfortable position and reposition frequently to release pressure. Use range-of-motion exercises, when allowed, to stimulate circulation. Monitor vital signs and laboratory studies to assess for changes and improvements in status. Encourage ambulation when the patient is off bed-rest, as tolerated, but provide for frequent rest periods to decrease cardiac workload. Discourage smoking to avoid vasoconstriction. Remove constricting clothing, and keep heavy bed linen from restricting peripheral circulation. Keep the patient's legs in an elevated position when he or she is not ambulating.

Give prescribed medications to reduce inflammation, prevent further thrombosis, and thus increase circulation. Discuss risk factors and preventive health-care measures with the patient. Explain lifestyle changes that will promote circulation and decrease the risk of further venous disorders (Highlight 10–10).

NDx: Impaired physical mobility
Assist the patient when he or she is allowed out of bed. The patient may be very weak after being on extended bedrest. Use durable medical equipment accessories, when appropriate, to assist the patient in maintaining mobility. Teach the patient to perform range-of-motion exercises to increase circulation and to maintain or improve strength and endurance.

Prepare a daily exercise schedule as soon as the patient is allowed to be mobile again, increasing the level as tolerated. Tell the patient to walk slowly and avoid stairs or inclines at first, if necessary, and to stop for a few minutes of rest when tired. Encourage the patient to persist in the exercise regimen, even if it must be moderated at times for lack of endurance. Praise the patient on achievements accomplished.

NDx: Impaired skin integrity
Handle the patient's legs and feet with care, especially if the skin is not intact. Use aseptic technique when bathing or dressing areas where the skin is broken to prevent infection. Keep linen off the extremities by using a bed cradle. Instruct the patient to avoid wearing constricting clothing. Keep the extremities warm and dry at all times.

Check peripheral circulation frequently. Observe for early signs of problems developing because of decreased circulation, such as pressure spots, absent pulses, coldness, and discoloration. Report any untoward signs. Have the patient change position frequently to stimulate circulation and prevent pressure ulcers. Use heel pads to prevent skin breakdown if the patient is in bed for long periods of time. Apply graduated compression stockings (30/40 mm Hg pressure gradient) during the acute phase to decrease venous stasis and promote venous return, thus preventing further skin problems. To promote healing and minimize tissue damage, promote a diet high in protein and vitamins.

NDx: Knowledge deficit: nature of the disease, complications of bedrest, treatments, and measures to reduce risk
Explain the cause, effects, and clinical course of thrombophlebitis to the patient. Allow opportunities for the

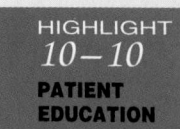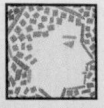

HIGHLIGHT
10-10
PATIENT EDUCATION

Discharge Instructions for the Patient with Thrombophlebitis

Upon discharge, instruct the patient with thrombophlebitis to do the following.
Prevent recurrence of the disorder by:

Avoiding crossing the legs when sitting or lying in bed.

Exercising the toes and feet frequently by dorsiflexion while sitting or lying in bed.

Participating in a walking exercise program to strengthen leg muscles and assist venous return.

Avoiding sitting with the legs in a dependent position.

Avoiding standing in place for long periods of time.

Ceasing smoking to prevent vasoconstriction.

Avoiding wearing tight, constricting clothing on the extremities.

Prevent complications of anticoagulant therapy by:

Understanding the dosage, actions, and side effects of the medication prescribed.

Avoiding over-the-counter medications without checking with the physician to prevent the potentiating or inhibiting effects of other medications.

Taking the anticoagulant medication at the same time each day to maintain the appropriate blood level.

Taking the medication until discontinued by a physician's order.

Returning to the physician's office as needed for medical and laboratory follow-up studies.

Notifying dentist and other medical personnel that an anticoagulant is being taken and bleeding precautions are necessary.

Carrying or wearing an identification card stating name and address, which anticoagulant is being taken, blood type, and physician's name and telephone number.

Being especially careful around sharp instruments or while shaving with a razor blade.

Avoiding contact sports or other rough physical activities.

Assess for signs and symptoms of excessive anticoagulation by:

Observing for petechiae, ecchymoses, bleeding gums when brushing teeth, and prolonged bleeding when cut or nicked while shaving.

Checking for blood in the urine or dark stools, which indicate occult blood.

(Notify the physician if any of these complications are apparent.)

---

patient to ask questions at any time. Provide appropriate literature about the disorder for the patient and family to review. Allow the patient to verbalize concerns and fears. Evaluate the discharge needs of the patient and family (see Highlight 10–10).

Alert the patient to signs and symptoms of thrombophlebitis and complications, such as impaired mobility, pain, skin breakdown, and infection of the extremities. Teach the patient to use safety measures or to ask for assistance when out of bed or ambulating. Teach exercises that the patient can perform after bedrest restrictions are removed to increase strength and endurance.

Teach the patient how to achieve comfort by frequent repositioning and padding bony prominences. Explain the use of a bed cradle to prevent pressure on joints and sensitive areas. Teach the patient how to apply the elastic graduated compression hose, which compresses superficial veins to enhance venous return and circulation to deep veins and de-

creases the chance of recurrence of the disorder (Highlight 10–11).

Teach the patient the dosage, route, time, frequency, side effects, and toxic effects of any medication prescribed. If the patient is on heparin and is being discharged with orders for coumadin therapy, explain the signs of bleeding to the patient and provide instructions on when to seek medical attention. Include the family in any of the teaching sessions when appropriate.

Compare the patient's status with the expected outcomes. If the outcomes are not met, reassess the patient and revise the plan.

CHRONIC VENOUS INSUFFICIENCY

Chronic venous insufficiency results from valve destruction, which occurs in chronic venous inflammation and venous stasis. Most patients in whom

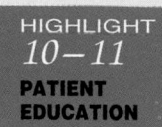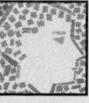

Application of Elastic Antiembolic Stockings to Prevent Venous Stasis

Instruct the patient with elastic antiembolic or graduated compression stockings prescribed to:

Apply the elastic stockings to both legs, even if only one is affected, to give support to the extremities and to increase circulation.

Wear rubber gloves to stroke the stockings on. Stroke the stockings up until they are smooth and wrinkle-free.

Be sure stockings feel tight but not constrictive to the extremities. If they feel too constrictive or if there is numbness in the feet or toes, they should not be worn, but instead returned for a better fitting pair.

Put the stockings on before getting out of bed in the morning. They may be removed for 30 minutes every 6 hours or as prescribed.

Observe the skin after removal for irritation, dryness, lesions, pressure areas, or discoloration.

Wash the stockings in a mild detergent without bleach to prevent skin irritation when reapplied. Have a second pair available for use when one pair is being washed.

chronic venous insufficiency develops have a history of deep venous thrombosis with repeated episodes of phlebitis.

The valves of the veins in the legs are unable to close completely because of thrombus formation, scarring, or fibrosis. Incompetency of the veins occurs from the prolonged high venous pressure in the extremities. As illustrated in Figure 10–9, the veins become weak, overstretched, and distended from the extensive pressure. The valve no longer closes completely, thus allowing the blood to flow back into the dilated veins. Venous stasis and increased venous pressure result in varicosities and venous ulcers.

Varicose Veins

Etiology and Pathophysiology
Abnormal dilatation of the veins as a result of venous insufficiency with valvular malfunction results in varicose veins. They may stem from congenital malformations of the vein walls and valves, repeated episodes of thrombophlebitis, or conditions that cause venous stasis, such as pregnancy or prolonged standing and sitting. A genetic predisposition to varicose veins is common in many people. Heavy lifting and obesity may also cause high venous pressure, resulting in varicosities. Deep venous thrombosis, obstruction, or inflammation may cause varicose veins through valvular destruction.

Some disease processes may also predispose a person to varicosities of veins in other parts of the body. Chronic liver disorders—such as cirrhosis, with its associated portal hypertension—cause varicose veins in the rectum, abdomen, and esophagus.

The veins are elongated, dilated, and tortuous as a result of increased venous pressure and venous stasis. Varicose veins develop in the superficial veins of the lower extremities, most commonly in the saphenous veins and branches.

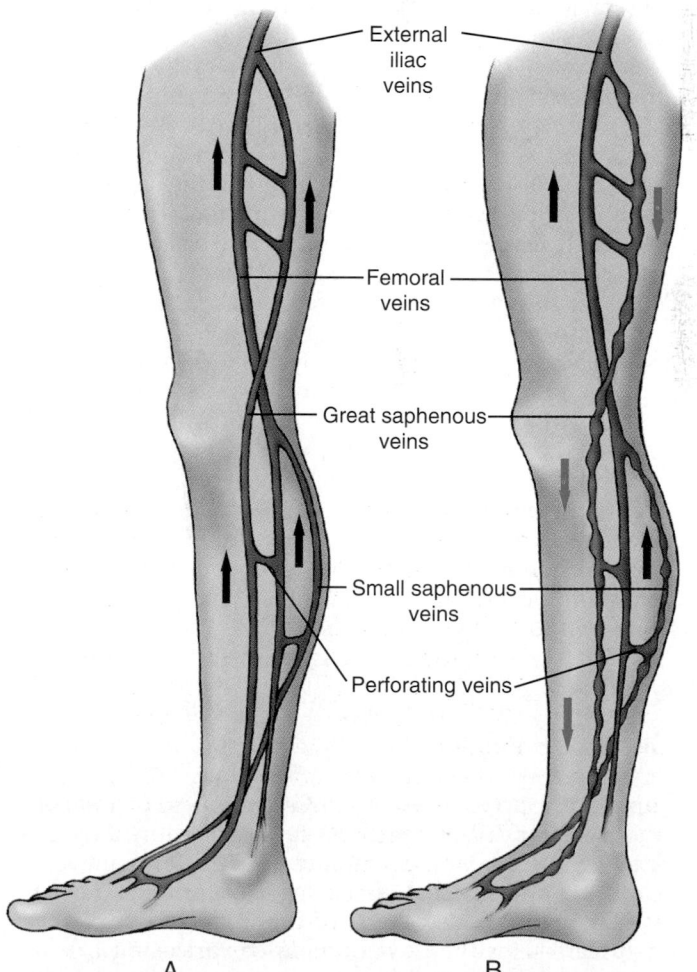

Figure 10–9

A, Normal (superficial and deep) venous flow. *B,* Venous flow in varicosities caused by incompetent valves.

Clinical Manifestations

Superficial, tortuous veins may be easily visible beneath the skin, especially in the upright position. Edema may occur from increased capillary pressure, which prevents fluids from being reabsorbed from the tissues. The patient with varicose veins may be asymptomatic or may experience a heavy feeling or fatigue in the legs. The pain and muscle fatigue result from lactic acid accumulation in the muscles. This is from the high venous pressure, which inhibits the removal of toxins and fluid from the tissues. Once the extremities are elevated, especially at night, cramps may occur as the waste products are removed.

Diagnosis

The diagnosis is based on inspection of the legs and on Doppler flow studies. Perthes' test and venography are used to assess the competency of the valves and the condition of the veins. (See Chapter 9 for a description of these tests.)

Management

Graduated compression elastic stockings (30/40 mm Hg) are prescribed to support the veins and promote venous return. Varicosities and incompetent veins may be removed surgically. This involves transection and ligation of the saphenous vein and stripping or removal of the superficial saphenous vein. The vein is ligated in the groin area while a wire is passed through the vein to the ankle. The vein is stripped as the wire is removed. The legs are elevated during surgery to minimize bleeding. Complications of the surgery include infection, thrombosis, and nerve damage. (Refer to Chapter 9 for discussion of peripheral vascular surgery.)

Small varicosities can be treated with sclerotherapy by aspirating the blood in the vein and injecting a sclerosing solution. This produces fibrosis and blocks the opening to the vein. Complications of sclerotherapy include phlebitis, tissue necrosis, and, rarely, infection. Treatment of any type will not prevent the recurrence of varicosities. Reducing risk factors, however, may help prevent further development of additional varicose veins.

NURSING PROCESS GUIDELINES
Varicose Veins

Assess the appearance of the extremities, comparing them bilaterally. Palpate for superficial, tortuous, dilated vessels beneath the skin. Assess for pain, discomfort, and edema in the legs. Determine the patient's medical history of thrombophlebitis or other risk factors for the development of varicosities.

Nursing interventions include teaching the patient about care of the extremities and preventive measures similar to those for thrombophlebitis, as described in Nursing Care Guide 10–2 (also see Highlight 10–10).

Postoperative care includes applying elastic bandages or compression stockings, checking the dressings sites, and assessing for bleeding. Observe for edema, discoloration, and decreased nerve sensation. Encourage ambulation as soon as prescribed to decrease edema and promote venous flow. Elevate the legs when the patient is sitting or lying in bed. Discourage standing in place or sitting with legs crossed.

Venous Stasis Ulcers
Etiology and Pathophysiology

Leg ulcers associated with chronic venous insufficiency occur from extensive damage to the integrity of the skin and subcutaneous tissues. This is the result of edema, decreased venous circulation leading to inadequate oxygen and nutrients in the area, and accumulation of toxic wastes. These changes usually occur in the lower leg near the ankle. Venous stasis ulcers are more common in elderly people with compromised circulation and limited mobility.

Clinical Manifestations

The clinical manifestations of venous stasis ulcers include:

* Hemosiderin deposits (visible in fair-skinned individuals as brownish skin pigmentation) from extravasated red blood cells from small vein rupture
* Dry, cracked skin from inadequate oxygen and nutrients to the area
* Infections from exposed skin breaks

Edema from vein dilatation and backup of venous flow from incompetent valves may also occur.

Diagnosis

The diagnosis is based on history and physical findings. Doppler ultrasonographic studies and venography are used to confirm the cause of the ulcerations.

Management

Venous stasis ulcers are treated with compresses of isotonic saline solution, aluminum acetate (Burow's solution), and silver sulfadiazine (Silvadene). Daily whirlpool therapy promotes circulation, comfort, and healing. A local corticosteriod can be used for dermatitis. Systemic antibiotics may be necessary to treat infectious organisms. Systemic rather than local antibiotics are preferred to prevent development of skin sensitivity, which impedes the healing process. To promote healing in large ulcers, it may be necessary to tie off the perforator veins before applying skin grafts. Débridement may be done to promote granulation. A semirigid boot (Unna's boot) may be applied to a noninfected leg to decrease the swelling and to promote venous return while compressing the superficial veins. This boot may help resolve dermatitis without topical steroids. The boot is left in place and changed every 1 to 2 weeks, depending

Nursing Care Guide 10–2
Patients with Varicose Veins

Assessment Findings: Patient complains of dull, aching pain in legs, especially after long periods of standing or sitting with legs in a dependent position; vein distention and dilatation are visible; some edema of ankles and feet is present.

Nursing Diagnosis: Pain related to effects of venous valvular insufficiency, venous stasis causing vein distention and blood pooling in the extremities

Patient Outcomes	Nursing Interventions	Rationale
Patient reports decrease in discomfort or absence of pain in legs and feet.	Give analgesics for leg aches as prescribed. Keep heavy linens elevated with a bed cradle.	Keeping pressure off the legs and administering pain medications as needed help relieve painful episodes.
Patient states methods to reduce or prevent pain in the legs and feet.	Teach the patient how to prevent effects of venous stasis by avoiding standing or sitting in one position for lengthy periods of time, elevating legs when sitting, wearing shoes that are comfortable and not too tight, massaging legs to promote venous return, unless contraindicated, and wearing graduated elastic support stockings.	An understanding of preventive methods may reduce the number of painful episodes the patient experiences.

Evaluation: Compare the patient's status with the expected outcomes. If the outcomes are not met, reassess the patient and revise the plan.

Assessment Findings: Patients ask questions about care of legs and feet, especially why there is so much edema and discomfort; seems anxious about managing effects of the disorder; is unsure about potential surgery for correction of the disorder; wants to know if self-care measures can prevent further effects of the disorder.

Nursing Diagnosis: Knowledge deficit: nature of disease and preventive care

Patient Outcomes	Nursing Interventions	Rationale
Patient states accurate information about the development of varicosities and preventive measures.	Explain the disease process to the patient in understandable terms. Give the patient appropriate literature about the disease to review. Explain the preventive measures. Tell the patient about the medications, time and route, and expected results. Teach the patient how to apply the support stockings. Allow time for questions and concerns to be voiced. Allow the patient's family to participate in the education sessions.	An understanding of the disorder and the events that exacerbate the condition may improve patient compliance with the management regimen.

(continued)

Nursing Care Guide 10–2
Patients with Varicose Veins (continued)

Patient Outcomes	Nursing Interventions	Rationale
Patient explains the surgical procedure and the risks and long-term implications of having surgery for varicose veins.	Find out whether the physician has explained to the patient about the surgical procedure for varicosities, the potential risks, and future implications. Assist the patient in clearing up any misconceptions about the procedure.	An understanding of the procedure may reduce the patient's fear and anxiety.

Evaluation: Compare the patient's status with the expected outcomes. If the outcomes are not met, reassess the patient and revise the plan.

Assessment Findings: Patient is unable to walk without assistance; legs are extremely edematous; patient complains of pain in extremities; physician orders bedrest.

Nursing Diagnosis: Impaired physical mobility related to exacerbation of effects of disorder and physician's response to patient's symptoms

Patient Outcomes	Nursing Interventions	Rationale
Patient reports decrease in pain when ambulating and is able to ambulate without aggravating effects of disorder.	Encourage range-of-motion exercises while on bedrest.	Exercises help venous return to reduce edema while maintaining muscle strength and endurance.
	Keep legs elevated above the patient's heart. Give diuretics and analgesics, as prescribed.	Elevating the legs reduces edema and aids in venous return.
Patient practices preventive measures when able to ambulate again, such as not standing or sitting for long periods of time and wearing graduated compression stockings.	Explain preventive measures that can prevent further episodes of acute exacerbation requiring bedrest.	An understanding of preventive measures may reduce the risk of complications.

Evaluation: Compare the patient's status with the expected outcomes. If the outcomes are not met, reassess the patient and revise the plan.

on the presence of edema and drainage from the ulcer.

NURSING PROCESS
Venous Stasis Ulcers

Assessment

Assess the affected area for discoloration, warmth, drainage, and edema. Ask the patient about pain, tenderness, or sensation in the affected limb. Note the color and amount of drainage.

Assess the patient's knowledge level regarding the disorder, the medications prescribed, and measures to prevent recurrence of the ulcerations. Observe the patient's activity level and note whether the ulcerations have impaired mobility. Review the patient's typical food choices to check for vitamin and protein content.

Nursing Diagnoses and Planning

Nursing diagnoses and related expected patient outcomes commonly applicable to patients with venous stasis ulcers include the following:

NDx: Impaired physical mobility related to bedrest and discomfort secondary to disease state

Planning: Patient Outcomes
1. Patient reports increased mobility, strength, and endurance.
2. Patient is able to perform activities of daily living.

NDx: Impaired skin integrity (in the extremities) related to immobility

Planning: Patient Outcomes
1. Patient's skin remains intact without evidence of infection, ulcerations, or gangrene.
2. Patient states appropriate skin-care measures to prevent impairment of skin integrity.

NDx: Knowledge deficit: nature of the disease, its complications, treatments, and measures to reduce risk

Planning: Patient Outcomes
1. Patient describes cause, effects, and risk factors associated with venous stasis ulcers.
2. Patient lists symptoms and treatments for the complications of the disorder, including how and when to apply graduated compression elastic hose (see Highlight 10–11) and care of the ulcerations at home.
3. Patient states the self-care needed to prevent risk or complications of venous stasis ulcers.
4. Patient chooses foods that promote health and healing.

Nursing Interventions and Evaluation

NDx: Impaired physical mobility
Assist the patient when he or she is allowed out of bed. The patient may be very weak after being on bedrest. Use durable medical equipment accessories, when appropriate, to assist the patient in maintaining mobility. Teach the patient to perform range-of-motion exercises to increase circulation and to maintain or improve strength and endurance.

Prepare a daily exercise schedule as soon as the patient is allowed to be mobile again, increasing the level as tolerated.

NDx: Impaired skin integrity
Maintain the patient on bedrest during the acute phase. Elevate the legs to decrease venous pressure. Culture any drainage from the ulcerations. Teach the patient to perform dorsiflexion while on bedrest to promote blood flow.

Cleanse the ulcerations daily with the prescribed solution. Use aseptic technique to prevent infection. Wet saline or Burow's solution compresses can be used to promote the healing process. Apply lotion to the surrounding skin to prevent dryness.

Reposition the patient frequently to prevent pressure areas. Use pads for heels and keep bed linen off the limbs by using a bed cradle.

Teach the patient measures to prevent recurrence of the ulcers, such as wearing graduated compression elastic hose and elevating the legs periodically to promote venous flow. Discourage standing in place or sitting with the legs in a dependent position for long periods of time. Encourage leg exercises, such as walking, to increase circulation to the distal limbs. Instruct the patient to avoid wearing constrictive clothing and extreme hot or cold temperatures.

Encourage the patient to eat a diet high in vitamin C, protein, and minerals to enhance healing and maintain tissue integrity. Seek dietary counseling if necessary.

NDx: Knowledge deficit: nature of the disease, its complications, treatments, and measures to reduce risk
Explain to the patient the cause, effects, and treatments for venous stasis ulcers. Allow opportunities for the patient to ask questions at any time. Allow the patient to verbalize concerns and fears. Evaluate discharge needs for the patient and family.

Alert the patient to the complications of ulcerations, such as impaired mobility, pain, and infection of the extremities. Teach the patient to use safety measures or ask for assistance when out of bed or ambulating. Teach exercises that the patient can use to increase strength and endurance after bedrest restrictions are removed.

Teach the patient how to achieve comfort by frequent repositioning and padding bony prominences. Explain the use of a bed cradle to prevent pressure on joints and sensitive areas. Teach the patient how to apply the graduated compression elastic hose, which compress superficial veins to enhance circulation to deep veins and decrease the chance that venous ulceration will recur (see Highlight 10–11). Explain how to apply the compresses if the patient will continue the dressings at home.

Teach the patient the dosage, route, time, frequency, side effects, and toxic effects of any medication prescribed. Explain the benefit of a diet high in vitamins and protein and give the patient lists of appropriate foods. Have a dietitian assist with the meal planning if needed. Include the family in the teaching sessions when appropriate.

Compare the patient's status with the expected outcomes. If the outcomes are not met, reassess the patient and revise the plan.

❖ Settings, Providers, and Collaboration for Care

Patients with venous vascular disorders may be treated in the hospital or in outpatient settings, such as the physician's office and the home. Patients with thrombophlebitis and patients undergoing surgery for varicosities may have a very short hospital stay and be discharged with instructions for home care and a follow-up visit to the physician. The nurse instructs the patient about medications, activity restrictions, and home care needed to prevent compli-

SOCIOCULTURAL PERSPECTIVES

Planning Self-Care for the Homeless Person

by Janice R. Ellis, PhD, RN

Homelessness confronts all of us when we walk the streets of our major cities. There we find people who sit begging on the sidewalks, walk aimlessly about, haul their belongings around in bundles and shopping carts, and look disheveled and dirty. Our responses to these people run the gamut. In our best moments, we feel compassion and may offer acts of kindness. In our worst, we feel outrage and disgust. In between, we feel powerless to help and simply turn a deaf ear to pleas for help. The homeless interfere with business, litter the streets, and even evoke fear—fear for our personal safety, and fear that somehow we could find ourselves in the same circumstances.

Some homeless people sleep and eat in official shelters. But many avoid shelters, opting instead for makeshift homes under bridges and in alleys. There, without showers and toilet facilities, conditions of filth and squalor begin to accumulate.

Homelessness is also hidden. Whole families sleep in their cars each night. They move from place to place to avoid being noticed. Children who are homeless may not attend school or may attend sporadically, lying about their lack of residence. Some homeless people move from home to home, staying with family, friends, and acquaintances until each welcome wears thin. We may never know that these people are homeless until some interaction forces them to disclose their status.

Who are the homeless in our society? Some people are homeless simply because they choose not to conform to society's expectations and roles. Often public policy is based on the assumption that all of the homeless fall into this category. However, there are many other reasons for homelessness. Some people are homeless because of drug and alcohol abuse that leaves them unemployable. Many of the homeless on our streets are mentally ill. The mental health reform movement succeeded in moving people out of large mental hospitals in the 1980s. However, an unforeseen result has been that many mentally ill people who were once institutionalized refuse outpatient treatment. Without treatment, these people sometimes become unable to work or manage their lives, and they end up on the streets. Elderly people whose small pensions have become inadequate to meet the costs of housing or whose savings were decimated by the cost of illness or other crises constitute another group of homeless. When entire families are homeless, it is most often because of the loss of a job or the desertion of one of the parents.

Homelessness brings with it a whole host of other problems. With limited money, and without cooking facilities, options for food become very limited. Hygiene for the homeless, when possible at all, takes place in shelters, public restrooms, and sometimes the homes of family, friends, and acquaintances. Clothing consists of what the person can carry, or perhaps store somewhere. Without money for a laundromat, and with perhaps only one set of clothes, it is nearly impossible to wash clothes, so the homeless person may wear one set of clothes until they are threadbare.

Health care is even more problematic. Only when problems become overwhelming do the homeless usually seek health care. When that happens, care may be sought in emergency rooms or street clinics. A few shelters have nurse-run clinics that provide limited health care services. But at these clinics there may not be adequate funding to support ongoing needs for the management of chronic illness. Imagine what kinds of problems nurses in these settings confront. Imagine how difficult they are to manage with their limited resources.

A common problem confronting the homeless person is the development of venous leg ulcers. Walking miles each day, often in poorly fitting shoes, falling, and bumping into obstructions—all of these factors contribute to the development of varicose veins and inadequate venous return in the legs. Swollen legs, bruises, and painful varicosities cause ongoing discomfort. The transition from a surface bruise to an ulcerated area on the leg occurs gradually. At first the person ignores the discomfort. After all, just getting shelter from the rain and cold and obtaining food constitute the challenges of each day.

When someone on a health-care team first sees a venous ulcer on a homeless patient, it is often far advanced, deep, and wide. A nurse practitioner or physician may diagnose the condition and prescribe medical treatment, but that does not address the real problem for the person. Someone must develop a relationship of trust with the homeless person. Someone must be willing to see beyond the exterior to the person in need, to develop an effective plan for self-care. This is often the role of the nurse.

How would you respond to such a homeless person? Can you remain sufficiently nonjudgmental and accepting that the person would begin to trust you? Do you have enough knowledge to help this person plan for self-care? What resources

(continued)

cations before discharge (see Highlight 10–10 and Highlight 10–11).

Patients with severe venous stasis ulcers may need nursing assistance in the home after discharge. The home health nurse (or institution nurse, if the patient is in a nursing home or residential care facility) makes visits to assess the patient's status, especially venous circulation and ulcer healing. The nurse may assist the patient and family with dressings and compresses prescribed for the extremities.

Careful attention must be paid to the patient's feet, since circulation is already compromised. A referral to a podiatrist may be necessary to treat the patient's feet and to trim the toe nails.

If the patient is alone or has problems with immobility or restricted mobility, the nurse makes a referral to a home meal service. In addition, a physical therapist can help the patient with mobility, since assistive walking aids may be necessary.

Common Lymphatic Disorders

The lymph system drains excess fluids and proteins from the interstitial spaces. It is important in maintaining control of tissue fluid volume. In lymphatic disorders, obstruction of the lymph vessels interrupts the control of tissue fluid volume, resulting in edema. Several factors may contribute to this process.

LYMPHANGITIS AND LYMPHADENITIS

Etiology and Pathophysiology
Lymphangitis and lymphadenitis are both inflammations of the lymph system. *Lymphangitis* refers to an inflammation of the vessels, usually caused by a bacterial infection. *Lymphadenitis* refers to inflammation of the lymph nodes. Both disorders may contribute to lymphedema. The bacteria invade the skin and spread to the lymph nodes through the lymphatic vessels.

Clinical Manifestations
The inflamed area may be only superficial, or an abscess may form. Red streaks appear along the pathway of the lymphatic vessels. Lymph nodes enlarge and become very tender. Local inflammation, pitting edema, and red discoloration in the extremity may occur as a response to the bacterial invasion. Cellulitis often occurs, causing throbbing pain in the affected part. The heart rate may be elevated to compensate for increased blood supply to the inflamed area. Fever, chills, malaise, anorexia, head-

ache, nausea, and vomiting may result as a systemic reaction to the infection.

Diagnosis

The diagnosis is based on history, present symptoms, and such laboratory studies as white blood cell count. Culture of the wound exudate determines the type of organism present.

Management

Systemic antimicrobial agents are administered on the basis of blood culture results. Penicillin is the usual drug prescribed for a streptococcal infection. Erythromycin or a cephalosporin may be ordered if the patient is allergic to penicillin.

If an abscess is present, fluid may be drained from the wound. Incision and drainage are avoided in the presence of cellulitis, however, to prevent spread of the infection. Early detection and treatment are important because the infection may progress rapidly and lead to septicemia or even death in rare cases. With treatment, the prognosis is excellent.

NURSING PROCESS GUIDELINES
Lymphangitis and Lymphadenitis

Observe the extremities for skin changes, such as discoloration, extreme warmth, and edema. Check for pain in the affected extremity. Palpate for pulses and tenderness. Assess vital signs for increased heart rate, fever, or respiratory difficulty, indicating systemic infection.

Promote healing of the affected extremity by preventing further trauma. Keep the extremity elevated to reduce edema. Apply warm compresses frequently to the site. Use aseptic technique when changing dressings. Provide for frequent rest periods to conserve energy. Keep the patient warm, and prevent drafts. After the inflammation has subsided, elastic support bandages or hose can be used to prevent further edema.

Give prescribed antibiotics and analgesics or antipyretics as needed. Teach the patient about the medications, frequency, amount, dosage, and side effects before discharge.

LYMPHEDEMA

Etiology and Pathophysiology

Lymphedema is defined as edema of the extremities from inadequate control of fluid volume in the tissues or interstitial spaces. Primary lymphedema (congenital lymphedema [Milroy's disease] or lymphedema praecox) is caused by obstructed lymph vessels. It may be visible at birth but is usually diagnosed later. Primary lymphedema is more common in females, ages 10 to 25, than it is in males.

Secondary lymphedema is caused by inflammation of the lymphatic vessels or obstruction of lymph flow as a result of pressure on the lymph nodes or vessels from neoplasms or other structures. Secondary lymphedema may result from a disruption of the lymphatic system that occurs postmastectomy or from varicose veins, phlebitis, or irradiation. Secondary lymphedema usually occurs after age 40 and may be found in either men or women. It is usually unilateral but may be bilateral depending on the cause.

Lymph accumulates distally because of the blockage of the lymph vessels or nodes. Lymphatic pressure rises in the periphery, causing incompetent valves and dilatation of the vessel walls. The edema is the result of accumulation of lymph in the interstitial spaces.

Clinical Manifestations

Clinical manifestations of lymphedema include fluid accumulation beginning in the distal limb. In the lower extremities, edema begins in the foot and extends proximally. Prolonged standing, extremely warm weather, obesity, and pregnancy may aggravate lower limb lymphedema.

Primary lymphedema is insidious in onset. It usually starts with bilateral, soft, pitting edema followed by firm, nonpitting edema. The skin is thick, and hair follicles are prominent. Pain is usually absent, but the patient may complain of a dull, heavy sensation in the affected extremities.

Secondary lymphedema is characterized by painless edema of the affected extremities. Pain appears if infection is present or if the edema is so severe that it stretches the skin and raises pressure in the affected limb. If the condition becomes chronic, the affected area is usually severely edematous, with thick, hard, woody skin resulting in deformity. The condition is severe lymphedema and resembles the changes in elephantiasis.

Diagnosis

The diagnosis is based on physical assessment, lymphangiography, and radioactive isotope studies.

Management

Treatment of lymphedema includes a low-sodium diet, oral diuretics (such as the thiazides), and use of an external pneumatic compressor to decrease edema. The patient should wear 40/50 mm Hg graduated compression hose when not using the compressor to keep the edema from returning. The extremity is kept elevated to prevent further edema. The underlying cause of secondary edema may also need to be treated. Antibiotics are prescribed for infection. The prognosis depends on the cause of the lymphedema, but it is usually very good. In most cases, the disorder can be controlled with treatment and graduated compression hose.

NURSING PROCESS GUIDELINES
Lymphedema

Review the patient's history, and assess present physical symptoms. Observe the extremities for color changes, pitting edema, and circulation states. Palpate for pulses in the extremities, checking presence, intensity, and regularity. Assess for pain or tenderness in the affected limb. Measure the circumference of the extremity daily to determine changes.

Nursing interventions include measures to relieve the edema, promote lymph drainage, and prevent infection. Elevate the extremity and wrap it with elastic bandages or apply graduated compression hose. Assist the patient in ambulation if necessary. Massage the affected extremity manually or mechanically to force lymph to drain toward the trunk of the body. Teach the patient how to use the mechanical device and compression stockings if they will be needed after discharge.

Explain the dosage, frequency, time, and side effects of prescribed medications. Encourage the patient to express feelings and concerns about the disorder, especially if it is chronic. The patient's self-image may suffer because of the appearance of the edematous extremity. Refer the patient to counseling if necessary.

The Elderly: Special Considerations

Physiologic changes of the aging process must be considered when caring for older people with vascular disorders. The blood vessel walls become thickened with age, leading to a decrease in elasticity of the smaller arteries. Vessels become dilated, elongated, and tortuous, and plaques collect in the inner vessel walls, resulting in vessel weakness. Inefficient heart valve function may decrease blood supply to the lower extremities. Most older adults experience some degree of atherosclerosis, which can be accentuated by changes in the cardiovascular system associated with disease processes. An older person may attribute discomfort in the lower limbs to "normal aging" and may thus delay seeking treatment for a vascular disorder. Pain sensation may be diminished from other disease processes that interfere with neurotransmission. Analgesic medication must be administered to older adults with caution because of their increased susceptibility to drug toxicity, interactions, and adverse effects.

Cardiac output may be decreased as a result of sclerosis in the endocardium and thickening of the left ventricular wall, which may cause myocardial hypertrophy and decreased blood flow to the extremities. Dependent edema may occur because of limited mobility, lack of exercise, and dilatation of the veins. Older adults can be encouraged to use support stockings or medically prescribed elastic stockings if they do not have arterial compromise or diabetes. Elevating the feet above heart level (unless they have arterial blockage) improves venous return and prevents dependent edema. Walking also helps to decrease edema because it contracts the calf muscles, which aids venous return.

The elderly patient may experience a variety of problems from arterial vascular occlusion. Skin changes resulting from decreased arterial blood flow may be superimposed on changes associated with aging and disease conditions. This complicates assessment of changes caused by arterial vascular disorders. Because thinning of hair is often part of the aging process, it is not a reliable symptom of arterial vascular disorders. The older adult experiences decreased sensation to extreme hot and cold temperatures and is more prone to burns or frostbite injuries. These injuries are aggravated by decreased circulation to the skin for healing.

Special considerations are taken into account when caring for the older person with hypertension. Because older patients may be hypersensitive to or less responsive to antihypertensive medications, they require close monitoring of changes in their medications. The goal of the therapy is to lower the blood pressure without reducing blood flow to the extremities or causing increased problems from side effects. Patients may be noncompliant with the hypertension regimen because of misconceptions, financial problems, lack of motivation, lack of understanding, or mental changes associated with disease processes or adverse medication effects.

The autonomic nervous system response in the aged is slowed, resulting in systolic hypertension or orthostatic hypotension. The nurse should assess all older adults for postural hypotension by recording the blood pressure with the patient in lying, sitting, and standing positions. Instruct the patient to move slowly when changing positions to avoid dizziness and falling. An adequate fluid intake and use of support stockings may reduce the risk of postural hypotension.

The older adult with a vascular disorder may need to follow a diet restricted in fat, sodium, calories, and cholesterol. Special care must be given to menu planning to facilitate compliance with the diet therapy. Diminished senses of smell and taste may contribute to poor dietary habits and noncompliance with the prescribed plan. A diet low in fat and cholesterol may not be palatable to an older adult who has eaten high-fat foods for years. Dietary planning should include the patient's preferences within the list of appropriate foods. Food preparation habits should be assessed to identify detrimental influences, such as deep-fat frying.

If bedrest is required for treatment of venous vascular disorders in the elderly, complications can develop rapidly. Impaired respiratory function increases the likelihood of respiratory complications, such as pneumonia. Increased fragility of the skin enhances the likelihood of skin breakdown, which can develop in just one or two days. Healing is slower because of poor nutrition, decreased circulation, and other complicating disorders.

Guidelines for ongoing care should be given verbally and in writing to promote understanding and to increase compliance. Family or friends can be included to assist the patient.

Chapter Review

1. How would you teach a patient Buerger-Allen exercises?
2. What relaxation strategies are important for the patient with vascular disorders to practice?
3. What instructions should be given to the patient with arterial blockage to prevent foot problems? How would they differ from instructions to a patient with venous problems?
4. What would happen to the patient with Raynaud's disease if some prevention and protection strategies are not instituted?
5. Which types of patients are at greatest risk for vascular disorders, and why?
6. What nutrition guidelines are important to teach the patient with atherosclerosis?
7. Which assessments should be made on patients with vascular problems or at risk for vascular problems?
8. What are common characteristics of the various types of aneurysms?
9. In what treatment settings might you deliver care to patients with vascular disorders?
10. What special considerations should be made when delivering care to an older adult with vascular problems?

Bibliography

Agency for Health Care Policy and Research. Acute pain management: Operative or medical procedures and trauma. AHCPR 92-0032. Rockville, MD: US Department of Health and Human Services, 1992.

Allen SL. Perioperative nursing interventions for intravascular stent placements. AORN J 1995; 61(4):689.

Allsup DJ. Use of the intermittent pneumatic compression device in venous ulcer disease. J Vasc Nurs 1994; 12(4):106.

Bloomfield R, Pearce K, Cross H. Hypertension: Choosing therapy when coexisting disease confounds the choice. Consultant 1993; 33(7):69.

Borriello SL, Siegel SC, Fishman RF. Directional coronary atherectomy: A new treatment for coronary artery disease. Heart Lung 1994; 23(3):199.

Czyrny JJ, Merrill A. Rehabilitation of amputees with end-stage renal disease: Functional outcome and cost. Am J Phys Med Rehabil 1994; 73(5):353.

Dimengo J. Commentary on tissue renin-angiotensin system in myocardial hypertrophy and failure. AACN Nurs Scan Crit Care 1993; 3(6):4. [Original article by Dzau appears in Arch Intern Med 1993; 153(8):937.]

Edwards LH. Commentary on homelessness as a determinant of health. Nurs Scan Administration 1993; 8(3):20. [Original article by Jackson appears in MCN 1982; 9(3):185.]

Flett R, Harcourt B, Alpass F. Psychosocial aspects of chronic lower leg ulceration in the elderly. West J Nurs Res 1994; 16(2):183.

Galindo-Ciocon D. Nursing care of the elders with leg edema. J Gerontol Nurs 1995; 21(7):7.

Galloway S, Bubela N, McKibbon A, et al. Symptom distress, anxiety, depression, and discharge information needs after peripheral arterial bypass. J Vasc Nurs 1995; 13(2):35.

Gardner AW, Skinner JS, Bryant CX, Smith LK. Stair climbing elicits a lower cardiovascular demand than walking in claudication patients. J Cardiopulm Rehabil 1995; 15(2):134.

Grace ML, Crosby FE, Ventura MR. Nutritional education for patients with peripheral vascular disease. J Health Educ 1994; 25(3):142.

Harley JR. Preventing diabetic foot disease. Nurse Pract 1993; 18(10):37.

Hatswell EM. Abdominal aortic aneurysm surgery: An overview and discussion of immediate perioperative complications. Part I. Heart Lung 1994; 23(3):228.

Hebdon B, Letourneau JG. Duplex sonography of extremity arteries and veins. Part 2. Appl Radiol 1994; 23(4):39.

Henderson LJ, Kirkland JS. Angioplasty with stent placement in peripheral arterial occlusive disease. AORN J 1995; 61(4):669.

Johnson M. Interactional aspects of self-efficacy and control in older people with leg ulcers. J Gerontol Nurs 1995; 21(4):20.

Kashyap A, Deshmukh N. Abdominal aortic aneurysms in females: A comparative analysis. J Womens Health 1994; 3(4):291.

Lacey KO, Meier GH, Krumholz HM, Gusberg RJ. Outcomes after major vascular surgery: The patient's perspective. J Vasc Nurs 1995; 13(1):8.

Lovell MB, Cameron D, Harris KA, et al. Peripheral aneurysms. J Vasc Nurs 1994; 12(2):44.

MacLean N, Fick GH. The effect of semirigid dressings on below-knee amputations. Phys Ther 1994; 74(7):668.

Maklebust J, Magnan MA. Risk factors associated with having a pressure ulcer: A secondary data analysis. Adv Wound Care 1994; 7(6):25.

Margolis S. Point/counterpoint. Chelation therapy is ineffective for the treatment of peripheral vascular disease. Alternative Ther Health Med 1995; 1(2):53.

McAbee R. Primary prevention of hypertension: A challenge for occupational health nurses. AAOHN J 1995; 43(6):306.

Orsted H. Physiology of venous leg ulceration. CAET J 1994; 13(3):6.

Phillips NA, Mate-Kole CC, Kirby RL. Neuropsychological function in peripheral vascular disease amputee patients. Arch Phys Med Rehabil 1993; 74(12):1309.

Plummer ES, Albert SG. Foot care assessment in patients with diabetes: A screening algorithm for patient education and referral. Diabetes Educ 1995; 21(1):47.

Podmore J. Leg ulcers: Weighing up the evidence. Nurs Stand 1994; 8(38):25.

Provan JL. Peripheral vascular disease: What's urgent, what's not. Med North Am 1993; 16(10):772.

Robertson C. Diabetes 2000: Chronic complications. RN 1995; 58(9):34.

Sabatino KA, Dougher MJ, Kee JC. Research: Conception to completion. J Vasc Nurs 1993; 11(4):110.

Sepka RS. Transcutaneous PO_2 measurement in peripheral vascular disease. Physician Assist 1993; 17(5):86.

Tosone NC, Marcley DM, Thielen JB, Vyhlidal SK. Discharge teaching for the directional coronary atherectomy patient. DCNN 1994; 13(4):208.

Waite LG. Commentary on circadian variations and possible external triggers of onset of myocardial infraction. AACN Nurs

Scan Crit Care 1993; 3(5):22. [Original article by Behar et al. appears in Am J Med 1993, 94(4):395.]

Waite LG. Commentary on cardiogenic shock complicating acute myocardial infarction in patients without heart failure on admission: Incidence, risk factors and outcome. AACN Nurs

Scan Crit Care 1993; 3(5):23. [Original article by Leor et al. appears in Am J Med 1993; 94(3):265.]

Wymelenberg S. Hit the road, Jack: Peripheral vascular disease. Harv Health Lett 1993; 18(10):4.

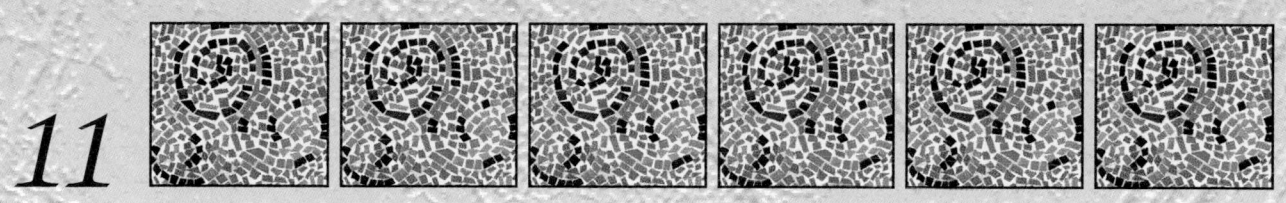

11

Knowledge Base for Patients in Shock

Study Outcomes

After studying this chapter, you should be able to:

1. Differentiate three types of shock according to etiology and pathologic alterations.
2. Contrast the clinical manifestations and laboratory findings present during compensatory and progressive stages of shock.
3. Outline definitive and supportive therapy for the three major types of shock.
4. Summarize the advantages and disadvantages of colloids and crystalloids in the management of shock.
5. Explain the beneficial and adverse effects of pharmacologic manipulation of the variables of cardiac output.
6. Explain the components of nursing assessment for the patient experiencing shock.
7. Correlate the hemodynamic parameter changes anticipated in the three types of shock.
8. Identify appropriate nursing diagnoses for the patient experiencing shock.
9. Formulate an appropriate nursing care plan for the patient in shock, including expected patient outcomes and nursing interventions.

Shock is a complex physiologic syndrome representing a diverse group of life-threatening circulatory conditions. Mortality rates from uncomplicated hemorrhagic shock are low, provided that the patient promptly receives adequate replacement of blood volume. However, despite advances in assessment and treatment, mortality rates from other forms of shock continue to range from 65 to 80%.

The three types of shock are hypovolemic, cardiogenic, and distributive. Hypovolemic shock results from low circulating blood volume, usually caused by hemorrhage or severe burn injuries. Cardiogenic shock occurs when the heart cannot pump an adequate blood volume to support body requirements. This usually relates to right or left ventricular failure, which may result from an underlying cardiac disorder. Distributive shock includes septic, neurogenic, and anaphylactic shock. Septic shock re-

sults from a massive systemic infection. Neurogenic shock is associated with injury or disease of the upper spinal cord or brainstem, or recent administration of general or spinal anesthesia. Anaphylactic shock is a hypersensitivity reaction to an antigen.

Shock may develop in any patient, in any setting. Its progression depends on the patient's physiologic state before the initial incident, the duration of the shock state, the response to therapy, and correction of whatever caused the shock. Early recognition of clinical signs and symptoms, and prompt initiation of therapeutic measures, may halt the progression of shock and reduce mortality. Therefore, nurses need a thorough understanding of the pathophysiology of shock to effectively recognize its manifestations and implement successful treatment.

For a successful outcome to be attained, patients who are in shock need prompt implementation of a collaborative treatment plan. These patients usually receive care in a hospital setting, commonly entering through the emergency department. Shock requires a team effort during the critical period, when its effects are life-threatening, and throughout the patient's stay in the hospital. Physicians, nurses, respiratory therapists, perfusion therapists, pharmacists, anesthesiologists, clergy, and others may all be involved in the patient's care.

Principles for Understanding Shock

Every cell in the body needs adequate tissue perfusion to provide the necessary supply of oxygen and nutrients and to remove metabolic byproducts. In shock, the blood flow becomes inadequate or the cells become unable to extract and use oxygen and substrates, or both. If left untreated, this functional impairment of cells, tissues, organs, and body systems progresses to multiple organ dysfunction and death.

HEMODYNAMIC PRINCIPLES

The circulatory system is composed of the heart, large blood vessels, and microcirculation (also called the peripheral or capillary circulation). These three components function interdependently to maintain cardiac output and tissue perfusion. Adequate blood flow depends on

- Adequate amounts of blood for the heart to pump
- Effective pumping ability by the heart
- The ability of blood vessels to constrict and dilate to maintain normal blood pressure

Shock results when one or more of these functions is disrupted.

Patients in shock may require placement of an arterial catheter and indwelling balloon-flotation pulmonary artery catheter and use of sophisticated bedside monitors to evaluate cardiac function, circulating blood volume, and physiologic response to treatment. From these measured pressures, various hemodynamic parameters can be obtained and used to assess the mechanisms that support normal cardiovascular function: cardiac output, preload, afterload, and systemic and pulmonary vascular resistance (Table 11–1).

Cardiac Output

Cardiac output reflects the amount of blood the heart pumps from the ventricles in 1 minute. It is expressed in liters per minute (L/min). Two major mechanisms that determine cardiac output (CO) include heart rate (HR) and stroke volume (SV): CO = HR × SV. Stroke volume is the amount of blood ejected by the ventricle with each heart beat. A de-

creased heart rate will decrease cardiac output if the amount of blood ejected from the ventricles (stroke volume) does not increase. Conversely, a decreased amount of blood ejected from the ventricles will lower cardiac output if the heart rate does not increase to compensate for the volume change. Thus, changes in either heart rate or stroke volume can change cardiac output.

As the body's metabolic needs change, the heart adjusts cardiac output by altering heart rate or stroke volume (Fig. 11–1). Normal resting cardiac output is 4 to 8 L/min. The large variation in cardiac output values reflects variations in body size.

To more accurately assess the heart's pumping ability, the cardiac index can be calculated. Cardiac index includes body size and is obtained by dividing cardiac output by the person's estimated body surface area. The result is expressed in square meters. The normal range for cardiac index (CI) is 2.5 to 4.5 L/min/m².

Heart Rate

Heart rate is influenced by the autonomic nervous system. Sympathetic innervation increases heart rate, whereas parasympathetic innervation decreases heart rate. Normally, the heart has the ability to increase its pumping capacity significantly above resting levels. In a healthy person, the heart can usually increase cardiac output by up to three times normal for short periods of time by increasing heart rate or stroke volume. However, sustained heart rates over 180 bpm significantly increase the work of the heart and decrease the duration of diastole, allowing less time for the ventricle to fill. The advantage of the increased heart rate is eventually negated as cardiac output begins to fall. The coronary

Table 11–1

Hemodynamic Terms and Normal Values

Pressure	Acronym	Normal Range	Definition
Cardiac output	CO	4–6 L/min	Volume of blood pumped by each ventricle each minute.
Cardiac index	CI	2.4–4.0 L/min/m²	CO divided by body surface area. Indexed to body surface area to adjust for differences in body size.
Central venous pressure	CVP	2–4 mm Hg	Pressure created by volume in the right side of the heart.
Stroke volume	SV	60–70 mL	Amount of blood ejected by the ventricle with each heartbeat.
Systemic vascular resistance	SVR	900–1400 dynes/sec/cm^{-5}	Resistance to blood flow created by the systemic vasculature (arteries and arterioles) against which the left ventricle must pump to eject its volume. As SVR increases, CO decreases.
Pulmonary vascular resistance	PVR	30–100 dynes/sec/cm^{-5}	Resistance to blood flow created by the pulmonary arteries and arterioles against which the right ventricle must pump to eject its volume.

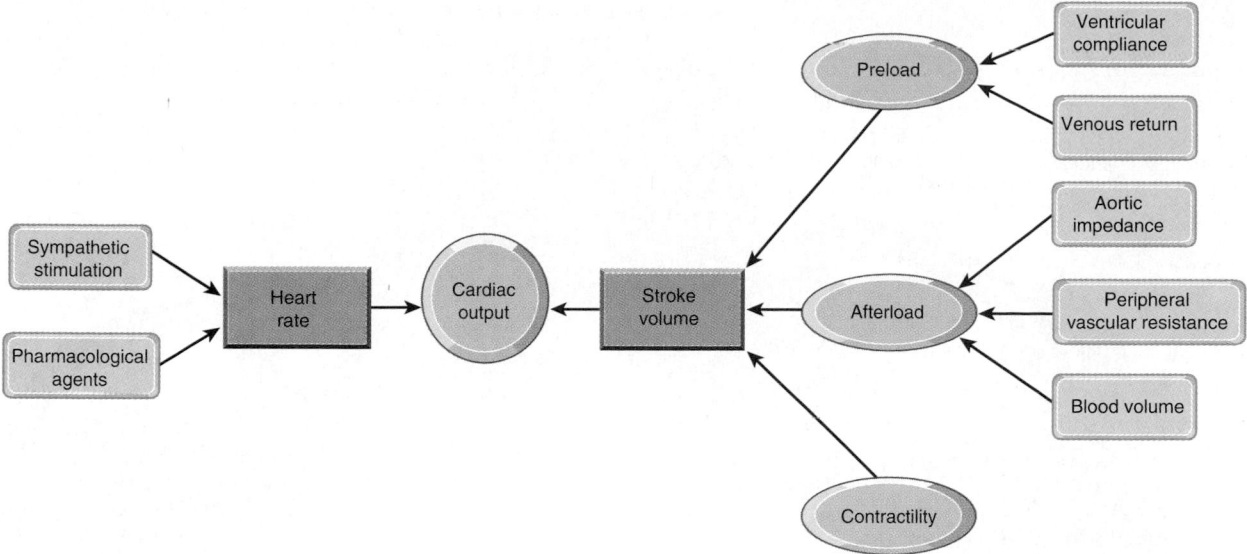

Figure 11-1

Determinants of cardiac output.

arteries are also perfused during this phase of the cardiac cycle. As heart rate increases, less time is available for the coronary arteries to be perfused. The heart muscle becomes ischemic when myocardial oxygen demand becomes greater than the myocardial oxygen supply.

Preload

The concept of preload was introduced independently by Otto Frank and Ernest Henry Starling, who found that as the amount of blood filling the ventricle during diastole increases, the force of contraction increases. A rubber band provides an analogous example. When a rubber band is stretched, the force of elastic recoil increases. The more the stretch, the greater the "pop." The Frank-Starling law of the heart, called also Starling's law, states that increasing the stretch of the myocardial fibers during diastole by increasing the volume will increase cardiac output, until it has reached a critical point at which further increases in volume actually decrease cardiac output (Fig. 11-2). Thus, preload is a function of the volume of blood filling the ventricle and the ability of the ventricle to stretch (ventricular compliance). Factors affecting the amount of blood volume returning to the ventricles, and factors affecting ventricular compliance, affect preload and subsequently cardiac output.

Measurement of right ventricular preload is by determination of central venous pressure. It has a normal range of 2 to 4 mm Hg. Measurement of left ventricular preload is not possible; therefore, it must be measured indirectly using a pulmonary artery catheter that has an inflatable balloon at the tip. As the balloon is inflated, it occludes pressure readings from the right side of the heart. During diastole,

when the mitral valve is open, there is a clear pathway between the tip of the pulmonary artery catheter and the left ventricle. In the absence of pulmonary hypertension, the pressure along this pathway is equal to left ventricular pressure. Pressure that registers at the catheter tip is identical to the pressure registered within the left ventricle. The left ventricular preload volume pressure is reflected as pulmonary artery wedge pressure (PAWP). It has a normal range of 5 to 12 mm Hg (Fig. 11-3).

Afterload

Afterload is defined as ventricular wall tension or stress during systolic ejection. It is increased by forces that oppose ejection of blood from the ventri-

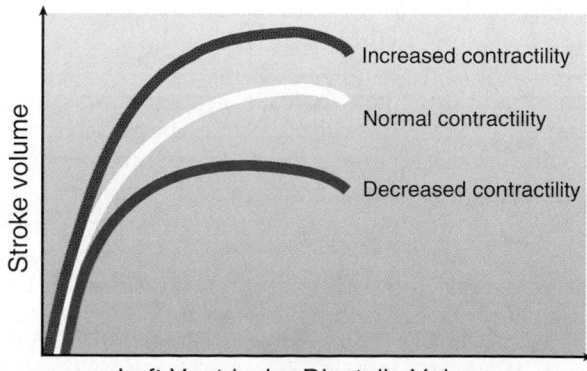

Figure 11-2

Frank-Starling law. As the amount of blood filling the ventricle during diastole increases, the force of contraction increases to a maximum point. After the maximum point has been reached, contractility and cardiac output decrease.

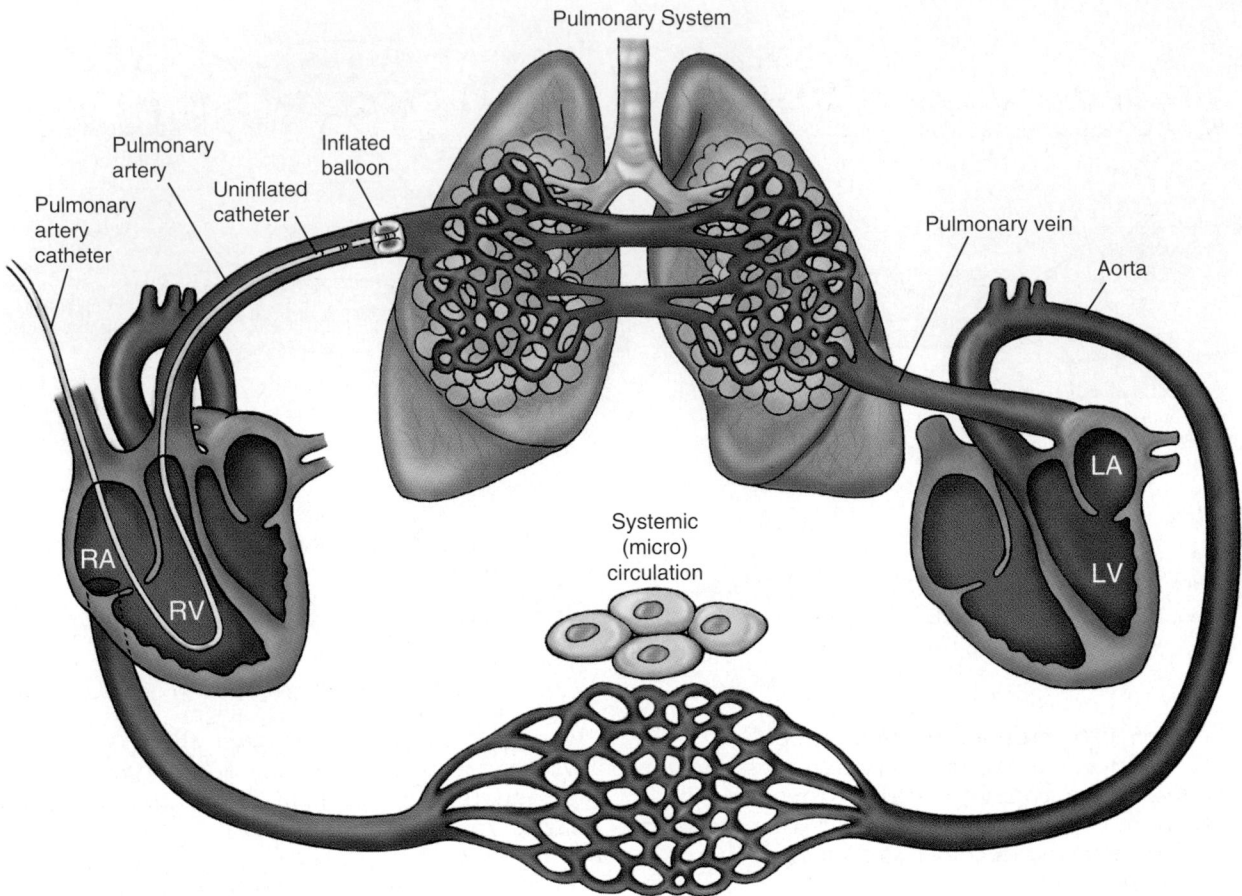

Figure 11-3

Pulmonary artery catheter position. When the balloon is deflated, pressures in the pulmonary artery can be measured. When the balloon is inflated, blood flow propels the catheter distally until the tip "wedges" in a small arterial branch. Pressure is normally transmitted from the left side of the heart through the pulmonary artery wedge pressure. LA, left atrium; LV, left ventricle; RA, right atrium; RV, right ventricle.

cle. The effect of an increased afterload is that the heart must work harder to pump blood from the ventricle. Afterload is increased

- In conditions that block aortic or pulmonary outflow, such as aortic stenosis or pulmonary stenosis.
- In conditions that obstruct the outflow tract, such as septal hypertrophy.
- In conditions that increase systemic or pulmonary vascular resistance, such as vasoconstriction.
- When blood volume or viscosity is increased.

As resistance to left ventricular ejection increases, the amount of blood ejected from the ventricle (stroke volume) decreases. This can lead to decreased cardiac output. The heart's ability to contract and respond effectively to alterations in preload and afterload allows maintenance of cardiac output. When the heart cannot effectively adapt to these alterations, cardiac output falls.

Afterload is calculated by a computerized bedside monitor system from information obtained from the pulmonary artery catheter. Systemic or arterial afterload is measured by systemic vascular resis-

tance, with normal values of 800 to 1400 dynes/sec/cm^{-5}. Resistance of the right side of the heart is measured by pulmonary vascular resistance, with normal values of 50 to 250 dynes/sec/cm^{-5}.

Contractility

Contractility refers to the heart's contractile force, or inotropy (*ino* = strength, *tropy* = enhancing). It results from many factors that have an impact on myocardial muscle function. Inotropy effects can be either positive, producing stronger contractions (as in the Starling mechanism or sympathetic nervous system stimulation), or negative, producing weaker contractions (as in acidosis and hypoxia). Contractility can also be altered by a variety of pharmacologic agents such as digoxin. This is especially true of drugs that mimic the sympathetic nervous system, such as sympathomimetics and adrenergics (Table 11-2). Increased contractility increases stroke volume and cardiac output by increasing ventricular emptying during systole. Decreased contractility can have a negative impact on cardiac output.

Table 11-2

Drugs Used to Increase Cardiac Output

Drug	Heart Rate	Preload	Afterload	Contractility
Dobutamine (Dobutrex)	No effect	Decreased	Decreased	Increased
Dopamine (Intropin)	Increased	Decreased at low doses	Decreased at low doses	Increased
Amrinone (Inocor)	No effect	Decreased	Decreased	Increased
Epinephrine (Adrenalin)	Increased	Decreased at low doses	Decreased at low doses	Increased
Norepinephrine (Levophed)	No significant effect	Increased	Increased	Increased

Control of Peripheral Circulation

Blood flow to individual vascular beds is intrinsically controlled through the response of arteriolar smooth muscles to metabolic byproducts, causing either vasodilatation or vasoconstriction. Other factors can also influence this balance, including local release of catecholamines, histamine, acetylcholine, serotonin, angiotensin, adenosine, and prostaglandins. These factors are released in response to tissue injury, hypoxemia, or hormones. Temperature and carbon dioxide can also influence the circulation locally.

Extrinsic control of peripheral blood flow is mediated by the central nervous system. The autonomic nervous system exerts dual antagonistic control over organ systems via sympathetic and parasympathetic fibers. Stimulation of the vasoconstrictor region in the medulla increases mean arterial pressure and heart rate by enhancing sympathetic nervous system outflow and inhibiting parasympathetic nervous system outflow. Sympathetic stimulation targets resistance vessels, causing vasoconstriction. Inhibition of these areas causes the opposite effect: vasodilatation. Sympathetic fibers causing vasoconstriction supply the arteries, arterioles, and veins. Veins also respond to sympathetic stimulation, but the effects are less apparent than they are in arterial vessels.

OXYGEN TRANSPORT PRINCIPLES

All forms of shock involve impaired delivery of oxygen to the tissues. Variables that influence oxygen transport include oxygen delivery, oxygen consumption, and the oxygen extraction ratio. These terms are defined in Table 11-3.

Oxygen delivery depends on blood flow (cardiac output), the amount of hemoglobin available to carry oxygen, and the percent of arterial oxygen hemoglobin saturation. The body normally delivers three to four times more oxygen to the tissues than they need for normal metabolism. Any condition that reduces cardiac output, hemoglobin availability, or hemoglobin saturation has an impact on the amount of oxygen delivered to tissues.

Oxygen consumption represents the body's demand for oxygen and is therefore a reflection of the body's total metabolism. Reduced oxygen consumption is common in all forms of shock and can create an imbalance between the amount of oxygen available to the tissues and the amount required to meet the increased need. In conditions with a decreased cardiac output, as in hypovolemic or cardiogenic shock, oxygen consumption at the tissue level is decreased. In the early stages of septic shock, when blood is distributed unevenly to the tissues, the tissues may not be able to extract all the oxygen they

Table 11-3

Oxygen Transport Terms

Term	Acronym	Definition
Oxygen delivery	DO_2	Amount of oxygen delivered to the tissues each minute. Reflects the ability of the circulatory system to supply oxygen to the tissues.
Oxygen consumption	VO_2	Amount of oxygen used by the tissues each minute. Reflects the body's total metabolism.
Oxygen extraction ratio	VO_2/DO_2	Ratio of oxygen consumption to oxygen delivery. Indicates the ability of the tissues to extract and use oxygen delivered.

need, even if oxygen is available. The magnitude of the oxygen consumption deficit in patients experiencing shock has been correlated with mortality rates.

Oxygen consumption and delivery can be measured using a specialized pulmonary artery catheter. The oxygen extraction ratio (VO_2/DO_2) provides an estimate of the balance between tissue oxygen demand (consumption) and oxygen supply (delivery). It also provides an indication of the ability of the tissues to extract and use the oxygen delivered.

Stages of Shock

The clinical syndrome of shock results from sustained, inadequate tissue perfusion leading to altered tissue metabolism and function at the subcellular, cellular, and organ-system levels. Untreated, the patient in shock will progress through a continuum of stages manifested by specific signs and symptoms that vary according to the patient's individual response and ability to compensate. The three stages of shock are compensatory, progressive, and irreversible (also called refractory).

THE COMPENSATORY STAGE

The compensatory stage of shock is characterized by an initial decrease in cardiac output and tissue perfusion. The resulting reduction in delivery of oxygen and nutrients at the cellular level decreases aerobic metabolism and increases anaerobic metabolism, resulting in the production of lactic acid. Compensatory mechanisms begin and, at least initially, maintain adequate cardiac output and tissue perfusion. No clinical manifestations are evident during this early stage of shock.

Initial compensatory mechanisms are complex and widespread, aimed largely at maintaining blood pressure within the low-normal to normal range, a level adequate to perfuse vital organs. The sympathetic nervous system is quickly activated when arterial blood pressure falls. Pressoreceptors in the walls of the aorta and carotid sinuses sense decreased pressure and transmit signals to the vasomotor center in the medulla. The autonomic nervous system signals sympathetic nerve fibers throughout the body to release norepinephrine. This release causes arterioles to constrict, which assists in increasing arterial pressure. The adrenal medulla is stimulated to release the catecholamines epinephrine and norepinephrine into the bloodstream. Stimulation of β_1-adrenergic receptors in the heart increases the rate and force of contraction. Stimulation of β_2-adrenergic receptors causes coronary artery vasodilatation and increased blood flow to the myocardium to meet the increased oxygen demand of the heart. Alpha-adrenergic receptor stimulation causes vasoconstriction. This results in blood's being shunted away from organs, including skeletal muscles, fat,

and skin. Arterioles in these areas constrict and shunt blood away from capillaries and through arteriovenous fistulas into the venous system. Arterioles in vital organs, such as the heart and brain, remain open and continue to receive blood flow.

Chemoreceptors in the aorta and carotid arteries respond to decreased arterial oxygen tension by sending signals to the respiratory center in the brain. The respiratory center responds by increasing the rate and depth of respirations, which results in a respiratory alkalosis.

Decreased cardiac output and vasoconstriction in the kidneys causes decreased renal perfusion. Resultant renal ischemia stimulates the release of renin by the juxtaglomerular apparatus. Circulating renin reacts with angiotensinogen produced in the liver, resulting in the production of angiotensin I. A converting enzyme in the lungs converts angiotensin I to angiotensin II. Angiotensin II, a potent vasoconstrictor, helps to increase blood pressure and venous return. It also stimulates release of aldosterone from the adrenal cortex, causing reabsorption of sodium and water and increased venous return to the heart. Reduced renal perfusion results in oliguria, with urinary output falling below 0.5 mL/kg/hour. Further reductions in cardiac output result in additional decreases in urinary output.

Catecholamine stimulation also causes contraction of the radial muscle of the iris, causing pupillary dilation. Vasoconstriction of the vessels in the skin and stimulation of the sweat glands cause the skin to be cool, pale, and moist. Decreased tissue perfusion in the liver stimulates breakdown of glycogen stores to increase availability of glucose for energy production. This results in increased blood glucose levels.

How long the body can maintain tissue perfusion and homeostasis depends on the patient's general health and reserves. Compensatory mechanisms may be able to maintain arterial blood pressure and tissue perfusion only briefly. If the underlying cause of shock is not managed, the patient will progress to the next stage.

Many of the clinical manifestations of compensated shock result from an excess of catecholamines and other vasoconstricting hormones and from increased sympathetic neural activity to the heart and vasculature. Manifestations of the compensatory stage of shock are summarized in Table 11–4. Sinus tachycardia is present, with heart rates exceeding 100 bpm. Respirations become deep and rapid. Blood gas analysis reveals respiratory alkalosis and hypoxemia. In most forms of shock the skin is cool, moist, and clammy, especially in the extremities. However, in patients with distributive forms of shock (septic, neurogenic, and anaphylactic), hypotension results from inappropriate vasodilatation, and the extremities may remain warm. Urine volume is reduced. An altered sensorium may be characterized by restlessness and agitation. The pupils are dilated. Blood glucose levels increase. The nurse must be aware that underlying disease states, such

Table 11–4

Manifestations of Shock

Parameter	Compensatory Shock	Progressive Shock	Refractory Shock
Heart rate	Increased	>150/min, commonly irregular	>150/min and irregular
Blood pressure	Adequate to perfuse vital organs Low-normal to normal pressure	No longer able to perfuse vital organs Systolic pressure <80–90 mm Hg	Pressure <80 mm Hg May not be audible
Arterial pulses	Rapid, weak, thready	Thready, weak, rapid May not be palpable	Weak, thready, or nonpalpable
Skin	Cool, moist, pale	Cold, cyanotic, mottled	Cyanotic, mottled
Respirations	Increased rate and depth	Rapid, shallow, crackles	Respiratory failure
Arterial blood gases			
PaO_2	Decreased	Decreased	Severely decreased
$PaCO_2$	Decreased	Increased	Increased
Arterial pH	Increased	Decreased	Severely decreased
Level of consciousness	Restlessness, agitation, lethargy, mental cloudiness and confusion Responds to verbal stimuli and follows simple commands	No longer responds to verbal stimuli Response to painful stimuli deteriorates from flexion and extension to flaccid	Flaccid
Pupils	Dilated Reactive to light	Dilated Response to light may deteriorate from sluggish to absent	May be fixed and dilated
Urine output	<0.5 mL/kg/hr	<0.5 mL/kg/hr	Anuria or negligible

$PaCO_2$, partial pressure of carbon dioxide; PaO_2, partial pressure of oxygen.

---

as diabetes, or the effects of such drugs as beta-blockers or vasodilators may mask the compensatory responses of tachycardia and vasoconstriction.

THE PROGRESSIVE STAGE

As shock progresses, compensatory mechanisms can no longer compensate for decreased cardiac output and fail to maintain blood pressure sufficient to perfuse the vital organs. Physiologic changes that initially helped shunt blood to vital organs become ineffective and organs begin to malfunction. The primary cause of the shock state must be corrected quickly or severe hypoperfusion of organs will lead to multi-system organ failure.

As cellular metabolism shifts from aerobic to anaerobic as a result of prolonged cellular hypoxia, production of adenosine triphosphate decreases, reducing metabolic cellular processes. The net result is decreased oxygen consumption. Glycolysis results in conversion of pyruvate to lactate. Increased lactate levels cause metabolic acidemia and promote cardiac dysrhythmias. The decrease in adenosine triphosphate availability also causes the sodium-potassium pump to malfunction. Active transport of sodium and potassium across the cell membrane diminishes. Sodium ions accumulate inside the cell, causing intracellular swelling. As organelles inside the cell begin to swell, their function deteriorates. Potassium collects outside the cell. Changes in the sodium-potassium ion concentration cause the resting membrane potential to become more positive, leading to development of dysrhythmias.

Bradykinin and myocardial depressant factor are important vasoactive polypeptides that appear to play a significant role in shock. Bradykinin produces vasodilatation, increased capillary permeability, smooth muscle relaxation, and infiltration of an area with leukocytes. Bradykinin is thought to have a major impact in later stages of shock and may be a factor in the development of associated pulmonary insufficiency. Myocardial depressant factor is released in response to splenic ischemia and appears to depress cardiac muscle contraction, further contributing to decreased cardiac output.

Metabolic acidosis worsens and causes precapillary sphincters to relax. Postcapillary vasoconstriction continues, however, creating increased resistance and decreased capillary flow rates. Capillary hydrostatic pressures increase, causing fluid to move out of the capillary beds into the interstitial space. Interstitial edema potentiates decreased blood return to the heart. As capillary flow rates decrease, microemboli can form, placing the patient at risk for disseminated intravascular coagulation.

As pulmonary capillary bed hypoperfusion persists, alveolar cells become ischemic and unable to produce surfactant. This causes alveoli to collapse, producing massive microatelectasis and reduced pulmonary compliance. Ischemia also increases pulmonary capillary permeability, allowing fluid to leave the pulmonary capillaries and producing interstitial and intra-alveolar edema. Pulmonary edema drastically reduces diffusion of oxygen and intensifies hypoxemia. Respiratory insufficiency and failure commonly develop in persistent shock states.

Prolonged kidney hypoperfusion potentiates development of acute tubular necrosis, progressing to renal insufficiency and acute renal failure. Toxic waste products cannot be excreted, leading to an increase in blood urea nitrogen (BUN) and serum creatinine levels.

Prolonged hypoperfusion of the liver reduces the organ's ability to perform important functions adequately, including drug and hormone metabolism and conjugation of bilirubin. Bilirubin accumulates in the blood and causes jaundice. The liver loses its ability to metabolize waste products, such as ammonia and lactic acid. As cellular damage occurs and death approaches, intracellular enzymes are released into the blood and can be observed as increases in serum glutamic-oxaloacetic transaminase, serum glutamic-pyruvic transaminase, and lactate dehydrogenase. Pancreatic hypoperfusion and ischemia result in release of the pancreatic enzymes amylase and lipase.

Clinical manifestations associated with the progressive stage of shock include decreased blood pressure with a narrow pulse pressure, decreased heart rate, decreased urine production, increased urine specific gravity, decreased creatinine clearance, and increased serum creatinine and BUN. Peripheral edema develops from altered capillary fluid dynamics.

Decreased cerebral blood flow further decreases the level of consciousness. As the persistent hypoperfusion state continues, more stimulation is required to elicit a response from the patient. Response to painful stimuli progressively decreases until the patient becomes flaccid (no response to painful stimuli).

Respiratory rate increases and the patient develops audible crackles as a result of interstitial pulmonary edema. Arterial blood gases demonstrate metabolic and respiratory acidosis with hypoxemia.

THE REFRACTORY STAGE

Irreversible or refractory shock is the final stage of shock. The body becomes refractory to all therapeutic measures. Multiple organ failure develops and produces signs and symptoms of cardiac, respiratory, neurologic, hepatic, gastrointestinal, pancreatic, and hematologic failure. Intractable circulatory failure develops as blood pressure and heart rate continue to decrease. The shock state is so profound and degree of cellular destruction so severe that death is imminent.

Types of Shock

Shock states can be classified by cause, by pathophysiologic process, or by clinical manifestations. Classifying the shock state by cause allows the nurse to focus on the pathophysiologic process and underlying disorder that must be treated to avoid irreversible impairment of cellular function. The major types of shock are hypovolemic, cardiogenic, and distributive.

HYPOVOLEMIC SHOCK

Etiology and Pathophysiology

Hypovolemic shock is the most common type of shock. It is caused by a loss of whole blood, plasma, or interstitial fluid in such quantities that the body's metabolic needs can no longer be met. The etiologic factors in hypovolemic shock are listed in Table 11–5.

Hypovolemic shock can develop from absolute or relative hypovolemia. Absolute hypovolemia results from an external loss of fluid from the body, as in external hemorrhage. Relative hypovolemia results from an internal shift of fluid from the intravascular space to the extravascular space. It may occur with increased capillary permeability, decreased colloidal osmotic pressure, or loss of intravascular integrity. Reduced intravascular blood volume leads to a decrease in the amount of blood

Table 11–5

Etiologic Factors in Hypovolemic Shock
Loss of blood volume (hemorrhage)
Internal
Hemoperitoneum
Hemothorax
Retroperitoneal hemorrhage
Ruptured aortic aneurysm
External
Gastrointestinal bleeding
Surgery
Trauma
Loss of plasma volume
Burns
Open or draining wounds or lesions
Loss of other body fluids
Gastrointestinal
Severe diarrhea
Severe vomiting
Renal
Adrenal insufficiency
Diabetes insipidus
Diabetic ketoacidosis
Diuretic therapy
High-output renal failure
Hyperosmolar nonketotic diabetes

returning to the heart (venous return). This, in turn, decreases the amount of blood received by the ventricles during diastolic filling (preload) and decreases the amount of blood available for ejection from the ventricle (stroke volume). As compensatory mechanisms begin to fail and can no longer maintain cardiac output, tissue perfusion to organ systems significantly decreases (Fig. 11–4).

Clinical Manifestations

Clinical manifestations of hypovolemic shock depend on the severity of fluid loss and the person's ability to compensate for the loss. Disease processes, age, amount of blood loss, rate of loss, and length of time over which the loss occurs all affect how quickly clinical manifestations of hypovolemic shock occur. The clinical presentation with various forms of hypovolemic shock is similar to the presentation of the individual experiencing hemorrhagic shock. Assessment findings for the different classes of hemorrhagic shock are listed in Table 11–6.

Class I hemorrhage represents a fluid loss of up to 15% and may be tolerated without any symptoms if compensatory mechanisms are effective in maintaining cardiac output.

Class II represents more significant volume losses of 15 to 30%. The body tries to initiate compensatory mechanisms to return to homeostasis. The heart rate increases to between 100 and 120 bpm in response to sympathetic nervous system stimulation. The patient's blood pressure remains normal but pulse pressure is narrowed. Urinary output ranges from 20 to 30 mL/hour. Capillary refill time is prolonged.

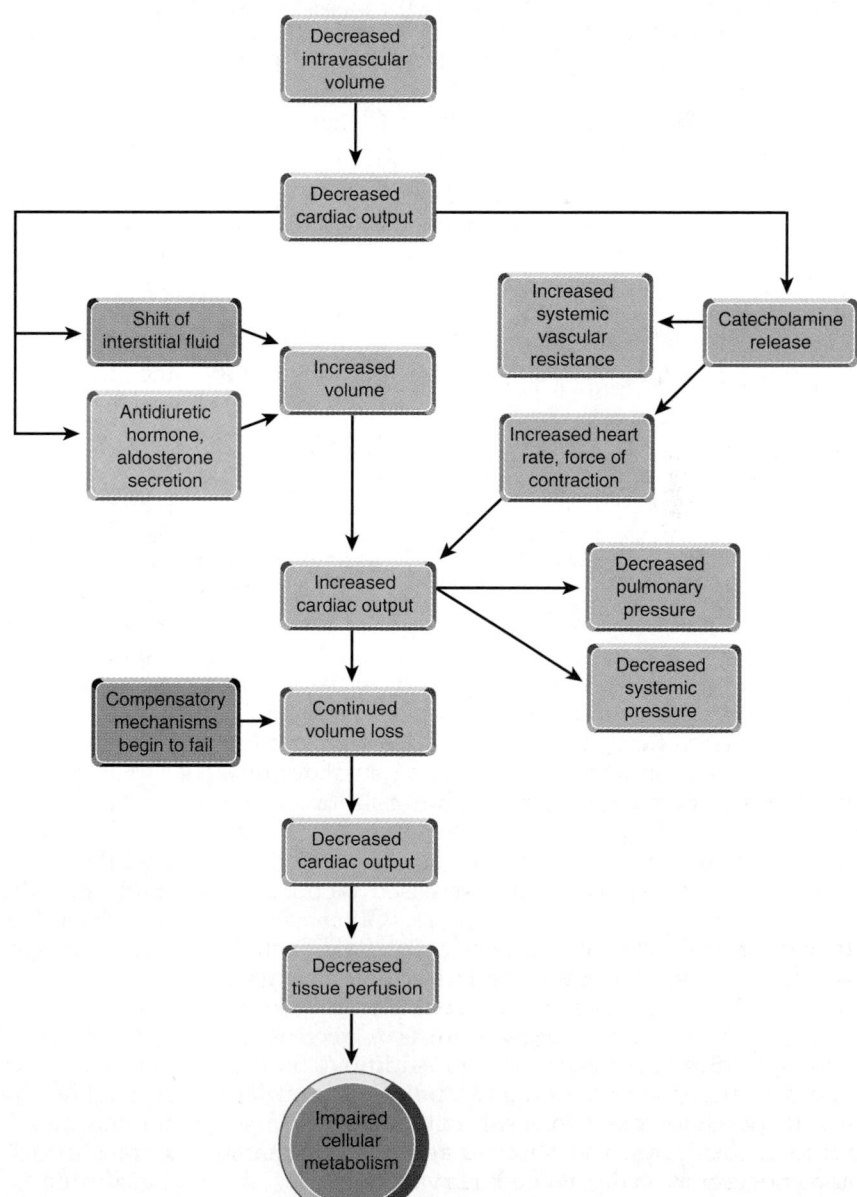

Figure 11–4
Pathophysiology of hypovolemic shock.

Table 11–6

Classification and Assessment of Acute Hemorrhage

Assessment Finding	Class I	Class II	Class III	Class IV
Blood loss				
Percent of body weight	15%	15–30%	30–40%	<40%
Volume	<750 mL	1000–1250 mL	1500–1800 mL	2000–2500 mL
Pulse rate	<100 bpm	>100 bpm	>120 bpm	>140 bpm
Respirations per minute	Normal	20–30	30–40	>35
Blood pressure	Normal	Normal or slightly increased	Decreased	Not palpable
Pulse pressure	Normal	Narrowed	Narrowed	Narrowed
Capillary refill	Normal	Prolonged	Prolonged	Prolonged
Skin	Pale, cool	Pale, cool	Pale, cold, moist	Cyanotic, cold, clammy
Level of consciousness	Slightly anxious	Mildly anxious	Anxious, confused	Confused, lethargic, or obtunded
Urine output	30 mL/hr or more	20–30 mL/hr	5–15 mL/hr	Negligible

Adapted with permission from American College of Surgeons, Committee on Trauma: Advanced trauma life support course for physicians. Chicago: American College of Surgeons, 1984.

Class III hemorrhagic shock occurs with major blood losses of 30 to 40% of total volume. The patient becomes increasingly anxious and progressively confused. Systolic blood pressure drops below 80 mm Hg and pulse pressure is narrowed. Respirations increase in rate and depth. Urine output falls to 5 to 15 mL/hour. Capillary refill continues to be prolonged.

Class IV hemorrhagic shock represents a severe blood loss of greater than 40% of the total volume. The patient develops severe hypotension. Heart rate may exceed 140 bpm and respirations may exceed 35 per minute. Urine output decreases to only negligible amounts. Peripheral capillary refill time is significantly greater than 3 seconds.

Diagnosis

The diagnosis of hypovolemic shock is based primarily on history and clinical manifestations. Patients with significant blood or fluid loss or a history of such loss, or with blunt chest or abdominal trauma, are considered at significant risk for having hypovolemic shock. Poor tissue perfusion is evidenced by decreased mentation and level of consciousness. Vital signs reveal decreased blood pressure and narrowed pulse pressure. Other clinical data that assist in establishing the diagnosis include decreased urinary output, faint peripheral pulses, peripheral vasoconstriction, and cool, clammy skin.

Hemodynamic monitoring reveals a decrease in cardiac output and cardiac index. Additionally, pulmonary artery pressures and pulmonary artery wedge pressures are decreased consequent to a reduced preload. Systemic vascular resistance increases as compensatory sympathetic innervation occurs.

Laboratory data that may be obtained include hemoglobin and hematocrit, platelet count, and co-

agulation profile. Additional laboratory tests may include serum electrolyte levels, BUN levels, serum osmolality, and lactic acid levels. Assessment of arterial blood gases reveals metabolic acidosis. Radiographic studies may be beneficial in cases of trauma, to assist in diagnosing a hemothorax. Depending on the underlying condition, other studies may be requested, including computed tomography and magnetic resonance imaging, to help locate the source of blood loss.

Management

The major goals in treating hypovolemic shock are to find and aggressively control the source of blood loss, and to reverse that loss with the administration of appropriate fluids to restore tissue perfusion. Fluid administration to replace intravascular volume may involve colloids, crystalloids, or both. The type of solution chosen usually depends on the type of fluid lost.

Colloid solutions (such as blood, blood components, dextran, hetastarch, and perfluorocarbons) increase serum colloid osmotic pressure within the vascular compartment. The net effect is to move fluid into the vascular compartment. Blood products, including whole blood, red blood cells, plasma, and platelets may be used to treat hypovolemic shock. A disadvantage to their use is that fluid leaks out of the vascular compartment into the interstitial space if the patient has increased capillary permeability. Autotransfusion may be especially useful in managing hypovolemic shock caused by chest trauma and hemorrhage. It involves collection and retransfusion of blood into the same patient. Autotransfusion is used to prevent or treat existing hypovolemia caused by chest trauma and hemorrhage following surgery.

Crystalloid solutions (such as Ringer's lactate and other balanced electrolyte solutions) contain electrolytes and help expand extracellular volume, reduce viscosity, and prevent sludging. Use caution when infusing lactated Ringer's solution, however. If the patient has poor perfusion during the shock episode, an accumulation of lactate only compounds the problem of acidosis.

Infusing 1 to 2 L Ringer's lactate or normal saline solution rapidly over 30 minutes can help in assessing the degree of blood loss. In Class I hypovolemic shock, in which there is no further blood loss, blood pressure will return to normal and stabilize after the infusion. In Classes III and IV, in which the patient continues to hemorrhage, the normalizing of blood pressure and pulse after infusion will be only temporary. Patients in Class IV have a poor prognosis without immediate surgical intervention.

In Classes I and II hemorrhagic shock, crystalloid solutions are administered at a replacement ratio of 1:1. In Classes III and IV, crystalloid solutions and blood products are administered at a replacement ratio of 3:1 or until the patient reaches hemodynamic stability.

In some trauma cases, a pneumatic antishock garment (PASG), also known as medical antishock trousers or MAST suit, may be beneficial as a circulatory assist device until the patient is transported to the emergency department. A pneumatic antishock garment is a one-piece suit with three individually controlled compartments, one for the abdomen and one for each leg. When inflated, the pneumatic antishock garment constricts the area to improve blood pressure and augment venous return to improve preload and cardiac output. The pneumatic antishock garment or MAST suit must be deflated slowly over several minutes before removal to prevent massive shock or cardiac arrest. When the suit is deflated and circulation returns, the patient may experience increased acidosis from accumulated lactic acid being released into the circulation.

As an alternative to a pneumatic antishock garment in cases of moderate shock, a modified shock position may be helpful. Position the patient with the lower extremities elevated about 45 degrees, the knees straight, the trunk horizontal, and the head positioned level with the chest. This position promotes venous return from the lower extremities without compressing the abdominal organs against the diaphragm. This modified shock position is not effective in cases of severe hypovolemia or cardiogenic shock, when the patient has circulatory overload.

Surgical intervention may be necessary to locate and control the source of bleeding in patients who develop hypovolemic shock after trauma or surgery. The most common bleeding sites postoperatively include the surgical wound, the site of operative dissection, and the upper gastrointestinal tract. Once bleeding has been controlled, interventions seek to restore adequate fluid volume.

CARDIOGENIC SHOCK

Etiology and Pathophysiology

Cardiogenic shock refers to a shock response generated when the heart's ability to pump blood becomes impaired. This impairment decreases cardiac output. If peripheral vascular resistance is not adequate to compensate for the decrease in tissue perfusion, the general shock response is stimulated (Fig. 11–5). Cardiogenic shock can be caused by dysfunction of the left ventricle, the right ventricle, or both. It may result from primary ventricular ischemia, structural problems, or dysrhythmias. Etio-

Figure 11–5
Pathophysiology of cardiogenic shock.

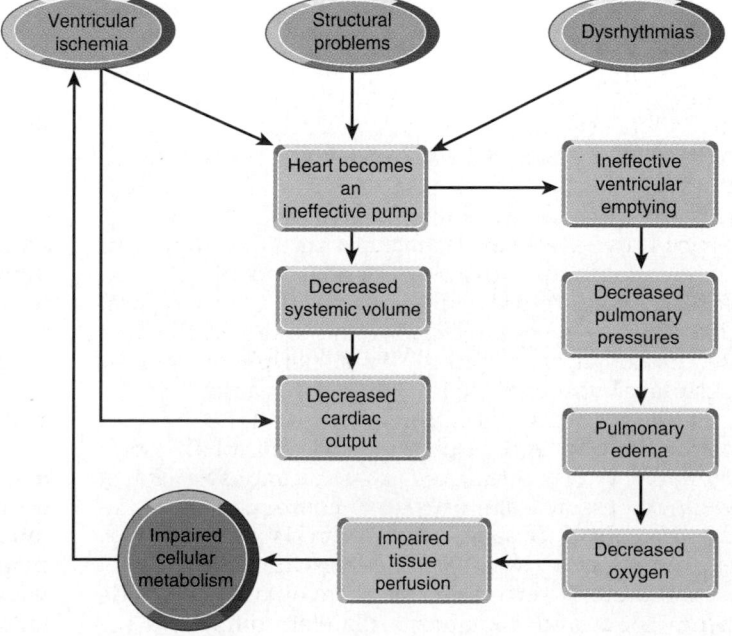

logic factors in cardiogenic shock are listed in Table 11–7. Mortality rates for cardiogenic shock are as high as 90%. Death results from cardiopulmonary collapse. Transient cardiogenic shock may develop following cardiac surgery, when the myocardium is depressed following hypothermia, cardioplegic arrest, and surgical incisions.

The most common cause of cardiogenic shock is a loss of contractile elements in the myocardial muscle. This usually results from ischemia related to acute myocardial infarction. Cardiogenic shock arises when 40% or more of the functional myocardium has been damaged, either from one massive myocardial infarction or from several smaller infarctions. Massive damage usually occurs in the anterior wall of the left ventricle.

Structural problems may cause cardiogenic shock as well, when forward motion of the blood is disrupted. Causes include papillary muscle rupture and septal rupture. Regurgitant or stenotic valve lesions also interrupt forward flow of blood through the heart and may result in an abrupt onset of congestive heart failure progressing to shock.

Dysrhythmias affecting heart rate can disrupt pump function and cause cardiogenic shock. Brady-arrhythmias can lower cardiac output, especially in patients unable to compensate by increasing stroke volume. Conversely, as the heart rate increases, diastolic filling time decreases, reducing stroke volume because the filling time is too short.

When the left ventricle is unable to pump blood forward adequately, three primary problems result. First, the amount of blood ejected from the ventricle with each heart beat (stroke volume) decreases. This subsequently decreases cardiac output, blood pressure, and tissue perfusion. Second, as blood pressure falls, coronary artery perfusion decreases. This subsequently decreases myocardial muscle perfusion. The increased workload and oxygen demand on the myocardium potentiate myocardial ischemia and predispose the patient to further muscle damage,

creating a vicious circle. Third, the amount of blood remaining in the left ventricle at the end of systole increases. If the primary problem involves the left ventricle, this increased end-systolic volume will eventually lead to increased ventricular filling pressure. Increased filling pressures are transmitted back to the left atrium and then to the pulmonary circulation. This increases pulmonary vascular pressure, causing fluid to move into the interstitial and intra-alveolar spaces, resulting in pulmonary congestion, hypoxia, and deteriorating blood gases. Increased pulmonary pressures are eventually reflected backward to the right ventricle, causing both left and right ventricular failure. As the ventricular pressures remain elevated, systemic manifestations of right-sided heart failure become evident.

Clinical Manifestations

Compensatory mechanisms may initially be able to maintain blood pressure and adequate tissue perfusion to vital organs. However, as compensatory mechanisms begin to fail, the patient shows a decrease in sensorium, systolic blood pressure falls to less than 90 mm Hg, and diastolic pressure increases, narrowing the pulse pressure. Heart rate increases above 100 bpm. A weak, thready pulse develops and heart sounds reveal a diminished S1 and S2 caused by decreased contractility. A summation gallop may be audible over the left apex from increased pressure in the left ventricle and decreased compliance. Skin becomes pale, cool, and moist from peripheral vasoconstriction. A variety of dysrhythmias may occur, depending on the underlying problem.

Urinary output progressively decreases to less than 30 mL/hr, and the urine becomes concentrated. Urinalysis shows increased osmolarity and specific gravity and decreased urine sodium. BUN and serum creatinine levels rise as waste products are no longer excreted effectively.

Respiratory rate and depth increase in an attempt to improve oxygenation. Arterial blood gases initially demonstrate respiratory alkalosis, but this progresses quickly to respiratory and metabolic acidosis with hypoxemia from alveolar hypoventilation. Auscultation of the lungs reveals crackles and wheezes.

Diagnosis

Diagnosis of cardiogenic shock is based on history, symptoms presented, laboratory studies, and diagnostic studies. In its initial stages, cardiogenic shock may be difficult to identify because sympathetic nervous stimulation increases the heart rate and force of contraction. During this phase, blood pressure and perfusion of vital organs may be maintained. However, as these compensatory mechanisms fail, systolic blood pressure falls and diastolic pressure remains increased because of the sympathetic simulation, narrowing the pulse pressure. The heart rate increases above 100 bpm. Peripheral vasoconstriction occurs, resulting in cool, clammy skin.

Table 11–7

Etiologic Factors in Cardiogenic Shock
Dysrhythmias
Bradydysrhythmia
Tachydysrhythmia
Structural problems
Cardiomyopathy
Papillary muscle rupture
Septal rupture
Valvular dysfunction
Ventricular aneurysm
Intracardiac tumor
Ventricular ischemia
Cardiac arrest
Open-heart surgery
Myocardial infarction

Monitoring of hemodynamic pressures with a flow-directed pulmonary catheter reveals a decreased cardiac output and cardiac index. A cardiac index less than 2.2 L/min/m² in a normovolemic patient is usually diagnostic. Because the left ventricle has difficulty contracting and effectively emptying blood with each contraction, the pulmonary capillary wedge pressure increases. An increase greater than 18 mm Hg causes fluid to shift from the vascular space to the interstitial and alveolar spaces, leading to pulmonary congestion. Systemic vascular resistance rises as a reflection of the vasoconstriction. Systolic blood pressure falls below 90 mm Hg, and the patient has a narrowed pulse pressure.

Arterial blood gas values initially reveal respiratory alkalosis from hyperventilation. However, this quickly progresses to metabolic and respiratory acidosis with hypoxemia as the patient's condition deteriorates.

Management

A patient with cardiogenic shock will receive pharmacologic and mechanical interventions. The goals of treatment are to decrease myocardial oxygen demands, increase myocardial oxygen delivery, and increase cardiac output. Interventions to increase oxygen supply include supplemental oxygen, respiratory support, and coronary vasodilatation. Vasodilating agents and diuretics are used to reduce preload and afterload. Pain medications and sedatives may also assist in decreasing myocardial demand. Antidysrhythmic agents are used to suppress or control dysrhythmias that decrease cardiac output. Positive inotropic drugs, such as dopamine and dobutamine, are used to increase contractility, cardiac output, and tissue perfusion.

Dopamine stimulates dopaminergic, β-receptor, and α-receptor sites. Activation of dopaminergic receptor sites increases mesenteric and renal blood flow. Stimulation of the β-receptor site increases myocardial contractility and heart rate. Alpha-adrenergic stimulation increases systemic vasoconstriction. Each of these effects is dose-dependent.

Dobutamine stimulates beta-adrenergic receptor sites and increases contractility of the heart but has little effect on heart rate or blood vessels. Dobutamine is used to improve myocardial contractility in patients who are not hypotensive.

Vasodilators are used to decrease the heart's work load by reducing systemic vascular resistance. Commonly used vasodilators include nitroglycerin and nitroprusside. Nitroglycerin dilates venous vessels and coronary arteries and increases coronary blood flow. It decreases pulmonary congestion by reducing venous return and left ventricular preload. Nitroprusside causes venous and arterial vasodilation, which reduces afterload by reducing systemic vascular resistance. Nitroprusside also increases cardiac output and decreases preload and myocardial oxygen demand. Continuous blood pressure monitoring during administration of nitroglycerin or ni-

troprusside is essential because either drug can cause hypotension. Amrinone, a phosphodiesterase inhibitor, decreases preload and afterload by increasing myocardial contractility and causes both arterial and venous vasodilatation.

Low doses of epinephrine may also be used to stimulate β-receptors to increase the force of myocardial contraction. In higher doses, it also stimulates α-receptors to constrict blood vessels, which raises systemic vascular resistance.

Counterpulsation with an intra-aortic balloon pump may be indicated for temporary circulatory assistance to restore hemodynamic stability in patients in cardiogenic shock. A polyurethane balloon is inserted percutaneously through the femoral artery and positioned just distal to the left subclavian artery (Fig. 11–6). The balloon is inflated during diastole and deflated in systole. The overall effects of counterpulsation are to increase coronary perfusion and improve cardiac output by decreasing preload and afterload. Intra-aortic balloon pump counterpulsation is an effective means of decreasing the work of the myocardium and decreasing oxygen consumption.

Invasive mechanical devices that have been used experimentally to improve the heart as a pump include ventricular assist devices and the artificial heart. These devices consist of electrically activated or pneumatic air-driven pumps that support the function of a single ventricle or the whole heart. Heart transplantation may be an option for patients who have severe myocardial damage due to cardiogenic shock.

DISTRIBUTIVE SHOCK

Distributive shock results from inadequate vascular tone that leads to massive vasodilatation. Although vascular volume remains normal during distributive shock, and the heart pumps blood adequately, the size of the vascular space increases. The result is a maldistribution of blood within the circulatory system. This disproportion between blood volume and capillary vessel size effectively decreases blood pressure. Distributive shock is frequently subdivided into three types: septic, neurogenic, and anaphylactic.

Septic Shock

Septic shock is a form of severe sepsis characterized by hypotension and altered tissue perfusion. The altered tissue perfusion results in a maldistribution of blood flow to the tissues, with some areas underperfused and others overperfused. Between 70,000 and 300,000 individuals become septic each year in the United States. Of those, about half develop septic shock. Mortality rates range from 40% to 95% and depend largely on the timeliness and aggressiveness of treatment. Despite advances in treating and man-

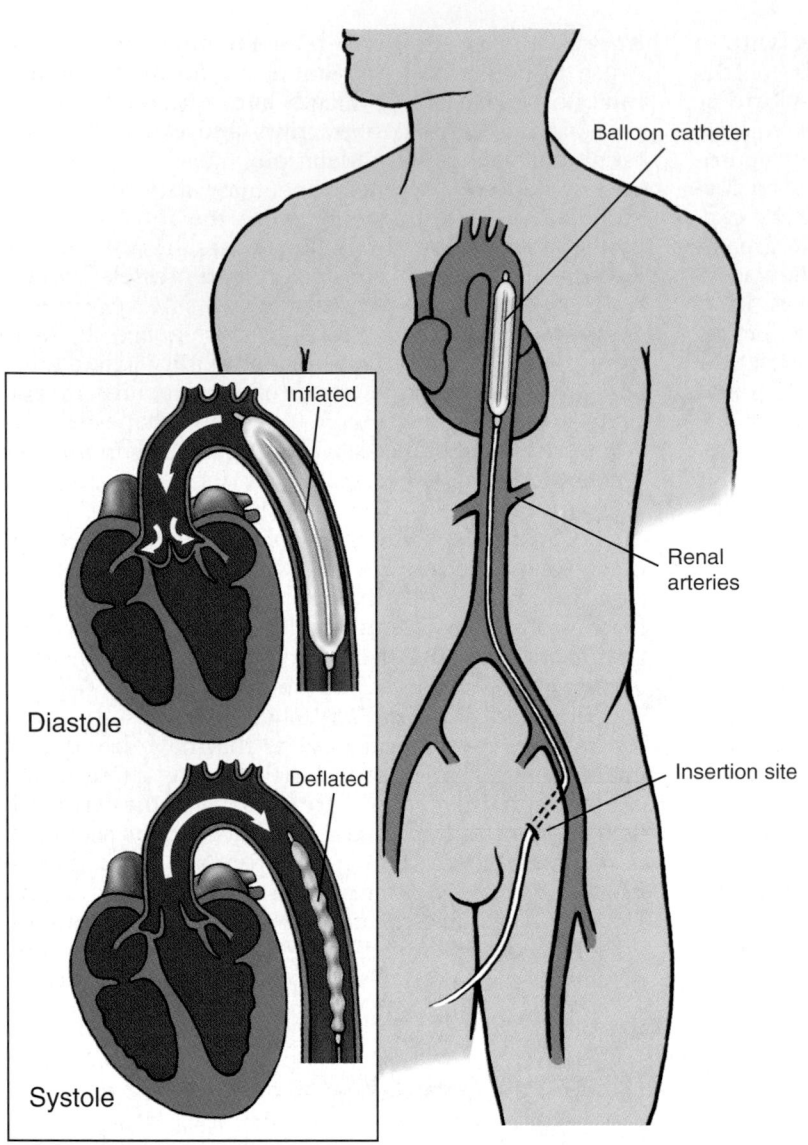

Figure 11-6

Placement of intra-aortic balloon pump catheter.

aging septic shock, it remains a major cause of death in critical care units.

Etiology and Pathophysiology

Sepsis stems from toxins produced by microorganisms. These toxins exert a harmful effect on the vascular, coagulation, and immune systems. Usually, sepsis is preceded by a bacteremia in which pathogens are circulating in the blood. Gram-negative bacteria account for more than half of all cases of septic shock, although gram-positive cocci and bacilli have also been implicated. Microorganisms implicated in sepsis and septic shock are listed in Table 11-8.

When gram-negative organisms are destroyed by the human immune system, endotoxins (lipoproteins) are released from the cell walls. These endotoxins produce adverse biochemical changes and trigger the release of various vasoactive mediators capable of interfering with normal regulation of arteriolar tone. Exotoxins capable of triggering the

body's immune response are released from gram-positive organisms while they are alive in the patient's body.

Once the organism enters the body, a set of complex humoral, cellular, and biochemical mediators are released, causing epithelial cell damage, peripheral vasodilatation, increased capillary permeability, initiation of coagulation and fibrinolysis, and myocardial depression. The immune system becomes so overwhelmed that the system designed initially to protect the body now works against it.

Four primary pathophysiologic changes occur in septic shock. They include myocardial depression, massive vasodilatation, maldistribution of the intravascular volume, and formation of microemboli. Myocardial depression occurs when the ventricular force of contraction decreases from biochemical mediators, including myocardial depressant factor, endotoxins, tumor necrosis factor, endorphins, complement products, and leukotrienes. Massive vasodilatation and increased capillary permeability re-

Table 11-8

Microorganisms Implicated in Septic Shock

Gram-negative bacteria
  Bacteroides spp
  Escherichia coli
  Enterobacter spp
  Haemophilus influenzae
  Klebsiella pneumoniae
  Pseudomonas aeruginosa
  Serratia marcescens
Gram-positive bacteria
  Clostridium spp
  Staphylococcus aureus
  Staphylococcus epidermidis
  Streptococcus pneumoniae
Fungi
Protozoa
Parasites
Rickettsiae
Spirochaeta spp
Viruses

duce the amount of blood returning to the heart (decreased preload). Afterload decreases as well, from massive vasodilatation that occurs secondary to the release of such mediators as bradykinin, endorphins, complement products, histamine, and prostaglandins. Although plasma volume is normal in the early phases of septic shock, it becomes maldistributed as shock progresses because of increased capillary permeability, selective vasoconstriction, and vascular occlusion. Increased capillary permeability allows protein and fluid to shift to the interstitial and intracellular compartments. However, not all vascular beds vasodilate. Stimulation of the sympathetic nervous system and prostaglandin and other biochemical mediators cause selective vasoconstriction in the pulmonary, renal, and splanchnic circulations.

Microemboli form in small blood vessels from neutrophil and platelet aggregation and activation of the clotting system. Some vascular beds receive more blood than they need, while others receive too little. The maldistribution of blood flow leads to hypoxia and lack of nutritional support to some areas, causing cellular dysfunction that ultimately ends in cell death.

The early stage of septic shock is characterized by a hyperdynamic or warm phase as compensatory mechanisms are activated. During this phase, massive vasodilatation occurs in venous and arterial beds. Venous dilatation decreases venous return to the heart and decreases preload. Dilatation of the arterial beds decreases afterload. The patient's blood pressure declines in response to reduced preload and afterload. Pulse pressure widens because of the vasodilatation. The skin becomes warm and flushed in appearance as a result of the massive vasodilatation. The heart rate increases to compensate for the hypotension and increased metabolic acidosis and

sympathetic nervous system stimulation and adrenal stimulation. A ventilation/perfusion mismatch occurs in the lungs as a result of pulmonary vasoconstriction. The respiratory rate increases to compensate for the hypoxemia. Crackles develop as increased pulmonary capillary membrane permeability leads to pulmonary edema.

As septic shock progresses, the patient will move into a hypodynamic phase in which cardiac output decreases and profound hypotension develops. These conditions result from ventricular failure caused by myocardial hypoxemia, release of myocardial depressant factor, acidosis, and the consequent rise in afterload. Tachycardia occurs as the body attempts to compensate for the decline in cardiac output and hypotension. Systemic vascular resistance increases through vasoconstriction, to compensate for the falling blood pressure. The patient's skin now is pale, cold, and clammy.

Clinical Manifestations

Clinical manifestations of septic shock vary according to whether the patient is in the hyperdynamic or hypodynamic phase (Table 11-9). The hyperdynamic phase is characterized by decreased blood pressure with widened pulse pressure. Cardiac output remains normal to high. Pulses are full and bounding. Respiratory rate increases and crackles develop as pulmonary edema begins. Arterial blood gas values reveal respiratory alkalosis, metabolic acidosis, and hypoxemia. Level of consciousness is altered and the patient becomes disoriented, confused, combative, or lethargic. The patient's temperature rises in response to the pyrogens released from invading microorganisms.

As the patient moves into the hypodynamic phase of septic shock, the cardiac output decreases and profound hypotension develops. Tachycardia and dysrhythmias develop. The patient's pulses are weak and thready. The respiratory rate remains high until respiratory fatigue occurs. Adventitious breath sounds are present. Arterial blood gases reveal severe hypoxemia and metabolic and respiratory aci-

Table 11-9

Clinical Manifestations of Septic Shock

Clinical Manifestation	Hyperdynamic Phase
Heart rate	Increased
Blood pressure	Decreased
Pulse pressure	Wide
Cardiac output (CO)	Increased
Systemic vascular resistance (SVR)	Decreased
Skin	Warm, flushed
Temperature	Increased
Respiratory rate	Increased
Level of consciousness	Decreased
Urine output	Decreased

dosis. The patient's level of consciousness continues to deteriorate until the patient no longer responds to painful stimuli.

As multiple organ failure occurs, laboratory data reflect progressive dysfunction. The patient's white blood cell count declines and BUN and serum creatinine levels are increased. Serum glutamic-oxaloacetic transaminase, serum glutamic-pyruvic transaminase, and lactate dehydrogenase levels rise. Patients who survive this stage of septic shock require prolonged and extensive rehabilitation.

Diagnosis

Diagnosis of septic shock is based primarily on history and clinical manifestations. Cultures from blood, sputum, urine, surgical or nonsurgical wounds, sinuses, and invasive lines may be helpful in identifying the invading microorganism. Computed tomographic scans may help in identifying sites of potential abscess formation. Chest and abdominal x-rays may reveal infectious processes. The white blood cell count is usually elevated but may decrease as shock progresses. Hyperglycemia may be evident in early stages of shock and progress to hypoglycemia in later stages.

The hemodynamic profile of the patient, along with clinical manifestations, help to establish the diagnosis. Systemic vascular resistance decreases from the massive peripheral vasodilatation. Although cardiac output increases in the early hyperdynamic phase of septic shock, it is not sufficient to maintain oxygen delivery to the tissues. The amount of blood ejected with each heart beat decreases and blood pressure falls. Pulmonary artery pressure and pulmonary artery wedge pressure decrease because of the reduced venous return to the heart. The patient is usually afebrile with pink skin that is warm to the touch. Arterial blood gases demonstrate respiratory alkalosis with mild hypoxemia. As shock progresses to the hypodynamic phase, cardiac output remains low. Peripheral vasoconstriction occurs from sympathetic stimulation and results in a narrowed pulse pressure. Severe hypotension results from the increased afterload produced by peripheral vasoconstriction and ineffective cardiac contractility. Pulmonary artery pressures and pulmonary artery wedge pressures become elevated. The skin becomes cool and clammy. Assessment of arterial blood gases reveal metabolic and respiratory acidosis with hypoxemia.

Management

Treatment of septic shock requires a multifaceted approach to control the infection, reverse the pathophysiologic responses, and provide metabolic support for the patient. Cultures and sensitivities can help identify the organism and establish the most effective antibiotic for treatment. Until culture reports are back from the laboratory, a broad-spectrum antibiotic is prescribed.

Crystalloid or colloid solutions are administered to restore adequate ventricular preload. It is imperative to monitor the patient's hemodynamic status to prevent fluid overload and congestive heart failure.

Vasoconstrictor agents are indicated during the hyperdynamic phase to reverse the effects of massive peripheral vasodilatation. Positive inotropic agents may be required to improve myocardial contractility. To optimize oxygenation and ventilation, mechanical ventilation may be required to maintain the patient's PaO$_2$ above 70 mm Hg and the pH within normal limits. Antipyretic agents and cooling measures may be necessary to control the patient's temperature. Nutritional therapy is crucial to promote wound healing, improve the immune response, maintain a positive nitrogen balance, and maintain the patient's overall nutritional status. As appropriate, the patient may require surgical intervention to débride infected or necrotic tissue or remove abscesses. This action facilitates removal of the septic source and, consequently, endotoxin or exotoxin production.

Experimental therapies being tested in septic shock include high-dose corticosteroids and naloxone administration. However, mixed results in clinical trials continue to make these agents controversial. Other investigational therapies include monoclonal antibodies that bind with the endotoxin and block activation of the immune response, pulmonary vasodilating prostaglandins, free radical scavengers, cyclooxygenase inhibitors, and anticomplement antibodies.

Neurogenic Shock

Neurogenic shock is characterized by massive vasodilatation from loss or suppression of sympathetic tone. It is a temporary condition associated with injury or disease of the upper spinal cord or brainstem or following administration of general or spinal anesthesia.

Etiology and Pathophysiology

Neurogenic shock can be caused by any condition that interrupts sympathetic nerve impulse transmission or blocks sympathetic outflow from the vasomotor center in the brain. Interruption of sympathetic activity occurs with trauma to the spinal cord or medulla, conditions that disrupt the supply of oxygen to the medulla, or conditions that deprive the medulla of glucose (such as an insulin reaction). Other causes of neurogenic shock include high-level spinal anesthesia, ganglionic- and adrenergic-blocking drugs, severe emotional stress, pain, depressive drugs, and drug overdoses.

The onset of neurogenic shock may occur within minutes of the injury, and the condition may last for days, weeks, or months, depending on the precipitating cause. Lack of sympathetic tone leaves a dominant parasympathetic nervous system, which results in massive vasodilatation. Neurogenic shock creates a relative hypovolemia in which the blood volume is distributed inappropriately. Vasodilatation decreases venous return and cardiac output, resulting in hypotension. Inhibition of the baroreceptor response results in the loss of compensatory reflex tachycardia, so the heart rate cannot increase in response to reduced blood pressure. Loss of vasomotor tone in cutaneous blood vessels disrupts thermoregulation, so the patient must depend on the environment for temperature regulation.

Clinical Manifestations

Patients with neurogenic shock have hypotension, bradycardia, hypothermia, and warm, dry skin. Bowel and bladder dysfunction and loss of sexual reflexes may occur from lost autonomic function.

Diagnosis

Assessment of hemodynamic parameters reveals a decrease in cardiac output and cardiac index. Venous vasodilatation results in a decreased preload, central venous pressure, and pulmonary artery wedge pressure. Arterial vasodilatation results in a decreased afterload, which is reflected in decreased systemic vascular resistance.

Management

Goals of therapy are to treat the cause, prevent cardiovascular instability, and promote optimal tissue perfusion. Fluid resuscitation is initiated if the patient has a systolic blood pressure lower than 90 mm Hg, urine output less than 30 mL/hour, or changes in mentation. The patient must be monitored carefully for fluid overload. Vasopressors may be required to maintain blood pressure and perfuse vital organs. Bradycardia may be treated with atropine, isoproterenol, and transvenous or external cardiac pacing to maintain cardiac output. The patient should be maintained in a normothermic state. Supplemental oxygen administration and ventilatory support may be required to treat hypoxemia and respiratory insufficiency.

Anaphylactic Shock

Anaphylaxis is a sudden, life-threatening hypersensitivity reaction to an antigen. It is characterized by massive vasodilatation and increased capillary permeability. Unless treatment begins immediately, the patient will quickly develop the general shock response.

Etiology and Pathophysiology

Anaphylaxis is mediated by immunoglobulin E (IgE) antibody. IgE is produced following the first exposure to an antigen. It binds to the surface of mast cells and basophils. During subsequent exposures, the antigen binds with the cell-bound IgE molecules. This binding of the antigen and antibody causes the mast cell or basophil to immediately release several biochemical mediators that cause widespread tissue responses. These chemical mediators include

- Histamine, which causes bronchial constriction, vasodilation, and increased capillary permeability
- Serotonin, which has similar effects
- Slow-reacting substance of anaphylaxis, which is a potent bronchoconstrictor that also causes smooth muscles of the internal organs to spasm and venules to dilate and increase in permeability
- Bradykinin, which causes vasodilatation and increases capillary permeability

The bronchoconstriction, vasodilatation, and increased capillary permeability caused by these chemical mediators produce most of the clinical manifestations of anaphylaxis. The severe hypotension and shock that can result make anaphylaxis a potentially life-threatening event. The most common triggers are drugs and insect stings.

Clinical Manifestations

Early recognition of anaphylaxis is crucial because, within minutes, it can progress to shock, respiratory arrest, and cardiovascular collapse. The earliest signs of systemic anaphylaxis include feelings of anxiety and uneasiness, flushing, diaphoresis, sneezing, and weakness. These are very quickly followed by nausea, dizziness, itching, and sometimes edema, especially of the face, hands, and feet. Severe respiratory distress from bronchospasm and laryngeal edema and severe hypotension from vasodilatation and increased capillary permeability quickly follow (Table 11–10).

Diagnosis

Anaphylaxis must be diagnosed rapidly based on the patient's signs and symptoms. There is virtually no time for laboratory tests because emergency interventions must be initiated immediately to save the patient's life. As the anaphylactic reaction progresses, hypotension and tachycardia develop from the massive vasodilatation and loss of circulating volume. Assessment of hemodynamic parameters reveals decreased cardiac output and cardiac index.

Table 11–10

Clinical Manifestations of Anaphylactic Shock

Body System	Manifestations
Cardiovascular	Hypotension
	Tachycardia
Cutaneous	Angioedema
	Erythema
	Pruritus
	Urticaria
Gastrointestinal	Diarrhea
	Nausea
	Vomiting
Neurologic	Apprehension
	Anxiety
	Decreased level of consciousness
	Feeling of impending doom
	Restlessness
Respiratory	Dysphagia
	Hoarseness
	Crackles
	Stridor
	Wheezes

CLINICAL ? THINKING

FLUSHING AND APPREHENSION AFTER CARDIAC CATHETERIZATION

A 58-year-old male patient admitted with unstable angina pectoris was wheeled back to the medical unit following cardiac catheterization with angiography. He was alert and oriented, with a regular heart rate of 82 bpm, respiratory rate of 18 per minute, blood pressure of 128/72, and temperature of 37°C (98.6°F). His skin was warm and dry, his color was good, his peripheral pulses were readily palpable, and his pressure dressing on the left groin was dry and intact. I instructed him to lie flat, keep his affected leg straight, minimize movement, and summon me with the call bell if he needed me.

Fifteen minutes later I returned to check the patient and noted that he was flushed, his skin was warmer than it had been, and he appeared apprehensive. He said he had a feeling that something was wrong and complained of feeling lightheaded and weak. He was moderately short of breath, said that he felt a "tightness" in his chest, and was starting to cough.

I immediately thought of all the possible life-threatening complications posed by cardiac catheterization, such as acute myocardial infarction, perforation, pulmonary embolism, cardiac tamponade, bleeding and hemorrhage, and anaphylaxis. With the exception of his flushed warm skin, the clinical picture he presented thus far could have indicated any of these conditions. Needing more information on which to base my clinical decisions and actions, I conducted a focused assessment.

The patient remained alert but I detected an increasing restlessness. His radial pulse was now up to 124 bpm and thready, respirations were 26 per minute and labored, and his blood pressure had fallen to 104/60. There was no evidence of bleeding or hematoma formation at the catheter insertion site, and no evidence of dysrhythmia. Auscultation of breath sounds revealed bilateral wheezing, and I noted a prolonged expiration.

The patient suddenly said the tightness in his chest had spread to his throat and that he was feeling "warm all over." Despite the patient's denial of allergic reactions to drugs, foods, or other substances before the procedure, this clinical presentation led me to eliminate the other potential complications and to suspect that the patient was experiencing an anaphylactic reaction to the contrast medium used in the cardiac catheterization. I inspected his trunk and discovered hives on his chest and abdomen. The sudden onset of respiratory distress and urticaria further confirmed my suspicion.

Recognizing that anaphylaxis can quickly lead to respiratory failure, shock, and death, I immediately implemented the following actions:

1. I called for help.
2. I asked another staff member to notify the physician and bring the crash cart to the bedside.
3. I placed the patient in a semi-Fowler's position to facilitate respirations.
4. I administered oxygen and started an IV (for administering medications and volume expanders) per hospital protocol.

(continued)

Reduced preload from vasodilatation results in decreased central venous pressure and pulmonary artery wedge pressures. Arterial vasodilatation decreases afterload, which is reflected in decreased systemic vascular resistance.

Management

Medical management of anaphylactic shock consists of drugs to help reverse the effects of the biochemical mediators, fluid replacement, and airway maintenance. Epinephrine is usually the first drug given. It helps raise the patient's blood pressure by causing vasoconstriction. Epinephrine also helps stop bronchospasm by causing bronchodilatation. Diphenhydramine HCl (Benadryl), an antihistamine, is given to help stop the effects of the histamine. Steroids may be given to help reduce capillary permeability, thus helping to maintain the intravascular volume. Steroids also help stabilize the mast cells so they stop releasing biochemical mediators. Dopamine or isoproterenol may be needed to help maintain the

patient's blood pressure. Intravenous aminophylline may be required to help relieve respiratory symptoms. Intravenous fluid replacement with normal saline or Ringer's lactate is used to help maintain the patient's blood pressure. Endotracheal intubation or tracheostomy may be necessary to maintain a patent airway. The patient may require additional oxygen to help maintain normal blood gas levels.

NURSING PROCESS
Shock

Assessment

Nursing management of a patient in shock is both complex and challenging. By remaining aware of the risk for shock in applicable patients, you may be able to recognize signs and symptoms that signal the onset of shock and correct them before they can progress. Assessment must be accomplished quickly,

CLINICAL ? THINKING

(continued)

5. I provided emotional support to the patient by reassuring him and explaining what was happening to him and what was being done to help him.
6. I attached a cardiac monitor and a pulse oximeter.

The physician arrived and ordered epinephrine, aminophylline, diphenhydramine, and corticosteroids, which I administered. No further diagnostic evidence was necessary. The patient's history of cardiac catheterization, along with his clinical manifestations, were enough to establish the diagnosis.

Additional nursing actions included:

7. I continued to assess the patient's airway, lung sounds, and respiratory rate and depth.
8. I continued to monitor his cardiovascular and neurologic status and his urinary output.
9. I monitored the patient's response to the medications.
10. I documented my findings and actions.

Approximately 20 minutes after treatment was initiated, the patient's condition began to improve. Within an hour, his breathing pattern was back to 18 per minute, with no dyspnea and no adventitious sounds. His other vital signs returned to baseline. Quick thinking and prompt nursing actions prevented this patient from getting into serious trouble and saved the patient's life.

Think Critically

Why was epinephrine the drug of choice? How does epinephrine act to reverse such life-threatening conditions as bronchospasm and hypotension? Why were corticosteroids administered?

What potential adverse effects of epinephrine should the nurse monitor the patient for?

What actions should the nurse have taken or anticipated if the patient's respiratory distress was not alleviated by the interventions listed above? Would an oral airway have been sufficient? Why or why not?

How might the scenario have changed if the patient had been severely hypotensive? Was placing the patient in a semi-Fowler's position the best action? What risks had to be considered by the nurse? When would having the patient sit up be contraindicated?

What was the rationale underlying the nurse's close monitoring of the patient's urinary output?

During his recuperation, the patient said, "I'll tell doctors I'm allergic to dye from now on, but I'm so glad I have nothing else to worry about." What would be the nurse's best response?

What education topics specific to this scenario should the nurse include in the teaching plan for this patient before discharge?

---

almost simultaneously with initiation of treatment. Assessment steps include watching for changes in clinical manifestations and monitoring hemodynamic parameters and laboratory values to detect subtle changes warning of progression of the shock state. Frequent nursing assessments are required, because the patient's condition can change significantly in minutes. Concise documentation should reflect the patient's condition and response to therapeutic interventions.

Hypovolemic Shock

It is essential to identify sources of fluid loss and estimate the amount lost. Assess quickly for abnormal gastrointestinal, skin, and renal losses; third-spacing or plasma-to-interstitial fluid shifts; or hemorrhage. If possible, correct this fluid loss immediately. Also perform a quick overview assessment to identify and treat any life-threatening problems. Monitor blood pressure, heart rate, and respiratory rate and depth closely. Assess the skin for

color and temperature. Check the patient's level of consciousness. Watch the patient's hydration and perfusion status by monitoring urine output, peripheral pulses, capillary refill time, condition of the mucous membranes, and presence of pallor or cyanosis.

Cardiogenic Shock

Rapidly assess the patient's level of consciousness and cardiopulmonary status. Check for a blood pressure less than 90 mm Hg, decreased sensorium, and reduced skin temperature. Monitor the patient for chest pain, dysrhythmias, a heart rate over 100 bpm, weak and thready pulses, and diminished heart sounds. As soon as the patient is stabilized, obtain a medical history and current data needed to detect diseases or medications that could cause or aggravate the shock syndrome. Observe for dyspnea, cyanosis, crackles or wheezes, rapid and shallow breathing, and chest expansion. Evaluate blood gas values for development of metabolic acidosis and hypoxemia. Assess for signs and symptoms of elevated right ventricular filling pressure. These may include neck vein distention, positive hepatojugular reflux, and increased central venous pressure. Monitor hemodynamic status via pulmonary artery catheter for a cardiac index of less than 2.2 L/min/m², increased pulmonary artery wedge pressures, and increased systemic vascular resistance. Observe for a urinary output less than 30 mL/hr.

Distributive Shock

Assess the patient's history and the nature of any recent invasive procedures that might predispose the patient to infection. Take note of severe respiratory infections, peritonitis, meningitis, recent spinal cord injury, endocrine disorders, or severe reactions to anesthetics, drugs, diagnostic agents, vaccines, or insect bites. Suspect anaphylactic shock if the patient has cutaneous effects (pruritus, generalized erythema, urticaria, and angioedema) or difficulty breathing, especially if you find inspiratory stridor or hoarseness or if the patient reports a sensation of fullness or a lump in the throat or dysphagia. Tachypnea is present in all early stages of distributive shock. As the shock state continues, however, and respiratory muscles tire, the respiratory rate will decline. Other assessment findings may include vomiting, diarrhea, cramping, abdominal pain, urinary incontinence, and vaginal bleeding. Assess for severe hypotension, but remember that pulse pressure is widened in the hyperdynamic stage of septic shock, and narrowed in the later stages of septic, neurogenic, and anaphylactic shock. Assess the patient's heart rate for tachycardia (bradycardia is a common finding in neurogenic shock). Examine the skin. In neurogenic shock, the skin may be warm and dry from pooling of blood in the extremities and loss of vasomotor control in surface vessels that normally control heat loss. Warm, flushed skin may also occur in the hyperdynamic stage of septic shock. However, as shock progresses, the skin will become pale, cool, and clammy.

Because changes in level of consciousness represent decreased cerebral perfusion, assess frequently for such changes. Assessment of hemodynamic parameters in anaphylactic and neurogenic shock reveals

- Decreased cardiac output and cardiac index
- Decreased central venous pressure and pulmonary capillary wedge pressures (from venous vasodilatation)
- Decreased systemic vascular resistance (from arterial vasodilatation)

Changes in hemodynamic parameters in the hyperdynamic phase of septic shock include increased cardiac output and cardiac index, decreased central venous pressure and pulmonary capillary wedge pressures, and decreased systemic vascular resistance. As the shock state progresses to the hypodynamic phase, cardiac output and cardiac index fall, central venous pressure and capillary wedge pressures increase, and systemic vascular pressures increase.

Nursing Diagnoses and Planning

Nursing diagnoses and related expected patient outcomes commonly applicable to patients in shock include the following:

NDx: Decreased cardiac output related to fluid volume deficit; changes in myocardial contractility, preload, and afterload; inadequate distribution of blood volume; or loss of systemic vasomotor tone

Planning: Patient Outcomes
1. The patient will demonstrate signs of hemodynamic stability as evidenced by:
   Heart rate <100 bpm
   Systolic blood pressure >110 mm Hg or within 10 mm Hg of baseline
   Cardiac output 4–8 L/min and cardiac index >2 L/min/m²
   Central venous pressure 0–8 mm Hg
   Pulmonary capillary wedge pressure 8–12 mm Hg
   Systemic vascular resistance 800–1400 dynes/sec/cm⁻⁵
   Warm extremities with capillary refill time <3 seconds
   Absence of dysrhythmias or presence of a hemodynamically stable dysrhythmia
   Normal sensorium

NDx: Fluid volume deficit or excess related to hemorrhage or fluid shifts associated with loss of plasma proteins (hypovolemic shock); increased levels of aldosterone and antidiuretic hormone secondary to reduced renal perfusion, and sodium retention (cardiogenic shock); distributional volume loss with fluid shifts to the interstitial space (distributive shock)

Planning: Patient Outcomes
1. The patient will:
   Maintain normal circulating blood volume and stable hemodynamic variables as listed above
   Maintain body weight within 5% of baseline
   Balance fluid intake and output
   Maintain urine output >30 mL/hr
   Maintain fluid and electrolyte balance as demonstrated by laboratory data within normal limits (electrolytes, hematocrit, hemoglobin, BUN and serum creatinine)
   Maintain normal body temperature
   Demonstrate adequate peripheral tissue perfusion (skin warm and dry; absence of cyanosis)

NDx: Altered tissue perfusion related to severely impaired myocardial contractility, reduced circulating blood volume, or fluid volume deficit

Planning: Patient Outcomes
1. The patient will:
   Demonstrate signs of hemodynamic stability as listed above
   Maintain adequate tissue perfusion

Be alert and oriented to person, time, and place
Demonstrate adequate peripheral tissue perfusion
   (skin warm and dry; absence of cyanosis)
Maintain urine output >30 mL/h
Have no dysrhythmias
Maintain arterial blood gases within normal
   limits

NDx: Impaired gas exchange related to reduced pulmonary perfusion (ventilation/perfusion mismatch) and changes in alveolar capillary membrane

Planning: Patient Outcomes

1. The patient will:
   Demonstrate signs of adequate cerebral oxygenation
   Be alert and oriented to person, time, and place
   Maintain optimal arterial blood gas values as
      listed below:
         pH 7.35–7.45
         PaO_2 >60 mm Hg
         $PaCO_2$ 35–45 mm Hg
         SaO_2 >90%
   Have breath sounds clear to auscultation

Nursing Interventions and Evaluation

NDx: Decreased cardiac output
Promptly assess cardiovascular function to determine the severity of the shock state and the efficacy of therapeutic interventions. Assess for signs and symptoms of progressive ventricular failure, including changes in cardiac output, cardiac index, heart rate, and blood pressure; development of third and fourth heart sounds, central or peripheral cyanosis, and dysrhythmias; and changes in sensorium, capillary refill time, and urinary output. Assess for signs and symptoms of hypoxemia and acidosis by monitoring arterial blood gas analysis.

Monitor respiratory status for development of crackles, bronchial wheezing, and dyspnea. Implement prescribed pharmacologic agents or standard protocols to improve myocardial contractility, increase preload, and decrease afterload or to reverse systemic vasoconstriction. If necessary, prepare the patient for insertion of an intra-aortic balloon pump or left ventricular device.

NDx: Fluid volume deficit or excess
Monitor fluid balance. Note urinary output, nasogastric drainage, or other measurable output loss. Assess for alterations in skin turgor and capillary refill time. Establish one or more large-gauge intravenous access sites for fluid and drug administration. For fluid volume deficits, administer prescribed fluid volume. Calculate and monitor fluid replacement as a cumulative and ongoing process. Monitor hemodynamic parameters for response to fluid, including arterial blood pressure, central venous pressure, pulmonary artery wedge pressure, and cardiac output and cardiac index. Assess for jugular venous distention. Closely monitor and document the patient's intake and output and urine specific gravity.

Closely monitor daily weights and serum electrolytes. Elevate the head of the bed 20 to 30 degrees.

Patients in cardiogenic shock should be weighed daily to monitor for gain or loss, establish a baseline for treatment, and evaluate diuretic therapy. Monitor for side effects of diuretic therapy (hypokalemia, hyponatremia, fatigue, muscle cramps, hypotension, tachycardia). Maintain accurate records of intake and output and urine specific gravity. Monitor fluid administration closely to prevent fluid volume overload. To help reduce cardiac workload, place the patient in a semi-Fowler's position (if blood pressure remains stable), and administer oxygen as needed.

In addition to the previously mentioned interventions, in patients experiencing anaphylactic shock, anticipate giving repeated doses of epinephrine, either subcutaneously or instilled directly into the endotracheal tube. This is usually followed by intravenous administration of epinephrine if no clinical improvement occurs.

Attempt to control the body temperature of any patient in septic shock. Monitor temperature every 2 hours while the patient is febrile, give antipyretic drugs as ordered, and apply hypothermia/hyperthermia blankets as prescribed to maintain a normothermic core temperature.

NDx: Altered tissue perfusion
In addition to assessments already discussed for decreased cardiac output, insertion of a Foley catheter may be necessary to monitor cardiovascular, neurologic, and renal function on an hourly basis. Notify the physician if urinary output falls below 30 mL/hr. Insert a nasogastric tube as ordered to decompress the stomach and prevent aspiration. Monitor oxygenation status and ventilator settings. Frequently auscultate the patient's lung sounds and record the rate, depth, and character of respirations. Administer oxygen as needed. Check neurologic status for changes in level of consciousness, restlessness, agitation, confusion, and somnolence. In cardiogenic shock, anticipate the use of mechanical circulatory assistance if therapeutic measures fail to restore tissue perfusion.

NDx: Impaired gas exchange
Perform an ongoing mental status assessment, noting confusion, restlessness, anxiety, stupor, and loss of consciousness. Monitor respiratory function, including rate and rhythm, and assess for presence of dyspnea, respiratory fatigue, cyanosis, and pallor. Auscultate lungs for adventitious sounds. Position the patient to facilitate lung expansion (30- to 40-degree supine head elevation or, if the patient is intubated, lateral recumbent position). Reposition hourly as tolerated to prevent atelectasis and areas of poor ventilation. Monitor arterial blood gases. Assist in initiating and maintaining oxygenation therapies, from nasal oxygen to endotracheal intubation. Implement strategies according to the physician's prescriptions or standing protocols to maintain adequate gas exchange.

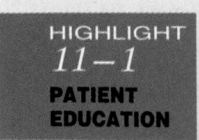 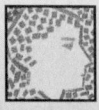

HIGHLIGHT
11-1
PATIENT EDUCATION   **Prevention of Anaphylaxis**

Explain to the patient:

What the precipitating factor was.

What happens in the body when exposure to the precipitating antigen occurs.

Identify with the patient:

Related substances that may cause a similar reaction.

Ways to avoid the antigen and related substances in the future.

Instruct the patient to:

Inform all health-care providers of the problem.

Carry or wear a MedicAlert tag or other identification that indicates the causative antigen and the response.

If the anaphylactic reaction was precipitated by a bee sting or other known allergen, also instruct the patient to keep an emergency kit containing Adrenalin available at all times and teach the patient or family how to administer the medication.

Additional Interventions

Once an anaphylactic patient is stable and out of danger, provide information on how to prevent further episodes (Highlight 11–1).

Compare the patient's status with the expected outcomes. If the outcomes are not met, reassess the patient and revise the plan.

The Elderly: Special Considerations

Older adults are more susceptible to shock because they have less physiologic reserve. Older adults with compromised renal, hepatic, respiratory, or cardiovascular function are even more at risk for shock because these disease-related conditions further diminish their ability to respond to physiologic stress. Because the progression of shock depends partly on the physiologic state before the initial incident, any condition that compromises physiologic function is likely to accelerate the progression of shock.

The earliest sign of shock in older adults may be a change in mental status. This is because age-related changes increase the sensitivity of brain tissue to physiologic imbalances. If the older adult already has impaired mental functioning, it may be more difficult to assess the mental changes and identify shock as a contributing factor. Thus, it is imperative to carefully assess any mental changes

and look for additional clues that might suggest the onset of shock.

During the treatment phase of shock, it is important to recognize that older adults are more sensitive to therapeutic and adverse medication effects. They may require lower doses and a longer duration between doses of medication. An important nursing responsibility is to assess the response of older adults to medications and to work with physicians so proper doses are administered. Keep in mind that mental changes may also be an early sign of adverse medication effects. If the older adult receives behavior-modifying medications (such as antianxiety agents) during the acute phase, it is important to reassess the need for these medications and discontinue them as soon as possible, because these medications are likely to interfere with functioning in an older person.

Recovery from shock may be prolonged in older adults because of their compromised ability to respond to physiologic stress. It is important to prevent complications that might be related to prolonged bedrest, such as pressure ulcers and impaired mobility. Physical therapy services might be helpful in assisting older adults regain strength, mobility, and independence as they recover from shock.

Chapter Review

1. How can the effectiveness of fluid resuscitation be assessed in a patient with hypovolemic shock?

2. Why is hemodynamic monitoring an important aspect of planning care for a patient in shock?

3. What is the meaning of pulmonary capillary wedge pressures >18 mm Hg in the patient in cardiogenic shock?

4. How can tissue perfusion best be assessed in a patient with shock?

5. What early signs and symptoms should be monitored for in patients at high risk for distributive shock?

6. How does the patient's physiologic state before the incident occurs that causes shock affect progression of the shock state?

7. What changes might be seen in blood gas studies in patients experiencing shock?

8. Why are vasoconstrictor medications useful in most types of shock?

9. Why might vasodilator medications be ordered for a patient in shock?

10. What nursing interventions are appropriate for patients experiencing a fluid volume deficit, common to most types of shock?

Bibliography

Astiz ME, Rackow EC. Assessing perfusion failure during circulatory shock. Crit Care Clin 1993; 9:299.

Astiz ME, Rackow, EC, Weil MH. Pathophysiology and treatment of circulatory shock. Crit Care Clin 1993; 9:183.

Berro EA, Bechler-Karsch A. A closer look at septic shock. Pediatr Nurs 1993; 19(3):289.

Blansfield J. Emergency autotransfusion in hypovolemia. Crit Care Nurs Clin North Am 1990; 2:167.

Brown KK. Septic shock: How to stop the deadly cascade. Part 1. Am J Nurs 1994; 94(9):20.

Brown KK. Critical interventions in septic shock. Part 2. Am J Nurs 1994; 94(10):20.

Burns KM. Vasoactive drug therapy in shock. Crit Care Nurs Clin North Am 1990; 2(2):167.

Coombs M. Haemodynamic profiles and the critical care nurse. Intensive Crit Care Nurse 1993; 9 (1):11.

Dahlen R, Robers SL. Nursing management of congestive heart failure. Part I. Intensive Crit Care Nurs 1995; 11(5):272.

Daleiden A. Physiology and treatment of hemorrhagic shock during the early postoperative period. Crit Care Nurs Q 1993; 16(1):45.

Epstein CD, Henning RJ. Oxygen transport variables in the identification and treatment of tissue hypoxia. Heart Lung 1993; 22:328.

Flavell CM. Combating hemorrhagic shock. RN 1994; 57(12):26.

Gates DM. Cardiac dysfunction in septic shock and multiple organ dysfunction syndrome. Crit Care Nurs Q 1994; 16(4):39.

Gorney DA. Arterial blood pressure measurement technique. AACN Clin Issues Crit Care Nurs 1993; 4(1):66.

Houston MC. Pathophysiology of shock. Crit Care Nurs Clin North Am 1990; 2(2):143.

Imm A, Carlson RW. Clinical trials of the pneumatic antishock garment in the urban prehospital setting. Ann Emerg Med 1993; 15:1410.

Keithley JK, Eisenberg P. The significance of enteral nutrition in the intensive care unit patient. Crit Care Nurs Clin North Am 1993; 5(1):23.

Laskowski-Jones L. Acute SCI: How to minimize the damage. Am J Nurs 1994; 93:23.

McCormac M. Managing hemorrhagic shock. Am J Nurs 1990; 90(2):22.

Misasi RS, Keyes JL. The pathophysiology of hypoxia. Crit Care Nurse 1994; 14(4):55.

Mohrman DE, Heller LJ. Cardiovascular physiology. New York: McGraw-Hill, 1991.

Moroney DA, Reedy JE. Understanding ventricular assist devices: A self-study guide. J Cardiovasc Nurs 1994; 8(2):1.

Nolan S. Current trends in the management of acute spinal cord injury. Crit Care Nurs Q 1994; 17(1):64.

Norris SO. Managing low cardiac output states: Maintaining volume after cardiac surgery. AACN Clin Issues Crit Care Nurs 1993; 4(2):309.

O'Neal PV. How to spot early signs of cardiogenic shock. Am J Nurs 1994; 94(5):36.

Ostrow CL, Hupp E, Topjian D. The effect of Trendelenburg and modified Trendelenburg positions on cardiac output, blood pressure, and oxygenation: A preliminary study. Am J Crit Care 1994; 3(5):382.

Phillips MC, Olson LR: The immunologic role of the gastrointestinal tract. Crit Care Nursing Clin North Am 1993; 5(1):107.

Rice V. Shock, a clinical syndrome: An update. II. The stages of shock. Crit Care Nurse 1991; 11(5):74.

Rice V. Shock, a clinical syndrome: An update. III. Therapeutic management. Crit Care Nurse 1991; 11(6):34.

Rice V. Shock, a clinical syndrome: An update. IV. Nursing care of the shock patient. Crit Care Nurse 1991; 11(7):28.

Ruppert SD, Kernicki JG, Dolan JT. Dolan's critical care cursing: Clinical management through the nursing process. 2nd ed. Philadelphia: FA Davis, 1996.

Schott KE. Intra-aortic balloon counterpulsation as a therapy for shock. Crit Care Nurs Clin North Am 1990; 2(2):187.

Shinn AE, Joseph D. Concepts of intraaortic balloon counterpulsation. J Cardiovasc 1994; 8(2):45.

Shoemaker WC. Monitoring and management of acute circulatory problems: The expanded role of the physiologically oriented critical care nurse. Am J Crit Care 1992; 1(1):38.

Shoemaker WC. Pathophysiology, monitoring, and therapy of acute circulatory problems. Crit Care Nurs Clin North Am 1994; 6(2):295.

Thelan LA, Davie JK, Urden LD, Lough ME (eds). Critical care nursing: Diagnosis and management. 2nd ed. St. Louis: Mosby-Year Book, 1994.

Verder A, Gallagher KJ, Severino R. The effect of nursing interventions of trancutaneous oxygen and carbon dioxide tensions. West J Nurs Res 1995; 17(1):76.

Vinsant GO, Fallon WF. General principles in the management of hemorrhagic shock: Lessons learned in the early care of the trauma patient. Trauma Q 1992; 8(4):28.

Von Rueden KT, Dunham CM. Sequelae of massive fluid resuscitation in trauma patients. Crit Care Nurs Clin North Am 1994; 6(3):463.

Yu M, Levy MM, Smith P, et al. Effect of maximizing oxygen delivery on morbidity and mortality rates in critically ill patients: A prospective, randomized, controlled study. Crit Care Med 1993; 21:830.

Unit III

Hematologic Dysfunction

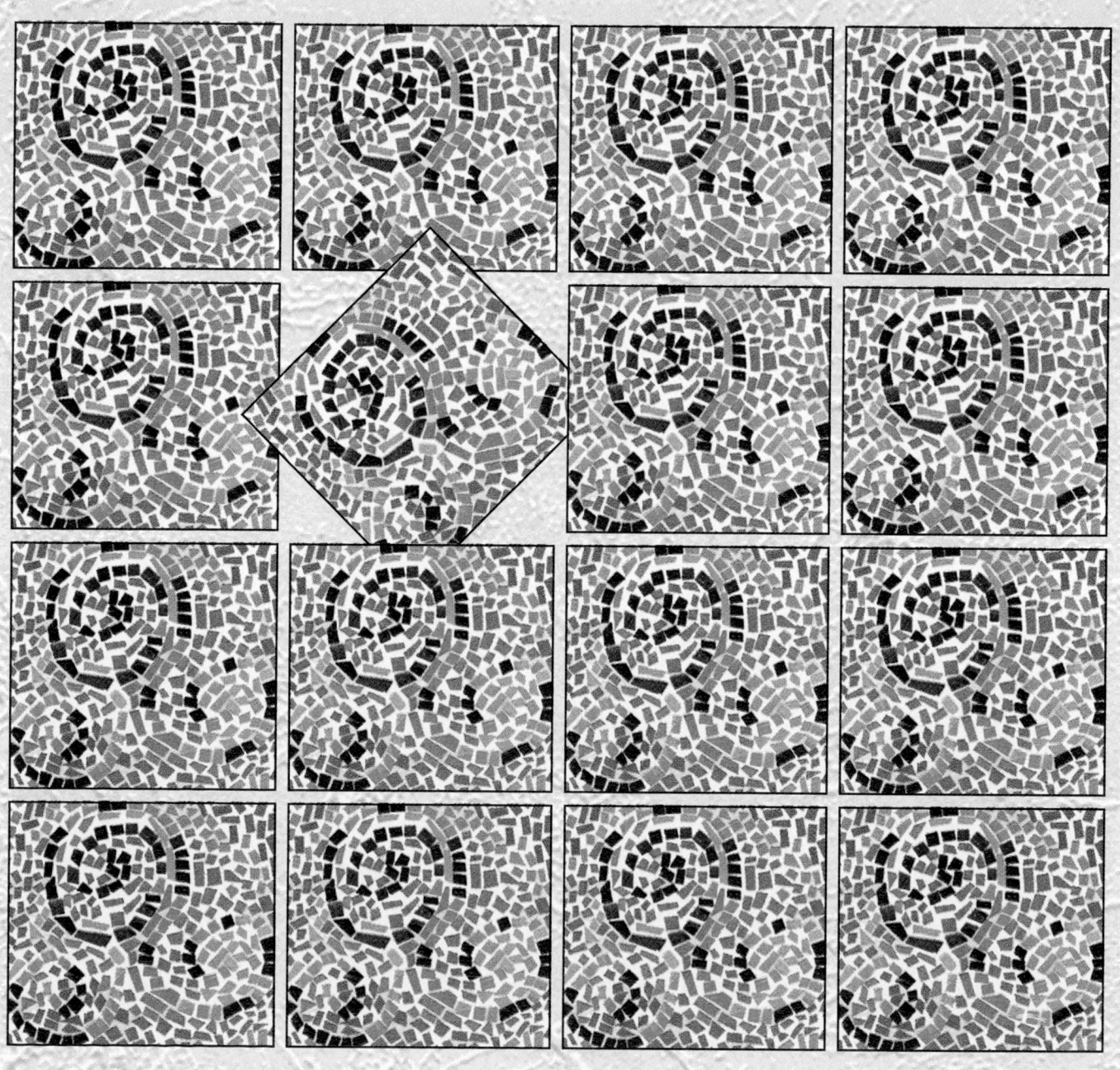

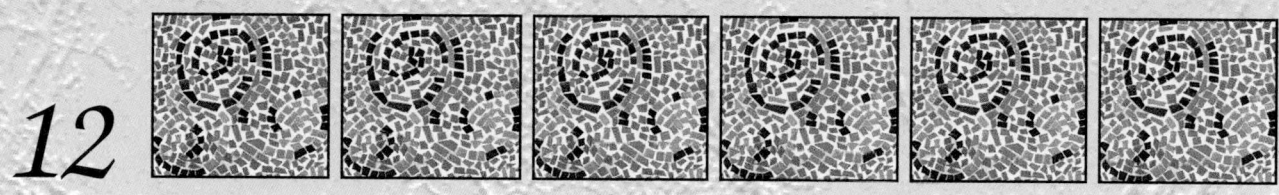

12

Knowledge Base for Patients with Hematologic Dysfunction

Study Outcomes

After studying this chapter, you should be able to:

1. Explain the normal anatomy and physiology of the blood and blood-forming organs.
2. Describe common clinical manifestations of hematologic dysfunction.
3. Describe the common laboratory tests used to confirm diagnoses of hematologic dysfunction.
4. Describe medical management and surgical procedures commonly used in the treatment of patients with hematologic disorders.
5. Identify disorders of the blood and blood-forming organs that have a genetic base.
6. Compare and contrast the use of blood and blood products for specific hematologic dysfunction.
7. Identify data essential to the assessment of patients undergoing treatment of hematologic disorders.
8. State nursing diagnoses and related expected patient outcomes commonly applicable to patients undergoing treatment of hematologic disorders.
9. Describe nursing interventions, with their rationales, commonly applicable to patients undergoing treatment of hematologic disorders.
10. Explain the basis for evaluation of nursing care provided to patients undergoing treatment of hematologic disorders.
11. Identify special considerations for the elderly patient with hematologic dysfunction.
12. Identify alternative treatment and care settings for patients with hematologic dysfunction and services related to community-based care.

The hematologic system is composed of the blood and blood-forming organs, which include the lymph nodes, bone marrow, the spleen, and the liver. This body system is responsible for producing healthy blood cells that are able to deliver nutrients and remove metabolic waste products from cells throughout the body. Naturally, disorders that affect the blood and blood-forming organs have the potential to cause serious and widespread problems. Diseases, dietary deficiencies, and drugs toxic to the hematologic system may also affect the respiratory, circulatory, integumentary, digestive, neurologic, and urinary systems.

Many of the laboratory tests and medical interventions needed by patients with hematologic dysfunction take place in outpatient settings. Such treatments as infusions of blood and coagulation factor concentrates may be administered in clinics, outpatient treatment areas of the hospital, or even, at times, in the patient's home.

Anatomy and Physiology

BLOOD

Blood transports oxygen to the cells and carries carbon dioxide from the cells to the lungs for removal from the body. It carries nutrients from the gastrointestinal tract to the tissues and removes waste products from the tissues and transports them to the lungs, kidneys, liver, and skin for excretion. Blood also transports hormones from the endocrine glands to various parts of the body and protects the body from harmful microorganisms by transporting leukocytes and antibodies to the sites of infection, injury, or inflammation. Finally, blood helps to regulate body temperature by transferring heat from deep within the body to small vessels near the skin. Here heat can be readily released into the environment.

Major characteristics of blood include:

- *Color.* Arterial blood is bright red from the effect of oxygen carried on hemoglobin (called *oxyhemoglobin*) in the red blood cells. Venous blood is dark red because oxygen has been lost from the hemoglobin (called *reduced hemoglobin*).
- *Volume.* An adult has about 70 to 75 mL of blood per kilogram of body weight, which makes for a total blood volume of about 5 to 6 L.

- *Viscosity.* Blood is three to four times more dense than water.
- *Reaction.* Blood has a slightly salty taste and an alkaline reaction, with a pH of 7.35 to 7.45.

Blood Components

Blood is composed of about 55% plasma and 45% formed elements, as shown in Figure 12–1. Plasma is a straw-colored fluid that contains mainly water, along with proteins and other substances. Formed elements include cellular suspended particles (erythrocytes and leukocytes) and non-nucleated cell fragments (platelets). Figure 12–2 shows the types of blood cells.

The process by which blood cells are formed is known as hematopoiesis. Blood cells develop from a common stem cell—an undifferentiated mesenchymal cell called a hemocytoblast—and go through many stages of maturation. Figure 12–3 depicts the development of a blood cell. Early in intrauterine life, blood cells are produced primarily by the liver. By the fifth month, the spleen becomes the dominant producer. By birth, however, both organs have stopped producing blood cells. This is because bone marrow begins to produce blood cells during the

fifth gestational month and continues in this role throughout life. The bone marrow produces blood cells in every bone at birth. With aging, blood cell production occurs only in flat bones. The inactive bone marrow becomes fatty tissue. As a result, the active areas of blood-cell production in the adult include the skull, ribs, sternum, vertebrae, humerus, femur, and pelvis. In the older adult, fatty areas increase in the bones, which reduces blood-cell production significantly.

PLASMA

Plasma, the liquid portion of blood, is straw colored and composed of 92% water, 7% proteins, and less than 1% other nutrients. Plasma proteins consist largely of albumin, globulin, fibrinogen, and prothrombin. Albumin, which is produced in the liver, regulates plasma volume and functions as a transport protein. Globulins consist of alpha, beta, and gamma fractions. The alpha and beta fractions include the transport globulins and clotting factors made in the liver. The gamma globulins, which consist largely of antibodies, are also known as immunoglobulins. These proteins, produced by the lymphocytes and plasma cells, are essential in the

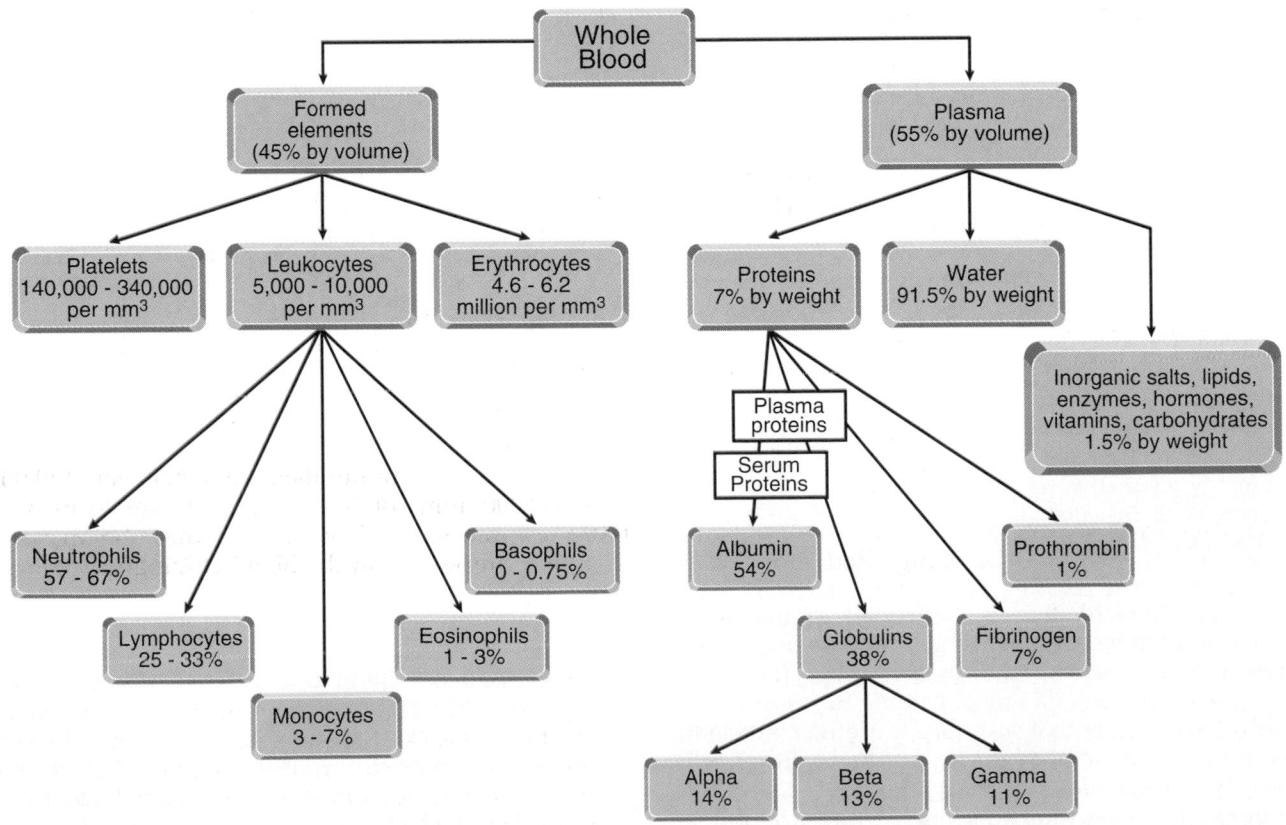

Figure 12–1

Composition of blood.

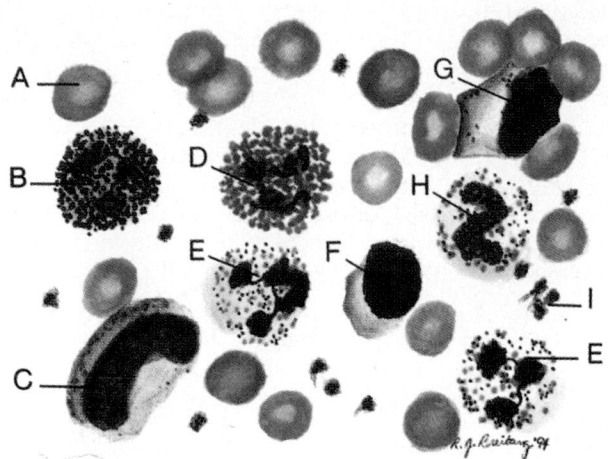

Figure 12–2

Human blood cells. *A,* Erythrocyte (red blood cell); *B,* basophil; *C,* monocyte; *D,* eosinophil; *E,* polymorphonuclear neutrophil; *F,* lymphocyte; *G,* large lymphocyte; *H,* band neutrophil; *I,* thrombocyte. (From Rodak BF. Diagnostic hematology. Philadelphia: WB Saunders, 1995.)

body's defense against microorganisms. Other plasma proteins produced in the liver include fibrinogen and prothrombin, which are essential for blood coagulation.

Serum differs from plasma in that the clotting factors have been removed. If plasma is clotted, the fibrinogen separates from the plasma and the remaining fluid is the serum.

FORMED ELEMENTS

The particles that travel suspended in the plasma are called the formed elements. These include red blood cells (erythrocytes), white blood cells (leukocytes), and platelets (thrombocytes).

Red Blood Cells

Red blood cells, or erythrocytes, transport oxygen from the lungs to the tissues. They are formed in the red marrow of bone by a process called erythropoiesis. Before reaching maturity, each red blood cell extrudes its nucleus, leaving a biconcave disk with a pliable membrane. This pliable membrane allows the cell to alter its shape so it can squeeze through the microcirculation without breaking. Red blood cells typically measure about 7 μ in diameter, but their size increases as blood pH decreases. Since venous blood has a lower pH than arterial blood, red blood cells are larger in venous blood than they are in arterial blood.

The life span of a red blood cell is about 120 days. Red blood cell production increases when oxygen to the tissues decreases. Likewise, red blood cell production decreases when oxygen concentration to tissues increases.

Hemoglobin, a part of the red blood cell, is im-

portant in transporting oxygen to the tissues. Hemoglobin is formed with the red blood cells in the red marrow of bone. It contains both iron and a globin fraction.

As red blood cells age, their membranes become more fragile. They are broken down and engulfed by macrophages in the liver, spleen, and tissues. Two to 10 million of them are destroyed and replaced each second, leaving the total count constant in the healthy person. When the red blood cells are broken down, hemoglobin is released. This is further broken down to bilirubin and iron. Bilirubin is excreted by the liver with bile, and the iron is used for continued production of red blood cells.

White Blood Cells   5 -10,000 normal

White blood cells, or leukocytes, help protect the body against invading microorganisms. Leukocytes can be differentiated from erythrocytes by the presence of a nucleus, their larger size, and different staining properties. The white blood cell count can rise as high as 500,000/mm³ in people with diseases like leukemia. *Leukocytosis* is the term used to describe a white blood cell count higher than 10,000/mm³, which usually indicates infection. *Leukopenia* is the term used to describe a white blood cell count below 5000/mm³, which occurs in people with certain viral disorders and as a reaction to certain drugs.

White blood cells are composed of 60% granulocytes and 40% mononuclear cells. Granulocytes have granular cytoplasm. They mature in the bone marrow and are then released into the blood stream. Their function is phagocytosis. Agranulocytes do not have granular cytoplasm. They are released into the blood stream earlier in their maturation. Their function is to recognize antigens and initiate the immune response. The granulocytes, also called polymorphonuclear cells, are formed in the bone marrow and are divided into three types: neutrophils, eosinophils, and basophils. Mononuclear cells are 30% lymphocytes and 5% monocytes. Lymphocytes are formed in the lymph nodes and the spleen. Monocytes are formed in bone marrow.

Platelets

Platelets (thrombocytes) are small particles in the blood plasma. Their numbers vary between 150,000 and 500,000/mm³ of blood. Platelets are formed in red bone marrow. They provide thrombokinase, a substance important in the blood-clotting process.

Blood Coagulation

Blood coagulation involves a process of platelet agglutination, blood vessel contraction, and blood components meshing to form a fibrin clot. Fibrin is formed from proteins in the plasma. The mechanisms of fibrin clot formation are depicted schematically in Figure 12–4.

Coagulation occurs when the blood vessels are injured or when blood leaves a vessel either by in-

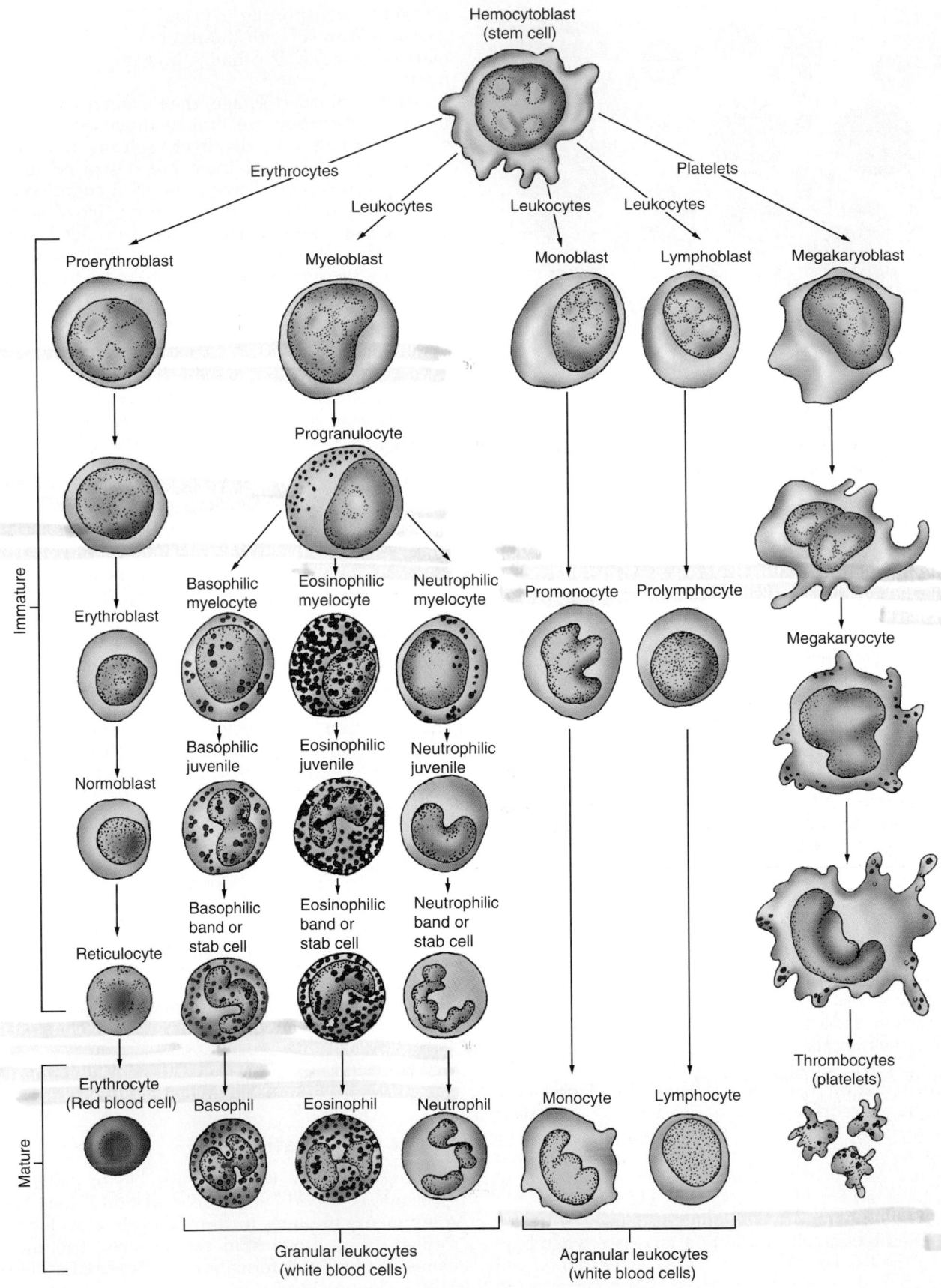

Figure 12–3

The development of blood cells.

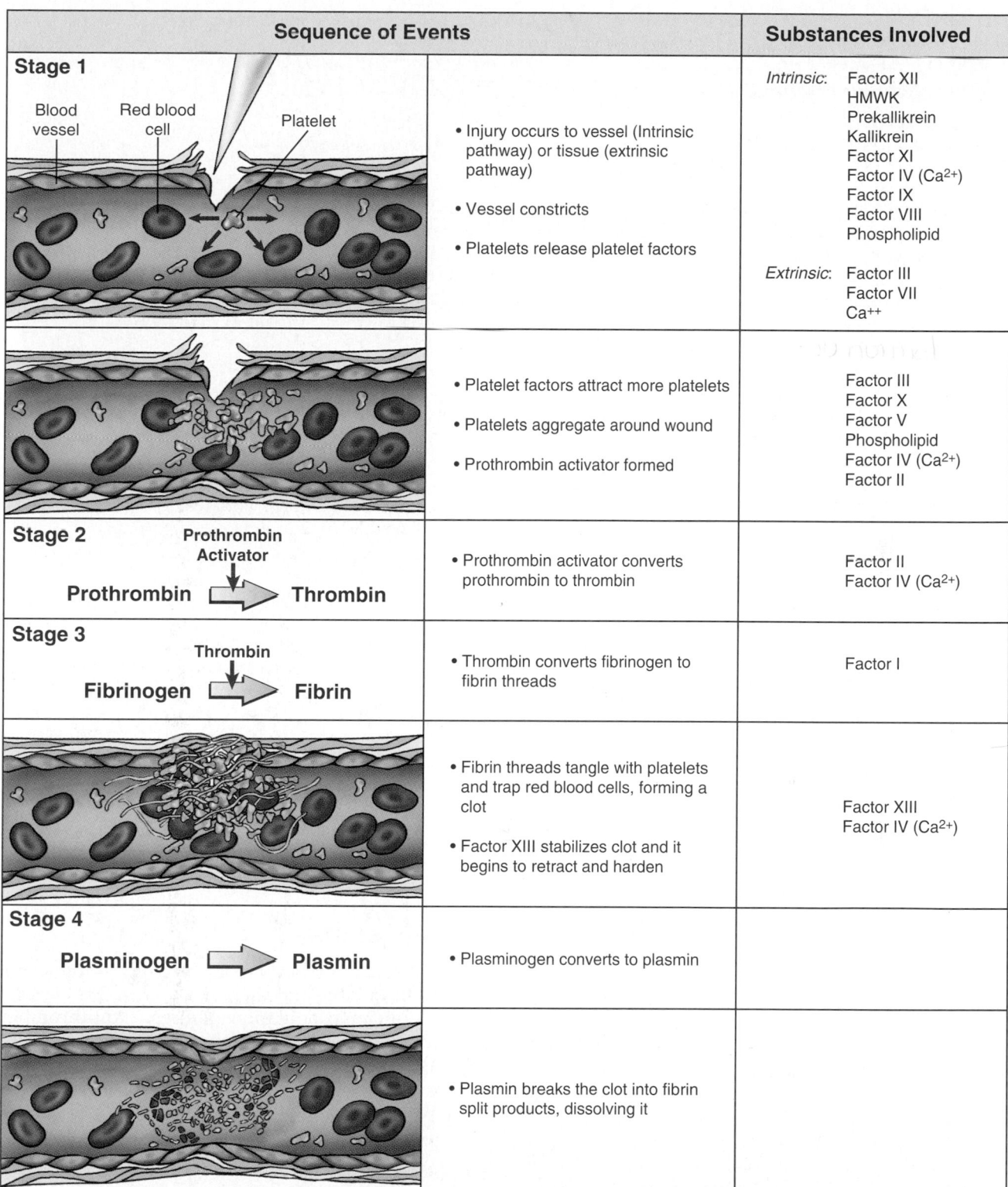

Sequence of Events		Substances Involved
Stage 1	• Injury occurs to vessel (Intrinsic pathway) or tissue (extrinsic pathway) • Vessel constricts • Platelets release platelet factors	*Intrinsic:* Factor XII HMWK Prekallikrein Kallikrein Factor XI Factor IV (Ca^{2+}) Factor IX Factor VIII Phospholipid *Extrinsic:* Factor III Factor VII Ca^{++}
	• Platelet factors attract more platelets • Platelets aggregate around wound • Prothrombin activator formed	Factor III Factor X Factor V Phospholipid Factor IV (Ca^{2+}) Factor II
Stage 2 **Prothrombin** → **Thrombin** (Prothrombin Activator)	• Prothrombin activator converts prothrombin to thrombin	Factor II Factor IV (Ca^{2+})
Stage 3 **Fibrinogen** → **Fibrin** (Thrombin)	• Thrombin converts fibrinogen to fibrin threads	Factor I
	• Fibrin threads tangle with platelets and trap red blood cells, forming a clot • Factor XIII stabilizes clot and it begins to retract and harden	Factor XIII Factor IV (Ca^{2+})
Stage 4 **Plasminogen** → **Plasmin**	• Plasminogen converts to plasmin	
	• Plasmin breaks the clot into fibrin split products, dissolving it	

Figure 12–4

The blood clotting process. This diagram represents the factors necessary to change blood into a solid clot and then dissolve it. The entire chain of reactions occurs at the site of injury.

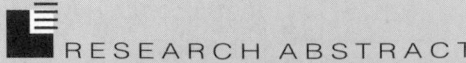

RESEARCH ABSTRACT

Does Aspirin Prevent Thrombotic Events in People With High Cholesterol?

Szczeklik A, Musial J, Undas A, et al. Inhibition of thrombin generation is blunted in hypercholesterolemia. Arterioscler Thromb Vasc Biol 1996;16(8):948.

Aspirin has been used for quite some time to inhibit thrombin generation, thereby preventing or reducing the incidence of thrombotic events. However, nurses have noticed that some patients who have been on long-term aspirin therapy still develop myocardial infarctions, strokes, and other thrombotic problems. Why is this? A recent study conducted by Szczeklik and colleagues may shed some light on this issue. Szczeklik and colleagues hypothesized that patients with known elevated cholesterol levels may not respond well to aspirin therapy.

The researchers therefore gathered a group of subjects and divided them into two subgroups. The first subgroup had cholesterol levels at 240 mg/dL or below. The second subgroup had values above this level.

Measurements were taken in both groups at two intervals: after a single 500 mg dose of aspirin and after 2 weeks of aspirin at a dose of 300 mg/day. The results were interesting. The research team found that in the subgroup with the lower cholesterol levels, "aspirin markedly prolonged the time at which thrombin reached its peak clotting activity" after only a single dose. After 2 weeks of aspirin therapy, "aspirin markedly depressed thrombin generation."

The findings for the subgroup with the elevated levels showed that after a single dose there was no change in clotting time. After 2 weeks of aspirin therapy in this subgroup, no changes were found in the clotting parameters measured.

The results show that in people with lower cholesterol levels, thrombin generation is depressed by aspirin ingestion. After extended aspirin therapy, the total amount of thrombin present is much lower than before.

This information has definite implications for patient care. Some patients may need higher doses of aspirin to reduce their risk of thrombotic events. Other patients may need an alternative antiplatelet drug. While the researchers did not make any specific recommendations, the use of aspirin as a therapy for patients who have known elevated levels of cholesterol may now be in question.

Questions to Consider

1. Do you think that patients should be told the results of this study? Why or why not?
2. If aspirin has a limited effect on thrombin suppression or generation, should its use be discontinued? Why? Why not?
3. Based on the results of this study, would you cease to recommend the use of aspirin as an antiplatelet agent? Why? Why not?
4. How many therapies can you list in which aspirin is prescribed?

tention or through injury. It involves the formation of thromboplastin, the conversion of prothrombin to thrombin, and the conversion of fibrinogen to fibrin. The clotting factors and their associated names are listed in Table 12–1. There are four progressive stages of clotting in which coagulation factors are involved. Stage I is divided into two phases. The first phase of stage I lasts 3 to 5 minutes and involves platelet activity. The second phase of stage I is the formation of thromboplastin. Moderate interference with stage I activity occurs with platelet counts of less than $1,000,000/mm^3$. Ninety percent of all coagulation disorders result from defects in stage I. Stage II, which lasts 8 to 15 seconds, involves the conversion of prothrombin (Factor II) in the presence of calcium. In stage III, which lasts 1 second, thrombin and fibrinogen interact to form a clot. At the end of this stage, Factor XIII acts to stabilize the clot. In stage IV, fibrinolysis removes the clot. Plasminogen is converted to plasmin, which breaks the clot into fibrin split products.

Anticoagulation

Coagulation in the absence of bleeding is prevented by antithrombins and heparin within the vessels. These are anticoagulation factors. Antithrombins prevent the release of thromboplastic substances unless injury is present. Heparin is produced by mast cells within the body and prevents thrombosis after normal clotting has occurred.

Blood Grouping

Blood classifications are designated by the antigen contained in red blood cells and the specific antibodies in the plasma. The major groups are ABO and Rh. Blood is typed as A, B, AB, and O. For each of these types, specific antibodies are present. Type A blood has A antigens and B antibodies. Type B blood has B antigens and A antibodies. Type AB blood has A and B antigens and no antibodies. Type O blood has no antigens and both A and B antibod-

Table 12-1

Clotting Factors and Names

Factor Number	Factor Name
I	Fibrinogen
II	Prothrombin
III	Tissue thromboplastin
IV	Calcium
V	Proaccelerin
VII	Proconvertin
VIII	Antihemophilic globulin (AHG)
	Antihemophilic factor (AHF)
IX	Plasma thromboplastin component (Christmas factor)
X	Stuart factor
XI	Plasma thromboplastin antecedent (PTA)
XII	Hageman factor
XIII	Fibrin stabilizing factor (FSF)

The factor numbers and names designate each clotting factor. The numbers indicate the order in which they were discovered.

NOTE: There is no Factor VI, because it is no longer considered to be a distinct part of coagulation.

ies. Each antigen type can be agglutinated (or clumped) by the corresponding antibody, also called the antiagglutinin. These relationships are shown in Figure 12-5.

The Rh grouping is based on 12 antigens. Of these, D is the most active antigen. Rh-positive blood refers to the presence of antigen D. Rh-negative blood does not contain antigen D.

BLOOD-FORMING ORGANS

Lymph Nodes

Lymph nodes are small, rounded bodies located along lymph vessels throughout the body. These nodes filter the passing lymph and may fight off pathogenic organisms draining from an infected part of the body. Lymph nodes produce lymphocytes and antibodies, which are added to the lymph fluid. In the adult, the only palpable lymph nodes are in the inguinal and the axillary regions. The cervical and supraclavicular nodes may be palpable during disease processes (Fig. 12-6).

Bone Marrow

Bone marrow accounts for 4 to 5% of total body weight, making it one of the body's larger organs. It is located inside spongy bones and in the central cavities of long bones. Bone marrow is either red or yellow. Active production of blood cells occurs in red marrow, the major blood-producing organ in the body. Yellow marrow does not actively produce blood elements and consists primarily of fat cells.

During childhood, most marrow is red and actively produces blood cells. With age, most of the marrow in the long bones changes into yellow marrow but retains the ability to convert back to blood-producing tissue if necessary. In the adult, red marrow is found mainly in such flat bones as the ribs, the skull, and parts of the pelvis.

Spleen

The spleen is the largest of the lymphatic organs. It is a soft, oval, highly vascular structure about 8 cm wide and 13 cm long located in the upper left quadrant of the abdominal cavity (Fig. 12-7). It weighs about 198 g. The spleen performs several functions, including:

- Protecting the body from various stressors through the purification process
- Storing large quantities of blood
- Producing lymphocytes, plasma cells, and antibodies
- Removing old or injured red blood cells and platelets
- Filtering microorganisms from the blood

Liver

The liver is the largest gland in the body and is an extremely complex organ. It is located in the upper right quadrant of the abdominal cavity. (See Chapter 25 for a thorough description of the liver and its functions.) The liver functions as a blood-forming organ only during intrauterine life. It plays a role in the coagulation process by producing prothrombin in the presence of vitamin K. The liver also forms most of the fibrinogen in circulating blood.

Clinical Manifestations of Hematologic Dysfunction

Disorders of the blood and blood-forming organs can affect any organ or tissue in the body, resulting in the diffuse clinical manifestations that characterize blood disorders. The signs and symptoms are commonly exaggerated in the very young and the aged.

FATIGUE, WEAKNESS, DYSPNEA, AND PALLOR

An insufficient blood supply, a decrease in erythrocytes, or a low hemoglobin level results in a

Recipient's Blood Group
(Plasma or serum tested)

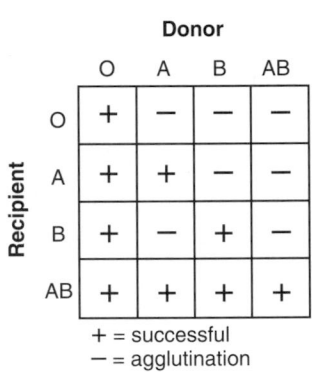

	O	A	B	AB
O	+	−	−	−
A	+	+	−	−
B	+	−	+	−
AB	+	+	+	+

+ = successful
− = agglutination

Figure 12–5

Cross-matching of blood types is necessary before blood from a donor can be administered to a recipient. If the two types are not compatible, agglutination, a serious or fatal reaction, may occur. (Redrawn from Jacob SW, Francone CA. Elements of anatomy and physiology. 2nd ed. Philadelphia: WB Saunders, 1989, p 171.)

① sided HF failure backs up to lungs

reduced oxygen-carrying capacity of the blood. Common signs and symptoms of a reduced oxygen-carrying capacity include fatigue, weakness, dyspnea, and pallor. These symptoms are usually found in patients with anemias, polycythemias, leukemias, and hemorrhagic disorders.

Fatigue may be manifested by a slow walk, drooping shoulders, and increased pulse rate. The patient may be completely exhausted and not feel like getting out of bed or bathing. Inability to perform activities of daily living may result. The patient may want to sleep continually. Weakness is manifested in the lack of strength to perform self-care or to ambulate. This can be extremely frustrating for the patient and family.

Dyspnea, with or without exertion, may arise from insufficient oxygen supply to the tissues. The skin, fingers, toes, and mucous membranes may grow pale. Cyanosis may develop. An increased respiratory rate, decreased vital capacity, and decreased respiratory reserve volume usually develop as the body seeks to make more oxygen available to the tissues. The heart rate increases and the blood vessels dilate. Venous return to the heart increases and, eventually, congestive heart failure may result.

NURSING PROCESS
Fatigue and Dyspnea

Assessment

Assess for tachycardia, tachypnea, and increased shortness of breath on exertion as indicators of the blood's decreased ability to carry oxygen. Observe the skin for pallor, which can result from decreased levels of hemoglobin. Check for cyanosis involving the lips, fingers, and toes, which indicates hypoxemia in cutaneous blood vessels. Review laboratory results.

Ask the patient about headaches, vertigo, visual disturbances, and confusion, which indicate some cerebral hypoxia. Assess the extremities for weakness, tingling, numbness, and paresthesia. Assess the patient's ability to complete activities of daily living.

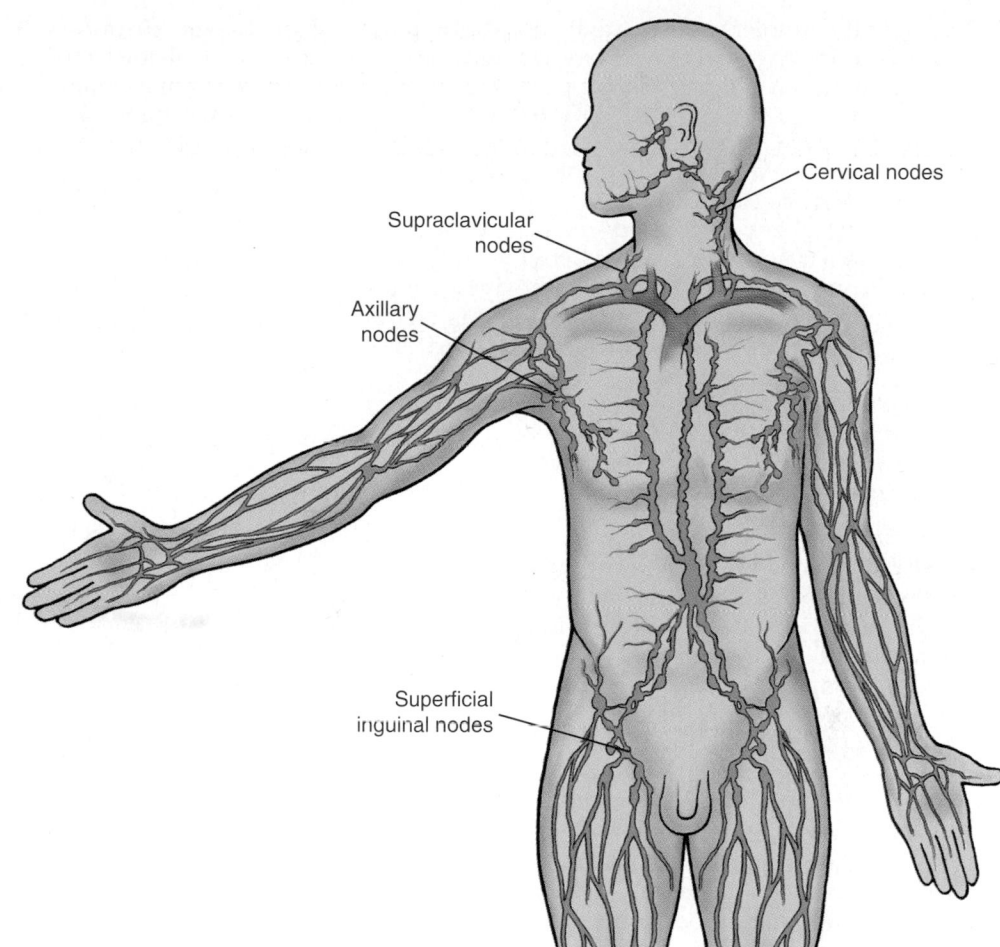

Figure 12–6
Palpable lymph nodes.

Ask whether the symptoms are intermittent or persistent. Check sleep and rest patterns. Assess self-esteem and feelings of guilt, depression, or resentment, which may occur because of the inability to take part in life's activities.

Nursing Diagnoses and Planning

Nursing diagnoses and related expected patient outcomes commonly applicable to patients with fatigue and dyspnea include the following:

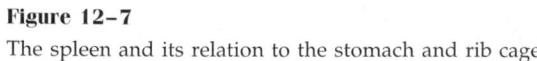

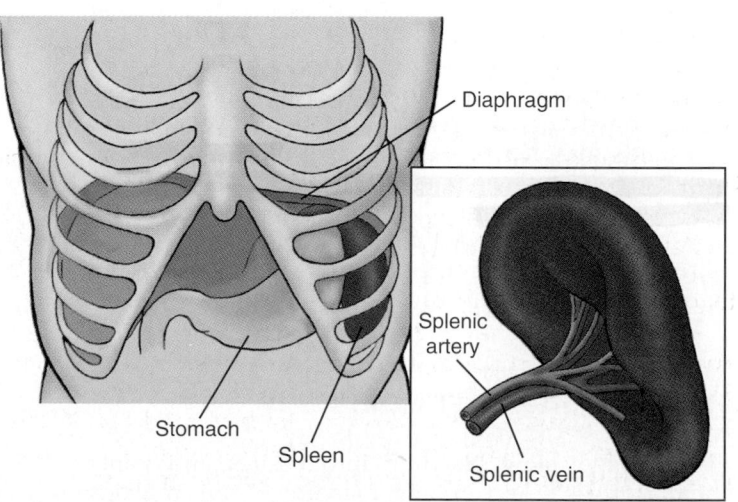

Figure 12–7
The spleen and its relation to the stomach and rib cage.

NDx: Activity intolerance related to fatigue and dyspnea secondary to decreased oxygen-carrying capacity of the blood

Planning: Patient Outcomes
1. Patient follows a regimen of planned activities and rest periods each day.
2. Patient verbalizes decreased feelings of fatigue and demonstrates an increased activity level.
3. Patient completes activities of daily living without signs of fatigue and dyspnea, such as tachycardia, tachypnea, shortness of breath, and cyanosis.
4. Patient's vital signs are within the normal ranges for the patient.

Nursing Interventions and Evaluation

NDx: Activity intolerance
Instruct the patient to develop a regimen of activity with frequent rest periods throughout the day. Encourage the patient to do range-of-motion exercises frequently while lying in bed to maintain muscle tone and strength. Note the times during the day when the patient seems most tired and allow for rest periods at those times. Provide and encourage frequent rest periods while delivering patient care. Prevent interruptions during rest periods and at night whenever possible. Reduce any disturbing noises and limit visitors as necessary.

Tell the patient to avoid sudden movements, such as getting out of bed quickly, since this decreases the blood supply to the brain, aggravating vertigo and disorientation. Have the patient practice deep-breathing exercises to increase oxygen and blood to the brain. Provide oxygen therapy if appropriate.

Teach the patient to practice energy-saving techniques to reduce fatigue and shortness of breath. Place frequently used articles within the patient's reach.

Encourage good nutrition to increase the patient's energy level. Offer four to six small meals per day. This is less tiring for the patient and prevents gastric overdistention. Assist the patient with feeding if necessary.

Recent research has shown that strategies such as doing something different during the day or talking to friends may help reduce fatigue. Short periods of exercise, such as a 10-minute walk, may also help increase energy levels.

Compare the patient's status with the expected outcomes. If the outcomes are not met, reassess the patient and revise the plan.

HEMORRHAGIC TENDENCIES

Hemorrhage, slow bleeding into tissues and joints (hemarthrosis), and minor bleeding from mucous membranes are common problems in patients with hematologic disorders. Hemorrhage results from a decreased platelet count, as seen in the purpuras, or from absence of one or more of the clotting factors, as in hemophilia. Slow bleeding into tissues or joints may also occur in leukemia, polycythemia, and disseminated intravascular coagulation.

NURSING PROCESS
Hemorrhagic Tendencies

Assessment

Assess for bruising, ecchymoses, petechiae, and purpura. Check the patient's oral cavity for bleeding in the mucous membranes. Look for retinal hemorrhages, which may occur in patients with severe anemia and decreased platelet count. Assess for bleeding in the gastrointestinal tract by noting any blood in vomitus and stools. Check for blood in urine. Review laboratory results of coagulation times. Assess for pain in joints, which may indicate hemarthrosis.

Also assess the patient's respiratory status. Look for cyanosis, shortness of breath on exertion, and inability to complete the tasks of daily living. Assess for tachypnea, tachycardia, dyspnea, and orthopnea and auscultate the chest for adventitious sounds.

Nursing Diagnoses and Planning

Nursing diagnoses and related expected patient outcomes commonly applicable to patients with hemorrhagic tendencies include the following:

NDx: Knowledge deficit: nature of disease and prevention of complication of hemorrhage

Planning: Patient Outcomes
1. Patient states accurate information about the nature of the disease and the resulting complication of hemorrhage.
2. Patient states the signs of bleeding and when to seek medical intervention.
3. Patient relates the measures necessary to reduce the risk of hemorrhage.
4. Signs of bleeding, such as petechiae, purpura, bruising, and dark stools, are absent.

NDx: Altered cardiopulmonary, peripheral, and cerebral tissue perfusion related to destruction of platelets or absence of clotting factors, causing excessive bleeding

Planning: Patient Outcomes
1. Patient's extremities are warm, color is adequate, and pulses are present.
2. Results from patient's laboratory studies are within normal ranges for the patient.
3. Patient denies headaches, confusion, or nausea.
4. Patient can perform activities of daily living without tachypnea, tachycardia, or dyspnea.

Nursing Interventions and Evaluation

NDx: Knowledge deficit: nature of disease and prevention of complication of hemorrhage

Instruct the patient about the clinical course of the disease and the complication of hemorrhage. Explain the signs of bleeding and tell the patient when to seek medical assistance. Tell the patient to avoid sharp objects, straight razors, contact sports, and injections and venipuncture whenever possible. Tell the patient to watch for discoloration of urine or stools.

Explain proper oral hygiene methods needed to prevent further irritation and ulceration of mucous membranes. Instruct the patient to use a soft toothbrush and to use mouth rinse frequently. Show how to inspect the oral cavity, checking the tongue and gums for early signs of irritation. Teach the patient to avoid extremely hot, spicy foods and acidic drinks to reduce oral and gastrointestinal irritation.

Tell the patient to carry an identification card containing the name of the blood disorder, the patient's name and address, the name of the patient's physician, the patient's blood type, and the name of a family member to call in an emergency.

Check the laboratory data for the bleeding times and platelet count. Be prepared for an emergency episode of bleeding. Tell the patient not to take aspirin or nonsteroidal anti-inflammatory drugs because they may extend the bleeding time.

NDx: Altered cardiopulmonary, peripheral, and cerebral tissue perfusion

Help the patient conserve oxygen by encouraging rest and limiting activities. Assist the patient with meals if needed. Administer oxygen if appropriate. Elevate the head of the bed to aid in chest expansion.

Keep the patient in a comfortable position and reposition frequently to release pressure. Use range-of-motion exercises to stimulate circulation, except in patients whose platelet count is less than 30,000. Monitor vital signs and laboratory studies to assess for changes and improvements in status. Encourage ambulation as tolerated but provide frequent rest periods to decrease cardiac workload. Assist the patient when ambulating because decreased cerebral circulation may cause disorientation and vertigo.

Discourage smoking to avoid vasoconstriction. Remove constricting clothing and keep heavy bed linens from restricting peripheral circulation. Keep the patient's legs in a nondependent position when the patient is not ambulating. Prevent any bleeding episodes if possible.

Compare the patient's status with the expected outcomes. If the outcomes are not met, reassess the patient and revise the plan.

ULCERATIVE LESIONS

Ulcerative lesions of the tongue, gums, or mucous membranes may occur as a result of abnormal changes in mucous membrane cells, poor nutrition, chemotherapy, and decreased gastric secretions. These lesions may be found in any of the hematologic disorders but are more common in severe anemias and leukemias. Bleeding from lesions in the mouth causes a foul taste, which may exacerbate poor nutrition and lead to halitosis. This may be further aggravated if the patient is receiving oxygen or is a mouth breather, which dries the mucous membranes.

Ulcerative lesions may also occur in the legs of patients with sickle-cell anemia because of the accumulation of sickled cells in the peripheral circulation.

NURSING PROCESS
Ulcerative Lesions

Assessment

Examine the oral cavity carefully. Note any bleeding, lesions, discolorations, and sore spots. Assess the tongue for coating, color, and lesions. Check the lips for dryness and cracks. Check the feet and between the toes for lesions and cracked skin.

Palpate the patient's peripheral pulses to assess circulatory status. Note the color of the legs. Check for early signs of breakdown, such as reddened areas and discolorations. Look for shearing, petechiae, cyanosis, and lesions.

Nursing Diagnoses and Planning

Nursing diagnoses and related expected patient outcomes commonly applicable to patients with ulcerative lesions from hematologic disorders include the following:

NDx: Impaired skin integrity related to abnormal changes in mucous membranes, effects of therapy, or insufficient peripheral circulation

Planning: Patient Outcomes
1. Patient states causes of ulcerative lesions and measures to prevent their occurrence or recurrence.
2. Patient demonstrates appropriate care of ulcerative lesions.
3. Patient's oral cavity and legs are free of ulcerative lesions.

Nursing Interventions and Evaluation

NDx: Impaired skin integrity
Teach the patient measures to prevent ulcerative lesions from developing. Avoid irritating the mouth with hot, spicy, or acidic foods and fluids. Provide soft or bland foods, especially when lesions are present. Keep the patient well hydrated. Use petrolatum on the lips to prevent cracking. Teach the patient good oral hygiene techniques. Have the patient use a mouth rinse of one part hydrogen peroxide to four parts water, or a commercial preparation,

frequently. A solution of 1 teaspoon of sodium bicarbonate in water may be soothing to the oral mucosa. Teach the patient to use a soft toothbrush to prevent irritation to the gums and mucous membranes. Have the patient inspect the oral cavity frequently and seek medical assistance for any breakdown or soreness.

Teach the patient to exercise, as tolerated, to promote circulation. Range-of-motion exercises should be done while the patient is on bedrest unless the platelet count is less than 30,000. Avoid exercising the affected joints in patients who have sickle-cell anemia. Turn the patient frequently and inspect pressure areas for early signs of breakdown. Keep heavy linens from constricting the peripheral circulation by using a bed cradle. Elevate the patient's legs when he or she is sitting in a chair. If ulcerations are present, use aseptic technique to cleanse them. Wear gloves during dressing changes. Teach the patient and family members the proper technique for dressing the legs. Keep the feet clean and dry. Moisturize the heels and soles of the feet with lotion daily. Inspect the areas between the toes for lesions or cracked skin daily.

Compare the patient's status with the expected outcomes. If the outcomes are not met, reassess the patient and revise the plan.

BONE AND JOINT PAIN AND DEFORMITIES

Bone and joint pain and deformities may be the result of bleeding into the joints, hyperactivity of bone marrow, gout, pathologic fractures, and invasion of malignancies into bone. Pain in the knees, wrists, or hands may indicate hemarthrosis, which frequently occurs with sickle-cell anemia and hemophilia. Aching bones often result from the pressure of expanding bone marrow, as seen in people with multiple myeloma and leukemias. In multiple myeloma, infiltration of malignancy into the bone causes both pain and fractures.

NURSING PROCESS
Bone and Joint Pain and Deformities

Assessment

Assess the patient for the extent of the pain—its location, duration, severity, and frequency—and for joint deformities. Look for swelling, redness, and warmth at the site of the pain. Assess for tenderness or pain when applying pressure over the bone or joint. Check the range of motion of the involved joint and the amount of flexibility or stiffness present. Note the patient's activity level and whether the pain restricts the patient's movements or ability to do self-care or to ambulate.

Nursing Diagnoses and Planning

Nursing diagnoses and related expected patient outcomes commonly applicable to patients with bone or joint pain include the following:

NDx: Pain related to bleeding into joints, invasion of malignancies into bone, and other effects of the hematologic disorder

Planning: Patient Outcomes
1. Patient reports that pain is controlled with analgesics.
2. Patient reports that comfort measures assist in controlling pain.
3. Patient utilizes coping measures to help relieve or tolerate pain.

Nursing Interventions and Evaluation

NDx: Pain
Place the patient in comfortable positions and reposition frequently. Use pillows to support bony prominences. Determine when the pain is most severe and allow the patient to rest during those periods. Give pain medications as ordered before activities so that the patient can better tolerate the movement.

Help the patient find alternative methods to alleviate or tolerate pain. Show the patient and family relaxation techniques and how to perform massage. Teach the patient how to use patient-controlled analgesia, if ordered.

Compare the patient's status with the expected outcomes. If the outcomes are not met, reassess the patient and revise the plan.

INCREASED SUSCEPTIBILITY TO INFECTION

Patients with disorders involving leukocytes, such as leukemia, leukopenia, and lymphomas, are especially prone to developing local and systemic infections. Patients with depressed immunity caused by such treatments as chemotherapy for malignancies of the hematologic system are also extremely susceptible to infections. When the tissues are hypoxic and there is a reduction in mature circulating leukocytes, fewer cells are available to effectively fight invading microorganisms and produce antibodies. Inadequate nutritional support may also contribute to the patient's overall poor health status, thus increasing the risk for infection.

NURSING PROCESS
Increased Susceptibility to Infection

Assessment

Assess the patient frequently for signs of infection. Note generalized signs, such as fever, malaise, and

Table 12–2

Standard Precautions

1. Wash hands before and after patient contact and immediately after contact with blood, body fluids, or human tissue.
2. Wear gloves when coming in contact with blood, body fluids, human tissue, or any contaminated surface.
3. Wear gowns or plastic aprons, masks, and goggles if blood may splatter.
4. Discard sharp objects, such as needles, in a puncture-resistant needle disposal box immediately after use. They should not be recapped, bent, or broken.
5. Clean up blood spills immediately with an agency-designated disinfectant solution.
6. Label blood or body fluid specimens as biohazardous.
7. Do not eat, drink, smoke, apply cosmetics or lip balm, or handle contact lenses in work areas where there is a likelihood of occupational exposure.
8. Do not keep food and drink in areas where potentially infectious materials are present.

fatigue. Look for increased respiratory rate, cough, dyspnea, chills, and shortness of breath. Auscultate the lungs for adventitious sounds. Check laboratory results, especially the white blood cell count and results of urinalysis.

Determine whether the patient experiences pain or burning on urination or low back pain, which could indicate a urinary tract infection. Note the color and consistency of the urine and the presence of dysuria, frequency, or urgency.

Assess the patient's mouth, looking for signs of infection from lesions. Note any ulcerative lesions on the patient's legs. Look for purulent drainage, redness, or swelling at the site of lesions. Assess the perirectal area for edema, redness, or localized pain and tenderness. Note nausea, vomiting, diarrhea or abdominal distention. Always use standard precautions (Table 12–2) to prevent the spread of infections.

Nursing Diagnoses and Planning

Nursing diagnoses and related expected patient outcomes commonly applicable to patients with increased susceptibility to infection include the following:

NDx: Risk for infection related to increased susceptibility secondary to compromised immunity

Planning: Patient Outcomes

1. Patient's vital signs are within normal ranges for the patient.
2. Signs of infection, such as fever, chills, tachycardia, tachypnea, or pain or burning on urination are absent.

3. Patient identifies early signs of infection and measures to prevent infections.

Nursing Interventions and Evaluation

NDx: Risk for infection
Keep the patient warm and avoid extreme changes in temperature in the room. Restrict visitors to prevent exposure to infections. Use protective isolation if appropriate.

Monitor the patient's vital signs frequently, observing subtle changes that may indicate early signs of infection. Report any changes noted. Promote good nutrition by serving meals in a relaxed, attractive atmosphere. Encourage a high-protein, high-vitamin diet. Provide oral hygiene frequently to prevent infection and promote better eating habits. Urge the patient to consume adequate fluids, especially water.

Keep the patient's lips well-lubricated to prevent skin breakdown. Encourage mouth cleansing every 2 hours with a nonirritating substance. Use a mixture of one part hydrogen peroxide and four parts water, especially when bleeding is present, to help prevent the growth of organisms. A solution of 1 teaspoon of sodium bicarbonate in water may be soothing to the oral mucosa (Highlight 12–1).

Teach deep-breathing exercises to keep the patient's lungs open and prevent atelectasis. Pulmonary infections can be prevented by mobilizing pulmonary secretions with coughing and deep-breathing exercises. Moving or turning the patient every 2 hours in bed will help prevent fluid buildup in the lungs.

Because early identification and treatment may limit the severity of the infection, teach the patient and family to observe continually for signs of devel-

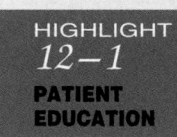 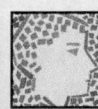

HIGHLIGHT
12–1
PATIENT EDUCATION   **Oral Hygiene**

Instruct the patient that oral hygiene is important to help prevent ulcerations and infection. The following guidelines are important in good oral hygiene:

- Remove dentures if they are irritating or if oral pain or ulcerations are present.
- Oral hygiene should be performed after each meal and at other times when needed.
- Mouth care should be performed every 2 hours if any irritation is present.
- Commercial mouthwashes and lemon-glycerine swabs should be avoided.
- Select soft, bland, nonirritating foods.

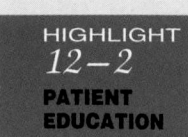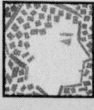

oping infection and to notify the physician if such signs appear. Refer to Highlight 12–2 for patient education regarding prevention of infection.

Compare the patient's status with the expected outcomes. If the outcomes are not met, reassess the patient and revise the plan.

JAUNDICE, PRURITUS, AND SKIN PROBLEMS

Bilirubin is a byproduct of red blood cell breakdown. In patients with hematologic disorders, red blood cells may break down so rapidly that the liver is unable to dispose of the bilirubin quickly enough. This leads to jaundice. Pruritus is a common manifestation of jaundice and can cause extreme discomfort for the patient. If the patient scratches the affected areas, skin breakdown may occur, leading to increased discomfort and infection.

Nursing care for the patient with jaundice includes promoting good skin care. Use nonirritating soaps and cool water for bathing and apply lotion frequently to prevent dry skin. Cut the patient's fingernails short to prevent skin breaks if the patient scratches. Have the patient soak in an oatmeal bath or commercially prepared bath additive to reduce pruritus. Dress area of skin breakdown with aseptic dressings to prevent infection. Keep the patient's environment cool and encourage loose-fitting clothing.

NUTRITIONAL DEFICIENCIES

Nutritional deficiencies commonly accompany hematologic dysfunction. These deficiencies may be the primary cause of the disorder, as in iron deficiency anemia or folic acid deficiency, or they may be secondary to the major disorder, as in leukemia and multiple myeloma. In these disorders, the nutritional deficiencies usually relate to the effects of the treatment instituted for the disorder.

Ulcerations of the mouth, nausea, and vomiting are common side effects of chemotherapy that interfere with the patient's ability to eat well. Other disorders cause gastrointestinal symptoms that may contribute to poor dietary intake. The extreme fatigue the patient experiences can also affect eating habits. Lack of knowledge about dietary deficiencies and proper diet planning may be a contributing factor to the nutritional deficiency. Refer to Highlight 12–3 for a list of the nutrients required for normal blood cell production.

NURSING PROCESS
Nutritional Deficiencies

Assessment

Assess the patient's typical dietary pattern. Note the types and amounts of foods consumed and the protein, vitamin, and caloric value. Assess for weight loss. Check for nausea, mouth soreness, diarrhea, constipation, vomiting, and gastric distention. Look for signs of dehydration. Assess the patient's energy level at meal times.

Nursing Diagnoses and Planning

Nursing diagnoses and related expected patient outcomes commonly applicable to patients with nutritional needs caused by hematologic disorders include the following:

NDx: Altered nutrition: less than body requirements related to disease process, dietary deficiencies, inability to eat, and complications of treatment

Planning: Patient Outcomes
1. Patient chooses appropriate foods to maintain a therapeutic nutritional status, replace deficiencies, and prevent gastrointestinal symptoms.
2. Patient tolerates the food served.
3. Patient eats at least 70 to 80% of the food served.
4. Patient relates accurate information about the disease and dietary deficiencies related to the disease or complications of treatment.

Nursing Interventions and Evaluation

NDx: Altered nutrition: less than body requirements
Help the patient maintain good nutritional status by providing high-protein and high-vitamin foods in an attractive atmosphere. Provide six to eight small meals per day to prevent distention, decrease gastric irritability, and increase the amount the patient can eat. Offer bland, soft foods if the patient has mouth lesions.

Assist with meals if the patient is extremely fatigued. Allow the patient to rest before meals. Encourage increased fluid intake. Avoid foods and fluids that are hot, spicy, acidic, or gas-producing to decrease mouth and gastric irritation.

Provide good oral hygiene after meals and between meals. Teach the patient to cleanse the mouth

HIGHLIGHT
12–3
NUTRITION

Requirements for Blood Cell Production

Nutrient	Food	Function
Protein (amino acid)	Meat	Builds strength and elasticity of plasma membrane Helps produce hemoglobin
Vitamin B$_{12}$	Meat and meat products	Helps produce DNA Facilitates folate metabolism.
Folic Acid	Liver, kidney, spinach, broccoli	Helps produce DNA and RNA Helps erythrocytes mature Helps produce white blood cells
Vitamin B$_6$ (pyridoine)	Muscle meat, vegetables, whole grain cereals	Helps produce the iron-containing portion of hemoglobin
Vitamin B$_2$ (riboflavin)	Milk and milk products, lean meat, eggs	Oxidative reactions
Vitamin C (ascorbic acid)	Citrus fruit, cabbage, green leafy vegetables, broccoli	Iron metabolism
Vitamin E	Egg yolks, cereal grains, green plants, butter	Helps produce iron-containing portions of hemoglobin Helps erythrocytes mature
Iron	Meat, legumes, whole grains, green vegetables	Helps produce hemoglobin
Copper	Organ meat, whole grains, shell-fish	Allows iron to move from tissue to plasma Helps produce hemoglobin
Vitamin K	Green leafy vegetables	Helps produce prothrombin and fibrin

frequently with a soft toothbrush and to use mouth rinse. Provide antiemetics before meals if the patient is nauseated.

Teach the patient about good nutritional habits. Provide examples of menus for the patient and family. If the patient has a specific dietary deficiency, such as iron deficiency anemia, provide specific instructions about foods high in the deficient nutrient.

Compare the patient's status with the expected outcomes. If the outcomes are not met, reassess the patient and revise the plan.

GASTROINTESTINAL SYMPTOMS

Several factors contribute to gastrointestinal symptoms experienced by the patient with a hematologic disorder. Abnormal changes in mucous membranes may result from the disorder or from treatments such as chemotherapy. Gastric secretions decrease in pernicious anemia, causing an irritable stomach.

Ulcerations in the mouth and extreme fatigue may reduce the desire to eat properly or may render the patient unable to eat. These factors may manifest in symptoms such as anorexia, nausea, vomiting, diarrhea, abdominal distention, flatulence, dehydration, and weight loss.

Nursing care for the patient with gastrointestinal symptoms is similar to that previously discussed under nutritional needs.

ENLARGED ORGANS

Hepatomegaly, splenomegaly, and hypertrophy of bone marrow may occur as a result of congestion in the tissue from overproduction of cells, as seen in polycythemia and leukemia. Splenomegaly may also occur as a result of an increased demand on the organ to destroy defective cells, as seen in hemolytic anemia.

Nursing care for the patient with enlarged organs includes assessing for symptoms resulting from the organ changes, such as increased bleeding tendency, decreased detoxification ability, abdominal discomfort, and ascites (see Chap. 25).

Assessment of the Hematologic System

Assessment of the hematologic system (blood and blood-forming organs) includes a thorough review of laboratory studies, radiologic studies, and presenting symptoms. Each of the structures of the hematologic system is also a component of another body system and is usually evaluated with that system.

The nursing assessment focuses on the clinical manifestations of hematologic disorders previously described in the chapter. Finally, assess the patient's understanding and compliance with health promotion and risk reduction measures related to the hematologic system (Highlight 12–4). For example, ask about bleeding tendencies, use of aspirin products (which prolong bleeding times), nutritional patterns, and any problems with repeated respiratory infections.

Diagnostic Procedures

A variety of diagnostic procedures can be used to diagnose hematologic disorders. Examination of the blood cells is important for all patients, regardless of disorder, but it is even more significant in determining dysfunction of the hematologic system. Abnormalities most commonly detected include anemia and leukocyte changes. Since hemostasis may be the primary problem or may be affected by disorders of the hematologic system, coagulation studies are also

necessary. Other tests used to evaluate function of blood-forming organs include biopsies, sonograms, and scans.

METHODS OF OBTAINING BLOOD

Blood can be obtained for examination by finger stick, venipuncture, and arterial puncture. The finger stick method is used to obtain capillary blood for peripheral blood smears. Venipuncture is used to obtain venous blood for most hematologic studies. Venous blood is usually drawn from the antecubital vein. Arterial puncture is used to obtain arterial blood for blood gas studies. Arterial blood is usually drawn from the radial or femoral artery. Universal precautions are necessary whenever exposure to blood is possible.

Because many patients with disorders of the hematologic system have hemorrhagic tendencies, bleeding episodes and hematomas (after venous or arterial sticks) are prevented by applying direct pressure with a sterile dressing to the site of the puncture. Pressure is applied for at least 5 minutes after arterial sticks.

BLOOD TESTS

Only disorders of the hematologic system related to each test are discussed in this chapter. It is important to keep in mind that laboratory values vary according to individual laboratory standards (Table 12–3).

Complete Blood Count

The complete blood count is the basic screening test for white blood cell (leukocyte) count, red blood cell (erythrocyte) count, differential white blood cell count, hematocrit, hemoglobin, red blood cell indices, stained red cell examination, and platelet count. Abnormal values in any of these may indicate dysfunction in the blood or blood-forming organs.

White Blood Cell Count

The white blood cell count is the total number of circulating white blood cells. Disease can be associated with either an increase or a decrease of white blood cells.

Leukocytosis is the term used to refer to a white blood cell count higher than 10,000/mm^3. This occurs in conjunction with infections, malignancies, tissue necrosis, hemorrhage, trauma, tissue injury, circulatory disease, and steroid therapy. Emotional stress, pain, moderate physical exercise, fever, prolonged exposure to cold, convulsions, and paroxysmal tachycardia may cause slight increases in the white blood cell count.

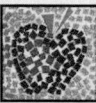

Table 12–3

Common Laboratory Tests for Diagnosing Dysfunction of Blood or Blood-Forming Organs

Test	Normal Results*	Measures
Complete blood count (CBC)		
White blood cells (WBCs)	4500–11,000/mm³	Total number
Red blood cells (RBCs)	4.2–5.4 million/mm³ (male)	Total number
	4.5–5.1 million/mm³ (female)	
Hematocrit (Hct)	40–54% (male)	Percentage of RBCs in whole blood
	37–47% (female)	
Hemoglobin (Hgb)	14–18 g/100 mL (male)	Amount of hemoglobin oxygen-carrying capacity in whole blood
	12–16 g/100 mL (female)	
Platelet count	50,000–350,000/mm³	Total number of platelets in whole blood
Coagulation studies		
Platelet aggregation	<5 minutes	Rate at which platelets adhere to one another
Prothrombin time (PT)	12–14 sec	Time for clotting to occur
Partial thromboplastin time (PTT)	20–35 sec	Detects stage 2 clotting deficiencies
Activated partial thromboplastin time (APTT)	16–25 sec	Detects stage 2 clotting deficiencies (a more sensitive test and less time consuming)
Leukocyte alkaline phosphatase (LAP) stain	30–130	Amount of enzyme alkaline phosphatase present in WBCs
Direct Coombs' test	Negative	Presence of antibody on RBCs or RBC sensitization
Serum iron	80–160 mg/100 mL (male)	Iron transported in blood serum
	50–150 mg/100 mL (female)	
Total iron-binding capacity (TIBC)	250–410 mg/100 mL	Total iron bound to transferrin, a transport protein in blood serum
Serum folic acid	5–21 mg/mL	Amount of folic acid in blood
Bone marrow aspiration	Normal percentage of cells and cell substances in bone marrow	Biopsy smear to determine whether bone marrow is producing normal RBCs, WBCs, and platelets
Urine studies		
Schilling	>7% excretion in urine	24-hour urine test to evaluate absorption of ingested vitamin B_{12} from gastrointestinal tract
Urobilinogen	0–4 mg in 24 hours excreted in urine	Amount of urobilinogen excreted in urine and feces
	50–300 mg in 24 hours excreted in feces	
Bleeding time (Ivy method)	2–9.5 min	Quality and quantity of platelets and ability of blood vessels to constrict
Hemoglobin studies		
Sickle cell	Absence of sickle-shaped cells	Detects presence of normal hemoglobin vs abnormal hemoglobin in RBCs
Heinz body	Occasional presence only when RBC ages	Detects presence of serrated granules containing denatured hemoglobin
Red blood cell studies		
Erythrocyte fragility	Hemolysis begins at 0.45–0.29%	Rate at which RBCs become fragile and rupture (hemolysis) in saline solution
	Hemolysis ends at 0.33–0.30%	
Erythrocyte sedimentation	0–15 mm/h (male)	Rate at which RBCs settle in uncoagulated blood
	0–20 mm/h (female)	
	Results vary greatly depending on test used	
Reticulocyte count	0.5–1.5% of total RBCs	Percentage of immature, non-nucleated RBCs

*Values vary depending on which laboratory method is used.

Leukopenia is the term used to refer to a white blood cell count lower than 4000/mm³. This occurs in conjunction with some viral infections, hypersplenism, bone marrow depression, radiation therapy, acute leukemia, agranulocytosis, pernicious anemia, aplastic anemia, and multiple myeloma.

Differential

The differential white blood cell count is the leukocyte count differentiated according to the type of cell and its functions, as described in Table 12–4. There are five types of white blood cells: neutrophils, eosinophils, basophils, lymphocytes, and monocytes. The differential count reflects a percentage of the total number of white blood cells. The number and type of cell and degree of change are important in diagnosing leukocyte disorders and other diseases. A *left shift* indicates an increased number of immature neutrophils or bands. This signals the presence of an acute infectious process. A *right shift* represents a greater number of mature neutrophils, as seen with pernicious anemia and following tissue breakdown.

Granulocytes are white blood cells that destroy bacteria. They are often affected in hematologic disorders and in the cytotoxic treatment used for malignancies. When there are less than 1000 circulating granulocytes, the risk of infection increases significantly. The risk of infection is also related to the duration of the decreased count and whether the count is decreasing or increasing. An absolute granulocyte count can be calculated by multiplying the total white blood cell count (WBC) by the percentage of bands and mature neutrophils (WBC × [% bands + % mature neutrophils] × 0.01).

Red Blood Cell Count

The red blood cell count reflects the total number of erythrocytes per cubic millimeter of blood. It takes 3 to 5 days for a red blood cell to mature, and it lives about 120 days. The reticulocyte is an immature red blood cell. The reticulocyte count is increased any time there is an accelerated production of red blood cells. It is decreased when the bone marrow has slowed production of red blood cells.

Increased red blood cell counts are seen with decreased cardiac output, impaired pulmonary gas exchange, steroid therapy, polycythemia vera, severe diarrhea, and dehydration. The higher the altitude, the greater the number of red blood cells. The decreased oxygen content of the air stimulates the production of red blood cells. Extreme exercise or excitement may produce a higher red blood cell count than in basal conditions.

Decreased red blood cell counts occur in people with B_6 and B_{12} vitamin deficiencies, iron deficiency, chronic infections, bone marrow depression, multiple myeloma, leukemia, hemolytic anemia, and pernicious anemia. There is a gradual decrease in the red blood cell count in the aged.

Hematocrit   37-47 females norm

The hematocrit measures the percentage of red blood cells in a volume of whole blood. The hematocrit value is approximately three times the hemoglobin value. The hematocrit value can be affected by changes in blood volume. The hematocrit value continues to decrease slightly after age 50.

Elevated hematocrit levels are seen in people with dehydration, pernicious anemia, and polycythemia. Immediately after an acute hemorrhage, the hematocrit value may be high because of the lower blood volume. A higher-than-normal hematocrit level is also seen in people who live at high altitudes.

A hematocrit level of 30% or less indicates moderate to severe anemia. Decreased values may also occur in leukemia, acute hemorrhage, iron deficiency anemia, and hemolytic anemias. The hematocrit can be as much as 10% lower in the evening than in the morning. Because hematocrit is measured as a proportion of red blood cells to a volume of blood, a decrease in fluid that makes up the blood can cause an increase in hematocrit level. Conversely, an increase in fluid can cause a decrease in the hematocrit level.

Hemoglobin

The hemoglobin (Hgb) level measures the amount of hemoglobin per 100 mL of blood. A normal hemoglobin level is necessary for transporting appropriate amounts of oxygen to the tissues of the body and helps to prevent significant changes in pH. Hemoglobin levels also vary slightly according to race, age, activity status, hydration status, and the time of day the measurement is taken. Hemoglobin measurements are significant in evaluating anemias. The amount of hemoglobin contributes to the size and color of the red blood cell. Too little hemoglobin makes the cell smaller than normal (microcytic) and pale in color (hypochromic).

Decreased hemoglobin values occur with decreased red blood cell volume, severe hemorrhage, decreased red blood cell oxygenation, malnutrition, iron deficiency anemia, and hemolytic anemia.

Increased hemoglobin values occur with increased red blood cell volume, dehydration, impaired pulmonary gas exchange, decreased cardiac output, and severe hemolysis. Drugs that may cause increased hemoglobin levels include gentamicin and methyldopa. The hemoglobin level may be elevated or normal immediately after acute hemorrhage. The hemoglobin level may also be elevated in individuals living in high altitudes.

Table 12–4

Differential White Blood Cell Count: Average Values, Functions, and Implications

Leukocyte Cell	Normal Value	Function	Increases in Patients with:	Decreases in Patients with:
Segmented neutrophils (segs)	3000–5800/mm³ (54–62%)	Phagocytosis	Pernicious anemia Acute infections Pathologic conditions Liver disease Myocardial infarction Burns Stress Steroid use Myelocytic leukemia	Acromegaly Agranulocytosis Aplastic anemia Folic acid deficiency Hypothyroidism
Band neutrophils (bands)	150–400/mm³ (3–5%)	Phagocytosis	Pharyngitis Acute infections Stress Steroid use Myelocytic leukemia	Iron deficiency anemia Chemotherapy Some viral infections Malnutrition
Eosinophils (EOS)	50–250/mm³ (1–3%)	Antigen-antibody reactions Phagocytosis Chemotaxis Microcidal	Addison's disease Autoimmune disease Allergies Asthma Cancer Hay fever Leukemia Pernicious anemia Rheumatoid arthritis Parasitic infection	Acromegaly Aplastic anemia Congestive heart failure Cushing's syndrome Infection Infectious mononucleosis Stress Corticosteroids
Basophils (BASO)	5–50/mm³ (0–0.75%)	Carry histamine and platelet-activating factors to inflamed areas Immunologic reactive and proliferative disorders	Allergic reactions Leukemia Hodgkin's disease Hypothyroidism Polycythemia vera Sinusitis granulocytosis Basophilic leukemia	Acute infection Anaphylaxis Cushing's syndrome Hyperthyroidism Stress Prolonged steroid therapy
Monocytes (monos)	300–500/mm³ (3–7%)	Tissue macrophages	Epstein-Barr virus Hodgkin's disease Leukemia Multiple myeloma Rheumatoid arthritis Tuberculosis Ulcerative colitis Bacterial parasitic infection	Aplastic anemia Leukemia
Lymphocytes (lymphs)	1500–3000/mm³ (25–33%)	Protect against microbial invasion Immune responses	Diverticulitis Hepatitis Infectious mononucleosis Leukemia Viral infections Chronic inflammations Autoimmune disease Thyrotoxicosis	Aplastic anemia Cushing's syndrome Hodgkin's disease Renal failure Systemic lupus erythematosus Infection with human immunodeficiency virus Steroid use Malignancy

Red Blood Cell Indices

The red blood cell indices are used to define the size and hemoglobin content of the red blood cell. The three red blood cell indices include the mean corpuscular volume, mean corpuscular hemoglobin, and mean corpuscular hemoglobin concentration. These tests are performed using the same blood sample used for hemoglobin, hematocrit, and red blood cell count.

The red blood cell indices assist in differentiating anemias and in determining whether red blood cells are normal in volume and hemoglobin content. Table 12–5 further describes the red blood cell indices and distinguishes anemias according to high and low values.

The mean corpuscular volume is the most significant index for classifying anemias. It indicates the volume of hemoglobin in each red blood cell. The mean corpuscular hemoglobin concentration is helpful in evaluating appropriate therapy for anemia because the two most accurate hematologic determinations (hematocrit and hemoglobin) are used in the calculation of this test. The mean corpuscular hemoglobin concentration is the proportion of hemoglobin contained in each red blood cell. It is an excellent indicator of the oxygen-carrying capacity of the individual red blood cell.

The mean corpuscular hemoglobin index is important in the diagnosis of severe anemia. But because the calculation of the mean corpuscular hemoglobin uses the often inaccurate red blood cell count, it is not as useful as the mean corpuscular hemoglobin concentration. The mean corpuscular hemoglobin is a measurement of the weight of hemoglobin in each red blood cell.

Stained Red Cell Examination

A stained red cell examination is a peripheral blood smear studied under a microscope to determine the characteristics of the red blood cells. This is the best method for determining abnormalities in red blood cell size, shape, structure, hemoglobin content, and staining properties. The examination is useful in diagnosing blood disorders such as anemia, thalassemia, and leukemia. It also serves as a guide to therapy and reveals harmful effects of chemotherapy and radiation treatments. Table 12–6 elaborates on the characteristics and disorders of abnormal red blood cells.

Platelet Count

The platelet count is useful in diagnosing and assessing the extent of bleeding disorders. It is also beneficial in evaluating the effects of anticoagulant therapy and in following the progress of disorders associated with bone marrow failure.

An increased platelet count (thrombocythemia) occurs in patients with cancer, some leukemias, polycythemia vera, iron deficiency anemia, posthemorrhagic anemia, acute infections, and hemolytic disorders, and after splenectomy. Platelets may also be increased at high altitudes, during cold weather, and after strenuous exercise.

A decreased platelet count (thrombocytopenia)

Table 12–5

Red Blood Cell Indices

Index	Measure	Ratio	Value	Disorders Associated with High Values	Disorders Associated with Low Values

Mean corpuscular volume (MCV)	Red blood cell volume	Hct/RBC	80–96 μm^3	Liver disease
				Alcoholism
				Antimetabolite therapy
				Macrocytic anemia:
				  Folic acid deficiency (infants)
				  Pernicious anemia
					Microcytic anemia:
					  Iron deficiency anemias
					Thalassemia major from spherocytic anemia
					Pernicious anemia
					Anemia from chronic blood loss

Mean corpuscular hemoglobin (MCH)	Hemoglobin per RBC	Hgb/RBC	26–34 picograms of Hgb/RBC	Macrocytic anemias (infants)	Microcytic anemias Pernicious anemia
Mean corpuscular hemoglobin concentration (MCHC)	Hemoglobin per 100 mL of packed RBCs	Hgb/Hct	32–36%	Spherocytosis	Macrocytic anemias

Table 12–6

Abnormalities of Red Blood Cells

Cell	Characteristics	Disorders
Poikilocytosis	Abnormal shape	Anemias
Target	Thin shape, small Hgb in center	Chronic anemias
		Thalassemia major
		Hgb C disease
Spherocyte	Small, round shape	Hereditary spherocytosis
		Congenital hemolytic anemia
Sickle	Crescent or sickle-shaped Hgb	Hemolytic anemia
	S present	Sickle-cell anemia
Schistocyte	Fragmented with unusual shapes	Hemolytic anemia
Hypochromic	Pale from decreased Hgb	Anemias
Basophilic stippling	Immature, non-nucleated	Pernicious anemia
		Leukemia
Polychromatophilia	Immature, non-nucleated	Hemolytic anemia
		Acute blood loss
Metarubricyte	Nucleated	Severe anemia
Megaloblasts	Nucleated, large with increased Hgb	Pernicious anemia
Anisocytosis	Abnormal size	Anemias
Microcyte	Small	Microcytic anemias:
		Iron deficiency anemia
		Thalassemia major
		Spherocytic anemia
Macrocyte	Large	Macrocytic anemias:
		Pernicious anemia
		Folic acid deficiency

occurs in people with idiopathic thrombocytopenia purpura, pernicious anemia, aplastic anemia, hemolytic anemia, and some leukemias, and after several blood transfusions. It may also occur after chemotherapy and in people with bone marrow depression disorders. A platelet count of 20,000/mm³ or lower may be associated with a tendency for spontaneous bleeding, a prolonged bleeding time, petechiae, and ecchymoses.

COAGULATION TESTS

Platelet Aggregation

The adherence of platelets to one another is defined as platelet aggregation. Platelets usually aggregate in less than 5 minutes. This test determines abnormalities in the rate and percentage of platelet aggregation. Increased platelet aggregation may occur after surgery, acute illness, venous thrombosis, and pulmonary embolism. Decreased platelet aggregation may occur in people with infectious mononucleosis, idiopathic thrombocytopenia purpura, acute leukemia, and von Willebrand's disease.

Prothrombin Time

Prothrombin, a protein formed in the liver, is also known as clotting Factor II. Sufficient intake and absorption of vitamin K is necessary for the formation of prothrombin. The prothrombin time (PT) detects a defect in Stage II of the clotting mechanism and is a useful screening test for deficiencies of Factors I, II, V, VII, and X. It is also used to monitor the effects of coumarin-derivative anticoagulant therapy.

The prothrombin time is elongated in people with prothrombin deficiency, vitamin K deficiency, hypervitaminosis A, malabsorption of fats, hyperprothrombinemia, disseminated intravascular coagulation, and liver disease, and in those undergoing anticoagulant therapy. An elongated prothrombin time may be considered therapeutic for the patient on anticoagulant therapy with warfarin sodium to prevent clotting, such as is used after myocardial infarction. For a patient in this situation, a prothrombin time of 1.5 to 2.5 times the normal value may be considered appropriate.

Drugs used for oral anticoagulant therapy have a narrow therapeutic index and must be carefully monitored. Periodic testing of prothrombin time has been used for this purpose. To help standardize their results, laboratories have adopted a reporting method called the International Normalized Ratio (INR). The INR is calculated using a nomogram that gives the relationship of the patient's prothrombin time to a normal control. (The control is a standard that is derived from the plasma of patients stabilized on a regimen of anticoagulant treatment for at least 6 weeks.) This allows anticoagulant control to be comparable at different laboratories and more accurate. The recommended INR range for oral anticoagulant therapy is 2.0 to 3.0, but this value may vary with the goals of therapy. For example, the recommended INR range for patients with mechanical heart prosthetic valves is 2.5 to 3.5, and for survivors of acute MI it is 2.5 to 3.5.

Partial Thromboplastin Time and Activated Partial Thromboplastin Time

The partial thromboplastin time (PTT) is a screening test for coagulation disorders that detects Stage II clotting deficiencies. Thromboplastin is clotting Factor III and is present in both blood and tissue. The PTT measures the time required for blood to clot after a reagent is added to it. The PTT is prolonged in heparin anticoagulant therapy and in defects of clotting Factors I (fibrinogen), II (prothrombin), V, VII, IX, X, XI, and XII. The therapeutic range for patients on anticoagulant therapy is 2.5 to 3.0 times the normal range.

The activated partial thromboplastin time (APTT) is essentially the same as the PTT but is considered slightly more sensitive and takes less time to perform. The APTT is indicated for the same conditions as the PTT, which includes monitoring of heparin therapy. The APTT is prolonged in conjunction with defects of the same factors as the PTT.

Bleeding Time (Ivy Method)

Bleeding time is a screening method used to differentiate disorders of primary hemostasis from disorders of coagulation defects. The duration of bleeding depends on the quality and quantity of platelets and the ability of the blood vessel wall to constrict. The Ivy method bleeding time is useful in diagnosing platelet disorders and von Willebrand's disease.

Table 12-7

Drugs that Delay Coagulation

Drug	Class or Usage
Alcohol	Nonmedicinal
Allopurinol	Hyperuricemia
Aspirin	Analgesic
Corticosteroids	Anti-inflammatory
Dextran	Plasma expander
Dipyridamole	Angina
Ibuprofen	Analgesic
Indomethacin	Anti-inflammatory
Methyldopa	Antihypertensive
Neomycin	Antibiotic
Phenylbutazone	Anti-inflammatory
Quinidine	Antiarrhythmic

To evaluate bleeding time by this method, a blood pressure cuff is applied to the upper arm and inflated to 40 mm Hg. Three small puncture wounds are made on the forearm. These areas are blotted with filter paper every 15 seconds until the bleeding stops. The time it takes for the bleeding to stop is recorded, and the time it takes a platelet clot to form is also noted. If the sites are still bleeding after 15 minutes, the test is discontinued and direct pressure is applied.

Bleeding time is prolonged when platelets are decreased or abnormal, as in thrombocytopenia, leukemia, aplastic anemia, von Willebrand's disease, and disseminated intravascular coagulation. Alcohol and a variety of drugs also extend the bleeding time (Table 12-7).

Coagulant Factor Assays

The coagulant factor assays determine genetic and acquired bleeding disorders. Deficiencies of all factors except III, IV, and XII are related to hemorrhagic disorders.

OTHER BLOOD COMPONENT TESTS

Hemoglobin Electrophoresis

The hemoglobin electrophoresis test detects the types of hemoglobin present in red blood cells and whether they are normal or abnormal. Abnormal hemoglobin can be found in several rare hematologic disorders and in sickle-cell anemia. Abnormal hemoglobins include Hgb S, Hgb C, Hgb H, Hgb D, and Hgb E. Hemoglobin electrophoresis is beneficial in diagnosing the exact problem in a Hgb S disorder. The test determines whether only sickled hemoglobin is present, which indicates sickle-cell anemia, or whether both sickled hemoglobin and normal hemoglobin are present, which indicates sickle-cell trait.

Sickle-Cell Test

The sickle-cell test, also called hemoglobin S test or Sickledex, is routinely used as a screening test for sickle-cell disorder. The test detects Hgb S, an inherited, recessive gene. The erythrocytes are examined for the presence of sickle-shaped forms characteristic of the sickle-cell trait or sickle-cell anemia.

The test involves oxygen removal from the red blood cells. In the normal red blood cell, the shape is retained, but in the red blood cell with Hgb S, the shape becomes sickled. The difference between sickle-cell trait and sickle-cell anemia is determined by hemoglobin electrophoresis.

A positive test indicates that large numbers of erythrocytes have assumed the typical sickle-cell look, or crescent shape. The test is 99% accurate. False-negative results may occur in patients with polycythemias or protein abnormalities and after transfusions of blood with sickled cells.

Heinz Body Test

Heinz bodies are serrated granules that contain precipitated denatured hemoglobin. They may be found in hemolytic anemias and glucose-6-phosphate dehydrogenase deficiency. Glucose-6-phosphate dehydrogenase deficiency is diagnosed if 40% or more of the cells contain five or more Heinz bodies. Some drugs may also interfere with the normal functioning of hemoglobin.

Heinz bodies are present after splenectomy in patients who had unstable hemoglobin syndromes or thalassemia prior to the surgery. Heinz bodies may also be present when red blood cells undergo normal aging.

Erythrocyte Fragility Test

The erythrocyte fragility test measures the rate at which erythrocytes become progressively fragile and finally rupture when suspended in hypotonic solutions of saline. Increased erythrocyte fragility is present in congenital hemolytic anemia and hereditary spherocytosis. Decreased erythrocyte fragility is present in thalassemia, sickle-cell anemia, iron deficiency anemia, and polycythemia vera and after splenectomy. Erythrocyte fragility is normal in patients with acquired hemolytic anemias.

Erythrocyte Sedimentation Rate

The erythrocyte sedimentation rate (ESR) determines the rate at which red blood cells settle in uncoagulated blood. The erythrocyte sedimentation rate is considered a nonspecific test, which means that it is not diagnostic of a specific disorder. It is, however, useful as a screening measure for determining whether a problem is present.

An elevated ESR occurs in conjunction with tissue or cell injury, inflammation, carcinoma, and severe anemia. The ESR is extremely elevated in the presence of malignant diseases such as multiple myeloma, lymphoma, and metastatic cancer. The presence of fibrinogen, globulins, and cholesterol may increase the ESR value.

Reticulocyte Count

The reticulocyte count indicates the percentage of immature, non-nucleated red blood cells. A reticulocyte count is used to distinguish between anemias related to bone marrow failure resulting from hemorrhage and anemias caused by erythrocyte destruction. The count is also used to determine the effectiveness of treatment for iron deficiency anemia, pernicious anemia, and the recovery of bone marrow function in aplastic anemia. It may be used to monitor the effects of radioactive substances on exposed individuals.

An elevated reticulocyte count indicates an increased rate of erythrocyte production with premature destruction of mature red blood cells. Increased reticulocyte levels occur in patients with hemolytic anemias, sickle-cell disease, metastatic carcinoma, leukemia, and hereditary spherocytosis and after hemorrhage (3–4 days), splenectomy, and treatment of anemias.

A decreased reticulocyte count indicates a reduction in erythrocyte production by the bone marrow. Decreased levels occur in people with iron deficiency anemia, aplastic anemia, untreated pernicious anemia, and chronic infections and in those undergoing radiation therapy.

Leukocyte Alkaline Phosphatase Stain

The enzyme alkaline phosphatase is present in leukocytes located in the bone and liver. Abnormal values in leukocyte alkaline phosphatase (LAP) are associated with disease states that affect bone and liver functions.

An elevated LAP level may be seen in patients with polycythemia vera, thrombocytopenia, and primary bone malignancies. Allopurinol and anticonvulsants may also increase the LAP value.

Decreased values may occur in patients with acute and chronic granulocytic leukemia, paroxysmal nocturnal hemoglobinuria, aplastic anemia, hereditary hypophosphatasia, and idiopathic thrombocytopenia purpura. Some medications such as oral contraceptives and fluorides may also decrease the LAP value.

Direct Coombs' Test

The direct Coombs' test, or direct antiglobulin test, detects the presence of antibodies against red blood cells, which increases the cell fragility or causes other cellular damage. The normal test result should be negative.

Positive results are reported on a +1 to +4 range. A positive direct Coombs' test result is seen in transfusion reactions and autoimmune hemolytic anemia and may also be found in patients receiving cephalothin therapy, penicillin, and some other drugs. Drug therapy may also cause a false-positive reading (Table 12–8).

Serum Iron

Iron is an essential component of hemoglobin. It aids in the transport of oxygen and can compromise red blood cell function if abnormal. The blood levels of iron are measured to determine iron deficiency.

Serum iron levels are elevated in patients with untreated drug-induced bone marrow failure, hereditary iron-loading anemia, pernicious anemia, and hemolytic anemia. Iron values may also be increased

Table 12-8

Drugs that Affect the Direct Coombs' Test

Drugs that cause a false-positive result on the direct
 Coombs' test include:
 Cephaloridine
 Cephalothin
 Chlorpromazine
 Diphenylhydantoin
 Isoniazid
 Levodopa
 Methyldopa
 Penicillin
 Procainamide
 Quinidine
 Rifampin
 Streptomycin
 Sulfonamides
 Tetracycline

in people with excessive iron intake, impairment of utilization of iron, and abnormal destruction of red blood cells.

Decreased levels of serum iron are found in people with dietary iron deficiency, absorption impairment, and hemorrhage. Low iron levels may also be seen in pregnant women, after prolonged heavy menstruation, and in elderly people.

Total Iron-Binding Capacity

Iron-binding capacity reflects the transferrin protein content of serum and the total amount of iron that can bind to transferrin present in the blood. Increased total iron-binding capacity values occur in people with iron deficiency anemia due to hemorrhage or inadequate intake, bone marrow damage, erythropoiesis, and polycythemia. When serum iron levels are low, the total iron-binding capacity is increased because there are more transferrin sites to bind with.

Decreased total iron-binding capacity values occur in people with iron overload, pernicious anemia, thalassemia, sickle-cell anemia, chronic infections, hepatic dysfunction, and cancer. Some interfering factors include altered protein balance, estrogen therapy, hormone imbalance, hydroxyurea, and adrenocorticotropic hormone therapy. When serum iron levels are high, total iron-binding capacity is decreased because the capacity of the transferrin to bind with iron is already saturated. About 30% of the total capacity of transferrin is usually bound to serum iron.

Serum Folic Acid

Folic acid is one of the B vitamins necessary for DNA and red blood cell production and growth. It is synthesized by bacteria in the small intestine and stored in the liver. Folic acid deficiency is frequently associated with dietary inadequacies because only a small amount of folic acid can be stored for future use.

Other than dietary deficiency, decreased serum folic acid levels may be associated with megaloblastic anemia, hemolytic disorders, liver disease, alcohol ingestion, and carcinomas. Several drugs may also decrease folic acid values. These are listed in Table 12-9.

NURSING PROCESS GUIDELINES
Diagnostic Blood Tests

Review the findings of studies and the interpretation of results. Assess the patient's hydration level, so that changes in hematocrit related to hypervolemia or hypovolemia can be noted. Assess the oxygenation of a patient whose oxygen-carrying capacity is affected by low hemoglobin and hematocrit levels. Look for cyanosis, tachypnea, tachycardia, dyspnea, pallor, and fatigue. If these symptoms are present, allow for frequent rest periods throughout the day while delivering care to the patient. Administer oxygen as needed. Keep the patient warm and prevent drafts.

Assess the nutritional pattern of a patient with a dietary deficiency. Provide patient education about foods containing the needed nutrients and meal-planning strategies to replace and maintain the level necessary.

Assess the patient's bleeding potential, because many patients subjected to the previously discussed tests may be diagnosed with a coagulation disorder. Look for petechiae, ecchymoses, bruising, and blood in the urine or stools. Teach the patient signs of bleeding and measures to prevent bleeding episodes.

The nursing diagnoses, expected patient outcomes, nursing interventions, and evaluation for patients undergoing diagnostic blood testing are specific to the disorder. Refer to Chapter 13 for application of the nursing process to specific hematologic system disorders. The following additional

Table 12-9

Folic Acid Antagonists

Drugs that may lower serum folic acid levels include:
 Ampicillin
 Chloramphenicol
 Estrogens
 Erythromycin
 Oral contraceptives
 Para-aminosalicylic acid
 Phenobarbital
 Phenytoin
 Tetracycline

interventions also apply to the care of patients undergoing diagnostic blood testing. Explain the scheduled diagnostic studies to the patient. Apply pressure to the site of the finger stick, venipuncture, or arterial puncture as needed. If the patient may have a bleeding disorder, it is extremely important to apply direct pressure to the puncture site for several minutes. For some studies, it may be necessary to withhold food and fluids after midnight on the test day. Check the institution's laboratory procedure manual for specific preparations.

OTHER TESTS SPECIFIC TO HEMATOLOGIC DISORDERS

Schilling Test

The Schilling test is a 24-hour urine study that indirectly measures intrinsic factor deficiency. It evaluates the body's ability to absorb ingested vitamin B_{12} from the gastrointestinal tract by tracking elimination of radioactive vitamin B_{12}. Normally, people absorb and excrete a large proportion of the radioactive vitamin B_{12}. An abnormally low excretion value, less than 7%, indicates the absence of the intrinsic factor.

The Schilling test is used to diagnose macrocytic and pernicious anemia. Factors that may interfere with test results include diabetes, hypothyroidism, enteritis, decreased renal function, and incontinence. Ingestion of laxatives during the test time is contraindicated.

The patient should refrain from food or fluid intake, except for water, for 12 hours before the test. A tasteless capsule of radioactive vitamin B_{12} is given orally. One hour later, the patient is given an intramuscular injection of vitamin B_{12}. Food and fluid intake is resumed at this time. The 24-hour urine collection is started; the appropriate collection container is used. The patient should increase his or her intake of fluids during the test periods to aid in the excretion of urine. The patient collects all urine excreted during the 24 hours in the appropriate receptacle until informed that the test has ended.

Urobilinogen Test

The urinary and fecal urobilinogen test determines the amount of urobilinogen excreted in urine or feces. Urobilinogen is produced when bilirubin is broken down by intestinal tract bacteria. Normally there is a small amount (1%, or 0 to 4 mg in 24 hours) of urobilinogen excreted in urine by the kidneys. Most of the urobilinogen (99%, or 50 to 300 mg) is excreted in the feces. Urinary and fecal urobilinogen both are elevated in people with hemolytic anemia and pernicious anemia as a result of excessive destruction of red blood cells and hemoglobin. Antibiotics and antibacterials may alter the results of the test.

TESTS TO EVALUATE BLOOD-FORMING ORGANS

Bone Marrow Aspiration and Biopsy

A bone marrow aspiration and biopsy determines the ability of the bone marrow to produce normal red blood cells, white blood cells, and platelets. It is an extremely important diagnostic tool for hematologic disorders. The results of the bone marrow smear indicate the cell ratios present. More than 25% lymphocytes or more than 15% monocytes is an abnormal finding. Abnormal cell ratio findings indicate specific diseases.

A bone marrow aspiration is useful in diagnosing aplastic anemia, pernicious anemia, leukemia, purpura, and agranulocytosis. A bone marrow study may also reveal:

- Deficiency states of vitamin B_{12}, folic acid, iron, and pyroxidine
- Bone marrow depression or destruction
- Neoplastic disease

Bone marrow aspiration is usually contraindicated in patients with hemophilia and other bleeding disorders. A bone marrow biopsy can be diagnostic for multiple myeloma. Refer to Chapter 32 for a description of the procedure and the application of the nursing process to the care of the patient having a bone marrow aspiration and biopsy.

Lymph Node Biopsy

A biopsy of lymph node tissue may be performed to diagnose Hodgkin's disease or leukemia. The most common sites for the biopsy are cervical, supraclavicular, and axillary nodes. The biopsy is usually performed by needle aspiration. The procedure and nursing care interventions are similar to those applicable to a bone marrow aspiration.

Ultrasonography

Ultrasonography is a noninvasive procedure for visualizing soft tissue structures of the body by monitoring the reflection of ultrasonic waves directed into the tissues. It is useful in determining spleen size and volume when splenomegaly is suspected, as in thrombocytopenia purpura. It can also be used to identify lymph node masses. Only when lymph nodes are enlarged, as in tumor invasion, are they visible on the ultrasonogram. The procedure takes only a few minutes to an hour and causes little, if any, discomfort.

Food and fluids are withheld, except water, for 12 hours before the test if the transducer is to be inserted into a body cavity or if it is an abdominal examination. The purpose of the test is explained to the patient, usually by the radiologist. The patient is reassured that the test is noninvasive, not painful, and easily tolerated.

Computed Tomography

Computed tomographic scans (also called computerized axial tomographic scans) provide three-dimensional views of soft body tissues with solid organs and bony structures that are projected onto film. The machine rotates around the body as small beams of x-rays pass through the organs. Photographs are taken of tissue density, and depth images are printed out by a computer. Total body scanning is useful in diagnosing Hodgkin's disease and other lymphomas.

Computed tomographic scanning is relatively safe but may be frightening because of the size and complexity of the machine. It delivers no more radiation than a conventional x-ray machine. Although the scanning does not cause discomfort, some individuals are uncomfortable lying on the table for long periods of time.

The procedure is explained to the patient. The patient may be cautioned not to eat or drink fluids 3 to 6 hours before the examination to prevent nausea if a contrast medium is to be used. The patient is reassured that it is a safe, noninvasive procedure.

Magnetic Resonance Imaging

Magnetic resonance imaging produces images similar to those of computed tomography, but with greater sophistication and refined accuracy. The patient is enclosed in a donut-shaped magnet. The surrounding magnetic field causes hydrogen atoms within the body to align in a position to emit radio signals that are received by an imaging system. The signals are converted by a computer into two-dimensional images that are portrayed on film or the video screen of the system's console. The images can be stored, recalled, and manipulated in a variety of ways, enabling detailed examination of the internal organs. It is a noninvasive diagnostic technique used for the hematologic system to analyze blood flow, detect malignant growths, and distinguish organ size.

$\mathcal{M}$anagement

Therapeutic goals for patients with hematologic dysfunction focus on diagnosing and correcting the underlying cause of the disorder. Medical treatment is either palliative or curative and may consist of bedrest with a prescribed regimen of exercise, nutritional support, oxygen therapy, protective isolation, transfusions of blood and blood components, radia-

tion therapy, and chemotherapy or other pharmacologic therapy. Surgical interventions include bone marrow transplants, tumor excision, and splenectomy.

NONSURGICAL MANAGEMENT

Bedrest and Exercise

Bedrest may be recommended to help reduce oxygen requirements and strain on the circulatory and respiratory systems. If the patient is allowed to ambulate and perform activities of daily living, frequent periods of rest are necessary to avoid extreme fatigue and respiratory distress. If the patient cannot actively exercise, passive range-of-motion exercises are performed to promote circulation, enhance joint mobility, and prevent skin breakdown. Application of the nursing process to the care of the patient with activity intolerance was discussed earlier in the chapter.

Nutritional Support

A diet high in protein, iron, and vitamins helps promote red blood cell production and prevent debilitation. Additional iron or vitamin supplements may also be ordered if the diet therapy is inadequate. Application of the nursing process to the care of the patient with nutritional deficiencies was discussed earlier in the chapter.

In cases in which complications of the disorder or treatments interfere with ingestion or digestion, enteral or parenteral support may be required. For the care of the patient receiving enteral or parenteral therapy, see Chapter 21.

Oxygen Therapy

The patient may require oxygen because of a deficiency in oxygen-carrying hemoglobin. Administration of oxygen helps prevent tissue hypoxia and decreases the heart's workload.

Protective Isolation

Protective isolation may be ordered to shield the patient with compromised immunity from microorganisms. This is frequently used for the patient with leukemia or bone marrow depression from a hematologic disorder or from treatment complications. The laminar air flow environment, or a similar system that uses sterilized air flow and sterile equipment, can be used to protect the patient from infection (see Chapter 32).

Blood Transfusions

Many components of blood are available for transfusion to patients with specific needs. A patient may receive whole blood, packed red cells, frozen red blood cells, platelets, granulocytes, plasma, albumin, coagulation factor concentrates, prothrombin complex, cryoprecipitate, or immune serum globulins. Blood for transfusion may be collected from donors (homologous blood), from the intended recipient (autologous blood), or from a donor designated by the recipient (designated [directed] blood).

Blood collected from a donor for transfusion to another individual is the most frequently used blood. Most of this blood is from volunteer donors. Risks associated with homologous blood transfusions include hemolytic and anaphylactic transfusion reactions and the transmission of malaria, hepatitis, syphilis, and human immunodeficiency virus.

Collection of blood from the intended recipient, also called self-donation or autologous, is becoming a common procedure before elective surgery. Autologous red blood cells can also be salvaged during surgery by automated cell-saver equipment or manual suction equipment. Postoperatively, autotransfusion can be instituted using a system designed to collect drainage from the operative site and reinfuse it to the patient with filtration of the blood. This procedure usually takes place while the patient is in an intensive care unit after extensive surgeries such as cardiothoracic surgery or a total hip replacement (Nursing Care Guide 12–1).

Autologous blood transfusions have become more widely used since the acquired immunodeficiency syndrome crisis raised public awareness about the risks associated with transfusions. Autologous transfusions eliminate the risks of immune transfusion reactions and transmission of viral diseases.

Designated (directed) blood is collected from a named donor who has been designated by the recipient. Compatibility testing must be completed before the transfusion, and the designated blood must be compatible with the recipient's blood. Risks are still high with this type of transfusion, because compatibility is a factor, and viral disease may be present in the donor.

WHOLE BLOOD

Whole blood contains cellular and noncellular plasma components, including:

Red blood cells
Plasma proteins
Stable clotting factors
An anticoagulant/preservative

Whole blood is used to treat acute hemorrhage, which requires the oxygen-carrying properties of red blood cells, and hypovolemic shock resulting from blood loss, which requires plasma expansion.

A unit of blood contains about 450 mL of blood with 63 mL of anticoagulant added. The adult dose varies with the patient's needs and symptoms. One unit of whole blood should raise the patient's he-

matocrit three percentage points and the hemoglobin 1 g/dL, if the patient is no longer hemorrhaging. Other than incompatibility, the major complication of whole blood transfusion is circulatory overload.

PACKED RED BLOOD CELLS

Transfusions of packed red blood cells (whole blood without the plasma) are usually preferred over whole blood because they are more economical and reduce the risk of fluid overload. Packed red blood cells are indicated for patients requiring an increase in the oxygen-carrying capacity of blood but without the need for volume expansion. Transfusions of packed red blood cells are ordered for patients with anemia, acute leukemia, or acute or chronic hemorrhage and before, during, and after surgical interventions. It is also the treatment of choice for patients with thalassemia major and may relieve the symptoms of sickle-cell anemia. In these disorders, monthly or bimonthly transfusions of packed red blood cells may be ordered if the hemoglobin level falls below 4 g/100 mL. Prophylactically, packed red blood cells may be administered every 15 days to maintain a hemoglobin level of 12 to 15 g/100 mL.

A unit of packed red blood cells is about 250 to 300 mL in volume. It is infused for 1 to 3 hours. The adult dose varies with patient need and symptoms or disease process. One unit of packed red blood cells should increase the hematocrit by three percentage points and the hemoglobin by 1 g/dL. Complications typically result from incompatibility reactions.

FROZEN RED BLOOD CELLS

When red blood cells are frozen, they can be stored for as long as 2 years. However, they must be used within 24 hours after thawing. Frozen red blood cells are less likely to cause an antigen reaction, because antigens are removed. Because frozen red blood cells are very expensive, their use is usually limited to patients with rare blood types or patients sensitized by previous transfusions.

PLATELETS

Plasma is first removed from whole blood, and then platelets are separated and pooled together in a collection bag. The patient may receive platelets from several different donors in one unit. Single donor platelet transfusions are available for patients who have developed antibodies to all blood products except those that are matched for transplantation antigen.

Platelets are indicated to control or prevent bleeding episodes in patients with platelet deficiencies associated with low number or dysfunction. They are also used prophylactically for platelet counts below 10,000 to 20,000/mm³. Platelet transfusions are not recommended for patients with immune thrombocytopenic purpura.

Patients Receiving an Autologous Blood Transfusion

Assessment Findings:	Patient presents symptoms of increased temperature, inflammation at wound site, and tachycardia; white blood cell count is elevated.
Nursing Diagnosis:	Risk for infection related to surgical intervention, open wound, and intravenous lines

Patient Outcomes	Nursing Interventions	Rationale
Patient's vital signs remain within normal limits for the patient.	Monitor vital signs every 2 hours. Notify physician if significant changes occur.	Vital sign changes may indicate complications.
Symptoms of infection, such as drainage at site, inflammation, and pain at site, are absent.	Maintain aseptic technique when handling transfusion system, changing dressings, or changing tubings. Monitor laboratory values. Check for early signs of infection. Culture any drainage.	Aseptic cleansing at the site and proper handling of the equipment prevents pyogenic infiltration.

Evaluation:	Compare the patient's status with the expected outcomes. If the outcomes are not met, reassess the patient and revise the plan.

Assessment Findings:	Patient displays signs of anxiety: tachycardia, increased blood pressure, nervousness, inability to rest; patient asks questions about the intensive care unit (ICU) and blood transfusion.
Nursing Diagnosis:	Anxiety related to fear and uncertainty about autologous transfusion and the ICU environment

Patient Outcomes	Nursing Interventions	Rationale
Patient verbalizes fears and concerns. Patient relates accurate information about the transfusion.	Allow the patient to verbalize fears and concerns and ask questions. Explain equipment, procedure, and necessity for the transfusion and the ICU environment.	Understanding the need for interventions reassures the patient and reduces anxiety.
Patient's anxiety decreases as evidenced by normal vital signs, patient's ability to rest and relax, and verbalization of less fear and concern.	Provide periods of undisturbed quiet and rest for the patient. Monitor vital signs and observe for other signs of anxiety.	Periods of quiet or rest may alleviate some of the patient's anxiety. Vital sign changes, such as increased pulse and respiratory rate, may indicate increasing anxiety.

Evaluation:	Compare the patient's status with the expected outcomes. If the outcomes are not met, reassess the patient and revise the plan.

(continued)

Nursing Care Guide 12–1
Patients Receiving an Autologous Blood Transfusion

Assessment Findings: Patient presents signs of hypovolemia such as decreased blood pressure, dry skin, decreased urine output, and thirst; patient is still losing blood from surgical intervention.

Nursing Diagnosis: Risk for fluid volume deficit related to blood loss

Patient Outcomes	Nursing Interventions	Rationale
Patient's laboratory values are within normal limits for the patient.	Maintain system for autologous transfusion as required, to keep adding blood volume as it is lost. Check laboratory values.	Replacement of deficient fluid returns the body to a homeostatic state.
Patient has no further blood loss.	Observe for signs of continued bleeding.	Although the nurse may not be able to prevent further blood loss, assessing for early signs of complications from that loss reduces trauma to the patient.
Clinical signs of hypovolemia, such as vital sign changes, dry skin, and oliguria, are absent.	Observe for early signs of hypovolemia. Notify physician if bleeding is greater than expected, or if vital signs change.	Vital sign changes may indicate continued fluid losses.

Evaluation: Compare the patient's status with the expected outcomes. If the outcomes are not met, reassess the patient and revise the plan.

Platelets are stored at room temperature in a device that rotates them to keep the cells from aggregating. They are administered as rapidly as is tolerated by the patient. The adult dose varies with the clinical situation. Transfused platelets may function effectively for as long as 5 to 6 days. The transfusions are given according to blood type, but cross-matching is not necessary because platelet concentrates contain few red blood cells. The patient's platelet count is increased by 5000 to 10,000/mm³ for each unit of platelets transfused. One unit of platelets is 50 to 70 mL in volume.

When a patient receives platelet transfusions over an extended period of time, antibodies to the platelets usually develop. If the patient's platelet count does not increase 1 hour after the transfusion is complete, then antibodies are present. If this situation occurs, platelets must be perfectly matched between the donor and recipient to provide adequate transfusions for therapeutic management of the patient's disorder. Adverse reactions to platelet transfusions are usually allergenic and treated with an antihistamine.

GRANULOCYTES

Granulocytes can be separated from whole blood and transfused, but they are rarely used. Granulocytes have a short survival time, making their effect only temporary. They are generally used only for treating life-threatening neutropenia. A unit is 200 to 400 mL in volume and must be administered over 1 to 4 hours. Adverse reactions may include fever and mild nonhemolytic allergic reactions.

PLASMA

Fresh frozen plasma contains approximately 91% water, 7% protein, and 2% carbohydrate. It contains all the clotting factors, which are then preserved by the freezing. Plasma transfusions are used to restore deficient coagulation factors in acquired or inherited bleeding disorders and to replace clotting factors in patients during hemorrhage. To permanently stop bleeding in patients with hemophilia, plasma is transfused to supply the antihemophilic factor (AHF) to the patient's plasma. The blood must be given within 6 hours after withdrawal from the donor, because AHF deteriorates rapidly.

One unit of plasma is about 200 to 250 mL in volume. It should be infused quickly for 30 to 45 minutes unless contraindicated. The adult dose is determined by the patient's clinical problem and symptoms. The effect of the transfusion is measured by monitoring coagulation times.

Plasma contains no red blood cells, so cross-matching is not necessary, but ABO typing is usually done. Plasma carries the same complications and risks as whole blood. Sensitization to AHF and the development of autoimmune anticoagulants occur in some cases.

In lieu of plasma, plasma substitutes may be ordered. These substitutes are not blood products but are used to expand plasma volume in emergency situations of massive blood loss. Refer to Highlight 12–5 for a list of plasma substitutes.

ALBUMIN

Plasma albumin is a large protein molecule considered free of all viral contaminants including hepatitis. Albumin is used to restore blood volume and protein for patients in shock from burns, trauma, infection, or surgery. It is not used for a particular hematologic disorder.

COAGULATION FACTOR CONCENTRATES

Factor VIII concentrate is prepared from donor plasma but does not carry the risk of disease of the plasma because of the process used to separate the factor. It is used to treat moderate Factor VIII deficiency (hemophilia A). It may also be used for patients lacking fibrinogen or Factor XIII and for those with von Willebrand's disease. The adult dose is calculated according to body weight and the level of anticoagulant activity desired. A level of 30 to 50% is the usual goal of the therapy. It is given as an intravenous push.

Factor IX concentrate is also prepared from donor plasma and does not carry risk of disease. It contains Factor IX in large quantities and small amounts of Factors II, VIII, and X. Factor IX concentrate is used to treat a Factor IX deficiency (hemophilia B), congenital Factor VIII deficiency, or Factor X deficiency and to treat hemophiliacs with Factor VIII inhibitors. The adult dose is calculated according to body weight and level of factor activity desired.

PROTHROMBIN COMPLEX

The prothrombin complex blood component contains:

Prothrombin
Factors VII, IX, and X
Part of Factor XI

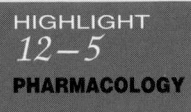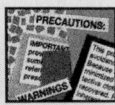

HIGHLIGHT 12–5 PHARMACOLOGY

Plasma Substitutes

Definition:

Dextran 70 (Macrodex)

Dextran 40 (Gentran 40, 10% LMD, Rheomacrodex)

6% Hetastarch (Hespan)

Action:

Dextran 70—High molecular weight, expands plasma volume.

Dextran 40—Low molecular weight, reduces blood viscosity.

Hetastarch—Expands plasma volume.

Uses:

Expand plasma volume in massive hemorrhage, fluid loss, and burns.

Side Effects:

Urticaria, fluid overload, nausea, vomiting, wheezing, increased bleeding time, and antigen-antibody reaction.

Interactions:

None

Nursing Implications:

Observe for fluid overload causing respiratory and cardiac distress, bleeding, dehydration, or other side effects. Check renal function. Assess for therapeutic results. Use aseptic technique in handling intravenous equipment and intravenous fluid (plasma substitute).

Transfusions of prothrombin complex are useful for treating bleeding disorders in patients with congenital or acquired deficiencies of these factors.

CRYOPRECIPITATE

Cryoprecipitate is prepared from whole blood and contains 80 to 120 U of Factor VIII, von Willebrand's factor, fibrinogen, and Factor XIII. Each unit is about 5 to 20 mL in volume. Cryoprecipitate is indicated for deficiencies of Factor VIII, Factor XIII, or fibrinogen, and for von Willebrand's disease. The average adult dose is calculated by plasma volume. Eight to 10 bags of cryoprecipitate supply enough fibrinogen for hemostasis, approximately 2 g. It is transfused at a rate of 1 to 2 mL/minute. Since cryoprecipitate contains no red blood cells, cross-matching is not required, but ABO compatibility is checked.

IMMUNE SERUM GLOBULINS

Immune serum globulins (ISG) are concentrated aqueous solutions of gamma globulin. Nonspecific ISG is indicated for passive immune protection and to treat hypogammaglobulinemia. Specific ISG is prepared from donors who have a high antibody titer. Some examples of specific ISG include the hepatitis B immune globulin, Rh immune globulin, and varicella-zoster immune globulin. The adult dose varies by the type of ISG. Patients with a history of allergic reactions to plasma should not receive immune globulins. They are given intramuscularly in most instances, but some preparations may be given intravenously. ISG is not generally used for hematologic disorders.

NURSING PROCESS
Transfusion of Blood or Blood Products

NURSING CARE BEFORE TRANSFUSION

Assessment

Assess the patient before administration of blood or blood products. Be sure an informed consent is obtained. Check baseline vital signs and record them. Notify the physician if the patient's temperature is elevated. Ask the patient about a history of transfusion reactions. Assess the patient's level of understanding about the procedure.

Nursing Diagnoses and Planning

Nursing diagnoses and related expected patient outcomes commonly applicable to patients receiving blood transfusions include the following:

NDx: Knowledge deficit: nature of procedure and signs of potential complications

Planning: Patient Outcomes
1. Patient relates accurate information about transfusions and the symptoms of a reaction.
2. Patient reports any unusual symptoms immediately.

Nursing Interventions and Evaluation

NDx: Knowledge deficit: nature of procedure and signs of potential complications
Describe the procedure, length of transfusion, potential for future transfusions, and expected outcomes in terms that are understandable to the patient. Explain the symptoms of a blood reaction and instruct the patient to report any unusual feeling immediately. Allow time for questions and expression of concerns.

Additional Interventions
Before administering blood, check that it has been typed and cross-matched and that the ABO group and Rh match that of the patient. The patient's information is usually on a special page in the chart. Observe for abnormal color or cloudiness, which indicate hemolysis. Check for the presence of gas bubbles, which indicate bacterial growth. Check the expiration date on the blood bag. Return outdated or abnormal blood to the blood bank.

Confirm with another nurse or physician that the patient's name, blood type, Rh factor, and identification number match what is listed on the blood bag before administering the transfusion. Document this confirmation with the signatures of both individuals. Check the same data with the patient's identification bracelet. Many institutions use a separate identification band for blood recipients. Verify this information and document the time, date, and confirmation of the match of data. Do not remove any identification information on the blood container until the transfusion is completed. Most institutions require that the blood container be returned to the laboratory upon completion of the transfusion.

Once the blood is unrefrigerated, begin administration within 1 hour to prevent hemolysis and bacterial growth. The rate of administration varies based on the patient's medical history and need, as well as on the blood product being administered. The physician may order the rate of administration if there are specific concerns related to the patient. Generally, the blood should be administered as rapidly as possible, especially in cases of hemorrhage. It should not take longer than 4 hours to administer 1 unit of blood.

Follow body substance precautions at all times when performing the venipuncture or handling blood products or blood equipment. Start the primary intravenous line with a 19-gauge or larger needle for adults. Use a Y-tubing blood administration set or other equipment as designated by hospital policy. Usually this intravenous tubing has a blood filter attached to screen out fibrin clots or other particles. Only normal saline should be used as the primary solution. The blood may be given without a primary solution, but in the case of a blood reaction, it is helpful to have a vein open when the blood is discontinued. Do not administer other products or drugs through this site while the blood is being infused. Document the date and time the infusion is started and any immediate reaction, if noted. The blood should infuse over 2 to 4 hours.

An electronic infusion device should be used only if recommended by the manufacturer. Follow the instructions for appropriate use. Blood warmers may be indicated to decrease the risk of arrhythmias or cardiac arrest associated with rapid transfusion of cold blood in situations of acute massive blood loss. Follow hospital policy and equipment directions when using the blood warmer.

Keep the recording sheet at the bedside for continued noting of the vital signs and symptoms throughout the transfusions. Check the values of the baseline data and compare for changes.

NURSING CARE DURING TRANSFUSION

Continue to assess the patient during the administration of the blood. Look for early signs of a reaction in the respiratory system, such as tachypnea, apnea, dyspnea, cough, wheezing, or crackles. Check for elevated temperature, chills, chest pain, muscle aches, headache, tingling, and numbness. Assess the cardiovascular system for bradycardia, tachycardia, change in blood pressure, cyanosis, skin temperature changes, and edema. Check the urine output. Look for urticaria, signs of itching, and diaphoresis. Note the patient's vital signs on the record sheet every 15 minutes.

Check the flow rate frequently during administration to be sure the blood is being infused as ordered. Tell the patient to notify the nurse if any unusual symptoms appear. The donor blood may contain viruses, bacteria, or parasites, which is rare, or the patient may be sensitive to leukocytes or platelets. If the blood is contaminated with microorganisms, fever and chills usually develop within 30 minutes after the start of the transfusion. Shock may ensue immediately. Sensitivity to leukocytes or platelets is common, especially in adults who have had previous transfusions or in women who have delivered infants. In sensitivity episodes, fever occurs, but not chills. This reaction is the most common blood transfusion reaction and is usually treated with an antipyretic.

The patient may be sensitive to plasma protein in the blood or to an allergen passed from the donor. To prevent this, people with multiple allergies are usually disqualified as donors. If the patient reacts to an allergen in the blood, the reaction is usually mild and treated with an antihistamine. Note any symptoms of a reaction, even if they are very mild. Severe respiratory distress or cardiac distress usually indicates that the patient has received incompatible blood from the donor. Incompatibility occurs when the red blood cells received from the donor blood clump together in the plasma of the recipient. Enzymes quickly break down the red blood cells, exceeding the liver's ability to detoxify the products of this process, resulting in damage to renal tubules. Although this type of reaction usually occurs within 10 minutes of the start of transfusion, observe the patient throughout the transfusion time for such signs of a severe reaction. Interventions must be started immediately.

In an unconscious patient, also take vital signs every 15 minutes, but observe the patient frequently, because an unconscious patient cannot warn the nurse of untoward symptoms. Look carefully for signs of a reaction in the unconscious patient, which might include a weak pulse, fever, tachycardia or bradycardia, hypotension, and oliguria.

Refer to Nursing Care Guide 12–2 for the care of the patient with a blood transfusion reaction.

NURSING CARE AFTER TRANSFUSION

Assessment

When the transfusion is completed, assess the patient's vital signs and record them along with the date and time. Look for any signs of a latent reaction. Document all pertinent information about the patient's symptoms during the transfusion and at the terminal point of the transfusion.

Remove the equipment, using body fluid precautions, and dispose of the transfusion equipment appropriately according to the institution's policy. Return the blood container to the blood bank. Assess the patient's knowledge level about the signs and symptoms of a delayed blood reaction and when to seek medical attention.

Nursing Diagnoses and Planning

Nursing diagnoses and related expected patient outcomes commonly applicable to patients after blood transfusions include the following:

NDx: Knowledge deficit: nature of delayed transfusion reaction, signs, and symptoms and when to seek medical intervention

Planning: Patient Outcomes
1. Patient relates accurate information about delayed transfusion reactions, the signs and symptoms, and when to seek medical intervention.
2. Patient observes for signs and symptoms of a blood reaction after discharge and seeks medical assistance if symptoms are evident.

Nursing Interventions and Evaluation

NDx: Knowledge deficit: nature of delayed transfusion reaction, signs, and symptoms and when to seek medical intervention
Teach the patient to observe for signs of infection, such as chills, fever, cough, respiratory distress, and circulatory changes. Explain to the patient that any symptoms of respiratory distress should be reported immediately to the physician. An anaphylactic reaction could be life-threatening, and the patient needs to seek assistance at the first signs of a reaction. Tell the patient that signs of a mild reaction may include a rash, itching, low-grade fever, or headache.

Allow the patient and family to ask questions and voice concerns. Have the patient verbalize the signs and symptoms of a reaction to verify understanding. Write the signs on a list for the patient or family to take home with them. Inform them that a reaction may not occur until 2 weeks after transfusion.

Nursing Care Guide 12–2
Patients with a Blood Transfusion Reaction

Assessment Findings: Patient experiences dyspnea, chest pain, feeling of tightness in chest, increased pulse and respirations, hypertension, chills, fever, facial burning within 15 minutes after transfusion begins, low back pain, headache or full feeling in the head, hematuria, anorexia, oliguria, apprehension, neck vein distention, and shock.

Nursing Diagnosis: Risk for injury related to antigen-antibody incompatibility

Patient Outcomes	Nursing Interventions	Rationale
Patient's vital signs are within normal range for patient. Patient indicates that chills, back pain, and headache are absent.	Monitor vital signs. If vital signs change or other untoward symptoms appear, discontinue blood transfusion. Also complete the following: Notify physician stat. Keep intravenous line open with saline. Draw client's blood for hemoglobin (Hgb), culture, and retyping; obtain urinalysis; and observe voidings. Return remaining blood and tubing to blood bank for repeat typing and culture. Reassure patient. Cover patient with blanket. Administer diuretics and colloids as ordered. If there is a history of previous reactions, may administer diphenhydramine (Benadryl) prophylactically.	Although the nurse may not prevent a transfusion reaction, appropriate nursing interventions are important to minimize the trauma of the reaction to the patient. The blood is rechecked for errors in typing and cross-matching.

Evaluation: Compare the patient's status with the expected outcomes. If the outcomes are not met, reassess the patient and revise the plan.

Assessment Findings: Patient experiences weakness, fatigue 1 to 2 weeks after transfusion, decreased Hgb, and positive Coombs' test results.

Nursing Diagnosis: Altered health maintenance related to lack of knowledge of delayed antigen-antibody incompatibility

Patient Outcomes	Nursing Interventions	Rationale
Patient states accurate information about the reaction and potential for a delayed reaction. Patient states the signs and symptoms of a delayed reaction.	Inform patient that this reaction is not dangerous and that subsequent transfusions may cause an acute hemolytic reaction. Instruct patient in signs and symptoms of a delayed reaction.	By knowing to expect a reaction, the patient will be alert to early signs of problems. A transfusion reaction can be delayed by up to 2 weeks after the infusion.

(continued)

Nursing Care Guide 12–2
Patients with a Blood Transfusion Reaction (continued)

Patient Outcomes	Nursing Interventions	Rationale
Patient verbalizes the need to contact medical personnel if symptoms of a reaction become apparent.	Instruct patient to notify the nurse or physician if signs or symptoms are evident. Check Hgb levels if patient experiences signs or symptoms.	Immediate intervention reduces the risk of complications.

Evaluation: Compare the patient's status with the expected outcomes. If the outcomes are not met, reassess the patient and revise the plan.

Assessment Findings: Patient is experiencing fever, chills, headache, flushing, tachycardia, palpitations, nausea, vomiting, diarrhea, malaise, and lumbar pain.

Nursing Diagnosis: Risk for infection related to bacterial pyogens transfused through blood

Patient Outcomes	Nursing Interventions	Rationale
Patient remains free of signs and symptoms of a pyogenic reaction. Patient's vital signs are within normal ranges for the patient.	Discontinue blood transfusion. Notify physician stat. Keep vein open with saline. Monitor vital signs. Reassure patient and family. Premedicate with antipyretic.	Appropriate nursing interventions reduce risk of further complications. Changes in vital signs may indicate complications.

Evaluation: Compare the patient's status with the expected outcomes. If the outcomes are not met, reassess the patient and revise the plan.

Assessment Findings: Patient is experiencing dyspnea, nausea, vomiting, urticaria, rash, itching, hives, facial flushing, wheezing, hypotension, shock, diarrhea, tight chest, and anxiety, but no fever.

Nursing Diagnosis: Risk for injury related to allergic reaction

Patient Outcomes	Nursing Interventions	Rationale
Patient remains free of signs and symptoms of an allergic reaction.	Discontinue transfusion. Keep vein open with saline. Notify physician stat. Resume transfusion slowly if the only symptoms are itching, hives, urticaria, rash, and anxiety.	Although the nurse may not prevent an allergic reaction, appropriate nursing interventions are important to minimize the trauma of the reaction.
Vital signs remain within normal range for patient.	Administer antihistamines and monitor vital signs.	Vital sign changes may indicate complications.

(continued)

Nursing Care Guide 12-2
Patients with a Blood Transfusion Reaction (continued)

Patient Outcomes	Nursing Interventions	Rationale
Patient indicates that symptoms of a reaction are absent.	If symptoms progress, discontinue transfusion, obtain urinalysis, draw patient's blood, notify blood bank, and return remaining blood and tubing. Administer diphenhydramine 15 to 20 minutes before the transfusion, as ordered, if the patient is suspected to have allergies. Give epinephrine, vasopressors, and crystalloids, if ordered.	The blood is rechecked for proper typing and cross-matching if the reaction continues.

Evaluation: Compare the patient's status with the expected outcomes. If the outcomes are not met, reassess the patient and revise the plan.

Assessment Findings: Patient is experiencing dyspnea; dry cough; rales in lungs; crackles at base of lungs; tightness in chest; bounding pulse; increased blood pressure; orthopnea; cyanosis; tachycardia; neck vein distention; anxiety; coughing of pink, frothy sputum; cold, clammy skin; and restlessness.

Nursing Diagnosis: Fluid volume excess related to circulatory overload from blood transfusion

Patient Outcomes	Nursing Interventions	Rationale
Patient's skin color remains pink, and skin is dry to touch.	Position patient upright. Check the skin for edema, color, and integrity, especially in the extremities.	Fluid pooling, especially in the extremities, is a sign of fluid overload.
Patient's vital signs remain within normal range for patient. Patient's lungs remain clear upon auscultation. Patient denies respiratory or circulatory distress. Peripheral and pulmonary edema are absent.	Monitor vital signs and venous pressure. Monitor lung sounds. Apply rotating tourniquets if ordered. Administer diuretics, oxygen, morphine, vasodilators, and aminophylline if ordered.	Vital sign changes, such as increasing pulse rate and blood pressure, may indicate fluid overload. Adventitious breath sounds may result from pulmonary edema from the fluid overload.

Evaluation Compare the patient's status with the expected outcomes. If the outcomes are not met, reassess the patient and revise the plan.

Compare the patient's status with the expected outcomes. If the outcomes are not met, reassess the patient and revise the plan.

TYPES OF TRANSFUSION REACTIONS

There are several types of transfusion reactions that a patient receiving donor blood may experience. An acute hemolytic reaction is caused by infusion of ABO-incompatible blood. This may occur in transfusions of whole blood, packed red blood cells, or blood components containing red blood cells (10 mL or more). Antigens from the donor's red blood cells react with the patient's antibodies, causing the clinical manifestations. This reaction may cause some of the most severe symptoms.

A febrile, nonhemolytic reaction is the most common type that blood recipients experience. It is caused by sensitization to the donor's platelets, proteins, or white blood cells. The reaction is usually treated symptomatically and the transfusion discontinued. Rarely is the reaction life-threatening.

A mild allergic reaction is caused by sensitivity to plasma proteins. The patient may experience a rash, some itching, and a low-grade fever. Antihistamines may be given, if needed.

An anaphylactic reaction is caused by the infusion of a specific protein to a patient who is deficient in the protein but has developed antibodies to it. The patient may experience mild to severe symptoms.

A circulatory overload is a rare transfusion reaction. It is caused by rapid fluid administration in a patient with a circulatory system unable to accommodate the volume. This may occur in the patient with a history of previous cardiac problems.

A septic reaction occurs when contaminated blood is transfused into the patient. The onset of symptoms is usually immediate. The patient experiences fever, chills, hypotension, and shock. It is treated with intravenous antibiotics and symptomatically.

A delayed transfusion reaction may occur several days to 2 weeks after the transfusion. Before discharge, the patient should be taught symptoms of a delayed transfusion reaction (Highlight 12–6) and told to seek medical intervention if any symptoms are evident. Delayed reactions can be caused by hemolytic reactions, hepatitis B, hepatitis C, human immunodeficiency virus infection, iron overload, or other infectious diseases in the donor blood. See Nursing Care Guide 12–2.

Management of Transfusion Reactions

Treatment instituted for a transfusion depends on the severity of the reaction. The administration of the blood is usually discontinued, but in cases of very mild reactions, administration can be continued with careful, continual monitoring of the patient's status. In life-threatening situations, emergency care is instituted immediately. Shock, respiratory distress, and cardiac arrhythmias are reversed with a variety of drugs and support interventions. Hypotension is treated with vasoconstrictors. Renal damage is prevented by administering intravenous colloids. Mannitol may be ordered as an osmotic diuretic. An indwelling catheter may be inserted to monitor urine output. If it is not adequate, acute renal tubular necrosis may have developed, and mannitol is contraindicated. The patient is then placed on fluid restriction, and dialysis may be necessary. In cases of mild reactions, antihistamines or antipyretics may be ordered.

Nursing Interventions

When a transfusion reaction occurs, follow the steps as listed below:

1. Stop the transfusion.
2. Keep the vein open with the primary solution.
3. Take vital signs, have a nurse stay with the patient, and document the symptoms.
4. Institute appropriate interventions if life-threatening symptoms appear.
5. Report the reaction to the physician and the blood bank.
6. Institute medical orders.
7. Send the blood container with attached labels to the blood bank.
8. Collect urine and blood samples and send to the laboratory.
9. Document the symptoms, treatment instituted, patient reaction, and follow-up care.
10. Explain the situation to the patient and family, reassure them, make the patient comfortable, and continue to observe for further symptoms.

SURGICAL MANAGEMENT

Splenectomy

In the adult patient, the spleen can be removed without complications, despite the organ's important role in the hematologic system. After splenectomy, the role of the spleen is taken over by the liver, lymph nodes, and bone marrow.

Uses

A splenectomy is performed for dysfunction of the organ as seen in many hematologic diseases, for

---

HIGHLIGHT
12–6

PATIENT EDUCATION

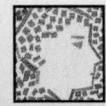

Signs and Symptoms of Delayed Transfusion Reactions

Teach the patient and family to observe for:

Respiratory system symptoms: tachypnea, dyspnea, apnea, wheezing, cyanosis, and rales.

Circulatory system symptoms: tachycardia, chest pain, palpitations, muscle aches, headache, chills, tingling, numbness, weakness, and fever.

Urinary system symptoms: oliguria and pain or burning with urination.

Integumentary system symptoms: itching, edema, cyanosis, rashes, and excessive perspiration.

rupture of the spleen due to trauma, and for tearing of the organ during abdominal surgery. Hypersplenism, a condition in which the spleen excessively destroys blood components, is another indication for a splenectomy. Splenomegaly, anemia, leukopenia, and compensatory increase in blood cell production by the bone marrow are all signs of hypersplenism. *Primary hypersplenism* describes overactivity of the spleen of unknown cause. *Secondary hypersplenism* describes overactivity of the spleen because of another disease. Primary hypersplenism is found in patients with idiopathic thrombocytopenia purpura and congenital spherocytosis. Secondary hypersplenism is found in patients with leukemia, lymphoma, and Hodgkin's disease.

The treatment of choice for primary hypersplenism is a splenectomy, which alleviates the disease in 60 to 80% of patients. In secondary hypersplenism, a splenectomy is only a palliative treatment for some of the symptoms of the disease. It does not change the major course of the disorder.

Procedure

A splenectomy is performed much like other abdominal surgeries under general anesthesia. Because the organ is very vascular and may be extremely enlarged as a result of overactivity, the surgery carries the risk of hemorrhage and can be quite difficult to perform. However, in most cases, the prognosis is excellent and the mortality rate is very low.

Patient Preparation

Preoperatively, the patient is informed about the procedure, risks, and postoperative course. After an informed consent is obtained from the patient, physical preparation begins. The patient's abdomen is prepped as designated by hospital procedure. A preoperative checklist is completed, and preoperative medication is administered.

Postoperative Course

If the patient does not have other disease complications, the postoperative course after a splenectomy is usually uneventful. Most patients are discharged in a few days with instructions for home care. Postoperatively, the patient is maintained on intravenous fluids until vital signs are stable and gastrointestinal function returns. A nasogastric tube may be inserted before or during surgery. The patient will have a sterile dressing on the abdomen, which is changed as needed. Prophylactic antibiotic therapy and analgesics may be ordered. Providing there are no other complicating factors, the patient is instructed about signs of bleeding and infection, how to change dressings, activity restrictions for a couple of weeks, and when to return to the physician for follow-up care. The patient is then discharged from the hospital. The patient with other interfering factors, such as a hematologic disease like leukemia, may be hospitalized for several days to weeks and may undergo many other treatment modalities instituted for the primary disease problem.

Complications

If the spleen is extremely enlarged, the surgery may be very difficult. Since it is a highly vascular organ, hemorrhage is the major risk during surgery. Postoperatively, the most common complications include infection, bleeding, and interference with healing from other complicating factors from the primary disease.

NURSING PROCESS
Splenectomy

PREOPERATIVE NURSING CARE

Assessment

Complete a physical assessment of the patient. Look for signs of respiratory distress, circulatory problems, and nutritional deficits and determine the patient's general health status to prepare for potential problems in the postoperative period. Assess the patient's understanding of the surgery, the postoperative course, and the self-care responsibilities after discharge.

Nursing Diagnoses and Planning

Nursing diagnoses and related expected patient outcomes commonly applicable to patients scheduled for splenectomy include the following:

NDx: Knowledge deficit: surgical procedure and postoperative course

Planning: Patient Outcomes
1. Patient states accurate information about the surgical procedure and expected results.
2. Patient describes the typical postoperative course.

Nursing Interventions and Evaluation

NDx: Knowledge deficit: surgical procedure and postoperative course
Explain to the patient about the surgical procedure, the recovery period, and the postoperative care required. Tell the patient about the intravenous therapy typically used, what discomforts to expect, and the preventive methods used to arrest respiratory problems after surgery. Allow time for questions and concerns from the patient and family.

Compare the patient's status with the expected outcomes. If the outcomes are not met, reassess the patient and revise the plan.

POSTOPERATIVE NURSING CARE

Assessment

Assess the patient's vital signs, orientation, and dressings and the intravenous solutions. Check for signs of discomfort and medicate accordingly. Check respiratory status and the patient's ability to cough and breathe deeply and auscultate the chest. Assess for patient's voiding within a reasonable time postoperatively. Look for abdominal swelling and drainage on or around the dressing.

Nursing Diagnoses and Planning

Nursing diagnoses and related expected patient outcomes commonly applicable after a splenectomy include the following:

NDx: Pain related to surgical incision and manipulation

Planning: Patient Outcomes
1. Patient states pain is relieved or is at a tolerable level.
2. Patient moves freely and is able to turn, cough, and breathe deeply without extreme discomfort.

NDx: Risk for infection related to abdominal wound, intravenous lines, and respiratory status

Planning: Patient Outcomes
1. Patient's vital signs are within normal range for the patient.
2. Patient's wound shows no signs of infection, such as purulent drainage or inflammation.

NDx: Knowledge deficit: self-care after discharge

Planning: Patient Outcomes
1. Patient relates accurate information about care needed after discharge.
2. Patient states the need for follow-up medical care.
3. Patient identifies signs of complications and the need to seek medical assistance if signs appear.

Nursing Interventions and Evaluation

NDx: Pain
Administer analgesics as ordered and needed. Encourage the patient to move frequently, to splint the abdomen when turning and coughing, and to request medication before the pain becomes intolerable.

NDx: Risk for infection
Have the patient frequently turn, cough, and breathe deeply. Explain the reason for this intervention and encourage the patient to perform the routine often while lying in bed. Get the patient up as soon as allowed. Encourage frequent position changes. Use aseptic technique when changing the abdominal dressing and when handling the IV equipment.

NDx: Knowledge deficit: self-care after discharge
Teach the patient how to care for the surgical wound and how to complete an aseptic dressing

change. Explain the signs and symptoms of complications and when to seek medical intervention. Tell the patient about any physical restrictions the physician has ordered and when to visit the physician's office for follow-up care.

Compare the patient's status with the expected outcomes. If the outcomes are not met, reassess the patient and revise the plan.

Other Surgical Procedures and Medical Treatments

BONE MARROW TRANSPLANT

Bone marrow transplantation is used to treat hematologic disorders such as aplastic anemia and leukemia and to treat severe bone marrow depression resulting from other therapeutic interventions. Refer to Chapter 32 for a description of bone marrow transplantation and nursing care applicable to the patient receiving a bone marrow transplant.

RADIATION THERAPY

The goal of radiation therapy for the patient with a hematologic disorder is usually to destroy malignant tissue growth with minimal damage to the normal tissue. Tissue cells more susceptible to radiation include hematopoietic cells of the bone marrow and lymphocytes. Radiation therapy is used to treat Hodgkin's disease, localized non-Hodgkin's disease, some leukemias, and multiple myeloma. Radioactive isotopes may be implanted internally to deliver direct radiation in polycythemia vera. Agranulocytosis is a major complication of radiation therapy. Refer to Chapter 32 for nursing care of the patient receiving radiation therapy.

CHEMOTHERAPY

Chemotherapy is the primary treatment used for patients with leukemia, multiple myeloma, and Hodgkin's disease. Chemotherapy may also be used to treat patients with polycythemia vera and nonlocalized Hodgkin's disease. The choice of chemotherapy, combinations of drugs, and frequency of therapy depends on the specific hematologic disease, its severity, and patient response to treatment. Refer to Chapter 34 for a description of chemotherapeutic agents and nursing care of the patient receiving chemotherapy. See Chapter 13 for the chemotherapeutic agents used for each specific hematologic disease.

The Elderly: Special Considerations

The older adult is prone to developing certain blood disorders. One reason for this is the decrease in the immunologic defense system, meaning the body's ability to protect against infections and malignancies is lowered. Anemia, one of the most common hematologic disorders of older adults, may develop secondary to disease conditions, poor eating habits, or other factors that interfere with adequate nutrition. Some types of leukemia are commonly found in the older adult. The older the person, the more likely that symptoms will be more severe and the progression of the disease more rapid.

In older adults, disorders of the blood-forming organs are usually caused by something other than hematologic problems. Cancer of the gastrointestinal system that metastasizes to the spleen, lymph, bone, or liver is common. Cancer of the liver as the primary site is also frequently found in older adults. Prostatic cancer may metastasize to the bone in older men. Interference with the production of blood clotting factors results in bleeding problems and reduced oxygen-carrying capacity.

Delayed wound healing associated with anemia may be exacerbated in the elderly as a result of reduced vascularity because of increased capillary fragility. Bruising may be associated with hematologic problems or with senile purpura. An increased risk of pressure sores is associated with deficiencies of protein, calories, and vitamins.

Chapter Review

1. What role does the liver play in blood formation and clotting?
2. How does a low hemoglobin and hematocrit value affect the patient's tolerance to exercise and why?
3. What signs might you note on assessment if the patient has a low platelet count?
4. What nursing interventions should be undertaken to prevent ulcerative lesions?
5. Why do patients with malignancies or other disorders involving the leukocytes have an increased susceptibility to infection?
6. What is important to include in your patient teaching plan when trying to prevent the dietary deficiencies seen in hematologic disorders?
7. What are differential white blood cells, and why are they important?
8. What nursing care is involved with patients undergoing a blood transfusion?
9. What would you include in a teaching plan for the patient about to undergo a splenectomy?
10. Why are the elderly more prone to develop certain hematologic disorders?

Bibliography

Bradbury M, Cruickshank JP. Blood and blood transfusion reactions: 1. Br J Nurs 1995; 4(14):814.

Burns JM, Tierney DK, Long GD, et al. Critical pathway for administering high-dose chemotherapy followed by peripheral blood stem cell rescue in the outpatient setting. Oncol Nurs Forum 1995; 22(8):1219.

Campbell J. Making sense of the technique of venipuncture. Nurs Times 1995; 90(31):29.

Carpenito LJ. Nursing care plans and documentation: Nursing diagnosis and collaborative problems. 2nd ed. Philadelphia: JB Lippincott, 1995.

Carroll PA. When a Jehovah's Witness refuses a transfusion. Nursing 1995; 25(8):60.

Dickson SL. Understanding the oxyhemoglobin dissociation curve. Crit Care Nurse 1995; 15(5):54.

Doenges ME, Moorhouse MF. Nurse's pocket guide: Nursing diagnoses with interventions. 5th ed. Philadelphia: FA Davis, 1996.

Duhadway N. Transfusion reaction. Home Healthc Nurse 1995; 13(6):73.

Esmon CT. Cell mediated events that control blood coagulation and vascular injury. Annu Rev Cell Biol 1993;9:1.

Gaedeke MK. Lab test tips: Evaluating serum ferritin levels. Nursing 1995; 25(10):67.

Gawlikowski J. White cells at war. Am J Nurs 1992; 92(3):45.

Goodnough LT. Current red blood cell transfusion practice. AACN Clin Issues Adv Pract Acute Crit Care 1996; 7(2):212.

Graydon JE, Bubela N, Irvine D, Vincent L. Fatigue-reducing strategies used by patients receiving treatment for cancer. Cancer Nurs 1995; 18(1):23.

Harovas J, Anthony H. Managing transfusion reactions. RN 1993; 56(12):32.

Higgins C. Full blood count (RBC, Hb, PCV, MCV, MCH and reticulocytes). Nurs Times 1995; 91(7): 38.

Higgins C. Deficiency testing for iron, vitamin B_{12}, and folate. Nurs Times 1995; 91(22):38.

Higgins C. Blood transfusions: Risks and benefits. Br J Nurs 1994; 3(19):986.

Higgins C. Haematology blood testing for anaemia. Br J Nurs 1995; 4(5):248.

Higgins VL. Leukocyte-reduced blood components: Patient benefits and practice application. Oncol Nurs Forum 1996; 23(4):659.

Hirsh J, Dalen JE, Deykin D, Poller L, Bussey H. Oral anticoagulants: Mechanism of action, clinical effectiveness, and optimal therapeutic range. Chest 1996; 108(4):2315.

Holder D. Psychosocial effects of bone marrow transplantation. Nurs Times 1994; 90(39):44.

Kessinger A. Utilization of peripheral blood stem cells in autotransplantation. Hematol Oncol Clin North Am 1993; 7(3):535.

Laxson CJ, Titler MG. Drawing coagulation studies from arterial lines: An integrative literature review. Am J Crit Care 1994; 3(1):16.

Levine TT. Blood transfusions: Playing it safe. Nursing 1996; 26(4):50.

Luchtman-Jones L, Broze GJ. The current status of coagulation. Ann Med 1995; 27(1):47.

Mannucci PM. Mechanisms, markers and management of coagulation activation. Br Med Bull 1994; 50(4):851.

Martin J. Red cell physiology. Biomed Instrum Technol 1995; 29(2):150.

Meagher RC, Herzig RH. Techniques of harvesting and cryopreservation of stem cells. Hematol Oncol Clin North Am 1993; 7(3):501.

Noureddine SN. Research review: Use of activated clotting time to monitor heparin therapy in coronary patients. Am J Crit Care 1995; 4(4):272.

Oertel LB. International normalized ratio (INR): An improved way to monitor oral anticoagulation therapy. Nurse Pract 1995; 20(9):15.

Rapaport SI. Blood coagulation and its alterations in hemorrhagic and thrombotic disorders. West J Med 1993; 158:153.

Speicher CE. The right test: A physician's guide to laboratory medicine. Philadelphia: WB Saunders, 1993.

Spencer KW. Medications that may increase tendency to bleed. Plast Surg Nurs 1995; 15(4):237.

Tiesinga LJ, Dassen TWN, Halfens RJG. Fatigue: A summary of the definition, dimensions, and indicators. Nurs Diagn 1996; 7(2):51.

Tranter J. Making sense of blood transfusion. Nurs Times 1995; 91(36):34.

United States Public Health Service. Put prevention into practice: Preventive care for anemia. J Am Acad Nurse Pract 1994; 6(6):267.

Walters MC, Abelson HT. Interpretation of the complete blood count. Pediat Clin North Am 1996; 43(3):599.

Watson J, Jaffe MS. Nurse's manual of laboratory and diagnostic tests. Philadelphia: FA Davis, 1995.

Weber MS. Clinical snapshot: Chemotherapy-induced nausea and vomiting. Am J Nurs 1995; 95(4):34.

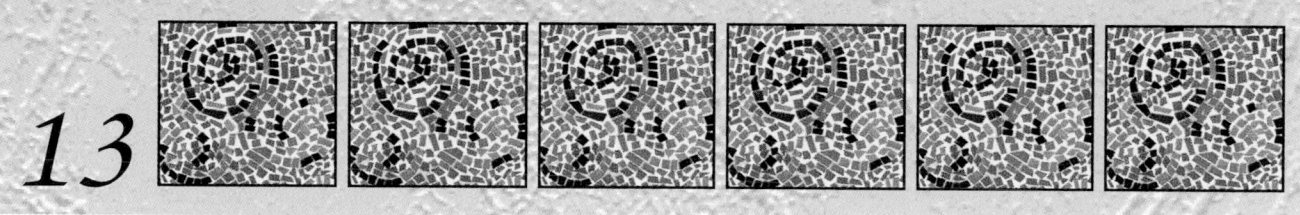

13

Nursing Care of Patients with Hematologic Disorders

Study Outcomes

After studying this chapter, you should be able to:

1. Describe the etiology, pathophysiology, clinical manifestations, diagnostic procedures, and management of common hematologic disorders.
2. Analyze pharmacologic therapies for the anemias and leukemias.
3. Identify information and physical examination data essential to the assessment of patients with common hematologic disorders.
4. State nursing diagnoses and related expected patient outcomes commonly applicable to patients with hematologic disorders.
5. Describe nursing interventions, with their rationales, commonly applicable to patients with hematologic disorders.
6. Explain the basis for evaluation of nursing care provided to patients with hematologic disorders.
7. Identify alternative treatment and care settings for patients with hematologic disorders and services related to community-based care.
8. Identify special considerations for the elderly patient with a hematologic disorder.

Hematologic disorders have many characteristics in common. Consequently, many different hematologic disorders require similar types of nursing assessments and interventions. In all cases, a thorough multisystem assessment and patient history are critical to effective nursing care. Long-term care is necessary for patients with many hematologic disorders because of the chronic nature of the disease. Patient and family education is important for continuing health maintenance. Referrals to other health-care professionals, such as home health nurses, psychologists, and nutritionists, may be required.

Disorders of the blood and blood-forming organs are treated in a variety of settings. Treatment most frequently takes place in outpatient settings such as doctor's offices or clinics. However, the patient may be hospitalized if the disease progresses to a critical stage, and the patient requires close observation or protection from infection.

*E*rythrocyte-Related Disorders

ANEMIAS

Etiology and Pathophysiology

Anemia is the medical term used to describe a low red blood cell count and a low hemoglobin or hematocrit level. Anemia results from bone marrow failure, excessive loss of red blood cells through hemorrhage or destruction, or a combination of these factors. Marrow failure may be caused by nutritional deficiency, toxic exposure, tumor invasion, or unknown factors. Loss of red blood cells may result from hemorrhage, decreased red blood cell production, or increased red blood cell destruction. Red blood cell lysis occurs predominantly in the liver and spleen.

Anemias can be classified by etiology or morphology. The etiologic classification system includes the following three groups.

ANEMIAS ASSOCIATED WITH BLOOD LOSS. In hemorrhagic anemias, the patient loses a large number of erythrocytes and experiences a severe decrease in blood volume and oxygen in the blood. The patient's prognosis depends on the rate and location of bleeding and on the volume of blood lost. Most people experience fewer effects when they lose blood slowly. In fact, slow loss of a large volume of blood may cause less trauma than rapid loss of even a small volume of blood. In the latter situation, the quick change in volume creates a major shock to the system. Acute hemorrhage may result from a severed blood vessel (as in a traumatic injury), rupture of an aneurysm, or tearing or erosion of an artery.

ANEMIAS ASSOCIATED WITH DECREASED RED BLOOD CELL PRODUCTION. In these hypoproliferative anemias, the red blood cell count declines because the bone marrow produces inadequate numbers of cells. This may result from damage to the marrow by drugs or chemicals, lack of erythropoietin (as in renal disease), or a lack of iron, vitamin B_{12}, or folic acid.

ANEMIAS ASSOCIATED WITH RED BLOOD CELL DESTRUCTION. Anemias resulting from hemolysis (called hemolytic anemias) may indicate red blood cell abnormality. This may occur in association with inherited hemolytic anemias, such as spherocytosis, sickle-cell anemia, thalassemia, and glucose-6-phosphate dehydrogenase deficiency. If the abnormality occurs in the plasma, it may be indicative of an acquired hemolytic anemia, such as immune hemolytic anemia.

The morphologic classification system includes these three groups:

NORMOCYTIC, NORMOCHROMIC ANEMIA. In this type of anemia, red blood cells are normal in size (normocytic) and normal in the amount of hemoglobin (normochromic). Anemias in this group include hemorrhagic anemia, anemia of chronic disease, and some forms of aplastic anemia.

MICROCYTIC, HYPOCHROMIC ANEMIA. In this type of anemia, red blood cells are small (microcytic) and contain low amounts of hemoglobin (hypochromic). Red blood cells may also have an abnormal shape. This group includes thalassemia, iron deficiency, renal failure, and sideroblastic anemia.

MACROCYTIC ANEMIA. In this type of anemia, red blood cells are larger than normal (macrocytic). This group includes some forms of aplastic anemia, megaloblastic anemia, and liver disease.

Clinical Manifestations

Anemia can produce a wide range of clinical manifestations. Perhaps the most common is pale skin, which develops as peripheral vessels constrict to maintain oxygen levels in essential organs. Also common is fatigue and a constant feeling of tiredness, particularly as hemoglobin levels drop to 9 or 10 mg/dL. Other common manifestations include weakness, lethargy, dizziness, or fainting. Later in the disorder, patients may become disoriented from cerebral anoxia and fever. Mucous membranes may become edematous or may bleed because a low oxyhemoglobin level decreases tissue oxygenation. Clubbing of the nails may develop from chronic hypoxia.

If red blood cells are being broken down, the patient's skin and sclerae will become discolored. This occurs because red blood cells release bilirubin as they break down. Discoloration occurs when bilirubin levels reach 1.5 mg/100 mL of blood. Free hemoglobin appears in the plasma and diffuses through the renal glomeruli into the urine. Cloudy or bloody urine and tarry stools may indicate bleeding from within.

A person with severe anemia usually experiences dyspnea, palpitations, irritability, headache, anorexia, and other gastrointestinal disturbances related to tissue hypoxia from red blood cell loss or marrow failure. Symptoms worsen after exercise. The person may also exhibit tachycardia, tachypnea, systolic heart murmur, and poor skin turgor.

Chills may occur if blood is shunted to major vessels or to areas of greater need. Thermoreceptors in the tissue may be dulled from oxygen deprivation. Elimination patterns may change from atrophy of the gastrointestinal mucosa.

Diagnosis

Anemia is diagnosed from the patient's medical and social history, physical assessment, and laboratory studies of red blood cell count, red blood cell indices, hemoglobin, hematocrit, and bone marrow. Analysis of blood gases may be needed if the patient has symptoms of hypoxia.

Management

Medical management for anemia depends on the cause and varies with the results of the patient's laboratory tests. Treatment for serious cases may include oxygen therapy and intravenous therapy, including blood transfusions. Epoetin alfa may be used to treat anemia related to chronic disease or chemotherapy (Highlight 13–1). Antipyretic medications are used to reduce fever. Analgesics and joint immobilization are used to reduce pain. Medications such as stool softeners, laxatives, and antidiarrheals may be used according to the patient's needs. Nutritional supplements to provide additional proteins, iron, vitamins, and calories may be used.

❖ Settings, Providers, and Collaboration for Care

Most anemias are detected and treated in the doctor's office or outpatient clinic. Patients may be hospitalized for treatment of the underlying cause of anemia or if the condition is severe enough that the patient needs close observation. Referrals to a home health nurse for nutrition assessment, education, and follow-up may be indicated.

NURSING PROCESS
Anemia

Assessment

Obtain the patient's medical history and conduct a physical examination. Because fatigue is one of the most common signs of anemia, assess the patient's level of physical activity, ability to perform the usual activities of daily living, and sleep and rest patterns. Check vital signs and observe for shortness of breath on exertion and elevated heart rate.

Check for signs of bleeding such as bruising, petechiae, and ecchymoses. Assess for bloody urine or tarry stools. It is important to determine the cause of anemia. If it is chronic blood loss, the site of bleeding should be determined and treated before the treatment of anemia will be effective.

Inspect the mouth, tongue, and gums for redness or pallor, soreness, and ulcers. Observe for disorien-

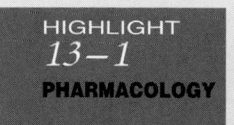 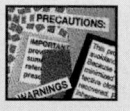

HIGHLIGHT
13–1
PHARMACOLOGY
Epoetin Alfa

Definition:

A glycoprotein used in the treatment of anemia associated with chronic disease or chemotherapy in cancer patients.

Commercial Preparations:

Procrit

Epogen

Supplied as single-dose vials. Keep refrigerated. Give IV or SC. Usual dose is 50–150 U/kg administered subcutaneously three times weekly.

Action:

Is a natural erythropoietin that stimulates red blood cell production.

Side Effects:

Generally well tolerated. Patient may experience a rise in blood pressure. Rarely, patient may experience flu-like symptoms, transient rash, urticaria, and seizures.

Interactions:

None known. Should not be administered with other medications because its stability and compatibility with other drugs is unknown.

Nursing Implications:

Remove from refrigerator about 30 minutes before administering and roll vial between hands to warm before administering. Do not use if medicine appears cloudy or discolored.

Once therapy is initiated, hematocrit should be evaluated weekly.

Patient should be educated about purpose and administration of the drug, as well as monitoring of therapy.

During therapy, monitor the patient for symptoms related to anemia.

Assess blood pressure before and during therapy.

Monitor serum iron and serum ferritin levels.

It may take 2 to 8 weeks for anemia symptoms to improve.

Most patients receiving epoetin alfa also require iron supplements to support erythropoiesis.

tation, cyanosis, and pallor in the face, conjunctivae, mouth, and nails caused by decreased hemoglobin levels.

Evaluate hydration by noting skin turgor, weight loss, sunken eyes, and dry skin. Check for pruritus by observing for signs of scratching, such as red marks, lesions, and scabs. Ask the patient about daily food and fluid intake. A dietary deficiency could be the major cause of the anemia.

Assess for abdominal distention, diarrhea, constipation, or flatus, which may be caused by the anemia, drug treatment, or fluid loss. Check for splenomegaly and hepatomegaly, because red blood cell lysis occurs in the spleen and liver.

Assess the patient's level of knowledge about the disorder, treatment, and care needed and instruct accordingly. Allow the patient to ask questions and verbalize concerns. Invite the family to participate when appropriate.

Nursing Diagnoses and Planning

Nursing diagnoses and related expected patient outcomes commonly applicable to patients with anemia include the following:

NDx: Activity intolerance related to decreased oxygen-carrying capacity of the blood

Planning: Patient Outcomes
1. Patient follows a regimen of planned activities and rest periods each day.
2. Patient states that he or she feels less fatigued and demonstrates signs of increased activity.
3. Patient is able to perform activities of daily living.
4. Patient's vital signs are within normal ranges for the patient.
5. Patient denies shortness of breath on mild exertion.

NDx: Knowledge deficit: nature of the disease, nutritional needs, treatment, and measures to prevent recurrence

Planning: Patient Outcomes
1. Patient describes cause, effects, and clinical course of anemia.
2. Patient lists symptoms of anemia and treatments.
3. Patient relates the nutritional therapy for anemia.
4. Patient describes the self-care needed to prevent recurrence or complications of anemia.

Nursing Interventions and Evaluation

NDx: Activity intolerance
Instruct the patient to develop a regimen of activity that includes frequent rest periods throughout the day. Encourage the patient to do range-of-motion exercises frequently while lying in bed to maintain muscle tone and strength. Tell the patient to avoid

sudden movements, such as getting out of bed quickly, because they decrease the blood supply to the brain, aggravating vertigo and disorientation. Have the patient practice deep-breathing exercises to increase oxygen and blood to the brain.

Teach the patient to practice energy-saving techniques to reduce fatigue and shortness of breath. Place frequently used articles within the patient's reach.

Provide and encourage frequent rest periods while delivering patient care. Prevent interruptions during rest periods and at night, whenever possible. Reduce any disturbing noises and limit visitors as necessary.

Provide warm clothes and blankets to prevent chilling. Avoid unnecessary exposure to drafts or extreme changes in temperature. Anemia leads to peripheral vasoconstriction. Therefore, the patient feels cool and is more susceptible to changes in temperature.

Encourage good nutrition to increase the patient's energy level. Offer four to six meals daily. This is less tiring for the patient and prevents gastric overdistention. Ask for a consultation with the dietitian.

NDx: Knowledge deficit: nature of the disease, nutritional needs, treatment, and measures to prevent recurrence

Explain the cause, effects, and clinical course of the disorder to the patient. Allow for questions from the patient at any time. Provide appropriate literature about anemia for the patient and family to review. Allow the patient to verbalize concerns and fears. Evaluate discharge needs of the patient and family.

Alert the patient to signs and symptoms of anemia, such as fatigue and disorientation from low levels of oxygen. Teach the patient to use safety measures or ask for assistance when out of bed or when ambulating. Stress the need for uninterrupted rest periods and 6 to 10 hours of sleep every night.

Instruct the patient about dietary modifications needed to reduce symptoms or prevent recurrence of the disorder. Explain the need for increases in dietary nutrients specific to the type of anemia present. Initiate counseling with a dietitian to assist with meal planning if needed (Highlight 13–2).

Teach the patient the signs of bleeding to observe for and when to seek medical assistance. Explain the need to avoid sharp objects, straight razors, contact sports, and injections and venipuncture whenever possible.

Explain proper oral hygiene methods necessary to prevent further irritation and ulceration of mucous membranes. Instruct the patient to use a soft toothbrush and to use mouthrinse frequently. Show how to inspect the oral cavity, checking the tongue and gums for early signs of irritation. Teach the patient to avoid extremely hot, spicy foods and

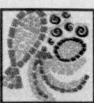

HIGHLIGHT 13–2
NUTRITION

Special Considerations for Patients with Iron Deficiency Anemia

Instruct patients with iron deficiency anemia to:

Increase dietary iron intake by eating foods such as meat, fish, and poultry.

Add fortified breads and cereals, dark green vegetables, and fruits (such as raisins, prunes, and apricots) to the diet.

Take iron supplements with food only if intolerable without food. Take iron with orange juice, because the juice may promote iron absorption. Refrain from taking iron supplements with milk or antacids, because they may reduce iron absorption.

Eat some high-fiber foods to prevent constipation, especially if taking iron supplements and increased dietary iron. Keep in mind, however, that a high-fiber diet may reduce iron absorption by moving food through the intestine more quickly.

Drink an increased amount of fluids daily to prevent constipation.

acidic drinks to lessen oral and gastrointestinal irritation.

Teach the patient how to achieve comfort by frequent repositioning and padding of bony prominences. Instruct the family to apply lotion to the skin to keep it supple and elastic. Tell the patient to avoid using heating pads, because thermoreceptors in the tissue may be dulled from oxygen deprivation. Explain the use of a bed cradle to prevent pressure on joints and sensitive areas.

Teach the patient the dosage, route, time, frequency, side effects, and toxic effects of any medication prescribed. Explain the diagnostic studies completed and the need for any follow-up studies after discharge. Include the family in the teaching sessions when appropriate.

Compare the patient's status with the expected outcomes. If the outcomes are not met, reassess the patient and revise the plan.

Anemia from Blood Loss

Etiology and Pathophysiology

Anemia may result from acute or chronic blood loss. During massive hemorrhaging, plasma and red blood cells decrease significantly in number and volume. Consequently, oxygen and iron stores in the blood are reduced.

Vasoconstriction occurs with a decrease in the volume of plasma, resulting in the accumulation of red blood cells. Laboratory values may show a falsely high red blood cell count within the first 48 hours after hemorrhage. Normal blood volume is restored by the movement of fluid into the circulating blood from interstitial compartments. The remaining dilute blood is deficient in red blood cells, and thus the oxygen-carrying capacity of the blood is reduced. This stimulates the bone marrow to increase production of red blood cells.

Clinical Manifestations

Clinical manifestations include changes in respirations, dyspnea, vertigo, rapid thready pulse, hypotension, pale skin, headache, restlessness, and disorientation resulting from the lack of oxygen supply to the tissues and major organs, such as the heart and brain. Bleeding causes the tissues to become edematous, which can be very painful.

Diagnosis

The medical diagnosis is based on history, physical findings, and laboratory studies. The red blood cell count and hemoglobin and hematocrit levels may demonstrate falsely high levels within the first 48 hours after hemorrhage before becoming significantly decreased.

Management

Immediate medical management includes replacing the blood that is lost with blood transfusions, administering intravenous fluids to increase the plasma volume, and treating for shock. Sedatives may be ordered if the patient is restless. Complications arise if treatment does not begin immediately, and the patient may die.

❖ Settings, Providers, and Collaboration for Care

If the blood loss is acute, the patient may be hospitalized for volume replacement with blood and intravenous fluids to avoid or treat shock. With chronic blood loss, the anemia may be treated on an outpatient basis. Tests need to be done to determine the cause of the blood loss. Follow-up care with a physician is important.

NURSING PROCESS
Anemia from Blood Loss

Assessment

Review the patient's history and medical management. Assess the patient for changes in vital signs, such as rapid and deep respirations, a rapid and thready pulse, hypotension, and fever, which may indicate continued bleeding or hypovolemia. Assess

for changes in consciousness and orientation, skin pallor, and cyanosis. Excessive thirst and diaphoresis may result from hypovolemia.

Bleeding may be obvious or occult. In either case, it is important to identify the cause. Observe for signs of bleeding such as bruising, petechiae, ecchymoses, and edema. Ask the patient about fatigue, changes in urine and stool color, and headaches.

Nursing Diagnoses and Planning

Nursing diagnoses and related expected patient outcomes commonly applicable to patients with anemia from blood loss include those previously described under anemias as well as the following:

NDx: Decreased cardiac output related to increased cardiac workload caused by reduced level of red blood cells and hemoglobin from hemorrhage

Planning: Patient Outcomes
1. Patient's vital signs and laboratory studies are within normal ranges for the patient.
2. Patient reports decreased fatigue, non-labored respirations, and increased activity tolerance, all indicative of increased cardiac output without increased workload.

Nursing Interventions and Evaluation

NDx: Decreased cardiac output
Nursing interventions for the patient with anemia from blood loss should focus on replacing lost volume with intravenous fluids. Fluids used for restoring blood volume include saline, dextrose, albumin, and plasma. The patient may receive a whole blood transfusion. Offer oral fluids as tolerated. Monitor vital signs and assess circulating fluid volume by arterial or venous pressures, urine output, and signs of overhydration or dehydration. Monitor laboratory studies and observe for signs of continued bleeding.

Since the patient may be hypovolemic initially, look for dry skin, sunken eyes, anuria, and decreased blood pressure. Symptoms vary with the type, location, and rate of blood loss. Also assess for hypervolemia, which may occur after fluid replacement therapy. Look for edema, increasing blood pressure, distention, pulmonary congestion, and scanty urine.

After the patient is stabilized medically, promote a diet high in iron, protein, vitamins, and fluids to replace losses and regain strength. Highlight 13–3 lists some high-protein, high-vitamin foods (also see Highlight 13–2). Assist the patient in conserving energy to reduce cardiac workload. Keep the patient warm by applying blankets and avoiding cold fluids and drafts.

Additional Interventions
In acute hemorrhagic anemia, continuing blood loss must be arrested. Nursing care focuses on replacing

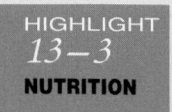 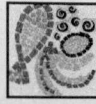

HIGHLIGHT
13–3
NUTRITION

Food Sources for High-Protein, High-Vitamin Diets

Certain foods contribute large amounts of protein and vitamins to the daily diet. Examples of high-protein foods include:

Food	Serving Size	Approximate Grams of Protein Provided
Cottage cheese (2%)	1 cup	31
Chicken	3 oz	26
Turkey	3 oz	26
Duck	3 oz	24
Tuna	3 oz	24
Veal	3 oz	23
Lamb	3 oz	22
Beef	3 oz	21
Shrimp	3 oz	21
Oysters	1 cup	20
Ham	3 oz	18
Evaporated whole milk	1 cup	17
Pork	2 oz	17
Peanut butter	2 Tbsp	9
Whole milk	1 cup	8
Skim milk	1 cup	8
Buttermilk	1 cup	8
Clams	3 oz	7
Swiss cheese	1 oz	7
American cheese	1 oz	6

Examples of high-vitamin foods include:

Vitamin A	Liver
	Whole milk
	Butter
	Cod liver oil
	Green, leafy vegetables
	Yellow or orange fruit
Vitamin B complex	Meat
	Milk
	Eggs
	Grains
	Green vegetables
Vitamin C	Citrus fruits
	Broccoli
	Potatoes
	Tomatoes
Vitamin D	Milk
	Eggs

Adapted from U.S. Department of Agriculture Bulletin: Nutritive Value of Foods, 1986.

fluids lost, assessing for continued blood loss, and preventing recurrence (Nursing Care Guide 13–1).

Compare the patient's status with the expected outcomes. If the outcomes are not met, reassess the patient and revise the plan.

Hypoproliferative Anemias

The hypoproliferative anemias result from a defect in production of red blood cells. Iron, vitamin B_{12}, folic acid, and protein are needed for erythropoiesis (red blood cell production). Inadequate intake, excessive loss, or deficient use of these nutrients by the body leads to a decreased production of red blood cells. Chemical or drug interference or renal disease may also reduce red blood cell production.

IRON DEFICIENCY ANEMIA

Etiology and Pathophysiology
Iron deficiency anemia is a depletion of iron stores in the body, resulting in deficient hemoglobin synthesis as a result of impaired absorption, loss, or low intake of iron. Red blood cells are small and pale from the hemoglobin deficit. This anemia is the most prevalent type. It occurs most frequently in women between 15 and 45 years of age as a result of blood loss during menstruation. Pregnant women and children are also vulnerable to iron deficiency anemia because of their increased need for iron and poor dietary supply. It is seen more frequently in countries where nutrition is poor and in tropical zones.

Inadequate iron absorption may also occur in chronic diarrhea states, in malabsorption syndromes, with a low intake of foods containing iron, and following a gastrectomy. Excessive blood loss from trauma, excessive menses, gastrointestinal bleeding, or blood donation can also result in iron depletion.

Clinical Manifestations
Patients typically develop fatigue and weakness from the decreased oxygen supply caused by a hemoglobin deficit. In severe cases of iron deficiency anemia, palpitations, vertigo, sensitivity to cold, brittle hair and nails, clubbing of the nails (spoon nails characterized by concave curves), dysphagia, mouth ulcerations, and an inflamed but smooth red tongue may be evident.

Diagnosis
The medical diagnosis of iron deficiency anemia is based on the patient's nutritional assessment, social history, and laboratory findings. Diagnostic laboratory tests would include bone marrow examination, platelet count, serum iron, total iron-binding capacity, red blood cell count, red blood cell indices, and hemoglobin level to detect defective red blood cell production and hemoglobin deficiency. A stained red blood cell examination is used to detect abnormally small red blood cells, which indicate iron deficiency anemia.

Nursing Care Guide 13–1

Patients with Acute Hemorrhagic Anemia

Assessment Findings: Patient experiences restlessness; dyspnea; and rapid, deep respirations followed by shallow respirations. Presence of cyanosis and pallor, clubbing of nails, and hypotension.

Nursing Diagnosis: Ineffective breathing pattern related to a reduction in the oxygen-carrying capacity of the blood; a decrease in red blood cells

Patient Outcomes	Nursing Interventions	Rationale
Patient exhibits a decrease in labored respirations, signs of cyanosis, and pallor.	Elevate head of bed and maintain the patient in this position as much as possible. Monitor vital signs.	This promotes expanded breathing by pulling diaphragm down and allows for better expansion of the diaphragm.
Patient's chest is fully expanded with respirations maintained between 12 and 16 per minute.	Tell the patient to breathe deeply, slow the respiratory pattern, and try to maintain a steady rate. Instruct patient to avoid gas-forming foods.	A relaxed, deep, full respiratory pattern is more efficient than a shallow, rapid pattern for good oxygen intake and exchange. Some foods produce large amounts of gas, which can lead to abdominal distention, interfering with respirations.
Patient completes activities of daily living without complaints of fatigue.	Plan rest periods throughout day for patient and provide quiet environment. Place frequently used objects within the patient's reach.	Frequent, planned rest periods help conserve strength and reduce oxygen needs.
Patient ambulates at least once every 8 hours for 5 to 15 minutes without respiratory distress.	Encourage ambulation on each shift for 5 to 15 minutes. Monitor blood levels. Administer oxygen as ordered.	Short, frequent periods of ambulation use less energy and oxygen.

Evaluation: Compare the patient's status with the expected outcomes. If the outcomes are not met, reassess the patient and revise the plan.

Assessment Findings: Patient experiences hypotension; weak, rapid, thready pulse; palpitations; fever; chills; cyanosis and pallor of face, skin, and nails; poor skin turgor; pruritus; and clubbing of nails.

Nursing Diagnosis: Fluid volume deficit related to excessive blood loss

Patient Outcomes	Nursing Interventions	Rationale
Patient remains free of fever and exhibits regular strong pulse rate and normal blood pressure. Patient maintains adequate blood volume with minimal blood loss as noted by normal results of blood studies.	Check vital signs frequently. Observe skin turgor. Check temperature. Administer blood transfusion as ordered. Initiate intravenous therapy. Monitor vital signs and laboratory data.	Adequate replacement of fluids may be evident in stability of vital signs and good skin turgor. Fluid replacement reduces the effects of the blood volume deficit.

(continued)

Nursing Care Guide 13–1
Patients with Acute Hemorrhagic Anemia (continued)

Patient Outcomes	Nursing Interventions	Rationale
Patient complies with directions and information given.	Instruct patient to avoid using heating pads.	Reduced circulation to the peripheral skin surfaces, with low blood volume, may decrease sensations, causing risk for burns.
	Instruct patient to avoid aspirin products.	Aspirin products may increase risk of bleeding, further aggravating blood volume deficit.

Evaluation: Compare the patient's status with the expected outcomes. If the outcomes are not met, reassess the patient and revise the plan.

Assessment Findings: Patient complains of disorientation, experiencing falls, bruises, extreme hot and cold sensations, vertigo, fever, and headache.

Nursing Diagnosis: Risk for injury related to changes in mental status and sensory perceptions

Patient Outcomes	Nursing Interventions	Rationale
Patient remains alert and oriented to time, place, and person. Patient denies vertigo, headaches, and disorientation.	Orient patient to time, place, and person. Assess patient's alertness. Assist patient when ambulating.	Checking the patient's orientation, reorienting the patient frequently, and assisting the unsure patient may decrease risk for injury due to decreased sensory perceptions.
Patient remains free of injury.	Instruct patient to take deep breaths when moving from supine to sitting position and to sit for a few minutes before rising. Instruct patient to avoid heating pads or extreme cold.	Vertigo may be exacerbated by sudden movements such as rising rapidly from a lying position. Decreased sensation to skin surfaces may increase risk for burns.

Evaluation: Compare the patient's status with the expected outcomes. If the outcomes are not met, reassess the patient and revise the plan.

Assessment Findings: Patient complains of nausea and vomiting; red, sore tongue; mouth ulcers; bleeding gums; diarrhea; constipation; abdominal distention; flatus; thirst; poor hydration; and anorexia.

Nursing Diagnosis: Altered nutrition: less than body requirements related to pain, mouth soreness, and fluid volume deficit

(continued)

Nursing Care Guide 13–1
Patients with Acute Hemorrhagic Anemia (continued)

Patient Outcomes	Nursing Interventions	Rationale
Patient's elimination patterns are adequate, without diarrhea or constipation.	Provide bland diet, low in roughage (with diarrhea) or high in roughage (with constipation).	A proper diet is essential to maintain normal intestinal function.
Patient's appetite improves.	Serve patient six to eight small meals per day. Serve foods the patient likes in an attractive manner free from offending odors.	The patient's appetite may improve with foods of choice served in an appealing way.
Patient's mouth remains free of ulcerations.	Offer bland, nonirritating foods.	Bland foods may eliminate some of the irritation of the oral mucosa.
Patient states which foods to consume and which to avoid.	Encourage 3000 mL fluid per day. Teach the patient about a nutritious diet, giving examples of meal plans.	Increased fluids help replace previous losses from diarrhea and increase motility of the intestinal tract.
	Administer diet high in proteins, vitamins, and calories. Avoid hot, spicy, and acid foods.	A high-protein, high-vitamin diet with increased calories helps replace deficiencies and prevent further nutritional disorders.
	Provide oral hygiene before and after meals.	Food is more palatable with proper oral hygiene. It also prevents further mouth problems.

Evaluation: Compare the patient's status with the expected outcomes. If the outcomes are not met, reassess the patient and revise the plan.

Assessment Findings: Patient and family ask questions about the disorder and the needs of the patient.

Nursing Diagnosis: Knowledge deficit: nature of illness, treatment, and prevention

Patient Outcomes	Nursing Interventions	Rationale
Patient verbalizes accurate information about diet, medications, and changes in activities of daily living.	Explain diagnostic tests and treatments to patient to allay anxiety and provide cooperation. Review all medications with patient. Explain dietary changes and provide meal-planning guides. Provide information on alterations in activities of daily living to promote adequate rest and relieve fatigue.	The more the patient understands about the disorder and the necessary treatment, the greater the chance for compliance with the prescribed care regimen.
Patient and family express confidence in their ability to cope with the health problems.	Allow time for questions and concerns from the patient and family. Correct any misunderstandings.	Explanation about diet, medications, and changes in lifestyle helps the patient cope with the disorder and eliminates misconceptions about the condition and health-care needs.

Evaluation: Compare the patient's status with the expected outcomes. If the outcomes are not met, reassess the patient and revise the plan.

Management

Management includes ferrous sulfate or ferrous gluconate, initially administered orally with food to decrease gastric irritation. After the patient develops a tolerance to the iron, it should be taken between meals. Iron is best absorbed on an empty stomach. Undiluted liquid preparations of iron salts are given through a straw to prevent the solution from staining teeth and gums. Encouraging good oral hygiene is necessary. Ferrous salts may be given with orange juice to promote absorption of the iron. Oral iron preparations are taken for as long as 2 to 3 months after the hemoglobin returns to normal. Iron may also be administered as an injection, called iron dextran.

❖ Settings, Providers, and Collaboration for Care

Iron deficiency anemia is most commonly detected and treated in outpatient settings. The patient may need diet instruction to increase iron intake. Injections or oral medication can be administered at home or in the doctor's office. Referral to a home health nurse for diet assessment and education and medication administration may be needed.

NURSING PROCESS
Iron Deficiency Anemia

Assessment

Obtain a social and dietary history from the patient to evaluate environmental and nutritional status. Review the medical history. Ask for a detailed typical daily diet plan. Note whether any of the foods on the list are high in iron. Ask whether the patient takes any dietary supplements.

Look for signs of general malaise, dyspnea, weakness, or vertigo, because the decreased oxygen level may precipitate these symptoms. Inquire about the patient's ability to perform activities of daily living. Inquire about sensitivity to cold. Look for pallor, nail clubbing, and cyanosis. Assess vital signs and any laboratory studies completed.

Check specifically for mouth irritation and ulceration. Review the patient's oral hygiene practices. Inquire about dietary changes brought about by mouth problems, if any.

Nursing Diagnoses and Planning

Nursing diagnoses and related expected patient outcomes commonly applicable to patients with iron deficiency anemia include those previously described under anemias as well as the following:

NDx: Altered nutrition: less than body requirements related to inability to provide for, or lack of knowledge about, needed dietary planning, or to mucous membrane soreness and irritation

Planning: Patient Outcomes
1. Patient chooses appropriate foods to replace dietary deficiencies (see Highlights 13–2 and 13–3).
2. Patient avoids irritating foods and fluids.

Nursing Interventions and Evaluation

NDx: Altered nutrition: less than body requirements
Help the patient maintain adequate nutrition by providing attractive meals in a pleasant atmosphere. Encourage the patient to eat foods high in iron, protein, and vitamins, such as red meat, liver, oysters, egg yolks, green leafy vegetables, carrots, whole wheat bread, dried fruits, raisins, and molasses. If these foods are taken with vitamin C, absorption will be enhanced. Provide six to eight small meals daily to prevent distention and reduce fatigue.

Instruct the patient to avoid foods that are gas forming, because they cause abdominal distention, which may decrease the appetite and interfere with respiratory efforts. Provide a diet low in roughage. Avoid hot, spicy foods and acidic fluids to decrease gastrointestinal irritation. Encourage increased fluid intake to prevent constipation and promote adequate hydration. Monitor the patient's intake and output.

If the patient receives iron injections in addition to dietary alterations to increase iron stores, observe and report any adverse reactions, such as pain at the injection site, headache, urticaria, and changes in vital signs. Instruct the patient to take oral iron supplements (if needed) on an empty stomach if possible, or with orange juice to enhance absorption. Milk should be avoided because it interferes with iron absorption (Highlight 13–4). Warn patients that oral iron preparations will cause their feces to be black and tarry. They may also cause constipation or diarrhea.

Review the cause, symptoms, nutritional implications, treatment, and prevention of iron deficiency with the patient and family. Allow time for questions and verbalization of concerns and misunderstandings.

Compare the patient's status with the expected outcomes. If the outcomes are not met, reassess the patient and revise the plan.

PERNICIOUS ANEMIA

Etiology and Pathophysiology

Pernicious anemia is caused by impaired vitamin B_{12} absorption through the small intestine as a result of a deficiency in the intrinsic factor. This deficiency results from gastric fundus atrophy. The cause of the gastric atrophy is unknown but is thought to be autoimmune and related to genetic predisposition. It also can be caused by chronic gastritis and gastrectomy. Vitamin B_{12} deficiency alters DNA synthesis, resulting in defective red blood cells, white blood cells, and platelets.

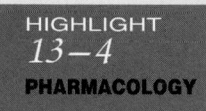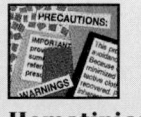

HIGHLIGHT
13–4
PHARMACOLOGY

Hematinics

Definition:

Iron salts used for replacement therapy in iron deficiency anemias. Available in oral, parenteral, and intravenous preparations.

Oral Iron Preparations:

Ferrous sulfate

Ferrous fumarate

Ferrous gluconate

Parenteral Intravenous Iron:

Iron dextran

Action:

Absorbed in the proximal portion of the small intestine. Important in the synthesis of hemoglobin.

Uses:

Replaces or supplements iron stores, which may be low from blood loss, poor diet, pregnancy, or lactation.

Side Effects:

Nausea, constipation, diarrhea, and anorexia. May stain mouth and teeth or color stools dark green or black. If given intramuscularly, pain at injection site, skin staining. If given intravenously, fever, rash, and local phlebitis.

Interactions:

Decreased absorption of tetracycline or penicillamine. Vitamin E may interfere with the effect of the iron therapy.

Nursing Implications:

Dilute liquid iron preparations in water or orange juice; use a straw to avoid staining teeth.

Take oral iron tablets with orange juice to promote absorption.

Avoid giving iron tablets with food because it slows absorption.

Check patient for constipation, nausea, and diarrhea.

Tell patient that iron supplements may turn stool black.

Do not give more than 2 mL at one intramuscular site because it may be painful or cause hematomas.

Use the Z-track injection method.

After intravenous administration of iron, flush vein with saline solution.

Instruct patient not to take oral iron preparations with milk or antacids because they may reduce iron absorption.

Geriatric Considerations:

Because iron preparations can be constipating, especially in the older adult, tell the patient to include more bulk in the diet and to drink increased amounts of fluids.

Only 0.1% of the population develops pernicious anemia. It is found primarily in people over age 50 who have a family history of the disorder. It occurs most commonly in blue-eyed persons of Scandinavian descent.

Clinical Manifestations

Clinical manifestations include changes in activity and strength that occur when red blood cell reduction leads to decreased oxygen in the blood. Patients may complain of weakness, light-headedness, a burning sensation of the tongue, weight loss, dyspnea, and orthopnea. Jaundice may result from rupture of large red blood cells in the blood and bone marrow. Gastrointestinal disturbances and changes in

elimination patterns occur from atrophy of the glandular mucosa of the fundus, resulting in decreased hydrochloric acid secretion. Gastrointestinal bleeding or obstruction from tumors may be present. Incidence of gastric carcinoma and benign gastric polyps is high in patients with pernicious anemia. Papillary atrophy and inflammation of the oral mucous membranes may occur.

Neurologic disturbances may arise from impaired vitamin B_{12} absorption and DNA synthesis and defective red blood cells, white blood cells, and platelets. Lack of vitamin B_{12} alters the structure and interferes with the function of the spinal cord, peripheral nerves, and brain. Patients are very sensitive to temperature changes and to pain from neurologic changes.

Diagnosis

The medical diagnosis of pernicious anemia is based on medical and social history, physical assessment, and laboratory findings. Laboratory studies include red blood cell count, stained red blood cell examination, red blood cell indices, hemoglobin count, white blood cell count, platelet count, glucose-6-phosphate-dehydrogenase level, serum iron level, lactate dehydrogenase level, bone marrow examination, bilirubin count, and gastric fluid analysis. A Schilling test is done to differentiate between dietary vitamin B_{12} deficiency and vitamin B_{12} malabsorption.

Management

Management includes parenteral vitamin B_{12} therapy, which must be continued for life. It is imperative that the patient continue therapy even when asymptomatic. Injections of vitamin B_{12} are initially administered daily and tapered to monthly. Most symptoms recede with treatment; however, spinal cord or brain damage usually is permanent. If the patient continues with adequate treatment for life, anemia does not recur.

Oral iron supplements may be ordered in addition to folic acid. Blood transfusions may be necessary in severe cases. Diagnostic tests are done to determine the presence of gastrointestinal polyps and carcinoma, because these disorders correlate highly with pernicious anemia. Delayed treatment in an elderly person can result in congestive heart failure and angina. Without treatment, the person will die.

❖ Settings, Providers, and Collaboration for Care

Pernicious anemia is usually detected and treated in a doctor's office or outpatient clinic. Iron supplements can be taken at home. Vitamin B_{12} injections can be administered at home by a home health nurse, or in the doctor's office. Hospitalization may be required if the illness is severe enough to require close observation.

NURSING PROCESS
Pernicious Anemia

Assessment

Review the medical history and complete a nutritional history. Keep in mind that strict vegetarians may suffer from a diet-based vitamin B_{12} deficiency. Observe for changes in oral mucous membranes, including a sore mouth and red, smooth tongue. Look for anorexia and weight loss, which indicate disturbances in the gastrointestinal tract. Assess for nausea, vomiting and restlessness, which may indicate gastric bleeding or obstruction from a tumor. Assess for constipation and diarrhea due to atrophy of the gastrointestinal mucosa.

Note any neurologic disturbances, including sensitivity to heat and pain, tingling, numbness of hands and feet, symptoms of gout, ataxia, vision changes, irritability, depression, and psychotic behavior caused by degeneration of the spinal cord and peripheral nerves.

Assess for clinical manifestations of diminished oxygen in the blood, as evidenced by dyspnea, weakness, fatigue, palpitations, and pallor. Assess skin color for jaundice resulting from hemolysis.

Identify the patient's knowledge level regarding pernicious anemia and vitamin B_{12} treatment. During initial vitamin B_{12} therapy, observe for signs of hypokalemia, as evidenced by muscle weakness, apathy, abdominal distention, paralytic ileus, anorexia, nausea, vomiting, thirst, arrhythmias, diminished tendon reflexes, and mental depression. Hypokalemia may occur because as vitamin B_{12} is administered, the body begins a normal process of erythropoiesis. This increases the use of potassium by the erythrocytes, possibly leading to hypokalemia. Observe for signs of anxiety, such as inability to follow instructions, crying, trembling, hyperventilation, tachycardia, and cold perspiration.

Nursing Diagnoses and Planning

Nursing diagnoses and related expected patient outcomes commonly applicable to patients with pernicious anemia include those previously described under anemias as well as the following:

NDx: Constipation or Diarrhea related to changes in the gastrointestinal mucosa

Planning: Patient Outcomes
1. Patient reports normal stool consistency without diarrhea or constipation.
2. Patient eats foods that promote adequate bowel elimination.
3. Patient eats small, frequent meals to prevent digestive problems.
4. Patient drinks adequate fluids to promote proper elimination.

NDx: Knowledge deficit: nature of disease, diet, and use of prescribed medications

Planning: Patient Outcomes
1. Patient states accurate information about relationship of vitamin B_{12} to symptoms of disorder.
2. Patient states dose, time, frequency, side effects, and toxic effects of prescribed medications.

Nursing Interventions and Evaluation

NDx: Constipation or Diarrhea
Help the patient maintain adequate bowel elimination. Encourage intake of eight glasses of water or other nonirritating fluids daily. Promote frequent moderate exercise and at least 8 hours of sleep each night.

Instruct the patient regarding a balanced diet high in protein, vitamins, and iron, including such foods as fish, red meat, milk, and eggs to increase the intake of vitamin B_{12}. Provide six to eight small meals daily, if tolerated, to conserve energy and decrease gastrointestinal distress.

Monitor the patient's bowel movements, noting the color, consistency, and amount. Provide stool softeners or antidiarrheal agents as prescribed.

NDx: Knowledge deficit: nature of disease, diet, and use of prescribed medications
Help the patient gain knowledge about the disorder by explaining the signs, symptoms, causes, and lifelong treatment needed to prevent complications. Discuss those complications with the patient and family. Explain the signs of hypokalemia and when to seek medical intervention.

Encourage the patient and family to ask questions and express concerns. Teach the patient about prescribed medications, including the dose, route, time, frequency, side effects, and toxic effects. Encourage the patient to continue with follow-up visits to the physician's office at least twice yearly.

Help the patient decrease stress levels to maximize coping mechanisms. Explain that irritability and depression are part of the disease process. Allow the patient and family to express feelings and concerns about lifelong therapy. Encourage relaxation exercises with deep, diaphragmatic breathing.

Compare the patient's status with the expected outcomes. If the outcomes are not met, reassess the patient and revise the plan.

FOLIC ACID DEFICIENCY

Etiology and Pathophysiology
A deficiency in folic acid results in defective red blood cell production. Folic acid deficiency is an extremely common disorder with an insidious onset. Increased metabolic needs, chronic malnourishment, and intestinal malabsorption can lead to folic acid deficiency.

Ingestion of anticonvulsants, antimetabolites, and certain oral contraceptives can impede the absorption of folic acid. Alcoholics often manifest a deficiency of folic acid, because alcohol interferes with folate metabolism and red blood cell production.

Alcoholics and the elderly living alone are more prone to develop folic acid deficiency as a result of dietary deficiencies and ingestion impairment. Folic acid deficiency may also develop in patients on prolonged intravenous feeding or hyperalimentation unless folic acid is given intramuscularly.

Clinical Manifestations
Clinical manifestations of folic acid deficiency are similar to those of pernicious anemia. Symptoms include those associated with anemia, combined with gastrointestinal disturbances and a beefy, red tongue. A deficiency of folic acid in pregnant women has been found to cause neural tube defects in infants.

Diagnosis
The diagnosis of folic acid deficiency is made on the basis of a history of dietary intake and laboratory studies of red blood cell count and red blood cell indices, serum folic acid level, and bone marrow examination. Absence of neurologic symptoms is important in differentiating folic acid deficiency from pernicious anemia.

Management
Daily oral doses of folic acid are prescribed. Parenteral doses are ordered if the patient has a malabsorption syndrome. The usual dose is 1 mg of folic acid daily, although alcoholics may require up to 5 mg daily. Vitamin C may be ordered with folic acid to promote erythropoiesis.

❖ Settings, Providers, and Collaborative Care
Folic acid deficiencies are most commonly detected and treated at home or in the doctor's office. Medications can be administered at home. Diet instruction may be needed to increase the patient's intake of folic acid.

NURSING PROCESS GUIDELINES
Folic Acid Deficiency

Review the patient's history and medical management. Assess for a smooth and reddened tongue, chills, and gastrointestinal disturbances. Note any fatigue, dyspnea, and weakness from oxygen deprivation. Check vital signs, auscultate the chest, and note any cardiac arrhythmias.

Ask about the patient's typical daily food intake. Look for dietary deficiencies. Monitor intake and output. Ask whether the patient is taking any anticonvulsants, antimetabolites, or oral contraceptives. Question the patient about alcohol ingestion.

The nursing diagnoses, expected patient outcomes, nursing interventions, and evaluation for patients with a folic acid deficiency include those described previously under anemias. The following additional interventions also apply to patients with folic acid deficiency. Help the patient achieve a balanced diet. Promote foods high in calories, proteins, and vitamins based on the patient's food preferences (see Highlight 13–3). Encourage the patient to eat foods high in folic acid, such as green and yellow vegetables, liver, citrus fruits, whole grains, yeast, and legumes. Discourage alcohol consumption. Provide six to eight small meals daily. Teach the patient good oral hygiene techniques to prevent mouth problems.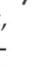

Maintain activity as tolerated. Use special safety measures if the patient is weak. Provide periods of rest between activities. Keep the patient warm and comfortable, free from chills and drafts. Teach the patient and family the importance of treatment and prevention of recurrence of the disorder.

APLASTIC ANEMIA

Etiology and Pathophysiology
Aplastic anemia is a rare condition that impairs red blood cell development in the bone marrow, thus

causing a deficiency of circulating red blood cells. Bone marrow failure may also result in concurrent agranulocytosis and thrombocytopenia. When all three conditions exist together, pancytopenia (deficiency of all blood elements) results.

The onset of aplastic anemia may be insidious, as in hereditary cases, or rapid, as when bone marrow failure develops after myelotoxic drug therapy. Tumor of the thymus is associated with this disorder. It may also be caused by autoimmune disease, renal failure, and exposure to radiation. Some drugs are known to cause aplastic anemia. A list of these drugs can be found in Table 13–1.

The cause of aplastic anemia is unknown in half of all affected individuals. More than 50% of individuals with pancytopenia die from hemorrhage or infection. Death occurs within a few months after the onset of anemia. Twenty-five percent of the 40 to 50% who survive die by the end of the third year after onset. The remaining 25% either completely recover or remain invalid for years.

Aplastic anemia can be staged according to prognostic features (Table 13–2). It is considered severe if the patient has three of the four features. In this case, median survival without treatment is approximately 3 months. Only 20% of patients survive 1 year. Aplastic anemia is classified as very severe if all of the prognostic features are present and the neutrophil count is less than 200/μL.

Clinical Manifestations
Clinical manifestations include decreased red blood cell and white blood cell counts and decreased number of platelets (thrombocytopenia). Infection and hemorrhage may result from pancytopenia and bone marrow failure. Prevalent symptoms include progressive weakness, fatigue, headache, dyspnea, hemorrhaging, and infection.

Diagnosis
The medical diagnosis of aplastic anemia is based on history, physical assessment, and laboratory findings. Laboratory studies include white blood cell count (especially granulocytes), red blood cell count,

Table 13–1

Drugs that Cause Aplastic Anemia

Chloramphenicol (Chloromycetin)
Sulfonamides
Phenytoin
Mephenytoin
Trimethadione (Tridione)
Phenylbutazone
Gold salts
Phenytoin
Carbamazepine
Tolbutamide
Quinacrine
Diphenylhydantoin

Table 13–2

Prognostic Features of Aplastic Anemia

Neutrophil count <500/μL
Platelet count <2,000/μL
Reticulocyte count 0.1%
Severe hypocellularity of the bone marrow

reticulocyte count, platelet count, and bone marrow examination. Tests are used to confirm whether the patient has been exposed to myelotoxic drugs. Prior use of myelotoxic drugs can predispose a person to aplastic anemia. Examples of these drugs include:

Antitumor agents
Antimetabolites
Antimicrobials
Anticonvulsants
Antithyroid drugs
Antidiabetic agents
Antihistamines
Analgesics
Sedatives
Insecticides

Management
Management may include replacement of deficient stem cells by bone marrow transplant, suppression of destructive immunologic processes, or identification and discontinuation of the causative agents. Bone marrow transplants and a splenectomy may be indicated. Bone marrow transplants are done in patients with severe aplastic anemia and a matched donor. Care of the patient undergoing a bone marrow transplant is discussed in Chapter 32, and care of the patient undergoing a splenectomy is discussed in Chapter 12. Medical management to improve blood counts temporarily includes transfusions of red blood cells and platelets, which may prevent symptoms from recurring. It is important to note that repeated transfusions may result in increased iron in the tissues and splenomegaly.

Myelotoxic drugs used for treating cancer can cause myelodepression. When patients are receiving myelotoxic drugs, blood cell counts are monitored to evaluate bone marrow function. If possible, the offending drug should be stopped. Immunosuppression through the use of drugs—such as antilymphocyte globulins and cyclosporins—reduces T-cell function and circulating lymphocytes. This treatment is most commonly used with patients over 40 years old who have no match for a bone marrow transplant. However, it may take months or years for hemoglobin, neutrophil, and platelet counts to return to normal. Recombinant hematopoietic growth factors are used to stimulate neutrophil growth and prevent infection in the early stages of treatment. These drugs do not increase numbers of other blood cell types.

❖ **Settings, Providers, and Collaboration for Care**

The detection and treatment of aplastic anemia may occur in the doctor's office or outpatient clinic. Blood cell counts are monitored closely in patients receiving myelotoxic agents. If blood cell numbers become very low, the patient may be hospitalized for transfusion and observation. Severe persistent pancytopenia can lead to hemorrhage or infection.

NURSING PROCESS
Aplastic Anemia

Assessment

Review the medical history for a cause of the anemia and conduct a physical examination. Note any dyspnea on exertion, fever, sore throat, pallor, weakness, and anorexia indicative of a respiratory infection. Assess for pain and burning on urination, which may suggest a urinary tract infection. Note the patient's urinary output for color, consistency, and amount. Assess for abnormal bleeding, wounds, and abrasions. Look for irritation or ulcers of the mucous membranes, which could be potential sites of infection.

Review the patient's nutritional intake. Check for recent weight loss. Observe the oral cavity for lesions, because mouth soreness may affect the patient's ability to eat well. Note the patient's bowel movements, checking for regularity and absence of constipation. Check for irritation or bleeding from hemorrhoids. Palpate for splenomegaly. Collect the blood specimens needed to monitor progress of the disease. Allow the patient and family time to voice their concerns and fears about the disorder and treatment. Help the patient find appropriate coping mechanisms.

Nursing Diagnoses and Planning

Nursing diagnoses and related expected patient outcomes commonly applicable to patients with aplastic anemia include those previously described under anemias as well as the following:

NDx: Anxiety related to poor prognosis, fear of death, or vulnerability to complications and prolonged therapy

Planning: Patient Outcomes
1. Patient relates concerns about illness to the nurse or other appropriate members of the health-care team.
2. Patient and family verbalize accurate information about the disorder, complications, and therapy.
3. Patient expresses feelings of reduced anxiety and fear.
4. Patient displays physical signs of decreased anxiety; vital signs are within normal ranges, and patient is resting well, appears calm, and eats well.

NDx: Risk for infection related to decreased body defenses against microorganisms

Planning: Patient Outcomes
1. Patient's vital signs are within normal ranges for the patient.
2. Patient's laboratory studies are within normal ranges for the patient.
3. Patient denies chills, sore throat, cough, shortness of breath, anorexia, or pain or burning on urination.

NDx: Knowledge deficit: nature of disease and prevention of complications

Planning: Patient Outcomes
1. Patient states accurate information about the nature of the disease.
2. Patient verbalizes the complications of aplastic anemia, such as bleeding, infection, and poor nutrition, and notes the signs and symptoms of each.
3. Patient relates strategies to avoid complications of the disease.
4. Patient states when it is appropriate to seek medical attention after observing signs of a complication of the disorder.

Nursing Interventions and Evaluation

NDx: Anxiety
Allow the patient to verbalize concerns about the disease, its effects on the patient and family, and fears about death. Help the patient and family find effective coping strategies to deal with anxiety. Allow time for questions from the patient and the family.

Seek assistance from clergy or other professional counselors when appropriate. Make referrals as needed to social service agencies.

NDx: Risk for infection
Keep the patient warm and avoid extreme temperature changes in the room. Restrict visitors to prevent exposure to infections. Use protective isolation if appropriate. Monitor the patient's vital signs frequently; watch for subtle changes that may indicate early signs of infection. Report any changes noted.

Promote good nutrition by serving meals in a relaxed, attractive atmosphere. Encourage a high-protein, high-vitamin diet. Provide oral hygiene frequently to prevent infection and promote better eating habits.

NDx: Knowledge deficit: nature of the disease and prevention of complications
Explain the causes, complications, treatment, and prevention of aplastic anemia to the patient and family. Allow the patient to vent feelings and ask questions about the information presented. Give the patient and family literature about aplastic anemia when appropriate. Use terminology that the patient can comprehend.

Teach the patient signs of bleeding to observe for and when to seek medical assistance. Explain the need to avoid sharp objects, straight razors, contact sports, and injections and venipuncture whenever possible (Highlight 13–5).

Explain oral hygiene methods needed to prevent further irritation and ulceration of mucous membranes. Instruct the patient to use a soft toothbrush and to use mouthrinse frequently. Show how to inspect the oral cavity, checking the tongue and gums for early signs of irritation. Teach the patient to avoid extremely hot, spicy foods and acidic drinks to lessen oral and gastrointestinal irritation.

Teach the patient to avoid constipation, because hard stools and straining can damage the rectal mucosa and cause bleeding. Obtain an order for a stool softener or laxative when needed.

Help the patient understand the signs of infection and how to prevent them. Tell the patient to stay warm and dry and to avoid extreme temperature changes. Encourage a diet high in protein and vitamins. Assist with oral care as needed to prevent mucous membrane breakdown, which would increase the potential for infection. Tell family mem-

bers to avoid contact with the patient when they have colds or other active infections.

Compare the patient's status with the expected outcomes. If the outcomes are not met, reassess the patient and revise the plan.

Hemolytic Anemias

In the hemolytic anemias, red blood cells have a shortened life span. It may result from intrinsic factors, such as plasma membrane defects or enzyme deficiencies, or extrinsic factors, such as infection or drugs. Hemolysis of red blood cells occurs more rapidly than erythropoiesis in these disorders. If the erythrocyte life span is less than 20 days, a hemolytic anemia is usually present.

HEREDITARY SPHEROCYTOSIS

Etiology and Pathophysiology
Spherocytosis is characterized by small, sphere-shaped red blood cells that swell from the accumulation of sodium and water. These spheres are rigid and thick. This rigidity prevents them from passing through the splenic microcirculation without being destroyed. Spherocytosis is found in all populations and is inherited as a dominant trait.

Clinical Manifestations
Clinical manifestations include anemia, painful splenomegaly, and jaundice resulting from red cell hemolysis in the spleen and large amounts of bilirubin in the blood. Gallstones are present from the increased level of bilirubin. Infection or chemical exposure may also cause hemolysis.

Diagnosis
The diagnosis of spherocytosis is based on family history, the presence of spherocytes in a blood smear, lowered red blood cell count and hemoglobin level, and elevated osmotic fragility. Serum bilirubin and urinary urobilinogen will also be elevated. Spherocytosis is often diagnosed during childhood, but mild cases may be discovered incidentally later in life.

Management
Management involves blood transfusions and a splenectomy. Splenectomy does not cure the disease, but it does eliminate the site of red blood cell destruction. Most patients who undergo splenectomy are free from symptoms but are not completely cured. Care of the patient undergoing splenectomy is discussed in Chapter 12.

❖ Settings, Providers, and Collaboration for Care
The detection and treatment of hereditary spherocytosis often occurs in a doctor's office or outpatient clinic. Blood transfusions can be given on an outpatient basis. Hospitalization is required if the patient needs a splenectomy.

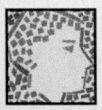

HIGHLIGHT
13–5
PATIENT EDUCATION

Self-Care for a Bleeding Disorder

Instruct the patient with a bleeding disorder that the risk of hemorrhage can be decreased by following these guidelines:

Exercise caution when using sharp objects.

Brush teeth with a soft toothbrush to prevent gingival irritation.

Use an electric razor rather than a razor blade for shaving.

Observe for signs of bleeding, such as bruising, petechiae, and black stools.

Ask for assistance, if needed, to avoid falls.

Avoid contact sports.

Apply direct pressure at the site of active bleeding.

Avoid intramuscular injections.

Take only medications that have been approved by the physician.

Carry identification stating the blood disorder, physician's name and phone number, patient's blood type, and name of significant other to notify in an emergency situation.

FATIGUE, WEAKNESS, AND DYSPNEA IN A PATIENT RECEIVING A BLOOD TRANSFUSION

Just 10 minutes after I started an infusion of packed red blood cells for a 27-year-old woman admitted with chronic hemolytic anemia and complaints of fatigue, weakness, and dyspnea, the patient reported that she felt "strange." Because I was keenly aware of the potentially dangerous risk associated with blood transfusions, I had very carefully checked the doctor's order, double-checked the patient's identity and the blood product with another nurse to ensure a proper match, checked the expiration date, and took baseline vital signs before starting the transfusion. I began the infusion slowly and planned to spend at least the first 15 minutes with the patient to watch for an adverse reaction.

Following her comment, I immediately took her vital signs again and found that her temperature was up to 101.6°F (up from 99.2°F), her pulse was 118 bpm, her respiratory rate was 28 per minute, and her blood pressure was 102/66 mm Hg (down from 120/82 mm Hg). She now appeared flushed and restless. She began to rub her lower back and complained of chills.

It was very clear to me that the patient was experiencing a transfusion reaction. I sought clues to the cause of the reaction and suspected that it was a hemolytic reaction—the most dreaded of all reactions. There was no evidence of rash or urticaria to indicate an allergic reaction. Although fever, hypotension, tachycardia, and tachypnea may indicate a hemolytic, febrile, or septic reaction, the early onset of symptoms and the presence of back pain and flushing pointed toward a hemolytic reaction.

A hemolytic reaction is a life-threatening situation that can lead to shock, disseminated intravascular coagulation (DIC), acute renal failure, and death. Less serious reactions can be potentially dangerous as well and, although medical interventions required may vary for each reaction, I knew that any blood transfusion reaction required the same immediate nursing interventions. I therefore performed the following actions:

1. I immediately stopped the blood transfusion.
2. I kept the IV line open with 0.9% sodium chloride solution.
3. I called for another staff nurse to notify the physician and the blood bank regarding the transfusion reaction and to bring the crash cart to the bedside.
4. I placed the patient in a semi-Fowler's position to facilitate breathing.
5. I administered oxygen according to hospital protocol.
6. I monitored the patient's vital signs every 5 minutes and noted further evidence of shock.

7. I explained what was happening to the patient and offered realistic reassurance.
8. I rechecked the patient's identification, ABO and Rh type, and transfusion identification number.
9. I drew blood samples and sent them to the blood bank together with the bag of blood and the tubing.
10. I obtained the first voided urine sample to be tested for hemoglobinuria.
11. I monitored the patient's urine output.
12. I documented my findings and actions.

The physician ordered mannitol, dopamine, and IV fluids, which I administered. I also inserted an indwelling urinary catheter, as ordered.

Despite the small amount of blood the patient had received, the laboratory results revealed hemolysis in the blood sample and hemoglobin in the urine. These findings confirmed my suspicion of a hemolytic reaction. The patient remained alert and oriented, and her vital signs stabilized after administration of the medications. She was transferred to the ICU for close monitoring of her renal and cardiovascular status and returned to the medical unit 24 hours later.

The final check for a possible mismatch between the patient and the blood product determined that no contradiction existed; rather, a clerical error had been made in labeling the blood. Even scrupulous nursing care before administering the blood was not sufficient to prevent a potentially fatal condition from developing. However, early detection and recognition of an adverse reaction, and rapid initiation of appropriate interventions, minimized the reaction and helped save the patient's life.

Think Critically

Should the nurse have stopped the transfusion sooner?

What medical interventions would the nurse have anticipated if the transfusion reaction had been an allergic, febrile, or septic one?

What additional nursing actions would the nurse have taken if the patient had lost consciousness?

Why did the nurse maintain the IV line with 0.9% sodium chloride solution?

What clinical manifestations of disseminated intravascular coagulation (DIC) should the nurse have assessed the patient for?

What was the rationale for sending a blood specimen, the remaining transfusion blood, and the tubing back to the blood bank?

Suppose the patient said to the nurse, "This hospital almost killed me. Do you think I should sue for malpractice?" What would the nurse's best response be?

NURSING PROCESS GUIDELINES
Hereditary Spherocytosis

Review the medical and family history and complete a physical assessment of the patient. Observe for jaundice, which will be apparent first in the mucous membranes in the roof of the mouth and then in the sclera, followed by generalized distribution. Check the patient for left upper quadrant fullness and abdominal pain, which indicate splenomegaly.

Ask the patient about complaints of generalized malaise, weakness, and inability to complete routine daily activities. Look for signs of infection, such as fever, cough, dyspnea, fatigue, and chills. Assess the patient's vital signs. Note the color, consistency, and amount of urine output. Check the skin for dryness, pruritus, and breakdown.

The nursing diagnoses, expected patient outcomes, nursing interventions, and evaluation for patients with hereditary spherocytosis include those described previously for anemias. The following additional interventions also apply to the care of patients with hereditary spherocytosis. Monitor the patient's vital signs and laboratory studies. Nursing care includes the administration of blood transfusions and preoperative and postoperative care if the patient undergoes a splenectomy. Make referrals for genetic counseling if the patient is planning to have children.

SICKLE-CELL ANEMIA

Etiology and Pathophysiology

Sickle-cell anemia is a chronic hereditary hemolytic disorder characterized by an abnormal hemoglobin S. Instead of the normal hemoglobin A in the blood, these abnormal red blood cells become crescent- or sickle-shaped in the presence of decreased oxygen content in the blood (Fig. 13–1). The elongated,

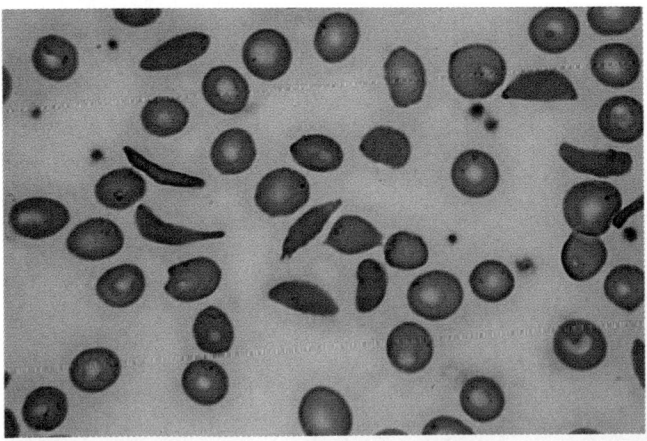

Figure 13–1

Cells from the peripheral blood smear of a patient with sickle-cell disease. Several characteristic sickle cells with pointed ends are shown. (From Rodak BF. Diagnostic hematology. Philadelphia: WB Saunders, 1995, p 257.)

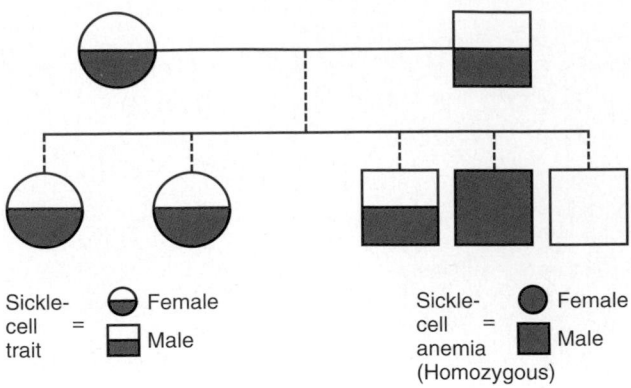

| Sickle-cell trait | = | ⬭ Female | ▢ Male | | Sickle-cell anemia (Homozygous) | = | ⬤ Female | ◼ Male |

Figure 13–2

Example of sickle-cell anemia heredity from a male and a female who are heterozygous for hemoglobin S.

rigid cells become lodged in small vessels, thus slowing or blocking peripheral blood flow or organ perfusion. The accumulation of damaged cells also causes the blood to become more viscous, which further decreases blood flow.

High stress levels, caused by such factors as work, exercise, anorexia, pregnancy, infection, and dehydration may precipitate a sickle-cell crisis. Sickle-cell symptoms may also be precipitated by exposure to low oxygen tensions, as in mountain climbing or flying in a nonpressurized aircraft.

Sickle-cell anemia primarily affects Africans, African-Americans and, to a lesser degree, Mediterraneans, Caribbeans, and Arabs. Sickle-cell trait occurs in about 8% of African-Americans in the United States and is present in those who are heterozygous for sickle-cell hemoglobin. These individuals usually have no symptoms. Figure 13–2 illustrates the probabilities of children inheriting sickle-cell anemia and sickle-cell trait from parents heterozygous (only one recessive gene) for hemoglobin S. People with sickle-cell trait have about 25 to 40% hemoglobin S, whereas those who are homozygous (two recessive genes for a characteristic) for hemoglobin S or those with sickle-cell anemia have about 80 to 100% hemoglobin S. Early detection and treatment are important (Highlight 13–6).

Clinical Manifestations

The clinical picture may vary from a person with mild, asymptomatic disease to one with severe hemolytic anemia and recurrent severe painful crises. Sickle-cell anemia does not affect only one body system but often causes a variety of clinical crises. Clinical manifestations include tachycardia, cardiomegaly, fatigue, dyspnea, joint pain, and ischemic leg ulcers. Painful leg ulcers develop when sickled cells block blood vessels, resulting in peripheral anoxia. As anoxia increases, thrombosis and infarction develop, resulting in tissue necrosis. Tenderness and enlargement of the liver, spleen, and penis occur from the pooling of sickled red blood cells, which

HIGHLIGHT
13–6

HEALTH PROMOTION & RISK REDUCTION

Sickle-Cell Anemia

Although sickle-cell disease cannot be prevented, early detection is important. The following guidelines should be followed to prevent complications and mortality:

All infants of African-American background should be screened for sickle-cell disease. (The U.S. Department of Public Health recommends that all infants be screened for sickle-cell disease to reduce morbidity and mortality.)

Parents of a child with sickle-cell disease should be educated about the disease and should obtain genetic counseling.

Infants with sickle-cell disease should receive standard well-baby care, including immunizations.

Twice-daily doses of penicillin are given prophylactically.

causes the blood to thicken. It is common for male patients to experience a sudden, painful, persistent penile erection.

Poor oxygenation and tissue ischemia lead to a very painful vaso-occlusive crisis. The pain occurs as bone, abdominal, central nervous system, or pulmonary vessels are occluded. This pain is progressive in severity and may last for several days. The most vulnerable organs are the brain, kidney, heart, lung, skin, bone marrow, and spleen. The gallbladder may also be affected, as demonstrated by tenderness and pain from elevated bilirubin levels and gallstones.

Sickled cells in the pulmonary circulation may result in pulmonary congestion and infection. A decrease in arterial oxygen from sickling cells results in tachycardia and decreased cardiac output. Cardiac dysrhythmias may occur. Joint pain and limited movement are present because of occlusion of the circulatory system. Kidneys are less able to concentrate urine because of the obstructed glomerular capillaries.

Changes in vision or eye pain occur from sickled cells trapped in blood vessels of the eye. Osteoporosis may develop from the rapid growth of bone marrow. The femoral head or vertebrae may collapse, leading to compression and deformities. The spleen is nonfunctioning in the patient with sickle-cell anemia because of the increased hemolysis. The spleen normally is important in fighting infection. So, infection is a common cause of death. Infections are most commonly caused by the *Pneumococcus*, *Meningococcus*, *Salmonella*, and *Haemophilus influenzae*.

Diagnosis

The diagnosis of sickle-cell anemia is based on history, physical assessment, and laboratory findings. Laboratory tests include a red blood cell count, stained blood smear, Sickledex test to detect sickle-cell hemoglobin, and a hemoglobin electrophoresis test to distinguish sickle-cell anemia from sickle-cell trait. All African-American infants should be screened for sickle-cell disease. (The US Department of Public Health recommends that all infants be screened for sickle-cell disease to reduce morbidity and mortality.)

Management

Patients with sickle-cell anemia begin penicillin prophylaxis by the age of 2 months. This helps prevent infection, the most serious complication of sickle-cell anemia. Medical management may also include surgery to treat gallstones and fractures, transfusions of packed red cells to treat anemia, antipyretics to reduce fever, IV fluids to maintain hydration, and localized heat and analgesics to promote joint comfort. Skin grafts may be needed to treat leg ulcers. The primary goal is to prevent complications of cerebral hemorrhage, shock, and uremia leading to renal failure and even death.

People with the disease or trait are offered genetic counseling to help them decide whether or not to have children. All siblings of those with sickle-cell anemia should be screened for the disorder. Life span is usually approximately 60 years, depending on the frequency of complications.

❖ Settings, Providers, and Collaboration for Care

Sickle-cell anemia is detected and treated most frequently on an outpatient basis. Medications can be administered at home. Supportive treatment, continued assessment, and education can be given by a home health nurse or may require visits to the physician's office or clinic. Patients and family members can be taught to manage some crises at home. Hospitalization is required for an acute, life-threatening crisis, such as splenic sequestration or acute chest syndrome.

NURSING PROCESS
Sickle-Cell Anemia

Assessment

Review the medical and family history and complete a physical assessment of the patient. Assess for chest pain, dyspnea, fever, cough, tachypnea, use of accessory muscles, and splinting, which may indicate pulmonary congestion and infection. Check for headache, nausea, and confusion.

Observe for jaundice, pallor, and dry skin. Assess for excessive thirst, poor skin turgor, diarrhea, and fatigue, which are indicative of dehydration. Palpate the liver and spleen for tenderness and enlargement. Assess the level of hydration and urine output to determine renal function. Large amounts of urine may be expected initially owing to interference in renal concentration.

Observe for and prevent high stress levels, anorexia, and malaise, which could aggravate a sickling crisis. Assess for changes in vision or eye pain caused from accumulation of sickled cells in the blood vessels of the eye.

Pain should be thoroughly assessed (Table 13–3). Sickle-cell patients often appear stoic and have become accustomed to having pain. They may not react to pain in the same way as other patients. Assess for pain in the extremities and reddened, warm, or inflamed skin resulting from inadequate circulation and infection. Assess for ulcers in the lower extremities, a common complication caused by impaired circulation. Check all peripheral pulses.

Assess the patient for joint pain, especially in the knees and elbows, caused by circulatory occlusion from the sickling. Monitor pain location, duration, and type. Observe the patient's activities. Look for limited movements and inability to move freely or to ambulate without assistance. Pain in weight-bearing bones may be indicative of osteoporosis. Look for signs of guarding or facial grimacing during ambulation.

Nursing Diagnoses and Planning

Nursing diagnoses and related expected patient outcomes commonly applicable to patients with sickle-cell anemia include those previously described under anemias as well as the following:

NDx: Pain related to venous stasis and occlusion from sickled cells

Planning: Patient Outcomes
1. Patient reports relief from pain.
2. Patient gradually moves freely without groaning, guarding, or grimacing.
3. Patient completes activities of daily living without interference from severe joint pain.

NDx: Altered cardiopulmonary, cerebral, and pe-

ripheral tissue perfusion related to decreased arterial oxygen saturation from sickled cells and decreased cardiac output from increased workload

Planning: Patient Outcomes
1. Patient's extremities are warm, color is adequate, and pulses are present.
2. Patient's laboratory studies are within normal ranges for the patient.
3. Patient denies headaches, confusion, or nausea.
4. Patient is able to perform activities of daily living without tachypnea, tachycardia, and dyspnea.

NDx: Risk for infection related to increased susceptibility from the systemic effects of the disease

Planning: Patient Outcomes
1. Patient's vital signs are within normal ranges for the patient.
2. Patient's laboratory studies are within normal ranges for the patient.
3. Patient denies chills, sore throat, cough, shortness of breath, anorexia, or pain or burning on urination.
4. Patient denies pain in joints and legs (long bones).

Nursing Interventions and Evaluation

NDx: Pain

Help the patient experience minimal joint pain by using pillows to support joints and bony prominences. Reposition the patient frequently. Bedrest may be required to decrease pain. Use passive and active range-of-motion exercises on the unaffected extremity to keep muscles in tone and to retain flexibility. Cleanse and dress leg ulcers carefully. Use a bed cradle to keep the bed linen off the painful area. Give analgesics as prescribed. Remove constricting clothing.

NDx: Altered cardiopulmonary, cerebral, and peripheral tissue perfusion

Help the patient conserve oxygen needs by encouraging rest and limiting activities. Assist the patient with meals, if needed. Encourage increased intake of fluid to decrease blood viscosity and prevent dehydration. Elevate the head of the bed to aid in chest expansion. Initiate oxygen therapy, if needed.

Keep the patient in a comfortable position and reposition frequently to release pressure. Utilize range-of-motion exercises to stimulate circulation. Monitor vital signs and laboratory studies to assess for changes and improvements in status. Encourage ambulation as tolerated, but provide for frequent rest periods to decrease cardiac workload. Assist the patient when he or she is ambulating, because decreased cerebral circulation may cause disorientation and vertigo.

Discourage smoking to avoid vasoconstriction. Remove constricting clothing and keep heavy bed linens from restricting peripheral circulation. Keep

Table 13–3

Assessment of Pain in the Sickle-Cell Patient

1. Where is the pain located? Have you experienced pain in this location previously?
2. What is the character of the pain? Is the character similar to pain you have experienced before?
3. What is the severity of the pain? Rate the pain on a scale of 0 to 10 with 0 being pain-free and 10 being the worst pain you have ever felt.
4. Is anything in particular associated with the onset of the pain? Does anything help the pain?
5. How long have you had the pain?

the patient's legs in a nondependent position when he or she is not ambulating.

NDx: Risk for infection

Reposition the patient frequently to stimulate circulation. Tell the patient to cough and take deep breaths, using maximum chest expansion. Monitor the patient's vital signs frequently, observing subtle changes that may indicate early signs of infection. Report any changes noted. Watch for an increasing white blood cell count on laboratory data. Prophylactic antibiotics are given to most patients with sickled cells on a long-term basis to decrease the risk of infection.

Culture any wounds on legs. Look for signs of purulent drainage. Use aseptic dressing changes (Highlight 13–7).

Promote good nutrition by serving meals in a relaxed, attractive atmosphere. Encourage a high-protein, high-vitamin diet (see Highlight 13–3). Provide oral hygiene frequently to prevent infection and promote better eating habits. Encourage increased fluid intake. Keep the patient warm and avoid extreme changes in temperature in the room. Restrict visitors to prevent exposure to infections. Use protective isolation if appropriate.

Compare the patient's status with the expected outcomes. If the outcomes are not met, reassess the patient and revise the plan.

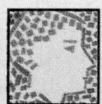

HIGHLIGHT
13–7
PATIENT EDUCATION

Methods to Prevent Infection in Leg Ulcers Related to Sickle-Cell Crisis

Instruct the patient with leg ulcers resulting from sickle cell complications to:

Utilize aseptic dressing changes to prevent infection.

Use gloves when handling dressings.

Remove dressings carefully to prevent further trauma.

Apply prescribed medications to legs before reapplying dressings.

Dispose of dressings in separate plastic bag.

Not rewrap dressings too tightly. Check feet for circulation by observing color and temperature.

Not exercise legs if they are swollen or ulcerations are severe.

Rest legs in a nondependent position.

THALASSEMIA

Etiology and Pathophysiology

Thalassemia is an inherited, chronic hemolytic anemia predominantly affecting individuals with Greek, Italian, and Southern Chinese ancestry. It also affects African-Americans and people from central Africa. This anemia is characterized by thin, fragile red blood cells known as target cells. Thalassemia minor is a mild anemia and occurs in heterozygotes, whereas thalassemia major or Cooley's anemia is more severe and occurs in homozygotes.

Clinical Manifestations

Patients with thalassemia minor may have a mild microcytic anemia that is not clinically significant. Clinical manifestations of thalassemia major include a mongoloid appearance caused by increased bone marrow activity, which results in thickening of the cranial bones. Cholelithiasis, splenomegaly, and jaundice are present as a result of hemolysis of abnormal cells. Leg ulcers may also be present. Cardiomegaly and fatigue result from increased cardiac workload.

Diagnosis

The diagnosis of thalassemia is based on history, physical assessment, and laboratory studies, including red blood cell count, serum electrophoresis, serum bilirubin, fecal and urinary urobilinogen, and hemoglobin studies.

Management

Patients with thalassemia minor require no treatment. Medical management of thalassemia major involves semi-monthly, monthly, or bimonthly blood transfusions of packed red blood cells. These patients may also receive folate supplements. Complications can occur from excessive blood transfusions. These include cardiac dysrhythmias and elevated iron levels. They are treated with antiarrhythmics and chelating agents, respectively. A splenectomy may be necessary if the spleen is destroying the transfused cells. Life expectancy is very poor for patients with thalassemia major.

❖ Settings, Providers, and Collaboration for Care

Thalassemia is most frequently detected and treated on an outpatient basis. Medications can be administered at home. Patients with thalassemia major may be admitted to the hospital for blood transfusion. Hospitalization will be required if a splenectomy is necessary. Referral to a genetic counselor for the patient and family is encouraged.

NURSING PROCESS GUIDELINES
Thalassemia

The assessment, nursing diagnoses, expected patient outcomes, nursing interventions, and evaluation for patients with thalassemia are similar to those described previously for patients with other anemias. In addition, because patients with thalassemia undergo marked changes in appearance and lifestyle, nursing care includes offering the patient and family support throughout the course of the disease. Help them find coping strategies to deal with the changes in appearance and lifestyle. Make referrals for additional counseling as needed.

GLUCOSE-6-PHOSPHATE DEHYDROGENASE DEFICIENCY

Etiology and Pathophysiology

Glucose-6-phosphate dehydrogenase deficiency is an inherited sex-linked disorder involving a deficiency of glucose-6-phosphate dehydrogenase enzyme, which is important in glucose metabolism by red blood cells and in membrane stability. The deficiency is carried by women and affects men. Hemolysis occurs most frequently when the red cells are affected by certain pharmacologic agents.

The disease affects more than 100 million people worldwide. In the United States, approximately 15% of African-Americans and 2% of whites are affected. It is also common among Greeks, Italians, and Arabs.

Like all cells, red blood cells need glucose for energy. When exposed to oxidative foods and drugs, or following a fever, red blood cells must metabolize an increased amount of glucose. In patients with glucose-6-phosphate dehydrogenase deficiency, the red blood cells cannot metabolize adequate amounts of glucose, resulting in hemolysis.

Clinical Manifestations

Patients are usually healthy without chronic anemia or splenomegaly. Clinical manifestations occur as a result of oxidative stress. Clinical manifestations include acute intravascular hemolysis that lasts up to 2 weeks. Generalized anemia, pallor, and jaundice are usually present. Hemoglobin is found in the urine and in higher-than-normal levels in the blood.

Diagnosis

The diagnosis of glucose-6-phosphate dehydrogenase deficiency is based on history and physical assessment. Laboratory findings may be normal except during episodes of hemolysis. During hemolysis, hemoglobinemia, hemoglobin in the urine, high serum bilirubin level, reticulocytosis, and Heinz bodies in red blood cells are present. High-risk populations should be routinely screened for glucose-6-phosphate dehydrogenase deficiency.

Management

Management includes removing the food or drug that precipitates the disorder (Highlight 13–8). Blood transfusions may be required.

❖ **Settings, Providers, and Collaboration for Care**

Detection and treatment of glucose-6-phosphate dehydrogenase deficiency occurs on an outpatient ba-

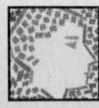

HIGHLIGHT
13–8
PATIENT EDUCATION

Prevention of Acute Attacks of Glucose-6-Phosphate Dehydrogenase Deficiency

Certain drugs initiate hemolysis of red blood cells. These attacks can be avoided by eliminating drugs known to cause the problem, including the following:

Sulfonamides

Aspirin

Thiazide diuretics

Oral hypoglycemics

Chloramphenicol

Antimalarial agents

Vitamin K derivatives

Persons not exposed to these agents may remain asymptomatic indefinitely.

sis in homes, doctor's offices, and clinics. Patient teaching is needed so that food and drugs precipitating the disorder can be avoided. Referral to a genetic counselor may be indicated.

NURSING PROCESS GUIDELINES
Glucose-6-Phosphate Dehydrogenase Deficiency

The assessment, nursing diagnoses, expected patient outcomes, nursing interventions, and evaluation for patients with glucose-6-phosphate dehydrogenase deficiency are similar to those described previously for patients with other anemias. In the acute phase of the disease, promote frequent rest periods, increased fluid intake, and good nutrition to maximize the patient's health status. Inform the patient and family about the clinical course of the disease and the treatment by reinforcing the physician's instructions and answering any questions the patient and family may have. Explain which drugs to avoid to reduce the risk of severe manifestations of the disease.

IMMUNE HEMOLYTIC ANEMIA

Etiology and Pathophysiology

Immune hemolytic anemia is caused by the lysis of red blood cells. In this case, lysis occurs when red blood cells combine with antibodies, which then may react with foreign cells (as in a blood transfusion) or with host cells. The red blood cell breakdown that occurs may be severe. The antibodies cover the red blood cells, which are then removed by the spleen. Undestroyed cells are reintroduced into the blood stream as spherocytes, which have a reduced life span.

The disorder may be caused by or may follow a variety of disorders, such as infection, systemic disease, transfusion reaction, snakebite, or fetal-maternal blood exchange. The resulting anemia may range from mild anemia to severe hemolysis and hyperbilirubinemia.

Clinical Manifestations

Clinical manifestations include fatigue, dyspnea, jaundice, splenomegaly, and cardiac arrhythmias. Anemia occurs with a rapid onset. Patients may present with angina or congestive heart failure. The disorder may be minor enough to produce no apparent symptoms, or extremely severe, resulting in a life-threatening state of shock.

Diagnosis

The diagnosis is based on physical findings, history of causative factors, and laboratory studies. Hematocrit levels may be less than 10%. Reticulocytosis is present with spherocytes seen on blood smear. The indirect bilirubin is increased and the direct Coomb's test is positive.

Management

The cause of the disorder is determined and removed if possible. Treatment consists of blood transfusions in severe cases or steroid therapy in mild cases. As the hemolysis decreases, drug treatment is reduced or discontinued. A splenectomy may be necessary if other interventions are not successful in reducing the red blood cell hemolysis.

❖ Settings, Providers, and Collaboration for Care

Detection and treatment of immune hemolytic anemia most frequently occurs on an outpatient basis. Medications can be administered at home or in the clinic. Hospitalization will be required for splenectomy or for close observation during transfusion.

NURSING PROCESS GUIDELINES
Immune Hemolytic Anemia

The assessment, nursing diagnoses, expected patient outcomes, nursing interventions, and evaluation for patients with immune hemolytic anemia are similar to those described previously for patients with other anemias.

POLYCYTHEMIAS

The polycythemias are a group of disorders characterized by an increase in circulating red blood cells and hemoglobin concentration. Polycythemia is grouped into three types: primary, secondary, and familial. Primary polycythemia is the most common type and is also known as polycythemia vera.

Polycythemia Vera

Etiology and Pathophysiology

Polycythemia vera is characterized by overproduction of erythrocytes, leukocytes, and thrombocytes. This results in increased blood viscosity and volume and congestion of all tissues and organs. Polycythemia vera is most common among the middle-aged and among Jewish men. The cause of the disease is unknown.

Clinical Manifestations

Clinical manifestations include splenomegaly and hepatomegaly as a result of an increase in red blood cells, white blood cells, platelets, and blood volume. Skin changes such as redness, pruritus, petechiae, ecchymoses, and hematomas occur from distended blood vessels. Blood pressure, pulse, and respirations are elevated owing to the increased blood volume and viscosity. Headaches, tinnitus, and epistaxis may occur because of increased blood pressure and distended vessels. The increased cardiac workload may result in respiratory and circulatory impairment, fatigue, and weakness.

Complications include cerebral vascular accident, thrombosis, myocardial infarction, and hemorrhage resulting from the high blood viscosity and distended blood vessels. Gastrointestinal bleeding and gangrene may occur from impaired circulation. Peptic ulcers are often the result of the high levels of gastric secretions. Increased red blood cell destruction results in high uric acid levels and in gout.

Diagnosis

The diagnosis of polycythemia vera is based on physical assessment and diagnostic procedures, including complete blood count, especially the red blood cell count and hematocrit, and bone marrow biopsy.

Management

Management involves administration of oxygen, radioisotope therapy, or chemotherapeutic agents such as chlorambucil, cyclophosphamide, busulfan, and nitrogen mustard to suppress bone marrow growth. Diet therapy includes foods low in sodium to reduce fluid accumulation. Emergency management includes removing 500 to 2000 mL of blood to decrease the hematocrit level to 45%. Phlebotomies are done initially one to three times per week until the hematocrit level is less than 45%. Once the hematocrit is decreased, the phlebotomies can be repeated every 2 to 3 months.

❖ Settings, Providers, and Collaboration for Care

Polycythemia vera is most frequently detected and treated on an outpatient basis. Medication can be administered at home or in the clinic. Phlebotomies can be performed in the laboratory or clinic. The disease may increase in severity over time. Hospitalizations may be required for more intensive therapies. Regular follow-up visits to the physician are important to keep the disorder in control.

NURSING PROCESS
Polycythemia Vera
Assessment

Check the patient's history and laboratory findings and complete a thorough physical assessment. Look for changes in skin color and appearance. Ask whether the patient has experienced epistaxis due to congested capillaries and increased blood pressure. Assess for vertigo, headache, tinnitus, blurred vision, shortness of breath, dyspnea, neck vein distention, orthopnea, edema, and fatigue to determine circulatory and respiratory status. Auscultate breath sounds. Observe for nausea, vomiting, or anorexia. Palpate for enlarged liver and spleen caused by tissue congestion. Note signs of thrombus formation such as edema, pain, and changes in skin color.

Assess for blood in the urine and stools, which indicate distended or ruptured vessels. Ask whether the patient has experienced any abdominal pain or heartburn, which indicate increased gastric secretions. Check for signs of elevated uric acid levels, as evidenced by edematous and painful joints. Note the big toe, which is frequently the first joint affected. Assess the level of knowledge about the disease, its manifestations, and treatment.

Nursing Diagnoses and Planning

Nursing diagnoses and related expected patient outcomes commonly applicable to patients with polycythemia vera include the following:

NDx: Fatigue related to increased metabolic requirements and circulatory changes

Planning: Patient Outcomes
1. Patient acknowledges increased energy levels.
2. Patient demonstrates interest in surroundings, appears energetic, and is less irritable.
3. Patient completes daily activities without complaints of fatigue.

NDx: Altered cardiopulmonary and peripheral tissue perfusion related to increased arterial pressure and interruption of arterial and venous blood flow

Planning: Patient Outcomes
1. Patient presents stable vital signs, palpable pulses, and appropriate level of consciousness.
2. Patient's urine output is adequate, with no apparent signs of blood.
3. Patient's skin is warm and dry, with no evidence of pallor.
4. Patient performs moderate activities without dyspnea, tachypnea, or tachycardia.

NDx: Knowledge deficit: nature of the disease, treatment, and potential alteration in lifestyle needed

Planning: Patient Outcomes
1. Patient relates accurate information about the cause, effects, and clinical course of the disorder.
2. Patient lists strategies to cope with the disorder and the adjustments in lifestyle that both the patient and family can achieve.
3. Patient chooses a diet low in sodium and avoids gas-producing and highly acidic foods and fluids.

Nursing Interventions and Evaluation

NDx: Fatigue

Instruct the patient to note fatigue levels, when the fatigue is most severe, when the peak energy level occurs, and what activities are performed at those times. Assist the patient in creating a schedule of daily activities that capitalizes on the patient's ability to function well at certain times and allows for rest during times of exhaustion. Review the activities in the patient's daily routine and prioritize them with the patient. Help the patient look for ways to delegate tasks and reduce energy-using activities. Tell the patient to ask for assistance with self-care or other activities of daily living when fatigued.

Identify coping strategies with the patient and family. Explain the effects of stress on energy levels. Teach the patient about the benefits of moderate exercise and assist with the planning of a realistic program of daily exercise with frequent rest periods. Stress the need for uninterrupted sleep periods.

Provide time for the patient and family to discuss their feelings and concerns about the disease, its effect on the patient, and the potential alterations in lifestyle needed.

NDx: Altered cardiopulmonary and peripheral tissue perfusion

Help the patient conserve oxygen needs by encouraging rest and limiting activities. Elevate the head of the bed to aid in lung expansion. Initiate oxygen therapy if needed. Assist the patient with activities of daily living, if needed, to conserve energy.

Keep the patient in a comfortable position and reposition frequently to release pressure. Utilize range-of-motion exercises to stimulate circulation. Monitor vital signs and laboratory studies to assess for changes and improvements in status. Encourage ambulation as tolerated but provide for frequent rest periods to decrease cardiac workload. Discourage smoking to avoid vasoconstriction. Discuss strategies to reduce stress, which could cause increased blood pressure. Remove constricting clothing and keep heavy bed linen from restricting peripheral circulation. Keep the patient's legs in a nondependent position when he or she is not ambulating.

Provide a low sodium diet to reduce fluid retention. Instruct the patient to avoid gas-forming and highly acidic foods and fluids. Give prescribed medications to promote increased circulation and diuresis as needed. Monitor laboratory studies to assess pulmonary, circulatory, and renal function.

NDx: Knowledge deficit: nature of the disease, treatment, and potential alteration in lifestyle
Explain the disease to the patient and family in understandable terms. Allow for questions and discussion about concerns, fears, and misunderstandings. Tell the patient that medical care must continue throughout his or her lifetime. Explain the need for phlebotomies every 2 to 3 months, or more frequently, to reduce the volume of circulating blood. Describe all prescribed medications, noting the dose, time, frequency, side effects, and toxic effects. Write out specific instructions for the patient and family to take with them upon discharge.

Teach the patient about diet modifications appropriate to reduce some of the complications of the disease. Give examples of menu plans incorporating low-sodium, low-gas-producing, and low-acid foods. Ask for consultation from a dietitian.

Teach the patient the signs and symptoms of complications of the disease, such as bleeding, and when to seek medical intervention. Advise the patient to avoid stimulants and to stop smoking to reduce vasoconstriction, which may increase blood pressure.

Teach strategies to reduce stress and how to balance rest with exercise. Demonstrate range-of-motion exercises to promote good circulation. Discuss the lifestyle changes necessary to cope with the complications of the disease, such as fatigue and circulatory problems. Find ways the family can assist the patient. Seek assistance from clergy or professional counselors if appropriate.

Compare the patient's status with the expected outcomes. If the outcomes are not met, reassess the patient and revise the plan.

Leukocyte-Related Disorders

AGRANULOCYTOSIS

Etiology and Pathophysiology

Agranulocytosis is characterized by a reduced number of leukocytes (leukopenia) and neutrophils (neutropenia) in the blood. The cause of agranulocytosis is usually a drug toxicity or hypersensitivity to phenothiazines, antithyroid drugs, sulfonamides, or other drugs. High doses of chemotherapeutic drugs and extended radiation therapy also cause neutropenia. The disorder is more common in women than in men. The incidence increases with age.

Antibiotics (handwritten annotation)

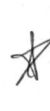

Clinical Manifestations

The primary clinical manifestation of agranulocytosis is infection, which produces symptoms of fever, chills, fatigue, and ulcerations of mucous membranes. Because the number of the patient's granulocytes is significantly reduced, the body's defense against infection is impaired. A variety of disorders other than anemias and infections—such as tuberculosis, typhoid fever, malaria, and uremia—are also associated with agranulocytosis.

Diagnosis

The diagnosis is based on history of exposure to a causative agent, physical assessment, and laboratory studies, including white blood cell count; throat, blood, urine, and stool cultures; and a bone marrow examination.

Management

Management includes removing the causative agent, treating infections with antibiotics, and reducing fever with antipyretics. Sedatives for sleep may also be necessary. Human granulocyte colony-stimulating factor can be given in the form of a drug known as filgrastim (Highlight 13–9). Agranulocytosis can be fatal without immediate treatment. With treatment, the production of granulocytes resumes.

❖ Settings, Providers, and Collaboration for Care

Detection and treatment of agranulocytosis occurs most frequently in the doctor's office or ambulatory clinic. The causative agent can be removed and infections can be treated without hospitalization. Hospitalization may be required for reverse isolation during severe neutropenia.

NURSING PROCESS
Agranulocytosis

Assessment

Review the history and potential cause of the disorder and perform a physical examination. Ask the patient what medications, if any, have been or are presently being taken. Observe for toxic signs if the patient is taking drugs known to increase the risk of agranulocytosis.

Check the skin and mucous membranes for redness. Assess the lungs for adventitious sounds. Assess for anorexia, severe fatigue, weakness, persistent cough, sore throat, ulcerations of the mouth or throat, and dysphagia. Also check for prostration, fever, dehydration, diaphoresis, weak, rapid pulse, and severe chilling. Any of these may indicate the presence of infection. Palpate for enlarged lymph nodes. Ask about problems with elimination such as constipation.

Nursing Diagnoses and Planning

Nursing diagnoses and related expected patient outcomes applicable to patients with agranulocytosis may vary with the cause (such as specific drugs). Those commonly applicable in all cases of agranulocytosis include the following:

NDx: Risk for infection related to decreased body defenses against microorganisms

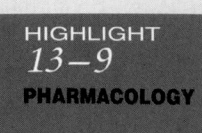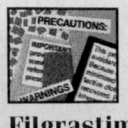

HIGHLIGHT
13–9
PHARMACOLOGY

Filgrastim

Definition:

Human granulocyte colony-stimulating factor produced by recombinant DNA

Commercial Preparations and Dosage:

Neupogen

Dosage ranges from 1 μg/kg/day to 6 μg/kg/day given by subcutaneous bolus, continuous subcutaneous infusion, or continuous intravenous infusion.

Peak serum levels will be reached 2 to 8 hours after subcutaneous or intravenous administration.

Treatment should be continued until the absolute neutrophil count reaches 10,000/mm^3.

Action:

Promotes the growth of neutrophils and enhances the function of mature neutrophils.

Side Effects:

Abnormal ST segment depression

Bone pain

Thrombocytopenia

Drug fever

Gastrointestinal distress

Dyspnea

Nursing Implications:

Dilute only with 5% dextrose in water (D$_5$W) when giving intravenously.

Store in refrigerator. Should be discarded if exposed to room temperature for more than 6 hours.

Do not shake the solution.

Monitor for side effects.

Monitor laboratory data.

Observe for leukocytosis.

Notify physician about temperatures >38°C (101°F)

Assess respiratory status and skin daily.

Teach patient and family infection control precautions.

Planning: Patient Outcomes
1. Patient's vital signs are within normal limits for the patient.
2. Patient's laboratory studies are within normal limits for the patient.
3. Patient denies cough, chills, fever, ulcerations, or other signs of infection.

NDx: Knowledge deficit: nature of the disorder and prevention of complications

Planning: Patient Outcomes
1. Patient states the cause and effects of the disorder.
2. Patient recognizes early signs of infection.
3. Patient verbalizes strategies to prevent infection.
4. Patient states the importance of avoiding self-medicating without a physician's approval.
5. Patient recognizes when to seek medical intervention.

Nursing Interventions and Evaluation

NDx: Risk for infection
Assist the patient in remaining infection-free by using protective isolation. Restrict visitors and pre-vent personnel with colds from caring for the patient.

Encourage increased fluid intake to prevent dehydration. Offer six to eight small meals daily that are high in protein and vitamins to promote energy and improve the patient's nutritional status. Soft, bland foods may be ordered if the patient is experiencing a sore mouth or throat. Give meticulous mouth care. Encourage warm saline irrigations of the throat every hour to prevent bacterial accumulation.

Assist the patient in bowel elimination by diet and fluid therapy and the addition of stool softeners if necessary. Tell the patient not to strain with defecation because tearing of the rectal mucosa could lead to infection. Enemas may be harsh and should also be avoided. Avoid taking the patient's temperature rectally because it may lead to a rectal abscess.

Encourage active and passive range-of-motion exercises every hour as tolerated. Turn the patient and encourage him or her to cough and breathe deeply to prevent hypostatic pneumonia. Encourage adequate rest periods and even bedrest, if necessary, to minimize oxygen requirements and conserve energy. Relieve fever with tepid baths but prevent chilling.

NDx: Knowledge deficit: nature of the disorder and prevention of complications

Teach the patient and family about the nature of the disease, possible causes, and preventive measures. Allow time for questions and verbalization of concerns. Give the patient literature about agranulocytosis, as appropriate, to refer to in the future. Speak in terms the patient and family can understand.

Inform the patient about the importance of avoiding infections. List signs and symptoms of infections for the patient and explain the need for early medical intervention if any symptoms appear. Tell the patient not to take any medications without the approval of the physician.

Explain the importance of good nutrition, moderate exercise, and frequent rest periods to prevent infections. Tell the patient to avoid drafts, extreme changes in temperature, and chilling.

Compare the patient's status with the expected outcomes. If the outcomes are not met, reassess the patient and revise the plan.

NEOPLASIA

Leukemias

Etiology and Pathophysiology

Leukemia is the term used to categorize a group of disorders in which a neoplastic growth of white blood cells occurs in the bone marrow. The leukemic cells multiply while suppressing bone marrow functions, resulting in decreased production of red blood cells, platelets, and other types of granulocytes. The spleen and lymph nodes are also involved. The etiology of leukemia remains unknown; however, studies indicate some genetic predispositions and viral implications. Leukemia has a high incidence in people previously exposed to excessive radiation and chemical agents. Leukemia occurs in eight to nine people per 100,000 per year. It is a common cause of death among children.

Leukemias are classified according to their onset, cell maturity, and prognosis. Each type affects a different age group. Acute leukemia has a rapid onset and involves blood-forming organs. The leukocytes produced are immature cells. Acute leukemia is usually fatal within days to months if untreated. It occurs most frequently in children and young adults. Chronic leukemia has an insidious onset. The cells produced are more mature and differentiated white cells. Most patients affected by chronic leukemia are between 25 and 60 years old at onset and survive 5 years or more.

Leukemias are also classified according to white blood cell type and tissue involved, such as lymphocytes, myelocytes, or monocytes. They are then further delineated as acute or chronic.

There are six primary categories of leukemias.

- Acute lymphocytic leukemia
- Acute myelocytic (granulocytic) leukemia
- Acute monocytic leukemia (rare)
- Chronic lymphocytic leukemia
- Chronic myelocytic (granulocytic) leukemia
- Chronic monocytic leukemia (rare)

About 60% of all leukemias are acute, 25% are chronic lymphocytic, and 15% are chronic myelocytic. Four of the most common types are discussed here.

ACUTE LYMPHOCYTIC LEUKEMIA. Acute lymphocytic leukemia is characterized by malignant growth of lymphoblasts in the marrow and peripheral tissues that spreads to surrounding organs. Hepatosplenomegaly and lymphadenopathy are present in 70 to 80% of patients with acute lymphocytic leukemia. Bone or joint pain occurs in approximately 25% of these patients. Eighty percent of those affected by acute lymphocytic leukemia are children. The peak incidence in children is between 2 and 4 years old, with a significant decrease at age 10. Acute lymphocytic leukemia rarely occurs after age 15.

Acute lymphocytic leukemia is usually treated with a variety of drugs, including vincristine, L-asparaginase, prednisone, daunorubicin, and doxorubicin. These and other chemotherapeutics can be used individually or in combination.

Acute lymphocytic leukemia has the best prognosis of all the leukemias. With chemotherapy, the median survival time is about 5 years. If untreated, the survival time is 4 to 6 months. When treated, about half of the children with acute lymphocytic leukemia are considered cured. In adults, only 10 to 15% are considered cured following treatment. In children, a complete remission rate of 80 to 95% can be expected, whereas in adults the rate is 50 to 70%. The older the patient, the lower the remission rate.

ACUTE MYELOCYTIC LEUKEMIA. Acute myelocytic leukemia is characterized by immature myeloblasts in bone marrow that infiltrate various organs. It most commonly occurs in adolescence and after age 55. If untreated, the median survival rate is about 2 to 4 months.

Chemotherapies frequently used include vincristine, prednisone, daunorubicin, cytarabine, and other drugs given singularly or concurrently. With chemotherapy, complete remission occurs in 50 to 75% of all patients. The median survival rate is approximately 2 to 3 years. Approximately 20% of treated patients are in complete remission after 5 years.

CHRONIC LYMPHOCYTIC LEUKEMIA. Chronic lymphocytic leukemia is characterized by a slow growth of lymphoid cells within the lymph nodes, bone marrow, liver, and spleen. It can occur at any age but is most common between ages 50 and 70. It is three times more common in men. Chronic lymphocytic leukemia occurs in about three people per 100,000 annually. The average survival time for a person with chronic lymphocytic leukemia without treatment is 4 to 6 years. With treatment, it is 7 years. Chemotherapeutic agents used for patients with chronic lymphocytic leukemia include chlorambucil, COP (Cytoxan, Oncovin, prednisone), or other similar drugs.

CHRONIC MYELOCYTIC LEUKEMIA. Chronic myelocytic leukemia is characterized by a slow, abnormal growth of granulocytic cells. It is associated with a chromosomal abnormality called the Philadelphia chromosome. Primary symptoms include long-bone pain due to bone marrow engorgement, anemia, and massive splenomegaly. Chronic myelocytic leukemia occurs in approximately one person per 100,000 per year. It occurs at any age but is most common in persons between 40 and 60 years old. It is more common in men. The average survival time for people with chronic myelocytic leukemia is 3 to 4 years. Chemotherapy does not increase the life span but does produce prolonged asymptomatic periods. Drugs used to arrest chronic myelocytic leukemia include busulfan, hydroxyurea, DAT

(daunorubicin, ara-C, thioguanine), and others in combination with these.

A comparison of the cellular changes, age of onset, signs and symptoms, treatment, and prognosis of the different categories of leukemia can be seen in Table 13–4.

Clinical Manifestations

Clinical manifestations of the leukemias include respiratory complications caused by an increased metabolic rate from the overproduction of leukocytes and increased susceptibility to infections, anemia, and bleeding tendencies from decreased red blood cells, low hemoglobin levels, and thrombocytopenia. Malnutrition may be evident, with anorexia, nausea, and vomiting. Mouth soreness also contributes to the anorexia. Infiltration into the central nervous system, meninges, and cranial nerves may cause headaches, visual problems, nausea, vomiting, tinnitus, and vertigo. Fatigue and weakness are present from hypoxia.

Table 13–4

Types of Leukemia

	Acute Lymphocytic Leukemia	Acute Myelocytic Leukemia	Chronic Myelocytic Leukemia	Chronic Lymphocytic Leukemia
Cellular Changes	Begins in bone marrow stem cell; affects growth of lymphoblasts	Mild proliferation of immature blast cells	Slow, abnormal growth of granulocytic cells	Slow abnormal growth of lymphoid cells
Age of Onset	Less than 15 years old; peaks between ages 2 and 4	Adolescence and after age 55	Any age, but most common between ages 40 and 60	Most common between ages 40 and 60
Symptoms	Abrupt onset of malaise, fever, lymphadenopathy, hepatosplenomegaly, pallor, fatigue, cutaneous and nasal bleeding, anemia, decreased platelets, increased susceptibility to infection	Abrupt onset of anemia, thrombocytopenia purpura, epistaxis, splenomegaly, increased susceptibility to infection	Long-bone pain, anemia, splenomegaly, malaise, fatigue, heat intolerance	Weight loss, anemia, splenomegaly, malaise, fatigue, enlarged lymph nodes
Treatment	Chemotherapy, such as vincristine, L-asparaginase, prednisone, daunorubicin, and doxorubicin	Chemotherapy, such as vincristine and prednisone	Chemotherapy with busulfan, hydroxyurea, and DAT (daunorubicin, ara-c, thioguanine)	Chemotherapy with chlorambucil, COP (Cytoxan, Oncovin, prednisone)
Prognosis	Good; 50% of all treated children are considered cured	20% of treated patients are in remission after 5 years	Average survival time is 3 to 4 years	Average survival time with treatment is 7 years

Systemic or local infections with fever develop as a result of an increased susceptibility to invading microorganisms. Pus is usually absent because of the low white blood cell count. Infections may also cause mouth and throat ulcerations to appear. These ulcers, along with some of the effects of the therapies, contribute to anorexia.

Splenomegaly, hepatomegaly, enlarged lymph nodes, and engorged bone marrow occur as a result of tissue distention from an increase in white blood cells. Abdominal pain and distention are also complications of tissue distention. Gradually leukemic cells invade all tissues and organs in the body.

Joint, sternum, bone, and nerve pain occur from deposits of blast cells in chronic myelogenous leukemia and from the pressure of enlarged lymph nodes, usually more common in chronic lymphocytic leukemia.

Uric acid levels are increased because of purine metabolism and chemotherapy destroying the white blood cells. When abnormal white blood cells invade the kidneys, uremia and renal failure result. Neurologic changes occur as well.

Diagnosis

The diagnosis of leukemia is based on history, physical assessment, and laboratory studies of white blood cell count, differential leukocyte count, presence of blast cells in the blood, and a bone marrow examination for the presence of abnormal cells. Blood, wound, throat, urine, and stool cultures are obtained to determine which organisms are present.

Management

Chemotherapy is the primary treatment for patients with acute leukemias. (See Chapter 34 for discussion on the care of the patient receiving chemotherapy.) Radiotherapy may be used in patients who are drug resistant, especially those with chronic myelocytic leukemia. A splenectomy may be indicated. (See Splenectomy, Chapter 12.) Autografting and bone marrow transplantation may be conducted in patients with chronic myelocytic leukemia. (See Bone Marrow Transplant, Chapter 32.)

Medical management includes analgesics for mild pain. Narcotics and tranquilizers may be ordered for severe pain and to enhance other drug actions. Nonaspirin antipyretics are used to control fever. Aspirin and nonsteroidal anti-inflammatory drugs should be avoided because they interfere with platelet function.

Stool softeners are ordered to promote bowel elimination. Allopurinol, potassium acetate or citrate, and sodium bicarbonate are ordered to alkalinize the urine and to prevent gout. The patient is hydrated with 3 to 4 L of intravenous fluids per day if uric acid levels are elevated.

Antibiotics are ordered to treat infections, which are a major cause of death in the leukemic patient. Studies are being conducted on the development of specific antibiotics to treat leukemic cells. Chest x-rays may be used to diagnose pneumonia and determine the degree of disease involvement.

Red blood cells and platelets are transfused, when necessary, to treat severe anemia or to prevent or treat acute hemorrhage. The use of leukapheresis (lymphocyte removal from the blood) is under investigation.

❖ Settings, Providers, and Collaboration for Care

Leukemia may be treated in outpatient settings. The first cycle of treatment may be given in the hospital because of the risk for infection and bleeding. Hospitalization may be required during crisis stages or immunosuppression. A central line may be inserted to give medications and draw blood at home. Home health care should be included in discharge planning and is needed for care of the central line and for patient and family education at home. If a splenectomy is required, the patient will be hospitalized. During the terminal stages of illness, the patient may be treated at home with the help of hospice personnel.

NURSING PROCESS

Leukemia

Assessment

Review the patient's history and laboratory findings and perform a physical examination. Ask whether the patient has had recent exposure to chemicals, chemotherapy, or radiation. Look for signs of infection, bleeding of the gums, ecchymoses, or pain.

Observe for fatigue, weakness, malaise, cyanosis, dyspnea, tachycardia, and weight loss from increased metabolic rate. Assess for petechiae, purpura, bruising, pallor, shortness of breath, headache, weakness, and tachycardia indicative of anemia.

Note any tender, reddened areas on mucous membranes. Assess for fever, ulcerations, and bleeding gums, which indicate a localized mouth infection. Also assess for systemic infections that may be manifested by changes in vital signs.

Ask about burning, pain, and frequency of urination, which may indicate an infection. Assess the color and consistency of the urine. Observe for elimination patterns. Check the stool for blood. Note any constipation or diarrhea episodes.

Check for anorexia, nausea, vomiting, and sore throat and mouth, which may interfere with nutritional intake. Ask whether the patient has been experiencing gastric irritation.

Assess for tenderness, pain, or enlargement of the liver, spleen, and lymph nodes. Note changes in degree and site of pain. Observe for muscle weakness and edema, which can further aggravate pain levels. Assess for joint, bone, or nerve pain. Subcutaneous lumps due to proliferating deposits of blast cells may be present in advanced stages of chronic myelocytic leukemia. Pain may be caused by pressure from enlarged lymph nodes. In chronic lymphocytic leukemia, lymph nodes are smooth, mobile, discrete, and nontender and vary in size (Nursing Care Guide 13–2).

Observe for presence of gout as manifested by heat, redness, or tenderness in one or more peripheral joints, especially the great toe. Assess for blood levels of uric acid. Check the diet for a high level of purine foods.

Assess for headaches, confusion, restlessness, changes in vision, retinal hemorrhages, and papilledema, which indicate abnormal white blood cell infiltration into the central nervous system.

Observe for crying episodes, withdrawal, inability to concentrate, loss of appetite, insomnia, irritability, depression, and threats of suicide, which indicate a high stress level. Assess the patient's and family's coping mechanisms. See which strategies seem to be most functional. Note any support systems.

Assess the patient's level of knowledge about leukemia. Find out whether the patient and family understand the effects of the disease and the treatments used to arrest the course of the disease.

Nursing Diagnoses and Planning

Nursing diagnoses and related expected patient outcomes commonly applicable to patients with leukemia include the following:

NDx: Risk for infection related to the compromised immune response

Planning: Patient Outcomes
1. Patient's vital signs and results of laboratory studies are within normal limits for the patient.
2. Patient denies cough, chills, fever, sore throat, ulcerations of the mouth, or burning on urination.
3. Patient identifies signs of infections and measures to prevent them.
4. Patient is in protective isolation.

NDx: Altered nutrition: less than body requirements related to anorexia secondary to sore mouth, chemotherapy, or radiation sickness

Planning: Patient Outcomes
1. Patient eats well-balanced meals, choosing high-protein and high-vitamin foods (see Highlight 13–3).
2. Patient chooses nonirritating foods.
3. Patient eats six to eight small meals daily to conserve energy and avoid distention.
4. Patient increases fluid intake to keep well hydrated.

NDx: Sensory/perceptual alterations (visual, auditory, and kinesthetic) related to malignant infiltration into the central nervous system

Planning: Patient Outcomes
1. Patient reports decrease in or absence of headaches, visual impairment, vertigo, nausea, and vomiting.

2. Patient requests assistance as needed when ambulatory to prevent injury.
3. Patient is alert and oriented to time, place, and person.

NDx: Pain related to enlarged nodes, chemical treatments, and bone infiltration

Planning: Patient Outcomes
1. Patient reports that pain is controlled with analgesics.
2. Patient utilizes comfort measures to help relieve pain.
3. Patient utilizes coping measures to help relieve or tolerate pain.

NDx: Activity intolerance related to weakness, poor nutrition, and depressed energy stores from anemia, complications of treatment, and stress

Planning: Patient Outcomes
1. Patient reports increased ability to perform activities of daily living.
2. Patient demonstrates no shortness of breath upon mild exertion.
3. Patient reports less weakness with increased tolerance for activity.
4. Patient sleeps 6 to 10 hours per night without difficulty.

NDx: Anxiety related to health status, fear of death or treatment outcomes, and complications of the disease

Planning: Patient Outcomes
1. Patient's anxiety is lessened as evidenced by stable vital signs, relaxed appearance, and calm, positive attitude.
2. Patient states strategies to cope with the disease manifestations.
3. Patient verbalizes fears and concerns.

NDx: Knowledge deficit: nature of illness and complication of bleeding related to thrombocytopenia

Planning: Patient Outcomes
1. Patient reports accurate information about the nature of the disease.
2. Patient states accurately the signs of bleeding and when to notify the physician.
3. Patient presents no signs or symptoms of bleeding such as petechiae, ecchymoses, epistaxis, dark stools, and so on.
4. Patient verbalizes the preventive measures necessary to prevent bleeding (see Highlight 13–5).

Nursing Interventions and Evaluation

NDx: Risk for infection
Keep the patient warm and avoid extreme changes in temperature in the room. Restrict visitors to prevent exposure to infections. Use protective isolation if appropriate.

Monitor the patient's vital signs frequently, observing subtle changes that may indicate early signs of infection. Report any changes noted.

Nursing Care Guide 13–2
Patients with Chronic Lymphocytic Leukemia

Assessment Findings: Patient complains of fatigue, weakness, hypoxia, dyspnea, tachycardia, malaise; exhibits decreased levels of hemoglobin and red blood cells and thrombocytopenia.

Nursing Diagnosis: Activity intolerance related to overall weakness and an increased metabolic rate from the overproduction of leukocytes

Patient Outcomes	Nursing Interventions	Rationale
Patient completes activities of daily living without fatigue or weakness.	Allow for frequent rest periods. Provide a quiet environment and encourage energy-saving techniques.	Adequate rest periods throughout the day prevent extreme fatigue, save energy stores, and decrease oxygen demands.
Patient states that he or she is free of insomnia and sleeps well at night.	Offer sedatives as indicated. Encourage at least 8 hours of sleep every night. Provide quiet without interruptions.	Increasing sleep periods restores energy and reduces fatigue.
Patient is free from labored respirations; vital signs are within normal ranges.	Elevate head of bed and monitor vital signs. Auscultate lungs every shift. Encourage patient to fully expand chest with respirations.	Changes in vital signs may indicate increasing problems of oxygen deficiency or other complications.

Evaluation: Compare the patient's status with the expected outcomes. If the outcomes are not met, reassess the patient and revise the plan.

Assessment Findings: Patient complains of fever; mouth ulceration; respiratory distress; bleeding gums; hypertrophy of mouth, throat, and gums; vital sign changes; tender, reddened areas; elevated white blood cell count; burning or pain with urination, frequency of urination, odor or dark amber coloration of urine; perirectal abscess; blood in urine and stool; diarrhea; constipation; signs of septicemia; and pneumonia.

Nursing Diagnosis: Risk for infection related to increased susceptibility from inadequate primary and secondary defenses

Patient Outcomes	Nursing Interventions	Rationale
Patient's temperature and vital signs are within normal limits.	Monitor temperature. Apply ice packs; use hypothermia units or cool body sponging and nonaspirin antipyretics.	Keeping the patient's temperature within normal limits is important to prevent complications of hyperthermia.
Patient identifies actions taken to prevent infections and reduce risk of contamination.	Encourage 3000 to 4000 mL of fluid daily to prevent dehydration. Tell the patient to refrain from association with people with respiratory infections.	The patient with insufficient defenses against secondary infections needs increased awareness of methods to prevent infections.

(continued)

Nursing Care Guide 13–2
Patients with Chronic Lymphocytic Leukemia (continued)

Patient Outcomes	Nursing Interventions	Rationale
	Instruct patient to avoid venipunctures and injections when possible to prevent organisms from entering the blood stream.	Multiple venipunctures may increase the patient's risk of septicemia or a localized infection.
	Place patient in reverse isolation (ie, laminar air flow).	Reverse isolation protects the patient from external contaminants. This may be particularly necessary during acute exacerbations of the disease.
	Obtain blood, throat, urine, stool, and/or wound culture to determine type of organism present.	
Patient denies pain or burning with urination, frequency of urination, and odor and dark coloration of urine.	Provide and encourage increased fluids.	Continual flushing of the urinary tract decreases risk of an infection.
Patient experiences adequate bladder and bowel elimination.	Offer the urinal or bedpan frequently, or assist the patient to the restroom.	
	Provide stool softeners to reduce irritation.	Eliminating straining with bowel movements may prevent breakdown and abscesses around the anal area.
	Inspect skin for reddened areas, lesions, and so on.	
Patient maintains skin integrity.	Promote good hygiene.	The patient with decreased immune function is at increased risk for skin breakdown and infection when on bedrest.
	Offer sitz baths to promote circulation and healing.	
	Turn the patient frequently and massage reddened areas.	Stimulating circulation to the skin surfaces helps alleviate some of the potential problems.

Evaluation:	Compare the patient's status with the expected outcomes. If the outcomes are not met, reassess the patient and revise the plan.

Assessment Findings:	Patient experiences nausea, vomiting, anorexia, diarrhea, constipation, abdominal distention, flatus, and sore mouth from ulcers.
Nursing Diagnosis:	Altered nutrition: less than body requirements related to anorexia, secondary to a sore mouth and radiation sickness

Patient Outcomes	Nursing Interventions	Rationale
Patient's appetite improves.	Promote good oral hygiene.	Appropriate nutrition is essential for healing, maintenance of normal body functions, and prevention of infections.
Patient consumes foods high in calories, protein, and vitamins.	Offer six to eight small meals a day.	
	Encourage diet high in calories, protein, and vitamins.	
	Encourage high fluid intake.	
	Monitor fluid intake and output.	
Patient maintains appropriate weight level.	Weigh patient daily on same scale with similar clothing.	Positive reinforcement encourages the patient to continue to progress.
	Commend the patient for achieving the appropriate weight as recommended.	

(continued)

Nursing Care Guide 13–2
Patients with Chronic Lymphocytic Leukemia (continued)

Patient Outcomes	Nursing Interventions	Rationale
Patient relates adequate knowledge regarding proper food intake.	Teach patient about appropriate diet and hygiene habits. Allow time for questions and concerns about the nutritional needs.	An understanding of the type of nutrition intake necessary may prevent future problems for the patient. Having the patient restate the information reinforces the learning and allows for corrections if there are misunderstandings.
	Have the patient reiterate the directions provided by the physician and nurse. Note bowel elimination pattern.	With inadequate nutrition, the patient may experience altered elimination patterns.
Patient's elimination patterns are adequate.	Offer stool softeners as needed. Encourage increased fluid intake.	

Evaluation: Compare the patient's status with the expected outcomes. If the outcomes are not met, reassess the patient and revise the plan.

Assessment Findings: Patient complains of red, sore tongue; mouth ulcers; sore throat; bleeding gums; anorexia; thirst; and dry mouth.

Nursing Diagnosis: Altered oral mucous membrane related to disease or treatment

Patient Outcomes	Nursing Interventions	Rationale
Patient states food intake does not irritate mouth.	Offer six to eight small meals of soft, bland food per day to reduce irritation to the mouth. Encourage 3000 to 4000 mL of fluids per day.	Small amounts of bland food at frequent intervals are less irritating to the oral mucosa.
Patient states mouth discomfort has subsided.	Instruct patient that mouth lesions will subside when remission is achieved.	Exacerbations of the disorder and the treatments initiated increase the susceptibility to oral mucosal breakdown.
	Encourage oral hygiene every 2 hours using a soft cotton-tipped applicator. Keep lips well lubricated.	Frequent oral hygiene helps reduce infections and breakdown within the oral cavity.
Patient's oral cavity is free from ulcers, bleeding, and lesions.	Have patient rinse mouth with hydrogen peroxide and water and gargle before eating.	Hygiene before meals makes foods more palatable.
	Offer cold foods high in protein (eg, ice cream, chilled fruit, vegetable juices). Avoid hot or spicy foods and acidic juices.	Cold foods are more soothing to the oral mucosa. Spicy foods may feel as if they are burning the mucosa if lesions are present.

(continued)

Nursing Care Guide 13–2
Patients with Chronic Lymphocytic Leukemia (continued)

Patient Outcomes	Nursing Interventions	Rationale
	Inspect mouth three times daily. Ensure that oral hygiene regimen is being completed every 2 to 3 hours throughout the day and every 6 hours during the night.	Continued proper oral hygiene prevents further mouth problems.

Evaluation: Compare the patient's status with the expected outcomes. If the outcomes are not met, reassess the patient and revise the plan.

Assessment Findings: Patient experiences joint, bone, or nerve pain; muscle weakness; edema; and heat, redness, or tenderness in joints, especially toes, ankles, knees, hands, and elbows, demonstrating gout. Enlarged, smooth, mobile, discrete, nontender subcutaneous nodes causing pain.

Nursing Diagnosis: Pain related to tissue distention, muscle wasting, edema, or chemotherapy

Patient Outcomes	Nursing Interventions	Rationale
Patient moves without signs of severe pain, such as grimacing, moaning, or guarding.	Investigate complaints of discomfort. Encourage relaxation exercises and deep diaphragmatic breathing. Position patient for comfort. Support joints and extremities with pillows.	Relaxation exercises may help reduce pain. Keeping bony prominences padded eliminates pressure to the area and increased discomfort.
Patient reports that pain is relieved or controlled.	Offer analgesics for mild pain, and narcotics for severe pain. Offer tranquilizers to enhance drug actions. Encourage patient's coping mechanisms. Massage areas of pain.	

Evaluation: Compare the patient's status with the expected outcomes. If the outcomes are not met, reassess the patient and revise the plan.

Assessment Findings: Patient exhibits behaviors of crying, withdrawal, inability to concentrate, loss of appetite, insomnia, irritability, depression, and threats of suicide.

Nursing Diagnosis: Anxiety related to diagnosis and concerns of death or dying

Patient Outcomes	Nursing Interventions	Rationale
Patient verbalizes fears and concerns.	Allow patient to vent feelings regarding disease and treatment process in a nonjudgmental environment.	Free verbalization of anxiety helps relieve some of the fear and concerns.

(continued)

Nursing Care Guide 13–2
Patients with Chronic Lymphocytic Leukemia (continued)

Patient Outcomes	Nursing Interventions	Rationale
Patient and family demonstrate reduced anxiety and fear.	Encourage family to participate. Reassure patient and family that feelings of fear, anxiety, and depression are very common. Allow for friends and clergy to visit. Maintain eye contact with patient.	Encouraging family or other significant others to participate helps provide support systems for the patient.
Patient exhibits coping mechanisms to deal effectively with problems.	Offer professional counseling referrals. Assist patient and family in identifying coping strategies.	Appropriate coping with the trauma of disease is important to the healing process.

Evaluation:	Compare the patient's status with the expected outcomes. If the outcomes are not met, reassess the patient and revise the plan.

Assessment Findings:	Patient asks questions when in doubt; states that he or she does not understand disease process, prevention techniques, and treatment.
Nursing Diagnosis:	Knowledge deficit: nature of disease, treatment, and prevention of complications

Patient Outcomes	Nursing Interventions	Rationale
Patient verbalizes accurate information about disease, treatment, and self-care.	Explain disease process to patient. Provide literature. Provide information about nutritional requirements, fatigue prevention, and comfort measures. Instruct patient to avoid contact sports, razors, aspirin, and alcohol intake to prevent or minimize bleeding.	Explanation of the disorder and typical treatment plan reinforces the physician's information and helps the patient understand the disease and health care needs. Explain to patient that aspirin should be avoided because it interferes with platelet functions and may enhance bleeding.
Patient relates the importance of reporting signs and symptoms of infection to the health-care team. Patient exhibits health-promotion behaviors such as choosing proper foods, inspecting mouth and gums, and so on.	Encourage patient and family to observe and report signs of developing infection. Provide a list of signs and symptoms of infections for the patient. Explain that early detection and treatment may limit the severity of infection. Discuss the importance of preventing constipation and rectal pain and bleeding. Teach the patient good oral hygiene techniques.	Having the patient relate information for preventions given provides opportunity to assess the patient's understanding of the disorder and to correct any misunderstandings. Having the family involved gives additional support to the patient. Compliance is more likely if the patient and family understand the importance of prevention of complications.

(continued)

Nursing Care Guide 13-2
Patients with Chronic Lymphocytic Leukemia (continued)

Patient Outcomes	Nursing Interventions	Rationale
Patient relates the side effects of therapy and coping strategies to minimize them. Patient states names, dosage, action, and side effects of medication.	Inform patient of common side effects of antileukemic therapy (eg, gastrointestinal disturbances, diarrhea). Explain treatment of chemotherapy or radiotherapy if applicable. Explain importance of taking antibiotics on schedule. Explain that platelet and white blood cell transfusions are routine in treatment. Red blood cells may be transfused in patients with anemia, and platelets may be used to treat hemorrhage. Teach patient some strategies for coping with or alleviating the side effects of therapy.	Information about the side effects alerts the patient to be prepared for them and to attempt to prevent their occurrence. Knowledge of the medications and therapy used is important to prevent additional problems and to promote patient participation in the treatment regimen.
Evaluation:	Compare the patient's status with the expected outcomes. If the outcomes are not met, reassess the patient and revise the plan.	

Promote good nutrition by serving meals in a relaxed, attractive atmosphere. Encourage a high-protein and high-vitamin diet. Provide oral hygiene frequently to prevent infection and promote better eating habits.

Encourage mouth cleansing every 2 hours with a nonirritating substance. Keep the patient's lips well lubricated to prevent skin breakdown. Have the patient use antimicrobial mouthrinse to help prevent the growth of microorganisms. One teaspoon of sodium bicarbonate in water is soothing, especially when bleeding is present.

Explain the importance of preventing constipation, because it can cause irritation, bleeding, and infection of the rectal mucosa. Use stool softeners when indicated. Diarrhea caused by chemotherapy is treated by careful cleaning of the rectal area after each episode. Give antidiarrheal medications as prescribed.

Since early identification and treatment may limit the severity of the infection, teach patients and their families to continually observe for signs of developing infection upon discharge and to notify the physician if such signs appear.

NDx: Altered nutrition: less than body requirements
Encourage the patient to eat a diet high in calories, protein, and vitamins (see Highlight 13–3). Offer six

to eight small meals per day of soft, bland foods to reduce irritation and trauma to the mouth and gastrointestinal tract.

Serve the meals in an attractive manner. Allow the patient time to eat and assist with eating if necessary. Provide rest periods prior to eating so that the patient will not be too fatigued to eat.

NDx: Sensory/perceptual alterations (visual, auditory, and kinesthetic)
Teach the patient to use safety measures at all times. Explain to the family the need for their assistance to the patient to prevent injury. Have the patient request assistance when getting out of bed and ambulating. Keep the bed rails up and place frequently used articles within the patient's reach.

Check the patient frequently for orientation to time, place, and person. Speak loudly if auditory problems are evident. Decrease the external stimuli and provide periods of rest. Give analgesics as prescribed to control headaches.

NDx: Pain
Place the patient in comfortable positions and reposition frequently. Use pillows to support bony prominences. Assess when the pain is most severe and allow the patient to rest during those periods. Give pain medications as ordered prior to activity

periods so that the patient can better tolerate the movement. An around-the-clock dosing schedule of analgesics may be needed for the patient with chronic severe pain.

Help the patient find alternate methods to alleviate or to be able to tolerate the pain. Show the patient and family relaxation techniques and how to perform massage. Teach the patient the use of patient-controlled analgesia if ordered.

NDx: Activity intolerance

Instruct the patient to develop a regimen of activity with frequent rest periods throughout the day. Encourage the patient to do range-of-motion exercises frequently while lying in bed to maintain muscle tone and strength. Tell the patient to avoid sudden movements, such as getting out of bed quickly, because this decreases the blood supply to the brain, aggravating vertigo and disorientation. Have the patient practice deep breathing exercises to increase oxygen and blood to the brain. Teach the patient to practice energy-saving techniques to reduce fatigue and shortness of breath. Place frequently used articles within the patient's reach.

Provide and encourage frequent rest periods while delivering patient care. Prevent interruptions during rest periods and at night, whenever possible. Reduce any disturbing noises and limit visitors as necessary.

Provide warm clothes and blankets to prevent chilling. Avoid unnecessary exposure to drafts and extreme changes in temperature.

Encourage good nutrition to increase the patient's energy level. Offer four to six meals daily. This is less tiring for the patient and prevents gastric overdistention.

NDx: Anxiety

Allow the patient to verbalize concerns about the disease, its effects on the patient and family, and fears about death. Help the patient and family find coping strategies that are effective to deal with their anxiety level. Allow time for questions from the patient and the family.

Teach the patient relaxation techniques to help reduce the anxiety. Explain how stress can aggravate the complications of the disease. Tell the patient to rest frequently during the day. Provide comfort measures, both physical and emotional, to the patient and family.

Explain the disease process, the treatments, and potential results so that the patient has a better understanding of the disease and its progression. Allow time for the patient and family to be alone when needed. Seek assistance from clergy or other professional counselors when appropriate. Make referrals as needed to social service agencies.

NDx: Knowledge deficit: nature of disease and complication of bleeding

Instruct the patient about the clinical course of leukemia and the complication of hemorrhage. Teach the patient signs of bleeding to observe for and when to seek medical assistance. Explain the need for avoiding sharp objects, straight razors, contact sports, and injections and venipuncture whenever possible. Tell the patient to watch for discoloration of urine or stools.

Explain proper oral hygiene methods necessary to prevent further irritation and ulceration of mucous membranes. Instruct the patient to use a soft toothbrush and to use mouthrinse frequently. Show how to inspect the oral cavity, checking the tongue and gums for early signs of irritation. Teach the patient to avoid extremely hot, spicy foods and acidic drinks to lessen oral and gastrointestinal irritation (Highlight 13–10).

Compare the patient's status with the expected outcomes. If the outcomes are not met, reassess the patient and revise the plan.

Hodgkin's Disease

Etiology and Pathophysiology

About half of all lymphomas are Hodgkin's disease, a chronic, malignant disorder of unknown etiology that originates in the lymphatic system and spreads to other organs and structures in later stages. Hodgkin's disease is characterized by large atypical tumor cells or abnormal histiocytes called Reed-Sternberg cells. These cells invade the lymph nodes, spleen, and liver. As they multiply, they replace normal cells and cause necrosis and fibrosis. Hodgkin's disease is classified by stages (Table 13–5) according to lymph node involvement, appearance, severity, and prognosis. The incidence of Hodgkin's disease peaks at the ages of 20 to 24 and again at 60 to 65 years of age. It is twice as likely to occur in men as in women.

Prognosis varies by stage at the time of diagnosis. Ninety-five percent of patients with localized Hodgkin's disease can be cured or have a 10-year survival without recurrence when treated early. Patients in Stages I and II are usually cured with radiation treatment if the disease has not spread to the lymph node chains, spleen, and nasopharynx. Patients in Stages III and IV cannot be cured but usually experience symptomatic relief when treated

Table 13–5

Stages of Hodgkin's Disease

Stage I	Involvement of a single lymph node region or lymphoid structure
Stage II	Involvement of two or more lymph node regions on the same side of the diaphragm
Stage III	Involvement of lymph node regions on both sides of the diaphragm
Stage IV	Diffuse or disseminated involvement of one or more distant extranodal organs

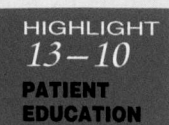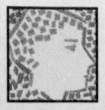

HIGHLIGHT 13–10

PATIENT EDUCATION

Self-Care for Prevention of Leukemia Complications

To prevent complications associated with leukemia, give patients these instructions:

Prevent infection by:

- Avoiding contact with persons who have coughs, colds, and fevers.
- Developing good hygiene practices, such as frequent hand washing, careful wound or abrasion cleaning, and good oral care.
- Recognizing early signs of infection and seeking treatment immediately.
- Avoiding sharp instruments, razors, injections, and venipunctures to prevent breaks in the skin that could provide entry for microorganisms.
- Getting adequate rest and eating properly to maintain general resistance levels.

Prevent bleeding by:

- Avoiding razor blades for shaving, using sharp instruments, having injections or venipunctures, and participating in contact sports.

Promote good nutrition and prevent irritation by:

- Eating a diet high in calories, protein, and vitamins.
- Eating six to eight small meals of soft, bland foods daily.
- Rinsing the mouth every 2 hours with a mixture of hydrogen peroxide and water.
- Avoiding hot, spicy foods.
- Drinking up to 4000 mL of fluids daily.
- Avoiding high-purine foods, such as liver, kidneys, sweetbreads, brains, sardines, and anchovies.

Prevent pain by:

- Understanding the usage, dosages, and side effects of medication prescribed for pain by the physician.
- Using relaxation methods.
- Developing comfort measures to be used at home.

---

with both radiotherapy and chemotherapy or combination chemotherapy. Eighty percent of patients undergoing combination chemotherapy experience complete remissions. Untreated patients have a 5-year life expectancy.

Clinical Manifestations

The first sign of Hodgkin's disease is a painless, superficial adenopathy. Other early clinical manifestations include pruritus, weakness, night sweats, and intermittent fever. Respiratory changes, edema, and cyanosis result from enlarged lymph nodes pressing on the superior vena cava. Pressure on the nerves and esophagus may result in laryngeal paralysis and dysphagia.

Infection occurs from immunodeficiency, the result of chemotherapy, and the invasion of the malignancy into the viscera. High- and low-grade fevers are common. Pneumonia, septicemia, and urinary infections are the most frequently acquired infections.

Renal impairment is present as a result of invasion of the kidneys by abnormal leukocytes. Gout may be present because of the increased production of uric acid in the blood as a result of increased cell production. The central nervous system may be affected as a result of infiltrating abnormal white blood cells. Dehydration may result from fever and diaphoresis.

Anemia is present as a result of red blood cell destruction. Prolonged lymphatic obstruction results in accumulation of fluid in the lungs and abdomen, usually present in later stages of the disorder.

Low blood counts indicate that the bone marrow and spleen are affected. Lymph nodes are painless and enlarged from the massive growth of abnormal cells. Splenomegaly and hepatomegaly are present, indicating organ involvement. Jaundice is present with liver damage and bile duct obstruction. Bilirubin is present in the blood.

Bone or mediastinal pain lasting as long as 1 hour occurs when alcohol is ingested. The cause of this symptom is unknown. Nerve pain resulting from nerve root compression may be present. If the spinal cord is compressed, paralysis occurs. Fractures or vertebral compression may occur if the disorder has spread to the bone.

Diagnosis

The diagnosis of Hodgkin's disease is based on history, physical assessment, and laboratory findings. Lymph node biopsy with the presence of Reed-Sternberg cells and a chest x-ray or computed tomographic scan to determine mediastinal involvement are the primary diagnostic tests. Blood tests are done to determine the presence of anemia. A staging laparoscopy is used to determine visceral involvement.

Management

Management for Stages I and II includes high-dose radiation therapy for 4 to 6 weeks. Stages III and IV are treated with radiation and chemotherapy combined. The most common chemotherapy combinations are the MOPP regimen, which includes mechlorethamine (Mustargen), vincristine (Oncovin), procarbazine, and prednisone, and the ABVD regimen, which is Adriamycin, bleomycin, vinblastine, and dacarbazine. Other chemotherapy combinations can be used if the treatment is for a recurrence following initial remission. Disease management may involve surgical removal of a large pressure-causing tumor. Antipyretics are ordered to reduce fever, and transfusions are given when anemia is present. (See Chapter 34 for care of the patient receiving chemotherapy.)

Complications of treatment include mouth and throat ulcers, anemia, and immunodeficiency following chemotherapy. Thrombocytopenia leading to hemorrhage may result from decreased levels of red blood cells and hemoglobin. Complications from radiation include hypothyroidism and radiation pneumonitis. Radiation toxicity may result from the high-dose radiation therapy. Side effects of radiation vary, depending on the area that is included in the treatment field.

❖ Settings, Providers, and Collaboration for Care

Hodgkin's disease is usually treated on an outpatient basis. The patient can visit the radiation therapy department and return home. Chemotherapy can be administered in a clinic, doctor's office, or sometimes in the home by a home health nurse. The patient and family need education on prevention of complications related to chemotherapy and radiation.

NURSING PROCESS
Hodgkin's Disease

Assessment

Review the history and conduct a physical examination. Question the patient about a recent history of pruritus, fever, and weakness. Assess for dyspnea, cough, stridor, chest pain, cyanosis, and pleural effusion, which indicate pulmonary involvement. Check the results of the laboratory studies.

Observe for facial and neck edema and cyanosis resulting from enlarged lymph nodes. Assess the patient's speech and swallowing for changes caused by pressure.

Observe for high fever alternating with prolonged low-grade fever, indicative of infection. Assess for night sweats, extreme fatigue, weight loss, and malaise, which are indicative of anemia. Assess for changes in urine output, which indicates spread of the disease to the urinary system.

Assess for complications from radiation or chemotherapy as manifested by dysphagia, dry mouth, fatigue, nausea, vomiting, skin rashes, hair loss, and myelosuppression. Palpate for painless enlargement of lymph nodes, especially on the sides of the neck, the axillae, and the groin.

Check the patient's dietary pattern. Observe for signs of inadequate intake, such as poor skin turgor and weight loss. Monitor fluid intake and output. Observe for signs of fatigue from malnutrition.

Look for edema of the extremities from pressure on the veins. Palpate for an enlarged spleen and liver, which indicates possible spread of the disease to those organs. Assess for vertebral compression and fractures, which indicate spread of the disease to bone. Observe for paralysis, which is indicative of spinal cord compression.

Assess for anxiety as evidenced by crying, withdrawal, lack of concentration loss of appetite, insomnia, irritability, depression and threats of suicide.

Nursing Diagnoses and Planning

Nursing diagnoses and related expected patient outcomes commonly applicable to the patient with Hodgkin's disease include the following:

NDx: Ineffective breathing pattern related to tracheobronchial obstruction from enlarged lymph nodes and pleural effusion

Planning: Patient Outcomes
1. Patient's vital signs are within normal ranges for the patient, with no signs of cyanosis, dyspnea, tachypnea, or tachycardia.
2. Patient uses good lung expansion techniques.
3. Patient is able to perform activities of daily living without respiratory distress.
4. Patient's blood gas levels are within normal ranges for the patient.

NDx: Risk for infection related to immunodeficiency, effects of chemotherapy, and the invasion of malignant cells into viscera

Planning: Patient Outcomes
1. Patient denies cough, dyspnea, sore throat, or mouth ulcers.
2. Patient denies pain or burning with urination.
3. Patient identifies actions needed to prevent infections.
4. Patient's vital signs are within normal ranges for the patient.

NDx: Altered nutrition: less than body requirements related to anorexia from treatments, fatigue, and complications of disease

Planning: Patient Outcomes
1. Patient chooses appropriate foods to replace dietary deficiencies.
2. Patient avoids irritating foods and fluids.

NDx: Activity intolerance related to reduced energy stores, decreased oxygen from ineffective breathing pattern, and inadequate nutrition

Planning: Patient Outcomes
1. Patient follows a regimen of planned activities and rest periods each day.
2. Patient reports feeling less fatigued and demonstrates signs of increased activity.
3. Patient is able to perform activities of daily living.
4. Patient's vital signs are within normal ranges for the patient.
5. Patient denies shortness of breath on mild exertion.

NDx: Anxiety related to inability to cope with the manifestations of the disease, fear of treatments, and threat of death

Planning: Patient Outcomes
1. Patient relates concerns about illness to the nurse or other appropriate member of the health-care team.
2. Patient and family verbalize accurate information about the disorder, complications, and therapy.
3. Patient expresses feelings of reduced anxiety and fear.
4. Patient displays physical signs of decreased anxiety: vital signs are within normal ranges and patient is resting well, appears calm, and eats well.

Nursing Interventions and Evaluation

NDx: Ineffective breathing pattern
Have the patient turn, cough, and breathe deeply hourly while awake to prevent respiratory infection and increase oxygen intake. Teach the patient to use full chest expansion. Elevate the head of the bed to assist with chest expansion and free movement of the diaphragm.

Encourage good nutrition with increased fluid intake for maintenance of health and hydration. Provide a diet high in protein, vitamins, and calories (see Highlight 13–3). Allow time for meals and provide rest periods prior to eating to prevent poor eating habits due to fatigue and respiratory difficulty. Assist the patient with eating if necessary.

Remove tight clothing to maximize respiratory efforts and promote circulation. Administer oxygen as needed. Have emergency equipment by the bedside for airway and respiratory support.

NDx: Risk for infection
Keep the patient warm and avoid extreme changes in temperature in the room. Restrict visitors to prevent exposure to infections. Use protective isolation if appropriate.

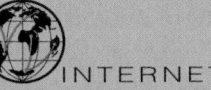
INTERNET CONNECTIONS
Hematologic Disorders

General
Bloodline—The Online Hematology Resource
http://www.cjp.com/blood/
An information resource for physicians, other health-care professionals, and patients. This site provides original reviews, forums, and a wide variety of links to other sites, including sites covering specific diseases.

Leukemia and Related Disorders
Leukemia Society of America
http://www.leukemia.org/
An authoritative site that includes specific information on leukemia as well as lymphomas, multiple myeloma, and Hodgkin's disease.

ONCOLINK
http://cancer.med.upenn.edu
This site, sponsored by the University of Pennsylvania Cancer Center Resource, provides links to a wide variety of sites, including:

Adult Leukemias
http://cancer.med.upenn.edu/disease/leukemia1/
This well-written site provides information, journal articles, and links to other sites.

Hemophilia
World Federation of Hemophilia
http://www.wfh.org/
This authoritative site provides updated family and medical news, a resource library, and links to other sites.

Promote skin integrity by avoiding sun exposure, shaving, or use of lotions, which may irritate the treatment area. Keep skin clean and dry.

Monitor the patient's vital signs frequently, watching for subtle changes that may indicate early signs of infection. Report any changes noted. Ask the patient to report any signs of infection, such as cough, dyspnea, sore throat, or pain or burning with urination.

NDx: Altered nutrition: less than body requirements
Help the patient maintain adequate nutrition by providing attractive meals in a pleasant atmosphere. Encourage patient to eat foods high in protein, vitamins, and calories. Provide six to eight small meals daily to prevent distention and reduce fatigue. Provide oral hygiene frequently to prevent infection and promote better eating habits. The patient may

require analgesics for discomfort related to esophagitis. Ask for a consultation with the dietitian.

Instruct the patient to avoid foods that are gas-forming, because they cause abdominal distention that may decrease the appetite and interfere with respiratory efforts. Avoid hot, spicy foods and acidic fluids to decrease gastrointestinal irritation when present. Encourage increased fluid intake to prevent constipation and promote adequate hydration. Monitor the patient's fluid intake and output.

NDx: Activity intolerance

Instruct the patient to develop a regimen of activity with frequent rest periods throughout the day. Encourage the patient to do range-of-motion exercises frequently while lying in bed to maintain muscle tone and strength. Tell the patient to avoid sudden movements, such as getting out of bed quickly, because this decreases the blood supply to the brain, aggravating vertigo and disorientation. Have the patient practice deep breathing exercises to increase oxygen and blood to the brain. Teach the patient to practice energy-saving techniques to reduce fatigue and shortness of breath. Place frequently used articles within the patient's reach. Provide and encourage frequent rest periods while delivering patient care. Prevent interruptions during rest periods and at night whenever possible. Reduce any disturbing noises and limit visitors when necessary.

Provide warm clothes and blankets to prevent chilling. Avoid unnecessary exposure to drafts or extreme changes in temperature. Encourage good nutrition to increase the patient's energy level. Offer four to six meals daily. This is less tiring for the patient and prevents gastric overdistention.

NDx: Anxiety

Allow patient to verbalize concerns about the disease, its effects on the patient and family, and fears about death. Help the patient and family find effective coping strategies to deal with their anxiety level. Allow time for questions from the patient and family. Seek assistance from clergy or other professional counselors when appropriate. Make referrals as needed to social service agencies.

Compare the patient's status with the expected outcomes. If the outcomes are not met, reassess the patient and revise the plan.

Non-Hodgkin's Lymphomas

Etiology and Pathophysiology

The incidence of non-Hodgkin's lymphoma has been rising 3 to 4% annually over the past few decades. It usually occurs in people between 50 and 60 years old. Non-Hodgkin's lymphomas consist of several lymphoid malignancies with varying histopathologies, clinical disease courses, and treatment responses. Generally, the abnormal lymphocytes infiltrate lymph nodes, organs, bone marrow, and peripheral blood. The cause of the lymphomas is unknown. Patients with renal transplant are at greater risk. Risk factors include exposure to certain viruses, immunosuppressive states, family history, and certain occupations with high exposure to herbicides and pesticides.

Non-Hodgkin's lymphomas are categorized into lymphocytic, histiocytic, and mixed cell types, each being nodular or diffuse on microscopic examination. These are further categorized as favorable or nonfavorable histology, depending on their response to treatment. Usually, a nodular cell structure has a more favorable prognosis than a diffuse cell structure, and a lymphocytic cytology is more favorable than a histiocytic cytology. Table 13–6 demonstrates the classifications of non-Hodgkin's lymphomas.

Clinical Manifestations

Clinical manifestations are similar to those of Hodgkin's disease, with some exceptions. Individuals with non-Hodgkin's lymphomas have involvement

Table 13–6

Stages of Non-Hodgkin's Lymphoma

Stage	Characteristics	Types
Low-grade lymphoma	Incurable but long survival	Small lymphocyte Follicular, small-cleaved Follicular, mixed small and large
Intermediate-grade lymphoma	May be curable but short survival in those who don't respond to treatment	Diffuse large cell Follicular large cell Diffuse mixed small and large Diffuse cleaved cell
High-grade lymphoma	Progresses rapidly May be curable but short survival in those who don't respond to treatment	Lymphoblastic Burkitt's Immunoblastic
Other		Cutaneous T-cell Adult T-cell leukemia/lymphoma T4 lymphocytosis

Table 13–7

Chemotherapy for Non-Hodgkin's Lymphomas

COP	Cyclophosphamide (Cytoxan)
	Vincristine (Oncovin)
	Prednisone
CHOP	Cytoxin
	Doxorubicin *Hydrochloride* (Adriamycin)
	Vincristine (Oncovin)
	Prednisone
COPP	Cytoxin
	Vincristine (Oncovin)
	Procarbazine
	Prednisone
MOPP	Nitrogen Mustard (Mustargen)
	Vincristine (Oncovin)
	Procarbazine
	Prednisone

of several sites early in the course of the disease rather than involvement of only one site, as is typical in Hodgkin's disease. Frequent sites of lymph node enlargement include cervical, axillary, inguinal, and femoral chains.

Initial painless lymphadenopathy usually occurs on one side of the body only. Abnormal cells spread to the bone marrow and eventually to the liver and spleen, causing hepatomegaly and splenomegaly. Gastrointestinal disturbances and nervous system changes are evident. Pressure on these areas creates pain and numbness, leading to paralysis. Anemia, fever, weight loss, weakness, and anorexia result from red blood cell destruction and infections.

Diagnosis

The diagnosis of non-Hodgkin's lymphoma is based on history, physical assessment, and laboratory findings. Lymph node biopsies; bone, chest, and abdominal x-rays and scans; and blood studies are the commonly used tests.

Management

Management involves a lower dose of radiotherapy for localized non-Hodgkin's lymphoma than for Hodgkin's disease because the bone marrow is involved and is more sensitive. Chemotherapy is given for nonlocalized non-Hodgkin's lymphoma.

The prognosis varies for non-Hodgkin's lymphomas. The chemotherapy combination COP (Cytoxan, Oncovin, and prednisone) produces some response in 90% of patients and complete response in 60 to 70% of patients. Cytoxan taken orally results in complete remission in 55% of patients, with a median survival time of more than 5 years. See Table 13–7 for common chemotherapeutic regimens used in non-Hodgkin's lymphomas.

In patients with diffuse histiocytic lymphoma, combination chemotherapy is preferred over single agents. COP, COPP (COP and procarbazine), MOPP,

CHOP (COP and Adriamycin), and other regimens result in complete responses in 40 to 50% of patients, whose median survival time is more than 3 years. Patients with nodular lymphocytic and histiocytic lymphoma have had complete responses with single agents, and 50 to 70% of patients treated with COP, COPP, MOPP, and other regimens have experienced a median survival time of 4.5 years for those who attained a complete response and 13 months for those with a partial response.

❖ Settings, Providers, and Collaboration for Care

Non-Hodgkin's lymphoma is treated on an outpatient basis. Radiation therapy and chemotherapy can both be given without hospitalization. Referral to a home health nurse for the drug administration is needed. Education may be needed to help the patient avoid complications related to anemia and chemotherapy. Hospitalization may be required during acute phases of illness or periods of neutropenia related to chemotherapy.

NURSING PROCESS GUIDELINES
Non-Hodgkin's Lymphoma

The assessment, nursing diagnoses, expected patient outcomes, nursing interventions, and evaluation for patients with non-Hodgkin's lymphomas are similar to those described previously for patients with Hodgkin's disease (Nursing Care Guide 13–3).

Multiple Myeloma

Etiology and Pathophysiology

Multiple myeloma is a malignant disease characterized by the growth of plasma cells, invading bone marrow, lymph nodes, liver, spleen, and kidneys. The cause of the disease is unknown. Multiple myeloma develops slowly over a period of time and occurs in older clients at a median age of 60 years. It is twice as common in men as in women. It accounts for 1% of all malignancies in whites and 2% of all malignancies in African-Americans. Usually, bone marrow is 5% plasma cells, but in multiple myeloma, bone marrow is 30 to 95% plasma cells, most of which are immature and malignant.

Clinical Manifestations

Clinical manifestations include the development of pneumonia, anemia, thrombocytopenia, and vascular insufficiency. Anemia, hemorrhage, renal failure, bone pain, and infection may occur as a result of impaired production of red blood cells, white blood cells, and platelets, resulting from replacement of bone marrow with plasma cells.

Neurologic complications may result from the tumor pressing on the spinal cord, causing paraplegia. Skeletal changes may occur from osteoporosis, pathologic fractures, and bone deformities.

Nursing Care Guide 13–3
Patients with Lymphomas

Assessment Findings: Patient complains of dyspnea, chest pain, hoarseness, cyanosis, and nonproductive cough.

Nursing Diagnosis: Ineffective airway clearance related to tracheobronchial obstruction, enlarged nodes, airway edema, or superior vena cava syndrome

Patient Outcomes	Nursing Interventions	Rationale
Patient exhibits a decrease in labored respirations without signs of pallor or cyanosis.	Assess respiratory status, rate, and rhythm. Observe for dyspnea, cyanosis, pallor, and cough. Auscultate chest.	Changes in respiratory pattern may indicate an airway problem.
Patient's chest is fully expanded, with respiratory rate maintained within normal range.	Teach patient how to maximize chest expansion. Administer oxygen as needed.	Maximizing chest expansion increases effectiveness of inspiratory pattern.
Patient completes activities of daily living without signs of respiratory difficulty or complaints of fatigue.	Promote rest and relaxation. Identify energy-saving techniques. Provide a quiet environment. Assist patient with activities of daily living. Administer cough suppressants as indicated.	Increased rest periods decrease fatigue and respiratory efforts.

Evaluation: Compare the patient's status with the expected outcomes. If the outcomes are not met, reassess the patient and revise the plan.

Assessment Findings: Patient experiences anorexia, dysphagia, unexplained weight loss, and edema.

Nursing Diagnosis: Altered nutrition: less than body requirements related to enlarged nodes, pressure on esophagus, or anorexia.

Patient Outcomes	Nursing Interventions	Rationale
Patient's appetite improves.	Encourage frequent small meals. Serve attractive meals of patient's choice of foods.	Frequent small meals served attractively help promote a better nutritional intake.
Patient verbalizes information regarding proper food intake.	Tell the patient to eat a diet high in calories, protein, and vitamins. Use soft or puréed foods if dysphagia persists.	Proper nutrition is necessary for general health maintenance and promotion of healing.

Evaluation: Compare the patient's status with the expected outcomes. If the outcomes are not met, reassess the patient and revise the plan.

Assessment Findings: Patient exhibits behavior of crying, irritability, withdrawal, anger, and fear; threatens harm to self.

Nursing Diagnosis: Anxiety related to diagnosis and fear of dying

(continued)

Nursing Care Guide 13–3

Patients with Lymphomas (continued)

Patient Outcomes	Nursing Interventions	Rationale
Patient verbalizes fears and concerns.	Encourage patient to verbalize concerns, fears, and questions regarding disease process and prognosis. Refrain from making judgments about the patient's fears.	Verbalization in a nonthreatening environment alleviates some of the distress and allows for free expression.
Patient and family demonstrate reduced anxiety and fear.	Encourage the family to participate.	Including the family gives support to the patient and allows them to freely express their concerns.
Patient exhibits coping mechanisms to deal effectively with problems.	Reassure patient that the fears are common and are experienced by most patients. Seek professional counseling assistance. Invite friends and clergy to visit. Identify coping strategies in patient and family.	Finding effective coping strategies is important to alleviate the anxiety. At times, professional assistance is necessary.

Evaluation: Compare the patient's status with the expected outcomes. If the outcomes are not met, reassess the patient and revise the plan.

Assessment Findings: Patient asks questions about disease process and treatment; expresses concerns about self-care.

Nursing Diagnosis: Knowledge deficit: nature of disease, treatment, and health care needed

Patient Outcomes	Nursing Interventions	Rationale
Patient verbalizes accurate information about disease, treatment, and self-care.	Explain the disease process, treatments, and health-care needs the patient will experience. Give patient written information when possible.	An understanding of the disease and its treatment and prognosis is important to increase the patient's compliance and prevent complications.
Patient relates the importance of health maintenance and complication prevention.	Have the patient reiterate the information provided by the physician and the nurse. Include family or significant others in the education sessions. Teach patient self-care health behaviors. Describe complications of the disease and prevention methods.	Reinforcement of information helps ensure understanding and allows corrections to be made if misinformation is present. Including the family adds additional reinforcement and provides support for the patient.
Patient states names and dosages of the medications and the side effects of each.	Inform patient of the medications used, side effects, and dosages.	Knowledge of the medications may decrease medication problems such as misuse or incorrect dosage once the patient is at home.

(continued)

Nursing Care Guide 13–3
Patients with Lymphomas (continued)

Patient Outcomes	Nursing Interventions	Rationale
Patient relates the treatment strategies, coping mechanisms to assist in reducing side effects, and self-care necessary.	Discuss the importance of preventing infections, maintaining adequate nutrition, and getting maximum rest. Teach patient how to employ coping mechanisms to reduce stress, pain, and other side effects.	Increased knowledge of self-care and prevention of complications decreases patient's risk of problems.
Evaluation:	Compare the patient's status with the expected outcomes. If the outcomes are not met, reassess the patient and revise the plan.	

Increased bilirubin and sedimentation rates and low sodium and chloride levels occur because of an increased susceptibility to infection as a result of impaired antibody formation. This is caused by plasma cell abnormalities in the bone marrow. Folate deficiency is present when the tumor absorbs the folate or the individual consumes a low amount of dietary folate.

Hypercalcemia, uremia, and renal stones may be present owing to inactivity and calcium and phosphorus lost in damaged bones. Bence Jones protein may be present in urine. These particles of protein are produced by malignant plasma cells in the bone tumors and may block convoluted tubules, resulting in renal disorders or failure. Osteolysis occurs if the tumor cells cause the marrow cavity to expand. Osteoporosis, backache, or bone pain results from skeletal involvement. Skeletal deformities occur in the sternum and ribs. Lytic lesions can be detected in the skull. The spine may be shortened. Multiple osteolytic lesions in the skull may be present.

Amyloidosis occurs in approximately 10% of all patients. Symptoms depend on the organ involved.

Diagnosis
The diagnosis of multiple myeloma is based on history, physical assessment, and laboratory studies, including serum electrophoresis and Bence Jones protein in urine. Skull x-rays are ordered to detect lesions. Bone marrow aspirations and biopsy are repeated every 6 to 12 months. Serum electrophoresis and urine protein electrophoresis are completed with each course of therapy and every 2 to 3 months during remission to determine the progress of the disorder.

Management
Management involves chemotherapy to reduce pain and bone tumor size and growth, and also supportive care for complications. Melphalan (Alkeran) and cyclophosphamide (Cytoxan) are two common alkylating agents used to treat patients with multiple myeloma. Alkeran, the most successful drug, has side effects of bone marrow depression and pancytopenia. Cytoxan has side effects of leukopenia, nausea, alopecia, and hemorrhagic cystitis. Blood counts are monitored weekly to determine the occurrence of myelosuppression.

Radiotherapy is used to treat spinal cord compression and pain unrelieved by chemotherapy. However, its use is limited because it may suppress marrow, which would limit the use of chemotherapy. Research suggests that interferon also has antitumor activity against multiple myeloma.

Anemia is treated with transfusions of packed red blood cells, and infections are treated with broad-spectrum antibiotics. Hypercalcemia, nausea, vomiting, and bone pain are treated with diuresis, prednisone, and mithramycin to help increase the secretion and catabolism. Allopurinol is used to treat and prevent hyperuricemia. Pain is also treated with a variety of analgesics. Allogenic bone marrow transplantation may be a curative treatment for patients under 55 years of age with a matching sibling donor.

The median survival time for untreated patients is less than 1 year. For treated patients, it is 20 to 30 months. Fewer than 10% of patients survive more than 5 years.

❖ Settings, Providers, and Collaborative Care
Multiple myeloma can usually be treated on an outpatient basis. Chemotherapy can be administered in a doctor's office or clinic. It may also be administered by a home health nurse in the patient's home. Education for the patient and family may also be done in the home. Hospitalization may be required to treat bone pain or complications, such as hypercalcemia.

NURSING PROCESS
Multiple Myeloma
Assessment
Review the history and complete a physical assessment. Assess for diminished or absent breath sounds over the involved areas. Listen for inspiratory wheezes and decreased resonance over areas of infiltration. Check for pallor, dry skin with poor turgor, nostril-flaring cyanosis, use of accessory muscles, elevated temperature, rapid pulse, and tachypnea.

Observe for symptoms related to the presence of renal stones and changes in urinary output. Monitor the laboratory data for the presence of Bence Jones protein in the urine. Check for signs of dehydration resulting from poor intake and vomiting caused by chemotherapy.

Observe for somnolence, polydipsia, anorexia, peripheral neuropathy, and constipation, which are indicative of hypercalcemia or uremia. Assess for dilated and tortuous retinal veins, papilledema, retinal hemorrhages, and epistaxis. Check the laboratory studies for the presence of calcium in blood or urine.

Observe for changes in activity and ambulation. Assess the patient for pathologic fractures of the ribs and weight-bearing bones and compression fractures of the spine due to osteoporosis. These may be evidenced by sudden, severe pain usually related to lifting or bending. Other clinical signs include kyphosis and loss of height. Check for changes in the pelvis, spine, and ribs that worsen with movement. Dysrhythmias, ecchymoses, peripheral nerve involvement, and gastrointestinal disturbances are common symptoms of amyloidosis, a complication of the disease.

Assess the patient's level of anxiety regarding the disease and prognosis. Check for an understanding of the treatment necessary and the complications.

Nursing Diagnoses and Planning
Nursing diagnoses and related expected patient outcomes commonly applicable to patients with multiple myeloma include those previously described under Hodgkin's disease and the following:

NDx: Pain related to malignant infiltration into bone

Planning: Patient Outcomes
1. Patient reports that pain is controlled with analgesics.
2. Patient states comfort measures to help relieve pain.
3. Patient states coping measures to help relieve or tolerate pain.

Nursing Interventions and Evaluation
NDx: Pain
Place the patient in comfortable positions and reposition frequently. Use pillows to support bony prominences. Assess when the pain is most severe and allow the patient to rest during those periods. Give pain medications as ordered prior to activity periods so that the patient can better tolerate the movement. Patients with bone involvement will require around-the-clock analgesia.

Help the patient find alternate methods to alleviate or to be able to tolerate the pain. Show the patient and family relaxation techniques and how to perform massage. Teach the patient the use of patient-controlled analgesia if ordered.

Additional Interventions
Assist the patient in counteracting calcium overload by promoting increased fluid intake to as much as 4000 mL/day. Record intake and output and note the color and consistency of the urine.

Prevent the complications of hypercalcemia and osteoporosis. Encourage ambulation and range-of-motion exercises as tolerated, as well as the use of canes, crutches, or a brace if necessary. Assist the patient with ambulation.

Promote good safety measures. Keep the side rails up. Use a trapeze for easier patient movement. Place personal items within reach of the patient.

Provide comfort by repositioning frequently and using pillows for support. Give good skin care without using harsh soap or rough towels. Use lotion on dry skin. Massage easily but frequently.

Compare the patient's status with the expected outcomes. If the outcomes are not met, reassess the patient and revise the plan.

Infections

INFECTIOUS MONONUCLEOSIS
Etiology and Pathophysiology
Infectious mononucleosis is a benign, self-limiting disease with mild, widespread effects throughout the body. It is caused by a herpes-like virus called the Epstein-Barr virus. The incubation period can be as long as several weeks. Mononucleosis commonly occurs in young adults with impaired body defenses and low resistance. It is estimated that 50 to 80% of the world's population is infected with the Epstein-Barr virus, but only those with antibodies to the virus develop infectious mononucleosis.

Infectious mononucleosis is most common in children between 3 and 5 years old and in persons between 15 and 30 years of age. The exact mode of transmission is unknown.

Clinical Manifestations
Symptoms include the presence of lymphocytosis, headache, sore throat, fever, chills, malaise, and generalized weakness and fatigue. Painful enlargement of the cervical, axillary, and groin lymph nodes is

common. The acute phase may last as long as a month, followed by an extended recovery period.

Splenomegaly may cause pain in the left upper quadrant. Hepatomegaly may indicate rare liver involvement. The nervous system may be affected by the increase in mononuclear leukocytes and pressure of enlarged organs or nerves.

Diagnosis

The diagnosis of infectious mononucleosis is based on history, physical assessment, and laboratory studies such as white blood cell count, positive heterophile agglutination test results (which demonstrate the presence of the Epstein-Barr virus), and increased mononuclear leukocytes.

Management

Infectious mononucleosis is usually self-limiting. The primary management is symptomatic. Bedrest is recommended. Salicylates are prescribed to reduce the fever, and antibiotics are used to suppress infection. The prognosis is excellent, and recovery usually occurs in 2 to 4 weeks. Rarely, a splenic rupture may occur from increased lymphocytes in the spleen. This may be evidenced by abdominal pain and shock. Emergency surgery is required to treat a splenic rupture.

❖ **Settings, Providers, and Collaboration for Care**

Infectious mononucleosis can be treated without hospitalization. The patient can remain on bedrest and take salicylates at home. Hospitalization is required only if major complications arise.

NURSING PROCESS GUIDELINES
Infectious Mononucleosis

Check the history and complete a physical examination of the patient. Observe for a sore throat, increased nasal secretions, generalized aches, and symptoms typical of influenza. Palpate for an enlarged liver and lymph nodes predominantly in the posterior cervical, axillary, and groin regions. Assess for left upper quadrant pain, which indicates splenic enlargement. Look for the presence of a macular rash. Check the nutritional status of the patient. Assess for headaches and vertigo, which indicate nervous system involvement. Observe for activity level changes such as weakness and inability to perform activities of daily living owing to extreme fatigue.

The nursing diagnoses, expected patient outcomes, nursing interventions, and evaluation for patients with infectious mononucleosis are similar to those described previously for patients with anemia. The patient with infectious mononucleosis is rarely hospitalized for treatment unless there are complicating factors present such as other infections or debilitation and extreme fatigue from long-term poor

nutrition. If this is the case, also focus on the specific manifestations of the complications.

*B*leeding Disorders

Bleeding disorders are classified as either purpuras—extravasation of a small amount of blood into the tissues and mucous membranes—or coagulation disorders. Purpuras are further divided into vascular purpuras or purpuras due to platelet disorders. Coagulation disorders include disseminated intravascular coagulation, acquired hypoprothrombinemia, and hemophilia. Major deficiencies underlying bleeding disorders include:

Weak, damaged vessels prone to rupture
Platelet deficiency (thrombocytopenia)
Impairment or lack of one of the clotting factors
Impaired fibrinolysis

PURPURAS

Etiology and Pathophysiology

Purpuras are either vascular, resulting from vessel damage or rupture, or thrombocytopenic, resulting from platelet deficiency. In vascular purpuras, bleeding into the tissues occurs when pressure on the small blood vessels causes tearing. This can result from exposure to chemicals and drugs, allergies, uremia, infections, injuries, and malnutrition.

Spontaneous bleeding into surrounding tissues may occur when the platelets are less than 100,000/mm³. This low platelet count is referred to as thrombocytopenic purpura. There are two types of thrombocytopenic purpura: primary idiopathic and secondary. Primary idiopathic thrombocytopenic purpura exists in an acute form and a chronic form.

In idiopathic thrombocytopenic purpura, platelets are destroyed prematurely by antiplatelet antibodies. The cause is unknown but is thought to be an autoimmune reaction in which patients make an antibody directed against the surface of their own platelets. Children tend to acquire acute idiopathic thrombocytopenic purpura after a viral infection; it is self-limiting. Adults, usually women, acquire chronic idiopathic thrombocytopenic purpura without a preceding viral infection. Unlike idiopathic thrombocytopenic purpura, secondary thrombocytopenic purpuras result from drug sensitivity or from a primary disorder.

Clinical Manifestations

Clinical manifestations of purpuras include small amounts of bleeding into the tissues and mucous membranes, resulting in petechiae and ecchymoses. Epistaxis and prolonged oozing from small wounds are common. Other common types of bleeding are from the oral mucosa, menorrhagia, purpura, and petechiae. Hepatomegaly, splenomegaly, and hematuria may be present because of increased blood loss and the body's compensatory mechanisms.

Diagnosis

The diagnosis is based on history, physical assessment, and laboratory studies, including platelet count, bleeding time, capillary fragility, partial thromboplastin time, prothrombin time, and fibrinogen level. The hallmark is a thrombocytopenia which may be less than 10,000 per liter. Anemia may also be present.

Management

Management for purpuras in general includes removing the causative agent and administering platelet transfusions. Steroid therapy, such as prednisone, is used to reduce bleeding tendencies and to elevate the platelet count. Bleeding usually ceases within 2 days with steroid therapy, and platelet counts rise within a week. Once the platelet count is above 50,000 per liter, a low dose of prednisone can be maintained.

A splenectomy may be required, which results in remission in 60 to 80% of patients (see Splenectomy, Chapter 12). Immunosuppressive drugs can be used if the splenectomy does not correct the problem.

Complications include hemorrhaging of the gastrointestinal tract and cerebral vessels. Nerve pain is evident by numbness and tingling of extremities. Paralysis may occur if a hematoma presses on a nerve or on brain tissue. Acute renal failure may be caused by a severe complication. Prognosis for recovery without medical management is 10 to 20% for adults. With treatment, the prognosis is excellent.

❖ **Settings, Providers, and Collaboration for Care**

Medications can be administered on an outpatient basis to patients with purpura. However, hospitalization is required if a splenectomy is needed or if complications arise.

NURSING PROCESS
Purpuras

Assessment

Check the patient's history for the cause of the disorder and complete a physical assessment. Assess for bleeding into the joints by checking for pain or edema. Look for other signs of bleeding such as ecchymoses, petechiae, hematomas, or epistaxis. Check the urine and stools for blood. Note the duration and severity of the bleeding. Check the laboratory studies for abnormal bleeding times and platelet counts.

Observe for faintness, tachycardia, hypotension, confusion, and air hunger indicative of hemorrhage. Check cardiopulmonary status. Monitor vital signs. Check peripheral pulses. Assess the level of consciousness and orientation to person, time, and environment.

Ask whether the patient has recently taken anticoagulants, aspirin, nonsteroidal anti-inflammatory drugs, or drugs that suppress bone marrow function such as chloramphenicol or antineoplastic drugs. Assess for jaundice and palpate the liver and spleen for enlargement.

Ask for the patient's history of any bleeding episodes or familial bleeding tendencies. Check the patient's level of understanding about bleeding disorders and prevention of hemorrhaging.

Nursing Diagnoses and Planning

Nursing diagnoses and related expected patient outcomes commonly applicable to patients with purpuras include the following:

NDx: Altered cardiopulmonary, cerebral, and peripheral tissue perfusion related to destruction of platelets causing excessive bleeding

Planning: Patient Outcomes
1. Patient's extremities are warm, color is adequate, and pulses are present.
2. Patient's laboratory studies are within normal ranges for the patient.
3. Patient denies headaches, confusion, or nausea.
4. Patient performs activities of daily living without tachypnea, tachycardia, and dyspnea.

NDx: Knowledge deficit: nature of disease and prevention of complication of hemorrhage

Planning: Patient Outcomes
1. Patient relates accurate information about the bleeding disorder, its clinical course, and the complication of hemorrhage.
2. Patient accurately states the signs of bleeding and when to notify the physician.
3. Patient remains free of signs and symptoms of bleeding such as petechiae, ecchymoses, epistaxis, or dark stools.
4. Patient verbalizes the measures necessary to prevent bleeding (see Highlight 13–5).

Nursing Interventions and Evaluation

NDx: Altered cardiopulmonary, cerebral, and peripheral tissue perfusion
Help the patient conserve oxygen by encouraging rest and limiting activities. Assist the patient with meals, if needed. Administer oxygen as needed. Elevate the head of the bed to aid in chest expansion.

Keep the patient in a comfortable position and reposition frequently to release pressure. Utilize range-of-motion exercises to stimulate circulation. Monitor vital signs and laboratory studies to assess for changes and improvements in status. Encourage ambulation as tolerated but provide for frequent rest periods to decrease cardiac workload. Assist the patient when ambulating, because decreased cerebral circulation may cause disorientation and vertigo.

Discourage smoking to avoid vasoconstriction. Remove constricting clothing, and keep heavy bed linen from restricting peripheral circulation. Keep the patient's legs in a nondependent position when he or she is not ambulating. Prevent any bleeding episodes if possible.

NDx: Knowledge deficit: nature of disease and prevention of complication of hemorrhage

Instruct the patient about the clinical course of the disease and the complication of hemorrhage. Teach the patient signs of bleeding to observe for and when to seek medical assistance. Explain the need for avoiding sharp objects, straight razors, contact sports, and injections and venipuncture whenever possible. Tell the patient to watch for discoloration of urine or stools (see Highlight 13–5).

Explain proper oral hygiene methods necessary to prevent further irritation and ulceration of mucous membranes. Instruct the patient to use a soft toothbrush and to use mouthrinse frequently. Show how to inspect the oral cavity, checking the tongue and gums for early signs of irritation. Teach the patient to avoid extremely hot, spicy foods and acidic drinks to lessen oral and gastrointestinal irritation.

Tell the patient to carry an identification card listing the blood disorder, patient's name and address, the name of the physician, patient's blood type, and the name of a family member to call in an emergency.

Check the laboratory data for the bleeding times and platelet counts. Be prepared for an emergency episode of bleeding. Tell the patient not to take aspirin or nonsteroidal anti-inflammatory drugs because they may increase the bleeding time.

Compare the patient's status with the expected outcomes. If the outcomes are not met, reassess the patient and revise the plan.

COAGULATION DISORDERS

Coagulation disorders may be hereditary or acquired and result from a decrease or absence of one or more clotting factors. The hereditary disorders are labeled as hemophilia A, B, or C, and von Willebrand's disease. The most common acquired disorders are hypoprothrombinemia and disseminated intravascular coagulation.

Hemophilias

Etiology and Pathophysiology

The hemophilias, hereditary coagulation disorders, consist of four major types:

Hemophilia A (classic hemophilia)
Hemophilia B (Christmas disease)
Hemophilia C (Rosenthal's disease)
Von Willebrand's disease

Hemophilia A is caused by an inherited deficiency of factor VIII. Hemophilia B is caused by an inherited deficiency of factor IX. Both occur in all ethnic groups and geographic areas. They are sex-linked recessive disorders transmitted by females, usually occurring in males and rarely in homozygous females. An example of the hereditary pattern of hemophilia is demonstrated in Figure 13–3. Hemophilia A occurs predominantly in children. Almost 80% of all hemophilias are hemophilia A. It occurs in equal frequency in all ethnic groups and geographic areas.

Hemophilia C, an extremely rare type of hemophilia, is transmitted as an autosomal dominant trait. It is a deficiency of clotting factor XI. Only 2% of the hemophilias are hemophilia C.

Von Willebrand's disease is a bleeding disorder occurring in both males and females equally. It is caused by an inherited deficiency of factor VIII and impaired platelet function. It is different from hemophilia A in that it is transmitted as an autosomal dominant trait in both sexes.

Clinical Manifestations

Clinical manifestations of hemophilia include severe bleeding episodes from minor injuries. Coagulation time in hemophilia A and B is prolonged, whereas the bleeding time is normal. In von Willebrand's

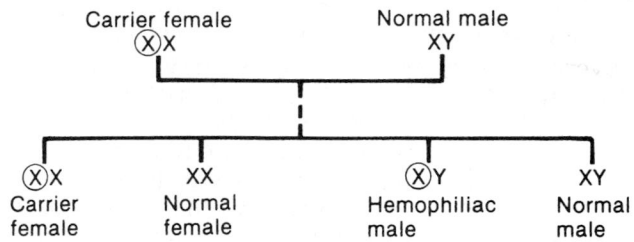

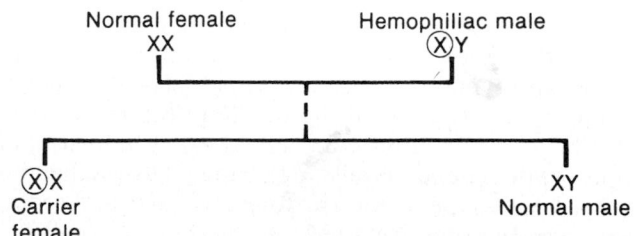

XY = Normal male
XX = Normal female
Ⓧ Y = Defective X chromosome in male (Hemophiliac)
Ⓧ X = Defective X chromosome in female (Hemophiliac carrier)

Defective gene is located in X chromosome.

Figure 13–3

Hemophilia heredity pattern.

disease, both coagulation and bleeding times are prolonged, with decreased platelet adhesiveness.

Repeated bleeding into the joints (hemarthrosis) is the hallmark of hemophilia. It impedes movement of the extremities while causing severe pain. The nose, gums, and mouth may bleed with the slightest irritation because the clotting factor is absent. Minor trauma may result in slow, prolonged bleeding. On the other hand, the patient may experience a cut that does not bleed initially but begins to bleed days later. Hematuria, gastrointestinal bleeding, or bleeding into the central nervous system may result from spontaneous bleeding or from increased intra-abdominal or intracranial pressure. It is important to note that even the slightest injury may result in massive hemorrhaging because no mechanism for clotting is present.

Diagnosis

The diagnosis of hemophilia is based on history, physical assessment, and laboratory studies of coagulation and bleeding times, fibrinogen levels, presence of factor VIII, IX, or XI, and platelet adhesiveness.

Management

Management includes administering the deficient clotting factors, parenteral administration of plasma, cryoprecipitate, whole blood, or commercially prepared antihemophilic factor as outlined in Highlight 13–11.

Joint pain and edema are controlled with analgesics and corticosteroids. Blood may be aspirated from the joint to alleviate pain. If bleeding into the joints is untreated, permanent damage is likely.

Complications include permanent joint deformity from hemarthrosis and permanent nerve damage with paralysis from hematomas that compress the nerves.

❖ Settings, Providers, and Collaboration for Care

Patients with hemophilia may be hospitalized for transfusions but are typically treated at clinics or even at home. Factor VIII can be administered by rapid intravenous injection prophylactically two to three times weekly at home. Referral to a home health nurse is necessary for drug administration and patient and family teaching. Hospitalization may be necessary for treatment of acute bleeding episodes or complications.

NURSING PROCESS GUIDELINES
Hemophilia

Check the patient's history for the type of hemophilia, the treatment instituted, and the frequency of bleeding episodes. Complete a physical assessment. Note any signs of bleeding, joint pain, hematomas, and limited movement. Assess the patient's level of

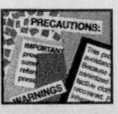

**HIGHLIGHT
13–11
PHARMACOLOGY**

Hemostatics

Definition:

Agents used to stop the flow of blood whenever excessive bleeding is or has been occurring. Hemostatics may be applied topically or systemically. Common hemostatics include aminocaproic acid, antihemophilic factor, thrombin, and Factor IX complex.

Action:

Promote the clotting of blood by affecting various components in the clotting cycle or replacing missing components.

Uses:

To stop excessive bleeding during surgery or after trauma, or to replace clotting factors in various types of hemophilia.

Side Effects:

Increased blood pressure and pulse rate. May also cause tingling, fever, chills, or headache.

Interactions:

May produce increased risk of thrombosis if used with aminocaproic acid.

Nursing Implications:

Monitor coagulation times; check patient's vital signs frequently. Report any significant changes.

understanding of the clinical course of the disease and prevention of complications.

The nursing diagnoses, expected patient outcomes, nursing interventions, and evaluation for patients with hemophilia are similar to those described previously for patients with purpuras. Focus nursing interventions on preventing further bleeding, promoting comfort, and teaching the patient and family about the disease, the necessary lifelong treatment, signs and symptoms of complications, and preventive measures (see Highlight 13–5).

Stop any bleeding immediately by direct pressure. In hemarthrosis, pack the joints in ice to control the bleeding and edema. Assist the patient in preventing injury by promoting safety measures and avoiding the use of sharp objects around the patient. Teach the patient how to prevent bleeding. Promote a diet high in iron to replace losses from hemorrhage (see Highlight 13-2).

The National Hemophilia Foundation serves as a resource for individuals with hemophilia and their families. Refer the patient to this organization for further assistance and information about the disease. Have the patient carry an identification card, noting the disease, physician, and blood type, at all times.

Acquired Hypoprothrombinemia

Etiology and Pathophysiology
In this disorder, there is a deficiency of prothrombin in the blood caused by either lack of vitamin K or excessive coumarin anticoagulants.

Clinical Manifestations
Clinical manifestations include ecchymosis and epistaxis resulting from minor trauma. Hematuria, gastrointestinal bleeding, postoperative hemorrhage from an incision, and prolonged bleeding from a venipuncture site may also be present.

Diagnosis
The diagnosis of acquired hypoprothrombinemia is based on history, physical assessment, and prothrombin time.

Management
Management involves oral or parenteral administration of vitamin K and discontinuation of the anticoagulant. Vitamin K may be administered intravenously for acute hemorrhage.

❖ Settings, Providers, and Collaboration for Care
Hypoprothrombinemia is usually detected and treated in a doctor's office or clinic. Medications can be administered in the clinic or at home.

NURSING PROCESS GUIDELINES
Acquired Hypoprothrombinemia

The assessment, nursing diagnoses, expected patient outcomes, nursing interventions, and evaluation for patients with acquired hypoprothrombinemia are similar to those described previously for patients with other bleeding disorders.

Disseminated Intravascular Coagulation

Etiology and Pathophysiology
Disseminated intravascular coagulation is characterized by widespread coagulation in the arterioles and capillaries throughout the body. This coagulation results in disseminated fibrin deposits and microthrombi formation in the microcirculation, with subsequent depletion of clotting factors. Circulatory impairment results in infarcts and necrosis of tissues and organs. Renal failure associated with obstruction of the renal capillaries is especially common.

With the depletion of clotting factors, prolonged bleeding may occur spontaneously from mucous membranes or internal tissues or organs, or result from minor trauma or venipunctures. Bleeding episodes may vary from minimal oozing to massive hemorrhage.

Although the exact cause of disseminated intravascular coagulation is unknown, it is usually associated with serious illness. Among the conditions that may predispose to disseminated intravascular coagulation are metastatic cancer, acute leukemias, hemolytic transfusion reactions, massive tissue trauma, septicemia, abruptio placentae, septic abortion, surgery, and shock. Any individual with a predisposing condition who develops purpura, bleeding tendencies, or signs of renal failure should be evaluated for disseminated intravascular coagulation.

Clinical Manifestations
Clinical manifestations include both bleeding and thrombosis. The patient may experience petechiae and ecchymoses, hematuria, and bleeding from any body orifice or venipuncture site. Gastrointestinal bleeding, oliguria, acute renal failure, convulsions, coma, and death may result from internal hemorrhage. Thrombosis is most commonly seen in digital ischemia and gangrene.

Diagnosis
The diagnosis is based on history, physical assessment, and laboratory studies of prothrombin time, partial thromboplastin time, thrombin time, platelet count, and fibrinogen levels.

Management
Management involves correcting the underlying condition, controlling the bleeding, and slowing the widespread coagulation. Severe hemorrhage is treated by transfusions of platelet concentrate, fresh frozen plasma, cryoprecipitate, and red blood cell concentrates. Heparin therapy may be used in combination with transfusions when thrombosis is present, but its use is controversial.

❖ Settings, Providers, and Collaboration for Care
Disseminated intravascular coagulation is detected and treated in the hospital setting. Since it usually occurs secondary to another serious illness, the patient will already be in the hospital when disseminated intravascular coagulation is detected. Treatment requires close observation and careful monitoring.

NURSING PROCESS GUIDELINES
Disseminated Intravascular Coagulation

Assess the patient at risk for bleeding tendencies, internal bleeding, pain caused by pressure from hematomas, oliguria, and altered level of consciousness. Look for changes in vital signs indicating shock from hemorrhage. Watch laboratory data for changes in bleeding times and platelet counts. Prepare to deal with an acute hemorrhage.

The nursing diagnoses, expected patient outcomes, nursing interventions, and evaluation for patients with disseminated intravascular coagulation are similar to those described previously for patients with other bleeding disorders.

The Elderly: Special Considerations

In contrast to younger adults, older adults with hematologic disorders are at higher risk of developing complications of the disease or the treatments. Also, older adults may have alterations in their response to treatments. For example, if the older adult undergoes surgery for a hematologic disorder, the risk is significantly increased compared with the risk for a young or middle-aged adult. Chemotherapy or radiation therapy is often the choice for medical intervention in leukocyte disorders, and older adults may not tolerate chemotherapy and radiation therapy as well as younger adults. Older adults are at higher risk for drug interactions, adverse drug effects, and altered therapeutic effects.

Anorexia is a major side effect of several therapeutic interventions for leukocyte disorders. It becomes a nursing challenge to improve the nutritional status of the older patient receiving treatment for hematologic disorders. Mouth problems resulting from treatments, the disease process, and poor dentition are common. For example, dry mouth is a common problem in older adults, and this may exacerbate problems with mucous membranes. Older adults with nutritional deficits resulting in hematologic disorders require additional nutritional supplements because vitamin and mineral absorption is diminished. Nutritional supplements and soft, bland foods may be necessary if the patient has mouth problems that contribute to a malnourished state. It is important to identify food preferences and try to incorporate preferred foods into the dietary plan.

When assessing the older adult for hematologic disorders, observe for fatigue or any mental changes that may be associated with decreased oxygen-carrying capacity of the blood. Find out what the older adult's normal baseline temperature is and observe for any deviations. Because the baseline temperature of the older person is usually subnormal, a slight increase in temperature may be significant. The white blood count may not be elevated in older people who have infections, as is typical in younger adults.

It is extremely important to listen to the elderly patient, make astute observations, and review the patient's history to accurately diagnose and care for problems associated with the hematologic system. The older adult affected by disorders of the blood or blood-forming organs may be in a life-threatening

state. Nursing interventions must be specific to the disorder as well as to the person's needs and desires. When planning care for the older adult with a hematologic disorder, consider the person's lifestyle, living arrangements, educational level, financial status, nutritional patterns, support systems, and transportation resources.

Chapter Review

1. How is nursing care of a patient with iron deficiency anemia the same as and different from the nursing care of the patient with aplastic anemia?
2. Describe ways that a nurse can help a patient with anemia to conserve energy so that cardiac workload is reduced.
3. What is the physiologic rationale for the occurrence of fatigue in the patient with polycythemia vera?
4. How can the effectiveness of treatment be evaluated in the patient with agranulocytosis?
5. Compare and contrast the four most common types of leukemia.
6. Why are some of the symptoms the same for the different types of leukemia?
7. Why is it important for patients with leukemia to eat diets high in protein and vitamins?
8. Differentiate Hodgkin's disease from non-Hodgkin's lymphoma.
9. Why are patients with Hodgkin's disease and non-Hodgkin's lymphoma at risk for infection?
10. Patients with hematologic disorders often experience anorexia. What are some possible solutions to this problem?

Bibliography

Alleyne J, Thomas VJ. The management of sickle cell crisis pain as experienced by patients and their carers. J Adv Nurs 1994; 19:725.

Andreoli TE, Bennett JC, Carpenter CCJ, et al. Cecil essentials of medicine. 4th ed. Philadelphia: WB Saunders, 1997.

Anemia: Knowledge for practice . . . part 1. Nurs Times 1995; 91(5 Prof Dev):1.

Anemia: The role of the nurse . . . part 2 of this Professional Development unit. Nurs Times 1995; 91(6 Prof Dev):5.

Anemia: Revision notes . . . final part of our Professional Development unit . . . part 3. Nurs Times 1995; 91(7):9.

Ball RA. Sickle cell . . . a patient's hell: What you need to know. JEMS 1993; 18(6):33.

Borson R, Loeb V. Acute and chronic leukemias in adults. CA 1994; 44(6):323.

Burns JM, Tierney K, Long GD, et al. Critical pathway for administering high-dose chemotherapy followed by peripheral blood stem cell rescue in the outpatient setting. Burns 1995; 22(8):1219.

Campbell K. The causes and incidence of haematological malignancies. Nurs Times 1995; 91(31):25.

Carpenito LJ. Nursing diagnosis: Application to clinical practice. 6th ed. Philadelphia: JB Lippincott, 1995.

Cook JD, Skikne BS, Baynes RD. Iron deficiency: The global perspective. Adv Exp Med Biol 1994; 356:219.

Devine SM, Larson RA. Acute leukemia in adults: Recent developments in diagnosis and treatment. CA 1994; 44(6):326.

Dickson CJ. Does folic acid harm people with vitamin B_{12} deficiency? Q J Med, 1995; 88:357.

Doenges ME, Moorhouse MF. Nurses' pocket guide: Nursing diagnoses with interventions. 5th ed. Philadelphia: FA Davis, 1996.

Erickson JM. Update on Hodgkin's Disease. Nurse Pract 1994; 19(11):63.

Fajardo LL. Hodgkin's disease in adults, part 1. Invest Radiol 1993; 28(8):737.

Gerhartz HH. Chemotherapy dose and survival in advanced Hodgkin's disease. Acta Haematol 1993; 89:137.

Huston CJ. Disseminated intravascular coagulation. AJN 1994; 94(8):51.

Kajs-Wyllie M. Thrombotic thrombocytopenic purpura: Pathophysiology, treatment, and related nursing care. Crit Care Nurse 1995; 15(6):44.

Kolic G, Scharnweber K. Recombinant human granulocyte colony-stimulating factor: An overview. J Intravenous Nurs 1993; 16(4):234.

Kurtz A. Disseminated intravascular coagulation with leukemia patients. Cancer Nurs 1993; 16(6):456.

Leitgeb C, Pecherstorfer M, Fritz E, Ludwig H. Quality of life in chronic anemia of cancer during treatment with recombinant human erythropoietin. Cancer 1994; 73(10):2535.

Lundquist DM, Stewart FM. An update on non-Hodgkin's lymphoma. Nurse Pract 1994; 19(10):41.

Maher DW, Leschke GJ, Green M, et al. Filgrastim in patients with chemotherapy-induced febrile neutropenia: A double-blind, placebo-controlled trial. Ann Intern Med 1994; 121(7):492.

McCance KL, Huether SE. Pathophysiology: The biological basis for disease in adults and children. 2nd ed. St. Louis: Mosby, 1994.

Messinezy M, Pearson T. Polycythemias. Practitioner 1995; 237:355.

Miller C. The role of transfusion therapy in the treatment of sickle cell disease. J Intravenous Nurs 1994; 17(2):70.

Payton RG, White PJ. Primary care for women: Assessment of hematologic disorders. J Nurse Midwife 1995; 40:120.

Preisler HD. The leukemias. Disease A Month 1994; 40(10):525.

Purandare L. Caring for patients with chronic leukemia. Nurs Times 1995; 91(31):27.

Rieger PT, Haeuber D. A new approach to managing chemotherapy-related anemia: Nursing implications of epoetin alfa. Oncol Nurs Forum 1995; 22(1):71.

Roberts HR, Eberst ME. Current management of hemophilia B. Hematol Oncol Clin North Am 1993; 7(6):1269.

Sickle Cell Disease Guideline Panel. Sickle cell disease: Screening, diagnosis, management, and counseling in newborns and infants. Clinical Practice Guidelines No. 6. AHCPR Pub. No. 93-0562. Rockville, MD: Agency for Health Care Policy and Research, Public Health Service, U.S. Dept. of Health and Human Services, April 1993.

Stevens R. Hemophilia and haemorrhagic disorders. Practitioner 1993; 237:350.

Tierney LM, McPhee SJ, Papadakis MA. Current medical diagnosis and treatment. 35th ed. Stamford, CT: Appleton & Lange, 1996.

Vose JM. Cytokine use in the older patient. Semin Oncol 1995; 22(1):6.

Vose JM, Armitage JO. Clinical application of hematopoietic growth factors. J Clin Oncol 1995; 13(4):1023.

Warne I. Chemotherapy for acute monoblastic leukemia. Nurs Times 1994; 90(17):43.

Waters J. Pain from sickle-cell crises. Nurs Times 1995; 91(16):29.

Young NS. Agranulocytosis. JAMA 1994; 271(12):935.

Young NS, Barnett AJ. The treatment of severe acquired aplastic anemia. Blood 1995; 85(12):3367.

Unit IV
Respiratory Dysfunction

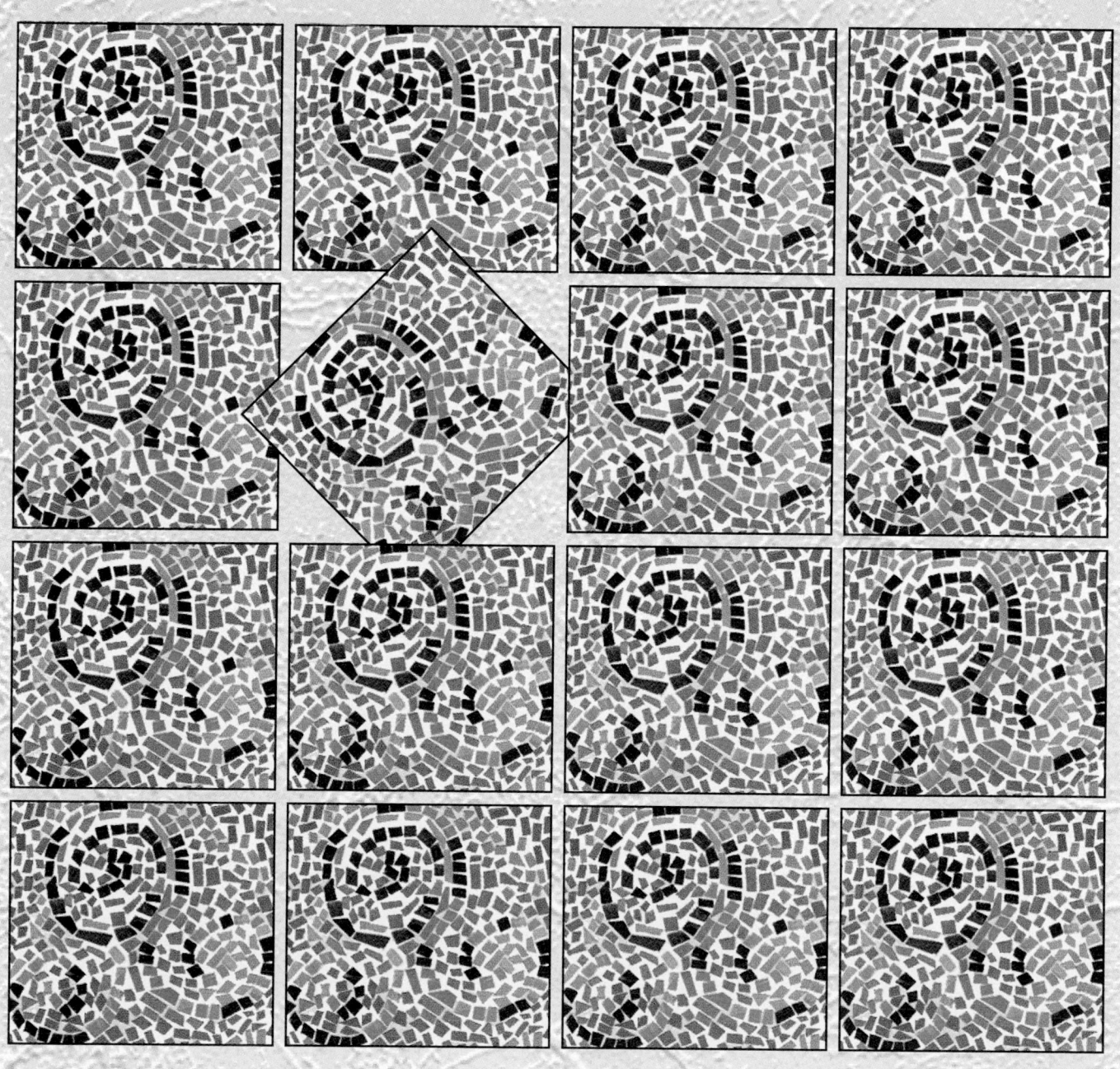

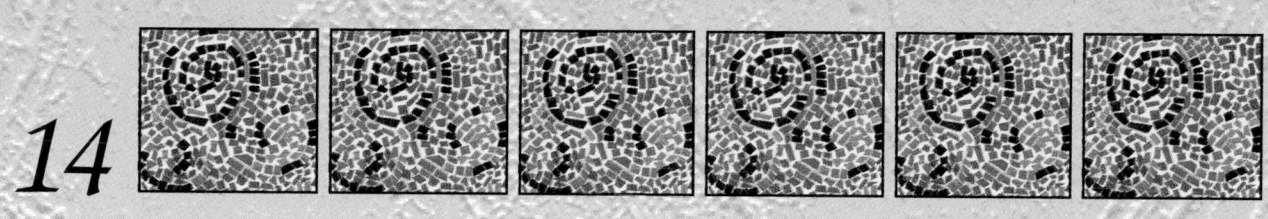

14

Knowledge Base for Patients with Respiratory Dysfunction

Study Outcomes

After studying this chapter, you should be able to:

1. Explain the normal anatomy and physiology of the respiratory system.
2. Describe common clinical manifestations of respiratory dysfunction.
3. Identify information and physical examination data essential to the assessment of respiratory status.
4. Describe basic diagnostic tests and treatment modalities (respiratory therapy, oxygen therapy, artificial airways, mechanical ventilation) used in the collaborative management of patients with respiratory disorders.
5. Describe basic surgical procedures (pneumonectomy and lobectomy) used in the treatment of patients with respiratory disorders.
6. Identify data essential to the assessment of patients undergoing treatment of respiratory disorders.
7. State nursing diagnoses and related expected patient outcomes commonly applicable to patients undergoing treatment of respiratory disorders.
8. Describe nursing interventions, with their rationales, commonly applicable to patients undergoing treatment of respiratory disorders.
9. Explain the basis for evaluation of nursing care provided to patients undergoing treatment of respiratory disorders.
10. Identify alternative treatment and care settings for patients with respiratory dysfunction and the services related to community-based care.
11. Identify special considerations for the elderly patient with altered respiratory function.

Respiratory function is complex and integral to the function of all other body systems. It is also directly related to the overall quality of an individual's life. To provide a foundation for studying the nursing care of patients with respiratory disorders, this chapter reviews the basic anatomy and physiology of the respiratory system and presents the major clinical manifestations of respiratory disease. It discusses assessment of respiratory status, diagnostic tests specific to problems of respiratory function, and surgical and nonsurgical modes of treatment

that are common to the management of many different respiratory disorders.

Anatomy and Physiology

The respiratory system has several complex functions. The primary function is gas exchange, which involves delivery of oxygen to the tissues and removal of carbon dioxide waste. Other functions include synthesis of surfactant and other chemicals, metabolism and detoxification of drugs and toxins, and defense against infection.

Traditionally, the respiratory system is divided into two parts: the upper respiratory system, which includes the nasal cavity, the sinuses, the mouth, the pharynx, and the larynx (Fig. 14–1), and the lower respiratory system, which includes the trachea and the lungs, which lie within the thoracic cavity. An alternative division is made on the basis of function. Functionally, the respiratory system has three main divisions: the conducting airways, the respiratory zone, and the accessory structures, such as the interstitium of the lung and the bones and muscles of the thorax.

THORAX

The bony thorax houses the lungs and the mediastinum, which contains the heart and the major blood vessels. It is primarily composed of the sternum, the thoracic portion of the vertebral column, and 12 pairs of ribs. The first 7 pairs of ribs are called "true" ribs because they attach posteriorly to the vertebral column and anteriorly to the sternum via the costal cartilages. Ribs 8 to 10 are called "false" ribs because they attach to the rib above them rather than directly to the sternum. Ribs 11 and 12 are referred to as "floating" ribs because they have no direct anterior skeletal attachment. The spaces between the ribs are called intercostal spaces. The angle between the xiphoid process of the sternum and the costal cartilages is the costal angle.

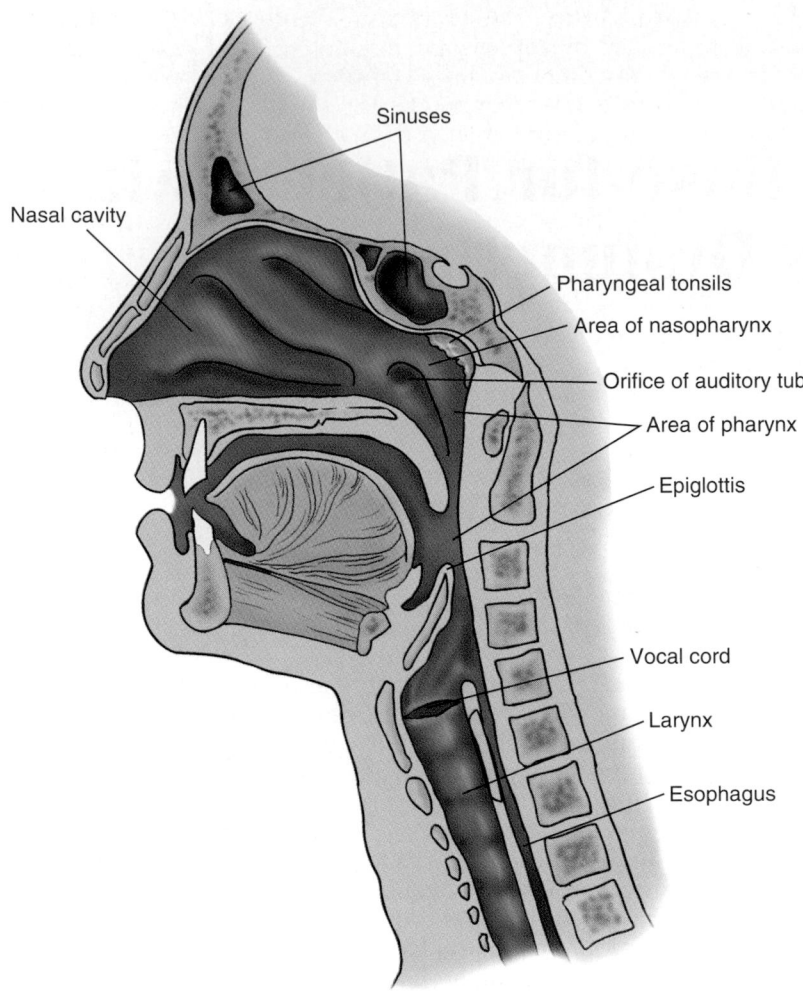

Sinuses

Nasal cavity

Pharyngeal tonsils

Area of nasopharynx

Orifice of auditory tube

Area of pharynx

Epiglottis

Vocal cord

Larynx

Esophagus

Figure 14–1
Structures of the upper respiratory system.

The diaphragm, which is the major muscle of respiration, separates the thoracic cavity from the abdominal cavity. Muscles of the thoracic wall, which also play a role in respiration, include the external intercostal muscles, which elevate the ribs and thus facilitate inspiration, and the internal intercostal muscles, which are accessory muscles of expiration. The thorax as a whole has a natural compliance that tends to cause it to spring outward and to expand.

LUNGS

The lungs, the chief organs of respiration, are paired, spongy, and cone-shaped. The right lung is thicker, wider, and shorter than the left lung because of the height of the liver, which lies beneath the diaphragm on the right side. This lung is divided into three lobes: upper, middle, and lower. These lobes further subdivide into 10 segments. The left lung is longer and more narrow than the right

lung because of the space in the left thorax occupied by the heart. This lung is divided into two lobes: upper and lower. These two lobes in turn are divided into eight segments.

The rounded, uppermost part of each lung is called the apex (plural: apexes or apices). The concave lowermost portion is called the base. The surface of the lung adjoining the thoracic cage is the costal surface. The surface facing the mediastinum is the mediastinal surface. The cardiac notch is a concavity in the mediastinal surface that accommodates the heart. The major bronchi, blood vessels, nerves, and lymphatic vessels enter each lung through the hilum.

The lungs are covered with two thin but tough layers of serous membrane. The inner layer is called the visceral pleura. This layer follows the contour of the lung and is virtually inseparable from it. The outer layer is called the parietal pleura. It lines the thoracic wall, covers the diaphragm, and is reflected over mediastinal structures. There is a small amount of lubricating fluid between the two layers in an airtight region known as the pleural space. This is a potential space and can be seen only when air or fluid collects in it, such as occurs with a pneumothorax or hemothorax. Normally the two layers are in constant, immediate contact during all phases of respiration.

CONDUCTING AIRWAYS

The conducting airways extend from the nose to the terminal bronchioles and are primarily tubes that transport air to its ultimate destination: the respiratory units. The conducting airways can be divided into two principal parts: the upper airways and the lower airways.

Upper Airways

The upper airways, like the traditional definition of the upper respiratory system, include the nasal cavity, sinuses, mouth, pharynx, and larynx (see Fig. 14–1).

Air in the atmosphere consists of approximately 21% oxygen and 78% nitrogen, with a small amount of other trace gases. When it is inhaled, it must be warmed to body temperature and completely saturated with water vapor to prevent drying of the respiratory mucosa. Air that is at body temperature and pressure and that is saturated with water vapor is referred to as body temperature pressure saturated. It is primarily the function of the nasal cavity to warm, filter, and humidify the air.

The pharynx consists of three sections: the naso-pharynx, the oropharynx, and the laryngopharynx. The nasopharynx contains the adenoids and the openings of the eustachian tubes. These tubes connect the pharynx to the middle ear, which is why middle-ear infections are common complications of upper respiratory tract infections. The oral cavity and oropharynx, or throat, contain the tongue. The tongue is the most common cause of airway obstruction in an unconscious person because, as a person loses muscle tone, the tongue can fall back on the oropharynx. The palatine tonsils are also located in the oropharynx.

The larynx, which connects the pharynx to the trachea, consists of nine cartilages. The epiglottis is a leaf-shaped, flexible cartilage that sits above the opening to the vocal cords. It closes over the larynx during swallowing and prevents aspiration of foreign bodies into the lower airway. Although phonation is its chief function, the larynx is also responsible for a strong cough and spasm reflex to protect against foreign substances entering the lower airways.

Lower Airways

The lower airways consist of the trachea, bronchi, and bronchioles (Fig. 14–2) and are normally sterile. The trachea, which sits directly in front of the esophagus, consists of 16 to 20 C-shaped cartilage rings opened to the posterior. At about the level of the space between the second and third ribs, it splits at the carina into right and left main-stem bronchi. The main-stem bronchi lead to each lung. The right main-stem bronchus is shorter, wider, and at a

Figure 14–2

Structures of the lower airways. Note that the right lung has three lobes and the left has two. Note also that the right main bronchus is shorter, wider, and more in line with the trachea than the left main bronchus.

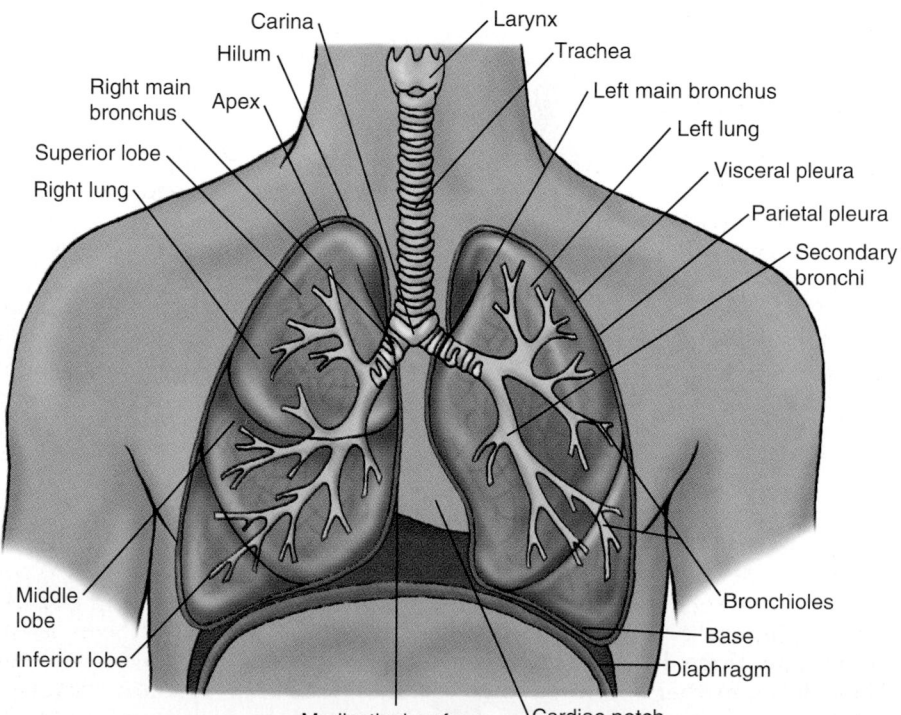

straighter angle than the left. Consequently, any aspirated foreign material usually enters the right lung. The main-stem bronchi divide into the lobar bronchi, which branch into segmental bronchi and then subsegmental bronchi. The conducting airways continue to branch into smaller and smaller divisions, resembling an inverted tree, hence the term *tracheobronchial tree.* Airways smaller than 2 mm in diameter are referred to as bronchioles. The terminal bronchioles are the last of the purely conducting airways. The lower airways, which expand and contract with inspiration and expiration, are referred to as anatomical dead space because they contain about 150 mL of air that never reaches the respiratory zone where gas exchange occurs.

The lower airways are lined with a specialized mucous membrane sometimes referred to as the mucociliary escalator. This respiratory mucosa is composed of pseudostratified columnar epithelium lined with small hairlike structures known as cilia. A layer of mucus sits on top of the cilia to trap dirt and debris. The cilia beat in a constant upward motion and transport the mucus to the pharynx, where it is swallowed. This mechanism is normally highly effective in keeping the lungs clear. The ciliated mucosa is, however, very sensitive to a variety of substances, such as smoke and pollutants, which can paralyze the cilia and erode the mucous membrane, rendering it nonfunctional. Anesthesia, alcohol, administration of high oxygen concentrations, poor tissue oxygenation, dehydration, and infection are some of the other irritants that can similarly impair the protective function of the respiratory mucosa.

Under the mucosal layer is smooth muscle, which gives the airway tone, and cartilage, which provides support. As the branches become progressively smaller, the smooth muscle, the supporting cartilage, and other tissues of the airway wall thin out.

RESPIRATORY ZONE

The respiratory bronchioles mark the transition from the conducting airways to the respiratory zone. Gas exchange begins with the respiratory bronchioles, which lead into the alveolar ducts, alveolar sacs, and ultimately the alveoli, the lumens of which are

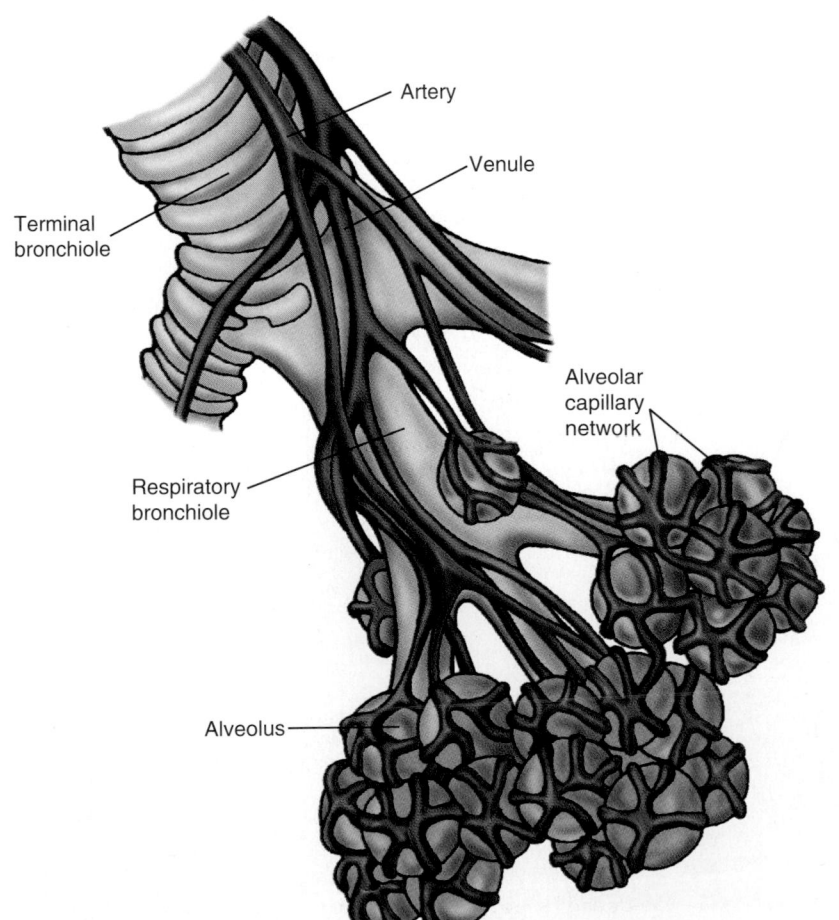

Figure 14–3

The respiratory bronchiole feeds the alveolus, or alveolar sac, which is surrounded by a capillary plexus. It is here that oxygen diffuses into the blood that returns to the heart through the pulmonary artery.

called alveolar spaces (Fig. 14–3). Adult lungs contain about 300 million alveoli, surrounded by a vast network of pulmonary capillaries that provide an extremely large and effective surface area for gas exchange. The alveolar epithelium consists of several types of cells. Type I cells line most of the alveolar surface. Type II cells produce surfactant, a phospholipid that alters surface tension to provide mechanical stability to the alveoli. On expiration, it reduces surface tension and prevents alveolar collapse, and on inspiration, it decreases surface tension and helps limit expansion. Alveolar macrophages are phagocytic cells that destroy any bacteria or other foreign particles that escape the mucociliary escalator.

Between the alveoli lies the interstitium, which contains pulmonary capillaries, lymphatic channels, and nerves. The interstitium also contains elastic connective tissue, which gives the lungs their elastic recoil (ie, the ability to return to resting position after stretching). Elastic and collagen fibers also enable the lung to expand or distend, a property known as compliance. In diseases such as emphysema, the walls between the alveoli break down, decreasing the surface area for gas exchange. The lung loses its elastic recoil and becomes hyperinflated. In pulmonary fibrosis, the connective tissue becomes replaced with scar tissue, making the lung stiff, noncompliant, and difficult to expand.

MECHANICS OF VENTILATION

Ventilation is the bulk movement of air in and out of the respiratory tract. Effective ventilation requires air to reach the alveoli so gas exchange can occur. To accomplish this, the airway must be patent, and the thoracic cage, lung, and muscles of respiration must be intact and functioning. Respiration is the exchange of gases. External respiration occurs in the respiratory units of the lung; internal respiration occurs at the tissue level throughout the body. Effective respiration requires adequate ventilation.

The process of ventilation takes place as a result of pressure gradients between the alveoli and atmospheric air. Atmospheric pressure is normally about 760 mm Hg. The intrathoracic pressure, and consequently the intrapleural pressure, is always slightly below atmospheric pressure. The natural compliance of the lungs and thorax results from opposing forces that are balanced to create these normal resting pressures. Inspiration is the active phase of ventilation. As the diaphragm contracts, it flattens and moves downward and out, expanding the thoracic cage in both the anteroposterior and transverse diameters (Fig. 14–4). As the volume in the chest increases, the pressure in the thoracic cavity decreases even further. This is a function of the physical principle known as Boyle's law, which states that pres-

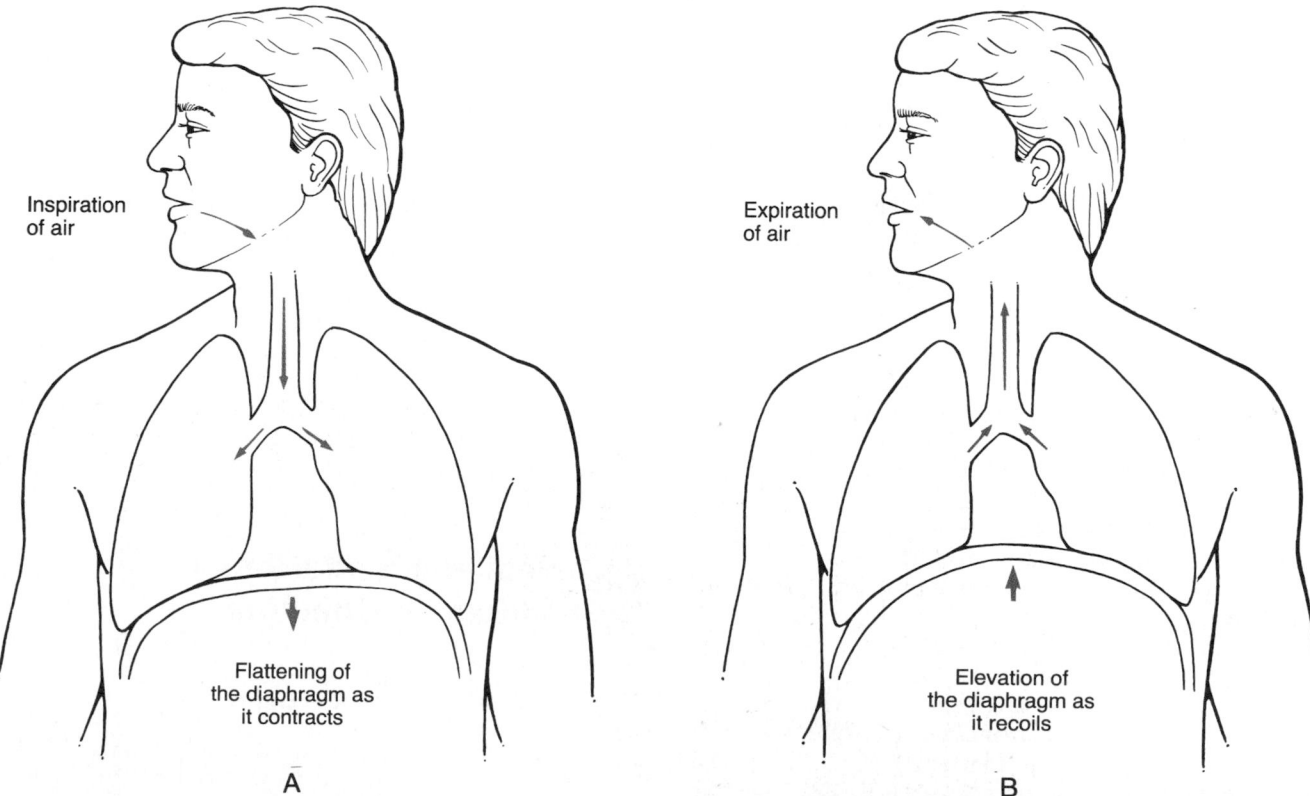

Figure 14–4

A, During inspiration, the diaphragm flattens as it contracts, and the chest cavity is lengthened. *B,* During expiration, the diaphragm recoils, and the chest cavity shrinks.

sure and volume are inversely proportional. As the airway pressure decreases below atmospheric pressure, air moves into the lungs.

Expiration is normally passive. As the muscles relax and the lung recoils to its normal position, the volume decreases. In turn, the airway pressure increases above atmospheric pressure, causing air to move out.

Ventilation is controlled by several mechanisms. The respiratory centers are located in the medulla. These central chemoreceptors are sensitive to carbon dioxide and hydrogen ion concentrations in the cerebrospinal fluid. Slight increases in either substance stimulate an increase in ventilation. Arterial carbon dioxide tension is the primary stimulus to breathe in a normal person. To a lesser extent, oxygen deficiency can also affect ventilation. The peripheral chemoreceptors located in the carotid and aortic bodies are stimulated when the partial pressure of oxygen in the arterial blood (PaO_2) falls below the normal of 100 mm Hg, with maximal response at a PaO_2 of less than 50 to 60 mm Hg. This serves as a back-up emergency system in a patient with respiratory dysfunction. Several types of lung receptors, such as pulmonary stretch receptors (Hering-Breuer reflex), irritant receptors, and J receptors, also play a role, although one not completely understood, in controlling ventilation. They may also be responsible for the sensation of dyspnea or labored breathing.

GAS EXCHANGE

Diffusion, or transfer of a substance from an area of higher concentration or pressure to one of lower concentration or pressure, occurs at both the alveolocapillary membrane level (external respiration) and the tissue level (internal respiration). Diffusion depends on the pressure gradients across the alveolocapillary membrane. Partial pressure of oxygen in the alveoli is approximately 100 mm Hg, whereas venous oxygen pressure is about 40 mm Hg. Therefore, oxygen moves from the alveoli into the pulmonary capillary blood. Carbon dioxide is 20 times as diffusible as oxygen and therefore requires less pressure gradient, going from venous blood at a pressure of 46 to 48 mm Hg to the alveoli at a pressure of 40 mm Hg.

Gas exchange also depends on a matching distribution of air in the lungs and blood flow in the pulmonary capillaries. This ventilation/perfusion matching is somewhat gravity dependent. In a normal upright individual, both ventilation and perfusion are greater at the bases of the lungs than in the apices. This condition changes as body position changes. In patients with unilateral lung conditions, the healthy lung should usually be placed in the gravity-dependent position to maximize ventilation/perfusion matching. If ventilation is present without perfusion, no gas exchange can occur, and the ventilated area that has no perfusion is referred to as dead space. In the conducting airways where no

pulmonary capillaries exist, anatomical dead space is normally present. In disorders such as pulmonary embolism and emphysema, physiologic dead space is created. Conversely, if capillaries are perfused but no ventilation is present, gas exchange cannot take place. This condition is referred to as a shunt. Atelectasis, pneumonia, and adult respiratory distress syndrome are examples of shunt-producing conditions.

TRANSPORT OF GASES

Oxygen is transported in the blood in two ways. A small portion is carried in dissolved form in the plasma; the major portion is chemically combined with hemoglobin in red blood cells. Normal arterial oxygen saturation of hemoglobin is 94 to 100%. It can be less than 100% because of several anatomical shunts that dump unoxygenated blood directly back into the arterial system. As oxygen is released to the tissues, carbon dioxide diffuses into the plasma and eventually into the red blood cells for transport back to the lungs, where it is eliminated. See the sections Gas Exchange and Transport of Gases.

WORK OF BREATHING

Normally a healthy person uses less than 5% of total body energy for normal, quiet breathing. This percentage can increase to 30% or more during exercise or for a person with a pulmonary disorder.

Several factors affect the work of breathing. The work that must be done to breathe depends on the pressures needed to overcome the forces opposing ventilation. These forces include the airway resistance and the elastic forces, or compliance, of the lung and chest wall. Airway resistance depends mostly on the radius of the airways and, to a lesser extent, the flow rate or speed of gas flow. The faster the breathing rate, the more resistance is created. Airways narrowed by mucus, bronchospasm, or edema significantly increase resistance to breathing. When the lungs are stiff and noncompliant, greater pressure gradients are required to cause expansion. This can occur as a result of a loss of surfactant, fibrosis, atelectasis, and edema.

Clinical Manifestations of Respiratory Dysfunction

LOCAL MANIFESTATIONS

Cough

Cough is a protective mechanism for clearing the lower airways. When persistent (lasting longer than 2 to 3 weeks), it may indicate the presence of a serious pulmonary disease.

A cough can be described as chronic, paroxysmal, dry, or productive. A chronic cough is commonly associated with irritation of the airway. Smoking is the most common cause, although allergies, sinus infections, chronic upper respiratory tract infections, and inhalation of polluted air can also produce a chronic cough. A paroxysmal cough is a spasmodic type that is difficult to stop. It is commonly observed in patients with asthma or chronic bronchitis. A dry cough is one not accompanied by the production of sputum, whereas a productive cough is associated with the production of sputum. Expectoration of sputum generally occurs with a productive cough. However, since patients may swallow sputum, its absence noes not necessarily indicate a nonproductive cough.

Excessive Nasal Secretions

Infection of the upper respiratory tract, irritants, or allergens that induce an allergic response produce congestion of the nasal mucosa. Allergic states produce a pale mucosa with a thin, watery discharge. With infection, the nasal mucosa is very reddened (hyperemic) and the discharge is purulent.

Excessive nasal secretions are common in persons exposed to very dry air in artificially heated environments or to smoke, dust, or fumes. Excessive nasal secretions drain into the back of the throat as a postnasal drip. This may produce coughing, frequent throat clearing, or, in extreme cases, gagging (the vomit reflex).

Expectoration of Sputum

Sputum production is related to irritation of the lower respiratory tract. This irritation stimulates the mucus glands to produce increased amounts of mucus, which is coughed up as sputum. Normally the respiratory tract produces about 100 mL of mucus daily. When respiratory passages are irritated, this amount can be increased to as much as 1000 mL daily.

Sputum is described as mucoid, purulent, mucopurulent, rusty, or blood-tinged. Mucoid sputum is white and clear. Purulent sputum may be yellow or greenish because of the presence of mucus and pus. Mucopurulent means there is more mucus than pus in the sputum. Rusty sputum is exudate containing traces of blood from capillary destruction. Blood-tinged mucus occurs in certain diseases such as bronchiectasis, tuberculosis, pulmonary infarct, and carcinoma. Blood in the sputum (hemoptysis) may be a presenting sign of either tuberculosis or carcinoma. It is commonly bright red and frothy and has an alkaline pH reaction. Because mucus is normally 95% water, thick sputum may indicate a need for hydration.

Pain

Lung tissue is insensitive to pain. Pain occurs when the muscles of the chest wall or the pleura are affected by disease. Three different types of chest pain—pleuritic, intercostal, and generalized—can occur as a result of respiratory dysfunction. Pleuritic pain is a catching, transient type produced when the thorax is moved. It is usually intensified when the person is breathing deeply and is felt unilaterally. There is often tenderness in the area of the pain. Intercostal pain is produced when coughing or straining causes compression of the intercostal muscles.

Dyspnea

Labored or difficult breathing (dyspnea) is a common clinical manifestation of respiratory dysfunction. The patient may present with:

- Rapid, audible, labored breathing
- Marked use of the accessory muscles of respiration
- Dilated nostrils
- Tachycardia
- Anxious expression
- Gasping
- A bluish or gray color to the skin (cyanosis)

SYSTEMIC MANIFESTATIONS

The main function of the lungs is the regulation of arterial oxygenation and carbon dioxide elimination. Because of its significant functional reserve, the respiratory system can regulate and maintain arterial blood gases (ABGs) despite pathologic conditions. When the functional reserve is exceeded, however, impairment of oxygenation and carbon dioxide elimination results in systemic manifestations of respiratory dysfunction.

Hypoxemia and Hypoxia

Hypoxemia is insufficient oxygenation of the blood and commonly refers to decreased PaO_2 or saturation below normal levels. Hypoxia is inadequate tissue oxygenation. Anoxia or the absence of oxygen is an extreme degree of hypoxia. Ventilation/perfusion mismatching is the most common cause of hypoxemia and hypoxia. Other causes are high altitude, inadequate oxygen in inspired air, anemia or abnormal types of hemoglobin preventing normal transport, circulatory impairment (such as hypotension or low cardiac output), and inability of the cells to use oxygen (such as with cyanide poisoning). ABGs are the most reliable indicator of hypoxemia. Most symptoms of hypoxemia are not present unless it is severe.

Cyanosis is the commonly accepted sign of hypoxemia. The slightly blue-gray discoloration of the skin and mucous membranes results from abnormal amounts of reduced hemoglobin or other hemoglobin compounds in the capillary blood. True cyanosis, which develops when 5 g of hemoglobin is reduced, can be differentiated from deposition of certain pigments by pressing over the discolored area. Cyanotic skin blanches; pigmented skin does not.

The presence of other hemoglobin compounds in the capillary blood is an uncommon cause of cyanosis. Cyanosis caused by unoxygenated blood in the capillaries is common.

The presence of cyanosis does not necessarily indicate arterial hypoxemia. Capillary blood flow and extraction of oxygen by the tissues determine how much hemoglobin is deoxygenated while in the capillaries. For example, a marked decrease in capillary blood flow permits enough oxygen extraction by the tissues for cyanosis to appear despite adequate arterial oxygenation. This is observed in the finger tips during very cold weather.

Conversely, the absence of cyanosis does not necessarily rule out arterial hypoxemia. Anemic patients may have a very low arterial blood oxygen level without cyanosis, because they do not have enough reduced hemoglobin to become visible.

Early signs of hypoxia include restlessness, tachycardia, tachypnea, irritability, and unexplained apprehension. Later signs include combativeness, retraction, and cyanosis. The brain is the organ most sensitive to the lack of oxygen. Acute cerebral hypoxia results in clumsiness, impaired judgment, headache, and a decreased level of consciousness. If severe and continued, cerebral hypoxia will lead to confusion, coma, and death. Chronic hypoxia results in fatigue, apathy, drowsiness, and muscular twitching.

Hypoxemia affects the cardiac system by increasing the heart rate and cardiac output. Cardiac dysrhythmias are commonly observed in people with severe hypoxemia.

Hypoxemia is also an important respiratory stimulant through its effect on the body's peripheral chemoreceptors. If a patient has long-standing carbon dioxide retention, administration of inappropriately large amounts of oxygen may result in respiratory depression by removing the hypoxemic ventilatory drive.

Severe hypoxemia causes metabolic acidosis. Inadequate tissue oxygenation causes anaerobic metabolism (metabolism in the absence of oxygen) to take place. The end products of such metabolism include lactic acid, the accumulation of which results in metabolic acidosis.

Hypercapnia

Hypercapnia, or hypercarbia, is a state of abnormally increased amounts of carbon dioxide in the arterial blood. Hypercapnia indicates that alveolar ventilation is inadequate for proper elimination of carbon dioxide. Common causes of hypercapnia are respiratory depression, pneumonia, pulmonary edema, and obstructive lung disease.

As carbon dioxide accumulates, hydrogen ion concentration increases into acidosis. Increased pulse rate, blood pressure, dizziness, headaches, and mental clouding occur. Severe hypercapnia may result in loss of consciousness.

Hypocapnia

Hypocapnia is an abnormally low amount of carbon dioxide in the arterial blood. It occurs when ventilation increases out of proportion to the metabolic production of carbon dioxide (too much carbon dioxide is blown off). This excessive alveolar ventilation is known as hyperventilation and can result from anxiety, improper mechanical ventilation, fever, anemia, and salicylate intoxication. Clinically, hypocapnia can be determined only by ABG studies.

Hypocapnia can result in respiratory alkalosis. Symptoms include lightheadedness, fatigue, inability to concentrate, irritability, tingling, muscle twitching, and impaired consciousness. The most common cause of hyperventilation is an anxiety reaction.

RESPIRATORY FAILURE

Respiratory failure is a nonspecific clinical diagnosis denoting the inability of the respiratory system to supply the body with needed oxygen and rid it of carbon dioxide waste. In terms of ABG values, it can be arbitrarily defined as:

$$PaO_2 \leq 50 \text{ mm Hg, or}$$

$$PaO_2 \geq 50 \text{ mm Hg and pH} \leq 7.25$$

(McCance and Heuther, 1994).

Respiratory failure may be acute or chronic and, depending on its cause, can be classified as ventilatory failure or oxygenation failure.

Ventilatory failure, the chief characteristic of which is alveolar hypoventilation with resultant hypoxemia, has many causes. These include upper airway obstruction, depression of the respiratory center in the medulla, impaired transmission of nerve impulses from the respiratory center to the muscles of respiration, and mechanical abnormalities of the lung or the chest wall. Depression of the respiratory center may occur after drug overdose, anesthesia, head trauma, specific types of cerebrovascular accidents, brain tumors, meningitis, encephalitis, hypoxia, or hypercapnia. Impaired transmission of nervous impulses to the muscles of respiration may result from a lesion at the cervical level of the spinal cord or to a disorder of the involved nerves or neuromuscular junctions. Thus, ventilatory failure occurs in patients with polyneuritis, poliomyelitis, muscular dystrophy, Guillain-Barré syndrome, multiple sclerosis, and myasthenia gravis. Conditions that interfere with lung expansion include pleural effusion, pneumothorax, hemothorax, and flail chest.

Ventilatory failure is also a risk after surgery, particularly after upper abdominal or thoracic procedures and after extensive trauma. Smokers are at particular risk of ventilatory failure if chronic obstructive lung disease is present.

In oxygenation failure, hypoxemia is most often the result of ventilation/perfusion mismatching or physiologic shunting. Disorders associated with oxygenation failure include pneumonia, adult respiratory distress syndrome, atelectasis, severe pulmonary edema, and pulmonary embolism.

Management of respiratory failure includes oxygenation, ventilation, or both, along with treatment of the underlying disorder.

Assessment of the Respiratory System

PATIENT HISTORY

Obtain a thorough patient history as a basis for individualizing care. Question the patient about the predominant complaint. It is usually this complaint that has caused the patient to seek medical attention and, by dealing with it right away, you can convey a sense of acceptance and understanding, which helps establish a trusting relationship. Use open-ended questions to determine the onset of the present problem and the patient's perception of it.

Review the patient's health history, including illnesses since birth. Elicit information about the frequency of illnesses and treatments, with particular attention to colds, pneumonia, allergies, sinus problems, tuberculosis, and asthma. Note the date of the last chest x-ray, tuberculin skin test, and any pulmonary function tests.

Review the family history. Include information about the health status or causes of death of immediate family members. If the patient has reported any hereditary diseases, review the family history for similar problems.

As part of the history, obtain information about smoking and the occupational and geographic environment. Ascertain how many years the patient has smoked and how many packs per day. If the patient states he or she does not smoke, follow up by asking whether he or she has ever smoked. Some people will say they do not smoke or have stopped, when in fact they just stopped a few days ago.

Because many respiratory dysfunctions are associated with occupational pollutants (such as chemicals, fumes, asbestos, beryllium, coal, magnesium silicate, and organic dust materials such as moldy wheat and hay), question about the type of employment and location of home to provide clues to possible exposure to these hazards. If the patient was in the armed forces, ask about possible exposure to Agent Orange or other carcinogens.

Direct the interview toward specific clinical manifestations of respiratory dysfunction, including cough, nasal secretions, pain, dyspnea, and fatigue.

Question about cough. If cough is present or reported by the patient, determine its frequency and duration. Coughs lasting longer than 2 or 3 weeks may indicate serious respiratory dysfunction. Ask the patient to describe the type of cough: productive, nonproductive, or paroxysmal. If the cough is productive, ascertain the quantity, color, consistency, and odor of the expectorate.

If nasal secretions are present, ask about frequency and duration. Ask whether they are present when the patient is indoors or outdoors. Question the patient about the environment as it relates to the presence or absence of secretions.

Ask about pain. If present, is it associated with deep breathing or coughing? Is it transient or steady? Does it radiate? What self-treatment has the patient used to control the pain? Carefully assess respiratory rate and depth when a patient is experiencing painful breathing because this is often associated with shallow respirations as a result of an attempt to limit movement of the chest.

Question about dyspnea. Remember that persons with normal respiratory function experience dyspnea with strenuous activity, such as running up stairs. Determine the level of activity that brings on the dyspnea. For example, can the patient do light housework or mow the lawn without experiencing dyspnea? Question the patient about other related symptoms, such as cough. Ask whether the dyspnea occurs at night or during the day. Does the patient use one or two pillows for sleeping?

Ask about fatigue and correlate it with the level of activity. The patient who experiences fatigue after light activity, such as personal grooming or light housework, might be hypoxic.

Do a general review of other body systems to help the patient remember all signs and symptoms. Also assess the patient's understanding of and compliance with risk reduction and health promotion information related to the respiratory system (Highlight 14–1). Record all pertinent information.

PHYSICAL EXAMINATION

The next step of respiratory assessment is the physical examination. Proceed in a stepwise manner through inspection, palpation, percussion, and auscultation (Table 14–1). Draw standard imaginary lines through the thorax to localize and record assessment findings (Fig. 14–5). Perform the physical examination in a private, warm, well-lit, and quiet room. Absence of background noise makes it easier to hear breath sounds.

Inspection

Begin this part of the physical examination with a general observation of the patient during the inter-

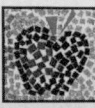

Optimal Respiratory System Function

To assist the patient in maintaining a healthy respiratory system:

Encourage the patient to engage in a physical fitness program or perform exercises that incorporate cardiorespiratory endurance and diaphragmatic breathing.

Provide information on risks associated with smoking and on smoking cessation programs.

Instruct patients who work in an environment where there are respiratory irritants (such as asbestos, solvents in paint and varnishes) to wear protective masks or other devices.

Explain how good nutrition decreases the risk of respiratory infection.

Instruct the patient to avoid close contact with persons who have a respiratory infection, to decrease the risk of contracting it.

Explain to obese patients that weight loss will promote optimal respiratory function.

---

view. Note the patient's overall condition, including nutritional status. Observe the patient's posture to obtain clues about general respiratory condition. Persons with respiratory problems frequently as-

Table 14–1

Respiratory Physical Assessment

INSPECTION:	Posture, contour, movement, dimensions of chest, flared nostrils, use of accessory muscles, skin color, and rate, depth, and rhythm of respirations
PALPATION:	Respiratory excursion, tactile fremitus, masses, and tenderness
PERCUSSION:	Flat, dull, tympanic, resonant, and hyperresonant sounds; diaphragmatic excursion
AUSCULTATION:	Breath sounds (vesicular, bronchial, bronchovesicular), voice sounds (bronchophony, egophony, whispered pectoriloquy), adventitious sounds (crackles, wheezes)

sume positions that facilitate breathing, such as sitting upright with arms supported on a table. During the interview, observe whether the patient can speak a full sentence without pausing for breath.

Ask the patient to disrobe to the waist and sit upright. Observe for flared nostrils, gasping, open mouth, pursed-lip breathing, and the use of accessory muscles. These signs indicate respiratory distress. Inspect the skin for lesions, color, and evidence of loss of subcutaneous tissue. When inspecting for color changes in persons with dark skin, inspect the least pigmented areas, such as nail beds, lips, mucous membranes, conjunctivae, palms, and soles. Remember that pallor may appear as a yellow-brown tinge in brown-skinned patients and as ashen-gray in black-skinned people. Cyanosis, which is a more subtle change to identify in dark-skinned patients, manifests as a gray hue on the lips and tongue and as a bluish tinge in the nail beds, palms, and soles.

Assess respiratory rate, depth, and rhythm during inspection. Do this without the patient's knowledge to avoid altering the normal respiratory pattern. Keep in mind that the normal respiratory rate in adults is 12 to 20 per minute. An increased respiratory rate (tachypnea) may indicate hypoxia. A decreased rate (bradypnea) may be seen when the respiratory center in the medulla is depressed, such as with head injury or drug overdose.

Observe the depth of respirations to obtain important information concerning alveolar ventilation. An increase in the depth of respirations is called hyperpnea. Hyperventilation refers to abnormally prolonged and deep respirations. Kussmaul's respirations are abnormally deep respirations with a rate of greater that 20 per minute. They are a labored respiration typical of air hunger and are seen in metabolic acidosis. A shallow breathing pattern fails to provide air to the alveoli or to remove carbon dioxide from the lungs. This pattern can result in hypercapnia, hypoxemia, and eventually hypoxia. Patients experiencing painful breathing frequently have this pattern.

Respiratory rhythm usually indicates the status of neurologic control of breathing. In the presence of brain damage, Biot's breathing may occur. These are respirations that vary in depth with irregular periods of apnea (cessation of breathing). Cheyne-Stokes respiration is a cycle of apnea and hyperpnea. See Figure 14–6 for schematic representations of these and other common breathing patterns.

Observe the duration of inspiration and expiration. Expiration, the passive process, is normally 1.5 times as long as inspiration, which requires energy. Prolonged expiration is associated with emphysema resulting from air trapping, which makes it difficult to move air out of the lungs.

Assess the muscles used for breathing. In thin persons, a slight retraction (drawing in of the spaces between the ribs) is normal during quiet breathing. More than slight retraction, however, indicates the

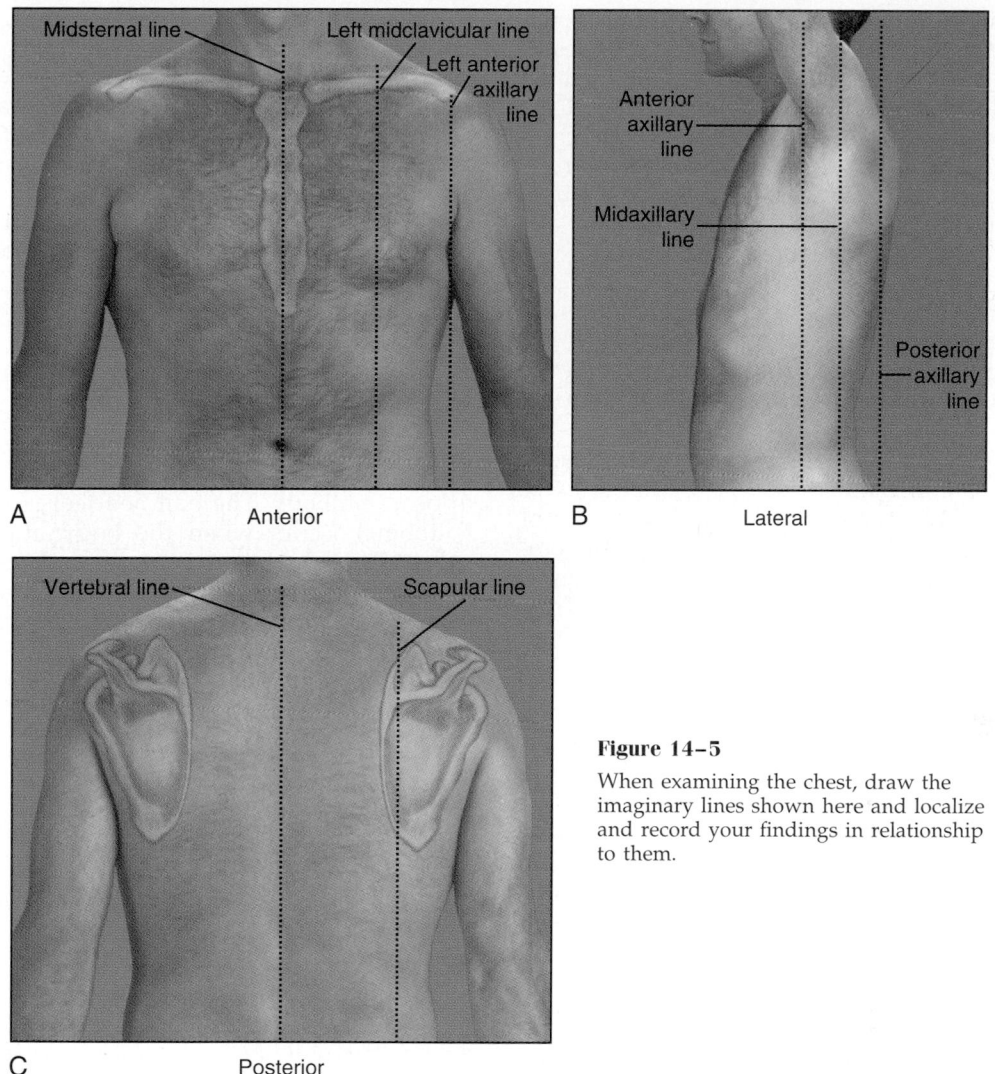

Figure 14–5

When examining the chest, draw the imaginary lines shown here and localize and record your findings in relationship to them.

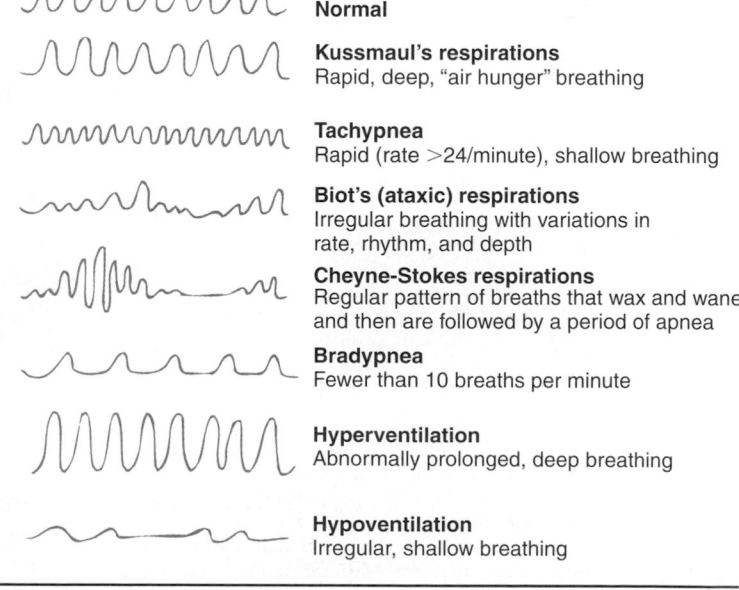

Figure 14–6

Schematic representation of abnormal breathing patterns.

Normal

Kussmaul's respirations
Rapid, deep, "air hunger" breathing

Tachypnea
Rapid (rate >24/minute), shallow breathing

Biot's (ataxic) respirations
Irregular breathing with variations in rate, rhythm, and depth

Cheyne-Stokes respirations
Regular pattern of breaths that wax and wane and then are followed by a period of apnea

Bradypnea
Fewer than 10 breaths per minute

Hyperventilation
Abnormally prolonged, deep breathing

Hypoventilation
Irregular, shallow breathing

use of accessory muscles. If breathing is difficult, you may observe the use of the accessory muscles of respiration, such as the neck and shoulder muscles—the scalenes, the sternocleidomastoids, and the trapezius—to assist ventilation. Marked retraction during inspiration, particularly if asymmetric, may indicate blockage of a branch of the respiratory tree. Bulging during expiration implies obstruction of airflow, as in emphysema or pleural effusion.

Note symmetry of the chest wall. Inspect the slope of the ribs and the costal angle. Normally the ribs are curved at an oblique angle of about 45 degrees. In chronic obstructive diseases, they may be fixed in a more rigid, linear position and appear horizontal.

Observe the contour of the chest wall closely. Normally the lateral diameter of the thorax is twice as large as the anteroposterior diameter, or a ratio of 1:2 (Fig. 14–7A). In infants and patients with emphysema, this ratio may be 1:1. Some of the abnormalities commonly encountered on inspection of the thorax are:

- Funnel chest (pectus excavatum), a congenital condition in which the sternum is abnormally depressed and the anteroposterior diameter is decreased (see Fig. 14–7B).
- Pigeon breast (pectus carinatum), an abnormal prominence of the sternum with an increase in the anteroposterior diameter (see Fig. 14–7C).
- Barrel chest, in which the chest appears rounded and the sternum pulled forward, is associated with emphysema or normal aging (see Fig. 14–7D).
- Kyphosis (hunchback), an exaggerated curvature of the thoracic spine associated with injury, osteoporosis, and congenital abnormality (see Fig. 14–7E).
- Scoliosis, a lateral deformity of the spine commonly identified in early adolescence (see Fig. 14–7F).

Observe for finger clubbing, which is a significant finding. Inspect the angle between the nail bed and the digit (Fig. 14–8). Normally this angle is 20 degrees. A flattened angle is an indication of early clubbing. In advanced clubbing, the nail is rounded over the end of the finger and the distal phalange appears bulbous. The nail bed feels soft and spongy. Clubbing occurs when the body attempts to compensate for chronic hypoxia and develops collateral circulation to areas of impaired oxygenation. Clubbing is associated with pulmonary disease, particularly chronic obstructive pulmonary disease. It is also seen in patients with congenital heart conditions and heart disease.

Palpation

With the pads of your fingers, palpate the anterior, posterior, and lateral portions of the chest for pain, tenderness, and masses. Also palpate to assess respi-

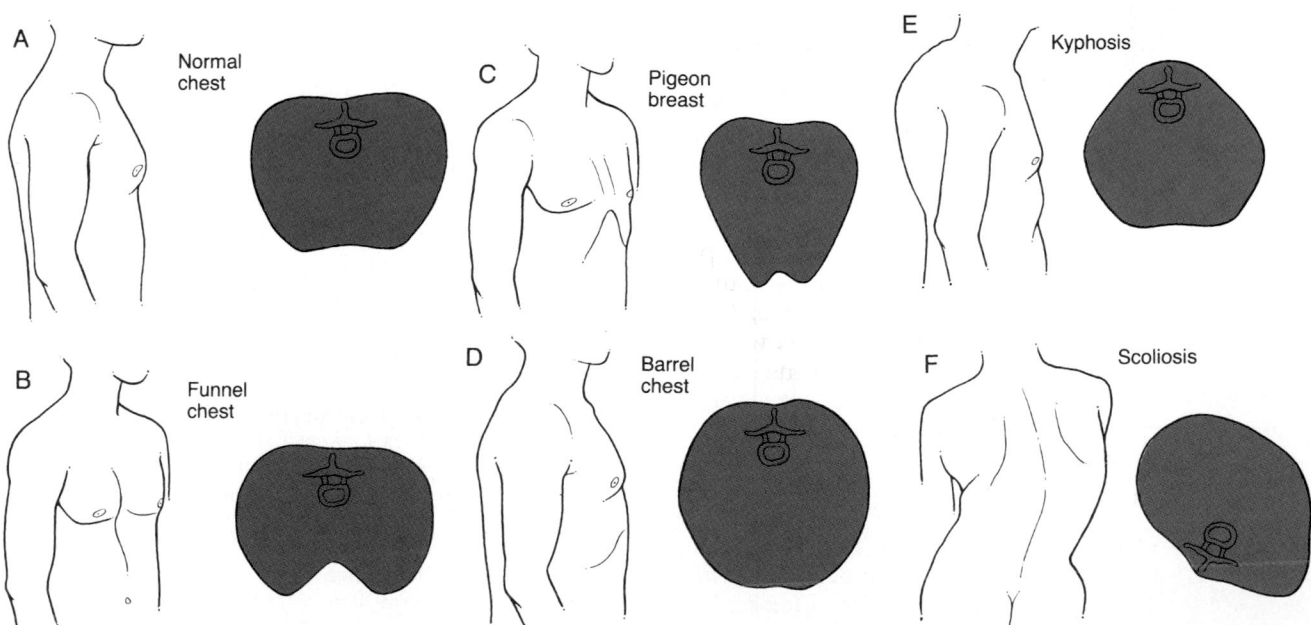

Figure 14–7

Common abnormalities of the chest. *A,* Normal chest. Elliptic shape with anteroposterior diameter roughly half the transverse diameter. *B,* Funnel chest. Depression of the sternum starting at the second intercostal space and most marked at the xiphoid process. Exaggerated on inspiration. *C,* Pigeon breast. Protrusion of the sternum with depressions at the costochondral junctions and backward sloping of the ribs. *D,* Barrel chest. Anteroposterior diameter enlarged to equal the transverse diameter. Ribs are horizontal rather than downward-sloped. *E,* Kyphosis. Exaggerated posterior curvature of the thoracic spine. *F,* Scoliosis. Lateral S-shaped curvature of the thoracic and lumbar spine.

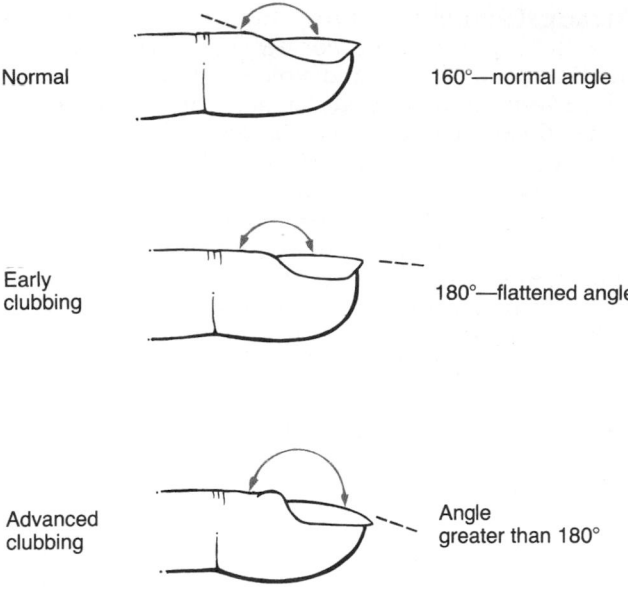

Figure 14–8

Clubbing of the fingers.

ratory excursion (estimation of thoracic expansion). With your thumbs about 2 inches apart, place your palms at the level of the tenth rib laterally on the posterior thorax. Slide the thumbs medially about 1 inch to raise loose skin folds between the thumbs, which are now about 1 inch apart. Ask the patient to take a deep breath, and observe the chest movement. Observe for normal flattening of the skin fold, and feel for symmetric movement of the thorax. A lag or impairment of thoracic movement indicates underlying disease of the lung.

The capacity to feel sound on the chest wall is known as tactile or vocal fremitus. Palpable vibrations are transmitted through the bronchial tree to the chest wall when the patient speaks. Fremitus is felt most easily over a thin, healthy patient. It is influenced by the thickness of the chest wall, especially by muscle thickness. Lower-pitched sounds travel better through the normal lung tissue; thus, fremitus is more pronounced in men than in women because of the deeper male voice. The intensity and pitch of the voice, the size of the thorax, the presence of lung disease, and the patient's body build all cause the vibrations in fremitus. It is more pronounced over the large bronchi and becomes less so over the periphery of the lungs. Fremitus can be increased in conditions in which lung consolidation is exaggerated, such as lobar pneumonia in which the sound waves hit a dense surface. Fremitus is decreased or absent when the voice is decreased, the bronchus is obstructed, or the pleural space is occupied by fluid, air, or solid mass.

Use the palmar surface of your fingers and hands or the ulnar aspect of your extended hands placed on the thorax to elicit vocal fremitus. Use only one hand to facilitate comparison. Ask the pa-

tient to repeat the word *ninety-nine* each time you move your hands.

Percussion

Percussion involves listening to the sounds produced by gently striking the chest wall. This technique sets the chest wall and underlying tissue into motion, producing audible sounds and palpable vibrations. Percussion helps to determine whether underlying tissues are air filled, fluid filled, or solid. Place the index or middle finger of one hand firmly on the chest wall, and strike the stationary finger with the middle finger of the other hand close to the tip near the distal interphalangeal joint (Fig. 14–9). Percuss downward, interspace by interspace.

Describe the quality of percussed sounds in relation to their pitch, intensity, and duration. The pitch is the number of vibrations per second. Intensity is the amplitude of the sound wave. Duration is the length of time the sound is heard. The five types of sounds detected by percussion are:

Flat
Dull
Tympanic
Resonant
Hyperresonant

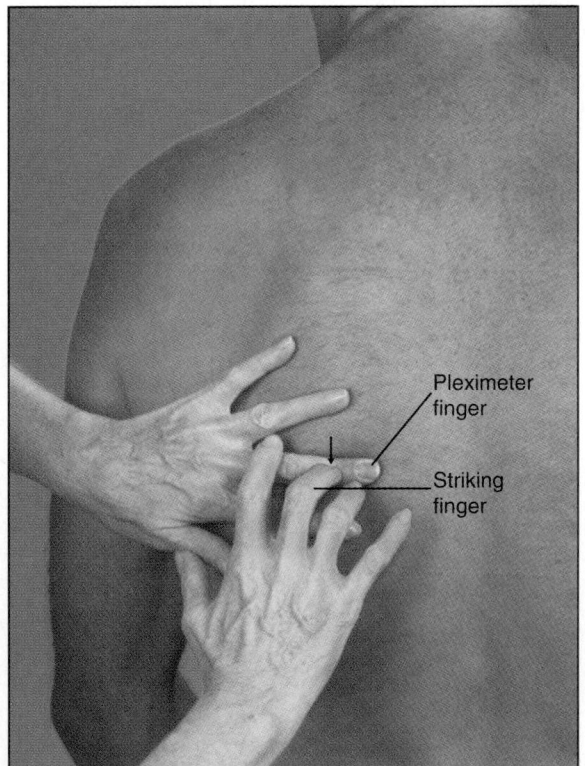

Figure 14–9

To perform percussion, place the index or middle finger of one hand on the patient's chest wall (this is the pleximeter finger). Strike the pleximeter finger with the middle finger of the other hand (this is the striking finger) near the interphalangeal joint.

A flat sound (high pitch, very little intensity, decreased duration) is heard when a solid area is percussed. This sound may imply the presence of a pleural effusion or mass. Dull sounds (higher pitch, low intensity, very short duration) are heard when there is no air or fluid in the lung, such as with consolidation or compression atelectasis. Tympanic sounds (high pitch, loud intensity, long duration) are normally heard over the stomach and bowel and below the left hemidiaphragm. Tympany over the chest is considered abnormal. Resonant sounds (low pitch, hollow, moderately loud) are normal. They are produced over the greater part of the lung and are usually of long duration. Hyperresonant sounds (low pitch, booming) are abnormal. They occur when free air exists in the thoracic cavity, such as in emphysema. Perform percussion, like palpation, in an organized manner, as shown in Figure 14–10.

Determine the excursion of the diaphragm. Hold the pleximeter finger above and parallel to the expected border of diaphragmatic dullness. Ask the patient to hold the breath after forced inspiration. Percuss downward to determine where the resonant sounds end at the margin of the diaphragm and mark this spot. Repeat this procedure after a forced expiration. For maximum accuracy, measure the space between the marks with a ruler. Normally diaphragmatic excursion is 5 to 7 cm. A much greater than normal excursion may indicate pleural effusion, ascites, or an abnormally high location of the diaphragm, as seen in pregnancy or paralysis. Diaphragmatic excursion may decrease in patients with emphysema.

Auscultation

Assess breath sounds and voice sounds. Also assess for adventitious sounds when auscultating the lungs. Breath sounds have characteristic changes related to specific disease processes. Ask the patient to take slow, deep breaths through the mouth while you listen with the diaphragm of the stethoscope. While auscultating, keep pulmonary anatomy in mind to determine what portion of the lung is being assessed. Because you may need to listen to two full respirations at each anatomical location, be sure to ask the patient to tell you whether he or she feels dizzy or lightheaded. Allow the patient to rest and breathe normally once or twice during the respiratory examination, if needed, to avoid these symptoms of hyperventilation.

Ideally, the patient should be sitting upright for this examination. If the patient is not able to assume the upright position, turn the patient side to side and auscultate the lung on the upper side of the body. Do not auscultate the lung in the dependent position.

Breath sounds are heard as a result of the transmission of vibrations produced by the movement of air in the respiratory passages from the larynx to the alveoli. Adventitious sounds are abnormal sounds superimposed over the breath sounds.

Normal breath sounds are described as vesicular, bronchial, and bronchovesicular. Keep in mind, during the examination, the locations at which each sound is normal. Vesicular breath sounds are quiet, low-pitched sounds with a long inspiratory phase and a short expiratory phase. They are heard over

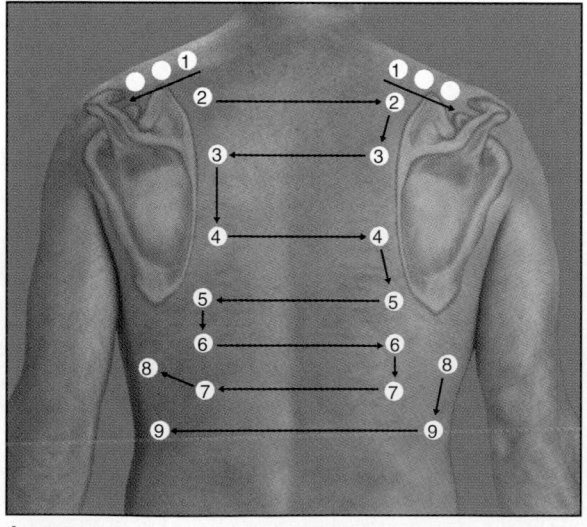
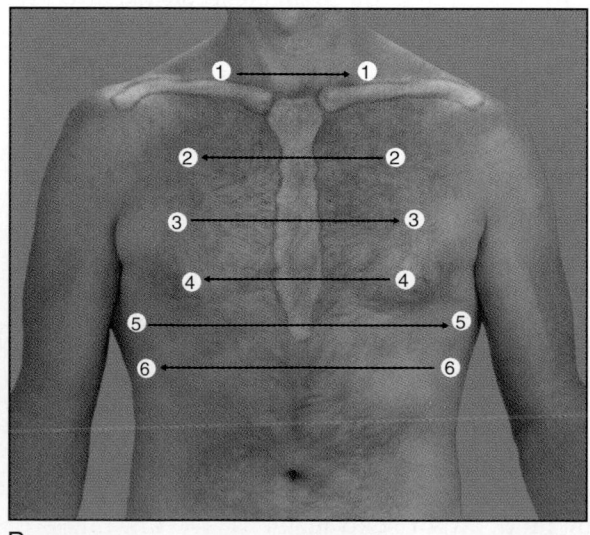

A   B

Figure 14–10

Sequence of percussion and auscultation, moving from side to side on the posterior thorax (*A*) and on the anterior chest (*B*).

most of the lung field except over the sternum and between the scapulae. Vesicular sounds are produced by air movement in the bronchioles and alveoli.

Bronchial breath sounds are high-pitched, very loud, and normally heard over the trachea. Bronchial breath sounds have a louder and longer expiratory phase. Make careful note of any bronchial sounds heard over any other portion of the lung, because this indicates respiratory dysfunction.

Bronchovesicular sounds are of medium pitch and are heard between the trachea and peripheral lung. Decreased breath sounds are present when there is fluid, air, or increased tissue in the pleural space that interferes with the transfer of the vibrations to the chest wall. Diminished breath sounds are present when there is obstruction. Patients with severe barrel chest have diminished breath sounds because of torso configuration.

Voice sounds are vibrations produced by the spoken voice that are transmitted to the chest wall via the tracheobronchial tree. During this process, the sounds are diminished in intensity so that syllables are no longer distinguishable. There are three abnormal voice sounds: bronchophony, egophony, and whispered pectoriloquy.

With bronchophony, vocal resonance is increased in intensity and clarity. Check for this by placing the diaphragm of the stethoscope over various sites on the chest wall and asking the patient to speak in a normal voice, repeating the word *ninety-nine*.

Egophony is a condition in which the spoken voice has a nasal or bleating sound. To check for egophony, ask the patient to repeat the letter *e* as you listen with the stethoscope. If you hear an *a* sound rather than an *e* sound, the presence of consolidation, usually pleural effusion, is indicated.

To auscultate whispered pectoriloquy, ask the patient to whisper "one, two, three" repeatedly. Normally, these sounds are very muffled. In the presence of very dense consolidation, transmission of high-frequency components of sounds is so enhanced that even whispered words are heard with unusual clarity.

Bronchophony, egophony, bronchial breathing sounds, and an increase in vocal fremitus all indicate an airless or solid consolidation. Therefore, any abnormality detected during percussion or palpation should be more fully assessed during auscultation. Conversely, if normal breath sounds are auscultated in all lung fields, voice sounds need not be routinely assessed.

Adventitious breath sounds, or superimposed sounds in the lungs, indicate the presence of an abnormal condition that affects the bronchial tree and alveoli. In the past, a wide variety of terms has been used to describe these added lung sounds. Today there are two classifications for adventitious breath sounds: discrete, noncontinuous sounds called crackles, and continuous musical sounds of greater duration called wheezes.

Crackles, also referred to as rales or crepitations, are discrete, noncontinuous sounds that result from delayed reopening of deflated airways. They are heard during inspiration as a series of tiny explosions as the deflated airways are reinflated. Fine crackles are heard at the end of inspiration and originate from the alveoli. This sound can be reproduced by rubbing together several strands of hair next to one's ear. Coarse crackles are audible early during inspiration and have a gross, moist sound. The presence of crackles may indicate pneumonia, bronchitis, bronchiectasis, or heart failure. Loud gurgling sounds during inspiration and expiration are produced by secretions in the trachea and large bronchi. They are heard in association with fulminating pulmonary edema and in moribund patients who cannot cough up their secretions. This sound is sometimes referred to as the "death rattle."

Friction rub (pleural rub) is heard during inspiration and expiration over a relatively small portion of the chest wall. It is a crackling, grating sound caused by the jerky movement of pleural surfaces that are inflamed. Friction rubs resemble crackles acoustically. This sound can be imitated by rubbing the thumb and index finger together next to one's ear.

Wheezes, also called rhonchi, are continuous musical sounds of greater duration. These sounds are produced by air flowing through airways that are narrowed or partially filled with fluid or mucus. Wheezing is most typical during expiration but may occur in both inspiration and expiration. When recording these findings, note whether it was an inspiratory or expiratory wheeze, or both. If the obstruction causing the wheeze is secretions, the wheezing may be cleared with coughing.

When wheezes originate in the smaller bronchi and bronchioles, they may be high pitched. Obstruction in the larger bronchi produces a lower pitched, sonorous sound. Wheezing is most common in patients with emphysema and asthma.

Diagnostic Procedures

PULMONARY FUNCTION STUDIES

Pulmonary function studies measure the functional ability of the lungs by comparing the patient's lung volumes and capacities with those of other people of the same age, sex, height, and race.

There are four basic lung volumes: inspiratory reserve volume, tidal volume, expiratory reserve volume, and residual volume. Together these volumes represent the maximum volume to which the lungs can be expanded. When evaluating the pulmonary cycle, it is sometimes necessary to consider two or more volumes together. These combinations are called pulmonary capacities (Fig. 14–11).

Lung volumes and capacities can vary with age, sex, height, and weight. They can also vary with body position. Most volumes and capacities decrease when a person lies down and increase when a person stands. This is caused by two factors. First, in the supine position, there is a tendency for the abdominal contents to press upward against the diaphragm. Second, there is an increase in the pulmonary blood volume in the supine position, which correspondingly decreases the space available for air.

Volumes and capacities used in pulmonary function studies are described in Table 14–2.

Uses

Pulmonary function tests are used to diagnose specific types of lung abnormalities and to assess the risk of respiratory complications in surgical patients. They are also used to monitor the course of pulmo-

nary diseases over time, to evaluate the effectiveness of prescribed medications, and to determine the need for mechanical ventilation.

Procedure

Pulmonary function studies may be performed in a pulmonary function laboratory, in a physician's office, or at the patient's bedside. They should not be done immediately after a meal, when the stomach is distended and pressing on the diaphragm. Medications that may affect respiration—such as sedatives, narcotics, and bronchodilators—are omitted unless specifically ordered to be given. A spirometer with an attached recording device (kymograph) that produces a graphic record is used for all pulmonary function tests.

The patient sits or stands and seals the lips around the mouthpiece of the spirometer. A nose clip prevents air leakage from the nostrils. The patient is instructed to breathe normally through the mouth. When the patient is comfortable breathing

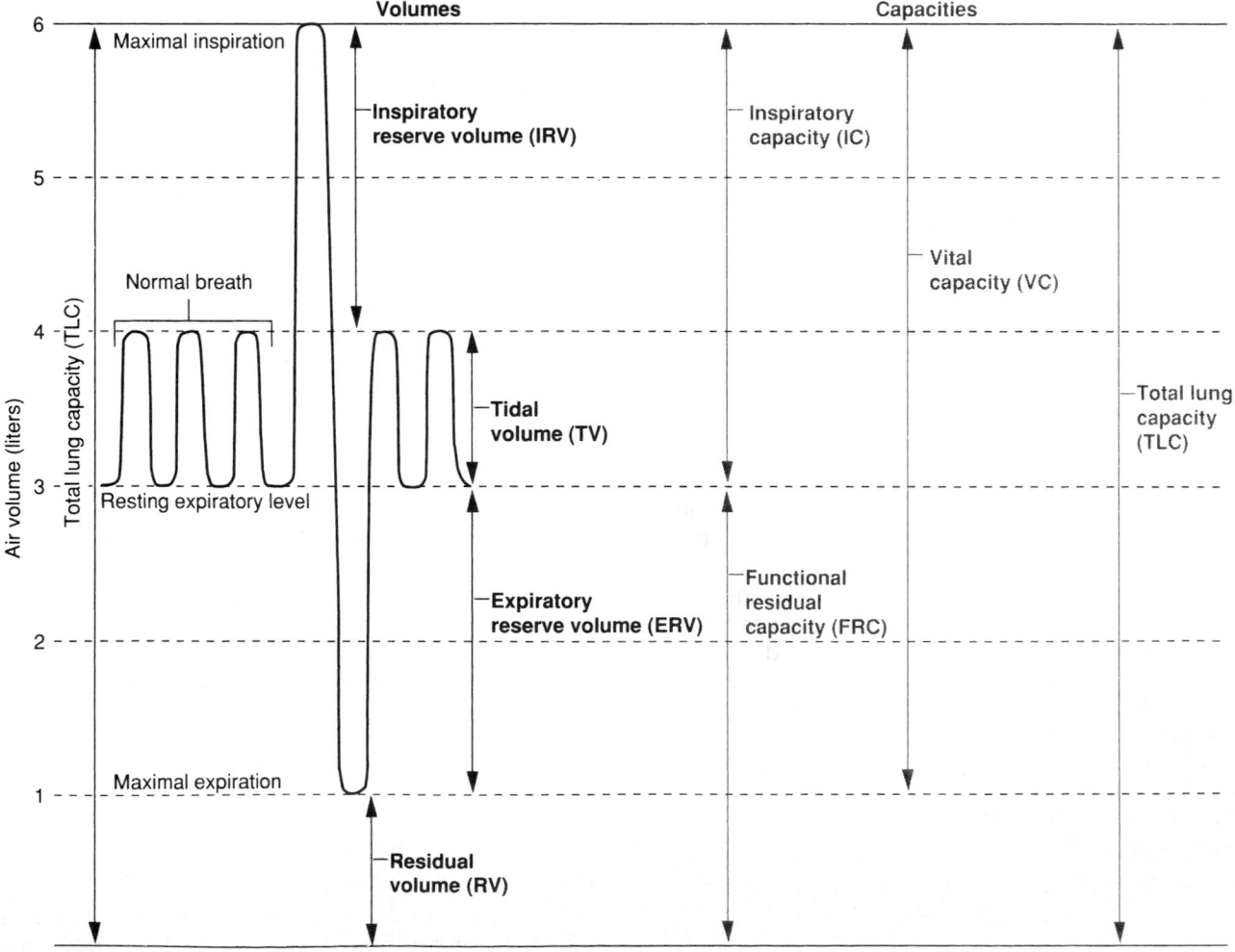

Figure 14–11

Schematic representation of pulmonary volumes and capacities.

Table 14–2

Pulmonary Function Tests

Term	Symbol	Description
LUNG VOLUMES		
Tidal volume	TV or V_t	Volume of air inspired and expired with a normal breath
Inspiratory reserve volume	IRV	Maximum volume that can be inspired from the end of a normal inspiration
Expiratory reserve volume	ERV	Maximum volume that can be exhaled by forced expiration after a normal respiration
Residual volume	RV	Volume of air left in lung after maximal expiration
Minute ventilation	MV or V_e	Volume of air inspired and expired in 1 minute of normal breathing
LUNG CAPACITIES		
Vital capacity	VC	Maximum amount of air that can be expired after a maximal inspiration
Forced vital capacity	FVC	Vital capacity performed with a maximally forced expiration
Forced expiratory volume	FEV_1 (subscript indicates the time interval in seconds)	Amount of air expelled in a specified time of the FVC maneuver
Ratio of timed forced expiratory volume to FVC	FEV_1/FVC	Amount of air forcefully expelled in 1 second compared with total amount forcefully expelled
Maximum expiratory flow rate	$FEF_{200-1200}$	Mean forced expiratory flow after the first 200 mL
Maximum midexpiratory flow	$FEF_{25-75\%}$	Average rate of flow during middle half of FVC
Maximal voluntary ventilation	MVV	Amount of air exchanged per minute with maximal rate and depth of respiration
Inspiratory capacity	IC	Maximum amount of air that can be inhaled after a normal respiration
Functional residual capacity	FRC	Amount of air left in the lungs after a normal expiration
Total lung capacity	TLC	Maximum amount of air the lungs and respiratory passages can hold after a forced inspiration

through the mouthpiece, testing begins. The patient is directed to perform various inspiratory and expiratory maneuvers.

Some spirometric tests can be done during exercise. Methods of exercise include using a bicycle ergometer or stepping up and down a raised platform for several minutes. ABG values can also be measured with the patient at rest and after exercise.

A primary nursing responsibility is to provide the patient with information about the procedures to allay anxiety and promote cooperation. The patient should know the following:

• The array of complex equipment used in the pulmonary function laboratory may appear frightening, but the test itself is relatively simple.
• Extensive testing can cause fatigue.
• For those patients with compromised pulmonary function, feelings of suffocation may occur when the nose clips are in place.

• Loose clothing should be worn.
• Usual measures aimed at mobilizing and removing secretions are performed before the tests. If this includes intermittent positive pressure breathing treatment, bronchodilators will be withheld for 4 hours before testing so that test results reflect the patient's usual status.

BLOOD STUDIES

Arterial Blood Gases

ABG analysis determines the actual levels of oxygen and carbon dioxide circulating in a sample of arterial blood. It provides direct information about ventilation and diffusion of gases between the alveoli and the blood. Interpretation of ABGs also provides data about overall acid-base balance.

An ABG analysis includes determination of the partial pressure of oxygen in arterial blood (PaO_2), the oxygen saturation level of hemoglobin in arterial blood (SaO_2), the partial pressure of carbon dioxide in arterial blood ($PaCO_2$), the degree to which arterial blood is acid or alkaline (pH), and the level of bicarbonate present in arterial blood (HCO_3^-). See Table 14–3 for normal ABG values.

Uses

ABGs are used to evaluate respiratory functioning in an individual and to help determine the need for and the effectiveness of therapeutic interventions such as the administration of supplemental oxygen.

ABG assessment can indicate the presence of hypoxemia (inadequate oxygen in the arterial blood as measured by PaO_2), hypoxia (inadequate oxygenation at the cellular level), hypercapnia (excessive carbon dioxide in the arterial blood as measured by $PaCO_2$), acidosis or alkalosis (as measured by pH), and the presence of the body's compensatory efforts to reduce an acid-base imbalance.

Physiologic Basis of ABG Use and Interpretation

DIFFUSION OF OXYGEN AND CARBON DIOXIDE. Oxygen and carbon dioxide are gases that diffuse from areas of greater concentration to areas of lesser concentration. For example, oxygen diffuses from the alveoli into the blood when the concentration of oxygen in the alveoli is greater than the concentration of oxygen in the blood. The partial pressure of a gas is defined as the pressure exerted by a particular gas when it is in a mixture of gases.

Inspired air is composed of 21% oxygen, and the partial pressure of atmospheric oxygen is 160 mm Hg (total pressure of atmospheric air is 760 mm Hg at sea level). The partial pressure of oxygen falls to about 100 mm Hg in the alveoli after it is exposed to vapors and air occupying the dead spaces in the lung. After normal ventilation with inspired air, the oxygen concentration in the deoxygenated blood circulating to the lung from the right side of the heart (partial pressure of 40 mm Hg) is significantly lower than the concentration of oxygen in the alveoli (about 100 mm Hg). Oxygen therefore diffuses into the blood before it returns to the left side of the heart. The partial pressure of well-oxygenated blood ranges from 75 to 100 mm Hg. Oxygen also diffuses from arterial blood into the tissues through the peripheral capillaries, where oxygen tension is significantly lower (partial pressure of 40 mm Hg).

Carbon dioxide diffuses from deoxygenated blood brought from the right side of the heart (partial pressure of carbon dioxide is 46 to 48 mm Hg) into the alveoli (partial pressure of carbon dioxide is 40 mm Hg). The $PaCO_2$ falls within the range of 35 to 45 mm Hg. At the cellular level, carbon dioxide diffuses from the tissues into the blood, which contains a lower concentration of this gas.

OXYGEN TRANSPORT. Oxygen is transported throughout the body in two forms. About 2% of the total oxygen in the blood exists in an unbound, dissolved form. This dissolved gas is the only oxygen that is available for immediate utilization in cell metabolism because it is the only form capable of crossing the cell membrane. The amount of oxygen that exists in the blood in this dissolved form is reflected by, and is directly proportional to, the partial pressure of oxygen (oxygen tension). The partial pressure of oxygen exerted in arterial blood is, therefore, a measurement of the amount of dissolved oxygen in arterial blood and is represented by the PaO_2.

About 98% of the oxygen circulating and transported in the blood exists in a bound form and is not available for immediate utilization. This oxygen is chemically bound to the hemoglobin molecule within red blood cells. This union of oxygen and hemoglobin forms the oxyhemoglobin molecule. The SaO_2 is a measurement of the amount of available hemoglobin that is actually bound with oxygen compared with the total capacity of the available hemoglobin for binding. It is expressed as a percentage. The oxygen saturation level of well-oxygenated arterial blood ranges from 94 to 100%.

OXYHEMOGLOBIN DISSOCIATION CURVE. The amount of oxygen that exists in the dissolved state is approximately 0.3 mL per 100 mL of blood. On the basis of an average hemoglobin level of 15 g per 100 mL of blood, the average amount of oxygen carried in the bound state is 20.1 mL of oxygen per 100 mL when oxygen saturation is 100%. (Each gram of hemoglobin is capable of carrying 1.34 mL of oxygen.)

The amount of oxygen that exists in the dis-

Table 14–3

Arterial Blood Gases

Symbol	Description	Normal Values
pH	Expression of hydrogen ion concentration; represents acidity or alkalinity of the blood	7.35–7.45
PaO_2	Partial pressure of oxygen in arterial blood	75–100 mm Hg
$PaCO_2$	Partial pressure of carbon dioxide in arterial blood	35–45 mm Hg
HCO_3^-	Bicarbonate	23–29 mEq/L
SaO_2	Percentage of oxygen carried in hemoglobin	>94%

solved state is insufficient to meet the body's metabolic needs and must therefore be continuously replenished. The chemical bond between oxygen and hemoglobin is a loose one and is easily reversible. The hemoglobin molecule releases oxygen into the plasma in response to cellular metabolic requirements. This released oxygen quickly dissolves and becomes available for utilization by the cells. As dissolved oxygen is used, PaO_2 levels decrease. Hemoglobin molecules respond by releasing oxygen, which in turn decreases SaO_2 levels. The hemoglobin molecule is capable of releasing all of its oxygen; however, hemoglobin saturation usually falls only from a range of 94 to 100% in arterial blood leaving the heart to about 70% in the venous circulation.

A definite and complex relationship exists between the partial pressure of oxygen in arterial blood (dissolved oxygen, or PaO_2) and the volume of oxygen that will combine with hemoglobin (SaO_2). Oxygen's affinity for hemoglobin and its ability to be released vary. Higher SaO_2 levels reflect a greater affinity of oxygen for hemoglobin, with greater ease of binding and greater difficulty with being released. Lower SaO_2 levels reflect lower affinity of oxygen for hemoglobin, with less binding capacity and greater ease of release. The PaO_2 is the critical determinant of oxygen's affinity for hemoglobin and, therefore, of SaO_2 levels. The greater the PaO_2 levels, the greater the SaO_2 (hemoglobin saturation percentage). In other words, the more oxygen dissolved and available for use (PaO_2), the more oxygen one can "store" and bind with hemoglobin (SaO_2). With decreased levels of dissolved oxygen available, less oxygen is bound to hemoglobin, and oxygen is more readily released for consumption. Oxygen uptake by blood in the lungs and oxygen release to tissues in the peripheral capillaries depend on this relationship.

The graphic representation of this relationship between the percentage of hemoglobin saturation (SaO_2) and the PaO_2 is known as the oxyhemoglobin dissociation curve (Fig. 14–12). This curve demonstrates the binding capacity of oxygen and hemoglobin and the ease with which they separate, as the partial pressure of oxygen in arterial blood (PaO_2) varies. Greater or lesser quantities of oxygen become available for consumption by the tissues as the hemoglobin saturation levels (SaO_2) vary. Because hemoglobin saturation levels vary in relation to PaO_2, more oxygen is available (less is bound) when PaO_2 levels are lower, and less oxygen is released (more is bound) when PaO_2 levels are high. A low PaO_2 of 40 mm Hg, such as that encountered in the peripheral capillaries, is accompanied by a hemoglobin saturation level of about 75%. Oxygen is readily released by hemoglobin molecules for tissue consumption at this point. A PaO_2 of 75 to 100 mm Hg, such as that encountered in the lungs, is accompanied by a high hemoglobin saturation level of approximately 94 to 100%. Minimal oxygen is released from hemoglobin molecules at this point because ad-

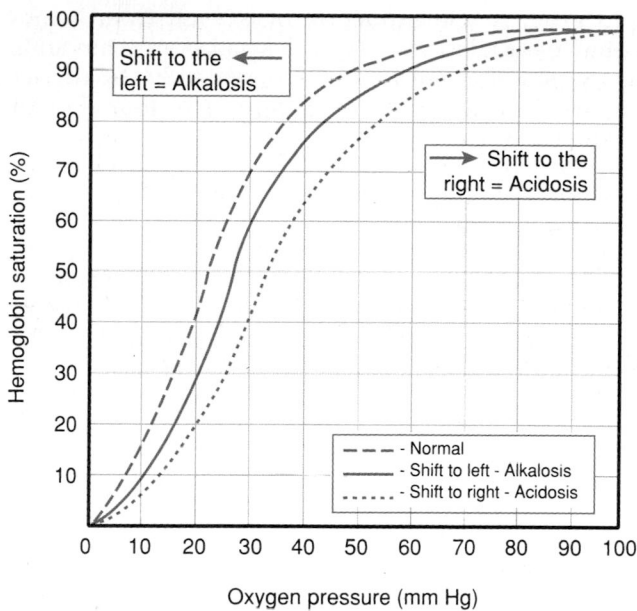

Figure 14–12

Oxyhemoglobin dissociation curve.

equate dissolved oxygen exists. These relationships are represented by the following formulas:

$$\uparrow PaO_2 \rightarrow \uparrow SaO_2 \rightarrow \uparrow O_2 \text{ binding} + \downarrow O_2 \text{ release}$$

$$\downarrow PaO_2 \rightarrow \downarrow SaO_2 \rightarrow \downarrow O_2 \text{ binding} + \uparrow O_2 \text{ release}$$

This relationship is not linear, however, and it is not unlimited. The relationship is depicted by a diphasic, or S, curve rather than a straight line and exists only up to a PaO_2 of 150 mm Hg (above normal). At this level, hemoglobin is 100% saturated and is not capable of combining with any more oxygen. A PaO_2 greater than 150 mm Hg would not result in a greater saturation of hemoglobin. A PaO_2 less than 150 mm Hg lowers the hemoglobin saturation percentage. The normal PaO_2 of 80 to 100 mm Hg results in an SaO_2 of 94 to 100%.

Changes in the PaO_2 are not accompanied by equivalent or proportional changes in SaO_2. Examination of the flat portion of the curve reveals that relatively large decreases in PaO_2 levels result in only a small drop in SaO_2 levels. This portion of the curve reflects oxygen uptake in the pulmonary capillaries, where normal PaO_2 levels of 80 to 100 mm Hg result in high SaO_2 levels. A large drop in PaO_2 is required in this portion of the curve before a significant drop in SaO_2 occurs. This serves to protect the individual because it ensures the availability of adequate oxygen to the tissues even if mild hypoxemia exists. The steep portion of the curve, on the other hand, illustrates sharp drops in SaO_2 as the PaO_2 decreases. This portion of the curve reflects PaO_2 levels encountered in the peripheral tissue capillaries. The lower levels of dissolved oxygen found here promote the extraction of oxygen from hemoglobin molecules as SaO_2 levels fall. Large amounts of oxygen are released with relatively small decreases in PaO_2. This ensures peripheral tissues of an adequate oxygen supply.

With normal respiration, the oxyhemoglobin dissociation curve represents the normal binding and releasing of oxygen by hemoglobin. Efficient tissue oxygenation depends on the ability of hemoglobin to bind with oxygen in the lung and to transport it to the tissues, where it releases oxygen as necessary and on demand to maintain tissue oxygenation. The curve can be further examined in terms of three levels of oxygen sufficiency as determined by an individual's PaO_2 levels. PaO_2 levels greater than 80 mm Hg in the blood as it leaves the heart represent normal oxygenation. The portion of the curve between a PaO_2 of 45 and 80 mm Hg represents relative safety (mild to moderate hypoxemia). The portion of the curve that represents a PaO_2 of less than 45 mm Hg (severe hypoxemia) endangers life because inadequate oxygen is available to meet the needs of tissues (hypoxia).

A number of factors other than PaO_2 affect hemoglobin's affinity for oxygen. Certain conditions shift the entire oxyhemoglobin dissociation curve to the right or to the left. Acidosis, hypercapnia, and an elevated temperature shift the curve to the right. A shift in this direction reduces hemoglobin's affinity to bind with oxygen and facilitates the release of oxygen from the oxyhemoglobin molecule to the tissues. These conditions represent an increase in tissue metabolism and a concomitant increase in the need for oxygen. An individual with an altered pH that falls within the acidotic range releases more oxygen for tissue consumption and maintains a lower SaO_2 than an individual with the same PaO_2 and a normal arterial blood pH. An increase in 2,3-diphosphoglycerate, which is found in red blood cells and may be seen in people with anemia and prolonged hypoxia, also causes a shift to the right.

Alkalosis, hypocapnia, and decreased temperature shift the curve to the left. A shift in this direction increases hemoglobin's affinity for oxygen and makes it more difficult to release oxygen to the tissues. These conditions represent a decrease in tissue metabolism. A person with an altered pH in the alkalotic range releases less oxygen and maintains a higher SaO_2 than an individual with the same PaO_2 and a normal pH.

The influence of arterial blood pH on hemoglobin's affinity to bind with oxygen is further illustrated by changes in carbon dioxide levels at various points of the respiratory cycle. Carbon dioxide levels play a major role in determining the pH of the blood, with elevated carbon dioxide levels resulting in acidosis, and below-normal levels of carbon dioxide resulting in alkalosis. As blood circulates through the pulmonary capillaries, excess carbon dioxide is released from the blood to the lungs. This raises the pH of the blood and produces a more alkaline environment. This, in turn, facilitates formation of oxyhemoglobin in the lungs and results in high SaO_2 levels. In the peripheral tissue capillaries, carbon dioxide levels are increased because of cellular metabolism. This increase in carbon dioxide levels lowers the pH of the blood and creates an acidic environment. This in turn facilitates release of oxygen from blood to tissues and promotes adequate oxygenation at this level. The following formulas represent the shifts created by these various factors:

$$\left.\begin{array}{l} \downarrow \text{pH} \\ \uparrow CO_2 \\ \uparrow \text{temperature} \end{array}\right\} \quad \downarrow O_2 \text{ binding} + \uparrow O_2 \text{ release}$$

$$\left.\begin{array}{l} \uparrow \text{pH} \\ \downarrow CO_2 \\ \downarrow \text{temperature} \end{array}\right\} \quad \uparrow CO_2 \text{ binding} + \downarrow O_2 \text{ release}$$

Two additional factors that affect oxygen transport are hemoglobin level and cardiac output. Hemoglobin levels must be within normal limits to ensure adequate oxygen transport. People who are anemic may have inadequate tissue oxygen delivery despite normal PaO_2 and SaO_2 levels. Those with decreased cardiac output are also at risk of inadequate tissue oxygenation despite normal PaO_2 and SaO_2 levels.

CARBON DIOXIDE TRANSPORT. Carbon dioxide is transported from the tissues back to the lungs in three forms. Most carbon dioxide enters red blood cells, where about 23% combines with hemoglobin to form carbaminohemoglobin. The remainder of the carbon dioxide that enters the red blood cells (70%) combines with water within the cells and then exits and is carried as bicarbonate ions (HCO_3^-) in the plasma ($CO_2 + H_2O \rightarrow H^+ + HCO_3^-$). A very small percentage (7%) of carbon dioxide remains in a dissolved form in the plasma. ABGs measure this dissolved form of carbon dioxide as the $PaCO_2$. This value gives information about the cellular production of carbon dioxide through metabolic processes and the removal of it from the body via the lungs. Normal levels of $PaCO_2$ range from 35 to 45 mm Hg. Changes in the $PaCO_2$ are regulated by the respiratory system. Hyperventilation is the term used when an individual is exhaling greater than normal amounts of carbon dioxide, resulting in a $PaCO_2$ of less than 35 mm Hg. Alveolar ventilation that exceeds the body's metabolic activity results in hypocapnia ($PaCO_2 <35$ mm Hg). Hypoventilation refers to the retention of greater than normal amounts of carbon dioxide, resulting in a $PaCO_2$ of greater than 45 mm Hg. Alveolar ventilation in this case is insufficient to meet the body's metabolic needs and results in hypercapnia ($PaCO_2 >45$ mm Hg).

The dissolved carbon dioxide becomes a source of carbonic acid in the blood. Because carbon dioxide combines with water to form carbonic acid, with resultant hydrogen ions (H^+), an increase in $PaCO_2$, as in hypoventilation, increases the formation of carbonic acid and in turn increases blood acidity. If more carbon dioxide is blown off, as in hyperventilation, there is a decrease in carbonic acid formation and the blood tends toward alkalinity. The $PaCO_2$ levels thus play a major role in determining acid-base balance.

Acid-Base Balance

The pH of the blood reflects the degree of acidity or alkalinity of the blood. It is a measurement of hydrogen ion concentration. Increased hydrogen ions result in increased acidity. ABGs measure the pH of arterial blood and express it as a negative logarithm (as hydrogen ion concentration rises, pH decreases, and vice versa). Under normal circumstances, acid-base balance must be maintained within a very narrow range (7.35–7.45). Deviations above 7.45 (alkalemia) and below 7.35 (acidemia) represent conditions that endanger life.

Regulation of acid-base balance refers to the maintenance of hydrogen ion concentration in the body within the normal range. This is accomplished by maintaining the proper ratio of bicarbonate to dissolved carbon dioxide, which is 20:1. (See Chapter 5 for a detailed discussion of acid-base balance.) The respiratory system and kidneys function together to maintain hydrogen ion concentration, and therefore pH, within normal limits.

The lungs adjust ventilation according to metabolic needs by increasing or decreasing the rate of respiration. This in turn increases or decreases $PaCO_2$ levels and the resulting hydrogen ion levels. The kidneys regulate the bicarbonate concentration in the body by retaining or excreting HCO_3^-. Bicarbonate is a base that plays a major role in the buffering system and therefore in acid-base balance. ABGs measure the amount of bicarbonate in the blood, with normal values ranging between 23 and 29 mEq/L.

When respiratory, kidney, or buffering mechanisms are unable to maintain acid-base balance, abnormal conditions of acidosis (pH < 7.35) or alkalosis (pH > 7.45) arise. If the increase or decrease in pH is from a respiratory problem, the imbalance is considered to be respiratory in origin. All other acid-based imbalances are considered to be metabolic in origin.

Accurate interpretation of ABGs can quickly reveal the source of the imbalance. In addition, ABGs can reflect the presence of any compensatory measures initiated by the body, which are aimed at reversing the imbalance.

Acidosis of respiratory origin is a result of hypoventilation, where insufficient carbon dioxide is blown off. This can be secondary to numerous respiratory diseases, infection, obstructive lung disease, drug overdose, neuromuscular diseases, and cardiopulmonary diseases. With hypoventilation, $PaCO_2$ levels increase above 45 mm Hg and acidosis results. Metabolic responsibility for acidosis results from an imbalance of any of the body's metabolic acids or bases with the exception of carbon dioxide.

There is either a loss of bases or an excess of acids. It can be due to diabetic ketoacidosis, diarrhea, or renal failure and is reflected by a decreased level of HCO_3^- (below 23 mEq/L).

Respiratory alkalosis develops as a result of hyperventilation, where too much carbon dioxide is blown off. This can be secondary to anxiety, hypermetabolic states as in fever, or improper management of a patient on a ventilator. ABGs in respiratory alkalosis reflect a $PaCO_2$ level below 35 mm Hg. Metabolic alkalosis stems from an imbalance of the body's acids and bases with the exception of carbon dioxide. A loss of acids or a gain of bases occurs. It can be secondary to sodium bicarbonate ingestion, vomiting, or nasogastric suctioning. ABG values in metabolic alkalosis reflect HCO_3^- (levels above 29 mEq/L).

When respiratory acidosis occurs, the kidneys attempt to compensate by retaining bicarbonate to balance the excessive hydrogen ions. With such attempts at compensation, ABGs reflect elevated HCO_3^- and pH values (compensatory) along with the elevated $PaCO_2$ value (causative). When respiratory alkalosis occurs, the kidneys excrete above-average amounts of bicarbonate to compensate for the lack of hydrogen ions. In an individual with respiratory alkalosis with compensation, ABGs reflect lowered levels of HCO_3^- (compensatory) along with below-normal levels of $PaCO_2$ (causative).

Metabolic acidosis is compensated for by the respiratory system. Respirations increase in rate and depth in an attempt to blow off carbon dioxide and to reduce the individual's acidotic state. Compensation of this type is reflected in the ABGs by a lowered level of $PaCO_2$ (compensatory) along with a below-normal level of HCO_3^- (causative). In metabolic alkalosis, the lungs compensate for the imbalance by decreasing ventilatory efforts. This retains carbon dioxide in an attempt to replace the metabolic acid lost or to balance the excess metabolic base. ABG interpretation in metabolic alkalosis with compensation reveals an increased $PaCO_2$ value (compensatory) along with an increased bicarbonate level (causative).

The procedure for interpretation of ABGs relative to acid-base balance is presented in Table 14–4.

Procedure

Blood specimens used for ABG analysis can be obtained from an arterial catheter or from percutaneous puncture of the femoral, radial, or brachial arteries. The specimen must be collected in a heparinized syringe, placed on ice, and sent to the laboratory immediately. Precautions must be taken to prevent contamination of the specimen with room air. The sample should be appropriately labeled and should include the time of collection, the patient's temperature, whether the patient was breathing room air or receiving oxygen therapy, whether or not mechanical ventilation was used, and ventilator settings.

Table 14–4

Steps in Interpreting Arterial Blood Gases Relative to Acid-Base Balance

1. Determine whether pH is normal, above normal, or below normal.
   a. If it falls between 7.35 and 7.45, the patient is within normal limits.
   b. If it is below 7.35, the patient is acidotic.
   c. If it is above 7.45, the patient is alkalotic.
2. Determine the origin of the imbalance by examining the partial pressure of arterial carbon dioxide ($PaCO_2$).
   a. If the patient is acidotic and the $PaCO_2$ level is above normal (above 45 mm Hg), the origin of the acidosis is respiratory. If the $PaCO_2$ is normal or below 35 mm Hg, the lungs could not possibly be the source of the excess acid; the origin must therefore be metabolic.
   b. If the patient is alkalotic and the $PaCO_2$ is below normal (below 35 mm Hg), the origin of the alkalosis is respiratory. If the $PaCO_2$ is normal or above 45 mm Hg, the lungs could not possibly be responsible for the deficiency of acid; the origin must therefore be metabolic.
3. Look for evidence of compensation by examining the bicarbonate ion (HCO_3^-) along with the $PaCO_2$. When compensation has occurred, the value that is causing the imbalance and the value that is compensating for the imbalance will both be abnormal in the same direction (ie, both will be elevated or both will be below normal levels).
   a. A patient with respiratory acidosis with compensatory efforts will have elevated $PaCO_2$ levels and elevated HCO_3^- levels as well.
   b. A patient with respiratory alkalosis with compensatory efforts will have decreased $PaCO_2$ levels and decreased HCO_3^- levels as well.
   c. A patient with metabolic acidosis with compensatory efforts will have decreased HCO_3^- levels and decreased $PaCO_2$ levels as well.
   d. A patient with metabolic alkalosis with compensatory efforts will have elevated HCO_3^- levels and elevated $PaCO_2$ levels as well.
Hint: When arrows are used to reflect the direction of deviation for each value including pH, $PaCO_2$, and HCO_3^-, the following rules apply:
   a. Examine the pH to determine whether the patient is acidotic or alkalotic.
   b. When the pH and $PaCO_2$ point in opposite directions, the origin of the imbalance is respiratory.
   c. When the pH and $PaCO_2$ point in the same direction, the origin of the imbalance is metabolic.
   d. When compensatory efforts are present, the $PaCO_2$ and the HCO_3^- will always point in the same direction.

$$pH \downarrow \quad PaCO_2 \uparrow \quad HCO_3^- \uparrow \; = \text{respiratory acidosis}$$

$$pH \uparrow \quad PaCO_2 \downarrow \quad HCO_3^- \downarrow \; = \text{respiratory alkalosis}$$

$$pH \downarrow \quad PaCO_2 \downarrow \quad HCO_3^- \downarrow \; = \text{metabolic acidosis}$$

$$pH \downarrow \quad PaCO_2 \uparrow \quad HCO_3^- \uparrow \; = \text{metabolic alkalosis}$$

Postprocedure Course

After the procedure, manual pressure is applied to the puncture site for at least 5 minutes, longer if coagulation time is altered. This is followed by application of a sterile dressing. The patient is monitored for bleeding and hematoma formation and for adequate peripheral circulation in the extremity.

Pulse Oximetry

Pulse oximetry is the measurement of SaO_2 with a device called a pulse oximeter. It is a painless, noninvasive procedure that requires no calibration and allows continuous monitoring even during patient transport because the oximeter can be operated by battery. The oximeter is frequently used

- During the perioperative period
- In intensive care units, emergency rooms, and obstetric practice
- In patients undergoing pulmonary function tests
- In patients with chronic respiratory problems and sleep apnea

The pulse oximeter measures the amount of infrared light absorbed by oxyhemoglobin compared with the amount of red light absorbed by reduced hemoglobin. A probe is attached to the patient over a pulsating vascular bed such as that found in the fingers, toes, nose, ear lobes, and forehead. One side of this probe has two light-emitting diodes that transmit the infrared and red light through the pulsating arterial blood to a photodetector on the other side. The photodetector receives the nonabsorbed light and converts it to an electrical signal. This signal is then sent to a microprocessor, and a digital display of the percentage of oxyhemoglobin compared with total functional hemoglobin (SaO_2) is produced (Fig. 14–13).

Placement of the probe over a pulsating vascular bed is critical to proper functioning of the oximeter. During systole, there is an influx of oxyhemoglobin, which results in an increase in the absorption of

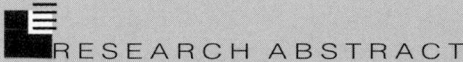

RESEARCH ABSTRACT

Are Oximetry Probe Sheaths Effective?

Gerber D, Santarelli R, Scott W, Kern M, DuBois J. Evaluation of a protective sheath for disposable oximetry probes. Respir Care 1996; 41(3):197.

The 1990s have been a decade of change in health care. Everywhere we look, we see the outcomes of these changes—cost containment, downsizing, and corporate takeovers. With these changes has come the use of standardized equipment—the result of centralized purchasing of large quantities to reduce costs. In facilities where such standardized equipment is used, nurses sometimes complain that the equipment available to them is not as effective as other equipment that they have used or that the equipment is difficult to use. Sometimes, the equipment available is truly *not* effective and must be replaced several times, increasing costs in the long run. However, many health-care facilities do not use product evaluation teams or committees to study a product for actual cost savings. These problems may therefore go on unresolved.

The investigative team led by Gerber, which was associated with the Robert Wood Johnson Medical School, sought to begin to address this problem. The team evaluated the use of a protective sheath for disposable oximetry probes. If this sheath worked as advertised, it would allow for longer use of the probes, so that the probes would not have to be replaced, or at least not as often. The group wanted to see whether the use of the sheath would cause significant changes in oximetry readings. The team found that there was *no* significant difference in readings with or without the sheath and that patient care would not be compromised if the sheath was used. The savings to both the hospital and patients were potentially significant. When a sheath was used, either with a disposable probe or with a nondisposable probe, the savings were noteworthy.

Product evaluation teams or committees like these are useful for the evaluation of savings to both inpatient and outpatient health-care facilities and to consumers.

Questions to Consider

1. What types of products does your clinical facility use with pulse oximeters?
2. Do you know what the costs are to the facility for the equipment used? To the patient?
3. Does your clinical facility have a team or committee to evaluate proposed new products? If so, what is the makeup of the committee?
4. List the criteria you would use to evaluate a new product if you were responsible for evaluating it. Defend your list.

---

infrared light; during diastole, there is a decrease in the amount of oxyhemoglobin and hence in the absorption of infrared light. The amount of light absorbed by venous blood, bone, and fat, on the other hand, is the same at all times. The signal resulting from the latter serves as the baseline with which the signal generated from the arterial blood is compared. Thus, inaccurate oximeter readings may result when the pulsatile signal is poor. This can occur as a result of inappropriate placement of the probe, hypotension, presence of a blood pressure cuff, administration of vasoconstricting drugs, or any other factor that causes hypoperfusion. Intravascular dyes, jaundice, patient movement, elevated carboxyhemoglobin levels (carbon monoxide bound to hemoglobin), hypothermia, and presence of nail polish are additional factors that may interfere with accurate results. There is also the possibility of inaccurate readings caused by the effect of bright external light such as fluorescent or surgical lights, sunlight, and bilirubin lights. For this reason, covering the probe with an opaque material is often recommended. A discrepancy of 2 to 3% between pulse oximetry readings and laboratory-reported SaO_2 levels may occur. Thus, pulse oximetry is better for monitoring changes in oxyhemoglobin levels than for determining baseline oxyhemoglobin levels.

Pulse oximetry is used to provide continuous monitoring and to decrease the need for blood gas analysis. Therapeutic interventions may be implemented and evaluated based on this continuous assessment.

Other Blood Studies

A venous specimen can be drawn for a complete blood count. An excess of red blood cells, polycythemia, which is an abnormal finding, may indicate respiratory dysfunction because chronic hypoxemia causes stimulation of red blood cell production. Chronically elevated blood carboxyhemoglobin levels, as seen in heavy smokers of cigarettes and cigars, are also known to cause secondary polycythemia.

SPUTUM STUDIES

Sputum can be examined for the presence of malignant cells and for organisms that cause infection.

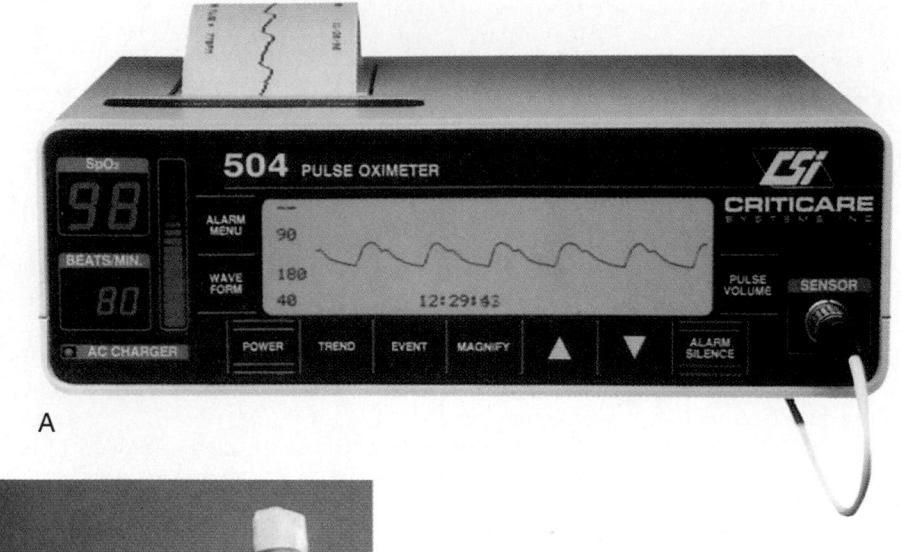

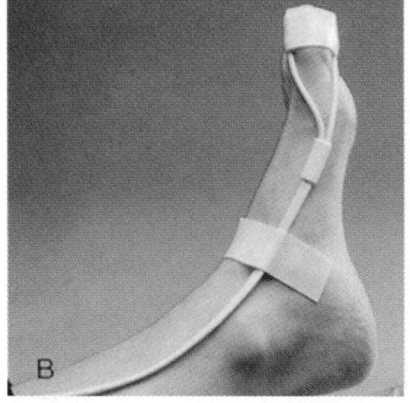

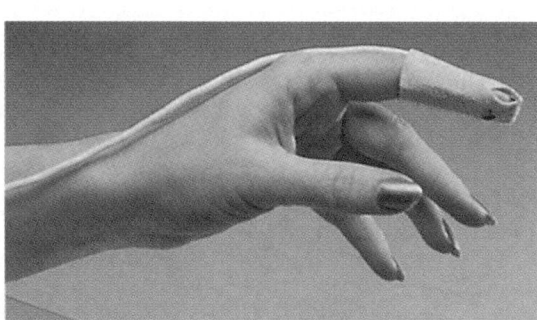

Figure 14–13

A, Pulse oximeter. *B*, Reusable sensor in place on toe, disposable sensor in place on finger. (Courtesy of Criticare Systems, Waukesha, WI)

Sputum culture and sensitivity studies are done to identify the causative organism and the corresponding antibiotics to which the organism is susceptible. A "cytologic" examination of sputum is done if carcinoma is suspected.

Collection of a Sputum Specimen

STANDARD METHOD

Sputum specimens are best collected as soon as the patient awakens in the morning because secretions accumulate in the bronchi during the night, and a few deep coughs usually bring this sputum to the back of the throat. In addition, the first sputum in the morning usually contains the most organisms. Have the patient brush the teeth or rinse the mouth to decrease contamination with oral flora. Provide the patient with a sterile, wide-mouth container, and instruct him or her to take several deep breaths, cough, and expectorate into the container provided. Remember that when not properly instructed, patients often expectorate saliva rather than sputum.

Collect initial specimens for culture and sensitivity before starting antibiotic treatment. Send speci-

mens directly to the laboratory. If there is any delay, refrigerate the specimen.

SALINE INHALATION METHOD

The saline inhalation method of collecting sputum is used for patients having difficulty raising secretions. Inhalation of a heated saline solution causes the heated vapor to condense on the surface of the tracheobronchial mucosa and thus stimulates production of secretions. Instruct the patient to breathe deeply and cough before the procedure. The mouth is then placed over, but not sealed around, the nebulizer. The vapor is inhaled for a few minutes until coughing is stimulated.

Some patients may become overly tired and should be encouraged to rest between periods of inhaling and coughing. If lightheadedness or dizziness occurs as a result of the hyperventilation, instruct the patient to relax and breathe normally for a few minutes. If the patient complains of nausea, discontinue the procedure.

GASTRIC WASHING METHOD

Many patients swallow sputum when coughing in the morning or during sleep. In the gastric washing method, gastric aspiration is used to collect gastric contents that contain this swallowed sputum.

A nasogastric tube is inserted, and a large syringe is used to gently withdraw a specimen of the stomach contents. The nasogastric tube is then removed. The specimen is obtained early in the morning, and breakfast is withheld until after the procedure. A microscopic examination and culture media test are performed by the laboratory, just as with other sputum samples. A gastric washing is usually done when the suspected diagnosis is tuberculosis.

RADIOGRAPHIC STUDIES

Chest X-Rays

Chest x-rays show the size, shape, position, and symmetry of the lungs, heart, diaphragm, and rib cage. Usually posterior and anterior (Fig. 14–14) views are taken; however, lateral or oblique views may be obtained from either the left or the right side. Chest x-rays can be used for screening or diag-

nosis. Comparison of previous and current x-rays also assists in determining the progress and development of disease.

There is no special preparation for flat films of the chest, and there is no discomfort during the procedure. The patient is asked to remove clothing from the waist up and any jewelry worn around the neck. The patient is also asked to hold his or her breath briefly while the x-ray is taken. Female patients who are pregnant or who suspect they may be should be instructed to inform the technician. Children and adult patients who need repeated x-rays should be shielded with a lead apron as a precautionary measure.

Fluoroscopy

Fluoroscopy is an x-ray technique in which the image of internal structures is projected on a screen, allowing movement to be viewed and evaluated.

Fluoroscopy allows expansion and contraction of the lungs and the diaphragm to be observed. It is used to diagnose the location of a tumor or a lesion

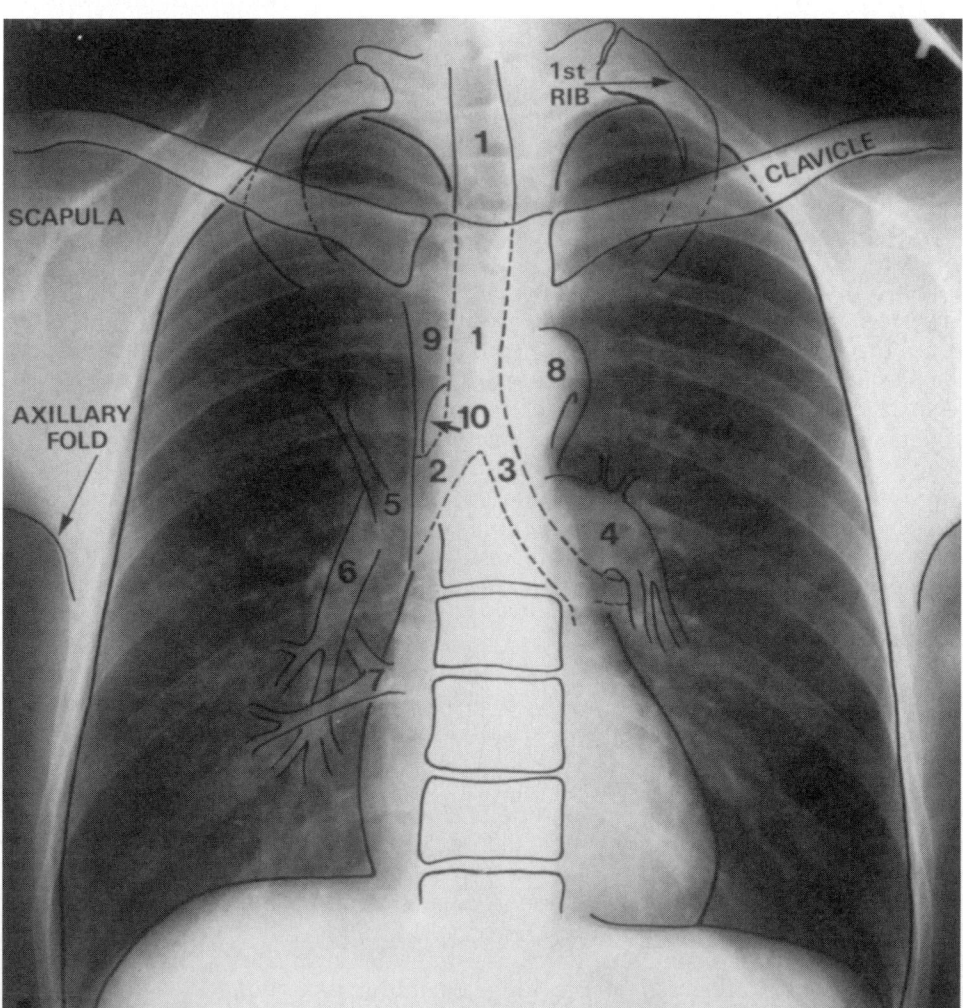

Figure 14–14

Normal chest x-ray, anterior view: *1*, trachea; *2*, right main bronchus; *3*, left main bronchus; *4*, left pulmonary artery; *5*, right upper lobe pulmonary vein; *6*, right interlobar artery; *7*, right lower and middle lobe vein; *8*, aortic knob; *9*, superior vena cava; *10*, azygos vein.

more precisely than can be done with x-ray film. Fluoroscopy is also used as an adjunct to other procedures to allow visualization of catheters or needles as they are advanced to various areas in the body. The procedure, which is not painful, is performed in a darkened room and persons accompanying the patient must wear a lead apron.

Tomography

Tomograms, or planigrams, are sequential films of the lungs taken in horizontal or vertical planes at different measured depths. These films allow detailed visualization of thoracic structures, including the trachea, bronchi, and hilar lymph nodes. They are valuable in the identification and evaluation of solid lesions, vascularity surrounding a lesion, and changes within a lesion.

When tomography is done, two x-ray tubes suspended over the x-ray table swing rapidly and abruptly in converging and then diverging paths above the patient. This rapid swooping action of the x-ray machine must be described before the test or the patient may be frightened.

Lung Scans

There are two types of lung scans: ventilation and perfusion. A ventilation scan uses a radioisotope and a scanning machine to demonstrate patterns of air movement and air distribution in the lungs. A perfusion scan uses a radioisotope and a scanning machine to determine patterns of blood flow through the lungs.

Uses

The primary use of ventilation and perfusion scans is in the diagnosis of pulmonary embolism. Since they lack specificity, results are reported as low, intermediate, or high in probability of pulmonary embolism. These scans are also used in diagnosing lung cancer, chronic obstructive pulmonary disease, and pulmonary edema. They are valuable diagnostic tools because they can demonstrate abnormalities in a specific region of the lung before results of other measures of respiratory function are affected.

Procedure

With the patient in a supine position and breathing normally, a radionuclide is administered intravenously. Shortly thereafter, scanning of the thorax is begun. During scanning, the patient is directed to assume various positions and otherwise to remain still and quiet. The result is an outline of the pulmonary blood vessels through which the radionuclide passes.

For a ventilation scan, the patient inhales a radioactive gas such as a mixture of xenon 133 and oxygen through a spirometer, which assists in delivering the gas to all areas of the lung. Scanning is then done, and an outline of alveoli into which the radioactive gas entered is obtained.

Radiation exposure is less during a lung scan than during the usual x-ray examination.

Pulmonary Angiography

Pulmonary angiography is the x-ray visualization of the pulmonary vasculature after injection of a contrast medium.

Uses

Pulmonary angiography is used to detect pulmonary emboli, lung tumors, and congenital or acquired lesions of the pulmonary vessels.

Procedure

After the patient is asked about sensitivity to contrast media, a catheter is introduced into an arm vein and threaded through the right atrium and ventricle into the pulmonary artery under surgically aseptic conditions and local anesthesia. Radiopaque material is then rapidly injected, and x-rays are taken to show its distribution. This injection may cause a warm, flushed sensation and evoke the urge to cough. Injections of the contrast medium and subsequent film recording may be repeated several times.

When the scan is completed, the catheter is withdrawn and the small incision through which the catheter was introduced is sutured and, if necessary, bandaged. Following the procedure, the patient rests in bed for 2 to 4 hours. During this time, peripheral pulses are checked, the site is observed for signs of inflammation or hematoma formation, and the patient monitored for numbness, tingling, or pain in the affected extremity.

ENDOSCOPIC STUDIES

Bronchoscopy

Bronchoscopy is a procedure in which the walls of the trachea, the main-stem bronchus, and the major subdivisions of the bronchial tubes are directly visualized by means of a bronchoscope.

Uses

Bronchoscopy may be used for diagnosis, treatment, or evaluation of disease progression or effectiveness of therapy. It can be used to determine location and extent of lesions (such as tumors and bleeding sites) and to obtain a biopsy, a bronchial brushing, or a bronchial washing. It is also used to destroy and remove lesions and to clear the airway when retained secretions or a foreign body causes persistent atelectasis (a collapsed or airless condition of the lung).

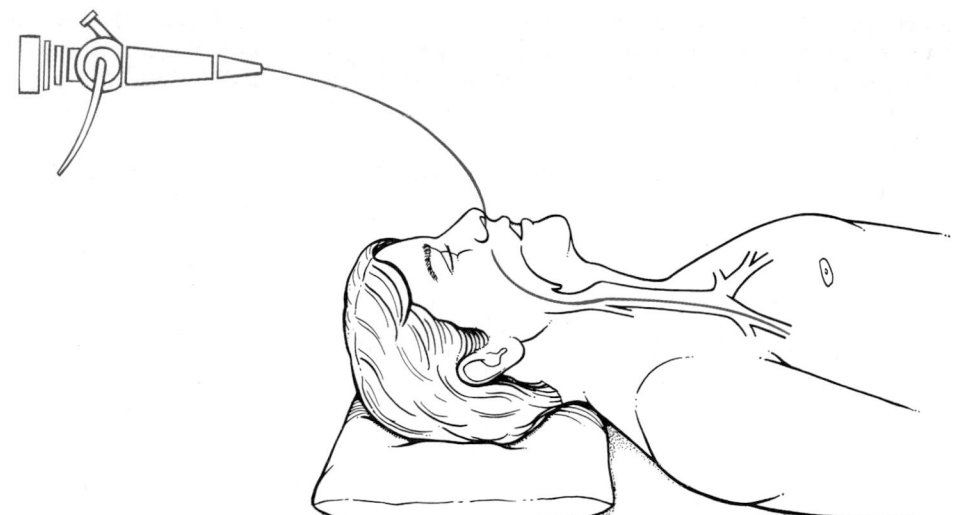

Figure 14–15
Bronchoscopy using a flexible
fiberoptic bronchoscope.

Physical Preparation of the Patient

The patient abstains from food and fluids for 6 hours before a bronchoscopic examination to decrease the risk of aspiration while the gag reflex is suppressed. Signed consent is obtained, and dental prostheses are removed. The patient is premedicated, usually with atropine and either a sedative or a narcotic to depress the vagus nerve, stimulation of which can cause bradycardia, dysrhythmias, and hypotension.

Procedure

A bronchoscopic examination can be performed with either a flexible or a rigid bronchoscope. The most frequently used is the flexible fiberoptic bronchoscope (Fig. 14–15) because it allows access to more areas of the airways, including the right upper lobe. It also provides better control of the patient's airway if respiratory distress develops. It can be used at the bedside and can be inserted through an endotracheal or tracheostomy tube. The rigid bronchoscope is a hollow metal tube with a light at the end. It is used almost exclusively for removal of foreign bodies or thick secretions, examination in the presence of massive hemoptysis, and endobronchial surgery.

Bronchoscopy is usually done under local anesthesia. An anesthetic such as lidocaine is sprayed on the patient's pharynx to suppress the cough and gag reflexes. The bronchoscope is then inserted through the mouth and into the airways, and examination is begun. When a flexible bronchoscope is used, the patient may remain in a sitting position if the physician so chooses, and insertion may be through the nose.

Complications

Complications that can occur as a result of bronchoscopy include bronchospasm, hypoxemia, bleeding, perforation, aspiration, cardiac dysrhythmias, and infection. When local anesthesia is used, a reaction to it may also occur.

NURSING PROCESS
Bronchoscopy

Assessment

Before bronchoscopy, assess the patient's understanding of the procedure. Also assess the patient's anxiety level and ability to cooperate with instructions if local anesthesia is used. Monitor the patient's pulse during the procedure. When completed, check for return of the swallow and cough reflexes. Also check for signs of complications: cyanosis, dyspnea, stridor, hemoptysis, hypotension, tachycardia, and dysrhythmias.

Remember that if a biopsy was performed, blood-streaked sputum is expected for several hours, but frank blood is indicative of hemorrhage. Assess elderly patients for confusion and lethargy if lidocaine was used for local anesthesia.

Nursing Diagnoses and Planning

Nursing diagnoses and related expected patient outcomes commonly applicable to patients undergoing a bronchoscopy include the following:

NDx: Anxiety related to the impending procedure and its outcome

Planning: Patient Outcomes
1. Patient's facial expression and body movements appear relaxed.
2. Patient attends to information and directions.
3. Patient verbalizes an understanding of the procedure.

NDx: Risk for aspiration related to suppression of swallow and cough reflexes

Planning: Patient Outcomes
1. Respirations are quiet and easy.
2. Respiratory rate is within patient's normal range.
3. Breath sounds are clear.

NDx: Pain related to throat irritation secondary to passage of the bronchoscope

Planning: Patient Outcomes
1. Patient swallows saliva and orally ingested liquids.
2. Patient states that throat discomfort is relieved.
3. Patient describes pain relief measures to be used at home.

Nursing Interventions and Evaluation

NDx: Anxiety
Tell the patient what to expect before, during, and after the bronchoscopy. Include information on food and fluid restrictions and the expected effect of premedications. Stress that premedications may cause feelings of drowsiness, euphoria, or floating but do not induce sleep. If local anesthesia is to be used, acknowledge that some discomfort may be felt, including a transient sense of gagging and inability to breathe when the local anesthetic is applied. Explain that during the procedure the patient will be asked to keep hands at the sides and to breathe through the nose. Explain also that vital signs will be taken frequently after the procedure and that a sore throat is to be expected. Allow the patient to verbalize concerns, and encourage the use of relaxation techniques such as slow, deep breathing and imagery.

NDx: Risk for aspiration
Position the patient who is not fully conscious in a flat, side-lying position to prevent aspiration.

Position the conscious patient in a flat or semi-Fowler's, side-lying position and instruct him or her to let saliva drain out of the corner of the mouth into a basin or tissues.

Keep the patient on a nothing by mouth (NPO) order until the swallow, gag, and cough reflexes return, usually in 2 to 8 hours.

NDx: Pain
Discourage talking, clearing the throat, coughing, and smoking to avoid further irritation of the throat. Apply an ice collar to ease discomfort. When the swallow and cough reflexes have returned, give warm, soothing liquids, gargles, and throat lozenges. Instruct patients who return home following the procedure to continue these comfort measures and to progress to a soft diet as tolerated, returning to a regular diet in 24 hours.

Additional Interventions
Make certain that any specific preprocedure laboratory data required (eg, hematocrit, coagulation studies, or platelet studies) are complete and that results are recorded in the patient's chart.

Compare the patient's status with the expected outcomes. If the outcomes are not met, reassess the patient and revise the plan.

Laryngoscopy

Laryngoscopy is direct visualization of the larynx via a laryngoscope for diagnostic or therapeutic purposes. Diagnostically, it is used to obtain tissue for biopsy, to evaluate laryngeal function (eg, to check for vocal cord paralysis), and to detect the presence of inflammation. Therapeutically, it is used to remove lesions or foreign bodies and to dilate laryngeal strictures.

Laryngoscopy is usually performed under local anesthetic because vocal cord motility can be viewed only when the patient is awake and able to phonate (make a voiced sound).

Before the procedure, a medication such as atropine may be given to reduce secretions.

NURSING PROCESS GUIDELINES
Laryngoscopy

The assessment, nursing diagnoses, expected patient outcomes, nursing interventions, and evaluation for patients undergoing a laryngoscopic examination are similar to those described previously for patients undergoing a bronchoscopic examination.

Mediastinoscopy

Mediastinoscopy is performed by passing a mediastinoscope through an incision made between the laryngeal prominence and the sternum under local or general anesthesia. It allows for visualization and biopsy of lymph nodes.

Mediastinoscopy is commonly used to detect metastasis of carcinoma of the lung or related structures to the lymph nodes. This procedure is done in an operating room equipped to deal with potential complications that include cardiac dysrhythmias, myocardial infarction, bleeding, pneumothorax, and vocal cord paralysis.

THORACENTESIS

Thoracentesis is the aspiration of fluid or air from the pleural space (Fig. 14–16).

Uses
Thoracentesis may be performed for diagnostic or therapeutic purposes. As a diagnostic procedure, it is used to obtain a specimen of fluid from the pleural space (normally there is no fluid in this space) for examination.

When fluid is aspirated for diagnostic purposes, it can be subjected to a variety of examinations. Gross appearance, which may be bloody (associated

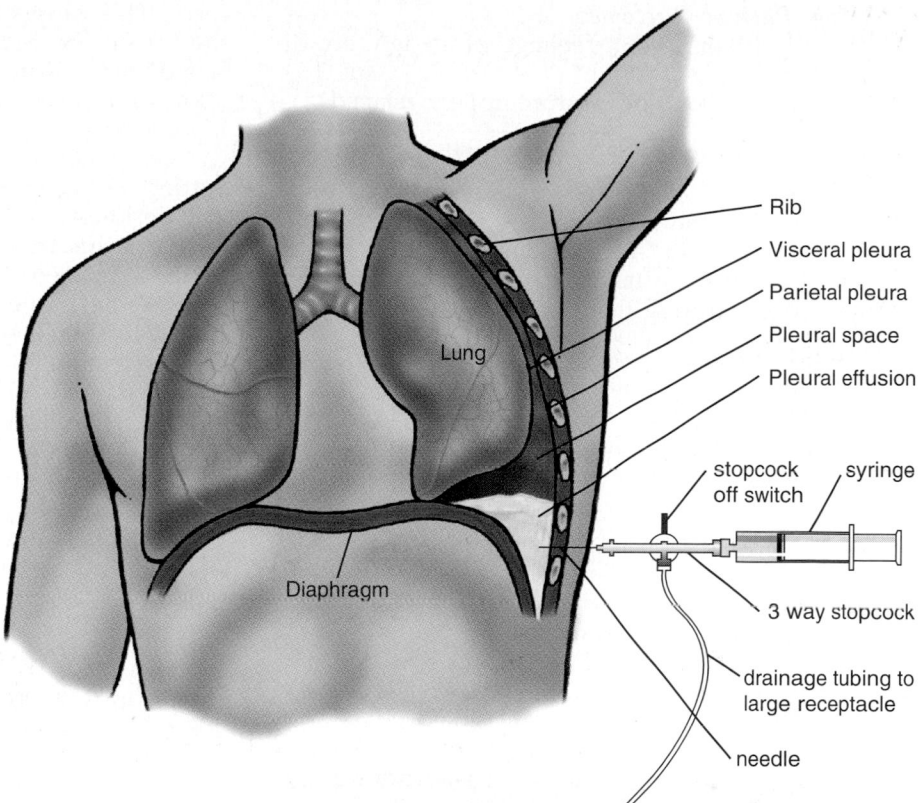

Figure 14–16
Thoracentesis.

with pleural trauma or advanced malignancy), serous (associated with malignancy, inflammatory disorders, or heart failure), or purulent (associated with infection), is noted. Specific gravity is measured. The fluid may also be biochemically analyzed for glucose, amylase, protein, and lactic dehydrogenase and a red and white blood cell count can be done. In addition, cytologic and bacteriologic studies, including smears and cultures for acid-fast bacilli, may be ordered.

Therapeutically, thoracentesis may be done to relieve respiratory distress or to instill medication into the pleural space. When fluid is drained, the amount is usually limited to 1 to 2 L at one time to avoid mediastinal shift and impaired venous return.

Procedure

A thoracentesis is done at the bedside or in a treatment room. A specialized needle, a three-way stopcock, sterile specimen containers, and a large sterile receptacle are used. The patient is assisted to a comfortable sitting position, with the feet dangling over the side of the bed or examining table. A pillow is placed on an over-bed table on which the patient can rest his or her arms and head. The arms may be crossed to allow maximal exposure of the intercostal spaces. If the patient cannot sit upright, he or she is placed in a side-lying position with the unaffected side down. The site of thoracentesis, which is determined by x-ray examination and percussion, is dis-

infected, and a local anesthetic is injected. The thoracentesis needle is then introduced, and fluid is removed with a syringe or via a tube connected to a sterile drainage container. When drainage of fluid is completed, an adhesive strip is placed over the needle insertion site and the patient is placed on bed rest. In some cases the patient is instructed to lie on the unaffected side for 1 hour to promote expansion of the lung on the affected side. A chest x-ray is taken after the procedure to check for pneumothorax.

NURSING PROCESS
Thoracentesis

Assessment

Assess the patient's understanding of the thoracentesis procedure and anxiety level regarding it. Assess ability to assume the required position and comply with directions. Obtain baseline vital signs.

Nursing Diagnoses and Planning

Nursing diagnoses and related expected patient outcomes commonly applicable to patients undergoing a thoracentesis include the following:

NDx: Anxiety related to discomfort during thoracentesis

Planning: Patient Outcomes
1. Patient verbalizes that feelings of anxiety are diminished.
2. Facial expression and posture appear relaxed.

Nursing Interventions and Evaluation

NDx: Anxiety

Briefly describe the thoracentesis procedure to the patient so that he or she will know what to expect. Include the following information on sensations that normally occur during the procedure:

- A mild burning sensation occurs as the local anesthetic is injected into the skin.
- A sharp but quickly passing pain occurs as the parietal pleura is infiltrated with the anesthetic.
- A feeling of pressure occurs as the needle is inserted.
- A pulling sensation or desire to cough is felt as the needle is withdrawn and the lung responds.

Reassure the patient and provide support through touch and eye contact.

Additional Interventions

Obtain an informed consent before the procedure is begun. During the procedure, monitor pulse and respirations. Instruct the patient to remain still and not talk during the procedure to avoid displacement of the needle or perforation of the pleura. Direct the patient to avoid sudden movements, deep breathing, and coughing and to pant if an urge to cough is felt.

On completion, record the total amount of fluid withdrawn, noting its color and viscosity.

Monitor the patient for signs and symptoms of hemorrhage and pneumothorax, which are rare but potential complications. Check blood pressure, pulse, and respirations, and check the insertion site for swelling, which could be due to bleeding. Also be alert for faintness, vertigo, tightness in the chest, dyspnea, pain, uncontrollable cough, and blood-tinged, frothy mucus.

Compare the patient's status with the expected outcomes. If the outcomes are not met, reassess the patient and revise the plan.

LUNG BIOPSY

A lung biopsy, like any other biopsy, is done to obtain a specimen for examination and definitive diagnosis. The majority of lung biopsies are done to distinguish benign from malignant lesions.

There are several nonoperative closed techniques used to obtain a lung biopsy. These include transcatheter bronchial brushing, percutaneous needle biopsy, and transbronchial lung biopsy.

A transcatheter bronchial brushing is done with a fiberoptic bronchoscope under fluoroscopy. A small brush is attached to the end of a flexible wire, which is inserted through the bronchoscope to the area under suspicion. It is then brushed back and forth. This causes cells to slough off and adhere to the brush. The brush is removed from the bronchoscope, and a slide is made for cytologic study. This allows for examination of a lung lesion and specific identification of pathogenic organisms.

A percutaneous (through the skin) biopsy uses a cutting or aspiration needle with local anesthesia. The lesion is located under fluoroscopy, and the needle is inserted through the skin into the pleura while the patient holds the breath in mid-expiration. The needle is then guided into the lesion, and the biopsy is obtained. The aspiration needle permits syringe aspiration of a small tissue sample. A larger core of tissue is obtained with a cutting needle.

A transbronchial lung biopsy uses cutting forceps introduced via a fiberoptic bronchoscope. This procedure is done when a lung lesion is suspected and sputum samples and bronchoscopic washings are negative. Potential complications of closed-lung biopsy include pneumothorax, hemorrhage, and air embolism.

NURSING PROCESS GUIDELINES
Closed Lung Biopsy

The assessment, nursing diagnoses, expected patient outcomes, nursing interventions, and evaluation for patients undergoing a closed lung biopsy are similar to those described previously for patients having a bronchoscopy. In addition, when caring for any patient undergoing a lung biopsy, recognize that biopsy has a connotation of cancer for most people. Expect the patient to be anxious regarding this possibility and encourage verbalization of concerns and use of relaxation techniques if needed. Keep the patient informed and be certain that he or she knows when and from whom to expect the results of the biopsy. Monitor all patients for complications of the procedure and report signs of respiratory distress or hemoptysis of frank blood immediately.

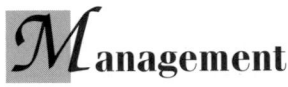

$\mathcal{M}$anagement

NONSURGICAL MANAGEMENT

Respiratory Therapy

BREATHING EXERCISES

The patient who is experiencing difficulty with breathing tends to increase respiratory rate and use the accessory muscles of respiration. This is a counterproductive response because it increases the work of respiration and hence the demand for oxygen. Controlled breathing techniques limit this response and enable the patient to breathe more efficiently to conserve energy. When used in combination with postural drainage, vibration, and percussion, they increase aeration and assist in the movement of secretions. The two main types of controlled breathing are pursed-lip breathing and diaphragmatic breathing.

Pursed-Lip Breathing

Pursed-lip breathing prolongs expiration and increases pressure in the lower airways, preventing collapse of bronchioles. This allows for more complete emptying of air rich in carbon dioxide from the alveoli on exhalation and permits more fresh air to enter the lungs with each inhalation. It is used in the management of respiratory diseases, such as chronic obstructive pulmonary disease, that are characterized by air trapping. For this breathing technique, air is inhaled through the nose with the abdominal muscles relaxed and exhaled slowly against lips pursed as though ready to whistle with the abdominal muscles contracted. To be effective, exhalation should be twice as long as inspiration. This technique can be practiced by blowing through a straw to make small bubbles in a glass of water, by blowing a Ping-Pong ball steadily across the table, or by blowing at a candle flame to bend it rather than extinguish it.

Diaphragmatic Breathing

Diaphragmatic breathing assists the patient in using the diaphragm rather than the accessory muscles to breathe. Because smaller muscles use more oxygen than large ones, this decreases the work of breathing. Diaphragmatic breathing also increases the volume of air exchanged with a normal breathing effort and enhances the distribution of the inhaled air.

To practice diaphragmatic breathing, the patient is asked to lie down and place the left hand on the rib cage just below the collarbone so that any motion of the rib cage can be felt. The right hand is placed in the area above the navel and just below the rib cage, with the palm down, the smallest finger reaching the navel, and the thumb resting on the sternum. The patient then takes deep breaths through the nose and at the same time allows the area under the palm of the right hand to rise. Pursed-lip breathing is used on expiration and timed to be twice as long as inhalation.

If diaphragmatic breathing is being done properly, the rib cage under the left hand does not move and the abdominal wall below the navel does not rise higher than the area under the right hand. If it does rise higher, the patient is using extra-abdominal muscles, which is unnecessary.

If needed, patients can be helped to master this breathing technique by placing a book on the upper abdomen and watching it rise and fall with inspiration and expiration.

Once the basic technique is learned, it should be practiced in the sitting position, which lowers the abdominal contents and allow easy descent of the diaphragm.

Diaphragmatic breathing requires more work than pursed-lip breathing alone, so acutely ill patients may be instructed to use pursed-lip breathing only. Otherwise, the combination of diaphragmatic breathing and pursed-lip breathing should be used while performing activities of daily living such as walking, standing, or climbing stairs. These techniques of controlled breathing should be practiced often so they are used automatically during acute episodes of breathlessness.

POSTURAL DRAINAGE

Postural drainage is a technique that uses gravity to assist in draining secretions from the lung. The various positions used relate to the entry angle of each segmental bronchus (Fig. 14–17). As specific segments of the lung are drained into the major bronchi and trachea, the patient is more likely to cough effectively and expectorate the excess secretions. Position depends on location of retained secretions, and duration of treatment depends on the patient's tolerance. If patients, particularly the elderly, have difficulty tolerating the required position, the duration of treatment may be gradually lengthened. Generally, treatments last from 5 to 15 minutes and are done two to four times daily, although in acute situations, frequency may be as often as every 1 to 2 hours. Postural drainage should not be done for at least 1 hour after a liquid meal and 2 hours after a solid meal. Scheduling postural therapy an hour before meals and at bedtime has the advantage of easing breathing for eating and sleeping. Oral hygiene should be provided if sputum drainage causes gagging or nausea.

Lung sounds are auscultated before and after the procedure to determine the areas that need drainage and the effectiveness of therapy. If prescribed, bronchodilators, saline, or water may be nebulized and inhaled before the procedure to reduce bronchospasm, decrease the viscosity of mucus, and combat edema of the bronchial walls. The patient is made as comfortable as possible and, if the prescribed position cannot be tolerated, repositioned as needed. Each time the position changes, the patient is instructed to inhale slowly through the nose and exhale through pursed lips several times and then cough and expectorate.

Postural drainage is contraindicated in patients with increased intracranial pressure, such as after head injury or craniotomy. It should also be avoided in patients with hypertension, cardiovascular compromise, and orthopnea.

PERCUSSION

Percussion (also known as cupping or clapping) is a manual technique used together with postural drainage to loosen secretions in the respiratory tract. The

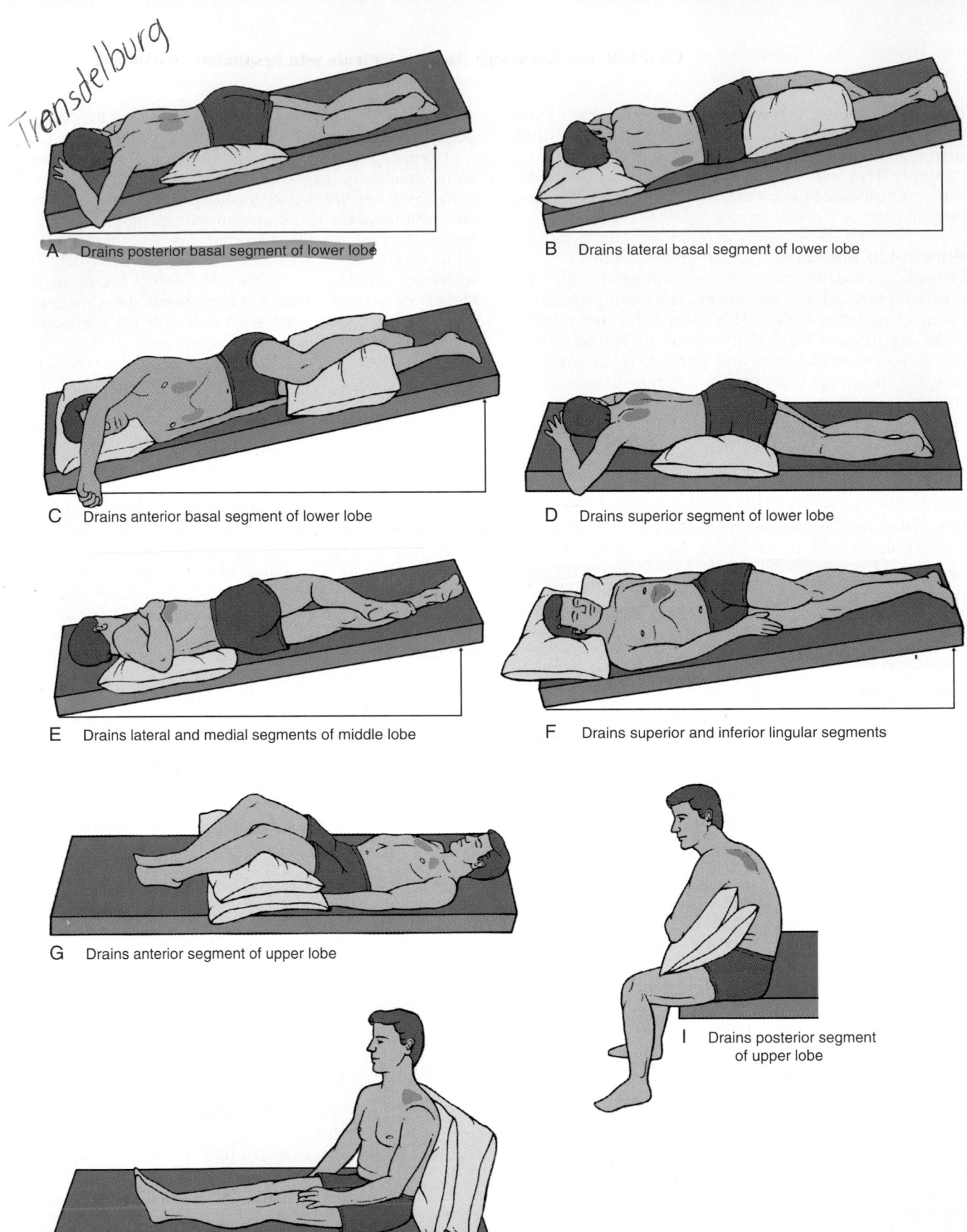

Trendelenburg (handwritten)

A   Drains posterior basal segment of lower lobe

B   Drains lateral basal segment of lower lobe

C   Drains anterior basal segment of lower lobe

D   Drains superior segment of lower lobe

E   Drains lateral and medial segments of middle lobe

F   Drains superior and inferior lingular segments

G   Drains anterior segment of upper lobe

I   Drains posterior segment of upper lobe

H   Drains apical segment of upper lobe

Figure 14–17

Postural drainage. The patient assumes various positions to facilitate the flow of secretions from various portions of the lung into the bronchi, trachea, and throat so that they can be expectorated. The drawing shows the various positions used to drain each segment of the lung.

patient is placed in the appropriate postural drainage position for treatment of the affected lung area. The skin is protected by a thin covering, such as a gown or a sheet. The nurse's hands are slightly cupped and facing downward with the fingers and thumbs together. Flexion and extension of the wrists are performed in a rhythmic manner, with a steady, even percussion maintained for 3 to 5 minutes over the affected area.

Percussion should not be done on bare skin, below the ribs, on the spine or scapulae, or over breast tissue. Areas of incision or severe pain should be avoided. Percussion is contraindicated in patients with hemoptysis, rib fractures, osteoporosis, pulmonary embolism, tuberculosis, and operable lung cancer. Possible complications include fractured ribs and hemoptysis.

If percussion is contraindicated, postural drainage may still be performed effectively.

VIBRATION

Vibration is the technique of applying manual compression and tremor to the chest wall during exhalation. This technique applies little or no pressure to the chest and is useful when other techniques are

Table 14-5

Common Methods of Oxygen Administration and Approximate Liter Flows and Fraction of Inspired Oxygen

Method	O$_2$ Delivery	Advantages	Disadvantages
Nasal cannula (nasal prongs)	Low concentrations dependent on rate and depth of breathing FLOWS 1 L = 24% O$_2$ 2 L = 28% O$_2$ 3 L = 32% O$_2$ 4 L = 36% O$_2$ 5 L = 40% O$_2$ 6 L = 44% O$_2$	Patient can move, talk, and eat without disrupting delivery of O$_2$	Easily dislodged; risk of necrosis to nostrils, cheeks, and ears; irritation of nasal mucosa; cannot be used for more than 6 L/min; must be humidified if used more than 4 L/min
Simple mask	Low to medium concentrations, 40–60%; must use liter flow greater than 5 L/min	Higher delivery of O$_2$ than with a cannula	Discomfort and risk of pressure necrosis caused by tight seal between face and mask; must be removed for eating, drinking, and oral medication
Partial rebreathing mask	Higher concentrations, 60–80%; must keep reservoir bag inflated at all times		Risk of pressure necrosis; not for long-term use
Non-rebreathing mask	Highest concentrations, 80–95%; must keep reservoir bag inflated at all times	Useful in emergency situations	Discomfort and risk of necrosis from snug fit; not for long-term use
Venturi mask	Delivers consistent F$_{IO_2}$ regardless of breathing pattern; concentration and liter flow marked on apparatus; 24–50% masks available	Useful when accuracy of delivery is essential	Discomfort and risk of skin irritation; must be removed for eating and oral medication
Tracheostomy collar	Delivers O$_2$ and humidification via tracheostomy; must be connected to a nebulizer; F$_{IO_2}$ is set on the nebulizer 24–100%	Adds humidity to liquefy secretions	Must drain condensation often; risk of nosocomial respiratory infection
T-bar (Brigg's adapter)	Delivers O$_2$ and humidification via tracheostomy; must be connected to a nebulizer; F$_{IO_2}$ is set on the nebulizer 24–100%	Adds humidity to liquefy secretions	Must drain condensation often; risk of nosocomial respiratory infection

F$_{IO_2}$, fraction of inspired oxygen; O$_2$, oxygen.

[Handwritten annotations: "Important placement humidify"; "increments of 4° per L"; "If having difficulty breathing"]

contraindicated. The nurse's hands are placed over the affected area of the patient's thorax. The nurse then contracts his or her own upper extremities isometrically. This results in muscle tension, which produces a fine vibration that is transmitted through the chest wall to the underlying pulmonary tissue. This procedure is continued for 5 to 10 deep breaths or until secretions are loosened and cleared by coughing. The precautions for and hazards of vibration are the same as for percussion.

Oxygen Therapy

Supplemental oxygen is administered when the patient has or is at risk for hypoxemia—when oxygen transport to body tissues is insufficient or likely to become so. Specific conditions that may require oxygen therapy include pneumonia, adult respiratory distress syndrome, chronic obstructive pulmonary disease, lung cancer, myocardial infarction, shock, and central nervous system disorders in which the respiratory center is depressed.

A variety of methods are used to administer oxygen (Table 14–5). The method used for a specific patient depends on the required concentration of inspired oxygen, the amount of humidification required, and the mental and physical conditions of the patient.

The flow rate at which oxygen is delivered is measured in liters per minute via a flowmeter. This rate varies depending on the condition of the patient and the route being used to administer the oxygen. More precise dosages are prescribed in percentage of inspired oxygen.

Oxygen is a medication, and its characteristics present a variety of hazards to the patient. Principles related to oxygen therapy and their implica-

Táble 14–6

Guidelines for Safe, Effective Oxygen Administration

Principle	Implications for Oxygen Administration
Anxiety activates the sympathetic nervous system and increases the body's need for oxygen.	Explain equipment and purpose of therapy to minimize anxiety.
Oxygen supports combustion. Combustion is extremely rapid in the presence of high concentrations of oxygen.	Prevent fire hazards where oxygen is in use. Avoid open flames. Post "No Smoking" signs. Check for faulty electrical equipment. Avoid wearing or using synthetic fibers, which build up static electricity. Avoid use of oil, which can ignite spontaneously in the presence of oxygen.
Oxygen is a dry gas and can remove normal moisture from respiratory passages.	Provide needed humidity through use of a bubble humidifier (bottle of water attached to oxygen source) or nebulizer.
Correct concentration of oxygen is necessary to maintain effective therapy and to prevent complications.	Check every 8 hours that the prescribed concentration of oxygen is being delivered.
Warm, moist environments support the growth of microorganisms.	Change masks and tubes daily.
Oxygen flow and pressure from a mask or cannula are irritating to the skin or nares. Aspiration of oil-based lubricant can cause oil pneumonia.	Wash and dry affected area thoroughly and gently and apply water-soluble lubricant to skin and nares.
High oxygen concentrations over a prolonged time can cause loss of elastic recoil and irritate the airways.	Monitor for signs of oxygen toxicity: nausea and vomiting, substernal pain, dyspnea, cough, and crackles.
Oxygen tanks used by many patients at home can cause serious accidents if patients fail to follow appropriate safety precautions.	Teach patient and family to keep tanks securely supported in a cylinder cart or base. Keep tanks away from heat sources, such as radiators, ovens, and heat ducts. Have a pressure-relief device fitted to the tanks at all times to allow gas to escape if pressure should suddenly increase.

tions for oxygen administration are presented in Table 14–6.

TRANSTRACHEAL OXYGEN (Tiny incision)

In transtracheal oxygen therapy, which is used for patients requiring long-term home oxygen therapy, oxygen is administered through a small catheter inserted directly into the trachea through the lower neck. This catheter, which is held in place by a flange, is attached to a tubing that runs under the clothing to a lightweight oxygen tank carried as an over-the-shoulder bag (Fig. 14–18).

There are many advantages of transtracheal oxygen over oxygen via nasal cannula or tracheostomy for the patient requiring long-term continuous therapy. Transtracheal oxygen is more efficient because oxygen is not lost to the environment and it decreases the work of breathing, thereby reducing dyspnea. Further, it does not interfere with coughing, speaking, eating, and shaving, and it does not cause nasal dryness, nosebleeds, sore throat, or changes in taste and smell, which lead to anorexia.

Transtracheal Catheters

Two types of transtracheal oxygen administration sets in use are the Heimlich Microtrach and the SCOOP. Both are inserted over a removable needle and guide wire, but the SCOOP, being a longer, wider catheter, requires a small incision, whereas the Microtrach is inserted through a needle puncture. Oxygen administration can be started immediately after insertion of a Microtrach, but in some cases the wound is first allowed to heal for a week to decrease the risk of subcutaneous emphysema (presence of air in subcutaneous tissue). With the SCOOP, a stent is inserted initially and is replaced with a SCOOP1 catheter at the end of 1 week. This catheter is suitable for low-flow oxygen administration of up to 2 L/minute. If the patient requires a higher flow, a SCOOP2 is inserted at 6 to 8 weeks.

Procedure

Insertion of a transtracheal catheter is an outpatient procedure. The patient is on NPO status for 6 to 8 hours and receives a sedative, a prophylactic antibiotic, and usually a cough suppressant. During the procedure, the patient sits with the head back or lies

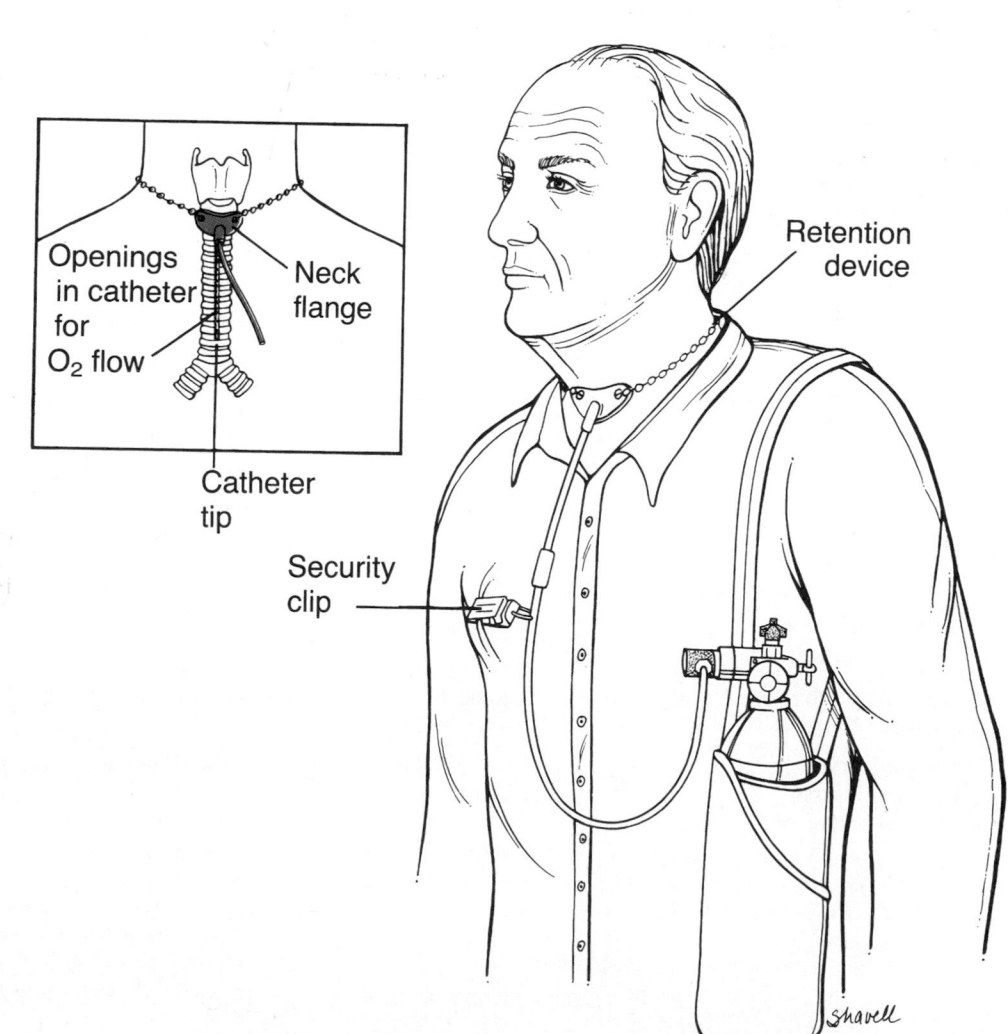

Figure 14–18

Transtracheal oxygen.

with a pillow under the shoulders to extend the neck; oxygen is administered by nasal catheter; and electrocardiogram and pulse oximetry monitoring are maintained. Once the skin is prepared, a local anesthetic is injected and the catheter is inserted according to the protocol for the type selected. A chest film is then obtained to verify the correct position of the catheter in the trachea and to rule out an accidental pneumothorax.

Transtracheal oxygen cannot be used for patients with respiratory failure or pleural herniation at the insertion site. It is used with caution in those with cardiac dysrhythmias, bleeding disorders, or poor mechanical pulmonary reserve.

NURSING PROCESS
Transtracheal Oxygen

Assessment

Assess for signs of respiratory distress for 2 to 3 hours after insertion of the catheter. Check ABGs and pulse oximetry readings. Inspect the insertion site for displacement of the catheter or for more than a few drops of bloody drainage. Note frequency and depth of coughing. Observe for large amounts of blood-stained sputum, which can be indicative of hemorrhage. Assess for pain and hoarseness.

Nursing Diagnoses and Planning

Nursing diagnoses and related expected patient outcomes commonly applicable to patients receiving transtracheal oxygen include the following:

NDx: Risk for altered health maintenance related to insufficient knowledge of self-care after transtracheal catheter insertion

Planning: Patient Outcomes
1. Patient describes self-care relevant to transtracheal oxygen therapy.

Nursing Interventions and Evaluation

NDx: Risk for altered health maintenance
Instruct the patient and significant others in self-care, as presented in Highlight 14–2.

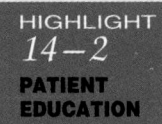 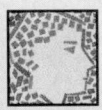

HIGHLIGHT 14–2
PATIENT EDUCATION
Transtracheal Oxygen Therapy

Instruct the patient to:

Adjust flow rate on basis of pulse oximetry readings when on transtracheal O$_2$.

Schedule follow-up for arterial blood gases to check adequacy of ventilation and oxygenation.

Cleanse skin surrounding catheter at least twice a day.
- Use cotton swab, water, and a mild soap such as Ivory if desired.
- Rinse thoroughly.
- Pat dry with a tissue.

Avoid use of skin products unless specifically prescribed.

Perform catheter care as appropriate for the type of catheter in use:
- Heimlich Micro-Trach
  Instill 0.5 to 1 mL sterile normal saline 2 to 3 times daily to stimulate cough and clear the lungs. Cleaning of Micro-Trach itself is not necessary.
  If the Micro-Trach is accidentally dislodged by coughing, wipe it with an alcohol swab and reinsert it. If difficult to reinsert, cover the insertion site loosely with a lint-free gauze square, begin nasal O$_2$, and call the physician.
  Replace in 6 months.
- SCOOP
  For 6 to 8 weeks, clean SCOOP twice daily in place using sterile saline and a special rod. Once the track is mature, remove and insert a new catheter. Wash the dirty catheter with the cleaning rod and antibacterial soap.
  Store in a clean, dry place.
  Replace every 3 months.

Take temperature orally twice daily for 7 days after insertion.

Report the following symptoms of complications immediately:
- Cough unrelieved by cough suppressant
- Increased sputum
- Increased dyspnea
- Cyanosis of the lips or nail beds
- Edema of the face or neck
- Marked pain or bleeding at the catheter site
- Fever of 37.5°C (99.5°F)

Additional Interventions

Give acetaminophen for pain and cough suppressants as ordered. Reassure the patient that coughing is a normal response to the presence of the catheter in the trachea but that the urge to cough will lessen in a few days. Also reassure the patient that hoarseness experienced right after the insertion procedure will disappear as the local anesthetic wears off.

Compare the patient's status with the expected outcomes. If the outcomes are not met, reassess the patient and revise the plan.

ARTIFICIAL AIRWAYS

In a healthy patient breathing room air, total airway obstruction will cause death from hypoxia in 5 to 10 minutes. To ensure adequate ventilation when a patient is threatened by an airway obstruction, an artificial airway may be necessary. Various types of artificial airways are depicted in Figure 14–19.

Oropharyngeal Airway

An oral airway holds the tongue away from the pharynx. It is easily inserted and is used for nasal obstruction or predisposition to epistaxis (bleeding from the nose). Selection of the correct size is critical, however, because obstruction may occur if the airway is too large. Size is correct if the airway when aligned on the side of the patient's face extends from the earlobe to the corner of the mouth. Proper insertion is also essential to ensure that the tongue is not pushed posteriorly, thus worsening the obstruction.

An oropharyngeal airway is inserted by pointing the tip toward the roof of the mouth and gently advancing it by rotating it 180 degrees. Another method is to hold down the tongue with a tongue depressor and guide the airway over the back of the tongue until it is in place. When the airway is in place, make certain the lips and tongue are not between the airway and the teeth and tape the top and bottom to the cheeks if desired.

Nasopharyngeal Airway

Nasopharyngeal airways are used to prevent airway obstruction after trauma to the lower face or after oral surgery. Use is contraindicated when a patient has a nasal obstruction, facial fracture, basilar skull fracture, or predisposition to epistaxis.

Nasopharyngeal airways are easily inserted and allow for suctioning without displacing the patient's nasal turbinates. On the negative side, they may kink or clog, obstructing the airway, or may cause pressure necrosis of the nasal mucosa. Selection of proper size is important because, like the oral airway, a size too large may cause obstruction. The correct length of nasopharyngeal airway is determined by measuring from the tip of the nose to the ear lobe and marking the distance on the tube to indicate the depth of insertion. The tube is lubricated with a water-soluble lubricant. The patient is placed in a supine position, and the tip of the nose

is pushed up. The larger nostril is selected and the airway is inserted and gently pushed along the floor of the nostril into the posterior pharynx until the predetermined mark or flange is flush with the nostril.

Correct position is checked by instructing the patient to exhale with the mouth closed. Air should be felt leaving the tube. A visual check can also be made by holding the patient's mouth open with a tongue depressor and looking for the tip of the tube just behind the uvula. If the length of airway inserted is too long, it may enter the esophagus, causing gastric distention and hypoventilation.

Endotracheal Tube

An endotracheal tube is a large-bore catheter inserted into the trachea through either the nose or the mouth. Endotracheal tubes are made of plastic or rubber. They contain a standard 15-mm adapter for attachment to a manual resuscitator bag or mechanical ventilator (Fig. 14–20) and have an inflatable balloon cuff. This cuff creates a seal in the trachea so air does not leak back around the tube when the patient is ventilated. The inflated cuff may also help to prevent aspiration of gastric contents into the lungs.

Like all artificial airways, endotracheal tubes are used to maintain a patent airway and are indicated when the patient needs mechanical ventilation because of impending respiratory failure or respiratory arrest. An endotracheal tube isolates the airway, provides access for suctioning secretions from the large airways of the pulmonary tree, and allows delivery of specific concentrations of oxygen up to 100%.

TYPES OF ENDOTRACHEAL TUBES. Orotracheal tubes are easily inserted and so are used in most emergency situations. They are also used for short-term intubation and mechanical ventilation when the patient has nasal obstruction or a predisposition to epistaxis. These tubes are often inserted with an oropharyngeal airway or bite block to protect them against being bitten or chewed. They increase oropharyngeal secretions and cannot be easily secured in place.

Nasotracheal tubes are more comfortable for the patient than orotracheal tubes, can be more securely held in place, allow for good oral hygiene, and cannot be bitten or chewed. However, they are more difficult to insert and cannot be used if the patient has a nasal obstruction, fractured nose, sinusitis, or predisposition to epistaxis. They also result in increased airway resistance and difficulty suctioning because of the small lumen size needed to fit nasal passages, and they may lacerate pharyngeal mucosa or the larynx during insertion. Pressure necrosis of the nasal mucosa, bleeding on removal, and maxillary sinusitis can also develop when a nasotracheal tube is used.

Double-lumen endotracheal tubes are used for independent lung ventilation for patients with single

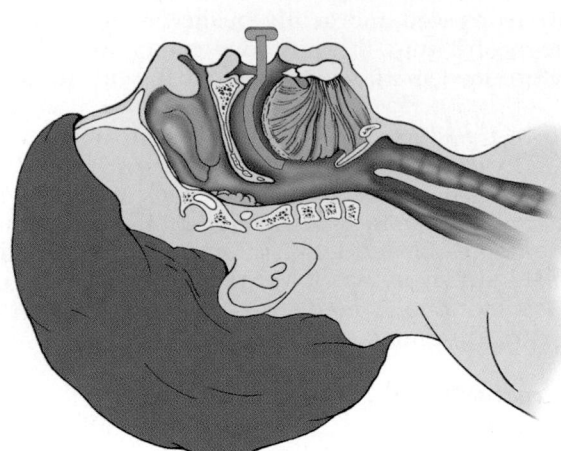

Oropharyngeal

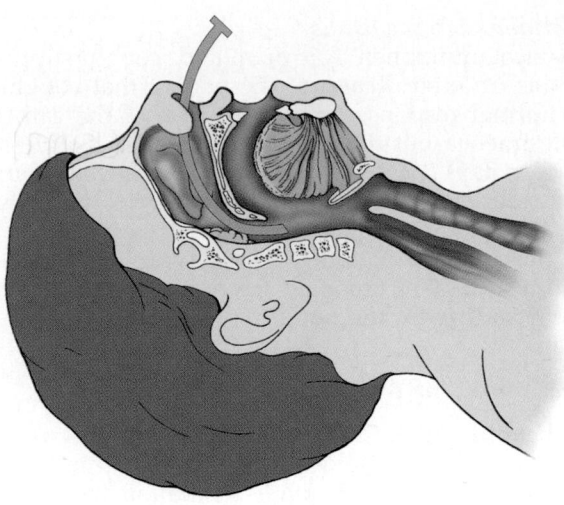

Nasopharyngeal

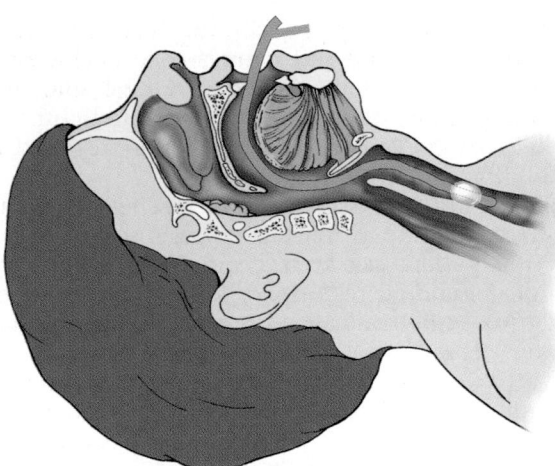

Oral endotracheal

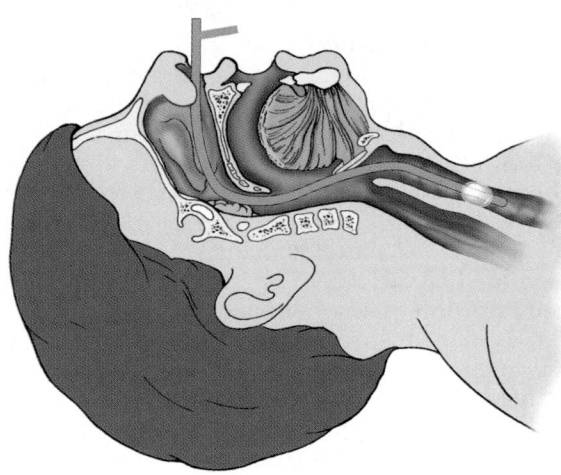

Nasal endotracheal

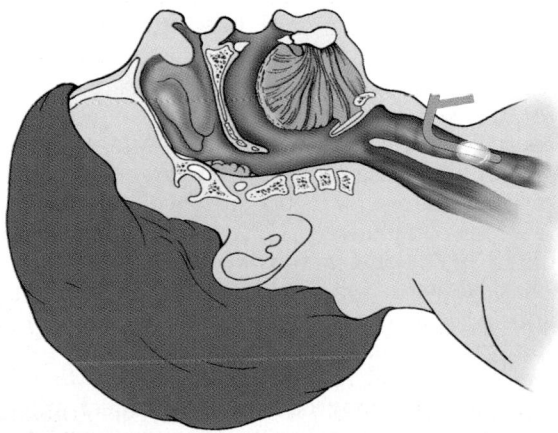

Tracheostomy

Figure 14–19
Types of artificial airways.

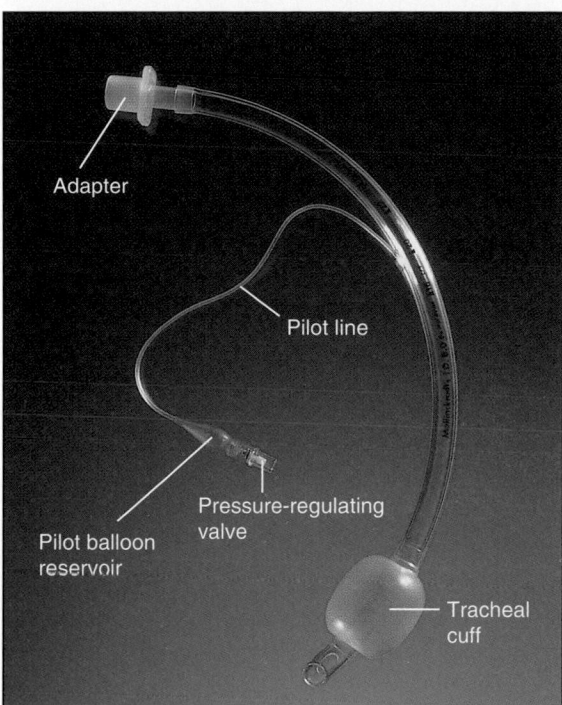

Figure 14–20

Components of an endotracheal tube. (Courtesy of Mallinckrodt Medical, St. Louis, MO)

lung disease. They consist of two tubes together with one lumen shorter than the other. When inserted, one lumen is positioned in a mainstem bronchus, and the other, shorter lumen is placed above the carina. A proximal cuff located in the trachea seals the trachea so that air cannot leak out during ventilation. A bronchial cuff separates the two lungs, allowing for unilateral lung diseases to be effectively treated by synchronous independent lung ventilation. Synchronous independent lung ventilation can be used to treat pulmonary contusion, aspiration pneumonitis, refractory atelectasis, unilateral lung disease, and bronchopleural fistula.

ENDOTRACHEAL TUBE INSERTION. Orotracheal tubes are inserted through the mouth via a laryngoscope, which allows direct visualization of the glottis, larynx, and trachea. For insertion, the patient is in a supine position, with the neck hyperextended and the mandible pulled forward. Nasotracheal tubes are inserted into the naris and then manipulated through the nasopharynx and larynx and into the trachea. Correct placement of the tube is initially checked by auscultating for breath sounds in both lungs, observing for symmetric chest movements, and feeling for warm, exhaled air at the end of the tube. Subsequently, correct placement of the tube at 3 to 5 cm above the carina (point of bifurcation of the mainstem bronchi) is confirmed by x-ray. Once in place, the cuff is inflated immediately to prevent aspiration, and the patient is suctioned and oxygenated. The tube is anchored in place to prevent it

from either being pulled out or moving downward into the right bronchus so that only the right lung is oxygenated. The tube is premarked at 2 cm intervals and the number of centimeters from the point at which it passes between the teeth or exits from the naris to the end of the tube is recorded. If the length of protrusion is more than 3 inches, the tube is cut back to eliminate the risk of bending from the weight of the ventilator circuit. Finally, ABGs are drawn to check oxygenation status. An endotracheal tube can be left in place for 5 to 7 days. If a patient continues to need an airway or mechanical ventilation, a tracheostomy is performed.

NURSING PROCESS
Endotracheal Tube

Assessment

Before intubation, perform a complete respiratory assessment. If the patient is conscious and the situation permits, also assess the patient's level of anxiety and understanding of the procedure.

When the endotracheal tube is in place, check its placement each shift and after adjusting or changing the tape or plastic anchoring device. This is done by auscultating for breath sounds in both lungs, observing for the symmetrical rise and fall of the chest wall, and checking the length of tube protrusion or, more dependably, by using a capnometer to measure the end-tidal partial pressure of carbon dioxide. Be alert for symptoms of partial obstruction such as choking, gagging, dyspnea, cough, wheezing, or stridor. Keep in mind that when the obstruction is minor, symptoms may be slight, but that prompt attention is necessary because partial obstruction can become complete obstruction very rapidly.

Observe the sides of the mouth for signs of irritation from orotracheal tubes and the naris for irritation from a nasotracheal tube. Inspect the underlying skin each time the anchoring tape is replaced for irritation or rash. Monitor cuff pressure with a manometer, keeping in mind that it should not exceed 20 mm Hg, because above this level stenosis and necrosis of the trachea may occur. If a ventilator is in use, check periodically that all connections to it remain secure.

Nursing Diagnoses and Planning

Nursing diagnoses and related expected patient outcomes commonly applicable to patients with an endotracheal tube include the following:

NDx: Anxiety related to the experience of intubation and the effect on other normal functions such as eating and speaking

Planning: Patient Outcomes
1. Facial expression and body posture are relaxed.
2. Patient attends to explanations and directions.

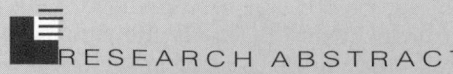

RESEARCH ABSTRACT

What Care of Endotracheal Tube Cuffs Is Provided in Clinical Practice?

Crimlisk J, Horn M, Wilson D, Marino B. Artificial airways: A survey of cuff management practices. Heart Lung 1996; 25(3):225.

Nurses and respiratory therapists alike have voiced concern over the management of cuffs on endotracheal tubes. How often are cuffs checked? How often are they deflated? What is the preferred method of cuff inflation? How often are cuff pressure measurements taken? Because there is wide variation in cuff management practices, because little research has been conducted to support cuff management recommendations, and because virtually all of the research has been carried out on adult populations, Crimlisk and colleagues sought to answer some of these questions.

The investigators developed a question-and-answer tool with which they surveyed a number of hospitals in the eastern United States. They found a wide variation in cuff management practices. Not only was there variation from one facility to the next, there was also variation *within* institutions. On the other hand, the team found no significant differences in cuff management practices between adult and pediatric units.

The researchers also discovered that only 41% of units deflated cuffs daily or more frequently. Furthermore, they found that most of the measurements are performed by respiratory therapists, because nurses are expected to assume more responsibility for patient care and management in other areas.

The research group identified a range of practices being carried out. The trend identified most often was that of no cuff care or minimal cuff care. The researchers said that the reason for this trend was the lack of a research base from which to develop guidelines or to provide consistent rationales for interventions.

Questions to Consider

1. What is the current practice for cuff deflation at your facility?
2. Why should cuffs be deflated?
3. What are the implications for patients if this intervention is not performed routinely?
4. Who is responsible for the management and documentation of airway care at your clinical facility?
5. Is there a difference between the way airways in adult patients are managed and the way airways in pediatric patients are managed? Should there be? Why or why not?

NDx: Risk for impaired tissue integrity related to pressure of the endotracheal tube on the trachea and mouth or naris

Planning: Patient Outcomes
1. Pressure in tube cuff is maintained at less than 20 mm Hg.
2. Tissues at the corners of the mouth or the naris are nonerythematous and intact.

Nursing Interventions and Evaluation

NDx: Anxiety
In nonemergency situations, prepare the patient for endotracheal intubation by providing brief factual information about the procedure. Explain the need for intubation. Tell the patient that sensations of gagging or suffocating may occur but provide reassurance that these sensations are normal and pass quickly. Explain that speaking will not be possible once the tube is in place, and plan with the patient some alternative means of communication such as blinking, paper and pencil, Magic Slate, or word, picture, or alphabet charts. Reassure the patient that

close observation will be provided and the call bell will be within reach at all times. Explain also that nourishment will be provided intravenously or by tube feeding because nothing can be taken by mouth.

NDx: Risk for impaired tissue integrity
Decrease the risk of erosion and necrosis of tracheal tissue and the development of a tracheoesophageal fistula by preventing traction on the endotracheal tube and carefully following guidelines for proper cuff inflation.

Keep the tube securely anchored and ascertain that swivel connectors and flexible tubing are used to connect it to the ventilator to prevent traction on it. Avoid unnecessary movement of the patient's head, and, when turning the patient, support both the head and the tube.

When inflating the endotracheal tube, a "minimal leak technique" is normally used. Inflate the cuff until a seal is established, that is, until no harsh sound is heard through a stethoscope placed over the trachea when the patient breathes in, but a slight leak on peak inspiration is present, and the patient cannot make a sound and no air is felt coming out of the patient's mouth. An alternative technique is known as "minimal occluding volume." Follow the procedure as just described but allow no air leak, even at peak inspiration. Keep in mind that the amount of air needed to inflate the cuff to the point of creating a seal varies with the size of the tube and the size of the patient's trachea. This amount is usually between 5 and 10 mL. If more air is required, it may be an indication that a larger size tube is necessary or that the trachea is becoming dilated.

Never overinflate the cuff. Maintain pressure within the cuff at less than 20 mm Hg to avoid exceeding capillary perfusion pressure in tracheal tissues. Higher pressures impair blood flow and damage tissues. When inflating a cuff, document the volume of air used and the pressure needed to obtain a seal. Check pressure at the end of inspiration if a pressure-limiting cuff is not used.

Periodic deflation of the cuff for 5 to 10 minutes has sometimes been suggested as a method to reduce potential tissue damage. However, the use of this method is of questionable value (Scanlan et al, 1995) and may in fact be hazardous because of the risk of aspiration and improper ventilation while the cuff is deflated.

Institute measures to protect against tissue damage to the mouth and naris. Apply water-soluble lubricant to the corners of the mouth and lips and provide good oral hygiene. Reposition orotracheal tubes in alternate sides of the mouth daily. Take extreme care to prevent inadvertent extubation. If scissors are used to cut the tape holding the tube in place, use caution to prevent accidentally cutting the cuff pilot tube (the small tube used to inflate and deflate the cuff). Use of endotracheal tube holders may prevent pressure necrosis and facilitate mouth care.

If a nasotracheal tube is in place, wash the naris gently and apply a water-soluble lubricant. Remove all anchoring tapes gently to avoid abrading the skin. Use hypoallergenic tape if rash or irritation appears.

Additional Interventions

If intubation is done at the bedside, make certain that an oxygen source is available, because, if intubation is not completed in a reasonable amount of time, the patient may need to be oxygenated with a manual resuscitator using 100% oxygen. Also make certain that a suction source and equipment are at the bedside.

Once intubation is accomplished, monitor equipment to ensure that the prescribed quantities of both oxygen and humidity are being delivered. Keep an extra endotracheal tube of the same size, a 10 mL syringe, and a manual resuscitator at the bedside at all times. If the patient is on a T-piece (provides oxygen and humidity, not mechanical ventilation), hyperinflate or "sigh" the patient every hour to open up atelectatic alveoli. This is not necessary if the patient is on a mechanical ventilator, because mechanical ventilators have a built-in sigh mechanism.

See Highlight 14–3 for nutritional guidelines in the care of the patient with an endotracheal tube.

Compare the patient's status with the expected outcomes. If the outcomes are not met, reassess the patient and revise the plan.

EXTUBATION OF AN ENDOTRACHEAL TUBE. The patient is extubated when clinical signs, ventilation tests, and ABGs indicate that a patent airway can be maintained and the patient can assume the work of breathing.

Endotracheal tubes are removed with the patient in a sitting position. The patient is hyperoxygenated, the trachea and oropharynx are suctioned, and the

---

HIGHLIGHT 14–3

NUTRITION

Special Considerations for Patients with Endotracheal Tubes, Tracheostomy Tubes, or Mechanical Ventilation

Weigh patient daily and maintain record of intake and output.

Provide frequent and meticulous mouth care because patient may experience loss of taste and decreased sense of smell.

Evaluate patient's ability to swallow.

Monitor closely for signs of dehydration and report same.

If patient is receiving tube feedings, follow established guidelines, being sure to check for tube placement in the stomach and residual before each feeding.

Replace residual and hold feedings if residual is greater than 100 mL.

If patient is eating and has a cuffed tracheostomy tube, inflate the cuff.

Provide high-calorie snacks.

Consult with nutritionist for planning of adequate calorie intake, serving of attractive meals to enhance appetite, and provision of some of patient's favorite foods. Remember carbohydrate intake is limited when carbon dioxide retention is a problem.

Always feed patient with head of bed elevated.

Assess and document patient's bowel sounds and activity.

and the patient is observed for stridor, pallor or cyanosis, and change in mental status. ABGs and pulse oximetry readings are also monitored to evaluate ventilation and oxygenation.

Tracheostomy

A tracheostomy is an artificial opening into the trachea created to establish an airway (Fig. 14–21). It may be temporary or permanent.

USES. Tracheostomies are done to provide a patent airway by bypassing complete upper airway obstruction as from pharyngeal tumors or laryngeal edema, by facilitating the removal of secretions, or by preventing aspiration of gastric contents. They are also used to allow for long-term mechanical ventilation and to decrease the work of breathing in paralyzed, weak, or critically ill patients by reducing the dead space in the respiratory tract.

TRACHEOSTOMY TUBES. A tracheostomy tube is a short, curved tube with a flange. The tubes are made of silver, stainless steel, or synthetic material and may be cuffed or uncuffed. As with endotracheal tubes, the cuff creates a seal in the trachea, preventing back-leaking of air during mechanical ventilation and aspiration of gastric contents. Most also have a removable inner cannula to facilitate cleaning the inside of the tube. Tracheostomy tubes are held in place by twill tape, which is attached to each side of the tube's flange and tied securely at the side of the neck.

Modifications of the basic tracheostomy tube include the fenestrated tube, cuffed speech-facilitating tubes, and the tracheostomy button. A fenestrated tracheostomy tube allows for air exchange between

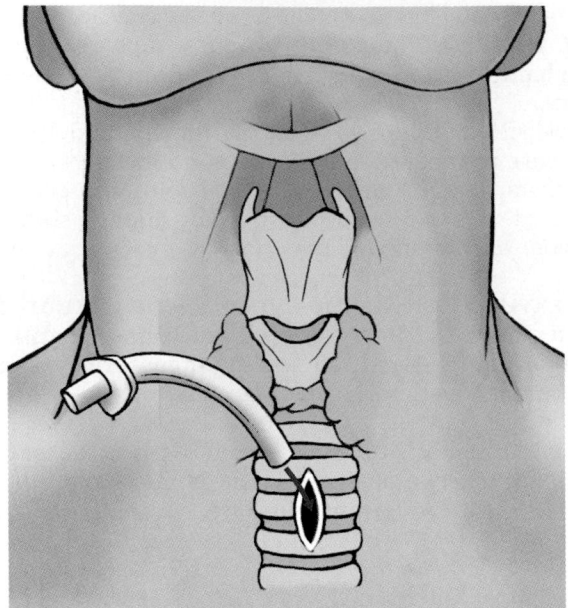

Figure 14–21

Tracheostomy. The diagram shows a vertical incision through tracheal rings three and four. As illustrated, the tracheostomy tube will be inserted through the incision.

cuff is deflated. The patient is then instructed to take a deep breath, the tube is withdrawn, and oxygen is given via a high-humidity face mask. The patient is observed for signs of hemorrhage, laryngeal spasm, and laryngeal edema. Respiratory rate, breath sounds, and chest excursion are monitored,

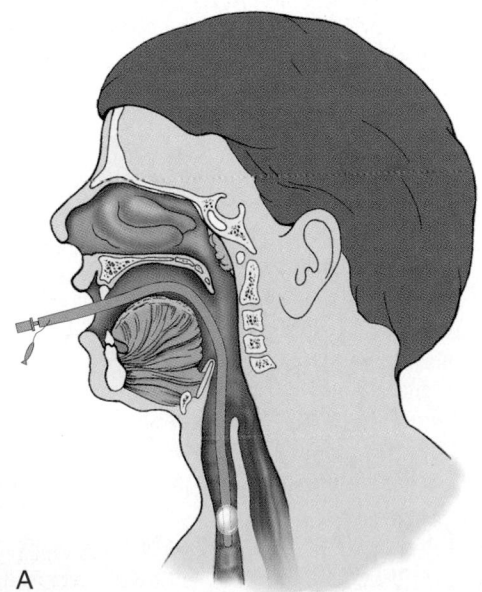
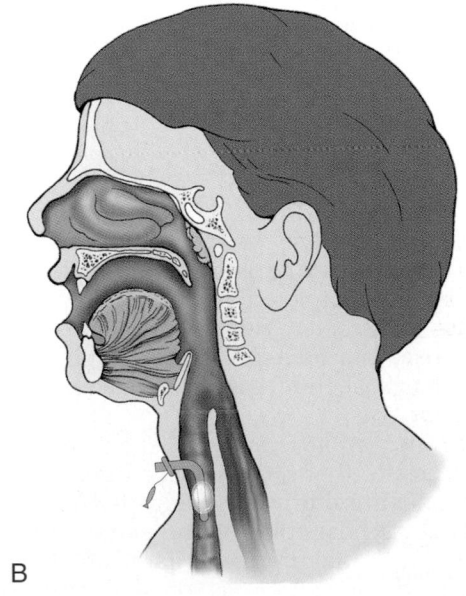

A   B

Figure 14–22

Tracheostomy tube compared with an endotracheal tube. *A*, Endotracheal tube. *B*, Tracheostomy tube.
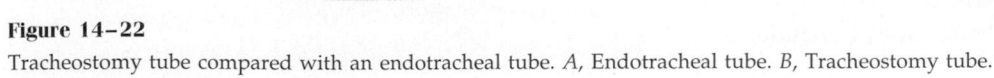

the lungs and the upper airway through an opening between the flange and the distal end of the tube. It permits the patient to talk when the tracheostomy tube is plugged or to be weaned from a mechanical ventilator.

Also available are cuffed tracheostomy tubes, which facilitate speech. These tubes work by directing an external air supply into the upper airway while the cuff is inflated.

The tracheostomy button fits into the tracheostomy opening extending from the opening to just inside the tracheal wall. It is used with uncuffed or fenestrated tracheostomy tubes and with cuffed tubes when cuffs are deflated. It facilitates talking, coughing, and normal breathing. It is often used in preparation for decannulation.

Tracheostomy tubes have significant advantages over endotracheal tubes. They are less traumatic because of their length and where and how they are inserted (Fig. 14–22). Tracheostomy tubes are easier to suction, are more comfortable, and allow the patient to swallow and eat.

PROCEDURE. Elective tracheostomy is a controlled procedure performed in an operating room. Under local anesthesia and with the neck hyperextended, a vertical incision is made in the trachea through the second and third tracheal rings. The trachea is incised, brought to the skin surface, and sutured. Then a tracheostomy tube of appropriate size is inserted with the aid of an obturator. The obturator is removed, and correct placement of the tube is confirmed by chest x-ray.

COMPLICATIONS. Complications that can occur as a result of tracheostomy surgery include left recurrent laryngeal nerve damage, hemorrhage, pneumothorax, and infection. There is also the risk of technical problems with the tube. These include airway obstruction caused by accidental displacement of the tube, underinflation or overinflation of the cuff, herniation of the cuff over the end of the tube, burst cuff, and blockage of the tube by secretions (Fig. 14–23). Long-term problems may include tracheal stenosis or necrosis and tracheoesophageal fistula.

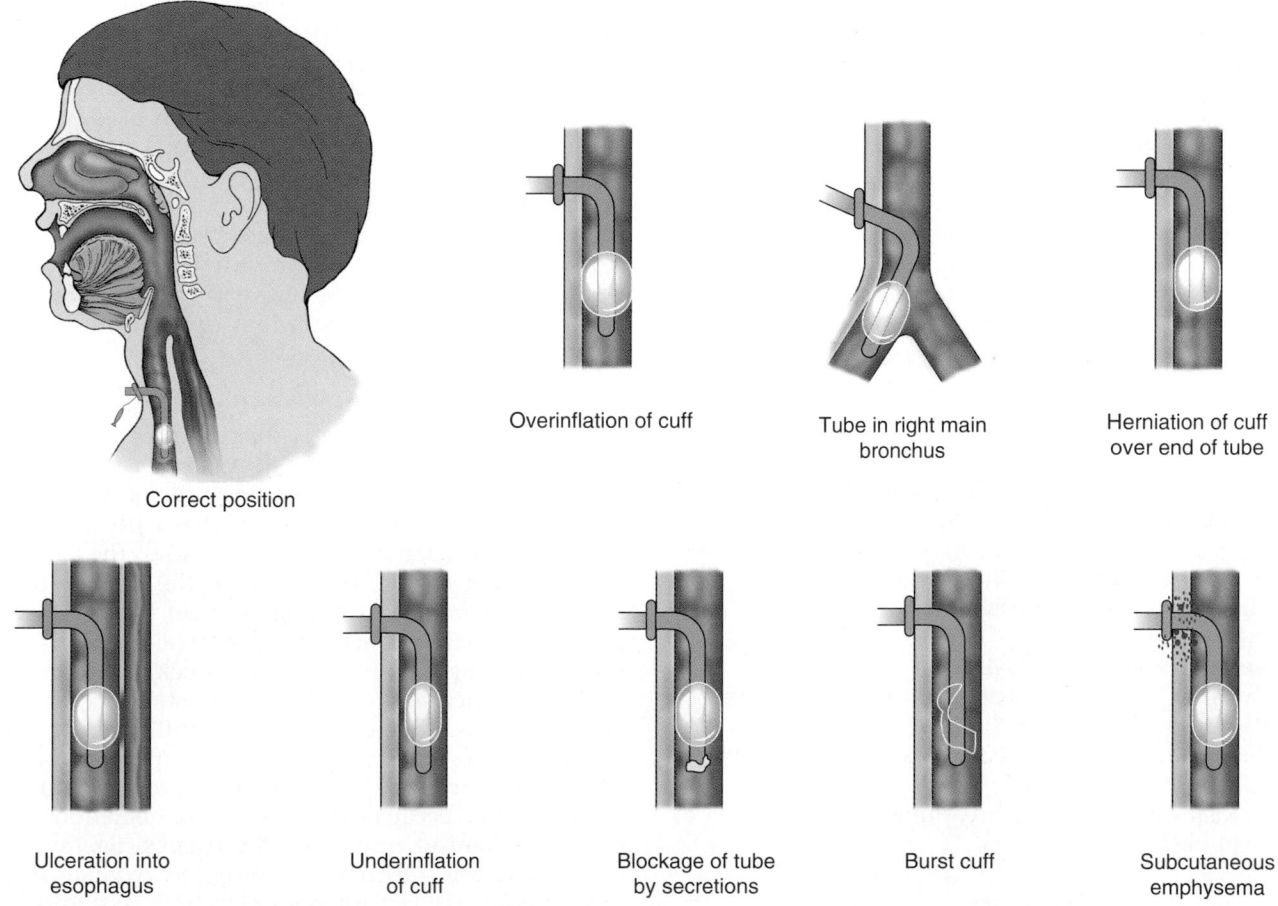

Correct position

Overinflation of cuff

Tube in right main bronchus

Herniation of cuff over end of tube

Ulceration into esophagus

Underinflation of cuff

Blockage of tube by secretions

Burst cuff

Subcutaneous emphysema

Figure 14–23

Selected complications of tracheostomy.

NURSING PROCESS
Tracheostomy

Assessment

Before the procedure, perform a complete respiratory assessment. If the situation permits, assess the patient's hearing, language ability, and writing ability in preparation for selecting alternative methods of communication after surgery. Determine the patient's understanding of the procedure and assess his or her level of anxiety.

After the procedure, note rate, rhythm, and depth of respirations. Note chest excursion, cough, amount and appearance of tracheal secretions, and frequency of the need for suctioning. Review ABG values if available. Check the placement of the tracheostomy tube and monitor the pressure in the cuff every shift by attaching a manometer to the cuff port. Note whether minimal occlusive volume is increased or decreased. Every 2 to 4 hours, check that the cuff is creating a good seal. Place a stethoscope over the trachea and listen for a harsh or gurgling sound during expiration. Feel for warm air from the mouth during expiration. Check the patient's ability to make sounds. Suspect a leak if any of these occur.

Observe the condition of the dressing and the tapes, and assess for signs of infection. Inspect the surgical site for bleeding, swelling, and purulent drainage. Check for fever and review laboratory reports for leukocytosis.

Assess also for the development of pneumothorax, pneumomediastinum, and cardiac tamponade. Be alert for cough, sharp chest pain, and tachycardia, which indicate pneumothorax. Also watch for dyspnea, crepitus, and edema of the face and neck, which indicate pneumomediastinum. Check for increased central venous pressure, narrowed pulse pressure, paradoxical pulse, hypotension, dyspnea, or decreased level of consciousness, which are symptoms of cardiac tamponade.

Nursing Diagnoses and Planning

Nursing diagnoses and related expected patient outcomes commonly applicable to patients with a tracheostomy include the following:

NDx: Anxiety related to the tracheostomy procedure and its effects on body function

Planning: Patient Outcomes
1. Facial expression and body posture are relaxed.
2. Patient is able to rest quietly.
3. Patient attends to explanations and directions.

NDx: Risk for ineffective breathing pattern related to tracheal obstruction

Planning: Patient Outcomes
1. Respiratory rate is 14 to 20 per minute.
2. Chest movement is smooth, symmetric, and of normal depth.

3. Breath sounds are clear.
4. Cyanosis is absent.

NDx: Risk for infection related to bacterial contamination of the tracheal wound

Planning: Patient Outcomes
1. Tracheostomy site is intact and without redness, edema, or drainage.
2. Purulent tracheal secretions are absent.
3. Patient is afebrile.

NDx: Impaired verbal communication related to interrupted flow of air between the lungs and the upper airway secondary to tracheostomy

Planning: Patient Outcomes
1. Patient uses nonverbal methods of communication.
2. Patient communicates needs effectively.

Nursing Interventions and Evaluation

NDx: Anxiety
Prepare the patient and the family for the tracheostomy by listening to their concerns, providing factual information, and answering questions. Ordinarily, the physician has provided an initial explanation of the procedure, so the focus is on reinforcing information. Be certain it is understood that slight discomfort is normal despite the local anesthesia, that speaking will not be possible with the basic tube in place, and that the tracheostomy will have to be suctioned because of the accumulation of secretions. Recognize that patients are often afraid of accidental suffocation when dependent on a tracheostomy to breathe. Reassure the patient in this regard. Remind the patient that tracheostomies are common, that close observation will be provided, and that a call bell will be readily available. Keep the patient physically comfortable and guide him or her in the use of relaxation exercises if needed.

NDx: Risk for ineffective breathing pattern
If the tracheostomy tube is dislodged after surgery, the opening can close over, leaving the patient unable to breathe. Therefore, keep a replacement tube and obturator at the bedside along with a curved hemostat that could be used to hold the trachea open. Do not change the tapes on the tracheostomy tube or deflate the cuff for the first 24 hours because of the risk of accidental dislodgement. Similarly, do not change the tube for at least a week.

Using strict sterile technique, suction the airway as often as needed to keep it patent. This may be every 5 to 10 minutes immediately after the procedure and later every 2 to 3 hours. Avoid suctioning unnecessarily because it can increase secretions and cause mechanical trauma to the tissues. Suction patients who are sensitive to decreased oxygen levels more frequently but for a shorter time to avoid hypoxemia or hypercapnia. Also hyperventilate them with 100% oxygen prior to, during, and after suctioning. Be sure to document time of suctioning, characteristics of secretions, respiratory status, and patient's response.

Keep a pair of scissors at the bedside to snip the tapes in the event the tracheostomy tube should become dislodged and the tapes tighten around the neck. Also keep a manual resuscitation bag with an adaptor mask at the bedside.

NDx: Risk for infection

Treat the tracheostomy as a surgical wound. Use all sterile equipment (eg, suction apparatus, gloves, dressings) and maintain strict sterile technique.

Cleanse the tracheostomy and the surrounding area to keep them free of secretions and bacterial contamination. Put on sterile gloves. Use sterile gauze to remove the inner cannula. If it is nondisposable, soak it in half-strength hydrogen peroxide solution. (Disposable inner cannulas are commonly used.) Suction the outer cannula and follow with deep breathing either by the patient or via a manual resuscitator bag. Remove the soiled tracheostomy dressing and use gauze and peroxide solution to remove secretions and crusts from around the tube. Use peroxide-soaked swabs to cleanse under the neck plate and the openings in its sides. Using a new pair of sterile gloves, thoroughly cleanse the inner cannula with a brush and pipe cleaners; rinse in sterile saline or water and dry thoroughly. Insert a disposable or a cleansed nondisposable inner cannula into the outer cannula. Proceed to change the tracheostomy tapes. Prepare the clean tapes before removing the soiled ones. To prepare, cut the tape, with about two thirds left on one side and one third on the other. Make a horizontal slit 1 inch from each end. Insert this slit end of the tie through the side opening of the outer cannula. Pull the opposite end through the slit and draw securely. Repeat this procedure and secure the other one-third piece to the opposite side of the cannula. Hold the tube while this is being done because the patient could easily cough the tube out, resulting in airway obstruction. Tie the tapes on the side of the neck to eliminate a knot at the back of the neck. Tracheostomy ties made of Velcro are also available. Finally, slip a 3 × 3 inch gauze pad folded into a V shape or a factory-made split sponge between the neck and the tracheostomy tube to provide padding and to absorb secretions. Never cut a gauze pad for this use because frayed threads can be aspirated. Dressings around the tracheostomy tube should be changed frequently if excessive secretions are present. Wet dressings promote infection by providing a warm, moist environment.

NDx: Impaired verbal communication

Before the tracheostomy, if possible, plan a method of communication for the patient to use once the tube is in place. Depending on the patient's physical and mental capacities, consider use of paper and pencil, Magic Slate, pictures, or an adjunct device such as the Passy-Muir valve, Olympic Trach-Talk, the Pitt speaking tube, and the Cyberset tone generator. Keep in mind that the selection of one of these devices depends on individual patient tolerance. Orient significant others to the planned method of communication to avoid creating confusion and frustration.

Compare the patient's status with the expected outcomes. If the outcomes are not met, reassess the patient and revise the plan.

REMOVAL OF A TRACHEOSTOMY TUBE. Removal of a tracheostomy tube is similar to that of an endotracheal tube. The patient is ventilated, oxygenated, and suctioned. The cuff is deflated, suctioning is repeated, and the tube is removed. A moist gauze pad is placed over the wound, which closes spontaneously in about 5 days.

Mechanical Ventilation Therapy

Mechanical ventilation therapy is used to overcome the patient's inability to ventilate or oxygenate adequately. It may be intermittent or continuous and short term or long term.

INTERMITTENT POSITIVE-PRESSURE BREATHING

Intermittent positive-pressure breathing is a mode of therapy used to deliver air or oxygen under a pressure greater than atmospheric pressure until a preset limit is reached. It improves the inspiratory phase of ventilation and promotes the flow of air to the alveoli. This form of therapy is both intermittent and short term.

Uses

The primary use of intermittent positive-pressure breathing is to deliver aerosol medications into the lower respiratory tract for patients unable to take a deep breath. It has also been used to promote alveolar ventilation and removal of secretions and to decrease the work of breathing but its value has been disputed, and some studies have shown that it is no more effective than good deep breathing and may, in fact, increase air trapping in chronic obstructive pulmonary disease.

Procedure

Treatments are usually administered for 15 to 20 minutes three to four times per day before meals. The patient is instructed to sit upright, to close the lips around the mouthpiece once a mist has formed, to maintain a slow respiratory rate, and to use diaphragmatic breathing during the treatment. The lungs are auscultated during inflation to make certain that all dependent areas are well ventilated and coughing is encouraged every few minutes. If a bronchodilator is administered as part of the treatment, vital signs, breath sounds, and simple bedside pulmonary function measures such as peak flow and vital capacity are recorded before and after it. The machine is turned off during coughing or other interruptions to prevent the loss of medications. The treatment is continued until the medication is finished.

Complications

Complications of intermittent positive-pressure breathing therapy are dizziness related to hyperventilation, which lowers carbon dioxide levels, exacerbation of hemoptysis, ruptured alveoli and pneumothorax, increased intracranial pressure, and cardiovascular problems. It may also cause nausea and vomiting if administered too soon after meals. Infection secondary to cross-contamination is another risk because medication or water left in the equipment serves as a medium for bacterial growth. To prevent this, careful cleansing techniques are followed and individual tubing, nebulizers, masks, mouthpieces, and filters are used. Intermittent positive-pressure breathing is contraindicated in the presence of untreated pneumothorax, impaired glottis function, and wound dehiscence. It is also contraindicated if the patient experiences a drop in blood pressure of more than 30 mm Hg during therapy.

MECHANICAL VENTILATION

If a patient is unable to ventilate enough to maintain proper levels of oxygen and carbon dioxide in the blood, mechanical ventilation by a respirator may be indicated.

Types of Ventilators

Many different types of ventilator models are available (Table 14–7). The models fall into two categories: negative-pressure ventilators and positive-pressure ventilators. Negative-pressure ventilators exert negative pressure on the chest and lung to expand them during inspiration. They are used in the care of patients with neuromuscular disorders, such as myasthenia gravis, multiple sclerosis, and muscular dystrophy. Positive-pressure ventilators exert positive pressure on airways to inflate alveoli during inspiration. They are used in the care of patients with chest and lung disorders, such as flail chest, chronic bronchitis, emphysema, and adult respiratory distress syndrome. The most widely used types today are pressure cycled and volume cycled; both are positive-pressure ventilators.

Table 14–7

Types of Ventilators

Classification	Remarks	Modes	Accessory Modes
NEGATIVE PRESSURE VENTILATORS			
Drinker respirator tank (iron lung)	No intubation required; reliable but cumbersome.		
Body wrap (raincoat or poncho ventilator)	Consists of rigid cage with a nylon wrap around abdomen and thorax; prone to leaks; causes musculoskeletal pain		
Chest cuirass	Rigid shell over chest; can be used in wheelchair; hard to fit; causes back pain		
POSITIVE PRESSURE VENTILATORS			
Pressure-cycled	Inspiration is terminated when a predetermined pressure is reached; volumes are inconsistent; used short term, such as in the PACU (Bird, PRII)	Control: assist/control	
Volume-cycled	Inspiration terminated when a preset volume is achieved regardless of pressure required; several modes available; most commonly used are the Ma-1, Bear, PB7200, and Servo*	Control: assist/control; IMV/SIMV; CPAP; pressure support	PEEP, sighs
Time-cycled	Inspiration is terminated at a predetermined time; this type is used chiefly in infants (Bear Cub)	Control: assist/control; IMV; CPAP	PEEP

*The classification of ventilators has been complicated by microprocessor technology. Several ventilators can be classified in different ways, and the distinction is not always readily apparent.

CPAP, continuous positive airway pressure; IMV, intermittent mandatory ventilation; PACU, postanesthesia care unit; PEEP, positive end-expiratory pressure; SIMV, synchronized intermittent mandatory ventilation.

The pressure-cycled ventilator is set to deliver a preset positive pressure for a specified length of time or until the preset pressure is reached. When the pressure is reached, the machine turns off and normal exhalation begins. The tidal volume (volume of gas) delivered is not necessarily constant because it depends on the resistance of the entire system, including the lung. Change in compliance or airway resistance, or both, can be caused by atelectasis, bronchospasm, mucous plug, or change in the patient's position. As a result, the pressure-cycled ventilators cannot be relied on to deliver consistent volumes for long-term mechanical ventilation. They are generally used for short-term, closely monitored situations, such as in a recovery room.

A volume-cycled ventilator delivers a constant volume of air with each breath regardless of the positive pressure necessary to attain that volume. There is a preset pressure-limiting valve that causes release of excessive pressure if the preset limit is reached. These pressure-limiting valves usually have an audible alarm. The limit can be set just slightly above the pressure required to ventilate the patient. The alarm then sounds when secretions accumulate or when the patient coughs or resists the machine.

Ventilation Modes

Whatever type of ventilator is used, various ventilator modes are adjusted to the individual patient's needs. They include the following.

ASSIST. This pattern means that the patient's respiratory effort triggers the machine and thereby controls the respiratory rate. The negative pressure required to trigger an assist breath is set on the machine. When the patient's inspiratory effort equals or exceeds this preset negative pressure, the machine responds with a positive-pressure breath. A disadvantage to this mode is that if the patient becomes apneic, ventilation will be inadequate. Both pressure-cycled and volume-cycled ventilators can be set with the assist mode.

CONTROL. This is inflation of the patient's lungs at a set interval and volume regardless of patient effort or breathing pattern. This is used if the patient is apneic or the respiratory rate is too low or if the patient is sedated with neuromuscular paralyzing agents. Since the patient cannot initiate breaths, asynchronous respiratory patterns may be observed if the patient tries to breathe faster than the set rate. This leads to agitation and increased work of breathing.

ASSIST-CONTROL. This is basically the assist pattern with a back-up control rate from the ventilator for minimum ventilation. The ventilator responds with a positive pressure breath at the preset tidal volume to every patient effort, and if the patient stops breathing, the machine automatically takes over ventilation at a preset rate and tidal volume. Hyperventilation is a complication of this pattern.

Advantages of this mode are that the patient has control of respiratory rate and makes an inspiratory effort, thus using respiratory muscles and preventing their atrophy.

SYNCHRONIZED INTERMITTENT MANDATORY VENTILATION. The synchronized intermittent mandatory ventilation mode allows the patient to breathe spontaneously but also delivers a mandatory but synchronized positive-pressure breath at a predetermined rate. The patient's own breaths are without positive pressure, and inspired oxygen is the same as with the ventilator-delivered breaths. This mode is used to wean patients from ventilators by gradually decreasing the number of breaths by the machine. The patient assumes a larger portion of the minute volume as the ventilator support is gradually removed. This mode offers the most patient comfort.

CONTINUOUS POSITIVE AIRWAY PRESSURE. In this mode, called continuous positive airway pressure, the intubated patient breathes spontaneously while the pressure in the airways is maintained above atmospheric pressure. This may be used as an alternate to T-piece weaning. When this continuous positive pressure on expiration is applied in combination with a mandatory ventilator breath, it is known as positive end-expiratory pressure.

A variation of continuous positive airway pressure for the nonintubated patient is referred to as bilevel continuous positive airway pressure (BiPAP). With this method, the patient wears a face mask or nose mask, and spontaneous respiration is augmented by maintained continuous positive pressure in the airway.

PRESSURE SUPPORT VENTILATION. In pressure support ventilation, the patient's spontaneous breath is augmented with a preset pressure. It does not provide the entire volume. The rate is not set by the machine but rather by the patient's spontaneous efforts.

There are other methods of manipulating or adjusting inspiration or expiration that are accessory modes, which may be used in conjunction with any of the primary modes previously described. These include the following:

POSITIVE END-EXPIRATORY PRESSURE. In this accessory mode, a positive pressure is maintained in the lungs at the end of exhalation. Its use increases the volume of air left in the lungs at the end of a passive expiration. Its primary purpose is to keep airways and alveoli from collapsing. The positive pressure allows more oxygen to diffuse across the alveolocapillary membrane, thereby improving oxygenation while decreasing oxygen supplementation. Possible complications of positive end-expiratory pressure include decreased cardiac output and hypotension caused by increased positive pressure on the thoracic vessels. Additional complications such as pneumothorax and other barotrauma are caused by high positive pressure rupturing lung tissue. Fluid retention is caused by inappropriate antidiuretic hormone secretion.

SIGHS. A normal person sighs six to 10 times per hour. Monotonous tidal volumes on mechanical ventilation can lead to microatelectasis. Although sighs are not always used, strong consideration should be given to providing a deeper than normal breath several times per hour. Some mechanical ventilators automatically cause the patient to sigh or can be adjusted to do so. If the type used does not have this ability, the patient can be caused to sigh manually with a bag-valve resuscitator to prevent atelectasis.

The ventilator used should have a regulator-controlled flow rate at which gas is delivered. It should also have the ability to regulate inspired concentrations of oxygen from 21 to 100%. An oxygen analyzer should always be used to ensure the accuracy of the delivered fraction of inspired oxygen (FIO_2). Basic ventilator characteristics necessary to ensure patient safety are as follows:

- Provision for heating (32.2–37.7°C [90–100°F]) and humidifying the inspired air.
- A reliable visible and audible alarm that sounds if there is a rise or fall in circuit pressure or if a patient disconnects within 15 seconds. *Note: Alarms should never be shut off.*
- Provisions for measurement of expired volumes to determine tidal and minute ventilations.
- Plugs and switches that are insulated and grounded.
- Breathing tubing and parts that are easily removed for sterilization or replacement.
- A fail-safe valve that opens at a few centimeters negative pressure. If there is electrical failure or machine malfunction, this allows the patient to draw in air to prevent suffocation.

NURSING PROCESS
Mechanical Ventilation

Assessment

Auscultate lung sounds every 2 hours and observe for symmetric chest expansion to determine whether both lungs are being ventilated. Assess need for suctioning because secretions increase with the use of mechanical ventilation. Check vital signs every 2 to 4 hours.

Because patients who are receiving positive pressure ventilation are at risk for ventilation/perfusion mismatch, assess the patient for signs of hypoxia, hypercapnia, and hypocapnia. Symptoms of hypoxia are restlessness, anxiety, tachycardia, increased respiratory rate, increased work of breathing, cyanosis, and confusion. Symptoms of hypercapnia are somnolence, lethargy, tachycardia, confusion, and headache. Symptoms of hypocapnia are muscle spasm, tetany, diaphoresis, light-headedness, tachypnea, and cardiac dysrhythmia. Assess the patient's synchrony with the ventilator. Check ABG values at regular intervals and whenever ventilator settings are changed.

In patients on positive end-expiratory pressure, observe for signs of decreased cardiac output. Be alert for weak peripheral pulses, hypotension, narrowed pulse pressure, slow capillary refill, decreased urinary output, restlessness, decreasing level of consciousness, pallor, fatigue, and chest pain. In patients with head trauma, be alert for signs of increased intracranial pressure. If settings for positive end-expiratory pressure are decreased, assess for signs of cardiac overload and pulmonary edema. If central venous pressure or pulmonary capillary wedge pressures are required, obtain all readings either with the patient connected or disconnected from the ventilator because the positive pressure alters the readings.

Assess nasogastric drainage or stool for frank and occult blood, because stress ulcers are a potential complication of mechanical ventilation. Review hematocrit values.

Observe the skin for redness and breakdown, because mobility of the patient on a respirator is limited. Also assess joint mobility and nutritional status. Determine the patient's emotional response to the ventilator. Be alert to signs of anxiety and to feelings of powerlessness.

Assess the endotracheal/tracheostomy tube every hour for proper placement and function. At the same time assess the ventilator for proper settings and working alarms.

Nursing Diagnoses and Planning

Nursing diagnoses and related expected patient outcomes commonly applicable to patients on a mechanical ventilator include the following:

NDx: Ineffective breathing pattern related to *(specify)* or Inability to sustain spontaneous ventilation related to *(specify)*

Planning: Patient Outcomes
 1. ABG values are within normal range.

NDx: Risk for ineffective airway clearance related to excessive secretions

Planning: Patient Outcomes
 1. Breath sounds are clear bilaterally.
 2. ABG values are within patient's normal range.

NDx: Risk for fluid volume excess related to blocked insensible water loss

Planning: Patient Outcomes
 1. Chest sounds are clear.
 2. Extremities are free of edema.
 3. Vital signs are within patient's baseline range.

NDx: Impaired physical mobility related to mechanical ventilation

Planning: Patient Outcomes
 1. Joints have patient's normal range of motion.
 2. Patient moves as directed.

NDx: Anxiety related to being on a mechanical ventilator

Planning: Patient Outcomes
1. Body posture appears relaxed.
2. Facial expression appears relaxed.

NDx: Risk for altered thought processes related to change in sensory input secondary to limited mobility

Planning: Patient Outcomes
1. Patient is oriented to time, place, and person.

Nursing Interventions and Evaluation

NDx: Ineffective breathing pattern or Inability to sustain spontaneous ventilation

Maintain the closed circuit of the ventilator system. Prevent accidental disconnection of the patient from the ventilator by leaving the alarm on at all times, even during suctioning. Keep a manual resuscitator bag at the bedside and manually ventilate the patient if power fails or the ventilator malfunctions. Respond immediately to any alarm; if the problem cannot be immediately identified and corrected, disconnect the patient and ventilate by hand while the problem is further investigated. Check settings on the ventilator every hour. Also check tubing for condensation and drain collected water to prevent aspiration.

If a patient is "fighting the ventilator," promote synchronization by slowly ventilating by bag for three to six breaths or by verbally coaching the patient as to when to inhale and exhale. Administer ordered analgesics or sedatives if pain or anxiety is the causative factor.

NDx: Risk for ineffective airway clearance

Direct the patient to cough and deep-breathe every 2 hours. Change the patient's position at least every 2 hours. If only one lung is affected, position the patient on the unaffected side or the back. Suction as needed. Maintain humidification, making certain that the water level is maintained in the ventilator reservoir. Also perform chest physiotherapy as ordered to help mobilize secretions. Administer prescribed intravenous or inhaled bronchodilators.

NDx: Risk for fluid volume excess

Measure intake and output. When interpreting these values, adjust for the fact that insensible water loss is blocked by the closed humidification system of the ventilator. Weigh patient daily to check for weight gain, which is indicative of fluid retention. Also monitor for edema, crackles, hyponatremia, and decreased hematocrit, which are additional symptoms of overload.

NDx: Impaired physical mobility

Change the patient's position and provide skin care every 2 hours. Perform active or passive range-of-motion exercises every 8 hours. Maintain the patient's position of function while the patient is on bedrest to prevent contractures and external hip rotation. Use supportive "booties" or have the patient wear high-top sneakers while in bed to prevent foot drop. Sit the patient up in a chair as soon as his or her condition allows. When permitted, walk the patient while ventilating with oxygen via a bag or while pushing the ventilator along.

NDx: Anxiety

Explain procedures and equipment to the patient and the family. Reassure them regarding the dependability of the machine and its built-in malfunction-detection system. Further reassure them that close supervision is provided by nursing and other health-care team personnel. Do not leave the patient unattended until he or she has anxiety under control and is comfortable with the ventilator.

Whenever possible, involve the patient in decision-making regarding care to provide a sense of having some control. Also encourage the use of relaxation exercises and tape-recordings as well as other stress-reduction techniques. Provide diversion suited to the patient's condition and personal preferences.

Remember that significant others are often as anxious as the patient, so facilitate discussion of concerns and provide information as needed. Also make certain to promote communication between the patient and the family.

NDx: Risk for altered thought processes

Speak frequently to the patient even though he or she cannot talk back. Call the patient by name and orient to day, date, time, and place as a part of routine care. Place a calendar and a clock within the patient's view. Dim lighting at bedtime to help distinguish day from night. Ask family members to bring in pictures or other personal items that can be placed in the patient's environment. If possible, provide the patient with a window view for light and sensory stimulation. Encourage diversionary activities and visits by significant others. To the extent possible, plan uninterrupted periods of rest and sleep.

Additional Interventions

Provide oral hygiene every 8 hours to increase comfort and to decrease the likelihood of bacterial contamination of the lower respiratory tract. Give antacids or other medication ordered to combat stress ulcers. Administer tube feedings or total parenteral nutrition solutions as ordered. Monitor bowel function.

Compare the patient's status with the expected outcomes. If the outcomes are not met, reassess the patient and revise the care plan.

Weaning from Mechanical Ventilation

Patients are weaned from dependence on a ventilator gradually over a period of time. Patients are

CLINICAL ? THINKING

RESTLESSNESS, CONFUSION, AND IRRITABILITY IN A PATIENT ON HOME VENTILATOR SUPPORT

As I entered the home of my last patient to be visited that day, I was met by the patient's husband and two sons. They appeared anxious and concerned as they described the change in the patient's condition over the past 24 hours. The patient, a 58-year-old female with a medical diagnosis of amyotrophic lateral sclerosis, had been maintained on home care for the past 8 months. Her treatment regimen was primarily supportive and included enteral feedings via a gastrostomy tube for long-term nutritional support, and continuous, positive-pressure mechanical ventilation via a tracheostomy for maintenance of an adequate breathing pattern. Regular visits by home health nurses were aimed at supporting and assisting the patient and family in meeting the many physical and psychosocial needs associated with this progressive neuromuscular disorder, to evaluate the effectiveness of her treatment, and to monitor the patient for complications.

The family's report revealed that the patient was experiencing nausea and vomiting of recent onset and was complaining of abdominal cramps and headaches. They also noted that she appeared irritable and hostile, was sleeping for longer periods of time, and had experienced a seizure that morning. Prior to this visit, the patient had been medically stable; however, it was immediately obvious to me that she had taken a turn for the worse.

I recognized that this change in the patient's condition could stem from any number of causes, including the onset of a new clinical problem, complications of the disease itself, or a wide range of complications associated with mechanical ventilation such as pneumothorax, infection, acid-base imbalance, cardiovascular, gastrointestinal and nutritional disturbances, and fluid and electrolyte imbalances. To gather additional clues to her status, I proceeded to conduct a thorough assessment of the patient.

I checked her neurologic status and found that although she was usually coherent, she was restless, disoriented to place and time, and was unable to follow simple commands. Her pupils were equal in size and reacted equally to light and accommodation. Next I checked her vital signs and cardiovascular and respiratory status and found that her blood pressure was 144/92 (about 20 mm Hg above her usual range), apical pulse was 100 bpm

and regular, temperature was 36.9°C (98.4°F), and she denied any chest pain or discomfort. All ventilator settings were correctly set and functioning as per medical orders, the respiratory rate was set at 14 per minute, and suctioning was not required at that time. Equal bilateral breath sounds were present, and crackles were noted over the bases upon auscultation. Her skin turgor was good and there was no evidence of peripheral or sacral edema. Physical assessment of her gastrointestinal and urinary tract revealed hyperactive bowel sounds heard on auscultation and no evidence of abdominal distention, bladder distention, or tenderness on palpitation. The family denied any change in the color or nature of her stool, but did state that her urinary output had decreased. A small urine specimen collected during my visit was concentrated and amber in color. As I proceeded with my assessments, the patient became increasingly more difficult to arouse.

The presence of confusion, restlessness, irritability, drowsiness, and tachycardia could be related to hypoxemia secondary to decreased cardiac output (from heart failure or the effects of positive-pressure ventilation), anemia (resulting from malnutrition), hypovolemia (from gastrointestinal bleeding), or hypoventilation. However, findings indicating adequate cardiac and peripheral perfusion, as well as an elevated blood pressure and bounding pulses, were not consistent with a decreased cardiac output; the rapid onset of her symptoms was not consistent with a nutritional anemia; her respiratory assessment including the absence of pallor and cyanosis was not consistent with hypoventilation; and despite the hyperactive bowel sounds, there was no evidence of gastrointestinal bleeding. Other possible complications such as sepsis and pneumothorax were eliminated as possibilities based on the absence of an elevated temperature and the presence of equal bilateral breath sound and chest excursions.

Although numerous clinical manifestations (headache, tachycardia, confusion, and restlessness) could have signified respiratory acidosis, these findings, in conjunction with the elevated blood pressure, bounding pulses, pulmonary crackles, decreased urinary ouput with increased concentration, and gastrointestinal symptoms (nausea, vomiting, cramps, and increased bowel sounds) led me to suspect that the patient had developed syndrome of inappropriate antidiuretic hormone related to mechanical ventilation. I knew that this complication of positive-pressure ventilation (which increases intrathoracic pressure, decreases

(continued)

CLINICAL ? THINKING

(continued)

venous return to the heart, and falsely stimulates stretch receptors and baroreceptors to trigger excessive release of antidiuretic hormone) results in excess fluid retention, hemodilution (hypo-osmolarity), dilutional hyponatremia, and water intoxication. The occurrence of a seizure, in conjunction with the patient's mental clouding and decreasing level of consciousness, strongly supported the likelihood of brain-cell swelling, cerebral edema, and increased intracranial pressure. The absence of peripheral edema despite fluid retention further supported my suspicion of syndrome of inappropriate anti-diuretic hormone precipitated by mechanical ventilation.

Because syndrome of inappropriate anti-diuretic hormone has a multisystem effect and can quickly progress to permanent neurologic damage, coma, and death if it is not appropriately addressed, I immediately implemented the following action:

1. I elevated the head of the bed to 30 degrees.
2. I instituted seizure and safety precautions.
3. I called the physician and informed him of my assessments.
4. I made arrangements to quickly transport the patient to the hospital.
5. I withheld all fluids and monitored the output.
6. I closely monitored the patient's neurologic and cardiopulmonary status.
7. I calmly explained what was happening to the patient and family, answered their questions, and provided emotional support.
8. I documented my findings and actions.

Following the patient's admission to the medical intensive care unit, the physician ordered a complete blood count, serum electrolytes, hemoglobin and hematocrit, serum and urine sodium and osmolarity studies, arterial blood gases, and a computed tomographic scan (to rule out a cerebral tumor or bleeding). The results of these laboratory tests confirmed my suspicion. Additional medical orders included a hypertonic saline IV infusion, the administration of demeclocycline and diuretics, hemodynamic monitoring for fluid volume and cardiac status, continuous electrocardiographic monitoring, fluid restriction, seizure precautions, input and output, measurement of urine specific gravity, and daily weights.

Within 48 hours, the patient's condition improved. She became lucid and was no longer irritable and disoriented; her blood pressure, fluid balance, and electrolytes returned to normal; she remained free of seizure activity and was discharged to her home on the fifth day following hospitalization. Although the clues of fluid imbalance precipitated by mechanical ventilation may be misleading, the possible lethal consequences of this hormonal imbalance were prevented by the nurse's early detection and appropriate interventions.

Think Critically

What specific laboratory results would the nurse expect upon admission?

Was elevating the patient's head the best action by the nurse? Why or why not?

Should the nurse have arranged for transport to the hospital sooner? Based on the family report alone?

A student nurse questioned the nurse regarding the absence of peripheral edema despite fluid retention and overload. What is the nurse's best response?

How would the home nurse's assessments and interventions have differed if the patient had diabetes insipidus?

What nursing assessments and interventions would be included in the patient's nursing care while in the intensive care unit? How would the effectiveness of treatment be evaluated?

What specific complications of hypertonic IV fluid administration in a patient with syndrome of inappropriate antidiuretic hormone should the nurse recognize and monitor for?

A family member asked if the seizure could be related to the pathophysiology of amyotrophic lateral sclerosis. What is the nurse's best response?

What nursing observations and actions should be implemented to prevent recurrences?

What nursing actions would be helpful in limiting fluid intake in the home?

What additional teaching should be included in the patient and family instructions prior to and following discharge?

What essential nursing diagnoses should be included in the patient's nursing care plan upon her return to home care?

Upon her return home, the patient told the nurse that she is considering the termination of mechanical ventilation. What is the nurse's best response? What legal and ethical dilemmas should the nurse consider?

judged ready to be weaned when their conditions are stable and the following criteria are met:

- Condition requiring mechanical ventilation has resolved or stabilized.
- Airway is patent.
- Chest wall is stable.
- Respiratory rate is between 12 and 25 per minute.
- Positive end-expiratory pressure is no higher than 5 cm of water.
- Vital capacity is greater than 10–15 mL/kg of body weight.
- Maximal inspiratory pressure is less than −20 cm H_2O.
- FIO_2 is less than 50% and PaO_2 is greater than 60 mm H_2O.
- Spontaneous tidal volume is greater than 4–5 ml/kg.
- Cough is strong and effective.
- Lungs are acceptably clear on auscultation and x-ray film.
- ABG values are within normal range.
- Cardiac output is adequate.
- Patient is afebrile.
- Nutritional status is satisfactory.

Weaning can be accomplished by several techniques used individually or in combination. These techniques include synchronized intermittent mandatory ventilation, pressure support, and use of a T-piece. When synchronized intermittent mandatory ventilation is used, the number of breaths delivered by the ventilator is gradually decreased, thus increasing the amount of spontaneous breathing done by the patient. Pressure support may be used to augment the spontaneous breaths. The positive pressure with this method is also gradually reduced until the patient is weaned from the ventilator. When a T-piece is used, the patient is disconnected from the ventilator and placed on the T-piece with humidified oxygen at an FIO_2 5 to 10% higher than when the patient is on the ventilator. Time spent off the ventilator begins with 5- to 10-minute intervals and is gradually increased on the basis of patient tolerance.

Whichever technique is used, the patient should be placed in a high Fowler's position and monitored carefully. Vital signs, vital capacity and negative inspiratory force, pulse oximetry readings, and ABGs should be obtained as often as necessary. Signs of intolerance to the weaning procedure may include tachypnea, dyspnea, tachycardia, dysrhythmia, diaphoresis, and change in mental status. Since weaning is an anxiety-provoking experience, reassurance and staying with the patient are important.

Pharmacologic Therapy

Drug therapy plays an important role in the medical management of disorders of the respiratory system. Major categories of drugs specific to the treatment of respiratory problems are nasal decongestants, anti-

---

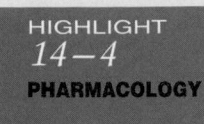 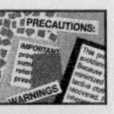

HIGHLIGHT 14–4 PHARMACOLOGY

Decongestants

Definition:

Drugs that reduce swelling of mucous membranes and relieve congestion.

Action:

Directly stimulate α-adrenergic receptors in the nasal mucosa and cause the release of norepinephrine, which in turn causes vasoconstriction with shrinking of the swollen mucous membranes and nasal drainage.

Uses:

Symptomatic relief of nasal congestion caused by rhinitis, coryza, and sinusitis.

Side Effects:

Nervousness, irritability, restlessness, and insomnia caused by central nervous system (CNS) stimulation; occasional nausea; palpitations; difficulty urinating; and dose-related hypertension caused by vasoconstriction and rebound congestion with repeated use. Side effects more likely with oral use as opposed to topical use.

Interactions:

Systemic decongestants (eg, ephedrine and phenylpropanolamine) interact with other sympathomimetics, resulting in increased CNS stimulation; inhibit action of adrenergic blocking agents; and interact with monoamine oxidase inhibitors and can cause severe hypertension.

Nursing Implications:

Counsel the elderly and those with hypertension, hyperthyroidism, cardiovascular disease, and prostatic hypertrophy to take with caution.

Caution patients not to use topical preparations for longer than 5 days because of rebound.

Instruct patients using drops to instill them with the head back and down to decrease the amount swallowed and to allow the solution to spread slowly over the nasal mucosa.

Suggest taking systemic decongestants a few hours before bedtime to decrease the risk of insomnia.

Caution patients not to break, cut, crush, or chew timed-release preparations.

histamines, antitussives, expectorants, mucolytics, and bronchodilators.

Nasal decongestants (Highlight 14–4) are drugs that reduce swelling of the mucosa and thereby promote drainage and relieve congestion. They are primarily over-the-counter drugs and are used to treat both allergic and nonallergic rhinitis (common cold).

Antihistamines are used to relieve sneezing, rhinorrhea, and nasal itching associated with allergic rhinitis. They are most effective when taken prophylactically.

Antitussives (Highlight 14–5) are cough suppressants. They are used to control nonproductive cough and allow the patient to rest. Antitussives should not be used indiscriminately because cough is a protective mechanism designed to remove excessive secretions and foreign matter from the respiratory tract. The most commonly used nonnarcotic antitussive is dextromethorphan, which is an over-the-counter drug with few side effects.

Expectorants (eg, terpin hydrate) are medications that make cough more productive by stimulating the flow of secretions, thus making them more liquid and easier to expectorate. It is questionable whether these drugs are any more effective than fluids, deep-breathing exercises, and position changes in promoting expectoration.

Mucolytics are medications that react with mucus to make it more watery and more easily expectorated. Two solutions used for this purpose are hypertonic saline and acetylcysteine. Both are administered by inhalation, and both can cause reflex bronchospasm.

Bronchodilators (Highlight 14–6) are medications that relax constricted airways. The two major groups of drugs used for their bronchodilator effects are the β_2-adrenergic agonists and the methylxanthines, also referred to simply as xanthines. Theophylline is the major xanthine used in the treatment of asthma. Aminophylline is a theophylline salt. It has identical pharmacologic actions to theophylline but is more soluble and is most often given intravenously.

Chest Drainage

Uses

The lungs are surrounded by the pleura. Under normal conditions, a negative pressure exists within the pleural space, which creates a vacuum that keeps the lungs adherent to the chest wall and permits expansion of the lung as the thorax expands during inspiration. If the integrity of the pleural membranes is disrupted, as in penetrating trauma to the chest wall, thoracic surgery, or open communication with alveoli (eg, ruptured emphysematous bleb), air enters the pleural space and the negative pressure is lost. This results in lung collapse. To remove air or fluid from the chest and thus restore negative pressure to re-expand the lung, a chest tube is inserted. A single chest tube is placed in the pleural space to remove air. To remove air and fluid, two tubes are

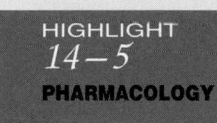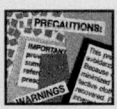

HIGHLIGHT
14–5
PHARMACOLOGY

Antitussives

Definition:

Medications that suppress cough; two major groups: opioids (eg, codeine) and nonopioids (eg, dextromethorphan).

Action:

Decrease the frequency and intensity of cough by directly inhibiting the response of the cough center in the medulla.

Uses:

Suppress cough that has no therapeutic purpose, such as raising secretions, and is causing throat irritation, discomfort, and loss of sleep.

Side Effects:

Side effects are rare at doses used in antitussives. Low risk of addiction and respiratory depression with codeine preparations, none with dextromethorphan. Toxic effects of opioid antitussives include miosis, bradycardia, tachycardia, hypotension, narcosis, seizures, circulatory collapse, respiratory arrest. Toxic effects of dextromethorphan include euphoria, hyperactivity, staggering gait, lethargy, uncoordinated movements, stupor, and shallow breathing.

Interactions:

Opioid antitussives potentiate the depressant effect of monamine oxidase (MAO) inhibitors, alcohol, and other central nervous system (CNS) depressants. Dextromethorphan can interact with MAO inhibitors to cause excitation and hyperpyrexia.

Nursing Implications:

Caution patient not to exceed recommended dose and not to mix with CNS depressants.

Instruct patient to report cough lasting longer than 1 week or changing from nonproductive to productive.

Give with caution to patients with a decreased respiratory reserve.

placed; one anteriorly through the second intercostal space and the other posteriorly through the eighth or ninth intercostal space in the midaxillary line to drain blood or fluid (Fig. 14–24).

Aminophylline toxic affect

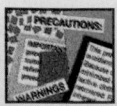

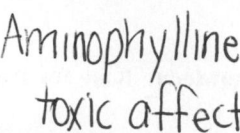

Bronchodilators

Definition:

Medications that relax constricted airways; two groups: β_2-adrenergic agonists (eg, terbutaline [Brethine]) and methylxanthines (eg, theophylline).

Action:

β_2-Adrenergic agonists are selective sympathomimetic drugs that relax the bronchial smooth muscle and result in bronchial dilatation. Methylxanthines also relax bronchial smooth muscles, possibly by blocking the receptors for adenosine.

Uses:

β_2-Adrenergic agonists are given by metered dose inhaler or nebulizer for quick relief of symptoms associated with an acute exacerbation of asthma. Long-acting β_2-agonists, inhaled β_2-agonist tablets, or sustained-release theophylline, are used for long-term control of symptoms in moderate and severe persistent asthma. In some cases, sustained-release theophylline may also be used for long-term control of mild persistent asthma, but it is not the preferred therapy because of its potential toxicity.

Side Effects:

β_2-Adrenergic agonists have minimal side effects when given by inhaler. With oral or parenteral administration, tremor, angina pectoris, and tachydysrhythmias can occur. Theophylline has few side effects at plasma levels below 20 mg/mL. At 20 to 25 mg/mL, nausea, vomiting, diarrhea, insomnia, and restlessness can de-

velop, whereas at levels greater than 30 mg/mL, severe dysrhythmias, convulsions, and death can occur.

Interactions:

β_2-Adrenergic agonist effects can be inhibited by β-adrenergic blocking agents such as propranolol. Theophylline levels can be lowered by marijuana, tobacco, and phenobarbital. They can be increased by oral contraceptives, cimetidine, erythromycin, and caffeine.

Nursing Implications:

β_2-Adrenergic agonist:
  Teach proper use of metered dose inhaler or nebulizer.
  Instruct the patient to wait at least 1 minute between puffs if two puffs or inhales are needed.
  Warn patient against exceeding recommended dosage

Systemic preparation:
  Instruct patient to report chest pain and changes in heart rate or rhythm.
  Administer with caution to patients with diabetes, hyperthyroidism, organic heart disease, hypertension or angina pectoris.

Theophylline:
  Instruct the patient not to break, crush, or chew enteric or timed-release preparations.
  Monitor plasma drug levels.
  Caution the patient to avoid ingestion of caffeine-containing foods or beverages.

Chest-Drainage Apparatus

A chest-drainage system consists of a chest tube attached to a valve mechanism designed to allow air or fluid to drain out of, but not into, the chest cavity. The chest tube is a large-bore catheter, usually a 34 or 36 French. The valve mechanism may be a one-way valve, a water-seal drainage system, or a water-seal drainage system with suction. A one-way valve is a simple unidirectional system in which the chest tube is made of soft material that collapses on inspiration and opens on expiration. Thus, the valve is open only when the pressure within the chest exceeds atmospheric pressure so air and fluid are removed from the chest.

The water-seal drainage system is the most common type in use. The Pleur-evac (Fig. 14–25), Thoraseal, and Medi-Vac systems are examples of water-seal, single-use, disposable, closed-drainage systems. Each of these systems has three chambers: the collection chamber, the water-seal chamber, and the suction control chamber. The collection chamber is where the chest tube from the patient connects to the system. Drainage from the tube drains into and collects in a series of calibrated columns in this chamber.

The second chamber provides a water seal, which establishes 2 cm of water pressure. If positive pressure in the pleural space is greater than 2 cm, air or fluid is expelled into the drainage system. The water seal allows for air to move from the pleural space into the drainage system but not back into the chest. In a properly functioning system, the water oscillates (moves up as the patient inhales and moves down as the patient exhales). Bubbling indicates an air leak from the lung or bronchus.

The third chamber provides the suction, which can be controlled to provide negative pressure to the chest. This may be necessary when there is a large air leak or large amount of fluid or when negative intrathoracic pressure must be re-established. The suction control chamber can be filled with various levels of water to achieve the desired level of suction. Suction is controlled in this manner because hospital suction pumps create large amounts of negative pressure. Without this control, lung tissue could be sucked into the chest tube. Bubbling in the suction control chamber indicates there is suction. It does not indicate that air is escaping from the pleural space. A water-seal drainage system can be used with or without a hospital suction pump attached.

Chest Tube Insertion

Chest tubes may be inserted at the time of surgery through an open thoracotomy incision or may be inserted via a closed thoracotomy procedure at the bedside. For the closed procedure, the patient either sits or lies down with the affected side up. After the area is prepared and local anesthetic injected, a

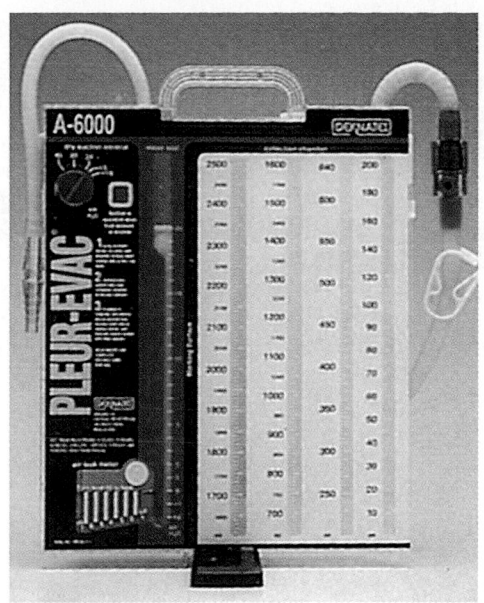

Figure 14–25

Pleur-evac disposable chest drainage system. (Courtesy of Deknatel DSP, Tucker, GA)

small incision is made into the chest wall. A clamp is then pushed through the incision into the intercostal space and into the pleural cavity. A chest tube marked for distance to be inserted and clamped at its free end is immediately inserted. Regardless of the method of insertion, the wound is closed and the tube is sutured to the chest wall. Its free end is then connected to the drainage system selected by the physician. All connections are securely taped to maintain an airtight system that re-establishes negative intrapleural pressure. An occlusive sterile dressing is applied to the insertion site, the first layer of which is usually a petrolatum jelly gauze. A chest x-ray is taken to check the position of the tube and to determine whether the lung has re-expanded.

NURSING PROCESS
Chest Drainage

Assessment

Assess the patient's respiratory status. Auscultate the lungs every 2 hours. Take vital signs every 4 hours. Note the quality of respirations, observe for abnormal chest movements, and check for cyanosis. Be alert to the possibility of an extended pneumothorax or hemothorax resulting from chest-drainage malfunction. Symptoms of extended pneumothorax are increased area of absent breath sounds and hyperresonant percussion note, increased tachycardia, increased respiratory distress, cyanosis, restlessness, sudden sharp chest pain, and confusion. Symptoms of hemothorax are diminished or absent breath sounds, dyspnea, and cyanosis.

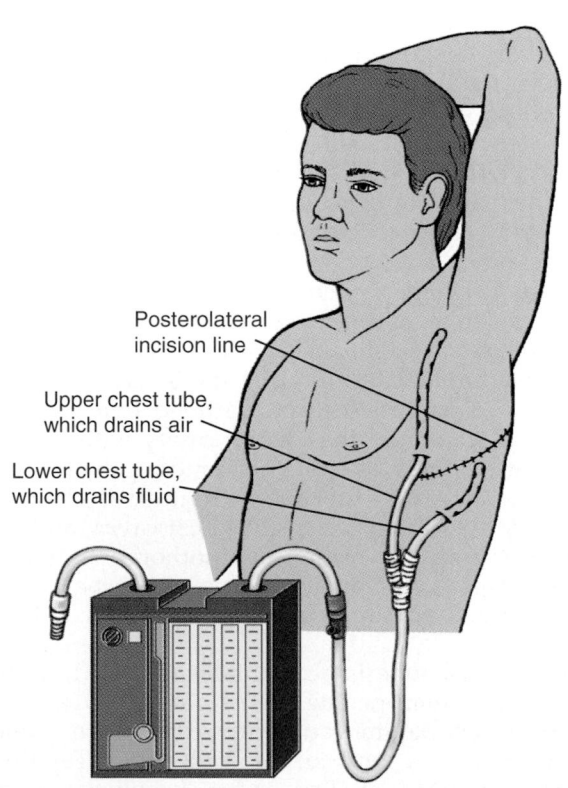

Posterolateral incision line

Upper chest tube, which drains air

Lower chest tube, which drains fluid

Figure 14–24

Placement of chest tubes for air and fluid drainage.

Assess the function of the chest drainage system hourly. Check that the drainage system is below the level of the patient's chest and is free of kinks, dependent loops, or other external obstruction. Check that all connections are secure. Note the color (serous, sanguineous, or serosanguineous) and amount of drainage since the previous check, keeping in mind that drainage should not exceed 200 mL/hour for 2 consecutive hours. Observe the chest-tube dressing. Note the amount and type of drainage and whether the taped connections are intact. Observe for fluctuation of the fluid level in the water-seal chamber, because its presence indicates a patent drainage system. Remember that, with normal breathing, the water level rises with inspiration and falls with expiration, whereas the opposite (falls with inspiration and rises with expiration) occurs when the patient is on positive pressure mechanical ventilation. Keep in mind too that fluctuation stops if the tube is obstructed, if a dependent loop exists, if the suction is not working properly, and if the lung has re-expanded. When observing for fluctuation, also look for bubbling in the water-seal chamber. If the patient has a known pneumothorax, intermittent bubbling is expected as air is drained from the chest, but constant bubbling is indicative of an air leak in the system. In the patient without a known pneumothorax, any bubbling in the water-seal chamber is suggestive of an air leak.

Assess the patient's anxiety level and his or her understanding of chest drainage. This is important because anxiety can increase the need for oxygen, and patients with conditions affecting the lungs are prone to anxiety because breathing is so essential to life. Be alert to verbal expressions of excessive anxiety as well as other indicators such as reluctance to move, frequent requests to check the drainage system, and inability to attend to information and directions.

Nursing Diagnoses and Planning

Nursing diagnoses and related expected patient outcomes commonly applicable to patients with chest drainage include the following:

NDx: Ineffective breathing pattern related to decreased lung expansion

Planning: Patient Outcomes
1. Breath sounds are normal.
2. Respirations are unlabored and occur at a rate of 16 to 20 per minute.
3. ABG values are approaching normal.
4. Lung re-expansion is seen on chest x-ray.

NDx: Anxiety related to perceived risk of chest tube dislodgement, system disruption, inability to breathe

Planning: Patient Outcomes
1. Patient realistically describes precautions to be observed relative to the chest-drainage system.
2. Patient describes expected drainage in terms of color and amount and describes normal fluctuation and bubbling in the system.

Nursing Interventions and Evaluation

NDx: Ineffective breathing pattern
Maintain an airtight, patent, functioning chest-drainage system. Retape all connections as needed. Retape chest-tube dressing if tape is loose. If the dressing becomes saturated with drainage, reinforce and tape securely or, if allowed, remove and replace wet gauze, being certain not to disrupt the petrolatum gauze seal. Keep the tubing free of loops, kinks, or other external pressure that could interfere with drainage or even force drainage back into the pleural space. Place a rolled towel under the chest tube when the patient is lying on the affected side to protect it from the body's weight.

Encourage the patient to cough and deep breathe frequently. This increases intrapleural pressure and promotes outflow of air and fluid through the chest tube and hence re-expansion of the lung. Change the patient's position frequently to promote both drainage and ventilation.

If fluctuation in the water-seal chamber ceases and the tubing is not kinked or otherwise obstructed, immediately ask the patient to cough or change position. If fluctuation does not begin, milk the tube in the direction of the drainage system. To do this, take hold of the tube close to the chest, squeezing it between the fingers and palm of the hand. Place the other hand around the tube just under the first hand and squeeze. Release the first hand, place it under the second hand, and squeeze. Repeat the length of the tube. This action briefly increases the negative pressure applied to the intrapleural space and moves drainage toward the drainage system. Do not milk a tube if an air leak exists unless specifically directed by a physician.

If fluctuation and free drainage still do not occur, notify the physician because tube replacement may be necessary.

If the drainage system is broken or interrupted, clamp the tube or place the end of the tube in a bottle of sterile saline held below the level of the chest and immediately replace the system. Remember that a chest tube can be clamped only momentarily if air can enter the pleural cavity with inspiration. This is because the air entering with each breath has no way to escape if the tube is clamped; therefore, it accumulates in the chest cavity and collapses the lung (a tension pneumothorax). Some institutional protocols require that a clamp be kept at the bedside at all times in case the system is interrupted.

If the chest tube is accidentally removed, immediately cover the opening in the chest wall with an occlusive, petrolatum gauze dressing, one of which should be kept at the bedside at all times. Tape this dressing in place on three sides. Leave the fourth side untaped so that if there is air leaking into the chest it can escape rather than causing a tension pneumothorax. In the event of an emergency, a gloved hand can become a nonocclusive dressing until supplies can be obtained.

NDx: Anxiety

Provide the patient with basic information about the chest-drainage system to allay anxiety. Explain that, although care must be taken not to exert pull on the tube, it is sutured in place at the chest wall and therefore moving in bed, sitting up, and walking will not cause it to be displaced. Do stress, however, that it is important that the tube not be kinked or compressed and that the drainage apparatus must be kept below chest level. Prepare the patient for the type and amount of drainage expected. For example, the patient should know that, after chest surgery, bright red drainage gradually decreasing in amount is normal for the first 72 hours. Also point out the normal fluctuation and bubbling in the system. Tell the patient about the frequent checks of the system so he or she is aware that this constitutes routine care and is not led to believe there is something wrong. Provide time for the patient to ask questions and express concerns. Reassure the patient that a staff member is nearby and provide easy access to the call bell or intercom.

Additional Interventions

Mark the amount of chest drainage in the collection chamber at 1- to 4-hour intervals. Do this by placing a piece of tape vertically on the container and drawing a line with date and hour noted each time the drainage is checked. This allows the change in the amount of drainage to be evaluated over time and, if the drainage is bloody, serves as a basis for blood replacement.

Notify the physician if there is constant bubbling in the water-seal chamber or if drainage becomes bright red or increases suddenly.

Compare the patient's status with the expected outcomes. If the outcomes are not met, reassess the patient and revise the plan.

Chest Tube Removal

Chest tubes are removed when x-ray films confirm the full re-expansion of the lung or when there is no fluctuation of fluid in the tubing. Thirty minutes before removal, the patient is usually given pain medication. When the medication has taken effect, the sutures are cut. A petrolatum gauze dressing is placed at the chest wall ready to occlude the opening so air does not enter the chest; the patient is asked to perform the Valsalva maneuver (take a deep breath, exhale, and bear down), the tube is quickly withdrawn, and an airtight dressing is taped in place. The pleura seals itself off, and the wound heals in less than a week.

After the dressing is removed, the patient is monitored for respiratory distress, and the dressing is checked for drainage.

Heimlich Valve

The Heimlich valve is a one-way valve that can be used in place of underwater chest drainage in selected patients. This valve consists of rubber flutter leaflets encased in a shell of clear hard plastic. These leaflets, which are compressed at their distal end, allow unidirectional flow of air, fluid, or blood clots out of the chest. The valve is connected to the chest tube or small-bore percutaneous thoracic catheter by means of a connecting tube that has a one-way stopcock at the end that attaches to the chest tube or thoracic catheter. If the tube is being used to treat a pneumothorax, the distal end of the valve is left uncovered. If it is being used to drain blood or fluid, a sterile drainage bag with a vent is attached to its distal end.

A major advantage of the Heimlich valve is that it allows for patient mobility because it is small and lightweight and does not have to be maintined below the level of the patient's chest to function. If needed, the distal end of the valve can be connected to suction or the connecting tube can be disconnected from the stopcock and a syringe attached that can be used to withdraw air of fluid or instill intrapleural analgesic or sclerosing agents. The valve can also be easily disconnected and the connecting tube attached to an underwater drainage system.

NURSING PROCESS GUIDELINES
Heimlich Valve

Make certain that the arrow on the valve is pointing away from the patient. This is critical because the arrow indicates the direction of flow, and, if the valve is reversed, air can flow into the pleural space, creating a life-threatening tension pneumothorax. Monitor tubing regularly to ensure that it is free of kinks and that all connections are airtight. Change dressing according to agency protocol. Between changes, check at regular intervals to make certian the dressing is intact. Expect to hear air exiting the distal end of the valve as the patient breathes and coughs if being used to treat a pneumothorax. Also expect to see the valve flutter as intrapleural pressure changes. Recognize, however, that although the absence of fluttering does not necessarily represent a problem, it can indicate that the system is blocked. This requires that the valve and tubing be carefully inspected. At the same time, the patient should be assessed for dyspnea, and the lung sounds should be auscultated.

If the patient is being discharged home with a Heimlich valve in place, explain how the valve works and the importance of keeping the dressing and tubing connections airtight. Teach the patient or family how and when to change the dressing; how to dispose of used dressings and drainage; and how to recognize a wound infection. Instruct the patient to check the integrity of all tubing connections if he or she becomes short of breath or develops chest pain or if the valve stops fluttering. If connections are not leaking and symptoms do not disappear, instruct the patient to contact a health-care provider immediately. Be certain to send a back-up valve home with the patient in the event the valve needs to be changed. When the valve is changed, the patient performs the Valsalva maneuver while the stopcock on the connecting tubing is turned to "off." The old valve is then disconnected, the new valve attached, and the stopcock reopened.

SURGICAL MANAGEMENT

Overview of Thoracic Surgery

Thoracic surgery refers to any operative procedure performed on a structure within the chest cavity or on the chest wall. It includes surgery on the heart, esophagus, and mediastinum as well as a variety of surgical procedures performed to maintain respiratory function and to treat lower respiratory tract disorders (Table 14–8). A special category of thoracic surgery is thorascopic surgery (also referred to as video-assisted thoracic surgery), which is performed endoscopically and is discussed separately.

Three basic incisions are used in conventional thoracic surgery: median sternotomy, anterolateral thoracotomy, and posterolateral thoracotomy. A median sternotomy incision is used primarily for cardiac and other surgery involving the mediastinum. An anterolateral thoracotomy incision is used for relatively simple thoracic procedures such as a lung biopsy. The third type of incision, the posterolateral thoracotomy, is used for the majority of complex procedures involving the lung because it allows good visualization and easy access.

After most thoracic surgery, one or more chest tubes are placed in the pleural space to drain air, blood, or other fluid; restore negative pressure; and allow re-expansion of the lung, which would have collapsed as a result of the change in intrathoracic pressure when the chest was opened. Chest tubes are not used after a pneumonectomy because there is no lung to reinflate, and fluid that ultimately solidifies is allowed to fill the remaining space in the thorax.

Patient Preparation for Thoracic Surgery

The respiratory and cardiac status of the patient is carefully assessed preoperatively because the success

Table 14–8

Thoracic Surgical Procedures Used in the Management of Respiratory Disorders			
Procedure	**Description**	**Usual Incision**	**Uses**
Pneumonectomy	Removal of an entire lung	Posterolateral	Primarily for cancer; sometimes for lung abscess, bronchiectasis, extensive unilateral tuberculosis
Radical pneumonectomy	Removal of a lung and anterior and posterior mediastinal and tracheobronchial nodes on affected side	Posterolateral	Lung cancer
Lobectomy	Removal of one lobe of lung	Posterolateral or anterolateral	Cancer, bronchiectasis, emphysematous bleb
Wedge resection	Removal of a small section of the lung	Anterolateral for upper and middle lobes, posterolateral for lower lobe	Used to remove small lesions located near the surface
Open-lung biopsy	Removal of small specimen of lung tissue	Anterolateral	Diagnostic tissue examination
Closed thoracotomy (thoracostomy)	Percutaneous insertion of chest tube through intercostal space into pleural cavity	Small incision in midclavicular line: over 2nd to 5th intercostal spaces to remove air; 6th to 8th intercostal spaces posteriorly to remove fluid	To remove blood, fluid, or air in cases of hemothorax, pleural effusion, pneumothorax, or acute empyema
Open thoracotomy (thoracostomy or partial rib resection)	Removal of part of rib(s) to establish continuous drainage	Posterolateral	Acute empyema

of the surgery is largely dependent on the function of these systems. Chest x-rays, lung scans, and an electrocardiogram are obtained. Pulmonary function tests are done to determine whether the proposed surgery will leave sufficient functioning lung tissue. ABGs are determined to provide an additional measure of pulmonary reserve and to provide baseline data for postoperative assessment. An exercise tolerance test may also be done preoperatively, especially when a pneumonectomy is being considered.

Other preoperative laboratory studies include blood glucose, electrolytes, coagulation studies, serum protein studies and a complete blood count.

Patients who smoke are encouraged to stop or at least cut down preoperatively to decrease secretions and to increase oxygen saturation. Antibiotics may be ordered to combat existing infection, and postural drainage may be used to remove excessive secretions.

Complications of Thoracic Surgery

Complications after thoracic surgery include atelectasis (most often caused by retained bronchial secretions), pneumonia, hemorrhage, cardiac dysrhythmia, and pulmonary edema secondary to hypervolemia from overinfusion of fluids. Other complications unique to surgery on the lung include bronchopleural fistula, empyema, persistent air leak, and subcutaneous emphysema.

A bronchopleural fistula is an abnormal opening between a bronchus and the pleural space. Symptoms of these fistulas that may develop during the first postoperative week are hemoptysis, fever, subcutaneous emphysema, and a severe air leak. Management usually involves surgical reclosure of the bronchial stump, although occasionally a pneumonectomy may be required.

Empyema is the presence of pus in the pleural cavity. It is characterized by fever, pleuritic pain, and dullness on percussion over the affected area. It is treated with chest drainage and systemic antibiotics.

A persistent air leak occurs when openings in the lung tissue fail to close spontaneously within 72 hours of surgery. An air leak is indicated by bubbling in the water-seal chamber of the chest-drainage apparatus. A persistent air leak can be treated by the injection of a sclerosing agent into the pleural cavity or by surgery.

Subcutaneous emphysema is the presence of air under the skin resulting from its escape from the respiratory tract. Subcutaneous emphysema can be due to a persistent air leak or a blocked chest tube. Symptoms are puffiness of the skin and crepitation (presence of a crackling sound like that produced by crumpling cellophane) when the area is palpated.

Respiratory failure and hypotension are also potential complications of thoracic surgery.

Pneumonectomy

Pneumonectomy is the surgical removal of an entire lung.

Uses

Pneumonectomy is performed to treat bronchogenic carcinoma, lung abscess, bronchiectasis, or extensive unilateral tuberculosis. It is done only when disease is so extensive that all involved tissue cannot be removed by a lobectomy.

Procedure

Most pneumonectomies are done through a posterolateral thoracotomy incision. Once the incision is made, the ribs are spread with a retractor, the pleura is entered, and the affected lung collapses because of the change in pressure that occurs when the pleura is opened. The bronchus is transected, the pulmonary artery and veins are ligated and severed, the lung is removed, and the bronchial stump is stapled. The phrenic nerve is severed or crushed. This paralyzes the diaphragm in an elevated position and decreases the size of the chest cavity on the operative side. During the procedure, the remaining lung is ventilated by means of an endotracheal tube and a mechanical ventilator. A chest tube is not generally inserted during a pneumonectomy; rather, the space is left to fill with serosanguineous fluid, which eventually solidifies.

Because pain after a thoracotomy is severe, a nerve block with a long-acting oral anesthetic may be performed just before the incision is closed.

Postoperative Course

After a pneumonectomy, there is relatively severe pain in the chest and shoulder because of the retraction of the ribs, transection of muscles and other tissues, and irritation of the intercostal nerves. This results in guarding of the operative area and a predisposition to hypoventilation and atelectasis. To prevent impaired mobility and its effects, breathing exercises and arm and shoulder exercises are begun in the immediate postoperative period. The patient is dangled on the evening of surgery and is ambulated on the first postoperative day. Oxygen is generally administered for the first 24 hours.

Intravenous fluids are administered until the patient is stable and oral intake is well established. The rate of administration may be as low as 10 mL per hour because of the risk of pulmonary edema resulting from the decrease in pulmonary vasculature. Oral fluids are begun as soon as the patient is alert, provided that the abdomen has not been opened and bowel sounds are present. Intake is then increased as tolerated, with a return to a normal diet by the third postoperative day.

The wound is covered with a light dressing at the time of surgery. Because little drainage is expected, it may be left open to the air after 24 hours. Sutures are removed in 1 week, but altered sensation, numbness, or tenderness may persist for months in the area surrounding the incision.

NURSING PROCESS
Pneumonectomy

PREOPERATIVE NURSING CARE

Assessment

Perform a complete respiratory assessment. Question about signs and symptoms related to the patient's respiratory problem. Ask about cough, expectoration, hemoptysis, chest pain, and dyspnea. Assess breathing pattern and determine the amount of exertion needed to produce dyspnea. Assess the patient's respiratory status while performing activities of daily living. Question about exposure to respiratory irritants and obtain a smoking history. Determine whether the patient currently smokes and how much. If the patient previously smoked, ask how much, for how long, and when he or she stopped.

Assess the patient's general physical status. Note general appearance, mental alertness, and apparent nutritional status. Question about any coexisting medical problems that may have implications for preoperative and postoperative care. List all medications taken by the patient, noting purpose and frequency of use, dose, and perceived effectiveness.

Observe the patient for signs of anxiety and assess the patient's understanding of the planned surgery and its expected outcome.

Nursing Diagnoses and Planning

Nursing diagnoses and related expected patient outcomes commonly applicable to patients scheduled for a pneumonectomy include the following:

NDx: Anxiety related to the surgical procedure and the postoperative course

Planning: Patient Outcomes
1. Patient verbalizes that feelings of anxiety are decreased.
2. Patient verbalizes an understanding of perioperative events.
3. Facial expression and body posture appear relaxed.
4. Vital signs are stable.

NDx: Risk for altered health maintenance related to insufficient knowledge of breathing exercises, effective coughing, wound splinting, arm and shoulder exercises

Planning: Patient Outcomes
1. Patient describes the role of breathing exercises, coughing, and arm and shoulder exercises in recovery.
2. Patient demonstrates breathing exercises and effective coughing.

3. Patient demonstrates methods of splinting the incision.
4. Patient demonstrates arm and shoulder exercises to be initiated in the early postoperative period.

Nursing Interventions and Evaluation

NDx: Anxiety
Provide the patient with basic information about the operative experience, such as preoperative preparation, the location of the incision, and what happens in the postanesthesia care unit. Prepare the patient for the presence of a central venous pressure catheter, arterial catheter, pulmonary artery catheter, urinary bladder catheter, and oxygen equipment. Avoid providing unnecessary detail that could add to the patient's anxiety rather than allay it. If the patient will be going to an intensive care unit, explain the environment or arrange a visit if possible.

Because one of the most common concerns of patients facing a pneumonectomy relates to the ability to breathe after surgery, explain the functional reserve of the respiratory system and reinforce that one of the purposes of many of the preoperative tests is to ensure that he or she is able to tolerate the removal of a lung. Also acknowledge pain as a concern and reassure the patient that, although significant pain is normal, analgesics will be given to control it.

Remember that significant others are often as anxious as the patient; therefore, provide the opportunity for them as well as the patient to ask questions and express their concerns.

NDx: Risk for altered health maintenance
Explain that deep-breathing and coughing help to clear secretions from the airways and facilitate good ventilation of the remaining lung. Acknowledge that it is not easy to cough and deep-breathe immediately after surgery but stress their importance. Reassure that discomfort will be minimized by splinting the incision and by the administration of pain medication. Explain, demonstrate, and have the patient practice diaphragmatic and pursed-lip breathing. Help the patient practice effective coughing as follows:

- Sit the patient upright with slightly flexed knees. If the patient is unable to sit upright, position him or her on the side with hips and knees flexed.
- Splint the incision site with the flat of your hands.
- Ask the patient to take two or three short breaths followed by a deep inspiration.
- Instruct the patient to contract (pull in) the abdominal muscles and cough forcefully with the mouth open.
- Explain that a folded blanket or sheet or a pillow can also be used to splint the incision, and demonstrate their use (Fig. 14–26).

Provide the patient with an incentive spirometer.

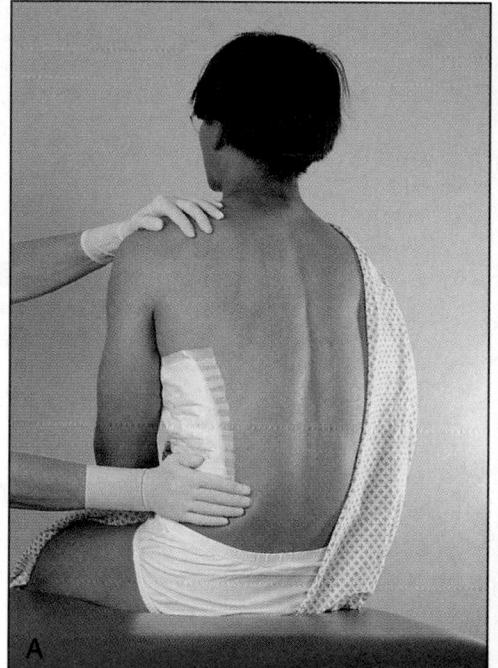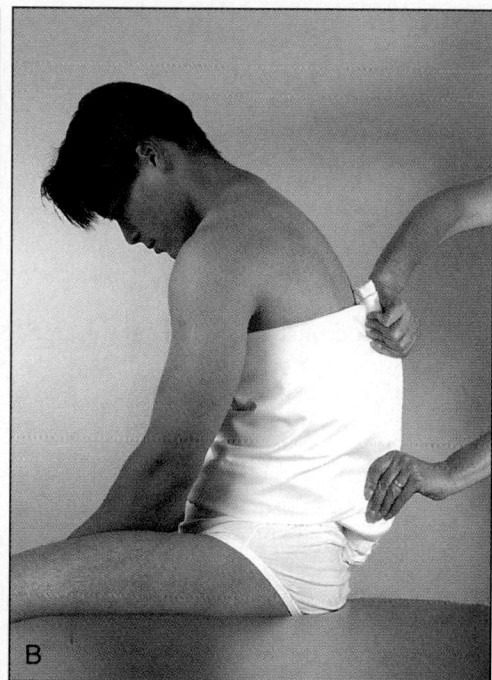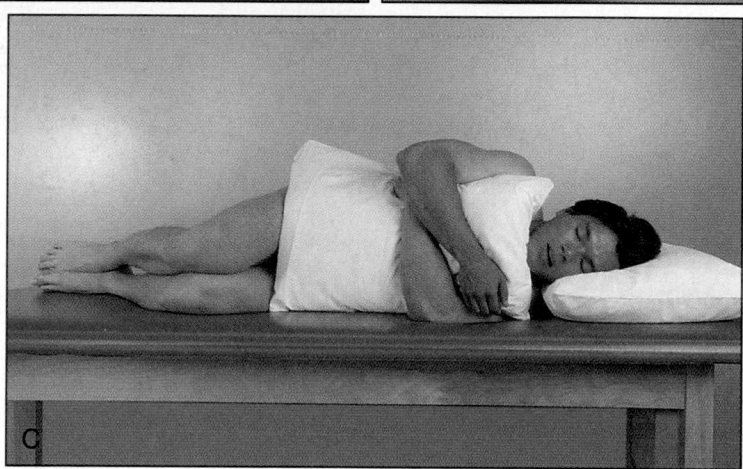

Figure 14-26

Methods of splinting a thoracotomy incision: *A,* with the flat of the hands; *B,* with a folded blanket; *C,* with a pillow.

Describe its use and encourage the patient to try it in preparation for postoperative use.

Describe to the patient the effect of the surgery on the movement of the chest and shoulder. Explain that passive range-of-motion exercises to the shoulder will be started immediately after surgery to prevent the development of stiffening, limited motion, and ultimately greater discomfort. Familiarize the patient with the range-of-motion exercises by performing them on his or her shoulder. Tell the patient that additional active exercises will be started as he or she progresses in the postoperative period. Explain that they help the patient regain muscle strength as well as maintain free movement of the joint and will have to be continued after the patient returns home.

Additional Interventions

Prepare the patient for preoperative diagnostic tests and institute measures to remove secretions and improve alveolar ventilation. Depending on the patient's condition and the physician's orders, these measures may include forced fluids, humidification to loosen secretions, administration of bronchodilators, chest percussion, and postural drainage.

Instruct all patients on the importance of avoiding exposure to cigarette smoke and other bronchial irritants. Ensure that the preoperative preparation is completed according to the surgeon's directions and that preoperative medications are given as ordered.

Compare the patient's status with the expected outcomes. If the outcomes are not met, reassess the patient and revise the plan.

POSTOPERATIVE NURSING CARE

Assessment

In the immediate postoperative period, assess return to physiologic stability. Pay particular attention to respiratory status and cardiac status. Check respiratory rate and observe for signs and symptoms of respiratory dysfunction every 15 minutes until stable and then every hour. Observe for slow, rapid, shallow, or irregular respirations; use of accessory muscles; orthopnea; duskiness or cyanosis; restlessness; irritability; confusion; and somnolence. Auscultate the chest for adventitious breath sounds and for diminished or absent breath sounds over areas of remaining lung tissue. Review ABG values and chest x-ray results.

Check heart rate and blood pressure every 15 minutes until stable and then every hour. Remember that continuous readings of blood pressure and pulmonary artery pressures are presented on oscilloscopes attached to a pulmonary artery catheter. Take central venous pressure readings every hour to assess right ventricular function. Measure pulmonary capillary wedge pressures every 1 to 2 hours if ordered to assess left ventricular function.

Take the patient's temperature every hour, because a change in temperature alters the metabolism and hence cardiac output. A temperature elevation is also indicative of fever.

Assess fluid and electrolyte status. Measure intake and output and observe for signs of overhydration or underhydration. Remember that a CVP reading below the normal range of 5 to 12 cm of water is suggestive of hypovolemia, whereas an elevated CVP reading suggests hypervolemia. Keep in mind that at least 30 mL of urine should be excreted per hour.

While a dressing is in place, check it for drainage, noting color and amount. Remember that bloody drainage is not expected. When the dressing is removed, assess the incision every 8 hours. Observe for signs of infection: redness, heat, induration, swelling, lack of approximation, and drainage.

Assess for signs of developing complications. Observe continuous electrocardiographic readings for dysrhythmias, because patients who have had a pneumonectomy are at particular risk. Keep in mind that the dysrhythmias most likely to occur are atrial fibrillation and atrial flutter. Observe for signs of pulmonary edema because the decrease in the pulmonary vascular bed places the patient who has had a pneumonectomy at high risk. Be alert for symptoms of pulmonary edema: severe dyspnea, tachycardia, dull percussion note over unoperated areas, adventitious breath sounds, persistent cough with frothy or blood-tinged sputum, cyanosis, and apprehension. Also observe for signs and symptoms of mediastinal shift, which is the movement of the mediastinum including the heart, trachea, esophagus, and great vessels to one side of the thorax and which is a risk after pneumonectomy because one side of the thorax is no longer occupied by a lung.

Symptoms of mediastinal shift include severe dyspnea, restlessness, agitation, rapid or irregular pulse, cyanosis, displacement of the trachea from the midline, and a change in the point of apical impulse.

Nursing Diagnoses and Planning

Nursing diagnoses and related expected patient outcomes commonly applicable to patients after a pneumonectomy include the following:

NDx: Ineffective breathing pattern related to unwillingness to breathe deeply secondary to pain and the depressant effects of anesthesia and analgesia

Planning: Patient Outcomes
1. Breath sounds and percussion note over the remaining lung are normal.
2. ABG values are within normal range.

NDx: Ineffective airway clearance related to increased secretions secondary to respiratory tract irritation and poor cough effort secondary to pain and the depressant effects of anesthesia and analgesia

Planning: Patient Outcomes
1. Respirations are easy and quiet at a rate of 12 to 20 per minute.
2. Breath sounds and percussion note over remaining lung are normal.
3. ABG values are within normal range.

NDx: Pain (chest and shoulder) related to surgical trauma to muscles, nerves, and other tissues

Planning: Patient Outcomes
1. Patient states pain is relieved.
2. Patient exhibits a relaxed body posture.
3. Facial expression is relaxed.
4. Patient coughs effectively.
5. Patient moves easily.

NDx: Impaired physical mobility related to transection of chest muscles, which move shoulder, and severe pain in the chest and shoulder

Planning: Patient Outcomes
1. Patient moves shoulder on affected side through usual active range of motion.
2. Patient uses affected arm in performing activities of daily living.
3. Patient exhibits an erect posture.

NDx: Body image disturbance related to loss of a lung and the accompanying change in respiratory function

Planning: Patient Outcomes
1. Patient realistically describes change in physical status related to loss of a lung.
2. Patient realistically identifies changes in lifestyle required by altered respiratory status.
3. Patient verbalizes acceptance of the change in respiratory status.

NDx: Risk for altered health maintenance related to insufficient knowledge of self-care after pneumonectomy

Planning: Patient Outcomes
1. Patient describes self-care after discharge as presented in Highlight 14–7.
2. Patient demonstrates arm and shoulder exercises to be done at home to regain muscle strength.

Nursing Interventions and Evaluation

NDx: Ineffective breathing pattern
Position the patient on the back or with the unoperated side up to promote maximum ventilation of the remaining lung and to help the fluid that accumulates in the pleural space remain below the level of the bronchial stump. Direct the patient in diaphragmatic and pursed-lip breathing and use of an incentive spirometer every 1 to 2 hours to prevent atelectasis. Assist the patient to splint the incision during these breathing exercises and coordinate them with the time when analgesic medications are exerting their peak effect.

Administer oxygen as ordered and monitor ABG values and oxygen saturation via pulse oximeter. Space patient care activities to provide for frequent rest periods and thus decrease demand on the respiratory system.

NDx: Ineffective airway clearance
Assist the patient to cough and deep-breathe and turn every 1 to 2 hours. For maximum effectiveness, assist the patient to a sitting position with the knees slightly flexed. If the patient is unable to sit upright, position the patient on the side with hips and knees flexed. Also assist the patient to splint the incision. Time the activity to correspond with the action of analgesic medications. Monitor breath sounds before and after each coughing and deep-breathing exercise. Record auscultatory finding as well as the amount, color, and viscosity of the expectorate. If the patient is unable to cough, use huffing rather than coughing to promote ventilation and raise secretions. Tell the patient to take a deep diaphragmatic breath and exhale forcefully in a rapid, distinct pant or huff. The effectiveness of huffing is enhanced if it is accompanied by a chest compression technique. To compress the chest, ask the patient to move the upper arms outward to a position midway between the shoulders and the chest. Then instruct the patient to move both upper arms briskly and firmly toward the chest as he or she exhales. Guide the patient in diaphragmatic breathing exercises and perform percussion, vibration, or postural drainage if ordered to facilitate the removal of copious secretions. Do not percuss or vibrate over the operative site. Administer humidification and mininebulizer therapy if ordered to moisten and thin secretions and to facilitate expectoration. Suction if secretions are present and are not being raised.

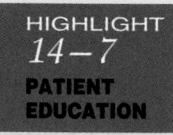 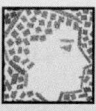

HIGHLIGHT
14–7
PATIENT EDUCATION

Discharge Instructions After Pneumonectomy

Instruct the patient to:

Perform breathing exercises as taught for the first 3 weeks at home.

Perform arm and shoulder exercises five times a day.

Practice standing fully erect in front of a mirror until normal posture is restored.

Expect soreness in the chest and shoulder for several weeks.

Use hot soaks or a heating pad to relieve chest or shoulder pain.

Take prescribed or recommended over-the-counter oral analgesics if additional relief is needed.

Expect altered sensation around the incision for several weeks.

Expect feelings of weakness and fatigue for the first 3 weeks after surgery.

Space activities to allow for frequent rest periods.

Avoid heavy lifting (more than 20 pounds) until muscles of the chest wall have healed completely in 3 to 6 months.

Build up tolerance to walking by using a moderate pace and by gradually increasing distance and duration.

Stop any activity that causes chest pain, shortness of breath, or excessive fatigue.

Stop or decrease smoking if a smoker.

Avoid exposure to smoke, fumes, aerosol sprays, and other respiratory tract irritants.

Avoid exposure to colds and other respiratory infections.

Obtain annual influenza vaccine and pneumonia vaccine as recommended by physician.

Report signs of respiratory infection: persistent fever, increased sputum production, shortness of breath, or increased discomfort or decreased mobility in affected arm and shoulder.

Return for follow-up evaluation of wound healing and respiratory function on *(specify date and time).*

NDx: Pain

Administer prescribed narcotic analgesics as needed around the clock for the first 24 hours postoperatively to keep the patient comfortable, to enable him or her to deep-breathe and cough effectively, and to keep the patient willing to turn, ambulate, and perform arm and shoulder exercises. Effective coughing, deep-breathing, turning, and moving are essential to good ventilation in the remaining lung. Arm and shoulder exercises are essential to return of full range of motion and use of the extremity. Administer analgesics before the pain becomes severe or 30 to 40 minutes before painful exercises are done. Be careful not to medicate the patient to the point at which respirations are depressed or the patient is too somnolent to effectively cough and deep-breathe, because this leads to poor ventilation and an increased risk of complications. After 48 to 72 hours, give oral analgesics such as codeine or acetaminophen as ordered to control pain. Thirty minutes after administering an analgesic ask the patient if the pain has been relieved. If effective pain relief has not been obtained, consult with the physician.

To prevent unnecessary pain, assist the patient to splint the incision with hands, folded sheet, or pillow when moving, coughing, or deep-breathing to reduce pull on inflamed tissues at the incision line. Similarly, support the affected arm and shoulder with pillows or a sling to reduce pull on transected muscles. Promote comfort and the use of relaxation exercises or guided imagery. Maintain a calm, quiet environment and provide diversions such as the radio or television in accordance with the patient's condition and preferences.

NDx: Impaired physical mobility

Perform passive range-of-motion exercises to the affected shoulder a minimum of two times every 4 to 6 hours for the first 24 hours postoperatively. Subsequently, instruct and guide the patient in active arm and shoulder exercises 10 to 20 times every 2 hours. There are many different active exercises that can be used, and some surgeons have a prepared regimen. Examples of exercises used are:

- Shoulder shrugs
- Wall climbing
- Reaching behind the back with the affected arm and trying to touch the opposite scapula
- Reaching over the chest and touching the opposite acromial process
- Extending the arm up and back, out to the side, and back and down at the side
- Placing the hands in the small of the back and pushing the elbows as far back as possible

In addition to scheduled exercises, structure the environment to encourage the use of the affected arm. Place frequently used articles to the patient's operative side to encourage reaching with the affected arm. Attach a rope to the foot of the bed and encourage the patient to pull on it with the affected arm to rise up to a sitting position. Also encourage the use of the affected arm in self-care activities. Recognize that use will vary depending on whether the patient's dominant side is involved. Be alert to the patient's posture and remind the patient as necessary to assume a fully erect position with the affected shoulder back and level with the unaffected one. Guide the patient in diaphragmatic breathing to mobilize the thorax.

NDx: Body image disturbance

Encourage the patient to verbalize feelings about the loss of a lung because confronting these feelings is the first step in coping. Recognize that the patient may feel angry, fearful, sad, or helpless and acknowledge the feelings as real and valid. Assist the patient to realistically identify the effect of the loss of the lung on respiratory status, physical stamina, and function. Review usual activities and lifestyle patterns with the patient and encourage identification of areas that will be unaffected by the surgery. Also help the patient to determine changes that are needed and to identify viable options. Facilitate discussion of changes and options between the patient and significant others and encourage sharing of mutual concerns. Make referrals to appropriate support groups or community resources such as the American Lung Association.

NDx: Risk for altered health maintenance

Instruct the patient in self-care after discharge (see Highlight 14–7).

Additional Interventions

Give fluids by mouth as soon as the patient is alert, and advance the patient to the regular prescribed diet as tolerated. Weigh the patient daily.

Report a temperature of 38.8°C (102°F) or higher to the physician. Also report a temperature of less than 36.6°C (98°F). A variation in temperature alters metabolism and increases the demand on the respiratory system. To protect the patient from this physiologic stress, antipyretics are given for temperatures of 38.8°C (102°F) or higher, a cooling mattress is used for temperatures of 40°C (104°F) or higher, and blankets and heating pads are used for hypothermia.

Notify the physician immediately if sputum is excessive or if it contains bright red blood.

Compare the patient's status with the expected outcomes. If the outcomes are not met, reassess the patient and revise the plan.

Lobectomy

A lobectomy is a surgical procedure in which a lobe of a lung is removed.

Uses

Lobectomy is performed to treat lung cancer and bronchiectasis or to remove emphysematous blebs. It is done when disease is limited to one lobe of the lung. It is preferred to pneumonectomy because it conserves the unaffected lobes of the lung and thus has a less profound effect on the patient's respiratory status.

Procedure

Depending on the lobe to be removed, either a posterolateral or an anterolateral thoracotomy incision is made and the ribs are spread with a retractor. The pleura is entered, and the lung on the affected side collapses. The bronchus is transected, the blood vessels to the lobe are ligated and severed, and the lobe is removed. Two chest tubes connected to water-seal drainage systems are placed for postoperative removal of air and fluid from the chest cavity. The upper tube drains air, whereas the lower tube drains the serosanguineous fluid that accumulates as a result of the operative procedure.

Postoperative Course

The postoperative course is essentially the same as that after a pneumonectomy.

NURSING PROCESS
Lobectomy

See Nursing Care Guide 14–1 for nursing care applicable to the patient undergoing a lobectomy.

Thoracoscopic Surgery

In thoracoscopic surgery, also referred to as video-assisted thoracic surgery, a thoracoscope and other endoscopic instruments are inserted through small incisions in the chest wall to diagnose or treat pulmonary and cardiac disease. The thoracoscope, which is equipped with a camera lens, allows the inside of the chest to be magnified and visualized on a video monitor.

Uses

Uses of thoracoscopic surgery include lung biopsy, staging lymph node biopsy, drainage of an empyema, pleural effusion or pericardial effusion, treatment of recurrent spontaneous pneumothorax, bilobectomy, and resection of mediastinal and peripheral pleural lesions. Because thoracoscopic surgery requires less anesthesia, less operating time, less tissue trauma, and less blood loss than conventional chest surgery, it can be used for patients who are considered at poor risk for thoracotomy.

Procedure

Thoracoscopic surgery is performed under general anesthesia after the patient has been NPO from midnight or, if done in the afternoon, with the patient NPO following a liquid breakfast.

The patient is mechanically ventilated. A double lumen endotracheal tube is used and the nonaffected lung is ventilated while the lung on the affected side is collapsed to allow better visualization. After a bronchoscopy is done to visualize the airways, a small incision is made in the lateral chest wall and the thoracoscope is inserted. Other required endoscopic instruments are inserted into the chest through additional small incisions. A laser is used for hemostasis and for excision of tissue. On the completion of the procedure, one or two chest tubes may be inserted through the existing incisions. Remaining incisions are sutured subcutaneously and paper strip closures are used to approximate the epidermis.

Complications

Complications are relatively rare and patients generally do not require a postoperative stay in a special care unit. When complications do occur, the most common is a prolonged air leak. Other potential complications are the same as for conventional thoracotomy.

Postoperative Course

On the evening of surgery, the patient is gotten up in a chair and if he or she does not have a chest tube may begin to ambulate independently. If chest tubes are in place, they are removed as early as the first postoperative day, depending on the reason for use. The chest tube wound is covered with a dry sterile dressing for 48 hours after the tube is removed, but dressings on the other incisions are generally removed on the first postoperative day. The incisions are then left open to the air unless there is serous drainage requiring a small dressing. Patients may shower as soon as the chest tubes are removed. Because there is little pain associated with thoracoscopic surgery, a mild analgesic such as acetaminophen may be all that is needed, unless there is pain associated with the underlying disease.

The length of hospital stay with thoracoscopic surgery varies with the underlying pathologic condition. It generally ranges from 1 to 5 days.

NURSING PROCESS GUIDELINES
Thoracoscopic Surgery

Provide preoperative care as for any surgical patient. Postoperatively, encourage coughing, deep-breathing, and the use of an incentive spirometer every hour while the patient is awake. Check incisions for bleeding and drainage and medicate the patient as needed for pain. Instruct the patient in self-care at home as follows:

Shower as desired.
Wash incisions daily with mild soap and water; pat dry. If paper strips are over your incision, peel off when the edges start to curl or allow them to fall off on their own.
Observe incisions daily for redness, swelling, or drainage.
Take Tylenol or other pain medication for incisional soreness as needed and as prescribed for 1 or 2 weeks after surgery.
Continue coughing and deep-breathing every hour while awake.
Exercise arm on affected side by doing arm circles and lifting the arm up over your head.

Text continued on page 596

Nursing Care Guide 14–1
Patient Undergoing a Lobectomy

Preoperative Care

Assessment Findings: Restlessness, tense facial expression, occasional trembling. Patient states, "I can't concentrate on anything. I'm just so worried about this whole thing."

Nursing Diagnosis: Anxiety related to the surgical procedure and the postoperative course

Patient Outcomes	Nursing Interventions	Rationale
Patient describes routine perioperative events. Patient reports decreased feelings of anxiety. Facial expression and body posture are relaxed. Vital signs are stable.	Provide basic information about the operative experience: preparation, location of incision, function of chest tubes, postanesthesia care unit routines, expected presence of a central venous pressure catheter, urinary bladder catheter, oxygen. Arrange a preoperative visit to the intensive care unit if the patient will be admitted there after surgery. If this is not possible, describe the unit to the patient. Encourage patient and significant others to verbalize concerns and ask questions. Reassure about the ability to breathe postoperatively by explaining the functional reserve of the respiratory system and the role of preoperative tests in determining the ability to tolerate removal of lung tissue. Acknowledge that there is significant pain after surgery, but that analgesics will be given to control it.	Familiarity with routines and equipment reduces anxiety. Identifies areas of concerns, provides perspective, permits a supportive relationship, and allows for clarification. Reassures the patient of the continued capability to perform the essential life function of breathing. Helps patient accept concerns as appropriate and provides positive facts on which to focus.

Evaluation: Compare the patient's status with the expected outcomes. If the outcomes are not met, reassess the patient and revise the plan.

Assessment Findings: Patient is scheduled for a lobectomy and has no prior knowledge of or experience with lung surgery.

Nursing Diagnosis: Knowledge deficit: breathing exercises, effective coughing, wound splinting, arm and shoulder exercises

(continued)

Nursing Care Guide 14–1
Patient Undergoing a Lobectomy (continued)

Patient Outcomes	Nursing Interventions	Rationale
Patient describes the role of breathing exercises, coughing, and arm and shoulder exercises in recovery.	Describe the importance of breathing exercises and effective coughing in clearing the airway and allowing for good ventilation.	Provides rationale that promotes compliance.
	Explain the effect of chest surgery on chest and shoulder muscles.	Understanding the reason for interventions promotes cooperation.
	Use the patient's arm to demonstrate the passive range-of-motion (ROM) exercises that will be done after surgery.	Learning is facilitated by involvement of the learner.
	Explain that additional active exercises will be taught postoperatively to maintain full ROM and to regain muscle strength.	Prepares the patient for the acceptance of new exercises during the postoperative period.
Patient demonstrates breathing exercises, effective coughing, and use of incentive spirometer.	Teach patient diaphragmatic and pursed-lip breathing, effective coughing technique, methods of splinting the incision, and use of an incentive spirometer.	The best time to learn is when the patient is free from pain and distraction. Teaching before surgery is more effective than teaching in the postoperative period.
	Encourage practice and obtain return demonstrations of those skills.	Practice improves technique, and return demonstration provides evidence that the patient can perform the required skills.

Evaluation: Compare the patient's status with the expected outcomes. If the outcomes are not met, reassess the patient and revise the plan.

Postoperative Care

Assessment Findings: Respirations are shallow at a rate of 28 per minute. Patient is guarding thoracotomy incision with both hands and states, "I can't let my chest move."

Nursing Diagnosis: Ineffective breathing pattern related to unwillingness to breathe deeply secondary to pain, fear of displacing chest tubes, or depressant effects of anesthesia and analgesics

Patient Outcomes	Nursing Interventions	Rationale
Breath sounds and percussion note over remaining lung tissue are normal within 4 postoperative days.	Monitor respiratory rate every 1 to 2 hours. Auscultate lungs every 2 to 3 hours.	Allows for early recognition of respiratory distress and provides information about effectiveness of interventions.

(continued)

Nursing Care Guide 14–1
Patient Undergoing a Lobectomy (continued)

Patient Outcomes	Nursing Interventions	Rationale
Blood gases are within normal range. Lung re-expansion is evident on x-rays.	Position patient on the back or with the operated side up for the first 48 hours.	Promotes expansion of remaining lung tissue.
	Monitor chest-tube drainage every 15 minutes immediately postoperatively and then at progressively longer intervals.	Promotes early recognition of tube blockage or bleeding.
	Report persistent chest drainage of more than 200 mL/hour.	Indicates bleeding and thus allows for medical intervention.
	Maintain chest drainage.	Removal of fluids and air from the pleural space allows for re-expansion of the lung.
	Keep patient elevated in semi-Fowler's position.	Facilitates coughing and allows air to rise and escape through the upper chest tube.
	Keep the chest-drainage system below the level of the patient's chest and free of leaks, dependent loops, and external pressure.	Maintains free gravity drainage.
	Monitor fluctuation of the fluid level in the water-seal chamber.	Fluid level should fluctuate with respirations if tube is not blocked.
	Monitor for excessive bubbling in the water-seal chamber.	Excessive bubbling can indicate an air leak within the set.
	Retape all connections in the system as needed to keep it airtight.	Negative pressure in the chest is required for re-expansion of the lung.
	Retape chest-tube dressing if needed to keep it airtight.	Prevents loss of negative pressure by air entering the chest.
	Reinforce or change gauze (not petrolatum gauze seal) of chest-tube dressing if saturated with drainage.	Maintains effectiveness of occlusive dressing.
	Place a rolled towel under the chest tube when patient is lying on the affected side.	Prevents pressure of body weight from occluding chest tube.
	Direct patient in diaphragmatic and pursed-lip breathing every 1 to 2 hours.	Promotes re-expansion of alveoli.
	Coordinate breathing exercises with time when pain medications reach their peak effectiveness.	Patient is more likely to cooperate with deep breathing when pain is eliminated or reduced.
	Instruct and assist patient in splinting the incision anteriorly and posteriorly to facilitate deep breathing.	Reduces strain on suture line and reassures patient that deep breathing will not damage suture line.
	Direct patient in use of the incentive spirometer every 2 to 3 hours.	Promotes ventilation.

(continued)

Nursing Care Guide 14–1
Patient Undergoing a Lobectomy (continued)

Patient Outcomes	Nursing Interventions	Rationale
	Administer oxygen (O$_2$) if ordered.	Improves oxygenation by providing greater amounts of O$_2$ in inspired air.
	Plan frequent rest periods.	Diminishes the body's O$_2$ requirements.
	Monitor arterial blood gas values, pulse oximetry values, or both.	Documents abnormalities and helps identify the need for and effectiveness of interventions.

Evaluation: Compare the patient's status with the expected outcomes. If the outcomes are not met, reassess the patient and revise the plan.

Assessment Findings: Respirations are shallow and noisy at a rate of 26 per minute. Wheezes are heard on auscultation of the chest. Patient coughs but does not raise and expectorate sputum.

Nursing Diagnosis: Ineffective airway clearance related to increased secretions secondary to respiratory tract irritation and poor cough effort secondary to pain and the depressant effects of anesthesia and analgesia

Patient Outcomes	Nursing Interventions	Rationale
Respirations are easy and quiet at a rate of 16 to 20 per minute. Breath sounds and percussion note over remaining lobes are normal within 4 postoperative days. Blood gas values are within normal range. Oxygen saturation is >90% on room air.	Assist patient to cough and deep-breathe every 1 to 2 hours. For most efficient coughing, place patient in a sitting position.	Helps clear secretions from the respiratory tract, allowing better gas exchange. Upright position allows better chest expansion and more forceful cough.
	Assist patient to turn every 1 to 2 hours because remaining in one position fosters retention of secretions in the lower areas of the lung.	Changes the area of the chest wall that is splinted, allowing better aeration of the lung and promoting drainage of secretions.
	Coordinate coughing, deep breathing, and turning with times when pain medication is at peak effectiveness.	When pain-free or in reduced pain states, the patient is more likely to cooperate in effective deep-breathing and coughing exercises.
	Instruct and assist the patient in splinting the incision anteriorly and posteriorly when coughing and moving.	Decreases strain on the incision, thus limiting discomfort and increasing patient willingness to cough and move.
	Monitor amount, color, and viscosity of expectorate.	Allows for early recognition of changes in amounts or types of respiratory secretions.
	Monitor breath sounds before and after each deep-breathing and coughing exercise.	Evaluates the effectiveness of coughing and deep-breathing.
	Monitor arterial blood gas values, pulse oximetry values, or both.	Evaluates effectiveness of interventions.

(continued)

Nursing Care Guide 14–1
Patient Undergoing a Lobectomy (continued)

Patient Outcomes	Nursing Interventions	Rationale
	Assist with diaphragmatic breathing and percussion, vibration, and postural drainage if ordered because of copious secretions. Do not percuss or vibrate over the operative site.	Helps aerate all lung tissue by removing secretions.
	Administer humidification and mini-nebulizer therapy as ordered.	Moistens and thins secretions to facilitate expectoration.
	Suction if secretions are present and are not being raised.	Mechanically removes respiratory secretions.
	Report immediately if expectorate is excessive or contains bright red blood.	Allows early medical intervention for complications.

Evaluation: Compare the patient's status with the expected outcomes. If the outcomes are not met, reassess the patient and revise the plan.

Assessment Findings: Patient is lying rigidly in bed with arms pressed against the area of the thoracic incision. Facial expression is drawn, and patient occasionally moans, "I can't breathe it hurts so much."

Nursing Diagnosis: Pain (chest and shoulder) related to surgical trauma to muscles, nerves, and other tissues

Patient Outcomes	Nursing Interventions	Rationale
Patient states that pain is relieved. Patient exhibits a relaxed body posture. Facial expression is relaxed. Patient coughs effectively. Patient moves easily.	Administer narcotic analgesics as ordered every 2 to 4 hours as occasion requires for 48 to 72 hours after surgery.	Narcotics alter awareness of pain.
	Give before the pain becomes severe or 30 to 40 minutes before painful exercises.	Administration before pain becomes severe increases effectiveness of the drug. Pain relief promotes coughing, deep-breathing, and turning.
	Avoid medicating to the point of respiratory depression or inability to cough effectively.	Overmedication suppresses respirations and diminishes the effectiveness of the cough.
	Administer oral analgesics as ordered after the first 48 to 72 hours.	Controls pain with decreased risk of suppressing respirations.
	Anchor chest tubes.	Minimizes movement of chest tubes, which is very painful.
	Assist the patient in splinting the incision with flat of hands, folded sheet or blanket, or a pillow when moving, coughing, or deep breathing.	Minimizes painful pull on the incision.

(continued)

Patient Undergoing a Lobectomy (continued)

Patient Outcomes	Nursing Interventions	Rationale
	Support the affected arm and shoulder with pillows or a sling.	Prevents painful pull on the surgically traumatized tissues.
	Promote comfort and relaxation with frequent position changes, backrubs, use of relaxation exercises, guided imagery, and diversional activities.	Reduces tension and promotes rest, which is conducive to healing.
	Maintain a calm, quiet environment.	Reduces stress and tension, allowing for rest and relaxation.

Evaluation: Compare the patient's status with the expected outcomes. If the outcomes are not met, reassess the patient and revise the plan.

Assessment Findings: Patient has a thoracotomy incision that required transection of muscles involved in shoulder movement.

Nursing Diagnosis: Impaired physical mobility related to transection of chest muscles affecting shoulder movement and severe pain in the chest and shoulder secondary to surgery

Patient Outcomes	Nursing Interventions	Rationale
Patient moves shoulder on affected side through usual active range of motion (ROM)	Perform ROM exercises to affected arm at least two times every 4 to 6 hours for 24 hours postoperatively.	Maintains ROM of affected arm.
	Instruct and guide patient in active arm and shoulder exercises 10 to 20 times every 2 hours thereafter.	Prevents atrophy of muscles from disuse.
Patient uses affected arm in performing activities of daily living.	Encourage use of affected arm in self-care activities (keep in mind whether patient is right- or left-handed).	Provides ROM exercise and maintains function of affected arm.
	Structure environment to foster use of affected arm (eg, place frequently used articles on affected side to encourage reaching with the affected arm).	Promotes movement of affected arm needed to maintain free range of joint motion and muscle strength.
	Guide patient in diaphragmatic breathing.	Mobilizes thorax.
Patient assumes an erect position.	Encourage patient to assume a fully erect position with the affected shoulder back and level with the unaffected one.	Prevents drooping of affected side.
	Suggest patient use a mirror to aid in correcting posture.	Allows patient to visualize posture to guide in positioning.

Evaluation: Compare the patient's status with the expected outcomes. If the outcomes are not met, reassess the patient and revise the plan.

(continued)

Nursing Care Guide 14–1
Patient Undergoing a Lobectomy (continued)

Assessment Findings: Patient has a thoracotomy incision and invasive lines.

Nursing Diagnosis: Risk for infection related to surgical incision, presence of invasive lines, and stress

Patient Outcomes	Nursing Interventions	Rationale
Patient is afebrile. Thoracotomy incision is intact and free of redness, edema, or purulent drainage. Chest tube incision site is free of redness, edema, or purulent drainage. Patient's white blood cell count is within normal limits.	Monitor skin integrity, IV lines, and incision site for abnormal redness and drainage every 8 hours. Change wound dressing as ordered by physician, usually day 2 and day 4 postoperatively. Monitor vital signs four times daily and as needed.	Allows for early detection of inflammation, infection, and skin changes.
		Detects changes in vital signs (eg, increase in temperature, pulse rate, and respiratory rate) that indicate infection.
	Adhere to IV or central venous line therapy protocols and change IV site according to hospital protocol.	Decreases risk of introduction and growth of microorganisms in the IV system and the IV site.
	Adhere to protocols for urinary drainage system.	Decreases risk of introducing microorganisms into the urinary tract.
	Maintain integrity of chest tube drainage system.	Decreases risk of introducing microorganisms into the chest tube drainage system.
	Report to the physician abnormal wound redness or purulent drainage, any temperature 38.3°C (101°F) or higher.	Allows for early medical intervention for complications.
	Monitor white blood cell counts.	Elevated white blood cell count is an early sign of infection.

Evaluation: Compare the patient's status with the expected outcomes. If the outcomes are not met, reassess the patient and revise the plan.

Assessment Findings: Two days after a left lower lobectomy, patient verbalizes negative feelings about his or her body and feelings of helplessness and hopelessness and is preoccupied with the loss of part of a lung.

Nursing Diagnosis: Body image disturbance related to loss of part of a lung and the accompanying change in respiratory function

(continued)

Nursing Care Guide 14-1
Patient Undergoing a Lobectomy (continued)

Patient Outcomes	Nursing Interventions	Rationale
Patient realistically describes changes in physical status caused by removal of part of a lung.	Encourage patient to verbalize perceptions and feelings about the altered respiratory status.	Allow any misconceptions to be identified and corrected.
	Acknowledge feelings of anger, fear, sadness, and helplessness as real and valid.	Communicates understanding and acceptance and encourages verbalization and "working through" of feelings.
	Assist patient in identifying the effect on respiratory status, physical stamina, and function.	Facilitates realistic self-assessment.
Patient realistically identifies changes in lifestyle required by altered respiratory status.	Encourage patient to review patterns of usual activities, identifying those unaffected by the surgery.	Provides a positive perspective to balance perception of negative changes.
	Help the patient identify areas of lifestyle in which change may be needed and list available options.	Promotes change in lifestyle to meet health needs. Identification of options provides a sense of control and increases the likelihood that changes will be made.
Patient verbalizes acceptance of the change in respiratory status.	Facilitate discussion of changes and options between the patient and significant others.	Support and encouragement from significant others increase the likelihood of compliance with lifestyle changes.
	Encourage sharing of mutual concerns between patient and significant others.	Changes affect significant others as well as the patient.

Evaluation: Compare the patient's status with the expected outcomes. If the outcomes are not met, reassess the patient and revise the plan.

Assessment Findings: Patient has no prior knowledge of self-care after lobectomy.

Nursing Diagnosis: Risk for altered health maintenance related to insufficient knowledge of self-care after lobectomy.

Patient Outcomes	Nursing Interventions	Rationale
Patient describes self-care after discharge as presented in Highlight 14-2.	Instruct the patient as described in Highlight 14-2.	Provides information necessary for self-care in the post-discharge period.
Patient demonstrates arm and shoulder exercises to be done at home to regain muscle strength.		

Evaluation: Compare the patient's status with the expected outcomes. If the outcomes are not met, reassess the patient and revise the plan.

(continued)

Nursing Care Guide 14–1
Patient Undergoing a Lobectomy *(continued)*

**Additional
Assessments and
Interventions**

Prepare the patient for preoperative diagnostic tests.
Ensure that prescribed measures to minimize secretions and promote alveolar ventilation are carried out. These
    measures may include increasing fluids and providing humidification, administration of bronchodilators,
    chest percussion, and postural drainage.
Prepare the patient for surgery according to the surgeon's orders.
Give oral fluids as soon as the patient is alert and progress to a regular prescribed diet as tolerated.
Monitor for signs of complications, such as pneumothorax, hemothorax, pulmonary edema, cardiac dysrhyth-
    mias, and mediastinal shift.

Resume normal activities but avoid heavy lifting
    for 1 month.
Return to work when approved by surgeon, usu-
    ally in 1 week.
Do not drive until approved by surgeon.
Report any shortness of breath, dyspnea, temper-
    ature over 38.3°C (101° F), or incisional red-
    ness or drainage.

❖ Settings, Providers, and Collaboration for Care

Patients with respiratory disorders are encountered
by nurses in hospitals, clinics, physicians' offices,
same-day surgery units, occupational settings, rehabilitation facilities, long-term care facilities, and in
the home.

Acute respiratory conditions are treated in hospitals typically by a team of physicians, nurses, and
respiratory therapists or technicians. Examples of
such conditions are lung cancer, chest trauma, acute
asthma attacks, and post-surgical states that require
ventilatory support. Nurses collaborate with physicians to manage the acute phase of diseases, to implement the dependent aspects of care, and to monitor changes in patient status.

In the acute-care setting, respiratory therapists
act as consultants to the nursing staff as well as
provide direct care in the form of nebulized medication treatments, intermittent positive-pressure
breathing treatments, percussion, and drainage and
suctioning. The respiratory therapy departments in
hospitals are generally responsible for ensuring that
oxygen delivery equipment is available for nursing
staff. In some cases, respiratory therapists will set
up the equipment, such as mechanical ventilation
equipment. In critical-care units, respiratory thera-

pists act to monitor patients and equipment as well
as deliver care and respond to emergency situations,
taking on the role of managing the airway and oxygen status of the patient.

In the long-term-care setting, patients may experience pulmonary pathology as a primary or secondary problem. As in the acute-care setting, nurses
collaborate with physicians to coordinate and deliver care to improve or maintain the respiratory
function of residents. In long-term-care facilities,
particularly where long-term ventilator-dependent
residents are cared for, respiratory therapists are
available as part of the care team. Residents are
cared for in these facilities unless their conditions
worsen to the extent that treatment in an acute-care
facility is required. Patients with pneumonia are also
treated in long-term-care facilities, provided that the
facility can provide intravenous therapy.

Increasingly, patients are discharged from the
hospital to home with the expectation that once a
respiratory condition is stabilized, the patient will be
cared for at home. In the home setting, the nurse
becomes the coordinator of care as well as a caregiver. The primary nurse calls for consultation with
the physician, respiratory therapist, and respiratory
nurse specialist as needed. The nurse also coordinates with respiratory therapy equipment and other
vendors to arrange for needed home care equipment
and supplies. In many cases, vendors have respiratory therapists available to instruct patients in the
maintenance and use of therapeutic equipment. The
nurse accesses this and other community resources
to provide for the education and support needs of
both patients and family members.

The Elderly: Special Considerations

Age-related changes make the respiratory system
less efficient, with less reserve capacity and less tol-

erance for exercise and stress. With increasing age, the cough reflex is weaker and less efficient. There is a loss of elastic tissue surrounding the alveoli and alveolar ducts. Skeletal changes associated with aging may accentuate the dorsal curve of the thoracic spine, producing kyphosis and an increased anteroposterior diameter of the chest. The respiratory muscles are weaker and the rib cage more rigid, and the older patient may not be able to cough or deep-breathe as well as a younger patient.

As the lungs undergo fibrosis, they inflate more easily but lose the ability to recoil. These changes result in a greater residual volume and less tidal volume. As alveolar membranes become thicker and larger, expiration requires more effort and is less automatic. The thickened alveolar membranes do not diffuse oxygen as quickly. Ventilation and oxygenation usually remain adequate to meet the demands of normal activity.

Chapter Review

1. In their quality, location, and cause, how do crackles differ from wheezes?
2. How can the nurse best assess a dark-skinned person for pallor or cyanosis?
3. What arterial blood gas values would indicate that the oxygen therapy the patient is receiving is effective?
4. How can hemoglobin level affect the clinical manifestations of arterial hypoxemia?
5. What assessment findings indicate the effectiveness of mechanical ventilation?
6. Why are intermittent sighs important for a patient on mechanical ventilation?
7. In their actions and uses, how do decongestants, expectorants, and antitussives differ?
8. What is the meaning of decreased oxygen saturation and increased respiratory rate in a post-pneumonectomy patient?
9. Why is maintaining an airtight system important when caring for a patient with chest tubes?
10. What are the similarities and differences between postoperative care of a patient with a lobectomy and that of a patient with a pneumonectomy?

Bibliography

Arbour R. Weaning a patient from a ventilator. Nursing 1993; 2: 52.

Badger J. Calming the anxious patient. Am J Nurs 1994; 5:46.

Bates B, Hoeckelman RA. A guide to physical examination and history taking. 6th ed. Philadelphia: JB Lippincott, 1995.

Bolton PJ, Kline KA. Understanding modes of mechanical ventilation. Am J Nurs 1994; 6:36.

Brooks-Brunn J. Postoperative atelectasis and pneumonia. Heart Lung 1995; 24(2):94.

Calianno C, Clifford D, Titano K. Oxygen therapy: Giving your patient breathing room. Nursing 1995; 25(12):33.

Campbell M. Managing terminal dyspnea: Caring for the patient who refuses intubation or ventilation. DCCN 1996; 15(1):4.

Carpenito LJ. Nursing diagnosis: Application to clinical practice. 7th ed. Philadelphia: JB Lippincott, 1997.

Carroll P. Nursing the thoracotomy patient. RN 1992; 55(6):34.

Carroll P. A med-surg nurse's guide to mechanical ventilation. RN 1995; 2:26.

Carroll P. Chest tubes made easy. RN 1995; 58(12):47.

Carson M, Barton D, Morrison C, Tribble C. Managing pain during mediastinal chest tube removal. Heart Lung 1994; 6:500.

Clement J, Buck E. Weaning from mechanical ventilation support. DCCN 1996; 15(3).

Clochesy JM, Breu C, Cardin S, Whittaker AA, Rudy EB. Critical care nursing. Philadelphia: WB Saunders, 1993.

Dabbs AD, Olsund L. The new alternative to intubation. Am J Nurs 1994; 8:42.

Flenley DC. Respiratory medicine. 2nd ed. Philadelphia: WB Saunders, 1990.

Fraser RG, Paré JAP, Paré PD, et al. Diagnosis of diseases of the chest. 3rd ed. Vol. 1. Philadelphia: WB Saunders, 1988.

Fraser RG, Paré JAP, Paré PD, et al. Diagnosis of diseases of the chest. 3rd ed. Vol. 2. Philadelphia: WB Saunders, 1989.

Fraser RG, Paré JAP, Paré PD, et al. Diagnosis of diseases of the chest. 3rd ed. Vol. 3. Philadelphia: WB Saunders, 1990.

Fraser RG, Paré JAP, Paré PD, et al. Diagnosis of diseases of the chest. 3rd ed. vol. 4. Philadelphia: WB Saunders, 1991.

Freichels TA. Orchestrating the care of mechanically ventilated patients. Am J Nurs 1993; 10:26.

Freichels TA. Cardiopulmonary effects of artificial ventilatory support. DCCN 1993; 1:67.

Gordon P, Norton J, Merrill R. Refining chest tube management: Analysis of the state of practice. DCCN 1995; 1:6

Guyton AC. A textbook of medical physiology. 9th ed. Philadelphia: WB Saunders, 1995.

Hayden, RA. What keeps oxygenation on track? Am J Nurs 1992; 92(12):32.

Jablonski RS. If ventilator patients could talk. RN 1995; 2:32.

Kaplow R, Bookbinder M. A comparison of four endotracheal tube holders. Heart Lung 1994; 1:59.

Karser LR, Daniel TM (eds). Thoracoscopic surgery. Boston: Little, Brown, 1993.

Kelly-Heidenthal P, O'Connor M. Nursing assessment of portable AP chest x-rays. DCCN 1994; 3:127.

Lee CL. Ventilator alarms: How to respond with confidence. Nursing 1995; 7:60.

Luce J, Tyler M, Pierson D. Intensive respiratory care. 2nd ed. Philadelphia: WB Saunders, 1993.

Macey BA, Landstrom LL. Replacing a chest tube drainage collection device. Am J Nurs 1993; 3:95.

Majors M. Nutritional support of the mechanically ventilated patient. Crit Care Nurs Q 1988; 11(3):50.

Mathews P. Laying the groundwork for successful intubation. Nursing 1995; 9:60.

Maxam V, Goedecke R. The development of an early extubation algorithm for patients after cardiac surgery. Heart Lung 1996; 25(1):61.

Mays L, Eckert S. Synchronous independent lung ventilation. DCCN 1994; 5:249.

McCance KL, Heuther SE. Pathophysiology: The biologic basis for disease in adults and children. St. Louis: Mosby, 1994.

Messina BA. Pulse oximetry: Assuring accuracy. J Post Anesth Nurs 1994; 4:228.

Murray JF, Nadel JA. Textbook of respiratory medicine. 2nd ed. Vols 1 and 2. Philadelphia: WB Saunders, 1994.

Nicholson C, Coleman C, Mack M. Are you ready for video thoracoscopy? Am J Nurs 1993; 3:54.

Querski N, Momin Z, Brandstetter R. Thoracentesis in clinical practice. Heart Lung 1994; 5:376.

Pierce JD, Wiggins SA, Plaskon CP, Glass C. Pressure support ventilation. DCCN 1993; 6:282.

Repasky TM. Tension pneumothorax. Am J Nurs 1994; 9:47.

Sabiston DC Jr. Textbook of surgery: The biological basis of modern surgical practice. 15th ed. Philadelphia: WB Saunders, 1996.

Sabiston DC, Spencer FC. Surgery of the chest. 6th ed. Philadelphia: WB Saunders, 1995.

Scanlan C, Spearman C, Sheldon R, Egan D (eds). Egan's fundamentals of respiratory therapy. 6th ed. St. Louis: Mosby, 1995.

Shawgo T. Thoracoscopic surgery: A new approach to pulmonary disease. Crit Care Nurse 1996; 16(2):76.

Smith RN, Fallentine J, Kessel S. Underwater chest drainage. Nursing 1995; 2:60.

Somerson S. Mastering emergency airway management. Am J Nurs 1996; 5:25.

Steismyer J. A four-step approach to pulmonary assessment. Am J Nurs 1993; 8:22.

Stringfield Y. Back to basics: Acidosis, alkalosis and ABGs. Am J Nurs 1993; 11:43.

Swartz M. Textbook of physical diagnosis. Philadelphia: WB Saunders, 1995.

Swartz M. Pocket companion to textbook of physical diagnosis. Philadelphia: WB Saunders, 1995.

Tasota F, Wesmiller S. Assessing ABGs: Maintaining the delicate balance. Nursing 1994; 5:34.

Thomas-Goodfellow L, Shelledy D, Rau J. A comparison of the effects of assist-control, SIMV and SIMV with pressure support on ventilation, oxygen consumption and ventilatory equivalent. Heart Lung 1995; 24(1):67.

Twomy CR. Preventing complications in double-lumen endotracheal tubes with independent lung ventilation. DCCN 1994; 6: 309.

Weilitz PB, Dettenmeier PA. Back to basics: Test your knowledge of tracheostomy tubes. Am J Nurs 1994; 2:46.

Weilitz PB, Lueckenotte A. Respiratory assessment of older adults: part II. Perspect Respir Nurs 1995; 6(2):1, 3.

Wilkins RL, Krider SJ, Sheldon RL. Clinical assessment in respiratory care. St. Louis: Mosby, 1995.

Yeaw EMJ. How position affects oxygenation. Good lung down? Am J Nurs 1992; 92(3):27.

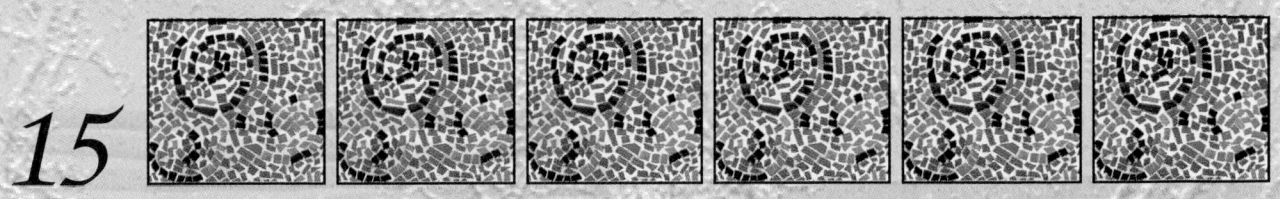

15

Nursing Care of Patients with Upper Respiratory Disorders

Study Outcomes

After studying this chapter, you should be able to:

1. Describe the etiology, pathophysiology, clinical manifestations, diagnostic procedures, and management of common upper respiratory disorders.
2. Identify information and physical examination data essential to the assessment of patients with common upper respiratory disorders.
3. State nursing diagnoses and related expected patient outcomes commonly applicable to patients with upper respiratory disorders.
4. Describe nursing interventions, with their rationales, commonly applicable to patients with upper respiratory disorders.
5. Explain the basis for evaluation of nursing care provided to patients with common upper respiratory disorders.
6. Identify alternative treatment and care settings for patients with upper respiratory disorders and the services related to community-based care.
7. Identify special considerations for the elderly patient with an upper respiratory tract disorder.

Upper respiratory tract diseases range in severity from a simple cold to life-threatening cancer of the larynx. The most common upper respiratory tract diseases are inflammations and infections, which include rhinitis, sinusitis, pharyngitis, and laryngitis. These disorders affect virtually everyone from time to time. They rarely require hospitalization and, in fact, are often self-treated. Thus, nurses play a major role in educating people who contract these disorders to ensure that they use over-the-counter preparations safely and that they obtain prompt medical attention if needed.

At the opposite end of the continuum is nursing care of patients with upper respiratory tract trauma or neoplasia. Patients with these disorders may be critically ill and require an advanced level of care, including maintenance of airway, nutrition, and effective communication as well as pain control and psychologic support.

Partly because of the varied nature of upper respiratory disorders, nurses may see these patients in many different settings both inside and outside the health-care network. All health-care providers must work in collaboration with the patient, the family, and other members of the team to meet the sometimes complex needs of these patients.

Infections and Inflammations

Upper respiratory tract infections and inflammations are among the most common forms of human illness. In most cases, they result in discomfort that is more annoying than disabling. Although they may interfere with normal activities of daily living, they are not life threatening, do not require hospitalization, may not require treatment, and do not usually lead to serious chronic disabilities. The focus of therapy is usually symptomatic. In many instances, symptoms disappear spontaneously; however, repeated infections and inflammations may lead to tissue damage, which can alter respiratory function. Upper respiratory tract infections and inflammations are responsible for roughly 50% of the total time lost from work by adults and about 70% of the time lost from school by children. Studies indicate that the average person among the general population has three to five episodes of respiratory infection each year. The frequency of occurrence, the economic loss, and the large number of people affected are sound reasons why even uncomplicated upper respiratory tract disorders deserve serious attention by health personnel.

RHINITIS

Rhinitis is an inflammation of the mucous membrane of the nose. Depending on cause and duration, it is classified as acute viral rhinitis, allergic rhinitis, vasomotor rhinitis, or chronic rhinitis.

Acute Viral Rhinitis

Etiology and Pathophysiology

Acute viral rhinitis (also known as the common cold and as coryza) is an infectious process of the upper respiratory tract. It usually results from infection with a rhinovirus, of which there are over 100 strains. Colds are highly communicable by inhalation of droplet nuclei and by direct contact. By themselves, they rarely require hospitalization; however, many other more serious illnesses begin with a cold or symptoms closely resembling those of a cold.

Clinical Manifestations

Colds can produce a wide variety of symptoms that include nasal congestion with erythematous (red), edematous (swollen) mucous membranes and a profuse, clear watery rhinorrhea (nasal discharge). Sneezing, watery eyes, coughing, low-grade fever, chills, and a dry or sore throat are also common. Symptoms usually appear suddenly, and full-blown infection may occur within 48 hours. Often as the cough develops it becomes productive. Other complaints, such as lethargy and vague pains in various limbs, may be reported. The major symptoms last 5 to 14 days. If a significant temperature elevation oc-curs with the cold, it may indicate a concurrent infection, such as sinusitis or otitis media. These infections (as well as pneumonia) may also follow the common cold, particularly if the patient is elderly or immunosuppressed.

Management

Usually, medical management is neither sought nor required for the common cold. If visited, the physician may prescribe decongestants for nasal congestion and an antitussive for cough. Antibiotics are not effective against viruses.

NURSING PROCESS GUIDELINES
Acute Viral Rhinitis

Nurses are not usually involved in the direct care of patients with a common cold. Most often, the nurse is simply asked informally for advice. If no symptoms exist other than those typical of a common cold, instruct or assist the person as described in Highlight 15–1. If a cough has been associated with high fever, purulent or blood-tinged sputum, or other symptoms that suggest serious disease, refer the patient to a primary care provider, nurse practitioner, or health clinic.

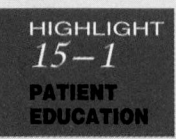 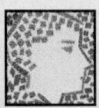

HIGHLIGHT 15–1
PATIENT EDUCATION

Care for the Common Cold

For a person with a cold, offer these instructions:

Rest, so your body will have energy to fight infection.

Increase fluid intake to help liquefy secretions.

Eat a balanced diet to provide energy and nutrients needed to fight infection.

Use a vaporizer to soothe mucous membranes and liquefy secretions.

When blowing your nose, open your mouth slightly and blow through both nostrils to equalize pressure and prevent infected material from being forced into the auditory tubes.

When using over-the-counter medications:
   Check dosages and follow them exactly. More is not necessarily better.
   Read instructions and do not take an over-the-counter medication if you have any of the chronic conditions listed as contraindications.
   Be alert to side effects and possible interactions with other medications, foods, or alcohol.

If using decongestant nose drops:
   Gently blow your nose before administration.

Either sit in a chair with your head tilted back or lie down with a pillow under your shoulders and your head tilted back.
Insert the dropper one-third of the way into each nostril and administer the correct number of drops. Avoid touching the dropper to the naris.
Remain in position with your head tilted back for several minutes.

If using decongestant nasal spray:
Sit with your head upright.
Place the tip of nozzle just inside each nostril, directed backward.
Sniff inward while squeezing the spray container. Use sufficient force to bring spray into contact with nasal membranes.
Limit use of nasal decongestants to every 4 hours for only 2 or 3 days. If used excessively, they can cause rebound vasodilatation and increased congestion. This is termed *rhinitis medicamentosa* and requires discontinuation of nasal decongestants.

Allergic Rhinitis

Allergic rhinitis is the single most common chronic disease. Thirty-five million Americans experience allergic rhinitis. One of every 40 doctor's office visits is prompted by this disease. It is caused by a hypersensitivity reaction to allergens. It may be acute and seasonal when caused by pollens from ragweed, grass, or trees (also called hay fever). It may be chronic and perennial when associated with such common allergens as dust, wool, foods, industrial chemicals, or animal dander. Cockroaches and dust mites are also a major source of perennial allergens. Symptoms commonly include:

Nasal obstruction
Sneezing
Watery eyes
Recurring thin, watery nasal discharge
Postnasal drip
Itchy eyes and nose
Headache

On physical examination, the turbinates appear pale and edematous.

The substance responsible for an allergy can often be identified through a careful and detailed history, skin testing, and the radioallergosorbent test. Management of allergic rhinitis may include avoidance of the offending antigen, desensitization, antihistamine and decongestant therapy, and suppression of the immune response. (See Chapters 32 and 33 for more on allergic rhinitis.)

People who have both seasonal and perennial rhinitis commonly develop nasal polyps, which may become serious enough to obstruct the airway and require removal. Further discussion of polyps appears later in the chapter, under nasal obstruction.

NURSING PROCESS GUIDELINES
Allergic Rhinitis

Obtain a personal and family history of allergy. Ask if the patient has been tested or treated for allergies in the past. Investigate factors that precipitate an attack. Ask whether symptoms occur in a particular season or throughout the year. Also ask about exposure to dust, animals, chemicals, or pollens from ragweed, grass, or trees. Urge the patient to avoid substances that trigger allergies when possible. Also mention that air conditioners effectively remove more than 99% of pollens from the air.

Vasomotor Rhinitis

When a person has a symptom complex similar to allergic rhinitis but no established allergic basis, *vasomotor rhinitis* is the term used to describe the disorder. Although the exact cause is unknown, it is thought to be the result of an instability in the autonomic nervous system resulting from stress, tension, or some endocrine disorder. Treatment is symptomatic.

Chronic Rhinitis

Chronic rhinitis refers to a chronic inflammation of the nasal mucous membranes caused by repeated infections, allergy, or vasomotor rhinitis. Clinically, chronic rhinitis presents with nasal obstruction and feelings of stuffiness and pressure in the nose. A nasal discharge (which may be serous, mucopurulent, or purulent) is always present. The patient may also complain of frontal headaches, sneezing, and vertigo.

The chronic nature of this condition leads to deposition of large amounts of connective tissue in the nasal mucosa, with resulting hypertrophy. Polyps frequently form. Eventually, mucous membranes, cartilage, and bones lining the nasal passages may atrophy. This creates a large, empty cavern in which an abundant exudate builds up on the walls, causing a highly offensive odor. This condition is known as *atrophic rhinitis* or ozena.

SINUSITIS

Sinusitis is an inflammation of one or more of the paranasal sinuses (Fig. 15–1). It may be a primary disorder or a complication of an upper respiratory tract infection. It may be either acute or chronic. It is frequently associated with allergies.

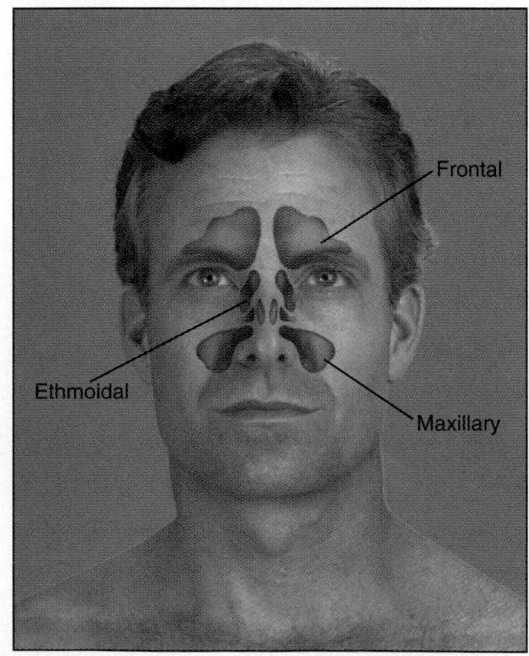

Figure 15–1

Paranasal sinuses include the frontal, ethmoidal, and maxillary.

Acute Sinusitis

Etiology and Pathophysiology

Acute sinusitis results from obstruction of the normal routes of sinus drainage. Obstruction can be caused by abscesses of the teeth that rupture into the maxillary sinuses, rhinitis, swimming, diving, nasal polyps, a deviated septum, direct trauma, or long-term nasotracheal or nasogastric intubation. As mucus collects in the obstructed sinus, it serves as an excellent medium for microbial growth. Common infecting organisms include viruses, streptococci, and staphylococci. Fungal infections may occur in immunocompromised patients.

Clinical Manifestations

Symptoms result from obstruction of drainage. When all the sinuses are involved, the condition is called *pansinusitis*. Clinical symptoms include fever as high as 40°C (104°F), chills, nasal congestion and discharge, and pain and tenderness over the involved sinuses. Recurrent headaches may develop that change in intensity depending on head position and may disappear as sinuses drain during the day. Frontal sinusitis is characterized by pain in the forehead when pressure is applied over the sinuses or on the lateral edge of the orbital ridges (Fig. 15–2). Swelling and tenderness in the anterior portions of the maxillae are common clinical manifestations of maxillary sinusitis. If the infection is severe, pain may refer to the upper teeth. Ethmoid sinusitis is characterized by pain in and around the eyes. Infection of the sphenoid sinuses (cavities in the sphenoid bones of the skull) causes pain over the mastoid bones and the occipital portion of the head. Patients may also complain of a sore throat from irritating secretions draining into the oropharynx.

Diagnosis

Diagnosis is based on history and physical findings. Radiologic examination of the sinuses by conventional x-ray or computed tomographic scan may be ordered to identify the specific sinus involved. Transillumination of the sinuses with a penlight will also reveal affected sinuses by showing them to be darker than normal. If the patient has nasal secretions, a culture and sensitivity test may be ordered.

Management

Medical management consists of a series of broad-spectrum antibiotics, such as penicillin or erythromycin. Oral or topical decongestants, such as phenylephrine (Neo-Synephrine) or pseudoephedrine, may be prescribed short-term to reduce edema and promote drainage. Steam can reduce discomfort. Cool Steroid nasal sprays are also used. In some cases, surgical intervention in the form of antral puncture and lavage (antral irrigation) may be necessary. In this procedure, saline solution is instilled into the maxillary sinus to irrigate and remove exudate.

Complications

Complications of sinusitis are related to the specific sinuses infected because they involve adjacent or contiguous structures. Rhinitis, pharyngitis, laryngitis, bronchitis, and bronchiectasis may all be associated with sinusitis. An acute suppurative infection (empyema) of a sinus may occur. If this empyema ruptures posteriorly, a brain abscess forms, which constitutes a rare but serious complication. Infection may also travel through the venous supply to the brain and cause meningitis or extradural abscess.

NURSING PROCESS GUIDELINES
Acute Sinusitis

Determine the location and duration of pain, as well as positions or activities that affect it. Ask about the amount, color, and consistency of nasal secretions. Inquire about other symptoms, such as sore throat

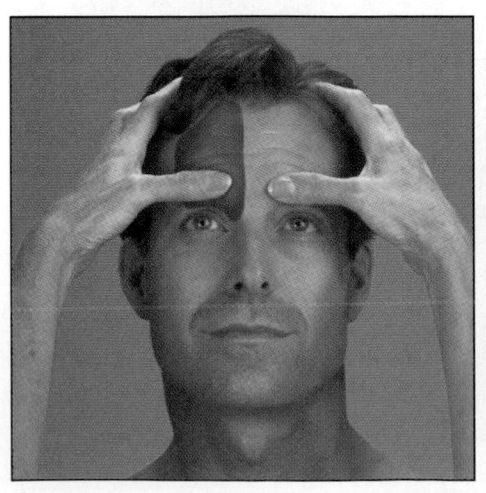
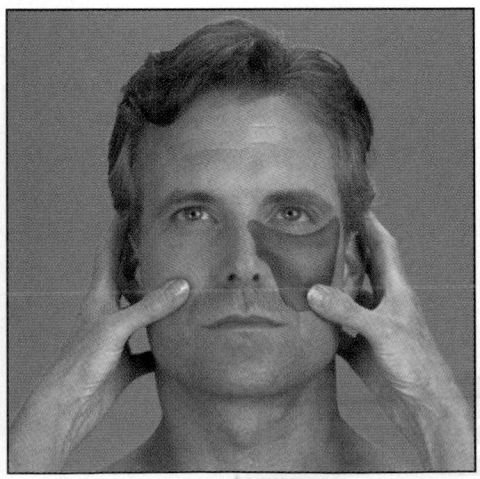

A   B

Figure 15–2

Palpating the frontal and maxillary sinuses for tenderness. *A*, Pressure applied to orbital ridge to check for frontal sinus tenderness. (Color indicates area of frontal sinus pain.) *B*, Pressure applied lateral to the naris to check for maxillary sinus tenderness. (Color indicates area of maxillary sinus pain.)

or cough. Monitor temperature. Check for tenderness over the sinuses. Palpate for enlarged cervical lymph nodes. Explain the use of prescribed medications and help the patient promote sinus drainage, increase comfort, and resolve the infection as explained in Highlight 15–2.

Chronic Sinusitis

Etiology and Pathophysiology

Chronic sinusitis is characterized by thickened mucous membranes and thickened sinuses as a result of prolonged, repeated irritation and infection. Although some cases of chronic sinusitis are related to persistent or repeated infection—as evidenced by repeated isolation of a pathogenic organism—many cases are related to such factors as irritating dust, gases, or excessive exposure to tobacco smoke.

Clinical Manifestations

Chronic sinusitis is characterized by a chronic, purulent nasal discharge, chronic cough related to postnasal drainage, and persistent headaches that are more pronounced on awakening in the morning. Fatigue, nasal stuffiness, anosmia (loss of smell), and mental dullness are common symptoms.

Diagnosis

Diagnosis of chronic sinusitis is made on the basis of the patient's history of symptoms, findings on physical examination, and radiologic examination of the sinuses, which shows thickening of the mucous membranes as well as diffuse cloudiness.

Management

Treatment for chronic sinusitis includes antibiotics if a causative organism is identified by culture and sensitivity test, antiallergic measures, and interventions aimed at promoting drainage. Decongestants can be prescribed, but the patient should be cautioned regarding overuse, particularly if they are applied topically to the nose.

If these interventions are not successful in managing chronic sinusitis, surgical treatment may be necessary. Endoscopic sinus surgery is effective for correction of structural obstructions and treatment of local disease. It may be performed in an outpatient, day-surgery department. Surgical procedures such as the Caldwell-Luc procedure and external sphenoethmoidectomy are done to remove advanced diseased tissues and create channels for aeration and drainage of sinuses. These procedures usually require hospitalization.

NURSING PROCESS
Chronic Sinusitis

The assessment, nursing diagnoses, expected patient outcomes, nursing interventions, and evaluation for patients treated nonsurgically for chronic sinusitis are similar to those described previously for patients with acute sinusitis. If sinus surgery is performed, nursing care is as follows.

PREOPERATIVE NURSING CARE

Basic preoperative nursing care is given as described in Chapter 6.

POSTOPERATIVE NURSING CARE

Assessment

Perform standard assessments as you would for any postanesthesia patient. Also, immediately after sinus surgery, observe for repeated swallowing because this may be the first indication of hemorrhage. Also make a gross check of visual acuity to assess for damage to the optic nerve, a risk with sinus surgery. Do this by simply holding up one or two fingers in front of the patient and asking how many fingers the patient sees. Monitor the patient's temperature every 4 hours and check for pain over the involved sinus to detect signs of postoperative infection or inadequate drainage.

Nursing Diagnoses and Planning

Nursing diagnoses and related expected patient outcomes commonly applicable to patients who have had surgery for chronic sinusitis include the following:

NDx: Pain related to surgical trauma

Planning: Patient Outcomes
1. Patient reports relief from pain.

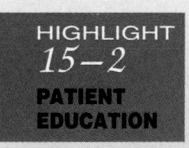
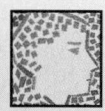

HIGHLIGHT
15–2
PATIENT EDUCATION

Nonpharmacologic Treatments for Sinusitis

To promote sinus drainage, comfort, and resolution of the infection, offer these instructions:

Apply heat in the form of hot, wet packs over the affected sinuses to promote comfort and help resolve the infection

Use a cool-mist vaporizer to help liquefy secretions and ease drainage.

Drink large amounts of fluids to help liquefy secretions.

Maintain a stable room temperature because significant changes in environmental temperature aggravate sinusitis.

Sleep with the head of the bed elevated to a 45-degree angle to promote drainage.

Lie on the unaffected side to promote drainage.

2. Patient demonstrates pain relief by relaxed facial expression and body positioning.

NDx: Risk for altered oral mucous membrane related to drying secondary to mouth-breathing

Planning: Patient Outcomes
1. Oral mucous membrane is moist and intact.
2. Patient performs frequent mouth care, avoiding use of drying agents.

NDx: Risk for altered health maintenance related to insufficient knowledge of factors that exacerbate sinusitis

Planning: Patient Outcomes
1. Patient lists factors that aggravate sinusitis.
2. Patient describes ways to avoid exacerbating factors.

Nursing Interventions and Evaluation

NDx: Pain
Apply ice compresses to the operative area to limit edema and relieve pain. Monitor pain level and administer analgesics as prescribed. Instruct the patient to continue the use of these pain relief measures at home according to the physician's directions.

NDx: Risk for altered oral mucous membrane
The patient will have packing in the nose for up to 48 hours after surgery and therefore will be breathing by mouth. This creates the potential for drying and cracking of the oral mucous membrane. To prevent this development, provide ice chips or sips of water frequently. Assist with oral hygiene as often as needed, avoiding the use of products that exert a drying effect, such as lemon-glycerine swabs. Keep the patient's lips lubricated with K-Y jelly or another water-soluble lubricant. Advance oral intake as soon as permitted and tolerated to improve hydration and stimulate salivation. Instruct the patient to continue with frequent fluid intake, oral hygiene, and lip lubrication as needed at home.

NDx: Risk for altered health maintenance
Explain that cold and dampness aggravate sinusitis and are therefore best avoided. This means turning on home heat, staying inside on cold and damp days, and avoiding overly chilled environments. Also explain the irritating effects of tobacco smoke and the importance of avoiding poorly ventilated areas.

Additional Interventions
The patient will have a piece of gauze folded and taped beneath the nose to absorb drainage. Change this nasal drip pad as necessary, and report excessive bloody drainage.

When the nasal packing is removed, instruct the patient to avoid blowing the nose, lifting heavy objects, or performing Valsalva's maneuver for 10 to 14 days. These activities increase local blood pressure, which could cause postoperative bleeding.

Compare the patient's status with the expected outcomes. If the outcomes are not met, reassess the patient and revise the plan.

PHARYNGITIS

Etiology and Pathophysiology
Pharyngitis is an inflammation of the throat. It commonly accompanies upper respiratory tract infections. It can be caused by several different viruses and bacteria; however, episodes caused by Group A beta-hemolytic streptococci are most serious because of the potential for dangerous cardiac and renal complications. Streptococcus may reside normally in the upper respiratory passages of some people without causing any symptoms of disease. These people are carriers and sources of spread of the organism. Pharyngitis is spread by droplet nuclei and is considered a contagious disease.

Clinical Manifestations
Streptococcal pharyngitis, the most commonly occurring upper respiratory tract infection of the streptococcal type, has a 2- to 4-day incubation period. This is followed by the sudden onset of sore throat accompanied by chills, fever, headache, and frequently severe dysphagia. A white or yellow patchy exudate may cover the tonsillar area. Foul breath odor and cervical lymph node enlargement may develop. Acute pharyngitis may precede other communicable diseases.

Diagnosis
Although pharyngitis usually is self-limiting, testing is done to determine if the causative organism is Group A beta-hemolytic streptococcus. Such tests as the Strep A optical immunoassay (OIA) and Biostar yield rapid identification of streptococcal infection in as little as 15 minutes. These tests can be performed in an outpatient clinic, physician's office, or laboratory. A standard 24-hour throat culture is usually done if results of a rapid identification test are negative to double-check that no streptococci are present.

Management
Early antibiotic treatment helps prevent the serious complications of hemolytic streptococcal infections. These complications include glomerular nephritis, rheumatic fever, otitis media, cervical adenitis, and mastoiditis. Penicillin is the drug of choice; erythromycin is recommended for penicillin-sensitive patients. Antibiotics are continued for 24 to 48 hours after visible throat inflammation subsides, which usually occurs after 7 to 10 days.

NURSING PROCESS
Pharyngitis

Assessment
Inspect the throat. Observe for redness, swelling, drainage, and lesions. Carefully note the presence of

white patches that characterize infection with Group A beta-hemolytic streptococcus. Palpate cervical lymph nodes for enlargement and tenderness.

Assess the location and extent of the patient's discomfort by asking the patient to describe the pain and noting whether the patient can swallow saliva, fluids, and soft foods without indications of distress. If swallowing is difficult, also check for signs of dehydration, which could result from decreased fluid intake and fluid loss related to fever. Take the patient's temperature and, if ordered, obtain a throat culture (Fig. 15–3). Check for any other symptoms, such as rash, that could indicate a disease other than simple pharyngitis.

If Group A beta-hemolytic streptococcus is the causative agent, assess the patient's understanding of the need to take all antibiotics prescribed and to have a follow-up culture.

Nursing Diagnoses and Planning

Nursing diagnoses and related expected patient outcomes commonly applicable to patients with streptococcal pharyngitis include the following:

NDx: Pain related to inflammation of the pharynx

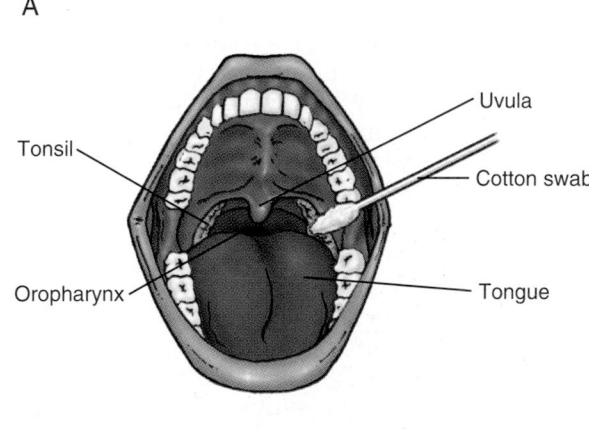

A

Uvula

Tonsil

Cotton swab

Oropharynx

Tongue

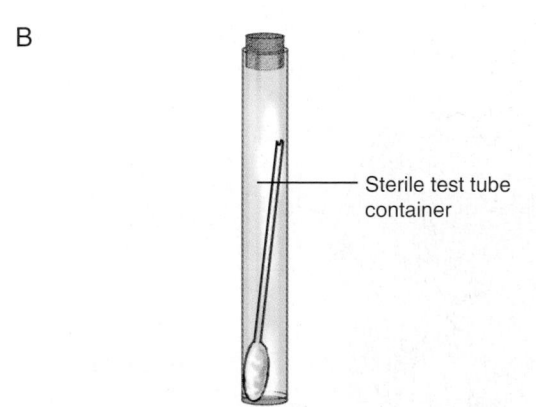

B

Sterile test tube container

Figure 15–3
Throat culture. *A,* Run a sterile cotton swab over areas of redness or exudate on the oropharynx to obtain a throat culture. *B,* Place the swab in a sterile container and send to the laboratory.

Planning: Patient Outcomes
1. Patient reports acceptable comfort level.
2. Patient can swallow saliva, fluids, and soft foods without complaints or facial expressions of discomfort.

NDx: Risk for fluid volume deficit related to decreased fluid intake secondary to pain on swallowing

Planning: Patient Outcomes
1. Patient denies thirst.
2. Mucous membranes are moist.
3. Skin turgor is normal.

NDx: Risk for altered health maintenance related to insufficient knowledge of prescribed antibiotic therapy, complications of strep throat, and follow-up care

Planning: Patient Outcomes
1. Patient states name and dose of antibiotic and the time, route, and frequency with which it should be taken.
2. Patient explains the role of antibiotics in preventing complications and the need to take all doses prescribed, even if symptoms have disappeared.
3. Patient explains the need for a follow-up throat culture to determine whether the infection has been eradicated and the risk of complications reduced.
4. Patient describes need to report worsening or recurring symptoms.

Nursing Interventions and Evaluation

Patients are not usually hospitalized for pharyngitis. Thus, the primary mode of nursing intervention usually involves giving directions to the patient for self-care rather than direct administration of physical care.

NDx: Pain
Instruct the patient in the correct administration of prescribed analgesics. Also instruct in the use of moist inhalations to relieve dryness of the throat and use of an ice collar for comfort. Encourage warm saline gargles every hour while the patient is awake to soothe the mucous membranes and remove irritating secretions. Advise the patient to avoid irritating foodstuffs as outlined in Highlight 15–3.

NDx: Risk for fluid volume deficit
Direct the patient to force fluids to a minimum of 2.5 L per day during the febrile stage of the disease. Advise that very hot or tart fluids may cause additional discomfort and should be avoided.

NDx: Risk for altered health maintenance
Review with the patient the dose, route, time, and frequency of the prescribed antibiotic. Stress that it must be taken as prescribed until the course is completed, even if all symptoms have disappeared. Explain that if only part of the antibiotic is taken,

Special Considerations for Patients with Pharyngitis and Tonsillitis

Instruct patients with pharyngitis or tonsillitis to do the following:

Consume cool, clear fluids, ice chips, or ice pops to soothe the painful throat during the acute stage of the disease.

Avoid citrus juices because they tend to irritate.

Avoid milk and milk products because they tend to increase mucus production.

Progress from clear liquids to full liquids to a pureed or soft diet depending on individual tolerance.

Avoid foods that are highly seasoned or irritating to the throat, such as crackers, potato chips, raw foods, or rough foods.

Drink 2000 to 3000 mL of fluid daily unless medically contraindicated.

some Group A streptococci may remain in the pharynx and cause reinfection or other complications. Explain the need for a follow-up throat culture and its importance in preventing complications. Also be certain the patient understands that worsening symptoms or development of new symptoms should be reported.

Additional Interventions
Instruct the patient to take his or her temperature in the morning and evening and advise bedrest while the temperature is elevated. Explain the importance of maintaining a balanced nutritional intake, and suggest that a liquid or soft diet may be tolerated better than a regular diet if dysphagia is present (see Highlight 15–3).

Compare the patient's status with the expected outcomes. If the outcomes are not met, reassess the patient and revise the plan.

TONSILLITIS

Tonsillitis is an inflammation of the tonsils. It most often affects the palatine tonsils, which are masses of lymphoid tissue located in depressions of the mucous membrane of the pharynx (Fig. 15–4).

Etiology and Pathophysiology
Tonsillitis can occur either as a primary bacterial infection or secondary to an upper respiratory viral infection. It can be caused by a variety of organisms. Group A beta-hemolytic streptococcus is a frequent causative agent and also one of the most important because of the associated risk of cardiac or renal sequelae.

Clinical Manifestations
A patient with tonsillitis has a severe, dry, scratchy sore throat usually accompanied by fever, chills, headache, muscle aches, and general malaise. On examination, the tonsils appear reddened and swollen. If the infection involves Group A beta-hemolytic streptococcus, white patches are present. Cervical lymph nodes are tender and swollen. If the infection travels to the ear, the patient may complain of otalgia (pain in the ear).

Diagnosis
A careful history is taken to rule out related conditions, such as allergy, asthma, and sinusitis. A culture is obtained from the tonsillar area to determine the presence of pathogens and the antibiotics to which they are most sensitive.

Management
Antibiotics form the cornerstone of treatment for tonsillitis. An appropriate agent is chosen based on results of the tonsillar culture and sensitivity. If the causative organism is Group A beta-hemolytic streptococcus, a full 10-day course of penicillin is prescribed and follow-up care is required. When other bacteria are the cause, the patient will probably take a 10-day course of erythromycin, 250 mg four times daily. For relief of throat discomfort, analgesics and throat irrigations may be ordered.

NURSING PROCESS
Tonsillitis

The assessments, nursing diagnoses, expected patient outcomes, nursing interventions, and evaluation for patients with tonsillitis are similar to those described previously for patients with pharyngitis.

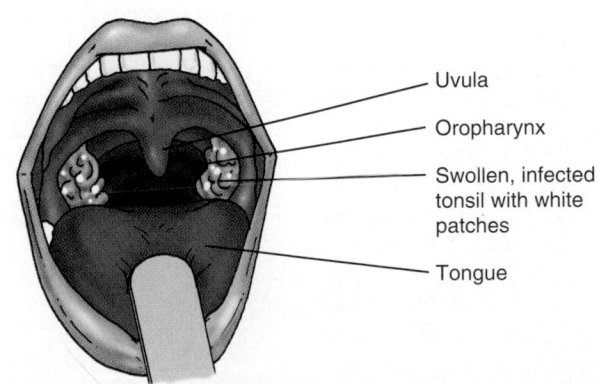

Uvula
Oropharynx
Swollen, infected tonsil with white patches
Tongue

Figure 15–4
Swollen, infected tonsils.

PERITONSILLAR ABSCESS

Etiology and Pathophysiology

Peritonsillar abscess (also called quinsy) is a secondary infection related to tonsillitis. It is an abscess that develops above the tonsil in the tissues of the anterior pillar and soft palate.

Clinical Manifestations

Peritonsillar abscess is manifested by sore throat, unilateral pain radiating to the ear on swallowing, and enlargement of the tonsil with redness and swelling of the adjacent soft palate. The uvula may also be swollen and deviated. Voice changes may occur. Often, the patient holds the head stiffly to the affected side. Swelling that may occlude the pharynx is the most serious symptom.

Diagnosis

Diagnosis is made on the basis of symptoms and physical findings.

Management

Treatment involves antibiotics to fight the infection and warm saline irrigations to relieve pain. If antibiotics and irrigations are not completely effective, surgical drainage by needle aspiration or incision and drainage may be necessary. A tonsillectomy (removal of the palatine tonsils) is performed after the surgical drainage or 6 weeks later.

TONSILLECTOMY. Tonsillectomy is not performed in the United States as often as it was in the 1970s and 1980s. It is still one of the most common operations, however, despite an ongoing debate over the indications for its use. Medical guidelines recommend that tonsils be removed only if they obstruct the air passages, interfere with breathing, or become infected more than three times in 1 year. Most tonsillectomies are performed on an outpatient basis. If hospitalized, the patient is admitted to the hospital either the day before or the morning of surgery, is maintained on a nothing-by-mouth (NPO) order from midnight the night before, and is discharged the evening of surgery or the day after. For adult patients, the procedure is usually done in a semi-sitting position under local anesthesia, usually procaine hydrochloride (Novocaine) 1% or lidocaine hydrochloride (Xylocaine) 1% with epinephrine, 1:100,000.

A major complication of tonsillectomy is immediate bleeding or bleeding that arises 5 to 10 days after surgery. Most often, this bleeding can be controlled by local pressure or vasoconstrictive drugs. Occasionally, resuturing is required to control early bleeding, and evacuation of a clot from the tonsillar depression is required to control late bleeding.

NURSING PROCESS
Peritonsillar Abscess

The assessment, nursing diagnoses, expected patient outcomes, nursing interventions, and evaluation for patients treated nonsurgically for peritonsillar abscess are similar to those for patients with pharyngitis. If a tonsillectomy is performed, nursing care is as follows.

PREOPERATIVE NURSING CARE

Basic preoperative assessments, nursing diagnoses, expected patient outcomes, nursing interventions, and evaluation discussed in Chapter 6 apply to the care of a patient scheduled for a tonsillectomy. In addition, because hemorrhage is a major risk associated with this procedure, be sure to assess pertinent laboratory reports, such as platelet count, clotting time, and hematocrit. Report any abnormalities to the surgeon.

POSTOPERATIVE NURSING CARE

Assessment

After a tonsillectomy, assess blood pressure and pulse every 15 minutes for 1 hour and then every 30 minutes for 2 hours. Monitor the patient's temperature every 4 hours, using the rectal or tympanic rather than the oral route to avoid possible trauma to the operative site. Carefully observe the patient for signs of postoperative hemorrhage. These signs include:

- Frequent swallowing
- Large amounts of bloody drainage
- Vomiting large amounts of bright red blood
- Gradually increasing pulse rate
- Restlessness
- Pallor
- Ultimately falling blood pressure

Nursing Diagnoses and Planning

Nursing diagnoses and related expected patient outcomes commonly applicable to the patient who has had a tonsillectomy include the following:

NDx: Risk for aspiration related to loss of the gag reflex as a result of anesthesia

Planning: Patient Outcomes
1. Respiratory secretions are clear.
2. Respiratory secretions are odorless.
3. Adventitious breath sounds are absent.

NDx: Pain related to surgical trauma of the throat

Planning: Patient Outcomes
1. Patient reports that throat is less sore.
2. Patient swallows liquids without difficulty.

NDx: Risk for tissue trauma related to mechanical, thermal, or chemical stress to the suture line

Planning: Patient Outcomes
1. Patient avoids coughing, clearing the throat, and blowing the nose in the immediate postoperative period.
2. Patient avoids irritating foods.
3. Patient is free of excessive bleeding from the operative site.

NDx: Anxiety related to bloody drainage or swallowing fluid and foods

Planning: Patient Outcomes
1. Patient states that bloody drainage is normal.
2. Patient demonstrates relaxed body posture and facial expressions.
3. Patient consumes fluids and soft foods as directed.

NDx: Risk for altered health maintenance related to insufficient knowledge of discharge instructions

Planning: Patient Outcomes
1. Patient explains discharge instructions (Highlight 15–4).

Nursing Interventions and Evaluation

NDx: Risk for aspiration
Immediately after surgery, place the patient in a side-lying position with an emesis basin placed to catch drainage and secretions until the patient is fully alert. Once fully conscious, elevate the head of the bed to 45 degrees.

NDx: Pain
Give analgesics according to the physician's order and apply an ice collar if allowed. To relieve pain, promote comfort, and help eliminate foul breath

odor, suction out viscous mucus and encourage warm gargles of saline or dilute hydrogen peroxide every 1 or 2 hours for 24 to 36 hours.

NDx: Risk for tissue trauma
To avoid bleeding and trauma to the operative area, instruct the patient not to cough, clear the throat, blow the nose, or use a straw for a few days postoperatively.

Begin oral intake with ice chips and cool, clear fluids as soon as the patient is alert. If these are tolerated well, progress to ice pops and other full fluids. Avoid red fluids because they may be confused with bleeding. Also avoid carbonated and citrus drinks. Instruct the patient to add other soft, nonirritating foods—such as custards and mashed potatoes—after 24 hours, as tolerated.

NDx: Anxiety
Reassure the patient that some anxiety is normal and encourage the patient to verbalize concerns. Reassure the patient that some bloody drainage may be expected and that nonirritating soft foods and fluids will not disrupt the wound. Forewarn the patient that stool may be black and tarry from swallowing bloody drainage. For day-surgery patients, explain that a nurse will call after discharge to check for problems. In addition, provide the patient with a telephone number to call should a problem arise.

NDx: Risk for altered health maintenance
Instruct the patient in self-care after tonsillectomy (see Highlight 15–4).

Compare the patient's status with the expected outcomes. If the outcomes are not met, reassess the patient and revise the plan.

LARYNGITIS

Laryngitis is an inflammation of the mucosa of the larynx (Fig. 15–5) that may be accompanied by edema of the vocal cords. It occurs in both acute and chronic forms.

Etiology and Pathophysiology
Acute laryngitis is most often caused by an upper respiratory tract infection or by abuse of the voice. *Chronic laryngitis* usually results from multiple factors, including irritation from smoking, repeated episodes of acute laryngitis, sinusitis, prolonged voice abuse, and allergies.

Clinical Manifestations
Clinical symptoms of acute laryngitis vary from slight hoarseness to complete loss of voice (aphonia), dry cough, and tenacious sputum. Chronic laryngitis is marked by persistent hoarseness that can leave the patient unable to speak for hours at a time.

Diagnosis
Diagnosis of laryngitis is based on history, presenting symptoms, and visual examination of the larynx.

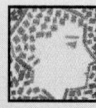

**HIGHLIGHT
15–4
PATIENT EDUCATION**

Discharge Instructions After Tonsillectomy

Instruct the patient to:

Advance diet from cool, clear liquids to full liquids.

Avoid hot fluids, carbonated beverages, milk, and milk products.

After 24 hours, add pureed foods or soft diet as tolerated.

Avoid rough foods, such as raw fruits, vegetables, potato chips, crackers, and acidic foods (such as orange juice) for 10 days to protect the scab over the operative area and to prevent bleeding.

Rest in bed or on a couch for 24 hours after the operation and then gradually resume full activity.

Avoid coughing, nose blowing, clearing the throat or using a straw for 2 to 3 days after surgery.

Report any heavy bleeding or a temperature higher than 38°C (100.4°F).

Return for a check-up in 1 week. Complete healing can take 3 weeks.

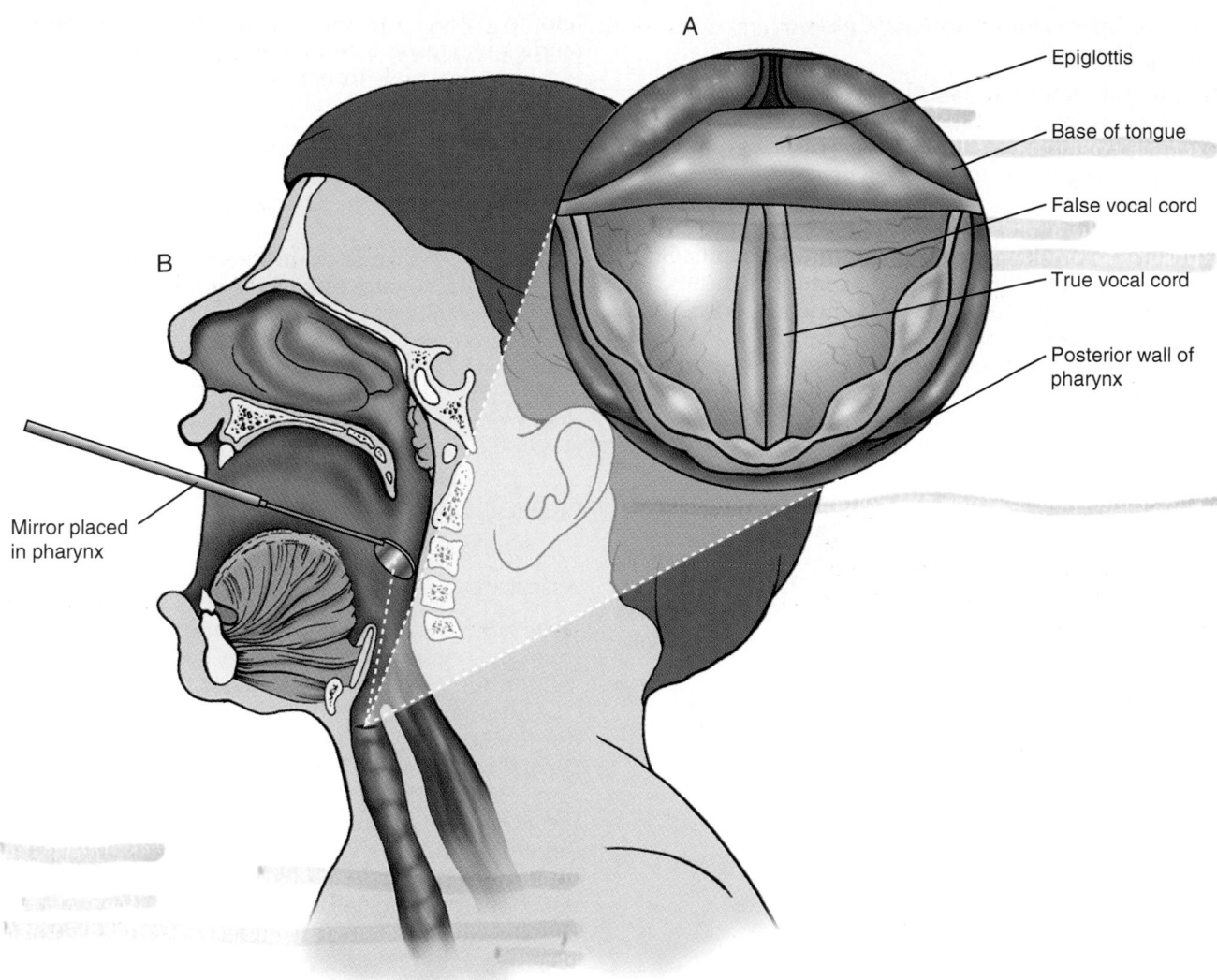

Figure 15–5

A, View of the vocal cords as seen in a mirror placed in the pharynx (indirect laryngoscopy). *B*, Their relationship to adjacent structures.

Management

Antibiotics are prescribed to treat any accompanying upper respiratory tract infection. Topical anesthetics in the form of throat lozenges or sprays and steam or aerosol inhalations are used to relieve laryngeal pain and irritation.

NURSING PROCESS
Laryngitis

Assessment

Obtain information about the onset and duration of hoarseness or voice loss, pain on speaking, and symptoms of an upper respiratory tract infection, such as fever, nasal congestion, postnasal drip, and cough. If the patient has severe hoarseness or pain, or cannot speak, obtain these data by having the patient write answers to specific questions or by having a significant other, knowledgeable about the problem, answer in the presence of the patient. This allows the patient to confirm or contradict answers with a shake of the head.

Nursing Diagnoses and Planning

Nursing diagnoses and related expected patient outcomes commonly applicable to patients with laryngitis include the following:

NDx: Pain on speaking related to inflammation of the vocal cords

Planning: Patient Outcomes
1. Patient speaks without discomfort.

NDx: Impaired verbal communication related to hoarseness or voice loss

Planning: Patient Outcomes
1. Patient demonstrates ability to use alternative communication techniques.

Nursing Interventions and Evaluation

NDx: Pain

Instruct the patient to rest the voice during the acute phase of the disease. Explain the use of analgesics or lozenges containing a topical anesthetic, as ordered. Instruct the patient to avoid whispering because it aggravates swelling and discomfort. Also instruct the patient to avoid nonproductive coughing and all exposure to smoke or other irritating inhalants. Suggest the use of a humidifier for comfort. In the case of chronic laryngitis, advise the patient to sleep in a side-lying position using a low pillow to prevent pharyngeal secretions from trickling into the larynx. In severe cases, the patient may need to move to a warmer climate or make a change in occupation.

NDx: Impaired verbal communication

Suggest alternate methods of communication such as a Magic Slate and a bell for attracting attention. Explain to significant others the need for the patient to avoid speaking and encourage them to phrase questions so the patient can answer them with a shake of the head or by pointing a finger whenever possible.

Compare the patient's status with the expected outcomes. If the outcomes are not met, reassess the patient and revise the plan.

Structural Disorders

EPISTAXIS

Etiology and Pathophysiology

Epistaxis, commonly known as a nosebleed, occurs in all age groups and results from disease or trauma. Some of the diseases associated with epistaxis include arterial hypertension, sclerosis of the blood vessels, acute rheumatic fever, purpura, and leukemia. Examples of local trauma include nose picking, allergies, forceful coughing or sneezing, low humidity, fracture, and abuse of such substances as cocaine.

Epistaxis may occur in the anterior or posterior region of the nose. The most common site of bleeding is Kiesselbach's area in the anterior septum. Epistaxis arising from the septum usually is more annoying than it is serious. Posterior bleeding typically is a more serious problem. It may involve up to 1 L of blood loss and systemic distress. Posterior epistaxis tends to occur in geriatric patients with cardiovascular disease, patients with hematologic disorders, and patients on anticoagulant drug therapy.

Management

Medical management is needed for significant epistaxis, in which case the aim is to control bleeding and to correct the underlying problem. Laboratory studies including a complete blood count, prothrombin time, partial thromboplastin time, and blood typing and cross-matching may be indicated.

Depending on the severity of bleeding, any of the following therapies may be used:

- Pressure on the nares
- Ice packs
- Cautery with silver nitrate or application of a local vasoconstrictive medication
- Nasal packing
- In rare cases, arterial ligation

Intravenous fluid replacement or supplementary doses of vitamins K and C may also be necessary.

NURSING PROCESS
Epistaxis

Assessment

Determine the amount and location of the bleeding (high or low in the right or left naris). Monitor vital signs, and note the patient's color.

Question the patient to determine whether this is the first episode of bleeding. If nosebleeds have occurred before, determine their frequency and duration. Ask the patient about any history of trauma to the nose, any recent oral or nasal surgery, allergies, hypertension, or blood disorders. Ask the patient about any medications taken—prescription or over-the-counter—to determine whether a drug affecting the clotting mechanism could be responsible for the bleeding. Also ask the patient what, if anything, has been done in an attempt to stop the bleeding. Report any abnormal laboratory results to the physician.

Nursing Diagnoses and Planning

Nursing diagnoses and related expected patient outcomes commonly applicable to patients with epistaxis include the following:

NDx: Anxiety related to bleeding and its cause

Planning: Patient Outcomes
1. Patient denies excessive anxiety.
2. Patient's body posture and facial expressions are relaxed.

NDx: Risk for altered health maintenance related to insufficient knowledge of cause of bleeding, follow-up care

Planning: Patient Outcomes
1. Patient states probable cause of bleeding episode.
2. Patient states the type of follow-up care required and the reason for it.
3. Patient describes self-care measures that help prevent bleeding from blood vessels close to the

skin surface and trauma to the nasal mucous membrane.

4. Patient states the correct actions to take if bleeding recurs.

Nursing Interventions and Evaluation

Loosen clothing around the neck to prevent pressure on the carotid arteries. Assist the patient to a sitting position, with the head tilted slightly forward, and apply pressure to the nares by pinching the nose toward the septum for 10 minutes. Apply ice packs to the nose and the forehead. If this is not successful in controlling the bleeding, apply an ice collar, administer a topical vasoconstrictive drug, or pack the nostrils, depending on the physician's orders. Provide an emesis basin for expectorated blood and estimate the amount of bleeding. Instruct the patient not to swallow blood to reduce the risk of nausea and vomiting.

NDx: Anxiety

Reassure the patient and encourage relaxation. Explain all procedures and measures taken to stop the bleeding. Maintain a quiet, calm environment. Encourage the patient to breathe slowly and deeply through the mouth.

NDx: Risk for altered health maintenance

Explain the cause of bleeding to the patient. If underlying disease is suspected, explain the need for further medical care and make certain the patient knows where and how to obtain it. If the cause of bleeding is simply drying and cracking of nasal mucosa that contains blood vessels close to the surface, suggest the use of a humidifier and nasal lubricant, such as K-Y jelly, to keep the membrane moist. Also instruct the patient to avoid hard nose blowing, picking the nose, and other nasal trauma. Tell the patient what to do if bleeding recurs.

Compare the patient's status with the expected outcomes. If the outcomes are not met, reassess the patient and revise the plan.

NASAL OBSTRUCTION

Nasal Polyps

Nasal polyps are smooth, pale, soft, edematous outpouchings of the nasal or sinus mucosa. These benign tumors are usually bilateral and freely moveable. Nasal polyps are a frequent complication of allergic rhinitis. As the polyps develop and mature, symptoms of nasal obstruction occur. Treatment may consist of steroidal nasal spray, injection of steroids directly into the polyp, or surgical removal called polypectomy (Fig. 15–6). The presence of polyps may cause great anxiety for the patient who fears they are malignant. Rarely, polypectomy (surgical removal of the polyps) is necessary. The proce-

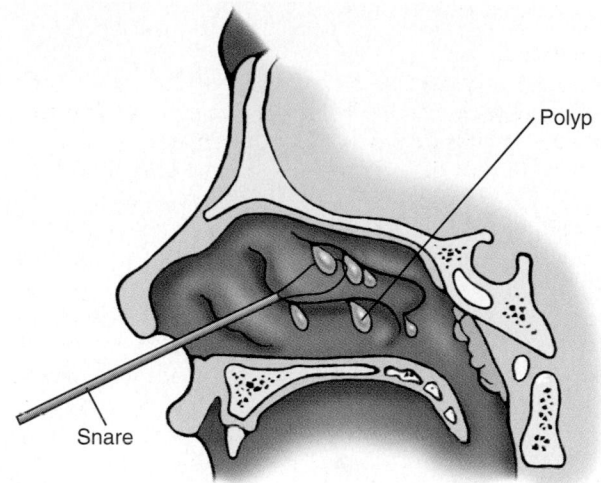

Figure 15–6

A nasal snare is used to remove nasal polyps. After the nose is anesthetized, the nasal snare is slipped around the polyp and the polyp is transected. Forceps are then used to remove the transected polyp.

dure, which may be done conventionally or with a laser, is performed under local anesthesia. Polyps are known to recur if the underlying allergy cannot be controlled.

Hypertrophied Turbinates

Hypertrophy of the turbinates is a complication related to chronic forms of rhinitis. The enlarged turbinates (three bony projections lined with mucous membrane) interfere with drainage and air passage, thereby contributing to nasal obstruction. Usually, astringent solutions or aerosolized corticosteroids are used to shrink the turbinates back against the side of the nose. A turbinectomy (removal of one of the turbinates) may be performed. However, surgeons are very cautious and selective in recommending this type of surgery because there is some evidence that it may lead to atrophic rhinitis years later.

Deviated Nasal Septum

The deviated nasal septum appears as rounded lumps or sharp projections that deflect from the midline of the nose (Fig. 15–7). It may also be bent to both sides (S-shaped curve). Deviations can be either in the vertical or horizontal plane. If these deviations or irregularities interfere with respiration by obstructing the airway, a submucous resection or a septoplasty is done. These procedures can be performed under local anesthesia and involve correction of the defect in the septum.

An operative procedure often done along with a repair of a deviated septum is a rhinoplasty. Rhino-

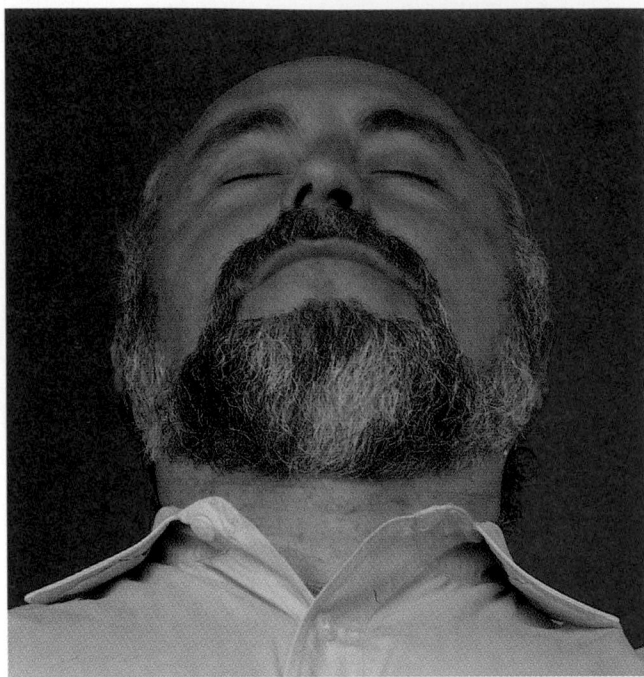

Figure 15–7
Deviated nasal septum seen protruding into the right naris and obstructing the airway.

plasty is the surgical reconstruction of the nose using local or distal tissues supplemented with alloplasty (use of inert plastic material) as needed. The purpose of this procedure is to cosmetically improve the patient's appearance, but it may also be done to remove an obstruction in the nasal airway resulting from a traumatic or developmental deformity.

Rhinoplasty is usually performed under local anesthesia. It involves restructuring the nasal bone and cartilage through an incision made at the end of the nose inside the nostril so that it will not be conspicuous. At the end of the procedure, the nares are packed, the nose secured with tape, and a nose splint applied. This maintains the shape of the nose, limits edema, and provides protection. The splint is left in place for about 1 week, when more tape may be applied to maintain the shape of the nose. Postoperative swelling and ecchymosis develop around the eyes and the nose.

Complications of this procedure include hemorrhage and infection.

NURSING PROCESS
Nasal Surgery

Nursing care of the patient having nasal surgery is presented in Nursing Care Guide 15–1.

Trauma

NASAL FRACTURE

Etiology and Pathophysiology
Fractures result from trauma to the nasal area. Fractures of the nasal bones or septum may be more common than generally supposed because, if there is no displacement of the nose or nasal obstruction, the person typically does not seek medical attention.

Clinical Manifestations
Nasal fractures can result in nasal pain, edema and ecchymosis of the soft tissues, nasal obstruction, and epistaxis. In some cases, bleeding may be copious both from the nostrils and back into the pharynx. In extensive fractures, cerebrospinal fluid, a thin, colorless liquid, may drain from the nares (rhinorrhea).

Diagnosis
Diagnosis is based on the history of trauma and the physical findings. Skull x-rays are taken to rule out skull fractures and to identify and locate any bone fragments.

Management
If the patient seeks medical care before edema develops, the fracture may be set at that time. Simple lateral displacements can be reduced by firm pressure on the convex side of the nose. If the nasal fracture requires repair of the bony structure and septum, general anesthesia is used. The fracture cannot be reduced until after the swelling has subsided (usually 2 or 3 days). After reduction, splinting may be used to stabilize the reduction until healing occurs.

If a nasal fracture causing misalignment is not set, deformity, obstruction, chronic rhinitis, or chronic sinusitis can occur.

NURSING PROCESS GUIDELINES
Nasal Fracture

Nursing care of the patient with a nasal fracture aims to maintain a patent airway, prevent complications, and provide relief of discomfort. If rhinorrhea occurs, instruct the patient not to blow the nose, cough, or perform Valsalva's maneuver. Place the patient on bedrest and monitor for evidence of meningitis. If surgical reduction is necessary, prepare the patient for surgery as described in Chapter 6. Postoperatively, elevate the head of the bed and apply ice compresses to minimize swelling.

LARYNGEAL TRAUMA

Etiology and Pathophysiology
The most common cause of laryngeal trauma is the neck striking the steering wheel during an automo-

Nursing Care Guide 15–1
Patients Undergoing Nasal Surgery

Preoperative Care

Assessment Findings: Patient asks questions about the surgical experience and aftercare. Patient makes incorrect statements about the surgery and its outcomes.

Nursing Diagnosis: Knowledge deficit: surgical procedure and its effects and perioperative care

Patient Outcomes	Nursing Interventions	Rationale
Patient describes surgery to be done and its expected effects accurately, at a level appropriate to his or her background.	Clarify or reinforce surgeon's explanation of the procedure, its purpose, and expected result. If surgery is cosmetic, be sure patient understands that result will not be seen until swelling disappears, which can take several weeks.	Allows identification of concerns and fears, which is essential to provision of information, clarification, and emotional support.
Patient states types of anesthesia to be used and what can be expected in the operating room.	If procedure is to be done under local anesthesia, explain this to the patient. Describe people, equipment, and routines that will be seen in the operating room.	Helps control anxiety for patient. Although some anxiety can be beneficial in preparing the body for the stress of surgery, excessive anxiety is detrimental.

Patient describes typical postoperative events for patient recovering from nasal surgery.	Prepare patient for postoperative routine.
	Explain the following:
	  Nasal packing will be in place, so breathing by mouth will be necessary.
	  Nasal pack and back of the throat will be inspected frequently and vital signs monitored.
	  There is only mild discomfort associated with nasal surgery, but pain medication will be administered as needed.
	  Patient will be on bedrest, with head elevated, for about 6 hours and then will be up and about.
	  A sucking noise may be heard on swallowing after surgery, but it will disappear when nasal pack is removed.
	  Oral intake will be resumed in 6 to 8 hours.
		Prepares patient for perioperative events, thus involving patient in plan of care, promoting cooperation, and decreasing risk of anxiety over routine measures.

Evaluation: Compare the patient's status with the expected outcomes. If the outcomes are not met, reassess the patient and revise the plan.

(continued)

Nursing Care Guide 15–1
Patients Undergoing Nasal Surgery (continued)

Assessment Findings: Patient states that he or she feels apprehensive, is afraid of the operation, and has a "dry mouth and a pounding heart." Patient is unable to sit still and is wringing the hands.

Nursing Diagnosis: Anxiety related to scheduled surgery

Patient Outcomes	Nursing Interventions	Rationale
Patient asks questions about the surgery. Patient attends to information and directions. Verbalization of feelings of overwhelming anxiety is absent. Nonverbal signs of excessive anxiety, such as pacing and hand-wringing, are absent.	Encourage patient to verbalize concerns by providing time, private environment, and an opening such as, "Tell me how you're feeling about tomorrow's surgery." Acknowledge that anxiety is normal before surgery. Answer questions simply and clearly.	Encourages the patient to share feelings and thus receive support. Provides emotional support and reassures patient that feelings are normal. Provides and clarifies information in a manner easily understood by the patient.

Evaluation: Compare the patient's status with the expected outcomes. If the outcomes are not met, reassess the patient and revise the plan.

Postoperative Care

Assessment Findings: Patient has nasal packing and external dressing in place. Patient complains of difficulty breathing by mouth and feels that he or she "can't get enough air."

Nursing Diagnosis: Risk for ineffective breathing pattern related to nasal obstruction secondary to nasal packing, external dressing, and swelling

Patient Outcomes	Nursing Interventions	Rationale
Respirations are of normal rate and depth. Complaints of dyspnea are absent. Blood gas values are within normal range.	Assist patient into Fowler's position. Apply ice to the nasal area. Remove constricting clothing or bedding to make patient feel it is easier to breathe. Encourage slow, rhythmic breathing and use of relaxation techniques. Encourage diversions, such as soft music or television.	Promotes lymphatic and venous drainage, decreases edema, and aids ventilation. Decreases edema. Restrictive clothing and bed covers interfere with chest expansion and increase the sense of difficulty in breathing. Increases gas exchange and decreases basal metabolic rate, thereby decreasing the rate of oxygen utilization. Helps reduce oxygen requirements by reducing stress, thereby slowing heart and respiratory rates.

Evaluation: Compare the patient's status with the expected outcomes. If the outcomes are not met, reassess the patient and revise the plan.

(continued)

Nursing Care Guide 15–1
Patients Undergoing Nasal Surgery (continued)

Assessment Findings: Patient is breathing by mouth, oral mucous membrane appears dry, and tongue is caked. Patient complains of a "dry, cracky feeling" in the mouth.

Nursing Diagnosis: Altered oral mucous membrane related to dryness secondary to breathing by mouth

Patient Outcomes	Nursing Interventions	Rationale
Oral mucous membranes are moist and smooth. Patient states that mouth feels better.	Give frequent, gentle oral hygiene. Irrigate mouth with sterile water, normal saline, or diluted hydrogen peroxide.	Keeps mucous membranes moist, thereby reducing risk of cracking.
	Avoid the use of lemon-glycerin swabs or other drying agents.	Dries mucous membranes and increases risk of cracking.
	Lubricate lips with water-soluble lubricant.	Adds to comfort and reduces cracking by maintaining tissue moisture.
	Force fluids when patient is able to resume oral intake.	Prevents dehydration and reduces drying and cracking of oral mucous membranes

Evaluation: Compare the patient's status with the expected outcomes. If the outcomes are not met, reassess the patient and revise the plan.

Assessment Findings: Patient has no previous experience with nasal surgery and asks questions about precautions to be taken and self-care in general.

Nursing Diagnosis: Risk for altered health maintenance related to insufficient knowledge of precautions to prevent new nasal bleeding, normal and abnormal signs and symptoms

Patient Outcomes	Nursing Interventions	Rationale
Patient lists precautions to be taken to prevent new nasal bleeding.	To prevent initiating new bleeding from the nose, instruct the patient in the following: Avoid touching the nose with hands, tissues, or any other objects. Avoid increasing pressure in the nose by doing the following: Using an extra pillow when lying down to keep the head elevated. Not bending over. Not blowing the nose, and if sneezing cannot be avoided, keeping the mouth open during the sneeze. Not straining during bowel movement. Avoiding heavy lifting. Avoid external pressure on the nose from eyeglasses. Avoid alcohol, aspirin, and cigarettes.	Provides information necessary for self-management after discharge.

(continued)

Nursing Care Guide 15–1
Patients Undergoing Nasal Surgery (continued)

Patient Outcomes	Nursing Interventions	Rationale
Patient states that edema and discoloration are normal and will disappear with time and that final result of cosmetic surgery may not be judged for several weeks.	Reinforce that edema and discoloration are normal and will disappear with time and the final cosmetic result of surgery cannot be judged for several weeks.	Helps control anxiety by increasing awareness of expected events during course of recovery.
Patient states that tarry stools may occur as a result of swallowed blood.	Explain that stools may appear tarry because of swallowed blood.	Helps prevent unnecessary anxiety over normal aspects of recovery course.
Patient lists symptoms to be reported to the surgeon.	Instruct patient to call the surgeon immediately if bleeding from the nose or throat, vomiting, or a temperature greater than 38.3°C (101°F) occurs.	Provides information necessary to recognize postoperative complications as well as appropriate patient responses.

Evaluation: Compare the patient's status with the expected outcomes. If the outcomes are not met, reassess the patient and revise the plan.

Additional Assessments and Interventions

Inspect the nasal packing and use a flashlight to observe the back of the throat for bleeding. Inspect and change the gauze pad (mustache dressing) beneath the nares as needed. Note the amount and color of drainage. The amount should gradually decrease and the color should turn from red to brown-tinged.

bile accident. Other causes are iatrogenic and include endoscopy and endotracheal intubation. Severe laryngeal trauma can cause death from respiratory obstruction unless a tracheostomy is performed immediately. Fracture of the thyroid cartilage can cause the mucosa and other soft tissue inside the larynx to be torn or a hematoma to form.

caused by physician.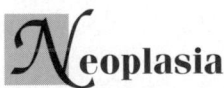

Clinical Manifestations
The patient with laryngeal trauma has a tender, swollen, ecchymotic neck. Stridor may also be present because of swelling of the airway tissues. Hoarseness, dysphagia, cyanosis, and hemoptysis may also occur.

Management
Endotracheal intubation or emergency tracheostomy is done, if necessary, to maintain a patent airway. Computed tomographic scanning may be ordered to determine the nature of the injury. Supportive care may include antibiotics to prevent infection and corticosteroids to control edema.

NURSING PROCESS GUIDELINES
Laryngeal Trauma

Symptoms of laryngeal injury may not be immediately present after neck trauma. Therefore, ongoing, frequent assessment is necessary. Keep equipment available for an emergency tracheostomy because edema or hematoma can develop rapidly. (See Chapter 14 for more information about tracheostomy.)

Neoplasia

CANCER OF THE LARYNX

Etiology and Pathophysiology
Cancer of the larynx is the most common upper respiratory tract malignancy. The incidence is some-

what higher in African-Americans than in whites, and also increases in the elderly. It occurs five times more often in men than in women. Heavy cigarette smoking and ingestion of alcohol are believed to be major factors in the development of this type of cancer. Recent statistics indicate that the incidence of laryngeal cancer is rising in the female population.

Cancer of the larynx is classified according to the site of the growth. Intrinsic tumors develop on the true vocal cords. They tend to be well differentiated and grow slowly. Extrinsic tumors develop above or below the true vocal cords. Their growth is more rapid, and there is usually early lymphatic involvement. These tumors are more difficult to treat.

Highlight 15–5 offers instructions to help patients reduce the risk of laryngeal cancer.

Clinical Manifestations

Intrinsic and extrinsic tumors produce markedly different symptoms. Tumors of the true cords (intrinsic tumors) cause hoarseness initially because they prevent the vocal cords from approximating correctly. As the growth spreads to the opposite cord, pain and coughing develop. Unchecked, the tumor continues to grow and becomes extrinsic.

Symptoms of extrinsic tumors do not occur until late in the disease. Initially, the patient may complain of feeling something in the throat, pain or burning of the throat when drinking hot liquids or orange juice, or pain radiating to the ear. In some cases, an enlarged lymph node in the neck may be the first indication of disease. Late symptoms include dysphagia (difficulty swallowing), dyspnea, hoarseness, weight loss, foul breath, and general disability.

Diagnosis

Tumors on and above the true vocal cords can be visualized by direct laryngoscopy, and tumors below the glottis can be visualized by indirect laryngoscopy. Diagnosis of malignancy is confirmed by biopsy. Specialized radiologic procedures, such as computed tomographic or magnetic resonance imaging scans and barium swallows, are done to determine the extent of disease. Laryngeal tumors are staged by the TNM staging system. Stage I tumors are confined to the site of origin and present with negative lymph nodes and no metastatic lesions. Depending on the degree of tumor extension and cord fixation, as well as nodal and metastatic involvement, tumors are progressively staged up to Stage IV.

Management

Management is determined by the stage of the tumor. Early intrinsic cancer of the larynx can be treated successfully by either surgery or radiation therapy. Types of surgical procedures performed on early intrinsic lesions, all of which leave the patient with a normal or hoarse voice, include transoral cordectomy (resection via a laryngoscope) and laryngofissure (incision into but not removal of the cord to remove a lesion). Excision may be done via laser. Radiation for early intrinsic tumors can be by either external beam or implanted iridium seeds. For more advanced tumors, laryngectomy may be necessary.

Laryngectomy

Three basic surgical procedures are used to treat cancer of the larynx: partial laryngectomy, conservation laryngectomy, and total laryngectomy. A radical neck dissection may be done with either a conservation or a total laryngectomy.

PARTIAL LARYNGECTOMY

A partial laryngectomy is used to treat tumors localized to a portion of the larynx. In this procedure, the malignant lesion is excised along with a surrounding lip of normal tissue. During surgery, a tracheostomy is also created to protect the patient from postoperative airway obstruction caused by edema or hemorrhage. Once this danger has passed, however, the tracheostomy tube is removed, usually in 2 or 3 days. Then the patient is allowed to begin whispering and then gradually to resume full use of the voice. Thus, after a partial laryngectomy, the patient has a normal airway and also retains the ability to speak.

Complications of this procedure include aspiration, bleeding, and subcutaneous emphysema.

CONSERVATION LARYNGECTOMY

A conservation (also called supraglottic) laryngectomy is used to treat selected extrinsic lesions located on the epiglottis or other nearby structures above the true vocal cords. The diseased portion of the larynx is removed and a temporary tracheotomy

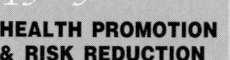
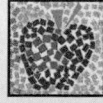

HIGHLIGHT
15–5

HEALTH PROMOTION & RISK REDUCTION   Laryngeal Cancer

To decrease the risk of laryngeal cancer, encourage the patient to:

Avoid cigarette smoking

Limit alcohol consumption

Avoid exposure to airborne carcinogens

Avoid vocal abuse

Schedule routine physical exams

Seek medical care for difficulty in swallowing, persistent hoarseness, enlarged lymph nodes in the neck, or unexplained weight loss

performed to protect against postoperative airway obstruction. As with a partial laryngectomy, the patient has a normal airway and normal speech after healing.

A major postoperative risk associated with this procedure is aspiration, because the epiglottis or other protective structures have been removed. The patient has to relearn the swallowing process, and intravenous therapy or nasogastric tube feedings are common for the first 2 or 3 weeks postoperatively. Additional information appears in Nursing Care Guide 15–2.

There is also a risk of bleeding, carotid rupture, or development of a fistula between the pharyngeal suture line and the skin. These latter problems are most likely to occur if a radical neck dissection has been done along with the laryngectomy and if the patient has had previous radiation therapy to the area.

TOTAL LARYNGECTOMY

A total laryngectomy is done for advanced lesions. In this procedure, the entire larynx, the hyoid bone, the pre-epiglottic space, the strap muscles, and one or more of the tracheal rings are removed. The trachea's pharyngeal opening is closed, and the distal portion of the trachea is formed into a permanent tracheostomy (Fig. 15–8). After this procedure, there is loss of normal speech, loss of normal ventilation through the nose and mouth, and olfactory changes secondary to the fact that air is no longer inhaled and exhaled through the nose and mouth (Fig. 15–9). Postoperatively, most patients have a laryngectomy tube in place. This is a wider, shorter version of a tracheostomy tube and requires the same care (see Chapter 14). It can be removed after 2 or 3 weeks when the stoma has healed completely or can be used permanently, depending on the individual

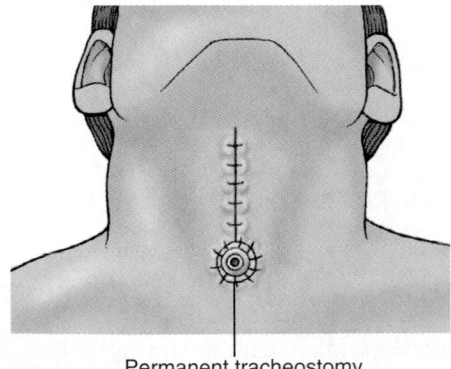

Permanent tracheostomy

Figure 15–8

Appearance of the surgical wound and permanent tracheostomy after total laryngectomy.

patient and physician. Wound drains may also be present to help remove air and fluid from the dead space where the larynx used to be. These drains are usually removed when drainage drops to less than 50 mL daily.

There is no danger of aspiration of materials from the oral cavity as with a conservation laryngectomy because there is no connection between it and the trachea. However, there is risk of bleeding, carotid rupture, and fistula formation, as previously mentioned. Lower respiratory tract infection is also a potential complication because the protective mechanisms of the upper respiratory tract are no longer functional.

The speech pathologist plays a critical role in the care of a patient undergoing total laryngectomy. This role begins before surgery, when the speech pathologist visits to answer questions the patient might have and to reinforce that oral communication is possible after the surgery.

Oral communication after total laryngectomy is possible by means of esophageal speech, an artificial larynx, or prosthetic voice-restoration surgery. *Esophageal speech* is generated when a person swallows air into the esophagus and "belches" it back up, creating a vibration at the junction of the esophagus and pharynx. This results in a deep tone, which can then be formed by the tongue and mouth into easily understandable words. Development of esophageal speech takes practice, and instruction may begin preoperatively when the patient is able to ask questions. For patients with severe emphysema or asthma, esophageal speech may not be possible.

The phrase *artificial larynx* describes a variety of devices used to generate sound that can be modified by oral structures into speech. One such device sends an electronically generated tone into the mouth by way of a tube that the patient inserts about 2 inches into the corner of the mouth (Fig. 15–10). This device, which can be used immediately after surgery, may be helpful for some patients to use in the interim, while mastering esophageal speech. Other patients use an artificial larynx as a permanent mode of speech. A second electronic device is held over the neck and produces a buzzing sound, which is transmitted through the tissues into the oral cavity, where it can be formed into words (Fig. 15–11).

Another device is a pneumatic one that directs air escaping from the stoma during exhalation through a funnel into a tube, the end of which is inserted into the mouth. This is an inexpensive device that produces relatively normal sound but, like the previous instrument, has the disadvantage of being obvious and requiring one hand to hold it.

Surgical procedures designed to allow speech production include creation of an opening between the esophagus and the trachea with insertion of a one-way valve prosthesis to prevent aspiration. This procedure is called a tracheoesophageal puncture. It

Text continued on page 626

Nursing Care Guide 15–2
Patients Undergoing Conservation (Supraglottic) Laryngectomy

Preoperative Care

Assessment Findings: Patient verbalizes fear of surgery, worry about the diagnosis of cancer, and apprehension about being able to breathe, eat, and speak postoperatively. Patient complains of dry mouth, trembling hands, and "heart palpitations." Patient is restless and unable to concentrate.

Nursing Diagnosis: Anxiety related to the diagnosis of cancer, the surgical experience, the effects of surgery on eating, breathing, speaking, appearance, work, and social activities

Patient Outcomes	Nursing Interventions	Rationale
Patient expresses concerns and fears. Patient attends to information given about the surgery and postoperative care. Patient asks questions about the surgery and its effects. Verbalization of feelings of overwhelming anxiety is absent. Nonverbal signs of excessive anxiety, such as constant pacing, hand-wringing, and trembling are absent.	Provide opportunity and environment conducive to expression of concerns and fears. Acknowledge that anxiety before this surgery is normal.	Encourages patient to share feelings and thus receive support. Encourages patient to share feelings and thus receive support by allaying fears of being perceived negatively because of anxiety.
	Explain postoperative course and routines (ie, recovery room, suctioning, humidification, coughing and deep breathing, intravenous fluids, tube feedings, and drains).	Prepares patient for postoperative events, thus promoting cooperation and decreasing the risk of anxiety over routine measures.
	Carefully describe how breathing will occur after surgery.	Helps control anxiety by providing patient with reassurance that breathing, which is essential to life, will be maintained despite the anatomic changes resulting from surgery.
	Discuss alternate modes of communication and, with the patient, select the mode that will be used.	Reassures patient that communication of needs will be possible and allows selection of a means acceptable and suitable to the patient, thus increasing the probability of its successful use.
	Reassure patient that assistance will be available at all times.	Reassures patient that he or she will not be alone, thus allaying anxiety and providing emotional support.
	Answer all questions clearly and simply.	Provides and clarifies information in a manner easily understood by the patient.
	Discuss patient's concerns about body image and also hopes for the future.	Verbalization provides perspective as well as the opportunity for clarification.

Evaluation: Compare the patient's status with the expected outcomes. If the outcomes are not met, reassess the patient and revise the plan.

(continued)

Nursing Care Guide 15–2
Patients Undergoing Conservation Laryngectomy *(continued)*

Assessment Findings: Patient verbalizes fear of not being able to cope with the tracheostomy, temporary voice loss, difficulty swallowing, and changes in physical appearance that will result from surgery.

Nursing Diagnosis: Risk for ineffective individual coping related to loss of normal breathing and swallowing patterns, inability to speak, and change in physical appearance

Patient Outcomes	Nursing Interventions	Rationale
Patient identifies sources of support that will be available postoperatively.	Assist patient in identifying available sources of support.	Provides objective evidence that assistance is available and thus helps build the patient's confidence in ability to deal successfully with the surgery and its outcomes.
Patient identifies effective coping patterns.	Explore with patient ways of coping that were effective in the past.	Because different people cope best in different ways, identification of coping methods encourages use of strategies proven effective for this person.
Patient expresses confidence in ability to cooperate and participate in postoperative care.	Work with patient to develop a plan for coping with current stress.	Provides patient with sense of control and promotes development of acceptable plan with which patient will cooperate, thus increasing its probability of success.
Patient expresses hope about the future.	Reassure patient that nursing staff and other health-care personnel will work with him or her toward recovery.	Provides patient with positive facts on which to focus and base hope for a successful surgical outcome.
	Arrange a meeting with a successfully rehabilitated laryngectomee.	Provides the patient with a positive role model at a time most likely to be acceptable to the patient.

Evaluation: Compare the patient's status with the expected outcomes. If the outcomes are not met, reassess the patient and revise the plan.

Postoperative Care

Assessment Findings: Patient has difficulty coughing and expectorating secretions. Secretions are heard during respiration and can occasionally be seen bubbling at tracheostomy stoma.

Nursing Diagnosis: Ineffective airway clearance related to increased secretions, impaired cough, and loss of humidification of air by upper airway

(continued)

Nursing Care Guide 15–2

Patients Undergoing Conservation Laryngectomy (continued)

Patient Outcomes	Nursing Interventions	Rationale
Airway is cleared of secretions by coughing or suctioning as they accumulate. Respirations are easy and quiet. Respiratory rate is within normal range. Complaints of dyspnea are absent. Lungs are clear on auscultation.	Maintain patient in mid-Fowler's position.	Decreases edema in neck and promotes ventilation because gravity pulls abdominal contents away frrom diaphragm, thus allowing greater chest expansion.
	Encourage patient to turn, cough, and deep breathe every hour.	Promotes expansion of airway and removal of secretions to allow for maximum gas exchange.
	Splint patient's neck by placing hands behind it when patient is turning and coughing.	Decreases pull on incision line.
	Have patient lean forward when coughing.	Promotes raising and expectoration of airway secretions.
	Suction the tracheostomy as occasion requires (PRN) to prevent obstruction of airflow.	Artificial means of secretion removal may be necessary to maintain a clear airway.
	Insert a few drops of saline into the stoma before suctioning if secretions are viscous and difficult to remove.	Thins secretions and thus aids their removal.
	Administer humidified air or oxygen as ordered.	Moisture liquefies secretions, thus facilitating airway clearance.

Evaluation: Compare the patient's status with the expected outcomes. If the outcomes are not met, reassess the patient and revise the plan.

Assessment Findings: Patient unable to speak because of temporary tracheostomy (about 1 week).

Nursing Diagnosis: Impaired verbal communication related to temporary inability to speak secondary to diversion of air passing in and out of lungs through a tracheostomy

Patient Outcomes	Nursing Interventions	Rationale
Patient uses alternative modes of communication such as a Magic Slate, flash cards, computer, mouthing of words for others to lip-read, and gestures. Patient successfully communicates wants, needs, and essential information.	Keep call bell within easy reach of patient at all times.	Provides a nonverbal means of communication with persons not in sight.
	Visit patient frequently and assure him or her that help is close by to meet needs.	Reduces sense of isolation.
	Provide equipment for alternative mode of communication, such as Magic Slate, computer, pencil and paper, flash cards.	Allows a means of communication.

(continued)

Patients Undergoing Conservation Laryngectomy *(continued)*

Patient Outcomes	Nursing Interventions	Rationale
	Ask questions that require only a short answer or yes or no signal. Do not ask patient to signal with a nod or a shake of the head because this motion is painful. Instruct in eye blink, hand, and finger signals instead.	Decreases patient frustration by reducing need for lengthy responses while maintaining communication.
	Allow time for patient to communicate. Do not complete patient's thoughts and do not put words in the patient's mouth.	Allows patient to accurately communicate needs and feelings and to feel comfortable in attempts to communicate.
	Post a sign on the door and on the intercom at the nurses' station to remind personnel that patient cannot speak.	Decreases patient frustration and reassures patient that health-care workers are aware of his or her needs.
	Try to anticipate patient needs.	Decreases patient frustration with impaired communication.
	Inform other health-care personnel and significant others of the communication systems being used by the patient.	Maximizes effective communication through consistent use of one system, decreases patient frustration, and reminds the patient that health-care workers are aware of his or her needs.

Evaluation: Compare the patient's status with the expected outcomes. If the outcomes are not met, reassess the patient and revise the plan.

Assessment Findings: Patient is observed having difficulty swallowing. Attempts to swallow are accompanied by coughing and choking.

Nursing Diagnosis: Impaired swallowing related to surgical trauma and removal of the epiglottis and false vocal cords

Patient Outcomes	Nursing Interventions	Rationale
Patient allows saliva to drain from mouth in early postoperative period.	Instruct patient to expectorate or allow saliva to drain out of mouth, not swallow it.	Prevents coughing, choking, and further injury to traumatized tissues.
	Keep patient's head turned to the side.	Promotes drainage of saliva from side of mouth.
	Provide basin and wipes for oral secretions.	Promotes cleanliness and comfort despite need to allow saliva to drain from side of mouth.
	When patient is resting, place a wick with one end in corner of mouth and the other in an emesis basin.	Removes oral secretions and maintains cleanliness and comfort without patient's active participation.

(continued)

Nursing Care Guide 15–2
Patients Undergoing Conservation Laryngectomy (continued)

Patient Outcomes	Nursing Interventions	Rationale
Patient practices swallowing food as directed when tube feedings are discontinued. Patient swallows soft foods and viscous fluids.	When tube feedings are discontinued and oral intake begins (about 2 weeks postoperatively), start the patient on soft, formed foods, such as ice cream, Jell-O, and mashed potatoes. Instruct patient to ingest them as follows: Hold the breath. Keep head flexed (chin on chest) and tilted toward unaffected side. Place small amount of soft food on back of tongue. Swallow Cough to expel any food that may have entered trachea.	Reduces risk of aspiration and helps patient relearn how to swallow foods and fluids.
	Provide privacy for eating to decrease embarrassment and stress.	Fears of others' reactions may decrease nutritional intake.
Patient eats a nutritionally balanced daily diet.	As patient relearns to swallow, add viscous fluids and other soft foods to the diet. Progress to other foods and fluids as tolerated.	Increases variety of food ingested to provide more appetizing and nutritionally balanced diet.

Evaluation:	Compare the patient's status with the expected outcomes. If the outcomes are not met, reassess the patient and revise the plan.

Additional Assessments and Interventions

Monitor vital signs every 15 minutes until stable, every 1 to 2 hours for the first 24 hours, and then every 4 hours.

Monitor breath sounds.
Administer intravenous fluids and tube feedings as ordered.

SEVERE DYSPNEA, TACHYPNEA, AND ANXIETY AFTER LARYNGECTOMY

Within 10 days of seeking medical attention for hoarseness that had lasted 5 weeks, a 58-year-old man with a history of heavy smoking and alcoholism was diagnosed with squamous cell carcinoma of the larynx. He underwent a conservation (supraglottic) laryngectomy with left-sided neck dissection. A course of postoperative radiation therapy was planned.

I was assigned to care for the patient on the evening of his second postoperative day. During report, I learned that the surgical procedure had been uneventful, as had his postoperative course to that point. A temporary tracheostomy for airway protection had been performed, through which he was receiving humidified oxygen via a tracheostomy collar. A small-bore weighted nasogastric tube was in place, through which he was receiving half-strength continuous enteral feedings at 60 mL per hour. Nasogastric suction had been discontinued and tube feedings had been initiated once bowel sounds had resumed that morning. The feedings had been well tolerated thus far. The patient had been out of bed in a chair, was receiving meperidine (Demerol) for pain, and was urinating adequate amounts without difficulty following removal of his indwelling urinary catheter and IV line.

My initial assessment of the patient revealed an alert, oriented, and cooperative patient in no acute distress. His vital signs were within normal limits according to his baseline data. There was no evidence of bleeding, as indicated by a dry and intact incisional dressing, small amounts of blood-tinged drainage from the surgical drain, the absence of hematoma formation, and his indicators of adequate peripheral circulation. He communicated with me via a Magic Slate and complained only of fatigue.

Knowing that the risk for impaired gas exchange and ineffective airway clearance were among the priority nursing diagnoses for the patient, I performed a focused assessment of his respiratory status. His respiratory rate was 22 breaths per minute, respirations were effortless, breath sounds included coarse gurgles over the large airways, and tracheal secretions could be heard during respirations. Chest excursions were equal bilaterally, and the color of his skin and mucous membranes was good.

Next, I checked the tracheostomy tube for patency and the presence of secretions and crusting. Some mucus was bubbling from the tracheostomy opening. Using sterile aseptic technique, I carefully suctioned the patient. No excessive secretions or encrustations were noted. I also checked the high-volume, low-pressure tracheostomy cuff for an adequate seal and the absence of an air leak, and the neck ties for both security and adequate space for edema formation.

Finally, I turned my attention to assessing the patient's gastrointestinal tract. The nasogastric tube was adequately secured to the right naris and did not appear to have migrated upward as indicated by the markings on the tube. The continuous enteral feeding was infusing according to medical orders. Assessment of the abdomen revealed no evidence of distention. Auscultation of all four quadrants revealed normal bowel sounds. The patient denied any nausea, abdominal cramping, or diarrhea.

Before leaving the patient, I encouraged him to cough and deep-breathe, and I performed oral suctioning and hygiene and complete tracheostomy care. I also validated the position of the nasogastric tube by instilling 10 mL of air into the tube and auscultating for the sound of air rushing in over the stomach. I aspirated and returned the residual gastric contents, then decided to continue the patient's feeding based on the small amount of residual and lack of any clinical findings to indicate sluggish gastrointestinal mobility. The acid pH of the aspirate supported proper tube placement as well. Finally, I positioned the patient comfortably with the head of the bed elevated to 30 degrees, placed the call bell within his reach, and reassured him that I would return to check on him within 30 minutes.

About 15 minutes later, his call light lit. I responded immediately both because of his high risk for a compromised airway, and because he couldn't speak. Upon entering his room, it was obvious that he was in acute distress. He appeared frightened and was frantically struggling to sit up. He was diaphoretic, his color was ashen and becoming cyanotic, and his respirations were rapid, shallow, and stertorous. He was gasping for air and demonstrating exaggerated chest movements with muscle retraction, use of accessory muscles or respiration, and nasal flaring. He coughed weakly, and I felt minimal airflow over the tracheostomy stoma.

The patient's symptoms of severe dyspnea, tachypnea, and anxiety clearly suggested a partial airway obstruction. I recognized that a number of possible causes could be responsible for this change in the patient's condition. They include development of a mucus plug, copious secretions and

CLINICAL ? THINKING

(continued)

accumulated encrustations in the tracheostomy tube, a dislodged tracheostomy tube, airway edema, anaphylaxis, the presence of formula in the respiratory tract secondary to a tracheoesophageal fistula, or aspiration of gastric contents. Because I had very recently completed tracheal suction and tracheostomy care, it seemed unlikely to me that a mucus plug or encrustation were the underlying cause. Although the inflated tracheostomy cuff offered some protection, and I had taken precautions to prevent the aspiration of gastric contents, the suddenness of the onset of the patient's clinical manifestations, his high risk for aspiration secondary to the surgical procedure itself, and the presence of an artificial airway led me to suspect that the patient had regurgitated or vomited and was choking on his gastric contents. The presence of a nasogastric tube and continuous feeding greatly increased the risk of aspiration and supported my suspicion. Closer examination of the patient revealed the presence of formula in the oral cavity which strongly supported the likelihood of a massive aspiration.

Because partial airway obstruction—regardless of etiology—can lead to complete obstruction of airflow, hypoxemia, acute respiratory failure, respiratory arrest, and cardiac arrest, and because clinical death can ensue within minutes, I responded to this threatening emergency by implementing the following immediate interventions:

1. I stopped the tube feeding.
2. I called for assistance and asked the responding nurse to notify the physician.
3. I raised the head of the bed to 45 degrees and turned the patient to the side.
4. I checked the tracheostomy tube for proper placement.
5. I initiated suctioning of the tracheostomy tube followed by oropharyngeal suctioning of the oral cavity.
6. I spoke to the patient in a calm and reassuring manner and told him that I would remain with him and help him re-establish his breathing.
7. I increased the flow of oxygen through the tracheostomy collar.
8. I attached a pulse oximeter.
9. I prepared to call a code if necessary.
10. I continued to monitor his respiratory status.
11. I monitored his vital signs and level of consciousness.
12. I documented my findings and actions.

The presence of formula and gastric contents in the secretions suctioned from the tracheostomy tube confirmed the suspicion of aspiration. The physician ordered a chest x-ray, arterial blood gases, oxygen therapy, IV fluids, bronchodilators, antibiotics, and intravenous steroids. The patient was transferred to the ICU for continuous monitoring and was scheduled for a bronchoscopy.

The health-care team succeeded in restoring a patent airway and in reversing the hypoxemia. Following rapid and effective action by a nurse, the patient's respiratory status began to improve and spontaneous independent respirations were maintained. The nurse's ability to skillfully respond without delay ensured adequate pulmonary gas exchange, saved the patient's life, and reduced the risk of aspiration pneumonia, sepsis, atelectasis, and acute respiratory distress syndrome.

Think Critically

Should the nurse have assessed the patient's breath sounds, pulse, and/or blood pressure before implementing the nursing interventions? Were these assessments essential? Might they have improved the patient outcome?

Could the nurse have implemented additional assessments and/or actions to prevent or minimize this complication of a supraglottic laryngectomy?

How does the maintenance of surgical asepsis when suctioning the patient's tracheostomy during an emergency compare with that during routine tracheal suctioning?

How might the nursing assessment and actions have differed if the patient's tracheostomy tube had become dislodged? If it was a mucus plug? If the nasogastric tube had become displaced?

Which clinical manifestations would lead the nurse to suspect that the patient had developed aspiration pneumonia? Atelectasis? Acute respiratory distress syndrome?

How would the scenario have differed if the patient had undergone a total laryngectomy? Would aspiration have been an issue?

What additional complications would the patient with a laryngectomy be at risk for in the immediate postoperative period? During hospitalization? Following discharge to the home? What plans to minimize these patient problems would be reflected in the nursing care plan?

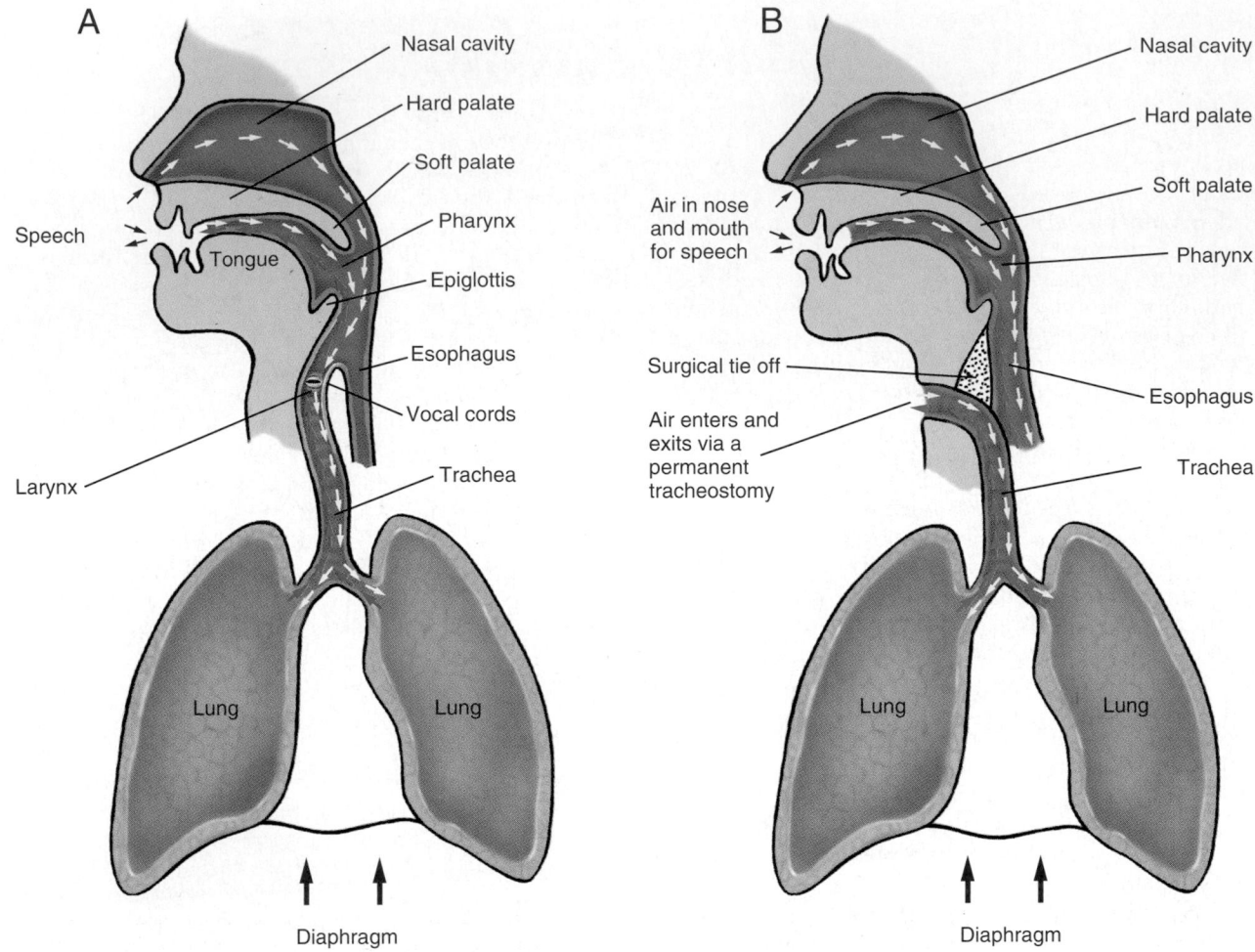

Figure 15–9

Pattern of air flow for respiration and speech before and after total laryngectomy. *A,* Before the laryngectomy, air passes in and out of the lungs through the nose and mouth, and speech is created as exhaled air passes through the larynx. *B,* After total laryngectomy, air passes in and out of the lungs through a permanent tracheostomy. Air in the nose, mouth, and pharynx is swallowed, enters the esophagus, and is expelled as a belch to create esophageal speech.

allows air exhaled from the lungs to pass from the trachea through the prosthesis into the esophagus. This air causes vibrations in the hypopharynx, which allow sound to be produced (Fig. 15–12). Laryngeal reconstruction using arm or leg tendons or rib cartilage has also been attempted.

NURSING PROCESS
Total Laryngectomy

PREOPERATIVE NURSING CARE

Assessment

The basic assessment required by any preoperative patient (see Chapter 6), as well as that required by

any patient diagnosed with cancer (see Chapter 34), applies also to the patient scheduled for a laryngectomy for cancer of the larynx. In addition, be certain to assess the patient's and significant other's understanding of and emotional response to the effects of surgery on breathing, swallowing, speech, and appearance.

Because speech will be impossible after surgery, assess the patient to determine which alternative forms of communication (eg, pad and pencil, flash cards, gestures) appear to be most suited to the patient's capabilities and temperament. For example, a Magic Slate would not be appropriate for a patient unable to write in English or one with tremors or paresis of the dominant hand that interferes with motor function. A laptop computer might be most appropriate for a patient accustomed to using a computer.

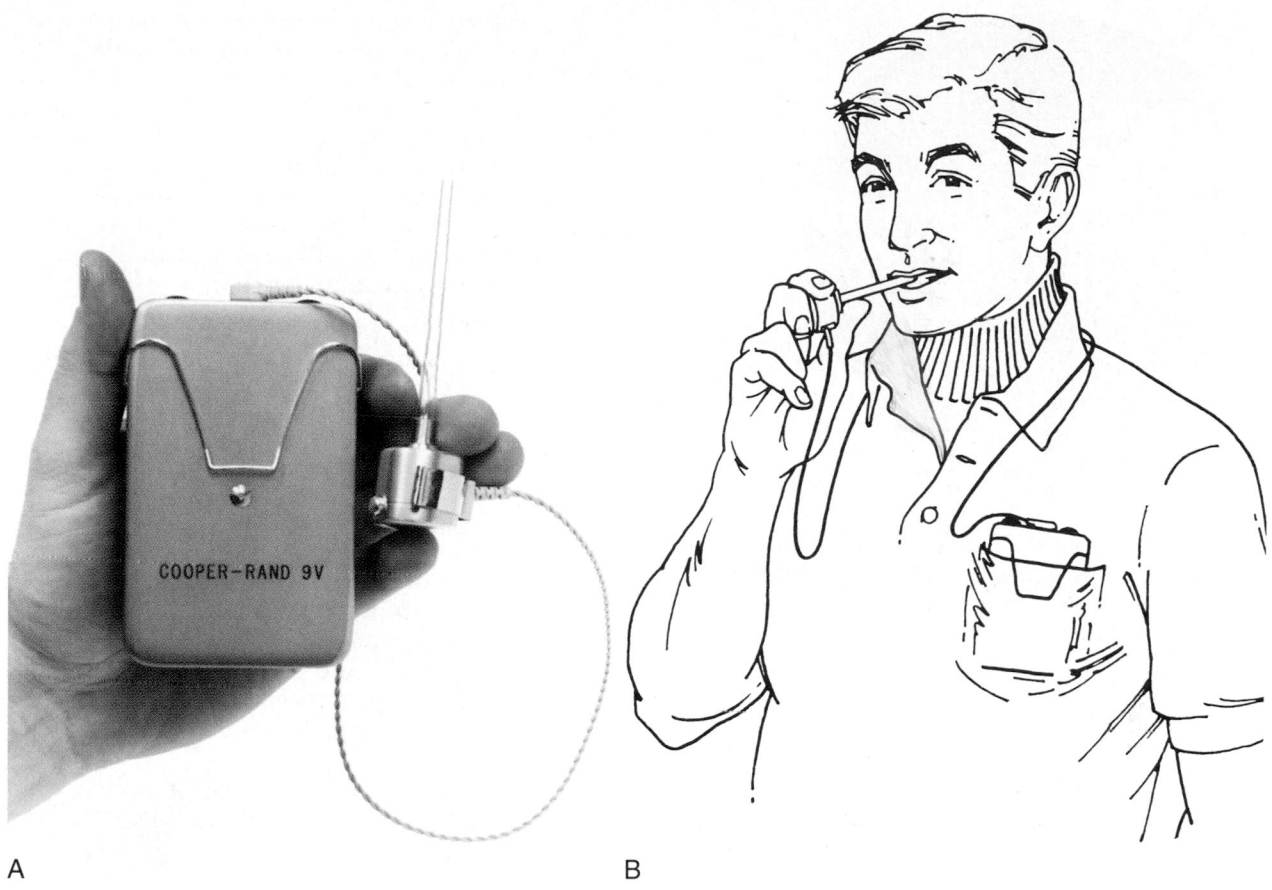

A   B

Figure 15–10

A, Cooper-Rand electronic speech aid. This device provides the vocal tone necessary for speech. Most patients can use it successfully immediately after surgery. *B,* Electronic speech aid in use. The patient inserts about 2 inches of the plastic tube into the corner of his mouth. The tip should be above the tongue and pointed toward the roof of the mouth to keep the end from being closed by the tongue. The patient presses the button on the tone generator and then speaks. Instruct the patient to speak slowly and distinctly, using the tongue and lips to form sounds just as before the laryngectomy. (Courtesy of Luminaud, Inc, Mentor, OH.)

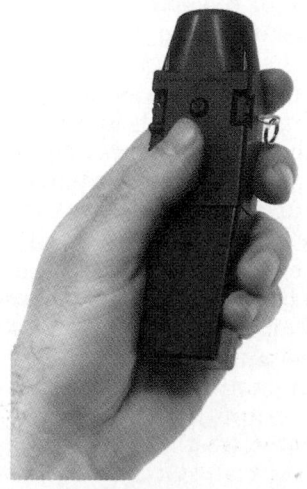

Figure 15–11

Example of artificial device used to create speech following total laryngectomy. The vibrating head is pressed firmly against the neck for use. (Courtesy of Luminaud, Inc, Mentor, OH.)

If the patient is scheduled for a total laryngectomy, assess his or her ability to learn and physically manage self-care postoperatively, including tracheostomy care, availability of support systems, and awareness of alternative methods of producing speech.

Nursing Diagnoses and Planning

Nursing diagnoses and related expected patient outcomes commonly applicable to patients scheduled for laryngectomy include the following:

NDx: Anxiety related to the diagnosis of cancer, the surgical experience, and the effects of surgery on eating, breathing, speaking, appearance, work, and social activities

Planning: Patient Outcomes
1. Patient attends to information given about the disease and surgery.
2. Patient asks questions about the surgery and its effects.

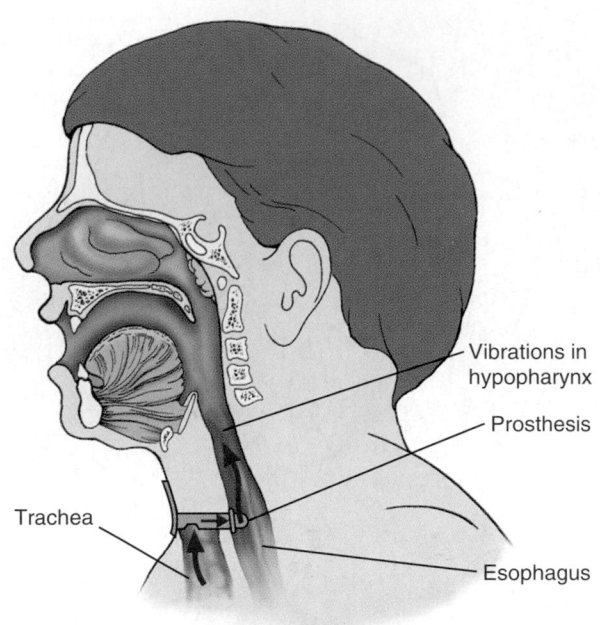

Figure 15–12
Tracheoesophageal opening with prosthesis in place. Exhaled air from the lungs moves through the trachea, prosthesis, and esophagus to create vibrations in the hypopharynx that allow production of sound.

3. Patient communicates feelings of concern and anxiety.
4. Nonverbal signs of excessive anxiety, such as constant pacing and refusing to let significant others leave, are absent.

NDx: Anticipatory grieving related to alteration in speech

Planning: Patient Outcomes
1. Patient acknowledges that feelings of grief are normal.
2. Patient expresses feelings of grief.
3. Patient verbalizes interest in speech rehabilitation.

NDx: Risk for ineffective individual coping related to the diagnosis of cancer, the surgical experience, and the effects of surgery on speech, appearance, interpersonal relationships, and employment

Planning: Patient Outcomes
1. Patient identifies effective and ineffective coping patterns.
2. Patient participates in the decision-making process.
3. Patient reacts with appropriate verbal and nonverbal responses applicable to the situation.

Nursing Interventions and Evaluation

NDx: Anxiety
Acknowledge that anxiety is normal before a laryngectomy and encourage the patient to verbalize concerns. Answer questions simply but clearly and describe the postoperative care routine. Tell the patient what tubes and dressings to expect and the reason for each. Be certain to carefully explain how breathing takes place after surgery. Emphasize that the patient will begin learning self-care the day after surgery. Reassure the patient that support and assistance will be available when needed. Arrange for consultation with a speech therapist to discuss alternate forms of oral communication.

NDx: Anticipatory grieving
Allow opportunities for the patient to express grief and encourage this expression. Provide a calm, private environment to facilitate patient and family grieving. Discuss with the patient and family the impact of this loss on the family unit and its functioning.

NDx: Risk for ineffective individual coping
Depending on the assessment of the individual patient's coping style, a visit from a well-adjusted laryngectomee (a person with a laryngectomy) may be arranged. Encourage the patient to express concerns about surgery, appearance, interpersonal relationships, and employment. Assist the patient in exploring available resources.

Compare the patient's status with the expected outcomes. If the outcomes are not met, reassess the patient and revise the plan.

POSTOPERATIVE NURSING CARE

Assessment

Priority assessments are those related to the effectiveness of ventilation. Monitor vital signs. Note the depth and effort of breathing, as well as the color of nail beds and mucous membranes. Assess the effectiveness of coughing. Observe the amount, color, and viscosity of secretions. Review arterial blood gas values and monitor oxygen saturation levels.

Observe the suture line and the tracheostomy for bleeding and later for signs of infection, such as redness, swelling, tenderness, and purulent drainage. If drains are inserted in the operative area, monitor the amount and character of the drainage. (Do not disconnect drains from suction to measure drainage without a specific order.)

Assess pain as well as difficulty swallowing. If a nasogastric tube is in place, check that it is functioning properly, observe the drainage, and inspect the patient's naris for irritation. When tube feeding or oral intake begins, assess the patient for nausea, vomiting, abdominal distention, and diarrhea. Measure intake and output and obtain daily weights.

Throughout the postoperative period, assess the patient's psychosocial status. Observe for signs of anxiety, withdrawal, or depression and note interest and cooperation related to self-care. Assess the ease and effectiveness of communication techniques being used and also the patient's response to staff members, other patients, and visitors.

Nursing Diagnoses and Planning

Nursing diagnoses and related expected patient outcomes commonly applicable to patients after laryngectomy include the following:

NDx: Ineffective airway clearance related to increased secretions, impaired cough, and loss of humidification and filtration of inhaled air by the upper airway

Planning: Patient Outcomes
1. Secretions are removed from the airway by suctioning or coughing.
2. No dust or other foreign matter enters the tracheostomy.
3. Respirations are easy and quiet.
4. Respiratory rate is within patient's normal range.
5. Complaints of dyspnea are absent.
6. Lungs are clear on auscultation.

NDx: Impaired verbal communication related to inability to speak secondary to diversion of air passing in and out of the lungs through a tracheostomy

Planning: Patient Outcomes
1. Patient uses alternative modes of communication such as Magic Slate, flash cards, computer, and gestures.
2. Patient successfully communicates wants, needs, and essential information.

NDx: Pain related to surgical trauma

Planning: Patient Outcomes
1. Patient reports pain relief.
2. Nonverbal indications of pain are absent.

NDx: Altered nutrition: less than body requirements related to surgical trauma and loss of sense of taste and smell

Planning: Patient Outcomes
1. Patient maintains weight.
2. Patient tolerates nasogastric tube feedings.
3. Patient gradually adds fluids, soft foods, and solid foods to the diet.

NDx: Risk for body image disturbance related to presence of tracheostomy and loss of voice

Planning: Patient Outcomes
1. Patient looks at tracheostomy.
2. Patient or significant other participates in care of tracheostomy.
3. Patient interacts with others using available means of communication.
4. Patient actively participates with speech therapist in learning esophageal speech or the use of a speech device.

NDx: Risk for altered health maintenance related to insufficient knowledge of self-care

Planning: Patient Outcomes
1. Patient or significant other demonstrates stoma care, suctioning, and oral hygiene.

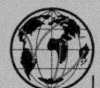

INTERNET CONNECTIONS
Upper Respiratory Disorders

Sinusitis
Med Facts/Sinusitis
The National Jewish Center for Immunology and Respiratory Medicine
http://www.njc.org/MFhtml/SIN_MF.html
A good patient-oriented source of basic information and answers to frequently asked questions related to sinusitis. This site includes descriptions of symptoms, diagnosis, and treatment (medications, surgery).

Cancer of the Larynx
Cancer of the Larynx: Information and Assistance
http://members.aol.com/fantumtwo/cancer1.htm
This unique site is produced by a laryngeal cancer survivor who provides a great deal of information in a readable format, including answers to frequently asked questions, referrals to authoritative sources of information, and links to relevant medical articles and resources.

Cancer of the Larynx
http://www.medicinenet.com/mainmenu/encyclop/ARTICLE/Art_L/larynC.htm
An article containing frequently asked questions and authoritative answers modified from information from the National Institutes of Health and the National Cancer Institute.

---

2. Patient describes precautions to be observed in regard to the tracheostomy.
3. Patient lists signs and symptoms to be reported to a health-care professional.
4. Patient identifies community resources that can assist with home maintenance and coping with effects of surgery and how to contact those resources.

Nursing Interventions and Evaluation

NDx: Ineffective airway clearance
Encourage the patient to turn, cough, and breathe deeply every 2 hours—more often if excessively large amounts of mucus are produced. Use a lint-free wipe to collect secretions discharged from the stoma during coughing. Have the patient lean forward to assist in expelling secretions. Remember that coughing can be difficult at first when the glottis is removed because the ability to increase intrathoracic pressure is impaired. Suction the tracheos-

tomy as needed to prevent obstruction of airflow. If secretions are viscous and not easily removed, insert a few drops of saline into the stoma before suctioning. During the initial postoperative period, administer humidified air or oxygen as ordered to help loosen secretions because normal humidification by the upper airways is lost.

While the laryngectomy tube is in place, clean and change it, as described in Chapter 14 in the discussion of tracheostomy care. When the tube is removed, keep a thin covering over the stoma (laryngectomy bib or scarf) to allow passage of air but prevent dust or other foreign matter from accidentally entering the tracheostomy. If dryness is a problem, saturate this cover with normal saline to provide some humidification.

NDx: Impaired verbal communication

For the patient unable to speak, it is of critical importance to feel that help is available at all times. Therefore, keep the call bell always within reach and frequently check on the patient's needs.

On the basis of the plan developed preoperatively, encourage the patient to use alternative methods of communication. Be certain to provide sufficient time for the patient to communicate needs and concerns by gesture, notes, beginning esophageal speech, or artificial device. Avoid acting hurried, and do not put words into the patient's mouth or complete what the patient appears to be trying to say.

Explain to significant others the importance of allowing the patient the time needed to communicate by an alternative method if the method is to be used with increasing facility and confidence.

NDx: Pain

Administer medication for pain if needed. Remember that opiates are contraindicated because of their potential for respiratory depression. However, this is generally not a problem because there is relatively little postoperative pain. Medications with the strength of opiates are rarely needed.

Enhance the effectiveness of nonopiate drugs by maintaining a quiet environment, making certain the patient is physically comfortable, and promoting the use of relaxation techniques and diversionary measures.

NDx: Altered nutrition: less than body requirements

Maintain patient on NPO status and on intravenous fluids in the immediate postoperative period. Administer enteral feedings when ordered. Resume oral intake with a soft diet. Provide mouth care before eating and privacy during early attempts at eating. Reassure the patient that choking or aspirating food is not a concern as there is no longer a connection between the esophagus and the trachea. If the patient has trouble swallowing, place a small amount of food on the back of the tongue, flex the head

forward and instruct the patient to consciously swallow. Provide small, frequent, attractively prepared meals. Monitor weight. Obtain a consultation with a dietician or a nutritionist.

NDx: Risk for body image disturbance

Provide an accepting, nonthreatening environment. Be sensitive to the patient's feelings and avoid comments or actions that could be construed by the patient as indicating distaste or pity for his or her condition. Be aware that, without speech, verbal expression of feelings is inhibited and may contribute to frustration manifested in nonverbal, angry behavior.

Acknowledge the patient's feelings and do not force the patient to look at the tracheostomy. When the patient does look at it, explain that the redness and swelling will decrease with time and provide other additional information needed to correct misconceptions.

Assist the patient as needed to maintain good grooming. Be certain the patient's hair is combed and that male patients are shaved. Encourage female patients to apply makeup, if usually worn. Help all patients get out of bed and dress as soon as they are able.

NDx: Risk for altered health maintenance

Health teaching, both for the patient and significant others, is also an integral part of care. It is best begun preoperatively and continued throughout the postoperative phase. Teach about suctioning and care of the tracheostomy and help the patient perform these tasks with the aid of a mirror. Later, teach the patient and significant others about self-care after discharge, as outlined in Highlight 15–6. As part of this teaching, be sure to show the patient the variety of stoma guards available, including metal, plastic, and nylon bibs.

Inform the patient and significant others about community support groups such as the Lost Chord Club and the Nu Voice Club and the availability of equipment and informational materials through the American Cancer Society. Provide telephone numbers and names of contact persons.

Additional Interventions

Position the patient with the head elevated to decrease edema, limit pull on the suture line, and promote pulmonary ventilation.

Provide frequent mouth care and suction oral secretions until the patient is able to swallow. Also suction the nares if needed because the patient is unable to blow the nose.

If wound drains are in place, observe and measure drainage. Record color and amount. Bring drainage of less than 50 mL daily to the attention of the surgeon, because it may be appropriate to remove the drain.

Compare the patient's status with the expected

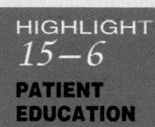 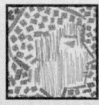

HIGHLIGHT 15–6

PATIENT EDUCATION

Discharge Instructions After Total Laryngectomy

Instruct the patient as follows:

Wash hands thoroughly before touching the stoma.

Wash the stoma daily with a well-wrung, warm washcloth.

Do not use soaps, cotton swabs, or tissue because they may obstruct the airway.

Do not use undiluted alcohol on the stoma because it is both drying and irritating.

Apply a thin layer of petrolatum to the skin surrounding the stoma to prevent cracking.

Wear a stoma guard, light scarf, or clothing with a high collar to protect the tracheostomy from cold, drying, and foreign bodies and to reduce its visibility.

Protect the stoma from water. Cover with a cupped hand when bathing, keep showers below neck level, wash hair by hanging the head over a tub or sink, and avoid water sports.

Keep powders and sprays used on the upper body (such as hair spray, deodorant sprays, and perfume) well away from the tracheostomy.

Place a guard and a towel over the stoma when shaving or having a haircut to prevent hairs from entering the stoma.

Use a nonaerosol shaving cream.

Use a humidifier in the home if excessive dryness is a problem.

Avoid air conditioning to protect from excessive coldness.

Check the stoma daily for redness, swelling, and purulent drainage and report to physician if present.

Clean teeth and mouth three times a day because halitosis may go undetected from loss of smell.

Wear a medical alert bracelet or chain indicating the presence of a tracheostomy and giving instructions to follow in an emergency.

---

outcomes. If the outcomes are not met, reassess the patient and revise the plan.

RADICAL NECK DISSECTION

Radical neck dissections are performed on patients with laryngeal (or oral pharyngeal) cancers known to metastasize to the cervical lymph nodes or when nodes are palpable at the time of surgery. In some cases, with a lower risk of metastasis, a modified (conservative or functional) dissection may be done, in which only the lymph nodes are removed.

In a radical neck dissection, the neck is opened between the jaw and the clavicle from its midline in the front to the interior border of the trapezius muscle on the side. Subcutaneous and soft tissue are removed, along with the sternocleidomastoid and other muscles, the jugular vein, and the spinal accessory nerve. A split-thickness skin graft is then placed as protection over the carotid artery, and the skin flaps are closed (Fig. 15–13). Because the accessory nerve (which innervates the trapezius muscle) is cut during this procedure, the trapezius muscle atrophies postoperatively and the affected shoulder droops. Because this surgery is extensive and has associated risks of airway obstruction, hemorrhage from carotid artery rupture, and skin flap necrosis, the patient is usually in the critical care unit.

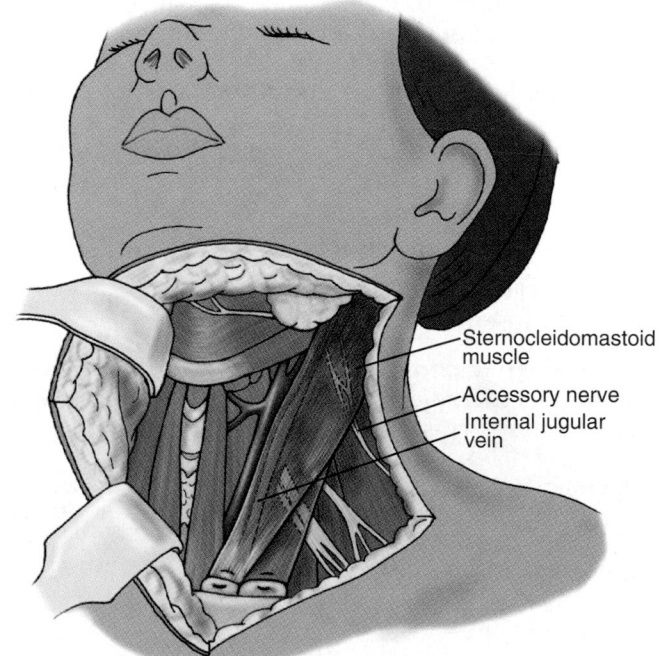

Figure 15–13

Radical neck dissection, in which the sternocleidomastoid muscle, the internal jugular vein, the accessory nerve, and other adjacent tissues are removed.

NURSING PROCESS GUIDELINES
Radical Neck Dissection

Assess the skin flap frequently throughout the postoperative period to detect evidence of necrosis. The flap should be pink and warm to the touch and have minimal edema. Position the patient in semi-Fowler's or high-Fowler's position to limit tension on the flap and to promote venous drainage. Monitor the amount and type of drainage from the surgical drains. Because tissues overlying and protecting the carotid artery have been removed, also monitor for signs of carotid artery rupture. These include sternal or high epigastric distress.

Assist the physical therapist and the patient in implementing the postoperative exercise regimen, which typically begins once the drains are removed, the suture line is intact, and edema has resolved (Fig. 15–14). Medicate for chest, shoulder, and neck pain before exercise sessions. Instruct the patient to follow these guidelines for several months after surgery:

- Maintain good posture, with shoulders pulled back
- Avoid lifting, pulling, or pushing with the affected arm
- Avoid carrying anything that weighs more than 3 pounds
- Expect pain and numbness in the neck, chest, and shoulder

Recognize that this is disfiguring surgery and assist the patient to identify and verbalize concerns about changes in body function and appearance. Encourage the patient to wear clothing with high necks and shoulder padding to improve appearance. Also encourage the use of accessories, such as hats, which can detract attention from the neck. See Nursing Care Guide 15–3 for further discussion of nursing care.

❖ SETTINGS, PROVIDERS, AND COLLABORATION FOR CARE

The patient undergoing a total laryngectomy, with or without a radical neck dissection, requires specialized care. This care is provided by a variety of health-care professionals in different treatment settings. An otolaryngologist performs the surgical procedure and the patient remains hospitalized for about 1 week. During this time, the nurse is assisted with administration of direct care by the respiratory therapist and the dietitian. Consultation with a speech therapist preoperatively is followed by postoperative speech rehabilitation. A physical therapist may be consulted for exercises to reduce shoulder droop and maintain range of motion if a radical neck dissection was performed. Discharge planners work to make the transition from hospital to home as smooth as possible. Arrangements for oxygen and suction equipment and other needed supplies, as well as a referral for home nursing care, must be made. The home health nurse may provide direct care or supervise and evaluate care given by the patient or family. A social worker may be needed to make financial arrangements and to assist the patient to cope with the surgery and its ramifications. The patient may continue to receive speech and physical rehabilitation as an outpatient. Some patients may require radiation therapy and others may need hospice care.

The Elderly: Special Considerations

Any upper respiratory tract infection or inflammation places the geriatric patient at risk for complications. Atrophy and weakness of respiratory muscles, coupled with decreased ciliary movement, make the cough reflex slower and less effective, thus interfering with airway clearance. Many older people have coexisting chronic illness, which further predisposes to complications.

Older persons should be referred to a physician if symptoms of a cold or other upper respiratory tract disease do not start to clear within 2 or 3 days. Encourage older adults to use local or topical rather than systemic over-the-counter products because the anticholinergic agents found in many cold preparations can cause mental changes and other adverse effects in older adults. Also, teach older adults to select the product with the fewest ingredients to reduce the chance of adverse effects and drug interactions. Encourage elderly patients to obtain a pneumonia vaccination and an annual influenza vaccination.

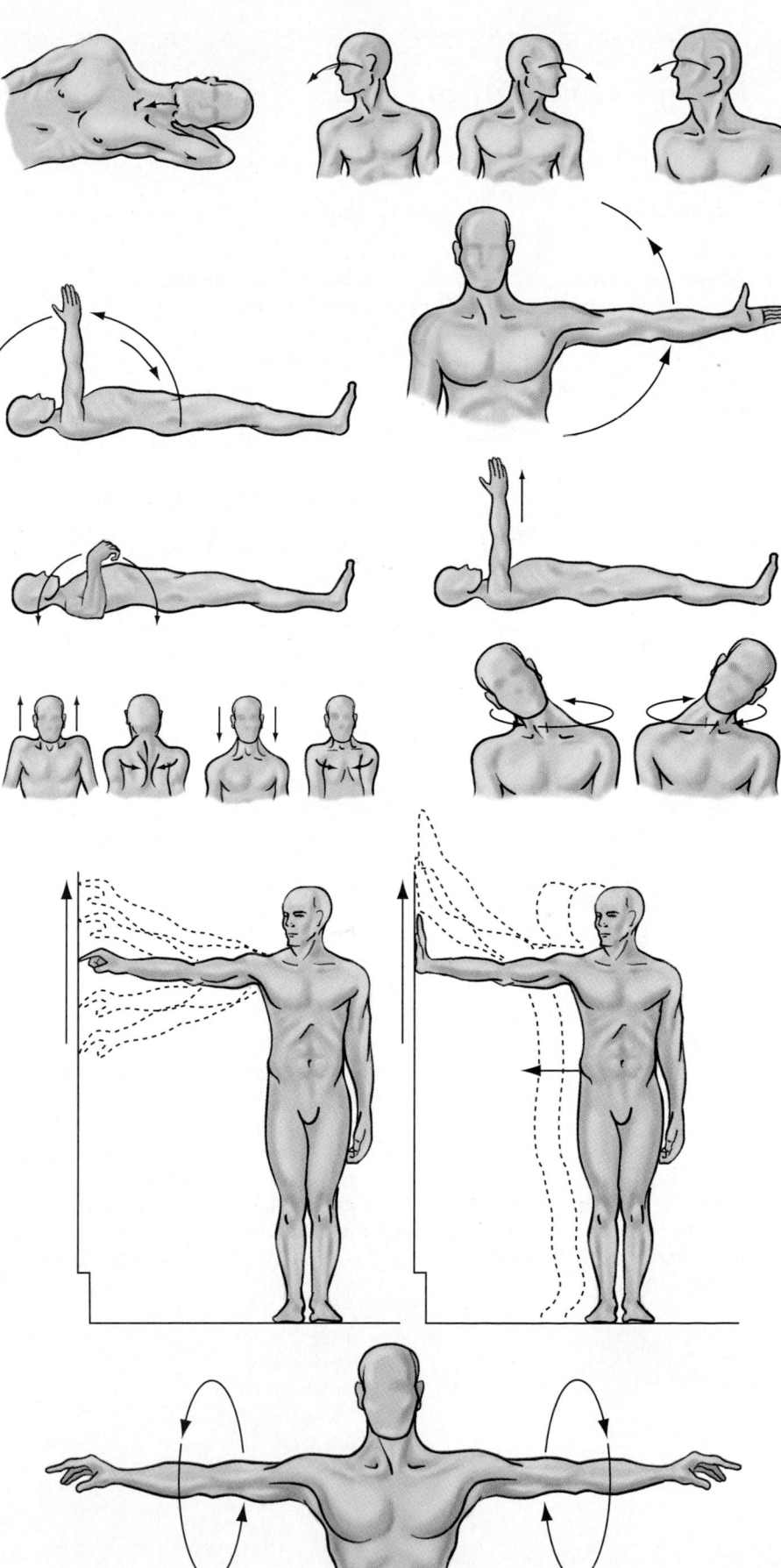

Figure 15–14

Neck exercises to be performed following radical neck dissection. (After J. L. Gluckman, M.D., University of Cincinnati Medical Center, Cincinnati, OH.)

Nursing Care Guide 15–3
Postoperative Patients with a Radical Neck Dissection

Assessment Findings: Patient complains of neck, chest, and shoulder pain. Patient grimaces on moving.

Nursing Diagnosis: Pain: neck, shoulder, and chest related to surgical trauma

Patient Outcomes	Nursing Interventions	Rationale
Patient states that pain is relieved. Patient moves and turns easily without groans, grimaces, or other nonverbal indications of pain.	Administer analgesics as ordered, remembering that narcotics are to be avoided because they depress respiration.	Provides pain relief by action specific to drug ordered.
	Keep the head of the bed elevated.	Decreases edema, thereby reducing pressure on surrounding tissues.
	Splint patient's neck when turning or moving.	Decreases pull on incision line.
	Maintain a quiet, restful environment.	Promotes relaxation, rest, and action of analgesics and sedative medications.
	Encourage use of relaxation techniques.	Reduces tension level of body, thereby decreasing strain on body tissues.
	Provide diversion, such as soft music.	Promotes relaxation, rest, and action of analgesic and sedative medications.

Evaluation: Compare the patient's status with the expected outcomes. If the outcomes are not met, reassess the patient and revise the plan.

Assessment Findings: Patient has had the tissues overlying the carotid artery removed and replaced with a split-thickness skin graft as part of a radical neck dissection.

Nursing Diagnosis: Risk for impaired tissue integrity (carotid artery) related to wound necrosis, infection, or tumor invasion

Patient Outcomes	Nursing Interventions	Rationale
Patient remains free of complications secondary to hemorrhage from the carotid artery	Monitor vital signs for indications of developing hypovolemic shock (increased pulse and respiratory rates, decreased blood pressure).	Early recognition allows early intervention and may prevent death, stroke, cardiac or other damage.
	Monitor wound drainage for signs of excess bleeding. Check for pooling of blood behind the neck.	Expected drainage is serosanguineous and up to 120 mL in the first 24 hours, gradually decreasing thereafter. Deviations may indicate excess bleeding.
	Monitor patient for high epigastric discomfort. Report immediately if it occurs.	Epigastric pain or discomfort is a sign of impending carotid rupture.
	Make certain that blood is available.	Blood replacement is essential to the management of a patient with a carotid artery rupture.

(continued)

Postoperative Patients with a Radical Neck Dissection (continued)

Patient Outcomes	Nursing Interventions	Rationale
	If carotid bleeding occurs, apply direct pressure on the artery. Maintain uninterrupted pressure until the patient is in the operating room and the surgeon takes over.	Pressure controls rapid blood loss.
	Call for a second person and direct that person to elevate the head of the bed and notify the surgeon stat.	Elevating the head of the bed helps maintain a patent airway. Control of hemorrhage from the rupture requires surgery.

Evaluation: Compare the patient's status with the expected outcomes. If the outcomes are not met, reassess the patient and revise the plan.

Assessment Findings: Patient has extensive suture lines and skin flaps secondary to radical neck dissection.

Nursing Diagnosis: Risk for impaired tissue integrity (extended) related to wound breakdown

Patient Outcomes	Nursing Interventions	Rationale
Wound heals free from complications.	Elevate head of bed 30 to 45 degrees.	Prevents stress on skin flaps and suture lines and promotes increased lymphatic and venous drainage, thus decreasing venous pressure in the skin flaps.
	Position patient with head slightly flexed.	Prevents stress on skin flaps and suture lines.
	Maintain functioning wound drainage system. Maintain suction. Milk tubing every 1–2 hours for 24 hours, then every 4 hours as needed.	Promotes drainage and prevents accumulation of drainage under flaps, which can result in hematoma requiring surgery or evacuation and re-establishment of drainage.
	Observe for air leaks.	Air leaking into the system prevents negative pressure and impairs drainage.
	Monitor wound for swelling or an ooze of dark red blood.	May indicate inadequate drainage and hematoma formation.
	Monitor color, capillary refill, and temperature of skin flaps.	Viable flaps are warm to the touch, have normal skin coloring, and have capillary refill less than 3 seconds. Decreased capillary refill, cool temperature, and pale color indicate inadequate circulation.

(continued)

Postoperative Patients with a Radical Neck Dissection *(continued)*

Patient Outcomes	Nursing Interventions	Rationale
	Avoid pressure or constriction (such as tight tracheostomy ties) on skin flaps.	Pressure or constriction impairs circulation and may decrease viability of skin flaps.
	Keep wound free of crusts and dry according to prescribed protocol.	Promotes healing.
	Monitor for signs of infection, such as redness, swelling, purulent drainage, areas of wound separation, fever, malaise, increased white blood cell count.	Early treatment of infection limits lymphatic and venous drainage thus decreasing venous pressure in the skin flaps.

Evaluation: Compare the patient's status with the expected outcomes. If the outcomes are not met, reassess the patient and revise the plan.

Assessment Findings: Patient has a large, disfiguring wound in neck and a shoulder that droops and is painful.

Nursing Diagnosis: Risk for body image disturbance related to changes in body appearance and alteration in body function

Patient Outcomes	Nursing Interventions	Rationale
Patient looks at wound. Patient communicates feelings about body changes.	Be sensitive to patient's need for acceptance.	Body image is closely tied to self-concept.
	Take care not to indicate shock or distaste for patient's condition by expression or comment.	Body image is derived in part from responses and opinions of others.
	Do not force patient to look at wound; wait until he or she is ready.	Allows time for acceptance of body-image changes.
	Expain that redness or swelling will decrease with time and then physical changes will not be as severe.	Provides realistic, positive expectations and promotes acceptance of appearance.
	Answer questions about changes in body and appearance honestly.	Promotes trust and provides realistic, positive expectations.
Patient participates in self-care.	Involve patient in self-care.	Promotes sense of control, self-confidence, and self-esteem.
Patient demonstrates an active interest in personal appearance.	Encourage attention to personal hygiene.	Promotes self-esteem.
Patient maintains relationships with significant others.	Encourage interaction with family and friends.	Prevents isolation, demonstrates that social interaction and acceptance are still possible, and provides source of emotional support.

Evaluation: Compare the patient's status with the expected outcomes. If the outcomes are not met, reassess the patient and revise the plan.

(continued)

Nursing Care Guide 15–3
Postoperative Patients with a Radical Neck Dissection *(continued)*

Assessment Findings: Patient asks questions about activities, limitations, and precautions to be taken after discharge.

Nursing Diagnosis: Risk for altered health maintenance related to insufficient knowledge of self-care after discharge

Patient Outcomes	Nursing Interventions	Rationale
Patient describes pain in shoulder over a period of months as expected and identifies measures to provide relief.	Explain that pain in the shoulder, neck, and chest will persist for months. Instruct the patient to use heat, massage, and liniment for relief.	Provides information about normal sequence of recovery and appropriate patient responses.
Patient describes need for precautions because of sensory loss in large area of chest, back, and shoulders.	Explain precautions that must be taken to guard against accidental injury because a large area of the shoulder, chest, and back will be numb.	Provides information necessary for self-management after discharge.
Patient describes and demonstrates neck, shoulder, and arm exercises to be performed after radical neck dissection.	Teach patient neck, shoulder, and arm exercises (see Fig. 15–14). Instruct patient to perform each exercise 10 times twice each day.	Increases range of motion on affected side.
Patient explains importance of avoiding exposure to smoke and, if a smoker, identifies a plan of action to stop smoking.	Reinforce importance of not smoking.	Smoking decreases gas exchange by altering lung structure and function.
Patient lists symptoms to be reported to physician.	Instruct patient to report fever, wound drainage, and increasing pain.	Provides information necessary to recognize postoperative complications after discharge.

Evaluation: Compare the patient's status with the expected outcomes. If the outcomes are not met, reassess the patient and revise the plan.

Chapter Review

1. What are possible solutions to the problem of allergies in a patient with rhinitis?
2. What are the advantages of a rapid throat culture test for a patient with pharyngitis?
3. Why is it important for a patient with streptococcal pharyngitis to take all antibiotics prescribed and to have a follow-up throat culture?
4. How is the care of a patient with tonsillitis similar to that of a patient with pharyngitis?
5. What could happen to a patient with laryngeal trauma if edema or hematoma develops rapidly?
6. How does the care of a total laryngectomy patient differ from that of a partial laryngectomy patient?
7. Why is it of critical importance to check frequently and keep the call bell within reach when caring for the total laryngectomy patient?
8. How would you communicate when caring for a patient who had a total laryngectomy?
9. Why is having suction apparatus available at the bedside important when caring for a patient who had a conservation laryngectomy?
10. Why is early medical treatment important for the geriatric patient with an upper respiratory tract infection?

Bibliography

Albanese AJ, Toplitz AD. A hassle-free guide to suctioning a tracheostomy. RN 1982; 45(4):24.

Al-Saden P. Anticoagulation-induced epistaxis. Nursing 1994; 24(12):33.

American Cancer Society. Cancer facts and figures—1995. New York: American Cancer Society, 1995.

Ballenger J, Snow J (eds). Otorhinolaryngology: Head and neck surgery. Baltimore: Williams and Wilkins, 1996.

Bartkiw TP, Pynn BR, Brown DH. Diagnosis and management of nasal fractures. Int J Trauma Nurs 1995; 1(1):11.

Bates B. A guide to physical examination. 6th ed. Philadelphia: JB Lippincott, 1995.

Benjamin B. A color atlas of otorhinolaryngology. Philadelphia: JB Lippincott, 1995.

Browning G. Updated ENT. Oxford: Butterworth-Heinemann, 1994.

Bryce J. Aspiration: Causes, consequences, and prevention. ORL Head Neck Nurs 1995; 13(2):14.

Calianno C. Guarding against aspiration complications. Nursing 1995; 25(6):52.

Clayman GL, Weber RS, Guillamondegui O, et al. Laryngeal preservation for advanced laryngeal and hypopharyngeal cancers. Archives of Otolaryngology Head Neck Surgery 1995; 121(2):219.

Cole P. The respiratory role of the upper airways: A selective clinical and pathophysiological review. St. Louis: Mosby Year-Book, 1993.

Crum R. Attachment of the adjustable tracheostoma valve and housing from the view of a laryngectomee. ORL Head Neck Nurs 1996; 14(1):15.

Cummings C (ed). Otolaryngology: Head and neck surgery. St. Louis: Mosby Year-Book, 1995.

Curtis LG. Common ear, nose, and throat problems: Disorders of the nose and throat, part 2. Physician Assistant 1990; 14(10):11.

Des Jardins T. Clinical manifestations and assessment of respiratory disease. St. Louis: Mosby Year-Book, 1995.

Dhillon R. Ear, nose, and throat, and head and neck surgery: An illustrated colour text. Edinburgh: Churchill Livingstone, 1994.

Douville L. Pharmacologic highlights: Management of acute sinusitis. Journal of the Academy of Nurse Practitioners 1995; 7(8):407.

Eibling DB, Snyderman CH, Weber PC, et al. Internal jugular vein reconstruction in bilateral radical neck dissection. Am J Otolaryngol 1995; 16(4):260.

Fishman A (ed). Pulmonary rehabilitation. New York: M. Dekker, 1996.

Gerchufsky M. Understanding upper respiratory infections. ADVANCE Nurse Pract 1995; 5:25.

Glavassevich M, McKibbon A, Thomas S. Information needs of patients who undergo surgery for head and neck cancer. Can Oncol Nurs J 1995; 5(1):9.

Hamaker RC, Hamaker RA. Surgical treatment of laryngeal cancer. Semin Speech Lang 1995; 16(Aug):221, 241.

Harding E. Preparing patients for the effects of laryngectomy. Nurs Times 1994; 90(32):36.

Harris R, Paine D, Wittler R, Bruhn F. Impact on empiric treatment of Group A streptococcal pharyngitis using an optical immunassay. Pediatrics 1995. 34(3):122.

Hirsch A (ed). Prevention of respiratory diseases. New York: M. Dekker, 1993.

Jarvis C. Physical examination and health assessment. Philadelphia: WB Saunders, 1995.

Kiselica D. Group A beta-hemolytic streptococcal pharyngitis: Current clinical concepts. Am Family Phys 1994; 49 (5);1147.

Krepsi Y. Laser practice report: Laser ablation of superficial tonsillar crypts. Clin Laser Mon 1994; 12(12):189.

Lee K (ed). Essential otolaryngology: Head and neck surgery. Norwalk, CT: Appleton and Lange, 1995.

Leiner S. Sore throats: Burning issues . . . recertification series. Physician Assist 1995; 19(3):19.

Lockhart JS, Bryce J. Restoring speech with tracheoesophageal puncture. Nursing 1993; 23(1):59.

Lucente FE, Sobol SM. Essentials of otolaryngology. 2nd ed. New York: Raven Press, 1993.

Mahler D (ed). Pulmonary disease in the elderly patient. New York: M. Dekker, 1993.

McCall M. Consultation forum. ORL Head Neck Nurs 1993; 11(4):9.

McCormick M. Facing disfigurement. Kai Tiaki Nurs NZ 1995; 1(2):13.

Murray J, Nadel J (eds). Textbook of respiratory medicine. Philadelphia: WB Saunders, 1994.

Nicklaus P, Herzon F, Steinle E. Short stay outpatient tonsillectomy. Arch Otolaryngol Head Neck Surg 1995; 121(5):521.

Niederman M. Respiratory infections: A scientific basis for management. Philadelphia: WB Saunders, 1994.

Norinkavich K, Howie G, Cariofiles P. Quality improvement study of day surgery for tonsillectomy and adenoidectomy patients. Pediatric Nursing 1995; 21(4):341.

Pasterkamp H, Sanchex I. Tracheal sounds in upper airway obstruction. Chest 1992; 102(3):963.

Pennington J (ed). Respiratory infections: Diagnosis and management. New York: Raven Press, 1994.

Practical Guidelines. Total laryngectomy. Society of Otorhinolaryngology and Head-Neck Nurses. ORL Head Neck Nurs 1994; 12(3):28.

Sasaki CT, Salzer SJ, Cahow CE, et al. Laryngopharyngoesophagectomy for advanced hypopharyngeal and esophageal squamous cell carcinoma: The Yale experience. Laryngoscope 1995; 105:160.

Schuller D. DeWeese and Saunders' otolaryngology: Head and neck surgery. St. Louis: Mosby Year-Book, 1994.

Schwartz R. The diagnosis and management of sinusitis. Nurse Pract 1994; 19(12):58.

Somerson SJ, Husted CW, Somerson SW, Sicilia MR. Mastering emergency airway management. Am J Nurs 1996; 96(5 Nurse Pract Extra Ed):24.

Stafford N. ENT. Edinburgh: Churchill Livingstone, 1994.

Stankiewicz JA, Newell DJ, Park AH. Complications of inflammatory diseases of the sinuses. Otolaryngol Clin North Am 1993; 26(4):639.

Understanding your laryngectomy [videotape]. University of Pittsburgh Medical Center. 1994

Watterson T, McFarlane S. The artificial larynx. Semin Speech Lang 1995; 16(3):205.

Weilitz P, Dettenmier P. Back to basics: Test your knowledge of tracheotomy tubes. Am J Nurs 1994; 94(2):46.

Wilkins R (ed). Respiratory disease: Principles of patient care. Philadelphia: FA Davis, 1993.

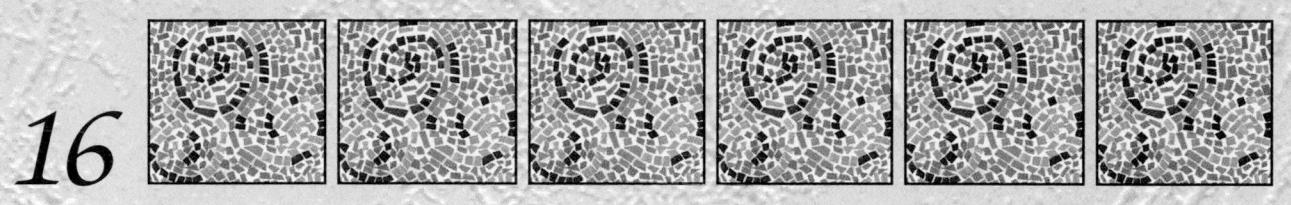

16

Nursing Care of Patients with Lower Respiratory Disorders

Study Outcomes

After studying this chapter, you should be able to:

1. Describe the etiology, pathophysiology, clinical manifestations, diagnostic procedures, and management of patients with lower respiratory disorders.
2. Identify physical examination data and information essential for the assessment of patients with lower respiratory disorders.
3. Identify nursing diagnoses and expected outcomes for patients with lower respiratory disorders.
4. List nursing interventions, and their rationales, for patients with lower respiratory disorders.
5. Explain the basis for evaluation of nursing care provided to patients with lower respiratory disorders.
6. Identify alternative treatment and care settings for patients with lower respiratory disorders and the services related to community-based care.
7. Identify special considerations for the older adult with lower respiratory disorders.

Lower respiratory tract disease is a major cause of morbidity and mortality in the United States. The incidence of chronic pulmonary disease (such as chronic bronchitis, emphysema, and asthma) is increasing. This may result from age-related changes in the population, environmental pollution, smoking, and an increased awareness and ability to diagnose the diseases.

Likewise, the incidence of lung cancer, the leading cause of cancer deaths in the United States, is on the rise, especially among teenagers and women. The influence of smoking, obesity, lack of regular exercise, and sedentary lifestyles predisposes patients to or exacerbates such conditions as lung cancer, chronic bronchitis, emphysema, and asthma.

Infectious lung disease is also on the increase. Opportunistic organisms are on the rise secondary to immunosuppression from chemotherapy for cancer, drug therapy after organ transplantation, and infection with the human immunodeficiency virus (HIV). The incidence of tuberculosis has increased dramatically in the past 10 years. The emergence of drug-resistant organisms—from inappropriate anti-

biotic use and the failure of patients to complete antibiotic regimens—has contributed to the increase in lower respiratory tract infections.

As the focus of the health-care system turns to health prevention and promotion, the role of the nurse shifts to more emphasis on patient and family education, including measures designed not only to promote health and prevent disease, but also to assist patients in managing chronic illness. In collaboration with other health-care team members (such as the dietitian, the pharmacist, the social worker, the physical therapist, and the physician), the nurse coordinates a team approach to dealing with a myriad of patient problems and needs.

*I*nfections and Inflammations

ACUTE BRONCHITIS

Acute bronchitis is an inflammation of the larger bronchi.

Etiology and Pathophysiology

Acute bronchitis results in diffuse inflammation of the mucosal lining of the bronchial tree and excess mucus production. Infectious agents (such as an influenza virus) or pyogenic organisms (such as various species of *Streptococcus, Pneumococcus, Staphylococcus,* and *Haemophilus*) can cause acute bronchitis. Infection is commonly preceded by a history of a cold, or it may occur secondary to other infectious diseases, such as measles or typhoid fever. Inhalation of such pollutants as smoke, dust, or chemical irritants may also cause acute bronchitis. Predisposing factors include exposure, getting chilled, fatigue, and malnutrition. Acute bronchitis is moderately common and usually results in little residual lung damage. Pneumonia may be seen as a complication, especially in the older adult.

Clinical Manifestations

Symptoms of acute bronchitis include fever that rarely exceeds 38.3°C (101°F), substernal burning discomfort caused by an associated tracheitis, and a cough that is at first dry, nonproductive, and painful, later becoming productive of large amounts of mucopurulent sputum. Paroxysmal attacks of coughing and wheezing may be present, especially during the night or associated with inhaled irritants.

Diagnosis

Physical findings include a history of nonproductive cough changing to productive, chest discomfort, wheezes or crackles on auscultation, low-grade fever, and general malaise. If a sputum culture is done, it may not reveal a predominant pathogen.

Management

Management is generally supportive because bronchitis is self-limiting. Bedrest, antipyretics for accompanying fever, and expectorants or antitussives may be included in the treatment plan. Antibiotics are not routinely prescribed unless sputum cultures indicate a suprainfection with a bacterial agent or the patient requires prophylaxis against a secondary infection because of a chronic respiratory disease or general debilitation.

❖ Settings, Providers, and Collaboration for Care

Most patients with acute bronchitis are diagnosed and treated in a physician's office or clinic setting and recuperate at home. Severely debilitated patients or those with advanced chronic obstructive pulmonary disease (COPD) may require hospitalization.

NURSING PROCESS
Acute Bronchitis

Assessment

Review the patient's history for predisposing or risk factors, such as asthma, emphysema, or cardiac disease. Question the patient about the cough and the amount and color of the expectorate. Assess respiratory status. Note rate and depth of respirations and auscultate breath sounds. Take the patient's temperature. Determine the patient's understanding of the therapeutic regimen and knowledge of how to prevent recurrence and spread of the disease.

Nursing Diagnoses and Planning

Nursing diagnoses and related expected patient outcomes commonly applicable to patients with acute bronchitis include the following:

NDx: Risk for altered health maintenance related to insufficient knowledge of self-care.

Planning: Patient Outcomes

1. Patient lists measures to be used to relieve respiratory symptoms.
2. Patient describes actions to prevent recurrent infection.
3. Patient identifies precautions to prevent the spread of infection to others.

Nursing Interventions and Evaluation

NDx: Risk for altered health maintenance

Since most persons with acute bronchitis are outpatients, the primary direct nursing intervention is health teaching. Instruct the patient on coughing and splinting techniques and in self-care (Highlight 16–1). Instruct other health-care providers and family members as necessary to promote support and implementation of these guidelines.

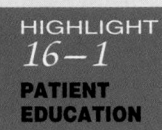 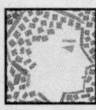

HIGHLIGHT *16–1* **PATIENT EDUCATION** **Managing Acute Bronchitis**

To provide relief of respiratory symptoms, instruct the patient to:

Use hot or cold inhalations to loosen and liquefy secretions and ease tracheal irritation.

Increase fluids to keep secretions liquid.

Cough and deep-breathe to mobilize secretions.

Sit up to allow most effective coughing.

Expectorate to clear secretions from the airways, thus decreasing the risk of progression to pneumonia.

Apply moist heat to the chest for soreness.

To promote uncomplicated resolution of the infection, instruct the patient to:

Take medication in the correct dose, route, and frequency, and for the prescribed length of time.

Report any symptoms of extension of the infection, such as persistent fever or dyspnea.

To prevent recurrent infection, instruct the patient to:

Avoid overexertion. Rest at regular intervals to conserve energy.

Avoid exposure to people with colds and flu.

Avoid exposure to environmental irritants, such as cigarette smoke and pollutants.

Dress warmly.

Eat a well-balanced diet.

To prevent spread of infection, instruct the patient to:

Wash hands thoroughly and often, especially after coughing, sneezing, or handling soiled tissues, and before handling food.

Cover mouth when coughing or sneezing.

Dispose of soiled tissues properly.

Avoid sharing drinking glasses or towels.

Compare the patient's status with the expected outcomes. If the outcomes are not met, reassess the patient and revise the plan.

PNEUMONIA

Pneumonia is an acute inflammation of the respiratory bronchioles, alveolar ducts, alveolar sacs, and alveoli. Pneumonia most often refers to an acute infectious process. However, it can also result from noninfectious causes, such as aspiration of gastric contents or a foreign body. In these cases, it is referred to as aspiration pneumonia.

Etiology and Pathophysiology

Infectious pneumonia is classified by its etiology as community-acquired, nosocomial (hospital-acquired), or opportunistic. It may also be divided into typical and atypical pneumonia based on its presenting symptoms and pattern of infiltrates on the chest x-ray.

The majority of community-acquired pneumonias are believed to be viral in origin. Frequently, they are not diagnosed because of their mild clinical presentation. Most viral pneumonias are caused by Type A virus. Cytomegalovirus is common in the adult immunosuppressed patient.

Less frequent but more serious are the bacterial pneumonias, of which pneumococci are the most common cause. Pneumonia caused by *Streptococcus pneumoniae* (group A β-hemolytic streptococci) is particularly common among older adults and is the type of community-acquired pneumonia most likely to require hospitalization. The next most common cause of community-acquired pneumonia is *Haemophilus influenzae*, a gram-negative bacillus. *H. influenzae* pneumonia occurs most often in patients with COPD and secondary to viral influenza, measles, or pneumonia. Pneumonia caused by *Moraxella catarrhalis* is increasing, especially among patients with cardiovascular disease.

Examples of atypical pneumonias include *Mycoplasma pneumoniae*, *Legionella pneumophila*, and *Pneumocystis carinii* pneumonia. *M. pneumoniae* is a frequent cause of community-acquired pneumonia in young persons. The organism shares both viral and bacterial characteristics. Its particle size is similar to that of a virus, but its enzyme systems are similar to those of bacteria. *M. pneumoniae* produces a characteristic rusty sputum.

Legionella pneumophila is a nonbacterial community-acquired pneumonia. It is a weakly organized gram-negative organism, identified after a convention of the American Legion, during which an outbreak of severe pneumonia occurred. This organism can result in multisystem failure. It affects males three times more often than females and occurs most frequently in older adults, smokers, and persons with predisposing chronic illness.

Nosocomial pneumonias are most often caused by gram-negative organisms, such as *Pseudomonas aeruginosa*, *Klebsiella pneumoniae*, and *Escherichia coli*. *Staphylococcus aureus* is the most common gram-positive coccus causing nosocomial pneumonia. The mortality rate for these hospital-acquired pneumonias is very high, as it is for pneumonias caused by other opportunistic organisms, such as cytomegalovirus, herpesvirus, *Candida* spp, *Aspergillus* spp, *Pneumocystis carinii*, and *Toxoplasma gondii* in immunocompromised patients.

Pneumonia-causing organisms can reach the alveoli in three ways: inhalation of droplets, aspiration of organisms from the nasopharynx or oropharynx, or seeding from the bloodstream. Viral and nonbacterial pneumonia result primarily from droplet inhalation. Bacterial pneumonias result primarily from aspiration of organisms from the pharynx. Seeding from the blood stream is the most infrequent source of organisms.

When pathogenic organisms reach the distal airways, an intense tissue reaction results. The intensity of the reaction depends on the virulence of the infectious organism and the immune response of the patient (host). An inflammatory reaction may result in an outpouring of exudates and cells into the interstitial tissue and alveolar spaces. White blood cells actively phagocytize the organism and release their enzymes and immunologic mediators, causing further inflammation. The body may or may not be able to prevent progression of the infection. If not, the infection continues to involve adjacent lung tissue and interalveolar spaces. As the lung fills with exudate and inflammatory cells, it becomes consolidated. When both the airways and lung parenchyma are involved, the condition is referred to as bronchopneumonia. If the adjacent pleura is also inflamed, pleural effusion may occur.

Inflammations caused by viruses and mycoplasma are predominantly in the interstitial tissue with alveolar wall infiltrates. Therefore, little or no exudate or consolidation results.

Physiologic changes associated with pneumonia result from reduced functional lung volumes and altered regional ventilation and blood flow. Arterial hypoxemia commonly seen in pneumonia results from ventilation/perfusion (V/Q) mismatching and intrapulmonary shunt.

Lung tissue typically returns to normal when the infection resolves. Occasionally there is significant destruction of the lung tissue, resulting in slow deposition of fibrous scar tissue and a measurable loss of lung function.

The host factor is important in the development of pneumonia. When there is significant impairment of the lungs' first line of defense mechanisms (filtration action of upper airways, reflexes closing the epiglottis and glottis, coughing, and mucociliary action), the distal airways and alveoli are at increased risk for contamination by pathogenic organisms. Further, impairment of blood supply, abnormally

Table 16-1

Risk Factors for Pneumonia

Community-Acquired Pneumonia
  Age over 65 years
  Chronic illness: chronic obstructive pulmonary disease, diabetes mellitus, heart failure
  Immunosuppressed state
  Depressed consciousness
  Chronic alcohol abuse
  Malnutrition
  Smoking
  Exposure to infectious organisms such as influenza
Hospital-Acquired Pneumonia
  Age over 65 years
  Abdominal or thoracic surgery
  Immobility
  Endotracheal/tracheal intubation
  Mechanical ventilation
  Nasogastric tube/enteral feeding
  Oxygen equipment
  Antibiotic therapy
  H$_2$ antagonist therapy
  Ineffective cough or gag reflex
  Underlying pulmonary disease or heart failure

low numbers of phagocytic and other cells involved in cellular immunity, lack of proper antibodies, and any alteration of other elements of the immunologic system can deprive the lungs of their second line of defense, thus placing the person at greater risk for pneumonia. Conditions associated with impaired respiratory defenses and predisposition to pneumonia include COPD, recent influenza, alcoholism, malnutrition, seizure disorders and other causes of altered consciousness, immunologic disorders, sickle-cell disease, malignant conditions and their treatments, major surgical procedures, diabetes, and advanced age (Table 16-1). Antibiotic and respiratory therapy predispose patients to nosocomial infections. Guidelines for preventing hospital-acquired pneumonia are presented in Highlight 16-2.

Clinical Manifestations

General signs and symptoms of pneumonia are fever, chills, productive cough, muscular chest wall discomfort from coughing, and general malaise. The exact clinical manifestations vary somewhat with the type of pneumonia. Bacterial pneumonia presents with an abrupt onset of symptoms, including copious sputum production, dyspnea on exertion and

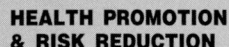

HIGHLIGHT
16-2

HEALTH PROMOTION & RISK REDUCTION

Guidelines for Prevention of Hospital-Acquired Pneumonia

Patient-Related Guidelines

Provide frequent, meticulous mouth care to minimize oropharyngeal colonization.

Turn and reposition from side to side every 2 hours.

Encourage frequent coughing, deep-breathing, and expectoration of sputum.

Ambulate or sit up in chair or bed as condition permits.

Perform chest physiotherapy as indicated.

Suction patients unable to bring up own secretions.

Keep head of bed elevated 30 to 45 degrees, especially when feeding.

Check breath sounds frequently.

Equipment-Related Guidelines

Use sterile water in respiratory equipment.

Change respiratory tubing every 48 hours.

Clean and dry medicine nebulizers between use.

Drain condensation in respiratory tubing.

Personnel- or Procedure-Related Guidelines

Wash hands between patients and before and after a dirty task is performed.

Wear gloves when appropriate.

Vaccinate staff with influenza vaccine.

If patient has a feeding tube:
  Check placement before each feeding.
  Check residual.
  Prepare feeding using strict aseptic technique.
  Elevate head of bed while feeding.

Use antibiotics prudently to avoid drug resistance.

Administer central nervous system depressants cautiously to avoid depressing respirations.

Take precautions with immunosuppressives to support the patient's immune system.

Be aware that patients receiving H$_2$ antagonists as prophylaxis for stress ulcers will increase their gastric bacterial colonization.

often at rest, hemoptysis, pleurisy, crackles and wheezes on auscultation, dullness to percussion over the involved area, and pleural effusion. Community-acquired, nonbacterial pneumonias usually present with severe, hacking cough, scant sputum production, and fine crackles on auscultation. In the older adult, symptoms may appear very gradually, and purulent sputum or a decreasing level of consciousness may be the only indication of disease.

Diagnosis

Diagnosis of pneumonia depends on a careful history, with special attention to recent respiratory infections, physical examination, and chest x-rays. The causative organism is suggested by a Gram stain of the sputum and confirmed by a sputum culture obtained before antimicrobial agents are given. The chest x-ray is used to confirm the presence and distribution of infiltrates, lung consolidation, and presence of pleural effusion.

Management

The treatment for pneumonia includes adequate hydration (increased oral fluids, intravenous fluids, or both) to thin secretions, supportive nutrition to provide nutrients needed to fight infection, supplemental oxygen to treat hypoxemia, analgesics to promote comfort and rest, and antibiotics, as appropriate, to destroy or disable the infecting organism. The choice of antibiotics is determined by bacterial studies. Table 16–2 lists antibiotics used in the treatment of pneumonia. Bedrest is frequently required because of the debilitating nature of pneumonia. Aerosolized and systemic bronchodilators and chest physiotherapy may be ordered if the patient is producing a large volume of sputum. Expectorants may be prescribed to help clear sputum. Cough suppressants may be prescribed to provide rest and conserve energy for the patient with an ineffective cough or excessive coughing.

Patients requiring hospitalization frequently receive intravenous therapy to replace fluid lost because of an elevated temperature and increased insensible water loss from an increased respiratory rate. Electrolytes are monitored and replaced as necessary. If respiratory failure occurs, the patient is intubated and placed on mechanical ventilation to improve oxygenation and ventilation and to promote secretion management.

❖ Settings, Providers, and Collaboration for Care

Patients with community-acquired pneumonia may require hospitalization and parenteral antibiotics if the causative organism is pneumococcus or there are coexisting medical conditions. Patients with nosocomial pneumonias usually require continued hospitalization with parenteral antibiotics and intensive respiratory, nutritional, and other supportive therapy. Collaboration with the respiratory therapist, the di-

Table 16–2

Organisms Causing Pneumonia and Common Drug Therapies

Pneumonia Type	Drug Therapy
COMMUNITY-ACQUIRED PNEUMONIAS	
Streptococcus pneumoniae	First- or second-generation cephalosporin
	Penicillin G
	Erythromycin
Haemophilus influenzae	Piperacillin
	Timentin
	Third-generation cephalosporin
	Trimethroprim & sulfamethoxazole (TMP-SMX)
Staphylococcus aureus	Nafcillin
	First-generation cephalosporin
	Vancomycin (if methicillin-resistant)
	TMP-SMX
Mycoplasma pneumoniae	Erythromycin
	Tetracycline
Legionella pneumophila	Erythromycin with or without rifampin
	TMP-SMX
Pneumocystis carinii	Trimethoprim
	Sulfamethoxazole
	Pentamidine
Anaerobic organisms	Third-generation cephalosporin
	Unasyn
	Clindamycin
HOSPITAL-ACQUIRED PNEUMONIAS	
Pseudomonas aeruginosa	Zosyn
	Timentin
	Tobramycin
	Third-generation cephalosporin
	Imipenem
Klebsiella spp	Third-generation cephalosporin
Enterobacter spp	Gentamycin
Proteus spp	Primaxin
Serratia spp	Aztreonam
Staphylococcus aureus	Nafcillin
	First-generation cephalosporin
	Vancomycin (if methicillin-resistant)
	TMP-SMX
Streptococcus spp	First- or second-generation cephalosporin
	Penicillin G
	Erythromycin

etitian, the social worker, and the physician is essential to developing and implementing a plan of care and a discharge plan, which may include home care services and home intravenous infusion.

■■■■■■▶
■ **Clinical Pathway for Pneumonia**

Patient Name _____   Date _____

DRG# _____   Expected LOS _____

	Day 1	Day 2	Day 3	Day 4
Medication	IV antibiotics Bronchodilators	IV antibiotics	IV antibiotics	IV antibiotics
Diagnostic Tests	Blood Cx x2 Sputum—Gram's stain Chest x-ray Pulse ox on room air Arterial blood gases if pulse ox <92% CBC, SMAC 20, PT, PTT, STS Electrocardiogram for man > age 45, woman > age 55	Complete blood count SMA 7	Chest x-ray	
Diet	Diet as ordered Encourage fluids	Diet as ordered Encourage fluids	Diet as ordered Encourage fluids	Diet as ordered Encourage fluids
Activity	Bedrest with bathroom privileges	Out of bed as tolerated	Ambulate with assistance	Ambulate ad lib
Treatments/Nursing Actions	IV fluids Intake and output VS q4h CPT or suction O_2 via NC to maintain $SaO_2 > 92\%$ R/A	IV fluids Intake and output VS q shift or as ordered Respiratory therapy O_2 to maintain $SaO_2 > 92\%$ R/A	IV fluids/Heplock Intake and output VS q shift or as ordered Respiratory therapy O_2 to maintain $SaO_2 > 92\%$ R/A	IV fluids/Heplock D/C'd Intake and output VS q shift or as ordered
Teaching/Discharge Planning	Instruct in coughing and deep-breathing, need for increased fluids, no smoking, disease process. Assess support systems and resources, need for social service consultation.	Assess need for home oxygen therapy, home IV infusion therapy, or home medication monitoring.	Instruct in need for rest, nutrition, medication regimen, and importance of compliance with regimen.	Instruct on follow-up date and time. Assess need for Pneumovax. Administer if needed.

NURSING PROCESS

Pneumonia

Assessment

Assessment focuses on four major areas:

- Factors that place the patient at risk for pneumonia and contribute to the severity of the disease
- Effects of the disease on respiration and other body functions
- Correct implementation and effectiveness of treatment measures
- The patient's understanding of health measures related to the prevention and cure of the disease

The development of pneumonia is associated with impaired first-line defenses in the respiratory system and aspiration of bacteria from the mouth. Therefore, when obtaining the history, ask about recent upper respiratory tract infections, smoking, alcohol use, patterns of oral hygiene, recent dental work, and existence of any predisposing illness, since these factors increase the risk of pneumonia.

Assess vital signs. Note respiratory rate and depth. Observe for the use of the accessory muscles, splinting of the chest, nasal flaring, and dyspnea.

Auscultate lung sounds. Inspect for cyanosis, specifically mucosal and circumoral. Question the patient about chest pain. Determine its type, location, and relationship to inspiration or expiration. Note characteristics of the cough, such as shallow or deep, dry or loose. Assess cough effectiveness and frequency, as well as amount, odor, consistency and color of sputum. Table 16–3 lists types of pneumonias commonly associated with certain colors of sputum.

Table 16–3

Sputum Colors Associated with Specific Pneumonias

Color*	Pneumonia Type
Colorless/clear mucoid	Noninfectious process
Creamy yellow	Staphylococcal pneumonia
Green	*Pseudomonas* pneumonia
"Currant jelly"	*Klebsiella* pneumonia
Rusty	Pneumococcal pneumonia

*Color alone is not diagnostic.

Assess fluid intake and output, skin turgor, and serum sodium levels because elevated temperature and increased insensible fluid loss from rapid breathing can lead to dehydration. Also assess the adequacy of the patient's caloric intake, since increased calories are needed to counteract the catabolism associated with the infection.

Monitor for signs of complications, such as lung abscess, empyema, pulmonary edema, and pleural effusion, to ensure early recognition and treatment. (Refer to the appropriate sections of this chapter for the signs and symptoms of each.)

Monitor oxygenation via pulse oximetry or arterial blood gas analysis. If the patient is receiving oxygen, check the flow rate, observe for proper position of the cannula or mask, and assess for potential skin breakdown associated with the delivery device.

Assess the patient's understanding of general health measures, such as covering the mouth when coughing, expectorating rather than swallowing raised secretions, and properly disposing of used tissues. Also assess understanding of the need for a balanced diet, increased fluid intake to keep secretions liquid, and adequate rest to foster the body's ability to combat the infection.

Nursing Diagnoses and Planning

Nursing diagnoses and related expected patient outcomes commonly applicable to patients with pneumonia include the following:

NDx: Ineffective airway clearance related to retained secretions

Planning: Patient Outcomes
1. Patient demonstrates effective coughing and deep-breathing techniques.
2. Secretions are thin, white, and watery.
3. Patient coughs and expectorates easily.

NDx: Impaired gas exchange related to V/Q mismatching and increased intrapulmonary shunt

Planning: Patient Outcomes
1. Patient states that dyspnea is absent.
2. Respiratory rate and depth are within normal limits.
3. Lungs are clear on auscultation.
4. Arterial blood gas (ABG) values are within normal limits.

NDx: Pain related to chest and lung expansion secondary to infection in the lung

Planning: Patient Outcomes
1. Patient demonstrates splinting techniques to reduce discomfort associated with coughing.
2. Patient states pain is diminished or relieved.
3. Patient remains pain free for periods of 4 to 6 hours.

NDx: Risk for fluid volume deficit related to increased insensible fluid loss secondary to fever and rapid respirations.

Planning: Patient Outcomes
1. Patient drinks 3 to 4 L of fluid per day (if not contraindicated by a coexistent medical condition).
2. Mucous membranes are moist.
3. Skin turgor is firm.
4. Urinary output is greater than or equal to 30 mL/hour.

NDx: Anxiety related to dyspnea, blood-tinged sputum, chest pain

Planning: Patient Outcomes
1. Patient denies being overly anxious.
2. Behavioral signs of excessive anxiety (restlessness, fear, need for frequent attention) are absent.

NDx: Risk for altered health maintenance related to insufficient knowledge of discharge instructions, risk of smoking, value of influenza vaccine

Planning: Patient Outcomes
1. Patient describes how he or she will carry out instructions for self-care after discharge.
2. Patient identifies risks of smoking and availability of smoking cessation programs.
3. Patient describes need for and benefit of influenza vaccine.
4. Patient describes need for and benefit of pneumococcal vaccine.

Nursing Interventions and Evaluation

NDx: Ineffective airway clearance
Encourage coughing and deep-breathing every 2 hours. Support thinning and raising of secretions by maintaining the fluid intake at 3 to 4 L daily. Humidification of the inspired air or oxygen may be helpful. Suction as necessary to provide adequate removal of secretions to maintain a patent airway. Time suctioning with bronchodilator treatments and postural drainage to increase secretion removal. Teach the patient and family breathing techniques and exercises to promote maximal ventilation and to raise secretions.

NDx: Impaired gas exchange
Position the patient to maximize oxygenation by placing the good lung down. This promotes drainage of the affected lung and increases blood flow and oxygenation of the good lung. Administer oxygen therapy as prescribed and monitor its effect via pulse oximetry or ABG analysis. Closely monitor the amount of delivered oxygen, especially in patients with a history of carbon-dioxide-retention COPD, since the ventilatory drive in these patients may be depressed by higher oxygen levels, leading to a respiratory crisis.

NDx: Pain
Give analgesics as needed and ordered for pain relief. Light analgesics, such as ibuprofen or acetaminophen, are usually sufficient to provide comfort. In the event an analgesic with a central nervous system depressant effect is needed, first assess the patient

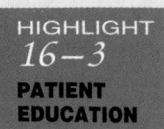 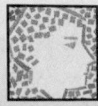

HIGHLIGHT
16–3
**PATIENT
EDUCATION**

Recuperating from Pneumonia

Instruct the patient to:

Increase activities gradually to avoid fatigue.

Obtain sufficient rest, eat a balanced diet, and avoid getting chilled to decrease susceptibility to infection.

Avoid exposure to people with colds or flu.

Report change or worsening of cough, change in color of sputum produced, shortness of breath, or recurrence of fever.

for evidence of cerebral hypoxemia, such as restlessness, confusion, and aggression. Position the patient comfortably and assist with splinting the chest during coughing and deep-breathing.

NDx: Risk for fluid volume deficit
Monitor fluid intake closely. Encourage intake of 3 to 4 L of fluids daily, if not contraindicated, to keep the patient well hydrated and to thin secretions. Accurately record intake and output to prevent fluid deficit or overload.

NDx: Anxiety
Because the patient with pneumonia is often anxious about feeling short of breath, about the presence of

chest pain, or about blood-streaked sputum, provide time for the patient to ask questions and express concerns. Explain expected symptoms, treatments, and procedures, and reassure the patient as appropriate about his or her condition.

NDx: Risk for altered health maintenance
Instruct the patient in self-care after discharge as specified in Highlight 16–3. Instruct cigarette smokers about their increased risk for lung disorders and inform them about American Lung Association or American Cancer Society smoking cessation programs. Teach high-risk patients about the benefits of the influenza and pneumococcal (Pneumovax) vaccine. Influenza immunizations are administered annually in the early fall. Pneumovax is administered only once. However, if the patient was immunized before 1984, when the vaccine was changed to include 21 rather than 14 pneumonia strains, readministration of the vaccine is recommended.

Additional Interventions
Although fever is a positive force in resolving infection, it does make energy demands on the body. Therefore, limit the patient's activity while his or her temperature is elevated. Promote bedrest and specifically plan for uninterrupted rest periods between times of turning, coughing, deep-breathing, and other treatments. Give tepid baths and provide frequent linen changes to keep the patient comfortable and to prevent chilling in the presence of elevated temperature and diaphoresis. Meet the nutritional needs of patients with pneumonia as specified in Highlight 16–4.

Collect sputum specimens from the patient as ordered. To obtain a satisfactory specimen, instruct the patient to perform the following:

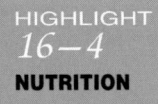 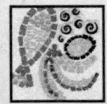

HIGHLIGHT
16–4
NUTRITION

Common Nutritional Problems and Interventions for Patients with Pneumonia

Problem	Nutritional Interventions
Fluid deficit secondary to fever and increased insensible fluid loss	Provide 3 L fluids daily. Keep water available at bedside. If oral intake cannot be maintained, intravenous administration may be necessary.
Increased metabolic demands secondary to infection and increased respiratory rate	Provide an intake of at least 1500 kcal daily. Ensure diet rich in protein. Aim for nitrogen balance for maintenance or a positive nitrogen balance to rebuild body tissue. Provide a liquid or blenderized diet if better tolerated in the beginning.
Dyspnea Anorexia secondary to decreased taste sensation caused by expectoration of sputum	Provide small, frequent feedings. Provide oral hygiene before meals.

- Rinse the mouth with water to minimize possible contamination with normal flora
- Breathe deeply several times
- Cough
- Expectorate into a sterile container

Compare the patient's status with the expected outcomes. If the outcomes are not met, reassess the patient and revise the plan.

ASPIRATION PNEUMONIA SYNDROME

Aspiration pneumonia results from aspiration of stomach contents, toxic materials, or a foreign body into the lower respiratory tract. It occurs most frequently when the patient is in an altered state of consciousness as a result of seizures, drugs, alcohol, anesthesia, acute infection, or shock. It also occurs in the presence of nasogastric tubes and tracheostomy tubes. In aspiration pneumonia, the aspirated substance triggers development of chemical injury within 48 to 72 hours.

NURSING PROCESS GUIDELINES
Aspiration Pneumonia Syndrome

For aspiration pneumonia, prevention is the best intervention. Place a high-risk patient in a side-lying position with proper pillow supports behind the back, between the knees, and in front of the chest. Give frequent mouth care and remove secretions as often as needed to prevent aspiration of organisms into the lower respiratory tract. When tube feedings are given, elevate the head of the bed at least 30 degrees during the feeding and for 1 hour after its completion. Check gag and cough reflexes before feeding as well as proper tube placement. If more than 100 mL are aspirated before feeding, withhold the feeding and consult the physician.

LUNG ABSCESS

A lung abscess is a localized collection of pus within the substance of the lung.

Etiology and Pathophysiology
Development of a lung abscess is a pathologic process that can occur during the course of any number of different inflammatory lung conditions. It results from a combination of suppuration (the process of pus formation) and tissue necrosis (death of areas of tissue). The most common cause of a lung abscess is a necrotizing infection of the parenchyma by a microorganism capable of destroying the tissue, such as staphylococcus, Friedländers bacillus, tubercle bacillus, and certain fungal infections, such as blastomycosis.

The precipitating event for this type of infection is usually aspiration. Another cause is a pulmonary infarct, which is a dead or devitalized area of lung tissue. These infarcts usually heal by fibrosis and scarring, but occasionally the area becomes necrotic and excavates, forming an abscess cavity. Pulmonary emboli, septic pulmonary infarction, and vasculitis are all possible causes of this type of lung abscess.

Cavitary malignancy abscess develops within the substance of a pulmonary neoplasm, which may be primary or secondary. The mechanism of development of this type of lung abscess is not fully understood. Theory suggests that certain malignancies grow faster than their blood supply, thus leading to necrosis of cells and an abscess in the center of the lesion.

Aspiration into the bronchi can also be followed by a lung abscess. Normally, the bronchial defenses are able to deal with nasopharyngeal and oral secretions that may be aspirated into the tracheobronchial tree during sleep. However, during anesthesia, traumatic shock, alcoholic stupor, coma, or postoperative shock, these defenses are impaired. Aspiration of vomitus, which is an irritating fluid, results in a diffuse lobular pneumonia with multiple abscesses. Aspiration of solid matter causes a localized abscess.

Abscesses in general are spherical in shape because of the pull of the surrounding healthy elastic parenchyma.

Clinical Manifestations
Cough, sputum production (moderate to copious, foul-smelling, sometimes bloody), and fever are present in all types of lung abscesses, unless the abscess is walled off without access to the bronchi. The duration of the episode and severity of clinical manifestations differ widely. The physical signs associated with lung abscess depend on the size of the abscess cavity, the degree of surrounding pneumonitis, and the distance from the chest wall. Signs and symptoms include dull chest pain, dyspnea, weakness, anorexia, and weight loss. If a febrile respiratory illness develops suddenly in a patient who has recently undergone a surgical procedure—especially one involving the mouth, nose, or throat—a lung abscess is suspected. Rupture of an abscess into a bronchus is associated with expectoration of a large quantity of foul-smelling green or brown sputum.

Diagnosis
A careful history seeking information about occupational exposure, pre-existing lung conditions, recent episodes of unconsciousness, or presence of periodontal disease provides important clues to the diagnosis of lung abscess. Diagnosis is confirmed by chest x-ray. The particular cause of the abscess is established by evaluating the results of laboratory tests, clinical tests, and x-rays. Sputum examination by a Gram stain and an acid-fast stain is important in identifying the responsible microorganism so appropriate initial antimicrobial therapy can be prescribed.

Management

The medical regimen has a twofold goal: first, to eradicate the underlying cause, and second, to alleviate the adverse consequences. Pyogenic bacterial infections are treated with antibiotics effective against the specific causative organism. High-dose intravenous antibiotics are required to penetrate the necrotic tissue and abscess fluid. The patient may be switched to oral antibiotics when signs of improvement begin to appear, such as normal temperature and return of the white blood cell count toward normal. The entire course of antibiotic therapy may extend from 6 to 12 weeks.

Postural drainage, aided by percussion, coughing, and breathing exercises, is ordered to promote drainage of the abscess. If these measures are not effective, a bronchoscopy may be performed to drain the abscess.

Rarely, surgical intervention in the form of a lobectomy may be necessary if the abscess fails to respond to more conservative treatment or when a major hemoptysis occurs. A thoracotomy tube inserted into the pleural space through the chest wall or some other form of surgical drainage may be used to treat the patient who cannot tolerate thoracic surgery.

❖ Settings, Providers, and Collaboration for Care

Most patients with a lung abscess are hospitalized initially. They can be discharged to home once their condition is stabilized and treatment regimen started. Often, they are discharged home on intravenous antibiotic therapy. An IV therapy nurse usually sees these patients in the home setting and instructs patients and families on how to administer the antibiotics. Home-care visits may also include dressing changes, reinforcement of patient and family education, and assistance with wound care. The patient may need to return to an outpatient clinic for treatments.

NURSING PROCESS
Lung Abscess

Assessment

Assess rate and depth of respirations, symmetry of chest expansion, characteristics of cough and expectorate, lung sounds, and pulse every 2 hours during the initial phase of hospitalization. Note the characteristics and amount of drainage from the pleural cavity resulting from postural drainage and observe the patient for response to antibiotic therapy.

Nursing Diagnoses and Planning

Nursing diagnoses and related expected patient outcomes commonly applicable to patients with lung abscess include the following:

NDx: Risk for ineffective airway clearance related to pain and ineffective coughing

Planning: Patient Outcomes
1. Sputum is expectorated.
2. Breath sounds are clear bilaterally.
3. Chest expansion is symmetric.

NDx: Risk for altered health maintenance related to insufficient knowledge of self-care

Planning: Patient Outcomes
1. Patient states name, dose, route, and frequency of prescribed antibiotics.
2. Patient explains the importance of taking antibiotics as prescribed.
3. Patient lists symptoms to be reported.

Nursing Interventions and Evaluation

NDx: Risk for ineffective airway clearance
Position the patient with the abscess area up to promote drainage. Teach coughing and deep-breathing exercises to mobilize secretions. Initiate chest physiotherapy in collaboration with the respiratory therapist. Perform postural drainage and percussion as ordered. Give prescribed analgesics if needed to promote comfort. Encourage fluids to keep secretions thin and stress the importance of expectoration. Ensure that the patient has easy access to tissues and a waste container.

NDx: Risk for altered health maintenance
Teach the patient about any prescribed antibiotics, including name, dose, route, and frequency. Explain the risk of a relapse if all the antibiotic is not taken. Also explain that a suprainfection can occur. Instruct the patient and family to report any diarrhea, vaginal discharge, recurrent fever, or other symptom of a new infection.

Additional Interventions
Instruct the patient in the importance of rest. Provide a high-calorie diet to support healing and reverse the catabolic state induced by chronic infection. Administer antibiotics as prescribed and monitor the patient's response by observing for signs of drug allergy, suprainfection, and failure to respond to medication.

If surgery was performed, change dressings frequently to prevent excoriation of the skin and an offensive odor. It may also be necessary to teach the family to change simple dressings because of the prolonged period of drainage before the wound closes completely.

Compare the patient's status with the expected outcomes. If the outcomes are not met, reassess the patient and revise the plan.

INFLUENZA

Influenza virus infections cause a nondistinctive syndrome that occurs in characteristic epidemic or pandemic patterns, usually in late fall, winter, or early spring. Because of these recognizable patterns, identifiable outbreaks of influenza have been noted as early as the year 1510.

Etiology and Pathophysiology

Influenza is caused by viruses that are divided into three major groups—A, B, and C—and their variants. These viruses frequently undergo changes in their chemical makeup, and infection with one type of influenza virus offers no immunity to subsequent infections with other types. Currently, influenza is the only epidemic disease in the United States that can affect a large enough proportion of the population to produce more deaths than otherwise expected (excess mortality). These deaths occur primarily among the very old and the very young and are mainly attributable to the Type A virus strain, which has a greater tendency to mutate than other viral types.

Type A virus causes pandemics and local epidemics, whereas Type B strains cause localized outbreaks and sporadic cases. Influenza is able to infect most surface epithelial cells of the respiratory tract and is transmitted principally by the aerosol route. Because it may infect the nasal mucosa, transmission by fomites is also possible.

Complications of influenza include primary influenza virus pneumonia, bacterial pneumonia, or both. Neurologic complications also may occur, such as Guillain-Barré syndrome, encephalitis, and acute sinusitis or exacerbation of pre-existing respiratory insufficiency. Complications occur most often in older adults, pregnant women, patients with compromised immune mechanisms, and patients with cardiovascular disease, pulmonary disease, diabetes mellitus, cirrhosis, or chronic renal disease.

Clinical Manifestations

After an incubation period of 1 to 3 days, illness starts with an abrupt onset of fever, sweating, headache, and muscular aches and pains. A nonproductive cough associated with conjunctival irritation and rhinitis is quickly followed by nasal obstruction. Other symptoms may include general malaise, sore throat, and laryngitis. The fever and cough are essential features of influenza and necessary for a clinical diagnosis. The infected patient is contagious for 2 to 3 days beginning with the onset of symptoms.

Diagnosis

During periods of local outbreak, a diagnosis of influenza may be based on clinical findings. It is also possible to identify Types A, B, and C in complement fixation and hemagglutination inhibition antibody tests. Serologic diagnosis is based on evidence of a fourfold rise in antibody titers when the acute and convalescent periods are compared 2 weeks apart.

Management

Uncomplicated influenza requires no treatment, although relief of symptoms may be obtained through prescription of decongestants, expectorants, antitussives, and analgesics. The patient is advised to rest and to force fluids. For patients with known underlying chronic respiratory or cardiac disease, close observation for extensive pulmonary involvement is needed, with supportive respiratory care as necessary. If a bacterial superinfection is documented by sputum Gram's stain, appropriate antibiotic treatment is initiated.

Amantadine hydrochloride (Symmetrel) can be given to high-risk people or groups as prophylaxis against influenza A virus infection when vaccination is contraindicated, not available, or not feasible. It can also be used in conjunction with the inactivated vaccine to protect at-risk people until a full antibody response has occurred. Although it can treat diagnosed cases of Type A virus, it is not widely used. It is effective only when started within 1 to 2 days of the onset of the illness, and very few patients are known to have laboratory-diagnosed Type A until after the illness has subsided.

The Immunization Practices Advisory Committee of the U.S. Public Health Service recommends annual influenza vaccination for all persons over age 65 and for those with chronic underlying illnesses. The effectiveness of the influenza vaccines has been variable. Problems include short duration of immunity, strain specificity, ineffectiveness against respiratory illnesses, and long lead time from production to distribution, making the inactivated vaccines useless for controlling epidemics resulting from new strains. Despite these problems, active immunization is the most effective prophylaxis against the influenza virus. After vaccination, people are less likely to be infected and, if infected, have milder courses of illness and shed less virus in their nasal secretions. The vaccine is a preparation of inactivated antigens that represent the influenza virus prevalent in a specific year. It takes about 6 to 8 weeks following the vaccine to develop a full antibody complement.

❖ Settings, Providers, and Collaboration for Care

Most patients with influenza are managed in the outpatient setting. Elderly patients may require hospitalization if they become dehydrated.

NURSING PROCESS GUIDELINES
Influenza

Nursing care of the patient with influenza is primarily supportive. Assess the patient for factors that may predispose to complications, such as a history of cardiac or respiratory disease. Assess the patient's symptom complex on an ongoing basis to determine whether the disease is resolving or worsening. Identify signs of complications as early as possible.

Encourage the patient to rest, force fluids, and eat nutritious, appetizing foods. Administer prescribed medications for symptomatic relief of fever, malaise, and headache. Instruct the patient in the purpose, indication, frequency, dosage, and side effects of each of the prescribed medications.

Nursing also has an important role in the prevention of influenza. Assess for persons at high risk (specifically, those older than 65 years and those with chronic diseases) and assess their knowledge of the disease, its mode of transmission, and immunizations available against it. When a knowledge deficit is found, instruct the patient as needed. Explain the relation of crowding and close contact with groups of people to the spread of influenza and thus the importance of avoiding theaters, shopping malls, and other crowded locations during an outbreak of influenza.

Provide information on the advantages of immunization and how it may be obtained. Monitor visitors in the hospital closely during epidemics to minimize the spread of influenza to patients.

TUBERCULOSIS

Tuberculosis is an infectious disease caused by the bacillus *Mycobacterium tuberculosis* and spread primarily by the airborne route. Although the most common site of tuberculosis is in the lungs, it can occur at any site in the body, or as disseminated disease. Infection occurs when tiny 1 to 5 μm droplet nuclei containing the bacteria, known as the tubercle bacilli, are inhaled into the alveolar surfaces of the lung. Clinically evident active disease occurs in 5 to 10% of those infected. This may be manifested by progression of the original infection (primary infection) or reactivation of the disease months or years after the initial infection (post-primary infection). Tuberculosis occurs most often in crowded, inner-city, economically disadvantaged environments and among people with other medical risk factors (Table 16–4). All suspected and diagnosed cases of tuberculosis must be reported to the local health department.

Tuberculosis was a major health problem in the early part of the 20th century. There was no treatment for the disease, which was associated with isolation, disability, and in many cases death. The advent of effective antibiotic therapy, combined with aggressive programs of prevention, detection, and treatment, brought the disease under control. The percentage of the population in developed countries infected with *M. tuberculosis* fell from about 60% in 1940 to 25% in 1975. This decline led to the projection that, by the year 2000, only 5% of these populations would ever become infected. Contrary to this projection, tuberculosis has re-emerged as a serious public health problem. Factors to which this resurgence is attributed are:

- The association of tuberculosis with the human immunodeficiency virus–acquired immunodeficiency syndrome (HIV/AIDS) epidemic

Table 16–4

Populations at High Risk for Tuberculosis Infection

Close contacts of patients with active disease (especially children)
HIV-infected patients
IV drug abusers
Immunocompromised patients
People with other medical risk factors, such as:
    Renal failure
    Diabetes mellitus
    Head and neck cancer
    Silicosis
    Gastrectomy
    Weight 10% below ideal
    Leukemia
    Lymphoma
Residents and employees of high-risk environments, such as:
    Prisons
    Long- and short-term health-care facilities
    Homeless shelters
    HIV residential settings
New immigrants from areas with a high incidence of tuberculosis, such as:
    Africa
    Asia
    Caribbean
    Latin America
People of low socioeconomic status (related to lack of health care and overcrowded housing)

- Immigration from areas such as Africa, Asia, the Caribbean, and Latin America, where tuberculosis is common
- Transmission of tuberculosis in congregate settings, such as health care facilities, homeless shelters, and correctional facilities
- A decline in public health screening and educational programs

The increase in multi-drug resistant tuberculosis has emphasized the need for new drug treatment regimens, and many are currently under study.

Etiology and Pathophysiology

Mycobacterium tuberculosis and three types of mycobacterial species (*M. bovis*, *M. africanum*, and *M. microti*) can cause tuberculosis. In the United States, *M. tuberculosis* causes the majority of cases. *M. tuberculosis* is an acid-fast aerobic bacillus that causes focal inflammatory reactions called granulomas. The centers of these granulomas commonly undergo necrosis. The organism multiplies slowly and can be killed by heat, sunshine, and ultraviolet light. It is resistant to drying and can remain viable for weeks in particles of dried sputum. It is not a highly contagious organism and usually requires close, frequent, prolonged contact for transmission.

Primary tuberculosis infection occurs when tubercle bacilli are inhaled into the lungs of a susceptible individual. Droplet nuclei are released into the air when an infected person talks, coughs, sneezes, or laughs. The inhaled bacilli lodge in the alveoli and give rise to a small area of gray-white inflammatory consolidation called the primary or Ghon's lesion. The tubercle bacilli multiply at this primary site, spread to the hilar lymph nodes, drain into the lymphatic system, enter the blood stream, and are carried throughout the body. The phrase *Ghon's complex* is used to refer to the combination of primary lesion and lymph node involvement.

The process of multiplication and spread of the tubercle bacilli is interrupted in about 2 to 10 weeks when the body's immune system begins to respond. Mycobacterium-specific lymphocytes attract macrophages to the foci of infection. Some of the macrophages are stimulated to a heightened mycobactericidal state. Others are stimulated to differentiate into fibroblasts that surround the primary lesion with a dense connective tissue enclosure. The resulting granuloma is the characteristic lesion of tuberculosis.

In most people, no symptoms arise during this initial infection, and the granulomatous lesion becomes fibrotic and calcified. At this stage of the infection, the tuberculin test is positive. Some of the bacilli remain dormant, however, and viable for many years in a period called *latent TB infection*. The potential for reactivation exists if specific and nonspecific host resistance decreases for any reason.

In the approximately 10% of patients whose defenses are not capable of controlling the growth and spread of *M. tuberculosis*, initial infection can progress directly to a granulomatous consolidation of multiple patchy lung areas. If the wall of a blood vessel is eroded, it can also progress to a miliary tuberculosis, which is extensive dissemination of the tubercle bacillus via the blood stream, or to tuberculous meningitis.

Secondary tuberculosis is infection in a person who has already had a primary lesion and an immune reaction to it. It may result from a new infection, although, in most cases, it involves reactivation of the initial infection. The course of secondary tuberculosis is different from the relatively silent primary infection because the person is already sensitized to the bacillus. The lesions of secondary tuberculosis occur most often in the apices of the lung and the regional lymph nodes. They tend to remain localized in the lung because of rapid phagocytosis and destruction of *M. tuberculosis* bacilli by activated macrophages. There is an acute local inflammation complicated by necrosis, with resulting ulceration of the infected lung tissue. As a result of developed sensitivity, local clusters of tubercles become surrounded by zones of inflammatory reaction. The surrounding alveoli become filled with exudate, and tuberculosis bronchopneumonia develops. The tuberculosis tissue gradually becomes caseous and ulcerates into a bronchus, causing a cavity (Fig. 16-1). The ulcerations heal, leaving considerable local scar tissue around the cavity. The pleura over the infected lobe, usually the upper lobe, becomes inflamed, thickened, and retracted by scar tissue. This cyclic process of inflammatory bronchopneumonia, ulceration, cavitation, and scarring—unless arrested—spreads slowly downward to the hilum and may later extend into adjacent lobes. This cavitation makes possible spread to other areas of the respiratory tract, as well as spread via the lymphatic vessels to other organs, such as the kidney and the bone. There may be long remissions of this disease process followed by periods of renewed activity.

Clinical Manifestations

Clinical manifestations of the pulmonary adult form of tuberculosis are insidious in onset. Nonspecific constitutional symptoms may develop before symptoms specific to lung disease do. Constitutional symptoms include low-grade fever, pallor, chills, night sweats, easy fatigability, anorexia, and weight loss. The first pulmonary inflammatory symptoms include a slight cough, usually each morning, and expectoration of a scant amount of mucoid sputum. As the disease progresses, the cough becomes more continuous throughout the day and night. If cavitation develops, sputum becomes purulent and blood stained. Dyspnea and chest pain are late symptoms that signify extensive lung involvement.

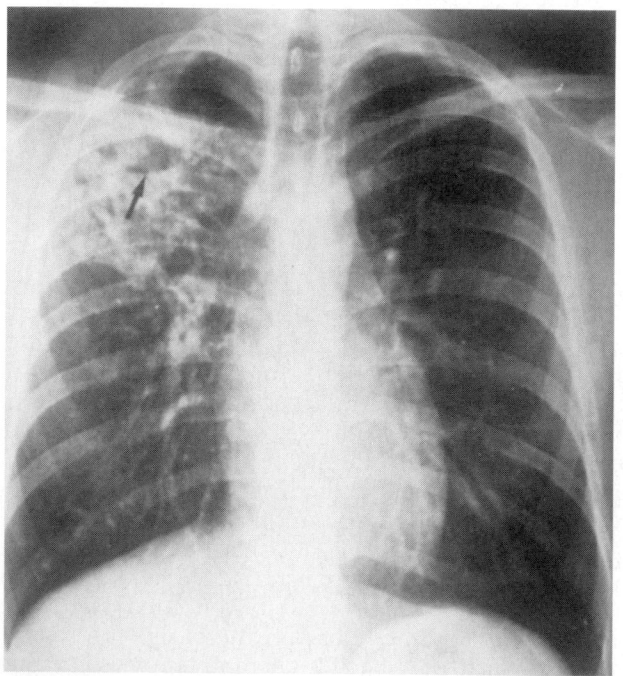

Figure 16-1

Cavitation in tuberculosis. (From Kersten LD. Comprehensive respiratory nursing: A decision making approach. Philadelphia: WB Saunders, 1989, p 146.)

Many patients with tuberculosis have other serious disorders, such as AIDS, alcoholism, renal failure, diabetes mellitus, and neoplastic disease. Often the signs and symptoms of tuberculosis are obscured by the signs and symptoms of the underlying diseases. Therefore it is important that health-care providers maintain a high level of suspicion when caring for patients in the high-risk groups.

Diagnosis
Presumptive diagnosis is made on the basis of a tuberculin skin test, a sputum smear that is positive for acid-fast bacteria, a chest x-ray, and histologic evidence of granulomatous disease on biopsy. Definitive diagnosis is confirmed through culture and isolation of *M. tuberculosis*.

Mantoux Test
Also called the tuberculin skin test or purified protein derivative (PPD), the Mantoux test is the standard method of identifying persons infected with tuberculosis. An injection of 0.1 mL of PPD tuberculin containing 5 tuberculin units is injected intradermally into the ulnar (medial) surface of the forearm. This should produce a discrete, pale elevation of the skin 6 to 10 mm in diameter. In sensitized individuals, this results in a reaction of palpable swelling and induration at the site of injection in 48 to 72 hours. The PPD is read by measuring the diameter of the induration. A reaction is considered positive if it is between 5 and 15 mm. A positive reaction does not mean that the patient has active tuberculosis. Further studies must be done to confirm active disease. Conversely, a negative reaction does not exclude tuberculosis in an immunosuppressed patient, since immunosuppression can be associated with anergy (the inability to react to specific antigens).

To test for anergy, two companion antigens to which most people have a positive reaction (usually *Candida* and tetanus toxoid) are administered intradermally with the PPD. If no reaction occurs to any of the antigens, the patient is considered to be anergic and additional diagnostic testing is required to check for tuberculosis infection.

Bacteriologic Studies
Diagnosis of tuberculosis is never certain without bacteriologic confirmation. Examination of a sputum smear for acid-fast bacilli is the most important laboratory test in the diagnosis of pulmonary tuberculosis. Freshly expectorated sputum must be obtained before the patient eats or drinks. If the patient cannot expectorate, sputum induction using a heated saline aerosol is tried. If not seen in a direct smear, organisms can be demonstrated after sputum or other suspected material is concentrated by one of several available methods. On the basis of a positive smear for acid-fast bacilli, chemotherapy is initiated and the patient's close contacts are examined. A sputum culture is done to differentiate *M. tuberculosis* from other acid-fast organisms and to determine the organism's susceptibility to antimicrobial therapy. It may also reveal the presence of *M. tuberculosis* when the number of bacilli is small. Sputum cultures are positive within 2 to 3 weeks of active disease but are not positive during the latent period.

The Tuberculosis Stat Test allows detection of *M. tuberculosis* in sputum or respiratory aspirate within 48 hours as opposed to the 3 to 6 weeks required for culture. This test is based on polymerase chain reaction technology, which amplifies DNA to allow direct detection of microorganisms. Because this test is very costly and cannot distinguish active disease from previous infection, it is used only in clearly defined situations, for quick diagnosis of a person in a high-risk group who has an abnormal chest x-ray.

Chest Radiography
The chest x-ray is the single most useful test for the diagnosis of tuberculosis. Primary tuberculosis in adults commonly appears as an infiltrate in the lower lobes. Reactivated infection usually produces an infiltrate or cavitation in the apical or posterior segment of the upper lobe and may include hilar involvement. Pleural effusion may also be seen.

Pleural Needle Biopsy
Tissue samples for histologic study may be obtained by pleural needle biopsy. However, even if positive for granuloma and for the presence of giant cells, indicating caseation necrosis, the diagnosis remains presumptive.

Management
A short hospital stay may be required for diagnostic studies, observation for effect of treatment and possible side effects of drugs, and isolation of the patient during the infective stage. During this time, the patient and family are taught about tuberculosis and the importance of adhering to long-term therapy.

In the acute-care setting, patients diagnosed with tuberculosis and high-risk patient populations with an unidentified pulmonary problem are isolated in a negative-pressure room (CDC, 1994). Air is drawn into the room and ventilated directly outside through a special filtering system. Air exchange takes place six to 12 times per hour. High-efficiency particulate filters, which enhance the existing ventilation system, can be used in older facilities where outside venting is impossible. Ultraviolet germicidal irradiation can also be used as a supplement to engineering controls and can be installed in air ducts or near the ceiling. Isolation is maintained until the patient has improved clinically and has three negative sputum acid-fast bacillus smears collected on 3 different days over a 2- to 3-week period. Patients can be discharged home while still infectious if there are no high-risk persons in the same home and appropriate discharge arrangements and assistance are confirmed.

Guidelines from the Centers for Disease Control recommend that an individually fitted disposable particulate respirator be worn by health-care providers when delivering direct patient care or when high-risk procedures such as endotracheal intubation or bronchoscopy are performed. An HIV test is recommended for all newly diagnosed patients with tuberculosis.

The cornerstone of medical treatment for tuberculosis is chemotherapy (Tables 16–5 and 16–6). The most important factor in drug therapy is adherence to the prescribed regimen. Adherence to drug therapy can be difficult because of the length of time medication must be taken and the cost of treatment. Properly selected drugs administered for an adequate period of time ensure a successful outcome in almost all patients with the common strain of tuberculosis. Four-drug therapy with isoniazid, rifampin, pyrazinamide, and either ethambutol or streptomycin is the initial regimen for treating tuberculosis in most patients. This drug regimen is necessary for the first 2 months to prevent the emergence of resistant organisms. When susceptibility studies become available, the regimen can be adjusted. For multi-drug resistant tuberculosis, consultation and collaboration with the Infectious Disease Department is recommended. In geographic areas where isoniazid resistance is below 4%, three-drug therapy may be adequate.

Intermittent drug therapy can be prescribed if the patient is on directly observed therapy, that is, the patient is directly observed while taking the medication. Most patients should be considered for directly observed therapy, because the major cause of drug-resistant tuberculosis and treatment failure is patients' not completing the prescribed treatment. Intermittent drug regimens decrease the number of drugs and the number of times a patient must meet with a health-care worker for medication administration. The local health department is closely involved in the treatment of all tuberculosis patients.

Sputum cultures and smears are monitored during drug therapy. Cultures and smears should be negative after 2 months of therapy. If they remain positive, the treatment regimen is re-evaluated and the patient's ability to complete the necessary treatment plan assessed. Surgical intervention for tuberculosis, thoracoplasty or lung resection, is rare.

Preventive measures for tuberculosis are the most effective "treatment." They include screening of high-risk populations, treatment of infected individuals and their contacts, and education of patients, families, and communities.

For persons at high risk of exposure to tuberculosis, such as a nurse on a respiratory unit or in a public health clinic, regular skin testing is recommended as often as every 3 months, especially if there contact is with multi-drug resistant tuberculosis patients.

Bacille Calmette-Guérin Vaccine
Bacille Calmette-Guérin is a vaccine used to prevent tuberculosis in high-risk infants and children in many countries of the world. It is usually not recommended in the United States because the risk of infection is low and the effects of the vaccine are variable. A bacille Calmette-Guérin vaccination may produce a PPD reaction that cannot be distinguished from a positive tuberculosis skin test reaction. However, a PPD test reaction greater than 10 mm can be attributed to tuberculosis infection in an adult who received bacille Calmette-Guérin as a child.

Chemoprophylaxis
Persons in the following risk groups who test positive to the tuberculin skin test after exposure to tuberculosis (ie, those with a latent tuberculosis infec-

Table 16–5

Recommended Therapy for Active Tuberculosis

Protocol	Initial Medications	Continuation

Standard therapy
  No risk factors for resistance
  Drug resistance <2% in area
	First 2 months:
	  Isoniazid
	  Rifampin
	  Pyrazinamide
		Next 4 months:
		  Isoniazid
		  Rifampin

Possible drug resistance
  No risk factors for resistance
  Drug resistance >2% in area
	Until cultures available:
	  Isoniazid
	  Rifampin
	  Pyrazinamide
	  Ethambutol or streptomycin
		If sensitive, continue as above.
		If resistant to isoniazid, continue other meds for 6 months.
		If resistant to rifampin, continue other meds for 12–18 months.

Multiple drug resistance probable
  High incidence of multiple drug resistance in area
  HIV infection
  Previous drug failure
	Until cultures available:
	  Isoniazid
	  Rifampin
	  Pyrazinamide
	  Ethambutol or streptomycin
	  Two meds recommended by infection control physician.
		Adjust meds according to sensitivity reports.
		Continue 18–24 months.
		Consult tuberculosis expert.

Table 16-6

Drug Therapy in the Treatment of Tuberculosis

Drug	Side Effects	Patient Management Considerations
Isoniazid	Peripheral neuritis: tingling, numbness, burning, or pain of the hands and feet, clumsiness, unsteadiness Hepatotoxicity	Pyridoxine effective as prophylaxis and treatment against isoniazid-induced paresthesias. Daily ingestion of alcohol increases risk of liver toxicity.
Rifampin	Hepatitis	Negates effect of oral contraceptives. Reduces effectiveness of coumarin derivatives, digitoxin, glucocorticoids, and methadone. Liver toxicity most likely in alcoholics and in cases of pre-existing liver disease. Colors urine, sweat, saliva, and tears red-orange. May stain soft contact lenses.
Pyrazinamide	Hepatotoxicity	AST and ALT levels obtained before start of treatment and every 2 to 4 weeks thereafter because elevation of these enzymes is first sign of liver damage.
Ethambutol	Optic neuritis: blurred vision, narrowed visual fields, impaired red-green color discrimination	Baseline vision test at start of treatment. Instruct patient to report any vision changes.
Streptomycin	Eighth cranial nerve damage Nephrotoxicity Facial paresthesias Rash	Risk of hearing loss is increased in the elderly. Used with caution in presence of renal disease. Must be given IM.
Aminosalicylic acid	Gastrointestinal upset: nausea, vomiting, diarrhea Hepatotoxicity Hypersenstivity	Given as a sodium salt so can produce significant sodium load.
Ethionamide	Gastrointestinal disturbance: anorexia, nausea, vomiting, diarrhea, metallic taste Hepatotoxicity Hypersensitivity	Baseline AST and ALT levels before start of treatment and periodically thereafter.
Cycloserine	Anxiety, depression, confusion, psychoses Seizures Rash	Used with caution in patients with impaired renal function.
Capreomycin	Nephrotoxicity Eighth cranial nerve damage: hearing loss, tinnitus, impaired balance	Give deep IM.
Kanamycin	Nephrotoxicity Eighth cranial nerve damage	

Abbreviations: AST, aspartate aminotransferase (formerly SGOT, serum glutamic oxaloacetic transaminase); ALT, alanine aminotransferase (formerly SGPT, serum glutamic pyruvic transaminase); PAS, para-aminosalicylate; GI, gastrointestinal; IM, intramuscular.

tion) are given prophylaxis (Table 16–7) unless contraindicated:

- Persons with suspected or diagnosed HIV or AIDS infection
- Close contacts of persons with tuberculosis
- Persons whose chest x-rays suggest previous tuberculosis
- IV drug abusers
- Health-care workers with recent PPD conversions

HIV/AIDS is one of the strongest risk factors for the progression of tuberculosis from infection to disease.

Other candidates for preventive therapy, if they test positive after an exposure, are persons with cancer of the head and neck, reticuloendothelial diseases, end-stage renal disease, intestinal bypass or gastrectomy, chronic malabsorption syndromes, and persons on corticosteroid therapy or other immunosuppressive drugs.

Table 16–7

Drug Therapy for Latent Tuberculosis Infection*

Indication	Duration of Treatment, mo	Medication
Persons <35 years old with no other risk factors†	6–12	Isoniazid
Health-care workers with risk factors for tuberculosis	6–12	Isoniazid
Patients infected with human immunodeficiency virus	12	Isoniazid
Persons exposed to multi-drug resistant tuberculosis	12	Multi-drug therapy determined by prevalence of resistant organism
Persons whose chest x-rays indicate silicosis or inactive fibrotic lesions	4 or 12	Isoniazid and rifampin or isoniazid

*Latent refers to recent purified protein derivative reaction but no active disease.

†People over age 35 with no other risk factors should have further screening. Potential drug hepatotoxicity should be weighed against the potential for developing tuberculosis. Liver function tests should be monitored carefully.

The usual therapy is isoniazid daily for 6 months to 1 year. Alternative therapy may be recommended after known exposure to a person with multi-drug resistant tuberculosis. Monthly liver function tests are necessary to monitor for adverse reactions, such as hepatitis, to the drug therapy.

❖ **Settings, Providers, and Collaboration for Care**

Patients with active tuberculosis require isolation during the initial detection and treatment period. This may be achieved in a variety of settings, such as acute-care, long-term health, and correctional facilities, provided that they are equipped with negative pressure flow rooms as required by the Occupational Safety and Health Administration (OSHA) and the Centers for Disease Control. Other patients may be treated at home with strict adherence to guidelines for preventing disease transmission.

Close collaboration among health-care providers and departments in health facilities is essential to ensure compliance with the treatment plan and prevent the spread of tuberculosis. Cooperation among the medical, nursing, and engineering departments is necessary to provide for immediate isolation in a negative-pressure room for each suspected active tuberculosis patient.

Discharge planning relies heavily on the Public Health Department's ability to provide follow-up care management until the patient is cured. Follow-up includes clinic appointments, visiting nurses, home health aides, social workers, and community outreach workers, especially those who are bilingual or bicultural. Prevention and detection education programs are necessary in all areas of the community and require the support of health-care and governmental agencies.

NURSING PROCESS
Tuberculosis

Assessment

When caring for the tuberculosis patient with clinical disease, monitor for temperature elevation associated with chills and night sweats. Assess lung sounds, cough, recent weight patterns, and eating habits.

Assess the patient's understanding of the disease, its prognosis, and the course of therapy. When a chemotherapeutic regimen has been prescribed, assess the patient's understanding of self-administration of the drugs and need for consistent long-term therapy. Assess the patient's willingness and ability to comply with the therapy. Determine the patient's understanding of disease transmission and methods for preventing its spread. Clear understanding is necessary to decrease the potential transmission of disease prior to control of the infection by antituberculosis drugs and to ensure that misconceptions concerning infectiousness do not result in unnecessary precautions that interfere with the patient's quality of life.

Tuberculosis still carries a social stigma and is perceived by many as a dread disease leading to isolation, disability, and death. Assess the patient's and family's reaction to the diagnosis and their emotional response. Older adults may perceive the diagnosis to be a death sentence based on their experiences before the development of the antimicrobial treatment.

Nursing Diagnoses and Planning

Nursing diagnoses and related expected patient outcomes commonly applicable to patients with active pulmonary tuberculosis include the following:

NDx: Knowledge deficit: mechanism of spread and precautionary measures

Planning: Patient Outcomes
1. Patient explains how tuberculosis is spread.
2. Patient describes measures to prevent the spread of tuberculosis to others.
3. Patient's contacts remain free of tuberculosis as evidenced by a negative tuberculin test.

NDx: Anxiety related to the disease, its prognosis, reaction of friends and relatives, effect on employment status, and/or possibility of transmitting it to others

Planning: Patient Outcomes
1. Patient expresses belief that drug therapy will effectively control the infection.
2. Patient verbalizes confidence in ability to carry out precautionary measures to prevent transmission to others.
3. Patient is realistic in discussing importance of the disease on social and work relationships.

NDx: Risk for altered health maintenance related to nonadherence to drug therapy secondary to duration, cost or lack of perceived importance

Planning: Patient Outcomes
1. Patient describes a plan for remembering to take the medication.
2. Patient states how and where one is able to obtain the medication.
3. Patient verbalizes importance of taking medication as prescribed and intent to comply.
4. On follow-up examination, sputum cultures are negative and chest x-rays improved.

NDx: Risk for altered health maintenance related to insufficient knowledge of disease and follow-up care

Planning: Patient Outcomes
1. Patient describes cause, treatment, and prognosis of tuberculosis.
2. Patient states name, dose, route, and frequency of prescribed medication.
3. Patient explains importance of taking medication consistently for as long as ordered.
4. Patient describes supportive self-care measures, need for medical follow-up, and symptoms that require prompt reporting.
5. Patient identifies community support services to assist with medication, necessary laboratory work, transportation, and follow-up care.

Nursing Interventions and Evaluation

NDx: Knowledge deficit: mechanism of spread and precautionary measures
Instruct the patient and family about how to prevent transmission of tuberculosis. Explain that the most important way to prevent the spread of tuberculosis is to cover the mouth and nose with double thickness tissue when coughing or sneezing and to take

the prescribed medication. Emphasize the importance of good handwashing after using tissues and proper disposal of used tissues. Provide specific instruction for preventing transmission of tuberculosis in the home-care setting (Highlight 16–5).

If hospitalization is required, maintain the patient in isolation, wear the prescribed respirator during all direct patient care, and assist other healthcare providers and visitors to comply with isolation requirements. Provide diversional activities, such as television, radio, books, or tapes because the patient must remain isolated.

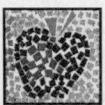

HIGHLIGHT
16–5

HEALTH PROMOTION & RISK REDUCTION

Preventing Tuberculosis Transmission in the Home-Care Setting

Keep the door to the patient's room closed.

Ventilate the room. If possible, open a window and use an exhaust fan.

Test all family members with purified protein derivative (PPD) and treat positive results prophylactically.

Instruct the patient and family members on the importance of taking medication as prescribed.

Arrange for DOT (direct observation of medication administration).

Limit visitors, especially those from high-risk groups and children, during the isolation period (usually 2 weeks of treatment).

Instruct the patient to cover the mouth with a fresh tissue when coughing and to dispose of the tissue immediately into a plastic bag.

Perform all cough-inducing procedures (to collect sputum) near an open window.

Instruct the patient to wear a surgical mask when entering other parts of the home.

Wear a fitted mask approved by OSHA when entering the home during the isolation period.

Recognize and manage noncompliant medication behavior:
  Perform routine pill counts.
  Note persistent pulmonary symptoms.
  Observe results of sputum smears (quantity of acid-fast bacilli should decrease with time).
  Observe urine. It should be orange if the patient is taking rifampin. A dipstick test can detect the presence of isoniazid.

NDx: Anxiety

Provide opportunity and encouragement for the patient to discuss feelings about the diagnosis. Recognize that in some circles, tuberculosis is associated with a degree of social stigma because of its prevalence among lower socioeconomic and minority groups. Tuberculosis can create fear because of its increased incidence and the development of drug-resistant strains. Many people remember when tuberculosis was a disease basically without treatment that devastated families and often caused early death. Distinguish between tuberculosis and multidrug resistant tuberculosis. Explain the effectiveness of drug therapy in controlling the disease and in preventing spread to families and close contacts. Encourage questions and always answer honestly and clearly.

NDx: Risk for altered health maintenance

The medication schedule must be followed strictly to cure tuberculosis. Stress the importance of this to both patient and family. Help the patient devise a way of remembering to take the medication, such as a monthly check-off chart of scheduled doses to be hung in a corner of the bathroom mirror. Inform the patient that antituberculosis drugs are available free of charge from most health departments, so financial concerns should not interfere with treatment. Instruct the patient in the importance of returning for follow-up tests as scheduled to protect both self and others.

NDx: Risk for altered health maintenance

Learn as much as possible about the patient: medical history, beliefs and attitudes, social supports, and whether there are any barriers to adherence to the treatment plan. Assess knowledge of the disease process. Using simple, nonmedical terms, reinforce accurate information and correct misconceptions. Explain what tuberculosis is, who gets it, and how it spreads. Use handouts when available. Provide written instructions the patient can refer to later, if needed.

Counsel the patient on the importance of plenty of rest and a nutritious diet high in protein and vitamins in supporting recuperation. Explain the importance of follow-up sputum cultures to determine the medication's effectiveness. Be sure the patient understands that recurrence of symptoms, hemoptysis, or pleuritic pain should be reported to the health-care provider immediately.

Teach the patient about the prescribed medications: name, dose, route, frequency, and expected action. Stress the importance of reporting any side effects from medications so that the regimen can be adjusted appropriately. Instruct the patient never to discontinue the prescribed medications unless specifically directed to do so by the health-care provider. Provide the patient with information related to community services available to facilitate compliance with the therapeutic regimen.

Additional Interventions

Collect sputum specimens in the morning, preferably when the patient first awakens. Have the patient cleanse the mouth and cough deeply to expectorate at least 1 teaspoon of mucus into a sterile, wide-mouthed cup. Replace the lid and put the container in a sealed plastic bag to avoid contamination of health-care workers. Specimens may be refrigerated for several hours if necessary.

Compare the patient's status with the expected outcomes. If the outcomes are not met, reassess the patient and revise the plan.

EMPYEMA

A collection of fluid in the pleural space is referred to as a pleural effusion. Empyema is a specific form of pleural effusion in which the fluid in the pleural space contains pus.

Etiology and Pathophysiology

A collection of pus in the pleural space may occur as a direct extension from adjacent structures in patients with a lung abscess, pneumonia, tuberculosis, fungal infection, bronchiectasis, or esophageal rupture. Empyema may also follow thoracic surgery or penetrating chest wounds and occurs quite often as a complication of staphylococcal pneumonia.

Empyema usually develops in the dependent part of the pleural space, usually in the lateral or posterior aspects. Initially the purulent fluid is thin, but it often becomes fibropurulent and may ultimately form a thick exudative membrane around the lung. If a large empyema remains untreated, septicemia commonly develops. Spontaneous evacuation of the pus may occur either by rupture through the lung into a bronchus (bronchopleural fistula) or by extension through the thoracic wall. Treatment of chronic, recurrent empyema is difficult because the pleura becomes thickened and fibrous and the lung may adhere to the chest wall. The retracted lung and the displaced mediastinum are anchored, and the overlying thoracic cage is retracted and immobile. The multiloculated cavities within the pleural space fill with pus and are difficult to drain.

Clinical Manifestations

Clinical manifestations include fever, unilateral pleuritic chest pain, dyspnea, and anorexia. Physical examination discloses foul-smelling sputum, pleural friction rub, dullness to percussion, decreased lung sounds over the area of the pus, decreased vocal fremitus, and unequal chest expansion. With chronic empyema, weight loss, low-grade fever, and malaise may be present.

Diagnosis

Diagnosis is made on the basis of history, physical examination, chest x-ray—which usually shows unilateral pleural fluid with an associated lung lesion—

and laboratory examination, including culture and sensitivity of pleural exudate obtained by thoracentesis. Of special diagnostic value is the pH of the exudate. A pH less than 7.20 suggests empyema that necessitates chest-tube drainage.

Management

Treatment consists of draining the pleural space, administering large doses of antibiotics to control infection, encouraging coughing and deep-breathing to promote maximal ventilation, and lung expansion and other supportive measures, such as oxygen therapy and bedrest. If the area is small and localized and the fluid is thin, drainage is accomplished by thoracotomy. For more extensive involvement, closed-chest drainage is used, and, for patients not responding to tube drainage, surgical evacuation of the pleural space may be necessary.

❖ Settings, Providers, and Collaboration for Care

Most patients with empyema are managed in the inpatient setting. Collaboration among respiratory therapists, nursing staff, and the physician is necessary to develop and implement an effective plan of care.

NURSING PROCESS GUIDELINES
Empyema

The assessment, nursing diagnoses, expected patient outcomes, nursing interventions, and evaluation for patients with empyema are similar to those described previously for patients with lung abscess. Specific implications for care arise in relation to the long-term, sometimes recurrent nature of empyema and when chest drainage is required.

In regard to the long recovery period associated with empyema, inform the patient and family that the healing process may be slow and that repeated treatments, drainage, irrigation, and follow-up chest x-rays may be necessary. If empyema is a recurrent problem, teach the patient and family the signs and symptoms that should be reported for early treatment. These include:

Elevated temperature
Shortness of breath
Increased or foul-smelling sputum
Painful breathing
Loss of appetite

If the patient has chest tubes, provide care as described in Chapter 14, with special attention to monitoring the patency of the tubes, because purulent drainage can readily obstruct them.

PLEURITIS

Pleuritis, also called pleurisy, is an acute inflammation of the pleural surfaces.

Etiology and Pathophysiology

Inflammation of the pleura is almost always a secondary effect of underlying disease. Pulmonary disorders associated with pleuritis include tuberculosis, pneumonia, lung abscess, pulmonary embolism, bronchiectasis, lung cancer, and trauma, including thoracotomy. Nonpulmonary causes include rheumatic fever, disseminated lupus erythematosus, uremia, and systemic infections caused by bacteria or fungi.

In the acute stage of inflammation, the pleura is red, swollen, and covered with exudate composed of fibrin, lymph, and cellular elements. Pain occurs when the parietal pleura (which contains sensory receptors for pain, touch, and temperature) rubs against the visceral pleura during respiration. Lung expansion in a person with pleuritis is inhibited because of the pain on respiration and the pressure of effusion if present. If not corrected, this reduced lung expansion predisposes the patient to atelectasis (collapse of lung tissue) and to further infection. If the exudative reaction is profuse, fluid accumulates in the pleural cavity. This is called "wet" pleuritis or pleuritis with effusion.

Clinical Manifestations

The most distinctive symptom of pleuritis is chest pain, which is usually unilateral, well localized along intercostal nerve zones, and related to respiratory movements. The pain is variously described as achy, sharp, burning, a "catch," or a "stitch." It is aggravated by deep-breathing, coughing, sneezing, and body movements, such as turning or stooping. If the inflammation involves the diaphragmatic pleura, pain is referred to the shoulder and the throat via the phrenic nerve.

Movement of the chest on the affected side may be reduced, and the patient may hold the area or lie still on that side. If "wet pleuritis" or pleural effusion occurs, pain may lessen and dyspnea may develop. Patients with "dry" pleuritis may complain of a feeling of difficulty breathing because the pain calls attention to a process that normally occurs unnoticed.

A friction rub can be heard over the inflamed area on auscultation. The exception is in cases in which a pleural effusion has separated the pleural surfaces so no friction rub occurs.

Diagnosis

Diagnosis of pleuritis is based on history and clinical findings, such as characteristics of the pain and presence of a friction rub on auscultation of the chest. Pleuritis is usually not a primary disease; therefore, the underlying problem must also be identified. The speed of onset of the pleuritis suggests the causative disorder. Acute, immediate onset is associated with pulmonary embolism or pneumothorax. Onset over a few hours, especially in the presence of fever and cough, is associated with pneumonia. Onset over a period of weeks is associated with tuberculosis or malignancy. Specific diagnostic procedures include chest x-rays, examination of pleural fluid, and pleural biopsy.

Management
Local application of heat or cold, analgesic medications, nonsteroidal anti-inflammatory agents, or, in severe cases, procaine intercostal blocks are used to manage the pleuritic pain. The main goal of treatment is resolution of the primary disease.

NURSING PROCESS GUIDELINES
Pleuritis

Observe breathing patterns. Note rate, depth, and symmetry of respiration. Auscultate the chest for a friction rub. Assess for chest pain, noting the type, location, and relation to breathing and other body movement.

Assess the patient's emotional state, because breathing difficulty can produce great anxiety. Reassure the patient that anxiety is normal and encourage expression of concerns and questions. Encourage the patient to breathe deeply every 1 to 2 hours. Change the patient's position every 2 hours, and encourage high Fowler's position when awake to facilitate chest expansion. Consider administration of analgesic, nonsteroidal anti-inflammatory drugs 30 to 60 minutes before deep-breathing to help reduce discomfort.

*A*sthma

Asthma is a chronic inflammatory disorder of the airways that is the result of complex interaction between inflammatory cells, mediators, and the cells and tissue resident in the airways. Specifically, mast cells, eosinophils, macrophages, T lymphocytes, neutrophils, and epithelial cells interact to produce episodes of variable but often reversible airflow obstruction and an increase in bronchial hyper-responsiveness to various stimuli. The end result over time may be structural or functional damage in the lungs. The incidence of asthma is increasing, especially among children and adolescents. It occurs more often among African-Americans than among white Americans and tends to run in families. It is estimated that 1 of every 20 people experiences symptoms of asthma at some time, and most have a history of allergies. About one-fourth of people who develop asthma attacks in childhood stop having them after adolescence.

The severity of the disease varies from person to person and ranges from mild, for which no treatment is needed, to disease so severe that hospitalization with intensive, aggressive therapy is required. A large number of patients remain in a chronic state of mild asthma, with symptoms exacerbated during periods of exertion or emotional excitement. The fa-

tality rate from asthma is more than 5000 deaths annually, with the highest death rate occurring among African-Americans aged 15 to 24 years (CDC, 1996).

Etiology and Pathophysiology
The exact cause of asthma is not known. Neither is the reason for its increasing incidence. Potential causal factors include deteriorating air quality, increased environmental allergens, and increased occupational exposure to allergens. Asthma usually begins in childhood and is often associated with atropy, which is a genetic predisposition to produce immunoglobulin E in response to common allergens. In adult-onset asthma, allergens may continue to play an important role. The airway hyper-responsiveness that leads to the classic wheezing and dyspnea of asthma commonly follows exposure to an allergen, irritant, or viral infection. Some of the more common, well-recognized allergens are:

- Cold or dry air
- Air pollutants, such as cigarette and industrial smoke, ozone, sulfur dioxide, and formaldehyde
- Perfumes
- Allergens, such as feathers, animal danders, molds, pollens, dust mites, and cockroaches
- Enzymes, such as those in laundry detergents
- Chemicals, such as those found in solvents, paints, rubber, and plastic
- Wood dust
- Vegetable dusts, such as in flour, coffee, and tea
- Alcoholic beverages
- Foods, such as eggs and those containing sulfates (for example, wine, beer, salads, fresh and dried fruits, fruit juices, molasses, wine vinegar, instant potatoes, shellfish, and snack foods)
- Upper respiratory viral infection
- Stress
- Exercise
- The act of lying down, possibly because it results in gastroesophageal reflux, which stimulates the vagus nerve by gastric-acid-initiating reflex bronchoconstriction

Pathophysiologic events in the airway that accompany an asthma attack can be divided into the early response and the late response. The early response, which typically lasts 90 minutes or less, is characterized by bronchospasm. This occurs when an inhaled substance, an emotional reaction, or a reflex stimulates mast cells to release histamine and related substances, which in turn trigger contraction of the smooth muscle of the bronchi, edema of the bronchial mucous membrane, and secretion of large amounts of mucus into the bronchi.

The late response occurs 3 to 4 hours later and lasts up to 12 hours. The lungs' immune defense system is activated, and eosinophils moving to the membrane secrete prostaglandins, leukotrienes, major basic protein, and other substances that produce inflammation and promote immunity. Simultaneously, sensory nerves in the lungs produce substance P, neurokinin A, and calcitonin. The result is sustained inflammation of the bronchial mucosa and a hyper-responsiveness to the original trigger substance. Thus, with the next exposure to a trigger, both the early and late responses are magnified, creating a vicious circle resulting ultimately in structural change in the lung (Fig. 16–2).

Clinical Manifestations

The classic symptoms of asthma are dyspnea, paroxysmal attacks of coughing, wheezing, and tightness in the chest. In addition, thick tenacious mucus may be produced. A patient with uncomplicated asthma often has no symptoms between attacks, and, in about one-fourth of all cases beginning in childhood, the attacks cease spontaneously after adolescence. A large number of other patients, however, remain in a chronic state of mild asthma, with symptoms exacerbated during periods of exertion or emotional excitement. On physical examination, the signs are similar to those of diffuse partial airway obstruction. The lungs are hyperinflated, with a resulting hyper-resonant sound on percussion. Breath sounds are distant. Expiration is prolonged, with high-pitched wheezes throughout the lung, sometimes audible at a distance.

During an asthma attack, perspiration is common and cyanosis is sometimes present. If the attack is severe, tachycardia, tachypnea of more than 30 breaths per minute, and use of accessory muscles of respiration may occur.

There is wide variation in the duration and the severity of asthma attacks. Symptoms range from mild respiratory discomfort to life-threatening respiratory failure, and for the same patient each attack may be quite different. In "cough variant" asthma, the presenting symptom is a chronic cough that worsens on exertion or exposure to cold dry air, smoke, or perfume.

Asthmatics frequently have other atopic diseases, such as allergic rhinitis or eczema, and also have a family history of them.

Status asthmaticus is a severe asthma attack that lasts for hours or days and that does not respond to the usual forms of treatment. It can progress to respiratory failure and is a life-threatening emergency. In status asthmaticus, severe bronchospasm, mucus plugging, and inflammation of the airways cause increased airway resistance, greatly increasing the amount of work required to breathe. This results in increased oxygen consumption and a build-up of carbon dioxide. As alveolar ventilation decreases, hypoxemia occurs. The end result is carbon dioxide retention, respiratory acidosis, and further hypoxemia. This can cause cardiac dysrhythmias and respiratory failure. Signs and symptoms vary but usually include an audible wheeze, tachycardia, severely labored respirations, and diaphoresis.

Diagnosis

Diagnosis of asthma depends primarily on a history of recurrent, episodic attacks of wheezing and shortness of breath with symptom-free intervals. Other

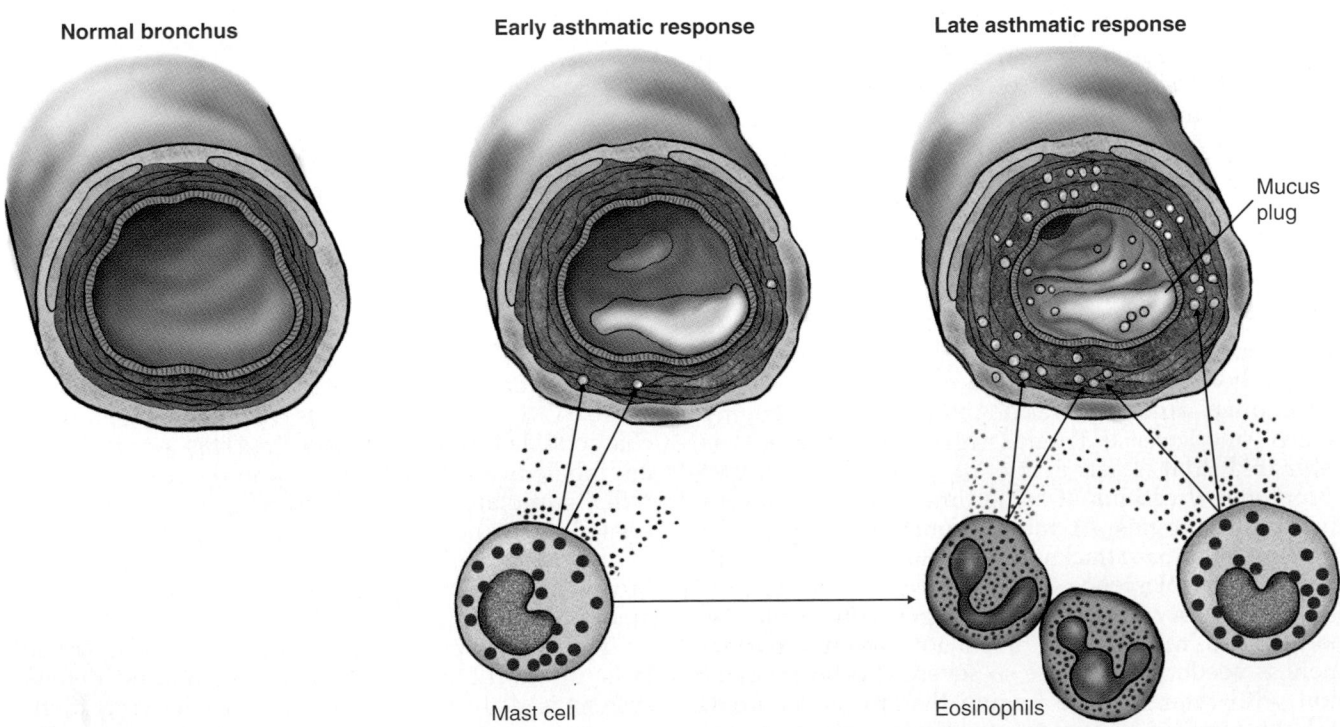

Normal bronchus   **Early asthmatic response**   **Late asthmatic response**

Mucus plug

Mast cell   Eosinophils

Figure 16–2

Cross sections of normal and asthmatic bronchi. Note that the asthmatic bronchi, both in the early and late response, have narrowed, thickened muscular walls invaded by inflammatory cells and have a collection of mucus in the lumen.

findings that support the diagnosis include decreased values on pulmonary function tests, such as forced expiratory flow volume and peak expiratory flow rate. An improvement in these measures following the administration of aerosolized bronchodilators is further confirmation of the diagnosis. Many patients also have an elevated eosinophil count.

Arterial blood gases or pulse oximetry are used to help determine whether hospitalization is required and to monitor the progress of the treatment plan.

Management

The goals of management are to prevent chronic and troublesome symptoms; maintain (near) normal pulmonary function; maintain normal activity levels, prevent recurrent exacerbations, and minimize emergency department visits or hospitalizations; provide optimal pharmacotherapy with minimal or no adverse effects; and meet patients' and families' expectations of and satisfaction with asthma care. If allergens to which the patient is sensitive are identified, then desensitization may be tried. Desensitization is not a cure, but an attempt to control symptoms induced by specific antigens. Avoidance of allergens can also be very helpful in controlling asthma. If an asthma attack is induced by infection, stress, exercise, or other factors not related to allergy, other ways must be found to manage these factors. Preventing asthma attacks is largely a product of self-management. Patients must be involved in their own treatment plans and know how to control their asthma.

The stepwise pharmacologic treatment of asthma is based on the severity classification (NAEPP-EPRII, 1997). This reflects the new awareness of chronic inflammation as the underlying disease process and represents a change from past therapy, which focused almost solely on episodic bronchodilation. The stepwise care approach to asthma treatment is represented in Table 16–8. It represents initiating higher level therapy at the onset of an attack to establish prompt control, and then stepping down.

Asthma medications are categorized into two general classifications: quick relief and long-term control. The quick relief medications are given for the symptoms of an acute exacerbation, whereas long-term control medications are taken on a daily basis to control persistent symptoms. Quick relief therapy begins with an inhaled β_2-agonist (albuterol, terbutaline). An anticholinergic may also be used, such as ipratropium bromide (Atrovent) which produces bronchodilatation with a minimum of the systemic side effects that usually accompany most anticholinergics. An anticholinergic may be the drug of choice if the patient cannot tolerate beta agonists because of cardiac disease. If the symptoms continue or worsen, anti-inflammatory medications are added to the regimen in the form of either a low-dose inhaled corticosteroid (beclomethasone) or a systemic steroid administered intravenously (hydrocortisone). The systemic steroids are used in the treatment of moderate to severe exacerbations to prevent the progression of symptoms, speed the recovery, and prevent early relapses. Treatment in children may include the use of inhaled cromolyn (Intal) or, in children over 12 years of age, nedocromil.

Long-term control includes daily doses of inhaled corticosteroid and a long-acting bronchodilator, either a β_2-agonist or a sustained-release theophylline (Theo-Dur, Slobid). The theophylline is not the preferred drug because of its potential toxicity. In mild persistent asthma, leukotriene modifiers (zafirlukast and zileuton) may also be added to improve lung function and reduce the dose of beta agonists. Zafirlukast (Accolate) blocks the action of leukotrienes (substances released by white blood cells in response to tissue injury, which induce bronchial constriction and increased muscus secretion) on target cells, thereby impairing the allergic response while zileuton prevents the synthesis of leukotrienes. Further study is needed to establish a more specific role for these drugs. In severe persistent asthma, an oral corticosteroid (prednisone, prednisolone) may be used.

To decrease the risk of side effects of long-term steroid therapy, such as osteoporosis, weight gain, peptic ulcers, diabetes, and infections, the steroids are administered directly to the airways by an inhaler with an attached spacer (Fig. 16–3). The spacer has the following functions:

- It prevents large droplets of medication from landing on the mucous membranes of the mouth or on the vocal cords, thus decreasing the chance of yeast infection.
- It dispenses the medication more uniformly and more deeply within the airways.

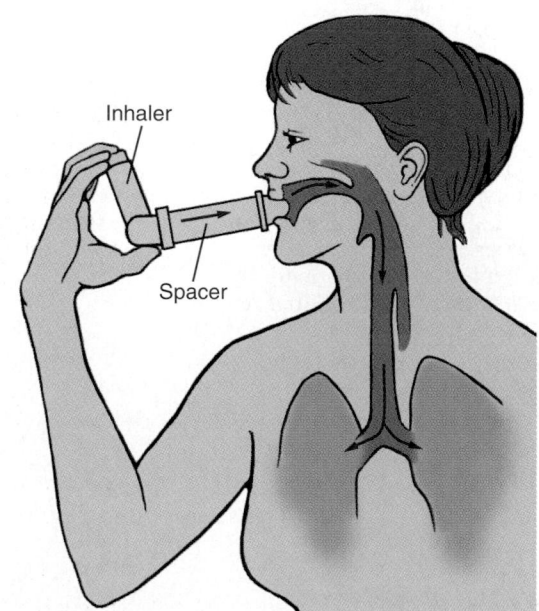

Figure 16–3

Metered-dose inhaler with attached spacer. The spacer is a molded plastic chamber attached to the inhaler and held in the mouth.

Table 16–8

Step-Care Approach to the Management of Asthma

Goals and expected outcomes of asthma treatment:
1. Patient maintains (near) normal pulmonary function.
2. Patient maintains normal activity levels (including exercise and other physical activity).
3. Recurrent exacerbations are prevented; the need for emergency treatment or hospitalization is minimized.
4. Patient participates in a pharmacotherapeutic regimen that controls all symptoms with minimal or no adverse effects.
5. Patient and family are satisfied with the management of the condition.

	Suggested Management	
Signs and Symptoms	*Short-Term/Quick Relief*	*Long-Term/Control Therapy*
STEP 1: MILD INTERMITTENT		
Brief episodes (lasting a few hours to a few days) occurring no more than twice weekly	Short-acting bronchodilator: β_2-agonist inhaler as needed for relief of symptoms	No daily medication needed
No symptoms and normal peak expiratory flows between episodes		
Nocturnal symptoms occurring no more than twice a month	If the inhaler is needed more than two times a week, long-term-control therapy may be indicated.	
Peak expiratory flow rates are more than 80% and vary less than 20%.		
STEP 2: MILD PERSISTENT		
Episodes with symptoms occurring more than twice a week but less than once a day	Short-acting bronchodilator: β_2-agonist inhaler as needed for relief of symptoms	Daily:
Activity may be affected.		• Anti-inflammatory: Either a low-dose inhaled corticosteroid or cromolyn or nedocromil
Nocturnal symptoms occurring more than twice a month.	If the inhaler is needed on a daily basis, long-term-control therapy may be indicated.	• Sustained-release theophylline to maintain a serum concentration of 5–15 μg/mL is an alternative but not preferred therapy.
Peak expiratory flow is more than 80% and may vary 20–30%.		• Zafirlukast or zileuton may be considered for patients older than 12 years of age, although the role of these agents is not fully established.
STEP 3: MODERATE PERSISTENT		
Symptoms occur daily.	Short-acting bronchodilator: β_2-agonist inhaler as needed for relief of symptoms	Daily:
Activity is affected.		• *Either* Anti-inflammatory: Inhaled corticosteroid (medium dose)
Episodes occur more than twice a week and may last for days	If the inhaler is needed on a daily basis or if its use is increasing, long-term-control therapy may be indicated.	*Or* Inhaled corticosteroid (low to medium dose) with a long-acting bronchodilator, especially for nocturnal symptoms: A long-acting β_2-agonist, sustained-release theophylline, or long-acting β_2-agonist tablets
Nocturnal symptoms occur more than once a week		• *If needed:* Anti-inflammatory: Inhaled corticosteroid (medium to high dose)
Peak expiratory flow is more than 60% but less than 80% but may vary more than 30%.		*And* Long-acting bronchodilator, especially for nocturnal symptoms: A long-acting inhaled beta-2 agonist, sustained-release theophylline, or long-acting beta-2 agonist tablets

Table 16–8

Step-Care Approach to the Management of Asthma *(continued)*

	Suggested Management	
Signs and Symptoms	*Short-Term/Quick Relief*	*Long-Term/Control Therapy*
STEP 4: SEVERE PERSISTENT Symptoms are present all the time. Physical activity is limited. Acute episodes occur frequently. Nocturnal symptoms occur frequently. Peak expiratory flow is less than 60% and may vary more than 30%.	Short-acting bronchodilator: β_2-agonist inhaler as needed for relief of symptoms If the inhaler is needed on a daily basis or if its use is increasing, long-term-control therapy may be indicated.	Daily: • Anti-inflammatory: Inhaled corticosteroid (high dose) *And* • Long-acting bronchodilator: A long-acting inhaled β_2-agonist, sustained-release theophylline, or long-acting β_2-agonist tablets *And* • Corticosteroid tablets or syrup long term (2 mg/kg/day, not to exceed 60 mg/day)

Information from Expert Panel Report II. Guidelines for the Diagnosis and Management of Asthma. National Asthma Education and Prevention Program. Atlanta: Centers for Disease Control and Prevention, February 1997.

• It reduces the importance of coordinating the use of the inhaler with breathing.
• It decreases the amount of medication used by reducing the required number and volume of puffs.

A device that is used as a basis for adjusting medication regimens is the peak flow meter (Fig. 16–4). This is an inexpensive, hand-held device that measures how fast air can be blown out of the lungs. Use of the peak flow meter reflects changes in the airways before clinical signs appear. Because decreased flow rate indicates an impending attack, early identification of the change allows for pharmacologic intervention designed to avert the attack.

Patients seek emergency medical help for severe asthma attacks when the attacks interfere with the patient's ability to eat, sleep, and perform normal daily activities. Patients usually require oxygen during a severe attack because hypoxemia is most often the underlying factor that brings them to the physician or hospital. Intravenous steroids are usually required to relieve bronchospasms if the inhaled beta agonists are not effective. Hydration is frequently needed as well, because asthmatics are often dehydrated by diaphoresis, hyperventilation, and the inability to drink. Breathing exercises, postural drainage, and aerosol therapy may be ordered to assist the patient in removing retained secretions.

Status asthmaticus requires aggressive emergency treatment with beta agonists and intravenous corticosteroids (hydrocortisone). Careful hydration may be required, and sodium bicarbonate may be used to correct respiratory acidosis. In some cases, mechanical ventilation may be necessary.

❖ **Settings, Providers, and Collaboration for Care**

While asthma may require occasional hospitalization for acute attacks, the treatment goal is to assist the

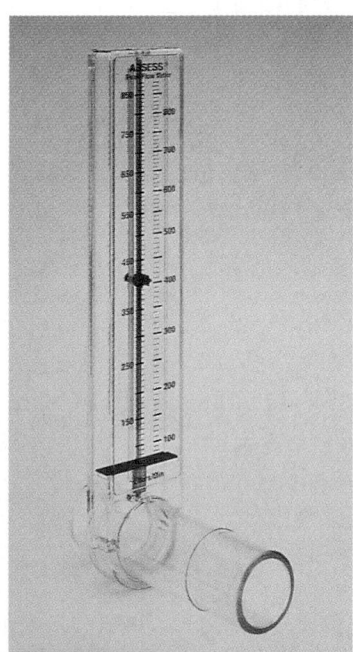

Figure 16–4

Peak flow meter, which provides objective measure of peak expiratory flow. Patient inhales as deeply as possible, places mouth firmly around the mouthpiece so lips form a tight seal, blows out as hard and fast as possible, and records the final position of the red indicator. (Courtesy of HealthScan Products Inc, Cedar Grove, NJ.)

patient in self-management of medications and lifestyle to avoid hospitalization. Patient education is important in helping manage triggers, emotions, and other lifestyle behaviors. Referrals to other healthcare providers may be very helpful to the patient learning to manage his or her lifestyle. A physical therapist may assist the patient in developing an exercise program to enhance pulmonary function. Counseling or biofeedback may also be helpful to the patient in managing stress that may exacerbate asthma attacks.

NURSING PROCESS
Asthma

Assessment

Obtain a nursing history that includes information about any family or personal history of allergy. Inquire about previous asthmatic episodes, including precipitating factors and treatment received. Assess the patient's understanding of the disease, prescribed medications, and factors known to precipitate an attack. Solicit the patient's emotional responses to the disease and the effect of the disease on the patient's lifestyle and activities. Obtain information about any coexisting medical problems and medications routinely taken. Assess respirations, including breath sounds, and observe the patient for signs of hypoxia, which include restlessness, tachycardia, confusion, hypotension, and cyanosis. Review results of laboratory tests, such as blood gas values.

If the patient is in acute distress, limit the history to immediately needed information. Determine the time of onset of the attack, any identifiable precipitating factor, and the name, dose, and time of any drug taken before admission. Obtain additional information from a significant other or from the patient once symptoms are under control.

Nursing Diagnoses and Planning

Nursing diagnoses and related expected patient outcomes commonly applicable to patients with asthma include the following:

NDx: Ineffective breathing pattern related to bronchial spasm and hypersecretion of mucus

Planning: Patient Outcomes
1. Respiratory rate returns to baseline.
2. Complaints of dyspnea are absent.
3. Audible expiratory wheeze is absent.
4. Cyanosis is absent.
5. Pulse oximeter values are within normal range.

NDx: Anxiety related to shortness of breath and recurrence of attacks

Planning: Patient Outcomes
1. Patient listens to what is being said.
2. Patient follows directions.

3. Behaviors such as grimacing, crying, or grabbing onto people are absent.

NDx: Risk for altered health maintenance related to insufficient knowledge of disease process; ways to avoid allergens; contributing factors, such as smoking, lack of sleep, and stress; medication regimen; and other self-care measures

Planning: Patient Outcomes
1. Patient identifies trigger factors.
2. Patient lists ways to eliminate or reduce exposure to trigger factors.
3. Patient states name, dose, route, time of administration, and use of prescribed medication.
4. Patient demonstrates correct use of metered dose inhaler medications.
5. Patient demonstrates use of peak flow meter.
6. Patient wears a Medic Alert emblem or similar device.
7. Patient describes the importance of informing health-care workers of the asthmatic condition.

Nursing Interventions and Evaluation

NDx: Ineffective breathing pattern
Administer medications as ordered to help the patient obtain relief from respiratory distress. Observe the patient for side effects, which include cardiac dysrhythmias, tremor, nervousness, nausea, and headaches. Assist the patient into a position that allows the greatest ease of respiration. Often this is a sitting position with the upper part of the body bent slightly forward. If so, use the over-bed table to provide necessary comfort and support. Keep the environment quiet and protect the patient from drafts and chills. If diaphoresis is present, change damp linens frequently.

Assist the patient with bronchial toilet as needed. This includes breathing exercises, postural drainage, and suctioning. Note and document the color, odor, quantity, and consistency of the expectorated sputum. Monitor fluid intake and output. If tolerated, give a minimum of 2 to 3 L of fluid per day to liquefy secretions.

NDx: Anxiety
Because most patients are anxious and exhausted during an acute asthma attack, treat them with a calm, caring manner. Assure them that they will not be left unattended and carefully explain each aspect of care. Since moderate to severe anxiety decreases the ability to comprehend, give explanations and instructions very slowly and repeat as necessary.

NDx: Risk for altered health maintenance
Health teaching is done to involve the patient in all aspects of self-management of this chronic disease. Explain what triggers the symptoms and what is happening in the lungs to cause the symptoms. Help the patient identify ways to avoid the antigen known to cause an attack. Once avoidance measures are identified, assist the patient in planning how to incorporate them into daily living. To make imple-

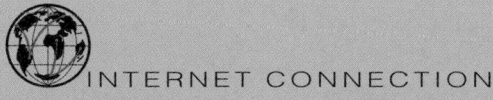

INTERNET CONNECTIONS
Lower Respiratory Disorders

General
The National Jewish Center for Immunology and Respiratory Medicine
http://www.njc.org/markethtml/NJCmore.html
This authoritative site describes the National Jewish Center for Immunology and Respiratory Medicine and provides links to information on a wide variety of respiratory disorders and related conditions, including asthma, chronic bronchitis, emphysema, tuberculosis, allergic conditions, interstitial lung disease, cystic fibrosis, chronic fatigue syndrome, vocal cord dysfunction, sleep-related breathing disorders, juvenile rheumatoid arthritis, lupus, and other autoimmune diseases.

University of Pittsburgh Medical Center Comprehensive Lung Center
http://www.clc.upmc.edu/
Although this site provides very little information in itself, it does provide links to more than 10 extremely useful sites, including the American Lung Association and sites addressing cystic fibrosis and lung cancer.

Tuberculosis
World Health Organization Global Tuberculosis Programme
http://www.who.ch/programmes/gtb/ GTB_Homepage.html
This comprehensive resource provides facts about tuberculosis as well as links to relevant web sites.

Asthma
Doctor's Guide to Asthma Information and Resources
http://www.pslgroup.com/ASTHMA.HTM

Directed to both health professionals and patients, this comprehensive site provides extensive coverage of asthma-related news, answers to frequently asked questions, drug information, discussion groups, and links to related sites.

Allergy and Asthma Rochester Resource Center
http://www.eznet.net/aarrc/
This site provides separate information and resources for health professionals and for patients, as well as links to sites sponsored by pharmaceutical companies, local Web sites, and search engines.

The American Academy of Allergy, Asthma and Immunology
http://www.aaaai.org
This authoritative resource provides information of general interest, health-care news, resources for further information, and links to other Web sites.

Lung Cancer
Lung Cancer
http://www.erinet.com/fnadoc/lung.htm
A Web site that provides patient-oriented information as well as links to other resources related to lung cancer.

ONCOLINK Lung Cancer
http://www.oncolink.upenn.edu/disease/lung1/
An authoritative site, part of ONCOLINK, which provides lung cancer information and link to other sites for both health professionals and patients.

---

mentation of these measures more acceptable to the patient, suggest that they be implemented on a trial basis for a month or so and then re-evaluated. This allows the patient time to see the benefit of the measures and begin to accept the need for them.

If assessment data indicate that emotional stress is a frequent cause of the patient's asthma attacks, recommend a stress management program to assist the patient in identifying ways to prevent a stressor from disrupting life or to lessen the degree of reaction. Relaxation training is one of the methods used in a stress management program. If the patient smokes, also recommend a smoking cessation program.

Teach patients the name of each medication, how much to take, when to take it, and how to take it. When medications are prescribed by inhaler, instruct the patient on how to use the metered dose inhaler correctly and have the patient demonstrate its use. Caution the patient not to exceed four to six inhalation treatments per day. Stress the importance of not discontinuing, increasing, or taking newly prescribed or over-the-counter medications without consulting the physician who is treating the asthma. This is critical because if, for example, steroids are discontinued abruptly, adrenal crisis from adrenal insufficiency can occur. Propranolol (Inderal) is not given to patients with asthma because of its potential to cause bronchoconstriction. Antihistamines and decongestants are to be avoided because of their drying effect on airway secretions, making expectoration more difficult. Table 16–9 lists medications to be avoided or used cautiously by the patient with asthma.

*S*OCIOCULTURAL PERSPECTIVES

Overcoming Language Barriers
by Janice R. Ellis, PhD, RN

In the United States, people whose primary language is not English are no longer found only in large coastal cities. Immigrants from Cambodia are found in Iowa. Vietnamese immigrants live in Texas. Immigrants from Mexico, although more numerous in the southern states, are also found in Maine. And these groups represent only a few of the languages found in the United States. For example, more than 60 different languages are spoken in the homes of children enrolled in the public school system in Seattle, Washington. Everywhere in the United States, we encounter people who have difficulty understanding, speaking, or reading English. In Canada, where the official languages are English and French, there are large groups of people whose primary language is *neither* English or French.

Receiving health care in an environment where you cannot be understood and you cannot communicate your needs can be very frightening. Have you ever talked with someone who spoke only English and became ill or injured while traveling in another part of the world? One woman who was in an automobile accident while visiting Seoul, South Korea, said she felt completely alone even when care providers were present. She was frightened and worried about what would happen next. The inability to ask questions only magnified her feelings of being helpless and controlled by others. In the United States, patients who do not speak English experience these same feelings; likewise, the Canadian patient who does not speak English or French may feel totally alone in a major urban medical center.

What is the impact of this phenomenon on health-care delivery? What are the responsibilities of health-care workers and institutions to meet the needs of people who do not speak the dominant language of the health-care system? As a nurse, you can take many different actions to overcome language barriers and improve health-care outcomes.

The most important action for you to take is to *identify* the person for whom language is a barrier. In a health-care setting, it may not immediately be apparent that a person's primary language is not the dominant language of the culture. People may nod agreeably when asked if they understand. Sometimes these people *do* understand—but only partially. In an attempt to cooperate and fit in, however, they hide the fact that their understanding is incomplete. If you suspect that a person with whom you are speaking does not understand you,

you can ask that the person restate your information in their own words. If you determine that language skills are limited, you can choose your own words carefully and stop for frequent explanations. When you do this, be sure to validate that understanding has occurred.

Using translators can also be valuable. In the United States, federal law requires that all institutions that receive payment through any federal program, such as Medicare or Medicaid, provide appropriate translation services for patients who do not speak English. However, the use of translators is not without problems. For example, the use of translators may mask differences in cultural attitudes about appropriate communication. With the use of a translator, you also have no way of ensuring that the information that the translator provided is adequate or accurate.

One important factor to consider when providing translation is the gender of the translator. In the Western world, we have grown very accustomed to the idea that health-care workers of either gender may ask personal questions. For people from other cultural backgrounds, however, this may not be true. The translator may need to be of the same gender as the patient to facilitate discussion of personal or intimate information. For example, an Islamic woman is likely to refuse to discuss care with a man as translator, whereas an Islamic man may refuse to discuss care with a woman as translator.

Another important factor to consider when providing translation is the age of the translator. In some cultures, very young people are not permitted to discuss personal issues or ask personal questions of their elders. One very young Chinese-American translator explained to the physician that she simply could not ask certain questions of an elderly Chinese patient. It would be so lacking in respect that the person would probably refuse to talk with her again. To overcome this barrier, the staff found an older Chinese-American woman who was able to provide culturally acceptable translation services.

In an attempt to find translators for some languages for which translators are scarce, a patient's children are often asked to translate for their parents. Although the children may speak the dominant language well, using children as translators is often very disruptive to family relationships. Respect for parents may be undermined when the child begins to see himself or herself as having power over the parent. Also, even if the child

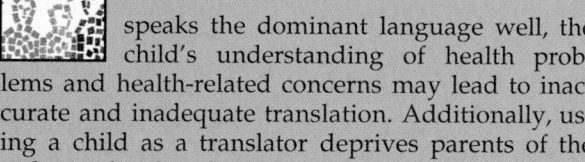

SOCIOCULTURAL PERSPECTIVES

Overcoming Language Barriers
(continued)

speaks the dominant language well, the child's understanding of health problems and health-related concerns may lead to inaccurate and inadequate translation. Additionally, using a child as a translator deprives parents of the right to decide what personal information to give the child.

Family members may also have a value system that supports protecting the patient from "bad" news. Therefore, while the health-care professional is carefully explaining all risks of a procedure to enable a patient to give informed consent, the family member who is translating may simply be saying, "Some problems are possible, but the doctor says this is important, so you should sign the form and not worry about it."

Lack of understanding of health and health problems may also extend to people who are not family members who serve as nonprofessional translators. In health-care institutions, janitors, clerks, and maintenance workers may sometimes be asked to translate. Think about all the health-care language you've learned since you began your nursing education. How would the person not trained in the health professions—even one quite fluent in two languages—successfully translate words and terms that are specific to health care? When the translator's understanding is partial or inadequate, the information conveyed to the patient may be incorrect.

To overcome translation problems, the use of professional health-care translators is increasing. These translators attend a course to learn medical terminology and the issues surrounding informed consent and honoring the patient's choices. Professional health-care translators are sometimes available over the telephone when in-person translation is not possible. A professional health-care translator is a partner in the provision of health care.

In many settings, however, professional translators are simply not available. In these instances, you will need to identify other interventions that may help the patient and family. For example, you might combine the use of picture boards with a makeshift form of sign language to meet simple needs for patient care. Sometimes nurses become quite creative in the use of body language and gestures to communicate. To meet some health-care needs, it might be safe to use family or nonprofessional translators. In these instances, you will need to use care with technical language. Ensure that the translator understands what you are saying. Also be sure that you understand the cultural concerns of the patient.

Clearly, language barriers are difficult to overcome, but they *must* be overcome to provide quality care. As a nurse, *you* can make a difference in creating successful health-care outcomes for people with language barriers.

If self-management is to be based on peak flow meter values, instruct the patient in the use of the peak flow meter and have the patient demonstrate its use. Review the physician's orders for changes in medication regimen based on peak flow values. Patients with severe asthma may require a portable nebulizer for respiratory treatments at home.

Discuss the importance of a good diet with plenty of fluids, avoidance of cigarette smoking, and follow-up for other medical problems. Explain the need to inform all health care providers about the asthma and the name and dose of medications currently being taken. Suggest the use of a Medic Alert bracelet or similar identification.

Additional Interventions

If the patient is unable to maintain an adequate nutritional intake because of shortness of breath, high-nutrient supplemental feedings may be necessary.

Encourage the asthmatic patient to lead as normal a life as possible. Stress that activities should

not be restricted. Encourage participation in exercise and sports. Explain that aerobic activities such as swimming, running, and brisk walking actually increase the efficiency of the body's use of oxygen.

Table 16–9

Drugs to be Avoided or Used Cautiously by Asthmatics

Drug	Reason for Caution
Antihistamines	Dry secretions make expectoration difficult
Sedatives	Depress respirations and aggravate hypoventilation
Cough suppressants	Impair clearance of secretions from the airways
Propranolol	Beta-blocker that causes significant bronchospasm

Stress that only those activities that precipitate an attack need to be avoided and that often a prophylactic dose of medication will allow participation in almost any activity. Explain that fatigue makes it more difficult for the asthmatic patient to handle stress and assist the patient in planning for sufficient rest.

Refer patients or families wanting additional information on asthma to organizations such as the Asthma and Allergy Foundation of America, the National Asthma Education Program, the National Jewish Center for Immunology and Respiratory Medicine, and the American Academy of Allergy and Immunology.

Compare the patient's status with the expected outcomes. If the outcomes are not met, reassess the patient and revise the plan.

*C*hronic Obstructive Pulmonary Disease

Millions of people in the United States suffer from some degree of chronic obstructive pulmonary disease (COPD), an impairment of expiratory airflow. Chronic bronchitis, emphysema, bronchiectasis, and sometimes asthma are classified as chronic obstructive pulmonary diseases.

Etiology and Pathophysiology
Airway obstruction results from inflammation of the mucosal lining of the airway, constriction of the muscles surrounding the airway, and/or excessive mucus production causing a narrowing of the airway.

Chronic airway obstruction primarily affects expiration, a passive process that is dependent on the elastic recoil of the lungs. The diaphragm and intracostal muscles are responsible for inspiration. When the patient inhales, the muscles are able to overcome atmospheric pressure easily to fill the lungs and move past the obstructions. On expiration, the elastic recoil of the lung is unable to force the air out. Because of structural changes in the terminal bronchioles, airways close early, trapping air in the alveoli. The patient must now work harder to exhale, resulting in the increased work of breathing. The expiratory phase of respiration becomes noticeably longer than the inspiratory phase.

The increased work of breathing results in a paradoxical problem. The inspiratory muscles, which are working harder to get air into the lungs, require help from the accessory muscles. When lung recoil is unable to move the air out, muscular assistance is again required to force expiration. All of this additional muscular activity uses up oxygen and thus, oxygen delivery may not meet oxygen demand.

Hypoxemia may result from fewer and fewer alveolar units effectively exchanging oxygen because of air trapping and loss of the alveolar-capillary membranes. Initially, the reserve of oxygen in the functional residual capacity (amount of air in the lung at end expiration) compensates for the ineffective gas exchange. However, as more and more of the lung becomes involved, there is less reserve. Oxygen desaturation may be noted initially as dyspnea on exertion, inability to climb stairs, or inability to walk as far or as fast. Over time, the patient experiences increased hypoxemia and a decreased oxygen level at rest. Chronic airway obstruction may also result in hypercapnia, an elevated carbon dioxide level.

Compensatory processes take place in the body in the presence of chronic obstructive airflow. The heart compensates for hypoxemia by increasing its output to make up for the blood's oxygen deficit. Pulmonary capillaries constrict around the insufficiently ventilated alveoli, diverting blood to more normal areas of the lung. As this chronic condition progresses, the area of involved lung increases so constriction becomes widespread, forcing the right side of the heart to pump harder to push blood through a vasculature blocked by constriction.

Prolonged hypoxemia causes the body to produce more red blood cells (polycythemia). The blood is more viscous than normal, making it more difficult to move through the vessels, increasing the work for the right side of the heart. Over time, pulmonary hypertension, high blood pressure in the pulmonary circulation, may occur. The pulmonary hypertension, coupled with the failure to adequately supply oxygen, produces cor pulmonale, hypertrophy, or failure of the right ventricle secondary to pulmonary disease.

Clinical Manifestations
Clinical manifestations of COPD (Table 16–10) include hypoxemia, hypercapnia, dyspnea on exertion and at rest, oxygen desaturation with exercise, use of accessory muscles of respiration, and a prolonged expiratory phase of respiration. Chest x-ray may reveal a hyperinflated chest and a flattened diaphragm, if the disease is advanced. Chronic hypoxia produces clubbing of the fingers. Many patients with COPD are underweight and all are malnourished, even if they are overweight. These patients tend to eat carbohydrates, which give them energy but provide little protein for muscle building and repair. In some patients, the added load of carbohydrates increases the retained carbon dioxide level.

CHRONIC BRONCHITIS

Chronic bronchitis is clinically defined as excess production of mucus, accompanied by a chronic cough lasting 3 months of the year for 2 consecutive years.

Etiology and Pathophysiology
Chronic bronchitis is usually caused by prolonged exposure to bronchial irritants, such as smoking, second-hand smoke, air pollution, toxic fumes, and dust. It is more prevalent in males over the age of 45 than in females, occurs more frequently in whites

Table 16–10

Clinical Manifestations of Chronic Obstructive Pulmonary Disease: Predominant Chronic Bronchitis Versus Predominant Pulmonary Emphysema

Manifestation	Predominant Chronic Bronchitis	Predominant Pulmonary Emphysema
Cough	Early, before onset of dyspnea	Late, after onset of dyspnea
Sputum	Copious, purulent	Scanty, mucoid
Weight loss	Absent or slight	Often marked
Dyspnea	Mild	Usually chief complaint
Chest x-rays results	Enlarged heart	Low, flat diaphragm
	Bronchoalveolar markings	Long, narrow cardiac silhouette
	Normal diaphragm position	
Carbon dioxide retention	Common	Uncommon
Cor pulmonale	Common	Rare

than nonwhites, and is more common in urban than in rural populations.

Airway obstruction associated with chronic bronchitis results from inflammation of the bronchi, with enlargement and hypersecretion of the mucus glands. Ventilation/perfusion mismatching develops because areas of inflammation and retained secretions do not occur uniformly throughout the lungs. Repeated infections with persistent obstruction can lead to scarring, damage of the mucociliary lining of the airway, necrosis, and destruction of small bronchioles.

Clinical Manifestations

Chronic bronchitis is characterized by repeated episodes of bronchial inflammation with a heavy, productive cough, particularly upon awakening. These episodes persist for months at a time and usually are worse during cold, damp weather. Cigarette smoking is the single factor that most exacerbates chronic bronchitis.

Chronic bronchitis has an insidious onset, developing over many years, with a long asymptomatic period. The patient frequently describes a "smoker's cough" as the first clinical manifestation. As the disease progresses, the cough becomes continuous, with production of large amounts of foul sputum. Dyspnea begins on exertion, but the condition progresses to dyspnea on very minimal activity, then to dyspnea at rest. Cyanosis occurs secondary to chronic hypoxemia and hypercapnia. Peripheral pedal edema may develop and worsen as right heart failure ensues. See Figure 16–5 for the classic appearance of a patient with chronic bronchitis.

Diagnosis

The diagnosis of chronic bronchitis is based on a patient history of repeated upper respiratory infections that linger and show a pattern over time. Pulmonary function test changes include a normal or decreased vital capacity, increased functional residual capacity, increased total lung capacity, increased reserve volume, and a decreased forced expiratory volume over 1 second. Chest x-ray may reveal early

signs of fluid overload with increased lung vascular markings and some infiltrates. In advanced disease, the heart may be enlarged and signs of right-sided heart failure evident.

EMPHYSEMA

Emphysema is progressive disease with enlarged air spaces distal to the terminal nonrespiratory bronchioles and destruction of the alveolar walls and supporting structures.

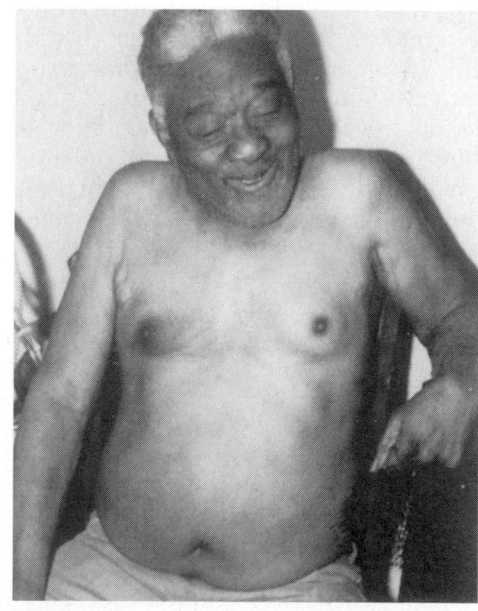

Figure 16–5

A man with chronic bronchitis and classic findings: stocky body build, no history of marked weight loss, onset of symptoms between ages 40 and 50, main complaint of sputum production, low PaO$_2$, high PaCO$_2$, cyanotic, dependent edema, episodes of right-sided heart failure, and variable clinical course. (From Kersten LD. Comprehensive respiratory nursing: A decision making approach. Philadelphia: WB Saunders, 1989, p 109.)

Etiology and Pathophysiology

Emphysema is the direct effect of cigarette smoking and may have a genetic component related to its development. Some research has shown an apparent failure of the connective tissue of the lungs to be protected against protein digestion from enzymes released from the alveolar macrophages and leukocytes. The theory suggests there are not enough enzyme inhibitors to control enzymes released from the macrophages and leukocytes. This results in lung tissue damage. A deficiency of alpha-antitrypsin, one of the main enzyme inhibitors, has been shown to produce emphysema in very young people.

Changes in the lung parenchyma involve the loss of elasticity of the lung. The elastic structure around the alveoli dissolves, stiffening the lung and decreasing compliance. Normally, each of the tiny alveolar walls offers resistance to stretching. As the lung expands during inspiration, these walls are stretched like tiny springs and each pulls back against the stretching. During relaxation of the inspiratory muscles at the end of inspiration, these combined pulls lower intrapleural pressure and draw the chest wall inward, facilitating expiration. At the end of expiration, the conflicting pulls of the lung inward and the chest wall outward balance each other, thus producing the normal configuration of the chest at rest.

In the presence of emphysema, expiration is weakened by the loss of lung recoil. Because less opposition is offered to the outward pull of the chest wall, the chest is partly expanded at the end of expiration. Over time this produces a visible "barrel chest."

Emphysema results in a hypoxic drive for respiration. Normally, changes in carbon dioxide levels in the blood trigger changes in respiratory patterns. In the patient with emphysema, a gradually increasing level of arterial carbon dioxide over time decreases the body's sensitivity to carbon dioxide, resulting in a decreased response by the respiratory center and a decreased rate. As a result, the primary stimulus to breathe comes from a decrease in oxygen rather than from an increase in carbon dioxide. The borderline or diminishing ventilatory drive may be further suppressed by increasing the arterial oxygen pressure (PaO_2) in the patient with documented carbon dioxide retention.

Emphysema is classified into two main types: centrilobular and panlobular. Centrilobular emphysema affects the central portion of the lung lobule close to the respiratory bronchiole. This type of emphysema is localized, and there may be unaffected units of lung tissue surrounding the affected areas. Centrilobular is the more common type and is more prevalent in males than in females. It is usually associated with chronic bronchitis and is very seldom found in nonsmokers.

Panlobular emphysema is the destruction and dilatation of the bronchioles and alveoli within a lobule in which the entire acinus is involved. This

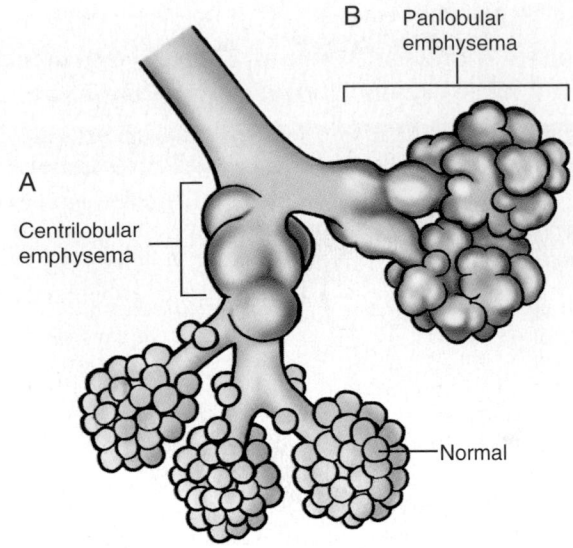

Figure 16-6

A, Centrilobular emphysema. The center of the pulmonary lobule at the level of the respiratory bronchiole is destroyed. *B*, Panlobular emphysema tends to be more diffuse, with the entire primary lobule involved and destruction and distention distal to the respiratory bronchioles.

type tends to be diffuse and is more severe in the lower lung areas. Panlobular emphysema occurs equally among males and females but is more frequent in older patients who do not have chronic bronchitis or clinical impairment of lung function. Panlobular and centrilobular emphysema, which are compared in Figure 16-6, may occur together or separately.

Clinical Manifestations

Emphysema unaccompanied by chronic bronchitis, bronchiectasis, or other chronic illnesses has an insidious onset of symptoms. Dyspnea worsening over time is the hallmark of emphysema. It initially presents with exertion, increasing with less and less exertional effort until the patient experiences dyspnea at rest. The patient with emphysema uses pursed-lip breathing and the accessory muscles of respiration (sternocleidomastoid, scalene, and trapezius) to aid in expiration. The expiratory phase of the respiratory cycle is prolonged. The chest is hyper-resonant to percussion with distant, absent, or dull breath and heart sounds from the chronic hyperinflation. Patients with emphysema have little appetite and lose weight, most likely because eating increases their oxygen consumption through digestion. In advanced emphysema, even the simple act of eating can result in severe breathlessness. The chronic malnutrition results in muscle mass wasting, including the mass of respiratory muscles, which further impairs the patient's ability to assist with expiration (Fig. 16-7).

During the later stages of emphysema, carbon dioxide retention can lead to carbon dioxide narcosis. This is the cause of the neurologic symptoms of

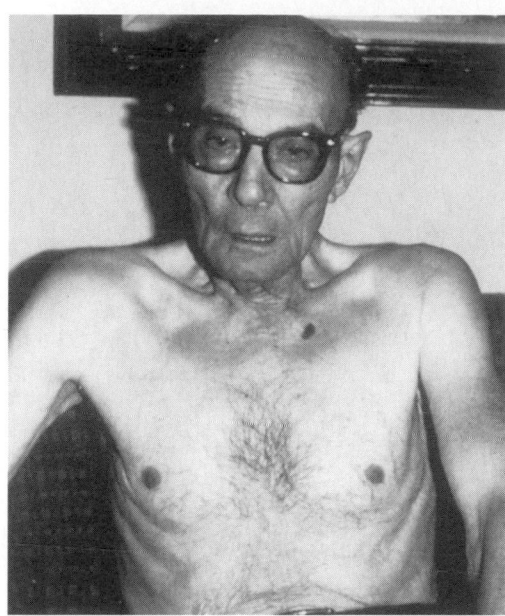

Figure 16–7

A man with emphysema and classic findings: cachectic appearance, history of weight loss, onset of symptoms between ages 50 and 75, main complaint of shortness of breath and cough, normal PaO_2 and $PaCO_2$, normal skin color, no edema, no history of right-sided heart failure, and persistent downhill course. Use of accessory muscles of respiration (intercostal, neck, and shoulder muscles) and the cachectic appearance reflect the patient's shortness of breath and the tremendously increased work of breathing needed to increase minute ventilation and maintain normal arterial blood gas levels. (From Kersten LD. Comprehensive respiratory nursing: A decision making approach. Philadelphia: WB Saunders, 1989, p 109.)

late emphysema: occipital headache, decreased ability to concentrate, and drowsiness. Other manifestations of carbon dioxide narcosis are a bounding pulse and arterial carbon dioxide ($PaCO_2$) levels greater than 75 mm Hg. Asterixis (flapping tremor), confusion, and coma may also occur.

This clinical picture of emphysema is usually complicated by symptoms of coexisting disease of the bronchial airways, such as chronic bronchitis, because emphysema rarely occurs alone. Thus the patient with emphysema generally has a history of cigarette smoking, dyspnea, chronic cough with wheezing, and frequent respiratory infections. On auscultation, inspirational coarse crackles at the base of the lungs are commonly heard.

Diagnosis

Emphysema is diagnosed and its severity determined by pulmonary function studies. Characteristic findings include decreased forced expiratory volume, prolonged expiration, decreased maximum voluntary ventilation, decreased forced vital capacity, increased total lung capacity, and increased residual volume.

Chest x-ray findings include an enlarged thoracic cage, a flattened diaphragm, an elongated and nar-

row cardiac silhouette, widened intercostal spaces, blebs and bullae in the apices and bases, and dilated bronchioles.

Management

Management of COPD employs measures to reverse airway narrowing, reduce mucus production, control symptoms, and maintain general health.

Bronchodilators, usually beta-adrenergic, are prescribed to treat bronchospasm and increase airway size (Table 16–11 and Highlight 16–6). Maintenance doses of theophyllines in amounts necessary to maintain a serum blood level of 10 to 20 mEq/mL, may also be prescribed to prevent exacerbations.

In some cases, corticosteroids, such as prednisone 20 to 40 mg daily, may be given for 3 to 4 weeks. If pulmonary function tests improve, the drug is slowly decreased to the lowest effective maintenance

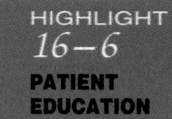
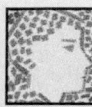

HIGHLIGHT 16–6

PATIENT EDUCATION

Prevention and Treatment of Respiratory Irritation and Infection in Patients with Chronic Obstructive Pulmonary Disease

To prevent irritation and infection of the airways, instruct the patient to:

Avoid exposure to cigarette, pipe, and cigar smoke as well as to dusts and powders.

Avoid the use of aerosol sprays.

Stay indoors when the pollen count is high.

Stay indoors when temperature and humidity are both high.

Use air conditioning to help decrease pollutants and control temperature.

Avoid exposure to persons known to have colds or other respiratory tract infections.

Avoid enclosed, crowded areas during cold and flu season.

Obtain immunizations against influenza and pneumococcal pneumonia.

To ensure prompt, effective treatment of a developing respiratory infection, instruct the patient to do the following:

Report any change in sputum color or character, increased tightness of the chest, increased dyspnea, or fatigue.

Call the physician if the ordered antibiotics do not relieve symptoms within 24 hours.

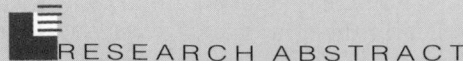

RESEARCH ABSTRACT

Are There Any Good Noninvasive Alternatives to Mechanical Ventilation in Chronic Obstructive Pulmonary Disease?

Boix J, Tejeda M, Alvarez F, Bataller A. Comparison of nasal positive-pressure ventilation to external high-frequency oscillatory ventilation in severe COPD. Respiratory Care 1996; 41(3):187.

The number of patients with chronic illnesses is growing dramatically, and the care of these patients is often a challenge. Some of the most frustrating patients are those with chronic obstructive pulmonary disease (COPD). It seems that most of these patients eventually require mechanical ventilation, and many times they develop complications that are a direct result of this invasive form of ventilation. Researchers are therefore beginning to investigate the use of noninvasive methods of ventilatory support during acute episodes of respiratory failure in patients with COPD.

An investigative team led by Dr. Boix explored and compared two such methods for managing patients with COPD during acute episodes of respiratory failure. The two methods studied were externally applied high-frequency oscillatory ventilation (which uses negative pressure and controls both inspiration and expiration) and noninvasive positive-pressure ventilation (using either a face mask or a nasal mask).

Both methods were well tolerated by patients. With both methods, patients experienced reductions in their $PaCO_2$ values and increases in their PaO_2 values. The best gains were seen in the patients who received noninvasive positive-pressure ventilation. However, these patients had to be coached in the use of this form of ventilation, and this form of ventilation required the cooperation of the patients. The researchers point out that such cooperation may not always be feasible, since not all patients who present with respiratory failure are able or willing to cooperate.

Although results with externally applied high-frequency oscillatory ventilation were comparable, it did not present the extra "edge" that noninvasive positive-pressure ventilation did. However, since externally applied high-frequency oscillatory ventilation controls both phases of respiration, active patient cooperation is not essential with this means of ventilation. In the research study, this made for easier use by members of the health-care team.

The researchers are quick to point out that these noninvasive methods of ventilation are not appropriate for every patient, but that they are very useful for patients in early respiratory failure. Moreover, they do not present the risk of complications often seen with invasive methods.

Questions to Consider

1. What is the pathophysiology associated with respiratory failure?
2. Why are patients with COPD so susceptible to respiratory failure?
3. You are assigned to care for a patient in respiratory failure. Would your plan of care be different for a patient receiving invasive versus noninvasive ventilatory support? If so, how?
4. List the risks and benefits of endotracheal intubation and positive-pressure ventilation. What are some risks and benefits of external ventilatory support?

dose. The patient is then placed on an inhaled steroid, which delivers the medication directly to the lung and helps decrease the side effects of prolonged systemic steroid use.

An influenza vaccine is given to protect patients from developing influenza, with its high risk of secondary bacterial respiratory infection. When bacterial infections occur, they are treated with antibiotics.

Measures to promote pulmonary hygiene include deep-breathing, coughing, chest percussion, vibration, and postural drainage and hydration. Some patients may need suctioning to help remove secretions and prevent airway plugging.

Oxygen therapy is administered to maintain a PaO_2 of at least 60 mm Hg. Research indicates that low-flow oxygen prolongs the life of patients with COPD, improves the quality of the patient's life, and decreases the frequency of hospitalizations. Long-term treatment may include low-flow oxygen (1–3 L/min) for 12 to 15 hours daily. This low-flow oxygen relieves pulmonary hypertension and polycythemia, increases exercise tolerance, and improves mental function by correcting hypoxemia. If the patient develops acute respiratory failure, mechanical ventilation is instituted to assist with respirations.

A program of exercise is prescribed unless a cardiac or other problem exists that contraindicates it. Exercise does not directly affect the underlying disease, but it does train the skeletal muscles to work more effectively and can increase the patient's ability for self-care and participation in household and social activities. Nutritional management is also essential. When all medical therapies have been exhausted, lung volume reduction surgery may be an option for patients with emphysema who meet the

Table 16—11

Speed of Onset and Duration of Action of Bronchodilators Used to Treat Chronic Obstructive Pulmonary Disease

Bronchodilator	Duration, h	Speed of Onset, min
FAST-ACTING		
Beta-antagonists* (metered dose inhalers)		
Albuterol (Proventil, Ventolin)	4–6	1–3
Bitolterol (Tornalate)	4–8	1–3
Isoetharine (Bronkometer, Bronkosol)	2–4	1–3
Isoproterenol (Isuprel)	1–2	1–3
Metaproterenol (Alupent, Metaprel)	4–6	1–3
Terbutaline (Brethaire)	4–6	1–3
SHORT-ACTING		
Theophylline (Elixophyllin)	4–8	30–60
Aminophylline (Truphylline)	4–8	30–60
Oxtriphylline (Choledyl, Brondecon)	6–10	30–60
SUSTAINED-RELEASE		
Theophylline (Slo-bid, Theo-Dur, Theo-Dur Sprinkle)	8–16	30–60
ULTRA-LONG SUSTAINED-RELEASE		
Anhydrous theophylline (Theo-24, Uniphyl)	16–24	30–60
ANTICHOLINERGIC		
Ipratropium (Atrovent)	3–4	15

*Oral beta-antagonists often take 1 hr to begin working, and the action of the drug does not last as long as that of the inhaled beta-antagonist. Taken orally, beta-antagonists also produce more side effects because of systemic absorption.

criteria. The hyperinflated portions of the lung, as much as 30%, are excised. This allows the chest wall and diaphragm to resume a more normal position, improves the mechanics of breathing, and enables patients to take deep breaths. Currently, Medicare does not provide reimbursement for this surgery.

❖ **Settings, Providers, and Collaboration for Care**

Patients with COPD are seen usually as outpatients in a clinic or private physician's office. As the disease progresses, hospitalizations become necessary during exacerbations of the disease. Home oxygen therapy, respiratory care, occupational therapy, and physical therapy are needed, and the nurse and physician must collaborate with these health-care providers to develop a plan to prevent exacerbations and complications and maintain the patient's functional status. For the plan of care to be effective, the patient and family must be an integral part of the planning process.

Patients with COPD may be referred to a pulmonary rehabilitation program. The program usually includes medical management integrated with patient and family education, teaching of coping skills, a progressive exercise program, and a support group. The exercise program is designed to improve endurance and strength. It teaches stretching exercises and provides support to patients with back problems caused by osteoporosis and spinal compressions that may be associated with prolonged steroid therapy. Techniques for activities of daily living, energy conservation, and self-care strategies are also included. The social worker assists the patient with home management, work environments, and community resources and often leads the support group. Because self-management is a major goal, the patient is considered the central member of the team (Fig. 16–8).

NURSING PROCESS
Chronic Obstructive Pulmonary Disease

Assessment

Obtain a thorough history. Include information about the patient's environment, work history, exercise and activity patterns, smoking habits, diet, and the onset and development of symptoms. Ask whether the symptoms are worse at any particular time of the year or whether they are aggravated by any particular activities. Symptoms of chronic bronchitis are usually worse in the cold weather, after

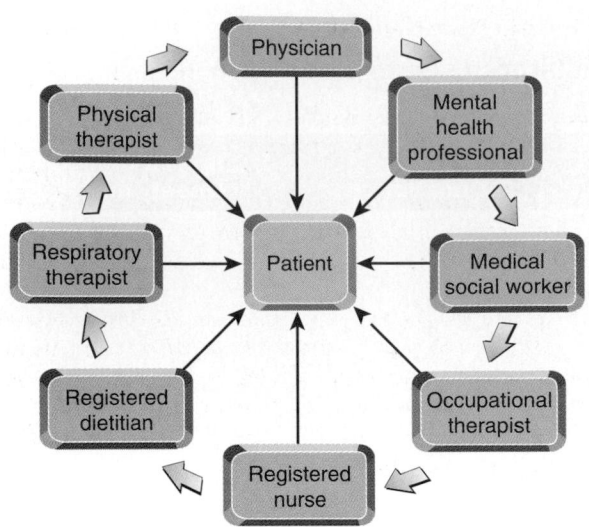

Figure 16–8
The pulmonary rehabilitation team.

intake of alcohol, or after talking for an extended time.

Question the patient about sleeping positions. This helps to differentiate cardiac dysfunction from emphysema. Because persons with cardiac disease have a greater total vital capacity in the sitting or standing position, they are more comfortable sleeping with the head of the bed elevated, whereas those with emphysema tend to be more comfortable sleeping in a flat position because their total vital capacity is greater in the supine position.

Review results of all diagnostic studies, such as arterial blood gases, pulmonary function tests, and x-rays.

On physical examination, observe for digital clubbing, distended neck veins on expiration, the presence of a large anteroposterior chest diameter, and a characteristic sinking of the tissues around the neck and supraclavicular spaces. Look for enlargement and active use of the accessory muscles of respiration. Note any outward flaring motion of the lower rib margins and widening of the subcostal angle. Observe for abdominal breathing, the use of pursed-lip breathing, and chest movements that are singular movements rather than rhythmic. Auscultate the chest and listen for musical wheezes characteristic of chronic bronchitis and for distant, dull, or absent heart sounds associated with moderately severe or severe emphysema.

Assess general physical status, because patients with advanced emphysema are often thin or even emaciated from a decreased appetite caused by breathlessness, excessive secretions, and coughing induced by eating.

Assess the patient's emotional response to the illness. Also assess available support systems, such as significant others and financial and community resources.

Nursing Diagnoses and Planning

Nursing diagnoses and related expected patient outcomes commonly applicable to patients with COPD include the following:

NDx: Ineffective airway clearance related to excessive, viscous secretions

Planning: Patient Outcomes

1. Patient uses nebulizer and medication as ordered.
2. Patient uses breathing exercise techniques during treatments.
3. Patient coughs productively after treatments.
4. Patient uses positioning techniques to help drain lungs after treatments.

NDx: Impaired gas exchange related to prolonged expiration and carbon dioxide retention

Planning: Patient Outcomes

1. Carbon dioxide levels range between 40 and 55 mm Hg (35–45 mm Hg is normal).
2. Arterial oxygen saturation remains greater than 92%.
3. Arterial oxygen level remains greater than 60 mm Hg (normal is 80–100 mm Hg).
4. Patient uses oxygen therapy equipment correctly and safely.
5. Patient lists signs of hypoxia and hypercapnia to be reported.

NDx: Ineffective breathing pattern related to increased work of breathing and oxygen consumption greater than oxygen delivery

Planning: Patient Outcomes

1. Patient demonstrates pursed-lip breathing technique.
2. Patient practices diaphragmatic breathing to strengthen the diaphragm, decrease work of breathing, and increase breathing efficiency.
3. Patient demonstrates positions used to relieve breathlessness.
4. Patient uses relaxation therapy techniques.

NDx: Activity intolerance related to muscular fatigue

Planning: Patient Outcomes

1. Patient participates in a program of aerobic exercise.
2. Patient describes four basic techniques of energy conservation.
3. Patient practices energy conservation techniques in daily living.

NDx: Risk for ineffective individual coping related to chronic disease, its effects, and its treatments

Planning: Patient Outcomes

1. Patient verbalizes anxieties and fears.
2. Patient identifies changes in lifestyle necessitated by the disease.
3. Patient describes a realistic plan for introducing lifestyle changes.

NDx: Risk for altered health maintenance related to insufficient knowledge of prevention, identification, and treatment of respiratory complications of COPD

Planning: Patient Outcomes
1. Patient lists ways to avoid irritation of the respiratory tract.
2. Patient identifies methods of avoiding respiratory tract infection.
3. Patient lists symptoms to be reported.
4. Patient acknowledges need for smoking cessation.

Nursing Interventions and Evaluation

NDx: Ineffective airway clearance

Essential to the improvement of ventilation and ease of the work of breathing are dilatation of the bronchi and removal of obstructing secretions. Administer oral, subcutaneous, intravenous, rectal or nebulized bronchodilator drugs as ordered. Nebulized aerosols relieve bronchospasm, decrease mucosal edema, and liquefy bronchial secretions and thus improve ventilatory function. Nebulized drugs can be delivered by pressurized aerosols, hand-bulb nebulizers, compressor-driven nebulizers, and ultrasonic nebulizers (Fig. 16–9). Teach the patient how to self-administer the drug and how to obtain equipment needed for home use. Instruct the patient to follow inhalation of bronchodilator aerosols with postural drainage, coughing, and moist inhalations as ordered to promote expectoration. The treatment should end with thorough oral hygiene. Instruct the patient to use the nebulizer before meals to improve lung ventilation and to reduce fatigue associated with eating. Also instruct the patient to use it before events known to precipitate symptoms.

Monitor for the therapeutic effect of the bronchodilator drugs, as well as for such side effects as tachycardia, cardiac dysrhythmias, and central nervous system excitation. Monitoring for therapeutic effect is particularly important because a guiding principle of bronchodilator therapy is to administer the minimum dose needed to relieve the patient's symptoms.

Increase fluids to 2 to 3 L daily (unless contraindicated) to replace fluid lost through mouth breathing and help keep secretions liquid. If needed, administer water via a nebulizer to humidify the bronchial tree and add water to the viscous sputum to make expectoration easier.

NDx: Impaired gas exchange

Administer oxygen as ordered and teach appropriate safety measures. If it has been determined during hospitalization that the patient has a low arterial oxygen level and continuous home oxygen therapy is required, explain to the patient and significant others the need for regular measurement of arterial oxygen levels. Explain the hypoxic drive to breathe in both chronic bronchitis and emphysema and caution about using the oxygen only as ordered by the physician, never increasing the flow unless directed to do so by the health-care provider.

Review the signs and symptoms of hypoxia and hypercapnia (increased shortness of breath, restlessness, lethargy, headache, confusion) with the patient and significant others. Stress the need to report them at once to the responsible health-care professional, because the appearance of these symptoms may indicate impending respiratory failure.

NDx: Ineffective breathing pattern

A combination of three breathing techniques promote good ventilation, ease the work of breathing, and assist in the control of dyspnea. These are control of the inspiratory-expiratory (I:E) ratio, diaphragmatic breathing, and pursed-lip breathing.

INSPIRATORY-EXPIRATORY CONTROL. I:E ratio control is used to decrease the work of breathing and to control dyspnea during stress and activity. During quiet breathing, the I:E ratio represents the efficiency of the breathing pattern. Normally, the exhalation phase of the breathing cycle is passive and longer than the inspiratory phase. In the COPD patient, however, expiration requires active muscular work because of the resistance to airflow, and the expiratory time of the respiratory cycle is lengthened. As demand on the respiratory system increases with activity or stress, the rate and depth of respiration increase and inspiration begins to take more time than expiration. This leaves the patient feeling short of breath as he or she struggles to inhale more air without leaving sufficient time for the air to be exhaled.

Severe uncontrolled dyspnea can be prevented if the patient can control the I:E ratio so that expira-

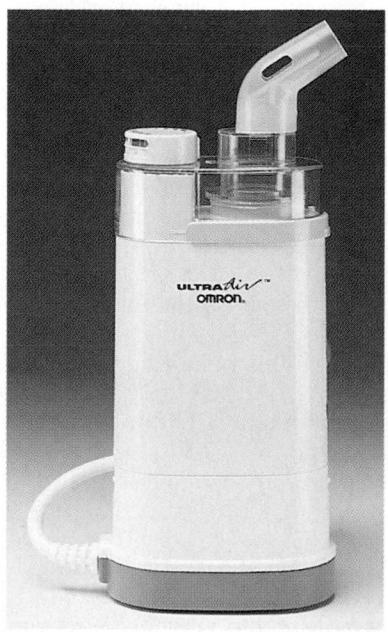

Figure 16–9
ULTRA-Air portable ultrasonic nebulizer. (Courtesy of Omron Healthcare Inc, Vernon Hills, IL.)

tion is three to four times longer than inspiration. Instruct the patient to practice timing the inhalation and exhalation portions of breathing patterns at rest. When the patient can do this easily at rest, have the patient practice consciously controlling the I:E ratio in various situations, particularly during shortness of breath. This type of practice not only allows the patient to prevent severe, uncontrolled shortness of breath but also aids the patient in regaining control of breathing patterns when shortness of breath does occur.

DIAPHRAGMATIC BREATHING. Diaphragmatic breathing helps the patient use the diaphragm rather than accessory muscles to breathe. Because smaller muscles use more oxygen than large ones, using the diaphragm decreases the work of breathing. Diaphragmatic breathing also increases the volume of air exchanged during a normal breathing effort and enhances distribution of the inhaled air. Several techniques for practicing diaphragmatic breathing are available. One of them is described here.

To practice diaphragmatic breathing, instruct the patient to lie down and place the left hand on the chest just below the collar bone to feel any motion of the rib cage. The right hand is placed on the area above the navel and just below the rib cage, with the palm down and the smallest finger reaching the navel and the thumb resting on the sternum (Figure 16–10). Next, tell the patient to take deep breaths through the nose and at the same time allow the area under the palm of the right hand to rise. Instruct the patient to use pursed-lip breathing on expiration, which should be timed at twice as long as inhalation.

If diaphragmatic breathing is being done properly, the rib cage under the left hand does not move and the abdominal wall below the navel does not rise higher than the area under the right hand. If it does rise higher, the patient is using unnecessary abdominal muscles. If needed, help the patient master this breathing technique by placing a book on the upper abdomen and watching it rise and fall with inspiration and expiration. Once the technique is perfected, it can be practiced when sitting, standing, walking, and running or during any activity that induces dyspnea. It is unlikely that the patient will ever use diaphragmatic breathing continuously; however, with practice it can be used to control dyspnea without fear.

PURSED-LIP BREATHING. Pursing the lips creates resistance to airflow, thereby slowing expiration and increasing positive pressure in the airways. This results in pressure greater than that in the alveoli, so the airways are supported in their open position, allowing for more complete emptying of the alveoli on exhalation. This leaves less trapped air and allows more fresh air to enter the lungs with each breath.

Instruct the patient to assume conscious control of the I:E ratio, use diaphragmatic breathing, and exhale through pursed lips (as if to whistle), maintaining a relaxed exhalation. Have the patient practice slow, relaxed, pursed-lip exhalations by blowing bubbles in a glass of water with a straw or by blowing a ping-pong ball steadily across a table.

NDx: Activity intolerance

A program of gradually increasing aerobic exercises (exercises that require a prolonged muscular effort and depend on inspired oxygen for energy) is used to train the skeletal muscles to work more efficiently and to increase the patient's tolerance for physical activity. The type and amount of exercise are recommended by the physician, and the program is carried out under the supervision of the respiratory therapist, physical therapist, or nurse. Common aerobic exercises used for COPD patients include upper extremity strengthening, treadmill or walking, stationary bicycle, stair climbing, and bouncing on a mini-trampoline. Typical exercise plans are 10 minutes a day, four to five times a week. It may take 2 to 6 weeks on an exercise program for the muscles to increase endurance and produce more work with less effort.

Review the purpose of the exercise program with the patient and emphasize the benefits of participation. Explain that the beneficial effects of the exercise program last only as long as the program is continued. Point out that within 6 weeks of not exercising, more than 50% of the gains are lost. Stress that exercise plans are progressive and should start with small steps at a speed that allows comfortable breathing.

Because patients with COPD need assistance with conserving energy, explore methods of energy conservation with them. Review stress-management techniques and help eliminate possible sources of tension in daily life. Teach physical and mental relaxation techniques for use in stress-producing situa-

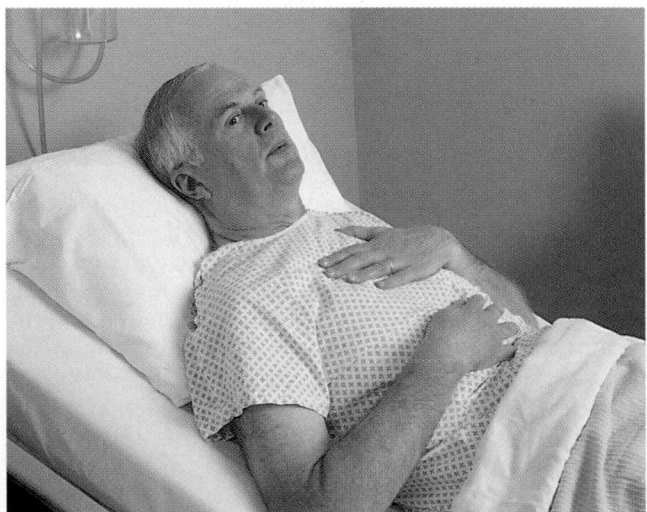

Figure 16–10
Position of patient practicing diaphragmatic breathing.

tions. Help the patient identify work-simplification strategies (ways to perform tasks at minimal energy cost) and measures to promote restful sleep. Overall, encourage the patient to consciously adopt a slower pace of living, to periodically assume a basic resting position (Fig. 16–11), and to space activities around these periods of rest.

NDx: Risk for ineffective individual coping
Although some patients adjust to chronic disease

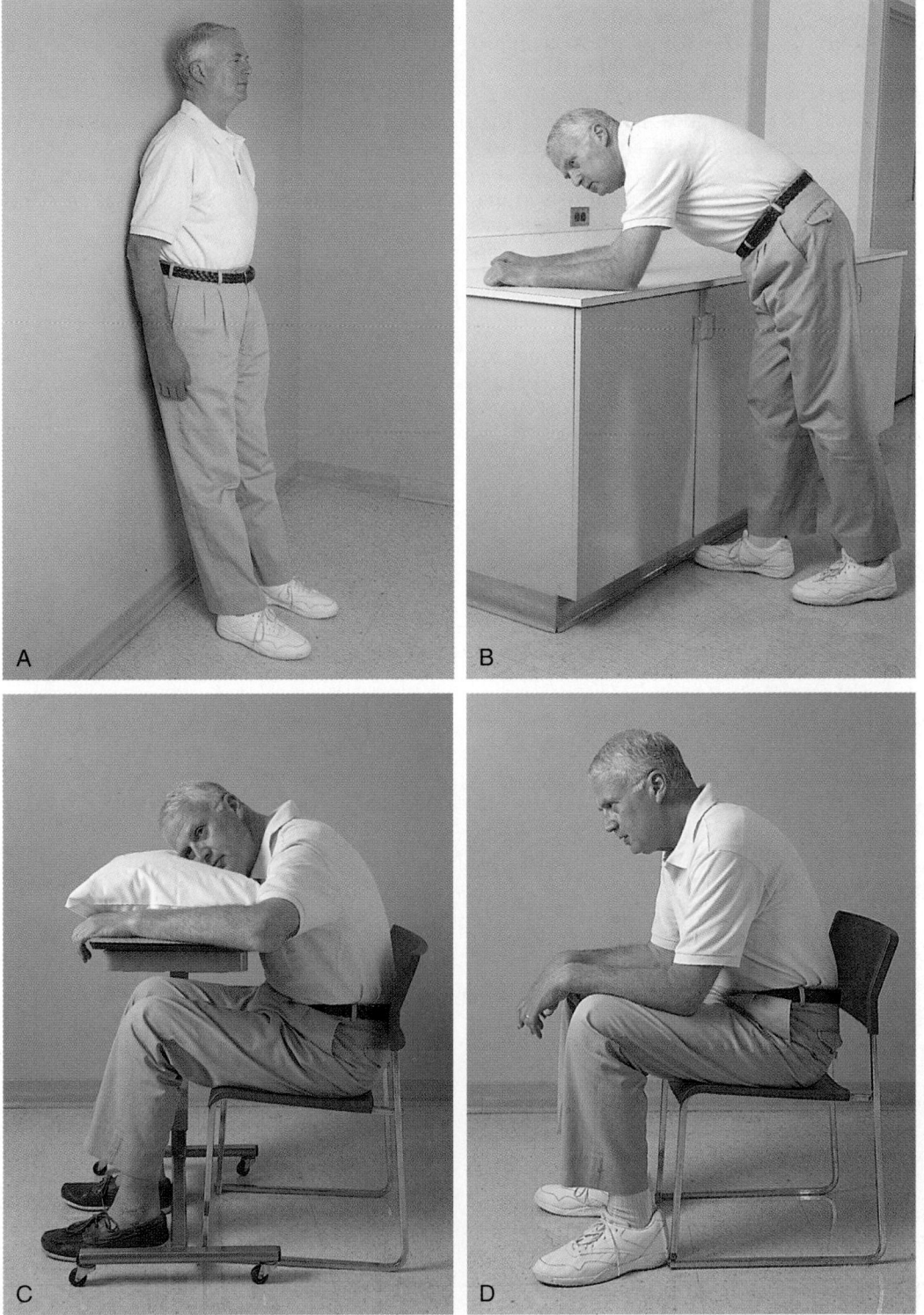

Figure 16–11
Basic positions of rest to avoid fatigue and dyspnea.

and cooperate with all modalities of treatment, many display denial and repression, resentment, anger, and anxiety. Depression is common and, in many instances, psychologic and emotional problems affect the patient's response to the overall treatment program. Be aware of these responses and acknowledge the feelings of these patients. Answer all questions honestly, listen attentively, and provide clear, concise information about the condition. Through understanding of the condition and management of symptoms, patients will be better able to cope with chronic respiratory disease.

If a change in job status is necessitated, refer the patient to a vocational counselor. In some instances, it may not be necessary to change jobs. It may be possible simply to alter the job description to accommodate the new level of functioning. The Americans with Disabilities Act requires employers to assist employees with adaptations that can maximize their work effectiveness and give them the necessary tools to perform the essential function of their jobs.

If it is not possible for the patient to return to gainful employment, it is important that the health-care team launch a major effort to achieve maximal self-care and minimize dependence on the patient's family and the community.

NDx: Risk for altered health maintenance

Instruct the patient in the prevention and treatment of respiratory irritation and infection (see Highlight 16–6). If the patient is a smoker, explain the importance of quitting and provide information on smoking cessation programs. If possible, arrange for a meeting with another person with COPD who has successfully stopped smoking. Teach the patient to identify symptoms of infection. To monitor for the onset of right-sided heart failure, instruct the patient to weigh himself or herself daily and to report a gain of 2.5 kg (5.5 lb) or more because this could indicate fluid retention.

Additional Interventions

A nutritional program designed to meet the needs of the particular patient is necessary if systemic complications are to be avoided (Highlight 16–7).

Compare the patient's status with the expected outcomes. If the outcomes are not met, reassess the patient and revise the plan.

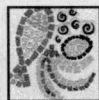

HIGHLIGHT
16–7
NUTRITION

Special Considerations for Patients with Chronic Obstructive Pulmonary Disease

Instruct patients with chronic obstructive pulmonary disease to:

Use a microwave oven to help decrease preparation time and conserve energy.

Sit at a table with elbows supported when preparing food to help conserve energy.

Use convenience foods, if appropriate. (Note: Many patients require sodium restrictions and must be instructed to read labels carefully.)

Plan rest periods for 30 minutes before eating to decrease dyspnea.

Avoid exercise and treatments at least 1 hour before and after eating.

Consume liquid, blenderized, or commercial foods to help avoid a "full" stomach, because a full stomach puts pressure on the diaphragm and decreases lung movement.

Avoid large meals and gas-forming foods, which contribute to abdominal distention.

Plan for fluid intake of at least 3 L daily unless contraindicated.

Space fluid intake between meals to prevent abdominal distention.

Maintain ideal weight or a weight slightly below ideal, because restricted activity limits calories required and extra weight may aggravate condition.

Instruct patients on theophylline or antipyrine therapy to:

Maintain regular eating patterns, because high-protein intake decreases the half-lives of these drugs and high-carbohydrate intake increases half-lives.

Avoid caffeine-containing products (coffee, tea, soft drinks), because theophylline-like derivatives contained in them may compound drug effects.

Use caution with charcoal-broiled foods, because they increase theophylline elimination and may reduce its half-life by up to 50%.

Instruct patients who require more protein and calories than normal to divide their high-protein, high-calorie diet into several small meals.

Bronchiectasis

Bronchiectasis is a disease characterized by permanent abnormal dilatation and distortion of the bronchi or bronchioles (Fig. 16–12). These structural changes may be in an isolated segment or widespread throughout the bronchi.

Etiology and Pathophysiology

Bronchiectasis may be congenital or acquired. It is associated with various hereditary immunodeficiency diseases and disorders that impair movement of cilia. Diffuse bronchiectasis is seen in patients with cystic fibrosis, asthma, and bronchitis. Localized disease is seen in patients with lung tumor and foreign bodies in the respiratory tree. In most cases, it appears that an obstruction in the lung prevents clearance of the airway and leads to infection in the wall of a bronchus or bronchiole, which causes changes in normal tissue structure. Smooth muscle and elastic tissue are impaired, and ciliated columnar epithelium is replaced with nonciliated cuboidal epithelium or fibrous tissue. These changes result in dilated, distorted areas of the bronchial tree, which in turn make airway clearance even more difficult and predispose to more infection, causing further structural damage.

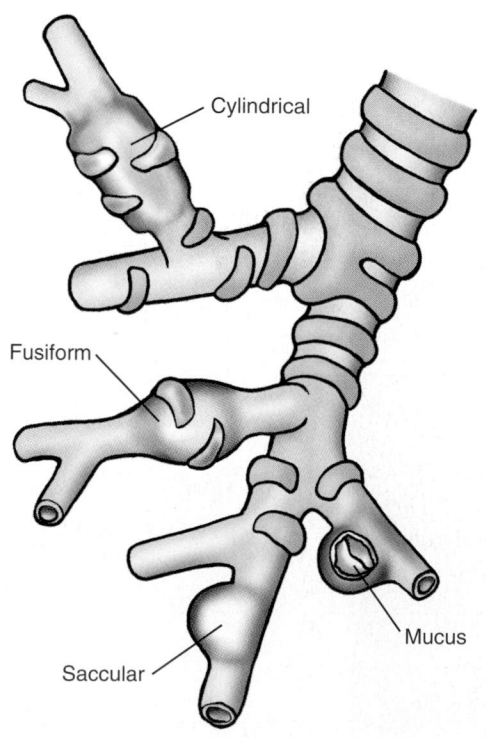

Cylindrical

Fusiform

Saccular

Mucus

Figure 16–12

Varieties of bronchiectasis based on type of dilatation of the bronchi. In the saccular form of bronchiectasis, secretions are caught and remain stagnant.

Clinical Manifestations

There are no clinical manifestations caused by bronchial dilatation itself. Rather, symptoms result from associated recurrent infection and hypersecretion of mucus.

A cough that produces large amounts of mucopurulent sputum, particularly in the morning, is characteristic. The sputum is unique in two ways. First, it has a rather sweet odor from being trapped in the dilated areas of the bronchial passages, where microorganisms grow freely. Second, on standing in a container, it visibly settles into three distinct layers: cloudy on top, clear saliva in the center, and heavy, thick, purulent matter at the bottom.

Other symptoms that may present include hemoptysis that may be profuse, malaise, fatigue, and exertional dyspnea, which in advanced disease may progress to cor pulmonale. Anorexia and weight loss may also occur.

Diagnosis

Diagnosis of bronchiectasis is suggested by a history of persistent cough with copious expectoration and presence of moist, coarse crackles over the affected area. Diagnosis is confirmed by a computed tomographic scan of the bronchi, which shows the dilated airways.

Management

Management of bronchiectasis is aimed at controlling infection, removing secretions, and avoiding irritants. Antimicrobial drugs are used to control infection. Postural therapy and adequate hydration are used to promote removal of secretions. Oxygen is given as needed. Bronchoscopy may be employed to remove thickened secretions.

NURSING PROCESS GUIDELINES
Bronchiectasis

The assessment, nursing diagnoses, expected patient outcomes, nursing interventions, and evaluation for patients with bronchiectasis are similar to those described previously for patients with chronic bronchitis and emphysema. Assess respiratory function carefully and determine the extent to which it is capable of supporting the patient in carrying out usual activities. Be sure to observe for hemoptysis. Patient education should stress the importance of avoiding respiratory irritants and sources of infection, and the need for vaccination against influenza.

Atelectasis

Atelectasis is a loss of volume in a segment or lobe of the lung from collapse of alveoli that previously were expanded (Fig. 16–13). It is common and occurs in association with many different diseases of the lower respiratory system.

Etiology and Pathophysiology

A major cause of atelectasis is obstruction in the bronchi or lower air passages, which blocks the movement of air in and out of the distal area of the lung. This may be caused by a mucous plug or aspiration of a foreign body. The result is that the air trapped in the affected portion of the lung is absorbed into the blood stream over a period of a few hours and the lung segment collapses.

Atelectasis may also result from compression of the lung by marked elevation of the diaphragm, a large pneumothorax, a pleural effusion, or an intrathoracic tumor. Lung volume declines to the point at which the airway closes, air is reabsorbed, alveolar size is reduced, and finally complete emptying and collapse occur. In other cases, atelectasis is associated with alveolar instability, as in respiratory distress syndrome, or with fibrotic changes in an area of lung tissue, which decrease the normal elastic recoil of the tissue and result in shrinkage of the area rather than complete lack of air.

Factors that increase the risk of atelectasis include a supine position, limited turning and moving, splinting the chest, respiratory depression from medication or anesthesia, muscle weakness, or any other factor that decreases chest excursion.

Clinical Manifestations

If atelectasis occurs rapidly and a large area of lung tissue is involved, then marked dyspnea and signs of hypoxemia develop. The patient sits upright, struggles for air, appears highly anxious, and exhibits tachycardia and cyanosis. Chest excursion on the affected side is markedly decreased or absent.

Basilar crackles heard in the posterior chest offer an early sign of mild to moderate amounts of slowly developing atelectasis. Otherwise, there are few symptoms except those of the underlying disease. After major surgery, dyspnea, cough, fever, and chest discomfort may indicate atelectasis. For patients on mechanical ventilation, an increasing requirement for oxygen and increased airway pressures indicate advancing atelectasis.

Diagnosis

Atelectasis is diagnosed by chest x-ray. If it appears to result from an obstruction in the airway, a bronchoscopy may be done to identify the specific cause.

Management

Management depends on the cause of the atelectasis. When caused by a foreign object, neoplasm, or other known obstruction, the obstruction is removed by the appropriate technique, such as withdrawal of air or fluid from the pleural cavity, resection of the neoplasm, or removal of secretions by suctioning or bronchoscopy. Inadequate lung expansion related to pain, sedation, mental obtundation, and similar factors is treated with periodic deep breathing, coughing, turning, ambulation, and the use of incentive breathing devices.

Measures to prevent atelectasis include coughing and deep breathing, postural drainage, and adequate humidification.

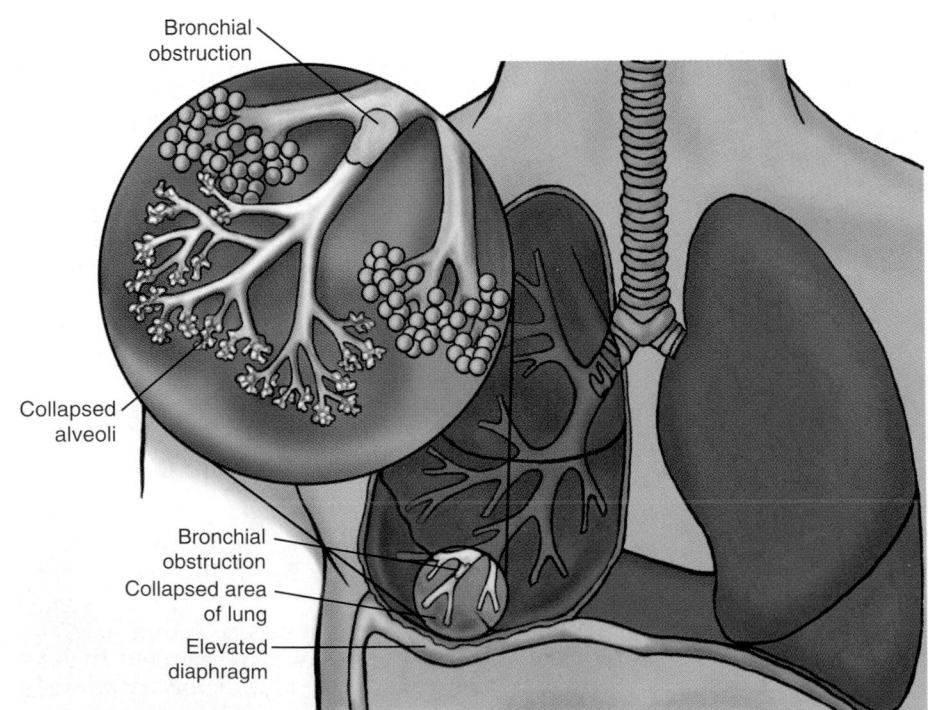

Bronchial obstruction

Collapsed alveoli

Bronchial obstruction

Collapsed area of lung

Elevated diaphragm

Figure 16–13

Atelectasis of the right lower lobe caused by bronchial obstruction.

NURSING PROCESS GUIDELINES
Atelectasis

Carefully assess patients at risk for the signs and symptoms of atelectasis. When atelectasis has occurred, institute measures to improve ventilation and remove secretions. If bronchial obstruction is the cause, encourage coughing and deep-breathing. Use an aerosol ultrasonic nebulizer, postural drainage, and chest percussion as ordered. Turn patients on bedrest frequently and position them to support maximal chest expansion to assist in mobilizing secretions. Encourage ambulation as soon as it is permitted.

Disorders of the Pulmonary Circulation

PULMONARY EMBOLISM

Pulmonary embolism is an occlusion of the pulmonary artery or one or more of its branches by matter carried in the blood stream from a vein or the right side of the heart to the lung. This disorder, which can occur in apparently well individuals, has an incidence of 500,000 each year in the United States, with a mortality rate of 50,000 (Murray, 1994).

Etiology and Pathophysiology
The most common type of pulmonary emboli are detached portions of venous thrombi originating in the deep veins of the lower extremities or pelvis. This is called deep vein thrombosis. Such thrombi also occasionally originate in the right atrium. Other types of emboli consist of amniotic fluid, fat, air, bone spicules, or fragments of organs. These latter types constitute a very small percentage of all pulmonary emboli.

Three factors, known as Virchow's triad, that predispose to thrombus formation and hence pulmonary embolism are:

• Damaged venous endothelium
• Venous stasis
• Hypercoagulability of the blood, which may result from increased platelets or the release of tissue thromboplastin after surgery or other injury

Persons at greatest risk are immobilized patients. These may include those with heart failure, multiple injuries, or long-bone fractures and those who have undergone thoracic, pelvic, or abdominal surgery. Other factors that place a patient at risk for venous thrombosis are pregnancy, use of oral contraceptives, varicose veins, carcinoma, obesity, polycythemia vera, and other blood diseases, such as sickle-cell anemia.

A pulmonary embolism obstructs the flow of blood to the area of the lung beyond it. This, along with vasoconstrictive substances released from the clot, results in a V/Q mismatch because ventilation is essentially normal. The V/Q mismatch, with its concomitant hypoxemia, stimulates an increase in respiratory rate, causing a drop in the $PaCO_2$ as large amounts of carbon dioxide are exhaled. This drop in turn increases vasoconstriction and bronchoconstriction, compounding the problem. Occurring simultaneously with these respiratory changes are changes in the circulatory system. Obstruction to blood flow in the lung decreases the total functional size of the pulmonary vascular bed and increases the resistance to blood flow within it. This in turn increases pressure in the pulmonary artery and consequently the amount of force required for the right ventricle to pump blood into the artery. When the force needed to pump blood into the artery exceeds the force the right ventricle can generate, cardiac output decreases, blood pressure drops, and shock ensues.

Clinical Manifestations
The clinical manifestations of pulmonary embolism are extremely variable. Increased respiratory rate and tachycardia are the most common signs.

Clinical presentation is determined by the size of the embolus and how much of the pulmonary vasculature is obstructed. If an embolus is small and obstructs a tiny vessel supplying a very limited area of the lung, there may be no symptoms at all. In the case of multiple tiny emboli lodging in arterioles, symptoms can mimic bronchopneumonia or heart failure. If a medium-size artery has been occluded, the patient may present with tachypnea, dyspnea, tachycardia, generalized chest discomfort, and pleuritic-type chest pain that has developed within a few hours. Fever, cough and hemoptysis, and a pleural friction rub may occur over several hours or days. A pleural effusion may also develop in some patients.

Massive embolism occurs suddenly. A large thrombus blocking a bifurcation of the pulmonary artery causes severe dyspnea, crushing substernal chest pain, tachycardia, hypotension, shock, syncope, and virtually instantaneous death. Respirations are rapid, shallow, and gasping and the arterial pulse is rapid and weak. If awake, the patient may express feelings of impending doom.

Diagnosis
Diagnosis of pulmonary embolism is difficult and requires that other disorders that can produce similar symptoms be ruled out. Thus, the diagnostic workup includes a chest x-ray, electrocardiogram (ECG), peripheral vascular tests, impedance plethysmography, ABG analysis, V/Q scans, and pulmonary arteriography.

Arterial blood gases are unreliable indicators of pulmonary emboli. The values show marked hypoxemia, with PO_2 levels ranging from 60 to 65 mm Hg and normal or decreased PCO_2, findings not unique to pulmonary embolism. If the PaO$_2$ is above 80 mm Hg on room air, a pulmonary embolism is less likely.

In 20% of pulmonary embolism patients, consolidation may be seen on the chest x-ray. Other significant findings include atelectasis, pleural effusion, elevated diaphragm, and a prominent pulmonary artery. The chest x-ray may be inconclusive within the first few hours after the development of the pulmonary embolism.

The ECG may be normal, with sinus tachycardia or right ventricular strain. In an extensive pulmonary embolus, the ECG shows right axis deviation, transient right bundle-branch block, ST segment depression, T-wave inversion in leads V$_1$ and V$_4$, and tall peaked P waves in lead II, III, and aVF. If the embolus is massive, the ECG may show electromechanical dissociation.

A V/Q scan that shows mismatched ventilation and perfusion is usually consistent with pulmonary embolism. However, other lung conditions need to be ruled out. A peripheral vascular test and impedance plethysmography are performed to detect the presence of a lower extremity thrombus (deep vein thrombosis). A definite diagnosis of pulmonary embolism is made by pulmonary angiography.

Management

Prevention of deep vein thrombosis is the best treatment. Basic preventive measures that increase venous return from the lower body and hence prevent venous stasis are early ambulation, leg elevation, active leg exercises, elastic stockings, graduated pressure stockings, electrical calf muscle stimulation, and intermittent pneumatic calf compression (Fig. 16–14). Keeping the patient well hydrated is also essential because dehydration predisposes to clotting.

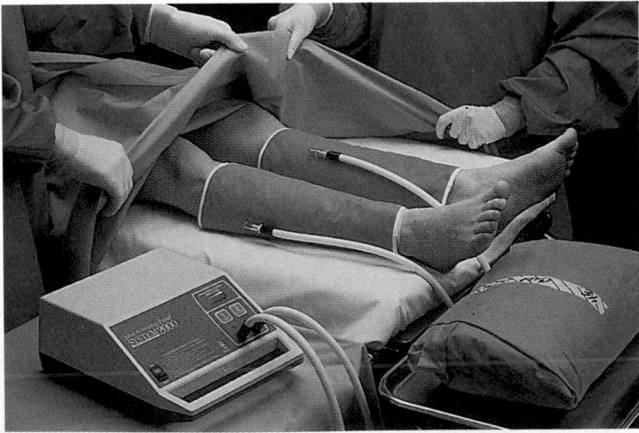

Figure 16–14

Intermittent calf compression. By applying pneumatic compression to the lower extremities using different cycle times and pressures, this procedure empties the deep calf veins of blood and increases pulsatile flow in the femoral veins. (Courtesy of Beiersdorf-Jobst, Charlotte, NC.)

Pharmacologic prophylaxis may be based on aspirin to prevent platelet aggregation or on low-dose heparin therapy and oral anticoagulants. Pharmacologic prophylaxis is commonly used for patients with normal hemostasis who are having major abdominal or thoracic surgery. When low-dose heparin therapy is used, it is usually administered subcutaneously 2 hours before surgery and then every 8 to 12 hours postoperatively until discharge.

When embolism occurs, management depends in part on its severity. Immediate stabilization of cardiorespiratory status is a priority because most deaths occur within 2 hours. Immediate management includes oxygen to correct hypoxemia, establishment of an IV line, ECG monitoring for right ventricular failure, and such diagnostic tests as ABGs, electrolytes, perfusion scans, and hemodynamic measurements. If the patient is hypotensive, dobutamine or dopamine is given by slow infusion and urinary output is monitored by indwelling catheter. Volume-controlled mechanical ventilation support is provided if needed. Other pharmacologic support includes cardiac glycosides, antiarrhythmics, and diuretics.

Treatment is also initiated to return pulmonary blood flow to normal and to prevent recurrence. To accomplish this, heparin is given for 7 to 10 days in the dose needed to keep the activated partial thromboplastin time at 1.5 to 2 times the control. This is followed by 12 weeks of warfarin therapy adjusted to maintain the prothrombin time at 1.5 times the control. Thrombolytic agents, such as streptokinase or urokinase, which hasten the lysis of clots in peripheral veins or pulmonary arteries, may be given, but they are not a substitute for anticoagulation therapy. Thrombolytic therapy resolves thrombi or emboli more quickly than heparin therapy but has a significant risk of bleeding. Therefore, it is used mainly for patients with massive pulmonary emboli or thrombi in the deep veins of the thigh or pelvis. It is also used if anticoagulant therapy is ineffective or contraindicated. During infusion of thrombolytic agents, all invasive procedures are avoided except for essential ABG studies, after which pressure is applied manually to the puncture site for at least 30 minutes, the patient is maintained on bedrest, and vital signs are checked every 2 hours. If uncontrolled bleeding occurs, the infusion is immediately discontinued. Tissue plasminogen activator has also been used to treat acute massive pulmonary embolism. It may be administered intravenously or by intrapulmonary infusion. It carries the same significant risk for bleeding as urokinase and therefore is used only for the same high-risk patients. Following thrombolytic therapy, anticoagulant therapy is prescribed.

Occasionally, surgical intervention is used in managing the patient with pulmonary embolism. A pulmonary embolectomy may be performed if initial stabilization is impossible because of massive obstruction of pulmonary blood flow. Transvenous embolectomy is a variation of this procedure, in which a vacuum-cupped catheter is advanced through the femoral vein, the inferior vena cava, the right heart, and into the pulmonary artery. Once in the area of the thrombus, suction is applied to pull the thrombus into the cup, and the catheter is withdrawn while suction is maintained. In cases in which emboli recur despite medical therapy or in which anticoagulant therapy cannot be used safely, blood flow through the vena cava may be surgically interrupted to prevent thrombi from the legs or pelvis from reaching the lung. This can be done by ligating the vena cava, using clips to divide it into smaller channels, or inserting a filtering device. The filtering device is a perforated umbrella-shaped device that can be inserted into the inferior vena cava by way of either the internal jugular vein or the common femoral vein. When in position, the umbrella is opened. Perforations allow blood to flow through but prevent the passage of thrombi. This device may be inserted at the time a transvenous embolectomy is done.

NURSING PROCESS
Pulmonary Embolism

Assessment

Be alert to the possibility of pulmonary embolism and carefully assess at-risk patients. Check for a positive Homans' sign (calf pain when the foot is dorsiflexed), which can indicate a deep vein thrombosis. Observe for sudden onset of dyspnea, chest pain, tachypnea, cough, hemoptysis, and unexplained apprehension. When an embolism has occurred, make ongoing assessment of the cardiorespiratory status, including characteristics of both pulse and respirations, presence or development of cyanosis, oxygen desaturation, hypoxemia, cough, and hemoptysis. Review ECG readings and ABG values. Assess anxiety level and understanding of the problem and its treatments.

Nursing Diagnoses and Planning

Nursing diagnoses and related expected patient outcomes commonly applicable to patients with pulmonary emboli include the following:

NDx: Impaired gas exchange related to increased dead-space ventilation

Planning: Patient Outcomes
1. Respirations are of normal rate and depth.
2. Complaints of dyspnea are absent.
3. Cyanosis is absent.
4. Blood gas values are within normal range.

NDx: Ineffective breathing pattern related to alveolar hypoventilation

Planning: Patient Outcomes
1. Respirations are unlabored.

2. Patient takes sigh breaths.
3. ABG values are within normal limits.

NDx: Anxiety related to difficulty breathing, outcome of the problem, treatment, possibility of recurrence

Planning: Patient Outcomes
1. Signs of anxiety are absent.
2. Patient controls breathing pattern.
3. Patient expresses confidence in the outcome of therapy.

NDx: Risk for decreased cardiac output related to right ventricular failure

Planning: Patient Outcomes
1. Cardiac output is at baseline.
2. Patient is free of weight gain.
3. Signs of pulmonary hypertension are absent.
4. Patient remains normotensive.
5 Jugular venous distention is at expected level.

NDx: Risk for inability to sustain spontaneous ventilation related to increased dead space and decreased alveolar ventilation

Planning: Patient Outcomes
1. Patient maintains spontaneous respirations.
2. Patient maintains adequate ventilation and $PaCO_2$.
3. Patient maintains positions designed to maintain maximum ventilation and perfusion.

NDx: Risk for altered health maintenance related to insufficient knowledge of anticoagulant therapy, prevention of recurrence

Planning: Patient Outcomes
1. Patient states name, dose, route, and frequency of prescribed medications.
2. Patient explains precautions required by anticoagulant therapy.
3. Patient states importance of promptly reporting bruising, prolonged or excessive bleeding, and tarry stools.
4. Patient describes measures to prevent venous stasis.
5. Patient explains importance of follow-up care.

Nursing Interventions and Evaluation

Carry out the prescribed medical regimen of anticoagulant or thrombolytic therapy, intermittent calf compression, or electrical calf stimulation. Monitor respiratory status, including lung sounds, ABGs, prothrombin time, and partial thromboplastin time. Check the patient for signs of bleeding. Apply antiembolic stockings and perform range-of-motion exercises as prescribed.

NDx: *Impaired gas exchange*
Place the patient in a semi-Fowler's position to facilitate breathing and administer oxygen as ordered. Facilitate ventilation and perfusion by placing patient in positions that do not result in oxygen desat-

CLINICAL ? THINKING

DYSPNEA, CHEST PAIN, AND ANXIETY AFTER PELVIC SURGERY

On the third day after pelvic surgery for ovarian cancer, a 62-year-old woman summoned me via the call light. When I entered the room, I noticed immediately that the patient was alert but short of breath, pale, and apprehensive. The patient complained of chest pain, which she said began suddenly after she walked to the bathroom. The patient's health history included hypertension, obesity, and type II diabetes mellitus of recent onset. Before this episode, the patient's recovery from surgery had been uneventful.

The patient's signs and symptoms (dyspnea, chest pain, and anxiety) clearly represented an acute change in health status. That much was obvious. The cause of the change was less obvious. I knew that dyspnea, chest pain, and anxiety could result from any of a number of clinical situations, ranging from an anxiety attack to a heart attack. For example, these signs and symptoms could indicate pericarditis, acute myocardial infarction, pulmonary embolism, pleuritis, pneumonia, or a gastrointestinal problem.

Because some of these potential causes were life-threatening, I immediately conducted a focused assessment. First, I took the patient's vital signs. Her pulse was 114. Respirations were 28 per minute. Blood pressure was 138/86 mm Hg. Temperature was 37.3°C (99.2°F). Next, I assessed the pa-

tient's respiratory status. I found crackles in the right lower lobe and noted rapid, labored, shallow breathing. The patient was pale, coughing nonproductively, and using her accessory muscles to breathe. I also checked the patient's cardiac status. Although her rhythm was regular, she was tachycardic and had a capillary refill of less than 3 seconds. I then checked her neurologic status. Although the patient was alert and oriented, she was restless. Finally, I asked about the nature and character of her chest pain. She described it as a stabbing pain exacerbated by inspiration. The pain did not radiate.

Because of the nature of the patient's chest pain, its onset after ambulation, the presence of crackles and a nonproductive cough, and the patient's shortness of breath, I suspected that the patient had suffered a pulmonary embolism—a life-threatening emergency.

Suspecting that the patient had dislodged a deep-vein thrombosis (DVT), sending a blood clot to her lungs, I immediately assessed for signs and symptoms of DVT. I checked for pain or tenderness in the calves, edema and erythema in the legs, and Homan's sign. The patient did have tenderness and edema in the right calf, supporting my suspicion of DVT. I also considered the patient's history. Her history of ovarian cancer, pelvic surgery, obesity, and diabetes mellitus further supported my suspicion.

At this point, I believed that I could tentatively

uration. Monitor oxygen saturation with pulse oximetry.

NDx: Ineffective breathing pattern
Promote effective breathing patterns through positioning, coaching for breathing patterns, and administering medication to reduce anxiety and decrease pain. Pain accompanying pulmonary embolism is usually pleuritic; therefore, analgesics may be used to facilitate ventilation.

NDx: Anxiety
Acknowledge that anxiety is normal and indicate understanding and willingness to help the patient deal with it. Stay with the patient during periods of severe dyspnea. Reassure the patient that someone is close by and will respond quickly if called. Keep the patient informed about his or her condition and prescribed tests and treatments.

NDx: Risk for decreased cardiac output
Monitor blood pressure, pulse rate and quality, and skin temperature. Maintain adequate hydration. Monitor jugular veins for increased venous distention.

NDx: Risk for inability to sustain spontaneous ventilation
Monitor the patient's respiratory pattern, ABGs, and fatigue level. Promote increased ventilation and perfusion by positioning, decreasing anxiety levels, and rest.

NDx: Risk for altered health maintenance
Instruct the patient in self-administration of prescribed anticoagulant medications, related precautions, symptoms to be reported, and prevention of recurrences.

Compare the patient's status with the expected

CLINICAL ❓ THINKING

(continued)

rule out conditions other than pulmonary embolism stemming from DVT because the patient's description of her chest pain, the evidence of DVT, the patient's health history, and her presenting risk factors were inconsistent with the other possible diagnoses.

Believing, as I did, that the patient's condition was life-threatening, I implemented the following interventions immediately:

1. I stat-paged the attending physician.
2. I placed the patient in semi-Fowler's position to facilitate respiration.
3. I administered oxygen and started an IV, following hospital protocols.
4. I called for another staff member to gather emergency equipment while I stayed with the patient.
5. I reassured the patient by explaining what was being done and by staying with her.
6. I continued to monitor the patient's respiratory, cardiovascular, and neurologic status.
7. I documented my findings and actions.

When the attending physician arrived, she ordered a chest x-ray, arterial blood gas (ABG) analysis, an electrocardiogram, a complete blood count, coagulation studies, cardiac enzymes, a ventilation-perfusion scan, and a pulmonary angiogram. She also ordered anticoagulant and thrombolytic therapy, which I administered.

Administration of thrombolytic agents successfully resolved the pulmonary embolism without any evidence of bleeding. By that evening the patient appeared calm and reported that she was free of chest pain. Her vital signs were stable and breath sounds were clear. Before discharge, patient instructions included home-care management of continued anticoagulant therapy.

Prompt and accurate recognition and treatment of this potentially fatal medical condition resulted in the patient's complete recovery.

Think Critically

Why did the nurse stay with the patient rather than going herself for the emergency equipment?

Why did the nurse call the physician first rather than immediately positioning the patient and starting oxygen therapy to facilitate breathing? Was calling the physician first the best thing to do?

How might the scenario have changed if the patient had been experiencing crushing substernal pain radiating to the left arm rather than a stabbing chest pain exacerbated by inspiration?

What patient teaching must be included in the discharge plans for this patient?

---

outcomes. If the outcomes are not met, reassess the patient and revise the plan.

PULMONARY HYPERTENSION

Pulmonary hypertension is defined as any condition that raises the resistance to blood flow in the pulmonary vascular bed, thereby increasing the pulmonary artery systolic blood pressure above normal. In the resting, healthy adult, the pulmonary artery systolic pressure range is 20 to 30 mm Hg and the pulmonary artery diastolic pressure is less than 12 mm Hg. A pulmonary artery pressure of 30/16 mm Hg or greater is defined as pulmonary hypertension.

Etiology and Pathophysiology
The most common causes of pulmonary hypertension are conditions of sustained hypoxemia, such as emphysema or chronic bronchitis. The reduced vascular bed and increased pulmonary artery resistance caused by hypoxemia contribute to the pulmonary hypertension. Other causes of pulmonary hypertension include pulmonary vasculitis or occlusion by pulmonary emboli. Elevation of left atrial pressure, increased pulmonary blood flow, as with ventricular septal defects, and mitral valve disease are examples of disorders that cause "postcapillary" pulmonary hypertension.

Clinical Manifestations
Dyspnea is the cardinal symptom of pulmonary hypertension. Other symptoms vary depending on the underlying disease.

Diagnosis
Differential diagnosis is made by establishing the presence of lung disease through pulmonary function studies. Cardiac catheterization studies are used to determine the presence of any cardiac defects.

Lung scanning and angiography may be done to detect pulmonary emboli.

Management

Management is aimed at the specific underlying disorder once it has been determined.

NURSING PROCESS GUIDELINES
Pulmonary Hypertension

The immediate aim of nursing care for the patient with pulmonary hypertension is provision of adequate oxygenation for respiratory needs. Specific nursing interventions vary with the cause of the hypertension.

ADULT RESPIRATORY DISTRESS SYNDROME

Adult respiratory distress syndrome (ARDS) is a life-threatening condition manifested by severe hypoxemia and decreased lung compliance. It is frequently referred to as noncardiogenic pulmonary edema—pulmonary edema not due to heart failure. The incidence of ARDS appears to be increasing as technologic advances allow the survival of more critically ill patients. Despite advanced technology and skill in caring for the patient with ARDS, the mortality rate remains above 50% (Dantzker & McIntyre, 1995).

Etiology and Pathophysiology

ARDS develops in response to a direct or indirect injury to the lung that causes increased pulmonary capillary permeability. The origin of ARDS is unclear, although the range of potential causes has been narrowed since the syndrome was first identified. Factors that place patients at risk for developing ARDS include:

Trauma
Oxygen toxicity
Drug overdose
Disseminated intravascular coagulation
Complications of coronary artery bypass grafting
Inhalation of noxious gases
Sepsis
Multiple blood transfusions
Shock
Hemolytic disorders
Cerebrovascular accident
Brain tumor
Sudden increase in intracranial pressure

Many mechanisms and mediators have been identified in the pathogenesis of ARDS, including neutrophil activation, platelet activation, alveolar macrophage stimulation, complement activation, and release of humoral vasoactive substances. Normally, the pulmonary capillary allows only small amounts of fluid to leak into the interstitial compartment that is readily drained by the pulmonary lymphatic system. In ARDS, capillary leakage results in a tremendous loss of fluid from the vascular space. This results primarily from loss of vascular proteins that pull large amounts of fluid into the pulmonary interstitial space, overwhelming the pulmonary lymphatic drainage capability and causing alveolar flooding, impaired oxygen transfer, and severe hypoxemia. Terminal airways become compressed and obliterated, resulting in decreased lung volume and compliance. Gas exchange is impaired, and extensive shunting of blood in the lung occurs.

Clinical Manifestations

The clinical presentation of ARDS can be divided into four stages. During the initial, or latent, stage, structural damage occurs at the walls of cells in the alveoli. Clinically, the precipitating or primary disorder responsible for triggering the ARDS response dominates. Unless the underlying process is pulmonary, there may be no evidence of respiratory distress.

In the second, or interstitial edema, stage, alveolar distensibility is reduced. The patient complains of breathlessness and is tachypneic. The patient may express a feeling of impending doom and demonstrate increasing restlessness and apprehension. This most likely results from increasing hypoxemia and respiratory alkalosis.

The third, or acute intra-alveolar edema, stage is characterized by excessive fluid accumulation in the interstitium. Lymph channels become compressed and fluid floods the alveoli. Gas exchange is severely compromised as perfusion continues to flooded, airless alveoli. The patient is extremely dyspneic and is using the accessory muscles of respiration. Intercostal retraction may be evident as the patient labors to breathe. Advancing hypoxemia results in agitation and depressed mental status. Diffuse fine crackles and diminished breath sounds are heard on auscultation.

The fourth stage is the chronic, or fibrotic, stage. In this stage, fibrotic changes and diffuse scarring occur in the lung. The patient remains hypoxemic despite aggressive oxygen and mechanical ventilation.

Diagnosis

Diagnosis is based on the patient's history, clinical signs of increasing respiratory failure, and worsening hypoxemia refractory to oxygen therapy. Early chest x-rays may appear normal. As the lung injury progresses, the chest x-ray initially shows fine infiltrates that progress to a ground-glass appearance of diffuse alveolar and interstitial infiltrates.

Arterial blood gases show a progressive deterioration of oxygenation with a falling arterial PaO_2. As oxygenation worsens, and the patient is unable to maintain an increased respiratory rate, arterial CO_2 begins to rise. Other oxygenation measures show an increasing V/Q mismatch, increasing shunt, falling oxygen delivery, and decreasing oxygen consumption.

Pulmonary artery catheter measurements show a normal, increased, or decreased cardiac output and cardiac index; normal central venous pressure; increased pulmonary vascular resistance; normal, increased or decreased systemic vascular resistance; normal or low pulmonary capillary wedge pressure; and a normal or increased pulmonary artery systolic and diastolic pressure.

Management

Successful management of ARDS begins with early detection and initiation of treatment. The primary goal is to support the patient's vital functions while identifying and treating the precipitating problem.

Oxygenation management aims to reduce oxygen consumption. Interventions include reducing fever and preventing hypothermia and alkalosis. Oxygenation and ventilation are maintained through supplemental oxygen, intubation, and mechanical ventilation with positive end-expiratory pressure or pressure controlled inverse ratio ventilation. Neuromuscular blockade may be used to reduce muscle activity and reduce excessive oxygen consumption. Supplemental oxygen at an FIO_2 of 50% or less is given to limit development of oxygen toxicity. Adequate cardiac output is maintained through administration of intravenous fluids to combat hypovolemia, which can result from loss of fluid into the interstitial spaces of the lung and through the use of inotropic or vasopressor drugs.

Pulmonary artery catheters are inserted to guide fluid administration. It is critical but difficult to maintain volume without contributing to overload. The pulmonary capillary wedge pressure is maintained as low as possible to limit additional increases in lung water while maintaining an adequate cardiac output to meet metabolic needs.

Crystalloids are used to decrease the alveolar edema resulting from albumin crossing the capillary membrane and drawing fluid into the alveoli. Colloids are used to increase circulating albumin and create a gradient that, theoretically, will draw fluid from the interstitium to the capillaries. The use of crystalloids or colloids remains controversial and depends primarily on what results in the best outcome for the patient. If the pulmonary capillary wedge pressure becomes elevated, diuretics and β-adrenergic agonists may be used to remove excessive fluid.

Other therapies used to treat alveolar damage include antioxidants, arachidonic acid metabolite inhibitors, antiendotoxins, monoclonal antibodies, anticytokines, and cycloxygenase inhibitors. Nonsteroidal anti-inflammatory drugs, antifungal agents, exogenous surfactant, prostaglandins, nitric oxide therapy, and corticosteroids may be used in later stages. In some centers, extracorporeal membrane oxygenation is used to treat severe hypoxemia; however, it is not yet widely available. Another therapy under investigation for the support of tissue oxygenation is extracorporeal carbon dioxide removal.

Nutritional needs are met via enteral or parenteral nutrition.

❖ Settings, Providers, and Collaboration for Care

Patients with ARDS are managed in the intensive care unit of the acute-care setting. Collaboration with physicians, respiratory therapists, physical therapists, social workers, and others is necessary to develop and implement an effective plan of care. Pastoral care may be needed to assist the patient and family with the possibility of death or long-term disability. Home health nursing and oxygen therapy may be needed following discharge.

NURSING PROCESS
Adult Respiratory Distress Syndrome

Assessment

Identify patients at risk for ARDS. Carefully assess oxygenation, respiration, and cardiac function. Review laboratory data.

Nursing Diagnoses and Planning

Nursing diagnoses and related expected patient outcomes commonly applicable to the patient with ARDS include the following:

NDx: Impaired gas exchange related to oxygenation and ventilation failure and increased oxygen consumption

Planning: Patient Outcomes
1. Arterial oxygen level remains equal to or greater than 60 to 70 mm Hg.
2. Arterial oxygen saturation remains equal to or greater than 90%.
3. Arterial carbon dioxide level remains equal to or less than 45 to 50 mm Hg.

NDx: Inability to sustain spontaneous ventilation related to increased intrapulmonary shunt and decreased V/Q ratio

Planning: Patient Outcomes
1. Patient maintains spontaneous ventilation.
2. Intrapulmonary shunt is improved.
3. V/Q ratio is improved.

NDx: Risk for infection related to artificial airway, immobility, impaired pulmonary defense mechanisms, and retained secretions

Planning: Patient Outcomes
1. White blood cell count is within normal limits.
2. Patient is afebrile.
3. Signs of infection are absent.
4. Secretions are managed and removed.

NDx: Impaired verbal communication related to intubation and mechanical ventilation

Planning: Patient Outcomes
1. Patient communicates effectively with health-care providers and family.

Nursing Interventions and Evaluation

NDx: Impaired gas exchange

Position the patient to promote oxygenation and ventilation. Limit activities and care measures to decrease the risk of oxygen depletion. Monitor arterial oxygen saturation level for desaturation. Pace activities to conserve oxygen delivery and consumption.

NDx: Inability to sustain spontaneous ventilation

Respirations are supported with mechanical ventilation and supplemental oxygen. Monitor breathing pattern, respiratory rate, and cardiac function. Monitor airway pressures for decreasing lung compliance.

NDx: Risk for infection

Suction the airway to remove secretions, which not only contribute to airway resistance but provide a good medium for bacterial growth. Use strict aseptic technique and maintain a clean environment. Monitor temperature and administer antibiotics as ordered.

NDx: Impaired verbal communication

Provide paper and pencil, alphabet or picture board, or electronic communication board. Be patient when trying to understand what the patient is communicating. Assist family members with communication methods.

Compare the patient's status with the expected outcomes. If the outcomes are not met, reassess the patient and revise the plan.

Occupational Lung Diseases

Pneumoconiosis refers to a fibrous inflammation or chronic induration of the lungs resulting from inhalation of dust. It is a general term used in relation to occupational lung diseases such as silicosis, asbestosis, or coal workers' pneumoconiosis.

SILICOSIS

The term silicosis refers to a disease produced by exposure to silica. Working without proper protection in occupations involved with quarrying, chipping, grinding, and polishing silica-containing rock is a factor in the development of this disease. Coal miners often contract this disease from mining and tunneling in such rock as quartz and sandstone, which are almost pure silica.

The chief symptom of silicosis is shortness of breath. The characteristic pathologic changes in silicosis are silicotic nodules, which are densely packed fibrotic lesions scattered unevenly throughout the lungs, mostly in the upper lobes. Such lesions have been frequently attributed to concurrent tuberculosis.

ASBESTOSIS

Asbestos is a generic name applied to a family of fibrous hydrated silicates widely used in industry. Asbestos has been used for more than 100 years; however, the potential risk was recognized only in the 1960s. Mining and milling of asbestos are obvious sources of asbestos-related disease. Occupational exposure to asbestos also occurs in insulation work, construction, ship building, and building demolition.

The parenchymal reaction to inhalation of asbestos is production of pleuropulmonary lesions involving mostly the lower part of the lung fields, accompanied by fibrous pleural thickening. Pulmonary fibrosis, bronchogenic carcinoma, pleural effusion, and pleural fibrosis are some of the common pulmonary complications of asbestosis.

Symptoms vary from none in early and mild cases to severe respiratory incapacity in advanced disease. Commonly, 20 to 30 years may elapse before clinical symptoms occur, of which dyspnea is the most common.

COAL WORKERS' PNEUMOCONIOSIS

Coal workers' pneumoconiosis is commonly referred to as "black lung" disease. Unlike silicosis, this disease results from prolonged exposure to coal dust. In essence, the clearance mechanisms of the lung are overwhelmed and coal dust accumulates in terminal air spaces. Severity and duration of exposure are the major factors determining the pathologic changes caused by coal dust. The area at which coal is cut, known as the coal face, is the dustiest part of the mine for workers. These workers are therefore exposed to the highest concentration of coal dust and are at greatest risk for the disease.

In simple coal workers' pneumoconiosis, the coal macule is the characteristic lesion. Coal macules, which appear as black dots on the lung, consist of macrophages filled with coal dust, fibroblasts, and cellular debris. Sometimes there is also a dilatation of the respiratory bronchioles called focal centrilobular emphysema.

The complicated form of coal workers' pneumoconiosis is characterized by large, black areas of fibrotic tissue with cores of dust, collagen, and other insoluble proteins.

Simple coal workers' pneumoconiosis is symptom-free, but the complicated form is characterized by dyspnea on exertion and may progress to severe respiratory insufficiency with obstructive lung disease, cor pulmonale, and pulmonary hypertension.

Clinically, evidence of small airway obstruction is demonstrated on pulmonary function studies.

Chest x-rays may show nodules that are small and not well defined. Large shadows of 1 cm or more in diameter indicate complicated pneumoconiosis.

❖ SETTINGS, PROVIDERS AND COLLABORATION FOR CARE

Patients with occupational lung diseases are managed in the outpatient setting until the disease reaches end stage. At that time, the patient may require hospitalization for support of oxygenation and ventilation.

NURSING PROCESS
Occupational Lung Disease

Assessment

Begin the assessment with a detailed occupational and environmental history, which includes information on the type and duration of the patient's exposure to dust and the development of symptoms in relationship to the work pattern. Obtain information about the patient's smoking habits, activity tolerance, and recent respiratory infections. Auscultate all lung fields and observe the patient for dyspnea, cough, and expectoration.

Occupational lung diseases, similar to COPD in presentation and treatment, are chronic disorders associated with permanent disability. Therefore, it is important to determine the patient's understanding of the disease course and to assess available support systems.

Nursing Diagnoses and Planning

Nursing diagnoses and related expected patient outcomes commonly applicable to patients with occupational lung disease include the following:

NDx: Impaired gas exchange related to ineffective ventilation secondary to fibrosis of the lung

Planning: Patient Outcomes
1. Patient describes measures to facilitate ventilation.
2. Patient uses oxygen correctly.
3. Arterial blood gas values are within normal limits.

NDx: Activity intolerance related to decreased oxygenation

Planning: Patient Outcomes
1. Patient describes how to avoid excessive demands on the respiratory system by spacing activities to allow for rest and recuperation of energy.
2. Patient demonstrates use of relaxation techniques.
3. Patient is able to perform activities of daily living.

NDx: Anxiety related to shortness of breath, outcome of disease, and inability to work

Planning: Patient Outcomes
1. Patient verbalizes feelings and concerns.
2. Patient demonstrates use of relaxation techniques.
3. Patient expresses confidence in ability to adapt to lifestyle changes necessitated by the disease.

NDx: Risk for altered health maintenance related to lack of knowledge about the disease, its progress, and its treatment

Planning: Patient Outcomes
1. Patient describes ways to avoid respiratory infection and airway irritants, such as wearing a protective mask, hood, or respirator.
2. Patient with asbestosis explains the importance of routine physical examinations.
3. Patient with asbestosis lists the warning signs of cancer.

Nursing Interventions and Evaluation

NDx: Impaired gas exchange
Explain measures that facilitate ventilation, such as the use of Fowler's or semi-Fowler's position, coughing, deep breathing, and adequate hydration to keep secretions liquid and movable. Instruct the patient and significant others in the use of oxygen and related precautions if needed.

NDx: Activity intolerance
Help the patient to plan activities so that time is provided between activities for energy to be restored. Discuss work-simplification techniques and assist the patient in implementing them.

NDx: Anxiety
Remain with the patient during episodes of breathlessness. Provide a calm, quiet environment and guide the patient in the use of relaxation exercises. Allow the patient to discuss concerns and provide reassurance and information on available resources as appropriate.

NDx: Risk for altered health maintenance
Teach patients and the general public about the hazards associated with exposure to industrial products such as silica, coal dust, and asbestos. Teach about the critical need for proper ventilation of work areas, use of wet techniques, and use of protective masks, hoods, and respirators.

Explain to patients the need to avoid environmental airway irritants outside the workplace, to take measures to protect themselves from respiratory infections, and to seek prompt medical treatment if an infection should occur.

Since patients with asbestosis have been found to be at increased risk for cancer, stress the need for routine physical examination and teach the warning signs and symptoms of cancer.

Compare the patient's status with the expected

patient outcomes. If the outcomes are not met, reassess the patient and revise the plan.

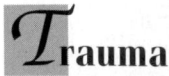rauma

Thoracic trauma is injury resulting from penetrating, crushing, or blunt force to the chest. Penetrating or open-chest trauma results from gunshot wounds, stab wounds, or other penetrating objects. Motor vehicle accidents are responsible for the majority of blunt or crushing chest trauma. In the United States, trauma is a leading cause of death. About 75% of traumatic deaths involve chest injury.

Chest injuries are always considered serious because of the potential for acute respiratory failure from damage to the chest wall or lower respiratory tract structures, and for shock caused by damage to the great vessels. Thus, a priority of treatment is to establish a patent airway and support cardiopulmonary function as needed.

FRACTURED RIBS

Etiology and Pathophysiology
Rib fractures, the most common type of chest injury, occur primarily as a result of blunt or crushing injury to the chest. Most often fractured are ribs 5 through 9, which are least protected and therefore more susceptible to trauma.

Fractures can range in severity from a simple crack to a splintered, displaced bony segment. If the broken edge of the bony segment is driven inward, it may injure the lungs or other underlying structures. Complications with rib fractures include hemothorax, pneumothorax, and lacerations of the lung, liver, or spleen.

Clinical Manifestations
Basic symptoms of an uncomplicated rib fracture are pain that increases with coughing, deep breathing, or movement; point tenderness at the site of the break; and muscle spasm on the affected side of the chest. Splinting and shallow breathing secondary to the pain also occur.

Diagnosis
Rib fracture is suggested by a history of chest trauma and the symptoms presented by the patient. It is confirmed by chest x-ray. Serial blood gas values are obtained to check for lung injury.

Management
Medical management of an uncomplicated rib fracture is aimed at relieving pain to promote effective ventilation. Narcotics are avoided whenever possible because of their depressive effect on respirations and cough. In some cases, an intercostal nerve block may be done to decrease pain and muscle spasm. Healing usually takes 3 to 6 weeks.

NURSING PROCESS
Fractured Ribs

Assessment

Take vital signs, paying particular attention to rate, depth, and symmetry of respiration. Note the patient's color. Assess pain level. Closely observe the patient for signs of any other injury.

Nursing Diagnoses and Planning

Nursing diagnoses and related expected patient outcomes commonly applicable to patients with uncomplicated fractured ribs include the following:

NDx: Pain related to chest wall and rib cage movement

Planning: Patient Outcomes
1. Patient states pain is relieved.
2. Patient's respirations are of normal rate and depth.
3. Patient states name, dose, route, and frequency of medication to be taken at home for pain.

NDx: Risk for ineffective breathing pattern related to pain on chest movement

Planning: Patient Outcomes
1. Respirations are of normal rate and depth.
2. Patient explains need for coughing and deep-breathing exercises.
3. Patient demonstrates coughing and deep-breathing correctly.

Nursing Interventions and Evaluation

Because the patient with an uncomplicated fractured rib is not hospitalized, the primary nursing intervention is patient teaching.

NDx: Pain
Give the patient medication for pain as ordered. Teach the patient the name, dose, route, and frequency of medication to be taken at home for pain relief. Be sure to specify when the patient should take the first dose.

NDx: Risk for ineffective breathing pattern
Explain the importance of coughing and deep breathing in maintaining good ventilation and preventing complications such as pneumonia. Instruct the patient in effective coughing and deep-breathing techniques and ask the patient to demonstrate them. Stress the importance of coordinating deep-breathing and coughing with the time when pain medication reaches peak effect to maximize comfort and effectiveness.

Additional Interventions
If the patient has past knowledge of treatment of a fractured rib, explain, if necessary, that the chest is no longer tightly wrapped or strapped, because it has been found that these interventions inhibit chest expansion and increase the risk of complications.

Compare the patient's status with the expected

patient outcomes. If the outcomes are not met, reassess the patient and revise the plan.

FLAIL CHEST

Etiology and Pathophysiology
Flail chest occurs when three or more adjacent ribs are fractured in two or more places, resulting in several free-floating rib segments. These free-floating segments cause paradoxic movement of the chest because they move inward during inspiration and outward with expiration. This action negates some of the chest expansion brought about by the anteroposterior and diaphragmatic movement, thus abolishing the pressure gradients essential for inspiration. Movement of air is diminished. Respiratory depth is decreased, and the patient cannot cough effectively. The result is increased secretions and fatigue.

Clinical Manifestations
The flail segment may not be immediately obvious because of intense spasm of the chest wall musculature overlying the fractures. However, as the muscles tire, the paradoxical movement of the affected chest wall segment appears (Fig. 16–15). The patient is in respiratory distress with hypoxemia, marked overbreathing, asymmetric chest movements, tachypnea, restlessness, and cyanosis.

Diagnosis
Diagnosis is based on current history of trauma, observation of the chest, and chest x-rays.

Management
If the area of flail is small, management may simply involve provision of pain relief and good pulmonary hygiene to promote lung expansion. Pain relief may be achieved by intercostal nerve block, high thoracic epidural block, or intrapleural or intravenous narcotics if not contraindicated by a concurrent head injury. Management of more severe cases of flail chest involves pain relief, administration of supplemental oxygen, and stabilization of the chest wall. Initially this is done by exerting firm but gentle pressure on the segment with either the palm of the hand or sandbags. Supplemental oxygen and pain medication (if not contraindicated by a concurrent head injury) are given.

Subsequently, the chest is more effectively stabilized either internally or operatively. Internal stabilization, the procedure of choice, involves endotracheal intubation and the use of a volume-controlled mechanical ventilator, sometimes accompanied by positive end-expiratory pressure (PEEP). Operative stabilization can be achieved through intramedullary pinning of the ribs, sternum, and costal cartilages.

Regardless of method, it is important that treatment be started as early as possible to prevent changes in the lung from compression, such as pulmonary congestion, atelectasis, and pulmonary hemorrhage. Stabilization of the chest wall also promotes more effective bone healing.

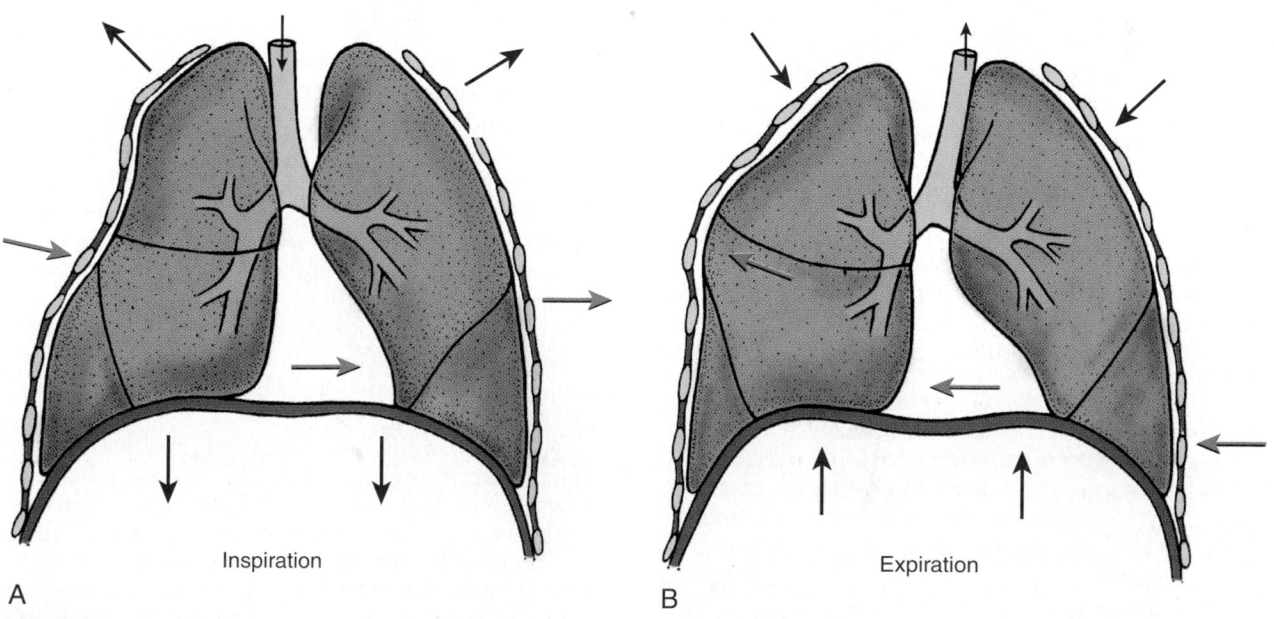

Inspiration

A

Expiration

B

Figure 16–15

Flail chest. *A,* The flail area of the chest wall sucks in on inspiration. Note that air flows from the lung on the affected side into the opposite lung, thus compromising ventilation of the lung on the flail side. Note also the movement of the mediastinum to the side opposite the flail. *B,* The flail area of the chest wall balloons outward on expiration, and a portion of exhaled air from the lung on the unaffected side passes into the lung on the flail side, again impairing ventilation.

❖ **Settings, Providers, and Collaboration for Care**

All patients with flail chest should be admitted to a trauma unit or critical care unit, where continued close observation is possible. This is important because patients with chest trauma of this magnitude are likely to have significant injuries of other organs that may or not have been obvious initially.

NURSING PROCESS

Flail Chest

Assessment

In addition to assessing pain and respiratory and cardiac status, assess the abdomen, extremities, and neurologic function because flail chest is associated with significant trauma.

Nursing Diagnoses and Planning

Nursing diagnoses and related expected patient outcomes commonly applicable to patients with flail chest include the following:

NDx: Ineffective breathing pattern related to flail chest

Planning: Patient Outcomes
1. Restlessness, cyanosis, and dyspnea are absent.
2. Arterial blood gas values are within normal limits.
3. Paradoxical chest wall movement is decreased or absent.

NDx: Risk for ineffective airway clearance related to ineffective coughing and pain

Planning: Patient Outcomes
1. Patient coughs and expectorates.
2. Lungs are clear on auscultation.

Nursing Interventions and Evaluation

NDx: Ineffective breathing pattern
Administer oxygen and give analgesics as ordered to relieve pain and encourage chest expansion. Reassure the patient and maintain a calm environment to alleviate the patient's anxiety and to lower the demand for oxygen.

NDx: Risk for ineffective airway clearance
Encourage the patient to cough and deep-breathe to mobilize secretions from the respiratory tract. If unable to move secretions in this way, suction as needed. Be sure the patient is always well hydrated to keep secretions liquid unless fluid is restricted because of underlying pulmonary contusion.

Additional Interventions
Other nursing interventions depend in part on the type of medical treatment prescribed. Nursing care of the patient who is intubated and on mechanical ventilation is discussed in Chapter 14 and applies to the patient whose chest is stabilized in this way. Note, however, that a patient being ventilated for flail chest is on controlled, not assisted, ventilation. Paralyzing agents may be ordered to prevent the patient from "fighting" the ventilator, and to decrease overall oxygen consumption by blocking neuromuscular activity.

Compare the patient's status with the expected patient outcomes. If the outcomes are not met, reassess the patient and revise the plan.

Pneumothorax

Pneumothorax is a condition in which air or gas exists in the pleural space.

Etiology and Pathophysiology

There are two major types of pneumothorax: open and closed. An open pneumothorax is one in which a hole in the chest wall allows atmospheric air to flow into the pleural space (Fig. 16–16A). This may result from a penetrating injury (such as a stab or gunshot wound), a therapeutic procedure (such as a thoracotomy or thoracentesis), or insertion of a central venous catheter or a pulmonary artery catheter.

In a closed, or spontaneous, pneumothorax, air enters the pleural space from the lung (Fig. 16–16B). If this occurs in the absence of disease, it is called a simple, spontaneous pneumothorax. This type occurs most often in men between ages 20 and 40 and results from the rupture of blebs on the apex of the lung (small vesicles of unknown cause). If a closed pneumothorax results from trauma or pulmonary disease, it is referred to as secondary, or complicated, pneumothorax. Trauma that causes secondary pneumothorax consists of blunt injuries to the chest, such as sudden compression of the thoracic cavity at the height of inspiration with the glottis closed, causing rupture of the alveoli from excessive pressure and perforation of the lung by the end of a fractured rib. The disease most often associated with secondary pneumothorax is widespread emphysema.

In each of these types of pneumothorax, the air in the pleural space causes increased intrapleural pressure, resulting in partial or total collapse of the lung.

A unique type of pneumothorax is a tension pneumothorax (Fig. 16–17). This occurs when injury allows air to leak into the pleural space during inspiration, but it is prevented from leaking out during expiration. With each inspiration, then, the amount of air continues to increase, causing pressure within the pleural space to rise above atmospheric pressure. This results not only in collapse of the lung but also in a shift of the mediastinum to the opposite side. This shift, in turn, causes pressure on the great vessels returning blood to the heart and impairs venous return.

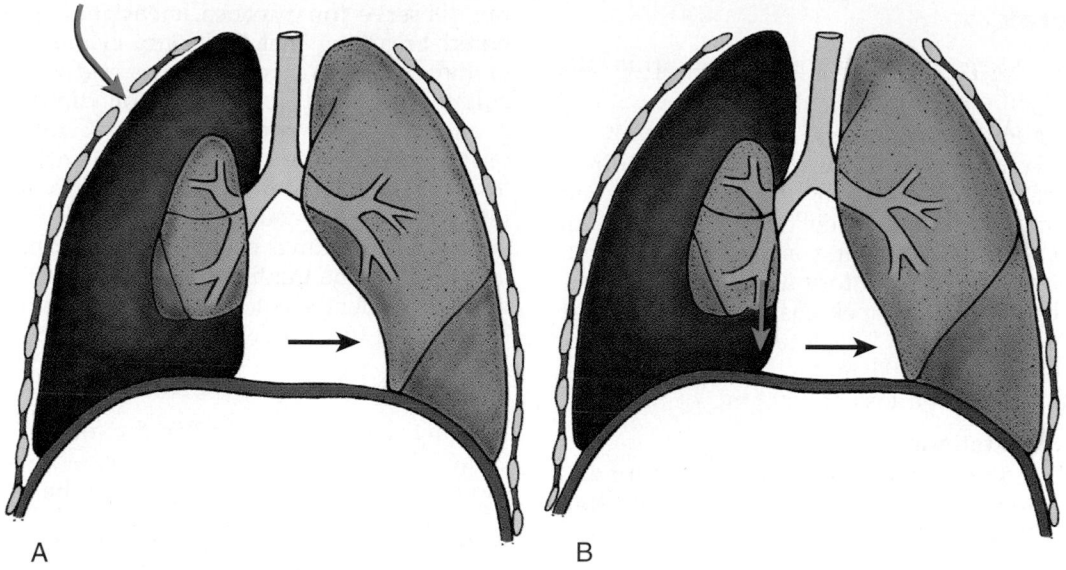

Figure 16–16

A, Open pneumothorax. Note the opening in the chest wall through which air enters the pleural space on inspiration. *B,* Closed pneumothorax. Note the tear in the lung through which air enters the pleural space during inspiration.

Clinical Manifestations

The patient with an open pneumothorax has a history of some event that has caused penetration of the chest wall. A sucking sound is audible on inspiration as the chest wall rises, and varying degrees of respiratory distress are present depending on the size of the pneumothorax.

The basic symptoms of a closed pneumothorax are shortness of breath and chest pain; however, the exact clinical signs depend on the size of the pneumothorax. A larger pneumothorax may present with tachypnea, cyanosis, diminished breath sounds, and subcutaneous emphysema. There may also be hyperresonance on the affected side.

A tension pneumothorax presents with clinical signs only as the positive pressure on the affected side increases. There is neck vein engorgement secondary to the pressure on the superior vena cava, progressive dyspnea, paradoxical movement of the chest, deviated trachea, cyanosis, distant breath sounds, hyper-resonance on the affected side, and cardiogenic shock.

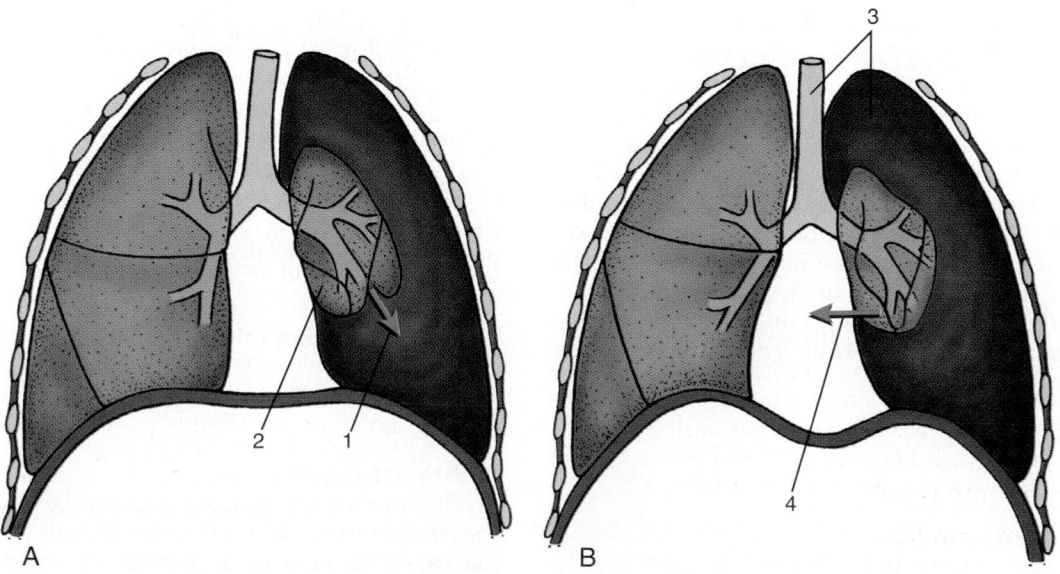

Figure 16–17

Tension pneumothorax. *A,* On the side of the damaged lung, air accumulates with each respiratory cycle causing (1) collapse of the injured lung as the pressure builds up, (2) deviation of the trachea, and (3) mediastinal shift, which compresses the opposite lung (4).

Hemothorax

Hemothorax is an accumulation of blood in the pleural space.

Etiology and Pathophysiology

A hemothorax is caused by bleeding of the pulmonary parenchyma and vessels, the intercostal and internal mammary arteries, the heart, the aorta, or the great vessels. The bleeding is usually self-limiting but, if it persists, respiratory and cardiac impairments and hypovolemic shock ensue because a large amount of blood is lost. The total accumulation of blood can range from 300 mL to a much more severe hemothorax with a loss of 1500 mL of blood.

Clinical Manifestations

The clinical findings for hemothorax are the same as for open or tension pneumothorax, with the addition of tachycardia, hypotension, dullness on chest percussion, pallor, and anxiety.

Diagnosis

Diagnosis of pneumothorax, hemothorax, or pneumohemothorax (combination of pneumothorax and hemothorax) is made on the basis of chest x-ray and arterial blood gas values.

Management

Medical management consists of insertion of a chest tube to re-establish the intrapleural pressure (see Chapter 14 for chest tube insertion and care). In the case of a tension pneumothorax, which always requires immediate intervention, a large-bore needle (16 to 18 gauge) is inserted either anteriorly at the midclavicular line between the second and third intercostal spaces or at the midlateral line between the fifth and sixth intercostal spaces. The patient's condition improves markedly once the needle is inserted.

An open pneumothorax should be immediately covered to prevent further entry of air into the chest. In an emergency, anything available is used, but in the hospital, petrolatum jelly gauze is used. Three sides are taped, and the fourth is left open to permit air to exit the pleural space and to prevent a tension pneumothorax.

The treatment for hemothorax may require a thoracotomy if the initial chest-tube drainage is greater than 1500 mL, persistent bleeding occurs at a rate greater than 500 mL per hour, increasing hemothorax is identified on chest x-ray, or the patient's condition remains unstable despite adequate blood replacement.

NURSING PROCESS
Pneumothorax or Hemothorax

Assessment

A comprehensive respiratory assessment is important for patients with a pneumothorax or hemothorax. Observe for dyspnea, tachypnea, retractions, labored breathing, nasal flaring, cyanosis, asymmetry of the chest wall, restlessness, and confusion. Auscultate the chest for distant or diminished breath sounds and for vocal fremitus or hyper-resonance on the affected side. Palpate for tracheal deviation and subcutaneous emphysema, and note the characteristics of any cough or sputum. Assess cardiac status by checking blood pressure and heart rate, auscultating the quality of the heartbeat, and observing the patient's color. Measure urinary output to check renal function.

Nursing Diagnoses and Planning

Nursing diagnoses and related expected patient outcomes commonly applicable to patients with a pneumothorax or a hemothorax include the following:

NDx: Impaired gas exchange related to collapse of an area of the lung

Planning: Patient Outcomes
1. Respiratory rate and depth are within normal limits.
2. Arterial blood gas values are within normal range.

NDx: Anxiety related to dyspnea, treatment, or both

Planning: Patient Outcomes
1. Patient states rationale for treatment and procedures.
2. Patient rests without behavioral signs of excessive anxiety.

Nursing Interventions and Evaluation

NDx: Impaired gas exchange
Place the patient in a semi-Fowler's position to facilitate breathing and encourage coughing and deep-breathing to remove secretions and enhance ventilation. Monitor ABGs, electrolytes, and blood counts to identify problems with oxygenation and bleeding.

Administer oxygen therapy and medications as ordered. If an occlusive dressing has been used for an open pneumothorax, observe the patient for signs of tension pneumothorax. If the patient is on mechanical ventilation or if a chest tube is inserted, provide care as discussed in Chapter 14.

NDx: Anxiety
Explain all procedures and the overall treatment plan to the patient. Be calm and reassure the patient about the condition, as appropriate. Encourage the use of relaxation techniques.

Additional Interventions
If a hemothorax is present, monitor for hypovolemic shock as required. Carry out fluid- and blood-replacement therapy as in anemia.

Compare the patient's status with the expected patient outcomes. If the outcomes are not met, reassess the patient and revise the plan.

PULMONARY CONTUSION

Crushing and bruising of the lung is known as pulmonary contusion.

Etiology and Pathophysiology
Pulmonary contusion can result from a severe blow to the chest, with or without rib or sternal fracture. Lung contusion leads to atelectasis and airway obstruction because bronchioles become plugged with blood and edema fluid. Ventilation is also impaired because of a reduction in lung compliance.

Clinical Manifestations
With a mild contusion there may be no symptoms. With more extensive lung contusion, however, there is a progression of atelectasis and a decrease in lung compliance, with a resulting low V/Q ratio. This leads to hypoxemia, and the patient exhibits dyspnea, cough, hemoptysis, increasing hyperpnea, tachypnea, chest pain, and restlessness.

Diagnosis
Diagnosis is based on current history of a blow to the chest. As complications occur, chest x-rays may reveal areas of atelectasis.

Management
Management depends largely on the area affected. In mild cases, supplemental oxygen and close observation may be sufficient. In more severe cases, fluids are restricted and broad-spectrum antibiotics given. Fluids are restricted because there is damage to the pulmonary capillary bed, which can lead to pulmonary fluid overload. Antibiotics are given to prevent septicemia, which is a complication of lung contusion.

NURSING PROCESS GUIDELINES
Pulmonary Contusion

Carefully assess respiratory status and vital signs to monitor for impending complications. Whenever possible, place the patient in a high Fowler's position to facilitate breathing. Suction if the patient is unable to raise secretions because of pain. Give oxygen and pain medication as ordered, and have the patient do deep breathing exercises every 1 to 2 hours.

SUBCUTANEOUS EMPHYSEMA

Subcutaneous emphysema is a potential complication of any injury affecting the integrity of the lower respiratory system. In this condition, air that has escaped from the lung has entered the subcutaneous tissue. Because the air can travel quite a distance, it may be present in the neck, thorax, and face. It can also involve the abdomen, the scrotum, and even the lower extremities. It is easily recognized by the classic crepitations (crackling sounds) heard when palpating the skin.

The presence of subcutaneous emphysema suggests the need for thorough x-ray examination and close observation to determine the extent of the intrathoracic injury. Once the underlying problem is resolved, the air is spontaneously reabsorbed, a process that can be hastened by administration of high concentrations of oxygen. In very severe cases of subcutaneous emphysema, a tracheotomy may be needed to keep the airway patent until the air has been reabsorbed.

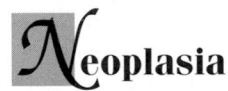

Neoplasia

LUNG CANCER
Etiology and Pathophysiology
The exact cause and pathogenesis of cancer in general remain unknown; however, there is strong evidence to suggest a relationship between prolonged inhalation of air pollutants and the occurrence of lung cancer. Smoke is the most common of these pollutants. Ninety percent of all patients with lung cancer are cigarette smokers. The risk of lung cancer diminishes with smoking cessation. In fact, some authorities believe that 15 years of abstention from smoking places the former smoker in the same risk category as a person who has never smoked. An increased risk for lung cancer is also believed to be associated with exposure to second-hand cigarette smoke.

A second major pollutant associated with the development of lung cancer is radon. Radon is a colorless, odorless radioactive gas that is a product of the breakdown of uranium in soil, rock, and water. In areas where uranium is present in significant amounts, it can enter homes through cracks and other openings in the foundation. It can also enter well water and be released into the air when the water is used. Any exposure to radon is associated with the risk of lung cancer, but levels of 4 picocuries (pCi/L) or higher in the lowest lived-in level of a home indicates the need for radon reduction measures. The outdoor level of radon is 0.4 pCi/L, and this is the long-term goal set by the United States Congress for all indoor areas.

Other factors associated with lung cancer are industrial exposure to certain inorganic and synthetic substances, asbestos dust, and radioactive substances.

The four major types of lung cancer are squamous cell carcinoma (also referred to as epidermoid), adenocarcinoma, large-cell carcinoma, and small-cell carcinoma.

Squamous cell carcinomas are central in origin; that is, they arise from the major bronchi or their immediate subdivisions. These tumors grow slowly, often into the lumen, thus obstructing the airways. They sometimes cavitate. Poorly differentiated squamous cell carcinomas of the lung tend to metastasize to the small bowel, whereas well-differentiated lesions primarily spread within the thorax. Prognosis is poorest for this type of lung cancer.

Adenocarcinomas, the most common type of lung cancer, tend to arise in the lung periphery. They are often quite large when discovered, having spread in a patchy distribution resembling an infectious process throughout one lobe or an entire lung. Adenocarcinomas frequently invade the pleura, resulting in a pleural effusion containing malignant cells. They metastasize early, most often to the brain, although the other lung, the liver, the adrenal glands, and bone may also be sites of metastases.

Bronchioalveolar carcinomas are a common subtype of adenocarcinoma that originate in the terminal bronchioalveolar regions. They tend to grow on the surfaces of the airways and are associated with copious sputum production. They do not tend to spread by invasion of local tissues but rather by dissemination through the airways.

Large-cell carcinomas tend to arise in peripheral bronchi and do not exhibit the well-defined patterns of other cell types. They usually present as a bulky tumor mass and metastasize early, usually to the central nervous system. They are very similar to the adenocarcinomas.

Small-cell carcinomas, also known as oat-cell carcinomas, are the most malignant of the lung cancers. They generally arise centrally in the bronchus region and metastasize through the blood stream and lymphatic vessels early in the disease process. Common metastatic sites are the mediastinum, liver, bone and bone marrow, central nervous system, adrenal glands, pancreas, and other endocrine organs. Hypersecretion of antidiuretic hormone by the tumor cells in small-cell lung cancer is very common. This leads to a condition known as syndrome of inappropriate antidiuretic hormone and will produce hyponatremia.

The main sites of metastases from all primary lung tumors are the liver, brain, bone, kidney, and adrenal glands.

Clinical Manifestations

Signs and symptoms depend on the location and size of the tumor mass. Localized symptoms include cough (usually mistaken for smoker's cough), dyspnea, hemoptysis, stridor or wheeze, and signs of obstructive pneumonitis. Expectoration of blood-tinged sputum is common. This is caused by the sputum becoming streaked with blood as it passes over the ulcerated tumor surface. Recurring fever may also be present because of an area of persistent pneumonitis.

In some cases, symptoms do not occur until the tumor has spread to adjacent thoracic structures and is putting pressure on nerves, or until it has invaded the chest wall or mediastinum. Symptoms depend on the area of spread and organs and nerves affected.

As the tumor spreads to the outside surface of the lung, fluid accumulates with resulting pleural effusion. This causes chest pain and difficulty breathing. If the tumor invades the mediastinum, there is obstruction of the superior vena cava, with resulting head and neck edema and possible pericardial effusion with cardiac tamponade. If the left recurrent laryngeal nerve is involved, hoarseness or left vocal cord paralysis may be the presenting symptom. Late in the course of the disease, weakness, anorexia, weight loss, and anemia appear, as well as symptoms caused by any distant metastases.

Diagnosis

The diagnosis of bronchogenic carcinoma is suggested by the patient's clinical history and the findings on physical examination, chest x-ray, computed tomographic scan, or magnetic resonance imaging. The diagnosis is confirmed by sputum cytology or by biopsy obtained during bronchoscopy.

If metastasis is suggested by presenting symptoms, physical examination, or results of standard blood chemistries, additional tests are done, such as bone, liver, and brain scans. If surgery is considered, tests of cardiac function and pulmonary function are done to determine the patient's ability to tolerate the physiologic stress of surgery.

Management

Management of lung cancer depends on the type of cancer, the stage of the cancer, and the patient's general condition. There are three basic forms of treatment: surgery, radiation therapy, and chemotherapy. One, two, or all three methods may be used.

Surgery is usually performed when the tumor is localized with no evidence of metastasis. The surgery may be a lobectomy or a pneumonectomy with resection of involved mediastinal lymph nodes. Palliative surgery is not advisable because symptoms can be alleviated by other forms of treatment (for example, a thoracentesis may be done to alleviate pain or shortness of breath caused by pleural effusion).

Radiation therapy is used as a definitive treatment for localized intrathoracic lung cancers. It is also used for small-cell and epidermoid tumors that cannot be resected. It is used to decrease tumor size and relieve pressure on vital organs and nerves. Relief of symptoms can last from a few weeks to many months and helps to improve the quality of life for these patients.

Because metastasis occurs in 90% of patients with lung cancer, chemotherapy is widely used. The small-cell cancers have been shown to be most responsive to this form of therapy. The drug of choice depends on the growth of the tumor cell and the specificity of the drug for a cell cycle phase. The chemotherapeutic regimen usually involves cyclophosphamide, methotrexate, vincristine, doxorubicin hydrochloride, and procarbazine in varying three- or four-drug combinations concurrently. Unfortunately, the results of chemotherapy are poor; often, it does not extend the patient's life significantly.

Management of the syndrome of inappropriate antidiuretic hormone, if present, is aimed at restoring normal fluid balance and osmolality. Fluid restriction alone may be useful. If this is unsuccessful, 5% saline solution may be given intravenously. If cardiac problems (such as heart failure) develop, diuretics are used to promote diuresis. This form of syndrome of inappropriate antidiuretic hormone is chronic in nature when associated with tumors. In some cases, demeclocycline 900 to 1200 mg daily may be given, which causes a nephrogenic diabetes insipidus.

❖ Settings, Providers, and Collaboration for Care

The patient having surgery for lung cancer is hospitalized. If radiation therapy or chemotherapy is a part of the treatment plan, it is given on an outpatient basis or, in the case of chemotherapy, may be given in the home. Home oxygen therapy may also be needed. Persons involved in the delivery of care vary with the stage of the disease and the plan of treatment. Home health-care nurses, nutritionists, respiratory therapists, social service workers, and ultimately hospice personnel all have a role in providing effective care.

NURSING PROCESS
Lung Cancer

Assessment

Carefully assess the patient's respiratory function. Obtain information about cough patterns, wheezing, chest tightness, hemoptysis, blood-tinged sputum, dyspnea, and hoarseness. Question the patient about shoulder and arm pain, headache, unsteady gait, fatigue, weight loss, edema of the head and neck, and anorexia. Note the time of onset, the pattern of progression, and current status.

Appraise the patient's overall physical condition, noting whether the patient appears nourished or emaciated. Review the patient's history to identify concurrent medical problems. Obtain information on any medications being taken.

Once the diagnosis is made, assess the emotional response of the patient and family as well as their understanding of the diagnosis, diagnostic procedures, and therapeutic interventions.

Nursing Diagnoses and Planning

Nursing diagnoses and related expected patient outcomes commonly applicable to patients with lung cancer include the following:

NDx: Impaired gas exchange related to decreased functional lung tissue secondary to tumor growth

Planning: Patient Outcomes
1. Dyspnea is absent.
2. Cyanosis is absent.
3. Arterial blood gas values are within normal limits.

NDx: Ineffective breathing pattern related to chest pain and/or depressant effects of narcotic analgesics

Planning: Patient Outcomes
1. Respirations are of normal rate and depth.
2. Arterial blood gas values are within normal limits.

NDx: Risk for fluid volume excess related to chronic syndrome of inappropriate antidiuretic hormone

Planning: Patient Outcomes
1. Patient's weight is stable.
2. Intake and output are balanced.
3. Serum sodium and osmolality levels are within normal limits.

NDx: Anxiety related to diagnosis, its treatment, and its outcomes

Planning: Patient Outcomes
1. Patient freely expresses anxiety about the diagnosis.
2. Patient discusses concerns and feelings with family or significant other.
3. Patient practices relaxation techniques daily.
4. Patient identifies available support systems.
5. Patient states telephone number of a mental health professional or support group representative to contact if needed.

NDx: Risk for altered health maintenance related to insufficient knowledge of lung cancer, its treatment and prognosis, and self-care.

Planning: Patient Outcomes
1. Patient verbalizes realistic perceptions about diagnosis and treatments.
2. Patient describes plan of follow-up care.
3. Patient lists general goals of self-care, describing methods of achieving them.

Nursing Interventions and Evaluation

NDx: Impaired gas exchange
Place the patient in high Fowler's position to facilitate chest expansion. Administer oxygen as ordered. Limit activity to decrease cardiac and respiratory workload. Because anxiety increases oxygen demands, act to put the patient at ease. Keep the environment calm and quiet, reassure the patient that you are available when needed, and prepare the patient for all aspects of care.

NDx: Ineffective breathing pattern
Give analgesics for chest pain to make the patient

comfortable and eliminate the need to splint the chest and take shallow breaths. Instruct the patient to breathe deeply, cough, and use an incentive spirometer every 2 hours. Assist with postural drainage, percussion, and vibration if ordered.

NDx: Risk for fluid volume excess

Monitor for and report signs and symptoms of syndrome of inappropriate antidiuretic hormone, including sudden weight gain, intake greater than output, irritability, lethargy, confusion, peripheral edema, headache, weakness, nausea, abdominal cramping, and seizures.

NDx: Anxiety

Provide frequent, private opportunities for the patient to express anxieties. If the patient indicates inability or reluctance to discuss concerns with significant others, promote discussion of these feelings and, if deemed appropriate, help the patient find the right words and approach through role playing. Guide the patient in the use of relaxation techniques and provide a diversion of the patient's choice. Work with the patient to identify available support systems and provide the patient with information needed to contact a support group or mental health professional if needed.

NDx: Risk for altered health maintenance

Clarify and reinforce information given by the physician to the patient and family. Review information on chemotherapy or radiation therapy if planned. Answer questions clearly, and refer to additional sources of information as appropriate.

Explain the rationale, side effects, and dosage schedules of prescribed medications. Review chest physiotherapy techniques, such as postural drainage, percussion, and vibration. Teach the use of any prescribed equipment, such as oxygen, nebulizer, metered dose inhaler incentive spirometer, or humidifier, and obtain a return demonstration.

Include the family or significant others in the teaching sessions to promote compliance. Provide a written summary of treatments, procedures, diet, medications, and follow-up appointments.

Provide information about community resources available to assist with home management, such as the American Cancer Society, Visiting Nurse Association, Meals on Wheels, Hospice, and I Can Cope. Instruct the patient in self-care as specified in Highlight 16–8.

Additional Interventions

Other nursing interventions relate directly to the type of medical treatment the patient receives. For example, if the patient is undergoing surgery, nursing care of the patient having chest surgery applies (Nursing Care Guide 16–1 and Chap. 14). If the patient is having radiation or chemotherapy, the care related to these respective treatments applies (see Chap. 34).

Compare the patient's status with the expected patient outcomes. If the outcomes are not met, reassess the patient and revise the plan.

TUMORS OF THE MEDIASTINUM

Mediastinal tumors are found adjacent to vital structures and have an unpredictable manner of growth. Lesions of the mediastinum are usually classified according to their location in the anterior, middle, or posterior mediastinal compartments. Some of the more common types are thymic tumors, mesodermal tumors, neurogenic tumors, and endocrine tumors.

Etiology and Pathophysiology

The exact cause of the various mediastinal tumors is unknown. They are usually neoplastic but may be congenital, traumatic, infectious, or degenerative in nature. Tumors that originate in the neck, chest wall, or diaphragm may extend or grow into the mediastinum and simulate a primary mediastinal mass.

Clinical Manifestations

Symptoms vary depending on which area of the intrathoracic region receives pressure from the tumor. They include chest pain, orthopnea, cardiac palpitation, anginal attacks, cyanosis, superior vena cava syndrome (swelling of the face, neck, and upper extremities), distention of the neck veins, and dysphagia caused by pressure on the esophagus.

Diagnosis

X-rays of the chest and mediastinal region and computed tomographic scanning are used to detect and define mediastinal masses. Sputum examinations are routinely done to rule out tuberculosis.

Management

Management of mediastinal tumors includes surgery, radiotherapy, and chemotherapy. If the tumor is benign and operable, surgery may be the only treatment necessary.

NURSING PROCESS GUIDELINES
Mediastinal Tumor

The assessment, nursing diagnoses, expected patient outcomes, nursing interventions, and evaluation for patients with mediastinal tumors are similar to those described for patients with tumors elsewhere in the chest who are treated with surgery, radiation, or chemotherapy (see Chaps. 14 and 34).

The Elderly: Special Considerations

All types of lower respiratory tract disease occur in the elderly. COPD, influenza, and pneumonia are among the most common. In older adults, lower

Text continued on page 707

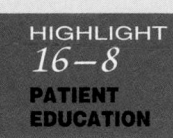 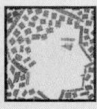

HIGHLIGHT
16–8
PATIENT EDUCATION

Managing Lung Cancer

To promote maximum respiratory efficiency, instruct the patient in the following:

Avoid respiratory irritants:
  Stop smoking.
  Avoid exposure to second-hand smoke.
  Avoid fumes from household chemicals.
  Avoid extremes of hot and cold temperatures.

Decrease risks of respiratory infection:
  Avoid persons with respiratory infections.
  Avoid crowds.
  Maintain good oral hygiene.
  Carefully cleanse all respiratory equipment.
  Drink at least 10 glasses of liquid daily.

Follow prescribed chest physical therapy routines.

Take medications as ordered.

To control chronic syndrome of inappropriate antidiuretic hormone (SIADH), instruct the patient in the following:

Take medications as prescribed.

Follow prescribed dietary modifications:
  Increased sodium intake
  Increased potassium intake

Report any new or worsened symptoms of SIADH:
  Lethargy, confusion
  Weakness
  Headache
  Sudden weight gain
  Nausea
  Abdominal cramping
  Intake consistently more than output
  Seizures

To promote adequate nutrition, instruct the patient in the following:

For loss of appetite:
  Eat small meals frequently.
  Keep snacks handy for nibbling.
  Rely on favorite foods during not-hungry times.
  Prepare foods attractively (eg, garnished, varied colors).
  Snack at bedtime.
  Try milk shakes, frozen yogurt, eggnog, or ice cream mixed with favorite soft drinks.

For change in taste:
  Try chicken, turkey, fish (avoid strong-smelling fish; cook on barbeque), cheese, eggs

  Add bacon bits, sliced almonds, or ham strips to vegetables for added flavor
  Use tart foods to enhance flavors (eg, vinegar, lemon or orange juice, pickles)
  Try marinating meats
  Use more and stronger seasonings, such as basil, oregano, rosemary, tarragon
  Try eliminating strange taste in the mouth by drinking more liquids, such as water, tea, and ginger ale, or eating foods that leave their own tastes, such as fresh fruits or hard candies
  Be sure to have dental checkup to rule out dental problems as the source of the change in taste

For feeling of fullness after eating only a little:
  Chew foods slowly.
  Limit greasy foods, butter, and rich sauces.
  Eat smaller, more frequent meals.
  Be sure liquids taken have nutritional content.
  Limit fluids at mealtime.

For feeling too tired to eat:
  Rely on frozen meals made during "well" times.
  Use convenience foods.
  Try canned cream soups with fish or chicken and fresh fruit to make well-balanced and quickly prepared meals.
  Accept offers of help from family and friends.
  Contact community service groups (eg, Meals on Wheels).

To allow for continuing care as needed, instruct the patient in the following:

Report the following symptoms:
  Increased symptoms of SIADH (see earlier section)
  Difficulty swallowing
  Increased fatigue, weakness, or shortness of breath
  Pain in shoulder, arm, or neck
  Swollen, painful joints
  Signs and symptoms of hypercalcemia: nausea, vomiting, muscle weakness, confusion, and increased thirst and urination
  Fever that persists
  Increasingly productive cough (purulent, foul-smelling, blood-stained sputum)
  Excessive depression or difficulty coping with the diagnosis

Nursing Care Guide 16–1
Patients Undergoing Pneumonectomy for Cancer of the Lung

Preoperative Care

Assessment Findings: Patient states "I'm afraid of anesthesia, I'm afraid of the surgery, and I'm afraid the cancer has spread, so there is nothing that can be done." Patient paces in room and wrings hands. Patient seems "lost in own world."

Nursing Diagnosis: Anxiety related to the diagnosis of cancer and the surgical experience

Patient Outcomes	Nursing Interventions	Rationale
Patient expresses concerns freely. Patient attends to information and directions. Pacing, hand-wringing, and other behaviors indicative of excessive anxiety are absent.	Provide opportunity and environment conducive to expression of anxiety. Listen to the patient. Acknowledge that anxiety over the diagnosis of lung cancer and surgery is normal. Reassure patient regarding safety of modern anesthetic and surgical techniques and the ability and concern of all the people involved in his or her care. Describe the close supervision given during each stage of the operative experience.	Allows for feedback, provides perspective, and permits a supportive relationship. Verbalization is therapeutic; listening allays patient concerns about being judged negatively because of anxiety. Provides the patient with positive facts about the operative procedure on which to focus and base hope for a successful surgical outcome.

Evaluation: Compare the patient's status with the expected outcomes. If the outcomes are not met, reassess the patient and revise the plan.

Assessment Findings: Patient has no prior experience with surgery. Patient asks questions about perioperative care.

Nursing Diagnosis: Knowledge deficit: perioperative care

Patient Outcomes	Nursing Interventions	Rationale
Patient describes preoperative preparations, postanesthesia care unit (PACU) routines, and expected postoperative course and treatments.	Explain perioperative care. Provide information on preparation for and transport to the operating room, the PACU and its routines, and the expected postoperative apparatus such as chest tubes (if used by the surgeon), intravenous fluids, oxygen, central venous pressure catheter, pulmonary artery catheter, urinary catheter, and surgical dressing.	Prepares patients for perioperative events; promotes compliance with perioperative care; and decreases the risk of anxiety over routine perioperative events.

(continued)

Nursing Care Guide 16–1
Patients Undergoing Pneumonectomy for Cancer of the Lung
(continued)

Patient Outcomes	Nursing Interventions	Rationale
	Tell the patient that chest pain is expected after surgery, that medication will be available, and that he or she should not hesitate to ask for it.	Provides information about normal experiences as well as appropriate patient response.
Patient explains importance of turning, coughing, and deep-breathing postoperatively. Patient demonstrates coughing and deep-breathing techniques.	Instruct the patient in the importance and technique of turning, coughing, and deep-breathing.	Learning is best accomplished when patient is in a pain-free, low-anxiety state before surgery.
Patient demonstrates use of a pillow or folded towel to splint the area of the incision.	Show the patient how the incision will be splinted with the nurse's hands or pillow or folded towel during turning, coughing, and deep-breathing.	Familiarity with procedures promotes cooperation.
Patient demonstrates exercises to maintain full range of motion in the affected shoulder.	Instruct the patient in exercises to maintain range of motion in the shoulders: Reach behind head and neck with affected arm and hand and try to touch top of shoulder blade on affected side. Reach across chest with affected arm and hand and touch outer edge of unaffected shoulder. Reach behind the middle of the back with affected arm and hand and touch lower edge of the shoulder blade on unaffected side.	Provides information that will be needed in the postoperative period at a time conducive to learning.

Evaluation:	Compare the patient's status with the expected outcomes. If the outcomes are not met, reassess the patient and revise the plan.

Postoperative Care

Assessment Findings:	Rapid, noisy respirations, crackles audible on auscultation, complaints of dyspnea, cough without expectoration
Nursing Diagnosis:	Ineffective airway clearance related to excessive secretions and shallow breathing

(continued)

Nursing Care Guide 16–1

Patients Undergoing Pneumonectomy for Cancer of the Lung

(continued)

Patient Outcomes	Nursing Interventions	Rationale
Airway is cleared of secretions by coughing or suctioning. Respirations are quiet and easy. Crackles are absent on auscultation.	Change position every 1 to 2 hours.	Position in bed splints the chest wall, decreasing aeration of tissues. Changing positions changes the section of the lung tissue splinted. Position changes also help drain secretions so that they can be removed from the lungs.
	Turn patient on back and to operative side only.	Keeps fluid in pleural space below the bronchial stump.
	Elevate head of bed approximately 30 degrees when blood pressure is stable to promote ventilation.	Gravity pulls the intestines away from the diaphragm, facilitating increased lung expansion.
	Instruct the patient to cough and deep-breathe every hour for the first 24 hours after surgery.	Promotes good ventilation and airway clearance.
	Splint the incision to limit discomfort.	Pain decreases patient's willingness to cough and breathe deeply.
	Assist with postural drainage if ordered.	Assists in removal of secretions to maintain oxygenation.
	Encourage fluid intake to 1500–2000 mL daily unless contraindicated.	Fluids thin respiratory secretions so that they can be cleared.

Evaluation:	Compare the patient's status with the expected outcomes. If the outcomes are not met, reassess the patient and revise the plan.
Assessment Findings:	Complaints of dyspnea, elevated pulse and respiratory rate, restlessness
Nursing Diagnosis:	Impaired gas exchange related to decreased functional lung tissue and hypoventilation

Patient Outcomes	Nursing Interventions	Rationale
Vital signs are within normal range. Cyanosis is absent. Arterial blood gas values are within normal range.	Administer humidified oxygen as ordered.	Increases/maintains PO_2 despite diminished lung tissue.
	Do not position patient on unoperated side.	Prevents bed from splinting the chest, interfering with maximal ventilation of the remaining lung tissue.

(continued)

Nursing Care Guide 16–1
Patients Undergoing Pneumonectomy for Cancer of the Lung
(continued)

Patient Outcomes	Nursing Interventions	Rationale
	If the patient does not have a chest tube or if it is clamped most of the time, monitor for mediastinal shift with decreased ventilation secondary to compression of the remaining lung and decreased cardiac output secondary to impaired venous return to the heart. This is manifested by dyspnea, cyanosis, nasal flaring and intercostal retraction, severe chest pain, agitation, and tachycardia.	Accumulation of blood or fluid increases pressure on operative side, causing mediastinal shift and compromise of functioning tissue.

Evaluation: Compare the patient's status with the expected outcomes. If the outcomes are not met, reassess the patient and revise the plan.

Assessment Findings: Patient complains of chest pain. Patient occasionally moans. Patient grimaces and groans on moving.

Nursing Diagnosis: Pain related to chest surgery

Patient Outcomes	Nursing Interventions	Rationale
Patient states that pain is relieved. Patient moves and turns easily without grimacing, groaning, or other behavioral indications of pain.	Administer narcotic analgesics as ordered and needed in the early postoperative period, often every 3 hours. Observe for resultant respiratory depression. Be certain to give pain medication 30 minutes or so before exercises or other painful treatments.	Early analgesic administration provides more effective pain relief. Pain relief encourages compliance with postoperative procedures such as coughing, deep-breathing, and turning, which improve oxygenation.
	If patient-controlled analgesia pump is in use, monitor doses of medication used and their effectiveness.	Because narcotics have a depressant effect on respirations, care should be taken in their administration to the patient whose respiratory status is compromised. Administration 30 minutes before exercise allows medication to reach its maximum effectiveness.
	Splint patient's chest and avoid moving the chest tube when turning or moving.	Reduces pain and increases compliance with turning or moving.
	Maintain a calm, quiet environment.	Tension-reducing environment promotes relaxation and rest.
	Give back care and reposition frequently.	Reduces muscle tension and promotes rest and relaxation.

(continued)

Nursing Care Guide 16–1
Patients Undergoing Pneumonectomy for Cancer of the Lung
(continued)

Patient Outcomes	Nursing Interventions	Rationale
	Encourage the use of relaxation techniques.	Reduces tension level and diverts attention from pain.
	Provide diversion such as soft music in accordance with the patient's wishes.	Reduces muscle tension, promoting rest and relaxation.

Evaluation: Compare the patient's status with the expected outcomes. If the outcomes are not met, reassess the patient and revise the plan.

Assessment Findings: Patient says, "I feel like I'm tied up in knots. I feel like something awful is going to happen." Patient also complains of dry mouth and heart palpitations. Voice is tremulous, and patient cries easily. Patient has obvious restlessness and difficulty concentrating.

Nursing Diagnosis: Anxiety related to outcome of treatment, effects of cancer on family and lifestyle, possible recurrence, and death

Patient Outcomes	Nursing Interventions	Rationale
Patient expresses anxieties openly to nurse and significant other.	Schedule regular opportunities for the patient to discuss and vent anxieties in an unhurried manner.	Demonstrates concern, facilitates a supportive relationship, and promotes open communication.
Patient asks relevant questions about prognosis, treatments, and self-care.	Give the patient information in clear, simple terms regarding anticipated treatments and their effects.	Promotes effective communication.
	Encourage the patient to ask questions. Avoid false reassurance.	Encouraging the patient to ask questions and avoiding false reassurances promotes a positive interpersonal relationship and provides an environment conducive to sharing of feelings.
Patient expresses confidence in ability to cope.	Arrange for patients to meet with a cancer patient who has had successful surgery for cancer of the lung.	Provides a credible source of hope and information.
	Encourage the patient to join a support group and facilitate contact with the group.	Support groups provide an environment conducive to sharing of feelings as well as resources and problem-solving actions.
Signs of excessive anxiety, such as inability to attend to directions or conversation, shaking, and hand-wringing, are absent.	If needed and ordered, administer anti-anxiety medications.	Pharmacologically reduces anxiety, allowing patient to focus on positive feelings and actions.

Evaluation: Compare the patient's status with the expected outcomes. If the outcomes are not met, reassess the patient and revise the plan.

(continued)

Nursing Care Guide 16–1
Patients Undergoing Pneumonectomy for Cancer of the Lung
(continued)

Assessment Findings: Patient has a thoracotomy incision, which affects the trapezius, rhomboideus major, serratus anterior, and latissimus dorsi muscles. Spontaneous movements of the arm on the operative side are limited.

Nursing Diagnosis: Risk for impaired physical mobility related to surgical trauma affecting muscles that control shoulder movement

Patient Outcomes	Nursing Interventions	Rationale
Patient participates in arm and shoulder exercises as directed. Patient regains usual range of motion in the shoulder on the operative side.	Give passive range-of-motion exercise to the affected shoulder during the early postoperative period.	Maintains free range of joint motion.
	Once the patient is out of bed, begin active range-of-motion and arm and shoulder exercises, taught preoperatively, four times daily.	Maintains free range of joint motion, increases muscle strength, and promotes muscle tone.
	Continue to stress the importance of following the exercise routine if shoulder stiffness, limitation of movement, and loss of muscle strength are to be prevented.	Provides incentive to maintain exercise regimen.

Evaluation: Compare the patient's status with the expected outcomes. If the outcomes are not met, reassess the patient and revise the plan.

Assessment Findings: Patient and various family members describe the family as normally working well as a unit and supportive of its members. The patient's illness is described as creating a great deal of stress for family members.

Nursing Diagnosis: Risk for altered family processes related to one of its members being diagnosed with cancer of the lung and undergoing surgery

Patient Outcomes	Nursing Interventions	Rationale
Family members express thoughts and feelings regarding effects of cancer to each other and to health-care professional.	Speak with each family member regarding his or her own stress.	Allows each individual to realize that his or her feelings are important, reducing individual stress and promoting family interaction.
Family affirms by words and deeds that the patient is a valued family member. Family members work together to attack problems and share responsibility.	Discuss ways of constructive coping with the family such as use of humor, respect of individuality, mutual reliance and support, sharing thoughts and feelings, and shared decision-making.	Promotes use of constructive coping techniques.
	Facilitate freer family communication patterns by clarifying ambiguous messages.	Reduces miscommunication, thereby improving relationship among family members.

(continued)

Nursing Care Guide 16–1
Patients Undergoing Pneumonectomy for Cancer of the Lung
(continued)

Patient Outcomes	Nursing Interventions	Rationale
	Stress that crises carry potential for positive change.	Helps individual family members recognize the positive as well as the negative side of a crisis and helps them mobilize for effective coping.
Family uses community services and referrals as needed.	Make referrals as needed to community research groups such as the American Cancer Society.	Community resources help patients and families meet their needs.

Evaluation: Compare the patient's status with the expected outcomes. If the outcomes are not met, reassess the patient and revise the plan.

Assessment Findings: Patient has no previous experience with chest surgery and asks questions about self-care after discharge.

Nursing Diagnosis: Risk for altered health maintenance related to insufficient knowlege of self-care after discharge

Patient Outcomes	Nursing Interventions	Rationale
Patient explains need to regularly perform arm and shoulder exercises to prevent a limitation of mobility.	Review the importance of regular arm and shoulder exercises as done in the hospital to prevent limitations of mobility.	Reminds the patient of the need for continued exercise to improve range of motion and strength.
Patient demonstrates ability to perform arm and shoulder exercises without ongoing direction.	Instruct the patient to:	Provides information necessary for self-maintenance in the post-discharge period.
Patient explains instructions for self-care after discharge.	Continue with coughing exercises, deep-breathing, and other breathing exercises for 3 to 4 weeks after discharge. Apply heat and take oral analgesics as ordered for pain in the chest wall. Expect muscle weakness in affected side and avoid lifting heavy objects for at least 3 months after surgery.	
Patient describes need for follow-up care. Patient states date and location of next scheduled health-care visit.	Explain the importance of follow-up care. Inform patient of the purpose and date of the next health-care appointment. Be certain the patient knows the category and location of health-care practitioner to be seen.	Promotes compliance by providing rationale for follow-up care and information necessary to comply.

Evaluation: Compare the patient's status with the expected outcomes. If the outcomes are not met, reassess the patient and revise the plan.

(continued)

Nursing Care Guide 16–1
Patients Undergoing Pneumonectomy for Cancer of the Lung
(continued)

Additional Assessments and Interventions

Take vital signs every 15 minutes for 2 hours and then every hour. Decrease frequency as the patient stabilizes and progresses through the postoperative period.

Assess carefully for cardiac dysrhythmias, which are common after pneumonectomy and are most likely to occur from the second to the sixth postoperative days in patients older than age 50.

Check chest dressing for bleeding. Report bleeding if present because drainage on thoracic dressings is not expected.

Monitor fluid and electrolyte status. Obtain daily weights and check central venous pressure every hour for indication of hypervolemia (more than 12 cm H_2O) or hypovolemia (less than 5 cm H_2O). Check that urinary output is at least 30 mL/hour.

Give fluids by mouth when alert and progress to the patient's usual diet over 72 hours.

respiratory tract diseases are more likely to be superimposed on age-related changes and coexisting disease and medication regimens. This results in greater severity, increased risk of complications, and a highly variable presentation and course. The earliest manifestation of lower respiratory disorders in older adults is often a change in functioning, particularly a change in mental status.

Pneumonia in the elderly can be very serious and, with influenza, is the leading infectious cause of death among this age group. Placing the patient at risk for pneumonia are the loss of elasticity in the lung, weakened respiratory muscles, decreased effectiveness of the mucociliary escalator, decreased forced vital capacity, decreased effectiveness of immune function, and, in some cases, the coexistence of chronic pulmonary disease.

Although the potential causative organisms are the same as in other age groups, older adults have a greater incidence of gram-negative disease, which is associated with a higher mortality rate. The clinical presentation of pneumonia is frequently atypical. An insidious deterioration in overall health status and mental changes often are the first manifestations. In some cases, an unexplained delayed recovery from another health problem or the sudden worsening of a coexistent problem constitutes the initial sign of disease. Fever, cough, and purulent sputum—the classic signs of pneumonia—may be absent, although increased respiratory rate and leukocytosis with a left shift are commonly seen. Other symptoms that may arise are chills, lethargy, vomiting, dyspnea, and stabbing chest pain. Thus, the early recognition of pneumonia in the elderly requires as-

tute observation and a high degree of clinical suspicion. Because of weakened cough and frequency of dehydration, obtaining a sputum specimen for identification of the causative organism can be difficult.

Tuberculosis is another disease for which the elderly, particularly those in institutional settings, are at risk. Many of today's elderly people were exposed to family members or friends with tuberculosis during childhood. Because prophylactic medication was not available until the 1950s, many of these people are now at risk for active disease, particularly in light of age-related impairments in immunity. Like pneumonia, the presentation of tuberculosis in the elderly is frequently atypical. Thus, it should be considered a possibility in any patient with unexplained cough or low-grade fever. Information on past exposure as well as tuberculin test results should be included in all patient histories.

Older adults should be encouraged to have annual influenza immunizations and a one-time pneumonia vaccination. Tuberculin testing is often performed upon admission to a nursing home or other institutional setting.

Chapter Review

1. What are the differences between hospital-acquired and community-acquired pneumonias in terms of cause, risk factors, treatment, and prognosis?

2. What information should be given to a 66-year-old patient who asks about the influenza vaccine?

3. What is the meaning of a positive tuberculin test?

4. Why is strict compliance with antitubercular drug therapy essential?

5. In what ways are emphysema and chronic bronchitis similar?

6. How does pursed-lip breathing assist in control of dyspnea?

7. How does a large pulmonary embolism place a patient at risk for right ventricular failure?

8. What signs developing in a patient with an open pneumothorax covered with an occlusive dressing indicate that the dressing must be removed?

9. What symptoms might be reported by a patient with chronic syndrome of inappropriate antidiuretic hormone?

10. What are the reasons for the similarities and differences in nutritional teaching for a patient with lung cancer and a patient with COPD?

Bibliography

Ahrens TS. Changing perspectives in the assessment of oxygenation. Crit Care Nurse 1993; 13(4):78.

Aloi A, Burns SM. Continuous airway pressure monitoring in the critical care setting. Crit Care Nurse 1995; 15(2):66.

American Thoracic Society. Guidelines for the initial management of adults with community-acquired pneumonia: Diagnosis, assessment of severity, and initial antimicrobial therapy. Am Rev Respir Dis 1993; 148:1418.

Blair JE, Conner BH, Huss K, et al, the Nurses' Asthma Education Working Group: Nurses: Partners in asthma care. Bethesda, MD: National Institutes of Health, National Heart, Lung, and Blood Institute, 1995. NIH Publication No 95-3308.

Centers for Disease Control. Asthma mortality and hospitalization among children and young adults—United States 1990–1993. MMWR Morb Mortal Wkly Rep 1996; 45:350.

Centers for Disease Control. Asthma—United States 1989–1992. MMWR Morb Mortal Wkly Rep 1995; 43:952.

Centers for Disease Control. Screening for tuberculosis and tuberculosis infection in high risk populations: Recommendations of the Advisory Council for the Elimination of Tuberculosis. MMWR 1995; 44(RR-11):19.

Centers for Disease Control. Guidelines for preventing the transmission of *Mycobacterium tuberculosis* in health care facilities. MMWR 1994; 43(RR-13):1.

Centers for Disease Control. Guidelines for prevention of nosocomial pneumonia. Am J Infect Cont 1994; 22:247.

Clochesy J, Breu c, Cardin S, Whittaker AA, Rudy EB. Critical care nursing. 2nd ed. Philadelphia: WB Saunders, 1996.

Dantzker D, MacIntyre N, Bakow E. Comprehensive respiratory care. Philadelphia: WB Saunders, 1995.

Dickson SL. Understanding the oxyhemoglobin dissociation curve. Crit Care Nurse 1995; 15(5):54.

Fein AM. Pneumonia in the elderly. Med Clin North Am Sept 1994; 78(5):1015.

Fraser RS, Paré JAP, Fraser RG, Paré PD. Synopsis of disease of the chest. 2nd ed. Philadelphia: WB Saunders, 1994.

Garvey C. Tuberculosis management in the home care setting. Caring 1994; XIII(8):12.

Hammer J. Challenging diagnosis: adult respiratory distress syndrome. Crit Care Nurse 1995; 15(5):46.

Higgins MW. Chronic airway disease in the United States: Trends and determinants Chest 1996; 238

Howland WA. Defending your patient against nosocomial pneumonia. Nursing 1995; 25(8):62.

Iseman M. Treatment of multidrug-resistant tuberculosis. N Engl J Med 1993; 329(11):784. [Published erratum appears in N Engl J Med 1993;329(19):1435.

Jardins T, Burton G. Clinical manifestations and assessment of respiratory diseases. 3rd ed. St. Louis: CV Mosby, 1995.

Lasater-Erhard M. The effect of patient position on arterial oxygen saturation. Crit Care Nurse 1995; 15(5):31.

Laskowski-Jones L. Meeting the challenge of chest trauma. Am J Nurs 1995; 95(9):23.

Kim MJ, McFarland GK, McLane AM. Pocket guide to nursing diagnosis. 7th ed. St. Louis: Mosby-Year Book, 1996.

Middleton AD. Managing asthma: It takes teamwork. Am J Nurs 1997; 97(11):39.

Misasi RS, Keyes JL. Matching and mismatching ventilation and perfusion in the lung. Crit Care Nurse 1996; 16(3):23.

Murry J, Nadel J. Textbook of respiratory medicine. 2nd ed. Philadelphia: WB Saunders, 1994.

National Heart, Lung, and Blood Institute (NHLBI). National asthma program, expert panel report: Guidelines for the diagnosis and management of asthma. J Allergy Clin Immunol 1991; 88:421.

National Heart, Lung, and Blood Institute and World Health Organization. Global initiative for asthma. Publication no. 95-3659. Bethesda, MD: National Institutes of Health, 1995.

Ortiz C, LaForce MF. Prevention of community-acquired pneumonia. Med Clin North Am Sept 1994, 78(5):1173.

Rachelefsky GS. Asthma update: new approaches and partnerships. J Pediatr Health Care 1995; 9:12.

Rakel RE (ed). Conn's current therapy. Philadelphia: WB Saunders, 1995.

Reichman LB. Multidrug-resistant tuberculosis: Meeting the challenge. Hosp Pract 1994; 29(5):85.

Rom W, Garay S. Tuberculosis. Boston: Little, Brown, 1996.

Ruggles L. Auto-Peep: Measurement issues and nursing interventions. Crit Care Nurse 1995; 15(2):30.

Saunders C, Ho M (eds). Current emergency diagnosis and treatment. 4th ed. Stamford, CT: Appleton & Lange, 1992.

Sinski A, Corbo J. Surfactant replacement in adults and children with ARDS. An effective therapy. Crit Care Nurse 1994; 14(6):54.

Stamp D, Arnold M. Tuberculosis in home care: Complying with OSHA. Caring 1995; XIV(2):16.

Thompson R. Prevention of nosocomial pneumonia. Med Clin North Am Sept 1994, 78(5):1185.

Tierney LM, McPhee SJ, Papadakis MA (eds). Current medical diagnosis and treatment. 35th ed. Connecticut: Appleton and Lange, 1996.

Urban NA, Greenlee KK, Krumberger JM, Winkelman C. Guidelines for critical care nursing. St. Louis: Mosby-Year Book, 1995.

Unit V

Neurologic Dysfunction

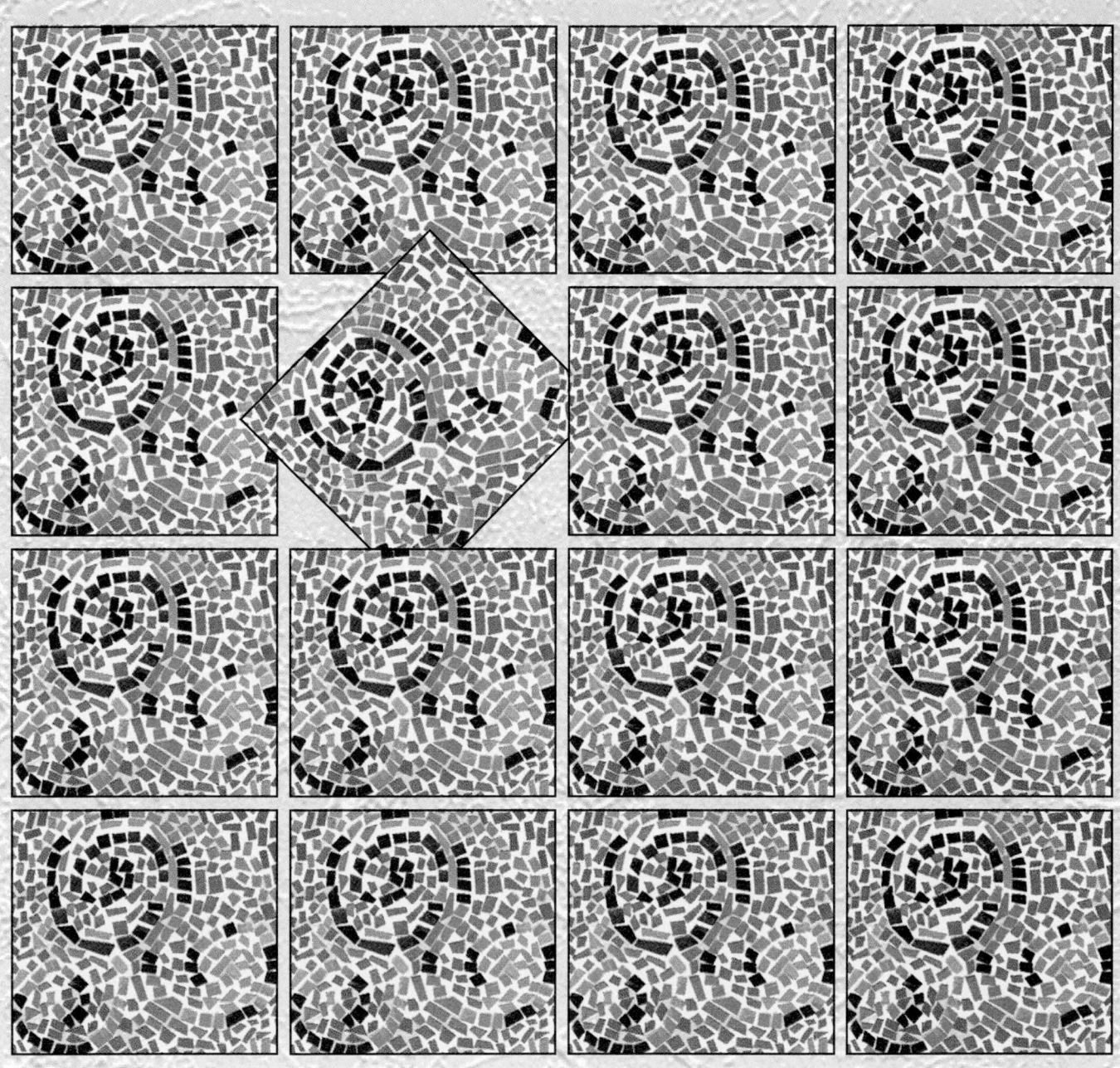

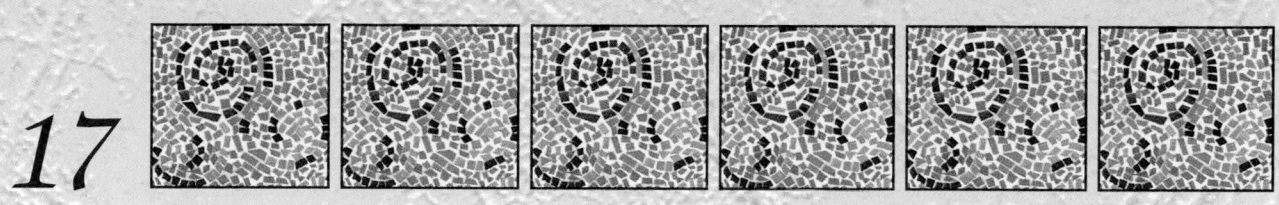

17

Knowledge Base for Patients with Neurologic Dysfunction

Study Outcomes

After studying this chapter, you should be able to:

1. Explain the normal anatomy and physiology of the nervous system.
2. Describe common clinical manifestations of neurologic dysfunction.
3. Identify information and physical examination data essential to the assessment of the nervous system.
4. Describe basic diagnostic tests and modalities of medical management used in the treatment of patients with neurologic dysfunction.
5. Describe basic intracranial and spinal surgery as used in the treatment of patients with neurologic dysfunction.
6. Identify data essential to the assessment of patients undergoing treatment of neurologic dysfunction.
7. State nursing diagnoses and related expected patient outcomes commonly applicable to patients undergoing treatment of neurologic dysfunction.
8. Describe nursing interventions, with their rationales, commonly applicable to patients undergoing treatment of neurologic dysfunction.
9. Explain the basis for evaluation of nursing care provided to patients undergoing treatment of neurologic disorders.
10. Identify special considerations for the elderly patient with altered neurologic function.
11. Identify alternative treatment and care settings for patients with neurologic dysfunction, and the services related to community-based care.

The nervous system is a communication network that provides for a constant relay of information to and from the environment. The ability of the central nervous system (CNS) to interpret incoming messages from the environment and then formulate and transmit a response via the peripheral nervous system (PNS) enables ongoing and evolving interaction between individual and environment.

The CNS underlies the ability to reason, to entertain abstract concepts such as past and future, and to experience emotion. In other words, it is the basis of function as a human being.

In preparation for the study of the nursing care of patients with disorders of this complex system, this chapter begins with a review of the anatomy and physiology of the system. Next, clinical manifestations common to many types of nervous system dysfunction, basic assessment of nervous system function, and frequently used diagnostic tests are discussed. The chapter then proceeds to a discussion of the general care required of patients having cranial or spinal surgery and ends with a section on special considerations relative to the care of the elderly.

Nursing care for patients undergoing testing for neurologic dysfunction may occur in the hospital, clinics, outpatient centers, or even the home. Treatments common to many neurologic disorders, such as those discussed in this chapter, may be completed in a variety of settings. It is becoming more common for patients to undergo neurologic testing as an outpatient rather than as an inpatient, unless there are complicating disorders or the patient is seriously ill.

Anatomy and Physiology

The nervous system is composed of the CNS and the PNS. The CNS includes the brain and spinal cord. The PNS includes the 12 pairs of cranial nerves, 31 pairs of spinal nerves, and the autonomic nervous system. It is the PNS that connects the CNS with organ systems, skin, and muscles.

CELLULAR STRUCTURE

Two main types of cells are found within the nervous system: neurons and neuroglia. Neurons are the basic functioning units, whereas neuroglial cells are viewed as providing assistance and support to the neurons.

Neurons

The basic function of neurons is to conduct impulses toward or away from the CNS. *Afferent* neurons conduct impulses toward the CNS. *Efferent* neurons conduct impulses away from the CNS. A neuron (Fig. 17–1) consists of a cell body, in which metabolic activities are carried out, dendrites, which conduct impulses to the cell body, and axons, which conduct impulses away from the cell body.

Nerve cell bodies primarily form the gray matter of the CNS. Nerve cell bodies grouped outside the CNS are known as ganglia.

The white matter of the CNS is made up of the myelinated axons of the neurons. Myelin is a white substance made up of lipids and proteins that encases many axons. Most long axons are myelinated, whereas shorter axons tend not to be.

Only peripheral nerves can recover from neuron trauma or injury. Peripheral nerves regenerate at the rate of 1.5 mm/d. The degree of recovery is based on severity of the injury and proximity to the cell body and distal and proximal ends.

Neuroglia

The neuroglial cells provide assistance, support, nutrition, and protection to neurons in the CNS. There are four types of neuroglial cells (Fig. 17–2):

- Oligodendroglia, which form myelin and surround axons and dendrites
- Astrocytes, which have a star-shaped appearance and provide nutrition and a protective barrier for neurons

- Microglia, which are known as phagocytic cells
- Ependymal cells, which line the cerebral ventricular system and aid in the production of cerebrospinal fluid (CSF)

NERVE IMPULSE TRANSMISSION

Neurons transmit impulses through the propagation of action potentials along conductive fibers. Action potentials are rapid changes in the membrane potential and consist of three stages: resting, depolarization, and repolarization.

In the resting stage, the neuron has a negative membrane potential (ie, inside the nerve fiber is more negative than the potential of the intercellular fluid outside the fiber). Because of this large negative difference, the membrane is said to be polarized. In the depolarization stage, the membrane becomes permeable to sodium. The resultant flow of sodium across the membrane causes the negative potential to be lost and a positive potential to occur. This is followed almost instantly by the repolarization stage, in which the sodium channels close and the potassium channels open wider, leading to an influx of potassium and restoration of the negative resting potential (Fig. 17–3).

Membrane depolarization, which can be initiated by chemical, mechanical, electrical, or thermal

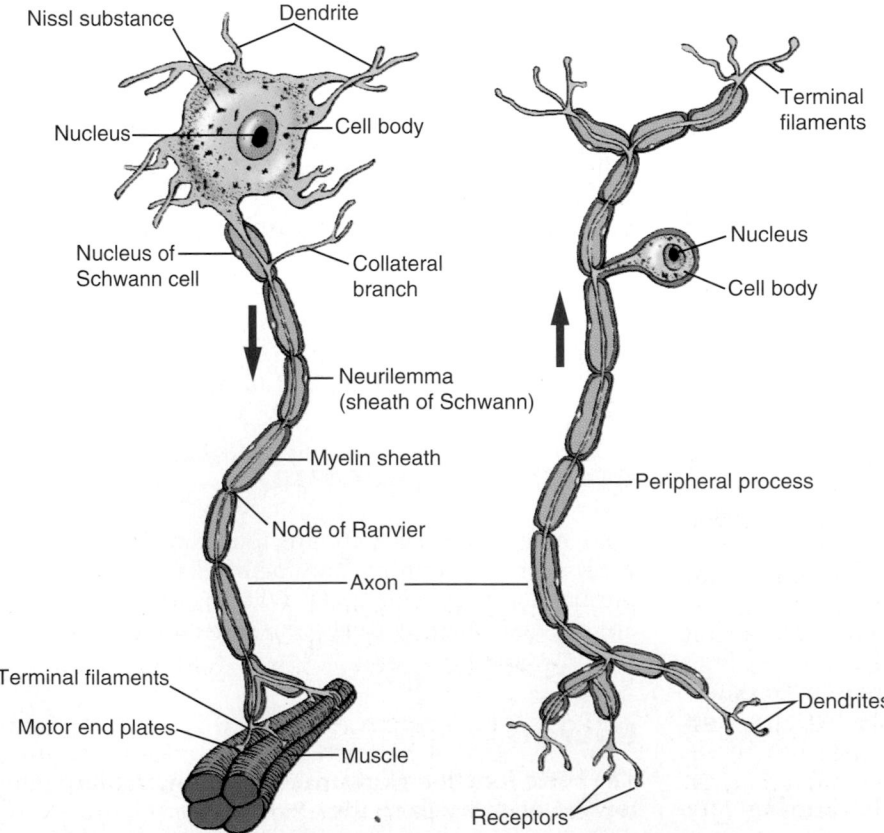

Effector Neuron   **Receptor Neuron**

Figure 17–1

Diagram of a motor (effector) neuron and a sensory (receptor) neuron. Arrows indicate the direction of impulse conduction.

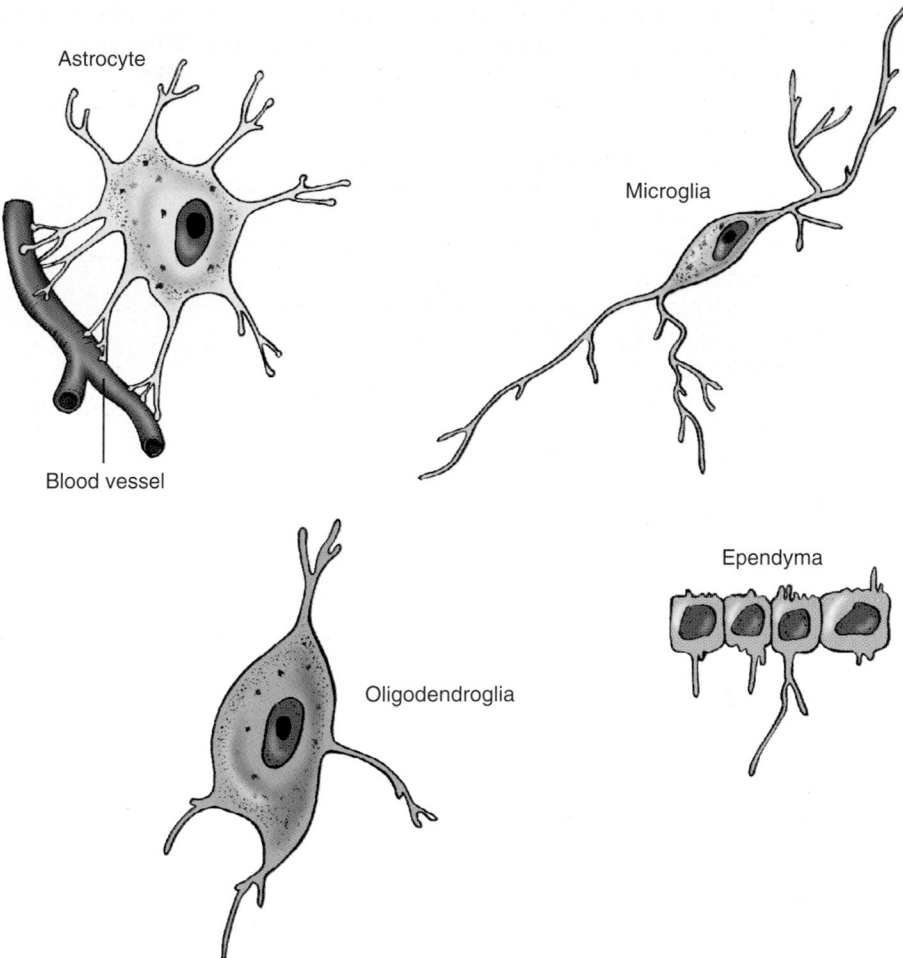

Figure 17-2
The four types of neuroglial cells, which provide support, nutrition, and protection to neurons in the central nervous system.

means, extends from one neuron to another, resulting in impulse transmission.

The synapse is where nerve impulses are transmitted from neuron to neuron. Nerve transmission at the synapse involves a chemical process. Each axon contains presynaptic neurotransmitters. As the impulse travels down the axon, away from the cell body, neurotransmitters are released at the terminal end and are taken up by the dendrites of the postsynaptic neuron. Neurotransmitters can be excitatory (eg, dopamine, serotonin, acetylcholine) or inhibitory (eg, gamma-aminobutyric acid). Neurotransmitters that are excitatory cause the postsynaptic neuron to depolarize, allowing nerve impulse transmission to occur, whereas neurotransmitters that are inhibitory tend not to allow the postsynaptic neuron to depolarize, inhibiting nerve impulse transmission.

Neuromuscular transmission occurs when the nerve impulse is transmitted from nerve to muscle. This takes place at the neuromuscular junction. As the nerve impulse travels down to the end of the axon, acetylcholine is released into the synaptic cleft. The acetylcholine travels across the synaptic cleft and binds with the postsynaptic receptor sites on the muscle, increasing its permeability to sodium

and potassium. An action potential results, calcium ions are released, and proteins bind together, formulating the contractile motion of the muscle. An enzyme known as acetylcholinesterase, found in the synapse, inactivates the acetylcholine milliseconds after its release. This returns the muscle fiber to its resting position, ready for the next stimulus.

PROTECTIVE COVERINGS OF THE BRAIN AND SPINAL CORD

Skull and Vertebral Column

The purpose of the bones of the skull and vertebral column (Fig. 17-4) is to protect the most sensitive and vulnerable structures of the body: the brain and the spinal cord.

The skull is composed of the 8 bones of the cranium and the 14 bones of the face. The cranium is the portion of the skull that forms the cranial vault, the protective covering for the brain.

The vertebral column is made up of 33 vertebrae: 7 cervical, 12 thoracic, 5 lumbar, 5 sacral, and 4

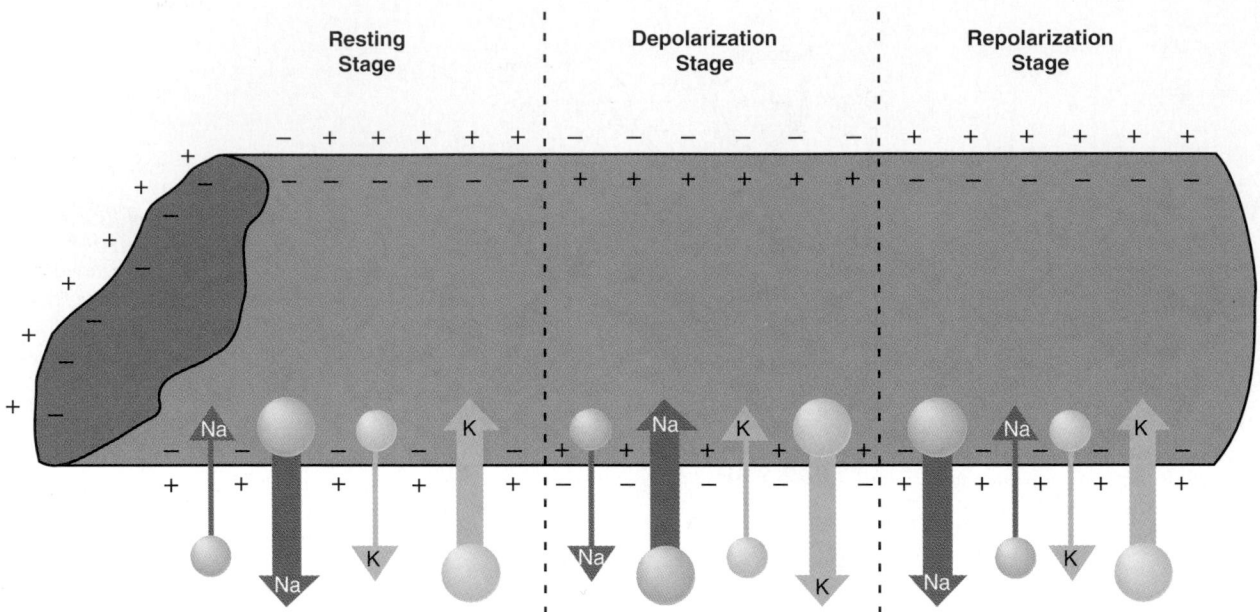

Figure 17–3
Successive stages of the action potential: resting stage, depolarization stage, repolarization stage.

coccygeal. Each vertebra is stacked on another, forming a flexible column that protects the spinal cord. Intervertebral disks of varying shape and size can be found between the individual vertebrae. They act as a cushion for vertebral column movement.

Meninges

There are three membranes, or meninges, that cover the brain and spinal cord: the dura mater, the arachnoid, and the pia mater (Fig. 17–5). The function of these membranes is to provide support and protection.

The dura mater is the dense, fibrous, outermost covering. It has a rich blood supply fed by the middle meningeal branch of the external carotid artery. The dura folds in four locations to form compartments within the cranial vault: the falx cerebri, tentorium cerebelli, falx cerebelli, and diaphragma sellae. The falx cerebri forms a vertical fissure that separates the cerebral hemispheres of the brain. The sagittal venous sinuses are formed between the two layers of dura at this location. The tentorium cerebelli forms the roof of the posterior fossa, separating the cerebellum from the occipital lobes. The transverse venous sinus is located between the layers of dura in this area. The falx cerebri attaches to the midline of the tentorium. The falx cerebelli forms a posterior cerebellar notch dividing the cerebellum into lateral hemispheres. The diaphragma sellae forms the roof of the sella turcica, where the pituitary gland is located.

The arachnoid is the second meningeal layer, located under the dura. It is a delicate, vascular membrane that loosely surrounds the brain and spinal cord. Arachnoid villi granulations are clusters of arachnoid and can be found projecting into the sagittal venous sinuses, allowing CSF to pass from the subarachnoid space into the venous sinus.

The pia mater is the most delicate meningeal layer. It adheres closely to the surface of the brain and spinal cord. The spinal cord pia mater is thicker, firmer, and less vascular than that of the brain.

Three meningeal spaces are formed by the meninges: the epidural, subdural, and subarachnoid. The epidural space is located between the outer layer of dura and the skull. The subdural space is located below the inner layer of dura and the arachnoid. The subarachnoid space is located between the arachnoid and the pia mater.

BLOOD SUPPLY AND CIRCULATION

Blood flows at a rate of 750 mL/min in the adult brain, carrying vital supplies of oxygen and glucose. The brain consumes 20% of the body's oxygen supply to oxidize glucose for energy. Without this supply, the brain suffers irreversible damage literally within minutes.

Cerebral Circulation

ARTERIAL BLOOD SUPPLY

Arterial blood is supplied to the brain through the internal carotid arteries and the basilar artery. The

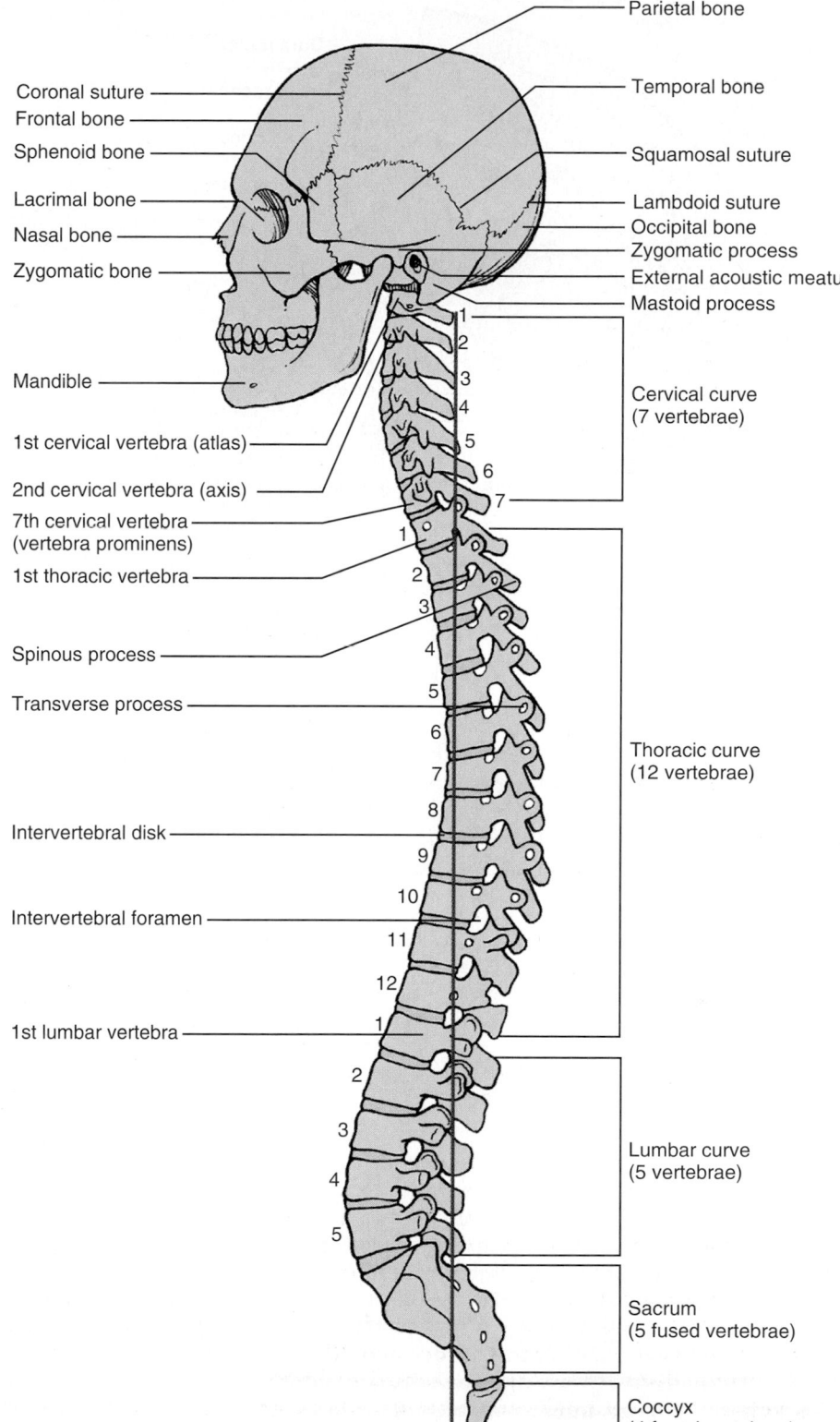

Parietal bone
Coronal suture
Frontal bone
Sphenoid bone
Temporal bone
Squamosal suture
Lacrimal bone
Nasal bone
Lambdoid suture
Occipital bone
Zygomatic bone
Zygomatic process
External acoustic meatus
Mastoid process
Cervical curve
(7 vertebrae)
Mandible
1st cervical vertebra (atlas)
2nd cervical vertebra (axis)
7th cervical vertebra
(vertebra prominens)
1st thoracic vertebra
Spinous process
Transverse process
Thoracic curve
(12 vertebrae)
Intervertebral disk
Intervertebral foramen
1st lumbar vertebra
Lumbar curve
(5 vertebrae)
Sacrum
(5 fused vertebrae)
Coccyx
(4 fused vertebrae)

Figure 17–4

Bony structure of the skull and vertebral column.

internal carotid artery originates as the common carotid, which branches from the aorta and subdivides into the internal and external carotid arteries. The basilar artery originates as two vertebral arteries that branch from the subclavian artery and then merge at the level of the pons to form the basilar artery (Fig. 17–6).

The internal carotid arteries and the basilar ar-

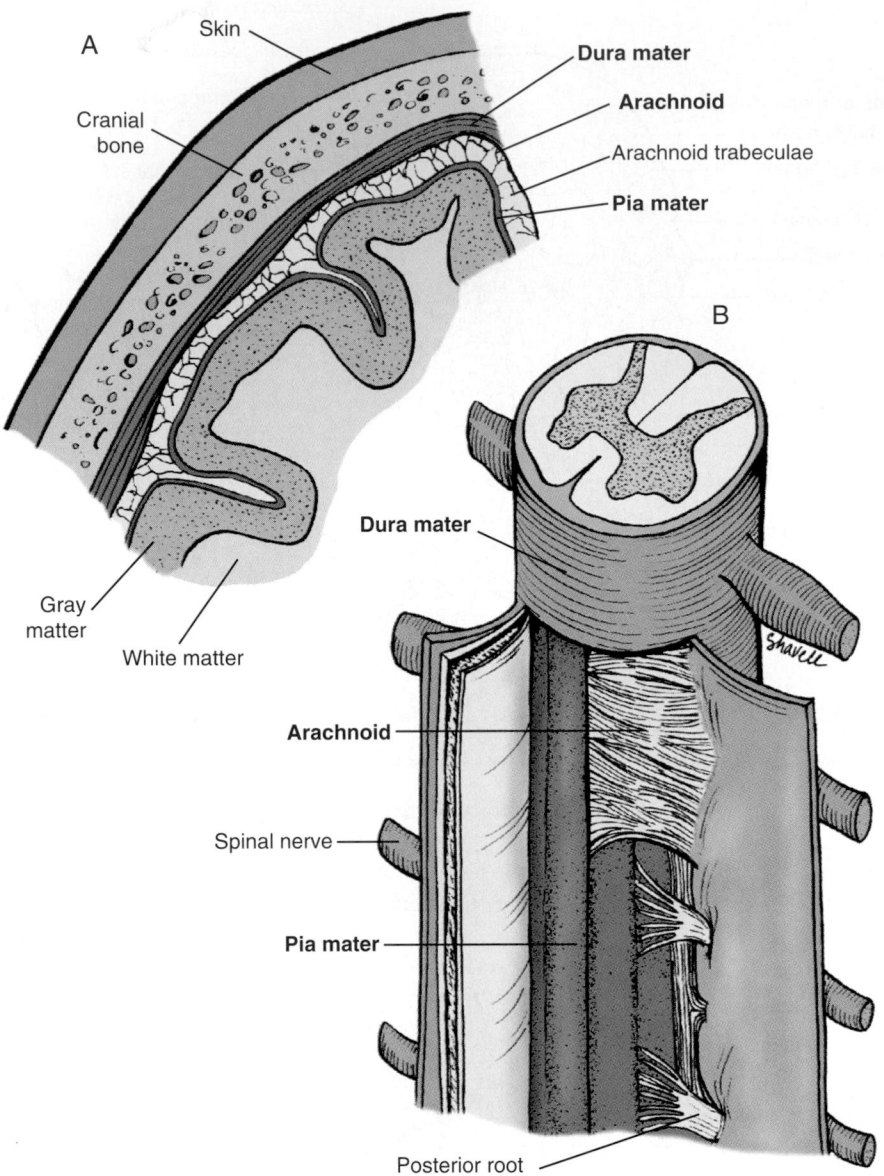

A

Skin

Cranial
bone

Dura mater

Arachnoid

Arachnoid trabeculae

Pia mater

Gray
matter

White matter

B

Dura mater

Arachnoid

Spinal nerve

Pia mater

Posterior root

Figure 17–5

The three meninges, or membranes, that cover the brain (*A*) and spinal cord (*B*). The dura mater is of leathery consistency and is the outermost of the three membranes. The arachnoid, which is loose, vascular, and like a spider web, is the middle membrane. The pia mater is thin, delicate, and closely adherent to the brain and spinal cord.

tery join the circle of Willis, which is located at the base of the skull. There are three major pairs of arterial branches from the circle of Willis that deliver blood to the brain: the anterior, middle, and posterior cerebral arteries (*see* Fig. 17–6).

The anterior cerebral artery supplies the medial surface of the frontal and parietal lobes and adjacent cortex. The middle cerebral artery supplies the lateral surface of the cerebral hemispheres and accounts for 60% of the cerebral circulation. The posterior cerebral artery supplies the inferior and medial surface of the temporal and occipital lobes and choroid plexus.

VENOUS DRAINAGE

The cerebral venous drainage is composed of dural venous sinuses. Venous sinuses are located and formed by vascular canals between the two layers of

the dura mater. There are no valves. Blood is drained from these sinuses into the internal jugular veins. Three major venous sinuses are the sagittal sinus at the convexity of the brain, the cavernous sinus at the inferior surface, and the transverse sinus at the lateral surface.

Spinal Circulation

The spinal cord primarily receives its arterial blood supply from the spinal arteries, which originate from the vertebral arteries. One anterior spinal artery supplies two-thirds of the spinal cord with arterial blood as it runs anteriorly the full length of the cord. Two posterior spinal arteries, each of which runs the full length of the cord, supply the posterior one-third of the cord with arterial blood. In addition, feeder vessels support blood supply to the cord.

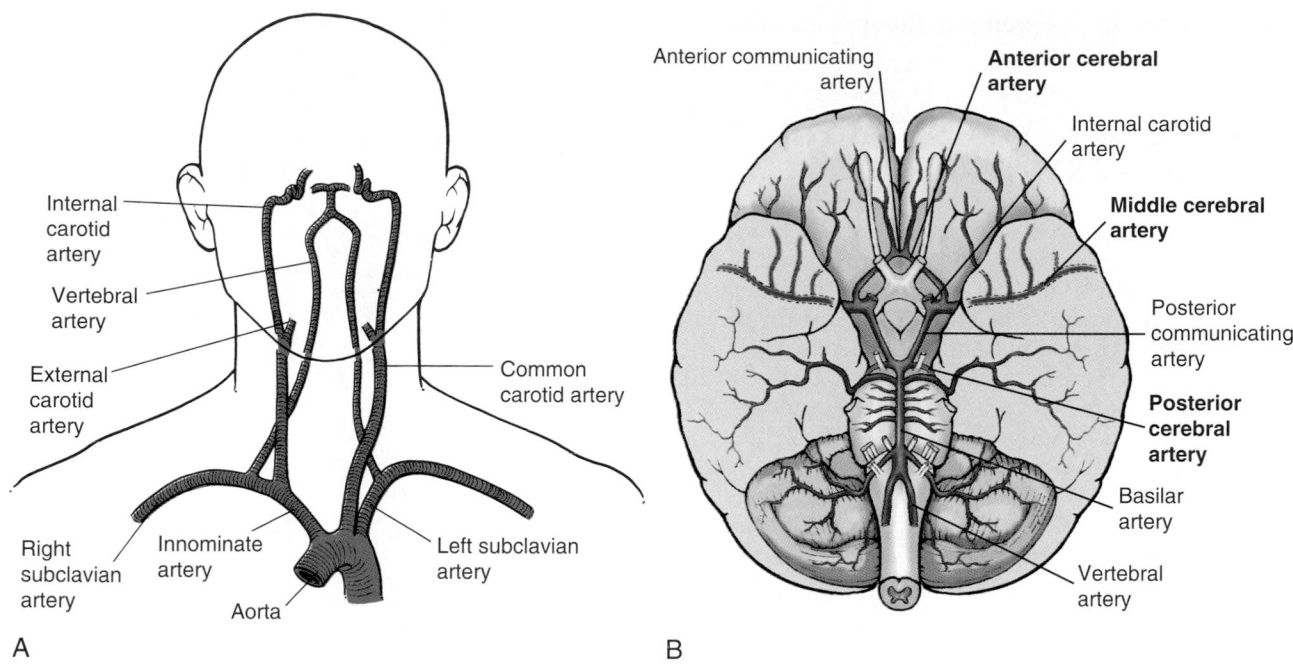

Figure 17-6

A, Major arteries supplying blood to the brain. *B,* The circle of Willis. Note the anterior, middle, and posterior cerebral arteries, which are the major pairs of arteries supplying the cerebrum.

BLOOD-BRAIN BARRIER

The blood-brain barrier is composed of capillary epithelium and an astrocyte membrane close to the neurons. Because of the tight junction formed at this site, a barrier is formed. This barrier selectively permits substances to pass from the blood into the neurons. Many medications are prohibited from pene-

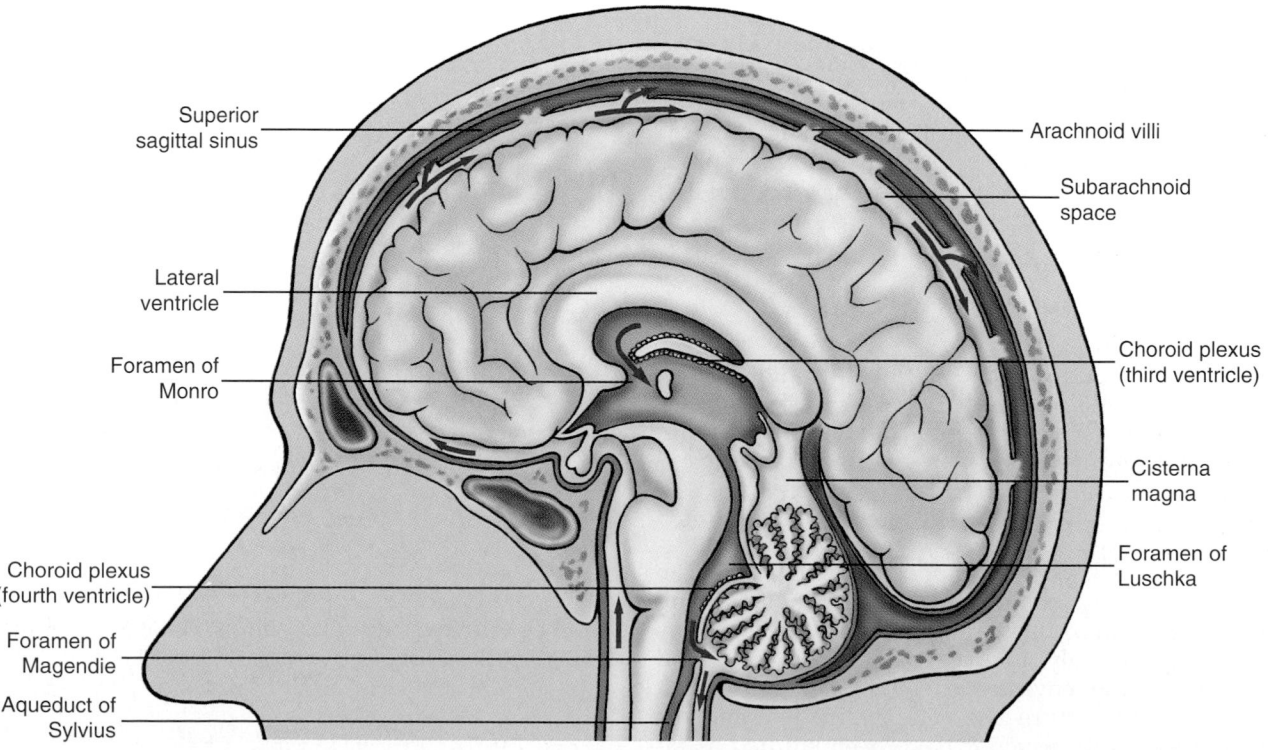

Figure 17-7

Cerebral spinal fluid circulation. Cerebrospinal fluid is produced by the choroid plexus in the lateral ventricles and flows around the brain and spinal cord until it reaches the arachnoid villi, from which it is absorbed into the venous circulation. Arrows indicate the major pathway of cerebrospinal fluid flow.

trating this barrier, preventing them from affecting the CNS.

CEREBROSPINAL FLUID AND THE CEREBRAL VENTRICULAR SYSTEM

Cerebrospinal fluid is a colorless, odorless fluid that fills the cerebral ventricles and subarachnoid spaces to provide a "cushion" for the CNS. This helps to prevent undue injury from sudden or abrupt movements. There is approximately 145 mL of CSF in the adult: 25 mL in the cerebral ventricles, 30 mL in the subarachnoid space, and 90 mL in the lumbar subarachnoid cistern. The pressure of CSF, while the patient is in a recumbent position, is normally less than 200 mm H_2O.

Cerebrospinal fluid is formed primarily in the choroid plexus, a structure found in the lateral ventricles. CSF is excreted constantly at a rate of 25 to 30 mL/h.

CSF flows in a closed, one-way system (Fig. 17–7). As the CSF is formed in the lateral ventricles, it passes through the foramen of Monro into the third ventricle. It then passes through the aqueduct of Sylvius into the fourth ventricle, exiting through the foramina of Luschka and Magendie into the subarachnoid spaces of the brain and spinal cord.

Enlarged areas of the subarachnoid space that contain a quantity of CSF are known as cisterns. The cisterna magna is located between the medulla and cerebellum, and the lumbar cistern is located at the base of the spinal cord at the L-2 to S-1 vertebral levels.

CSF is reabsorbed constantly into the body's venous system. It passes from the subarachnoid space through the arachnoid villi, which are one-way valve projections into the dural venous sinuses. This allows for a direct pathway for CSF and waste products to enter the venous system and to be excreted by the body.

CENTRAL NERVOUS SYSTEM

The CNS, composed of the brain and spinal cord, accounts for approximately 2% of overall body weight (Fig. 17–8). This equates to a volume of approximately 1400 to 1500 mL.

Brain

The brain is a highly developed structure and can perform the most complicated activities. It is composed of the cerebrum, brain stem, and cerebellum. The brain not only interprets impulses from and responds to the environment but also stores that information for future use. The brain, its function, and its relation to behavior have been studied as far back as 3000 B.C. Today, it is possible to identify specific localization of function and begin to under-

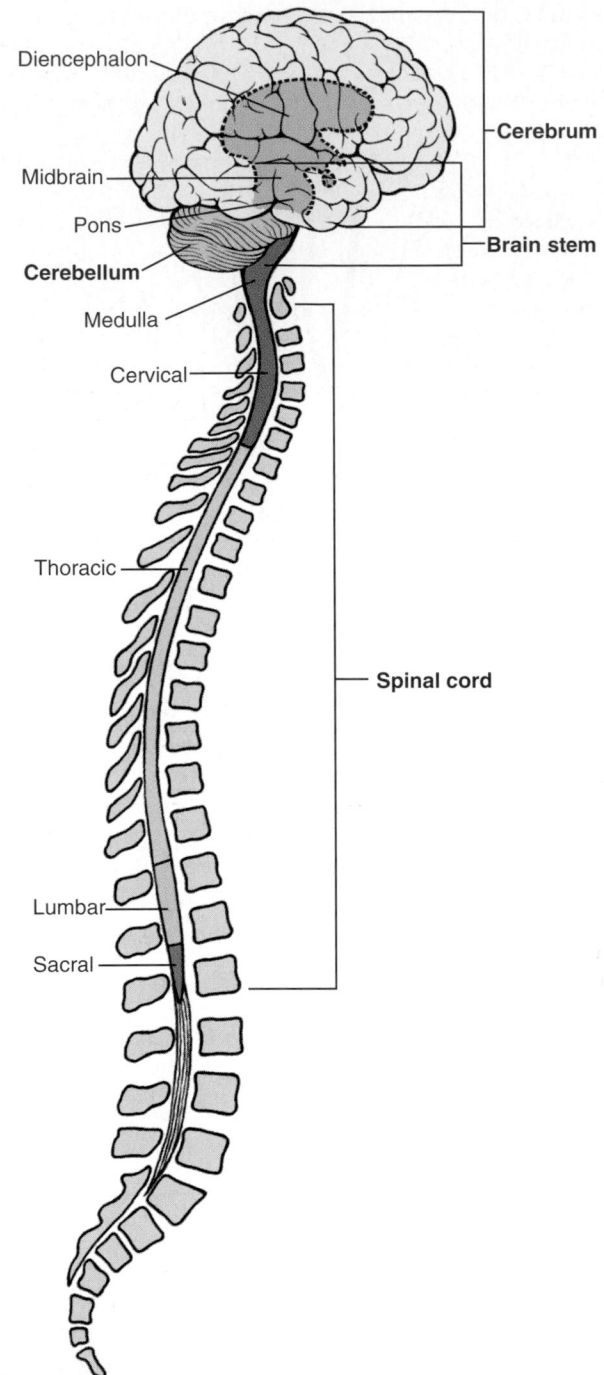

Figure 17–8
Lateral view of the central nervous system, showing its main divisions.

stand the brain-behavior relationship. The cerebrum can be further divided into the cerebral hemispheres, diencephalon, and basal ganglia.

CEREBRAL HEMISPHERES

The cerebral hemispheres have a convoluted surface with many peaks, known as gyri (singular, gyrus), and valleys or indentations, known as sulci (sulcus). The hemispheres are connected by a structure known as the corpus callosum. This a thick structure of nerve fibers that directly connects corresponding areas of each hemisphere to one another.

The cerebral hemispheres are subdivided into the lobes of the brain: frontal, temporal, parietal, and occipital. There are corresponding lobes on each cerebral hemisphere. Each lobe has areas of specialized function (Fig. 17–9).

The frontal lobes make up approximately one-third of the mass of the cerebral hemispheres and are thought to be the seat of the highest cognitive functions (abstract thinking, judgment, emotion). Motor function is also localized in front of the central sulcus on the cerebral motor cortex. The specific areas for motor control can be configured in a topographic scheme (Fig. 17–10). Motor speech (Broca's area) is also located in the frontal lobe of the dominant hemisphere.

The temporal lobes are located on the lateral aspects of the cerebral hemispheres. Much of the temporal lobes is concerned with perception of verbal material (Wernicke's area, dominant hemisphere), memory, behavior, and emotions.

The parietal lobes are strategically located between the frontal, occipital, and temporal lobes. The anterior border is formed by the central sulcus. The posterior border is formed by the parieto-occipital sulcus. The parietal lobe is considered the sensory associative area of the brain. The primary sensory cortex is located in the parietal lobe posterior to the central sulcus. It is arranged in a topographic scheme similar to that of the cerebral motor cortex (see Fig. 17–10). The primary purpose is to analyze gross aspects of deep sensation and cutaneous sensations of touch, position, pressure, and vibration. It is also responsible for spatial-perceptual abilities.

The primary visual cortex is located in the occipital lobe in the most posterior portion of the cerebral hemispheres. Its major functions include vision and visual interpretation.

Although no two human brains are exactly alike, all normally developed brains share basic characteristics and qualities. There are highly specialized locations related to behavior and function as well as lateral symmetry of function between the hemispheres.

The most obvious functional difference between the hemispheres is that the left hemisphere, in approximately 93% of persons, is responsible for language (ie, provides the ability to speak and understand the spoken word). For this reason, the left hemisphere is considered to be dominant. The left hemisphere is the primary mediator of verbal function. Wernicke's area, responsible for the reception of verbal input, and Broca's area, responsible for motor phonation, are also located in the left hemisphere.

The right hemisphere, however, does not lie dormant. It is responsible for the processing of information that does not readily lend itself to verbalization. The primary function involved here is the perception of spatial orientation and perspective.

BASAL GANGLIA

The basal ganglia structure is located deep in the cerebral hemispheres. It is composed of gray matter.

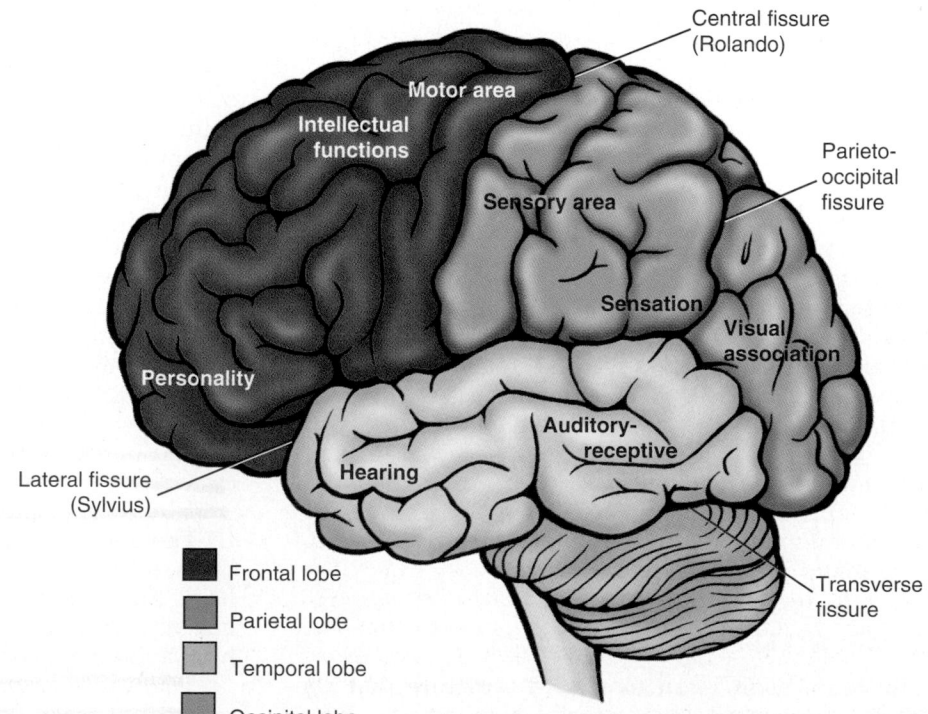

Figure 17–9

Lobes of the cerebral hemispheres and specialized functions of the lobes.

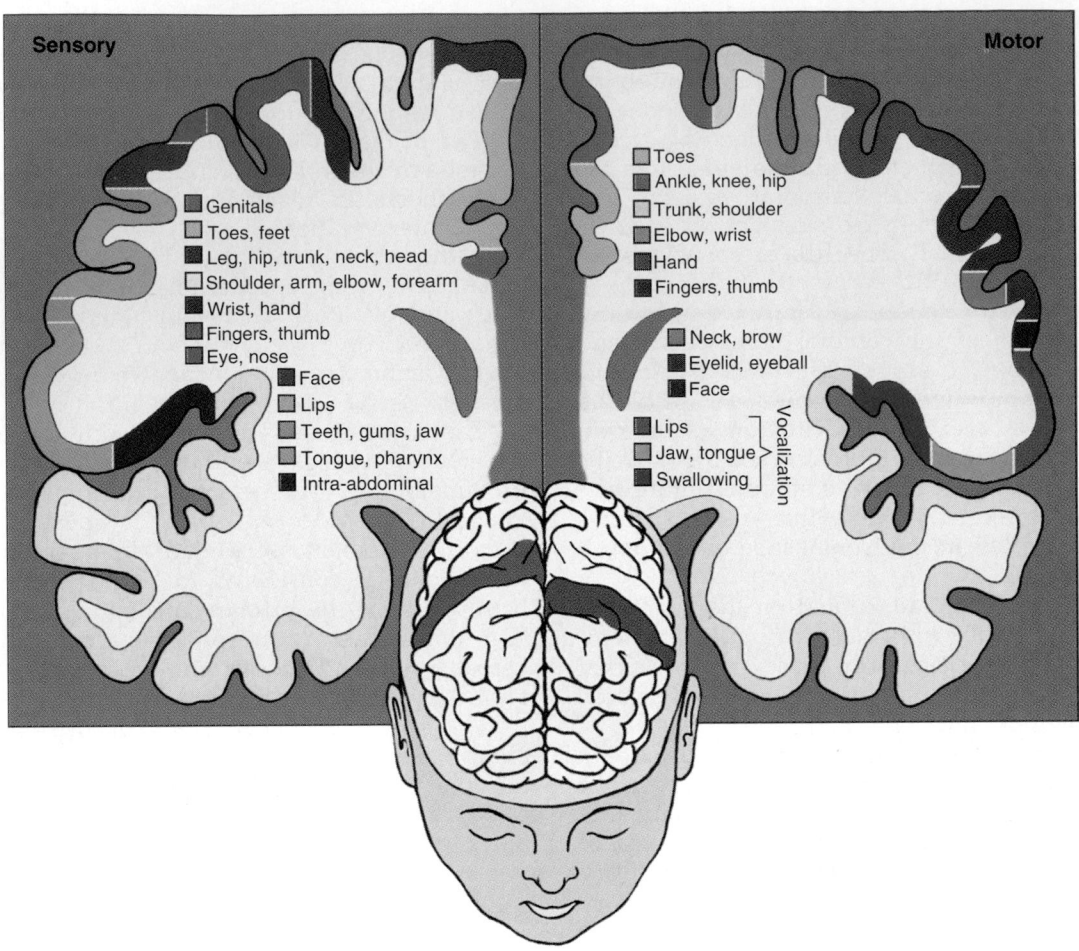

Sensory

☐ Genitals
☐ Toes, feet
■ Leg, hip, trunk, neck, head
☐ Shoulder, arm, elbow, forearm
■ Wrist, hand
■ Fingers, thumb
☐ Eye, nose
   ■ Face
   ☐ Lips
   ■ Teeth, gums, jaw
   ■ Tongue, pharynx
   ■ Intra-abdominal

Motor

☐ Toes
■ Ankle, knee, hip
☐ Trunk, shoulder
■ Elbow, wrist
■ Hand
■ Fingers, thumb
   ■ Neck, brow
   ■ Eyelid, eyeball
   ■ Face
☐ Lips ⎫
☐ Jaw, tongue ⎬ Vocalization
☐ Swallowing ⎭

Figure 17–10

Areas in the cerebral cortex that control voluntary motor activity of specific body parts and areas that receive sensory input from specific body parts. The diagram is of a frontal section of the cerebrum through the postcentral (sensory) gyrus and the precentral (motor) gyrus, respectively.

Its function has been linked with the cerebellum in the coordination and control of fine motor activity.

DIENCEPHALON

The diencephalon, also located deep within the cerebral hemispheres, houses two important structures: the thalamus and the hypothalamus. The thalamus plays a role in one's sleep-wakefulness state, conscious awareness of pain, and relay of ascending impulses to the sensory cerebral cortex. The hypothalamus lies at the base of the diencephalon and is responsible for global actions of body systems (ie, heart rate, body temperature, water-electrolyte balance, appetite). The hypothalamus works with the autonomic nervous system and influences the pituitary gland in its release of hormones.

BRAIN STEM

The brain stem is an elongated structure that connects superiorly to the cerebral hemispheres, inferi-orly to the spinal cord, and posteriorly to the cerebellum. It houses nerve fibers that form the reticular formation. Motor and sensory neurons gather information regarding muscle activity, and the reticular formation relays motor impulses from the hypothalamus to the autonomic nervous system and from the extrapyramidal system to voluntary muscles. In addition, sensory impulses ascend through the reticular formation to the cerebral sensory cortex to activate it. This is called the reticular activating system and is responsible for a person's state of wakefulness.

The brain stem has become known as the "life center" of a person. It is divided into the midbrain, pons, and medulla oblongata.

The midbrain is the uppermost portion of the brain stem. Cranial nerves III and IV are located here. The midbrain functions as a relay station for impulses among the cerebral hemispheres, cerebellum, and spinal cord.

The pons is located between the midbrain and medulla. Cranial nerves VI, VII, and VIII are located here. In addition to providing relay transmission of impulses through the pons, respiratory centers are localized here. These centers control the rate and pattern of respirations.

The medulla oblongata is located at the inferior portion of the brain stem, adjacent to the foramen magnum (base of the skull). Cranial nerves IX, X, XI, and XII are located here. The medulla controls and regulates vital centers responsible for swallowing, vomiting, respiration, and vasomotor activities.

CEREBELLUM

The cerebellum is located in the posterior fossa, posterior to the pons and medulla, and below the tentorium cerebelli. Its functions involve the coordination of movement, fine motor activities, equilibrium, and orientation in space (proprioception).

Spinal Cord

The spinal cord (Fig. 17–11) is a cylinder-shaped mass, approximately 43 cm in length, and weighing 35 g in the adult. The spinal cord is continuous with the medulla oblongata, so that a specific line of demarcation between structures is not evident. The spinal cord lies within the vertebral canal with the conus medullaris (caudal end of the spinal cord) extending to the L-1 to L-2 vertebral column level. The three meningeal layers surround the spinal cord to provide protection.

Two enlargements are found in the spinal cord. The first is at the C-5 to T-1 level and is known as the cervical or brachial enlargement. It is formed from the volume of motor cells that innervate the upper extremities. The second is at the L-3 to S-2 level and is known as the lumbosacral enlargement. It is the result of the large number of motor cells that innervate the lower extremities.

The internal structures of the spinal cord consist of gray matter and white matter. The gray matter has an H-shaped configuration. The gray color is due to the neuronal cell bodies and synapses found there. The white matter contains ascending and descending pathways, which are mostly made up of myelinated axons. Ascending pathways carry sensory impulses to the brain, whereas descending pathways carry motor impulses from the brain (Fig. 17–12).

Motor and sensory pathways are configured in tracts and are named after the tract in which they travel, the location of the origin of the impulse, and the location of impulse termination.

MAJOR SENSORY (ASCENDING) PATHWAYS

The ascending pathways transmit sensory impulses from the spinal cord to the brain for interpretation. Three major sensory pathways are responsible for the transmission of pain and temperature, proprioception, and light touch.

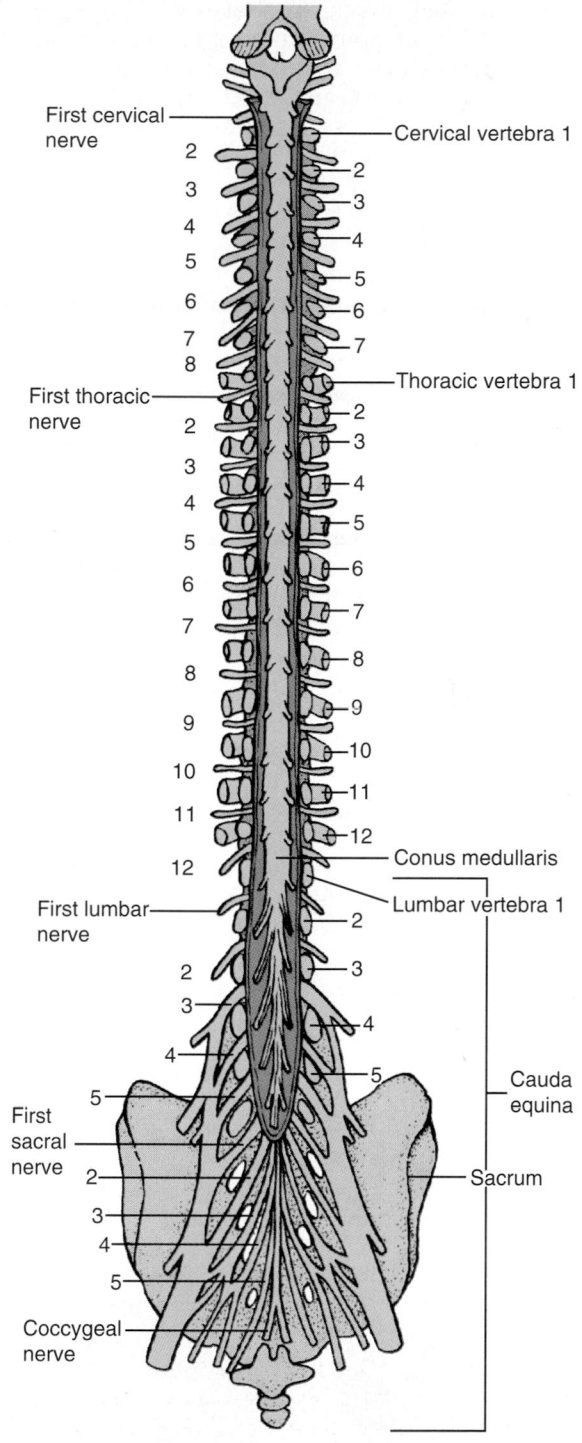

Figure 17–11

Spinal cord and spinal nerves in relation to the vertebral column.

The lateral spinothalamic tract is the sensory pathway for pain and temperature. Sensory impulses enter the spinal cord and cross almost immediately to the lateral spinothalamic tract, where the impulse is carried upward to the thalamus.

The posterior columns are the pathways for proprioception, deep touch, pressure, and vibration. As impulses enter the spinal cord, they ascend the posterior columns of the spinal cord and cross over at the area between the spinal cord and brain stem.

The ventral (anterior) spinothalamic tract is the pathway for light touch. When the sensory impulse enters the spinal cord, a combination of events occur. The impulse ascends the ipsilateral anterior tract and crosses over to the contralateral anterior tract and also ascends this tract.

Each of these sensory tracts crosses over (decussates) the spinal cord and ends in the thalamus. The thalamus then interprets the impulse and sends it to the corresponding area of the sensory cerebral cortex.

MAJOR MOTOR (DESCENDING) PATHWAYS

The major motor descending pathways transmit motor impulses from the brain to the spinal cord. The impulse is generated in the motor cerebral cortex, descends via the internal capsule (a band of motor fibers from the motor cortex, which synapses with motor pathways in the spinal cord), crosses over at approximately the junction of the brain stem and spinal cord, and travels to the desired spinal level. Thus, motor activities are contralateral to where the specific impulse is generated.

The corticospinal (pyramidal) tract is responsible for voluntary motor movement. The corticospinal tract synapses in the anterior horn of the gray matter before exiting the spinal cord to the PNS. Motor neurons located between the cerebral motor cortex and the anterior horn are known as upper motor neurons, whereas motor neurons located below the level of the anterior horn to the PNS are known as lower motor neurons.

The extrapyramidal tract, composed of the descending motor pathways excluding the pyramidal tract, functions in conjunction with the basal ganglia and cerebellum to ensure coordination, accuracy, and smoothness of muscle movement.

PERIPHERAL NERVOUS SYSTEM

Cranial Nerves

There are 12 pairs of cranial nerves that are part of the PNS. The cranial nerves arise from the brain stem. The specific name and function of each are presented in Table 17–1.

Spinal Nerves

There are 31 pairs of spinal nerves (*see* Fig. 17–11) that are a part of the PNS. They are symmetrically arranged and exit adjacent to the corresponding level of the vertebral column: 8 cervical, 12 thoracic, 5 lumbar, 5 sacral, and 1 coccygeal. As mentioned previously, the conus medullaris (caudal end of the spinal cord) ends at the L-1 to L-2 level of the vertebral column. Subsequently, the lumbar and sacral spinal nerves develop long roots and are often called the cauda equina or "horse's tail."

Each pair of spinal nerves has a dorsal and a ventral root. The dorsal root carries sensory input

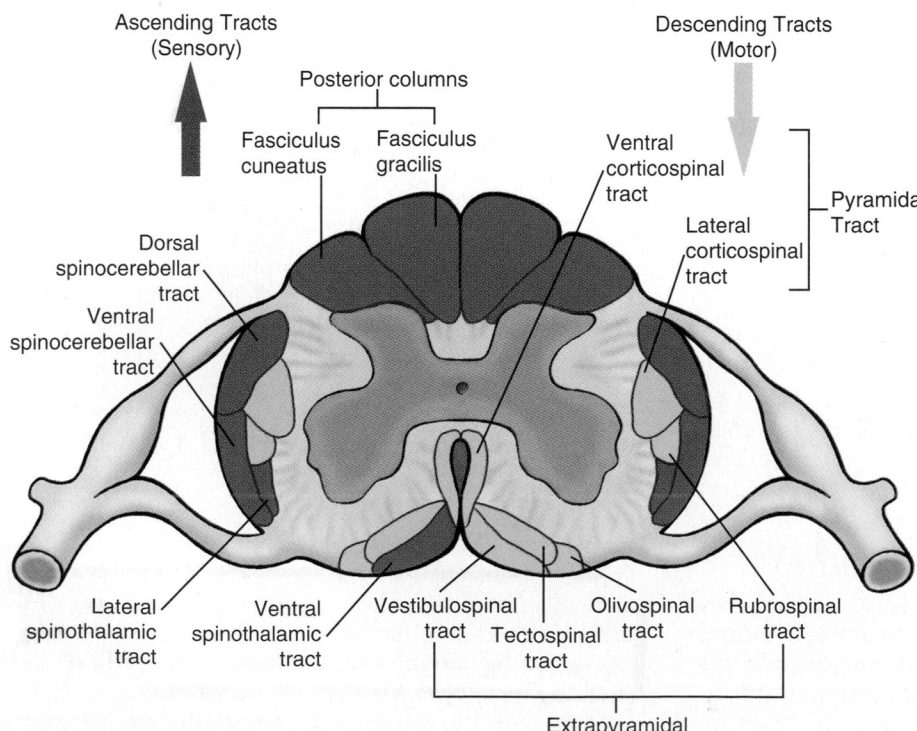

Figure 17–12

Cross-section of the spinal cord showing the major ascending (sensory) pathways and the major descending (motor) pathways.

Table 17–1

Cranial Nerves: Function and Assessment*

Number	Name	Function	Assessment
I	Olfactory	Olfactory sense (sense of smell)	Patient's eyes are closed. Test one nostril at a time to differentiate odors (spices, peppermint, cloves).
II	Optic	Vision	Assess visual acuity with an eye chart. Using a small object (finger, penlight), test visual field by moving object in from periphery to central vision. Examiner uses own vision to compare results.
III	Oculomotor	Movements of the eyeball and upper eyelid; size of the iris (ie, constriction and dilation of pupil to regulate amount of light admitted); control of ciliary muscle to regulate degree of refraction by lens	Assess pupil size and shape. Check for ptosis of eyelid. Using a small object (penlight), assess ability for eye movement in all quadrants.
IV	Trochlear	Movement of eyeball by superior oblique muscles	Assessment is the same as for oculomotor nerve.
V	Trigeminal (largest cranial nerve; has three sensory divisions: ophthalmic, maxillary, and mandibular)	*Motor function:* movement of muscles of mastication *Sensory function:* pain, touch, temperature of face, nose, teeth, mouth	Ask patient to clench jaw. Touch face with fingertips or cotton swab; have patient close eyes.
VI	Abducens	Movement of eyeball by lateral rectus muscle	Test ability for lateral movement of each eye.
VII	Facial	*Motor function:* contraction of facial and scalp muscles (facial expression); secretion of saliva by submaxillary and sublingual glands *Sensory function:* taste (from anterior two-thirds of tongue)	Ask patient to frown, smile, raise eyebrows. Note symmetry of facial expressions.
VIII	Auditory (acoustic; has two divisions: vestibular, cochlear)	*Sensory function, vestibular branch:* equilibrium (position balance) *Sensory function, cochlear division:* sense of hearing	Ask patient to take a few steps. Note equilibrium. Assess ability for hearing: whisper a phrase, and ask patient to repeat it. Check one ear at a time.
IX	Glossopharyngeal	*Motor function:* swallowing; reflex control of blood pressure through connection with carotid pressoreceptors; salivary secretion by parotid glands *Sensory function:* taste and oral and pharyngeal sensations	Test gag reflex by placing applicator against pharynx. Assess ability to swallow.
X	Vagus (has very wide distribution)	*Motor function:* muscles of pharynx, larynx, thoracic, and abdominal viscera (eg, regulates gastrointestinal motility or peristalsis; influences cardiac rate); secretion by gastric, intestinal, and pancreatic glands *Sensory function:* sensations in pharynx, larynx, and thoracic and abdominal viscera	Test gag reflex by placing applicator against pharynx.

Table continued on following page

Table 17–1

Cranial Nerves: Function and Assessment* (continued)

Number	Name	Function	Assessment
XI	Accessory	Movement of shoulder and head by trapezius and sterno-cleidomastoid muscles	Assess muscle strength by asking patient to shrug shoulders and turn head from one side to the other against resistance.
XII	Hypoglossal	Movements of the tongue	Ask patient to stick out tongue. Note deviation from midline or abnormal movements.

*Most motor nerves are considered to also contain some sensory fibers, by which information as to the existing conditions in the muscles concerned (proprioceptive data) is transmitted into the central nervous system. The proprioceptive impulses result in appropriate motor responses to facilitate the required pattern of movement.

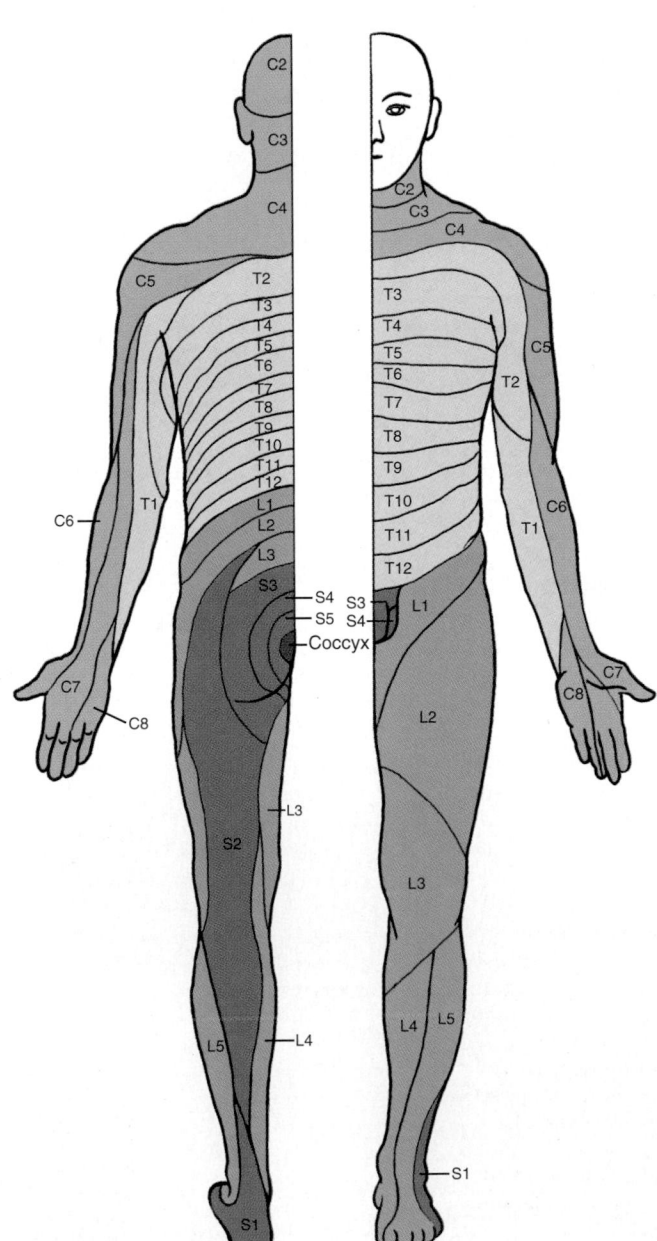

Figure 17–13
Skin areas innervated by spinal nerves (dermatomes).

(afferent impulses) from the skin and organs of the body to the spinal cord. The ventral root carries motor input (efferent impulses) from the spinal cord to voluntary striated muscles and smooth and cardiac muscles.

Superficial receptors of pain, temperature, and light touch are located throughout the skin in specific regions called dermatomes. Dermatome areas correspond to the level of the spinal cord at which

the spinal nerves innervating that region enter and exit (Fig. 17–13).

AUTONOMIC NERVOUS SYSTEM

The autonomic nervous system innervates and regulates the activities of the viscera: cardiac muscle, smooth muscle, and glands (Table 17–2). Its func-

Table 17–2

Functions of the Autonomic Nervous System

Structure or Activity	Parasympathetic Effects	Sympathetic Effects
EYE		
Pupil	Constricted	Dilated (β)
Ciliary muscle	Constricted	Slightly relaxed (β)
Lacrimal glands	Increased secretion	None
CIRCULATORY SYSTEM		
Rate and force of heartbeat	Decreased	Increased (β_1)
Blood vessels		
In heart muscle	Constricted (α)	Dilated (β_2)
In skeletal muscle	None	Dilated cholinergic, adrenergic (β_2)
		Constricted adrenergic (α)
In abdominal viscera and skin	None	Constricted (α)
Blood pressure	Decreased	Increased
RESPIRATORY SYSTEM		
Nasal glands	Copious secretion	Vasoconstriction and slight secretion
Bronchioles	Constricted	Dilated (β_2)
Rate of breathing	Decreased	Increased
DIGESTIVE SYSTEM		
Tone and peristaltic movements of digestive tube	Increased	Decreased (α and β_2)
Muscular sphincters of digestive tube	Relaxed	Contracted (most often) (α)
Secretion of salivary glands	Thin, watery saliva	Thick, viscid saliva (α)
Secretions of stomach, intestine, and pancreas	Increased	Vasoconstriction and slight secretion (α)
Conversion of liver glycogen to glucose	None	Increased (α and β_2)
Gallbladder and bile ducts	Contracted	Relaxed
GENITOURINARY SYSTEM		
Urinary bladder		
Muscular walls	Contracted	Relaxed (β)
Sphincters	Relaxed	Contracted (α)
Muscles of the uterus	Relaxed; variable	Contracted under some conditions; varies with menstrual cycle and pregnancy (α and β_2)
Blood vessels of external genitalia	Dilated	No direct effect
Penile function	Erection	Ejaculation (α)
INTEGUMENTARY SYSTEM		
Secretion of sweat	Sweating on palms	Copious secretion
Pilomotor muscles	None	Contracted (gooseflesh)
Secretion of apocrine glands	None	Thick, odoriferous secretion
MEDULLAE OF ADRENAL GLANDS	None	Secretion of epinephrine and norepinephrine
BLOOD		
Glucose	None	Increased
Lipids	None	Increased

tion is to maintain the internal homeostasis of the body. This is accomplished by the two antagonistic divisions that constitute the autonomic nervous system: the sympathetic nervous system and the parasympathetic nervous system.

The sympathetic nervous system is associated with the fight or flight response and is activated at the time of stress. It increases heart rate, blood pressure, and blood supply to the body. Noradrenalin is the neurotransmitter associated with this system. This chemical reaction promotes the energy expenditure associated with the sympathetic response.

The parasympathetic nervous system is associated with the conservation of energy, relaxation, and restoration of level of functioning (ie, decreased heart rate, blood pressure). Acetylcholine is the neurotransmitter associated with this system, which induces a cholinergic effect on the system.

Clinical Manifestations of Neurologic Dysfunction

ALTERED LEVELS OF CONSCIOUSNESS

Consciousness is defined as awareness of self and the environment. Physiologically, it is divided into two components: content and arousal. The content of consciousness encompasses the ability to think, communicate, and feel, which are functions of the cerebral hemispheres. Arousal refers to the state of wakefulness. Content and arousal are independent components of consciousness, and both can be affected by a variety of neurologic as well as systemic disorders.

Etiology and Pathophysiology

The ascending reticular activating system is responsible for the state of wakefulness. The ascending reticular activating system is a complex system of neurons with connections to many parts of the brain. The pathways originate in the lower brain stem (medulla), travel upward through the pons and midbrain to the thalamus, and are then dispersed throughout the cerebral cortex. Sensory information is relayed through the ascending reticular activating system to the cerebral cortex. Arousal and stimulation of cortical neurons occur, inducing a state of alertness. The excited cerebral cortex transmits impulses back through the ascending reticular activating system to the brain stem, thus establishing a feedback mechanism that maintains wakefulness and cerebral alertness. Consciousness is impaired when this circuit system is disrupted. The degree of impairment can vary from slight to complete. Alterations in consciousness can occur secondary to the following:

- Dysfunction in one or both cerebral hemispheres
- A localized abnormality in the brain stem affecting the ascending reticular activating system

- Global CNS dysfunction involving the brain stem and the cerebral hemispheres

Specific causes of alterations in consciousness are varied and can include metabolic disorders, systemic failure, toxins, infectious processes, fluid and electrolyte imbalance, structural lesions, and psychiatric disorders.

Clinical Manifestations

Table 17–3 presents the terms commonly used to describe altered levels of consciousness and their defining clinical characteristics.

In describing alterations in consciousness, the fo-

Table 17–3

Range of Levels of Consciousness	
Level of Consciousness	**Clinical Characteristics**
Full consciousness	Patient is awake and alert, appropriate in conversation. Patient is oriented to person, place, and time.
Confusion	Patient has short attention span and poor memory and demonstrates difficulty following commands. Patient experiences increased agitation at night and is disoriented first to time, then place, and possibly self.
Delirium	Patient is restless, agitated, and possibly combative. Patient is disoriented to time and place and is possibly hallucinating.
Obtundation	Patient rouses easily when stimulated and engages in simple but limited conversation and will sleep when undisturbed; lethargy, somnolence, and drowsiness are synonymous terms.
Stupor	Patient is very drowsy and appears unresponsive. When repeatedly and vigorously stimulated, patient will withdraw extremities purposefully and possibly speak incoherently.
Semicomatose	Patient is unresponsive to stimuli, although painful stimuli to the skin may result in moaning or stirring. Corneal, pupillary, and gag and tendon reflexes (called brain-stem reflexes) are intact.
Comatose	Patient is unarousable and does not stir or moan in response to painful stimuli. Most brain-stem reflexes are intact. Patient may exhibit decorticate or decerebrate posturing.
Deeply comatose	Patient is completely unarousable and unresponsive to all stimuli, including pain. Brain-stem reflexes are absent.

cus is on the behavior exhibited by the patient in response to a specific stimulus rather than on labeling the response with a term, because terms alone are subject to individual interpretation. The fully conscious person is awake, alert, appropriate in conversation, and oriented to person, place, and time.

The unconscious person is one who is unable to open the eyes, to obey commands, or to utter recognizable words. The person experiencing unconsciousness has lost the ability to interact effectively with his or her environment.

Diagnosis

A diagnosis of an altered level of consciousness is based on the presence of the clinical manifestations previously described. This is determined by means of complete neurologic assessment.

Management

Medical management consists of sustaining vital functions while the underlying problem is identified and treated. In the unconscious patient, the mechanisms essential for awareness and response to comfort, protection, and self-preservation are diminished or absent. The more severe and more prolonged the dysfunction causing the unconscious state, the less likely the recovery. The unconscious person's survival directly depends on the standard of care provided and on the measures taken to prevent complications that could interfere with rehabilitative potential as well as the quality of survival.

NURSING PROCESS
The Unconscious Patient

Assessment

The priority assessment for the unconscious patient is for a patent airway and management of the airway. Assess neurologic status using the Glasgow Coma Scale (Table 17–4). The Glasgow Coma Scale is a tool that allows for consistency in assessment and documentation. It is based on the assessment of three main components of behavioral response: eye-opening response, motor response, and verbal response. A numeric score is assigned to each response. The minimum score attainable is 3; the maximum is 15. A total score of 7 or less is commonly accepted as a definition of coma. In assessing the unconscious patient, observe the patient, then attempt to get a response by talking to the patient, touching the patient, and lastly by using pain. At each point observe for evidence of involuntary motor function, noting whether it is purposeful.

Check pupils for size, shape, equality, and reaction to light. Assess the corneal reflex, and note and report any decrease in response. Assess for patency of the airway. Note rate, rhythm, and depth of respirations. Auscultate the lung fields for the presence of adventitious breath sounds. Assess adequacy of circulatory function by checking pulse and blood

Table 17–4

Glasgow Coma Scale

Variable	Response	Scale No.
Eyes	Open spontaneously	4
	Open to verbal commands	3
	Open to pain	2
	No response	1
Best motor response	Obeys verbal command to painful stimulus	6
	Localizes pain	5
	Flexion withdrawal	4
	Flexion abnormal	3
	Extension	2
	No response	1
Best verbal response	Oriented and converses	5
	Disoriented and converses	4
	Inappropriate words	3
	Incomprehensible sounds	2
	No response	1
Total		3–15

pressure and noting any changes in rate, rhythm, and pattern. Measure temperature rectally to detect hyperpyrexia secondary to urinary tract or respiratory tract infections, wounds, or drug reactions. Assess the motor and sensory function. Check muscle tone, muscle size, and joint flexibility. Inspect the skin carefully whenever the patient is turned and positioned. Observe for redness, indicating possible tissue damage secondary to pressure. Note color, texture, and turgor of the skin. Assess for bowel and bladder function by recording urinary output and bowel movement characteristics and frequency. Palpate the abdomen to detect distention. Auscultate bowel sounds to determine gastrointestinal mobility. Review laboratory values, particularly serum electrolytes, to assess the patient's fluid and electrolyte status. Record all nutritional intake to determine the patient's daily caloric intake.

Nursing Diagnoses and Planning

Nursing diagnoses and related expected patient outcomes most commonly applicable to unconscious patients include the following:

NDx: Ineffective airway clearance related to inability to expectorate secondary to unconscious state

Planning: Patient Outcomes
1. Airway remains patent.
2. Patient is free of respiratory distress.

NDx: Risk for impaired skin integrity related to immobility

Planning: Patient Outcomes
1. Skin remains intact.

2. Redness or excoriation at pressure points is absent.

NDx: Altered nutrition: less than body requirements related to inability to swallow

Planning: Patient Outcomes
1. Patient's weight is maintained
2. Electrolytes and serum proteins are within normal limits

NDx: Self care deficit related to unconscious state

Planning: Patient Outcomes
1. Basic needs are met.
2. Patient's dignity is maintained.

NDx: Impaired physical mobility related to inability to participate in movement

Planning: Patient Outcomes
1. Joints remain freely mobile.
2. Extremities remain in correct alignment.

NDx: Total incontinence related to unconscious state

Planning: Patient Outcomes
1. Patient maintains urinary output of 30 mL/h.
2. Patient is free of urinary tract infection.

NDx: Constipation related to immobility

Planning: Patient Outcomes
1. Patient has bowel movement at least every other day.
2. Stool is soft and formed.

Nursing Interventions and Evaluation

NDx: Ineffective airway clearance
Assess airway and ventilation every 15 minutes to 4 hours depending on the patient's status. Because the unconscious patient cannot take deep breaths in response to instruction, initiate vigorous pulmonary toilet including percussion and postural drainage. Turn the patient from side to side after pulmonary toilet every 2 hours to prevent pooling of secretions in the dependent lung base. Avoid positioning the unconscious patient on his or her back to prevent the tongue from falling back and obstructing the airway, unless an airway is in place or the patient has undergone tracheostomy. Suction equipment should be readily available and accessible. Suction the patient's nasopharynx and oropharynx to remove pooled secretions. Oral airways may be used for the first 48 hours, although endotracheal tubes are generally inserted in the unconscious patient in the emergency department. Endotracheal tubes are left in place for 5 to 7 days. If an artificial airway is recommended for longer than 7 days, a tracheostomy is performed. Perform tracheostomy care according to hospital protocol. Monitor arterial blood gases. If the patient has undergone tracheostomy, suction after pulmonary toilet. Be certain to preoxygenate before suctioning, and limit suctioning to no more than 15 seconds to prevent hypercapnia and prevent increased intracranial pressure (ICP or IICP). Monitor and document color, consistency, and amount of sputum. Assess lung sounds before and after suctioning to determine if suctioning helped clear the secretions. Administer oxygen therapy as needed.

NDx: Risk for impaired skin integrity
The unconscious patient is at high risk for skin breakdown. Turn and position the patient every 2 hours to ensure proper circulation. Blood flow becomes restricted to any body part in which a bone is close to the skin surface if prolonged pressure is maintained. The greater the pressure, the less time that is needed to cause tissue compression and compromised blood flow. If the patient is extremely thin, with more noticeable bony prominences, turn and position him or her more often. Give special attention to ears, shoulders, hips, knees, and ankles. Remember that these areas are direct pressure points when the patient is in a side-lying position. Take care to equitably distribute weight. Place a pillow between the knees to maintain alignment and prevent pressure. Keep the heels from direct contact with the bed. Use lotion to prevent cracking and breakdown of dry skin. Gently massage pressure points to improve circulation. Place an air mattress or other pressure-relieving device on the bed. Avoid many layers of bed protectors and linen because excess bedding can inhibit airflow, limit the pressure-reducing property of the mattress, and trap moisture next to the skin. Keep bed linen free from wrinkles or ridges because wrinkled linen causes excess pressure on bony areas. Use a lifting sheet when moving the patient to avoid shearing force. If the patient is incontinent of urine or feces, gently cleanse the area and dry thoroughly. Constant moisture against the skin renders the tissues more fragile and increases the risk of skin breakdown. Keep the patient well hydrated, at least 2000 mL daily, unless the ICP is increased.

NDx: Altered nutrition: less than body requirements
The unconscious patient is allowed nothing by mouth (NPO status) because there is no gag or swallowing reflex. Administer intravenous fluids slowly. Administer tube feedings as ordered by the physician. A nasogastric or gastrostomy tube is placed. Elevate the head of the bed at 30 degrees during feeding and for 1 hour after bolus feedings. Monitor intake and output every shift. Bowel sounds must be present and the risk of paralytic ileus must be past before tube feedings are begun. Placement of the tube in the stomach is assessed according to hospital policy by aspirating stomach contents (if less than 30 mL, feeding can progress), instilling air through the tube while auscultating the stomach, or both. The feeding tube is flushed with 50 mL of water before and after each feeding or once a shift for continuous feedings. Feeding is administered at room temperature.

Total parenteral nutrition (TPN) may be needed if the patient is unable to absorb nutrients from the gastrointestinal tract. TPN must be administered through a central line, usually placed in the superior vena cava. Monitor calorie intake, blood urea nitrogen and electrolyte levels, weight, and intake and output.

NDx: Self care deficit

Because the unconscious patient cannot perform his or her own activities of daily living, provide basic hygienic care to maintain cleanliness. Bathe the patient daily and more often if the patient is incontinent. Provide mouth care to the tongue and gums every 3 to 4 hours using a sponge swab moistened with a nondrying mouthwash. Lubricate the lips with water-soluble lubricant to prevent drying and encrustation. Brush the teeth with a toothbrush and use a suction catheter to remove excess fluid from the mouth. Wash hair regularly at the bedside according to agency procedure. Inspect fingernails and toenails daily. File and clip nails as necessary to protect the patient from injury. Shave the male patient daily as a part of routine basic care. If the patient is receiving anticoagulant therapy, use an electric razor. Protect the patient at all times from unnecessary body exposure. Provide measures of comfort such as blankets in accordance with the patient's temperature and warmth of the skin.

If the patient has lost the blink reflex, apply and eye patch or tape the eyes closed. Be cautious to avoid corneal contact with the eye patch, which could result in corneal abrasion. Artificial Tears or saline drops are administered to eyes four times a day to prevent keratoses. Monitor the ears and nose for drainage. If drainage occurs, apply a small sterile dressing and test for glucose; if glucose is present, notify the physician. Secure the nasogastric tube if used. Tape the tube to the patient's forehead or directly to the nose to prevent irritation and erosion of nares.

Involve the family in the patient's care whenever possible. The family may wish to provide personal care items for the patient and participate in some activities of daily living (eg, washing the hair). Ascertain the family's coping strategies while observing their involvement with the patient.

NDx: Impaired physical mobility

The unconscious patient is unable to move spontaneously and thus is at risk for contractures, ankylosis, and muscle atrophy. The patient on bed rest who cannot bear weight can lose calcium from the bones, predisposing to conditions such as osteoporosis and urinary tract calculi.

Perform passive range-of-motion exercises for all joints every 4 hours to prevent joint stiffness and contractures. Position the patient properly in a side-lying position. Position the head in alignment with the spine. Avoid flexing the neck, which impedes venous drainage from the head. Place the upper-most hip joint slightly forward and support with a pillow so that it is slightly adducted. Flex the upper arm at the elbow and shoulder. Flex the upper leg slightly at the hip and knee. Support both the upper arm and the upper leg by pillows. Reposition the patient every 2 hours, maintaining correct body alignment. Remember that the unconscious patient is unable to express discomfort if position is misaligned. Support limbs with pillows or hands with a towel roll to prevent dependent edema. Use a footboard or high-top sneakers to prevent foot drop. Collaborate with the physical therapist if special splints or devices are being used for paralyzed extremities to ensure correct use and to establish a regular on-off use schedule. Teach family members to perform passive range-of-motion exercises. This allows them to actively participate in the patient's therapeutic regimen and allows for sensory stimulation of the patient through touch.

NDx: Total incontinence

Urinary incontinence may result from the unconscious patient's inability to communicate elimination needs or from overall nervous system dysfunction. An indwelling Foley catheter is inserted to manage incontinence and prevent skin breakdown. Assess the catheter for patency. Palpate the abdomen for bladder distention. A full bladder is palpable in the lower midline abdomen. Monitor intake and output. For the male patient, a condom-type catheter applied over the penis may be used.

Indwelling Foley catheters are a major source of infection. Monitor for signs and symptoms of urinary tract infection. Record urinary output every 8 hours. Notify the physician of output less than 30 mL/h. Monitor for odor, cloudy appearance of urine, and hematuria. Obtain urinalysis results and specimens for culture and sensitivity as necessary. Monitor temperature every 8 hours because fever may indicate a developing urinary tract infection. Secure the catheter to the inside of patient's thigh with nonirritating tape to prevent traction on the urethra and meatus. Report any drainage from urethral orifice. Removal of the catheter as soon as possible is strongly recommended.

NDx: Constipation

Because of immobility, the unconscious patient's peristaltic activity is diminished. Constipation and fecal impaction are complications of this decrease and of the lack of a normal diet that would stimulate peristalsis.

Check all stools for occult blood. Auscultate for hyperactive or hypoactive bowel sounds. Assess for abdominal distention. Administer stool softeners and mild laxatives or suppositories daily to facilitate elimination. Avoid enemas, which may increase ICP. Provide a fluid intake of at least 2000 mL daily, if not contraindicated, to provide hydration, facilitate digestion, and aid in the softening of stool.

Compare the patient's status with the expected

outcomes. If the outcomes are not met, reassess the patient and revise the plan.

INCREASED INTRACRANIAL PRESSURE

ICP (or IICP) is the pressure exerted within the cranial cavity by its contents, which normally consist of brain tissue, blood, and CSF. The ICP is not a constant—that is, it is a continuously fluctuating phenomenon within a normal range of 80 to 180 mm H_2O or 0 to 15 mm Hg. Activities that increase intrathoracic or intra-abdominal pressure, such as coughing, sneezing, or straining at stool (the Valsalva maneuver), cause a momentary increase in ICP. Activities such as sitting or standing up result in a momentary decrease in ICP. Whereas transient increases in pressure are benign, sustained increases in ICP can be life-threatening.

Etiology and Pathophysiology

Increased ICP can be caused by anything that takes up space within the intracranial compartment and changes the normal ratio of blood, brain, and CSF (Table 17–5). Thus, edema of the brain, blood clots, tumors, cysts, abscesses, and hydrocephalus can all cause increased ICP.

Table 17–5

Causes of Increased Intracranial Pressure

General Causes	Examples of Specific Pathology
Increase in brain volume	Tumor
	Cerebral edema secondary to trauma, surgical manipulation, tumor, tissue hypoxia, infarction
	Brain abscess
	Encephalitis
Increase in CSF volume	Decreased cerebrospinal fluid absorption as a result of meningitis or subarachnoidal hemorrhage
	Obstruction of cerebrospinal fluid flow because of hydrocephalus
	Tumors compressing the ventricles
	Trauma
Increase in blood volume	Aneurysms or arteriovenous malformations
	Intracranial hemorrhage secondary to hypertension or trauma
	Dilation of cerebral arteries as a result of hypoxemia or hypercapnia
	Obstruction of venous drainage as a result of compression of internal jugular vein, increased central venous pressure
	Hematomas

With increased pressure, brain tissue is compressed and lacks blood and oxygen. The end result is brain damage if treatment is not available. Increased blood pressure and decreased pulse are physiologic changes that occur in response to brain tissue being deprived of oxygen. Decreased level of consciousness is a clinical change that results from damage to brain tissue because of lack of nutrition or oxygen. Pupillary reactions change when brain tissue is forced through the uncus, resulting in pressure on the oculomotor nerve. This occurs because of the anatomic relationships of involved structures.

The tentorium is a fold of dura that serves as a shelf on which the cerebral cortex rests. A small space exists between the end of the tentorium and brain stem. This space is called the uncus. With increased ICP, brain tissue is forced through this small opening. This is called uncal herniation. As tissue is forced through the opening, it exerts pressure on the brain stem. It is exactly at this anatomic point that the third cranial nerve (oculomotor) exits from the brain stem. This causes unilateral changes in pupillary response because of compression of the oculomotor nerve. A fixed, dilated pupil is considered to be a late sign of increased ICP.

Clinical Manifestations

The classic symptoms of increased ICP are decreasing level of consciousness, which is the most sensitive indicator of increased ICP, increasing blood pressure, decreasing pulse, and pupillary changes. Changes in vital signs occur late. Respirations decrease and become irregular. Cheyne-Stokes respirations, characterized by waxing and waning of respiration with periodic apnea, occur. Body temperature increases in response to increased ICP. Motor changes may be present depending on the cause of the increased pressure.

As ICP increases, headache, nausea, restlessness, lethargy, and drowsiness as well as increasing systolic blood pressure and decreasing pulse may occur. Irritability and restlessness are subtle signs of impending change in a patient's level of consciousness due to increasing ICP. Unilateral motor weakness of the upper and lower extremities may or may not be present depending on the location and extent of the damage. The patient may experience seizures, projectile vomiting, visual disturbances, and papilledema.

Late signs of increased ICP are coma, apnea, unilateral pupil changes, high blood pressure, and slow pulse. If untreated, increased ICP causes death.

Diagnosis

A diagnosis of increasing ICP may be based on the patient's presenting signs and symptoms, history, diagnostic studies, and actual ICP. Monitoring may be performed by three different devices: a ventricular catheter, a subarachnoid screw, and an epidural sensor (Fig. 17–14). None of these devices is ideal. Rather, each has specific advantages and disadvantages.

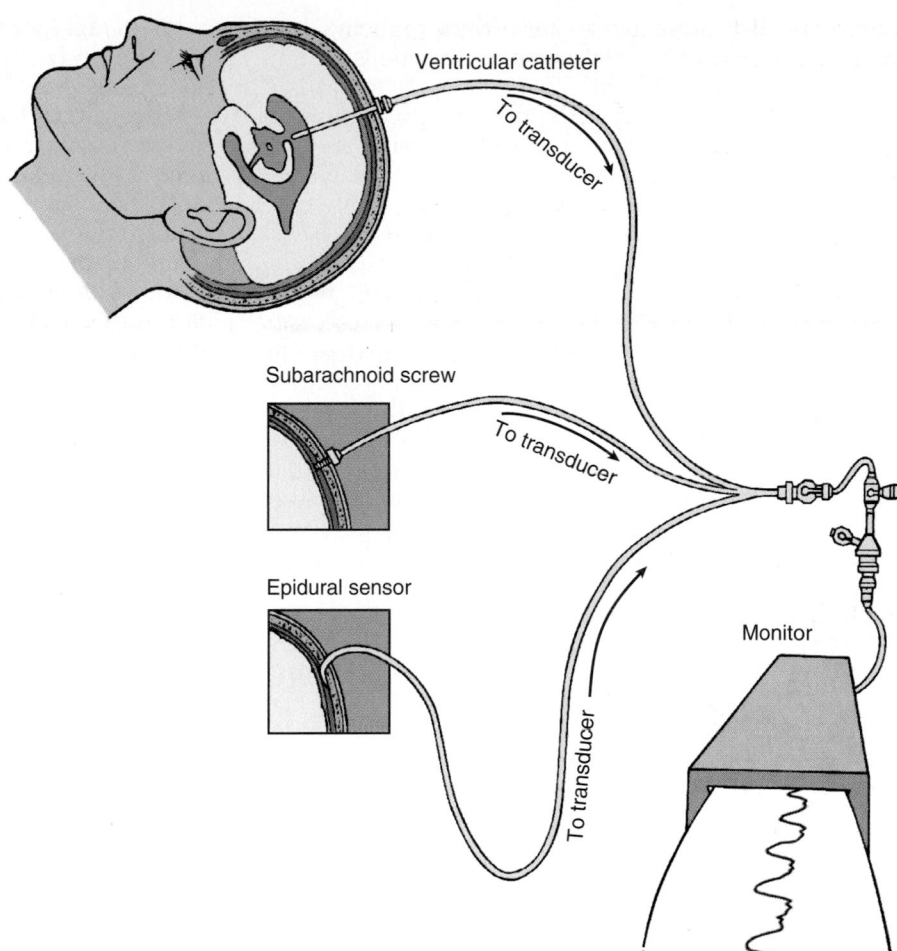

Figure 17–14

Devices used for monitoring intracranial pressure: a ventricular catheter, a subarachnoid screw, and an epidural sensor.

The ventricular catheter allows accurate, direct measurement of ICP and drainage of CSF and blood from the ventricles, but because it is placed via a burr hole through the cerebrum into a lateral ventricle, there is a risk of both infection and brain damage.

The subarachnoid screw, like the venous catheter, allows direct measurement of pressure and removal of CSF. There is still a risk of infection, although it is not as severe because the screw does not enter the brain tissue but remains in the subarachnoid space. There is also risk that the screw may become obstructed if the brain should swell.

The least invasive and therefore the safest device is the epidural sensor. Unfortunately, it is also the most unreliable because the pressure of the CSF is not measured directly but is measured via a fiberoptic sensor placed in the epidural space. Recent advances in fiberoptic technology have improved the accuracy of epidural sensors. Their use is rapidly becoming widespread. Drainage of CSF is not possible with this device.

Cerebral perfusion pressure is also measured. Cerebral perfusion pressure is the difference between ICP and systemic arterial pressure. As ICP increases, cerebral perfusion pressure falls. Normal cerebral perfusion pressure is 80 to 100 mm Hg. If cerebral perfusion pressure falls below 60 mm Hg, irreversible ischemia results. When cerebral perfusion pressure falls to zero there is no cerebral blood flow.

Apart from these devices, medical diagnosis is usually based on clinical assessment and computed tomography (CT). CT shows an area of increased density if a space-occupying lesion is present. A lumbar puncture is generally contraindicated because, by removing spinal fluid, the pressure differential is dramatically changed. This increases the chance of uncal herniation, brain damage, and even death.

Management

Medical management of increased ICP focuses on diagnosing the cause and intervening with appropriate pharmacologic, medical, and surgical therapies.

DRUG THERAPY. There are three general classes of medications most often used for patients with increased ICP: osmotic diuretics, glucocorticoids, and anticonvulsants. Barbiturates may be used in some cases.

Osmotic diuretics are drugs that are hyperosmolar. The high osmotic concentration of the drug causes water to be drawn from the edematous brain tissue into the vascular system, thus reducing ICP. The most commonly used osmotic diuretic is mannitol (Osmitrol) (Highlight 17–1). It is administered intravenously. It acts quickly, and its effect is short-term. Mannitol is particularly useful during surgical procedures or as an emergency measure when patients need to be transferred from one location to another for appropriate treatment. The dosage and rate of administration of mannitol vary, but the usual dose is 1.5 to 2 g/kg of body weight. Serum osmolarity levels must be monitored during its use. A Foley catheter should be inserted to assess the effectiveness of diuretic therapy.

Glucocorticoids are effective in reducing focal cerebral edema, particularly if caused by tumors or abscess. Intravenous dexamethasone (Decadron) is the most commonly used glucocorticoid. Large doses are given initially, followed by regular maintenance doses, usually every 4 to 6 hours. Steroid therapy can potentiate gastrointestinal bleeding, infection, and hyperglycemia.

Although anticonvulsants do not specifically treat cerebral edema, they control convulsive or seizure activity of the brain. This is particularly important because, during a seizure, ICP is dramatically increased. If the patient already has increased ICP, the additional pressure produced by the seizure may be incompatible with life.

The most commonly used anticonvulsant medication is phenytoin (Dilantin). The usual dosage is 100 mg three to four times daily. The method of administration may be intravenous or oral. Dilantin is poorly absorbed when given intramuscularly.

Barbiturate therapy may be used in instances of severe, uncontrolled ICP unresponsive to the usual treatment modalities. Sodium pentobarbital (Nembutal) or thiopental sodium (Pentothal) is administered by continuous intravenous infusion to induce a barbiturate coma. Although the actual mechanism of action is unclear, it is theorized that inducement of barbiturate coma decreases overall cerebral metabolism, glucose utilization, and oxygen demand, allowing brain tissue to better tolerate hypoxia and diminished cerebral perfusion. Barbiturate coma necessitates mechanical ventilation, arterial pressure monitoring, electrocardiogram (ECG) monitoring, and use of an ICP monitoring device in the intensive care setting.

SUPPORTIVE THERAPY. Maintaining the head of the bed continuously at a 30- to 40-degree angle promotes venous return and decreases cerebral blood volume. Hyperventilation reduces the partial pressure of arterial carbon dioxide ($PaCO_2$) levels and stimulates cerebral vasoconstriction, thus reducing cerebral blood flow and lowering ICP. As $PaCO_2$ levels rise, cerebral vasodilation occurs, thus increasing cerebral blood flow and increasing ICP. $PaCO_2$ levels are maintained between 25 and 30 mm Hg. Intubation and mechanical ventilation are usually required.

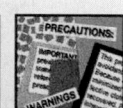

HIGHLIGHT 17–1 PHARMACOLOGY

Osmotic Diuretics

Definition:

These drugs assist in the management of increased intracranial pressure. Mannitol (Osmitrol) is one of the most commonly used.

Action:

Osmotic diuretics are hyperosmolar. The drug causes water to be drawn from the edematous brain tissue into the vascular system.

Uses:

Through decreasing the fluid in brain tissue and cerebrospinal fluid, the intracranial pressure is decreased.

Side Effects:

Marked diuresis, dehydration, electrolyte imbalances, dizziness, convulsions, hypotension, tachycardia, pulmonary congestion, nausea and vomiting.

Interactions:

Increases excretion of lithium. Mixing with whole blood may cause agglutination.

Nursing Implications:

Monitor vital signs, intracranial pressure, urinary output, central venous pressure and pulmonary artery pressures before administration and every hour during administration.

Assess for signs and symptoms of dehydration and electrolyte imbalance.

Monitor potassium, sodium, chloride, blood urea nitrogen, complete blood count, and serum creatinine.

Assess for pulmonary edema.

Monitor renal and neurologic function.

Medication should be administered with an in-line filter or drawn up with a filter needle.

Hypothermia decreases the metabolic demands of the brain and decreases cerebral blood flow and volume. Therapeutic hypothermia induced by a hypothermia blanket cools the body's surface and decreases cerebral metabolism by 35 to 40%. Shivering, which can increase the metabolic rate, is controlled with chlorpromazine (Thorazine).

SURGERY. As an emergency intervention, a small burr hole can be made in the skull for insertion of a ventricular drain. This allows for drainage of CSF and immediately reduces increased ICP. Surgical decompression of the skull (removal of a small segment of bone) may be necessary to relieve pressure. In cases of a space-occupying lesion documented by CT, such as an epidural hematoma compressing brain tissue, surgical removal is warranted via craniotomy.

NURSING PROCESS
Increased Intracranial Pressure

Assessment

Establish a baseline neurologic assessment on all patients with a neurologic problem. Perform frequent assessments on patients at risk for increased ICP. Be sure to document observations in measurable terms. For example, when documenting level of consciousness, state "Rouses easily to verbal stimuli and responds to questions appropriately."

Question the patient about headache, which can be a signal of gradually increasing ICP. Assess quality and type. Remember to report headaches, which occur with greater intensity on rising from sleep because the recumbent position decreases venous outflow and can precipitate an increase in ICP.

Because alteration in level of consciousness is an early sign of acutely increasing ICP, assess the patient for subtle behavioral changes, such as restlessness, irritability, drowsiness, confusion, or apathy. Check orientation to person, place, and time. Observe for any difficulties or hesitation in following simple commands or in verbalizing appropriately.

Assess proximal muscle strength by testing for arm drifts. A downward drifting of the extended arm or a pronation of the hand that was not present on baseline examination could indicate developing hemiparesis. Check handgrips and plantar flexion and dorsiflexion. Note strength and equality. Use a pin or dull needle to test for impaired sensory discrimination in the extremities.

When the patient's baseline level of responsiveness is minimal (ie, he or she does not follow commands), test motor response by applying a painful stimulus. Press your thumbnail against the patient's nail bed. The unconscious patient usually withdraws the stimulated extremity. Note the symmetry of the withdrawal response from one side of body to the other. An inappropriate response would be posturing. Posturing is a nonpurposeful motor reflex, indicating involvement of the brain stem or cerebrum. It is exhibited in one of two ways: decorticate and decerebrate (Fig. 17–15).

In decorticate posturing (abnormal flexion response), the patient has a rigid spine, flexed and adducted arms, and extended and externally rotated legs with plantar flexion. This state indicates dysfunction in the cerebrum.

In decerebrate posturing (abnormal extension response), the patient has a rigid and possibly arched spine, rigidly extended and pronated arms with the wrists flexed and the palms facing backward, and extended legs with plantar flexion. This state indicates brain stem dysfunction.

Assess the size and shape of both pupils, noting any deviation from the patient's baseline. Using a penlight, observe the response of each pupil to the light stimulus. Remember that a change in the reaction from brisk to sluggish can indicate increasing ICP and impending herniation. Also keep in mind that pupillary changes generally occur first ipsilaterally (on the same side as the cerebral hemisphere being compressed). Papilledema is observed with the ophthalmoscope, which denotes that pressure has increased in the brain. Then, as further swelling occurs, both pupils become fixed and dilated (nonresponsive and large), an indication of severe and probably irreversible brain damage.

Take blood pressure, pulse, and respirations because increasing systolic blood pressure, widening pulse pressure, or bradycardia indicates that the brain is beginning to decompensate. Observe for alterations in respiratory function, such as Cheyne-Stokes respiration, which can lead to respiratory arrest.

Nursing Diagnoses and Planning

Nursing diagnoses and related expected patient outcomes most commonly applicable to patients with increased ICP include the following:

NDx: Ineffective breathing pattern related to altered level of consciousness and increased ICP

Planning: Patient Outcomes
1. Respiratory rate is regular, between 12 and 24 breaths per minute.
2. Arterial blood gas levels are within normal range.

NDx: Altered cerebral tissue perfusion related to an increase in brain tissue, intracranial volume, or CSF volume

Planning: Patient Outcomes
1. Patient maintains baseline neurologic status.
2. ICP returns to normal range.

NDx: Risk for fluid volume deficit related to osmotic diuretic therapy or fluid restriction

Planning: Patient Outcomes
1. Serum electrolytes are within normal range.
2. Serum osmolarity is within normal range.
3. Urine specific gravity is within normal range.

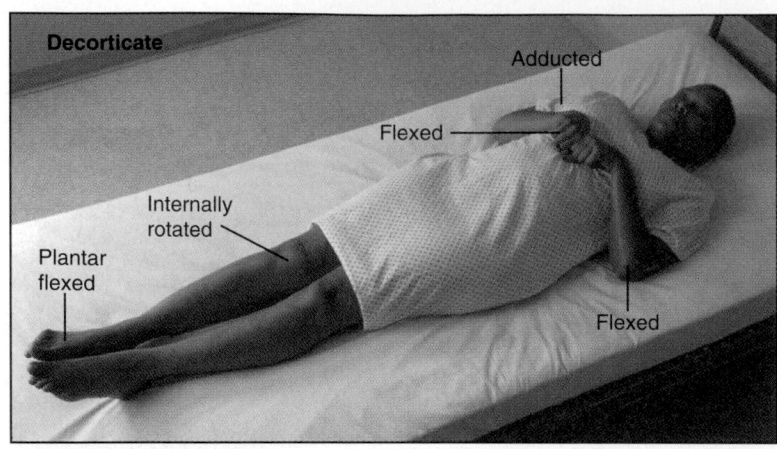

A

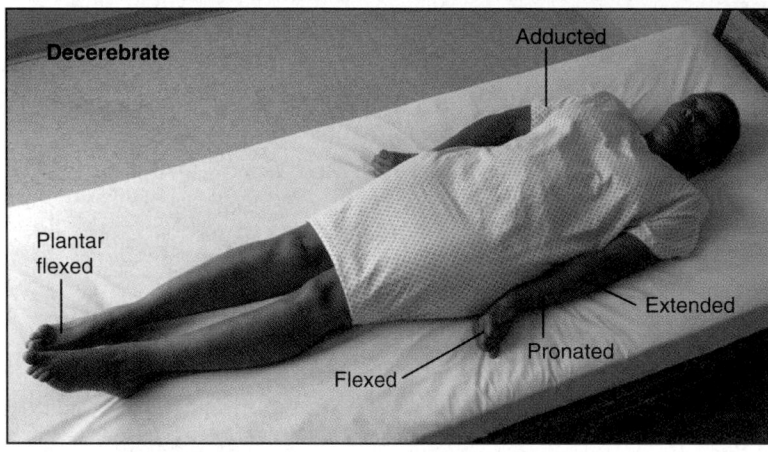

B

Figure 17–15
Types of posturing: decorticate and decerebrate.

NDx: Risk for impaired skin integrity related to immobility, hypothermia therapy

Planning: Patient Outcomes
1. Skin is free of redness.
2. Skin is intact.

NDx: Altered family processes related to actual or perceived loss of well-being of patient

Planning: Patient Outcomes
1. Family verbalizes feelings related to fears.
2. Family verbalizes acceptance of actual or potential altered abilities of patient.
3. Family verbalizes a plan for coping with the actual or potential altered abilities of patient.

Nursing Interventions and Evaluation

NDx: Ineffective breathing pattern
Maintain a patent airway to prevent hypoxia and hypercarbia. Use airway adjuncts as needed. Auscultate lung fields every 4 hours, and document findings. Administer oxygen therapy as ordered, and document effectiveness. Monitor trends in arterial blood gas values. Use hyperventilation techniques via manual resuscitation bag or via a mechanical ventilator to maintain $PaCO_2$ levels between 25 and

30 mm Hg and PaO_2 of 100 mm Hg. Hyperventilation produces respiratory alkalosis, which in turn produces cerebral vasoconstriction. Vasoconstriction decreases the amount of cerebral blood volume. A decrease in cerebral blood volume decreases ICP. This is the desired effect of hyperventilation. Monitor for Cheyne-Stokes respiratory pattern, indicative of increasing ICP affecting the respiratory center in the brain stem.

NDx: Altered cerebral tissue perfusion
Control and decrease of ICP is the focus of nursing care for altered cerebral tissue perfusion. Document accurate patient behavioral assessments every 1 to 2 hours. Report any deviation from baseline immediately. Maintain adequate venous drainage by elevating the head of the bed 30 to 40 degrees as ordered and by avoiding flexion of the neck. This promotes a decrease in cerebral blood volume, thereby preventing a further increase in ICP. Instruct the patient to refrain from activities that increase intrathoracic or intra-abdominal pressure such as straining at bowel movement, isometric exercises, coughing, sneezing, blowing the nose, and sitting in a high Fowler's position. A rise in intrathoracic or intra-abdominal pressure causes momentary compression

CLINICAL ? THINKING

HEADACHE AFTER A SKIING ACCIDENT

Forty-eight hours after his admission to the hospital with a fractured leg and a possible closed head injury, a 25-year-old man was preparing for discharge. The patient has been brought to the emergency department of a large medical center by ambulance after experiencing an unwitnessed fall while skiing. He had been discovered shortly after the incident by another skier, who reported that the patient had been conscious and coherent, but that the patient had no recollection of the accident itself. The patient's only significant medical history included asthma and atopic allergies since his preschool years. Theophylline had been discontinued 6 months previously. The patient was currently being treated with a regimen of corticosteroid and bronchodilator inhalers with good results. The patient denied any allergies to medications.

Physical examination of the patient in the emergency department revealed an alert and oriented, well-developed male with a closed fracture of the left tibia and multiple small abrasions and superficial lacerations of the head, left arm, and left leg. Blood work was drawn, skull and cervical spine fractures were ruled out by x-rays, and the results of cranial computed tomography (CT) were negative. No neurologic abnormalities or deficits were noted. His vital signs were: blood pressure 116/80; apical pulse 82 and regular; respirations 16 per minute, regular and unlabored; and temperature 98.2°F.

The tibial fracture was realigned with closed reduction and immobilized with a long leg plaster cast. The patient was admitted to the orthopedic unit for further evaluation and observation.

The nurse giving me the report stated that the patient's condition had remained stable since admission, and that he was to be discharged later that day. His Glasgow Coma Scale score remained at 15, and his neurologic status and vital signs had not deviated from his baseline. The patient had been instructed in weight-bearing and crutch-walking techniques.

Despite the patient's imminent discharge, I knew that the complications of head injury could still develop and that they could do so rapidly. I therefore performed a thorough physical assessment, which revealed no unusual respiratory, cardiovascular, or gastrointestinal findings. His cast was dry and intact with no rough edges, skin irritation, unusual odors, or evidence of drainage. Neurovascular evaluation of his left leg revealed no evidence of compartment syndrome. His toes were warm, capillary refill was less than 3 seconds,

he was able to move his toes, and he denied any paresthesias or pain.

The patient was alert and oriented to person, place, and time. He was able to move the three unaffected extremities on command and exhibited equal motor strength and sensory functioning on both sides. There was no evidence of weakness or paralysis. Examination of the patient's pupils revealed that they were equal in size and reacted equally and briskly to light. I checked for cerebrospinal fluid leakage from the patient's nose and ears and found none, and the patient denied a postnasal drip. Nor did I note any evidence of ecchymotic areas on the mastoid bone (Battle's sign) or the periorbital areas (raccoon eyes). Assessment for nuchal rigidity, papilledema, and a Babinski reflex also proved negative. The patient's vital signs were: blood pressure 120/82; apical pulse 80 and regular; respirations 18 per minute, regular and unlabored; and temperature 98.4°F.

I informed the patient that I would return shortly to review his discharge instructions. As I was leaving the room, the patient stated that perhaps going home would help rid him of his headache. I stopped and questioned him about this complaint, and I learned that the pain had started upon awakening that morning and had persisted.

Although I recognized that a headache, in the absence of any other positive findings, can be an innocuous complaint with no neurologic significance, its presence in a patient with a history of a recent head injury could signal a potential cerebral disaster. This change in the patient's condition, therefore, alerted me to watch him more carefully, and I decided to monitor his neurologic status more frequently.

When I returned to his room half an hour later to perform a quick, focused, neurologic check, the patient was lying in bed and appeared to be drowsy, lethargic, and confused. He was mumbling incoherently and was disoriented to time and place. I continued to perform some key assessments by asking him to grasp and push against my hand. He was able to follow commands but demonstrated some right-sided paresis. Next I evaluated his pupillary responses and noted that his left pupil was slightly dilated and sluggish to light. I checked his vital signs and found that they remained unchanged. I noted no papilledema or nuchal rigidity. The Babinski reflex remained negative. The patient denied any chest pain and showed no evidence of petechiae on the buccal mucosa or chest. As I completed my focused assessment, the patient vomited.

I was aware that the change in the patient's

(continued)

CLINICAL ? THINKING

(continued)

mental status could be the result of a number of complications of his orthopedic and neurologic condition. The possibilities included cerebral hypoxia secondary to bleeding, pulmonary embolism, fat embolism syndrome, or increased intracranial pressure (ICP). However, the absence of hypotension and tachycardia were not consistent with the possibility of hemorrhage and shock. The absence of chest pain, dyspnea, and tachycardia was not consistent with a pulmonary embolism. And the absence of tachycardia, dyspnea, fever, and petechiae was not consistent with fat embolism syndrome.

The classic findings of deterioration in level of consciousness, unilateral weakness, and unilateral pupillary changes were, on the other hand, a clear indication of intracranial injury with increasing ICP. The patient's complaint of headache and his vomiting further supported my suspicion. Although Cushing's triad (increasing systolic blood pressure, widening pulse pressure, and bradycardia) was absent, I recognized that this was a late sign of increased ICP and so did not necessarily rule out my hypothesis.

I knew that increased ICP can result after a head injury from intracranial bleeding in the form of an epidural hematoma, subdural hematoma, intracerebral bleed, or subarachnoid bleed, or from cerebral edema. I therefore considered the evidence and attempted to identify the underlying cause. A subarachnoid bleed was not likely because of the absence of nuchal rigidity. Nor was an epidural hematoma likely, because the rapid deterioration in the clinical picture of the patient with this condition typically occurs within the first 24 hours. The timing of this event (approximately 48 hours after the injury), and the findings of contralateral hemiparesis and ipsilateral pupillary changes, indicated the development of an acute subdural hematoma on the left side of the brain.

Regardless of the underlying cause, I knew that increased ICP was a neurologic emergency with a high morbidity and mortality rate. I also recognized that without immediate medical or surgical treatment, increased ICP reduces cerebral perfusion, resulting in cerebral hypoxia and infarction. It can also lead to the displacement of brain tissue and brainstem compression, herniation, permanent brain damage, coma, and death. I therefore took the following actions:

1. I checked the patency of the patient's airway and the adequacy of his ventilation.
2. I summoned another nurse, reported my assessments, and asked him to stat-page the physician while I remained with the patient.
3. I elevated the head of the bed to 30 degrees and placed the patient's head in the midline position.
4. I administered oxygen and established intravenous (IV) access as per hospital protocol.
5. I attached a pulse oximeter.
6. I initiated seizure precautions.
7. I instructed the patient not to cough, blow his nose, or perform the Valsalva maneuver.
8. I continued to monitor the patient's neurologic, cardiovascular, and respiratory status.
9. I provided emotional support by explaining what was happening and by offering realistic reassurance.
10. I documented my findings and actions.

Following the physician's arrival and examination of the patient, the patient was transferred to the neurologic intensive care unit (ICU) for continuous monitoring. Medical orders were written for stat cranial CT, arterial blood gases, oxygen therapy, hypertonic IV fluids, mannitol, glucocorti-

(continued)

---

of the internal jugular vein and increases cerebral blood volume. Administer medications such as stool softeners and analgesics as necessary, and monitor their effectiveness. Administer diuretics and steroids to draw fluid from the cranial structure as well as decrease cerebral edema, thereby decreasing ICP. Administer oxygen as needed and ordered. Monitor arterial blood gases. If hypothermic therapy is used, monitor the patient's temperature every 15 minutes rectally. Shivering may occur. This should be controlled with chlorpromazine because it increases ICP. Be alert for cardiac dysrhythmias as the body temperature lowers. Minimize the number and length of noxious or invasive nursing procedures, such as suctioning or venipuncture, whenever possible. Reduce stimulation. Organize nursing care to allow the patient optimal rest periods. Use restraints only when absolutely necessary because agitation increases ICP.

NDx: Risk for fluid volume deficit

Monitor and record intake and output and urinary specific gravity. Monitor pertinent laboratory data such as serum electrolytes, osmolality, and creatinine because administration of osmotic diuretics such as mannitol promotes diuresis and can deplete

CLINICAL ? THINKING

(continued)

coids, endotracheal intubation with hyperventilation via mechanical ventilation, nasogastric tube connected to continuous low suction, fluid restrictions and input and output measurements, and the insertion of an indwelling urinary catheter.

CT confirmed the presence of an acute left-sided subdural hematoma, and the patient was immediately taken to the operating room for evacuation of the hematoma via burr holes.

The patient tolerated the surgical procedure well, returned to the neurologic ICU with invasive intracranial pressure monitoring in place, and was transferred back to the medical-surgical unit 2 days later. The patient had survived the acute period and was then discharged without significant neurologic deficits. His prognosis for a complete recovery with no disabilities, following a potentially catastrophic head injury, was due in large measure to the nurse's anticipation of problems, vigilant monitoring, astute assessments, accurate clinical judgments, and quick interventions.

Think Critically

How much validity should be given to a nurse's "intuition"? What benefit does it afford the patient?

Should the nurse have reported the concern about the patient's headache sooner? Why? Why not?

Why did the nurse assess the patient's pupillary and motor responses before the patient's vital signs? Was this the best action? Why? Why not?

How did the assessment findings of ipsilateral pupillary changes and contralateral hemiparesis support the nurse's suspicion?

Is unequal pupil size always indicative of increased ICP? What else must be considered?

Was using the Glasgow Coma Scale the most appropriate check of neurologic functioning? Why? Why not? What parameters of cerebral perfusion are not measured by the Glasgow Coma Scale?

Should the nurse have reported the clinical findings directly to the physician? Why? Why not?

Was elevating the head of the bed the best action? Although it decreases ICP, it also decreases cerebral perfusion. Is this signficant?

What abnormal breathing patterns should the nurse have assessed the patient for if the patient's neurologic status had continued to deteriorate? How would these abnormal patterns exacerbate increased ICP? How would hyperventilation help?

The patient's mother asked why the patient was intubated and placed on mechanical ventilation prior to surgery when he was not having any difficulty breathing. What would be the nurse's best response?

A student nurse asked why hypertonic IV fluids and mannitol were ordered. What would be the nurse's best response?

What are the nursing implications and responsibilities when glucocorticoid therapy is implemented in the treatment of head injury?

What teaching and community referrals must be included in the discharge planning to help the patient and the family cope upon his return to the home and community? What possible short-term problems might the patient be faced with following a head injury? What long-term effects?

How might the outcome of this scenario have changed if the nurse had found Cushing's triad? What does the presence of an increasing systolic blood pressure, widening pulse pressure, and bradypnea signify?

---

electrolytes. Serum osmolality should not be allowed to exceed 320 mOsm to prevent oversaturation. Monitor vital signs every 1 to 2 hours for tachycardia and hypotension secondary to hypovolemia. Monitor skin turgor for signs of dehydration every 4 hours.

NDx: Risk for impaired skin integrity
Patients with increased ICP may exhibit a decrease in the level of consciousness, placing them at risk for skin breakdown while bed rest is maintained. Massage bony prominences every 2 hours to promote circulation. Use an air mattress to decrease

pressure to total body area. If hypothermia is used to decrease ICP, monitor peripheral circulation, color, and temperature of the skin every 2 hours. If using hypothermic therapy, give special attention to the digits and scrotum because they are at risk for compromised circulation.

NDx: Altered family processes
Increased ICP results in a deterioration in the patient's neurologic status and a threat to the patient's life. This may be a temporary condition and may have necessitated the patient's transfer to the intensive care unit. Recognize that the uncertainty of the

patient's prognosis and the stress of the event can interfere with the family's coping abilities. Explain all procedures to the family. Answer questions, and encourage verbalization of concerns. Provide privacy if needed, and make referrals to other personnel, such as clergy and physician, to assist the family in coping with the patient's condition. Involve the patient's family in care if they are willing. Family and staff should be aware that the sense of hearing is the last sense lost and the first sense regained. Assume the patient hears everything. Do not discuss the patient's status at the bedside.

Compare the patient's status with the expected outcomes. If the outcomes are not met, reassess the patient and revise the plan.

SPEECH AND LANGUAGE DYSFUNCTION

Aphasia is defined as a loss or impairment of language function. It can be used to refer to a variety of disturbances including dysfunction of spoken language, writing (agraphia), reading (alexia), or auditory comprehension. The specific dysfunction depends on the area in which brain injury has occurred. Thus a person rarely loses all abilities to communicate. Aphasia is often the result of cerebrovascular accident, tumor mass, hemorrhage, penetrating wounds, or trauma.

The three major types of aphasia syndromes are as follows:

> Expressive or motor aphasia, known as Broca's aphasia
> Receptive or sensory aphasia, known as Wernicke's aphasia
> Global aphasia, which is a combination of expressive and receptive aphasia

EXPRESSIVE APHASIA (BROCA'S APHASIA). Expressive aphasia is the result of injury to Broca's area, located in the frontal lobe of the dominant hemisphere (Fig. 17–16).

The patient demonstrates difficulty in expressing himself or herself through the spoken or written word. Speech is slow, nonfluent, and labored. Object naming is poor. Comprehension of written or verbal communication is intact.

Patients with Broca's aphasia are aware of their deficits. Often they become frustrated and at times depressed because they are not responding appropriately to their environment and have difficulty communicating their needs.

RECEPTIVE APHASIA (WERNICKE'S APHASIA). Receptive aphasia is the result of injury to Wernicke's area, located in the temporal lobe of the dominant hemisphere (see Fig. 17–16).

The patient experiencing receptive aphasia cannot comprehend written or verbal communication. Even though sounds are heard, the brain is unable to interpret or give meaning to the sound. The pa-

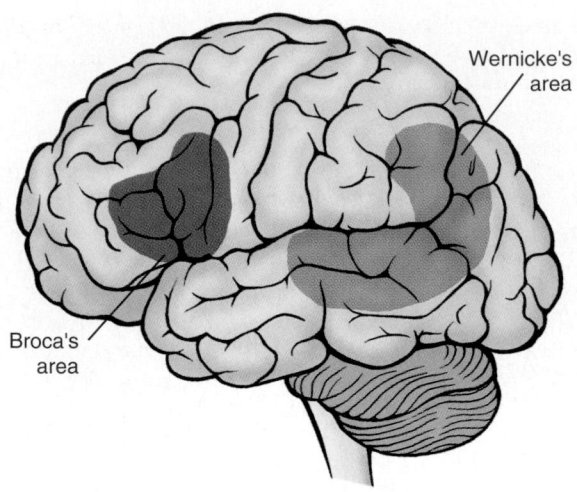

Figure 17–16
Speech areas of the dominant cerebral hemisphere: Broca's area (to the anterior) and Wernicke's area (to the posterior).

tient has fluent speech with normal rhythm and articulation. The patient conveys information poorly because of the use of empty or incorrect words. Repetition and object naming are poor.

Patients with receptive aphasia may not realize the nature of their deficit. These patients usually have a pleasant disposition and are not depressed.

GLOBAL APHASIA. Global aphasia is a combination of expressive and receptive aphasia. Little of the communication system is intact. These patients experience difficulty in interpreting the verbal or written word as well as expressing their own thoughts or needs by speaking or writing.

Global aphasia is the result of an extensive injury, encompassing both Broca's and Wernicke's areas. Prognosis for these patients is poor.

NURSING PROCESS
Speech and Language Dysfunction

Assessment

When a patient has sustained a brain insult, assessment of the speech and language system is a basic component of the neurologic baseline assessment. Specifically, assess for the presence of aphasia syndromes. Assess both expressive and receptive language centers through the testing of general behavior and mental status, auditory comprehension, verbal expression, reading, writing, motor speech skills, and verbal fluency. Note any alterations or disturbances in speech and language ability.

When establishing the patient's baseline functional level, be certain to identify and note factors that influence or affect the accuracy of the assessment. Factors to be identified include decreased level of consciousness that would decrease the ability for the patient to respond, visual or hearing deficits or loss, use of prosthetic devices such as dentures and eyeglasses, swallowing difficulties causing garbled speech, and language barriers.

Nursing Diagnoses and Planning

Nursing diagnoses and related expected patient outcomes most commonly applicable to patients with speech and language dysfunction include the following:

NDx: Sensory/perceptual alterations (auditory) related to receptive aphasia

Planning: Patient Outcomes
1. Patient communicates needs.
2. Patient demonstrates successful method of communication.
3. Patient uses alternative methods to understand and comprehend interaction with the environment.

NDx: Impaired verbal communication related to expressive aphasia

Planning: Patient Outcomes
1. Patient communicates needs.
2. Patient shares frustration when communicating with others.
3. Patient demonstrates alternative methods of communication.

Nursing Interventions and Evaluation

NDx: Sensory/perceptual alterations (auditory)
The patient with receptive aphasia can communicate through means other than comprehension of the spoken word. Therefore, promote communication through the use of alternative devices or techniques such as pad and pencil, touch, pointing, flash cards, pictures, and object communication boards. Face the patient. Establish eye contact to focus communication. Reduce external stimuli, speak slowly, and use simple commands and gestures when addressing the patient. Speak in a normal tone. The patient can hear. Increase the patient's ability to comprehend by having only one person try to communicate at a time. Provide an accepting environment in which the patient can practice communicating effectively.

NDx: Impaired verbal communication
The patient with expressive aphasia cannot accurately express needs. Encourage the patient to express thoughts and needs through the use of alternative communication devices and techniques such as pantomime, cueing, gestures, pointing, communication boards, or flash cards. Provide the patient with choices by asking questions in a "yes or no" format or by supplying two options. This alleviates the patient's frustration at trying to communicate with phrases that are often unintelligible. Engage the patient in conversation. Allow time for the patient to search for words. Disregard incorrect use of words. Allow the patient to express frustration. Provide an accepting atmosphere for him or her to learn and test communication skills.

Compare the patient's status with the expected outcomes. If the outcomes are not met, reassess the patient and revise the plan.

MOTOR SYSTEM DYSFUNCTION

Dysfunction of the motor system probably is the most marked of all clinical neurologic manifestations. Two major classes of motor system dysfunction are motor neuron disease and movement disorders.

Motor Neuron Disease
The motor system allows for voluntary motor movements by way of the pyramidal tract of the descending motor pathway, which transmits impulses from the cerebral cortex to the spinal cord and PNS. An alteration in this pathway, whether caused by trauma, infection, degenerative disease, vascular insult or hemorrhage, congenital disorder, or neoplasm, results in a disturbance of motor function and level of mobility. Such alterations are classified as either an upper motor neuron lesion or a lower motor neuron lesion (Table 17–6).

Upper motor neuron lesions can be located in the cerebral cortex, internal capsule, brain stem, or spinal cord. Characteristics of upper motor neuron lesions include loss of voluntary motor movement, muscle spasticity, hyper-reflexia, and atrophy of affected muscle groups related to disuse.

Lower motor neuron lesions are located in the anterior horn cells of the spinal cord or their axons. Characteristics of lower motor neuron lesions include muscle flaccidity, hyporeflexia or areflexia, atrophy of involved muscles related to denervation, and fasciculations.

Lack of voluntary motion in affected muscles is known as paralysis or plegia. Weakness of muscle strength is known as paresis. Hemiplegia or hemiparesis involves extremities on the same side of the body. Paraplegia or paraparesis involves both lower extremities. Quadriplegia or quadriparesis involves all four extremities. Paresis or paralysis is classified as either spastic or flaccid depending on whether there is upper motor neuron or lower motor neuron involvement.

Movement Disorders
Coordination, smoothness, and accuracy of motor movement is influenced by the intactness of the extrapyramidal tract of the descending motor pathway in conjunction with the basal ganglia and cerebellum. Neoplasms, degenerative disease, and infection commonly cause interference of motor impulse transmission within the extrapyramidal tract. As a result, the patient experiences movement disorders: bradykinesia (slowness of movement) and involuntary motor movements.

Patients with bradykinesia demonstrate extreme slowness in voluntary motor movement. This condi-

Table 17–6

Comparison of Paralysis due to Upper Motor Neuron Lesions and Lower Motor Neuron Lesions

Variable	Upper Motor Neuron Lesion	Lower Motor Neuron Lesion
Involvement	Muscle groups affected	Individual muscles may be involved
Tonus	Increased; muscles spastic; resist passive movement	Absent; muscles flaccid; no resistance offered
Reflexes *Normal*	Normal tendon reflexes exaggerated (hyperactive); abdominal reflex absent or diminished on affected side	Tendon reflexes absent; abdominal reflexes diminished if lesion is at thoracic level
Pathologic	Babinski's sign present (ie, dorsiflexion of toes, especially the great toe, in response to scratching sole of the foot) Hoffmann's sign present in hand (flexion of thumb and index finger after sudden release of terminal phalanx of middle finger after it has been flexed)	Babinski's sign absent; normal response (plantar flexion of toes) present Hoffmann's sign absent
Muscle atrophy	Only slight atrophy	Marked muscle wasting
Fasciculations (involuntary contractions of small groups of muscle fibers in a muscle)	Absent	May be present

tion is typically seen in patients who have a basal ganglia disorder, such as Parkinson's disease.

Common involuntary motor movements include tremor, dystonia, chorea, and dyskinesia. Tremor is a rhythmic, quivering, purposeless movement of the extremities or head. A tremor observed when the body part, usually the hand, is at rest is known as a resting tremor. Tremor observed when the patient initiates a movement is known as an intention tremor.

Dystonia is a condition in which there are involuntary twisting movements of the body and trunk. Torticollis is a form of dystonia characterized by the head being pulled to one side of the body as a result of neck muscle spasms. Dystonic movements often involve large muscle groups and produce bizarre movements and appearance.

Choreiform movements are irregular and variable and involve the extremities and facial muscles. Movements may occur at rest and increase when there is purposeful initiation of motor movement.

Dyskinesia is associated with adverse effects of psychotropic medications, such as phenothiazines. It is characterized by involuntary movements of the face, tongue, trunk, and extremities.

NURSING PROCESS
Motor System Dysfunction

Assessment

Assessment of the patient includes a history and physical examination. Ask the patient whether there is any family history of motor system dysfunction (movement disorders or motor neuron disease). Allow the patient to describe progression of motor dysfunction and how it affects ability to function.

Focus physical assessment on the cranial nerves influencing motor function: III, IV, V, VI, VII, IX, X, XI, and XII. Assess extraocular movements, chewing, swallowing, and facial movement. Assess the patient's ability to clear oral secretions. Also assess motor speech function, the muscle strength of the extremities and trunk, and respiratory muscle strength. Observe gait and ability to perform activities of daily living as well as coordination of movements.

Differentiate whether the motor system dysfunction involves the voluntary or involuntary motor movements of the patient. Determine the extent of dysfunction by asking questions such as "Is it limited to a specific area or muscle group?"

Determine whether the motor system dysfunction has had a psychosocial or emotional impact. Ask probing questions, such as the following:

"Has this condition changed your lifestyle?"
"Have you had to change what you do at home, at work, or with your friends?"
"Do you get upset or depressed about your condition?"

If the dysfunction has occurred recently and the patient has not had time to accept or accommodate the deficit, it would be better not to ask these questions. Also, these questions should be asked only in the rehabilitation setting because the patient is just beginning to comprehend the loss.

Nursing Diagnoses and Planning

Nursing diagnoses and related expected patient outcomes most commonly applicable to patients with motor system dysfunction include the following:

NDx: Impaired physical mobility related to muscle weakness

Planning: Patient Outcomes
1. Patient moves, transfers, and ambulates with or without assistance.
2. Patient remains free of complications of immobility.
3. Patient remains free of self-injury.

NDx: Self care deficit related to muscle weakness or uncontrolled motor movements

Planning: Patient Outcomes
1. Patient hygiene, nutrition, and elimination needs are met.
2. Patient participates in self-care within limitations.

NDx: Impaired gas exchange related to respiratory muscle weakness or uncontrolled motor movements

Planning: Patient Outcomes
1. Breath sounds are normal bilaterally.
2. Cyanosis is absent.
3. Patient remains free of aspiration and atelectasis.

NDx: Self esteem disturbance related to loss of motor function control

Planning: Patient Outcomes
1. Patient acknowledges motor dysfunction.
2. Patient willingly expresses feelings.
3. Patient performs activities of daily living within limitations of motor dysfunction.
4. Patient maintains personal and social relationships.

Nursing Interventions and Evaluation

NDx: Impaired physical mobility
To reduce complications related to immobility or subluxation of joints, provide active and passive range-of-motion exercises at least every 6 hours. Allow the patient to do as much for herself or himself (moving, transferring, bathing, eating, dressing) as possible.

Arrange for a trapeze to be placed on the bed to allow the patient to aid in positioning herself or himself. Maintain good body alignment. Eliminate undue pressure or rotation of joints. Consult with physical and occupational therapists to obtain supportive and assistive devices to be used by the patient for activities of daily living, such as a cane, wheelchair, eating utensils, splints, and slings.

Maintain a turning and positioning schedule every 2 hours. Provide good skin care. Use an air mattress or special bed as necessary. This care may vary if the patient is able to be up. Ensure that clothing and bed sheets are dry and clean.

Plan daily activities so there are rest periods between strenuous activities. Instruct the patient on recognizing signs of fatigue and organizing daily routine to provide optimal rest periods.

NDx: Self care deficit
Establish the patient's ability to meet own self-care needs of hygiene, dressing, eating, ambulating, and toileting. Encourage the patient to provide self-care within limitations. Provide assistance as necessary in the form of additional support and assistive devices to meet needs.

Because uncontrolled movements may inhibit the patient from feeding herself or himself and increase the risk of aspiration, feed the patient if necessary. Consult with the nutritionist and physician to initiate alternative methods to provide nutrition to patient, such as a gastrostomy tube if needed.

Intervene and assist the patient to prevent fatigue or frustration. Ensure that safety measures are followed to avoid injury. For example, instruct the patient to ambulate or transfer with assistance as necessary. Caution him or her not to perform beyond limitations.

Consult with physical and occupational therapists to promote self-care. Consult with social services to assist in discharge planning. Identify available community resources (eg, home health aide, family involvement).

NDx: Impaired gas exchange
Monitor respiratory status by auscultating lung fields and checking respiratory rate, rhythm, and breath sounds. Position the patient to facilitate drainage of secretions. Encourage the patient to be up if able.

Instruct the patient on deep breathing, coughing, and incentive spirometry exercises. Perform suctioning, postural drainage, and chest percussion as necessary.

Instruct the patient to eat in the upright position to avoid aspiration unless contraindicated. Provide foods of appropriate consistency for the patient to chew and swallow. Allow adequate time for meals.

NDx: Self esteem disturbance
Provide an accepting atmosphere in which the patient feels comfortable to discuss feelings and needs by planning time to spend together in a quiet, private area. Encourage the patient to discuss feelings of inadequacies or embarrassment, changes that need to be made in professional, family, and social activities.

Identify resources that are available for support and therapeutic intervention, such as self-help groups, church and community resources, and support groups specific to the type of dysfunction or disease process that the patient is experiencing (eg, multiple sclerosis patient group).

Encourage maintenance of professional, family, and social roles and interactions. Recognize the patient's need to be active and successful in endeavors to increase feelings of self-worth. Assist the patient in identifying effective coping mechanisms. Plan opportunities for the patient to role-play various responses to situations to increase his or her ability to use effective coping mechanisms in unpredictable situations. Always consider the patient's emotional readiness.

Compare the patient's status with the expected outcomes. If the outcomes are not met, reassess the patient and revise the plan.

SENSORY SYSTEM DYSFUNCTION

Sensory system dysfunction is not easily discernible. However, it has a dramatic impact on the functional level of a patient. Dysfunction of the sensory system manifests as a disturbance in vision, hearing, taste, smell, pain perception, touch sensation, temperature discrimination, or proprioception (awareness of the position of a body part in space).

Vision
Visual disturbances vary with the cause and disease process involved. The visual structures and visual sensory pathway are affected by neurologic conditions, including degenerative disease, neoplasms, infection, vascular disease, and hemorrhage. Nystagmus is a condition in which there is tremor-like, oscillating movement of the eyes. This often occurs in patients with cerebellar dysfunction, such as those with multiple sclerosis. Diplopia, also known as double vision, is caused by weakness of the ocular muscles. Scotomata are blind or absent gaps in the visual field. Patients may report alterations of visual acuity, such as blurred vision, clouded vision, or visual loss.

Visual field deficits occur when there is an interruption or lesion of the visual sensory pathway (Fig. 17–17). Patients with pituitary tumors in particular exhibit visual field deficits. As the tumor enlarges, it compresses the optic chiasm, which lies superior to the pituitary gland. Patients complain of hemianopia or loss of vision in one-half of their visual field.

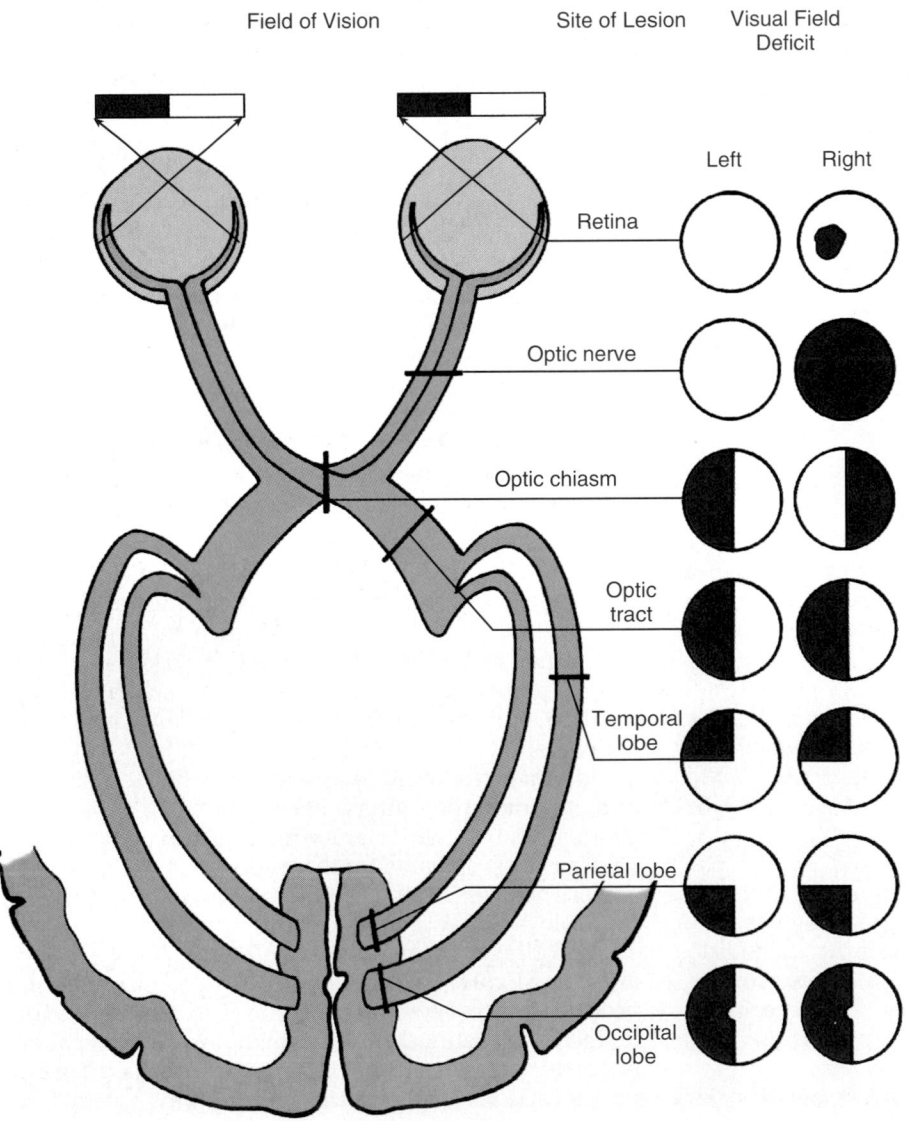

Figure 17–17

Visual field deficits resulting from interruptions of the visual pathways at various locations.

Hearing

Hearing disturbances range from diminished to total loss of hearing. Neoplasms, ototoxic medications, head injury, and meningitis are common causes of hearing disturbances. Acoustic neuromas are tumors that affect cranial nerve VIII, resulting in a hearing impairment or loss.

Tinnitus, conduction deafness, and nerve deafness are three common types of hearing disturbances. Tinnitus is a condition in which the patient complains of a ringing or buzzing in the ear when there is no external source for the sound. Conduction deafness is a hearing loss attributed to lack of sound transmission because of a structural problem in the cochlea or inner ear. Nerve deafness is a hearing loss resulting from a disturbance in the auditory pathway related to a neurologic disease or condition affecting cranial nerve VIII.

Pain, Temperature, Touch, and Proprioception

Disturbances of pain perception, temperature discrimination, proprioception, and touch sensation are caused by impulse transmission interference in the ascending sensory pathways of the spinal cord or the sensory cortex located in the parietal lobe. This interference can be related to varied pathology, such as trauma, neoplasms, hemorrhage, or degenerative changes affecting any portion of the sensory system.

When a complete spinal cord injury occurs, the patient loses all motor and sensory function below the level of injury (Fig. 17–18). There is no recovery of this loss.

When a hemitransection of the spinal cord occurs, the patient manifests what is known as the Brown-Séquard syndrome (*see* Fig. 17–18). This is characterized by ipsilateral (same side) loss of proprioception, ipsilateral paresis or paralysis, and contralateral (opposite side) loss of pain sensation and temperature discrimination.

Complete hemianalgesia results from a thalamic lesion, loss of sensation in the sacral area from a cauda equina lesion, and loss of pain and temperature sense across the upper chest from a central cord lesion (*see* Fig. 17–18).

The degree and extent of pain, temperature, proprioception, and touch dysfunction depend on the extent of injury. The clinical manifestations may range from paresthesia (abnormal or diminished sensations) to anesthesia (total loss of sensation).

NURSING PROCESS
Sensory System Dysfunction

Assessment

Obtain a patient history. Ask the patient to identify specific sensory alterations being experienced and to

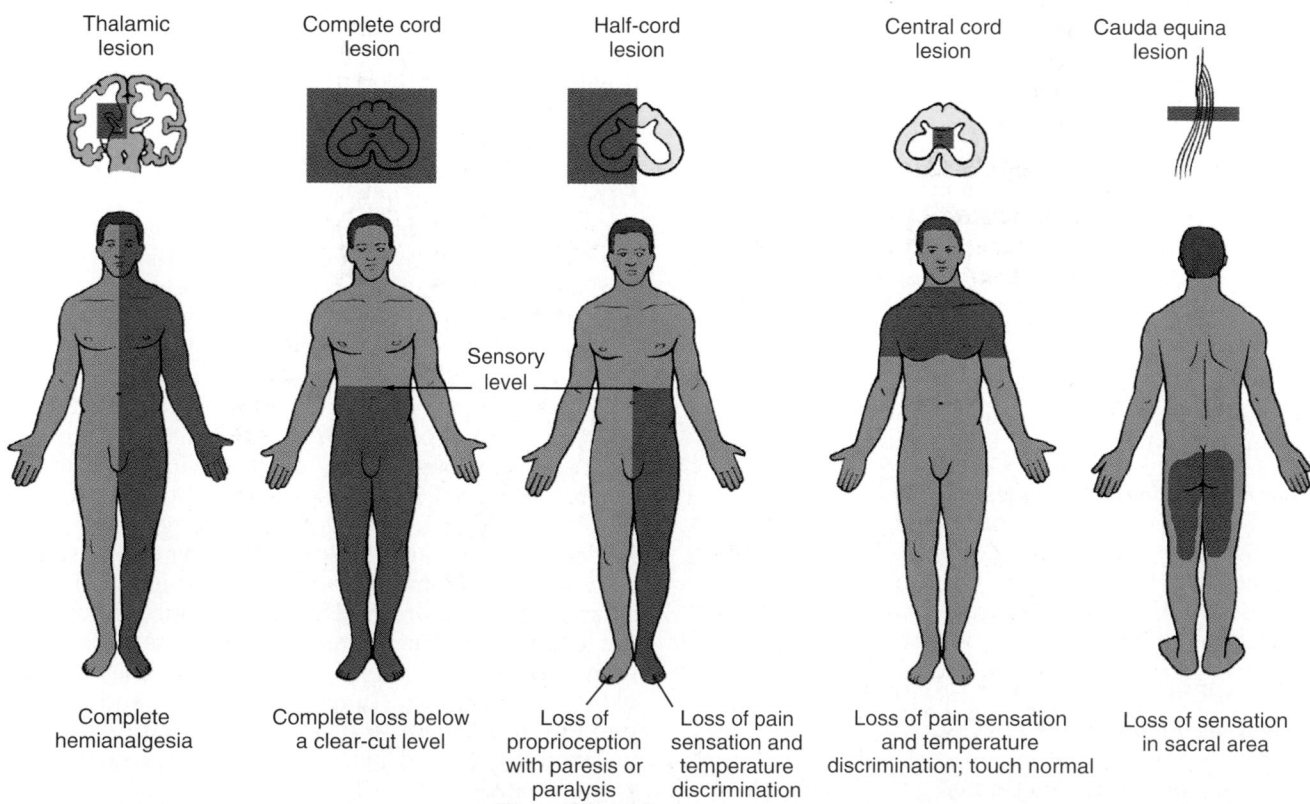

Figure 17–18

Patterns of altered sensation resulting from various spinal cord lesions.

describe their onset and progression. Inquire about any infectious process or other illnesses that may have caused or contributed to the sensory alteration. Determine what prescribed or over-the-counter drugs have recently been or are currently being taken. Review the patient's nutritional intake.

Focus physical assessment on the cranial nerves influencing sensory function, including cranial nerves I, II, V, VII, VIII, IX, and X. Assess visual acuity and visual fields. Assess the patient's hearing ability and pain, proprioception, temperature, and light-touch discrimination. Explore how the sensory alteration affects daily function. Observe the patient's ability to perform activities of daily living.

Assess the patient's risk for injury as a result of the following:

Visual deficits
Hearing alterations
Dysfunction of pain, temperature, or light-touch sensation, or proprioception

Ask probing questions, such as "Have you had any bruises or burns that you did not feel?" and "Do you find yourself doing tricks, such as squinting, visualizing body parts, or using devices, to help perform tasks or prevent you from hurting yourself?"

Nursing Diagnoses and Planning

Nursing diagnoses and related expected patient outcomes most commonly applicable to patients with sensory system dysfunction include the following:

NDx: Risk for injury related to sensory system dysfunction

Planning: Patient Outcomes
1. Patient remains free of injuries such as burns, falls, lacerations, and pressure injuries.
2. Patient uses assistive devices and techniques to compensate for sensory dysfunction.
3. Patient and family demonstrate safety precautions.

NDx: Self care deficit related to sensory system dysfunction (vision, touch, proprioception, temperature discrimination)

Planning: Patient Outcomes
1. Patient performs self-care using compensatory techniques and devices with or without assistance.
2. Patient's hygiene, nutrition, and elimination needs are met.

Nursing Interventions and Evaluation

NDx: Risk for injury
Sensory system deficits compromise a patient's ability to perform activities or tasks safely. The patient has to be protected through his or her own or others' efforts and taught how to meet needs safely.

Maintain a consistent environment within the acute-care setting and the home for the patient with a visual alteration. Place furniture out of the way so it does not present obstacles. Encourage the patient to use visual abilities to the fullest extent. Teach the patient to compensate for visual field deficits by scanning the environment. Encourage the patient to use eye wear (glasses or eye patches) as prescribed to increase visual acuity. Ensure that personal belongings (tissues, telephone) are within reach when the patient is confined to bed. Use side rails if needed to prevent the patient from falling off of the edge of the bed. Teach the patient and family members to keep the bed in the lowest position. Instruct the patient to use footwear with nonskid soles. Soft slippers should not be worn.

Modify the environment to compensate for hearing impairments. Explore with the patient assistive devices that increase awareness of the environment. Special sounding doorbells, telephones, and warning devices are available to augment the patient's ability to hear various tones.

Encourage the patient with an altered sensorium (touch, pain, temperature discrimination) to concentrate continuously on each step of activities performed. Instruct the patient that awareness and visualization of activities are essential to prevent injury. Teach the patient alternative safety measures, such as the use of a thermometer to establish the temperature of water or the use of protective clothing and gloves to shield skin.

When a patient is unaware of position sense (proprioception), instruct him or her to visualize the legs and extremities when walking, sitting, or lying down. Teach the patient to ensure that extremities are in proper body alignment to avoid subluxation of joints or undue pressure.

NDx: Self care deficit
Establish the patient's ability to meet his or her own self-care needs of hygiene, dressing, eating, ambulating, and toileting. Determine the level of additional support and assistive devices needed. Encourage the patient to provide self-care within limitations. Provide assistance to meet needs as necessary.

Encourage the patient to focus on performance of individual steps of self-care when alterations in proprioception, temperature discrimination, pain, or touch sensations are present. This helps to ensure that each step is carried out thoroughly to avoid inadequate self-care. Teach the patient to visualize steps of psychomotor activities to heighten self-awareness of actions and to avoid injury. Encourage the use of a thermometer to determine bath water temperature. Role-play everyday situations, such as using sharp objects (knives), the oven, and an iron to allow the patient to practice and predict the steps he or she needs to perform to accomplish the task without harm.

Compare the patient's status with the expected outcomes. If the outcomes are not met, reassess the patient and revise the plan.

BRAIN DEATH

Brain death is defined as an irreversible condition in which cerebral function is absent and the brain stem cannot maintain cardiovascular and respiratory vital functions. The heart fails to function within hours or weeks once a person is brain dead and supported on mechanical ventilation. Determination of brain death, as death of a patient, has been the source of moral, social, religious, medical, and legal controversy.

The Harvard University Ad Hoc Committee to Examine the Definition of Brain Death published its criteria for brain death determination in 1968. These criteria included unresponsiveness, total lack of reflexes, apnea, and lack of spontaneous movement of the person.

Findings that confirm brain death include the following:

• Pupils unreactive to light
• Apnea
• Absence of corneal, oculocephalic (doll's eyes), oculovestibular (caloric testing), and gag reflexes

Electroencephalography, CT, and cerebral blood flow studies have been used to document absence of brain function and to support the determination of death.

Confirmatory tests for diagnosis of brain death are repeated in 24 hours to document that the patient's status has not changed. This is critical to rule out the possibility that the patient may be in coma from a reversible event such as drug- or metabolic-induced CNS depression, hypothermia, or shock.

The physical care of the patient focuses on maintaining and supporting body functioning while the determination of brain death is in process. The patient does require mechanical ventilation to support respiratory function. The potential of the patient to be an anatomic gift donor needs to be assessed once the determination of death has been confirmed. The option of donation is then presented to the family for their consideration and decision.

Assessment of the Nervous System

Assessment of the nervous system is actually a three-part evaluative process that progresses from the history and description of the patient's complaints and symptoms (subjective data) to a physical examination of nervous system structures and their functions (objective data) to needed diagnostic testing.

Important information that provides a baseline of the patient's functional status is elicited during the data-collection and examination phases of the assessment. In addition, the patient's self-care needs can be identified and can serve as a basis for planning and evaluating progress toward maximizing capabilities.

PATIENT HISTORY

Obtain a careful health history before the physical examination of the nervous system. Allow the patient to describe, in his or her own words, the exact nature of the problem that has prompted a neurologic evaluation. Give special attention to eliciting a chronologic account of the presenting symptoms, noting in particular the nature of onset—sudden or insidious—as well as any circumstances surrounding the initial event. Explore specific details of the present illness in terms of intensity, improvements, or exacerbations. Directly question the patient regarding, such symptoms as numbness or tingling sensations, headaches, seizures, or syncopal episodes, as necessary.

Obtain a summary of the patient's medical and surgical history, including prescription and over-the-counter medications currently and previously used. Ask questions regarding family history of illness because many neurologic diseases are hereditary. Gather psychosociocultural data needed to provide key insights into the patient's and family's coping mechanisms and to serve as the basis for discharge planning. Include the patient's marital status, number and ages of children, past and present occupational status, ethnic background, type of housing, recreational interests, and any financial concerns or constraints. Assess the patient's understanding and compliance with health promotion and risk reduction measures related to the health of the neurologic system (Highlight 17–2). If the patient cannot provide accurate or complete information, obtain the data from a family member.

PHYSICAL EXAMINATION

Examination of the nervous system in the conscious adult generally follows a standardized approach, organized into the following components: mental status, speech and language, cranial nerves, motor system, sensory system, and reflexes. Equipment needed for a neurologic examination includes the following:

Cotton
Flashlight
Newspaper (or other printed material)
Ophthalmoscope
Otoscope
Reflex hammer
Safety pins
Snellen chart
Tape measure
Tongue depressor

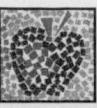
Tuning fork
Various objects of different shapes (key, marble, coin)
Vials (stoppered) containing the following:
  Peppermint, coffee (smell)
  Salt, vinegar (taste)
  Hot and cold water (temperature)

Mental Status

Although the mental status examination is delineated as a separate component of assessment, much of the evaluation of the patient's mental status is integrated throughout the whole interactive process of the neurologic examination. Valuable data are gathered during the interview phase. During this somewhat relaxed conversation, observe the patient's appearance and behavior. Note the overall state of awareness, ability to relax, manner of dress and personal hygiene, facial expressions, quality of speech patterns, and overall mood and thought processes.

Because assessment of a person's mental status is actually an evaluation of cerebral function, ask specific questions that test orientation, judgment, attention span and concentration, memory, intellectual ability, and abstract reasoning.

To assess orientation, ask the patient to correctly state his or her full name, the name of the hospital or facility, and the correct date, including day of week, month, and year. To assess judgment, note whether the patient can draw logical conclusions and express thoughts clearly in response to the question "What would you do if there was a fire in the wastebasket?" To assess attention and concentration abilities, ask the patient to repeat a series of five or six digits forward and then backward. Serial 7 testing can also be used. Instruct the patient to start at 100 and subtract 7, then subtract 7 again, and so on. Note the effort required and the speed and accuracy of the answers.

Test both recent and remote memory. Assess remote memory by asking straightforward questions about events in the past that can be validated, such as anniversaries or year of graduation from school. To test recent memory, ask the patient to recall a mutually known event that occurred earlier in the day. Assess immediate recall by giving the patient two or three common objects to remember. Ask the patient to list them after 5 or 10 minutes. Test underlying intelligence by asking general knowledge questions such as "Who is the president of the United States?", "What is the capital city of France?", "What are the four seasons of the year?", or other questions consistent with the patient's cultural and educational background. To assess the capacity to reason abstractly, ask the patient to explain a proverb, such as "A stitch in time saves nine" and to discuss why similar items are alike (eg, an orange and an apple, or a child and a dwarf).

Speech and Language Function

Language is a system in which symbols are used to convey meaning. It can be expressed as the spoken word or in writing. Speech is a mode of communication that uses sounds to represent that symbolic meaning. Speech and language function is a highly complex cerebral process involving coordination between parts of the temporal and frontal lobes of the dominant (usually the left) hemisphere and the occipital lobes. In addition, the muscles of the tongue, palate, pharynx, and lips are necessary for the articulation of speech. Any interference or disruption in the intricate inter-relationship of any of these areas results in impairment of communication.

Assessment of speech and language function requires the patient to produce spontaneous speech, repeat phrases, and identify objects. Assess the expressive component of speech by asking the patient to repeat one or two phrases. Note the clarity and fluency of speech as well as the ability to repeat the words without hesitancy or substitution. Show the patient at least five objects, and ask him or her to identify each by name. Note the patient's responses. Keep in mind that the object should not be described by its functional use. For example, a person with a language impairment might be unable to say "hairbrush" but could state that it is "something to use for my hair."

To assess the receptive component of speech, ask the patient to follow a simple one-step command such as "stick out your tongue." If the patient can follow simple instructions, give more complex commands involving two or three steps. Do not give the patient any visual cues. If the ability to perform complex commands without demonstration is unimpaired, the receptive portion of communication is intact.

To further assess language comprehension as well as the ability to express himself or herself in writing, give the patient a paper and pencil. Ask him or her to write his or her name, to draw a picture of a simple object, to write a dictated sentence, and to write a response to an open-ended question.

Cranial Nerve Function

Test the function of the cranial nerves as described in Table 17–1.

Motor Function

The motor system is composed of many intertwining pathways that allow movement to be synchronous, smooth, and coordinated. Assessment of the motor system therefore involves evaluation of gait and posture as well as muscle mass, size, tone, and strength.

Observe the patient's gait, if possible, while the patient is unaware of the observance. Note body posture, rhythm, symmetry of gait, and coordination of movement. For example, if hemiparesis (ie, weakness of one side of the body) is present, the normal rhythmic swinging of the arms is reduced on that side (when walking, the right arm should swing with the left leg). Request the patient to lie down in a relaxed manner to assess muscle mass, size, and tone. Inspect and palpate each muscle group, comparing the muscles on the left side of the body with the same ones on the right side. Investigate any suspicion of differences in muscle size by verifying size with a tape measure. Palpate muscle groups to help detect the presence of atrophy or wasting of the muscles.

Tone refers to the resistance detected when a joint is moved through its range of motion without any active or voluntary muscle contractions. Passively move each extremity through a full range of motion (flexion and extension) to detect hypotonia or hypertonia.

Assess muscle strength by asking the patient to move each of the muscle groups against your active resistance. Compare one side of the body with the same muscle group on the other side. Note symmetry and equality of strength. Test the flexors and extensors of the upper and lower arms and then the flexors and extensors of the upper and lower legs. To test the biceps, hold the patient's wrist and ask him or her to flex the arm as you pull on the wrist. To test the triceps, instruct the patient to extend the arm as you push against the wrist. Test other muscle groups similarly. When possible, assess both sides at the same time to enhance comparison. Grade motor strength against gravity and resistance on a scale of 0 to 5 (Table 17–7).

Use the formal testing methods previously described to establish a baseline of the patient's motor function. Make subsequent assessments quickly by using the techniques listed next.

ARM DRIFT. Have the patient extend both arms forward, palms up. Ask him or her to close the eyes and hold this position for 10 to 15 seconds. Observe for any downward drift of arms or pronation of hands.

HAND GRIP. Place the first two fingers of each of your hands in each of the patient's hands. Ask him or her to squeeze tightly and simultaneously. Note the strength and equality of grips.

STRAIGHT LEG RAISE. Ask patient to raise each leg individually as high as possible from a recumbent position without bending the knees. Note any inability of the patient to reach the maximum possibility of 90 degrees.

KNEE LIFTS. While the patient is still lying recumbent, place your hands above each kneecap and ask him or her to bend the knees simultaneously against your resistance. Observe for strength and equality of knee bends.

ANKLE DORSIFLEXION. Stand at the foot of the patient's bed. Ask the patient to pull the toes of both feet up toward the face and maintain this position. Place your hands on the dorsa of both feet and pull down simultaneously. Note the presence of decreased patient resistance.

ANKLE PLANTAR FLEXION. Ask the patient to pull the toes up toward the face again. Place the palms of your hands on the soles of the patient's feet and instruct him or her to push down simultaneously. Note any weakness or inability to perform plantar flexion.

Sensory Function

Assessment of the sensory system involves evaluation of light-touch sensation, pain sensation, temperature discrimination, position sense, and vibration sense. Because these sensory modalities travel on

Table 17–7

Grading Scale for Motor Strength

Grade	Description
5/5	Normal muscle strength (ie, full range of motion against examiner resistance)
4/5	Full range of motion of muscle but can be overcome with increased examiner resistance
3/5	Full range of motion of muscle against gravity only; is overcome with slight examiner resistance
2/5	Weak movement of muscle but insufficient to overcome gravity
1/5	Slight visible or palpable contraction of muscle noted but no movement results
0/5	Complete paralysis

distinct pathways in the nervous system, test each separately. Ask the patient to keep the eyes closed during this portion of the examination to avoid distraction of visual cues from the environment.

To assess light touch, use a wisp of cotton and stroke a section of the patient's skin. Ask the patient to identify the area touched and to describe what is felt. Repeat the procedure in the same area on the opposite side of the body, and compare results. Continue to test light-touch perception systematically (eg, begin with the upper arm and progress to the forearm, hand, torso, thigh, lower leg, and foot, remembering to stop and compare right side with left side as each area is tested).

Assess superficial pain sensation by gently touching the point of a pin against the skin in the same systematic manner used for light touch, occasionally substituting the pin's blunt end. Ask the patient to indicate whether the sensation felt is sharp or dull. Determine temperature sensitivity by touching a stoppered vial or test tube of hot water to the patient's abdomen for approximately 1 second. Repeat with the cold-water vial, requesting the patient to differentiate between hot and cold. Use the same technique to test other areas on the extremities. As-

sess position sense (proprioception) by moving one of the patient's digits up or down. Ask the patient to determine which way the digit has been moved. Check at least three to four digits on each extremity. Assess vibration sense by tapping a tuning fork on the heel of your hand to cause vibration and then placing the base of the fork firmly on the interphalangeal joint of the great toe. Ask the patient to describe what is felt. Repeat this procedure on the bony prominences of the wrists, shoulders, hips, ankles, shins, knees, and elbows. Assess stereognostic function by placing a small common object such as a key in the patient's right hand. Ask him or her to manipulate it in the hand and identify it. Repeat this procedure with a marble and a coin, and then test the left hand with the same objects.

Reflex Function

Assess the deep tendon reflexes with a reflex hammer. Reflexes are graded on a scale of 4 to 0:

4+   Very brisk, hyperactive
3+   More brisk than average
2+   Normal
1+   Diminished response
0   No response

Table 17–8 presents a guide to a quick neurologic assessment, which is useful in determining changes in neurologic baseline.

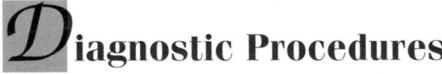

Diagnostic Procedures

SKULL X-RAY EXAMINATIONS

X-ray examinations of the skull are a painless, noninvasive radiographic diagnostic tool. They allow visualization of the skull bones and the cranial sinuses. Routine skull x-ray films are taken in the anteroposterior views.

The most frequent reason for an x-ray examination of the skull is to detect a fracture, usually related to a traumatic injury. Skull x-ray films can also detect calcifications and bone erosion.

It is necessary to remove dentures and all jewelry from the head and neck area to allow full visualization of the skull region.

SPINE X-RAY EXAMINATIONS

X-ray examinations of the spine allow for visualization of the cervical, thoracic, and lumbar spine. Lateral, anterior, and posterior views are routine. They are useful in the evaluation and detection of fractures, degenerative changes, displacement of the spinal cord, and spinal tumors. Which area of the spine

Table 17–8

Guide to Quick Neurologic Assessment

Parameter*	Assessment
Level of consciousness	Assess orientation to person, place, time
	Assess appropriateness of speech; note clarity and fluency
Cranial nerves	Assess pupillary response to light bilaterally (oculomotor nerve)
	Assess extraocular movements: oculomotor, trochlear, and abducens nerves
	Assess facial symmetry (facial nerve)
	Assess gag reflex (glossopharyngeal nerve)
	Assess tongue in midline when extended (hypoglossal nerve)
Motor function	Assess arm drifting
	Assess handgrip
	Assess straight leg raise
	Assess knee bends
	Assess ankle plantar flexion and dorsiflexion
Sensory function	Assess sensation to light touch and pinprick in extremities and on trunk, comparing right with left sides

*These parameters can be assessed quickly to determine changes in neurologic baseline.

is x-rayed depends on the type and extent of injury suspected.

If a fracture is suspected, undue manipulation is avoided. If a cervical collar is in place, it should not be removed until cervical injury is ruled out. Head hyperextension is avoided until cervical fracture is ruled out.

COMPUTED TOMOGRAPHY

CT is used to identify, evaluate, and follow-up abnormalities of cranial structures as well as other areas of the body.

This procedure uses an x-ray scanner, computer, and display mechanism to print images. Images of the brain are produced as narrow x-ray beams scan successive layers of the head. As x-ray beams are projected on various planes, they are absorbed or transmitted depending on the density of the tissue. There are different absorption coefficients for varying substances, such as bone, air, tissue, CSF, blood, and calcification. A computer calculates the absorption density of a selected region, and a display of the image is produced. The brightness or dullness demonstrated in the image is proportional to the x-ray absorption in that area. Lesions can be identified when comparing differences in densities with normal surrounding tissue.

For a brain CT scan, the patient lies in the supine position on an adjustable table with the head resting in a snug cap. The x-ray scanner rotates around the head in various cross sections, passing a narrow x-ray beam through the head from one side to the other. It is important that the head be secure and that the patient refrain from talking or purposefully moving the head, because movement can produce artifacts on the image produced. Extra support, such as sponges on either side of the head, may be used to decrease head movement. It is a painless procedure with no postprocedure care indicated.

In an enhanced scan, the patient receives an intravenous iodinated dye. Then the entire scanning procedure is repeated. Enhanced scans increase the detection of vascular lesion, detection of small lesions, and sharpness of lesion demarcations. A consent is needed if dye is used.

POSITRON EMISSION TOMOGRAPHY

Positron emission tomography (PET) is an imaging technique that uses radioactive tracers to produce images that measure physiologic and biochemical activities and functioning levels of the brain. PET can determine the rate at which the brain consumes glucose and oxygen. It also measures regional cerebral blood flow and volume.

The patient either inhales or is injected with a radioactive tracer (eg, carbon-11). The tracer passes through the blood-brain barrier. The positively charged tracer combines with electrons in the brain, thereby creating gamma rays. The scanning equipment, arranged in a circular array of detectors, records the presence of gamma rays. A computer measures the rays and produces an image that corresponds to specific regions of the brain and their cellular functioning.

PET has been useful in diagnostic assessment of patients with neurologic dysfunction. Specific indications include locating brain lesions that alter brain function, identifying metabolic changes such as in patients with Alzheimer's disease, measuring cerebral perfusion, and determining biochemical processes in patients experiencing behavioral disturbances (ie, depression, schizophrenia).

MAGNETIC RESONANCE IMAGING

Magnetic resonance imaging (MRI) is an advance in imaging techniques. MRI can reveal variations in cerebral structures that are subtle and often not seen with other diagnostic modalities. Unlike CT, MRI does not use x-ray beams. MRI uses a powerful magnet and radiofrequency signals to scan the head and body. Then a computer transforms these signals into images, or pictures (Fig. 17–19).

The patient is placed inside a giant, cylinder-shaped electromagnet, which aligns the hydrogen proton atoms found in the water of the cell bodies. The patient is kept immobilized. Temporary radiofrequency pulsations knock the protons out of alignment. Once the pulsation ends, excess energy is released as the protons return to their resting state (known as relaxation time). This excess energy can be decoded by a computer to give specific information in the form of an image. MRI does not involve exposure to ionized radiation or the use of contrast mediums.

MRI is used in the evaluation of patients with cerebral dysfunction as well as other bodily abnormalities. MRI is useful in its ability to do the following:

- Demonstrate changes in tissue water content associated with tumors
- Detect necrotic tissue and degenerative changes of the CNS
- Visualize the brain stem and the structures of the posterior fossa

Before the procedure, the patient must remove all metals that would be attracted by the magnet. This procedure is contraindicated for patients with metal implants that cannot be removed, such as a pacemaker, internal defibrillator, or internal metallic plate or clip.

CAROTID DOPPLER STUDIES

Carotid Doppler studies use a Doppler instrument, which emits ultrasound waves to evaluate carotid

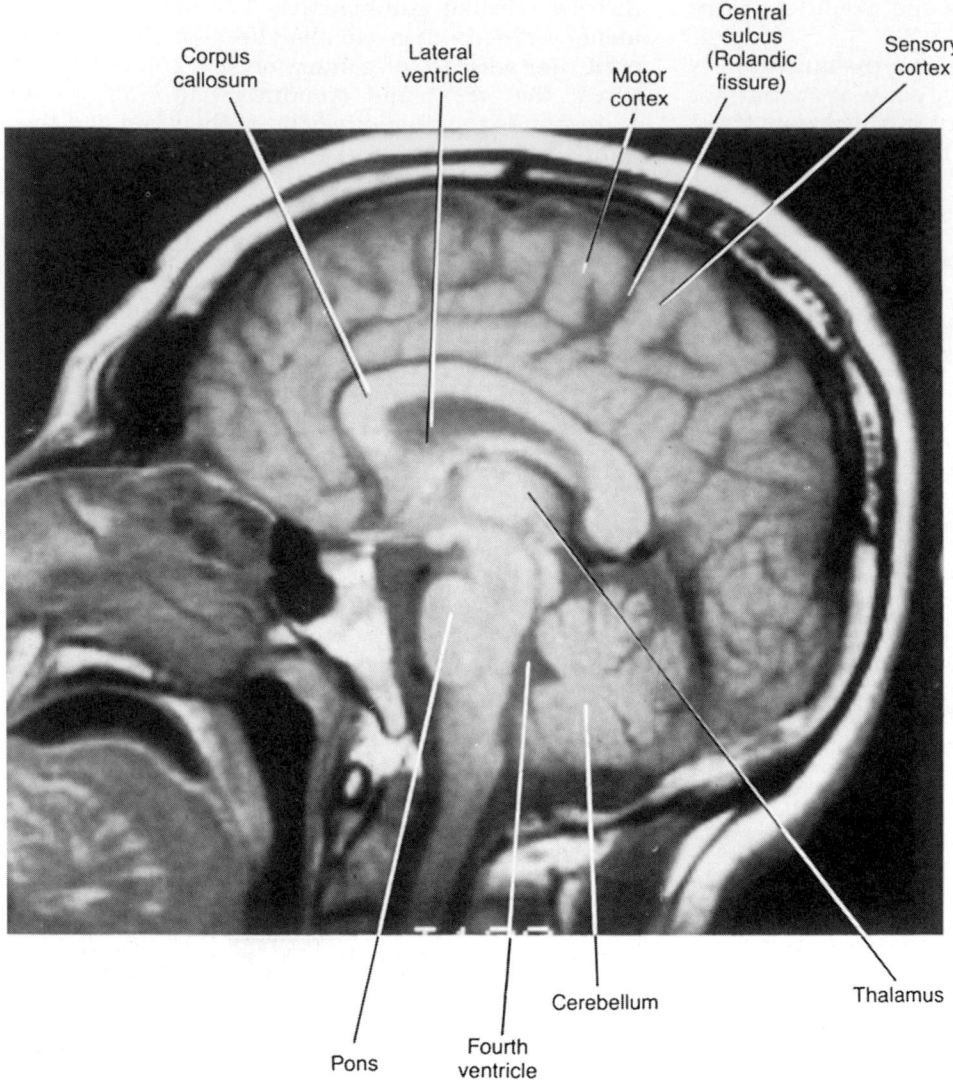

Corpus callosum · Lateral ventricle · Motor cortex · Central sulcus (Rolandic fissure) · Sensory cortex · Pons · Fourth ventricle · Cerebellum · Thalamus

Figure 17–19

Sagittal midline magnetic resonance image demonstrating the exquisite visualization of detail of discrete anatomic structures that is possible with this imaging technique. (From Marshall SB, Marshall LF, Vos HR, Chesnut RM. Neuroscience critical care: Pathophysiology and patient management. Philadelphia: WB Saunders, 1990, p 128.)

arterial blood flow. Ultrasound waves are reflected off moving red blood cells back to the Doppler instrument. The velocity of the blood flow influences reflection of the ultrasound waves. This is evidenced by a change in frequency in sound as recorded by the Doppler instrument.

The patient lies in the supine position. The Doppler instrument is placed over the neck in the area of the carotid artery (Fig. 17–20). It is moved over the common carotid artery to the bifurcation of the internal and external carotid arteries. As the Doppler instrument receives reflected ultrasound waves, an audible sound is heard and the blood flow velocity is recorded. In addition, the blood flow velocity is measured and reflected as a series of images. These images allow for visualization of the vessels and their lumen size.

Carotid Doppler studies aid in the detection of turbulent arterial blood flow and anatomic changes in the carotid vasculature, such as stenosis or occlusion. It is a noninvasive, painless, accurate, safe procedure requiring no preprocedure preparation or postprocedure management.

CEREBRAL ANGIOGRAPHY

Cerebral angiography is an invasive procedure that involves x-ray visualization of the cerebral vessels after the injection of a contrast material into the cerebrovascular circulation (Fig. 17–21).

Uses

Cerebral angiography is used to visualize the lumen of vessels and allows the identification of thrombus formation, stenosis, ulceration, occlusion, and spasms. It is also used to detect structural abnormalities, such as a vascular tumor, aneurysm, or arteriovenous malformation. It aids in the identification of space-occupying lesions, such as cysts, tumors, edema, herniation, hematoma, or hydrocephalus, which may cause vessel displacement. Angiography

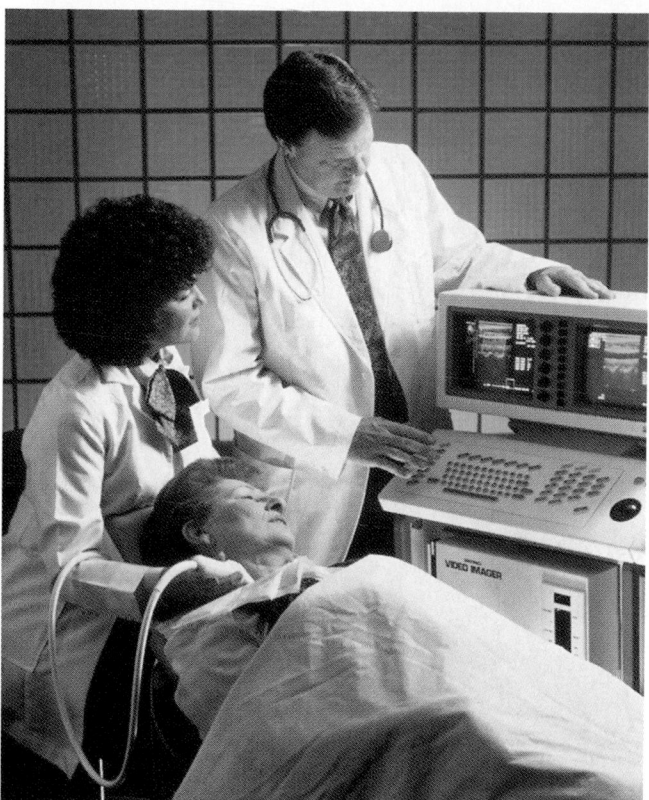

Figure 17–20

Patient undergoing a carotid Doppler study. (Courtesy of Diasonics, Milpitas, CA.)

also maps collateral circulation, shunting, or variances in blood flow. Angiography is contraindicated in pregnant women, patients with bleeding disorders, allergic reactions to contrast medium, and patients with renal or hepatic disease.

Patient Preparation

Ask the patient about allergies to the dye and give nothing by mouth (NPO status) for 8 hours before angiography. Blood clotting studies, ECG, and chest x-ray are performed prior to the procedure. The skin of the puncture site is usually shaved and prepared the night before or at the time of the procedure. Before the start of the procedure, complete a baseline neurologic assessment, and have the patient void and remove dentures and valuables. If an extremity is to be used for the puncture site, assess and document pulses distal to the site. Sedate the patient if ordered, provided the consent form for the procedure has been signed.

Procedure

Angiography is performed by a direct approach, with the contrast material injected into the carotid or vertebral artery, or by an indirect approach, with the contrast material injected into the femoral (most common approach), brachial, axillary, or subclavian artery with selective catheterization of the cerebral

vessels. As the radiopaque dye is injected and passes through the cerebral circulation, films are taken at timed intervals. Angiography is performed under local anesthesia or general anesthesia when it is a part of a surgical procedure.

Postprocedure Course

Monitor vital signs and do neurologic assessments frequently for the first 24 hours. Assess color, temperature, and pulse distal to the puncture site when it is in an extremity. If the carotid site was used, elevate the head of the bed slightly and assess the patient for neck edema, changes in respiratory status, and changes in swallowing and gag reflex. The puncture site is covered with a pressure dressing and is immobilized for approximately 8 hours to avoid excessive bleeding. Apply ice to decrease bleeding and edema.

Complications

Potential complications from cerebral angiography include allergic reaction to the radiopaque dye, vasospasm, thrombosis, hemorrhage, hematoma, embolism, or stroke. These complications may manifest as behavioral, motor, sensory, or language dysfunctions.

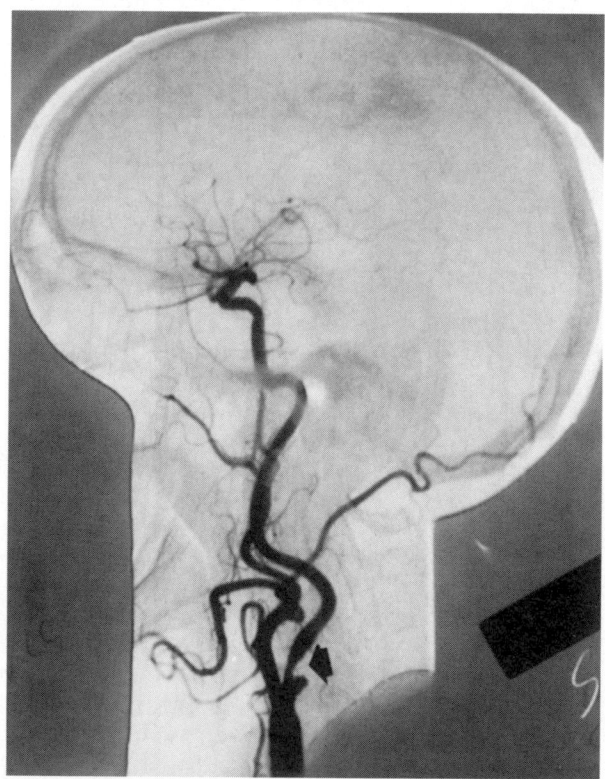

Figure 17–21

Cerebral angiogram showing stenosis and an ulcerated plaque (*arrow*) in the internal carotid artery of a patient with multiple transient ischemic attacks. (From Marshall SB, Marshall LF, Vos HR, Chesnut RM. Neuroscience critical care: Pathophysiology and patient management. Philadelphia: WB Saunders, 1990, p 135.)

NURSING PROCESS GUIDELINES
Cerebral Angiography

Before the procedure, identify any allergies that contraindicate the use of contrast dye by asking the patient about allergic or sensitive reactions to iodine or shellfish. Perform a neurologic assessment to establish baseline status, with particular attention to the motor and sensory function of the extremities. Assess peripheral circulation. Palpate peripheral pulses. Mark their location with a pen to guide postprocedure assessment. Note strength and presence of the pulses and the warmth and color of skin. Obtain baseline vital signs.

After the procedure, instruct the patient to lie supine for 8 hours and to refrain from bending joints in the extremity with the puncture site. Check vital signs, peripheral pulses, and color and temperature of the extremity distal to the puncture site every 15 minutes for 1 hour, then every half-hour for 1 hour, then every hour until stable. Notify the physician if peripheral pulses diminish or vital signs change. Monitor the puncture site for bleeding. Should bleeding occur, apply a pressure dressing and notify the physician.

Encourage the patient to drink fluids to decrease the concentration level of the dye in circulation. Notify the physician immediately if difficulty breathing, itching, rash, or another sign of an allergic reaction occurs to allow immediate intervention. If sutures are used, they are removed 1 week after the procedure.

MYELOGRAPHY

Myelography is the introduction of a contrast medium into the subarachnoid space via a lumbar puncture to diagnose alterations of the spinal cord structures by fluoroscopic and x-ray techniques. A myelogram can show one or all segments of the spinal cord.

Uses
Myelography is used in the diagnosis of herniated disk, bony changes, congenital lesions, spinal cord tumors, cysts, and compression (Fig. 17–22). Myelography is contraindicated in pregnancy, allergic reaction to iodine or iodinated contrast media, increased ICP, and chronic neurologic disease.

Patient Preparation
Discontinue monoamine oxidase inhibitors, major tranquilizers, and phenothiazine medications 48 hours before the procedure. Anticonvulsant medications may be continued in some instances.

Check for patient allergies and keep him or her

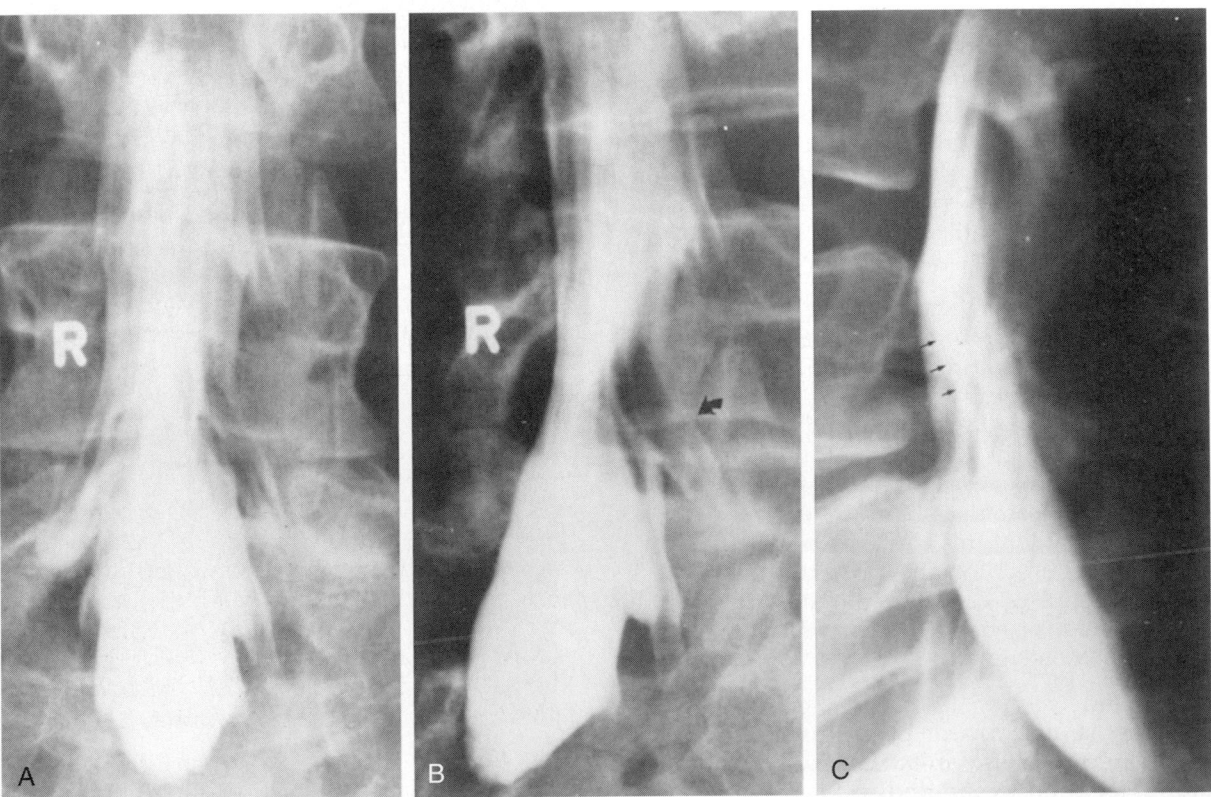

Figure 17–22
Lumbar myelogram, showing an L-4–L-5 herniated disk. *A,* Anteroposterior view. *B,* Oblique view. *C,* Lateral view. (From Resnick D. Diagnosis of bone and joint disorders. 3rd ed. Philadelphia: WB Saunders, 1995.)

on NPO status for a minimum of 6 hours before the procedure. Complete a baseline neurologic assessment, check vital signs, and have the patient void. Give preprocedure sedation, as ordered, provided the consent form has been signed. Shave the lumbar puncture area if needed.

Procedure

The patient is placed on an x-ray table that can be tilted. The lumbar puncture site is anesthetized by local injection. A spinal needle is inserted in the lumbar subarachnoid cistern (a puncture of the cisterna magna may be indicated if a cerebellopontine angle tumor is suspected). Approximately 10 to 15 mL of CSF is removed for laboratory studies, then the same amount of contrast medium is injected. The x-ray table tilts up and down to move the contrast material throughout the subarachnoid space. X-ray films that define the spinal cord, nerve entry roots, and bony structures are periodically taken.

Advances in myelography techniques have focused on the type of contrast medium used. Water-based mediums are absorbed by the body and excreted in the urine. The medium does not need to be removed manually from the patient after the procedure. If an oil-based medium is used, it is removed by aspiration after the procedure is completed and before the needle is removed.

Postprocedure Course

If a water-based medium was used, maintain the patient on bedrest with the head elevated 30 to 45 degrees for the first 6 to 8 hours and possibly as long as 24 hours, depending on the patient's condition and complaints. If an oil-based medium was used, keep the patient flat in bed for 6 to 24 hours. This prevents the contrast medium from entering and irritating the cranial structures. Encourage the patient to drink fluids to aid in the dilution and excretion of the contrast material. Adverse reactions include headache, nausea, vomiting, and seizures. Phenothiazine antiemetics (eg, chlorpromazine) are avoided because of a drug-dye interaction that potentiates seizure activity and other untoward reactions.

If nausea and dehydration occur, intravenous fluid hydration may be indicated. Frequently assess the neurologic status, vital signs, and puncture site for adverse reactions.

NURSING PROCESS GUIDELINES
Myelography

Before myelography, ask the patient about any known allergies or sensitivities. Review the patient's current medical status. Identify any medications such as phenothiazines that would be contraindicated when used with contrast dye. Perform a neurologic assessment to establish baseline status. Also assess the condition of the skin, noting any infec-

tions or the presence of a spinal anomaly that would prevent completion of the procedure. Assess the hydration status of the patient. Explain the importance of adequate hydration in reducing the concentration of contrast dye in the circulation. Instruct the patient to drink approximately 2 L of fluid the day before the procedure and every day for several days afterward unless contraindicated by a coexisting medical problem. Tell the patient that the injection of dye causes a burning sensation.

After the procedure, instruct the patient to lie flat or with the head elevated 30 degrees for 8 hours, depending on which medium was used. Check vital signs every 15 minutes for 1 hour, then every half-hour for an hour, and then hourly until signs are stable. Assess neurologic function for any changes from baseline status. Administer analgesics as ordered for headache, but do not administer phenothiazine medications. Instruct the patient to remain quiet and lie down if headache persists. Notify the physician of complaints of persistent or increased headache. Report any changes in vital signs or untoward reactions, such as seizure activity, nausea, vomiting, or nuchal rigidity, to the physician immediately to allow for immediate intervention and treatment.

LUMBAR PUNCTURE

Lumbar puncture is a procedure in which a sterile needle is inserted into the subarachnoid space at the L-4 to L-5 level. This landmark protects the integrity of the spinal cord because, in the adult, the spinal cord usually ends at the T-12 level but can extend to the L-1 or L-2 level.

Uses

A lumbar puncture is performed to determine CSF pressure and to obtain samples of CSF for laboratory analysis. CSF analysis usually includes color, red blood cell count, culture, pressure protein, glucose, and serology (Table 17–9). Test findings aid in the diagnosis of bacterial meningitis, subarachnoid hemorrhage, pseudotumor cerebri, neurosyphilis, multiple sclerosis, brain tumors, and normal pressure hydrocephalus.

Therapeutic uses of lumbar puncture include serial removal of CSF to reduce ICP and the introduction of spinal anesthetics and intrathecal medications. Medications are given by the intrathecal route when local rather than systemic administration is needed in order for them to exert the desired effect. Medications given by this route include some antibiotics and chemotherapeutic agents.

Procedure

Lumbar puncture is an invasive procedure performed in an outpatient setting or at the bedside. Care of the patient undergoing a lumbar puncture is described in Nursing Care Guide 17–1. There are no

Table 17–9

Cerebrospinal Fluid Analysis

Variable	Normal	Abnormal
Color	Clear	Cloudy (infection)
		Initially bloody (traumatic tap)
		Uniformly bloody (hemorrhage)
		Xanthochromic (red blood cell decomposition)
Red blood cell count	None	Presence (subarachnoid hemorrhage)
Culture	No organism	Positive (infection)
Pressure	Less than 200 mm H_2O	Above 200 mm H_2O (tumor, hemorrhage edema, obstruction)
Protein	15–45 mg/dL	Elevated values (tumor, infection)
Glucose	50–75 mg/dL	Lower values (tumor, infection)
Serology	Negative	Positive (venereal disease)

specific preparations or dietary restrictions for this procedure. The procedure takes approximately 30 minutes. The patient is placed in either a sitting or a lateral recumbent position and instructed to flex the neck and rest the chin on flexed knees. The puncture site is prepared with an antiseptic agent. The patient is draped. A local anesthetic is administered. The physician then introduces the spinal needle through the fourth and fifth lumbar interspace and enters the subarachnoid space while maintaining sterility of the equipment and field (Fig. 17–23). An opening pressure can be measured by connecting a manometer and a three-way stopcock to the lumbar puncture needle. Spinal fluid pressure in a bilateral recumbent position is normally 70 to 200 mm H_2O. Spinal fluid for specific laboratory analysis is then collected in sterile tubes. Before the spinal needle is removed, a closing pressure can be obtained by connecting a manometer and a three-way stopcock.

A bandage is placed over the puncture site. A record is maintained of the patient's tolerance of the procedure, opening and closing pressure, and color and characteristics of the CSF.

Contraindications

Lumbar puncture is not performed if there is evidence of high ICP that could result in a herniation syndrome. Other contraindications for lumbar puncture include presence of CSF pathway blockage above the puncture site, spinal anomalies that make puncture difficult or impossible, and skin infection at the puncture site.

Postprocedure Course

Instruct the patient to lie flat for 6 to 8 hours after the procedure. Monitor vital signs and neurologic signs. Medicate the patient as ordered. A mild analgesic such as propoxyphene (Darvon) or codeine may be ordered for discomfort. Hydrate the patient by forcing oral fluids or by intravenous fluid replacement.

Headache follows lumbar puncture in 10% of patients and is caused by leakage of CSF at the puncture site and traction on the meninges. It may occur a few hours to a few days after the lumbar puncture and may be mild or severe. It is typically described as a throbbing in the frontal or occipital area that is aggravated by sitting up or standing. It is not serious but can be disturbing to the patient.

CISTERNAL PUNCTURE

A cisternal puncture is similar to the lumbar puncture. A short, beveled needle is inserted into the cisterna magna at the C-2 level. A cisternal puncture has the same therapeutic and diagnostic indications as the lumbar puncture.

Cisternal puncture aids in the diagnosis and detection of upper level blockage of CSF circulation and cerebellopontine angle tumors.

ELECTROENCEPHALOGRAPHY

The electroencephalogram (EEG) measures the electrical impulses of the brain. These impulses, known as brain waves or brain impulses, are picked up by electrodes placed on the surface of the scalp.

Uses

An EEG is used to detect and localize abnormal activity of the brain. It is useful in the diagnosis and assessment of patients with seizures, brain tumors, infections, neurobehavioral disorders, abscesses, metabolic disorders, and other syndromes such as headaches, sleep disorders, and head injury. An EEG is also a vital diagnostic tool in the assessment of electrocerebral silence and confirmation of brain death.

Patient Preparation

Restrict medications and stimulants, as ordered, that influence brain impulses before an EEG. Anticonvulsants may be discontinued because they can mask electrical impulses in the brain. Stimulants, such as tea and coffee, are restricted to decrease artificial

Nursing Care Guide 17–1
Patients Undergoing Lumbar Puncture

Preprocedure Care

Assessment Findings: The patient is admitted with a temperature of 103.2°F, chief complaint is neck pain. A lumbar puncture is ordered. The patient appears anxious and nervous. The patient verbalizes fear and concern regarding the procedure and its risks.

Nursing Diagnosis: Anxiety related to fear about the procedure and potential risks

Patient Outcomes	Nursing Interventions	Rationale
Patient verbalizes feeling less fearful and appears relaxed. Patient states and demonstrates methods to relax.	Explain procedure to the patient and family. Provide a calm, quiet environment. Teach deep-breathing techniques and other relaxation strategies.	Having an understanding of the procedure and knowing what to expect lessens fear and anxiety. Relaxation techniques may decrease anxiety and allow the patient to facilitate the procedure.

Evaluation: Compare the patient's status with the expected outcomes. If the outcomes are not met, reassess the patient and revise the plan.

Assessment Findings: Patient seems concerned about the procedure, asking many questions about the procedure and what to expect.

Nursing Diagnosis: Knowledge deficit: nature of the procedure (lumbar puncture)

Patient Outcomes	Nursing Interventions	Rationale
Patient accurately describes the purpose of the procedure and what will occur during and after the procedure.	Explain to the patient and family that the procedure is done to check the pressure of cerebrospinal fluid and to obtain samples of cerebrospinal fluid for laboratory analysis. Explain the following to the patient: The patient will be asked to urinate before the procedure. The patient will be asked to lie in a lateral recumbent position and flex the neck and rest the chin on flexed knees. A local anesthetic will be injected into the site. A long thin needle will be inserted into the lumbar space in the lower back using sterile technique. It is important to stay very still during the procedure. The needle is removed, and a bandage is placed over the incision site.	Giving explanations allows the patient to know what to expect during and after the procedure.

(continued)

Nursing Care Guide 17–1

Patients Undergoing Lumbar Puncture (continued)

Patient Outcomes	Nursing Interventions	Rationale
Evaluation:	Compare the patient's status with the expected outcomes. If the outcomes are not met, reassess the patient and revise the plan.	

Postprocedure Care

Assessment Findings: Lumbar puncture completed, patient complains of slight tenderness at site and a mild headache.

Nursing Diagnosis: Pain related to lumbar puncture

Patient Outcomes	Nursing Interventions	Rationale
Patient reports relief of pain.	Instruct the patient to lie flat for at least 6 hours or for the amount of time ordered.	Lying flat will help decrease the chance of headache.
	Administer analgesics as ordered.	Will help relieve pain.
Patient's vital signs and neurologic signs remain stable.	Monitor vital signs and neurologic signs every 2 to 4 hours or as ordered for 24 hours.	May detect hemodynamic or neurologic changes. Changes in vital signs may reflect an increase in pain.
Patient remains well hydrated.	Push oral fluids. If patient is unable to take oral fluids, administer intravenous fluids as ordered.	Rehydrates the patient and helps prevent headache.
Puncture site is free of drainage and hematoma.	Monitor the puncture site.	Assess for any cerebrospinal fluid drainage or hematoma.
Evaluation:	Compare the patient's status with the expected outcomes. If the outcomes are not met, reassess the patient and revise the plan.	

influences on impulse tracings. Inform the patient that electrical activity is measured as it flows from the body and not into the body. Instruct the patient that this test is painless, noninvasive, and safe.

Procedure

Surface electrodes are applied with paste to various areas of the patient's scalp to detect electrical impulses, or brain waves. The patient is positioned in a chair or lies supine on a table. The electrodes are connected to the electroencephalograph, which measures the impulses and produces a continuous paper recording.

Brain waves are routinely recorded in four states. First, the patient is asked to lie quietly with eyes closed to establish a baseline recording at rest. The patient is then asked to hyperventilate by breathing through the mouth for 3 to 5 minutes. Recordings continue throughout this period and are maintained to determine the length of time required for the recording to return to baseline. Photic stimulation is the third state. The patient is asked to keep the eyes closed and then open them as a light is flickered in front of him or her. Seizure activity may be noted at this time.

Finally, the brain waves are recorded while the patient is asleep. If the patient cannot fall asleep, a hypnotic may be administered. However, the EEG is more accurate if no medications are administered. The procedure takes several hours.

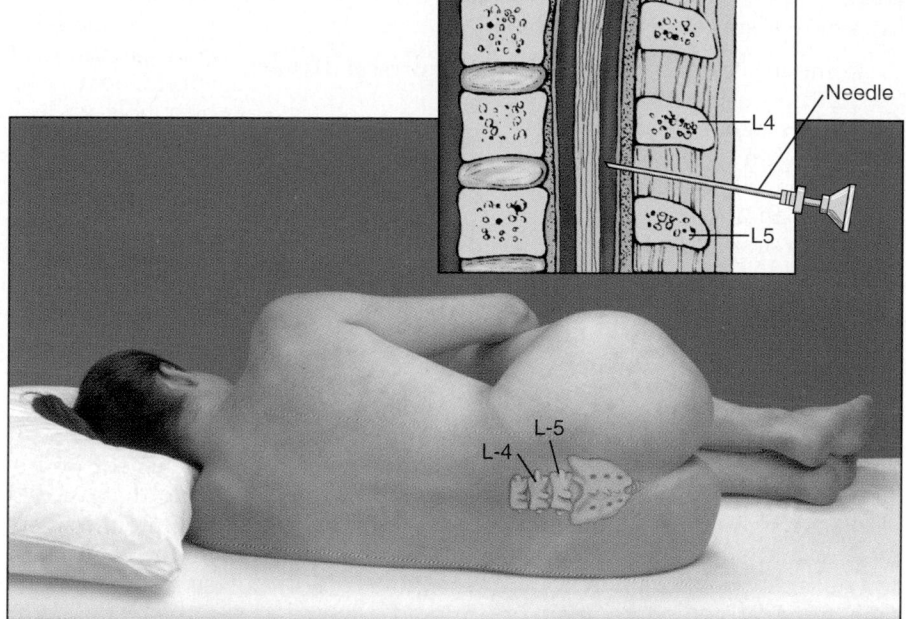

Figure 17–23

Lumbar puncture. With the patient in a flexed position to maximize the space between vertebrae, the lumbar puncture needle is inserted between L-4 and L-5 to gain entry to the subarachnoid space. During the actual procedure, the patient would be gowned and draped to protect privacy.

Postprocedure Course

No postprocedure management is required. The EEG paste can be removed with acetone or witch hazel and then by shampooing. The patient resumes routine activities and his or her usual medication regimen immediately.

EVOKED POTENTIAL STUDIES

Evoked potential studies measures the electrical responses in brain waves when various sensory stimuli are used. This includes auditory, visual, and somatosensory stimuli. Electrodes are placed on the scalp, and brain activity is measured. A stimulus is administered, and the brain wave is recorded.

This study is useful in diagnosing visual and auditory disorders. It can also differentiate between organic brain disorders and physiologic disorders.

ELECTROMYOGRAPHY

An electromyogram is the recording of electrical impulses of the muscle fibers and peripheral nerves. Teflon-coated needle electrodes are inserted into skeletal muscles. These electrodes detect electrical activity of skeletal muscle and send the impulse to an oscilloscope, which forms wave tracings. Recordings are made when the muscle groups are at rest and in contraction. When at rest, muscle fibers are silent. When they are active, muscle fibers have electrical activity.

Electromyograms aid in differentiating neural from muscular causes of muscular weakness. Therefore, neuromuscular diseases such as myasthenia gravis can be differentiated from disorders of the nerves supplying the muscle, such as amyotrophic lateral sclerosis.

No specific patient preparation or postprocedure management is indicated. The patient is told there may be some discomfort as the needle electrodes are placed on the specific muscle. Mild analgesics may be ordered to relieve discomfort after the procedure.

NERVE CONDUCTION STUDIES

Nerve conduction studies measure the velocity of conduction of motor and sensory peripheral nerves. The specific peripheral nerve area to be studied is identified. The nerve is stimulated. The time from nerve stimulation to muscular contraction is recorded by electrodes placed on the skin surface.

Nerve conduction studies evaluate the integrity of the myelin and axon of peripheral nerves. They are indicated in the diagnosis of peripheral neuropathies and neuromuscular disorders, such as Guillain-Barré syndrome.

Management

Intracranial Surgery

Conventional intracranial surgery involves opening the skull to perform a surgical intervention on or near any of the intracranial structures. Surgery performed on the cerebral hemispheres is called supratentorial. Surgery performed in the brain stem or cerebellar region below the cerebral cortex is called infratentorial.

Uses

Intracranial surgery is done to:

- Remove a neoplasm, a hematoma, or scar tissue that is causing seizures
- Clip or ligate an aneurysm
- Ligate an arteriovenous malformation or other vascular abnormality
- Drain an abscess
- Repair a skull fracture
- Remove a foreign object
- Obtain tissue samples for biopsy
- Redirect CSF via a shunt
- Relieve increased ICP

Patient Preparation

Obtain written consent for the procedure. Routine preoperative laboratory tests include a complete blood count, serum electrolytes, coagulation profile, blood typing and cross-matching, an ECG, and chest x-ray examination. As a prophylactic measure, anticonvulsants such as phenytoin and a glucocorticoid such as dexamethasone may be ordered preoperatively as a treatment for anticipated cortical irritation and cerebral edema. Shave and cleanse with antiseptic the area of the scalp to be incised. Complete a baseline neurologic assessment and offer emotional support to the patient and family.

Procedure

Craniotomy is the most common intracranial procedure. Craniotomy involves the making of an opening in the skull configured to form a bone flap. This is performed by making several burr holes in the skull in the configuration required for exposure. A special saw with a guidewire is inserted into one burr hole under the bone and is brought up through the second burr hole. The surgeon is able to cut through the skull by alternately pulling on each end of the saw, allowing the bone to be cut from the inside of the skull out, avoiding injury to brain tissue. This process is repeated through each burr hole until a bone flap is made (Fig. 17–24). The bone flap is replaced at the conclusion of the surgery. Craniectomy is removal of part of the skull. This may vary from a small burr hole to an area of several centimeters. This approach is used for surgery in the posterior fossa (brain-stem region). Cranioplasty is the placement of a synthetic plate or bone graft onto an area that is defective or opened. The incision for supratentorial surgery is made high on the forehead, in the tentorium and behind the hairline. The incision for infratentorial surgery is made just above the nape of the neck.

Postprocedure Course

The prognosis for recovery for a patient who has undergone craniotomy depends on the nature and location of the brain lesion. Occasionally patients have permanent physical and mental handicaps such as paralysis, aphasia, skull defects, personality changes, or severe depression. Residual disorders such as diplopia may be temporary.

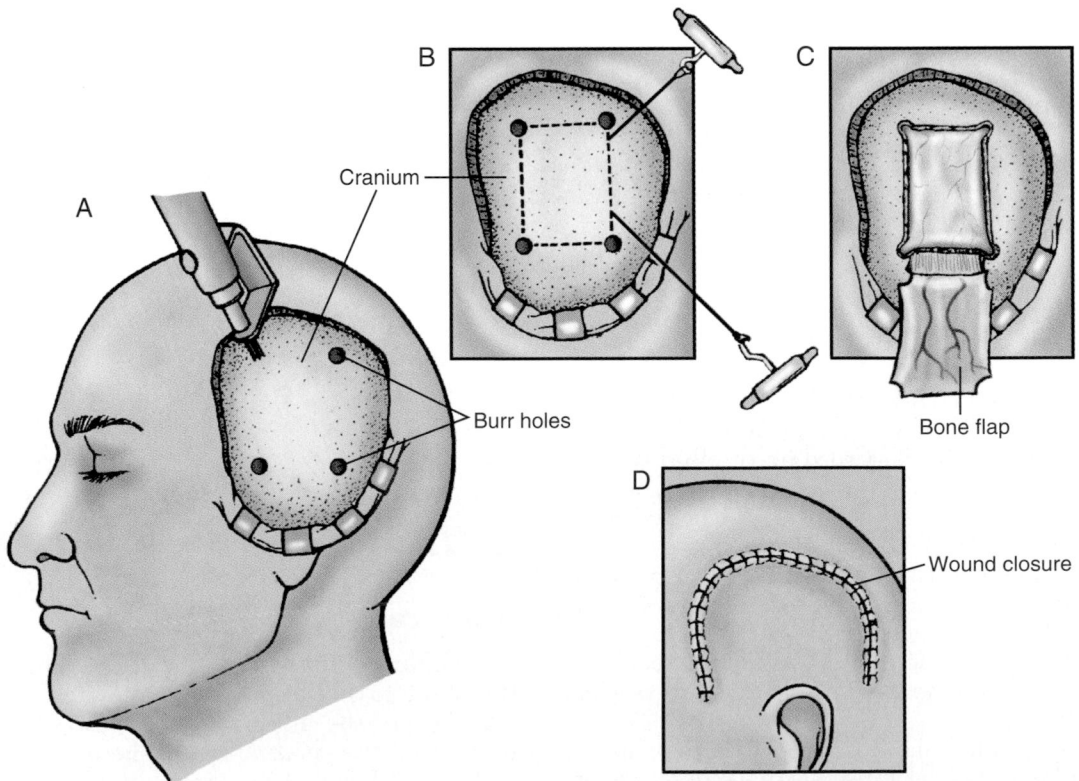

Figure 17–24

Craniotomy procedure. *A*, Burr holes are drilled into the skull. *B*, The skull is cut between the burr holes with a surgical saw. *C*, A bone flap is turned back to expose the cranial contents. *D*, After surgery, the bone flap is replaced and the wound is closed.

A patient who undergoes surgery for the removal of a brain tumor may have received a dye (fluorescein sodium) intravenously to aid in locating the lesion during surgery. The dye causes the skin and sclera of the patient to appear jaundiced for several days after surgery.

If supratentorial surgery was performed, the patient may have generalized facial edema and may be unable to open one or both eyes. Discoloration (ecchymosis) of the skin around the eyes may also be present. These conditions usually improve within 3 to 4 days postoperatively.

A catheter may be left in place in the lateral ventricle to drain excessive amounts of CSF and to prevent increased ICP. The catheter is usually removed by the neurosurgeon 24 to 48 hours after surgery. The head dressing with supratentorial surgery is caplike and covers the ears.

After infratentorial surgery, the head dressing may extend down to the shoulders to prevent movement of the head and neck. Sutures are usually removed by the surgeon on the fifth day after supratentorial surgery and on the seventh day after infratentorial surgery. When the final dressings are removed, the healed wound may be covered by a stockinet cap or scarf or left open to the air.

After infratentorial surgery, the gag and swallowing reflexes may be impaired. Therefore, the patient is kept on NPO status for 24 hours to prevent aspiration, and intravenous fluids are administered. These are given slowly to prevent increased ICP. If difficulty in swallowing persists, tube feedings may be necessary and are usually begun 48 hours after surgery. On the second day after supratentorial surgery, the diet is progressed as tolerated.

With supratentorial surgery, place the patient in a semi-Fowler's position postoperatively to decrease cerebral edema. Place the patient with infratentorial surgery flat on the side to prevent herniation of the brain downward into the space produced by tumor removal. Patients are generally not allowed out of bed until the third to fifth postoperative day after infratentorial surgery, but those who have undergone supratentorial surgery may be allowed to sit in a chair in 24 to 48 hours. See Table 17–10 for a comparison of supratentorial and infratentorial surgery.

Complications

Increased ICP may result from brain edema or intracranial bleeding after craniotomy. A progressive impairment of responsiveness, such as diminishing responses to stimuli, significant changes in vital signs, increased restlessness, paralysis of the extremities, changes in vision, dilated pupils, and increasing headaches, may indicate increased ICP.

Respiratory complications and hyperthermia or hypothermia may develop, especially after infratentorial surgery, because the incision is made adjacent to the medulla and vital centers. Close monitoring of respiratory status is imperative.

Convulsions are not uncommon after any form of intracranial surgery, but the risk is even greater after supratentorial surgery. The physician usually orders antiseizure medication to prevent their occurrence.

Other complications that may develop after craniotomy are meningitis and wound infection.

NURSING PROCESS
Intracranial Surgery

PREOPERATIVE NURSING CARE

Assess and document the patient's neurologic status, including level of consciousness, motor and sensory function, pupils, and cranial nerve function. Record vital signs and respiratory status to provide a baseline for intraoperative and postoperative comparisons.

Table 17–10

Comparison of Supratentorial Surgery and Infratentorial Surgery

Variable	Supratentorial	Infratentorial
Location of surgery	Cerebral hemispheres	Brain-stem or cerebellar region
Postoperative effects	Generalized facial edema	Impaired gag and swallow reflexes
	Inability to open one or both eyes	
	Ecchymosis around the eyes	
Common complications	Convulsions	Respiratory center impairment
		Hyperthermia
		Hypothermia
Dressing	Encircles head like a bathing cap	Encircles head and supports neck to prevent flexion
Activity	Out of bed in 24–48 h	Out of bed after 3–5 d
Diet	Fluids when alert	Nothing-by-mouth status for at least 24 h
	Regular diet as tolerated on second postoperative day	If dysphagia persists, tube feedings started after 48 h
Suture removal	Fifth postoperative day	Seventh postoperative day

Assess the patient's and family's understanding of the medical problem and the procedure to be performed. Be sure to ascertain whether expectations in regard to the patient's prognosis are realistic.

Recognize that anxiety and apprehension are expected in any patient facing surgery but are greatly intensified in the patient scheduled for brain surgery. The patient and family may be concerned about permanent disability, loss of cognitive abilities, and death. Encourage the patient and family to express their feelings by providing time and privacy and acknowledging a willingness to listen.

Explain in simple terms the preoperative routines. Provide information about the postoperative phase, including the possible need for respiratory support, intubation, and ventilation; routine monitoring equipment used; anticipated tubes, such as intravenous catheters and an indwelling urinary catheter; and a description of the head dressing. Instruct the patient in effective deep breathing, if he or she is able. Inform the patient that the scalp is shaved for surgery. Corticosteroids and antiseizure medications are often started preoperatively. With the supratentorial approach, the patient's eyes may be swollen shut and facial edema may be present. Instruct the patient that bedrest is strictly enforced immediately after surgery.

POSTOPERATIVE NURSING CARE

Assessment

The postoperative care of a patient after a craniotomy is complex and requires keen assessment skills. This care is generally provided in a critical care unit until the patient's condition stabilizes.

After craniotomy, begin assessment of the patient with the measurement of vital and neurologic signs: temperature, pulse, respirations, blood pressure, pupillary and other reflexes, level of consciousness, arm lifts, handgrips, leg lifts, and ankle plantar flexion and dorsiflexion.

Frequency of these assessments depends on the neurosurgeon's orders and the nurse's judgment of the patient's condition and may range from every 5 to every 30 minutes for the first 6 postoperative hours. As the patient's condition stabilizes, decrease the frequency of these assessments to every 2 to 4 hours. At all times, interpret these findings in view of the baseline data obtained preoperatively. Report any significant changes to the neurosurgeon immediately.

Carefully assess respiratory status. Because surgical trauma may impair the function of the respiratory center, observe the depth and pattern of respiration and check blood gas values. Because surgical trauma may also impair the function of the vagus and glossopharyngeal nerves and thus cause paralysis of the muscles involved with swallowing, carefully observe the unconscious patient for the accumulation of secretions, which can be aspirated. Remember that patients who have undergone infra-

tentorial surgery are at the greatest risk for these effects.

Inspect the patient's head dressing for signs of abnormal bleeding and for clear or yellowish drainage, which may indicate leakage of CSF. Because severe headache may occur during the first 2 postoperative days, assess for signs of restlessness and discomfort. Observe for seizures, which are most common after supratentorial surgery, although they can also follow infratentorial surgery. Also observe for signs of gastrointestinal or urinary tract involvement. When the head dressing is removed, inspect the incision for bulging, redness, drainage, or suture disruption.

Nursing Diagnoses and Planning

Nursing diagnoses and related expected patient outcomes most commonly applicable to patients who have undergone intracranial surgery include the following:

NDx: Pain related to surgical trauma of the scalp and cranial tissues

Planning: Patient Outcomes
1. Patient rests quietly.
2. Patient reports that pain is relieved or manageable.

NDx: Risk for impaired gas exchange related to postanesthetic state

Planning: Patient Outcomes
1. Patent airway is maintained.
2. Patient maintains regular respiratory pattern of 12 to 24 breaths per minute.

NDx: Risk for altered cerebral tissue perfusion related to postoperative cerebral edema

Planning: Patient Outcomes
1. Patient maintains or improves neurologic status.

NDx: Risk for infection related to break in skin integrity

Planning: Patient Outcomes
1. Patient is afebrile.
2. Incision is clean and approximated.
3. Purulent drainage is absent.

Nursing Interventions and Evaluation

NDx: Pain
Medicate the patient as ordered for head pain, keeping in mind that narcotics and most barbiturates are contraindicated after brain surgery because they can cause respiratory depression and mask signs of increasing ICP. To further promote comfort, keep the patient's environment dim and free of loud noise. Avoid sudden or jarring movement of the patient. Apply ice packs to the head if ordered. Report increasingly severe prolonged or newly occurring headache to the physician because it may indicate increasing ICP. Use the AHCPR (Agency for Health Care Policy and Research) Guidelines for Pain Con-

trol after Surgery to assist with acute pain management. Discuss pain control options with the patient and physician. Help the patient find alternative pain relief measures such as relaxation strategies.

NDx: Risk for impaired gas exchange

Suction the patient as needed to clear the airway of secretions. Keep in mind that general anesthetic agents may depress the cough reflex as well as cause residual relaxation of muscles in the immediate postoperative phase. Maintaining a patent airway provides adequate air exchange, preventing hypercarbia, which could potentiate an increase in ICP. Administer oxygen therapy as ordered. If the patient is conscious, coach him or her in deep breathing. Make certain to instruct the patient not to cough vigorously, however, because this can increase ICP. Turn the patient frequently to further promote adequate ventilation of all lung areas. Care of tracheostomy and ventilator may be indicated with patients needing airway and ventilatory support.

NDx: Risk for altered cerebral tissue perfusion

The patient who has undergone intracranial surgery is at risk for increased ICP secondary to cerebral edema. Position the patient who has undergone supratentorial craniotomy with the head elevated 30 to 45 degrees to promote venous and CSF drainage from the head, which reduces cerebral edema. Position the patient on the back or on the side opposite the incision. If the patient is unconscious, make certain the neck is not twisted or flexed because this also inhibits venous return and flow of CSF. Never position the patient with the head lowered, because the increased blood flow to the brain can cause an increase in ICP.

Instruct the patient to prevent intra-abdominal and intrathoracic pressure, which can lead to increased ICP. This includes avoiding straining, coughing, sneezing, and hip flexion. Also instruct the patient in seizure precautions, especially after supratentorial surgery, because the risk for seizures is greater.

If the patient has undergone infratentorial surgery, support the head with a small pillow and align carefully because the infratentorial incision disrupts the neck muscles, which support the head. Position the patient flat on the side postoperatively for 48 hours. This patient may also experience dizziness, hypotension, nausea, and cranial nerve edema.

Administer hypertonic urea, mannitol, or steroids as ordered to decrease postoperative edema. Monitor for both therapeutic and adverse effects. Also restrict fluids as ordered. Because metabolic disturbances, which cause a decrease in urinary output, may occur after intracranial surgery, record fluid intake and output. Also record bowel elimination, keeping in mind that cathartics and enemas are usually contraindicated after intracranial surgery because straining at stool and absorption of fluid can cause an increase in ICP. Alert the neurosurgeon to signs of fecal impaction. Periorbital edema usually occurs within 24 to 48 hours after supratentorial surgery. Apply cold or warm compresses around the eyes for relief.

NDx: Risk for infection

The surgical incision site presents an open break in the protective skin barrier and a potential site for normal flora to proliferate and enter the body, producing infection. Record temperature and report elevations. Administer prophylactic antibiotics as ordered. Wash hands thoroughly before and after patient contact. Use strict aseptic technique when handling drains at the operative site. Monitor the head dressing for unexpected drainage of blood or CSF. Report drainage to the physician immediately because moisture at the incision provides a medium for bacterial growth. When the dressing is removed, cleanse the operative site as directed by the neurosurgeon. Instruct the patient to keep the incision clean and dry once the dressing is removed and not to scratch the incision.

Additional Interventions

After supratentorial surgery, give nothing by mouth for 24 hours. Then give fluids as desired as soon as the patient is alert, provided there is no dysphagia or nausea. Progress to a regular diet as tolerated. Keep in mind that it is critical for the patient to avoid vomiting because it increases ICP. Antiemetics may be given to control nausea and vomiting. After infratentorial surgery, keep the patient on NPO status for at least 24 hours. Begin giving small amounts of fluid when swallow and gag reflexes return and bowel sounds are heard. Gradually progress the diet as tolerated. Provide assistance as needed with feeding because the patient may have problems with actions such as controlling the tongue and raising the arms as a result of the effects of surgery on the cranial nerves.

For the first 48 hours after surgery, provide total nursing care. Thereafter, provide care as required by the type of surgery and the patient's functional ability. Whenever possible, encourage the patient to participate in care, whether it be physical participation or making judgments in terms of timing and sequence of care, what to wear, or what to drink.

Compare the patient's status with the expected outcomes. If the outcomes are not met, reassess the patient and revise the plan.

Spinal Surgery

Uses

Spinal surgery is performed to remove spinal cord tumors, to correct fractures of the vertebrae secondary to trauma, to remove arteriovenous malformations from the spinal cord, and, most commonly, to remove a herniated or ruptured intervertebral disk.

Procedure

Laminectomy is the removal of all or part of the vertebral lamina to gain access to the spinal cord and nerve roots. In the case of a herniated or ruptured disk, this procedure allows the removal of protruding disk material pressing on the spinal nerve. Laminectomy is also performed to remove neoplasms of the spine. In this case, the amount of bony lamina removed is larger to allow for a wider exposure for tumor removal. Cervical laminectomy may be performed through either an anterior or a posterior approach. A spinal fusion is the union of two or three vertebrae, generally performed after a laminectomy, when indicated, to stabilize the vertebral column. A microdiskectomy is the excision of a herniated disk using a microscope. The incision is smaller than that required for a laminectomy, resulting in decreased postoperative pain, decreased blood loss during surgery, rapid recovery, and a shorter hospital stay.

Postprocedure Course

The postprocedure course varies with the specific surgical procedure performed and with the underlying medical problem. Whenever laminectomy is performed, maintenance of alignment of the spine is critical. Position is restricted, pain is usually significant, and movement is gradually resumed.

With microdiskectomy, there is little limitation on movement and little postoperative pain. The patient is out of bed on the evening of surgery and goes home on about the third postoperative day.

Complications

Complications of spinal surgery include respiratory failure as a result of cord compression and urinary retention caused by irritation of autonomic fibers. There is also the risk of hemorrhage and infection.

NURSING PROCESS
Spinal Surgery

PREOPERATIVE NURSING CARE

Nursing care for patients scheduled for spinal surgery is similar to that for any preoperative patient, with several considerations. Be sure to obtain data regarding the initial onset of symptoms, the precipitating event (if any), and the patient's degree of pain or discomfort. Determine whether the patient is taking medication for pain relief. Assess neurologic status, particularly motor and sensory function. Assess the presence of bowel or bladder involvement, particularly if the cause is related to neoplasm or trauma. Assist the patient to deal with preoperative anxiety, which is often high with spinal surgery. Instruct the patient to practice log rolling. (Also see Clinical Pathway for Lumbar Laminectomy with Fusion.)

POSTOPERATIVE NURSING CARE

Assessment

Postoperatively, assess neurologic status and note deviations from baseline. Keep in mind that upper-or lower-extremity weakness can be the first sign of cord compression and impending paralysis. If the patient has undergone cervical surgery, assess for sensation in the arms, upper back, shoulder, and neck. If the patient has undergone anterior cervical surgery, also assess for dysphagia resulting from esophageal edema secondary to esophageal trauma during surgery, as well as for hoarseness and the inability to cough because of laryngeal nerve trauma. Assess also for signs of respiratory difficulty as a result of airway compression from bleeding and aspiration. Inspect the neck for swelling, which can be indicative of hemorrhage. Observe the dressing for serosanguineous drainage, test for glucose, and observe for the "halo effect," which indicates that the drainage is CSF. This can indicate a dural leak and pose the threat of meningitis. Notify the physician immediately if CSF is present. Monitor vital signs for indications of hypovolemia or hyperpyrexia. If the patient has undergone lumbosacral surgery, check dorsalis pedis and posterior tibial pulses. Note the color and temperature of the legs. Check for sensation in the lower back, buttocks, legs, and toes. Determine the patient's level of comfort. Check the dressing for bleeding or CSF at frequent intervals. Assess for urinary retention. Assess the patient's ability to progress in ambulation. If bone was taken from the iliac crest or fibula for a fusion, monitor the donor site for hematoma formation. Assess the patient's pain at both the site of the spinal surgery and the donor site. Remember that the sudden reappearance of radicular pain can indicate extrusion of the graft.

Nursing Diagnoses and Planning

Nursing diagnoses and related expected patient outcomes most commonly applicable to patients who have undergone spinal surgery include the following:

NDx: Pain related to edema secondary to tissue trauma and muscle spasms secondary to intraoperative irritation of nerves

Planning: Patient Outcomes
1. Patient rests quietly.
2. Patient states that pain is relieved or manageable.

NDx: Risk for trauma related to displacement of the bone graft after spinal fusion

Planning: Patient Outcomes
1. Patient complies with positioning and activity instructions designed to protect the bone graft from extrusion.
2. Patient is free of radicular pain.

NDx: Risk for injury related to lightheadedness secondary to postural hypotension

Planning: Patient Outcomes
1. Patient resumes activities gradually.
2. Patient remains free of injury.

■■■■■■▶
■ Clinical Pathway for Lumbar Laminectomy with Fusion

Patient Name _____   Date _____

DRG _____ #24 _____   Expected LOS _____

	Day 1	Day 2	Day 3	Day 4
Medication	*Preoperative:* IV antibiotic *Postoperative:* Pain control IM analgesia PCA pump or epidural catheter IV antibiotics every 6 h × 48 h Continuous IV Stool softener TID	Continue pain management Stool softener TID IV @ TKO rate	Discontinue epidural catheter or PCA pump PO analgesia (narcotics) Stool softener IV to saline lock	Acetaminophen (Tylenol) PO PRN Discontinue IV Stool softener
Diagnostic tests	*Preoperative:* Chest x-ray, CBC with differential, electrolytes Type and screen, prothrombin and partial thromboplastin time, electrocardiogram if >40 years old, lumbar spine films, computed tomography, magnetic resonance imaging, myelogram	Hemoglobin and hematocrit	N/A	CBC with differential
Diet	*Preoperative:* NPO after 12 AM *Postoperative:* NPO, advance to clear liquids after 4 h	DAT	DAT	DAT
Activity	*Preoperative:* Bedrest with bathroom privileges *Postoperative:* Bedrest, lob roll after 2 h	OOB with lumbar brace Leg exercises	OOB with lumbar brace Ambulate as tolerated	OOB with lumbar brace Ambulate as tolerated
Treatment and nursing actions	*Preoperative:* Assessment, focus on neurologic status (neurovascular check list), weight, VS Document use of nonsteroidal anti-inflammatory agents *Postoperative:* VS and neurovascular check every 15 min × 4 h, then every 30 min × 2 h, then VS every 4 h and neurovascular check every 2 h Incentive spirometry every 2 h Systems and pain assessment Check incision and hemovac/JP for drainage and patency Elastic stockings Monitor for complications: paralytic ileus, CSF leak, muscle spasms, urinary retention, HA Maintain I&O	VS and neurovascular check every 4 h Systems assessment every 8 h Pain assessment Elastic leg stockings TCDB every 2 h Incentive spirometry every 2 h Check dressing for drainage Monitor for complications: paralytic ileus, CSF leak, muscle spasms, urinary retention, HA Maintain I&O	VS and neurovascular check every 4 h Systems assessment every 8 h Pain assessment Elastic leg stockings TCDB every 2 h Incentive spirometry every 2 h Check dressing for drainage Monitor for complications: paralytic ileus, CSF leak, muscle spasms, urinary retention, HA Maintain I&O Check incision for signs and symptoms of infection Assess ability to perform activities of daily life	VS and neurovascular check every 4 h Systems assessment every 8 h Pain assessment
Teaching and discharge planning	*Preoperative:* Orient to hospital and postoperative routine: TCDB and incentive spirometry, log rolling, activity restrictions and body mechanics, pain control management *Postoperative:* Review plan of care with patient and family Involve family in care routine Discuss activity and work restrictions Consider financial implications and other stresses for the patient and family	Instruct patient not to twist, flex, or hyperextend Consult with PT and OT Reinforce PT and OT exercises Obtain necessary assistive devices and instruct in their use	Instruct patient not to twist, flex, or hyperextend Consult with PT and OT Reinforce PT and OT exercises Obtain necessary assistive devices and instruct in their use Teach care of incision, signs and symptoms of infection, and when to notify the physician Reinforce activity restrictions	Instruct patient not to twist, flex, or hyperextend Consult with PT and OT Reinforce PT and OT exercises Obtain necessary assistive devices and instruct in their use Teach care of incision, signs and symptoms of infection, and when to notify the physician Reinforce activity restrictions Review all teaching with patient and family orally and give them written instructions Make follow-up appointment with physician Make referrals for continued assistance at home if needed

NDx: Risk for urinary retention related to effects of anesthesia, swelling at operative site, and reduced mobility

Planning: Patient Outcomes
1. Palpable bladder distention is absent.
2. Patient voids sufficient quantity of urine at 3- to 4-hour intervals.

NDx: Knowledge deficit: activity limitations and life-style modifications needed to decrease stress to spine

Planning: Patient Outcomes
1. Patient verbalizes activity limitations.
2. Patient expresses willingness and ability to comply with necessary lifestyle modifications.

Nursing Interventions and Evaluation

NDx: Pain
Surgical manipulation causes irritation to the nerves and local edema, which contribute to pain. Administer prescribed analgesics for pain and discomfort caused by the incision and muscle spasm as ordered and at least a half-hour before position changes. After a lumbar laminectomy, pain and spasms occur in the lower body, abdomen, or thighs. After a cervical laminectomy, pain and spasms occur in the upper back, shoulder, neck, or arms. If more than one analgesic is prescribed, determine the severity of the patient's pain, and select the appropriate analgesic to be administered. Monitor for untoward side effects of analgesics, such as respiratory depression, nausea, or constipation. Use the AHCPR guidelines for pain management as a resource for pain control strategies. Discuss the pain-management regimen with the patient. Encourage the use of alternate pain-relieving techniques such as the use of imagery and relaxation.

NDx: Risk for trauma
After spinal surgery, maintain correct spinal alignment at all times. For the first 48 hours after surgery, log-roll the patient for position changes. The bed is kept flat. The patient is placed in a side-lying position. Patients in whom a posterior approach has been used should be positioned on their backs. A fracture pan should be used for patient voiding—log-roll the patient onto the fracture pan. Place a pillow between the patient's knee when he or she is in a side-lying position to maintain correct alignment of the spine.

After cervical surgery, keep the cervical collar on the patient at all times to support the head in a neutral position, thus preventing flexion or extension, which could displace the graft. Place a small pad under the patient's head when he or she is in a side-lying position to maintain neck alignment and to protect the ears from pressure. Do not use pillows, which, because of their thickness, alter align-

ment of the spine. Encourage deep breathing, but do not encourage coughing, because it can lead to extrusion of the cervical bone graft. Frequently assess motor and sensory function. Changes from the baseline should be immediately reported to the physician.

NDx: Risk for injury
The patient who has undergone spinal surgery is required to remain on bed rest and in some cases has also been on bed rest before surgery. If the patient has been supine for an extended period, orthostatic changes may occur when he or she first attempts to sit up. Have the patient sit on the edge of the bed, dangle his or her feet, and breathe deeply for 5 minutes before standing. Check blood pressure while the patient is sitting. Compare it with the blood pressure obtained in the supine position. If the systolic pressure has fallen 10 mm Hg or more, consider the patient at risk for postural hypotension when standing. Have two persons provide support for the patient who is getting out of bed for the first time after spinal surgery. Institute fall precautions as per agency protocol.

If sensation is diminished, protect the involved area from injury. For example, instruct the patient to visually check the position and location of the affected extremity.

NDx: Risk for urinary retention
Retention of urine after spinal surgery may be due to the depressant effects of perioperative drugs or to sympathetic fiber stimulation during lumbar laminectomy, edema at the operative site, and reduced mobility. An indwelling urinary catheter may be used but is usually removed as soon as possible to minimize the risk of infection. Encourage fluid intake. Palpate the bladder for distention. Provide privacy for urination. Use a fracture pan for female patients after lumbar laminectomy. Offer the bedpan every 2 hours. Monitor intake and output. Obtain an order to straight-catheterize the patient if he or she is unable to void within 6 to 8 hours of removal of the catheter.

NDx: Knowledge deficit: activity limitations and lifestyle modification needed to decrease stress on the spine
Instruct patients who have undergone cervical surgery to wear the cervical collar as directed by the surgeon, usually for about 6 weeks. Instruct patients who have undergone lumbosacral surgery to schedule rest periods throughout the day. Activity must be increased gradually because it takes 6 weeks for the ligaments to heal. Suggest the use of warm, moist heat to relieve muscle spasms and to promote healing. Caution the patient to avoid activities that produce strain on the spine, such as driving and stair climbing. Tell the patient to avoid heavy work for 2 to 3 months. Instruct the patient in techniques to decrease the stress of the spine and promote

proper body mechanics. Objects should be carried close to the chest and should not exceed 10 lbs. Teach the patient to bend from the knees and not from the waist. The patient is to sleep on the side with slight knee-hip flexion. Place a pillow between the knees to relieve the stress on back muscles. Encourage the patient to strengthen abdominal muscles postoperatively as directed by the physician. If needed, advocate weight reduction.

Additional Interventions

Provide good skin care to prevent the development of pressure sores. Change the dressing immediately if it is contaminated with urine or feces to decrease the risk of infection. Report any bloody or CSF drainage on the dressing.

Encourage the patient to ingest a high-fiber diet and increase fluid intake, because constipation is a risk as a result of decreased activity and perioperative medications that decrease peristalsis.

If a donor site is present, check it regularly for bleeding or drainage. Keep the site covered with a dry, sterile dressing. Position the patient to prevent excessive pressure on the area.

Compare the patient's status with the expected outcomes. If the outcomes are not met, reassess the patient and revise the plan.

❖ Settings, Providers, and Collaboration for Care

Patients with neurologic dysfunction may be assessed, diagnosed, and treated at inpatient or outpatient settings, depending on the nature of the tests and the findings. Because of the clinical manifestations of neurologic dysfunction, many patients must be admitted to a hospital or rehabilitation center for initial treatment. Life-threatening problems may require intensive-care monitoring for several days to weeks for some patients. Acute problems (and surgery) are managed in the hospital, but once the patient is stable, discharge to a rehabilitation center, intermediate care facility, or the home is likely. The patient still needs medical intervention, nursing care, and support from other health professionals.

In the rehabilitation center, specialists assist the patient to regain lost function or to adjust to the change in lifestyle due to loss of motor or sensory function. The guiding principle is to assist the patient to be as independent as possible. A speech therapist may be necessary for patients with partial or complete loss of speech. An occupational therapist assists the patient to learn new skills for employment. The physical therapist helps the patient build strength in weakened muscles and use assistive devices to perform activities of daily living. A counselor may be needed to help the patient and family cope with the changes in lifestyle.

If the patient is discharged to the home, a home health nurse and physical therapist may be needed to assist the patient with postoperative care needs and mobility problems. The nurse assesses the patient's status, changes dressings, teaches the patient and family about medications prescribed and the care regimen, and monitors the patient's recovery. The physical therapist may teach the patient strength exercises, help the family modify the home environment to provide safety for the patient, and teach the patient how to use assistive mobility devices.

A nutritionist may also be consulted for assistance in meal planning if the patient has difficulty swallowing due to loss of motor function. If the patient is on liquid feedings, the nurse instructs the family in the management of the parenteral or enteral therapy.

Communication with the physician through the patient's recovery period is imperative. The patient usually makes several visits to the physician during the recovery or rehabilitation phase for evaluation. The rehabilitation nurse, case manager, or home health nurse may be the liaison among the various health professionals during this time.

The Elderly: Special Considerations

STRUCTURAL CHANGES RELATED TO AGING

An age-related loss of neurons occurs throughout the CNS. Neuronal loss is a gradual and variable process, occurring throughout the life span and accelerating in later adulthood. Neuronal losses influence brain weight, contributing to a 10 to 12% decrease in brain weight by very old age. Information about normal brain aging is limited because much of the research is performed on autopsied, rather than living, brain tissue. When changes have been identified in older brains, questions have been raised about whether they are age-related or disease-related. Some changes that were once thought to be age-related are now thought to be disease-related. Other changes are present to a small degree in non-diseased brains but to a greater degree and in different distributions in diseased brains. Some of the changes that have been identified in older brains are loss of neurons, diminished blood flow, accumulation of lipofuscin, reduction of brain weight, decline in synaptic function, changes in neurotransmitter activity, decreased utilization of glucose and oxygen, and the presence of senile plaques and neurofibrillary tangles.

Alzheimer's disease, a common neurologic disorder, is associated with specific pathologic brain changes. Neuritic plaques and neurofibrillary tangles are the specific pathologic changes that Alzheimer discovered in the early 1900s. Neuronal loss or degeneration is a another central feature of brain changes in Alzheimer's disease. Significant neuronal losses related to Alzheimer's disease are more highly concentrated in specific areas of the brain, such as the hippocampus, cerebral cortex, and nucleus basalis. Destruction of neurons has also been identified in the hypothalamus and brain stem. It is thought that the cognitive impairments and behavioral manifestations of Alzheimer's disease are caused by the resulting damage to particular parts of the brain.

FUNCTIONAL CHANGES RELATED TO AGING

Reaction time (ie, the lag between stimulation and the initiation of a response) increases with age. Age-related changes in some intellectual skills are noticed beginning around the age of 60 years, even in healthy adults. Noticeable age-related effects on cognitive abilities include a slight and gradual decline in some intellectual abilities, such as short-term memory. Older adults are as capable of learning new things as younger people are, but their speed of processing information is slower. Also, older adults may be more cautious in their responses and may make more errors of omission. Age-related cognitive changes are minor and do not interfere significantly with daily functioning, especially if compensatory interventions, such as memory aids, are used. Factors that influence cognitive abilities in older adulthood include chemical effects (eg, medications), personal characteristics (eg, educational level), and physical and mental health status (eg, sensory functioning). Any major decline in cognitive functioning is due to disease conditions, such as dementia, or other risk factors, such as adverse medication effects.

Sleep patterns may be altered in the older adult. The total amount of time of deep sleep decreases, and the older person tends to wake more during sleep time as well as stay awake more during the night. This is usually compensated for by taking a nap during the day.

CHANGES IN THE SPECIAL SENSES RELATED TO AGING

Normal age-related changes in vision include a decrease in visual acuity, diminished peripheral vision, increased sensitivity to glare, and difficulty adapting to dark and light. Hearing loss for high-frequency sound is an age-related change. Older persons may have difficulty in distinguishing words spoken too fast. There is a slight decline in taste perception and a moderate decline in olfactory sensation. Tactile sensation decreases with age, making it difficult to discriminate temperature and perform fine motor tasks.

Chapter Review

1. What are the three meninges, where are they located, how do they differ, and what purpose do they serve?
2. Name the lobes of the cerebrum, identify their location, and what type of deficits would occur if a lobe were injured.
3. How is level of consciousness best assessed in a patient with a head injury?
4. What is the relationship of brain tissue, blood, and CSF to ICP?
5. Explain the relationship of arterial carbon dioxide ($PaCO_2$) levels and ICP.
6. Compare and contrast expressive, receptive, and global aphasia.
7. Describe how to assess mental status.
8. How is the care of the patient undergoing intracranial surgery different from that of the patient undergoing spinal surgery?
9. What nursing diagnosis would be appropriate for the patient undergoing spinal surgery and why?
10. Describe age-related changes in the nervous system and their nursing implications.

Bibliography

Adams RD, Victor M. Principles of neurology. 5th ed. New York: McGraw-Hill, 1993.

Adams RD, Victor M. Principles of neurology companion handbook. 5th ed. New York: McGraw-Hill, 1994.

Asbury AK, McKhann GM, McDonald WI. Diseases of the nervous system: Clinical neurobiology. 2nd ed. Philadelphia: WB Saunders, 1992.

Carpenito LJ. Nursing diagnosis: Application to clinical practice. 6th ed. Philadelphia: JB Lippincott, 1996.

Dolan JT. Critical care nursing: Clinical management through the nursing process. 2nd ed. Philadelphia: FA Davis, 1991.

Gilroy J. Basic neurology. 3rd ed. New York: McGraw-Hill, 1996.

Grossman RG, Hamilton WJ (eds). Principles of neurosurgery. New York: Raven Press, 1991.

Gunderson CH. Essentials of clinical neurology. New York: Raven Press, 1991.

Guyton AC. Basic neuroscience: Anatomy and physiology. 2nd ed. Philadelphia: WB Saunders, 1991.

Hickey J. The clinical practice of neurological and neurosurgical nursing. 4th ed. New York: JB Lippincott, 1996.

Lee BY, Ostrander L, Cochran G, Shaw W (eds). The spinal cord injured patient: Comprehensive management. Philadelphia: WB Saunders, 1991.

Lemke DM. Defining assessment parameters in dual injuries: Spinal cord injury and traumatic brain injury. SCI Nurs 1995; 12(2):40–47.

Lertz A. Neuroanatomy made easy and understandable. 4th ed. Rockville, MD: Aspen Systems, 1991.

Lower J. Rapid neuro assessment. Am J Nurs 1992; 92(6):38.

Schinner KM, Chisholm AH, Grap MJ, et al. Effects of auditory stimuli on intracranial pressure and cerebral perfusion pressure in traumatic brain injury. J Neurosci Nurs 1995; 27(6): 348–354.

Way C, Segatore M. Development and preliminary testing of the neurological assessment instrument. J Neurosci Nurs 1994; 26(5):278–287.

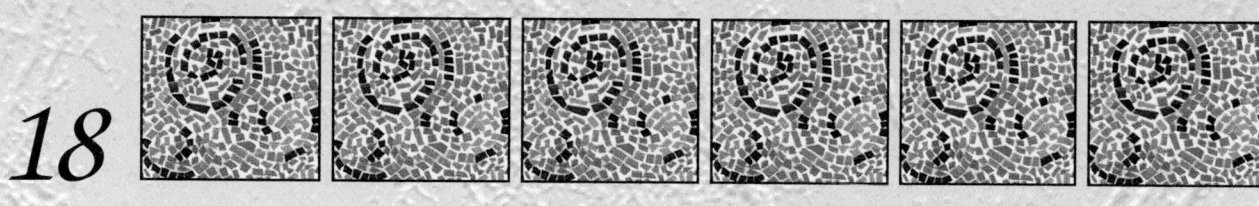

18

Nursing Care of Patients with Neurologic Disorders

Study Outcomes

After studying this chapter, you should be able to:

1. Describe common neurologic disorders in terms of etiology and pathophysiology, clinical manifestations, diagnostic procedures, and management.
2. Identify information and physical examination data essential to the assessment of patients with common neurologic disorders.
3. State nursing diagnoses and related expected patient outcomes commonly applicable to patients with neurologic disorders.
4. Describe nursing interventions, with their rationales, commonly applicable to patients with neurologic disorders.
5. Explain the basis for evaluation of nursing care provided to patients with common neurologic disorders.
6. Identify special considerations for the elderly patient with a neurologic disorder.
7. Identify alternative treatment and care settings for patients with neurologic disorders and the services related to community-based care.

Disorders of the nervous system can be insidious in onset, presenting with symptoms that are characteristic of many systemic diseases. Neurologic disorders also directly affect function as a human being—that is, the ability to think, to feel, to communicate, and to move. Many neurologic disorders, whether acute or gradual in onset, are chronic and often characterized by progressive deterioration of function. Because the brain cannot regenerate and suffers irreversible damage in a matter of minutes if its supply of oxygen and nutrients is impaired, many neurologic disorders also carry the threat of sudden death. Thus, accurate assessment and rapid intervention paired with sensitivity to the needs of both the patient and significant others are essential to nursing care of patients with neurologic disorders.

Patients with neurologic disorders may be cared for in a variety of settings. The setting depends on the disorder, clinical manifestations, prescribed medical regimen and nursing care, and the patient's response to the regimen and care. These settings may include the critical care unit, acute care unit, rehabilitation unit, long-term care facility, health-care clinic, or the home, including home care and hospice care. To provide nursing care in these varied settings, the nurse must possess a strong knowledge base of neurologic disorders and how to utilize the nursing process.

Infections and Inflammations

MENINGITIS

Meningitis is defined as an inflammation of the meninges of the brain. Two types of meningitis exist: bacterial and viral. The most frequently occurring type of meningitis is bacterial.

Bacterial Meningitis

Etiology and Pathophysiology

The causative organisms responsible for bacterial meningitis are many. The most common ones include the following:

> *Staphylococcus, Streptococcus,* and *Diplococcus pneumoniae* (gram-positive cocci)
> *Escherichia coli, Klebsiella* species, and *Pseudomonas* (gram-negative rods)
> *Haemophilus influenzae* (gram-negative cocci)
> *Neisseria meningitidis* (gram-negative diplococci)

Staphylococcus, Streptococcus, Diplococcus, N. meningitidis, and *H. influenzae* are normal inhabitants of the oral and nasal cavities. Because of the close proximity to the sinuses, conditions such as sinusitis, otitis media, upper respiratory tract infection or pneumonia, and direct trauma to the ears, nose, or sinuses predispose to entry of these organisms into the central nervous system. *E. coli, Klebsiella, Pseudomonas,* and others can be inadvertently introduced into the central nervous system during neurosurgical procedures, lumbar puncture, and spinal anesthesia or may be introduced secondary to trauma.

Entry of organisms into the central nervous system occurs predominately via the blood stream. The pia mater and arachnoid layers of the meninges as well as the subarachnoid space containing cerebrospinal fluid are affected. The purulent exudate spreads quickly via the free-flowing cerebrospinal fluid. Inflammatory lesions caused by the accumulation of exudate can form, particularly around the base of the brain. The blood vessels of the meninges can become engorged secondary to the inflammatory changes. Thrombosis or rupture may occur. Early treatment of the infectious process is critical to prevent adhesions and scarring, resulting in hydrocephalus.

Clinical Manifestations

The signs and symptoms manifested by the patient with bacterial meningitis occur in response to the bacterial invasion and are not particular to any one organism. The exception to this is meningococcal meningitis, caused by *N. meningitidis,* in which 50% of patients acquire a petechial rash, purpuric lesions, or ecchymosis.

The patient with bacterial meningitis usually presents with symptoms related to increasing intracranial pressure, such as headache and fever. The headache is generally severe and is usually the initial symptom. Variations in level of consciousness may be present in the early stage. These include poor attention span, irritability and restlessness, disorientation, and hallucinations. The patient's level of responsiveness may fluctuate and may decrease with progression of the illness.

Signs of meningeal irritation are also present. These include nuchal rigidity and Kernig's and Brudzinski's signs (Fig. 18–1). Nuchal rigidity, or stiff neck, is manifested by the patient's tendency to keep the neck extended and immobile. Attempts to flex the neck forward cause pain. Kernig's sign is the inability to extend the leg from a position of 90% flexion at the hip. If attempts to extend the leg cause pain and spasms in the hamstrings, the sign is considered positive. A positive Brudzinski sign is when passive flexion of the head and neck onto the chest results in a flexion response of the thighs and legs.

Other signs and symptoms that can occur include photophobia, cranial nerve dysfunctions, and generalized seizures secondary to the irritation of the cerebral cortex.

Diagnosis

A careful history and physical examination are necessary to obtain pertinent information to aid in the diagnosis of meningitis. A history of any preceding infections, particularly involving the ears, sinuses, or

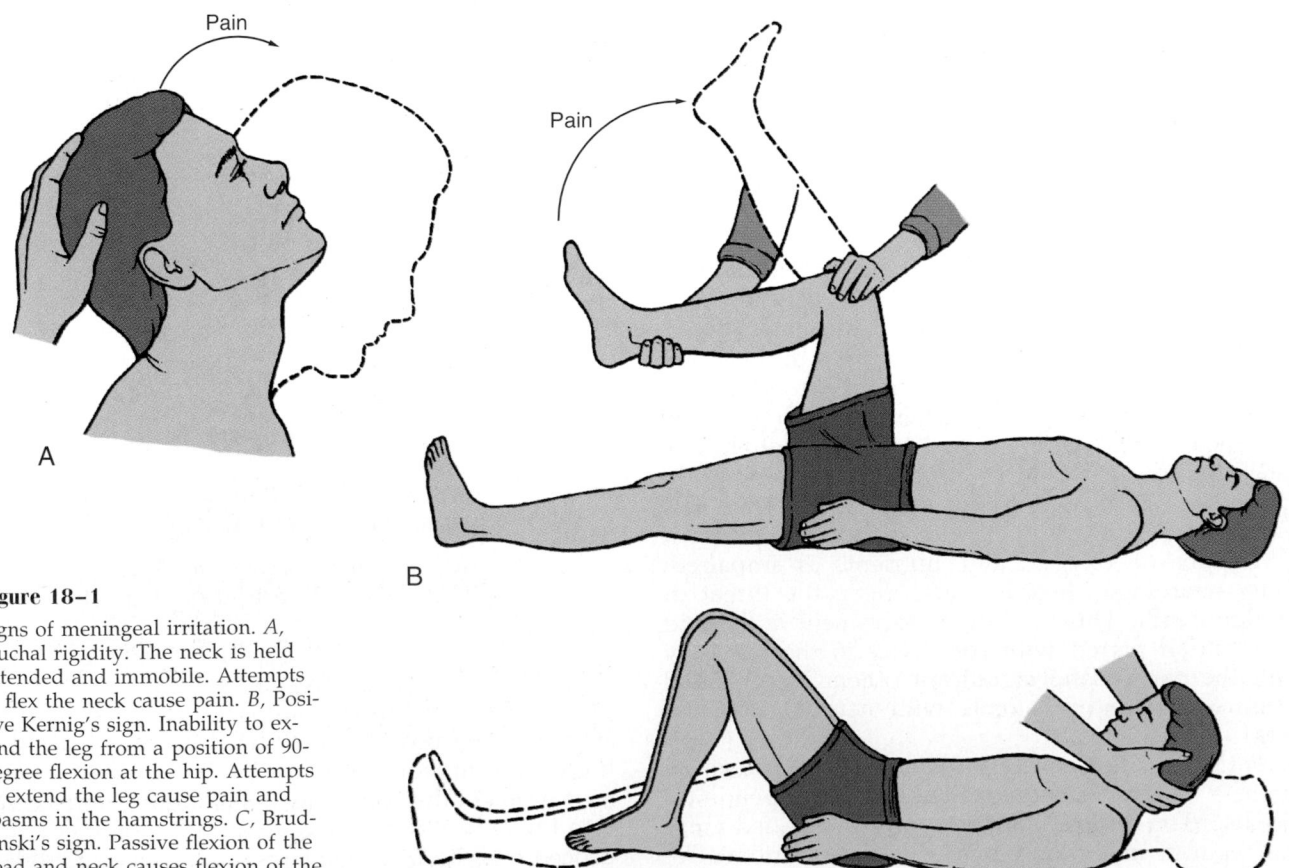

Figure 18–1

Signs of meningeal irritation. *A,* Nuchal rigidity. The neck is held extended and immobile. Attempts to flex the neck cause pain. *B,* Positive Kernig's sign. Inability to extend the leg from a position of 90-degree flexion at the hip. Attempts to extend the leg cause pain and spasms in the hamstrings. *C,* Brudzinski's sign. Passive flexion of the head and neck causes flexion of the thighs and legs.

respiratory tract, as well as any evidence of recent exposure to persons known or suspected to have meningitis, further supports the diagnosis. The presence of headache, fever, and meningeal irritation on physical examination also suggests meningitis.

The definitive diagnostic measure is the lumbar puncture. Data that indicate bacterial meningitis include turbid, cloudy fluid, a markedly increased white blood cell count and protein content, and a decreased glucose content. The opening pressure on lumbar puncture is also elevated (>180 mm H_2O). Gram's stain and culture reports indicate the causative organism. Other laboratory findings that may be significant include skull and sinus x-ray films as well as cultures of the nose, throat, blood, and any other infected sites.

Management

The focus of medical management of the patient with bacterial meningitis is prompt initiation of intravenous antibiotic treatment with broad-spectrum antimicrobials before obtaining the culture reports. Once the causative organism is known, drug therapy is continued for at least 10 days, using the most effective drug or drugs specific to that bacteria. Steroids and osmotic diuretics may be used to decrease cerebral edema. Anticonvulsants are used if seizures are present.

Isolation procedures are not routinely required for the patient with bacterial meningitis. However, respiratory isolation until the patient has received antibiotic therapy for 24 hours is generally adhered to. Universal precautions and the individual institution's policies on infection control should be followed.

❖ Settings, Providers, and Collaboration for Care

The patient with bacterial meningitis is usually hospitalized and treated with intravenous antibiotics. If the patient's condition is severe, admission to the critical care unit may be necessary. Follow-up care is managed through a clinic or physician's office. Contacts should be made with all persons who were in contact with the patient. The public health department should be notified. Representatives from this department are usually responsible for tracking the contacts and recommending any treatment if needed.

Viral Meningitis

Etiology and Pathophysiology

Viral meningitis, also called aseptic meningitis, almost uniformly occurs as a complication of a primary viral infection outside the central nervous system. The most common viruses are the enteroviruses, mumps virus, herpesvirus, and arboviruses. The most frequent portals of entry of these viruses are the oral, fecal-oral, or respiratory pathways.

Once the virus enters the body, it replicates and spreads to the brain via the blood stream.

Clinical Manifestations

Viral meningitis usually begins with abrupt onset of fever, headache, stiff neck, and occasional vomiting. Mental status changes, such as irritability or slight lethargy, may be present. Confusion and severe lethargy are rare. It is often difficult to distinguish between bacterial and viral meningitis on the basis of symptoms alone.

Diagnosis

The diagnosis of viral meningitis is based on the history and physical examination as well as laboratory data from a lumbar puncture and cerebrospinal fluid analysis. In viral meningitis, the protein content of the cerebrospinal fluid is normal or slightly increased, and the glucose content is normal. No bacteria are reported on Gram's stain or cultures.

Management

The management of the patient with viral meningitis focuses on supportive care and is based on the presenting symptoms. Because symptoms are generally influenza-like, antipyretics and analgesics may provide relief. No drug therapy is effective against the virus itself. Viral meningitis is treated in an outpatient setting, unless complications occur.

ENCEPHALITIS

Encephalitis is defined as inflammation of the brain. It is generally classified according to cause. The inflammation associated with encephalitis may be secondary to viruses, bacteria, fungi, or parasites. Viruses are the most common offending organisms.

Viral Encephalitis

Etiology and Pathophysiology

Several types of viral encephalitis are known:

> Arbovirus encephalitis transmitted by mosquitoes, such as western and eastern equine encephalitis
> St. Louis encephalitis
> California virus encephalitis
> Venezuelan equine encephalitis
> Japanese B encephalitis

Tick-transmitted arboviruses include those that cause Colorado tick fever, Russian tick-borne encephalitis, and Far Eastern encephalitis. Several of these viruses are endemic to certain geographic regions as well as to seasons of the year. Less frequent causes of viral encephalitis include the following:

> Vaccines for smallpox, measles, mumps, and rabies
> Viral infections such as measles, mumps, infectious mononucleosis, and rubella

Toxins from ingested substances such as lead and arsenic

Herpes simplex encephalitis is the most common form of nonepidemic encephalitis in the United States.

Viruses require a living host to reproduce. Viruses gain access to the central nervous system through the systemic circulation or through the cranial and peripheral nerves. The virus "takes over" the normal activities of brain cells to reproduce and maintain itself. This process causes inflammation without exudate in the cells of the cortex, resulting in degenerative changes. Widespread edema, compression of blood vessels, hemorrhage, cavitation, and necrosis can occur in a scattered pattern throughout the brain.

Herpes simplex encephalitis can affect all age groups. It is caused by herpes simplex virus 1 or 2. Herpes simplex virus 1 is associated with the common cold sore and is present in a dormant state in most people. It can produce acute encephalitis in the adult through reactivation of the latent virus. Although the mechanisms for this reactivation are unclear, fever, emotional stress, and infectious diseases may play a role.

Herpes simplex virus 2 is associated with the sexually transmitted genital disease. It can cause encephalitis only in neonates who acquire it during passage through the birth canal of an infected mother. In adults, herpes simplex virus 2 causes aseptic (viral) meningitis in association with recent genital herpes simplex infections.

The herpes simplex virus attacks the brain, particularly the temporal lobes, and causes destruction and necrosis of neurons. Pronounced cerebral edema occurs, resulting in increased intracranial pressure and possibly a herniation syndrome. It is unclear how the virus enters the central nervous system, but it is postulated that the probable routes of entry are the blood stream and the peripheral nerves. Herpes simplex encephalitis is associated with a 70% mortality rate if untreated.

Clinical Manifestations

The onset of symptoms is usually gradual, initially manifested by fever, malaise, headache, listlessness, joint pain, nausea, and vomiting. Within a few days, neurologic symptoms appear. These may include alterations in level of consciousness, such as confusion and stupor, ataxia, photophobia, stiff neck, and possibly tremors and convulsions, hemiparesis, and abnormalities of cranial nerves. The symptoms can be similar to those seen in meningitis, but the severity is somewhat lessened in the initial stages. Stupor progressing to coma may occur secondary to increased intracranial pressure and diffuse cerebral edema. The mortality rate dramatically increases if progression to a comatose state occurs.

Diagnosis

Diagnosis of viral encephalitis is based primarily on the history and the physical examination. A history of a preceding viral infection or of recent travel to an area where ticks and mosquitoes are prevalent can be significant to the diagnosis. Laboratory findings are of little to no significant value because they are frequently normal in viral infections. Brain biopsy and tissue culture can aid in identification of a particular virus, provided there is accessibility to laboratories capable of performing these sophisticated analyses. Lumbar puncture may be performed to obtain cerebrospinal fluid for laboratory analysis. Protein and white blood cell count are elevated. Computed tomography (CT) as well as electroencephalograms (EEGs) may also be ordered.

Management

Specific drug therapy is not available for the treatment of viral encephalitis. Steroids may be used to decrease cerebral edema. Anticonvulsants aid in preventing seizures. Antipyretics and analgesics combat hyperthermia and assist in relieving headaches. The focus of treatment is supportive and is aimed at prevention of complications secondary to encephalitis. Herpes simplex encephalitis may be treated with antiviral agents that interfere with DNA synthesis. These agents include acyclovir (Zovirax) and vidarabine (ara-A, Vira-A). This treatment regimen with antivirals is questionable because effectiveness is not clear. Treatment must be initiated in the early stages of the inflammatory process. Controversy exists because the definitive diagnosis by brain biopsy takes time, and the potency and side effects of the drug therapies pose risks to the patient. Other treatment modalities include glucocorticoids, such as dexamethasone (Decadron), to reduce edema and anticonvulsants to treat seizure activity. Intracranial pressure monitoring may be instituted.

❖ Settings, Providers, and Collaboration for Care

Patients with encephalitis are usually very ill and are treated in the critical care unit and the acute care unit. Upon discharge, the nurse gives instructions to the patient and family about continued follow-up at the physician's office and the medications prescribed. The public health department should be notified since investigation of contacts and the epidemiology of the case may be necessary.

BRAIN ABSCESS

Etiology and Pathophysiology

A brain abscess is the result of an infectious process either outside or within the central nervous system. Organisms from the infectious process migrate directly to brain tissue, forming a lesion, usually in the white matter of the brain. This lesion is filled with suppurative material and has the ability to enlarge and, therefore, behave as a space-occupying lesion within the cranium. This predisposes not only to the systemic effects of the inflammatory process but to the serious consequences of increased intracranial pressure.

The precipitating factors leading to the formation of a brain abscess are the presence of organisms and the ability of these organisms to gain entry into the brain tissue. Approximately 40% of all brain abscesses extend into the brain directly from middle-ear and mastoid infections. Sinus infections and direct trauma to the brain, allowing for immediate access, are responsible for another approximate 10%. The remaining 50% are the result of infections in other sites within the body that cause septic emboli to travel via the blood stream to the brain. Common sources of septic emboli include the following:

Lungs (lung abscesses)
Heart (bacterial endocarditis or congenital heart disease)
Pelvis (pelvic abscesses)
Skin infections

Clinical Manifestations

The signs and symptoms exhibited depend on the location of the lesion. Initially, the patient exhibits the general symptoms associated with an acute infectious process, such as chills, fever, malaise, anorexia, and myalgias. Because brain abscess formation generally occurs secondary to a previously existent infection, these signs may be considered by the patient to be an exacerbation of that illness. As the abscess enlarges, focal neurologic signs may develop, such as headache, nuchal rigidity, and vomiting. The patient continues to experience these symptoms but with increasing severity and persistence. Confusion, drowsiness, seizures, and signs of increased intracranial pressure or cranial nerve palsies may develop as the abscess continues to enlarge and compress surrounding structures. Fever may or may not be present.

Diagnosis

Diagnosis of a brain abscess can present some difficulties because of the lack of definitive symptoms and the somewhat confusing clinical picture. A careful history specifically geared to the presence of a previous infection is helpful in suggesting the presence of a brain abscess. X-ray films of the chest, skull, and sinuses may help identify a primary source of infection. Lumbar puncture reveals a markedly elevated pressure (200 to 300 mm H_2O), with protein content and white blood cell count dramatically elevated. Glucose content is normal. The culture and sensitivity results are negative because the bacteria are contained within the abscess and have not invaded the cerebrospinal fluid. CT, magnetic resonance imaging (MRI), or arteriography assist in localizing the lesion and determining its size as well as ascertaining the presence of multiple abscesses.

Management

Prompt initiation of antibiotic therapy is the primary focus of the medical management of the patient with a brain abscess. Anaerobic streptococci and bacteroids are the most common bacteria causing brain abscess formation. Penicillin G and chloramphenicol administered intravenously in divided doses are the usual choices to treat these organisms. In addition, steroid therapy with dexamethasone is given to combat cerebral edema.

Surgical intervention may be necessary. If the abscess is well encapsulated, it may be removed in its entirety. Aspiration and drainage of the abscess is another option. Antibiotics may be directly injected into the sac once aspiration is completed.

❖ Settings, Providers, and Collaboration for Care

Patients with brain abscess are treated initially in the hospital for intravenous medication and possible surgical intervention. Depending on residual symptoms the patient may need long-term care or home care. Follow-up should take place in an outpatient setting. Occupational and physical therapy should be consulted as needed. The type of intervention needed from these professionals depends on the patient's condition, prognosis, and needs at the time of discharge. A home health agency may be contacted for specific nursing needs as well as basic hygiene needs if the patient has residual effects from the disease. If the patient is still receiving nutritional therapy by the parenteral route, a home intravenous (IV) care agency should be contacted to set up the equipment in the home and teach the family the maintenance routine needed.

NURSING PROCESS
Meningitis, Encephalitis, or Brain Abscess

Assessment

The first priority when assessing the patient with meningitis, encephalitis, or brain abscess is to establish a baseline of the patient's neurologic function. Assess the level of consciousness, pupils and cranial nerves, movement, and sensation. Altered levels of consciousness can lead to airway obstruction. Note the presence and severity of meningeal signs. Assess the vital signs as part of the neurologic assessment. Observe the patient's sleep-wake cycle, noting any patterns or trends of increased or decreased restlessness in relation to environmental stimuli. Assess skin integrity, color, and turgor. Note whether diaphoresis, dryness, or pallor is present. Test the patient's ability to swallow. Assess the gag reflex. Obtain the patient's weight. Determine the patient's level of comfort on the basis of either subjective complaints of headache, stiff neck, or joint pain or observation of increased irritability in relation to stimulation. Discuss the illness with the patient and the family to assess their level of comprehension of the disease process and anticipated outcome.

Nursing Diagnoses and Planning

Nursing diagnoses and related expected patient outcomes most commonly applicable to patients with meningitis, encephalitis, or brain abscess include the following:

NDx: Pain: headache and neck pain related to meningeal irritation

Planning: Patient Outcomes
1. Patient exhibits ability to rest.
2. Patient states that pain is decreased.

NDx: Risk for injury related to restlessness, disorientation, seizure activity

Planning: Patient Outcomes
1. Patient remains free from injury.

NDx: Risk for altered nutrition: less than body requirements related to anorexia, fatigue, nausea and vomiting, and inability to swallow

Planning: Patient Outcomes
1. Weight is maintained within 1 to 2 lb of baseline.
2. Patient is free of symptoms of dehydration.
3. Nausea and vomiting episodes are reduced or eliminated.

NDx: Risk for impaired skin integrity related to immobility, dehydration, and diaphoresis

Planning: Patient Outcomes
1. Skin remains intact.
2. Irritation and redness are absent.

NDx: Altered family processes related to critical nature of situation and uncertain prognosis

Planning: Patient Outcomes
1. Family members acknowledge difficulty in accepting the illness.
2. Family members identify positive coping patterns.

Nursing Interventions and Evaluation

NDx: Pain
The patient with meningeal irritation often experiences hyperalgesia and hyperirritability. Minimize unnecessary stimulation by consolidating nursing care activities when feasible. Maintain a quiet environment: Keep the room darkened, and keep environmental noise at a low level. Speak in a quiet voice to avoid startling the patient. Administer analgesics as ordered and monitor for effectiveness. Provide cool compresses to the head. Offer gradual position changes and back massages as needed.

NDx: Risk for injury
The patient with meningitis or encephalitis may exhibit a fluctuating level of consciousness as a result of the diffuse inflammation throughout the central nervous system. Seizures are not uncommon. Institute measures to protect the patient from injury during restless or disoriented episodes or during seizure activity. Maintain the bed in the lowest position when the patient is not under observation. Keep the side rails up. Place pads or bumpers along the side rails to prevent the patient from striking the extremities against the sides of the bed. Protect intravenous catheters and other tubes such as nasogastric tubes or indwelling urinary catheters from dislodgment. Cautiously use restraints when necessary. Institute seizure precautions, and administer anticonvulsant medications as ordered. Monitor laboratory data for therapeutic serum levels of the drug prescribed. Administer sedation if ordered. Remember that sedation may not be prescribed despite restless or agitated behavior because of the potential for an altered level of consciousness secondary to the medication. This may interfere with determination of true changes in mentation versus the effects of sedation.

NDx: Risk for altered nutrition: less than body requirements
The patient's nutritional status is at risk secondary to fluctuating levels of consciousness and inability to tolerate oral intake. The infectious process and associated fever increase the body's metabolic and nutritional needs. If the patient is unable to take fluids by mouth because of nausea and vomiting or because of a reduced level of alertness, which poses a risk of aspiration, intravenous fluids will be necessary. Confer with the dietitian to determine the patient's daily caloric requirements. Supplemental feedings by nasogastric tube or total parenteral nutrition (TPN) may be indicated to ensure that an adequate calorie intake is maintained. Monitor intake and output every 8 hours. Weigh the patient every 3 days. If the patient has persistent vomiting, daily weighings are necessary. Monitor laboratory values such as blood urea nitrogen (BUN), creatine, and albumin levels. Administer antiemetics as needed.

NDx: Risk for impaired skin integrity
Bed rest and immobility imposed by the acuteness of the infectious process predispose the patient to skin breakdown. In addition, diaphoresis causes the skin to be moist and prone to irritation and ischemic changes, particularly over pressure-sensitive areas. Change the linen frequently to avoid wetness against the skin. Minimize covers and blankets to avoid excess moisture. Turn and position the patient every 2 hours if he or she is unable to shift position without assistance. Inspect the bony prominences for signs of redness or pressure. Protect the heels and elbows. Remember that irritation of these areas occurs quickly, particularly if the patient is restless.

NDx: Altered family processes
In the acute phase of meningitis, encephalitis, or brain abscess, the patient exhibits changes in mentation and level of consciousness. The patient may be restless, irritable, and possibly unable to recognize family members. Realize that this is a frightening experience for the family and that helplessness and anxiety regarding the prognosis may interfere with coping abilities. Encourage the family to express their feelings of fear, anger, and concern. Offer ex-

planations of the disease process and relate patient behaviors and symptoms to the course of the illness. Help the family to identify their strengths as well as behaviors that may be interfering with their abilities to be supportive. Facilitate interaction with the social worker and spiritual counselor if needed.

Compare the patient's status with the expected outcomes. If the outcomes are not met, reassess the patient and revise the plan.

GUILLAIN-BARRÉ SYNDROME

Guillain-Barré syndrome is an acute, rapidly progressive inflammation and demyelination of nerve endings of the peripheral nervous system that predominately affects motor function. It is also known as acute idiopathic polyneuritis or postinfectious polyneuritis.

Etiology and Pathophysiology

The cause of Guillain-Barré syndrome is unknown. The most widely accepted theory is that it is an autoimmune response. Current research has linked *Campylobacter jejuni* as a chief precipitant of the syndrome. *C. jejuni* is the most common cause of diarrheal illness in developed countries. Sixty to seventy percent of patients with Guillain-Barré syndrome report a mild febrile illness, usually respiratory or gastrointestinal, 1 to 3 weeks before the onset of symptoms. This precipitating illness is believed to be the stimulus for an immune reaction to occur in the body against the body's own peripheral nerves. Guillain-Barré syndrome is nonseasonal and nonepidemic, occurring in the adult population and more frequently between 30 and 50 years of age. There is an equal distribution among both sexes. Viral illnesses and vaccines have also been suggested as causative factors.

The insulatory covering of the axons of nerve fibers, called myelin, is broken down and in some instances destroyed by the inflammatory process associated with Guillain-Barré syndrome. This demyelination process results in slowed or blocked nerve impulse conduction, generally affecting the cranial nerves, the ventral and dorsal roots of the spinal nerves, and the entire length of peripheral nerves. The muscles innervated by these nerves undergo progressive paralysis. Respiratory failure is the chief cause of death secondary to paralysis of respiratory muscles. Remyelination and regeneration of axons occurs spontaneously and completely in approximately 80% of cases.

Clinical Manifestations

Approximately 1 to 3 weeks after an influenza-like illness, paresthesias—that is, numbness, tingling, or burning sensations—occur in the hands and feet and progress upward to involve the arms, legs, and trunk. This is quickly followed by weakness of the muscles, again affecting the distal areas of the hands and feet and ascending upward. The weakness may

rapidly progress to total paralysis, including the respiratory muscles, necessitating mechanical ventilatory support. The patient may appear to be unconscious but is mentally alert. Bilateral facial paralysis and difficulty swallowing occur secondary to involvement of the cranial nerves. The severity of the symptoms varies from patient to patient.

In all instances, there is an initial progressive phase, lasting anywhere from a few days to 2 weeks, in which the sensory and motor symptoms occur in a progressive and ascending manner. This is followed by a plateau phase, during which symptoms become maximal. This phase generally lasts several days to 2 weeks. The final phase is the recovery, in which there is a progressive return of motor and sensory function, which occurs in a descending pattern. This phase can last from several months to 2 years. Approximately 20% of patients with Guillain-Barré syndrome are left with residual deficits, such as mild motor weakness or diminished reflexes in the lower extremities.

Diagnosis

The diagnosis of Guillain-Barré syndrome is based primarily on the physical examination and history. An acute onset, rapid progression of weakness and paralysis, lack of reflexes, absence of muscle atrophy in the limbs, and a precipitating febrile illness of either respiratory or gastrointestinal origin are significant. Lumbar puncture for cerebrospinal fluid analysis indicates an increase in the protein count without a significant increase in the cell count. Nerve conduction studies show slowing initially, and abnormalities are seen several weeks after the onset of symptoms.

Management

There is no known cure for Guillain-Barré syndrome. Treatment focuses on supportive therapy and the prevention of complications, such as pneumonia and respiratory failure secondary to respiratory paralysis and cardiovascular complications resulting from paralysis and immobility. Glucocorticoids, such as prednisone and dexamethasone, are often used because of their anti-inflammatory properties, but their efficacy is not clearly documented.

Plasmapheresis may be used. This plasma-exchange treatment is thought to remove antibodies in the blood stream that are destructive to peripheral nervous system tissue. Treatment should be initiated within the first 2 weeks after the onset of symptoms to be effective.

❖ Settings, Providers, and Collaboration for Care

The patient is initially treated in the critical care unit and moved to a medical floor when the patient's condition permits. Follow-up assessment should take place in a physician's office or outpatient clinic. Physical therapy should be consulted if the patient has residual motor problems. The therapist may prescribe strength exercises or help the patient use assistive devices for motor control.

NURSING PROCESS
Guillain-Barré Syndrome

Assessment

During the acute, initial phase of Guillain-Barré syndrome, obtain a baseline neurologic assessment. Assess motor strength of the extremities, and check for absence of sensation, numbness, tingling, and weakness in the hands and feet. Compare subsequent evaluations to the baseline assessment to determine ascending progression of sensory loss and weakness. The severity of symptoms varies from patient to patient. Assess for cranial nerve involvement, which results in difficulty swallowing, chewing, and speaking. The gag and cough reflexes may be absent. Assess respiratory function. Observe for dyspnea and confusion. Cyanotic nail bed color may be present. Obtain arterial blood gas levels and vital capacity measurements. Assess cardiovascular status through measurement of blood pressure, heart rate, and peripheral pulses. Cardiac arrhythmias may be present if the vagus nerve is affected. Check baseline temperature. Obtain the patient's weight.

Because of progressive paralysis the patient may appear to be unconscious but is mentally alert and aware. Assess the patient's anxiety level. Note any expressed verbalizations of fear or anger as the weakness and paralysis progress. Observe the patient and family interaction to determine coping abilities.

Nursing Diagnoses and Planning

Nursing diagnoses and related expected patient outcomes most commonly applicable to patients with Guillain-Barré syndrome include the following:

NDx: Risk for ineffective breathing pattern related to respiratory muscle paralysis

Planning: Patient Outcomes
1. Gas exchange with assistance of mechanical ventilator is maintained.
2. Patient is free of cyanosis and other signs of hypoxia.
3. Arterial blood gas levels are within normal limits for the patient.

NDx: Impaired physical mobility related to muscle dysfunction and weakness

Planning: Patient Outcomes
1. Patient actively or passively participates in physical activity.
2. Joint mobility is maintained.

NDx: Risk for impaired skin integrity related to immobility

Planning: Patient Outcomes
1. Skin remains intact.
2. Pressure areas are free of nonblanching erythema.

NDx: Self care deficit: feeding, bathing/hygiene, dressing/grooming, toileting related to paralysis

Planning: Patient Outcomes
1. Patient acknowledges need for assistance with care.
2. Patient performs self-care activities to the extent possible.
3. Patient accepts assistance with self-care.

NDx: Impaired verbal communication related to cranial nerve paralysis or tracheostomy

Planning: Patient Outcomes
1. Effective means of communication are established.
2. Patient expresses needs nonverbally with minimal frustration.

NDx: Powerlessness related to inability to control progression of weakness and paralysis

Planning: Patient Outcomes
1. Patient identifies factors contributing to a sense of powerlessness.
2. Patient participates in decision-making regarding the plan of care.

Nursing Interventions and Evaluation

NDx: Risk for ineffective breathing pattern
Monitor the patient's respiratory rate, rhythm, and depth of respirations at least every hour in the acute phase. Changes in the pattern of respiration may develop quickly. The patient may require emergency intubation or tracheostomy if weakness and paralysis interfere with effective gas exchange. Mechanical ventilation may be required to ensure adequate oxygenation and lung expansion. If the patient requires an artificial airway, such as a tracheostomy, keep the head of the bed elevated to reduce pressure on the diaphragm and to promote chest expansion. Suction the airway, maintaining sterile technique, every 2 hours and as needed to prevent respiratory tract infections. Note the color, amount, and consistency of secretions. Provide pulmonary toilet and position changes every 2 hours to prevent atelectasis. Monitor arterial blood gas levels for acid-base abnormalities and decreased oxygen saturation.

NDx: Impaired physical mobility
The weakness associated with Guillain-Barré syndrome often progresses to a flaccid paralysis, which may lead to atrophy and the development of contractures. Reposition the patient or encourage position change every 2 hours. Maintain therapeutic body alignment of shoulders, hips, and extremities. Perform passive range-of-motion exercises every 2 to 4 hours. Support the extremities in functional ana-

tomic positions. Consult with the physical therapist for structured bedside exercises and for the use of splints or other protective devices, if necessary.

NDx: Risk for impaired skin integrity

The paralysis and paresthesias associated with Guillain-Barré syndrome place the patient at risk for skin breakdown. Monitor the patient's skin for intactness, presence of redness, temperature, and turgor every 2 hours. Massage the skin and bony prominences to promote circulation after position changes every 2 hours. Maintain wrinkle-free bed linen. Institute the use of a pressure prevention aid, such as an air or egg-crate mattress. Use lotion or cream if the skin appears dry.

NDx: Self care deficit: feeding, bathing/hygiene, dressing/grooming, toileting

The patient in the progressive and plateau phases of Guillain-Barré syndrome lacks the motor ability to perform activities of daily living (ADLs) at an optimally functional level. If paralysis is present, the patient completely depends on others for feeding, bathing, and toileting. Provide basic hygienic care for the patient daily. Involve the patient in planning a schedule for such activities as hair washing and nail trimming. Feeding needs vary with the patient's ability to swallow. Assess gag and swallow reflexes. Assess for paralytic ileus. Bowel sounds must be present before administering food. Remember that even if the patient is able to swallow without the risk of aspiration, some degree of weakness in the upper extremities is likely, so provide assistance as needed. If the patient is unable to swallow, nasogastric feedings may be necessary. Bowel and bladder sphincter control remains surprisingly intact despite diffuse involvement of other sympathetic nerve fibers throughout the nervous system. However, the patient is generally unable to toilet himself or herself because of the motor weakness and paralysis, so assist with toileting as needed.

NDx: Impaired verbal communication

Paralysis of the facial muscles alters the patient's ability to communicate. If tracheostomy is required to maintain the airway, an additional barrier to verbal communication exists. Explain to the patient why he or she is unable to speak. Ask questions that can be answered by a "yes" or "no" response. Establish an individual pattern of simple communication, if necessary, such as eye blinks. Use flash cards or an alphabet board to facilitate two-way communication. Try to anticipate the patient's needs. Acknowledge the patient's frustration, and provide positive reinforcement when barriers to communication are overcome.

NDx: Powerlessness

Recognize that the immobility imposed by the weakness and paralysis associated with Guillain-Barré syndrome as well as the barriers to communication can contribute to feelings of lack of control and influence over the immediate environment. Encourage the patient to express his or her feelings of powerlessness over the disease progression itself as well as the limitations imposed by the symptoms. Include the patient in decision-making as it pertains to the care routine. Provide explanations and rationales for all care provided and for any treatments or procedures. Establish a trusting relationship with the patient through consistency of care providers if possible.

Compare the patient's status with the expected outcomes. If the outcomes are not met, reassess the patient and revise the plan.

Degenerative Disorders

AMYOTROPHIC LATERAL SCLEROSIS

Amyotrophic lateral sclerosis is a progressive degeneration and loss of both upper and lower motor neurons. This is the most common motor neuron disease in adults and is often called Lou Gehrig's disease, after the baseball player with this condition. The incidence of amyotrophic lateral sclerosis is 1.5 per 100,000 persons in the United States. It affects males three times more often than females. Five thousand new cases are diagnosed each year.

Etiology and Pathophysiology

The cause of amyotrophic lateral sclerosis remains unclear. A current hypothesis reports a vulnerability of motor neurons by glutamate (an amino acid metabolized by the brain) with possible genetic predisposition or environmental causes. Premature aging and autoimmune response are additional suggested causes currently under investigation. Whatever the cause, motor neurons in the brain stem and spinal cord atrophy and die, resulting in progressive motor dysfunction. Estimated survival time after the onset of symptoms is 3 to 5 years. Approximately 10% of amyotrophic lateral sclerosis is familial.

Clinical Manifestations

The onset of amyotrophic lateral sclerosis is insidious. The symptoms experienced by a patient with amyotrophic lateral sclerosis include muscle weakness, muscle atrophy, hyper-reflexia, fasciculations, spasticity, and cramping. No sensory dysfunction is noted. Cognitive dysfunction is rare.

Weakness usually begins in the upper or lower extremities. There is progressive atrophy and wasting of muscle groups, with absent reflexes in the affected muscle groups and hyper-reflexia noted distal to affected areas. As the brain stem is affected, patients present with bulbar signs, which include slurred speech, difficulty swallowing, and inability to clear oral secretions. The respiratory muscles are eventually compromised. Aspiration and respiratory arrest are often the immediate cause of death in these patients. Although mental status is unaffected, the patient is unable to speak or move. Often patients report feeling like prisoners in their own bodies.

Diagnosis

Currently there are no specific diagnostic tests for amyotrophic lateral sclerosis. A complete history and neurologic examination are performed to identify patterns of motor system involvement with the absence of sensory system dysfunction. CT, MRI, and cerebrospinal fluid analysis are performed to rule out other disorders or causative factors. Serum creatine phosphokinase levels are checked because findings of slightly elevated levels correlate with muscle atrophy. An electromyogram is performed to document diminished muscle contraction and fibrillations.

Management

Medical management focuses on supportive and palliative interventions to maintain the patient's highest functional level. Medication is used to control symptoms. Muscle relaxants (such as diazepam [Valium], baclofen [Lioresal], and dantrolene [Dantrium]) are used to control muscle spasticity. Anticholinergics are used to eliminate or reduce oral secretions and sialorrhea (excessive salivation). Gabapentin (Neurontin), an antiseizure medication with possible antiglutamate properties, is also prescribed. Quinine is beneficial in relieving muscle cramps. Rilutek (Riluzole) was approved by the FDA in 1996. It is the first drug proven effective in the treatment of amyotrophic lateral sclerosis. Rilutek extends survival time.

Use of supportive measures is discussed and decided with the patient. Supportive measures include enteral feedings and mechanical ventilation. The goal of the decision-making is to retain meaning and value in the patient's life.

❖ Settings, Providers, and Collaboration for Care

The patient with amyotrophic lateral sclerosis may be cared for in the home and treated in a physician's office as long as the patient's condition permits. As the patient's condition deteriorates, treatment may take place in the hospital, long-term care facility, or in the home. The case manager works with several other health-care workers to meet the patient's needs during exacerbations of the disease.

Home health care is needed to assist the patient with basic hygiene and even feedings in many cases. The home health nurse also assesses the patient's condition, directs the care in the home, and communicates with the physician as needed. Physical therapists, social workers, and hospice workers may also be consulted. The physical therapist works with the patient to maintain strength and mobility. The therapist also helps the patient learn to safely use assistive devices as problems with immobility gradually worsen. The social worker works with the patient

and family to find supportive resources for financial burdens and other health-care needs.

NURSING PROCESS
Amyotrophic Lateral Sclerosis

Assessment

The assessment of the patient includes a history and neurologic examination. Explore any family history of muscle weakness or dysfunction. Ask the patient to review in detail the onset of the current problem. Allow the patient to describe the progression of muscle weakness and how it affects ability to function. Focus physical assessment on the cranial nerves, determining ability to swallow, speak, chew, and maintain a clear airway, and on motor system function, determining the presence of muscle weakness and atrophy, cramps, and the possibility of joint subluxation.

Explore the psychosocial and emotional impact of the condition. Assess the patient's level of anxiety, and be alert to feelings of hopelessness, anger, and poor self-esteem. Assess the effect of the illness on family functioning.

Nursing Diagnoses and Planning

Nursing diagnoses and related expected patient outcomes most commonly applicable to patients with amyotrophic lateral sclerosis include the following:

NDx: Impaired physical mobility related to muscle weakness and atrophy

Planning: Patient Outcomes
1. Patient participates in ADLs.
2. Patient ambulates, transfers, or moves himself or herself with or without assistance.
3. Patient avoids complications of immobility: deep venous thrombosis, pulmonary embolism, decubitus formation.

NDx: Altered nutrition: less than body requirements related to dysphagia and inability to chew

Planning: Patient Outcomes
1. Patient remains free of aspiration.
2. Patient ingests adequate volume of food and fluids to meet nutritional needs.
3. Patient maintains optimal body weight.

NDx: Impaired gas exchange related to bulbar and respiratory muscle weakness and inability to clear secretions

Planning: Patient Outcomes
1. Arterial blood gas levels are within normal range.
2. Breath sounds are normal bilaterally.
3. Cyanosis is absent.
4. Complications of respiratory insufficiency, such as atelectasis, pneumonia, aspiration, and respiratory arrest, are absent.

NDx: Hopelessness related to irreversible terminal condition

Planning: Patient Outcomes
1. Patient acknowledges and shares feelings of hopelessness.
2. Patient and family use resources and support systems available.
3. Patient effectively moves through anticipatory grieving process.

Nursing Interventions and Evaluation

NDx: Impaired physical mobility
To reduce complications related to immobility and subluxation of joints, provide range-of-motion (passive and active) exercises at least every 6 hours. Stretching exercises also help to maintain muscle strength. Allow the patient to do as much for himself or herself (eg, moving, bathing, dressing) as possible. Maintain good body alignment. Eliminate undue pressure or rotation of joints. Consult with the physical and occupational therapist to obtain supportive and assistive devices to be used by the patient for ADLs, such as a cane, wheelchair, eating utensils, splints, and slings. Maintain a turning and positioning schedule every 2 hours. Provide good skin care, use sheepskin pads, and provide an air mattress or special bed as necessary.

Arrange for an evaluation of the home for installation of assistive devices, such as tub rails, a raised toilet seat, and a railing by the toilet. Plan daily activities so there are rest periods between strenuous activities. Instruct the patient how to recognize signs of fatigue and organize his or her daily routine to provide optimal rest periods. Muscle degeneration eventually impairs patients speech. Provide an alternative method of communication: yes and no questions, blinking system, or communication board with pictures. If gross motor function is intact, computers, letter boards, and keyboards are available options.

NDx: Altered nutrition: less than body requirements
Deterioration in the patient's nutritional status can result from shortness of breath, fear of aspiration, muscle weakness, and fatigue. Initially weigh the patient and determine optimal body weight. Then weigh the patient at least weekly. Determine dietary requirements for the patient. Encourage foods high in protein, carbohydrate, and calories. Select foods that are soft and easy to chew. Instruct the patient to hold the chin in a flexed position to facilitate swallowing. Consult the dietitian as necessary. Count calories and monitor intake and output. Provide the patient with approximately 3000 mL of fluids daily. Plan for smaller, frequent meals to allow the patient rest periods and to prevent undue fatigue. Place the patient in a 45-degree to upright position when eating to prevent aspiration. Provide suctioning to prevent aspiration when the patient is unable to swallow, chew, or handle secretions or fluids. Supplemental and enteral feedings may be necessary when the patient cannot ingest optimal calories to maintain body weight.

NDx: Impaired gas exchange
Monitor the patient's respiratory status. Aspiration pneumonia is a common complication with amyotrophic lateral sclerosis patients, especially as the disease progresses. Auscultate the lung fields and check respiratory rate, rhythm, and breath sounds. Instruct the patient on deep breathing, coughing, and incentive spirometry exercises. Provide chest percussion and postural drainage as necessary. Instruct the patient to suction herself or himself to clear secretions that pool in the mouth area. Keep the patient in an upright position (45 degrees) to increase lung expansion and to prevent aspiration or place the patient on his or her side to facilitate drainage of oral secretions.

Have intubation and suction equipment available to support ventilatory efforts if respiratory compromise occurs. If the patient experiences respiratory insufficiency and requires long-term mechanical ventilatory support, provide suctioning to maintain a clear airway. Check ventilator equipment frequently to ensure that it is in proper working order.

NDx: Hopelessness
Provide the patient and family with support to develop effective coping mechanisms. Provide an accepting atmosphere to allow for expression of anxiety, hopelessness, and other emotions. Identify support groups and resources available, such as other people with amyotrophic lateral sclerosis, the National Amyotrophic Lateral Sclerosis Foundation, hospice, respite care, home care, and clergy. Allow the patient and family to express feelings about the terminal condition, and assist and support in preparation for and acceptance of impending death. Assist the patient to plan realistically for the future. Living wills and health-care proxies can be filled out in order to ensure that the patient's wishes are carried out.

Compare the patient's status with the expected outcomes. If the outcomes are not met, reassess the patient and revise the plan.

MULTIPLE SCLEROSIS

Multiple sclerosis is a progressive neurologic condition characterized by the demyelination and scarring of sites along the central nervous system. Patients with multiple sclerosis experience a variety of alterations of sensory, motor, visual, and emotional functions. The onset is insidious, occurring between 15 and 30 years of age. Multiple sclerosis is more common in females. The average life expectancy is 30 to 40 years after onset of symptoms with varying disability.

Etiology and Pathophysiology
The cause of multiple sclerosis is uncertain. Suggested causes include an autoimmune reaction, an

infection by a virus with a long incubation period (known as a slow virus), and a genetic predisposition. Current research has focused on genetic control and the function of the immune system, which supports the theory of an autoimmune-associated dysfunction. Multiple sclerosis is not believed to be an infectious or inherited condition. However, familial traits have been identified.

Demyelination and plaque formation occur throughout the central nervous system, predominately affecting the white matter (Fig. 18–2). An inflammatory process occurs and results in edema of the axons. The clinical course of this condition is random and can be silent. Patients experience exacerbations of symptoms that are unpredictable and vary in duration and severity.

Clinical Manifestations

Because demyelination and plaque formation occur throughout the brain and spinal cord, a wide variety of symptoms can be manifested by patients with multiple sclerosis. Symptoms may initially present alone or in combination with other symptoms. As repeated exacerbations occur, severity of symptoms and residual deficits may increase.

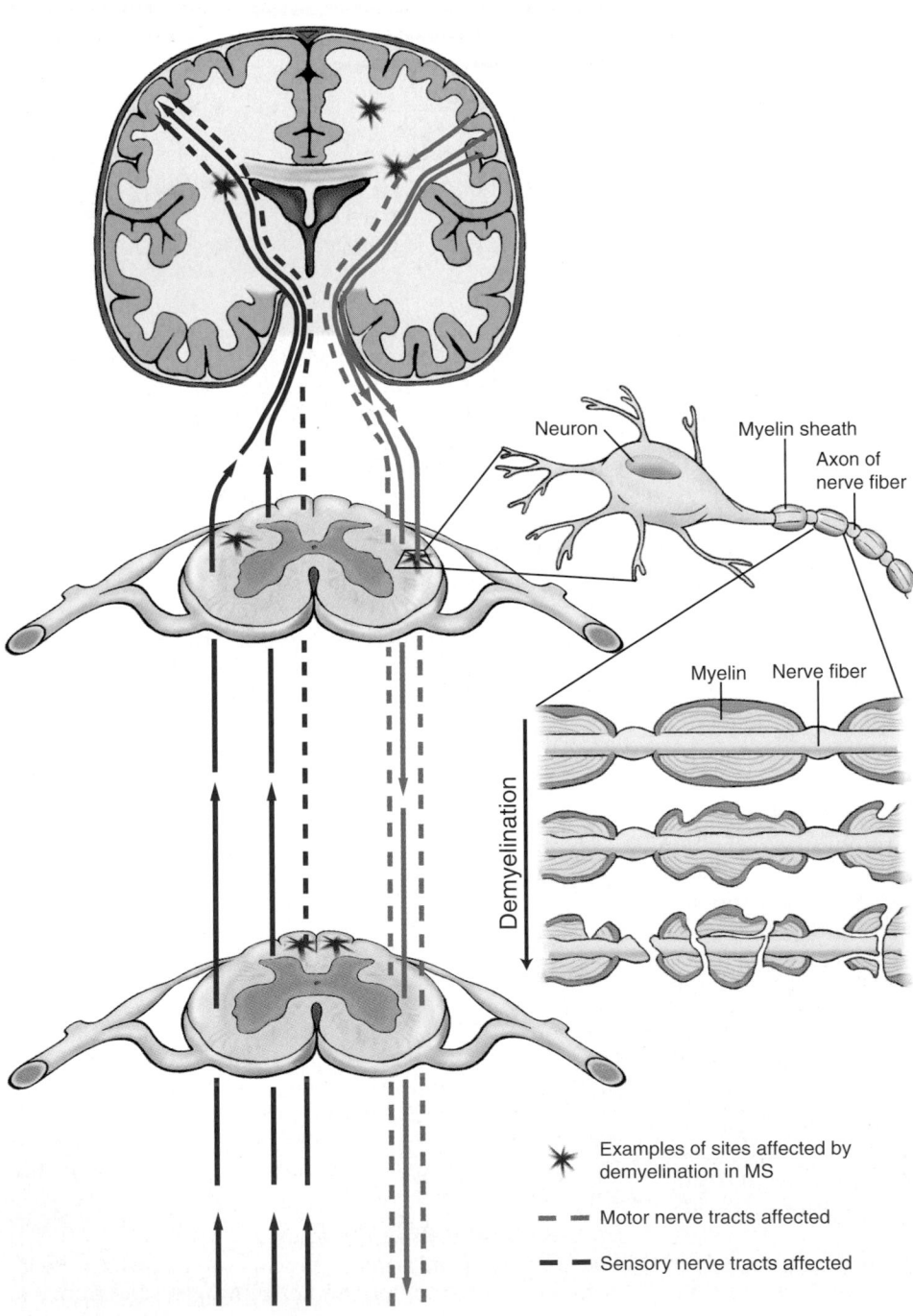

Neuron

Myelin sheath

Axon of nerve fiber

Myelin   Nerve fiber

Demyelination

Figure 18–2

The lesions in multiple sclerosis: location and effects.

✱   Examples of sites affected by demyelination in MS

– –   Motor nerve tracts affected

▪ ▪   Sensory nerve tracts affected

Patients with multiple sclerosis may present clinically with any of the following alterations:

- *Visual:* Diplopia, scotomata, nystagmus, blindness
- *Sensory:* Paresthesia, numbness, tingling, pain, altered position and temperature sense
- *Motor:* Incoordination, ataxia, falling, intention tremor, fatigability, muscle spasms, contractures, spastic paraplegia, dysphagia, impaired speech, bladder/bowel retention/incontinence
- *Emotional:* Euphoria, depression, inappropriate affect, mental deterioration, impaired judgment

Diagnosis

A history is obtained to identify previous episodes of neurologic dysfunction and evidence of more than one lesion. An extensive physical and neurologic examination is conducted to detect visual, motor, sensory, and emotional alterations. Lumbar puncture with cerebrospinal fluid analysis is performed to establish presence of oligoclonal (immunoglobulin G) bands, which is diagnostic of multiple sclerosis. Evoked potential studies (visual, somato-sensory, and auditory) and electromyograms are performed to evaluate peripheral nervous system functioning and help to identify clinically silent lesions. CT and MRI are performed to visualize plaques and cerebral atrophy and identify other pathology.

Management

Multiple sclerosis has no known cure. Medical management is symptomatic and supportive. Antineoplastic and immunosuppressive drugs prevent the destruction of nervous system tissue by suppressing the immune system and decreasing inflammation. Cyclophosphamide (Cytoxan) and corticosteroids (prednisone [Deltasone, Solu-Medrol]) are the drugs of choice. Interferon beta-16 (Betaseron) is a recently approved medication that possesses antiviral and immunoregulatory action. It is used to decrease the frequency and severity of relapses and exacerbations of multiple sclerosis. Another recently approved drug is glatiramer acetate (Copaxone) used for cases of relapsing multiple sclerosis. There is, however, no

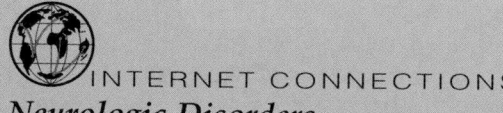

INTERNET CONNECTIONS
Neurologic Disorders

Multiple Sclerosis
The International Federation of Multiple Sclerosis Societies
http://www.ifmss.org.uk
This international resource provides answers in French, German, Italian, and Spanish to frequently asked questions. In addition, it provides links to current research in multiple sclerosis and to other resources.

National Multiple Sclerosis Society
http://www.nmss.org
An authoritative resource for both health professionals and patients. This site features general information as well as information on medications, other treatments, information in Spanish, information especially for health professionals, publications, and reports on current research.

Multiple Sclerosis Society of Canada
http://204.92.87.160
Highlighting the high rates of multiple sclerosis found in Canada, this authoritative resource provides medical updates, information on national publications addressing multiple sclerosis, lists of services, and general information.

Alzheimer's Disease
Alzheimer's Association
http://www.alz.org
This authoritative resource provides general information about Alzheimer's disease, as well as updates on new research, medical information, and information for caregivers. This site also provides links to other sites related to Alzheimer's disease.

Alzheimer's Disease Web Page
Bedford Geriatric Research Education Clinical Center
http://med-amsa.bu.edu/Alzheimer/home.html
This site provides resources for both health professionals and family caregivers as well as links to other Internet resources related to neurologic disease and neuropathology.

Seizure Disorders
Epilepsy Foundation of America
http://www.efa.org/index1.htm
An excellent resource that includes answers to frequently asked questions, new medical information, and general information about what the Epilepsy Foundation does. This site also allows the user to search for articles based on a particular subject, word, or phrase.

restoration of deficits in neurologic functioning. Medical intervention focuses on managing the four common symptoms presented by these patients: muscle spasticity, neurogenic bladder, paresthesias, and cerebellar ataxia.

Muscle spasticity impedes the patient's ability to perform routine tasks and ADLs. Physical therapy focused on performance of self-grooming, ambulation, gait training, and feeding is prescribed to promote optimal muscle function. In addition, muscle relaxants, such as diazepam or baclofen, are prescribed to control the level of spasticity.

Patients with multiple sclerosis manifest an autonomic disturbance of the bladder characterized by incontinence and recurrent urinary retention. This condition is known as neurogenic bladder. Interventions focus on preventing urinary tract infections and establishing a bladder-emptying regimen. Medications such as bethanechol chloride (Urecholine), propantheline bromide (Pro-Banthine), or baclofen are prescribed to promote bladder muscle control. Intermittent catheterization is used to ensure that the bladder is emptied at scheduled intervals, thus decreasing the incidence of urinary stasis.

The control of paresthesias primarily involves pharmacologic management. Medications that have proven useful in the management of paresthesias are carbamazepine (Tegretol), baclofen, and phenytoin (Dilantin). However, the exact mechanisms of action of these agents are not fully understood.

To control cerebellar ataxia, short courses of steroids are prescribed to decrease the inflammatory process in the cerebellum. Medications such as clonazepam (Klonopin) are given to provide increased muscle control. To control depression and insomnia, amitriptyline (Elavil) is often prescribed. Factors such as heat (both internal and external), infection, stress, fatigue, and child-bearing can exacerbate symptoms of multiple sclerosis.

❖ **Settings, Providers, and Collaboration for Care**

Most patients with multiple sclerosis can be treated in an outpatient setting. As the condition worsens, treatment may be in the hospital, long-term care facility, or the home. Physical and occupational therapy should be consulted as needed to assist the patient to maintain maximal functioning as long as possible. As the patient becomes more immobile or has complicating problems, a home health nurse may assist the patient and family with hygienic care, evaluation of health status, medication administration, and plans for long-term care. The nurse can provide for the safety of the patient and assist the family in adapting the home environment to the patient's needs. A social worker or case manager may coordinate the various needs of the patient, including physical, spiritual, psychosocial, and financial.

NURSING PROCESS
Multiple Sclerosis

Assessment

Assessment of the patient includes a history, neurologic examination, and determination of current level of safety and function. Ask the patient about his or her symptoms, and obtain a description of their onset and progression. Inquire specifically about urinary pattern and bladder function. Ask the patient whether he or she has had any urinary tract infections or feels as though there is a problem emptying the bladder on urination. Assess the patient for the clinical presence of visual, motor, sensory, and emotional alterations.

Assess the social and emotional impact of multiple sclerosis on the lifestyle and self-concept of the patient. Ask the patient about problems with lifestyle activities:

"What do you have difficulty doing for yourself?"
"Is there anything you used to do that you cannot do any more?"
"Are you injuring or hurting yourself (eg, burns, bruises)?"

Question about any sexual alteration. Explore the impact of the disease on self-image. Determine strengths and weaknesses as well as effective coping and defense mechanisms.

Nursing Diagnoses and Planning

Nursing diagnoses and related expected patient outcomes most commonly applicable to patients with multiple sclerosis include the following:

NDx: Sensory/perceptual alterations (visual, kinesthetic, tactile) related to progressive disease process

Planning: Patient Outcomes
1. Patient identifies behaviors that compensate for sensory-perceptual alterations.
2. Patient performs ADLs without injury.

NDx: Impaired physical mobility related to muscle spasticity, contractures, and ataxia

Planning: Patient Outcomes
1. Patient maintains motor function.
2. Patient maintains range of motion of joints.
3. Patient remains free from injury.

NDx: Fatigue related to progressive disease process

Planning: Patient Outcomes
1. Patient plans balanced rest and exercise periods.
2. Patient schedules daily activities relative to energy levels to avoid exhaustion.

NDx: Risk for altered urinary elimination related to neurogenic bladder

Planning: Patient Outcomes
1. Patient is continent.
2. Patient empties bladder completely.
3. Patient is free of urinary tract infections.

NDx: Risk for ineffective individual coping related to presence of a chronic disease with effects on multiple areas of physical and psychosocial functioning

Planning: Patient Outcomes
1. Patient expresses confidence in ability to cope.
2. Patient adjusts lifestyle according to physical limitations.
3. Patient maintains independence in ADLs.
4. Patient recognizes emotional alterations as a component of multiple sclerosis.

Nursing Interventions and Evaluation

NDx: Sensory/perceptual alterations (visual, kinesthetic, tactile)
Establish the patient's degree of visual alteration (ie, diplopia, blurred vision, narrowing of visual fields). Encourage the patient to wear eyeglasses if prescribed. Instruct the patient on the use of an eye patch to diminish diplopia when present.

Establish the level of impairment in touch sensation, temperature perception, and position sense, and protect the patient from injury associated with these deficits. Because skin impairment is a risk resulting from impaired sensation and immobilization, provide good skin care and encourage the patient to move and ambulate as much as possible. Instruct the patient to use an air mattress and paddings to decrease pressure on joint and bony prominences. Keep the patient off reddened areas and, if needed, establish a turning and positioning schedule every 2 hours.

Instruct the patient to visualize extremities to ensure proper alignment and freedom from injury. Tell the patient: "Look where your arms and legs are to make sure you are not injuring them or placing undue pressure on them." Instruct the patient and family that extremes in temperature, both internal and external, can exacerbate symptoms of multiple sclerosis. Have the patient regulate bath water using a thermometer. Also have the patient use caution with cooling and heating devices, use fever reducing agents as needed, and avoid restrictive clothing. Teach the patient to use visual cues to overcome alteration in position and sense of touch.

NDx: Impaired physical mobility
Encourage the patient to be as physically independent as possible in ADLs. Provide active and passive range-of-motion exercises at least every 6 hours. Maintain proper body alignment. Consult with the physical therapist to establish an exercise program, including progressive and resistive exercises, and to evaluate the need for supportive and assistive devices (ie, brace, walker, devices for reaching, eating utensils). Administer ordered muscle relaxants and antispasmodics as necessary. Instruct the ambulatory patient to use a wide-based gait and to watch his or her feet if sense of position is a problem.

NDx: Fatigue
Identify high- and low-energy periods of the day. Assist the patient in developing a realistic schedule of activities with rest periods. Perform daily tasks during high-energy times. Divide complicated tasks into steps, allowing for rest between steps. Assist the patient in identifying physical limits. Patients should not push to exhaustion, because doing so can exacerbate the disease process. Instruct the patient on the signs of fatigue (ie, weakness, tired feeling).

NDx: Risk for altered urinary elimination
Maintain a schedule for bladder training. Monitor intake and output. Check for a postvoid residual urine (have the patient void, then catheterize him or her to check how much urine is left in the bladder) to determine whether the patient has urinary retention. Establish an appropriate bladder regimen, such as intermittent catheterization and opportunity to void five times daily.

Instruct the patient on the importance of emptying the bladder. Multiple sclerosis patients are susceptible to urinary tract infections secondary to urinary retention. Signs and symptoms of urinary tract infection are frequency, burning sensation, hematuria, odor, cloudy urine, urgency, and elevated temperature. Instruct the patient to drink 2 to 3 L of fluids per day. Administer medications (such as propantheline and bethanechol, which promote bladder muscle control) as ordered to establish bladder regimen. Teach the patient intermittent self-catheterization technique for long-term management.

NDx: Risk for ineffective individual coping
Monitor the social and emotional impact of multiple sclerosis on the lifestyle and self-concept of the patient. Encourage expression of feelings and fears. Patients may experience depression and insomnia. Organic changes may cause forgetfulness and emotional lability. Encourage the patient to record appointments and write down important information. Maintain a supportive and accepting environment in an attempt to reduce stress. Explore resources available to the patient and family. Facilitate contact with another person with multiple sclerosis, a local support group, or the Multiple Sclerosis Society. Encourage self-care and physical and social activity within physical limitations. The frequent mood changes, from depression to euphoria, as well as inappropriate decision-making can be a cause of concern and stress for families, friends, and coworkers. Support groups can and should be utilized by significant others to increase understanding of the disease process.

Compare the patient's status with the expected outcomes. If the outcomes are not met, reassess the patient and revise the plan.

MYASTHENIA GRAVIS

Myasthenia gravis is a progressive neuromuscular condition characterized by generalized weakness and fatigue of the skeletal muscles of the body. Exacerbations and remissions occur. Symptoms vary from patient to patient.

Myasthenia gravis is not believed to be an inherited condition, although familial tendencies do exist. Females appear to be afflicted three times more frequently than males. The peak onset in women is between 20 and 40 years of age. In men, peak onset is at 40 years of age or older.

Etiology and Pathophysiology

In patients with myasthenia gravis, the acetylcholine released at the neuromuscular junction appears not to be effective in producing an action potential in the muscle group. The exact cause is unclear. However, several theories are under consideration. One theory suggests an autoimmune mechanism, because antibodies to acetylcholine receptors have been found in 60 to 90% of patients with myasthenia gravis. Other theories suggest decreased release of acetylcholine, excessive cholinesterase in the synapse, reduced numbers of postsynaptic folds, a widened synaptic space, and decreased numbers of acetylcholine receptors (Fig. 18–3). The end result of each of these theorized mechanisms is the same. There is weakness and inability to perform activity because of lack of an action potential in the muscle group.

Clinical Manifestations

Patients with myasthenia gravis present with weakness that is abnormally increased by continued or repeated use of the muscles at any one time. Weakness is partially relieved by a short period of rest or inactivity of the muscle group. Specific signs and symptoms include ocular muscle weakness (eg, ptosis, diplopia), skeletal muscle weakness (facial weakness, dysphagia, difficulty supporting the head in the upright position, generalized muscle weakness), and respiratory muscle weakness (inability to maintain adequate gas exchange, shallow respirations). The classic symptom is fatigue with continued or repeated use of the muscle group.

Progression of symptoms is varied and unpredictable. Periods of remission and exacerbations occur. The range of severity of the condition is as follows:

- *Mild ocular:* Involves one or more ocular muscle group; no mortality
- *Mild to severe:* May involve ocular, bulbar, and skeletal muscle groups, sparing respiratory muscles; low mortality
- *Acute, severe:* Involves ocular, bulbar, skeletal, and respiratory muscles; high mortality rate
- *Chronic, late severe:* Severe symptoms with marked bulbar involvement; high mortality rate

Myasthenic and cholinergic crises in a patient with myasthenia gravis occur when there is an inability to maintain respirations that allow for gas exchange. Some cases involve total respiratory arrest. A myasthenic crisis occurs when there is too little acetylcholine available at the neuromuscular junction and, therefore, no action potential is generated for respiratory muscles to maintain adequate respirations. This is often the result of too little anticholinesterase medication, infection, stress, or trauma. A cholinergic crisis occurs when there is too much acetylcholine available at the neuromuscular junction. In cholinergic crisis, the patient experiences total fatigue of respiratory muscles from the con-

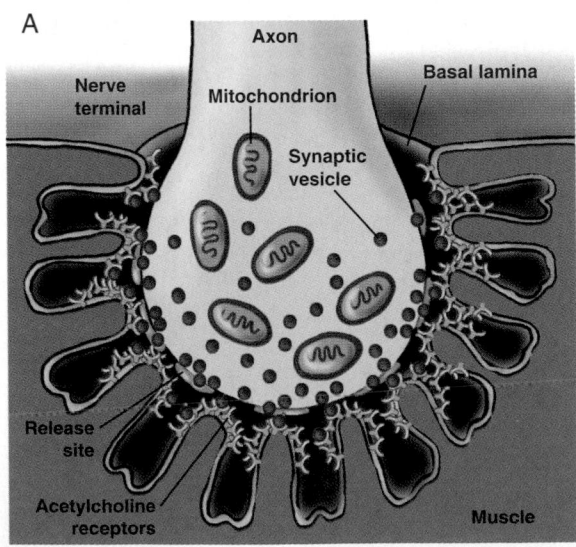
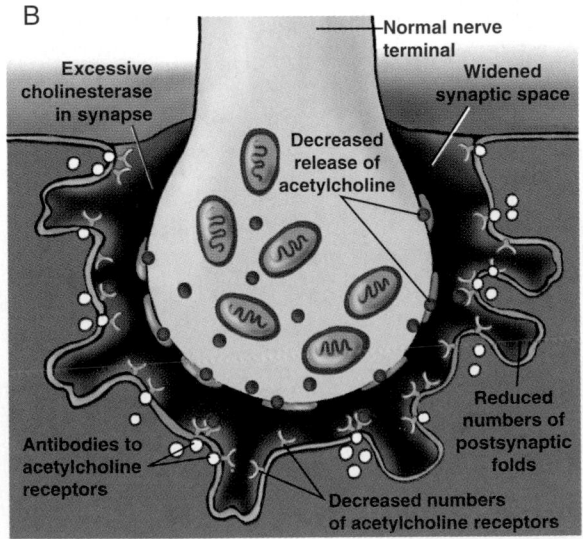

Figure 18–3

Pathophysiology of myasthenia gravis. *A,* Normal neuromuscular junction. *B,* Possible changes in the neuromuscular junction in a patient with myasthenia gravis.

stant action potential generated. This results from the administration of an excessive amount of anticholinesterase medication. Each crisis, although having opposing physiology, manifests with the identical outcome ranging from muscle weakness, respiratory compromise, and respiratory arrest.

Both types of crises are medical emergencies due to the potential for respiratory failure. Edrophonium (Tensilon IV) is given to differentiate the causes of the crisis. In myasthenic crisis, the patient's condition improves with edrophonium. In cholinergic crisis, the patient temporarily worsens and atropine sulfate (an anticholinergic), an antagonist for edrophonium, is given.

Diagnosis

A history and complete physical and neurologic examination are performed to determine symptoms of muscle weakness and the extent of progression. Serum laboratory studies include acetylcholine receptor antibody, lupus erythematosus cells, electrophoresis of serum proteins, and thyroid function tests to determine level of or alteration in autoimmune function. Chest x-ray examination and CT are performed to identify the presence of thymoma (tumor of the thymus gland). Electromyogram and nerve conduction studies are performed to document abnormal muscle action potentials. Findings include rapid reduction in amplitude with repetitive stimulation. In addition, drug challenge studies diagnostic of myasthenia gravis are performed, such as the edrophonium test or neostigmine (Prostigmin) test. Two to 10 mg of edrophonium is injected intravenously. In the myasthenic patient, an increase in muscle strength is noted. This is the result of increasing the amount of available acetylcholine at the neuromuscular junction. If the patient does not have myasthenia gravis, or if the level of acetylcholine at the neuromuscular junction is decreased, increased weakness occurs, with the potential for respiratory arrest. Emergency equipment should be at the bedside.

Management

Medical management of patients with myasthenia gravis focuses on maintaining optimal respiratory function and muscle strength. Use of anticholinesterase medications (pyridostigmine [Mestinon]) is the most common treatment modality. Anticholinesterase medications, also called cholinesterase inhibitors, maintain an effective chemical balance of acetylcholine and cholinesterase at the neuromuscular junction, allowing for optimal respiratory function and muscle strength. Therefore, timing of anticholinesterase medication is critical. Patients and health-care workers need to be instructed to administer this medication on time, not before or after the time when it is due, to maintain an effective chemical balance at the neuromuscular junction (Highlight 18–1).

Other treatment modalities include the use of steroids, immunosuppressives, plasmapheresis, and

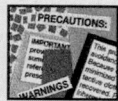

HIGHLIGHT
18–1
PHARMACOLOGY

Cholinesterase Inhibitors (Anticholinesterase Agents)

Definition:

These drugs prevent the breakdown of acetylcholine by cholinesterase at the neuromuscular junction. Two widely used drugs in this class are neostigmine (Prostigmin) and pyridostigmine (Mestinon).

Action:

Inhibit destruction of acetylcholine by cholinesterase, thereby enhancing transmission of impulses across the neuromuscular junction.

Uses:

Maintain chemical neurotransmitter balance to optimize muscle strength, respiratory function, and adequate and effective gas exchange in patients with myasthenia gravis.

Side Effects:

Side effects are dose related and include respiratory distress and myasthenic crisis (blurred or double vision, shortness of breath, increased weakness, rapid heartbeat, twitching, dizziness). Other side effects include abdominal cramps, diarrhea, nausea, vomiting, salivation, and sweating.

Interactions:

Atropine inhibits the effect of cholinesterase inhibitors.

Nursing Implications:

Assess patient's ability to swallow before administering oral preparations.

Administer drug on time.

Monitor patient for improvement of symptoms within 30 minutes after drug is administered.

Monitor patient for side effects.

Notify physician if signs of respiratory deterioration (vital capacity below 1 L) or distress occur.

thymectomy. Steroids (corticotropin and corticosteroids) have proved effective in preventing the progression and severity of symptoms. Plasmapheresis cleanses the blood stream of the anti–acetylcholine receptor antibodies. Plasmapheresis is a temporary method to control symptoms. However, it is useful in predicting the patient's response to thymectomy (surgical removal of the thymus gland). The thymus produces antibodies, including the anti–acetylcholine receptor antibody. Thus, thymectomy decreases levels of these antibodies.

❖ Settings, Providers, and Collaboration for Care

Most patients with myasthenia gravis are treated in an outpatient setting unless the disease warrants a more acute care treatment center. As the condition worsens, treatment may take place in the hospital. Patients who experience a crisis or respiratory failure are treated in the critical care unit. A physical therapist may be needed to teach the patient strengthening exercises. Respiratory therapy is needed to maintain maximum respiratory function. The specific type of therapy is specific to the severity of the disease and the patient's needs.

NURSING PROCESS
Myasthenia Gravis

Assessment

Assess for ocular, bulbar, skeletal, and respiratory muscle group involvement and generalized weakness, level of deterioration, and degree of fatigability. Identify functional limitations affecting mobility, self-care, respiratory ability, and activity intolerance.

Assess the extent of ocular muscle weakness. Ask whether the patient has double vision. Observe for facial symmetry and ptosis of the eyelid.

Assess the patient for dysphagia. Explore particular patterns associated with the ability to swallow (ie, types and consistencies of foods). Ask the patient, "Do you find yourself drooling because you are unable to swallow oral secretions?" "Do you choke or cough during meals"?

In assessing motor function, determine the level of physical mobility. Ask the patient if he or she tires or fatigues easily after slight exertion or with repetitive movement. Ask to what extent he or she can perform ADLs:

- "Do you need someone to assist in performing personal hygiene, feeding, toileting, moving, and ambulating?"
- "Do you find you can perform tasks most easily with the use of assistive devices, such as special eating utensils?"
- "Are there periods of the day when you feel more energetic than others?"

Note whether the patient is able to support the head in an upright position with or without assistance. Assess for skin integrity. Note alterations related to undue pressure points.

Assess respiratory status. Ask the patient whether breathing is effortless. Assess the rate and rhythm of respirations. Auscultate the lung fields to assess breath sounds on inspiration and expiration. Determine the effectiveness of respiratory function by measuring vital capacity (forceful exhaled volume after a maximal inspiration on a spirometer). Ask the patient the following questions:

- "Are there any activities or times of the day that make it more difficult for you to breathe?"
- "Do you feel stronger and better able to breathe after you take your anticholinesterase medication?"

Assess for a weak, nasal-sounding voice and dysarthria due to impairment of muscles essential for the production of speech. Stress can also cause exacerbation of myasthenia gravis. Assess the patient for infections, temperature extremes (climate), injuries, emotional upset, and erratic schedule, as well as for menses in females.

Nursing Diagnoses and Planning

Nursing diagnoses and related expected patient outcomes most commonly applicable to patients with myasthenia gravis include the following:

NDx: Ineffective breathing pattern related to disease process and myasthenic or cholinergic crisis

Planning: Patient Outcomes
1. Respiratory rate and rhythm are within normal limits.
2. Patient maintains optimal tidal volume with or without the support of mechanical ventilation.
3. Breath sounds are normal bilaterally.

NDx: Impaired physical mobility related to weakness of voluntary muscle groups

Planning: Patient Outcomes
1. Patient performs ADLs.
2. Patient ambulates and transfers with or without assistive devices.
3. Patient maintains muscle strength.

NDx: Fatigue related to repetition of muscle stimulation

Planning: Patient Outcomes
1. Patient plans daily schedule with periods of activity and rest.
2. Patient recognizes the signs of fatigue.
3. Patient reports success in controlling or preventing fatigue with scheduling of activities.

NDx: Risk for aspiration related to dysphagia

Planning: Patient Outcomes
1. Patient avoids aspiration.
2. Patient clears oral secretions effectively.
3. Breath sounds are normal bilaterally.
4. Patient is afebrile.

Nursing Interventions and Evaluation

NDx: Ineffective breathing pattern

Establish baseline vital capacity and monitor periodically by measuring exhaled volume on a spirometer. Call the physician immediately if vital capacity falls below baseline or 1 L. This indicates that the patient is in crisis and needs immediate intervention.

Monitor effectiveness of anticholinesterase medications in maintaining strength of respiratory muscles (ie, Is the patient able to take a deep breath? Are respiratory rate and rhythm within normal limits?). Instruct the patient to perform coughing and deep-breathing exercises. Provide chest physiotherapy and postural drainage if the lung fields are congested to decrease risk of infection. Provide suction when necessary to clear oral and tracheal secretions.

Notify the physician immediately if vital capacity falls or if the patient exhibits signs of increased secretions or respiratory distress. Ensure that intubation, oxygen, suction, and mechanical ventilation equipment are readily available if the patient experiences a respiratory crisis or arrest.

NDx: Impaired physical mobility

Monitor and record patient's motor strength and high- and low-energy periods throughout the day. Schedule activities during high-energy periods. Administer anticholinesterase medications as prescribed and precisely on time. A delay in medication administration can result in an inability to swallow oral medication, requiring intramuscular injection. Monitor for effectiveness of medication regimen. Timespan pyridostigmine can be used to avoid the need to take medication during the night and eliminate extreme muscle weakness in the morning. Consult physical and occupational therapists as necessary to develop exercise program and to obtain supportive and assistive devices. Encourage the patient to be as independent as possible in activities, ranging from ambulation to turning and repositioning herself or himself.

NDx: Fatigue

Encourage the patient to perform activities during high-energy periods. Assist in identifying limits of physical activity. Instruct the patient on signs of fatigue (tired, increasing weakness). Do not push beyond physical limits. Allow rest between daily activities.

NDx: Risk for aspiration

Monitor the patient's ability to clear secretions and swallow. Suction as occasion requires to maintain clear airway. Encourage the patient to eat small bites of food at a time. Teach the patient to eat with his or her head at a 30-degree angle or greater to assist in swallowing food. Supervise during meal periods. Provide and instruct the patient on the use of suction and oral catheters to decrease the risk of aspirating by removing pooled oral secretions and food that cannot be swallowed, which is gagging or choking the patient. A nasogastric or gastric tube may be used for feedings.

Compare the patient's status with the expected outcomes. If the outcomes are not met, reassess the patient and revise the plan.

MUSCULAR DYSTROPHY (LIMB-GIRDLE)

Muscular dystrophy is a broad classification of specific hereditary neurologic conditions characterized by progressive degeneration and weakness of the voluntary muscles. Although the majority of persons afflicted with muscular dystrophy are children, clinical presentation may occur at any point throughout the life span. Limb-girdle muscular dystrophy is the condition that presents clinically in young adulthood. The earlier the clinical symptoms appear, the more rapid the progression and severity of the disease process.

Etiology and Pathophysiology

Limb-girdle muscular dystrophy has a clinical onset anywhere from birth to the twenties. This is an autosomal recessive disease. Therefore, both parents need to carry the defective gene for their child to inherit this condition. When both parents carry the defective gene, their children have a 25% chance of being afflicted with the disease, a 50% chance of passing along the defective gene to their offspring, and a 25% chance of being free of the disease. Males and females are affected equally.

Clinical Manifestations

Clinical onset initially involves the proximal muscles of the pelvic and shoulder girdle. The patient appears to have a forward-stooped appearance. Progression of muscular weakness varies. When progression is slow, the patient may live a normal life span.

Diagnosis

A complete history and physical and neurologic examination are performed to substantiate muscle weakness. The history focuses on family history, incidence of muscular dystrophy, patient perception of onset of symptoms, and severity of weakness. The physical and neurologic examination focuses on differentiation of the muscle group involvement. A muscle biopsy is performed to demonstrate abnormal characteristics. In addition, an electromyogram, creatine kinase, and serum enzyme tests are performed to substantiate the diagnosis and to rule out any underlying pathology.

Management

There is no known cure for limb-girdle muscular dystrophy. Medical management focuses on supportive and palliative interventions to maintain the patient's highest level of functioning. Physical, occupational, and respiratory therapies are prescribed to keep unaffected muscles functioning and to delay development of contractures and skeletal deformities.

❖ **Settings, Providers, and Collaboration for Care**

Patients with muscular dystrophy are treated in the home and in outpatient clinics. If complications arise they are treated in a hospital. A physical therapist and respiratory therapist should be consulted. The patient may visit the physical therapist frequently for evaluation and treatment to delay development of contractures. Because of the skeletal deformities, respiratory function may be compromised. The respiratory therapist assesses the patient's respiratory functioning and gives the patient strategies to maintain an appropriate breathing pattern.

NURSING PROCESS
Limb-Girdle Muscular Dystrophy

Assessment

Patient assessment includes a history and neurologic examination. Inquire about any family history of muscle weakness or dysfunction. Ask the patient to describe the onset of his or her muscle weakness, including how and when it was first noticed and how it affects the ability to carry out tasks and activities. Focus the neurologic assessment on the motor system function. Identify the muscle groups involved. Observe the patient for gait disturbances and a forward-stooped appearance. Assess severity of motor system dysfunction. Establish whether the patient is at risk for injury. Determine whether the patient uses any assistive devices, such as a wheelchair or cane, for mobility. Ask whether falling occurs because of any increase in muscle weakness. Assess the patient for presence of contractures or skeletal deformities. Inspect the extremities and have the patient go through a range of motion.

Assess the psychosocial and emotional impact of this progressive degenerating condition on the patient. Ask questions such as "How are you coping with your illness?" Once a rapport is developed with the patient, ask questions such as "Do you find there is any disruption in your relationships at work, with your family, or with your friends?"

Nursing Diagnoses and Planning

Nursing diagnoses and related expected patient outcomes most commonly applicable to patients with limb-girdle muscular dystrophy include the following:

NDx: Impaired physical mobility related to progressive muscular weakness, contractures, and skeletal deformities

Planning: Patient Outcomes
1. Patient performs ADLs within limitations.
2. Patient maintains range of joint motion.

NDx: Powerlessness related to progressive muscular deterioration

Planning: Patient Outcomes
1. Patient expresses feelings of powerlessness.
2. Patient identifies areas over which he or she does have control.
3. Patient makes choices in areas over which he or she has control.
4. Patient and family acknowledge and use resources and support systems available.

Nursing Interventions and Evaluation

NDx: Impaired physical mobility
Perform range-of-motion exercises every 6 hours to maintain joint motion and to prevent development of contractures. Allow the patient to do as much for himself or herself as possible (ambulation, feeding, toileting, grooming). Encourage the patient to perform activities using varied muscle groups so that muscles that are still functioning remain healthy. Consult with physical and occupational therapists to obtain supportive devices to be used by the patient for ADLs, such as a wheelchair, bathroom lifts, walkers, and braces or supports.

Monitor the patient for any change in motor system function and increased risk of falling. Instruct the patient on signs of weakness and the importance of not pushing beyond limits to prevent self-injury. Encourage the patient to use assistive devices for ambulation when gait is unsteady.

Consult with the social worker for discharge planning. Encourage the patient and family members to actively participate in this process. Because the home environment needs to be prepared to support the optimal functioning level of the patient, equipment such as a bed, bathroom equipment, and ramps may have to be purchased.

NDx: Powerlessness
Encourage the patient to express fears and feelings of powerlessness. Provide for an accepting atmosphere to allow for expressions of anxiety, powerlessness, and other emotions. Acknowledge to the patient and family that their feelings are legitimate and that it is difficult not to have control over what is happening physically. Reassure that feelings of loss and grieving are normal. Identify and facilitate contact with support groups and resources, such as other persons with muscular dystrophy, clergy, social workers, therapists, and the Muscular Dystrophy Association.

Additional Interventions
Allow the patient and family to express feelings about the irreversible condition and assist and support in preparation and acceptance of impending death when imminent.

Compare the patient's status with the expected outcomes. If the outcomes are not met, reassess the patient and revise the plan.

PARKINSON'S DISEASE

Parkinson's disease is a progressive neurologic disorder characterized by degenerative changes in the basal ganglia, primarily in the area known as the substantia nigra. Parkinson's disease affects men and women equally, with symptoms presenting between the ages of 40 and 70 years. Approximately 1% of the population older than 50 years has Parkinson's disease.

Etiology and Pathophysiology

The cause of Parkinson's disease is unknown. Possible causes include viral agents, genetic disposition, and premature aging.

Dopamine, a major neurotransmitter, is manufactured and stored in the area of the brain known as the basal ganglia. Dopamine acts to provide a homeostatic balance of inhibitory and excitatory actions. The degenerative changes associated with Parkinson's disease interfere with the production and storage of dopamine. The symptoms classic of Parkinson's disease (tremors, muscle rigidity, and bradykinesia) reflect the imbalance of inhibitory and excitatory actions. This can be directly related to the reduction of available dopamine in these patients.

Clinical Manifestations

The symptoms experienced by a patient with Parkinson's disease include resting tremors, a pill-rolling motion of the hands when at rest; slowness and rigidity of movement; flexion posture; "stooped" appearance; shuffling propulsive gait; loss of automatic, coordinated movement; fatigue; an expressionless, masklike face with fixed gaze; drooling; oily skin; dysphagia; urinary hesitancy; depression; and heat insensitivity (Fig. 18–4). Patients are alert but slow to respond and irritable. The patient does not experience any loss of mental functioning, although depression is common. Onset is gradual, beginning with unilateral involvement and progressing slowly to total dependence. Symptoms increase in severity as the disease progresses.

Diagnosis

Overall history and clinical findings substantiate the diagnosis of Parkinson's disease. Because the progression of symptoms is slow, the diagnosis of Parkinson's disease may not be made initially. Electromyography, EEG, CT, and MRI may be ordered to rule out other pathology. The patient's urine and cerebrospinal fluid are tested to document decreased levels of homovanillic acid, a metabolite of dopamine.

The Unified Parkinson Disease Rating Scale, developed by an international group of neurologists, is used to classify patients with Parkinson's disease. This scale is as follows:

0 = no sign of disease
1 = unilateral disease
2 = bilateral disease without impairment of balance

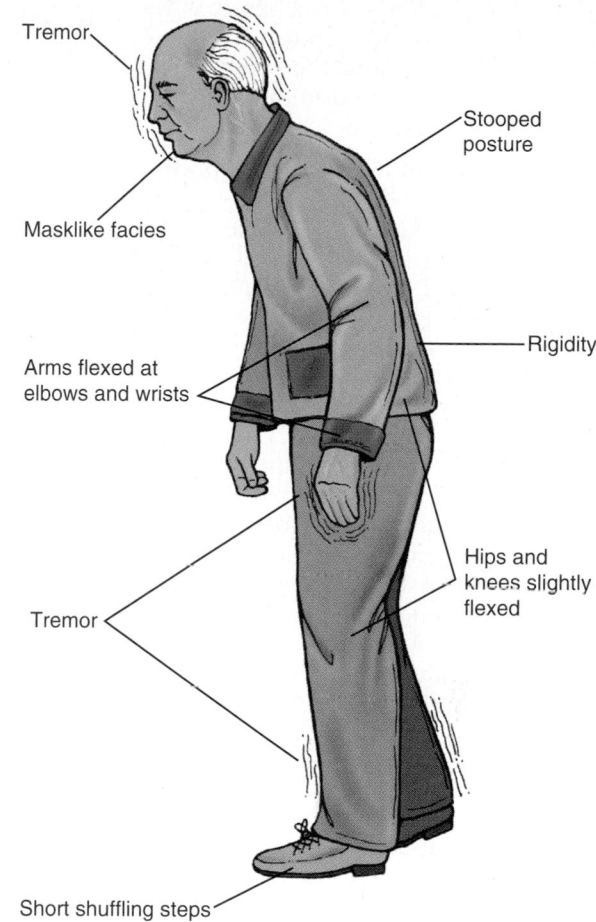

Figure 18–4

Clinical manifestations of Parkinson's disease.

3 = mild to moderate bilateral disease with postural instability, still physically independent
4 = severe disability, still able to stand and walk
5 = wheelchair-dependent or bedridden

Management

Medical management focuses on the use of drug therapy to control a patient's symptoms. It is established that decreased levels of dopamine cause the symptoms exhibited by the patient with Parkinson's disease (tremors, muscle rigidity, and bradykinesia). Amantadine (Symmetrel), bromocriptine, levodopa, and carbidopa (Sinemet) are drugs that, once metabolized, break down to the precursor: dopamine. When these drugs are used in various combinations, therefore, the amount of available dopamine at the neuromuscular junction increases and the patient displays decreased or controlled symptoms. Anticholinergics (trihexyphenidyl [Artane], ethopropazine [Parsidol], benztropine [Cogentin]) are used when levodopa is ineffective or in conjunction with levodopa to increase available dopamine as well as to reduce drooling. Selegiline (Eldepryl) is also used as adjunct therapy in patients receiving levodopa/carbidopa but who have experienced a deteriorating response to treatment. Investigations into alternative treatment are currently underway involving fetal tissue transplantation into the brain of Parkinson's patients as well as pallidotomy for relief of muscle rigidity and tremors.

❖ Settings, Providers, and Collaboration for Care

Patients with Parkinson's disease are treated in their homes and outpatient settings until their disease warrants further treatment. As the condition worsens, treatment may take place in the hospital or long-term care facility. Collaboration occurs among the case manager, nurse, social worker, speech, physical and occupational therapists, and physician. Depending on the severity of the disease and the success of the medical regimen, the patient may need only minor assistance from these health professionals. The patient with more severe manifestations of the disease may need assistance with mobility, speech, self-care, and safety precautions. Patients with severe problems from Parkinson's disease are frequently admitted to long-term care facilities for continued treatment.

NURSING PROCESS
Parkinson's Disease

Assessment

Obtain a complete history of the current problem, including symptoms, time of onset, and progression. Proceed to assess current status beginning with motor system functioning. Observe posture and gait. Note muscle rigidity. Check strength. Look for characteristic resting tremors. Note the ability to swallow and to clear secretions. Assess mental status. Question about depression and altered thought processes. Observe for signs of depression. Determine the patient's ability to communicate. Observe for masklike face, dysarthria, and a monotone, whispering voice. Assess for alterations in autonomic system function, such as oily skin and urinary hesitancy. Assess for drooling and possible dehydration.

Ask the patient about what medication regimens have been used. Note the name and dose of all medications. Question the patient about their effectiveness in controlling symptoms. Ask the patient whether any specific practices are used to ensure that medications are taken at the right time or intervals.

Assess ability for self-care and the ability to perform ADLs. Note the extent and type of assistance required by the patient.

Ask the patient how he or she feels: "How has this condition affected the way you live?" Assess the social and emotional impact of Parkinson's disease on the lifestyle and self-concept of the patient. Allow the patient to describe how Parkinson's disease has affected the ability to meet work and family obligations.

Nursing Diagnoses and Planning

Nursing diagnoses and related expected patient outcomes most commonly applicable to patients with Parkinson's disease include the following:

NDx: Impaired physical mobility related to muscular rigidity, bradykinesia, muscle tremors, and loss of postural reflexes

Planning: Patient Outcomes
1. Patient performs ADLs.
2. Patient maintains current level of mobility with or without assistance.
3. Patient remains free from accidental injury.

NDx: Self esteem disturbance related to physical limitations and changes in appearance

Planning: Patient Outcomes
1. Patient verbalizes positive feelings about himself or herself.
2. Patient adjusts lifestyle according to physical limitations.
3. Patient maintains social interactions with family and friends.
4. Patient participates in ADLs.

NDx: Impaired verbal communication related to dysarthria and monotonous, whispering speech

Planning: Patient Outcomes
1. Patient communicates without frustration.
2. Patient uses alternative methods of communication as necessary.

NDx: Risk for altered health maintenance related to insufficient knowledge of self-care

Planning: Patient Outcomes
1. Patient and family describe self-care measures presented in Highlight 18–2.
2. Patient and family verbalize willingness and ability to follow the guidelines presented in Highlight 18–2.

Nursing Interventions and Evaluation

NDx: Impaired physical mobility
Encourage the patient to be as physically independent as possible in ADLs. Provide active and passive range-of-motion exercises at least every 6 hours. Allow sufficient time to perform ADLs by establishing a schedule or routine. Provide for periods of activity and rest. Avoid rushing, which can result in falls.

Administer medications as prescribed to reduce and control muscle rigidity, tremors, and bradykinesia. Evaluate the patient for tolerance of medication. Determine the degree of symptom control and side effects experienced by the patient, such as nausea, vomiting, orthostatic hypotension, dry mouth, dizziness, and "on-off" phenomenon, in which there is periodic loss of symptom control. Instruct the patient to decrease intake of vitamin B_6, multivitamins,

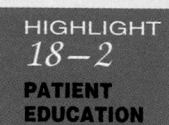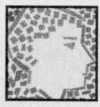

HIGHLIGHT
18–2
PATIENT EDUCATION

Coping with Parkinson's Disease

Instruct the patient and/or family to:
Adapt home environment to minimize the risk of injury and to facilitate independence.

- Provide good lighting in all living areas.
- Remove all loose or scatter rugs.
- Remove doorsills that are easily stumbled over.
- Place sharp pointed tables or other objects out of the traffic pattern, so that if the patient should fall, the likelihood of injury from striking a sharp object is decreased.
- Arrange patient's living quarters on one floor if possible.
- Install sturdy stair rails on both sides if stairs are unavoidable.
- Install handles on walls adjacent to doorknobs to provide the patient with a secure source of support while he or she opens doors.
- Facilitate getting in and out of a chair by using chair with sturdy arms and a slightly forward tip. The forward tip can be arranged by having a carpenter lengthen the back legs or by placing secure 2- to 4-inch blocks under them.
- Facilitate getting in and out of bed by placing a heavy piece of furniture next to the bed for support or by tying a loop of rope or a sheet with a knot in the end to the bottom of the bed to use to pull self into a sitting position.
- Install bars on either side of the toilet to facilitate getting on and off the toilet.
- Buy or make a toilet seat that is elevated 2 inches above the bowl to allow patient to remain seated while wiping self.
- Keep home temperature slightly above normal to eliminate the need for layers of clothing that are difficult for the patient to put on and that increase the difficulty of moving.

Select or adapt clothing and other personal use items so that they are easy to manipulate and therefore conserve energy and allow maximum independence.

- Use elastic shoelaces or wear shoes with Velcro fasteners to avoid having to tie shoes or tripping over untied laces.
- Use Velcro patches to fasten clothing; maintain proper appearance by sewing buttons on the top surface.
- Leave neckties knotted; slip over the head and tighten to wear.
- Choose raglan rather than set-in sleeves.
- Contact a rehabilitation center or support group for information about companies in your area that carry especially designed "easy to get in and out of" clothes.

Keep active to prevent physical disability due to disuse and to promote a positive outlook.

- Perform daily home exercises as taught.
- Participate in a formal exercise program once or twice a week; this may be an individual session or a group session offered through a Parkinson patient self-help group.
- Remember that overdoing exercises can be counterproductive, so follow physician's guidelines carefully.
- Remain involved in family and social activities.
- Drive if able, but consider staying in low-traffic areas and having another driver with you to allow breaks if needed.
- Be aware that there is no need to restrict travel, although having a companion along is desirable.

Eat a balanced diet sufficient to prevent weight loss.

- Eat 1500 to 2000 calories per day.
- Eat small, frequent meals because problems with chewing, swallowing, and handling food items make eating a slow, difficult process.
- Reduce dietary protein moderately because proteins reduce the absorption of levodopa; do not drastically reduce protein unless specified by your physician.
- Use an electric warming tray if needed to keep foods warm and palatable during the time it takes to eat.
- Select foods that are easy to handle, chew, and swallow, such as mashed potatoes and other vegetables, meat loaf, and stew.
- Remember that semisolid foods are easier to swallow than liquids or solids and that a commercial product (Thick-It) is available that can be used to thicken fruit juice and carbonated beverages.

Institute measures to cope with sleep pattern disturbances (early to sleep, with awakening in about 3 hours followed by several hours of wakefulness before returning to sleep) that predispose to episodes of nocturnal confusion due to sensory deprivation.

- Keep a light on at night.
- Keep a radio playing softly.
- Consult with the physician if serious sleep pattern disturbance effects persist, because a change in medication may be helpful.

Recognize that caregivers need intervals of relief from responsibilities and plan for respite care accordingly.

and high-protein foods (eg, milk, eggs, meat) because they facilitate the destruction of dopamine in the liver, thereby decreasing levels of available dopamine.

Consult with the physical and occupational therapists to assist the patient in mobility and to provide assistive devices (ie, cane, walker). Instruct the patient about safety hazards and how to maintain a safe environment. Explain the importance of removing scatter rugs, maintaining good lighting, avoiding rushing, and allowing time for movements. Instruct the patient to walk erect and use a wide base marching gait (heel-toe gait) and swing arms. Warm baths help to relieve rigidity associated with muscle spasm.

NDx: Self esteem disturbance

Allow the patient to verbalize fears and feelings about loss of function. Inform the patient about the resources available such as support groups and the Parkinson's Disease Foundation. Explore strengths and weaknesses as well as effective coping and defense mechanisms. Assist the patient in setting realistic short-term goals. Discuss patient symptoms (eg, drooling, tremors) and their impact on self-image. Support self-care and physical and social activities within physical limitations. Patients are slow and untidy when eating. Instruction in the use of self-help devices for feeding and dressing are beneficial in improving self-esteem.

NDx: Impaired verbal communication

Provide an accepting environment for the patient to communicate, whether attempts are successful or not. This can be accomplished by providing a private, unrushed atmosphere. Decrease external distractions, such as noise from the television or radio, and move close when communicating with the patient. This allows for whispers to be heard. Ask questions simply by supplying two options or in a "yes or no" format. Recognize the patient's frustrations when efforts to communicate are unsuccessful. Instruct the patient to perform face and tongue exercises to maintain optimal muscle strength, such as raising eyebrows, wrinkling the forehead, opening the mouth widely, blowing out cheeks, whistling, and wiggling the nose. Consult with a speech therapist to evaluate the patient. Develop an individualized program or provide or suggest alternative methods of communication when necessary. Instruct the patient in the importance of making his or her feelings known because nonverbal communication (monotone speech and lack of facial expression) may impede their intended message.

NDx: Risk for altered health maintenance

Instruct the patient and family in self-care measures, as presented in Highlight 18–2.

Compare the patient's status with the expected outcomes. If the outcomes are not met, reassess the patient and revise the plan.

ALZHEIMER'S DISEASE

Alzheimer's disease is a chronic progressive neurodegenerative condition characterized by marked cognitive dysfunction. Its peak onset is between 45 and 65 years of age. Alzheimer's disease is a prominent dementing illness.

Etiology and Pathophysiology

The exact cause of Alzheimer's disease is unknown. Theories of cause include genetic tendency, autoimmune reaction, slow virus, and dysfunction of neurotransmitters. Alzheimer's disease is not considered a hereditary disease. However, familial tendencies have been noted. Recent research has revealed that small strokes increase the chances of Alzheimer's disease, so stroke-prevention measures may reduce the risk of developing the disorder.

Cerebral atrophy is noted primarily in the frontal and temporal lobes. Degenerative neuronal changes occur, involving the development of neurofibrillary tangles, formation of senile plaques, and loss of neurons. Symptoms manifested by these degenerative changes progress from confusion and memory loss to dementia.

Clinical Manifestations

Alzheimer's disease has been classified into three stages (Table 18–1). Each stage is characterized by progressive mental and physical dysfunction. Initially, the patient may be forgetful. However, this progresses to memory loss, wandering behavior, and an eventual lack of awareness of the environment, with custodial care required. Death usually occurs in the last stage as a result of aspiration pneumonia.

Diagnosis

A history and neurologic examination are performed to ascertain the level of deterioration of mental and physical functioning. Neurodiagnostic studies include CT to demonstrate cerebral atrophy and enlarged ventricles, positron emission tomography to identify glucose utilization of the brain, and EEG to identify slowing patterns of brain impulses. In some cases, a brain biopsy is performed.

Management

Medical management of patients with Alzheimer's disease is symptomatic and supportive. No known treatment plan alters progression of the condition or functioning level of the patient. Medications such as vasodilators (papaverine [Pavabid], ergoloid mesylates [Hydergine]), or psychostimulants (methylphenidate [Ritalin]) are prescribed in an attempt to improve mental status.

❖ Settings, Providers, and Collaboration for Care

Patients with Alzheimer's disease are usually treated in their home and should be seen regularly in a physician's office. It is difficult to manage all the care necessary for the patient with Alzheimer's dis-

Table 18–1

Stages of Alzheimer's Disease

EARLY STAGE (2–4 YEARS)

Forgetfulness (may be subtle and patient may try to cover up using lists and notes)

Declining interest in environment, people, and present affairs

Vague uncertainty and hesitancy in initiating actions

Poor performance at work by the end of this stage; may be dismissed from job

MIDDLE STAGE (2–12 YEARS)

Progressive memory loss

Hesitates in response to questions; shows signs of aphasia

Has difficulty following simple instructions or doing simple calculations

Has episodic bouts of irritability

Becomes evasive, anxious, and physically active

Wanders, particularly at night

Becomes apraxic for many basic activities

Loses important papers

Loses way home in familiar surroundings or loses way in own home

Forgets to pay bills; lets household chores slip and newspapers pile up; does not dispose of garbage; does not take medications

Loses possessions and then claims they were stolen

Neglects personal hygiene (bathing, shaving, dressing)

Loses social graces; behavior can be a major embarrassment to family and friends; usually ends in social isolation of the family and patient

FINAL STAGE (UP TO A YEAR)

Marked loss of weight because of lack of eating; becomes emaciated

Unable to communicate verbally or in writing

Does not recognize family

Incontinent of urine and feces

Possibility of major seizures

Grasping, snout, and sucking reflexes are readily elicited

Finally loses the ability to stand and walk and becomes bedridden

Death is usually from aspiration pneumonia

ease as the manifestations of the disorder become more severe. The families struggle to provide all the care needed for the patient in the home setting. A nurse assistant may help with the patient's hygienic needs. A visiting nurse assesses the patient's status, teaches the family about the medication regimen, and consults with the physician as needed.

A social worker may help with a variety of family and patient needs, such as finding resources for financial burdens, transportation requirements, respite care, and meal delivery to the home. As their condition deteriorates, patients are frequently admitted to long-term care facilities.

NURSING PROCESS
Alzheimer's Disease

Assessment

Patient assessment includes a history and neurologic examination. Assess for progressive deterioration in mental and physical abilities. Determine the limitations of cognitive function and self-care. Assess the risk of injury or self-harm. Also assess the impact of the disease on family members.

Begin with an assessment of the level of cognitive function, determining orientation to time, place, and person and presence of delusions. Check for loss of recent and remote memory and the ability to retain new information. Assess for errors in judgment, abstract thinking, and loss of insight. Also assess for the presence of aphasia syndromes and difficulty in comprehension.

Assess for behavioral and affective disturbances. Observe for signs of hyperactivity, restlessness, wandering, antisocial behavior, emotional outbursts, paranoia, diminished motivation, and depression.

Determine the level of motor function. Note gait disturbances, seizure activity, and muscle twitching. Assess the ability to carry out purposeful tasks or movements. Identify the ability to perform self-care and ADLs. Determine the level of supervision and assistance required to complete tasks.

Explore the impact on family functioning. Ask family members the following questions:

"How have your lives changed?"
"Are you able to socialize with friends and meet your work responsibilities?"
"Do you feel as though you have enough time for yourself?"
"Do you find yourself getting frustrated, edgy, or irritable?"

Nursing Diagnoses and Planning

Nursing diagnoses and related expected patient outcomes most commonly applicable to patients with Alzheimer's disease include the following:

NDx: Altered thought processes related to cognitive decline

Planning: Patient Outcomes
1. Displays of behavioral dysfunction are minimal.

NDx: Chronic confusion related to effects of progressive cerebral degeneration

Planning: Patient Outcomes
1. Participate to maximum level in ADLs.
2. Frustrations are decreased when environmental stressors are reduced.

NDx: Self care deficit: feeding, bathing/hygiene, dressing/grooming related to cognitive decline

Planning: Patient Outcomes
1. Patient performs self-care within limits of ability.
2. Patient wears clean, neat clothes during daytime.

3. Patient maintains acceptable personal hygiene.
4. Family or significant other identifies personal and community resources that can provide support and assistance.

NDx: Risk for injury related to cognitive decline

Planning: Patient Outcomes
1. Patient remains free from injury.

NDx: Ineffective family coping related to constant, total care of family member with Alzheimer's disease

Planning: Patient Outcomes
1. Family describes strategies to manage behavioral alterations of the patient.
2. Family identifies personal and community sources of support.

Nursing Interventions and Evaluation

NDx: Altered thought processes
Provide a consistent, structured environment for the patient. Allow the patient to have familiar objects around (eg, pictures, furniture). Establish daily routines. Avoid any variations in day-to-day activities. Do not expect the patient to function or respond beyond his or her capabilities. Anticipate the patient's needs. Eliminate any stress associated with meeting those needs. Eliminate undue noise or disruption of physical surroundings.

NDx: Chronic confusion
Promote communication by talking in simple sentences, presenting one idea at a time, asking questions the patient can answer, and using good eye contact. Attempt to identify fears and frustrations that are associated with combative episodes that Alzheimer patients often exhibit. Keep the environment simple and uncluttered. Plan and maintain a consistent routine. Focus on the patient's ability. Be alert to increasing fatigue and anxiety.

NDx: Self care deficit: feeding, bathing/hygiene, dressing/grooming
Monitor the patient's level and ability to perform ADLs. Ensure that the patient attends to daily personal hygiene, wears clean clothing, and eats an adequate diet. Allow the patient to maintain self-care activities as long as possible. Encourage the patient to complete self-care. Supervise the patient, when necessary, to ensure completion of the steps involved in each task. Provide direct care when the patient cannot adequately perform self-care. Consult with the nutritionist as necessary to determine nutritional needs. Ensure that the patient is fed and groomed and that hygiene is attended to on a daily basis.

NDx: Risk for injury
Monitor the patient's cognitive function. Identify changes that increase the risk for patient injury, such as wandering, behavioral outbursts, and inattention to what is going on in the environment.

Provide a consistent, familiar environment with good lighting for the patient. Remove obstacles and hazards from the environment (ie, scatter rugs, candles). Supervise the patient if he or she has a tendency to wander or has the potential to inflict self-harm. Ensure that the patient carries identification.

NDx: Ineffective family coping
Support the family in developing effective coping mechanisms. Provide for an accepting environment to allow for expression of anxiety, fear, hopelessness, and other emotions. Allow family members or significant others to express feelings without placing value or judgment on what they say. Ensure that a private area is available to meet with family members or significant others.

Identify support groups and resources available, such as the Alzheimer's Disease and Related Disorders Association. Teach the family strategies that are effective in managing the patient's behavioral alterations (ie, consistent environment, reduction of stress in environment, consistent manner to handle outbursts and other behaviors). Monitor the family's reaction to caring for the patient. Identify increased periods of stress or difficulty coping with situations. Reinforce with the family their need for respite and support. Encourage family members to meet their own personal needs and not to extend beyond their physical or emotional limitations. Refer to day-care centers and respite centers.

Compare the patient's status with the expected outcomes. If the outcomes are not met, reassess the patient and revise the plan.

DISK HERNIATION

Etiology and Pathophysiology
The intervertebral disk lies between two adjacent vertebrae. Its function is to absorb shock and permit motion. Traumatic incidents, such as lifting heavy objects without proper body mechanics or falling, can precipitate a herniation or rupturing of disk material into the spinal canal, where it can impinge on a spinal nerve root (Fig. 18–5). Degenerative changes in the supporting ligaments predispose to herniation, and in many cases no specific precipitating event can be identified.

The cervical and lumbar spines are the most flexible and therefore the most susceptible to stress and injury. Herniation of an intervertebral disk in the cervical spine usually takes place between the fifth and sixth or sixth and seventh cervical vertebrae. Herniation of a lumbosacral disk most often occurs between the fourth and fifth lumbar vertebra and results in irritation and compression of the fifth lumbar root. Herniated disks in the thoracic area are rare.

Clinical Manifestations
The clinical manifestations of a herniated disk vary with the location of the affected disk and the degree

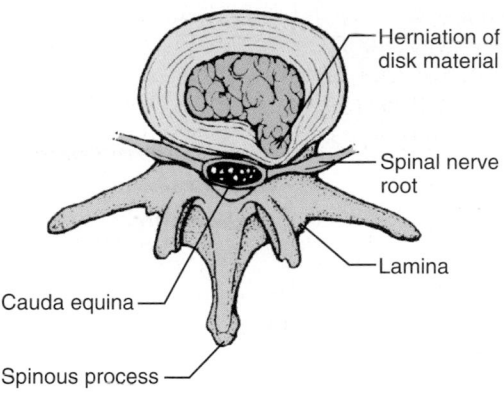

Figure 18–5
Herniation of an intervertebral disk.

of herniation. A small protrusion of a cervical disk causes a stiff neck accompanied by shoulder pain, which radiates down the arm.

Clinical manifestations associated with herniation of lumbar disks include low back pain with muscle spasms and pain radiating down the leg, change in posture, and limited motion of the spine. The back pain associated with herniation of a lumbar disk is generally relieved by lying supine on a firm surface with the head slightly elevated and the hips and knees slightly flexed or by lying on the unaffected side with the affected leg flexed at the hip and knee.

Table 18–2

Clinical Manifestations of Nerve Root Compression Secondary to Disk Herniation

Compressed Nerve Root*	Clinical Manifestations
Sixth cervical	Paresthesias and sensory loss in the dorsum of the head Weakness of the biceps Decreased biceps reflex
Seventh cervical	Paresthesias and sensory loss in third and fourth fingers Slight weakness of the triceps Decreased triceps reflex
Fifth lumbar	Pain and paresthesias in the hip, groin, posterolateral thigh, lateral calf, top of the foot to the great and second toes
First sacral	Pain and paresthesias in the midgluteal area, posterior thigh, calf, heel, bottom of the foot to the fourth and fifth toes
Fourth lumbar	Pain in the lower back extending down the anterior surface of the leg to the great toe

*Compressed nerve roots are listed in order of frequency of occurrence.

The pain is aggravated by sitting, standing, bending, coughing, sneezing, and straining.

Larger herniations, whether cervical or lumbar, can compress the nerve root and cause more extensive pain and paresthesias, as described in Table 18–2.

Diagnosis

The diagnosis of herniated disk disease is suggested by the symptoms elicited through the history and physical examination. It is confirmed by CT and myelogram. Electromyography may be performed to localize affected nerve roots. The use of MRI, a non-invasive test that provides clear images of spinal cord anatomy, is also being increasingly used. Spinal x-ray films can indicate narrowing of an intervertebral disk but may not show a herniated disk or spinal cord lesion.

Management

Medical management of a herniated disk can consist of conservative or surgical treatment. Conservative treatment consists of the following:

Enforced bedrest
Use of a firm mattress
Avoidance of any activity involving flexion of the spine
Use of supportive devices such as a corset, brace, or cervical collar
Use of halter traction (cervical disk)
Physiotherapy treatments
Medications to relieve pain and decrease muscle spasm

Surgery is indicated for those patients who do not respond to conservative treatment or whose symptoms warrant immediate surgical intervention. Refer to Chapter 17 for a discussion of laminectomy.

❖ **Settings, Providers, and Collaboration for Care**

The patient with a herniated disk can be treated in a physician's office when treatment is conservative. The patient may also be referred for physical therapy. The therapist may use exercises, ultrasound therapy, massage therapy, traction, or a combination thereof to treat the condition. If surgical treatment is necessary, the patient is hospitalized.

NURSING PROCESS
Disk Herniation

Assessment

Assess the patient's discomfort. Ask the patient to describe the type of pain experienced (eg, aching, burning, tearing), its severity, its location, any identifiable precipitating factors, such as sitting for a long period of time or writing at a desk, and any pattern to the pain such as an exacerbation in the morning. Ask also about associated symptoms, including limitation of movement, and paresthesias.

Explore when the current problem began as well as any history of a similar problem. Determine what treatment measures, if any, have been used and their effectiveness. Observe for changes in posture that suggest that the patient is trying to prevent pain or to protect a painful area. Check range of motion, muscle strength, and reflexes in the affected areas.

If this is a recurrent problem, assess the patient's understanding of the cause of the pain and of measures that limit stress on the spine. Also assess the psychosocial effects of the problem on the patient. Explore the patient's ability to work and to participate in household, social, and recreational activities. Assess the patient's feelings about himself or herself in relationship to the disorder and the patient's ability to cope and the style of doing so.

Nursing Diagnoses and Planning

Nursing diagnoses and related expected patient outcomes most commonly applicable to patients with a herniated disk include the following:

NDx: Pain related to nerve irritation and muscle spasm

Planning: Patient Outcomes
1. Patient restricts movement as directed.
2. Patient reports that pain is manageable and decreasing.
3. Patient performs allowed activities without exacerbated pain.

NDx: Risk for altered tissue perfusion related to impaired venous blood flow secondary to thrombophlebitis or pulmonary embolism

Planning: Patient Outcomes
1. Patient performs foot and leg exercises as directed.
2. Calves are free of heat, redness, and swelling.
3. Homans' sign (pain in calf on strong, passive dorsiflexion of foot) is negative.

NDx: Risk for altered health maintenance related to insufficient knowledge of measures to reduce stress on the cervical or lumbar spine

Planning: Patient Outcomes
1. Patient explains measures to reduce stress on the lumbar spine, as presented in Highlight 18–3.
2. Patient expresses willingness to comply with measures to reduce stress on the lumbar spine.
3. Patient expresses confidence in the ability to comply with measures to reduce stress on the lumbar spine.

Nursing Interventions and Evaluation

NDx: Pain
Maintain the patient with herniation of a cervical disk on bed rest with continuous traction while pain is acute. Subsequently, keep the neck immobilized with a collar. Apply traction intermittently as di-

---

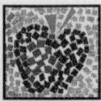

HIGHLIGHT
18–3
HEALTH PROMOTION & RISK REDUCTION

Measures to Reduce Stress on the Lumbar Spine

Instruct the patient to:

Maintain good posture: back straight, shoulders back, abdomen and neck tucked in.

Exercise regularly during asymptomatic periods to strengthen the muscles of the back and abdomen. Perform flexion or isometric exercise routine prescribed by the physician.

Sit in a straight-back chair with feet on footstool so knees are flexed above level of hips.

Avoid extended periods of sitting or driving.

Sleep on the back or side, never on the stomach.

Sleep on a mattress with firm support. Use bed board if necessary, but avoid placing the mattress on the floor, because getting up and down may further injure the spine.

Avoid rotating or extending the spine.

Carry objects close to the chest.

Bend at the hips and knees, not at the waist.

Face objects to be lifted directly.

Avoid lifting while bending.

Avoid lifting anything heavier than 10 pounds.

Wear a lumbar corset to protect the back during strenuous activities.

Reduce activity at the first sign of pain.

Use a firm backrest in the car.

Stop and walk at least every 2 hours while riding.

Maintain or regain recommended body weight.

---

rected by the physician. (Refer to Chap. 19 for the care of the patient in cervical traction.)

Maintain patients on bed rest to control pain and muscle spasm during the acute phase of lumbosacral disk herniation. Make certain that the mattress provides firm support. Use a bed board if necessary. Place the patient in a supine position with the head elevated 30 degrees and the hips slightly flexed to minimize intradisk pressure. Explain to the patient that attempting to get up or sitting for even a short time can cause the disk to protrude further and result in another attack. Use a pull sheet, which goes from under the shoulder to midthigh, and a pillow between the legs to move the patient while maintaining correct alignment. Instruct the patient not to move without assistance. Caution the patient not to raise himself or herself by pulling on the side rails, not to stretch to reach for anything, and not to write, do handwork, or hold a book or magazine to read while lying flat because all these activities place further stress on the spine. Also instruct the patient to avoid coughing and sneezing when possible. To facilitate compliance with these instructions, keep the call bell and personal items within easy reach, and provide a reading rack and prism glasses to allow the patient to read or watch television. Give cough suppressants and allergy medications as ordered to control coughing or sneezing.

Administer analgesics every 3 to 4 hours for the first 48 to 72 hours, and have the patient wear a lumbar corset if ordered to immobilize the spine and provide proper alignment. Apply hot, moist packs as ordered every 1 to 2 hours for up to 30 minutes. Administer muscle relaxants and anti-inflammatory medications as ordered.

Change the patient's position to a side-lying one with knees flexed and the upper knee resting on a pillow when permitted. Recognize that this is often the position of comfort for the patient with leg pain.

Use a fracture pan to meet patient's elimination needs. Place a small pillow on the bed just above the upper edge of the pan to support the spine. Log-roll the patient on and off the pan. Caution the patient not to use toilet paper or get off the pan without assistance. Encourage the patient to increase water and roughage in the diet to prevent straining at stool. Administer stool softeners as ordered.

Guide the patient in the progressive exercise program prescribed by the physician. When allowed, provide instruction on how to get out of bed with the least amount of strain on the back. Instruct the patient to turn on the side with the knees flexed and slide (or be moved on a pull sheet) to the edge of the bed. Have the patient next push himself or herself up with the hands while keeping the spine straight and easing the feet and legs over the side of the bed. Instruct the patient to select a straight chair with arm rests and to sit with the back flat against the chair and the knees flexed higher than the hips. Remind the patient to resume activities slowly according to the physician's directions and to sit a maximum of 30 minutes at one time.

NDx: Risk for altered tissue perfusion
Begin foot and leg exercises to promote venous circulation as soon as the acute pain subsides. Instruct the patient to flex the hip and the knee and to slide the heel of the foot along the mattress to the top of the incline created by the knee gatch and then down. Have the patient perform this exercise five times with each leg every 2 to 3 hours while awake. Apply antiembolic stockings if prescribed.

NDx: Risk for altered health maintenance
Instruct the patient in self-care measures to reduce stress on the lumbar spine, as presented in Highlight 18–3.

Compare the patient's status with the expected outcomes. If the outcomes are not met, reassess the patient and revise the plan.

Functional Disorders

SEIZURE DISORDERS

Seizure disorders are chronic conditions characterized by a change in a person's motor or sensory system functioning and behavior. The specific symptoms manifested and their magnitude depend on the area of cerebral tissue involved. This change in functioning and behavior results from an uncontrolled excessive discharge of neurons in the cerebral tissue. The period between seizure episodes varies and can range from minutes to days to months to years.

Etiology and Pathophysiology
Seizure disorders are caused by factors affecting the cortex of the brain. These factors include genetic disorders, metabolic or electrolyte imbalances, infection, trauma, vascular disease, congenital malformations, encephalopathies, neoplasms, degenerative diseases, and alcohol or barbiturate withdrawal.

During a seizure episode, there is an uncontrolled excessive discharge of neurons in the brain. This is accompanied by an increase in the oxygen consumption of the brain and body, an increase in the blood pressure and pulse, and a decrease in the blood oxygen tension level. During the recovery phase between seizure episodes, the body regains homeostasis and no residual brain damage occurs.

Status epilepticus is a state of recurrent seizure activity without recovery between seizures. Without a recovery period, hypoxia results and brain damage is imminent. Status epilepticus is a neurologic emergency and requires immediate intervention. Adults often present in status epilepticus as a result of their noncompliance to a prescribed anticonvulsant medication regimen. It may also be a symptom of an underlying structural abnormality (ie, lesion, tumor mass).

Clinical Manifestations
The clinical manifestations of the patient during a seizure episode depend on the part of the brain from which the abnormal neuron discharge originates, the number of neurons excited, and the extent to which there is spread of activity.

Seizures are often classified into two categories: focal or partial (involving a particular area of the brain) and generalized (involving the entire brain, no focus identified). See Table 18–3 for the characteristics of partial and generalized seizures.

Diagnosis
A complete history and neurologic examination are performed to establish the focal or general character-

Table 18–3

Characteristics of Partial and Generalized Seizures

Type	Duration	Seizure Symptoms	Postictal Symptoms
PARTIAL SEIZURES			
Simple partial	30 sec	Symptoms vary: sudden jerking, sensory phenomena	No loss of consciousness
Complex partial	1–2 min	May have aura Staring Automatism (eg, lip smacking, picking at clothes, fumbling) Unaware of environment May wander	Amnesia for seizure events Mild to moderate confusion
GENERALIZED SEIZURES			
Absence (petit mal)	2–15 sec	Staring Fluttering of eyes	Amnesia for seizure events No confusion Able to resume activity
Generalized tonic-clonic (grand mal)	1–2 min	A cry Fall Tonicity (rigidity) Clonicity (jerking) May have cyanosis	Amnesia for seizure events Confusion Deep sleep

istics of the seizure disorder. Laboratory serum tests are performed to establish baseline parameters and to identify any metabolic or electrolyte imbalance that could induce seizure activity (glucose, sodium, BUN, calcium). An EEG with simultaneous video recording is performed to document abnormal electrical discharge of the brain in conjunction with visual monitoring of actual seizure. When temporal lobe involvement is suspected, a sleep EEG may be performed. CT, MRI, and lumbar puncture with cerebrospinal fluid studies may also be performed to rule out other underlying pathology.

Management

The first step in planning appropriate medical management for persons with a seizure disorder is to determine the cause. If the seizure disorder is related to a space-occupying lesion, metabolic imbalance, or infectious process, the underlying cause is the focus of treatment.

Anticonvulsant drug therapy (Highlight 18–4) is the most common treatment mode for patients with seizure disorders. Anticonvulsant therapy is a symptomatic treatment, not a cure for seizure disorders. Certain drugs are more effective for specific types of seizure activity than others. For example, phenytoin, primidone (Mysoline), carbamazepine, divalproex (Depakote), and phenobarbital tend to be more effective for partial and generalized tonic-clonic seizures. Ethosuximide (Zarontin), divalproex, and clonazepam tend to be more effective for absence and generalized (non–tonic-clonic) seizures. Diazepam, phenobarbital, phenytoin, and paraldehyde tend to be more effective for status epilepticus. Lamotrigine is indicated for adjunct therapy for partial seizures, but has a potentially fatal side effect, a life-threaten-

ing rash. A recently FDA-approved antiseizure medication, topiramate (Topimax), is also an add-on therapy for partial seizures in adults.

Anticonvulsants are introduced gradually while serum blood levels are monitored to establish the therapeutic dose for seizure control. Monotherapy is the goal of most anticonvulsant treatment regimens, but occasionally drugs are used in combination to decrease the potential for toxic effects associated with single-drug therapy.

Just as anticonvulsant drugs are introduced gradually, withdrawal of therapy is also gradual, using tapered dosages. Sudden withdrawal of anticonvulsants precipitates seizure activity or even status epilepticus.

In certain instances, surgical intervention may be indicated to control seizure activity. These include situations in which medications cannot control seizure activity or a surgical procedure would not risk neurologic deficit (the language center is not involved). The corpus callosum has been surgically divided in patients with severe generalized seizures.

❖ Settings, Providers, and Collaboration for Care

The patient who experiences seizures may be treated initially in the emergency department. The patient may then be diagnosed in the hospital or in an outpatient setting. Medical management usually occurs in an outpatient setting such as a clinic or physician's office. The nurse instructs the patient and family about the medication regimen and how to care for the patient during and after a seizure. Frequent physician office visits may be necessary for follow-up monitoring and treatment.

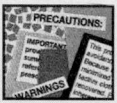

HIGHLIGHT
18—4
PHARMACOLOGY

Anticonvulsants

Definition:

These drugs prevent or decrease seizure activity. Major classes of anticonvulsants are barbiturates (eg, phenobarbital), benzodiazepines (eg, clonazepam), hydantoins (eg, phenytoin), oxazolidinedione derivatives (eg, trimethadione), and succinimides (eg, ethosuximide).

Action:

Anticonvulsants act on the central nervous system (CNS) in a variety of ways to reduce seizure activity. For example, barbiturates depress impulse transmission across synapses, whereas hydantoins alter the passage of sodium ions across membranes and thus affect impulse generation.

Uses:

Barbiturates are generally effective against generalized tonic-clonic and absence seizures, hydantoins against generalized tonic-clonic and complex partial seizures, and oxazolidinediones and succinimides against absence seizures. However, each anticonvulsant is used for specific types of seizures, so indications for individual drugs should be checked.

Side Effects:

Side effects vary with the individual drug. Common side effects for a drug from each of the major classes of anticonvulsants are as follows:

Barbiturates (phenobarbital): drowsiness, lethargy, nausea, vomiting, rashes, nerve, muscle or joint pain, inflammation

Benzodiazepines (clonazepam): drowsiness, ataxia, behavioral disturbances, increased salivation

Hydantoins (phenytoin): ataxia, slurred speech, confusion, nausea, vomiting, hyperplasia of the gums, dermatitis, nystagmus, double vision, agranulocytosis

Oxazolidinediones (trimethadione): drowsiness, malaise, exfoliative dermatitis, agranulocytosis, aplastic and hypoplastic anemia

Succinimides (ethosuximide): drowsiness, fatigue, dizziness, euphoria, nausea, vomiting, epigastric and abdominal pain, agranulocytosis, aplastic anemia

Interactions:

Interactions vary with the individual drug. Common examples of interactions are as follows:

Phenobarbital: taken with alcohol, narcotic analgesics, other CNS depressants, or monoamine oxidase inhibitors can result in excessive CNS depression; taken with primidone or valproic acid may result in excessive blood levels of phenobarbital; taken with rifampin may have a decreased effect

Clonazepam: None of significance

Phenytoin: taken with alcohol, folic acid, or loxapine results in a decreased effect; taken with oral anticoagulants, antihistamines, chloramphenicol, diazepam, cimetidine, diazoxide, isoniazid, phenylbutazone, salicylates, and sulfamethoxazole results in an increased and potentially toxic effect

Trimethadione: None of significance

Ethosuximide: None of significance

Nursing Implications:

For all anticonvulsants, instruct the patient to do the following:

Avoid activities that demand mental alertness and coordination until the response to the drug is determined.

Call physician immediately if side effects occur.

Never stop taking the drug without consulting the physician because such action can precipitate increased seizure activity.

Additional nursing implications are as follows:

Phenobarbital: Observe for signs of toxicity: wheezing, cyanosis, clammy skin, hypotension, coma.
  Instruct patient to avoid use of alcohol.
  Explain that full therapeutic effect may not occur for 2 to 3 weeks.
  If ordered intravenously, give drug slowly and monitor respiratory status closely.

Clonazepam: Observe for oversedation.
  Explain need for complete blood count (CBC) and liver function tests.

Phenytoin: Instruct the patient to do the following:
  Carry an identification card indicating that phenytoin is taken and the dose.
  Avoid heavy use of alcohol because it may interfere with effectiveness of the drug.
  Do not change drug brands once stabilized on a drug because untoward effects may occur.
  Explain (1) that drug may color urine pink, red, or reddish brown; (2) the importance of good oral

(continued)

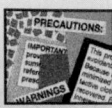

hygiene and regular dental checkups; (3) need for CBC and serum calcium levels every 6 months.

If ordered intravenously, do not mix with dextrose 5% in water; do not use cloudy solution; administer over 30–60 minutes when possible; begin infusion within 1 hour of mixing and discard after 4 hours.

Trimethadione: Explain the need for CBC, liver function tests, and urinalysis before starting drug and monthly thereafter.

Instruct the patient to (1) report immediately skin rash, alopecia, sore throat, fever, bruises, or nosebleeds; (2) wear sunglasses if vision blurs in bright light and report to physician.

Ethosuximide: Explain the need for a CBC every 3 months.

NURSING PROCESS
Seizure Disorders

Assessment

Assessment of the patient includes a history and neurologic examination. Ask the patient to describe how the seizure started. Also ask the following questions:

- "Were there any physical symptoms, such as the head or eyes turning to one side, arm or leg rigidity or shaking movements, or incontinence?"
- "Were there any warning signs or auras?"
- "How did the seizure progress?"
- "How long did the seizure last?"
- "Did you sleep after the seizure was over?"
- "Do you remember anything that was said during the seizure?"

When the patient cannot give complete information, ask a family member or significant other to provide the history and other information.

Ascertain whether anyone else in the family has similar complaints, symptoms, or known seizure disorders. Identify medical or social conditions that would influence or precipitate seizure activity, such as alcohol or drug ingestion, adherence to medication regimen, trauma at birth, cerebrovascular accident (CVA), neoplasm, and surgical procedures involving the brain.

Allow the patient to discuss the emotional and psychosocial impact of this condition on himself or herself and family functioning. Ask the patient the following questions:

- "Have you changed how you act or what you do when you are at home or at work?"
- "Is there anything you refuse to do because you feel you may get hurt or that it may put you into

an embarrassing situation if you were to experience a seizure episode?"

Assess the patient's level of safety, compliance with therapeutic plan, alteration of lifestyle, and emotional status.

Nursing Diagnoses and Planning

Nursing diagnoses and related expected patient outcomes most commonly applicable to patients with seizure disorders include the following:

NDx: Risk for injury related to uncontrolled movements during seizure episode

Planning: Patient Outcomes
1. Patient remains free from injury.
2. Patient avoids activities or jobs that could cause injury to herself or himself or to others (operating powerful machinery, mountain climbing, driving).
3. Patient adheres to prescribed anticonvulsant medication regimen.

NDx: Risk for altered oral mucous membrane related to effects of drug therapy on oral tissue

Planning: Patient Outcomes
1. Patient performs mouth care daily.
2. Gum hyperplasia is absent.

NDx: Self esteem disturbance related to unpredictable nature of seizures, and embarrassment

Planning: Patient Outcomes
1. Patient actively engages in social and job-related activities.
2. Patient expresses feelings of anxiety and concerns.
3. Patient expresses confidence in ability to cope with necessary alteration of lifestyle and family functioning.

NDx: Risk for aspiration related to seizure activity

Planning: Patient Outcomes
1. Patient maintains clear airway.
2. Arterial blood gas values are within normal range.
3. Patient remains afebrile.
4. Patient remains free from aspiration of secretions during seizure episode.

NDx: Impaired gas exchange related to status epilepticus

Planning: Patient Outcomes
1. Patient avoids irreversible cerebral damage or hypoxia.
2. Arterial blood gas values remain within normal range.

NDx: Risk for altered health maintenance

Planning: Patient Outcomes
1. Patient and family describe self-care measures, as presented in Highlight 18–5.
2. Patient and family verbalize willingness and ability to comply with the self-care measures presented in Highlight 18–5.

Nursing Interventions and Evaluation

NDx: Risk for injury
Provide a safe environment for the patient. Keep the bed in the lowest position. Ensure that bed side rails are in working order, and pad side rails for patients with known motor seizures. Instruct the patient to promote his or her own safety by lying down when an aura is experienced. Do not restrain a patient during seizure activity. Place the patient in a side-lying position to promote drainage of secretions. Protect the patient's head from hitting a hard surface, such as the floor, by placing a pillow or blanket under the head or by holding it. Call for help. Do not leave the patient. Loosen clothing and provide privacy if possible. If present at the onset of a seizure, place an oral airway in the mouth when the patient is in a relaxation phase to maintain airway and allow for suctioning as necessary. After the seizure, reorient the patient, perform neurologic assessment, and monitor postictal effects. Take vital signs and provide the patient with a place to sleep.

Encourage normal daily activities. Discuss with the patient activities that could result in injury or harm and that should be avoided (eg, operating hazardous machinery, mountain climbing). Conduct an environmental safety review of the home (eg, hard floors that could be carpeted) and suggest improvements or changes. Explain that a driver's license is granted only with evidence of seizure-free activity between 1 and 3 years, depending on individual state laws.

Encourage the patient to wear a MedicAlert bracelet. Instruct the patient on the importance of adherence to anticonvulsant medication regimen. Caution the patient not to stop or skip doses of

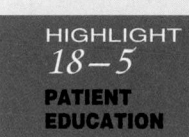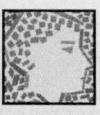

HIGHLIGHT 18–5
PATIENT EDUCATION
Self-Care Related to Seizures

Instruct the patient and/or family to:

Maintain a diary/journal of all seizure activity.

Note time of onset, duration, and description of seizures.

Take all antiseizure medications on time.

Report any side effects of medication (ie, dizziness, unsteady gait, cognitive impairment, visual changes, nausea, or vomiting).

Practice good oral hygiene.

Wear medical alert identification.

Protect the patient from harming self during a seizure.

Refrain from restraining patient, and never place objects in the patient's mouth.

Call emergency services if seizure lasts longer than 5 minutes.

Avoid driving and operating heavy equipment.

Wear a helmet while bike riding.

Swim only under close supervision.

Avoid cigarette smoking.

Keep regularly scheduled health care appointments.

medications if no seizure activity is noted or if he or she feels better. Avoid the use of alcohol and limit caffeine to decrease the risk of seizure activity. Instruct the patient about factors that can lower the seizure threshold such as fever, stress, fatigue, hypoglycemia, and menstruation.

NDx: Risk for altered oral mucous membrane
Instruct the patient on the importance of good oral hygiene. Allow the patient to redemonstrate steps of oral hygiene to ensure understanding and performance. Explain to the patient that gum hyperplasia is a side effect of some anticonvulsant medications such as phenytoin. If soreness or bleeding of the gums is noticed, inform the physician.

NDx: Self esteem disturbance
Ask the patient how this condition has affected the ability to carry out daily activities. Support the patient, and encourage sharing of fears, feelings, and anxieties. Assist the patient in identifying strengths and weaknesses, and encourage the use of effective coping mechanisms to manage alterations in lifestyle. Set expectations for social, family, and work

interactions. Provide the patient with resources for support, such as the Epilepsy Foundation, other persons with seizure disorders, and support groups.

NDx: Risk for aspiration
Place an oral airway at the patient's bedside. Ensure proper working order of suction equipment for emergency use. When a patient is having a seizure, place an oral airway in the mouth during initiation or relaxation phase of seizure activity. Do not force the airway into the mouth when the teeth are clenched. Turn the patient on his or her side to allow for drainage of secretions. Administer oxygen. Suction patient as necessary to maintain a clear airway.

NDx: Impaired gas exchange
Ensure that properly working oxygen and suction are maintained at the patient's bedside for emergency use. Obtain access to emergency medications used to treat patients in status epilepticus: dextrose 50%, diazepam, phenytoin, and phenobarbital injectables.

When a patient is in status epilepticus, call for help, do not leave the patient, maintain a patent airway (position the head, insert the oral airway, suction as needed), administer or give oxygen via nasal cannula, call for the physician, prepare intravenous catheter and medications to be administered to interrupt status epilepticus, assist the physician, and maintain the safety of the patient.

NDx: Risk for altered health maintenance
Instruct the patient and the family in self-care measures as presented in Highlight 18–5.

Compare the patient's status with the expected outcomes. If the outcomes are not met, reassess the patient and revise the plan.

HEADACHE

Headache is probably the most prevalent of complaints and varies in intensity, duration, and frequency.

Etiology and Pathophysiology
The symptom of headache may be caused by an organic factor (intracranial, extracranial lesions, mass, or hemorrhage), stress or muscle tension, vasodilation, or a combination of these. The majority of patients presenting with headache as a chief complaint do not have an underlying neurologic cause for the headache.

Clinical Manifestations
Clinical manifestations of a patient experiencing a headache depend on the type of headache. The most common types of headache include vascular (cluster and migraine) and tension.

CLUSTER HEADACHES. Cluster headaches are a type of vascular headache. Alcohol ingestion can be a precipitating factor. The headaches occur in clusters: They could occur 8 times a day and even more than 30 times each week. The attacks may be seasonal and even may awaken the patient from sleep. The duration of cluster headaches varies from 30 minutes to hours. Males seem to experience cluster headaches more frequently than females. Patients may also complain of nasal congestion, drooping eyelid (ptosis), tearing of the eyes (lacrimation), and feeling flushed.

MIGRAINE HEADACHES. Migraine headaches are also a type of vascular headache. They are considered a hereditary condition and are precipitated by vasodilation and increased cerebral blood flow. Females seem to experience migraine headaches more frequently than males. Patients complain of a throbbing sensation, unilateral head pain, nausea, vomiting, photophobia, blurred vision, and nasal congestion.

TENSION HEADACHES (MUSCLE CONTRACTION HEADACHES). Tension headaches are also known as muscle contraction headaches. Anxiety and tension are usually the precipitating factors for this type of headache. Common complaints from patients with tension headaches include tightness around the forehead area, dizziness, tenderness in the neck and scalp, and bilateral involvement.

Diagnosis
A history and physical and neurologic examination are performed to determine the type of headache and the underlying cause. The history focuses on familial patterns and the patient's own history of headaches. The physical and neurologic examination focuses on assessment of the body systems to rule out or identify underlying pathology. In addition, neurodiagnostic tests, such as CT, MRI, and EEG, are performed to rule out a neurologic cause.

Management
Medical management of the patient with a headache focuses on the symptomatic relief of pain. The management of vascular headaches (migraine, cluster) includes a combination of drug therapy and awareness and control of precipitating factors. Drug therapy includes the prescription of sumatriptan succinate (Imitrex), isometheptene mucate (Midrin), ergotamine tartrate (Gynergen), ergotamine with caffeine (Cafergot), or dihydroergotamine for immediate relief of vascular headache. Isometheptene and ergotamine have a vasoconstrictive action and are used primarily for treatment of headaches. Other drugs that are useful as a means of prophylactic treatment of vascular headaches include methysergide (Sansert), propranolol (Inderal), and clonidine (Catapres), which inhibit vasodilation of blood vessels.

The management of tension and muscle contraction headaches includes a combination of anxiety and tension relief and drug therapy. Drug therapy includes analgesics and sedatives to relieve anxiety and tension. Analgesics may include the following:

> Butalbital, aspirin, and caffeine (Fiorinal)
> Oxycodone hydrochloride, oxycodone terephthalate, and aspirin (Percodan)
> Propoxyphene, aspirin, and caffeine (Darvon)

Sedatives may included diazepam, phenobarbital, and meprobamate. Biofeedback techniques are used to promote reduction of anxiety and tension.

❖ Settings, Providers, and Collaboration for Care

Most headaches are diagnosed and treated on an outpatient basis. If the headache is severe, the patient may seek treatment in an emergency department.

NURSING PROCESS
Headache

Assessment

Assessment of the patient with headache includes a history and a physical and neurologic examination. The history is extensive and includes a general history, a familial history, and a history of headaches. Ask the patient probing questions such as the following:

- "Have you had any significant injuries, medical conditions, or diseases, such as sinusitis, surgery, infections, or trauma?"
- "Does anyone else in your family complain of headaches?"
- "Are there any members of your family with long-standing medical problems such as seizure disorders, a neurologic condition, allergies, or psychiatric illness?"

Allow the patient to describe the onset of the headaches, their extent, and their duration. Ask the patient questions such as "Is there anything you can do to decrease or eliminate your headache, such as lying down in a dark, quiet room or even trying to calm yourself down from feeling anxious or stressed?" Elicit any patterns that seem to coincide with headaches, such as menstruation in women, argument with a family member or significant other, or stress in the work setting. Focus the physical and neurologic examination on identifying abnormal findings that may be attributed to underlying pathology. Assess for the presence of motor or sensory dysfunction, such as ptosis and photophobia.

Identify any psychosocial or work stress that could precipitate headache. Allow the patient to describe work, family, and social settings. Ask the patient what he or she does for relaxation (ie, hobbies, sports, activities). Determine whether the people whom the patient is around complain of headaches at the same time to identify an environmental factor as a potential causative agent.

Nursing Diagnoses and Planning

Nursing diagnoses and related expected patient outcomes most commonly applicable to patients with headache include the following:

NDx: Pain related to headache

Planning: Patient Outcomes
1. Patient identifies factors that precipitate headaches.
2. Patient performs daily activities without limitations.
3. Headache pain is absent.

NDx: Anxiety related to incidence of headache

Planning: Patient Outcomes
1. Patient verbalizes anxiety and concerns.
2. Patient states that anxiety is manageable.

NDx: Ineffective individual coping related to recurrent headache

Planning: Patient Outcomes
1. Patient uses effective coping strategies.
2. Patient describes knowledge of available resources and supports.

Nursing Interventions and Evaluation

NDx: Pain
Monitor the level of discomfort that the patient is experiencing by using a visual analogue scale (scale from 1 to 10, with 10 being the worst pain ever experienced). Encourage the patient to discuss the pain. Monitor and observe for a trend as to how the patient reacts to pain and his or her tolerance to pain. Administer prescribed analgesics and other medications promptly. Observe the patient for relief of headache pain.

NDx: Anxiety
Monitor the patient for signs of anxiety and stress. Explore with the patient feelings of anxiety and circumstances that precipitate an anxious feeling. Encourage the patient to verbalize fears, past experiences, and perceptions of pain. Explain to the patient that anxiety and stress can cause headaches. Explain the relationship of stress and its effect on physiologic functioning (irritability, tension, stomach upset, and headache). Explore with the patient typical work, family, and social situations that elicit anxiety. Identify strategies to control or decrease anxiety. Role-play difficult or confrontational situations to allow the patient to practice responding. Encourage the patient to remove himself or herself from a situation in which he or she has no control over reducing the anxiety level.

NDx: Ineffective individual coping
Establish a trusting relationship with the patient. Provide an accepting environment that allows the

patient to express himself or herself freely. Accomplish this by maintaining privacy and a nonjudgmental approach to the patient. Encourage the patient to describe various personal situations and how he or she felt and responded. Explore with the patient alternative responses to the same situation that may have produced a more positive outcome or that allowed him or her to maintain, or even increase, control over personal feelings and actions. This enables the patient to gain insight into circumstances in which he or she may not have coped effectively and to increase awareness of effective coping mechanisms. Role-play to provide the patient with an opportunity to practice responding effectively in difficult and conflicting situations.

Compare the patient's status with the expected outcomes. If the outcomes are not met, reassess the patient and revise the plan.

Structural Disorders

HYDROCEPHALUS

Hydrocephalus is a clinical syndrome involving an increase in the volume of cerebrospinal fluid in the cerebroventricular system.

Etiology and Pathophysiology
Hydrocephalus is related to a dysfunction in the production, circulation, or reabsorption of cerebrospinal fluid. There are three types of hydrocephalus: communicating, noncommunicating, and normal-pressure.

In communicating hydrocephalus, there is interference in the reabsorption process of cerebrospinal fluid through the subarachnoid villi into the venous blood circulation. This often occurs in patients who have had a subarachnoid hemorrhage or meningitis, in which the subarachnoid villi become blocked or occluded from blood, exudate, or other particles. This may be a transient or permanent blockage.

Noncommunicating hydrocephalus, also known as obstructive hydrocephalus, occurs when a blockage exists within the cerebroventricular system. The most significant causes of this obstruction are tumors of the third and fourth ventricles (pinealomas, medulloblastomas). These tumors create a blockage within the ventricles and impinge on the aqueducts and incisural edge of the tentorium, restricting cerebrospinal fluid circulation and flow to the subarachnoid villi for reabsorption.

Normal-pressure hydrocephalus frequently occurs in adults older than 60 years. There is no known cause. The volume of cerebrospinal fluids increases, causing enlargement of the cerebral ventricles. However, no increased cerebrospinal fluid pressure or signs of increased intracranial pressure are noted.

Clinical Manifestations
The clinical manifestations of patients with communicating and noncommunicating hydrocephalus are related to increased intracranial pressure. Initial headache, restlessness, and irritability progress to severe headache, projectile vomiting, decreased level of consciousness, blurred vision, diplopia, papilledema, and eventually neurologic deterioration resulting in death if the patient is not treated.

Patients experiencing normal pressure hydrocephalus manifest a classic triad of symptoms: gait disturbance, dementia, and urinary incontinence. Gait disturbance is often the presenting symptom. The patient may be forgetful and have impaired memory function. With treatment, mental functioning can be improved.

Diagnosis
A complete history and neurologic examination are performed to identify onset and progression of symptoms and underlying pathology. CT is used to demonstrate enlarged ventricles. A lumbar puncture is performed to document increased or normal cerebrospinal fluid pressure. MRI and myelogram may be indicated to demonstrate cerebrospinal fluid pathways as well as identify underlying pathology.

Management
The most common method of treatment for hydrocephalus is ventricular shunting, which re-establishes normal routes of cerebrospinal fluid circulation and thus alleviates hydrocephalus. The two types of ventricular shunts are internalized shunts and externalized shunts.

Internal Ventricular Shunts
Ventriculoperitoneal internal shunts are used to treat adults with hydrocephalus (Fig. 18–6). Insertion of the shunt is a major surgical procedure that takes 1 to 2 hours.

PATIENT PREPARATION. The patient's hair is washed two times with an antiseptic shampoo. Once in the operating room, general anesthesia is administered. To decrease the risk of infection, the head area where the shunt will be inserted is shaved, and the scalp and abdomen are scrubbed with an antiseptic solution.

PROCEDURE. Two incisions are made: one in the head and one in the abdomen. The shunt tube is passed beneath the skin in the fatty tissue. A burr hole is made in the skull. The ventricular shunt catheter tip is passed through the brain into the frontal horn of the lateral ventricle. This is a direct, uncomplicated approach, ensuring accuracy of shunt catheter tip placement. The distal end of the catheter is placed in the peritoneal cavity. The shunt has a standardized, one-way flow valve unit that allows for the outward flow of cerebrospinal fluid from the cerebral ventricles into the peritoneal cavity, where it can be reabsorbed.

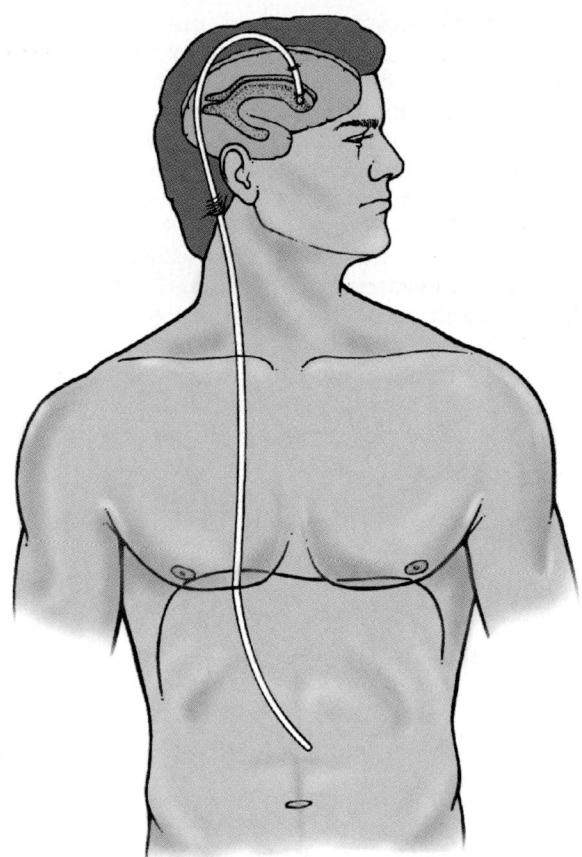

Figure 18–6
Ventriculoperitoneal internal shunt.

POSTOPERATIVE COURSE. The physician determines the progress in activity level after the procedure. The patient initially is on bed rest with the head of the bed flat or minimally raised. The patient then slowly increases activity over the following days. This allows the patient's body to adjust to the changes in pressure and return of normal cerebrospinal fluid circulation and reabsorption. Patients are usually out of bed and mobile in about 1 to 2 days.

COMPLICATIONS. Common complications of an internal shunt include infection and shunt failure. Shunt failure may be related to the following:

Blockage of the system by debris, blood, or cells
Misplacement of catheter tip end
A break in the integrity of shunt components

Shunt failure requires surgical revision of the shunt, whereas infection may necessitate externalization (an exit-site incision is made in the neck area through which the distal portion of the shunt is removed and attached to an external cerebrospinal fluid collection device to maintain outflow of cerebrospinal fluid from ventricles to collection device) of the shunt temporarily and initiation of antibiotic treatment regimen. Contamination during the operative placement of the ventricular shunt or infection

at the insertion incisional sites increases the risk of tract infections, meningitis, and peritonitis.

External Ventricular Shunts
External ventricular shunts allow for temporary regulation of intracranial pressure and control of cerebrospinal fluid flow. The external shunt is used during operative procedures and during treatment for an infected internal shunt that had to be removed. Complications and risks of external shunts include infection, overdrainage of cerebrospinal fluid resulting in cortical decompression, and underdrainage of cerebrospinal fluid resulting in increased intracranial pressure. External systems are maintained for up to 5 days. Then they are internalized to reduce the risk of infection.

NURSING PROCESS
Ventricular Shunt

Assessment

Patient assessment includes a history and neurologic examination. Check for signs of increased intracranial pressure to establish a baseline. Assess frequently thereafter for subtle changes, informing the physician immediately of progression of symptoms or complaints. Assess respiratory function by auscultating the lung fields, breath sounds, and respiratory pattern. Observe chest movements. Monitor respiratory pattern and rate. Observe for subtle changes in level of consciousness that may precipitate alteration of respiratory function.

Assess the patient frequently for signs of potential complications: increasing intracranial pressure resulting from underdrainage of cerebrospinal fluid and signs of shock resulting from overdrainage of cerebrospinal fluid.

Assess the incisional sites used for shunt placement for signs of infection. Observe for redness, swelling, and purulent drainage. Note pain or tenderness at the incisional sites and in the peritoneal area. Check the patient's temperature daily. Ask the patient about the presence of chills or other discomfort.

If the patient has an externalized ventricular shunt, assess the character and color of the cerebrospinal fluid in the drainage system. Cerebrospinal fluid is normally colorless and clear. Inspect the drainage system to ensure that the system is closed and intact. Inform the physician immediately of any complications.

Nursing Diagnoses and Planning

Nursing diagnoses and related expected patient outcomes most commonly applicable to patients after a ventricular shunting procedure include the following:

NDx: Risk for ineffective breathing pattern related to increased intracranial pressure secondary to shunt malfunction

Planning: Patient Outcomes
1. Respirations are regular and of normal rate and depth.
2. Cyanosis and other signs of hypoxia are absent.

NDx: Risk for infection related to surgical placement of cerebroventricular shunt

Planning: Patient Outcomes
1. Patient is afebrile.
2. Redness, swelling, and purulent drainage of shunt placement incisional sites are absent.
3. Signs and symptoms associated with meningitis and peritonitis are absent.

Nursing Interventions and Evaluation

NDx: Risk for ineffective breathing pattern
For patients with an external shunt, the regulation of cerebrospinal fluid flow is critical to prevent increased intracranial pressure or herniation syndrome. The external shunt has a pressure valve that helps regulate flow. However, both patient activity and changes in the patency of the drainage system can result in inappropriate outflow of cerebrospinal fluid.

Check the physician's orders for activity level, head gatch, and placement level of drainage system collection chamber. Instruct the patient regarding activity level (ie, bed rest) and limitations. Unplug electric beds to eliminate the risk of altering head gatch and placement level of the collection chamber.

Monitor the system at least once per hour for intactness and patency. Ensure that the system allows for downward flow from the externalization site to the collection chamber. Check the drainage valve every 1 to 2 hours. Inform the physician immediately if drainage is not within ordered parameters (eg, 15 mL/h).

Be aware that activities such as suctioning, turning, defecating, and chest physiotherapy increase intrathoracic pressure and therefore indirectly increase intracranial pressure, which can lead to increased cerebrospinal fluid drainage. To control the volume to be drained, plan patient care to minimize the potential of increasing intracranial pressure, and temporarily clamp tubing to prevent overdrainage of cerebrospinal fluid when indicated. Educate both the patient and visitors about the need for limitations on activities to promote compliance. Monitor respiratory status. Notify the physician immediately of any change.

Ensure that oxygen and suction equipment are at the patient's bedside and in working order. Make intubation and mechanical ventilation support equipment accessible in case a crisis arises (eg, the patient herniates and respiratory function is compromised).

NDx: Risk for infection
For patients with internal or external shunts, inspect the patient's skin at the incision sites (neck, chest, and abdomen) every 8 hours. Monitor for signs of infection: redness, swelling, and purulent drainage. Take the patient's temperature daily and when the patient complains of being uncomfortable and shivering. Keep incisional sites dry and clean. Protect them with a sterile dressing. Palpate for abdominal tenderness and check for nuchal rigidity.

Infection is the major complication of external ventricular shunts. Remember that it is critical that the system remain closed and sterile because it is an extension of the circulatory system of the patient's cerebrospinal fluid. Maintain the integrity of the system by keeping all connections secure and intact, not introducing any fluids into the system, and covering the externalization site with a sterile dressing. Monitor the color and character of the patient's cerebrospinal fluid, keeping in mind that cloudy fluid with sediment indicates an infectious process. Inform the physician of any signs of infection. Administer prophylactic antibiotics as ordered.

Compare the patient's status with the expected outcomes. If the outcomes are not met, reassess the patient and revise the plan.

CEREBROVASCULAR ACCIDENT

CVA is a broad term used to describe a condition in which blood flow to the brain is interrupted. As a result, there is temporary or permanent dysfunction of a patient's motor, sensory, perceptual, emotional, or cognitive abilities. Symptoms vary depending on the part of the brain affected.

CVA is the third leading cause of death. It afflicts 500,000 people in the United States each year. There is no gender preference, although its incidence is slightly higher in African-Americans. Incidence increases sharply with age. However, it may be preventable in some cases.

Etiology and Pathophysiology
CVA is an interruption of blood flow to the brain as a result of occlusive disease of the cerebral arteries and vessels (Fig. 18–7). This is caused by a thrombosis or an embolism. Hemorrhage, either intracerebral or subarachnoid, is also a cause of CVAs (Fig. 18–8).

A thrombotic CVA is the most common type. The thrombosis or clot develops within the vascular system in the neck or brain (ie, the internal carotid arteries). This type of CVA develops more slowly than other causes. The lumen of the artery narrows obstructing the flow of blood. A thrombotic CVA can be preceded by a transient ischemic attack.

An embolic CVA occurs when a substance or a blood clot is carried from a location in the body to the brain, where it obstructs an artery. Frequently, this embolic CVA is due to a blood clot that can result from any disease process affecting the left side of the heart. Risk factors include myocardial infarction, rheumatic heart disease, mitral valve disease, atrial fibrillation, and pacemaker failure.

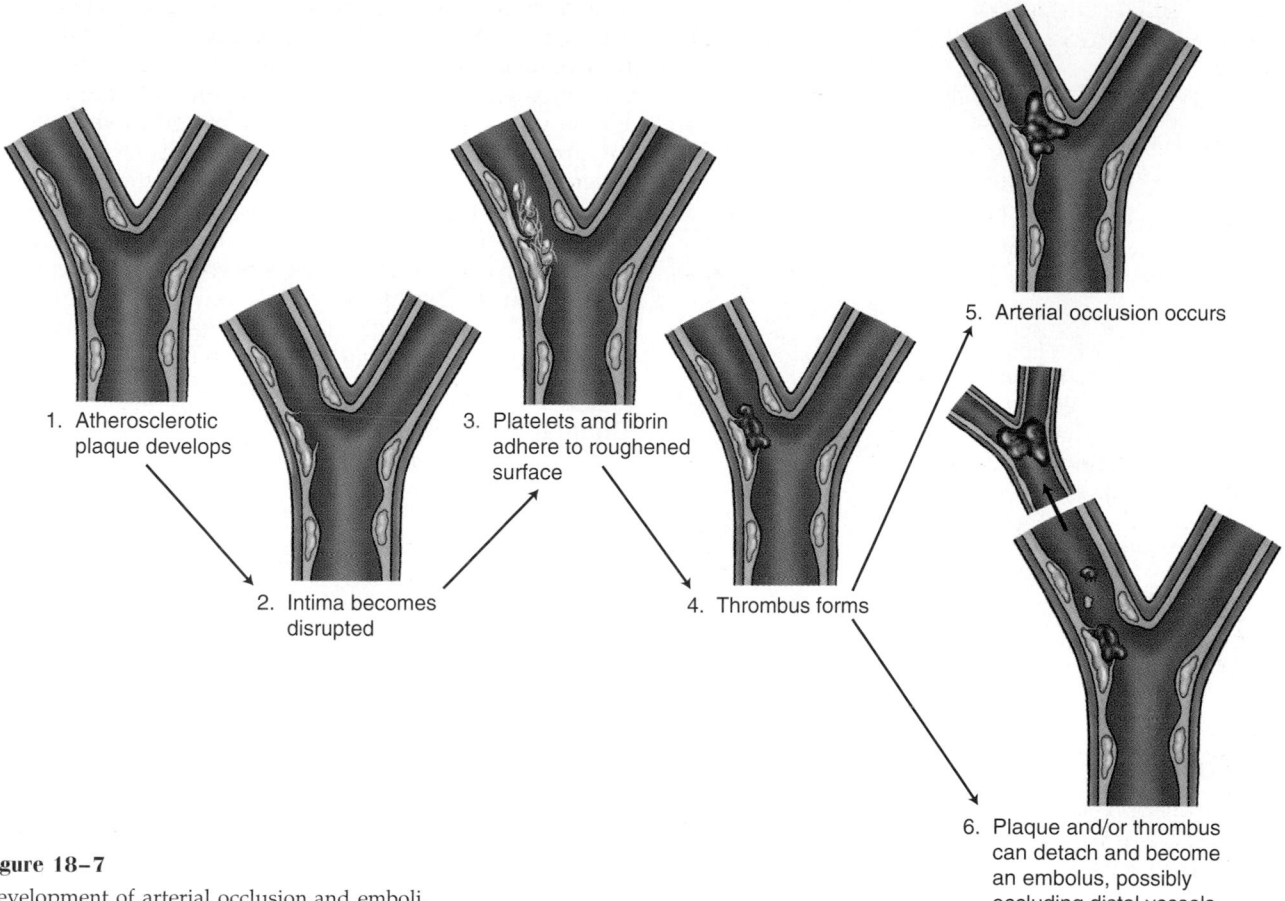

1. Atherosclerotic plaque develops

2. Intima becomes disrupted

3. Platelets and fibrin adhere to roughened surface

4. Thrombus forms

5. Arterial occlusion occurs

6. Plaque and/or thrombus can detach and become an embolus, possibly occluding distal vessels

Figure 18–7

Development of arterial occlusion and emboli.

Hemorrhagic CVAs account for approximately 15% of strokes. This includes hemorrhages that occur in the space surrounding the brain or hemorrhage within the brain itself (intracerebral). Common causes include aneurysm, hypertension, arteriovenous malformations, and hemorrhagic disorders (eg, leukemia, thrombocytopenia, anticoagulant therapy overdose).

The risk factors that predispose one to sustaining a CVA include history of hypertension, heart dis-

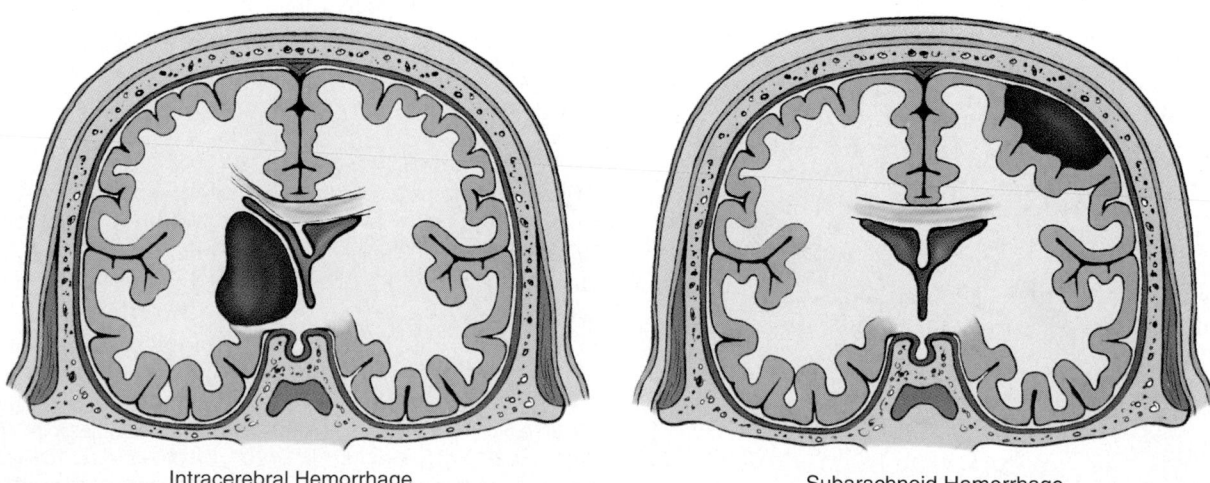

Intracerebral Hemorrhage

Subarachnoid Hemorrhage

Figure 18–8

Hemorrhage either within the brain itself (intracerebral) or in the space surrounding the brain (subarachnoid) is a cause of cerebrovascular accident or stroke.

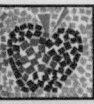

**Measures to Reduce
the Risk of
Cerebrovascular
Accident**

- Reduce or control weight
- Decrease sodium and fat in the diet
- Decrease alcohol consumption
- Control hypertension
- Comply with the medical regimen
- Cease smoking
- Control diabetes (if present)

ease, atherosclerosis, obesity, stress, smoking, hypercholesterolemia, hypercoagulopathies, polycythemia, and diabetes mellitus (Highlight 18–6).

Regardless of specific cause, the interruption in blood flow results in decreased oxygen available to an area of cerebral tissue. This leads to anaerobic glycolysis and loss of function. Cerebral ischemia, infarction, and edema may then follow.

There are four major classes of CVAs. They are transient ischemic attack, reversible ischemic neurologic deficit, progressive stroke, and completed stroke. The defining characteristics, duration, and type of deficit associated with each of these major classes of CVAs are presented in Table 18–4.

Clinical Manifestations

Neurologic symptoms are related to the severity of blood interruption and cerebral artery involved. Table 18–5 lists the clinical manifestations associated with interruption of blood flow in each of the major cerebral arteries.

Table 18–4

Classification of Cerebrovascular Accidents

Type	Defining Characteristics	Duration	Type of Residual Deficit
Transient ischemic attack	Onset and disappearance of neurologic deficit within 24 h, caused by a temporary disturbance of the blood supply to the brain	Brief episode of focal neurologic deficit Attacks sometimes occur with considerable frequency, 5–20 times daily; these should be considered as warnings of impending neurologic catastrophe Attacks typically last several minutes to 2–3 h but can last up to 24 h	No residual deficit noted
Reversible ischemic neurologic deficit	Onset and disappearance of focal neurologic deficit within 12 h, up to days Associated with cerebral emboli	Neurologic deficit persisting longer than 12–24 h	Minimal to no residual deficits
Progressive stroke	Usually severe, caused by cerebrovascular disease Results from hemorrhagic infarction, with edema or progressive thrombosis of a major cerebral vessel	Symptoms persist beyond 24 h, with an associated progressive deterioration of neurologic status	Residual neurologic deficits, most likely related to failure of collateral brain circulation
Completed stroke	Severe related to cerebrovascular disease	Condition stabilizes and neurologic deficit remains	Optimal recovery has ensued; however, a static deficit persists—the deficit is assumed to be permanent

Table 18–5

Clinical Manifestations of Interrupted Blood Flow in Major Cerebral Arteries

Artery	Clinical Manifestations
Middle cerebral artery	Contralateral hemiplegia Paralysis of the face alone or limb alone Numbness Hemianopia Dysphasia Agnosia
Anterior cerebral artery	Numbness in opposite lower limb Cognitive decline Impaired judgment and insight Bowel and bladder incontinence
Posterior cerebral artery	Alexia Mental change with memory impairment Hemianopia Cranial nerve III palsy
Internal carotid artery	Monocular blindness, fleeting or permanent
Vertebral basilar artery	Dizziness, syncope, vertigo Loss of muscle coordination Drop attacks Weakness Diplopia Vomiting Impairment of touch sense on face

The right and left hemispheres of the brain are not mirror images. Therefore, the clinical presentation of the patient with a CVA is also related to hemispheric involvement (Fig. 18–9). Left hemispheric involvement is characterized by

Dysfunction of language and speech in 95% of patients
Slow and cautious behavioral style
Motor paralysis of the right side

In right hemispheric involvement, speech and language are usually unaffected. Paralysis occurs on the left side, and there is left-sided neglect (patient ignores left side of body, unaware that it belongs to him or her). Behavioral style is quick and impulsive. The most significant recovery from a CVA occurs during the first 6 weeks after the event.

Diagnosis

A complete history and neurologic examination are performed to identify baseline functioning. Serum blood tests are performed to determine hemoglobin, hematocrit, electrolyte, and cholesterol levels to identify risk and causative factors. CT or MRI is performed to differentiate a hemorrhagic from an occlusive cerebrovascular event. Doppler studies may be performed to establish patency of blood flow. An electrocardiogram may be indicated to establish any cardiac origin of CVA.

Management

Medical management for a patient experiencing a CVA involves treatment of predisposing conditions, such as heart disease and diabetes mellitus; control of hypertension; anticoagulant or antiaggregation therapy in nonhemorrhagic events; and possibly surgical intervention.

Control of hypertension is maintained through the use of antihypertensive agents. This decreases the risk for extension of hemorrhagic stroke and promotes adequate cerebral perfusion to the brain.

Anticoagulant therapy is the treatment of choice for patients with an embolic or thrombotic cerebral ischemic event. Heparin is quick-acting and of short duration and prolongs blood clotting time by interfering with the conversion of thrombin to fibrinogen and of prothrombin to thrombin. Heparin is initiated immediately and administered intravenously with a goal therapeutic activated partial thromboplastin time value 2 to $2\frac{1}{2}$ times the control. Warfarin (Coumadin) is long-term therapy after heparin. Warfarin produces a deficiency of prothrombin and interferes with the conversion of prothrombin to thrombin. The goal therapeutic prothrombin time value is $1\frac{1}{2}$ times the control. Patients are usually on warfarin for 3 months and then maintained on aspirin. New research has presented evidence that aspirin therapy may reduce the risk of stroke by reducing inflammation in vessels rather than preventing coagulation.

Platelet antiaggregation therapy inhibits the ini-

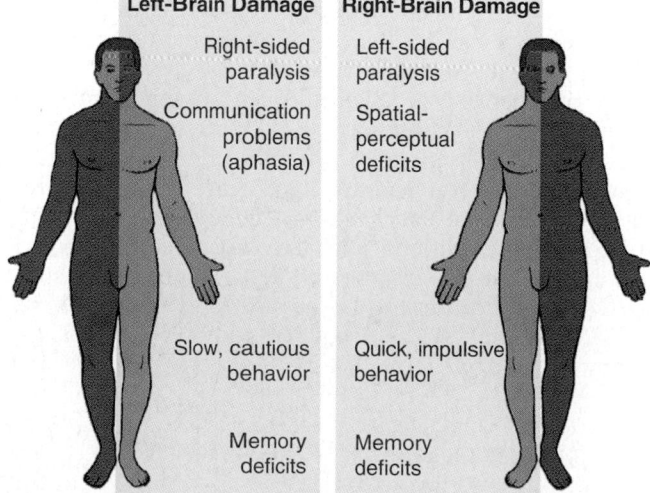

Figure 18–9

Clinical manifestations of cerebrovascular accidents affecting the left or right hemisphere of the brain.

tial step of thrombus formation. The two common medications that are effective are aspirin and dipyridamole (Persantine).

Surgical intervention may be indicated in certain cases. A carotid endarterectomy is the removal of the lining of the carotid artery. This is performed to remove a thrombus that totally or partially obstructs the carotid artery. A microvascular bypass procedure may be performed to provide an alternative route in order to supply blood, oxygen, and nutrients to an infarcted area.

❖ Settings, Providers, and Collaboration for Care

The patient who experiences a CVA is hospitalized in the critical care unit or a medical floor, depending on how extensive the damage is. Treatment continues in a transitional care or rehabilitation setting. If the patient does not progress, treatment continues in a long-term care facility or the home. Care of the CVA patient involves a multidisciplinary approach. A social worker, physical therapist, occupational therapist, speech therapist, dietitian, and possibly hospice worker should be consulted. The case manager may coordinate the care provided by the various professionals. Some of these health-care workers may begin to see the patient while he or she is still hospitalized. The social worker may help the family make financial arrangements and find resources for other needs.

In the home, the nurse evaluates the patient's progress, assists with direct care, and teaches both the patient and family about the care regimen. The patient may receive speech therapy in the home or at an outpatient clinic. The physical therapist works with the patient to increase strength, retain present function, and develop motor skills in affected extremities. The home health nurse continues to evaluate the patient's progress and encourages the patient to continue the exercise regimen. The nutritionist assists the patient and family with special dietary needs as prescribed by the physician and dictated by the patient's complications.

If the patient is admitted to a long-term care facility, the speech therapist and physical therapist usually see the patient in the institution. Staff nurses may continue the therapy and care regimen prescribed by them. A hospice agency may be consulted for the patient who is comatose or deemed terminal because of the CVA. The hospice staff works with the nursing home staff and the family to provide the special care needed for the terminal patient.

NURSING PROCESS
Cerebrovascular Accident

Assessment

Obtain a history of the onset of the present problem from the patient or significant others. Determine what the initial symptoms were, when they began, and how they progressed. Inquire about any history of similar problems. Question about the presence of risk factors such as hypertension, heart disease, smoking, and history of transient ischemic attack. Perform a complete physical assessment. Check for the following impairments:

- *Language:* Aphasia syndromes, agnosia, alexia, hemiplegia
- *Motor:* Paresis, ataxia, bowel or bladder dysfunction, dysphagia, syncope, vertigo, spasticity, nuchal rigidity
- *Sensory:* Numbness, paresthesia, spatial-perceptual dysfunctions, one-sided neglect, hemianopsia
- *Behavioral:* Impaired judgment, memory impairment, emotional instability

Symptoms of a CVA vary greatly depending on the location and extent of blockage or ischemia. The patient may experience headache, nausea and vomiting, seizures, a change in vital signs, and a change in level of consciousness.

Assess the impact of neurologic dysfunction on other body system functioning, particularly respiratory. Note any difficulty in clearing secretions, intactness of the gag reflex, breath sounds, and respiratory rate and pattern.

Assess the patient's ability to perform ADLs, to be free from injury, to communicate wants and needs, and to maintain appropriate social interaction. Observe the patient. Note any lack of completeness of tasks or unawareness of missed steps. Determine whether the patient is interpreting communication from others and responding appropriately. Assess the extent of supervision or assistance needed. Assess the need for assistive devices to facilitate self-care.

Nursing Diagnoses and Planning

Nursing diagnoses and related expected patient outcomes most commonly applicable to patients with CVAs include the following:

NDx: Risk for ineffective breathing pattern related to muscle weakness and immobility

Planning: Patient Outcomes
1. Cyanosis is absent.
2. Arterial blood gas values are within patient's normal range.
3. Bilateral breath sounds are clear.

NDx: Risk for aspiration related to dysphagia

Planning: Patient Outcomes
1. Patient avoids aspiration.
2. Mouth and airway are free of secretions.
3. Cyanosis and fever are absent.
4. Breath sounds are normal bilaterally.

NDx: Impaired physical mobility related to paralysis

Planning: Patient Outcomes
1. Patient participates in ADLs.
2. Patient ambulates, transfers, or moves self with or without assistance.
3. Complications of immobility—deep venous thrombosis, pulmonary embolism, decubitus formation, subluxation of joints—are absent.

NDx: Self care deficit: feeding, bathing/hygiene, dressing/grooming, toileting related to paralysis

Planning: Patient Outcomes
1. Patient meets self-care needs with or without assistance.
2. Patient is well groomed.

NDx: Risk for altered nutrition: less than body requirements related to dysphagia

Planning: Patient Outcomes
1. Patient maintains optimal body weight.
2. Skin turgor is good.

NDx: Unilateral neglect related to behavioral alteration caused by interruption in blood supply to right hemisphere of brain

Planning: Patient Outcomes
1. Patient acknowledges the existence of the sensory perceptual impairment.
2. Patient describes protective measures for the affected side.
3. Patient demonstrates behaviors consistent with concern for the affected side.

NDx: Risk for injury related to perceptual loss secondary to interruption of blood flow to left hemisphere

Planning: Patient Outcomes
1. Patient uses alternative strategies to compensate for sensory-perceptual loss.
2. Patient performs tasks in appropriate sequence of steps.
3. Patient remains free from injury.

NDx: Risk for constipation related to immobility

Planning: Patient Outcomes
1. Stools are soft and formed.
2. Patient passes stool regularly.
3. Patient defecates without straining.

NDx: Altered urinary elimination related to motor system dysfunction

Planning: Patient Outcomes
1. Patient is continent.
2. Patient empties bladder completely.
3. Patient is free from urinary tract infections.

NDx: Impaired verbal communication related to aphasia syndromes

Planning: Patient Outcomes
1. Patient uses effective alternative communication strategies.
2. Patient successfully communicates needs.

Nursing Interventions and Evaluation

NDx: Risk for ineffective breathing pattern
Monitor respiratory function by auscultating lung fields for breath sounds and noting respiratory pattern. Observe chest movements. Obtain vital signs. Position the patient at a 30-degree head elevation to facilitate respiratory effort. Suction the airway as necessary. Perform chest physiotherapy as needed. Encourage and teach the patient to perform cough and deep-breathing exercises every 2 hours. Provide the patient with an incentive spirometer and instruct in its use. Review the patient's arterial blood gas values.

Monitor the patient for respiratory distress and decreased level of consciousness. Administer oxygen as ordered or when patient is in respiratory crisis (shortness of breath, cyanosis). Have emergency intubation and mechanical ventilation readily available to be used in a respiratory arrest.

NDx: Risk for aspiration
Monitor the patient's ability to clear secretions from the airway and intactness of the gag reflex. Maintain working suction equipment at bedside. Elevate the patient at a 30-degree angle to facilitate drainage of secretions. Suction the patient as needed to maintain a clear airway.

Monitor patient during feeding. Suction the airway as needed to prevent aspiration. Encourage the patient to eat semisolid, soft foods, such as boneless chicken, custard, and mashed potatoes. Avoid solid and liquid foods that are difficult for the patient with dysphagia to swallow and that increase the risk for aspiration.

NDx: Impaired physical mobility
During the acute phase of care for a patient with a CVA, positioning is a major concern. Place the patient in a semiprone position with the head of the bed elevated 30 degrees to decrease intracranial pressure. Avoid positioning the patient on the affected side because of altered sensory perception. Maintain body alignment with the use of splints, trochanter rolls, and pillows.

Decrease the risk of immobility problems with range-of-motion exercises every 6 hours. Exercises should progress from passive to active. The patient needs to build strength in preparation for walking. Position the patient flat in bed and prone for 30 minutes each day to prevent flexion deformities of extremities.

Up to 70% of patients who have suffered strokes report severe shoulder pain on the affected side. Shoulder subluxation can occur. When performing range-of-motion exercises to the affected side, be careful not to overstretch the joint. When the patient is sitting, place the flaccid arm on a pillow on a table. Elevating the arm prevents edema. Encourage the patient to wear an arm sling if ordered. When transferring, never lift a patient by the affected shoulder.

CLINICAL ? THINKING

DECREASED LEVEL OF CONSCIOUSNESS IN A 74-YEAR-OLD WOMAN

The husband of a 74-year-old woman had awakened to discover that it was difficult to awaken his wife, that her speech was slurred, and that she was confused. He dialed 911 for help. The patient, accompanied by her husband, arrived in the emergency department by ambulance 45 minutes later.

In the emergency department the patient was unresponsive and pale but breathing spontaneously. As I helped transfer her to the examining table (a stretcher in the examining cubicle) and loosened the patient's night clothes, I attempted to gather as much data as possible related to her medical history and this recent event from the spouse.

He reported that the woman had been sad and withdrawn and was having difficulty sleeping since the death of her brother 5 months ago. A bottle of sodium secobarbital (Seconal) was found open and spilled near her bed. However, the husband could not estimate whether or not she had taken more than the prescribed dose, based on the number of pills remaining. The patient was not currently under any psychiatric care and had no history of suicide attempts. Her medical history did include hypertension, high cholesterol and triglyceride levels, obesity, and two transient ischemic attacks (TIAs), which occurred 18 months and 1 month ago. The husband was not aware of any cardiac, respiratory, endocrine, or seizure disorders, nor of any recent falls or infections. The patient seldom drank alcohol. Current pharmacologic therapy included Tenormin for hypertension, Mevacor for hypercholesterolemia, and secobarbital for sleep problems.

I identified numerous common medical conditions that might be responsible for a decreased level of consciousness (LOC) in a person the age of this patient. They included dehydration, hypoglycemia, diabetic ketoacidosis, hyperglycemic hyperosmolar nonketotic syndrome, myxedema coma, sepsis, cerebrovascular accident (CVA), and medication overdose. However, the patient's medical history led me to consider two likely possibilities: a drug overdose or a thrombotic CVA.

As with any patient with a compromised LOC, my priority assessment focused on the ABCs—airway, breathing, and circulation. I began my assessment by focusing on the patient's respiratory status. Her airway was clear; respirations were 12 per minute, stertorous and regular; and breath sounds were clear to auscultation. I noted no unusual breath odor. Because the patient was unre-

sponsive, I decided to maintain an open airway by inserting an oral artificial airway and by positioning her with her head to the side to facilitate drainage. Because barbiturate toxicity depresses the central nervous system and in turn leads to possible respiratory depression, and because a CVA damages cerebral tissue, leading to possible respiratory distress, I planned to re-evaluate the patient's breathing frequently. Despite her seeming lack of awareness, I explained to the patient in simple terms what I was doing, in case she could hear and understand me.

Next I checked her blood pressure (which was 172/98), apical pulse (which was 92 and regular), and temperature (which was 37°C [98.6°]). Her peripheral circulation was adequate, as evidenced by strong peripheral pulses, warm extremities, and capillary refill of less than 3 seconds. Assessment of her abdomen was unremarkable, with normal bowel sounds on auscultation. However, I did note moderate distention of the urinary bladder. At this point, the patient vomited. I initiated oral suctioning. The patient's airway remained clear. I found no evidence of pills.

Because both barbiturate toxicity and a CVA directly affect neurologic function, I next turned my attention to her nervous system. Knowing that all future neurologic monitoring would indicate improvement or deterioration, I established a baseline assessment of her neurologic status.

I began by assessing her LOC. The patient responded to loud verbal stimuli (ie, calling her name loudly) by opening her eyes and then immediately closing them again. She did not attempt to answer any of my questions and did not follow simple commands. I continued to assess her LOC further by using tactile stimuli (ie, shaking her lightly while calling her name). Again, she opened her eyes briefly but gave no verbal response. To determine her level of motor and sensory responsiveness, I progressed to painful stimuli. Using the eraser tip of a pencil, I applied pressure to the nail bed of her right thumb. She showed no response. However, when I compressed the left thumb nail, she withdrew from the pressure in a normal, purposeful manner. To validate this response, I applied pressure to the patient's supraorbital ridge. There was no motion on the right side, but her left hand reached up toward the painful site. I observed facial grimacing and noted that the right side of the patient's face appeared to be drooping. In addition, her right cheek puffed out with each respiration.

I noted spontaneous movements on the left side only, and the patient's right leg was externally ro-

CLINICAL ❓ THINKING

(continued)

tated. There was no evidence of nuchal rigidity. Upon auscultation, I heard a bruit over the left carotid artery.

Next, I evaluated the patient's pupillary reactions and extraocular movements. Her left pupil was slightly smaller than the right. Both pupils were sluggish to respond to light. I lifted both eyelids and observed that both eyes were pointing in the same direction and tended to gaze toward the left side (conjugated deviation). The doll's eye (oculocephalic) reflex was present. There was no evidence of nystagmus.

Based on my assessment of the patient to this point, I strongly suspected that she had suffered a thrombotic CVA. A significantly decreased LOC, slurred speech, and a risk of hypoventilation and respiratory insufficiency are possible findings in both a CVA and drug toxicity. However, the patient's hypertension, good peripheral perfusion, pallor, pupillary changes, absence of nystagmus, doll's eye reflex, normal temperature, and normal bowel sounds were not consistent with barbiturate overdose. On the other hand, the presence of lateralizing signs such as hemiparesis/hemiplegia of the patient's extremities, facial drooping and ballooning out of one cheek, and pupillary changes and conjugate deviation, along with the presence of a bruit, dysarthria, and hypertension, strongly supported my suspicion of a thrombotic CVA of the left hemisphere. The patient's risk factors included her age, lipid profile, and obesity. Her history of hypertension and TIAs further supported my suspicion. Finally, the development of thrombotic CVAs during sleep is common.

As I waited for the emergency department resident to examine the patient, I planned to continue assessing her neurologic status. I decided, however, to complete another check of her respiratory status first. I found that her respirations had fallen to 8 breaths per minute and were shallow. She was pale and cyanotic around the lips. As I began to auscultate for breath sounds, the patient stopped breathing altogether. There was no movement of her chest or abdomen and no airflow from her mouth or nose.

Regardless of whether the patient was experiencing respiratory depression secondary to cerebral ischemia associated with a CVA, or central nervous system depression associated with barbiturate toxicity, the treatment of her respiratory arrest was the same, and it was urgent. Recognizing that respiratory arrest is a medical emergency in which hypoxemia, hypercapnia, respiratory acidosis, metabolic acidosis, cardiac arrest, and death could

develop, and recognizing that my actions could mean the difference between life and death, I immediately implemented the following measures:

1. I called the physician and another nurse, who were nearby.
2. I checked for the patient's carotid pulse, which was present.
3. I placed a manual Ambu resuscitation mask over the patient's mouth and nose and maintained ventilation.
4. I asked the other nurse to prepare for intubation and to call respiratory therapy to set up a mechanical ventilator.
5. I assisted the physician with the endotracheal intubation.
6. I initiated oxygen therapy and established intravenous access as per verbal orders.
7. Once the endotracheal tube was inserted, I checked its placement, established correct cuff pressure, and maintained ventilation with the Ambu resuscitation bag without the mask until the ventilator was set up.
8. I raised the head of the bed to 30 degrees.
9. I attached a pulse oximeter.
10. I instituted seizure precautions.
11. I spoke to the patient to decrease her anxiety, in case she could hear and understand me.
12. I continued to monitor the patient's respiratory, cardiovascular, and neurologic status.
13. Later, I offered emotional support to her husband by explaining what had occurred and encouraging him to verbalize and ask questions.

Resuscitation efforts were successful, and the patient was transferred to the neurologic intensive care unit. The resident ordered a complete blood count, serum electrolytes, serum glucose, coagulation studies, blood and urine toxicology screens, arterial blood gases, intravenous fluids, oxygen therapy, a 12-lead electrocardiogram followed by continuous electrocardiographic monitoring, insertion of an indwelling urinary catheter, and computed tomography. Computed tomography confirmed a left hemispheric thrombotic CVA, which was treated with diuretics, anticoagulants, antihypertensives, cerebral vasodilators, and steroids.

The patient began to regain consciousness approximately 72 hours after admission and was able to respond to "yes or no" questions by blinking, nodding her head, or both. Although she was stable and improving neurologically, the prognosis regarding the extent of her recovery was uncertain at the time of her transfer to the medical-surgical unit. Further assessment and evaluation was neces-

(continued)

CLINICAL ❓ THINKING

(continued)

sary before her chances for a good recovery with moderate neurologic deficits and moderate disability could be predicted.

Think Critically

Based on the nurse's assessment of the patient upon admission, was inserting an artificial oral airway the best action? Why? Why not?

Based on the nurse's assessment in this scenario, what score would the nurse have given the patient on the Glasgow Coma Scale? How many points for each area? Why?

Was taking the time to speak to, and explain things to, the unresponsive patient the best action by the nurse? Why? Why not?

What would have been the nurse's interpretation if the patient had demonstrated posturing in response to painful stimuli?

A student nurse observing in the emergency department expresses concern over the use of painful stimuli to assess the patient's LOC. What would be your best response?

Which means of eliciting a response to painful stimuli are appropriate? Which are inappropriate? Why?

What is the significance of the doll's eye reflex? When might the assessment of this reflex be contraindicated? Why?

What additional neurologic assessments might the nurse have completed if the patient had not suffered respiratory arrest?

Could any nursing assessments or actions have prevented the onset of respiratory arrest? Should the nurse have acted sooner?

How would the nurse's actions have differed if the respiratory arrest had occurred on the medical-surgical floor rather than in the emergency department? In the community?

Was elevating the head of the bed to 30 degrees the best action? Why? Why not? How does the nurse decide between reducing increased ICP and increasing cerebral perfusion?

Shortly after the respiratory arrest, the patient's husband states, "Who knows how long she will be unconscious. . . . What she will be like if she wakes up? Maybe she would have been better off if you hadn't put her on that breathing machine." What would be the nurse's best response?

How would the treatment and follow-up of the patient have differed if the patient had ingested an excessive amount of barbiturate?

What additional immediate and long-term neurologic deficits and complications would the nurse anticipate that the patient will experience as she recovers?

With which health care disciplines would the nurse expect to collaborate when planning for the patient's rehabilitation?

What information would the nurse include in the teaching plan in order to prevent another CVA?

How would the nurse support the patient and family through the complicated process of recovery and rehabilitation in the hospital? In a rehabilitation or long-term care facility? In the home and community?

What considerations must be included when planning for the patient's discharge to the home and community following such a catastrophic illness? What community referrals would be made?

What assessments and adjustments in the home would be required in preparation for the patient's return?

Prepare the patient for ambulation by teaching standing balance and standing pivot. Encourage the patient to look at his or her extremities and assess their position prior to moving. Instruct the patient to lean toward the unaffected side.

General principles followed for patients with CVAs are as follows:

Bear weight on the unaffected side.

Always move toward the unaffected side for easiest and safest transfers.

Position the chair or wheelchair on the unaffected side and pivot to the chair on the unaffected leg.

Consult with occupational and physical therapy to obtain supportive and assistive devices.

Provide good skin care. Use an air mattress or special bed as necessary to prevent injury from immobility. Apply thigh-length antiembolic stockings to prevent venous pooling in extremities and to decrease the risk of deep venous thrombosis. Inspect the lower extremities daily for an increase in calf circumference or redness, and check for Homans' sign. Notify the physician of any change in the patient's condition.

NDx: Self care deficit: feeding, bathing/hygiene, dressing/grooming, toileting

Encourage the patient to participate actively in self-care (feeding, bathing/hygiene, dressing/grooming, and toileting). Allow the patient to perform activities to the limit before actively intervening to complete the task. Support and guide the patient in self-care attempts, but be careful to avoid overfatigue. Explore alternative strategies for the patient to meet self-care needs. Determine the level of additional support and assistance that is needed. Obtain devices to assist in the completion of self-care (eg, eating utensils, devices to assist with getting in and out of the bathtub, reaching devices).

Assess the patient's ability to recognize and see objects on the affected and unaffected side. Assess for hemianopsia. Place all equipment on the unaffected side to facilitate the patient's ability to perform activities.

To facilitate dressing, suggest that the patient use clothing one size larger than normal, use stretch fabrics, and provide a mirror to dress. This increases the patient's awareness of the affected side of the body.

Consult with social services to assist in discharge planning and identifying available resources. This allows for preparation of the home environment to promote optimal patient functioning. Special equipment (eg, commode, wheelchair, ramp, bed) may need to be purchased. In addition, the family will have the support and knowledge they require to assist the patient in caring for himself or herself at home.

NDx: Risk for altered nutrition: less than body requirements

Obtain a calorie count to establish the relationship of intake to nutritional requirements. Monitor and record intake and output. Weigh the patient initially to obtain baseline weight. Then weigh the patient weekly and note variations. Monitor the ability to tolerate feedings and intactness of the gag reflex. Place food tray on the nonaffected side of the patient. Teach the patient to chew on the nonaffected side of the mouth. Ensure that the patient is positioned at a 30-degree angle or higher during feeding. Educate the patient regarding the importance of a low-salt, low-cholesterol diet.

Consult with the nutritionist regarding patient diet, needs, and ability to ingest required calories. Identify the need for supplemental feedings or enteral feedings when the patient cannot tolerate oral feedings. Monitor the patient's tolerance of oral and enteral feedings. Notify the physician regarding intolerance and the need for parenteral or peripheral nutrition.

NDx: Unilateral neglect

Neglect of the affected side occurs more often with patients experiencing left hemiparesis with right hemisphere injury. Assess the patient's pain, touch, and temperature sensation in the affected side, as well as posture and position sense. Document any deficits noted. Approach the patient from the unaffected side and instruct the patient to scan the full visual field by turning the head toward the affected side. Place furniture, bed table, eating tray, and personal items on the non-neglected side of the patient. Sit, stand, and talk to the patient on his or her non-neglected side. Reorient the patient to the affected side. Give feedback to the patient about the neglected limb and environment. Use verbal cues, pictures, and repetitive learning opportunities. Teach the patient sitting and balancing exercises. Encourage activities that cause the patient to pass his or her midline, such as placing an object on the patient's affected side and having the patient pick it up using the unaffected hand. Encourage the patient to touch and make conscious effort to care for the affected side. Use a mirror during ADLs to draw attention to the neglected side. Place the call bell on the unaffected side when leaving the patient unattended.

NDx: Risk for injury

Monitor the impact of perceptual loss on the patient's ability to perform tasks. For example, consider whether the patient misjudges distance and hence is at risk for falling, spilling hot liquids, and the like. Encourage the patient to think through steps before initiating tasks and activities. This allows the patient to focus attention on each step of the task to decrease the risk of injury from performing the task incorrectly or impulsively. These patients are at risk for cuts, burns, bruises, and falls secondary to sensory-perceptual deficits. Establish the extent to which the patient can verbalize and perform ADLs without risk of injury or harm. If the patient is unable to verbalize or perform steps of activities, recognize that direct supervision of the patient is required. Eliminate obstructing hazards from the environment such as scatter rugs, electrical cords, and furniture.

Teach the patient alternative strategies, such as visual cues and assistive devices for ambulation, to compensate for sensory-perceptual alterations. Give one direction at a time. Break tasks into simple, one-step commands. Keep objects on the unaffected side. Approach the patient from the unaffected side. Encourage the patient to scan the entire visual field completely. Teach the patient sitting and balancing exercises.

NDx: Risk for constipation

Establish a bowel regimen acceptable to the patient that is based on the patient's usual pattern of elimination. Be aware of risk for fecal impaction. Administer stool softeners, suppositories, and laxatives as per regimen. Educate the patient regarding necessary daily roughage and fluid intake in the diet.

NDx: Altered urinary elimination

During the acute phase of care for a patient who has experienced a CVA, an indwelling Foley catheter may be inserted. Provide catheter care, monitor intake and output, and observe for signs and symptoms of urinary tract infection. The patient who is not catheterized may experience incontinence and be embarrassed by this. Initiate a bladder training regimen as soon as possible. Offer the opportunity for bladder elimination five times daily. Administer medications such as bethanechol and propantheline as prescribed to increase bladder muscle control. Check the volume of postvoid residual. Implement straight catheterization protocol if needed. Ensure a fluid intake of 2500 mL daily. Limit fluid intake after 8:00 PM.

NDx: Impaired verbal communication

Monitor the type and extent of communication deficit. The patient with left hemisphere injury is affected by aphasia, which may be temporary or permanent. Receptive aphasia (Wernicke's or sensory aphasia) is characterized by the patient's inability to comprehend the spoken word. This patient often responds to nonverbal cues. Attempt to communicate with the patient using alternative forms of communication. Written messages bypass spoken language and allow communication. Body language and gesture also improves the patient's understanding.

Expressive aphasia (Broca's or motor aphasia) is characterized by an inability to produce language. The patient understands the spoken word, knows what the response should be, but is unable to express their thoughts verbally. Expressive aphasia is frustrating to the patient. It is the most common form of aphasia. Speech boards as well as laptop computers that produce speech help the patient to respond.

Global aphasia is a combination of expressive and receptive aphasia. This patient has difficulty with interpreting verbal and written communication as well as expressing thoughts, both verbally and in writing. Injury has occurred to Broca's and Wernicke's areas of the brain.

When communicating with a patient with aphasia, reduce environmental distractions. Turn off televisions and radios. Limit environmental noise such as the conversations of others. Communicate with the patient during all contacts. Use a normal tone of voice. Face the patient and establish eye contact. Speak slowly and clearly, using simple language. Phrase questions so they can be answered with "yes" or "no." Allow the patient time to process messages and respond. Give the patient one direction at a time.

Provide a relaxed, accepting environment in an attempt to reduce the patient's stress. Be nonjudgmental and avoid labeling the patient. Use a positive and calm attitude.

Speech therapy is actively involved with the rehabilitation of the patient with aphasia. Interdisciplinary team work enhances the patient's care and improves the patient's communication. Consult with the speech therapist as needed.

Compare the patient's status with the expected outcomes. If the outcomes are not met, reassess the patient and revise the plan.

SUBARACHNOID HEMORRHAGE

Subarachnoid hemorrhage accounts for 10% of deaths from cerebral hemorrhage. Peak incidence is between the ages of 35 and 65 years.

A high mortality rate is associated with subarachnoid hemorrhage. Approximately 30% of patients die from the initial bleed, and 30% of patients rebleed within the first 2 weeks. Of the latter, only about 50% survive.

Etiology and Pathophysiology

The subarachnoid space lies between the pia mater and the arachnoid, two of the protective membranes of the brain. Cerebrospinal fluid fills the subarachnoid space to provide the protective cushion for the brain and spinal cord. A subarachnoid hemorrhage occurs when blood escapes from a cerebral artery into the subarachnoid space. Causes of subarachnoid hemorrhage include head trauma, ruptured cerebral aneurysm, hypertension, and arteriovenous malformations.

ANEURYSM. A cerebral aneurysm is an outpouching or dilation of an arterial vessel, usually found at one of the major bifurcations of the circle of Willis (Fig. 18–10).

Several types of aneurysms have been classified:

- *Berry, saccular:* Most common; congenital anomaly; has a neck to aneurysm
- *Fusiform:* Occurs in conjunction with atherosclerosis; rarely ruptures
- *Mycotic:* Embolus originates from bacterial endocarditis; as embolus lodges in cerebral vessel, inflammatory process develops and vessel wall weakens and dilates
- *Giant:* Large in diameter (greater than 3 mm); mimics a space-occupying lesion; usually has ill-defined neck

An aneurysm is often a congenital weakness in the wall of the artery. Cerebral aneurysms are usually asymptomatic until they rupture. Twenty percent of persons with a ruptured aneurysm are found to have other aneurysms.

ARTERIOVENOUS MALFORMATION. Arteriovenous malformations are congenital anomalies in which there is an entangled, ill-defined network of arterial, venous, and capillary vessels. The feeding and draining vessels of the arteriovenous malformation become tortuous and distended (Fig. 18–11).

Arteriovenous malformations are often seen in the parietal and occipital regions of the brain, but they can be found elsewhere also. They often present with symptoms of a space-occupying lesion and seizure. Seventy-two percent of arteriovenous malformations rupture by the time the afflicted person is 40 years of age.

Clinical Manifestations

The clinical manifestations in a patient experiencing a subarachnoid hemorrhage range from minor to severe neurologic deficits. The severity and extent of the deficit depend on the type of pathology, the area and extent of bleeding, and the presence and degree of vasospasm and increased intracranial pressure.

The "classic" complaint of patients with a subarachnoid hemorrhage is "All of a sudden I had the worst headache of my life." Other signs and symp-

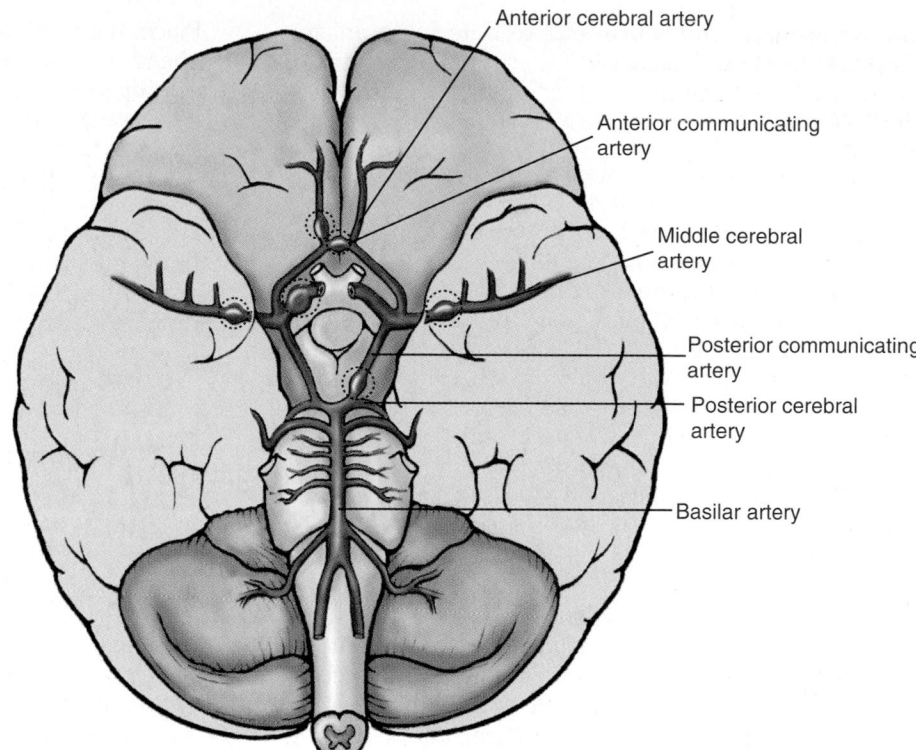

Figure 18-10
Common sites of cerebral aneurysms.

toms associated with subarachnoid hemorrhage are altered levels of consciousness (alert to drowsy), restlessness, irritability, photophobia, nuchal rigidity, nausea and vomiting, and focal neurologic deficits (eg, weakness, speech and language dysfunction, sei-

zures, sensory alterations, diplopia, hemiparesis, visual loss).

A grading system of the patient's condition has been established by Hunt and Hess. It is used to direct and determine appropriateness of medical treatment and intervention:

Grade I: Asymptomatic, minimal headache, slight nuchal rigidity
Grade II: Moderate to severe headache, nuchal rigidity, cranial nerve III dysfunction
Grade III: Drowsy to confused, nuchal rigidity, minimal focal deficits
Grade IV: Stupor, mild to severe hemiparesis, possibly early decerebrate posturing
Grade V: Deep coma, decerebrate posturing, moribund appearance

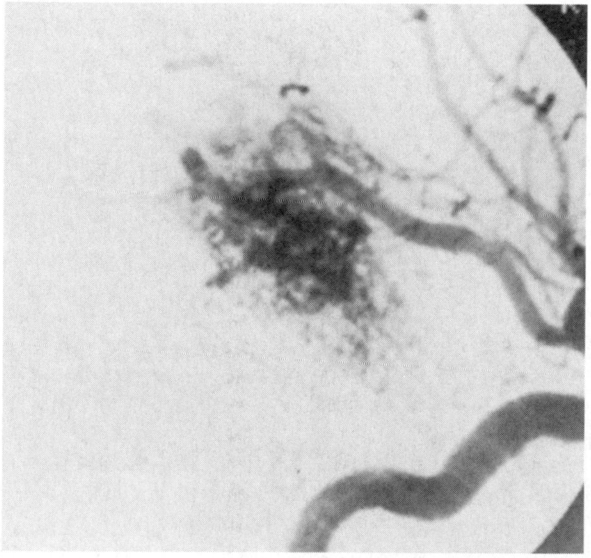

Diagnosis

A complete history is taken and a neurologic examination performed to establish baseline function. CT is performed to demonstrate the presence of a subarachnoid hemorrhage versus an intracerebral hemorrhage or infarction. A lumbar puncture is performed to confirm the diagnosis of subarachnoid hemorrhage by verifying increased opening pressure, presence of blood on a nontraumatic tap, presence of erythrocytes in cerebrospinal fluid, or xanthochromic appearance of cerebrospinal fluid.

Angiographic studies may be performed to differentiate the cause of aneurysm or arteriovenous malformation. The angiogram defines location, size, extent, and feeding vessels to the pathology. An angiogram is performed before surgical intervention to

Figure 18-11
Right internal carotid arteriogram, lateral view, showing an arteriovenous malformation supplied by a temporal branch of the right posterior cerebral artery. Arteriovenous malformations are characterized by dilated, tortuous veins and arteries that extend wedge-like into brain tissue. Blood is shunted rapidly and under high pressure through the arteriovenous malformation, leaving ischemic and necrotic areas on the adjoining cortex. (Courtesy of Grant Hieshima, MD, Radiology Department, University of California, San Francisco.)

fully investigate the cause and to determine an appropriate treatment plan.

Management

In recent years there has been a more aggressive approach to the management of patients with subarachnoid hemorrhage. It is believed that, because the mortality rate is high, prompt intervention and treatment are needed to prevent cerebral ischemia from vasospasm and death from rebleed.

Modes of medical management include the use of volume expanders, blood pressure control, antifibrinolytic therapy, and calcium channel blocking agents. Surgical interventions involve clipping or wrapping aneurysms, carotid ligation to reduce the size of or obliterate an aneurysm, and removal or induced thrombosis of arteriovenous malformations. Surgery is usually performed when the patient is graded in the Hunt and Hess system as I, II, or possibly III.

Environmental precautions for the patient with subarachnoid hemorrhage include the administration of stool softeners to prevent straining, avoidance of rectal treatments, and limitation of activities to prevent stress, elevated blood pressure, and elevating intracranial pressure.

❖ **Settings, Providers, and Collaboration
for Care**

The patient with subarachnoid hemorrhage is treated in a critical care unit. As the patient progresses, treatment takes place on a surgical floor with transfer to a transitional care or rehabilitation unit if needed. Follow-up care should be in the physician's office. If deficits remain, a speech therapist, physical therapist, and occupational therapist should be consulted. Comatose patients or patients with severe deficits may be admitted to a long-term care facility.

NURSING PROCESS GUIDELINES
Subarachnoid Hemorrhage

Complete a neurologic assessment frequently. Focus the assessment on onset, duration, and progression of symptoms, including headache, nuchal rigidity, decreased level of consciousness, motor and sensory alterations, speech difficulties, visual changes, hemiparesis, nausea and vomiting, and pupillary responses and changes. Obtain a baseline assessment of cardiac and respiratory function, and monitor for ensuing changes. Also monitor for subtle changes in level of consciousness or an increase in headache that may indicate rebleed, increasing intracranial pressure, or herniation syndrome. Notify the physician of any such changes. Ensure that oxygen and suction equipment is at the patient's bedside and in working order. Make intubation equipment and mechanical ventilation equipment accessible in case the patient herniates and sustains respiratory crisis.

Place the patient on bedrest immediately with the head of the bed elevated 30 degrees or flat, depending on the attending physician. Any activity that increases intracranial pressure is contraindicated. No enemas are permitted. Stool softeners and laxatives are ordered to prevent straining with defecation. Keep the lights dim because of photophobia. Keep stimuli to a minimum. Institute seizure precautions and administer antiseizure medication as ordered. Calcium channel blockers are administered to prevent vasospasm.

Trauma

HEAD INJURY

Trauma is the leading cause of death in persons younger than 40 years. Head trauma accounts for a significant number of these fatalities. Statistical evidence indicates that most head injuries occur in the 16- to 25-year age group, with twice as many occurrences among males as females. Vehicular accidents are the most common cause of head injury. Next most common are the following:

- Head traumas associated with alcohol and drug ingestion
- Violent acts such as gunshot wounds, stab wounds, and other blunt trauma secondary to assaults
- Sports-related injuries and falls

Recovery from head trauma is directly correlated to the type and severity of the injury sustained and the age and premorbid health of the injured person. Severe head injuries can result in a wide spectrum of disabilities for the patient, ranging from mild cognitive effects to severe functional deficits. The psychologic and financial impact for the patient and family can be devastating.

Head injury refers to an injury to the scalp, the cranium, or the brain. Frequently, the injury involves all three. The major concern in head injury is the extent of injury to the brain itself. Such injury can occur directly or secondary to other injuries.

Scalp Injury

Etiology, Pathophysiology, and Clinical Manifestations

Injuries to the scalp usually occur as abrasions, contusions, or lacerations. An abrasion of the scalp results in a scraping away of the top layer of the scalp. It is generally considered a minor injury, with minimal bleeding. A contusion of the scalp is a bruise to the scalp. The integrity of the skin remains intact. Effusion of blood into the subcutaneous layer may occur. A scalp laceration is an actual tear in the tissue of the scalp. Scalp lacerations tend to bleed

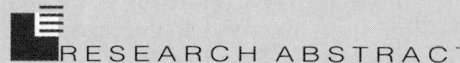

RESEARCH ABSTRACT

Does Cognitive Screening Help Prevent Disability in Young Patients with Mild Brain Injuries?

Veltman R, VanDongen S, Jones S, et al. Cognitive screening in mild brain injury. J Neurosci Nurs 1993; 25(6):367.

One of the greatest contributors to disability in young adults is motor vehicle trauma. When we think of disability resulting from motor vehicle accidents, however, we usually think of serious disability, such as that resulting from major head trauma. But each year, many young people suffer from mild disability due to trauma that requires little intensive follow-up but that nevertheless contributes to cognitive disability in the workplace.

These victims of mild traumatic brain injury sometimes fall through the cracks of the U.S. healthcare system. Because of the mild nature of their injury, they are often returned to home and work, but are unable to function. Complaints of young people with such mild disability range from headaches to inability to concentrate to slowed response time for many cognitive functions. Veltman and colleagues contend that some of this difficulty could be spared if these patients had been screened during the acute episode of their injury and if they had received appropriate follow-up care.

Veltman and colleagues therefore studied the efficacy of inpatient cognitive screening in early identification of those patients who were most likely to have cognitive difficulties after discharge from the hospital. The researchers point out that, without this screening, patients often do not discover their cognitive difficulties for 3 or more months, and that this delay extends the recuperative period and contributes to financial problems for the patients. According to the research team, early detection and intervention could help these patients return to employment and activities of daily living more rapidly and with much less disability than those who had no early intervention. The early intervention program would also help make families aware of the potential problems that may occur, so that families are not left floundering.

The investigative team concluded, "Early identification of deficits, patient and family education, reassurance, and further intervention when indicated are all imperative if persons with mild traumatic brain injury are to cope with cognitive and emotional changes and return to a productive role in society."

Questions to Consider

1. Do you think that patients with some mild form of brain injury should be screened for cognitive problems? Why or why not? Who should be doing the screening?
2. Who do you think should be involved in setting up a screening program if the hospital did not have one? Would a rehabilitation unit (referral or on-site) support such a program?
3. Imagine that you are a nurse working in a clinic. One of your patients today is complaining of headaches and inability to concentrate, leading to problems at work. You learn that the patient had been involved in a motor vehicle accident 10 months ago but that no serious problems had been diagnosed at the time. How would you handle this patient?
4. Conduct a mini-investigation of patients at a rehabilitation center to see how many are having difficulties due to a mild traumatic brain injury. Are there any? What do the staff think should be done to deal with these types of patients?

profusely because of the scalp's extensive vascularity.

Diagnosis

Injuries to the scalp are diagnosed by direct visual inspection. If underlying cerebral damage such as a skull fracture is suspected, x-ray films of the skull are obtained.

Management

No intervention is necessary for scalp abrasions. For a scalp contusion, ice applied soon after injury aids in the prevention of hematoma formation. Profuse bleeding from a scalp laceration can usually be controlled by direct pressure, but suturing of the wound may be necessary in more serious injuries. When suturing is required, the surrounding hair is shaved and the wound cleansed thoroughly with copious amounts of saline to ensure removal of any dirt or foreign material. The wound is débrided if necessary. Prophylactic antibiotic therapy is often ordered.

Skull Fractures

Etiology, Pathophysiology, and Clinical Manifestations

Skull fractures are identified as a break in the continuity of the bone in the skull. Skull fractures occur

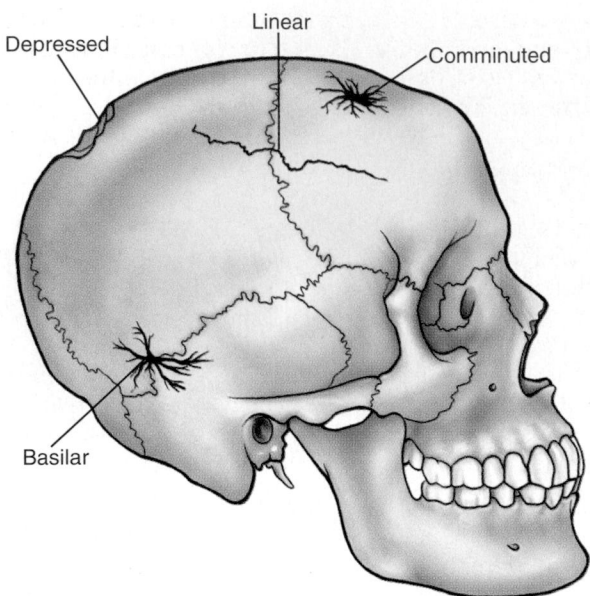

Figure 18–12

Types of skull fractures.

in approximately 7% of head injuries. Skull fractures are classified into one of four major categories: linear, comminuted, depressed, or basilar (Fig. 18–12).

Linear skull fractures account for 70 to 80% of all skull fractures. Sometimes called a simple fracture, a linear fracture resembles a single line or crack in the skull. There is no displacement of bone.

A comminuted fracture is one in which the bone is broken or crushed into small pieces. A depressed skull fracture is an inward depression of bone fragments, resulting in an indentation in the contour of the skull. Depressed skull fractures are classified as open or closed, depending on the presence or absence tears in the dura.

A basilar skull fracture occurs at the base of the skull, frequently involving the frontal and temporal bones. The dura can be torn in this type of fracture, resulting in the leakage of cerebrospinal fluid from the nose, called rhinorrhea, or from the ear, called otorrhea. Bilateral periorbital ecchymosis, called raccoon's eyes, occurs if the fracture is in the anterior portion of the base of the brain. Ecchymosis over the mastoid bone, called Battle's sign, is another clinical indication of a basilar skull fracture.

Diagnosis

CT and MRI are the diagnostic tools of choice when diagnosing skull fractures. CT allows visualization of the fracture as well as hemorrhaging and changes within the brain. Linear fractures are easily seen on x-ray film. Depressed skull fractures can generally be visualized. Basilar skull fractures are extremely difficult to visualize by radiography. The diagnosis is generally based on the clinical picture. The presence of rhinorrhea or otorrhea raises suspicion of a basilar skull fracture. Skull x-ray films or CT may disclose the presence of air in the frontal sinuses,

indicating the presence of a tear in the dura, which allows air to enter the sinus. Otoscopic examination may reveal the presence of blood or fluid behind the tympanic membrane.

Management

The treatment of a skull fracture depends on the type of fracture and the location. Skull fracture may be only one of several head injuries.

A simple linear fracture generally requires no treatment other than bed rest and close observation for underlying brain tissue injury. Depressed skull fractures require surgical intervention, usually within 24 hours of the injury, to débride the wound completely and remove any bone fragments, which may become imbedded in brain tissue or cerebral blood vessels. The depressed bone is elevated and the dura is closed if possible. Cranioplasty with insertion of acrylic bone may be performed at this time or postponed for 3 to 6 months if cerebral edema is present or if concern exists regarding infection. Dexamethasone is administered to reduce cerebral edema. Prophylactic antibiotic therapy is used for 24 to 48 hours postoperatively.

Skull fracture patients with a dura tear are closely monitored for signs and symptoms of encephalitis and meningitis. Leakage of cerebrospinal fluid indicates dura tears. All drainage is assessed for glucose. Cerebrospinal fluid is positive for glucose.

The focus in managing basilar skull fracture centers on preventing both further tears in the dura and infection, such as meningitis or brain abscess. Because activities that cause transient increases in intracranial pressure, such as the Valsalva maneuver, coughing, sneezing, and blowing the nose, may cause further tears in the dura, the patient is instructed to refrain from these activities. In addition, any procedure that requires invasion of the nasal cavity or ear canal is contraindicated. Antibiotic therapy is prescribed to prevent infection. The head of the bed is elevated 30 degrees or kept flat, depending on physician orders. Most cerebrospinal fluid leaks from dural tears resolve spontaneously in 7 to 10 days. If leakage of fluid persists, craniotomy may be necessary to surgically repair the tear.

Brain Injury

Brain injury can result from a closed head injury or from direct penetration of the cranium and brain. Brain injury can occur with any head trauma causing an interruption in the cerebral blood flow. Neurons become damaged and do not regenerate.

CLOSED BRAIN INJURY

Etiology and Pathophysiology

A closed head injury is a nonpenetrating injury to the head, usually the result of blunt trauma. There is no break in the integrity of the barrier between the intracranial cavity and the outside environment. Examples of blunt trauma include the head striking a windshield, a fall resulting in hitting or bumping the head, and a blow to the head such as occurs in assaults.

Concussion and contusion can be the result of closed head trauma. Concussion is a transient, temporary neurologic dysfunction secondary to head injury.

Contusion is an area of brain tissue into which bleeding has occurred. It differs from intracerebral hemorrhage in that the blood is dispersed rather than concentrated in one area of tissue. Contusion is the result of trauma that causes the brain to strike the internal surface of the skull. Areas of bruising or contusion directly beneath the site of trauma are described as coup injuries. Contrecoup injuries are those that occur in an area of the brain opposite the site of impact (Fig. 18–13). Contrecoup injuries are always accompanied by a coup injury but may be significantly greater. Coup and contrecoup injuries frequently follow acceleration-deceleration trauma such as occurs in automobile accidents.

Clinical Manifestations
Concussion can be classified as mild or severe. There is no structural damage. Recovery is complete. In mild concussion, there is a temporary neurologic dysfunction without loss of consciousness. Confusion and disorientation occur but clear within seconds to minutes. The patient often complains of dizziness and sees spots before his eyes.

Severe concussion, also called classic cerebral concussion, is characterized by temporary neurologic deficit associated with a brief loss of consciousness usually lasting less than 24 hours, headache, vomiting, and irritability. Recovery of consciousness is usually associated with a period of confusion and disorientation. Retrograde amnesia occurs, rendering the patient unable to recall the injury as well as the events immediately preceding the injury.

The clinical presentation of the patient with a cerebral contusion is more severe than concussion. It depends on the area of the brain that is involved and the extent of the bruising or damage. There is a loss of consciousness, with stupor and confusion and focal deficits corresponding to the area involved. Ipsilateral pupil changes, shallow respirations, weak pulse, incontinence, and cerebral edema may also occur.

Diagnosis
The diagnosis of concussion and contusion is based on the history and neurologic examination. CT is performed to rule out the presence of any underlying injury such as a hematoma.

Management
The patient who has sustained a closed head injury requires close observation for the development of symptoms of increased intracranial pressure. Observe the patient with a concussion for headache, dizziness, vomiting, confusion, and weakness. The patient is instructed to resume ADLs at a slow pace. Monitor the patient with a contusion for changes in vital signs, signs and symptoms of increased intracranial pressure, and changes in level of consciousness. Patients regain consciousness and experience residual headache, vertigo, and possibly cerebral damage resulting in impaired mental abilities and seizures. Management of the patient is individualized to the clinical picture presented. Dexamethasone may be administered to help reduce cerebral edema during the acute phase of care.

PENETRATING BRAIN INJURY

Missile injuries result in penetration of the cranium and brain tissue. Missile injuries result most often from gunshot wounds to the head. The extent of injury depends on the caliber and velocity of the bullet and the direction and action of the bullet within the cranial space.

The damage caused by a bullet includes contusion and laceration of brain tissue, hemorrhage, and cerebral edema. These effects can be localized or can occur diffusely within the brain. The consequences can be fatal. Immediate surgical intervention is necessary on arrival at the emergency room if the patient has survived the initial insult.

Complications of Head Injury: Hematomas

Head injury may be complicated by the development of intracranial hematomas. These hematomas may develop at initial injury or later. Epidural, sub-

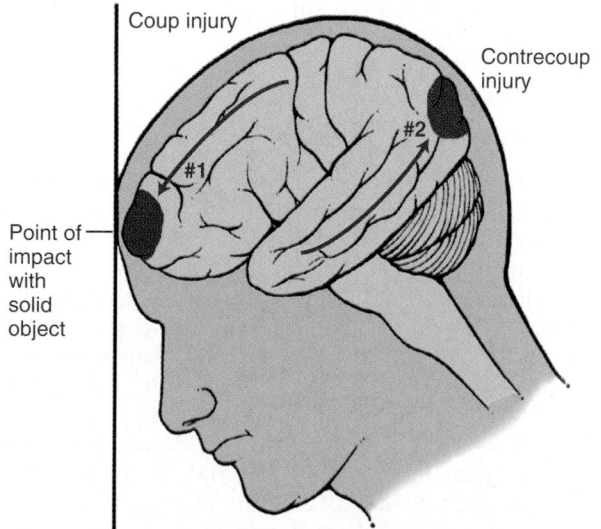

Figure 18–13

Coup and contrecoup injuries. When the forehead impacts a solid surface, the brain moves forward and the frontal lobes hit the inside of the skull and are bruised (coup injury). The brain then bounces backward, causing the occipital area to hit the inner skull and become bruised (contrecoup injury).

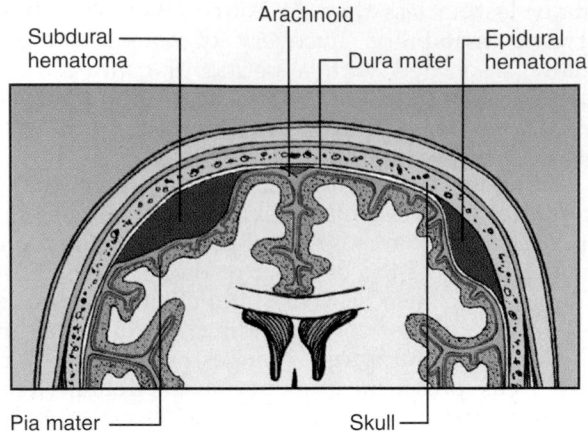

Figure 18–14

Epidural hematoma and subdural hematoma.

dural, and intracerebral hematomas are three types of intracranial hemorrhages.

EPIDURAL HEMATOMA

Etiology and Pathophysiology
An epidural hematoma refers to bleeding between the skull and the dura in the epidural space (Fig. 18–14). This creates pressure on the brain. Epidural hematomas are usually arterial in origin with rapid formation of a clot and are most frequently associated with fractures in the temporoparietal bones. An epidural hematoma constitutes a medical emergency.

Clinical Manifestations
The patient with an epidural hematoma may be unconscious at the time of the initial injury, become lucid and alert for a few hours or even 1 to 2 days, and then quickly deteriorate in level of consciousness. Headache and vomiting occur followed by ipsilateral (same-side) pupil dilation. Contralateral (opposite-side) motor paralysis with an increase in tendon reflexes, positive Babinski's sign, coma, and decerebrate posturing indicative of a herniation syndrome is an ominous sign (refer to discussion of increased intracranial pressure in Chap. 17).

Diagnosis
Emergency CT establishes the location of the hematoma. It further indicates the presence and amount of associated cerebral edema. Craniotomy may be necessary for direct visualization of the brain in order to stop intracranial hemorrhage often involving the meningeal artery.

Management
Immediate surgical evacuation is necessary. Burr holes are made. The clot is evacuated. Prognosis is considered to be better with early detection and intervention.

SUBDURAL HEMATOMA

Etiology and Pathophysiology
A subdural hematoma is bleeding between the dura and the arachnoid in the subdural space, which is venous in nature and develops more slowly than arterial hematomas (see Fig. 18–14). Subdural hematomas are categorized as acute, subacute, and chronic. Acute subdural hematomas are those that are symptomatic within 48 hours of the initial injury. Subacute subdural hematomas are those that are symptomatic from 2 days to 2 weeks after the initial injury. Chronic subdural hematomas are those that are symptomatic from 2 weeks to months after the initial injury.

Clinical Manifestations
The most common symptoms of acute and subacute subdural hematoma include signs and symptoms of intracranial pressure, headache, drowsiness, and confusion, which insidiously worsen. Ipsilateral pupil dilation occurs. Chronic subdural hematomas develop more slowly. Headache, variable levels of consciousness, personality changes, and motor weakness are noted. The mortality rate is high with acute and subacute subdural hematomas.

Diagnosis
CT is the definitive diagnostic tool to localize the lesion. The slower progression of symptoms helps distinguish between acute and chronic subdural hematomas.

Management
If a subdural hematoma is small, it is generally absorbed. Large acute subdural hematomas require surgical intervention via burr holes to drain the hematoma. Surgical removal via craniotomy may be necessary to evacuate a solid clot.

❖ Settings, Providers, and Collaboration for Care

Treatment settings for a head injury vary with the severity of the injury. The patient may be seen in the emergency department and sent home for observation and follow-up in the physician's office for mild injury. The patient with a severe head injury is treated in the critical care unit. As the patient progresses, treatment takes place on a medical or surgical floor, then in a rehabilitation unit, then in the home. If the patient's injury is so severe that rehabilitation is not beneficial, treatment takes place in a long-term care facility or the home. A multidisciplinary approach is used. A case manager may visit the patient while he or she is still in the hospital and collaborate with the discharge planner to determine what the patient's ongoing care needs should be after discharge. The team of professionals working with the patient recovering from a head injury is similar to those working with the patient with a subdural hematoma or CVA. The need for services varies with the extent of injury and prognosis.

NURSING PROCESS
Head Injury

Assessment

Head-injured patients are immobilized and presumed to have a cervical spine injury until it is ruled out. Initial assessment of the head-injured patient occurs in the emergency room. The first priority involves assessment of the patient's airway. Note the rate and depth of respirations. Ascertain the patient's level of consciousness. Assess for vital-sign changes indicating increased intracranial pressure (increasing systolic pressure and decreasing respiratory rate). An injury with bleeding and shock may cause fluctuating vital signs. Compare these data to the information available from the scene of the injury. Obtain a description of the cause of injury. Inquire about the patient's use of alcohol or drugs. Perform a baseline neurologic assessment by checking pupils for size and reaction to light and checking motor function of all four extremities. Thoroughly inspect the nose and ears for the presence of blood or cerebrospinal fluid. Note the presence of bruises, lacerations, or abrasions on the scalp, skull, and face. Determine whether the patient lost consciousness at the scene of the injury. Carefully examine the entire patient to determine the presence of other injuries. Assess the patient's and family's emotional reaction to the injury. Because deviations from the patient's baseline neurologic status can indicate the development of hematomas or cerebral edema, re-evaluate neurologic function every 2 hours using the Glasgow Coma Scale. Be alert to the development of complications following head injury, such as pneumonia, urinary tract infection, septicemia, meningitis, brain abscess, wound infection, and osteomyelitis.

Nursing Diagnoses and Planning

Nursing diagnoses and related expected patient outcomes most commonly applicable to patients with a head injury include the following:

NDx: Risk for ineffective breathing pattern related to altered level of consciousness and inadequate respiratory function

Planning: Patient Outcomes
1. Respiratory rate and depth are within normal limits.
2. Cyanosis is absent.
3. Arterial blood gas levels remain within normal limits for the patient.

NDx: Acute confusion related to cerebral injury

Planning: Patient Outcomes
1. Patient has diminished episodes of confusion.

NDx: Risk for infection related to impaired integrity of the cranium

Planning: Patient Outcomes
1. Patient is afebrile.
2. Local signs of wound infection are absent.

NDx: Ineffective individual coping related to physical disabilities, memory loss, and dependence

Planning: Patient Outcomes
1. Patient and family verbalize feelings related to loss and grief.
2. Patient and family demonstrate effective coping patterns.

NDx: Risk for altered health maintenance related to insufficient knowledge of treatment and prognosis

Planning: Patient Outcomes
1. Patient and family demonstrate knowledge of patient's condition.
2. Patient and family verbalize realistic expectations of patient's rehabilitation potential.

   Refer to the sections on Increased Intracranial Pressure and Altered Levels of Consciousness in Chapter 17 for additional nursing diagnoses that might pertain to head-injured patients.

Nursing Interventions and Evaluation

Continuous assessment is imperative. Monitor the patient's neurologic status. Report any changes from baseline immediately. Record vital signs every 2 hours. Administer medications as ordered to decrease cerebral edema. Perform interventions to control the environmental stimuli in an attempt to minimize elevations in intracranial pressure.

NDx: Risk for ineffective breathing pattern
Hypoxia and hypercarbia increase carbon dioxide levels and potentiate an increase in intracranial pressure. Maintain the patient's position on the side to maintain a patent airway. Suction the patient as necessary. Obtain arterial blood gas values. Change the patient's position every 2 hours to prevent pooling of secretions.

NDx: Acute confusion
Assess for causative and contributing factors. Promote communication—speak with a low-pitched voice at a normal volume. Confused patients can hear. Orient the patient to person, place, and time. Encourage participation in ADLs when possible. Educate the family regarding the patient's confusion. Encourage conversation with the patient. Keep the side rails up at all times when the patient is in bed. Avoid restraints, which can lead to anxiety, therefore elevating intracranial pressure. Headaches and dizziness may persist for several months after the initial injury.

NDx: Risk for infection
Injuries such as scalp lacerations, depressed skull fractures, and basilar skull fractures increase the risk of introduction of organisms. If the dura mater has

been torn or if the sinuses have been involved, bacteria can enter the cerebrospinal fluid and cause meningitis or brain abscess. Monitor the patient's temperature every 4 hours. Monitor wounds for signs and symptoms of infection, such as redness or exudate. Maintain strict aseptic technique. Do not place gauze or packing into the nose or ears. If leakage of cerebrospinal fluid occurs, loosely apply sterile gauze over the patient's nose or ears to collect drainage, then notify the physician. Administer antibiotics as ordered and evaluate their effectiveness. Monitor the patient's white blood cell count.

NDx: Ineffective individual coping

The head-injured patient may have residual cognitive deficits, memory loss, or functional impairments. Deficits in cognitive abilities may not be apparent during the acute phase of care. In the postacute phase, the patient may express frustration and alarm as deficits become evident. The patient may experience aphasia, seizures, emotional instability, judgment impairment, personality changes, and a decreased capacity for processing information. Encourage the patient and family to express feelings of grief and loss and to openly discuss concerns. Assist the patient in relearning necessary aspects of ADLs. Encourage the patient to function at the maximum of his or her capability. Avoid fostering an unnecessary level of dependence. Discourage family members from performing tasks for the patient that he or she can do or can learn to do. Refer the patient and family to social service counseling as needed.

NDx: Risk for altered health maintenance

The unanticipated traumatic event that resulted in the patient's injury may interfere with the family's ability to focus on the reality of the patient's condition. Inform the family of the patient's daily progress, focusing on realistic expectations. Encourage verbalization and questions by the family. Provide support and assistance in the family's decision-making regarding discharge and long-term care needs. Suggest utilization of community resources, support groups, and home care services for the patient and the family.

Compare the patient's status with the expected outcomes. If the outcomes are not met, reassess the patient and revise the plan.

SPINAL CORD INJURY

Traumatic spinal cord injury affects 12,000 persons yearly. Statistics indicate that 62% of spinal cord injury victims are between the ages of 15 and 30 years. The causative factors include vehicular accidents, falls, sports injuries, and gunshot wounds. Advances in technology have increased the average expected life span after spinal cord injury to 30 to 40 years. The economic impact associated with spinal cord injuries is major.

Etiology and Pathophysiology

Trauma to the spinal cord is produced by compression of the spinal cord. Spinal cord injury can occur at any point along the spinal column and can vary in severity. Damage can range from concussion to complete transection of the cord.

Injuries involving cervical vertebrae above C-4 are prone to respiratory failure, and paralysis affects all four extremities. Injuries at C-3 and above are generally fatal injuries. Quadriplegia is defined as an injury to T-6 or above. All four extremities are affected by these injuries. Paraplegia is defined as an injury to T-7 or below. This injury affects the lower extremities.

Injuries to the spinal cord are usually the result of a force exerted on the vertebral column, which in turn affects the spinal cord. The areas of the vertebral column most vulnerable to injury are the cervical and lumbar areas. These injuries may or may not cause fractures of the vertebrae.

Closed Injuries

HYPERFLEXION INJURIES. Hyperflexion injuries are the result of extreme flexion of the spine beyond its normal range of motion (Fig. 18–15). Two common illustrations of this type of injury are (1) sudden deceleration in a head-on vehicular collision and (2) diving into shallow water. In flexion injuries, a wedge or compression fracture of the vertebral body is common. The fracture may be dislocated forward onto the lower vertebrae. The degree of damage to the spinal cord is determined by the extent of compression caused by the dislocated or fractured vertebrae. Hyperflexion injuries occur most often in the cervical and lumbar areas.

HYPEREXTENSION INJURIES. Hyperextension injuries are caused by extension of the head and neck, which stretches the spinal cord and causes contusion and ischemia (Fig. 18–16). As a general rule, no fractures or dislocations occur, but the contusion

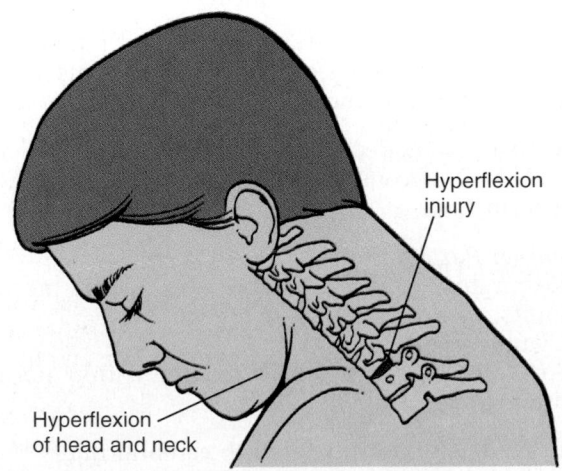

Hyperflexion injury

Hyperflexion of head and neck

Figure 18–15

Hyperflexion spinal injury.

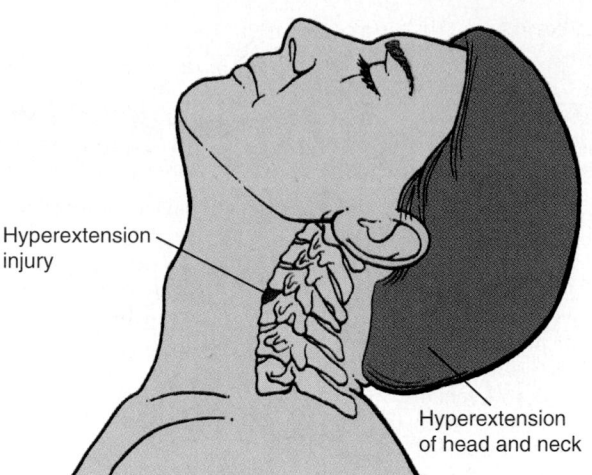

Figure 18–16
Hyperextension spinal injury.

and ischemia may produce severe damage to the spinal cord. Examples of this type of injury include falls that involve striking the chin and rear-end vehicular collisions. A less severe form of hyperextension injury is called a whiplash or acceleration injury in which there is stress and strain to the soft tissue but no vertebral or cord injury. Hyperextension injuries occur most frequently in the cervical area.

SUBLUXATION INJURIES. A subluxation deformity is a partial or incomplete dislocation of one vertebra over another. Injury to the spinal cord may or may not occur.

COMPRESSION INJURIES. Compression injuries may occur secondary to falling from a height and landing on the feet or buttocks (Fig. 18–17). There is compression of lower thoracic and lumbar vertebrae severe enough to produce a burst-type fracture. Fragments of the burst vertebra can compress a portion of the cord.

SPINAL CORD SYNDROMES. Several syndromes are often associated with spinal cord injuries. These syndromes are described in Table 18–6.

Open Injuries
Open or direct injuries to the spinal column may be caused by missile wounds (gunshot wounds) or stab wounds. Both these injuries may result in lacerations and transection or severing of the spinal cord. Direct injury to the spinal cord causes a loss of function below the level of the area injured.

The close anatomic relationship among the vertebrae, ligaments, intervertebral disks, and spinal cord predisposes injury in one of these structures to directly affect one or all of the other structures. Whenever injury has occurred, edema of the spinal cord occurs, similar to the response of injured tissue in other parts of the body. The functional ability of the spinal cord may be temporarily inhibited until the edema has resolved, at which time spinal cord func-

tion may return as long as irreversible damage has not occurred.

Clinical Manifestations
The symptoms exhibited by the patient with spinal cord injury depend on the type of injury sustained and, most importantly, the amount of compression or injury to the spinal cord. Transection of the spinal cord, either complete or incomplete, results in spinal shock, which is an immediate response to acute spinal cord injury. Spinal shock is a state of reflex suppression below the level of the injury, both visceral and somatic. Following the injury, impulses cannot descend below the injured site and impulses cannot ascend from the injured site to the brain. The result is flaccid paralysis of skeletal musculature and absence of sensation below the level of the lesion. Urinary and fecal retention occurs. Blood pressure is unstable and lowered as a result of the loss of vasomotor tone. Perspiration is absent below the level of injury. If the injury occurs above C-4, the muscles responsible for respirations are paralyzed. In males, priapism, an abnormal, painful, and continuous erection of the penis, may occur because of venous congestion.

The symptoms of spinal shock may last from a few days to months depending on the severity of the injury. Generally, spinal shock lasts for about 1

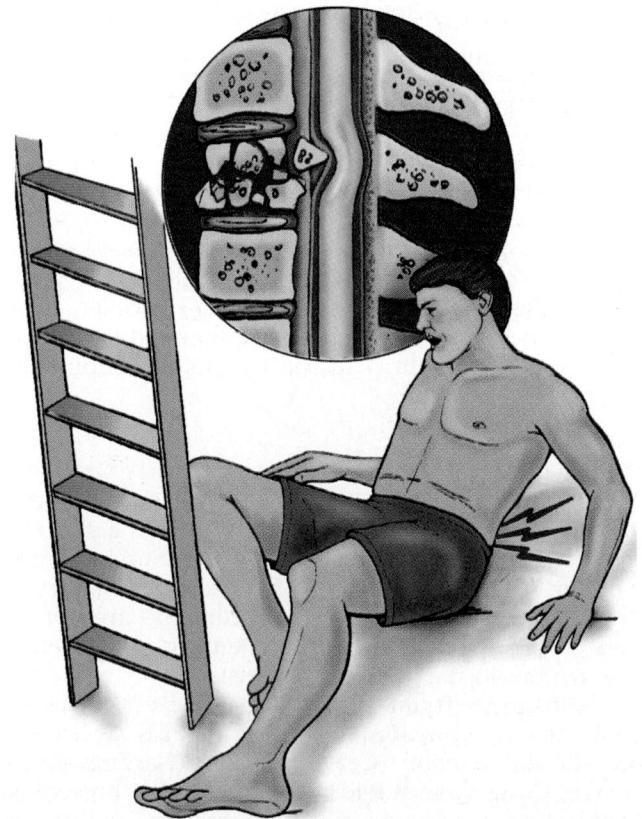

Figure 18–17
Compression spinal injury.

Table 18–6

Spinal Cord Syndromes

Syndrome	Cause	Clinical Manifestations	Treatment
Anterior cord syndrome	Herniated disk Hyperflexion injuries with fracture or dislocation	Loss of sensation, pain, and motor function below the lesion	Surgical decompression
Brown-Séquard syndrome (lateral cord syndrome)	Hemisection of the cord	Paralysis on the same side as the lesion, with loss of position and vibratory sense	Management of fracture and/or dislocation
Central cord syndrome	Hyperextension injuries	Motor and sensory loss, more severe on the upper extremities; bowel and bladder function variable	Mobilization Steroids
Horner's syndrome	Lesion involving the cervical sympathetic nerve trunk	Pupillary constriction, ptosis, and loss of sweating on the affected side of the face	

to 6 weeks. Recovery from spinal shock is a gradual process. There are two possible expected outcomes:

• Return of motor, sensory, and autonomic function
• Development of automatic spinal reflex activities, resulting in various degrees of spasticity

Patients may recover gradually and completely from spinal shock or have varying degrees of disabilities and paralysis secondary to the injury.

Diagnosis
The diagnosis of spinal cord injury is based on neurologic examination and x-ray films of the vertebral column. Special techniques may be necessary to view the cervical area. CT and myelography assist in defining specific areas of injury. However, these tests may not be feasible because they require movement of the patient, causing possible manipulation of the spinal column.

Management
The management of the patient with a spinal cord injury depends on the type of injury as well as any other associated injuries. Treatment may be surgical, nonsurgical, or a combination of both. Surgical intervention is indicated if bone fragments secondary to fractures need to be removed from the area of injury, if cord compression is evident, or if a penetrating wound to the spinal cord exists.

Nonsurgical treatment includes the use of immobilization and traction. Cervical fractures are treated by skeletal traction. Cervical tongs (Gardner-Wells, Vinke, Cone, Crutchfield) are used with a prescribed amount of weight to provide traction and to reestablish alignment of the vertebrae. The halo device

is used to provide skeletal fixation to the cervical area. The halo device may be used as skeletal traction, similar to cervical tongs, or it may be used with a body vest or jacket, which decreases the length of hospitalization because it allows the patient to be ambulatory. (See Chap. 19 for illustrations of these devices.)

❖ Settings, Providers, and Collaboration for Care
Treatment settings for a spinal cord injury vary with the severity of the injury. The patient may be seen in the emergency department and sent home for observation and follow-up in the physician's office for mild injury. The patient with a severe spinal cord injury is treated in the critical care unit. As the patient progresses, treatment takes place on a medical or surgical unit, then in a rehabilitation unit, then in the home.

Rehabilitation focuses on restoring the patient's motor function and helping the patient to maintain independence. If the patient's injury is so severe that rehabilitation is not beneficial, treatment takes place in a long-term care facility or the home. A multidisciplinary approach is used. A social worker, physical therapist, and occupational therapist should be consulted, depending on the particular needs of the patient. A home health service can provide assistance with the patient's personal care needs.

When the patient has a spinal cord injury with resulting paralysis, the emotional trauma for both the patient and the family is severe. Referral to a counselor or clergy may help the patient and family cope with the changes in lifestyle and the disabilities of the patient.

NURSING PROCESS

Spinal Cord Injury

Assessment

Initial assessment of the patient who has sustained a spinal cord injury occurs in the emergency room. The first priority is establishing immobilization of the spinal column. Gather information related to the exact nature of the traumatic incident. Ensure that the neck is securely immobilized and that the lower spine is in alignment. Never move the patient unless a physician is present and a sufficient number of trained staff members are available to transfer the patient correctly by log-rolling or lifting. Assess the patency of the airway and the rate and depth of respirations. Cervical injuries above C-4 can produce pulmonary complications. The patient may need ventilatory assistance. Assess the patient's neurologic function to establish a baseline for subsequent evaluations. Be alert to symptoms of deterioration in the patient's neurologic functioning. Observe motor strength, sensation, and reflexes. Assess vital signs. Note blood pressure, pulse, and elevation of temperature secondary to autonomic disruption. Assess for symptoms of spinal shock (falling blood pressure, loss of reflexes). Palpate the bladder for distention. Assess the patient's gastrointestinal status. Bowel sounds may be absent because of paralytic ileus.

Determine whether the patient ingested alcohol or other drugs. Assess the patient's level of anxiety and ability to comprehend the severity of the present circumstances. Note the patient's and family's emotional reaction to the injury.

Assessment of complications of spinal cord injury is ongoing. Autonomic dysreflexia can occur. This happens when a massive sympathetic discharge from the autonomic nervous system occurs in response to a stimuli. Norepinephrine is released, causing vasoconstriction. The patient experiences hypertension, bradycardia, and profuse sweating above the level of the injury. The patient may have cyanosis below the level of the injury because impulses cannot get by the level of the injury. The most frequent cause of autonomic dysreflexia is bowel distention, bladder distention, or both. Assessment of Foley tubing, palpation of the bladder, and assessment of the bowel are indicated. The patient may experience a CVA if autonomic dysreflexia goes untreated. Monitor the patient closely. If hypertension occurs, elevate the head of the bed to 90 degrees to lower the blood pressure. If the bowel is impacted, stool should be removed manually. Once the bowel is clear, place the patient on an aggressive bowel regiment to prevent recurrence. Other possible causes of autonomic dysreflexia include drafts, heat, cold, pain, and injury. Remove any stimuli that may cause or trigger autonomic dysreflexia.

Nursing Diagnoses and Planning

Nursing diagnoses and related expected patient outcomes most commonly applicable to patients with a spinal cord injury include the following:

NDx: Risk for ineffective breathing pattern related to impaired function of the diaphragm secondary to spinal cord edema

Planning: Patient Outcomes
1. Patient has clear bilateral breath sounds.
2. Arterial blood gas values remain within normal limits for the patient.
3. Patient remains free from pulmonary complications.

NDx: Risk for injury related to unstable vertebral column

Planning: Patient Outcomes
1. Baseline neurologic function is maintained.
2. Immobilization device is correctly maintained.

NDx: Impaired physical mobility related to motor and sensory deficits and spinal instability

Planning: Patient Outcomes
1. Joint flexibility is maintained.
2. Patient demonstrates ability to cope with limitations.

NDx: Risk for infection related to skeletal traction

Planning: Patient Outcomes
1. Signs of infection at pin sites are absent.

NDx: Reflex incontinence/Urinary retention related to bladder atony secondary to sensory motor deficits

Planning: Patient Outcomes
1. Patient empties bladder without residual and retention.
2. Patient remains free from urinary tract infection.

NDx: Constipation related to decreased peristalsis and decreased ability to defecate voluntarily

Planning: Patient Outcomes
1. Patient evacuates soft, formed stool at regular intervals.
2. Patient is free from impaction.

NDx: Anticipatory grieving related to anticipated losses secondary to sensory-motor deficits

Planning: Patient Outcomes
1. Patient verbalizes anger.
2. Patient verbalizes perceptions of loss as it relates to himself or herself.
3. Patient discusses concerns about sexuality.

Nursing Interventions and Evaluation

NDx: Risk for ineffective breathing pattern
Maintain a patent airway with proper positioning and suctioning as needed. Auscultate the patient's

breath sounds every 2 to 4 hours. Encourage coughing and deep-breathing exercises every 2 hours to mobilize secretions. Instruct the patient in the use of incentive spirometry. Obtain vital capacity measurements every 6 to 8 hours. Use an air mister or vaporizer to provide humidity and to assist in breaking up secretions. Administer oxygen as ordered. Obtain arterial blood gas values and pulse oximetry readings.

Patients who have sustained a cervical injury are at risk for development of pulmonary complications. Be alert to changes in respiratory status—prepare for possible intubation and ventilation support. Assess for possible pulmonary embolism. With a high-level injury, be aware that the patient may not experience chest pain (no sensation below the level of the injury). Assess for shortness of breath, tachycardia, and adventitious breath sounds. Report to the physician if symptoms of pulmonary embolism are present.

NDx: Risk for injury

Injury to the vertebral column can cause compression of the spinal cord if stabilization of the vertebral column is not adequate. Spinal cord compression results in worsening of any neurologic deficits. Traction is used to re-establish and maintain alignment. Cervical traction provides stability to the cervical spine. Maintain the traction weights at the ordered level. Ensure that they are free-hanging and not resting on the floor or the headboard. When positioning the patient on his or her side, log-roll the patient. Use adequate help to maintain proper alignment of the head and neck. Assess for skin breakdown. Report any deterioration in motor or sensory function immediately. Assess pins, bolts, and vest structure (with halo traction) for looseness. Do not attempt to tighten—notify the physician immediately. If the patient in a halo vest is ambulatory, caution the patient that the trunk of the body is limited in flexibility. The patient should wear rubber-soled shoes and use a walker until he or she develops a steady gait.

NDx: Impaired physical mobility

Immobilization of an unstable spinal column places the patient at risk for contracture deformities if motor function is severely impaired. The immobile patient whose activity is restricted is at risk for venous stasis. Maintain the patient in proper alignment at all times. Use supports such as hand rolls or trochanter rolls. Initiate passive range-of-motion exercises every 4 hours. Instruct the patient who is able to move the extremities independently in active range-of-motion exercises. Apply an antiembolic hose. Remove the hose every 8 hours to assess skin integrity and circulatory status. Apply posterior splints or high-top sneakers to lower extremities to prevent foot drop. Instruct the patient to avoid stimuli that trigger spasms, such as fatigue, anxiety, extremes in temperatures, and emotional stress.

NDx: Risk for infection

Inspect the skin around the pins of the cervical traction device or halo vest every 8 hours for redness or drainage. Cleanse the area daily according to the specified order for pin care. Maintain aseptic technique. Inspect the pins sites to ensure that they are secure.

NDx: Reflex incontinence/Urinary retention

Loss of bladder tone results from spinal shock, necessitating an indwelling Foley catheter. Once spinal shock has subsided, bladder function may become spastic, predisposing the patient to urinary tract infection.

Maintain accurate intake and output records. Force fluids to ensure an intake of 3000 mL in 24 hours to prevent the formation of urinary tract calculi. Obtain urinalysis, culture, and sensitivity samples as necessary. Spinal cord–injured patients are at risk for urinary tract infections. Provide catheter care twice a day. Tape the catheter to prevent traction on the meatus. If an intermittent catheter regimen is begun, maintain strict aseptic technique. Monitor the patient's temperature every 8 hours. Administer medications such as prophylactic sulfa drugs (sulfisoxazole [Gantrisin]) or internal acidifiers (vitamin C) if ordered. Instruct the patient to avoid caffeine in the diet. It may contribute to reflex incontinence and bladder spasms.

NDx: Constipation

Encourage fluids and foods high in fiber and roughage to stimulate peristalsis. Consult with the dietitian and the patient to determine what food the patient likes and dislikes. Administer stool softeners, bulk producers, and lubricants as ordered. A bowel-training regimen may be instituted once the patient is considered stable. This often includes daily use of a medicated suppository if necessary.

NDx: Anticipatory grieving

Encourage the patient to verbalize fears regarding loss of independence. Allow the patient to express anger. Decrease environmental stress by providing for continuity of care, privacy, and adequate rest periods. Allow the patient to grieve in his or her own way. Provide simple, concrete explanations. Encourage the patient to make choices and become involved in decision-making in care whenever feasible. Provide support and understanding when angry feelings are expressed. Perceived loss of sexual function can occur, resulting in grieving of the loss.

Spinal cord injuries often occur in young adults. Provide a supportive environment and encourage the patient to express concerns regarding sexuality. Male patients experience reflex erections but may not be able to ejaculate. Female patients may experience adductor spasm. Patients can be told that sexual expression is possible but different with spinal cord injury. Counseling is advised regarding modification in positions, techniques, alternative methods of gratification, and suggestions for managing common problems related to sex. The patient's sexual capabilities are generally known approximately 6 months after the injury.

Compare the patient's status with the expected outcomes. If the outcomes are not met, reassess the patient and revise the plan.

PERIPHERAL NERVE INJURY

Etiology and Pathophysiology
Peripheral nerve trauma can result from the following:

    Partial or complete severing
    Contusion
    Stretching
    Compression
    Ischemia
    Electrical, thermal, and radiation injuries
    Drug injection

A partially or completely severed nerve is usually the result of a sharp cutting instrument. Regeneration is possible in certain circumstances. Contusion to a nerve is the result of direct blows to the nerve, gunshot wounds, or fractures near the nerve. The nerve remains structurally intact, but complete functional ability is impaired. A stretch trauma to a nerve occurs secondary to extreme movement and excessive application of weight such as in orthopedic traction. Compression injury to a nerve is caused by extreme or prolonged pressure on a nerve. Examples include tumors, a herniated intervertebral disk, and narrowed, bony foramina, causing nerve entrapment. Ischemia deprives a nerve of an adequate blood supply. Electrical, thermal, and radiation trauma injuries occur if an electrical wire comes in contact with a peripheral nerve, causing burning and necrosis. An injection of a drug into or near a peripheral nerve causes necrosis and scarring. The sciatic and radial nerves are most commonly affected secondary to improper intramuscular injection techniques.

The most common traumatic syndromes affecting peripheral nerves include the following:

- Brachial plexus injury
- Upper-extremity injuries to the ulnar, radial, or medial nerves (carpal tunnel syndrome)
- Lower-extremity injuries to the femoral, sciatic, and common perineal nerve

When a nerve in the central nervous system is transected, the entire neuron degenerates because the cell nucleus has been injured. Scar tissue forms secondary to degeneration of the axon. However, if a peripheral nerve has been severed, self-repair is possible. In the proximal axon, tiny unmyelinated sprouts begin to form, enlarge, and join together. These joined sprouts grow at the rate of 1 to 4 mm per day to cross the gap to the distal axon (Fig. 18–18). If realignment is successful, remyelination occurs, growth of the severed axon continues, and eventually 80% of the nerve's former capacity may return.

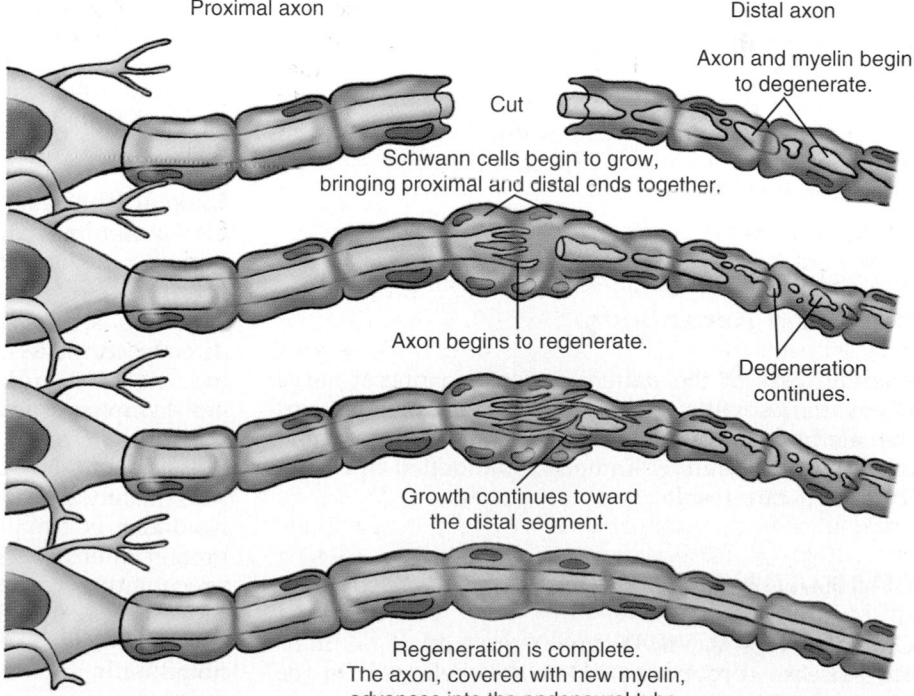

Figure 18–18
Example of nerve fiber regeneration after severing.

Proximal axon

Distal axon

Axon and myelin begin to degenerate.

Cut

Schwann cells begin to grow, bringing proximal and distal ends together.

Axon begins to regenerate.

Degeneration continues.

Growth continues toward the distal segment.

Regeneration is complete. The axon, covered with new myelin, advances into the endoneural tube.

Clinical Manifestations

The signs and symptoms of a peripheral nerve injury include flaccid paralysis or paresis of the muscles supplied by the nerve, loss of reflexes in the affected area, loss of muscle tone, and diminished or complete loss of sensation.

Diagnosis

Diagnosis of peripheral nerve injuries is based on the history and neurologic examination. Electromyography and nerve conduction studies aid in determining the intactness of the nerve. Tinel's sign also indicates nerve function. To elicit this sign, percussion is applied over the site of a divided nerve. A tingling or painful sensation is perceived at the distal end of the limb involved. This may indicate the beginning of regeneration of the nerve.

Management

Primary nerve repair is usually scheduled to take place 3 weeks after the injury. Anastomosis of a severed nerve requires the two nerve segments to be dissected to remove scar tissue and aligned so that the slow regeneration process can occur. This may require the patient to have the extremity positioned in exaggerated flexion by a cast or splint. Cable grafting with autologous nerve tissue is a newer surgical technique that may eliminate the need for the exaggerated flexion.

The recovery process is often long and tedious for the patient. The primary concern is joint stiffness and muscle atrophy, which begin almost immediately after injury. A vigorous physiotherapy program is necessary. Daily use of electrical stimulation to the affected muscles, instituted as soon as possible after injury, may facilitate the rehabilitation process.

❖ Settings, Providers, and Collaboration for Care

Treatment for peripheral nerve injuries is usually performed in an outpatient setting unless surgical intervention is required. Speech therapy may be consulted if needed.

NURSING PROCESS GUIDELINES
Peripheral Nerve Injury

Nursing care of the patient with a peripheral nerve injury varies with the specific nerve involved and the method of treatment. In most cases, movement of the affected limb is limited. Some deficit in mobility or self-care results.

CRANIAL NERVE DISEASE

Cranial nerves V, VII, IX, and X are subject to different disease processes. Most are believed to be caused by infection or trauma, but this is not established. Trigeminal neuralgia (tic douloureux), Bell's

palsy, Menière's disease, and glossopharyngeal neuralgia are described in Table 18–7.

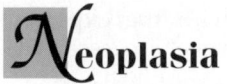

Neoplasia

BRAIN TUMORS

Intracranial tumors occur as either primary tumors or secondary (metastatic) tumors. Primary brain tumors arise or grow from brain tissue. Primary brain tumors occur in people of all ages but are statistically more prevalent in children and middle-aged adults.

Secondary or metastatic brain tumors arise from tissue elsewhere in the body and seed or spread to the brain. The most frequent sites of the primary malignancy are the lungs, breast, skin, gastrointestinal tract, and kidneys. Metastatic brain tumors are more commonly found in the adult population.

Etiology and Pathophysiology

The cause of primary brain tumors is unknown. Environmental agents, familial tendencies, viral implications, and others may be related.

A brain tumor, similar to any other tumor or neoplasm, is an abnormal mass resulting from the excessive multiplication of cells. Brain tumors can grow either as a spherical mass or in a diffusely infiltrating manner, invading surrounding brain tissue without any mass formation. Tumor growth results in compression and invasion of surrounding structures, causing pathophysiologic changes in the brain. Edema develops in the vicinity of the tumor. Signs of increased intracranial pressure are evident as the tumor expands.

Table 18–8 classifies brain tumors according to name, origin, and most frequent sites of development.

Clinical Manifestations

The symptoms exhibited by the patient with a brain tumor can be either focal or generalized. Focal symptoms result from direct compression of surrounding structures. The signs and symptoms are directly correlated to the location. Headache, vomiting, visual disturbances, and papilledema are general symptoms associated with most intracranial tumors.

Headache is the only presenting symptom in approximately 20% of patients with brain tumor. The headache is usually intermittent and presents with greater intensity in the morning. Vomiting without a precipitating cause is the initial symptom in about 10% of patients with a brain tumor. Vomiting indicates increased intracranial pressure. Papilledema, noted only by visualizing the optic disk with an ophthalmoscope, is present in about 70 to 75% of patients with brain tumors. The optic disk is blurred rather than sharply defined, indicative of an early rise in intracranial pressure.

Other signs and symptoms that may occur include personality changes, decrease in intellectual abilities, and seizures, which indicate irritation of the cerebral cortex.

Diagnosis

History and physical examination are the initial steps taken in diagnosing brain tumors. Important data are gathered that assist in ruling out diseases that present with similar symptoms. Skull x-ray film, CT, and MRI provide information regarding the size and location of the tumor as well as the presence of any bone erosion. Cerebral angiography indicates any displacement of cerebral blood vessels by the invading tumor. Chest films rule out carcinoma of the lung as a primary site. Specific diagnostic procedures are used if the presenting symptoms suggest localized areas of tumor growth. Examples include audiometric testing if an acoustic neuroma is suspected or endocrinologic studies if a pituitary tumor is suspected.

All patients should undergo funduscopic examination to assess for the presence of papilledema. Lumbar puncture should be avoided and may be contraindicated if intracranial pressure is increased.

Management

Once the diagnosis of brain tumor has been established, the medical management of the patient most often involves surgery, radiotherapy, or chemotherapy alone or in combination. Surgical intervention via a craniotomy approach is the recommended

Table 18–7

Cranial Nerve Disorders

	Trigeminal Neuralgia (Tic Douloureux)	Bell's Palsy	Menière's Disease	Glossopharyngeal Neuralgia
NERVE INVOLVED	Trigeminal	Facial	Acoustic (vestibular and cochlear branches)	Glossopharyngeal
ETIOLOGY	Unknown	Unknown—possibly due to viral or immune disease	Unknown	Unknown
CLINICAL MANIFESTATIONS	Attacks of intense, sudden pain in areas innervated by the trigeminal nerve: upper and lower jaw, teeth, cheeks, hard palate, tongue, paranasal and maxillary sinuses, forehead, nose, eyes, and temples There may be muscle spasms in the areas involved	Weakness of an entire half of the face Paralysis of the ipsilateral facial muscles Inability to close the eye on the affected side Pain, drooling, decreased taste, and increased tearing may occur	Tinnitus Vertigo Deafness Fullness May result in complete deafness	Sudden, intense pain in the back of the throat, tonsils, and middle ear
TREATMENT	Phenytoin (Dilantin) or carbamazepine (Tegretol) suppresses or shortens attacks Injection of the nerve with alcohol or phenol Surgery using radiofrequency percutaneous electrocoagulation to destroy small parts of the nerve	Oral corticosteroids (prednisone) 60–80 mg/d for 1 wk Analgesics Warm, moist heat	Bedrest during attacks Drugs to control vertigo, such as dimenhydramine (Dramamine) or meclizine (Bonine, Antivert) Mild sedatives may be used to control anxiety	Administering phenytoin (Dilantin) or carbamazepine (Tegretol) Spraying the throat with a topical anesthetic Intracranial surgery to divide the nerve (in severe cases)

Table continued on following page

Table 18—7

Cranial Nerve Disorders (continued)

	Trigeminal Neuralgia (Tic Douloureux)	Bell's Palsy	Menière's Disease	Glossopharyngeal Neuralgia
NURSING CARE	Provide psychosocial support in dealing with chronic pain Identify activities that trigger the pain and medicate at the first indication of pain Encourage activities of daily living with bouts of pain Instruct the patient to visit the dentist at least twice a year Assess nutritional status and assist the patient in planning a tolerable diet Teach the patient not to chew on the affected side Teach the patient about the disorder, the medical regimen, and the needed lifestyle alterations	Protect the affected eye by using patches, by using artificial tears 4 times daily, and by instructing the patient to close the eye manually from time to time Provide moist heat packs Instruct the patient to eat small, soft foods frequently Provide emotional support related to the change in self-image Reinforce the fact that 80% of patients recover completely	Provide a safe home environment Assess the efficacy of drug therapy Provide emotional support	Teach the patient to evaluate the response to the medication

treatment for benign primary tumors. Craniotomy is also performed on the patient with an encapsulated malignant brain tumor that is likely to be easily removed. Radiotherapy or chemotherapy is given postoperatively.

Stereotaxic surgery is rapidly gaining popularity as a method of treating grossly infiltrative tumors that present difficulty for conventional surgical removal. The procedure is usually performed under local anesthesia in the radiology department. The stereotaxic frame is attached to the patient. CT is used to obtain precise landmarks of the lesion. A burr hole is made and a biopsy obtained for pathology. This allows for prompt initiation of either chemotherapy or radiotherapy once the pathology of the tumor has been determined. The risks to the patient are markedly decreased compared with those of a craniotomy. Image-guided neurosurgery, with a keyhole approach, is making surgery possible for areas of the brain that were previously inoperable.

Radiotherapy is a treatment modality often used after craniotomy or stereotaxic biopsy. Astrocytomas, glioblastomas, oligodendrogliomas, sarcomas, and craniopharyngiomas are tumors that are often treated with a course of radiotherapy. The total tumor dose is usually from 4000 to 7000 rad administered over 4 to 8 weeks.

Chemotherapy is also used in the management of malignant brain tumors. Medulloblastomas and glioblastomas generally respond well to chemotherapy. The drugs used and the dosages depend on the tumor size, location, and general health of the patient.

❖ Settings, Providers, and Collaboration for Care

Treatment for a brain tumor may be in an outpatient setting. Surgical treatment, and some medical treatment, of a brain tumor requires hospitalization. Depending on the course of the illness, the treat-

Table 18–8

Classification of Brain Tumors

Name of Neoplasm	Origin	Most Frequent Sites of Development	Comments
Gliomas	Neuroglial tissue		Most common type of intracranial neoplasm; rate of growth varies with type of glioma
Astrocytoma	Astrocytes	*Adults:* cerebrum *Children:* cerebellum	Most common glioma; grows slowly; infiltrates surrounding tissue
Glioblastoma	Undifferentiated glial cells	Frontal, parietal, and temporal lobes	Highly malignant
Medulloblastoma	Undifferentiated glial cells	Cerebellum	Rapid extension; highly malignant
Ependymoma	Ependymal cells of the lining of the ventricles and aqueducts	Fourth ventricle	Rare; frequently papillomatous; may obstruct the flow of cerebrospinal fluid
Oligodendroglioma	Oligodendrocytes	Cerebral hemispheres	Rare; grows slowly; tends to calcify
Meningioma	Meninges	Along the course of the intracranial venous sinuses	Extracerebral, causing compression of brain tissue; usually encapsulated; grows slowly
Hemangiomas			
Angioma	Blood vessel wall	Middle cerebral artery	Not a true neoplasm; a congenital mass of tortuous, enlarged vessels; benign but may interfere with adjacent tissues
Angioblastoma	Blood vessel wall	Cerebellum	Tendency to form cysts
Pituitary adenomas			
Chromophobe adenoma	Adenohypophyseal glandular tissue	Anterior pituitary lobe (adenohypophysis)	Encapsulated; compresses pituitary gland tissue and the optic nerves, leading to hypopituitarism and impaired vision
Chromophilic adenoma (acidophilic adenoma)	Adenohypophyseal glandular tissue	Anterior pituitary lobe (adenohypophysis)	Seen less often than chromophobe adenoma; causes hypopituitarism (gigantism or acromegaly)
Craniopharyngioma	Embryologic defect in craniopharyngeal duct	Anterior to the pituitary stalk	Produces pressure on surrounding structures, interfering with their function
Acoustic neuroma	Eighth cranial (acoustic) nerve	Between pons and cerebellum	Encapsulated

ment may take place in a rehabilitation unit, a long-term care facility, or the home. The discharge planner or the case manager will contact other health-care services for the patient as needed upon discharge. A home health worker, social worker, physical therapist, occupational therapist, and hospice worker may be consulted for a particular patient.

NURSING PROCESS GUIDELINES

Brain Tumors

Nursing care for a patient with a brain tumor varies with the stage of the disease and the mode of treatment selected. For patients with terminal disease, the nursing care discussed in Chapter 3 applies. For patients receiving radiation therapy or chemotherapy, the care discussed in Chapter 34 applies. For patients undergoing surgery for a brain tumor, the care discussed in Chapter 17 applies. In all cases, periodic neurologic assessment and observation for worsening headache or vomiting, which can indicate increasing intracranial pressure, are essential.

The Elderly: Special Considerations

Some neurologic disorders occur more predominately in the elderly population and, in this age group, may differ in clinical presentation, clinical course, and method of treatment. Examples include dementia, delirium, subdural hematomas, CVAs, and normal pressure hydrocephalus.

DEMENTIA AND DELIRIUM

Organic brain syndrome is the phrase that has been used in reference to a deterioration in brain functioning that may occur in either an acute or a chronic form. However, "dementia" is currently the most accurate medical term for progressive impairments of cognitive functioning. Dementia is characterized as a persistent decline in two or more acquired intellectual functions in the presence of a stable level of consciousness. In addition, noncognitive manifestations, such as changes in personality and behavior, may be associated with dementia. Because dementia is not a single disease but a syndrome, the term refers to a unique combination of symptoms that indicate the need to look for an underlying cause. Dementia of the Alzheimer's type is the most common type of progressive dementing condition, accounting for 50 to 60% of the cases of dementia. Vascular disorders, such as transient ischemic attacks, are the second most common cause of dementia in older adults.

Delirium is an acute confusional state that is characterized by a diminished level of alertness and attention, along with deficits in thinking, memory, perception, psychomotor skills, and the sleep-wake cycle. Although this disorder can occur in people of any age, it is more common in older adults, particularly in older adults who have dementia. Hypoxia, trauma, infection, metabolic disorders, infectious processes, fluid and electrolyte imbalances, and adverse medication effects are common precipitating factors.

Particular problems arise when delirium occurs in older adults, because the manifestations are likely to be more subtle. If delirium occurs in older adults with dementia, the acute changes are superimposed on already existing cognitive deficits, and the recent changes may be attributed to dementia. Another complicating factor is that the manifestations of delirium may persist for months or years, even after underlying causes are detected and treated. Also, delirium in older adults often causes a severe and long-term decline in and loss of physical functioning.

In both dementia and delirium, nursing management focuses on developing an individualized plan of care. An essential component of assessment is the identification of any factors that may cause or contribute to the mental changes. Ensure that safety is maintained, provide orientation regularly, and use familiar objects in the environment whenever possible. Involve family members in care, allow time for discussion of anxieties and fears, and suggest support groups or community resources, such as the Alzheimer's Association, when planning for discharge.

CEREBROVASCULAR ACCIDENT

Neurologic deficits suffered as a consequence of a CVA, or stroke, are directly related to the type, location, and extent of damage to cerebral tissue. Aging is not a factor in this physiologic response. However, age may be a factor in the level of functioning that is attained after a stroke. The older stroke victim is more likely than a younger person to have multiple chronic illnesses. This may prolong the rehabilitation phase secondary to potential complications of those chronic illnesses.

SUBDURAL HEMATOMA

Mild atrophy of brain tissue is an age-related change that may slow the rate of bleeding into the subdural space that occurs after mild trauma. This may delay the presentation of symptoms. In the elderly, subdural hematomas often are chronic, and the symptoms of confusion, drowsiness, and cognitive impairment may be inaccurately attributed to the aging process.

Chapter Review

1. Why is the neurologic assessment important to the care of the patient with meningitis?
2. How does amyotrophic lateral sclerosis affect the neurons, and what signs and symptoms are produced?
3. What are the advantages of active and passive range of motion for a patient with multiple sclerosis?
4. How can the effectiveness of amantadine be evaluated when caring for the patient with Parkinson's disease?
5. Why is planning and maintaining a consistent routine important when planning care for a patient with Alzheimer's disease?

6. What questions are important to ask when assessing the patient with a seizure disorder?

7. What might happen to a patient with a CVA if the bed was in the flat position and the patient was maintained in the supine position?

8. How does hypertension affect the patient with a subarachnoid hemorrhage?

9. How does the nursing care of a patient with a brain tumor different from that of a patient with brain injury?

10. How might a patient with a spinal cord injury react to being told that he or she is now a quadriplegic?

Bibliography

Adams RD, Victor M. Principles of neurology. 5th ed. New York: McGraw-Hill, 1993.

Adams RD, Victor M. Principles of neurology companion handbook. 5th ed. New York: McGraw-Hill, 1994.

Agency for Health Care Policy and Research. Acute pain management: Operative or medical procedures and trauma. US Department of Health and Human Services. AHCPR Pub. No. 92-0032, 1992.

Ahlstrom G, Sjoden P. Assessment of coping with muscular dystrophy: A methodological evaluation. J Adv Nurs 1994; 20(2): 314.

Armstrong SL. Cerebral vasospasm: Early detection and intervention. Crit Care Nurse 1994; 14(4):33.

Asbury AK, McKhann GM, McDonald WI (eds). Diseases of the nervous system: Clinical neurobiology. 2nd ed. Philadelphia: WB Saunders, 1992.

Bell TE, Kongable GL. Innovations in aneurysmal subarachnoid hemorrhage: Intracisternal t-PA for the prevention of vasospasm. J Neurosci Nurs 1996; 28(2):107.

Blount M, Kinney AB, Stackhouse J. Myasthenia gravis: A manual for the nurse. New York: Myasthenia Gravis Foundation, 1991.

Carpenito LJ. Nursing diagnosis: Application to clinical practice. 6th ed. Philadelphia: JB Lippincott, 1996.

Chiocca EM. Emergency! Meningococcal meningitis. AJN 1995; 95(12):25.

Dzienkowski RC, Smith KK, Dillow KA, Yucha CB. Cerebral palsy: A comprehensive review. Nurse Pract 1996; 21(2):45.

Eisenhart K. New perspectives in the management of adults with severe head injury. Crit Care Nurs Q 1994; 17(2):1.

Fitzsimmons B, Bunting LK. Parkinson's disease: Quality of life issues. Nurs Clin North Am 1993; 28(4):807.

Frank J. The role of the nurse in seizure management. In Roth SP, Morse JS (eds). A life-span approach to nursing care for individuals with developmental disabilities. Baltimore: Paul H. Brookes, 1994.

Gauwitz DF. How to protect the dysphagic stroke patient. AJN 1995; 95(8):34.

Gibbon B. Stroke care and rehabilitation. Elderly Care 1995; 7(4): 25.

Gilroy J. Basic neurology. 3rd ed. New York: McGraw-Hill, 1996.

Gray M, Rayome R, Anson C. Incontinence and clean intermittent catheterization following spinal cord injury. Clin Nurs Res 1995; 4(1):6.

Guyton AC. Basic neuroscience: Anatomy and physiology. 2nd ed. Philadelphia: WB Saunders, 1992.

Hemmingway S. Rehabilitation of people with traumatic head injury. Ment Health Nurs 1995;15(3):9.

Hickey J. The clinical practice of neurological and neurosurgical nursing. 4th ed. Philadelphia: JB Lippincott, 1996.

Jacobs BB. Emergent neurological events. Crit Care Nurs Clin North Am 1995; 7(3):427.

Janowski MJ. A road map for stroke recovery. RN 1996; 59(3):26.

Kernich CA, Kamiski HJ. Myasthenia gravis: Pathophysiology, diagnosis and collaborative care. J Neurosci Nurs 1995; 27(4): 207.

Kloss D. Critical care extra: Caring for the patient with meningococcal meningitis. AJN 1996; 96(4):16.

Kolanowski A. Everyday functioning in Alzheimer's disease: Contribution of neuropsychological testing. Clin Nurse Spec 1996; 10(1):11.

Lemke DM. Defining assessment parameters in dual injuries: Spinal cord injury and traumatic brain injury. SCI Nurs 1995; 12(2):40.

Martinson IM, Muwaswes M, Gillis CL, et al. The frequency and troublesomeness of symptoms associated with Alzheimer's disease. J Community Health Nurs 1995; 12(1):47.

Meissner JE. Caring for patients with multiple sclerosis. Nursing 1994; 24(8):60.

O'Donnell L. Caring for patients with myasthenia gravis . . . Find out your role in assessing and managing this debilitating disorder. Nursing 1995; 25(3):60.

Parker CD. Fast action for subarachnoid hemorrhage. AJN 1995; 95(1):47.

Pieper DR, Valadka AB, Marsh C. Surgical management of patients with severe head injuries. AORN J 1996; 63(5):854.

Quinn AA, Barton JA, Magilvy JK. Weathering the storm: Metaphors and stories of living with multiple sclerosis. Rehabil Nurs Res 1995; 4(1):19.

Rusy KL. Rebleeding and vasospasm after subarachnoid hemorrhage: A critical care challenge. Crit Care Nurse 1996; 16(1): 41.

Schinner KM, Chisholm AH, Grap MJ, et al. Effects of auditory stimuli on intracranial pressure and cerebral perfusion pressure in traumatic brain injury. J Neurosci Nurs 1995; 27(6): 348.

Shaddinger DE. An acute spinal cord injury: My family's story. J Neurosci Nurs 1995; 27(4):236.

Smith K. Bringing epilepsy care into the 1990s: The epilepsy liaison service. Prof Nurse 1995; 10(4):255.

Teunissen LL, Rinkel GJ, Algra A, van-Gijn J. Risk factors for subarachnoid hemorrhage: A systematic review. Stroke 1996; 27(3):544.

Veltman R, Jones SJ. Nursing care for patients with mild brain injury. Int J Trauma Nurs 1995; 1(3):82.

Weber CE. Stroke: Brain attack, time to react. AACN Clin Issues Adv Pract Acute Crit Care 1995; 6(4):562.

Wertz E. On guard for meningitis. Emergency 1995; 27(8):36.

Woolf K. Intravenous methylprednisolone for exacerbations in multiple sclerosis. MEDSURG Nurs 1995; 4(3):207.

Ziemba SK. Seizures. AJN 1995; 95(2):32.

Unit VI

Musculoskeletal Dysfunction

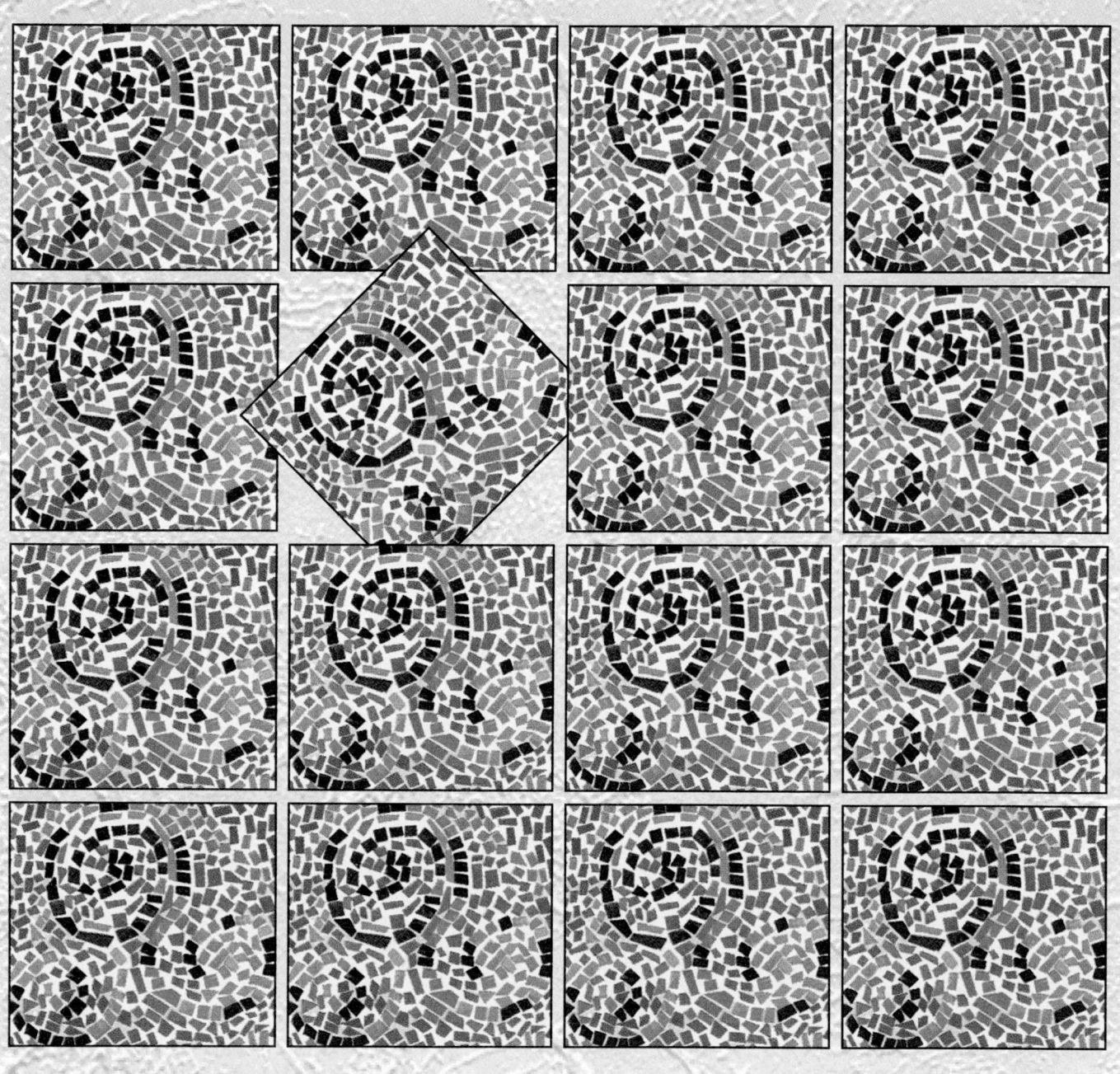

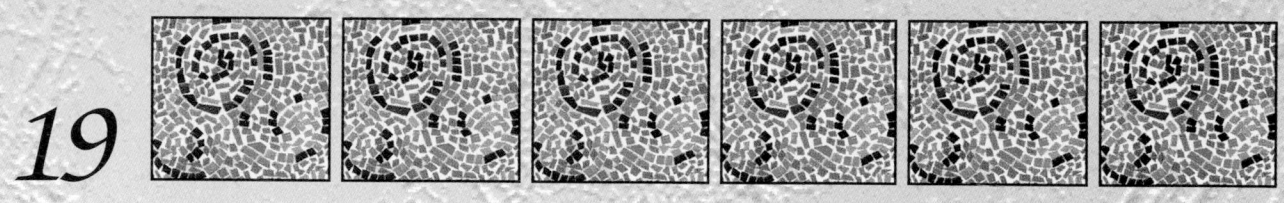

19

Knowledge Base for Patients with Musculoskeletal Dysfunction

Study Outcomes

After studying this chapter, you should be able to:

1. Explain the normal anatomy and physiology of the musculoskeletal system.
2. Describe common clinical manifestations of musculoskeletal dysfunction.
3. Identify information and physical examination data essential to the assessment of the musculoskeletal system.
4. Identify the most common laboratory and radiologic studies used to diagnose musculoskeletal dysfunction.
5. Describe the medical management and surgical procedures commonly used in the treatment of patients with musculoskeletal dysfunction.
6. Identify data essential to the assessment of patients undergoing treatment of musculoskeletal dysfunction.
7. State nursing diagnoses and related expected patient outcomes commonly applicable to patients undergoing treatment of musculoskeletal dysfunction.
8. Describe nursing interventions, with their rationales, commonly applicable to patients undergoing treatment of musculoskeletal dysfunction.
9. Explain the basis for the evaluation of nursing care provided to patients undergoing treatment of musculoskeletal dysfunction.
10. Identify special considerations for the elderly patient with altered function of the musculoskeletal system.
11. Identify alternative treatment and care settings for patients with musculoskeletal dysfunction and the services related to community-based care.

The musculoskeletal system is the supporting framework of the body. It is composed of bones, joints, cartilage, ligaments, muscles, and tendons. These components interact and connect to produce locomotion and to support and protect body structures. Disease or damage to any part of the system can cause pain, immobility, and disability. The musculoskeletal system is intricately related to the individual's overall sense of independence and wellbeing.

Patients with musculoskeletal dysfunction may be treated in the hospital, in outpatient clinics, and in the home setting. Since home maintenance management is a common problem, the home health nurse is frequently the caregiver for the patient along with family members. Physical and occupational therapists are also important health-care professionals who assist the patient with musculoskeletal dysfunction to regain maximum independence.

Anatomy and Physiology

SKELETAL SYSTEM

Consisting of 206 bones, the axial and appendicular skeletons form a rigid supporting framework for the human body. The axial or central skeleton is made up of the skull, sternum, ribs, and vertebral column. The appendicular skeleton consists of the bones in the shoulders, pelvis, and limbs. In addition to support, the skeletal system has the four other functions of body movement, protection, blood cell formation, and storage of minerals.

Bones and their joints, powered by contracting skeletal muscles, create body motion. Flat bones, such as the skull, ribs, and ileum, provide protection for vital organs. Bones also play a role in homeostasis by producing new blood cells (hematopoiesis) and by serving as a storage space for body minerals such as calcium, phosphorus, magnesium, and sodium. Approximately 99% of the total body calcium and 90% of total body phosphorus are stored in the bones.

Calcium is constantly being deposited in and resorbed (absorbed and removed) from the bones. This constant process is regulated by a number of factors, including local stress to the bone such as weight-bearing, adequate intake and absorption of vitamin D, and circulating blood levels of parathyroid hormone and calcitonin.

Microscopic Anatomy

Bone is a dynamic structure composed of 35% organic and 65% inorganic matter. It is continually being produced and absorbed. The organic substance, which consists of cells, blood vessels, and cartilaginous material, gives the bone elasticity. The inorganic substance, which provides hardness, is primarily composed of calcium, with some phosphorus, magnesium, and sodium chloride.

There are three different types of bone cells: osteoblasts, osteoclasts, and osteocytes. Osteoblasts are active bone-building cells that synthesize organic bone matrix or collagen. Osteoclasts are large multinucleated cells that resorb bone. Osteocytes are mature bone cells in a resting state and are positioned in small spaces called lacunae. Osteocytes become active osteoblasts during periods of bone growth or repair.

CLASSIFICATION OF BONE BY CELLULAR STRUCTURE

Bone is classified as cortical or cancellous depending on how the lacunae are organized. As illustrated in Figure 19–1, the hard outer layer of all bones is composed of compact cortical bone. The lacunae, tiny cavities in these bones, are organized in concentric rings or lamellae around haversian canals. The haversian canals contain blood vessels and lymphatic vessels. The lacunae are densely packed and are connected to one another and to the haversian

canals by tiny canaliculi, which together form a haversian system, or osteon. The osteon is the microscopic functioning unit of mature bone. Haversian canals run parallel to the length of the bone and are connected horizontally by Volkmann's canals (see Fig. 19–1). It is through Volkmann's canals that bone cells communicate with the inside and outside lining of the bone. This network of canals provides compact bone with a system of blood and lymphatic vessels.

In cancellous or spongy bone, the lacunae are laid out in loosely arranged sheets connected by canaliculi. The sheets of lacunae are arranged in irregular patterns that form open spaces between thin networks of bone and resemble the inside of a sponge. This pattern is organized to withstand compressive and tensile stresses applied to the bone. Cancellous bone is more porous than compact bone and has a rich blood supply. It forms the inside of flat bones and the ends of long bones.

OSSIFICATION

The process of bone formation is called ossification. Ossification is either intramembranous or endochondral. In intramembranous ossification, bone forms from within a membrane. During this process, a fi-

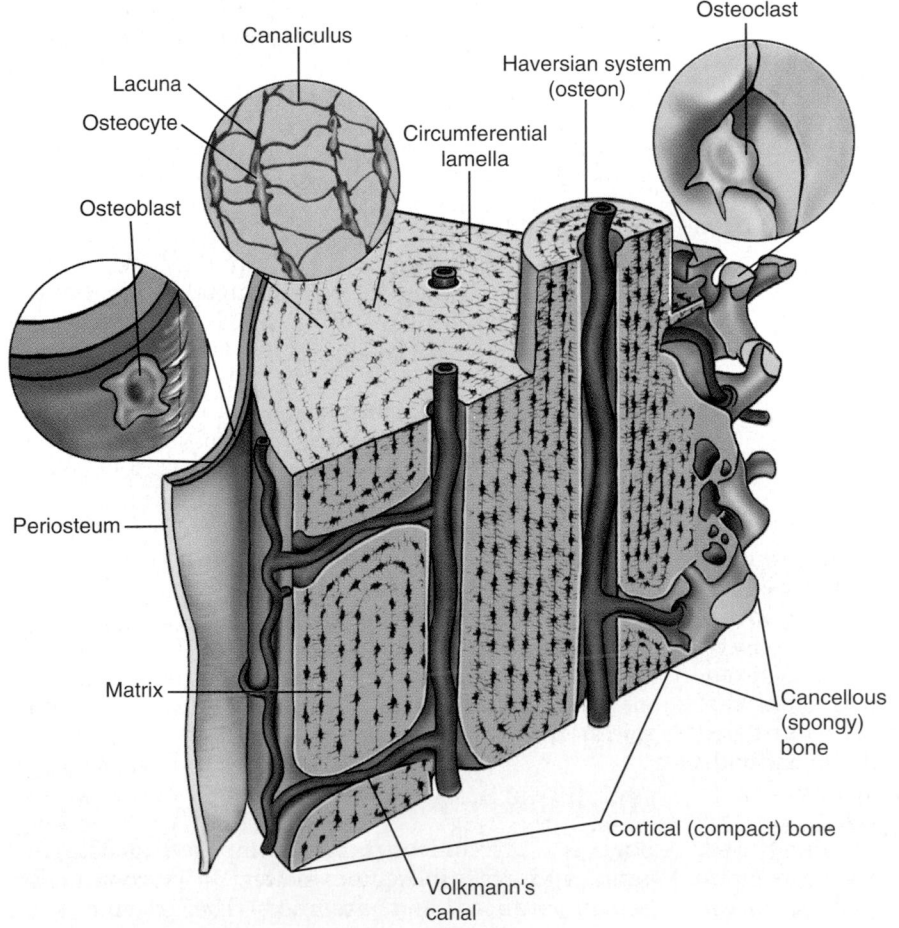

Figure 19–1
Microscopic anatomy of bone.

brous union occurs in which dense connective membrane is directly replaced by deposits of inorganic calcium salts. Flat bones such as the skull, sternum, and ribs are formed by this process.

In endochondral ossification, a cartilage framework exists first and is then resorbed and replaced by bone. Most bones in the body are formed, and fractured bones heal, by the process of endochondral ossification. When bone forms by endochondral ossification, the fibrous union is not created until the cartilage framework is replaced by bone.

By the end of puberty, axial skeletal growth, or growth in the length of the bones, is complete. Although the size of the skeleton in height and build is genetically determined, bone cell content and strength are determined by a counterbalance of resorption and deposit of bone tissue. Throughout life, the osteoblasts deposit newly formed bone while the osteoclasts resorb or thin the bone. Osteoblasts deposit bone on the outer surface while osteoclasts remove bone from the medullary side, so that bone grows in diameter but not in thickness. A balance of these two processes is essential for a strong, healthy skeleton.

Gross Anatomy

All bones, except the joint surfaces, which are covered by articular cartilage, are enclosed in a tough fibrous connective tissue called periosteum. The periosteum provides a supportive structure for blood vessels and nerve tissue and serves as the point of attachment to the bones for muscles, tendons, and ligaments. The periosteum is essential for nourishment, growth, repair, and resorption of bone. The endosteum is a thin membrane that lines the medullary cavity of long bones and the spaces in cancellous bones.

Within the bones there are two types of marrow: yellow and red. Yellow marrow consists mainly of fat cells and is found in the medullary canals of long bones in adults. Red marrow, which is actively involved in hematopoiesis, is found in the cancellous portion of flat bones and in the medullary cavity of growing children.

BLOOD AND NERVE SUPPLY

With its intricate internal microscopic network of vessels, bone is very vascular. Blood circulates to bone by several pathways. One-third of compact bone receives its blood from vessels in the periosteum. The medullary or nutrient artery penetrating the long bones supplies blood to the other two-thirds of the compact bone and to the cancellous bone. Blood vessels entering and leaving the capsular attachment at joints also supply cancellous bone with circulation. Nerves enter the bone through the periosteum and continue inside the bone along the medullary cavity. Since bone has sensation, pain

may arise from bone as well as from soft tissue in individuals with musculoskeletal dysfunction.

CLASSIFICATION OF BONES BY SHAPE

Bones may be classified by their shape as long, short, flat, or irregular. Long bones are those with a shaft and include the bones of the extremities, such as the femur, tibia, humerus, and radius. Short bones include the small bones in the hands and feet. Flat bones are those that cover or protect organs, such as the skull, sternum, ribs, and ileum. Irregular bones are those with irregular shapes, such as the vertebrae and the jaw bone. The external surfaces of most bones have grooves and prominences for the origin and insertion of muscles, which allow gliding of tendons over bone.

A typical long bone can be divided into specific structural components, as illustrated in Figure 19–2. The diaphysis, or shaft, is made up of compact bone around a central medullary canal. The portion of compact bone that flares out at the ends is the metaphysis. The epiphysis, or end of the bone, is made up of cancellous bone. The metaphysis and epiphysis are separated by a cartilaginous epiphyseal plate until full adult growth is achieved. The epiphyseal plate provides growth in length of the diaphysis and metaphysis. Its cartilage cells are converted to bone at the end of puberty. This process extends over several years.

Bone Repair

Bone, like other tissues in the body, may be damaged or injured as a result of trauma or disease process. The damage or injury may or may not involve tissue surrounding the bone and displacement of bone fragments, or pieces, from their anatomical location. After injury or damage, the process of bone healing or repair occurs in five stages. These stages are listed as they would occur after a fracture or break in the bone.

First, at the time of injury, there is bleeding from within the bone and from surrounding tissue. A clot or hematoma begins to form around the fracture site within 24 hours. Fibroblasts and capillaries invade the clot to form granulation tissue.

During the second stage of bone repair, there is a proliferation of cell formation where the periosteum is torn. Fibroblasts develop from the periosteal region as osteogenic cells from the periosteum and endosteum migrate to and proliferate at the site. The proliferating cells begin to form a callus or bridge across the damaged bone or fracture.

Once callus formation is complete, the third stage begins. During the third stage, the cells differentiate into bone or cartilage, depending on where they are located. Cells nearest the bone surface transform directly into osteoblasts. Less well vascularized cells form cartilage.

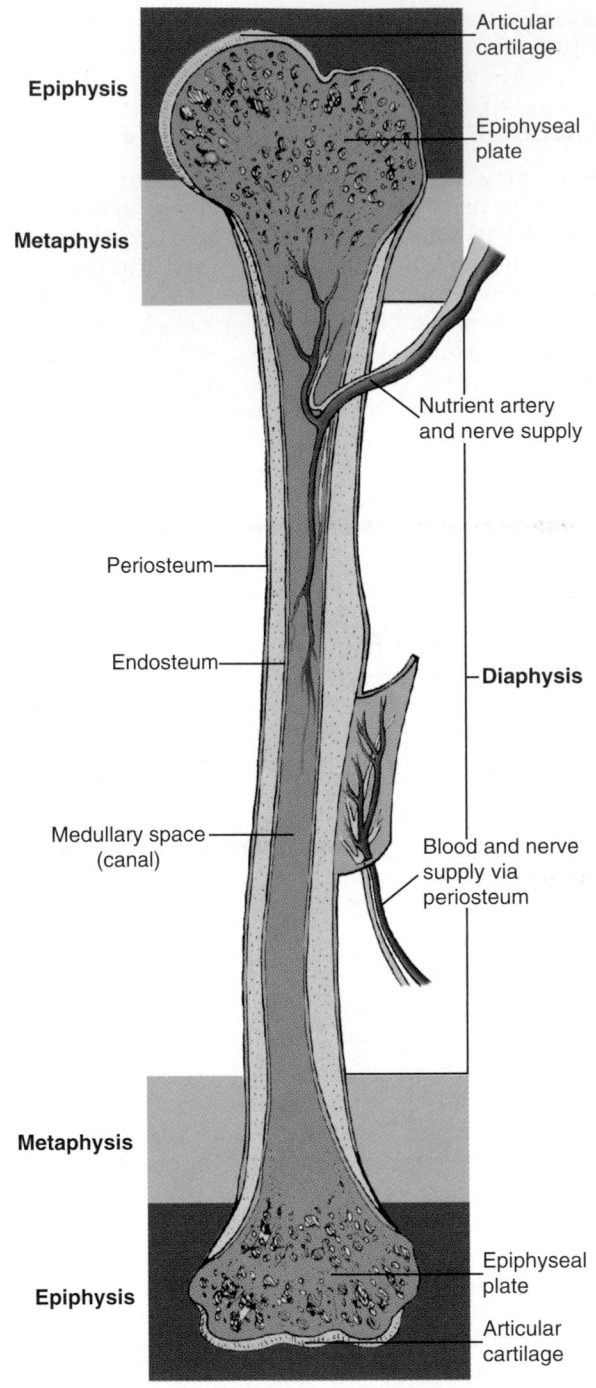

Figure 19–2
Structure of a long bone.

The fourth stage is the ossification stage. Inorganic salts are deposited in the new bone matrix to calcify the bone.

During the fifth and final stage of bone repair, consolidation and remodeling of the new bone gradually occurs. Cancellous trabeculae (bony spikes that form a meshwork of spaces for the bone marrow) are absorbed, new lamellae are formed, new haversian systems are developed, and the medullary canal

is re-established. Remodeling continues according to Wolff's law, which states that the structure, function, and shape of a bone are determined by the forces or stress applied to it. Thus, the new bone continues to be remodeled by the stresses placed upon it until it assumes the most efficient shape for its function.

A number of factors can affect how damaged bone heals. These factors include the following:

Age
General physical condition (eg, anemia, endocrine imbalance, dietary intake)
Type of injury (traumatic, degenerative)
Degree of displacement of bone fragments ·
Presence of infection (localized, systemic)
Immobilization after injury
Vascular sufficiency
Periosteal function

SKELETAL MUSCULAR SYSTEM

Skeletal Muscle

Skeletal muscle is sometimes called striated muscle because of its microscopic banded appearance. It is also termed voluntary muscle because its movement can be controlled by conscious effort. Individual muscles are covered and separated by a fibrous membrane called fascia. The fascia is similar to a compartment or envelope. In addition to providing support, the fascia allows skeletal muscle to move smoothly across bones, joints, and muscles and enhances the contractility of skeletal muscle.

Skeletal muscle is made up of bundles of cell fibers that are covered and held together in a parallel arrangement by connective tissue. Each muscle fiber contains several myofibrils. Each myofibril is composed of sliding protein filaments called sarcomeres. The sarcomeres are the contractile or working units of the myofibrils. As the sarcomere filaments slide across one another, they shorten or contract the muscle and lengthen or relax the muscle. This sliding action produces the elastic character of muscle tissue.

Skeletal muscle contracts in response to impulses from the central nervous system. These impulses produce the release of acetylcholine from the motor end plate of the motor neuron, or nerve cell, that innervates the muscle. In response to the presence of acetylcholine, calcium ions are released within the muscle cell fibers, and the sarcomeres contract.

The partially contracted quality of muscle fibers at rest produces muscle tone. Abnormal muscle tone is referred to as either flaccid (less than normal tone) or spastic (greater than normal tone). Groups of muscles in a continuous partially contracted state maintain skeletal posture.

There are two types of muscle contraction, isometric and isotonic. Isometric contraction produces tension within the muscle without change in muscle length, thus no joint movement is produced. Pushing against an immovable object such as a wall produces an isometric contraction. Isotonic contraction results in shortening of the muscle length without changing the tension within the muscle. Flexion of the arm at the elbow is an example of isotonic contraction.

Locomotion, or movement, is made possible by muscles working together with the bones and joints. To produce movement, muscles contract over bones.

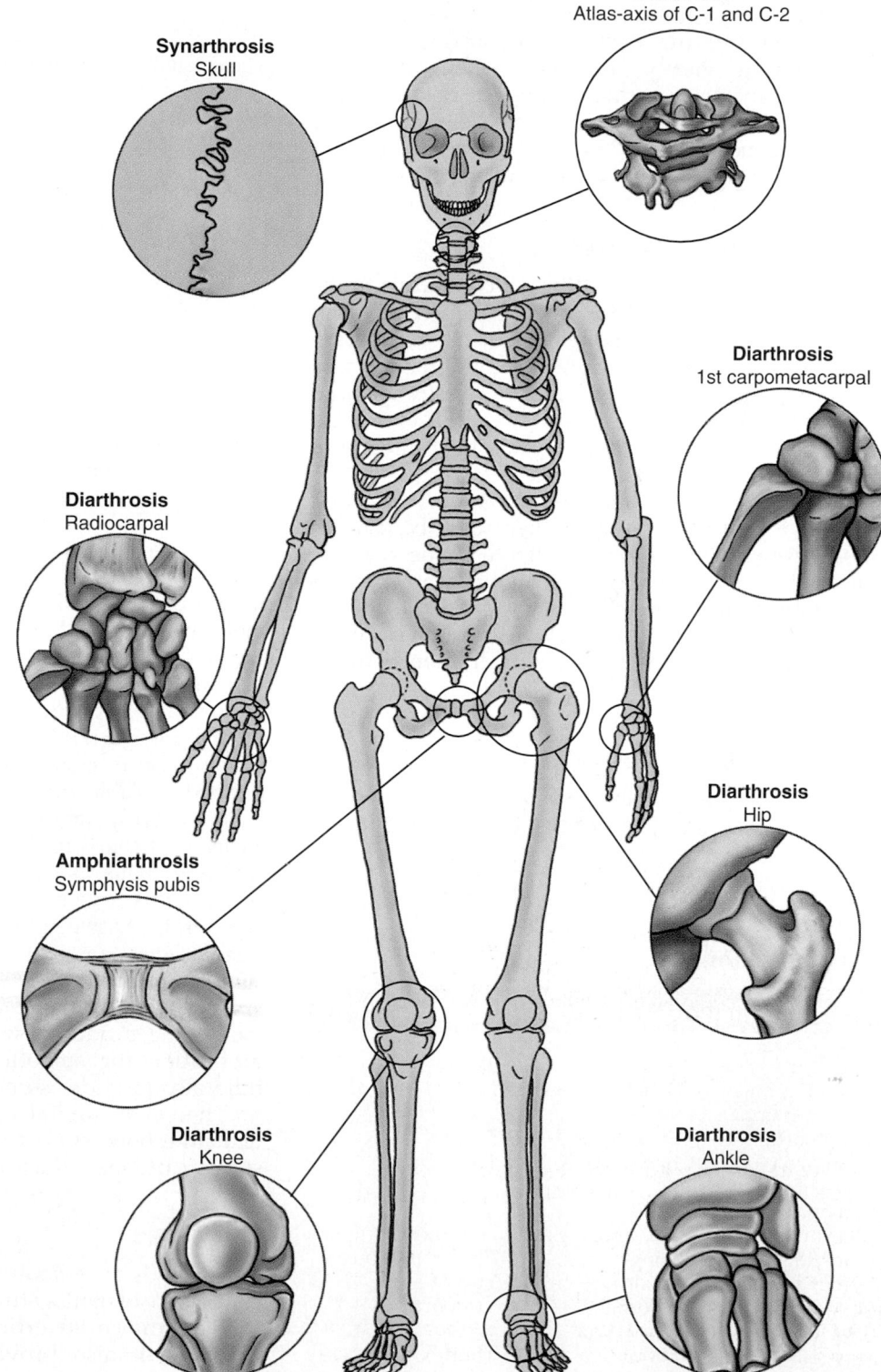

Figure 19–3

Classification of joints. Joints are classified as synarthroses, amphiarthroses, or diarthroses. Most joints in the body are diarthrodial joints. Diarthrodial joints allow free movement.

Through the contraction of a variety of muscles, the body is able to produce specific, deliberate movements.

Muscle activity or movement requires energy. The primary energy source for muscle activity and movement is the breakdown of adenosine triphosphate within the cell. Creatine phosphate is a secondary energy source that can be converted to adenosine triphosphate when needed. Since adenosine triphosphate is synthesized by glycolysis (an anaerobic process) and the Krebs cycle (an aerobic process), during heavy exercise when increased amounts of oxygen are unavailable for efficient functioning of the aerobic process, increased amounts of glucose are necessary. This is provided by the release of glycogen, which is stored in the cells.

Ligaments and Tendons

Ligaments are composed of fibrous connective tissue bands that bind bones to other bones. They may either limit or facilitate movement of the joint. Ligaments pass over bone joints, where they remain taut to provide joint stability. Tendons are strong, nonelastic fibrous connective tissue cords. They are an extension of the muscle sheath and attach muscle to the periosteum of the bone.

Where ligaments, tendons, muscle, bone, and skin move across one another there may be friction. Bursae are small sacs of connective tissue that are found where musculoskeletal structures move across one another under pressure. They are lined with a synovial membrane and filled with synovial fluid. Bursae act as cushions to decrease friction between body structures.

Joints and Articulations

A joint is the point where two or more bones meet. Joints are classified according to the amount of

Table 19–1

Types of Joints

Classification	Description	Example
Synarthrosis (allowing no movement)	Suture Synchondrosis	Skull Femur
Amphiarthrosis (allowing slight movement)	Symphysis Syndesmosis	Pelvis Tibiofibular
Diarthrosis (allowing free movement)	Ball and socket Hinge Pivot Gliding Condyloid Saddle	Hip and shoulder Elbow and knee Top of spine Vertebrae Wrist Thumb

Table 19–2

Movements of Diarthrodial Joints

Movement	Definition
Abduction	Movement away from and out to the side of the body
Adduction	Movement toward the body or across the midline of the body
Circumduction	Movement of the limb in a circular fashion from its pivotal point
Extension	Unfolding or movement from a flexed or bent position to a straight or neutral position
Flexion	Bending or folding movements going toward the center of the body
Hyperextension	Extension beyond a straight or neutral position in a direction away from the center of the body
Pronation	Movement of the palm so that the hand is turned downward or toward the posterior surface of the body
Rotation	Movement of a bone upon its own axis or pivoting
Supination	Movement of the palm so that the hand is turned outward with the palm facing the anterior surface of the body

movement they allow. Joints that allow no movement are classified as synarthrodial joints. Amphiarthrodial joints allow slight movement. Joints that allow free movement are diarthrodial joints. Examples of the different joints in the body are illustrated in Figure 19–3 and listed in Table 19–1. Terms describing the movements of the diarthrodial joints are defined in Table 19–2.

Most body joints are diarthrodial. The articular surfaces of diarthrodial joints are covered by hyaline cartilage. This cartilage decreases friction as the bones move against one another, but it does not regenerate. Between the two articulating surfaces is a small space or joint cavity. The entire diarthrodial joint is enclosed by a fibrous capsule of connective tissue that is lined with synovial membrane. This membrane produces synovial fluid, which provides lubrication for smooth joint motion. The synovial fluid also provides some nutrients to joint surfaces.

The synarthrodial joints have no cavity. The articulating bone surfaces are connected by fibrous tissue or cartilage, which prevents movement.

Cartilage

Cartilage is a smooth, resilient supporting tissue composed of collagen. It provides a smooth, low-friction surface for articulating bones. Because of its elasticity, it also provides a cushion that absorbs shock and reduces stress and strain on joint surfaces. The three types of cartilage in the body are hyaline, elastic, and fibrocartilage. Hyaline cartilage is the most prevalent and is found on the articular surfaces of bone. Hyaline cartilage has no blood vessels, lymph channels, or nerves. It receives nutrients from synovial fluid, adjacent tissues, or an occasional blood vessel passing through to other tissues. Elastic cartilage contains more elastic fibers and is more flexible than hyaline cartilage. It is found in the outer ear, epiglottis, and larynx. Fibrocartilage contains more collagen fibers and is very resilient. It forms the transitional tissue between hyaline cartilage and the connective tissue of capsules or ligaments and forms the attachment of tendons to bone. Fibrocartilage is also found in the symphysis pubis, the knee meniscus, and the intervertebral discs, where it functions as a shock absorber for the skeleton.

Clinical Manifestations of Musculoskeletal Dysfunction

The individual with an injury or a disease of the bones, muscles, ligaments, tendons, joints, or cartilage can be expected to present with alteration in movement of the affected body parts. The degree of immobility can vary from a change in the normal gait pattern to inability to ambulate. The presence of pain interferes with free joint movement and locomotion and may actually be the primary problem causing the musculoskeletal dysfunction. Fractures, trauma, and diseases affecting the musculoskeletal system produce specific clinical manifestations, which are covered in detail under each disorder in Chapter 20. The extent of musculoskeletal involvement determines how much limitation occurs in a person's ability to perform self care and other activities of daily living. Patients with musculoskeletal dysfunction may be treated in the hospital, in outpatient clinics, or in the home setting. Since home maintenance management is a common problem, the home health nurse and the family are caregivers for the patient with musculoskeletal dysfunction.

MOBILITY IMPAIRMENT

Symptoms the individual may experience include limitation in strength, function, and range of motion of the involved musculoskeletal structures. A deformity or change in shape and size of the involved area may be evident, as well as local soft tissue inflammation, pain, and edema.

Immobility and disuse resulting from injury or disease affect the entire musculoskeletal system. Muscles become weak and atrophy in a short time from lack of use. This is evident when a casted or splinted extremity has not been exercised. Joints develop stiffness and lose range of motion or develop contractures from immobility and improper positioning. The patient may be unable to perform activities of daily living as a result of weakness and fatigue. Without mobility and normal stresses of use and weight-bearing on the skeleton, bone destruction (osteoclastic activity) and bone resorption occur at a greater rate than bone production and repair. The calcium released from bone destruction can result in an alkaline urine, which may cause the development of kidney stones or urinary tract infection.

NURSING PROCESS
Mobility Impairment
Assessment

Complete a thorough movement assessment on the patient. Review past history and present mobility problems, including the patient's chief complaint and characteristics of the onset of signs and symptoms. Examine the impact of the musculoskeletal impairment on the patient's lifestyle and ability to perform activities of daily living. Ask the patient to demonstrate mobility of all major joints to evaluate strengths and limitations of movement. Note grip strength, weight-bearing ability, gait, and ability to move freely about the room, with or without assistance. Monitor the patient's respiratory system, noting shortness of breath after movement. Assess the cardiovascular system through vital signs and observation of peripheral edema and orthostatic hypotension. Look for signs of impaired circulation to extremities, weak or absent pulses, decreased capillary refill, and pallor. Check muscle tone and the patient's ability to repeat a strength exercise without tiring, such as standing on one foot or gripping an object. Ask the patient about symptoms of fatigue after mild exercise. Assess the relation of the symptoms to the patient's disorder or need for assistive devices for movement or locomotion. Observe the type of device used by the patient and its effectiveness. Ask the patient about interferences with movement caused by generalized pain or pain in specific body parts.

Assess the patient frequently for signs of respiratory infection, which is a complication of immobility. Look for increased respiratory rate, cough, dyspnea, fever, chills, and shortness of breath. Auscultate lungs for adventitious sounds. Check laboratory results, especially those of the white blood cell count and the urinalysis.

Assess the patient's understanding about the effects of immobility and how to prevent the complications that may occur. Ask the patient about present signs of problems related to immobility, which may include reduction in muscle size and strength or decrease in joint range of motion. Talk to the patient's family to determine their understanding of the symptoms associated with the hazards of immobility.

Determine whether the patient experiences any pain or burning on urination or low back pain indicative of a urinary tract infection. Note the color and consistency of the urine.

Assess the patient's extremities, looking for signs of infection from lesions or any areas of breakdown. Note any skin lesions and report them immediately. Look for purulent drainage from the areas of breakdown or around pin sites. Check distal pulses and the color, temperature, capillary refill, movement, and sensation in the extremity.

Note the patient's ability to perform self-care. Observe the patient's appearance, assessing for poor hygiene, improper dress, or lack of general grooming. Check whether the patient is able to eat without assistance. Ask whether toileting is a problem for the patient or whether assistance is necessary.

Nursing Diagnoses and Planning

Nursing diagnoses and related expected patient outcomes most commonly applicable to patients experiencing immobility problems include the following:

NDx: Activity intolerance related to fatigue and dyspnea secondary to decreased muscle tone and cardiovascular fitness from lack of exercise or interference with mobility from appliances, deformity, or pain

Planning: Patient Outcomes
1. Patient follows regimen of planned activities and rest periods each day.
2. Patient verbalizes decreased feelings of fatigue and demonstrates increased activity level.
3. Patient completes activities of daily living without signs of fatigue and dyspnea, such as tachycardia, tachypnea, shortness of breath, and cyanosis.
4. Patient is able to complete some activity, as prescribed, without pain or interference from appliance or in spite of deformity.

NDx: Knowledge deficit: nature of immobility problems and prevention of complications

Planning: Patient Outcomes
1. Patient states accurate information about the nature of the potential problems related to immobility.
2. Patient states the signs of complications of immobility and when to seek medical intervention.
3. Patient relates the measures necessary to lessen the risk of complications.
4. Patient is free of complications, such as extreme fatigue, inability to complete activities of daily living, deformities, skin breakdown, infection, or elimination problems.

NDx: Altered peripheral tissue perfusion related to complications of immobility; constriction from casts, traction, or other devices; or bedrest

Planning: Patient Outcomes
1. Patient's extremities are warm, color is adequate, and pulses are present.

2. Patient presents no evidence of edema, calf pain, inflammation, or venous distention.

NDx: Impaired skin integrity related to insufficient peripheral circulation from bedrest or restrictive devices, or related to direct injury from immobilizing devices

Planning: Patient Outcomes
1. Patient states causes of skin lesions and measures to prevent their occurrence or recurrence.
2. Patient relates appropriate knowledge about skin care.
3. Patient is free of interruptions in skin integrity, such as skin breakdown.

NDx: Risk for infection related to increased susceptibility secondary to bedrest, placement of internal fixation devices, pressure from restrictive devices, or compromised circulation

Planning: Patient Outcomes
1. Patient's vital signs are within normal ranges for the patient.
2. Patient is free of signs of infection, such as fever, chills, tachycardia, tachypnea, cough, dyspnea, or drainage from lesions or at pin sites.
3. Patient identifies early signs of infection and measures to prevent infections.

NDx: Self care deficit (feeding, hygiene, toileting, or other activities of daily living) related to impaired mobility

Planning: Patient Outcomes
1. Patient performs activities of daily living, using assistive devices if necessary.
2. Patient states alternative methods to complete tasks that are restricted by musculoskeletal dysfunction or immobilization.

Nursing Interventions and Evaluation

NDx: Activity intolerance
Determine the patient's baseline activity level. Instruct the patient to develop a regimen of activity with frequent rest periods throughout the day. Develop an exercise regime in conjunction with the physician, physical therapist, and occupational therapist as needed. Encourage the patient to do active range-of-motion exercises frequently while lying in bed to maintain muscle tone and strength, or complete passive range-of-motion exercises if necessary. Encourage isometric exercises to strengthen the abdominal, gluteal, and quadriceps muscles used in ambulation. Teach the patient to practice energy-saving techniques to reduce fatigue and shortness of breath. Place frequently used articles within the patient's reach for safety and to prevent overtiring. Assist the patient in establishing a realistic activity program and making necessary lifestyle changes. Discuss the relationship of the disease process or impairment to activity performance.

Provide and encourage frequent rest periods

while delivering patient care. Alternate the rest periods with a planned regimen of appropriate exercises to enable the patient to improve locomotion ability. Monitor the patient's response to activity and make necessary modifications.

NDx: Knowledge deficit: nature of immobility problems and prevention of complications

Instruct the patient about the effects of immobility and the signs of complications, such as elimination difficulty, urinary calculi, skin breakdown, diminished pulses, paresthesia, and the symptoms of infections. Teach the patient the signs and symptoms that require the patient to seek medical assistance. Explain the need for safety measures if locomotion is a problem. Consult with physical and occupational therapists for guidance.

Teach the patient to drink an increased amount of fluids daily to prevent urinary stasis. Instruct the patient to cough and deep-breathe and use the incentive spirometer to prevent pulmonary complications. Provide fiber foods to prevent constipation, especially if the patient is on extended bedrest.

Explain the proper methods necessary to prevent further irritation and ulceration of skin where pressure has occurred from bedrest, the appliance, or a cast, if present. Allow the patient to ask questions as needed. Include the family in the education sessions when appropriate. Assist the patient and family in identifying activity limitations imposed by the disease process and in making the modifications in lifestyle necessary to promote increased independence.

NDx: Altered peripheral tissue perfusion

Help the patient conserve oxygen needs by encouraging rest and limiting activities. Assist the patient with meals if needed. Administer oxygen and elevate the head of the bed to aid in chest expansion if appropriate.

Keep the patient in a comfortable position and reposition frequently. Use range-of-motion exercises to stimulate circulation. Explore the need for antiembolism hose or pneumatic compression devices to decrease venous pooling. Assess for signs and symptoms of thrombosis, such as absent or diminished peripheral pulses, delayed capillary refill, positive Homans' sign, edema, tenderness, redness, and warmth in the calf. Monitor vital signs and laboratory studies to assess for changes in status.

Discourage smoking to avoid vasoconstriction. Remove constricting clothing and keep heavy bed linen from restricting the peripheral circulation. Avoid the use of a knee gatch or pillows placed directly under the popliteal area. Tell the patient to notify the nurse if signs of compromised circulation from constricting bandages, casts, or other devices seem apparent, such as discoloration, pain, edema, paresthesia, or a temperature change in an extremity. Maintain the patient's legs in a nondependent position when he or she is not ambulating.

NDx: Impaired skin integrity

Teach the patient measures to prevent skin injury from developing. Avoid irritating sheets or garments. Protect the skin from rough edges of immobilizing devices. Have the patient inspect the skin frequently and seek medical assistance if any breakdown or soreness is noted.

Teach the patient to exercise, as tolerated, to promote good circulation. Range-of-motion exercises should be done while the patient is on bedrest. Turn the patient frequently and inspect pressure areas for early signs of breakdown. Avoid massaging areas of redness, as pressure from massage may cause further tissue damage. Keep heavy linen from constricting the peripheral circulation by using a bed cradle. Elevate the patient's legs when he or she is sitting in a chair. Inspect the areas distal to constrictive devices for signs of compromised circulation. If lesions are present, use aseptic technique to cleanse them. Wear gloves during the dressing changes. Teach the patient and family members the proper technique for dressing areas of breakdown.

NDx: Risk for infection

Keep the patient warm and avoid extreme changes in temperature in the room. Turn the patient as needed to stimulate circulation to prevent skin breakdown and skin infections. Have the patient deep-breathe and cough frequently to prevent respiratory infections, especially if the patient is on bedrest. Use incentive spirometry if appropriate. Monitor the patient's vital signs frequently, observing for subtle changes that may indicate early signs of infection. Report any changes noted.

Monitor intake and output and note the color and consistency of the urine. Assess for signs and symptoms of urinary tract infections. Encourage an increased fluid intake to prevent urinary infections, especially if the patient is on bedrest.

Promote good nutrition for proper healing by serving meals the patient will eat, in a relaxed attractive atmosphere. Encourage a high-protein and high-vitamin diet and high fiber content to prevent constipation. Provide skin care frequently, especially if areas of breakdown are present. Use aseptic technique to cleanse around pin sites, as ordered.

Early identification and treatment may limit the severity of an infection. Teach the patient and family to continually observe for signs of developing infection and to notify the physician if such signs appear.

NDx: Self care deficit (feeding, hygiene, toileting, or other activities of daily living)

Assist the patient with activities of daily living as needed. Seek alternative methods for the patient to be able to complete the activities when restricted by a disorder or immobilizing device. Teach the patient how to maneuver with the assistance of supportive aids. Explain how to use other extremities to complete a task, or how to move appropriately with the restrictive device in place, such as how to use crutches when the patient's leg is in an immobilizer or fixation device. Seek the assistance of physical therapists or occupational therapists when necessary for consultation or teaching sessions for the patient and family. Assess the need for home-care assistance and the use of medical equipment in the home (bathing chair, raised toilet seat).

Compare the patient's status with the expected outcomes. If the outcomes are not met, reassess the patient and revise the plan.

PAIN

A common manifestation of musculoskeletal dysfunction is pain in muscles, joints, and bones. The location and type of pain vary with each particular dysfunction. Typically, bone pain is a throbbing, nonlocalized, aching feeling. It may, however, be localized with a fracture or tumor. Pain in the joints may be associated with inflammation and may be more severe at different times of the day or with movement. Pain associated with inflammation of tendons may be increased during sleeping hours. Rest and anti-inflammatory agents may relieve the pain of inflammation. Muscle pain ranges from mild tenderness and aching to severe pain with movement

or pressure to the affected part. Quick movements may increase the sensation of pain in the muscle. Muscle spasms may also accompany the episodes of pain. Stiffness or decreased flexibility is not defined as pain. However, attempts to use a stiff body part may cause pain. Nonpharmacologic measures such as imagery, distraction, music, and relaxation techniques may be used to decrease the pain. Pain is treated with a variety of anti-inflammatory agents, analgesics, and skeletal muscle relaxants (Highlight 19–1).

NURSING PROCESS
Musculoskeletal Pain

Assessment

Assess the patient for the extent, location, duration, quality, intensity, and frequency of the pain. A pain assessment scale such as number, visual analogue, or verbal scale may be used to assess the pain. The patient's self report of the intensity of pain is the most reliable indicator of the pain. Aggravating and alleviating factors for the pain should be identified. Inspect for swelling, redness, and warmth at the site of the pain. Assess for tenderness or pain with pres-

---

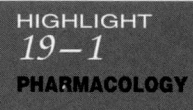 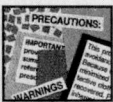

HIGHLIGHT
19–1
PHARMACOLOGY

Skeletal Muscle Relaxants

Definition:

Drugs that promote relaxation of muscles and some sedation.

Action:

These drugs depress the central nervous system in the brain stem, basal ganglia, and spinal cord without altering nerve conduction or muscle excitability.

Uses:

Used for relief of pain, spasticity, and stiffness in musculoskeletal disorders.

Side Effects:

Drowsiness, gastrointestinal distress, photosensitivity, weakness, sensitivity reactions, ataxia, visual or speech difficulties, and dry mucous membranes.

Interactions:

The drugs interact with alcohol products, antidepressants, and other depressants.

Nursing Implications:

Give the drugs with milk or food to decrease gastric irritation. Observe for signs of sensitivity reactions such as fever, rashes, or dyspnea. Tell the patient not to drive or perform tasks that require alertness. Teach the patient about the side effects and caution about taking the drugs with alcohol. Warn the patient against abrupt withdrawal after prolonged use.

Geriatric Considerations:

Drowsiness may be more severe in the elderly. Gastric irritation may also be more severe. Explain the need to take the medication with food and to refrain from participating in activities that require mental alertness while under the influence of the drug. Assess for drug interactions and toxic effects that are more likely in the elderly. Modify assessment techniques as necessary to determine the effects of the medication.

sure applied to the area over the bone or joint. (Palpation or range of motion should not be done if a fracture is suspected until cleared by x-ray examination.) Look for joint deformities and assess the range of motion of the involved joint and the amount of flexibility or stiffness present. Notice the activity level of the patient and whether the pain restricts the patient's movements or ability to do self-care or ambulate. Note the area distal to and around devices that may cause constriction of the extremities and thus cause pain.

Nursing Diagnoses and Planning

The nursing diagnosis and related expected patient outcomes most commonly applicable to patients with musculoskeletal pain are as follows:

NDx: Pain (acute/chronic) related to effects of the musculoskeletal disorder

Planning: Patient Outcomes
1. Patient reports that pain is controlled with analgesics or skeletal muscle relaxants (see Highlight 19–1).
2. Patient states nonpharmacologic measures to help relieve pain.
3. Patient states coping measures to help relieve or tolerate pain.

Nursing Interventions and Evaluation

NDx: Pain
Ask the patient to rate the degree of pain and pain relief measures. Place the patient in comfortable positions with proper alignment and support. Reposition frequently. Check traction to ensure proper alignment and appropriate weight of pull, if appropriate. Look for signs of pressure causing pain if the patient has a restrictive device applied, such as a cast or splint. Use pillows to support bony prominences.

Assess when the pain is most severe, and allow the patient to rest during those periods. Administer pain medications as ordered and before activity periods so that the patient can better tolerate the movement. Offer pain medications on a regular schedule, which will prevent a resurgence of pain as blood levels of the medication decrease. Teach the patient and the family about the effects of prescribed pain medications. Assess the patient for any side effects from the pharmacologic agents.

Teach the patient nonpharmacologic methods to alleviate or tolerate the pain. Demonstrate relaxation and massage techniques to the patient and family. Distraction and imagery techniques may also be taught to the patient and family.

Patient-controlled analgesia may be prescribed for a postoperative patient. Teach the patient the appropriate use of patient-controlled analgesia and reinforce the instructions as needed. Evaluate the effects of the pain medication. Teach the patient and the family how to use a transcutaneous electrical nerve stimulator if ordered. Heat or cold application may be ordered in different situations to reduce pain. Be sure the hot packs are at an appropriate temperature to prevent burning.

Inspect the skin and palpate pulses in distal areas for signs of compromised circulation or skin breakdown caused by constrictive devices that may be the cause of the pain. Tell the patient to report any signs of pain or paresthesia immediately.

Research indicates that many patients suffer considerable pain and distress with musculoskeletal disorders. Therefore, evaluation is a key to determine the effectiveness of pain interventions. Compare the patient's status with the expected outcomes. If the outcomes are not met, reassess the patient and revise the plan.

Assessment of the Musculoskeletal System

The assessment of the musculoskeletal system includes a review of the history of illness or problems with movement and an examination that includes inspection, palpation, measuring the range of motion of joints, grading muscle strength, observing gait, checking neurovascular status, and observing for alterations in activities of daily living.

PATIENT HISTORY

Ask the patient about symptoms of pain, joint stiffness, immobility, swelling, deformity, and any other obvious changes. Obtain detailed descriptions of the pain experienced by the patient. Note the location, duration, precipitating factors, and effective relief methods. Ask the patient whether any recent trauma or injuries have occurred. Check whether the patient has noticed a recent change in gait, ability to handle utensils, grip strength, posture, joint function, or overall movement ability.

Assess the patient for short- and long-term effects of the musculoskeletal dysfunction on lifestyle, activities of daily living, and potential rehabilitation. This information is elicited through scales or open-ended questions to the patient. Determine the patient's level of independence.

During the patient interview, ask questions that elicit a detailed past history and description of present symptoms. The client's age, sex, and occupation are also important demographic data to document. Muscle strength varies among individuals. Identify the family history of musculoskeletal problems. Question the patient about recreational physical activity and activity at the workplace. Ask about the location and type of residence (one-level versus stair access only). Obtain a detailed history of past and present use of prescribed and over-the-counter medications.

PHYSICAL EXAMINATION

During the assessment, note any abnormalities, and ask questions of the patient about the findings to determine the extent of the problem, its onset, and the potential interferences with activities of daily living. Document each of the responses.

Note the patient's ability to sit, change position, stand, bend over, grasp objects, or walk with ease. These activities are important to manage personal hygiene and grooming needs.

Inspect the patient for symmetry, size contour, and random movements on either side of the body. Be sure to compare one side with the other. Note any areas of swelling, discoloration, or obvious malalignment or deformity. Observe the patient in both a standing and a sitting position from the anterior, lateral, and posterior views. The normal spine is straight from the posterior view. Scoliosis is identified by a lateral curvature of the spinal column. From the lateral view, look for a normal forward concave curvature of the cervical spine, a convex curvature of the thoracic spine, and a concave curvature of the lumbar spine. Collapse of one or more vertebral bodies can cause an increased curvature of the involved spine and an overall shortening in height. Excessive convex curvature of the thoracic spine, common in the older adult, is known as kyphosis. Excessive concave curvature of the lumbar vertebral column is termed lordosis. Lordosis may be seen in conjunction with pregnancy, obesity, and hip deformities.

Observe the appearance of major muscles of the upper extremities and the lower extremities and compare bilaterally. Major muscles may be measured to confirm symmetry.

Palpate all major muscles and joints bilaterally. Note areas of swelling, unusual hardness, localized heat spots, muscle tone, and involuntary movement when palpated. Ask the patient to report the location, quality and intensity of the pain when present on examination. The patient may not voluntarily report pain and tenderness in an affected joint. Observe for nonverbal signs of discomfort such as wincing, contracting, or gasping. Note decreased sensation in any area assessed.

Assess the range of motion for the neck, waist, shoulder, elbows, wrists, fingers, hips, knees, ankles, and toes. Note the appropriate range of movement and direction for each. Table 19–3 lists the degrees of movement for each area of assessment. A goniometer is used to accurately measure the range of motion. Place the goniometer against the joint with the arms of the instrument parallel with the axis of each of the bones that connect to form the joint. The angle formed is calibrated on the instrument and represents the amount of flexion or extension of the joint being measured. Patients are also assessed for abnormal muscle movement. Observe the patient for tremors, spasms, fibrillations, and athetoid move-

Table 19–3

Degrees of Movement of Joints

Joint	Movement	Degrees
Neck	Flexion	45
	Extension	55
	Lateral bending (right and left)	40
	Rotation (right and left)	70
Spine/Waist/Hip	Flexion	75+
	Extension	30
	Lateral bending (right and left)	35
	Rotation (right and left)	30
Arms (from shoulder)	Flexion	180
	Extension	50
	Abduction	180
	Adduction	50
	Internal rotation	90
Elbows	Flexion	160
	Extension	0
	Supination	90
	Pronation	90
Wrists	Flexion	90
	Extension (dorsiflexion	70
	Radial deviation	20
	Ulnar deviation	55
Hip		
Straight knee	Flexion	90
	Hyperextension	15
	Abduction	45
	Adduction	30
	Internal rotation	40
	External rotation	45
Bent knee	Flexion	120
	Extension	0
Ankles/Feet	Plantar flexion	45
	Dorsiflexion	20
	Inversion	30
	Eversion	20

ments. Assess for alterations in muscle tone such as atony, hypertonicity, rigidity, and spasticity.

Test the patient's muscle strength by applying force to the extremity while the patient tries to hold it in position. Check facial, neck, arm, wrist, finger, hip, leg, ankle, and foot muscle strength. Compare the findings bilaterally. Note whether the patient exhibited no strength, slight strength, strength without force, or strength with force applied. Frequently a rating scale is utilized to document the data and any differences from one side to the other.

Have the patient walk across the room, turn, and

return. If possible, have the patient walk without assistive devices. Note the patient's balance and gait during this procedure. Look for irregular movements, unsteadiness, limping, or abnormal stride. Observe the position of the shoulders and pelvis in relation to the legs, knee joints, and feet.

Normal gait can be divided into two phases: the stance phase, when the leg bears weight, and the swing phase, when the non-weight-bearing leg is in motion. In the normal adult gait pattern, the distance between the heels is 5 to 10 cm (2–4 inches) and the length of stride is approximately 38 cm (15 inches). Pain, muscle weakness, instability of joints, and structural deformity are common causes of abnormal gait patterns. Changes in supporting structures, such as decreased elasticity of ligaments and physical changes in weight-bearing joints, can affect gait. The elderly tend to walk with a wide heel base and shorter strides because of structural changes of aging. Also have the patient stand first on one foot, then on the other foot. Note balance, change in posture, and any involuntary movements. Stand near the patient during this part of the assessment for support and to prevent a fall if the patient wavers or loses balance.

If the patient has a musculoskeletal dysfunction, assess the neurovascular status proximal and distal to the defect. Neurovascular assessment includes circulatory, nerve, and muscle function. This is done to establish a baseline for comparison. Neurovascular function is then monitored frequently to detect changes that may indicate potential neurovascular complications. Assess the position, color, proximal and distal pulses, capillary refill, motor function, sensation, edema, and temperature of the body part. Assess the pain level of the patient. Compromised neurovascular status is indicated by pain, paresthesia, pallor, edema, decreased temperature, or decreased pulse. Evaluation of the motor function indicates that the nerves controlling those muscles are also functioning. Diminished movement or altered sensation indicates altered neurovascular functioning. Evaluate and compare for symmetry on both sides of the body.

Be aware of the differences in expectations for the elderly patient in all areas of the assessment as compared with the average adult. Normal changes of aging may affect the posture, gait, range of motion, strength, and sensation in the older adult.

Assess the patient's understanding and compliance with health promotion and risk reduction measures related to the health of the musculoskeletal system (Highlight 19–2).

*D*iagnostic Procedures

Numerous diagnostic studies are used in a workup for musculoskeletal dysfunction. These may be classified as radiologic studies, laboratory studies, endoscopic studies, and other studies. The procedures, with nursing implications, are described in Table 19–4.

*M*anagement

Medical intervention to treat joint injury, immobilize a fracture, correct a deformity, or provide support for weak joints or muscles may include nonsurgical interventions, such as application of heat or cold, application of casts, and traction, or surgical interventions, such as application of fixation devices or amputation. In some instances, more than one therapy may be used concurrently. The type of medical management selected is determined by a number of factors, including the location of the injury, the type and severity of the injury (or defect), and the age and the general health of the patient.

NONSURGICAL MANAGEMENT

Application of Heat and Cold

Heat is applied to promote circulation, analgesia, and relaxation, to reduce muscle spasms, and to en-

---

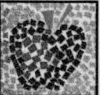

HIGHLIGHT
19–2

HEALTH PROMOTION & RISK REDUCTION

Optimal Musculoskeletal System Function

Patient strategies for promoting the health of and preventing problems or diseases of the musculoskeletal system include:

1. Having a regular periodic health examination by a physician that includes assessment of the musculoskeletal system
2. Participating in screening programs such as scoliosis screening
3. Maintaining the recommended immunization schedule
4. Being attentive to proper posture
5. Using proper body mechanics in lifting or carrying heavy objects
6. Practicing safety at home or work and on the road.
7. Maintaining a well-balanced diet with recommended amounts of calcium and vitamin D
8. Participating in a regular exercise program

Table 10-4

Common Diagnostic Tests for Musculoskeletal Function

Study	Description	Nursing Implications
RADIOLOGIC		
Arthrogram	X-ray film of a joint after a radiopaque dye or air has been injected into the joint cavity. It is used in the diagnosis of intrajoint and cartilaginous disorders.	Assess for allergies to the dye substance or iodine. Determine the patient's understanding of the test and provide necessary information. Obtain a signed consent if required. After the procedure, assess the site for pain or edema. Also observe for signs of latent allergic reactions.
X-ray examination	General roentgenographic studies of any bone or joint for diagnosis of suspected problems.	Determine the patient's understanding of the test ordered. Explain what is to be done. If the patient is in pain from an injury, give prescribed medication for pain because the affected area may be manipulated during the x-ray examination, causing more pain.
Bone scan	X-ray examination of skeletal bone using a gamma camera scanner after an injection of a radioactive substance. The dye is picked up in areas of increased metabolism. It is not collected in poorly perfused bone. It is used to diagnose cancer, osteomyelitis, fractures, and osteoporosis.	Assess whether the patient is pregnant or allergic to iodine, because it is contraindicated in these situations. Provide information about the test to the patient. Explain that the patient must remain immobile for the duration of the scan. Obtain a signed consent. Give the patient increased fluids prior to the test to aid in the excretion of the medium after the test. If pelvic bones are to be scanned, have the patient void prior to the test, because a full bladder may obscure pelvic bones. After the scan, observe for signs of an allergic reaction and encourage increased fluid intake.
Computed tomographic (CT) scan	Combines x-rays with computer technology to produce pictures of internal musculoskeletal structures. A contrast medium may be used. CT scan is used to identify tissue tumors, injuries to ligaments or tendons, or fractures.	Assess the patient's knowledge about the procedure and provide information. Because the machine used is often frightening to the patient, provide reassurance and allow the patient to ask questions and voice concerns. Explain that the patient will be lying flat while passing very slowly through a cylinder-type apparatus. Inform the patient about the importance of lying still and that the scan may take several minutes (20 minutes or more is common).
Gallium scan	Nuclear scan that utilizes gallium, a radionuclide, that is concentrated by areas of inflammation, infection, and tumors.	The procedure is contraindicated in pregnant patients. Assess the patient's knowledge and explain the procedure. The injection with gallium is followed by body scans performed at various intervals up to 72 hours following injection. Explain that there is no discomfort with the injection but that it may be uncomfortable to lie still on a hard table for the duration of the scan.
Arteriogram	Series of x-ray films taken of the arterial system after injection of a dye. The test is used to diagnose occlusion of blood vessels. Bones do not heal properly and osteomyelitis is more likely if the blood supply to an injured limb is compromised.	Assess the patient's knowledge about the procedure and provide information needed. Determine whether the patient has allergies to contrast dye. After the procedure, monitor the injection site for signs of hematoma, inflammation, or drainage.

Table 19–4

Common Diagnostic Tests for Musculoskeletal Function (continued)

Study	Description	Nursing Implications
LABORATORY		
Blood analysis	The complete blood count is used to determine possible infection and low hemoglobin level (due to hemorrhage). Blood chemistry is used to determine osteomalacia, some bone tumors, and muscle damage. Serium calcium, phosphorous, and alkaline phosphatase levels are monitored to determine bone activities such as resorption, destruction, and growth. Erythrocyte sedimentation rate detects inflammatory, neoplastic, and infectious processes.	Explain the tests to the patient. Reinforce the physician's report of the findings to the patient and family.
Urinalysis	Calcium levels in the urine may increase in some musculoskeletal conditions such as cancer of the bone. The urine may also be tested for bacteria because bladder infections may result from long-term immobility.	Explain why a urine sample is needed. Collect and send the sample to the laboratory according to the set procedure of the institution. Reinforce the results of the tests as reported to the patient by the physician.
Arthrocentesis	A needle puncture into the space of a joint to aspirate fluid. For diagnostic purposes, the fluid is sent to the laboratory for analysis. It is used to determine infection, hemorrhage, or other problems of the joint such as arthritis.	Explain the procedure to the patient. Obtain a signed consent. Assist the physician with the procedure if needed. Observe the puncture site after the test for inflammation, drainage, or swelling, indicative of an infection. An ice bag or compression bandage may be applied. Teach the patient to rest the joint for 8 to 24 hours.
ENDOSCOPIC		
Arthroscopy	Endoscopic examination of a joint for diagnostic or treatment purposes. It is most commonly used for knee disorders. It is performed under aseptic technique in an examining room, or operating room (if corrective), under local or general anesthetic. It is usually an outpatient procedure.	Preparation prior to the procedure may include teaching the individual to fast from midnight the night before. Explain the procedure to the patient and obtain a signed consent. If arthroscopy is done for diagnostic reasons only, local anesthesia is usually used, so the patient's preoperative preparation is limited. After the procedure, teach the individual to observe for pain, bleeding, drainage, or swelling at the site. Inform the individual that a normal diet may be resumed when desired. Reinforce the home-care instructions from the physician. Check dressings or wrap before the patient's discharge.
OTHER		
Magnetic resonance imaging (MRI)	Uses magnetic force to provide clear three-plane pictures of internal structures. No radiation or contrast medium is used. It is used for diagnosis of any musculoskeletal dysfunction that is not readily diagnosable by other means, but it is particularly valuable for viewing soft tissues.	Explain the procedure to the patient. Because the equipment is sometimes frightening to the patient, mild sedation may be used. Some patients become claustrophobic during the test. Have the patient remove all metal objects. Identify any patient who has internal metal objects such as a fixation device or prosthesis because MRI may cause it to migrate. The MRI is contraindicated for any patient with internal metal objects.

Table continued on following page

Table 19–4

Common Diagnostic Tests for Musculoskeletal Function *(continued)*

Study	Description	Nursing Implications
Electromyography (EMG)	Determines the electrical activity of skeletal muscle and its ability to respond to a stimulus. An oscilloscope records the activity of the muscle through needle electrodes inserted through the skin. EMG is used to differentiate between neurologic and muscular disorders.	Before the EMG, assess the patient's functional capacity involving specific muscles, such as gait, ability to do range-of-motion exercises, and sensory motor deficits. This is helpful in interpreting the results. Explain the test to the patient. Tell the patient that the test may be lengthy (sometimes up to 2 hours). Obtain a signed consent.
Thermography	An infrared camera is used to determine the amount of heat radiating from soft tissue. The photograph shows variations from cold (blue) to hot (red). It is used to evaluate inflammation of joints, damage to supporting structures, and muscle trauma.	Explain the test to the patient. Tell the patient it is noninvasive and painless. Expose the body part to be tested to room air for 15 minutes prior to the test. The room temperature should be between 20° and 20.9°C (68° and 70°F).

hance flexibility. Heat may be applied by radiation (light), conduction (hot pack or pad), or conversion (diathermy, ultrasound). The temperature of the heat application should not exceed 37.8°C (100°F). Heat may be applied intermittently as ordered, usually in 15- to 30-minute time periods.

The local application of cold immediately after an injury causes local vasoconstriction, prevents swelling, and aids in pain relief and muscle spasm. Cooling reduces the inflammatory response to tissue trauma. After the first 24 to 48 hours, heat may be applied to increase circulation and promote comfort. Ice bags or commercial cold packs can be used to apply cold to a specific area. Cold is applied intermittently to prevent reflex dilatation of blood vessels and frostbite injury. Cold is applied for 20 minutes or less, then removed for 10 to 15 minutes to allow capillary circulation to return to the affected area.

NURSING PROCESS
Application of Heat or Cold

Assessment

Before the prescribed application of heat or cold, assess the patient's skin for lesions or sensitive areas. Caution is necessary in patients with decreased peripheral circulation or decreased sensation because these patients may not feel an extremely hot or cold sensation until trauma to the tissue has occurred. During the treatment, question the patient about subjective sensations of extreme heat or cold, numbness, tingling, or increased pain. Assess for effects of the application such as comfort, relief of pain, or absence of swelling.

Nursing Diagnoses and Planning

The nursing diagnosis and related expected patient outcomes most commonly applicable to patients undergoing heat or cold application therapy are as follows:

NDx: Risk for injury (tissue trauma) related to the treatment regimen

Planning: Patient Outcomes
1. Patient denies sensation of extreme heat or cold at site of application.
2. Patient's skin remains intact without a burn or frostbite injury.

Nursing Interventions and Evaluation

NDx: Risk for injury
Apply all heat and cold therapy with caution, especially in the patient with decreased peripheral circulation or sensation, as in the elderly or a patient with peripheral vascular disease. Protect the skin from direct contact with the heat or cold source by placing a towel next to the patient's skin. To ensure maximum effectiveness, secure the heat or cold application loosely in the desired position. Leave the application on no longer than the prescribed time (usually 20 to 30 minutes at a time). Check the skin frequently for irritation. Tell the patient to report any increased pain, numbness, or burning sensations. Observe for signs of the effectiveness of the therapy, such as absence of edema or decreased edema and tenderness.

Compare the patient's status with the expected outcomes. If the outcomes are not met, reassess the patient and revise the plan.

Cast Therapy

A cast provides circumferential support and protection of an involved body part without prohibiting movement of the entire body. It may be applied to part of an extremity, an entire extremity, the entire body trunk, or part of the trunk. The purposes of a cast include immobilization, correction of deformities, realignment, support, and healing. Usually the cast encompasses the joint above and below the bone to be immobilized. If a joint is to be immobilized, then the cast encompasses the bone above and below the joint.

While in a cast, the body part is supported and fixed in one position. The cast is applied while the body part is maintained in a functional position with proper alignment of bone fragments. The cast must fit the specific body part correctly.

The body part to be immobilized, corrected, or rested determines the type of cast applied. Some of the common types of casts are described in Table 19–5.

CAST APPLICATION

A cast may be applied in an ambulatory clinic setting, an emergency room, or in a hospital. A cast is applied after abrasions have been cleaned and wounds dressed. The skin should be clean and dry and thoroughly inspected. The application procedure should be explained to the individual and the family. The body part is aligned and maintained in the position in which the cast will harden. If the patient cannot assist, the nurse maintains the position of the body part during cast application. The patient's clothing and bed linen are protected from water and cast residue by a drape during application of the cast.

A layer of tubular stockinette is applied next to the patient's skin. The stockinette may be made of cotton or polyester. Next, a layer of thin padding is applied in a circular fashion. Extra padding may be applied over bony prominences for added protection. The padding is made of cotton or a synthetic material. These coverings should fit smoothly since wrinkles can cause skin trauma and breakdown. The cast is then applied over the stockinette and padding.

Most casts are made of polyester, fiberglass, or thermoplastic material, but plaster of Paris casting material may be used in some instances. Each of the different casting materials requires an agent such as water or heat to prepare the substance for use. Plaster of Paris and polyester casting material are moistened with water. Fiberglass is moistened with water or a special agent. The thermoplastic materials are prepared using hot water or hot air. The various materials differ in characteristics and cost.

Casts made of synthetic materials are ready for weight-bearing within minutes after application. Plaster of Paris casts require several hours for drying of the material. A long leg cast of plaster can take 24 to 48 hours to dry completely and allow weight-bearing.

Synthetic casts weigh less and are more durable than plaster of Paris casts. Plaster of Paris disintegrates in water once it has hardened, but the synthetic materials are unchanged by water. Although the synthetic materials withstand dampening, they must be dried thoroughly to prevent irritation and maceration of the skin underneath the cast. With the use of a blow dryer on cool setting, it may take as long as 3 hours to completely dry all layers of a short arm synthetic cast. A dryer should not be placed too close or only on one area of the cast. A dryer should not be placed on an operative site without physician approval. Care must be taken not to burn the skin while using the dryer.

CAST REMOVAL

A cast is removed by an electric cast cutter. Most cast cutters use an oscillating circular blade that cuts through the cast material. These cutters produce a loud buzzing noise that may frighten a patient. The patient is informed in advance of what to expect and is cautioned to avoid moving the limb while the cast is being removed to prevent skin injury. Explain to the individual that a cast cutter should not cut skin. Once the cast is separated along the sides with the electric cutter, the padding and stockinette are cut with scissors. The cast is then removed, top piece first. This method of removal allows the bottom cast half to be used as a posterior splint for handling of the body part.

COMPLICATIONS OF CAST THERAPY

A cast that is too tight constricts circulation and causes pressure areas, skin lesions, and tissue necrosis. A cast may seem to fit properly when first applied but become too tight from edema that develops after the cast application. The assessment for impaired circulation includes changes in pulse, skin color, sensation, pain or function. Conversely, a cast applied to an edematous body part may become too loose when the edema subsides and may provide inadequate support for the affected part. Nerve damage from pressure where a nerve passes over a bony prominence may also be a complication from a cast. Changes in sensation, increasing pain, or motor weakness may indicate nerve pressure. In these situations, the cast must be altered or replaced to provide an appropriate fit.

The cast cutter is used to cut through the cast without removing it to release the pressure of a tight cast. Cutting the cast allows edematous soft tissues under the cast to expand without compromising neurovascular function. Once the edema has subsided, the cast is usually sealed and reinforced with an elastic wrap or additional casting material.

Casts, except preformed ones, are applied by lay-

Table 19–5

Some Common Types of Casts

Cast	Description	Potential Pressure Points
Short arm cast	Extends from the palmar crease of the hand to the elbow. It allows movement of the fingers and thumb and is used for stable fractures or conditions of the metacarpals, carpals, or distal radius. If the thumb is incorporated, the cast is called a gauntlet or thumb spica cast.	Radial and ulnar styloids; also the base of the thumb
Long arm cast	Extends from the palmar crease to the proximal humerus. The elbow is encompassed, and the cast is applied with the elbow flexed in a 90-degree functional position. It is used for unstable fractures of the carpals, stable fractures or conditions of the distal humerus, and fractures and conditions of the radius or ulna.	Radial styloid, olecranon, and lateral epicondyle
Short leg cast	Extends from the toes to just below the knee joint. It is used for stable fractures or conditions, such as fusions of the metatarsals, calcaneus, talus, and tarsal bones. It may be fitted with a wedge attached to the foot portion to allow walking and weight-bearing. The attachment may be applied with the initial cast or after complete drying.	Lateral and medial malleolus and fibular head. Pressure to the peroneal nerve may result in foot drop.
Long leg cast	Extends from the toes to the groin and includes the knee joint. It immobilizes the tibia, fibula, knee, and ankle joint and is used to treat stable injuries of the knee and distal femur. It is applied with the knee slightly flexed to relax the ligaments.	Lateral and medial malleolus and the fibular head
Spica cast	Encompasses one or more extremities and the body trunk.	Malleoli, fibular heads, and iliac crests for the hip spica casts. Care must taken to prevent pressure on the mesenteric artery from the lower trunk portion of the cast.

Table 19–5

Some Common Types of Casts (continued)

Cast	Description	Potential Pressure Points
One-half hip spica (single hip spica)	Encompasses one leg and the lower trunk. It restricts pelvis rotation and limits hip movement.	
One and one-half hip spica	Encompasses one whole leg, the lower trunk, and half of the other leg. It also restricts pelvic rotation and hip movement.	
Double hip spica	Encompasses both legs and the lower trunk. It immobilizes both hip joints. Hip spica casts are used to immobilize the pelvis, hip joints, femur, and knee after injuries or surgery. An abduction bar may be incorporated into the cast for support.	
Shoulder spica	Encompasses one arm and its shoulder and the upper trunk. It is used in unstable fractures of the shoulder girdle, humerus, and elbow joint, or conditions of the shoulder such as a fusion.	Iliac crest, ulnar styloid, lateral and medial epicondyle, and olecranon for the shoulder spica casts
Body cast	Encircles the trunk to immobilize the spine. The cervical, thoracic, or lumbar spine may be immobilized for repair of injuries or following operative procedures.	Superior mesenteric artery

ering the materials. Because of the multiple layers of material, any drainage from beneath the cast comes to the surface of the outside of the cast very slowly. This characteristic of casting material causes difficulty in determining the exact extent of drainage produced at a given time. It may take several days for a small amount of drainage to completely ooze to the outer layer of the cast. Circling and recording time of drainage noted on the surface of the cast, although a good practice in general, may not provide an accurate estimate of the current drainage occurring under the cast or the time it occurred. The patient's subjective sensations of wetness and an assessment of vital signs are the best indicators of hemorrhage under a cast.

Tissue necrosis or infection under a cast may also occur in cast therapy. The patient's indication of warmth in an area or a musty offensive odor may indicate necrosis or infection.

Application of a body cast may predispose the patient to a serious complication of cast therapy termed cast syndrome. It is characterized by anorexia, nausea, vomiting, and abdominal discomfort and distention. It may be caused by the compression of the mesenteric artery from hyperextension of the spine, which puts pressure on the duodenum, causing eventual obstruction. Treatment includes instillation of a nasogastric tube for decompression, intravenous fluids, and possibly, removal or readjustment of the cast. This syndrome may not develop until several weeks after the application of the body cast. It may be prevented by the use of a belly pad during application and the addition of a belly hole in the cast.

NURSING PROCESS
Cast Therapy

Assessment

Prior to the casting, assess the skin for lesions, areas of redness, swelling, and irritation. Check and document proximal and distal neurovascular function to establish a baseline. After the casting, check for proper cast fit by assessing the neurovascular status of the area involved every hour for 48 hours and every 8 hours thereafter. If distal pulses are covered by the cast, check capillary refill, color, and temperature of the extending part. Assess the area for swelling and ask the patient to describe sensation. Observe for skin irritation under and around the cast edge and on bony prominences. Assess for any drainage or foul odors, which may indicate lesions or infection of lesions under the cast. Assess the patient's knowledge about self-care and the care of the cast at home. Thorough assessment and prompt interventions are essential to prevent complications from a cast.

If the patient is in a body cast, observe for signs and symptoms of cast syndrome or restricted chest expansion. Auscultate breath sounds in exposed areas of the chest, if applicable, for early signs of respiratory problems. Observe the perineal area, noting any problems with fecal matter or urine on the cast.

After cast removal, observe the skin for dryness, irritation, or the presence of breakdown. Expect the skin to be somewhat dry, pale, flaking, and slightly irritated. Inspect the limb for atrophy, weakness, and loss of range of motion.

Nursing Diagnoses and Planning

Nursing diagnoses and related expected patient outcomes most commonly applicable to patients with a cast include the following:

NDx: Altered peripheral tissue perfusion related to constriction of circulation and possible nerve or vascular damage from the cast

Planning: Patient Outcomes
1. Patient's extremities are warm, color is adequate, and pulses are present.
2. Patient is free of complications from compromised circulation such as changes in color, temperature, movement, sensation, capillary refill, and edema.
3. Patient denies pain or decreased sensation in affected extremities.

NDx: Impaired skin integrity related to insufficient peripheral circulation and/or irritation from the cast over the skin and bony prominences

Planning: Patient Outcomes
1. Patient verbalizes factors associated with irritation and skin lesions and measures to prevent the occurrence or recurrence.
2. Patient relates appropriate knowledge about skin care.
3. Patient is free of skin complications.

NDx: Self care deficit related to physical limitations imposed by cast application

Planning: Patient Outcomes
1. Patient performs activities of daily living, using assistive devices as necessary.
2. Patient states alternative methods to complete tasks that are restricted by musculoskeletal dysfunction and cast therapy.

NDx: Pain related to pressure of the cast, itching, or inability to move freely

Planning: Patient Outcomes
1. Patient denies pain, itching, or other irritation from the cast.
2. Patient rests and sleeps well and appears relaxed and able to cope with wearing the cast.

NDx: Impaired home maintenance management related to self-care needs and care of the cast

Planning: Patient Outcomes
1. Patient states accurate information about self-care and cast care at home (Highlight 19–3).
2. Patient states the signs of complications of cast therapy and when to seek medical intervention.

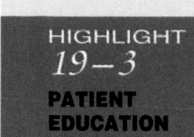
HIGHLIGHT
19-3
**PATIENT
EDUCATION**

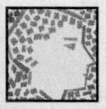

Discharge Instructions After Cast Application

Instruct the patient to:

Allow air to circulate around the cast until it has thoroughly dried from the inside out. (For plaster casts only.)

Refrain from using external heat sources to hasten the drying process, as this may result in burns under the cast. (For plaster casts only.)

Refrain from placing plastic or rubber materials around or under a fresh cast because the heat produced by the cast will be directed toward the skin and cause irritation or burns. (For plaster casts only.)

Use the palms of the hands, not the finger tips, when handling the wet cast, to prevent distortion of the cast. (For plaster casts only.)

Protect the wet cast from resting on hard surfaces that might cause distortion of the cast. (For plaster casts only.)

Keep the cast clean and dry. The cast may be wiped clean with a damp cloth. Extra care is needed if the cast extends to the perineal area.

Refrain from inserting sharp objects under the cast, or injury to the skin may result.

Cover rough edges of the cast with tape "petals" to prevent skin irritation and crumbling of the cast edges once it has dried completely.

Observe the cast for areas of softening or indentation and report observations to the attending physician.

Exercise the joints proximal and distal to the cast if not contraindicated to prevent muscle atrophy, weakness, and loss of joint motion.

Keep casted extremities elevated above the heart level for at least 24 to 48 hours to reduce swelling.

Avoid elevating the extremity, if compartment syndrome is suspected.

Report fever, foul odors, feelings of warmth, and drainage from under the cast.

Report edema, burning, numbness, coldness, discoloration of the skin, painful or decreased movement, decreased sensation, persistent pain, or tingling to the attending physician immediately. Pressure caused by swelling must be relieved by cutting the cast before irreversible damage occurs. Therefore, teach the patient to report these signs to the physician immediately.

Refrain from using emollient lotions on the skin around the cast because they may run down into the cast, causing dampness and becoming a potential site for bacterial growth.

Refrain from putting talcum powder down the cast because it tends to build up on the skin. Corn starch may be used for perspiration control.

Follow safety instructions for the use of any assistive devices, such as crutches or walkers, used for locomotion.

Rearrange the home environment to accommodate the ambulatory aid to prevent falls or other injuries.

Expect discomfort the first few times a casted extremity is placed in a dependent position.

---

3. Patient relates the measures necessary to lessen the risk of complications.
4. Patient shows no evidence of complications of cast therapy, such as inability to complete activities of daily living, deformities, skin breakdown, or infection.

Nursing Interventions and Evaluation

NDx: Altered peripheral tissue perfusion
Perform a neurovascular assessment of the casted extremity to determine peripheral circulation. The assessment should determine that peripheral pulses are palpable and equal in strength, with warm skin temperature and adequate capillary refill. The skin should demonstrate no cyanosis or pallor, with adequate sensation and movement of the extremities. A complication of compromised circulation is compartment syndrome, which can result in permanent

functional damage to the limb. Compartment syndrome can result from a tight cast that constricts circulation to a limb. Compartment syndrome may be exhibited by a change in the pain experienced by the patient and pain that is not controlled by the use of analgesics. Changes in skin color or diminished distal pulses is a late sign of the syndrome. The physician must be notified immediately of any compartment syndrome signs. A cast cutter must be available to remove the cast if peripheral circulation is compromised.

Additional nursing interventions for the patient with a cast include maintaining the patient in a comfortable position with frequent repositioning. Utilize range-of-motion exercises to stimulate circulation. Monitor vital signs to assess for changes and improvements in status. Encourage ambulation as allowed, but provide for frequent rest periods to decrease cardiac workload and prevent further compromised peripheral circulation.

Discourage smoking to avoid vasoconstriction. Remove constricting clothing and keep heavy bed linen from causing pressure. Teach the patient to notify the nurse if signs of compromised circulation from the cast are apparent, such as pain, swelling, discoloration, paresthesia, temperature change, or immobility of an extremity. Maintain the patient's extremities in a nondependent position when he or she is not ambulating.

NDx: Impaired skin integrity

Teach the patient measures to prevent skin breakdown from developing. Teach the patient to inspect the skin frequently around the edges of the cast. Instruct the patient to seek medical assistance if any signs of skin breakdown develop.

Keep the cast and skin around the cast clean and dry. If the cast extends to the perineal area, clean the patient thoroughly after urination or bowel movements. Teach the patient or family to do the same at home to prevent breakdown of the skin in the perineal area.

Teach the patient to exercise, as tolerated, to promote good circulation to the skin. Range-of-motion exercises should be done while the patient is on bedrest. Turn the patient frequently and inspect pressure areas for early signs of breakdown. If lesions are present, use aseptic technique to cleanse them according to agency policy. Teach the patient and family members the proper technique for dressing areas of breakdown.

NDx: Self care deficit

Assist the patient with activities of daily living as needed. Seek alternative methods for the patient to be able to complete these activities when restricted by the cast. Assist the patient as needed in cleaning the perineal area. Position the patient for maximum comfort for urination.

Teach the patient how to maneuver with the assistance of supportive aids. Explain how to utilize other extremities to complete a task or how to move appropriately with the restrictive device in place, such as how to use crutches when the patient's leg is in a cast. Develop an exercise regime to increase strength and endurance. Seek the assistance of physical therapists or occupational therapists when necessary for consultation or teaching sessions for the patient and family.

NDx: Pain

Instruct the patient how to move in bed using assistive devices such as an overhead trapeze or the side rails. Once the patient is able to be out of bed, assist with the changes in balance or weight-bearing, if applicable, when the patient is mobile. Help the patient change positions frequently to relieve pressure areas. Give pain medications as prescribed to reduce discomfort. Relieve pressure areas from the cast by cutting windows if ordered.

NDx: Impaired home maintenance management

Instruct the patient about the effects of immobility if the patient is in a full body cast and the effects of disuse of the affected extremity in the case of an arm or leg cast. (See Mobility Impairment in the section on Clinical Manifestations.) Teach the patient and family the signs of complications, such as elimination difficulty, discoloration of the skin, skin breakdown, diminished pulses, numbness, and the symptoms of infections. Tell the patient when to seek medical assistance if symptoms appear. Explain the need for safety measures if locomotion is a problem.

Teach the patient about cast care management as described in Highlight 19–3. Allow the patient to ask questions as needed. Include the family in the education sessions when appropriate.

Additional Interventions

Once the cast has been applied and until it is dry, provide firm support for the entire cast. Cleanse any excess casting material from the skin. A cast cutter should be available in case the cast needs to be removed quickly as a result of extreme swelling or just bivalved to release minor pressure from edema. Reposition the patient frequently, maintaining body and cast alignment. Initiate measures to promote comfort and combat itching, such as massaging the skin around the edges of the cast, directing cool air under the cast, or encouraging isometric exercises of the casted body part to increase blood flow and decrease itching, unless contraindicated.

Prepare the patient with a cast for the appearance of dry, scaly skin and lack of muscle strength and tone in the affected part upon the removal of the cast. Also, provide proper care of the body part after removal of the cast by washing the skin gently with a mild soap and water. Gently cleanse the area to remove dead skin. Apply lotion with lanolin as a protective emollient to the dry areas.

If the patient is in a body cast, assess for abdominal distention, nausea, and vomiting, which are symptoms of pressure on the mesenteric artery or abdomen. Place the patient in a prone or side-lying position if any abdominal symptoms occur and notify the attending physician. Encourage good nutrition to promote healing and to help maintain proper elimination patterns.

Physical and occupational rehabilitation may be indicated in some cases. Follow-up rehabilitation may be required to promote transition from a health-care agency to the home. The family and the patient may require teaching to promote this transition.

Compare the patient's status with the expected outcomes. If the outcomes are not met, reassess the patient and revise the plan.

Traction Therapy

Traction is a pulling force applied to a body part while countertraction pulls in the opposite direction. The pulling force is usually generated by a system of weights and pulleys attached to the patient's body. Countertraction is generated by the body's own weight, although it may also be applied by weights and pulleys. The traction or force applied to the body is classified by the direction of the pulling force and the way the force is applied. The direction is either straight or vectored. Straight traction pulls only in one direction, usually in line with the longitudinal axis of the involved bone. Vectored traction is the pulling force that results when traction is applied in two different directions.

Traction is used as a therapeutic intervention for a variety of musculoskeletal problems. Traction may be used to do the following:

- Reduce a fracture or return the pieces of bone to the original position and proper anatomical alignment
- Lessen muscle spasm and prevent muscle contractions that displace fractured bone fragments and create pain
- Maintain a reduction while the bone heals
- Prevent or correct a deformity by decreasing skin and muscle contractures around a joint or injured part—traction may be used alone or in conjunction with surgery for this purpose
- Lessen the chance of necrosis due to pressure on the articular surfaces of an injured joint and to rest the joint after a fracture within the joint capsule or joint dislocation

PRINCIPLES OF TRACTION

For any type of traction, to achieve the desired effect of rapid healing with optimal function, the basic principles of traction must be followed. The pull of the traction as well as the use of weights and counterweights, as ordered, must be set up and maintained in an appropriate manner. The principles of traction are detailed in Table 19–6.

TYPES OF TRACTION

Traction can be applied to the body by manual traction, skin traction, or skeletal traction. Manual traction is applied to a body part when someone, such as the physician, applies a temporary smooth and steady pull on the involved part. Manual traction is used to reduce a fracture or a dislocated joint. It is effective only as long as the pull is maintained by the individual applying the manual traction. For long-term application of traction, the pulling force is maintained by a system of weights, ropes, and pulleys attached to the patient's skin or skeleton.

Skin traction applies indirect pulling force to the skeleton. It is accomplished by attaching wide strips of adhesive or nonadhesive strapping to the skin, or by applying traction boots. Weights are then suspended by ropes and pulleys (Figs. 19–4 and 19–5). Belts and halters can be used when a pull is desired on the spine. Common types of skin traction are Buck's and Russell's traction.

Skin traction is used only for temporary manage-

Table 19–6

Principles of Traction

Principle	Nursing Implications
The line of pull must be maintained.	Center the patient in the bed and place in good body alignment.
The pull of traction must be continuous, unless specified otherwise by the attending physician.	Remove or add weights only by a physician's order. Discontinue or release the traction only on the physician's order.
The ropes and weights must be free of friction.	Keep the ropes from becoming entangled in the linen. Be certain the weights hang free at all times. Keep the ropes over the center of the pulley.
There must be sufficient countertraction maintained at all times.	Keep the patient from sliding to the foot of the bed. Keep the patient in side-arm traction in the center of the bed.

ment of fractures in adults because the skin cannot tolerate the weight for the long length of time required for healing. It is used temporarily in femur fractures to maintain alignment and prevent muscle spasm until surgical reduction can occur. The traction weights are usually limited to 2.3 to 3.6 kg (5–8 lbs).

Skin traction is contraindicated in the presence of skin abrasions or wounds, dermatitis, impaired circulation, varicose ulcers, and peripheral neuropathies. It is used with extra caution on individuals with diabetes mellitus because of the risk of skin and circulatory disorders in these patients. Skin traction does not control rotation of a body part.

Complications associated with skin traction include

- Allergic reactions to the adhesive or rubber
- Irritation of skin from belts, straps, or halters
- Peroneal nerve palsy from pressure over the lateral fibular head
- Pressure sores around malleoli and radial and ulnar styloids

Adhesive skin traction is applied to clean, dry skin that has had the hair removed for better adhesion. Hair is best removed by an electric shaver, clipping with scissors, or use of a commercial skin depilatory, because shaving with a razor blade can cut the skin. A nonirritating protective adhesive agent may be applied to the skin first. Adhesive strips or material with a hypoallergenic gummed surface that allows air to reach the skin is then applied. A spreader helps keep the pressure off the bony prominences and provides a connection for the rope. The adhesive strips are then wrapped with an

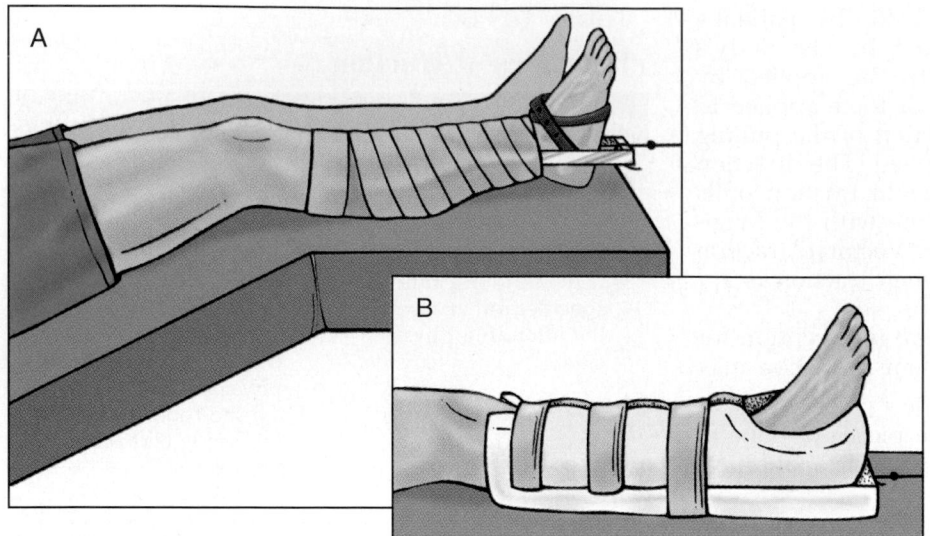

Figure 19-4

Skin traction: Buck's extension. The traction may be attached to the leg with wide strips of adhesive or non-adhesive strapping (*A*) or traction boots (*B*).

elastic bandage. The bandage is wrapped diagonally or in a modified figure eight. It should be snug but not tight or constricting. The adhesive is never applied to bony prominences or over superficial nerves. These areas can be protected with cast padding to prevent adhesion of the tape.

Some conditions may be treated by intermittent skin traction applied by commercial traction boots, belts, or nonadhesive straps. Intermittent skin traction allows removal of the weights for bathing and inspecting the skin, toileting, and some limited activity.

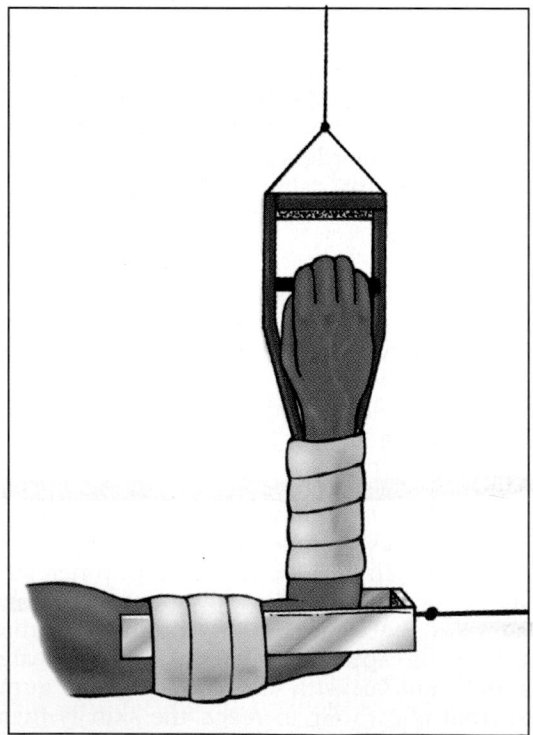

Figure 19-5

Skin traction: side arm.

Skeletal traction applies a pulling force directly to a body part by metal pins, screws, or tongs inserted into bone. The metal is made of nonferrous material and is generally placed into cancellous bone distal to the fracture or affected body part. The pins, screws, or tongs for skeletal traction are inserted in the operating room using surgical asepsis.

A small incision is made in the skin, and the metal piece is drilled by hand into the bone. The metal pins, screws, or tongs are then attached to a U-shaped bow or similar device. Either the Steinmann pin or Kirschner wire is commonly used in achieving skeletal traction (Fig. 19-6). They are both round stainless steel rods. The Kirschner wire is a thin wire (0.7–1.6 mm) while the Steinmann pin has a larger diameter (2–4.8 mm). Both come in various lengths and each has a holder or bow that is attached to the traction weights. The bow is connected by rope to weights via a free-hanging pulley system. Areas away from nerves and blood vessels are selected for insertion sites. Traction weights used can range from 2.3 to 18.1 kg (5–40 lbs). The amount of weight applied varies with the condition and part of the body being treated.

Skeletal traction is effective in reducing and maintaining alignment of fracture fragments because it provides control of rotation as well as longitudinal pull. Skeletal traction, applied by the use of Steinmann pins or a Kirschner wire, is used primarily for fractures or disorders of the pelvis, acetabulum, and femur. Skeletal traction is seldom used for upper extremity fractures except in the case of complicated distal humerus and elbow injuries or disorders.

Skeletal traction to an arm or leg may be combined with a splint to create a balanced suspension apparatus. The splint maintains suspension and alignment of the limb while other body parts move about freely. A Thomas (or Hodgen) splint is frequently used for balanced suspension to the lower extremity. The splint provides support for the thigh. A Pearson attachment may be clamped to the splint

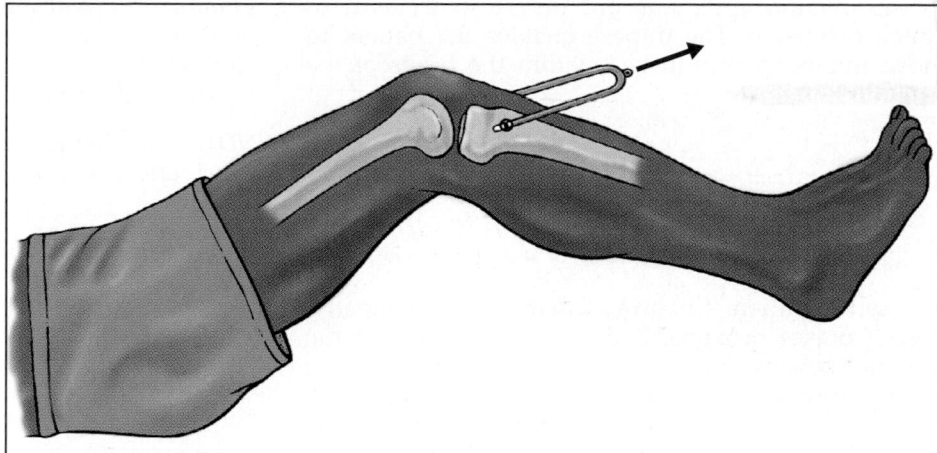

Figure 19-6

Skeletal traction: Steinmann pin. The pin is inserted through the bone and attached to a U-shaped bow. Traction is maintained with ropes, pulleys, and weights attached to the top of the bow. This immobilizes and maintains the alignment of the body part for extended periods.

at the level of the knee to permit flexion of the knee and movement of the lower leg. When the leg is suspended in this apparatus, the foot also needs support to prevent footdrop. Remove foot supports regularly for ankle exercise amd to inspect the skin. Elastic or rubber bands attached to a foot splint allow exercise without the splint's being removed.

Traction to the cervical spine is applied by inserting metal tongs into the parietal prominences of the skull. Some common types of tongs are Crutchfield, Vinke, Gardner-Wells, and Barton (Fig. 19-7). Screws and a ring or halo may also be used to immobilize the cervical spine. To prevent rotation of the spine, the halo apparatus is connected to a body jacket, vest, or cast (Fig. 19-8).

APPLICATION OF TRACTION

The physician prescribes the type and amount of traction to be applied. Who applies the traction varies according to the type of traction, specific orders of the physician, and agency standards and procedures. Skeletal traction is applied by the physician because of the pin insertion. A nurse or orthopedic technician may assist in the attachment of the weights, ropes, pulleys, slings, and splints. Adhesive

or nonadhesive skin traction and circumferential belts and halters may be applied by the nurse or orthopedic technician. Occasionally, a physician purposely sets up traction differently to achieve a special effect. The nurse documents in the patient's care plan the particulars of unusual traction applications to ensure the optimal result from treatment as well as continuity of care.

The patient in traction is placed in a bed with a firm mattress that allows connection of an overbed frame. This frame is primarily used to attach parts

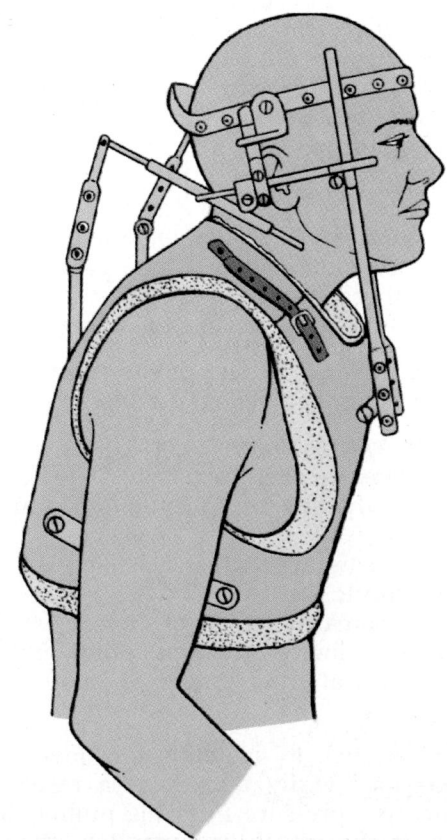

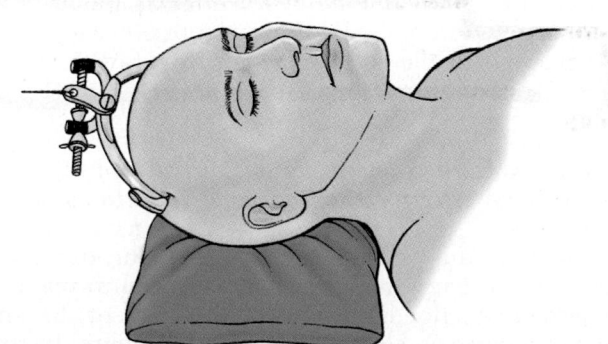

Figure 19-7

Cervical traction: Crutchfield skull tongs. This cervical traction apparatus is attached directly to the skull.

Figure 19-8

Halo traction apparatus with a body brace.

of the traction apparatus but may also be used to attach a trapeze. The trapeze enables the patient to move independently in bed within the limits of the traction apparatus.

NURSING PROCESS
Traction Therapy

Assessment

Assess the patient's neurovascular status frequently. Assess pulses proximal and distal to the site of the traction attachment. Note the color, texture, and temperature of the skin. Test capillary refill. Look for swelling, which may indicate constriction of the extremity. Ask the patient about pain, numbness, or tingling in the affected part. Compare assessment of both limbs. Document findings and notify the physician of any abnormalities.

Assess the traction equipment for proper alignment, attachment, weight, and countertraction. Note whether the ropes and weight hang freely. Assess the equipment in light of the principles of traction as listed in Table 19–6. Check whether the patient is positioned properly in the bed for the type of traction being maintained.

Observe for signs of pressure areas, such as on the elbows, back of the head, back, buttocks, and heels and under slings or wraps. Assess for signs of the hazards of immobility (see Mobility Impairment section earlier in this chapter). Note the amount of movement the patient is able to accomplish. Ask whether the patient is completing range-of-motion exercises of unaffected extremities at regular intervals. Check the positioning of the foot and watch for evidence of footdrop.

Nursing Diagnoses and Planning

Nursing diagnoses and related expected patient outcomes most commonly applicable to patients in traction include those described previously for patients with impaired mobility and the following:

NDx: Anxiety related to fear of the equipment, unknown recovery potential, and discomfort

Planning: Patient Outcomes
1. Patient denies anxiety, fear, or nervousness about the traction therapy and potential outcome of the therapy.
2. Patient appears relaxed and is able to rest at intervals and to sleep well.
3. Signs of increased anxiety, such as twitching, nervousness, increased respirations and pulse, and withdrawal from participation in care, are absent.

NDx: Pain related to inability to move well or change positions easily in bed as a result of the traction therapy, pressure from the pulling force or method of attachment of the apparatus, and/or irritation at the site of injury

Planning: Patient Outcomes
1. Patient denies pressure, pain, or discomfort.
2. Patient is able to exercise and move as is possible within the confines of the traction equipment.

NDx: Knowledge deficit: nature of traction equipment, effective traction, and limitations imposed by traction.

Planning: Patient Outcomes
1. Patient verbalizes understanding of type of traction and need to maintain effective traction.
2. Patient states limitations in activity while in traction.

Nursing Interventions and Evaluation

NDx: Anxiety
Explain the purpose of the traction equipment to the patient. Explain the necessity of maintenance of body and traction alignment. Prior to performing any procedure on the patient, explain the steps of the procedure and the reason for it. Allow the patient time to ask questions and relay concerns. Check vital signs and watch for changes that indicate increased anxiety. Teach the patient relaxation methods and strategies to cope with the fears of hospitalization. Have the patient practice range-of-motion exercises to help relieve discomfort from the static position and to maintain muscle tone and joint motion. Also, provide diversional activity for the patient to relieve the boredom and anxiety associated with bedrest.

NDx: Pain
Assess the patient's pain level for location, type and severity as necessary. Reposition the patient, as allowed, for comfort and release of pressure. Teach the patient how to move in the bed with the use of the overhead trapeze. Explain how much movement is allowed. Check complaints of pain or pressure areas for cause. Leg wrapping that is too tight causes increased discomfort in the extremities. Assess leg wrapping and neurovascular status at least every 8 hours. Give prescribed pain or sedation medications as needed and monitor their effectiveness. Give the medication for pain prior to performing procedures with the patient that cause increased discomfort. Be certain the traction equipment is in proper alignment, with the appropriate weight. Incorrect use of the equipment may aggravate the patient's discomfort as well as cause harm to the patient.

NDx: Knowledge deficit: nature of traction equipment, effective traction, and limitations of traction
Explain to the patient the type and purpose of the traction. Instruct the patient in the need to maintain effective traction. Encourage the patient to shift weight and turn slightly every 1 to 2 hours. Instruct the patient in the need for appropriate body alignment. Encourage the use of the trapeze and unaf-

Table 19-7

Pin-Site Care

Regardless of the type of pin, screw, or tong used to maintain traction or immobility of a body part, the care of the pin site is an important nursing responsibility. The nurse provides pin-site care every shift (or as otherwise prescribed in terms of the care routine and frequency):

1. Assess around the pin site for redness, swelling, increase in tenderness, and the presence of drainage.
2. Examine the pin for breakage, bending, or shifting.
3. Use a prescribed cleansing agent.
4. With gloved hands, clean from the pin site outward using sterile cotton-tipped applicators and the prescribed cleansing agent. Use a separate applicator for each site to eliminate possible cross-contamination.
5. Refrain from applying ointments to the site, unless specifically ordered, because they tend to occlude drainage and keep the site moist, which increases the potential for bacterial growth.
6. If drainage is evident, notify the physician, who will determine whether a culture of the drainage should be obtained and if sites are to be covered.
7. Instruct the patient to avoid touching the pin site.

fected extremities to pull up in bed. Discourage the patient from sitting up in bed.

Perform range-of-motion exercises four times a day to unaffected extremities to prevent muscle weakness and maintain normal range of motion. Instruct the patient to perform isometric exercises for affected and unaffected limbs. Encourage the patient to perform flexion and extension exercises of the ankles to prevent foot drop.

Additional Interventions

To prevent infection at the site of insertion of the pins, wires, or tongs, perform pin-site care as described in Table 19-7. Assess for the presence of deep vein thrombosis.

Compare the patient's status with the expected outcomes. If the outcomes are not met, reassess the patient and revise the plan.

SURGICAL MANAGEMENT

External Fixation Devices

Treatment of musculoskeletal disorders by simple casting or prolonged immobility in traction is not appropriate for all patients or all disorders. In some situations, an external fixation device may be used to stabilize the involved bone or joint.

An external fixation device consists of a metal frame with attached metal percutaneous pins that are held rigidly in place by the frame. The percutaneous pins are inserted into or through the bone above and below a fracture or defect in the bone or joint. The device is usually applied by the physician in the operating room under sterile conditions. An external fixation device is used to compress bone fragments and to maintain alignment for bone, joint, or soft tissue healing. External fixation devices are illustrated in Figure 19-9.

Indications for external fixation therapy include open fractures with nerve and vascular damage, open contaminated fractures with soft tissue damage and infection, severe comminuted fractures, leg lengthening, joints to be removed temporarily, and joint-fusions. Access to wounds for assessment of healing and neurovascular function, débridement, dressing changes, irrigations, skin grafting, and burn injury treatment are possible while stabilization of the bone is maintained. An external fixation device can also be used after skeletal traction to maintain alignment until there is complete bone or joint healing. This allows earlier ambulation and discharge, which decreases the risk of complications of immobility.

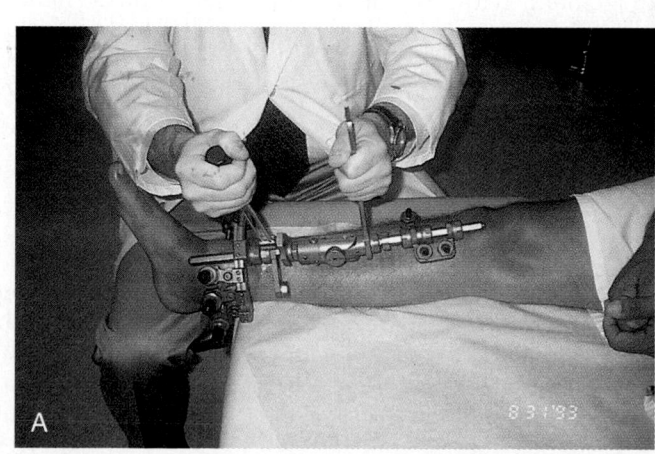
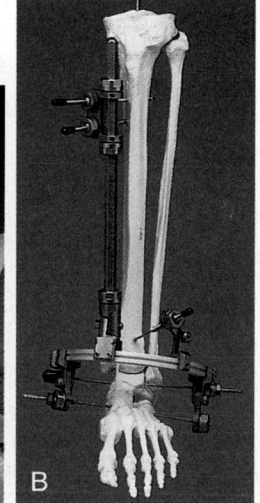

Figure 19-9

An external fixation device. *A,* Torus external fixator being applied to the lower leg. *B,* Internal attachment of pins into bones using the Torus external fixator. (Courtesy of Zimmer, Inc, Warsaw, IN.)

External fixation may be used for almost any bone. Situations for which external fixation therapy is frequently applied include:

fractures of long bones of the extremities
elbow, wrist, knee, and ankle disorders
unstable fractures of the pelvic ring

There are a number of different external fixation systems made by various manufacturers, but the principle of each system is similar.

In some situations, external fixation is used to stabilize a severely injured limb during treatment in an effort to avoid amputation. Despite these efforts, the patient may still lose the limb.

NURSING PROCESS
External Fixation Devices

Assessment

Assess the pin sites and the neurovascular status of the involved limb. Patients with external fixation often have extensive soft tissue, nerve, and blood vessel damage, and the potential for neurovascular deficit is high. Compare current findings with baseline data and elicit reports of changes by the patient. Check the stability of the frame and security of the pins at least once every 4 hours until discharge. Assess any wounds and soft tissue injuries for odor, drainage, inflammation, or necrotic areas. Assess the patient's knowledge about self care after discharge and about care of the pin site and fixation device. Encourage the patient to discuss feelings about the device and changes in body image.

Nursing Diagnoses and Planning

Nursing diagnoses and related expected patient outcomes most commonly applicable to patients with an external fixation device include the following:

NDx: Anxiety related to the appearance of the device and ability to manage self-care and maintain independence with the device in place

Planning: Patient Outcomes
1. Patient denies anxiety, fear, or nervousness about self care and management with the device in place.
2. Patient looks at the device with acceptance.
3. Patient verbalizes feeling relaxed, resting at intervals, and sleeping well.
4. Signs of increased anxiety, such as twitching, nervousness, and increased respirations and pulse, are absent.

NDx: Impaired home maintenance management related to the external fixation device, pin-site care, and mobility management

Planning: Patient Outcomes
1. Patient states appropriate information about care and management of the device and when to notify the physician if problems such as infection or loosening of pins become evident.

2. Patient demonstrates correct pin-site care.
3. Patient moves safely with the fixation device intact, using assistive devices if needed.

NDx: Risk for infection related to the pin sites and other soft tissue injuries

Planning: Patient Outcomes
1. Patient remains free from infection.
2. Patient's skin shows signs of healing, such as new granulation tissue and closure of wounds.
3. Patient verbalizes correct pin-site care.

Nursing Interventions and Evaluation

NDx: Anxiety
Reinforce the physician's explanation about the need for the external fixation device and how it will help the patient to become mobile. Prior to the application of the device, show a picture of it to the patient to reduce surprise, fear, and anxiety afterward. Allow time for questions or verbalization of concerns from the patient or family. Assist the patient in finding strategies that enhance effective coping. Encourage the patient to actively participate in care. Refer the patient to social services, physical therapy, or occupational therapy if needed for assistance with adjustment of lifestyle and maintenance of independence. Seek assistance of clergy or a professional counselor if appropriate.

NDx: Impaired home maintenance management
Teach the patient how to care for the fixation device and when to notify the physician if problems arise. Instruct the patient in how to assess the neurovascular status of the involved limb. Demonstrate pin-site care, as detailed in Table 19–7, to the patient, and allow time for the patient to practice it with supervision. Reinforce the physician's instructions about weight-bearing and manipulation of the device. Remind the patient not to use the fixation device as a handle to lift the limb. Inform the patient that the affected extremity and external fixation device must move as a unit. Discuss limitations, if any, and the use of the affected limb. Encourage the patient to continue with the prescribed exercises to maintain muscle and bone strength and range of motion of joints adjacent to the affected part. Instruct the patient that elevation of the affected extremity will help to decrease edema.

Teach the patient the appropriate use of the assistive device, if applicable, or refer the patient to physical therapy or occupational therapy. Provide for the patient's safety by assisting with movement until the patient can securely manage alone or with the assistive device. Have the patient perform a return demonstration using the assistive device to evaluate for independent and safe usage prior to discharge from the hospital. Discuss any obstacles that may interfere with the patient's safe mobility in the home setting. Help the patient plan modifications of the home environment if needed.

Provide the patient with suggestions on how to modify clothing to fit over the apparatus. Assist with preparations for self-care after discharge. Allow the patient to practice with self-help aids that may be needed to assist with daily hygiene and grooming tasks or other activities of daily living. Teach the patient about dosage, frequency of administration, and side effects of any analgesics or other medications prescribed.

NDx: Risk for infection

Teach the patient to watch for signs of localized infection, such as redness, swelling, increased pain or drainage at the pin sites, and signs of systemic infection, such as fever, increased pulse and respiratory rate, and general malaise. Be certain the patient understands aseptic pin site care. Tell the patient to report any signs of infection to the attending physician.

Compare the patient's status with the expected outcomes. If the outcomes are not met, reassess the patient and revise the plan

Internal Fixation Devices

Internal fixation devices are surgically inserted directly into or attached onto bone to provide support, to fill in a defect, or to achieve and maintain reduc-tion of fracture fragments (Fig. 19–10). Internal fixa-tion allows early ambulation by patients with muscu-loskeletal disorders and promotes more rapid healing.

Internal fixation devices are made of rigid, strong, biologically inert substances, such as poly-ethylene and nonferrous metal alloys, that can with-stand considerable amounts of stress. Although most internal fixation devices are implanted completely under the skin and muscle, some may protrude through the skin and be attached to casts, traction, or external fixation devices.

Internal fixation devices include both temporary and permanent pins, rods, nails, screws, plates, and wires. The type of device selected depends on the condition to be treated and the physician's prefer-ence. Intraoperative fluoroscopy and postoperative radiographic studies are used to ensure proper placement of the device and correct bone alignment.

Although internal fixation devices are of great benefit to most patients, there are possible complica-tions associated with their use. Patients with an in-ternal fixation device may develop an infection around the device. To prevent the complication of infection, prophylactic antibiotics are administered before and after surgery. Tissue reaction to a foreign substance in the body and breakage or migration of

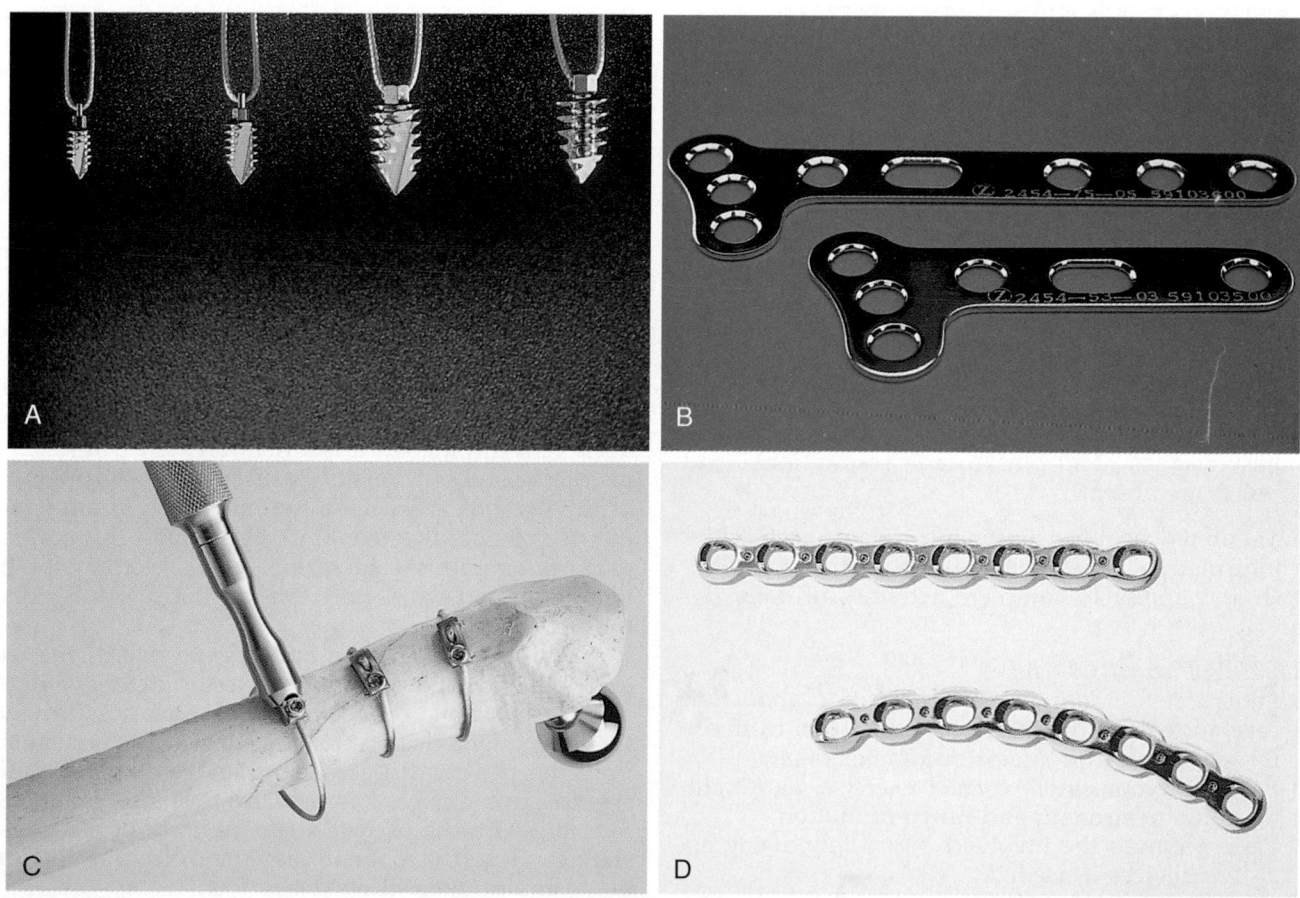

Figure 19–10

Internal fixation devices. *A*, Statak soft tissue attachment device; *B*, ECT internal fracture fixation device; *C*, Cable-Ready cable grip system; *D*, Zimmer reconstruction system. (Courtesy of Zimmer, Inc, Warsaw, IN.)

the device can also occur. Circulating bacteria from another source such as a decayed tooth or urinary tract infection can lodge on the surface of the device and multiply long after surgery. Intravenous antibiotic therapy and the removal of the device may be required.

NURSING PROCESS
Internal Fixation Devices

Assessment

Preoperatively, assess the neurovascular status of the affected body part and compare bilaterally as a baseline to detect changes in the postoperative period. Determine the patient's understanding about the surgery and the postoperative course. Ask the patient about feelings of anxiety or other concerns about the surgery. Observe for signs of anxiety, such as twitching, increased heart rate and respiratory rate, withdrawal, and crying.

Postoperatively, assess the neurovascular status of the affected body part. Monitor vital signs and observe the dressings for security and excessive drainage. Check the suture site for redness, swelling, purulent drainage, and bleeding. Assess the patient for pain and other discomforts. Assess knowledge about self care after discharge.

Nursing Diagnoses and Planning

Nursing diagnoses and related expected patient outcomes most commonly applicable to patients with an internal fixation device include the following:

NDx: Anxiety related to placement of a foreign substance in the body and the results of the intervention

Planning: Patient Outcomes
1. Patient denies anxiety, fear, or nervousness about the surgery and its potential outcome.
2. Patient verbalizes being relaxed, resting at intervals, and sleeping well.
3. Signs of increased anxiety, such as twitching, nervousness, and increased respirations and pulse, are absent.

NDx: Altered health maintenance related to the lack of information about self care, potential complications, and ability to complete activities of daily living

Planning: Patient Outcomes
1. Patient states appropriate information about self care, avoiding complications, and when to notify the physician if problems become evident.
2. Patient demonstrates correct exercise, as taught, to maintain strength and range of motion.
3. Patient moves the involved part safely, using assistive devices if needed.

NDx: Risk for infection related to the wound, surgical intervention, and foreign device

Planning: Patient Outcomes
1. Patient remains free from infection.
2. Patient's suture line shows signs of healing, such as new granulation tissue, and absence of drainage, swelling, or redness.
3. Patient states an understanding for the need to take prophylactic antibiotics prior to some invasive procedures and dental work.

NDx: Risk for injury related to premature weight-bearing and/or failure of the internal fixation device

Planning: Patient Outcomes
1. Patient denies problems with mobility or use of the affected part.
2. Patient remains free from injury.
3. Patient verbalizes understanding about prescribed weight-bearing progression.

NDx: Pain related to surgical intervention and muscle spasms from manipulation during placement of the device

Planning: Patient Outcomes
1. Patient denies discomfort or pain.
2. Patient's affected body part returns to an acceptable level of mobility.

Nursing Interventions and Evaluation

NDx: Anxiety
Reinforce the physician's explanation about the need for the internal fixation device and how it will help the patient to maintain mobility. Allow time for questions or verbalization of concerns from the patient or family. Assist the patient in finding strategies that enhance effective coping. Refer the patient to social services, physical therapy, or occupational therapy, if needed, for assistance prior to discharge. Seek assistance of clergy or a professional counselor if appropriate.

NDx: Altered health maintenance
Teach the patient how to care for the fixation device and when to notify the physician if problems such as compartment syndrome, respiratory distress, or deep vein thrombosis arise. Reinforce the physician's instructions about weight-bearing and manipulation of the involved part. Discuss limitations, if any, and the use of the affected limb. Encourage the patient to continue with the prescribed exercises to maintain muscle strength and range of motion of joints adjacent to the affected part.

Teach the patient the appropriate use of the assistive device if applicable, or refer the patient to physical therapy or occupational therapy. Provide for the patient's safety by assisting with movement until the patient can securely manage alone or with the assistive device. Discuss any obstacles that may interfere with the patient's safe mobility in the home setting. Help the patient plan modifications of the home environment if needed.

Assist with preparations for self-care after discharge, as described in Highlight 19–4. Teach the

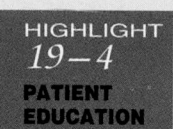 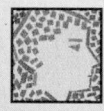

HIGHLIGHT 19–4
PATIENT EDUCATION

Discharge Instructions After Application of an Internal Fixation Device

Instruct the patient to:

Follow the physician's instructions regarding weight bearing, limitations of range of motion and use of the involved extremity, and the use of ambulatory aids to prevent problems with the device.

Maintain the physical therapy routine as prescribed.

Observe for signs of infection or reaction to the internal fixation device, such as pain, redness, swelling, or fever.

Observe for signs of migration of the device, such as sudden or continuous pain, protrusion at the site of insertion, and limitation of motion of the joint.

Report any signs of infection or problems immediately to the attending physician.

Wear a MedicAlert emblem to inform health-care personnel of the internal fixation device, because of the risk for long-term or latent infection of the device and because magnetic resonance imaging may loosen the placement of the device.

---

patient about dosage, frequency of administration, and side effects of any analgesics or other medications prescribed.

NDx: Risk for infection
Teach the patient to watch for signs of localized infection, such as redness, swelling, increased pain, or drainage at the suture line (see Highlight 19–4). Be certain the patient understands aseptic wound care if it is still necessary after discharge. Tell the patient to report any signs of infection to the attending physician. Explain about the need to take prophylactic antibiotics prior to undergoing an invasive procedure or dental work. Explain to the patient that bacteria circulating in the blood can lodge in the fixation device and multiply.

NDx: Risk for injury
Reinforce the information that the physician presented to the patient about the surgery and the typical postoperative course. Explain when weight-bearing is appropriate and how to manipulate the limb until that point in time. If an assistive device is needed, teach the patient how to use it safely. Ask a physical therapist or occupational therapist to work

with the patient for strengthening of muscles as well as ambulation. Teach the patient how to readjust in the home environment to maintain safety.

Tell the patient to report any untoward sign to the physician, such as sudden severe pain at the site, inability to bear weight at the appropriate time, or falls or other blows to the affected area that may occur. Demonstrate exercises that will help develop strength in preparation for weight-bearing.

NDx: Pain
Offer analgesics as prescribed, especially prior to physical therapy and other painful procedures. Position the patient for comfort and reposition frequently unless otherwise contraindicated. Support the affected part and maintain proper alignment with pillows or blankets until the patient is able to move independently. Avoid extreme adduction or abduction of the involved body part. Elevate the extremity for 48 hours postoperatively to reduce swelling and pressure, unless otherwise ordered.

Compare the patient's status with the expected outcomes. If the outcomes are not met, reassess the patient and revise the plan.

Total Joint Replacement

Total joint replacement or arthroplasty involves the surgical removal of deformed or diseased joint surfaces with replacement by smooth artificial surfaces made of metal and plastic. The implant pieces are held in place by a special bone cement called methyl methacrylate, or a special coating on the prosthesis pieces that allows bone growth into the surface of the implant. These biologic ingrowth joint prostheses have a special finish created by a sprayed- or baked-on metal surface that produces a porous finish that eliminates the need for cement. This porous surface allows new bone to grow into the artificial joint pieces and provides a strong bond between the implant and the bone.

Joint prostheses exist for most joints, but replacements for the knee, hip, shoulder, ankle, and wrist and Silastic implants for the phalanges of the fingers and toes are the most common. Numerous manufacturers produce a variety of replacement parts. Joint parts can also be custom made to fit the individual patient. Examples of hip joint prostheses are shown in Figure 19–11.

The purpose of joint replacement is to relieve pain and provide increased range of motion and function of the involved joint. The length of wear for an artificial joint is limited by cracking and loosening of the methyl methacrylate. An active person can expect the standard metal, plastic, and methyl methacrylate joints to last approximately 10 years. The coated or biologic ingrowth implants may provide longer wear.

All patients having a joint replacement should be aware of the potential complications and participa-

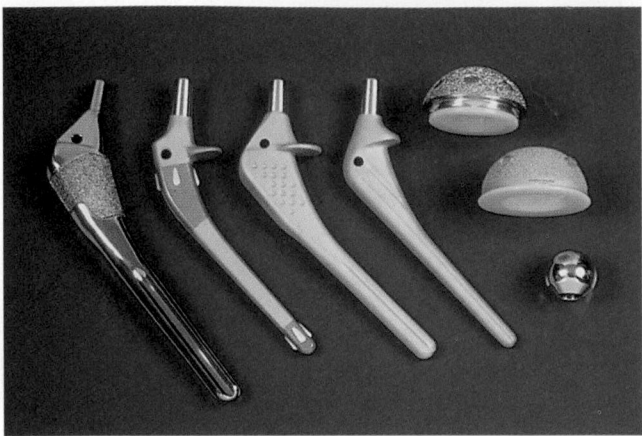

Figure 19–11

Hip joint prostheses. (Courtesy of Zimmer, Inc, Warsaw, IN.)

tion required for successful postoperative rehabilitation. Adverse effects of artificial joints include

- Injury to nerves, producing pain or numbness
- Infection of the incision or the new joint
- Thromboembolism
- Loosening of metal or plastic parts
- Limb length differences
- Dislocation of the new joint

Loosening and infection within the joint can lead to loss of the implant, and additional surgery, pain, and expense to the patient. Infection may occur several months after the surgical procedure and may require as much as 6 weeks of intravenous antibiotic therapy. If the joint cannot be corrected, or if another replacement is not an option because of either the patient's choice or physical condition, the joint may be removed or fused.

TOTAL HIP REPLACEMENT. With hip replacement, the femoral head and part of the femur neck are removed and the acetabulum is enlarged. The metallic femoral prosthesis is inserted into the femoral medullary canal and the acetabular component, which is composed of a polyethylene surface, is placed into the enlarged acetabular space. Positioning of the patient so that the head of the prosthesis remains within the acetabular cup is vital. Place the leg in abduction to prevent the dislocation of the prosthesis. Flexion is limited to 90 degrees or less. Weight-bearing limits are determined by the physician, but full weight bearing on the affected extremity may be avoided for 3 to 6 months.

Use pillows or an abductor splint to maintain legs in abduction. Assess for peroneal nerve irritation resulting from pressure of the abduction splint. Limit elevation of the head of the bed to 45 degrees. Note weight-bearing status. Encourage ankle pumps and quadriceps exercises to strength muscles. Discuss discharge needs related to need for extended care, home physical therapy, home care, and equip-

ment needs. Teach limitations on adduction, flexion, and hip rotation to prevent dislocation.

TOTAL KNEE REPLACEMENT. With knee replacement, the tibial, femoral, and patellar joint surfaces are replaced. Several types of knee prostheses can be used. Some prostheses compensate for weak ligaments while others rely on the ligaments to provide joint stability. After the implant has been completed, the knee is immobilized with a compression dressing to keep the leg in maximal extension. In uncomplicated cases, patients are frequently placed on a continuous passive motion device, which gently puts the knee through preset degrees of passive range of motion. The initial degrees of flexion and extension are set by the physician and are gradually increased until flexion reaches 90 degrees. This device is used to decrease joint stiffness and facilitate remobilization of the knee in the postoperative period. Weight-bearing limits depend on the use of cemented or cementless prostheses. Dislocation is a rare occurrence.

Apply ice to the knee as ordered to control edema and bleeding. Note limits of flexion and extension and properly place client on continuous passive motion if ordered. Encourage the use of analgesics prior to flexion exercises. Teach home use of continuous passive motion as needed. Assist with transfer and elevate the affected leg when the patient is sitting in a chair.

NURSING PROCESS
Total Joint Replacement

The assessment, nursing diagnoses, expected patient outcomes, nursing interventions, and evaluation for patients with a total joint replacement are similar to those described previously for patients with an internal fixation device. (Also see Nursing Care Guide 19–1.)

Amputation

An amputation is the removal of an extremity or part of an extremity. This may be either traumatic or therapeutic. Indications for a surgical amputation include circulatory disorders, traumatic injuries including severe thermal or crushing injuries, malignant tumors, uncontrolled infection, gangrene, and congenital deformities that result in nonfunctional disfigured limbs. An auto-amputation is a nonsurgical spontaneous separation of devitalized tissue. This may be seen in a patient with severe vascular disease (often due to diabetes mellitus).

LEVELS OF AMPUTATION. A limb may be amputated at any point along its length. The level of amputation depends on the extent of the disease process, circulation to the area, and optimal function of the residual limb or stump. The level of amputation is as distal as possible. The terminology used to

Nursing Care Guide 19–1
Patients Undergoing Total Joint Replacement

Preoperative Care

Assessment Findings: Patient appears nervous, withdraws from conversation, clenches hands; blood pressure, pulse, and respirations are slightly elevated for the patient; patient makes statements indicating concern about the procedure and results of the surgical intervention and potential problems with immobility and discomfort.

Nursing Diagnosis: Anxiety related to uncertainty about surgery, potential risk factors, discomfort, and fear of loss of mobility

Patient Outcomes	Nursing Interventions	Rationale
Patient reports feeling less nervous, seems relaxed, and is able to rest well.	Teach the patient relaxation techniques. Provide a quiet, calm environment with periods of rest during the delivery of nursing care. Ask for assistance from clergy or the patient's significant others.	Having an understanding of the procedure lessens fears and reduces anxiety. Telling the patient what to expect prior to initiating procedures for preoperative preparation reduces fear of the unknown.
Patient's vital signs are within normal ranges for the patient.	Check vital signs after the patient is rested and more relaxed and note any changes.	Changes in vital signs may reflect increasing or decreasing anxiety levels.
Patient states methods to relax and reduce tension.	Teach deep-breathing techniques and other relaxation strategies.	Practicing relaxation exercises may decrease anxiety and promote rest.

Evaluation: Compare the patient's status with the expected outcomes. If the outcomes are not met, reassess the patient and revise the plan.

Assessment Findings: Patient and family seem very concerned about the procedure; they ask several questions about the surgery, the preparation before surgery, the joint replacement device, the expectations of the intervention, and possible complications.

Nursing Diagnosis: Knowledge deficit: nature of prosthetic surgery, preoperative preparations, expected outcome, and possible complications

Patient Outcomes	Nursing Interventions	Rationale
Patient accurately describes the purpose of the surgery and the necessity for the prosthesis.	Explain the procedure to the patient and the expected outcomes. Give the patient literature explaining the procedure and showing what the prosthesis looks like.	Explanations of all the appropriate information about the surgery to the patient and family decreases the knowledge deficit.
Patient relates information about the procedure, complications, and expected results as presented to the patient by the physician.	Reinforce the information the physician presented to the patient. Have the patient relate what the physician has explained, and clear up any misunderstandings.	Having the patient repeat the information gives the opportunity to correct any misinformation.

(continued)

Nursing Care Guide 19–1
Patients Undergoing Total Joint Replacement (continued)

Patient Outcomes	Nursing Interventions	Rationale
Patient reports an understanding of the preoperative preparation necessary.	Explain the preoperative preparation and allow time for questions from the patient or the family.	Giving the patient and the family the opportunity to ask questions about the procedure reduces anxiety and may enhance compliance with the preparation.

Evaluation: Compare the patient's status with the expected outcomes. If the outcomes are not met, reassess the patient and revise the plan.

Assessment Findings: Patient complains of discomfort because of positioning for the traction and inability to move in bed; patient complains of pain in affected hip; patient grimaces frequently, seems apprehensive, and twitches in the bed.

Nursing Diagnosis: Pain related to injury to hip requiring joint replacement surgery, temporary traction, and/or immobility

Patient Outcomes	Nursing Interventions	Rationale
Patient states relief of pain and discomfort.	Utilize a pain rating scale (visual analogue, number scale, verbal scale) to determine level of pain and effectiveness of interventions. Explain the importance of the patient reporting pain. Administer analgesics as prescribed. Teach nonpharmacologic interventions such as relaxation, distraction, imagery. Reposition the patient as allowed in the bed. Teach the patient how to move by using the overhead trapeze.	Pain medication administered at regular intervals helps manage pain. Slight movement in bed releases pressure from bony prominences.

Evaluation: Compare the patient's status with the expected outcomes. If the outcomes are not met, reassess the patient and revise the plan.

Postoperative Care

Assessment Findings: Patient has incision site with dressings, an intravenous line, and a urinary catheter and is on bedrest.

Nursing Diagnosis: Risk for infection related to wound site, intravenous line, urinary catheter, and bedrest

Patient Outcomes	Nursing Interventions	Rationale
Patient's wound site remains free from symptoms of infection such as redness, purulent drainage, or excessive swelling.	Check the wound site and suture line for evidence for healing. Watch for signs of infection. Use aseptic technique for dressing changes.	Early diagnosis of complications increases potential for successful treatment. Aseptic technique decreases risk of infection.

(continued)

Nursing Care Guide 19–1
Patients Undergoing Total Joint Replacement (continued)

Patient Outcomes	Nursing Interventions	Rationale
Patient denies cough or respiratory distress.	Assess vital signs frequently. Have the patient cough and deep-breathe at regular intervals.	Coughing and deep-breathing help clear the respiratory system.
Patient's intravenous site remains free from infection.	Check the intravenous site at least each shift, looking for infiltration, redness, or swelling.	Continually assessing for problems allows for early intervention.
Patient remains free from a urine infection as noted by the urinalysis.	Observe the color, consistency, and amount of urine. Encourage increased fluid intake. Use aseptic cleansing around catheter area.	Increased fluid intake and aseptic care of the catheter decrease risk of a urinary infection.
Patient's vital signs are within normal limits for the patient.	Assess vital signs frequently; especially note an increasing respiratory and pulse rate. Also report and document a temperature increase.	Vital sign changes may indicate infection, such as in the respiratory system, if patient begins to present an increased respiratory rate and pulse rate and some respiratory distress.

Evaluation: Compare the patient's status with the expected outcomes. If the outcomes are not met, reassess the patient and revise the plan.

Assessment Findings: Patient grimaces, moans, and complains of discomfort at surgery site.

Nursing Diagnosis: Pain related to invasive surgical procedure with manipulation, muscle spasms, and previous injury

Patient Outcomes	Nursing Interventions	Rationale
Patient reports relief of pain and appears relaxed and comfortable as evidenced by a calm, relaxed manner and willingness to participate in the care.	Document patient's rating of pain. Use a rating scale. Give prescribed analgesics for control of postoperative pain. Monitor effects of analgesics given. Make patient comfortable, and provide a quiet atmosphere for rest after surgery.	Relief of postoperative pain allows patient to rest as needed and promotes healing.
	Check insertion site for signs of infection, which may increase pain at site.	Infection inflammation increases pain at the site.
	Tell the patient to practice relaxation techniques taught before surgery.	Practicing relaxation techniques may decrease some of the discomfort.
	Using the AHCPR guidelines, collaborate with the patient, and other health-care team members to plan strategies for maximal pain relief.	Getting input from a variety of specialists and the patient increases the chance of success with the pain control program.

Evaluation: Compare the patient's status with the expected outcomes. If the outcomes are not met, reassess the patient and revise the plan.

(continued)

Nursing Care Guide 19-1
Patients Undergoing Total Joint Replacement (continued)

Assessment Findings: Patient seems overly anxious and reluctant to listen to home-care instructions; patient is reluctant to work with ambulatory aid and to practice physical therapy; patient states concerns about providing self care, hygiene, grooming, and activities of daily living when home.

Nursing Diagnosis: Impaired home maintenance management related to inability to manage mobility problems, use of ambulatory aid, fear for safety, and suture line care (if needed)

Patient Outcomes	Nursing Interventions	Rationale
Patient relates accurate information about the home care required, signs of potential problems, and plans for follow-up care with the attending physician.	Describe the signs requiring immediate medical intervention, such as pain or discomfort at surgical site, fever, chills, dizziness, fainting, excessive fatigue, or shortness of breath.	Early diagnosis of potential problems by the patient at home and early medical intervention increase the chance for successful treatment.
Patient demonstrates appropriate use of ambulatory aid.	Assist the patient in practicing using the ambulatory aid. Seek assistance from a physical therapist.	Having the patient practice before discharge reinforces the instructions for use and enhances safety for the patient.
Patient states safety measures for the home environment to prevent falls or other injuries.	Help the patient find ways to increase safety measures in the home environment. Have the patient reiterate the information provided.	Having the patient relate information presented reinforces the information and allows for correction of misconceptions.

Evaluation: Compare the patient's status with the expected outcomes. If the outcomes are not met, reassess the patient and revise the plan.

describe common amputation procedures refers to the level of amputation and is listed in Figure 19–12.

TYPES OF AMPUTATIONS. After removal of the body part, the residual limb is either closed with flaps of muscle and tissue or left open. The open type, called a guillotine amputation, is used when infection is present and free drainage of infected material is necessary for healing. It may also result from traumatic amputation of a limb or an auto-amputation.

In a guillotine amputation, the soft tissue and bone are severed at the same level. Blood vessels are cauterized or tied. The wound requires meticulous aseptic wound care and close assessment for hemorrhage. Hemorrhage is more common after a guillotine procedure than after a flap closure. Additional débridement of necrotic tissue may be required. Once the infection is eradicated, the residual limb is surgically revised and the tissues closed to provide a functional residual limb.

PHANTOM LIMB SENSATION. A particularly stressful event unique to patients who have under-

gone an amputation is phantom sensation. Phantom sensation is a phenomenon in which the patient feels that the amputated appendicular parts are still present. The individual verbalizes awareness that the body part is gone but that sensations are still present as though the part is still there. Phantom sensations may include pain, tingling, numbness, itching, and temperature changes. This sensation is caused by stimulation along the pathway of a nerve whose sensory endings were in the amputated part. Phantom sensation usually develops soon after surgery or within a few months. This sensation usually ceases after several months but may persist for years in some individuals. When patients understand that phantom sensation is a normal occurrence, they are less disturbed by it.

Some patients experience not only the sensation of the presence of an amputated limb, but aching, knifelike, jabbing, throbbing, tearing, or burning pain. This is referred to as phantom pain and is not experienced by all amputees. It may result from stimulation of certain points in the extremities or other activities. Measures to help relieve phantom

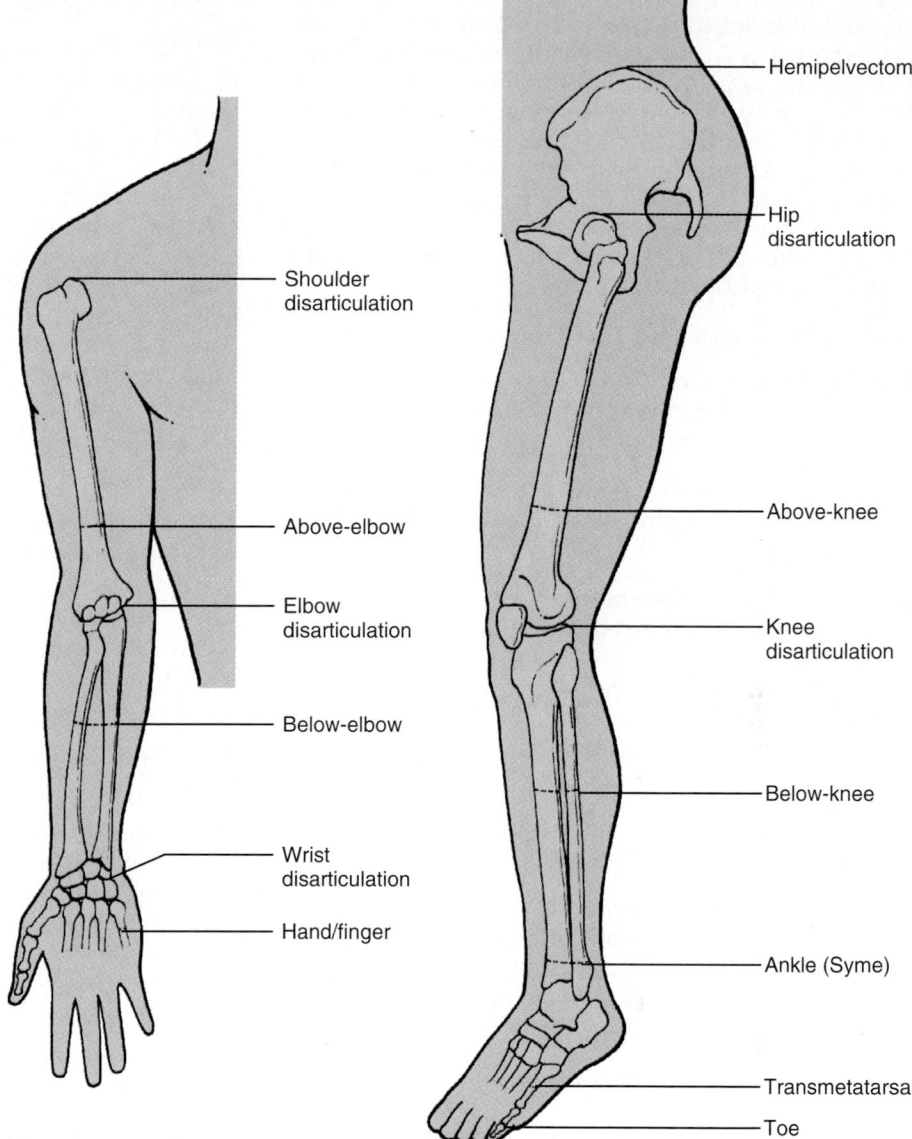

Figure 19–12
Levels of amputation for the upper and lower extremities.

pain include exercise of the residual limb, massaging the end of the residual limb, diversional activity, and pharmacologic agents such as beta blockers and anticonvulsant and antidepressant therapies. Additional interventions may include spinal or epidural analgesia. Carefully assess the residual limb to rule out infection, compromised circulation or pressure areas as a cause of the pain.

Preoperative preparation and acceptance of the need for the amputation may reduce phantom limb sensation and pain. Anxiety, stress, and depression may intensify but not cause phantom pain. Adequate pain management during the preoperative and postoperative period may decrease phantom sensation and pain.

In some instances after an amputation, severed nerve endings attempt to regenerate and form a neuroma. The neuroma produces a localized area of numbness and tingling. If discomfort becomes problematic for the patient, the neuroma is surgically removed.

NURSING PROCESS
Amputation

PREOPERATIVE NURSING CARE

Assessment

Perform a neurovascular assessment on the affected and the unaffected limb for baseline data. Assess the patient's physical and emotional reaction to the planned amputation. Check vital signs. Look for signs of increased anxiety, such as nervousness, crying, and increased pulse and respiratory rate. Observe the general physical condition and nutritional status of the patient, and the extent of other injuries sustained, if applicable. Determine what the patient and family have been told about the surgery and the postoperative plans. Observe their anxiety level and reaction to the situation. Determine the patient's coping mechanisms, support systems, resources, and the effect the amputation will have on the patient's lifestyle for postoperative planning.

Nursing Diagnoses and Planning

Nursing diagnoses and related expected patient outcomes most commonly applicable to patients scheduled for a surgical amputation include the following:

NDx: Anxiety related to the pre-existing condition, the surgery, and coping with the amputation postoperatively

Planning: Patient Outcomes
1. Patient appears relaxed and is able to rest and sleep well.
2. Patient expresses concerns and acknowledges relief of anxiety.
3. Patient's vital signs are within normal limits for the patient.

NDx: Knowledge deficit: nature of surgical intervention and preoperative preparation

Planning: Patient Outcomes
1. Patient relates accurate information about the surgery and preoperative preparation.
2. Patient states correct information presented by the physician about the perioperative course.

Nursing Interventions and Evaluation

NDx: Anxiety
Allow the patient to freely express concerns and ask questions about the surgery and preoperative preparation. Help the patient find relaxation methods that are effective to relieve anxiety, such as guided imagery, meditation and deep breathing. Use the assistance of the patient's support systems, such as family, friends, or clergy. Explain all procedures to the patient prior to performing them. Allow the patient time to rest and sleep as needed.

NDx: Knowledge deficit: nature of surgical intervention and preoperative preparation
Reinforce the information provided to the patient by the physician. Ask the patient to reiterate the information, and correct any misunderstandings. Tell the patient about preoperative plans, such as what treatments and diagnostic tests are to be performed. Allow time for questions and concerns from the patient. Include the family whenever possible.

Compare the patient's status with the expected outcomes. If the outcomes are not met, reassess the patient and revise the plan.

POSTOPERATIVE NURSING CARE

Assessment

In addition to the usual postoperative care, observe for hemorrhage or signs of infection in the affected limb. Postoperative dressings vary, including soft bandages, rigid dressings (casts), or air splints. The goal is to reduce edema and shape the stump to enhance prosthetic fitting. Note drainage through the dressings, especially the bottom and back of the dressing. Assess the patient for psychologic problems related to the absence of the limb. Ask the patient about pain in the residual limb and determine its intensity and duration and the effect of pain medication. As the residual limb heals, assess the patient's understanding of the instruction for skin care, care of the bandages or prosthesis, if applicable, and home care. Further discussion of the postoperative nursing care of patients with amputations occurs in the Clinical Pathway for Amputation.

Nursing Diagnoses and Planning

Nursing diagnoses and related expected patient outcomes most commonly applicable to patients after a surgical amputation include the following:

NDx: Body image disturbance related to the loss of a body part

Planning: Patient Outcomes
1. Patient relates feelings about changes in body image.
2. Patient participates in self care activities as tolerated.
3. Patient is able to look at self with positive realistic body image and acceptance.

NDx: Dysfunctional grieving related to loss of a body part

Planning: Patient Outcomes
1. Patient freely expresses feelings of grief and significance of the loss.
2. Patient verbalizes feelings of improved emotional status.
3. Patient begins to progress through the grief process and returns to daily activities as able.

NDx: Pain related to surgical intervention and postoperative phantom pain

Planning: Patient Outcomes
1. Patient denies pain in surgical area.
2. Patient states methods to decrease pain, such as use of relaxation strategies.
3. Patient states accurate information about the cause of phantom pain.
4. Patient reports effectiveness of the prescribed analgesics.

NDx: Impaired physical mobility (if lower limb) related to inability to manipulate ambulatory aid or prosthesis

■■■■■■▶
■
■ Clinical Pathway for Amputation

Patient Name _____   Date _____

DRG# _____   Expected LOS _____

	Day 1 (day of surgery)	Day 2 (1st postop day)	Day 3 (2nd postop day)	Day 4 (3rd postop day)	Day 5 (4th postop day)	Day 6 (5th postop day) to discharge
Medication	Analgesia as needed and ordered Home meds as ordered	Analgesia as needed and ordered	Analgesia as needed and ordered	Analgesia as needed and ordered	Analgesia as needed and ordered	Analgesia as needed and ordered
Diet	Intravenous therapy as ordered Clear liquid diet as ordered	Progress diet as ordered	Progress diet as ordered	Progress diet as ordered	Progress diet as ordered	Progress diet as ordered
Activity	Bedrest Head of bed as tolerated Turning and repositioning every 2 hours Elevate stump Overhead trapeze	Turn and reposition Chair transfer as tolerated No stump elevation 24 hours postoperatively Prone position as directed	Range of motion to stump as directed Stand at bedside Transfer to chair Promote activities of daily living	Range of motion to stump as directed Physical therapy with gait training and strength exercises Promote activities of daily living	Range of motion to stump as directed Physical therapy with gait training and strength exercises Promote activities of daily living	Range of motion to stump as directed Physical therapy with gait training and strength exercises Promote activities of daily living
Treatments/ Nursing Actions	Stump bandaging/wrapping as directed Maintain dressing without wrinkles/constrictions Prosthesis as directed Therapeutic communication about anxiety, anger, loss	Stump bandaging/wrapping as directed Maintain dressing without wrinkles/constrictions Prosthesis as directed Therapeutic communication about anxiety, anger, loss Allow privacy for grief	Stump bandaging/wrapping as directed Maintain dressing without wrinkles/constrictions Prosthesis as directed Allow privacy for grief Coordinate discharge planning, social services, home care, equipment, amputee clinic support group	Stump bandaging/wrapping as directed Maintain dressing without wrinkles/constrictions Prosthesis as directed Allow privacy for grief Coordinate discharge planning, social services, home care, equipment, amputee clinic support group	Stump bandaging/wrapping as directed Maintain dressing without wrinkles/constrictions Prosthesis as directed Allow privacy for grief Coordinate discharge planning, social services, home care, equipment, amputee clinic support group	Stump bandaging/wrapping as directed Maintain dressing without wrinkles/constrictions Prosthesis as directed Allow privacy for grief Coordinate discharge planning, social services, home care, equipment, amputee clinic support group
	Postoperative assessment for bleeding, edema, pulses, perfusion, pain, infection Support and teach family	Postoperative assessment for bleeding, edema, pulses, perfusion, pain, infection Support and teach family	Postoperative assessment for bleeding, edema, pulses, perfusion, pain, infection Support and teach family	Postoperative assessment for bleeding, edema, pulses, perfusion, pain, infection Support and teach family	Postoperative assessment for bleeding, edema, pulses, perfusion, pain, infection Support and teach family	Postoperative assessment for bleeding, edema, pulses, perfusion, pain, infection Support and teach family

(continued)

■ Clinical Pathway for Amputation *(continued)*

	Day 1 (day of surgery)	Day 2 (1st postop day)	Day 3 (2nd postop day)	Day 4 (3rd postop day)	Day 5 (4th postop day)	Day 6 (5th postop day) to discharge
	Use pharmacologic pain control measures	Acknowledge grief and provide support for patient and family	Acknowledge grief and provide support for patient and family	Acknowledge grief and provide support for patient and family	Acknowledge grief and provide support for patient and family	Acknowledge grief and provide support for patient and family
			Facilitate patient/family communication about loss, anxiety, and home care issues	Facilitate patient/family communication about loss, anxiety, and home care issues	Facilitate patient/family communication about loss, anxiety, and home care issues	Facilitate patient/family communication about loss, anxiety, and home care issues
	Protect stump from contamination	Protect stump from contamination	Protect stump from contamination	Protect stump from contamination	Protect stump from contamination	Protect stump from contamination
Teaching/ Discharge Planning	Review preoperative teaching to prevent complications	Support client in looking at stump	Explain the causes of phantom sensation and pain	Explain the causes of phantom sensation and pain	Explain the causes of phantom sensation and pain	Explain the causes of phantom sensation and pain
	Teaching positioning and exercise to prevent contractures and improve strength and endurance	Teaching positioning and exercise to prevent contractures and improve strength and endurance	Implement methods to alleviate phantom pain	Implement methods to alleviate phantom pain	Implement methods to alleviate phantom pain	Implement methods to alleviate phantom pain
			Teach stump care, hygiene, wrapping	Teach stump care, hygiene, wrapping	Teach stump care, hygiene, wrapping	Teach stump care, hygiene, wrapping
			Involve family in care as desired	Involve family in care as desired	Involve family in care as desired	Involve family in care as desired
			Teach signs of complications	Teach signs of complications	Teach signs of complications	Teach signs of complications

Planning: Patient Outcomes
1. Patient demonstrates ability to ambulate with assistance, assistive devices, or prosthesis.
2. Patient uses safety tips as presented by the therapist.
3. Patient uses the prescribed ambulatory aid correctly.
4. Patient demonstrates proper locomotion with the prosthesis in place.

NDx: Risk for impaired skin integrity related to improper healing or fit of the prosthesis or improper care of the residual limb

Planning: Patient Outcomes
1. Patient relates appropriate skin care as instructed.
2. Patient states signs of infection, skin breakdown, or improper prosthesis fit and when to seek medical intervention.
3. Patient states systematic method to assess condition of the stump.

NDx: Impaired home maintenance management related to inability to move freely, safety problems, lack of an extremity, and/or unsuitable home environment

Planning: Patient Outcomes
1. Patient relates accurate information about alterations in the home environment that are needed to move freely.
2. Patient verbalizes necessary safety measures.
3. Patient completes activities of daily living with the assistance of the ambulatory aid or prosthesis (upper or lower body).
4. Patient utilizes appropriate resources to increase independence at home.

Nursing Interventions and Evaluation

NDx: Body image disturbance
Spend time with the patient to encourage the patient to vent feelings about the loss of a limb. Provide information about self-help and support groups. Seek assistance from clergy or professional counseling. Provide diversional activities for the patient until he or she is allowed to ambulate. Involve support from the family and friends. Seek effective coping strategies for the patient. Assist the patient in find-

ing the positive aspects of life to focus on during periods of depression. Early in the postoperative period, when the patient is ready, encourage her or him to look at the stump. Have the prosthetist assist the patient with finding artificial parts that are cosmetically appealing. Facilitate the use of a prosthesis as soon as possible. Introduce the patient to others that have coped with similar amputations.

NDx: Dysfunctional grieving
Allow the patient to vent feelings about the surgery and limb loss. Facilitate open communication between patient and family regarding the loss. Have a professional counselor visit with the patient. Seek assistance from other amputees. Give the patient time to grieve because this process is much the same as losing a loved one. Offer support without making false claims to the patient about how good everything will be. Allow the patient and family to have time alone as needed.

NDx: Pain
Utilize a pain rating scale for assessing pain. Discuss pain management objectives with the patient and family using the AHCPR guidelines for pain control after surgery. Teach the patient about the use of patient-controlled analgesia if prescribed postoperatively. Administer prescribed medications and explain the dosage, frequency, side effects, and expected therapeutic effects of the medications. Utilize adjunctive therapies such as relaxation exercises and deep-breathing techniques. Consider diversion, imagery, biofeedback, hypnosis, or cutaneous stimulation. Explore the use of a transcutaneous electrical nerve stimulator device, which may be helpful. Explain phantom sensation and pain to the patient and family. Implement measures to manage phantom pain.

Evaluate the dressing for tightness each time a patient complains of pain. If circulation, sensation, or movement are impaired, notify the physician immediately. Reposition the patient or the affected limb every few hours. Handle the patient carefully when moving him or her in bed.

Place the patient with a leg amputation in the prone position for 30 minutes four to six times per day, as ordered, to prevent flexion contractures of the hip, which also increase the pain.

Explore body image, grief, and denial issues with the patient and family. Utilize therapeutic communication techniques to support the patient and family in dealing with surgical pain and phantom sensation or pain, and loss of the limb.

NDx: Impaired physical mobility
Teach the patient use of the overhead trapeze while still on bedrest to increase movement in bed, as allowed, to prevent complications of immobility. Reposition the patient frequently to stimulate circulation and prevent skin breakdown. Limit weight bearing until instructed. Institute range-of-motion exercises early, as directed. Teach appropriate muscle strengthening exercises to the patient. Demon-

strate each exercise and provide the patient with specific written directions, including the number of repetitions and frequency of exercise completion. Assess the patient's understanding with a return demonstration of each exercise. Assist the patient in locomotion, once he or she is able, to promote safe use of the ambulatory aid. Explain that the center of gravity and stance will be altered. Teach and support the patient during motion activities. Use the assistance of the physical therapist and prosthetist to instruct the patient and family about the device or prosthesis. Encourage the patient to perform exercises as described by the therapist. Give analgesics as needed to decrease pain levels that may interfere with the patient's ability to be mobile.

NDx: Risk for impaired skin integrity
Teach the patient to check the residual limb carefully every day, as described in Highlight 19–5. Teach the patient to watch for signs and symptoms of decreased circulation to the stump. Have the patient relate potential signs of infection, such as redness, tenderness, unusual warmth, purulent exudate, or sudden extreme pain. Teach the patient to wrap the residual limb, being careful not to pull the elastic bandages too tight or allow wrinkles. Have the patient move frequently in bed in the early postoperative course to prevent skin breakdown. Tell the patient to keep the residual limb clean and dry. Teach the patient the importance of a properly fitting prosthesis and signs of problems.

Encourage and provide a good, well-balanced meal plan to promote healing and prevent skin problems. Have the patient drink plenty of fluids to maintain good skin integrity and prevent dry, cracked skin.

NDx: Impaired home maintenance management
Provide information to the patient and family about the postoperative course and self-care interventions. Encourage the patient to ask questions and to express fears and concerns. Answer questions honestly, while reinforcing the positive aspects of the patient's life. Encourage and reinforce instructions in the use of medications, the prosthesis, and ambulatory aids. Discuss modification of the home environment that will help the patient maintain independence.

Teach the patient about wrapping the residual limb, as described in Figure 19–13, and care of the skin and prosthesis, as described in Highlight 19–5. Have the patient demonstrate the technique, and correct any misunderstandings about the care regimen.

Teach the patient about good nutrition to maintain health status and to continue to promote healing. Encourage a diet high in protein, vitamins, and minerals.

Additional Interventions
Residual limb care is an important part of the nursing care for a patient after an amputation. For the first 24 hours postoperatively, elevate the limb as

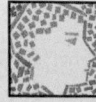

Care of the Skin and Prosthesis After an Amputation

Instruct the patient to:

Wash the stump daily with warm water and a mild soap to prevent irritation.

Rinse the skin and dry thoroughly to prevent macerated skin.

Wash the stump at night so it can air dry over night before being rewrapped.

Inspect the entire residual stump daily for reddened or open areas, dry skin, or other signs of irritation such as blisters or abrasions.

Use a hand mirror to view the back of the stump.

Contact the physician for treatment if lesions are present.

Avoid using topical antiseptics, because they may cause further irritation of the skin.

Avoid using lotions unless otherwise instructed by the physician, because they soften the skin and may predispose it to breakdown.

Keep the prosthesis, elastic bandages, and prosthetic socks clean and in good condition. Change prosthetic socks daily.

Follow the prosthetist's instructions for the care of the prosthesis, socks, and straps.

Contact the prosthetist if loosening or pressure from the prosthesis occurs.

Refrain from padding, taping, or altering the prosthesis without consultation with the prosthetist, because this may interfere with the proper fit or use of the device.

Discontinue use of the prosthesis until consultation if irritation develops.

Put the prosthesis on immediately when arising to prevent swelling. Consult with the prosthetist as directed.

chair with rolled towels or sand bags to prevent external rotation and abduction contractures.

The prescribed exercises for the residual limb and proximal joint help maintain the range of motion, prevent contractures, and assist in early conditioning of prosthesis fitting. Encourage the patient to practice the exercises as ordered.

Wrapping the residual limb with an elastic bandage helps prevent postoperative edema and, as healing progresses, helps shrink and shape the residual limb to ensure good fit of the prosthesis. Wrap the limb so that all the skin is covered. Instruct the patient to leave the wrap on. Remove and reapply the wrap every 4 to 8 hours unless otherwise advised, or whenever loosening occurs. Inspect the skin and assess circulation every time the residual limb is rewrapped. Refer to Figure 19–13 for a description of the wrapping process.

If the patient experiences throbbing or uncomfortable pressure, rewrap the residual limb. Check the finished wrap for smoothness and constriction and then secure the wrap.

Compare the patient's status with the expected outcomes. If the outcomes are not met, reassess the patient and revise the plan.

❖ SETTINGS, PROVIDERS, AND COLLABORATION FOR CARE

The amputation procedure is performed in an acute-care setting. Prosthetic fitting and ambulation training may continue in a rehabilitation facility. Continuity of care for the individual dealing with an amputation is essential. Therefore, discharge from a health-care setting does not mean the end of care. Interventions by a nurse in the home may help clients and families continue adjusting to the new situation of an amputation. Follow-up at the physician's office to check the healing process is also necessary. A physical therapist and an occupational therapist may assist the patient to maintain mobility or use of the limb (with a prosthesis) and continue employment. Initiate social service and home-care referral to help the patient use all resources available to provide financial assistance and to maintain independence. Provide the patient and family with the address and phone number of the National Amputation Foundation (12-45 150th Street, Whitestone, New York 11357; 212-767-0596). Inform the patient of any local support groups for amputees.

prescribed to decrease swelling and promote comfort. Stumps with compromised circulation may not be elevated. Elevation of the lower extremities is done at intervals because elevation for longer periods of time may cause flexion contractures of the hip. To prevent hip contractures, position the patient on the abdomen for 30-minute periods every 4 to 6 hours. Maintain a lower extremity residual limb in alignment while the patient is in the bed or in a

ASSISTIVE AND SUPPORTIVE DEVICES

There are a variety of assistive and supportive devices that patients with musculoskeletal disorders can use. These aids may be ambulatory devices, such as canes, walkers, and crutches, or protective devices, such as splints or braces. A limb prosthesis is an example of an assistive device for the patient with the loss of part or all of an extremity. Numer-

Below the knee - Have the patient sit in semi-Fowler's position with the limb raised and supported a few inches off the bed. Hold one end of an elastic wrap above the knee, as shown below. Then stretch and unroll the bandage diagonally down the front of the limb, around the stump, and diagonally up the front, crossing the original wrap. Extend the bandage across the back of the limb and continue down the front, making a "figure 8" pattern. Repeat the pattern until the stump and knee are covered, using more than one bandage if necessary. Secure the bandage with clips, safety pins, or tape.

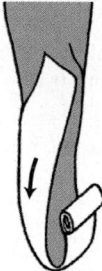 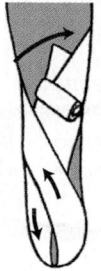 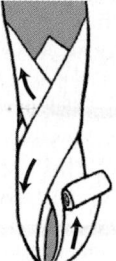 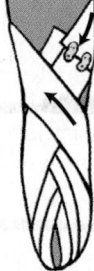

Above the knee - Have the patient stand (with assistance) or lie flat with the limb raised and supported a few inches off the bed. Wrap an elastic bandage around the patient's waist and diagonally down the limb, as shown below. Stretch and unroll the bandage around the stump and diagonally up the limb to the opposite side of the patient's waist, making a "figure 8" pattern. As an alternative, you can use a spiral pattern, as shown. Repeat either pattern until the stump and leg are covered. Then secure the bandage with clips, safety pins, or tape.

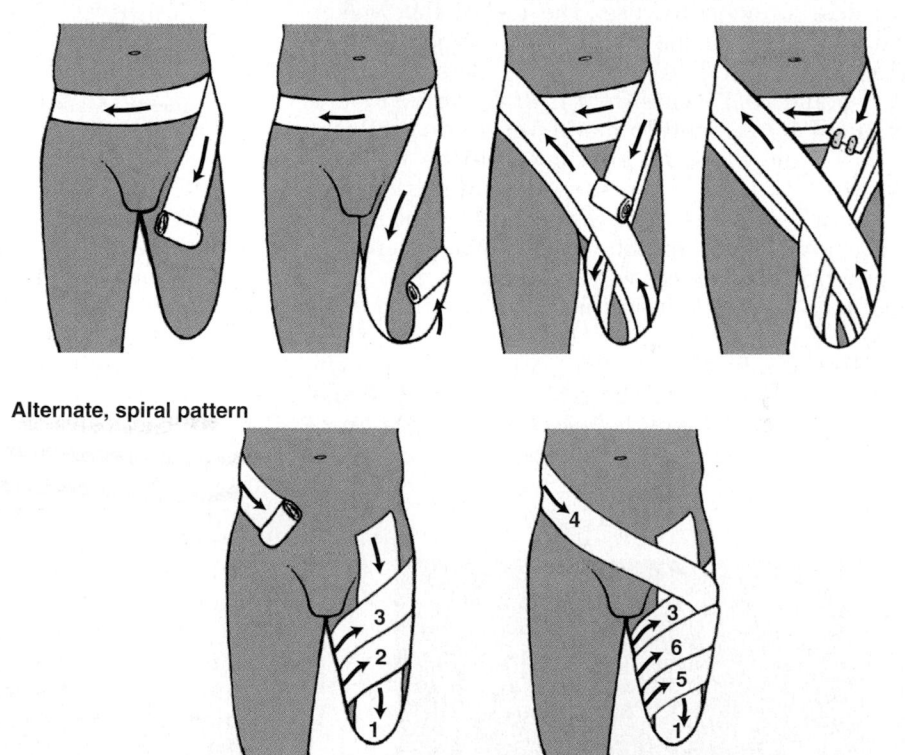

Alternate, spiral pattern

Figure 19–13
Wrapping a lower residual limb.

ous self-help devices exist to assist a person in adapting to almost any physical limitation.

Ambulatory Aids

In most health-care settings, the physician prescribes the ambulatory aid to be used. The patient is measured for and taught to use the device by a physical therapist. To be correctly measured for an ambula-

tory aid, the patient should be in a standing position on a flat surface, wearing the same style shoes that are worn for daily activity. Outside of the hospital, canes, walkers, and crutches are available for purchase from surgical supply stores and for rent from community agencies. Generally, no prescription is needed to obtain this equipment. However, third-party payers may not reimburse a patient for such equipment without consultation with a health-care professional, or the patient may not receive a proper fit or instruction in the use of the device.

A cane is an ambulatory aid used for balance and to promote a feeling of security. Canes provide only limited support and cannot be used unless the person can tolerate some weight on both lower extremities. The tip of the cane should have a thick, nonskid rubber surface for safety. The top curve or handgrip of the cane should be in line with the hip joint. The patient's elbow is slightly flexed when holding the cane correctly positioned at hip height.

Usually a cane is held on the uninvolved side. Thus, if the patient becomes weak or loses control of the involved extremity, the cane provides support on the uninvolved side to which the person will instinctively shift the weight to remain standing. With the cane held on the unaffected side, the typical gait pattern is to move the affected leg and cane forward together, then the unaffected leg.

Walkers provide four points of support, one on each of the four corners surrounding the ambulating patient (Fig. 19–14). They have a wide base, give the most security of all the ambulatory aids, and require less strength for use. The top of the walker should be level with the proximal thumb joints, with the elbow flexed at 25 to 30 degrees. The sides of the walker should be 6 inches from the side of the foot.

Walkers are difficult to maneuver in small places and must have a special attachment to be used on stairs. Most walkers are made of aluminum. Some have unique features such as anterior wheels for ease in moving and modified underarm extensions to accommodate persons with upper extremity limitations such as weak wrists or fingers or a broken bone.

Walkers create a slow gait pattern. The patient places the walker in front then steps forward. Walkers are primarily used by the elderly or by postoperative patients when they first begin ambulating.

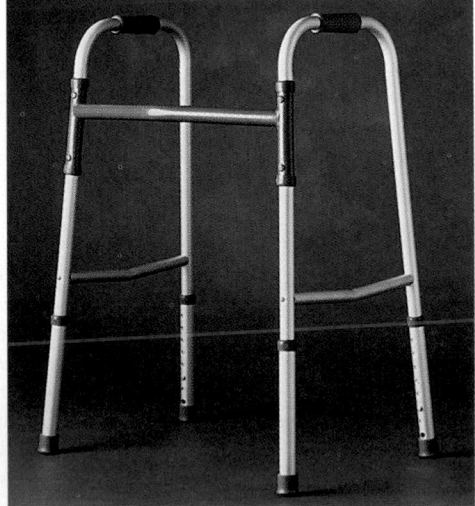

Figure 19–14

A rigid walker. (Courtesy of Invacare Corporation, Elyria, OH.)

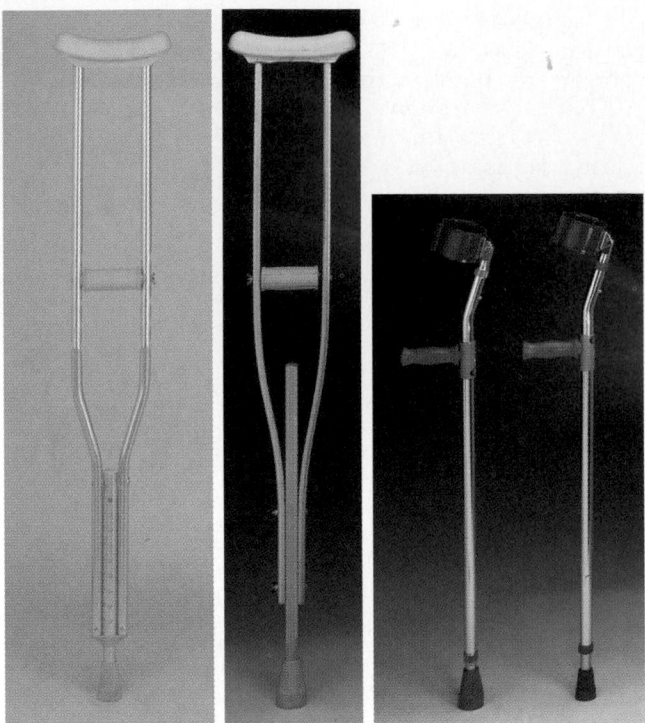

Figure 19–15

Some varieties of crutches. (Courtesy of Rubbermaid Health Care Products, Winchester, VA.)

To rise from a sitting position, the individual should not pull on the walker, but rise by using the arms of a chair or some other assistance. Once the patient is in a standing position, the weight of the upper extremities can be placed on the walker for balance and support.

Crutches can be used when no weight-bearing is allowed on one lower extremity or when weight-bearing is allowed on one or both lower extremities (Fig. 19–15). The patient must have upper body strength and arm control to use crutches. The patient's weight is supported on the wrists, hands and shoulders, not on the axillae. Pressure on the axillae can result in nerve damage. Crutches should be measured and fitted by a trained professional. The foam rubber underarm and handgrip pads provide patient comfort, and the thick nonskid tips promote safety.

Before ambulation, the patient is instructed in the proper gait. When ambulating with crutches, the body is kept in good alignment, with the head held high, shoulders back, and stomach and buttocks in. The gait pattern is determined by the physician or therapist. Certain gait patterns are used for specific circumstances. The two-point gait is used if the patient has good coordination and strength. It resembles normal walking and involves moving one leg and the opposite crutch forward, and following with the other leg and the other crutch. The three-point gait is used when weight-bearing is not allowed on one extremity. It is slower than the two-point gait and requires the use of both arms, the trunk, and one leg. There are three points of contact with the floor at any point in time. Both crutches are placed in front of the patient, and the patient bears weight on the crutches for half of the gait as the weight-bearing leg is advanced. The four-point gait is used for the weak patient with poor balance who can bear weight on both legs. It requires four points touching the floor as the patient moves forward. One crutch is moved forward, the opposite crutch is then placed forward, then one leg is brought forward, followed by the other leg.

Careful instruction and practice with supervision are necessary to ensure safety for the patient. If the patient has to climb stairs or manipulate in other difficult areas, special instruction sessions are planned with the therapist.

Splints and Braces

Splints immobilize or protect a specific body part while allowing motion of nonsplinted areas. They are not circumferential like casts and are usually removable. Splints such as the polyethylene foot-drop splint are also used to treat or prevent the formation of flexion contractures.

Braces serve as functional substitutes to provide support and allow movement of body structures. Lower-extremity spring braces provide stability for weight-bearing while allowing mobility for ambulation. Some braces provide anatomical correction as well as support and protection.

NURSING PROCESS
Assistive and Supportive Devices

Assessment

If the patient already uses an assistive or supportive device, identify which type the patient uses, why it is needed, and how well the patient maneuvers with the device. Note the patient's gait, balance, and ease of motion. Check whether the patient uses the device correctly. Determine the wearing schedule, fit, and effectiveness. If the patient does not already have an assistive or supportive device but has had one prescribed, determine the patient's knowledge about the device and ability to manipulate it correctly.

Nursing Diagnoses and Planning

Nursing diagnoses and related expected patient outcomes most commonly applicable to patients using assistive or supportive devices for musculoskeletal dysfunction include the following:

NDx: Risk for injury related to improper fit or misuse of the device

Planning: Patient Outcomes
1. Patient demonstrates safe use of the prescribed device.

2. Patient denies improper fit or problems with the device.
3. Patient relates safety measures to follow when using the device to prevent injury.

NDx: Impaired home maintenance management related to use of the device, ability to manipulate the device properly in the home, and how to perform activities of daily living while using the device

Planning: Patient Outcomes
1. Patient demonstrates proper use of the device.
2. Patient relates strategies for manipulating the device while performing necessary tasks in the home.

Nursing Interventions and Evaluation

NDx: Risk for injury
Teach the patient how to manipulate the device and have the patient demonstrate its use. Refer the patient to physical therapy for assistance with learning the safe use of the aid. Supervise the patient in the early stages of practice. Be certain the device is properly fitted. Discuss areas of the home that may be potentially hazardous for the patient using an assistive device. When possible, evaluate functioning in the home and involve the family in the sessions.

NDx: Impaired home maintenance management
Explain the use of the assistive or supportive device prescribed to the patient. Ask the physical therapist to assist in the instruction. Determine the patient's ability to maneuver with the device in an environment with furniture similar to the home setting. If the patient has difficulty, plan instruction to assist the patient in learning how to cope with this problem prior to discharge. Have the patient walk and stand with the equipment to assess proper gait and fit. Encourage the patient to do range-of-motion and strength exercises to build upper body strength, which will be beneficial if the patient is using a walker or crutches. Promote increased independence and encourage progression toward that goal. Also teach the patient proper maintenance of the device.

Compare the patient's status with the expected outcomes. If the outcomes are not met, reassess the patient and revise the plan.

EXTERNAL PROSTHESES

A prosthesis is a device that substitutes for a lost or nonfunctioning body part. Total joint replacement parts are permanent internal prostheses that replace diseased or damaged joints inside the body. External prostheses replace upper and lower extremities that have been lost as a result of congenital deformity, trauma, or disease process.

External prostheses (artificial limbs) are available in a variety of designs. They are made of wood, plastic, or lightweight synthetics such as polyurethane. The devices are attached to the body by straps, belts, or suction and may be functional or cosmetic. Functional prostheses may be powered by the individual's own muscles or by the use of levers, springs, cables, locks, gears, or hydraulic mechanisms (Fig. 19–16).

Proper selection and fit of an artificial limb requires close collaboration of health-care team members. The physician prescribes the prosthesis. A prosthetist (one knowledgeable and skilled in the construction and fit of the prosthesis) manufactures and fits the prosthesis. The physical therapist, occupational therapist, and nurse instruct the patient in its use and care. Each has a different but important role in the patient education process. A rehabilitation counselor is also a valuable team member in assisting with the establishment of long-range goals for the patient receiving a prosthesis. Because limb prostheses are custom-made, expensive, and require extensive teaching and follow-up, a social service referral is important and often necessary.

Factors considered in the selection of an appropriate prosthesis include the following:

- The general health of the individual and the presence of disorders that might prevent maximum use of the device
- The weight, strength, and coordination of the individual—excessive weight, lack of strength, or poor coordination could prevent the individual from safely using the prosthesis
- The lifestyle and activity level of the individual, which determine the choice between a cosmetic and a functional prosthesis
- The individual's ability to learn—the individual must be able to understand and follow instructions on the use and care of the prosthesis

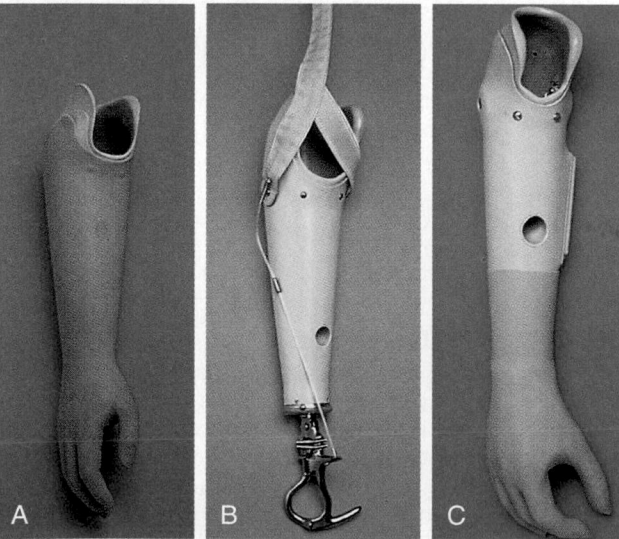

Figure 19–16

Three types of prostheses. *A*, cosmetic; *B*, cable-activated; *C*, myoelectrically controlled. (Courtesy of Otto Bock Orthopedic Industry, Inc, Minneapolis, MN.)

- The individual's potential for rehabilitation—the individual must be motivated to cooperate in the prescribed exercises and therapy, to care for the residual limb, and to maintain the prosthesis, and must also be willing to spend many hours practicing to obtain maximal use of a functional prosthesis.

A variety of prosthetic parts are available to match a particular patient's needs. There are artificial parts for the hand, forearm, upper arm, shoulder, foot, ankle, and legs. Temporary artificial parts may be used until a permanent one can be properly fitted or made for the patient.

Upper Extremity Prostheses

The forearm prosthesis is held in place by a strap or harness. There are various "hands," called terminal devices, available, depending on the desired use of the prosthesis or the occupation of the individual. The simplest terminal devices consist of a hook-type mechanism. The hook may be concealed within a cosmetic hand or be undisguised. Some forearm prostheses have several different terminal devices, each with its own function, which may be screwed into the prosthesis according to the individual's need at a given time.

The terminal device is controlled by a cable attached to the patient's muscles in the upper arm or opposite shoulder. Specific muscle movements made by the wearer can elicit motion in the terminal device (Fig. 19–17*A*).

The upper arm prosthesis has an artificial elbow joint and a cable attached to the shoulder or opposite extremity that controls movement of the elbow. Flexion and extension of the elbow maneuver the terminal device for functions such as eating, brushing teeth, and grooming (Fig. 19–17*B*).

With a shoulder prosthesis, there is no elbow or upper arm muscle to trigger movement. Control for the terminal device, the elbow, or for elevation of the prosthetic arm is achieved by cables attached to the muscle of the opposite extremity (Fig. 19–17*C*).

Lower Extremity Prostheses

A variety of foot and ankle prostheses are available. Foot and ankle prostheses include

- the Syme prosthesis, which is an artificial foot for an amputation at the ankle joint
- the two-way foot or articulating ankle
- the solid ankle/cushioned heel, or SACH, foot (Fig. 19–18)
- the Flexfoot, which allows flexibility for a more normal gait
- the Seattle foot, which has a specially designed heel with a plastic spring and mesh pad that provide a natural lift and forward thrust of the artificial limb. This allows for a more nor-

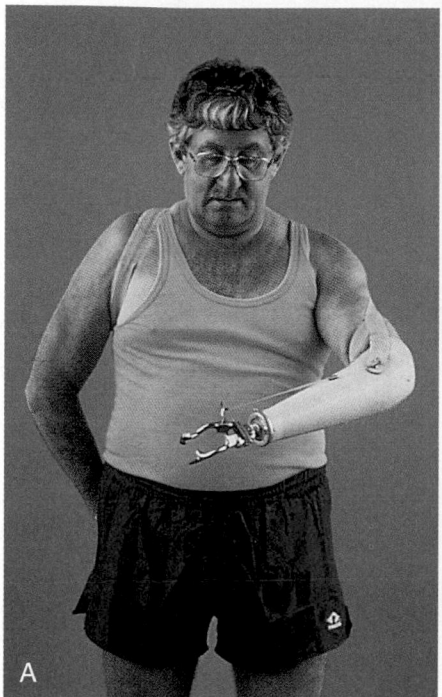 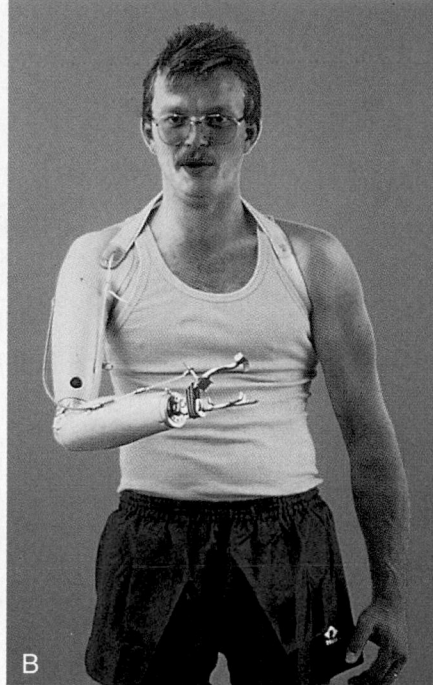 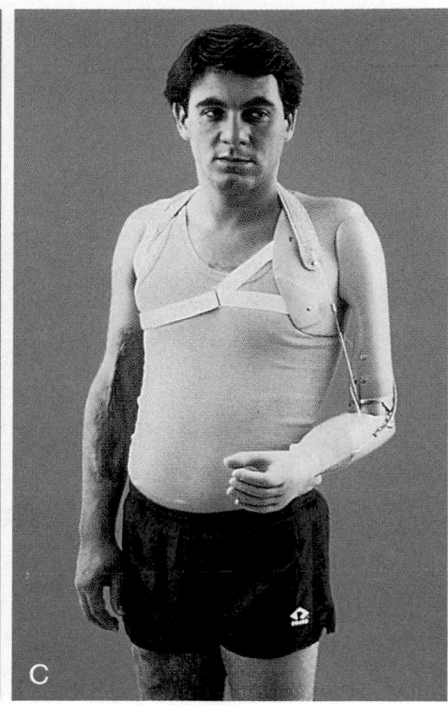

Figure 19–17

Upper extremity prostheses. *A*, Forearm (below-elbow) prosthesis with a hook as a terminal device; *B*, Upper arm (above-elbow) prosthesis with a hook as a terminal device; *C*, shoulder prosthesis (shoulder disarticulation prosthesis) with a polyethylene hand as a terminal device. (Courtesy of Otto Bock Orthopedic Industry, Inc, Minneapolis, MN.)

mal gait and running by the amputee. The outer covering of the Seattle foot is made to resemble the individual's other foot, including a sole and toes.

Below-the-knee prostheses replace the lower leg and foot following a below-the-knee amputation (Fig. 19–19). The individual must have an intact knee joint to use a below-the-knee prosthesis. A patellar tendon-bearing prosthesis is one type of artificial lower leg. It provides a smooth gait for the wearer and requires less energy to use than some of the other below-the-knee prostheses.

Above-the-knee artificial limbs have different types of knee joints (see Fig. 19–19). One type, a Bock safety knee, automatically locks whenever weight is applied to prevent the leg from buckling. This prosthesis is frequently used by elderly or weak persons with poor coordination. An above-the-knee prosthesis with a hydraulic knee provides a smooth gait but requires strength and coordination to use.

Temporary Prostheses

Artificial limbs are custom designed for each patient. Final fitting and adjustment of the prosthesis is not possible until all soft tissue has healed, the residual limb is free of edema, and the residual limb size is stable. From amputation to final application of the prosthesis can take 3 to 6 months. Often, a temporary prosthesis is used to prevent postoperative edema, provide support for early ambulation, prevent postoperative contractures of the residual limb, and encourage early rehabilitation and independence. One type of immediate prosthesis consists of a plaster base connected to a metal pylon that is attached to a shoe. Soon after surgery the amputee may begin gait training when directed. An air splint is another device used to decrease edema and assist in early ambulation after amputation. There are a number of commercial brands of air splints, and the

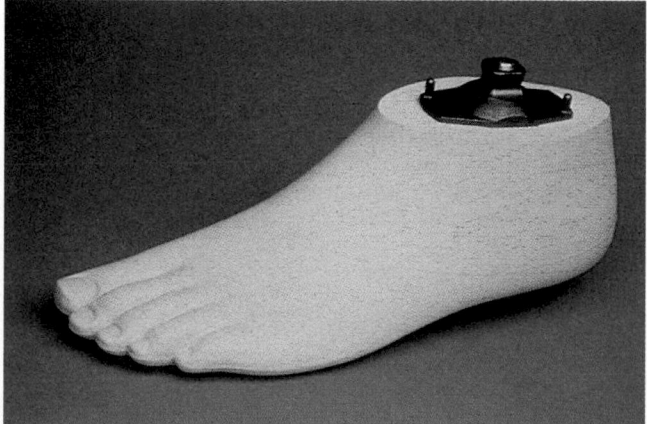

Figure 19–18

SACH foot prosthesis. (Courtesy of Otto Bock Orthopedic Industry, Inc, Minneapolis, MN.)

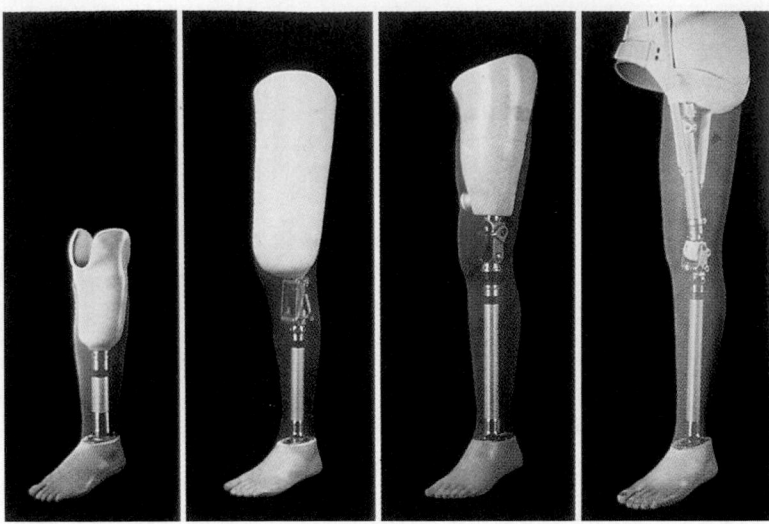

Figure 19–19

Lower extremity prostheses. The prosthesis shown at the far left is for a below-knee (transtibial) amputation. The other three prostheses are for above-knee amputations: knee disarticulation, transfemoral amputation, and hip disarticulation (from left to right). (Courtesy of Otto Bock Orthopedic Industry, Inc, Minneapolis, MN.)

instructions for use vary with each type. All types of air splints require frequent inspection of the skin and close monitoring of air pressure.

SELF-HELP DEVICES

A number of devices are available that assist individuals in safely completing self-care activities that they are no longer able to perform independently. The list is too extensive to discuss in detail here. However, be aware that such equipment is available and recognize the value of these devices to the patient with musculoskeletal limitations.

Elevated toilet seats, bath benches, and grab bars around toilets, tubs, and showers enable individuals with limited hip and knee range of motion to manage personal hygiene and toileting needs independently. Brushes, combs, and toothbrushes with long-handled extensions permit individuals with limited shoulder and arm strength and range of motion to function more independently in their own grooming. Reachers and dressing appliances such as hooks for zippers and Velcro fasteners assist the individuals with limited movement of multiple joints to dress themselves.

In most hospitals, the occupational therapist provides information on types of equipment available and how to obtain it and instructs the patient in the use of the equipment. During the initial history and assessment, or while observing the patient perform self care, identify the patient who could benefit from an occupational therapy referral. Also request a social service referral if the patient needs assistive equipment but cannot afford to buy it. Connect the patients with the resources necessary to maximize their potential for independent self-care.

The Elderly: Special Considerations

Age-related changes may cause some limitation of range of motion, but they do not cause pain, discomfort, or significant impairments. Common chronic conditions, such as arthritis, may cause the older person to experience discomfort, disability, and deformity. Joint pain, swelling, stiffness, loss of flexibility, and an increased susceptibility to injury, falls, and fractures are common problems associated with musculoskeletal diseases in older adults.

When assessing the geriatric patient for strength, sensation, motor function, and range of motion, assist the patient as needed to support the joints being evaluated. This prevents pressure from interconnecting joints from affecting the findings. The assessment often takes more time with the older adult than with a middle-aged or younger adult because the older patient may be slower in moving through the steps of gait evaluation and range of motion. Allow time for the patient to rest at intervals during the examination.

Although strength in the lower extremities may be slightly diminished, the strength in both lower extremities should be equal. If extremities are of equal strength and joints bilaterally have the same range of motion, determine the patient's ability to carry out normal activities of daily living. Assessment of function is more important than assessment of strength or range of motion. Limited hip flexion may cause difficulty in sitting in certain chairs, rising from a sitting position, or dressing the lower extremities. Similarly, limited strength may interfere with the patient's ability to lift heavy objects.

Older adults affected by musculoskeletal problems may lose some of their ability to function independently. An increase in dependency may lead to significant lifestyle changes and may have an impact on the person's self-esteem. Decreased ability to carry out normal activities of daily living can challenge the older adult's coping skills.

Older adults who are hospitalized with musculoskeletal problems may have difficulty adjusting to treatments and therapies such as casts, traction, or orthopedic surgery. Time must be allowed for reinforcement and learning of new skills. The use of assistive devices or walking with a prosthesis may require patience and encouragement from the nurse.

A teaching plan for the geriatric patient with musculoskeletal dysfunction includes instruction on a well-balanced diet to promote healing and to preserve strength and well-being. Teach older patients about their increased susceptibility to fractures. Identify fall risks and provide a safe environment.

Extended use of traction therapy is usually not the treatment of choice for the older adult because of the negative consequences of immobility. However, short-term traction is commonly used. When skin traction is applied, proper alignment of the body or affected part is an important measure in preventing contractures. Because older adults are more sensitive to changes in room temperature, they may need extra blankets. If necessary, use a bed cradle to keep the blankets from restricting the traction device. Assess skin temperature, observe the color of the nail beds, and tell the patient to notify the nurse if they feel cold or chilled.

Short-term traction for a fractured hip, and side-arm or overhead traction for fractures of the humerus, require a supine position with the head of the bed flat. This position may impair respiratory function and predispose older patients to pneumonia. Maintain adequate ventilatory capacity by frequent coughing and deep-breathing exercises and the use of incentive spirometry. The potential for skin breakdown associated with bedrest for traction therapy is also aggravated by the patient's age. Use special care to prevent skin irritation and breakdown when the elderly patient's mobility is limited.

Older patients are more prone to the complications of immobility. Plan strategies to prevent these complications and maintain maximum musculoskeletal function. Aging is not synonymous with dependency. Encourage the older adult to participate in self care and to remain as mobile and independent as possible.

Chapter Review

1. Why is pain control important in the nursing care of patients with musculoskeletal disorders?
2. Compare the effects of heat and cold when utilized in musculoskeletal disorders.
3. How is circulation assessed in a patient with a cast?
4. What is the meaning of decreased movement in an extremity of a patient with a cast?
5. What are possible solutions to the problem of impaired mobility in a patient in traction therapy?
6. How is the care of a patient with internal fixation different from that of a patient with external fixation?
7. How does positioning affect the nursing care of a patient with a total hip replacement?
8. What evidence supports the therapeutic effect of pin-site care as part of the nursing care plan for a patient with external fixation?
9. What are possible interventions for the problem of phantom pain in a patient with an amputation?
10. What would you teach about self care when caring for a patient who has an amputation?

Bibliography

Armstrong R, Bolding F. Septic arthritis after arthroscopy: The contributing roles of intraarticular steroids and environmental factors. Am J Infect Control 1994; 22(1):16.

Bates B, Bickley L, Hoekelman R. A guide to physical examination and history taking. 6th ed. Philadelphia: JB Lippincott, 1995.

Bennett JC, Plum F. Cecil textbook of medicine. 20th ed. Philadelphia: WB Saunders, 1996.

Brander VA, Stulberg SD, Chang RW. Rehabilitation following hip and knee arthroplasty. Joint Dis 1994; 5(4):815.

Buck M, Paice J. Pharmacologic management of acute pain in the orthopaedic patient. Orthop Nurs 1994; 13(6):14.

Bullock BL. Pathophysiology: Adaptations and alterations in function. 4th ed. Philadelphia: JB Lippincott, 1996.

Camp N, Iyer P. Patient outcomes in medical-surgical nursing. Springhouse, PA: Springhouse Corporation, 1995.

Carpenito L. Nursing diagnosis: application to clinical practice. 6th ed. Philadelphia: JB Lippincott, 1995.

Deathe A, Hayes K, Winter DA. The biomechanics of canes, crutches, and walkers. Crit Rev Phys Rehabil Med 1993; 5(1): 15.

Doyle W, Goldstone J, Kramer D. The Syme prosthesis revisited. J Prosthet Orthot 1993; 5(3):95.

Dykes PC. Minding the five Ps of neurovascular assessment. Am J Nurs 1993; 93(6):38.

Eliopoulos C. Gerontological nursing. 3rd ed. Philadelphia: JB Lippincott, 1993.

Fischbach F. A manual of laboratory and diagnostic tests. 5th ed. Philadelphia: JB Lippincott, 1996.

Fuller J, Schaller-Ayers J. Health assessment: A nursing approach. 2nd ed. Philadelphia: JB Lippincott, 1994.

Gulanick M, Klopp A, Galanes S, Gradishar D, Puzas MK. Nursing care plans. 3rd ed. St. Louis: Mosby Year-Book, 1994.

Ham R, deTrafford J. Patterns of recovery for lower limb amputation. Clin Rehabil 1994; 8(4):320.

Hayes K. Heat and cold in the management of arthritis. Arthritis Care Res 1993; 6(3):156.

Hazzard W, Bierman E, Blass J, Ettinger Jr W, Halter J. Principles of geriatric medicine and gerontology. 3rd ed. New York: McGraw-Hill, 1994.

Holloway N. Medical surgical care planning. 2nd ed. Springhouse, PA: Springhouse Corporation, 1993.

Iyer P, Taptich B, Bernocchi-Losey D. Nursing process and nursing diagnosis. 3rd ed. Philadelphia: WB Saunders, 1995.

Jones-Walton P. Orthopaedic health promotion 2000. Orthop Nurs 1994; 13(3):29.

Kaul M, Herring S. Superficial heat and cold. Physician Sportsmed 1994; 22(12):65.

Kee JL. Laboratory and diagnostic tests with nursing implications. 4th ed. Norwalk, CT: Appleton & Lange, 1995.

Kuhn MA. Pharmacotherapeutics: A nursing process approach. 3rd ed. Philadelphia: FA Davis, 1994.

Lankford T. Foundations of normal and therapeutic nutrition. Albany, NY: Delmar, 1994.

Lehne R. Pharmacology for nursing care. 2nd. ed. Philadelphia: WB Saunders, 1994.

Lichtenstein R, Semaan S, Marmar E. Development and impact of a hospital-based perioperative patient education program in a joint replacement center. Orthop Nurs 1993; 12(6);17.

Lyth H. Invisible problem. Nurs Times 1995; 91(19):38.

Maher AB, Salmond SW, Pellino TA. Orthopaedic nursing. Philadelphia: WB Saunders, 1994.

Mallory TH. Total hip replacement in the 90's: The procedure, the patient, the surgeon. Orthopedics 1992;15(4):427.

Mayers M, Pankratz C (eds). Clinical care plans: Medical surgical nursing. New York: McGraw-Hill, 1995.

Mikulaninec C. An amputee critical path. J Vasc Nurs 1992; 10(2): 6.

Moriarty L, Rothman NL. Transitional home care after joint arthroplasty. Home Healthc Nurse 1994; 12(1):31.

Mourad L, Droste M. The nursing process in the care of adults with orthopaedic conditions. 3rd ed. Albany, NY: Delmar, 1993.

Neff JA, Kidd RS. Trauma nursing: The art and science. St. Louis: Mosby Year-Book, 1993.

Pontieri-Lewis V. Focus on wound care therapeutic beds: An overview. Medsurg Nurs 1995; 4(4):323.

Reiss B, Evans M. Pharmacological aspects of nursing. 4th ed. Albany, NY: Delmar, 1993.

Rothman NL, Moriarty L, Rothman RH, et al. Establishing a home care protocol for early discharge of patients with hip and knee arthroplasties. Home Healthc Nurse 1994; 12(1):24.

Rounseville C. Phantom limb pain: The ghost that haunts the amputee. Orthop Nurs 1992; 11(2):67.

Shu Y. A study on functioning for independent living among the elderly in the community. Public Health Nurs 1995; 12(1):31.

Steadman JR. Transitional home care after joint arthroplasty. Home Healthc Nurse 1994; 12(1):31.

Styrcula L. Traction basics: Part I. Orthop Nurs 1994; 13(2):71.

Styrcula L. Traction basics: Part II. Traction equipment. Orthop Nurs 1994; 13(3):55.

Styrcula L. Traction basics: Part III. Types of traction. Orthop Nurs 1994; 13(4):34.

Styrcula L. Traction basics: Part IV. Traction for lower extremities. Orthop Nurs 1994; 13(5):59.

United States Department of Health and Human Services. Clinical practice guideline. Acute pain management: Operative or medical procedures and trauma. (AHCPR Pub. No. 92-0032). Rockville, MD: Agency for Health Care Policy and Research, 1992.

United States Department of Health and Human Services. Pressure sores in adults: Prediction and prevention. (AHCPR Pub. No. 92-0047). Rockville, MD: Agency for Health Care Policy and Research, 1992.

Walker J. Caring for elderly people with persistent pain in the community: A qualitative perspective on the attitudes of patients and nurses. Health Soc Care Community 1994; 2(4):221.

Yandrich T. Preventing infection in total joint replacement surgery. Orthop Nurs 1995; 14(2):15.

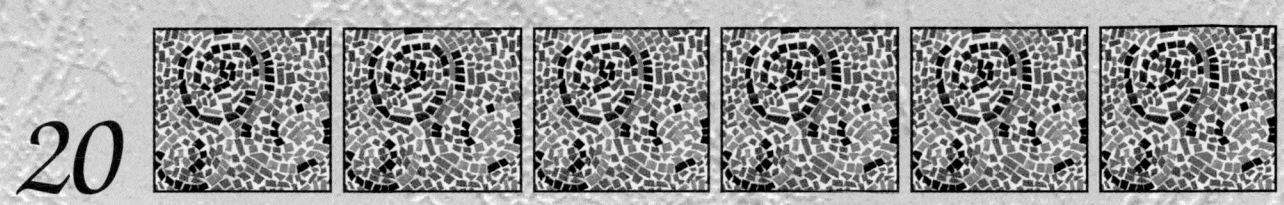

20

Nursing Care of Patients with Musculoskeletal Disorders

Study Outcomes

After studying this chapter, you should be able to:

1. Describe common musculoskeletal disorders in terms of etiology, pathophysiology, clinical manifestations, diagnostic procedures, and medical management.
2. Compare and contrast the various types of fractures in terms of cause, risk factors, treatment, and nursing interventions.
3. Identify common pharmacologic agents used to treat musculoskeletal disorders.
4. Explain the effects of osteoporosis, osteoarthritis, and rheumatoid arthritis.
5. Describe the health-care teaching appropriate for the patient who is at risk for musculoskeletal disorders.
6. Identify information and physical examination data essential to the assessment of patients with common musculoskeletal disorders.
7. State nursing diagnoses and related expected patient outcomes commonly applicable to patients with musculoskeletal disorders.
8. Describe nursing interventions, with their rationales, commonly applicable to patients with musculoskeletal disorders.
9. Explain the basis for evaluation of nursing care provided to patients with common musculoskeletal disorders.
10. Identify special considerations for the elderly patient with a musculoskeletal disorder.
11. Identify alternative treatment and care settings for patients with musculoskeletal disorders and the services related to community-based care.

The musculoskeletal system provides support and protection for the body. Disorders of the system are often multifaceted and have a variety of underlying causes. The disorders may affect all age groups in the adult population and are particularly common in the older adult. Musculoskeletal disorders affect bones, joints, muscles, tendons, ligaments, and bursae. A major manifestation of musculoskeletal problems is immobility, which, in turn, has an adverse effect on many other body systems.

Many of the disorders of the musculoskeletal system are debilitating. This presents specific impli-

cations for nursing care. The elderly, in particular, are prone to musculoskeletal disorders, many of which are due to the natural aging process. Long-term care planning, home care instructions, and follow-up care are important facets of nursing interventions. Referrals to other agencies outside the hospital for continued care may be necessary for certain individuals because of immobility and safety problems associated with musculoskeletal disorders. The home health nurse and the physical therapist are key personnel who collaborate with the physician to assist patients with musculoskeletal disorders to maintain independence.

Infections and Inflammations

OSTEOMYELITIS

Etiology and Pathophysiology

Osteomyelitis is an infection of the bone that may result in necrosis of bone and marrow tissue. It weakens the bone and places it at risk for spontaneous pathologic fractures or fractures with minimal trauma. Osteomyelitis may be caused by bacteria, virus, tubercle bacilli, *Treponema pallidum*, fungi, or the presence of contaminated foreign material such as a bullet or a joint prosthesis. *Staphylococcus aureus* and *Streptococcus pyogenes* are the organisms most frequently associated with osteomyelitis. The pathogens may enter the bone by direct contamination from an open fracture, may spread to the bone from another infected body part, or may be present in the blood stream and travel into and lodge in the bone or marrow. Osteomyelitis can be acute or chronic. Both forms have the same pathologic process but may vary in causative agent, progression, and symptoms.

Osteomyelitis involves infection of the haversian canals, bone marrow, and subperiosteal spaces. Initially, bone tissue and blood vessels are destroyed by proteolytic enzymes released by the pathogens. Because of diminished blood flow, removal of debris from the infected area is impaired. As the infection spreads through the bone and subperiosteal spaces, the necrotic debris accumulates. ~~It separates from the rest of the bone and forms a substance known as sequestrum~~. The sequestrum becomes a reservoir for more bacterial growth.

Damage to the bone and periosteum stimulates osteoblastic activity, and new bone tissue, called involucrum, forms around the sequestrum. Formation of the involucrum and separation of the sequestrum further impair circulation to the diseased bone.

Acute Osteomyelitis

Acute osteomyelitis is a condition seen more in children than in adults. It occurs four times more often in males than in females. The prime causative organism is *S. aureus*.

Clinical Manifestations
Clinical manifestations depend on the extent of the infection and route of contamination. When acute osteomyelitis develops directly from bacteremia, the patient experiences a sudden onset of fever and a rapid pulse, with limited movement and severe pain in the involved body part caused by spasms of surrounding muscles. Erythema, heat, and swelling around the affected bone may also be present. Osteomyelitis contracted by direct contamination of the bone or by spread from another body part presents fewer systemic effects, but muscle spasms and tenderness over the bone are present.

Diagnosis
Laboratory data include elevated leukocyte count and sedimentation rate. Radiographic, tomographic, and imaging changes may not be seen for 1 to 3 weeks after the onset of infection. X-ray films then reveal a localized area of destruction surrounded by a zone of decalcified bone. The sequestrum appears as dense areas on x-ray films. Identification of the causative organism is made by blood cultures and aspiration of subperiosteal pus for culture and sensitivity testing.

Management
The goal of medical management is to rid the body of the infectious organism and prevent spread of the infection to surrounding tissues. Treatment includes débridement of necrotic tissue and large doses of parenteral, then oral, antibiotics until the organism is eradicated. Combinations of antibiotics to prevent the growth of resistant organisms may be administered for up to 1 year.

Because the sequestrum and involucrum impair circulation to the infected bone, they must be removed before antibiotic therapy can be effective. Surgical débridement or a closed irrigation system to low suction with normal saline or antibiotic solution can be used to flush away necrotic tissue.

Complications of acute osteomyelitis include septicemia, meningitis, tenosynovitis, and thrombo-phlebitis. Acute osteomyelitis may also become a chronic infection if inadequately treated.

Chronic Osteomyelitis

Chronic osteomyelitis is characterized by the gradual progressive development of multiple bone cavities with sequestrum and involucrum throughout the bone.

Clinical Manifestations
The patient with chronic osteomyelitis experiences episodes of pain, caused by the inflammatory activity, and symptom-free periods when the inflammatory activity is decreased. Pain is usually more intense at night. Involved areas are swollen, reddened, warm, and tender. Other symptoms may include deformed bone, dusky skin, atrophied muscles of the involved area, and the development of draining sinuses.

Diagnosis
X-ray films show multiple dense areas of sequestrum. Drainage from sinus tracts and aspirated fluid is cultured to identify the causative organism. Sensitivity studies determine the antibiotic therapy.

Management
Treatment involves the surgical removal of involved tissue, continuous closed suction wound drainage, laser débridement, and combination antibiotic therapy. A windowed cast that allows access for wound care may be applied to support the weakened bone. A splint may be applied to provide comfort and support for the involved extremity. For cases involving particularly resistant or difficult-to-eradicate organisms, a muscle flap transfer that increases blood supply to the involved bone may be performed. Bone grafting may also be required. Hyperbaric oxygen has also been effective in treating some patients. When all conservative measures to control osteomyelitis are unsuccessful, amputation may be required.

Complications of chronic osteomyelitis include muscle contractures, septic arthritis or osteoarthritis, decreased rate of bone growth, nonunion of fractures, and pathologic fracture through the involved bone.

Tuberculous Osteomyelitis

Infection of bone tissue and joints by the tubercle bacillus *Mycobacterium tuberculosis* occurs secondary to tubercle lesions elsewhere in the body. Like active tuberculosis, it is more likely to occur in malnourished and physically compromised individuals. Currently there is a rise in the incidence of active tuberculosis in the United States, which may cause an increase in tuberculous osteomyelitis.

Tuberculosis of the bone precipitates the same response in bone tissue as in the lung. The tubercle bacillus invades the bone, and the body's natural immune response encases the organisms within the bone, causing a cavity. The bacillus becomes reactivated when the patient's immune system is weakened.

Clinical Manifestations

The onset of bone tuberculosis is slow and secondary to other organ lesions. The involved areas are warm and tender. The patient may report pain and muscle spasm, muscle atrophy, and stiff joints. The spine and lower extremities are most often affected. The involved vertebrae may collapse, giving the patient a hunchbacked appearance. Abscesses and draining sinuses may develop. Neurologic dysfunction from spinal cord compression or inflammation may result in muscular weakness and paralysis. Systemic symptoms include a low-grade fever that is higher at night or in the late afternoon, anorexia, malaise, and weight loss.

Diagnosis

Diagnostic x-ray films show altered bone structure, collapsed vertebrae, and compression deformities. Tuberculin skin test results are positive. Acid-fast tubercle bacilli are identified in sputum cultures, joint fluid, or tissue biopsy. Laboratory studies reveal an elevated leukocyte count and an increased sedimentation rate.

Management

Treatment includes the administration of combinations of antitubercular agents to control the infection. Isoniazid, ethambutol, streptomycin, rifampin, and pyrazinamide are drugs of choice.

Other Forms of Osteomyelitis

Other causative organisms of osteomyelitis include *T. pallidum,* fungi, and *Salmonella* spp. Syphilis osteomyelitis, caused by *T. pallidum,* affects the bone in the tertiary stage of the disease. It is characterized by a "moth-eaten" appearance of the bone on x-ray film. The patient may complain of bone pain and experience pathologic fractures. Penicillin is used to treat the infection.

Fungal or mycotic osteomyelitis is caused by blastomycetes and *Coccidioides immitis.* Bone involvement usually begins after respiratory infection. The fungus invades cancellous bone and produces well-defined areas on x-ray film. Amphotericin B is administered to treat the infection.

Salmonella organisms produce an acute form of osteomyelitis. Individuals with sickle-cell disease are at risk for this condition. Treatment consists of administration of chloramphenicol or high doses of penicillin or ampicillin.

❖ Settings, Providers, and Collaboration for Care

Management of osteomyelitis can occur in the hospital and in outpatient settings. The nurse teaches the patient and the family about the nature of the disease, its symptoms, and the length of treatment. A physical therapist may be involved in the hospitalization of a patient with osteomyelitis to prevent complications of immobility such as contractures.

Long-term antibiotic therapy may be implemented in the home or community setting with proper follow-up, education, and supervision. Home nursing visits may be implemented to administer intravenous antibiotics in a home setting. The patient and family should be instructed on the management of antibiotic therapy. Follow-up evaluation visits are scheduled at the physician's office.

NURSING PROCESS
Osteomyelitis

Assessment

Review the patient's history, presenting symptoms, and results of diagnostic studies. Complete an assessment, observing for outward signs of infection in the affected area. Look for redness, warmth, swelling, and pain. Ask the patient about the severity and duration of the pain and what relief methods have been successful. Check vital signs. Look for additional signs of fever such as flushing, night sweats, and chilling. Determine the patient's understanding of the disease and the treatment regimen.

Nursing Diagnoses and Planning

Nursing diagnoses and related expected patient outcomes most commonly applicable to patients with osteomyelitis include the following:

NDx: Pain related to infection and inflammation

Planning: Patient Outcomes
1. Patient denies pain in affected part.
2. Patient states methods to decrease pain, such as using relaxation strategies and reducing swelling and trauma to the affected part.

NDx: Knowledge deficit: nature of disease, treatment, and prognosis

Planning: Patient Outcomes
1. Patient states accurate information about the cause of the disease and methods to reduce complications.
2. Patient discusses concerns about the disease and states an understanding of the prognosis and treatment regimen.

NDx: Risk for infection (recurrent or spreading) related to knowledge deficit

Planning: Patient Outcomes
1. Patient states local and systemic signs of infection.
2. Patient states knowledge of when to alert healthcare providers.

Nursing Interventions and Evaluation

NDx: Pain

Administer prescribed analgesics and nonsteroidal anti-inflammatory drugs. Explain the dosage, frequency, side effects, and expected therapeutic effects of the medications. Schedule activity when the medication is most effective. Instruct and support the patient in nonpharmacologic pain control methods. Caution the patient not to perform tasks that require mental alertness while taking pain medication. Teach the patient to elevate and provide support to the involved body part, which will reduce swelling and pain. Caution the patient about weight-bearing if contraindicated, because weight-bearing might increase the pain significantly. Teach the patient to avoid exercise and heat application, which increase circulation. Maintaining proper alignment and position changes may promote comfort. When directed, use support devices such as a cast or a splint.

NDx: Knowledge deficit: nature of disease, treatment, and prognosis

Teach the patient about the disease, the cause, methods of prevention of injury to the affected part, and appropriate treatment. Explain that increased swelling, redness, discoloration, or decreased sensation in the affected part may be signs of complications and that the physician should be notified. Reinforce the physician's instruction about weight-lifting (if shoulder, arm, or hand is affected) or weight-bearing (if knee, leg, ankle, or foot is affected). Teach the patient about the therapeutic effects and side effects of the prescribed antibiotics, as well as the dosage and frequency. Emphasize the importance of adherence to a long-term antibiotic regimen and keeping follow-up appointments.

NDx: Risk for infection (recurrent or spreading)

Teach the patient about signs and symptoms of local and systemic infection and the need to inform a health-care provider of these findings. Provide written material for reinforcement. When necessary, provide for continuity through referral to a home- or community-nursing service.

Compare the patient's status with the expected outcomes. If the outcomes are not met, reassess the patient and revise the plan.

ARTHRITIS

The general term *arthritis* is defined as inflammation of a joint. It is associated with swelling and pain and can include changes in the structure of involved musculoskeletal tissue. There are more than 100 types of arthritis, each differing somewhat in etiology, pathophysiology, and method of treatment. More than 23 million people in the United States are affected by some form of arthritis that is severe enough to require medical attention.

Arthritis is a leading cause of mobility limitation. It can make activities such as dressing, opening a jar, climbing stairs, or getting out of a chair difficult and painful tasks. People suffering from arthritis may need more time to perform everyday activities and may also be more dependent on other people. Arthritis has an impact on the physical, psychologic, and social functioning of a patient and his or her family in the health-care setting and in the home. The most prevalent forms of arthritis are rheumatoid arthritis and osteoarthritis.

Rheumatoid Arthritis

Rheumatoid arthritis is the most serious form of arthritis in terms of its potential for chronic disability. Rheumatoid arthritis is a chronic systemic disease characterized by inflammation of the joints and extra-articular manifestations. When it occurs in persons older than 60, it tends to be severe and rapidly progressive.

Etiology and Pathophysiology

The cause of rheumatoid arthritis is unknown, but it is believed to be an autoimmune disorder. A combination of factors, such as genetic predisposition, may cause rheumatoid arthritis. The condition affects more than 6 million people in the United States.

In rheumatoid arthritis, antibodies produced by the immune system, which usually protect the body, become destructive agents that attack and destroy joint structures. The antibodies first attack the synovium of the joint, causing the joint to become inflamed and swollen with excess synovial fluid. Gradually the articular cartilage and surrounding tendons and ligaments are involved. Chronic congestion and thickening of the synovium produce granulation tissue called *pannus*, which is Latin for "cloth." The pannus causes further erosion of the articular cartilage and invades the joint capsule. As the disease progresses, underlying bone and adjacent connective tissues are damaged. Tough fibrous connective tissue replaces the pannus and fills the joint space. As the fibrous tissue calcifies, the joint becomes ankylosed, or fused. The patient is left with a joint that is painful and often deformed and has a very limited or no range of motion.

Rheumatoid arthritis is more prevalent among females than males and affects all racial and ethnic groups. The prevalence among black and white Americans is similar.

Clinical Manifestations

Rheumatoid arthritis is characterized by remissions, or periods of improvement of symptoms, and exacerbations, or periods of an increase in the severity of symptoms. Exacerbations may be aggravated by emotional or physical stress and illness. Patients usually appear anemic, are anorexic, look and feel ill, have a low-grade fever, and are likely to be underweight. Muscle aching may also occur.

Joint involvement is symmetrical. The joints are swollen, shiny, reddened, and painful. The joints of the hands and wrists, with the exception of the distal interphalangeal joints, are commonly affected first (Fig. 20–1). The patient has a weakened grip. Diarthrodial joints are more frequently affected, but any joint of the body may be involved. Pathologic changes in the hand joints commonly result in subluxation of the fingers, hand, and wrist. Classic deformities such as a swan-neck deformity (hyperextension of the proximal interphalangeal joint with fixed flexion of the distal interphalangeal joint), a boutonniere deformity (persistent flexion of the proximal interphalangeal joint with hyperextension of the distal interphalangeal joint), and ulnar deviation of the fingers occur, leaving the hands painful and nonfunctioning. Chronic joint pain of varying intensity, which is more severe upon rising in the morning, is experienced by most patients.

Systemic manifestations include

- Muscle atrophy
- Vasculitis of the smaller peripheral vessels, which can lead to cutaneous ulceration
- Inflammation of tissue overlying the sclera of the eye
- A decrease in salivary and lacrimal secretions (Sjögren's syndrome)

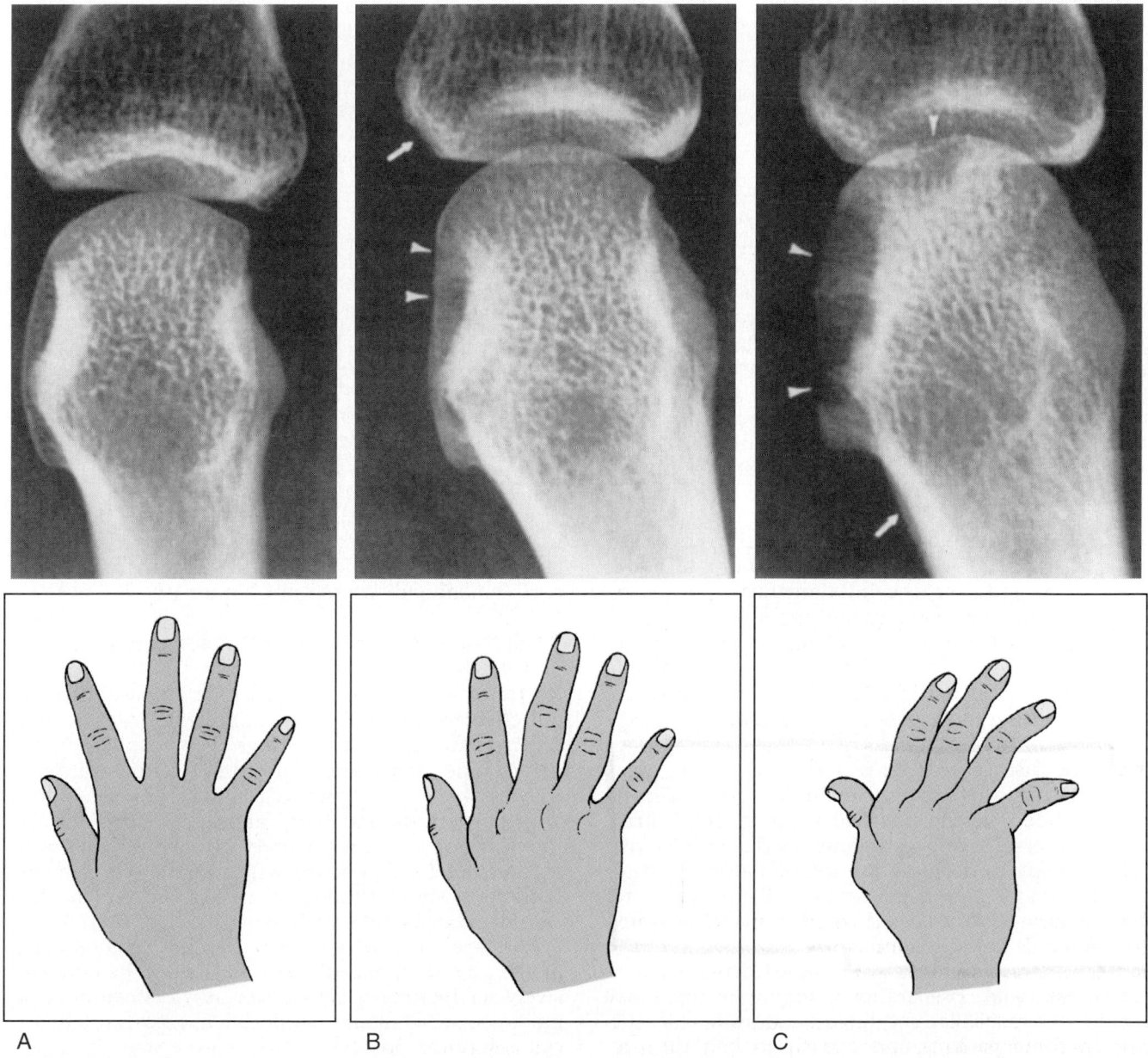

Figure 20–1

Structural changes in the hand from rheumatoid arthritis. *A*, Early stage; *B*, moderate stage; *C*, advanced stage. (Photographs from Resnick D. Bone and joint imaging. 2nd ed. Philadelphia: WB Saunders, 1996, p 213.)

- Carpal tunnel syndrome
- Pulmonary nodules and pulmonary fibrosis

Rheumatoid nodules, which are painless subcutaneous moveable skin nodules near bony prominences, may occur anywhere on the body.

Diagnosis

Diagnosis is made on the basis of history and radiologic studies. X-ray films reveal clouding of fluid spaces, fraying of inner joint margins, and gradual lessening of joint space.

Although specific blood values are usually abnormal in rheumatoid arthritis, none are considered diagnostic. Laboratory studies show a normal red blood cell count in the early stages of the disease, then a decreasing red blood cell count as the disease progresses. Also present are

- an increased white blood cell count
- an elevated erythrocyte sedimentation rate, which rises with the severity of the disease
- an elevated platelet count

The rheumatoid factor, an immunoglobulin that reacts with antibodies produced by lymphocytes in the synovial fluid, is present in 40 to 50% of patients with rheumatoid arthritis in the early stages of the disease, and in 80 to 90% of patients with advanced disease. Because the rheumatoid factor may be present in other inflammatory diseases, it is not considered diagnostic for rheumatoid arthritis. Levels of antinuclear antibodies and C-reactive proteins may also be elevated. A genetic marker, HLA-Dw4, is present in 50% of patients. Synovial fluid has a high white blood cell count and poor viscosity.

Management

Since there is no cure for rheumatoid arthritis, efforts are directed at improving the general health of the patient, reducing the inflammatory process, relieving pain, and maintaining mobility of the affected joints. This requires lifelong treatment by numerous health-care specialists. Patient understanding and participation and family support are essential factors affecting the course of the disease.

Early management involves educating the patient about the disease process, providing adequate nutrition, having the patient maintain good general health while avoiding physical stress, giving instruction in stress control techniques, and administering drug therapy to decrease the inflammatory reaction. Medications used to decrease the inflammatory process include enteric-coated aspirin in large doses, nonsteroidal anti-inflammatory drugs (Highlight 20–1), and systemic steroids. Other drugs such as parenteral gold preparations, immunosuppressive agents, and penicillamine have been used with success in some patients and appear to halt the progression of the arthritis. Investigational treatments include the use of alkylating or antineoplastic drugs, sulfonamide, fish oils, cyclosporine, and cytotoxic

agents. Total lymph node irradiation is also being studied.

Local heat and cold applications may be used to relieve pain. The patient is instructed in their proper use at home. Although thermal applications do not decrease synovial proliferation and swelling, they provide temporary comfort by decreasing muscle spasms and altering the pain threshold. Generally, cold is used for acute joint pain, and heat is used for chronic joint pain. Cold can be applied by massage with an ice pack until numbness is achieved. Heat can be applied by moist heat packs, paraffin baths, diathermy, ultrasound, or whirlpools.

Another method for controlling chronic pain is the use of transcutaneous electrical nerve stimulation (TENS) to a body part by electrodes attached to the skin. The system is portable and patient-controlled. A TENS unit relieves pain and reduces the need for analgesics. Theories to explain how it works suggest that TENS promotes the release of endorphins or blocks the passage of pain impulses from the local area to the central nervous system.

When conservative treatment is not adequate, surgery is sometimes used to relieve pain and correct deformities. The types of surgery performed for rheumatoid arthritis are synovectomy, osteotomy, arthrodesis, and arthroplasty, or total joint replacement. A synovectomy is the removal of hypertrophied synovium. It is done to delay the destructive process within the joint. Synovectomies are most commonly performed on the elbow, wrist, fingers, and knees. An osteotomy is the cutting and removal of bone to change joint alignment. This procedure reduces stress on the involved joint, and improved function often results. Arthrodesis is fusion of a joint. Although it causes permanent immobilization of the joint, the joint is more stable and less painful. The joints that are most frequently surgically fused are the wrist and ankle. Arthroplasty with total joint replacement is discussed in Chapter 19.

❖ Settings, Providers, and Collaboration for Care

Rheumatoid arthritis is a chronic disease that requires interventions by the entire health-care team in a variety of health-care settings. The hospital, outpatient, home, and community-health settings provide treatment, support, and education for rheumatoid arthritis patients and their families. Support groups provide assistance in a variety of ways for the family and patient diagnosed with rheumatoid arthritis. Long-term care includes referrals to several health-care personnel and a variety of modes of therapy.

A social service referral is usually initiated early in the course of the disease because of its progressively debilitating nature. Social services can provide guidance in available support resources and financial assistance.

Occupational therapists teach the patient how to conserve energy and maintain joint alignment. They also provide splints to protect and support involved

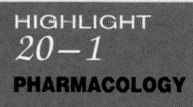 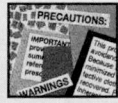

Nonsteroidal Anti-Inflammatory Drugs (NSAIDs)

Definition:

An important class of drugs used for analgesic, antipyretic, anti-inflammatory effects in arthritis management. They are classified as salicylates or nonsalicylates.

Generic and Trade Names:

Diclofenac (Voltaren), diflunisal (Dolobid), ibuprofen (Motrin, Advil), indomethacin (Indocin), naproxen (Naprosyn), piroxicam (Feldene), oxaprozin (Daypro), ketorolac (Toradol), acetylsalicylic acid (Aspirin).

Action:

They produce anti-inflammatory, analgesic, and antipyretic effects, probably through the inhibition of prostaglandin synthesis. Some suppress platelet aggregation.

Uses:

They are used primarily for osteoarthritis and rheumatoid arthritis but may also be prescribed for ankylosing spondylitis, bursitis, or tendinitis.

Side Effects:

Drowsiness, irritability, headache, tinnitus, indigestion, nausea, gastrointestinal bleeding, colitis, pruritis, rashes.

Interactions:

Interactions vary with specific NSAIDs. Interactions may occur with anticoagulants, oral hypoglycemic agents, aspirin, digoxin, antacids, probenecid, barbiturates, antihypertensive agents, beta blockers, diuretics, angiotensin-converting enzyme inhibitors. The patient should consult the physician and health-care provider regarding these medication interactions.

Toxic Effects:

Nephrotoxicity and hepatotoxicity.

Nursing Implications:

Teach the patient the correct dose and frequency as well as the side effects and therapeutic effects of the NSAID.

NSAIDs are contraindicated for patients with a history of severe hypersensitivity.

NSAIDs should be used with extreme caution by patients with peptic ulcer disease and bleeding disorder.

Watch for gastric distress and signs of gastrointestinal bleeding, such as dark stools.

Observe for bruising, petechiae, or excessive bleeding from mucous membranes or small skin lesions.

NSAIDs should be avoided by children and adolescents with chickenpox or influenza.

NSAIDs should be discontinued 1 week prior to elective surgery.

~~Administer the drug with food, milk, or water to reduce gastric irritation.~~

~~Food will delay absorption rate but not alter absorption.~~

Instruct patients not to chew enteric-coated or sustained-release formulations.

NSAIDs can increase the risk of bleeding in patients taking oral anticoagulants.

Explain that a patient should not consume alcohol with NSAIDs.

Instruct the individual to contact a physician with any symptoms of tinnitus, sweating, gastrointestinal distress, and dizziness.

Watch for, document, and report side effects or apparent interactions.

Geriatric Considerations:

Caution is needed when treating elderly individuals with NSAIDs. The drug can cause renal impairment. Therefore, monitor the weight, urine output, and elevation of serum creatinine and blood urea nitrogen. The drug can also cause liver failure, so the patient should be monitored for elevated serum bilirubin, aspartate transaminase, alanine transaminase, prolonged coagulation studies, alkaline phosphatase, and lactate dehydrogenase (LDH). Caution should be used when administering NSAIDs to patients with congestive heart failure, alcoholism, and pre-existing renal or liver dysfunction. Dosages may need to be reduced or eliminated if nephrotoxicity or hepatotoxicity is identified.

joints. Resting splints may be used for night wear and functional splints for protection and support while the patient is working.

Physical therapists play an important role in the care of the patient with rheumatoid arthritis. They provide assistive devices to protect weight-bearing joints and assist with ambulation. Physical therapy includes exercises to prevent stiffness and slow loss of joint motion and to maintain muscle size and strength. Passive, active, and stretching exercises may be recommended. During acute exacerbations, joints may remain at rest with only limited exercise.

Nurses providing home care are significant health-care team members. Promoting home safety, lifestyle modifications, health maintenance, and patient education are important nursing interventions. Assessment of the patient and family's ability to physically and psychosocially manage the chronic illness in the home is a key nursing role. Follow-up care by the home health nurse can reinforce the prescribed regimen and previous nursing interventions with the patient. The patient may be seen routinely in the physician's office for further evaluation or for treatment of exacerbations or complications of the disease.

NURSING PROCESS
Rheumatoid Arthritis

Assessment

Review the patient's history and current physical problems. Because pain is one of the most significant and chronic problems in arthritis, assess the patient's pain tolerance and its debilitating effects. Check which joints are most severely affected. Determine the patient's perception of the pain experienced, what time of day it is most severe, and what precipitates it. Emotional stress has been associated with exacerbations of rheumatoid arthritis. Ask the patient which, if any, medications have been beneficial in relieving pain, stiffness, or inflammatory reactions.

Examine the affected joints, observing for redness, edema, crepitation, deformity, subluxation, dislocation, ankylosis, and muscle contractions. Look at the affected limbs, noting atrophy, decreased subcutaneous fat, and the presence of subcutaneous nodules. Note mobility problems and difficulties with hand motions.

Assess the psychologic and social impact of the arthritis on the patient and family. Determine the patient's and family's understanding of the disease and its progression. Identify coping strategies used by the patient and the family to manage the illness. Ask the patient and family about effective coping mechanisms used in the past and what personal support systems are available.

Nursing Diagnoses and Planning

Nursing diagnoses and related expected patient outcomes most commonly applicable to patients with rheumatoid arthritis include the following:

NDx: Pain related to joint or muscle deformity and inflammation

Planning: Patient Outcomes
1. Patient denies pain in affected part.
2. Patient states methods to decrease pain, such as rest and relaxation therapies and alternating rest and activity.
3. Patient states appropriate use of analgesics or anti-inflammatory agents and the TENS unit, if prescribed.

NDx: Impaired physical mobility related to the rheumatoid disease process and pain

Planning: Patient Outcomes
1. Patient demonstrates ability to tolerate physical mobility.
2. Patient performs measures to regain and maintain joint range of motion.
3. Patient maintains mobility and self-care with the assistance of an ambulatory aid or assistive device.

NDx: Self esteem disturbance related to change in appearance from deformities and inability to move freely

Planning: Patient Outcomes
1. Patient relates feelings of self-worth.
2. Patient demonstrates increased confidence in ability to deal with illness.
3. Patient is able to look at self with acceptance.

NDx: Ineffective individual coping related to chronic effects of the disorder on the life of the patient and family

Planning: Patient Outcomes
1. Patient demonstrates positive coping measures in dealing with the effects of the disorder.
2. Patient uses available resources in coping with effects of the disorder.
3. Patient uses problem-solving techniques and skills in dealing with the disorder.

NDx: Self care deficit: bathing, dressing, or grooming related to decrease in strength and deformities of joints with restricted movement

Planning: Patient Outcomes
1. Patient cares for self with little assistance from others.
2. Patient uses assistive devices to provide support for self-care.
3. Patient practices exercises to maintain joint mobility to allow continued independence.

NDx: Risk for injury: falls related to mobility problems secondary to joint deformity and pain, and improper use of ambulatory aids

Planning: Patient Outcomes

1. Patient remains free from injury.
2. Patient demonstrates safe use of ambulatory aid device.
3. Patient states accurate information about the causes of injuries and methods to prevent injury.

NDx: Knowledge deficit: nature of disorder, its progression, and self-care interventions

Planning: Patient Outcomes

1. Patient relates accurate information about the disorder.
2. Patient repeats instructions as issued by the physician for home care.
3. Patient has list of referral services and support networks available.

Nursing Interventions and Evaluation

NDx: Pain

Help the patient deal with the chronic pain by using alternatives to pain medication, such as relaxation exercises, deep-breathing techniques, imagery, and distraction. Pain may be exacerbated by anxiety and depression. Group education and counseling may help the patient cope with the pain of the disorder.

When pain is acute, give prescribed analgesics and anti-inflammatory agents. Explain the dosage, frequency, side effects, and expected therapeutic effects of the medications. Caution the patient not to perform tasks that require mental alertness while taking pain medication. Handle the patient carefully when moving him or her in the bed. Caution the patient about weight-bearing on affected joints without assistance when the disease is in a stage of exacerbation, because weight-bearing might cause the pain to increase significantly. Maintain rest and support of affected inflamed joints.

Apply prescribed heat or cold to decrease muscle spasms and promote pain relief. Advise the patient that a warm bath or shower may be helpful in relieving morning pain and stiffness. During acute inflammation, prolonged or deep heat should be avoided. Cold is used to reduce the effects of inflammation and also relieve pain. Range of motion or activity after heat application may reduce stiffness and pain.

Teach the use of the TENS unit in managing pain. The use of splints may reduce swelling and help control pain.

NDx: Impaired physical mobility

An exercise program promotes and maintains skeletal and joint function. The nurse, physician, and physical therapist should collaborate regarding the type of exercise program for the patient with rheumatoid arthritis. An individualized exercise program may be developed to improve flexibility and strength. The amount of rest and activity varies with the patient's disease and limitations. Regularly scheduled rest periods are alternated with activity throughout the day. Total bedrest and immobility are avoided, to prevent joint stiffness and immobility complications. Localized rest for the involved joint may be more effective than complete bedrest.

Teach the patient who is on bedrest to increase movement in the bed by using the overhead trapeze, as allowed, to prevent complications of immobility. Reposition the patient frequently to stimulate circulation and prevent skin breakdown. Gentle range-of-motion exercises may help the patient maintain mobility.

Application of moist heat to affected joints may relieve stiffness. For example, a morning shower or tub bath may increase mobility by decreasing stiffness.

Authorities differ on the use of active or passive range of motion during acute swelling of arthritis. Gentle range-of-motion exercises are usually completed daily to maintain functional joints.

An important part of the exercise program for the patient with rheumatoid arthritis includes protection of the joints from stress. Excessive joint exercise can increase inflammation and pain. Therefore, any exercise must be balanced with rest to avoid fatigue. Assist the patient in reducing joint use during acute inflammation. The patient's pain and fatigue must be monitored closely during exercise. The exercise may be excessive if joint pain persists for a period of time after the patient has completed the exercise.

Positioning, range-of-motion, and stretching exercises may prevent the complication of contractures. Teach the patient and family the safe use of exercise and ambulatory aids. Administer analgesics as needed to decrease pain levels that may interfere with the patient's mobility. Instruct the patient and family in a diet to avoid obesity, which would place extra stress on joints.

NDx: Self esteem disturbance

Spend time with the patient to provide an opportunity for venting feelings about the disorder. Teach the patient and family skills to enhance their communication about loss, role changes, and needs associated with arthritis. Provide information about self-help groups. When appropriate, seek assistance from clergy or professional counseling. Provide the patient with diversional activities when activity is decreased during disease exacerbations. Involve support from family and friends. Seek effective coping strategies for the patient. Assist the patient in finding the positive aspects of life to focus on during periods of depression. Provide anticipatory guidance to prepare for arthritis treatments and interventions. Assist the patient in the organization of daily tasks and the home environment to promote the accomplishment of goals.

NDx: Ineffective individual coping
Provide the patient with a list of resources and support systems. Do not offer false reassurance but help the client set realistic goals. Support the family in adjusting to the strain and changes within the family brought about by the disorder. Allow the family to express feelings about the impact of the illness on the family. Use problem-solving techniques to cope with the stresses associated with the chronic nature of arthritis. Spend time with the patient to allow him or her to vent feelings of loss, anger, powerlessness, uncertainty, and dependency. Involve the patient and family in the planning process. Support and reinforce actions of independence, control, and acceptance of losses.

NDx: Self care deficit: bathing, dressing, or grooming
Provide assistance for the patient during bathing and grooming. Grooming aids may be used to help with shaving, hair combing, and oral care. Adaptive aids are also available to assist in holding and carrying objects. Elevated seats on the toilet may be helpful in promoting self-care with independence. Explain to the family that clothing with Velcro attachments may be easier for the patient to use. Tell the patient to avoid pain and fatigue by frequently resting while performing self-care activities.

NDx: Risk for injury
If the physical therapist recommends an ambulatory aid, help the patient learn how to use it properly. Provide assistance during ambulation until the patient becomes adept at using the device. Be sure the patient wears well-fitting shoes with gripper soles while ambulating. Teach the patient's family about safe use of the ambulatory aid and explain how to make the home environment safer for the patient while he or she is using it.

NDx: Knowledge deficit: nature of the disorder, its progression, and self-care interventions
Provide information to the patient and family about the disease, its progression, the planned treatment, and self-care interventions. Encourage the patient to ask questions and to express fears and concerns. Answer questions honestly while reinforcing the positive aspects of the patient's life. Encourage and reinforce instructions in the use of medications, splints or braces, and ambulatory aids. Discuss modification of the home environment to help the patient maintain independence.

Teach the patient about good nutrition to maintain health status. Encourage a diet high in protein, vitamins, and minerals, with increased fiber to prevent constipation during periods of inactivity.

Initiate social service referrals to help the patient use available resources and obtain financial assistance. Social service resources may help the patient maintain role performance and independence. Inform the patient of the local and national arthritis support groups. The Arthritis Foundation is a voluntary national organization that provides a number of services, including research support, training of specialists, and public and patient information services. The local address is usually found in the yellow pages of the telephone directory. For information on the national organization and the National Arthritis/Musculoskeletal and Skin Diseases Information Clearinghouse, see the appendix.

Compare the patient's status with the expected outcomes. If the outcomes are not met, reassess the patient and revise the plan.

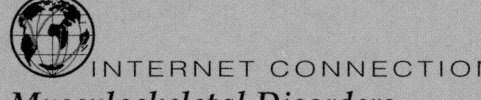

INTERNET CONNECTIONS
Musculoskeletal Disorders

Arthritis
American College of Rheumatology
http://www.rheumatology.org
An authoritative site geared toward physicians and other health-care professionals. This site includes frequently asked questions and other patient-oriented topics as well as the opportunity to perform literature searches of all issues of *Arthritis & Rheumatism* since 1959.

Arthritis Foundation
http://www.arthritis.org
A comprehensive, authoritative resource for arthritis information for health-care professionals, patients, and families.

Osteoporosis
Doctor's Guide to Osteoporosis Information and Resources
http://www.pslgroup.com/OSTEOPOROSIS.HTM
A resource providing extensive information related to osteoporosis for health-care professionals and patients, including a file of frequently asked questions and links to relevant sites.

National Osteoporosis Foundation
http://www.nof.org/
An authoritative resource geared to both health-care professionals and patients, including general information, risk factors, prevention tips, treatment suggestions, medical news, and clinical guidelines.

Bone Cancer
ONCOLINK/Bone Cancer
http://oncolink.upenn.edu/disease/bone1/
This authoritative site provides both professional and patient-oriented information, as well as links to other helpful resources, including the National Cancer Institute. Particular areas of focus include Ewing's sarcoma and osteosarcoma.

Osteoarthritis

Osteoarthritis (also called degenerative joint disease) is the most common form of arthritis. It is a slow, progressive, noninflammatory, destructive, nonsystemic disorder confined to the joint. Osteoarthritis causes degenerative changes in the joint surfaces of weight-bearing joints, such as the spine, hips, knees, and in the frequently used joints of the hands. A person can have both rheumatoid arthritis and osteoarthritis. The prognosis for osteoarthritis is much more positive than that of rheumatoid arthritis because treatment can slow joint destruction, and not all joints are involved.

Etiology and Pathophysiology

There are two types of osteoarthritis: primary and secondary. Primary osteoarthritis is attributed to a genetic predisposition to deterioration of articular cartilage. Primary osteoarthritis is more prevalent in women, and onset may occur as young as 40 years of age. Theories suggest that the predisposition is the result of either an abnormal chemical structure of the articular cartilage or the presence of joints that do not fit together properly and thus develop early wear.

Secondary osteoarthritis, the result of excessive "wear and tear" or trauma of affected joints, is more common after the age of 50. Obesity with continuous excessive stress on joints from excess weight and repeated joint injuries from athletic or work activities are factors identified as predispositions to secondary osteoarthritis. The accumulated effects of daily stress and wear can also result in secondary arthritis as age advances. X-ray films of most persons older than age 65 reveal some joint deterioration.

In both forms of osteoarthritis, as the articular cartilage deteriorates, the surface becomes rough, and malacia (soft spots) develop. As the softened cartilage is worn away, the joint space narrows and bone surfaces begin to rub against each other. New subchondral bone forms to heal the damaged joint surfaces. As new bone repeatedly forms and is rubbed off, bone spurs, bone cysts, and extended joint margins called osteophytes develop. These abnormal bone growths create joint deformity and pain on motion. Fusion of the joint does not occur.

Clinical Manifestations

Osteoarthritis is characterized by the presence of a dull aching pain in the affected joints. Unlike with rheumatoid arthritis, systemic manifestations are absent and joint involvement is not symmetric. Crepitus, or a grating sound, may be heard and felt on joint movement. Enlargement of the joint and limitation of motion progress over time. The involved fingers often develop painless bony nodules on the dorsolateral surface of the interphalangeal joints. Nodules on the distal interphalangeal joints are called Heberden's nodes. Those on the proximal interphalangeal joints are called Bouchard's nodes.

Stiffness and joint pain increase as joint deterioration progresses. Stiffness also increases with lack of activity. It is usually more severe early in the morning and may be aggravated by cold damp weather or a falling barometric pressure. The presence of constant pain and stiff joints leads to fatigue and loss of coordination.

Diagnosis

X-rays may show lessening of joint space and extension of joint margin. However, radiologically apparent changes are not always consistent with the degree of pain and limitation of motion a patient is experiencing.

No specific laboratory findings are useful in diagnosing osteoarthritis. The patient may have a normal or slightly elevated sedimentation rate.

Management

The management of osteoarthritis is planned to meet the individual patient's needs as determined by the patient's lifestyle and general health. Enteric-coated aspirin or nonsteroidal anti-inflammatory agents are prescribed to relieve pain (see Highlight 20–1). These agents are usually prescribed on a regular basis and in larger than usual doses. These pharmacologic agents reduce pain, swelling, and stiffness. Parenteral steroids are injected into an acutely inflamed joint. If the patient is overweight, a weight reduction diet may be recommended.

Exercises to preserve joint strength and range of motion, as well as heat or cold applications to relieve pain and relax muscles, are implemented as needed. Joint protection to prevent further joint damage may include avoidance of strenuous activities that create excessive stress on affected joints and the use of assistive devices such as canes, walkers, and crutches to reduce weight-bearing.

A TENS unit may be prescribed to reduce joint pain. Orthotic devices and splints may also be utilized to provide benefit to patients with osteoarthritis.

In situations in which extensive damage of involved joints is present, arthroplasty or total joint replacement may be done to decrease pain and improve function.

❖ Settings, Providers, and Collaboration for Care

Patient and family education related to osteoarthritis is an important nursing intervention in the home and other health care settings. The nurse teaches the patient and family about osteoarthritis and management of the disorder. The nurse also assists the patient and family in implementing strategies for chronic disease management. The nurse and therapists explain safety measures in the home and work environment to the patient. The use of assistive devices may also be implemented to promote safety. Physical therapists may use splints to stabilize painful joints.

NURSING PROCESS GUIDELINES
Osteoarthritis

The assessment, nursing diagnoses, expected patient outcomes, nursing interventions, and evaluation for patients with osteoarthritis are similar to those described previously for patients with rheumatoid arthritis. In addition, discharge instructions for patients with osteoarthritis are discussed in Highlight 20–2.

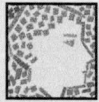

HIGHLIGHT
20–2
PATIENT EDUCATION

Discharge Instructions for Patients with Osteoarthritis

Instruct the patient to:

Take prescribed analgesics and/or anti-inflammatory agents as scheduled and before activities that may precipitate episodes of pain.

Maintain the affected joints in a non-flexed, well-aligned position to prevent flexion contractures.

Apply heat or cold packs, as preferred, to decrease muscle spasms and promote pain relief.

Take a warm bath or shower to help relieve morning stiffness.

Perform relaxation techniques, as demonstrated, to help reduce muscle spasms and relieve pain.

Follow prescribed exercise program to maintain range of motion of involved joints.

Refrain from exercising joints beyond the point of pain or fatigue because further injury can occur.

Follow dietary recommendations for weight loss (if overweight) to decrease stress on weight-bearing joints.

Use ambulatory aids or assistive devices, as prescribed, to decrease stress on joints.

Follow safety instructions while using the ambulatory aids.

Avoid activities that increase stress on involved joints or that may cause additional trauma to the joints.

Maintain good posture and proper body mechanics to reduce stress on joints.

Avoid forceful repetitive movements that may precipitate pain and injury.

Maintain safety in the home by prevention strategies such as removing scatter rugs, providing hand rails, and installing proper lighting.

Ankylosing Spondylitis

Also called Marie-Strümpell disease, ankylosing spondylitis is chronic, progressive, inflammatory arthritis of the spine and sacroiliac joint. It is characterized by spondylosis and fusion of the vertebrae. It is actually a distinct type of systemic arthritis.

Etiology and Pathophysiology

Ankylosing spondylitis has a strong familial tendency, but the exact cause is unknown. It occurs more frequently in families with a history of the disorder and is usually diagnosed in early adulthood. This disorder is more common in males. There is a lower incidence in the nonwhite population in the United States.

Ankylosing spondylitis begins in the sacroiliac joints and spreads up the spine. As it spreads, succeeding joints become inflamed and fibrotic. As the costovertebral joints and disk spaces deteriorate, they are replaced by bony growth. The spine becomes rigid and ankylosed. Thoracic kyphosis develops, with compensating hip flexure, and the ribs, shoulder, neck, and temporomandibular joint become involved. Ocular and cardiac involvement can also occur.

Clinical Manifestations

The disease follows an insidious pattern of exacerbations and remissions. Some patients have experienced complete spontaneous remission. The patient usually has a long history of low back pain that is worse at night and upon rising in the morning. The pain radiates from the buttocks to the thigh. Although the pain pattern resembles that of sciatica, it does not extend below the knee as sciatic pain does. Pain during rest or sleep may cause fatigue in the patient. Involvement is asymmetric and slow in onset. The patient may also experience fever, malaise, stiffness, and back muscle spasms. Physical examination may reveal a decrease in chest expansion caused by costovertebral involvement.

Untreated patients can develop a rigid kyphosis that results in the complication of thoracic organ compression. Patients who develop iritis or other ocular complications are referred to an ophthalmologist. Cardiac dysrhythmias, valve disease, and pulmonary fibrosis may also occur.

Diagnosis

A genetic marker, the human leukocyte-associated antigen with a *B27* gene (HLA-B27), is present in 90% of the patients with ankylosing spondylitis. Rheumatoid factor and rheumatoid nodules are absent. The erythrocyte sedimentation rate and levels of alkaline phosphatase and creatine phosphokinase are usually elevated.

X-ray films show fusion of intervertebral bodies with possible calcification on the anterior and posterior longitudinal ligaments of the spinal column. This appearance of the spinal column is referred to as "bamboo spine."

Management

Medical management focuses on providing relief from pain, decreasing the inflammatory process, and preventing and correcting deformity. Pain and inflammation are treated with heat applications and nonsteroidal anti-inflammatory agents. Indomethacin and phenylbutazone have been particularly successful in relieving the symptoms of ankylosing spondylitis. Steroids are sometimes successful in inducing remission.

Rest may be prescribed for acute episodes of inflammation. Spinal extensor strengthening exercises to promote back extension and breathing exercises to maintain chest expansion are recommended. Physical therapy related to spinal mobility and physical fitness may prove effective in dealing with spondylitis. Instruct the patient to maintain an erect posture when sitting or standing to prevent flexion contractures. Wearing special orthotic back braces, sleeping in the prone position on a firm mattress without a pillow, and sitting in chairs with a high back and firm support help prevent further deformity. Surgical intervention to correct flexion deformities or total hip replacement of ankylosed hip joints may be indicated.

NURSING PROCESS GUIDELINES
Ankylosing Spondylitis

The assessment, nursing diagnoses, expected patient outcomes, nursing interventions, and evaluation for patients with ankylosing spondylitis are similar to those described previously for patients with rheumatoid arthritis.

GOUT

Etiology and Pathophysiology

Gout is a painful metabolic bone disorder in which an inflammatory joint reaction is caused by accumulation of uric acid crystals in the involved joint and soft tissues. These chalky nodular deposits are known as tophi (Fig. 20–2). The base of the large toe (the first metatarsal phalangeal joint) is primarily affected, but the insteps, ankles, knees, elbows, and hands may also be affected.

Gout is caused by a buildup of uric acid in the blood, which leads to urate crystal deposits in the joints. Primary gout results from a genetic error in purine metabolism, which leads to overproduction or retention of uric acid. Although purines are present in high concentrations in protein and alcohol, high dietary intake of these substances alone does not cause hyperuricemia. However, their ingestion may precipitate an acute episode of gout in a person who already has the disorder.

More than 90% of the individuals who have primary gout are men older than age 30. Few women suffer from primary gout. Those who do are usually

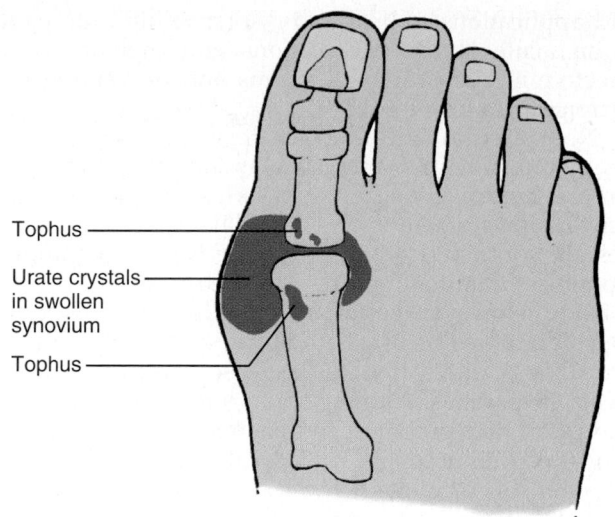

Figure 20–2
Gouty joint.

postmenopausal or older than age 50. Prolonged fasting or excessive alcohol intake increases uric acid in the blood by decreasing excretion through the kidney and can cause secondary gout. Hypertension, obesity, and lead exposure are also factors that increase the risk of gout.

Clinical Manifestations

Initial episodes of acute gout usually involve one joint. The joint becomes red, warm, shiny, swollen, and extremely sensitive to the slightest touch. The patient may have an elevated temperature of 38° to 39.5°C (100–103°F). Blood pressure is sometimes elevated, possibly because of the pain response. Tophi may be present around the fingers or ear lobes in individuals with chronic severe hyperuricemia. Episodes of acute inflammation usually last less than 10 days. Repeated inflammation may result in joint deformity. Patients are forced by extreme pain to rest the joint and most seek medical attention early in an acute episode.

Diagnosis

Diagnosis of gout is made on the basis of the clinical manifestations, hyperuricemia, and the presence of uric acid crystals in the synovial fluid of the inflamed joint. Blood studies show an increased serum uric acid level of more than 7 mg/100 mL. The erythrocyte sedimentation rate and white blood cell count may be elevated during an acute episode. Twenty-four-hour urine uric acid levels are elevated. X-ray films may show urate deposits in the joints or tophi.

Management

The goals of medical management are to relieve pain and inflammation, prevent permanent joint damage, and eliminate further acute episodes. Rest and applications of heat and cold may alleviate pain in an acute attack. Medications and diet are very effective in alleviating symptoms and preventing recurrent episodes of gout.

Nonsteroidal anti-inflammatory agents such as phenylbutazone indomethacin (Indocin), and ibuprofen are used to treat acute episodes. Glucocorticoids may be prescribed if nonsteroidal anti-inflammatories are contraindicated. Colchicine is effective in decreasing inflammation if given early in the acute episode. However, serious toxic side effects warrant consideration. The uricosuric drug allopurinol (Zyloprim), is administered to decrease serum uric acid levels in patients with chronic gout. Sulfinpyrazone (Anturan) and probenecid (Benemid), also uricosuric drugs, can be used prophylactically to prevent reabsorption of uric acid by the kidneys (Highlight 20–3). Aspirin inactivates uricosurics and therefore should be avoided by persons with a history of gout. Weight reduction is recommended for overweight individuals.

NURSING PROCESS
Gout
Assessment

Review the patient's history and presenting symptoms. Examine the affected joint for the classic manifestations of an acute episode of gout. Determine the extent of pain and interference with mobility. Question the patient about precipitating events such as trauma, changes in diet, or the use of medications that inhibit the excretion of uric acid.

Nursing Diagnoses and Planning

Nursing diagnoses and related expected patient outcomes most commonly applicable to patients with gout include the following:

NDx: Pain related to joint inflammation

Planning: Patient Outcomes
1. Patient denies acute pain in affected joint.

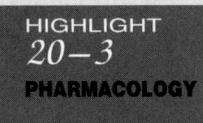 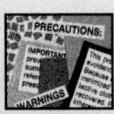

HIGHLIGHT 20–3 PHARMACOLOGY

Uricosuric Drugs

Definition:

A class of drugs effective for controlling serum urate levels.

Generic and Trade Names:

Colchicine, probenecid (Benemid), sulfinpyrazone (Anturane), allopurinol (Zyloprim)

Action:

The agents increase urinary excretion of uric acid by preventing the reabsorption of uric acid in the renal tubules.

Uses:

The drugs are used to control hyperuricemia to prevent attacks of gout.

Side Effects:

Headache, dizziness, hypotension, anorexia, nausea, gastric distress, urinary frequency, renal colic, fever, and flushing.

Interactions:

The drugs may interact with salicylates. Some of the drugs can also enhance the effects of hypoglycemic agents and warfarin and decrease indomethacin excretion.

Nursing Implications:

Tell the patient to avoid alcohol because it increases the urate level.

Inform the patient to avoid all medications that contain aspirin.

Encourage increased fluid intake to maintain an adequate urine output. This helps prevent hematuria, renal colic, and stone development.

Administer the drug with milk or meals to prevent gastric distress.

Teach the patient to limit high purine foods as listed in Highlight 20–4.

Explain the importance of adherence to the medication regimen.

Encourage weight loss to avoid additional joint stress.

Geriatric Considerations:

Increased gastric irritation may be present as a result of decreased gastrointestinal motility in the older adult. Give the drug with food and fluids.

2. Patient is able to tolerate some discomfort without decreasing mobility.

NDx: Ineffective management of therapeutic regimen (individuals) related to lack of knowledge about the disease, its cause, prognosis, and information regarding medications and diet therapy

Planning: Patient Outcomes
1. Patient relates accurate information about the disease, its cause, and prognosis.
2. Patient states correct information about the drug and diet therapy.
3. Patient chooses food low in purine as listed in Highlight 20–4.

Nursing Interventions and Evaluation

NDx: Pain

Focus on supportive care for the affected joint and effective pain management. Teach the patient about the therapeutic effects, side effects, and interactions of prescribed pain medications (see Highlight 20–3). Administer prescribed analgesics and anti-inflammatory agents. Instruct the patient to avoid using the affected joint until the acute episode subsides.

NDx: Ineffective management of therapeutic regimen (individuals)

Inform the patient about the disorder, its clinical manifestations, and treatment regimens. Allow the patient to ask questions and voice concerns. Instruct the patient about prescribed diet therapy to reduce weight and reduce amount of ingested purines (see Highlight 20–4). Teach the patient about the drug therapy to continue at home. Explain the side effects of the agents and inform the patient to notify the physician of untoward effects.

Compare the patient's status with the expected outcomes. If the outcomes are not met, reassess the patient and revise the plan.

LYME DISEASE

Etiology and Pathophysiology

Lyme disease is a chronic inflammatory disease that is transmitted by the bite of a tick. The causative agent is the tickborne spirochetal bacterium *Borrelia burgdorferi.* The disease was first identified in the 1970s, although similar disorders were recognized in Europe in the early 1900s. The ticks primarily responsible for transmission are the bear and deer tick *Ixodes dammini.* However, other ticks of the same family may also transmit the disease.

Lyme disease is most prevalent during seasons of warm weather, when ticks are most numerous. It was named after Lyme, Connecticut, where the first epidemic occurred. The incidence has been reported in 40 states but is more common in the northeast, northern midwest, and far west regions of the United States.

Clinical Manifestations

The disease usually progresses in three stages. Clinical manifestations include the development of a macule at the site of the tick bite within 20 to 30 days. The macule then forms a larger lesion. This fades over a period of weeks, and the individual may not realize it was present. Some patients have several lesions or a rash, which may be primary or secondary. The primary lesions are usually asymptomatic. The secondary lesions often present symptoms of pruritus, malaise, headache, fever, and chills. Nausea, vomiting, and sore throat may also accompany the influenza-like symptoms.

The second stage of the disease occurs as the organism spreads through the body. Cardiac and neurologic manifestations occur at this time. The problems range from cardiac dysrhythmias to complete heart block. Neurologic complications include meningitis, encephalitis, and neuritis. The seventh cranial nerve is most frequently involved. Other nerves are also commonly involved, so the symptoms may vary from some weakness to pain and dysesthesia.

In the third stage, neurologic complications persist but the major manifestation is musculoskeletal involvement, typically arthritis. This begins approximately 4 weeks after the skin lesions appear. The joints, especially the knees, become swollen, warm, and painful. Destruction of the joint may occur from erosion of cartilage and bone.

HIGHLIGHT
20–4
NUTRITION

High-Purine and Low-Purine Foods

High Purine Content	Low Purine Content
Anchovies	Bread (white)
Bouillon	Butter
Broth	Cookies
Gravies	Cereals
Heart	Custard
Kidney	Eggs
Liver	Fruits
Mincemeat	Ice cream
Mussels	Most vegetables (except
Sardines	peas, spinach, aspara-
Scallops	gus, and beans)
Sweetbreads	Milk
Yeast (brewer's	Nuts
and baker's)	Oils
	Popcorn
	Pudding
	Rice

Diagnosis

The diagnosis is made by assessment, history, and serologic testing. Immunoglobulin antibodies can be detected after approximately 6 weeks. The patient has an elevated erythrocyte sedimentation rate, but this is not specific to the disease. Skin biopsies may isolate the spirochete. A detailed history, with an analysis of the presenting symptoms and the exclusion of other disorders, is the most common diagnostic tools.

Management

Lyme disease is treated by a variety of regimens, depending on the extent and severity of symptoms and the stage of the disease. However, exacerbations of the disease are common. Oral antibiotics are used early in the disease process. Cardiac rhythm problems are treated with medications specified for the conduction disorder. Patients are hospitalized and monitored until stable. Steroids may be prescribed, especially if the patient has severe cardiac involvement. The musculoskeletal problems are treated symptomatically. Intravenous antibiotics are used in later stages of the disease. Ceftriaxone therapy is beneficial in treating Lyme arthritis.

Prognosis is good for patients treated in the early stages. Patient and family education about prevention is an important health issue in areas where the disease is prevalent (Highlight 20–5).

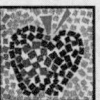

HIGHLIGHT
20–5

HEALTH PROMOTION & RISK REDUCTION

Preventing Lyme Disease

Instruct individuals in endemic areas to take the following precautions:

Avoid areas of dense foliage and high grasses.

Wear clothing that covers the extremities completely.

Tuck pants legs into socks or boots.

Inspect the skin and clothing for ticks after being outside.

Inspect pets frequently for ticks.

Remove any ticks found on the individual or pets immediately. Be sure to remove the entire tick and dispose of it.

Use repellants such as diethyltoluamide (DEET) or permethrin, which are effective against the ticks and safe to use on the skin. Be sure to reapply after bathing or swimming.

BURSITIS

Bursitis is inflammation of bursae, such as those located between muscles or tendons and bones. It most commonly occurs in the elbow (tennis elbow), the knee (housemaid's knee), or the shoulder. Bursitis is diagnosed by assessment, history, and x-ray examination to eliminate musculoskeletal conditions. It is treated by rest, immobilization, heat therapy, and medication. Oral medications used include aspirin or nonaspirin analgesics and nonsteroidal anti-inflammatory agents. The affected joint may also be injected with cortisone or a local anesthetic agent to relieve symptoms and pain.

TENOSYNOVITIS

Tenosynovitis is the inflammation of a tendon or its sheath. It is a common cause of acute shoulder pain. Calcific tendinitis, a form in which calcium deposits occur in the tendon, causes pain when the arm is abducted 50 to 130 degrees. Treatment of tenosynovitis is directed at decreasing the pain and inflammation. Immobility may be used to relieve the pain.

*S*tructural Disorders

Musculoskeletal structural disorders include metabolic conditions in which bone structure is altered, causing pain, deformity, or fracture. The cause of the disorder may be unknown or may result from diet or a combination of factors. In any case, potential for injury is significant, and safety becomes an important factor in the care and education of the patient while in the hospital and in the home or rehabilitation, long-term-care, or intermediate-care facility.

OSTEOMALACIA

Etiology and Pathophysiology

Osteomalacia is a metabolic bone disorder characterized by a decrease in calcium and phosphorus deposits in new bone matrix. This results in structurally weak bone mass. Osteomalacia is a condition of adults. In children, whose epiphyseal plates have not closed, the same disorder is known as rickets. The condition in children results in deformed bones, characterized by bowing, and a decrease in skeletal height. Osteomalacia is caused by lack of vitamin D, which is essential for the mineralization of bones.

A number of factors can cause a decrease in vitamin D and result in osteomalacia. A lack of dietary intake of vitamin D is one cause, but this is extremely rare in the United States. Most cases in this country are the result of malabsorption of vitamin D secondary to hepatobiliary disease. A lack of sunlight, chronic pancreatitis, and nontropical sprue are conditions that can lead to osteomalacia.

Clinical Manifestations

The patient with osteomalacia presents with complaints of weakness and vague aches and pains. The bones may be tender to palpation. Vertebral collapse results in kyphosis. The curvature or bowing of the long bones frequently seen in children with rickets may also be found in prolonged cases in adults.

Diagnosis

Diagnosis is made on the basis of x-ray films, which show diffuse erosion of the subperiosteal bone. There may be areas resembling fractures that appear as zig-zagging bands of decalcification with callus formation on each side of the bone. These false fractures are known as Looser's zones and occur in areas where fractures are not commonly seen. Serum calcium and phosphorus levels are low, and the alkaline phosphatase level is elevated.

Management

Medical management focuses on treating the underlying cause of the disorder. Supplements of vitamin D, calcium (Highlight 20–6), and phosphorus may be prescribed. The disorder responds dramatically to administration of vitamin D. Exercises are helpful in stimulating bone reformation. The patient is counseled to consume a diet of foods high in vitamin D, calcium, and phosphorus and to follow a prescribed program of progressive exercises and weight-bearing to promote recalcification of the bones.

NURSING PROCESS
Osteomalacia

Assessment

Review the patient's history and presenting symptoms. Complete a physical assessment, noting deformities and areas of weakness. Ask the patient about pain and its onset, intensity, and duration. Look for abnormal curvature of the spine and bowing of the long bones. Assess the patient's nutritional pattern. Determine the intake of vitamin D, calcium, and phosphorus. Ask whether the patient takes supplemental minerals and vitamins. Determine the patient's understanding of the disorder and the treatment program.

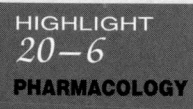 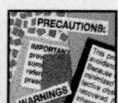

HIGHLIGHT
20–6
PHARMACOLOGY

Oral Calcium Supplements

Definition:

This group of drugs includes a variety of prescription and nonprescription calcium products such as calcium carbonate, calcium lactate, calcium gluconate, calcium phosphate, Alka-Mints, Chooz, Tums, Rolaids, Calcium Rich, Cal-600, and others.

Action:

Calcium supplements are indicated for prevention of hypocalcemia, osteomalacia, and osteoporosis, and for other disorders of the bone caused by lack of calcium.

Side Effects:

Side effects include constipation, gastric irritation, chalky taste, nausea, and gastric bleeding.

Interactions:

The supplements may interact with oxalic acid, phytic acid, and phosphorus, causing decreased absorption of the calcium.

Nursing Implications:

Most supplements should be taken on an empty stomach to promote absorption. If gastric irritation develops, food may be necessary.

Tell the patient to refrain from taking the supplements with rhubarb, spinach, bran, or whole-grain cereals. These foods may decrease the absorption of the calcium.

Calcium carbonate should not be given with milk.

Tell the patient to take only the dosage prescribed because overdosing could precipitate formation of calcium stones.

Teach patients that calcium reduces the absorption of tetracycline. Calcium and tetracycline administration should be separated by at least 1 hour.

Teach patient taking calcium supplements to drink water, which will prevent renal stones.

Nursing Diagnoses and Planning

Nursing diagnoses and related expected patient outcomes most commonly applicable to patients with osteomalacia include the following:

NDx: Pain related to structural changes in bones and deformities in limbs

Planning: Patient Outcomes
1. Patient denies discomfort or extreme pain in limbs.
2. Patient relates accurate information about analgesics prescribed.

NDx: Knowledge deficit: nature of the disorder, its treatment, and prevention

Planning: Patient Outcomes
1. Patient states accurate information about the disorder, its prognosis, and treatment measures.
2. Patient demonstrates exercises that promote increased bone growth and performs them as prescribed.
3. Patient states accurate information about the appropriate diet and medication therapy.

Nursing Interventions and Evaluation

NDx: Pain

Administer prescribed analgesics and teach the patient about their frequency, dose, side effects, and therapeutic effects. Talk with the patient about relaxation strategies to reduce pain. Tell the patient to refrain from weight-bearing during painful episodes. Pad bony prominences when the patient is in bed. Assist with ambulation to reduce weight-bearing.

NDx: Knowledge deficit: nature of the disorder, its treatment, and prevention

Teach the patient about the cause and symptoms of the disease and treatment regimens to be undertaken. Tell the patient about the proper use of prescribed medications. Be sure the patient understands the need to take the supplements continually to help reverse the effects of the disorder and to prevent further damage (see Highlight 20–6). Demonstrate the prescribed exercises and encourage the patient to practice them frequently because they promote increased bone recalcification and formation.

Review a diet plan with the patient that contains food high in vitamins, calcium (Highlight 20–7), and phosphorus. Teach the patient how to read labels for food content. Note which food the patient chooses from the daily hospital menu and reinforce good choices.

Compare the patient's status with the expected outcomes. If the outcomes are not met, reassess the patient and revise the plan.

OSTEOPOROSIS

Etiology and Pathophysiology

Osteoporosis is a metabolic bone disorder characterized by thinning, less dense, or porous bone mass.

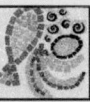

HIGHLIGHT 20–7
NUTRITION

Calcium Content of Some Common Foods

Food	Calcium (mg)
Dairy Products:	
1 cup whole milk	291
½ cup canned evaporated milk	318
⅓ cup dry nonfat milk	293
1 cup skimmed milk	302
1 cup yogurt, low-fat	294
1 cup custard	297
1 oz Swiss cheese	272
1 oz cheddar cheese	130
1 oz American cheese	174
½ cup ice cream	88
8 oz cream cheese	141
1 cup cottage cheese	212
Vegetables:	
1 cup beet greens	144
½ cup collard greens	179
½ cup turnip greens	134
½ cup spinach	100
½ cup rhubarb	106
1 cup asparagus	30
1 cup cooked cabbage	64
1 cup chopped broccoli	136
Meats, Beans, Nuts:	
1 cup almonds	304
1 cup soybeans, cooked	131
1 cup navy beans, cooked	95
3 oz sardines	371
3 oz salmon	165

The chemical composition of the bone tissue remains the same, but there is less bone matter present within the bone, resulting in fragile bones that are susceptible to fractures.

Bone production is a dynamic process of constant bone formation and bone resorption. Individuals achieve peak bone mass by approximately 30 years of age. After this time, there is normally a gradual decline in bone mass. It is not known whether the decreased bone mass is due to less new bone being produced, an increase in bone breakdown, or both.

Normal bone loss with aging is referred to as osteopenia. More severe bone loss that is age-related is called primary or senile osteoporosis. Osteoporosis affects more than 25 million people in the United States. Many individuals with osteoporosis develop spontaneous pathologic fractures or experience fractures associated with minimal trauma. Factors placing individuals at risk of developing osteoporosis include increasing age in white females, low dietary intake of calcium, diminished physical activity, and estrogen depletion (surgical or biologic menopause). Additional factors to be considered are a positive family history of osteoporosis, alcoholism, cigarette smoking, and an excessive protein intake.

Secondary osteoporosis is loss of bone caused by drugs or disease. Medications that can cause osteoporosis include tetracyclines, corticosteroids, aluminum-containing antacids, and some anticonvulsants, diuretics, and thyroid medications. Diseases involving catabolic hormone excess, such as hyperthyroidism and Cushing's disease, can also produce osteoporosis.

Evidence supports the theory that a person may have a genetic predisposition to osteoporosis. In the United States, whites and Asians are affected more often than blacks. Differences in peak bone masses among various races or people may account for the differing incidence. A northern European background also increases the incidence of osteoporosis. A decreased incidence in males may be explained by the fact that they have more bone mass to begin with and do not normally experience a sudden loss of hormones. Petite, thin women or small framed men who do not exercise are at greater risk because they have less bone to lose than those with a larger frame and more body weight. Osteoporosis occurs in about one-fourth of the elderly population.

Idiopathic postmenopausal osteoporosis is the term used to describe the bone loss in women that can be directly related to a decrease in exercise and a decrease in estrogen level. Bones most affected by idiopathic postmenopausal osteoporosis are the femoral neck, wrists, vertebrae, and humeral neck.

Clinical Manifestations

Clinical manifestations of osteoporosis are localized low-back or mid-thoracic pain from vertebral involvement and collapse. The pain increases on sitting and standing. Pain may also be found in other affected parts of the body but seems to be more common in the low back. The patient may develop kyphosis, referred to as dowager's hump, and lumbar lordosis. With collapse of vertebrae, there is also a decrease in height (Fig. 20–3). Involvement of the jaw can result in a loss of teeth. Pathologic fracture of the femoral neck, wrist, or humeral neck is common.

Diagnosis

Early diagnosis of osteoporosis has been difficult in the past because patients are asymptomatic until significant bone loss has occurred. X-ray films show bone loss only after 30% loss has occurred. X-ray films of the hand, wrist bones, and radius at this time reveal diffusely reduced bone density with cortical thinning.

Bone densitometry is a noninvasive diagnostic test with minimal radiation exposure, which can detect bone loss of less than 3%. Some physicians rec-

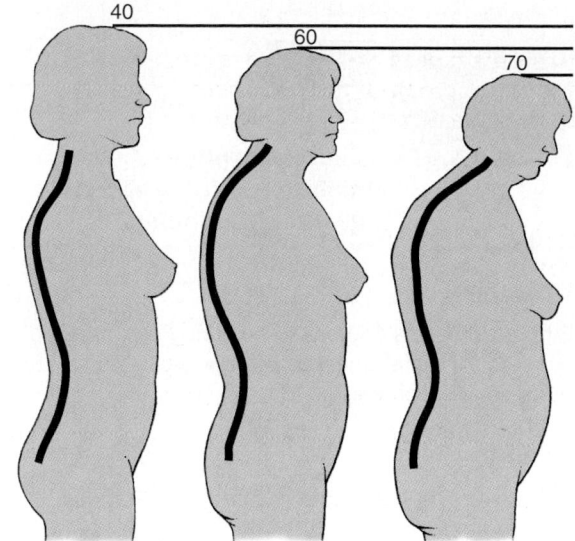

Figure 20–3

Changes in height and posture associated with osteoporosis and the process of aging.

ommend routine bone densitometry for patients older than age 35 who are at risk, to identify and treat early osteoporosis and decrease the risk of pathologic fractures. Laboratory values for serum calcium, phosphorus, and vitamin D are normal with osteoporosis, but their evaluation may help rule out other conditions.

Management

The goals of medical management are protection from pathologic fracture and prevention of further bone loss. Good body mechanics decreases the risk of pathologic fractures. The patient is taught to avoid lifting heavy objects, straining to open windows, and bouncing in a car over bumps or potholes and to practice safety in the home to prevent slips and falls. A back brace or corset may protect the vertebrae and help relieve back pain.

Calcium and vitamin D supplements may be prescribed to maintain bone mass. The recommended dietary allowance (RDA) of calcium for adults is 1000 mg. Some research studies recommend that postmenopausal women receive 1500 mg per day. The RDA of vitamin D is 400 IU per day. Estrogen hormone replacement, unless contraindicated, may be prescribed to reduce the rate of bone loss. Estrogen replacement therapy has beneficial effects for 10 to 15 years after menopause. Inhibitors of osteoclasts or bone resorption such as calcitonin may be administered in patients who are not candidates for estrogen therapy. Alendronate sodium (Fosamax), a biphosphonate, may be prescribed in the management of osteoporosis to inhibit osteoclast bone resorption. Highlight 20–8 gives the information about alendronate sodium that should be taught by the nurse. An intermittent cyclical regime of etidronate disodium (Didronel), a biphosphonate, may be used in the management of osteoporosis. The use of sodium

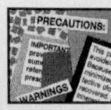

Bone Resorption Inhibitors: Biphosphonate-Alendronate Sodium

Definition:

Biphosphonate-alendronate sodium (Fosamax) is used for the treatment of osteoporosis in post-menopausal women.

Action:

Decreases the faster rate of bone loss that occurs after menopause.

Reduces the activity of osteoclast cells that cause bone loss.

Uses:

Fosamax is used to increase the density of bone and reverse the progression of osteoporosis and Paget's disease.

Side Effects:

Side effects include abdominal pain, nausea, heartburn, esophageal irritation, vomiting, difficulty swallowing, constipation, diarrhea, flatulence. Muscle/bone pain, headache, or an altered sense of taste may also be experienced.

Interactions:

Calcium supplements, antacids, and oral medications decrease the absorption. Food significantly decreases absorption.

Nursing Implications:

Teach the patient to take the drug in the morning with a full glass of plain water and not with coffee, tea, juice, or mineral water.

Teach the patient to not lie down for at least 30 minutes after the drug is taken to help avoid esophagus irritation.

Teach the patient to take the drug on an empty stomach. The drug should be taken at least 30 minutes before the first meal, beverage, or another medication, including antacids, calcium supplements, and vitamins.

The drug is contraindicated in a patient with severe kidney disease or hypocalcemia.

Advise female patients to notify the physician or health-care provider if pregnancy is planned or suspected or if she is breastfeeding.

---

fluoride and anabolic steroids is experimental in the treatment of osteoporosis.

Because immobility predisposes a person to bone resorption, planned regular physical activity is important in the prevention of bone loss. Weight-bearing activity, if possible, is often recommended because it increases bone formation. To maximize bone mass, aerobic exercise at least three times a week is recommended.

A diet that includes the RDAs in all food groups to supply adequate vitamins and minerals is important for normal bone growth and development throughout the life span and for the prevention of osteoporosis. Alcohol and caffeine consumption and cigarette smoking have been linked to excess bone loss. The elimination of these substances is recommended in the prevention of osteoporosis. Health promotion and risk reduction are important aspects of the management of osteoporosis. Health promotion aspects that are taught by the nurse are described in Highlight 20–9.

❖ Settings, Providers, and Collaboration for Care

There may be no evidence of osteoporosis until a fracture occurs. The physician may manage the fracture and evaluate the osteoporosis in an inpatient or outpatient setting. The physical therapist develops an individualized physical therapy program and makes recommendations regarding assistive devices to promote the patient's rehabilitation. The occupational therapist assists the patient to modify work and home activities to decrease the risk of a fracture. The dietitian teaches the patient strategies to minimize the progression of the osteoporosis. The nurse collaborates with the physical and occupational therapist regarding the exercise program. The nurse teaches the patient and family about the disease, management techniques, pharmacologic agents, and measures to avoid the complications of osteoporosis. The nurse reinforces the dietary teaching and evaluates the need for continuing care in the home or extended care facility. The home health nurse may be used to promote patient and family understanding of the disease and its management.

NURSING PROCESS
Osteoporosis

Assessment

Review the patient's history, physical findings, and diagnostic studies. Evaluate the lifestyle of the patient, including dietary intake and exercise. Assess the patient's pain, noting intensity, location, duration, precipitating factors, and relief methods. Ask the patient about any structural changes noticed, such as diminishing height. Complete a musculoskeletal system assessment, noting deformities, strength, and range of motion. Observe the patient's ability to move freely. Assess the patient's knowl-

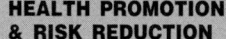
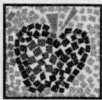

HIGHLIGHT 20–9
HEALTH PROMOTION & RISK REDUCTION
Osteoporosis

Strategies for prevention or alleviation of osteoporosis include:

Explaining that weight-bearing exercises on a daily basis during the years before peak bone mass is formed (approximately age 30) will promote bone development.

Explaining the benefits of continuous moderate exercise in maintaining bone density.

Teaching that the recommended daily allowance of calcium is 1000 mg in premenopausal women and 1500 mg in postmenopausal women. Emphasize the importance of calcium intake in the years before peak bone mass is reached.

Teaching the calcium content of foods. Promote the recognition that nonfat dairy food contains the same amounts of calcium as higher fat dairy products (see Highlight 20–7).

Recommending avoiding smoking and high caffeine and high protein intake.

Recommending that menopausal women consult the physician or health-care provider regarding estrogen replacement.

Promoting the awareness that plain roentgenograms are not effective in identifying osteoporosis, since 30 to 50% of bone mass must be lost before osteoporosis detection is possible.

Teaching that the recommended dietary allowance of vitamin D is 400 IU per day for women and children and 300 IU for adult males.

Explaining that vitamin D supplements may be needed for individuals who do not receive an adequate amount of sunlight. Monitor individuals taking antiseizure medications (phenobarbital and phenytoin) and digoxin with vitamin D closely for adverse interactions.

Teaching individuals about calcium supplements (see Highlight 20–6).

---

edge of the disorder, its manifestations and treatment, and prevention methods. Ask the patient whether falls have been a problem. Determine the safety of the patient's environment.

Nursing Diagnoses and Planning

Nursing diagnoses and related expected patient outcomes most commonly applicable to patients with osteoporosis include those previously discussed for the patient with osteomalacia and the following:

NDx: Risk for injury: falls related to lack of bone integrity, causing weakness and fractures

Planning: Patient Outcomes
1. Patient states methods to promote safe mobility.
2. Patient uses ambulatory aids properly.
3. Patient requests assistance when needed to prevent falls.

NDx: Impaired physical mobility related to pain, fractures, and limited range of motion

Planning: Patient Outcomes
1. Patient is able to perform activities of daily living.
2. Patient maintains maximum mobility of extremities.
3. Patient states methods to compensate for limited mobility.

NDx: Altered nutrition: less than body requirements related to lack of calcium intake

Planning: Patient Outcomes
1. Patient states recommended dietary intake of calcium.
2. Patient states calcium content in various foods.
3. Patient develops a meal plan for 3 days that includes adequate amounts of calcium.

Nursing Interventions and Evaluation

NDx: Risk for injury
Teach the patient and family about injury prevention. Help them plan strategies to make the home environment safer for the patient. To prevent a fall, tell the patient to ask for assistance if needed when ambulating. Teach the patient how to use ambulatory aid devices. Observe the patient while using the device, checking for proper handling. Refer the patient to a physical therapist for assistance.

NDx: Impaired physical mobility
Assist the patient in locomotion as needed. Encourage ambulation to prevent the problems of disuse. Use the assistance of a physical therapist to instruct the patient and family about the prescribed ambulatory aid and to reinforce its safe use. Give analgesics as needed to decrease pain levels that may interfere with the patient's ability to be mobile. Encourage participation in a daily exercise program to maintain strength and joint mobility.

NDX: Altered nutrition: less than body requirements
Educate the family (parents, young children, and adolescents) that the peak bone mass before the age of thirty is an important factor in the development of osteoporosis. Teach the importance of calcium intake in the prevention and management of oseoporosis (see Highlight 20–9). Explain how to maintain a diet rich in calcium (see Highlight 20–7). Assist the patient in planning menus that include recommended calcium intake. Emphasize the importance of decreasing caffeine and alcohol intake. Refer to a dietitian as needed.

Compare the patient's status with the expected outcomes. If the outcomes are not met, reassess the patient and revise the plan.

PAGET'S DISEASE

Etiology and Pathophysiology

Also called osteitis deformans because of the bone deformity resulting from the disease, Paget's disease is a chronic, progressive metabolic bone disease of unknown cause. It is characterized by excessive bone resorption with replacement by structurally abnormal bone. The bones most frequently involved are the pelvis, spine, sacrum, skull, femur, and humerus.

Osteoclastic resorption in the initial lesion is followed by increased osteoblastic activity. This results in the formation of bone that is normal in mineral content but is structurally thickened and of poor quality. The new bone has a mosaic pattern, which causes it to be weaker and more prone to fracture. Pagetic bone is also more vascular.

Paget's disease occurs in 3% of the population older than age 40 and is more common among males. It mainly affects individuals of Anglo-Saxon descent and occurs less frequently in African, Asian, and Scandinavian people.

Clinical Manifestations

Clinical manifestations are few and vague in the early stages of the disease. The patient usually seeks medical attention for fractures or bone deformities in later stages of the disease process. Paget's disease may also be detected by laboratory results or radiologic examinations performed during a routine physical examination or treatment for another disorder.

In later stages, bone deformity can cause pain and create pressure on nerves. Bones with increased vascularity also feel warm, and pressure on the periosteal lining stimulates pain. The pain experienced is generally a dull aching discomfort. Involvement of spinal vertebrae causes kyphosis and loss of the lumbar curve. Compression fractures of the vertebrae result in a decrease in height and pain from pressure on the spinal nerve roots.

Skull deformity may be identified early and confirmed by x-ray examination. The patient may have noticed an increase in hat size. Skull involvement results in headaches, osteosclerotic hearing loss, tinnitus, and vertigo because of an increase in perfusion of blood and pressure on the cranial nerves in the skull. Maxillary and mandibular involvement can cause a change in facial features and loss of teeth. Long-bone deformity and bowing are common with progression of the disease. The increased vascularity of pagetic bone can cause stress on the heart by increasing the demand on cardiac output.

The development of sarcoma in pagetic bone is 40 times greater than in normal bone. However, only 1% of patients with Paget's disease develop sarcoma. Some patients develop secondary osteoar-thritis as a result of bone deformity adjacent to the joint. Gout is also more common among individuals with Paget's disease.

Diagnosis

Diagnosis is made on the basis of radiologic examination and blood and urine studies. Affected bones have a "cotton wool" appearance in thickened areas such as the skull. X-ray films also reveal a punched-out or mosaic appearance in the bone structure. The bones are more dense than normal, with cortical thickening. New bone is not laid down along lines of stress. A bone scan can reveal the extent of Paget's disease and eliminate the need for numerous skeletal x-ray films.

The serum alkaline phosphatase level is elevated, indicating increased osteoblastic activity. Increased osteoclastic activity is indicated by elevated levels of urinary hydroxyproline, as measured in a 24-hour urine specimen.

Management

The goals of medical management are relief of symptoms, protection from pathologic fracture, and prevention of further bone deformity. Nonsteroidal anti-inflammatory agents are generally effective in pain relief. Aspirin, ibuprofen, and indomethacin may also be used as analgesics. Structural changes, especially in the hip, may require surgical correction by a total hip replacement. Spinal changes can be diminished by a supporting corset or brace. Changes in posture require patient education on good body mechanics and safe ambulating techniques. Assistive devices may be necessary for locomotion. Hearing loss may be improved by a hearing aid or referral to a hearing therapist to learn communication skills such as lip-reading.

Administration of antipagetic medications can retard the progress of the disease and bring about temporary remission. Calcitonin is used to inhibit osteoclastic bone resorption and produce pain relief. Because calcitonin must be administered subcutaneously for several doses to be effective, the nurse must teach the patient or another reliable person to administer the injection. Biphosphonates such as etidronate disodium can be administered to slow the rate of bone resorption and the formation of new bone and to reduce bone vascularity. Teach the patients the administration schedule, expected actions, and side effects of these medications. Lifetime medical follow-up is necessary.

NURSING PROCESS GUIDELINES
Paget's Disease

The assessment, nursing diagnoses, expected patient outcomes, nursing interventions, and evaluation for patients with Paget's disease are similar to those described previously for patients with osteoporosis.

DISORDERS OF THE WRIST AND HAND

Carpal Tunnel Syndrome

Carpal tunnel syndrome results from compression of the median nerve at the wrist within the carpal tunnel (Fig. 20–4). It is the most common nerve entrapment syndrome. Compression causes sensory motor changes in the hand in sites affected by the median nerve, which includes the thumb, index finger, middle finger, and radial side of the ring finger. Females are affected more than males. The syndrome occurs most frequently in the summer months in individuals between 30 and 60 years of age. It occurs in conditions that cause swelling in the carpal tunnel, which places pressure on the median nerve in the wrist. Rheumatic disorders, tenosynovitis, tumors, tuberculosis, myxedema, and wrist sprain may be causative factors. Carpal tunnel syndrome is aggravated by repetitive or strenuous wrist and hand motions. Knitting, driving, sewing, and work-related tasks such as those of a computer operator, grocery checker, or cosmetologist may contribute to carpal tunnel syndrome.

Clinical manifestations include pain, numbness, and tingling. The paresthesia affects the thumb, forefinger, and middle fingers. The pain may radiate up the arm. An inability to grasp objects or clench the fist may also be present. Carpal tunnel syndrome is diagnosed on the basis of assessment, history, a compression test, and electromyography, which detects a median nerve conduction delay. Treatment includes rest of the affected wrist and hand, immobilization with a splint to provide neutral extension, and correction of the underlying cause. Steroid injections into the carpal tunnel may be used. However, adverse effects may occur with this technique. Ice packs and NSAIDS may decrease the inflammation.

Because occupation is a contributing factor either to the cause or to increasing the distress of the disorder, the patient may be counseled to seek other employment. If the condition persists or is unrelieved by conservative treatment, surgical decompression may be necessary. Endoscopic carpal tunnel release is being used in some health-care settings.

Dupuytren's Contracture

Dupuytren's contracture is a deformity of the hand in which the ring finger and little finger contract. Because of the shortening of the palmar fascia, the affected fingers cannot extend and bend into the palm. The flexion disorder occurs more frequently in older men who are of Scandinavian origin. Treatment consists of finger-stretching exercises and a surgical fasciectomy.

Ganglion

A ganglion is a cystic mass that develops overlying or adjacent to a wrist joint or tendon. It develops through a defect in the tendon sheath or capsule. Ganglions are more common in young women than in men. Pain is the chief symptom of a ganglion. Treatment includes aspiration of the ganglion, injection of corticosteroids, and the administration of nonsteroidal anti-inflammatory drugs. Surgical excision may be necessary if symptoms persist and range of motion is impaired.

NURSING PROCESS
Wrist and Hand Disorders

Assessment

Review the patient's history and presenting symptoms. Determine the patient's ability to use the af-

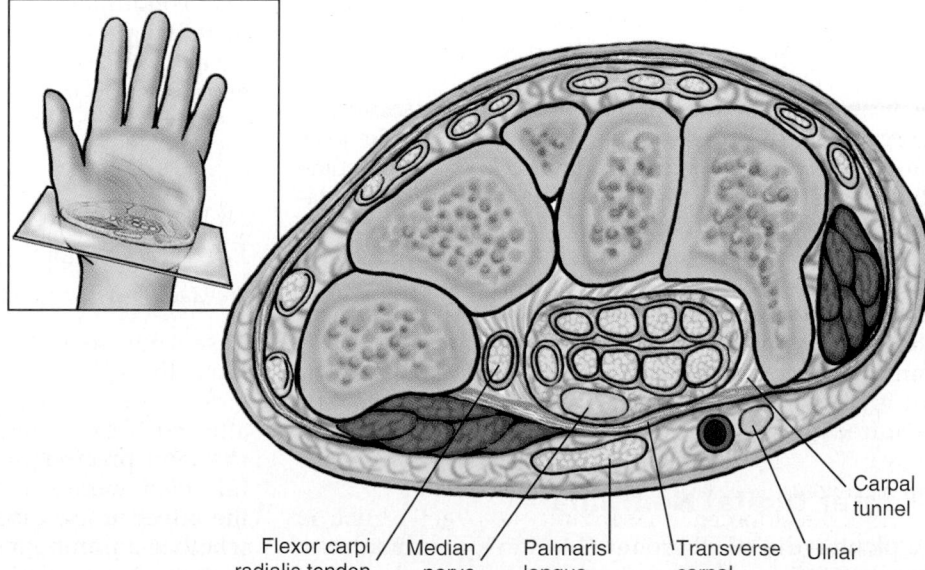

Figure 20–4

The carpal tunnel in the wrist.

Flexor carpi radialis tendon   Median nerve   Palmaris longus tendon   Transverse carpal ligament   Ulnar nerve   Carpal tunnel

fected hand. Ask about the effect of the problem on the patient's employment. Check whether the patient's occupation may be a contributing factor to the problem. Determine the patient's ability to perform self-care with the affected extremity.

Nursing Diagnoses and Planning

The nursing diagnosis and related expected patient outcomes most commonly applicable to patients with a disorder of the wrist or hand are as follows:

NDx: Self care deficit: grooming, bathing, hygiene and activities of daily living related to the deformity or pain

Planning: Patient Outcomes
1. Patient maintains maximum use of the affected extremity.
2. Patient adapts to the deformity by using assistive devices or the other extremity.
3. Patient performs activities of daily living and personal self-care tasks.

Nursing Interventions and Evaluation

NDx: Self care deficit: grooming, bathing, hygiene, and activities of daily living
Assist the patient, as needed, to perform self-care tasks. Teach the patient how to use assistive devices to perform activities that were previously too difficult to perform as a result of pain or the deformities. Have the patient practice using the opposite hand to perform self-care tasks. Administer analgesics as prescribed to relieve pain that may be inhibiting the patient's ability to use the affected extremity. Seek assistance from family members when the patient cannot complete activities.

Compare the patient's status with the expected outcomes. If the outcomes are not met, reassess the patient and revise the plan.

DISORDERS OF THE FEET

Hallux Valgus (Bunion)

Hallux valgus, commonly known as a bunion, is a progressive disorder in which the great toe deviates laterally (Fig. 20–5A). There is also a bony (osseous) enlargement of the medial aspect of the first metatarsal joint and a fluid-filled cavity called a bursa. The cause of a bunion may be arthritis, improperly fitting shoes, or heredity. Pain, redness, and edema are the typical symptoms presented. The treatment depends on the severity of the discomfort and deformity. A correctly fitting or open-toed shoe may be all that is necessary, or surgical excision may be required.

Plantar Digital Neuroma

A plantar digital neuroma (Morton's neuroma) is a swelling of the plantar nerve caused by ischemia of

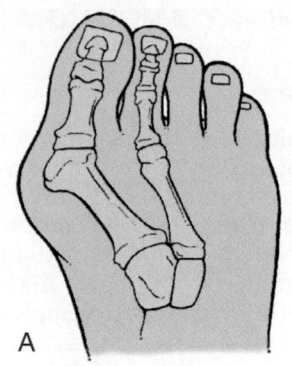
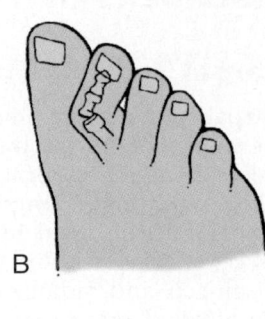

Figure 20–5
Disorders of the foot. *A,* Hallux valgus (bunion); *B,* hammer toe.

the nerve. Loss of the transmetatarsal arch may also cause the swelling. The most common symptom is a throbbing pain between the third and fourth digits in the foot. The pain may subside with rest. It is treated with local cortisone or anesthetic injections or, if necessary, by surgical excision or reconstruction of the arch.

Hammer Toe

Hammer toe is a flexion deformity of the interphalangeal joint (see Fig. 20–5B). The condition is usually an acquired disorder from prolonged wearing of ill-fitting shoes. The toe or toes are pulled up, with the ball of the foot pushed downward. Corns usually form on the top of the toes. Treatment consists of exercises, wearing open-toed or well-fitting shoes, and protecting the joints with pads.

Pes Planus

Pes planus, commonly called flatfoot, is an abnormal lowering and flatness of the transmetatarsal arch. The condition causes pain in the foot or leg and may interfere with normal foot functioning. It may be an acute or chronic problem. Treatment consists of arch supports, or in severe cases, surgical intervention.

NURSING PROCESS
Foot Disorders

Assessment

Assess the severity of the patient's disorder. Determine the effect on mobility and the ability to provide self-care. Ask the patient about pain in the affected area. Determine the onset, duration, intensity, and precipitant factors of the pain, and successful relief methods. Watch the patient walk, noting the effect of the disorder on basic movement. Check whether an ambulatory device is necessary for locomotion. Assess the patient's footwear, observing for too-tight fit and nonskid soles. Determine the patient's knowledge about the condition, progression, and potential treatment modalities.

Nursing Diagnoses and Planning

Nursing diagnoses and related expected patient outcomes most commonly applicable to patients with a foot disorder include the following:

NDx: Pain related to structural changes in bones and deformities in feet

Planning: Patient Outcomes
1. Patient denies discomfort or extreme pain in feet.
2. Patient relates accurate information about analgesics prescribed.
3. Patient wears well-fitting shoes.

NDx: Altered health maintenance related to lack of knowledge about the disorder, its progression, and treatment

Planning: Patient Outcomes
1. Patient states accurate information about the disorder, its progression, and treatment measures.
2. Patient wears shoes with appropriate fit for the deformity.

NDx: Risk for injury: falls related to deformities and/or improper use of ambulatory aids

Planning: Patient Outcomes
1. Patient states methods to promote safe mobility.
2. Patient uses ambulatory aids properly.
3. Patient requests assistance when needed to prevent falls.
4. Patient wears shoes with nonskid soles.

NDx: Impaired physical mobility related to pain, deformities, and limited range of motion

Planning: Patient Outcomes
1. Patient is able to perform activities of daily living.
2. Patient maintains maximal mobility of extremities.
3. Patient states methods to compensate for inability to move freely.

Nursing Interventions and Evaluation

NDx: Pain
Administer prescribed analgesics and teach the patient about the frequency, dosage, side effects, and therapeutic effects. Talk with the patient about relaxation strategies to reduce pain. Tell the patient to refrain from weight-bearing during painful episodes. Assist with ambulation to reduce weight-bearing. Teach the patient about wearing properly fitted shoes to reduce constriction, which causes pain.

NDx: Altered health maintenance
Teach the patient about the disorder, explaining its cause, symptoms, progression, and treatment regimens. Teach the patient about the proper use of prescribed medications. Assist the patient in determining the type of shoes for best fit and mobility.

NDx: Risk for injury
Teach the patient and family about injury prevention and strategies to make the home environment safe. Tell the patient to ask for assistance if needed when ambulating. Teach the patient how to use the prescribed ambulatory aid. Observe the patient using the device and check for proper handling. Refer the patient to a physical therapist for further assistance. Be sure the patient wears nonskid shoes when ambulating.

NDx: Impaired physical mobility
Assist the patient in locomotion as needed. Encourage ambulation to prevent the problems of disuse. Use the assistance of the physical therapist to instruct the patient and family about the prescribed ambulatory aid and to reinforce its safe use. Administer analgesics as needed to decrease pain levels that may interfere with the patient's ability to be mobile. Encourage participation in a daily exercise program to maintain strength and joint mobility.

Compare the patient's status with the expected outcomes. If the outcomes are not met, reassess the patient and revise the plan.

❖ SETTINGS, PROVIDERS, AND COLLABORATION FOR CARE

Wrist, hand, and foot disorders are most often managed in the out-patient setting. Patients may be hospitalized if surgical repair is needed. The hospitalization often includes day surgery. The occupational therapist or physical therapist may be consulted regarding occupational changes needed to manage wrist, hand, or foot disorders. The home health nurse can maintain safety in the home and change dressings for the patients with wrist, hand, and foot disorders.

LOW BACK PAIN

Low back pain is a common problem affecting musculoskeletal function. Back pain occurs in men and women and is a significant cause of lost working hours in the United States. The lumbar or sacral areas of the back are involved in acute or chronic low back pain.

Etiology and Pathophysiology
Risk factors associated with low back pain include tension, smoking, obesity, poor physical fitness, and poor posture. A job that requires prolonged sitting and standing, repetitive heavy lifting or vibrations, or extended periods of driving is also a major risk factor. The causes of low back pain include lumbosacral strain, osteoarthritis of lumbosacral vertebrae, and intervertebral disk degeneration or herniation.

Acute low back pain is usually associated with an activity that causes stress on tissues of the lower back. The causes of chronic back pain may include degenerative disk disease, structural abnormalities, lack of physical exercise and obesity. Herniated disk disease is described in Chapter 18.

Clinical Manifestations

Symptoms of low back pain include pain in the back, buttocks, or legs. The pain may be associated with walking, turning, or straining. Numbness or tingling in the extremities may also occur with low back pain. Physical assessment symptoms may include tenderness or tenseness in paravertebral muscles and decreased range of motion of the spine.

Diagnosis

The diagnosis of acute low back pain is based on neurologic and musculoskeletal clinical manifestations. Diagnostic studies include radiologic studies, myelography, magnetic resonance imaging, and computed tomography. Assessments of neurologic reflexes and motor function may indicate lumbar disc herniation. A straight-leg-raise test may be positive if there is herniation of an intervertebral disc. A positive test is indicated by back or leg pain that occurs when the patient in a supine position raises a leg and flexes the foot at 90 degrees.

Management

Many patients with acute low back pain require only a short-term treatment regimen, including short-term rest, application of heat or cold, and medications. Pharmacologic agents prescribed may include analgesics, nonsteroidal anti-inflammatory drugs, and muscle relaxants. Short-term bedrest to limit muscle spasms may be implemented. Intermittent application of heat or ice may be used to minimize pain and spasms, and a corset or brace may be used to limit lower back movement.

A rehabilitation program that provides education for the client is essential. Back school is a rehabilitation program that teaches the techniques to manage and prevent episodes of acute back pain. Patients are also taught about the negative impact that excess body weight and weak abdominal muscles have on the lower back.

Surgical interventions may be required in the management of acute low back pain. Chapter 18 discusses the management of herniated disk and spinal surgery.

NURSING PROCESS
Low Back Pain

Assessment

Review the physician's history and physical examination. Ask the patient about the history of the pain, precipitating factors, and relief measures. Have the patient describe the pain and exact location. Observe the patient's posture, ability to complete range of motion, lifting techniques, and general leg strength. Check for abnormal curvature of the spine. Check calcium levels and other laboratory data collected.

Nursing Diagnoses and Planning

The nursing diagnoses and related expected patient outcomes most commonly applicable to patients with low back pain are as follows:

NDx: Pain related to specific problems such as muscle spasms and ineffective comfort measures

Planning: Patient Outcomes
1. Patient reports that pain is manageable and decreasing.
2. Patient performs activities as prescribed with manageable pain.

NDx: Impaired physical mobility related to pain, muscle spasms, or therapeutic regimen

Planning: Patient Outcomes
1. Patient performs activities as prescribed.
2. Patient demonstrates techniques that enable resumption of activities as tolerated.
3. Patient maintains strength and function of neurologic and musculoskeletal system.

NDx: Ineffective management of therapeutic regimen (individuals) related to lack of knowledge regarding body mechanics, posture, lifting techniques, positioning, and therapeutic measures.

Planning: Patient Outcomes
1. Patient explains movements that reduce stress on the back.
2. Patient demonstrates proper techniques to decrease back pain.
3. Patient identifies necessary lifestyle changes to decrease back strain.

Nursing Interventions and Evaluation

NDx: Pain

Promote short-term bedrest to decrease muscle spasms. Be certain the call bell and necessary items are within easy reach. Keep the head of the bed elevated 20 degrees with knee flexion. Administer prescribed analgesics and muscle relaxants. Reinforce proper turning, transfer, and positioning techniques. Use log-rolling technique for position changes. Teach and reinforce nonpharmacologic measures to manage pain. Apply prescribed heat or cold to reduce pain and muscle spasms. Evaluate effectiveness. Instruct patient and family about methods of pain control such as heat, cold, and TENS. Assist the patient in identifying activities that increase pain and make the necessary modifications. Assess reports of pain. Ask the patient to rate the pain and to evaluate the effectiveness of pain interventions.

NDx: Impaired Physical Mobility

Explain the rationale for bedrest and avoidance of bending, sitting, or lifting. Teach the patient range-of-motion and muscle-strengthening exercises. Assist with passive and active range-of-motion exercises. Provide good skin care. Promote progressive ambulation as prescribed. Assist the patient in developing changes in lifestyle that increase pain and decrease mobility.

NDx: Ineffective management of therapeutic regimen (individuals)

Review the injury process, prognosis, and activity restrictions. Assess body mechanics and teach proper body mechanics, posture, and lifting techniques. Teach about the positive effect of a firm mattress, small pillow, and sleeping in a side-lying position with knees flexed. Discuss the side effects of the medications. Reinforce the physical therapist's teaching about low back exercises. Collaborate with the dietitian to teach weight reduction measures if needed. Teach what symptoms need to be further evaluated, for example, sharp pain, paresthesia, loss of function. Reinforce the need for continued follow-up and evaluation. Discuss recommended lifestyle changes related to work, recreation, and driving that will minimize back strain and pain.

Compare the patient's status with the expected outcomes. If the outcomes are not met, reassess the patient and revise the plan.

Trauma

Musculoskeletal trauma can involve any of the body's bones, articular cartilage, muscles, ligaments, or tendons. The degree of soft tissue damage and associated nerve, vascular, or organ damage varies with each injury. It is estimated that three-fourths of all musculoskeletal trauma involves the appendicular skeleton. Falls, accidents involving motor vehicles, and sports injuries account for most musculoskeletal trauma. Many of the musculoskeletal injuries can be avoided by following various injury prevention strategies as described in Chapter 19. The nurse can play an important role in injury prevention through teaching and counseling about these strategies.

MINOR MUSCULOSKELETAL INJURIES

Minor musculoskeletal injuries are those that do not usually require medical intervention for readjustment or repair of the injured part. Although there may be considerable pain present, the affected part usually heals in time, especially if care is taken not to re-injure it until the healing has occurred.

Contusions and Strains

Etiology and Pathophysiology

Soft-tissue trauma with no damage to musculoskeletal structures is a contusion. It is usually the result of a blow or blunt force. A strain is injury of a muscle that has been stretched beyond its capacity. Small blood vessels in the affected muscle rupture, causing inflammation of surrounding soft tissue structures.

Clinical Manifestations

Clinical manifestations of a contusion include swelling and tenderness and localized hemorrhage, with discoloration and ecchymosis from damage to superficial blood vessels in the skin and subcutaneous tissue. Contusions can cause restriction in the range of motion of a joint because of localized tenderness and swelling, but there is no loss of joint stability. With a strain, the area also becomes swollen, tender, and ecchymotic. Painful muscle spasms may occur.

Diagnosis

Diagnosis of contusions and strains is made on the basis of examination, history of incident, and the ruling out of a fracture, dislocation, or ligament injury. Computed tomography and magnetic resonance imaging can be used to localize the strain injury in cases of acute muscle strain.

Management

Treatment involves prevention of further trauma, bleeding, or swelling. Surgery may be needed if rupture of the tendon-bone interface has occurred. The involved body part is elevated, and ice is applied to prevent or reduce swelling as well as to reduce discomfort. An elastic wrap may be applied to protect it from further damage, relieve pain, and promote comfort. Teach the patient how to apply and remove the wrap. If numbness, tingling, or swelling occurs distal to the elastic wrap, it is too tight. Have the patient demonstrate application of the wrap. Instruct the patient that an elastic wrap provides protection but little support of an affected joint. Encourage the patient to avoid overactivity as tissue is healing.

Sprains

Etiology and Pathophysiology

A sprain refers to an injury of a joint. The joint is stretched beyond its normal range of motion, and tearing of the ligaments, capsule, or synovium of the joint results. The most common joints affected are the ankle, knee, and wrist.

Clinical Manifestations

The clinical manifestations depend on the severity of damage to joint structures. Assessment findings may include swelling, pain, ecchymosis, and limited joint mobility. With severe sprains, the person may complain that the joint feels unstable and may describe the occurrence of a "snapping" sound at the time of injury.

Diagnosis

Diagnosis is made on the basis of assessment, history of incident, and x-ray examinations.

Management

Treatment of a sprain also depends on the severity of damage to joint structures. Minor sprains, those with minimal ligament injury, are treated by application of cold, elevation, and an elastic wrap to provide protection and decrease swelling. Use of the joint is restricted for a prescribed period of time to prevent further damage and to allow healing.

Joint weakness and abnormal motion are present when the ligament is torn halfway through. These sprains require restricted use of the joint or immobilization for up to 4 weeks, in addition to the ice, elevation, and wrap.

Major sprain injuries involve complete tearing of the ligament. They are treated by surgical repair of the torn ligament, followed by rigid immobilization in a splint or cast. A tear of the anterior cruciate ligament of the knee is a common sports injury. The cruciate ligaments are the main stabilizing ligaments of the knee. At the time of injury, the patient experiences a snapping sensation. The individual immediately experiences pain, swelling, and instability of the joint. Immediate treatment involves the application of ice, compression through wrapping, and splinting. The ligament tear is repaired by arthroscopic surgery, usually on an outpatient basis. A full leg immobilizer is worn for up to 4 weeks after the repair (Fig. 20–6). Specific leg exercises are prescribed to restrengthen the affected part.

The individual with a sprained knee or ankle needs crutches for ambulation to maintain non-weight-bearing or limited weight-bearing on the involved joint. In some instances, when surgical intervention is not necessary, controlled, passive movement of the involved joint is prescribed to decrease loss of joint function, prevent muscle atrophy, and maintain the strength of other supporting structures during healing. Prescribed passive exercises can be provided by the nurse, a physical therapist, or a joint exercise machine.

Many types of passive joint exercise machines are available today. The most popular machines are used to flex and extend the knee following an injury or surgical repair of a joint. Passive joint movement exercise devices may also be used after total joint replacements as described in Chapter 19. With each type of machine, the physician prescribes the degree of flexion and extension, speed (movements per minute), and length of time for therapy. The extent of movement is usually increased gradually.

Meniscal Tears

Etiology and Pathophysiology

The meniscus is a fibrocartilaginous semicircular structure within the knee joint. There are two menisci in each knee, one each on the lateral and medial aspects of the joint. They act as a cushion between adjacent articular cartilage and provide stability from rotational forces. One or both of these structures may be injured by knee trauma. Meniscal tears are often associated with moderate or severe knee sprains. Only the outer one third of the meniscus has a limited blood supply so healing is often very slow.

Clinical Manifestations

Manifestations include a popping or tearing sensation at the time of injury, swelling, and an inability to fully extend the knee, caused by movement of loose pieces of cartilage.

Diagnosis

Diagnosis of a torn meniscus is made on the basis of a history of injury, physical examination of the knee, loss of knee stability, radiographic studies to rule out fracture, and arthroscopic examination.

Management

Treatment is a partial or total meniscectomy by arthroscopy or arthrotomy.

❖ Settings, Providers, and Collaboration for Care

Treatment for minor musculoskeletal injuries is usually performed on an outpatient basis at the physician's office, in a free-standing surgical clinic, or in the outpatient surgical department of the hospital. If surgery is required, postoperative nursing interventions include assessment of proximal and distal neurovascular function, cold applications, and elevation of the leg for 48 hours. Teach the patient prescribed weight-bearing restrictions and strengthening and range-of-motion exercises. Reinforce in-

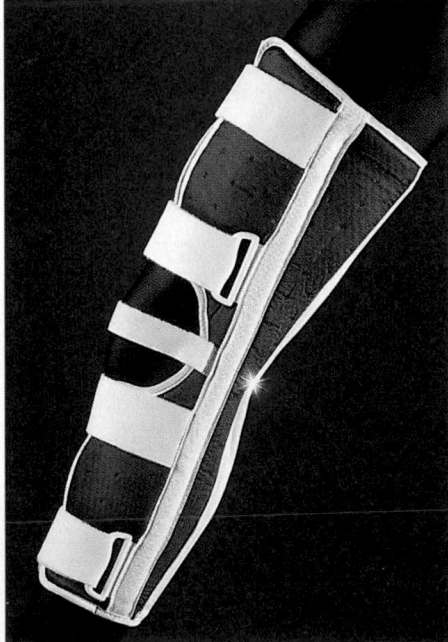

Figure 20–6

Knee immobilizer used after knee injury or operative knee repair. (Courtesy of Zimmer, Inc, Dover, OH.)

structions, usually provided by the physical therapist, in the use of crutches or an immobilization device as needed.

MAJOR MUSCULOSKELETAL INJURIES

Major musculoskeletal injuries are those that include severe injury to the bone, joint, tendon, or ligament. These injuries require medical intervention for adequate repair or readjustment of the injury.

Subluxations and Dislocations

Etiology and Pathophysiology
A subluxation is the partial separation of adjacent joint surfaces. A dislocation occurs when normally adjacent joint surfaces become completely separated from one another. Dislocations often occur in combination with fractures of the bone within or near the joint. A subluxation or dislocation may also cause damage to the surrounding ligaments, joint capsule, synovial lining, and the articular cartilage, as well as soft tissue, nerves and blood vessels.

Clinical Manifestations
Clinical manifestations include minimal deformity of the joint in a subluxation and marked deformity of the joint with a dislocation. The actual degree of deformity may be masked by the presence of swelling of the injured joint. The joint may be painful, or if major nerves are injured, it may become numb. The length of the affected extremity may change. Loss of joint function varies from slight to complete loss of range of motion. Ecchymosis may result from tearing of adjacent blood vessels. Neurovascular function distal to the injury may be impaired as a result of pressure from displaced joint structures or edema.

Diagnosis
Diagnosis of a subluxation or dislocation is made on the basis of history of an injury or pathologic condition, physical examination, and radiographic studies of the involved area. If distal circulation is impaired, arteriography may be performed. However, the dislocation is reduced immediately to restore circulation. During diagnostic procedures, the examiner should support and handle the affected body part carefully to protect it from further injury.

Management
Cold applications and immobilization with protective elastic wraps or a sling may be prescribed before x-ray examination. Once diagnosis is established by x-ray examination, the joint is reduced or returned to anatomical alignment. In a closed reduction, the physician is able to return the joint structures to anatomical alignment by manipulation and manual traction. The patient is usually sedated during a closed reduction procedure if the injury is recent.

An open reduction requires hospitalization for surgery under general anesthesia. Following reduction, the joint is immobilized by application of a splint or cast for approximately 3 to 6 weeks. Weight-bearing is avoided for this period of time.

❖ **Settings, Providers, and Collaboration
   for Care**
Treatment of subluxations and dislocations generally occurs in a clinic or a hospital outpatient unit such as the emergency room. Untreated dislocation of a longer duration, however, may require general anesthesia for reduction, which may necessitate admission to an outpatient surgical unit. The patient needs someone to drive him or her home after recovery from the anesthesia. The nurse and physician give the patient instructions for further care prior to discharge.

NURSING PROCESS
Subluxations and Dislocations

Assessment

Assess the patient's affected part for pain, swelling, discoloration, or malalignment. Check the neurovascular status proximal and distal to the injury by palpating for pulses, feeling for warmth of the part, and assessing for decreased sensation. Ask the patient about numbness or tingling in the extremity. Review how the injury occurred, and note what treatment was instituted, if any, at the time of the occurrence. Determine the patient's understanding of the injury and the necessary treatment.

Nursing Diagnoses and Planning

Nursing diagnoses and related expected patient outcomes most commonly applicable to patients with musculoskeletal injuries include the following:

NDx: Pain related to joint trauma, pressure from edema, and immobilization

Planning: Patient Outcomes
  1. Patient denies pain in affected part.
  2. Patient states methods to decrease pain by reduction of swelling and keeping immobilizer properly applied.

NDx: Altered health maintenance related to lack of knowledge about the injury, management of immobilization device, exercises to perform, and prevention of re-injury

Planning: Patient Outcomes
  1. Patient states accurate information about the cause of the injury and methods to prevent re-injury.
  2. Patient demonstrates proper application of the immobilizer device and states when it is to be in place, how much weight-lifting or weight-bearing is allowed, and when the device may be removed.

3. Patient demonstrates exercises, as taught, to maintain strength and range of motion of the joint.

Nursing Interventions and Evaluation

NDx: Pain

Administer prescribed analgesics and explain the dosage, frequency, side effects, and expected therapeutic effects of the medications. Caution the patient not to perform tasks that require mental alertness while taking pain medication. Teach the patient to check for tightness of the immobilizer and signs of swelling or diminished sensation in the distal part of the affected extremity. Teach the patient to elevate the extremity to reduce swelling and pain. Caution the patient about weight-bearing if contraindicated, because that might increase the pain significantly.

NDx: Altered health maintenance

Teach the patient about the injury, the cause, methods of prevention of re-injury, and appropriate treatment. Explain how to apply the immobilizer or wrap to the affected part and have the patient redemonstrate the process. Check to see that it is not too tight and tell the patient how to check for improper fit. Explain that increased swelling, discoloration, and decreased sensation in the affected part may be signs of improper fit of the device and that prolonged pressure could cause severe problems if not relieved. Reinforce the physician's instruction about weight-lifting (if shoulder, arm, or hand is affected) or weight-bearing (if knee, leg, ankle, or foot is affected). Demonstrate prescribed exercises to the patient, and encourage participation in the exercise regimen to prevent loss of strength and joint motion.

Compare the patient's status with the expected outcomes. If the outcomes are not met, reassess the patient and revise the plan.

Fractures

A fracture is a crack or break in the continuity of a bone. A fracture may or may not involve damage to tissues or organs surrounding the bone.

Etiology and Pathophysiology

Fractures may be caused by a direct blow or trauma to the bone, a sudden strong muscle contraction that bends the bone to the breaking point, continuous extreme stress on the bone, or pathologic conditions that cause demineralization of the bone. Demineralization of bones that occurs with prolonged bedrest, decreased weight-bearing, and the aging process increases the risk of bone fracture with minimal stress or trauma.

There are many types of fractures. Some of the more common types are illustrated in Figure 20–7. Fractures can be further described by the part of the bone involved and the transverse, linear, or oblique direction of the fracture line.

A closed fracture is one in which the bone is broken but there is no external injury. A closed fracture is not considered a life-threatening injury unless it is an unstable fracture that may damage vital organs or major blood vessels or unless it is associated with internal hemorrhage, shock, or both.

A compound or open fracture is one in which the bone fragments have broken through or penetrated the skin. Because this type of fracture is usually associated with severe tissue damage and blood loss, as well as a risk of infection, a compound fracture is considered a life-threatening injury.

Clinical Manifestations

In the case of a fracture in which the fragments are displaced or are no longer in their normal alignment, the bone either lies in an abnormal position with angulation where no joint exists or appears as a shortened or abnormally rotated extremity. In a nondisplaced fracture, the bone remains in normal alignment. Nondisplaced fractures are more difficult to diagnose without radiologic examination.

The degree of pain can vary from tenderness over the fracture site to extreme pain and muscle spasms of the involved body part. Pain may limit motion and use of a fractured bone or adjacent joints. In the case of some closed nondisplaced fractures, however, the patient may still have use of the affected body part. Crepitus, a grating sound created by bone fragments scraping against one another, may be heard or felt on movement.

Swelling and ecchymosis of the soft tissue surrounding the injury always occur. This is caused by bleeding (which may be considerable) at the fracture site from damage to soft tissue. However, discoloration may not be seen on the skin surface for several days. A decrease in hematocrit and hemoglobin levels indicates the degree of blood loss but may not do so for up to 72 hours after injury. A break in the skin over the fracture site indicates an open or compound fracture. Bone may or may not be visible in the wound.

Injury to nerves and blood vessels near the fracture site is caused by direct trauma from a dislocated joint or fracture fragments at the time of injury. Stretching, tearing, or compression of a nerve or blood vessel is common. Localized swelling, discoloration, and hemorrhage may occur. Numbness in the affected extremity is frequently experienced. The danger of further soft tissue damage continues until the injured part is immobilized.

Organ damage can result from direct trauma at the time of injury or from a laceration or puncture caused by the displaced bone fragments. Common organ injuries include

Cardiac contusions
Lung punctures

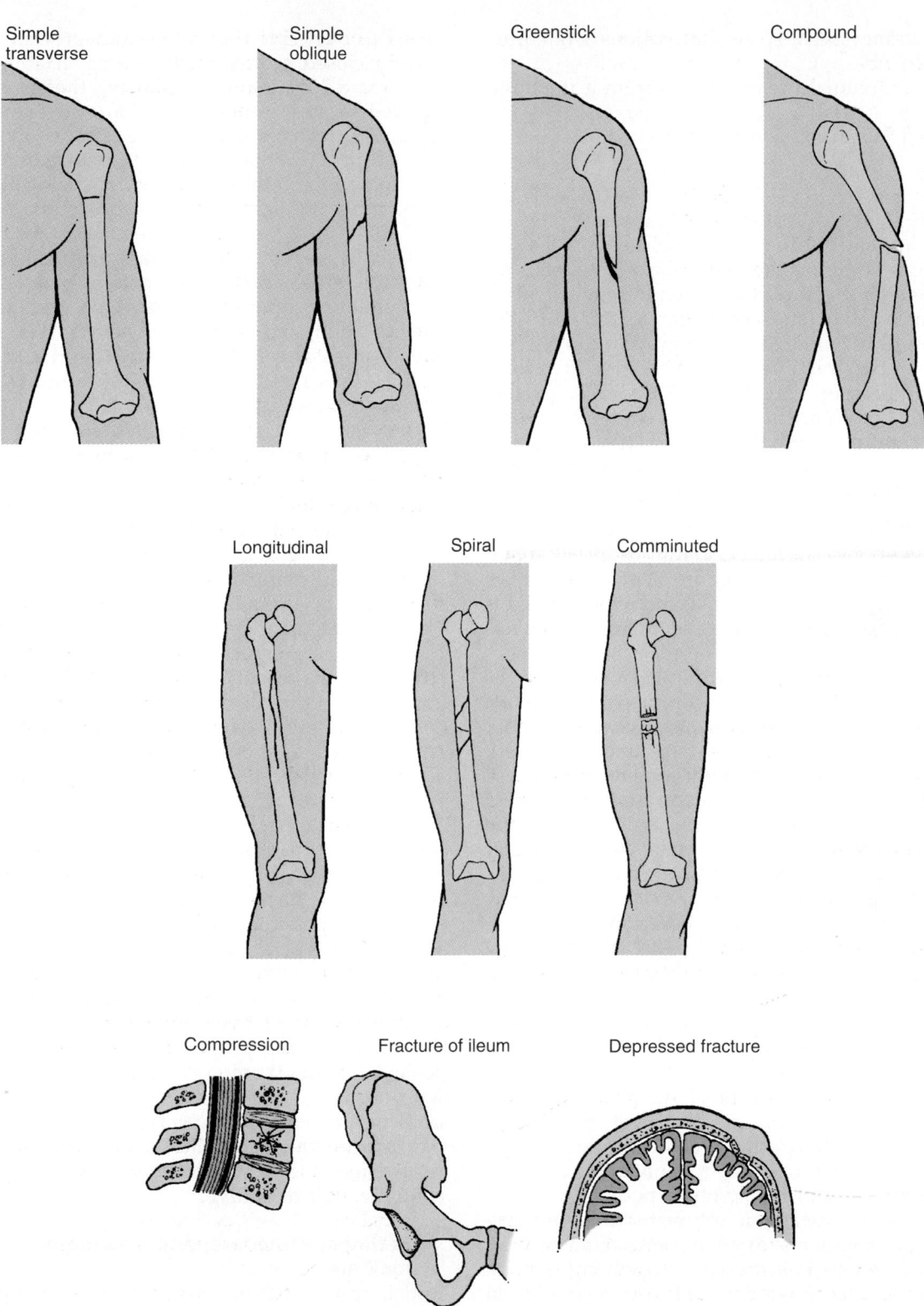

Figure 20–7
Types of fractures.

Liver, kidney, and spleen lacerations from fractured ribs

Lower abdominal organ injuries from a fractured pelvis

Brain injuries from skull fractures

Diagnosis

Diagnosis of a fracture is made on the basis of history of an injury or pathologic condition, physical examination, and radiographic studies of the involved area. Computed tomographic (CT) scans can be used to identify the exact location and extent of skull, spinal, pelvic, and acetabular fractures. If distal circulation is impaired, arteriography can be performed, but the fracture is reduced first to restore circulation. During diagnostic procedures, protect the affected body part from further injury by splinting and careful handling. Explain the diagnostic procedure to the patient and administer prescribed analgesics as needed for patient comfort.

Management

Protect known or suspected fractures from further injury until medical intervention is possible. Cover open wounds with sterile or clean, white or light-colored, lint-free material to prevent further contamination.

Splint extremities by the application of bandages or well-padded improvised or commercial splints. If the injured part is in a deformed position, do not attempt to realign the limb or correct the deformity because movement of the bone fragments may cause further damage to soft tissues, nerves, and blood vessels. Instead, splint the involved part in the shape of the deformity. Assess distal neurovascular function before and after splinting. Stabilize the patient with known or suspected spinal or pelvic injuries with sandbags on a firm board before movement or transport. After injured parts are adequately splinted, position the patient for comfort for transport to an appropriate health-care facility.

Medical management depends on the type of fracture sustained, the amount of blood lost, and the severity of associated soft-tissue injuries as well as the patient's general condition. Treatment of all fractures includes reduction of displaced bone fragments, immobilization for bone healing and repair of supporting structures, and rehabilitation and restoration of function of the involved body part.

REDUCTION. Reduction is restoration of displaced bone fragments to their normal anatomical position. Reduction is achieved by applying traction or pull to the bone fragments until the pieces are in proper alignment. Closed reduction can be achieved by manual traction or can be gradually achieved by applying skin or skeletal traction.

In some instances, the bone must be reduced surgically to properly position and stabilize the bone fragments and surrounding structures. Situations that require open reduction include interposition of soft tissue between the bone fragments and strong muscle pull or spasms that cause the bone fragments to over-ride each other and prevent stabilization by closed reduction. If internal fixation devices are used to maintain alignment, the procedure is referred to as an open reduction with internal fixation. The primary disadvantage of an open reduction is that it converts a closed fracture into an open one and subjects the patient to the additional potential complications of a surgical procedure and infection.

Usually, open fractures are surgically cleaned, débrided, and reduced. The patient may receive tetanus immune globulin or toxoid on admission. Parenteral antibiotics are administered preoperatively and postoperatively to prevent wound and bone infection. Prescribed analgesics are administered before and after reduction.

IMMOBILIZATION. Dislocated fracture fragments must be immobilized and maintained in proper alignment to allow complete healing of the bone and surrounding tissue. Bone repair and the use of casts, skin and skeletal traction, external fixation, and internal fixation for immobilization and healing were discussed in Chapter 19. The length of time the fracture must be immobilized depends on the type of fracture, the degree of displacement of the bone fragments, the injuries to surrounding soft-tissue structures, the presence of infection, and the age and general condition of the patient. A fractured bone is considered healed when the aligned bone fragments have formed a strong enough union, or callus, to allow gradual resumption of function and weight-bearing.

REHABILITATION. Rehabilitation of the involved body part with restoration of function begins early. Prescribed use of the part and exercise under supervision of the physical therapist or nurse are begun as early as possible. Isometric exercises may be prescribed postoperatively following open reduction and internal fixation or for a limb in a splint, cast, traction, or an external fixation device.

Passive and active movement of joints is prescribed as healing progresses. Once the fracture has achieved a solid union, exercise is increased along with use of the part and weight-bearing on the part until optimal function returns. Patients with multiple fractures and complicated musculoskeletal injuries require lengthy rehabilitation programs that continue after discharge.

❖ Settings, Providers, and Collaboration for Care

Initial treatment usually occurs in an emergency department or trauma center. Fractures requiring a surgical correction necessitate either an inpatient or an outpatient surgical unit, depending on the extent of the injury and the surgical treatment needed. A patient may use a long-term-care or rehabilitation center to complete rehabilitation after a fracture. If the patient is discharged home, a referral to a home-care agency and guidance for the family may be needed to promote the safety of the patient.

Rehabilitation requires a multidisciplinary team approach to restore the optimal level of function. The exercise program is prescribed by the physician, implemented and taught by the physical therapist, and reinforced and encouraged by the nurse. Support services and specialized training may also be provided by an occupational therapist, social service workers, and dietary and mental health practitioners.

NURSING PROCESS
Fracture

Assessment

After the immediate care to stabilize the patient has been provided, continue to assess the patient's affected part for pain, swelling, discoloration, or malalignment. Look for signs of continued bleeding. Check the neurovascular status proximal and distal to the injury by palpating for pulses, feeling for warmth of the part, and assessing for decreased sensation. Assess vital signs, noting changes reflective of ensuing shock, such as decreasing blood pressure and rapid weak pulse rate with increased respiratory effort. Ask the patient about numbness or tingling in the extremity. Obtain an accident history to help identify other potential injury sites.

After the patient's fracture has been treated medically, continue to assess neurovascular status of the affected part. Look for signs of decreased tissue perfusion caused by constriction from the immobilization device or edema. In the case of forearm fractures and lower leg fractures, assess for symptoms of compartment syndrome, a limb-threatening complication.

Assess the patient's level of anxiety and available support network. Determine the patient's understanding of the injury and the necessary treatment. Assess the patient's ability to perform self-care and to be mobile if a lower extremity is affected.

Nursing Diagnoses and Planning

Nursing diagnoses and related expected patient outcomes most commonly applicable to patients with a fracture include those previously discussed under musculoskeletal injuries and the following (also refer to Nursing Care Guide 20–1 and the discussion of care of patients with a cast, patients in traction, and patients with fixation devices in Chapter 19):

NDx: Altered peripheral tissue perfusion related to the interruption of blood flow secondary to the trauma, edema, thrombus formation, or pressure from the attached device (wrap, cast, traction, or immobilizer)

Planning: Patient Outcomes
1. Patient's affected part has adequate color, and sensation and pulses are present, with no signs of compromised circulation.

2. Patient denies numbness, tingling, or decreased sensation in the affected part.

NDx: Impaired skin integrity related to bedrest, constriction from immobilization device, edema, and internal altered circulation

Planning: Patient Outcomes
1. Patient states causes of skin breakdown and measures to prevent the occurrence or recurrence.
2. Patient relates appropriate knowledge about skin care.
3. Patient is free of skin complications.

NDx: Risk for infection related to increased susceptibility secondary to bedrest, placement of internal or external fixation devices, pressure from restrictive devices, or compromised circulation

Planning: Patient Outcomes
1. Patient's vital signs are within normal ranges for the patient.
2. Signs of infection, such as fever, chills, tachycardia, tachypnea, or pain or burning on urination, or drainage from lesions or at pin sites or under the cast are absent.
3. Patient identifies early signs of infection and measures to prevent infections.

NDx: Self care deficit: feeding, hygiene, toileting, or other activities of daily living requiring mobility related to interference from immobilization of affected part

Planning: Patient Outcomes
1. Patient performs activities of daily living, using assistive devices if necessary.
2. Patient states alternative methods to complete tasks that are restricted by musculoskeletal dysfunction.

NDx: Risk for fluid volume deficit related to blood loss and fluid shifts to the injured area

Planning: Patient Outcomes
1. Skin turgor is firm.
2. Urine output is greater than 30 mL/hour.
3. Mucous membranes are moist.

Nursing Interventions and Evaluation

NDx: Altered peripheral tissue perfusion
Help the patient conserve oxygen needs by encouraging rest and limiting activities. Administer oxygen if appropriate. Elevate the head of the bed to aid in chest expansion. Assess for signs of compromised circulation and document findings. Relieve pressure to the affected part by cutting a window in the cast and padding bony areas. Prevent edema by elevating the extremity unless there is concern that compartment syndrome is developing.

Keep the patient in a comfortable position and reposition frequently to release pressure. Utilize range-of-motion exercises to stimulate circulation.

Text continued on page 923

Nursing Care Guide 20–1

Patients Undergoing Surgery for a Fractured Femur

Preoperative Care

Assessment Findings: Patient appears nervous, withdraws from conversation, clenches hands; patient states fear about the impending surgery; blood pressure, pulse, and respirations are slightly elevated for the patient; patient makes statements about potential problems with immobility and pain; patient seems concerned about preoperative traction therapy.

Nursing Diagnosis: Anxiety related to fears about surgery, preoperative traction equipment, potential risk factors, pain, and fear of loss of mobility

Patient Outcomes	Nursing Interventions	Rationale
Patient reports feeling less fearful, seems relaxed, and is able to rest well.	Explain all preoperative procedures to the patient. Provide a quiet, calm environment with periods of rest during the delivery of nursing care. Ask for assistance from clergy or the patient's significant others.	Having an understanding of the procedure lessens fears and reduces anxiety. Telling the patient what to expect prior to initiating procedures for preoperative preparation reduces fear of the unknown.
Patient's vital signs are within normal ranges for the patient.	Check vital signs after the patient is rested and more relaxed and note any changes.	Changes in vital signs may reflect an increase or decrease in anxiety.
Patient states methods to relax and reduce tension.	Teach deep-breathing techniques and other relaxation strategies.	Relaxation exercises may decrease anxiety and promote rest.
Patient uses coping mechanisms that are effective.	Explore previous successful coping mechanisms and encourage the patient to use them.	Using previously tried, effective coping methods may help relieve the anxiety and stress present at this time.

Evaluation: Compare the patient's status with the expected outcomes. If the outcomes are not met, reassess the patient and revise the plan.

Assessment Findings: Patient seems very concerned about the surgery; patient asks questions about the surgery, the preparation for surgery, the fixation device or cast to be used, the expectations of the intervention, and possible complications.

Nursing Diagnosis: Knowledge deficit: nature of surgery for reduction of the fracture, preoperative preparations, and possible complications

Patient Outcomes	Nursing Interventions	Rationale
Patient accurately describes the purpose of the surgery and the necessity for the traction preoperatively and the immobilizing device postoperatively.	Explain the procedure to the patient, the usual preoperative preparation, and the expected outcomes.	Giving explanations of all the appropriate information about the surgery helps decrease the "unknown" for the patient.

(continued)

Nursing Care Guide 20–1
Patients Undergoing Surgery for a Fractured Femur (continued)

Patient Outcomes	Nursing Interventions	Rationale
Patient relates information about the procedure, complications, and expected results as presented to the patient by the physician. Patient reports an understanding of the preoperative procedures necessary.	Have the patient relate what the physician has explained, and clear up any misunderstandings. Discuss potential complications with the patient. Allow time for questions from the patient or the family. Give the patient literature explaining the procedure and showing what the prosthesis looks like	Reinforcing the previous information from the physician decreases the knowledge deficit and confirms what the physician stated. Having the patient repeat the information gives opportunity to correct any misinformation.

Evaluation: Compare the patient's status with the expected outcomes. If the outcomes are not met, reassess the patient and revise the plan.

Assessment Findings: Patient reports discomfort because of positioning and force of the traction and inability to move freely in bed; patient complains of pain in affected leg; patient grimaces frequently, seems apprehensive, and has an increased pulse and respiratory rate.

Nursing Diagnosis: Pain related to fracture of leg, temporary traction, and/or immobility

Patient Outcomes	Nursing Interventions	Rationale
Patient reports relief of pain and discomfort.	Administer analgesics as prescribed. Reposition the patient as allowed in the bed. Teach the patient how to move by using the overhead trapeze. Check the traction equipment and patient for alignment.	Pain medication administered at regular intervals helps keep pain levels low and vital signs in normal limits. Slight movement in bed releases pressure from bony prominences. Keeping the traction and patient in proper alignment prevents unnecessary extrapulling forces.
Patient's vital signs are within normal limits for the patient, and no nonverbal signs of pain such as grimacing, guarding, restlessness in bed are present.	Watch for nonverbal signs of pain or discomfort. Assess vital signs. Check the patient frequently for pressure areas.	Changes in vital signs may reflect increasing pain levels.

Evaluation: Compare the patient's status with the expected outcomes. If the outcomes are not met, reassess the patient and revise the plan.

Postoperative Care

Assessment Findings: Patient has incision site with dressings and a cast or external fixation device attached to the affected leg.

Nursing Diagnosis: Risk for impaired skin integrity related to wound site, pin sites, or irritation and pressure from cast

(continued)

Patient Outcomes	Nursing Interventions	Rationale
Patient's wound site and/or pin sites remain free from symptoms of infection such as redness, purulent drainage, or excessive swelling.	Check the wound site and suture line for evidence of healing. Watch for signs of infection. Use aseptic technique during dressing changes. Perform pin care as ordered.	Early diagnosis of complications increases potential for successful treatment. Aseptic technique decreases risk of infection.
Patient's skin around and within cast (if applicable) remains intact and free from breakdown.	Tell patient not to put anything into the cast. Check the cast for proper fit.	Putting objects into the cast may cause skin breakdown.
Patient's neurovascular signs are adequate in the affected leg, and vital signs are normal.	Check the neurovascular status proximal and distal to the cast or fixation device. Assess vital signs frequently.	Pressure from a cast that is too tight may cause tissue breakdown. Vital sign changes may indicate infection, especially a systemic one, or compromised circulation in the extremity.

Evaluation: Compare the patient's status with the expected outcomes. If the outcomes are not met, reassess the patient and revise the plan.

Assessment Findings: Patient grimaces, moans, and complains of discomfort at surgery site; patient's blood pressure, pulse, and respiratory rate are elevated.

Nursing Diagnosis: Pain related to invasive surgical procedure with manipulation and application of external fixation device or cast

Patient Outcomes	Nursing Interventions	Rationale
Patient reports relief of pain; patient appears relaxed and comfortable without signs of distress.	Give prescribed analgesics for control of postoperative pain. Make patient comfortable, and provide a quiet atmosphere for rest after surgery.	Relief of postoperative pain allows patient to rest as needed and assists in keeping vital signs within normal limits.
	Check insertion site for signs of infection, which may increase pain at site.	Infection with inflammation increases pain at the site.
	Tell the patient to practice relaxation techniques taught prior to surgery, such as deep breathing and muscle group relaxation exercises.	Relaxation may reduce anxiety and pain.

Evaluation: Compare the patient's status with the expected outcomes. If the outcomes are not met, reassess the patient and revise the plan.

Assessment Findings: Patient seems worried about discharge to the home with crutches and self-care instructions for management of the cast or fixation device; patient is reluctant to work with the physical therapist and to practice exercises and locomotion on crutches; patient states concerns about providing self-care, hygiene, grooming, and activities of daily living when home.

(continued)

Nursing Care Guide 20-1
Patients Undergoing Surgery for a Fractured Femur (continued)

Nursing Diagnosis: Altered health maintenance related to inability to manage mobility on crutches, fear for safety, and self-care, skin care, cast care, or external fixation device care

Patient Outcomes	Nursing Interventions	Rationale
Patient relates accurate information about the home care required and signs of potential problems. Patient demonstrates correct care of skin and pin sites or cast, as described in Chapter 19. Patient states plans for follow-up care with the attending physician. Patient demonstrates appropriate use of crutches and states safety measures for the home environment to prevent falls or other injuries.	Describe the signs requiring immediate medical intervention, such as severe pain or discomfort at surgical site, fever, chills, dizziness, fainting, excessive fatigue, or shortness of breath. Teach the patient the proper care of the skin and pin sites and/or the cast. Assist the patient in practicing using the crutches. Help the patient find ways to increase safety measures in the home environment. Make appropriate referrals for assistance in the home if necessary.	Early diagnosis of potential problems by the patient at home and early medical intervention increase the chance for successful treatment. Having the patient relate information presented reinforces the information and allows for correction of misconceptions. Having the patient practice under supervision allows for a check on the patient's progress and safety practices before discharge.

Evaluation: Compare the patient's status with the expected outcomes. If the outcomes are not met, reassess the patient and revise the plan.

Monitor vital signs and laboratory studies to assess for changes and improvement in status.

Discourage smoking to avoid vasoconstriction. Remove constricting clothing, and keep heavy bed linen from restricting peripheral circulation. Tell the patient to notify the nurse if signs of compromised circulation seem apparent, such as discoloration, pain, swelling, or numbness of an extremity. Keep the patient's legs in a nondependent position when he or she is not ambulating.

NDx: Impaired skin integrity
Teach the patient measures to prevent skin lesions from developing. Avoid irritating sheets or garments. Have the patient inspect the skin frequently and to seek medical assistance if any breakdown or soreness is noted.

Teach the patient to exercise, as tolerated, to promote good circulation. Range-of-motion exercises should be done while the patient is on bedrest. Turn the patient frequently and inspect pressure areas for early signs of breakdown. Keep heavy linen from constricting the peripheral circulation by using a bed cradle. Elevate the patient's legs when he or she is sitting in a chair. Inspect the areas distal to constrictive devices for signs of compromised circulation. If lesions are present, use aseptic technique to cleanse them. Wear gloves during the dressing changes. Teach the patient and family members the proper technique for using and positioning orthopedic devices and for dressing areas of breakdown.

NDx: Risk for infection
Keep the patient warm and avoid extreme changes in temperature in the room. Turn the patient as needed to stimulate circulation to prevent skin breakdown and skin infections. Have the patient deep-breathe and cough frequently to prevent respiratory infections, especially if the patient is on bedrest. Monitor the patient's vital signs frequently, observing subtle changes that may indicate early signs of infection. Report any changes noted.

Encourage a diet high in protein and vitamins to promote healing and high in fiber to prevent constipation. Provide skin care frequently, especially if areas of breakdown are present. Utilize aseptic technique to cleanse around pin sites as ordered. Teach the patient and family to continually observe for signs of infection and notify the physician if signs appear.

NDx: Self care deficit: feeding, hygiene, toileting, or other activities of daily living requiring mobility
Assist the patient with activities of daily living as

needed. Seek alternative methods for the patient to be able to complete the activities when restricted by a cast or immobilization device. Teach the patient how to maneuver with the assistance of supportive aids. Explain how to use other extremities to complete a task, or how to move appropriately with the restrictive device in place, such as how to use crutches when the patient's leg is in a cast, immobilizer, or fixation device. Consult physical therapists or occupational therapists for patient and family teaching sessions.

NDx: Risk for fluid volume deficit

Assess skin turgor, mucus membranes, and vital signs. Record intake and output, including blood loss from drains or wounds. Assess the patient's hemoglobin and hematocrit values. Maintain fluid replacement as ordered by the physician. Ensure that infusion systems are intact and monitor for adverse reactions.

Compare the patient's status with the expected outcomes. If the outcomes are not met, reassess the patient and revise the plan.

Fractures Common in Geriatric Patients

Physical changes accompanying aging, such as changes in posture, a broader-based shuffling gait, poor vision, slower reflexes, and weaker muscles make the elderly individual more prone to falls. In addition, the bone structure of the geriatric patient is osteoporotic, or more porous and brittle than the bone structure of younger adults. Osteoporotic bone is more likely to fracture with minimal trauma. Bones heal more slowly. Slowing the osteoporotic changes in aging bone with diet, vitamins, and exercise and preventing the number of injuries by identifying individuals at increased risk for falls are measures that could help lower the number of fractures in the geriatric population. Some fractures are more common in the elderly patient than in other age groups. The most frequent fractures are those of the hip and the wrist.

HIP FRACTURES

Etiology and Pathophysiology

Fractures of the hip with complications compete with heart disease, cancer, and stroke as a leading cause of mortality in the elderly. Most hip fractures occur from falls that involve only slight trauma and would cause little injury in a young adult.

A hip fracture refers to a fracture of the proximal end of the femur. The three types of hip fractures are fractures of the femoral neck, intertrochanteric fractures, and subtrochanteric fractures.

Femoral neck fractures occur within the hip joint capsule. They have a high incidence of improper healing and avascular necrosis because the medullary vessels in the femoral neck are torn as the bone fragments shift when the neck is fractured.

Intertrochanteric fractures are extracapsular or outside of the hip joint capsule. Occasionally the fracture line extends into the capsule, and circulatory problems can develop.

Subtrochanteric fractures are extracapsular. These are rarely associated with circulatory impairment or healing problems.

Clinical Manifestations

With nondisplaced intracapsular fractures, the individual may still be able to walk. The involved limb may be of normal length and position, or lateral rotation and shortening of the extremity may be present. Pain is usually felt in the groin and may extend to the knee. It is exacerbated by movement of the hip.

Limbs with intertrochanteric fractures appear shortened and externally rotated. These fractures produce more pain than intracapsular fractures. The history of injury usually includes a direct blow to the trochanter.

Subtrochanteric fractures result from a significant force and create an externally rotated, shortened extremity. Because subtrochanteric fractures can involve blood loss of as much as 1500 mL, the risk of hypovolemic shock is high.

Diagnosis

The diagnosis of a hip fracture is made on the basis of history, physical assessment, and x-ray or CT studies.

Management

Most hip fractures are treated by surgical insertion of an internal fixation device. An open reduction with internal fixation is the most common procedure for displaced fractures. The surgery is usually performed under general or spinal anesthesia. It is important to remember that elderly patients are at increased risk for complications of anesthesia, such as paralytic ileus, disorientation, cardiac dysrhythmias, fluid and electrolyte imbalance, and thromboembolism.

The selection of internal fixation device and postoperative care depends on whether the fracture is intracapsular or extracapsular, and whether the fracture is a stable nondisplaced fracture or an unstable displaced fracture. (See Clinical Pathway.)

Extracapsular fractures may be treated with nails, a nail and plate, multiple pins, or a compression screw device. Intracapsular fractures of the neck are usually treated with a femoral head replacement such as an Austin Moore or Thompson prosthesis or, in complicated fractures, a total hip replacement. Some nondisplaced intracapsular fractures with good circulation may be treated with pins. (Refer to the discussion of internal fixation devices in Chapter 19.)

Rarely are elderly patients treated by traction for an extended period of time because of their increased risk for complications from prolonged immobility. Intracapsular fractures can take 24 weeks

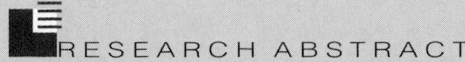

RESEARCH ABSTRACT

What Is It Like to Care for a Friend or Family Member Recovering from a Hip Fracture?

Williams MA, Oberst MT, Bjorklund BC, Hughes SH. Family caregiving in cases of hip fracture. Rehabil Nurs 1996; 21(3):124.

Hip fractures are unexpected events that result in a prolonged recovery period. With health care moving more and more out of hospital settings, family and friends are increasingly being called upon to actively support the recovery of loved ones. Caregivers may be spouses, adult children of patients, or significant family friends. The support that they give may be provided directly in the home or as a supplement to care provided in a nursing home. Some families are able to give the time needed for such physical and emotional support; others, however, must rely on the health-care system to meet these needs.

The ability of nurses to prepare caregivers for the extended recovery experience requires an understanding of the types of demands caregivers are likely to face. To this end, Williams and colleagues studied the experience of adults who were designated as caregivers for people recovering from hip fractures. Their prospective descriptive study included 57 men and women caregivers, with an average age of 60.6 years. The subjects all cared for women patients, with an average age of 78 years, who were recovering from hip fractures after treatment in an acute care setting. The researchers used a combination of written self-report instruments and open-ended interview questions to explore the experience of caregiving over a 6-month period.

As might be expected, caregiving needs varied by the location of the patient and the caregiver. People who cared for patients in the same residence reported higher levels of physical demands than those whose loved ones were in a different residence or nursing home. On the other hand, the self-reported emotional demands were highest for those caregivers whose loved one was recovering in a nursing home. These differences in caregiving demand point to the need for individualizing the preparation of caregivers rather than assuming that they will all have the same experience.

Two months following the fractures, caregivers rated patient progress as worse than expected in the areas of mood, mobility, and pain. The researchers point out that such perceptions may be based on an expectation that the early, rapid rate of recovery that they saw initially would continue rather than slow down. According to the researchers, these expectations may not have been realistic for such elderly patients. The researchers therefore recommend that caregivers be counseled to gauge their expectations of recovery based on the achievement of long-term goals over an extended period, perhaps up to a year.

During interviews with the researchers, caregivers most frequently gave the following advice to future caregivers: have patience, give moral support and encouragement, and encourage independence.

The researchers caution against generalizing their results too broadly, since the characteristics of the sample are not representative of all caregivers and people recovering from hip fractures.

Questions to Consider

1. In your clinical facility, how are the abilities of caregivers to meet the emotional and physical needs of people recovering from hip fractures assessed prior to discharge?
2. In your clinical facility, what instruction or training do caregivers receive to help them meet the emotional and physical needs of people recovering from hip fractures?
3. What referral sources are available in your area to help families meet the emotional and physical needs of people recovering from hip fractures?
4. What community support systems are available in your area for caregivers of people recovering from hip fractures?
5. What information about goals for recovery is shared with families in your clinical facility?
6. How might caregivers be better prepared to assume responsibility for meeting at least some of the recovery needs of the person who has had a hip fracture?

to heal, and extracapsular fractures at least 12 weeks. Buck's skin traction may be used on a short-term basis for preoperative comfort and immobilization. Skeletal traction may replace the Buck traction if surgery is delayed because of existing medical conditions or other circumstances that prohibit surgery.

❖ Settings, Providers, and Collaboration for Care

Patients with hip fractures are most generally admitted to inpatient surgical units or trauma centers for treatment. Rehabilitation after repair may occur in an inpatient facility or on an outpatient basis, depending on the patient's needs and complicating

■ ■ ■ ■ ■ ■ ▶

■ Clinical Pathway for Open Reduction and Internal Fixation of a Hip Fracture

Patient Name _____   Date _____

DRG# _____   Expected LOS _____

	Day 1 (day of surgery)	Day 2 (1st postop day)	Day 3 (2nd postop day)	Day 4 (3rd postop day)	Day 5 (4th postop day)	Day 6 (5th postop day to discharge)
Activity	Bedrest	Physical therapy as ordered ————————————————————→				
	Maintain legs in abduction	Up in chair	Begin assisted ambulation ————————————→			
				Progressive activity as ordered ——————→		
Medication	IV as ordered	IV TKO if tolerating fluids and afebrile				
	Analgesia as needed and ordered ————————————————————————————————→					
	Prophylactic intravenous antibiotics as ordered ————————→			Oral antibiotics as ordered ————————————→		
		Laxatives/stool softeners ————————————————————————→				
		Home meds resumed ————————————————————————→				
Diet	Nothing by mouth	Clear liquid; advance to full liquids	Diet as tolerated ————————————————→			
Treatments/ Nursing Actions	Drainage device ————————→					
	Foley catheter ————————→					
	Incentive spirometer ————————————————————————————————→					
	Ankle pumps/quadriceps exercises ————————————————————————→					
	Ted hose/sequential compression devices as ordered ——————→					
	Apply abduction pillow or splint ————————————————————→					
	Turn every 2 hours as allowed by physician.					
	Assess, measure, and document drainage q8 h	Note weight bearing status ————————————————————→				
	Intake and output ————————————————————→			Discuss discharge needs: extended care, home physical therapy, home care, and equipment needs ————————→		
	Assess vital signs and neurovascular status as needed ——————→					
	Cough & deep-breathe q1–2 h ————————————————————————→					
	ROM of unaffected limbs ————————————————————————————→					
	HOB to 45 degrees	D/C Foley catheter				
Teaching/ Discharge Planning	Pain management	Review preoperative teaching to prevent complications ————————→				
		Teach activity limitations, exercise regimen, and safe use of ambulatory aids ——→				
			Teach signs and symptoms of infection and wound care if needed ————————→			
			Encourage family to visit PT/OT before discharge ————————————————→			

factors. The older adult patient may need more assistance upon discharge than other patients, so a referral to a home health agency may be necessary. The rehabilitation team works with the patient and family to preserve the patient's independence, improve or restore mobility and protect the patient's safety. The home health nurse continues the treatment plan from the physical therapist and physician and assists the patient with care and safety needs in the home.

NURSING PROCESS

Hip Fractures

Assessment

Assess for signs and symptoms of complications as discussed under care of the patient with a fracture in the previous Nursing Process section. This includes looking for signs of compromised circulation, impaired skin integrity, and infection. All these problems may be more common in the older adult. Also assess the patient's extent of immobility and ability to perform self-care activities. Investigate the patient's knowledge about the treatment, self-care needs, care of the surgical site, use of ambulatory aids, and prevention of further injury.

Nursing Diagnoses and Planning

Nursing diagnoses and related expected patient outcomes most commonly applicable to geriatric patients with a hip fracture include those already discussed under fractures and the following:

NDx: Impaired physical mobility related to pain, inability to bear weight, and immobilization device

Planning: Patient Outcomes
1. Patient moves in bed with the assistance of nursing intervention and an overhead trapeze.
2. Patient denies pain or discomfort in affected part.
3. Patient is mobile with the assistance of an ambulatory aid.

NDx: Risk for injury: falls related to weakness from immobility and improper use of ambulatory aids

Planning: Patient Outcomes
1. Patient demonstrates proper use of a prescribed ambulatory aid.
2. Patient states measures to provide for safe locomotion in the home and community.
3. Patient performs prescribed exercises to maintain strength and joint motion.
4. Patient remains injury-free.

Nursing Interventions and Evaluation

NDx: Impaired physical mobility
Teach the patient how to use the overhead trapeze while still on bedrest to increase movement in bed,

as allowed, to prevent complications of immobility. Reposition the patient frequently to stimulate circulation and prevent skin breakdown. Assist the patient in locomotion, once he or she is able, to provide safe use of the ambulatory aid. Use the assistance of physical therapy to instruct the patient and family about the device and to reinforce its safe use. Give analgesics as needed to decrease pain levels that may interfere with the patient's ability to be mobile.

NDx: Risk for injury
Provide assistance during locomotion, as necessary, until the patient becomes skillful with the ambulatory aid. Reinforce the information about the use of the device that was presented by the therapist. Teach the family about safe use of the ambulatory aid. Be sure the patient wears well-fitting shoes with gripper soles while ambulating. Explain how to make the home environment safer for the patient using the ambulatory aid. (Also see Nursing Care Guide 20–1.)

Compare the patient's status with the expected outcomes. If the outcomes are not met, reassess the patient and revise the plan.

WRIST FRACTURES

Etiology and Pathophysiology

The distal radius and ulnar styloid are common sites for osteoporotic fractures in the elderly. A fractured wrist, or Colles' fracture, usually occurs as the individual attempts to break a fall with extended arms and dorsiflexed hands. This type of fracture is extremely common in the elderly and occurs most frequently when the older adult slips and falls on an ice-coated walkway or wet floor.

The injury produces an obvious deformity, described as a dinner-fork deformity, with a proximal depression and a fullness in the distal aspect of the wrist. If the median nerve and flexor tendons are involved, sensation and function of all the fingers in the limb may be affected. The elbow and clavicle should also be inspected for possible injury, because force is often transferred along the skeleton.

Clinical Manifestations
Patients with a Colles' fracture present with pain, swelling, tenderness at the point of fracture, and the dinner-fork deformity.

Diagnosis
The diagnosis is made on the basis of physical examination, history, and radiographic studies.

Management
Medical management usually consists of reduction by closed manipulation and immobilization in a short-arm cast. If there is comminution of the fracture and extensive swelling or soft tissue involve-

CONFUSION, TACHYCARDIA, AND TACHYPNEA AFTER A FRACTURED HIP

After sustaining a fall while visiting her daughter, an 83-year-old woman was admitted to the orthopedic surgical unit with a medical diagnosis of an intertrochanteric fracture of the right hip. She was placed in Buck's extension with 5 lbs of traction to immobilize the joint and to decrease muscle spasm and pain. Her previous medical history included osteoporosis, rheumatoid arthritis, hypertension, hypercholesterolemia, and a vaginal hysterectomy. Vital signs upon admission were: BP 146/92, apical pulse 90 bpm and regular, respiratory rate 18 per minute and unlabored, and temperature 37°C (98.6°F).

An open reduction internal fixation was performed under general anesthesia 2 days after admission, and her recovery thus far had been uncomplicated. During report on the third postoperative day, it was noted that the patient's condition remained stable. The patient was reported to be alert and oriented, vital signs were stable, and her neurovascular status was good. The prophylactic antibiotic and Hemovac drain had been discontinued the previous evening. The patient continued to be medicated with Demerol for pain, which she reported to be a 7 on a scale of 1 to 10. Anticoagulant therapy with coumadin and the application of antiembolic stockings continued as well. The patient had been out of bed in a chair for brief periods limited only by pain, and she needed repeated encouragement to perform deep-breathing and incentive spirometry exercises.

During my morning rounds, I noticed that the patient appeared to be slightly confused and was taking rapid, shallow breaths. Her vital signs were: BP 150/96, apical pulse 116 bpm and regular, respiratory rate 32 per minute, and temperature 38.3°C (101°F). These findings represented a change in the patient's condition. Although vague, these clinical manifestations (confusion, tachycardia, tachypnea) could indicate any number of possible complications related to the patient's past medical history or her recent surgery. I recognized that confusion, particularly in the elderly, along with tachycardia and tachypnea, may be associated with the following;

Decreased cardiac output from heart failure or acute myocardial infarction
Hypoxemia from a pulmonary embolism, fat embolism, atelectasis, or pneumonia
Sepsis
Side effects of medications
Dehydration
Pain

The elevated blood pressure supported the possibility of hypoxemia, sepsis, or pain. The elevated temperature, although slight, could represent an infectious process in an elderly patient.

In light of the report of the patient's limited activity and reluctance to participate in breathing exercises and the current clinical picture, I began to suspect that the patient had developed a hospital-acquired pneumonia. Because additional information was critical to help identify the problem, I continued my assessment.

Questions about the presence of chest pain revealed occasional discomfort that was sharp and stabbing, increased with deep-breathing and coughing, and did not radiate. The patient's skin was pink, warm, and dry. Peripheral pulses were bounding. Capillary refill was less than 3 seconds. There was no evidence of deep vein thrombosis, petechiae on the upper torso, jugular vein distention, or dependent edema. The dressing was dry and intact, and the wound was free of the clinical manifestations of infection.

A comprehensive respiratory assessment revealed decreased breath sounds and scattered crackles over the bases of both lungs upon auscultation. There was also dullness over both bases upon percussion. Sporadic coughing produced scanty amounts of purulent sputum.

The evidence of an adequate cardiac output (elevated blood presure, strong peripheral pulses, capillary refill within normal limits, and the color and temperature of the extremities), and the absence of any evidence of deep vein thrombosis and petechiae did not support the likelihood of a cardiogenic event, pulmonary embolism, or fat embolism.

Despite the absence of the classic signs of pneumonia (high fever and shaking chills), the original assessments (altered mentation, tachycardia, and tachypnea), accompanied by pleuritic pain associated with breathing and coughing, the presence of a cough and purulent sputum, and the changes in the patient's breath sounds, strongly supported my suspicion of pneumonia. The likelihood of this complication was further supported by the existing risk factors, which included the patient's age, immobility, use of analgesics, and recent anesthesia.

I knew that hospital-acquired pneumonia is a serious disease that requires immediate intervention. I also knew that high mortality rates in the elderly result from complications of pneumonia, such as pleural effusion, pneumothorax, sepsis, acute respiratory distress syndrome, and respiratory failure. I therefore took the following immediate steps:

CLINICAL ? THINKING

(continued)

1. I placed the patient in semi-Fowler's position.
2. I called the physician and reported my assessments.
3. I administered oxygen and established an IV line for access, as per hospital policy.
4. I attached a pulse oximeter.
5. I continued to monitor the patient's vital signs and level of consciousness for signs of hypoxemia.
6. I provided the patient with emotional support and clear explanations of all procedures.
7. I documented my findings and actions.

The physician ordered a STAT chest x-ray, arterial blood gases (ABGs), a 12-lead electrocardiogram, high-concentration oxygen therapy, IV fluids, a complete blood count, and blood and sputum specimens for culture. Intravenous antibiotic therapy was ordered and initiated following the collection of the culture specimens. The chest x-ray and ABGs confirmed my suspicion of pneumonia.

The pneumonia resolved, and the patient recovered without further incident following antibiotic, respiratory, and supportive therapy. Thorough assessments and sound clinical judgments by the nurse saved the patient from worsening hypoxemia, respiratory failure necessitating intubation and mechanical ventilation, and possibly death.

Think Critically

What additional nursing interventions might have prevented the development of the pneumonia?

How did each of the patient's risk factors contribute to the development of pneumonia?

Was placing the patient in semi-Fowler's position the best action by the nurse? How would the nurse's action have differed if the patient had undergone a total hip replacement?

What similarities and differences would the nurse have noted if the patient had developed a pulmonary embolism? Fat embolism? How would the nurse's actions have differed?

What deviations from normal limits would the nurse anticipate when evaluating the patient's ABGs?

What was the rationale for collecting the culture specimens prior to the initiation of antibiotic therapy?

What nursing interventions would be implemented to improve the patient's respiratory status?

What realistic short-term expected outcomes might the nurse include in the nursing care plan once the suspicion of pneumonia was confirmed?

What specific drug-related nursing actions would be implemented once antibiotic therapy was ordered and initiated?

Under which conditions would the nurse question a medical order for high-concentration oxygen therapy?

The patient's daughter asks how the pneumonia could have developed if the patient was on an antibiotic following surgery. What is the nurse's explanation?

Following the initiation of antibiotic therapy the patient stated, "I'm on medication now and that should be enough; it hurts too much to cough and deep-breathe." What is the nurse's best response?

What teaching should be included in the discharge plan for the patient in order to prevent the recurrence of pneumonia at home?

---

ment, percutaneous pinning, open reduction with internal fixation, or an external fixation device may be used for immobilization.

❖ **Settings, Providers, and Collaboration for Care**

Treatment of wrist fractures can be performed in an outpatient emergency room or clinic unless internal or external fixation is warranted. This type of treatment requires short-stay hospitalization. Upon discharge, the nurse provides instructions to the patient for care at home and when to return for a follow-up visit.

NURSING PROCESS
Wrist Fractures

Assessment

Assess the patient's affected wrist for pain, swelling, discoloration, or malalignment. Check the neurovascular status proximal and distal to the injury by palpating for pulses, feeling for warmth of the part, and assessing for decreased sensation. Ask the patient about numbness or tingling in the wrist, hand, or even in the entire arm. Review how the injury occurred and note what treatment was instituted at the time of the occurrence. Be sure to assess the entire patient, because other injuries could have easily occurred in the older patient during the fall. Determine the patient's understanding of the injury and treatment necessary.

Nursing Diagnoses and Planning

Nursing diagnoses and related expected patient outcomes most commonly applicable to geriatric patients with a wrist fracture include the following:

NDx: Pain related to joint trauma, pressure from edema, and immobilization

Planning: Patient Outcomes

1. Patient denies pain in affected part.
2. Patient states methods to decrease pain by reduction of swelling and keeping immobilizer properly applied.

NDx: Ineffective management of therapeutic regimen (individuals) related to lack of knowledge about the injury, management of cast or immobilization device, exercises to perform, and prevention of re-injury

Planning: Patient Outcomes

1. Patient states accurate information about the cause of the injury and methods to prevent re-injury.
2. Patient demonstrates proper application of the immobilizer device or care of the cast, how much weight-lifting or weight-bearing is allowed, and when the device may be removed, if applicable.
3. Patient demonstrates proper care of pin sites, if applicable, and signs of infection.
4. Patient demonstrates exercises, as taught, to maintain strength and range of motion of joints.

NDx: Self care deficit: grooming and hygiene related to inability to use wrist or hand of the affected arm

Planning: Patient Outcomes

1. Patient demonstrates use of assistive devices if necessary to aid in self-care activities.
2. Patient is able to use opposite arm, wrist, or hand to perform self-care.

Nursing Intervention and Evaluation

NDx: Pain

Administer prescribed analgesics and explain the dosage, frequency, side effects, and expected therapeutic effects of the medications. Caution the patient not to perform tasks that require mental alertness while taking pain medication. Teach the patient to check for tightness of the cast or immobilizer, looking for signs of swelling or diminished sensation and movement in the distal part of the affected extremity. Tell the patient to elevate the arm to reduce swelling and thus reduce pain.

NDx: Ineffective management of therapeutic regimen (individuals)

Teach the patient about the injury, how to prevent falls, methods of prevention of further injury to the

wrist, and appropriate treatment. Explain how to apply the immobilizer or wrap to the affected part (if not casted) and have the patient perform a return demonstration. Check to see that it is not too tight, and tell the patient how to check for improper fit. Explain that increased swelling, discoloration, and decreased sensation in the affected part may be signs of improper fit of the device or a cast that is too tight, and that prolonged pressure could cause severe problems if not relieved. Reinforce the physician's instruction about weight-lifting with the hand. Teach the patient and family proper pin care, if applicable, and signs of infection to observe for at the pin site. Demonstrate prescribed exercises to the patient and encourage participation in the exercise regimen to prevent loss of strength and joint motion.

NDx: Self care deficit: grooming and hygiene

Assist the patient in performing activities of self-care. Explain how assistive devices may aid the patient in performing self-care. Help the patient learn to use the other hand to complete tasks. Teach the family what they need to do to assist the patient during the healing process.

Compare the patient's status with the expected outcomes. If the outcomes are not met, reassess the patient and revise the plan.

Traumatic Amputations

A traumatic amputation refers to any injury that cuts off an appendage or body projection. The body part, if it can be recovered, is saved for possible reattachment. It is placed in a plastic bag, which is then put in a container of crushed ice. The amputated part is transported with the patient to the emergency room for continued care. Fingers, toes, arms, hands, and other body parts have been successfully reattached. The patient is stabilized as quickly as possible with intravenous fluids, treatment to other affected areas, and medications. Once this has occurred, the patient is taken to surgery for the microvascular anastomosis of the amputated body part. If reimplantation is not possible, débridement and closure of the residual body part occur. Prognosis varies, depending on the time since the injury, access to an institution performing microsurgery, degree of damage to the amputated part, and the patient's stability, age, and health status prior to the incident.

NURSING PROCESS
Traumatic Amputation with Reattachment Surgery
Assessment

After the patient has been stabilized, assess the patient's awareness of the situation and knowledge of the impending surgery. Continue to check vital signs. Assess the patient's pain, noting the intensity, whether analgesics have been given, and the patient's response. Determine whether the patient has significant others available for assistance and emotional support. Because the time between the presentation of the patient to the hospital and the initiation of surgical intervention is extremely limited, most nursing interventions, other than the emergency care, occur in the postoperative period.

In addition to the usual postoperative care, as described in Chapter 6, assess the patient's neurovascular status proximal and distal to the surgical site. Palpate pulses and check color, sensation, and edema of the part. If the entire limb is bandaged, assess the bandages for tightness and ask the patient about sensation in the part. It is expected that there may be no sensation for some time. Check for drainage on the bandages.

Assess the patient's anxiety level, coping ability, and understanding of the incident and the treatment regimen. Note the availability of support systems for the patient.

Assess pain and general discomfort. Check whether the patient is able to rest and sleep at intervals.

Nursing Diagnoses and Planning

Nursing diagnoses and related expected patient outcomes most commonly applicable to patients with a traumatic amputation undergoing reattachment surgery include the following:

NDx: Anxiety related to traumatic injury, potential permanent loss of limb, and pain

Planning: Patient Outcomes
1. Patient denies anxiety, fear, or nervousness about the surgery and potential outcome of the surgery.
2. Patient appears relaxed and is able to rest at intervals and to sleep well.
3. Patient does not display signs of increased anxiety, such as twitching, nervousness, or increased respirations and pulse.

NDx: Pain related to trauma, manipulation during surgery, and usual postoperative physiologic events

Planning: Patient Outcomes
1. Patient denies pressure, pain, discomfort, or alteration in sensation.
2. Patient is able to exercise and tolerate mobility (of unaffected body parts) without interference from acute pain episodes.

NDx: Risk for infection related to original injury and surgical intervention

Planning: Patient Outcomes
1. Patient's vital signs are within normal ranges for the patient.
2. Signs of infection, such as fever, chills, tachycardia, tachypnea, pain or burning on urination, or drainage from suture lines or at intravenous site are absent.

3. Patient identifies early signs of infection and measures to prevent infections.

NDx: Impaired home maintenance management related to lack of knowledge about postoperative expectations, potential for rehabilitation and ability to manage self-care, and resources available for assistance

Planning: Patient Outcomes
1. Patient states accurate information about the surgical intervention and expected postoperative course as explained by the physician.
2. Patient demonstrates adapted methods for providing self-care.
3. Patient demonstrates exercises for maintenance of mobility of nonaffected extremities and any prescribed for the affected area.
4. Patient recalls resources available for assistance if necessary.

Nursing Interventions and Evaluation

NDx: Anxiety
Explain the purpose of all treatments to the patient. Teach the patient how to reposition in the bed. Prior to performing any procedure on the patient, explain the steps of the procedure and the reason for it. Allow the patient time to ask questions and relay concerns. Reinforce information from the physician to the patient. Give support without offering unrealistic reassurances.

Check vital signs and watch for changes that indicate increased anxiety. Teach the patient relaxation methods and strategies to cope with the fears of hospitalization and medical interventions. Have the patient practice range-of-motion exercises to help relieve discomfort from the static position and to maintain muscle tone and joint motion of unaffected extremities, as allowed. Also, provide diversional activity for the patient to relieve the boredom and anxiety from bedrest.

NDx: Pain
Place the patient in comfortable positions and reposition frequently. Check the affected extremity to ensure proper alignment and positioning. Look for signs of pressure causing pain, such as from the bandages or positioning of the extremity. Use pillows to support bony prominences.

Administer analgesics as prescribed. Assess when the pain is most severe, and allow the patient to rest during those periods. Administer pain medications prior to activity periods so that the patient can better tolerate the movement.

Help the patient find alternate methods to alleviate or to be able to tolerate the pain. Show the patient relaxation techniques. Teach the patient the use of patient-controlled analgesia if ordered.

Inspect the skin and palpate pulses in distal areas for signs of compromised circulation or skin breakdown caused by constrictive bandages, which may be the cause of the pain. Tell the patient to report any signs of pain, numbness, or temperature changes immediately.

NDx: Risk for infection

Keep the patient warm and avoid extreme changes in temperature in the room. Turn the patient as needed to stimulate circulation to prevent skin breakdown and skin infections. Massage bony prominences. Have the patient deep-breathe and cough frequently to prevent respiratory infections, especially while the patient is on bedrest. Monitor the patient's vital signs frequently, observing for subtle changes that may indicate early signs of infection. Report any changes noted.

Promote good nutrition for proper healing by serving meals the patient will eat, in a relaxed attractive atmosphere. Encourage a high-protein, high-vitamin diet. Use aseptic technique when changing bandages and cleaning the suture line, as ordered. Check the intravenous site for signs of infection and use aseptic technique when cleaning around the insertion site. Because early identification and treatment may limit the severity of the infection, teach the patient and family to continually observe for signs of developing infection and to notify the physician if such signs appear. Stress the importance of taking antibiotics as prescribed.

NDx: Impaired home maintenance management

Explain all interventions to the patient. Tell the patient about the expectations postoperatively. Reinforce the physician's information about recovery and rehabilitation.

Teach the patient about the prescribed medications. Explain the correct dosage, frequency, side effects, and therapeutic effects. Tell the patient when to notify the physician if any problems become evident. Teach the patient signs of complications such as extreme pain, discoloration, intense swelling, temperature changes, and decreased sensation after normal sensation has returned to the affected part. Teach the patient to avoid factors that would increase vasoconstriction such as nicotine, caffeine, or cold for about 2 weeks postoperatively.

Assist the patient with activities of daily living as needed. Seek alternative methods for the patient to be able to complete the activities when restricted by the affected extremity. Teach the patient how to maneuver with the assistance of supportive aids if the affected part was a lower extremity. Explain how to use other extremities to complete a task, or how to move appropriately, such as how to use crutches when weight-bearing is not allowed on the reattached extremity. Seek the assistance of physical therapists or occupational therapists when necessary for consultation or teaching sessions for the patient and family.

Rehabilitation may be necessary for an extended period of time. Provide a list to the patient and family of possible resources for assistance in the community. Make appropriate referrals prior to the patient's discharge.

Compare the patient's status with the expected outcomes. If the outcomes are not met, reassess the patient and revise the plan.

COMPLICATIONS OF MUSCULOSKELETAL INJURIES

A number of complications can result from major trauma to the musculoskeletal system. Immediate complications may occur following the trauma or up to 3 days thereafter. Delayed complications arise secondary to the initial injury and can develop as long as 6 months to 1 year after the injury. Although all complications are not preventable, early detection and treatment lessen their severity and long-term effects. Thrombophlebitis, deep vein thrombosis, and pulmonary embolism are complications of musculoskeletal injuries that usually occur early in the postinjury course.

Immediate Complications

SHOCK

Loss of blood, either internally from a fracture of the pelvis, femur, ribs, or vertebrae or from an open compound fracture, can result in hypovolemic shock. Hypovolemic shock usually develops immediately or within the first 48 hours after injury. The patient becomes restless, thirsty, agitated, and confused, followed by a decrease in the level of consciousness. The pulse becomes weak and thready as the blood pressure falls. A narrowed pulse pressure is indicative of shock. Respirations are rapid, and the patient's skin becomes cool and clammy.

Immediate splinting of suspected fractures prior to transport helps prevent excess blood loss. If profuse external bleeding is apparent, pressure is maintained on the site. If paramedic aid is available, parenteral fluids are started at the scene of the injury. Otherwise, intravenous fluid replacement is initiated immediately upon arrival at the health care facility. Shock and internal bleeding must be treated before the fracture can be reduced and immobilized.

COMPARTMENT SYNDROME

Etiology and Pathophysiology

Compartment syndrome is an increase in the pressure within a fascial muscle compartment. A rise in intracompartmental pressure may occur after a closed-fracture injury, crushing injuries, burns, application of a dressing or cast that is too tight, or when a muscle swells after exercise. The forearm and lower leg are most commonly affected by this syndrome. As the pressure within the muscle compartment exceeds diastolic blood pressure, circulation to the muscle is impaired or interrupted completely and necrosis results. Tissue damage can occur within 30 minutes. Elevated pressures for more than 4 hours can result in irreversible damage and limb loss.

Clinical Manifestations

A major clinical manifestation is severe or increased pain in the affected area that is not relieved by narcotics. The pain increases on passive stretching of the muscle. The muscle feels tense and swollen on palpation. The patient may experience numbness and tingling in and distal to an involved muscle as a result of nerve compression. Decrease in movement, strength, and sensation may occur. Paralysis may then follow. Loss of the distal pulse is a late sign of compartment syndrome.

Diagnosis

Diagnosis is made on the basis of physical symptoms and measurement of the muscle compartment pressure. Intracompartment pressure is measured by inserting a needle into the muscle compartment. The needle is connected to a saline-filled tube, which is, in turn, connected to a manometer. The specialized monitoring device can provide a constant read-out of compartment pressure.

Management

When compartment syndrome is suspected, dressings or constrictive coverings should be removed and the extremity should not be higher than the heart. If relief of compartment syndrome is not evident, abnormal pressure within the muscle compartment is released by fasciotomy, a surgical incision of the fascia. A monitored intracompartment pressure of 30 mm Hg or higher is considered sufficient to impair blood flow. A fasciotomy may be performed at lower compartment pressures in hypotensive patients. Diligent nursing assessment and early diagnosis are the most important steps in treating compartment syndrome to prevent a functionless extremity and limb loss. The complications of compartment syndrome include infection, amputation, contractures, loss of extremity function, and renal failure.

FAT EMBOLISM

Etiology and Pathophysiology

Fat embolism is a potentially fatal complication of long-bone fractures and multiple trauma. Theories differ as to where the fat globules that form the emboli originate. The mechanical theory hypothesizes that the fracture of the bone releases fat globules from the marrow cavity into the blood stream. The physiochemical theory identifies the stress response of the body and the release of catecholamines by the sympathetic nervous system at the time of injury as the cause. The catecholamines alter the metabolism of fatty acids, which leads to accumulation of fat globules in the blood. Once the fat globules enter the circulation, they cause platelets to clump and form fat emboli. Pulmonary fat emboli damage the alveolar capillary membranes and obstruct capillary blood flow, similar to the effects of a pulmonary embolus of vascular origin. Disruption of the exchange of oxygen and carbon dioxide across the capillary membrane results in pulmonary insufficiency, pulmonary infarct, and alveolar collapse. Fat emboli can also lodge in vessels in the heart, brain, kidneys, and other tissues and organs of the body, causing circulatory insufficiency, tissue infarcts, and sudden death.

Clinical Manifestations

The symptoms of fat embolism occur within the first 72 hours after injury. Headache, drowsiness, irritability, memory loss, confusion, rapid pulse, and fever may occur. Pulmonary symptoms include tachypnea, dyspnea, use of accessory muscles, and wheezing caused by blockage of air passages. Inspiratory stridor is caused by obstruction of the upper airways from copious thick white sputum. Petechiae may appear on the neck, upper chest, shoulder, axillae, buccal membranes, and conjunctiva in a small percentage of patients. The petechiae, which result from intravascular thromboses secondary to decreased oxygenation, are characteristic of fat emboli and help differentiate fat embolism from a blood clot embolism and adult respiratory distress syndrome.

Diagnosis

Medical diagnosis is made on the basis of history of a long-bone fracture, diagnostic data, and presenting symptoms. Blood gas values usually indicate a decrease in PaO_2 to lower than 60 mm Hg, a $PaCO_2$ value higher than 50 mm Hg, and acidosis. Blood lipase and sedimentation rate are elevated.

Management

The goals of medical management are to improve oxygenation and prevent further deterioration. Oxygen in high concentrations is administered. Coughing and deep-breathing or positive end-expiratory pressure mechanical breathing, or both, improve ventilation. Low-molecular-weight dextran and intravenous fluids are carefully titrated to prevent both shock and an increase in pulmonary congestion. Steroids are administered to decrease lung inflammation and the cerebral edema associated with hypoxemia. Heparin may be administered to prevent new emboli from forming. Some physicians believe that steroids and heparin should be used prophylactically in high-risk patients, whereas others advocate the use of aspirin. Patients are placed on bedrest to prevent the chance of movement of the bone fragments and the release of additional fat globules.

Delayed Complications

JOINT STIFFNESS AND CONTRACTURES

Joint stiffness is a common sequela of musculoskeletal injuries that involve a diseased or older joint. Contracture formation may occur with a joint fracture or dislocation that causes a loss of range of motion. Careful positioning, early passive exercises, and progressive active and resistive exercises are the key to preventing joint stiffness and contractures. Once intra-articular adhesions occur, manipulation under anesthesia and aggressive physiotherapy may be required to reverse them. Nonsurgical treatment of contractures includes the use of casts, splints, and traction. Intra-articular structures that have been fractured are also at risk for the development of early osteoarthritis.

INFECTION

A bone infection is called osteomyelitis. Direct contamination of a bone by bacteria may occur as a result of an open fracture, during open reduction of a fracture, or from infection of a superficial wound or surgical incision. Infection of the bone interferes with the process of fracture healing and can result in permanent disability.

Gas gangrene, from gram-positive *Clostridium perfringens*, or tetanus may also develop in grossly contaminated open fractures. Callus formation and union of the fracture fragments may be prevented by the presence of bacteria. Wound infections may aggravate overall healing even though the bone may continue to heal and allow weight-bearing. Wound infections also increase the risk for development of bone infections.

Symptoms of osteomyelitis include pain in the affected area, local erythema, a draining tract, and fever. Local symptoms of gas gangrene include cellulitis engorged with gas bubbles and a foul-smelling watery exudate. The patient may also appear anemic, have a decreased pulse rate, and if untreated, develop septic shock. Symptoms of a wound infection include

Redness, swelling, and warmth at the site
Purulent drainage
Low-grade temperature elevation

HEALING PROBLEMS

MALUNION. A fracture that heals in a position of deformity is referred to as a malunion. This complication leaves a limb at a mechanical disadvantage and may be a severe problem in lower extremities. A malunion is identified on x-ray examination, usually during routine follow-up.

If complete union has not yet occurred, the deformity may be treated by manipulation and recasting. If fracture repair is complete, refracture and alignment or an osteotomy may be necessary.

DELAYED UNION. A delayed union is identified when the expected average time for a fracture to heal has passed without consolidation of the fracture. The age, nutritional status, and general health of the individual are considered in the expected time for bone healing. A delayed union is evident

on x-ray film. If a cause can be determined, treatment is focused on correcting the cause of the delayed union. A delayed union may progress to a nonunion.

NONUNION. Nonunion is diagnosed when a fracture has failed to heal within the expected time and x-ray films show sclerosed fracture ends, a fluid gap between fragments, or a fibrocartilaginous union. Causes of nonunion include infection, excessive movement of the bone fragments, interposed soft tissue, inadequate blood supply, failed internal fixation, and concurrent pathologic disorders such as metastatic cancer and osteoporosis. As many as 10% of all fractures become delayed unions or nonunions. The distal one-third of the tibia is the most common site for delayed union and nonunion healing problems.

Symptoms of nonunion include local pain and instability of the fracture. A nonunion is diagnosed on the basis of assessment, history, and x-ray examination. The goals of medical management are identification and correction of causative factors and promotion of bone healing. Treatments instituted to promote formation of a healthy fibrous union may include bone grafts and use of an electrical bone stimulator. Bone grafts may be autogenous (using the patient's own bone), homogeneous (using bone from another person), or heterogeneous (using a synthetic calcium substance). Autografts are frequently taken from the iliac crest, greater trochanter, or fibula. Surgical incisions at both the donor and graft sites require meticulous wound care to prevent further complications such as osteomyelitis.

An electrical bone stimulator may be used to promote bone healing instead of, or in addition to, bone grafts. Healthy bone possesses a positive electrical potential, which increases with mechanical stress. Fractured bone develops a negative charge. Although scientists are uncertain how it works, electrical stimulation produces an electromagnetic field around the fracture site that promotes new bone growth.

The bone stimulator's electrical current is one thousand times weaker than that of a cardiac pacemaker. Three types of electrical bone stimulators are available:

- An implantable device similar to a battery in appearance, which requires surgery for insertion and an incision for removal
- A semi-invasive device with percutaneous pins that is inserted into the fracture site under fluoroscopy and has an external battery pack
- A noninvasive apparatus that the patient wears around the fracture site

The external noninvasive device consists of electrical coils within a pack that is wrapped externally around the fracture site. It is worn for 10 to 12 hours a day until healing is complete.

The success rate for all types of electrical bone stimulators is 75 to 85%. The average time for healing is 16 weeks. The decision on the type of device to use is determined by physician preference and patient compliance.

REFLEX SYMPATHETIC DYSTROPHY

Reflex sympathetic dystrophy is a complication of unknown etiology that occurs in conjunction with severe sprains and fractures of the wrist and ankle. The hand or foot becomes swollen and painful, and range of motion is impaired. X-ray films reveal patchy osteoporosis. The skin over the area appears glossy, reddened, and swollen. Medical management involves aggressive physical therapy and pain management.

PATHOLOGIC OSSIFICATION

Pathologic ossification (also called myositis ossificans) develops in fractures in which the periosteum is stripped from the bone during injury. Ossification extends into the hematoma, soft tissue, and muscle around the fracture site. Fractures of the elbow frequently develop this complication. The symptoms are painful and limited motion of the involved area. Medical management consists of controlled exercise of the involved area and sometimes surgical removal of abnormal bone growth.

AVASCULAR NECROSIS

Necrosis of bone and intra-articular structures can occur from a lack of circulation to the tissue following injury as a result of malalignment, thrombus, or constriction from an immobilizing device or wrap. The ischemic bone becomes necrotic and collapses. Frequent sites of avascular necrosis are the femoral head, the body of the talus bone in the ankle, and the carpal scaphoid bone and lunate bone in the wrist. This complication is most prevalent in the femoral head because the circulatory supply to the intracapsular tissue is disrupted in fractures of the neck of the femur and in hip dislocations posteriorly.

The patient with avascular necrosis experiences increasing pain, limb instability, and decreasing function of the involved area. Diagnosis is confirmed by x-ray films, bone scan, and CT scan that show a collapsing, necrotic bone structure.

Initial medical management attempts to prevent further osteonecrosis. Treatment differs depending on the stage or extent of the necrosis. Protective non-weight-bearing and removal of a core of the cancellous bone through a drill hole in the metaphysis to decrease pressure may halt the degenerative process. When conservative efforts fail to prevent progression of necrosis, a bone graft, bone prosthesis, joint fusion, joint replacement, or amputation may be necessary.

❖ Settings, Providers, and Collaboration for Care

Complications of musculoskeletal injuries often require hospitalization during the acute phase of the complication. During hospitalization collaboration occurs among nurses, physicians, physical therapists, occupational therapists, dietitians, and social workers to plan and treat the patient's needs. Discharge from the hospital following a musculoskeletal complication often requires follow-up by the home health nurse for assessment, dressing changes, patient teaching, and continuation of the medical treatment plan and physical therapy regimen.

Neoplasia

A neoplasm is any abnormal cell growth that serves no useful purpose and derives its nutrition from, and often destroys, healthy surrounding tissues. Bone tumors are neoplasms that may be either osteoblastic (bone-forming) or osteolytic (bone-destroying). The exact cause of the formation and growth of bone tumors is not known. Bone tumors can be classified by the type of tissue they arise from. Osteogenic tumors arise from osseous or bone tissue. Chondrogenic tumors arise from cartilage. Collagenic tumors arise from connective tissue such as tendons or ligaments. Myelogenic tumors arise from the bone marrow. Table 20–1 describes common types of bone tumors.

Bone tumors can cause pain, deformity, weakening of the bone structure, and pathologic fractures. Bone necrosis may develop secondary to disruption of vascular supply by pressure from the growing tumor mass or actual destruction of blood vessels. Bone tumors may be further classified by their destructive capacity and cellular activity as either benign or malignant.

BENIGN BONE TUMORS

Etiology and Pathophysiology

Most benign bone tumors occur in children and young adults. They grow slowly and do not metastasize or spread through the blood or lymphatic system to other body parts. The benign tumor can weaken bone structure through compression and displacement of adjacent normal bone tissue. Some benign bone tumors are described in Table 20–1.

Clinical Manifestations

Clinical manifestations of benign bone tumors include deformity, swelling over the involved area, and restricted motion. Pain is persistent and may increase with weight-bearing. If the bone structure is weakened or necrosis has developed as a result of impaired circulation, pathologic fractures following minimal or no trauma may occur.

Table 20–1

Common Types of Bone Tumors

Type	Description
BENIGN TUMORS	
Osteochondroma	A common tumor that appears on x-ray film as a bone spur or projection with a cartilage cap. It usually develops near an epiphyseal growth plate during adolescence. The tumor may stop growing with skeletal maturation. Symptoms include a palpable nodule and mild pain.
Compact osteoma	Growth of dense bone from the outer surface of bones of the facial sinuses and skull. It may be painful and cause facial deformity.
Osteoid osteoma	Osseofibrous tumor usually found in the long bones of the femur and tibia, but can grow in any bone of the body. Tissue is reddish gray and granular in appearance. Occurs most frequently in adolescent and young adult males and causes severe, localized pain. May present as a painful scoliosis with vertebral involvement.
Cyst	A unicameral (single-chamber) cyst arises from bone tissue. It contains blood or amber or clear fluid. An aneurysmal bone cyst arises from vascular tissue. It consists of large spaces filled with blood and looks like a bubble on x-ray film.
Giant cell tumor	A tumor characterized by large "giant cells" with many nuclei. The tumor looks like soap bubbles on x-ray film. Although it is a benign tumor, it is aggressive, destroys some surrounding tissue, and has the potential to become malignant. It is usually painful. The tumor occurs most frequently in the distal femur, proximal tibia, and distal radius. Females are affected more often than males.
Enchondroma	An oval tumor of hyaline cartilage. It usually develops on the small tubular bones of the hands and feet. The inside of the tumor is pale and bluish.
Hemangioma	A highly vascular cavernous tumor filled with red blood cells. It may appear anywhere on the body but is frequently found on the face, skull, or neck.
MALIGNANT TUMORS	
Osteosarcoma	This is the most common malignant bone tumor, characterized by extreme pain, rapid growth, and metastasis. It is more common in young males than other populations. Treatment usually involves resection and chemotherapy.
Chondrosarcoma	The tumor arises from chondroblasts (cartilage tissue). The incidence is highest among middle-aged males. It primarily affects the bones in the trunk, pelvis, and proximal femur. It is slow-growing and produces persistent dull pain. The lesions show osseous destruction with the presence of scattered areas of ringlet calcification on x-ray film. This tumor tends to be radioresistant and thus is treated with surgery and chemotherapy.
Fibrosarcoma	The tumor arises from fibrous connective tissue. These tumors are slow-growing and can occur at any age. They are found more frequently in males than females. Treatment includes surgical excision with radiotherapy.
Malignant fibrous histiocytoma	The tumor arises from fibrous connective tissue. It grows rapidly and is destructive to adjacent bone. Lesions can occur at any site but are primarily seen in the long bones. The overlying skin is usually fixed to the tumor. There is no correlation between the occurrence of this tumor and age and gender of affected people. Treatment is similar to that for osteosarcoma.
Ewing's sarcoma	This is a rare, highly malignant tumor that originates in the marrow and metastasizes early in its course. It occurs mainly in long bones or the flat bones of the pelvis and ribs. It is more common in young males. Pain is frequently extreme. It is treated with chemotherapy or radiation and surgery, or both.
Multiple myeloma	This is a primary tumor arising from plasma cells in the bone marrow. It is most common in middle to old age, with a higher incidence in males. It is rarely diagnosed before bone destruction and metastasis have occurred. Pain is the most common symptom.

Diagnosis

Preliminary diagnosis of a benign bone tumor is made on the basis of history and physical examination. X-ray films, bone scans, arteriography, and surgical biopsy are used for differential diagnosis. Blood values are usually normal with benign tumors.

Management

The goals of medical management are pain relief and prevention of complications such as pathologic fracture. Surgery is not necessary if tumor growth has stopped, if there is little or no deformity, and if the patient is free of pain.

When surgery is indicated, curettage or resection of the lesion is performed. If the defect from a resected tumor is large, bone grafts may be required. The involved area is protected by splints or casts until the bone heals. Internal fixation may also be used depending on the size and location of the lesion. Ambulatory aids are used if a lower extremity is involved. To relieve pain, analgesics are prescribed, and the affected area is handled and positioned carefully. Prophylactic antibiotics and aseptic wound care are routine to prevent osteomyelitis. Periodic re-evaluation after treatment for a benign bone tumor is important because recurrence of benign lesions is common and malignant tumors may develop.

NURSING PROCESS
Benign Bone Tumors

Assessment

Review the patient's history, results of diagnostic studies, and presenting symptoms. Determine the patient's and family's understanding of the diagnosis. Evaluate the site for symptoms of pain, swelling, deformity, or restricted motion. Ask the patient about problems with mobility of the affected part. Note the patient's anxiety level and what coping mechanisms are in place.

Nursing Diagnoses and Planning

Nursing diagnoses and related expected patient outcomes most commonly applicable to patients with a benign bone tumor include the following:

NDx: Anxiety related to diagnosis, potential permanent loss of limb, and pain

Planning: Patient Outcomes
1. Patient denies anxiety, fear, or nervousness about the diagnosis, therapy, and potential outcome of the therapy.
2. Patient appears relaxed and is able to rest at intervals and to sleep well.
3. Signs of increased anxiety such as twitching, nervousness, increased respirations and pulse, or withdrawal from self-care activities are absent.

NDx: Pain related to effects of the tumor, swelling, and deformity

Planning: Patient Outcomes
1. Patient denies pain in affected part.
2. Patient states methods to decrease pain by reduction of swelling, relaxation strategies, and appropriate use of analgesics.

NDx: Knowledge deficit: nature of disorder, prognosis, management, and prevention of injury of weakened part

Planning: Patient Outcomes
1. Patient states accurate information about the cause of the tumor, prognosis, treatment, and methods to prevent injury.
2. Patient reports an understanding of the disorder and the information presented by the physician for management of the condition.

Nursing Interventions and Evaluation

NDx: Anxiety
Explain the purpose of all treatments to the patient. Before performing any procedure on the patient, explain the steps of the procedure and the reason for it. Allow the patient time to ask questions and relay concerns. Reinforce information from the physician to the patient. Give support without offering unrealistic reassurances.

Assess vital signs and watch for changes indicating increased anxiety. Teach the patient relaxation methods and strategies to cope with the fears of hospitalization and medical interventions. Provide diversional activities for the patient to relieve the boredom and anxiety associated with bedrest.

NDx: Pain
Administer prescribed analgesics and explain the dosage, frequency, side effects, and expected therapeutic effects of the medications. Caution the patient not to perform tasks that require mental alertness while taking pain medication. Teach the patient to elevate the affected part to reduce swelling and thus reduce pain. Caution the patient about weight-bearing, if contraindicated, because that might increase the pain significantly.

NDx: Knowledge deficit: nature of disorder, prognosis and management, and prevention of injury of weakened part
Teach the patient about the tumor, the prognosis, methods of prevention of injury, and appropriate treatment. Explain that increased swelling, discoloration, and decreased sensation in the affected part may be signs of complications or increased tumor growth and that the physician should be notified.

Reinforce the physician's instructions about weight-bearing because the bone structure may be weakened or necrosis may have developed. Weight-bearing on the weak structure may cause increased pain or fracture. Demonstrate prescribed exercises to the patient and encourage participation in the exercise regimen to prevent loss of strength and joint motion.

Compare the patient's status with the expected outcomes. If the outcomes are not met, reassess the patient and revise the plan.

MALIGNANT BONE TUMORS

Etiology and Pathophysiology

Malignant bone tumors grow rapidly, metastasize to other parts of the body through the blood or lymphatic system, and destroy surrounding tissue. Malignant tumors are further described as primary tumors, which arise directly from musculoskeletal tissue, or secondary metastatic tumors, which spread to the bone from a malignancy in some other part of the body. Primary bone tumors include osteosarcomas, Ewing's sarcomas, chondrosarcomas, fibrosarcomas, and malignant fibrous histiocytomas.

Malignant primary bone tumors account for less than 1% of all malignancies. They affect predominantly the young, aged 10 to 30 years old. The prognosis and treatment depend on the type and size of the tumor and a staging system based on site and metastatic activity of the tumor.

Clinical Manifestations

Clinical manifestations of malignant tumors include deformity, pathologic fractures, swelling, pain, malaise, fever, and unexplained weight loss. Pain is persistent and usually increases with activity of weight-bearing. Numbness or paresthesias may be present in the distal portion of an involved extremity if the tumor presses on nerves or blood vessels. A palpable soft tissue mass may be present.

Diagnosis

X-ray films, bone scans, CT scans, or magnetic resonance imaging (MRI) are used to find bone lesions. The bone may have a "moth-eaten" appearance, with many areas of destruction. In multiple myeloma, the formation of an abnormal globulin, called a Bence Jones protein, occurs in the urine.

Management

At one time, the prognosis for patients with bone malignancies was only 10 to 20% survival, even with radical surgery. Technologic advances in nuclear detecting methods, chemotherapy, radiation, and newer surgical procedures such as limb salvage account for improved statistics.

Patients with malignant bone tumors may experience changes in blood coagulation as a result of interference with cell production in the marrow. Thus, they are at risk for hematologic complications with surgery.

❖ Settings, Providers, and Collaboration for Care

Treatment at a comprehensive cancer center with coordination of pathology, radiology, medical and surgical oncology, and rehabilitation services is generally considered to be ideal for the treatment of malignant bone tumors. Patients may need long-term care at rehabilitation facilities or in the home, depending on the treatment needed.

Osteosarcoma

Etiology and Pathophysiology

Osteosarcoma, or osteogenic sarcoma, is the most common of the malignant bone tumors. It is characterized by rapid growth and metastases. The highest incidence is in adolescent males, but osteosarcoma can also occur in older people with Paget's disease or people who have undergone bone irradiation. The epiphyseal plate and metaphysis of the long bones are the common sites of osteosarcoma. Today the survival rate for osteogenic sarcoma is 80 to 85% after 5 years after diagnosis. Early metastasis to the lung is common and increases the risk for a poor prognosis.

Clinical Manifestations

The main symptom of osteosarcoma is debilitating pain that is unrelieved by analgesics. It frequently is so severe that it causes the patient to awaken at night. Because of the rapid growth of the tumor, the involved area is noticeably larger than normal. Joint motion may also be restricted. The patient has a history of fatigue, lethargy, and weight loss.

Diagnosis

Diagnosis requires radiologic and pathologic examination. X-ray films show the tumor as destructive lesions that extend through the medullary cortex. Soft tissue involvement creates a "sunburst" appearance around the lesions. For suspected lesions, a biopsy is performed in such a way as to allow for complete removal of the biopsy scar and its track if further surgery is indicated. Once a diagnosis is confirmed, full lung tomograms, to detect early metastasis to the lung, and bone scans are performed to stage the disease and plan treatment. Positive blood studies show an increase in the serum alkaline phosphatase level.

Management

Surgical intervention, excision either through a limb-sparing procedure or amputation, in conjunction with radiation and chemotherapy is the treatment of choice. Surgery usually includes wide resection from 7 to 10 cm beyond any involved tissue. Postoperative care depends on the extent of surgery and the need for additional chemotherapy or radiation. Chemotherapy may be administered preoperatively to reduce the size of the tumor and postoperatively to prevent micrometastases.

Because of the risk of tumor recurrence, long-term medical follow-up with repeated x-ray examinations, bone scans, and physical assessment is necessary (Nursing Care Guide 20–2).

Text continued on page 942

Nursing Care Guide 20–2
Patients Undergoing Surgery for Osteosarcoma

Preoperative Care

Assessment Findings: Patient appears nervous, withdraws from conversation, clenches hands; blood pressure, pulse, and respirations are slightly elevated for the patient; patient makes statements indicating concern about the procedure and results of the surgical intervention, and potential problems with mobility and discomfort following the surgery and the loss of the limb.

Nursing Diagnosis: Anxiety related to uncertainty about surgery, potential risk factors, discomfort, and fear of loss of mobility

Patient Outcomes	Nursing Interventions	Rationale
Patient reports feeling less nervous, feeling relaxed, and resting well.	Teach the patient relaxation techniques. Provide a quiet, calm environment with periods of rest during the delivery of nursing care. Ask for assistance from clergy or the patient's significant others.	Having an understanding of the procedure lessens fears and reduces anxiety. Telling the patient what to expect prior to initiating procedures for preoperative preparation reduces fear of the unknown.
Patient's vital signs are within normal ranges for the patient.	Check vital signs after the patient is rested and more relaxed, and note any changes.	Changes in vital signs may indicate changes in level of anxiety.
Patient states methods to relax and reduce tension.	Teach deep-breathing techniques and other relaxation strategies. Allow the patient to voice concerns about the loss of the extremity.	Relaxation exercises may decrease anxiety and promote rest.

Evaluation: Compare the patient's status with the expected outcomes. If the outcomes are not met, reassess the patient and revise the plan.

Assessment Findings: Patient and family seem very concerned about the procedure; they ask several questions about the surgery, the preparation prior to surgery, the expectations of the intervention, and possible complications.

Nursing Diagnosis: Knowledge deficit: nature of amputation surgery, preoperative preparations, expected outcome, and possible complications

Patient Outcomes	Nursing Interventions	Rationale
Patient accurately describes the purpose of the surgery and the necessity for the amputation and relates information about the procedure, complications, and expected results as presented to the patient by the physician.	Explain the procedure to the patient, the usual preoperative preparation, and the expected outcomes. Have the patient relate what the physician has explained, and clear up any misunderstandings.	Explanations of all the appropriate information about the surgery to the patient and family and reinforcement of the information the physician has provided decrease the knowledge deficit and better prepare the patient for the postoperative period.

(continued)

Nursing Care Guide 20–2
Patients Undergoing Surgery for Osteosarcoma (continued)

Patient Outcomes	Nursing Interventions	Rationale
Patient reports an understanding of the preoperative procedures necessary.	Allow time for questions from the patient or the family. Give the patient literature explaining the procedure and showing which prosthesis may be used to provide mobility.	Having the patient repeat the information gives you an opportunity to correct any misinformation.

Evaluation: Compare the patient's status with the expected outcomes. If the outcomes are not met, reassess the patient and revise the plan.

Postoperative Care

Assessment Findings: Patient has incision site with dressings, an intravenous line, and is on bedrest.

Nursing Diagnosis: Risk for infection related to wound site, intravenous line, and bedrest

Patient Outcomes	Nursing Interventions	Rationale
Patient's wound site remains free from symptoms of infection such as redness, purulent drainage, or excessive swelling.	Check the wound site and suture line for evidence of healing. Watch for signs of infection. Use aseptic technique during dressing changes.	Early diagnosis of complications increases potential for successful treatment. Aseptic technique decreases risk of infection.
Patient's vital signs are within normal limits for the patient, and the patient denies cough or respiratory distress.	Assess vital signs frequently. Have the patient cough and deep-breathe at regular intervals.	Vital sign changes may indicate infection, such as in the respiratory system if patient begins to present an increased respiratory rate and pulse rate and some respiratory distress.
Patient's intravenous site remains free from infection.	Check the intravenous site at least each shift, looking for infiltration, redness, and swelling.	Checking the intravenous site frequently may prevent complications or allow for early intervention if a problem is evident.

Evaluation: Compare the patient's status with the expected outcomes. If the outcomes are not met, reassess the patient and revise the plan.

Assessment Findings: Patient grimaces, moans, and complains of discomfort at surgical site and in the absent extremity (phantom pain); patient's blood pressure, pulse, and respiratory rate are elevated.

Nursing Diagnosis: Pain related to invasive surgical procedure with manipulation, muscle spasms, and/or contractures

(continued)

Nursing Care Guide 20–2
Patients Undergoing Surgery for Osteosarcoma (continued)

Patient Outcomes	Nursing Interventions	Rationale
Patient reports relief of pain and reports feeling relaxed and comfortable.	Give prescribed analgesics for control of postoperative pain. Make patient comfortable, and provide a quiet atmosphere for rest after surgery. Check insertion site for signs of infection, which may increase pain at site. Explain to the patient about the phenomenon of phantom pain.	Relief of postoperative pain allows patient to rest as needed and assists in keeping vital signs within normal limits. Infection with inflammation increases pain at the site.

Evaluation: Compare the patient's status with the expected outcomes. If the outcomes are not met, reassess the patient and revise the plan.

Assessment Findings: Patient cries frequently and withdraws from conversations; patient states fear of returning to social life; patient is concerned about the future without the limb and potential mobility problems; patient seems very depressed and refuses to participate in care.

Nursing Diagnosis: Dysfunctional grieving related to loss of lower extremity

Patient Outcomes	Nursing Interventions	Rationale
Patient voices concerns about loss of limb, looks at surgical area, and states feelings about the care necessary.	Allow patient to voice concerns. Be supportive without making false reassurances about the prognosis.	Free expression of grief is therapeutic. Having the patient look at self is important so that the patient will be able to perform self-care and to help the patient get over problems with body image.
Patient returns to social activities and participates in self-care.	Encourage participation in activities with others. Teach the patient to care for the residual limb.	Getting involved in social activities assists the patient in returning to a healthy lifestyle.
Patient talks freely to others about the diagnosis and surgical intervention.	Have the patient visit with other amputees for support.	Talking with other amputees gives the patient strategies to cope with the loss.

Evaluation: Compare the patient's status with the expected outcomes. If the outcomes are not met, reassess the patient and revise the plan.

Assessment Findings: Patient seems overly anxious and reluctant to listen to home care instructions; patient is reluctant to work with ambulatory aid and to practice physical therapy; patient states concerns about providing self-care, hygiene, grooming, and activities of daily living when home.

Nursing Diagnosis: Impaired home maintenance management related to inability to manage mobility problems, use of ambulatory aid, fear for safety, and suture line care (if needed)

(continued)

Nursing Care Guide 20–2
Patients Undergoing Surgery for Osteosarcoma (continued)

Patient Outcomes	Nursing Interventions	Rationale
Patient relates accurate information about the home care required and signs of potential problems. Patient states plans for follow-up care with the attending physician.	Describe the signs requiring immediate medical intervention, such as pain or discomfort at surgical site, fever, chills, dizziness, fainting, excessive fatigue, or shortness of breath.	Early diagnosis of potential problems by the patient at home and early medical intervention increase the chance for successful treatment. Having the patient relate information presented reinforces the information and allows for correction of misconceptions.
Patient demonstrates appropriate use of ambulatory aid and states safety measures for the home environment to prevent falls or other injuries.	Assist the patient in practicing using the ambulatory aid. Help the patient find ways to increase safety measures in the home environment.	Having the patient practice under supervision allows for evaluation of patient's ability to practice safe use of ambulatory aids.

Evaluation: Compare the patient's status with the expected outcomes. If the outcomes are not met, reassess the patient and revise the plan.

Ewing's Sarcoma

Etiology and Pathophysiology

A rare but highly malignant bone tumor, Ewing's sarcoma originates in the marrow and metastasizes early. It can occur in major long bones or the flat bones of the pelvis and ribs. Pulmonary involvement is common. Ewing's sarcoma is more prevalent in young males in their early teens to early twenties.

Clinical Manifestations

The clinical manifestations of Ewing's sarcoma are similar to those of osteosarcoma, with the pain more incapacitating, and the malaise, lethargy, and weight loss more pronounced. Pathologic fracture through the lesion is common.

Diagnosis

The diagnosis is made on the basis of history, physical examination, and radiographic studies.

Management

Treatment of Ewing's sarcoma has been most successful with systemic chemotherapy, which includes combinations of two or more drugs, followed by radiation or surgery. The most effective neoplastic agents and the duration of therapy vary among patients. Surgery usually follows chemotherapy or radiation, or both. Because Ewing's sarcoma has a high incidence of recurrence, surgery alone is of little value. Some pelvic masses, inaccessible to radiation and surgery, are treated by chemotherapy alone.

NURSING PROCESS
Malignant Bone Tumors

Assessment

Review the patient's history, results of diagnostic studies, and presenting problems. Assess the affected area, noting any swelling, deformity, or pain. Perform a neurovascular assessment of the affected limb. Ask the patient about range-of-motion and mobility problems. Determine whether there is pain and when it is most significant. Note problems with weight-bearing and changes in ability to perform activities of daily living.

Determine the patient's and family's understanding about the diagnosis and possible treatment alternatives. The patient's reaction to the diagnosis of malignancy is important to the care planning. Assess the patient's coping strategies and their effectiveness. Ask about support systems that are available to the patient, such as relatives and friends.

Nursing Diagnoses and Planning

Nursing diagnoses and related expected patient outcomes most commonly applicable to patients with a malignant bone tumor include those discussed previously for patients with a benign bone tumor and the following (also see Chapter 34 for care of the patient with cancer):

NDx: Self esteem disturbance related to deformity, effects of chemotherapy, or amputation

Planning: Patient Outcomes
1. Patient relates feelings of self-worth.
2. Patient maintains social activity.
3. Patient is able to look at self with understanding and acceptance.

NDx: Fear related to forthcoming treatments, prognosis, and uncertain future

Planning: Patient Outcomes
1. Patient appears relaxed and is able to rest and sleep at intervals.
2. Patient denies extreme fear about the diagnosis or prognosis and the future.
3. Patient freely expresses concerns about the diagnosis and prognosis.
4. Patient states acceptable coping mechanisms to deal with the fear.

Nursing Interventions and Evaluation

NDx: Self esteem disturbance
Allow the patient to vent feelings about the diagnosis. Involve support from the family and other friends. Provide information about cancer support groups. Seek effective coping strategies for the patient. Assist the patient in finding the positive aspects of life to focus on during periods of depression. Provide diversional activities for the patient when he or she is bedridden as a result of exacerbations from the disease or the treatment regimen. Seek assistance from clergy or professional counseling. Help the patient deal with the altered appearance by suggesting methods of concealment such as the use of appropriate clothing, makeup, or natural-looking prosthetic devices.

NDx: Fear
Help the patient cope with the diagnosis and uncertain future. Provide referral to professional counseling services. Assist the patient in the identification of support systems. Talk with clergy and significant others about support for the patient. Explain and reinforce all information provided by the physician regarding the diagnosis and treatment modalities. Allow time for questions and concerns from the patient and family. If appropriate, provide opportunity for the patient and family to talk with others who have successfully faced similar circumstances. Inform the patient about organizations such as the American Cancer Society that provide psychologic support, educational services, and other assistance for patients and families.

Compare the patient's status with the expected outcomes. If the outcomes are not met, reassess the patient and revise the plan.

Metastatic Bone Tumors

Etiology and Pathophysiology
A metastatic bone tumor is cancer of the bone that arises from a primary tumor in another part of the body and metastasizes to bone. The tumor cells me-

tastasize through the circulatory system or lymphatic system. Metastatic bone tumors commonly originate from primary lesions of the breast, kidney, lung, prostate, and thyroid. These tumors can be osteolytic or osteoblastic.

Clinical Manifestations
The most common clinical manifestations are pain in the involved bone and pathologic fracture.

Diagnosis
Diagnosis of a metastatic bone tumor is made on the basis of x-ray examination, bone scan, CT scan, biopsy, and elevated blood levels of alkaline phosphatase and serum calcium.

Management
Treatment is palliative rather than curative. The goals of medical management and nursing care are pain relief and prevention of complications such as pathologic fractures. The secondary bone tumor may be treated in conjunction with the primary lesion using chemotherapy or radiation, or both. Treatment of pathologic fractures with braces, splints, or internal fixation is often necessary. Another palliative treatment to relieve pain is the administration of strontium-89 chloride. Strontium-89 is a beta emitter and behaves much like calcium. Uptake of strontium by bone occurs more readily in areas where active osteogenesis is occurring. Strontium-89 chloride can selectively irradiate metastatic bone lesions resulting in decreased pain.

The Elderly: Special Considerations

Age-related alterations in stature and posture occur, especially in older women. This is caused by compression of the spinal column. Other changes in bone mass, metabolism, and musculature occur in later adulthood. Some loss of agility and flexibility is common. These alterations may compound the effects of many musculoskeletal disorders. The changes also increase the risk for some musculoskeletal problems such as arthritis, osteoporosis, and hip fractures. These conditions were discussed earlier in the chapter.

Degenerative joint diseases can be debilitating for the older adult. Painful or immobile joints may interfere with self-care activities and the ability to maintain locomotion, resulting in a loss of independence.

Nursing interventions for the older adult with musculoskeletal disorders are focused on maintenance of safety, mobility, and independence. Exercise programs may be beneficial in maintaining or increasing strength, flexibility, and function. Weight-bearing exercises are most helpful in preventing osteoporosis. Other exercises, such as stretching, and moderate weight-lifting regimens can be helpful in improving and maintaining overall musculoskeletal function.

Safety may be a major problem for older adults with musculoskeletal disorders because of their loss of mobility and the difficulty of using ambulatory aids. Patients are taught safe use of the assistive devices. The older adult also needs information on making the home environment safe, especially when using an ambulatory aid. The patient may benefit from an in-home assessment by a physical or occupational therapist. These assessments can be provided through home-care agencies and they may be covered by Medicare if the person is homebound. Even if on-going therapy is not necessary, an initial assessment and one or two follow-up visits may be helpful in assisting older people to modify their environments for safety and improved functioning.

Dietary evaluation and education may be needed to provide an appropriate meal plan for healing and health maintenance and to prevent other musculoskeletal disorders. The need for increased vitamins, calcium, and other minerals is stressed.

Medication education is also necessary. Pain management may be complicated in older adults, especially if they are taking other medications. A medication regimen that achieves adequate pain control yet avoids side effects and drug interactions needs to be established. The geriatric patient may react to drug therapy differently than the middle-aged or younger adult. Teach the patient the dosage, frequency, therapeutic effects, and side effects of all prescribed medications and when to notify the physician. Because gastrointestinal irritation is a common side effect of analgesics, tell the patient to take the medications with milk or meals unless otherwise advised.

Chapter Review

1. What patient teaching is required when nonsteroidal anti-inflammatory drugs are prescribed for a patient with arthritis?
2. What are the therapeutic effects of activity and exercise for a patient with rheumatoid arthritis?
3. What teaching interventions are appropriate for the patient with gout?
4. What interventions are important in the nursing care plan for a patient with osteoporosis?
5. What are common psychologic and social problems in individuals with musculoskeletal disorders?
6. What does numbness indicate in a patient with a fracture?
7. How does open reduction affect the nursing care of a patient with a fracture?
8. What neurovascular assessments are important in caring for patients with musculoskeletal injury?
9. How do you think a patient with osteosarcoma would perceive surgical intervention?
10. How is the care of a patient with an open reduction and internal fixation of a fractured hip similar to the care of a patient with a total hip replacement?

Bibliography

Almekinders L. Osteomyelitis: Essentials of diagnosis and treatment. J Musculoskeletal Med 1994; 11(11):31.

Arthur V. Nursing care of patients with rheumatoid arthritis. Br J Nurs 1994; 3(7):325.

Barlow J, Macey S, Struthers G. Health locus of control, self-help and treatment adherence in relation to ankylosing spondylitis patients. Patient Educ Counsel 1993; 20(2/3):153.

Beare B. Endoscopic carpal tunnel release techniques. ACORN J 1994; 7(4):23.

Bennett JC, Plum F. Cecil textbook of medicine. 20th ed. Philadelphia: WB Saunders, 1996.

Beutler A, Schumacher H. Gout and pseudogout. Postgrad Med 1994; 95(2):103.

Boggins-Magill M. Carpal tunnel release: Scoping out the carpal tunnel. Todays OR Nurse 1994; 16(3):27.

Brown S. Women's experiences of rheumatoid arthritis. J Adv Nurs 1995; 21(4):695.

Broy SB. A "whole patient" approach to managing osteoporosis. J Musculoskeletal Med 1996; 13(2):15.

Calin A. Managing hyperuricemia and gout: Challenges and pitfalls. J Musculoskeletal Med 1995; 12(2):42.

Camp N, Iyer P. Patient outcomes in medical-surgical nursing. Springhouse, PA: Springhouse Corporation, 1995.

Childs SA. Musculoskeletal trauma: Implications for critical care nursing practice. Crit Care Nurs Clin North Am 1994; 6(3): 483.

Deloach E, DiBenedetto R, Womble L, Gillery J. The treatment of osteomyelitis underlying pressure ulcers. Decubitus 1993; 5(6): 32.

DeNuccio M. Recognizing gout and pseudogout in hospitalized patients. J Musculoskeletal Med 1994; 11(10):38.

El-Choufi L, Nelson J, Kleerekoper M. Therapeutic options in osteoporosis. J Musculoskeletal Med 1994; 11(10):15.

Eliopoulos C. Gerontological nursing. 3rd ed. Philadelphia: JB Lippincott, 1993.

Escalante A. Ankylosing spondylitis. Postgrad Med 1993; 94(1): 153.

Fleischer E, LeBel L. Fat embolism syndrome. Nurse Anesth 1993; 4(1):18.

Fuller J, Schaller-Ayers J. Health assessment: A nursing approach. 2nd ed. Philadelphia: JB Lippincott, 1994.

Galsworthy TD, Wilson PL. Osteoporosis: It steals more than bone. Am J Nurs 1996; 96(6):26.

Goldberg V. Surgical treatment of osteoarthritis. J Musculoskeletal Med 1994; 11(12):13.

Gordon N. Arthritis: Your complete exercise guide. Champaign, IL: Human Kinetics Publishers, 1993.

Gray M. Osteoporosis medications: What's your source of information? Orthop Nurs 1994; 13(5):55.

Gray M. Antigout medications. Orthop Nurs 1993; 12(4): 53.

Gulanick M, Klopp A, Galanes S, et al. Nursing care plans. 3rd ed. St. Louis: Mosby Year-Book, 1994.

Gulli B, Templeman D. Compartment syndrome of the lower extremity. Orthop Clin North Am 1994; 25(4):677.

Hayes K. Heat and cold in the management of arthritis. Arthritis Care Res 1993; 6(3):156.

Hazzard W, Bierman E, Blass J, et al. Principles of geriatric medicine and gerontology. 3rd ed. New York: McGraw-Hill, 1994.

Hidding A, VanderLinden S, Boers M, et al. Is group physical therapy superior to individualized therapy in ankylosing spondylitis? 1993; 6(3):117.

Holloway N. Medical surgical care planning. 2nd ed. Springhouse, PA: Springhouse Corporation, 1993.

Iyer P, Taptich B, Bernocchi-Losey D. Nursing process and nursing diagnosis. Philadelphia: WB Saunders, 1995.

Ismeurt R, Wilson L, Long C. Lyme disease: An emerging infection with home health care implications. Home Healthc Nurse 1995; 13(3):28.

Jones-Walton P. Orthopaedic health promotion 2000. Orthop Nurs 1994; 13(3):29.

Kan MK. Palliation of bone pain in patients with metastatic cancer using strontium-89 (Metastron). Cancer Nurs 1995; 18(4): 286.

Kee JL. Laboratory and diagnostic tests with nursing implications. 4th ed. Norwalk, CT: Appleton & Lange, 1995.

Kuhn MA. Pharmacotherapeutics: A nursing process approach. 3rd ed. Philadelphia: FA Davis 1994.

Lankford T. Foundations of normal and therapeutic nutrition. Albany, NY: Delmar, 1994.

Lehne R. Pharmacology for nursing care. 2nd ed. Philadelphia: WB Saunders, 1994.

Mader J, Landon G, Calhoun J. Antimicrobial treatment of osteomyelitis. Clin Orthop Related Res 1993; 295:87.

Mayers M, Pankratz C (eds). Clinical care plans: Medical surgical nursing. New York: McGraw-Hill, 1995.

McCue F III, Mayer V. Carpal tunnel syndrome: How you can help your patient. Consultant 1994; 34(2):240.

McCue F III, Mayer V. Carpal tunnel syndrome: When to suspect and how to make the diagnosis. Consultant 1993; 33(12):40.

McKeon V. Hormone replacement therapy: Evaluating the risks and benefits. JOGNN 1994; 23(8):647.

Miller B. Carpal tunnel syndrome: A frequently misdiagnosed common hand problem. Nurse Pract 1993; 18(12):52.

Miller-Blair D, Robbins D. Rheumatoid arthritis: New science, new treatment. Geriatrics 1993; 48(6):28.

Minor M, Sanford M. Physical interventions in the management of pain in arthritis. Arthritis Care Res 1993; 6(4):197.

Newcomer K, Jurisson M. Rheumatoid arthritis: The role of physical therapy. J Musculoskeletal Med 1994; 11(11):14.

Nicholas J. Physical modalities in rheumatological rehabilitation. Arch Phys Med Rehabil 1994; 75:994.

Patzakis M, Abdollahi K, Sherman R, et al. Treatment of chronic osteomyelitis with muscle flaps. Orthop Clin North Am 1993; 24(3):505.

Pontieri-Lewis V. Focus on wound care therapeutic beds: An overview. Medsurg Nurs 1995; 4(4):323.

Preisinger E, Alacamlioglu Y, Pils K, et al. Therapeutic exercise in the prevention of bone loss. Am J Phys Med Rehabil 1995; 74(2):120.

Prestwood K, Raisz L. Using estrogen to prevent and treat osteoporosis. J Musculoskeletal Med 1994; 11(5):17.

Reed L, Keegan M. Fat embolism syndrome: A complication of trauma. Crit Care Nurse 1993; 13(3):33.

Reiss B, Evans M. Pharmacological aspects of nursing. 5th ed. Albany, NY: Delmar, 1996.

Schnitzer T. Osteoarthritis treatment update. Postgrad Med 1993; 93(1):89.

Shu Y. A study on functioning for independent living among the elderly in the community. Public Health Nurs 1995; 12(1):31.

Sipos D. Carpal tunnel syndrome. Orthop Nurs 1995; 14(1):17.

Skinner J. Exercise testing and exercise prescription for special cases: Theoretical basis and clinical application. 2nd ed. Philadelphia: Lea & Febiger, 1993.

Spencer-Green G. Drug treatment of arthritis. Postgrad Med 1993; 93(7):129.

Star V, Hochberg M. Gout: Steps to relieve acute symptoms, prevent further attacks. Consultant 1994; 34(12):1697.

Steere A. Current understanding of Lyme disease. Hosp Pract 1993; 28(4):37.

Wetherbee L. Caring for the client with arthritis. Home Healthc Nurse 1994; 12(1):13.

Williams R, Westmorland M. Occupational cumulative trauma disorders of the upper extremity. Am J Occup Ther 1994; 48(5):411.

Unit VII

Gastrointestinal Dysfunction

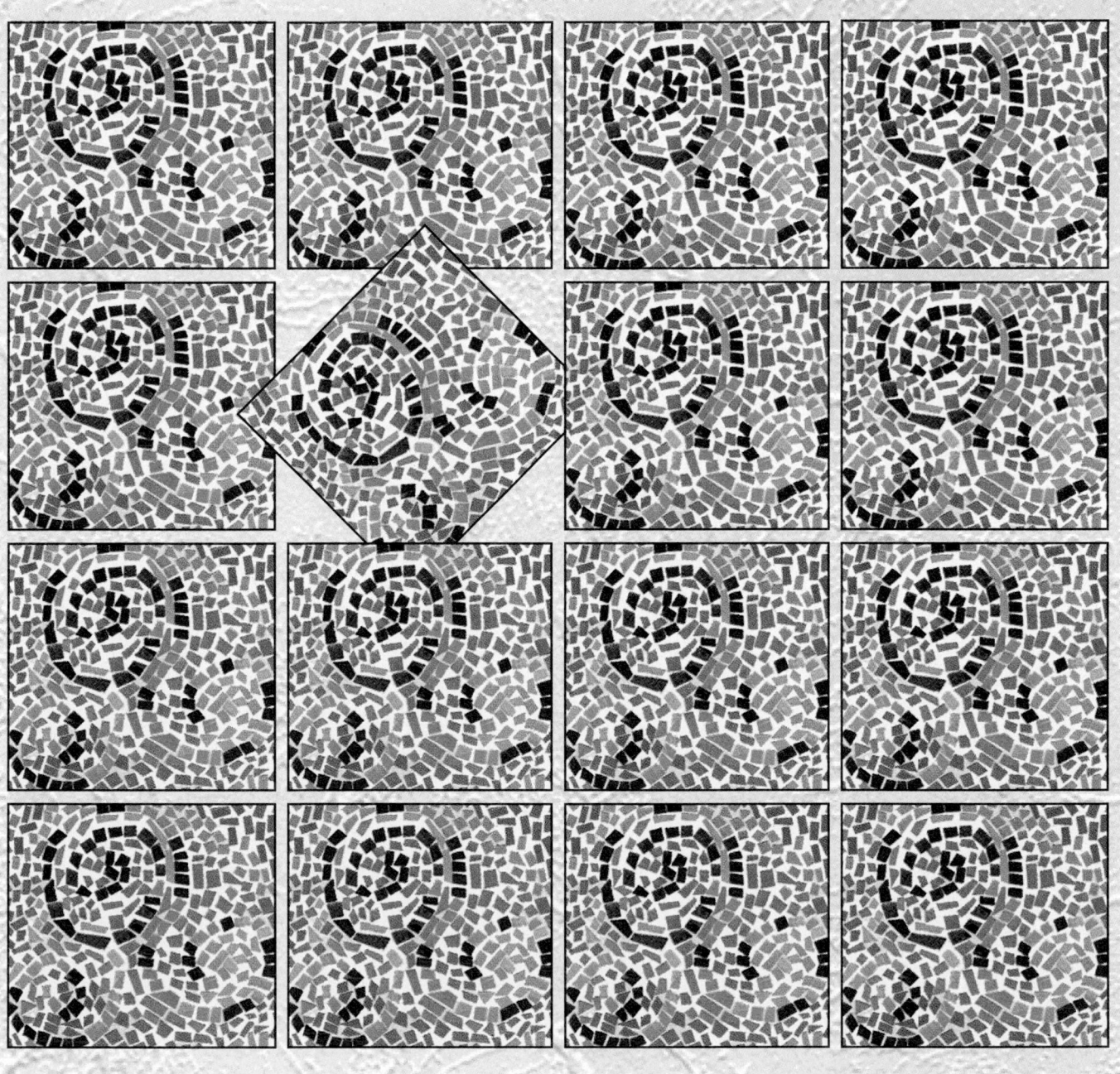

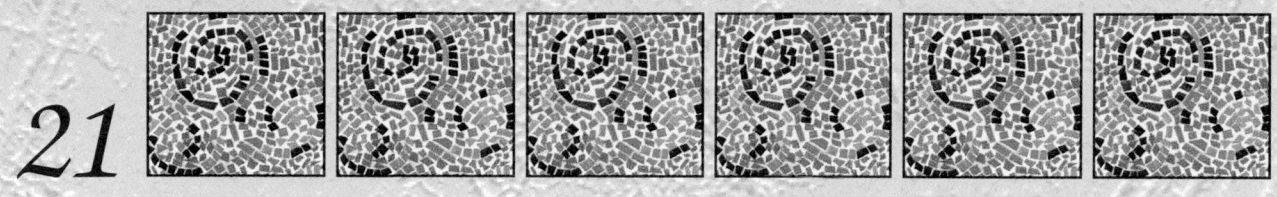

21

Knowledge Base for Patients with Gastrointestinal Dysfunction

Study Outcomes

After studying this chapter, you should be able to:

1. Explain the normal anatomy and physiology of the digestive system and its accessory organs.
2. Describe common clinical manifestations of gastrointestinal dysfunction.
3. Identify information and physical examination data essential to the assessment of gastrointestinal status.
4. Describe basic diagnostic tests and methods of medical management used in the treatment of patients with gastrointestinal dysfunction.
5. Describe basic surgical procedures used in the treatment of patients with gastrointestinal dysfunction.
6. Identify data essential to the assessment of patients undergoing treatment for gastrointestinal disorders.
7. State nursing diagnoses and related expected patient outcomes commonly applicable to patients undergoing treatment for gastrointestinal dysfunction.
8. Describe nursing interventions, with their rationales, commonly applicable to patients undergoing treatment for gastrointestinal dysfunction.
9. Explain the basis for evaluation of nursing care provided to patients undergoing treatment for gastrointestinal dysfunction.
10. Identify alternative treatment and care settings for patients with gastrointestinal dysfunction, and the services related to community-based care.
11. Identify special considerations for the elderly patient with altered gastrointestinal function.

The gastrointestinal (GI) tract is responsible for ingestion, digestion, and absorption of nutrients essential for life and growth, as well as for excretion of solid waste from the body. Patterns of GI function vary both within and among individuals. People have varying patterns of intake, abilities to tolerate wide-ranging food types, and patterns of elimination. Likewise, a person's intake, tolerance of foods, and pattern of elimination vary from time to time such that transient episodes of anorexia, distention, flatulence, or stool that is dryer or looser than normal are considered normal alterations. This fact presents a challenge to the health-care provider because these same differences can represent disease.

Many types of abnormalities can occur in this complex body system, from simple indigestion to cancer affecting several organs. Thus, a clear understanding of the anatomy and physiology of the GI tract, as well as the pathophysiology underlying major clinical manifestations of GI disease, is essential to accurate assessment and effective intervention.

Patients with GI complaints may present and be treated at clinics, emergency rooms, and physician's offices. More complex problems require hospital admission and possibly ambulatory or inpatient surgery. More and more GI disorders are being treated outside the hospital. For example, since the advent of acid-suppressing medications, most patients with ulcer disease are hospitalized only when they manifest complications. Because patients with chronic diseases, and especially the elderly, often experience GI disturbances, health-care professionals working in nursing homes and hospices need to pay particular attention to the functioning of this system.

Anatomy and Physiology

The GI tract is a continuous tube of varying diameter about 9 m (30 ft) long. It begins with the mouth and extends through the pharynx, esophagus, stomach, small intestine, and large intestine to the anus (Fig. 21–1). Accessory organs of digestion include the teeth, tongue, salivary glands, gallbladder, pancreas, and liver.

The primary function of the GI tract is to convert complex food substances into simpler compounds that can be absorbed into the blood stream and used by the cells of the body. It also excretes solid waste from the body.

BASIC STRUCTURE AND FUNCTION OF THE GASTROINTESTINAL TRACT

From the lower third of the esophagus to the anus, the GI tract is composed of four layers of tissue:

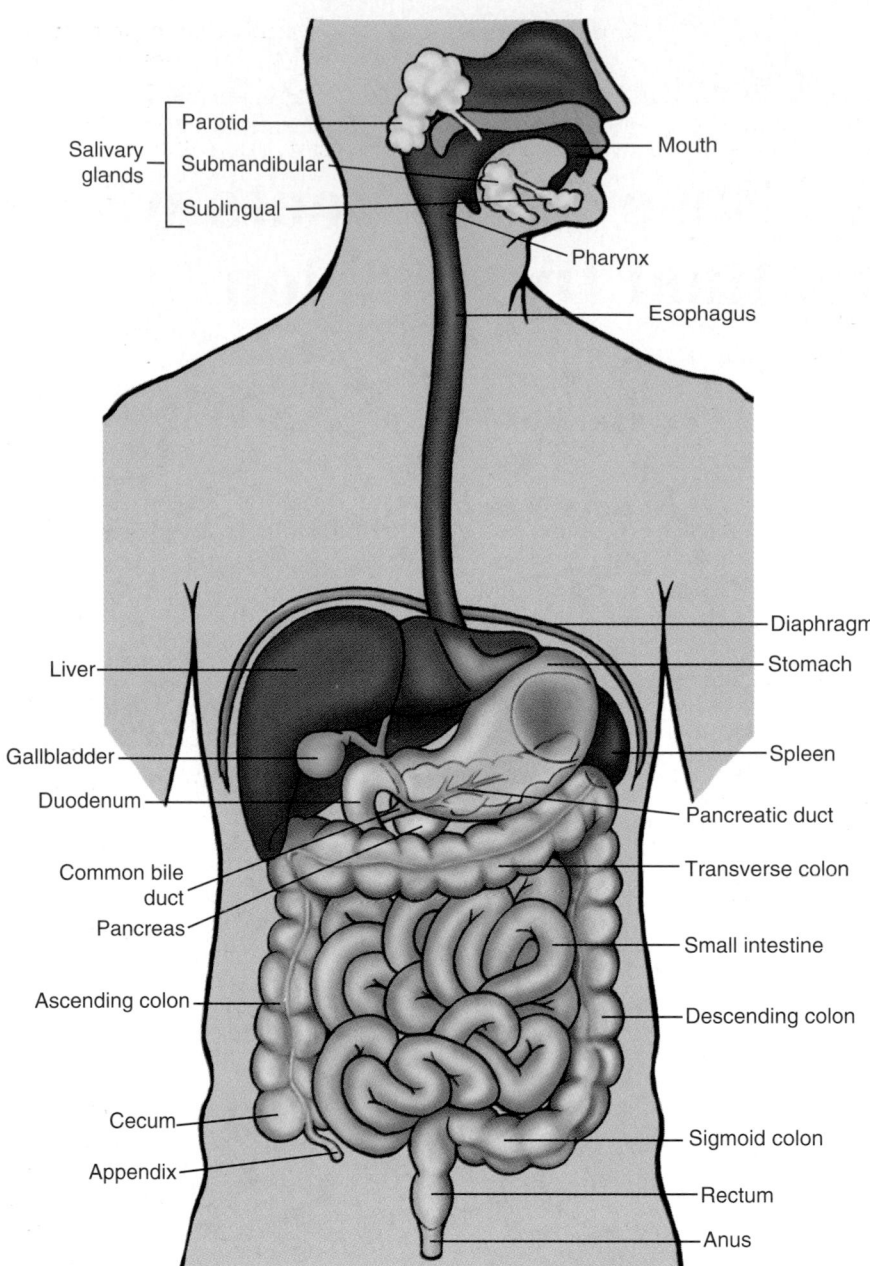

Figure 21–1
Basic anatomy of the gastrointestinal tract.

Mucosa, or inner layer
Submucosa
Muscularis
Serosa, or outer layer

The mucosa is composed of a surface layer of epithelium, a layer of loose connective tissue rich in blood and lymphatic vessels called the lamina propria, and a thin layer of smooth muscle. Mucus and digestive juices are secreted by the cells of the mucosa.

The submucosa is composed of loose connective tissue. It connects the mucosa to the underlying muscularis and allows for movement and size changes in the tract.

The muscularis is composed of smooth muscle arranged in two layers. An inner circular layer of fibers surrounds the tube. An outer layer of longitudinal fibers runs parallel with its long axis. Each of these layers provides a specific type of motility necessary for maximal efficiency of digestion and absorption. Contraction of the longitudinal muscles causes a motion called peristalsis. Peristalsis primarily propels nutrients down the tube. Contraction of the circular muscles causes segmentation. This helps mix food and digestive juices and forces food close to the mucosal lining, thus facilitating absorption.

The outer layer, or serosa, consists of epithelial and connective tissue. The serosa is also called the visceral peritoneum.

PERITONEUM

GI organs located below the esophagus are in the abdominal cavity and are covered with peritoneum, the largest serous membrane of the body. The peritoneum is composed of two layers. The parietal layer lines the walls of the abdominal cavity. The visceral layer covers some of the organs within the cavity. Between the parietal and visceral portions of the peritoneum is a potential space called the peritoneal cavity, which contains serous fluid. The peritoneum contains several large folds that pass between the viscera of the abdomen and pelvis. These folds connect the organs to one another and to the walls of the cavity. They also contain blood vessels, lymph vessels, and nerves that supply the abdominal organs.

MOUTH

The mouth is the structure through which food enters the GI tract. Inside the mouth are the tongue with its taste receptors, the teeth, and the salivary glands.

The mouth is bounded laterally by the cheeks and anteriorly by the lips. The hard palate forms the anterior portion of the roof of the mouth. The soft palate forms the posterior portion. The tongue, along with its associated muscles, forms the floor of the mouth.

Mucous membrane lines the oral cavity. It contains many small glands, called buccal glands, which secrete small amounts of saliva. Three pairs of salivary glands secrete the bulk of saliva. They include the parotid, submandibular, and sublingual glands. Each of these pairs supplies different proportions of ingredients to saliva. The parotid glands secrete serous fluid that contains the enzyme salivary amylase. The sublingual glands secrete mucus, which is a thicker fluid and contains a small amount of enzyme. The submandibular glands secrete both mucus and serous fluid.

The process of digestion begins in the mouth with chewing or mastication. Chewing mechanically breaks up large food particles and mixes food with saliva. This not only facilitates swallowing but initiates the first phase of chemical digestion, which is the breakdown of starches by salivary amylase (ptyalin) in saliva.

Swallowing, or the act of deglutition, is the process by which chewed food, now called a bolus, moves from the mouth to the stomach. This process has three distinct stages:

Oral phase
Pharyngeal phase
Esophageal phase

In the oral phase, which is under voluntary control, the bolus is moved by the tongue into the oropharynx. There, the process becomes involuntary.

Impulses are sent to the swallowing center in the medulla oblongata. Returning impulses cause the epiglottis to cover the tracheal opening to prevent aspiration of food into the lung, and the bolus passes through the pharynx into the esophagus. During the esophageal phase, the bolus is forced through the esophagus by involuntary peristaltic waves.

PHARYNX

The pharynx, or throat, is a musculomembranous tube about 13 cm (5 in) long. It extends from the base of the skull to the esophagus and lies in front of the cervical vertebrae. The pharynx has openings that communicate to the ears, nose, mouth, larynx, and esophagus. It is divided into three parts:

Nasopharynx
Oropharynx
Laryngopharynx

The nasopharynx is situated behind the posterior nares and above the soft palate. It connects with the posterior nares and allows the passage of air during breathing. It also contains the openings of the auditory tubes through which air enters the middle ear. The oropharynx extends from the soft palate to the hyoid bone, and the laryngopharynx extends from the hyoid bone to the esophagus. The oropharynx and the laryngopharynx serve as a passageway for both the digestive and the respiratory tracts.

ESOPHAGUS

The esophagus is a muscular tube about 24 cm (9 in) long that lies behind the trachea. It extends from the distal portion of the pharynx, passes through the mediastinum in front of the vertebral column, penetrates the diaphragm through an aperture called the esophageal hiatus, and terminates in the upper portion of the stomach.

Peristaltic waves move down the esophagus to transport food and fluids from the oral cavity to the stomach. To facilitate this process, esophageal glands secrete mucus, which lubricates the food bolus and helps prevent damage to the esophageal wall. Passage of liquids and very soft foods from the mouth to the stomach takes about 1 second. Semisolid or solid foods pass through in about 4 to 8 seconds.

Just above the diaphragm and 1 to 2 inches above the esophageal-gastric junction, nutrients pass through the lower esophageal sphincter. The lower esophageal sphincter (Fig. 21–2) is an area of the esophageal smooth muscle that remains tonically constricted except when it relaxes as part of the swallowing reflex to permit passage of a bolus into the stomach. Its primary purpose is to prevent re-

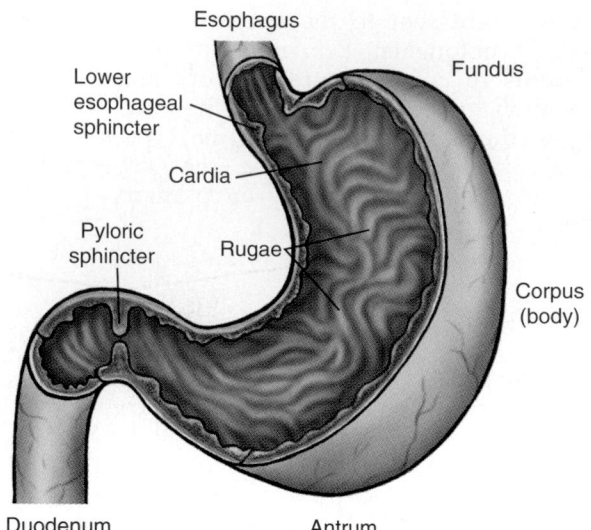

Figure 21–2

Physiologic anatomy of the lower esophagus and the stomach. Note the location of the lower esophageal sphincter and the regions of the stomach.

flux of gastric contents—which are highly acidic and contain protein-digesting enzymes—into the upper esophagus during contractions of the stomach.

Also preventing reflux of gastric contents is a physiologic valve-like mechanism at the end of the esophagus just under the diaphragm. This is a pressure-controlled closure whose action stems from the fact that three-fourths of the esophagus is in the thoracic cavity under negative pressure, whereas the one-fourth distal to the diaphragm is in the abdominal cavity under positive pressure. This pressure difference forces the lower end of the esophagus closed, thus preventing high pressure in the stomach from forcing gastric contents back into the esophagus. This is less efficient than a true valve would be, and any compromise of the diaphragmatic opening can result in incompetence and development of related pathology.

STOMACH

The stomach is the dilated portion of the GI tract. It lies in the left upper part of the abdomen, directly under the diaphragm. The upper part of the stomach communicates with the distal portion of the esophagus. The lower part communicates with the duodenum. The size and shape of the stomach vary according to the volume of stomach contents, the stage of digestion, the condition of the muscular wall, and the status of adjacent intestines.

The stomach is divided into several anatomic parts, including the cardia, the fundus, the body, the antrum, and the pylorus (see Fig. 21–2). The cardia is the upper area of the stomach that surrounds the

lower esophageal sphincter. The fundus is the rounded portion above and to the left of the cardia. The body, or corpus, is below the fundus and is the central portion of the stomach. The pylorus is the narrow, inferior portion of the stomach, the first part of which is sometimes called the antrum. A ringlike muscle in the pyloric opening forms the pyloric sphincter, which controls the opening between the stomach and duodenum. The pyloric sphincter is a true anatomic valve and remains closed at rest.

The major functions of the stomach include the start of digestion by hydrochloric acid and pepsin, storage of nutrients, and controlled passage of the altered food bolus into the duodenum. The bolus, altered by gastric secretions, is now called chyme. These functions are carried out by specialized secretory and motility mechanisms made possible by unique structural adaptations found in the gastric wall.

The surface epithelium of the gastric mucosa is composed of columnar cells dotted with deep, narrow gastric pits into which gastric glands empty their secretions. Gastric glands in different regions of the stomach contain different types of secretory cells and hence produce different secretions. The four main types of secretory cells are:

Chief cells
Parietal cells
Mucous cells
Enteroendocrine cells

Chief cells secrete pepsinogen, precursor of the protein-digesting enzyme pepsin. Parietal cells secrete hydrochloric acid, which creates the acidic environment needed to convert pepsinogen into pepsin. Parietal cells also secrete intrinsic factor, which is essential for absorption of vitamin B_{12} in the terminal ileum. Mucous cells secrete a sticky, alkaline mucus that adheres to the epithelial surface and helps protect the gastric wall from damage by acid gastric secretions. The secretions of the chief, parietal, and mucous cells are collectively called gastric juice and total about 3000 mL per day. Enteroendocrine cells secrete a variety of hormone and hormone-like substances involved in the regulation of gastric secretion, motility, and emptying (Table 21–1). These include gastrin, histamine, and serotonin.

The glands in the cardiac area of the stomach primarily secrete mucus, whereas those in the fundus and the body of the stomach secrete almost all the hydrochloric acid, pepsinogen, and intrinsic factor. The pyloric glands secrete mucus and the hormone gastrin.

Secretion of gastric glands is under both nervous and hormonal control and occurs in three phases:

Cephalic
Gastric
Intestinal

Table 21-1

Hormone and Hormone-Like Substances Involved in Regulating Gastric Secretion, Motility, and Emptying

Hormone	Source	Stimulus	Function
Gastrin	Enteroendocrine cells in gastric mucosa	Partially digested proteins, caffeine, and other chemicals in food present in stomach	Increases secretion of hydrochloric acid, pepsinogen by gastric glands Relaxes ileocecal valve
Serotonin	Enteroendocrine cells in gastric mucosa	Presence of food in the stomach	Contracts gastric muscles
Histamine	Enteroendocrine cells in gastric mucosa	Presence of food in the stomach	Stimulates secretion of hydrochloric acid by parietal cells
Somatostatin	Enteroendocrine cells in gastric mucosa	Presence of food in the stomach	Inhibits gastric secretion, motility, and emptying Inhibits pancreatic secretion Inhibits absorption in the small intestine by decreasing blood flow
Intestinal gastrin	Duodenal mucosa	Presence of acidic, partially digested food in the duodenum	Stimulates secretion by gastric glands
Secretin	Duodenal mucosa	Acid chyme, irritants, or partially digested protein in chyme, hypertonic fluids, or hypotonic fluids	Inhibits gastric secretion during gastric phase Increases production of bicarbonate ion-rich pancreatic juice Stimulates increased production of bile
Cholecystokinin (CCK)	Jejunal mucosa	Presence of fats in the intestinal contents	Stimulates gallbladder to contract and eject bile Simultaneously relaxes sphincter of Oddi and stimulates release of pancreatic juice
Gastric inhibitory peptide (GIP)	Duodenal mucosa	Presence of fats in the duodenum and, to a lesser degree, presence of carbohydrates	Decreases motor activity of the stomach and slows emptying of gastric contents into the duodenum

In the cephalic phase, gastric secretion is stimulated by the sight, smell, taste, or thought of food. This is a reflex response mediated by the vagus nerve. It serves to prepare the stomach for the arrival of foods requiring digestion.

In the gastric phase, several factors initiate secretion of gastric juice. The most significant factor is the hormone gastrin. Gastric distention also prompts secretion of gastric juice, as does histamine produced by enteroendocrine cells in the gastric mucosa. Gastrin-secreting (enteroendocrine) cells are directly activated by foods, such as partially digested proteins and caffeine. The gastrin secreted then directly stimulates other gastric secretory cells to increase production of gastric juice. The greatest effect is on the hydrochloric acid–producing parietal cells. Gastrin secretion is controlled by a negative feedback mechanism based on the pH of the stomach contents. When protein, which acts as a buffer, enters the stomach, pH rises and gastrin and hydro-

chloric acid are secreted. As protein digestion occurs and pH falls to 2, secretion is inhibited.

The intestinal phase of gastric secretion begins when partially digested food enters the duodenum. This stimulates release of a hormone called intestinal gastrin, which stimulates continued gastric secretion. Later, as chyme reaching the duodenum becomes more acidic, gastric secretion is inhibited.

In addition to its specialized secretory cells, the stomach wall differs from the rest of the GI tract in that the muscularis contains an innermost oblique layer of smooth muscle beneath the longitudinal and circular layers. This allows gastric contents not only to be propelled through the stomach but to be churned and pummeled to effectively mix and liquefy the bolus of food. It also contributes to the great distensibility of the stomach.

As a bolus of food enters the stomach, peristaltic movements pass over the stomach every 15 to 25 seconds. These movements macerate the bolus and mix it with the gastric secretions to form a thinner substance called chyme. As digestion continues, more forceful movements begin in the body of the stomach and increase as they reach the pylorus. When the chyme reaches the pylorus, a small amount is forced through the pyloric sphincter into the duodenum with each peristaltic movement. The remaining chyme is forced back into the stomach, where further mixing occurs (Fig. 21–3). Another wave pushes the chyme forward again, and a little more is squirted into the duodenum. This forward and backward movement of stomach contents accounts for most of the mixing in the stomach.

Like gastric secretion, gastric motility is under both hormonal (see Table 21–1) and nervous control. Parasympathetic stimulation via the vagus and its branches results in increased secretion and mobility, whereas sympathetic stimulation has an inhibiting effect on GI function.

Chemical digestion in the stomach consists of the breakdown of proteins into smaller molecules called peptides through the action of pepsin. Digestion of starches, which began in the mouth, ceases as salivary amylase is inactivated by the highly acid gastric environment. Basic nutrients are not absorbed in the stomach. Substances that are absorbed include water, alcohol, and weak acids such as aspirin.

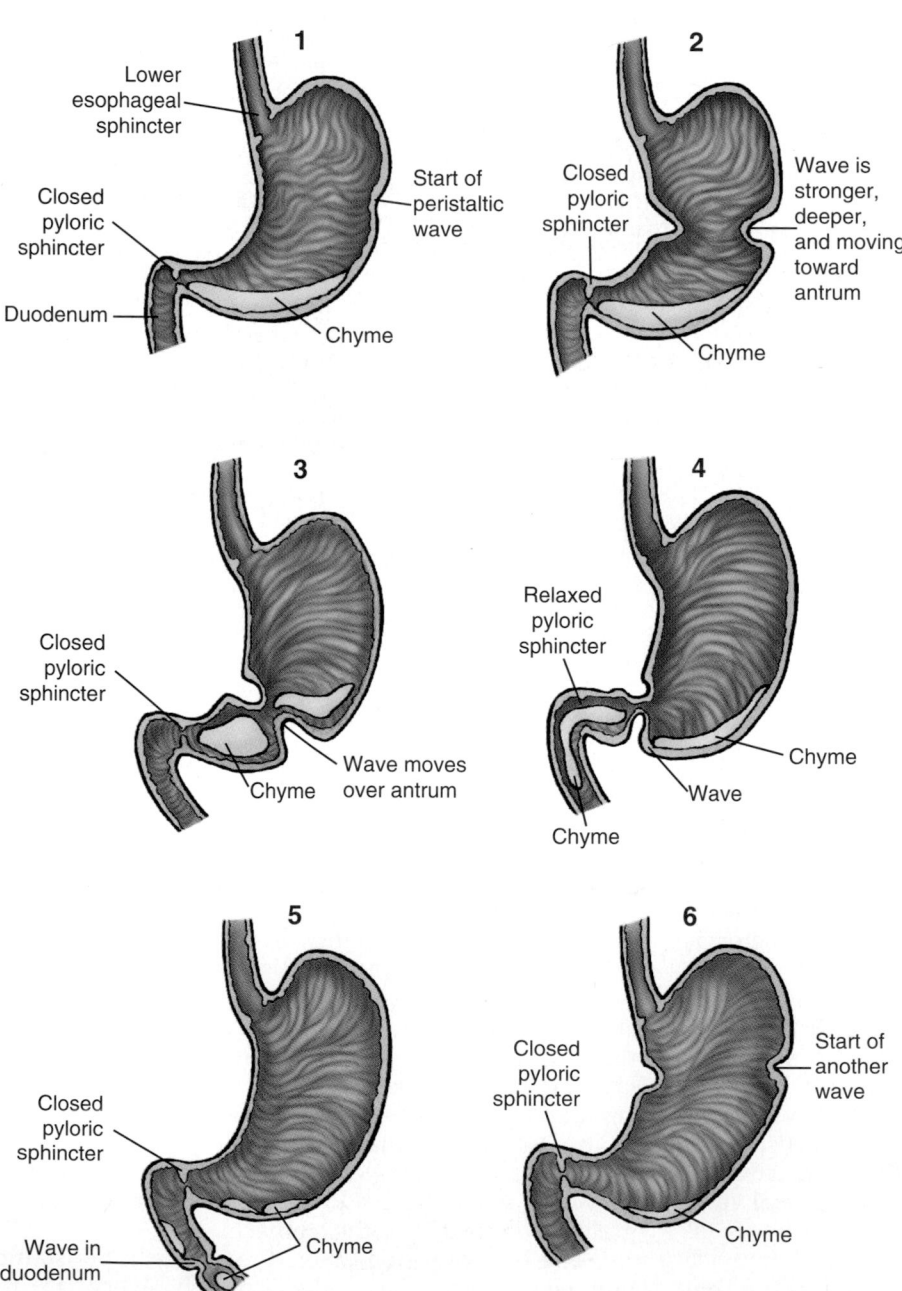

Figure 21–3

With each peristaltic wave passing over the stomach, chyme is forced toward the pyloric sphincter, a small amount is squirted into the duodenum, and the remainder is forced back into the stomach, where further mixing occurs.

SMALL INTESTINE

The small intestine is about 7 m (23 ft) long and 2.5 cm (1 in) in diameter. It is divided into three segments: duodenum, jejunum, and ileum. The duodenum, the shortest of the three, begins at the pyloric valve of the stomach and continues about 25 cm (10 in) until it unites with the jejunum. The pancreatic and bile ducts, joined at the common bile duct, empty into the duodenum through the sphincter of Oddi. The jejunum, the middle segment, is about 2.5 m (8 ft) long and merges with the ileum, which is about 3.5 m (12 ft) long. The ileum connects with the large intestine at the ileocecal valve, which guards the entrance to the cecum. This valve, which is usually closed to increase absorption time and prevent movement of bacteria from the large intestine into the small intestine, opens to allow passage of chyme into the cecum.

The small intestine is the principal organ of digestion and absorption. Structural adaptations in the form of plicae circulares, villi, and microvilli have developed to support these functions (Fig. 21–4).

The plicae circulares are deep, permanent circular folds in the mucosa and submucosa that force chyme to move in a spiral direction. This enhances mixing with digestive juices and slows forward movement of the chyme, prolonging contact time

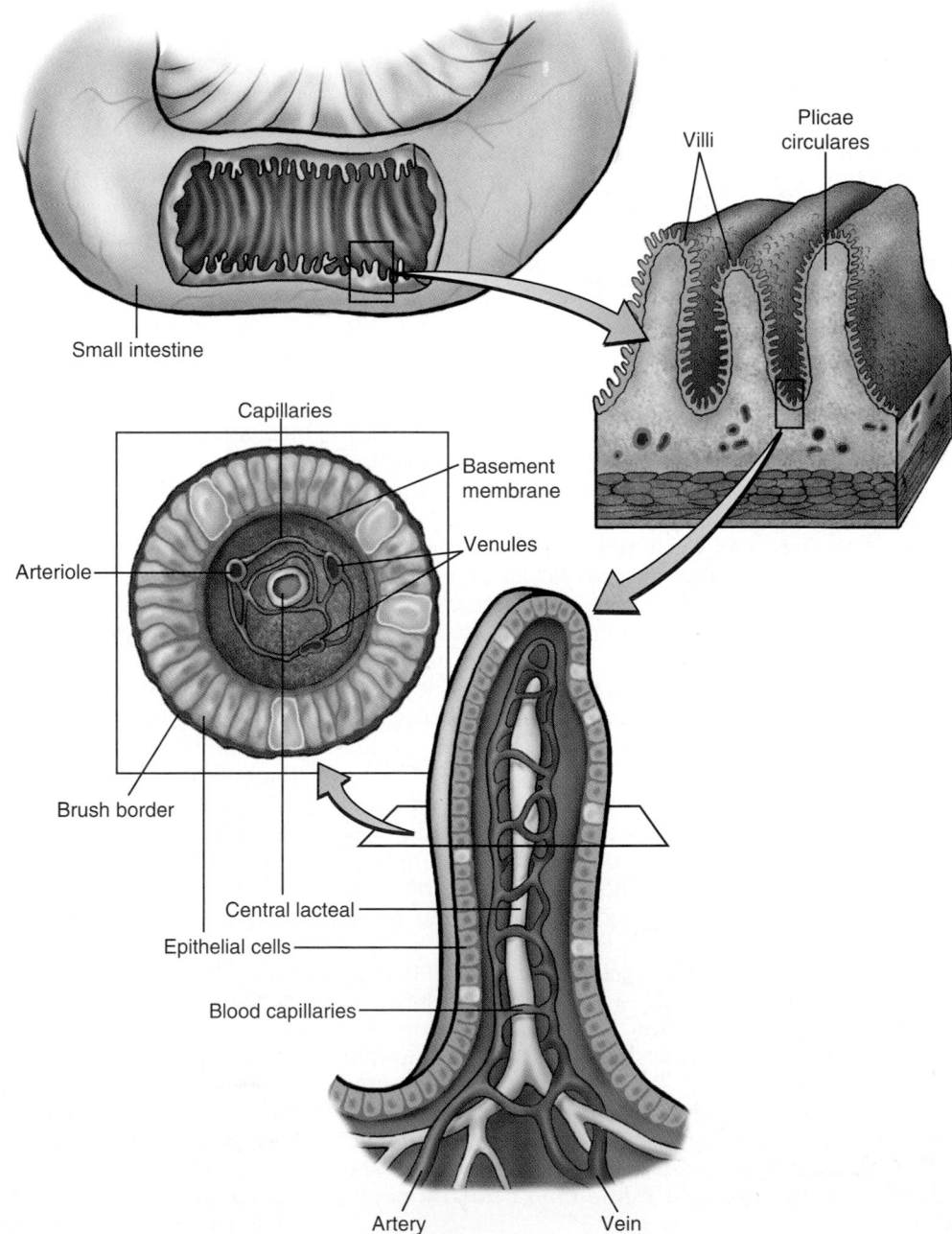

Figure 21–4

Adaptations in the wall of the small intestine assist digestion and absorption of foods. Note the plicae circulares covered with villi, the capillary bed and central lacteal in each villus, and the brush border of microvilli.

with both intestinal enzymes and the absorptive surface of the mucosa. Villi are finger-like projections clustered over the entire mucosa. They give the small intestine the texture of velvet. Each villus is about 1 mm long and contains a dense capillary bed and a modified lymphatic vessel called a lacteal. Villi absorb digested nutrients and transport them via the capillary bed or the lacteal into the blood stream. Microvilli are minute projections of the plasma membrane of mucosal absorptive cells that increase the absorptive surface. Microvilli form the "brush border" on the absorptive cells; they also contain digestive enzymes.

Between the villi, the mucosa is dotted with pits that lead into the crypts of Lieberkühn (intestinal crypts). These glands secrete both intestinal juice and hormones. The number of crypts and the size and number of plicae, villi, and microvilli decrease toward the end of the small intestine.

Brunner's glands are located in the submucosa of the duodenum. These glands secrete an alkaline mucus that protects the wall of the small intestine from the action of the digestive enzymes and assists in neutralizing the acid chyme as it enters from the stomach.

As previously described, movement of chyme from the stomach into the small intestine is a slow process carefully controlled by the pyloric valve. It is essential for two reasons that only small amounts of chyme enter the duodenum at one time. First, chyme is usually hypertonic, and large amounts would pull water by osmosis into the intestine and could seriously decrease blood volume. Second, chyme from the stomach is highly acidic, and the pH must be raised for the digestive enzymes in the small intestine to function.

Once in the small intestine, chyme is subjected to two types of movement: segmentation and peristalsis. Segmentation involves alternate contractions of the circular muscle fibers. It mixes the chyme with digestive juices and brings it into contact with the villi. Peristaltic waves then move the chyme forward in the small intestine. Both movements are initiated by distention of the intestine and controlled by the autonomic nervous system.

Chyme that enters the small intestine contains partially digested carbohydrates, partially digested proteins, and for the most part, undigested lipids. The completion of the digestion of these nutrients is a combined effort of bile, pancreatic juice, and intestinal juice.

Starches entering the small intestine are hydrolyzed by pancreatic amylase into disaccharides, which in turn are broken down into absorbable monosaccharides by disaccharases in the intestinal juices and on the brush border. Similarly, proteoses (protein fragments) that enter the duodenum are split into peptides by trypsin, chymotrypsin, and other proteases found in the pancreatic juice. The peptides in turn are split into amino acids by peptidases.

Fats entering the small intestine are emulsified by bile to prepare them for the action of pancreatic lipase, which breaks them down into fatty acids and glycerides. Bile then renders the fatty acids water-soluble so they can be absorbed across the intestinal mucosa.

LARGE INTESTINE

The large intestine is about 1.5 m (5 ft) long and 6.5 cm ($2\frac{5}{8}$ in) in diameter. It extends from the ileum to the anus and is divided into four parts:

Cecum
Colon
Rectum
Anal canal

The cecum is a blind pouch about 6 cm ($2\frac{3}{8}$ in) long. Attached to the lower portion of the cecum is a narrow coiled tube called the vermiform appendix. The opening from the ileum into the cecum is protected by a large fold of mucous membrane called the ileocecal valve, which allows digestive byproducts from the small intestine to pass into the large intestine.

The colon extends from the cecum to the rectum and is divided into the ascending, transverse, descending, and sigmoid colon. The ascending colon passes upward on the lower right side of the abdomen to become the transverse colon at the hepatic flexure. The transverse colon crosses the mid-abdomen, bends downward at the splenic flexure on the left side, and becomes the descending colon. At the level of the iliac crest, the colon curves like the letter S and is called the sigmoid colon, which terminates at the rectum. The rectum continues from the sigmoid colon and ends at the anal canal. The terminal portion of the large intestine, or the anal canal, is about 2 to 3 cm (1 in) long. The opening of the anal canal to the exterior, called the anus, is guarded by an internal and an external sphincter. These sphincters remain closed except during the act of defecation, when the residue of digestion is expelled.

The mucosa of the large intestine differs from that of the small intestine in that it does not have villi or circular folds. It does, however, contain simple columnar epithelium with numerous goblet cells that absorb water and secrete mucus to lubricate the residue as it passes through the colon.

The muscularis of the colon is also unique in that it does not completely surround the colon but rather forms three bands called the taeniae coli. These bands, when contracted, gather the colon into a series of pouches called haustra, giving it a puckered appearance.

Movement in the large intestine consists of peristalsis, which is mild and slow, haustral churning, and mass movements. Haustral churning refers to the action of smooth muscle in individual haustra. As chyme passes through the ileocecal valve, it fills and distends the first haustrum in the cecum. This distention causes the smooth muscle in the haustrum to contract and thus mixes and propels the chyme to the next haustrum.

Mass movements are long, slow, strong waves of muscular contraction that start in the transverse colon and propel colonic contents into the rectum. They occur three or four times daily, usually during or just after eating, as a result of the gastrocolic and gastroduodenal reflexes. These reflexes result from the presence of food in the stomach or duodenum, which stimulates mass peristalsis in the colon. These mass movements become stronger as the amount of bulk in the diet is increased.

The large intestine reabsorbs water and electrolytes, particularly sodium and chloride, and stores feces until defecation. No enzymes are produced in the colon, and no digestion occurs. However, any remaining carbohydrates or amino acids are metabolized by colonic bacteria, releasing gases such as hydrogen, carbon dioxide, and methane, which contribute to fecal odor.

Colonic bacteria also produce vitamin K and some B vitamins. These are absorbed by the colon along with water and electrolytes. Finally, they provide bulk and help propel the stool into the rectum.

The defecation reflex is stimulated by distention of the rectum. The internal and external sphincters involuntarily relax when this happens, but an overriding central nervous system control allows the person to voluntarily suppress the urge to defecate by contracting the external sphincter.

Nearly 10 L of fluid pass through the GI tract of the average adult every 24 hours. This includes 1 to 2 L of saliva, 3 L of gastric fluid, 0.5 L of bile, 1 L of pancreatic juice, and 2 L of intestinal secretions in addition to the average 1 to 2 L that is ingested. Evacuated feces contain about 150 mL of water.

LIVER

The liver is the body's largest internal organ. It has multiple functions that affect many different body systems (see Chap. 25). These functions include storage and metabolism of nutrients that have been digested and absorbed, detoxification of noxious substances, and production of bile.

Bile, which is continuously produced by the liver, prepares lipids to be broken down by the enzyme lipase. This is done by the bile salts, mainly cholic acid and chenodeoxycholic acid, which emulsify fats (break them into small droplets and distribute them throughout the watery chyme). The result is a large surface area on which lipase can act. Bile salts also facilitate fat and cholesterol absorption and, with lecithin, make cholesterol soluble.

The pigment chiefly responsible for the greenish-yellow color of bile is bilirubin. Bilirubin is metabolized by bacteria in the small intestine, and a breakdown product, urobilinogen, gives feces their characteristic brown color. Without urobilinogen, feces are pale gray to white.

GALLBLADDER

The gallbladder is a pear-shaped muscular sac located below the liver. It is about 8 cm (3 in) long and 2.5 cm (1 in) wide. Its major function is to store and concentrate bile secreted by the liver. The liver secretes bile continuously, but the sphincter of Oddi, through which bile passes into the duodenum, is closed when bile is not needed for digestion. At these times, bile backs up into the gallbladder to be stored until fats enter the duodenum and stimulate release of cholecystokinin. This intestinal hormone stimulates the gallbladder to contract and eject bile into the cystic duct, from which it flows into the common bile duct, through the sphincter of Oddi, and into the duodenum (Fig. 21–5). Cholecystokinin simultaneously stimulates release of pancreatic juice and relaxes the sphincter of Oddi.

PANCREAS

The pancreas is the primary producer of digestive enzymes. It is a large gland about 15 cm (6 in) long and 2.5 cm (1 in) wide and is divided into the head, the body, and the tail. The pancreas lies behind the stomach, with its head lying in the curve of the duodenum and its tail reaching to the spleen.

The pancreas is both an endocrine and an exocrine gland. Its endocrine cells secrete insulin and glucagon (see Chap. 28), and the exocrine (or acinar) cells secrete a high-bicarbonate solution and enzymes specific to the digestion of each of the three basic nutrients.

The watery, very alkaline solution with a high sodium bicarbonate content is produced by specialized cells in the head of the pancreas. This solution neutralizes acid chyme and raises the pH to the level needed for effective action of pancreatic and intestinal enzymes. It is secreted in response to stimulation by the hormone secretin, which is released when hydrochloric acid enters the small intestine.

The secretion of enzyme-rich pancreatic fluid is stimulated by cholecystokinin, the same hormone that stimulates the gallbladder to contract. Intestinal cholecystokinin is released when proteoses, peptones, or fats are present in the upper small intestine. Pancreatic fluid contains the following enzymes:

- Pancreatic amylase, which hydrolyzes starch into maltose and chains of glucose molecules
- Pancreatic lipase, which breaks emulsified fats into fatty acids and monoglycerides
- Trypsin, chymotrypsin, and other proteases, which split proteoses into peptides

The last three all are secreted in inactive form to prevent digestion of the pancreatic cells themselves.

Pancreatic juice leaves the pancreas through the pancreatic duct, which enters the duodenum near the common bile duct. A summary of the digestive secretions, including their source, pH, daily volume,

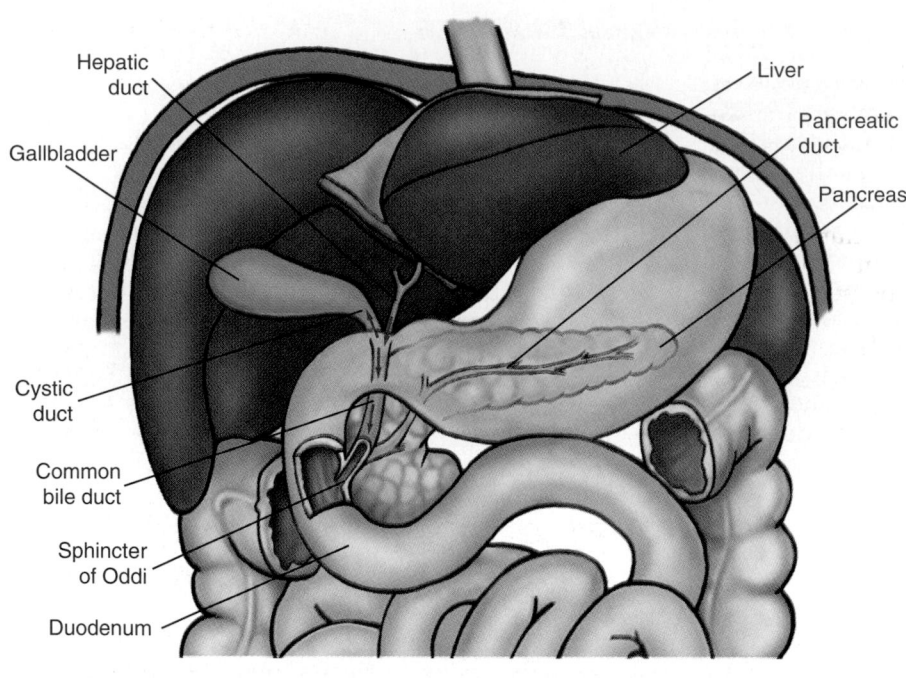

Hepatic duct
Gallbladder
Cystic duct
Common bile duct
Sphincter of Oddi
Duodenum
Liver
Pancreatic duct
Pancreas

Figure 21–5

Anatomical relationships of the liver, gallbladder, pancreas, and duodenum. Arrows indicate the path of bile flow.

component enzymes, and role in chemical digestion is presented in Table 21–2.

Clinical Manifestations of Gastrointestinal Dysfunction

ANOREXIA

Anorexia is the absence of desire to eat despite the physiologic need for food or a situation in which the desire for food is normally expected. This lack of appetite can be episodic and transient, or it can be chronic.

Appetite is a complex phenomenon controlled by the interplay of bilateral feeding and satiety centers in the hypothalamus. Because these centers are affected by a wide variety of sensory, metabolic, and hormonal factors, anorexia can have both physical and psychologic causes. Physical causes include GI and liver disorders that disturb normal metabolic processes or produce edema or decreased muscle tone in the tract, inflammatory disorders, severe pulmonary disease, uremia, congestive heart failure,

Table 21–2

Summary of Digestive Secretions and Enzymes

Secretion	Volume per Day	pH	Enzyme	Source	Action and Products
Saliva	1–1.5 L	6.8	Salivary amylase	Salivary glands	Hydrolyzes starch to maltose
Gastric juice	1.5–2.5 L	2–4	Pepsin	Gastric mucosa	Breaks down protein into proteoses, peptones, and polypeptides
Pancreatic juice	600–800 mL	8–8.4	Trypsin	Pancreas	Splits proteins into amino acids and polypeptides
			Chymotrypsin	Pancreas	Splits proteins
			Pancreatic amylase	Pancreas	Splits starch into maltose
			Pancreas lipase	Pancreas	Hydrolyzes fats into fatty acids and monoglycerides
Intestinal juice	2–3 L	7–9	Intestinal lipase	Intestinal glands	Splits fats into fatty acids and glycerol
			Peptidase	Intestinal glands	Splits polypeptides into amino acids
			Enterokinase	Duodenal mucosa	Activates trypsin
			Maltase Sucrase Lactase	Intestinal glands	Split disaccharides into monosaccharides

and cancer. Anorexia is also associated with poor oral hygiene, abdominal distention, and such drugs as amphetamines. Psychologic causes of anorexia include fear, anxiety, depression, and offensive sights, odors, and conversations, as well as the association of eating or particular foods with unpleasant experiences.

Prolonged anorexia can lead to malnutrition and ultimately to life-threatening fluid and electrolyte imbalance. Medical management is focused on treating the underlying condition and correcting nutritional deficiencies. The latter may include supplemental feedings, total parenteral nutrition, or both.

NURSING PROCESS
Anorexia

Assessment

Begin assessment of the anorexic patient with a dietary history. Determine the types and amounts of foods usually eaten. Compare this with the patient's report of current dietary intake. Determine when the anorexia began, and explore its relationship to any other symptoms, environmental factors, or life events.

Assess the patient's general nutritional status. Check current weight and determine whether weight loss has occurred and over what period of time. Observe for signs of malnutrition, such as dull, thin, brittle hair; tired, apathetic facial expression; dry skin and nails; and muscle wasting. Review laboratory values—such as albumin levels, lymphocyte counts, and serum electrolyte levels—for changes that suggest malnutrition (albumin level <3.5 g/dL, lymphocyte count <1500 mm³).

Ask about foods and fluids the patient likes and dislikes. Then determine which are tolerated well and which not well. Find out times during the day when the patient usually eats, and times when the patient is usually most hungry. Assess the patient's understanding of dietary requirements, nutritional value of foods, and methods of food preparation.

Nursing Diagnoses and Planning

Nursing diagnoses and related expected patient outcomes commonly applicable to patients with anorexia include the following:

NDx: Altered nutrition: less than body requirements related to lack of appetite

Planning: Patient Outcomes
1. Patient eats a *(specify for individual)* calorie diet per day.
2. Patient consumes *(specify for individual)* grams of protein per day.
3. Patient maintains current weight.

NDx: Altered health maintenance related to insufficient knowledge of dietary requirements, nutritional value of specific foods, or methods of adjusting food preparation or service to make the food more appetizing

Planning: Patient Outcomes
1. Patient describes his or her daily dietary requirements.
2. Patient identifies nutritional value of specific foods relative to his or her dietary needs.
3. Patient describes ways to make foods more appetizing.

Nursing Interventions and Evaluation

NDx: Altered nutrition: less than body requirements
Offer the patient foods that are well liked and that meet the patient's nutritional needs. Avoid offering foods that will fill the patient up but have little nutritional value. Urge the family to provide favorite foods if not otherwise available.

Encourage the patient to eat at the time of day when he or she is most hungry. Before serving food, be sure that the patient does not need to go to the bathroom. Check that hands, face, and mouth are clean. Confirm that he or she is positioned appropriately and is as comfortable as possible. Provide small portions attractively served. Make sure that utensils are spotlessly clean and that cold foods are cold and hot foods hot. Keep the environment calm, neat, and free of odors or offensive sights and sounds. Explore the possibility of communal dining or guest trays for visitors to enhance the social quality of dining.

Discuss with the patient and significant others strategies that can improve appetite at home or when eating out. For example, a nutritious appetizer can be ordered in a restaurant and served when others receive their main course.

NDx: Altered health maintenance
Explain the patient's individual dietary needs so that they are clearly understood by the patient and any significant other who has a key role in food selection and preparation. Describe the nutrient value of various foods and identify those best suited to the patient's needs. Discuss methods of preparation that maximize nutritional value and tend to be appetizing. Explain the importance of personal comfort, a clean, stress-free environment, and attractively served food in promoting appetite. Arrange for teaching by a dietitian whenever necessary.

Compare the patient's status with the expected outcomes. If the outcomes are not met, reassess the patient and revise the plan.

NAUSEA AND VOMITING

Nausea is a disagreeable feeling of revulsion usually accompanied by symptoms of altered autonomic nervous system activity, such as diaphoresis, increased salivation, pallor, tachycardia, dizziness, and faintness. Nausea usually precedes the act of vomiting, which is the expulsion of upper GI contents through the mouth as a result of reverse peristalsis and relaxation of the lower esophageal sphincter.

Two centers in the medulla are involved with vomiting: the vomiting center and the chemoreceptor trigger zone. The vomiting center is stimulated directly by the autonomic nervous system. Such stimulants as GI distention, irritants and toxins, injury to the viscera, pain, and even emotional upheaval can cause nausea and vomiting in this direct way. The vomiting center can also be directly stimulated by the local pressure that occurs with increased intracranial pressure.

Indirect stimulation of the vomiting center occurs when an emetic agent stimulates the chemoreceptor trigger zone, which in turn causes the vomiting center to respond. Emetic agents include such drugs as morphine, meperidine (Demerol), ergot derivatives, and digitalis preparations, as well as metabolic substances resulting from uremia, infection, and radiation. Motion in the semicircular canals of the ears is also believed to cause nausea and vomiting through the indirect trigger zone route.

A specific type of vomiting is projectile vomiting, which is associated with increased intracranial pressure and pyloric obstruction. It occurs without warning and is so forceful that the emesis is projected a distance from the mouth. Retching is contraction of the stomach as in vomiting but without emesis because the stomach is empty.

The medical management of nausea and vomiting focuses both on treating the underlying disorder and on removing the precipitating cause of the reflex. For example, gastric lavage or suction may be used to remove irritating substances from the stomach. A nasogastric tube may be inserted to reduce gastric distention. Drugs known to stimulate the chemoreceptor trigger zone are discontinued. Metabolic disorders that result in circulating "toxins" that stimulate the chemoreceptor trigger zone are corrected. Antiemetic drugs may be ordered to depress the sensitivity of the chemoreceptor trigger zone.

The major complication of vomiting is fluid and electrolyte imbalance. Gastric acid contains large amounts of potassium and chloride as well as hydrogen ions. Excessive losses of these substances can result in metabolic alkalosis and hypokalemia as well as dehydration.

A second serious complication of vomiting is aspiration of vomitus into the lungs, which can cause asphyxia, atelectasis, or pneumonitis.

NURSING PROCESS
Nausea and Vomiting

Assessment

Question the patient about the occurrence of nausea and vomiting. Ask about times of onset, duration, precipitating factors, associated symptoms, and types of remedies tried as well as their effectiveness in providing relief. Also ask about the appearance, amount, and odor of vomitus. When possible, inspect vomitus for the presence of undigested food, which can indicate gastric irritation so acute that food is immediately vomited. Check for mucus, which can indicate chronic gastritis or rhinopharyngitis. And check for parasites or foreign bodies. Note also the color of the vomitus. If it is black or has a coffee-ground appearance, it probably contains old blood. Red vomitus may indicate recent bleeding. Green vomitus contains bile and indicates that it came from the duodenum beyond the entrance of the bile duct. Brown vomitus may contain feces, indicating that the vomitus has come from the large intestine.

Nursing Diagnoses and Planning

Nursing diagnoses and related expected patient outcomes commonly applicable to patients with nausea and vomiting include the following:

NDx: Risk for fluid volume deficit related to loss of fluids from the GI tract secondary to vomiting

Planning: Patient Outcomes
1. Skin turgor is firm.
2. Oral mucous membranes are moist and shiny.
3. Serum electrolyte levels remain in normal range.

Nursing Interventions and Evaluation

NDx: Risk for fluid volume deficit
Avoid exposing the patient to stimuli likely to produce or worsen nausea, which in turn can precipitate vomiting and concomitant fluid loss. Maintain a calm, quiet environment. Limit visitors if necessary. Avoid moving the patient suddenly or unnecessarily. Encourage the patient to take deep breaths when feeling nauseated. Apply cold compresses to the forehead if these comfort the patient.

Keep the room well ventilated and free of strong or disagreeable odors. Discard vomitus and remove soiled clothing or linens immediately. Assist the patient in rinsing and cleansing the mouth after each episode of vomiting.

Administer antiemetics and intravenous fluids as ordered. Measure all vomitus. Maintain a careful record of all fluid intake and output.

When oral intake is resumed, give clear fluids, such as water or ginger ale, in small amounts (eg, 20 mL every 30 minutes). If this is tolerated, gradually increase amounts, adding foods such as gelatin, tea, and consommé. Progress to small, frequent meals of toast, cereal, chicken, and other easily digested bland foods. Encourage the patient to take fluids an hour before or after a meal but not with it, because fluids with meals distend the stomach and can precipitate vomiting.

Avoid giving foods high in fat and those that are known to stimulate peristalsis, such as orange juice. Caffeine and high-fiber foods should also be avoided.

If foods high in potassium are needed for replacement, include tea, bananas, dry whole milk, and cheese in the diet as tolerated.

Additional Interventions

Position the patient in a side-lying or semi-Fowler's position to prevent aspiration. Remove dentures. If necessary, remove vomitus from the mouth of comatose, anesthetized, or otherwise impaired patients.

Compare the patient's status with the expected outcomes. If the outcomes are not met, reassess the patient and revise the plan.

INTESTINAL GAS

Symptoms caused by intestinal gas are eructation, abdominal distention, pain, and excessive flatus. Eructation, commonly known as belching, is the escape of gas from the GI tract through the mouth. This can result from disease (eg, gastric dilatation) or outlet obstruction but most often results from swallowed air.

Abdominal distention or bloating is caused by abnormal motility of the intestine. It is not from excessive amounts of gas. In some areas of the intestine, motility is increased, whereas other areas are in spasm. When gas being propelled through the intestine more rapidly than normal encounters areas of resistance due to spasm, the proximal bowel dilates, stretching the smooth muscle, and distention and cramping result.

Flatus is gas passed through the rectum. Seven to 10 L of gas ordinarily enter the large intestine daily. Part of this gas comes from swallowed air and part results from bacterial action in the large intestine. Of this, only 0.6 L is normally expelled. The remainder is absorbed.

Increased flatus can result either from excessive production of gas or from impaired absorption of gas. Excessive gas production occurs with ingestion of gas-forming foods, such as beans, cabbage, onions, cauliflower, and corn, many of which contain nonabsorbable carbohydrates that serve as a medium for bacterial growth. Impaired absorption occurs when intestinal motility increases and gases pass through the large intestine so quickly that there is insufficient time for absorption. This may result from ingestion of irritating foods.

CONSTIPATION

Constipation is the passage of hard, dry stool—less often than occurs with the person's normal pattern of defecation. Stool becomes hard and dry when it spends an abnormally long time in the large intestine, where water is constantly removed. This prolonged transit time can result from a disorder, such as a stricture or partial obstruction of the intestinal lumen by a tumor. In most cases, however, constipation relates to personal habits. Specific factors that contribute to constipation include lack of adequate dietary fiber, inadequate fluid intake, lack of exercise, and irregular bowel habits (eg, suppressing the urge to defecate because of inopportune time or fear

of discomfort, as with hemorrhoids). Constipation can also result from a weakened ability to raise intra-abdominal pressure, as with emphysema or poor abdominal muscle tone. It may also occur as a side effect of medications, such as anticholinergics, tranquilizers, morphine derivatives, and aluminum-containing antacids. It can also result from progressive weakening of reflexes involved in defecation secondary to prolonged use of laxatives.

Symptoms that often accompany constipation are a feeling of pressure or fullness in the rectum, back pain, headache, anorexia, and malaise. Streaks of blood may appear in the stool from irritation of the rectal and anal mucosa as the hard stool passes. If an incomplete obstruction of the bowel is causing the constipation, loose stool seeps around it and the patient passes a colored, watery mucus. Occasionally, constipation may become so severe that a fecal impaction forms. This is a condition in which exceedingly hard feces block the rectum. When this occurs, the impaction may need to be mechanically removed with a gloved finger. Prolonged constipation may result in a true obstruction of the colon, a pathologic state that is discussed in Chapter 23.

Medical treatment of constipation aims to eliminate the cause. Laxatives (Highlight 21–1) and enemas are prescribed only when all natural efforts have failed, because these agents decrease muscle tone and mucus production, and they do not resolve the underlying problem. Stool softeners may be used for patients at risk for constipation, such as the bedridden or those taking narcotics on a long-term basis.

NURSING PROCESS
Constipation

Assessment

Obtain a bowel history to serve as a baseline for assessment. Ask the patient how often bowel movements normally occur and obtain a description of the stool's color, amount, and consistency (formed, mushy, frothy, or liquid). Determine the time of day that defecation usually occurs and any associated events, such as drinking hot coffee, eating, or smoking. Keep in mind that bowel pattern varies from person to person such that two bowel movements per day may be normal for one patient, whereas one bowel movement every 3 days may be normal for another.

Ask about any symptoms related to defecation, such as abdominal distention, cramping, straining, or bleeding. Determine current bowel status, noting time of last bowel movement, type of stool, and any accompanying distress. Explore personal habits and lifestyle characteristics that could affect bowel function. Obtain information about diet, exercise, and use of medications, including laxatives. Auscultate bowel sounds, noting frequency and pitch. Gently palpate and percuss for abdominal distention. In-

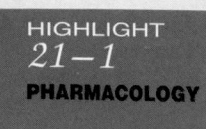 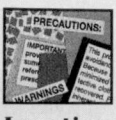

HIGHLIGHT
21–1
PHARMACOLOGY

Laxatives

Definition:

Drugs used to facilitate or stimulate passage of feces

Classified by action into bulk formers, surfactants, contact laxatives, saline laxatives, and miscellaneous

Classified by effect into the following categories:

Group I—act in 2 to 6 hours and produce watery stool

Group II—act in 6 to 12 hours and produce semi-fluid stool

Group III—act in 1 to 3 days and produce soft, formed stool

Action:

Bulk Formers—These nondigestible, nonabsorbable substances swell with water to form a gel that softens and enlarges the fecal mass, thus stretching the intestinal wall and stimulating reflex peristalsis (eg, psyllium [Metamucil])

Surfactants—Soften stool by lowering its surface tension, allowing absorption of water; also inhibit fluid absorption by intestinal wall and stimulate secretion of water and electrolytes into lumen (eg, docusate sodium [Colace]).

Contact Laxatives—Promote secretion of water and electrolytes into the intestine, and decrease their absorption, softening feces and stimulating peristalsis (eg, bisacodyl [Dulcolax], castor oil)

Saline Laxatives—Pull water into intestine by osmotic action, swelling and softening feces and stimulating peristalsis (eg, magnesium hydroxide [milk of magnesia])

Miscellaneous—Mineral oil lubricates feces and inhibits water absorption

Uses:

Bulk Formers—Temporary treatment of constipation; symptomatic relief of diarrhea in patients with a colostomy or ileostomy—also used in irritable bowel syndrome and diverticulosis

Surfactants—Used to prevent straining at stool in postoperative cardiac patients and those with anal or rectal diseases

Contact Laxatives—Few therapeutic uses other than preparing the bowel for diagnostic tests.

Saline Laxatives—High-dose therapy used for bowel preparation, to eliminate ingested poisons, or to remove dead parasites after treatment with antihelmintic agents

Side Effects:

Repeated laxative use depresses the reflexes involved in defecation, leading to further dependence on laxatives. It can also cause dehydration, electrolyte imbalance, and colitis.

Interactions:

None with stimulant, bulk-forming, or hyperosmolar agents. Mineral oil can interfere with absorption of fat-soluble vitamins, oral contraceptives, and anticoagulants. Also interferes with the anti-infective action of nonabsorbable sulfonamides.

Nursing Implications:

Administer bulk-forming laxatives with a full glass of water or juice to prevent esophageal obstruction. Also give a full glass of water with surfactant and saline laxatives.

Make castor oil more palatable by chilling and giving with juice.

Instruct patients in regard to bowel function:

- Individuals have different elimination patterns.
- Quality of stool is more important than quantity or frequency.
- The urge to defecate should not be ignored.
- Dietary fiber, as found in fruits, vegetables, and bran, is needed for proper bowel function.
- Daily exercise promotes good bowel function.
- Laxatives should be taken only when absolutely necessary and in the smallest effective dose.

---

spect the anal area for hemorrhoids, fissures, or irritation. Inspect stool specimens when available.

Nursing Diagnoses and Planning

Nursing diagnoses and related expected patient outcomes commonly applicable to patients with constipation include the following:

NDx: Constipation related to lifestyle factors, lack of knowledge about normal bowel function, or both

Planning: Patient Outcomes
1. Patient passes soft, formed stool at regular intervals.
2. Patient reports absence of uncomfortable straining at stool.

Nursing Interventions and Evaluation

NDx: Constipation

Explain to the patient the relationship of fluids and dietary fiber to normal bowel function. Stress the need for 8 to 10 glasses of fluid per day, and teach about good sources of dietary fiber, such as fruits, vegetables, grain products, and nuts. Suggest adding bran to cereal to increase dietary fiber. Instruct the patient to begin with a small amount of added bran and to gradually increase the amount as tolerated until 2 g have been added.

Explain the importance of exercise, and encourage walking and abdominal exercises (eg, leg-lifts and sit-ups) when possible. Encourage bedridden patients to move frequently, do range-of-motion exercises, leg raising, or bicycle exercises as their condition allows.

To facilitate defecation, provide privacy and assist the patient to the most normal position possible. Take time to help the patient to the bathroom or to a commode rather than onto a bedpan, which should be used only as a last resort. Support the patient's usual schedule of evacuation, and encourage defecation when the gastrocolic reflex is most active (following a meal, particularly breakfast).

Compare the patient's status with the expected outcomes. If the outcomes are not met, reassess the patient and revise the plan.

DIARRHEA

Diarrhea is an abnormally liquid stool passed more often than normal for the patient's usual pattern of defecation. It results from excessive water in the intestinal contents, from changes in intestinal motility, or—as is often the case—a combination of the two. Abnormally large amounts of water in the intestinal contents can result from impaired absorption or from increased secretion of electrolytes and water by cells of the intestinal wall in reaction to toxins (eg, the salmonella enterotoxin) or to hormones (eg, serotonin), as occurs in malignant carcinoid syndrome. It may also result from substances that pull water into the intestine by osmosis. Such substances may be poorly absorbable solutes that have been ingested (eg, bran), products of maldigestion, or a dietary nonelectrolyte (eg, glucose) that has failed to be transported into the cells.

Changes in intestinal motility most often contribute to diarrhea by increasing peristalsis and thus the speed with which intestinal contents pass through the tract. This decreases the time that intestinal contents are in contact with the cells of the intestinal wall, decreasing water absorption. Increased peristalsis may result from abnormal bowel contents, intrinsic irritability of the bowel, or inflammation of the bowel. Examples of disorders that produce diarrhea because of one or more of these mechanisms are irritable bowel syndrome, enteritis, ulcerative colitis, and Crohn's disease.

Symptoms that commonly accompany diarrhea include the following:

- Abdominal cramping
- Presence of mucus, blood, or fat in unformed stool
- Urgency, such that stool may be expelled involuntarily if there is any delay in reaching the toilet
- Tenesmus (painful straining to empty the bowel without evacuation of feces)
- Perianal discomfort
- A feeling that the rectum has not been completely emptied

Uncorrected diarrhea can lead to severe fluid and electrolyte imbalance. Water loss as high as 10 L in 24 hours—accompanied by loss of sodium, potassium, and bicarbonate—can lead to dehydration, electrolyte imbalance, metabolic acidosis, and malnutrition. Irritation and breakdown of the anal area can result from contact with the diarrheal stool.

In addition to identifying and treating the cause of diarrhea, a major concern of medical management is preventing or treating fluid and electrolyte imbalances and acidosis. In cases of moderate to severe diarrhea, fluids are administered intravenously. Potassium is added once adequate renal function is established.

NURSING PROCESS
Diarrhea

Assessment

Assess the patient as described under Constipation. Be certain to question the patient about urgency and anal discomfort. Assess for signs and symptoms of dehydration and electrolyte imbalance, and review related laboratory values. If the diarrhea may be infectious in origin, question the patient about exposure to persons with similar symptoms. Ask about foods eaten in the last 24 to 48 hours. Determine whether the patient has traveled recently.

Nursing Diagnoses and Planning

Nursing diagnoses and related expected patient outcomes commonly applicable to patients with diarrhea include the following:

NDx: Diarrhea related to (*specify*)

Planning: Patient Outcomes
1. Patient passes formed stool at regular intervals.
2. Patient reports decrease in frequency and liquidity of stools.

NDx: Fluid volume deficit related to excessive water loss in the stool

Planning: Patient Outcomes
1. Skin turgor is firm.
2. Mucous membranes are moist.
3. Urinary output is at least 50 mL/h.

4. Urine specific gravity is within normal range.

5. Serum electrolyte levels are within normal range.

NDx: Risk for impaired tissue integrity related to irritation of the anal area by diarrheal stool

Planning: Patient Outcomes

1. Anal skin and mucous membrane are free of erythema.
2. Anal skin and mucous membrane are intact.
3. Patient denies tenderness or burning in the anal area.

Nursing Interventions and Evaluation

NDx: Diarrhea

Recognize that diarrhea embarrasses most people, especially when accompanied by urgency and possible loss of control. Be sensitive to the patient's need for privacy. Ensure that the room is well ventilated and odor-free. Maintain easy access to the bedpan or toilet. If the patient needs assistance, respond as quickly as possible. Maintain a quiet, stress-free environment and encourage bedrest because activity stimulates peristalsis.

Administer prescribed antidiarrheal medications (Highlight 21–2). Limit oral intake according to physician's orders because ingestion of food or fluids stimulates peristalsis. In cases of mild diarrhea, the patient is typically allowed nothing by mouth (NPO status) for at least 4 hours. When oral intake is resumed, offer small amounts of liquids, such as weak tea, bouillon, Jell-O, and then thin-cooked cereal, which replaces lost electrolytes but does not stimulate the intestine. Progress as tolerated to a low-residue diet that includes such foods as tender beef, veal, chicken, boiled or steamed rice, and hard-boiled eggs. Avoid cold liquids, caffeine, and concentrated sweets.

NDx: Fluid volume deficit

Administer intravenous fluids as ordered. Maintain a record of fluid intake and output, being certain to measure liquid stool and count it as output. Check urine specific gravity and weigh the patient daily. Monitor laboratory values for indications of fluid and electrolyte balance, such as increased serum osmolality, increased hematocrit, and hypokalemia.

NDx: Risk for impaired tissue integrity

After every bowel movement, wipe the anal area with soft toilet tissue, then wash gently with warm water and gentle soap, rinse thoroughly, and pat dry. Apply a protective salve such as petroleum jelly. If irritation develops or persists despite this routine, try washing and drying with warm water and absorbent cotton. Also eliminate the use of ointments, because they restrict perspiration and may contribute to irritation in some cases.

Give sitz baths for 10 minutes two or three times daily to promote healing and comfort. Apply witch hazel–soaked soft pads, such as Tucks, as an additional comfort measure if needed.

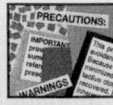

HIGHLIGHT 21–2 PHARMACOLOGY

Nonspecific Antidiarrheal Agents

Definition:

Drugs used in the treatment of diarrhea. Specific antidiarrheal drugs are used to treat the underlying cause of the diarrhea. Nonspecific antidiarrheals act on or within the bowel to relieve diarrhea without regard to its cause.

Action:

Opioids, the most effective nonspecific antidiarrheal agents, stimulate receptors in the gastrointestinal tract that suppress peristalsis and promote absorption of water and electrolytes (eg, diphenoxylate [Lomotil], loperamide [Imodium]).

Uses:

Decrease the fluidity of feces and the frequency of defecation.

Side Effects:

When used in cases of infectious diarrhea, lengthen the time the infecting organisms remain in the gastrointestinal tract and can prolong the infection. No other side effects at dose used to treat diarrhea.

Interactions:

Can decrease absorption of digoxin if given at the same time. Kaolin and pectin mixtures decrease the absorption of lincomycin if given 2 hours before or 3 to 4 hours after it.

Nursing Implications:

Monitor frequency, amount, and appearance of stool. Monitor for related systemic manifestations: fever, pain, dehydration, and electrolyte imbalance. Caution against excessive use because morphine-like side effects can occur.

If leaking fecal matter is a problem, place a piece of absorbent cotton over the anus and hold the cotton in place with snug underwear. This allows air circulation to the area and is easily replaced as frequently as required.

Compare the patient's status with the expected outcomes. If the outcomes are not met, reassess the patient and revise the plan.

PAIN

Pain from the viscera and the peritoneum is mediated by the sympathetic nervous system. It is usually due to anoxia, inflammation, or stretching of smooth muscle or organ capsules.

Pain from hollow viscera is called visceral pain. It begins in the midline and is perceived as dull regardless of the specific organ involved. Subsequently, as inflammation or ischemia progresses, it localizes at a site specific to the affected organ (Table 21–3). For example, the pain of appendicitis starts in the periumbilical region and, over a period of hours, localizes to the lower right quadrant.

Quality of pain also differs according to the tissues affected. Pain related to stretching of the smooth muscle of the intestinal tract or the common bile duct is colicky and unaffected by movement. Pain from peritoneal irritation, in contrast, is described as sharp and severe and is exacerbated by jarring or moving. This can be an important factor in assessing a patient in whom the GI tract may have been perforated, allowing the contents to spill into the peritoneum.

BLEEDING

Bleeding can occur in any part of the GI tract. Upper GI bleeding originates in the esophagus, stomach, or duodenum. Lower GI bleeding originates in the jejunum, ileum, colon, or rectum. Multifocal GI bleeding originates from lesions throughout the tract.

GI bleeding may be acute or chronic. Acute bleeding occurs in minutes to hours and may be massive (>1000 mL blood loss) or discrete (⟨100 mL blood loss). Chronic bleeding occurs over a period of weeks or months and may be recurrent, intermittent, or persistent. Recurrent bleeding resumes after stopping completely. Intermittent bleeding occurs at regular or irregular intervals. Persistent bleeding is continuous or ongoing.

Etiology and Pathophysiology

GI bleeding results when the mucosa is irritated and its blood vessels are disrupted. This can result from inflammation, as occurs secondary to ingestion of alcohol or irritating medications. It can result from mechanical trauma, as seen in Mallory-Weiss syndrome, wherein the esophagus tears from forceful vomiting and retching. It can result from erosion by an expanding neoplasm. It can result from corrosion by gastric acid or pepsin, as in peptic ulcer disease. It can also be related to a vascular defect (eg, esophageal varices, which are dilated veins prone to rupture and hemorrhage), systemic disease (eg, nonthrombocytopenic purpura), or toxic reaction (eg, antibiotic-induced colitis).

Clinical Manifestations

Clinical characteristics vary with the magnitude and

Table 21–3

Locations of Pain from Organs of the Gastrointestinal Tract

Source of Pain	Perceived Location of Pain
Esophagus	Over the site of the lesion
	Occasionally, lower esophagus pain is felt at the suprasternal notch or neck or, if severe, in the back
Stomach and duodenum	Right epigastric or midepigastric
Jejunum and ileum	Periumbilical
Distal ileum	Periumbilical or lower right quadrant
Colon	Lower abdomen, often poorly localized
Rectum	Posterior, over the sacrum
Gallbladder and common bile duct	Right upper quadrant or epigastric
Pancreas	Midepigastric or left epigastric, radiating to midline of upper back
	Pain in tail of pancreas may be referred to shoulder
Diaphragmatic pleura	Trapezius ridge of the shoulder

location of the bleeding. Bleeding may be occult or may present as melena, hematochezia, rectorrhagia, or hematemesis.

Occult bleeding is not visible to the naked eye but is detected by chemical test (eg, guaiac test or Hematest). It indicates chronic GI bleeding and can originate anywhere from the mouth to the anus. It is often identified as part of a routine examination or as a result of diagnostic studies on a patient with iron deficiency anemia. Occult blood can be found in the stool for as long as 3 weeks after bleeding has occurred.

Melena is the passage of black, tarry, sticky, foul-smelling stool that contains a large amount of digested blood. It occurs with bleeding from the upper GI tract or from lesions in the jejunum or ileum.

Hematochezia, or the passage of obviously bloody stools, usually indicates lower GI bleeding. Blood mixed with stool is characteristic of inflammatory bowel disease, whereas blood on the surface of the stool suggests the presence of polyps or a malignant tumor. Blood that appears after the passage of formed stool is characteristic of hemorrhoids. Hematochezia may also occur with upper GI bleeding if it is massive and rapid, because such bleeding can increase intestinal motility.

Rectorrhagia is the passage of red blood from the rectum in the absence of feces. It usually indicates anorectal disease.

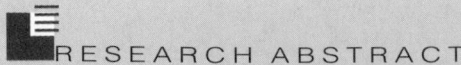

RESEARCH ABSTRACT

How Common Is Gastrointestinal Bleeding in ICU Patients With Strokes?

Davenport R, Dennis M, Warlow C. Gastrointestinal hemorrhage after acute stroke. Stroke 1996; 27(3):421.

It is well known that patients admitted to an intensive care unit (ICU) are at risk of developing stress ulcers. For this reason, many patients in ICUs are medicated prophylactically for stress ulcers.

Davenport and colleagues therefore wondered whether there might be an increased incidence of gastrointestinal bleeding among ICU patients recovering from strokes. They conducted a retrospective review of the frequency of gastrointestinal bleeding in patients who had suffered strokes.

Although the researchers found that the incidence of gastrointestinal bleeds in patients recovering from strokes was not *excessively* high, they did find that a significant number of the patients had developed gastrointestinal bleeds. The research team speculated that the antiplatelet and anticoagulant medications administered to stroke patients contributed to these bleeds. The researchers found that several of the patient charts included notations indicating that the patients had suffered hematemesis or melena, but that these problems had not been investigated because the patients had not suffered drops in hemoglobin levels. This finding led the researchers to surmise that the actual incidence of gastrointestinal bleeding may have been higher than indicated in the patients' charts, but that the bleeding had not been considered serious and so had not been investigated. In a small percentage of the patients, the bleed had been severe enough to contribute to death.

This research suggests that it is important for nurses to call instances of bleeding to the attention of the physician, so that complicating sequelae can be avoided or minimized. This is especially important if the patient is receiving some type of anticoagulant therapy.

Questions to Consider

1. Are H_2 blockers prescribed routinely for ICU patients at your clinical facility? If not, why not?
2. What are the clinical manifestations of gastrointestinal bleeds?
3. What types of patients are at risk of developing gastrointestinal bleeds?
4. What interventions would you expect to be carried for a patient with a gastrointestinal bleed or hemorrhage?

Hematemesis, or the vomiting of blood, ordinarily results from upper GI bleeding. The vomitus may contain frank red blood or appear dark red, brown, mahogany, or black. Because color darkens with exposure to gastric secretions, the longer the blood has been in the stomach, the darker it tends to be. If blood has clotted in the stomach and the clots have begun to be digested, vomitus looks something like coffee grounds.

In cases of acute, massive bleeding of more than 500 mL, nausea, thirst, diaphoresis, orthostatic hypotension, and syncope develop. If the blood loss continues, hypovolemic shock ensues, manifested by pallor, cold and clammy skin, hypotension, and tachycardia.

Management

The first priority in managing GI bleeding is to assess blood loss and return the patient to hemodynamic stability. Focus then turns to identifying the bleeding source and diagnosing and treating the underlying disorder.

Blood loss estimates can be based on vital signs, physical assessment data, and laboratory data. If a normotensive patient's systolic blood pressure drops to less than 90 mm Hg in the upright position, suspect a 25 to 50% volume loss. Postural changes of 10 mm Hg or more, a heart rate above 120, or both suggest volume losses of 20 to 25%. Remember that elderly patients exhibit postural changes with a much smaller blood loss. It is important also to have some idea of the patient's baseline blood pressure.

Hemoglobin and hematocrit values are also analyzed, although blood loss is not reflected in these values for 12 to 24 hours after the onset of bleeding. A persistent decrease in these values indicates a continuous loss of blood.

To stabilize a patient with acute bleeding, normal saline or Ringer's lactate is given until blood pressure rises, signs of peripheral vasospasm disappear, and urinary output returns to 30 mL/h. When shock is severe, plasma expanders are given until typed and cross-matched blood is available for transfusion. A central venous pressure line (or, for patients with cardiac compromise or the need for massive fluid replacement, a Swan-Ganz line) is inserted to monitor circulatory volume. The patient is placed in a head-down left lateral position to increase cerebral blood flow and prevent aspiration. Volume of urinary output and urine specific gravity are monitored via an indwelling catheter. Oxygen may be administered.

Measures to locate the site of bleeding begin with insertion of a nasogastric tube to check for blood or clots in the stomach. Other diagnostic tests are then used as indicated. These may include upper and lower flexible endoscopy to attempt to directly visualize the lesion, air contrast studies, arteriography to demonstrate extravasation of blood into the GI lumen or alterations in the vasculature, and radioisotopic scintigraphy.

Treatment of bleeding varies with the cause and the location. Gastric lavage provides immediate treatment of gastric bleeding because upper GI bleeding usually stops, regardless of cause, when acid-blood contents are removed from the stomach and replaced by a neutral solution. Cool saline is the solution of choice for this procedure, although tap water is sometimes used. Water breaks up large clots more readily than saline but is more likely to contribute to electrolyte imbalance. The cool solution is instilled 50 to 100 mL at a time, left for a short interval, and then aspirated. This volume is small enough to prevent distention but sufficient to cause vasoconstriction from the cold. If the bleeding is from esophageal varices, a Sengstaken-Blakemore tube may be used to directly compress the varices and promote hemostasis. See Chapter 26 for discussion of the special needs of the patient with this tube.

Pharmacologic agents that reduce gastric acidity, such as antacids and H$_2$-receptor antagonists, are given to treat bleeding from inflammatory, erosive, or ulcerative upper GI lesions (Highlight 21–3). Other drugs used, regardless of the source of bleeding, include antifibrinolytic agents. Vasoconstrictive medications may be therapeutic in controlling active bleeding from esophageal varices. Embolization therapy (injection of a natural or synthetic clot into the bleeding vessel), endoscopy with electrocoagulation or laser photocoagulation, and surgery for uncontrolled hemorrhage are other treatment options.

NURSING PROCESS GUIDELINES
Bleeding

Nursing care of the patient with GI bleeding varies with the severity and location of the bleeding and the method of treatment. Thus, it may include measures discussed under care of the patient in shock,

---

HIGHLIGHT
21–3
PHARMACOLOGY

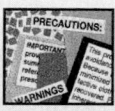

Antacids

Definition:

Over-the-counter alkaline compounds that neutralize gastric acid

Action:

React with gastric acid to produce neutral or low acidity salts, thereby raising pH and inactivating pepsin at pH of 5 or higher

Uses:

Decrease destruction of gut wall in peptic ulcer disease, provide prophylaxis against stress ulcers, and provide symptomatic relief of heartburn due to reflux esophagitis

Side Effects:

Altered bowel function: constipation or diarrhea—antacids causing constipation include aluminum hydroxide and calcium carbonate; those causing diarrhea include magnesium hydroxide and magnesium carbonate

Antacids with high sodium content may induce fluid retention and exacerbate hypertension and congestive heart failure

Hypermagnesemia, which can lead to respiratory or mental depression and coma, can develop in patients with renal failure taking magnesium compounds; similarly, hyperaluminemia and hypophosphatemia may occur

Interactions:

Affect dissolution and absorption of many drugs as a result of raising the gastric pH; also interfere with the action of the local antiulcer drug sucralfate

Nursing Implications:

Teach patients to combine use of constipating and diarrhea-producing antacids to counteract effect of each and maintain normal bowel function.

Shake liquid preparations well before administering.

Instruct patient to chew antacid tablets thoroughly and follow with a full glass of water.

Allow 1 hour between the administration of antacids and other medications to minimize drug interactions.

Explain that stools may appear white or speckled as a result of antacid therapy.

Instruct patients with a sodium or potassium restriction to check label on antacids for amounts of these ions.

care of the patient with ruptured esophageal varices, care of the patient who has undergone gastrectomy, or care of the patient who has undergone intestinal resection. Regardless of cause or treatment, basic assessment data for any patient with acute bleeding include level of consciousness, vital signs, color, appearance of neck veins, capillary refill, and condition of the abdomen (presence or absence of bowel sounds, distention, and guarding).

Assessment of the Gastrointestinal System

PATIENT HISTORY

Obtain a diet history. Have the patient describe his or her usual diet. Ask about the amount and types of foods eaten and daily pattern of intake. For example, does the patient eat three meals daily? Does the patient snack throughout the day? Does the patient skip breakfast and eat lunch, dinner, and a bedtime snack? Ascertain which, if any, foods or food groups are not eaten. Ask if the patient takes vitamin, mineral, or other supplements and, if so, the amount and frequency.

Inquire about the condition of the patient's teeth, and note the date of the last dental examination. Find out whether the patient has dentures and whether they are comfortable and worn regularly. Ask about the usual pattern of bowel elimination, noting frequency, color, and consistency of stool. Be certain to note measures used to promote bowel function, such as daily bran or routine use of laxatives. Obtain specific data about any GI symptoms. Ask about difficulty chewing, difficulty swallowing, soreness of the mouth, anorexia, nausea, vomiting, belching, indigestion, abdominal distention, abdominal pain, diarrhea, flatulence, constipation, pencil-shaped stools, straining at stool, painful defecation, and blood in the stool or from the rectum. If symptoms are reported, determine their onset, duration, and severity. Explore the relationship of symptoms to specific foods, use of alcohol, or specific activities or events. Also determine what measures or over-the-counter drugs have been used to treat symptoms, the frequency of their use, and their effectiveness.

Review the patient's medical history. Ask specifically about previous GI disorders and abdominal surgery, noting date of occurrence, treatment, and results. Inquire about previous diagnostic tests, including the most recent rectal examination and testing of stool for occult blood. Note the patient's general health status, other current medical problems, and all medications being taken. This last factor is particularly important because so many medications have side effects related to GI function.

PHYSICAL EXAMINATION

Ask the patient to remove any dental appliances. Then examine the mouth and pharynx using a flashlight and tongue blade to ensure good visibility of all areas. Note the condition of the lips, including color, moistness, suppleness, symmetry, and the presence of any lesions, such as cracks, cold sores caused by the herpes simplex virus, or areas of leukoplakia. Using a tongue blade to move the tongue aside and a flashlight for good visibility, inspect the teeth and gums. Note the absence of teeth or presence of loose teeth. Assess for caries and plaque. Note the color of the gums, gum recession or hypertrophy, and any evidence of bleeding gums. Look for ulcerated areas and other signs of poorly fitted dentures.

Keep in mind that, normally, the mucosa of the gums is light pink and may be shiny and thin in older people. Also remember that gum recession is normal with age. Observe the mucous membranes in the mouth, including those under the tongue. Look for areas of redness or swelling, as well as for lesions—such as ulcerations, white patches of thrush or leukoplakia, and nodules. Observe the color and condition of the tongue. Keep in mind that a smooth, red tongue may indicate nutritional deficiency. A thickly coated tongue may indicate inadequate oral hygiene.

Using the tongue blade to depress the tongue, inspect the pharynx and tonsils for redness, swelling, and exudate. Finally, note the odor of the patient's breath, which may indicate recently ingested substances (eg, alcohol or garlic), poor oral hygiene, local infection (foul odor), or systemic disease, such as diabetic acidosis (acetone odor) or liver disease (ammonia odor).

Next examine the abdomen. Assist the patient into a supine position with arms at sides, and uncover the abdomen from the xiphoid process to the symphysis pubis. In good light, inspect the abdomen. Note the color and texture of the skin, contour (flat, hollow, rounded, or protuberant), and whether or not it is symmetric. Note the presence and location of scars, striae, visible vasculature, or other abnormalities. Examine the umbilicus for signs of inflammation or hernia. Observe for peristaltic waves, keeping in mind that, except for slow waves in very thin people, peristalsis is not normally visible. Auscultate all four quadrants for bowel sounds and note their frequency and character. Normal bowel sounds, clicking, and gurgling noises, which occur 5 to 34 times per minute, are usually loudest in the right lower quadrant of the abdomen. Remember always to auscultate first and then proceed to percussion and palpation.

Percuss all four quadrants of the abdomen to determine areas of tympany and dullness. Tympany is normal over most of the abdomen because of the small amount of air in the bowel. Dullness is heard over bowel filled with stool, over areas of ascites, over organs (eg, the liver), and over solid or fluid-filled masses. Dullness in the suprapubic area may be from a full bladder or an enlarged uterus. After percussion, proceed to palpate the abdomen. Perform light palpation using the pads of the fingertips to check for muscle tenderness and resistance, as well as for superficial masses. Palpate gently with the fingers together in each quadrant. If the patient has localized abdominal pain, palpate the painful area last. If the abdomen is involuntarily rigid or boardlike (rigid on expiration despite the patient's breathing through the mouth with the jaw dropped open), stop the examination and notify the physician, because this may indicate acute peritonitis. Follow light palpation with deep palpation to check for deeper masses and areas of tenderness. Perform

deep palpation only if trained in the technique, however, because it is not a routine part of basic nursing care.

The lower edge of the normal liver is usually palpable under the costal margin at the midclavicular line. It is normally felt as soft, clearly defined, regular, and smooth. To palpate for it, place your dominant hand on the right side of the abdomen at the midclavicular line below the level of percussed liver dullness. Press the fingers gently inward and upward as you instruct the patient to take a deep breath. Feel for the edge of the liver striking your finger as it is moved downward by the flattening of the diaphragm on inspiration. When the liver is felt, raise your fingers slightly to let the liver slip beneath them and thus allow palpation of its anterior surface.

Finish assessment of the GI tract with examination of the anal region. Inspect the perianal area for hemorrhoids, fissures, ulcerations, or other lesions. Note any drainage, abnormal odor, or change in skin color. If the rectum is to be examined, insert a gloved and lubricated finger gently through the anal sphincter. Palpate for nodules and note presence of stool. Upon withdrawing the gloved finger, observe for blood or mucus and note color of any stool.

Assess the patient's understanding of and compliance with health promotion and risk reduction measures related to GI health (Highlight 21–4).

Diagnostic Procedures

While many diagnostic examinations of the GI tract are complex, all can be accomplished in an outpatient setting. Educating patients to assure adequate preparation for these tests is extremely important to the accuracy of results.

GASTRIC ANALYSIS

Gastric analysis is a procedure in which stomach contents are examined. It is usually done to determine whether hydrochloric acid is present and in what amount, although it can also demonstrate the presence of occult blood, malignant cells, bacteria, and parasites. It is useful in diagnosing ulcer disease, which is characterized by high gastric acidity. It is also useful in diagnosing pernicious anemia, in which gastric acid is absent. It also aids in evaluating the effects of a vagotomy (cutting the vagus nerve to decrease production of gastric acid) and in diagnosing malignant tumors of the stomach.

Patient Preparation
The evening before a gastric analysis, the patient receives a light meal or clear fluids. After midnight, the patient is placed on NPO status. Smoking is not allowed on the morning of the test because it can

---

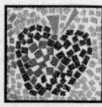

HIGHLIGHT
21–4

HEALTH PROMOTION & RISK REDUCTION

Optimal Gastrointestinal System Function

The American Cancer Society recommends the following preventive measures:

Maintain a diet that limits fat to 20 to 25% of total calories, and include 25 to 30 g of fiber per day. Bran cereals, beans, legumes, and many vegetables and fruits are high in fiber.

Report any episodes of bleeding, habitual gas, or gastrointestinal distress to the physician.

Be aware of symptoms and have a yearly checkup if at increased risk for colorectal cancer:

- 40 years old, with incidence doubling every decade until age 80
- History of such bowel conditions as ulcerative colitis and familial polyposis
- First-degree relative with colorectal cancer
- High-fat, low-fiber diet
- Colon cancer is more common among women (2 : 1 ratio)
- Rectal cancer is more common among men (3 : 2 ratio)

Reduce stressful events and use relaxation strategies frequently.

Undergo stool examinations for occult blood yearly for those over 50.

Undergo digital rectal examinations yearly for those over 40.

Undergo sigmoidoscopy every 3 to 5 years for those over 50, based on the advice of a physician.

stimulate production of gastric acid and affect test results.

Procedure

A nasogastric tube is inserted through the mouth or nose into the stomach and is taped in place. Gastric contents are withdrawn with a syringe and gentle suction. When hydrochloric acid production is being measured, this initial aspiration provides a baseline level. Subsequent aspirations of secretions are obtained at 15- to 20-minute intervals for 1 to 2 hours. A stimulus in the form of a carbohydrate meal of dry toast and tea, 50 mL of alcohol or caffeine, or an injection of histamine is usually given to stimulate gastric secretion.

Complications

Nausea and vomiting may occur during ingestion of the stimulus or following the procedure. If histamine is used as a stimulus, an allergic reaction may occur.

NURSING PROCESS GUIDELINES
Gastric Aspiration

Make sure the patient understands the limitations required on diet and smoking before the test. Just before the procedure, explain that a tube will be passed into the stomach to obtain gastric secretions and that the patient will be asked to swallow while the tube is being inserted. Explain about any stimulus to be given and, in the case of histamine, warn the patient to be prepared for a hot, flushing sensation and for frequent measurements of pulse and blood pressure. Assess each patient for a history of allergies because this may contraindicate the use of histamine.

Monitor the patient immediately after the procedure for any discomfort, nausea, or vomiting. Give mouth care using a toothbrush or mouthwash to remove any dried secretions from the oral mucosa. Instruct the patient to resume a normal diet as tolerated.

UPPER GASTROINTESTINAL SERIES

An upper GI series is an x-ray examination of the esophagus, stomach, and duodenum. Barium sulfate—a white, chalky, radiopaque substance—is used to allow x-ray visualization of the structures. This procedure is used to detect esophageal tumors, esophageal varices, gastric ulcers, and gastric tumors. It also allows visualization of any esophageal strictures or swallowing disorders. As the barium progresses through the small intestine, obstructions, inflammations, or diverticula can be identified (Fig. 21–6).

If only the esophagus is examined, the procedure is called a barium swallow. If the jejunum and ileum

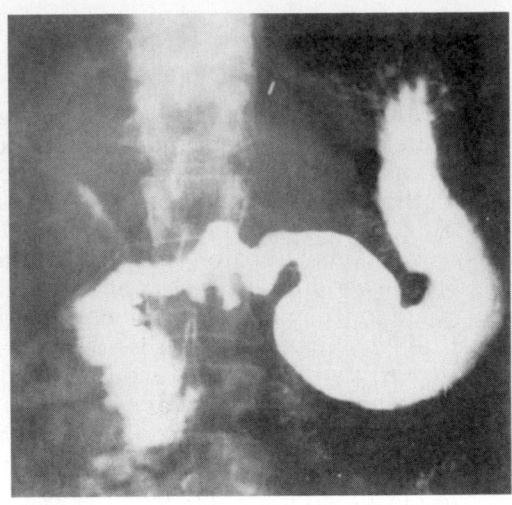

Figure 21–6

Upper gastrointestinal series showing barium in the lower end of the esophagus, stomach, and small intestine. (From Sleisinger MH, Fordtran JS. Gastrointestinal disease: Pathophysiology/diagnosis/management. 4th ed. Philadelphia: WB Saunders, 1989, p. 956.)

are also visualized, it is an upper GI series with a small bowel examination.

Patient Preparation

Basic preparation for an upper GI series consists of keeping the patient on NPO status after midnight before the examination. In some instances, a low-residue diet is followed for 2 to 3 days, and narcotic and anticholinergic drugs are avoided for 24 hours so that bowel motility will be normal.

Procedure

The patient takes an upright position behind a fluoroscopic screen and swallows the contrast medium. X-rays are taken with the patient tilted in various positions on a tilt table as the barium progresses through the upper GI tract. For visualization of the jejunum and ileum, additional barium is swallowed and films are taken at 30-minute intervals.

Postprocedure Course

Because barium sulfate is a constipating substance that can obstruct the GI tract if not eliminated, cathartics are ordered after the procedure. Patients commonly take 30 mL of milk of magnesia or half a bottle of magnesium citrate.

Complications

A major complication of an upper GI series is perforation of the stomach or intestine. If this occurs, barium can escape into the peritoneum and peritonitis can result.

If cathartics are not taken as ordered after the test, severe constipation, impaction, or intestinal obstruction may occur in 1 to 2 days. Occasionally, nausea occurs from swallowing the barium.

NURSING PROCESS GUIDELINES
Upper Gastrointestinal Series

Assess the patient's understanding of the procedure. Make sure the patient understands the restrictions on diet and medications to be observed before the test. Explain that the patient will be asked to drink a thick, chalky substance at the beginning of the test, that she or he will be tilted on a table into various positions so that all areas of the upper GI tract can be seen and x-rayed, and that the procedure can take 1 to 2 hours or longer. If you identify a knowledge deficit, provide information as needed.

Following a barium swallow, assess the patient's tolerance of the procedure and note any nausea. Encourage the patient to rest and to resume food and fluids as ordered and tolerated. Because of the potential for constipation from the barium, instruct the patient on the use of cathartics and basic measures to promote bowel function, such as keeping adequate amounts of fiber and water in the diet. Tell the patient to expect white stools for 48 to 72 hours and, if an outpatient, to report the development of constipation. With inpatients, check for the passage of barium and chart it in the patient's record.

BARIUM ENEMA

A barium enema is a radiologic examination of the rectum and colon. It is used to diagnose problems in the large intestine, such as tumors, polyps, and diverticula. It can also identify filling defects that could be ulcerative, as in Crohn's disease and ulcerative colitis.

A barium enema should precede an oral barium study because it takes several days for swallowed barium to pass completely out of the GI tract and any residual barium can distort the results of a barium enema.

Patient Preparation
The bowel is prepared before the procedure to cleanse it of feces, which interfere with the test and produce inaccurate results. For a basic bowel preparation, oral intake the day before the examination is limited to clear fluids. That evening the patient should undergo tap-water enemas until the return is clear and take an oral cathartic such as magnesium sulfate. On the morning of the examination, a suppository and an enema are taken.

Alternative bowel preparation better suited to the outpatient consists of Fleet enemas or the use of an osmotic solution such as GoLYTELY that induces diarrhea. With GoLYTELY, only clear liquids are allowed the day before the examination. Then the patient drinks 240 mL (8 ounces) of GoLYTELY every 10 to 15 minutes until a clear diarrhea develops. This takes about 2 or 3 hours. No food or fluids are taken after midnight, and on the morning of the examination, Fleet enemas may be administered. If a patient is on daily medication, it may be taken with a small amount of fluid on the morning of the examination provided the physician gives permission. Patients may also be instructed to avoid taking aspirin for 10 days before the examination to decrease the risk of bleeding.

Procedure
Barium is instilled into the large intestine through the rectum. If needed, a rectal tube with an inflatable balloon can be used to help the patient retain the barium during the examination. The progress of the barium is followed on a fluoroscopy screen, and x-rays are taken with the patient in different positions. When this is completed, the patient is allowed to expel the barium, and additional films are taken of the entire lower GI tract.

Postprocedure Course
After a barium enema, an oral cathartic such as magnesium sulfate or an oil retention enema is ordered to aid in elimination of the barium and prevent bowel impaction.

Complications and Contraindications
The major complications of a barium enema are severe constipation and impaction of barium in the bowel. The test is usually contraindicated in patients with toxic megacolon or a perforated or obstructed GI tract.

NURSING PROCESS GUIDELINES
Barium Enema

Assess the patient's understanding of the procedure, and provide information as needed to enable the patient to describe the test and its preparation accurately in general terms. Also assess the patient's ability to tolerate the extensive bowel preparation necessary for this examination. This includes checking hydration and electrolyte status, sphincter control, and ability to get to the bathroom. Ensure that the preparation is completed as ordered and evaluate its effectiveness by checking that enema returns are clear on the morning of the test.

After the test, encourage the taking of oral fluids and give cathartics or enemas as ordered to prevent constipation or impaction due to the barium. Tell the patient that stools will be white for 24 to 72 hours. Document passage of barium in the patient's record.

ORAL CHOLECYSTOGRAM

An oral cholecystogram is an x-ray visualization of the gallbladder. It is used to evaluate gallbladder function and aids in diagnosing gallstones or other gallbladder disease.

Patient Preparation

Normal dietary intake of fat should be maintained during the days preceding the test in order to empty bile from the gallbladder. The evening before the test, the patient has a fat-free supper and takes several tablets containing the contract substance. The fat-free supper prevents contraction of the gallbladder and allows accumulation of the contrast substance needed for x-ray visualization. After midnight, the patient is placed on NPO status.

Procedure

An oral cholecystogram hinges on successful completion of several sequential metabolic steps:

1. Absorption of orally ingested radiopaque dye tablets from the small intestine
2. Removal of dye from blood by the liver
3. Excretion of dye with bile from the liver
4. Concentration of bile and dye in the gallbladder
5. Excretion of bile and dye through the common bile duct in response to a fatty meal

The dye tablets are taken early (about 7 PM) on the evening before the test. The most commonly used tablets are Telepaque, which come in a 500 mg form. Because the dose is calculated on body weight, six or more tablets may be needed. To minimize nausea, tablets are given 5 minutes apart with small sips of water.

On the following day, initial films are taken to determine the position of the gallbladder and to ensure that it has opacified. After the gallbladder is visualized, a fatty meal is given to stimulate contraction and emptying of the gallbladder. This takes 15 to 20 minutes, after which additional x-rays are taken. If gallstones are seen on the first x-ray, no fatty meal is given and no additional films are taken. If the gallbladder cannot be visualized, it indicates biliary obstruction or inappropriate preparation, and the test may be repeated the next day.

Complications

Severe diarrhea and vomiting with subsequent dehydration can be caused by the Telepaque tablets. A severe anaphylactic reaction can occur if the patient is allergic to iodine, which is present in the dye. Liver and kidney damage can occur if the dye is not properly excreted.

NURSING PROCESS GUIDELINES
Oral Cholecystogram

Assess the patient's understanding of the oral cholecystogram. The patient should be able to say why it is being done, state the dietary restrictions involved, and describe the procedure in general. The patient should know that the procedure is performed in the x-ray department and takes about 1 hour.

Assess the patient for allergy to iodine. Explore the patient's history to determine whether other tests using iodine-based dye have been performed and, if so, whether any adverse reactions occurred. Also determine whether the patient ever had an adverse reaction to eating shellfish.

Administer the dye tablets, taking care to give them as scheduled to ensure that the dye has adequate time to be absorbed before the test. Then assess for nausea, vomiting, abdominal cramps, and dysuria, which may occur as side effects of the Telepaque. If vomiting or diarrhea occurs, inspect the vomitus or stool for Telepaque tablets. Whether tablets can be identified or not, notify the x-ray department and the physician, because expulsion would affect uptake of the dye and could result in an inaccurate test.

When planning care for a patient scheduled for an oral cholecystogram, check to see whether the patient will undergo any other tests that involve iodine. If so, schedule them before the oral cholecystogram. Schedule any tests using barium after the cholecystogram, or the gallbladder will not be accurately visualized.

After the test, assess the patient's hydration status. Monitor urinary output and check skin turgor. Also assess for nausea and vomiting. Instruct the patient to resume the prescribed diet when GI function appears stable.

CHOLANGIOGRAM

A cholangiogram is an x-ray examination in which a contrast medium is used to outline the hepatic, cystic, and common bile ducts. In intravenous cholangiography, dye is given slowly into a vein, and x-rays are taken as the dye is excreted by the liver. In some cases, a fatty meal is then ingested and additional x-rays are taken to show contraction of the gallbladder. In operative and postoperative cholangiography, dye is injected into the common bile duct via a drainage tube. Percutaneous transhepatic cholangiography involves injection of the dye through the skin of the abdomen into the liver. In endoscopic retrograde cholangiography, the contrast medium is instilled via a cannula inserted through the ampulla of Vater by means of a flexible fiberoptic duodenoscope.

Cholangiography takes about 4 hours and is contraindicated by severe liver disease or jaundice. For an intravenous cholangiogram, the patient is assessed for allergy to shellfish or contrast media, is placed on NPO status after midnight, and is given a laxative or enema to cleanse the bowel. The patient is also told to expect a brief burning sensation when the dye is injected. After the procedure, rest is promoted, fluids are encouraged, and diet is resumed as tolerated.

ENDOSCOPY

Endoscopy is the visualization of the inside of a body cavity by means of a lighted tube. Most endoscopic examinations of the upper and lower GI tract are performed with a flexible fiberoptic scope, which can provide an undistorted image of the body cavity even when completely bent. Illumination is provided by an external light source. The scope is designed to allow passage of instruments so that pictures can be taken, biopsies obtained, polyps and foreign objects removed, and bleeding areas cauterized. The scope varies in length, depending on the area in which it is used (Fig. 21–7).

Esophagogastroduodenoscopy

Esophagogastroduodenoscopy is the direct visualization of the esophagus, the stomach, and the beginning of the duodenum by means of an endoscope passed through the patient's mouth (Fig. 21–8).

This upper GI endoscopy is performed primarily as an adjunct to x-ray evaluation or as an emergency procedure in patients with acute upper GI bleeding. It is used in diagnosing hiatus hernia, esophageal varices, esophagitis, ulcer disease, polyps, strictures (eg, achalasia), and malignant tumors. It is also used to identify areas of bleeding in the upper GI tract, to obtain biopsy specimens, and to detect small or surface lesions that do not show up on x-ray film.

Patient Preparation
Unless the procedure is performed on an emergency basis, all food, fluids, and antacids are withheld for 8 hours before the examination to ensure optimal visualization and prevent aspiration. If the procedure is performed on an emergency basis, stomach contents are aspirated beforehand through a nasogastric tube.

Usually a sedative, such as midazolam (Versed), is given intravenously with or without meperidine (Demerol) at the onset of the procedure to decrease anxiety. The dose is titrated to achieve the degree of sedation required. Occasionally, atropine is also given to decrease salivary and gastric secretions.

Procedure
The throat is anesthetized either by swabbing it or by having the patient gargle with a local anesthetic. When the gag reflex has disappeared, the patient is placed in a lateral recumbent position and the endoscope is guided through the mouth to the hypopharynx. The patient is instructed to swallow, and the scope is further advanced to the anatomic area to be examined. Because the patient must lie perfectly still during the procedure, a general anesthetic may be necessary for patients unable to cooperate. Visualization is optimized by insufflating air through the scope to distend the area being examined. Photographs of lesions, biopsy specimens, and brushings for cytologic examination are taken when indicated.

Postprocedure Course
The patient rests until the sedation has worn off and then may return to usual activity. Foods and fluids are resumed when the gag reflex returns, which is usually in 1 to 2 hours.

Complications
The major complication is perforation of the GI tract, with the possibility of excessive bleeding and subsequent infection. Aspiration is a risk if food and fluids have not been withheld before the procedure.

NURSING PROCESS GUIDELINES
Esophagogastroduodenoscopy

Assess the patient for ability to swallow, for presence of GI symptoms (eg, nausea, vomiting, pain,

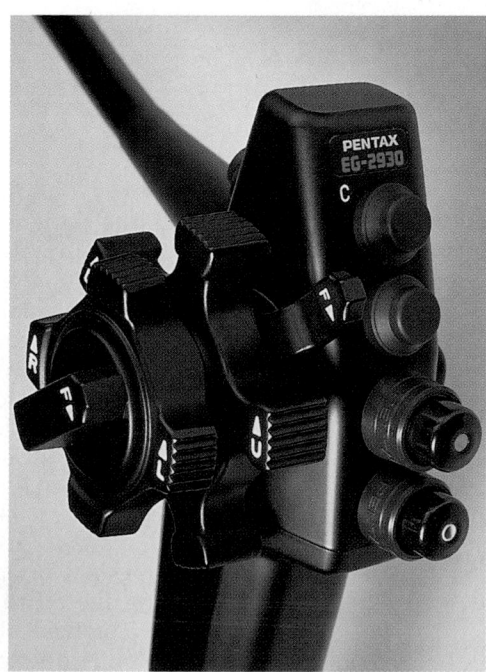
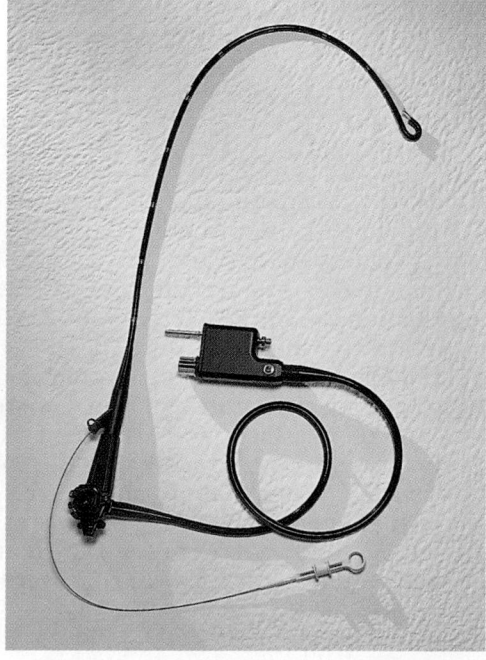

Figure 21–7

Upper gastrointestinal flexible endoscope. (Courtesy of Pentax Precision Instrument Corporation, Orangeburg, NY.)

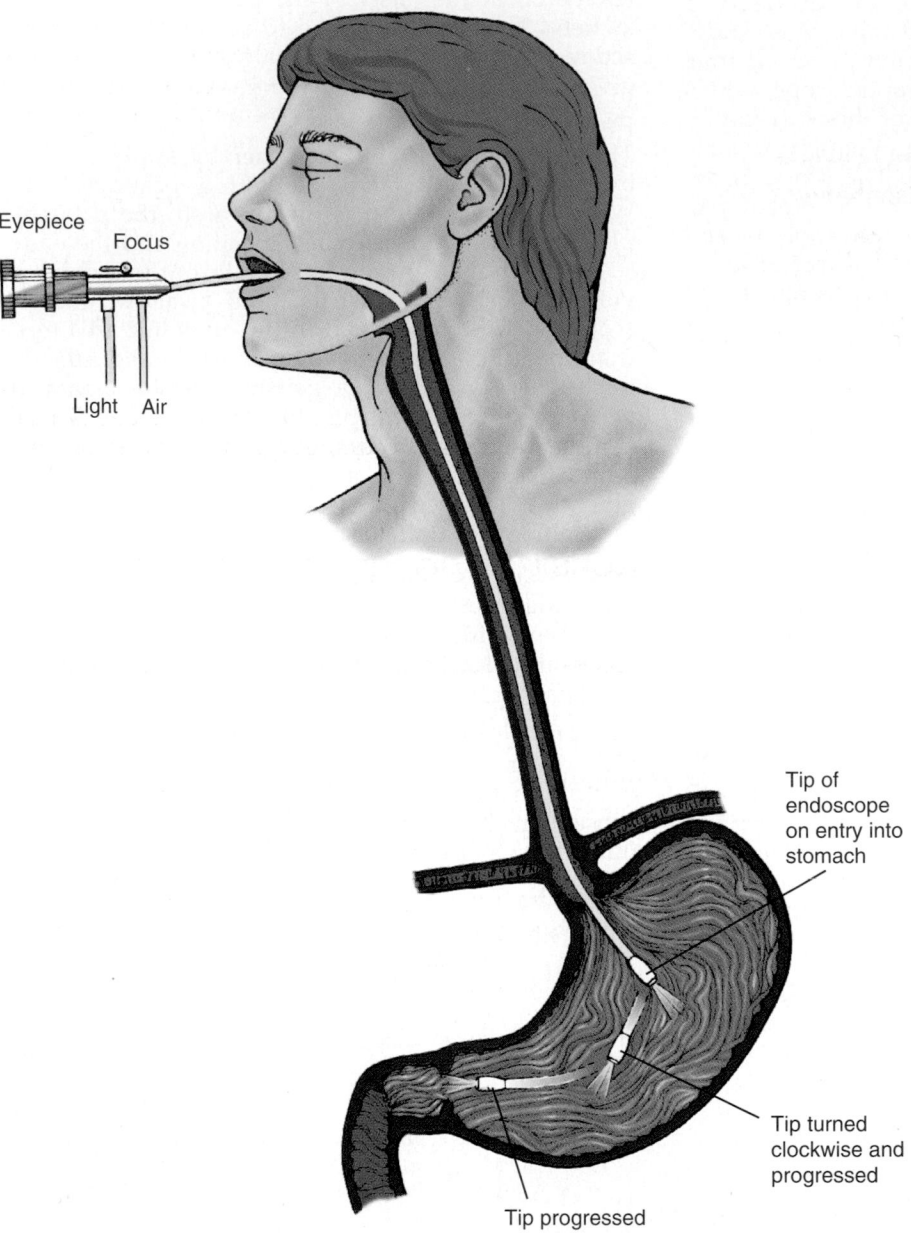

Eyepiece

Focus

Light   Air

Tip of
endoscope
on entry into
stomach

Tip turned
clockwise and
progressed

Tip progressed
to within antrum

Figure 21–8

Flexible endoscope shown passing
through the mouth and the esophagus to
the stomach. Dotted lines show how the
endoscope is moved to allow visualization of all areas of the stomach.

abdominal distention, and GI bleeding), and for understanding of the procedure. In assessing the patient's understanding and providing needed information, make certain that the patient knows the
information presented in Highlight 21–5.

Following the procedure, assess the patient's
physiologic stabilization by monitoring vital signs
and checking for return of the gag reflex. Assess
level of consciousness and keep side rails raised until the patient is fully alert. Assess the patient for
bleeding and pain. Report and record immediately
any complaints of sharp, intense pain in the abdomen or chest. Also report immediately a sudden rise
in temperature and tachycardia, because these are
symptoms of perforation.

Give food and fluids when the gag reflex returns,
and instruct the patient in the use of lozenges and
gargles for a sore throat.

If the upper GI endoscopy is being performed on
an outpatient basis, make certain someone is available to escort the patient home after it is completed
and the sedation has worn off. Provide instruction
about resumption of food and fluids and about
symptoms that should be reported to the health care
professional.

Colonoscopy

A colonoscopy is a procedure in which the lining of
the large intestine all the way to the ileocecal valve
is directly visualized through a fiberoptic colonoscope. A colonoscopy can help distinguish inflam-

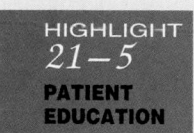 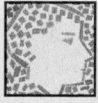

HIGHLIGHT
21–5
PATIENT
EDUCATION

Information for the Patient Undergoing an Esophago-gastroduodenoscopy

Explain to the patient that:

The procedure is uncomfortable and very tiring but not painful.

Food and fluids must not be taken for at least 8 hours before the procedure.

Dentures, eyeglasses, and jewelry will be removed before the procedure.

A sedative will be given to promote relaxation (but not sleep) before the procedure begins.

The procedure will be done in the _____. *(endoscopy suite, treatment room on the unit, or outpatient department)*

The throat will be anesthetized, and this can make the tongue and throat feel swollen.

The gag sensation will be lost, but swallowing is unimpaired.

It is important to remain perfectly still during the examination.

She or he will be told to swallow to help pass the tube. If air is insufflated, a feeling of fullness, bloating, or cramping may occur.

After the procedure, vital signs will be taken and activity limited until the sedation has worn off.

Food and fluids will be withheld until the gag reflex has returned, usually 1 to 2 hours.

The throat may be sore after the procedure.

The procedure takes 15 to 60 minutes.

---

matory from neoplastic diseases. It is indicated when the patient has a history of undiagnosed constipation and diarrhea, anorexia, persistent rectal bleeding, or lower abdominal pain. It is also used to check for recurring polyps or malignant tumors.

Patient Preparation

A bowel preparation as described previously under Barium Enema is performed to allow proper inspection of the colon. In some cases, the patient may also be kept on NPO status for 8 hours. Medication such as meperidine, midazolam, or diazepam (Valium) may be given intravenously at the onset of the procedure to promote comfort and relaxation.

Procedure

With the patient in left Sims' position, a digital rectal examination is performed to dilate the rectum

and rule out obstruction. The colonoscope is inserted into the rectum, and a small amount of air is insufflated to distend the bowel lumen. The scope is then advanced through the rectum and into the sigmoid colon, past the splenic flexure, and on through the transverse colon and the cecum to the ileocecal valve. The scope is then slowly withdrawn for detailed visualization. If needed, suction is used to remove blood or secretions obstructing the view. Biopsy and cytology specimens may be obtained, polyps excised, and photographs taken if required.

Complications

Infrequent but possible complications of a colonoscopy are bleeding and perforation of the bowel wall. If either of these occurs, surgical intervention may be necessary.

NURSING PROCESS GUIDELINES
Colonoscopy

Assess the patient's understanding of the colonoscopy as a procedure and as a diagnostic test. If a knowledge deficit is identified, provide information as needed. Make sure the patient understands the prescribed preparation. This is particularly important when the test is performed on an outpatient basis and the patient is responsible for following the instructions accurately. Also make sure that the patient understands the purpose of the test and the procedure itself—that it permits examination of the large intestine, that a flexible instrument is passed through the anus and may cause a feeling of needing to have a bowel movement or a cramping sensation, and that the test takes from 30 to 60 minutes.

After the procedure, assess the patient for signs of perforation, including sudden temperature elevation, tachycardia, or abdominal pain. Observe stools for red blood and take vital signs every 2 hours until stable. Instruct the patient to expel all air from the rectum. Encourage rest for 30 to 60 minutes. Give food and fluids once the patient has passed flatus.

When the test is performed on an outpatient basis, be sure the patient has arranged to be driven home. Sedatives used during the procedure may temporarily impair the ability to drive. Also provide instructions for self-care as presented in Highlight 21–6.

ULTRASONOGRAPHY

Ultrasonography is a noninvasive procedure that uses high-frequency, inaudible sound waves to form images of internal structures. Sound waves are directed at the area to be studied by a transducer that is rubbed slowly on the lubricated skin surface. As the sound waves hit internal organs, they are re-

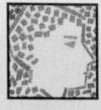

HIGHLIGHT 21-6 PATIENT EDUCATION

Self-Care After a Colonoscopy

Instruct the patient to:

Avoid driving or operating any power-related machinery if medication was received before or during the procedure.

Avoid making important decisions for 24 hours if medication was received before or during the procedure.

Resume oral intake gradually, starting with a light meal and progressing to a regular diet.

Remember that feelings of gassiness or bloatedness are caused by the air that is instilled in the bowel during the procedure.

Remember that abdominal tenderness may occur as a result of stretching of the abdominal muscles during the procedure.

flected back and converted to an image on a screen. Photographs of these images can be taken as desired.

Ultrasonic examination of the gallbladder and biliary system helps diagnose cholelithiasis (gallstones) and cholecystitis when results of the cholecystogram are inconclusive. Liver ultrasonography can detect metastasis, abscesses, and hematomas. Pancreatic ultrasound studies aid in diagnosing pancreatitis, pseudocysts, and pancreatic cancer. Abdominal sonograms can detect tumor masses in the abdominal cavity.

Minimal preparation is required for ultrasonic studies of the GI tract. The patient is instructed to avoid carbonated beverages and large amounts of carbohydrates for 48 hours before the test to help decrease intestinal gas. Ascites and extreme obesity interfere with ultrasonic studies, as does barium. For this reason, ultrasonography should be scheduled before tests using barium.

The test is painless. All that is required of the patient is to lie still and hold his or her breath for 20- to 30-second intervals as directed.

COMPUTED TOMOGRAPHY

Computed tomography (CT) of the abdomen produces three-dimensional images of abdominal tissues. It is used to identify tumors and other diseases of the abdominal organs, including the gallbladder, biliary ductal system, pancreas, and peritoneum. A contrast medium may be used to visualize the biliary tract or to highlight differences in pancreatic tissue density.

The patient is placed on NPO status for 8 to 12 hours before an abdominal CT scan and is assessed for allergies to shellfish and contrast media. During the scan, which takes 45 minutes to 1 hour, a supine position must be maintained.

Because barium can interfere with the CT scan, barium studies should be scheduled after the scan or at least 4 days before it.

MAGNETIC RESONANCE IMAGING

Magnetic resonance imaging (MRI) produces cross-sectional images of tissue. It can be used to study blood flow in the abdomen as well as to identify areas of infection or malignancy. The procedure takes 1 to $1\frac{1}{2}$ hours and requires that the patient lie still. Contraindications to MRI include pregnancy and the presence of a pacemaker, a metallic implant, or an infusion pump.

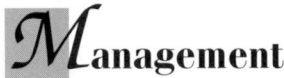

Management

GASTROINTESTINAL INTUBATION

GI intubation refers to the insertion of a tube into the stomach or intestine. This may be for the purpose of removing toxic substances by suction, removing fluids and gas by suction or gravity drainage, instilling irrigating solutions (lavage) or medications, controlling bleeding, or administering enteral feeding. Different types of tubes are used for different purposes (Fig 21–9). Tubes may be inserted through the nose or via a surgical stab wound into the abdomen.

Intubation for Decompression and Drainage

Intubation is performed to remove contents of the stomach or intestines when the GI tract cannot properly propel and absorb secretions, such as when an obstruction develops or peristalsis is greatly reduced from the effects of anesthesia and surgery. Patients are also intubated after surgery on the stomach or intestines to remove gas and secretions from the area of the suture line until healing takes place. Another indication for use is treatment of a drug overdose.

Types of Tubes Used for Decompression and Drainage

Nasogastric or short tubes are used to intubate the stomach. Examples of short tubes used for decom-

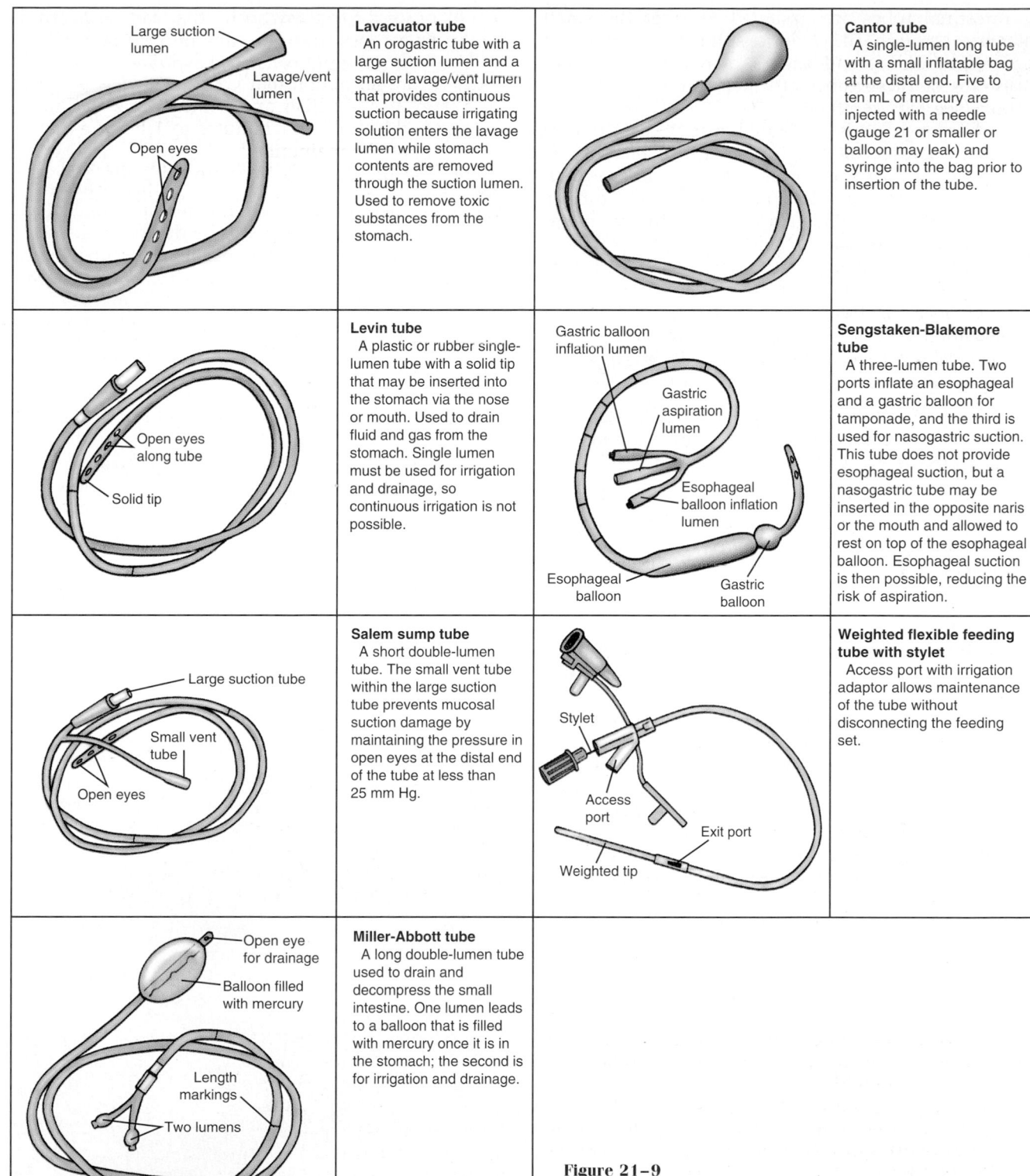

Lavacuator tube
   An orogastric tube with a large suction lumen and a smaller lavage/vent lumen that provides continuous suction because irrigating solution enters the lavage lumen while stomach contents are removed through the suction lumen. Used to remove toxic substances from the stomach.

Cantor tube
   A single-lumen long tube with a small inflatable bag at the distal end. Five to ten mL of mercury are injected with a needle (gauge 21 or smaller or balloon may leak) and syringe into the bag prior to insertion of the tube.

Levin tube
   A plastic or rubber single-lumen tube with a solid tip that may be inserted into the stomach via the nose or mouth. Used to drain fluid and gas from the stomach. Single lumen must be used for irrigation and drainage, so continuous irrigation is not possible.

Sengstaken-Blakemore tube
   A three-lumen tube. Two ports inflate an esophageal and a gastric balloon for tamponade, and the third is used for nasogastric suction. This tube does not provide esophageal suction, but a nasogastric tube may be inserted in the opposite naris or the mouth and allowed to rest on top of the esophageal balloon. Esophageal suction is then possible, reducing the risk of aspiration.

Salem sump tube
   A short double-lumen tube. The small vent tube within the large suction tube prevents mucosal suction damage by maintaining the pressure in open eyes at the distal end of the tube at less than 25 mm Hg.

Weighted flexible feeding tube with stylet
   Access port with irrigation adaptor allows maintenance of the tube without disconnecting the feeding set.

Miller-Abbott tube
   A long double-lumen tube used to drain and decompress the small intestine. One lumen leads to a balloon that is filled with mercury once it is in the stomach; the second is for irrigation and drainage.

Figure 21–9

Comparison of design and function of selected gastrointestinal tubes.

pression and drainage are the Levin and Salem sump tubes (see Fig. 21–9). The Levin tube is a single-lumen tube about 91 cm (3 feet) long with a solid tip and holes along the sides. The Salem sump is a double-lumen tube (a tube within a tube). In the Salem sump, the small air vent tube within the larger tube prevents suction damage to the gastric mucosa by preventing greater than 25 mm Hg of pressure at the openings in the distal end of the tube.

Intestinal tubes are designed to enter the small intestine through the pyloric sphincter because of the weight of a small bag of mercury at the end. Examples of these tubes are the Cantor and Miller-Abbott (see Fig. 21–9).

A Cantor tube is a single-lumen, 3-m (10-foot) tube with a reservoir for 5 to 10 mL of mercury at its tip below the level of the drainage holes. With this tube, the mercury is inserted before the tube is passed through the patient's nose, making it an uncomfortable procedure.

A Miller-Abbott tube is a rubber tube with two lumens. One leads to a bag into which mercury is instilled once the tube is in the stomach. The other is the lumen used for irrigation and drainage. Before a Miller-Abbott tube is inserted, 5 to 10 mL of water are injected into the lumen leading to the balloon to check for leaks.

Intubation Procedure

Most tubes have markings that indicate the distance to the tip of the tube. Before insertion, the length of tube required to reach the desired placement location is estimated. This is performed as follows:

- To estimate the length of tube needed to extend from the naris into the stomach, measure the distance from the tip of the patient's nose to the ear lobe and from the ear lobe to the xiphoid process.
- To estimate the length of tube needed to extend from the naris to the intestine, add 5 cm (2 inches) to the measurement obtained in the previous step.

In preparation for insertion, the patient sits upright with the head hyperextended if possible. If the patient is unconscious or unable to sit up, the bed is raised to Fowler's position. Rubber tubes are iced so that they are stiff, because this eases insertion. The first 2.5 to 10 cm (1–4 inches) of all the previously mentioned tubes are lubricated with a water-soluble lubricant. The tube is then inserted into the naris. (Some tubes need only be wet with water, so be sure to check package directions.) When the tube reaches the pharynx, the patient is encouraged to lower the head slightly, swallow, and—if allowed— take sips of water to help passage of the tube. Coughing, choking, and the inability to talk or hum in an otherwise unimpaired patient indicate that the tube is entering the trachea and must be withdrawn and repassed.

When the estimated length of tube has been passed into the nose, placement of the tube is checked. The most reliable means to determine this is radiology. Bedside methods for checking tube placement include the following:

- Aspirating gastric juice with a 50 mL syringe
- Instilling 10 to 20 mL of air into the tube while auscultating just to the left of the tip of the xiphoid process for a "swoosh" that can be heard as the air escapes from the tube into the stomach
- Measuring the pH of gastric aspirate

The method of placing the end of the tube in water to check for bubbling is no longer recommended because lack of bubbling does not prove that the tube is in the stomach. Recent research indicates that the each of these methods has drawbacks. The ideal method for verifying feeding tube placement at the bedside has yet to be determined.

When placement of the nasogastric tube in the stomach has been confirmed, it should be securely anchored to the patient's nose in a manner that avoids trauma to the nares (Fig. 21–10). The point of entry into the naris is then marked on the tube with a permanent-ink pen.

When an intestinal tube reaches the stomach, the patient is positioned on the right side until the tube passes the pyloric sphincter. Movement of the tube is monitored by x-ray examination because the tube is radiopaque. Because long intestinal tubes are moved through the intestine by peristalsis to the desired location, these tubes are not taped at the time of insertion.

When GI tubes are attached to suction, it may be continuous or intermittent, with a pressure not exceeding 25 mm Hg. The specific pressure and the intervals are ordered by the physician.

If a tube is needed for an extended period, it is

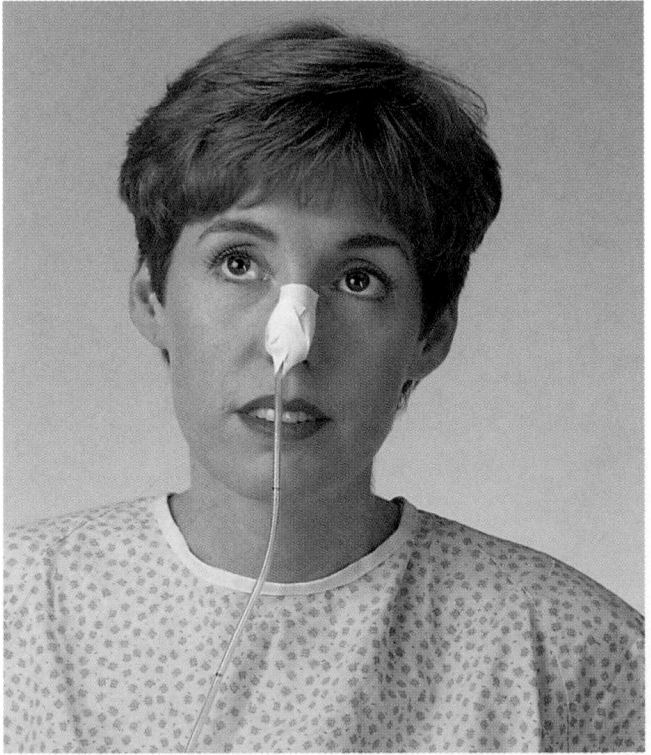

Figure 21–10

Method of taping a nasogastric tube to the nose, which anchors it securely but avoids trauma to the nares.

changed every 2 to 3 weeks, alternating nares if possible.

NURSING PROCESS
Intubation for Removal of Gastric Contents

Assessment

Assess the function of a GI tube every 4 hours. If it is functioning well, there should be drainage in the collection apparatus and the patient should not feel full or nauseated. Irrigate the tube with normal saline to determine patency if needed.

Note amount, color, and consistency of drainage as well as any changes in these parameters. Normal gastric secretions are yellow-green. If blood is present from previous bleeding, drainage is dark brown and resembles coffee grounds because of the action of hydrochloric acid on hemoglobin. Immediately report the presence of bright red blood because it indicates frank, current bleeding. Be alert for the passage of flatus or feces. If either occurs, report it to the physician, because this may indicate that the tube is no longer needed.

Assess the patient for signs of fluid, electrolyte, and acid-base imbalance, which can occur because of excessive losses from the GI tube. Record fluid intake and output, including amounts of irrigating solutions instilled and returned. Measure body weight, check skin turgor, and monitor serum electrolytes.

Also assess the patient for redness, bleeding, and discomfort of the nares, where the tube may exert pressure, and for a sore throat because the pharynx is irritated by the tube.

Nursing Diagnoses and Planning

Nursing diagnoses and related expected patient outcomes commonly applicable to intubated patients include the following:

NDx: Altered oral mucous membrane related to mouth breathing and limitation on oral intake

Planning: Patient Outcomes
1. Oral mucous membrane is pink and moist.
2. Lips are supple, moist, and free of cracks.
3. Patient denies soreness or dryness of mouth and lips.

NDx: Risk for fluid volume deficit related to drainage rather than reabsorption of GI secretions

Planning: Patient Outcomes
1. Skin turgor is firm.
2. Mucous membranes are moist.
3. Urinary output is at least 50 mL/h.
4. Urine specific gravity is between 1.003 and 1.035.
5. Serum electrolyte levels and acid-base parameters are within normal range.

NDx: Risk for impaired tissue integrity related to mechanical irritation from the nasogastric or nasointestinal tube

Planning: Patient Outcomes
1. Skin and mucous membranes of the nares are free of erythema.
2. Skin and mucous membranes of the nares are intact.
3. Bleeding from the nares is absent.

Nursing Interventions and Evaluation

NDx: Altered oral mucous membrane
Because most intubated patients breathe through the mouth, meticulous mouth care is essential for comfort and protection of the mucous membrane. Assist the patient in brushing the teeth and rinsing the mouth every 4 hours while awake. Use a soft toothbrush to avoid accidental trauma. Avoid lemon and glycerin swabs as well as commercial mouthwashes containing alcohol because these further dry the mucous membrane. If the patient is unconscious, clean the mouth with saline or diluted hydrogen peroxide–moistened swabs four to six times each day. Apply a water-soluble lubricant to the lips to keep them supple and prevent cracking.

When permitted, allow the patient to "mist" the mouth with a spray bottle of water or offer gum, small amounts of Gatorade, warm saline gargles, or anesthetic throat lozenges to help wet mucous membranes of the mouth and soothe an irritated pharynx. Do not allow the patient to swallow sips of water or suck on ice chips unless specifically ordered because these small amounts of hypotonic fluid can add up rapidly and contribute to significant fluid and electrolyte imbalance.

NDx: Risk for fluid volume deficit
Monitor laboratory data, skin turgor, and condition of mucous membranes for signs of dehydration. Remember that oral mucous membrane reflects changes caused by mouth breathing and restricted oral intake as well as by dehydration. Administer replacement fluids and electrolytes as ordered. Maintain an accurate and complete fluid intake and output record, always being certain to subtract any fluids given by mouth or tube from the total amount of GI drainage. Obtain daily weights and monitor central venous pressure or other hemodynamic parameters to ensure adequate but not over-replacement of fluid.

NDx: Risk for impaired tissue integrity
Cleanse the area around the nares gently using warm water or saline. Gently remove any crusts that have resulted from increased nasal secretions secondary to irritation from the tube. Apply a protective water-soluble lubricant.

Question the patient about discomfort from the tube and adjust accordingly. To prevent pull on the tube, loop an elastic band around it, then loop the tube above the elastic around the patient's ear, and use a safety pin inserted through the elastic band to pin the tube to the patient's gown or pajamas. Inspect both the naris and the skin behind the ear frequently for signs of irritation. If present, reinsert the tube through the opposite naris or change the position of the tube over the ear.

The skin beneath the anchoring tape becomes oily with time, loosening the tape and creating a risk of dislodging the tube. To reduce this risk, remove the tape anchoring the tube in place daily, being careful to avoid stripping the epidermis. Wash the area thoroughly, wipe with an alcohol swab, shave male patients, and apply new tape. If skin irritation is a problem, use a transparent, moisture- and vapor-permeable dressing such as Op-Site, which can remain in place for as long as 7 days.

Additional Interventions

Explain the purpose of intubation and describe what to expect during insertion to help allay the patient's anxiety. Provide ongoing explanations about intubation and related treatments as needed. This is especially important for the patient with a long intestinal tube who is constantly being x-rayed and repositioned.

Mark the tube at the end of the naris right after insertion so it is possible to tell later whether the tube's position has changed.

Irrigate GI tubes as ordered to maintain patency. Use the type and amount of solution specified by the physician. If the tube is in place to protect a suture line in the GI tract, follow strict sterile technique during the procedure. Instill irrigating fluid manually, and then reattach the tube to suction. Monitor returns and be certain to record the irrigating fluid as intake. Keep in mind that a clogged tube can result in gastric distention, which can lead to shock if unrelieved.

If the tube has a mercury weight, record the amount of mercury instilled in the patient's record. When the tube is removed, follow institutional procedure for collection and disposal of the mercury, which is a toxic substance. If mercury escapes into the GI tract, it is allowed to pass normally because it is not absorbed and is therefore not toxic to the patient.

Compare the patient's status with the expected outcomes. If the outcomes are not met, reassess the patient and revise the plan.

Removal of Gastrointestinal Tubes

Before removal of a GI tube that has been inserted for decompression and drainage, assess GI function. Auscultate bowel sounds. Assess the abdomen for distention. Ask the patient whether flatus has been passed. Note the patient's tolerance of ice chips, clamping of the tube, or both. Also note the volume of drainage, which should have decreased before removal of the tube.

For removal of the tube, raise the patient to a semi-Fowler's position and place a towel across the chest. Tell the patient that some gagging, sneezing, or nasal discomfort may occur, and provide tissues. While wearing gloves, flush the tube with 10 mL of normal saline to cleanse it of debris and move it away from the mucosa. Next, clamp the tube by folding it in the hand. Tell the patient to take a deep breath and exhale slowly. Withdraw the tube during exhalation. When the tube is removed, place it in the towel and remove it from the immediate environment. Withdraw long intestinal tubes slowly, a few inches at a time, because rapid withdrawal can cause vomiting. Provide mouth care, and document the procedure in the patient's record. Subsequently, assess the patient for nausea, vomiting, and abdominal distention.

ENTERAL AND PARENTERAL NUTRITION

Adults ordinarily need 1500 to 2000 calories and 0.5 g/kg of protein per day for normal activity. If the patient is acutely ill, as with serious infection or major surgery, requirements can increase to as much as 10,000 calories and 4 g/kg of protein. This increased need is complicated by the fact that the patient may not be able to maintain minimal nutrition because of lack of appetite or physical impediments to eating. Enteral feedings and hyperalimentation are two methods that provide supplemental nutrition to patients unable to meet their needs through oral feedings.

Enteral Nutrition

Enteral nutrition is another term for tube feeding. It is used to maintain weight in patients with severe anorexia or increased metabolic needs and in patients who cannot eat by mouth because of dysphagia or obstruction of the upper GI tract, decreased level of consciousness, surgery of the GI tract or the head and neck region, malabsorptive syndromes such as Crohn's disease, or anorexia nervosa.

Enteral therapy requires a functional GI tract. It is contraindicated when conditions such as persistent vomiting, upper GI bleeding, obstruction, or inflammatory bowel disease are present.

TYPES OF TUBE FEEDINGS

Feedings are primarily absorbed in the upper small intestine and require minimal digestion. Most enteral feedings provide 1 kcal/mL of feeding. Between 2000 and 3000 mL can be given within 24 hours. An important factor to consider in enteral therapy is osmolarity. Feedings should be as close to the normal body osmolarity of 340 mOsm/L as possible to avoid the shifting of fluid from one body space to another.

Tube feedings can be made by blenderizing various foods until they are thin enough to pass through the tube. Although this type of feeding is nutritious and less expensive, the convenience and standardization of commercial products far outweigh the possible economic savings for most people. Commercial products are consistently smooth and easy to administer, there is minimal chance of contamination, and the contents are clearly stated on the label. They also have the advantage of not requiring refrigeration until opened, and they can be stored for long periods of time.

Commercial products may be divided into two categories. First are nutritionally complete formulas that provide all recommended dietary allowances for vitamins and minerals if given in adequate volume (1 to 2 L every 24 hours). They are available in two formulas: polymeric and defined. Polymeric formulas contain nutrients in complex forms and require some digestive and absorptive capabilities to be useful. They provide 1 to 2 kcal/mL and come in a range of osmolality, so it is important to check the label before administering. Some come with added fiber. Examples of polymeric formulas are Sustacal and Magnacal.

Defined formulas are usually hyperosmolar and therefore must be diluted before administration. If they are not diluted, the body shifts intracellular fluid to achieve iso-osmolarity, possibly causing diarrhea. These formulas contain nutrients in simpler forms and require little digestive and absorptive ability. Most defined formulas provide 1 kcal/mL. Examples are Vital and Vivonex, powdered products that must be dissolved before administration.

Another category of commercial nutritional preparation is the disease-specific formula. Not all of these are nutritionally complete. There are specialized formulas for patients with renal, hepatic, or pulmonary diseases, as well as specific products for patients with acquired immunodeficiency syndrome (AIDS).

METHODS OF DELIVERY

Tube feedings may be given by bolus or by intermittent or continuous drip. In bolus feedings, 300 to 400 mL of formula is infused for several minutes every 4 to 6 hours, usually through an Asepto syringe or a funnel. This type of feeding is usually not well tolerated and therefore is used least often.

Intermittent feedings can be given either by gravity drip or by pump infusion. They are usually given five to eight times daily over a few hours.

Continuous feedings are given by pump at a slow, constant rate in amounts of 75 to 150 mL/h. They are given when large amounts of formula cannot be tolerated at one time. They are used for patients with nasointestinal or jejunostomy tubes as well as for selected patients with nasogastric or gastrostomy tubes.

The type of delivery method selected is based on the needs of the individual patient. Factors considered in selecting a method include the patient's physical and nutritional status, tolerance of the feedings, mobility, comfort, and psychologic wellbeing.

ROUTES OF DELIVERY

Feedings may be given directly into the stomach by nasogastric or gastrostomy tube, into the esophagus by esophagostomy tube, or into the small intestine by nasointestinal or jejunostomy tube. Types of feeding tubes and their placement and advantages are outlined in Table 21–4.

Table 21–4

Feeding Tubes: Types, Placement, and Advantages

Type of Tube	Placement	Advantages
Nasogastric tube	Passed via nose into stomach	No surgical wound
Nasogastric tube	Passed via nose into intestine	Placement beyond pyloric sphincter is thought to reduce backflow
		No surgical wound
Esophagostomy tube	Passed directly into the esophagus through a surgically created opening in the cervical area	Decreased risk of aspiration
		Bypasses operative area in patients who have had head and neck surgery, while allowing maximal normal function of the gastrointestinal tract
Gastrostomy tube	Passed directly into the stomach through an opening created in the abdominal wall	Good for long-term use
		Prevents pharyngeal irritation
		Decreased risk of aspiration
		Is not immediately visible
Jejunostomy tube	Passed into the jejunum through an opening created in the abdominal wall	Good for long-term use
		Bypasses pathology of the upper gastrointestinal tract
		Decreases risk of aspiration

Nasogastric Feeding

Nasogastric tubes are inserted through the nose and passed down the esophagus into the stomach. Nasogastric feeding requires intact gag and swallow reflexes, a competent lower esophageal sphincter, and the capacity to handle a high-osmotic load. An intermittent feeding schedule is preferred whenever possible because the stomach normally functions as a reservoir for food injected at intervals.

Nasointestinal Feeding

Nasointestinal tubes are inserted through the nose and passed down the esophagus and stomach into the duodenum (nasoduodenal) or the jejunum (nasojejunal). Nasointestinal feeding is used when the potential for aspiration is high, when there is dysfunction of the gastric outlet, or when digestive processes are impaired so that a simple nutrient formula is required.

Feedings are administered on a continuous schedule via a nasointestinal tube because the intestine normally receives nutrients from the stomach in slow peristaltic waves.

Gastrostomy

In a gastrostomy, a tube is passed directly into the stomach through the abdominal wall. It provides permanent access and hence is excellent for long-term enteral nutrition. The two major types of gastrostomy are the traditional surgical gastrostomy and the newer percutaneous gastrostomy.

SURGICAL GASTROSTOMY. Surgical gastrostomy is performed with the patient under general anesthesia and involves a laparotomy. A permanent stoma is created by suturing the stomach wall to the abdominal wall. A large-diameter tube is inserted.

Postoperative ileus is usually present for 24 to 48 hours following the procedure. Enteral feeding cannot be started until peristalsis has resumed.

PERCUTANEOUS ENDOSCOPIC GASTROSTOMY. A percutaneous endoscopic gastrostomy is a procedure in which an endoscope is inserted into the stomach, the light from which shines against the abdominal wall and allows visualization of the tube placement site. A large-gauge needle and suture are passed through the abdominal and stomach walls. A snare or biopsy forceps is used to bring the inner end of the suture up through the endoscope into the patient's mouth. The percutaneous endoscopic gastrostomy tube is tied to the suture and is then pulled through the mouth down into the stomach and out through the abdominal wall (Fig. 21–11). The tube is held in place by an anchor system, such as an internal and external rubber bumper or an internal retention balloon and outer disk. In several weeks a fibrous track forms between the gastric wall and the exit site.

Percutaneous gastrostomy has several advantages over surgical gastrostomy. There is less risk because it is performed while the patient is under intravenous sedation rather than general anesthesia. Recovery is faster. The patient is more comfortable because laparotomy has not been performed. Feeding can be started within 24 hours (as soon as bowel sounds return). Finally, the procedure can be performed in the endoscopy suite or at the bedside, so it is less costly.

In preparation for percutaneous endoscopic gastrostomy, the patient is kept on NPO status for 24 hours to empty the stomach and decrease the risk of aspiration. If the patient was receiving tube feedings

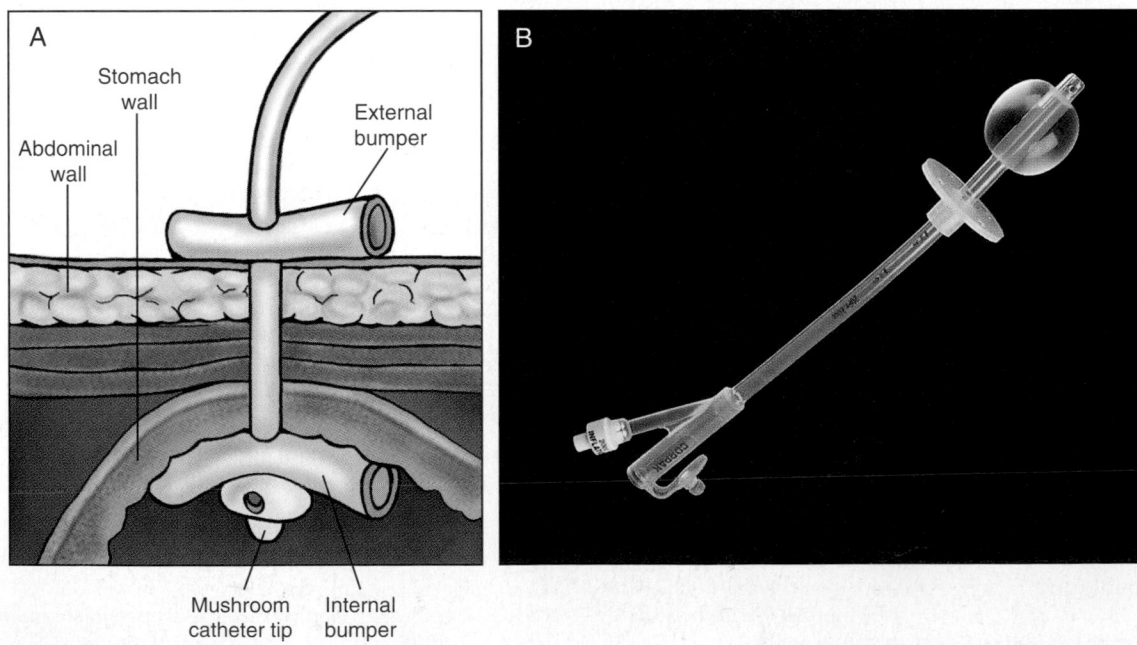

Figure 21–11

A, Percutaneous endoscopic gastrostomy tube in place. *B,* Gastrostomy tube designed for initial placement during a surgical gastrostomy as well as for replacement of a percutaneous endoscopic gastrostomy tube. (Courtesy of CORPAK MedSystems, Wheeling, IL.)

before the procedure, feedings are withheld for 8 hours. During the procedure, vital signs, color, and level of consciousness are monitored. Suctioning is used as necessary because secretions can accumulate in the mouth. Complications of gastrostomy include aspiration, peritonitis, accidental tube removal, and wound cellulitis.

Jejunostomy

In jejunostomy, a tube is passed into the jejunum through an opening in the abdominal wall. As with gastrostomy, a surgical or a percutaneous approach may be used. Percutaneous endoscopic jejunostomy is an extension of percutaneous endoscopic gastrostomy. A small tube is passed through a percutaneous endoscopic gastrostomy tube and guided via an endoscope into the duodenum. The tube is then propelled by peristalsis into the jejunum.

Jejunostomy tubes must be of very small diameter because of the small size of the jejunum. Therefore, they can easily become clogged. They can also be moved back into the stomach by vomiting, in which case the tube must be repositioned under endoscopy.

Feedings must be given continuously because the small size of the tube and because the jejunum is not normally a reservoir for nutrients. Because no residual feeding is present in the jejunum, placement can be confirmed by x-ray only after injection of a contrast medium.

DELIVERY SYSTEMS

Feeding Tubes

Nasoenteric tubes in use today for enteric feedings are predominantly small bore, made of Silastic, and flexible. The majority are weighted, usually with tungsten or silicone. Many are inserted and removed with a stylet. The stylet is designed to assist passage of these newer, soft flexible tubes. Wire stylets or guidewires are stiff and straight and provide easy insertion. However, they are associated with a risk of perforation. Plastic stylets do not have this risk but coil easily and may be difficult to insert into the feeding tube. The stylet is removed once the tube is inserted. The stylet is stored in a plastic bag or other container labeled with patient identification information in case the tube must be reinserted.

Most feeding tubes are coated with a water-activated lubricant. Therefore, they are moistened rather than lubricated before insertion. These tubes usually are comfortable, are unaffected by contact with digestive juices, help prevent reflux esophagitis, and allow oral intake while in place. Disadvantages of these tubes include a tendency to clog if not routinely irrigated, the need for very slow administration, and the need for a feeding pump because of the small lumen.

Feeding Administration Sets

Administration sets consist of a container to hold formula and tubing to connect to the feeding tube itself. The basic container is an open system: a plastic bag with attached tubing, which can be filled with feeding and when empty may be washed and refilled for a 24-hour period. Some of these bags, such as the Kangaroo (Fig. 21–12), have an outside pocket designed to hold a Polar pack of ice to keep the formula cool and discourage bacterial growth. A second type is a closed administration set featuring a disposable prefilled bottle used with a spike set. A spike set has tubing attached to a spike that perforates the formula container when put in place. Bottles are replaced when empty. Spike sets are replaced every 24 to 36 hours.

Feeding Pumps

Infusion pumps are used to provide constant slow administration of formula, which helps prevent symptoms such as feelings of excessive fullness, ab-

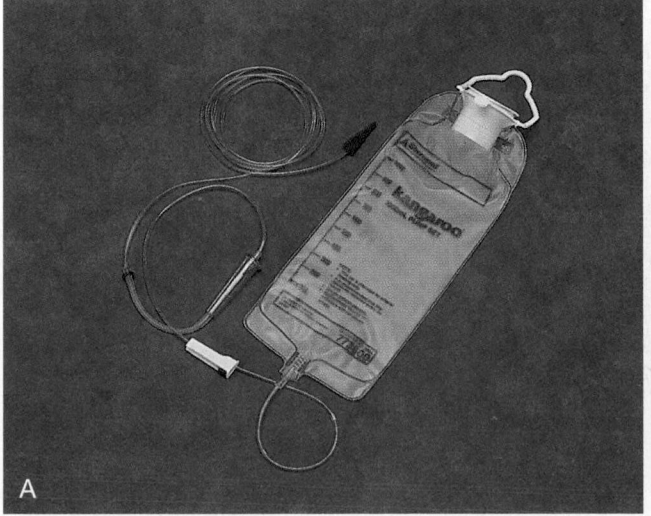
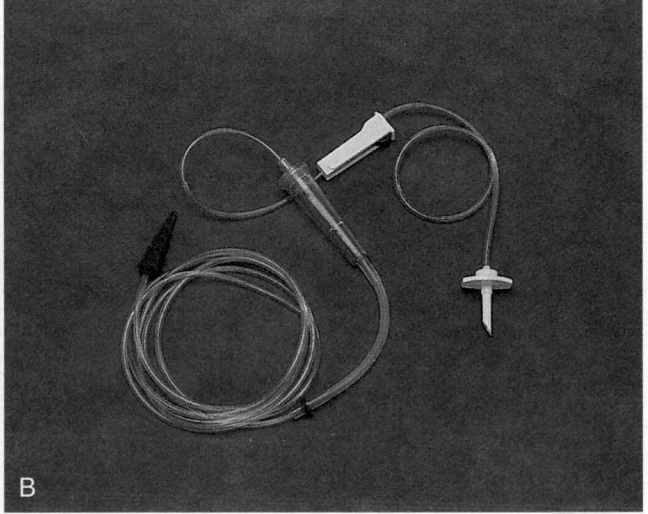

Figure 21–12

Feeding administration sets. A, Kangaroo refillable pump set. B, Spike set. (Courtesy of Sherwood Medical, St. Louis, MO.)

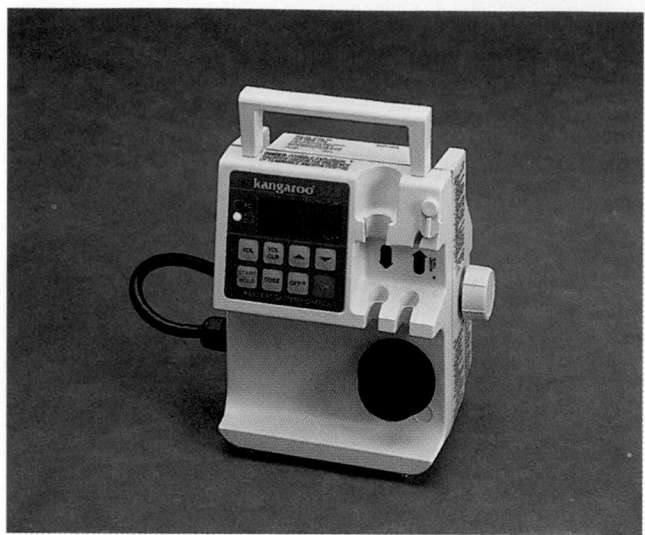

Figure 21-13

Kangaroo 324 pump. (Courtesy of Sherwood Medical, St. Louis, MO.)

dominal cramping, and diarrhea. Use of a pump also permits administration of thicker-consistency feedings than would pass through a small-bore tube by gravity alone.

A variety of pumps are available. All feature a mechanism to set the drop rate in milliliters per hour and an alarm that signals an empty feeding bag or occlusion of the tube. Many also have an alarm that signals a change in flow rate. Most can be operated by battery for some time interval and indicate when battery charge is low. All are small and easy to use, simply requiring that the drip rate be set, the tubing primed and threaded around the drive, and a button pushed to start (Fig. 21-13).

NURSING PROCESS
Enteral Feedings

Assessment

Assess the patient's nutritional status in response to therapy. Observe for physical signs of improved nutrition, such as weight gain and better condition of hair, nails, and skin. Also look for increased energy and subjective statements of feeling stronger.

Auscultate for bowel sounds, and check feeding tube placement before each intermittent feeding and every 4 hours during continuous feeding to ensure delivery to the intended area and to prevent aspiration. Remember that the small intestine is not a reservoir, so no residual formula can be aspirated. The only way placement in the duodenum or jejunum can be checked is by x-ray after injection of a contrast medium.

Assess for tolerance of feedings. Be alert to complaints of nausea or cramping, and observe for ab-

dominal distention, vomiting, or diarrhea. Check respirations and airway clearance to assess for aspiration. Assess for hyperglycemia by:

- Observing for thirst, polyuria, and confusion
- Testing urine for glucose and acetone
- Checking blood glucose levels daily

Observe for signs of dehydration, which can result from inadequate fluid intake or excess fluid loss. Check for reduced skin turgor, thirst, changes in mentation, rapid weight loss, and urine specific gravity greater than 1.018. Inspect the condition of the area around the tube insertion site. Look for signs of infection or irritation, such as redness, excoriation, bleeding, or purulent drainage. If the patient has undergone percutaneous endoscopic gastrostomy or has a percutaneous endoscopic jejunostomy tube, expect a small amount of drainage for about a week from the tissue reaction to the tube, which is a foreign body. When assessing the wound, slide the outer bumper about half an inch away from the skin to check for redness and breakdown. Gently press around the tube to check for drainage. Also inspect the tube for signs of wear.

Assess the patient's psychologic reaction to the feeding system. If the patient is to be discharged home with it, assess both the patient's and any significant other's understanding of and ability to manage and cope with this therapy. Also assess the need for follow-up visits by a home health nurse.

Nursing Diagnoses and Planning

Nursing diagnoses and related expected patient outcomes commonly applicable to patients on enteral feedings include risk for impaired tissue integrity and altered oral mucous membrane previously described in the sections on intubation. Other diagnoses include the following:

NDx: Altered nutrition: less than body requirements related to inadequate intake or absorption of nutrients

Planning: Patient Outcomes
1. Patient maintains weight or shows slow, steady weight gain.
2. Patient is in positive nitrogen balance.
3. Serum electrolyte and protein levels are within normal range.

NDx: Risk for aspiration related to enteral feeding

Planning: Patient Outcomes
1. Abrupt coughing and gagging are absent.
2. Respirations are silent and easy.
3. Lungs are clear on auscultation.

NDx: Diarrhea related to intolerance of formula administered

Planning: Patient Outcomes
1. Patient passes formed stool at regular intervals.
2. Patient denies abdominal cramping.

NDx: Constipation related to enteral feeding formula

Planning: Patient Outcomes

1. Patient passes soft, formed stool at regular intervals.
2. Patient denies uncomfortable straining at stool.

Nursing Interventions and Evaluation

NDx: Altered nutrition: less than body requirements

Administer enteral feedings according to physician's order. Record fluid intake and output. Weigh the patient daily at the same time of day on the same scale, wearing the same amount of clothing. Report any rapid weight gain or loss to the physician. This is important because rapid weight gain may indicate that the patient is retaining fluid and is overhydrated. Rapid loss may indicate dehydration. Give additional water throughout the day in the amount needed to have daily intake exceed output by 500 mL.

If you must decrease the administration rate because of lack of tolerance, calculate the patient's daily caloric intake at the new rate (calories per milliliter of formula × number of milliliters given per hour × number of hours of administration per day). Compare this with the caloric intake ordered. Record the change on the patient's chart and, if the patient is receiving significantly fewer calories per day because of the decrease in administration rate, notify the physician.

NDx: Risk for aspiration

Patients at greatest risk for aspiration of tube feedings are the unconscious, the confused, the seriously debilitated, the elderly, those with tracheostomies or large-bore feeding tubes, and those whose gag reflexes are impaired or who cannot sit upright. Protect the patient from aspiration by keeping the head elevated at least 30 degrees during feeding and for 1 hour thereafter. If this is not possible, position the patient on the right side.

Check placement of the feeding tube before every intermittent or bolus feeding and every 4 hours during continuous feeding. If you question tube placement, delay feeding until correct placement is confirmed. Also check for gastric residual, because overloading the stomach predisposes to reflux and regurgitation. Check before each intermittent or bolus feeding and every 2 to 4 hours during continuous feeding. If the residual is more than 30 mL, discontinue the feeding for 30 to 60 minutes and then recheck. If a residual still exceeds 30 mL, notify the physician. Remember that malposition of the tube in the GI tract makes it difficult to check for residual. For example, if the plunger on the syringe cannot be withdrawn, the end of the tube may be lodged against the stomach wall. If only air can be aspirated, the tube may be curled up in the esophagus or in the stomach above the level of the gastric contents. Attempt to reposition the tube by rotating it, advancing it a few inches, pulling it back

slightly, changing the patient's position, or injecting a little air to push the tube away from the stomach wall if this is the problem. Try again to obtain a residual. If nausea or vomiting occurs, discontinue the feeding and notify the physician.

NDx: Diarrhea

Diarrhea is usually the result of feedings that are too rapidly administered, too high in lactose, or incompatible in osmolality. It may also be due to bacterial contamination of the feeding.

Build the patient's tolerance to feedings by initially administering slowly over long periods of time and then gradually increasing the rate and the time between feedings (Fig. 21–14).

Dilute formulas with water if needed for tolerance. This is often necessary at the start of enteral therapy. Hypertonic formulas generally need to be diluted by half with water, but even full-strength isotonic feeding may not be tolerated initially by patients who have been ill for some time and have become malnourished. Increase diluted formulas to full strength gradually. Do not attempt to increase rate and strength of feeding at the same time. Focus first on developing the patient's tolerance to full-strength formula because diluted formula provides fewer calories per milliliter, placing the patient at risk for receiving inadequate daily caloric intake. Be sure to administer all feedings at room temperature because cramping occurs when feedings are too cold.

Protect the patient from diarrhea caused by bacterial contamination of the feeding by careful handwashing before and meticulous aseptic technique during handling of equipment. Change the feeding bag and tubing completely every 24 hours. Mark each new set with the patient's name, room number, date, and time so that time for replacement is easily and accurately known. Never let formula hang longer than the time recommended by the manufacturer, and never store formula in the refrigerator for longer than 24 hours. If refillable bags are used, never add new formula to that remaining in the bag. Rather, rinse the bag and tubing with warm water, then fill with new formula. Remember that diarrhea can result from viral disease or a change in medication, as with any other patient. Report persistent diarrhea.

NDx: Constipation

Patients receiving tube feedings, particularly those on tube feedings for a long time, are at risk for constipation. Guard against this by ensuring adequate fluid intake and exercise when possible. If changes in bowel habits begin to suggest constipation, explore with the physician the possibility of switching to a fiber-containing formula.

Additional Interventions

Prevent clogging of the feeding tube by flushing with 30 mL of water every 3 to 4 hours during continuous feedings and both before and after inter-

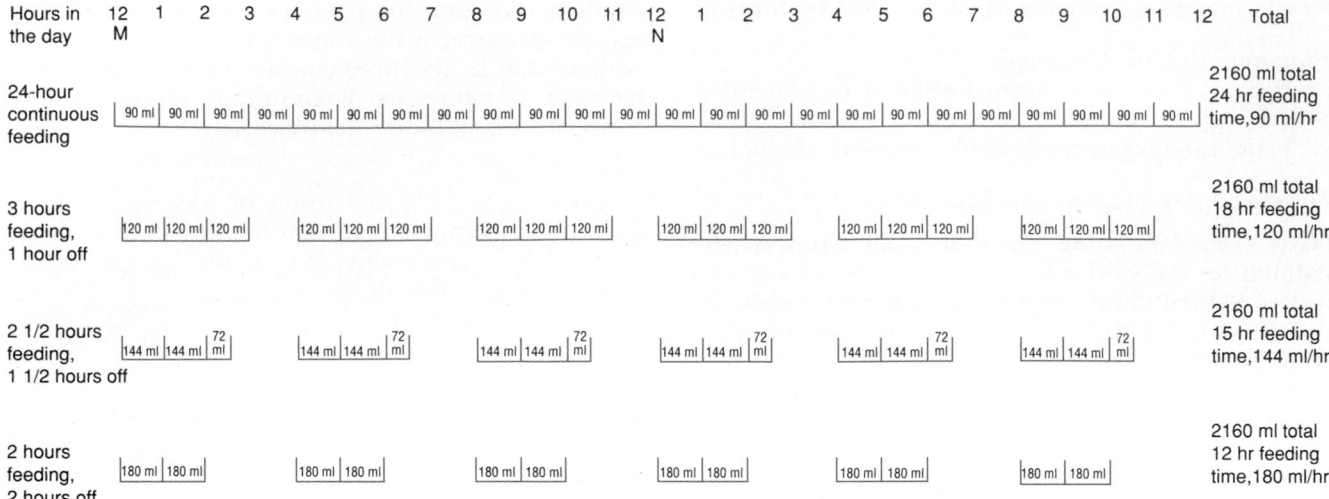

Hours in the day	12 M	1	2	3	4	5	6	7	8	9	10	11	12 N	1	2	3	4	5	6	7	8	9	10	11	12	Total
24-hour continuous feeding	90 ml	90 ml	90 ml	90 ml	90 ml	90 ml	90 ml	90 ml	90 ml	90 ml	90 ml	90 ml	90 ml	90 ml	90 ml	90 ml	90 ml	90 ml	90 ml	90 ml	90 ml	90 ml	90 ml	90 ml	90 ml	2160 ml total 24 hr feeding time, 90 ml/hr

Figure 21–14

Graphic representation of gradually increasing the rate and time between enteral feedings while maintaining a constant daily caloric intake.

mittent or bolus feedings. Do not flush with fruit juice because this merely curdles the formula. Cola is sometimes used to discourage clogging. If this is done, immediately flush with water to remove the stickiness. If formula is thick, squeeze or shake the container at intervals.

Attempt to unclog a blocked feeding tube by aspirating formula behind the clog. If this is not successful, flush the tube with warm water. Use at least a 30 mL syringe, because anything smaller could build up pressure and rupture the tube.

When administering medications via a feeding tube, request the liquid form when possible. If pills or tablets must be given, crush thoroughly (remember that some medications cannot be safely crushed) and mix with a small amount of water. Pull the mixture up in a syringe and feed it into the tube. Flush the feeding tube with 5 mL of water between each medication and with 25 mL of water when the last medication is given. When giving medications directly into the jejunum, dilute with 50 to 100 mL of water to prevent mucosal damage. Never give bulk-forming agents via the tube.

Protect against damage to the naris and the oral mucous membranes caused by nasogastric or nasointestinal tube as described previously. If the patient has a gastrostomy or jejunostomy tube, cleanse it daily with diluted hydrogen peroxide, being certain to move the outer bumper on a percutaneous endoscopic gastrostomy or percutaneous endoscopic jejunostomy tube away from the skin surface. Dry thoroughly, replace the bumper if present, and leave exposed to the air. Cover the area with a dressing only immediately following the ostomy because dressings tend to hold moisture to the skin and thus support maceration and bacterial growth. Change any dressing in use at least once a day and immedi-

ately if wet, noting date and time on tape. Never place a dressing under a percutaneous endoscopic gastrostomy or percutaneous endoscopic jejunostomy bumper.

Many patients maintain enteral feedings when at home. Along with teaching about the administration of feedings, be certain that the patient and significant others know how to troubleshoot when problems arise and have an identified resource to contact in case of a problem. They should be aware of the location for purchase of supplies. Refer the patient to home health care and community resources as needed.

Compare the patient's status with the expected outcomes. If the outcomes are not met, reassess the patient and revise the plan.

Total Parenteral Nutrition

Total parenteral nutrition, also called intravenous hyperalimentation or simply hyperalimentation, is the intravenous administration of nutrients in amounts needed to produce a state of anabolism. It is used when a person's nutritional needs cannot be met satisfactorily through the GI tract. Thus, it is used in a wide variety of clinical conditions, such as inflammatory bowel disease, pancreatitis, trauma, extensive burns, acute renal failure, and following extensive bowel surgery.

SOLUTIONS

Basic components of total parenteral nutrition solutions include the following:

- Synthetic, highly usable essential and nonessential amino acids

- Large amounts of dextrose to provide protein-sparing calories
- Electrolytes
- Vitamins
- Minerals
- Trace elements

To some degree, these components can be modified to meet the needs of individual patients. For example, additional sodium or potassium can be added. Insulin can be added. For patients with renal failure, all protein may be in the form of essential amino acids.

ADMINISTRATION

Because solutions are highly concentrated and hypertonic, they must be administered into a wide-diameter vessel with a rapid blood flow so that they are diluted quickly before they can cause sclerosis of the vessel. The only veins into which the catheter tip can be safely placed are the innominate, the intrathoracic subclavian, and the superior vena cava. The middle of the superior vena cava is the most ideal site. Insertion of a catheter for total parenteral nutrition is most often through the subclavian vein.

Another option is a peripherally inserted central catheter. This procedure can be performed at the bedside but involves strict surgical asepsis. During insertion of the inside-the-needle catheter, when the needle is open to the air and while the catheter is being threaded into position, the patient is instructed to take a deep breath, hold it, and bear down slightly. This Valsalva maneuver increases central venous pressure and thus protects against air embolism. Once the catheter is in place, the needle is withdrawn and covered with a plastic guard to prevent inadvertent puncture of the catheter. A single suture anchors the catheter at the insertion site to prevent accidental dislodgment or back-and-forth movement, which could contaminate the wound with microorganisms from the skin. A dressing is applied and a chest x-ray taken immediately at the bedside to confirm accurate catheter placement. An isotonic intravenous solution is run at a rate sufficient to keep the catheter open until placement is verified, and then the infusion is begun.

COMPLICATIONS

Complications of total parenteral nutrition occupy two categories: those associated with catheter insertion and those related to ongoing infusion.

Major complications of insertion include pneumothorax from accidental pleural puncture, hemothorax from damage to the subclavian or nearby vessels, and hydrothorax from the catheter passing through the vein and infusing solution into the chest. Symptoms of these complications are sharp chest pain and decreased breath sounds. Treatment varies with the severity of the condition. In some cases insertion of a chest tube may be necessary.

Inadvertent arterial puncture can also occur during catheter insertion. If not noted at the time of occurrence, symptoms that develop include a rapidly expanding hematoma, signs and symptoms of tracheal compression, and respiratory distress. Treatment consists of direct pressure on the artery for a minimum of 5 minutes.

Major complications of ongoing total parenteral nutrition include infection, hyperglycemia, and hypoglycemia. Infection is the most serious complication because it can lead to sepsis. It can occur from in-line contamination or from migration of organisms along the catheter from the insertion site. Infection typically presents as a low-grade fever of several days' duration, which then becomes a high fever. In some cases, however, glycosuria or a dramatic spike in temperature may be the first symptom to develop. Whenever fever occurs, a history is taken and physical examination is performed, and cultures not only of the invasive line site but of urine, sputum, feces, and any wound drainage are obtained. When temperature spikes suddenly, the intravenous lines are changed, new solution is hung, and the discontinued materials are sent for culture. The catheter itself may have to be removed to prevent sepsis.

Glucose imbalance is the most common metabolic complication of total parenteral nutrition. Hyperglycemia occurs when the glucose load in the total parenteral nutrition solution exceeds the body's ability to metabolize it. Symptoms include nausea, weakness, excessive thirst, excessive urination, and headache. This may be a transient state at the beginning of total parenteral nutrition because beta cells in the pancreas are not yet producing the increased amount of insulin demanded by the glucose load. When this is the case, treatment simply involves slowing the rate of infusion to give the pancreas time to adjust. At other times, hyperglycemia may relate to actual compromised glucose tolerance caused by factors such as old age, diabetes, stress, shock, sepsis, hepatic or renal failure, starvation, or medication (eg, some diuretics and tranquilizers). In these cases, exogenous insulin is added to the total parenteral nutrition solution. It is administered in this way to achieve a more constant serum level than is possible with intermittent, subcutaneous injections. Progressive hyperglycemia can result in osmotic diuresis with dehydration and electrolyte imbalance, which can lead to coma and death.

Hypoglycemia can result from the body's overproduction of insulin in response to the increased glucose load or from sudden interruption of therapy. It occurs because serum insulin levels stay high for a period of time after serum glucose drops. The infusion can be interrupted accidentally because the tubing becomes kinked or bent as the patient changes position. Symptoms of hypoglycemia are weakness, headache, chills, tingling in the mouth or extremities, thirst, hunger, diaphoresis, and apprehension.

Air embolism is a potential complication of total parenteral nutrition therapy because it can occur whenever the central venous system is open to air. Thus, there is a risk of air embolism during insertion, during tubing changes, during infusion if the line accidentally disconnects, and through the track left after removal of the catheter. To protect against air embolism, the patient is positioned in a Trendelenburg or flat position and asked to perform Valsalva's maneuver whenever the catheter will be open to the air. In addition, all junctures in the line are taped, and when the catheter is removed, an airtight dressing is immediately put in place and left for 48 hours to allow full closure of the track.

If an embolism does occur, symptoms include dyspnea, apnea, hypoxia, disorientation, tachycardia, hypotension, and precordial murmur. Symptoms vary with the severity of the embolism. The immediate treatment is to place the patient on the left side, with the feet higher than the head. This traps air in the right atrium, from where it can be removed by direct intracardiac aspiration if necessary.

The risk of complications related to the administration of total parenteral nutrition are greatly reduced by using a volumetric infusion pump that can detect occlusions and air.

NURSING PROCESS
Total Parenteral Nutrition

Assessment

Assess the patient's baseline condition before the start of total parenteral nutrition. Review the patient's medical history and determine current status in relationship to symptoms and treatment of the problem underlying the need for total parenteral nutrition. Note the patient's weight and observe for signs of nutritional deficiency and fluid and electrolyte imbalance. Assess the patient's understanding of total parenteral nutrition therapy and level of anxiety regarding it.

Once total parenteral nutrition is begun, assess for signs of complications. Immediately after catheter insertion, assess for sharp chest pain and decreased breath sounds, which can indicate pneumothorax, hemothorax, or hydrothorax. Observe also for signs of a rapidly expanding hematoma, tracheal compression, and respiratory distress, which may indicate accidental arterial puncture.

Assess for infection. Check temperature every 4 hours and observe for malaise. When changing the dressing, assess the insertion site for erythema, edema, skin ulceration, and drainage. Make ongoing assessments of fluid and electrolyte status and acid-base balance. Be alert to signs of vitamin and trace element deficiency or toxicity.

Assess carefully for signs of glucose imbalance because this is the most common metabolic complication. Check serum glucose every 4 to 6 hours

using bedside glucose monitoring. Observe for diuresis, dry skin, and thirst, which may indicate hyperglycemia. Also observe for weakness, diaphoresis, and pallor, which may indicate hypoglycemia.

Assess for therapeutic responses to total parenteral nutrition therapy. Weigh the patient daily. Review laboratory data, and watch for signs of improved healing.

Nursing Diagnoses and Planning

Nursing diagnoses and related expected patient outcomes commonly applicable to patients receiving total parenteral nutrition include the following:

NDx: Anxiety related to the total parenteral nutrition procedure

Planning: Patient Outcomes
1. Patient describes the procedures involved with total parenteral nutrition.
2. Patient attends to instructions.
3. Patient states that anxiety is under control.
4. Overt signs of excessive anxiety are absent.

NDx: Altered nutrition: less than body requirements related to inability to take in needed amounts of nutrients via the GI tract

Planning: Patient Outcomes
1. Patient is in positive nitrogen balance.
2. Patient gains *(specify amount)* of weight per week.

NDx: Risk for infection related to in-line contamination or migration of organisms along the catheter from the insertion site

Planning: Patient Outcomes
1. Patient is afebrile.
2. Insertion site is free of erythema, edema, and drainage.
3. Skin around insertion site is intact.

Nursing Interventions and Evaluation

NDx: Anxiety
Tell the patient what to expect during catheter insertion. Tell the patient that the physician will wear a mask, gown, and gloves and that other persons at the head of the bed will wear masks to guard against infection. Explain that the Trendelenburg position is used to distend the vein and facilitate positioning of the catheter. Tell the patient that a small towel roll will be placed under the back to hyperextend the neck and raise the collar bone and that the face will be turned to the side and loosely covered. Assure the patient that there will be no difficulty breathing or seeing.

Describe the preparation with acetone, iodine, and alcohol to cleanse the skin of microorganisms. Explain that a local anesthetic will be given to numb the shoulder and that it can feel like a bee sting until it starts to work. Tell the patient to expect a strange feeling of pressure or even pain within the chest as the catheter is introduced, and stress that this is normal. Show the patient the tubing and point out how thin it is. Reassure the patient that removal of the catheter is a quick, simple, painless procedure, not anything like the insertion procedure.

If the patient is highly anxious despite explanation and reassurance, indicate this to the physician and suggest an order for an antianxiety agent.

Following insertion of the catheter, keep the patient informed about his or her care and progress. For example, explain that the chest x-ray taken after insertion is standard procedure to check catheter placement and not an indication of a problem. Also explain dressing and tubing change procedures and inform the patient of positive responses to therapy, such as weight gain or signs of improved healing.

NDx: Altered nutrition: less than body requirements

Administer total parenteral nutrition solutions according to physician's orders. Check labels on all solution containers carefully for accuracy. Maintain a constant rate of infusion around the clock, keeping in mind that initially solution is infused slowly, at a rate of 60 to 80 mL/h for the average adult. The rate is then increased by 25 mL/h/d to allow time for the pancreatic beta cells to increase insulin production to meet the need created by the total parenteral nutrition solution. Use a mechanical controller or pump. Check the rate every 30 minutes and reset as necessary. Remember that too-rapid administration can cause a hyperglycemic reaction or even hyperosmotic, nonketotic coma. Never adjust the rate to compensate for past increases or decreases. Mark the container in hourly amounts to aid in assessing the accuracy of the flow rate.

Maintain accurate fluid intake and output records, and weigh the patient daily at the same time, on the same scale, and in the same clothing.

NDx: Risk for infection

Infection as a complication of total parenteral nutrition may be caused by in-line contamination or by migration of organisms along the catheter from the site of insertion. Guard against in-line contamination by keeping all prepared total parenteral nutrition solutions refrigerated until used. When hanging a new container, examine it carefully for cracks or small punctures. Also inspect the solution against a bright light to check for turbidity or particulate matter, which can indicate bacterial contamination. Change intravenous tubing and filters every 24 hours using strict aseptic technique. Do this at the same time the solution container is changed because each time the line is disconnected there is a risk of contamination. Do not use the total parenteral nutrition line for central venous pressure monitoring, drawing blood, or administering medications.

Decrease the risk of infection originating at the site of insertion by meticulous cleansing and dressing of the area while maintaining strict aseptic technique. This is so important in the prevention of sepsis that some agencies have a special team responsible for maintaining catheter dressings. Others require staff nurses to be "certified" before assuming this responsibility. Such certification typically consists of an in-service program, assigned readings, demonstration, and satisfactory performance of a supervised dressing change. Although precise protocols for dressing changes vary somewhat among agencies, most are based on the technique developed by Grant and Dudrick, outlined here.

Change the dressing over the catheter insertion site every 48 hours or three times per week and whenever wet or contaminated. If the airtight seal of the dressing is broken, do not reinforce the dressing. Change it.

Using sterile gloves and a sterile clamp to hold the swabs, scrub the catheter site with acetone to defat the skin. Scrub until the sponges come away clean. Follow with tincture of iodine, which has an antifungal and antibacterial effect. Apply for a full 2 minutes, allow to air dry, and then use alcohol to remove the iodine because it can irritate or burn if left on the skin. Again air dry. Do not fan or blow. Throughout this procedure, be certain to work in concentric circles going from clean to dirty areas (from the site of insertion outward). Also be certain to clean the catheter and all its parts. After cleansing, apply a topical antimicrobial ointment to the insertion site and cover with two small gauze sponges. Apply a skin protectant on exposed skin to protect against breakdown and cover with an occlusive dressing, being certain not to touch the side of the dressing being placed against the patient's skin. Place a slit piece of tape under the catheter for occlusion while allowing easy access for tubing changes. Seal all edges of the dressing with tape or cover with a product such as Op-Site, a thin transparent waterproof dressing that allows vapor to escape while maintaining sterility. Also tape all tubing junctions to protect against accidental separation. Anchor the filter to the dressing to eliminate pull on the insertion site (Fig. 21–15). Central line dressing change kits are available that greatly simplify this procedure.

Monitor the condition of the insertion site with each dressing change. Notify the physician if drainage or skin irritation is noted, and obtain cultures as ordered.

Take the patient's temperature every 6 hours and report an increase to the physician. Keep in mind that certain drugs and disease states inhibit the fever response, so although an oral temperature of higher than 37.7°C (100°F) should always be reported, judge each patient individually. If the temperature rises suddenly, culture and change the intravenous tubing and hang new solution immediately. If new solution is unavailable, hang 20% dextrose with insulin if ordered.

Additional Interventions

Keep the patient lying flat when changing the tubing. Also instruct him or her to perform a Valsalva maneuver when the catheter is open to the air to further protect against an air embolism.

Compare the patient's status with the expected outcomes. If the outcomes are not met, reassess the patient and revise the plan.

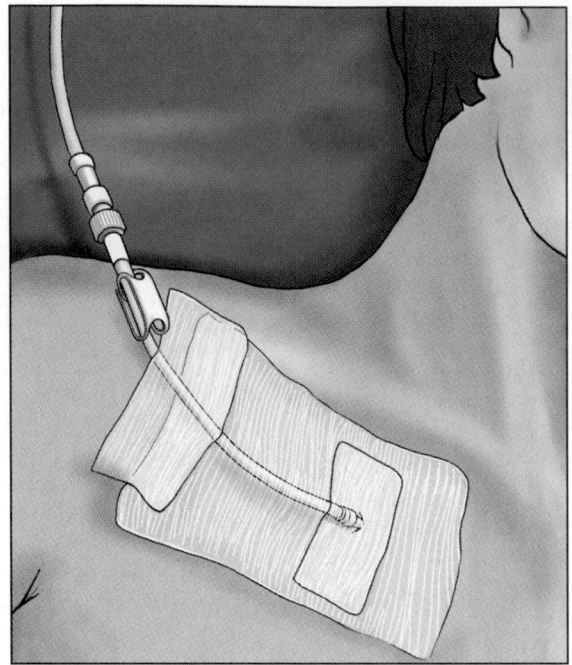

Figure 21–15

Method of dressing the exit site of a total parenteral nutrition catheter using tape and a transparent waterproof dressing.

INTRAVENOUS LIPIDS

Fats are needed to prevent or treat essential fatty acid deficiency, which is characterized by poor wound healing, dry and scaling skin, thin hair, thrombocytopenia, and liver function changes. Fat is also a major source of calories, generating 9 kcal/g, as opposed to the 4 kcal/g generated by carbohydrates. Fats may be given alone or simultaneously with the basic total parenteral nutrition solution through a Y-connector just proximal to the catheter hub.

If fat is used as a major source of calories, the amount of glucose in the total parenteral nutrition solution is decreased and administration through a peripheral vein is possible. A pump must be used if the solution is still hypertonic, however. Ten-percent fat emulsions are isotonic and can also be administered via a peripheral vein.

When administering lipids, do not keep the solution refrigerated. However, before hanging the bag, do examine the emulsion carefully for signs of separation or an oily appearance. Check recommendations for the type of tubing to be used, because conventional tubing contains a plasticizer that can be extracted by fat-containing fluids unless specifically stated to the contrary on the package insert.

Add nothing to fat solutions because the stability of the emulsion may be disturbed. Do not use a filter, because it clogs or disturbs the emulsion. Never store or reuse a partially used container, and never leave a container hanging more than 12 hours.

Maintain flow rate strictly within the manufacturer's guidelines, remembering that initial rate is very slow and the patient must be observed for adverse reactions. These include nausea and vomiting, headache, flushing, perspiration, insomnia, vertigo, chills, and fever. Never exceed the maximum daily dose.

Necessary fats may also be provided through use of a total nutrient admixture that contains carbohydrates, proteins, and fats in a single solution. These solutions are potentially unstable because emulsion can be disrupted by commonly used additives such as magnesium.

TOTAL PARENTERAL NUTRITION AT HOME

Many patients who require total parenteral nutrition over long periods are now taught to administer the solution at home. Some even can tolerate cyclic rather than continuous feedings. When this is the case, the solution is generally run at night, leaving the patient free during the day to carry on with usual lifestyle activities. Home total parenteral nutrition is administered either through a long catheter tunneled subcutaneously to an exit point easily accessible to the patient (Fig. 21–16) or through an implantable infusion device.

The two basic catheters used for home total parenteral nutrition are the Broviac catheter, which has

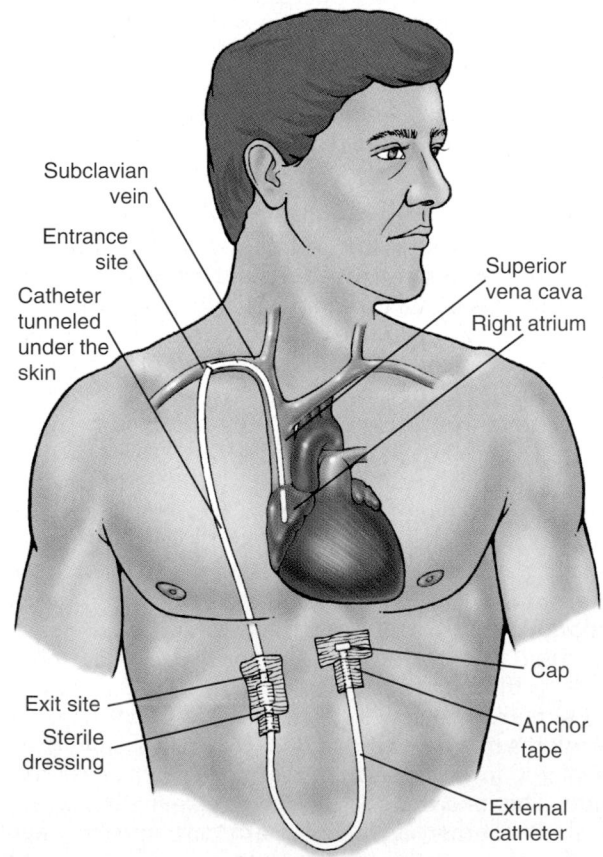

Figure 21–16

Placement of a long tunneled tube for total parenteral nutrition therapy.

WEAKNESS, HEADACHE, THIRST, AND NOCTURIA IN A PATIENT ON TOTAL PARENTERAL NUTRITION

As a community health nurse caring for a patient discharged with total parenteral nutrition (TPN), I remained in close contact with the nutritional support nurse at the local hospital for follow-up and consultation. Before my third visit to the home of a 31-year-old male patient with acquired immunodeficiency syndrome (AIDS), I reviewed my notes and prepared for the visit.

Following positive human immunodeficiency virus (HIV) testing 4 years ago, and an episode of *Pneumocystis carinii* pneumonia 13 months ago, the patient had developed oral and esophageal candidiasis and cryptosporidiosis. He had no significant medical history and was currently being treated with aerosolized pentamidine every 4 weeks, fluconazole, and supportive therapy. Difficulty eating secondary to mouth and throat discomfort, and frequent episodes of nausea, vomiting, and watery diarrhea, had led to significant weight loss, loss of muscle and fat, debilitation with subsequent inability to eat, and the dangerous cycle of malnutrition and wasting.

Attempts to improve his nutritional status with small frequent feedings and oral liquid supplements proved unsuccessful, and the patient was placed on enteral feedings. Nasogastric tube feedings were initiated but poorly tolerated. Intractable diarrhea and continued nausea and vomiting, with its concomitant risk for aspiration, necessitated an alternative method of feeding. Although percutaneous endoscopic gastrostomy or jejunostomy were possibilities, the decision to initiate TPN was strongly considered. TPN would not directly alter the course of HIV infection and AIDS, but perhaps this method of complete nutritional support would prolong his survival, reduce the frequency and length of hospital stays, reduce the number of opportunistic infections, and improve his quality of life and overall health. The patient was both willing and highly motivated; and the absence of any evidence of dementia or active intravenous drug abuse made him an acceptable candidate.

The patient was hospitalized for stabilization of his condition, percutaneous insertion of a Hickman catheter into the superior vena cava via the subclavian vein, initiation of TPN, adjustment of the formula to approximate his needs, evaluation of his response, and instruction on home care. Following an uneventful procedure and hospital stay, the patient was discharged to his home with continuous TPN feedings and referrals for direct and close supervision of his health care beginning with the day of discharge.

My initial visit was spent helping the patient get settled and organized, and assisting him with the preparation and administration of his feeding. Nursing goals established for my second visit included the following:

- Reinforcing patient teaching done before discharge regarding home intravenous nutrition and maintaining a central line
- Evaluating the patient's competency in performing necessary skills and managing aseptic technique
- Evaluating the patient's understanding of potential imbalances and complications of TPN, knowledge of assessments to be made and reported, and emergency procedures to be followed
- Assessing the patient's physical condition and psychosocial needs
- Modifying the home environment to facilitate his care
- Identifying any immediate problems

The patient, who lived alone, demonstrated adequate knowledge and proficiency to maintain his feedings and expressed confidence in his ability to manage alone. His physical condition appeared stable. Assessment findings were consistent with those noted in the discharge summary.

Upon entering the patient's home the next day for my third visit (the patient's 8th day of TPN), I noticed a marked change in the patient's condition. He complained of weakness, headache, and thirst, and stated that he had been up much of the night urinating. Although he recognized me, he was confused about when he had seen me last and couldn't recall events from the previous day. The patient's eyes appeared to be sunken in. His face was flushed. Before assisting the patient back to bed, I weighed him and noted a weight loss of 1.5 lbs in the past 24 hours.

Next I assessed the patient's vital signs. His blood pressure was 112/72, down from 124/80 the previous day. Apical pulse was 110 and regular, up from 88 the previous day. Respiratory rate was 22 breaths per minute and unlabored, with no evidence of Kussmaul breathing or fruity odor to the breath. This was only slightly changed from his rate of 20 breaths per minute the previous day. Temperature was 100°F, up from 98.6°F the previous day.

Lung sounds were clear to auscultation. The patient's skin and mucous membranes were dry. I noted decreased skin turgor. Peripheral pulses were palpable but weak. Capillary refill was less than 3 seconds. The patient requested the urinal and voided 150 mL of pale urine with a dilute

(continued)

CLINICAL **?** THINKING

(continued)

appearance. It tested 4+ for glucose (up from previous readings of 1+) and negative for ketones. I performed a fingerstick for a blood glucose reading and noted a blood glucose of 400 mg/dL plus. The patient denied any pain, but did report an increase in the number of episodes of diarrhea.

I recognized that the patient was at risk for developing any number of complications related to the TPN therapy, AIDS, and its accompanying opportunistic infections. The complications associated with TPN included mechanical complications related to the catheter, infection and sepsis, electrolyte imbalances, and metabolic disturbances including hyperglycemic hyperosmolar nonketotic syndrome. Dehydration related to the cryptosporidiosis was a possible complication as well, because weight loss and dehydration (dry, flushed skin and mucous membranes, sunken eyes, and poor skin turgor) were consistent with this condition. Glycosuria was not consistent with it, however.

The patient's clinical picture—which included an altered level of consciousness, elevated temperature, tachycardia, flushing, and glycosuria—pointed to hyperosmolar nonketotic syndrome, sepsis, or both as possible explanations. Knowing that a patient with AIDS was at particularly high risk for infection related to TPN, I focused my assessment on the possibility of an infection and the presence of sepsis by examining the insertion site for evidence of redness, warmth, swelling, tenderness, or drainage. I found none. The patient denied experiencing any muscle aches or chills.

Although an altered level of consciousness, elevated temperature, tachycardia and glycosuria were consistent with sepsis secondary to TPN, the lack of signs and symptoms of local and systemic infection did not support the likelihood of sepsis. In addition, the early stage of sepsis in which flushing may be evident is not consistent with a drop in blood pressure. Nor are the findings of thirst, excessive urination, weight loss, and dehydration consistent with sepsis.

The presence of polydipsia, polyuria, hyperglycemia, glycosuria, altered level of consciousness, tachycardia, weight loss, and dehydration led me to strongly suspect that the patient had developed hyperosmolar nonketotic syndrome. The additional evidence of headache, lethargy, and decreased blood pressure supported this suspicion. Although hyperosmolar nonketotic syndrome most commonly develops secondary to diabetes mellitus or certain medications, I believed that this condition had developed secondary to the glucose load in the TPN formula. However, it could have been

related to sepsis instead of or in addition to the glucose content of the formula and would have to be ruled out.

Because hyperosmolar nonketotic syndrome is a life-threatening emergency which, if left untreated, can lead to osmotic diuresis, severe dehydration, cardiovascular collapse, central nervous system depression, convulsions, hyperosmolar coma, and death, I took the following actions:

1. I explained to the patient that a complication had developed and provided him simple explanations and emotional support. I asked if there were any significant others to notify.
2. I called the patient's primary physician and reported my assessments.
3. I discontinued the TPN infusion and performed the appropriate catheter care.
4. I called for an ambulance to transport the patient to the hospital.
5. I continued to assess the patient's cardiovascular and mental status for evidence of deterioration.
6. I documented my findings and actions.

The patient was met and examined by the primary physician in the emergency room. A complete blood count, serum electrolytes, serum glucose and ketones, serum bicarbonate level, free fatty acids, blood urea nitrogen, and urine osmolality were ordered and confirmed the presence of hyperosmolar nonketotic syndrome. Blood cultures were also ordered and obtained, and later proved to be negative.

Intravenous insulin therapy was initiated, and intravenous fluid replacement of half-strength normal saline with potassium supplement was initially infused at 250 mL/h. The patient's blood glucose level was closely monitored and, when it reached 300 mg/dL, the insulin was discontinued and 5% dextrose added to the intravenous fluids.

Despite the high mortality rate associated with hyperosmolar nonketotic syndrome, the patient recovered, TPN was reinitiated with the proper adjustment made to glucose content, and the patient was once again discharged to his home with home care nursing supervision and follow-up. Accurate interpretation of the clues, sound clinical judgment based on knowledgeable nursing assessments, and prompt and appropriate nursing interventions prevented further complications and improved the patient's chance of survival.

Think Critically

What psychologic and social considerations associated with not eating would the nurse recog-

CLINICAL ? THINKING

(continued)

nize? What nursing interventions would be implemented?

What long-term physical and psychosocial needs should the nurse anticipate for the patient receiving TPN at home?

What nursing diagnoses and expected outcomes would be included in the nursing care plan for a patient receiving TPN at home?

What are some of the financial considerations when TPN is administered in the home? What information would the nurse need? What resources might the nurse identify as possible sources of funding for meeting home TPN expenses?

How does caring for the patient at home differ from the controlled environment of the hospital? What nursing responsibilities are unique to the nurse practicing in the home care setting? What are the advantages of the delivery of home care? What are the disadvantages?

How would the home care nurse assist the patient receiving TPN in obtaining community resources for emotional support as well as for the maintenance of home equipment and supplies?

With which other members of the health care team would the home care nurse collaborate to best meet the physical and psychosocial needs of the patient receiving TPN at home?

What criteria would the nurse recognize as essential when considering the selection of candidates for home TPN?

A student nurse accompanying the home care nurse on the home visit expresses concern regarding the risk of contracting HIV infection when administering TPN to an AIDS patient. How should the home care nurse respond? Do infection control procedures differ in the home as compared with those in the hospital?

What are some of the mechanical complications associated with TPN? Why didn't the nurse consider these as possibilities?

What potential risks associated with sudden discontinuation of TPN would the nurse recognize? Was this the best nursing action? Should the nurse have questioned the doctor's order?

Was obtaining a fingerstick blood sample to test the patient's serum glucose level the best action? Why didn't the nurse obtain a blood sample directly from the Hickman catheter?

What potential complications of fluid replacement and insulin therapy would the nurse recognize? What nursing assessments would be made?

How would nursing actions have differed if the nurse suspected that the patient in this scenario was septic? Experiencing an electrolyte imbalance? A mechanical complication?

Following this episode, the patient stated, "I'm going to end this misery. I'm going to kill myself before this disease kills me." What would be the nurse's best response? What nursing actions would be taken?

What potential precipitating factors of hyperglycemia would the nurse identify in the patient receiving TPN? Could this episode have been prevented? What additional patient teaching would be included to prevent a recurrence?

Consider the time, effort, and finances involved in successfully managing a home TPN program. Should patients receive TPN if there is no possibility for recovery from the underlying medical condition? Is the length of time a patient is likely to live a factor? Once initiated, is termination of TPN similar to terminating mechanical ventilation? Why? Why not?

---

a narrow lumen, and the Hickman, which has a larger bore size through which blood can be withdrawn or medications administered. Newer catheters, double- and triple-lumen, represent the fusion of the two and have the advantage of allowing one port and line to be maintained for administration of total parenteral nutrition solution only. These long catheters are usually inserted with the patient under general anesthesia. Then continuous or cyclic infusion via volumetric pump begins immediately. Volumetric pumps must be used to maintain flow because of the long length and small diameter of these catheters. The pump used must be a low-pressure one to guard against rupture of the catheter and resultant embolism and contamination.

GASTROINTESTINAL SURGERY

Abdominal Incisions

Laparotomy is the surgical opening of the abdomen. Of the many types of incisions that can be used to open the abdomen, the specific one used depends on the organ or area to undergo surgery, the type of procedure, ease of entry, ease of making the incision larger if the need arises, ease of closure, and postoperative wound strength. Table 21–5 describes and illustrates common abdominal incisions.

Patients with abdominal incisions usually experience short-term, acute pain at the incision site, especially when attempting to cough, breathe deeply, or

Table 21-5

Common Abdominal Incisions

Incision	Diagram	Primary Uses	Comments
Upper midline		Gastrectomy	Simple, fast, good exposure of upper abdomen Wound weak High incidence of dehiscence
Lower midline		Genitourologic procedures	Simple, fast, good exposure of sigmoid colon and other pelvic organs High incidence of dehiscence
Upper paramedian (upper rectus)	Right	Biliary surgery	Fast entry, slow but strong closure Little bleeding No nerve injury
	Left	Gastrectomy Vagectomy Repair of hiatus hernia	
Lower paramedian (lower rectus)	Right	Appendectomy Small bowel resection	Fast entry, slow but strong closure Little bleeding No nerve injury
	Left	Sigmoid colon surgery	

Table 21–5

Common Abdominal Incisions (continued)

Incision	Diagram	Primary Uses	Comments
Subcostal	Right	Biliary surgery	Oblique incision Very strong wound but very painful postoperatively
	Left	Operations on spleen and pancreas	
Gridiron (McBurney)		Appendectomy	
Upper transverse		Transverse colostomy or colon resection Pancreatic procedures	
Pfannenstiel		Gynecologic procedures	

ambulate. The goal of pain management is to maintain a tolerable level of discomfort at all times. The Agency for Health Care Policy and Research recommends that, during the first 36 to 48 hours postoperatively, analgesics be administered on a regular time schedule rather than as requested by the patient. Patient controlled analgesia, in which the patient self-administers small doses of intravenous opioids via a regulated pump, may be an appropriate choice for some patients during this period.

Complications

Patients undergoing surgery of the GI tract are at risk for a number of complications. These include infection, wound dehiscence, paralytic ileus, atelectasis, and urinary retention.

INFECTION. For an unknown reason, the abdominal wall is particularly susceptible to infection. In addition, the GI tract is not sterile, so when the lumen is opened, organisms can spill into the abdomen. Infection is a greater risk with intestinal surgery than with gastric surgery because fewer microorganisms are found in the acid environment of the stomach.

WOUND DEHISCENCE. Abdominal suture lines are subjected to stress from breathing, coughing, and straining during movement or defecation. This stress predisposes to dehiscence. To help prevent dehiscence, as well as to protect against impaired blood clotting and impaired liver tolerance to anesthesia, the patient's fluid, electrolyte, and nutritional status is carefully assessed preoperatively, and measures are instituted to correct any imbalances or deficiencies. Adequate protein and vitamin C are particularly important to support wound healing. A nasogastric tube is used postoperatively to prevent distention, which also creates stress on the suture line and can contribute to dehiscence.

ILEUS. Handling of the GI tract, along with the effects of preoperative medications and anesthesia, results in some degree of paralytic ileus in almost all patients. Paralytic ileus is the impaired movement of intestinal contents through the intestine because of reduced or absent peristalsis. For this reason, all patients are placed on NPO status until peristalsis returns, as indicated by the presence of normal bowel sounds and the passage of flatus.

ATELECTASIS. Because breathing is difficult and painful, particularly with an upper abdominal incision, the patient may tend toward shallow respirations and chest splinting. Secretions may pool in the lungs, bronchi can be clogged with mucus, and atelectasis and pneumonia can result.

URINARY RETENTION. The pain of an abdominal incision, along with the effects of medications and anesthesia, can result in the inability to empty the urinary bladder.

Gastrectomy

Gastrectomy is the surgical excision of the stomach. In total gastrectomy, the entire stomach is removed and the esophagus is sutured to either the duodenum or the jejunum (Fig. 21–17). In subtotal gastrectomy, part of the stomach is removed.

Uses

Total or subtotal gastrectomy is performed to remove a benign or malignant tumor of the stomach or to remove a chronic peptic ulcer. It may also be performed to stop hemorrhage from a perforating ulcer.

Procedure

Two procedures involving subtotal gastrectomy are the Billroth I and the Billroth II (see Fig. 21–17). In the Billroth I procedure, the pyloric portion of the stomach is removed and the remaining stomach is anastomosed to the duodenum (gastroduodenostomy). In a Billroth II procedure, the pylorus is removed, the proximal end of the duodenum is sutured closed, and the remaining portion of the stomach is anastomosed to the jejunum (gastrojejunostomy). The Billroth II is preferable in treating

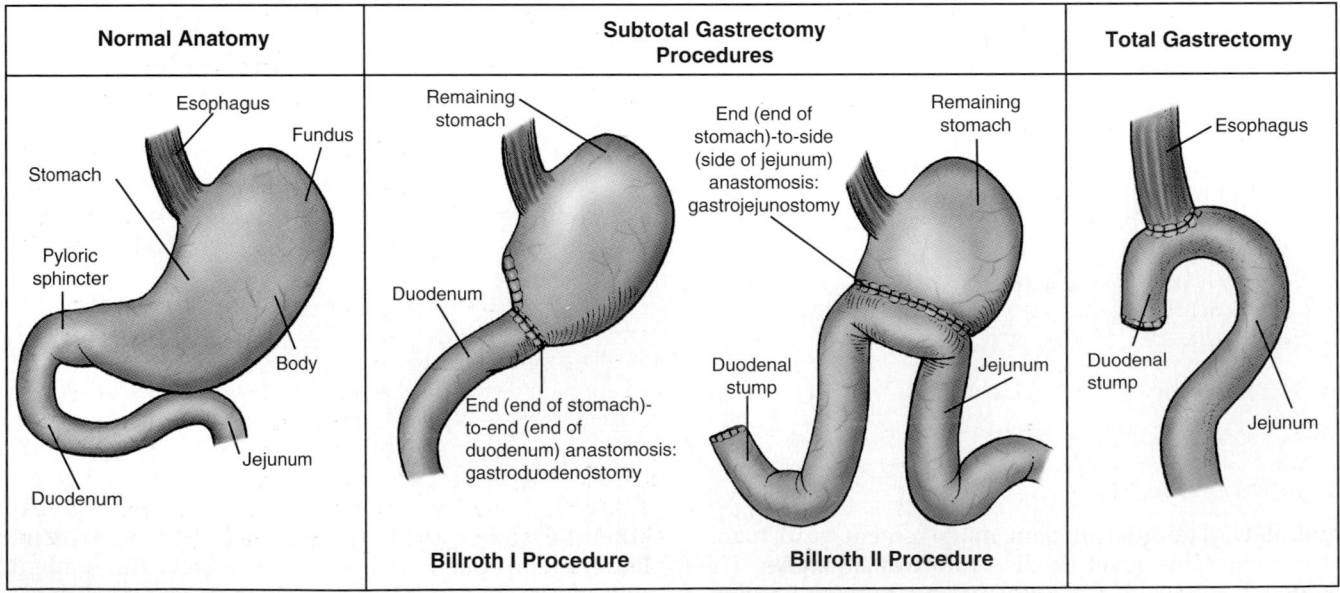

Figure 21–17

Normal anatomy, total gastrectomy, and subtotal gastrectomy procedures (Billroth I and Billroth II).

duodenal ulcers because it reduces the chance of reulceration.

Patient Preparation

Fluid and electrolytes are given as needed to make up for deficiencies caused by the underlying disease and losses from preoperative tests. In some cases, total parenteral nutrition is used for protein replacement and vitamins K and C are administered to promote clotting and wound healing. The patient is usually on a fluid diet for 24 hours and then placed on NPO status after midnight before surgery. The abdomen is prepared from nipple line to symphysis pubis.

Postoperative Course

On the evening of surgery, the patient is gotten out of bed and is progressively ambulated. The patient remains on NPO status and is maintained on intravenous fluids until bowel sounds return and the nasogastric tube, which is inserted to remove secretions and prevent distention and vomiting, is removed. Oral intake is then begun, usually with sips of warm tea because cold liquids tend to cause distress. Intake is gradually increased until the patient is eating six small, bland meals daily and drinking 120 mL of fluid in between.

Table 21–6 presents potential complications of gastrectomy, as well as their causes, symptoms, and treatment.

NURSING PROCESS
Gastrectomy

PREOPERATIVE NURSING CARE

Assessment

Question the patient about symptoms related to the underlying disease process (eg, nausea, vomiting, heartburn, anorexia, bleeding). Determine whether they affect immediate care needs. Assess nutritional status. Review the patient's usual dietary patterns, and ask about any weight loss. Examine for signs of dehydration. Review laboratory data such as serum electrolyte and serum albumin levels, which indicate nutritional status.

Explore the patient's understanding of the disease and the planned surgery. Be alert to signs of excessive anxiety or ineffective coping.

Nursing Diagnoses and Planning

Nursing diagnoses and related expected patient outcomes commonly applicable to patients scheduled for gastrectomy include the following:

NDx: Anxiety related to anesthesia and surgery

Planning: Patient Outcomes
1. Patient practices relaxation as instructed.
2. Patient reports feeling more relaxed.

3. Patient expresses an optimistic view about the surgical outcome.
4. Patient rests quietly.

NDx: Knowledge deficit: preoperative preparation, postoperative course

Planning: Patient Outcomes
1. Patient describes preoperative preparation.
2. Patient describes usual postoperative procedures and course.
3. Patient describes importance of coughing, deep-breathing, and leg exercises in the prevention of complications.
4. Patient demonstrates coughing and deep-breathing.
5. Patient demonstrates postoperative leg exercises.

Nursing Interventions and Evaluation

NDx: Anxiety

Reassure the patient that some anxiety before surgery is normal and in fact helps prepare the body for stress and promotes recovery. Offer reassurance about the success of surgery, as appropriate. Depending on the individual situation, you might reassure the patient about his or her general state of health and fitness for surgery, mention the frequency of the procedure and its success rate, or describe the professionals who participate in surgery, noting their roles in protecting the patient and their competency. Keep in mind that many times the patient's concerns stem from misconceptions about normal anatomy and physiology, so the patient may be unable or too embarrassed to ask questions.

Review relaxation techniques with the patient, or provide the patient with a relaxation tape and orient the patient to its use. Maintain a quiet, calm environment and administer sedatives as ordered.

NDx: Knowledge deficit: preoperative preparation, postoperative course

Review preoperative events with the patient. Explain that many tests, including a physical examination, x-ray examinations, and blood tests, will be performed to determine general state of health and identify any problems that need special consideration. Reassure the patient that the specific nature and purpose of each test will be explained before it is performed.

Describe the preoperative preparation. Explain that the GI tract must be empty during the operation, so only liquids will be allowed for 24 hours before surgery and a bowel preparation will be taken the day before surgery to clean out the large bowel. Explain that the abdomen will be shaved and scrubbed from nipple line to symphysis pubis to remove as many bacteria as possible. Emphasize that the incision will be much smaller than the area prepared.

If the patient will receive intravenous fluids or hyperalimentation therapy to make up nutritional deficiencies before surgery, describe these to the pa-

Table 21–6

Complications of Gastrectomy

Complication	Cause	Symptoms	Treatment
Hemorrhage *Early*	Splenic injury Slipped ligature	Persistent bloody drainage from nasogastric tube	Saline gastric lavage Blood replacement Reoperation Cool saline lavage
7th to 10th day	Sloughing at anastomosis	Recurrence of bloody gastric drainage	
Acute gastric dilation	Swallowed air distends stomach, stimulating gastric secretions, which can lead to dehydration and a fall in plasma volume	Epigastric pain, feeling of fullness, hiccoughs, gagging, tachycardia, and hypertension	Nasogastric suction Fluid replacement to restore plasma volume
Alkaline reflux gastritis	Reflux of intestinal contents including bile salts injures gastric mucosal barrier	Persistent pain and epigastric "burning" that is worse after meals; nausea and vomiting	Semi-Fowler's position Antacid or histamine blocker therapy
Dumping syndrome	Rapid entry of large amounts of hypertonic chyme into the small intestine causes fluid to move into bowel lumen, decreasing plasma volume and causing vasomotor symptoms; resultant distention of intestine causes gastrointestinal symptoms	Tachycardia, palpitations, fainting, hypertension, flushing, diaphoresis, bloating, cramping, diarrhea, and nausea occurring with eating 1–3 wk postoperatively Disappears in 1 hour Usually resolves in 3–6 mo postoperatively	Avoid drinking fluid with meals Eat six small meals per day of dry foods Avoid concentrated carbohydrates Lie down for 30–60 min after eating Avoid very hot and very cold foods Anticholinergic drugs taken 30 min before eating
Postprandial hypoglycemia	Increased insulin release following carbohydrate ingestion	Weakness, faintness, perspiration, hunger, nausea, anxiety, tremors, and palpitations occurring 2–3 h after eating	Ingestion of sugar or hard candy relieves symptoms More frequent meals low in sugar prevent attacks
Impaired absorption of iron	Deficiency of gastric acid, which is needed to increase solubility of iron for absorption to occur	Anemia	Iron taken orally, with recumbent position after ingestion to promote absorption
Impaired vitamin B_{12} absorption	Lack of intrinsic factor caused by atrophy of gastric mucosa	Pernicious anemia	Parenteral administration of vitamin B_{12}
Impaired calcium absorption	Deficiency of gastric acid, which is needed to increase solubility of calcium for absorption to occur	Osteoporosis	
General nutritional deficiency	Reduced capacity of stomach causes a feeling of satiation after ingesting small amounts of food Malabsorption from decreased gastric acid or pancreatic enzymes	Failure to gain or maintain weight	Small meals six times daily

tient. Also explain if a nasogastric tube is to be inserted before surgery to empty the stomach, as in cases of pyloric obstruction.

Prepare the patient for postoperative events. Inform the patient that there will be a tube going from the stomach out through the nose to drain stomach secretions into a bottle on the wall and that the drainage may be red initially. Explain that because the purpose of the tube is to keep the stomach empty to promote healing of the suture line, no foods or fluids will be given by mouth for the several days that the tube is in place. Assure the patient that the tube does not cause pain, although the nostrils may feel a bit sore and the mouth dry, symptoms that will be eased by salves and mouth rinses.

Intravenous fluids will be given until peristalsis returns, the nasogastric tube is removed, and oral intake is re-established. Oral intake will begin with clear fluids once bowel function has returned, as indicated by the presence of bowel sounds and passage of flatus. Full fluids and then bland foods will be added as tolerated. Eating patterns will be altered. A return to former eating habits will be slow and perhaps impossible.

Compare the patient's status with the expected outcomes. If the outcomes are not met, reassess the patient and revise the plan.

POSTOPERATIVE NURSING CARE

Assessment

Monitor and record vital signs every 4 hours or more frequently if necessitated by the patient's condition. Assess for pain. Check the dressing for drainage, and inspect the suture line for signs of infection and dehiscence.

Check the patency of the nasogastric tube, and observe and record the amount and character of drainage from it. Normally, drainage is bloody for 24 hours postoperatively and then changes to brown-tinged and then to yellow or clear. Remember that, if total gastrectomy has been performed, gastric drainage is less than that with subtotal gastrectomy because the stomach is no longer present to produce secretions or to hold them and that the amount of secretions decreases as peristalsis returns.

Note the odor of the gastric aspirate, because a fecal smell can indicate regurgitation of the contents of the large intestine into the operative area.

Auscultate for bowel sounds and question the patient about passage of flatus to determine when peristalsis has resumed and oral intake may be begun. Measure abdominal girth to detect development of distention. Once bowel function has returned and oral intake is resumed, assess tolerance of food and fluids. Note nausea, vomiting, diarrhea, and other signs of dumping syndrome (see Table 21–6). Record all intake and output and assess overall nutritional status, because the reduced size and functional capacity of the stomach can cause decreased appetite and difficulty gaining weight.

Nursing Diagnoses and Planning

Nursing diagnoses and related expected patient outcomes commonly applicable to patients who have undergone gastrectomy include the following:

NDx: Pain related to trauma from surgery and irritation of the nostril by the nasogastric tube

Planning: Patient Outcomes
1. Patient moves without loud moans, complaints

of severe pain, or signs of severe pain, such as pallor and tachycardia.
2. Patient states that abdominal pain is relieved.
3. Patient appears relaxed (eg, lips are not pressed together, face does not appear drawn).
4. Patient denies nostril discomfort.

NDx: Risk for ineffective airway clearance related to shallow breathing secondary to diaphragmatic splinting accompanying upper abdominal surgery

Planning: Patient Outcomes
1. Patient moves, coughs, and breathes deeply as directed.
2. Lung sounds are clear on auscultation.

NDx: Risk for injury (internal suture line) related to gastric distention, vomiting, or movement of the nasogastric tube

Planning: Patient Outcomes
1. Patient is afebrile.
2. Abdomen is soft.
3. Patient states that pain is decreasing.

NDx: Risk for altered oral mucous membrane related to mouth breathing and NPO status

Planning: Patient Outcomes
1. Oral mucous membrane is pink and moist.
2. Lips are free of cracks.
3. Patient reports that mouth and lips feel soft and supple.

NDx: Risk for infection related to contamination of the abdominal wound

Planning: Patient Outcomes
1. Wound is odorless and free of purulent drainage.
2. Wound edges are approximated.

NDx: Altered nutrition: less than body requirements related to postoperative dietary restrictions, early satiety, or dumping syndrome

Planning: Patient Outcomes
1. Patient ingests a nutritionally balanced diet.
2. Patient achieves and maintains recommended weight.

NDx: Risk for altered health maintenance related to insufficient knowledge of need for follow-up care

Planning: Patient Outcomes
1. Patient lists symptoms to be reported to the physician.
2. Patient states when to return for follow-up.

Nursing Interventions and Evaluation

NDx: Pain
Administer pain medication as ordered. Keep the head of the bed elevated to decrease pull on the incision. Splint the incision with a pillow when the patient is turning, coughing, or deep-breathing. Apply a binder as ordered to support the incision when the patient is moving.

Encourage the patient to relax. Play soft music, and prompt the patient to concentrate on slow, even breathing or contemplate a calm, pleasant scene permeated by a relaxing color.

Clean the nostril through which the nasogastric tube passes with applicators dipped in water. Apply water-soluble lubricant.

NDx: Risk for ineffective airway clearance
Have the patient turn, cough, and deep-breathe every 2 hours while on bedrest. Splint the incision to decrease pain when the patient is turning, coughing, and deep-breathing. Ambulate the patient as ordered.

NDx: Risk for injury (internal suture line)
Keep the nasogastric tube connected to suction, as ordered, to drain secretions and prevent gastric distention and vomiting. Irrigate the tube gently with normal saline as ordered to keep it patent. Reinforce or replace the tape anchoring the tube as needed. Be careful not to move the tube when adding or changing tape. Notify the physician if abdominal girth increases.

NDx: Risk for altered oral mucous membrane
Assist the patient in brushing and flossing the teeth after eating. Assist the patient in rinsing the mouth frequently. Offer throat lozenges or gum if allowed. Apply water-soluble lubricant to lips to prevent drying and cracking.

NDx: Risk for infection
Caution the patient against touching the abdominal dressing or the surrounding area. Use strict aseptic technique when caring for the wound. Reinforce the dressing as needed unless it is wet with predominantly bloody drainage. In this case, it should be changed.

NDx: Altered nutrition: less than body requirements
Administer intravenous fluids and electrolytes as ordered (usually for about 4 days). When bowel motility has returned, give clear fluids, preferably beginning with sips of warm tea, because cold liquids tend to cause distress. Gradually introduce full fluids and progress to a bland diet as tolerated. Give iron and vitamin supplements as ordered. Give six small feedings per day. Give liquids before or after but not with feedings to combat early satiety.

To combat dumping syndrome, instruct the patient to:

- Avoid high-carbohydrate foods, including fluids such as fruit nectars
- Assume low-Fowler's position during meals
- Lie down for 30 minutes after eating to delay gastric emptying
- Avoid drinking fluids with meals
- Take antispasmodics as ordered to aid in delay of gastric emptying

NDx: Risk for altered health maintenance
Instruct the patient to report continuous epigastric distress that increases after eating because it may indicate alkaline reflux gastritis. Also stress the need to report persistent fatigue because it may be related to iron or vitamin B_{12} deficiency.

Compare the patient's status with the expected outcomes. If the outcomes are not met, reassess the patient and revise the plan.

Intestinal Resection

An intestinal resection is a procedure in which a part of the small intestine or large intestine is excised.

Uses
Intestinal resection is used in treating such problems as intestinal malignancy, obstruction, inflammatory bowel disease, perforated diverticulum, and ischemic or traumatic injury.

Patient Preparation
To ensure that the bowel is clean and empty of stool, the bowel is prepared extensively. The patient is placed first on a low-residue diet and then, for 24 hours before the operation, on a liquid diet so that stool does not accumulate in the bowel. To empty the bowel of any stool already present, an oral preparation—such as GoLYTELY or Colyte—and a series of enemas are taken. To decrease bacteria in the bowel and help prevent postoperative infection, oral anti-infectives are taken. The anti-infective must be nonabsorbable, so it passes through the entire intestinal tract, where its action is needed. Anti-infectives that can be used for this purpose include neomycin, erythromycin, kanamycin sulfate (Kantrex), and succinylsulfathiazole (Sulfasuxidine).

Fluids and electrolytes are ordinarily given preoperatively to make up losses from dietary restrictions, preparation for preoperative diagnostic tests, and the operation itself, as well as for deficiencies that may have resulted from the disease process and its symptoms. Often, it is necessary to give vitamins C and K parenterally to ensure amounts adequate for blood clotting and wound healing. For some patients, total parenteral nutrition may be needed for protein replacement.

On the day of surgery or during surgery, a nasogastric tube is inserted. This removes gastric secretions and prevents vomiting until GI function returns. If an intestinal (long) tube is used in place of a nasogastric tube, it may be inserted 24 to 48 hours before the operation, to allow time for it to pass into the intestine. In addition to removing secretions from the operative area, an intestinal tube also causes the intestine to "gather up on it," resulting in more operative space.

An indwelling catheter is also inserted because urinary retention is common after intestinal surgery, particularly on the distal colon or rectum. The catheter keeps the bladder empty during surgery, thereby giving more space in the surgical field and decreasing the chance of accidental injury to it.

■■■■■■▶
■
■ **Clinical Pathway for Colon Resection**

Patient Name _____   Date _____

DRG# _____   Expected LOS _____

	Day 2 (PO#1)	Day 3 (PO#2)	Day 4 (PO#3)	Day 5 (PO#4)	Day 6 (PO#5)
Medication	Parenteral analgesia as ordered	Parenteral analgesia as ordered	Parenteral analgesia as ordered	Begin PO pain medication	PO pain medication
	Heparin 5000 units SQ q 12 hrs	Heparin 5000 units SQ q 12 hrs	Heparin 5000 units SQ q 12 hrs	Heparin 5000 units SQ q 12 hrs	Heparin 5000 units SQ q 12 hrs
	IV ATB as ordered	Complete IV ATB			
Diagnostic Tests	CBC, Chem 6 in PM	CBC, Chem 6			
Diet	NPO, IVF as ordered	NPO, IVF, may have ice chips	IVF, clear liquids (if NG tube D/C)	D/C IVF, advance to soft diet	Advance to general diet
Activity	Dangle at bedside in PM	Up in chair, ambulate with assistance	Ambulate TID	Ambulate ad lib	Ambulate ad lib
Treatments/ Nursing Actions	Assess VS q 2–4 hrs	VS q 4 hrs	VS q 4 hrs	VS q shift	VS q shift
	Assess pain status q 2–4 hrs	Assess pain status q 2–4 hrs	Assess pain status q 2–4 hrs	Assess pain status q 2–4 hrs	Assess pain status q 4 h while awake
	Incentive spirometer q 1–2 hrs while awake	Incentive spirometer q 1–2 hrs while awake	Incentive spirometer q 1–2 hrs while awake	Incentive spirometer q 1–2 hrs while awake	Incentive spirometer q 1–2 hrs while awake
	Cough and deep-breathe 1–2 hrs while awake	Cough and deep-breathe 1–2 hrs while awake	Cough and deep-breathe 1–2 hrs while awake	Antiembolism hose, leg exercises when in bed	Antiembolism hose
	Antiembolism hose, leg exercises	Antiembolism hose, leg exercises when in bed	Antiembolism hose, leg exercises when in bed	Assess wound daily	Assess wound daily
	Monitor voiding in 6–8 hrs	Assess wound (dressing changed by MD)	Assess wound open to air	D/C I & O	Assess for bowel movement
	Assess dressing	Assess bowel activity	Assess bowel activity		
	Assess NG tube functioning	Assess NG tube functioning	Remove NG tube if ordered		
Teaching/ Discharge Planning	Reinforce incentive spirometer, cough, deep-breathe	Reinforce incentive spirometer, cough, deep-breathe	Reinforce incentive spirometer, cough, deep-breathe	Reinforce incision care, diet, medications, activity upon discharge.	Reinforce incision care, diet, medications, activity for discharge in AM.
					Follow-up visit to physician

Procedure

The preferred type of resection is one in which the diseased part of the bowel is removed and the two remaining ends are anastomosed (surgically joined together). This restores the continuity of the bowel and preserves normal defecation. In a second type of resection, the diseased part of the bowel is removed and the functioning end of the remaining intestine is brought out onto the surface of the abdomen, forming an ostomy. Subsequently, it is through this artificial opening that fecal matter exits from the GI tract. The opening is called an ileostomy when the ileum is brought to the abdominal surface and a colostomy when the colon is brought to the abdominal surface.

Postoperative Course

The nasogastric or nasointestinal tube remains in place attached to low intermittent suction until bowel sounds return and the suture lines have begun to heal. During this time, usually about 5 days, the patient is maintained on intravenous fluid and electrolytes and in some cases on total parenteral nutrition. After the tube is removed, oral intake is resumed, beginning with clear fluids and progressing to full fluids and a regular diet as tolerated.

Ambulation is begun 8 to 24 hours postoperatively because thrombophlebitis and pulmonary embolism are potential complications, particularly between postoperative days 7 and 10.

Various difficulties can accompany the resumption of oral intake, depending on the location and extent of the resection. For example, resection of the jejunum results in malabsorption of fluids, electrolytes, fat, and the fat-soluble vitamins (A, D, E, K). Resection of the ileum results in malabsorption of fat and vitamin B_{12}. Resection involving the ileocecal valve often results in diarrhea.

Postoperative weight loss follows almost all bowel resections. Weight and strength are slowly regained over a period of months.

NURSING PROCESS
Anastomosed Intestinal Resection

PREOPERATIVE NURSING CARE

The assessment, nursing diagnoses, expected patient outcomes, nursing interventions, and evaluation for patients scheduled for an anastomosed intestinal resection are similar to those described previously for patients scheduled for gastrectomy, with the following consideration. Review the patient's normal bowel habits to provide a baseline for postoperative assessment of bowel function.

POSTOPERATIVE NURSING CARE

Assessment

Postoperatively, assess physiologic stabilization by monitoring vital signs and observing the wound for bleeding. Assess the patient for pain and note its location, type, and intensity. Check the nasogastric or intestinal tube every 4 hours for patency. Note the amount of drainage, which should decrease during the first 24 to 48 hours. Also note the color and consistency of the drainage and observe it for the presence of blood. Question the patient about nausea and check for abdominal distention, both of which indicate a malfunction in the GI suction that, if not corrected, can injure the suture line.

Assess fluid and electrolyte status. Measure fluid intake and output. Observe for signs and symptoms of dehydration or overhydration. Review serum electrolyte values.

Carefully assess respiratory status because hypoxia secondary to ineffective ventilation is a potential complication of an intestinal resection. Observe for normal chest excursion, note color, and auscultate the lungs every 4 hours for the first 72 hours postoperatively. Also assess for signs of thrombophlebitis. Observe for redness and swelling and check for heat and pain in the calf. Check for a positive Homans' sign. Be alert to signs of urinary tract infection. Note the color and clarity of urine. Question the patient regarding pain.

Check temperature throughout the postoperative period. Keep in mind that elevation in the evening with a return to normal by morning is a characteristic of infection. When this occurs early in the postoperative period, aspiration pneumonia or urinary tract infection is likely. Fever that occurs 4 to 7 days after surgery suggests a leak at the anastomosis or a wound abscess. As the postoperative period progresses, assess the patient for return of bowel function. Listen for bowel sounds every 4 hours and question the patient about the passage of flatus and then the passage of feces.

Obtain daily weights. When oral intake is resumed, monitor food intake and assess the patient's tolerance of it. Check for singultus, nausea, vomiting, abdominal distention, diarrhea, or other GI distress.

Nursing Diagnoses and Planning

Nursing diagnoses and related expected patient outcomes commonly applicable to patients who have undergone intestinal resection with anastomosis include the following:

NDx: Pain related to surgical trauma to the abdomen

Planning: Patient Outcomes
1. Patient moves without signs of severe pain, such as moaning, pallor, and tachycardia.
2. Patient rests quietly without signs of discomfort, such as clenched hands, groaning, and crying.
3. Patient reports pain relief.

NDx: Risk for ineffective breathing pattern related to shallow breathing secondary to incisional pain on deep breathing

Planning: Patient Outcomes
1. Patient coughs and breathes deeply as directed.
2. Cyanosis is absent.
3. Arterial blood gas levels are within normal range.

NDx: Risk for altered oral mucous membrane related to NPO status and presence of a nasogastric or nasointestinal tube

Planning: Patient Outcomes
1. Oral mucous membrane is moist and free of cracks.
2. Lips are supple, moist, and free of cracks.
3. Patient denies dryness of the mouth.

NDx: Risk for altered nutrition: less than body requirements related to inadequate intake or malabsorption

Planning: Patient Outcomes
1. Patient maintains expected weight.
2. Patient resumes oral intake of a nutritionally balanced diet.
3. Patient takes nutritional supplements as directed.

NDx: Risk for infection related to surgical incision of the skin and opening of the peritoneal cavity and bowel

Planning: Patient Outcomes
1. Wound is approximated and free of erythema and drainage.
2. Abdomen is soft and nondistended.
3. Patient is afebrile.

NDx: Risk for altered peripheral tissue perfusion related to thrombophlebitis secondary to venous stasis

Planning: Patient Outcomes
1. Patient does foot and leg exercises as directed.
2. Calves and upper thighs are free of redness, swelling, heat, and pain.
3. Homans' sign is negative.

NDx: Risk for altered health maintenance related to insufficient knowledge of discharge instructions

Planning: Patient Outcomes
1. Patient explains instructions for self-care at home.
2. Patient lists symptoms to be reported to the physician.
3. Patient states time of follow-up appointment.

Nursing Interventions and Evaluation

NDx: Pain
Give prescribed analgesics as often as needed. Assist the patient into semi-Fowler's position to relieve stress on the suture line. To relieve gas pains associated with the return of peristalsis, encourage ambulation and use a rectal tube to remove flatus as needed.

NDx: Risk for ineffective breathing pattern
Teach the patient to splint the abdomen with pillows. Assist the patient in turning, coughing, and deep-breathing every 2 hours for 72 hours after surgery. Instruct in the use of an incentive spirometer. Reassure the patient that coughing and deep-breathing, despite the fact that they may hurt, do not damage the incision. When the patient is able, ambulate him or her at least three times daily.

NDx: Risk for altered oral mucous membrane
Assist the patient in brushing the teeth at least three times daily. Encourage frequent mouth rinses, but avoid the use of solutions that dry the mucous membranes. Apply a water-soluble lubricant to the lips to keep them supple and prevent cracking.

NDx: Risk for altered nutrition: less than body requirements
Administer total parenteral nutrition if ordered. When oral intake is resumed, give small amounts of clear fluids of the patient's choice. If these are tolerated without singultus, nausea, vomiting, or other discomfort, gradually progress to full fluids and then to a regular diet. Give nutritional supplements as ordered, and alert the physician to any weight loss promptly.

NDx: Risk for infection
Monitor for signs of peritoneal irritation caused by leaking of the suture line. Use strict aseptic technique when performing wound care. Reinforce or change the dressing when wet to prevent transfer of microorganisms from the environment by capillary action.

NDx: Risk for altered peripheral tissue perfusion
Guide the patient in foot and leg exercises, 10 times each, every 2 hours while on bedrest. Apply antiembolic stockings or Ace bandages to further support venous return. Avoid gatching the bed to elevate the knees, using pillows under the knees, or exerting any other form of pressure in the popliteal space. Assist the patient out of bed, and begin ambulation as ordered 24 to 48 hours after surgery. Instruct the patient to avoid crossing the legs or sitting for long periods.

NDx: Risk for altered health maintenance
Review the physician's instructions on caring for the incision, diet, and limitations on activities after discharge. Be certain that the patient understands that although stool softeners may be used to prevent constipation and straining, laxatives must be avoided because of their irritating effects on the bowel. Instruct the patient to report bleeding, abdominal distention, abdominal rigidity, or fever, and to return for a follow-up appointment at the designated time.

Compare the patient's status with the expected outcomes. If the outcomes are not met, reassess the patient and revise the plan.

Colostomy

A colostomy is a surgically created opening between the colon and the abdominal wall through which fecal matter is expelled. Depending on its location in the colon, it is called an ascending, transverse, descending, or sigmoid colostomy. The fecal output from an ascending colostomy is predominantly liquid because it passes through only a small portion of water-absorbing large bowel before exit. From a transverse colostomy, fecal output is mushy. From a descending colostomy, it is semiformed. From a sigmoid colostomy, it is almost identical to that which would be evacuated from the rectum.

Uses
Temporary colostomies are performed to divert fecal matter from diseased or injured intestine in order to rest the affected area of the bowel and allow healing. Conditions that can require a temporary colostomy include diverticulitis, ischemia of the bowel, volvulus, perforation of the bowel, and gunshot or stab wounds.

Permanent colostomies are performed when the distal bowel must be removed or is obstructed and inoperable. Colorectal cancer is the most common indication for permanent colostomy.

Patient Preparation

The physical preparation of a patient for colostomy is the same as for an anastomosed intestinal resection but with one addition. With colostomy, the stoma site may be identified and marked on the abdomen preoperatively by either an enterostomal therapist or the surgeon. When this is performed, the abdomen is inspected with the patient lying supine, sitting up, and standing so that all folds, creases, scars, and bony prominences are avoided.

Procedure

Colostomy involves surgical construction of an end colostomy, a double-barrel colostomy, or a loop colostomy. An end colostomy (Fig. 21–18) is one in which there is a single stoma on the abdomen created from the end of the proximal bowel (that section of bowel that remains connected to the upper GI system and through which intestinal contents will pass). This end is brought out through an opening in the abdominal wall, folded on itself in a cuff, and sutured to the skin. Thus, the surface of the stoma is actually the mucosal lining of the bowel. The distal portion of the bowel (that section of bowel connected only to the rectum) may be removed or left in place within the abdominal cavity. An end colostomy is usually a permanent procedure that may be necessitated by a malignancy in the large bowel, abdominal trauma, or another pathologic condition in which the distal colon is nonfunctional.

A double-barrel colostomy (see Fig. 21–18) is one in which two separate stomas are created on the abdominal wall. The proximal stoma is the end of the functioning colon that is continuous with the upper GI tract. The distal stoma, also called a mucous fistula, opens into the nonfunctioning section of colon that is continuous with the rectum. Most often, this is a temporary colostomy that is performed to rest an area of bowel and will be closed at a future time.

As the name suggests, a loop colostomy is performed by bringing a loop of bowel through an incision in the abdominal wall. A glass rod or rubber tube is slipped under the loop to hold it in place outside the abdomen until sufficient healing has occurred to maintain it in this position. An incision is made in its anterior wall, which results in an opening leading to the proximal bowel and an opening leading to the distal bowel within the single stoma (see Fig. 21–18). This opening of the bowel may be performed in the operating room but is often performed several days later in the patient's room. This delay decreases the chance of infection by allowing the wound to seal off before the contaminated bowel is opened. Bleeding is minimal with this procedure because electrocautery is used. It is also pain-free because the bowel wall has no sensory innervation. There is, however, an odor of burning tissue, and good ventilation should be provided during and after the procedure. Within 7 to 10 days, adhesions form that prevent retraction of the stoma into the abdomen, allowing the supporting glass rod or rubber tube to be removed. Loop colostomy is often performed as a temporary emergency procedure to divert the fecal stream from an area of bowel that is obstructed or perforated.

Postoperative Course

For 24 to 48 hours after surgery, there is mucous and serosanguineous drainage from the stoma. As peristalsis returns, large amounts of malodorous flatus are passed, followed by fecal drainage, usually within 72 hours. Initially the feces are liquid, but their consistency changes when the patient starts to

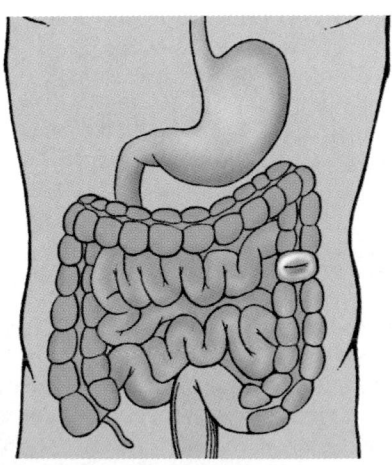
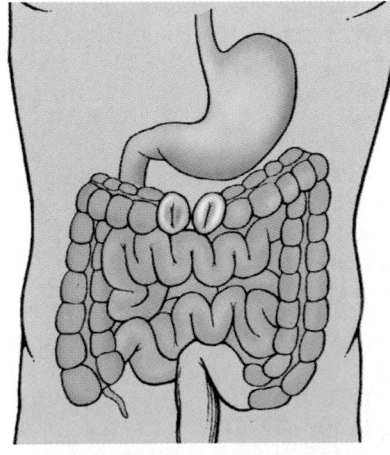
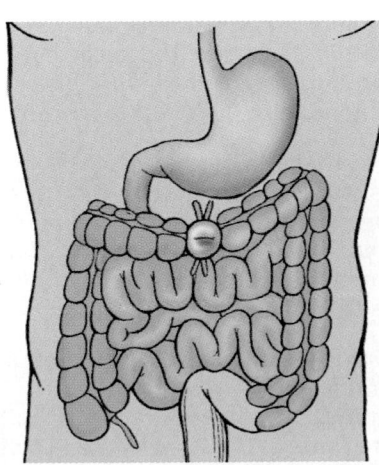

End colostomy   Double-barrel colostomy   Loop colostomy

Figure 21–18

Types of colostomy.

ingest solid foods. Fecal output from a sigmoid colostomy generally resumes the form and consistency of normal stool within a few weeks. Feces from a transverse colostomy eventually have the consistency of toothpaste but continue to drain several times per day.

The nasogastric or nasointestinal tube is removed. The patient is started on clear fluids when bowel function has completely returned. Intravenous fluids are discontinued when oral intake is tolerated well. The diet is gradually progressed to a full low-residue diet. After 4 to 6 weeks, a high-carbohydrate, high-protein general diet is taken as tolerated. The patient is ambulated in 8 to 24 hours and discharged in 5 to 10 days.

Complications

Potential complications of colostomy include infection, hemorrhage, obstruction, and stomal problems, such as necrosis, retraction, stenosis, prolapse, and mucocutaneous separation.

Stomal necrosis can result from impaired circulation. It begins as a dusky, dark discoloration of the stoma, usually appearing 24 to 72 hours postoperatively. If the necrosis extends below the level of the fascia, the stoma is surgically revised to prevent perforation and peritonitis. Otherwise the affected area of the stoma is débrided and subsequently evaluated.

Stomal retraction is a condition in which the stoma does not protrude from the abdomen (Fig. 21–19). This can develop at any time from poor surgical technique or significant weight gain. Stomal retraction complicates pouching and maintenance of the peristomal skin. In some cases, surgical revision may be required.

Stenosis of the stoma is a narrowing of the opening at either the level of the skin or the fascia. Typically, the patient complains of constipation and a sense of pressure when stool is passed and, although the stoma may appear normal, a tight band is felt on digital examination. Treatment of stomal stenosis varies with its severity and the patient's condition. Temporary relief measures include stool

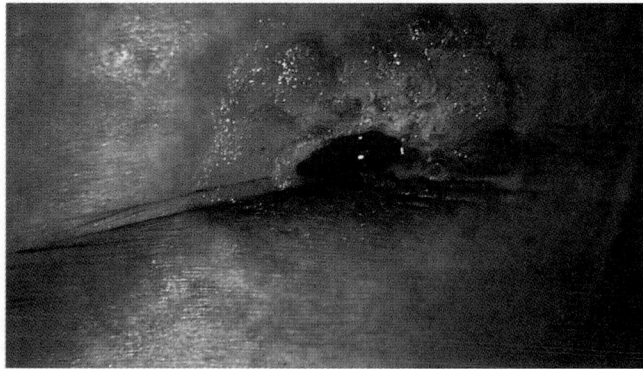

Figure 21–19

Stomal retraction. (Courtesy of Convatec, Princeton, NJ.)

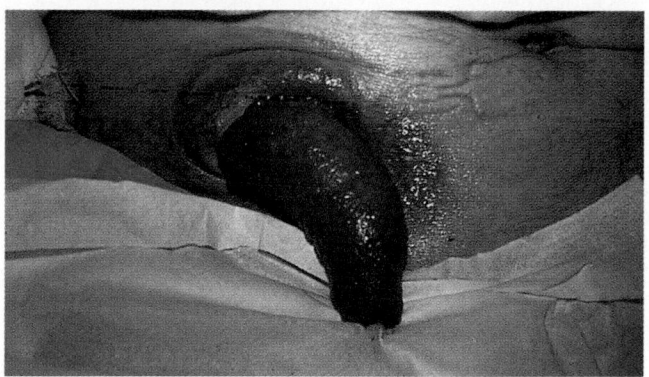

Figure 21–20

Stomal prolapse. (Courtesy of Convatec, Princeton, NJ.)

softeners, irrigations, and stomal dilation. The only long-term corrective measure is surgical revision.

Prolapse of the stoma is a condition in which all layers of the bowel protrude through the stoma, which appears swollen and elongated (Fig. 21–20). Protrusion occurs after discharge and is painless. It occurs most frequently following a loop colostomy and when the bowel was distended during surgery. If circulation to the stoma is unimpaired, the patient may be taught to manually reduce the protrusion and to wear a binder or abdominal support belt. Other cases require surgical correction.

Mucocutaneous separation is a disruption of the suture line at the base of the stoma with a resultant open wound. This occurs early in the postoperative period and is often preceded by red skin around the base of the stoma. Once the separation has occurred, the patient complains of pain or burning when the effluent (drainage) from the ostomy comes in contact with the wound. Treatment varies with the extent of the wound. Shallow wounds are filled with paste or solid skin barrier. Deep, draining wounds are irrigated and packed. All wounds are left to heal by secondary intention.

NURSING PROCESS
Colostomy

PREOPERATIVE NURSING CARE

Assessment

When assessing a patient scheduled for colostomy, include those assessments that apply to any surgical patient and those for the patient undergoing intestinal resection with an anastomosis. In addition, thoroughly assess the patient's ability to accept and deal with ostomy.

Assess the patient's emotional reaction to the scheduled surgery. Keep in mind that the alteration in body function and structure that occurs with this surgery can precipitate an intense emotional response. Observe for signs of anxiety and manifestations of grieving such as denial, anger, depression, and withdrawal.

Question the patient about any previous experience with ostomy. Determine whether the patient has ever seen the results of colostomy, knows what it is and how it works, or knows anyone who has undergone colostomy. If so, what are the patient's perceptions of colostomy based on this experience? Are there any misconceptions based on type of ostomy, changes in surgical procedures, available appliances, or methods of care?

Assess the patient's perception of the effects of colostomy on his or her lifestyle. Is the patient aware that colostomy will require certain adjustments in the pattern of daily living, that supplies will be needed, and that time will be required for its care? Can the patient imagine incorporating colostomy into a daily routine and expect that life will resume a usual pattern?

Assess sources of support available to the patient. Keep in mind that the closest relative or other seemingly obvious source of support is not always the person most acceptable or best able to help the patient.

Nursing Diagnoses and Planning

Nursing diagnoses and related expected patient outcomes commonly applicable to patients scheduled for colostomy include the following:

NDx: Anxiety related to the outcome of the surgery and ability to live with and manage colostomy

Planning: Patient Outcomes
1. Patient expresses confidence in the decision to have the surgery.
2. Patient cooperates with preoperative preparation.
3. Signs of excessive anxiety—such as trembling, inability to direct attention, tachycardia, and dry mouth—are absent.

NDx: Knowledge deficit: appearance and function of colostomy results, need for an appliance, and need for learning self-care measures

Planning: Patient Outcomes
1. Patient describes what the stoma will look like, where it will be, how the colostomy will function, and what kind of appliance will be in place after surgery.
2. Patient asks questions about care of the colostomy or states that care procedures will have to be learned.

Other nursing diagnoses that may apply to the patient depending on the underlying intestinal disorder include the following: fluid volume deficit related to disease symptoms such as diarrhea, vomiting, and anorexia or dietary restrictions for diagnostic tests and surgery; and altered nutrition; less than body requirements, related to effects of the disease process or dietary restrictions for diagnostic tests and surgery.

Nursing Interventions and Evaluation

NDx: Anxiety
Provide time, privacy, and encouragement for discussion of the patient's concerns. Acknowledge that feelings of anxiety are normal and expected when facing colostomy. Do not give false reassurance, but do stress the expected beneficial effects of the surgery and the competence of the persons responsible for patient care. Assure the patient that undergoing colostomy does not dramatically change the quality of life and that most activities—work, personal and recreational—can be resumed. Offer to arrange a visit from an ostomate (a person who has undergone colostomy, adjusted well to it, and acts as a volunteer in helping others adjust before and after surgery). Guide the patient in relaxation exercises, and provide diversion, such as radio, television, or reading materials, as appropriate to the patient's condition.

Remember that the prospect of colostomy can be as upsetting to significant others as to the patient. Be sure to provide significant others with the opportunity to ventilate their feelings and concerns so that they can support the patient's coping process.

NDx: Knowledge deficit: appearance and function of colostomy, need for an appliance, and need for learning self-care measures
Provide the patient with basic information about the planned colostomy and its function. Include a simple description of the normal structure and function of the GI tract, illustrated by an uncomplicated drawing. Explain how colostomy is undertaken and its effect on bowel function. Define pertinent terms, such as stoma, appliance, and pouch. Describe the location and appearance of the stoma, as well as the characteristics of drainage. If there is a doll set up for teaching ostomy procedures, let the patient see and handle the equipment to reduce fear of the unknown. Explain that daily routines of self-care that will be necessary, that they will be taught, and that with time they become part of everyday living, like taking a bath or shaving. Show the patient the type of collection pouch that will be in place after surgery, and let him or her examine it if desired.

Adjust the information given to the needs of the individual patient. Add more depth and detail when desired by the patient, but avoid providing unnecessary, unwanted material that will only increase the patient's anxiety. If reading materials are given to the patient, make sure they contain only information pertinent to the patient, to avoid confusion and anxiety. Also be certain to arrange a follow-up discussion so that any questions or concerns can be addressed.

Additional Interventions
When possible, check for sensitivity to colostomy care products—such as skin barriers and sealants to be used postoperatively—by performing a patch test. Apply small amounts of these products to the

skin of the upper back and cover with an airtight dressing. Remove the dressing in 48 hours, leave the area exposed to the air for 30 minutes, and then inspect for signs of a skin reaction.

Compare the patient's status with the expected outcomes. If the outcomes are not met, reassess the patient and revise the plan.

POSTOPERATIVE NURSING CARE

Assessment

Make postoperative assessments as described for the patient following an anastomosed intestinal resection. In addition, make assessments related to ostomy structure and function, stoma care, and patient acceptance.

Assess the condition of the stoma. Observe its shape, which may be perfectly round or somewhat irregular, depending on its surgical construction. Note its color and consistency. Keep in mind that it should feel soft or slightly firm to the touch and be deep pink to red, shiny, and moist, like the mucous membrane inside the mouth. A dark red or purple color indicates poor circulation. Light pink indicates either poor circulation or anemia.

Inspect for signs of bleeding. Note the amount of edema. In the immediate postoperative period, expect to see small amounts of pinpoint bleeding on the stoma as a result of the high vascularity of the intestine. Also expect significant edema, which should disappear gradually over 4 to 6 weeks.

Examine the collection pouch to determine the amount and characteristics of the drainage from the stoma. Remember that mucous and serosanguineous drainage are expected for the first 24 to 72 hours after surgery.

Assess for the return of bowel function. Listen for bowel sounds. Check for the passage of flatus. When the colostomy begins to function, note the color, consistency, and amount of fecal drainage. Inspect the peristomal skin for signs of impaired circulation, irritation, and excoriation. Also check that the skin surrounds the stoma closely about its entire circumference.

Continue to assess the response of the patient and significant others to the colostomy, as well as the patient's readiness for teaching related to colostomy care. Remember that a person in shock and disbelief, who has not looked at the stoma, is not ready for teaching. Remember also that teaching will not be effective when the patient is angry or depressed. Be alert to questions from the patient about the colostomy or related care, because these are generally good indicators of readiness for learning.

Nursing Diagnoses and Planning

Nursing diagnoses and related expected patient outcomes commonly applicable to patients following colostomy include those previously described under the care of the patient who has undergone anastomosed intestinal resection and the following:

NDx: Bowel incontinence related to colostomy and loss of rectal function

Planning: Patient Outcomes
1. Patient uses the selected pouching system effectively to collect fecal drainage.
2. Patient identifies factors, such as change in diet and times of eating, that affect the pattern of colostomy function.

NDx: Risk for impaired skin integrity related to irritation of the peristomal skin from contact with ostomy output, from removal of adherent appliances, or from sensitivity to adhesives and other materials

Planning: Patient Outcomes
1. Peristomal skin is free of erythema and blisters.
2. Peristomal skin is intact.

NDx: Risk for altered nutrition: less than body requirements related to omission of foods with essential nutrients from the diet because of flatulence, odor, or diarrhea

Planning: Patient Outcomes
1. Patient describes components of a nutritionally balanced diet.
2. Patient is able to select a nutritionally balanced diet from foods that are tolerated well.
3. Patient identifies specific foods that are likely causes of flatulence, odor, or diarrhea.

NDx: Risk for body image disturbance related to loss of bowel control, presence of the stoma, release of fecal material onto abdomen, passage of flatus, odor, and need for an appliance

Planning: Patient Outcomes
1. Patient verbalizes acceptance of self with the colostomy results.
2. Patient identifies his or her own strengths.
3. Patient expresses pleasure at visits from relatives and friends.
4. Patient discusses resumption of work, household, and social activities from a positive perspective.

NDx: Altered sexuality patterns related to fear of rejection because of the presence of a stoma or an appliance

Planning: Patient Outcomes
1. Patient discusses concerns about the effects of the colostomy on sexual function.
2. Patient verbalizes confidence in ability to participate in a satisfying sexual relationship.

NDx: Altered health maintenance related to insufficient knowledge of care of the stoma, effect on lifestyle, and support services

Planning: Patient Outcomes
1. Patient demonstrates correct appliance application.
2. Patient identifies symptoms that should be reported to the health care professional.

3. Patient correctly demonstrates cleaning and deodorizing of the appliance.
4. Patient identifies potential effects of the colostomy on lifestyle without exaggeration or denial.
5. Patient describes available support services, including how to contact the United Ostomy Association.

Nursing Interventions and Evaluation

Carry out basic postoperative interventions as for the patient who has undergone intestinal resection with an anastomosis.

Encourage the patient to cough and breathe deeply every 2 hours to enhance lung expansion and decrease the risk of pulmonary congestion and pneumonia. Guide the patient in foot and leg exercises every hour while the patient is awake and on bed rest to foster venous return and help prevent thrombus formation and pulmonary embolism. Begin ambulation 8 to 24 hours after surgery.

NDx: Bowel incontinence

Use a colostomy appliance to collect feces expelled involuntarily from the stoma. In most cases, a collection pouch, usually translucent plastic, is placed over the stoma at the completion of the operation. Monitor this pouch for accumulation of flatus and drainage. Empty or change it as necessary. Do not allow the pouch to get too full because back pressure can damage the suture lines and disrupt the pouch seal.

Help the patient select a collection system for daily use that is suited to his or her needs. Various types of colostomy equipment are available. Selection of the appliance system appropriate to the individual patient is essential if problems with leaking and skin irritation are to be prevented (Fig. 21–21). Factors that influence the appropriateness of specific systems include the location of the stoma, abdominal size and shape, physical and mental capabilities, and personal preference of the patient. If the patient cannot perform self-care and will depend on a spouse or significant other for assistance, include that person in the selection process as well.

Appliances are either disposable or reusable and come as one- or two-part systems. (A two-part system includes both a collection pouch and a skin barrier.) Collection pouches come in clear or opaque plastic and can be odorproof. Pouch covers of soft material that make the pouch more comfortable to wear can be purchased or made.

Appliances must be sized to fit the stoma. Because of the progressive decrease in postoperative edema, check the size after 3 weeks and determine final stoma size at 3 to 4 months after surgery.

Once a system is selected, use it consistently to eliminate confusion for the patient and make learning the required care skills easier. Similarly, if caring

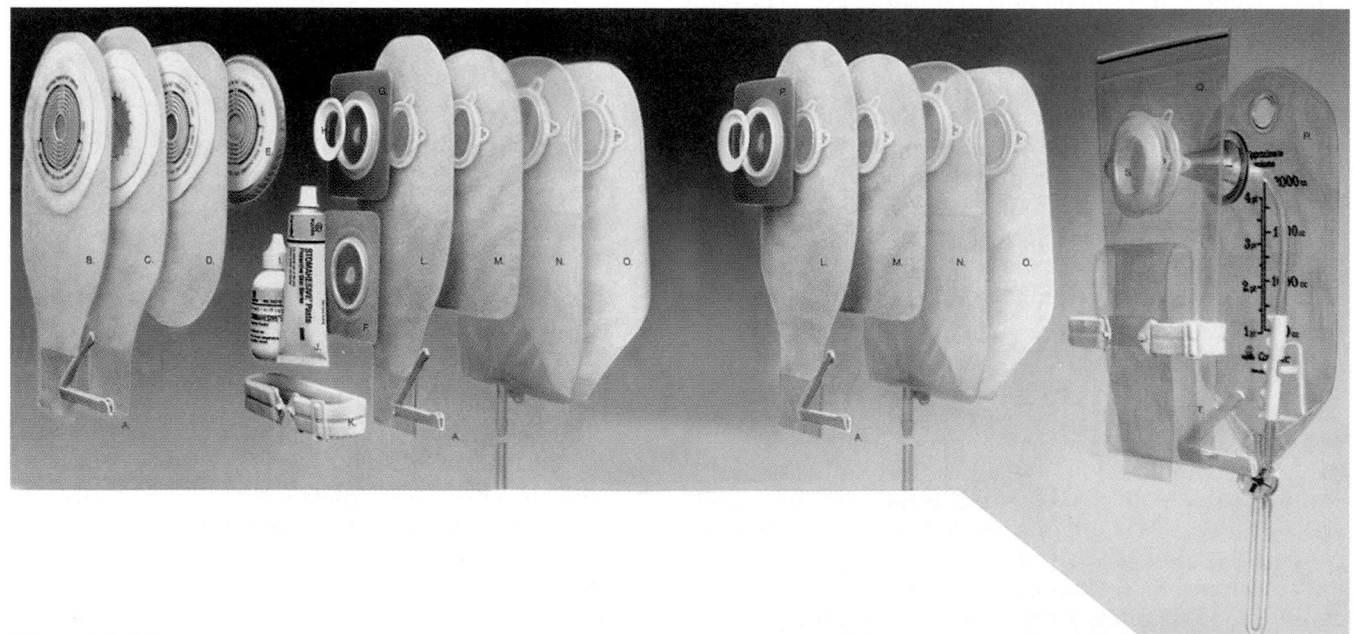

Figure 21–21

Examples of the various types of colostomy equipment patients may use: *A,* Active Life/Sur-Fit Tail Closure; *B,* Active Life One-Piece Drainable Custom Pouch; *C,* Active Life One-Piece Drainable Pouch with pre-cut openings; *D,* Active Life One-Piece Closed-End Pouch; *E,* Active Life One-Piece Stoma Cap; *F,* Sur-Fit Flexible; *G,* Stomahesive Wafer with Sur-Fit Flange; *H,* Sur-Fit Disposable Convex Insert; *I,* Stomahesive Protective Powder; *J,* Stomahesive Paste; *K,* Adjustable Belt; *L,* Sur-Fit Drainable Pouch; *M,* Sur-Fit Closed-End Pouch; *N,* Sur-Fit Urostomy Pouch; *O,* Sur-Fit Urostomy Pouch with Accuseal Tap; *P,* Durahesive Wafer with Flange; *Q,* Sur-Fit Irrigation Sleeve; *R,* Visi-Flow Irrigation System; *S,* Sur-Fit Adapter Faceplate; *T,* Sur-Fit Irrigation Sleeve Tail Closure. (Courtesy of Convatec, Princeton, NJ.)

for a patient with a pre-existing stoma, follow the patient's usual method of care. Make suggestions if appropriate, but do not try to force change if the existing system is effective.

Inform patients who have undergone sigmoid or descending colostomy that control over fecal expulsion maybe gained in time by means of a regular diet or periodic colostomy irrigation, although the latter method is seldom used today. Explain that if control is achieved, a collection pouch will not be necessary all of the time because something as simple as a gauze pad covered with Saran Wrap over the stoma is sufficient. Some people choose to continue with a small, lightweight collection appliance for security. In assisting patients to establish control, instruct him or her in basic dietary considerations as presented in Highlight 21–7 and in the importance of maintaining a regular pattern of eating and exercise.

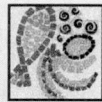

HIGHLIGHT
21–7
NUTRITION

Special Considerations for Patients with a Colostomy

Instruct patients with a colostomy to:

Eat a low-residue diet for 4 to 6 weeks after surgery.

Progress to a high-carbohydrate, high-protein general diet after this 4- to 6-week period.

Add new foods one at a time to determine their effect.

Try each food at least three times before eliminating it from the diet.

Consider the effects of specific foods on the gastrointestinal system when selecting the diet.

Constipating foods: cheese, nuts, chocolate, corn, raisins

Laxative foods: prunes, fresh fruits, broccoli, spinach, green beans, liver, highly spiced foods, beer

Gas-forming foods: nuts, cabbage, sauerkraut, corn, cauliflower, broccoli, spinach, peas, beans, apples, avocados, watermelon, cucumbers, carbonated beverages

Odor-causing foods: alcohol (particularly beers), onions, beans, cabbage, turnips, asparagus, mushrooms, radishes, cucumbers, eggs, fish, highly spiced foods

Deodorizing foods: parsley, beet greens, spinach, buttermilk, yogurt

Remember that many adults tolerate milk and milk products poorly; they should be limited.

NDx: Risk for impaired skin integrity

Peristomal skin irritation and breakdown can result from contact with fecal drainage containing enzymes, exposure to constant moisture, sensitivity to substances applied to the skin, and removal of pouch adhesives from the skin. Risk of irritation from enzymes in the fecal drainage varies with the location of the stoma. It is highest with ascending colostomy, less with transverse colostomy, and slight with sigmoid colostomy. Good skin care is critical to successful adaptation to colostomy. If skin irritation and breakdown occur, the result is discomfort and additional time and money spent on treatment—all of which are greater intrusions on lifestyle. Nursing interventions to protect the integrity of the peristomal skin are as follows.

Remove mucus or feces with a tissue and thoroughly wash the peristomal skin to remove all traces of intestinal discharge. Rinse carefully to remove all soap residue. Dry gently and completely. If the patient is an elderly person whose skin tends to be dry, omit the soap and wash with warm water only. Do not use oily soaps or emollients, because they interfere with adherence of the collection pouch. Spray on "no-rinse" commercial products are available that are effective cleansers and require minimal contact of cloth or gauze to the skin.

Use a skin barrier to protect the $\frac{1}{8}$ inch of exposed skin between the stoma and the pouch opening from exposure to fecal drainage. Most appliances today are already treated with a skin barrier substance.

If the patient has undergone colostomy in a difficult location, powders and pastes are available to fill creases and folds to obtain a better and longer-lasting pouch seal. Apply a skin sealant to the peristomal skin area where adhesive will be applied to hold the collection pouch in place. Skin sealants are sprays, liquids, gels, or wipes that coat the skin with a clear film so that, when the adhesive substance is removed, the protective film is torn off rather than the epidermis.

Apply the pouch snugly and monitor routinely for leaking. Change the pouch immediately if it leaks. When removing the pouch, follow carefully the directions accompanying it to ensure the least traumatic removal.

If needed, remove hair from the peristomal skin regularly to decrease the risk of folliculitis caused by trauma of the hair follicles. Use an electric or straight razor according to personal preference, but avoid depilatories because of the risk of sensitivity to them.

If skin irritation does occur, institute immediate treatment. When the skin around the stoma is reddened, change the appliance every 1 to 2 days. Wash the area with warm water or special cleansing products for ostomates. Allow to dry. Apply a skin barrier carefully patterned to the stoma and a collection appliance.

If the skin around the stoma is broken, change

the collection appliance daily. Wash the skin and apply a protective preparation such as Orabase to broken areas. Reapply a skin barrier and appliance. Do not use antacids on the skin because they raise the pH and predispose to infection. Also avoid aluminum paste because it decreases adhesion of the pouch and is hard to remove.

Monitor carefully for signs of yeast infection, which is most often caused by *Candida albicans.* Observe for the characteristic irregular patches of deep erythema with papular lesions and the appearance of dry, scaling areas of skin as the process progresses.

NDx: Risk for altered nutrition: less than body requirements

Review basic principles of nutrition with the patient. Discuss the components of a nutritionally balanced diet, the use of the basic food groups in planning a balanced diet, and the need for at least 2500 mL of fluid per day. Explain to the patient that there are no specific dietary restrictions following colostomy. Some patients can eat anything, whereas others find that specific foods cause constipation, diarrhea, odor, or excessive flatus. Teach the patient which foods are most likely to cause these effects (see Highlight 21–7). Stress, however, that food tolerance is an individual issue and that desired foods should be tried one at a time, at least three times, before being eliminated from the diet.

NDx: Body image disturbance

Acknowledge to the patient that negative feelings about the colostomy are normal and that it takes time to accept and adjust to this body change. Recognize that patients typically experience fear of rejection, disgust, or shame. Be certain, therefore, that facial expressions and other nonverbal behaviors convey acceptance, not revulsion, distaste, or pity, which would reinforce the patient's distress. Recognize too that denial is common after ostomy surgery. Allow the patient to experience denial while gently fostering acceptance of the reality. Do this not by forcing the patient to look at the stoma or participate in care, but by using the terms colostomy and stoma and by describing their appearance and giving brief, matter-of-fact explanations of the colostomy care being given. Touch the stoma to show that it does not hurt, is not easily damaged, and is not revolting. Provide an opportunity for the patient to look at or touch the stoma, as by leaving it uncovered while supplies are obtained. Be alert to comments and questions that suggest the patient has looked at the stoma. Encourage discussion of related feelings and concerns.

Protect the patient from unnecessary embarrassment about the stoma by ensuring privacy for discussion, teaching, and colostomy care, and by controlling odor. Empty the collection pouch of malodorous flatus or fecal drainage before meals and visiting hours. Provide good ventilation, and deodorize the room immediately. Do not put pin holes in the disposable plastic pouch to allow flatus to escape in the early postoperative period, because this results in unpredictable, uncontrolled odor. In helping the patient select an appliance for long-term use, recommend one that is odor-free except when emptying or if the outlet is not cleaned. Such an appliance may cost somewhat more initially, but the subsequent need to purchase deodorizers is eliminated.

Encourage the patient to be well groomed. Stress that, with some attention to the style of clothing purchased, the ostomy and the pouch cannot be noticed. Suggest a visit from an ostomate as one way of demonstrating this fact. Throughout the recovery period, foster the patient's sense of control. Involve the patient in decision-making. Help the patient identify personal strengths. Encourage the family to treat the patient normally and to engage in a frank discussion of feelings.

NDx: Altered sexuality patterns

Encourage the patient to discuss resumption of sexual activity, and provide basic information in this regard. Affirm that sexual intercourse, conception, and pregnancy are all possible following colostomy. If a collection appliance is worn, suggest that it be emptied before intercourse, and recommend different positions if needed to accommodate the appliance.

Acknowledge that concerns about sexual activity are normal, and encourage the patient to discuss them openly with the spouse or significant other. Provide privacy and time for such discussion. Provide access to written material, such as "Sex and the Male Ostomate," published by the United Ostomy Association. Refer to an enterostomal therapist or sex therapist if needed.

NDx: Altered health maintenance

Begin teaching the patient to care for the colostomy as soon as possible postoperatively. It is true that learning occurs best when teaching coincides with the time that the patient is most ready to learn, but this is not always possible when patients may be discharged in as few as 5 or 6 days because of changes in reimbursement. As a result, teaching must sometimes take place while the patient is still struggling to accept the reality of the ostomy and to express feelings about it. The importance of written material to supplement teaching is especially important in these situations. Keep in mind that, although the challenge of effective teaching is increased, learning self-care can lead to a sense of control and confidence in the ability to cope that can help overcome negative feelings about the ostomy.

Given the possibility that teaching time may be limited, it is important to identify critical learning topics. Teach the patient first to care for the colostomy. This involves:

Identifying needed supplies
Emptying the pouch

Changing the pouch
Controlling odor
Cleaning the appliance
Caring for peristomal skin

Adapt the teaching to the patient's needs within the confines of the situation. For example, if time permits, consider initially teaching the patient to use the clamp on the pouch and to empty the pouch and allowing the patient to simply observe a pouch change and skin care. Subsequently, when teaching the patient to change the pouch, recognize that the pouch may have to be changed every day, regardless of need, to ensure that the patient will have sufficient opportunity to learn the procedure before discharge. When teaching colostomy care, also be certain to have the patient do it in the manner best done after discharge (eg, have the patient sit on the toilet to empty the bag) because the initial method learned tends to remain the patient's preference.

Be sure to tell the patient to empty the pouch when it is one-third full and at bedtime. Suggest that, for a few days after discharge, an alarm clock be set to ensure that the patient is awakened in time to empty the pouch. Stress the importance of always using one hand to support the skin while lifting adhesive with the other when changing the pouch. For maximum convenience and ease, suggest changing the pouch first thing in the morning, before eating or drinking, because the stoma usually is not functioning at this time. Instruct the patient to dispose of pouches in plastic bags, first wrapping them in aluminum foil if it is desired to disguise the contents.

Explain that odor is best controlled by the use of an odorproof pouch but that, if necessary, deodorant substances such as Nilodor or baking soda may be put in the bag. Instruct the patient to wash reusable appliances with soap and water and expose them to fresh air, not only to clean them and prolong their use, but to keep them odor-free. If odor persists, instruct the patient to soak the appliances in a commercially available deodorizer.

Inform the patient that any type of clothing can be worn, including girdles and panty hose. Also inform the patient that physical activities are unrestricted. Showers and tub baths may be taken, and swimming, tennis, and exercise programs may be resumed, usually within 8 weeks after surgery. Explain that there is no restriction on travel. It is simply necessary to carry supplies for colostomy care so they are easily accessible. Remind the patient to wear seat belts above or below the stoma, not directly on it.

Describe to the patient ostomy clubs and support groups available in the community, and give information as to how to contact them. Explain that the United Ostomy Association has meetings in every city to provide ostomy patients with assistance and psychologic support.

Provide the patient with written instructions regarding care upon discharge. This is important because information given in stressful situations is often forgotten or confused, and review is necessary. In addition, when making referrals for follow-up care in the home, be certain to specify the type of appliance system being used and carefully describe what the patient has been taught.

Compare the patient's status with the expected outcomes. If the outcomes are not met, reassess the patient and revise the plan.

Ileostomy

Ileostomy is the surgical creation of an opening between the ileum and the abdominal wall through which fecal matter is expelled. The major difference between ileostomy and colostomy is the type of fecal output. The output from an ileostomy is a malodorous, enzyme-rich, caustic, yellow, green, or brown liquid. Exactly how liquid output is, and therefore its volume, depends on where in the ileum the stoma is. Because the terminal ileum begins to take over the water-absorbing function of the colon, the closer the ileostomy is to the junction of the large bowel, the less liquid the output.

Uses
Ileostomies are most often used in treating cancer of the colon and ulcerative colitis, an inflammatory disease of the colon.

Patient Preparation
The preparation of the patient is the same as for colostomy. If an ileal pouch-anal anastomosis is to be performed, a more extensive medical workup is performed up to 1 month before the scheduled surgery in order to ascertain the status of the rectal mucosa. This usually includes a flexible sigmoidoscopy and anorectal manometry. Preoperative preparation in this situation involves the same procedure for bowel cleansing described for intestinal resection. Steroids or sulfasalazine may also be given preoperatively for the anti-inflammatory effect.

Procedure
The three types of ileostomy are the standard end (Brook's) ileostomy, ileal pouch-anal canal anastomosis, and continent ileostomy or Kock pouch.

Conventional ileostomy is performed in a manner similar to that of end colostomy. The proximal end of the ileum is pulled through the right abdominal wall. It is then cuffed to form a stoma that protrudes about an inch beyond the skin surface to decrease the risk of effluent coming in contact with the skin and causing irritation. The distal ileum may either be removed or left in place with the end sutured closed.

An alternative method to the standard end procedure is loop ileostomy. In this case, the intact ileum is pulled through the right abdominal wall. A rod is inserted through the loop to support the ileum in this position. The top portion of the loop is

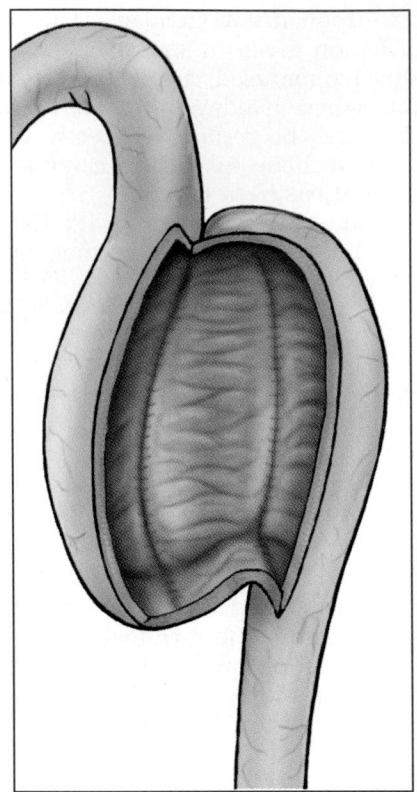

Figure 21–22

Creation of an S-pouch for ileal pouch-anal anastomosis.

then incised to allow drainage. This is a temporary procedure used to divert fecal matter from an unhealed anastomosis between the distal ileum and the anus.

The ileal pouch-anal canal anastomosis is being used more often in the surgical management of chronic ulcerative colitis. It involves resection of the

cecum, the colon (including the ileocecal valve), the rectum, and the proximal anal canal. Next a J or S pouch (Fig. 21–22) is created using loops of terminal ileum. The end of the pouch (or in the case of the S pouch, the distal end of the ileum) is pulled through the rectal stump and anastomosed to the anus.

Gowns and gloves are then changed. A loop ileostoma is created through a predetermined site in the abdominal wall (Fig. 21–23A). The abdominal wound is closed, and an ileostomy appliance is placed. Usually the patient has the temporary loop ileostomy for 2 to 3 months. A second operation to close the ileostoma and restore bowel continuity is performed (Fig. 21–23B). After this second operation, stool is once again passed via the rectum and no collection appliance is needed.

In continent ileostomy, an internal pouch to hold stool is created by suturing two loops of ileum together. A nipple valve is then constructed by intussuscepting the ileum (Fig. 21–24). This controls the passage of feces and gas, because as the pouch fills, pressure forces the valve to close. The pouch initially holds 100 to 600 mL but gradually stretches with use up to a capacity of 1000 mL in about 6 months. This procedure is designed to eliminate the need for an external collection appliance. It cannot be used for patients with short bowel syndrome or Crohn's disease, nor can it be used when patients are obese, on high doses of steroids, or unable to perform the required self-care.

Postoperative Course

Ileostomies result in the expelling of flatus and then dark-green odorless liquid in 12 to 72 hours, with stomas just proximal to the ascending colon taking the longest. Initially, the amount of effluent is between 1000 and 2000 mL daily. With resumption of oral intake, volume decreases noticeably and the effluent turns dark-green to yellow to brown. It also develops a distinctive odor. In 3 to 6 months, as the

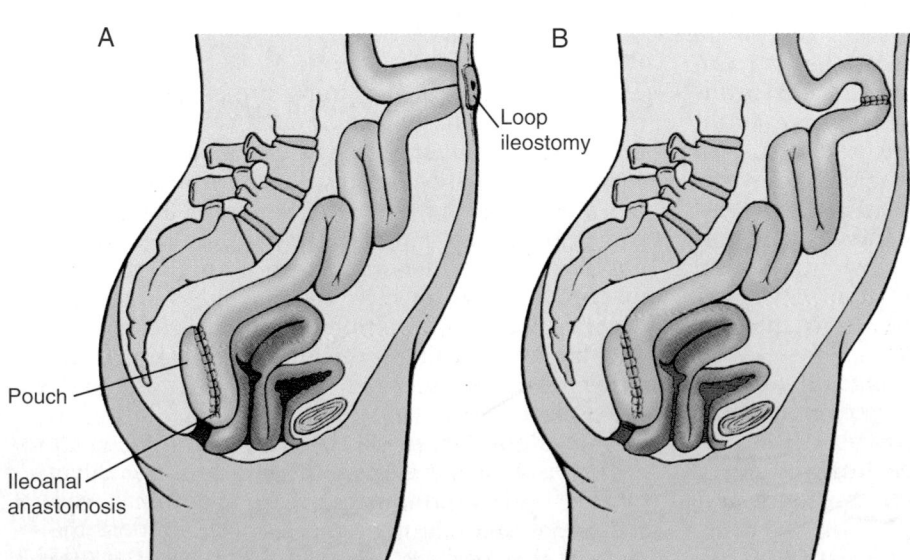

Figure 21–23

Ileal pouch-anal anastomosis. *A,* Anatomical relationships of the lower gastrointestinal organs following initial surgery. *B,* Anatomical relationships of the lower gastrointestinal organs following closure of the ileostomy.

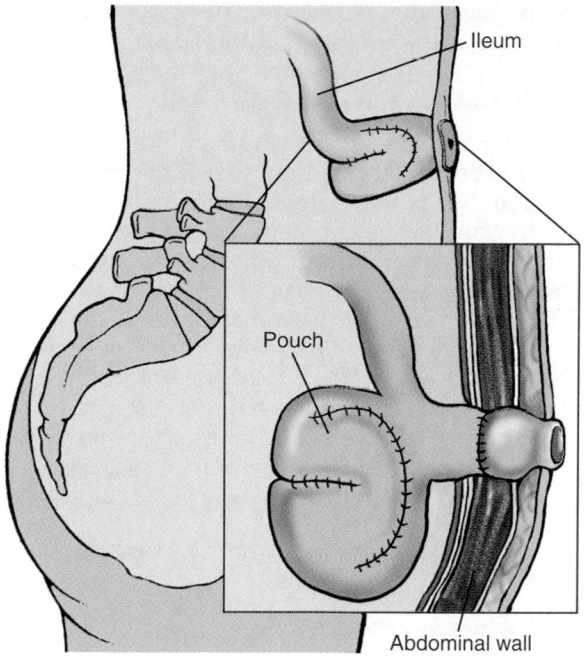

Figure 21–24

Continent ileostomy, or Kock pouch. The pouch to hold fecal matter is created surgically from a loop of ileum folded back on itself.

ileum begins to absorb more water, the effluent becomes like a fluid paste.

With conventional or loop ileostomy, the amount of fecal discharge usually is greatest 4 to 6 hours after meals, but discharge does occur in smaller amounts at unpredictable intervals. As a result, the patient must wear an appliance (pouch) at all times to collect the fecal output. One type of appliance is an open-ended bag that can be emptied every 4 to 6 hours or whenever the patient urinates. This type of bag is changed after 3 to 4 days, or if leakage occurs around the stoma.

Patients with an anal-pouch anastomosis ultimately have nearly normal digestive function, with about six to eight small, soft bowel movements per day. About half of patients experience some incontinence at night, decreasing to 25% after 4 years.

With a continent ileostomy (Kock pouch), a catheter is inserted into the internal pouch at the time of surgery. It is attached to suction to keep the pouch empty until the suture lines have healed.

During this time, the catheter is irrigated with 10 to 20 mL of normal saline every 3 hours to keep it patent. The saline is usually instilled with a syringe; return is by gravity drainage. The catheter is removed in 10 to 14 days. Subsequently, a catheter is reinserted to drain the pouch every 3 to 4 hours. The interval is gradually increased until catheter insertion is performed not more than three times daily. Eventually, the patient becomes aware of

pressure in the pouch and begins to drain it as needed.

Because mucus is expelled from the ileostomy, an absorbent dressing is needed, although an external pouch is not.

Other aspects of the postoperative course parallel those following colostomy.

Complications

A major problem following ileostomy is the potential for fluid and electrolyte imbalance. Because the output is high in fluid and electrolyte content, the ileostomy patient risks dehydration, potassium and sodium deficiencies, and acidosis as a result of the loss of bicarbonate. These problems can occur quickly, particularly if diarrhea develops, whether from illness, dietary changes, or in response to medications (eg, antibiotics) that alter flora in the ileum. Laxatives are never given to these patients, nor is the ileostomy irrigated. If a bowel preparation is required, the patient simply adheres to a liquid diet for 24 hours.

Malabsorption of fat, iron, folate, and vitamin B_{12} may occur, and there is the risk of infection, hemorrhage, or obstruction. Other complications that can occur with end or loop ileostomy include skin excoriation from contact with the caustic effluent and stomal problems as described under Colostomy.

Complications of an anal-pouch anastomosis are postoperative intestinal obstruction and nonspecific inflammation in the ileal pouch. These are usually managed satisfactorily by medical or surgical intervention. In addition, there is the risk that the primary disorder will recur in the rectal stump, creating the need for conventional ileostomy.

Complications of a continent ileostomy include incontinence caused by valve malfunction, difficult intubation, perforation, and pouchitis from bacterial overgrowth.

NURSING PROCESS GUIDELINES
Ileostomy

PREOPERATIVE NURSING CARE

Preoperative assessment, nursing diagnoses, expected patient outcomes, nursing interventions, and evaluation for patients undergoing ileostomy are similar to those described previously for patients undergoing colostomy.

Because ileostomy often is performed for uncontrollable inflammatory bowel disease, it is more likely that patients undergoing ileostomy will need longer, more intensive fluid, blood, and protein therapy preoperatively to make up for existing deficiencies. Be certain, therefore, to assess for signs of fluid and electrolyte imbalance, particularly hypokalemia, hyponatremia, and fluid deficit. Maintain accurate fluid input and output records at all times.

If the patient is undergoing ileal pouch-anal

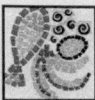

Strategies for Reducing the Risk of Complications Following an Ileostomy

Eat foods such as clear soups, cottage cheese, dry cheese, liver, lean meat, rice, tea, and coffee during the initial period of adjustment to the ileostomy.

Resume ingestion of high-fiber foods one at a time after ileostomy function has stabilized to allow tolerance of them to be evaluated.

Try each new food three times before deciding that it cannot be tolerated.

Record problem foods in a food diary for future reference.

Prevent obstruction:
Chew all foods well.
Avoid foods such as corn, popcorn, celery, Chinese food, peanuts, coconut, and skins of raw fruits, which could block the stoma.
Add salt to the diet if the ileostomy output is too dry.

Prevent fluid and electrolyte imbalances:
Drink six to eight glasses of water daily to guard against dehydration because the water-absorbing surface of the intestine is decreased.
Ingest electrolyte replacement solutions, such as Gatorade, in the summer or at other times of heavy perspiration.

Prevent diarrhea and skin irritation:
Decrease the amount of dietary fiber if the ileostomy output is too liquid.
Eat pasta, boiled rice, or low-fat cheese to thicken stool.

anastomosis, make certain that he or she fully understands that this is a two-stage procedure and has a realistic expectation regarding ultimate bowel function (eg, although the need for a collection appliance is eliminated, the pattern of bowel function will not be the typically normal one). It is important to remember that patients with intractable ulcerative colitis experience 30 to 50 bowel movements a day as part of their disease process, so this bowel pattern will be an improvement important to the patient's lifestyle. Also recognize that, given the extent and location of the surgery, patients may have concerns about its effect on sexual and bladder function. If such fears are expressed, reassure the patient that the risk of impotence or bladder dysfunction is slight because the autonomic nerves in the pelvic region are not disturbed with this type of procedure.

POSTOPERATIVE NURSING CARE

Postoperative assessment, nursing diagnoses, expected patient outcomes, nursing interventions, and evaluation for patients who have undergone ileostomy are similar to those described previously for patients who have undergone colostomy. Nutritional considerations, patient teaching information, and health promotion information specific to the patient who has undergone ileostomy are presented in Highlights 21–8 and 21–9 (also see Highlight 21–7). If the patient has been on long-term steroid therapy for ulcerative colitis before surgery, monitor for signs of adrenal insufficiency during the period of gradual steroid withdrawal. These include weak-

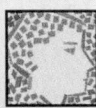

Self-Care After Ileostomy

Instruct the patient to:

Expect the ileostomy to be noisy initially as a result of tissue edema but be assured that this will decrease with time.

Expect undigested foods such as seeds and kernels to pass through the stoma.

Give meticulous care to the skin surrounding the stoma because this is more critical with an ileostomy than with a colostomy owing to the increased danger of skin excoriation from enzymes in the effluent.

Make ongoing assessments of self for signs of dehydration, hypokalemia, and hyponatremia.

Ingest a mixture of 1 tsp of table salt, 1 tsp of baking soda, and 1 quart of water as ordered by the physician if diarrhea occurs to correct acidosis secondary to the loss of bicarbonate.

Avoid laxatives.

Treat blockage of the ostomy lumen by a mass of undigested high-fiber foods as follows:
Assume knee-chest position.
Gently massage area below the stoma.
Call physician if lumen remains blocked, because a lavage by bulb syringe with 30 to 50 mL of normal saline may be required.
Adjust pouch, because stoma swells with blockage.
Increase fluid intake after removal to compensate for the resultant diarrhea.
Expect abdominal pain around the stoma for 3 to 5 days.

ness, headache, fever, falling blood pressure, diarrhea, and increased fecal output.

Following an ileal pouch-anal anastomosis, keep the patient in a semi-Fowler's position during the first postoperative day. This reduces tension on the ileoanal anastomosis and is critical to the success of the surgery.

Patients may have as many as 20 loose bowel movements daily during the first week after closure of the ileostomy, and three to eight bowel movements daily and one at night thereafter. In some cases, it is necessary to intubate the anus to drain it for 6 to 16 months. In others, medications or bulk formers are needed to provide acceptable control. Anal function usually normalizes in 6 months to a year, although the patient may experience some nocturnal fecal leakage during deep sleep. Following closure of the ileostomy, instruct the patient in self-care (see Highlights 21–8 and 21–9).

In recent years, the use of laparoscopy to create a diverting ileostomy or colostomy has been documented extensively in the literature. These procedures reduce the amount of patient discomfort, incidence of complications, and length of hospital stay.

The Elderly: Special Considerations

Age-related changes occur throughout the GI tract. In the mouth, taste sensation is diminished, gingival tissue is resorbed, and teeth are typically missing. Dry mouth is a common problem associated with disease processes and adverse medication effects. Slowed esophageal and gastric emptying may cause early satiety and a predisposition to esophageal reflux. Gastric symptoms may predispose the person to using antacids and other medications, which may, in turn, further alter GI motility. For instance, magnesium-based antacids have a laxative effect, and aluminum-based antacids have a constipating effect. Antacids also may contribute to electrolyte imbalance. For example, calcium carbonate can cause milk-alkali syndrome, which involves hypercalcemia, renal impairment, and metabolic alkalosis. A decrease in intestinal motility may contribute to increased flatulence.

Older adults are predisposed to constipation because of the age-related slowing of intestinal motility. However, in the absence of additional factors, a healthy nonmedicated older adult does not necessarily have problems with constipation. The factors that most commonly cause or contribute to constipation in older people include the following:

• Diminished activity and mobility
• Lack of dietary fiber, bulk, and fluid
• Adverse medication effects, including long-term laxative abuse

When caring for an older adult, carefully assess age-related changes as well as contributing factors. Identify any problems with digestion and the elimination of digestive wastes. Encourage regular dental care, daily flossing and brushing, and the use of mouthwash that does not contain alcohol. If appropriate, suggest small, frequent meals and the use of nonsodium spices as flavor enhancers. Also suggest that the person remain in an upright position after eating to facilitate digestion. To promote bowel elimination, encourage fluid intake of at least 2500 mL daily (unless contraindicated by a disease process), inclusion of fiber in the diet, and daily exercise. Teach about the proper use and avoidance of laxatives, antacids, bulk-forming agents, and other over-the-counter products that affect GI function.

Just as changes in the digestive system may have implications for the care of older people, changes in other areas of function may affect the care of the geriatric patient with a GI disorder. For example, perception of abdominal pain may be diminished, and abdominal muscles may not display the true rigidity characteristic of peritoneal irritation. This complicates assessment of the abdomen. Disorders such as dementia may interfere with the person's ability to report the chronology and character of the pain. Use questions that are specific and related to other activities, such as "What happens to the pain when you turn on your side?" Allow enough time for an unhurried approach.

Frail older people with a reduced functional reserve may have difficulty maintaining homeostasis. Thus, geriatric patients undergoing extensive diagnostic or surgical procedures may be at high risk for complications. Physiologic status must be closely monitored. Actions to support homeostasis must be aggressively pursued. In the case of diagnostic tests, preparation may be adjusted to the patient's tolerance or alternative tests selected. Expected progress following surgery may also be different for the geriatric patient. For example, start of drainage from a stoma is not as rapid as in a younger person because of decreased peristalsis and mucus production.

Chapter Review

1. What can be learned by careful assessment of the amount, color, characteristics and odor of a patient's vomitus?
2. What considerations would have to be made for an elderly patient with nausea and vomiting whose intravenous fluids were running too slowly?
3. How can hemodynamic status best be assessed in a patient experiencing a GI bleed?
4. How would the care of an elderly patient undergoing a bowel preparation differ from that of a young person?
5. How would you evaluate the therapeutic effect of enteral feedings for a patient?
6. Why would total parenteral nutrition be more appropriate than enteral tube feed-

ings for a patient with severe inflammatory bowel disease?

7. How would you respond to a patient who asked if it was possible to eliminate the use of an ileostomy appliance?

8. What are possible solutions to the problem of constipation in a patient who has undergone colostomy?

9. What is the difference between the effect of excessive diarrhea on the skin of a patient who has undergone ileostomy and one who has undergone sigmoid colostomy?

10. What are the advantages of ileostomy for a patient with intractable ulcerative colitis?

Bibliography

Bates B. A guide to physical examination and history taking. 6th ed. Philadelphia: JB Lippincott, 1995.

Becker JM. Ileal pouch-anal anastomosis: Current status and controversies. Surgery 1993; 113(6):599.

Billings JA. Anorexia. J Palliat Care 1994; 10(1):51.

Blaylock B. Factors contributing to protein-calorie malnutrition in older adults. MEDSURG Nurs 1993; 2(5):351.

Byers PH, Ryan PA, Regan MB, et al. Effects of incontinence care cleansing regimens on skin integrity. J WOCN 1995; 22(4):187.

Calkins E, Ford AB, Katz PR. The practice of geriatric medicine. 2nd ed. Philadelphia: WB Saunders, 1992.

Carnevali D. Nursing management for the elderly. 3rd ed. Philadelphia: JB Lippincott, 1993.

Davis AE, Arrington K, Fields-Ryan S, Pruitt J. Preventing feeding-associated aspiration. MEDSURG Nurs 1995; 4(2):111.

Department of Health and Human Services. (1992). Acute pain management in adults: Operative procedures (AHCPR Publication No 92-0091). Rockville, MD: Department of Health and Human Services.

Doughty B, Jackson D. Gastrointestinal disorders. St. Louis: CV Mosby, 1993.

Fater K. Determining nasoenteral feeding tube placement. MEDSURG Nurs 1995; 4(1):27.

Fuhrman GM, Ota DM. Laparoscopic intestinal stomas. Dis Colon Rectum 1994; 37(5):444.

Govoni LE, Hayes JE. Drugs and nursing implications. 8th ed. Norwalk, CT: Appleton & Lange, 1995.

Hall GR, Karstens M, Rakel, B, et al. Managing constipation using a research-based protocol. MEDSURG Nurs 1995; 4(1):11.

Harald EA, Kaufman K. Understanding the gastrointestinal system. Part 1. Nursing 1994; 24(7):71.

Harald E, Kaufman K. Understanding the gastrointestinal system. Part 2. Nursing 1994; 24(8):84.

Jess LW. Acute abdominal pain. Nursing 1993; 23(9):34.

Kelly KA. Approach to the patient with ileostomy and ileal pouch. In Yamada T (ed). Textbook of gastroenterology. Philadelphia: Lippincott, 1995, pp 881–893.

Keithley J, Kohn C. Nutrition. In Brozenec S, Russell S (eds). Core curriculum for medical-surgical nursing. Pitman, NJ: Jannetti Publications, 1994, pp 37–54.

Khoo RE, Cohen MM, Chapman GM, et al. Loop ileostomy for temporary fecal diversion. Am J Surg 1994; 167(5):519.

Lieberman D. Gastrointestinal bleeding: Initial management. Gastroenterol Clin North Am 1993; 22(4):723.

Lyerly HK, Mault JR. Laparoscopic ileostomy and colostomy. Ann Surg 1994; 219(3):317.

Marcello PW, Robers PL, Schoety DJ, et al. Long-term results of the ileoanal pouch procedure. Arch Surg 1993; 128(5):500.

Meeker M, Rothrock J. Alexander's care of the patient in surgery. 10th ed. St. Louis: CV Mosby, 1995.

Omura Y, Anazawa S. Outcome of peristomal skin management by long-term use of skin barrier. J WOCN 1994; 21(6):251.

Quigley M. Upper gastrointestinal hemorrhage. In Parrillo J (ed). Current therapy in critical care medicine. Philadelphia: BC Decker, 1991, pp 279–283.

Ross Laboratories. (1994). Caring for a gastrostomy. Nursing 24(8):48–59.

Sabiston DC (ed). Textbook of surgery: The biological basis of modern surgical practice. 15th ed. Philadelphia: WB Saunders, 1996.

Saunderlin G. Mechanical bowel preparation in review. MEDSURG Nurs 1995; 4(4):267.

Sleisenger MH, Fordtran JS. Gastrointestinal disease: Pathophysiology, diagnosis, management. 5th ed. Philadelphia: WB Saunders, 1993.

Surratt S, Ryan A, Hallenbeck P, et al. Troubleshooting a sump tube. Am J Nurs 1993; 93(1):42.

Sweed MR, Guenter R, Jones S. Nursing implications for the adult patient receiving nutritional support. MEDSURG Nurs 1995; 4(2):99.

Taylor P. Colostomy irrigation: A safe practice? J Clin Nurs 1995; 4(3):203.

Vonfrolio LG, Noone J. Understanding GI disorders. Nursing 1995; 25(4):32.

Weinstein S. Plumer's principles and practice of intravenous therapy. 5th ed. Philadelphia: JB Lippincott, 1993.

Williams SR. Nutrition and diet therapy. 7th ed. St. Louis: Mosby, 1993.

Zuidema GD (ed). Shackelford's surgery of the alimentary tract. 4th ed. Philadelphia: WB Saunders, 1996.

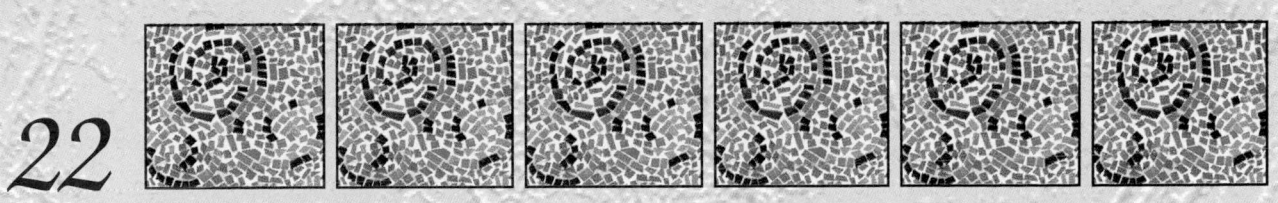

22

Nursing Care of Patients with Disorders of the Upper Gastrointestinal System

Study Outcomes

After studying this chapter, you should be able to:

1. Describe the etiology, pathophysiology, clinical manifestations, diagnostic procedures, and medical management of common upper gastrointestinal disorders.
2. Identify information and physical examination data essential to the assessment of patients with common upper gastrointestinal disorders.
3. State nursing diagnoses and related expected patient outcomes commonly applicable to patients with upper gastrointestinal disorders.
4. Describe nursing interventions, with their rationales, commonly applicable to patients with upper gastrointestinal disorders.
5. Explain the basis for evaluation of nursing care provided to patients with common upper gastrointestinal disorders.
6. Identify special considerations for the elderly patient with an upper gastrointestinal tract disorder.
7. Identify alternative treatment and care settings for patients with upper gastrointestinal disorders and the services related to community-based care.

Upper gastrointestinal disorders are among the most common health problems of adults and range in severity from simple cold sores to gastric cancer. Normal ingestion and digestion of nutrients are affected regardless of the specific problem, creating the potential for nutritional imbalance, for pain, and sometimes for life-threatening complications.

Patients with disorders of the upper gastrointestinal tract are commonly diagnosed and treated in the hospital. Depending on the severity of the problem, however, patients may be treated in a physician's office, an employee health center, a freestanding clinic, or an emergency room, as well as in inpatient settings. Additionally, the chronic nature of many upper gastrointestinal disorders indicates a need for follow-up care in the home. The nurse must be able to provide appropriate patient or family teaching, provide support for an extended period of time, and act as liaison between such resources as the community health nurse, the physician, and the pharmacist.

Infections and Inflammations

ORAL INFECTIONS

There are many different types of oral infection. Generally, they result from interacting factors, such as poor oral hygiene, poor nutritional habits, and stress. In some instances, however, oral infections may be related to a systemic disorder. For the most part, they simply cause discomfort and are a nuisance. However, if they are not cared for properly, more serious complications can occur.

The etiology, pathophysiology, clinical manifestations, medical diagnosis, and medical management of the most common oral infections are presented in Table 22–1. Although these problems may be treated in a primary physician's office, they may also commonly be cared for in outpatient settings such as an employee health center or a walk-in treatment center.

NURSING PROCESS
Oral Infection

Assessment

When assessing a patient with an oral infection, wear a mask and gloves. Begin with careful inspection of the mouth. Use a penlight and tongue blade to visualize all areas of the mouth, including under the tongue and inside the lips, which can be retracted with the tongue blade. Examine the lips for color, hydration, and lesions, especially in the angles. Check the gums for retraction, inflammation, edema, bleeding, and lesions. Note the odor of the breath, and question the patient about any unusual tastes or areas of soreness in the mouth.

Review the patient's usual pattern of oral hygiene. Explore recent activities or stresses that may have prompted development of an oral infection. Ask if the patient has a history of oral infections.

Assess the patient's general nutritional status. In-

Table 22–1

Common Infections of the Mouth

Type of Infection	Etiology and Pathophysiology	Clinical Manifestations	Medical Diagnosis	Medical Management
Herpes labialis (cold sores)	Caused by herpes simplex virus. Latent virus appears to be activated by an external factor such as cold or fever. Vesicles form scab, and heal in 1 to 3 weeks without scarring. Wide variation in individual susceptibility.	Clear vesicles, most often located at the mucocutaneous junction of the lips and face, which scab.	Based on clinical appearance and history.	No specific treatment available. Symptomatic relief is provided by topical anesthetics.
Aphthous ulcers (canker sore or ulcerative stomatitis)	Cause is unknown, although hereditary predisposition and involvement of Ig-E–bearing lymphocytes appear to be involved. Occur more often in women.	Painful, shallow, pseudomembranous covered ulcers with a ring of erythema, occurring on the oral mucosa.	Based on clinical appearance and history.	Topical anesthetics such as viscous lidocaine or the antihistamine diphenhydramine held in the mouth provide symptomatic relief, as do bland washes and mild analgesics. Antibiotic suspensions such as tetracycline, 250 mg/mL, held on ulcers for 2 minutes four to five times per day, promote healing. Short courses of corticosteroids (eg, 40 mg prednisone q.d., 2–3 days) control severe symptoms.
Acute gingivitis (acute necrotizing ulcerative gingivitis, trench mouth, or Vincent's disease)	Noncontagious, acute infection of the gums, often associated with fusiform bacilli or a spirochete. No epidemiologic pattern is seen. Malnutrition, stress, fatigue, and poor oral hygiene appear to be predisposing factors.	Foul taste in the mouth. Malaise. Occasional fever and lymphadenopathy.	Based on clinical symptoms and response to treatment.	Good oral hygiene. Hydrogen peroxide mouthwashes. Balanced diet. Penicillin or erythromycin, 250 mg PO q.i.d., if fever or lymphadenopathy is present.
Chronic gingivitis	Related to poor mouth care, irritating fillings, or poorly fitting dentures.	Often asymptomatic, although gums may be reddened and edematous and may be painful and bleed after brushing or flossing.	Based on history and physical findings.	Improved oral and dental care.

Table 22–1

Common Infections of the Mouth *(continued)*

Type of Infection	Etiology and Pathophysiology	Clinical Manifestations	Medical Diagnosis	Medical Management
Moniliasis (thrush)	Infection with the fungus *Candida albicans*, which is part of the normal flora of the mouth. Often associated with dentures, poor oral hygiene, diabetes mellitus, and the use of antibiotics. Apparently noncontagious.	Creamy white patches of fungus on the mucous membranes that resemble mild curds and are surronded by erythematous mucosa.	Based on smear or culture showing the fungus.	Nystatin suspension, chewable tablets, or lozenges, 100,000 units three to four times q.d.

q.d., every day; PO, by mouth; q.i.d., four times a day.

quire about any dietary changes necessitated by the oral infection. If these changes are significant and prolonged, review the current diet for nutritional adequacy and check for weight loss and signs of nutritional deficiency.

Also assess for any misconceptions related to the infection, particularly its contagion and cause.

Nursing Diagnoses and Planning

Nursing diagnoses and related expected patient outcomes commonly applicable to patients with oral infections include the following:

NDx: Pain related to irritation of ulcerated areas in the mouth when eating or speaking

Planning: Patient Outcomes
1. Patient uses pain medication or topical anesthetic as needed.
2. Patient avoids irritating foods and fluids.
3. Patient states mouth is less sore.
4. Lesions are decreasing in size and number.

NDx: Risk for altered health maintenance related to insufficient knowledge of nature of the infection, treatment, and measures to prevent recurrence

Planning: Patient Outcomes
1. Patient describes the infection, stating cause, usual duration, and degree of contagion.
2. Patient explains treatment regimen to be followed at home.
3. Patient describes relationship of oral hygiene, nutrition, and stress to the development of oral infections.
4. Patient demonstrates good oral hygiene.

Nursing Interventions and Evaluation

NDx: Pain
Minimize discomfort and aid healing by administering mild analgesics and topical anesthetic preparations, such as viscous lidocaine (viscous Xylocaine), as prescribed. Instruct the patient in the use of mouth rinses, which can be medicated solutions or simply quarter-strength hydrogen peroxide and water, used every 1 to 2 hours. Limit the diet to soothing foods, such as Jell-O, pudding, eggnogs, cool drinks, and custards.

NDx: Risk for altered health maintenance
Explain the cause, expected course, usual duration, and contagion of the infection to the patient. Review the treatment regimen, making certain that the patient understands the importance of taking antibiotics on a consistent schedule and taking all doses ordered, even if symptoms have disappeared.

Instruct the patient and family on the value and technique of good oral hygiene, the importance of good nutrition, and the control of stress in the prevention of recurrences.

Compare the patient's status with the expected outcomes. If the outcomes are not met, reassess the patient and revise the plan.

ESOPHAGITIS

Etiology and Pathophysiology
Esophagitis is an inflammation of the esophagus. As with any inflammation, esophagitis may be triggered by a variety of thermal, chemical, physical, and mechanical factors. These include:

- Smoking
- Intake of alcohol or spicy foods
- Ingestion of caustic agents (such as lye or ammonia)
- Reflux of acidic gastric contents into the esophagus from gastroesophageal reflux disease
- Friction from the movement of a sliding hiatal hernia
- Prolonged gastric intubation
- Bacterial or viral invasion of the esophageal wall

Of these, reflux of gastric contents is most often the causative factor.

Clinical Manifestations

The onset of symptoms of esophagitis may be sudden or gradual. Classic symptoms include:

- Burning
- Retrosternal discomfort (pyrosis, usually called heartburn)
- Pain on swallowing, which may radiate into the arms, neck, back, or jaw
- Eructation (belching) or acid regurgitation

The effects of the inflammatory process on the esophagus range from a local area of hyperemia to edema, necrosis, and ulceration, depending on the nature of the causative agent and the amount and duration of exposure to it. With prolonged or recurrent inflammation, the esophageal wall may become thickened and fibrotic. If the esophageal lumen is narrowed from edema or fibrosis, dysphagia for solid foods may develop. In severe cases involving mucosal erosion, bleeding may develop, manifested as hematemesis or melena.

Diagnosis

Diagnosis of esophagitis is based on symptoms, history of recent exposure to irritating factors, and, if needed, direct examination of the mucosa with an esophagoscope.

Management

Treatment of esophagitis aims to eliminate the causative factor and promote an environment conducive to healing within the esophagus. For patients with simple esophagitis, management usually includes a bland diet, elimination or reduction of smoking, and antacids to be taken at bedtime and when pain occurs (Highlight 22–1).

If gastroesophageal reflux disease is the cause of esophagitis, drugs are prescribed to suppress acid secretion, such as ranitidine (Zantac) or omeprazole (Prilosec). Additionally, drugs that increase lower esophageal pressure, such as metoclopramide (Reglan), and prokinetic agents that increase gastric emptying, such as cisapride (Propulsid), may be ordered (Highlight 22–2). Treatment must be continued until the esophagus is completely healed and not merely until symptoms are relieved. Early discontinuation of treatment is a common cause of recurrence.

Surgical resection of the esophagus is indicated if obstruction, perforation, or hemorrhage occurs, or if severe pain persists. When gastroesophageal reflux disease is the problem, a procedure such as Nissen fundoplication may be required. This procedure will be discussed under Hiatus Hernia, a common condition in which gastroesophageal reflux occurs.

❖ **Settings, Providers, and Collaboration for Care**

Patients with simple esophagitis may be treated in a physician's office or an outpatient setting, such as a walk-in clinic or employee health department. If complications arise, such as obstruction or bleeding, hospitalization may be required.

NURSING PROCESS
Esophagitis

Assessment

Inasmuch as pain is the most prominent symptom of any esophageal disorder, determine the type, severity, and location of pain experienced by the patient. Question the patient about odynophagia (painful swallowing), pyrosis (heartburn), and diffuse epigastric pain. Also investigate the relationship between the onset or aggravation of pain and such factors as meals, ingestion of specific foods, eating at particular times, smoking, body position, or activity. Also question the patient about related symptoms, such as eructation, dysphagia, regurgitation, and hematemesis.

Assess the patient's current nutritional status. Identify the normal daily diet, and explore any changes in eating patterns necessitated by the presence of symptoms. An example of the latter would be the elimination of specific foods from the diet that the patient previously enjoyed. Nonprescription remedies may cause undesirable side effects, such as the acid rebound effect and potential for metabolic acidosis associated with the use of bicarbonate of soda as an antacid. Therefore, elicit the frequency of their use and their effects.

When the medical diagnosis has been made and treatment prescribed, assess the patient's level of understanding. Assess for other factors likely to promote or prevent compliance with the treatment regimen. These include economic factors, home and family situation, and psychologic response to the disorder and the treatment.

Nursing Diagnoses and Planning

Nursing diagnoses and related expected patient outcomes commonly applicable to patients with esophagitis include the following:

NDx: Pain related to esophageal inflammation

Planning: Patient Outcomes
1. Patient explains proper self-administration of antacids (see Highlight 22–1).
2. Patient describes the potential for aggravation of the pain by alcohol and nicotine.

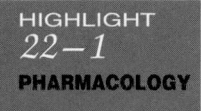
HIGHLIGHT
22–1
PHARMACOLOGY

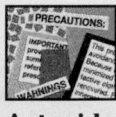
Antacids

Definition:

Over-the-counter medications that neutralize gastric acid. Most in current use are nonabsorbable and are bases of magnesium, aluminum, or calcium.

Action:

Antacids that are weak bases combine with hydrochloric acid in the stomach to form salts and water and thus raise gastric pH and decrease the proteolytic action of pepsin.

Uses:

Treatment of peptic ulcer disease, esophagitis due to reflux, gastritis, and symptomatic relief of pyrosis.

Side Effects:

Increase of gastric pH with predisposition to gastrointestinal infection is a side effect of all antacids. Other side effects are specific to the type of antacid used. Those containing magnesium can cause diarrhea, dehydration, and in patients with renal insufficiency, hypermagnesemia with neurologic, muscular, and cardiovascular changes. Those containing aluminum can cause constipation, impaction, and, with long-term use, hypophosphatemia, which can cause osteomalacia and myopathy. Calcium carbonate can cause acid rebound and milk-alkali syndrome.

Interactions:

Antacids are capable of interacting with virtually all other drugs through effects on their absorption owing to chemical binding, a change in gastric pH, or a change in gastric emptying time. Drugs whose absorption is impaired by antacids include tetracyclines,

anticholinergics, cardiac glycosides, phenothiazides, indomethacin, isoniazid, and phenylbutazone. Drugs whose absorption is accelerated include weak bases and enteric-coated preparations.

Nursing Implications:

Shake liquid preparations well, and follow with a small amount of water. If given by nasogastric tube, flush with at least 60 mL of water to prevent caking on the sides of the tube and subsequent blockage.

Instruct patients to chew chewable tablets thoroughly and follow with a full glass of water.

Give other medications 2 to 3 hours before or after antacids.

Instruct patients taking aluminum- or calcium-based antacids to drink at least 2500 mL of fluid per day to prevent constipation. Instruct those taking magnesium preparations to add bananas, rice, applesauce, and tea to the diet to combat diarrhea.

Instruct all patients to report persistent problems with bowel function as well as symptoms of electrolyte imbalance.

Warn patients that antacid therapy may cause stools to be white or speckled in appearance.

Geriatric Considerations:

The elderly are at risk for hypermagnesemia and other fluid and electrolyte imbalances when taking magnesium-containing antacids.

The elderly, especially those with dehydration, decreased bowel motility, or renal disease, are at risk for severe constipation and impaction when taking calcium- or aluminum-containing antacids.

---

3. Patient states that discomfort has decreased.
4. Patient reports absence of discomfort when swallowing nonirritating foods and fluids.

NDx: Risk for constipation or diarrhea related to use of antacids (*specify*)

Planning: Patient Outcomes
1. Patient describes effects of antacids on bowel activity.
2. Patient lists measures to promote normal bowel activity.
3. Patient reports regular passage of soft, formed stool.

NDx: Risk for altered health maintenance related to insufficient knowledge of the disorder, dietary modifications, measures to limit gastric reflux, and use of prescribed medications

Planning: Patient Outcomes
1. Patient describes the causes, effects, and usual clinical course of esophagitis.
2. Patient lists symptoms to be reported, such as hematemesis and melena.
3. Patient lists foods to be avoided.
4. Patient describes benefit of small, frequent feedings.

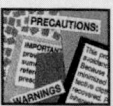

Drugs That Decrease Gastric Acid Secretion

HISTAMINE$_2$-RECEPTOR ANTAGONISTS

Definition:

Drugs that block the histamine H$_2$-receptor sites as opposed to H$_1$-receptor sites blocked by traditional antihistamines.

Action:

Block the H$_2$-receptor sites on the gastric parietal cells, inhibiting the secretion of hydrochloric acid (HCl). Also decrease HCl secretion in response to other chemical and nervous stimuli. Have no significant cardiovascular effects at the doses used to treat gastric disease.

Uses:

Treatment of peptic ulcer disease, Zollinger-Ellison syndrome and other hypersecretory disorders, and gastrointestinal reflux. Prevention of stress ulcers.

Side Effects:

Infrequent with cimetidine and ranitidine.

Cimetidine—Occasional mild diarrhea, nausea, dizziness, rash, and muscle aches. May also cause impotence, decreased sperm count, and gynecomastia in males and galactorrhea in females because of antiandrogenic effects.

Ranitidine—Headache, nausea, and constipation.

Famotidine—Headache, diarrhea, dizziness, and constipation.

Interactions:

Antacids decrease the absorption of H$_2$-receptor antagonists.

Cimetidine mildly inhibits the cytochrome oxidase system of the liver and thereby increases the half-life of drugs such as diazepam, flurazepam, warfarin, and theophylline; also beta-blockers, phenytoin, salicylates, and quinidine.

Cimetidine plus morphine can cause muscle twitching, confusion, and apnea.

Cimetidine can decrease serum levels of dioxin, decrease absorption of ketoconazole, and increase effects of carbamazepine and procainamide.

Nursing Implications:

Give H$_2$ blockers at least 1 hour before or after antacids.

Do not dilute with sterile water for injection; use a compatible solution as listed on the label.

Observe elderly patients on cimetidine for confusion.

Monitor fluid intake and output of elderly patients and those with impaired renal function. Instruct patients to take with meals so that the peak effect coincides with the time of maximum secretion of gastric acid; avoid cigarette smoking because it impairs the effect of H$_2$ blockers; not self-dose for pain—take prescribed doses only; and report persistent or worsening side effects.

Explain the need for periodic blood counts and tests of renal and hepatic function when taking H$_2$ blockers for longer than 4 weeks.

Geriatric Considerations:

Mental confusion, agitation, depression, and hallucinations may occur in the elderly. These effects are most common with cimetidine and are usually associated with decreased renal function.

PROTON-PUMP INHIBITORS

Definition:

Drugs that block the "proton pump" on the lumen side of the parietal cell.

Action:

Block the enzyme K$^+$H$^+$-ATPase on the parietal cells of the stomach, preventing final transport of hydrogen ions into the gastric lumen.

Uses:

Approved by the Food and Drug Administration for short-term therapy in ulcer disease.

Side Effects:

As for H$_2$-receptor antagonists, less than 1% exhibit headache, diarrhea, nausea and vomiting when used in short-term therapy.

Interactions:

May increase effects of phenytoin, diazepam, and warfarin, may interfere with absorption of drugs requiring acidic gastric pH.

Nursing Implications:

Do not crush, open or chew capsules—they should be given whole.

Patients should be instructed to take medication for the full course of treatment, even if they begin to feel better.

Therapy should be limited to 4 to 8 weeks.

5. Patient states plan for implementing dietary changes.
6. Patient verbalizes the importance of and a realistic plan for reducing or eliminating smoking.
7. Patient explains relationship of tight clothing and body positions to reflux of gastric contents into the esophagus.
8. Patient identifies name, use, dose, time, route of administration, and side effects of each prescribed drug.

Nursing Interventions and Evaluation

NDx: Pain
Administer or teach the patient to self-administer antacids prescribed for pain (see Highlight 22–1). Encourage use of relaxation techniques to assist the patient in handling the pain. Caution the patient against smoking or drinking alcohol in an attempt to relax and relieve the pain, because these activities can in fact aggravate the condition.

NDx: Risk for constipation or diarrhea
Explain to the patient that aluminum- or calcium-based antacids have a tendency to cause constipation and magnesium-based antacids can cause diarrhea. If the patient is taking an aluminum- or calcium-based antacid, review the importance of plenty of fluids and roughage in the diet, as well as the value of regular exercise, in preventing constipation. If the patient is taking a magnesium-based antacid, advise the patient to avoid large amounts of fresh fruits, vegetables, and other foods that stimulate bowel function, such as licorice. In all cases, instruct the patient to report uncomfortable constipation or diarrhea, because it is possible to use antacids in combination and thus control these side effects.

NDx: Risk for altered health maintenance
Explain the causes, effects, and usual clinical course of esophagitis to the patient at a level he or she can understand. Describe the role of gastric reflux as a causative or exacerbating factor. Alert the patient to symptoms—such as hematemesis and melena—that should be promptly reported.

Instruct the patient and family about dietary modifications that facilitate healing and help prevent recurrence. Stress the need to avoid alcohol, caffeine, and any food that causes pain. Because gastric reflux is a factor in the vast majority of cases of esophagitis, recommend small, frequent meals to help reduce secretion of gastric acid. Initiate a consultation with a dietitian to assist the patient with meal planning, if needed. To further aid in preventing gastric reflux, instruct the patient to avoid eating for 2 to 3 hours before bedtime, to remain in an upright position for 2 to 3 hours after eating, and to avoid bending and wearing tight clothes.

Teach the patient the dose, route, time, frequency, expected side effects, and signs of toxic effects of all prescribed medications.

Compare the patient's status with the expected outcomes. If the outcomes are not met, reassess the patient and revise the plan.

ACUTE GASTRITIS

Acute gastritis is a self-limiting inflammation of the stomach mucosa. It may be diffuse or localized. In the diffuse form, all areas of the stomach are affected. In the localized form, only a specific area is involved.

Etiology and Pathophysiology
Acute gastritis can result from any chemical, thermal, bacterial, or mechanical factor that injures the gastric mucosa. Examples of these factors include:

- Drugs, such as aspirin, digitalis, and steroids
- Alcohol
- Excessive amounts of irritating foods such as tea, coffee, pepper, and other spices
- Foods that are very rough, very hot, or contaminated with *Staphylococcus*
- Corrosive substances
- Exposure to radiation

Acute gastritis may also develop in association with severe medical problems, such as acute respiratory failure, sepsis, renal failure, advanced carcinomatosis, hypovolemic shock, and extensive trauma.

Regardless of the specific precipitating factor, the involved mucosa exhibits vascular congestion, edema, petechial hemorrhages, and areas of erosion and superficial ulceration. All of these are reversible, although healing time varies with the cause.

Clinical Manifestations
Acute gastritis is often asymptomatic. When symptoms do occur, they include one or more of the following: epigastric pain, abdominal tenderness, nausea, vomiting, and eructation. If the gastritis is of the hemorrhagic type, as caused by aspirin or stress, hematemesis or melena also occurs, accompanied by decreased hematocrit and elevated blood urea nitrogen.

Diagnosis
The diagnosis of acute gastritis is based on endoscopy or biopsy.

Management
Acute gastritis is treated only when symptoms are present. Treatment consists of removing the precipitating factor when possible, giving antiemetics to control nausea and vomiting, or initiating antacid and H_2-antagonist therapy to decrease gastric secretions that can further irritate inflamed areas. In cases of acute hemorrhagic gastritis, parenteral fluid, blood replacement, and nasogastric lavage may also be required.

❖ **Settings, Providers, and Collaboration for Care**

Like esophagitis, uncomplicated acute gastritis may be treated in a variety of outpatient settings, such as a clinic, employee health service, or physician's office. Patients may look to their local pharmacist for advice about antacids or over-the-counter histamine receptor antagonists.

NURSING PROCESS
Acute Gastritis

Assessment

History and the subjective description of symptoms are critical to the assessment of the patient with gastritis. Carefully question the patient regarding location, onset, and duration of pain in addition to factors that relieve or aggravate pain. Collect information about changes in appetite and eating habits as well as data about eructation, weight changes, and color and character of stool. If emesis is reported, question the patient about its characteristics, such as the presence of red blood, "coffee grounds," or bile, as well as its relationship to nausea. Elicit information related to possible precipitating factors. Ask the patient about use of prescription or over-the-counter medications; ingestion of alcoholic beverages, tea, and coffee; and types of foods included in the usual daily diet.

Assess the patient's understanding of and reaction to the problem and its treatment. Keep in mind that anxiety over the meaning of the symptoms is common, especially in patients with hematemesis.

During physical examination, check for upper abdominal tenderness and signs of dehydration. Also observe for signs of systemic disease that might be related to the gastritis.

Nursing Diagnoses and Planning

Nursing diagnoses and related expected patient outcomes commonly applicable to patients with acute gastritis include the following:

NDx: Pain related to inflammation of the gastric mucosa

Planning: Patient Outcomes
1. Patient states that pain is decreased or absent.
2. Behavioral signs of pain, such as moaning and holding the upper abdomen, are absent.

NDx: Risk for fluid volume deficit related to vomiting and limited fluid intake

Planning: Patient Outcomes
1. Skin turgor is firm.
2. Mucous membranes are moist.
3. Urinary output is at least 50 mL/hour or 1500 mL/day.

4. Serum electrolyte levels are within normal range.
5. Symptoms of electrolyte imbalance are absent.

NDx: Risk for altered health maintenance related to insufficient knowledge of causes and prevention of acute gastritis

Planning: Patient Outcomes
1. Patient names any identified causative factors.
2. Patient describes how to avoid causative factors in the future.
3. Patient lists irritating substances that can contribute to gastritis.
4. Patient identifies changes in eating habits necessary to avoid irritating food substances.
5. Patient identifies substitute foods or food seasonings for those to be avoided as well as correct methods of food preparation.

Nursing Interventions and Evaluation

NDx: Pain
Administer prescribed antacids to neutralize gastric acid and raise gastric pH. Administer H_2- antagonists to inhibit gastric acid secretion. Encourage the patient to avoid cigarette smoking because nicotine increases gastric acidity. Provide restful diversion, such as soft music, and encourage the use of controlled breathing or other relaxation techniques.

NDx: Risk for fluid volume deficit
Initiate interventions to control vomiting. Keep the patient on NPO status, administer antiemetics as ordered, and maintain a quiet environment. Monitor intravenous fluids. Maintain an accurate record of fluid intake and output. Review electrolyte values daily.

When the acute phase has passed, start the patient on clear fluids and progress to a full bland diet divided into several small feedings, as tolerated.

NDx: Risk for altered health maintenance
Explain the causative factor to the patient if a specific one, such as a drug or contaminated food, is identified. Provide information needed to enable the patient to avoid exposure to it in the future. For example, if aspirin is involved, explain that aspirin is found in many over-the-counter medications, such as Alka-Seltzer. Instruct the patient to read labels or consult with the pharmacist before using new products. If contaminated food was responsible, review the patient's knowledge of proper food storage and preparation techniques. In all cases, explain the role of irritating foods, and assist the patient in identifying desirable changes in his or her daily diet. When indicated, initiate a consultation with a dietitian.

Additional Interventions
Maintain the patient on bedrest during the acute phase, and check all emesis for signs of bleeding.

Compare the patient's status with the expected outcomes. If the outcomes are not met, reassess the patient and revise the plan.

CHRONIC GASTRITIS

Chronic gastritis is a long-term progressive disease. It affects women more commonly than men, and its overall frequency increases with advancing age.

Etiology and Pathophysiology

Most cases of chronic gastritis are one of two types. Type A is an autoimmune disorder associated with pernicious anemia. Autoantibodies against the intrinsic factor that causes pernicious anemia also infiltrate the gastric mucosa, resulting in decreased parietal cells and atrophy of the mucosa. This type of gastritis usually occurs in the body of the stomach.

Type B chronic gastritis primarily involves the antrum of the stomach. The bacterium *Helicobacter pylori* has been found universally in type B chronic gastritis.

Chronic gastritis begins as superficial gastritis, in which inflammatory changes are limited to the upper portion of the mucosa. As the process invades the mucosa more deeply, it is referred to as atrophic gastritis. In this stage, the mucosa becomes thin, and parietal and chief cells are absent. The progressive decrease in gastric acid secretion results in altered digestion.

Gastric cancer occurs more often in patients with chronic gastritis than in the general population. However, no causal relationship has been confirmed.

Clinical Manifestations

Chronic gastritis is often asymptomatic. When symptoms do occur, they resemble those of peptic ulcer disease or gastric cancer. Epigastric fullness, burning or pain, nausea, vomiting, and flatulence may occur, especially following large meals. Anorexia, weight loss, and symptoms of anemia also develop.

Diagnosis

Definitive diagnosis of chronic gastritis is based on endoscopy with gastric biopsy. Because the disease process may be localized, several biopsies from different areas of the stomach are required.

Management

There is no specific treatment for chronic gastritis. Symptomatic relief is typically obtained with antacid therapy and a bland diet taken in small, frequent feedings throughout the day. Patients are monitored for development of pernicious anemia, which requires monthly injections of vitamin B_{12} for life, as well as for the occurrence of gastric cancer.

❖ Settings, Providers and Collaboration for Care

Chronic gastritis, as its name suggests, is a disorder requiring treatment over a long period of time. Follow-up visits to the physician, along with repeated diagnostic testing, is imperative. Consultation with a dietitian may be indicated. Complications (such as severe bleeding) require treatment in an emergency department and possibly admission to the hospital.

NURSING PROCESS GUIDELINES
Chronic Gastritis

The assessment, nursing diagnoses, expected patient outcomes, nursing interventions, and evaluation for patients with chronic gastritis are similar to those described previously for patients with acute gastritis, with the following considerations.

Because patients with chronic gastritis commonly fail to receive follow-up care, be sure to stress the importance of physical examination on a regular basis. Discuss the relationship of chronic gastritis to pernicious anemia and gastric cancer. Explain the importance of observing for and reporting stomatitis, glossitis, and symptoms of vitamin B_{12} deficiency (Fig. 22–1).

Structural and Functional Disorders

PEPTIC ULCER DISEASE

Peptic ulcer is a general term that refers to a sharply defined break in the muscularis mucosae in any part of the gastrointestinal tract that is exposed to gastric secretions that contain acid and pepsin (Fig. 22–2). Thus, a peptic ulcer can occur in the distal esophagus, the stomach, the duodenum, or any part of the intestinal tract that has been surgically connected to the stomach. When referring to an ulcer, it is necessary to identify it by location—for example, a gastric ulcer or a duodenal ulcer—because there are differences in incidence and etiology.

Ulcer disease is a common disorder. Some 5 to 10% of persons in the United States suffer from peptic ulcer disease during their lifetimes. Peak incidence of duodenal ulcers is between ages 30 and 50 although the disorder is not uncommon in 20-year-

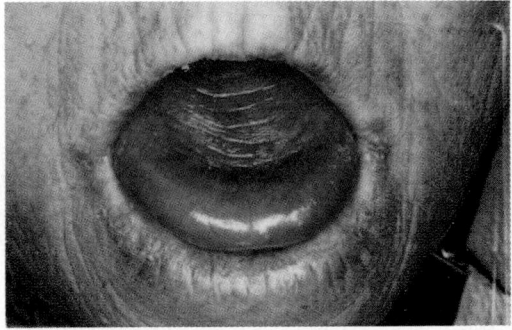

Figure 22–1

Severe atrophic glossitis. The tongue is painful, smooth, shiny, and bright red as a result of the atrophy of papillae. (From Sleisenger MH, Fordtran JS. Gastrointestinal disease: Pathophysiology/diagnosis/management. 5th ed. Philadelphia: WB Saunders, 1993.)

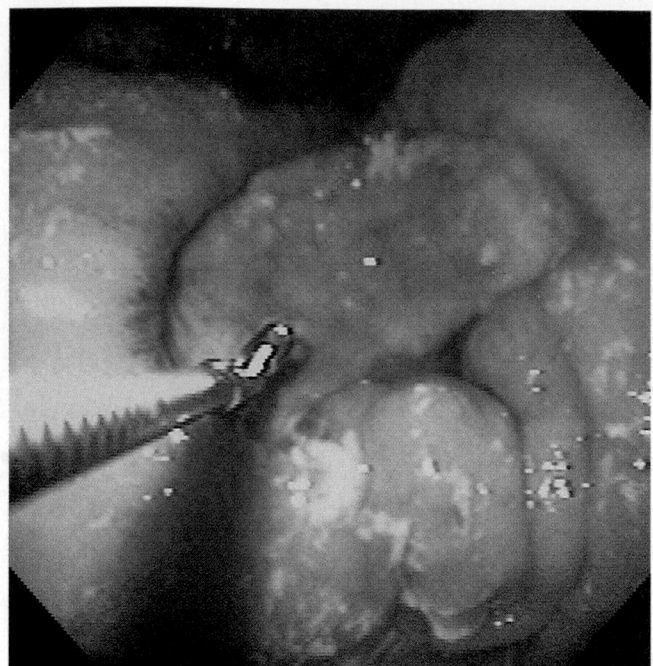

Figure 22–2

Large, deeply excavated peptic ulcer. (From Wilcox CM. Atlas of gastrointestinal endoscopy. Philadelphia: WB Saunders, 1995.)

olds. Gastric ulcers, in contrast, are more common in persons between ages 50 and 70. Both types of ulcer can occur in the same person. In fact, they occur together 20 times more often than would be expected.

Etiology and Pathophysiology

Ulceration of the gastrointestinal mucosa is believed to result from an imbalance between the resistance of the mucosa to injury and the amount of gastric secretions. Although the precise determinants of these two variables are unknown, many factors have been implicated. The finding that duodenal ulcers are more common in those with type O blood suggests a hereditary or genetic relationship. Use of nonsteroidal anti-inflammatory drugs, such as salicylates, indomethacin, ibuprofen, and the glucocorticoids, correlates highly with development of gastric ulcers. Smoking is associated with increased incidence of gastric and duodenal ulcers, more complications, and slower healing—possibly because smoking inhibits bicarbonate secretion from the pancreas. Personality characteristics, such as compulsive "Type A" behavior, as well as life stressors are no longer considered to be important in the development of ulcers. It remains true, however, that the effect of the autonomic nervous system on gastric blood flow continues to be an important factor in the healing of existing ulcers.

The recent discovery of the role of the bacterium *Helicobacter pylori* in ulcer disease has added a new dimension to the understanding and treatment of peptic ulcer disease. This organism has been found in 80% of patients with gastric ulcers and nearly all

of those with duodenal ulcers. The organism may be transmitted via the fecal-oral route, much like the hepatitis A virus. Studies indicate that 40 to 50% of persons in developed countries are infected with this bacterium, with much larger numbers in developing nations. The organism secretes the enzyme urease, which results in production of ammonia and the subsequent inflammatory response.

Recurrence of ulcers that have healed has always been a treatment problem. Some sources indicate a 50 to 80% recurrence within one year of healing, even with maintenance treatment. Recent studies on the importance of *H. pylori* in ulcer disease indicate that eradication of the bacteria is essential in preventing recurrence of lesions.

In the person with a gastric ulcer, gastric secretion is normal or even reduced, and gastric emptying time is unchanged. There is, however, an impairment of the mucosal barrier of the stomach, which normally prevents back-diffusion of hydrochloric acid. Possible causes of such damage include reflux of bile acids into the stomach, decreased blood flow to the gastric mucosa, and the inflammatory response initiated by *H. pylori*.

In the person with a duodenal ulcer, mucosal resistance is normal, but numbers of parietal cells in the stomach are increased, as is the volume of gastric acid. Plus, stomach contents empty more rapidly into the duodenum. The effect of these changes is that the duodenal mucosa is exposed to an abnormally low pH for an extended period of time. Although the gastric mucosa is the natural habitat of *H. pylori*, it is thought that the cells lining the duodenum undergo metaplasia, resulting in gastric-like cells in the duodenum. This change, plus increased acid secretion by the stomach, allows the organism to migrate to the duodenum and colonize there.

Regardless of type or cause, progressive ulceration can result in massive hemorrhage if the wall of a large blood vessel erodes. Or it can result in peritonitis if the wall of the stomach or intestine is perforated. If an ulcer is in the narrow pyloric area, associated edema can result in partial or total obstruction of the gastrointestinal tract.

Clinical Manifestations

The major symptom of uncomplicated peptic ulcer is pain. Associated symptoms include a change in appetite and weight, and very rarely nausea and vomiting. Ulcer pain may be described as a feeling of pressure, burning, heaviness, or hunger. The pain, which can vary from mild to severe, is sharply localized near the midline of the epigastrium in an area that the patient can usually point to with one finger.

Usually, the onset of pain relates directly to gastric activity, with pain occurring a few hours following meals, at bedtime, and in the middle of the night, when gastric activity is high and there is no food to act as a buffer. Because the patient with duodenal ulcers has increased acidity and gastric emptying time, food usually relieves the pain—a pain-food-relief pattern. Therefore, these patients commonly have good appetites and may even gain weight.

With gastric ulcer, the pain has no clear pattern because the gastric mucosa is sensitive to any acid secretion. Some patients have relatively constant pain. These patients tend to be anorexic, fearful of the effect of food on the pain, and usually experience weight loss.

Ulcer pain may worsen under conditions of emotional stress, tension, fatigue, or exposure to cold. See Table 22–2 for a summary of ulcer disease.

Diagnosis

The diagnosis of peptic ulcer disease is suggested by the patient's history of pain and confirmed by endoscopy. Barium studies are of little value because they cannot locate the exact lesion or determine the extent of mucosal damage. Similarly, physical examination yields few significant data. The presence of *H. pylori* can be established by biopsy of tissue taken during endoscopy or by serology tests for antibodies to the organism. The advantages of the serology test are that it is noninvasive and has a high degree of sensitivity and specificity. However, serology tests are not useful in monitoring a treatment protocol because they stay positive for an indefinite period of time.

Management

Medical management is designed to relieve symptoms, promote mucosal healing by controlling gastric acid, prevent or detect complications, and prevent recurrence by eradicating *H. pylori*. The treatment is similar regardless of the ulcer's location and is based on a program of dietary modification, rest, and medications.

Diet

Dietary therapy for the patient with an ulcer today is much more flexible than in the past. The traditional ulcer diet used to involve elimination of all potentially irritating food and ingestion of large amounts of milk and cream. Because research failed to support the effectiveness of this regimen, dietary modification now hinges on the patient's tolerance of specific foods. If a food causes pain, it should be reduced or eliminated from the diet. Substances likely to fit this category include heavily spiced foods, fresh fruits, and alcohol. Caffeine is also restricted because it stimulates gastric acid secretion.

In addition to avoiding pain-producing foods, patients may be encouraged to eat smaller, more frequent meals to create a more continual neutralization of gastric acid. All these dietary factors are determined individually for each patient. Absence of pain indicates manageable acid levels and is the best guide to determining diet changes.

Drug Therapy

Medications used to treat ulcer disease include antacids, drugs that reduce production of stomach acid, drugs that protect the gastric mucosa, and antibiotics effective against *H. pylori*.

Antacids (see Highlight 22–1) neutralize acid in the stomach and thereby relieve pain. Antacids do not heal the ulcer, but they do provide an environ-

Table 22–2

Differential Features of Peptic Ulcers

Type	Incidence	Pathophysiology	Clinical Features
Duodenal ulcer	75% of peptic ulcers M:F 3:1 20–50 years	Normal to reduced parietal cell mass Normal to reduced acid secretion Normal to reduced gastrin levels *Helicobacter pylori* nearly always present Associations: COPD, cirrhosis, pancreatitis	Rhythmic, periodic pain Pain-food-relief pattern Sometimes asymptomatic
Gastric ulcer	M:F about equal 50–70 years	Normal to reduced parietal cell mass Normal to reduced acid secretion Normal to reduced gastrin levels *Helicobacter pylori* present in about 80% of non-NSAID cases Incompetent gastric mucosa Associations: chronic gastritis, drugs	Variable pain Pain-food-relief or food-pain pattern Weight loss Anorexia
Stress ulcer	Studies find gastric lesions in nearly all patients at risk No gender difference	Head injuries: marked acid hypersecretion Others: gastric mucosa ischemia, acid back-diffusion *Helicobacter pylori* not present Associations: sepsis, burns, trauma, head injuries	Few actual clinical symptoms Unexpected slight or severe bleeding 2–10 days following trauma

COPD, chronic obstructive pulmonary disease; M:F, male-to-female ratio; NSAID, nonsteroidal anti-inflammatory drug.

ment conducive to healing. They are usually taken at bedtime and 1 to 3 hours after meals because the presence of food in the stomach delays gastric emptying and prolongs the time the antacid is in the stomach. Their effects last only 30 to 60 minutes, so they may be required much more frequently by some patients. If the patient is awakened by pain during the night, antacids may be taken routinely about 1 hour before the time at which pain usually occurs.

The histamine H_2-receptor antagonists (see Highlight 22–2) such as cimetidine (Tagamet) and ranitidine (Zantac) decrease basal secretion of gastric acid to almost zero and food-induced secretion of acid by 75%. This decrease in gastric acid reduces further irritation to the mucosa and thus facilitates healing. Duration of action is 6 to 7 hours for cimetidine and 10 to 12 hours for ranitidine. However, because studies have failed to show that ulcers heal faster in response to treatment with histamine H_2-receptor antagonists as opposed to antacids, the main reason for their use is convenience. Because they are effective for 6 to 12 hours, the patient can take one tablet two or four times daily instead of four or more 30 mL doses of liquid antacid.

Proton-pump inhibitors, such as omeprazole (Prilosec), inhibit gastric acid secretion by blocking final transport of hydrogen ions into the gastric lumen. These new drugs also assist in eradicating *H. pylori*.

Also used in the treatment of peptic ulcer disease is sucralfate (Carafate). This drug promotes healing by coating the ulcer, thus protecting it against further damage from acid and pepsin. Sucralfate is not absorbed, has minimal side effects, and neither neutralizes acid nor decreases acid secretion. Another drug that functions by coating the gastric mucosa is bismuth subsalicylate (Pepto-Bismol).

Antibiotic therapy protocols for eradicating *H. pylori* include amoxicillin (Amoxil), metronidazole (Flagyl), and clarithromycin (Biaxin). Interestingly, bismuth subsalicylate has also been found to be bacteriocidal for *H. pylori*, and is part of many treatment protocols for eradicating the organism. The most recent protocols involve two antibiotics and a proton-pump inhibitor for 1 to 2 weeks.

To further control acid secretion, patients with ulcer disease are advised to reduce or quit smoking. This is because nicotine reduces the bicarbonate content of pancreatic secretions and therefore decreases the degree of gastric acid neutralization. Because alcohol and aspirin are directly absorbed across the gastric mucosa, they should be avoided too, although many physicians allow small amounts of wine or alcohol with meals.

Sedatives or tranquilizers may be prescribed to promote physical and psychologic rest.

Surgery

When a complication (hemorrhage, obstruction, or perforation) occurs, or in cases where conservative treatment is unsatisfactory, surgery is performed.

Among the most common surgical procedures for peptic ulcer disease are gastric resection, vagotomy, and pyloroplasty.

In a gastric resection or subtotal gastrectomy done for peptic ulcer disease, the distal portion of the stomach, including the antrum and the pylorus, is removed. The remaining stomach is then attached either to the duodenum via an end-to-end anastomosis as in a Billroth I procedure, or to the jejunum via an end-to-side anastomosis as in a Billroth II procedure (see Chap. 21). This procedure involves removal of the ulcer and a large portion of the parietal cells that produce hydrochloric acid, as well as the antrum of the stomach, where gastrin is secreted. Because gastrin is the hormone that stimulates secretion of hydrochloric acid and pepsinogen, future hypersecretion of damaging secretions is limited. A Billroth II procedure is usually preferred for treating duodenal ulcers because gastric contents bypass the duodenum, resulting in a lower incidence of reulceration.

Vagotomy, or cutting of the vagus nerve, is done to eliminate parasympathetic stimulation of gastric secretion (Fig. 22–3). If the vagus nerves are cut as they enter the stomach (truncal vagotomy), gastric secretion is decreased, but intestinal motility is also decreased and gastric emptying delayed. The latter effects are sometimes avoided by a selective vagotomy in which only those branches of the vagus nerve that innervate the parietal cells are cut. Vagotomy is commonly done in conjunction with other surgical procedures for ulcers to ensure continued reduction of acid secretion and to reduce the potential for reulceration.

A pyloroplasty is a procedure in which the pylorus is incised and resutured to relax the muscle and

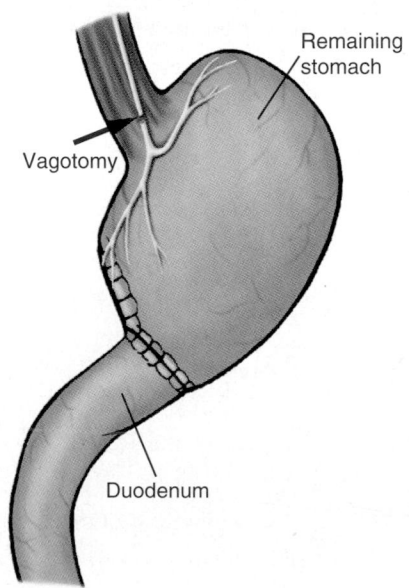

Figure 22–3

Billroth I with vagotomy.

enlarge the opening from the stomach to the duodenum to increase the rate of gastric emptying. It is done to relieve or prevent obstruction in the pylorus caused by the effects of vagotomy or the presence of scar tissue. See Chapter 21 for more details on gastric surgery.

Complications

The three major complications of peptic ulcer disease are hemorrhage, gastrointestinal obstruction, and perforation.

Hemorrhage

Hemorrhage occurs when the wall of a large blood vessel is eroded through (Fig. 22–4). It is manifested by vomiting of frank blood, by the presence of coffee-ground material in emesis or nasogastric drainage, or by melena. The preferred treatment is nonsurgical because the bleeding patient is a poor surgical risk. One treatment approach involves continuous gastric lavage with cool saline. A second approach is transendoscopic treatment, such as sclerotherapy, topical therapy with tissue adhesives or coagulative agents, electrocoagulation, or laser photocoagulation. Once the bleeding is controlled, ulcer medication and diet regimen are slowly reinstated. Care of the patient with gastrointestinal bleeding is discussed in Chapter 21.

Obstruction

Obstruction occurs secondary to edema or scarring, most often in the narrow pyloric region. Its primary symptoms are a sensation of fullness followed by vomiting of partially digested gastric contents, and abdominal distention. Conservative treatment includes maintenance of fluid and electrolyte balance through intravenous therapy, and nasogastric suction of stomach contents until healing occurs.

Perforation

Perforation occurs when the ulcerative process has extended through the gastric or duodenal wall, creating an opening through which gastrointestinal contents may spill into the peritoneal cavity. The result of such spillage is an immediate chemical peritonitis and subsequent bacterial peritonitis caused in most cases by *Escherichia coli*, staphylococci, or streptococci. Posterior perforations may self-seal or manifest as an abscess.

Symptoms of perforation depend on the size and location of the defect. Acute gastric perforation is characterized by sudden, sharp, intolerably severe pain beginning in the midepigastric area and spreading over the abdomen, which becomes rigid and boardlike. Referred pain to the shoulder may also occur via the phrenic nerve from irritation of the diaphragm. Nausea is common and occasionally accompanied by vomiting. Peristalsis decreases and paralytic ileus develops. Respirations are rapid and shallow, with minimal movement of painful abdominal muscles. Hypovolemic shock occurs, and the patient develops tachycardia, pallor, cold clammy skin, and decreased blood pressure. Progression of peritonitis is very rapid and may result in death within 72 hours. With duodenal perforation, symptoms are usually similar, but vital signs may remain within normal range.

In cases of very small perforations that close almost immediately by adhering to adjoining tissues and therefore are accompanied by little or no spillage of gastrointestinal contents, the immediate symptoms are similar to those previously listed but quickly subside. Abscess formation may follow in some cases, however.

Immediate treatment of perforation involves gastrointestinal suction by nasogastric tube to prevent further spillage of gastrointestinal contents into the peritoneal cavity; fluid and electrolyte replacement; and antibiotic therapy to resolve or prevent peritonitis. With this treatment, small perforations heal completely. Larger defects require emergency surgical closure.

❖ Settings, Providers, and Collaboration for Care

Most people with ulcer disease are treated in an outpatient setting, such as a physician's office or freestanding clinic. Consultation with a dietitian may be necessary. The dietitian assists the patient and significant others with food selection and preparation. The nurse may instruct the patient about the medication regimen. Hospitalization is required only for treatment of complications, such as surgery for obstruction or gastrointestinal hemorrhage.

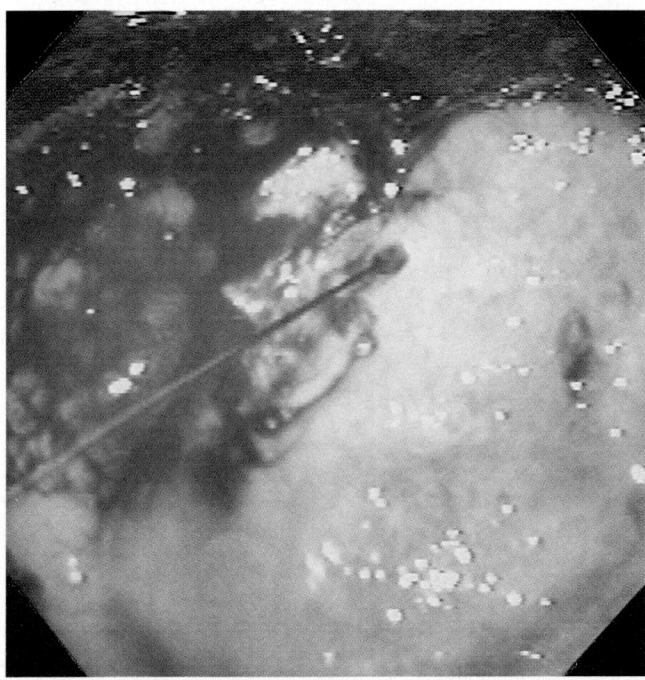

Figure 22–4

Close-up of a bleeding ulcer. (From Wilcox CM. Atlas of gastrointestinal endoscopy. Philadelphia: WB Saunders, 1995.)

CLINICAL ❓ THINKING

"INDIGESTION" AFTER A LARGE MEAL

After 4 hours of unrelieved "indigestion," a 50-year-old male was admitted to the emergency room. Despite differences in the onset, nature, and location of the pain, the patient thought his usual antacids would be sufficient to relieve the pain. He reported that the pain began as a "feeling of pressure" in his chest just after a large dinner, that it was located behind his sternum, and that it radiated to his left shoulder and arm.

The patient's blood pressure was 132/84. His apical heart rate was 88 and regular. Respirations were 18 and unlabored. Temperature was 36.7°C (98°F). He denied experiencing any other symptoms, and his pain was relieved by sublingual nitroglycerin administered in the emergency room. Serial electrocardiograph (ECG) readings and cardiac enzyme levels were not consistent with a myocardial infarction. The patient was admitted to the telemetry unit with a medical diagnosis of angina pectoris and was scheduled for a cardiac work-up.

The patient had no previous history of anginal episodes or coronary artery disease. His medical history included rheumatoid arthritis and bilateral multiple joint replacements, most recently a left shoulder replacement one year ago. He was currently being treated with nonsteroidal anti-inflammatory drugs, methotrexate, and corticosteroids during exacerbations of the disease. He also took aspirin occasionally for the pain.

The patient admitted to frequent episodes of gastrointestinal distress relieved by food or antacids, but denied any history of gastrointestinal disorders. During the nursing history, the patient stated that he had smoked about one pack of cigarettes each day for the past 30 years. He drank one or two alcoholic beverages and three or four cups of coffee each day. He also revealed that he was in the midst of changing jobs and moving his family to another state.

Shortly after report the next morning, I entered the patient's room and noted that he appeared pale, alert, and comfortable. He denied having chest pain and reported his appetite at breakfast had been good. His vital signs remained stable. At 11:30 AM, the patient summoned me via the call bell. Before leaving the nurse's station, I checked his ECG reading on the monitor and noted normal sinus rhythm with no evidence of myocardial ischemia. He stated that he was experiencing some indigestion and requested an antacid. He also reported feeling lightheaded and fatigued when he got up to go to the bathroom.

This change in the patient's condition warranted further nursing assessment, which revealed the following information about his vital signs. The patient's blood pressure was 134/80. His apical heart rate was 96 and regular. His respiratory rate was 18 and unlabored, and his temperature was 37°C (98.6°F). He remained alert and oriented. His skin was warm, dry, and pale. Peripheral pulses were palpable, with capillary refill less than 3 seconds. Breath sounds were clear to auscultation and percussion.

The patient told me that this pain was "different" from the pain he experienced at admission. He described it as a gnawing, burning pain that did not radiate. He pointed to the epigastric area. His abdomen was soft. I auscultated increased bowel sounds. Palpation revealed localized epigastric tenderness slightly right of midline.

Although the clinical findings of pallor, fatigue, and dizziness might have related to the patient's cardiovascular status, the stability of his vital signs and ECG, along with the absence of chest pain, dyspnea, and restlessness, led me to investigate further. The postprandial nature and location of the pain and the epigastric tenderness upon palpation suggested that the patient might have peptic ulcer disease. In light of this possibility, I began to suspect that the pallor, fatigue, and dizziness could indicate slow upper gastrointestinal bleeding. To help identify the problem, I asked the patient about recent vomiting or changes in the color or consistency of his stool. He denied any vomiting, but reported that he had noticed occasional black, soft stools in the past few days, but thought it was related to his diet. I also assessed the patient for orthostatic hypotension by checking his blood pressure in both the lying and sitting positions. I found that his systolic reading decreased by 10 mm Hg in the sitting position. This finding (which often indicates blood loss), together with the hyperactive bowel sounds and the patient's report of melena (which usually indicates upper gastrointestinal blood in the stool), strongly supported my suspicion.

Next, I checked the patient's admitting labora-

CLINICAL ?THINKING

(continued)

tory data and noted that both the hemoglobin (Hgb) level and hematocrit (Hct) were below the normal range. The presence of anemia and the patient's history of smoking, alcohol and caffeine consumption, and stress further supported my suspicion of upper gastrointestinal bleeding related to a peptic ulcer.

Although no objective signs of active bleeding were evident, and the amount and rate of blood loss did not appear to be life-threatening, I recognized that the origin of the bleeding must be determined and treated. Because any gastrointestinal bleeding has the potential for rapidly developing into acute hemorrhage, hypovolemic shock, and possibly death, I implemented the following nursing actions:

1. I instructed the patient to remain in bed and placed the call bell within reach.
2. I instructed the patient to call if he felt light-headed or restless.
3. I instructed the patient to remain NPO (nothing by mouth).
4. I instructed the patient regarding the need to save all stool specimens.
5. I increased the rate of flow of the patient's existing KVO (keep vein open) intravenous infusion.
6. I notified the physician about the patient's change in condition.
7. I continued to monitor the patient's vital signs for signs of hemorrhage or hypovolemia.
8. I monitored the patient for hematemesis and melena.
9. I provided the patient with clear explanations and the opportunity to express his anxiety.
10. I documented my findings and actions.

Upon her arrival, the physician examined the patient and ordered a STAT Hgb and Hct, complete blood count, serum electrolytes, blood urea nitrogen, coagulation studies, type and cross-match for two units of packed red blood cells, arterial blood gases, IV fluids, and a nasogastric tube connected to low suction. The patient was scheduled for a fiberoptic esophagogastroduodenoscopy.

The nasogastric aspirate tested positive for occult blood, and the endoscopic examination con-

firmed the presence of a duodenal peptic ulcer, which was treated with laser photocoagulation. In addition, a biopsy specimen was taken to test for *Helicobacter pylori* infection.

The patient remained free of any evidence of further bleeding. His Hct remained stable, no blood transfusions were required, and he was started on diet and pharmacologic therapy that included a histamine H_2-receptor antagonist and antacids. The nurse's keen assessment skills, ability to recognize and interpret the clues, and appropriate and timely response led to the early recognition and successful management of a potentially dangerous condition.

Think Critically

Should the nurse have initiated oxygen therapy? Why? Why not?

What was the nurse's rationale for increasing the IV flow rate? Was this the best action? What potential complications should the nurse monitor for?

What was the rationale for the nursing action to maintain the patient NPO? Was this the best action?

What medical regimen should the nurse anticipate if the biopsy is positive for the *H. pylori* bacillus?

What teaching topics would the nurse include in the discharge plan to promote healing and minimize the risk of recurrence?

How might the nurse support the patient in his efforts to modify his lifestyle? In his coping skills? To comply with the medical regimen?

The patient stated, "I'll have to prove that I was the best choice for this new job." What is the nurse's best response?

What additional potential complications of peptic ulcer disease would the nurse consider when planning care for the patient?

The patient asked, "Does this diagnosis mean that I will eventually need surgery?" What is the nurse's best response?

How would the scenario have been different if the patient experienced hematemesis of large amounts of "coffee-ground" material? Bright red hematemesis?

NURSING PROCESS
Peptic Ulcer Disease

Assessment

Obtain a comprehensive history of the patient's pain. Include type, location, time of onset, precipitating factors, and remedies employed—such as taking an antacid or eating food—and their effectiveness. Question the patient about other symptoms, such as nausea, vomiting, and change in appetite and weight.

Obtain information about any family history of ulcer disease as well as lifestyle factors known to be associated with its development. Question the patient about smoking, use of prescription and non-prescription drugs, and use of alcohol. Explore the patient's dietary patterns and eating habits. Ask the patient to name favorite types of foods and beverages and to describe the number and schedule of meals and snacks per day. Have the patient validate this information by listing the time, amount, and type of foods eaten during the past 48 hours.

Explore sources of stress and the patient's coping mechanisms. Investigate the patient's perception of the amount of stress and the effectiveness of coping.

Assess the patient's and the family's knowledge of the disease and its treatment. Also assess the probability of compliance with treatment.

Assess the patient hospitalized with ulcer disease on an ongoing basis for intolerance to specific foods, response to therapy, and development of complications. Changes in the character of pain, the presence of bloody or coffee-ground emesis or nasogastric drainage, and melena are classic indications that a complication may have occurred.

Nursing Diagnoses and Planning

Nursing diagnoses and related expected patient outcomes commonly applicable to the patient with uncomplicated peptic ulcer disease include the following:

NDx: Pain related to the irritating effects of gastric acid on injured tissue

Planning: Patient Outcomes
1. Patient lists prescribed medications aimed at reducing pain, stating name, dose, route, and frequency of each.
2. Patient describes dietary modifications conducive to pain reduction.
3. Patient selects or plans nutritionally balanced meals that exclude pain-producing foods.
4. Patient reports that pain is relieved.
5. Patient sleeps through the night without pain.

NDx: Risk for altered health maintenance related to insufficient knowledge of disease process, aggravating factors, promotion of physical and psychologic rest, and need for follow-up care

Planning: Patient Outcomes
1. Patient describes the relationship of gastric acidity, mucosal damage, and symptomatology.
2. Patient lists substances known to aggravate the disease process.
3. Patient describes the relationship of stress to the disease process.
4. Patient describes a plan to reduce stress and promote physical rest.
5. Patient lists symptoms to be reported.

NDx: Risk for noncompliance related to dietary modifications, reduction of smoking, or medication regimen

Planning: Patient Outcomes
1. Patient reduces smoking.
2. Patient adheres to dietary and medication regimen.
3. Complications are absent.

Nursing Interventions and Evaluation

NDx: Pain
Teach self-administration of antacids, histamine antagonists, or other prescribed medications, adhering strictly to the ordered schedule to promote healing. Many protocols for *H. pylori* eradication involve several medications at once. Be sure the patient understands the importance of completing the prescribed doses. Encourage the patient to avoid cigarette smoking and foods that commonly exacerbate ulcer pain. These include highly spiced foods and those that contain caffeine, such as cola, tea, coffee, and chocolate. Explain that pain-causing foods vary from person to person. Instruct the patient to keep a daily record of foods eaten and the amount of pain experienced so that problem foods can be identified and avoided. If needed, enlist the dietitian to help the patient select and plan a well-balanced diet based on foods that are tolerated well.

Instruct the patient to eat small, frequent meals to help keep gastric acid neutralized and to drink six to eight glasses of water daily to dilute it. Also instruct the patient to eat slowly and to chew foods thoroughly, because large chunks of food are associated with increased secretion of hydrochloric acid.

Stress the importance of physical and psychologic rest. For the hospitalized patient, provide the physical care needed to keep the patient comfortable. Maintain a quiet environment, which may mean limiting visitors and telephone calls. When attempting to create a restful atmosphere, consider not only how much activity the patient can tolerate but how much inactivity can be tolerated. It may be less stressful to the patient if some phone calls and some work is allowed than if they are prohibited entirely.

NDx: Risk for altered health maintenance
Teach the patient basic pathophysiology of ulcer disease and the relationship of gastric acidity, mucosal damage, and symptoms. Explain the effect of smoking, caffeine, and drugs containing aspirin, and the

need to avoid them. Discuss the importance of psychologic and physical rest, and explore with the patient ways to reduce stress and organize activities to leave time for rest periods. Instruct the patient in the importance of follow-up care. Stress the need to report promptly severe abdominal pain, nausea, vomiting, abdominal distention, or persistence of original symptoms despite compliance with treatment.

NDx: Risk for noncompliance
Allow the patient to express feelings about limitations on diet, need to avoid smoking, and the need for daily medication. Stress that the patient is taking control of his or her life when the decision is made to adopt lifestyle changes to promote healing as opposed to being controlled by these changes. Identify with the patient factors seen as interfering with compliance and explore ways of dealing with them. Involve the family or significant others in planning for self-care and recommend counseling or support groups as needed.

Compare the patient's status with the expected outcomes. If the outcomes are not met, reassess the patient and revise the plan. See Nursing Care Guide 22–1 for care of the patient undergoing a subtotal gastrectomy for duodenal ulcer disease.

ACUTE STRESS ULCERS

Acute stress ulcers are a form of peptic ulcer disease that occur in patients who have suffered a major physiologic insult. They are distinct from chronic peptic ulcer in pathophysiology and in clinical presentation.

Etiology and Pathophysiology
Many kinds of physiologic stress are associated with development of acute stress ulcers. These include acute respiratory insufficiency, sepsis, renal failure, advanced carcinomatosis, and severe traumatic injuries. Stress ulcers also occur following burn injuries, brain injury, trauma, or cerebrovascular accident. Stress ulcers following burn injury are sometimes called Curling's ulcers, and those following brain injury are called Cushing's ulcers.

Acute stress ulcers are multiple superficial lesions that occur primarily in the gastric fundus, commonly in the middle of an area affected by acute gastritis. Although the exact pathophysiology of their development is not known, it is believed that the intensive stress response causes mucosal ischemia, which results in backflow of hydrogen ions and deficiency of mucus that normally coats the stomach wall. Stress ulcers following brain injury or lengthy cranial surgery (Cushing's ulcers) are thought to be caused by hypersecretion of gastric acid. It is known that, although it is not the cause, gastric acid must be present for stress ulcers to develop. Reflux of bile salts and pancreatic enzymes from the duodenum into the stomach may also contribute to the process.

Clinical Manifestations
The only symptom of stress ulcers is painless hemorrhage, indicated by hematemesis or melena, occurring 2 to 10 days following the physiologic insult (see Table 22–2).

Diagnosis
Diagnosis of acute stress ulcers depends on visualization of the lesions during gastroscopy. This requires that the patient's stomach be lavaged with cool water before the procedure to remove clots that could obscure the lesions. Radiologic studies are of no value in diagnosing stress ulcers because they are too superficial to be identified.

Management
The most effective treatment of stress ulcers is prevention. The mainstay for prophylaxis has been routine antacids via a nasogastric tube, intravenous H_2-receptor antagonists, or both. Recent literature indicates that an increase in gastric pH over time may cause other complications, such as nosocomial pneumonia, and suggests use of drugs that protect the gastric mucosa, such as sucralfate.

Although studies indicate a high incidence of gastric lesions in patients suffering from massive trauma, only a small proportion of them bleed. If bleeding does occur, there is a 50% mortality rate. Because bleeding is from several lesions in the gastric mucosa, it must be treated aggressively as a medical emergency. This may involve the standard technique of gastric lavage medication or may involve electrocoagulation during endoscopy.

❖ **Settings, Providers, and Collaboration for Care**
Development of stress ulcers, and administration of treatment for them, nearly always occurs in an intensive care setting. Care requires the efforts of the physician and the nursing staff to plan and implement the appropriate care regimen.

NURSING PROCESS GUIDELINES
Stress Ulcers

Identify patients at risk for stress ulcers and observe for hematemesis, blood, coffee-ground material in gastric drainage, and melena. Other assessments and interventions relate to the prescribed regimen for preventing stress ulcers as well as to the patient's primary medical problem. A bleeding patient will require intensive observation of hemodynamic status along with standard interventions for a hemorrhagic emergency.

HIATUS HERNIA

A hiatus hernia is a protrusion of part of the stomach into the thoracic cavity through the opening in the diaphragm where the esophagus passes. It

Text continued on page 1041

Patients Undergoing Subtotal Gastrectomy for Duodenal Ulcer Disease

Preoperative Care

Assessment Findings: Patient states, "I hope everything goes all right tomorrow. I'll sure be glad to be rid of my ulcer, but it makes me really nervous to think about being put to sleep and opened up." Patient also complains of feeling jittery and not being able to sit still.

Nursing Diagnosis: Anxiety related to experience of anesthesia and surgery

Patient Outcomes	Nursing Interventions	Rationale
Patient reports feeling more relaxed.	Reassure patient that some anxiety prior to surgery is normal and in fact helps prepare the body for the stress and promotes recovery.	Encourages patient to share feelings and thus receive support by allaying fears of being negatively perceived because of anxiety.
Patient expresses an optimistic view about the surgical outcome.	Offer reassurance about the success of surgery as appropriate. Possible examples include: reassure patient about his or her general state of health and therefore fitness for surgery; mention the frequency of the procedure and its success rate; describe the professionals that participate in surgery, noting their roles in protecting the patient and their competency.	Provides the patient with positive facts on which to focus and base hope for a successful surgical outcome.
Patient practices relaxation as instructed.	Review relaxation techniques with the patient and/or provide patient with a relaxation tape and orient patient to its use.	Helps control anxiety.
Patient rests quietly.	Maintain a quiet, calm environment.	Facilitates relaxation, rest, and action of sedative medications.
	Administer sedatives as ordered.	Promotes rest and relaxation.

Evaluation: Compare the patient's status with the expected outcomes. If the outcomes are not met, reassess the patient and revise the plan.

Assessment Findings: Patient says, "Tell me what to expect; I've never had surgery before except to have my tonsils out when I was 4, and I really don't remember very much. Am I going to have a lot of pain when I wake up? Will I be able to eat? Will I have a lot of tubes?"

Nursing Diagnosis: Knowledge deficit: preoperative preparation, postoperative course.

(continued)

Nursing Care Guide 22–1
Patients Undergoing Subtotal Gastrectomy for Duodenal Ulcer Disease (continued)

Patient Outcomes	Nursing Interventions	Rationale
Patient describes preoperative preparation. Patient describes usual postoperative procedures and course. Patient describes importance of coughing, deep breathing, and leg exercise in the prevention of complications.	Explain to the patient that: • Many tests, including a physical examination, x-rays, and blood tests, will be done before surgery to determine general state of health and identify any problems that need special consideration. • The specific nature and purpose of each test will be explained before it is done. • It is important that the gastrointestinal tract be empty when the operation is done, so only liquids will be allowed for 24 hours before surgery, and enemas may be given the day before surgery to clean out the bowel. • The abdomen will be shaved and scrubbed from nipple line to symphysis pubis to remove as many bacteria as possible, but the incision will be much smaller than the area prepared. (If the patient is to receive intravenous fluids or hyperalimentation therapy to make up nutritional deficiencies before surgery, explain this to the patient.) • After surgery, there will be a tube going from the stomach out through the nose to drain stomach secretions into a bottle on the wall. Drainage may be red initially. Because the purpose of the tube is to keep the stomach empty to promote healing of the suture line, no foods or fluids will be given by mouth for the several days that the tube is in place. The tube does not cause pain, although the nostrils may feel a bit sore and the mouth dry—symptoms that will be eased by salves and mouth rinses.	Prepares the patient for perioperative events, thus involving the patient in the plan of care, promoting cooperation, and decreasing the risk of anxiety over routine measures.

(continued)

Patients Undergoing Subtotal Gastrectomy for Duodenal Ulcer Disease (continued)

Patient Outcomes	Nursing Interventions	Rationale
	• Intravenous fluids will be given until peristalsis returns, the nasogastric tube is removed, and oral intake is reestablished.	
	• Coughing, turning, and deep-breathing will be encouraged every 2 hours while on bedrest in order to promote lung expansion, clear secretions from the airways, and prevent respiratory infection.	
	• Leg exercises should be done five times every 1 to 2 hours to promote movement of blood in the veins and discourage formation of blood clots.	
	• Ambulation usually begins on the first postoperative day.	
	• Oral intake will begin with clear fluids once bowel function has returned as indicated by the presence of bowel sounds and passage of flatus; full fluids and then bland foods will be added as tolerated.	
Patient demonstrates coughing and deep-breathing.	Demonstrate, and have the patient practice, turning, coughing, and deep-breathing with a pillow used to splint the abdomen.	
Patient demonstrates postoperative leg exercises.	Demonstrate leg exercises.	

Evaluation: Compare the patient's status with the expected outcomes. If the outcomes are not met, reassess the patient and revise the plan.

Postoperative Care

Assessment Findings: Patient states, "I have so much pain. It hurts when I lie still, but it's even worse when I move." Patient moans softly on moving. Face appears tense and strained. Patient also complains of nostril discomfort and asks if the nasogastric (NG) tube can be removed.

Nursing Diagnosis: Pain related to trauma from abdominal surgery and irritation of the nostril by the NG tube

(continued)

Nursing Care Guide 22–1
Patients Undergoing Subtotal Gastrectomy for Duodenal Ulcer Disease (continued)

Patient Outcomes	Nursing Interventions	Rationale
Patient moves without loud moans, complaints of severe pain, or signs of severe pain such as pallor and tachycardia.	Administer pain medication.	Pain relief promotes rest, which facilitates the healing process.
Patient states abdominal pain is relieved.	Keep the head of the bed elevated. Splint the incision with a pillow when turning, coughing, deep-breathing.	Decreases pull on the incision line. Decreases discomfort by reducing pull on incised tissues.
Patient appears relaxed (ie, lips are not pressed together, face does not appear drawn).	Encourage the patient to relax. Play soft music, and prompt the patient to concentrate on slow, even breathing or to contemplate a calm, pleasant scene permeated by a relaxing color.	Relaxation decreases muscle spasm.
Patient denies nostril discomfort.	Clean the nostril through which the tube passes with applicators dipped in water, and apply water-soluble lubricant.	Removes secretions, which can form crusts and irritate the nares. Lubricant protects area from contact with irritating secretions, decreases friction, and keeps tissues moist and supple.

Evaluation: Compare the patient's status with the expected outcomes. If the outcomes are not met, reassess the patient and revise the plan.

Assessment Findings: Patient has had a gastric resection with anastomosis of the remaining stomach to the small intestine.

Nursing Diagnosis: Risk for trauma (internal suture line) related to gastric distention, vomiting, or movement of the NG tube

Patient Outcomes	Nursing Interventions	Rationale
Signs of leakage at the anastomosis are absent. Patient is afebrile. Increased pain is absent. Abdomen is soft.	Keep the NG tube connected to suction as ordered.	Gastric distention and vomiting place stress on the suture line and can lead to disruption of the anastomosis and leakage of gastric contents into the abdominal cavity.
	Do not reposition the NG tube. Irrigate the tube gently with normal saline as ordered to keep it patent.	Maintains drainage, thereby preventing stress on the anastomosis from gastric distention. Gentle irrigation protects the suture line from disruption. Normal saline is isotonic and therefore maintains osmotic pressure and minimizes loss of electrolytes from the stomach.

(continued)

Patients Undergoing Subtotal Gastrectomy for Duodenal Ulcer Disease (continued)

Patient Outcomes	Nursing Interventions	Rationale
	Reinforce or replace the tape holding the tube in position as needed. Be careful not to move the tube when adding or changing tape.	Prevents movement of the NG tube, which could lead to trauma to the anastomosis.

Evaluation: Compare the patient's status with the expected outcomes. If the outcomes are not met, reassess the patient and revise the plan.

Assessment Findings: Patient has had major abdominal surgery and was intubated for general anesthesia. Respirations are shallow and secretions can be heard in the large airways.

Nursing Diagnosis: Ineffective airway clearance related to shallow breathing secondary to diaphragmatic splinting accompanying upper abdominal surgery

Patient Outcomes	Nursing Interventions	Rationale
Patient moves, coughs, and breathes deeply as directed. Lung sounds are clear on auscultation.	Turn, cough, and deep-breathe every 2 hours while on bed rest.	Promotes elimination of inhalation anesthetics in the immediate postoperative period. Also promotes aeration of alveoli, and moves secretions into larger respiratory passages for expectoration.
	Splint incision to decrease pain and anxiety when turning, coughing, and deep-breathing.	Minimizes discomfort and promotes willingness to turn, cough, and breathe deeply.
	Ambulate patient as ordered.	Promotes maximum lung expansion and movement of secretions.

Evaluation: Compare the patient's status with the expected outcomes. If the outcomes are not met, reassess the patient and revise the plan.

Assessment Findings: Patient is mouth breathing because of the NG tube in the nose and is on nothing by mouth (NPO) status.

Nursing Diagnosis: Risk for altered oral mucous membrane related to mouth breathing and NPO status

Patient Outcomes	Nursing Interventions	Rationale
Oral mucous membranes are pink and moist.	Assist the patient in brushing and flossing the teeth.	Cleanses the mouth and provides feeling of freshness and comfort.
Patient states mouth and lips feel moist and free of discomfort.	Assist the patient in rinsing the mouth frequently.	Moistens mucous membranes of the mouth.
	Offer throat sprays, lozenges, or gum if allowed.	Increases saliva, thereby relieving dryness of the oral mucous membranes.
Lips are supple and intact.	Apply water-soluble lubricant to lips.	Helps keep the lips moist, supple, and free of cracks.

(continued)

Nursing Care Guide 22–1

Patients Undergoing Subtotal Gastrectomy for Duodenal Ulcer Disease (continued)

Evaluation: Compare the patient's status with the expected outcomes. If the outcomes are not met, reassess the patient and revise the plan.

Assessment Findings: Patient has an upper abdominal wound.

Nursing Diagnosis: Risk for infection related to contamination of the abdominal wound

Patient Outcomes	Nursing Interventions	Rationale
Wound is odorless and free of purulent drainage. Wound edges are approximated.	Caution patient against touching the abdominal dressing or the surrounding area.	Protects against introduction of pathogens from the patient's hands to the area of the surgical wound.
	Use strict aseptic technique when caring for the wound.	Protects against contamination of the wound with pathogens.
	Reinforce/change dressing as needed. If dressing is wet with predominantly bloody drainage, notify the physician.	Excessive bloody drainage is indicative of bleeding from a large vessel, and needs immediate attention.

Evaluation: Compare the patient's status with the expected outcomes. If the outcomes are not met, reassess the patient and revise the plan.

Assessment Findings: Patient has had part of the stomach removed, is on NPO status, and is at risk for early satiation and dumping syndrome on resumption of oral intake.

Nursing Diagnosis: Altered nutrition: less than body requirements related to dietary restrictions related to surgery, early satiety, or dumping syndrome

Patient Outcomes	Nursing Interventions	Rationale
Patient ingests a nutritionally balanced diet. Patient achieves and maintains recommended weight.	Administer intravenous fluids and electrolytes as ordered (usually for about 4 days).	Replaces fluids and electrolytes lost through nasogastric drainage, wound drainage, and normal elimination processes, because patient is on NPO status after surgery and only gradually resumes oral intake once bowel motility has resumed.
	Give clear fluids when bowel motility has returned.	Clear fluids are easiest to digest and absorb and least likely to cause nausea and vomiting.
	Gradually introduce full fluids, and progress to a bland diet as tolerated.	Gastric capacity is significantly decreased because of the partial gastrectomy. Nausea and vomiting can occur from oral intake that is "too much, too fast."

(continued)

Nursing Care Guide 22–1
Patients Undergoing Subtotal Gastrectomy for Duodenal Ulcer Disease (continued)

Patient Outcomes	Nursing Interventions	Rationale
	Give iron and vitamin supplements as ordered.	Prevents deficiency due to insufficient oral intake.
	Give six small feedings per day and liquids before or after but not with feedings.	Decreases risk of early satiation.
	To combat dumping syndrome: • Avoid hypertonic liquids and high-carbohydrate foods. • Position patient in low Fowler's position during meals. • Instruct patient to lie down for 30 minutes after eating to delay gastric emptying. • Avoid fluids with meals. • Take antispasmodics as ordered to aid in delay of gastric emptying.	Rapid entry of large amounts of hypertonic chyme into the small intestine precipitates dumping syndrome.

Evaluation: Compare the patient's status with the expected outcomes. If the outcomes are not met, reassess the patient and revise the plan.

Assessment Findings: Patient has no previous experience with surgery.

Nursing Diagnosis: Risk for altered health maintenance related to lack of knowledge of prevention of recurrence, need for follow-up care

Patient Outcomes	Nursing Interventions	Rationale
Patient describes importance of avoiding aspirin products, alcohol, and cigarette smoking.	Instruct the patient to avoid aspirin-containing over-the-counter drugs such as Excedrin and Alka-Seltzer, use of alcohol, and cigarette smoking.	Decreases the risk of ulcer recurrence.
Patient identifies sources of stress.	Help the patient identify sources of lifestyle stress.	Sources of stress must be identified before strategies to reduce stress can be planned.
Patient identifies ways of relieving or coping with stress.	Explore with the patient methods of decreasing or lowering stress.	Stress is associated with exacerbation of peptic ulcer disease, although its role as a causative factor remains in question.
	Refer to stress reduction groups or other professional help as necessary.	In some cases, external support is needed to help the patient plan and carry through with stress-reducing strategies.
Patient lists symptoms to be reported to the physician.	Instruct the patient to report: • Continuous epigastric distress that increases after eating. • Persistent fatigue.	Continuous epigastric distress may indicate alkaline reflux gastritis. Persistent fatigue may indicate iron or vitamin B_{12} deficiency.

(continued)

Nursing Care Guide 22–1
Patients Undergoing Subtotal Gastrectomy for Duodenal Ulcer Disease (continued)

Evaluation:	Compare the patient's status with the expected outcomes. If the outcomes are not met, reassess the patient and revise the plan.

Additional Assessments and Interventions

Monitor and record vital signs every 4 hours or more frequently if necessitated by the patient's condition.

Observe and record the amount and character of the drainage from the NG tube. Normally, drainage is bloody for 24 hours postoperatively, then changes to brown-tinged and then to yellow or clear. Amount of secretions decreases as peristalsis returns.

Note odor of gastric aspirate, because a fecal smell can indicate regurgitation of large intestine contents into the operative area.

Auscultate for bowel sounds and question the patient about passage of flatus to determine when peristalsis has resumed and oral intake may begin.

Record all intake and output.

---

occurs more often in women than in men and is the most common pathologic condition of the upper gastrointestinal tract.

Etiology and Pathophysiology

Normally, the opening (or hiatus) in the diaphragm through which the esophagus passes encircles the esophagus tightly and prevents the stomach from ascending into the thoracic cavity. A congenitally short esophagus, trauma, or weakening of the diaphragmatic muscle around the hiatus can permit movement of the lower esophagus and upper stomach into the chest cavity. Weakening of the diaphragmatic muscle may be congenital, with symptoms occurring later in life, or it may be the result of aging. The major contributing factor in the development of hiatus hernia is increased intra-abdominal pressure. This can result from bending, straining, lifting heavy objects, coughing, vomiting, obesity, pregnancy, and so on.

Ninety percent of hiatus hernias are classified as "sliding." That is, the top of the stomach enters the thoracic cavity when the person is supine but slides back into the abdomen when the person assumes a vertical position (Fig. 22–5). Mechanical irritation caused by friction, along with reflux regurgitation of acidic gastric contents into the lower esophagus, results in esophagitis. The pain and swelling of esophagitis can lead to aspiration and malnutrition.

Another type of hiatus hernia is a paraesophageal or "rolling" hernia (see Fig. 22–5). In this type, a portion of the stomach other than that directly adjoining the esophagus moves up through the diaphragmatic opening and protrudes into the thoracic cavity. If this protruding portion of the stomach becomes incarcerated, circulation can be impaired and ulceration or tissue necrosis can result.

Clinical Manifestations

Hiatus hernia is commonly asymptomatic and may remain undetected unless discovered by chance. When symptoms do occur, the most frequent is heartburn. With the common sliding hernia, pyrosis (heartburn) and acid regurgitation occur from reflux of acidic gastric contents into the esophagus. If this leads to air swallowing, eructation (belching) and flatulence also occur. Dysphagia (difficulty swallowing) appears if irritation of esophageal tissue leads to scarring and decreased motility. Symptoms are aggravated by any increase in intra-abdominal pressure.

Diagnosis

Diagnosis of hiatus hernia is suggested by the patient's history and presenting symptoms. It is confirmed by such diagnostic tests as a barium swallow or esophagoscopy.

Management

Treatment of hiatus hernia is usually conservative, with surgery reserved for severe cases in which symptoms cannot be adequately controlled. Conservative treatment consists of:

- A bland diet taken in small, frequent feedings
- Positioning in a semi-Fowler's position after eating to promote movement of ingested foods

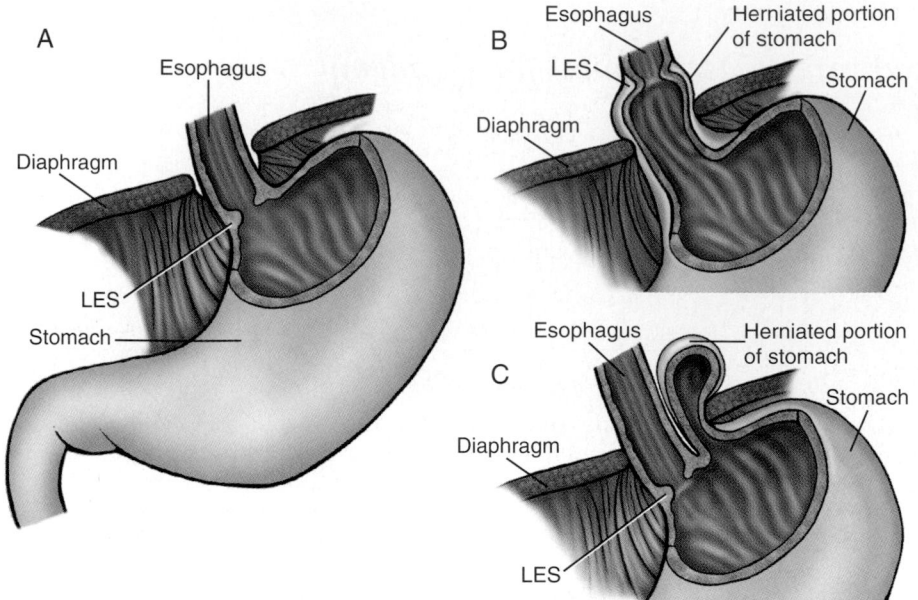

Figure 22–5

A, Normal relationship of esophagus, diaphragm, and stomach. *B*, Sliding hiatus hernia. Note top of the stomach above the diaphragm in the thoracic cavity. *C*, Rolling (paraesophageal) hiatus hernia. Note part of the stomach other than that adjoining the esophagus in the thoracic cavity. (LES, lower esophageal sphincter.)

into the stomach and to discourage esophageal reflux

- Raising the head of the patient's bed at home on 6-inch blocks to reduce reflux during the night
- Antacids for symptomatic relief of pyrosis
- Commonly, histamine-receptor–blocking agents to reduce the amount of acid in the stomach

If surgical intervention is required, a procedure such as a Nissen fundoplication is done (Fig. 22–6). In this operation, the fundus of the stomach is wrapped around the lower esophagus, creating a one-way valve to control the flow of upper gastrointestinal contents. As with any major surgery, there is a postoperative risk of hemorrhage, infection, and pulmonary embolus. Other complications that can

occur because the surgery specifically involves the esophagus are postoperative dysphagia, esophageal obstruction, esophageal perforation, and esophageal fistula. A less complex variation of this procedure is now being performed using a laparoscopic approach.

❖ Settings, Providers, and Collaboration for Care

Unless surgical repair is indicated, patients with hiatus hernias may be treated on an outpatient basis, with medication and continued diagnostic assessment. The expertise of a dietitian may be helpful in assisting the patient with the selection of a diet that does not exacerbate symptoms. The dietitian may

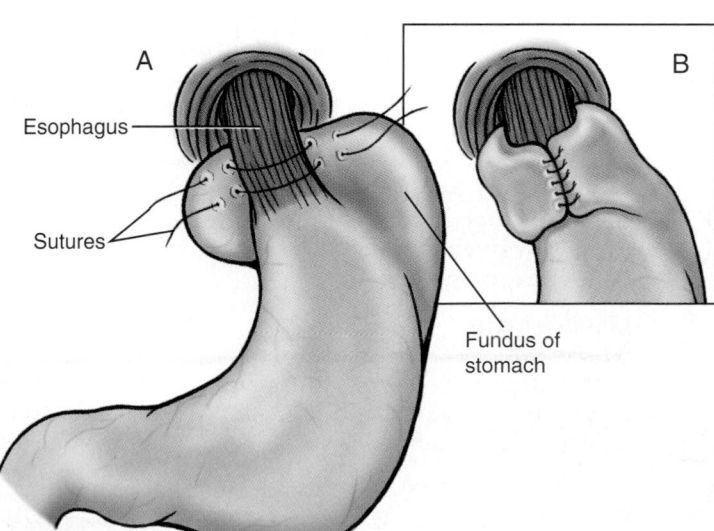

Figure 22–6

Nissen fundoplication. *A*, Fundus of the stomach has been brought up in preparation for being wrapped around the esophagus. *B*, Fundus is sutured in place around the lower esophagus.

also teach family members how to plan and prepare meals to meet the patient's needs.

NURSING PROCESS
Nonsurgical Treatment for Hiatus Hernia

Assessment

Assess the type and extent of the patient's discomfort and its relationship to meals, to ingestion of specific foods, or to specific activities. Examples of such relationships are pyrosis occurring after eating spicy food or after eating a large meal and then lying down. Identify remedies that the patient uses for relief of symptoms. Determine the frequency of their use as well as their effectiveness. Assess the patient's general nutritional status and identify dietary changes made because of discomfort.

Because medical management is not completely effective in relieving symptoms, it is also important to identify the patient's understanding of the disease process and expectation of treatment.

Nursing Diagnoses and Planning

Nursing diagnoses and related expected patient outcomes commonly applicable to patients undergoing nonsurgical treatment for a hiatus hernia include the following:

NDx: Pain related to esophageal irritation secondary to reflux of acidic gastric contents

Planning: Patient Outcomes
1. Patient describes the proper use of antacids.
2. Patient reports that pain is relieved.

NDx: Risk for altered health maintenance related to insufficient knowledge of nature of the disorder and prevention and control of symptoms

Planning: Patient Outcomes
1. Patient describes the basic pathology of hiatus hernia.
2. Patient describes measures to reduce the severity of symptoms.
3. Patient reports that pyrosis occurs no more than twice daily.

Nursing Interventions and Evaluation

NDx: Pain
Instruct the patient in the use of antacids for pain (Highlight 22–3). Warn against the use of alcohol for pain relief because it reduces pressure in the lower esophageal sphincter and thus worsens the problem. Instead, encourage use of relaxation measures and diversion to cope with discomfort.

NDx: Risk for altered health maintenance
Describe what a hiatus hernia is, how it produces symptoms, and how changes in diet, activities, and personal habits can aid in preventing or controlling symptoms.

Instruct the patient in food selection and other

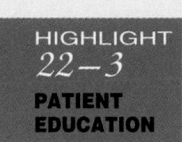 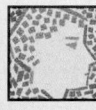

HIGHLIGHT 22–3
PATIENT EDUCATION
Use of Antacids

To promote safe, effective self-administration of antacids, instruct the patient to:

Shake all liquid antacids well before taking.

Chew chewable tablets thoroughly and take with a full glass of water because antacid must be in liquid form in order to work.

Check the expiration date on the bottle and discard outdated medication because antacids become less effective as they age.

Adhere to the prescribed schedule of doses.

Always measure the antacid dose; do not drink from the bottle.

Consult with the physician or pharmacist before changing antacids because different antacids contain different ingredients, some of which may be contraindicated for particular patients.

Check with the physician or the pharmacist about the scheduling of other medications while taking antacids because antacids alter the gastric pH and can affect the absorption of many medications, including antibiotics, cardiac glycosides, and enteric-coated tablets. As a general rule, medications should be taken 2 to 3 hours before or after an antacid.

Drink at least 2500 mL of fluids per day to help prevent constipation and impaction if taking antacids that contain calcium or aluminum.

dietary considerations (Highlight 22–4). Also tell the patient to avoid activities that increase intra-abdominal pressure, such as bending, lifting, wearing clothing that constricts the abdomen, straining at stool, and vigorous coughing. Suggest that the patient sleep on the right side and elevate the head of the bed 6 inches on blocks so that gravity can aid in preventing reflux. Discourage eating close to bedtime. Also discourage smoking, which increases gastric secretion.

Compare the patient's status with the expected outcomes. If the outcomes are not met, reassess the patient and revise the plan.

NURSING PROCESS GUIDELINES
Surgical Treatment for Hiatus Hernia

Nursing care of a patient having surgery for a hiatus hernia involves the general preoperative and

HIGHLIGHT 22–4
NUTRITION

Special Considerations for Patients with Hiatus Hernia

Patients with a hiatus hernia should be instructed to:

Eat small, frequent meals to prevent distention of the stomach, which increases acid secretion.

Eat a high-protein diet because protein stimulates gastrin secretion and increases lower esophageal sphincter pressure.

Avoid fat in the diet because fat decreases pressure in the lower esophageal sphincter.

Avoid substances such as tea, coffee, cola, and chocolate that contain caffeine, which stimulates gastric acid secretion.

Avoid irritating foods such as citrus fruits and tomato products.

Drink water after eating to cleanse the esophagus.

Promote the passage of food into the stomach by gravity by not lying down for 2 to 3 hours after eating, eating slowly, and chewing food well.

Lose weight if overweight to improve posture and general body mechanics.

---

postoperative measures required by any major surgery (see Chap. 6), with the following considerations.

Because the operative area is in close proximity to the diaphragm, postoperative coughing and deep breathing are commonly difficult and painful. This puts the patient at risk for pulmonary complications. Preoperative assessment of respiratory status and patient teaching about the need for and technique of postoperative turning, coughing, and deep breathing are of critical importance. If the patient smokes, stress the importance of decreasing or eliminating cigarettes for at least a few days prior to surgery.

Postoperatively, assessment of respiratory status continues to be critically important, and a nursing diagnosis of "risk for infection related to inadequate airway clearance" is applicable to all patients. Assist the patient in turning, coughing, and deep breathing until he or she is ambulatory to promote good ventilation, move secretions, and prevent respiratory infection. Consider these interventions effective if the lungs are clear to auscultation, no purulent sputum is produced, and body temperature remains within normal range.

Because eructation can also be difficult postoperatively from the proximity of the operative area and

the diaphragm, assess for postoperative distention. Also assess for dysphagia, which may occur temporarily from edema of the distal esophagus. When gastric suction is discontinued, start the patient on a liquid diet and progress to a full diet as tolerated. Encourage the patient to eat slowly to keep from swallowing air. Avoid carbonated beverages and gas-producing foods as the diet is progressed.

ACHALASIA

Etiology and Pathophysiology

Achalasia is a motor disorder of the lower two-thirds of the esophagus in which peristalsis is decreased or absent, the lower esophageal sphincter fails to relax and allow swallowed food to pass into the stomach, and the esophagus above the sphincter dilates (Fig. 22–7). The cause of achalasia is unknown, but a disturbance of the intrinsic innervation of the smooth muscle appears to be involved.

Clinical Manifestations

Symptoms of achalasia are odynophagia and dysphagia. Odynophagia (painful swallowing) typically occurs 5 to 8 seconds after swallowing and can range from mild discomfort to severe pain described as sharp and crushing. It is commonly substernal and often radiates to the back, neck, jaw, and arms. Dysphagia associated with achalasia may be inter-

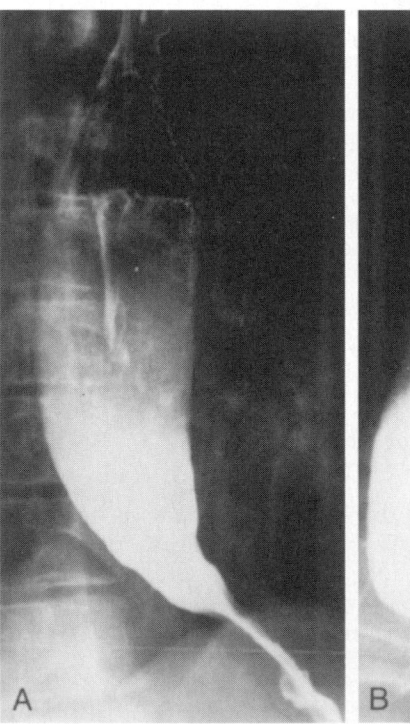
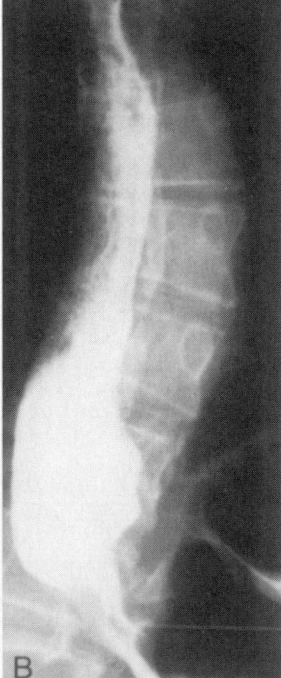

Figure 22–7

A, Achalasia with a narrowed, elongated esophagogastric junction (rat-tail sign). *B,* Widening of the esophagogastric junction in a patient with achalasia following balloon dilation. (From Zuidema GD [ed]. Shackelford's surgery of the alimentary tract. 4th ed. Vol 1. Philadelphia: WB Saunders, 1996.)

mittent or continuous. It may occur with ingestion of solids and liquids. Regurgitation, which can lead to aspiration, may also occur. Symptoms appear to worsen with emotional stress, rapid eating, and ingestion of large amounts of very hot or very cold foods.

Diagnosis
Diagnosis of achalasia is based on radiologic and manometric studies. Dilatation of the esophageal body, and a narrowed distal end, can be seen during a barium swallow. Manometry directly measures pressure and function of the lower esophageal sphincter, as well as esophageal motility. With achalasia, there is a high resting pressure at the sphincter, little or no relaxation of the sphincter on swallowing, and absence of peristalsis in the lower two-thirds of the esophagus.

Management
Medical management of achalasia aims to alleviate the obstruction at the lower end of the esophagus caused by the aperistaltic esophagus and failure of the lower esophageal sphincter to relax. The three basic management options are esophageal dilatation, drug therapy, and surgery.

Pneumatic dilatation is the most effective nonsurgical intervention. In this procedure, a balloon-tipped dilator is passed through the mouth and positioned in the lower esophageal sphincter under radiologic guidance. It is then abruptly inflated to partially rip the muscle of the sphincter. After dilatation, the patient remains on nothing by mouth (NPO) status for about 6 hours and is monitored for signs of esophageal perforation, which is the major risk associated with the procedure. Because an emergency thoracotomy is required if perforation occurs, this procedure is not done on elderly patients or on those with significant cardiovascular, renal, or pulmonary disease. Because dilatation does not restore normal esophageal motility, the procedure often needs to be repeated over time. If dilatation is unsatisfactory, a myectomy may be done. This involves direct cutting of the muscle of the lower esophageal sphincter to enlarge the opening into the stomach so that food can pass through more readily. A myectomy may be done through either an abdominal or a thoracic incision.

Anticholinergic agents and calcium antagonists, such as nifedipine (Procardia), are sometimes used to decrease the tone and contraction of the esophageal smooth muscle. Their use is usually limited to patients who are poor surgical risks or who have had esophageal dilatation with less than the desired effect.

NURSING PROCESS
Achalasia

Assessment
Explore the patient's symptoms, including severity, frequency, and relationship to any specific factor, such as type of food eaten or a stressful situation. Assess the patient's nutritional status and usual daily diet. Identify changes in diet necessitated by symptoms, including changes in the size and timing of meals, consistency of foods, foods avoided, or foods newly included in the diet. Determine the effect of such changes, as well as of any other home remedies used.

In preparation for patient teaching, assess the patient's understanding of the disorder, the proposed treatment, and its expected result. Also assess the resources available to the patient that could support compliance with the treatment program.

Nursing Diagnoses and Planning
Nursing diagnoses and related expected patient outcomes commonly applicable to patients with achalasia include the following:

NDx: Impaired swallowing related to motor dysfunction of the esophagus

Planning: Patient Outcomes
1. Patient identifies measures to aid swallowing.
2. Patient describes both the plan and its importance for reducing stress.
3. Patient ingests a nutritionally balanced diet composed of a variety of foodstuffs without stated or other overt signs of discomfort.

NDx: Pain related to swallowing

Planning: Patient Outcomes
1. Patient reports that pain on swallowing is decreased.
2. Signs of discomfort such as posturing are absent.

Nursing Interventions and Evaluation

NDx: Impaired swallowing
Instruct the patient in measures to facilitate swallowing (Highlight 22–5). Explain the relationship of stress to exacerbation of symptoms. Discuss sources of stress to the patient, and help the patient identify ways of coping with or reducing it. Particularly emphasize the importance of avoiding stress at meal times.

NDx: Pain
Intervene as described for difficulty swallowing. Instruct the patient to elevate the head of the bed to help prevent nocturnal regurgitation and tracheal aspiration.

Compare the patient's status with the expected outcomes. If the outcomes are not met, reassess the patient and revise the plan.

NURSING PROCESS GUIDELINES
Surgical Treatment for Achalasia

Nursing care of the patient undergoing an esophageal myectomy for relief of achalasia combines the care required by any patient undergoing major surgery, that necessitated by opening the thoracic or

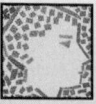

Self-Management for Dysphagia

To facilitate swallowing, instruct the patient to:

Sit up straight when eating. Keep the head upright and tilted slightly forward.

Allow sufficient time for meals and eat slowly.

Take small bites of solid foods and small sips of liquids.

Eat textured foods that need to be chewed.

Avoid sticky foods such as bananas, mashed potatoes, and peanut butter.

Avoid very hot or cold foods.

Take fluids to wash down solid food.

---

abdominal cavity (depending on the approach used), and that necessitated by the effects on the esophagus.

Because gastric reflux may develop after the surgical procedure, be sure to assess the patient for related symptoms. If they occur, institute nursing interventions related to diet, position, and avoidance of factors that increase intra-abdominal pressure, as described in Nursing Process: Nonsurgical Treatment for Hiatus Hernia.

*T*rauma

Many types of traumatic injury can affect the mouth and other organs of the upper gastrointestinal tract (Table 22–3). These include abrasions, lacerations, penetrating injuries, blunt force injuries, and chemical or thermal injuries. They can be minor, requiring little or no treatment, or severe, potentially life-threatening events that require intensive, prolonged therapy.

FRACTURE OF THE MANDIBLE

Etiology and Pathophysiology
Most fractures of the mandible, or lower jaw, result from a blow to the face or chin. They may be simple fractures without bone displacement or, in severe accidents, there may be both marked displacement and loss of tissue. Occasionally the mandible is fractured as part of a planned surgical correction of a deformity.

Clinical Manifestations
Symptoms of a fractured mandible are pain on movement, abnormal mobility of the lower jaw, malocclusion, and irregularity of the dental arch.

Diagnosis
The diagnosis of mandibular fracture is suggested by palpation and confirmed by x-ray.

Management
Simple fractures of the mandible can be managed by intermaxillary fixation. In this procedure, wires are placed around the upper and lower teeth on both sides of the fracture. Then, using these wires as sources of attachment, wires or rubber bands are applied, holding the top teeth to the bottom teeth and thus firmly holding the lower jaw against the upper jaw (Fig. 22–8). If teeth or bone are lost or displaced, alternative means of immobilization—such as metal arch bars in the mouth or pins into the bone—are used.

The patient is usually out of bed on the first postoperative day and discharged in 2 to 3 days. The jaw remains immobilized for 6 to 8 weeks.

❖ Settings, Providers, and Collaboration for Care
The patient with a fractured mandible may be treated initially in an emergency department, followed by hospitalization or frequent return visits to an outpatient clinic. These patients may also require home care services, including the expertise of a dietitian. The dietitian monitors the patient's caloric and nutrient intake, and teaches the patient how to manage the nutritional regimen. For elderly patients or patients without assistance at home, a home health nurse may visit the patient to assess healing status. The nurse also reinforces nutritional instruction provided by the dietitian and teaches the patient about safety measures, such as use of wire cutters, potential complications, when to notify the physician, and communication strategies.

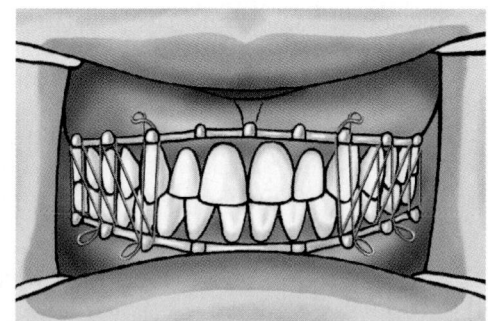

Figure 22–8

Intermaxillary fixation. Note wires surrounding tops of upper and lower teeth and the bands attached to them, holding the lower jaw firmly in place against the upper jaw.

Table 22–3

Selected Types of Upper Gastrointestinal Trauma

Type of Trauma	Etiology	Clinical Manifestations	Treatment
Esophageal damage from medication	Lodging of medications—such as tetracycline, doxycycline, quinidine, and ascorbic acid—in the esophagus causes localized, shallow mucosal ulcer	Steady burning chest pain and odynophagia 4 to 6 hours after taking medication	Symptomatic with antacids and soft, bland diet. Healing occurs in about 1 week. Teach prevention: Take capsules in an upright position and with a large glass of water.
Chemical burns	Accidental ingestion of strong acid or base such as lye Suicide attempt	Acute pain, possible respiratory distress secondary to pharyngeal edema or mucus block, fever, shock	Emergency treatment for respiratory distress and shock. If these are not present, sips of water to dilute chemical. Do not induce vomiting. Analgesics for pain. Nasogastric tube to keep esophagus patent. Corticosteroids to decrease inflammatory response. Antibiotics to combat infection. Tube feedings, daily dilation with a bougie, starting about 1 week after the insult.
Esophageal obstruction by a foreign body	Accidental ingestion of pins, fishbones, tooth, or a large bolus of meat or other food Suicide attempt	Pain, dysphagia, and possible dyspnea	Remove with an esophagoscope. Bolus of meat may be dissolved with proteolytic enzymes.
Esophageal perforation	Stab or bullet wounds, accidental perforation with a surgical instrument, spontaneous rupture with vomiting	Retrosternal pain followed by dysphagia, hyperpnea, cervical tenderness, subcutaneous emphysema, fever, leukocytosis, and sometimes severe hypotension	Semi-Fowler's position and nasogastric tube to limit reflux. Patient is placed on NPO status with hyperalimentation. Broad-spectrum antibiotics to combat mediastinitis. Chest tubes to drain the chest, and if a large perforation, surgical repair.

NPO, nothing by mouth.

NURSING PROCESS
Mandibular Fracture

PREOPERATIVE NURSING CARE

Give basic preoperative care as discussed in Chapter 6. Remember that, in most cases, fixation of the mandible represents emergency rather than elective surgery. Be sure the patient understands what will be done and how it will look. Reassure the patient that he or she will be able to breathe and swallow after the fixation. Explain that speech may be difficult at first but within a few days should be understandable. Plan for an alternative means of communication during the first postoperative days.

POSTOPERATIVE NURSING CARE

Assessment

Make assessments as for any postoperative patient. Pay particular attention to respiratory status. Assess amount of secretions and the need for suctioning.

Use a tongue blade and flashlight to inspect accessible areas of the mouth for cleanliness and for irritation from the wires. Observe and record the patient's intake and response to the blenderized diet. Question the patient about constipation and passage of excessive flatus.

Nursing Diagnoses and Planning

Nursing diagnoses and related expected patient outcomes commonly applicable to patients with a fractured mandible include the following:

NDx: Risk for ineffective airway clearance related to inability to open mouth and clear throat effectively

Planning: Patient Outcomes
1. Respiratory rate is within normal limits.
2. Respirations are silent and easy.
3. Lungs are clear on auscultation.

NDx: Risk for aspiration related to inability to open mouth and clear throat effectively

Planning: Patient Outcomes
1. Signs of regurgitation are absent.
2. Signs of respiratory distress are absent.

NDx: Risk for infection related to break in the oral mucous membrane and limited ability to clean the oral cavity

Planning: Patient Outcomes
1. Patient denies areas of irritation from the wires.
2. Gums are pink and smooth.
3. Breath is free of offensive odor.

NDx: Impaired verbal communication related to inability to open mouth

Planning: Patient Outcomes
1. Patient uses alternative communication techniques.
2. Patient's needs are understood.

NDx: Risk for altered nutrition: less than body requirements related to inability to eat other than by sucking liquids through a straw or from a spoon

Planning: Patient Outcomes
1. Patient experiences minimal weight loss.

NDx: Risk for constipation related to a liquid, high-carbohydrate diet

Planning: Patient Outcomes
1. Patient describes interventions to combat constipation.
2. Patient has soft, formed bowel movement at least every third day.
3. Patient denies excessive flatus.

NDx: Risk for altered health maintenance related to insufficient knowledge of self-care after discharge

Planning: Patient Outcomes
1. Patient describes measures to prevent airway obstruction, including how and when to cut wires or bands.

2. Patient describes the selection and preparation of a high-protein, high-calorie, liquid diet.
3. Patient demonstrates oral hygiene.
4. Patient lists signs and symptoms to report.
5. Patient states date of follow-up visit.

Nursing Interventions and Evaluation

NDx: Risk for ineffective airway clearance
Keep wire cutters (or scissors if rubber bands are used) taped to the head of the bed and suction equipment at the bedside. Maintain the patient in a side-lying position with the head elevated until fully awake. Wearing gloves, suction the nose with a small catheter to remove secretions as needed. To suction the mouth, move the cheek away from the teeth with a tongue blade. Gently run the suction catheter in the space created, and insert it into the oral cavity itself either through a space between teeth or around the back of the third molar. If the patient is able, teach him or her to self-suction as needed.

If the patient is in respiratory distress and suctioning is not effective, cut the wires or bands to clear the airway. Note that, if wires need to be cut, the patient will have to return to surgery to have them replaced.

NDx: Risk for aspiration
Give ordered antiemetics as needed to prevent vomiting. If vomiting occurs, tilt the patient's head forward or to the side and use suction to remove the vomitus. If there is a nasogastric tube, keep it patent and attached to low suction.

NDx: Risk for infection
Maintain meticulous oral hygiene. Give warm alkaline mouthwashes or oxygenating rinses every 2 hours and after eating. Cleanse the teeth with a soft toothbrush if permitted, or use an oral syringe to irrigate between the teeth and along the outer gum line. A Water-Pik may be used if the water flow is very gentle. Lubricate the lips with a water-soluble lubricant to prevent cracking.

NDx: Impaired verbal communication
Provide the patient with pencil and paper, chalkboard, Magic Slate, or other means of communication during the first few postoperative days, when speech is difficult to understand. Respond to the patient's call signal in person rather than by intercom during this time.

NDx: Risk for altered nutrition: less than body requirements
Start the patient on clear fluids through a straw. Progress as tolerated to a full blenderized diet. Give foods that can be sucked from a spoon, such as Jell-O or custard, as desired. Administer protein supplements as ordered. Follow each feeding with water.

Before discharge, arrange for the patient to see a dietitian for help in planning a high-calorie, high-protein blenderized diet with variation in taste. This is very important because the patient will be on the diet for 6 to 8 weeks. The risk of inadequate nutrition is great because eating a blenderized diet through a straw becomes boring. Weight loss of 10 to 20 pounds is not unusual in patients with wired jaws.

NDx: Risk for constipation
Tell the patient about the potential for excessive flatus and constipation because of the liquid, high-carbohydrate diet and intake of air when sucking through a straw or from a spoon. Encourage ambulation and exercise to promote good bowel function. If needed, provide prune juice and give a bulk-forming laxative as ordered.

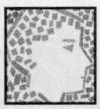

HIGHLIGHT 22–6 PATIENT EDUCATION

Discharge Instructions After Intermaxillary Fixation

Instruct the patient to:

Protect against airway obstruction.

- Keep a wire cutter (or if rubber bands were used, a scissors) with him or her at all times.
- Avoid carbonated beverages because their foam can be difficult to clear from the throat.
- Avoid alcoholic beverages because they depress the reflexes needed to keep the airway clear.
- Do not swim because it can be difficult to remove water from the throat.

Prevent oral infection.

- Brush teeth regularly if permitted.
- Rinse mouth with water, mouthwash, dilute hydrogen peroxide, or saline after eating and at bedtime.
- Use a Water Pik or oral syringe as desired to cleanse the mouth, but keep the stream of solution gentle.
- Apply paraffin to the ends of the wires to avoid injury to the mouth.

Maintain a balanced nutritional intake.

- Blenderize foods.
- Select foods high in protein and carbohydrate.
- Select a variety of foods.
- Drink at least 2500 mL of fluid per day.

Obtain necessary follow-up care.

- Report any irritation, swelling, or unusual pain.
- Report to the physician immediately if the wires or bands are cut.
- Return for scheduled visits.

NDx: Risk for altered health maintenance
Instruct the patient in self-care after discharge (Highlight 22–6).

Additional Interventions
If an appliance is in place outside the mouth, alert the patient to its presence and caution against turning over onto it.

Compare the patient's status with the expected outcomes. If the outcomes are not met, reassess the patient and revise the plan.

Neoplasia

ORAL CANCER

Cancer of the oral cavity is primarily a disease of the elderly. Its incidence increases between ages 50 and 70, and it is more common in men. It can occur on the lip, the tongue, or inside the mouth.

Etiology and Pathophysiology
Two clearly identified causes of oral cancer are the use of tobacco and the use of alcohol, which are thought to interfere with local defense mechanisms. Tobacco use includes smoking cigarettes, pipes, and cigars, and the use of chewing tobacco and snuff. Irritation from prolonged exposure to sun and wind or from a hot pipe stem contributes specifically to the development of cancer of the lip. Other factors believed to contribute to development of cancer of the mouth include poor oral hygiene, with subsequent bacterial invasion, and physical trauma as from jagged teeth or improperly fitting dentures. Malnutrition, syphilis, and cirrhosis have also been found in large numbers of patients with this disease.

The majority of oral malignant lesions are squamous cell carcinomas. Most commonly these tumors occur on the lips, the lateral aspects of the tongue, or the floor of the mouth, although any part of the oral cavity—including the pharynx and sinuses—can be affected.

Cancer of the mouth spreads primarily by local extension and via the regional lymph nodes of the head and neck. Cancer of the lip has a good prognosis because it is well localized and is easily detected before extensive tissue involvement occurs.

Cancers of the tongue and the floor of the mouth have a poorer prognosis because the tumors are not as readily noticeable in their early stages. In addition, the extensive vascular and lymphatic supply of the mouth facilitates metastasis.

Clinical Manifestations
Malignant lesions of the lip tend to arise in areas of leukoplakia. These are white, nodular, patchy areas on the mucosa that cannot be easily rubbed off (Fig. 22–9). Often, these lesions are found in areas of constant irritation, such as loose dentures or the

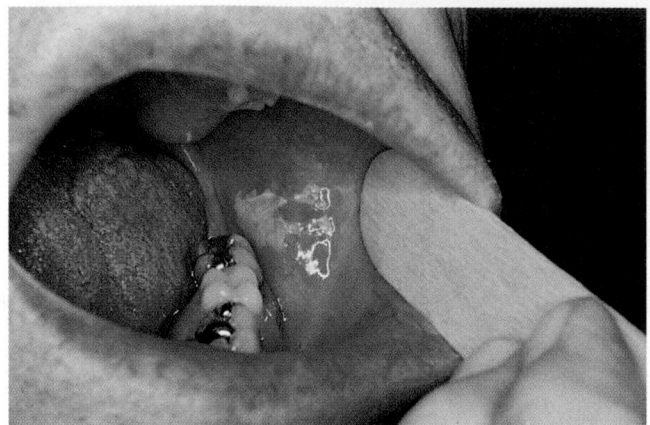

Figure 22–9

Leukoplakia. (From Callen JP, Greer KE, Hood AF, et al. Color atlas of dermatology. Philadelphia: WB Saunders, 1993.)

place where a pipe is most often held. The cancer may appear as a blister, as a nonhealing sore that crusts and bleeds, or as a painless, hard, white, fixed mass. As tumor growth progresses, secondary infection occurs, resulting in ulceration, tenderness, edema, and surrounding erythema.

Malignant lesions of the mouth and tongue usually are white or yellowish ulcerated lesions, although in their earliest stages they may appear simply as a red or white surface patch. Initially the lesions are asymptomatic, although patient may be aware of feeling a roughened area with the tongue, depending on the location of the lesion. As the tumor enlarges, symptoms develop that vary with the location and extent of spread. With cancer of the anterior, mobile portion of the tongue, pain or soreness can occur when eating hot or spicy foods. As tongue mobility becomes impaired, speech can become slurred. Swallowing is painful. As neighboring structures are affected, pain can arise in the area of the temporomandibular joint and the outer ear, along with increased salivation and blood-tinged sputum. With tumors of the base of the tongue, odynophagia, unilateral sore throat, and salivary changes occur.

Diagnosis

Any oral lesion that does not heal within 3 weeks should be evaluated as a possible oral malignancy. Oral exfoliative cytology, in which the suspicious lesion is scraped and the cells examined microscopically, can support the diagnosis of cancer. However, only a biopsy provides a definitive benign diagnosis. Submental, submaxillary, and cervical nodes are palpated to determine metastases. Malignant lesions of the mouth are commonly found by the patient's dentist during a routine dental examination.

Management

Treatment depends on the location, type, size, and lymphatic spread of the tumor. Nonmetastasized cancers of the lip are effectively treated either by external beam radiation or by simple surgical excision, usually under local anesthesia. If metastasis to the lymph nodes has occurred, surgical resection is combined with postoperative radiation therapy.

Small tumors located on the anterior portion of the tongue may be treated by either radiation or surgical excision. Larger tumors require partial glossectomy (removal of part of the tongue) and subsequent radiation. If tumor involves the floor of the mouth near the lower jaw, removal of the mandible (mandibulectomy) and a radical neck dissection may also be required. This surgery is also followed by radiation and then by reconstructive procedures because removal of the mandible results in a noticeable cosmetic deficit.

For tumors on the base of the tongue, surgical treatment involves a total glossectomy and a laryngectomy, with follow-up radiation and chemotherapy. Because this is extremely disfiguring and incapacitating surgery accompanied by a high incidence of tumor recurrence, radiation alone may be elected in some cases. A radical neck dissection is performed in conjunction with surgical treatment of tumors at the base of the tongue, with follow-up radiation and chemotherapy if lymph node metastasis has occurred.

❖ Settings, Providers, and Collaboration for Care

Patients in the early stages of oral cancer may be treated in a physician's office or outpatient clinic. If extensive surgical treatment is required, a long hospitalization, including an intensive care setting, may be necessary. Upon discharge, home care assistance may be in order. The home health nurse instructs the patient and family about the prescribed care, assists with dressing changes, assesses the patient's progress, and assists with nutritional needs. A dietitian may also provide counseling to the patient about meal planning. Follow-up care is in the physician's office.

For patients with extensive facial disfigurement, referral to a counselor may be necessary to help the patient maintain a positive self-concept and to develop coping strategies. The home health nurse also assists the patient and family in developing coping mechanisms and encouraging their use.

NURSING PROCESS
Oral Cancer

PREOPERATIVE NURSING CARE

Assess the patient's readiness for surgery as described in Chapter 6. Pay particular attention to the patient's nutritional, fluid, and electrolyte status because oral cancer causes soreness and difficulty swallowing that typically interfere with eating. Check for weight loss. Review recent patterns of dietary intake. Review laboratory data related to nutrition as well as fluid and electrolyte balance. Carefully assess respiratory status because the patient is at risk for problems with airway clearance postoperatively.

Assess the patient's understanding of the proposed surgery and his or her psychologic response to it. This is critical because oral surgery can result in unconcealable disfiguration and impairment in the basic functions of speaking, swallowing, and eating. If the patient will be unable to speak, discuss alternative forms of communication. Review with the patient expected postoperative procedures, such as oral suctioning, nasogastric suction, and wound care.

With extensive surgery, such as total glossectomy and removal of the palate and mandible, prostheses of the palate and jaw may be constructed to replace portions of tissues that have been resected. If prostheses are to be made, impressions will be taken preoperatively. Be sure to explain this process to the patient.

Institute nutritional support measures as ordered. These may involve supplemental feedings, vitamin supplements, or hyperalimentation therapy to maximize the patient's nutritional status for surgery.

Cleanse the patient's mouth, and ensure that other preoperative preparations are carried out as ordered.

POSTOPERATIVE NURSING CARE

Assessment

Make usual postoperative assessments as outlined in Chapter 6. If the parotid gland has been resected, assess the function of cranial nerve VI by asking the patient to raise his or her eyebrows, frown, smile, show teeth, and pucker the lips. Assess for nutritional problems when oral foods and fluids are reinstated. Also assess the psychologic response to the surgery. Be alert for signs of reluctance to interact with other people. Watch for anxiety about resuming personal responsibilities, about the prognosis, or about self-care. Also watch for any other nonadaptive response. Explore the patient's coping mechanisms and available support systems.

Nursing Diagnoses and Planning

Nursing diagnoses and related expected patient outcomes commonly applicable to patients who have had surgery for a neoplasm of the oral cavity include the following:

NDx: Risk for ineffective airway clearance related to edema, difficulty swallowing or handling secretions

Planning: Patient Outcomes
1. Patient coughs and deep breathes as directed.
2. Respirations are easy, quiet, and symmetric.
3. Lungs are clear on auscultation.

NDx: Pain related to surgical tissue trauma

Planning: Patient Outcomes
1. Patient reports being at least fairly comfortable.
2. Behavioral signs of pain, such as grimacing or moaning, are absent.
3. Patient reports decreasing pain throughout postoperative course.

NDx: Risk for altered nutrition: less than body requirements related to inability to ingest foods and fluids orally

Planning: Patient Outcomes
1. Patient's daily calorie intake meets basic requirements as identified by the dietitian.
2. Serum albumin and albumin-globulin ratio are within normal limits.
3. Patient maintains weight.

NDx: Impaired verbal communication related to removal of oral tissues and postoperative restrictions on mouth movement

Planning: Patient Outcomes
1. Patient uses alternative communication techniques.
2. Patient's needs are understood.

NDx: Risk for body image disturbance related to changes in appearance secondary to surgery

Planning: Patient Outcomes
1. Patient looks in the mirror.
2. Patient indicates interest in appearance.
3. Patient welcomes visitors.
4. Patient interacts with other patients.

NDx: Risk for infection related to the location of the surgical incision

Planning: Patient Outcomes
1. Purulent drainage from wound is absent.
2. Foul odor from the wound is absent.
3. Patient is afebrile.

NDx: Risk for altered health maintenance related to insufficient knowledge of self-care after discharge

Planning: Patient Outcomes
1. Patient demonstrates care of the wound.
2. Patient demonstrates self-examination for facial and oral cancer.

Nursing Interventions and Evaluation

NDx: Risk for ineffective airway clearance
Immediately after surgery, place the patient in a side-lying position to facilitate drainage. When the patient is alert, assist him or her into Fowler's position if desired. Suction the mouth as needed, or allow saliva and other drainage to flow into an emesis basin via a gauze wick. Turn the patient frequently and assist with coughing and deep breathing every 2 hours. If a tracheostomy was done to facilitate breathing, provide care as described in Chapter 14.

NDx: Pain

Administer prescribed pain medication as needed. This can range from viscous lidocaine to anesthetize a painful area of the mouth after removal of a small, localized malignancy to systemic analgesics like meperidine hydrochloride (Demerol) for severe, generalized pain after extensive surgery. Use the Agency for Health Care Policy and Research pain (postsurgical) guidelines to provide strategies for pain relief. Have the patient practice relaxation exercises and provide diversional therapy. Avoid any trauma to the mouth during oral hygiene.

NDx: Risk for altered nutrition: less than body requirements

Because a high-protein, high-calorie diet is needed to promote healing, supplemental tube feedings may be given. In some cases, hyperalimentation therapy may be ordered. When oral intake is allowed, place small amounts of bland fluids on the back of the tongue with an Asepto syringe or a soft feeding tube. As the patient's tolerance permits, increase the diet to include nonirritating foods, such as Jell-O, pudding, custard, and pureed foods. Avoid acidic foods and very hot and very cold foods.

Teach the patient to eat slowly, take small sips or bites of food, eat small amounts frequently, avoid using a fork, and drink water after eating to clear the mouth of food particles. Provide privacy, sufficient time, and a comfortable upright position so the patient can succeed in learning how to manage food and fluids.

NDx: Impaired verbal communication

If the patient cannot speak because of a tracheotomy or restricted mouth movement, use an alternative form of communication, such as a Magic Slate or flash cards, as discussed preoperatively. Keep the patient's call light within reach at all times, and alert all members of the health care team to the fact that the patient cannot speak.

When speech is possible, encourage the patient to speak slowly. Maintain an unhurried, undemanding atmosphere, and provide for privacy as the patient "relearns" to speak. Initiate referral to speech therapy as necessary.

NDx: Risk for body image disturbance

Provide an accepting, nonthreatening environment. Be sensitive to and acknowledge the patient's feelings. Be straightforward about the patient's appearance, but avoid comments or actions that could be construed as indicating distaste or pity. Do not force the patient to look at the wound. When the patient does look at it, remind the patient that it is not yet healed and still has swelling and inflammation.

Assist the patient with grooming. Be sure that hair is combed and male patients are shaved. Encourage makeup for female patients. Get patients up and dressed as soon as allowed.

NDx: Risk for infection

To cleanse the oral cavity and promote wound healing and comfort, irrigate the oral area with sterile water, dilute hydrogen peroxide, or soda bicarbonate solution. Use a cotton-tipped applicator to cleanse the teeth and gums if needed, but do not use any commercial toothbrush because it may cause tissue damage. Avoid commercial mouthwashes and lemon-glycerin swabs because of their drying effect on mucous membranes.

Meticulous care of the incision lines is important. Use a cotton-tipped applicator to gently clean the incision with dilute hydrogen peroxide. If an antibiotic ointment such as bacitracin is ordered, apply it lightly to the incision line. If the patient has a wound suctioning device to facilitate drainage, monitor every 4 hours for proper functioning and amount and character of drainage.

NDx: Risk for altered health maintenance

Instruct the patient in self-care after discharge. Keep in mind that each patient has specific teaching needs based on the type of surgical procedure done. If needed, provide instructions for wound care (Highlight 22–7). Instruct all patients in self-examination for facial and oral cancer and in the need for medical follow-up (Highlight 22–8). A patient with one of these cancers is at great risk for developing another.

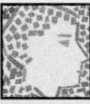

HIGHLIGHT 22–7
PATIENT EDUCATION
Wound Care After Surgery for Oral Cancer

Instruct the patient to:

Mix equal amounts of hydrogen peroxide and sterile saline in a sterile container. Always mix new solution each time wound care is done. Discard remaining solution when finished.

Place several cotton applicator sticks into the container. Do not touch any part of the applicator beyond the end of the stick.

Beginning at the top of the wound, gently cleanse the incision with a damp applicator. Do not go back over any area that has been touched. Use a new applicator as needed.

Go over an area with a dry applicator as needed if the peroxide has caused a lot of bubbling.

Apply a *thin* layer of any prescribed ointment to the incision with a dry applicator. Use the same technique as with cleansing—do not retrace areas already touched and use a new applicator as needed. When squeezing the ointment onto the applicator, do not let the tip of the applicator touch the tube itself.

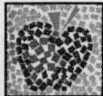

Self-Examination for Facial and Oral Cancer

Instruct the patient to use a mirror and good light and examine himself or herself monthly for signs of facial or oral cancer as described here:

Examination of the Face and Neck

Inspect your face and neck for any differences in shape between the right side and the left side.

Observe the skin on the face and neck for changes in color, changes in a mole, lumps, or sores. Be certain to remove glasses and inspect the skin around the eyes and on the bridge of the nose.

Press along the sides and front of the neck with your finger tips, feeling for tender areas or lumps.

Examination of the Mouth

Remove dentures and partial plates in preparation for examination of the inside of the mouth.

Pull the lower lip down, and inspect for sores or color changes. Palpate for lumps.

Pull the top lip up and back. Inspect for sores or color changes, and palpate for lumps.

Grasp the upper lip on one side of the mouth with one hand and the lower lip on the same side with the other. Pull out and to the side to expose the inside of the cheek.

Observe for discoloration and sores. Repeat with other cheek.

Check for lumps and tenderness in the cheek. Put your thumb on the inside of the cheek and your index finger on the outside. Gently compress the tissue between them. Repeat with other cheek.

Open your mouth and tilt your head back. Inspect the roof of the mouth for discoloration, raised areas, sores, or swelling.

Open your mouth wide and touch the roof of the mouth with the tip of your tongue. Look for discoloration and raised areas or sores on the floor of the mouth and the bottom of the tongue.

Press the floor of the mouth with your fingers to detect lumps or tender areas.

Stick the tongue out and look at its top surface for discoloration or sores.

Grasp the tongue with a piece of gauze or tissue. Pull it forward and to each side in turn. Inspect for discoloration, raised areas, sores, or other lesions.

Additional Interventions

If drooling is a problem, encourage the patient to consciously swallow more often. Keep tissues and a disposal bag readily available to the patient at all times. Administer anticholinergics, such as atropine or belladonna compounds as ordered, to decrease salivation.

Compare the patient's status with the expected outcomes. If the outcomes are not met, reassess the patient and revise the plan.

NURSING PROCESS GUIDELINES
Supportive Treatment for Oral Cancer

If the patient with oral cancer is not having surgery, nursing care is primarily planned to make the patient comfortable, to maintain oral intake for as long as possible, and to cope with a terminal illness. Provide food, fluids, and oral hygiene as described previously. Give medication for pain as needed in accordance with the physician's orders. Provide psychologic support by allowing time and opportunity to verbalize feelings and facilitating visits by family, chaplain, or hospice worker.

CANCER OF THE ESOPHAGUS

The incidence of cancer of the esophagus varies greatly throughout the world. In the United States, it occurs most often in males 60 to 80 years old, with African-American, Chinese, and Japanese men affected more frequently than white American men.

Etiology and Pathophysiology

The wide variation in geographic distribution suggests that environmental factors have a definite role in the development of esophageal carcinoma. Implicated factors are smoking, alcohol abuse, poor oral hygiene, and poor nutritional habits. Esophageal cancer also appears to be related to untreated achalasia and the presence of strictures caused by ingestion of lye.

Two types of cancer primarily affect the esophagus: squamous cell carcinoma and adenocarcinoma. Squamous cell carcinoma, by far the more common of the two, usually involves the upper or middle third of the esophagus. Adenocarcinoma, in contrast, most commonly arises in the stomach and extends secondarily into the esophagus.

The tumor appears as an ulcerating mass that projects into the lumen. It tends to extend around the total inner circumference as well as up and down the esophagus. As it enlarges, the normal distensibility of the esophagus is overcome, and the passage of ingested food past the tumor is progressively obstructed. Unfortunately, by the time obstruction is sufficient to cause symptoms, spread of the cancer has usually occurred into lymph nodes and adjacent tissues. For this reason, the prognosis is very poor.

The pattern of spread is specific to the location of the original tumor. Tumors of the upper third of the esophagus spread to the cervical nodes, trachea, larynx, and thyroid gland. Middle third tumors spread to the lymph nodes of the lungs. Lower tumors spread to the lungs and the liver. With advanced disease, extensive mediastinal or pericardial involvement can occur as well as tracheoesophageal fistula or aortic erosion with exsanguinating hemorrhage.

Clinical Manifestations

Esophageal cancers tend to be asymptomatic until relatively far advanced. When symptoms do occur, the most common is dysphagia, which develops when the mass begins to occlude the esophageal lumen. Over a period of 6 to 8 months, the dysphagia progresses from difficulty with solid foods to difficulty with liquids and finally with saliva. The dysphagia is insidious in that the patient eliminates foods that are difficult to swallow one by one over a period of time and commonly does not realize the extent of the problem until the diet is essentially liquid. Occasionally, dysphagia is accompanied by vague substernal discomfort or a feeling of fullness after ingestion of only a small amount of food.

As the disease advances, halitosis, anorexia, weight loss, and emaciation occur. Nausea and vomiting of undigested food occur if obstruction is complete, and cough occurs if a tracheoesophageal fistula or other tracheal involvement is present. A steady, boring pain on swallowing, hoarseness, or both develop with extensive mediastinal involvement.

Diagnosis

Diagnosis of esophageal carcinoma is based on an x-ray esophagram with barium swallow. This demonstrates the tumor by showing a narrowing of the esophagus in the area of the mass. The pathologic type of the malignancy is determined by esophagoscopy with biopsy and cytologic brushings. Subsequently, the patient is scheduled for a variety of procedures, the results of which are needed to stage the disease and plan therapy. These procedures include bronchoscopy, organ scanning, liver function tests, chest x-ray, and computed tomography scan for mediastinal spread.

Management

Treatment of esophageal cancer varies with the location of the tumor, the overall condition of the patient, and the stage of the disease.

Surgical Resection or Bypass

When possible, surgical resection is the treatment of choice for esophageal cancer because the obstruction is removed and the continuity of the gastrointestinal tract and ability to swallow are restored. Two types of resection are esophagogastrostomy and esophagectomy with interposition of colon. Esophagogastrostomy, sometimes referred to as a *gastric pull-up*, is done for tumors of the distal esophagus, and involves bringing the stomach up into the thoracic area for anastomosis to the remaining esophagus. Esophagectomy with interposition of a section of colon is used when such a large segment of the esophagus is removed that a conduit between the remaining esophagus and the stomach is needed. Interposition of colon is usually done as a second-stage procedure following recovery from the esophagectomy.

In esophageal bypass surgery, the stomach or colon is anastomosed to the esophagus above the tumor, thus bypassing the obstruction and restoring the ability to swallow.

Intensive preparation for surgery is necessary because most patients with esophageal cancer are poor surgical risks from malnutrition and the resulting decreased blood volume, protein depletion, fluid and electrolyte imbalances, and loss of resistance to infection.

Postoperatively, the patient is kept on NPO status for about 5 days. A nasogastric tube is in place to prevent pressure on the suture line for about 1 week. If the thoracic cavity is opened, a chest tube is inserted to re-expand the lungs. In some cases, a tracheostomy may also be done to manage airway clearance.

Postoperative complications include respiratory infection and leaking at the anastomosis. The patient is prone to respiratory infection from the location of the incision and related difficulty in coughing and deep breathing to clear the airways of secretions. The patient is also at risk for aspiration pneumonia secondary to reflux of gastric contents.

Leaking of the anastomosis is a major, frequently fatal, development that occurs more often in the esophagus than in any other part of the gastrointestinal tract. It can result from tension on the suture line, poor healing, or impaired blood supply. Symptoms include low-grade fever, substernal pain, elevated pulse and respiratory rates, and shock. Occasionally, subcutaneous emphysema or symptoms mimicking pulmonary embolism occur. Treatment consists of draining accumulated fluid from the thoracic cavity or, in some cases, repeat surgery for reanastomosis.

Radiation

For tumors of the upper or middle esophagus, preradiation and postradiation therapy are commonly combined with surgery. When surgery is not an option because of the size of the tumor and existing metastases, radiation alone may be used to shrink the tumor and provide symptomatic relief. Side effects of radiation to the upper and middle thirds of the esophagus include retrosternal discomfort, pain on swallowing, increased salivation, and nausea.

Laser Palliation

Laser therapy may be used in place of or together with surgery or radiation to reduce tumor size, maintain a patent esophageal lumen, and reduce dysphagia and discomfort. With the patient under local anesthesia, a laser passed through an endoscope is used to vaporize the obstructing tumor mass. This is a long procedure, and treatments are usually scheduled on alternating days until a patent lumen is established. A temporary increase in dysphagia and discomfort occurs immediately after therapy but an oral diet can be gradually resumed within a few days after the last treatment.

Major advantages of this treatment are that it can be repeated an unlimited number of times, it has no undesirable systemic effects, and it can be used regardless of where the tumor is located in the esophagus. Potential complications of laser palliation include aspiration, bleeding, and perforation of the esophagus.

Prosthetic Intubation

When other measures fail, a pliable tube may be inserted into the esophagus to keep the lumen open and allow the patient to eat fairly normally for a period of time. A tube prosthesis may also be inserted to bypass a tracheoesophageal fistula and prevent aspiration of ingested food. An example of a tube prosthesis is the Celestin tube, which is semirigid and held open by a wire coil. Under fluoroscopy, with the patient heavily sedated, it is pulled into place in the esophagus from below through an opening into the stomach. A prosthetic tube may also be placed in the esophagus via endoscopy. The difficulty with this procedure is that the prosthesis tends to slip.

The swallowing reflex is unaffected by a tube prosthesis, but swallowing is initially uncomfortable and difficult. Patients start with sips of water and gradually add other fluids and foods as they learn how much can be swallowed at one time.

A major problem associated with tube prostheses is reflux of gastric contents and subsequent aspiration pneumonia. This occurs because the tube interferes with normal peristalsis in the esophagus, leaving only the effect of gravity to prevent reflux. Thus, patients with a tube prosthesis can never lie flat but must keep the head elevated even at night.

Gastrostomy

As a last recourse, a gastrostomy tube is inserted as a means of maintaining nutrition. In some cases, a surgical gastrostomy is done in which the anterior wall of the stomach is sutured to the abdomen, creating a permanent fistula that allows the tube to be easily inserted and replaced. The percutaneous endoscopic gastrostomy, however, has increasingly become the procedure of choice.

❖ Settings, Providers, and Collaboration for Care

Although many of the palliative and diagnostic procedures involving cancer of the esophagus can take place in an outpatient setting, treatment usually involves extensive hospitalization and long-term follow-up care in the home. Referral to a home health agency is commonly needed. The home health nurse continues the treatment regimen started in the hospital. The nurse assesses the patient's status and progress, teaches the patient and family about the medication and nutritional plan, and assists with their psychoemotional needs. The patient may also need assistance with feedings and, depending on the particular need, a home enteral therapy nurse or dietitian may be indicated.

Collaboration with a social worker and psychologist may be necessary. The patient may need help finding resources for financial support and continued care. The psychologist or counselor assists the patient and family to cope with the trauma of the condition and the future prognosis.

NURSING PROCESS
Surgery for Esophageal Cancer

Nursing care of patients having surgery for esophageal cancer combines the basic care of any operative patient, the care of the patient who has had chest surgery, and the care of any patient with a diagnosis of cancer.

PREOPERATIVE NURSING CARE

Assessment

Perform a complete assessment of the patient scheduled for surgery for esophageal cancer, as for any patient having major surgery. Pay particular attention to assessment of nutritional status and fluid and electrolyte balance because surgery is commonly preceded by a long period of dysphagia, during which foods and fluids in the diet are progressively eliminated or decreased. Question the patient about changes in appetite and food intake. Check for weight loss. Review laboratory studies for electrolyte imbalances, decreased serum albumin level, decreased total protein level, and decreased serum transferrin level or iron-binding capacity.

Assess the patient's pulmonary function. Because the surgical procedure may involve opening the thoracic cavity and manipulation in the area of the diaphragm, postoperative coughing and breathing will be painful and the patient will have an increased risk of respiratory complications.

Observe the patient for signs of infection because malnutrition secondary to progressive dysphagia reduces the number of inflammatory and immune cells that normally fight infection.

Because cancer of the esophagus is usually far advanced at the time of diagnosis, and surgery is therefore palliative rather than curative, carefully assess the emotional response of the patient and family, their usual coping mechanisms, and available support systems.

Nursing Diagnoses and Planning

Nursing diagnoses and related expected patient outcomes commonly applicable to patients scheduled for esophageal resection for carcinoma include the following:

NDx: Knowledge deficit: operative procedure and its expected outcome, postoperative course, and treatments

Planning: Patient Outcomes
1. Patient describes the operative procedure and its expected effect in general terms.
2. Patient verbalizes understanding of postoperative equipment and treatments.
3. Patient demonstrates coughing and deep breathing.
4. Patient describes how nourishment will be maintained after surgery.

NDx: Anxiety related to the surgical experience and the resulting report on the extent of disease and its prognosis

Planning: Patient Outcomes
1. Patient expresses concerns about the surgical experience and its effect on body functions.
2. Patient cooperates with preoperative preparation.
3. Signs of excessive anxiety—such as trembling, crying, and pacing—are absent.

NDx: Altered nutrition: less than body requirements related to inability to swallow foods or fluids before surgery

Planning: Patient Outcomes
1. By the time of surgery, patient's weight approximates ideal body weight.
2. Nitrogen balance is positive.
3. Serum electrolyte values, albumin level, and albumin-globulin ratio are within normal limits.

Nursing Interventions and Evaluation

NDx: Knowledge deficit: operative procedure and its expected outcome, postoperative course, and treatments
Clarify the patient's understanding of the surgery and its expected outcomes. Explain the usual postoperative procedures. Prepare the patient for the presence of a nasogastric tube and chest tube. Explain that blood transfusions are commonly given and that intravenous fluids can be expected for about a week. Discuss how and when oral intake will be resumed.

INTERNET CONNECTIONS
Upper Gastrointestinal System Disorders

General
American Gastroenterological Association
http://www.gastro.org/
This authoritative resource provides links to other sites for medical professionals. It also includes links to more specific information, for example to peptic ulcer; links to publications; and links to medical news.

Peptic Ulcer
MedicineNet/Peptic Ulcer Disease
http://www.medicinenet.com/mainmenu/encyclop/ARTICLE/Art_P/PEPULC.htm
An encyclopedia-style article providing up-to-date patient-oriented information about peptic ulcer disease.

Oral Cancer
MedicineNet/Oral Cancer
http://www.medicinenet.com/mainmenu/encyclop/ARTICLE/Art_O/ORALC.htm
This web site provides extensive patient-oriented information about oral cancer, including its causes, symptoms, diagnosis, and treatment, and information on clinical trials.

Cancer of the Esophagus
ONCOLINK/Esophageal Cancer
http://oncolink.upenn.edu/disease/esophageal/
This authoritative site provides both health professional- and patient-oriented information as well as links to other helpful resources, including CancerNet from the National Cancer Institute.

Gastric Cancer
ONCOLINK/Gastric Cancer
http://oncolink.upenn.edu/disease/gastric/
This ONCOLINK site provides information for health professionals and for patients. In particular, it offers links to other helpful resources, including CancerNet from the National Cancer Institute.

Teach techniques of coughing and deep breathing, and describe the use of incentive spirometers and intermittent positive pressure breathing. Explain their importance in preventing postoperative respiratory infection and promoting a rapid recovery. Encourage deep abdominal breathing every 2 hours while awake in preparation for surgery. Discourage smoking.

NDx: Anxiety

Acknowledge that anxiety over the surgery and disease prognosis is normal. Encourage the patient and family to verbalize concerns and ask questions about the surgery. Seek to identify specific worries, such as ability to eat after surgery, ability to breathe with the nasogastric tube in place, or risk of acquired immunodeficiency syndrome (AIDS) or hepatitis associated with blood transfusion. Correct any misconceptions, and provide reassuring information when possible.

Maintain a calm environment. Suggest the use of relaxation techniques. Administer sedatives as ordered.

NDx: Altered nutrition: less than body requirements

Carry out measures to restore nutritional, fluid, and electrolyte balance as ordered. These usually include administration of intravenous solutions; vitamin supplements (particularly vitamins B, C, and K); high-protein, high-caloric feedings; and even hyperalimentation therapy. Record all intake and output.

Additional Interventions

Thoroughly cleanse the mouth. Brush and floss the teeth. Clean dentures. Use a swab or gauze to scrub the tongue and other areas in the mouth. Use milk of magnesia and mineral oil or the equivalent to remove crusts.

Compare the patient's status with the expected outcomes. If the outcomes are not met, reassess the patient and revise the plan.

POSTOPERATIVE NURSING CARE

Assessment

Assess the patient's return to physiologic stability. Check vital signs, color, skin temperature, responsiveness, wound drainage, and fluid intake and output. Assess the function of both the chest tube and the nasogastric tube. Note the amount and color of drainage from each. In the early postoperative period, when the stomach is still atonic, observe carefully for signs of reflux and aspiration.

Assess the patient for pain, and note the response to pain medication. Check respiratory status frequently. Note the rate, depth, and symmetry of respirations, and listen for abnormal breath sounds. Observe for signs of dehydration, and review laboratory data related to fluid and electrolyte balance as they become available. If the patient is on intermittent positive pressure breathing, note pulse rate, color, chest expansion, and amount and character of expectorate, as well as the patient's general reaction to each treatment.

Assess for signs of leaking at the anastomosis. Question the patient about substernal pain. Check for fever, increased pulse or respiratory rate, and signs of shock. Be alert for subcutaneous emphysema or symptoms mimicking those of a pulmonary embolism.

When oral intake begins, assess tolerance of various food substances. Note development of nausea, vomiting, or any other distress. Be alert to signs of nutritional deficiency, such as negative nitrogen balance and weight loss.

Nursing Diagnoses and Planning

Nursing diagnoses and related expected patient outcomes commonly applicable to patients after esophageal resection for carcinoma include the following:

NDx: Pain related to thoracic/upper abdominal surgery

Planning: Patient Outcomes
1. Patient reports that pain is relieved.
2. Patient coughs, breathes deeply, and moves without moaning, crying out, or exhibiting pallor or other sign of distress.

NDx: Risk for ineffective airway clearance related to splinted respirations secondary to thoracic and epigastric pain, presence of chest tube, and poor cough effort

Planning: Patient Outcomes
1. Respirations are easy, silent, and symmetric.
2. Lungs are clear on auscultation.

NDx: Altered nutrition: less than body requirements related to inability to ingest foods or fluids orally

Planning: Patient Outcomes
1. Patient's intake is nutritionally adequate.
2. Patient maintains weight.
3. Electrolyte values, albumin level, and albumin-globulin ratio are within normal limits.

NDx: Risk for infection related to the surgical incision or leaking of the esophageal anastomosis

Planning: Patient Outcomes
1. External incision line is clean and approximated.
2. Foul wound drainage is absent.
3. Patient is afebrile.
4. Pulse, respiration, and blood pressure are within normal limits.
5. Patient denies substernal pain.

Nursing Interventions and Evaluation

NDx: Pain

Medicate for pain as ordered. Avoid overmedicating and depressing the cough reflex and respiratory center. Pay careful attention to positioning and other basic comfort measures. Use the Agency for Health Care Policy and Research postsurgical guidelines to find strategies to help the patient with pain relief. Provide a quiet environment, and encourage the use of breathing, visualization, and other relaxation techniques.

NDx: Risk for ineffective airway clearance

Assist the patient to a semi-Fowler's position to encourage lung expansion. Turn, cough, and deep breathe every 2 hours. Encourage use of the incentive spirometer. If the patient is receiving intermittent positive pressure breathing treatments, ensure that each treatment is followed by supervised coughing. Otherwise, its effectiveness is lost.

NDx: Altered nutrition: less than body requirements
When oral intake is initiated, usually on the fifth or sixth day after surgery, give small sips (about 5 mL) of water every 15 to 30 minutes. Over the next few days, increase the amount taken at one time to 10 or 15 mL, and give plain tea in addition to water. Subsequently, give other bland fluids and, by the end of 2 weeks, allow the patient a soft diet as tolerated. Teach the patient to swallow only small amounts at a time. To prevent reflux and aspiration, instruct the patient to avoid lying down after eating and to keep the head of the bed elevated at night.

If the patient has had a pliable tube prosthesis inserted into the esophagus, swallowing can be very difficult, although the swallowing reflex is intact. Start oral intake with small sips of water until the patient learns how much can be swallowed at one time without difficulty. Add other fluids and soft foods to the diet as tolerated. Because pneumonia resulting from reflux and aspiration of gastric secretion is the primary problem associated with pliable tube prostheses, do not allow the patient to lie flat, and monitor for signs of aspiration. Also monitor the patient for obstruction of the prosthesis, which can be caused by blockage with solid food, pills, or mucosal prolapse.

NDx: Risk for infection
Cleanse the mouth thoroughly and frequently with dilute hydrogen peroxide to decrease oral bacteria. Tape the nasogastric tube securely to the nose. Do not reposition or manipulate it because this could traumatize the anastomosis. Use meticulous aseptic technique in caring for the patient's wounds.

Additional Interventions
Position the patient in semi-Fowler's position to discourage reflux of gastric secretions. Keep the nasogastric tube patent.

Compare the patient's status with the expected outcomes. If the outcomes are not met, reassess the patient and revise the plan.

GASTRIC CANCER

Gastric cancer is seen throughout the world but, like esophageal cancer, exhibits a wide variation in its occurrence. Its incidence is greatest among men in their late sixties who belong to a low socioeconomic group. The incidence of gastric cancer has been steadily decreasing in the United States, although it still remains one of the leading causes of cancer deaths. Table 22–4 lists risk factors for gastric cancer.

Table 22–4

Risks for Gastric Cancer

The following factors represent increased risk:
  Males > females
  Blood group A increases risk by 20%
  50 years old and over
  History of precancerous lesions, pernicious anemia, gastric polyps, chronic gastritis
  Helicobacter pylori infection increases risk 3 to 6 times over risk of general population
  Some correlation with a diet of smoked, highly salted, spiced food, as well as ingestion of nitrites used in preserving foods

Note: The survival rate for early gastric cancer restricted to mucosal and submucosal layers is 85%. This statistic drops to 30% once the tumor has invaded the muscle wall. This is the stage at which gastric tumors are most commonly diagnosed in the United States. Once the lymph nodes are involved, survival rate decreases to 5%. Gastric cancer in early stages is typically asymptomatic. Consequently, screening for gastric cancer is imperative for those at risk.

Etiology and Pathophysiology
The cause of gastric cancer is unknown, but many factors may influence its development. Some are dietary, such as smoked foods, reuse of cooking fats that contain many carcinogens, foods preserved with nitrites, and ingestion of few fresh fruits and vegetables. Other correlations include a history of chronic gastritis or pernicious anemia, and infection with *H. pylori*. Heredity may be a factor as well, because gastric cancer occurs significantly more often in people with type A blood.

Most gastric carcinomas occur in the pyloric region of the stomach, in the area adjacent to the antrum. All are adenocarcinomas, and most present as a bulky mass projecting into the gastric lumen with a deep central ulcer. The remaining tumors appear either as an infiltrating lesion that narrows the lumen, a polypoid mass with or without a stalk, or a diffuse lesion that spreads superficially over the mucosa.

Gastric carcinoma spreads by direct invasion of adjacent tissues, such as the lower esophagus, pancreas, transverse colon, and peritoneum, and by way of the lymphatics to the pancreas and the liver. Late in the disease, hematogenous spread occurs to bone, brain, and lung.

Clinical Manifestations
Early gastric cancer is asymptomatic. When symptoms do occur, they consist of anorexia, weight loss, fullness, and vague epigastric discomfort. This discomfort most often occurs after eating and is unrelieved by antacids. As the disease progresses, bloating, dysphagia, boring epigastric pain, and vomiting caused by obstruction occur. Because gastric tumors

tend to bleed, anemia with its accompanying weakness and fatigue is also a frequent finding. In a few instances, a palpable abdominal mass and ascites are the first noticeable sign.

Diagnosis

Typically, gastric cancer is suggested by barium studies and confirmed by gastroscopy, biopsy, and cytologic studies.

Management

The only curative treatment for gastric cancer is surgery. The type of surgery done depends on the location, type, and extent of the tumor mass. Effectiveness depends on how early the diagnosis is made. Gastrectomy, either partial or complete (see Chap. 21), is the usual procedure. Total gastrectomy is the procedure of choice for a large cancer.

If surgery is contraindicated because of advanced disease, chemotherapy may be used to relieve symptoms. As indicated, gastric cancers are commonly not diagnosed until too late for any effective results from surgery.

❖ Settings, Providers, and Collaboration for Care

Inasmuch as surgery is the main intervention for gastric cancer, treatment for this disorder requires hospitalization for some period of time. Diagnostic and palliative treatment may be administered in an outpatient setting. The discharge planner organizes any follow-up care and physician office visits needed. Before discharge, the nurse instructs the patient and family about continued care needs in the home. If the patient is debilitated or lives alone, a home health nurse may be consulted to assist the patient for a few days after discharge. A dietitian can help the family provide necessary nutrition for the patient. The type of nutritional plan the patient needs depends on the type of surgery. After a total gastrectomy, the patient may need additional evaluation and emotional support from the nurse to maintain a healthy state. Referral to a counselor or psychologist may also be indicated for patients and families not coping well with changes in the patient's health status.

NURSING PROCESS GUIDELINES
Gastric Cancer

Nursing care of patients with gastric cancer varies with the stage of the disease and the type of treatment prescribed. Individualize care given to these patients based on careful assessment of each person's needs. Assess the current physical and psychologic status of all patients. Explore current symptoms and carefully assess nutritional status. Question the patient about changes in appetite and food intake. Check for weight loss. Review laboratory studies for electrolyte imbalances, decreased serum albumin level, decreased total protein level, and decreased serum transferrin level or iron-binding capacity.

Review the patient's history. Note when the cancer was diagnosed, what treatments were given, and the patient's subsequent course. Assess the patient's response to the current hospitalization. Determine the patient's expectations, the patient's and family's understanding of the disease and treatment prescribed, and the support systems available to them.

The Elderly: Special Considerations

Gastrointestinal disorders are a common source of chronic distress among the elderly. Nonetheless, there are no gastrointestinal diseases that are unique to the aged, nor are diseases of the gastrointestinal tract more prevalent in older people than in the rest of the population. The incidence of certain diseases of the upper gastrointestinal system increases with age, and some gastrointestinal symptoms in older people are associated with diseases of the cardiovascular or central nervous system, whose functions affect that of the gastrointestinal system.

Perhaps the most marked oral change in the aged is the loss of teeth. Because older adults have not benefited from recent improvements in dental care, about half the people in the United States age 65 or older wear dentures. This may contribute to a decrease in chewing efficiency and an increased risk of gingivitis and oral cancer.

In the esophagus, age changes give rise to a condition called presbyesophagus. This is a condition in which the intensity of propulsive waves decreases and the frequency of nonpropulsive waves increases. Because these motility changes are generally asymptomatic, complaints of difficulty swallowing or pain on swallowing cannot be attributed to solely to age changes.

Esophageal diseases whose incidence increases with age include hiatus hernia, esophageal diverticula, and esophageal cancer. Hiatus hernias are caused by weakening of the diaphragmatic musculature. The presence of diverticula appears to be associated with weakening of the muscular layer of the esophagus.

Symptoms of esophageal disorders are not always similar to those seen in other age groups. At times, typical symptoms are absent and the presence of disease is indicated by malnutrition or repeated episodes of aspiration pneumonia caused by dysphagia. When pain occurs, it must be carefully differentiated from cardiac pain. Findings consistent with esophageal pain include onset with lying down and relief following administration of antacids.

With increased age, there is a decreased secretion of hydrochloric acid due to atrophy of the gastric mucosa. These changes may contribute to chronic gastritis and pernicious anemia.

The onset of peptic ulcer disease occurs after age 60 in a significant number of patients. Contributing factors include decreased blood flow to the gastric mucosa and increased use of such drugs as aspirin and steroids for arthritic conditions. Symptoms in older adults may be insidious, atypical, or even absent. The first sign of disease might be an episode of upper gastrointestinal bleeding.

Chapter Review

1. Nonsteroidal anti-inflammatory drugs are commonly prescribed for treating arthritis. What are possible solutions to the problem of gastric ulcer formation in these patients?

2. What is the meaning of emesis that looks like coffee grounds in a patient who just had a partial gastrectomy for ulcer disease?

3. How is the care of a patient with ulcer disease similar to that of a patient with acute gastritis?

4. What could happen to a patient after surgery for esophageal cancer if he or she were given oral fluids too soon?

5. How is the care of a patient with a hiatus hernia different from that of a patient with achalasia?

6. Why is monitoring of the red blood cell count, hemoglobin, and hematocrit important for a patient with chronic peptic ulcer disease?

7. What are possible solutions to the problem of dumping syndrome after gastrectomy?

8. How does smoking affect the pain of a patient with gastric ulcer disease?

9. What is the meaning of diarrhea when seen in a patient taking antacids frequently for acute esophagitis?

10. Why would intramuscular vitamin B_{12} supplements be ordered for a patient with chronic gastritis?

Bibliography

Agency for Health Care Policy and Research. Acute pain management: Operative or medical procedures and trauma. AHCPR 92-0032. Rockville, MD: US Department of Health and Human Services, 1992.

Anderson M. *Helicobacter pylori* infection: When and in whom is treatment important? Postgrad Med 1994; 96(6):40.

Ateshkadi A, Lam N, Johnson C. *Helicobacter pylori* and peptic ulcer disease. Clin Pharm 1993; 12:34.

Bates B. A guide to physical examination and history taking. Philadelphia: JB Lippincott, 1995.

Bezarro ER. Changing perspectives of H_2 antagonists for stress ulcer prophylaxis. Crit Care Nurs Clin North Am 1993; 5(2): 325.

Carnevali D, Patrick M (eds). Nursing management of the elderly. 3rd ed. Philadelphia: JB Lippincott, 1993.

Carvajal SH, Mulvihill SJ. Postgastrectomy syndromes: Dumping and diarrhea. Gastroenterol Clin North Am 1994; 23(2):261.

Chase SL. Rx-to-OTC switches: Two H_2 antagonists. RN 1995; 58(9):71.

Drossman D (ed). The functional gastrointestinal disorders: Diagnosis, pathology and treatment. Boston: Little, Brown, 1994.

Fennerty M. Helicobacter pylori. Arch Intern Med 1994; 154(7): 721.

Fitzgerald M, Berg-Gulcher L. Diagnosis and treatment of *Helicobacter pylori* infection in peptic ulcer disease. J Am Acad Nurse Pract 1995; 7(5):233.

Geisinger K. The enigma of achalasia. Am J Gastroenterol 1995; 90(8):1354.

Hall MR, MacLennan WJ, Lye MD. Medical care of the elderly. 3rd ed. New York: John Wiley and Sons, 1993.

Jamieson GC, Debas HT. Surgery of the upper gastrointestinal tract. 5th ed. London: Chapman and Hall, 1994.

Labenz J, Borsch G. Evidence for the essential role of *Helicobacter pylori* in gastric ulcer disease. Gut 1994; 35(1):19.

Lilley LL, Guanci R. Adverse effects of NSAIDs. Am J Nurs 1995; 95(8):17.

Malseed RT, Goldstein FJ, Balkon N. Pharmacology, drug therapy and nursing considerations. 4th ed. Philadelphia: JB Lippincott, 1995.

Mamel JJ. Clinical pharmacology of commonly used drugs in GI practice. Part I. Gastroenterol Nurs 1993; 15(3):114.

Mamel JJ. Clinical pharmacology of commonly used drugs in GI practice. Part II. Gastroenterol Nurs 1993; 15(4):156.

Mathewson M. Pharmacotherapeutics: A nursing process approach. 3rd ed. Philadelphia: FA Davis, 1994.

McKernan JB, Champion JK. Laparoscopic antireflux surgery. Am Surg 1995; 61(6):530.

Meeker MH. Alexander's care of the patient in surgery. 10th ed. St. Louis: CV Mosby, 1995.

Mohamed H, Chiba N, Wilkinson J, Hunt R. Eradication of Helicobacter pylori: Meta-analysis. Gastroenterology 1994; 106(4): A142.

Navab F, Steingrub J. Stress ulcer: Is routine prophylaxis necessary? Am J Gastroenterol 1995; 90(5):708.

National Institutes of Health Consensus Development Panel. *Helicobacter pylori* in peptic ulcer disease. JAMA 1994; 272(1):65.

Norris TE. Upper gastrointestinal problems. Kansas City, MO: American Academy of Family Physicians, 1995.

Parent K. Acid reduction in peptic ulcer disease. Postgrad Med 1994; 96(6):53.

Parsonnet J. *Helicobacter pylori* and gastric cancer. Gastroenterol Clin North Am 1993; 22(1):89.

Shoemaker WC, Ayres S, Grenvik A, et al. Textbook of critical care. 3rd ed. Philadelphia: WB Saunders, 1995.

Sleisenger MH, Fordtran JS. Gastrointestinal disease: Pathophysiology/diagnosis/management. 5th ed. Philadelphia: WB Saunders, 1993.

Sloane R, Cohen H. Common-sense management of *Helicobacter pylori*-associated gastroduodenal disease. Gastroenterol Clin North Am 1993; 22(1):199.

Stanley M, Beare P (eds). Gerontological nursing. Philadelphia: FA Davis, 1994.

Swonger AK, Burbank PM. Drug therapy and the elderly. Boston: Jones and Bartlett, 1995.

Troch P, Jansen H. Laparoscopic Nissen fundoplication: A minimal access alternative. Can Oper Room Nurs J 1994; 12(3):13.

U.S. Public Health Survice, Oral Health Coordinating Committee. Toward improving the oral health of Americans: An overview of oral health status, resources, and care delivery. Public Health Rep 1993; 198:657.

Wastell C, Nyhus LM, Donahue PE. Surgery of the esophagus, stomach and small intestine. Boston: Little, Brown, 1995.

Weant CA. Easing the pain of esophageal surgery. RN 1995; 58: 26.

Williams SR. Nutrition and diet therapy. 7th ed. St. Louis: Mosby–Year Book, 1993.

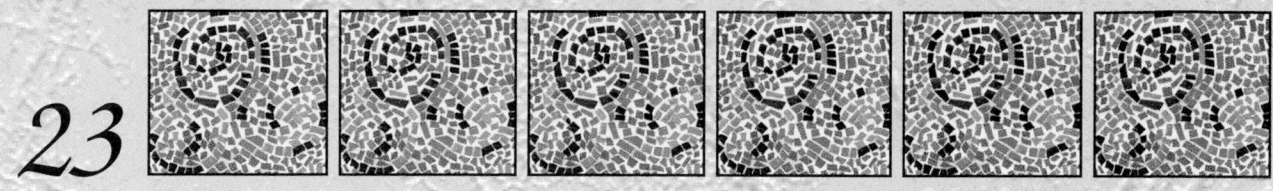

23

Nursing Care of Patients with Disorders of the Lower Gastrointestinal System

Study Outcomes

After studying this chapter, you should be able to:

1. Describe the etiology, pathophysiology, clinical manifestations, diagnostic procedures, and medical management of common lower gastrointestinal disorders.
2. Identify information and physical examination data essential to the assessment of patients with common lower gastrointestinal disorders.
3. State nursing diagnoses and related expected patient outcomes commonly applicable to patients with lower gastrointestinal disorders.
4. Describe nursing interventions, with their rationales, commonly applicable to patients with lower gastrointestinal disorders.
5. Explain the basis for evaluation of nursing care provided to patients with common lower gastrointestinal disorders.
6. Identify alternative treatment and care settings for patients with lower gastrointestinal disorders and the services related to community-based care.
7. Identify special considerations for the elderly patient with a lower gastrointestinal tract disorder.

The major work of the gastrointestinal (GI) system takes place in the small and large intestines. Digestion and absorption of nutrients take place primarily in the small intestine. The colon functions mainly in excretion of waste products.

Disorders of the lower GI system present a challenge to nurses for several reasons. Many of these diseases are obstructive in nature, their signs and symptoms vague and difficult to define. This commonly delays diagnosis of a problem until it is too late for effective treatment. Other disorders, such as the inflammatory bowel diseases, continue to elude efforts to determine their cause, thus thwarting efforts to prevent them or detect them early in their development. Finally, some lower GI disorders are uncomplicated in themselves but become difficult to manage when present in the elderly. Appendicitis,

for example, is a relatively minor problem in a young adult that can be very dangerous in a geriatric patient.

Many lower GI disorders are familial and require frequent assessment to be detected in the early stages. This ongoing assessment may take place in a physician's office or outpatient clinic. Some lower intestinal surgical procedures, such as hernia repairs and hemorrhoidectomies, can take place in a freestanding surgery center or ambulatory surgery department. Other treatments for lower intestinal disorders require extensive hospitalization, including intensive care, and home health services after discharge.

*I*nfections and Inflammations

PERITONITIS

Peritonitis is an inflammation of the peritoneum, which is the thin membrane that lines the abdominal cavity and covers the abdominal organs.

Etiology and Pathophysiology

Bacterial infection is the most common cause of peritonitis. Specific causative organisms include *Escherichia coli*, α-hemolytic and β-hemolytic streptococci, *Staphylococcus aureus*, enterococci, and gram-negative rods. These organisms enter the peritoneal cavity by escaping from the intestinal tract through an opening in its wall or by extension of an infection through the wall of a hollow organ. Thus, conditions that can lead to bacterial peritonitis include:

- Appendicitis
- Perforated peptic ulcer
- Perforated diverticulum

- Necrosis of the intestine secondary to obstruction, infection, or malignancy
- Acute salpingitis
- Continuous ambulatory peritoneal dialysis

Peritonitis also may occur as a result of chemical irritation secondary to introduction of GI secretions into the peritoneal cavity. This can occur with acute hemorrhagic pancreatitis. It also occurs from leakage of an internal suture line at the liver, pancreas, or stomach.

A classic inflammatory reaction—characterized by vascular dilatation, increased capillary permeability, and a serous or slightly turbid exudate—occurs after bacterial or chemical invasion of the peritoneal cavity. Subsequently, the exudate becomes fibrinous and purulent and may be copious. In some cases, it remains localized as abscesses or pockets of pus. In others, it becomes generalized and involves the entire peritoneal cavity.

Generalized peritonitis stimulates the sympathetic nervous system, decreasing peristaltic activity and causing a condition called paralytic ileus, discussed later in the chapter. Loss of large amounts of fluid from the bowel lumen and peritoneal cavity leads to hypovolemia and hemoconcentration, which can lead to shock and oliguria or even to acute tubular necrosis. Septicemia is another dangerous complication, in which the organism causing the peritonitis enters the general circulation.

Resolution of peritonitis takes different forms in different people. In some, the exudate disappears without residual effects. In others, walled-off abscesses remain that either eventually heal or serve as the source of a new infection. In still others, the exudate forms fibrous adhesive bands called adhesions that bind abdominal tissues together and interfere with normal function.

Clinical Manifestations
The primary symptom of peritonitis is severe abdominal pain localized to the involved area and intensified by movement. The abdomen is rigid. The patient experiences nausea, vomiting, and a sudden spike in temperature. Leukocytosis develops. Oliguria, tachycardia, hypotension, sweating, and pallor develop in severe cases of generalized peritonitis as shock ensues secondary to hypovolemia and sometimes to septicemia.

Diagnosis
The diagnosis of peritonitis is usually based on the presenting symptoms coupled with a history of a predisposing event. Diagnosis can be difficult in the elderly and in patients taking corticosteroids, because symptoms can be masked or suppressed. In such cases, tachycardia or unexplained hypotension may be the only early symptom. Definitive diagnosis may depend on x-ray demonstration of free air in the peritoneal cavity, or on paracentesis to confirm the presence of polymorphonuclear leukocytes and bacteria.

Management
Initially, large doses of broad-spectrum intravenous antibiotics are given to combat the infection. If necessary, the antibiotic regimen is adjusted later, based on results of peritoneal fluid cultures.

Fluid, electrolyte, and colloid replacement begins immediately. Nasogastric suction is instituted to help relieve abdominal distention. An indwelling urinary catheter is inserted to allow accurate monitoring of urinary output. If ventilation is impaired because of pressure on the diaphragm from fluid in the abdominal cavity, oxygen is given and, if needed, assisted ventilation with a tracheostomy is instituted.

Eliminating the cause of the problem is also an essential part of management. Thus, a ruptured appendix is excised, a suture line repaired, an abscess drained, a perforation repaired, or an intestine resected. In cases of intestinal pathology, a temporary ostomy may be the initial procedure of choice. Usually, surgery is done as quickly as possible. In selected cases, such as when the patient is a poor operative risk, medical treatment to encourage localization may be used, with surgical drainage performed at a later date.

❖ Settings, Providers, and Collaboration for Care
Peritonitis is a complication of another gastrointestinal problem and is treated in an inpatient setting on either a general unit or an intensive care unit. Initial assessment and treatment may occur in an emergency department, with the patient presenting with signs and symptoms of peritonitis after discharge from the hospital.

NURSING PROCESS
Peritonitis

Assessment
If peritonitis is a potential problem, closely monitor the patient's pain for changes in location and character. Report severe, well-localized abdominal pain, especially if it changes suddenly from the previous pain pattern. Palpate the abdomen for tenderness and rigidity, observe for abdominal distention, and check for diminished or absent bowel sounds every 2 to 4 hours. Check temperature and other vital signs every hour. If peritonitis has been diagnosed, assess vital signs and bowel sounds at least every 2 to 4 hours.

Assess for fluid and electrolyte imbalance by reviewing laboratory values, checking skin turgor, and monitoring intake and output carefully. Be sure to include nasogastric drainage. If a surgical drain is in place, note the color and consistency of the drainage and include the amount on the intake and output record.

Nursing Diagnoses and Planning

Nursing diagnoses and related expected patient outcomes commonly applicable to patients with peritonitis include the following:

NDx: Pain related to inflammation of the peritoneum

Planning: Patient Outcomes
1. Patient states that abdominal pain is relieved.
2. Signs of severe pain, such as pulled-up knees, are absent.
3. Patient rests quietly.

NDx: Risk for altered oral mucous membrane related to mouth breathing and nothing-by-mouth (NPO) status

Planning: Patient Outcomes
1. Oral mucous membranes are pink and moist.
2. Lips are smooth and free of cracks.

NDx: Fear related to treatment and prognosis

Planning: Patient Outcomes
1. Patient acknowledges and discusses fears.
2. Patient verbalizes accurate knowledge of the situation.
3. Patient rests quietly.

Nursing Interventions and Evaluation

NDx: Pain
Position the patient in a semi-Fowler's position to minimize discomfort and promote localization of the infection in the abdominal area. Give analgesics as ordered. Keep in mind, however, that these may need to be given sparingly because of the risk of masking symptoms. Consequently, the use of non-pharmacologic pain control methods is critical. Keep the environment quiet and calm. Keep the bedding clean and free from wrinkles. Provide comfort measures frequently, such as a back rub, change in position, or a fluffed pillow.

NDx: Risk for altered oral mucous membrane
Assist the patient in brushing teeth and cleaning and rinsing the mouth frequently. Avoid using lemon and glycerine swabs and commercial mouthwashes that contain alcohol, because these further dry the mucous membrane. Apply a water-soluble lubricant to the lips to prevent drying and cracking.

NDx: Fear
Acknowledge the patient's fear and give permission for feelings to be expressed. Allow sufficient time for the patient to express feelings. Clarify the patient's understanding of the situation so that groundless fears can be eliminated. Provide opportunities for questions, and give honest answers. Allow the patient to make decisions about care when possible. Explain procedures at a level the patient can understand and within the boundaries of what he or she wants to know.

Additional Interventions
Maintain bedrest and administer intravenous antibiotics as ordered. Monitor the patient for side effects and for expected therapeutic responses. Indications that antibiotics are effectively eliminating the infection include softening of the abdomen, return of bowel sounds, passage of flatus, defecation, and return to normal body temperature.

Replace fluids, electrolytes, and plasma expanders as ordered. Administer oxygen as ordered. If a nasogastric tube is in place, keep it taped securely to the nose and maintain its function. Apply water-soluble lubricant to the nares as needed to prevent irritation and discomfort. When peristalsis returns, start the patient on clear fluids as ordered. Progress as tolerated in accordance with the prescribed diet.

Compare the patient's status with the expected outcomes. If the outcomes are not met, reassess the patient and revise the plan.

APPENDICITIS

Appendicitis is an acute inflammation of the vermiform appendix. It is a common disorder, with a peak incidence between ages 20 and 40.

Etiology and Pathophysiology
Obstruction of the appendix appears to be the precipitating factor in appendicitis. Possible causes of obstruction include calculi (fecaliths) in the appendix, parasites, lymphoid hyperplasia secondary to viral infection, twisting of the appendix by adhesions, and malfunction of a valve system at the appendiceal opening.

Obstruction increases intraluminal pressure, which in turn may collapse the blood vessels in the wall of the appendix and predispose to invasion by local bacteria, such as *E. coli*, enterococci, and β-hemolytic streptococci.

In early acute appendicitis, there is scant neutrophilic exudation throughout the wall, the subserosal vessels are congested, and the serosa becomes a dull, granular red. Subsequently, neutrophilic exudation increases, a suppurative exudate covers the serosa, abscesses form within the wall, and ulcerations and areas of necrosis appear in the mucosa. If unchecked, large areas of hemorrhagic ulceration develop in the mucosa, areas of gangrenous necrosis develop in the wall, and rupture occurs.

Complications of appendicitis include perforation with generalized peritonitis, paralytic ileus, pylephlebitis and thrombosis of the portal veins, septicemia, and subphrenic, pelvic, or lumbar abscess. Table 23–1 shows how to recognize and manage some of these complications.

Table 23–1

Recognition and Management of Appendicitis Complications

Complication	Symptoms	Management
Perforation with generalized peritonitis	Severe pain Fever of 37.7°C (100°F) or higher Abdominal rigidity Vomiting Tachycardia	IV electrolyte and amino acid solutions Nasogastric suction Antibiotics Surgical drainage when localized

Abscess
  Subphrenic
  Lumbar
  Pelvic
	Chills, fever, diaphoresis
	Tachycardia
	Anorexia
	Diarrhea with a pelvic abscess
	Increased leukocytosis
		Parenteral antibiotics to help localize infection
		Surgical drainage
		Appendectomy in 6 weeks

Paralytic ileus	Absent bowel sounds	Nasogastric suction IV fluids and electrolytes

Clinical Manifestations

The principal symptom of appendicitis is persistent pain. In the classic presentation, pain begins as a vague, mild discomfort over the epigastric or periumbilical areas. Over about 4 hours, it increases in intensity, becomes colicky, and usually localizes in the right lower quadrant (Fig. 23–1). This pattern does not occur in all patients, however. Variations include diffuse pain, pain in the lower abdomen, pain referred to the right thigh or testicle if the appendix is behind the cecum, or even pain in the left lower quadrant. If the appendix ruptures, pain may be suddenly relieved, only to be followed by pain resulting from localized or generalized peritonitis.

In addition to pain, anorexia and nausea with or without vomiting are the most frequent symptoms of appendicitis. Occasionally, constipation occurs, but diarrhea is rare. Temperature is usually between 38° and 38.5°C (100.4°–101.4°F) unless the appendix has ruptured, in which case it is higher. Dysuria is not common.

Physical examination findings vary with the age of the patient and the stage of the inflammation. The most significant finding is tenderness when pressure is applied over McBurney's point, which is located midway between the umbilicus and the right anterior iliac spine. Other frequent findings are rigidity of the right rectus muscle, rebound tenderness (pain when deep pressure on the abdomen is released), exacerbation of pain associated with coughing, right lower quadrant pain triggered by palpation of the left lower quadrant, and leukocytosis (12,000/mm^3 or more) with an elevated neutrophil count.

Diagnosis

The diagnosis of acute appendicitis is not easy given the variability of presenting symptoms and the large number of other conditions that can cause an acute abdomen. The diagnosis is especially difficult in the very young and in the elderly. It requires expert clinical judgment based on the patient's history, physical findings, and laboratory and x-ray studies.

Management

The patient who presents with a question of appendicitis is kept on NPO status. No analgesics are given until the decision to operate is made, because they may mask symptoms needed for differential diagnosis. No cathartics or enemas are given because the resultant stimulation of peristalsis irritates the already inflamed area and can precipitate perforation. Intravenous antibiotics are begun, and an ap-

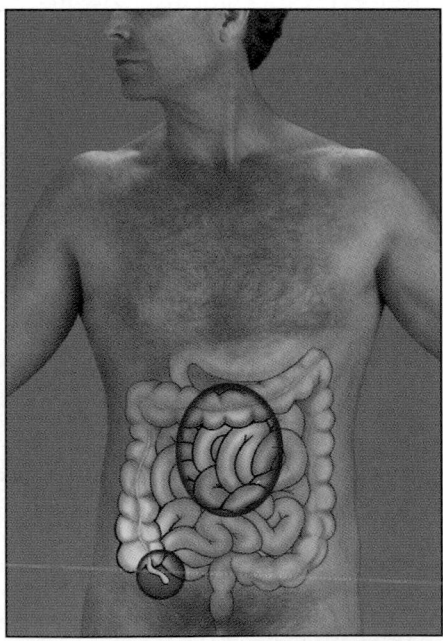

Figure 23–1

Sites of pain in classic appendicitis. The pain usually begins in the epigastric or periumbilical region and, within 4 hours, localizes in the lower right quadrant at McBurney's point, the midpoint between the umbilicus and the right anterosuperior iliac spine.

pendectomy is performed as soon as possible because the longer the duration of symptoms, the greater the likelihood of perforation.

An appendectomy is the surgical removal of the vermiform appendix. The appendix is removed through a lower right quadrant incision and may be done under general or local anesthesia. The laparoscopic approach is also used to remove the appendix in uncomplicated situations.

Patient Preparation

An intravenous infusion is started, and prophylactic antibiotics are given. In some cases, aspirin is also given to reduce fever. A nasogastric tube is inserted if paralytic ileus is suspected; the patient is asked to void; the abdomen is shaved and scrubbed; and preoperative medications are administered.

Postoperative Course

In an uncomplicated appendectomy, oral fluids may be given as soon as the patient is awake, and the patient is progressed to a regular diet as soon as tolerated. If the temperature is normal and discomfort is not excessive, the patient may return home on the day of operation, although a hospital stay of 2 to 3 days is usual. Sutures are removed at a follow-up visit between the fifth and seventh postoperative days. Physically stressful activities need to be avoided for several weeks until the wound is completely healed. If the appendectomy was performed through the laparoscopic approach, discharge is in 1 to 2 days, with return to normal activities within 8 to 10 days.

❖ **Settings, Providers, and Collaboration for Care**

Appendicitis is almost always treated surgically. Although a simple procedure, the patient is usually hospitalized for 1 or 2 days following operation to ascertain that no infection or peritonitis has taken place. Upon discharge, the nurse instructs the patient about any follow-up care needed. An appointment is made for a postoperative visit to the physician's office.

NURSING PROCESS
Appendectomy

PREOPERATIVE NURSING CARE

Because an appendectomy is usually an emergency procedure, the time for preoperative nursing care is limited. Nonetheless, make certain to assess the patient for coexisting physical problems that have implications for nursing care. For example, observe for signs of respiratory infection and question the patient or significant other about any chronic disease and routine use of medication.

Make the patient as comfortable as possible through positioning. Keep in mind that bending the right knee on the abdomen often provides relief. Administer analgesics when prescribed. When pain

medication is not allowed, be certain to explain to both the patient and significant others that the medication may mask symptoms and thus interfere with correct diagnosis. Keep all instructions brief and to the point, as the patient is usually too uncomfortable for long explanations.

Anxiety regarding surgery is generally not a major problem for the patient because it is seen as "the way out of the pain."

POSTOPERATIVE NURSING CARE

Assessment

Make usual postoperative assessments: Take vital signs, measure intake and output, and check the dressing for intactness and for drainage. Also assess for pain and for good respiratory excursion and airway clearance. Check bowel sounds and assess the patient's tolerance of oral intake when resumed.

Nursing Diagnoses and Planning

Because of the lack of time for preoperative teaching, the nursing diagnosis and related expected patient outcomes most commonly applicable to patients who have had an appendectomy are as follows:

NDx: Risk for altered health maintenance related to lack of knowledge of operative procedure, postoperative activities, and discharge instructions

Planning: Patient Outcomes
1. Patient coughs, deep-breathes, splints the incision, and ambulates as directed.
2. Patient states that questions regarding the surgery have been answered satisfactorily.
3. Patient describes self-care at home.

Nursing Interventions and Evaluation

NDx: Risk for altered health maintenance
Explain the importance of coughing and deep-breathing after general anesthesia and guide the patient in performing these activities correctly. Show the patient how to splint the incision with the hands or with a pillow to make coughing and moving easier. Explain how oral intake and ambulation will be resumed.

Ask the patient whether these are any questions about the surgery. Provide the requested information or tell the patient how to acquire it.

Instruct the patient in self-care after discharge (Highlight 23–1).

Additional Interventions
Place the patient in a Fowler's position after recovery from anesthesia. Have the patient cough and deep-breathe every 2 hours. Give oral fluids when desired, and progress the patient to a regular diet as tolerated. Medicate for pain every 3 or 4 hours as prescribed. Get the patient out of bed and beginning to ambulate when he or she is alert and in stable condition.

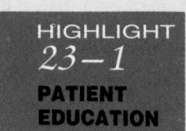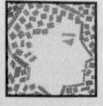

HIGHLIGHT
23–1

PATIENT EDUCATION

Self-Care After Appendectomy

Instruct the patient to:

Gently wash the incision with soap and water daily, and pat dry.

Be aware that if Steri-Strips are in place, they will eventually fall off by themselves. This is expected.

Inspect the incision daily and report any incisional redness, swelling, or drainage.

Avoid clothing that places pressure on the incision line, such as bikini underwear and pantyhose.

Avoid heavy lifting and strenuous exercises. Resume normal activities gradually over 2 to 3 weeks.

Eat small, frequent, high-calorie meals and gradually increase as tolerated.

Report any chills, fever, or increased pain.

Return for follow-up visit on *(specify date and place)*.

Compare the patient's status with the expected outcomes. If the outcomes are not met, reassess the patient and revise the plan.

INFLAMMATORY BOWEL DISEASE

Inflammatory bowel disease is a chronic, inflammatory condition affecting the small intestine, the large intestine, or both. Inflammatory bowel disease is characterized by remissions and exacerbations. It involves several clinical disorders, but the two most common are Crohn's disease and ulcerative colitis. These two syndromes have overlapping characteristics, but they should be considered as two clinically and pathologically distinct disorders.

Crohn's Disease

Crohn's disease is a form of inflammatory bowel disease that is chronic and characterized by exacerbations and remissions. Incidence is highest in adults ages 20 to 40, and it occurs in males and females alike. It is prevalent in the Jewish population and occurs infrequently in African-Americans.

Etiology and Pathophysiology

The cause of Crohn's disease is unknown, although immunologic dysfunction, allergy to such foods as cow's milk or other specific proteins, and heredity are all postulated to contribute to its development. Infection may be an etiologic factor or a secondary effect, because intestinal bacteria counts increase in conjunction with Crohn's disease, fever is a common symptom, and antibiotics and parenteral nutrition (both of which decrease intestinal bacteria), can be effective treatment. Psychogenic factors, for many years thought to cause the disease, are now seen as merely contributing to exacerbations.

Crohn's disease most often involves the terminal ileum and the adjacent right colon, although any part of the GI tract can be affected. Inflamed areas occur randomly in the affected section, producing a patchy distribution of lesions (Fig. 23–2). The affected areas of the bowel are swollen and hyperemic, with ulcerations and longitudinal fissures. Adhesions develop between loops of bowel, and the serosal surface has deposits of mesenteric fat. The mesentery itself is thickened, with engorged lymphatic vessels and enlarged lymph nodes.

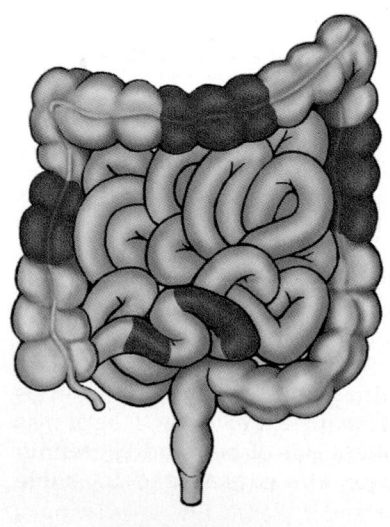

Crohn's Disease

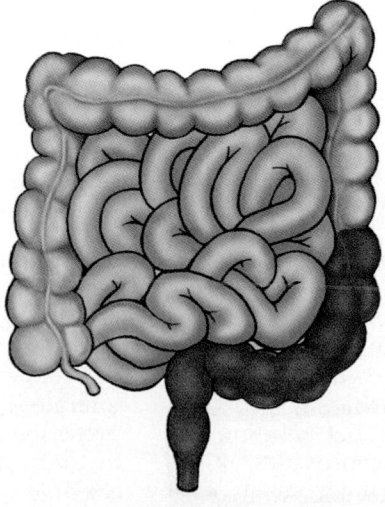

Ulcerative Colitis

Figure 23–2

Regions of the intestine affected by Crohn's disease (left) and ulcerative colitis (right). Crohn's disease most often involves the terminal ileum and the small and large intestine in a segmental manner, with areas of involvement adjacent to undiseased areas. Ulcerative colitis usually starts in the rectum and continues proximally, involving the sigmoid and descending colon.

As the disease progresses, deep ulcers and fissures extend into the muscle layers of the wall. These lesions, which surround small islands of mucosa, give rise to the characteristic "cobblestone" appearance of advanced disease. The lesions of Crohn's disease are transmural, affecting all layers of the intestine. Consequently, fistulas often develop into adjacent segments of the intestine, into other abdominal organs (such as the gallbladder, urinary bladder, and uterus), or through the abdominal wall. Ultimately, the intestinal wall becomes permanently fibrosed, thickened, and narrowed. Absorption is impaired, and small-bowel obstruction may result.

Clinical Manifestations

Crohn's disease affecting the region of the terminal ileum is characterized by episodes of abdominal pain most often occurring after eating and accompanied by fever and mild, usually non-bloody diarrhea (not more than four or five stools daily). Over time, these episodes increase in frequency, duration, and severity. The pain eventually localizes in the right lower quadrant. Weight loss and a history of recurrent oral aphthous ulcers are common, accompanied in some cases by persistent right lower quadrant tenderness or a palpable mass. Weight loss is more profound and pain more diffuse when the jejunum is affected, whereas diarrhea and crampy abdominal pain predominate when primarily the colon is involved.

Weakness, fatigue, anorexia, anemia, and other symptoms of malabsorption and protein-losing enteropathy occur with advanced disease. Perirectal and perianal fistulas are common.

Complications of Crohn's disease can occur outside the GI system, including:

- Erythema nodosum, which manifests as raised, dull red, painful lesions on the legs
- Sacroiliitis, painful inflammation in the sacroiliac joints
- Spondylitis
- Arthritis of the large peripheral joints
- Hepatobiliary disorders, such as cirrhosis and gallstones
- Kidney stones
- Conjunctivitis
- Iritis

Diagnosis

The diagnosis of Crohn's disease is suggested by the patient's history and supported by identification of characteristic changes in upper and lower GI barium studies. These changes include segmental narrowing of the bowel, absence of the normal mucosal pattern, presence of intestinal fistulas, and the "string sign" (ie, narrowed terminal ileum seen when the disease is localized to the terminal ileum and adjacent colon). Proctosigmoidoscopy and colonoscopy may be performed to determine the extent of involvement. In a few cases, intestinal biopsy may be necessary to confirm the diagnosis.

Management

Treatment is palliative because there is no known cure for Crohn's disease. It is aimed at restoring and maintaining normal nutritional status, suppressing inflammation, preventing complications, and minimizing the discomforts of pain and diarrhea.

Nutritional management depends on the severity of the patient's condition. During periods of relatively mild disease, a low-fiber, low-fat diet is prescribed to help control cramping and diarrhea. If lactase deficiency exists, high-lactose foods are eliminated. During acute stages of the disease, enteral feedings with a low-residue defined formula or total parenteral nutrition (TPN) is usually required.

Pharmacologic therapy also varies somewhat with the severity of the disease. Corticosteroids in the form of corticotropin (ACTH), prednisone, or hydrocortisone are used to suppress inflammation in acutely ill patients. These drugs are then tapered off and discontinued when the acute symptoms subside. Parenteral anti-infectives, such as metronidazole, are also given in acute cases. Despite the fact that no causative infective organism has been identified, the use of anti-infectives is sometimes associated with clinical improvement. Similarly, oral antimicrobials may be prescribed in milder cases. Sulfasalazine (Asulfidine), an anti-infective with anti-inflammatory properties, is also often used. Other drugs that may be used in the treatment of Crohn's disease are immunosuppressant and antidiarrheal agents.

Surgery is not ordinarily a part of the treatment plan for patients with Crohn's disease because the disease almost always recurs in the remaining bowel. It is done only when absolutely essential, such as when obstruction, perforation, or a fistula has developed. It is also done in selected cases of intractable disease, in which the patient is so incapacitated by intestinal or systemic symptoms that an acceptable quality of life is not possible. When surgery is essential, the procedure most often performed for Crohn's disease is total proctocolectomy (excision of the rectum and the colon) with ileostomy, although a total colectomy with an ileosigmoid, ileorectal, or ileoanal anastomosis may also be done.

❖ Settings, Providers, and Collaboration for Care

Inflammatory bowel disease is a chronic, progressive disorder that usually requires a variety of treatment settings during its course. Patients with Crohn's disease may need hospitalization for fluid and electrolyte imbalances, malnutrition, or fistula repair. The majority of treatment, however, is managed through a clinic or physician's office, where continued assessment and modification of the treatment plan can occur. Referral to a dietitian may be indicated for nutritional instruction. If a patient is on continuous TPN treatment, home health services will be required. The nurse assists the patient and family to cope with the disease and teaches them to manage the parenteral therapy regimen.

NURSING PROCESS
Crohn's Disease

Assessment

Obtain a history and description of the patient's symptoms. Ask about abdominal pain and note its type, location, severity, duration, and relationship to eating, stress, or other identifiable factors. Question the patient about diarrhea. Determine the number of stools per day, their color, consistency, and odor. Ask specifically about whether the patient has seen any blood in the stool.

Assess the patient's nutritional status. Check for weight loss. Question the patient about anorexia and explore the patient's usual diet both before and after the onset of symptoms. Assess for signs of fluid and electrolyte imbalance. Gently palpate the abdomen for tenderness or a mass. Take the temperature, and inspect the perineal area for irritation, skin breakdown, and fistula formation.

Assess also for signs of extraintestinal complications. Inspect the legs for the dull, red, raised nodules of erythema nodosum. Question the patient about stiffening of the spine and joint pain and observe for movement limitations. Inspect the conjunctiva for signs of inflammation and look for redness in the iris. Question the patient about pain on pupil dilation (pain that is worse in the dark), which is characteristic of iritis. Question about a family history of Crohn's disease and about any known allergies, particularly to milk.

Explore sources of stress in the patient's life and the relationship of episodes of stress to exacerbations of the disease. Identify the person's mode of handling stress, as well as sources of support.

Nursing Diagnoses and Planning

Nursing diagnoses and related expected patient outcomes commonly applicable to patients with Crohn's disease include the following:

NDx: Pain related to inflammation of the intestinal wall

Planning: Patient Outcomes
1. Patient reports that pain has decreased.
2. Patient exhibits no nonverbal signs of abdominal pain.

NDx: Diarrhea related to impaired absorption of sodium and water secondary to mucosal inflammation

Planning: Patient Outcomes
1. Patient passes no more than three stools daily.
2. Stools are formed.

NDx: Risk for impaired skin integrity related to perianal irritation secondary to diarrhea

Planning: Patient Outcomes
1. Patient denies perirectal soreness.
2. Perirectal skin is free of redness.
3. Perirectal skin is intact.

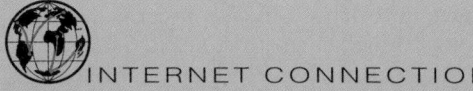
NDx: Risk for altered nutrition: less than body requirements related to limited intake of nutrients as a result of anorexia and fear of exacerbating symptoms and malabsorption

Planning: Patient Outcomes
1. Patient describes appropriate nutritional guidelines.

2. Patient is in positive nitrogen balance.
3. Patient maintains or regains normal weight.

NDx: Ineffective individual coping related to the unpredictable nature of the disease and the inability to manage the stress of changes, common situational crises, and general life demands

Planning: Patient Outcomes

1. Patient identifies ineffective coping behaviors.
2. Patient identifies personal strengths.
3. Patient identifies effective methods of coping.
4. Patient identifies available resources to support coping ability.

Nursing Interventions and Evaluation

NDx: Pain

Encourage the patient to report abdominal pain and accept medication. Administer analgesics and antispasmodics as prescribed and monitor their effectiveness. Position the patient with knees flexed and apply heat to the abdomen if allowed. Encourage deep-breathing and other relaxation exercises.

NDx: Diarrhea

Maintain the patient on bedrest during severe exacerbations to decrease peristalsis. Keep a bedpan and toilet tissue readily available for the patient because episodes of diarrhea are sudden. Place a deodorizer in the room and empty the bedpan immediately to control odor. Administer prescribed antidiarrheal agents. Document the frequency, color, and consistency of stools. Keep the patient on NPO status or give small, frequent, low-residue meals.

NDx: Risk for impaired skin integrity

Monitor for perianal skin irritation and fissures. Wash the area well after each bowel movement. Use tap water for irritated areas and mild, soapy water for surrounding areas. Rinse and pat dry thoroughly. Apply an emollient or topical anesthetic for comfort.

NDx: Risk for altered nutrition: less than body requirements

Administer intravenous fluid and electrolytes, TPN, or nutritional supplements as prescribed. Administer prescribed anticholinergics 30 minutes before meals to decrease bowel motility.

Encourage the patient to avoid smoking because it increases peristalsis. Record intake, output, and weight daily. Instruct the patient in nutritional guidelines (Highlight 23–2).

NDx: Ineffective individual coping

Encourage the patient to discuss fears and feelings related to the disease. Remember that the attacks are unpredictable and can be exhausting and incapacitating, forcing the patient to be out of work and unable to make plans. Acknowledge understanding of these difficulties and provide a private, unrushed environment for discussion of them.

Help the patient identify measures to be used at home to limit the disruptive effect of the disease.

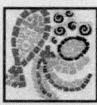

HIGHLIGHT
23–2
NUTRITION

Special Considerations for Patients with Crohn's Disease

Instruct patients with Crohn's disease to:

Eat foods high in protein (eggs, meat, cheese) and calories to promote healing.

Limit fat intake, especially if steatorrhea (fatty stools) is present, by avoiding all fried foods and most dairy products except skim milk.

Eat a low- or minimum-residue diet to reduce fecal output. Avoid raw fruits and vegetables, dried fruit and beans, whole-grain breads and cereals, bran, seeds, and nuts.

Avoid foods that stimulate intestinal peristalsis, such as prune juice, coffee, and carbonated beverages.

Take note of foods that cause discomfort or diarrhea, because individual food intolerances are common. Eliminate these foods from the diet.

Ensure adequate intake of vitamins and minerals, especially vitamin C (found in citrus fruits and juices), folic acid (found in green, leafy vegetables), and zinc (found in red meat). If foods high in these substances are not tolerated in the diet, take supplements as directed.

Promote a restful environment while eating.

Eat slowly and chew foods well.

For example, suggest buying a bedpan or commode if getting to the bathroom is a problem during acute attacks. If time spent in the bathroom is distressing, help the patient identify activities, such as sewing or reading, that can be done during this time.

Support the patient in evaluating lifestyle and in identifying sources of stress. Explore with the patient his or her usual method of coping with stress caused by change, situational crises, or general life demands. Assist the patient in identifying coping mechanisms that have been effective and those that have not. Encourage the patient to devise new strategies to reduce stress. Identify what can be changed and what cannot. Discuss the importance of obtaining adequate rest and avoiding fatigue in relation to coping ability. Help the patient identify and select among available resources, such as support groups. Refer to an appropriate support group or, if indicated, to professional therapy.

Compare the patient's status with the expected outcomes. If the outcomes are not met, reassess the patient and revise the plan.

Ulcerative Colitis

Ulcerative colitis is a form of inflammatory bowel disease that involves only the mucosal and submucosal layers of the colon. It occurs primarily in young adults, although a significant number of cases develop between ages 55 and 60. The disease is much more common among whites than African-Americans. It is also more prevalent among females and those of Jewish descent.

Etiology and Pathophysiology

The cause of ulcerative colitis is unknown. However, the same factors implicated in Crohn's disease are thought to play a role in the development of ulcerative colitis. These include immunologic dysfunction, allergy to specific proteins, viral or bacterial infection, and heredity.

Ulcerative colitis most often begins in the rectum and spreads proximally (see Fig. 23–2). In most cases, spread is limited to the sigmoid and descending colon, although involvement of the transverse and ascending colon can occur. The disease is characterized by diffuse continuous inflammation of the bowel mucosa, which becomes engorged, red, and friable. Multiple small hemorrhages appear, as do scattered yellowish spots—microabscesses in the mucous membrane. These abscesses subsequently develop into larger, multiple, irregular, open ulcerations that give the mucous membrane a moth-eaten appearance. As the disease progresses, these ulcers join to form large, denuded areas where the lining of the colon has been destroyed (Fig. 23-3).

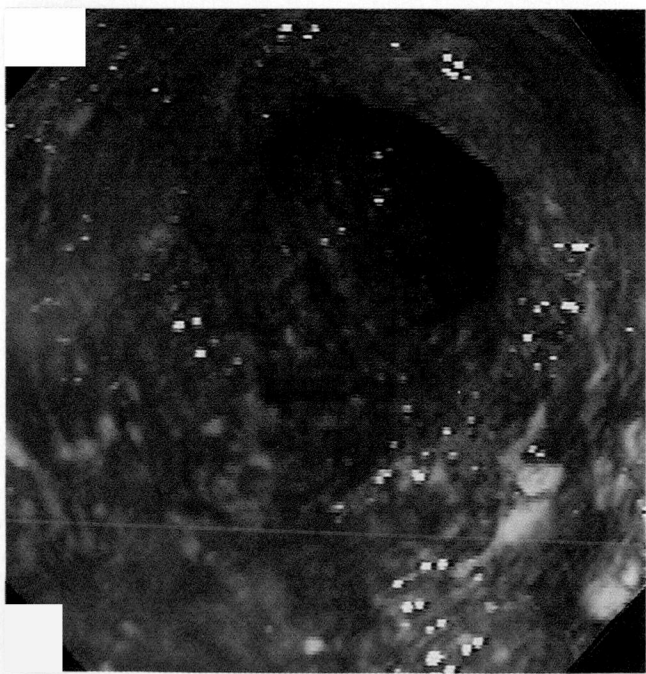

Figure 23–3

Severe ulcerative colitis. (From Wilcox CM. Atlas of clinical gastrointestinal endoscopy. Philadelphia: WB Saunders, 1995, p 218.)

As a result of these changes in the mucosa, sodium and water absorption is impaired, leading to watery diarrhea. Potassium resorption is also impaired and can lead to significant loss, because intestinal juices are high in potassium. In addition, protein is lost through the damaged areas, and hypoalbuminemia results. Iron deficiency anemia eventually develops because of blood loss from the hemorrhagic mucosa.

With repeated attacks of inflammation, the bowel becomes fibrosed, the muscularis mucosae becomes hyperplastic, and the haustrations disappear. This results in a narrowed, shortened bowel with a smooth, tubular appearance. In severe cases, the inflammation also leads to perforation or to dilatation and thinning of the bowel wall. Cancer of the colon has been found to occur in direct proportion to the duration of ulcerative colitis and the extent of colonic involvement.

Clinical Manifestations

Symptoms of ulcerative colitis may develop gradually or have a sudden, acute onset, which sometimes follows a stressful event, minor infection, or even antibiotic therapy. The most frequent symptoms are rectal bleeding, diarrhea, abdominal pain, weight loss, and fever. Other symptoms are those associated with anemia from chronic blood loss in the stools, dehydration and electrolyte imbalance from loss of fluid and electrolytes in the diarrhea, and nutritional problems related to chronic malabsorption of specific nutrients.

Depending on the symptoms, the disease is classified as mild, moderate, or severe (fulminant). In mild ulcerative colitis, symptoms occur gradually and include more frequent bowel movements, rectal bleeding, lower abdominal discomfort, and malaise. With moderate disease, onset is more abrupt, with four or five loose, bloody stools daily and abdominal cramps severe enough to wake the patient from sleep. Low-grade fever, fatigue, and extraintestinal manifestations may occur, such as erythema nodosum on the legs, back pain and stiffening, arthritis in the large peripheral joints, inflammations of the eye, and kidney stones. Severe ulcerative colitis is characterized by profuse diarrhea, rectal bleeding, rectal urgency, high fever, anorexia, and weight loss. Pallor, tachycardia, hypertension, and even shock are not uncommon.

Diagnosis

The diagnosis of ulcerative colitis is based on the patient's history of symptoms, visualization of inflammation on proctoscopy or sigmoidoscopy, negative stool cultures, and absence of parasites on stool examination.

Colonoscopy is contraindicated in moderate to severe cases because of the risk of perforation and hemorrhage. Barium enema is also contraindicated because of the bowel preparation involved and its effects on the inflamed mucosa.

Management

Medical management of ulcerative colitis is similar to that of Crohn's disease. Mild to moderate cases are controlled by a low-roughage diet without milk or milk products, anticholinergics to decrease peristalsis and GI secretion, antidiarrheal drugs to reduce the frequency of bowel movements, and anti-infective drugs such as sulfasalazine. In addition, corticosteroids and immunosuppressive drugs may be prescribed.

For treatment of severe disease, anti-infectives and corticosteroids are used in conjunction with intravenous fluids and electrolytes, blood transfusions, and a nasogastric tube attached to low suction.

Surgery is indicated for unremitting disease and for such complications as perforation or hemorrhage. The most common surgical treatment of ulcerative colitis is a total colectomy with ileostomy (Fig. 23–4). If the rectum is severely involved, proctocolectomy with ileostomy may be performed. Two alternatives to this procedure are the continent ileostomy, or Kock pouch, and an ileoanal anastomosis with or without an ileal reservoir.

Table 23–2 compares Crohn's disease and ulcerative colitis.

❖ Settings, Providers, and Collaboration for Care

Treatment of ulcerative colitis occurs in settings similar to that of Crohn's disease. Mild to moderate presentations may be managed through an outpatient clinic or physician's office. Of course, surgical treatment (ileostomy) requires hospitalization, with long-term home health needs.

NURSING PROCESS GUIDELINES
Ulcerative Colitis

Assessment, nursing diagnoses, expected patient outcomes, nursing interventions, and evaluation for patients with ulcerative colitis are similar to those described previously for patients with Crohn's disease. When a total colectomy with ileostomy is done, provide care as presented later in this chapter.

ANORECTAL ABSCESS

An anorectal abscess is a localized infection with a collection of pus in the anorectal area.

Etiology and Pathophysiology

Rectal abscesses begin as inflammations of the rectal crypts. Later, cysts form that extend into the submucosal layer. Abscess formation occurs secondary to infection with normal rectal flora such as *E. coli*, *Proteus*, staphylococci, or streptococci. An anorectal fistula (Fig. 23–5) may develop as a complication of an anorectal abscess (Table 23–3). Persons with Crohn's disease and immunodeficiency disorders are at risk for anorectal abscess.

Clinical Manifestations

A classic symptom of anorectal abscess is constant, throbbing pain aggravated by sitting and by defecation. Other symptoms are tenderness and swelling in the area of the abscess, foul-smelling and purulent drainage, and fever.

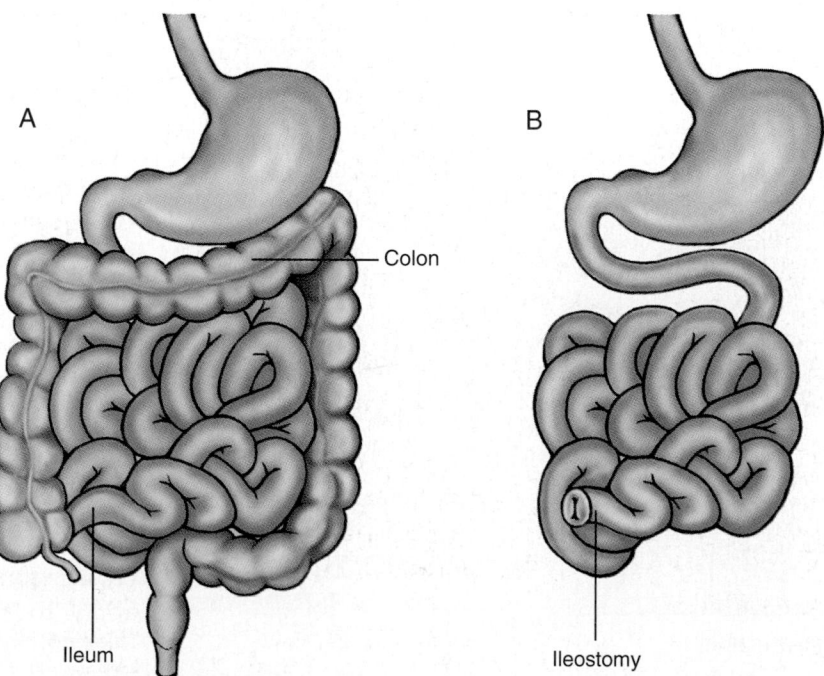

Figure 23–4

A, Lower gastrointestinal tract before total colectomy. *B*, Lower gastrointestinal tract after total colectomy with ileostomy.

Table 23—2

Comparing Crohn's Disease and Ulcerative Colitis

ETIOLOGY	*Both.* Cause is unknown. Similar factors are postulated to contribute to both: heredity, immunologic dysfunction, allergy.
PATHOPHYSIOLOGY	*Crohn's disease.* Can affect any area of the gastrointestinal tract and is characterized by segmental involvement, linear ulcers, cobblestone appearance, and fistulas. *Ulcerative colitis.* Affects primarily the lower colon and is characterized by continuous symmetric inflammation and engorged, friable mucosa with a moth-eaten appearance because of multiple, large, irregular, open ulcers.
CLINICAL MANIFESTATIONS	*Crohn's disease.* Mild diarrhea accompanied by right lower quadrant abdominal pain but without rectal bleeding and a palpable abdominal mass. *Ulcerative colitis.* Diarrhea, often severe, with rectal bleeding. *Both.* Extraintestinal complications, including erythema nodosum, spondylitis, arthritis in the large joints, cirrhosis, cholelithiasis, kidney stones, conjunctivitis, and iritis.
MEDICAL DIAGNOSIS	*Crohn's disease.* Diagnosis depends on characteristic findings on upper and lower intestinal contrast studies. *Ulcerative colitis.* Diagnosis depends on visualization of diffuse inflammation during proctosigmoidoscopy and negative stool cultures and examination for parasites. *Both.* Diagnosis of both diseases is suggested by the patient's history. Occasionally, a biopsy is necessary to confirm either diagnosis.
MEDICAL MANAGEMENT	*Crohn's disease.* Surgery is not a treatment of choice because of almost certain recurrence in the remaining bowel. *Ulcerative colitis.* Colectomy is considered curative. *Both.* Palliative management includes low-fiber, low-fat diet (also low in lactose if lactase deficiency exists); enteral feedings with a low-residue defined formula or total parenteral nutrition if needed; corticosteroids to suppress inflammation; anti-infectives, sulfasalazine, immunosuppressive or antidiarrheal therapy.

Diagnosis

A diagnosis of anorectal abscess is suggested by characteristic rectal pain. It is confirmed by digital palpation of the abscess externally or internally or, in some cases, by visualization during proctoscopy.

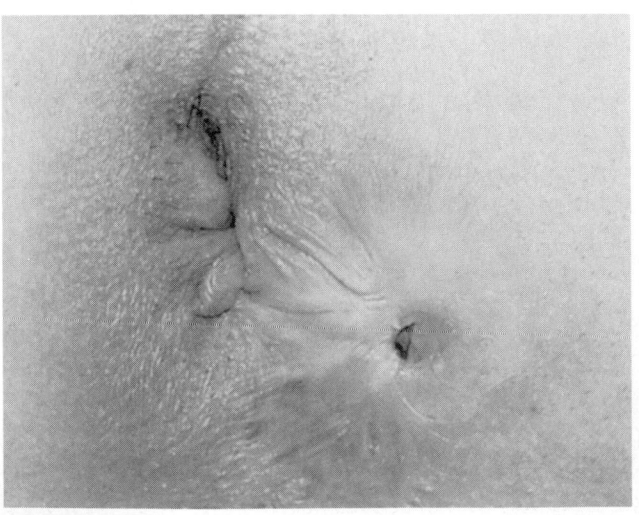

Figure 23–5
Anorectal fistula. (From de los Ríos Magriñá E. Atlas of therapeutic proctology. Philadelphia: WB Saunders, 1984, p 106.)

Management

Treatment of an anorectal abscess involves incision and drainage, followed by antibiotic therapy. Often the wound is packed with Vaseline gauze and allowed to heal by granulation.

❖ Settings, Providers, and Collaboration for Care

Usually, an anorectal abscess is treated as a day-surgery procedure or in a standing clinic or physician's office. In some cases, the patient may require admission to an acute care hospital for a 1- or 2-day stay.

NURSING PROCESS
Incision and Drainage of a Rectal Abscess

PREOPERATIVE NURSING CARE

Preoperative nursing care of a patient scheduled for incision and drainage of an anorectal abscess involves the basic assessments and interventions that apply to any surgical patient. The patient should take nothing by mouth after midnight, and a bowel preparation should be done. Be sure the patient understands what will be done, its expected effect, and

Table 23–3

Anorectal Fissures, Fistulas, and Cysts

	Anal Fissure	Anorectal Fistula	Pilonidal Cyst
DESCRIPTION	Ulcer or crack in lining of anal wall	Hollow tract connecting anal canal or rectum with perianal skin	Cyst lined with dermoid tissue and hair found at the base of the spine about 5 cm (2 in) above anus
ETIOLOGY	Anal trauma, such as passage of a hard, large stool	Rupture or incision and drainage of anorectal abscess, cancer, radiation therapy, Crohn's disease	Congenital defect
CLINICAL MANIFESTATIONS	• Severe, burning pain on defecation • Small amount of bleeding • Painful spasms of anal sphincter • Constipation from fear of pain on defecation	• Constant irritating drainage of blood, pus, mucus, and sometimes stool	• Asymptomatic unless infected, in which case pain, swelling, and drainage.
MEDICAL MANAGEMENT	• Comfort measures, such as local anesthetics, sitz baths, and stool softeners until healed • Chronic cases may require surgical excision	• Fistulotomy (opening of the tract) or fistulectomy (excision of the tract) • Wound is packed with gauze and allowed to heal by granulation • Treatment of underlying disorder	• Incision and drainage • Wound either closed or packed and left to heal by granulation • Sitz baths
NURSING CARE	Same as for hemorrhoidectomy	Same as for hemorrhoidectomy	Same as after incision and drainage of anorectal abscess

the usual postoperative course. Provide additional explanation as needed.

POSTOPERATIVE NURSING CARE

Assessment

Assess the patient's return to physiologic stability after surgery. Make ongoing assessments of the patient's discomfort. Inspect the operative area for bleeding and drainage, being careful not to dislodge any rectal packing inserted during surgery. Note the amount, color, and odor. Measure urinary output and check the frequency and consistency of bowel movements, because some degree of urinary retention and constipation is likely to occur. If the patient's surgery took place in a surgicenter or ambulatory surgery department, assess the understanding of the patient or significant other of the signs and symptoms of complications and the ability to reach health care if needed.

Nursing Diagnoses and Planning

Nursing diagnoses and related expected patient outcomes commonly applicable to patients who have

had incision and drainage of an anorectal abscess include the following:

NDx: Pain related to surgical trauma in the anorectal area

Planning: Patient Outcomes
1. Patient states that he or she is comfortable.
2. Patient tolerates a sitting position 24 hours postoperatively.

NDx: Risk for infection (recurrent) related to contamination and poor healing of the wound

Planning: Patient Outcomes
1. Pink granulation tissue is evident in the wound.
2. Wound is free of odor and purulent drainage.
3. Patient is afebrile.

NDx: Knowledge deficit: self-care in the home

Planning: Patient Outcomes
1. Patient verbalizes normal appearance and odor of drainage from wound site.
2. Patient demonstrates ability to assess wound dressings.
3. Patient verbalizes that wound packing is not to be removed until the physician does so.

Nursing Interventions and Evaluation

NDx: Pain

Administer prescribed analgesics as needed, usually every 4 hours in the immediate postoperative period and, after the immediate postoperative period, before dressing changes and bowel movements. Keep the patient in a side-lying position for the first 24 hours to prevent pressure on the surgical area. Thereafter, allow the patient to sit for short periods of time and provide a flotation pad or foam doughnut cushion for comfort. Give sitz baths, or apply warm, moist compresses as ordered.

Provide a high-fiber diet and encourage the patient to drink large amounts of fluids daily to promote passage of soft, formed stools. Give bulk-forming stool softeners as ordered to prevent constipation and trauma to the operative area from the passage of hard stool.

NDx: Risk for infection

Use a binder to anchor a dressing over the wound while drainage persists. If packing is in place, it is ordinarily changed daily. Remove packing gently after soaking it loose with saline or half-strength hydrogen peroxide or soaking in a sitz bath. Use strict sterile technique when caring for the wound. Explain to the patient the importance of careful cleansing of the area after defecation. Instruct the patient to take a sitz bath after each bowel movement.

NDx: Knowledge deficit: self-care in the home

Before discharge, teach the patient how to care for the wound at home. Stress the need to avoid any potential contamination to the area and to report signs of recurrent infection, such as increased pain, purulent drainage, or fever.

Compare the patient's status with the expected outcomes. If the outcomes are not met, reassess the patient and revise the plan.

Functional Disorders

MECHANICAL OBSTRUCTION

Mechanical obstruction is a condition in which movement of intestinal contents through the intestine is impaired by an identified obstructing source.

Etiology and Pathophysiology

Mechanical obstruction can result from problems outside the intestine, within the wall of the intestine, or within the lumen of the intestine. Problems outside the intestine that can cause mechanical obstruction include adhesions, tumors on adjacent organs, and hernias. Problems within the intestinal wall include stricture, hematomas, and intramural tumors. Foreign bodies, intussusception, volvulus (twisting of the bowel), and epithelial tumors are examples of problems within the intestinal lumen (Fig. 23–6).

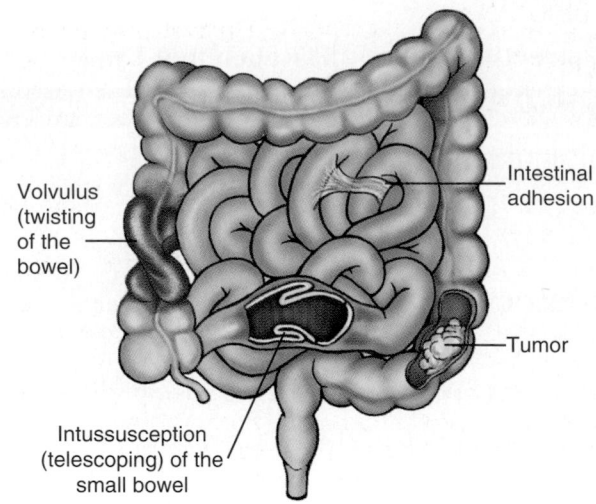

Figure 23–6

Causes of mechanical intestinal obstruction. Illustrated here are volvulus (twisting of the bowel), adhesion, tumor, and intussusception (telescoping of the bowel).

Movement of air, food, and secretions in the direction of the rectum ceases. The bowel proximal to the obstruction dilates, and the distal bowel tends to collapse. Absorption is diminished and intestinal secretion increases. Intraluminal pressure increases and ultimately results in ischemia and necrosis of the bowel. Bacteria multiply.

Fluid and electrolyte imbalances that occur include hyponatremia and the loss of hydrogen ions and chloride from vomiting gastric contents, metabolic alkalosis, and hypochloremia. In unresolved intestinal obstruction, large amounts of extracellular fluid become sequestered in the intestine and plasma weeps into the peritoneal cavity. Hypovolemia and shock can ensue.

Clinical Manifestations

The predominant symptoms of mechanical ileus are vomiting, cramping, abdominal pain, distention, and inability to pass stools or flatus. When the obstruction is high in the intestine, vomiting is marked and abdominal distention limited. Conversely, when the obstruction is low, the patient has marked distention but little vomiting. Bowel sounds are high-pitched, frequent, and rushing (periodic loud bursts). Sometimes they disappear late in the course of the obstruction. With loss of extracellular fluid into the intestine and vomiting, symptoms of dehydration and hypovolemia occur.

Diagnosis

Diagnosis of mechanical bowel obstruction or ileus is based on the history and physical findings. It can be confirmed by plain x-rays of the abdomen, which show air or fluid levels in the obstructed bowel. Once obstruction is confirmed, diagnostic measures to determine its cause can begin.

Management

Initial treatment of mechanical bowel obstruction is supportive. The patient is on NPO status, and a nasogastric or intestinal tube is inserted to decompress the intestine and prevent vomiting. Intravenous fluids and electrolytes, and in some cases TPN, are given as needed to maintain homeostasis. Antibiotics are given to combat infection. Analgesics may be given for pain. Once the underlying condition is diagnosed and the patient stable, surgical correction is performed.

❖ **Settings, Providers, and Collaboration for Care**

Mechanical bowel obstructions are a complication of some other problem. Persons experiencing signs and symptoms may present in an emergency department or may already be hospitalized for treatment of the original disorder. Usually, patients with mechanical obstructions are hospitalized for several days.

NURSING PROCESS
Mechanical Ileus

Assessment

Assess symptoms and their time of onset. Assess for abdominal pain. If present, note the type, location, and severity. Ask about vomiting and determine the amount, color, odor, and consistency of the vomitus. Listen for bowel sounds and check for abdominal distention. Determine when the patient last had a bowel movement and passed flatus.

Observe for signs of dehydration and hypovolemia. Inspect oral mucous membranes for dryness and check skin turgor. Take vital signs to check for increased temperature, a rapid and weak pulse, rapid respirations, and hypotension. Check urinary output, and review laboratory values of hematocrit and serum electrolytes.

Palpate the abdomen gently for rigidity and be alert to increasing pain, fever, or leukocytosis, which could indicate peritonitis.

Once the nasogastric or intestinal tube is in place and attached to suction, assess its function and note the amount and character of the drainage. Inspect the naris for signs of irritation, and question the patient about nasal discomfort.

Assess the patient's understanding of the supportive treatment being given and the diagnostic procedures ordered. Once the underlying problem is diagnosed, assess the patient's understanding of it and of the planned surgical intervention.

Nursing Diagnoses and Planning

Nursing diagnoses and related expected patient outcomes commonly applicable to patients with a mechanical ileus include the following:

NDx: Risk for fluid volume deficit related to sequestering of ECF in the intestine, weeping of plasma into the peritoneal cavity, and vomiting

Planning: Patient Outcomes
1. Blood pressure, pulse, and respirations are within the patient's normal range.
2. Urinary output is 50 mL or more per hour.
3. Serum electrolytes and osmolarity are within normal limits.

NDx: Pain related to increased intraluminal pressure

Planning: Patient Outcomes
1. Patient states that pain is relieved.
2. Patient rests without verbal or nonverbal signs of pain.

NDx: Risk for altered health maintenance related to insufficient knowledge of supportive treatment, diagnostic tests, diagnosis, and surgical intervention

Planning: Patient Outcomes
1. Patient states reasons for supportive treatment, such as NPO status and nasogastric suction.
2. Patient states purpose of ordered diagnostic tests.
3. Patient describes simply but accurately the diagnosis underlying the disorder.
4. Patient describes the surgical procedure and its expected effect.

Nursing Interventions and Evaluation

NDx: Risk for fluid volume deficit

Administer intravenous fluid and electrolytes prescribed to replace lost water, sodium, chloride, and potassium. These might consist of isotonic sodium chloride alternating with 5% dextrose and water with up to 40 mEq of potassium. Monitor central venous pressure to ensure adequate replacement and prevent overload.

NDx: Pain

Monitor function of the nasogastric suction and give analgesics as ordered for pain. Change the patient's position frequently for comfort. Maintain a quiet, calm environment.

Apply water-soluble lubricant to the naris to prevent irritation from the nasogastric or nasointestinal tube.

NDx: Risk for altered health maintenance

Explain to the patient the reason for treatments. Describe ordered diagnostic tests and explain their purpose. When the underlying problem and a plan of surgical intervention have been identified, clarify and reinforce the physician's explanation to ensure that the patient and the family understand. Encourage questions and allow time for expression of concerns.

Compare the patient's status with the expected outcomes. If the outcomes are not met, reassess the patient and revise the plan.

PARALYTIC ILEUS

Paralytic ileus, also called adynamic ileus, is the impaired movement of intestinal contents through the intestine because of reduced or absent peristalsis.

Etiology and Pathophysiology

Paralytic ileus can result from severe physiologic stress such as:

Abdominal surgery
Burns
Peritonitis
Blunt traumatic injury to the abdomen
Intra-abdominal vascular accident
Severe electrolyte imbalance

Abdominal surgery is by far the most common cause of paralytic ileus. In fact, it is said that ileus occurs to some extent in every patient who has had an abdominal operation.

Excessive sympathetic nervous system activity is believed to cause the decrease or absence of peristalsis, which, in turn, causes the intestine to become flaccid and functionally obstructed. Fluid accumulates in the bowel lumen because intestinal secretion is normal but absorption and motility are impaired. There is little increase in intraluminal pressure, however, because the fluid is evenly distributed throughout the tract; hence, there is little risk of ischemia of the intestinal wall. There is a risk of dehydration, which can lead to shock and renal failure as a result of fluid loss from the intestine by vomiting or suction if fluid and electrolytes are not replaced.

Clinical Manifestations

The major symptoms of paralytic ileus are decreased to absent bowel sounds, abdominal distention, and vomiting or increased nasogastric drainage. If dehydration results, oliguria, tachycardia, poor skin turgor, and dry mucous membranes may present. Tenderness or pain is minimal or absent unless the ileus is associated with peritonitis, although patients will often complain of severe abdominal gas pain.

Diagnosis

Paralytic ileus is diagnosed primarily on the patient's history and presenting symptoms (decreased or absent bowel sounds, failure to pass flatus, emesis, or excessive GI tube drainage). A plain abdominal x-ray showing uniform distention of the intestinal lumen throughout the small and large bowel substantiates the diagnosis.

Management

Paralytic ileus resolves spontaneously in an average of 3 to 5 days. Therefore, symptomatic treatment consisting of nasogastric suction for intestinal decompression, and fluid and electrolyte replacement is provided while waiting for the parasympathetic nervous system to override the sympathetic nervous system and allow return to normal function. Ambulation is encouraged if possible because it promotes bowel function. Rarely, drugs that stimulate the parasympathetic nervous system are given.

❖ Settings, Providers, and Collaboration for Care

Paralytic ileus is a complication of physiologic stress and is treated in the setting of the original care.

NURSING PROCESS
Paralytic Ileus

Assessment

Assess all postoperative patients, especially those who underwent abdominal procedures, for signs and symptoms of paralytic ileus. Check bowel sounds every 4 to 8 hours and check the abdomen for distention. Note vomiting because, although some emesis is not unusual after general anesthesia, profuse vomiting indicates paralytic ileus. Observe the amount and quality of any GI tube drainage every 4 hours. Question the patient about the presence and passage of flatus and assess the frequency of bowel movements.

Nursing Diagnoses and Planning

Nursing diagnoses and related expected patient outcomes commonly applicable to patients with paralytic ileus include the following:

NDx: Risk for fluid volume deficit related to vomiting or excessive GI drainage

Planning: Patient Outcomes
1. Patient's intake approximates output.
2. Patient's skin turgor is good.
3. Patient's mucous membranes are moist and pink.

NDx: Anxiety related to meaning of vomiting, distention, insertion of a nasogastric tube, and prolonged NPO status

Planning: Patient Outcomes
1. Patient describes paralytic ileus as a basically benign response to surgery that disappears with time.
2. Patient states the reason for a nasogastric tube and NPO status.
3. Patient expresses confidence that the ileus will resolve without negative sequelae.

Nursing Interventions and Evaluation

Although there is no specific treatment for paralytic ileus, interventions that diminish existing distress and promote peristalsis are used. Encouragement of ambulation is especially important.

NDx: Risk for fluid volume deficit
Administer intravenous fluids as ordered. Record intake and output, including emesis and nasogastric drainage. Monitor laboratory data, skin turgor, and condition of mucous membranes for signs of dehydration.

NDx: Anxiety
Explain paralytic ileus to the patient. Stress that it is a common response to abdominal surgery and that normal intestinal function returns spontaneously, usually within a week. Explain the need for nasogastric drainage and being NPO.

Additional Interventions
If allowed, encourage the patient to move about and walk. Explain that these activities promote normal

bowel function. Maintain NPO status until peristalsis returns, then give small amounts of fluid, and progress the diet as tolerated in accordance with the physician's order.

Compare the patient's status with the expected outcomes. If the outcomes are not met, reassess the patient and revise the plan.

MALABSORPTION SYNDROME

Malabsorption syndrome refers to the signs and symptoms that result from impaired passage of proteins, carbohydrates, fats, vitamins, and minerals across the intestinal wall and into the circulation. In its full-blown form, absorption of all of these major nutrients is impaired. In less severe cases, impaired absorption is limited to one or more of the nutrients.

Etiology and Pathophysiology

The causes of malabsorption are many. Any factor that interferes with chemical or mechanical digestion, and thus affects the condition or the length of time during which nutrients are presented to the intestinal wall for absorption, can result in malabsorption. Examples of these conditions are pancreatic insufficiency, deficiency of conjugated bile acids, and gastrectomy.

Any conditions that alter the intestinal mucosa or decrease the absorptive surface can also cause malabsorption. These conditions include gluten-induced enteropathy, Crohn's disease, and intestinal resection. Additional causes of malabsorption are obstruction to the intestinal lymphatic system (as can occur with lymphoma), tuberculosis, infections, disease of the distal ileum, and such drugs as cholestyramine, colchicine, kanamycin, bacitracin, polymyxin, neomycin, and irritant laxatives.

For unknown reasons, malabsorption can also accompany thyroid disorders and diabetes mellitus.

Clinical Manifestations

The clinical manifestations of malabsorption vary with the nutrients affected and the severity of the problem (Table 23–4). The classic symptoms of full-blown malabsorption syndrome are weight loss, muscle wasting, bloating, borborygmus, and passage of frequent bulky, gray, greasy, foul-smelling stools, which are indicative of steatorrhea.

In cases in which malabsorption is less severe or intermittent, the primary symptoms may be chronic fatigue, lack of drive, and depression.

Diagnosis

The diagnosis of malabsorption and identification of the underlying cause require extensive diagnostic testing. Diagnostic findings compatible with malabsorption syndrome are decreased serum albumin, carotene, calcium, cholesterol, potassium, magnesium, vitamin B_{12} and folic acid, elevated prothrombin time, and an increase in stool fat based on the chemical analysis of a 72-hour stool collection obtained while the patient is ingesting 80 to 100 g of fat per 24 hours.

Other diagnostic tests include tolerance tests for

Table 23–4

Manifestations of Nutritional Deficiency in Malabsorption Syndrome

Malabsorbed Nutrient	Clinical Manifestations
Protein	Weight loss, muscle wasting, alopecia, peripheral edema
Carbohydrate	Weight loss, diarrhea, flatulence, abdominal distention
Fat	Weight loss, diarrhea, steatorrhea, dermatitis
Vitamin A	Epithelial keratinization, follicular hyperkeratosis, skin and mucous membrane infections
Thiamin (B_1)	Anorexia, constipation, fatigue, depression, apathy, neuritis in the legs, cardiac failure
Riboflavin (B_2)	Glossitis, cheilosis, dermatitis, photophobia
Folic acid	Macrocytic and megaloblastic anemia, glossitis, cheilosis, dermatitis
Niacin	Dermatitis, weakness, anorexia, diarrhea, apathy, depression, mental confusion
Pyridoxine	Nervous irritability, weakness, hypochromic and microcytic anemia, seborrhea-like skin lesions
Vitamin B_{12}	Pernicious anemia, glossitis, cheilosis, peripheral neuropathy, paresthesias
Vitamin D	Softening of the bones, bone deformity, bone pain, fractures, muscle weakness, tetany
Vitamin K	Bruising, bleeding, hematuria, hypoprothrombinemia, prolonged clotting time
Calcium	Positive Trousseau's and Chvostek's signs, tetany, osteoporosis, osteomalacia, bone pain, fractures, hypertension
Iron	Brittle nails, anemia, glossitis, cheilosis, stomatitis, decreased resistance to infection
Sodium	Muscle cramps, weakness
Zinc	Dermatitis
Potassium	Muscle flaccidity, weakness, decreased tendon reflexes, cardiac dysrhythmias
Magnesium	Neuromuscular dysfunction, muscle spasms, tremors, tetany, anorexia, nausea, decreased tendon reflexes, apathy, personality changes, cardiac dysrhythmias
Phosphate	Osteomalacia
Water	Dehydration

d-xylose, glucose, lactose, sucrose, and vitamin B_{12}; breath tests for fat absorption and bacterial overgrowth; ultrasonography, computed tomographic scans, and x-rays to identify abnormalities in the GI tract; and, in some cases, biopsies of the intestinal mucosa.

Management

Medical management depends on the specific underlying cause. Measures to restore fluid, electrolyte, and nutritional balance are an essential part of the management of all patients.

❖ Settings, Providers, and Collaboration for Care

Malabsorption syndromes are treated in a variety of settings, depending on the cause. Usually, long-term malabsorption problems are treated on an outpatient basis. Hospitalization may be required when severe fluid and electrolyte imbalances or nutritional deficits occur. If the underlying cause is treated surgically, hospitalization is required. The expertise of a dietitian may be needed to assist with meal planning.

NURSING PROCESS GUIDELINES
Malabsorption Syndrome

Nursing care of patients with malabsorption syndrome varies with the medical management of the underlying cause. In all cases, however, thoroughly assess nutritional status, and administer replacement or supplementary fluids, electrolytes, and nutrients as ordered.

GLUTEN-INDUCED ENTEROPATHY

Gluten-induced enteropathy is a disorder of absorption also referred to as nontropical sprue or celiac sprue. It varies in severity and occurs more often in females than in males.

Etiology and Pathophysiology

As the name suggests, gluten-induced enteropathy is caused by an immunologic sensitivity to the protein gluten. Large amounts of gluten are found in wheat and rye. Smaller amounts are found in oats and barley.

In sensitive persons, gluten causes atrophy of the intestinal mucosa and flattening of the villi (Fig. 23–7). The result is impaired absorption as a result of decreased uptake and transport of proteins, fats, carbohydrates, and often the fat-soluble vitamins, vitamin B_6, vitamin B_{12}, iron, folate, and trace elements.

In some cases, a temporary intolerance to lactose (milk sugar) also occurs. This results from a deficiency of the enzyme lactase, which develops from changes in the intestinal mucosa.

Clinical Manifestations

Gluten-induced enteropathy presents with the classic symptoms of malabsorption, which vary in degree

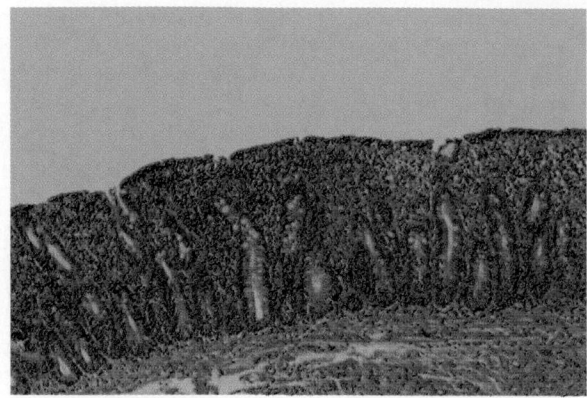

Figure 23–7

Gluten-induced enteropathy. This biopsy specimen from the second part of the duodenum shows the characteristic flattened mucosa. (From Owen DA, Kelly JK. Atlas of gastrointestinal pathology. Philadelphia: WB Saunders, 1994, p 76.)

with the severity of the disorder. GI and other symptoms include:

- Frothy, gray, foul-smelling, bulky stools that float in the toilet bowl because of their gas content, indicative of steatorrhea
- Abdominal distention
- Crampy abdominal pain
- Anorexia
- Sometimes diarrhea
- Chronic fatigue
- Weight loss
- Anemia

In delayed diagnosis and severe disease, additional symptoms may include muscle wasting, edema, bleeding, hypotension, and symptoms of hypocalcemia.

Diagnosis

There is no diagnostic text specific for gluten-induced enteropathy. An intestinal biopsy showing atrophy of the villi is considered essential to the diagnosis but does not exclude other possible disorders. Definite diagnosis requires a demonstrated remission of the disease in response to the elimination of dietary gluten.

Management

Management of gluten-induced enteropathy involves elimination of gluten from the diet. Such a gluten-free diet requires avoidance of all cereal grains except for rice and corn. This diet must be followed for life because, even though the intestinal mucosa returns to normal when the diet is followed, reexposure to gluten causes a reactivation of the pathology. A therapeutic response to the gluten-free diet is seen as early as in a week and, in the majority of patients, in no more than 8 weeks.

In the initial period of treatment, a high-calorie, high-protein diet with vitamin and mineral supplements is often given to help the patient regain normal nutritional status. If lactose intolerance is a problem, milk and milk products are limited until improvement occurs.

Corticosteroids may be used temporarily in patients who are critically ill or in long-term patients who are unresponsive to a gluten-free diet.

❖ Settings, Providers, and Collaboration for Care

Gluten-induced enteropathy is treated in an outpatient setting unless severe complications occur. Consultation with a dietitian about foods appropriate to a gluten-free diet should be considered, especially for the primary food shopper.

NURSING PROCESS
Gluten-Induced Enteropathy

Assessment

Assess the patient for symptoms of malabsorption. Explore the patient's symptoms. Question the patient about bowel elimination patterns. Note the frequency of bowel movements and the characteristics of stool. Ask specifically about the occurrence of frothy, foul-smelling, bulky stools that float, because these are characteristic of steatorrhea. Also ask the patient about abdominal pain, cramping, and distention. Obtain current weight. Determine whether weight loss has occurred and over what period of time. Question the patient about anorexia. Obtain a diet history that includes types and amounts of foods usually eaten. Compare this with the patient's report of current dietary intake, and explore the relationship of eating to symptoms. Also question about fatigue, and check for signs of anemia. Observe for muscle wasting and note the condition of the skin, hair, and nails. Assess for signs of vitamin deficiency and fluid and electrolyte imbalance.

Once gluten-induced enteropathy is diagnosed, assess the patient's understanding of the disorder and its treatment. Also assess the patient's motivation and ability to comply with the therapeutic diet.

Nursing Diagnoses and Planning

Nursing diagnoses and related expected patient outcomes commonly applicable to patients with gluten-induced enteropathy include the following:

NDx: Risk for altered health maintenance related to insufficient knowledge of cause, prognosis, and treatment of the disorder

Planning: Patient Outcomes
1. Patient describes the disorder as caused by a sensitivity to the protein gluten.
2. Patient explains that if gluten is eliminated from the diet, symptoms will disappear, but that symptoms will return any time gluten is eaten.
3. Patient lists foods to be avoided and allowable substitutes.

NDx: Risk for noncompliance related to gluten-free diet

Planning: Patient Outcomes
1. Patient verbalizes intent to comply with the diet.
2. Symptoms have regressed by the time of follow-up.

Nursing Interventions and Evaluation

NDx: Risk for altered health maintenance
Clarify and reinforce the patient's understanding of the relation between the ingestion of gluten, changes in the intestine, and resulting symptoms. Stress that elimination of gluten results in a rapid improvement in symptoms, but that a gluten-free diet must be followed for life or symptoms will return. If needed, use an example familiar to the patient to illustrate this fact. One such example might be the skin reaction to poison ivy that occurs in response to each exposure to the oil of the plant.

Also clarify and reinforce the patient's understanding of the requirements of a gluten-free diet (Highlight 23–3). Explain that, because many of the grains permitted on this diet are refined and unenriched, supplementary multivitamins with minerals are recommended.

NDx: Risk for noncompliance
Explain the importance of maintaining a gluten-free diet not only to the patient but also to the family or significant others to encourage them to support the patient's compliance with the diet rather than to discourage it.

To further facilitate compliance with the diet, provide the patient with a basic list of foods to be avoided and foods that are allowed, as well as recipes for preparing gluten-free meals. Also make certain that the patient is familiar with gluten-free products, such as soy flour and rice flour, and knows where to purchase them. Refer the patient to resources for additional recipes, and explain that lists of gluten-free products can be obtained from the major food companies.

Compare the patient's status with the expected outcomes. If the outcomes are not met, reassess the patient and revise the plan.

LACTASE DEFICIENCY

Lactase deficiency is a condition marked by low levels or absence of the enzyme lactase in the intestine. It is so prevalent among certain ethnic groups as to be almost considered normal for them. These groups include the Japanese, Filipinos, African-Americans, Native Americans, and Greenland Eskimos.

Etiology and Pathophysiology
Lactase deficiency occurs as a primary or a secondary disorder. Primary lactase deficiency occurs in rare instances as a congenital disorder but predominantly develops for unknown reasons in late adolescence or early adulthood. Secondary lactase deficiency accompanies disorders such as inflammatory bowel disease, gastroenteritis, and gluten-induced enteropathy, which damage the intestinal mucosa.

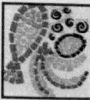

HIGHLIGHT 23–3
NUTRITION

Special Considerations for Patients with Gluten-Induced Enteropathy

Instruct patients with gluten-induced enteropathy to:

Eliminate from the diet all foods containing wheat, rye, oats, and barley.

When cooking, substitute soybean flour, corn flour, cornmeal, potato flour, or rice flour for wheat flour.

Remember that cereal grains are used in many processed foods including:

    creamed soups and vegetables
    ice cream
    cakes, cookies, breads
    pasta
    processed cheese
    commercial salad dressing
    hot dogs and luncheon meats
    beer and ale
    malted milk

Read the list of ingredients on all food labels carefully to check for cereal, starch, flour, thickening agents, emulsifiers, gluten, and stabilizers.

Avoid foods that list hydrolyzed vegetable protein because this may be soybeans, corn, wheat, or a combination of these.

Avoid foods that list vegetable protein because this can be soybeans, corn, wheat, rye, oats, or barley.

Avoid foods that list starch as long as they are made in the United States, because this refers to cornstarch.

Lactase is the enzyme that breaks down lactose, the predominant disaccharide in milk and milk products, into galactose and glucose as part of the digestive process. Without sufficient lactase, lactose remains undigested and is fermented by bacteria in the intestine into lactic and other organic acids. Water is then pulled into the intestinal tract by the osmotic pressure of these substances.

Lactase deficiency has no known effect on the absorption of protein, fat, calcium, or other nutrients.

Clinical Manifestations

Symptoms of lactase deficiency include bloating, loud bowel sounds (borborygmus), cramping abdominal pain, flatulence, and diarrhea. These symptoms can develop from 30 minutes to several hours after ingesting lactose. Anorexia or significant weight loss is rare. Symptoms vary with the amount of lactose consumed; only 20 to 30% of lactose-deficient people develop symptoms in response to the lactose load found in 240 mL (8 oz) of milk. Development of symptoms also varies with the type of dairy food eaten. Because cottage cheese, ice cream, and yogurt contain less lactose than milk and hard cheese, these foods cause fewer symptoms. Symptoms are also reduced by eating dairy foods in conjunction with other foods that delay emptying of the stomach.

Diagnosis

The diagnosis of lactase deficiency is suggested by a rise in blood sugar of less than 20 mg/dL after oral administration of lactose and a normal rise in blood sugar after oral administration of an equal amount of glucose and galactose. Diagnosis can be confirmed by low lactase activity in a jejunal biopsy specimen.

The simplest diagnostic test is a hydrogen breath test. This test is based on the fact that hydrogen is a product of the metabolism of unabsorbed carbohydrate by bacteria in the colon. Thus, in the person with lactase deficiency, ingestion of lactose that cannot be absorbed increases hydrogen in the breath two to eight times the normal level.

Management

Lactase deficiency is managed by decreasing the amount of lactose in the diet to a level that can be tolerated by the patient or by using a commercially available enzyme to predigest lactose or supplement the body's lactase, thereby increasing tolerance.

Enzymes (called LactAid) can be purchased over the counter in the form of drops or caplets. The drops are added to milk and allowed to incubate for 24 hours. The caplets are taken just before meals and are effective for a lactose challenge equal to 240 mL (8 oz) of milk. Enzyme-supplemented, low-fat and nonfat ready-to-drink milk is also available in supermarket dairy cases.

NURSING PROCESS
Lactase Deficiency

Assessment

Obtain a complete description and history of the patient's symptoms. Question carefully about anorexia and weight loss. Review the patient's diet and explore relationships between diet and the onset of symptoms. Have the patient keep a log of foods eaten and symptoms experienced if needed.

Nursing Diagnoses and Planning

Nursing diagnoses and related expected patient outcomes commonly applicable to patients with lactase deficiency include the following:

Special Considerations for Patients with Lactase Deficiency

Instruct patients with lactase deficiency to do the following:

Eliminate milk and milk products from the diet until symptoms have disappeared. Then reintroduce these products gradually as tolerated.

Resume intake of fermented dairy products—such as yogurt, cottage cheese, buttermilk, sour cream, and hard cheeses—first because they contain bacteria that break down lactose.

Use whole milk rather than skim milk, or substitute soy milk if necessary.

Drink milk only with meals, because this is when it is best tolerated.

Limit milk consumption to one glass at a time.

Read labels on drug and food products carefully because lactose can be used as a filler in such foods as breads, pastries, candy, liquid diet aids, instant cocoa mix, french fries, hot dogs, sausages, artificial sweeteners, puddings, gravies, and powdered eggs. Look for such terms as "milk fat solids," "nonfat milk solids," and "whey."

Try using LactAid, a commercially available enzyme that breaks down lactose, with milk to increase tolerance.

Maintain an adequate supply of calcium for the body despite limited amounts of dairy products in the diet by eating other high-calcium foods, such as salmon, sardines, spinach, rhubarb, and Tang beverages, or by taking calcium supplements.

NDx: Risk for altered health maintenance related to insufficient knowledge of the disorder and its treatment

Planning: Patient Outcomes
1. Patient describes relationship between lactose and symptoms.
2. Patient identifies sources of lactose.
3. Patient explains self-care measures.

Nursing Interventions and Evaluation

NDx: Risk for altered health maintenance
Reinforce the patient's understanding of the relationship between ingestion of lactose and development of symptoms, and identify sources of lactose. Explain that lactose intolerance varies in severity and

that dairy products can often be tolerated to some degree depending on type and amount. Instruct the patient in dietary guidelines (Highlight 23–4).

Compare the patient's status with the expected outcomes. If the outcomes are not met, reassess the patient and revise the plan.

Structural Disorders

DIVERTICULAR DISEASE

Diverticula are outpouchings of mucosa through the muscular wall of the intestine (Fig. 23–8). They can occur in any part of the intestine but are most common in the sigmoid colon. Diverticulosis is one form of diverticular disease. It is characterized by the presence of noninflamed diverticula and in many cases is asymptomatic. Diverticulitis is a form of diverticular disease in which there is inflammation of a diverticulum.

Diverticular disease is the most common pathologic condition of the colon in the United States. Its incidence increases with age, beginning at about age 35. It is estimated that about one-third of the population is affected by 60 years of age.

Etiology and Pathophysiology
Diverticula appear to be caused by increased pressure within the lumen of the bowel, which forces herniation of the mucosa through weak areas of the

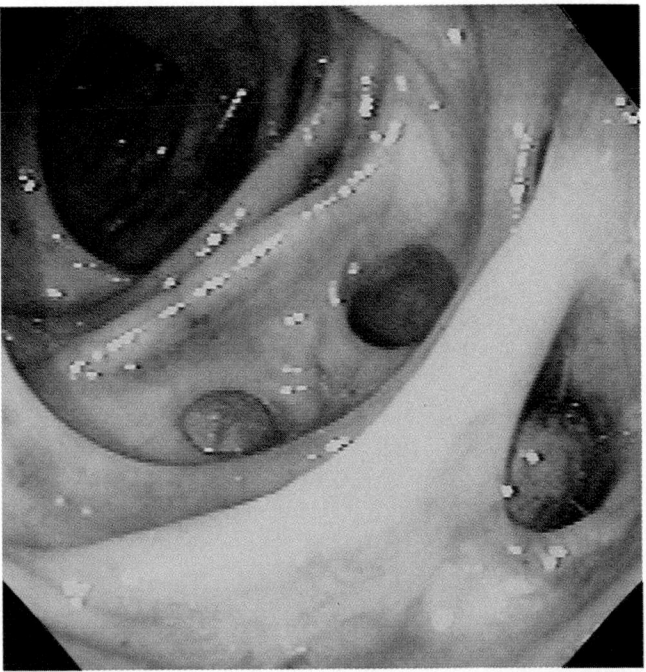

Figure 23–8

Diverticular disease. (From Wilcox CM. Atlas of clinical gastrointestinal endoscopy. Philadelphia: WB Saunders, 1995, p 229.)

muscular wall. Such weak areas occur naturally at points where blood vessels penetrate or may develop as a result of the atrophy of the intestinal muscle, which occurs with aging. Increased intraluminal pressure is believed to result from small, scant stools, which increase the force and alter the mechanical characteristics of the peristaltic waves needed to propel them. This change in peristalsis causes hypertrophy of the muscle such that the muscular ridges thicken and almost touch during contractions, producing temporary obstruction and increased pressure in the affected segment of bowel (Fig. 23–9).

Diverticular disease is rare in cultures where high-residue diets are the norm, as in Africa, for example. Therefore, lack of fiber in the diet, which leads to low-bulk stools and prolonged transit time in the intestine, is considered a prime precipitating factor in this sequence of events.

Inflammation in a diverticulum is believed to occur when increased pressure results in microperforation or macroperforation of the mucosal pouch. The inflammation spreads around the diverticulum into the pericolic fat and can cause fibrosis of the colonic wall. If the perforation is large, pericolic abscesses, fistula formation into the bladder or vagina, or generalized peritonitis may occur.

Clinical Manifestations

Clinical manifestations of both symptomatic diverticulosis and diverticulitis include:

- Left quadrant pain, which typically begins as intermittent crampy pain and, in the case of diverticulitis, subsequently becomes constant and may radiate to the back
- Constipation sometimes alternating with diarrhea
- Abdominal distention
- Palpation of a sausage-shaped mass in the lower left quadrant

Symptoms unique to diverticulitis are fever and leukocytosis.

Bleeding may accompany both diverticulosis and diverticulitis. Many times it is occult. However, it can also occur in significant amounts in otherwise asymptomatic patients, especially among the elderly.

Diagnosis

Diverticular disease is usually diagnosed by colonoscopy or barium enema, although the latter is not done during the acute stage of diverticulitis because of the danger of massive perforation. In many asymptomatic or mild cases, diverticula are found by chance during examination for another reason. Cancer of the colon must be ruled out as part of the diagnostic process because the presenting symptoms are so similar.

Management

Management of diverticulosis aims to increasing stool bulk and prevent constipation and increased intraluminal pressure in the bowel. Thus, a high-

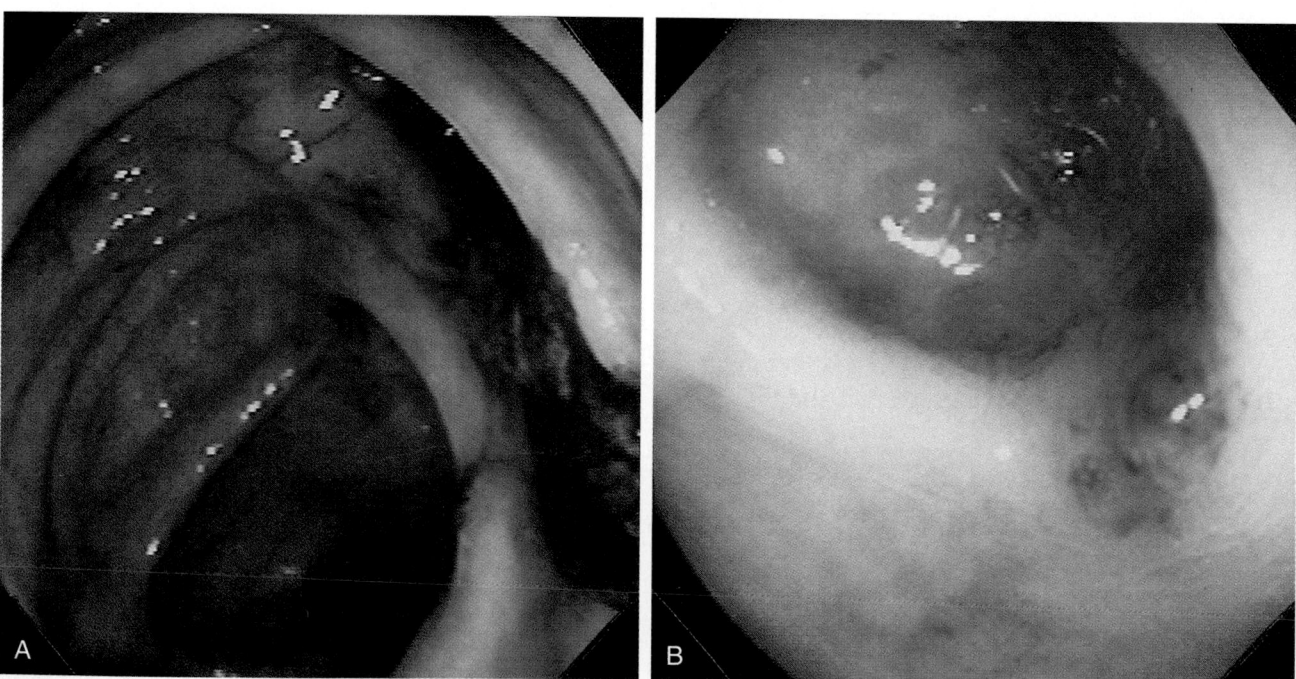

Figure 23–9

A, A large blood clot just proximal to the ileocecal valve. *B,* After irrigation, a small amount of blood appears in the diverticulum near a visible vessel at the entrance to the diverticulum. (From Wilcox CM. Atlas of clinical gastrointestinal endoscopy. Philadelphia: WB Saunders, 1995, p 231.)

fiber diet and bulk-forming laxatives such as Metamucil are prescribed. Stool softeners (such as dioctyl sodium sulfosuccinate) or a suppository (such as bisacodyl) may be used to prevent straining at stool. Spasmolytic anticholinergics, such as propantheline bromide, are taken before meals and at bedtime. Nonopiate analgesics are given for pain. Narcotic analgesics are avoided because they increase intraluminal pressure.

Patients with uncomplicated diverticulitis are treated with clear fluids to rest the bowel and parenteral antibiotics, such as gentamycin and clindamycin. With high fever and signs of abscess formation, the patient is NPO, has nasogastric suction, and is on intravenous fluids.

Surgical intervention, such as a bowel resection and sometimes a temporary colostomy, is required when complications occur, such as perforation, hemorrhage, obstruction, or abscess formation. When a colostomy is formed, the distal bowel stump may be oversewn or exteriorized as a mucous fistula.

❖ Settings, Providers, and Collaboration for Care

Patients with diverticulitis may require hospitalization to stabilize fluid and electrolyte balance and manage pain. Surgical repair may also be necessary. Once a definitive diagnosis is made and a satisfactory treatment regimen established, the patient will require assessment and modification of treatment through a physician's office or outpatient clinic. If a colostomy is necessary, the expertise of an enterostomal therapist would be appropriate.

NURSING PROCESS
Diverticular Disease

Assessment

Assess the patient's pain. Ask about its onset, type, location, and intensity. Check for abdominal distention and question the patient about bowel function. Determine the usual elimination pattern. Ask about the appearance, size, and consistency of stool. Ask whether the patient strains at stool, and about rectal bleeding. Ask about the use of laxatives or enemas.

Review the patient's usual diet. Ascertain the types and amounts of foods ingested, as well as the pattern of eating.

Check for fever and review the white blood cell count and sedimentation rate values for indications of infection. Also check for abdominal rigidity and tenderness, tachycardia, and hypotension, which can indicate perforation.

Nursing Diagnoses and Planning

Nursing diagnoses and related expected patient outcomes commonly applicable to patients with symptomatic diverticulosis include the following:

NDx: Pain related to increased pressure within an area of the intestine

Planning: Patient Outcomes
1. Patient reports decrease in pain.
2. Signs of abdominal discomfort, such as pressing on abdomen or flexing legs on abdomen, are absent.

NDx: Constipation related to scant stool with prolonged transit time in the intestine

Planning: Patient Outcomes
1. Patient passes soft, formed stool of normal size.
2. Straining at stool is absent.

NDx: Risk for altered health maintenance related to insufficient knowledge of prevention or recurrence

Planning: Patient Outcomes
1. Patient describes self-care measures to prevent recurrence of symptoms.
2. Patient states time of any follow-up visit.

Nursing Interventions and Evaluation

NDx: Pain
Administer or teach the patient to self-administer analgesics and spasmolytics as prescribed. Encourage rhythmic deep-breathing and use of progressive relaxation exercises to promote pain relief.

For patients with diverticulitis, give clear fluids or a low-residue diet as ordered to rest the bowel. If a nasogastric tube is in place, keep the patient on NPO status and monitor the suction apparatus for proper function.

NDx: Constipation
Explain the role of diet, fluid intake, exercise, and a schedule for eating and defecation in promoting good bowel function. Teach the patient about a high-fiber diet and fluid intake (Highlight 23–5). Administer or teach the patient to self-administer prescribed bulk-forming laxatives and stool softeners. Caution the patient against the use of other types of laxatives.

NDx: Risk for altered health maintenance
Instruct the patient in self-care measures to prevent recurrence of symptoms (Highlight 23–6). Be certain the patient knows when to return for any needed follow-up.

Additional Interventions
Administer intravenous fluid and antibiotics as ordered. Maintain function and placement of the nasogastric tube, and keep the patient NPO. Give frequent mouth care. Apply water-soluble lubricant to the naris. When oral intake resumes, give clear liquids, progressing to a low-residue diet as ordered. Be certain to explain to the patient that these dietary restrictions are designed to rest the bowel and allow the inflammation to subside. If the patient is on bedrest, encourage frequent turning, as well as foot and leg exercises, to prevent skin breakdown and

in intestinal obstruction by causing angulation (folded on itself), torsion (twisting), or constriction of the bowel.

Clinical Manifestations

The patient with adhesions presents with the signs and symptoms of moderate to severe obstruction, depending on the degree of luminal narrowing. Abdominal distention, decreased or absent bowel sounds, and sometimes vomiting and abdominal cramping occur.

Diagnosis

Diagnosis of adhesions is based on presenting signs and symptoms, a history of recent abdominal surgery or infection, and absence of other causes of obstruction. A distended bowel is seen on abdominal x-rays.

Management

Medical management aims to relieve the obstruction. A long intestinal tube, such as a Miller-Abbott tube, may be used to treat small adhesions because the weighted end may be enough to dilate the constricted area and relieve the obstruction. If this is unsuccessful or if the adhesion is large, surgical release (lysis) or excision is performed.

NURSING PROCESS GUIDELINES
Intestinal Adhesions

The assessment, nursing diagnoses, expected patient outcomes, nursing interventions, and evaluation for patients with adhesions that are obstructing the

Text continued on page 1093

venous stasis. Encourage periodic coughing and deep-breathing if the patient is at risk for respiratory complications.

Compare the patient's status with the expected outcomes. If the outcomes are not met, reassess the patient and revise the plan.

See Nursing Care Guide 23–1 for the care of the patient who has had a temporary colostomy for diverticular disease.

INTESTINAL ADHESIONS

Intestinal adhesions are bands of fibrous tissue that develop as a result of trauma or infection within the peritoneal cavity.

Etiology and Pathophysiology

Adhesions develop as part of the healing process. They form when fibrin, which is deposited near the wound after injury, becomes organized with an ingrowth of capillaries and fibroblasts rather than being absorbed. Most adhesions result from abdominal surgery, but they can also occur secondary to intraabdominal inflammatory disease. Adhesions result

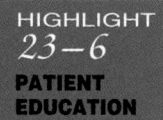
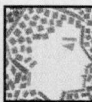

Nursing Care Guide 23–1
Patient Care After a Temporary Colostomy for Diverticular Disease

Assessment Findings: Patient complains of abdominal pain and grimaces and groans on moving.

Nursing Diagnosis: Pain related to surgical trauma to the abdomen

Patient Outcomes	Nursing Interventions	Rationale
Patient moves without signs of severe pain such as moaning, pallor, and tachycardia.	Give prescribed analgesics every 3–4 hours for 72 hours.	Early analgesic administration provides more effective pain relief.
Patient rests quietly without signs of discomfort such as clenched hands, groaning, and crying.	Place the patient in semi-Fowler's position.	Decreases stress on the suture line.
	Encourage ambulation.	Stimulates return of bowel function and relief from gas pains.
Patient states pain is relieved.	Use a rectal tube to remove flatus.	Decreases distention and relieves associated pain.

Evaluation: Compare the patient's status with the expected outcomes. If the outcomes are not met, reassess the patient and revise the plan.

Assessment Findings: Patient is restless, and face appears tense. Patient states he or she feels apprehensive, inadequate, and helpless.

Nursing Diagnosis: Anxiety related to prognosis and ability to live with and manage the colostomy

Patient Outcomes	Nursing Interventions	Rationale
Physical signs of high anxiety such as trembling, tachycardia, and dry mouth are absent. Patient attends to directions and information. Patient expresses confidence in ability to cope with the colostomy and its care.	Provide time, privacy, and encouragement for discussion of the patient's concerns. Arrange for a visit from an ostomate if desired. Provide desired information about prognosis, reason for surgery, and function and care of the colostomy.	Allows for feedback, provides perspective, and permits a supportive relationship. Patient may have had limited preoperative preparation because of the emergency nature of the surgery and lack of knowledge predisposes to anxiety.
	Acknowledge that feelings of anxiety are normal and expected after emergency colostomy surgery.	Allays patient concerns about being judged negatively because of anxiety.
	Guide the patient in relaxation techniques if needed.	Reduces tension level and diverts patient's attention. Provides the patient with concrete evidence that a normal lifestyle can be maintained despite the presence of a colostomy. It also allows for sharing of realistic, practical answers to concerns and questions.

Evaluation: Compare the patient's status with the expected outcomes. If the outcomes are not met, reassess the patient and revise the plan.

(continued)

Nursing Care Guide 23–1

Patient Care After a Temporary Colostomy for Diverticular Disease (continued)

Assessment Findings: Patient has had a resection of the large bowel and formation of a descending colostomy.

Nursing Diagnosis: Bowel incontinence related to the formation of a colostomy and loss of rectal function

Patient Outcomes	Nursing Interventions	Rationale
Patient uses the selected pouching system effectively to collect fecal drainage.	Monitor the collection pouch placed over the colostomy at the time of operation for the accumulation of flatus and drainage.	Indicates functional status of the bowel.
Patient identifies factors such as change in diet and times of eating that affect pattern of colostomy function.	Empty or change the pouch when it is no more than half full.	Back pressure can damage suture lines and disrupt the pouch seal.
	Assist the patient in selecting a collection system for daily use that is best suited to his or her needs after discharge. If the patient is unable to perform self-care, include a significant other in the selection process.	Eliminates unnecessary frustration and thus promotes adaptation and correct self-management.
	Use the selected system consistently.	Assists the patient in mastering self-care and adapting to the demands of the colostomy.
	Explain to the patient that some control over fecal expulsion may be obtained eventually by means of a regular dietary intake and irrigations.	Provides the patient with a positive but realistic fact on which to focus.
	Irrigate the colostomy if ordered.	Promotes bowel emptying.

Evaluation: Compare the patient's status with the expected outcomes. If the outcomes are not met, reassess the patient and revise the plan.

Assessment Findings: Patient has a descending colostomy and uses a collection system that is applied to the abdomen with adhesive.

Nursing Diagnosis: Risk for impaired skin integrity related to irritation of the peristomal skin from contact with fecal matter, removal of collection systems, or sensitivity to adhesives or other materials

Patient Outcomes	Nursing Interventions	Rationale
Peristomal skin is free of erythema and blisters.	Remove mucus and feces from the stoma with a tissue.	Prepares area for washing.
Peristomal skin is intact.	Wash the peristomal skin to remove all traces of drainage.	Removes substances that can irritate the skin.
	Avoid use of oily soaps and emollients.	Oily substances interfere with adherence of the collection system.

(continued)

Patient Care After a Temporary Colostomy for Diverticular Disease (continued)

Patient Outcomes	Nursing Interventions	Rationale
	Omit soap, and wash with water only if the patient is elderly with a tendency for dry skin.	Soap dries the skin.
	Rinse thoroughly and dry gently.	Removes all irritating soap residue and avoids irritation from friction.
	Fit the appliance to the stoma so that there is 1/8 in of skin between the pouch opening and the stoma.	Prevents loosening of appliance due to moisture from stoma.
	Use a skin barrier between the pouch opening and the stoma.	Protects the skin from contact with fecal drainage.
	Apply a skin sealant to the area of skin that will be covered with adhesive when collection system is applied.	Prevents damage to the epidermis when the appliance is removed.
	Apply the pouch snugly.	Helps prevent leakage of irritating material onto the skin.
	Monitor the pouch for leaking, and change immediately if it occurs.	Prevents prolonged contact between irritating drainage and the skin.
	Institute a vigorous treatment regimen immediately if peristomal skin irritation does occur.	Irritation can progress rapidly to skin breakdown.

Evaluation: Compare the patient's status with the expected outcomes. If the outcomes are not met, reassess the patient and revise the plan.

Assessment Findings: Respirations are shallow. Patient states that "it hurts to take a deep breath."

Nursing Diagnosis: Ineffective breathing pattern related to incisional pain on deep breathing

Patient Outcomes	Nursing Interventions	Rationale
Patient coughs and deep-breathes as directed. Cyanosis is absent.	Teach the patient to splint the abdomen with pillows.	Pain decreases patient's willingness to turn, cough, and deep-breathe.
Arterial blood gases are within normal range.	Assist patient in turning, coughing, and deep-breathing every 2 hours for 72 hours postoperatively.	Promotes good ventilation and airway clearance.
	Reassure the patient that coughing and deep-breathing, although they may hurt, will not harm the incision.	Promotes cooperation with the therapeutic plan by allaying fear of injury.
	Ambulate the patient at least three times a day (tid) as soon as able.	Promotes good ventilation and airway clearance.

Evaluation: Compare the patient's status with the expected outcomes. If the outcomes are not met, reassess the patient and revise the plan.

(continued)

Nursing Care Guide 23-1

Patient Care After a Temporary Colostomy for Diverticular Disease (continued)

Assessment Findings: Patient is under nothing by mouth orders (NPO), has a nasogastric or nasointestinal tube in place that is connected to low suction, and is mouth-breathing.

Nursing Diagnosis: Risk for altered oral mucous membrane related to NPO status and presence of a nasogastric or nasointestinal tube

Patient Outcomes	Nursing Interventions	Rationale
Oral mucous membrane is moist and free of cracks.	Assist patient to brush teeth at least tid.	Cleanses and moistens the mouth.
Lips are supple, moist, and free of cracks.	Encourage frequent mouth rinses.	Moistens oral mucous membranes.
Patient denies dryness of the mouth.	Avoid use of rinses that are drying.	Helps prevent drying and cracking.
	Apply water-soluble lubricant to the lips.	Keeps lips supple and reduces cracking by maintaining tissue moisture.

Evaluation: Compare the patient's status with the expected outcomes. If the outcomes are not met, reassess the patient and revise the plan.

Assessment Findings: Patient has had abdominal surgery under general anesthesia and is on bedrest.

Nursing Diagnosis: Risk for altered peripheral tissue perfusion related to thrombophlebitis secondary to venous stasis

Patient Outcomes	Nursing Interventions	Rationale
Calves are free of redness, swelling, heat, and pain.	Guide the patient in foot and leg exercises 10 times every 2 hours while on bedrest.	Muscle contraction promotes venous return by its squeezing action on the veins and thus reduces the risk of thrombus formation.
	Apply antiembolic stockings or Ace bandages.	Supports venous return by enhancing the squeezing action of the muscles on the veins.
	Avoid use of knee Gatch or any other source of pressure on the popliteal space.	Eliminates obstruction to venous return as a result of bending or compressing veins and thus decreases stasis, which predisposes to thrombus formation.
	Ambulate the patient as soon as ordered.	Muscle contraction promotes venous return by its squeezing action on the veins and thus reduces the risk of thrombus formation.
	Instruct patient to avoid crossing legs or sitting for long period of time.	Eliminates obstruction to venous return caused by bending or compressing veins and thus decreases stasis, which predisposes to thrombus formation.

(continued)

Nursing Care Guide 23–1
Patient Care After a Temporary Colostomy for Diverticular Disease (continued)

Evaluation:	Compare the patient's status with the expected outcomes. If the outcomes are not met, reassess the patient and revise the plan.
Assessment Findings:	Patient may have had the bowel surgically opened without standard bowel preparation.
Nursing Diagnosis:	Risk for infection related to surgical incision of the peritoneal cavity and bowel

Patient Outcomes	Nursing Interventions	Rationale
Suture line is approximated and free of erythema and purulent drainage. Abdomen is soft and nondistended. Patient is afebrile.	Monitor for signs of peritoneal irritation: muscle rigidity and rebound tenderness. Use strict aseptic technique when doing wound care. Reinforce or change dressing when wet.	Muscle rigidity and rebound tenderness are early signs of peritonitis. Protects against wound infection as a result of cross-contamination. Microorganisms can travel through wet dressings by capillary action.

Evaluation:	Compare the patient's status with the expected outcomes. If the outcomes are not met, reassess the patient and revise the plan.
Assessment Findings:	Patient has a new colostomy and verbalizes negative feelings about it and fear of negative reaction from family and friends, stating "This thing is disgusting. No one is going to want to come near me."
Nursing Diagnosis:	Body image disturbance related to loss of bowel control, presence of the stoma, release of fecal material onto abdomen, passage of flatus, odor, need for a collection system

Patient Outcomes	Nursing Interventions	Rationale
Patient verbalizes acceptance of self with a colostomy.	Acknowledge to the patient that negative feelings about the colostomy are normal and that it takes time to accept and adjust to this body change. Be certain facial expressions and other nonverbal behaviors convey acceptance not revulsion, distaste, or pity. Touch the stoma to show it does not hurt, is not easily damaged, and is not revolting.	Reassures patient that his or her negative feelings are not abnormal and that feelings will ease with time. Nonverbal communication can contradict and "speak more loudly" than verbal communication. Negative nonverbal communication acts to reinforce patient's negative perceptions of self. Allays patient's fears and connotes acceptance.

(continued)

Nursing Care Guide 23–1
Patient Care After a Temporary Colostomy for Diverticular Disease (continued)

Patient Outcomes	Nursing Interventions	Rationale
	Provide opportunity for the patient to look at the stoma and express feelings about it.	Looking at the stoma and verbalizing feelings about it are essential to accepting and caring for the colostomy.
	Provide privacy for care and teaching.	Protects the patient from embarrassment.
Patient expresses pleasure at visits from relatives and friends.	Empty the pouch of malodorous fecal drainage or flatus before meals, visiting hours, and the like.	Prevents embarrassment, promotes socialization, and prevents anorexia that may result from unpleasant odor.
Patient discusses resumption of work, social activities, and so on in a positive way.	Provide good ventilation and deodorize the room as needed.	Prevents embarrassment as a result of odor.
	Do not put pinholes in a plastic pouch to allow release of flatus.	This creates unpredictable, uncontrollable odor.
Patient verbalizes interest in grooming.	Encourage good grooming.	Promotes patient's sense of wellbeing.
	Stress that, with a little attention to style, the pouch is not visible beneath clothing.	Guides the patient in strategies for minimizing effect of colostomy on appearance and preventing unnecessary embarrassment.
	Help the patient to identify personal strengths.	Helps place feelings about the negative effect of the colostomy on self in perspective.
	Include patient in decision making.	Fosters a sense of control.
	Encourage frank discussion of feelings with significant others.	Allows for validation of feelings and a supportive relationship.

Evaluation: Compare the patient's status with the expected outcomes. If the outcomes are not met, reassess the patient and revise the plan.

Assessment Findings: Patient states, "I suppose this is the end of good eating. No more fresh fruits and vegetables, gravy, spices, and other good things."

Nursing Diagnosis: Risk for altered nutrition: less than body requirements related to omission of foods because of flatulence, odor, or diarrhea

Patient Outcomes	Nursing Interventions	Rationale
Patient describes components of a nutritionally balanced diet.	Review basic principles of nutrition with the patient.	A nutritionally balanced diet is needed to heal the wound and maintain overall state of health. In adjusting to a new colostomy, patients are at risk for inadvertently adopting a nutritionally imbalanced diet.

(continued)

Nursing Care Guide 23–1

Patient Care After a Temporary Colostomy for Diverticular Disease (continued)

Patient Outcomes	Nursing Interventions	Rationale
Patient is able to select a nutritionally balanced diet from foods that are tolerated well.	Discuss the use of the food pyramid in planning a balanced diet.	The food pyramid is one of the simplest methods available for selecting a generally balanced diet. Because of its simplicity, it is easily complied with and is suitable for virtually all patients.
Patient identifies specific foods that are likely causes of flatulence, odor, or diarrhea.	Explain the importance of drinking at least 2500 mL daily.	Extra fluid intake is needed because more fluid is lost through a colostomy than is lost with normal stool passing through the rectum.
	Provide the patient with a list of foods likely to cause flatulence, odor, or diarrhea.	Allows patient to minimize problems by avoiding these foods until colostomy is well established.
	Instruct the patient initially to avoid high-roughage foods such as nuts, popcorn, and raw celery.	High-fiber foods stimulate bowel activity and increase the volume of stool. In some cases, fiber can accumulate and block the stoma.
	Instruct the patient to try new foods one at a time and at least three times before eliminating them from the diet.	Allows the patient to accurately determine effects of individual foodstuffs on the gastrointestinal tract.

Evaluation: Compare the patient's status with the expected outcomes. If the outcomes are not met, reassess the patient and revise the plan.

Assessment Findings: Patient states, "I may have to learn how to care for this bag but I guess I don't have to worry about birth control while I have this thing."

Nursing Diagnosis: Risk for altered sexuality patterns related to fear of rejection because of the presence of a stoma and a collection system

Patient Outcomes	Nursing Interventions	Rationale
Patient discusses concerns about the effects of the colostomy on sexual function.	Acknowledge that concerns about sexual activity after a colostomy are normal.	Helps put the patient at ease with his or her concerns and thus helps make the patient feel comfortable in discussing them.
Patient verbalizes confidence in ability to participate in a satisfying sexual relationship.	Encourage the patient to discuss sexual concerns openly with spouse or significant other.	Allows for mutual support and problem solving.
	Provide privacy and time for discussion of sexual concerns.	This establishes an environment conducive to open communication.

(continued)

Patient Care After a Temporary Colostomy for Diverticular Disease (continued)

Patient Outcomes	Nursing Interventions	Rationale
	Explain that sexual intercourse, conception, and pregnancy are all possible after a colostomy.	Provide factual information to combat misconceptions about functional changes resulting from a colostomy.
	Recommend that the collection pouch be emptied before intercourse.	Protects against spillage as a result of accidental disruption of the seal and contributes to comfort.
	Suggest positions that accommodate the collection pouch.	
	Provide access to written materials about sex and a colostomy such as the pamphlets published by the United Ostomy Association called "Sex and the Male Ostomate" and "Sex and the Female Ostomate."	Allows the patient to review information when desired in a private and comfortable environment of choice.
	If possible, have an individual with a colostomy visit with the patient. Refer to a sex therapist if needed.	Provides a source of additional help if other coping strategies prove insufficient.

Evaluation: Compare the patient's status with the expected outcomes. If the outcomes are not met, reassess the patient and revise the plan.

Assessment Findings: Patient is newly postoperative from colostomy surgery, has no previous knowledge of colostomy function or care, and asks questions regarding it.

Nursing Diagnosis: Risk for altered health maintenance related to insufficient knowledge of care of the colostomy and effects on lifestyle

Patient Outcomes	Nursing Interventions	Rationale
Patient identifies supplies needed for colostomy care and where to obtain them. Patient empties, changes, and cleans the pouch effectively. Patient demonstrates peristomal skin care. Patient states guidelines for performing colostomy care.	Teach the patient to care for the colostomy as soon as possible postoperatively. Include information on needed supplies and on emptying and changing the pouch, cleaning the pouch, controlling odor, and caring for the peristomal skin.	Provides a sense of control and allows independence, both of which are essential to adjusting to the colostomy and resuming a normal lifestyle.
	Instruct the patient to empty the pouch when it is one-third full and at bedtime.	Guards against back pressure, which can disrupt the suture line and the pouch seal.
Patient describes the effect (or lack thereof) of the colostomy on day-to-day activities.	Suggest that an alarm clock be set the first few nights after discharge to wake the patient to empty the bag.	Ensures that the patient awakes to empty the bag.

(continued)

Nursing Care Guide 23-1
Patient Care After a Temporary Colostomy for Diverticular Disease (continued)

Patient Outcomes	Nursing Interventions	Rationale
	Suggest changing the pouch first thing in the morning before eating or drinking.	Allows maximum convenience and ease because the colostomy usually does not function at this time.
	Explain that physical activities are unrestricted and can be resumed in full usually within 8 weeks after surgery.	Provides patient with lifestyle guidelines for self-care after discharge.
	Be certain to stress that showers and baths may be taken, any type of clothing may be worn, including girdles and pantyhose, and that travel is possible as long as supplies are kept available and seat belts are worn above the stoma.	
Patient identifies services available from the United Ostomy Association.	Inform the patient about the services available through the United Ostomy Association.	Makes patient aware of community resources and how to access them.
	Provide the patient with written instructions regarding self-care.	Provides a ready reference for use after discharge because information learned during periods of stress is not generally retained in full.
Evaluation:	Compare the patient's status with the expected outcomes. If the outcomes are not met, reassess the patient and revise the plan.	

bowel are similar to those described previously for patients with mechanical ileus. Pay particular attention to the patient's anxiety level and need for knowledge. This is important because many of these patients have a history of serious illness and extensive abdominal surgery and attribute the current symptoms to further critical disease with poor prognosis.

INTESTINAL HERNIAS

An intestinal hernia is a protrusion of peritoneum, omentum, and intestine out of the abdominal cavity through an abnormal opening in the muscle of the abdominal wall. On the basis of location, hernias are classified as inguinal, femoral, or ventral (umbilical). Inguinal hernias are most common and occur in males more often than females (Fig. 23–10).

Etiology and Pathophysiology

The basic defect underlying the development of an intestinal hernia is a congenital or acquired weakness of the abdominal wall. Actual herniation occurs from the effect of prolonged increased intra-abdominal pressure on the weakened area. Such increased intra-abdominal pressure can result from obesity, pregnancy, chronic or strenuous coughing, heavy lifting, straining, or an enlarging tumor. In males, anatomical passage of the vas deferens through the abdominal wall presents a likely location for later herniation.

The peritoneum pouches out through the weakened abdominal wall, forming the hernial sac. In early stages, tissues such as omentum and intestine enter the sac when the patient stands or strains. They spontaneously re-enter the abdominal cavity when the patient sits and intra-abdominal pressure declines. Once formed, hernias tend to enlarge.

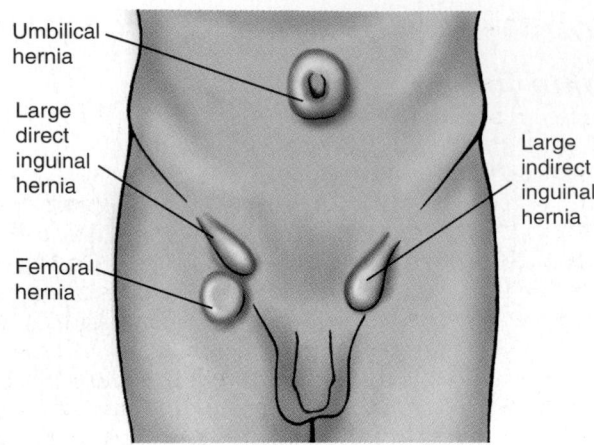

Figure 23–10
Types of hernias.

Soon, tissues remain in the hernial sac all the time. If the herniated tissues can be replaced in the abdominal cavity by manual manipulation, the hernia is referred to as reducible. If they cannot be replaced in the abdominal cavity, the hernia is called irreducible or incarcerated. A hernia is strangulated when twisting or swelling of the tissues in the sac, or constriction of the ring of tissue through which the sac protrudes, blocks blood flow to the intestine and obstructs passage of materials through it (Fig. 23–11). Such acute obstruction leads to necrosis and gangrene.

Clinical Manifestations
An uncomplicated hernia presents as a bulge that may only be apparent or that may increase in size on exertion. The bulge is soft to the touch and typically tender. Symptoms of a strangulated hernia are those of an acute intestinal obstruction: severe pain, nausea, vomiting, distention, and fever.

Diagnosis
Diagnosis of hernia is based on the patient's history and visualization or palpation of the hernia on physical examination. When examining for an inguinal or femoral hernia, the patient is asked to strain downward to increase intra-abdominal pressure and cause a reducible hernia to enter the hernial sac, where it can be seen or palpated. Similarly, when an incisional or umbilical hernia is suspected but not visible, the patient is asked to raise the head and shoulders off the examining table because this maneuver usually causes the hernia to bulge.

Management
The treatment of choice for incisional, inguinal, and femoral hernias is surgical repair because it eliminates the risk of strangulation. In rare cases—for example, when a patient must be stabilized medically before surgery is possible—a truss or girdle may be used to prevent protrusion of the hernia after manual reduction. A truss is a pad placed over the hernia that is held in place with a belt. It should be worn as consistently as possible, and activities that increase intra-abdominal pressure should be avoided. Potential complications of a truss are skin irritation and strangulation of the hernia.

Herniorrhaphy is the permanent surgical reduction of a hernia. It is most often an elective procedure but is a surgical emergency in cases of incarceration and strangulation. The surgical approach varies depending on the location and severity of the problem. Often, the hernia can be reduced by laparoscopy, or the hernia sac may need to be opened via an abdominal incision for repair to take place. Closure with either approach is sometimes reinforced with synthetic mesh. If the herniated portion of the intestine is necrotic, an intestinal resection may be necessary. Inguinal herniorrhaphy may be done as an overnight or day surgery procedure with spinal or local anesthesia.

Complications of herniorrhaphy, although uncommon, can occur. They include infection, hemorrhage, and compromise of the vas deferens or impaired blood supply to the testes in men. Infection is signaled by soreness in the operative area and fever. It is treated with antibiotics, warm compresses, and incision and drainage.

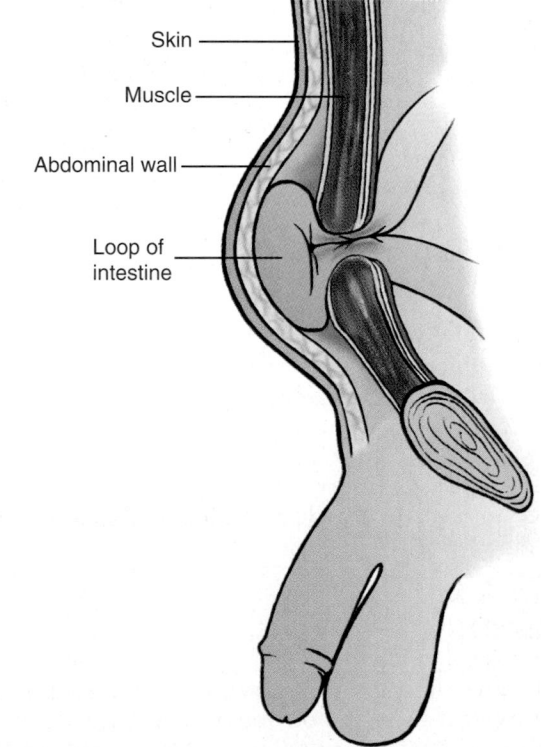

Figure 23–11
Strangulated hernia. Note compression of the herniated loop of intestine by the ring of tissue through which it passes.

❖ **Settings, Providers, and Collaboration for Care**

Most hernias are treated surgically, usually a simple procedure than can be performed in a surgicenter or ambulatory surgery setting. More complicated hernias may require admission for the surgery, followed by a 1- to 3-day postoperative course. Before discharge, the nurse instructs the patient about continued care at home and when to return for a follow-up evaluation.

NURSING PROCESS
Herniorrhaphy

PREOPERATIVE NURSING CARE

Assessment

Assess the patient's physical status as before any surgical procedure. Assess carefully for respiratory infection, chronic cough, or allergies. Because postoperative coughing or sneezing can disrupt the repair, the procedure may be postponed or palliative medications such as antihistamines prescribed.

Assess the patient's understanding of the surgical procedure and the expected postoperative course, as well as the psychologic response to the scheduled surgery. This is particularly important when the patient is a male with an inguinal hernia because the potential exists for misunderstanding and anxiety about the effect of the surgery on sexual activity.

Nursing Diagnoses and Planning

Nursing diagnoses and related expected patient outcomes commonly applicable to patients scheduled for herniorrhaphy include the following:

NDx: Knowledge deficit: surgical procedure, perioperative routines, and usual postoperative course

Planning: Patient Outcomes
  1. Patient describes perioperative events.
  2. Patient describes expected postoperative discomforts.

Nursing Interventions and Evaluation

NDx: Knowledge deficit: surgical procedure, perioperative routines, and usual postoperative course
Describe the surgical procedure and perioperative routines in accord with the type of anesthesia to be used and the expected length of hospitalization. Explain that urination may be difficult right after surgery and that pain and scrotal swelling may last for 24 to 48 hours.

Compare the patient's status with the expected outcomes. If the outcomes are not met, reassess the patient and revise the plan.

POSTOPERATIVE NURSING CARE

Assessment

Assess return to physiologic stability. Take vital signs and inspect the dressing for drainage.

Assess the patient's ability to empty the bladder, particularly in men who have had an inguinal hernia repaired, because difficulty voiding is not uncommon, especially in the first 8 postoperative hours. Measure intake and output. Observe and palpate the suprapubic area for signs of bladder distention. Also observe for scrotal edema.

Assess patients for pain as well as for coughing, sneezing, or other strenuous movements.

If the patient is returning home shortly after the procedure, assess the patient's understanding of the signs and symptoms of complications and his or her ability to obtain help if needed.

Nursing Diagnoses and Planning

Nursing diagnoses and related expected patient outcomes commonly applicable to patients who have had a herniorrhaphy include the following:

NDx: Pain related to surgical trauma to the groin

Planning: Patient Outcomes
  1. Patient states that pain is relieved.
  2. Patient moves without grimaces or other behavioral signs of pain.
  3. Scrotal swelling is decreased or absent.

NDx: Risk for urinary retention related to effects of anesthesia and surgical trauma

Planning: Patient Outcomes
  1. Patient voids adequate amounts (200–300 mL) within 8 hours.
  2. Urinary bladder distention is absent.

NDx: Risk for impaired tissue integrity related to stress on the wound secondary to increased intra-abdominal pressure

Planning: Patient Outcomes
  1. Patient splints incision if coughing is necessary.
  2. Patient describes ways to avoid increasing abdominal pressure, such as sneezing with mouth open.
  3. Straining at stool is absent.

NDx: Risk for altered health maintenance related to insufficient knowledge of self-care after discharge

Planning: Patient Outcomes
  1. Patient describes limitations on activity.
  2. Patient explains good body mechanics.
  3. Patient identifies measures to prevent constipation.
  4. Patient lists symptoms to be expected and those to be reported.

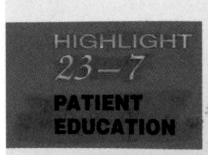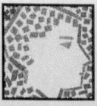

**HIGHLIGHT
23-7**

**PATIENT
EDUCATION**

Self-Care After a Herniorrhaphy

Instruct the patient to:

Expect pain and scrotal swelling for 24 to 48 hours.

Resume nonstrenuous activities gradually over 5 to 7 days.

Use good body mechanics.

Avoid heavy lifting and sexual activities for 6 to 8 weeks or in accordance with surgeon's instructions.

Avoid straining at stool.
- Eat a high-residue diet.
- Drink at least 2000 mL of fluid per day.
- Take stool softeners as ordered.

Report immediately incisional soreness or drainage, fever, or difficult urination.

Nursing Interventions and Evaluation

NDx: Pain
Follow the AHCPR guidelines for strategies to relieve pain in the postoperative patient. Administer prescribed analgesics as needed. Elevate the scrotum and apply ice packs while the patient is in bed to decrease pain and swelling. Apply a scrotal support when the patient is out of bed.

NDx: Risk for urinary retention
Assist the patient to a standing position to void. Use inducements, such as running water, as needed. Report bladder distention to the surgeon because catheterization will probably be required.

NDx: Risk for impaired tissue integrity
Encourage the patient to turn and deep-breathe. Do not encourage coughing. Instruct the patient to splint the incision with hands or a pillow if coughing is unavoidable. Instruct the patient to sneeze with the mouth open if sneezing is unavoidable. Explain the importance of not straining at stool and assist the patient to limit pull on the incision when moving.

NDx: Risk for altered health maintenance
Instruct the patient in self-care after discharge (Highlight 23–7). Remember that restrictions on activities vary from surgeon to surgeon, with some imposing no limitations whatsoever.

Compare the patient's status with the expected outcomes. If the outcomes are not met, reassess the patient and revise the plan.

HEMORRHOIDS

Hemorrhoids are dilated, swollen rectal veins. Internal hemorrhoids protrude within the anal canal and are covered with mucous membrane. External hemorrhoids protrude at the anal opening and are covered with anoderm and perianal skin (Fig. 23–12).

Etiology and Pathophysiology
Stasis in the anal venous system is believed to play a principal role in the development of hemorrhoids. Thus, straining at stool, prolonged sitting on the toilet, heavy lifting, pregnancy, infiltrating cancer, and portal hypertension secondary to liver disease are predisposing factors.

Clinical Manifestations
Symptoms of internal hemorrhoids are pain and bleeding on defecation. Bleeding is more red than dark and is often slight, appearing as red streaks on the stool or toilet tissue. It is chronic, however, and over time can be sufficient to cause iron deficiency anemia.

External hemorrhoids appear as lumps of pink to red tissue at the anus. If they are thrombosed, they are very tender, tense, and blue. Rectal itching is common with external hemorrhoids.

Diagnosis
External hemorrhoids are diagnosed by visual examination. Internal hemorrhoids are diagnosed through history, rectal examination, and visualization through an anoscope.

Management
Treatment of uncomplicated hemorrhoids is symptomatic. Sitz baths and topical preparations such as dibucaine ointment and witch hazel are used to shrink mucous membranes and relieve pain. A high-

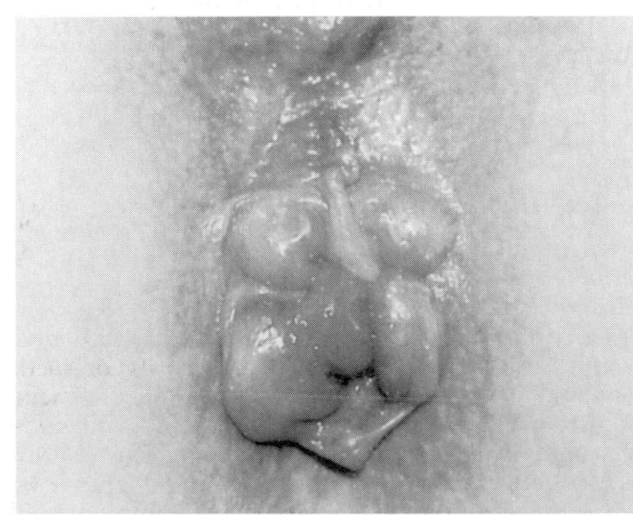

Figure 23–12

External hemorrhoids. (From de los Ríos Magriñá E. Atlas of therapeutic proctology. Philadelphia: WB Saunders, 1984, p 37.)

fiber diet, 2000 mL of fluid per day, and stool softeners or mild laxatives are used to prevent constipation and to keep the stool soft and formed.

Internal hemorrhoids are sometimes treated with a sclerosing agent or rubber band ligation. In the former, a sclerosing agent—such as 5% phenol in oil—is injected into the subcutaneous tissue between and around the internal hemorrhoids, causing the tissue to fibrose and shrink, reducing the size of the mass. This is done on an outpatient basis but requires one to four injections 5 to 7 days apart.

Rubber band ligation is also done on an outpatient basis and requires multiple visits, depending on the number of hemorrhoids present. In this procedure, rubber bands are put around the base of internal hemorrhoids that bleed or are prolapsed. This results in ischemia followed by necrosis and sloughing in about a week. No anesthesia is required for this procedure, and subsequent discomfort is readily controlled with non-narcotic analgesics such as aspirin. Neither injection of a sclerosing agent nor rubber band ligation is used for external hemorrhoids because of the pain that would occur as a result of the sensory innervation of the area.

Other approaches to the treatment of hemorrhoids include:

- Cryosurgery—injection of liquid nitrogen to freeze hemorrhoids and cause necrosis
- Infrared photocoagulation—use of an infrared light beam to cause necrosis
- Bipolar diathermy—use of high-frequency current
- Electrocoagulation—use of low voltage current.

For patients with multiple prolapsed or thrombosed hemorrhoids and severe symptoms, hemorrhoidectomy is the treatment of choice. In this procedure, which may be done under regional anesthesia, the anal canal is first dilated and inspected with an anoscope. Each hemorrhoid is then grasped and excised and the base sutured. When all hemorrhoids are removed, petrolatum gauze packing may be placed in the anal canal and a dressing and T-binder applied.

NURSING PROCESS
Hemorrhoids

Assessment

Question the patient about rectal pain, itching, and bleeding. Note the frequency and severity of each. Determine the type and effectiveness of treatment measures used to relieve symptoms. Assess for lifestyle factors—such as prolonged standing on the job, heavy lifting, or frequent pregnancy—that may contribute to the development or worsening of hemorrhoids.

Obtain information about bowel habits, because constipation, straining at stool, and sitting on the toilet for long periods of time contribute to anal venous stasis. Explore the patient's usual diet and type of exercise, because these factors affect bowel function and can cause straining.

Nursing Diagnoses and Planning

Nursing diagnoses and related expected patient outcomes commonly applicable to patients with hemorrhoids include the following:

NDx: Risk for altered health maintenance related to insufficient knowledge of self-management of hemorrhoids

Planning: Patient Outcomes
1. Patient describes measures to obtain symptomatic relief of hemorrhoids.
2. Patient explains relationship of constipation and other activities to hemorrhoids.
3. Patient lists symptoms that require medical evaluation.

Nursing Interventions and Evaluation

NDx: Risk for altered health maintenance
Review with the patient measures usually effective in providing symptomatic relief of hemorrhoids, such as sitz baths, cold witch hazel compresses, and such preparations as dibucaine cream. Discuss constipation, straining at stool, and such activities as heavy lifting and prolonged standing as aggravating factors. Explain the importance of dietary fiber, large amounts of fluid, and daily exercise in preventing constipation.

Instruct the patient to obtain medical care if excessive pain, bleeding, or prolapse of hemorrhoids occurs.

Compare the patient's status with the expected outcomes. If the outcomes are not met, reassess the patient and revise the plan.

NURSING PROCESS
Post-Hemorrhoidectomy

Assessment
Check vital signs and assess the patient's discomfort. Inspect the rectal area for bleeding every 2 to 4 hours during the first 24 hours after surgery. Measure urinary output because difficulty voiding is not unusual. Assess for anxiety over defecation. Assess the patient's ability to determine signs and symptoms of complications and the accessibility of health care if needed.

Nursing Diagnoses and Planning

Nursing diagnoses and related expected patient outcomes commonly applicable to patients who have had a hemorrhoidectomy include the following:

NDx: Pain related to surgical trauma to the anal area

Planning: Patient Outcomes
1. Patient reports that pain is relieved by analgesics.
2. Patient moves freely without verbal or nonverbal signs of pain.

NDx: Risk for constipation related to fear of pain on defecation

Planning: Patient Outcomes
1. Patient passes soft, formed stool at regular intervals.

NDx: Risk for altered health maintenance related to insufficient knowledge of self-care after hemorrhoidectomy

Planning: Patient Outcomes
1. Patient describes or demonstrates measures to promote healing.
2. Patient lists measures to decrease the risk of recurrence.
3. Patient describes signs and symptoms of complications during the first 24 hours after surgery.

Nursing Interventions and Evaluation

NDx: Pain
Do not underestimate the extent of the patient's discomfort, because hemorrhoidectomy, although not major surgery, is very painful. The patient should take analgesics as often as needed. A flotation pad or soft ring cushion to use when lying supine or sitting will relieve pressure. Sitz baths promote comfort and healing by helping keep the area clean and reducing edema.

The patient should not be alone during the first sitz baths because dilatation of the pelvic veins can cause hypotension during the early postoperative period. Limit sitting to short periods of time. If ordered, ice packs, warm compresses, or analgesic ointments may be used.

As recommended in the AHCPR guidelines for postoperative pain, discuss with the patient which strategies work best for pain relief. Design a plan incorporating relaxation methods along with prescribed pain medication to help the patient remain pain free.

NDx: Risk for constipation
Be alert to anxiety over having a bowel movement. Explain that some discomfort will occur but that it is expected. The patient should take stool softeners as ordered to keep the stool easy to pass. If enemas are ordered, the patient should take pain medication in advance, and the enema tip should be well-lubricated and gently inserted into the rectum.

NDx: Risk for altered health maintenance
Instruct the patient in self-care measures to promote uncomplicated healing and to decrease the risk of recurrence (Highlight 23–8).

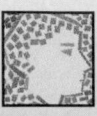

HIGHLIGHT 23–8
PATIENT EDUCATION
Self-Care After a Hemorrhoidectomy

Instruct the patient to:

Report symptoms of complications such as bleeding, increased pain, purulent drainage, or fever.

Take sitz baths after bowel movements for 1 to 2 weeks for cleanliness and comfort.

Prevent constipation.
• Take stool softener as ordered.
• Eat high-fiber diet.
• Drink at least 2000 mL/day.
• Exercise regularly.

Avoid prolonged sitting or standing.

Lose weight if obese.

Additional Interventions
Help the patient out of bed to void. If difficulty voiding persists, give a sitz bath. Use a dressing held in place with a binder to absorb drainage if needed.

Compare the patient's status with the expected outcomes. If the outcomes are not met, reassess the patient and revise the plan.

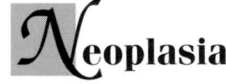eoplasia

POLYPS OF THE COLON

Etiology and Pathophysiology
Although polyps are the most common benign tumor of the bowel, their cause is unknown. Polyps arise from the mucosa of the bowel and project into its lumen (Fig. 23–13). They may be single or multiple and hyperplastic, pedunculated (on a stalk), or flat (sessile).

Polyps are usually considered to be associated with some risk of cancer. This risk is greatest when polyps are multiple, larger than 2 cm in diameter, and histologically of the villous type. The risk is further increased with a family history of cancer. In familial polyposis, a rare genetic disorder in which there are multiple polyps along the intestine, there is a 100% association with cancer by the age of 40 years.

Clinical Manifestations
Polyps are usually asymptomatic, although rectal bleeding and symptoms of iron deficiency anemia

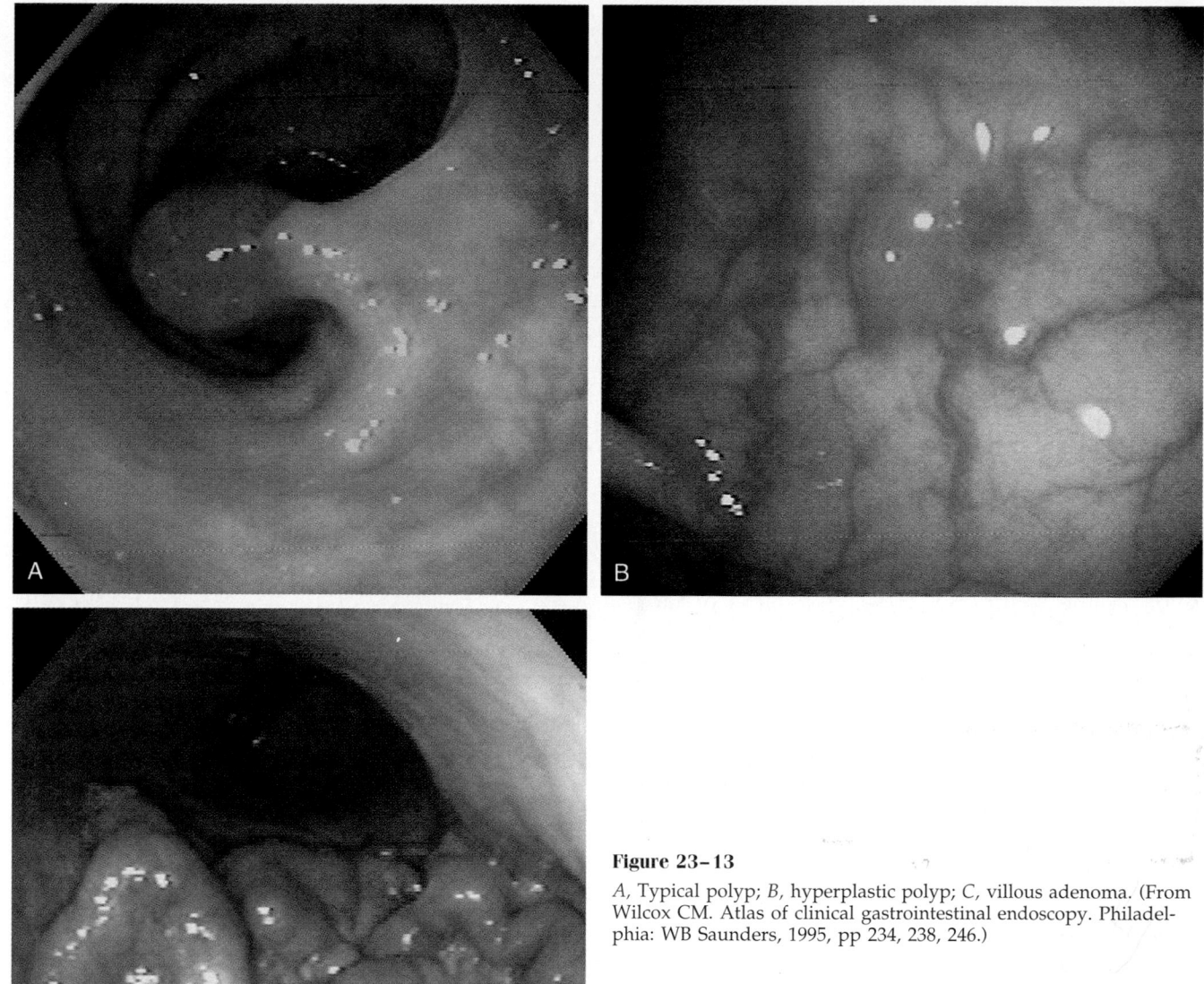

Figure 23–13

A, Typical polyp; *B*, hyperplastic polyp; *C*, villous adenoma. (From Wilcox CM. Atlas of clinical gastrointestinal endoscopy. Philadelphia: WB Saunders, 1995, pp 234, 238, 246.)

occasionally occur. Very large polyps can partially obstruct the colon and cause abdominal pain.

Diagnosis

Polyps are most often diagnosed by sigmoidoscopy or barium studies of the colon. A biopsy is usually done in conjunction with sigmoidoscopy to rule out cancer. Small polyps in the rectal area can be diagnosed by digital rectal examination.

Management

Removal is the treatment of choice for polyps because of their malignant potential. In most cases, polyps can be removed by cautery snare through a colonoscope. Surgical excision may be used for large, sessile polyps. After endoscopic polypectomy, a repeat colonoscopy is done 1 year later and then at least every 3 years.

❖ Settings, Providers, and Collaboration for Care

Polyps may be treated in a physician's office if colonoscopic abilities are present. If surgical excision is necessary, it may be performed in a surgicenter, ambulatory surgery department, or inpatient setting.

The patient is usually discharged shortly after the surgery. A follow-up visit to the physician's office is scheduled. The nurse instructs the patient about the care regimen before discharge.

NURSING PROCESS GUIDELINES
Polyps of the Colon

Nursing care of the patient with polyps of the colon primarily involves patient education. Explain the relationship between polyps and cancer of the colon. Be alert for signs of excessive anxiety on the patient's part about this risk. Stress the effectiveness of follow-up rectal examinations and colonoscopies in identifying early malignant changes that can be effectively treated.

CANCER OF THE COLON AND RECTUM

Most cancers originating in the GI tract occur in the colon or the rectum. Of these, two-thirds or more arise in the rectosigmoid area, with a significant portion within reach of the finger on rectal examination. The incidence of cancers of the colon and rectum is equal in men and women and is highest between ages 50 and 65. The cure rate for persons with early, localized colon cancers is 92%, with a reduction to about 50% once the cancer spreads to adjacent organs or the lymph system. Unfortunately, in many cases, the patient does not seek treatment until the cancer is too far advanced for successful treatment.

Etiology and Pathophysiology

The cause of colorectal cancer is unknown. However, it occurs most often among populations with diets low in fiber, high in refined carbohydrates, high in fats, and high in meat. Thus, it is suggested that prolonged transit time for stool in the intestine may predispose to carcinogenic changes.

Other risk factors associated with development of colorectal cancer are a familial history of the disease, familial polyposis, rectal polyps, and active inflammatory bowel disease of at least 10 years' duration. Highlight 23–9 outlines strategies to reduce the risk of colorectal cancer.

Colorectal cancers are primarily adenomas and develop from the epithelial lining of the intestine (Fig. 23–14). The tumor may project into the lumen of the bowel or encircle the bowel, causing stenosis, ulceration, or perforation. Spread occurs by invasion through the bowel wall into adjacent organs such as the small intestine and uterus. It also occurs by metastasis via the lymphatic vessels and the portal vein. The liver is the most common metastatic site, although metastases to the lungs, kidneys, and bones also occur. The survival rate is proportional to the depth of the lesion and the number of lymph nodes involved at the time of surgery.

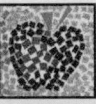

Strategies for Reducing the Risk of Colorectal Cancer

I. Dietary modification:
 High in insoluble fiber—wheat bran, cellulose (carrots, celery)
 Low in animal fats
 Many studies indicate that calcium, vitamins C and E, and carotene are chemopreventive for colon cancer.

II. Screening:
 Men and women over 40: Yearly digital rectal examination
 Men and women over 50: Yearly stool test for occult blood
  Sigmoidoscopy every 3 to 5 years

III. Studies indicate that the effect of NSAIDS on prostaglandin synthesis plays a positive role in colon cancer prevention

Those at risk for colorectal cancer should be especially vigilant.

Risk factors for colorectal cancer include:
 Family history of colorectal cancer
 Previous history of colorectal cancer
 History of breast cancer (women)
 Familial polyposis
 Colorectal polyps
 Chronic inflammatory bowel disease

Clinical Manifestations

Colorectal cancer is frequently asymptomatic in its early stages. When symptoms do occur, they vary somewhat according to the location of the tumor. The first symptoms of left colon tumors are changes in bowel function that often go unnoticed as significant by the patient. These changes consist of constipation or diarrhea along with the gradual development of flat, ribbon-like, or pencil-shaped stools. Other symptoms of left colon tumors are crampy gas pains, bright red blood in the stool, and ultimately progressive abdominal distention and vomiting as obstruction becomes more complete.

Characteristic symptoms of right colon tumors include vague, dull abdominal pain exacerbated by walking, and dark red or mahogany blood mixed in the stool. Symptoms of rectal cancer are straining at stool, a feeling of incomplete evacuation, a mucous discharge, bright red bleeding and, with advanced disease, pain.

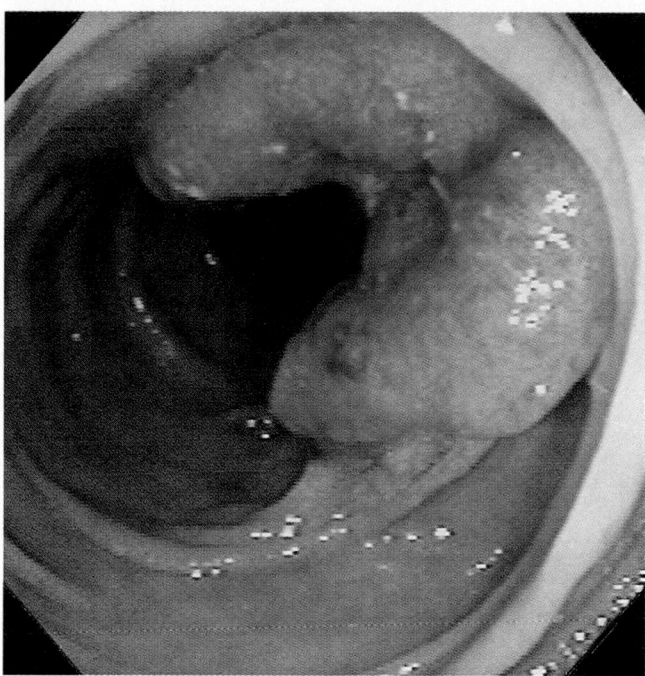

Figure 23-14

Adenocarcinoma of the sigmoid colon. (From Wilcox CM. Atlas of clinical gastrointestinal endoscopy. Philadelphia: WB Saunders, 1995, p 257.)

Late symptoms of any colorectal cancer are weakness, anorexia, weight loss, and anemia. Once metastasis has occurred, signs of liver, respiratory, or renal failure may develop or back pain may develop because of possible bone involvement.

Diagnosis

The diagnosis of colorectal cancer is suggested when a patient presents with a combination of these symptoms. To establish the diagnosis, a rectal examination, barium studies, and colonoscopy are done. Liver function tests, an intravenous pyelogram, and other studies are done to detect metastases and stage the disease.

Management

Medical management depends on the location of the tumor and the stage of the disease. Surgery is the treatment of choice because it is most effective. When possible, the section of bowel containing the tumor, along with a section of bowel on either side, is excised to eliminate the area of immediate lymphatic spread. The remaining bowel is then rejoined in an end-to-end anastomosis. Thus, for a tumor of the right colon, a right colectomy with an ileotransverse anastomosis is done, whereas for a tumor of the descending colon, a left colectomy is done with the transverse colon anastomosed to the sigmoid colon. For tumors low in the sigmoid or in the rectum where reanastomosis of the bowel is impossible, an abdominal perineal resection is done (see later discussion).

In some cases of widespread disease, palliative surgery is done. For example, when symptoms of obstruction are present, the involved area may be resected or bypassed or, if necessary, a colostomy created proximal to the obstructed bowel.

Radiation may be given preoperatively to shrink the size of the tumor. Chemotherapy is occasionally given postoperatively to patients with extensive invasion or metastases. Radiation and chemotherapy are also used for palliation when tumors are inoperable.

Late in the disease, treatment simply consists of comfort measures and nutritional support. This may include continuous analgesic infusion via implantable pump and tube feedings or TPN given in the home, hospital, or hospice.

Abdominal Perineal Resection

An abdominal perineal resection is a procedure in which a colostomy is created and the distal sigmoid colon, rectum, and anus are removed (Fig. 23-15).

PATIENT PREPARATION. Fluid and electrolyte imbalances are corrected. Nutritional status is improved through a high-calorie diet or TPN depending on the patient's condition. Iron supplements or blood transfusions are given to correct anemia.

To reduce the risk of contamination at the time of operation, the bowel is emptied and cleansed. The patient is on a low-residue diet and then, for 2 to 3 days before surgery, a liquid diet to prevent accumulation of feces. Laxatives and enemas are given to empty the bowel. Intestinal anti-infectives, such as neomycin or kanamycin, are administered to decrease the bacteria in the bowel.

A nasogastric tube is inserted for decompression, as is an indwelling urinary catheter to keep the bladder empty during surgery.

Because formation of a colostomy is part of the surgical procedure, preparatory sessions with the enterostomal therapist are also an essential part of the patient's preparation.

PROCEDURE. An abdominal perineal resection is a two-step procedure. First the abdomen is opened, the sigmoid colon cut above the level of the tumor, and the proximal end of the sigmoid brought out through a stab wound in the abdominal wall to form a colostomy. After closure of the abdominal incision, a perineal incision is made and the lower sigmoid, rectum, and anus, along with the skin, muscle, fat, and lymphoid tissue in the area, are removed. The perineal wound is then (1) closed completely with a suction drainage tube in place in the wound through incisions made on either side of it, (2) partially closed with a Penrose drain in place in the midline, or (3) left open and packed to heal by granulation. Usually the first method is preferred except in cases of contamination or active infection.

POSTOPERATIVE COURSE. Immediately after surgery, profuse serosanguineous drainage from the perineal wound is expected. Suction drainage tubes are left in place attached to low, continuous suction

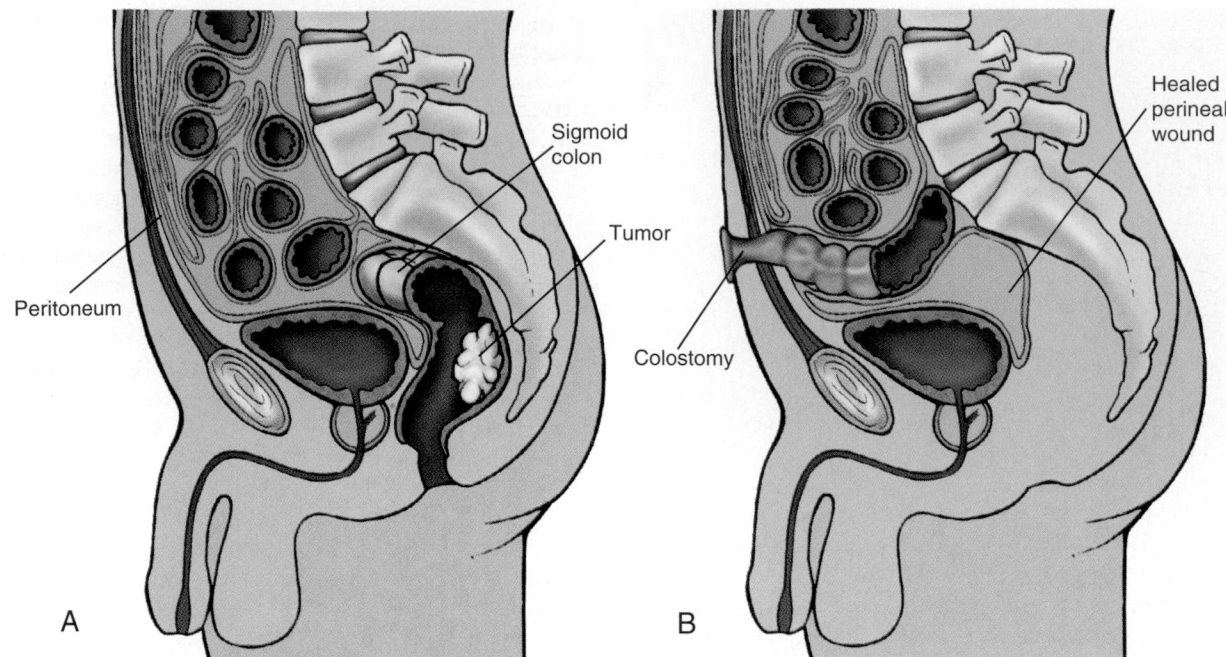

Figure 23-15

Abdominal perineal resection. *A*, Anatomy before surgery; *B*, anatomy after surgery.

or to a portable suction apparatus such as a Hemovac until drainage is less than 50 mL per 24 hours, usually 3 to 5 days. Both Penrose drains and packing are removed gradually over a period of 5 to 7 days. An indwelling catheter is in place for 5 to 7 days to prevent urinary retention and pressure of a full bladder on the perineal wound. It also helps keep the perineal dressing dry.

The patient is on NPO status and receives intravenous fluid and electrolytes until bowel function returns and stool is passed through the colostomy, which is usually in 5 to 7 days.

Parenteral nutrition may also be given during this time if the patient's nutritional status needs improvement.

The patient is ambulatory in 24 to 48 hours and is usually discharged in 10 to 12 days. The perineal wound can heal in 2 to 4 months, although 6 to 8 months is not uncommon.

After hospitalization, the patient is monitored closely for signs of recurrence of the malignancy. This often includes repeated tests for carcinoembryonic antigens, antigens normally present in the fetus but which, when found in the adult, are thought to be specific for cancerous tumors. A drop in the level of carcinoembryonic antigens after surgery is consistent with complete tumor removal. No decrease or an increase is indicative of residual tumor or spread.

COMPLICATIONS. Complications of abdominal perineal resection are many. They include hemorrhage, infection, impaired wound healing, persistent draining perineal sinus tract, urinary dysfunction, and impotence.

❖ Settings, Providers, and Collaboration for Care

Surveillance of colorectal cancer can be carried out in an outpatient setting, such as a physician's office with x-ray and sigmoid and/or colonoscopic capabilities, or a clinic with the same machinery. Hospitalization is required for surgical excision of the cancer. The extent of hospitalization depends on the type of procedure required. Patients may receive chemotherapy, radiation therapy, or both as part of the treatment plan in outpatient settings. As mentioned, there are implications for home-health or hospice care for these patients. The expertise of an enterostomal therapist is appropriate for the patient treated with an abdominal perineal resection. The enterostomal therapist may visit the patient in the hospital and after discharge to the home or other care facility. The home health nurse and the enterostomal therapist collaborate to meet the patient's self-care and education needs. In many cases, the therapist teaches the family to assist with the stomal care. A nutritionist may also consult with the nurse and the patient to assist in the appropriate meal planning for the patient. A counselor or psychologist may be indicated to help the patient and family cope with the traumatic surgery and change in body image.

NURSING PROCESS
Abdominal Perineal Resection

PREOPERATIVE NURSING CARE

Preoperative nursing care of a patient scheduled for an abdominal perineal resection involves the basic assessments and interventions that apply to any surgical patient. Pay particular attention to GI and nutritional status, ability to tolerate the preoperative tests and bowel preparation, and the propensity for a successful surgical outcome.

POSTOPERATIVE NURSING CARE

Assessment

Assess the patient's return to physiologic stability. Check blood pressure, pulse, and respirations at least every 15 minutes and then at increasing intervals. Inspect the stoma for signs of hemorrhage. Remember that a small amount of oozing is expected; frank bleeding is not. Also assess the adequacy of the blood supply to the stoma by observing its color, which should be a moist, deep pink to red. Note the degree of edema, keeping in mind that significant edema is normal as a result of surgical trauma. It should decrease progressively over time.

Inspect the abdominal dressing for drainage. Later, when the dressing is changed or removed, observe the wound for approximation of the suture line, redness, edema, and drainage. Also check for abdominal distention, which can lead to dehiscence of the incision.

Inspect the perineal wound. If it is a closed wound, check the amount and color of drainage in the collection container. Observe the wound itself for signs of separation or infection. If it is a semiclosed or packed wound, examine for bleeding, excessive drainage, or unusual odor. Be certain to note any signs of necrosis.

Assess the patient for abdominal and perineal pain. Remember that perineal discomfort is worsened by sitting, so be certain to assess the amount of discomfort at this time. Also question about perineal itching because this is a common problem after perineal resection.

Assess for a return of peristalsis. Listen for bowel sounds and check for the passage of flatus. When the colostomy begins to function (usually within 72 hours after surgery, although it may take up to 5 days), note the color, consistency, and amount of stool. Be certain to also inspect the peristomal skin for signs of irritation or excoriation.

Assess fluid, electrolyte, and nutritional status. Measure intake, output, and daily weight. Review serum electrolyte data, and observe for signs of dehydration. Assess function of the urinary tract. Observe for signs of infection. Note the color of the urine and its clarity. When the catheter is removed, check for retention and, in men, for incontinence, which can occur as a result of the surgery.

Throughout the postoperative period, assess the patient's emotional reaction to the surgery and coping ability. Note his or her willingness to speak about the surgery and its effects and whether or not the patient looks at the wounds and the stoma or asks questions about them. Note the degree of patient cooperation with and participation in care as well as the patient's outlook toward the future.

Nursing Diagnoses and Planning

Nursing diagnoses and related expected patient outcomes commonly applicable to patients who have had an abdominal perineal resection include the following:

NDx: Pain related to surgical trauma to the abdomen and perineum

Planning: Patient Outcomes
1. Patient moves without signs of severe pain, such as moaning, pallor, and tachycardia.
2. Patient rests quietly without signs of discomfort, such as clenched hands, groaning, and crying.
3. Patient reports that pain is relieved.

NDx: Risk for ineffective breathing pattern related to shallow breathing secondary to incisional pain on deep breathing

Planning: Patient Outcomes
1. Patient coughs and deep breathes as directed.
2. Lung sounds remain clear to auscultation.
3. Arterial blood gases are within normal range.

NDx: Impaired tissue integrity related to presence of large perineal wound

Planning: Patient Outcomes
1. Drainage is serosanguineous and decreases progressively over 4 to 5 days.
2. Suture line of a closed wound is approximated.
3. Granulation tissue forms in open wounds.

NDx: Bowel incontinence related to the formation of a colostomy and loss of rectal function

Planning: Patient Outcomes
1. A selected pouching system is used effectively to collect fecal drainage.
2. Patient identifies factors, such as change in diet and times of eating, that affect the pattern of colostomy function.

NDx: Risk for altered nutrition: less than body requirements related to inadequate intake of nutrients, impaired absorption, or both

Planning: Patient Outcomes
1. Patient maintains expected weight.
2. Patient resumes oral intake of a nutritionally balanced diet.
3. Patient takes nutritional supplements as directed.

NDx: Risk for impaired skin integrity related to irritating effects of colostomy drainage and removal of adhesives on the peristomal skin

Planning: Patient Outcomes
1. Peristomal skin is intact.
2. Peristomal skin is free of erythema.
3. Patient denies burning or soreness of the peristomal skin.

NDx: Risk for altered oral mucous membrane related to NPO status and presence of a nasogastric or nasointestinal tube

Planning: Patient Outcomes
1. Oral mucous membrane is moist and free of cracks.
2. Lips are moist, supple, and free of cracks.
3. Patient denies dryness of the mouth.

NDx: Risk for altered peripheral tissue perfusion related to thrombophlebitis secondary to venous stasis

Planning: Patient Outcomes
1. Patient does foot and leg exercises as directed.
2. Calves and upper thighs are free of redness, swelling, heat, and pain.
3. Homans' sign is negative.

NDx: Body image disturbance related to loss of bowel control, presence of a perineal wound and a stoma, release of fecal material onto the abdomen, passage of flatus, odor, need for an appliance

Planning: Patient Outcomes
1. Patient verbalizes self-acceptance with the colostomy and the perineal wound.
2. Patient identifies personal strengths.
3. Patient expresses pleasure at visits from relatives or friends.
4. Patient verbalizes interest in grooming and appearance.

NDx: Risk for sexual dysfunction related to the effects of the abdominal and perineal surgery

Planning: Patient Outcomes
1. Patient discusses sexual concerns openly.
2. Patient describes potential effects of the surgery on sexual function.
3. Patient verbalizes optimism about resuming a sexual relationship.

NDx: Risk for altered health maintenance related to insufficient knowledge of self-care after discharge

Planning: Patient Outcomes
1. Patient demonstrates wound care and colostomy care.
2. Patient describes dietary regimen.
3. Patient lists prescribed medications, giving name, purpose, dose, route, time, and side effects.
4. Patient identifies community resources.

5. Patient lists symptoms to be immediately reported.

Nursing Interventions and Evaluation

NDx: Pain
Use the AHCPR postoperative pain control guidelines to assist with planning for pain relief. Give prescribed analgesics every 3 to 4 hours for 72 hours. Remember that the patient will have a great deal of pain not only from the abdominal incision but also from the perineal incision. Keep the patient physically comfortable to aid in the effectiveness of the analgesics. Place the patient in a side-lying position with the knees flexed to reduce stress on the incision line. Have the patient change position every 2 hours. Avoid the dorsal recumbent position, which is uncomfortable because of pressure on the perineal wound and may interfere with drainage and healing.

Teach the patient to splint the abdominal incision when turning, coughing, and deep breathing. Time wound care to coincide with the peak effects of analgesics. Give sitz baths and apply antipruritics for discomfort from perineal itching, a common occurrence as the wound begins to heal. When the patient is out of bed, encourage short walks rather than sitting in a chair. When sitting is necessary, provide a soft foam ring to increase comfort.

If "phantom" rectal pain is a problem, explain that it occurs because the sympathetic nerves, which used to control the rectum, are still intact even though the rectum was removed. Reassure the patient that it is not an indication of a complication and should disappear with time.

NDx: Risk for ineffective breathing pattern
Teach the patient to splint the abdomen with pillows. Assist in turning, coughing, and deep-breathing every 2 hours for 72 hours after surgery. Instruct the patient in the use of an incentive spirometer. Reassure the patient that coughing and deep-breathing, despite the fact that they may hurt, will not damage the incision or the ostomy. When the patient is able, he or she should ambulate at least three times daily.

NDx: Impaired tissue integrity
Reinforce and change the perineal dressing as often as needed to keep the area dry. Cleanse the rectal area frequently to prevent odor and skin irritation. Use a binder or similar device to hold the dressing in place without using adhesive tape.

If the perineal wound is closed with drains attached to suction, monitor the function of the apparatus. Record the amount and color of the drainage. Expect the drains to be removed when drainage has decreased to less than 50 mL per 24 hours, which is usually in 3 to 5 days.

Provide sitz baths three times per day to promote comfort and healing both before and after the drains are removed. If the perineal wound is semi-closed with Penrose drains in place, start sitz baths after the drains are removed.

Irrigate open wounds as ordered at least four times daily after the packing is removed, 3 to 4 days postoperatively. Use a hand-held shower device or an Asepto syringe. Irrigate gently, because too much force can damage granulation tissue and increase the risk of introducing bacteria. Hold the tip several inches from the wound and irrigate with a normal saline, hydrogen peroxide, or antibiotic solution according to the surgeon's orders. Apply streptokinase or streptodornase if ordered to débride the wound chemically.

NDx: Bowel incontinence

Use a colostomy appliance to collect feces expelled involuntarily from the colostomy. In most cases, a clear plastic, open-ended collection pouch is placed over the colostomy at the time of surgery. Monitor this pouch for accumulation of flatus or drainage and empty or change as necessary. Subsequently, assist the patient in the selection of a collection system for daily use that is best suited to his or her needs. If the patient is unable to perform self-care and will depend on a spouse or significant other for assistance, include that person in the selection process. Once a system is selected, use it consistently to eliminate confusion and facilitate the patient's learning of self-care.

Explain that control over fecal expulsion may be gained in time by means of a regular diet or periodic irrigation and that a collection pouch may not be needed all the time. To assist the patient in achieving control, instruct the patient in basic dietary considerations and in the importance of maintaining a regular pattern of eating and exercise.

NDx: Risk for altered nutrition: less than body requirements

If the patient is vomiting, give antiemetics as prescribed. Maintain the TPN schedule if ordered. When oral intake resumes, give small amounts of clear fluids of the patient's choice. If these are tolerated without singultus (hiccups), nausea, vomiting, or other discomfort, gradually progress to full fluids and then to a regular low-residue diet. Give nutritional supplements as ordered. Promptly alert the physician to any weight loss.

NDx: Risk for impaired skin integrity

Remove mucus or feces with a tissue and thoroughly wash the peristomal skin. Rinse carefully to remove all soap residue. Dry gently and completely. Omit the soap if dry skin is a problem, but do not use oily soaps or emollients because they interfere with the adherence of an appliance. Use a skin barrier to protect the eighth-inch of exposed skin between the stoma and the pouch opening from exposure to fecal drainage. Apply a skin sealant to the peristomal skin areas where adhesive will be used and position the collection pouch snugly in place. Monitor for leaking from the pouch, and change the pouch immediately should it occur. If skin irritation develops, institute immediate treatment as described in Chapter 21.

NDx: Risk for altered oral mucous membrane

Assist the patient to brush the teeth at least three times daily. Encourage frequent mouth rinses with dilute mouthwash or saline solution. Avoid the use of solutions with a drying effect on mucous membranes. Apply water-soluble lubricant to the lips to keep them supple and prevent cracking.

NDx: Risk for altered peripheral tissue perfusion

Guide the patient in foot and leg exercises, 10 times each, every 2 hours while he or she is on bedrest. Apply antiembolic stockings or sequential compression devices as ordered to further support venous return. Avoid the use of the knee gatch, pillows under the knees, or any other form of pressure in the popliteal space. Assist the patient out of bed and in beginning ambulation as ordered in 24 to 48 hours after surgery. Instruct the patient to avoid crossing the legs or sitting for long periods of time.

NDx: Body image disturbance

Acknowledge to the patient that ambivalent feelings about the surgery are normal because on the one hand it is a potentially life-saving procedure, yet on the other hand it involves a change in both body appearance and function. Recognize that patients often experience fear of rejection, disgust, or shame, and be certain that comments, facial expressions, or other nonverbal behaviors convey acceptance and not revulsion, distaste, or pity.

Recognize that denial is a common reaction to this surgery and permit its use while also promoting acceptance. Describe the appearance of the stoma and the perineal wound, and refer to them by name when giving care. Also offer to provide a mirror for the patient to view the wounds if desired. Do not force the patient to look at the wounds, but be certain to indicate that there is nothing abnormal in wanting to see the effects of the surgery on the body.

Protect the patient from undue embarrassment by providing privacy during care, discussions, and teaching and by taking steps to keep the patient and the environment odor free.

Encourage the patient to be well groomed and discuss how the ostomy and pouch are not visible under clothing if styles are selected with a bit of care. Foster a sense of control by allowing the patient to make decisions whenever possible and assisting the patient to incorporate colostomy care into the daily routine.

Promote communication of feelings between the

patient and significant others, and encourage family and friends to treat the patient normally.

NDx: Risk for sexual dysfunction

Encourage the patient to express feelings and ask questions about sexual function and, whenever possible, include the spouse in the discussion. Make certain that the male patient understands that, although sexual dysfunction is a potential complication of this surgery, erection, ejaculation, and orgasm involve different nerve pathways so that sexual dysfunction, if it occurs, is not necessarily complete. Also inform the patient that, if impotence should occur and persist for more than 3 months, a penile implant could be considered. If appropriate, have another ostomate come and talk to the patient and family about this and other topics relating to the ostomy.

NDx: Risk for altered health maintenance

Instruct the patient in the care of the abdominal wound, the perineal wound, and the colostomy. Begin teaching as soon as the patient's condition allows postoperatively. Provide the information the patient needs and requests, but avoid unnecessary detail, which may create anxiety or confusion. Encourage participation of family members who will be assisting with the patient's care or purchasing supplies and equipment. Repeat information as needed and provide written care instructions because what is explained under stress tends to be easily forgotten. Teach the patient to change the appliance, do peristomal skin care, take sitz baths, and eat a balanced diet while avoiding foods that cause constipation or diarrhea. Also teach the patient about the action, purpose, side effects, and administration of prescribed drugs. Inform him or her about available community resources such as the United Ostomy Association and the American Cancer Society, which offer information, counseling, and other support services.

Instruct the patient to report stenosis, prolapse, or retraction of the stoma, irritation of the peristomal skin, bleeding, abdominal distention or rigidity, and persistent diarrhea. Also instruct the patient to weigh him or herself weekly and to report the loss of more than 2 pounds (1 kg).

Compare the patient's status with the expected outcomes. If the outcomes are not met, reassess the patient and revise the plan.

The Elderly: Special Considerations

There is no lower GI disorder unique to the aged, nor is the overall prevalence of these disorders greater among the elderly than the rest of the population. Nonetheless, lower GI diseases are an important cause of both morbidity and mortality among the aged.

With aging, there is atrophy of the muscle and the mucosa throughout the small and large intestines. However, motor and secretory function do not undergo significant change. There does appear to be some decrease in absorption, particularly in the absorption of fats and vitamin B_{12}, however, because of the decrease in intestinal epithelial cells.

Malabsorption syndromes in the elderly differ from those in the younger adults in the presenting symptoms. Diarrhea is the most common symptom among the younger groups, whereas symptoms caused by the secondary effects of malabsorption such as fatigue from anemia or bone pain from osteomalacia predominate in the elderly.

Diverticular disease occurs with increasing frequency as age advances, affecting about 40% of the world's population of persons older than 70 years. It is thought that the increase in duodenal diverticula found in the aged contributes to the development of bacterial overgrowth, which in turn can cause malabsorption.

Ischemia of the small intestine can occur in the elderly because of acute occlusion of the mesenteric vessels, thrombosis of the mesenteric vessels, or a decrease in cardiac output secondary to shock, myocardial infarct, or sepsis. Symptoms of intestinal ischemia resulting from an acute embolism are abdominal pain, distention, and fever. When ischemia is widespread, diarrhea, which may be bloody, leukocytosis, and hemoconcentration also occur. Ischemia caused by thrombosis, on the other hand, develops over a number of hours or days and is characterized by nonspecific abdominal pain. Management of these mesenteric vascular disorders consists of replacement of intravascular volume, correction of acidosis, and surgical resection of the intestine with or without vascular bypass or endarterectomy.

Another form of intestinal ischemia that occurs in the elderly is abdominal angina. This is a chronic disease caused by atherosclerosis of the mesenteric vessels. It is characterized by severe, crampy pain occurring 20 to 30 minutes after eating and is often accompanied by diarrhea, steatorrhea, and marked weight loss. It is diagnosed by angiography and is treated with small, frequent feedings or surgical revascularization.

Inflammatory bowel disease is also a problem in the elderly. A significant number of cases of ulcerative colitis develop after the age of 60 years. In many of these, the initial attack is more severe than when the disease develops at a younger age, and there is a greater incidence of recurrence of an earlier problem. The immediate precipitating factor is often chronic constipation, but multiple pregnancies and years of work requiring one to stand on the feet are common predisposing factors.

Appendicitis is an example of a disorder that is usually minor in younger patients but can be very serious in the elderly. Its occurrence is rare in the older population because of the tendency for lymphoid atrophy, which obliterates the lumen of the appendix. When it does occur, however, there are two major problems. First, the reduced lymph tissue, which normally prevents infections, makes systemic infection more likely. Second, the reduced blood flow to this area of the colon means that appendicitis in the elderly is often associated with gangrene. In addition, the initial signs and symptoms of appendicitis may be absent or atypical in the older patient, but a rapid, severe course may follow. Peritonitis readily develops, and world mortality rates are 12% in those older than 60 years and 30% in those older than 70 years.

Chapter Review

1. How is the care of a patient with ulcerative colitis similar to that of a patient with Crohn's disease?
2. What are the advantages of outpatient or ambulatory surgery for a patient diagnosed with internal hemorrhoids?
3. How would you assist with ambulation when caring for a patient who has had an abdominal perineal resection for colon cancer?
4. Why is abdominal assessment important when planning care for a patient with appendicitis?
5. What would happen to a patient with peritonitis if he or she were given large amounts of fluid by mouth?
6. What is the meaning of steatorrhea when seen in a patient with malabsorption syndrome?
7. How can the effectiveness of bowel rest be evaluated when caring for a patient with diverticulitis?
8. Why is nutrition important when planning the care of a patient with Crohn's disease?
9. What evidence supports the effect of a high-fiber, low-fat diet when planning the care for a patient with intestinal polyps?
10. How would you manage the discomfort of a patient who has undergone drainage of an anorectal abscess?

Bibliography

Agency for Health Care Policy and Research. Acute pain management: Operative or medical procedures and trauma. Rockville, MD: US Department of Health and Human Services. AHCPR 92-0032, 1992.

Arullani A, Cappello G. Diagnosis and current treatment of hemorrhoidal disease. Angiology 1994; 45(96):560.

Bates B. A guide to physical examination and history taking. 6th ed. Philadelphia: JB Lippincott, 1995.

Carethers JM, McDonnell WM. Extraintestinal manifestations of Crohn's disease. N Engl J Med 1994; 330(26):1870.

Cox J. Inflammatory bowel disease: Implications for the medical-surgical nurse. Medsurg Nursing 1995; 4(6):427.

Deckmann RC, Cheskin LJ. Diverticular disease in the elderly. Journal of the American Geriatrics Society 1993; 40:986.

Dolan MMB, Robinson JH, Roberts S. When the doctor delays pain relief. Nursing 1993; 23(4):46.

Doughty BD. What you need to know about inflammatory bowel disease. Am J Nurs 1994; 94(7):24.

Doughty BD, Jackson DB. Gastrointestinal disorders. St. Louis: Mosby Year-Book, 1993.

Fitzsimmons ML, Fales L. Colon cancer prevention update. Semin Oncol Nurs 1993; 9(3):163.

Fulton JS. Chemotherapeutic treatment of colorectal cancer: Rationale, trends, and nursing care. J WOCN 1994; 21(1):12.

Gonzalez-Cortez SB, Procuniar CE. Laparoscopic inguinal herniorrhaphy. AORN J 1994; 60(3):419.

Grant J, Chapman G, Russell M. Malabsorption associated with surgical procedures and its treatment. Nutr Clin Pract 1996; 11(2):43.

Hale J. Detecting colorectal cancer. Nurs Times 1994; 90(43):32.

Handerhan B. Investigating peritoneal irritation. Am J Nurs 1994; 94(4):71.

Hastings GE, Weber RJ. Inflammatory bowel disease: Part I. Clinical features and diagnosis. Am Fam Physician 1993; 47(3):598.

Hastings GE, Weber RJ. Inflammatory bowel disease: Part II. Medical and surgical management. Am Fam Physician 1993; 47(4):811.

Kinash RG, Fischer DG, Lukie BE, Carr TL. Inflammatory bowel disease impact and patient characteristics. Gastroenterol Nurs 1993; 15(4):147.

Kirsner J, Shorter RG (eds). Inflammatory bowel disease. 3rd ed. Baltimore: Williams and Wilkins, 1995.

Landercasper J, Cogbill T, Merry W, Stolee R, Strutt J. Long-term outcome after hospitalization for small-bowel obstruction. Arch Surg 1993; 128(7):765.

Ludwig K, Cattey R, Henry L. Initial experience with laparoscopic appendectomy. Dis Colon Rectum 1993; 36(5):463.

MacRae HM, McLeod RS. Comparison of hemorrhoidal treatment modalities. A meta-analysis. Dis Colon Rectum 1995; 38(7):687.

Malseed RT. Pharmacology, drug therapy and nursing considerations. 4th ed. Philadelphia: JB Lippincott, 1995.

Marchiondo K. When the diagnosis is diverticular disease. RN 1994; 57(2):42.

Mathewson M. Pharmacotherapeutics: A nursing process approach. Philadelphia: FA Davis, 1994.

Mazier W. Hemorrhoids, fissures, and pruritus ani. Surg Clin North Am 1994; 74(6):1277.

McConnell EA. Loosening the grip of intestinal obstruction. Nursing 1994; 24(3):34.

McConnell EA. Managing a nasoenteric-decompression tube. Nursing 1994; 24(3):18.

McConnell EA. Myths & facts. Nursing 1995; 25(4):17.

Meeker MH, Rothrock J. Alexander's care of the patient in surgery. 10th ed. St. Louis: Mosby Year-Book, 1995.

Misiewicz JJ, Pounder RE, Venables CW (eds). Diseases of the gut and pancreas. Baltimore: Blackwell Scientific, 1994.

Nathens A, Rotstein O. Therapeutic options in peritonitis. Surg Clin North Am 1994; 74(3):677.

Ogorek CP, Fisher RS. Differentiation between Crohn's disease and ulcerative colitis. Med Clin North Am 1994; 78(6):1249.

Pfenninger JL, Surrell S. Nonsurgical treatment options for internal hemorrhoids. Am Fam Physician 1995; 52(3):821.

Roberts PL, Veidenheimer MC. Current management of diverticulitis. Advanced Surg 1994; 27:189.

Schoetz DJ. Uncomplicated diverticulitis: Indications for surgery and surgical management. Surg Clin North Am 1993; 73(5):965.

Shoji BT, Becker JM. Colorectal disease in the elderly patient. Surg Clin North Am 1994; 74(2):2993.

Sleisenger MH, Fordtran JS. Gastrointestinal disease: Pathophysiology, diagnosis and management. 4th ed. Philadelphia: WB Saunders, 1993.

Spiro CM, Grant EG, Gilly MT. Diverticular disease: Surgical options, patient management. AORN J 1994; 59(3):625.

Spiro H. Clinical gastroenterology. 4th ed. New York: McGraw Hill, 1993.

Steel, G. Colorectal cancer. In Murphy G, Lawrence W, Lenhard R (eds). American Cancer Society textbook of clinical oncology. Atlanta: American Cancer Society, 1995.

Swonger AK, Burbank PM. Drug therapy and the elderly. Boston: Jones and Bartlett, 1995

Targon S, Shanahan F (eds). Inflammatory bowel disease: From bench to bedside. Baltimore: Williams & Wilkins, 1994.

Wastell C, Nyhus LM, Donahue PE. Surgery of the esophagus, stomach and small intestine. Boston: Little, Brown, 1995.

Williams SR. Nutrition and diet therapy. St. Louis: Mosby, 1993.

Witt ME. Current management of adults with colorectal cancer. Medsurg Nursing 1993; 2(2):105.

Zighelboim J, Talley NJ. What are functional bowel disorders? Gastroenterology 1993; 104(4):196.

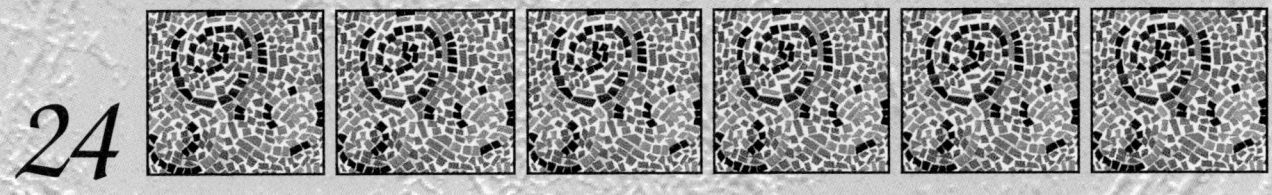

24

Nursing Care of Patients with Disorders of the Accessory Organs of Digestion

Study Outcomes

After studying this chapter, you should be able to:

1. Describe the etiology, pathophysiology, clinical manifestations, diagnostic procedures, and medical management of common disorders of the accessory organs of digestion.
2. Identify information and physical examination data essential to the assessment of patients with common disorders of the accessory organs of digestion.
3. State nursing diagnoses and related expected patient outcomes commonly applicable to patients with disorders of the accessory organs of digestion.
4. Describe nursing interventions, with their rationales, commonly applicable to patients with disorders of the accessory organs of digestion.
5. Explain the basis for evaluation of nursing care provided to patients with common disorders of the accessory organs of digestion.
6. Identify alternative treatment and care settings for patients with disorders of the accessory organs of digestion and the services related to community-based care.
7. Identify special considerations for elderly patients with disorders of the accessory organs of digestion.

The exocrine pancreas and the gallbladder are accessory gastrointestinal organs that play a role in the normal digestive process. The exocrine pancreas secretes the enzymes amylase, lipase, and protease, which break down carbohydrates, fats, and proteins, respectively. The gallbladder stores bile, which emulsifies fat, stimulates pancreatic secretion, and activates pancreatic lipase. Because their functions relate directly to the gastrointestinal system, diseases of the pancreas and gallbladder typically manifest as changes in the digestive process. Similarly, management of these disorders typically includes measures to promote a return to normal digestion.

Disorders of the pancreas and gallbladder are commonly treated in an inpatient setting because surgical repair is often the focus of treatment. Patients with acute pancreatitis or other acute problems of the accessory organs, such as severe pain, may present at an emergency department.

*I*nfections and Inflammations

CHOLECYSTITIS

Etiology and Pathophysiology
Cholecystitis, or inflammation of the gallbladder, is almost always associated with cholelithiasis. Cholelithiasis refers to the presence of stones in the gallbladder, cystic duct, or common bile duct (Fig. 24–1). The exact cause of stone formation is unknown; however, bile stasis, imbalances in cholesterol metabolism, and infection seem to be precipitating factors (Highlight 24–1). Once formed, stones may remain in the gallbladder or migrate to the cystic or common bile duct, causing inflammation and obstruction. Cholelithiasis is a very common disorder; 10 to 15% of adults in the United States have gallstones.

Clinical Manifestations
Most patients with gallstones remain asymptomatic. Early symptoms of cholecystitis include intolerance to fatty foods, nausea with or without vomiting, flatulence, elevated temperature, and right upper quadrant discomfort. In acute episodes, right upper quadrant pain is intense and may radiate to the right scapula and shoulder. If the flow of bile is obstructed, jaundice, clay-colored stools, and dark-colored urine also develop.

Diagnosis
Laboratory data indicative of cholecystitis include an elevated white blood cell count, alkaline phosphatase, aspartate aminotransferase (formerly serum glutamic oxalo-acetic transaminase), and lactate dehydrogenase. If biliary obstruction is present, serum bilirubin levels are also elevated.

Diagnosis of cholelithiasis is confirmed by the visualization of gallstones. The availability of high-resolution ultrasonography has changed the course of gallbladder imaging, and is now the gold standard for diagnosis. Still, nuclear imaging and intravenous or oral cholecystography have a role in some

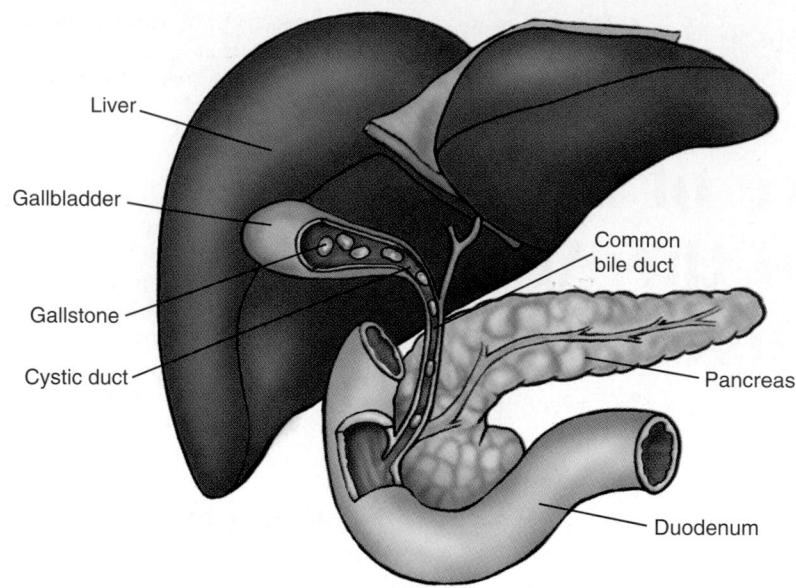

Figure 24–1
Common locations of stones in the biliary tract.

**Primary Prevention of
Gallstone Formation**

Strategies to reduce risk of gallstone formation:

Eliminate obesity (decreases excessive cholesterol synthesis and mobilization)

Eat a high-fiber, high-calcium diet (diminishes input of deoxycholic acid)

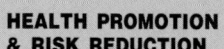 Lower intake of saturated fatty acids (diminishes nucleation of supersaturated bile)

Ingest meals at regular intervals (diminishes gallbladder storage)

Participate in vigorous exercise (allows frequent meals with decreased caloric uptake)

Risk factors for cholelithiasis:

Female sex

History of pregnancy

Age >40

Obesity

Familial tendency

Native American heritage

Mexican American heritage

clinical situations. Endoscopic retrograde cholangio-pancreatography may also be employed.

Management

Supportive treatment for acute cholecystitis includes the control of pain through the administration of analgesics and anticholinergic drugs and the control of infection through intravenously administered antibiotics. If nausea and vomiting are present, the patient is maintained on a nothing-by-mouth (NPO) order and has a nasogastric tube with suction in place. Fluid and electrolyte balance is maintained through replacement therapy. When tolerated, oral intake begins with a low-fat, clear-liquid diet or minimal-fat, full-liquid diet, which is progressed gradually to a restricted soft diet (Highlight 24–2).

Asymptomatic cholelithiasis is usually not treated because many people never experience problems. The treatment of choice for most symptomatic gallstones is surgical removal of the gallbladder. Other, nonsurgical approaches have been developed for patients who are poor surgical risks or who do not consent to surgery.

Gallstone Dissolution Therapy

ORAL BILE ACIDS. Chenodeoxcholic acid (chenodiol) and ursodeoxycholic acid are bile acids. They facilitate the gradual dissolution of cholesterol gallstones by decreasing the amount of cholesterol in the bile and increasing cholesterol solubility. Oral dissolution therapy is most effective in treating small stones (<5 mm in diameter) with a high cholesterol content in a functioning gallbladder. This situation represents about 15% of patients with gall-

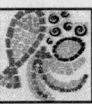

HIGHLIGHT
24—2
NUTRITION

Special Considerations for the Patient with Cholecystitis

Instruct patients with chronic cholecystitis and those for whom gallbladder surgery is planned in the following:

To achieve a general decrease in dietary fat:

Avoid fatty meats, sauces, and gravies.

Avoid cream and rich desserts.

Avoid fried and other fatty foods.

To limit total fat intake to a specific number of grams while not totally eliminating specific foods from the diet:

Use a Fat Portion Exchange List to select type and amount of foods in the daily diet.

Remember that the specified amount of each food item on the list provides 5 g of dietary fat and is equal to one fat portion.

Select the number of portions per day that equals the total amount of fat allowed in the daily diet. Example: For a daily diet containing 50 g of fat, select 10 portions.

---

stones. These drugs are taken by mouth, and 6 to 12 months of therapy with monitoring is necessary.

Side effects of bile acid therapy include:

- Diarrhea, which in most cases can be controlled by reducing the dose
- Gastritis, which can lead to gastric ulcers
- Liver damage characterized by elevated liver enzymes
- Reduced effectiveness of oral contraceptives

When therapy is discontinued, gallstones may recur. Because chenodiol is hepatotoxic and ursodeoxycholic acid is relatively free from side effects, the latter drug is used more extensively. Oral bile acid therapy is contraindicated for patients with gastric ulcers, liver disease, or atherosclerosis, and in women who are pregnant.

CONTACT SOLVENTS. Contact solvents are substances that, on contact, chemically react with cholesterol gallstones and cause them to dissolve. The most commonly used agent is methyl tert-butyl ether (MTBE). An agent called monoctanoin is used less often. MTBE is instilled via a percutaneous transhepatic catheter inserted into the gallbladder by a radiologist. Once the stones are dissolved (about 7

hours) the agent is withdrawn. This treatment has a high success rate, but it does require the expertise of a radiologist, and the agent is flammable and potentially explosive.

Monoctanoin has been used primarily for dissolution of bile duct stones retained after cholecystectomy. Catheters are placed in the duct (either intraoperatively or percutaneously), and the agent is perfused over a period of days.

Anorexia, nausea, vomiting, and abdominal pain are potential side effects of this therapy. To help prevent them, the infusion is stopped during meals. In addition, the patient may be placed on a bland diet. When gastric upset occurs despite these measures, the infusion rate is slowed and antiemetics or antidiarrheals are given if necessary. Care of the patient who has had a transhepatic catheter inserted is similar to that following a liver biopsy (see Chap. 25).

Mechanical Litholysis of Common Bile Duct Stones
Mechanical litholysis is the endoscopic removal of stones from the common bile duct via endoscopic retrograde cholangiopancreatography. In this procedure, the endoscope with an attachment is inserted into the duct. The stone is trapped in the basket device and is crushed into small fragments, which can be extracted or expelled into the duodenum (Fig. 24–2). Sphincterotomy, in which the opening of the duct is widened, may or may not be done. In some cases, follow-up oral bile acid therapy may be prescribed.

Preprocedure and postprocedure care for a patient undergoing mechanical lithotripsy is the same as for an esophagogastroduodenoscopy, described in Chapter 21.

Extracorporeal Shock Wave Lithotripsy
Extracorporeal shock wave lithotripsy refers to the crushing of a stone using high-pressure or high-energy sound waves. Its use on gallstones is a logical extension of its original use on kidney stones. Although the procedure is used throughout Europe and Canada, it is not yet approved by the Food and Drug Administration for clinical use in the United States. Stone clearance by this method may require successive treatments and the later removal of debris by endoscopic or surgical means. There is a low mortality (0.5%), and the post-treatment course is relatively uncomplicated, which is especially important in the elderly and other high-risk patients. Most clinicians believe that extracorporeal shock wave lithotripsy should be combined with oral dissolution therapy.

Entry in most protocols is limited to symptomatic patients with one to three noncalcified stones, 30 mm or less in diameter, and a functioning gallbladder. Of all patients with symptomatic gallstones, about 16% would fit into this category. The efficacy of this treatment for larger, single stones and multiple stones is poor. Another point to consider is that

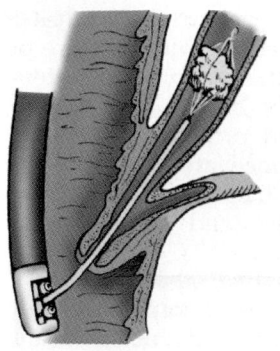
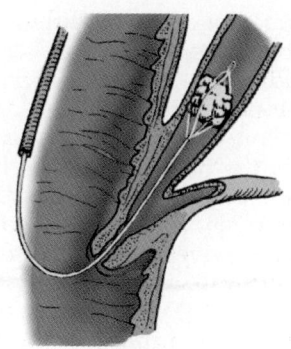
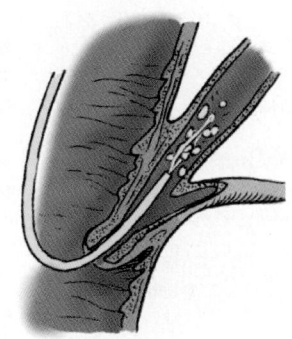

Figure 24–2

A basket contained in a flexible cord spring sheath is used to trap a stone and crush it. (After Siegel JH, Ben-Zvi JS, Pullano WE. Mechanical lithotripsy of common duct stones. Gastrointest Endosc 1990; 36(4):353. © American Society of Gastrointestinal Endoscopy.)

extracorporeal shock wave lithotripsy is not as cost-effective as a cholecystectomy.

All lithotriptors generate waves in a liquid medium. These waves can then be propagated through living tissue because of its high water content, provided that the body is in contact with (or "coupled" with) the water medium in which the shock wave was generated. With "wet" lithotriptors, coupling is accomplished by placing the patient in a shallow pool of water or via a porthole in the lithotriptor table that opens to the fluid medium. With a dry lithotriptor (Fig. 24–3), the patient is coupled by being placed on a flexible membrane, which in turn is in contact with the water medium. A gel, such as is used for ultrasonography, is placed on the surface of the membrane to couple it with the patient's body.

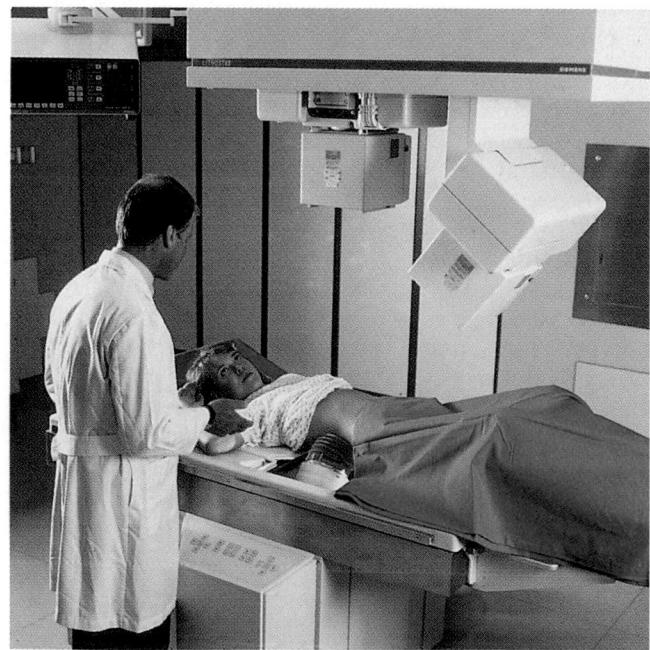

Figure 24–3

Patient positioned on a dry lithotriptor. Note that the patient is lying on a flexible membrane that is in contact with the liquid medium in which the shock waves are generated. (Courtesy of Siemens Medical Systems, Inc, Iselin, NJ.)

PATIENT PREPARATION. Patients should be on NPO status for at least 12 hours before the procedure, and the physician may order a laxative or enema the night before. Because intestinal gas interferes with shock waves, 80 mg of simethicone is taken after each meal, at bedtime, and on awakening in the morning beginning 24 hours before the procedure.

PROCEDURE. An IV infusion is started to allow the administration of drugs, if necessary. The lower chest and abdomen are exposed, and the patient is coupled to the lithotriptor. Because electrocardiogram, blood pressure, and oxygen saturation are monitored throughout the procedure, electrocardiographic leads, a blood pressure cuff, and a pulse oximetry monitor are put in place. The gallbladder is then imaged on an ultrasonogram so that the stones can be targeted (to visualize stones in the common bile duct, a contrast medium must be introduced) and application of shock waves is begun. About 1500 shocks are given during a period of 1 to 2 hours. The shock waves are synchronized with the heart rate to avoid triggering a dysrhythmia. As each is generated, a popping sound is heard, and as it is propagated, the patient may feel fluttering or a mild blow.

Lithotripsy is basically a painless procedure, although toward the end of the procedure some discomfort may result from lying in one position for an extended length of time and from passage of stone fragments through the common bile duct. Because sudden movements and muscle tension can interfere with the procedure, a short-acting analgesic such as alfentanil is often given IV to maintain the patient's comfort.

POSTPROCEDURE COURSE. Because lithotripsy usually does not require general anesthesia or sedation, patients may return home and resume full activity as soon as the effects of any analgesic have worn off. Others may require admission to an observation unit until the next morning. Transient gross hematuria may occur after treatment, and the patient may experience episodes of right upper quadrant pain for 2 to 3 months as fragments of stone pass through the common bile duct. Adjuvant oral bile acid therapy begins immediately, and the patient returns in 6 weeks for a follow-up examination. At this time, an ultrasonogram is obtained to check the size of remaining stone fragments, and liver function tests are performed to check for liver damage secondary to the oral bile acid therapy. Subsequent follow-up examinations are at 3-month intervals. Administration of oral bile acids is continued until the patient is free of stone fragments on two successive follow-up visits. Patients are instructed to report fever, severe nausea and vomiting, jaundice, abdominal pain, and persistent hematuria.

COMPLICATIONS. Potential complications of extracorporeal shock wave lithotripsy include accidental damage to the gallbladder and surrounding tissues, acute cholecystitis, bile duct obstruction by stone fragments, pancreatitis, and stone recurrence.

Surgical Intervention

A variety of surgical procedures are performed in the treatment of cholelithiasis and cholecystitis. These include:

- Cholecystectomy—the surgical removal of the gallbladder
- Cholecystotomy—the opening of the gall bladder for decompression and drainage
- Choledochostomy—the creation of an opening into the common bile duct
- Choledocholithotomy—the removal of a stone from the common bile duct

Of these, cholecystectomy is the procedure most often performed. The two basic types of cholecystectomy are open cholecystectomy and laparoscopic cholecystectomy. It is estimated that about 80% of cholecystectomies are performed through the laparoscopic approach.

PATIENT PREPARATION. Preoperative preparation for patients undergoing a cholecystectomy includes restriction of foods and fluids, cleansing enemas, and nipple-to-groin surgical skin preparation. If nausea and vomiting are present, a nasogastric tube attached to suction is used for gastric decompression. Patients with obstructive jaundice have their prothrombin time monitored and, if needed, receive vitamin K before surgery. Before laparoscopic cholecystectomy, a urinary drainage catheter and a nasogastric tube are inserted for decompression to decrease the risk of accidental puncture of the bladder or the stomach when the trocar (a sharp-pointed instrument equipped with a cannula) is inserted. The urinary catheter and nasogastric tube usually are inserted in the operating suite and removed in the recovery area.

LAPAROSCOPIC CHOLECYSTECTOMY. Although a laparoscopic cholecystectomy is less invasive than an open cholecystectomy, it still requires general anesthesia for about the same length of time. There is minimal postoperative pain, the procedure is done on an outpatient or overnight basis, and recovery time is shorter. The procedure is contraindicated in cases in which the gallbladder is so inflamed that it could rupture, and when multiple adhesions are present.

PROCEDURE. A long, narrow, cylindrical laparoscope is inserted through a 1 cm incision in the abdomen (usually in the lower aspect of the umbilicus) after insufflation with carbon dioxide. This scope visualizes the internal organs and projects their image onto a video monitor, which the surgeon watches while performing the procedure. Three smaller incisions are made, through which other instruments are inserted for dissection, coagulation, irrigation, and suction. The excised gallbladder is removed through the umbilical incision. When a laser is used for incision and cauterization, the

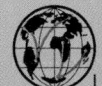

INTERNET CONNECTIONS

Disorders of the Accessory Organs of Digestion

General

Patient Information Documents on Digestive Diseases

http://www.niddk.nih.gov/DigestiveDocs.html

A U.S. government-sponsored site that provides access to patient information related to a wide variety of digestive diseases, including gallstones and pancreatitis. The site also includes a listing of digestive disease organizations for health-care professionals as well as disease statistics.

Cholecystitis

Gallstones and Laparoscopic Cholecystectomy

gopher://gopher.nih.gov/00/clin/cdcs/individual/90.gall

Intended as information for health-care professionals, this site provides the text of a National Institutes of Health Consensus Development Conference Statement from 1992.

Gallstones

http://www.niddk.nih.gov/Gallstones/Gallstones.html

A brief encyclopedia-style article for patients from The National Institute of Diabetes and Digestive and Kidney Diseases.

Cancer of the Pancreas

Pancreatic Cancer

http://cancer.med.upenn.edu/disease/pancreas/

An ONCOLINK site that provides links to a wide variety of sources related to pancreatic cancer. Useful for both patients and health-care professionals.

procedure is called a laser laparoscopic cholecystectomy or laser endoscopic cholecystectomy.

COMPLICATIONS. Potential complications of laparoscopic cholecystectomy include accidental bowel or bladder puncture and uncontrolled bleeding. There is also a higher incidence of common bile duct injury than with open cholecystectomy. Incomplete reabsorption of the carbon dioxide can result in irritation of the diaphragm and respiratory distress.

CONVENTIONAL OPEN CHOLECYSTECTOMY

PROCEDURE. Through a high right subcostal incision, the cystic duct is ligated and the gallbladder excised. A Penrose drain is inserted in the wound to prevent accumulation of drainage in the operative area. This drain exits through a stab wound on the abdominal wall close to the incision. If the patient is suspected of having stones in the bile duct, a choledocholithotomy, or incision into the common bile duct and removal of stones, is performed. Following this, a T-tube is placed in the duct to ensure its patency until edema produced by the procedure subsides. The T-tube also prevents narrowing of the tube secondary to healing. Because the T-tube does not completely occlude the duct, some bile flows around the T-tube into the duodenum, and some flows into the drainage collection system (Fig. 24–4).

POSTOPERATIVE COURSE. Breathing tends to be shallow postoperatively because of the effect of anesthesia and the patient's reluctance to breathe deeply as a result of the pain, which is caused by the proximity of the incision to the diaphragm.

A sterile dressing covers the right upper quadrant incision. Serosanguineous drainage with a small amount of bile is expected from the Penrose drain for the first 24 hours. Drainage then decreases and the Penrose drain is removed, usually in 48 hours. If a T-tube was inserted during surgery, the end of the tube leading to the drainage collection system is se-

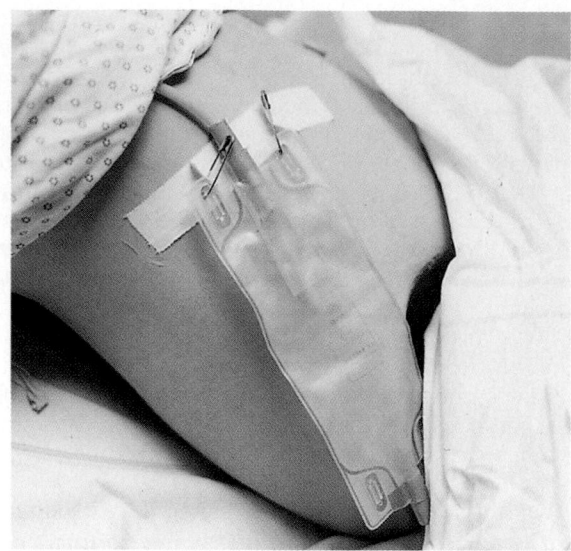

Figure 24–5
Bile drainage bag in place. Note tape on the abdomen, which allows the bag to be pinned in a way that prevents the tube from being dislodged.

curely fastened to the dressing (Fig. 24–5). Drainage that is initially bloody and then turns green-brown is measured as output, with the amount ranging from 500 to 1000 mL per day. Excess bile drainage may be returned to the patient via the nasogastric tube to prevent electrolyte imbalance. As an alternative, replacement with synthetic bile salts may be ordered. When drainage diminishes, cholangiography is performed to confirm the patency of the common bile duct. The surgeon then removes the T-tube. Before this, the T-tube may be clamped for 1 hour before and after meals to allow bile to flow into the duodenum and to determine the patient's tolerance to elimination of external drainage. If distress develops, the tube is immediately unclamped and the surgeon is notified.

Fluids are administered intravenously for 24 to 48 hours. The patient's diet is then progressed as tolerated from clear fluids to soft, regular foods. Because bile flows continuously into the duodenum after removal of the gallbladder rather than periodically in response to fat intake, a few patients may be temporarily unable to tolerate large amounts of fat. For these patients, fat intake may need to be limited for up to a month. Fried food may need to be avoided by all patients despite an otherwise normal diet.

Usually, the patient is ambulated 8 hours after surgery. Return to work is generally in about 4 weeks.

Some ambulatory surgical centers are performing uncomplicated conventional cholecystectomies on selected patients. In these cases, patients can be discharged to the care of family members as soon as 4 hours after surgery. They are instructed to remain

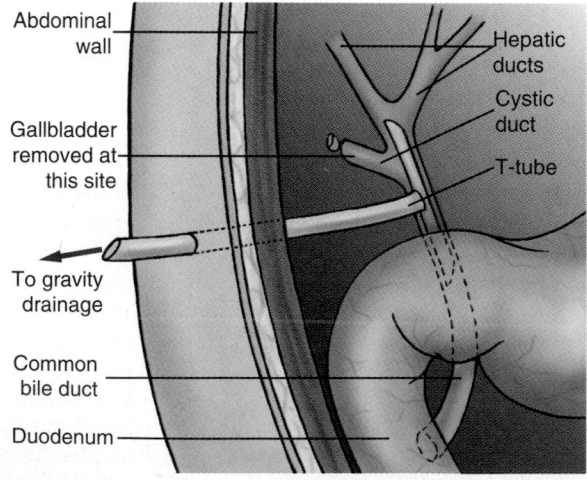

Abdominal wall

Hepatic ducts

Cystic duct

Gallbladder removed at this site

T-tube

To gravity drainage

Common bile duct

Duodenum

Figure 24–4
Placement of a T-tube following cholecystectomy.

■■■■■■▶
■
■ Clinical Pathway for Open Cholecystectomy

Patient Name _____   Date _____

DRG# _____   Expected LOS _____

	Day 1	Day 2 (PO#1)	Day 3 (PO#2)	Day 4 (PO#3)
Medication	• Parenteral analgesia as ordered • Heparin 5000 units SQ q 12 hrs • IV ATB as ordered	• Parenteral analgesia as ordered • Heparin 5000 units SQ q 12 hrs	• Begin PO pain medication • Heparin 5000 units SQ q 12 hrs	• PO pain medication • Heparin 5000 U SQ q 12 hrs
Diagnostic Tests	CBC, Chem 6 in PM	CBC, Chem 6		
Diet	NPO, IVF as ordered	IVF, clear liquids to soft diet, D/C IV if tolerated	Advance to general diet	General diet
Activity	Dangle at bedside, up in chair in PM	Ambulate with assistance	Ambulate ad lib	Ambulate ad lib
Treatments/Nursing Actions	• Assess VS q 2-4 hrs • Assess pain status q 2-4 hrs • Incentive spirometer q 1-2 hrs while awake • Cough and deep-breathe 1-2 hrs while awake • Antiembolism hose, leg exercises • Monitor voiding in 6-8 hrs • Assess dressing • Assess function of T-tube, drains if present • Assess skin around T-tube for excoriation from bile	• VS q 4 hrs • Assess pain status q 2-4 hrs • Incentive spirometer q 1-2 hrs while awake • Cough and deep-breathe 1-2 hrs while awake • Antiembolism hose, leg exercises when in bed • Assess wound (dressing changed by MD) • Assess function of T-tube, drains • Assess skin around T-tube for excoriation	• VS q 4 hrs • Assess pain status q 2-4 hrs • Incentive spirometer q 1-2 hrs while awake • Cough and deep-breathe 1-2 hrs while awake • Antiembolism hose, leg exercises when in bed • Assess wound/dressings, T-tube, drain sites. • Assess for discomfort if T-tube ordered to be clamped	• VS q shift • Assess pain status q 2-4 hrs • Incentive spirometer q 1-2 hrs while awake • Antiembolism hose • Assess wound • Assess for bowel movement
Teaching/Discharge Planning	Reinforce incentive spirometer, cough, deep-breathe, splinting	Reinforce incentive spirometer, cough, deep-breathe, splinting	Reinforce incentive spirometer, cough, deep-breathe, splinting	Reinforce incision care, diet, medications, activity, tube care if indicated, for discharge in AM. Follow-up visit to physician

on bedrest with bathroom privileges and a clear liquid diet for 24 hours, after which both activity and diet can be gradually increased. Follow-up is with a home health nurse and a visit to the surgeon in 1 or 2 days.

COMPLICATIONS. Potential complications of gallbladder surgery include respiratory problems because of the location of the incision, wound infection, peritonitis, and abscess or fistula formation. Usually, however, patients experience an uncomplicated postoperative course and are discharged 3 to 5 days after surgery. Sometimes patients are discharged with the T-tube clamped, to be removed later.

OPEN LASER CHOLECYSTECTOMY. Laser cholecystectomy is a variation on the conventional open cholecystectomy. After laser surgery, patients seem to have less discomfort and may be ready to resume usual activities more quickly. In one study, patients were typically discharged on the second postoperative day, resumed normal at-home activities in 10 to 14 days, and returned to work in 15 to 17 days.

❖ **Settings, Providers, and Collaboration for Care**

Gallstone dissolution therapy may be received in an outpatient setting. Endoscopic or laparoscopic procedures may be performed in a surgicenter or ambulatory surgery department, although laparoscopic cholecystectomies commonly involve overnight hospitalization. The more complex surgeries require 3 to 5 days' hospitalization, especially if the common bile duct is explored. The expertise of a dietitian may be appropriate to assist the patient and significant others in selecting foods low in fat. The nurse (discharge planner) instructs the patient about home care and sets a follow-up appointment with the physician.

NURSING PROCESS GUIDELINES
Laparoscopic Cholecystectomy

Nursing care for patients undergoing laparoscopic cholecystectomy is similar to that for any patient undergoing surgery under general anesthesia. The patient is usually discharged the day after surgery. A nursing diagnosis unique to the patient who has had a laparoscopic cholecystectomy is pain (referred right shoulder) related to pressure from insufflated carbon dioxide on the phrenic nerve. To relieve this pain, place the patient in Sims' position (left side with right knee and thigh drawn up toward the chest and left arm along the back). Also encourage ambulation to increase the body's absorption of the gas. Administer or teach self-administration of oral analgesics, as prescribed, for 24 to 48 hours. Instruct the patient to gradually resume normal activities over a 3-day period, but to avoid heavy lifting for about 10 days. Instruct the patient to observe the puncture sites and notify the physician if redness, swelling, or bile-colored drainage appears. The patient may shower on the second postoperative day.

NURSING PROCESS
Conventional Open Cholecystectomy

PREOPERATIVE NURSING CARE

The assessment, nursing diagnoses, expected patient outcomes, nursing interventions, and evaluation for patients scheduled for a cholecystectomy are similar to those for any other preoperative patient (see Chap. 6), with several considerations. After cholecystectomy, breathing tends to be shallow because deep-breathing is painful as a result of the location of the incision. Therefore, assess respiratory status and teach prophylactic measures, such as coughing and deep-breathing, carefully. Keep in mind that respiratory complications occur more frequently among patients who smoke.

In patients with obstructive jaundice, monitor the serum prothrombin level, because a decrease in prothrombin increases the usual risk of postoperative bleeding.

POSTOPERATIVE NURSING CARE

Assessment

After a cholecystectomy, assessments are those required by any patient who has had major surgery. Take vital signs, measure intake and output, observe wound drainage for color and amount, monitor fluid intake, and observe the IV site for signs of infiltration and irritation.

Assess respiratory excursion every hour for the first 6 hours, then every 2 to 4 hours for the remainder of the first 24 hours postoperatively. Auscultate the lungs every 4 hours for the next 2 to 3 days.

Note shallow or guarded breathing, weak cough, and decreased or adventitious breath sounds.

Check for displacement of the T-tube. Every 2 hours, check for patency of the T-tube, and note the amount, color, consistency, and odor of the drainage. Keep in mind that drainage is initially bloody but changes to green-brown, that 500 to 1000 mL of drainage is expected in 24 hours, and that little or no drainage may indicate duct obstruction by a retained stone. Check the T-tube exit site for signs of infection and for bile drainage, which may indicate dislodgement of the tube.

Observe the color and amount of drainage from the Penrose drain. Inspect the suture line for signs of infection and the surrounding skin for signs of irritation caused by drainage from the Penrose drain.

Inspect the sclerae for jaundice, and review white blood cell counts for elevation over $10,000/mm^3$. If a nasogastric tube is in place, check the amount and characteristics of drainage. Auscultate for bowel sounds and palpate for abdominal distention, because a return of bowel sounds and a soft, nondistended abdomen indicate that oral intake may be resumed.

Nursing Diagnoses and Planning

Nursing diagnoses and related expected patient outcomes commonly applicable to patients after cholecystectomy include the following:

NDx: Risk for impaired gas exchange related to shallow breathing secondary to pain on deep breathing

Planning: Patient Outcomes
1. Rate and depth of respirations are within patient's normal range.
2. Lungs are clear to auscultation.
3. Arterial blood gas values are within patient's normal limits.

NDx: Risk for impaired skin integrity related to copious drainage from the T-tube site

Planning: Patient Outcomes
1. Skin is free from excoriation.
2. Dressing remains dry and intact.

NDx: Risk for altered peripheral tissue perfusion related to obstruction in venous return

Planning: Patient Outcomes
1. Patient wears elastic stockings or a sequential compression device as instructed.
2. Patient performs foot and leg exercises as instructed.
3. Patient ambulates with assistance.
4. Calves and thighs are free of redness, tenderness, and heat.

NDx: Risk for altered health maintenance related to insufficient knowledge of self-care after discharge

Planning: Patient Outcomes
1. Patient lists signs and symptoms that should be reported to a health-care professional.
2. Patient demonstrates care of the wound.
3. Patient states date of follow-up appointment.

Nursing Interventions and Evaluation

NDx: Risk for impaired gas exchange

Medicate the patient every 3 to 4 hours for the first 24 to 48 hours after surgery because respiratory excursion is painful as a result of the location of the incision. Expect to administer an analgesic such as meperidine hydrochloride (Demerol) rather than morphine sulfate because the opiate drugs may increase biliary duct spasm. Thereafter, administer a milder analgesic as ordered to provide relief. Splint the incisional area while encouraging the patient to cough and deep-breathe every hour in the early postoperative period. Place the patient in a low Fowler's position while he or she is in bed to reduce pressure on the diaphragm. Turn the patient every 2 hours and help him or her to ambulate as soon as allowed.

NDx: Risk for impaired skin integrity

Change dressings frequently for the first 24 hours if a Penrose drain is in place, because the drainage contains bile that is very irritating to the skin. Use Montgomery straps to minimize skin irritation from frequent removal of tape. Cleanse the suture line and around the T-tube site with a sterile solution of normal saline or an antiseptic at each dressing change.

Avoid altering the position of the T-tube during dressing changes because if it becomes dislodged, surgical replacement may be required.

NDx: Risk for altered peripheral tissue perfusion

Apply antiembolic stockings or a sequential compression device to help prevent thrombosis. Remind the patient to do foot and leg exercises every hour while awake as taught preoperatively. Encourage ambulation when permitted, and instruct ambulatory patients to avoid sitting or standing in one position for a long time.

NDx: Risk for altered health maintenance

Instruct the patient in self-care after discharge as presented in Highlight 24–3. Be certain to explain the principles of asepsis as well as the ordered protocol for care of the wound and of the T-tube if present. Allow the patient to practice with supervision. Correct the patient's technique and answer questions as needed. Provide instruction to significant others and initiate a referral to a home-care agency if needed.

Additional Interventions

Attach the T-tube to the patient's gown to prevent pull on the tube from the weight of the drainage bag. Keep the tubing free of kinks and the bag below the level of the suture line to prevent reflux of bile. Position the patient off the tube to maintain

---

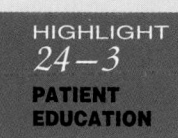
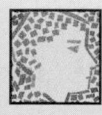

HIGHLIGHT 24–3
PATIENT EDUCATION

Discharge Instructions after Conventional Cholecystectomy with T-Tube Insertion

Instruct the patient to:

Keep the T-tube drainage bag below the level of the T-tube.

Prevent pull on the tube by coiling the drainage tubing and securing to the abdomen with tape or other fastener.

Avoid tight-fitting clothing, which can irritate the wound or put pressure on the T-tube.

Expect possible bile leakage, and select clothing that can be washed in a solution of detergent, bleach, and baking soda if staining occurs.

Open the drain spout and empty the T-tube drainage bag each day at the same time. Be sure to note the amount of drainage in the bag so that changes in the amount of drainage can be identified.

Change the dressing around the T-tube daily. While holding the tube in place, remove the old dressing, wipe skin area around the tube with an antiseptic, apply a clean precut dressing, and tape in place.

Take showers, not tub baths, to help prevent bacteria from entering the wound.

Avoid strenuous activities, which could place strain on the wound.

Report increased, purulent, or foul-smelling drainage; redness, swelling, warmth, or pain at the incision line; oral temperature greater than 37.7°C (100°F); abdominal pain; nausea or vomiting.

Return for a follow-up cholangiogram on *(specify date, time, and place)*.

---

free flow of drainage. Never irrigate, aspirate, or clamp a T-tube. The resulting back pressure could disrupt the suture line.

Report T-tube drainage of more than 1000 mL per day. If ordered, return excess bile to the patient via the nasogastric tube. Also report purulent or foul-smelling drainage or a sudden increase in drainage after it has diminished. Such an increase can indicate an obstruction below the T-tube.

Keep the patient on NPO status and maintain the nasogastric tube to suction as ordered until peristalsis returns. Administer antiemetics as ordered for episodes of postoperative nausea. When peristalsis is re-established and the nasogastric tube removed, give clear fluids as tolerated. Progress gradually to a full diet.

Compare the patient's status with the expected outcomes. If the outcomes are not met, reassess the patient and revise the plan.

ACUTE PANCREATITIS

Acute pancreatitis is a diffuse inflammation of the pancreas caused by activation of pancreatic enzymes within the organ itself, which precipitates a process of pancreatic autodigestion. It is a serious disorder with a significant mortality risk.

Etiology and Pathophysiology

Acute pancreatitis can be associated with:

- Excessive use of alcohol, thiazide diuretics, steroids, acetaminophen, or oral contraceptives
- Biliary tract disease
- Abdominal surgery or other trauma
- Penetrating duodenal ulcer
- Metabolic disorders
- Mumps
- Bacterial infection

Nonetheless, the precise reason for activation of pancreatic enzymes in the pancreas rather than in the intestine is unknown. Obstruction of the pancreatic ducts and reflux of duodenal contents into the pancreas through a dilated sphincter of Oddi may be significant factors. Regardless of cause, the basic factor in the onset of acute pancreatitis is the presence of activated trypsin within the pancreas. Trypsin is thought to initiate pancreatic digestion and activate elastase, kinins, and phospholipase.

Elastase dissolves the elastic fibers of the blood vessels within the pancreas, resulting in blood loss or hemorrhage. Activated kinins cause systemic vasodilation and increased vascular permeability, thus predisposing the person with acute pancreatitis to hypovolemic shock. The activity of phospholipase A results in pancreatic parenchymal and fat necrosis.

Acute pancreatitis often resolves without residual damage, although in some cases it may progress to the chronic form of the disease.

Clinical Manifestations

Sudden onset of intense left upper quadrant abdominal pain radiating to the mid back or left shoulder is the most outstanding symptom of acute pancreatitis. Onset of pain is often acute and frequently occurs 24 to 48 hours after a heavy meal or heavy use of alcohol. The pain is unrelieved by antacids and is usually accompanied by nausea and vomiting and in some cases by symptoms of circulatory shock. Examination of the abdomen reveals muscle guarding and rigidity with rebound tenderness. If there is seepage of bloody exudate from the pancreas, periumbilical bruising (Cullen's sign) and bruising of the flanks (Turner's sign) may occur. Respiratory distress may also occur.

Diagnosis

A serum amylase level of more than 500 U/dL (normal is 60 to 160 U/dL), an elevated urinary amylase level, and an elevated serum lipase level are diagnostic of acute pancreatitis. The WBC, serum glucose, blood urea nitrogen, and lactate dehydrogenase levels are also usually elevated.

Management

The course of acute pancreatitis can range from a mild, self-limiting disease to a critical emergency. Prognostic tools are used to help determine which patients are at greater risk for development of more severe forms of pancreatitis. One example of these tools is the Ranson scale, composed of 11 risk factors that are evaluated on admission and 48 hours later.

During the critical stage, pancreatic activity is diminished by keeping the patient on NPO status, administering anticholinergic drugs, and instituting nasogastric suction, which relieves abdominal distention and removes hydrochloric acid before it can enter the duodenum and stimulate the pancreas. Pain is usually controlled by meperidine in combination with the anticholinergics. Morphine is avoided because it can cause spasm in the sphincter of Oddi.

If hypovolemic shock develops, volume replacement is initiated immediately with Ringer's lactate solution followed by administration of whole blood, packed cells, or plasma expanders. Central venous pressure or pulmonary capillary wedge pressure is used to monitor the response to fluid replacement, and urinary output is measured hourly.

Blood gases are monitored and, if hypoxemia occurs, oxygen therapy and even intubation and ventilation are used, if necessary.

Antibiotic therapy is usually instituted to defend against secondary infections, and in some cases, exudate is removed from the peritoneal cavity by peritoneal dialysis. Insulin is given if hyperglycemia develops.

When the critical phase is over, oral intake can begin. Clear fluids are given first, followed by carbohydrate foodstuffs or elemental protein feedings, which do not stimulate pancreatic secretion. Gradually, a bland, low-fat diet is introduced with six daily feedings. If glucose tolerance is impaired, the amount of carbohydrate in the diet is restricted.

NURSING PROCESS
Acute Pancreatitis

Assessment

Assess the patient's response to prescribed pain medication. Keep in mind that the patient with

CLINICAL ❓ THINKING

ABDOMINAL PAIN, PALLOR, AND DIAPHORESIS IN A MAN WITH GALLBLADDER DISEASE

A 55-year-old male employee arrived in the Health Services suite of a large corporation complaining of acute abdominal pain. He stated that he wanted to leave work and go directly home, but his coworkers had urged him to see the nurse instead. He was perspiring profusely, appeared pale, and reported that the pain, which was located in the upper abdominal region, had started suddenly that morning. It was tolerable at first, but was steadily increasing in intensity. He had one episode of vomiting before arriving at work and was currently nauseous.

Although not all instances of abdominal pain indicate a potentially serious disorder, I knew that the patient's acute distress and the accompanying symptoms of nausea, vomiting, pallor, and diaphoresis could be caused by a variety of life-threatening conditions. These included cardiovascular emergencies, such as an acute myocardial infarction or a ruptured abdominal aortic aneurysm, and a number of gastrointestinal disorders, including intestinal obstruction, appendicitis, peritonitis, perforated peptic ulcer, and acute pancreatitis. Other conditions that might have required immediate medical attention included cholecystitis, renal colic, and acute diverticulitis.

The patient's level of consciousness and absence of respiratory distress afforded me some time to perform a focused assessment to help differentiate the possible causes and determine the best course of action. I anticipated clinical decisions that would result in administering emergency care in the employee health service, arranging for transportation to the Emergency Room, or a referral to the patient's primary health-care provider.

I began by exploring his previous medical history and by asking some key questions about the pain, including its nature, character, precipitating factors, and exact location. He stated that he had gallbladder disease, which had been treated medically with diet and anticholinergic medication for the past 2 years. He had occasional "flare-ups," and was planning to undergo a cholecystectomy "when time permitted." His medical history also included hyperlipidemia and surgical repair of a herniated vertebral disk. He denied any cardiovascular, pulmonary, or renal disease, abdominal surgery, and any recent trauma to the abdomen. He reported that he drank alcohol socially and stopped smoking 15 years ago. He had attended a wedding the previous day and had eaten a large quantity of restricted foods.

He described the pain as piercing and persistent, identified the left upper quadrant and midepigastrium when asked to point to the painful area, and stated that it radiated to the back. His blood pressure was 102/60, apical pulse was 110 and regular, respirations were 26 per minute and shallow, and oral temperature 38.1°C (100.6°F). Radial pulses were palpable but weak and thready. Capillary refill was 3 seconds. The patient denied chest pain or discomfort and denied difficulty breathing. Despite his tachypnea, I noted no adventitious sounds on auscultation. His skin was warm and pale with no evidence of jaundice. His skin turgor was poor.

Upon inspection, his abdomen was rounded, symmetrical, and appeared slightly distended. Neither Turner's nor Cullen's sign appeared. During auscultation, I noted decreased bowel sounds and the absence of a bruit. On palpation, the patient exhibited direct and rebound tenderness, guarding, and rigidity. He had no pulsating mass. Percussion of the abdomen revealed no ascites and no enlargement of the liver and spleen. Facial expressions observed during physical assessment of the abdomen confirmed left upper quadrant and midepigastric tenderness. The patient reported having a normal bowel movement that morning and denied any change in his bowel habits or the color or consistency of his stool.

The patient remained oriented but grew increasingly agitated during the examination. He stated that the pain was becoming more acute, and vomited a small amount of green liquid. The vomitus appeared free of blood and fecal odor. He denied any relief following this episode of vomiting, and assumed a forward leaning position to help reduce the pain.

Several of my assessment findings—such as acute abdominal pain, nausea, vomiting, abdominal distention, guarding, rigidity, and an elevated temperature—could point to a number of potential disorders. However, these clinical findings, in conjunction with the location, radiation, and intensifying and relentless nature of the pain, the hypoactive bowel sounds, the lack of relief following vomiting, the position assumed by the patient, and the signs and symptoms of hypovolemia (hypotension, tachycardia, tachypnea, poor skin turgor, and weak pulses) suggested that the patient had developed acute pancreatitis.

Although hypotension, tachycardia, tachypnea, and weak peripheral pulses could also indicate decreased cardiac output secondary to an acute myo-

(continued)

(continued)

cardial infarction, the absence of chest pain and the early elevation of the patient's temperature helped me eliminate this possibility. The absence of an abdominal mass, bruit, and evidence of bleeding in the gastrointestinal tract helped me rule out peptic ulcer disease and a ruptured or leaking abdominal aortic aneurysm as likely possibilities. The decreased bowel sounds, continuous nature of the pain, lack of pain relief following vomiting, lack of fecal odor to the vomitus, and reported bowel movement that day were not consistent with the likelihood of an intestinal obstruction. The location of the pain was not consistent with appendicitis.

My suspicion that the patient was suffering from acute pancreatitis was reinforced by his history of biliary tract disease, hyperlipidemia, and his ingestion of a large, heavy meal the previous day.

Although the patient continued to express a desire to go home, I recognized the urgent need for further clinical and laboratory evaluation of his acute abdomen and for stabilization of his condition. I knew that acute pancreatitis could have detrimental consequences if untreated, including infection, acute respiratory distress syndrome, hyperglycemia, pseudocysts, shock, multisystem organ failure, and death. So I took the following steps:

1. I arranged for immediate transportation to the hospital.
2. I implemented comfort measures for the non-pharmacologic relief of pain, including helping the patient assume a sitting, forward-leaning position of comfort, and teaching the patient deep-breathing and relaxation techniques.
3. I reduced the patient's anxiety by explaining the need for immediate hospitalization and medical attention, by enabling the patient to verbalize his fears and concerns, and by offering to notify family members.
4. I maintained the patient NPO.
5. I continued to monitor his vital signs and level of consciousness and for hypovolemia and shock.
6. I documented my findings and actions.

Upon arrival at the Emergency Room, the physician examined the patient, concurred with my suspicion of acute pancreatitis, and ordered a complete blood count with differential, hemoglobin, hematocrit, electrolytes, cardiac enzymes, serum and urine amylase levels, serum lipase, serum bilirubin, serum glucose, serum calcium, liver enzymes, chest and abdominal x-rays, a 12-lead electrocardiogram, a computed tomographic scan, and continuous cardiac monitoring.

Additional orders included IV fluid and electrolyte replacement, meperidine for pain, insertion of a nasogastric tube with low continuous suction, intake and output, antibiotics, and complete bedrest with bathroom privileges.

Following admission to a medical unit, laboratory and diagnostic tests confirmed the diagnosis. The patient had a favorable response to treatment, remained free of complications, and was discharged to the care of his primary care provider for further treatment and follow-up. The nurse's ability to use a problem-solving approach, sort out evidence, distinguish a minor from a serious abdominal problem, make sound clinical judgments, and implement an appropriate plan of care in a timely fashion were vital to the patient's successful outcomes.

Think Critically

What was the rationale underlying use of an oral thermometer when assessing the patient's temperature?

Was delaying pharmacologic pain relief the best action for the nurse to take? Why? Why not?

Was maintaining the patient NPO before arriving at the hospital the best action for the nurse to take in light of the suspected hypovolemia? Why? Why not?

What information regarding the patient's dietary restrictions and allowances would the nurse include in the discharge teaching plan to prevent a recurrence?

How would the nurse's assessments and interventions have differed if the patient in this scenario had an acute small bowel obstruction? Appendicitis?

The patient asked the nurse, "Will I have to live with this disease for the rest of my life?" What would be the nurse's best response?

How would the nurse have interpreted the presence of Turner's and/or Cullen's signs? Would the nurse's actions or clinical decisions have differed?

How might the assessment findings have differed if alcoholism, rather than biliary tract disease, played a role in the development of the acute pancreatitis? How would nursing responsibilities related to discharge planning and teaching differ?

CLINICAL ? THINKING

(continued)

What nursing interventions would be included in "resting the pancreas"? Is complete bedrest the best intervention?

What would the nurse identify as the priority goals of treatment upon admission to the hospital?

Under what circumstances would the nurse anticipate that the patient would undergo endoscopic retrograde cholangiopancreatography?

Was allowing the patient to assume a position of comfort the best action? What alternative positions might the nurse have considered? What if the patient demonstrated the clinical manifestations of hypovolemic shock?

What physiologic explanations to hypovolemia re-lated to acute pancreatitis did the nurse consider?

Was auscultating the patient's abdomen before palpating and percussing the best action by the nurse? Why? Why not?

What nursing interventions should be included in the nursing care plan when monitoring for potential complications of acute pancreatitis?

What type of follow-up care would the occupational health nurse implement when the patient returns to his home, job, or community?

Following this acute episode, what medical or surgical treatment does the nurse anticipate if biliary tract disease was the primary etiologic factor?

---

acute pancreatitis is in persistent, intense pain and often assumes the fetal position in an attempt to minimize it.

Assess vital signs, hemodynamic status, and urinary output every hour because the patient is prone to hypovolemic shock as a result of vomiting, blood loss, systemic vasodilation, and increased vascular permeability. Measure all intake and output, including nasogastric drainage. Weigh the patient daily and observe for the appearance of ascites. Measure abdominal girth daily if ascites is suspected.

Observe for signs of sodium, chloride, and potassium deficits resulting from vomiting, gastric suctioning, and fluid shifts. Observe also for signs of hypocalcemia because serum calcium levels decrease in acute pancreatitis, possibly from fat necrosis that results in binding of calcium with free fatty acids. Report signs of muscle twitching, tremors, and irritability immediately. Have intravenous calcium gluconate on hand in case it is needed to prevent tetany.

Inspect the oral and nasal mucosa for dryness and cracking. This is important because the patient is on NPO status, has nasogastric suction, and is receiving anticholinergic drugs, which decrease salivary and respiratory secretions.

Assess for signs of respiratory infection because the patient's breathing is typically shallow and guarded from peritoneal irritation. Auscultate the lungs and record the patient's temperature every 4 hours.

Auscultate the abdomen for bowel sounds every 4 hours. Remember that they will initially be diminished or absent from peritoneal irritation and gastric suctioning. When oral intake is resumed, monitor the patient's response to foods and fluids. Also ascertain the patient's understanding of dietary restric-tions and willingness and ability to comply with them.

Nursing Diagnoses and Planning

Nursing diagnoses and related expected patient outcomes commonly applicable to patients with acute pancreatitis include the following:

NDx: Pain related to the inflammatory process in the abdomen

Planning: Patient Outcomes
1. Patient reports diminished pain.
2. Patient assumes a high-Fowler's position without verbal or nonverbal signs of discomfort.

NDx: Risk for fluid volume deficit related to vomiting, gastric suction, and activation of pancreatic enzymes

Planning: Patient Outcomes
1. Skin turgor is normal.
2. Mucous membranes are moist.
3. Capillary refill is within normal limits.
4. Vital signs are within patient's baseline ranges.
5. Fluid intake approximates fluid output.

NDx: Altered oral mucous membrane related to drying effects of NPO status and anticholinergic drugs

Planning: Patient Outcomes
1. Oral mucous membranes are moist and supple.
2. Oral mucous membranes are free of cracks.

NDx: Risk for ineffective airway clearance related to shallow, guarded respirations

Planning: Patient Outcomes
1. Patient coughs and deep-breathes as directed.
2. Lungs are clear on auscultation.

NDx: Risk for altered health maintenance related to insufficient knowledge of self-care after discharge

Planning: Patient Outcomes
1. Patient describes dietary and other lifestyle adjustments to be followed after discharge.
2. Patient verbalizes intent to comply with lifestyle adjustments.

Nursing Interventions and Evaluation

NDx: Pain
Medicate the patient as ordered for pain before it becomes severe enough to render the medication relatively ineffective. Maintain a calm, quiet environment. Give back rubs. Assist the patient in changing position to further promote comfort. Guide the patient in relaxation exercises and provide background distraction in the form of soft music if appropriate.

NDx: Risk for fluid volume deficit
Monitor vital signs every hour, or more frequently if necessary, until fluid volume is stable. Monitor the amount of nasogastric tube drainage, and check it and the stool for signs of bleeding. Measure urinary output hourly. Maintain the patency of the IV line and administer IV solutions as ordered. Monitor laboratory data related to fluid and electrolyte status.

NDx: Altered oral mucous membrane
Encourage the patient to rinse his or her mouth every 1 to 2 hours while awake. Avoid using glycerin or commercial mouthwash because they contain drying agents. Apply water-soluble lubricant to the lips as needed to keep them soft and supple.

NDx: Risk for ineffective airway clearance
Maintain the patient in Fowler's position to promote respiratory expansion. Turn the patient frequently, and encourage coughing and deep-breathing every 2 hours when awake to decrease the risk of atelectasis and pooling of secretions.

NDx: Risk for altered health maintenance
Explain to the patient and family that this serious illness has a prolonged recovery period. Stress that the patient will need rest. Only with time will the patient regain strength and resume former activities.

Reinforce to both the patient and significant others the relationship of alcohol to pancreatitis and the necessity of avoiding it completely. If this is likely to be a problem for the patient, provide information on community resources, such as Alcoholics Anonymous. If appropriate, also explain the relationship of particular medications to pancreatitis. In all cases, reinforce the patient's understanding of the therapeutic diet (Highlight 24–4) and its effect in preventing recurrence.

Additional Interventions
Apply water-soluble lubricant to the naris to reduce irritation from the nasogastric tube. When bowel sounds have returned to normal, give small frequent feedings as ordered.

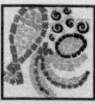

HIGHLIGHT 24–4
NUTRITION

Special Considerations for Patients with Pancreatitis

Instruct patients with pancreatitis to:

Avoid large meals.

Eat small amounts of food high in carbohydrates (450 g) and proteins (120 g).

Eat only small amounts of fats (30 g) until there is no evidence of steatorrhea.

Limit fiber intake because this may increase steatorrhea.

Eliminate coffee, tea, and spices from the diet because they stimulate pancreatic secretion.

Avoid alcohol completely because it stimulates the pancreas and can precipitate acute attacks of pancreatitis.

Report as directed for vitamin B_{12} injections.

Take prescribed enzyme replacements with or immediately after meals, being certain to swallow them whole and not disrupt their protective coating with hot foods or liquids.

Compare the patient's status with the expected outcomes. If the outcomes are not met, reassess the patient and revise the plan.

CHRONIC PANCREATITIS

Etiology and Pathophysiology
The causes of chronic pancreatitis are similar to the causes of acute pancreatitis, except that it does not occur in association with biliary tract disease. Some 70 to 80% of the cases of chronic pancreatitis in the United States are associated with chronic alcoholism.

There are three fundamental pathologic changes in the pancreas with chronic pancreatitis. One is the formation of protein plugs in the ducts, some of which are calcified. The second is a decrease in the number of acinar cells, which produce digestive enzymes. The third is fibrosis of the pancreatic tissue. These changes lead to obstruction of the ducts, a decrease in digestive enzymes, and hence malabsorption and nutritional deficiencies. Eventually, the islet cells are affected and diabetes mellitus results. Chronic pancreatitis is complicated by the development of pseudocysts, abscesses, and external fistulas.

Clinical Manifestations
Chronic pancreatitis is characterized by acute attacks of upper abdominal and back pain, often accompa-

nied by vomiting. These attacks increase in frequency and duration over time. The pain accompanying each attack becomes progressively more severe, even to the point at which opiates are ineffective in relieving it.

Another prominent symptom is weight loss. Early in the disease, this may result from inadequate nutritional intake secondary to anorexia or fear that eating will precipitate an attack. Late in the disease, it results from malabsorption and is accompanied by vitamin deficiencies and the frothy, foul-smelling stools indicative of steatorrhea.

Diagnosis

Patients with chronic pancreatitis usually seek medical help when they are experiencing an acute exacerbation of the disease. Diagnosis is based primarily on the presenting symptoms and the patient's history. Laboratory tests confirming chronic pancreatitis include increased alkaline phosphatase, increased serum glucose, and a secretion-challenging test that reveals decreased secretion of pancreatic juices. A glucose tolerance test is done to evaluate islet cell function.

Management

Treatment of chronic pancreatitis attempts to prevent severe episodes by minimizing the work of the pancreas. A low-fat, high-carbohydrate, high-protein, bland diet with abstention from alcohol and caffeine is instituted. If there is insufficient enzyme production, oral pancreatic enzymes (Highlight 24–5) are prescribed to be taken with meals. Anticholinergic drugs, antacids, and gastric acid inhibitors are also given to decrease gastric acid, which stimulates pancreatic function. Because the absorption of vitamin B_{12} is impaired in many cases, parenteral administration may be necessary. Patients with hyperglycemia are treated with insulin or, if the islet cells can be stimulated, with oral hypoglycemic agents.

Pain control is the most difficult part of managing chronic pancreatitis. Because of the chronic nature of the disease and the nature of the pain, the risk of opiate tolerance is high. Thus, nonopiate pain control measures are usually used, with limited success. Surgery is indicated when pain becomes intractable, or when complications, such as abscesses and fistulas, compromise the patient's quality of life. The goal of surgery is to provide drainage of pancreatic secretions into the intestine. To this end, a variety of procedures, including pancreaticojejunostomy, revision of the sphincter of Oddi, and even pancreatectomy, are performed. However, the results are commonly unsuccessful because of a high morbidity and mortality rate associated with the procedures and recurrence of symptoms from progression of the disease.

❖ **Settings, Providers, and Collaboration for Care**

As with any chronic disorder, chronic pancreatitis may be treated in varied settings and may involve

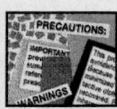

HIGHLIGHT 24–5 PHARMACOLOGY

Pancreatic Enzymes

Definition:

Classified as digestants, oral pancreatic enzymes are usually derived from pork pancreas.

Action:

Pancreatic enzymes aid in the digestion and absorption of carbohydrates, fats, and proteins.

Uses:

These enzymes replace or supplement exocrine pancreatic secretions in malabsorption syndrome precipitated by acute and chronic pancreatitis, cancer of the pancreas, and cystic fibrosis.

Side Effects:

Holding tablets in the mouth may cause ulceration. Nausea, diarrhea, and hyperuricemia may occur with high dosage.

Interactions:

None are known.

Nursing Implications:

Direct patient to take medication with meals unless otherwise advised. Instruct patient to report loss of appetite or constipation because these may be signs that the dosage is too high. Check for pork allergy and, if present, arrange for a bovine preparation. Do not crush enteric-coated tablets.

various health-care workers. Maintenance is usually managed in the physician's office or an outpatient clinic. Exacerbations of the disease often require hospitalization. Collaboration with dietitians, social workers, diabetes specialists, and, possibly, mental health professionals may be appropriate in individual situations.

NURSING PROCESS
Chronic Pancreatitis

Assessment

Assess the location and intensity of pain. Determine the time of onset, and ask for the name of any pain medication taken at home and the frequency with which it is taken. Assess the effectiveness of the pain medication and ask about any other interventions used successfully to reduce pain. Ask the patient about nausea and vomiting and obtain a description of stools. Question specifically about frothy, bulky, foul-smelling stools. Ask what the patient had to eat and drink in the 48 hours preceding the attack, because dietary intake usually correlates with the development of pain and distressing abdominal symptoms.

Obtain the patient's weight and assess general nutritional status. When the patient is able, obtain a complete history of attacks and their treatment. Assess the patient's understanding of the disease and the dietary restrictions needed for its control (see Highlight 24–4). Determine whether oral pancreatic enzymes are prescribed and the patient's understanding of their use. Assess the patient's compliance with the treatment regimen and seek to identify factors that affect it negatively.

Assess blood and urinary glucose levels, because patients with chronic pancreatitis frequently acquire diabetes mellitus. Ascertain the patient's knowledge about diabetic diets and medication if a diagnosis of diabetes mellitus has already been made.

Nursing Diagnoses and Planning

Nursing diagnoses and related expected patient outcomes commonly applicable to patients with chronic pancreatitis include the following:

NDx: Pain related to the inflammatory process in the abdomen

Planning: Patient Outcomes
1. Patient states that abdominal pain has diminished.
2. Patient moves without groans, grimaces, or other signs of discomfort.

NDx: Risk for noncompliance related to medication regimen and diet therapy

Planning: Patient Outcomes
1. Patient self-administers oral pancreatic enzymes and antacids as prescribed.
2. Patient describes dietary regimen.
3. Patient chooses low-fat, bland foods and decaffeinated coffee from the regular hospital menu.
4. Patient reports intent to avoid alcoholic beverages because alcohol can exacerbate symptoms.

NDx: Altered nutrition: less than body requirements related to decreased intake or malabsorption

Planning: Patient Outcomes
1. Patient eats foods served at mealtime.
2. Patient takes vitamin supplements as prescribed.
3. Patient maintains weight or gains a specified amount.

Nursing Interventions and Evaluation

NDx: Pain
Acknowledge the severity of the patient's pain and give prescribed medications as necessary. Discuss with the patient other methods of relieving pain (such as focusing, biofeedback, relaxation techniques, and diversional activities). Explain that the pain is related to digestive activity and that diet and gastric-related medications help limit discomfort.

NDx: Risk for noncompliance
Review with the patient the prescribed medication regimen and diet program (see Highlight 24–4). Explain the reason for taking the prescribed pancreatic enzymes (see Highlight 24–5) and antacids. Ask the patient to monitor the response to the regimen. Tell the patient to note whether abdominal discomfort declines and whether stools return to normal. Compliance improves when the patient associates treatment with a lessening of symptoms. Obtain a written order allowing the patient to self-administer oral pancreatic enzymes and antacids as prescribed while hospitalized. Self-care begun in the hospital is more likely followed-up after discharge. Be certain to observe that the patient takes the medication as prescribed.

Include the family in discussions about medication and diet therapy. Family support facilitates compliance with the long-term therapeutic regimens that patients with chronic pancreatitis are required to follow.

NDx: Altered nutrition: less than body requirements
Because anorexia is frequently a problem, enhance the patient's feelings about food by ensuring a clean, quiet environment for eating and providing foods of the patient's choice when possible. Acknowledge that some people fear eating because it might trigger an acute attack. Reassure the patient that all foods being offered are on the prescribed diet. Also stress that adequate nutrition is necessary to prevent health from deteriorating further. Stress the importance of taking pancreatic enzymes as prescribed and receiving parenteral vitamin B_{12} if needed.

Compare the patient's status with the expected outcomes. If the outcomes are not met, reassess the patient and revise the plan.

Structural Disorders

PANCREATIC FISTULA

Etiology and Pathophysiology
Pancreatic fistulas most commonly result from pancreatic abscesses that develop secondary to acute pancreatitis. Once a pancreatic abscess has formed, an abnormal tract or tunnel develops, connecting the

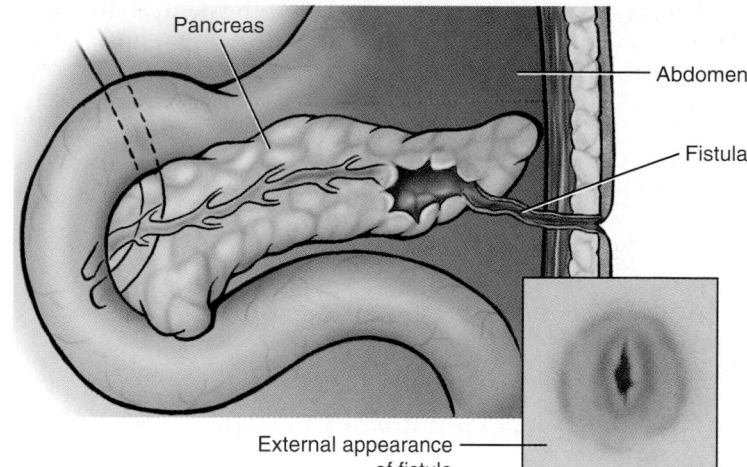

Figure 24–6
Internal view of a pancreatic fistula.

internal abscess site with the abdominal wall (Fig. 24–6). The fistula or tunnel ultimately erodes through the abdominal wall and begins to drain. Very quickly, the opening enlarges, and copious amounts of purulent drainage appear (Fig. 24–7).

Clinical Manifestations
The patient with a pancreatic fistula appears acutely ill and has an elevated temperature. If the fistula has not yet broken through the abdominal wall, examination discloses a small, reddened area that is warm to the touch. If it has broken through, the fistula opening as well as purulent, foul-smelling drainage is evident.

Diagnosis
Diagnosis is based on examination of the wound. Sonography and computed tomographic scan may be used to define the source of the fistula. The white blood cell count is elevated.

Management
The offending organism is identified by wound culture, and appropriate IV antibiotic therapy is instituted. The wound may be irrigated with half-strength normal saline and hydrogen peroxide several times daily. Because the fistula should heal from the inside out, the wound is sometimes packed with sterile gauze after each wound irrigation. Acetaminophen is given for discomfort as well as for fever.

❖ **Settings, Providers, and Collaboration for Care**
The development of a pancreatic fistula is a serious complication of pancreatic disease. Treatment requires hospitalization initially. Once the drainage is manageable and the healing process well-established, the patient may be followed in the physician's office or an outpatient clinic. The nurse instructs the patient about caring for the fistula, dressing changes, and follow-up appointments as needed. The discharge planner may make a referral to a home health agency. The home health nurse:

• Assesses the patient's status and progression toward healing.
• Reinforces hospital-based teaching about caring for the fistula and application of drainage appliance.
• Checks the skin integrity and observes for signs of complications.

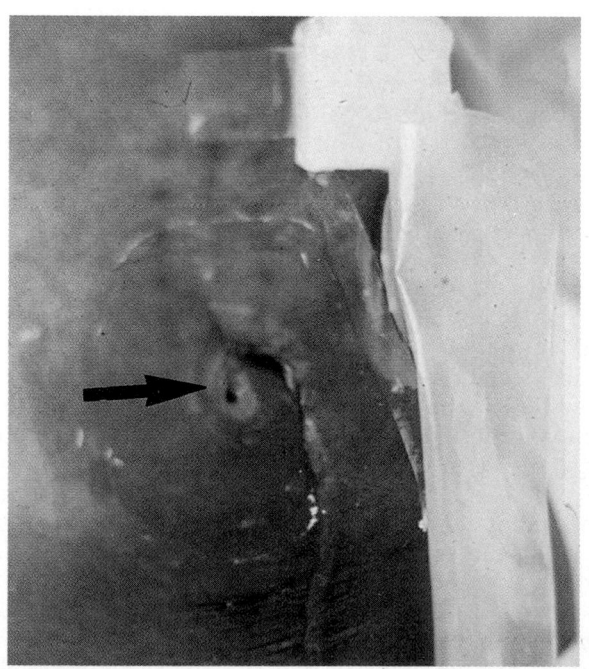

Figure 24–7
External appearance of a pancreatic fistula.

- Assists the patient and family in coping with the change in health status and the home care needed.

NURSING PROCESS
Pancreatic Fistula

Assessment

Take vital signs every 4 hours because an elevated temperature and pulse rate accompany pancreatic fistulas. Observe the amount and character of the drainage and obtain a culture of it before administering antibiotics. Assess the condition of the abdominal skin, because it is prone to excoriation from the drainage. Because a secondary fistula tract sometimes develops, either to a hollow organ or to the body surface, gently palpate the abdomen for signs of increased tenderness. Auscultate bowel sounds and observe for signs of urinary tract infection.

Nursing Diagnoses and Planning

Nursing diagnoses and related expected patient outcomes commonly applicable to patients with a pancreatic fistula include the following:

NDx: Risk for impaired skin integrity related to irritating wound drainage

Planning: Patient Outcomes
1. Skin surrounding fistula opening is intact.
2. Skin surrounding fistula opening is free of erythema.

NDx: Risk for fluid volume deficit related to loss of pancreatic fluid through the fistula

Planning: Patient Outcomes
1. Skin turgor is normal.
2. Mucous membranes are moist.
3. Capillary refill is within normal limits.
4. Vital signs are within patient's baseline ranges.
5. Fluid intake approximates fluid output.

NDx: Risk for altered health maintenance related to insufficient knowledge of wound care

Planning: Patient Outcomes
1. Patient demonstrates wound irrigation.
2. Patient demonstrates care of skin around fistula site.
3. Patient demonstrates proper application of dressing.

Nursing Interventions and Evaluation

NDx: Risk for impaired skin integrity
Irrigate the fistula with the prescribed irrigant. Note the color and odor of drainage. Cleanse the area around the fistula with normal saline and pat dry. Keep skin surrounding the fistula dry and free of drainage because purulent drainage can cause excoriation. If prescribed, pack the fistula tunnel with sterile gauze to hasten inside-out healing and to minimize leakage of drainage onto surrounding skin. Use Montgomery straps if drainage is copious and if dressing changes are frequent to prevent skin irritation from frequent use of tape. Instruct the patient to notify the nurse when the dressing seems damp or wet. An ostomy-type appliance may be used to contain the drainage and protect the skin.

NDx: Risk for fluid volume deficit
Monitor vital signs frequently until fluid volume is stable. Monitor the amount of fistula drainage and replace the amount with IV fluids if ordered. Maintain the patency of the IV line and administer IV solutions as ordered. Monitor laboratory data related to fluid and electrolyte status.

NDx: Risk for altered health maintenance
Because the patient will most likely be discharged before the fistula has completely closed, wound irrigation and dressing must be taught. Explain that irrigating the wound is necessary to facilitate healing, and show the patient how to do it. Have the patient demonstrate irrigating the wound several times before discharge. Similarly, teach proper dressing technique and have the patient demonstrate the procedure.

Compare the patient's status with the expected outcomes. If the outcomes are not met, reassess the patient and revise the plan.

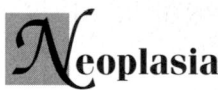

Neoplasia

CANCER OF THE PANCREAS

Cancer of the pancreas is increasing in incidence and ranks second to colon cancer as the most common cause of death from cancers of the gastrointestinal tract. It is twice as common in men as in women and has its peak incidence between 50 and 70 years of age.

Etiology and Pathophysiology

The cause of cancer of the pancreas is unknown, but genetic and environmental factors may play a role in its development. Positive associations have been identified with ingestion of a high-fat diet, meat and carbohydrate consumption, cigarette smoke, and occupational exposures to carcinogens.

Pancreatic cancers are usually adenocarcinomas that originate from the epithelial lining of the duct areas of the organ. Sixty to 70% of the time, they originate in the head of the pancreas. As the tumor mass grows, it blocks the ducts and frequently extends into nearby structures, such as the stomach, liver, intestines, and lymph nodes. The tumor usually grows rapidly and quickly metastasizes to the liver, lungs, or bones. Hence, it typically has a poor prognosis.

Clinical Manifestations

Many symptoms of pancreatic cancer are nonspecific and late in onset, thus contributing to the fact that the disease is often far advanced at the time of diagnosis. Symptoms include anorexia, vague abdominal discomfort, upper or midabdominal pain, boring pain in the middle back, nausea, and vomiting. There is also weight loss and, in 80 to 90% of patients, jaundice that indicates impairment of liver or biliary function. Weight loss is rapid and progressive, and, in most cases, the reason the patient seeks medical help. Fluid and electrolyte imbalances, steatorrhea, bleeding tendencies caused by vitamin K deficiency, and ascites also occur. If the islet cells are involved, diabetes may be the first indication of the malignancy, with glycosuria, hyperglycemia, and abnormal glucose tolerance presenting. Because of the location of the pancreas, the tumor is not usually palpable. However, the liver may enlarge during the course of disease, as may the gallbladder.

Diagnosis

The diagnosis of cancer of the head of the pancreas is strongly suggested by the appearance of painless jaundice and unexplained weight loss. Ultrasonography and tomography help differentiate between enlargement of the pancreas from inflammation and enlargement from a tumor. Also useful in diagnosis are cholangiography, endoscopic retrograde cholangiopancreatography, and angiographic visualization showing engorgement of the small arteries of the pancreas, which suggests cancer. Percutaneous fine-needle aspiration biopsy may be performed to confirm the diagnosis and to guide in selecting the surgical approach to be used for patients who are scheduled for surgery.

Management

The usual treatment for cancer of the pancreas is surgical. If the head of the pancreas is involved and there is no evidence of distant metastasis, a radical pancreatoduodenectomy (Whipple's procedure) is performed.

In patients with cancer of the body or tail of the pancreas, a curative operation cannot be performed because of the location of the tumor and probable extensive metastasis. Thus, the treatment goal is palliation of symptoms through a combination of a simple surgical procedure such as a cholecystojejunostomy (Fig. 24–8), radiation, and chemotherapy.

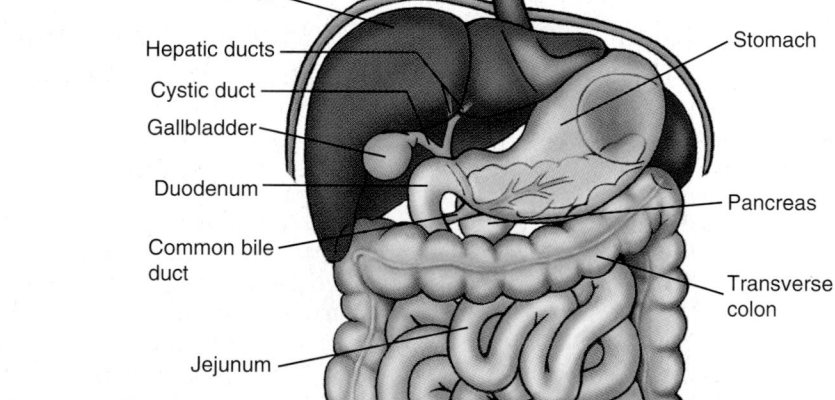
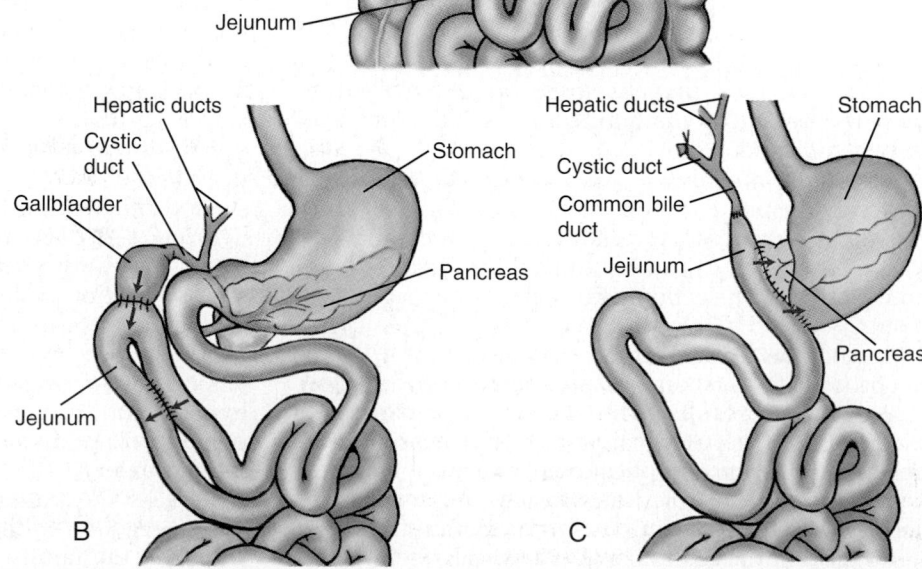

Figure 24–8

A, Normal relationship of upper abdominal organs. B, Cholecystojejunostomy. Note the anastomosis between the gallbladder and the jejunum, which allows bile to flow directly into the intestine, bypassing obstruction caused by an inoperable tumor of the head of the pancreas. C, Upper abdominal contents following a Whipple procedure. Note the removal of the proximal pancreas, duodenum, lower half of the stomach, and gallbladder.

Chemotherapy and radiation therapy have little or no influence on the primary tumor but can relieve the pain of tumor pressure as the disease advances. Other aspects of palliative treatment include pain control, nutritional support, and control of complications.

Radical Pancreatoduodenectomy

A radical pancreatoduodenectomy (Whipple's procedure) is a very extensive surgical procedure involving removal of the proximal pancreas, the duodenum, the lower half of the stomach, and the gallbladder. The pancreatic duct is implanted into the jejunum, as are the remaining stomach and hepatic duct (see Fig. 24–8). The purpose of this procedure is to allow gastric, hepatic, and pancreatic secretions to empty into the jejunum so that reasonably normal digestion can take place. This procedure once carried a high mortality rate and a low 5-year survival rate after the operation. However, recent advances in surgical technique and treatment protocols have improved both of these statistics. It remains the mainstay of the curative management of cancer of the head of the pancreas.

PATIENT PREPARATION. Preparation for a Whipple procedure is intensive and often requires a long period of time because of the extensiveness of the procedure and the fact that the patient usually is malnourished and in poor physical condition. The patient is hydrated and usually given parenteral nutrition. Blood transfusions are commonly used to correct anemia, and vitamin K is given to correct prothrombin deficiency. Because postoperative infection is a major risk, antibiotics such as kanamycin or neomycin are typically started 3 to 4 days before surgery.

POSTOPERATIVE COURSE. After surgery, the patient is usually admitted to a surgical critical care unit. IV fluids and electrolytes are administered, and transfusions may be given to replace blood lost during the operation. An arterial catheter is in place to monitor arterial pressure. An indwelling urinary catheter is in place to monitor urinary output. To minimize pancreatic secretion and to decompress the stomach and thus prevent stress on internal suture lines, the patient is maintained on NPO status with nasogastric suction.

Parenteral nutrition is continued, with oral intake gradually resumed when bowel function has fully returned. Vasopressor drugs are used to combat hypotension, which can occur during the first 48 hours after pancreatic resection. Prophylactic antibiotics are given.

COMPLICATIONS. Major complications of a Whipple procedure are hemorrhage, necrosis, fistula formation (which results from the action of pancreatic enzymes) and hepatorenal failure and vascular collapse. Pulmonary complications—such as pneumonia, atelectasis, and pleural effusion—also are prevalent, given the proximity of the operative area to the diaphragm and the chest. The incidence of complications is high not only because of the extent of the surgery but also because patients tend to be at increased risk from a history of alcohol or drug abuse, diabetes, and malnutrition.

❖ Settings, Providers, and Collaboration for Care

Patients with pancreatic cancer may be treated on an outpatient basis through their physician or a clinic. Usually, however, they require some hospitalization, especially if surgery is part of the treatment plan. Often, extended home care or hospice care is necessary.

After surgery, the discharge nurse or case manager assists the patient and family members with preparation for home care. Depending on the patient's specific needs, the home health nurse assesses the patient's progress, teaches the patient and family about continued care needed, and instructs them about the medication regimen. The nurse may assist with hygienic care, dressing changes, nutritional planning, and other prescribed treatments. A dietitian may also be consulted to help maintain the patient's nutritional status. Because of the traumatic nature of the diagnosis and surgical intervention, a counselor, psychologist, or cleric may be necessary to help the patient and family cope with the situation.

NURSING PROCESS
Whipple's Procedure

PREOPERATIVE NURSING CARE

Assessment

Assess the patient's symptoms. Assess pain and determine what measures are used to control it and how effective they are. Assess nutritional status and fluid and electrolyte balance. Note height and weight. Question about anorexia, nausea, and vomiting. Determine what the patient's intake has been before hospitalization. Observe the condition of oral mucous membranes and check skin turgor. Review laboratory data.

Observe the skin and sclerae for jaundice. Check the color of stools and urine. Observe for ecchymosis and other signs of bleeding because prothrombin deficiency secondary to a lack of vitamin K is likely. If the appearance of the abdomen suggests ascites, measure abdominal girth.

Obtain repeated measures of blood pressure to obtain a good baseline against which to compare postoperative pressure. This is important because hypotension can occur after pancreatic resection, perhaps from division of the sympathetic fibers to the mesentery.

Assess the patient's and family's understanding of and reaction to the impending surgery. Assess the ability of the family or significant others to meet the patient's expected home-care needs, including nutritional support and pain control.

Nursing Diagnoses and Planning

Nursing diagnoses and related expected patient outcomes commonly applicable to patients scheduled for a Whipple procedure include the following:

NDx: Pain related to pressure on and destruction of intra-abdominal structures from carcinoma

Planning: Patient Outcomes
1. Patient states that pain is reduced to at least a bearable level with use of medication or other pain-control strategies.
2. Patient rests quietly without groaning or moaning.

NDx: Altered nutrition: less than body requirements related to anorexia and malabsorption

Planning: Patient Outcomes
1. Patient maintains or increases body weight.

NDx: Knowledge deficit: preoperative preparation, surgical procedure, postoperative course

Planning: Patient Outcomes
1. Patient states reasons for preoperative procedures.
2. Patient describes planned surgery as an extensive gastrointestinal operation.
3. Patient acknowledges awareness of the various equipment that will be used in postoperative treatment.
4. Patient practices deep-breathing and coughing exercises.
5. Family and patient discuss home-care options.

Nursing Interventions and Evaluation

NDx: Pain
Medicate the patient for pain according to medication orders. Position the patient carefully. Remember that pain from pancreatic cancer is sometimes worsened by lying supine and is relieved by sitting hunched forward. Use a foam pad or other pressure-distributing device under the patient in bed to provide maximal comfort and to protect bony prominences.

NDx: Altered nutrition: less than body requirements
Administer parenteral fluids, electrolytes, and nutrients as prescribed. Combat nausea and vomiting by ensuring that the patient's environment is clean and odor-free and by administering antiemetics as ordered. If oral intake is allowed, offer the patient small amounts of high-nutrition foodstuffs of his or her choice. Report any changes in factors that affect metabolic rate and therefore nutritional needs. These include increased temperature, increased gastrointestinal drainage, signs of infection, and increased stress.

NDx: Knowledge deficit: preoperative preparation, surgical procedure, postoperative course
Review preoperative procedures, the surgical procedure, and the postoperative course with the patient and family. Be sure to explain that the surgical procedure takes several hours to complete, because frequently a family equates extended time in the operating room with occurrence of serious complications. Also begin discussing preparation for discharge. This focuses the patient and family on a positive goal and allows the family time to mobilize the resources that will be required on discharge.

Keep in mind that the patient is critically ill and may not have the physical energy or mental concentration to follow lengthy explanations. Remember also that both the patient and family are likely to be very anxious over the outcome of the surgery and may have difficulty attending to and remembering information.

Compare the patient's status with the expected outcomes. If the outcomes are not met, reassess the patient and revise the plan.

POSTOPERATIVE NURSING CARE

Assessment

Take vital signs and measure urinary output every hour. Read the operative report. Check placement of all drainage tubes. Make certain they are free of stress or kinks and that they are in a dependent position. Note the characteristics and amount of drainage from each. Keep in mind that serosanguineous drainage is normal and that clear, bile-tinged, or bloody drainage can indicate disruption of an anastomosis. Carefully assess functioning of the nasogastric suction because removal of gastrointestinal drainage and secretions is necessary to prevent stress on the anastomosis sites. As with the drains, check for pull or binding. Also check suction gauge at regular intervals.

Observe for signs of fluid and electrolyte imbalance because patients lose large amounts of protein and fluid into the peritoneal cavity and the intestinal tract. Measure all intake and output. Monitor serum electrolytes, serum albumin, serum and urine osmolality, hematocrit levels, arterial blood gas levels, and pH. Monitor for signs of the third-spacing phenomenon: increase in weight, fluid in the lungs, pitting edema in the extremities, and dependent edema in the back and over the sacrum. Check blood sugar levels because removal of islet cells may necessitate administration of insulin to prevent hyperglycemia.

Assess the patient's pain and note the effectiveness of medication and other comfort measures. When analgesics are given that depress the central nervous system, assess for any depressant effect on the respiratory system that would increase the risk of complications in this area.

Observe the wound for signs of hemorrhage. Monitor prothrombin levels because of the potential for impaired coagulation. Observe both the wound and the entry site of the total parenteral nutrition catheter for signs of infection: redness, purulent drainage, and foul odor. Also check for signs of peritonitis by watching for a sudden increase in temperature and by palpating the abdomen for rigidity. Observe skin areas in contact with pancreatic drainage for excoriation.

Assess general nutritional status. Obtain daily weights. Listen for the return of bowel sounds and observe for passage of flatus and stool. When oral intake is resumed, observe for signs of malabsorption, such as steatorrhea and diarrhea, and assess for dumping syndrome. Inspect the skin for signs of breakdown, for which the patient is at risk because of bedrest and impaired nutrition.

Assess the patient's emotional status. Look for signs of depression, anger, and anxiety. Explore coping mechanisms for both the patient and the family.

Nursing Diagnoses and Planning

Nursing diagnoses and related expected patient outcomes commonly applicable to patients who have had a Whipple procedure include the following:

NDx: Risk for impaired gas exchange related to lengthy anesthesia and location of surgical trauma

Planning: Patient Outcomes
1. Rate and depth of respirations are within patient's normal range.
2. Lungs are clear on auscultation.
3. Arterial blood gas values are within baseline limits.

NDx: Pain related to surgical trauma and irritation of the naris by the nasogastric tube

Planning: Patient Outcomes
1. Patient reports that pain is relieved to at least a bearable level after medication.
2. Patient performs routine postoperative exercises without complaints or signs of severe pain, such as pallor and tachycardia.
3. Patient denies nostril discomfort.

NDx: Risk for fluid volume deficit related to effects of pancreatic surgery, presence of multiple drainage tubes, and limited oral intake

Planning: Patient Outcomes
1. Hourly urinary output is 50 mL or more.
2. IV intake approximates urinary and nasogastric tube output.
3. Skin turgor is good.
4. Serum electrolyte levels are within normal limits.

NDx: Risk for altered nutrition: less than body requirements related to inadequate intake of nutrients or malabsorption

Planning: Patient Outcomes
1. Patient maintains or gains weight.
2. Patient is in positive nitrogen balance.

NDx: Risk for trauma to the internal suture lines related to gastrointestinal distention

Planning: Patient Outcomes
1. Nasogastric suction is functioning.
2. Abdomen is soft.
3. Patient states that pain is decreasing over time.

NDx: Risk for altered oral mucous membrane related to mouth breathing secondary to the nasogastric tube and NPO status

Planning: Patient Outcomes
1. Oral mucous membranes are pink and moist.
2. Lips are free of cracks.
3. Patient states that lips are supple and pain-free.

NDx: Risk for infection related to contamination of the abdominal wound or catheter site or to contamination or disruption of an internal anastomosis, presence of a parenteral nutrition catheter

Planning: Patient Outcomes
1. Patient remains afebrile.
2. Patient's white blood cell count is within normal limits.
3. Wound drainage is nonpurulent.
4. Abdomen is soft to palpation.
5. TPN catheter site is nonreddened and free of foul odor or purulent drainage.

NDx: Risk for altered health maintenance related to insufficient knowledge of self-care after discharge

Planning: Patient Outcomes
1. Patient demonstrates sterile dressing change.
2. Patient describes signs and symptoms to be reported to physician.

Nursing Interventions and Evaluation

NDx: Risk for impaired gas exchange
Place the patient in semi-Fowler's position to promote lung expansion and reduce pull on the suture line. Establish and maintain a consistent pulmonary hygiene routine that includes turning, coughing, deep-breathing, ambulation, and use of an incentive spirometer.

NDx: Pain
Use the AHCPR guidelines for pain management to develop strategies with the patient for pain relief. Medicate the patient for pain as often as prescribed. Assist the patient to splint the incisional area when moving, coughing, or deep-breathing. When the patient is ambulatory, plan to get him or her out of bed while pain medication is effective. Encourage relaxation and provide a calm, quiet environment. Use other pain-relieving strategies, such as imaging and distraction, as appropriate. Find out which pain medication the patient will use after discharge. Instruct the patient and family about the administration and side effects of the drug.

To prevent or ease nasal discomfort from the nasogastric tube, wash the nostril with applicators wet with water and apply a water-soluble lubricant. Make certain that the tube is taped in place in a manner that does not exert pressure on the naris.

NDx: Risk for fluid volume deficit
Administer fluids as ordered. Monitor urinary output. Report an output of less than 25 mL hourly to the physician. Record all intake and output.

NDx: Risk for altered nutrition: less than body requirements
Administer parenteral nutrition as prescribed. When oral intake is allowed, advance the patient's diet, as tolerated, to a full high-carbohydrate, high-protein, high-vitamin diet as ordered. Administer prescribed vitamin and mineral supplements as well as any prescribed pancreatic enzymes.

NDx: Risk for trauma
Keep the nasogastric tube free of kinks and connected to suction, as ordered, to drain secretions and to prevent distention. Irrigate the tube gently with normal saline (usually 10 to 20 mL) as ordered to keep it patent. Reinforce or replace the tape holding the tube in place as needed. Avoid moving the tube when adding or moving tape. Keep the patient on NPO status until bowel function has completely returned to avoid distention and vomiting.

NDx: Risk for altered oral mucous membrane
Give mouth care frequently. Encourage the patient to rinse his or her mouth with water often when able.

NDx: Risk for infection
Administer prophylactic antibiotics as ordered. Use strict aseptic technique when doing wound care and handling catheters and related equipment. Reinforce the dressing as needed unless it becomes wet with predominantly bloody drainage, in which case it should be changed. Institute a skin-care protocol before signs of irritation from drainage develop. Use paste or salve to prevent contact between drainage and the skin surface.

Change the dressing at the total parenteral nutrition catheter site regularly, using strict technique as described in Chapter 21. Caution the patient against touching the abdominal dressing or the dressing at the catheter site.

NDx: Risk for altered health maintenance
Because the patient will most likely be discharged before the surgical wounds are completely healed, demonstrate to the patient and the family techniques to be used for wound care and dressing changes. Observe as the patient or a family member performs wound care and one or more dressing changes. Teach the patient and family about signs of wound infection, and instruct them to notify the physician at the first sign of infection.

Additional Interventions
Support the patient's and family's coping mechanisms. Use additional sources of support, such as social services and pastoral care, as needed. Make referrals as needed to ensure care at home.

Compare the patient's status with the expected outcomes. If the outcomes are not met, reassess the patient and revise the plan.

The Elderly: Special Considerations

The incidence of gallstones increases with advancing age. The associated clinical manifestations may be atypical, however, with symptoms of septic shock being the first sign of disease. When surgery is required, it is ideally performed as an elective procedure. This allows thorough patient preparation and thus decreases the risk of complications from coexisting disease.

Pancreatic disease is also common among the elderly, and pancreatic enzyme replacement is often needed. When such replacement is ordered for an elderly patient who has difficulty swallowing, be sure to request the powdered form. Mix it well with applesauce or other fruit, but do not mix with foods containing protein. Do not let the enzymes stay on the lips or the skin because tissue breakdown can occur. Never crush enteric-coated tablets.

Chapter Review

1. How does the care of a patient with acute pancreatitis differ from that of a patient with chronic pancreatitis?
2. What are the advantages of a laparoscopic cholecystectomy for an elderly patient with gallstones?
3. Why is attention to respiratory assessment especially important in caring for a patient following an open cholecystectomy?
4. Why is fluid volume deficit an important nursing diagnosis for a patient following a Whipple procedure for pancreatic cancer?
5. What are possible solutions to the problem of skin excoriation in a patient with a pancreatic fistula?
6. How can the effectiveness of oral bile acid medications be evaluated when caring for a patient with gallstones?
7. How would you treat abdominal pain when caring for a patient following laparoscopic cholecystectomy?
8. Why is compliance with medication regimens especially important for the patient with chronic pancreatitis?
9. How can pain best be assessed in a patient with acute pancreatitis?
10. What could happen to a patient following a Whipple procedure if the nasogastric tube became dislodged?

Bibliography

Agency for Health Care Policy and Research. (1992) Acute pain management: Operative or medical procedures and trauma. Rockville, MD: US Department of Health and Human Services. AHCPR 92-0032.

Calleja GA, Barkin JS. Acute pancreatitis. Med Clin North Am 1993; 77(5):1037.

Cameron JL. Long-term survival following pancreaticoduodenectomy for adenocarcinoma of the head of the pancreas. Surg Clin North Am 1995; 75(5):939.

Conlon KC, Klimstra DS, Brennan FF. Long-term survival after curative resection for pancreatic ductal adenocarcinoma. Ann Surg 1995; 223(3):273.

Cappuccino H, Cargill S, Nguyen T. Laparoscopic cholecystectomy. Surg Laparoscop Endoscop 1994; 4(3):213.

Claussen DW. Orally administered gallbladder therapeutic agents, Part II (UDCA). Gastroenterol Nurs 1993; 15(6):254.

Cotton PB. Endoscopic retrograde cholangiopancreatography and laparoscopic cholecystectomy. Am J Surg 1993; 165(4):474.

Drossman DA (ed). The functional GI disorders: Diagnosis, pathology and treatment. Boston: Little, Brown, 1994.

Doughty BD, Jackson DB. Gastrointestinal disorders. St. Louis: Mosby-Year Book, 1993.

Ghoulson CF, Sittig K, McDonald JC. Recent advances in the management of gallstones. Am J Med Sci 1994; 307(4):293.

Goldschmid S, Brady PG. Approaches to the management of cholelithiasis for the medical consultant. Med Clin North Am 1993; 77(2):413.

Hofman AF. Primary and secondary prevention of gallstone disease. Am J Surg 1993; 165(4):541.

Holt S. Management of chronic pancreatitis. Compr Ther 1994; 20(1):24.

Jaffe PE. Gallstones. Who are good candidates for nonsurgical treatment? Postgrad Med 1993; 94(6):45.

Kleinbeck SV, Hoffart N. Outpatient recovery after laparoscopic cholecystectomy. AORN J 1994; 60(3):394.

Kohn CL, Brozenec SA, Foster PF. Nutritional support for the patient with pancreatobiliary disease. Crit Care Nurs Clin North Am 1993; 5(1):37.

Krumberger JM. Acute pancreatitis. Crit Care Nurs Clin North Am 1993; 5(1):185.

Marshall JB. Current options in gallstone management. What to do when symptoms are mild or absent. Postgrad Med 1994; 95(5):115.

Meeker MH, Rothrock JC. Alexander's care of the patient in surgery. 10th ed. St. Louis: Mosby Year-Book, 1995.

Misiewicz JJ, Pounder RE, Venables CW (eds). Diseases of the gut and pancreas. Baltimore: Blackwell Scientific Publishers, 1994.

Moody FG. Lithotripsy in the treatment of biliary stones. Am J Surg 1993; 165(4):479.

Murphy D, Berry D. Mechanical lithotripsy. Gastroenterol Nurs 1994; 16(5):204.

Nahrwold DL. Gallstone lithotripsy. Am J Surg 1993; 165(4):431.

NIH Consensus conference. Gallstones and laparoscopic cholecystectomy. JAMA 1993; 269(8):1018.

Noone J. Acute pancreatitis: An Orem approach to nursing assessment and care. Crit Care Nurse 1995; 15(4):27.

Ondrusek RS. Cholecystectomy: An update. RN 1993; 56(1):28.

Reber HA, Ashley SW, McFadden D. Curative treatment for pancreatic neoplasms. Surg Clin North Am 1995; 75(5):905.

Schoenfield LJ, Marks JW. Oral and contact dissolution of gallstones. Am J Surg 1993; 165(4):427.

Senzatimore S, Barkin JS. Chronic pancreatitis and pancreatic cancer. Am J Gastroenterol 1994; 89(9):1593.

Shaw MJ. Current management of symptomatic gallstones. Postgrad Med 1993; 93(1):183.

Sleisenger MH, Fordtran JS. Gastrointestinal disease: Pathophysiology, diagnosis and management. 4th ed. Philadelphia: WB Saunders, 1993.

Stillman A. Laparoscopic cholecystectomy. AORN J 1993; 57(2): 429.

Swonger AK, Burbank PM. Drug therapy and the elderly. Boston: Jones and Bartlett. 1995.

Tait N, Little JM. The treatment of gallstones. Br Med J 1995; 311(7):99.

Thompson C. Managing acute pancreatitis. RN 1992; 55(5):9.

Wietlispach-Clausen D. Orally administered gallbladder therapeutic agents, Part I (CDCA). Gastroenterol Nurs 1993; 15(5):208.

Williams SR. Nutrition and diet therapy. 7th ed. St. Louis: Mosby, 1993.

Yeo CJ. Management of complications following pancreaticoduodenectomy. Surg Clin North Am 1995; 75(5):913.

Unit VIII

Hepatic Dysfunction

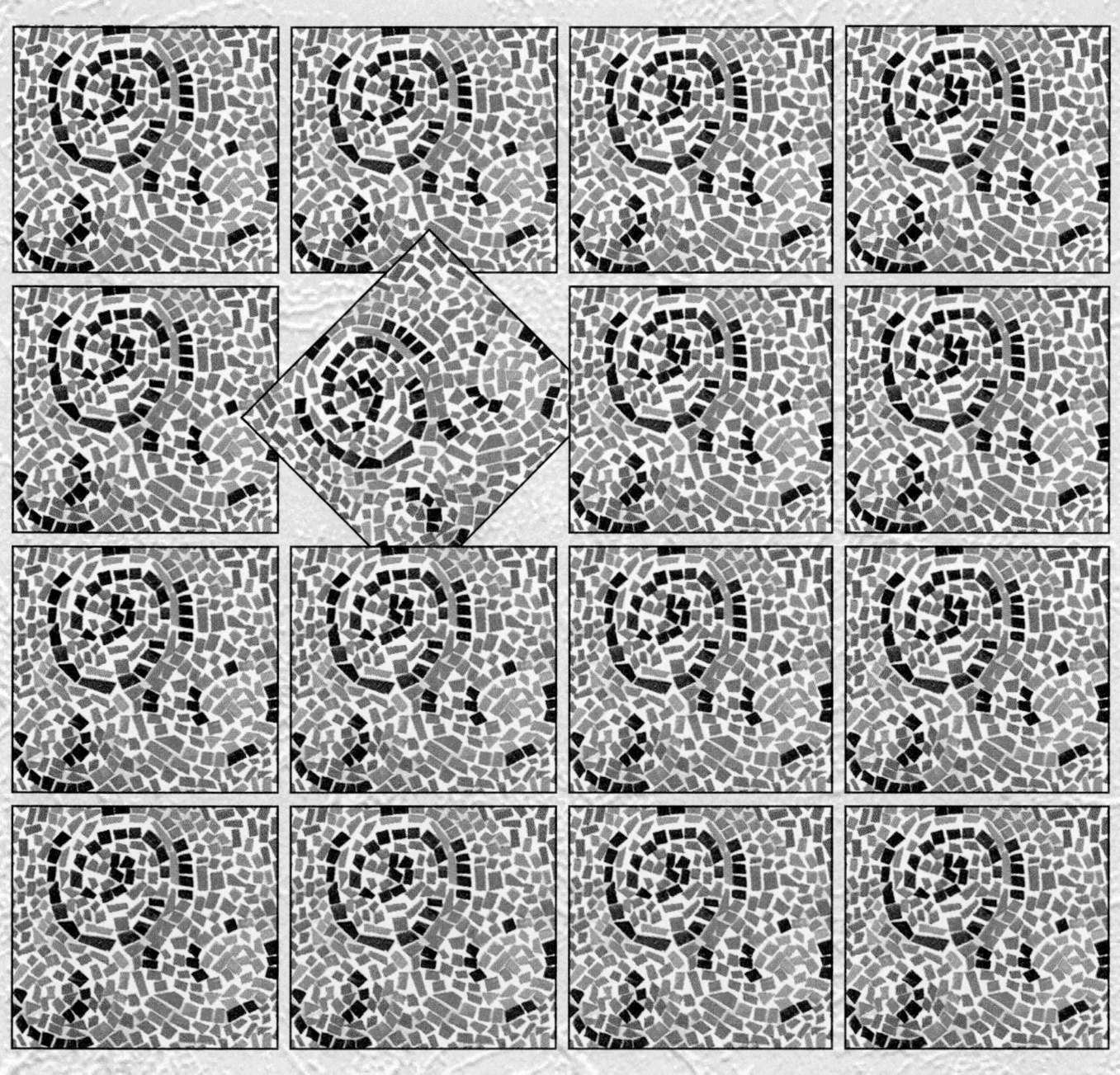

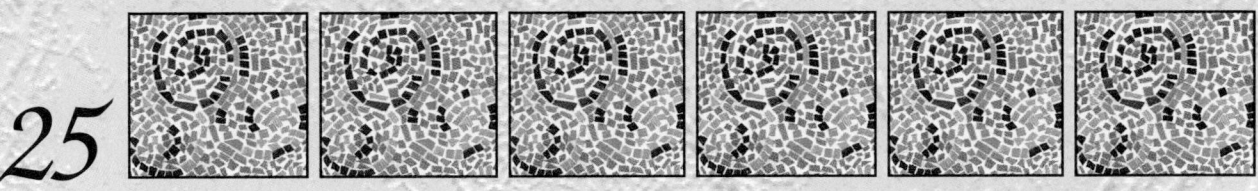

Knowledge Base for Patients with Hepatic Dysfunction

Study Outcomes

After studying this chapter, you should be able to:

1. Explain the normal anatomy and physiology of the liver.
2. Describe common clinical manifestations of liver dysfunction.
3. Identify information and physical examination data essential to the assessment of liver status.
4. Describe basic diagnostic tests and treatment modalities used in the collaborative management of patients with liver disorders.
5. Describe basic surgical procedures used in the treatment of patients with liver disorders.
6. Identify data essential to the assessment of patients undergoing treatment of liver disorders.
7. State nursing diagnoses and related expected patient outcomes commonly applicable to patients undergoing treatment of liver disorders.
8. Describe nursing interventions, with their rationales, commonly applicable to patients undergoing treatment of liver disorders.
9. Explain the basis for evaluation of nursing care provided to patients undergoing treatment of liver disorders.
10. Identify special considerations for elderly patients with altered liver function.

The liver—the body's largest internal organ—performs a host of functions related to the digestion, absorption, metabolism, and storage of nutrients. Interference with the liver's normal function may result in serious or even life-threatening illness. Common clinical manifestations of liver dysfunction include jaundice, ascites, portal hypertension, bleeding, hepatic encephalopathy, and nutritional deficiencies.

A sound understanding of liver function and dysfunction is essential for providing timely and accurate nursing care for patients with hepatic problems. Depending on the severity of the condition, patients may receive care in a variety of settings, including a physician's office, an acute inpatient facility, an ambulatory center, or a long-term or home-health setting.

Anatomy and Physiology

The liver of an adult human weighs about 1500 g (3.5 lbs). It is the body's largest internal organ and performs the greatest number of diverse functions. The liver is located in the right upper quadrant of the abdomen and extends across the midline to the left upper quadrant. It extends upward beneath the ribs by 6 to 12 cm at the right midclavicular line and by 4 to 8 cm at the midsternal line.

The liver is composed of two major lobes: a large right lobe and a smaller left lobe. These lobes are separated by the falciform ligament, a fold of visceral peritoneum that fastens the liver to the anterior abdominal wall. Two smaller lobes are present on the posterior surface of the liver. They include the quadrate lobe near the gallbladder and the caudate lobe near the inferior vena cava. A dense layer of connective tissue called the capsule of Glisson covers the entire organ. Figure 25–1 illustrates the anterior surface of the liver.

Each lobe is composed of 50,000 to 100,000 hepatic lobules, the functional units of the liver. Lobules, as shown in Figure 25–2, are made up of layers of hepatocytes (hepatic cells) only one or two cells thick that radiate outward from a central vein. The portal vein brings about 75% of the blood supply to the liver. This blood is rich in nutrients from the intestine and flows to the hepatic sinusoids, large capillaries that separate the layers of hepatocytes. This venous pathway through the liver is known as the hepatic portal system. The remaining 25% of the blood supply to the liver is delivered via the hepatic artery. This blood is rich in oxygen and mixes with the portal blood in the sinusoids. Some 1450 mL of mixed arteriovenous blood flows through the liver each minute. From the hepatic sinusoids, blood flows to the central vein of each lobule and through a series of merging vessels into the hepatic vein. The hepatic vein empties into the inferior vena cava. Although there are two sources for blood flow into the liver (the portal vein and the hepatic artery), all blood leaves the liver via the

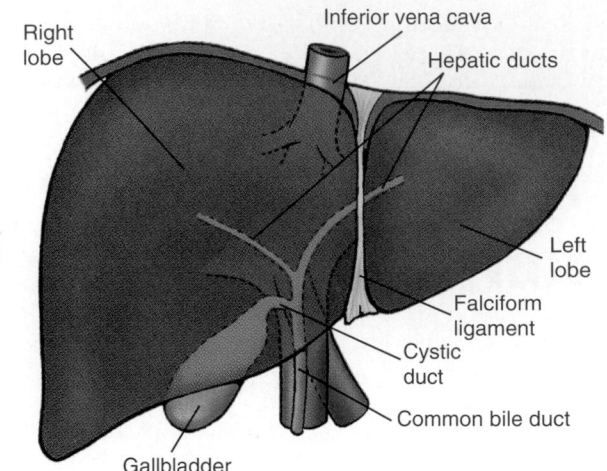

Figure 25–1
Anterior view of the liver.

same route: the hepatic vein to the inferior vena cava.

Each hepatic lobule also has specialized bile ducts called canaliculi, which drain bile produced by the hepatocytes. The canaliculi flow into the larger hepatic ducts, which then empty into the common bile duct. The cystic duct, a branch of the common bile duct, carries bile to the gallbladder, where it can be stored.

The liver plays a vital role in the digestion, absorption, metabolism, and storage of nutrients. The functions of the liver are summarized in Table 25–1. In addition to the metabolizing carbohydrates, lipids, and proteins, the liver manufactures and secretes bile; filters blood; detoxifies drugs, toxins, and hormones; and serves as a storage depot for glycogen, fat-soluble vitamins, copper, and iron.

CARBOHYDRATE METABOLISM

In carbohydrate metabolism, the liver is especially important in maintaining normal blood glucose levels. When blood glucose levels are within normal range, glucose from digested food sources is transported from the intestines to the liver via the portal circulation, where it is converted to glycogen. This process, called glycogenesis, prevents large amounts of glucose from entering the blood stream when it is

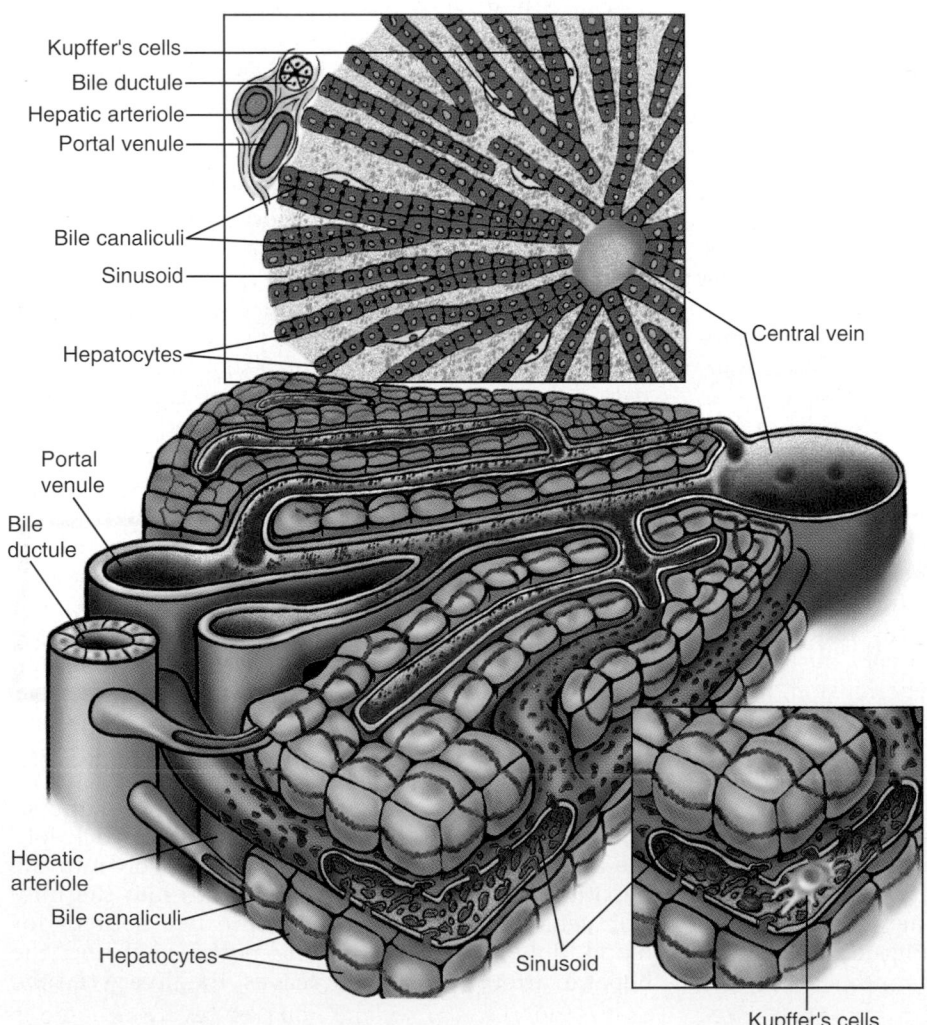

Figure 25–2
Structures of a hepatic lobule.

Table 25–1

Liver Functions

Function	Description
Metabolism	
Carbohydrate	Converts glucose to glycogen for storage (glycogenesis)
	Breaks down glycogen into glucose for energy (glycogenolysis)
	Converts protein and fat to glucose for energy (gluconeogenesis)
Lipid	Oxidizes fatty acids and glycerol for energy
	Reforms triglycerides
	Produces cholesterol and ketones
Protein	Synthesizes new amino acids, albumin, alpha and beta globulins, fibrinogen, prothrombin, and clotting factors V, VII, VIII, and X
	Converts ammonia to urea
Secretion	Produces and secretes bile needed for fat digestion
Filtration	Removes foreign substances from the blood, including bacteria and aged red blood cells
Detoxification	Chemically modifies drugs, toxins, and hormones and makes them more suitable for excretion
Storage	Stores glycogen; vitamins A, D, B_{12}, K_1, and K_2; folic acid; iron; manganese; copper; and zinc

not needed. Glycogen is stored in the liver for future use. When energy demands increase and available blood glucose levels are inadequate, the liver converts the glycogen to glucose through the process of glycogenolysis and returns glucose to the blood stream. When glycogen stores are exhausted, nonglucose sources, such as protein and fat, are converted by the liver to glucose in a process called gluconeogenesis. Through these processes, a relatively constant blood glucose level is maintained in the body.

Patients with liver disease may experience hypoglycemia or glucose intolerance. This occurs because of diminished glycogen stores, decreased liver response to glucagon, decreased gluconeogenesis, and poor oral intake.

LIPID METABOLISM

The liver serves as the major regulator of lipid metabolism. Dietary fat, primarily in the form of triglycerides, is digested in the small intestines under the influence of pancreatic lipase and bile salts. Fatty acids, the end-products of dietary fat digestion, are transported to the liver, where they are oxidized to produce energy when glucose is not available. If glucose is available, they are used to reform triglyc-

erides or to produce cholesterol and ketones. Cholesterol is important in the synthesis of liver cell membranes, for the production of bile salts that aid fat digestion, and for the production of various sex hormones and hormones produced by the adrenal glands. Ketones, in the form of acetoacetic acid, are transported to peripheral tissues, where they are used for energy. When glucose is not available and fat is used for energy, ketones are formed in large quantities, resulting in the accumulation of ketones in the blood. This occurs with prolonged fasting or starvation and in uncontrolled diabetes mellitus. If not treated, ketosis leads to a lowering of the pH of body fluids (metabolic acidosis), which can be fatal.

Persons who ingest large amounts of alcohol frequently have an accumulation of triglycerides in the liver. This condition, called fatty liver, causes an enlarged liver and abnormal liver function.

PROTEIN METABOLISM

Amino acids are the end products of the digestion of protein in the small intestine. They are transported via the portal vein to the liver, where they are used to form new compounds and new amino acids. These substances are delivered into the systemic circulation for use by body tissues. The liver uses amino acids to produce:

- Albumin, needed to maintain blood osmotic pressure
- Alpha and beta globulins, needed to transport lipids and fat-soluble vitamins
- Fibrinogen, prothrombin, and clotting factors V, VII, VIII, and X, major factors in blood coagulation.

Vitamin K, a fat-soluble vitamin, is needed for production of prothrombin and clotting factors V, IX, and X. Ammonia is formed as an end product of protein metabolism in the liver, as well as by the action of bacteria on proteins in the intestine. This potentially toxic substance is removed from the blood almost entirely by conversion to urea in the liver. Urea enters the circulation, travels to the kidney, and is excreted from the body in urine.

In hepatic disorders, liver protein metabolism is disrupted and blood ammonia levels rise, affecting acid-base balance and brain function. Decreased plasma proteins reduce intravascular fluid volume resulting in edema formation. Bleeding problems develop from decreased production of clotting factors and the inability to use fat-soluble vitamin K. Fatigue and muscle-wasting occur from decreased amino acid production and utilization, which prevents adequate tissue building and repair.

BILE PRODUCTION AND BILIRUBIN CONJUGATION

Bile, a yellowish-green fluid, is continually manufactured and secreted by the hepatocytes. In a 24-hour period, 700 to 1200 mL are produced. In addition to water, bile contains bile salts, bile pigments including bilirubin, cholesterol, sodium, chloride, and other electrolytes.

Bile salts, formed in the hepatocytes from cholesterol, are used to emulsify fat in the intestinal tract. Large fat molecules are broken down into minute molecules, which can be acted on by pancreatic enzymes. Bile salts also aid in the absorption of fatty acids, cholesterol, and the fat-soluble vitamins A, D, E, and K. Bile salts are reabsorbed in the small intestine, returned to the liver, and once again excreted into the bile. This recycling path from the liver to the systemic circulation and back to the liver is known as enterohepatic circulation. With liver disease, bile salts may be deficient, and steatorrhea (excess fat in the stool) may develop. The normal 2 to 5 g of fat excreted in the stool daily may increase to as much as 60 g. Deficiencies of the fat-soluble vitamins A, D, E, and K also occur.

Bile pigments, composed principally of bilirubin and biliverdin (an oxidized form of bilirubin), are responsible for the color of bile. Bilirubin is produced from hemoglobin when red blood cells are destroyed by the spleen, bone marrow, and Kupffer's cells in the liver. Kupffer's cells are large, mononuclear phagocytic cells that line the hepatic sinusoids and cleanse the blood of bacteria and toxins as it circulates through the liver (see Fig. 25–2). The bilirubin attaches to a plasma protein, primarily albumin, and circulates in the plasma until it reaches the liver and is absorbed by the hepatocytes. Bilirubin loosely bound to protein is called unconjugated bilirubin and is insoluble in plasma. Once bilirubin enters the liver and is absorbed by the hepatocytes, it is separated from the albumin and conjugated with glucuronide transferase, which makes it soluble in aqueous solutions. It is then excreted into the bile. The conjugated bilirubin is transported to the small intestine, where it is converted into urobilinogen. Part of the urobilinogen is excreted in the feces, and the remainder returns to the liver (enterohepatic circulation), where it is removed from the blood. Traces of urobilinogen not removed from the blood by the liver are carried to the kidneys and excreted in the urine. Figure 25–3 summarizes bilirubin metabolism.

Unconjugated bilirubin levels rise with increased destruction of red blood cells or hemolytic disease. Both unconjugated and conjugated bilirubin levels rise in liver disease.

BLOOD FILTRATION

As blood flows through the intestinal capillaries, many intestinal bacteria are picked up by Kupffer's cells. Less than 1% of bacteria from the intestine succeed in passing to the systemic circulation. In addition to bacteria, Kupffer's cells also phagocytize aged erythrocytes. Through a series of enzyme reactions, amino acids and iron from the erythrocytes are salvaged and reused, and the heme portion of the erythrocyte is used to produce bilirubin.

DETOXIFICATION

The liver chemically modifies a wide variety of drugs, toxins, and hormones. Under normal conditions, the liver inactivates these substances or alters

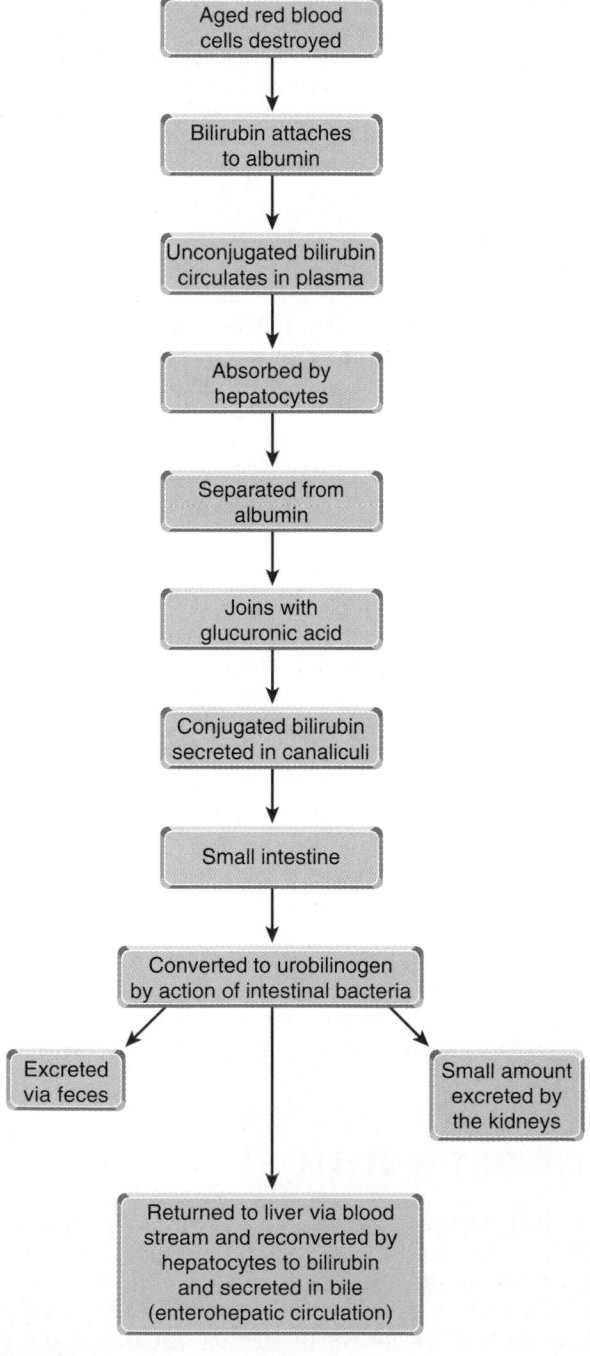

Figure 25–3
Bilirubin metabolism.

them to make them more suitable for excretion. When hepatic disorders are present, the liver's ability to chemically modify substances may be impaired. As a result, sensitivity to certain drugs, such as sedatives and hypnotics, may increase. The effects of hormones may be enhanced. For example, conversion of androgens to estrogens may increase, resulting in gynecomastia. Toxins usually metabolized and excreted via the liver may be returned to the circulatory system, as in increased ammonia levels, which affect acid-base balance and brain function.

STORAGE

About 450 mL of blood, or 10% of total blood volume, is normally circulating through the liver at a given time. During periods of hypotension and shock, the liver is capable of shunting extra blood to the systemic circulation. Because the liver is highly vascular, it has the capability of storing as much as 1 L of blood if the total blood volume rises above normal and pressure increases in the vena cava.

In addition to glycogen and amino acids, the liver stores vitamins A, D, and B_{12}, folic acid, and iron. Manganese, copper, and zinc, although found in other body tissues, are most concentrated in the liver. Vitamin K_1, found in foods that are ingested,

and vitamin K_2, produced by bacteria in the intestine, are stored to a limited degree in the liver. In the presence of liver disease, many of these stored substances may be depleted.

Clinical Manifestations of Hepatic Dysfunction

The major clinical manifestations associated with hepatic dysfunction are jaundice, portal hypertension and ascites, clotting disorders, hepatic encephalopathy, and nutritional deficiencies. Patients experiencing liver failure will usually exhibit all of these manifestations, which are summarized in Table 25–2.

JAUNDICE

Jaundice, also known as icterus, is a yellow discoloration of the skin, sclerae, and mucous membranes caused by elevated bilirubin levels in the blood. Jaundice is classified as hemolytic (prehepatic), hepatocellular (hepatic), or obstructive (intrahepatic or extrahepatic).

Table 25–2

Clinical Manifestations of Hepatic Dysfunction

Clinical Manifestation	Etiology	Nursing Assessment
Jaundice	Elevated blood bilirubin levels	Assess for yellow discoloration of skin, sclerae, and mucous membranes; dark urine; light or clay-colored stools; scratch marks or scratching.
Portal hypertension and ascites	Blood flow through liver obstructed, leading to elevated pressure in the portal system, which forces plasma filtrate into the peritoneal cavity	Monitor for weight gain, increased abdominal girth, dyspnea, and edema. Assess for taut skin over abdominal area. If patient has had a peritoneojugular shunt, monitor hematocrit levels, urinary output, and lung sounds.
Clotting disorders	Production of clotting factors in the liver may be decreased with liver disease, or impaired fat metabolism may cause interference with vitamin K utilization	Assess body surfaces for evidence of bleeding: purpura, spider angiomas, ecchymoses, petechiae. Assess stool and urine for presence of blood. Monitor prothrombin time.
Hepatic encephalopathy	Liver is unable to metabolize toxic substances produced in the intestines; exact pathophysiology unknown	Assess for change in mental status. Monitor blood ammonia levels and precipitating factors, especially diuretic therapy, excessive ingestion of protein and gastrointestinal bleeding Assess for fetor hepaticus and asterixis.
Nutritional deficiencies	Liver unable to metabolize, produce, or store essential nutrients	Assess for symptoms shown in Table 25–5.

Pathophysiology

Hemolytic jaundice occurs when red blood cells are destroyed at a rate that exceeds the liver's ability to remove bilirubin from the blood. A higher-than-normal amount of unconjugated bilirubin is present in the blood stream. Hemolytic jaundice is seen in pernicious anemia, in sickle-cell anemia, and in transfusion reactions.

In hepatocellular jaundice, liver cells are unable to metabolize bilirubin because of infection, chemical or drug toxicity, or hepatocyte necrosis. The uptake, conjugation, and excretion of bilirubin are usually impaired. When hepatocytes are damaged, intracellular enzymes are released into the circulation. Alanine aminotransferase and aspartate aminotransferase are sensitive indicators of liver cell injury and will be elevated when hepatocellular jaundice occurs. The level of both these enzymes is determined to differentiate between hemolytic jaundice and jaundice caused by liver disease. Hepatocellular jaundice is seen with hepatitis, cirrhosis, and liver cancer.

Obstructive jaundice occurs when the flow of bile is obstructed. The obstruction can be intrahepatic or extrahepatic. Intrahepatic obstructive jaundice involves obstruction of bile ductules within the liver. It can result from pressure created by inflammatory processes, as seen in cirrhosis and hepatitis. Both unconjugated and conjugated levels of serum bilirubin are elevated. Extrahepatic obstructive jaundice results from obstruction of bile flow through the common bile duct. Elevated conjugated bilirubin levels are seen with this form of jaundice. Elevated serum alkaline phosphatase levels are also found in obstructive jaundice because this enzyme, produced by the liver, is normally excreted with bile.

Clinical Manifestations

The patient with jaundice has a yellow discoloration of the skin and mucous membranes. In light-skinned people, the first site of yellow discoloration is usually the sclerae of the eye. This is an area rich in elastin, which has a special affinity for bilirubin. General skin color may range from a light yellow tint to a deep bronze color. In dark-skinned persons whose sclerae normally have a yellow tinge, jaundice is best identified by yellow discoloration of the hard palate. Pruritus occurs when bile salts, which are an irritant, are deposited in the skin.

Because bile cannot enter the intestine in normal quantities, the stool is lighter in color, progressing to a clay color in the absence of bile. Urine becomes a deep orange color and foams when shaken because bile is now excreted through the kidney.

Management

Because jaundice is a symptom of an underlying disorder, no specific medical interventions are used to treat it in the adult. Bile acid sequestrants, described in Highlight 25–1, may be prescribed to relieve pruritus.

NURSING PROCESS
Jaundice

Assessment

Monitor skin, urine, and stool color daily. Diminished evidence of jaundice in the skin, a decrease in the color intensity of the urine, and a return of color to the stool indicate an improved clinical status. Note evidence of scratching. Increased scratching indicates an increase of bile salt deposits in the skin, which accompanies an increased level of circulating unconjugated bilirubin. Because jaundice changes the physical appearance, these patients may withdraw or verbalize negative feelings. Observe the patient for evidence of decreased interpersonal relationships or decreased involvement in self-care activities.

Nursing Diagnoses and Planning

Nursing diagnoses and related expected patient outcomes commonly applicable to patients with jaundice include the following:

NDx: Risk for impaired skin integrity related to pruritus secondary to bile salt accumulation

Planning: Patient Outcomes
1. Patient's skin remains intact with no evidence of scratch marks.
2. Patient verbalizes a decrease in pruritus.

NDx: Body image disturbance related to altered skin pigmentation

Planning: Patient Outcomes
1. Patient verbalizes an acceptance of self in present condition.
2. Patient takes an active part in grooming activities.

Nursing Interventions and Evaluation

NDx: Risk for impaired skin integrity
Administer cool-water baths, with a water temperature of 32° to 37.8°C (90–100°F). Keep the room cool, apply lightweight bedding, and advise the patient to wear lightweight clothing. Warmth increases blood flow and results in increased bile salt deposits, leading to increased pruritus. Use a mild soap, such as castile or lanolin, or a soap substitute for bathing. Apply lotion gently to the skin every 8 hours. The alkalinizing effects of soap dry the skin, which intensifies pruritus. Lotion minimizes dryness and has a cooling effect. If prescribed, cornstarch, oatmeal powder, and baking soda baths have a soothing effect on the skin, which decreases pruritus. However, caution patients that bathing more than once a day may increase pruritus because of the drying effects of water. At all times, pat the skin dry rather than rubbing. Rubbing stimulates nerve endings and increases discomfort.

Trim and file nails to prevent injury to the skin. Mittens or white socks can be worn on the hands to

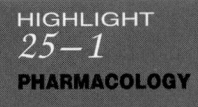 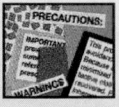

HIGHLIGHT 25–1 PHARMACOLOGY

Bile Acid Sequestrants

Definition:

Drugs that bind bile acids (resin) in the gastrointestinal tract. Colestipol hydrochloride (Colestid).

Action:

Bind with bile acids to form an insoluble complex that is excreted in the feces; they also increase cholesterol excretion.

Uses:

Relieve pruritus associated with elevated levels of bile acids and lower the cholesterol level in patients at risk for heart disease who do not respond to dietary treatment.

Side Effects:

Constipation, nausea, and abdominal discomfort.

Interactions:

May bind with oral drugs concurrently administered and prevent their absorption. They decrease the absorption of fat-soluble vitamins A, D, E, and K.

Nursing Implications:

Administer other drugs 1 hour before or 4 hours after to prevent drug binding. Must not be taken in dry form; esophageal irritation or blockage may result. Put dose on top of 4 to 6 oz of water, milk, or juice and let stand for 1 to 2 minutes. Stir and have patient drink medication while it is suspended in solution; will not dissolve in fluid. Supplemental vitamin therapy may be necessary. Monitor bowel movements. Constipation occurs in 20% of patients. Encourage high-bulk diet and adequate fluid intake (2500–3000 mL/day) if allowed. A stool softener may be required.

Geriatric Considerations:

The elderly are at increased risk for constipation and are more likely to develop a fecal impaction.

---

help prevent scratching. Administer bile acid sequestrants, if prescribed.

Provide diversional activities. Television, radio, books, board games, or other activities of interest help to distract the patient and lessen awareness of the pruritus.

NDx: Body image disturbance
Reinforce positive progress. Inform the patient when bilirubin levels are decreasing, urine color is less intense, and stool color is returning. Explain that these are indications that normal bile flow is returning and jaundice will be decreasing. Clarify any misconceptions that the patient may have. If the patient's liver dysfunction has a favorable prognosis, explain that jaundice will not remain after the underlying cause is treated. Provide reliable, accurate information to establish a trusting nurse-patient relationship.

Assist the patient with grooming activities to improve personal appearance. Encourage the patient to wear his or her own pajamas rather than a hospital gown. Assist the patient in choosing clothing colors that do not accentuate the jaundice. Assist the patient with grooming activities. These interventions allow the patient to maintain control and can help minimize social isolation.

Compare the patient's status with the expected outcomes. If the outcomes are not met, reassess the patient and revise the plan.

PORTAL HYPERTENSION AND ASCITES

Pathophysiology

Portal hypertension is elevated pressure within the portal venous blood vessels of the liver. This condition is usually associated with cirrhosis or cancer of the liver, although it can occur in some hematologic and cardiovascular diseases. In liver disease, portal hypertension develops when blood flow through the liver is obstructed because of destruction of hepatocytes, fat deposits, and fibrous tissue formation.

As portal blood flow through the liver becomes obstructed, collateral blood vessels and portal branch vessels enlarge as venous blood seeks an alternate route to the systemic circulation that bypasses the liver. Enlarged collateral channels develop between the portal and systemic veins that supply the esophagus, stomach, spleen, and rectum, and in the umbilical veins of the falciform ligament. The collateral vessels dilate because of high intravascular pressure caused by the shunting of blood from the portal vessels. They become tortuous and may rupture, as seen in esophageal varices, a complication of portal hypertension. Management of esophageal varices is discussed in Chapter 26. An enlarged spleen (splenomegaly) results from splenic vein congestion caused by high pressure in the portal system.

Ascites, the accumulation of fluid in the peritoneal cavity, occurs when elevated portal vessel pressure in the liver increases resistance to blood flow and forces protein-rich plasma filtrate into the hepatic lymphatic vessels. This filtrate oozes from the liver surface into the peritoneal cavity because the lymphatic vessels are unable to absorb the large quantity of filtrate.

The amount of ascitic fluid is further increased because the damaged hepatocytes are unable to produce albumin, which is essential for maintaining oncotic pressure within the circulatory system. Decreased albumin levels (hypoalbuminemia) cause decreased oncotic pressure, which results in a loss of fluid from the circulating blood volume and hemoconcentration. Fluid leaves the plasma and enters the peritoneal cavity and the interstitial spaces. Fluid in the interstitial spaces results in tissue edema.

In response to decreased circulating volume, the kidneys release renin, which increases secretion of aldosterone from the adrenal cortex and antidiuretic hormone from the hypothalamus. As a result, so-

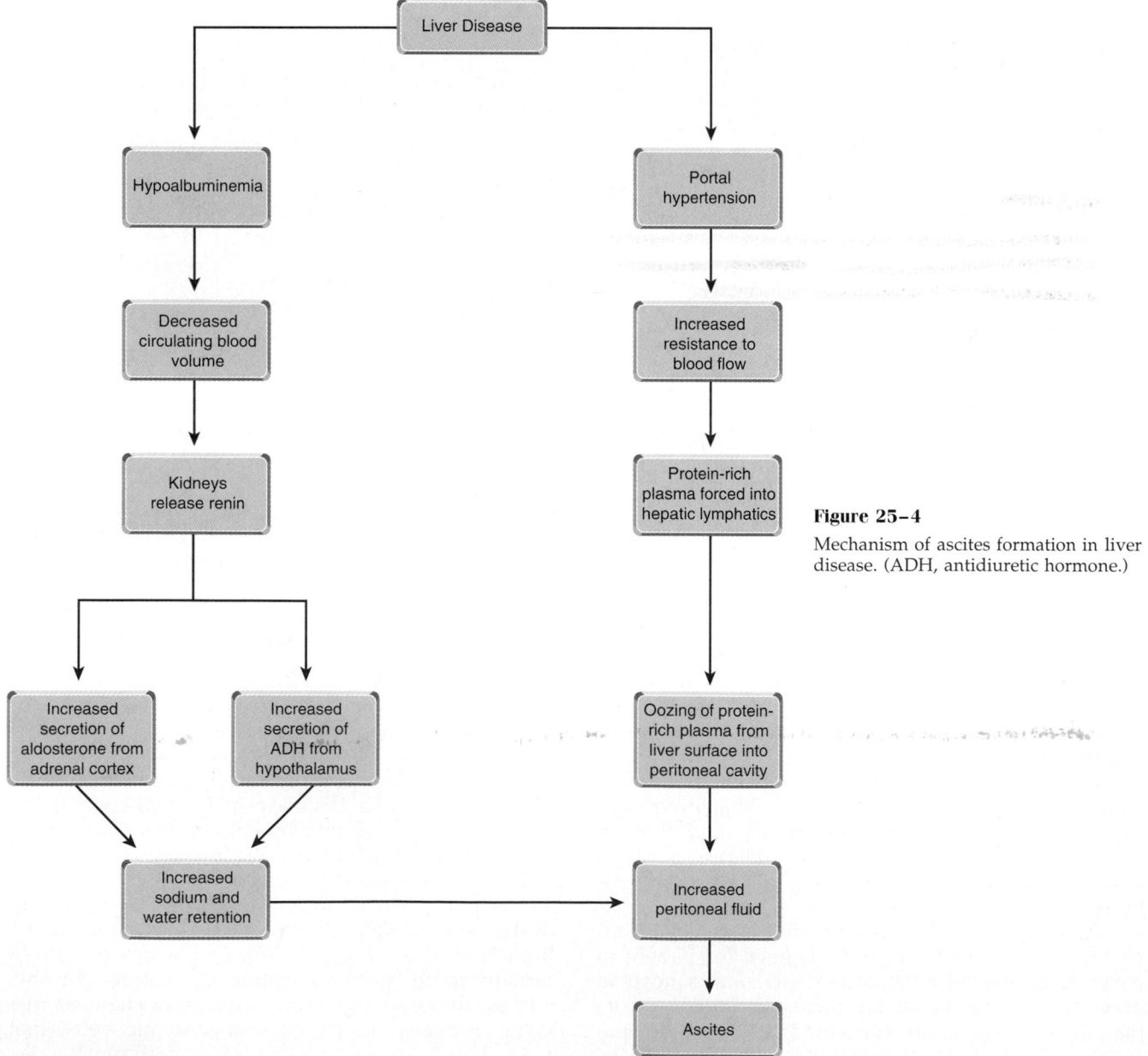

Figure 25–4

Mechanism of ascites formation in liver disease. (ADH, antidiuretic hormone.)

dium and water are retained. This further increases both ascites and edema. Figure 25–4 illustrates the mechanism of ascites formation in the presence of liver disease.

Clinical Manifestations

Portal hypertension will not be evident unless the patient has visibly dilated abdominal blood vessels (caput medusae), bleeding from collateral blood vessels, or ascites.

Ascites is suspected when a patient reports increased abdominal girth, unexplained weight gain, or both. As the amount of fluid increases in the peritoneal cavity, the abdomen becomes distended and the umbilicus may evert because of the pressure exerted by the fluid. When fluid accumulation approaches 1000 mL, a dull sound is heard when the patient is in the supine position and the abdomen is percussed over the fluid-filled area. If the patient is turned on the side, fluid shifts with gravity and a dull sound is percussed in the dependent area. Distended abdominal veins and striae (stretch marks) may also be present.

Fluid accumulation and displacement of the intestines in the peritoneal cavity may cause respiratory difficulty from pressure on the diaphragm. The lungs are unable to expand completely, resulting in shallow respirations.

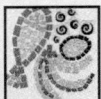

HIGHLIGHT
25–2
NUTRITION

Sample Daily Food Allowance for a 1000 mg Sodium-Restricted Diet

No salt is added during the preparation of foods or at meals.

Group	Daily Allowance	Sodium (mg)
Milk	2 cups	240
Meat, fish, or poultry (fresh or frozen)	5 oz	125
Egg	1 medium (1 oz meat may replace egg)	60
Whole-grain or enriched cereal (no sodium added)	1 serving (includes puffed wheat, puffed rice, shredded wheat, farina; no quick-cooking cereals or dry cereals with more than 5 mg sodium per serving)	0.5–5
Whole-grain enriched bread	6 slices	480
Potato, pasta, rice	1 medium potato or 1 cup cooked pasta or rice	2–6
Vegetables	1 cup (no carrots, kale, beet greens, chard, spinach, frozen peas, frozen lima beans, beets, celery, or white turnips; no vegetables packaged with added sodium)	2
Fruit	3–5 servings (includes 1 serving citrus fruit)	0–1
Butter, margarine	2 tsp	100

Foods that must be avoided:

Vegetable salts and flakes, such as garlic, onion, or celery salt; celery and parsley flakes

Salted foods, such as potato chips, popcorn, and pretzels

Prepared condiments, relishes, Worcestershire sauce, catsup, pickles, soy sauce, mustard, and olives

Prepackaged frozen foods, packaged mixes for sauces, gravies, and casseroles

Salt-preserved foods such as salted or smoked meats (bacon, corned beef, frankfurters, ham, kosher meats, luncheon meats), salted or smoked fish (herring, anchovies, frozen fish fillets), and sauerkraut

Canned soups

Meat extracts, bouillon cubes, and meat sauces

All canned meats and vegetables unless prepared without sodium

Cheese and peanut butter unless prepared without sodium

Packaged baking mixes or flour mixes unless prepared without sodium

Sherbet and flavored gelatins

Management

Treatment of portal hypertension requires identification of the underlying cause. Medical management of ascites may include bedrest with sodium and fluid restriction, pharmacotherapy with diuretic agents, administration of albumin, paracentesis, and surgical intervention.

DIETARY INTERVENTION. Ascitic fluid accumulation occurs when patients are in positive sodium balance as a result of excess aldosterone secretion. Therefore, sodium restriction decreases or stops the accumulation of ascitic fluid. A diet containing 1000 to 2000 mg of sodium is usually prescribed. Highlight 25–2 describes the daily food allowance for a patient on a 1000 mg sodium-restricted diet. A fluid restriction of 1000 to 1500 mL daily is maintained when patients have decreased blood serum sodium levels (hyponatremia), which usually reflects excess body water rather than decreased sodium levels.

PHARMACOTHERAPY. If there is no decrease in ascitic fluid accumulation with sodium restriction alone, diuretics are added to the treatment plan. Diuretics cause a loss of fluid from the plasma, which is replaced by the reabsorption of ascitic or edema fluid. Spironolactone (Aldactone) is the diuretic of choice for patients with mild to moderate sodium retention. This medication blocks the action of aldosterone and promotes sodium loss and potassium retention. If spironolactone does not produce adequate fluid loss within 1 week, furosemide (Lasix) is prescribed in combination with spironolactone. Highlight 25–3 summarizes patient information related to the use of diuretic therapy.

ALBUMIN THERAPY. Salt-poor human albumin is administered to increase plasma colloid osmotic pressure and to promote reabsorption of ascitic fluid. Because this therapy is very expensive and the results are only temporary, it is not a therapy of choice.

PARACENTESIS. Paracentesis is a procedure that removes fluid from the peritoneal cavity. It is performed either for diagnostic or palliative purposes. When ascitic fluid is requested for diagnostic study, only a small amount of fluid (50–100 mL) is usually aspirated. For the patient with large-volume ascites that interferes with eating and breathing, as much as 20 L of fluid may need to be removed (Runyon, 1993). Large-volume paracentesis may also be performed when fluid interferes with diagnostic visualization studies such as x-rays or abdominal ultrasonography.

Fluid removed from the peritoneal cavity contains large amounts of albumin, sodium, and potassium. Because this fluid rapidly reforms in the peritoneal cavity after removal, paracentesis is not a practical treatment for most patients with ascites. Intravenous administration of salt-poor albumin, which may be ordered during or after a therapeutic paracentesis, may help to slow the reaccumulation of ascitic fluid.

Paracentesis can be performed using a sterile 22-gauge, 1.5-inch needle for a diagnostic tap and an 18-gauge, 1.5-inch needle for a palliative tap. Following local anesthesia to the skin site, the needle, which is attached to a syringe, is inserted below the umbilicus. If a large amount of fluid is to be drained, tubing will be connected to the syringe to allow fluid to flow slowly over a period of 30 to 60 minutes.

This procedure may be carried out in a physician's office, ambulatory care setting, or at the bedside. Table 25–3 describes the nurse's role before, during and after a paracentesis.

LEVEEN SHUNT. Patients who have severe and incapacitating ascites that does not respond to dietary and diuretic therapy are candidates for a surgical procedure that drains ascitic fluid from the

---

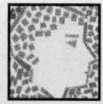

HIGHLIGHT
25–3

PATIENT EDUCATION

Self-Management of Diuretic Therapy

Diuretics are a class of drugs that increase water and electrolyte elimination via the kidneys. The mechanism of action varies depending on the medication prescribed. With all diuretics, except the potassium-sparing diuretics, potassium is excreted in addition to sodium. When a potassium-sparing diuretic is prescribed with other diuretics, potassium balance is usually maintained.

Instruct the patient to do the following:

Except if taking a potassium-sparing diuretic, eat foods high in potassium, such as whole-grain cereals, bananas, apricots, oranges, raisins, and potatoes.

Take the medication early in the day to avoid the need to urinate during the night.

Report vomiting, leg cramps, or muscle weakness. These may indicate a potassium level less than 3.5 mEq/L.

Report signs of dehydration: thirst, altered mental status, decreased urine output, and decreased skin turgor.

Notify physician if vomiting or diarrhea occurs that lasts longer than 1 day. This can cause electrolyte imbalances.

Check weight at least three times a week.

If the patient switched to a potassium-sparing diuretic or is taking a potassium-sparing diuretic in addition to another diuretic, caution the patient to omit all potassium supplements that may have been ordered previously. Hyperkalemia can result.

Table 25–3

Paracentesis

Nursing Actions	Rationale
BEFORE PROCEDURE	
Obtain written consent.	Invasive procedure
Have patient void immediately before procedure.	Prevents accidental puncture of the bladder
Position patient upright in a chair or on edge of bed with feet and back supported.	With patient in upright position, air inside the intestines allows them to float away from needle insertion site
Assess vital signs.	Baseline data for comparison
Cleanse skin below umbilicus with antiseptic solution.	Removes surface organisms to reduce risk of infection
DURING PROCEDURE	
Remain with patient.	Nurse's presence provides support
Monitor vital signs.	Close observation detects complications early; vascular collapse is preceded by increased pulse and decreased blood pressure
AFTER PROCEDURE	
Record the color and amount of fluid collected.	Color of fluid may indicate infection or bleeding; provides an accurate record of output.
Apply sterile pressure dressing to site and allow patient to assume a comfortable position.	A break in the skin is a potential site for infection; pressure reduces risk of bleeding
Monitor vital signs every 15 minutes for 1 hour, every 30 minutes for 2 hours, every hour for 2 hours, and then every 4 hours for 24 hours. Monitor dressing site for leakage of ascitic fluid each time vital signs checked.	Patient is monitored for evidence of delayed complications; hypovolemic shock can result from shift of fluid from circulatory system to peritoneum to replace aspirated fluid

peritoneal cavity into the superior vena cava. The LeVeen peritoneojugular shunt is a silicone catheter inserted and positioned surgically, as illustrated in Figure 25–5. One end of the catheter is implanted in the peritoneal cavity, and the other end is channeled through the subcutaneous tissue to the superior vena cava, where the end is implanted. A one-way, pressure-sensitive valve regulates the flow of ascitic fluid. When the patient inhales, the diaphragm descends and pressure in the peritoneal cavity increases. This causes the valve to open and fluid is transported to the superior vena cava. During exhalation, the valve closes and prevents backflow. Diuretic therapy is usually prescribed in conjunction with the LeVeen shunt.

The Denver shunt is a modification of the LeVeen shunt and is usually used when ascites results from malignancy. Malignant ascites contains particulate matter that may block flow of ascitic fluid through the tubing. The Denver shunt has a subcutaneous pump that can be compressed manually to irrigate the tubing and maintain patency.

The emptying of large amounts of fluid into the superior vena cava may additionally benefit the patient by producing hemodilution, an increase in cardiac output, improved renal blood flow, and a decrease in serum aldosterone level. Complications of the shunting procedure include infection, occlusion of the shunt, leakage of peritoneal fluid, and disseminated intravascular coagulation. As a result of endotoxins and coagulant precursors in the ascitic

fluid, some degree of disseminated intravascular coagulation develops in more than half of these patients. When this occurs, normal clotting factors are depleted, anticoagulants are released, and bleeding may occur. In most patients, the degree of bleeding is insignificant. However, if excessive bleeding occurs, the shunt is removed.

Although the shunt procedure provides patients with temporary relief from the symptoms of ascites, it does not correct the underlying problem. Usually, a shunt remains patent for a few days to 3 years. About half are patent after 1 year.

NURSING PROCESS
Ascites

Assessment

Assess for changes in weight, abdominal girth, and degree of edema. Increasing weight, abdominal girth, and edema indicate fluid retention. Note the appearance of taut, shiny skin over the abdomen, caused when fluid accumulates in the peritoneal cavity and stretches the skin. Observe the patient for difficulty in breathing. Ascites presses on the diaphragm and prevents total lung expansion. Examine all skin surfaces for evidence of redness or breakdown. Fluid accumulation in the tissues places the patient at risk for skin breakdown. Imposed bedrest increases the risk even further.

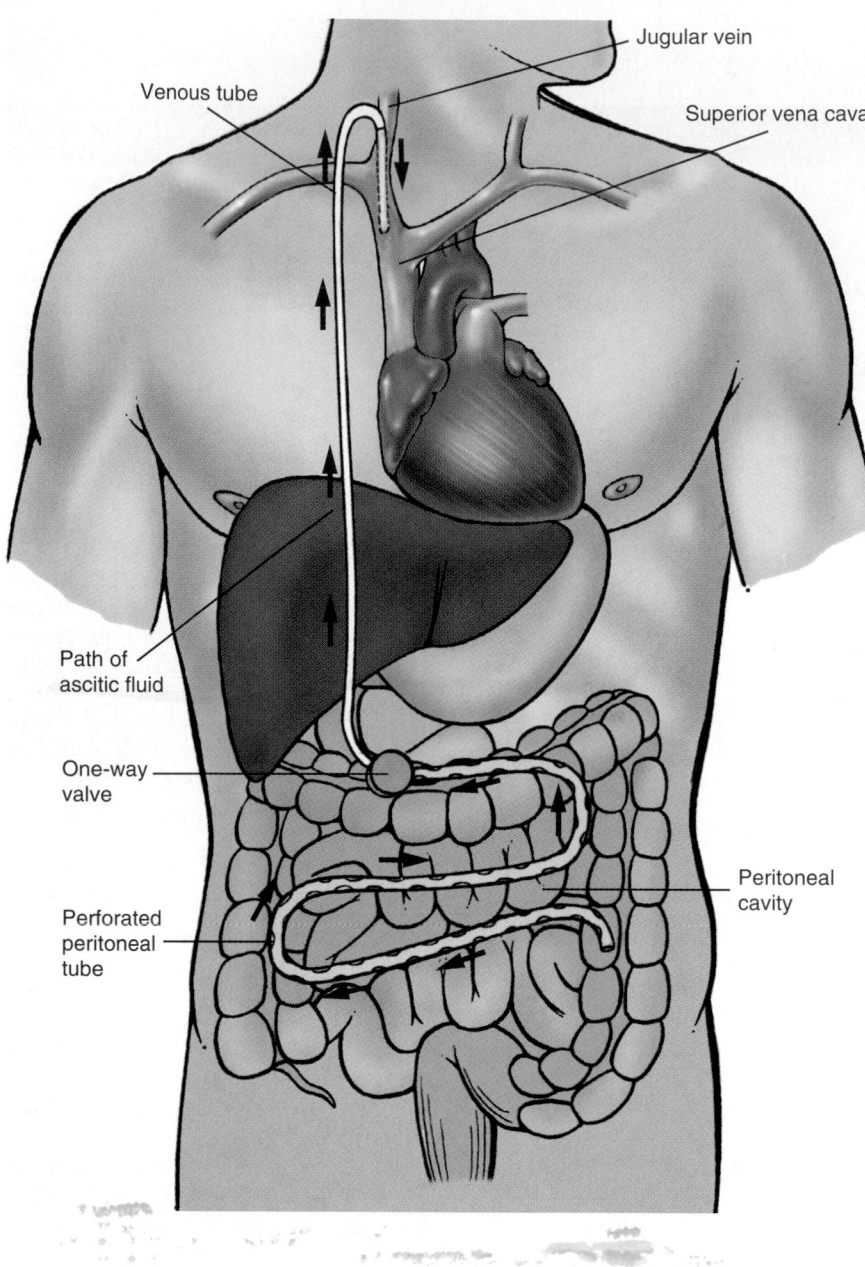

Jugular vein

Venous tube

Superior vena cava

Path of ascitic fluid

One-way valve

Perforated peritoneal tube

Peritoneal cavity

Figure 25–5

LeVeen shunt. Arrows show direction of flow of ascitic fluid out of the peritoneal cavity, through the shunt, into the superior vena cava.

Assess the postoperative patient who has had a peritoneojugular shunt to determine shunt function. Assess abdominal girth, body weight, hematocrit level, and urinary output to establish a baseline for comparison with later measurements. A decrease in girth, body weight, and hematocrit level and an increase in urinary output indicate that the shunt is operating effectively.

Also observe the patient for early signs of disseminated intravascular coagulation. These signs include bleeding of the mucous membranes, hematuria, oozing of blood from intravenous or puncture sites, and changes in mental status. Coagulation studies will indicate a decreased platelet count, low levels of fibrinogen, increased fibrin-split products,

and prolonged prothrombin times and partial thromboplastin times. Report these findings immediately to the physician.

Observe the dressing site for evidence of peritoneal fluid leakage, which may predispose the patient to infection.

Nursing Diagnoses and Planning

Nursing diagnoses and related expected patient outcomes commonly applicable to patients with ascites include the following:

NDx: Ineffective breathing pattern related to pressure on the diaphragm from ascites

Planning: Patient Outcomes
1. Patient's respiratory rate remains between 12 and 20 per minute.
2. Patient has full chest expansion with each respiration.
3. Patient verbalizes ability to breathe with less difficulty.

NDx: Fluid volume excess related to the accumulation of fluid in the peritoneal cavity and dependent areas of the body

Planning: Patient Outcomes
1. Patient's abdominal girth decreases daily until reaching baseline girth.
2. Patient's body weight decreases daily until reaching baseline weight.

NDx: Risk for impaired skin integrity related to ascites and edema

Planning: Patient Outcomes
1. Patient's skin remains intact.

Nursing diagnoses and related expected patient outcomes most commonly applicable to patients who undergo a peritoneojugular shunt procedure include the following:

NDx: Risk for fluid volume excess (LeVeen shunt) related to too rapid removal of fluid from the peritoneal cavity to the superior vena cava

Planning: Patient Outcomes
1. Patient's electrolyte values remain within normal limits.
2. Patient's lungs remain clear.
3. Patient's vital signs remain stable.

NDx: Risk for altered health maintenance (LeVeen shunt) related to lack of knowledge of signs of shunt failure

Planning: Patient Outcomes
1. Patient states intent to weigh self daily.
2. Patient demonstrates ability to weigh self accurately.
3. Patient lists situations that require physician notification.

NDx: Risk for ineffective management of therapeutic regimen (individuals) related to lack of knowledge of causes of ascites, pharmacologic therapy, nutritional requirements, and need for alcohol restriction

Planning: Patient Outcomes
1. Patient, family member, and/or significant other verbalizes basic understanding of the cause, treatment plan, and need to initiate lifestyle changes.

Nursing Interventions and Evaluation

NDx: *Ineffective breathing pattern*
Position the patient in a semi-Fowler's or high Fowler's position as tolerated to promote maximal chest expansion by decreasing pressure from ascitic fluid and internal organs on the diaphragm. Instruct the patient to deep-breathe every 2 hours to promote maximal lung expansion. Auscultate the lungs for diminished breath sounds every 4 hours. Compare the right upper and lower lobes with the left upper and lower lobes. Diminished breath sounds, especially in the lower lobes, indicate inadequate chest expansion. Monitor vital signs every 4 hours to identify early indications of oxygen deficit. Manifestations of hypoxemia include

> Restlessness
> Confusion
> Rising, bounding pulse
> Rising systolic blood pressure
> Rapid respirations

NDx: *Fluid volume excess*
Weigh the patient daily before breakfast but after he or she has urinated. Have the patient wear similar clothes and use the same scale each day to ensure consistency. A change of 1 kg (2.2 lbs) is equivalent to 1 L of fluid. As much as 2.7 to 3.6 kg (6–8 lb) can be gained before physical signs of ascites or edema are evident. Measure the abdominal girth daily. Mark the abdomen with ink to indicate the point at which the measurement is taken to ensure consistent comparison with previous measurements. Abdominal girth decreases as ascites decreases.

Monitor fluid intake and output daily. Fluid intake exceeding output may indicate fluid retention. Limit fluids to the prescribed amount, spread out over a 24-hour period, with the greatest amount of fluid given during patient's waking hours. Allow the patient choices in oral fluid intake, thus providing a sense of control. Administer prescribed diuretics. Notify the dietary department and determine how much fluid will be served with meals. Subtract this from the total fluid allowance to prevent excess intake. Remember that fluids given with medications are included in the daily fluid intake. Provide the patient with mouthwash for oral hygiene every 4 hours to decrease thirst. Do not use lemon-glycerin swabs to moisten the mouth. Glycerin is an astringent and has a drying effect on mucous membranes.

NDx: *Risk for impaired skin integrity*
Inspect the patient's skin daily for evidence of redness or skin breakdown, especially in dependent body areas. These include the sacral area for a patient on bedrest, and the lower extremities for a patient out of bed. Edema causes pressure on the blood vessels and impedes blood flow to peripheral vessels. Obstructed capillary blood flow leads to tissue ischemia and necrosis. Use pressure-relieving pads on the bed and chair to provide more even weight distribution. Teach the patient the importance of changing position every 2 hours. Provide a bed trapeze if the patient is capable of using it. The trapeze bar allows the patient to lift rather than pull the body when repositioning and therefore decreases shearing force, a major contributor to skin break-

down. A footboard to prevent the patient from sliding down in bed further minimizes shearing force. If the patient is permitted out of bed, limit time in the chair to no more than 2 hours unless the patient can shift his or her weight unassisted.

Avoid injections when possible. If injections must be administered, inspect injection sites carefully. Do not administer injections in sites that are edematous. Absorption of drugs is decreased in these areas because of fluid accumulation and decreased blood supply. In addition, drugs injected into edematous areas can act as irritants and predispose to skin breakdown.

Keep bed linens and the patient's clothing dry. Moisture increases the incidence of skin breakdown fivefold. Keep the skin dry and apply a thin layer of lotion daily. Moisture, like excessive dryness, decreases the skin's resistance to infection. Application of lotion massages the skin and increases blood supply to the area.

NDx: Risk for fluid volume excess

Monitor serum sodium, serum osmolarity, urine specific gravity, and hematocrit every 4 hours during the immediate postoperative period to identify early signs of excess hemodilution. Monitor respiratory rate and auscultate the lungs for crackles (rales) every 2 hours. Excess hemodilution, dyspnea, tachycardia, or crackles may indicate that fluid is being removed too quickly from the peritoneal cavity. To slow the rate of fluid flow from the peritoneal cavity, place the patient in a sitting position. This action increases the difference in pressures between the peritoneal and thoracic cavities, thus interrupting the flow of peritoneal fluid into the superior vena cava. Exhaling against a closed glottis also decreases flow. Monitor intake and output. Examine skin and mucous membranes daily. Decreased skin turgor and dry mucous membranes indicate fluid depletion.

NDx: Risk for altered health maintenance

Instruct the patient to weigh himself or herself each morning before eating breakfast but after urinating to monitor fluid volume status. Observe the patient carry out the procedure without assistance to determine accuracy and evaluate learning. Teach the patient to notify the physician if clothing becomes tight at the waist, weight rises more than 0.45 kg (1 lb) per day or 1.4 kg (3 lb) per week, urinary output decreases, or breathing becomes difficult. Highlight 25–4 provides self-care guidelines for the patient with a LeVeen shunt.

NDx: Risk for ineffective management of therapeutic regimen (individuals)

Teach the patient and family about the formation of ascites, its cause, and its treatment.

Use a diagram such as Figure 25–4 to illustrate the formation of ascites and thus facilitate learning. Explain the prescribed diuretic therapy, making sure the patient or family knows the name, dose, side

---

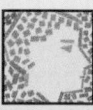

HIGHLIGHT 25–4

PATIENT EDUCATION

Self-Management of a LeVeen Shunt

Instruct the patient to do the following:

Use strict aseptic technique when caring for the incision.

Examine the wound daily for signs of infection, including redness, edema, purulent discharge, increasing tenderness.

Perform deep-breathing at frequent intervals during the day to maintain shunt patency.

Measure abdominal girth daily.

Record weight obtained each day before breakfast but after voiding.

Report the following symptoms to the physician immediately: increased weight, increased abdominal girth, decreased urinary output, respiratory distress, edema, signs of wound infection.

Keep appointments for follow-up evaluations with the physician.

---

effects, and frequency of medication to be taken. Provide important information on self-management of diuretic therapy in writing so the patient and the family can refer to it later as needed (see Highlight 25–1).

Explain any dietary sodium restrictions prescribed to reduce ascites. Give the patient literature describing the sodium content of common food items and stress the need to adhere to the prescribed diet. Instruct the patient to eat frequent, small meals to avoid gastric distention. Refer the patient to a dietitian for assistance with meal planning if needed.

Explain the need for fluid restriction if ordered. With patient participation, plan a schedule for taking fluids during the waking hours. Use household equivalents rather than the metric system. Remind the patient that any fluid taken with meals and medications must be included as part of the amount allotted. Advise the patient to rinse the mouth with mouth wash or brush teeth frequently to decrease thirst. Stress the importance of being weighed twice weekly and the need to report a gain of more than 1 kg (2.2 lbs) to the physician promptly.

Instruct the patient to abstain from alcoholic beverages and explain that alcohol will increase irritation of the liver and interfere with recovery. Help the patient understand the adverse effects of drinking and make appropriate lifestyle changes. If necessary, counsel the patient to seek assistance from Alcoholics Anonymous or others who help individuals recover from alcohol abuse.

Compare the patient's status with the expected outcomes. If the outcomes are not met, reassess the patient and revise the plan.

CLOTTING DISORDERS

Pathophysiology

A healthy liver synthesizes a number of clotting factors, including factors V, VII, IX, and X, fibrinogen, and prothrombin. With liver disease, production of these factors may decline. Altered fat metabolism also interferes with the utilization of vitamin K, which further decreases synthesis of clotting factors.

Clinical Manifestations

Bleeding is frequently seen in patients with hepatic dysfunction. Bleeding may be noted from the gums after brushing the teeth, from the nose after forceful blowing, as petechial hemorrhages of the eye, or as skin or mucous membrane lesions that result from spontaneous rupture of small blood vessels. The most common lesions are:

- Petechiae: pinhead-size, purplish hemorrhagic areas
- Purpura: larger hemorrhagic areas up to 1 cm in diameter
- Ecchymoses: large irregularly shaped hemorrhagic areas
- Spider angiomas: small hemorrhagic areas with numerous dilated vessels radiating outward.

Though not always visible, blood may also be present in the urine and stool.

Management

A parenteral aqueous solution of vitamin K is prescribed when prothrombin production is decreased because of obstruction of bile flow. Parenteral vitamin K is absorbed in the absence of bile and can be used for the production of prothrombin. If the liver has ceased to produce clotting factors because of hepatocyte damage, fresh plasma or packed red blood cells may be indicated.

NURSING PROCESS
Risk for Bleeding

Assessment

Observe all body surfaces and mucous membranes daily to identify bleeding sites, precipitating factors, and amount of bleeding. Monitor prothrombin time, platelet count, and other clotting factors. Monitor all body fluids and stool for the presence of blood. Observe for excessive menstrual bleeding.

Nursing Diagnoses and Planning

Nursing diagnoses and related expected patient outcomes commonly applicable to patients at risk for bleeding include the following:

NDx: Risk for injury related to interference with the clotting mechanism

Planning: Patient outcomes

1. Patient avoids activities that increase the risk of bleeding.

Nursing Interventions and Evaluation

NDx: Risk for injury

Instruct the patient to avoid all substances and activities that may precipitate bleeding. These include alcohol, all nonprescription drugs containing aspirin, coarse foods, and large meals. Gastrointestinal bleeding is precipitated when the gastrointestinal tract is irritated. Forceful coughing, straining at stool, and heavy lifting are also contraindicated. Excessive pressure within the thoracic or abdominal cavities may cause bleeding. Test all urine, stool, and emesis for occult blood because small amounts of bleeding may not be visible to the naked eye. Provide a soft toothbrush to minimize gum bleeding while brushing, and substitute foam swabs if bleeding continues. Male patients should shave with an electric razor. Take oral or tympanic temperatures to minimize irritation to blood vessels in the rectal area. If the patient is confused or agitated, pad the side rails to decrease the risk of injury.

Because frequent diagnostic blood studies are required with hepatic disorders, group the patient's tests to limit the number of venipunctures needed and use the smallest gauge needle possible. Apply pressure to all venipuncture sites for at least 3 minutes or until bleeding stops. Coagulation may require up to 10 minutes.

Compare the patient's status with the expected outcomes. If the outcomes are not met, reassess the patient and revise the plan.

HEPATIC ENCEPHALOPATHY

The term *hepatic encephalopathy* is used to describe a group of manifestations of impaired neurologic function that are experienced by patients with advanced liver disease. The syndrome is frequently referred to as hepatic coma.

Pathophysiology

The exact pathophysiology of hepatic encephalopathy is unclear. However, it is known that the liver's inability to metabolize and cleanse the blood of ammonia and mercaptans (toxic substances produced in the intestines) is a major contributor to the problem. Ammonia is produced by intestinal bacteria as an end-product of protein metabolism. Mercaptans are produced when sulfur-containing compounds are metabolized in the intestine. These substances alter metabolism in the central nervous system, possibly by interfering directly with brain carbohydrate metabolism, or indirectly by causing formation of other neurotoxic substances. Actual blood ammonia levels do not always correlate directly with the se-

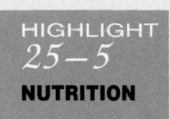
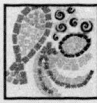

HIGHLIGHT 25–5

NUTRITION

Sample Daily Food Allowances for a 40 g Protein-Restricted Diet

Food Source	Protein Supplied
1 cup milk	8 g
2 eggs or	12 g (eggs)
2 oz of meat	19–20 g (meat)
3 slices of bread	6 g
½ cup of cereal (cooked)	1.5 g
1 potato	5 g
1 cup of vegetables	1–2 g
2 servings of fruit	2 g
2 tbsp of cream	5 g
Butter	Trace
Jelly	Trace
Sugar	0
Nonprotein foods to supply caloric requirements	0

In a restricted-protein diet, the protein source should be primarily from animal food sources containing high-quality proteins: meat, eggs, dairy products, poultry.

If the patient cannot take food by mouth, enteral feedings of Hepatic-Aid II Instant Drink or Travasorb Hepatic Diet may be substituted.

thought processes, and slurred speech. Determine orientation to person, place, and time. Assess for changes in psychomotor function. Request a handwriting sample for comparison with later samples. Assess for asterixis and fetor hepaticus. Note blood ammonia levels and potassium levels. Increasing ammonia or decreasing potassium may indicate development of hepatic encephalopathy. Assess for the presence of treatable precipitating factors, such as diuretic therapy, gastrointestinal bleeding, and surgical procedures that place the patient at increased risk for hepatic encephalopathy. Assess family members' understanding of hepatic encephalopathy. Family members may not be prepared to deal with the rapid deterioration in mental function.

Nursing Diagnoses and Planning

Nursing diagnoses and related expected patient outcomes commonly applicable to patients with hepatic encephalopathy include the following:

NDx: Risk for injury related to altered thought processes secondary to impaired liver function

Planning: Patient outcomes
1. Patient remains free of injury.

NDx: Altered family processes related to family member with hepatic encephalopathy

Planning: Patient outcomes
1. Family members verbalize their concerns to nursing staff.

NDx: Risk for ineffective management of therapeutic regimen (individuals) related to lack of knowledge of pharmacologic therapy, nutritional plan, and signs and symptoms of neurologic impairment secondary to hepatic encephalopathy

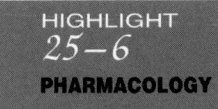
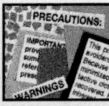

HIGHLIGHT 25–6

PHARMACOLOGY

Neomycin Sulfate

Definition:

Aminoglycoside antibiotic; anti-infective.

Action:

Destroys bacteria by inhibiting protein synthesis; broad-spectrum antibacterial activity.

Uses:

Reduces the number of ammonia-producing organisms in the intestine.

Side Effects:

Ototoxicity and nephrotoxicity. Mild laxative effect; diarrhea, nausea, vomiting.

Interactions:

Increased risk for ototoxicity when administered with loop diuretics (furosemide and ethacrynic acid).

Nursing Implications:

Monitor for evidence of ototoxicity: diminished hearing, tinnitus, vertigo, loss of balance, or altered gait in ambulatory patients. Monitor urinary output. Notify physician if output decreases. Provide adequate hydration. Test urine for evidence of cells or casts. Compare baseline and periodic audiometric and renal studies for early detection of toxicity. Be aware that neomycin can cause suprainfection of the bowel and intestinal malabsorption syndrome.

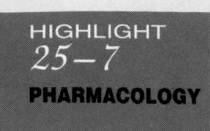
HIGHLIGHT
25—7
PHARMACOLOGY
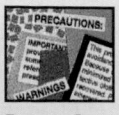

Lactulose

Definition:

Colonic acidifier; hyperosmotic laxative.

Action:

Acidifies colonic contents, resulting in the retention of ammonia in the colon as ammonium ion. Because the colon is more acidic that the blood, ammonia migrates from the blood to the colon to form ammonium ion. The laxative action of lactulose then expels the trapped ammonium ion from the colon.

Uses:

Reduces blood ammonia level in hepatic encephalopathy by 25 to 50%.

Side Effects:

Cramps, borborygmi, distention, flatulence, and diarrhea; hypernatremia due to water loss.

Interactions:

Nonabsorbable antacids inhibit desired effect of lactulose.

Nursing Implications:

Assess patient's mental status frequently during therapy. Improvement usually occurs within 24 to 48 hours. Monitor stools for diarrhea, which indicates that the dose should be decreased until the patient has two or three soft stools per day. Lactulose enemas may be used when oral administration is contraindicated because of the danger of aspiration or if the patient is intubated. 300 mL of lactulose and 700 mL of water are administered rectally and must be retained for 30 to 60 minutes.

Geriatric Considerations:

The elderly are at increased risk of hypernatremia because of reduced capacity to adjust to fluid loss.

Planning: Patient outcomes
1. Patient and/or family verbalizes a basic understanding of factors involved in the development of hepatic encephalopathy, the treatment plan, and signs and symptoms of increasing neurologic impairment.

Nursing Interventions and Evaluation

NDx: Risk for injury

Monitor level of consciousness, orientation, rate of speech, and response time every 4 hours. Ask the patient to state his or her name and the date and month and to identify present location. Request a daily sample of handwriting, either a short sentence or the patient's name. A decreasing level of consciousness, disorientation, slurred speech, prolonged response time, and difficulty writing indicate that the patient's condition is deteriorating. Monitor for the irregular, jerking movements of asterixis every 4 hours. This is the most common sign of impending coma. Restrict protein intake and administer neomycin or lactulose, or both, as prescribed. Decreased ammonia levels correlate with improvement in the patient's condition. Provide increased carbohydrates for energy and to spare protein from being broken down. Monitor daily serum potassium levels. De-

creased potassium levels, which may occur with diuretic therapy, can precipitate coma. The use of potassium-sparing diuretics minimizes this risk.

Keep side rails up and the bed in low position at all times. If the patient is disoriented or comatose, continue to identify yourself on entering the room and explain all procedures. Keep a night-light on during sleeping hours.

NDx: Altered family processes

Provide an explanation of hepatic encephalopathy in understandable terms. Keep the family informed of the patient's progress on a daily basis. Allow family members to visit with minimal interruption. Include the family in care if they desire to take part. Provide a private place, away from the patient's room, for family to ask questions and discuss progress. Include the family in nursing care conferences when possible. Illness of one family member affects the family unit. Successful coping strategies require that the family, with the support of the professional health-care team, acknowledge the problem, accept it, and adjust to its consequences.

NDx: Risk for ineffective management of therapeutic regimen (individuals)

Teach the patient and caregiver about factors contributing to the development of hepatic encephalopathy. Stress the importance of avoiding alcohol, sedatives, and high-protein foods to prevent further neurologic changes.

Be certain to modify teaching to the degree of the patient's neurologic impairment. For example, if the patient is in a stuporous state and is being discharged home, instruct the caregiver on activities of daily living skills such as bathing, dressing, and toileting the patient. Also stress the importance of safety, the need for a hospital bed with side rails elevated, and round-the-clock supervision.

Instruct the patient and caregiver about any protein restriction ordered to prevent further neurologic deterioration. Discuss the need for extra carbohydrate (unless contraindicated) to spare protein breakdown, thus reducing ammonia production. Collaborate with the dietitian in making sure the patient and caregiver understand the prescribed diet (which may also include a sodium restriction) before discharge.

Explain the purpose of bowel-cleansing medication and make sure the patient or caregiver knows the name, dose, side effects, and frequency of the prescribed medication. Inform the patient and caregiver to expect two to three soft bowel movements daily and to promptly notify the health care provider if constipation develops.

Instruct the caregiver to observe for and immediately report any change in neurologic function, such as asterixis, disorientation, or lethargy. Refer the patient to the local community health nurse to monitor compliance with the therapeutic regimen as well as for the provision of emotional support.

Compare the patient's status with the expected outcomes. If the outcomes are not met, reassess the patient and revise the plan.

NUTRITIONAL DEFICIENCIES

Because the liver performs so many varied functions, hepatic disorders can affect digestion, absorption, metabolism, and storage of nutrients.

Pathophysiology
Anorexia, the absence of hunger, is frequently seen with hepatic disorders. Regulation of food intake is controlled by feeding centers at separate sites in the hypothalamus. The satiety centers are stimulated by high blood levels of glucose and free fatty acids after a meal and cause a decreased desire for food. Although the exact cause of anorexia is unknown, the slowed metabolism of fatty acids may be a factor that causes a feeling of "fullness" and, therefore, a lack of appetite. Nausea and vomiting, also seen in the patient with hepatic dysfunction, may result from slowed or incomplete metabolism of body wastes by the liver. The presence of anorexia, nausea, and vomiting presents a challenge to health-care providers because nutrients are essential for regeneration of hepatocytes. When intake is inadequate to

meet the body's needs, stored nutrients are depleted.

The most pronounced nutritional deficiencies are seen in patients with alcohol-related liver disease. In the liver, alcohol is converted to acetaldehyde, with excessive amounts of hydrogen resulting from this reaction. Acetaldehyde is toxic to the liver and causes inflammation and hepatocyte necrosis. The hydrogen replaces fatty acid as a fuel, and fat accumulates in the liver. Because this fat occupies most of the volume of the hepatocytes, normal cell functions are interrupted. When alcohol consumption is stopped, fat deposits disappear within 3 to 6 weeks.

In addition to the problems caused directly by alcohol intake, the chronic alcoholic is usually malnourished because of inadequate nutrient intake. Alcohol replaces food in the diet. When nutrients are ingested, there is malabsorption of thiamine, vitamin B_{12}, folic acid, and ascorbic acid as a result of inflammation of the gastrointestinal tract. Because hepatocytes are inflamed, they cannot activate vitamin D, vitamin B_6, and thiamine. To metabolize the alcohol, increased amounts of the B vitamins are needed by the body, and liver stores are depleted.

Regardless of the cause, all patients with liver disease are at risk for nutritional deficiencies when hepatocytes cannot perform normal functions. Protein synthesis is impaired. Stored proteins are exhausted, which results in muscle wasting and inability to repair and regenerate damaged tissues. Also, decreased levels of the plasma protein albumin result in fluid imbalance from reduced intravascular oncotic pressure. Interference with carbohydrate metabolism depletes glycogen stores. Proteins are used for energy, further depleting protein stores. Hypoglycemia results when both glycogenolysis and gluconeogenesis are no longer possible. Inadequate production of bile salts causes malabsorption of fats and fat-soluble vitamins. Fats that cannot be absorbed are excreted in the stool (steatorrhea) and deprive the body of substantial calories, which contributes to weight loss and malnutrition. Because calcium binds to fatty acids, calcium is excreted in the stool and calcium deficits occur.

Clinical Manifestations
Patients with nutritional deficiencies exhibit a wide variety of signs and symptoms. Table 25–5 summarizes the major clinical characteristics of nutrient deficiencies associated with hepatic disorders.

Management
A high-protein, moderate-fat, high-carbohydrate diet is recommended for patients with liver disease to promote positive nitrogen balance, correct undernutrition, replenish plasma protein, and promote regeneration of functioning liver tissue to minimize the risk of hepatic encephalopathy. Protein is restricted when hepatic encephalopathy is present. Sodium restriction is required if ascites and edema are present.

A vitamin supplement containing vitamin B com-

Table 25–5

Clinical Characteristics of Nutritional Deficiencies Associated with Hepatic Disorders

Deficient Nutrient	Clinical Characteristics
Protein	Muscle wasting
	Impaired tissue repair
	Decreased synthesis of plasma proteins
Carbohydrate	Hypoglycemia
Fat	Steatorrhea
Vitamin A	Overgrowth of epidermal cells
Vitamin D	Osteomalacia (bone softening)
Calcium	Osteomalacia
Vitamin K	Clotting disorder
Thiamine	Dermatitis, neuritis, neuropathy
Niacin	Muscle weakness, anorexia
Folic acid	Anemia
Vitamin B$_{12}$	Anemia, neuritis, glossitis
Vitamin C	Anemia, weakness, decreased appetite, inflamed gums, delayed wound healing
Iron	Anemia

plex, especially folic acid and thiamin, is recommended. Water-soluble forms of vitamins A, D, and E are given if steatorrhea is present. Vitamin K is administered if prothrombin time is prolonged. Antiemetic agents may be prescribed to relieve symptoms of nausea and vomiting, thereby increasing the potential for improvement in appetite.

NURSING PROCESS
Nutritional Deficiencies

Assessment

Obtain a complete dietary history to determine dietary patterns. One method to assess nutritional intake is to ask the patient to recall all intake for the previous 3-day period. Include between-meal and bedtime snacks as well as meals. Determine drinking habits, including how long the patient has consumed alcohol, how often consumption occurs, the amount consumed, and the type of alcoholic beverage. Assess for the clinical manifestations of specific nutrient deficiencies (see Table 25–5).

Nursing Diagnoses and Planning

Nursing diagnoses and related expected patient outcomes commonly applicable to patients with nutritional deficiencies include the following:

NDx: Altered nutrition: less than body requirements related to nausea, vomiting, anorexia, or inadequate dietary intake

Planning: Patient outcomes
1. Patient eats 75 to 100% of all meals.
2. Patient has a steady weight gain with no evidence of fluid retention.
3. Patient outlines a 3-day meal plan.
4. Patient verbalizes the importance of avoiding alcohol.

Nursing Interventions and Evaluation

NDx: Altered nutrition: less than body requirements
If the patient is vomiting, administer the prescribed antiemetic agent 30 to 45 minutes before meals. Most antiemetic drugs require at least 20 to 30 minutes to reach effective levels. Provide mouth care before each meal to remove unpleasant tastes and stimulate a desire for food. Offer clear liquids (gelatin, tea without milk, ginger ale, or apple juice), 60 mL/hour, to the patient who cannot tolerate solid food. Gradually increase the amount as tolerated by the patient.

Provide five or six small meals rather than three large meals when anorexia is present. Large meals are unappealing during anorexia and may discourage the patient. Consider the patient's food preferences in planning meals. Arrange to have foods with the highest caloric intake served at the time the patient feels most like eating. This increases the potential of the patient eating adequate amounts of protein and calories. Offer fruit juices between meals. Juices have a protein-sparing effect, providing vitamins and extra calories.

As the patient's condition improves, explain his or her nutritional needs and assist in choosing meals for the next day. Provide the patient with written information describing the prescribed diet and the food pyramid. Review materials with the patient daily. When the patient can outline the prescribed diet, ask him or her to outline a 1-day meal plan for home use. If successful, ask him or her to outline a 3-day plan. Explain the risks of alcohol ingestion, informing the patient that alcohol is toxic to the liver. Also, because of its "empty calorie" effect, it decreases appetite.

Compare the patients' status with the expected outcomes. If the outcomes are not met, reassess the patient and revise the plan.

Nursing care for the patient experiencing major clinical manifestations of hepatic dysfunction is presented in Nursing Care Guide 25–1.

*A*ssessment of Liver Status

PATIENT HISTORY

When collecting a history, determine whether the patient has any complaints related to the clinical manifestations of liver disease. Areas to focus on are

Text continued on page 1158

Nursing Care Guide 25–1

Patients with Major Clinical Manifestations of Liver Dysfunction

Assessment Findings: Patient with ascites complains of "feeling tired almost all the time." Shortness of breath is noted after walking more than a few steps. Respirations are 26 per minute and shallow. Abdominal girth has increased 10 cm and the abdomen is dull to percussion.

Nursing Diagnosis: Ineffective breathing pattern related to pressure on the diaphragm from ascites

Patient Outcomes	Nursing Interventions	Rationale
Patient's vital signs remain within normal limits, with respirations between 12 and 20 per minute with full chest expansion.	Elevate the head of the bed 45 to 90 degrees.	Promotes maximum chest expansion and relieves pressure from ascites.
	Instruct patient to deep-breathe every 2 hours.	Encourages maximum chest expansion.
	Monitor vital signs and auscultate lungs every 4 hours.	Facilitates early identification of decreased air exchange and oxygen deficit.
	Use pulse oximetry to check O_2 saturation every 4 hours.	

Evaluation: Compare the patient's status with the expected outcomes. If the outcomes are not met, reassess the patient and revise the plan.

Assessment Findings: Patient indicates pants are tight around the waist and a 4.5 to 5.5 kg (10–12 lbs) weight gain has been noticed over the past 2 weeks. Abdomen is distended, shiny, and taut, with striae. Edema of both ankles is present.

Nursing Diagnosis: Fluid volume excess related to accumulation of fluid in the peritoneal cavity and dependent areas of the body

Patient Outcomes	Nursing Interventions	Rationale
Patient's abdominal girth and weight decrease daily.	Monitor intake and output.	Fluid intake that exceeds output from all sources over 24 hours indicates fluid retention.
	Administer prescribed diuretics.	Diuretics increase fluid excretion.
	Restrict fluids as ordered. Plan to include fluids given with medications when calculating allotted fluids.	Restriction limits fluid accumulation. The largest amount of fluid is given during waking hours. The majority of the total allowance will be allocated to meals.
	Provide oral hygiene every 4 hours; *do not* use lemon–glycerin swabs.	Mouth care decreases thirst. Glycerin dries mucous membranes.
	Weigh the patient daily before breakfast but after he or she has voided.	Weight loss or gain may indicate fluid loss or gain.
	Measure abdominal girth daily. Mark point at which girth is measured.	Decreasing girth indicates a decrease in ascitic fluid. Measuring at the same point ensures accuracy.
	Restrict dietary sodium intake as ordered.	Restrictions of dietary sodium aids in reducing fluid volume excess.

(continued)

Patients with Major Clinical Manifestations of Liver Dysfunction

(continued)

Evaluation:	Compare the patient's status with the expected outcomes. If the outcomes are not met, reassess the patient and revise the plan.
Assessment Findings:	Patient indicates loss of appetite and reports frequent vomiting after eating. Patient has not finished a "full meal" in the past 3 weeks.
Nursing Diagnosis:	Altered nutrition: less than body requirements related to anorexia, vomiting, and inadequate dietary intake

Patient Outcomes	Nursing Interventions	Rationale
Patient eats 75–100% of each meal.	Arrange to have food with the highest protein and calorie content served at the time of day the patient is most likely to eat.	Increases the likelihood of the patient consuming adequate amounts of protein and calories.
Patient demonstrates steady weight gain with no evidence of fluid retention.	Provide five or six small meals during the day.	Small portions are more appetizing and better tolerated.
	Provide oral hygiene before meals.	Refreshes mouth and stimulates appetite.
	Administer antiemetics 30–45 minutes before meals if ordered.	Most antiemetics require 20–30 minutes to reach effective levels.
	Maintain a low-sodium diet.	Decreases risk of fluid retention.
	Offer juice of patient's choice between meals.	Juice provides calories and vitamins.
	Monitor dietary intake by carrying out a calorie count for at least 3 days.	Provides data regarding actual intake of nutrients.

Evaluation:	Compare the patient's status with the expected outcomes. If the outcomes are not met, reassess the patient and revise the plan.
Assessment Findings:	On the third day of hospitalization, the patient's skin, mucous membranes, and sclerae are light yellow. Patient is observed scratching upper arms and abdomen; reports feeling "kind of itchy." Urine is darker than usual and has a strong odor. Spider angiomas are noted on upper torso, and multiple ecchymotic areas are visible on arms and legs.
Nursing Diagnosis:	Risk for impaired skin integrity related to pruritus, ascites, edema, and interference with clotting mechanisms

Patient Outcomes	Nursing Interventions	Rationale
Patient's skin is free of scratch marks.	Administer baths with cool water and use lightweight bed clothing. Keep room cool.	Warmth increases blood flow and increases bile salt deposits on skin.
Patient states itching is relieved.	Use a mild soap or soap substitute.	The alkalinizing effects of soap dry the skin.
	Pat skin dry. *Do not* rub.	Rubbing stimulates nerve endings and increases pruritus.
	Gently apply emollient lotion to the skin every 8 hours.	Lotion has a cooling effect and minimizes dryness.

(continued)

Patients with Major Clinical Manifestations of Liver Dysfunction
(continued)

Patient Outcomes	Nursing Interventions	Rationale
	Trim and file nails. Apply white socks or mittens to hands at night.	Prevents injury from scratching.
	Administer bile acid sequestrants as prescribed.	Relieves pruritus by decreasing bile acid deposits on the skin.
	Provide diversional activities: television, books, magazines, and so on.	Activities lessen awareness of pruritus.
Patient experiences no excessive bleeding.	Use a soft toothbrush. Do not use floss.	Minimizes risk of bleeding from gums.
	Use electric razor for shaving.	Protects from facial cuts.
	Monitor oral or tympanic temperature.	Rectal irritation may develop when rectal route is used. Hemorrhoids may be present due to portal hypertension.
	Group venipunctures, and apply pressure for at least 3 minutes after venipunctures. Use smallest gauge needle possible for injections and venipuncture.	Decreases the number of skin punctures and potential bleeding sites. Direct pressure promotes coagulation.
Patient's skin remains intact during hospitalization.	Inspect surfaces daily for lesions or open areas.	Early detection and intervention minimizes skin damage.
	Do not administer injections in edematous sites.	Drugs act as irritants when not absorbed.
	Teach patient to reposition self every 2 hours in bed or chair.	Frequent position changes relieve pressure and increase local blood flow.
	Place trapeze over bed and teach patient to use it to lift the body during position changes.	Lifting the body off the bed prevents injury from shearing force.
	Keep bed linens dry.	Moisture predisposes to skin breakdown.

Evaluation: Compare the patient's status with the expected outcomes. If the outcomes are not met, reassess the patient and revise the plan.

Assessment Findings: On the fourth day of hospitalization, patient is apathetic and responds slowly to questions. Speech is slurred. Patient answers appropriately when asked name but cannot identify location or month of the year. Handwriting is difficult to read, whereas admission writing sample is clear and distinct. Irregular, jerking movements are noted when arms are extended. Serum potassium level is within normal limits. Blood ammonia level is elevated.

Nursing Diagnosis: Risk for injury related to altered thought processes secondary to impaired liver function.

(continued)

Patients with Major Clinical Manifestations of Liver Dysfunction
(continued)

Patient Outcomes	Nursing Interventions	Rationale
Patient remains free of injury.	Monitor blood ammonia levels when ordered. Place samples on ice and transport to the laboratory immediately.	Ammonia is a central nervous system toxin. Samples stored at room temperature may produce inaccurate results.
	Monitor level of consciousness, orientation, rate of speech, and response time every 4 hours.	Changes in level of consciousness, orientation, speech, and response time indicate a change in condition.
	Monitor for asterixis every 4 hours.	Most common sign of impending coma due to hepatic encephalopathy.
	Obtain daily writing sample.	Difficulty writing indicates deterioration in condition.
	Restrict protein intake as prescribed.	Reduces ammonia production by intestinal bacteria.
	Monitor serum potassium level.	Decreased potassium levels can precipitate hepatic coma.
	Administer neomycin and lactulose as prescribed.	Lower blood ammonia levels.
	Keep bed in low position, with side rails up and call bell in reach.	Minimizes risk of injury.
	Administer sedatives, narcotics, and anti-anxiety agents with extreme caution.	Many of these agents are metabolized in the liver and may precipitate non-nitrogenous hepatic coma.
Evaluation:	Compare the patient's status with the expected outcomes. If the outcomes are not met, reassess the patient and revise the plan.	

reports of increased fatigue, shortness of breath, changes in skin color, bruising, itching, recent weight gain, and changes in stool or urine color. Ask specifically about tightness of clothing, especially at the waistline, or pain or discomfort in the abdomen. Determine whether there has been any change in eating, sleeping, or elimination patterns. Determine the patient's present and former use of alcohol. Specifically ask the amount of alcohol consumed daily. Ask whether, in the course of a typical week, any prescribed medications, over-the-counter medications, or recreational drugs are used. Review any past hospitalizations and the reason for admission. Ask whether the patient has received blood or blood products, as these can transmit viral hepatitis. Ask the female patient if she has noted menstrual irregularities. Question the male patient about enlargement of breast tissue or change in body hair

distribution because impaired liver function may interfere with hormone metabolism. Also assess the patient's understanding of and compliance with risk reduction and health promotion guidelines related to the liver. These are presented in Highlight 25–8.

PHYSICAL EXAMINATION

Examine the skin, sclerae, and mucous membranes for jaundice. Remember that, in dark-skinned people, jaundice is best identified by observing the hard palate. Inspect the skin for evidence of scratching, petechiae, purpura, ecchymosis, and spider angiomas. These are seen most often on the shoulders and upper trunk. Note breast enlargement in the male. Measure abdominal girth. Examine the abdomen for prominent veins caused by obstructed por-

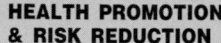
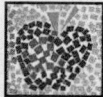

HIGHLIGHT
25-8

HEALTH PROMOTION & RISK REDUCTION

Guidelines for Maintaining a Healthy Liver

To aid in maintaining a healthy liver, instruct the patient to:

Avoid taking unnecessary over-the-counter medications.

Take all prescribed medications in strict accordance with instructions.

Limit drinking of alcoholic beverages.

Eat a balanced diet moderate to high in protein, moderate in carbohydrate and fat, and with adequate vitamins.

Avoid drinking any nutritional products unless advised to do so by a physician or a nutritionist.

Take the following precautions to protect against contracting hepatitis A:

- Wash hands thoroughly after using the toilet because spread occurs by fecal contamination and hand-to-mouth contact.
- Avoid drinking, rinsing the mouth with, or brushing the teeth with potentially contaminated water.
- Avoid eating fresh fruits and raw vegetables that may have been washed in contaminated water.
- Cook shellfish sufficiently to kill the hepatitis A virus, which can be present if the shellfish were harvested from a contaminated bed.

Obtain a hepatitis A vaccination if you:

- travel or relocate to an area where hepatitis A is endemic (Africa, Asia except Japan, the Mediterra-

nean basin and Eastern Europe, Middle East, Central and South America, Mexico and parts of the Caribbean)
- are a member of a geographic or ethnic group, such as native Alaskans or native Americans, that experiences cyclic outbreaks of hepatitis A
- are employed in a child daycare center or as a caretaker in a facility for the developmentally challenged
- handle live hepatitis A virus in a laboratory or you contact primates who may harbor the virus
- are exposed to a family member or friend with hepatitis A

Obtain a hepatitis B vaccination if you:

- travel to, or adopt a child from, an area where hepatitis B is prevalent
- work in a high-risk occupation such as medicine, nursing, laboratory technology, dentistry, criminal justice, fire-fighting, undertaking, or embalming
- have more than one sexual partner in 6 months
- use illicit injectable drugs
- undergo hemodialysis
- require large amounts of blood or blood products to treat a health problem
- have sexual contact with a hepatitis B patient or carrier
- share a household with a person exposed to hepatitis B patients or carriers

---

tal blood flow and for a glistening, taut appearance caused by stretching of the skin with ascites. Note the presence of striae and abdominal distention.

Percuss the abdomen with the patient in a supine position to detect fluid laterally. The abdomen is normally tympanic on percussion; fluid produces a dull sound. Turn the patient on the left and right sides and percuss again. Fluid shifts to the dependent side, causing bulging and shifting dullness. As shown in Figure 25–6, percuss the liver starting at an area below the umbilicus at the midclavicular line. Continue percussing upward until dullness over the liver is noted. Then start at the fourth intercostal space, midclavicular line, and percuss downward until dullness is noted. The vertical span of liver dullness should be 6 to 12 cm ($2\frac{1}{2}$ to $4\frac{1}{2}$ inches). If midclavicular percussion indicates liver enlargement, percuss the liver in the midsternal line, where

it is normally 4 to 8 cm ($1\frac{1}{2}$ to 3 inches) and note span.

Palpate the abdomen to determine the size and location of the liver. To palpate, place your left hand under the patient at the eleventh and twelfth ribs and lift upward toward the abdominal wall, as shown in Figure 25–7. Place your right hand on the abdomen so that the tips of the fingers rest on the right midclavicular line below the level of dullness. Fingers may point toward the head or be positioned slightly oblique to the midclavicular line. Press your right hand in and up as you instruct the patient to take a deep breath. Usually the liver is not felt. In some thin people and with liver enlargement, it may be felt as a firm, smooth, even, nontender mass that slides under the fingers of the right hand.

Observe and palpate for muscle wasting. Muscle tone should be firm, not doughy. Test muscle

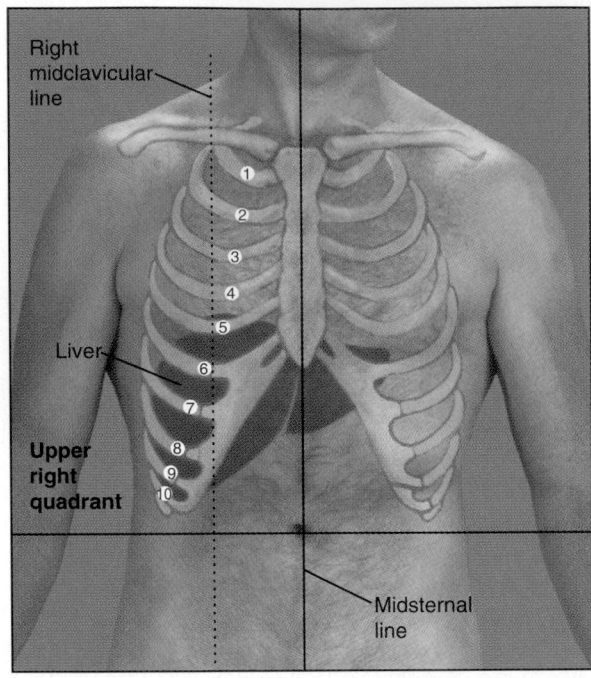

Figure 25–6

Anatomic landmarks for percussion of the liver.

strength in the upper and lower extremities by asking the patient to flex a limb and then resist you when you apply opposing force against the flexion. Instruct the patient to extend the arms to test for asterixis.

To assess cognitive abilities, ask the patient to describe the similarities between two objects, such as a peach and a pear. Provide a series of four or five numbers, and ask the patient to repeat them to test recent memory. Have the patient write a short sentence or his or her name or draw a picture to test coordination.

Diagnostic Procedures

Hepatic function is evaluated by:

- Blood studies to assess metabolic function
- Urine and fecal examinations
- Noninvasive procedures, such as ultrasonography, computed tomographic scans, and magnetic resonance imaging
- Liver biopsy, an invasive procedure

All blood tests and invasive procedures place the patient at risk for bleeding because of altered clotting mechanism. Application of the nursing process to the care of the patient at risk for bleeding was discussed earlier in this chapter under Clotting Disorders. Common diagnostic studies used to assess liver function are summarized in Tables 25–6 and 25–7.

BLOOD STUDIES

Liver Enzymes

Enzymes are intracellular protein catalysts that enhance chemical reactions. They are released in response to cellular damage. Consequently, elevated enzyme levels in a specific organ are useful indicators of cellular damage to that organ. Aspartate aminotransferase, formerly known as serum glutamic-oxaloacetic transaminase, is found in the largest quantities in cardiac, liver, and skeletal muscle, and

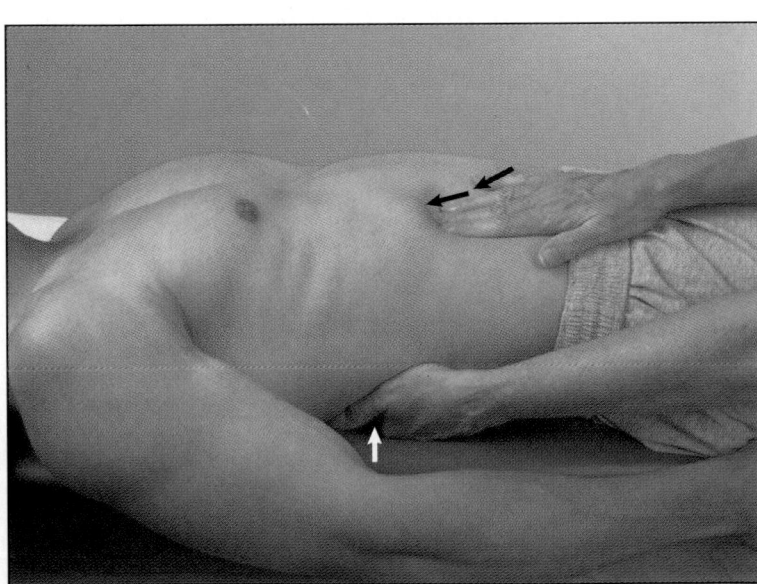

Figure 25–7

Palpation of the liver. As the patient inhales, the examiner presses in and up at the midclavicular line to feel for the edge of the descending liver.

Table 25-6

Common Diagnostic Studies of Liver Function

Study	Normal Value	Procedure/Interpretation
SERUM ENZYMES		
Aspartate aminotransferase (AST)	10–30 U/L	5 mL venous sample obtained; elevated with acute hepatitis, active cirrhosis, and hepatic necrosis
Alanine aminotransferase (ALT)	5–30 U/mL	5 mL venous sample obtained; high concentration of this enzyme normally found in the liver is more specific than AST for liver disease
Lactate dehydrogenase (LDH) Isoenzymes	100–190 U/L	5 mL venous sample obtained
LDH_4	3–10% of total	Liver contains high concentrations of LDH_4
LDH_5	2–9% of total	and LDH_5, isoenzymes of LDH; both levels are elevated with liver disease
Alkaline phosphatase	20–90 U/L	10 mL venous sample obtained; levels increased with extrahepatic and intrahepatic obstructive disease
Isoenzymes AP-1, Alpha-2	>30% of total	Elevated with hepatic carcinoma and intrahepatic biliary obstruction
5'-Nucleotidase	0–1.6 U	Elevated with liver metastasis and cirrhosis
Gamma glutamyl trans-peptidase	6–37 U/L	5 mL venous sample obtained; elevated with cirrhosis, metastatic liver tumors, and chronic hepatitis
BILIRUBIN METABOLISM		
Total serum bilirubin	0.3–1.2 mg/dL	5 mL venous sample, with 4-hour fast before sample
Direct (conjugated)	0.1–0.4 mg/dL	
Indirect (unconjugated)	0.3–1.1 mg/dL	Elevated unconjugated bilirubin associated with increased destruction of red blood cells; elevated conjugated bilirubin seen with most liver disease
Urine bilirubin	Negative	Examine urine within 1 hour of sample collection; should be performed on every routine urinalysis; early indicator of liver disease
Urine urobilinogen	1–4 mg/24 hr	Usually a 24-hour urine collection; increased in any condition that causes increased bilirubin and any disease that prevents removal of reabsorbed urobilinogen from the portal circulation
Fecal urobilinogen	40–200 mg/24 hr	Stool specimen obtained; decreased or absent when normal amounts of bilirubin are not excreted into intestinal tract; decreased values seen with severe liver disease
PROTEIN METABOLISM		
Total serum protein	6.0–8 g/dL	5 mL venous sample obtained; decreased total protein with insufficient protein intake or decreased formation in the liver
Serum albumin	3.5–5.5 g/dL	Decreased albumin levels occur with hepatocellular disease
Serum globulin	2.0–4.2 g/dL	Elevated levels in advanced cirrhosis and chronic active hepatitis
Serum protein electrophoresis	Total protein: Albumin, 52–68% Globulin, 32–48% alpha₁ globulin, 2.0–3.5% alpha₂ globulin, 5.0–10.6% beta globulin, 7.0–14% gamma globulin, 8.0–18%	5 mL venous blood sample; percentage of alpha₁, alpha₂, beta, and gamma globulin is determined; total percentage of globulin increases as a result of increased levels of these immunoglobulins when infections and diffuse inflammatory liver disease are present; occurs with chronic hepatitis and advanced cirrhosis

(continued)

Table 25-6

Common Diagnostic Studies of Liver Function *(continued)*

Study	Normal Value	Procedure/Interpretation
Blood ammonia	15–49 μg/dL	Fasting 3 mL arterial or venous sample obtained and packed in ice; elevated levels occur when liver cannot convert ammonia to urea for excretion from the body; elevated levels seen in liver failure
LIVER METABOLISM		
Total cholesterol	Varies with age and diet; desirable level <200 mg/dL	Fasting venous blood sample; decreased levels associated with liver disease
Cholesterol esters	60–75% of total cholesterol	Percentage of cholesterol esters decreases with liver disease as a result of a decrease of lecithin cholesterol acryl transferase, an enzyme needed to esterize cholesterol
CARBOHYDRATE METABOLISM		
Serum glucose	70–115 mg/dL	Fasting 5 mL venous sample; hypoglycemia (40–60 mg/dL) occurs with 50% of patients who have acute viral hepatitis; caused by depleted glycogen stores, decreased gluconeogenesis, and poor intake
COAGULATION STUDIES		
Prothrombin time (PT)	Males: 9.6–11.8 sec Females: 9.5–11.3 sec	7 mL venous sample; PT is prolonged when liver is unable to use vitamin K or form protein; because patient may have a coagulation disorder, apply pressure to the puncture site for 3–5 minutes after needle is withdrawn
TUMOR MARKER		
Alpha-fetoprotein (AFP)	<30 ng/mL	5 mL venous sample; levels of 10,000–100,000 ng/mL are seen with hepatic carcinoma or metastatic lesions involving liver; successful treatment response causes immediate drop in levels; with recurrence of hepatic carcinoma, levels rise 1–6 months before symptoms occur

Normal values and procedures are guidelines. Reported reference ranges may vary depending on the method used for testing as well as the population tested. Contact the laboratory performing the test for absolute values, interfering substances, specimen preservation, and specific collection procedures.

in kidney cells. Damage to any one of these organs will result in elevated blood levels. Alanine aminotransferase, formerly known as serum glutamic-pyruvic transaminase, occurs in relatively high levels in liver tissue and low levels in other organs. Therefore, an elevated alamine aminotransferase level is a more specific indicator of liver damage than an elevated aspartate aminotransferase level. Decreasing levels can be monitored to determine improvement in liver function.

Alkaline phosphatase is found in the liver, bone, and intestine. When this enzyme is elevated and no clinical symptoms indicate the source of the elevation, isoenzyme studies are indicated. Isoenzymes are forms of an enzyme characteristic of a specific tissue. 5'-Nucleotidase (5'-N) and AP-1, Alpha 2 (two isoenzymes of alkaline phosphatase) are found in greatest concentrations in hepatobiliary tissue. Lactate dehydrogenase (LDH), widely distributed in the body, exists in five isoenzymes. Elevated levels of LDH_4 and LDH_5 are associated with liver damage. Gamma glutamyl transpeptidase found in liver, kidney, spleen, and prostate tissue, is used to assess for liver cell dysfunction, alcohol ingestion, and alcohol-induced liver disease. In the presence of an elevated alkaline phosphatase level, assessment of gamma glutamyl transpeptidase may be more useful in differentiating liver pathology from bone disease, since gamma glutamyl transpeptidase is not present in bone.

Table 25-7

Visualization Procedures to Evaluate Liver Function

Study	Purpose/Description
Liver scan	Determines size, shape, position, and function of the liver. A tracer dose of a radioactive material, usually technetium, is given intravenously 30 minutes before the scan. The procedure takes about 60 minutes and causes no patient discomfort. Pregnancy contraindicates the procedure because of fetal exposure to the isotope. Pregnant health-care personnel should not care for patients who have had a scan for 48 hours after the procedure. In the normal liver, technetium uptake is uniform. "Cold" spots, areas with decreased uptake of the isotope, indicate lesions. Use of this procedure is decreasing because of improved results with ultrasonography, computed tomography (CT), and magnetic resonance imaging (MRI).
Abdominal ultrasonography	Harmless, high-frequency sound waves differentiate tissues in the abdominal cavity, including the liver. Fluid-filled structures in the liver, such as cysts, transmit ultrasound waves easily. Solid tumors transmit poorly. Ascites, even in small quantities, can be identified. A conductive gel is placed on the abdomen, and the patient must lie still for about 30 minutes.
Computed tomography (CT)	Computer processing of x-ray images provides cross-sectional views of the liver. An intravenous iodinated contrast agent may be used to enhance results. Before the procedure, question the patient about allergy to shellfish or iodine. CT is useful for identifying tumors, cysts, and abscesses.
Magnetic resonance imaging (MRI)	MRI produces a cross-sectional image of tissues in the body by generating a magnetic field between the machine and hydrogen atoms in the body. MRI is the most sensitive study for detecting lesions. The major disadvantages of MRI are the long time required for scanning (more than an hour in many cases) and the need for the patient to remain absolutely still during the procedure. Patients with cardiac pacemakers, surgical clips, and metal prostheses cannot have MRI because of the magnetic field.
Endoscopy Esophagoscopy	An endoscope is inserted via the oral cavity to visualize the esophagus and identify esophageal varices. Patient is kept on NPO status for 8 hours before the procedure. A local anesthetic in the form of a gargle or spray is administered to prevent gagging during tube insertion. The examination takes about 20 to 30 minutes. Assess patient for return of gag reflex before allowing oral food or fluids after the procedure.
Peritoneoscopy	A laparoscope is introduced through an incision in the abdominal wall. The patient usually receives a sedative before the procedure, and local anesthetic is used at the insertion site. Direct visualization of the liver is possible. Procedure is most commonly done to obtain samples of liver tissue. Total examination time is about 1 hour. Patient usually has a small dressing over the incision site. Monitor site for bleeding or discharge.

NPO, nothing by mouth.

Bilirubin Levels

Bilirubin is produced by the cells of the reticuloendothelial system. It circulates loosely bound to protein (unconjugated or direct bilirubin) and is removed from the body by the liver, where it is conjugated with glucuronide transferase and excreted into the bile. If the total bilirubin level is elevated or if jaundice is present, both conjugated and unconjugated levels of bilirubin are determined. Elevated levels of unconjugated bilirubin are usually associated with increased destruction of red blood cells. Elevated levels of conjugated bilirubin are seen with most liver diseases.

Protein Studies

Protein studies are done to determine the liver's ability to carry out protein metabolism. Albumin and globulin, synthesized in the liver, comprise most of the plasma protein and can be measured separately or together as total protein. In the presence of liver dysfunction, the formation of one or both of these proteins usually decreases. Thus, serum protein is widely used to assess liver function. Serum protein electrophoresis, a process that separates and quantifies albumin and globulin according to their electrical charge, may be ordered if the serum protein analysis is inconclusive for a specific

verity of hepatic encephalopathy, but decreasing ammonia levels are associated with successful treatment.

The most common factors that precipitate hepatic encephalopathy in the patient with liver disease are the excessive ingestion of protein and gastrointestinal bleeding. The metabolism of blood protein in the intestine results in ammonia production. Other causes include overzealous use of chlorothiazide diuretics, which can cause potassium depletion. In this instance, the diuretic causes hypokalemic metabolic alkalosis and increased absorption of ammonia from the renal tubules and gastrointestinal tract. This ultimately increases the amount of ammonium hydroxide that enters the brain. When the potassium level is maintained within normal limits, this problem does not occur.

Factors unrelated to ammonia levels may also be associated with hepatic encephalopathy. These include severe infection, operative procedures, and the use of sedatives, tranquilizers, or narcotics.

Clinical Manifestations

Hepatic encephalopathy must be suspected in any patient with liver disease who experiences abnormal neurologic signs and symptoms. Initial signs are apathy, restlessness, and a shortened attention span. The patient picks at the bedclothes and has a dazed look, slowed thought processes, and slurred speech. Simple tasks become difficult. Sometimes, the patient's breath may take on a sweet, musty odor (fetor hepaticus) from the breakdown of mercaptans. The most common and reliable sign that hepatic encephalopathy is developing is the presence of asterixis, often referred to as liver flap or hepatic tremor. Asterixis is irregular flapping movements of the fingers and wrists when the hands and arms are outstretched, with the palms down, wrists bent up, and fingers spread. Jerking muscle tremors can also be seen in the feet and the tongue. Progression to deep coma can occur gradually or suddenly. Table 25–4 summarizes the stages of hepatic encephalopathy.

Diagnosis

Altered neurologic signs, advanced liver disease, and the exclusion of other causes of neurologic impairment are sufficient to arrive at a diagnosis of hepatic encephalopathy.

Management

Precipitating factors that can be corrected, such as hypokalemia or gastrointestinal bleeding, are addressed by the physician. If neurologic function does not improve after these are corrected, treatment includes dietary restriction of protein and bowel cleansing.

DIETARY INTERVENTION. To reduce ammonia production in the early stages of hepatic encephalopathy, protein intake is restricted to 15 to 40 g daily with sufficient carbohydrate to provide 2000 kcal/day. Vitamin and mineral supplements are also

Table 25–4

Stages of Hepatic Encephalopathy

Stage	Characteristics
1. Prodromal	Shortened attention span, slowed thought processes, apathy, or euphoria present; mild confusion, slight tremor may be noted; picking at bedclothes and yawning common; reversal of usual sleep pattern
2. Impending coma	Disorientation, asterixis, peculiar musty odor to breath (fetor hepaticus), sleeping most of time but easily aroused, incontinent
3. Stupor	Deep sleep but can be aroused, incoherent speech
4. Coma	Stage 4A: patient responds to painful stimuli Stage 4B: no response

prescribed. Protein is eliminated if the patient is in an advanced stage of hepatic encephalopathy. As neurologic signs and symptoms resolve, protein intake can be increased by 10 to 15 g each week. If neurologic manifestations recur, protein is once again decreased. Highlight 25–5 illustrates the daily intake for a patient on a 40 g protein-restricted diet.

BOWEL CLEANSING. The purpose of bowel cleansing is to decrease enteric organisms, which produce ammonia when they break down nitrogenous substances. Bowel cleansing can be achieved in a number of ways. Neomycin, a poorly absorbed antibiotic excreted in the stool, can be administered orally, 1 to 2 g every 6 hours, to reduce ammonia-forming bacteria in the intestine. Neomycin enemas containing 4 g of the drug can be administered to cleanse the lower bowel. Lactulose, a nonabsorbable disaccharide, can be used to decrease bowel ammonia absorption. Lactulose is metabolized by colonic bacteria to organic acids, which prevent diffusion of ammonia through the intestinal mucosa. Lactulose syrup, 30 to 45 mL three to four times daily, can be administered until diarrhea develops. The dose is then decreased to the amount necessary to produce two to three soft stools per day. Lactulose and neomycin can be prescribed together. Highlights 25–6 and 25–7 describe neomycin and lactulose.

NURSING PROCESS
Hepatic Encephalopathy

Assessment

Assess the patient for changes in mental function. Note the presence of apathy, restlessness, slowed

liver disorder. In some liver diseases, such as cirrhosis, total serum protein levels may remain normal despite altered liver function. With this disorder, protein electrophoresis may reveal a decreased albumin level with an increased alpha$_1$ globulin.

Ammonia, an end product of protein metabolism, is converted to urea in the liver and excreted by the kidneys. With impaired hepatocellular function, ammonia levels rise, placing the patient at risk for hepatic encephalopathy.

Lipid Studies

Cholesterol, a lipid, is synthesized by the liver. Hepatocyte damage interferes with synthesis, causing a decreased blood cholesterol level.

Alpha-Fetoprotein

Alpha-fetoprotein is the major serum protein during fetal life. It is produced in large quantities by the liver until about the 32nd week of gestation. Only small quantities are produced after the first year of life. Rapidly multiplying liver cells resume production of alpha-fetoprotein. Elevated levels are seen when patients have hepatocellular carcinoma or metastatic lesions that affect the liver. Although levels may rise to thousands of times their normal level, 30 to 50% of patients with hepatocellular carcinoma do not have elevated alpha-fetoprotein levels. When levels are elevated, successful treatment of hepatic carcinoma results in an immediate drop in alpha-fetoprotein levels.

Prothrombin

The prothrombin time represents the time required for a firm fibrin clot to form after coagulation factor III and calcium are added to a blood sample. Prothrombin, a vitamin K–dependent protein necessary for blood coagulation, is formed by the liver. Any condition that impairs the liver's ability to use vitamin K or to form proteins will prolong the prothrombin time and increase the risk of bleeding.

URINE AND FECAL STUDIES

Bilirubin metabolism is also assessed by examining urine and stool samples. Under normal circumstances, no bilirubin is excreted in the urine, and only a small amount of urobilinogen is present. Bilirubin appears in the urine when increased amounts of conjugated bilirubin enter the blood stream.

Urobilinogen, normally secreted into the intestine with bile, appears in feces. When bilirubin metabolism is impaired, urobilinogen levels are decreased in the feces and increased in the urine. Because blood and urine samples are easier to obtain, fecal urobilinogen levels are measured infrequently.

VISUALIZATION PROCEDURES

Liver scan, ultrasonography, computed tomographic scan, magnetic resonance imaging, esophagoscopy, and peritoneoscopy are useful diagnostic tools that provide a pictorial image of the liver (see Table 25–7).

LIVER BIOPSY

Liver biopsy, usually performed at the bedside, is used to obtain a specimen of liver tissue for examination. After local anesthesia is administered to the skin site, a special needle is inserted through the right intercostal space between the sixth and seventh or eighth and ninth ribs. A liver tissue sample is then aspirated. Biopsy may also be done by direct visualization via laparoscopy. Ultrasonography or computed tomographic scan may be used to identify specific sites to undergo biopsy. Direct visualization is the preferred method because tissue samples can be taken from specific areas of the liver. This is important when isolated lesions are present, such as in the early stage of hepatic carcinoma.

Although the procedure is relatively safe, complications can occur. Improper placement of the biopsy needle upward into the chest cavity can result in pneumothorax. Laceration of a bile duct causes leakage of bile into the peritoneal cavity, resulting in peritonitis. Puncture of a blood vessel within or surrounding the liver can cause hemorrhage. Elevated clotting times and the highly vascular nature of liver tissue can also predispose patients to hemorrhage.

Table 25–8 explains nursing responsibilities before, during, and after a liver biopsy.

NURSING PROCESS
Diagnostic Studies of Hepatic Function
Assessment

Before all diagnostic procedures, question the patient to determine familiarity with the procedure. Also assess for a history of allergies, especially to contrast dyes. Observe the patient for physiologic and emotional signs and symptoms of anxiety. These include diaphoresis, trembling, restlessness, difficulty sleeping, crying, inability to concentrate, and elevated blood pressure and pulse.

Nursing Diagnoses and Planning

Nursing diagnoses and related expected patient outcomes commonly applicable to patients undergoing diagnostic studies of hepatic function include the following:

NDx: Anxiety related to lack of knowledge of diagnostic procedures

Table 25-8

Liver Biopsy

Nursing Actions	Rationale
BEFORE PROCEDURE	
Obtain written consent.	Invasive procedure
Verify that coagulation studies are within normal limits.	Bleeding tendencies may be present as a result of liver disease
	Complications requiring surgery can occur
Preferably, patient is maintained on NPO status for 6 hours before procedure.	
Assess vital signs.	Baseline data for comparison
Administer prescribed medications 30–60 minutes before procedure.	Medication to calm an anxious patient requires time to act
Position patient in supine or left lateral position with right arm extended above the head.	Widens the intercostal spaces and fully exposes the hepatic area
DURING PROCEDURE	
Stand on the patient's left side, hold patient's left hand, and place one hand lightly on right arm	Nurse's presence provides support and distracts patient during procedure; touching right arm allows nurse to quickly restrain it from movement during the procedure
When the physician is ready to insert biopsy needle, instruct patient to inhale deeply, exhale fully, and hold breath on exhalation while specimen is obtained.	On exhalation, the diaphragm ascends and risk of pneumothorax and liver laceration is minimized
AFTER PROCEDURE	
Place sterile dressing over needle insertion site, and position patient on right side with folded towel under costal margin for 6–8 hours; bedrest remaining 24 hours decrease risk of bleeding.	This position compresses the liver capsule against the chest wall, minimizing leakage of blood or bile
Monitor vital signs every 15 minutes for 1 hour, every 30 minutes for 2 hours, and then hourly until stable.	Bleeding or bile peritonitis causes change in vital signs
Assess patient for pain.	Some pain in RUQ and right shoulder is common because of leakage of small amounts of bile, blood, or both from biopsy site; it pain is severe, notify physician immediately

NPO, nothing by mouth; RUQ, right upper quadrant.

Planning: Patient outcomes
1. Patient describes the procedure.
2. Patient explains the purpose of the procedure.
3. Patient verbalizes concerns related to procedure.
4. Patient verbalizes decreased anxiety after teaching.

Nursing Interventions and Evaluation

NDx: Anxiety
Provide a quiet environment. Excess stimulation can increase anxiety. Encourage the patient to verbalize concerns about the diagnostic test. Explain the procedure and post-procedure care using terminology the patient can understand. Provide time for the patient to ask questions and to repeat the information provided. When possible, provide the patient with written material explaining the procedure. Return to the patient after 20 to 30 minutes and answer any additional questions. Repeated explanations may be necessary because anxiety can interfere with learning. Acknowledge the patient's fears and anxiety regarding the procedure. Inform the patient that some anxiety is normal. Remain with the patient during liver biopsy and paracentesis to ensure safety and provide emotional support and comfort.

Compare the patient's status with the expected outcomes. If the outcomes are not met reassess the patient and revise the plan.

The Elderly: Special Considerations

With normal aging, the liver's size, weight, and blood flow decreases. However, liver function tests remain normal with the exception of serum albumin levels, which tend to decline very slightly. This may result from decreased albumin synthesis or decreased protein intake.

The most consistent finding associated with the aging process is a decrease in liver enzymes vital for drug metabolism and detoxification. Smaller doses of all drugs are recommended for elderly patients. Drug interactions and cumulative drug effects occur with higher frequency in the aged.

A number of factors contribute to a prolonged recovery time for elderly patients with liver disease. As the liver ages, regeneration of this organ takes longer. Delayed diagnosis is another factor. Because the symptoms are similar, liver disease is sometimes mistaken for gallbladder disease or biliary obstruction, conditions common in the elderly person. Days or weeks may be spent treating biliary conditions before the correct diagnosis of liver disease is made. Early signs of hepatic encephalopathy are often overlooked when forgetfulness and confusion are attributed to the normal aging process. In addition, although the precise mechanism is not known, elderly patients have a decreased immunologic response to many infectious and inflammatory disorders. Thus, symptom development is delayed. Even with prompt diagnosis and treatment, the chronic health problems experienced by many elderly people—such as diabetes mellitus, heart failure, hypertension, and malignancy—can prolong the recovery time for patients with concurrent liver disease.

Normal aging changes in other body systems can also affect the elderly patient with liver disease and can intensify symptoms. Thinning of epidermal skin layers, decreased subcutaneous fat, and decreased sebum production contribute to dry skin and make the skin more prone to trauma. When jaundice is present, itching is intensified and skin injury from scratching is more likely. Diminished salivary flow and changes in the sense of smell may decrease appetite. Anorexia, experienced by many patients with liver disease, becomes even more problematic to treat in the elderly. Finally, the toxic effects of alcohol on the liver are increased by the physiologic changes of aging. Therefore, alcohol use (and abuse) in the elderly is a priority concern, placing the elderly at increased risk for liver dysfunction.

Chapter Review

1. What is the meaning of deep orange foamy urine when seen in a patient with jaundice?
2. What evidence supports the therapeutic effects of cornstarch or baking soda baths as part of the nursing care plan for a patient with jaundice?
3. How does accumulation of peritoneal fluid affect the respiratory system of a patient with ascites?
4. What are the advantages of a sodium-restricted diet for a patient with ascites?
5. How can fluid volume excess best be assessed in a patient with ascites?

6. Why is it necessary to limit venipunctures when planning care for the patient with liver disease?
7. How does excessive protein ingestion and gastrointestinal bleeding affect the central nervous system in a patient with hepatic encephalopathy?
8. How can the effectiveness of neomycin and lactulose be evaluated when caring for a patient with hepatic encephalopathy?
9. What evidence supports the therapeutic effects of a restricted-protein diet as a part of the nursing care plan for a patient with hepatic encephalopathy?
10. What liver function test results would you review if you were caring for an elderly patient who presents with confusion and forgetfulness?

Bibliography

Abrams W, Beers H, Berkow R, Fletcher M (eds.). The Merck manual of geriatrics. 2nd ed. Whitehouse Station, NJ: Merck & Co, Inc. 1995.

Carpenito LJ. Nursing care plans and documentation. 2nd ed. Philadelphia: JB Lippincott, 1995.

Carpenito LJ. Nursing diagnoses: application to clinical practice. 6th ed. Philadelphia: JB Lippincott, 1995.

Cohen A. Liver disease. In Copstead LE. Perspectives on pathophysiology. Philadelphia: WB Saunders, 1995, pp 758–777.

Coy D, Blei A. Portal hypertension. In Haubrick W, et al (eds). Gastroenterology. 5th ed. Philadelphia: WB Saunders, 1995, pp 1955–1987.

Davis J, Sherer K. Applied nutrition and diet therapy for nurses. 2nd ed. Philadelphia: WB Saunders, 1994.

Deglin JH, Vellerand AH. Davis drug guide for nurses. 5th ed. Philadelphia: FA Davis, 1997.

Eliopoulos C. Gerontological nursing. 3rd ed. Philadelphia: JB Lippincott, 1993.

Ferenci P. Hepatic encephalopathy. In Haubrick W, et al (eds). Gastroenterology. 5th ed. Philadelphia: WB Saunders, 1995, pp 1988–2003.

Fishbach FT. A manual of laboratory diagnostic tests. 5th ed. Philadelphia: JB Lippincott, 1995.

Friedman S. Cirrhosis of the liver and its major sequelae. In Bennett JC, Plum F (eds). Cecil textbook of medicine. 20th ed, Vol 1. Philadelphia: WB Saunders, 1992, pp 786–796.

Giger J, Davidhizer R. Transcultural nursing: Assessment and intervention. 2nd ed. St. Louis: Mosby Year-Book, 1995.

Guyton AC, Hall J. Textbook of medical physiology. 9th ed. Philadelphia: WB Saunders, 1996.

Kuhn MA. Pharmacotherapeutics: A nursing process approach. 3rd ed. Philadelphia: FA Davis, 1994.

Lehne R, Pharmacology for nursing care. 2nd ed. Philadelphia: WB Saunders, 1994.

Lutz C, Przytulski K. Nutrition and diet therapy. Philadelphia: FA Davis, 1994.

Ockner RK. Clinical approaches to liver diseases. In Bennett JC, Plum F (eds). Cecil textbook of medicine. 20th ed. Philadelphia: WB Saunders, 1996, pp 752–753.

Pagana KD, Pagana TJ. Mosby's diagnostic and laboratory test reference. 2nd ed. St. Louis: Mosby Year-Book, 1995.

Peckenpaugh N, Poleman C. Nutrition: Essentials and diet therapy. 7th ed. Philadelphia: WB Saunders, 1995.

Podlosky D, Isselbacher K. Alcohol related liver disease and cirrhosis. In Isselbacher K, et al (eds). Harrison's principles of internal medicine. 13th ed. New York: McGraw-Hill, 1994, pp 1444–1448.

Porth CM. Pathophysiology: Concepts of altered health states. 4th ed. Philadelphia: JB Lippincott, 1994.

Runyon B. Ascites and spontaneous bacterial peritonitis. In Sleisenger M, Fordtran J. (eds). Gastrointestinal disease: Pathophysiology/diagnosis/management. 5th ed. Philadelphia: WB Saunders, 1993, pp 1962–2003.

Runyon B. Ascites. In Schiff L, Schiff E (eds). Diseases of the liver. 7th ed. Philadelphia: JB Lippincott, 1993, pp 990–1015.

Schaffner F. Jaundice. In Haubrich W, Schaffner F, Berk JE (eds). Gastroenterology. 5th ed. Philadelphia: WB Saunders, 1995, pp 129–139.

Scharschmidt BF. Acute and chronic hepatic failure and hepatic encephalopathy. In Bennett JC, Plum F (eds). Cecil textbook of medicine. 20th ed. Philadelphia: WB Saunders, 1996, pp 797–800.

Seeley R, Stephens T, Tate P. Anatomy and physiology. 3rd ed. St. Louis: Mosby Year-Book, 1995.

Sherlock S. Diseases of the liver and biliary system. 9th ed. Cambridge, MA: Blackwell Scientific, 1993.

Stanley M, Beare P. Gerontological nursing. Philadelphia: FA Davis, 1995.

Ulrich S, Canale S, Wendell S. Nursing care planning guides (medical-surgical). 3rd ed. Philadelphia: WB Saunders, 1994.

Watson J, Jaffe M. Nurse's manual of laboratory and diagnostic tests. 2nd ed. Philadelphia: WB Saunders, 1995.

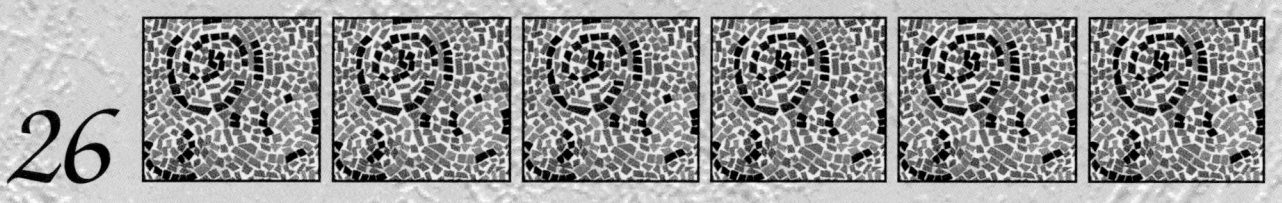

26

Nursing Care of Patients with Hepatic Disorders

Study Outcomes

After studying this chapter, you should be able to:

1. Describe the etiology, pathophysiology, clinical manifestations, diagnostic procedures, and management of patients with hepatic disorders.
2. Identify physical examination data and information essential for the assessment of patients with hepatic disorders.
3. Identify nursing diagnoses and expected outcomes for patients with hepatic disorders.
4. List nursing interventions and their rationales for patients with hepatic disorders.
5. Explain the basis for evaluation of nursing care provided to patients with hepatic disorders.
6. Identify alternative treatment and care settings for patients with hepatic disorders and the services related to community-based care.
7. Identify special considerations for the older adult with a hepatic disorder.

Patients with hepatic disorders have signs and symptoms that reflect alterations in normal liver functions. The major hepatic disorders include infectious and inflammatory conditions, structural abnormalities, trauma, and neoplasms.

*I*nfections and Inflammations

Viral hepatitis and liver abscess are the most common hepatic infectious processes. Inflammation results when a person ingests, inhales, or receives parenteral substances that have a toxic effect on the liver.

VIRAL HEPATITIS

Etiology and Pathophysiology

Acute viral hepatitis is characterized by inflammation and necrosis of hepatic cells. Although the major forms of hepatitis differ from one another with regard to incubation period, route of transmission, antigenic properties, and progression to chronicity, they all produce an inflammatory response in the liver. All forms of viral hepatitis are characterized by liver cell necrosis, inflammation, and cell regeneration. The regular organizational pattern of the hepatocytes is disrupted by the inflammatory process and cellular damage. Bile flow is impaired by inflammation involving the hepatic cells and bile canaliculi. Liver cell necrosis occurs in a spotty, piecemeal manner. Hepatocytes adjacent to blood vessels show the first evidence of damage. Even as cell necrosis is occurring, previously destroyed cells are regenerating. During the recovery period, hepatocytes regain their normal appearance and function. The most commonly occurring hepatitis viruses are compared in Table 26–1.

Hepatitis A

Hepatitis A virus (HAV) is found worldwide and is almost exclusively spread by the fecal-oral route. It occurs sporadically from close person-to-person contact or epidemically from the ingestion of water, milk, or food (especially shellfish) contaminated with infected human waste. HAV infection can be spread from one family member to another, via food handlers in restaurants, and from resident to resident in an institutional setting. Lack of toilet training and hand-to-mouth contact can lead to outbreaks of hepatitis A in preschool settings.

HAV is endemic in underdeveloped countries and is related to overcrowding and poor sanitation. In addition, 90% of the population of Taiwan and Israel have serologic evidence of previous exposure to hepatitis A by age 50 (Spiro, 1993). Sexual transmission of HAV is also seen in cases of oral-anal-genital contact.

Hepatitis B

Hepatitis B virus (HBV) is distributed worldwide and is increasing in frequency. This is attributed to increased intravenous drug use and sexual activity with multiple partners. The parenteral route is the major route of transmission. Groups at risk for infection via the parenteral route include IV drug users

Table 26–1

Comparison of Hepatitis Viruses

	Hepatitis A	Hepatitis B	Hepatitis D	Hepatitis C	Hepatitis E
CAUSATIVE AGENT	Hepatitis A virus (HAV)	Hepatitis B virus (HBV)	Hepatitis D virus (HDV)	Hepatitis C virus (HCV)	Hepatitis E Virus (HEV)
OTHER NAMES	Infectious hepatitis	Serum hepatitis	Delta agent hepatitis	Post-transfusion hepatitis; parenterally transmitted non-A, non-B hepatitis	Enterically transmitted non-A, non-B hepatitis
INCUBATION PERIOD	15–50 days; mean, 28–30 days	45–160 days; mean, 60–90 days	30–180 days (mean, 60–90 days); HBV must be present	15–180 days; mean, 6–9 weeks	15–64 days; mean, 26–42 days
MODE OF TRANSMISSION	Fecal-oral route; may be sexually spread	Infected blood or body fluids; sexually spread	Infected blood or body fluids; sexually spread	Infected blood or body fluids; sexual spread rare	Fecal-oral route
SOURCES OF INFECTION	Direct contact with infected persons; poor sanitation; infected food handlers; contaminated food, especially shellfish, water, milk; persons with subclinical infections	Contaminated needles and syringes; blood products; sexual contact; perinatal transmission; asymptomatic carriers	Same as hepatitis B	Same as hepatitis B	Direct contact with infected persons; contaminated water; poor sanitation; infected food handlers and food (rare in United States)
HIGH-RISK GROUPS	Preschoolers, family members, homosexual males	Intravenous drug users, recipients of commercial blood transfusions, health-care workers, dialysis patients	Same as hepatitis B	Same as hepatitis B	Persons living in underdeveloped countries

and persons coming into contact with blood or blood products.

HBV is found in sweat, tears, vaginal secretions, semen, and saliva in addition to blood. Two nonparenteral routes of transmission include sexual contact and perinatal transmission. Persons at risk for infection via the nonparenteral route include spouses and sexual contacts of those with active hepatitis B, family members of chronically infected patients, and residents and staff of institutions for the developmentally delayed.

Perinatal transmission, rare in the United States but common in the Far East and in developing countries, occurs in infants born to healthy carrier mothers or mothers who have acute hepatitis B during the third trimester of pregnancy. It is unclear whether mother-to-infant infection occurs in utero or at the time of delivery. Hepatitis B infection is not related to breast feeding.

Hepatitis D

The hepatitis D virus (HDV), or delta agent, occurs only in persons infected with hepatitis B, and is transmitted through the percutaneous route. The hepatitis B surface antigen must be present for the HDV to replicate. It is most common among drug users, hemodialysis patients, and recipients of multiple transfusions.

HDV has a worldwide distribution and is endemic in Mediterranean countries (Northern Africa, Southern Europe, and the Middle East) where HBV is prevalent. Hepatitis D will be reduced and possi-

Table 26–1

Comparison of Hepatitis Viruses (continued)

	Hepatitis A	Hepatitis B	Hepatitis D	Hepatitis C	Hepatitis E
LABORATORY CONFIRMATION	HAV-Ab/IgM	HB_sAg, HB_cAb	Delta antigen in serum	HCV-Ab	Elimination of other forms of hepatitis
MORTALITY	<0.6%	1–2%	Concurrent HDV infection increases risk of fulminant HBV infection	Rare	Unknown; 20% in pregnant women in the third trimester
PROPHYLAXIS	Good sanitation, hygiene; immune serum globulin; HAVRIX vaccine	HBIG; hepatitis B vaccine; alpha interferon	HBIG; hepatitis B vaccine (hepatitis D occurs only if HBV present)	Alpha interferon	Good sanitation, hygiene; immune serum globulin not effective
GERIATRIC CONSIDERATIONS	Most fatalities in the aged population	More severe clinical course, greater progression to chronicity, higher mortality rate	Same as hepatitis B	Same as hepatitis B	Uncommon in elderly
POSTRECOVERY CONSIDERATIONS	No carrier or chronic state; lifelong immunity to HAV reinfection	5–10% develop carrier state or chronic hepatitis; chief cause of cirrhosis and hepatocellular cancer in United States; lifelong immunity to HBV reinfection	Higher incidence of chronic active hepatitis and cirrhosis than with HBV alone	Frequent carrier state and chronic hepatitis; increased risk of cirrhosis and hepatocellular cancer; reinfection possible	No evidence of chronic or carrier state

Special precautions for all types: Blood, tissue, organ, and sperm donations cannot be made by persons with a history of hepatitis.
Ab, antibody; HB_cAb, antibody to hepatitis B core antigen; HB_sAg, hepatitis B surface antigen; HBIG, hepatitis B immune globulin; IgM, immunoglobulin M.

bly eradicated wherever universal vaccination for hepatitis B is implemented.

Hepatitis C
Hepatitis C (HCV), commonly referred to as post-transfusion hepatitis, is the leading cause of chronic hepatitis in the United States, Japan, and Europe (Boyer and Reuben, 1993). HCV is transmitted primarily by contact with contaminated blood and blood products, either through transfusion or percutaneously. HCV is present in 1% of the blood donor population worldwide. With the adoption of routine screening of all blood donors in the United States since the mid 1990s, the risk of transfusion HCV infection has been reduced to less than 1% per patient (Newman, 1994). Other persons at risk for contacting HCV include IV drug users, persons exposed to contaminated blood and blood products, and transplant recipients. Occasionally, perinatal transmission of HCV occurs in utero, at birth, or shortly after delivery.

Chronic hepatitis C is one of the most common indications for liver transplantation in adults.

Hepatitis G
Hepatitis G virus (HGV) is a recently isolated blood-borne infectious agent transmitted by needlesticks and blood transfusions. Hepatitis G infection has a worldwide distribution and has been found as a coinfection in some patients with hepatitis C. In the United States, it is estimated that HGV is present in 1 to 2% of the blood donor population (Hospital

Infection Control, 1996) After transmission, hepatitis G infection appears to persist for at least 12 months. In some patients recovery is uncomplicated, and in others chronic hepatitis ensues (Bowden, 1996). At present, there is no antibody test for HGV.

Hepatitis E

The hepatitis E virus (HEV), formerly enterically transmitted non-A non-B hepatitis, is transmitted via the enteric route and has characteristics similar to those of HAV. Hepatitis E is a leading cause of acute viral hepatitis in young to middle-aged adults in developing countries, including those in Asia, Africa, and Central America. The mortality rate for infected pregnant women is close to 20%. There is no evidence of a chronic form. Diagnosis depends on exclusion of other forms of hepatitis, especially HAV. At present, there is no serologic test for HEV.

Clinical Manifestations

The period of time between infection and actual symptoms (the incubation period), and the severity of viral hepatitis depend on the organism responsible for the infection.

Hepatitis A has an incubation period of 15 to 50 days. It is characterized by an acute onset that produces a mild illness lasting about 6 weeks. Infection with HAV does not produce a carrier state and does not lead to chronic liver disease. The mortality rate for HAV is less than 0.6%.

Hepatitis B has an incubation period of 45 to 160 days. The clinical course is usually more prolonged than that of hepatitis A, and it is more likely to cause serious illness in the elderly and the debilitated. Infection with HBV can cause chronic hepatitis and lead to a carrier state, and may also increase the risk of liver cancer. Simultaneous infection with HBV and the delta agent does not increase the risk of chronic hepatitis. However, when a patient is chronically infected with HBV and has an acute infection with the delta virus, the condition usually results in chronic active hepatitis. Acute delta infection can result in liver failure. The mortality rate for people with hepatitis B is approximately 2%.

The incubation period for HCV ranges from 2 to 26 weeks, with an average of 6 to 9 weeks. A carrier state can occur, and more than 25% of patients with HCV develop chronic hepatitis. For most patients, however, it is mild and symptoms disappear after a year. Hepatitis C increases the incidence of primary liver cancer.

The incubation period for HEV is 15 to 64 days; incubation for HDV ranges from 30 to 180 days with a mean of 60 to 90 days.

From the onset of infection, clinical and biochemical recovery from uncomplicated viral hepatitis takes about 6 months. The earliest symptoms are usually nonspecific and often mistaken for influenza or an upper respiratory tract infection. Although some patients experience no further symptoms, the usual course of hepatitis includes the preicteric, icteric, and posticteric phases.

Preicteric Phase

The preicteric phase is characterized by nonspecific complaints of fatigue, anorexia, nausea, pharyngitis, cough, coryza, abdominal discomfort, and joint pain. They begin 1 to 3 weeks before jaundice appears. During the final 1 to 5 days of the preicteric phase, the patient may note that urine is becoming darker and stools are lighter in color. Laboratory results indicate elevated enzyme levels—especially aspartate aminotransferase and alanine aminotransferase—and elevated urine bilirubin levels.

Icteric Phase

The icteric phase begins with the appearance of jaundice. Laboratory tests show elevated levels of direct bilirubin. Because of obstructed bile flow, decreased urobilinogen is excreted in the feces, resulting in a lighter stool color. Increased excretion of urobilinogen in the urine causes its color to darken. Symptoms seen in the preicteric phase subside, but appetite remains poor. Right upper quadrant pain is common from the enlarged liver. Pruritus is associated with worsening jaundice and increased bile salt deposits in the skin. Clinical manifestations associated with decreased production of clotting factors are rare, but a few spider angiomas may be seen. The icteric phase usually lasts from 2 to 6 weeks.

Posticteric Phase

The recovery period is characterized by decreasing jaundice and, in uncomplicated cases, lasts from 2 to 12 weeks. Stool and urine color return to normal and appetite improves. Patients may continue to complain of fatigue.

Table 26–2 summarizes the clinical manifestations and laboratory data commonly seen in each phase.

Diagnosis

The diagnosis of viral hepatitis is based on information obtained from the patient's history, physical examination, and laboratory findings, including specific serologic tests. If viral hepatitis is suspected, the patient is questioned regarding possible sources of the virus. This includes contact with jaundiced individuals, recent travel to countries where hepatitis is endemic, injections, IV drug use, tattooing, dental treatments, blood transfusions, and shellfish ingestion. Physical examination confirms a tender, palpable liver with hepatomegaly and splenomegaly.

Laboratory indicators include:

- Elevated liver enzyme levels resulting from hepatocyte necrosis
- Elevated erythrocyte sedimentation rate from hepatic inflammation
- Leukopenia associated with viral infections
- Elevated serum bilirubin levels, especially conjugated bilirubin, in the presence of jaundice
- In severe cases, prolonged prothrombin time from the liver's inability to produce clotting factors

Table 26–2

Clinical Manifestations and Laboratory Data Associated with the Preicteric, Icteric, and Posticteric Phases of Hepatitis

Phase	Manifestations	Laboratory Findings
Preicteric (occurs 1 to 3 weeks before onset of jaundice)	Fatigue Anorexia Nausea Vomiting Abdominal discomfort Joint pain Pharyngitis Cough Coryza	Elevated enzyme levels (especially AST and ALT), elevated urine bilirubin levels
Icteric (may last from 2 to 6 weeks)	Jaundice appears Appetite remains poor Right upper quadrant pain Stool color lightens Urine color darkens Pruritus	Same as preicteric phase with addition of elevated serum levels of direct bilirubin
Posticteric (lasts from 2 to 12 weeks)	Jaundice subsides Stools return to normal color Urine returns to normal color Appetite improves Fatigue may continue	All laboratory values return to normal

ALT, alanine aminotransferase; AST, aspartate aminotransferase

Specific serologic tests are available to identify HAV, HBV, HCV, and the delta antigen, although serologic identification of the delta antigen is not widely used. A diagnosis of HEV is made by excluding HAV, HBV, and HCV and the patient's history of probable risk factors.

To differentiate hepatitis A and hepatitis B, the first marker tested is the antibody to HAV, which is immunoglobulin-M specific (designated HAV-Ab/IgM). This is present 4 to 6 weeks after infection and indicates an acute stage of hepatitis A infection. The remaining two markers are the B surface antigen and the B core antibody. The HBV surface antigen (HB_sAg) is detected 2 to 8 weeks before the onset of jaundice. It may appear before liver enzymes rise and clinical symptoms appear, and it remains detectable during and beyond the icteric phase of acute hepatitis B. Shortly after the surface antigen appears, the hepatitis B core antibody (HB_cAb) appears and is detectable for 6 to 14 weeks. HCV-Ab is the serologic marker for hepatitis C. It appears 5 to 12 months after infection.

Tests to identify serologic markers that indicate resolution of the infection may be ordered after symptoms subside. These include the HAV antibody, which is specific to immunoglobulin G (designated HAV-Ab/IgG) and indicates previous exposure and immunity to hepatitis A, and the hepatitis B surface antibody (HB_sAb), which appears 2 to 10 months after infection and indicates previous exposure and permanent immunity to hepatitis B.

Table 26–3 summarizes the significance of the various hepatitis markers commonly used to diagnose and monitor a patient's progress.

Management

Rest is advised, but strict bedrest is not necessary. The amount of activity the patient can tolerate is usually dictated by the patient's level of fatigue. No specific dietary interventions are necessary provided the patient can tolerate and receives a well-balanced diet. A low-fat, high-carbohydrate diet is often more tolerable to a patient with anorexia and nausea. If vomiting is present and the patient cannot tolerate oral feedings, IV fluid replacement and small doses of antiemetic agents may be prescribed. Alcoholic beverages are contraindicated during the course of the illness.

Integral to the management of hepatitis is prevention of its spread. Prophylactic measures are available for hepatitis A and B.

Hepatitis A

Administration of immune serum globulin provides temporary immunity (passive) to hepatitis A for people who are planning travel to the tropics and developing countries where the incidence of hepatitis A is high. Protection is afforded for up to 3 months. Repeat immunization is required for longer stays. ISG can also be given to close contacts of patients diagnosed with hepatitis A. It should be administered within the first few days of exposure. Casual work or school contacts do not require ISG

Table 26-3

Common Hepatitis Markers and Their Significance

Type	Appearance	Implications
HEPATITIS A		
HAV-Ab/IgM	4–6 weeks after infection	Indicates current acute infection with HAV
HAV-Ab/IgG	8–12 weeks after infection	Indicates previous exposure and immunity to HAV
HEPATITIS B		
HB_sAg	4–12 weeks after infection	Present in most cases of acute and chronic infection with HBV
HB_eAg	4–12 weeks after infection	Indicates "highly infectious" state
HB_cAb	6–14 weeks after infection	Indicates past infection with HBV
HB_sAb	2–10 months after infection	Indicates previous exposure and immunity to HBV
HEPATITIS C		
HCV-Ab	5–12 months after infection	Present in up to 90% of patients with chronic post-transfusion hepatitis C. Found in 1% of normal volunteer blood donors as well as patients with hepatocellular carcinoma

Ab, antibody; HAV, hepatitis A virus; HB_cAb, antibody to hepatitis B core antigen; HB_sAb, antibody to hepatitis B surface antigen; HB_eAg, hepatitis B e antigen; HB_sAg, hepatitis B surface antigen; HBV, hepatitis B virus; HCV, hepatitis C virus; IgG, immunoglobulin G; IgM, immunoglobulin M.

unless there is mutual handling of food and beverages or if hygiene practices are poor.

Vaccines for hepatitis A using live activated and inactivated virus have been tested and seem safe and effective. Havrix, a vaccine containing the inactive virus of hepatitis A, is available and may replace gamma globulin for travelers. A single dose of this vaccine is given intramuscularly. For maximum antibody titer, a booster dose is recommended 6 to 12 months after the initial injection.

Hepatitis B

Hepatitis B immune globulin provides passive immunity to hepatitis B. Because the cost is extremely high—$250 to $300 for the recommended two doses 4 weeks apart—it is usually administered only under select circumstances, such as:

- Inoculation of material known to be contaminated with HBV, such as an accidental cut or puncture with a contaminated needle or instrument from an HB_sAg-positive patient
- Splashing of HB_sAg-positive material into the eye or onto an open skin wound
- Ingestion of HB_sAg material during laboratory procedures using pipettes

The use of hepatitis B immune globulin requires that the source of the virus be known and that the recipient of hepatitis immune globulin actually be at risk. The usual procedure is to test blood for HB_sAg from both the source and the exposed person. If the exposed person is already positive for HB_sAg or immune, there is no reason to administer hepatitis immune globulin.

Active immunity to hepatitis B is provided by the hepatitis B vaccine (Engerix-B, Recombivax HB).

It is recommended for all adults at high risk for hepatitis B and for all infants and children. Those in high-risk categories include travelers to countries where hepatitis B is endemic, clients and staff of institutions for the mentally retarded, health-care workers, hemodialysis patients, homosexually active males, and household and sexual contacts of HBV carriers. The vaccine is administered three times over a period of 6 months. The second dose follows the first by 1 month; the third dose is given 6 months after the first dose.

Complications

Previously healthy individuals in whom hepatitis develops usually recover completely with no complications. However, elderly patients, the chronically malnourished, and those with chronic medical problems (heart failure, diabetes mellitus, malignancy) may have a prolonged recovery. After complete recovery, second episodes of the same type of hepatitis are rare, although the possibility of infection with another hepatitis virus does exist. Drug addicts, because of poor hygiene practices and the use of dirty needles and syringes, experience a higher incidence of repeat occurrences, most frequently HCV. The major complications associated with hepatitis infection are chronic hepatitis and fulminant hepatitis.

Chronic Hepatitis

Chronic hepatitis is possible in patients who have had HBV or HCV hepatitis. There are two types of chronic hepatitis: chronic persistent hepatitis and chronic active hepatitis.

Chronic persistent hepatitis is characterized by inflammation of the portal tracts with no hepatocyte necrosis. In chronic persistent hepatitis, there is a delayed convalescent period marked by fatigue, ano-

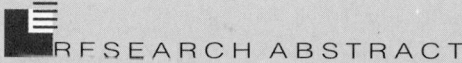
RESEARCH ABSTRACT

What Hepatitis B Immunization Regimen Is Safe and Effective for Elderly Adults?

Bennett RG, Powers DC, Remsburg RE, Scheve A, Clements ML. Hepatitis B virus vaccination for older adults. J Am Geriat Soc 1996; 44(6):699.

According to the US Preventive Services Task Force, hepatitis B infection affects an estimated 200,000 to 300,000 people each year. Hepatitis B infection can lead to such serious complications as cirrhosis, liver failure, and liver cancer. The Advisory Committee on Immunization Practices (ACIP) and others therefore recommend that in addition to immunizing all infants against hepatitis B infection by the age of 18 months, people in high-risk groups should also be immunized. Such groups include

- Health-care workers
- Hemophiliacs
- Hemodialysis patients
- Household contacts of people who test positive for hepatitis B or who live in an area where the disease is endemic
- Injection drug users
- Sexually active homosexual or bisexual males
- Heterosexual males or females with more than one partner in the past 6 months or a recent sexually transmitted disease
- Prisoners
- Institutionalized people with developmental disabilities and the staff who care for them

Vaccination schedules involving three injections (one each at 0, 1, and 6 months) are usually effective in stimulating a protective response in immune-competent people. However, older adults have less of an immune response to vaccinations than younger people. As part of a multicenter study of the effectiveness of a newly developed hepatitis B vaccine, Bennett and colleagues therefore examined an alternative immunization schedule of four injections in older adults. Their goal was to see whether older adults who had a poor response to the standard three-injection schedule would have a better immune response to a four-injection schedule and thus be protected in the event of a hepatitis B exposure. The researchers found that a fourth injection resulted in adequate levels of anti-body to hepatitis B to protect the recipients from the disease. No systemic or major adverse effects of a fourth injection were reported by any of the 19 subjects.

According to the researchers, a larger clinical trial is needed before four injections are recommended as the preferred immunization schedule for older adults. They also note that their subjects include only healthy adults over 50 years of age without any active chronic disease conditions. Results with other groups of older adults might differ.

Another question that needs to be examined is how long a recipient's active acquired immunity to hepatitis B will last. Since widespread vaccination to hepatitis B is relatively recent, it will be some time before studies can measure long-term effects. In the meantime, immunization should not substitute for limiting high-risk behaviors and using Standard Precautions as additional protective measures.

As members of a high-risk group, nurses should keep up with recommendations of such groups as APIC.

Questions to Consider

1. How is the vaccination status of patients assessed and recorded in your clinical setting?
2. What is the setting's policy and procedure for ensuring that members of high-risk groups, including health-care workers, are vaccinated against hepatitis B?
3. What types of illness prevention interventions, such as immunizations, are covered by health maintenance organizations and other insurance providers in your area?
4. What immunizations are provided by the local health department?
5. What is the procedure in your clinical facility for protecting nurses against hepatitis B when they have suffered a blood exposure incident?
6. Are you fully immunized?

---

rexia, hepatomegaly, and right upper quadrant pain. Moderate increases in serum enzyme levels and bilirubin occur. Symptoms may persist for 10 years or longer. Usually, no specific treatment is indicated. However, recombinant alpha interferon has been approved for the treatment of chronic hepatitis. Prognosis is favorable because no further liver damage occurs.

Chronic active hepatitis is a more serious form of chronic hepatitis because it may progress to cirrhosis and liver failure. About one-third of the patients acquire postnecrotic cirrhosis, and one-fifth die of liver failure within 4 years. Active hepatocellular necrosis occurs. Diagnosis requires liver biopsy. Although research findings are contradictory, there is some agreement that corticosteroids should be used to treat chronic active hepatitis to suppress the inflammatory response seen on biopsy.

Fulminant Hepatitis

Fulminant hepatitis is seen in less than 1% of patients with viral hepatitis. Massive cell necrosis occurs, and the liver is unable to regenerate functional tissue. There is rapid liver decompensation within a few weeks after the onset of hepatitis. The patient enters Stage III or IV of hepatic encephalopathy and may die within a week.

❖ Settings, Providers, and Collaboration for Care

Patients with acute viral hepatitis are usually followed in the physician's office or ambulatory care setting. Referral to home care may be needed to monitor management of the treatment plan and to assess for developing complications. Acute hospitalization is reserved for patients with an uncertain diagnosis, those with a delayed recovery, and those who are critically ill.

NURSING PROCESS
Hepatitis

Strict adherence to standard precautions is essential when caring for the patient with hepatitis to prevent transmission via blood and body fluids. Standard precautions include the use of gloves when handling blood or body fluids, gowns when clothing may be contaminated, and face shields or goggles and masks when blood or body fluids could splash or splatter. If the patient with hepatitis A is incontinent or has poor hygiene practices, contact precautions are instituted and a private room is required to prevent spread of the virus to other patients.

Assessment

Question the patient about known or possible exposure to contaminated food, water, needles, surgical equipment, blood transfusions, or persons with hepatitis. Assess for the clinical manifestations of hepatitis. Palpate and percuss the liver to identify hepatomegaly and tenderness or pain. Question the patient about activity level, appetite, and nausea or vomiting.

Nursing Diagnoses and Planning

Nursing diagnoses and related expected patient outcomes commonly applicable to patients with hepatitis include the following:

NDx: Risk for altered health maintenance related to insufficient knowledge of viral hepatitis disease process and transmission

Planning: Patient Outcomes
1. Patient explains the cause of viral hepatitis.
2. Patient describes precautions to prevent transmission of the disease.
3. Patient verbalizes an understanding of the treatment plan.

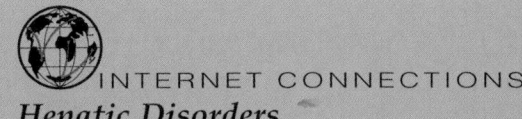

INTERNET CONNECTIONS
Hepatic Disorders

General
American Liver Foundation
http://sadieo.ucsf.edu/alf/alffinal/
homepagealf.html
An authoritative site that provides information for patients and for health-care professionals. Information ranges from a list of clinical trials of treatments and reports on recent medical research to answers to 100 frequently asked questions and listings of regional chapters and support groups.

Hepatitis
The Hepatitis Information Network
http://www.hepnet.com/
This site, intended for health-care professionals, includes updates on patient care issues, news releases, quizzes, survey results, answers to frequently asked questions, and links to relevant professional sites.

Five Million Americans Have Hepatitis. Do You?
http://www.hep-help.com/
A patient-oriented site sponsored by Schering-Plough. This site includes information about risk factors, symptoms, and treatment for hepatitis A, B, C, and G.

Cirrhosis
MedicineNet/Cirrhosis
http://www.medicinenet.com/mainmenu/encyclop/
article/Art_c/cirrho.htm
This patient-oriented encyclopedia-style article could also be useful to health-care professionals. It includes a discussion of the causes, symptoms, diagnosis, and treatment of cirrhosis.

NDx: Activity intolerance related to fatigue

Planning: Patient Outcomes
1. Patient participates in activities of daily living without experiencing fatigue.
2. Patient increases ambulation distance daily.

NDx: Body image disturbance related to altered skin pigmentation

Planning: Patient Outcomes
1. Patient verbalizes acceptance of self in present condition.
2. Patient takes part in grooming activities.

Nursing Interventions and Evaluations

NDx: Risk for altered health maintenance

Explain the mode of transmission to the patient and significant others. For HAV and HEV, explain that the virus is passed in stool and spreads to others when the patient fails to wash his or her hands adequately, then touches food, dishes, glasses, or other items that could transmit the virus. Explain the purpose of contact precautions to the patient, family members, or significant others, and the importance of hand washing to remove the organism. Teach correct hand-washing procedure. For HBV, HCV, and HDV, explain that blood, semen, and saliva can spread the disease, and teach the patient and significant others how to prevent transmission. Also assist the patient in identifying close contacts who may have been exposed to the hepatitis virus. Immune serum globulin or hepatitis B immune globulin may be indicated to provide these people with passive immunity.

Instruct the patient to refrain from kissing and sexual contact until liver enzyme tests return to normal. Caution the patient to refrain from consuming alcohol and using all drugs, unless prescribed by the physician. Explain that because alcohol and drugs are metabolized by the liver, use of these substances can lead to further liver damage. Stress the importance of rest, exercise, and a well-balanced diet. Provide written dietary instructions if needed.

Explain to the patient that blood, tissue, sperm, and organ donations cannot be made by persons who have a history of hepatitis.

NDx: Activity intolerance

Explain that activity should not exceed what the patient is comfortable doing. Fatigue is a normal response to hepatic cellular damage, and activity tolerance will increase as liver inflammation subsides. Provide rest periods between activities. Allow 60 to 90 minutes for rest between meals and hygiene or other activities. Explain to the patient and family that visitors are important during illness, but that they must not interfere with sleep and rest. If bedrest is not prescribed, encourage the patient to ambulate short distances each day. Provide a rest period before ambulation. Increase the distance walked by 10 to 20 feet each succeeding day. Monitor pulse rate before and after ambulation to determine the effect of ambulation on the cardiovascular system.

NDx: Body image disturbance

Explain the pathophysiologic basis for jaundice, stressing that it is temporary and will diminish as condition improves. Inform the patient of signs of improvement, such as decreasing bilirubin levels and improved stool and urine color. Encourage the patient to use his or her own clothing and select colors that do not accentuate the jaundice. Assist the patient as needed with grooming. Encourage the patient to discuss feelings and concerns. Facilitate communication between the patient and significant others.

Refer to the discussion of jaundice in Chapter 25 for other nursing diagnoses, expected patient outcomes and nursing interventions applicable to the patient with hepatitis during the icteric phase.

Compare the patient's status with the expected outcomes. If the outcomes are not met, reassess the patient and revise the plan.

TOXIC AND DRUG-INDUCED HEPATITIS

Etiology and Pathophysiology

Toxic hepatitis is an inflammatory condition caused by ingestion, inhalation, or parenteral administration of substances that have a poisonous effect on the liver. Table 26–4 illustrates some common hepatotoxins and their sources. These agents produce liver damage with predictable regularity.

Drug-induced toxic hepatitis is usually an idiosyncratic response. The patient may have a unique susceptibility to the medication or an immunologic response. Drugs are responsible for 2 to 5% of all hospital admissions for jaundice in the United States. Certain drugs account for 20 to 50% of the cases of fulminant hepatic failure. Table 26–5 presents the medications most commonly associated with drug-induced toxic hepatitis and their potential hepatotoxic effect.

The specific liver changes associated with toxic hepatitis depend on the offending agent. Exposure to vinyl chloride over many years leads to sclerosis of the portal venules and subsequent portal hypertension. Ingestion of poisonous mushrooms causes massive cell destruction. Drug-induced liver disease is classified as cytotoxic, cholestatic, or mixed. Cyto-

Table 26–4

Common Hepatotoxins and Their Sources	
Toxin	**Source**
Carbon tetrachloride	Dry-cleaning fluid
Trichloroethylene	Cleaning fluid (often sniffed by adolescents)
Toluene	Glue (often sniffed by adolescents)
Chlorophenothane	Insecticide
Vinyl chloride	Used in the production of synthetics
Muscarine	Poisonous mushrooms
Arsenic	Garden and household pesticides, Fowler's solution used in the treatment of psoriasis
Yellow phosphorus	Rat poison, firecrackers

Table 26–5

Drugs Commonly Associated with Hepatotoxicity

Drug	Toxic Effect
Acetaminophen (Tylenol)	Has a predictable, dose-dependent effect; causes liver cell necrosis; acute liver failure and death in doses >10–15 g at one time; cell necrosis may also occur at therapeutic doses of 3–8 g/day; cellular injury reversed if drug discontinued
Acetylsalicylic acid (Aspirin)	Elevated liver serum enzyme levels and abnormal liver function tests with doses >3 g/day; mechanism of liver injury not known; reversible if drug discontinued
Chlorpromazine (Thorazine)	Impaired secretion of bile with cellular inflammation and cell necrosis
Erythromycin estolate (Ilosone)	Impaired secretion of bile and liver cell necrosis; documented cases of patients who had unnecessary gallbladder surgery on basis of presenting signs and symptoms
Isoniazid (INH)	Symptoms mimic viral hepatitis infection; seen in approximately 1% of patients taking drug as prophylaxis against tuberculosis; of this group, 10% may have fatal reaction; incidence exceeds 2% in those older than 50 years; usually occurs 2–3 months after starting drug but can occur up to 12 months later; elevated enzyme levels seen in 10–20% of patients taking isoniazid, although no actual symptoms are present
Phenobarbital (Luminal)	Lowers serum bilirubin levels by inducing increased production of glucuronyl transferase; increases excretion and flow of bile salts; altered liver function and jaundice more common with long-term use
Diazepam (Valium)	Long-term use alters liver function by unclear mechanism, manifested by jaundice
Oral contraceptives	May interfere with bile secretion and flow, cause hepatic vein thrombosis and predisposition to cholesterol gallstone formation; symptoms and effects resolve if drug discontinued

toxic injury causes damage to hepatic cells. Cholestatic injury causes arrested bile flow. Mixed injury has simultaneous characteristics associated with both cytotoxic and cholestatic injury. Isoniazid, used as a prophylactic agent in patients with a positive tuberculin test, produces liver necrosis in susceptible individuals. If isoniazid is administered in combination with rifampin for treatment of active tuberculosis, the patient is at even greater risk for liver damage. Chlorpromazine produces cholestasis in 1 to 2% of patients receiving the drug. Phenobarbital and diazepam produce mixed injury.

Clinical Manifestations
The person with toxic hepatitis experiences signs and symptoms similar to those of viral hepatitis. Initially, gastrointestinal and influenza-like symptoms appear. Depending on the toxic agent, the degree of exposure, and the extent of liver damage, jaundice, hepatomegaly, and other signs of hepatic necrosis may be present.

The onset of symptoms depends on the type of reaction experienced. Drug-induced liver disease may develop within days of exposure to a known hepatotoxic agent. It may take several weeks for symptoms caused by a hypersensitivity or drug allergy to appear. Weeks or months often pass before manifestations of metabolic idiosyncratic reactions to drugs appear.

Diagnosis
If symptoms of chronic active hepatitis are present, but serologic tests for viral hepatitis are negative, a complete history of exposure to hepatotoxins is obtained. Liver biopsy may be performed to identify the extent of liver damage.

Management
Treatment of toxic hepatitis requires removal of the suspected hepatotoxin. In most cases of drug-induced hepatitis, hepatic damage will resolve if the offending agent is discontinued.

❖ **Settings, Providers, and Collaboration for Care**
Depending on the severity of this type of hepatitis, care may be given in the physician's office, in an ambulatory care setting for liver biopsy, or through acute hospitalization.

NURSING PROCESS GUIDELINES
Toxic Hepatitis

Nursing assessment of the person with toxic hepatitis includes close observation for the clinical manifestations of hepatitis previously mentioned. Obtain a complete list of all medications taken currently and within the past 3 months, including over-the-counter medications. Ask specifically about any past exposure to hepatotoxic agents. Nursing diagnoses reflect the patient's response to the clinical manifestations and the need to teach the patient to avoid exposure to the hepatotoxic agent or use of the hepatotoxic drugs.

LIVER ABSCESS

Etiology and Pathophysiology
A pyogenic liver abscess is a collection of pus within the liver that results from bacterial infection. The organisms most commonly associated with this condition are the enteric flora *Escherichia coli*, *Klebsiella pneumoniae*, and *Staphylococcus aureus*. In areas of the world where sanitation is poor, liver abscess may be caused by the ameba *Entamoeba histolytica*. This ameba invades the intestinal mucosa, causing a colitis, and may travel via the blood stream to the liver. In about two-thirds of cases, multiple bacterial species are present. Anaerobic bacteria are present in half or more of cases. Since the introduction of antibiotics, the incidence of liver abscess is low.

Organisms reach the liver in a number of ways. The most common source is biliary tract disease, such as acute cholecystitis. Other sources of liver abscess include:

- Infections in areas drained by the portal system, such as the appendix and diverticulum
- Direct extension from an adjacent structure, such as a subphrenic abscess
- Organisms introduced from outside the body as a result of a gunshot or knife wound
- Organisms introduced via the hepatic artery as a result of bacteremia

The mortality rate for patients with a pyogenic abscess ranges from 10 to 60%. Multiple abscesses that cannot be surgically drained, advanced age, underlying malignancy, and spread of the organism to other locations adversely affect the prognosis. Uncomplicated amebic liver abscess has a mortality rate of less than 1%.

Clinical Manifestations
The clinical manifestations of liver abscess are usually those of a systemic infectious process. Fever may precede other symptoms. Abdominal pain, weight loss, and anorexia are the characteristic complaints. Jaundice is present in up to 20% of the cases and usually indicates biliary tract disease. On physical examination, 50% of the patients have hepatomegaly with right upper quadrant pain or tenderness.

Diagnosis
Laboratory data indicate the presence of leukocytosis, but liver function test results may be only slightly altered if the abscess is confined to a small area of the liver. Most commonly, alkaline phospha-

tase levels are elevated. Blood cultures are positive in more than 50% of cases.

X-ray examination of the chest reveals elevation of the right hemidiaphragm in about half the patients with liver abscess. Ultrasonography and computed tomographic (CT) scan are ordered to visualize abscess formation. They reveal single or multiple collections of pus encased in fibrous tissue. Ultrasonography is most useful in differentiating liver abscess from neoplasms, hematomas, and cysts. CT has the advantage of being able to reveal abscesses high up in the right lobe that may be missed by ultrasonography. When amebic abscess is suspected, contents of the abscess can be aspirated, guided by ultrasonogram or CT scan.

Management
Initial treatment for patients with liver abscess includes combination intravenous antibiotic therapy. An aminoglycoside or third-generation cephalosporin is prescribed to destroy gram-negative organisms. Clindamycin may be prescribed to destroy anaerobic organisms, and ampicillin to destroy gram-positive organisms. Specific antibiotic therapy is instituted when blood and abscess cultures are complete. Antibiotic therapy may need to be continued for up to 16 weeks. Oral preparations are usually prescribed after the third week. When etiologic factors indicate an amebic liver abscess, metronidazole (Flagyl) is prescribed for 5 to 7 days. Metronidazole is described in Highlight 26–1.

Percutaneous closed drainage may be used for bacterial liver abscess. It is used for amebic liver abscess only if the patient fails to respond to oral medication. A catheter is inserted into the abscess under radiologic guidance and remains in place for 3 to 20 days for drainage. Surgical incision and drainage may be required when additional disease, such as bile duct obstruction, is present.

❖ Settings, Providers, and Collaboration for Care
The initial care setting for these patients is usually acute hospitalization. As the patient's condition improves, care may take place in a physician's office, an ambulatory care setting, or at home.

NURSING PROCESS GUIDELINES
Liver Abscess

Assess the patient for pain and note changes in its severity. Monitor vital signs, especially temperature, to determine the response to antibiotic therapy. Administer antibiotics at prescribed intervals to maintain therapeutic blood levels. Because patients may think they can stop taking the medication when their physical condition improves, teach them the rationale of long-term antibiotic therapy and the importance of continuing therapy for the prescribed length of time.

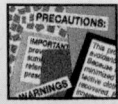

HIGHLIGHT
26–1
PHARMACOLOGY

Metronidazole (Flagyl)

Definition:

Antiprotozoal agent.

Action:

Metabolized by anaerobic organisms to products that disrupt DNA synthesis.

Uses:

Drug of choice for treating acute intestinal amebiasis and for liver abscess caused by *Entamoeba histolytica*. It is also used for the treatment of anaerobic bacterial infections of the abdomen, bones or joints, lower lung, and central nervous system.

Side Effects:

Previously unrecognized *Candida* infections may present more prominent symptoms and require treatment. Nausea, dry mouth, headache, and dizziness may occur. Toxicity may precipitate seizures, and peripheral neuropathy may occur. The appearance of abnormal neurologic signs requires discontinuation of the drug.

Interactions:

Potentiates the anticoagulant effect of warfarin and other oral anticoagulants, resulting in a prolonged prothrombin time. Simultaneous administration of phenytoin or phenobarbital causes lower plasma levels of metronidazole. Alcohol consumption during therapy and for 1 day after therapy causes abdominal cramps, nausea, vomiting, headache, and flushing. Disulfiram should be discontinued 2 weeks before therapy begins.

Nursing Implications:

Instruct the patient to avoid all alcoholic beverages during and immediately after therapy. Caution against use of hazardous equipment if dizziness ocurs. Notify the physician immediately if seizures or abnormal neurologic signs are present. Instruct the patient to report evidence of numbness or paresthesia of an extremity. Patients with edema may not be able to tolerate the 28 mEq of sodium in each gram of metronidazole.

Structural Disorders

CIRRHOSIS

Cirrhosis of the liver is a chronic, degenerative process that follows hepatocellular necrosis. It is characterized by nodule formation and generalized liver fibrosis. Three forms of cirrhosis are commonly identified: Laënnec's, primary biliary, and postnecrotic. Although each type has a different cause, the ultimate outcome is essentially the same. The major types of cirrhosis are compared in Table 26–6.

Etiology and Pathophysiology
Laënnec's Cirrhosis
Laënnec's cirrhosis—also known as alcoholic, portal, or fatty cirrhosis—is the most common type of cirrhosis in North America, South America, and Western Europe. It usually results from excessive alcohol (ethanol) ingestion over a long period of time. However, cirrhosis does not develop in all alcoholics and can occur in nonalcoholic patients.

Several studies have shown that the disorder develops in about 20% of persons who consumed an average of 160 g of ethanol per day, equivalent to two six-packs of beer or a pint of whiskey, for more than 10 years. However, women appear to develop Laënnec's cirrhosis with lesser amounts of alcohol than men, suggesting that hormonal factors may play a role in susceptibility. Poor nutrition is also implicated as a possible reason for the development of Laënnec's cirrhosis. Frequently, alcoholics do not maintain a balanced diet and consume only the calories supplied by the alcoholic beverage. However, Laënnec's cirrhosis develops in many alcoholics even in the presence of a balanced diet.

The incidence of Laënnec's cirrhosis is disproportionately high in African-Americans, Hispanics, and Native Americans, and disproportionately low in Asian-Americans. Because conflicting evidence does not support one specific cause for this type of cirrhosis, it is believed that genetic, nutritional, and environmental factors may all play a role in its development.

The first indication of liver damage as a result of alcohol use is fatty infiltration of the liver. Large droplets of fat gradually occupy most of the volume of the hepatocyte cells. Patients at this stage rarely have symptoms. These cellular changes usually resolve within 3 to 6 weeks if alcohol is withdrawn and the patient consumes a diet with adequate protein, calories, and vitamins. If alcohol intake contin-

Table 26-6

Comparison of Major Types of Cirrhosis

	Laënnec's	Primary Biliary	Postnecrotic
OCCURRENCE	Most common type in North America and Western Europe	No specific distribution	Most common form worldwide
CAUSE	Most commonly alcohol consumption	Unknown	Previous viral hepatitis, toxic drug or chemical reaction, autoimmune disease, and unknown (10%)
SEX AFFECTED	Males most often, but females seen more frequently as drinking habits change	Women 30–65 years of age	Men and women equally
OTHER NAMES	Alcoholic cirrhosis Fatty cirrhosis Micronodular cirrhosis	Cholangitic or obstructive cirrhosis	Toxic cirrhosis Cryptogenic cirrhosis Coarsely nodular cirrhosis
MAJOR CLINICAL FEATURES	Muscle wasting Jaundice Portal hypertension Ascites	May be asymptomatic for years; pruritus earliest symptom; eventually portal hypertension, ascites, and jaundice occur	Usually resembles active hepatitis in early stage and Laënnec's cirrhosis in late stage

ues, toxic hepatitis may develop. This condition, an acute liver inflammation, is often a precursor of Laënnec's cirrhosis.

Primary Biliary Cirrhosis

Primary biliary cirrhosis, also known as cholangitic or obstructive cirrhosis, is reported in all races and in most geographic areas of the world. More than 90% of the patients are women, and the typical age of onset is between 30 and 65. The cause of primary biliary cirrhosis is unknown. However, it is frequently associated with certain autoimmune disorders, such as Raynaud's phenomenon and Sjögren's syndrome. A genetic factor may be important because the disease has been reported in mothers and daughters, siblings, and twins.

Primary biliary cirrhosis starts in the medium and small bile ducts with obstruction of bile flow (cholestasis). Gradual scarring and destruction of hepatocytes occur, and bands of fibrous tissue extend to adjacent structures in the liver.

Postnecrotic Cirrhosis

Postnecrotic cirrhosis, also known as cryptogenic, toxic, or macronodular cirrhosis, is a type of advanced liver injury of both specific and unknown (cryptogenic) causes. Liver tissue is replaced with small to large nodules of fibrous tissue. It is believed that most cases represent the end-stage of a previously active hepatitis B or C, or a chronic active hepatitis of the autoimmune type. Some cases

have been linked to a toxic drug or chemical response. Patients with postnecrotic cirrhosis can remain asymptomatic for years. Cirrhotic changes may be detected during evaluation for an unrelated problem or when there is a progression of symptoms resulting from the original liver disorder.

Regardless of the type of cirrhosis, the end result is extensive destruction of hepatocytes and interference with liver function. Destroyed hepatocytes are replaced with dense, fibrous scar tissue and nodules. The nodules impede portal blood flow, and portal hypertension occurs. This leads to development of ascites, varices, and splenomegaly. The thin-walled varices, especially in the mucosa of the gastric fundus and esophagus (Fig. 26-1), may bleed slowly or may rupture, causing massive and possibly fatal hemorrhage. Decreased hepatic synthesis of coagulation factors and decreased platelets as a result of splenomegaly further complicate the control of bleeding. The pathophysiology of portal hypertension is discussed in Chapter 25.

Clinical Manifestations

In many patients with Laënnec's cirrhosis, the symptoms are insidious in onset, usually developing after 10 or more years of excessive alcohol intake. Most patients seek medical care because of ascites or jaundice. Complaints of generalized weakness and nonspecific gastrointestinal symptoms are common, such as anorexia, nausea and vomiting, indigestion, flatulence, and possibly right upper quadrant pain made

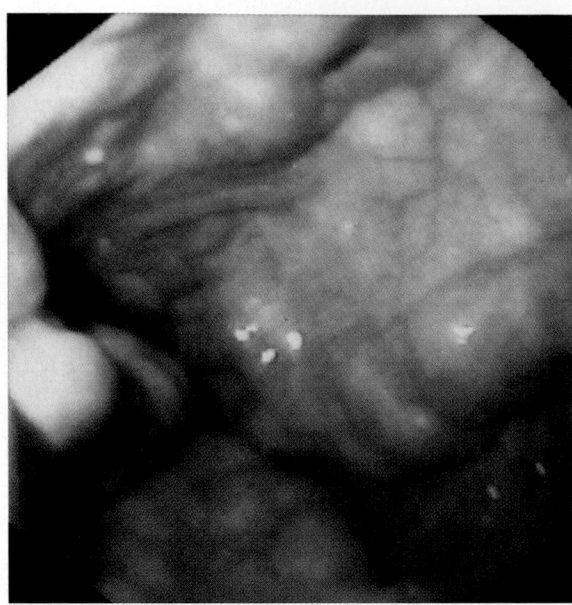

Figure 26–1

Multiple, large, tortuous esophageal varices as seen through an endoscope. (From Gitlin N, Strauss RM. Atlas of clinical hepatology. Philadelphia: WB Saunders, 1995.)

worse by sitting up or leaning forward. Peripheral edema may be present before ascites, but frequently they appear together. Weight loss is common but, because of fluid retention, it is not apparent. Some patients do not seek medical attention until massive gastrointestinal hemorrhage from ruptured esophageal or gastric varices occurs.

Table 26–7 presents the major clinical manifestations of cirrhosis and corresponding pathophysiology. The severity and number of manifestations are generally proportional to the extent of liver damage. Because of the many and varied functions of the liver, every body system is affected in some way. The clinical manifestations and medical and nursing management of jaundice, ascites, and hepatic encephalopathy are discussed in detail in Chapter 25.

Diagnosis

A diagnosis of cirrhosis is based on presenting clinical manifestations, patient history, liver function tests, visualization studies, and liver biopsy.

In Laënnec's cirrhosis, the patient is usually anemic from the direct toxic effect of alcohol on bone marrow; a nutritional deficiency of folic acid, pyridoxine and vitamin B_{12}; and the possibility of chronic gastrointestinal blood loss. Leukopenia may also be present from bone marrow depression caused by alcohol. Liver function studies indicate

Table 26–7

Clinical Manifestations of Cirrhosis

Clinical Manifestation	Pathophysiology
Gastrointestinal symptoms	Venous congestion of gastrointestinal tract
Palpable liver	Fatty infiltration of liver cells causes liver enlargement and nodule formation
Fever (low grade)	Hepatic inflammation and necrosis
Weakness, fatigue, and muscle wasting	Interference with synthesis of tissue proteins and utilization of nutrients
Bleeding tendencies	Decreased absorption of vitamin K or decreased production of clotting factors, especially prothrombin
Ascites and edema	Portal hypertension, decreased serum albumin level, decreased ability of liver to metabolize aldosterone
Striae	Stretching of abdominal skin because of ascites
Jaundice and pruritus	Failure of liver cells to metabolize and excrete bilirubin
Spider angiomas	Arterial lesions formed by dilation of groups of small blood vessels believed to be caused by high estrogen levels
Gynecomastia; scant hair on chest, pubic area, and axilla	Inability of liver to detoxify estrogen
Palmar erythema (liver palms)	Bright red palms and soles of feet believed to be caused by high estrogen levels
Distended abdominal blood vessels	Obstructed liver blood flow, leading to formation of collateral blood vessels
Impaired neurologic function (hepatic encephalopathy): shortened attention span, slurred speech, asterixis, hyperactive muscle reflexes, grimacing, blinking, appearance of sucking and grasp reflexes, loss of consciousness. Table 27–4 lists additional characteristics of impaired neurologic function.	Formation of toxic products, most notably ammonia and mercaptans, which interfere with brain metabolism

decreased serum albumin levels and elevated alkaline phosphatase, aspartate aminotransferase, alanine aminotransferase, and bilirubin levels. Prothrombin time is prolonged, and blood ammonia levels may be increased because portal hypertension shunts blood around the liver. Ultrasonography and CT scan confirm the presence of fibrous tissue and impaired hepatic blood flow. An endoscopy or upper gastrointestinal barium study verifies the presence of varices. A liver biopsy confirms a diagnosis of cirrhosis but may be contraindicated if the patient has a coagulation disorder.

Management

Management depends on the stage of the disease and the presenting clinical manifestations. Abstinence from alcohol in all types of cirrhosis is of the utmost importance. Continued alcohol use with Laënnec's cirrhosis reduces the 5-year survival rate to about 40%.

No dietary restrictions are imposed unless ascites or hepatic encephalopathy is present. Patients are encouraged to consume a well-balanced diet of 2500 to 3000 calories daily. At least 1 g of protein per kilogram of body weight is recommended to promote regeneration of hepatocytes. Vitamin supplements are usually prescribed because of malabsorption of the fat-soluble and B-complex vitamins. Supplements include vitamin K injections, folic acid, thiamin, and pyridoxine. If symptoms of hepatic encephalopathy occur, protein is restricted. With ascites, sodium is restricted.

Complications

Bleeding from esophageal varices is a major, life-threatening complication of portal hypertension. The varices, usually located in the lower third of the esophagus, may extend into the stomach. Slow bleeding can occur, but hemorrhage is more common. The exact cause of bleeding from esophageal varices remains controversial. The theory that bleeding results from esophageal irritation caused by eating solid foods, which cause trauma to the thin-walled vessels, has been abandoned. It is now believed that a combination of factors, including increased portal hypertension and thinning of the walls of the varices, leads to rupture.

The most common manifestation of ruptured esophageal varices is hematemesis with rapid development of hemorrhagic shock and severely compromised blood flow to vital organs. Hemorrhagic shock is treated with parenteral fluid replacement and blood transfusions as described in Chapter 11. Bleeding from ruptured varices stops spontaneously in 60% of patients, but recurrent episodes are common. There is no way to identify those patients in whom bleeding will spontaneously stop and those who, without treatment, will continue to bleed.

Initial treatment to control bleeding usually consists of pharmacologic therapy and insertion of a large-bore nasogastric tube to aspirate blood from the stomach. As discussed in Chapter 25, breakdown of blood in the gastrointestinal tract places the patient at risk for elevated serum ammonia levels and hepatic encephalopathy. The nasogastric tube may also be used for gastric lavage (gentle irrigation of the stomach) with room-temperature normal saline or tap water to facilitate complete removal of blood and blood clots. Use of iced saline or water to promote vasoconstriction of bleeding varices is controversial. The benefits are questionable, especially if the bleeding is esophageal rather than gastric.

Once the gastric aspirate clears with lavage, or at least shows partial clearing of clots, immediate endoscopy is performed to confirm the diagnosis and rule out other sources of bleeding. Patients with cirrhosis frequently bleed from nonvariceal causes, such as hemorrhagic gastritis and peptic ulcers. When bleeding from varices is confirmed, treatment may include injection sclerotherapy and possibly balloon tamponade. Long-term control of bleeding may require additional sclerotherapy or surgical intervention.

Pharmacologic Therapy

Pharmacologic therapy is initiated early in a bleeding episode. Vasopressin (Pitressin) or octreotide (Sandostatin) may be ordered to lower the portal venous pressure in an acute variceal bleed. Vasopressin, a potent vasoconstrictor, decreases portal pressure by constricting splanchnic arterioles, thus decreasing portal blood flow. It is administered either intravenously via an infusion pump or through a catheter placed in the superior mesenteric artery under fluoroscopy. Temporary control of bleeding is achieved in approximately 80% of patients; however, rebleeding within 24 to 48 hours after vasopressin therapy is discontinued occurs in as many as 45%. Vasopressin must be used with caution in patients who have coronary artery disease because its vasoconstrictive effects can induce angina or even a myocardial infarct in these patients. It can also induce cardiac dysrhythmias and can cause abdominal pain because of decreased blood flow to abdominal organs. Sandostatin, reported to be as effective as vasopressin but without its cardiac side effects, is administered either intravenously or subcutaneously. Since it causes gastrointestinal side effects such as nausea, vomiting, and abdominal pain, it is administered between meals and at bedtime when possible.

Nitroglycerin, a potent systemic vasodilator, is often administered via the IV or sublingual route in combination with vasopressin. Nitroglycerin causes vasodilation of the portosystemic collateral blood vessels. It enhances portal pressure reduction and reduces side effects associated with vasopressin alone. Studies indicate that combination therapy is effective in controlling acute bleeding in 64% of patients.

Propranolol or nadolol, beta-blocking agents, is used to prevent initial and recurrent variceal hemorrhage, but they are not widely used for acute variceal bleeding because of their potential impairment

CLINICAL ❓ THINKING

COFFEE-GROUND VOMITUS IN AN ALCOHOLIC PATIENT

A 58-year-old male came to the emergency room at 2 AM saying that, in the past 24 hours, he had twice vomited small amounts of a substance that looked like coffee grounds. Also in the past week, he had developed an upper respiratory infection with a dry, hacking cough. He denied any previous episodes of hematemesis as well as any history of gastrointestinal disorders, significant medical history, previous hospitalizations, and use of medications. His blood pressure was 108/70 and apical pulse rate was 98 bpm. He had regular, unlabored respirations with a rate of 20 per minute. His temperature was 98.8°F.

Peripheral intravenous therapy was initiated and a nasogastric tube inserted. About 150 mL of coffee-ground aspirate was returned and tested positive for blood. Blood specimens were drawn for type and cross-match and chemistry and coagulation studies. He was admitted to a medical-surgical unit and scheduled to undergo endoscopic evaluation that afternoon for determination of the cause of the gastrointestinal bleeding.

Upon arrival on the unit, the patient appeared comfortable, alert, and oriented. The nasogastric tube, attached to low intermittent suction, was draining small amounts of coffee-ground aspirate. My initial physical examination of the patient revealed the following assessments: blood pressure 112/72, apical pulse rate 94 and regular, respiratory rate 20 per minute and unlabored, temperature 99.2°F. Lungs were clear to both auscultation and percussion. The patient's skin was pale, warm, and dry. Peripheral pulses were palpable, with capillary refill time less than 3 seconds. Slight pitting edema (+1) was noted in the lower extremities. Abdominal assessment revealed hyperactive bowel sounds and hepatic and splenic enlargement with no evidence of abdominal tenderness or ascites. Upon further examination, I noted the presence of spider angiomas on the patient's neck, shoulders, and chest, as well as marked gynecomastia.

In response to focused questions, the patient reported that each episode of vomiting was precipitated by coughing, and that although he did not experience any epigastric or abdominal discomfort, he had been experiencing a loss of appetite, flatulence, weight loss, and fatigue over the past few months. He denied any change in his bowel habits or nature of his stool, but did complain of discomfort from hemorrhoids of recent onset. He denied any alcohol abuse in recent years, but reported a history of "heavy drinking" previously.

The patient's history of hematemesis and alcoholism, reports of anorexia, fatigue, weight loss, flatulence, and hemorrhoids—coupled with physical findings that included hepatomegaly, splenomegaly, peripheral edema, spider angiomas, and gynecomastia—led me to suspect the development of cirrhosis, portal hypertension, and esophageal varices. Although upper gastrointestinal bleeding can be associated with gastritis, peptic ulcer disease, Mallory-Weiss syndrome, or esophageal varices, I suspected that esophageal varices had ruptured, secondary to increased intra-abdominal pressure from coughing, and were the origin of the bleeding.

Twenty minutes after I left his room, I was summoned back by his shouts for help. He was lying down, coughing and vomiting large amounts of bright red blood with clots around the nasogastric tube. Based on the patient's history and a quick assessment of his nares and the nature of the blood, I eliminated epistaxis and hemoptysis as possible sources of bleeding. Because the patient was at risk of airway obstruction and aspiration of the vomitus, I turned the patient on his side and prepared the suction equipment should it become necessary. The patient remained alert, but was pale and diaphoretic. His blood pressure had fallen to 80/56, his pulse rate had increased to 124 bpm and was weak and thready, his respiratory rate was 30 per minute. His skin was cool and clammy, peripheral pulses were weak and capillary refill time was greater than 3 seconds. The patient was extremely restless, anxious, and alarmed by the bleeding.

These findings represented a significant change in the patient's clinical status. The changes in vital signs (hypotension, tachycardia, tachypnea) in the presence of bright red bloody hematemesis, prompted me to suspect decreased circulatory volume and the onset of hypovolemic shock from gastrointestinal bleeding. The presence of additional classic signs of shock—including pale, cool, clammy skin; weak peripheral pulses; and increased capillary refill time—supported my suspicion. The abrupt onset of profuse gastrointestinal bleeding in the absence of pain further supported the likelihood of esophageal varices as the origin.

Bleeding esophageal varices constitute a life-threatening emergency and are associated with high mortality rates. Because blood loss is rapid, hypovolemic shock, inadequate perfusion of vital organs, and sudden death can occur. I therefore immediately implemented the following measures:

1. I continued to ensure a patent airway.
2. I remained with the patient, called for help, and asked another nurse to notify the physician.

CLINICAL ? THINKING

(continued)

3. I asked another staff member to bring the crash cart to the bedside.

4. I placed the patient in a modified shock position with the head of the bed slightly elevated.

5. I increased the flow rate in the existing intravenous line.

6. I inserted a second IV line with a large-bore peripheral venous catheter, and initiated O_2 therapy according to hospital protocol.

7. I irrigated the patient's nasogastric tube.

8. I attached a pulse oximeter to the patient.

9. I attached a cardiac monitor to the patient and monitored for dysrhythmias.

10. I monitored and documented the patient's intake and output.

11. I continued to frequently monitor the patient's cardiovascular and neurologic status.

12. I placed an additional blanket on the patient.

13. I provided psychologic support to the patient by providing realistic reassurance, clear explanations, and an opportunity to verbalize his fears.

14. I asked another nurse to check that the previously ordered blood was available.

15. I asked another staff member to obtain supplies for gastric lavage with saline and for insertion of a Sengstaken-Blakemore tube.

16. I documented my findings and actions.

Admitting laboratory results reflected abnormal liver function tests and provided further evidence for the likelihood of bleeding esophageal varices secondary to liver disease. The physician arrived and ordered the infusion of IV fluids and 2 units of packed red blood cells, a STAT complete blood count, hemoglobin, hematocrit, serum electrolytes, blood urea nitrogen, serum creatinine, serum ammonia, liver function tests, coagulation studies, arterial blood gases, and type and cross-match for an additional 4 units of packed red blood cells. Oxygen therapy, a 12-lead electrocardiogram, and insertion of an indwelling urinary catheter were also ordered. To accomplish hemostasis, the physician ordered gastric lavage with saline, IV vasopressin therapy, and preparation of the patient for the insertion of a Sengstaken-Blakemore tube.

Following transfer to the intensive care unit, the acute esophageal hemorrhage was temporarily controlled by the IV vasopressin therapy and esophageal tamponade with the Sengstaken-Blakemore tube. Following hemostasis and stabilization of vital signs, endoscopic injection sclerotherapy was performed. The patient remained alert and hemodynamically stable and was transferred back to the medical-surgical unit for continued observation and monitoring.

During my afternoon rounds on the third day following the bleeding episode, I noted that the patient was confused and agitated and that his speech was slurred. These changes in his mental status and speech pattern indicated yet another change in the patient's condition. Although I recognized that these symptoms might be associated with conditions such as transient ischemic attack or cerebrovascular accident, these findings in a patient with liver disease following a massive gastrointestinal bleed may be manifestations of early hepatic encephalopathy. The patient's vital signs were stable and additional signs and symptoms, such as asterixis, were absent. Because this condition is reversible if treated but can potentially progress to cerebral intoxification, coma, and death, I notified the physician immediately. The development of hepatic encephalopathy was confirmed by the patient's ammonia levels. Treatment with enemas, lactulose, and neomycin was initiated to clear the gastrointestinal tract of blood and reduce ammonia formation.

The patient's condition improved over the next 36 hours, his mental status returned to normal, and he remained stable with no further evidence of encephalopathy or bleeding. Before planning his discharge, the patient was scheduled for a medical workup to determine the extent of hepatic dysfunction and an appropriate treatment plan to impede the progress of the disease.

Although the patient encountered two critical and potentially fatal complications, the nurse prevented further deterioration of the patient's condition by carefully assessing the patient, anticipating problems, recognizing the need for immediate medical treatment, and quickly and skillfully intervening. Expert nursing care and sound clinical judgments reversed the life-threatening course of both episodes.

Think Critically

Was positioning the patient in a modified shock position with the head of the bed slightly elevated the best action? Why? Why not?

What changes in the hemoglobin and hematocrit levels would the nurse expect to find immediately following the bleeding episode? Why? Following fluid replacement therapy? Why?

Was increasing the rate of flow of the IV line the best action? Why? Why not? What complications specific to rapid volume expansion in a patient with esophageal varices must the nurse recognize and monitor for?

(continued)

CLINICAL ? THINKING

(continued)

How would the nurse's assessments and actions have differed if the source of the gastrointestinal hemorrhage had been peptic ulcers? Mallory-Weiss syndrome?

What clinical manifestations of electrolyte imbalance secondary to blood loss should the nurse monitor the patient for?

What complications of IV vasopressin therapy would the nurse recognize and monitor for?

What complications of treatment with the Sengstaken-Blakemore tube would the nurse recognize and monitor for?

During the course of vasopressin therapy the patient complained of chest pain and asked, "Am I having a heart attack?" What would be the nurse's best response?

How would this scenario have differed if the medical treatment described had been insufficient? What additional medical approaches would the nurse anticipate?

The patient's wife asked the nurse about his prognosis. What would be the nurse's best response?

What specific information regarding medications, diet, symptoms to report, emergency procedures and modification of lifestyle should the nurse include in the discharge teaching plan?

When planning for discharge, with which other members of the health-care team should the nurse collaborate? Why?

What psychosocial aspects of care should be included in planning for the patient's discharge?

What community resources and/or agencies should be included in planning for the patient's discharge?

What community resources and/or agencies should be included in the nurse's referrals?

What specific interventions would be implemented by the nurse during the insertion of and treatment with the Sengstaken-Blakemore tube?

---

of cardiovascular response to hemorrhage. These drugs reduce portal pressure by reducing portal and collateral blood flow.

Sclerotherapy
Endoscopic sclerotherapy is the procedure of choice for long-term control of actively bleeding esophageal varices. In this procedure after baseline vital signs are obtained, the patient is sedated with an agent such as diazepam (Valium) or midazolam hydrochloride (Versed) and a local anesthetic is sprayed on the throat in preparation for insertion of the endoscope. When the varices are visualized, a sclerosing agent such as sodium tetradecyl is injected directly into them until they are obliterated. The sclerosing agent that causes thrombosis and eventual hardening should stop bleeding in 2 to 5 minutes. If bleeding does not stop, a second injection below the bleeding site is administered. In some cases, nonbleeding varices may also be injected as a prophylactic measure. Sclerotherapy requires a high degree of skill and is effective in stopping bleeding in 75 to 90% of patients. Complications of the procedure include esophageal perforation, esophageal ulceration, and aspiration with subsequent pneumonia and pleural effusion.

Following sclerotherapy, vital signs are monitored because the procedure is usually done on a patient who is bleeding. Chest discomfort for 1 to 2 days is expected and is treated with mild analgesics, but severe pain characteristic of esophageal perforation must be reported immediately to the physician.

Follow-up endoscopies are recommended at 6-month intervals to monitor for recurrence of varices. Prophylactic sclerotherapy, performed before any bleeding episodes, remains highly controversial. Some studies indicate that the procedure may actually increase the risk of bleeding.

Balloon Tamponade
The Sengstaken-Blakemore tube, illustrated in Figure 26–2, controls bleeding from esophageal varices by exerting direct pressure on bleeding sites. It is a triple-lumen tube with ports for gastric aspiration, inflation of a gastric balloon, and inflation of an esophageal balloon. The gastric balloon applies pressure at the cardioesophageal junction. This decreases blood flow to the esophageal varices and directly compresses gastric varices. The esophageal balloon directly compresses the esophageal varices. Balloon tamponade is used when sclerotherapy cannot be performed because of excessive bleeding or when pharmacotherapy is ineffective. It stops bleeding in approximately 78% of patients, but up to 50% rebleed after the tube is removed.

The Sengstaken-Blakemore tube is passed via the nares into the stomach. The gastric balloon is inflated with air, clamped, and pulled tightly against the cardiac portion of the stomach to tamponade bleeding sites. Traction is applied to maintain the gastric balloon snugly in place. One method for maintaining traction is to use a pulley system with a 0.5 kg weight (500 mL of saline in a plastic bottle). Another method is fitting the patient with a football

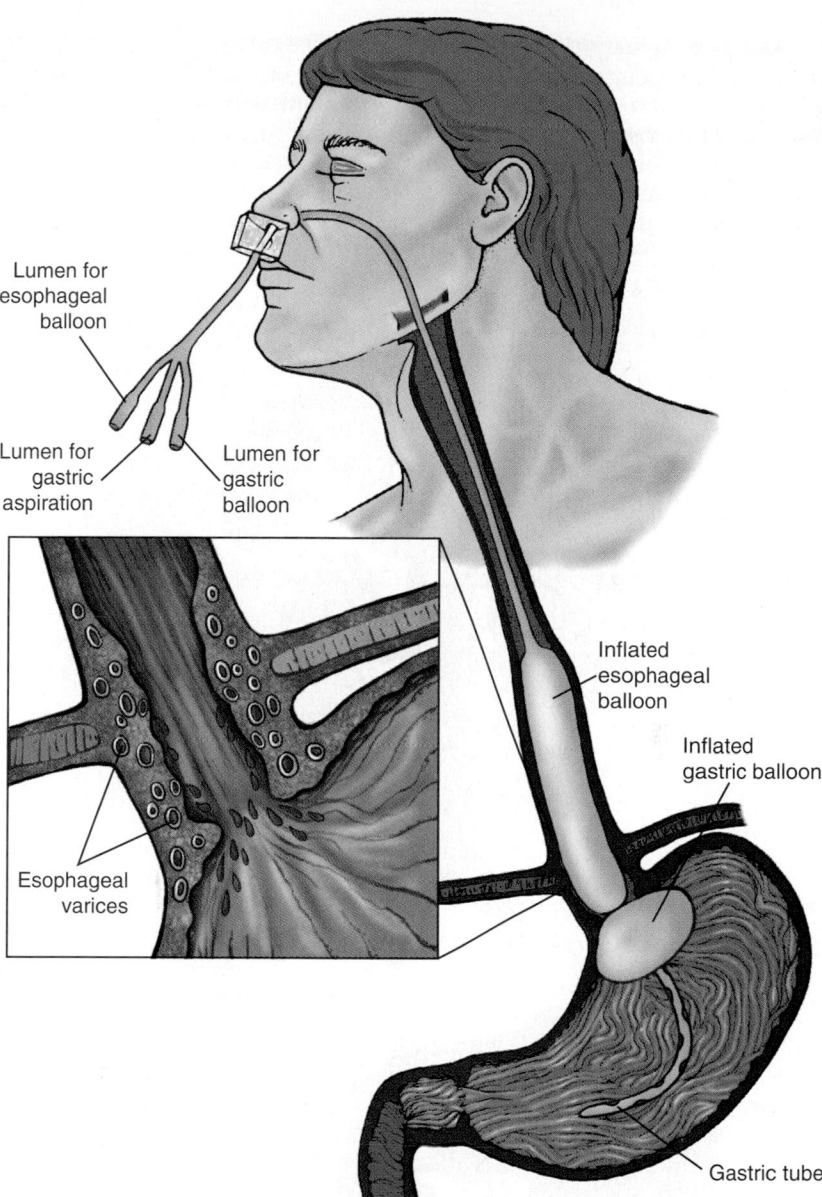

Figure 26–2
Sengstaken-Blakemore tube.

helmet and taping the tube to the chin guard under tension. If bleeding does not stop with inflation of the gastric balloon, the esophageal balloon is inflated to 25 to 45 mm Hg. Inflation pressure is constantly monitored by manometer to prevent esophageal necrosis from overinflation. X-ray examination of the upper abdomen and chest using portable equipment confirms balloon placement. Gastric contents and blood are aspirated by gastric lavage or intermittent suction via the gastric aspiration port.

When the esophageal balloon is inflated, the patient cannot swallow. Secretions accumulate above the level of the balloon and place the patient at risk for pulmonary aspiration. To minimize the risk, a nasogastric tube is inserted in the opposite naris, passed to the level of the esophageal balloon, and connected to intermittent suction to aspirate esophagopharyngeal secretions. If a Salem sump tube is used, it is connected to low, continuous suction. Stuporous or comatose patients may require endotracheal intubation to prevent aspiration.

The Minnesota esophagogastric tamponade tube, a four-lumen balloon tube, is a modification of the Sengstaken-Blakemore tube. The Minnesota tube has an additional lumen for aspirating esophagopharyngeal secretions. When this tube is used, an additional nasogastric tube is unnecessary. The Linton tube has only one balloon for gastric tamponade and esophageal and gastric ports for suctioning. Studies show no specific superiority or lower complication rate with the use of any particular tamponade tube.

In addition to pulmonary aspiration, major complications associated with balloon tamponade therapy are mechanical airway obstruction and esophageal perforation. If the gastric balloon ruptures or deflates, the entire tube moves upward and may obstruct the airway. Esophageal necrosis resulting from prolonged esophageal tube pressure may cause

esophageal perforation. Most experts recommend that esophageal balloon tamponade therapy be discontinued in 24 hours; however, the gastric balloon tamponade may be maintained for 48 to 72 hours. Some authorities recommend deflating the esophageal balloon for 30 to 60 minutes every 8 hours, but this practice is not universal.

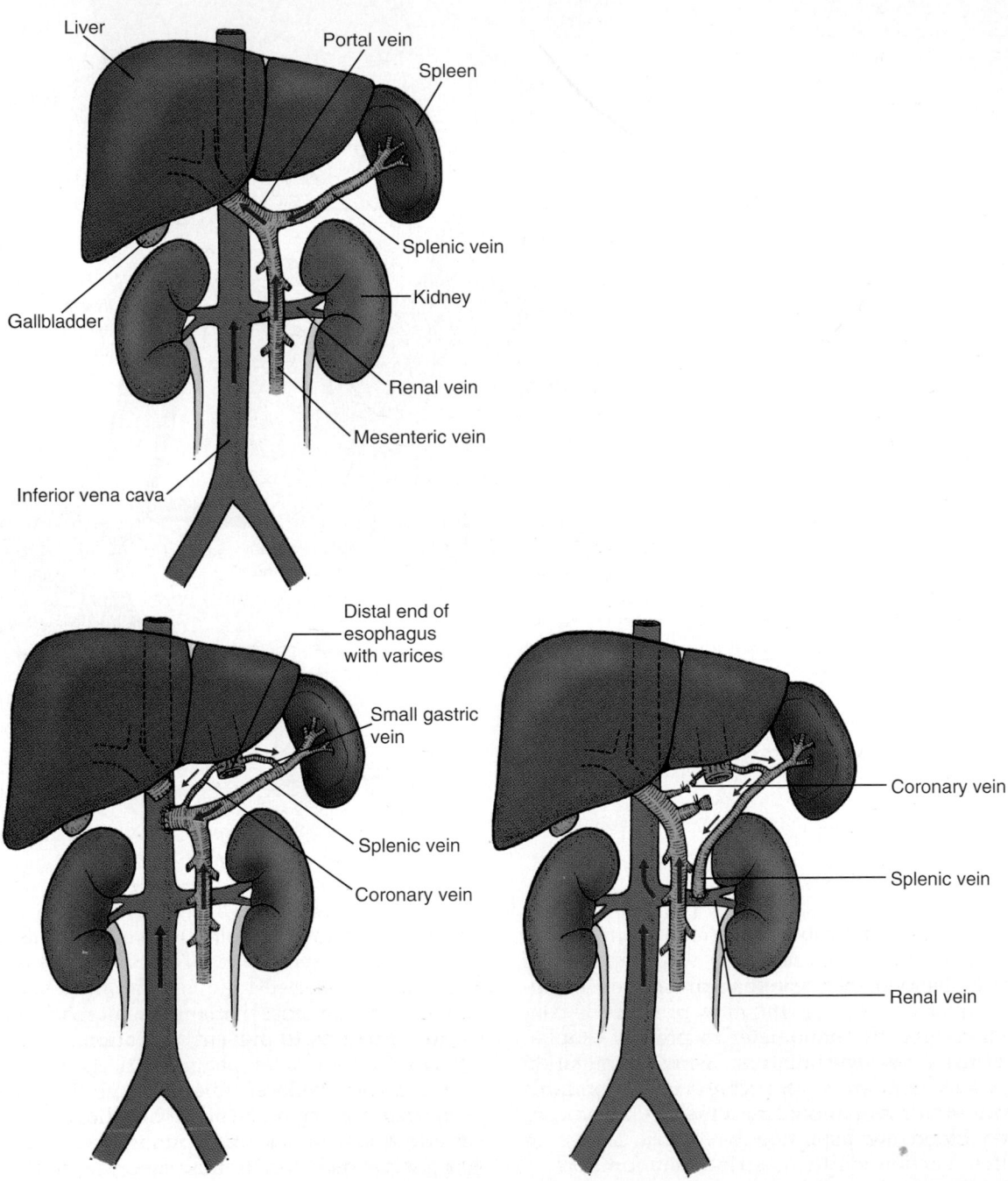

Figure 26-3

Normal portal system and selected surgical shunts. Illustration at top shows the normal portal system. Bottom left shows an end-to-side portacaval shunt. Portal hypertension is reduced and gastroesophageal varices are decompressed by improving blood flow through the small gastric vein and coronary vein and anastomosing the portal vein to the inferior vena cava. Bottom right shows a distal splenorenal shunt. The coronary vein is ligated to reduce portal hypertension, and gastroesophageal varices are decompressed by anastomosing the splenic vein to the renal vein.

Surgical Procedures

Surgical shunt procedures, which reduce portal pressure by diverting blood away from the portal circulation, may be used to decrease the incidence of variceal bleeding when sclerotherapy, pharmacologic interventions, and balloon therapy are ineffective. However, these procedures may place the patient at increased risk for hepatic encephalopathy and remain quite controversial. Even when the patient is in the best possible physical condition, the shunt procedure controls bleeding, but the long-term survival rate is not improved.

Two types of shunt procedures are done: the selective shunt procedure and the nonselective shunt procedure. Selective shunt procedures decompress only the varices; nonselective shunt procedures decompress the entire portovenous system.

Numerous variations of selective and nonselective shunt procedures are performed. However, the most widely recommended shunt procedure is the selective distal splenorenal shunt. This procedure causes minimal disruption of normal hepatic blood flow and has a lower incidence of hepatic encephalopathy. In this procedure, the distal end of the splenic vein is anastomosed to the side of the left renal vein. Blood is diverted from the high-pressure varices to the low-pressure renal vein. The portocaval shunt is the most common nonselective shunt procedure. It creates an anastomosis between the portal vein and the inferior vena cava. This procedure results in total loss of portal blood flow to the liver and is associated with an increased incidence of hepatic encephalopathy. The portocaval shunt is usually used in emergency situations when all other nonsurgical treatment options have failed. Figure 26–3 illustrates the normal portal system, the distal splenorenal shunt, and the portocaval shunt.

The transjugular intrahepatic portosystemic shunt is a nonsurgical percutaneous procedure for the treatment of acute and recurrent variceal hemorrhage in patients unable to withstand surgery or awaiting a liver transplant. It is a painful procedure with the risk of serious complications such as rupture of a major blood vessel, liver or kidney failure, and myocardial infarction. In this procedure, done under intravenous conscious sedation, the right internal jugular vein is accessed and a metallic, flexible stent is inserted into a new pathway created by balloon dilation of the tissue between the hepatic vein and the portal vein in the liver. This artificial shunt creates a new pathway for unobstructed blood flow and results in reduced portal venous pressure and decompression of esophageal varices. Periodic portal venograms confirm patency of the shunt.

❖ **Settings, Providers, and Collaboration for Care**

Patients with cirrhosis receive care in a variety of settings depending on the stage of the disease. These may include the physician's office, ambulatory care setting, and long-term care setting. Patients receiving balloon tamponade are assigned to a critical care unit. In the terminal stage of the disease, hospice care may be used. Implementation of a successful treatment plan requires collaboration with a nutritionist and a pharmacist, as well as with a social worker and representatives of community resource groups, which may be needed to help cope with any coexisting psychosocial problems such as alcohol abuse.

NURSING PROCESS GUIDELINES
Cirrhosis

Nursing Care Guide 26–1 presents nursing management of a patient with cirrhosis. Nursing care for patients with jaundice, ascites, hepatic encephalopathy, and nutritional deficiencies is described in Chapter 25. Assessments, nursing diagnoses, expected patient outcomes, and nursing interventions specific to the care of a patient with esophageal varices follow.

NURSING PROCESS
Esophageal Varices

Assessment

Question the patient about the use of alcohol, including type, amount, and length of use. Examine the patient to detect the presence of jaundice, ascites, and edema. Assess mental status to determine the presence of hepatic encephalopathy. Question the patient regarding hematemesis or black, tarry stools, which indicate blood in the stool. Test for occult blood in the stool.

If pharmacologic therapy with vasopressin is instituted, assess for side effects related to vasoconstriction and cardiotoxicity. These include dysrhythmias, hypertension, and chest pain. Assess fluid and electrolyte balance, since vasopressin may cause water intoxication (dilutional hyponatremia).

With active variceal bleeding, assess vital signs for evidence of hypovolemic shock. The patient in shock is restless and has cool, clammy skin, a decrease in blood pressure, tachycardia, and a decrease in urinary output. Note the frequency and amount of hematemesis and blood in the stool. Frank blood in the stool may indicate massive bleeding from varices.

If balloon tamponade therapy is instituted, frequent respiratory assessment is indicated to identify accumulation of secretions above the level of the esophageal balloon. Monitor rate and quality of respirations. Auscultate the lungs for evidence of aspiration. Esophageal perforation caused by balloon tamponade is suspected if the patient complains of back pain or upper abdominal pain or if shock is evidenced. Perforation requires immediate surgical intervention.

Nursing Care Guide 26–1
Patients with Cirrhosis

Assessment Findings:	Patient is admitted to the hospital for the third time in the last 18 months with a diagnosis of cirrhosis. Patient has gained 10 lbs over the past 3 days. Abdomen is distended. Patient complains of difficulty breathing. Respirations are 26 per minute and shallow.
Nursing Diagnosis:	Ineffective breathing pattern related to pressure on the diaphragm from ascites

Patient Outcomes	Nursing Interventions	Rationale
Patient's vital signs remain within normal limits with respirations between 12 and 20 per minute with full chest expansion.	Elevate the head of the bed 45 to 90 degrees.	Gravity helps to pull ascitic fluid down away from the diaphragm, thereby promoting full chest expansion.
	Instruct patient to deep breathe every 2 hours.	Encourages maximum chest expansion.
	Monitor vital signs every 4 hours.	Identify early indicators of oxygen deficit.
	Auscultate lungs every 4 hours. Use pulse oximeter to check O$_2$ saturation every 4 hours.	Identify respiratory problems in early stage.

Evaluation:	Compare the patient's status with the expected outcomes. If the outcomes are not met, reassess the patient and revise the plan.

Assessment Findings:	Abdominal girth increased 4 inches since last admission. A 10 to 12 lb weight gain has been noticed over the past 2 weeks. Abdomen is shiny and taut with striae. Lower extremities are edematous.
Nursing Diagnosis:	Fluid volume excess related to the accumulation of fluid in the peritoneal cavity and dependent areas of the body

Patient Outcomes	Nursing Interventions	Rationale
Patient's abdominal girth and weight decrease daily.	Monitor intake and output.	Fluid intake that exceeds output from all sources over 24 hours indicates fluid retention.
	Administer prescribed diuretics.	Diuretics promote loss of fluid.
	Restrict fluid as ordered, including fluids given with medication and meals. Discuss with dietitian regarding this order.	Limits fluid accumulation. Largest amount of fluid is given during waking hours to minimize thirst.
	Provide mouth care every 4 hours. Do *not* use lemon-glycerin swabs.	Decreases thirst. Glycerin dries mucous membranes.
	Weigh the patient daily before breakfast with bladder empty and similar clothes each time.	Weight loss or gain may indicate fluid loss or gain. 1 kg equals 1 L of fluid.

(continued)

Patients with Cirrhosis (continued)

Patient Outcomes	Nursing Interventions	Rationale
	Measure abdominal girth daily. Mark point at which girth is measured.	Decreasing girth indicates a decrease in ascitic fluid. Measuring at the same point ensures accuracy.
	Restrict dietary sodium as ordered.	Sodium restriction will aid in reducing fluid volume excess.

Evaluation: Compare the patient's status with the expected outcomes. If the outcomes are not met, reassess the patient and revise the plan.

Assessment Findings: Sacral edema is present with ascites.

Nursing Diagnosis: Risk for impaired skin integrity related to ascites and edema

Patient Outcomes	Nursing Interventions	Rationale
Patient's skin remains intact during hospitalization.	Inspect skin surfaces daily for lesions or open areas.	Early intervention minimizes skin damage.
	Do not administer injections in edematous sites.	Drugs act as irritants when not absorbed.
	Teach patient to reposition self every 2 hours in bed or chair.	Frequent position changes increase blood flow.
	Place trapeze over bed.	Prevents injury from shearing force.
	Keep bed linens dry.	Moisture predisposes to skin breakdown.

Evaluation: Compare the patient's status with the expected outcomes. If the outcomes are not met, reassess the patient and revise the plan.

Assessment Findings: Patient vomits large volume of blood. Blood pressure decreases from 136/86 mm Hg to 102/64 mm Hg. Pulse increases from 78 to 106 per minute. Sengstaken-Blakemore tube is inserted.

Nursing Diagnosis: Risk for aspiration related to retained secretions or balloon rupture

Patient Outcomes	Nursing Interventions	Rationale
Patient's respirations remain within normal limits with no evidence of respiratory distress.	Suction esophagus every 15–30 minutes or more often if indicated.	When Sengstaken-Blakemore tube is in place, patient cannot swallow and secretions accumulate above the esophageal balloon or can be aspirated.
	Monitor respirations. Auscultate lungs every 15–30 minutes.	Aspiration can occur as a result of loss of swallowing ability.
	Monitor patient closely. Keep scissors at bedside.	Airway obstruction is a major danger. All balloon lumens must be cut immediately and tube removed if respiratory distress occurs.

(continued)

Nursing Care Guide 26–1
Patients with Cirrhosis (continued)

Evaluation:	Compare the patient's status with the expected outcomes. If the outcomes are not met, reassess the patient and revise the plan.

Assessment Findings:	Bleeding is controlled, and the Sengstaken-Blakemore tube is removed. Patient becomes apathetic. Patient responds slowly to questions, and speech is slurred. Patient answers appropriately when asked name but cannot identify location or month of year. Handwriting is difficult to read, but admission sample is legible.
Nursing Diagnosis:	Risk for injury related to altered thought processes secondary to impaired liver detoxification (hepatic encephalopathy)

Patient Outcomes	Nursing Interventions	Rationale
Patient remains free from injury.	Monitor orientation, rate of speech, and response time every 4 hours.	Changes in level of orientation, speech, and response time indicate a change in patient condition.
	Monitor for asterixis every 4 hours.	Most common sign of impending hepatic coma.
	Obtain daily handwriting sample.	Deterioration indicates deterioration in patient's condition.
	Restrict protein intake, as prescribed.	Reduces ammonia production.
	Monitor potassium level.	Decreased potassium levels can precipitate hepatic coma.
	Administer neomycin and lactulose, as prescribed.	Lower blood ammonia levels.
	Keep bed in low position, side rails up, and call bell in reach.	Minimizes risk of injury.

Evaluation:	Compare the patient's status with the expected outcomes. If the outcomes are not met, reassess the patient and revise the plan.

Assessment Findings:	Family members are standing in hall outside patient's room pacing back and forth. Patient's sister is crying intermittently. Patient's brother is heard raising his voice in response to questions or comments by other family members.
Nursing Diagnosis:	Altered family processes related to family member with impending hepatic encephalopathy

(continued)

Nursing Care Guide 26–1
Patients with Cirrhosis (continued)

Patient Outcomes	Nursing Interventions	Rationale
Family members verbalize concerns to nursing staff.	Explain hepatic encephalopathy in terms family can understand.	Family must face the diagnosis and its implications if successful coping is to be achieved.
	Keep family informed of patient's progress and arrange a specific time for family members to meet with health-care team to discuss concerns.	Open communication between family and health-care team facilitates adjustment to the illness and prognosis.
	Allow family members to assist with care, if they desire.	Promotes self-esteem of individual family members and continued contact with patient.
	Refer family to community and social services agencies for emotional, financial, and home-care assistance as needed.	Additional resources may be needed to help with home management.

Evaluation: Compare the patient's status with the expected outcomes. If the outcomes are not met, reassess the patient and revise the plan.

Assessment after a surgical shunt procedure is similar to that of a patient undergoing abdominal surgery, as discussed in Unit 7. In addition, the patient is assessed for signs of hepatic encephalopathy and thrombus formation at the anastomosis site. Pain, fever, distention, and nausea indicate thrombus formation.

Nursing Diagnoses and Planning

Nursing diagnoses and related expected patient outcomes commonly applicable to patients with esophageal varices who are undergoing balloon tamponade therapy include the following:

NDx: Risk for aspiration related to retained secretions or balloon displacement secondary to balloon tamponade therapy

Planning: Patient Outcomes
1. Patient's respirations remain between 12 and 20 per minute with no evidence of respiratory distress.
2. Lungs are clear on auscultation.

Nursing Interventions and Evaluation

NDx: Risk for aspiration
Constant nursing observation is necessary when balloon tamponade therapy is in progress. Monitor respirations and auscultate the lungs every 15 to 30 minutes. Maintain intermittent suction to nasogastric tube or esophagopharyngeal port of Minnesota tube, if used. Maintain low, continuous suction if a Salem

sump tube is used. Suction esophagopharyngeal secretions every 15 to 30 minutes if the Sengstaken-Blakemore tube is used without an accompanying nasogastric tube. Retained secretions lead to aspiration and occlude the airway. Observe the patient for sudden respiratory distress, which occurs if the gastric balloon ruptures and the entire tube moves upward. Gasping, dyspnea, and cyanosis will be evident. If this occurs, immediately cut all balloon lumens and remove the tube. Keep scissors at the patient's bedside at all times for this purpose. Supply the patient with tissues to expectorate oral secretions.

To provide comfort, remove dried blood from the nares and mouth with a solution of equal parts hydrogen peroxide and normal saline. Apply a water-soluble lubricant to the nares to protect the skin.

Compare the patient's status with the expected outcomes. If the outcomes are not met, reassess the patient and revise the plan.

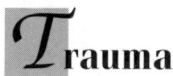

$\mathcal{T}$rauma

BLUNT AND PENETRATING INJURIES

Etiology and Pathophysiology
Liver trauma usually results from an automobile accident, fall, stab wound, or gunshot wound. Blunt or

nonpenetrating hepatic injuries result from direct blows, compression between the lower right ribs and spine, or shearing secondary to rapid deceleration. Blunt hepatic injuries are common in victims of motor vehicle accidents. Unrestrained drivers and front-seat passengers involved in frontal collisions are especially at risk. Stab wounds or gunshot wounds below the right nipple or in the right upper abdominal quadrant are most likely to cause penetrating hepatic injuries.

Liver trauma may result in hepatic contusions, simple lacerations, or small intrahepatic hematomas. More serious injuries include hemorrhage resulting from major hepatic lacerations as well as damage to the hepatic veins or retrohepatic vena cava.

Clinical Manifestations

The diagnosis of liver trauma is difficult to make if physical signs are minimal. After a serious accident, obvious injuries are often treated first, and "hidden" injuries may not be immediately diagnosed.

Fractured lower right ribs, bruising, and pain in the right upper quadrant or posteriorly may indicate liver trauma. Because the liver is highly vascular, severe internal hemorrhage is possible. Restlessness, decreasing blood pressure, and tachycardia indicate hypovolemic shock as a result of blood loss. If blood and bile leak into the peritoneal cavity, peritonitis occurs. This is suspected if the patient has abdominal tenderness, rebound tenderness, and decreased or absent bowel sounds. In some cases, the presence of blood in peritoneal lavage is the only sign of liver trauma.

Diagnosis

When a patient is admitted with known right upper quadrant trauma, abdominal distention, and profound hypotension only temporarily responsive to blood and fluid administration, immediate surgical intervention is indicated. The diagnosis of liver trauma is confirmed in the operating room. In hemodynamically stable, asymptomatic or minimally symptomatic patients, diagnosis is based on peritoneal lavage to detect bleeding into the peritoneal cavity and CT scan to detect the presence and magnitude of the injury.

Management

Small lacerations or intrahepatic hematomas with no evidence of active bleeding require nonoperative management. Repeat CT examinations document healing. Hemorrhage caused by minor injury is treated by simple suture and drainage. Deeper lacerations and damage to the intrahepatic vessels require blood vessel ligation and deep sutures. Severe liver trauma may require hepatic segmentectomy (removal of a portion of the liver).

Complications

The most common complications after surgical intervention for hepatic injury are intrahepatic abscess formation, recurrent hemorrhage, sepsis, pneumonia, and renal failure. Injuries to the hepatic veins or retrohepatic inferior vena cava are almost always fatal.

❖ Settings, Providers, and Collaboration for Care

Patients with liver trauma are admitted to an acute care facility with the specific setting being dictated by the severity of the trauma. Care is typically initiated in the emergency room, followed by a transfer to a critical care unit for close observation and hemodynamic monitoring. If surgery is performed, the patient will be admitted to intensive care and monitored for persistent bleeding.

NURSING PROCESS GUIDELINES
Liver Trauma

Monitor vital signs hourly, strictly monitor intake and output, and review laboratory results of hemoglobin, hematocrit, and electrolyte levels to detect changes in hemodynamic status. Assess for abdominal pain, tenderness, and presence of bowel sounds to detect changes in gastrointestinal function. Nursing care of postoperative patients is discussed in detail in Chapter 6, and nursing care after gastrointestinal surgery is discussed in Unit 7.

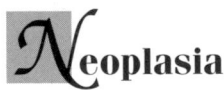 **eoplasia**

BENIGN HEPATIC TUMORS

The most common benign hepatic tumor is the hemangioma. This tumor, found most often in women up to 50 years of age, is usually discovered incidentally during surgery or at autopsy. When manifestations of an abdominal mass are present, surgical resection is performed.

Benign hepatic adenomas, although rare, are also found almost exclusively in women during the childbearing years. Hormonal factors are believed to influence adenoma development. The incidence of this disorder increases with the use of oral contraceptives. If oral contraceptives are discontinued, the lesions usually regress.

Although hepatocellular adenoma is not considered premalignant, hepatocellular carcinoma has developed in a small number of patients. Symptoms of adenoma include abdominal pain with a palpable mass, leukocytosis, and fever. Intra-abdominal hemorrhage develops in approximately one-third of patients, with a mortality rate of approximately 20%. Complete surgical excision is usually performed when the tumor is identified. However, if a patient is taking oral contraceptives and the tumor has not ruptured, a trial period during which the drugs are discontinued may be indicated. Visualization studies, usually a liver scan, are performed to monitor tumor regression.

MALIGNANT HEPATIC TUMORS

Etiology and Pathophysiology

Primary hepatic malignancies are hepatocellular carcinoma (arising in the liver cell), cholangiocellular carcinoma (arising in the bile duct cell), or a combination of both. Primary hepatocellular carcinoma is the most common type, but it remains relatively uncommon in the United States and Western Europe. It is one of the most frequently encountered malignancies in other areas of the world, including sub-Saharan Africa, Japan, and Greece. In China, people are found to be at risk for cancer of the liver that is believed to be associated with an intake of fermented and moldy foods, as well as nitrosamines contained in corn, bran, and pickled vegetables. (Chang, 1995)

Although primary hepatocellular carcinoma occurs infrequently, the liver is a major site for metastatic lesions. Only cirrhosis surpasses metastatic carcinoma of the liver as a cause of fatal liver disease.

Primary hepatocellular carcinoma is four times more common in men and frequently develops in a cirrhotic liver. Development of hepatocellular carcinoma is higher in patients with chronic HBV and HCV infection. Other factors linked to the development of hepatocellular carcinoma include exposure to carcinogens and the use of androgenic steroids.

The rich blood supply and lymphatic flow in the liver make it a prime site for the growth of cancerous cells originating elsewhere in the body. Liver metastasis is common for tumors originating in the stomach, colon, pancreas, lung, oropharynx, and bladder.

Malignant cells multiply randomly and invade liver tissue. Normal liver functions are compromised. In cases in which cirrhosis is present, the growth of malignant cells further compromises a failing liver. Nodules are usually present in advanced stages of the disease.

Clinical Manifestations

The most common complaint associated with primary or metastatic hepatic carcinoma is abdominal pain localized in the upper abdomen or right upper quadrant. An abdominal mass may be present. Hepatomegaly is evident in two-thirds of patients and weight loss is noted. A friction rub or vascular bruit is heard over the liver.

Diagnosis

Liver function studies commonly reveal elevated alkaline phosphatase and serum enzyme levels, but these tests are not specific for carcinoma. An increased or progressively rising alpha-fetoprotein level strongly suggests hepatocellular carcinoma, but many patients have only a low-level elevation, which is nonspecific.

Scanning techniques, ultrasonography, CT scan, and magnetic resonance imaging are used to identify a liver mass and localize the area for liver biopsy. A definitive diagnosis is made via biopsy.

Management

The results of treatment for both primary and secondary hepatocellular carcinoma are poor. Most patients die within 3 to 6 months of diagnosis.

Treatment for hepatic carcinoma includes hepatic resection, liver transplantation, radiation therapy, and chemotherapy. For many patients, there is no appropriate treatment because the lesion is discovered in an advanced stage of the disease. Supportive care is provided.

If a solitary tumor is located, hepatic resection is possible. Because the liver has excellent regenerative abilities, up to 90% can be removed. Liver transplantation may be performed in some patients. However, the survival rate for both procedures is poor unless the tumor is detected at an early stage.

External radiation therapy is occasionally used, but success rates are extremely poor because of the liver's low tolerance for radiation. Chemotherapy with doxorubicin (Adriamycin) and 5-fluorouracil administered individually, as well as combination therapy with multiple agents, yields similarly poor results. Although chemotherapy produces tumor regression, the survival rate is not improved. Sometimes, combined radiation and chemotherapy may increase the survival rate.

Chemotherapeutic agents may be administered intravenously, via hepatic artery infusion, or through the use of an external or internal pump. Hepatic artery infusion requires the placement of a catheter into the hepatic artery either percutaneously or via laparotomy. The catheter is brought out of the abdomen via a stab wound and attached to an external pump, which administers the chemotherapeutic agent at a prescribed rate directly into the liver. Complications include sepsis, hemorrhage, and thrombosis. This technique usually requires hospitalization and may limit the patient's activities.

The internal implantable pump also delivers a continuous flow of cytotoxic drugs to the liver. This device is implanted under the skin on the chest or abdominal wall. An outlet catheter is surgically implanted inside the hepatic artery. Drugs are instilled by injection through the skin into a chamber in the center of the pump. Heparin is used to maintain pump patency when chemotherapy is not being administered. The pump is usually filled every 1 to 2 weeks. Patients have fewer complications and increased independence when an internal implantable pump is used.

Patients with hepatic neoplasias require the same support and nursing care as patients with other oncologic disorders described in Chapter 34.

❖ Settings, Providers, and Collaboration for Care

Treatment settings for the patient with a tumor of the liver vary depending on the extent of the liver involvement and whether it is a benign or malignant process. If the disease is considered terminal, care may be provided either in the home using hospice services or in a long-term facility. As for any patient with cancer, collaboration among physicians (eg, medical oncologist, radiation oncologist, surgeon, internist), nurses, pharmacists, social workers, family members, and others involved in the patient's care is essential.

Orthotopic Hepatic Transplant

Orthotopic hepatic transplant is removal of the liver and replacement with a donor liver. The first hepatic transplant was performed in 1963, but the procedure remained experimental until 1983. Increased use of the procedure at major medical centers is possible because of better preservation techniques for donor organs, revised criteria for recipients, improved surgical techniques, better control of complications, and the use of improved immunosuppressive therapy to prevent organ rejection by the liver recipient. Although figures vary among transplant centers, the 1-year survival rate is about 85% and the 4- to 5-year survival rate is about 60%.

SELECTION CRITERIA FOR RECIPIENTS

Each transplant center develops specific criteria for choosing liver transplant recipients. These criteria are based on the outcomes of previous transplant surgeries. Although some differences may exist, criteria generally include several common factors. The candidate for liver transplant must be in the final stage of hepatic disease. If the cause of liver failure is alcohol related, the patient must be free from alcohol use for a period determined by the transplant center.

Factors that contraindicate hepatic transplant include bacterial or fungal infections outside the hepatobiliary system, malignancies outside the hepatobiliary system, advanced cardiac disease, psychologic instability, and lack of adequate support systems. These factors have been found to increase significantly the risk of death after transplant surgery. For patients with advanced renal disease, combined liver-kidney transplants are performed at many major transplant centers.

SELECTION CRITERIA FOR DONORS

Generally, liver donors must be between the ages of 3 months and 60 years with no history of liver disease, drug or alcohol abuse, malignancy, syphilis, tuberculosis, or acquired immunodeficiency syndrome. Ideally, the donor's height and weight approximate that of the recipient for a proper "fit." However, the increasing use of "pared-down livers" allows the use of larger donor organs.

Typical donors present with head injuries or cerebral vascular accidents or are victims of homicide or suicide. Brain death must be diagnosed and documented. The donor must be ventilator-dependent with no evidence of sepsis.

The donor liver is removed during a surgical procedure that takes 3 to 4 hours. The liver is placed in a University of Washington (UW) preservative solution containing high-molecular-weight sugar molecules, which is kept on ice at 40°C. The UW solution has extended the period of safe liver storage time up to 36 hours with improved liver function after transplantation.

SURGICAL PROCEDURE

Liver transplantation is a long and complex procedure, taking anywhere from 8 to 22 hours to complete. The recipient's liver is removed at a time that coincides with the arrival of the donor liver. With removal of the diseased organ, the splanchnic and vena cava circulations are occluded and a venous bypass system may be used. Heparinized shunts are placed in the femoral vein and the axillary vein to shunt blood back to the heart through the axillary system. The donor liver is flushed with cold solution to remove the preservative solution and any air bubbles. The portal venous system, hepatic artery, and biliary systems are anastomosed. A removable T-tube for bile drainage is brought out through the abdominal wall. Prompt outflow of bile through the T-tube is an early indicator of proper function of the transplanted liver.

During the surgical procedure, the patient is placed on a heating blanket to prevent hypothermia. Fluids and blood products are administered as needed. An arterial catheter, nasogastric tube, and indwelling urinary catheter are in place. After surgery, immunosuppressive drug therapy, usually begun in the preoperative period, is continued. Cyclosporine, prednisone, and azathioprine (Imuran) are the pharmacologic agents most often used in combination to prevent organ rejection. Highlight 26–2 describes cyclosporine, the most commonly used maintenance drug. If acute organ rejection occurs, monoclonal antibody OKT-3 (orthoclone) or the polyclonal antibody (antilymphocyte globulin ALG) is usually administered.

POSTOPERATIVE COMPLICATIONS

After surgery, hepatic transplant recipients require close observation and monitoring by critical care nurses. Signs of organ rejection, which usually occur within 4 to 10 days postoperatively, must be recognized early (Table 26–8). Other possible complications in the postoperative period include:

  Gastrointestinal bleeding
  Biliary leaks and strictures
  Fluid and electrolyte imbalances

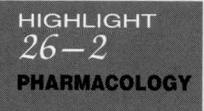 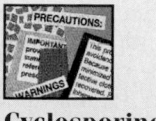

HIGHLIGHT
26—2
PHARMACOLOGY

Cyclosporine

Definition:

Immune suppressant.

Action:

Inhibits cell-mediated immune reactions, specifically T lymphocytes. Bone marrow function is not affected.

Uses:

Protects transplanted organs from rejection by the host. It is often used in combination with prednisone for liver transplant recipients.

Side Effects:

The major reactions seen with this therapy are tremor, hypertension, hirsutism, gum hyperplasia, and renal dysfunction, which is dose dependent. Gastrointestinal symptoms may include diarrhea, nausea, and vomiting. Natural defenses against bacterial, viral, fungal, and other types of infections are lowered. Patients are at risk for infection from all causes.

Interactions:

Medications causing nephrotoxicity should not be administered concurrently. Rifampin, phenytoin, and phe-

nobarbital increase the metabolism of cyclosporine and decrease its plasma levels. Plasma concentrations are increased with high doses of methylprednisolone, erythromycin, and antifungal agents.

Nursing Implications:

Caution patient to avoid hazardous equipment if tremor develops. Monitor blood pressure and teach patient and family members to monitor at home. Inspect mouth and gums at frequent intervals. Teach patient importance of oral hygiene, including brushing, flossing, and regular dental checkups. Monitor weight, intake, and output. Assess blood urea nitrogen and serum creatine levels for evidence of nephrotoxicity. Instruct patient to report any sign of infection immediately, including fever, sore throat, increased fatigue, urinary frequency or dysuria, coughing or chest congestion, and skin eruptions. Stress the importance of avoiding exposure to persons with infections. Review hand-washing technique with patient and family.

Pulmonary problems
Thrombosis of the hepatic artery
Infection
Some degree of renal failure caused by cyclosporine's nephrotoxicity

NURSING PROCESS GUIDELINES
Orthotopic Hepatic Transplant

Nursing care for patients who have had an orthotopic liver transplant is similar to that described previously in Unit 7 for the patient who has had abdominal surgery. In addition, the nurse monitors for signs of biliary obstruction, rejection, and infection.

A T-tube is inserted at the time of surgery. Thick, dark-green bile drainage indicates good liver function. A sudden drop in amount or a change in color to light yellow suggests liver dysfunction. The T-tube usually remains in place for several months, but it is clamped after 2 or 3 weeks. If fever, abdominal pain, or cramping develops within 24 hours after the tube is clamped, the T-tube is reconnected

to drainage, and evaluation for biliary infection or obstruction begins.

Because liver transplant patients receive large doses of steroids and immunosuppressants to prevent liver rejection, the patient is at increased risk for infection, especially of the lungs, liver, colon, and oral mucous membrane. Suppression of antibodies prevents rejection of the implanted liver but

Table 26–8

Clinical Manifestations of Acute Rejection of a Transplanted Liver

Fever
Jaundice
Right upper quadrant pain
Diminished bile flow through the T-tube
Elevated levels of serum bilirubin, alkaline phosphatase, aspartate aminotransferase, alanine aminotransferase, and lactate dehydrogenase
Prolonged prothrombin time

also puts the patient at risk for bacterial, fungal, and viral infection. Symptoms of infection are masked by the immunosuppression therapy and complicated by possible rejection of the organ. Use aseptic technique with all invasive procedures and dressing changes. Assess the oral mucous membrane at least once every 8 hours for signs of infection including the redness, cheesy white plaques, and dysphagia indicative of candidiasis. Provide gentle mouth care after meals and at bedtimes, using an alkaline-based mouthwash and soft tooth brush. Nystatin mouthwash may be ordered if candidiasis is suspected.

Rejection and infection result in fever, decreased quantity and quality of bile, jaundice, elevated results of liver function tests, loss of appetite, and right upper quadrant pain. To determine the cause of the problem, liver biopsy, CT scan, ultrasonography, blood, sputum, urine, and drainage cultures, and chest x-ray examinations may be performed. If rejection is identified, the dose of immunosuppressive drugs is increased. If infection is the problem, less immunosuppressive drug is given, and antibiotic therapy is instituted. Because immunosuppressive therapy is lifelong, patient education related to drug therapy and recognition of complications is instituted early in the postoperative period.

Patients who undergo liver transplant experience a great deal of stress both before and after the procedure. A long waiting period for a donor liver, followed by the realization that the transplanted organ may be rejected, leaves the patient in need of ongoing support by a multidisciplinary team. It is essential that patients understand the importance of lifelong drug therapy and follow-up visits.

The Elderly: Special Considerations

Older people who have undergone numerous surgical procedures and received a number of blood transfusions are at increased risk for hepatitis B and hepatitis C. In geriatric patients, both hepatitis B and hepatitis C are associated with a more severe clinical course, a greater progression to chronicity, and a higher mortality rate.

Hepatitis infection in the elderly may be misdiagnosed as gallstones or malignancy. Because symptoms of hepatitis are often delayed or subtle in older adults, the condition is usually not diagnosed or treated in the early stages. In addition, the hospital stay of older patients may be prolonged and complicated if the person has concomitant diseases.

Older people are at greater risk for drug-induced hepatitis because they take more medications. Because of the decreased production of liver enzymes vital for drug metabolism, the older person may experience a prolonged effect from drugs that are metabolized in the liver. The potential for toxicity and cumulative effects of medications and toxins increases with aging. Geriatric patients should be monitored carefully for signs of drug-related hepatic impairment.

Cirrhosis in elderly patients is frequently of unknown origin. Individuals in whom cirrhosis develops in the middle years, most often related to alcohol abuse, usually do not survive into old age. When cirrhosis does occur in the elderly, the complications are similar to those in the younger population, but hepatic encephalopathy occurs with greater frequency and the prognosis is worse.

A condition known as cardiac cirrhosis is seen in elderly patients; however, many authorities do not consider this a true cirrhosis. Severe, prolonged right-sided heart failure leads to hepatic congestion, which results in cellular necrosis and fibrosis. Often the hepatic damage is overshadowed by the cardiac problem and resulting symptoms. Hepatic damage can be reversed if the heart failure is controlled.

Chapter Review

1. What is the meaning of the marker HAV-Ab/IgM in the patient with hepatitis A?
2. What is a solution to the problem of fecal incontinence in a patient with hepatitis A?
3. What evidence supports the therapeutic effect of rest as a part of the nursing care plan for a patient with viral hepatitis?
4. How is the care of a patient with hepatitis A similar to that of a patient with hepatitis B?
5. What is the meaning of an elevated bilirubin level in the patient with cirrhosis of the liver?
6. How can ascites best be assessed in the patient with cirrhosis of the liver?
7. What would happen to a patient with a Sengstaken-Blakemore tube in place if the gastric balloon deflates?
8. Why is oral suctioning important when planning care for the patient with a Sengstaken-Blakemore tube in place?
9. What is the meaning of an elevated serum creatinine level in a liver transplant patient who is receiving cyclosporine?
10. What is the meaning of a decrease in blood pressure and tachycardia in a patient who has experienced blunt trauma to the liver?

Bibliography

Abrams W, Beers M, Berkow R, Fletcher M (eds). The Merck manual of geriatrics. 2nd ed. Whitehouse Station, NJ: Merck & Co, Inc, 1995.

Anglucci P. TIPS for controlling bleeding. Nursing 1995; 25(7):43.

Atkins C, Bender P, Rippert L. Transplantation. In Dossey B, Guzzetta C, Kenner CV, et al (eds). Critical care nursing. 3rd ed. Philadelphia: JB Lippincott, 1992, pp 909–961.

Bouley G, Grimshaw K, Lindewall D, Kiernan L. Transjugular intrahepatic portosystemic shunt: An alternative. Crit Care Nurse 1996; 96(16):23.

Bowden DS, Moaven LD, Locarnini, SA. New hepatitis viruses: Are there enough letters in the alphabet? Med J Aust 1996; 164:87.

Boyer JL, Reuben P. Chronic hepatitis. In Schiff L, Schiff E (eds). Diseases of the liver. 7th ed. Philadelphia: JB Lippincott, 1995, pp 586–637.

Carpenito LJ. Nursing care plans and documentation. 2nd ed. Philadelphia: JB Lippincott, 1995.

Carpenito LJ. Nursing diagnoses: Application to clinical practice. 6th ed. Philadelphia: JB Lippincott, 1995.

Chang K. Chinese Americans. In Giger JN, Davidhizar RE (eds). Transcultural nursing: Assessment and intervention. 2nd ed. St. Louis: CV Mosby, 1995, pp 395–414.

Cohen A. Liver disease. In Copstead LE. Perspectives on pathophysiology. Philadelphia: WB Saunders, 1995, pp 758–777.

Copstead L. Perspectives on pathophysiology. Philadelphia: WB Saunders, 1995.

Coy D, Blei A. Portal hypertension. In Haubrich W, Schaffner F, Berk JE (eds). Bockus gastroenterology. 5th ed. Philadelphia: WB Saunders, 1995, pp 1955–1987.

Davis G, Johnson Y. Hepatitis. In Haubrich W, Schaffner F, Berk JE (eds). Bockus gastroenterology. 5th ed. Philadelphia: WB Saunders, 1994, pp 2082–2133.

Davis J, Sherer K. Applied nutrition and diet therapy for nurses. 2nd ed. Philadelphia: WB Saunders, 1994.

Deglin J, Vellerand A. Davis drug guide for nurses. 5th ed. Philadelphia: FA Davis, 1997.

Dienstag J, Isselbacher K. Acute hepatitis. In Isselbacher K, Braunwald E, Wilson J, et al (eds). Harrison's principles of internal medicine. 13th ed. New York: McGraw-Hill, 1994, pp 1458–1477.

Dienstag J, Isselbacher K. Chronic hepatitis. In Isselbacher K, Braunwald E, Wilson J, et al (eds). Harrison's principles of internal medicine. 13th ed. New York: McGraw-Hill, 1994, pp 1479–1483.

Doherty MM, Carver DK. Transjugular intrahepatic portosystemic shunt: New relief for esophageal varices. Am J Nurs 1993; 93(4):58.

Eliopoulos C. Gerontological nursing. 3rd ed. Philadelphia: JB Lippincott, 1993.

Evan G (ed). Hepatitis G discovery raises new worries. Hosp Infect Control 1996; 5:62.

Ferenci P. Hepatic encephalopathy. In Haubrich W, Schaffner F, Berk JE (eds). Bockus gastroenterology. 5th ed. Philadelphia: WB Saunders, 1995, pp 1988–2003.

Fishbach F. A manual of laboratory diagnostic tests. 5th ed. Philadelphia: JB Lippincott, 1995.

Friedman S. Cirrhosis of the liver and its major sequelae. In Bennett JC, Plum F (eds). Cecil textbook of medicine. 21st ed, Vol 1. Philadelphia: WB Saunders, 1995, pp 788–796.

Garner JS and the Hospital Infection Control Products Advisory Committee, Public Health Service. Special communication: CDC isolation guidelines part I—Guidelines for isolation precautions in hospitals—and part II—Recommendations for isolation precautions in hospitals. Am J Infect Cont 1996; 24(1):24.

Giger J, Davidhizar R. Transcultural nursing: Assessment and intervention. 2nd ed. St. Louis: Mosby Year-Book, 1995.

Gregory PB. Acute hepatitis. In Dale DC, Federman DD (eds). Scientific American medicine 4: Gastroenterology. New York: Scientific American Inc, 1995, pp 11–12.

Gregory PB. Cirrhosis. In Dale, DC, Federman DD (eds). Scientific American medicine 4: Gastroenterology. New York: Scientific American Inc, 1995, pp 1–18.

Guyton AC, Hall J. Textbook of medical physiology. 9th ed. Philadelphia: WB Saunders, 1996.

Herreid JA. Hepatitis C: Past, present, and future. Medsurg Nurs 1995; 4(3):179.

Hoofnagle J. Hepatitis B. In Haubrich W, Schaffner F, Berk JE (eds). Bockus gastroenterology. 5th ed. Philadelphia: WB Saunders, 1994, pp 2062–2079.

Hsu H, Feinstone S, Hoofnagle J. Acute viral hepatitis. In Mandell G, Bennett J, Dolin R (eds). Principles and practice of infectious diseases. 4th ed. New York: Churchill Livingstone, 1995, pp 1136–1153.

Jackson M, Rymer T. Viral hepatitis: Anatomy of a diagnosis. Am J Nurs. 1994, 94(1):43.

Keeffe EB. Acute hepatitis. Scientific American medicine 4: Gastroenterology VII. New York: Scientific American Inc, 1997, pp 1–12.

Koff R. Viral hepatitis. In Schiff L, Schiff E (eds). Diseases of the liver. 7th ed. Philadelphia: JB Lippincott, 1993, pp 492–560.

Krawczynski K. Hepatitis E. In Haubrich W, Schaffner F, Berk JE (eds). Bockus gastroenterology. 5th ed. Philadelphia: WB Saunders, 1994, pp 2129–2138.

Kuhn MA. Pharmacotherapeutics: A nursing process approach. 3rd ed. Philadelphia: FA Davis, 1994.

Lehne R. Pharmacology for nursing care. 2nd ed. Philadelphia: WB Saunders, 1994.

Lutz C, Przytulski K. Nutrition and diet therapy. Philadelphia: FA Davis, 1994.

McMahon B, Shapiro C, Robertson B, et al. Hepatitis A. In Haubrich W, Schaffner F, Berk JE (eds). Bockus gastroenterology. 5th ed. Philadelphia: WB Saunders, 1994, pp 2044–2056.

Messner J. Liver cancer. Nursing 1996; 26(1):52.

Newman R. Adverse reactions to blood transfusions. In Rakel RE (ed). Conn's current therapy 1997. Philadelphia: WB Saunders, 1997, pp 432–437.

Ockner RK. Clinical approaches to liver diseases. In Bennett JC, Plum F (eds). Cecil textbook of medicine. 20th ed. Philadelphia: WB Saunders, 1996, pp 752–753.

Pagana KD, Pagana TJ. Mosby's diagnostic and laboratory test reference. 2nd ed. St. Louis: Mosby Year-Book, 1995.

Peckenpaugh N, Poleman C. Nutrition: Essentials and diet therapy. 7th ed. Philadelphia: WB Saunders, 1995.

Physician's Desk Reference. 51st ed. qv Hepatitis A vaccine inactivated. Havrix. Montvale, NJ: Medical Economics Co, 1997, p. 2663–2665.

Podlosky D, Isselbacher K. Alcohol-related liver disease and cirrhosis. In Isselbacher K, Braunwald E, Wilson J, et al (eds). Harrison's principles of internal medicine. 13th ed. New York: McGraw-Hill Inc, 1994, pp 1444–1448.

Porth CM. Pathophysiology: Concepts of altered health states. 4th ed. Philadelphia: JB Lippincott, 1994.

Reed S. Amebiasis and infection with free-living amebas. In Isselbacher K, Braunwald E, Wilson J, et al (eds). Harrison's principles of internal medicine. 13th ed. New York: McGraw-Hill, 1994, pp 884–886.

Rizetto M, Ferruccio B, Verme G, et al. Hepatitis D (delta). In Haubrich W, Schaffner F, Berk JE (eds). Bockus gastroenterology. 5th ed. Philadelphia: WB Saunders, 1994, pp 2115–2128.

Runyon B. Ascites and spontaneous bacterial peritonitis. In Sleisenger M, Fordtran J (eds). Gastrointestinal disease: Pathophysiology/diagnoses/management. 5th ed. Philadelphia: WB Saunders, 1993, pp 1962–2003.

Runyon B. Ascites. In Schiff L, Schiff E (eds). Diseases of the liver. 7th ed. Philadelphia: JB Lippincott, 1993, pp 990–1015.

Schaffner F. Jaundice. In Haubrich W, Schaffner F, Berk JE (eds). Bockus gastroenterology. 5th ed. Philadelphia: WB Saunders, 1995, pp 129–139.

Scharschmidt BF. Acute and chronic hepatic failure and hepatic encephalopathy. In Bennett JC, Plum F (eds). Cecil textbook of medicine. 20th ed. Philadelphia: WB Saunders, 1996, pp 797–800.

Seeley R, Stephens T, Tate P (eds). Anatomy and physiology. 3rd ed. St. Louis: Mosby Year-Book, 1995.

Sherlock S, Sherlock S, Dooley J (eds). Diseases of the liver and biliary system. 10th ed. Cambridge, MA: Blackwell Scientific, 1993.

Spiro H (ed). Clinical Gastroenterology. 4th ed. New York: McGraw-Hill, 1993, p 1105.

Stanley M, Beare P. Gerontological nursing. Philadelphia: FA Davis, 1995.

Ulrich S, Canale S, Wendell S. Nursing care planning guides (medical-surgical). 3rd ed. Philadelphia: WB Saunders, 1994.

Watson J, Jaffe M. Nurse's manual of laboratory and diagnostic tests. 2nd ed. Philadelphia: WB Saunders, 1995.

Unit IX

Endocrine Dysfunction

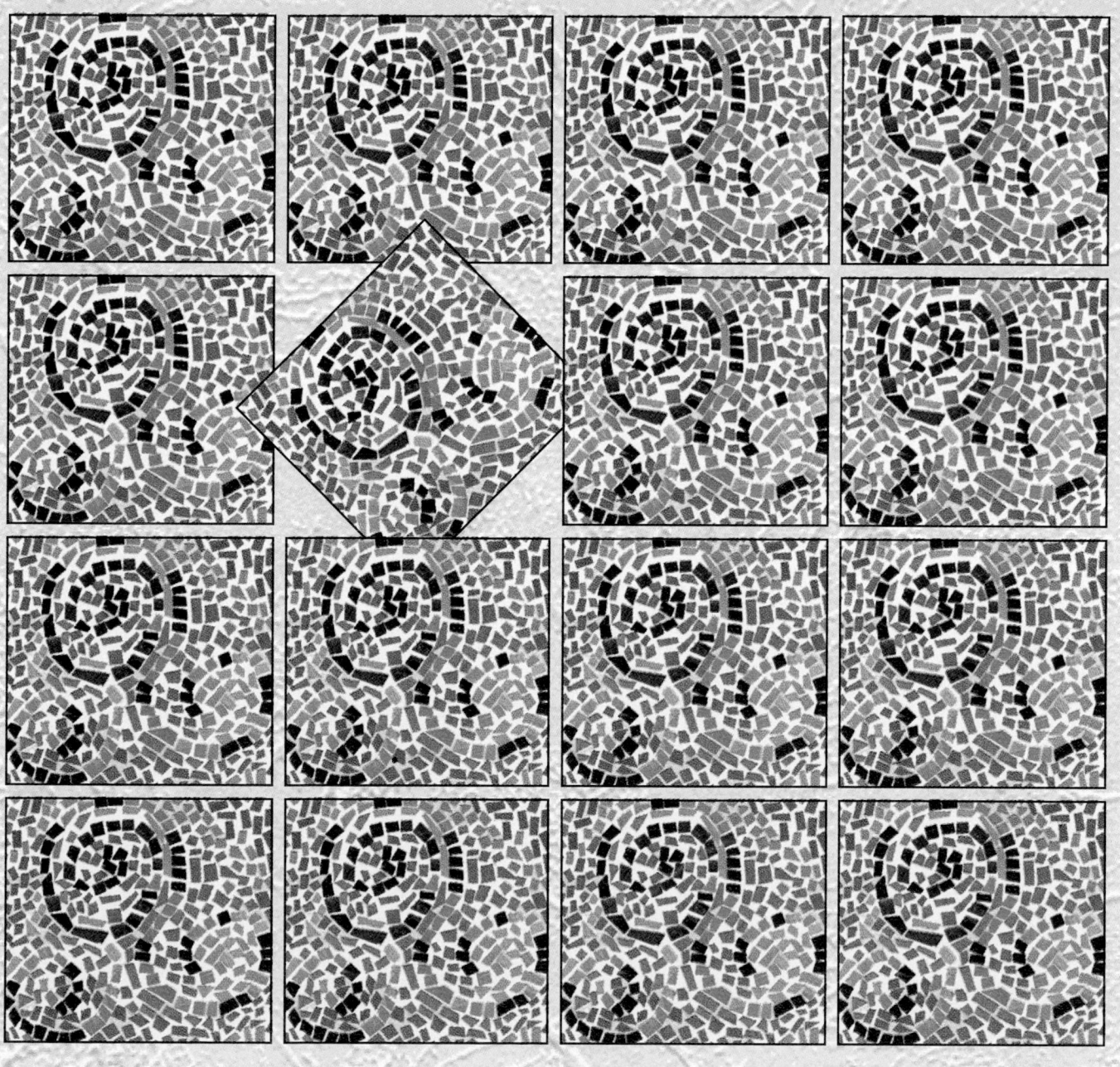

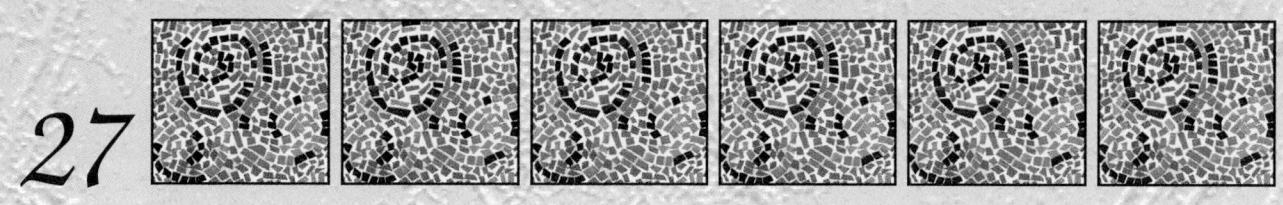

27

Knowledge Base for Patients with Endocrine Dysfunction

Study Outcomes

After studying this chapter, you should be able to:

1. Explain the function of the endocrine system and hormone receptors.
2. Describe regulation of hormone secretion.
3. Identify the endocrine glands and the hormones they secrete.
4. Explain the three common types of endocrine dysfunction.
5. Identify physiologic and psychologic alterations commonly assessed in patients with endocrine dysfunction.
6. Describe guidelines for application of the nursing process to the care of patients with endocrine dysfunction.
7. Identify alternative treatment and care settings for patients with endocrine dysfunction and the services related to community-based care.
8. Identify special considerations for the elderly patient with endocrine dysfunction.

The endocrine system is a group of ductless glands and tissues that produce and secrete chemical substances called hormones, which regulate cell functions. These hormones are discharged directly into the blood or lymph system. They circulate throughout the body. Settings in which endocrine dysfunction may be diagnosed and treated vary with the particular type of endocrine problem involved. The assessment of the system, or any particular gland, is usually completed in an outpatient setting or the physician's office.

Anatomy and Physiology

As illustrated in Figure 27–1, endocrine glands are located throughout the body. Although the locations and functions of these glands vary widely, the endocrine system acts as an interrelated whole. Secretion by one gland commonly affects other glands in the body. Table 27–1 summarizes the endocrine glands, the hormones they secrete, and their effects.

Each hormone of the endocrine system may affect a specific organ or tissue, called a target organ or target tissue, or it may have a general effect on the entire body. The complex interactions between hormones and their target organs (hormone receptor sites) are controlled by the endocrine system and the nervous system. The ever-changing balance achieved in the body is called homeostasis.

HORMONE RECEPTORS

Most hormones belong to one of three categories:

- Proteins and polypeptides
- Steroids
- Amines and amino acid derivatives

As a group, hormones have diverse molecular structures and physiologic properties. Each one may affect a target organ or the entire body through a relationship with hormone receptors. The cells of target tissues contain receptors that recognize and bind strongly with specific hormones. They also reject inappropriate substances. Hormone receptor sites may be on the cell membrane or in the interior of the cell. A cell does not respond to a hormone unless it has receptor sites for that hormone. Some hormones increase the number of receptors for other hormones. For example, estrogen can increase the number of receptors for the hormone progesterone. Also, if a hormone receptor is abnormal, or if it is absent for some reason, the target cell will reject the receptor site's hormone. This, in turn, could trigger a disease process. This effect can be seen in some obese patients. In obesity, a decrease in the number of insulin receptors may occur in response to abnormal levels of circulating insulin.

Cell Membrane Receptors

Protein and peptide hormones, and most amine and amino acid derivative hormones, are water soluble

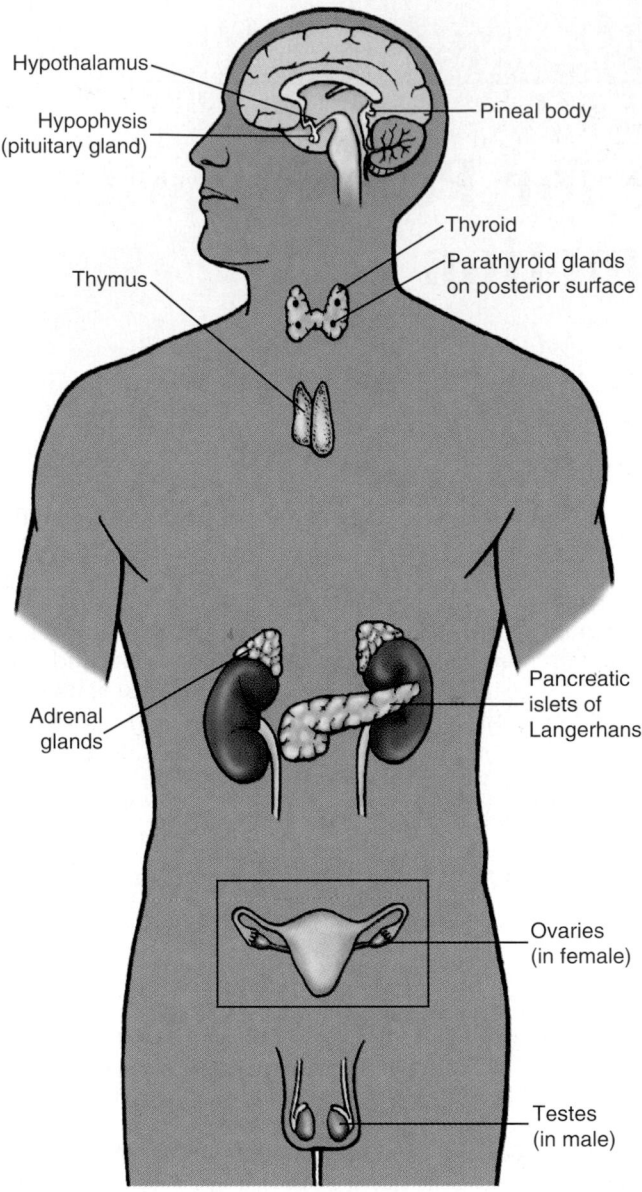

Figure 27–1

Anatomical locations of the endocrine glands.

and cannot readily penetrate the lipid barrier of the cell membrane. As illustrated in Figure 27–2, they interact first with receptors on the surface of the cell, activating the enzyme adenyl cyclase in the cell membrane. The adenyl cyclase enzyme then causes cytoplasmic adenosine triphosphate to convert into short-acting cyclic adenosine monophosphate inside the cell. Once formed, cyclic adenosine monophosphate acts as an intracellular hormonal messenger. It also diffuses throughout the cell and alters cell function to produce hormonal effects inside the cell. This response can occur almost instantly, requiring only a few seconds or minutes to complete.

Intracellular Receptors

Because of their smaller size and chemical composition, the lipid-soluble steroid hormones readily penetrate the cell membrane to bind directly with intracellular protein receptors (Fig. 27–3). These combined hormone-receptor molecules diffuse into the cell nucleus and activate specific genes within the nuclear DNA to produce messenger RNA. The messenger RNA diffuses out of the nucleus into the cytoplasm, where it promotes synthesis of a specific protein within the cell. This protein alters cell function, growth, or differentiation. This response takes about 45 minutes to begin, and several hours or days for the full effect to occur.

REGULATION OF HORMONE SECRETION

Hormone secretion by the endocrine glands may be affected by the nervous system, by chemical substances in the blood, or by other hormones. Because hormones are very potent substances, their concentration in the blood must be maintained at a relatively constant level. One way this is accomplished is through negative feedback control, which is illustrated in Figure 27–4. As the hormone concentration in the blood or the concentration of a substance affected by a hormone rises, further secretion of that hormone is inhibited. When blood levels fall, hormone production is stimulated. Besides negative feedback control, secretion of hormones by the pineal gland, adrenal medulla, posterior pituitary, and hypothalamus can be affected directly by neurologic stimuli.

THYMUS GLAND

The thymus gland consists of two flattened lobes of lymphoid tissue located in the mediastinal cavity just below the clavicle. Its principal secretion is thymopoietin, which stimulates development of mature immunologic lymphocytes called T cells. The thymus gland is important in the development of the immune response in newborns and the maintenance of immunologic competence in adults.

PINEAL GLAND

Sometimes called the pineal body, the pineal gland is a small pinecone-shaped structure located in the cranial cavity behind the midbrain and the third ventricle. It produces and secretes melatonin, and possibly other hormones that interact with the hypothalamic-pituitary system to affect and respond to the circadian release of many endocrine hormones. In sighted people, pineal gland activity fluctuates

Table 27–1

The Endocrine Glands

Gland	Hormones	Primary Hormonal Functions	Effects of Excess	Effects of Deficit
Hypothalamic neurosecretory cells	Releasing hormones Inhibiting hormones	Control secretion of specific hormones from the anterior pituitary gland	Pituitary dysfunction Tertiary target gland dysfunction	Pituitary dysfunction Tertiary target gland dysfunction
Anterior pituitary (adenohypophysis)	Somatotropin (STH) or growth hormone (GH)	Stimulates growth of cells, bones, muscles, and soft tissue Insulin antagonist	Gigantism in children Acromegaly in adults Glucose intolerance	Pituitary dwarfism in children Insulin sensitivity
	Thyrotropin or thyroid-stimulating hormone (TSH)	Regulates secretory activity of the thyroid gland	Secondary hyperthyroidism	Secondary hypothyroidism
	Adrenocorticotropic hormone (ACTH)	Stimulates secretion of hormones from the adrenal cortex	Cushing's disease	Adrenal hypoplasia
	Gonadotropic hormones Luteinizing hormone (LH)	Induces ovulation and development of the corpus luteum in women Stimulates testosterone secretion in men	Precocious sexual development Hirsutism Altered secondary sex characteristics	Delayed sexual development Altered secondary sex characteristics Infertility Scant menses or amenorrhea in women Impotence in men
	Follicle-stimulating hormone (FSH)	Stimulates graafian follicle growth and estrogen secretion in women		
	Prolactin	Stimulates mammary gland development and lactation Suppresses secretion of gonadotropin-releasing hormones	Suppression of gonadal function Depressed libido Infertility Amenorrhea Persistent lactation (galactorrhea) in women Impotence in men	Mammary involution Failure to lactate postpartum
	Melanocyte-stimulating hormone (MSH)	Stimulates melanin synthesis	Hyperpigmentation	Depigmentation
Posterior pituitary (neurohypophysis)	Antidiuretic hormone (ADH)*	Regulates osmolality of extracellular fluids by increasing reabsorption of water from the renal tubules Vasopressive effect	Syndrome of inappropriate antidiuretic hormone (SIADH)	Diabetes insipidus
	Oxytocin*	Stimulates uterine contraction Initiation of breast-milk expression (let-down reflex) in women Increases ejection of sperm into the semen during ejaculation in men	(Under investigation)	Prolonged labor Inability to breast-feed Decreased sperm count

Table continued on following page

Table 27–1

The Endocrine Glands *(continued)*

Gland	Hormones	Primary Hormonal Functions	Effects of Excess	Effects of Deficit
Thyroid	Thyroxine (T_4) Triiodothyronine (T_3)	Regulate metabolism, energy production, and growth and development	Primary hyperthyroidism Graves' disease	Primary hypothyroidism Myxedema Juvenile hypothyroidism Cretinism in infants
	Calcitonin	Increases the rate at which calcium is deposited into bones	Increased bone density Hypocalcemia	Osteoporosis Hypercalcemia
Parathyroids	Parathormone, or parathyroid hormone (PTH)	Regulates serum calcium and phosphate levels Promotes resorption of calcium from bones	Hyperparathyroidism Hypercalcemia, osteoporosis	Hypoparathyroidism Tetany Hypocalcemia
Adrenal medulla	Epinephrine (Adrenalin)	Instantaneous stress reaction Fight-or-flight response Raises metabolism, blood glucose levels, cardiac output	Pheochromocytoma Severe hypertension	No known disease or effect
	Norepinephrine	Generalized vasoconstriction		
Adrenal cortex	Glucocorticoids Cortisol Cortisone Corticosterone	Mediate the stress response Promote protein and fat catabolism to raise blood glucose levels Promote sodium and water retention, potassium excretion Suppress ACTH secretion	Inhibit the inflammatory response Cushing's syndrome	
	Mineralocorticoids Aldosterone Deoxycorticosterone (DOC)	Promote sodium and water retention, potassium excretion	Primary aldosteronism	Addison's disease
	Sex hormones Androgens Estrogen	Development and maintenance of secondary sex characteristics and libido Source of testosterone in women, estrogen in men	Virilism	
Pancreas Beta cells	Insulin	Regulates fat, protein, carbohydrate metabolism Lowers blood glucose levels by promoting glucose transport into the cells	Hyperinsulinism Hypoglycemia	Diabetes mellitus

Table 27-1

The Endocrine Glands (continued)

Gland	Hormones	Primary Hormonal Functions	Effects of Excess	Effects of Deficit
Alpha cells	Glucagon	Raises blood glucose levels by promoting hepatic glycogenolysis Promotes glyconeogenesis (gluconeogenesis) Insulin antagonist	Glucose intolerance and hyperglycemia	(Under investigation; probable hypoglycemia)
Delta cells	Somatostatin†	Inhibits diverse endocrine functions Inhibits the release of insulin, glucagon, and somatotropin (STH)	Hyperglycemia	(Under investigation)

Gonads
  Ovaries
    (female)
	Estrogen
	Progesterone
		Development, maturation, and cyclic function of the reproductive system
		Development of breasts and secondary sex characteristics
			Infertility
			Altered menstrual cycle
			Altered secondary sex characteristics
				Amenorrhea
				Infertility
				Spontaneous abortion
				Regression of secondary sex characteristics
				Decreased libido

Testes (male)	Testosterone	Development, maturation, and function of the reproductive system and secondary sex characteristics Stimulates growth of skeletal muscles, bones, skin, and hair Stimulates closure of the epiphyseal plates at puberty	Suppresses gonadotropic activity, thereby causing testicular atrophy, infertility, impotence Precocious sexual development Premature epiphyseal closure in children	Impotence Infertility Cryptorchidism in children
Thymus	Thymopoietin	Development of the immune response in the newborn Maintenance of immunologic response in the adult	(Under investigation)	Immunodeficiency disorders
Pineal	Melatonin	Influences and responds to the body's circadian rhythms	(Under investigation)	(Under investigation)

* Antidiuretic hormone and oxytocin are produced in the hypothalamus, but stored in and secreted from the posterior pituitary.

† Somatostatin is also produced in the hypothalamus, many regions of the central and peripheral nervous system, retina, thymus, adrenal medulla, placenta, and delta cells of the stomach and intestine. It may also function as a neurotransmitter in the central nervous system.

with cycles of light and darkness and with the wavelength (color) of light. Melatonin levels are highest during daily periods of darkness. Some research indicates that melatonin may affect the sleep-wake cycle by inducing drowsiness. In blind people, melatonin levels fluctuate in a 24.7-hour cycle.

Although the effects of melatonin on the human reproductive cycle are unclear, the amount of mela-

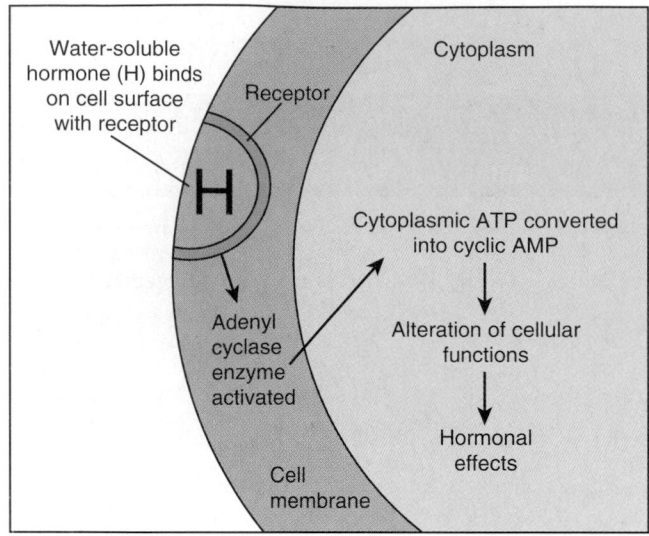

Figure 27–2

Mechanism by which water-soluble hormones alter the cellular function of target cells to produce short-term hormonal effects. (AMP, adenosine monophosphate; ATP, adenosine triphosphate.)

tonin in the circulation has been shown to vary with the phases of the menstrual cycle. Melatonin levels rise during the days just preceding menstruation.

HYPOTHALAMUS

The hypothalamus region of the brain lies beneath the thalamus and forms the floor and part of the lateral walls of the third ventricle. Special neurose-

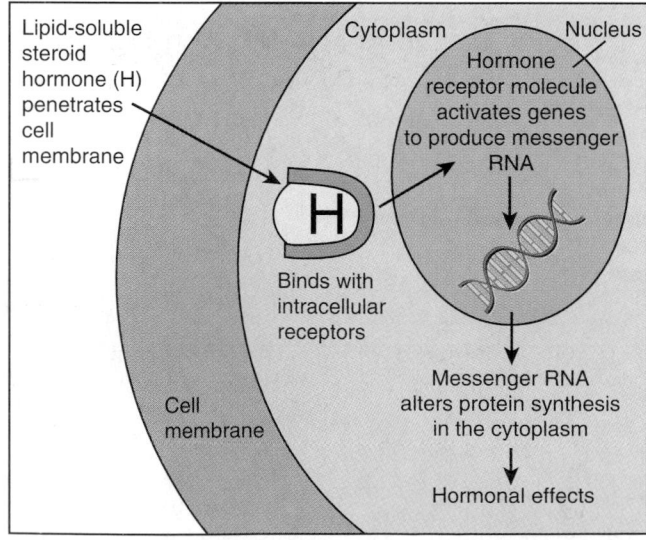

Figure 27–3

Mechanism by which lipid-soluble steroid hormones alter the cellular function of target cells to produce long-term hormonal effects.

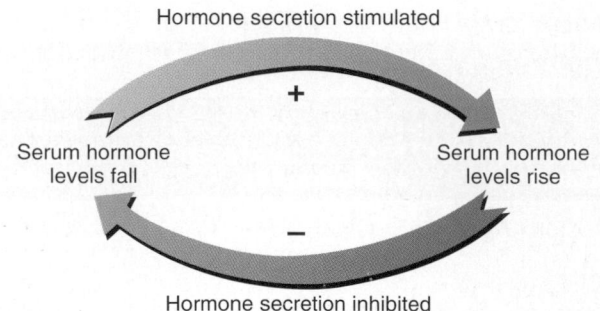

Figure 27–4

Negative feedback mechanism that controls blood serum hormone levels. As the endocrine gland secretes its hormone, serum levels rise and inhibit further secretion from the gland.

cretory cells in the hypothalamus synthesize and secrete hypothalamic hormones, which regulate the secretory functions of the anterior pituitary gland. Hypothalamic hormones that stimulate pituitary secretions are called releasing hormones. Those that inhibit pituitary secretions are called inhibiting hormones. These hormones are transported via the hypothalamic-hypophyseal portal vessels to the anterior lobe (adenohypophysis) of the pituitary, which is located just below the hypothalamus and connected to it by the pituitary stalk. Figure 27–5 illustrates the anatomic relationship of the hypothalamus

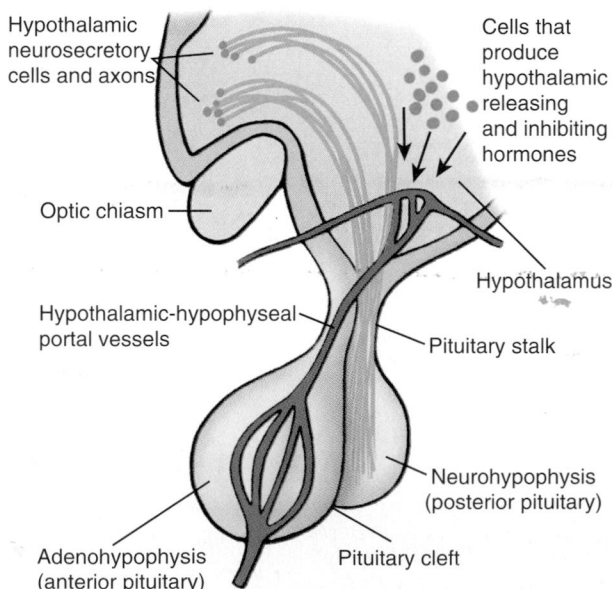

Figure 27–5

Anatomical relationship of the hypothalamus and the pituitary gland, with vascular and neurologic connections. Hypothalamic releasing and inhibiting hormones enter the hypothalamic-hypophyseal vessels for transport to the adenohypophysis (anterior pituitary). Antidiuretic hormone and oxytocin produced by hypothalamic neurosecretory cells pass down the axons to the neurohypophysis (posterior pituitary).

and pituitary gland. A partial list of hypothalamic secretions and their effects on pituitary function appears in Table 27–2.

Other neurosecretory cells in the hypothalamus produce two hormones: antidiuretic hormone and oxytocin. These two hormones pass down the cell axons to the posterior pituitary, where they are stored. Later, they are released in response to neurostimulation of the posterior pituitary by the hypothalamus. Another example of neuroregulation of hormone secretion by the hypothalamus is the secretion of epinephrine and norepinephrine from the adrenal medulla in response to impulses transmitted via a direct nerve pathway that connects the adrenal medulla to the hypothalamus.

The hypothalamus constantly monitors the body's homeostasis by analyzing input from nerve circuits connecting it to almost all parts of the brain, and from information carried in the blood passing through it. Through the dynamic processes of feedback and regulation, almost all of the endocrine system is controlled by either hormonal secretions or nervous signals from the hypothalamus.

PITUITARY GLAND

The pituitary gland, or hypophysis, is a complex structure composed of many independently functioning units, each of which is regulated by the hypothalamus. It is anatomically and physiologically divided into two functioning lobes (see Fig. 27–5): the adenohypophysis (anterior lobe) and the neurohypophysis (posterior lobe).

The posterior lobe of the pituitary gland is neural in origin. Its functioning unit is composed mainly of axons that originate in the hypothalamus and pass down the hypothalamic-hypophyseal tract in the pituitary stalk (or infundibulum) to terminate in the neurohypophysis. The posterior pituitary stores and secretes antidiuretic hormone and oxytocin, which are produced in the hypothalamus.

The anterior lobe, which accounts for about 80% of the pituitary, is glandular in structure. It is composed of several cell types, each of which functions as an almost independent unit in response to hypothalamic stimulation to secrete its own hormone or hormones. Table 27–3 identifies the cell types, the hormones they secrete, and the targets they affect.

A pituitary hormone can produce its effect either by altering the physiologic function of its target cells or tissue, or by altering the secretory function of other endocrine glands. Pituitary hormones that directly affect the secretory functions of other endocrine glands are called tropic hormones. A tropic hormone stimulates the target gland to secrete its hormone or hormones. For example, the tropic hormone thyrotropin (thyroid-stimulating hormone [TSH]) stimulates the thyroid gland to secrete thyroxine (T_4) and triiodothyronine (T_3). When the tropic hormone is no longer present, secretion from the target gland stops. If pituitary dysfunction causes hyposecretion or hypersecretion of a tropic hormone, the affected person shows clinical signs of a corresponding alteration in secretion from the dependent target gland. Thus, if the person has hypersecretion of TSH from the pituitary gland, the

Table 27–2

Hypothalamic Secretions and Their Functions

Hypothalamic Secretion	Function
Somatostatin (SS) or growth hormone–inhibiting hormone	Inhibits secretion of somatotropin (STH)
Growth hormone–releasing hormone (GH-RH)	Stimulates growth hormone (GH) secretion
Thyrotropin-releasing hormone (TRH)	Stimulates thyroid-stimulating hormone (TSH) secreted by thyrotrope cell
Corticotropin-releasing hormone (CRH)	Stimulates adrenocorticotropic hormone (ACTH) secreted by corticotrope cell
Luteinizing hormone–releasing hormone (LH-RH)*	Stimulates secretion of luteinizing hormone (LH) secreted by gonadotrope cell and follicle-stimulating hormone (FSH) secreted by gonadotrope cell
Follicle-stimulating hormone–releasing hormone (FSH-RH)	Stimulates FSH secretion secreted by gonadotrope cell
Prolactin-releasing hormone (PRH)	Stimulates secretion of prolactin secreted by lactotrope cell
Prolactin-inhibiting hormone (PIH)	Inhibits secretion of prolactin
Melanocyte-stimulating hormone–releasing hormone	Stimulates melanocyte-stimulating hormone (MSH) secreted by corticotrope cell
Melanocyte-stimulating hormone–inhibiting hormone	Inhibits secretion of MSH

* These two releasing hormones are sometimes grouped and called gonadotropin-releasing hormone (Gn-RH).

Table 27–3

Cell Types, Hormones, and Targets of the Anterior Pituitary Gland

Cell Type	Hormone Secreted	Target
Somatotrope	Somatotropin (STH, growth hormone)	Body cells
Thyrotrope	Thyrotropin (TSH)	Thyroid gland
Corticotrope	Adrenocorticotropic hormone (ACTH)	Adrenal cortex
	Melanocyte-stimulating hormone (MSH)	Melanocytes
Gonadotrope	Luteinizing hormone (LH)	Ovaries
	Follicle-stimulating hormone (FSH)	
Lactotrope	Prolactin (PRL)	Mammary glands

thyroid gland may over-secrete thyroxine and triiodothyronine.

Secretion of all anterior pituitary hormones is monitored by the hypothalamus and regulated by negative feedback control. As illustrated in Figure 27–6, a stimulus monitored by the hypothalamus indicates an alteration in the homeostasis of the body. The hypothalamus responds by secreting a releasing hormone. The releasing hormone stimulates one of the secretory cell types in the anterior pituitary to secrete its tropic hormone. The tropic hormone is released into systemic circulation and stimulates secretion by its target gland. As the target gland secretes its hormone, physiologic changes occur that are monitored by the hypothalamus. These changes may include a rising serum level of the hormone secreted by the target gland or other physiologic alterations initiated by the effect of the target gland hormone. The physiologic effects are then monitored by the hypothalamus, either directly through the blood, or through impulses transmitted to it by the central nervous system. When the desired physiologic changes have occurred, the hypothalamus stops secreting the releasing hormone or starts secreting an inhibiting hormone. Secretion of the tropic hormone from the anterior pituitary ceases.

Dysfunction of the hypothalamus, although rare, can result in pituitary dysfunction. A number of other disorders can also alter pituitary function. Most common among these are secreting and nonsecreting tumors of the gland itself, pressure from tumors in adjacent tissues, genetic disorders, iatrogenic disorders, and trauma. At the same time, because of its influence on other endocrine glands, pituitary disorders can have wide-ranging and serious effects on the body.

Pituitary disorders are grouped according to the pituitary lobe involved, the dysfunction that results, and the specific hormone affected. They are further classified as primary (caused by a dysfunction within the gland itself) or secondary (caused by either dysfunction of the hypothalamus or some other factor outside the gland).

THYROID GLAND

The thyroid gland is a highly vascular, butterfly-shaped organ that consists of two lobes of tissue situated on either side of the trachea. The lateral

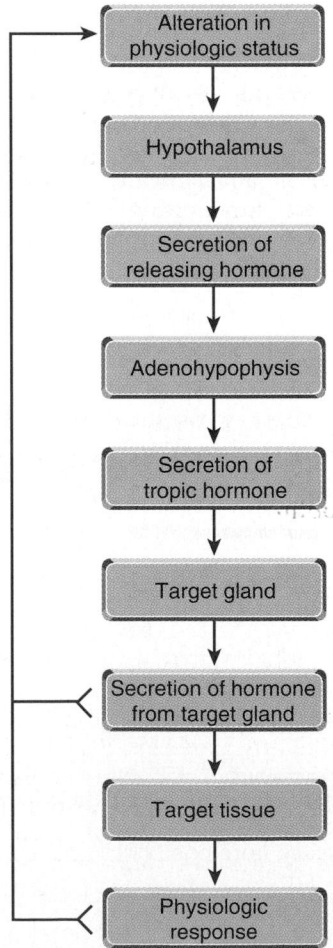

Figure 27–6

Negative feedback regulation of anterior pituitary endocrine secretion.

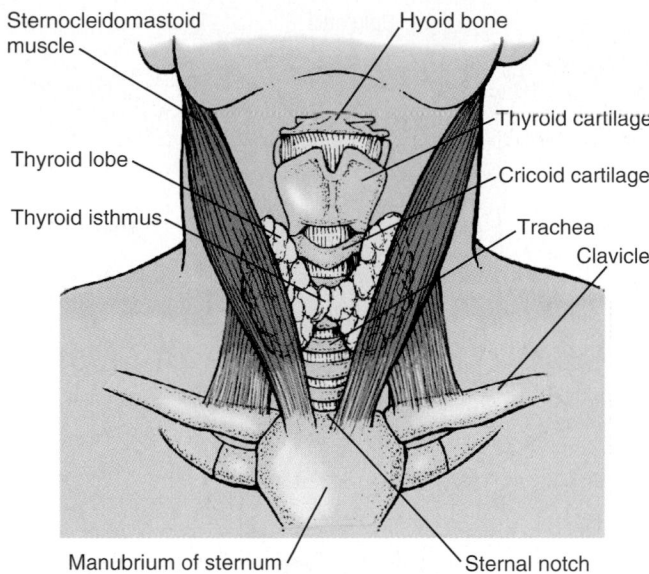

Figure 27–7

Anterior view of the thyroid gland anatomy and surrounding structures.

lobes are connected by a narrow isthmus of thyroid tissue lying over the anterior surface of the trachea (Fig. 27–7).

The lobes of the thyroid gland are composed of two types of cells: follicular and parafollicular. Three hormones are produced and secreted by these cells: thyroxine, triiodothyronine, and calcitonin.

Thyroxine and Triiodothyronine

The follicular cells form tiny, closely packed sacs called follicles or acini. Inside the follicles is a gelatinous iodine-containing colloid and large molecules of thyroglobulin. Thyroxine and triiodothyronine, the primary thyroid hormones, are produced within the thyroglobulin molecules by a process of iodine metabolism and biosynthesis. The hormones are then stored in the follicles, bound to thyroglobulin, until they are released into the circulation. This large reservoir of stored hormone is unique among the endocrine glands and can provide up to 100 days of normal thyroid hormone secretion if thyroid synthesis is interrupted.

In the blood, thyroxine and triiodothyronine are almost entirely bound to circulating plasma proteins. Most of the hormone is bound to thyroxine-binding globulin (TBG). Small amounts bind to albumin and prealbumin. Only the free, unbound hormone in the plasma is biologically active and available for use by body tissues.

About 15% to 20% of the triiodothyronine used by the body is released from the thyroid gland. The rest is produced by a process of monodeiodination of thyroxine (removal of one iodine molecule from

thyroxine) that converts thyroxine to triiodothyronine after thyroxine binds with cell receptor sites in peripheral tissues.

Adequate dietary intake of iodine and protein is necessary for the synthesis of thyroxine and triiodothyronine. The recommended daily intake of iodine is 0.15 mg/day, or about 1 mg a week. In the United States, the use of iodized salt and commercial bread products made with iodine-containing dough conditioners has greatly reduced the risk of inadequate iodine intake.

REGULATION OF SECRETION

The production and secretion of thyroxine and triiodothyronine by the thyroid gland are controlled by secretion of TSH, also called thyrotropin, from the anterior pituitary gland. Secretion of TSH is initiated by low circulating levels of thyroid hormone and by secretion of thyrotropin-releasing hormone (TRH) from the hypothalamus. Thyrotropin-releasing hormone is secreted in response to the body's metabolic needs and emotional reactions. TSH secretion is inhibited primarily by increased thyroxine and triiodothyronine levels in the circulation. This feedback mechanism, illustrated in Figure 27–8, maintains an almost constant level of free thyroxine and triiodothyronine in the circulation. TSH secretion may also

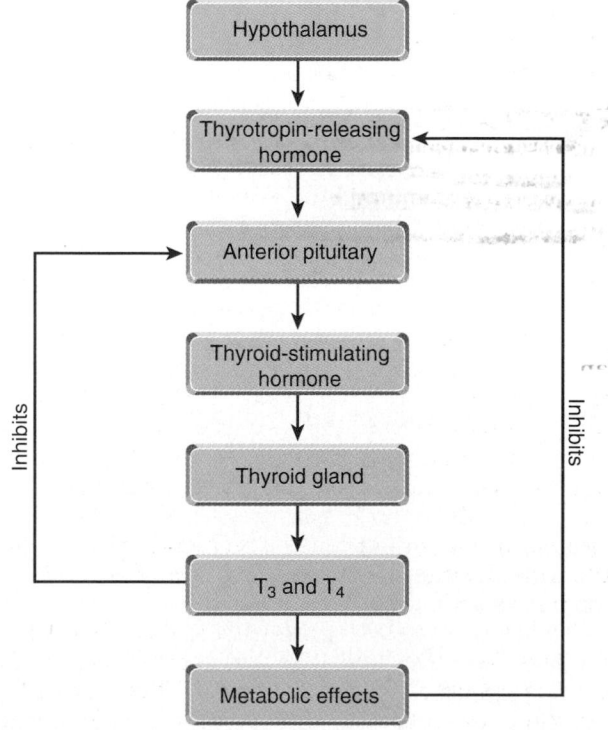

Figure 27–8

Regulation of thyroid hormone secretion by negative feedback control.

be inhibited by increased levels of somatostatin, dopamine, corticotropin (adrenocorticotropic hormone), and glucocorticoid hormones. It is stimulated by growth hormone and estrogen.

FUNCTIONS OF THYROXINE AND TRIIODOTHYRONINE

The primary function of thyroxine and triiodothyronine is to regulate cell metabolism and energy production. They also influence growth and development and affect cell differentiation in the fetus. The functions of thyroxine and triiodothyronine are detailed in Table 27–4.

In healthy people, serum thyroxine (T_4) is present in much larger amounts than triiodothyronine (T_3). In fact, the T_4:T_3 ratio is about 7–10:1. Triiodothyronine is more potent and more biologically active than thyroxine, but its effects last a shorter time. Triiodothyronine is secreted in increased amounts during severe stress and times of high energy need. Because thyroxine and triiodothyronine have similar functions, they are frequently referred to collectively as thyroid hormone.

Calcitonin

The parafollicular cells (C cells) are interspersed in clusters between the follicles. They produce and se-

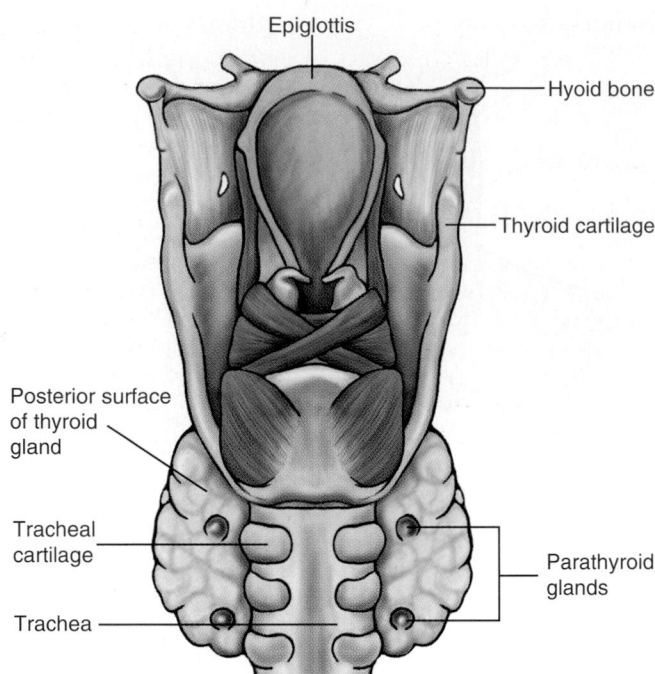

Figure 27–9

The parathyroid glands are positioned on the posterior surface of the thyroid gland. Although the parathyroids may be located anywhere on the posterior surface of the thyroid, one parathyroid gland is usually located in the upper half and one in the lower half of each thyroid lobe.

Table 27–4

Physiologic Effects of Thyroxine (T_4) and Triiodothyronine (T_3)

Increase basal metabolic rate
Increase metabolic activity of most body tissues (except brain, retina, spleen, testes, and lungs)
Increase oxygen utilization
Increase rate and depth of respiration
Increase heart rate, contractility, and cardiac output
Increase pulse pressure
Increase cardiac sensitivity to catecholamine secretion (epinephrine and norepinephrine)
Increase utilization of food for energy
Increase protein synthesis and catabolism
Stimulate all aspects of carbohydrate metabolism
Stimulate all aspects of fat metabolism
Increase vitamin metabolism
Stimulate conversion of carotene to vitamin A in the liver
Stimulate mental processes
Stimulate neuromuscular responses
Increase muscle tone
Stimulate red blood cell production
Stimulate activity of other endocrine glands
Promote growth and development in fetuses and children
Promote growth and development of the central nervous system in the fetus and during the first few years of life
Maintain normal reproductive function

crete calcitonin. Calcitonin lowers serum calcium levels by increasing calcium deposition in the bones. Calcitonin is an antagonist to parathyroid hormone. Secretion of calcitonin is controlled by serum calcium levels. Increased serum calcium levels stimulate calcitonin secretion. Decreased levels inhibit its secretion.

PARATHYROID GLANDS

The parathyroid glands secrete parathyroid hormone. Most people have four ovoid parathyroid glands imbedded on the posterior surface of the thyroid gland (Fig. 27–9). However, some people may have as few as two or as many as eight parathyroid glands. Ectopic glands have been found in the mediastinum and in the neck above the thyroid gland. Each gland is about the size of a match head and weighs about 30 to 40 mg.

The primary function of parathyroid hormone is to regulate serum calcium and phosphate levels by maintaining extracellular ionic calcium concentrations. Parathyroid hormone has a half-life of only a few minutes. Therefore, it must be secreted constantly to maintain serum calcium levels within a very narrow margin of homeostasis. A serum calcium fluctuation as small as 0.5 mg/dL outside a person's normal range may alter body functions. Serum calcium levels rise as parathyroid hormone is secreted. Because there is an inverse relationship between serum calcium and serum phosphorus concentrations, as serum calcium increases, serum phosphorus decreases.

Parathyroid hormone raises serum calcium levels by acting on three target sites in the body: the bones, the kidneys, and the gastrointestinal tract. In the bones, parathyroid hormone stimulates osteoclast activity, causing bone breakdown and increased resorption of calcium from the bones. The action of parathyroid hormone on the bones is counterbalanced by the effect of calcitonin.

In the kidneys, parathyroid hormone acts directly on the renal tubules to increase reabsorption of calcium and promote excretion of phosphate. In the intestines, parathyroid hormone activates vitamin D, which acts directly on the intestinal mucosa to increase absorption of dietary calcium. Adequate intake of vitamin D is necessary for intestinal absorption of dietary calcium and its use by the body. Although there are few natural food sources of vitamin D, it is synthesized in the skin during exposure to ultraviolet light. In many countries, it is added to pasteurized milk.

Parathyroid hormone secretion is regulated by negative feedback control in response to the serum concentration of free calcium ions. Free calcium ions, or serum ionized calcium, is the physiologically active form of calcium in the body. A drop in serum ionized calcium stimulates the parathyroid glands to rapidly secrete parathyroid hormone (Fig. 27–10). Secretion of parathyroid hormone decreases within seconds once serum calcium rises to normal physiologic levels.

ADRENAL GLANDS

The two pyramid-shaped adrenal glands lie embedded in fat on the upper pole of each kidney. Each gland measures about $5 \times 2 \times 1$ cm and weighs about 4 g. Each of the adrenal glands consists of two distinct endocrine glands: the adrenal cortex and the adrenal medulla. The adrenal cortex is the larger outer structure that surrounds the central adrenal medulla (Fig. 27–11). Each of these structures differs in cellular composition, function, and regulatory mechanism.

Adrenal Cortex

The adrenal cortex secretes a group of steroid hormones called corticosteroids, which mediate the body's response to stress and affect metabolism, fluid and electrolyte balance, and secondary sex characteristics.

The adrenal cortex is composed of three distinct layers. The zona glomerulosa, which secretes miner-

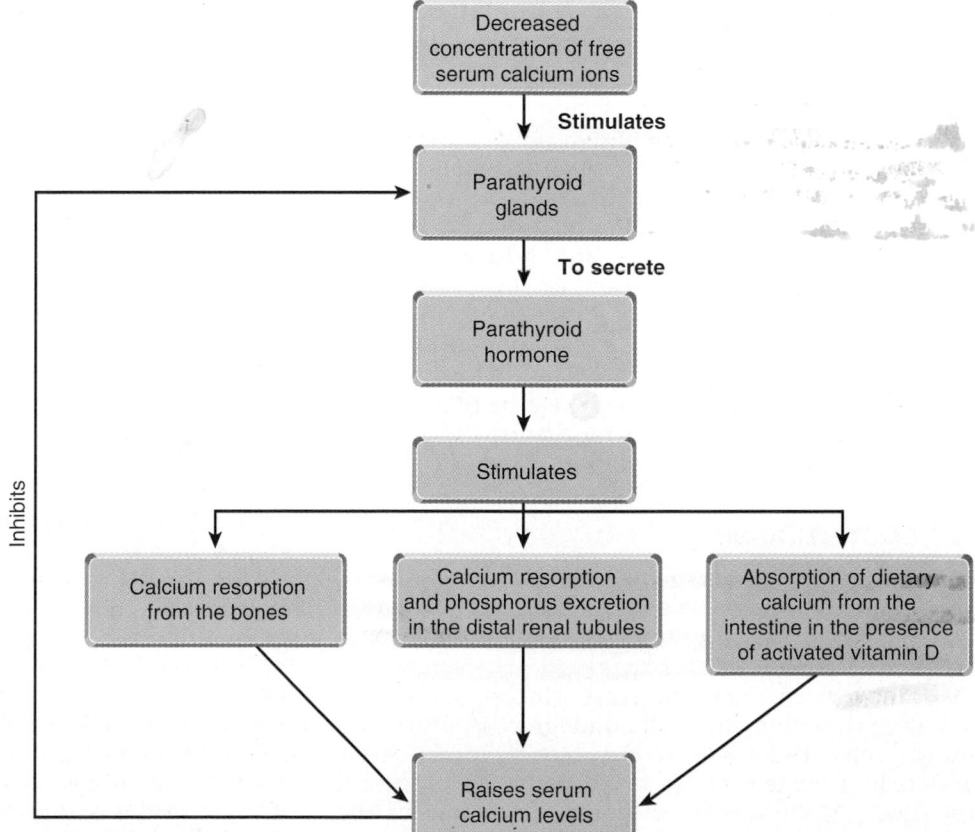

Figure 27–10

Regulation of parathyroid hormone secretion by negative feedback control.

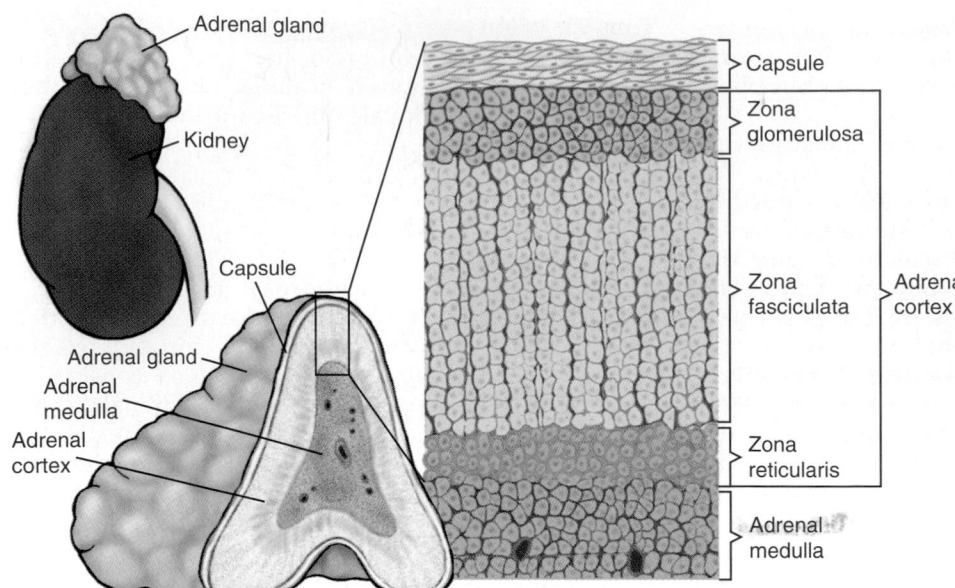

Figure 27–11

Structures of the adrenal gland. The central adrenal medulla constitutes about 20% of the glandular structure and secretes epinephrine and norepinephrine. The inset box shows the cellular structure of the adrenal gland with the three zones of the adrenal cortex. The zona glomerulosa secretes mineralocorticoids. The zona fasciculata and zona reticularis secrete glucocorticoids and sex steroid hormones.

alocorticoids, functions independently of the zona fasciculata and zona reticularis, which secrete glucocorticoids and sex steroid hormones (see Fig. 27–11). The adrenal cortex is the body's only source of mineralocorticoids and glucocorticoids. They are essential for life. Death occurs within 2 weeks after loss of these adrenocorticoid hormones.

MINERALOCORTICOIDS

Mineralocorticoids promote sodium retention and potassium excretion in the distal renal tubules. Therefore, they are primary factors in maintaining extracellular fluid volume and electrolyte balance in the body. Aldosterone is the principal mineralocorticoid secreted by the adrenal cortex. It is secreted in response to increased serum potassium levels, decreased serum sodium levels, and release of renin-angiotensin into the circulation in the presence of hypovolemia or hypotension. Pituitary adrenocorticotropic hormone also has a weak stimulatory effect on aldosterone secretion. Figure 27–12 illustrates the secretion of aldosterone in response to renin-angiotensin release, an important mechanism in homeostatic fluid and electrolyte balance.

GLUCOCORTICOIDS

The glucocorticoids are important in the regulation of carbohydrate, protein, and fat metabolism. Glucocorticoids stimulate gluconeogenesis by the liver and mobilize amino acids from the tissues for conversion into glucose. They also decrease glucose and amino acid transport into the cells and glucose utilization by the cells. These effects raise blood glucose levels and reduce protein stores in all body tissues except the liver. Mobilization of amino acids out of the cells results in decreased protein synthesis and increased protein catabolism. In the presence of de-

creased glucose transport into the cells, fatty acids are mobilized from adipose tissue for energy production, raising serum fatty acid levels. These metabolic effects help maintain blood glucose levels and supply energy for vital tissues between meals and during periods of starvation and fasting. The glucocorticoids also influence cognitive functions and help maintain emotional stability and the ability to respond to stress. In supraphysiologic amounts, the glucocorticoids exert a strong anti-inflammatory effect, suppress the immune system, and decrease the number of eosinophils and lymphocytes in the blood.

Glucocorticoid secretion is controlled almost entirely by adrenocorticotropic hormone secretion from the anterior pituitary gland. Secretion of adrenocorticotropic hormone is initiated by secretion of corticotropin-releasing hormone from the hypothalamus. Corticotropin-releasing hormone is secreted in response to circadian rhythms, physiologic need, and the increased energy demands of acute stress. Corticotropin-releasing hormone secretion is inhibited by elevated serum cortisol levels and relief of stress. Regulation of glucocorticoid secretion by this negative feedback cycle is illustrated in Figure 27–13.

Although glucocorticoid secretion varies constantly in response to circadian rhythms, serum levels are usually lowest during sleep, peak near awakening, rise again about 4 to 6 hours later, and then gradually drop through the rest of the day. Because this secretion pattern is characterized by periods of increased production during the daytime, it is referred to as a diurnal secretion pattern. It takes about 48 hours for the cyclic secretion of the glucocorticoids to adjust to changes in daily sleeping habits, one of the reasons for jet lag and excess fatigue in people who work different shifts on successive days.

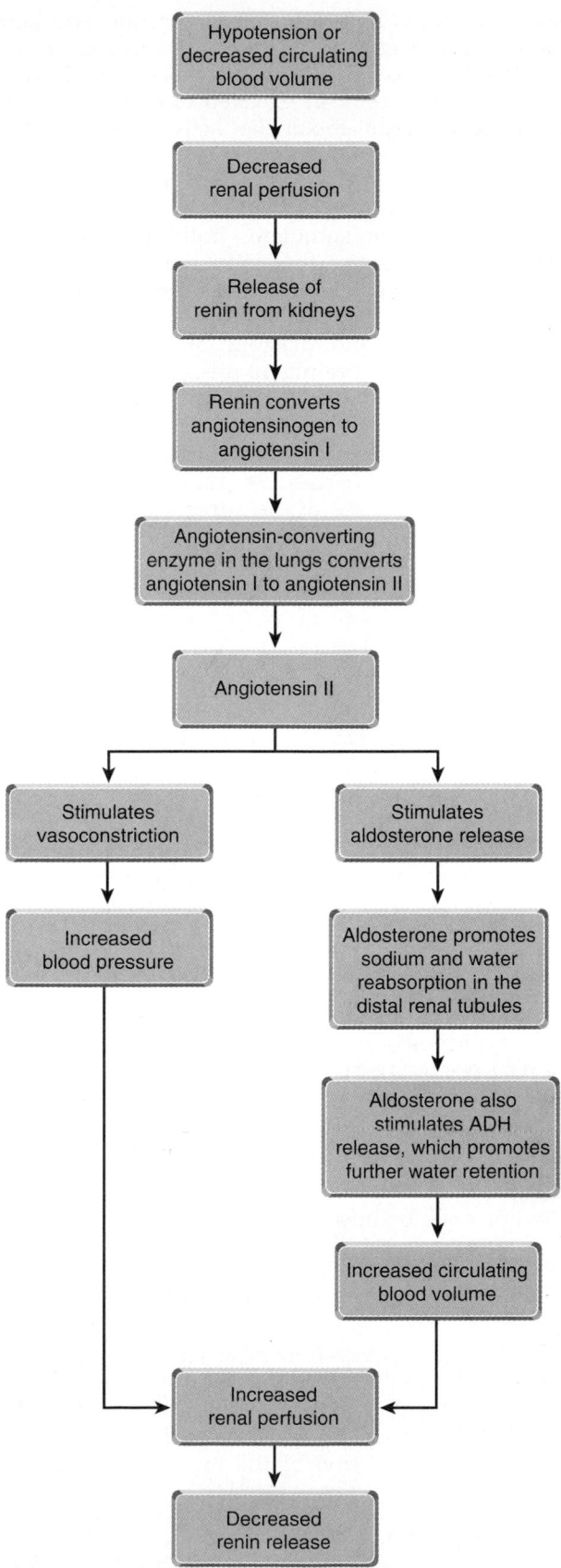

Figure 27–12

Secretion of aldosterone from the adrenal cortex in response to renin-angiotensin release. Restoration of blood pressure and circulating blood volume inhibits further renin release, completing the negative feedback cycle. (ADH, antidiuretic hormone.)

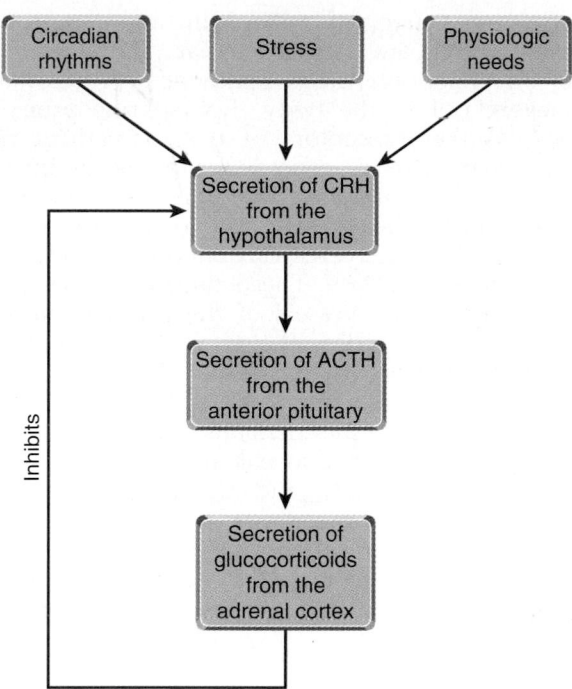

Figure 27–13

Regulation of glucocorticoid secretion by the corticotropin-releasing hormone (CRH)–adrenocorticotropic hormone (ACTH) negative feedback cycle.

Cortisol, also known as hydrocortisone, is the primary glucocorticoid secreted by the adrenal cortex. Cortisol plays a major role in the body's use of carbohydrates, fats, and proteins. For example, cortisol mobilizes the movement of amino acids from muscle and plasma so the liver can make new glucose. Cortisol also stimulates myocardial contractility.

Adrenal Medulla

The adrenal medulla and the sympathetic nervous system both develop from the ectodermal tissue of the fetal neural crest. Cells from the ectodermal tissue differentiate to form chromaffin cells and sympathetic ganglion cells. The adrenal medulla is a specialized glandular structure composed of chromaffin cells within the sympathetic nervous system. Any stimulus that activates the sympathetic nervous system can stimulate the adrenal medulla and elicit secretion of medullary hormones. The adrenal medulla functions in conjunction with the sympathetic nervous system to support and prolong the effects of sympathetic stimulation in the body. Because the adrenal medulla is an extension of the sympathetic nervous system, it is not essential for life.

The chromaffin cells of the adrenal medulla secrete two catecholamines: epinephrine and norepinephrine. The adrenal medulla is the primary source of epinephrine in the body. In normal people, epinephrine constitutes about 80% of the medullary secretions. Norepinephrine is the principal catecholamine secreted by sympathetic neurons outside the adrenal medulla.

The major effects of epinephrine and norepinephrine secretion are cardiovascular and metabolic. They affect not only the sympathetic nervous system but every cell in the body. Epinephrine primarily stimulates the β-receptors of the sympathetic nervous system, causing constriction of the peripheral, renal, and gastrointestinal vascular beds. Epinephrine also increases the rate and force of heart contractions, which increases cardiac output and raises systolic blood pressure. These cardiovascular effects shunt blood to the vessels of the heart, brain, and active skeletal muscles, the vital organs necessary for the fight-or-flight response. Stimulation of the sympathetic nervous system by epinephrine also dilates the pupils, inhibits peristalsis, increases sphincter tone, stimulates the sweat and apocrine glands, and increases the rate and depth of respirations while dilating the bronchi.

Epinephrine's metabolic effects can raise the body's metabolic rate to twice normal. Oxygen consumption and body temperature increase as the metabolic rate rises. Insulin secretion declines, whereas glycogenolysis (the conversion of stored glycogen to glucose) in the liver and muscles rises. These activities result in elevated blood glucose levels. The increased metabolic activity and rise in blood glucose levels contribute to the increased mental alertness and muscle strength associated with secretion of epinephrine.

Norepinephrine stimulates both the α-receptors and the β-receptors of the sympathetic nervous system, but predominantly affects the alpha-adrenergic receptors. It causes generalized vasoconstriction and increases systolic and diastolic blood pressures by greatly increasing peripheral resistance. The metabolic and cardiac effects of norepinephrine are not as pronounced as those of epinephrine.

The effects of epinephrine and norepinephrine on the body are summarized in Table 27–5. It is the effects of mass release of the adrenal catecholamines that cause the cold sweat, pounding heart, rapid and deep respirations, tremulousness, and feeling of wide-eyed alertness that occurs in extremely stressful situations.

Table 27–5

Physiologic Effects of Epinephrine and Norepinephrine

Substance	Physiologic Effect
Epinephrine	Heart rate increases
	Force of heart contractions increases
	Cardiac output increases
	Peripheral vascular bed constricts
	Renal blood vessels constrict
	Gastrointestinal vascular bed constricts
	Systolic blood pressure rises
	Metabolic rate increases to 100% above normal
	Oxygen utilization increases
	Body temperature rises
	Liver and muscle glycogenolysis increases
	Insulin secretion inhibited
	Blood glucose levels rise
	Peristalsis slows
	Sphincter tone increases
	Sweat and apocrine gland activity increases
	Respirations increase in rate and depth
	Bronchi dilate
	Pupils dilate
	Mental alertness increases
	Muscle strength increases
Norepinephrine	Generalized vasoconstriction
	Greatly increased peripheral vascular resistance
	Moderate cardiac stimulation
	Greatly increased systolic and diastolic blood pressures
	Mild metabolic effects

Endocrine Dysfunction

Endocrine dysfunction arises from the effects of an imbalance in the production of one or more hormones or from the effects of an alteration in the body's ability to use the hormones produced. Endocrine dysfunction can originate at almost any point in the production-secretion-feedback-regulation cycle. Dysfunction of one endocrine gland is likely to affect the function of one or more of the others.

PRIMARY ENDOCRINE GLAND DYSFUNCTION

Primary endocrine gland dysfunction implies that an endocrine gland is secreting either too much or too little hormone because of a defect in the gland itself. Secretion of excessive amounts of hormone is called hypersecretion. Secretion of inadequate amounts of hormone is called hyposecretion or hormone deficiency.

Primary hypersecretion from an endocrine gland usually results either from a secreting benign or malignant tumor, or from idiopathic hyperplasia. Idiopathic hyperplasia is an increase in the size of the gland and proliferation of the number of active secreting cells from unknown causes.

Primary hyposecretion by an endocrine gland can result from anything that destroys glandular tissue or interferes with the gland's ability to function. Common causes of glandular hypofunction include a destructive benign or malignant tumor, an inflammatory or infectious process, a destructive autoimmune response, and mechanical damage to the gland.

SECONDARY ENDOCRINE GLAND DYSFUNCTION

Secondary endocrine gland dysfunction implies that a gland is secreting too much or too little hormone secondary to factors outside the gland itself. Depending on the cause of the dysfunction and how long it has been present, secondary glandular dysfunction may be temporary or permanent. If the gland is structurally sound, normal function may return once the causative factor is corrected.

INABILITY TO USE HORMONE PRODUCED

Inability of the body to use a hormone may produce clinical manifestations of glandular hyposecretion when the endocrine gland is actually producing normal or even increased amounts of hormone. Two common causes of inability to use a hormone produced are production of a biologically inactive hormone and production of autoantibodies that destroy a specific hormone or hormone receptors.

*A*ssessment of the Endocrine System

Because each hormone affects numerous functions throughout the body, a person with endocrine dysfunction may have many health problems and nursing needs. Accurate assessment, reporting, and documentation of clinical manifestations, changes in condition, and response to treatment are especially important in caring for these patients because they commonly experience rapid fluctuations in physical and emotional status. As a group, endocrine disorders commonly produce alterations in the function of multiple body systems (Table 27–6). The focus of the physical examination of a patient with an endocrine disorder varies with the specific gland involved and is discussed in Chapters 28 and 29.

In collecting a history from a patient with an endocrine disorder, it is sometimes helpful to solicit input from someone familiar with the patient because altered cognitive function caused by the disorder may cause the patient to misunderstand questions or give vague or inaccurate answers. Assess alertness, mental processes, and speech patterns while collecting the history. The patient history should include the following information:

Biographic data, including family history
Presence and type of endocrine dysfunction in family history

Previous diagnosis of endocrine dysfunction
Current plan of care, including medications and other therapies
Growth or developmental disorders in the family
Coexisting conditions
Related care activities
The patient's chief concerns
Description of symptoms, especially unusual fatigue or lethargy
Presenting signs and symptoms, including date of onset, sudden or gradual, duration, and current status
Pattern of symptoms (steady progression or cyclic, with remission and exacerbation)
Precipitating factor or event related to the symptoms
Aggravating or alleviating factors
Psychosocial history, including patient's perception of symptom severity, impact on activities of daily living, and perception of emotional stress level
Intervention history, including measures implemented in response to endocrine dysfunction
Patient's knowledge of and compliance with health promotion and risk reduction measures related to the health of the endocrine system (Highlight 27–1)

Determine whether the patient has noted any changes characteristic of endocrine disorders (see Table 27–6). Collect information on the patient's usual coping patterns and support systems because endocrine disorders commonly require surgical intervention and usually require lifelong self-management and follow-up care. Physical assessment of each endocrine gland's functioning, as applicable, is discussed in Chapter 28 and 29.

NURSING PROCESS GUIDELINES
Endocrine Dysfunction

Diagnostic procedures to evaluate endocrine gland function are initially determined by the patient's history and clinical manifestations. Patients are often acutely ill during the diagnostic phase. Nursing care is planned to provide physical and emotional support while facilitating accurate and timely collection of specimens and rapid completion of diagnostic procedures. Specimens must be collected and preserved correctly for results to be accurate. Many diagnostic procedures for endocrine disorders are timed and require special preparation and specimen collection for a period of hours or days. Patient teaching and cooperation are essential.

Emotional support and teaching about lifelong adjustments in lifestyle, medications, and indications of impending hormonal imbalance are probably the most important nursing functions for helping a person live successfully with an endocrine disorder. Important topics to include in the patient teaching plan are identified in Highlight 27–2. Ample opportunity

Table 27–6

Alterations Commonly Assessed in Patients with Endocrine Dysfunction

System/Area	Alteration
Body structure and function	Fatigue or lethargy
	Altered rest and activity patterns
	Altered growth and development patterns
	Changes in appearance and body characteristics
	Atypical skin pigmentation and/or texture
	Changes in hair texture and/or distribution
	Disturbances in sexual function and reproduction
	Changes in secondary sex characteristics
Psychosocial	Changes in body image and role performance
	Changes in cognitive function
	Personality changes
	Emotional lability
	Disturbances in coping mechanisms and support systems
	Anxiety or fear
Nutrition and elimination	Changes in appetite and fluid intake
	Weight loss or gain
	Changes in bowel elimination pattern
	Changes in urinary pattern and/or quantity
	Deficiencies or excesses of nutritional elements
Gaseous transfer	Altered cardiac output
	Fluid and electrolyte imbalances
	Dependent edema or anasarca
	Changes in pulse rate and/or blood pressure
	Changes in peripheral circulation
	Anemia
	Altered respiratory rate or pattern
Body defenses	Elevated or subnormal body temperature
	Decreased resistance to inflammation and infection
	Impaired wound healing and recovery from illness
	Impaired stress response
Sensorimotor function	Bone and joint abnormalities
	Muscle wasting and atrophy
	Altered balance and gait
	Tetany, paresthesias, and muscle cramps
	Visual disturbances
	Headaches

must be provided for the patient and family to share concerns and to discuss perceptions of the effects the condition will have on lifestyle and responsibilities. Success is determined by the patient's ability to achieve short-term goals and hormonal balance while in the hospital, and the ability to continue to maintain hormonal balance after discharge while adapting to required lifestyle changes.

❖ Settings, Providers, and Collaboration for Care

Diagnosis and care of the patient with an endocrine dysfunction may be provided in the acute care setting when initial problems are identified or surgical interventions conducted. It may take place in outpatient clinics and physician offices as ongoing care is monitored. It may also take place in the home as the patient and family increasingly participate in the planning and implementation of care. Providers of care may include the acute care nurse, community health nurse, physician, surgeon, physical therapist, social worker, and pharmacist. Because of the complexity of endocrine dysfunction, a comprehensive plan of care often necessitates long-term participation of the different health care providers in a cooperative program for optimal health maintenance.

The Elderly: Special Considerations

The aging process is accompanied by changes in the function of the endocrine glands. With advancing years, the amount of hormones secreted by many of the endocrine glands changes. One age-related change is a diminished ability to respond to physiologic stress. This response is mediated by hypothalamic-pituitary-adrenal gland interactions. Pancreatic and thyroid secretions also diminish, altering digestion and metabolism. Thyroid function should be evaluated as a routine part of an annual physical examination for all geriatric patients. Normal gonadal secretions diminish, altering secondary sex characteristics and contributing to osteoporosis.

The incidence of many endocrine dysfunctions increases with age. With replacement therapy and dietary adjustment, these chronic disorders are manageable and not life-threatening.

The geriatric patient with an endocrine disorder presents many nursing care challenges. Common manifestations associated with endocrine disorders are more difficult to assess in older people because of diminished skin turgor and ongoing alterations in fluid and electrolyte status. Many elderly people have chronic cardiovascular problems that make it difficult to determine the cause of changes in cardiovascular status. These conditions, along with problems related to sight, hearing, mobility, elimination, and nutritional intake, can make it more difficult to diagnose and manage endocrine disorders in older adults.

Liver and kidney functions decline with increased age. This may alter the metabolism and

---

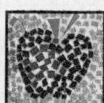

HIGHLIGHT *27–1*

HEALTH PROMOTION & RISK REDUCTION

Optimal Endocrine System Function

To maintain the health of the endocrine system and reduce risk of endocrine dysfunction, instruct your patient to practice these healthy behaviors:

Maintain adequate intake of calcium or supplement dietary intake with calcium tablets.

Maintain adequate intake of iodine and protein. Use iodized salt, bread with iodine-containing conditioners, or both.

Keep weight within appropriate limits for age and body structure.

Have blood pressure checked regularly.

Have blood glucose screening done yearly, especially with family history of diabetes mellitus.

Report symptoms of extreme lethargy, fatigue, chilling, or weight gain.

Report symptoms of extreme restlessness, weight loss, or hot flashes.

Have a yearly checkup at a physician's office, especially with family history of endocrine dysfunction or apparent symptoms.

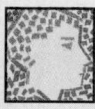

HIGHLIGHT *27–2*

PATIENT EDUCATION

Self-Management of Endocrine Dysfunction

Instruct the patient in the following:

The correct medical term for the diagnosis

Pathophysiology, disease progression, and patient prognosis

Prescribed therapeutic regimen, its rationale, and expected results

Self-administration of medications and/or treatments and schedule

Expected action and side effects of medications

Dietary alterations

Alterations in lifestyle and activities

What to do if unable to follow prescribed regimen because of illness

Self-monitoring of the effectiveness of treatment

Symptoms of a recurrent hormone imbalance

Symptoms that should be reported to the physician

Need to carry or wear emergency medical information and identification

Plans for follow-up care

Information on community and national support groups

Referral to community agencies

---

elimination of replacement hormones, placing the older patient at greater risk for developing adverse effects to medications. Target organs may lose the ability to respond to hormones. Hormone replacement therapy for the elderly must be initiated cautiously and the dosage increased slowly, with close assessment of the therapeutic and potential adverse drug effects.

Chapter Review

1. Which endocrine glands are essential to life and why?
2. How does negative feedback work with the endocrine glands?
3. How do each of the endocrine glands regulate hormone secretion?
4. What is the function of hormones and what are the affected target organs?

5. What effect does dysfunction in one endocrine gland have upon other endocrine glands?
6. What are the three types of endocrine dysfunction and how does each affect the system as a whole?
7. How is endocrine gland dysfunction assessed?
8. What physiologic alterations are common in endocrine gland dysfunction?
9. What changes are seen in elderly patients with endocrine dysfunction?
10. In what settings would you typically find patients with endocrine dysfunction being assessed and treated?

Bibliography

Abrams AC. Clinical drug therapy: Rationales for nursing practice. 4th ed. Philadelphia: JB Lippincott, 1995.

Aranow WS. The heart and thyroid disease. Clin Geriatr Med 1995; 11(2):219.

Baxter MA. Acromegaly and transsphenoidal hypophysectomy: A case report. AANA J 1994; 62(2):182.

Boulanger BR, Gann DS. Management of the trauma victim with pre-existing endocrine disease. Crit Care Clin 1994; 10(3):537.

Bruton-Maree N, Maree SM. Acute adrenal insufficiency: A case report. CRNA 1993; 4(3):128.

Burke MM, Walsh MB. Regulation: Endocrine, temperature, and infection in gerontologic nursing: Care of the frail elderly. Mosby-Year Book 1992, 167-196.

Caraceni P, Fagiuoli S, Gurakar A, et al. Liver disease: Clues from the hematologic, gastrointestinal, and endocrine systems. Consultant 1994; 34(3):427.

Carpenito LJ. Nursing diagnosis: Application to clinical practice. 6th ed. Philadelphia: JB Lippincott, 1995.

Cassel CK, Walsh JR (eds). Geriatric medicine. 3rd ed. New York: Springer-Verlag, 1996.

Cella JH, Watson J. Nurse's manual of laboratory tests. 2nd ed. Philadelphia: FA Davis, 1995.

Coffland FI. Endocrine disorders affecting the cardiovascular system. Crit Care Nurs Clin North Am 1994; 6(4):735.

Cooper JAD, Pappas PG (eds). Cecil review of general internal medicine. 6th ed. Philadelphia: WB Saunders, 1996.

Counsell CM, Gilbert M, Snively C. Challenging diagnosis. Management of the patient with a pituitary tumor resection. DCCN 1996; 15(2):75.

Curtis P, Dworkin H. Nuclear medicine and the thyroid gland: A retrospective review. J Nucl Med Technol 1995; 23(Suppl 4): 8S.

Daniels GH. Thyroid function tests: The pivotal role of sensitive TSH measurements. Consultant 1995; 35(2):209.

Dean E. Bedrest and deconditioning. Neurol Rep 1993; 17(1):6.

DeGroot LJ (ed). Endocrinology. 3rd ed. Philadelphia: WB Saunders, 1994.

Doenges M, Moorhouse M. Nurse's pocket guide: Nursing diagnoses with interventions. 5th ed. Philadelphia: FA Davis, 1996.

Dranov P. Tired? Wired? It could be your thyroid. Am Health 1995; 13(4):90.

Dudek SG. Nutrition handbook for nursing practice. 2nd ed. Philadelphia: JB Lippincott, 1993.

Eliopoulos C. Gerontological nursing. 4th ed. Philadelphia: JB Lippincott, 1996.

Figlewicz DP, Schwartz MW, Seeley RJ, et al. Endocrine regulation of food intake and body weight. J Lab Clin Med 1996; 127(4):328.

Fischbach F. A manual of laboratory diagnostic tests. 5th ed. Philadelphia: JB Lippincott, 1996.

Gambert SR. Hyperthyroidism in the elderly. Clin Geriatr Med 1995; 11(2):181.

Gordon M. Nursing diagnosis: Process and applications. 3rd ed. St. Louis: CV Mosby, 1993.

Greenspan FS. Basic and clinical endocrinology. 4th ed. Norwalk, CT: Appleton & Lange, 1994.

Griffin J, Ojeda S (eds). Textbook of endocrine physiology. 3rd ed. New York: Oxford University Press, 1996.

Guyton AC. Textbook of medical physiology. 9th ed. Philadelphia: WB Saunders, 1995.

Hart IR. Management decisions in subclinical thyroid disease. Hosp Pract 1995; 30(1):43.

Healy PF. Self-test. Caring for patients with endocrine disorders. Nursing 1995; 25(9):22.

Kee JL. Handbook of laboratory and diagnostic tests with nursing implications. 2nd ed. Norwalk, CT: Appleton & Lange, 1994.

Kessenich CR, Rosen CJ. Vitamin D and bone status in elderly women. Orthop Nurs 1996; 15(3):57.

Lawler DA. Hormonal response in sepsis. Crit Care Nurs Clin North Am 1994; 6(2):265.

Lehne RA. Pharmacology for nursing care. 2nd ed. Philadelphia: WB Saunders, 1994.

Malseed RT, Harrigan G. Textbook of pharmacology and nursing care: The nursing process. 4th ed. Philadelphia: JB Lippincott, 1995.

Managing thyroid troubles. Health News 1994; 12(1):1.

Matteson MA, McConnell ES. Gerontological nursing: Concepts and practice. 2nd ed. Philadelphia: WB Saunders, 1996.

Maugeri D, Russo MS, Carnazzo G, et al. Altered laboratory thyroid parameters indicating hyperthyroidism in elderly subjects. Arch Gerontol Geriatr 1996; 22(2):145.

Miller M, Gold GC. Acute endocrine emergencies. Clin Geriatr Med 1994; 10(1):161.

Mundy GR. Evaluation and treatment of hypercalcemia. Hosp Pract 1994; 29(6):79.

Nimmagadda U. Anesthesia and the parathyroid gland. Curr Rev Nurse Anesth 1994; 16(21):183.

North American Nursing Diagnosis Association. NANDA nursing diagnoses: Definitions and classifications, 1997–1998. Philadelphia: Author, 1996.

Novak S, Greenwood R. Patterns of urine flow and electrolyte excretion in patients following traumatic brain injury. Clin Rehabil 1995; 9(4):331.

Perry HM, Miller DK, Morley JE, et al. A preliminary report of vitamin D and calcium metabolism in older African Americans. J Am Geriatr Soc 1993; 41(6):612.

Piziak VK, Gilliland PF. Pituitary tumors: Look for early signs and symptoms. Emerg Med 1993; 25(7):124.

Roberts A. Systems of life: Endocrine system—an overview. Nurs Times 1995; 91(15):33.

Roberts A. Growth hormone and prolactin. Nurs Times 1995; 91(28):33.

Roberts A. Systems of life: The thyroid gland 2. Nurs Times 1995; 91(41):33.

Roberts A. Systems of life: The adrenal glands. Nurs Times 1995; 91(45):34.

Roberts A. Systems of life: The adrenal gland 2. Nurs Times 1995; 91(50):31.

Rutecki GW, Whittier FC. Hyponatremia: Cause of hypotonicity directs management. Consultant 1994; 34(5): 705.

Shannon MT, Wilson BA. Govoni & Hayes drugs and nursing implications. 8th ed. Norwalk, CT: Appleton & Lange, 1994.

Siconolfi LA. The forgotten system: Endocrine dysfunction during multiple system organ dysfunction. Crit Care Nurs Q 1994; 16(4):16.

Smith-Rooker JL, Garrett A, Hodges LC. Case management of the patient with pituitary tumor. MEDSURG Nurs 1993; 2(4):265.

Sticco SL. Clinical case conference. Anesthesia and the endocrine system. CRNA 1996; 7(1):57.

Thyroid tests: Who needs them? University of California at Berkeley Wellness Letter 1996; 12(8):2.

Toto KH. Endocrine physiology: A comprehensive review. Crit Care Nurs Clin North Am 1994; 6(4):637, 655.

Toto KH. Nonsteroidal anti-inflammatory drugs: A pharmacologic update. Physician Assist 1994; 18(9):31, 36, 46.

Ulrich SP, Canale SW, Wendell SA. Nursing care planning guides: A nursing diagnosis approach. 3rd ed. Philadelphia: WB Saunders, 1994.

Vague symptoms may signal thyroid disease. University of Texas Lifetime Health Letter 1993; 5(10):1, 6.

Willensky D. How it works: The endocrine system. Am Health 1996; 15(3):92.

Wyngaarden JB, Smith LH, Bennett JC (eds). Cecil textbook of medicine. 20th ed. Philadelphia: WB Saunders, 1996.

Ziomek R. Commentary on endocrine responses to the stress of critical illness. AACN Nurs Scan Crit Care 1993; 3(1):17.

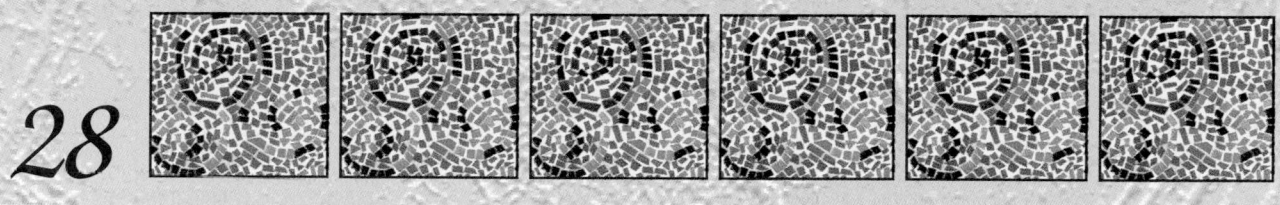

28

Nursing Care of Patients with Diabetes Mellitus

Study Outcomes

After studying this chapter, you should be able to:

1. Explain the normal physiology of insulin and the hormonal regulation of blood glucose levels.
2. Describe the classifications, etiology, pathophysiology, clinical manifestations, diagnostic procedures, and medical management of diabetes mellitus.
3. Identify information and physical examination data essential to the assessment of patients with diabetes mellitus.
4. State nursing diagnoses and related expected patient outcomes commonly applicable to patients with diabetes mellitus.
5. Describe nursing interventions, with their rationales, commonly applicable to patients with diabetes mellitus.
6. Explain the basis for evaluation of nursing care provided to patients with diabetes mellitus.
7. Describe the etiology, pathophysiology, clinical manifestations, diagnostic procedures, medical management, and prevention of the acute complications and long-term degenerative changes of diabetes mellitus.
8. Identify alternative treatment and care settings for patients with diabetes mellitus, and the services related to community-based care.
9. Identify special considerations for the elderly patient with diabetes mellitus.

Diabetes mellitus is a chronic disorder of altered carbohydrate, fat, and protein metabolism caused either by a relative or absolute lack of insulin, or by the inability of tissues to respond to insulin. Diabetes mellitus is characterized by persistent hyperglycemia, impaired leukocyte activity, and long-term vascular and neurologic degeneration. It is one of the oldest diseases known to humans and was recorded as early as 1500 BC. The name is derived from the Greek verb *diabetes*, meaning "to run through." Mellitus is from a Latin word meaning "honey," because physicians noticed that these patients had polyuria and that their urine was sweet.

Patients diagnosed with diabetes mellitus are usually managed throughout the course of the disease and treatment regimen in outpatient clinics and in the home. Many patients with minor complications of the disease or education needs are routinely assessed and cared for by the home health nurse. Hospitalization may be necessary when the patient develops serious complications or is in an uncontrolled state of the disease.

*H*ormonal Regulation of Blood Glucose Levels

INSULIN

Insulin is a hormone secreted by beta cells in the islets of Langerhans in the pancreas. It is a small protein composed of two amino acid chains that are connected to each other by disulfide linkages. The primary function of insulin is to transport glucose into muscle and fat cells to be used for energy. Insulin affects carbohydrate, fat, and protein metabolism and lowers blood glucose levels. Table 28–1 presents a glossary of terms frequently used in discussion of insulin and diabetes mellitus.

Carbohydrate Metabolism

The effects of insulin on carbohydrate metabolism are to increase the rate of glucose metabolism, decrease blood glucose concentration, and increase glycogen stores. Insulin binds with the cell's receptor sites, causing rapid uptake, storage, and use of glucose by most cells in the body. Insulin promotes transport of glucose across the cell wall by a process known as facilitated diffusion, thereby providing the body with energy. After a meal, insulin promotes storage of excess glucose in the liver by converting glucose into glycogen, a process called glycogenesis. Between meals, when blood glucose levels fall, the liver converts glycogen back into glucose, a process called glycogenolysis.

Table 28–1

Terms Frequently Used In Nursing Care of the Patient with Diabetes Mellitus

Term	Definition
Anabolism	Synthesis of complex molecules from simple molecules
Catabolism	Breakdown of complex molecules to simple molecules with the release of energy
Diffusion	Means by which molecules or solutes move across a selectively permeable membrane from an area of higher concentration to an area of lower concentration
Facilitated diffusion	Means by which glucose crosses a membrane; it combines with a carrier substance, insulin, to cross the cell membrane
Glycogen	A polysaccharide formed from glucose and stored in the liver and muscle cells
Glycogenesis	Synthesis of glycogen from glucose
Glycogenolysis	Breakdown of glycogen to glucose
Gluconeogenesis	Conversion of fat or protein to glycogen and then to glucose in the liver
Lipogenesis	Conversion of glucose and triglycerides into fat for storage
Lipolysis	Breakdown of fat to glucose

Fat Metabolism

Insulin promotes fatty acid synthesis by converting glucose into fatty acids. These fatty acids are subsequently deposited as fat in adipose tissue. Although most of this synthesis occurs in the liver, a small amount occurs in the fat cells themselves. The conversion of glucose into fatty acid is called lipogenesis.

Protein Metabolism

Insulin promotes the entry of amino acids into cells and inhibits catabolism of protein. Insulin also decreases the rate at which amino acids are released from cells, especially muscle cells. Insulin inhibits the rate of gluconeogenesis by decreasing the activity of enzymes that promote it.

REGULATION OF INSULIN SECRETION

Insulin normally is secreted at a continuous basal rate, with increased secretion in response to food. At the normal fasting blood glucose level, insulin secretion is minimal. Insulin secretion in response to glucose stimulation is rapid and occurs within minutes. This rise in insulin allows transport of glucose into muscle, liver, and other cells, thereby reducing the blood glucose concentration. The reduced blood glucose level then causes decreased secretion of insulin. Between meals and overnight, insulin and glucose levels fall. If the period of fasting is prolonged, stored glucose is released from the liver, protein is released from muscle, and fat is released from adipose tissue to provide energy for the cells.

COUNTER-REGULATORY HORMONES

Blood glucose concentrations are also influenced by counter-regulatory hormones, all of which oppose the action of insulin and are therefore also known as insulin antagonists. These counter-regulatory hormones are glucagon, epinephrine, cortisol, growth hormone, and somatostatin (growth hormone–inhibiting hormone).

Glucagon is secreted by the alpha cells of the islets of Langerhans in the pancreas. It increases blood glucose concentration by causing glycogenolysis and by increasing gluconeogenesis. Glucagon is essential for recovery from hypoglycemia and is the primary counter-regulatory hormone. The effect of epinephrine on blood glucose concentration is similar to that of glucagon, although not quite as strong.

Cortisol increases the blood glucose concentration by increasing the rate of gluconeogenesis and decreasing glucose utilization by the cells. More information on the physiologic effects of epinephrine and cortisol appears in Chapter 29.

Growth hormone (somatotropin) is secreted by the anterior pituitary gland. Long-term growth hormone excess limits glucose transport into cells and results in elevated blood glucose levels.

Somatostatin is a hormone secreted by the hypothalamus. It inhibits release of somatotropin from the anterior pituitary gland and also of certain hormones, such as glucagon and insulin.

ABSENCE OF INSULIN

The absence of insulin results in hyperglycemia (elevated blood glucose) by impairing glucose uptake in the cells, especially in muscle and liver cells. Cells starve despite elevated blood glucose levels because glucose transport into the cells is impaired. Impaired protein synthesis and excessive protein catabolism also occur, causing an increase in glucogenic amino acids. This leads to increased hepatic glucose production and causes further increase in blood glucose levels.

In severe insulin deficiency, lipolysis occurs. Lipolysis is the formation of excessive amounts of glycerol and free fatty acids through the hydrolysis of triglycerides. Glycerol increases hepatic glucose production, causing a higher level of hyperglycemia. At the same time, in an attempt to provide energy, ketone bodies are formed in the liver from the free fatty acids.

Hyperglycemia causes osmotic diuresis, which leads to fluid losses, dehydration, and electrolyte depletion. The presence of ketone bodies causes ketoacidosis, an acute complication of type 1 (insulin-dependent) diabetes mellitus. Figure 28–1 compares the normal physiologic response to the ingestion of food with the pathophysiologic response in diabetes mellitus.

Diabetes Mellitus

According to the American Diabetes Association (ADA), roughly 7 million people have been diagnosed with diabetes. However, it is estimated that almost as many people have *not* been diagnosed. The actual number of people with diabetes may be as high as 14 million. The annual incidence of diagnosed diabetes is about 29 cases per 10,000 people. Some 725,000 new cases are diagnosed annually, with most being type 2 (formerly called non-insulin-dependent) diabetes mellitus.

The effects of diabetes mellitus are both physical and economic. Diabetes is a major chronic health care problem and the seventh leading underlying cause of death in the United States. Each year, about 150,000 people die from diabetes and its complications. It is the leading cause of new cases of blindness in adults between ages 20 and 74. It accounts for 30% of new cases of end-stage renal disease, 50 to 60% of adult deaths from coronary heart disease, and 40 to 50% of nontraumatic amputations for foot or ankle ulcers. In 1992, health care expenditures for diabetes totaled about $105.2 billion—14.6% of total U.S. health care expenses. Per capita annual health care expenditures for diabetics averaged $9943 in 1992, compared with $2604 for nondiabetics.

The impact of diabetes on the health care system can be directly affected by how the diabetes patient manages the disease and maintains control of blood glucose levels. In 1993, a 10-year study in the Diabetes Control and Complications Trial showed that tight control of blood glucose can delay or prevent development of long-term complications (ADA, 1995). These findings support what health professionals have said for many years. In fact, the findings were so clear-cut that the 10-year study was halted a year early so results could be shared with health care providers and with diabetics.

It is now recommended that diabetics switch to an intensive treatment program, individually tailored for that person, to maintain blood glucose levels as close to normal levels as possible. Most people can accomplish this at home by learning to check their own blood glucose levels. By learning how to interpret the results and working closely with the physician and other members of the health care team, these patients can adjust their insulin injections, food intake, and exercise program. Ultimately, this helps preserve their quality of life.

ETIOLOGY AND PATHOPHYSIOLOGY

Progress in the fields of molecular biology, virology, protein chemistry, genetics, and immunology has helped increase knowledge of the etiology of diabetes. Although some controversy exists, most research indicates that type 1 diabetes (formerly called insulin-dependent diabetes mellitus) is an autoimmune disease. Studies have shown that in more than 90% of patients with type 1 diabetes mellitus, antibodies are directed against their own islet cells. These autoantibodies bind to a substance inside the islet cells, destroying the cells and making the pancreas unable to produce insulin. Further, these autoantibodies have been found in diabetic patients long before the symptoms of diabetes appear, suggesting that they play a role in causing the disease. However, the mechanism that triggers the immunologic attack is still unknown. Studies of people with type 1 diabetes mellitus have revealed human leukocyte antigen molecules on chromosome 6.

Researchers have also made progress in searching for genes that determine susceptibility to diabetes. People at risk for diabetes mellitus are as follows:

- Those with a strong family history of diabetes
- Those of African-American, Hispanic, or Native American descent
- Those who are obese
- Those who have a morbid obstetric history or a history of delivering infants weighing more than 9 lb

It has long been known that among identical twins wherein one twin has type 1 diabetes, there is a 50% chance of the disease developing in the other twin. Twin studies of type 2 diabetes show a 90% concordance. This has led to the search to identify which genes determine susceptibility to diabetes.

The ability to prevent the onset of diabetes mellitus in high-risk people is becoming a reality. Clinical trials are underway to test for the presence of islet cell antibodies. The immunosuppressant drug azathioprine (Imuran) has been used successfully in preventing diabetes from developing in some patients.

When diabetes does develop, it manifests as the body's inability to produce adequate insulin in response to rising blood glucose levels or inability to utilize the insulin produced. As shown in Figure

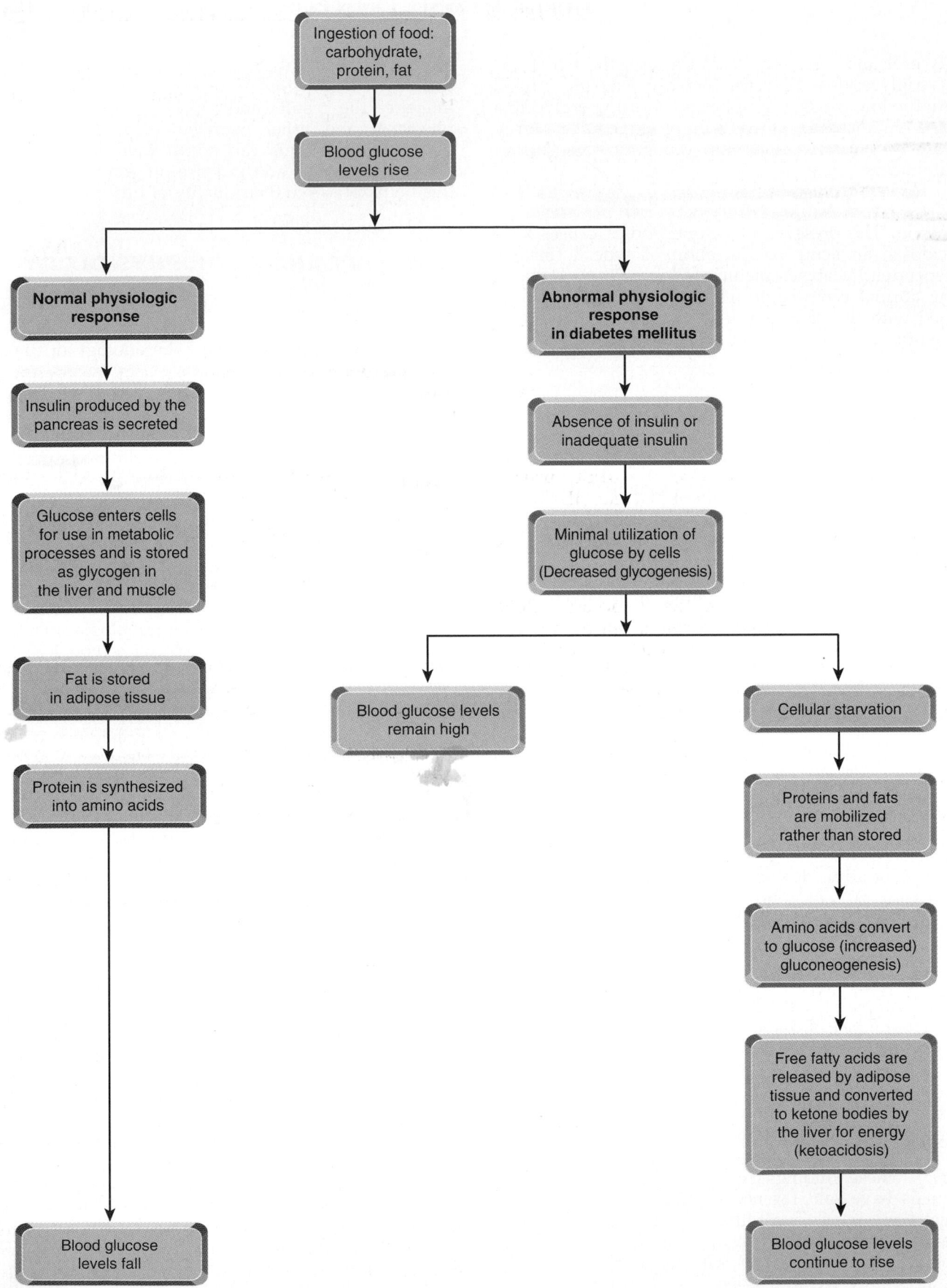

Figure 28–1

Comparison of the physiologic response to food ingestion in the nondiabetic person (normal physiologic response) and the diabetic person (abnormal physiologic response).

28–1, when a nondiabetic person eats a meal, the beta cells in the pancreas produce just the right amount of insulin to maintain normal blood glucose levels. When blood glucose levels start to fall, such as between meals, the pancreas decreases the amount of insulin it produces. This is an ongoing, continuous process to maintain normal blood glucose levels.

When a person has diabetes mellitus, the beta cells of the pancreas either do not produce insulin or the insulin they produce is ineffective. This, in turn, causes decreased utilization of glucose by the cells and increased blood glucose levels (as high as 800 mg/dL). It also causes increased mobilization of fats from fat storage areas, resulting in abnormal fat metabolism and deposits of lipids in vascular walls, causing atherosclerosis. Finally, it results in loss of protein from tissues in the body.

As blood glucose levels rise, glucose enters the kidney tubules and spills into the urine, usually when glucose levels reach about 180 mg/dL. This is called the *renal threshold* and varies somewhat from person to person. The increase in blood glucose levels dehydrates tissue cells, because glucose cannot diffuse through the cell wall without insulin. As the osmotic pressure increases in the extracellular fluid, there is an osmotic transfer of water out of the cells. The loss of glucose in the urine causes diuresis, because the osmotic effect of glucose in the tubules of the kidney prevents tubular reabsorption of fluids. The overall effect is dehydration associated with hypovolemia.

As the body shifts from metabolizing carbohydrates to metabolizing fats for energy, there is an increase in the production of ketones, resulting in ketosis. These ketones decrease sodium concentration because they combine with sodium derived from extracellular fluid for excretion in the urine. Hydrogen ions replace the sodium, increasing the acidosis. Metabolic acidosis occurs, leading to Kussmaul's respirations, which is deep and rapid breathing with increased expiration of carbon dioxide. There is a marked decrease in the bicarbonate level of extracellular fluid and, as a compensatory mechanism to correct the acidosis, chloride ions are excreted by the kidneys. In diabetic ketoacidosis, coma and death can occur within hours.

TRANSCULTURAL CONSIDERATIONS

Diabetes is found in epidemic proportions among Native Americans and is a major risk factor for cardiovascular disease, according to the results of The Strong Heart Study. This study was performed to estimate prevalence rates of diabetes and impaired glucose tolerance among this population. The results showed diabetes is more prevalent in Native American women, but rates of impaired glucose tolerance were similar to those of the rest of the U.S. population. The type of diabetes diagnosed is almost exclusively type 2 diabetes mellitus. Risk fac-

tors found to predict the onset of diabetes are age, diet, obesity, genetic markers, and parental diabetes. These results point to the need to develop screening and prevention programs for the Native American population.

African-American and Hispanic men and women also have a higher prevalence of type 2 diabetes mellitus than non-Hispanic whites.

CLASSIFICATION OF DIABETES MELLITUS

In 1997, the National Diabetes Data Group of the National Institutes of Health changed the classification system for diabetes based on etiology and pathogenesis. Diabetes mellitus is currently classified as follows:

   Type 1 diabetes, formerly known as insulin-dependent diabetes mellitus
   Type 2 diabetes, formerly known as non-insulin-dependent diabetes mellitus
   Gestational diabetes
   Other types of glucose intolerance

Type 1 Diabetes

Type 1 diabetes was formerly known as insulin-dependent diabetes mellitus, or juvenile diabetes. Type 1 diabetes occurs mostly in people younger than the age of 40 but can also occur in older adults—thus the change in name from juvenile diabetes to type 1 diabetes. Type 1 diabetes involves a marked decrease in the number of beta cells in the pancreas, leading to a lack of insulin and elevation of blood glucose level. Therefore, the person with type 1 diabetes (insulin-dependent diabetes mellitus) must have daily insulin injections to control blood glucose concentration and depends on exogenous insulin.

Type 2 Diabetes

Type 2 diabetes, formerly known as non-insulin-dependent diabetes mellitus, is the most prevalent form of diabetes in the United States. It usually occurs in adults over age 40. The major characteristic of type 2 diabetes is insulin resistance. The amount of endogenous insulin produced by the pancreas may be normal, decreased, or even increased. The problem is that available insulin cannot bind with cell receptor sites to promote transport of glucose into the cells for use or storage. This has been attributed to a defect at the cell's receptor site, in the number of receptor sites, or at the postreceptor site located inside the cell. Insulin injections usually are not necessary to treat type 2 diabetes (non-insulin-dependent diabetes mellitus) but at times may be required to control blood glucose levels. Patients with type 2 diabetes mellitus who receive insulin injections are known as insulin-requiring diabetics rather than insulin-dependent diabetics.

Gestational Diabetes

Gestational diabetes arises during pregnancy and usually disappears after delivery. It is associated with increased fetal morbidity and requires tight control to maintain normal blood glucose levels. The woman with gestational diabetes usually monitors her blood glucose four to six times a day and takes multiple injections of insulin. Women with gestational diabetes are at increased risk of developing diabetes later in life.

Other Types of Glucose Intolerance

Included in this grouping are disorders of temporary carbohydrate and glucose intolerance that are associated with, or secondary to, other physical or mechanical problems. Examples include the following:

• Pancreatic disease or pancreatectomy
• Various endocrine disorders, such as acromegaly, Cushing's syndrome, and pheochromocytoma
• Administration of medications or hormones, such as cortisone preparations, that cause hyperglycemia

Also included in this group is impaired glucose tolerance. A diagnosis of impaired glucose tolerance is made when plasma glucose levels are higher than normal but not high enough to diagnose as diabetes. The terms *chemical, latent, borderline, subclinical,* and *asymptomatic* diabetes were formerly used to identify this condition, but these terms have been discontinued. Because about 25% of patients with impaired glucose tolerance eventually develop diabetes, these patients should be re-evaluated frequently.

CLINICAL MANIFESTATIONS

The clinical manifestations of type 1 diabetes (insulin-dependent diabetes mellitus) and type 2 diabetes (non-insulin-dependent diabetes mellitus) differ. The patient with type 1 diabetes usually has a sudden onset of polyuria (frequent urination), polydipsia (extreme thirst), and polyphagia (hunger). In addition, the patient loses weight despite increased food intake, suffers extreme fatigue, and experiences pruritus and vaginal itching. The patient is usually thin and under age 40. Patients with type 1 diabetes are prone to developing ketosis during episodes of hyperglycemia and must take daily insulin injections. Ketoacidosis results from excess circulating ketone bodies and is manifested by Kussmaul's respirations; loss of sodium, potassium, chloride, and water; and continued catabolism of fat stores, cellular protein, and liver glycogen.

The patient with type 2 diabetes (non-insulin-dependent diabetes mellitus) may initially have none of the classic symptoms of the disease. If symptoms of polyuria, polydipsia, or polyphagia do occur, they are less severe than in type 1 diabetes. However, vaginal itching from vaginitis is a more common clinical manifestation in type 2 diabetes. Patients with type 2 diabetes rarely experience ketosis except during periods of stress or illness. Their blood glucose levels usually can be controlled by diet and exercise. Oral antidiabetic agents may be prescribed for better control, but patients may also be prescribed insulin. These patients are usually over age 30 and obese. Table 28–2 compares the major characteristics of type 1 and type 2 diabetes.

Additional clinical manifestations that may be

Table 28–2

Comparing Type 1 and Type 2 Diabetes

Characteristic	Type 1 Diabetes	Type 2 Diabetes
Incidence	20%	80%
Endogenous insulin production	None	Normal, decreased, or increased
Clinical manifestations	Polyuria Polydipsia Polyphagia Pruritus Vaginal itching Weight loss Dehydration Ketosis Fatigue	Classic symptoms of polyuria, polydipsia, and polyphagia are usually absent
Characteristics	Usually younger than age 40 at onset Prone to ketosis	Usually older than age 40 at onset Not prone to ketosis
Treatment	Insulin Diet Exercise	Oral antidiabetic agents Diet Exercise Insulin if blood glucose levels cannot be controlled with diet, oral antidiabetic agents, and exercise

present in type 1 or type 2 diabetes include blurred vision; tingling, numbness, or pain in the extremities; and slow-healing skin infections.

DIAGNOSIS

Diabetes mellitus is diagnosed by the presence of hyperglycemia and the classic symptoms of diabetes: polyuria, polydipsia, polyphagia, and weight loss. Patients with these symptoms usually have fasting plasma glucose levels higher than 140 mg/dL and random plasma glucose levels higher than 200 mg/dL. When the fasting plasma glucose level is lower than 140 mg/dL, the diagnosis is confirmed by an oral glucose tolerance test.

The criteria for diagnosis of diabetes mellitus in nonpregnant adults, gestational diabetes, and impaired glucose tolerance, established by the Expert Committee on the Diagnosis and Classification of Diabetes Mellitus, are summarized in Table 28–3.

Fasting Blood Sugar

The fasting blood sugar test measures the amount of glucose in the blood after fasting for 10 hours. It is performed both as a diagnostic test and to measure the glucose levels of the already diagnosed diabetic to monitor control. Venous blood is usually used in laboratories and hospitals. Capillary blood is used by patients testing their own blood glucose at home with a glucose meter.

The patient is instructed to have nothing to eat or drink for 10 hours before the test. If the fasting blood glucose level is higher than 140 mg/dL on more than one occasion, diabetes mellitus can be diagnosed. If the fasting blood glucose level is normal or near normal, an oral glucose tolerance test must be performed to confirm the diagnosis. Factors that cause glucose to rise in the absence of diabetes include stress, illness, trauma, and some drugs.

Oral Glucose Tolerance Test

The oral glucose tolerance test is performed to diagnose diabetes when the fasting plasma glucose is at or below 140 mg/dL.

PROCEDURE

A blood sample is drawn to obtain a fasting blood glucose level. Next, the patient drinks 75 g of glucose solution. Pregnant women drink 100 g of solution. Children drink 1.75 g/kg of ideal body weight (not to exceed 75 g). Blood samples are obtained at 30 minutes, then every hour for up to 5 hours.

NURSING IMPLICATIONS

The oral glucose tolerance test is considered a sensitive test for diabetes mellitus. However, if preparation and procedure guidelines are not followed strictly, erroneous results could occur. The test is performed in the morning before any other activities. The patient is instructed to have nothing to eat or drink for the previous 10 hours. During the test, the patient is instructed to sit or lie quietly and not to smoke or to drink any liquid except water.

For 3 days before the test, medications should be discontinued when possible. The diet should contain at least 150 g of carbohydrate daily. Patients who have undergone gastric surgery should undergo an intravenous glucose tolerance test rather than an oral glucose tolerance test, because the oral glucose quickly passes into the small intestine and is rapidly absorbed, giving an abnormal result. Nonhospitalized patients may need written instructions for the test to ensure adequate preparation.

Diabetes mellitus in the nonpregnant adult is diagnosed when the 2-hour plasma glucose level is 200 mL/dL or higher *and* either the $\frac{1}{2}$ hour, 1 hour, or $1\frac{1}{2}$ hour glucose level is greater than 200 mL/dL.

Table 28–3

Criteria for Diagnosis of Diabetes Mellitus

Criteria for Diagnosis of Diabetes Mellitus

- Symptoms of diabetes plus casual plasma glucose concentration of 200 mg/dL or higher (11.1 mmol/L). Casual is defined as any time of the day without regard to time since last meal. The classic symptoms of diabetes include polyuria, polydipsia, and unexplained weight loss *OR*
- Fasting plasma glucose level of 126 mg/dL or higher (7.0 mmol/L). Fasting is defined as no caloric intake for at least 8 hours *OR*
- Two-hour plasma glucose level of 200 mg/dL or greater during an oral glucose tolerance test. The test should be performed as described by WHO using a glucose load containing the equivalent of 75 g anhydrous glucose dissolved in water.

Confirmation should be obtained on the subsequent day for each of the above methods.

Criteria for Diagnosis of Gestational Diabetes

Following an oral glucose load of 100 g of glucose, two venous plasma glucose levels must be equal to or higher than the following values: Fasting, 105 mg/dL; 1 hour, 190 mg/dL; 2 hours, 165 mg/dL; 3 hours, 145 mg/dL.

Criteria for Impaired Fasting Glucose in Nonpregnant Adults

- Fasting plasma glucose level of at least 110 mg/dL but less than 126 mg/dL signifies impaired glucose tolerance.
- Fasting plasma glucose level of 126 mg/dL or greater signifies a provisional diagnosis of diabetes.
- Oral glucose tolerance test 2-hour plasma glucose level of at least 140 mg/dL but less than 200 mg/dL signifies impaired glucose tolerance.
- Oral glucose tolerance test 2-hour plasma glucose level of 200 mg/dL or greater signifies a provisional diagnosis of diabetes.

From The Expert Committee on the Diagnosis and Classification of Diabetes Mellitus. Report of the Expert Committee on the Diagnosis and Classification of Diabetes Mellitus. Diabetes Care 1997; 20(7):1183.

SOCIOCULTURAL PERSPECTIVES

Cultural Competence in Nursing Care

By Janice R. Ellis, PhD, RN

Have you looked closely at the people walking the streets of your community? Do you observe the foods available in your local supermarket? Do you listen to the voices of people in stores and restaurants? Have you seen retail signs in languages you do not understand? If you pay attention, you will note that the diversity found in all our communities has been increasing rapidly. Faces are of every hue. People wear garments as different as the head coverings of Muslim women and the black leather of heavy-metal devotees. From business suits to body-piercing, the variety is staggering.

The variety of foods available in a typical Western supermarket is also astonishing. Vegetables once considered exotic are now standard fare. Many varieties of rice and other grains are available. A global array of ethnic restaurants—Thai, Greek, Vietnamese, Korean, German, Chinese, Mediterranean, and others—can be found in most medium to large communities.

The kaleidoscope of ethnic and cultural backgrounds in the United States and Canada has changed dramatically over the past 20 years. Although the immigrants of the 19th and early 20th centuries came from many different countries, most were from European countries that shared much in background, custom, and appearance. Today's immigrants to the United States and Canada come from all parts of the globe. With them they bring religious beliefs, cultural practices, and value systems that are uniquely their own. This diversity presents a special challenge to nurses as they seek to provide nursing care to individuals and families.

"Cultural competence" is therefore becoming an important key to effective health care. The culturally competent nurse responds to diversity with respect based on accurate knowledge, an accepting attitude, and a belief in the value of every individual.

Specific cultural knowledge is gained in many ways. Books and magazine articles focus on specific cultural groups and their patterns of life, including such factors as religious beliefs and practices, dietary patterns, family relationships, and values. Workshops, videos, and classes can provide a wealth of information. Of course, talking personally with individuals from different backgrounds is one of the best ways to build bridges of mutual understanding.

What areas of knowledge will be important to you as you work to become a more culturally competent nurse? Think about the factors in your own life that affect your health, your health choices, and your attitudes about health care. One factor is your religious background. Another is your ethnic origin. A third is your skin color. Still another are the patterns from your family of origin. All of these factors interact with your *personal* beliefs and values to make you a unique individual. The more knowledge you gain about different ethnic groups—their religious beliefs, their dietary patterns, their attitudes about health, family, and individual choices, and their life experiences—the more effective you can be as a nurse. However, you must always balance an understanding of group patterns against assessment of individuals. Be careful not to act based on generalities. Instead, use your general knowledge to more effectively focus individualized assessment and planning.

Learning about different religions and their approaches to health and illness will help you be alert to the possible influence of religious beliefs on interactions between patients and the health-care system. For example, Islam puts great emphasis on prayer at specific times throughout the day. Although Muslims who are ill may be excused from some of these obligations, many do not wish to be excused and would prefer to receive assistance in meeting them. Knowledge of the practice of anointing the sick, which is a sacrament to Roman Catholics and an important practice to some Protestants, may lead you to ask a Christian patient if he or she desires anointing by an appropriate person. Accurate knowledge about a group can facilitate individualized assessment and nursing care.

Adapting diets for people of different ethnic and cultural backgrounds is one way in which your cultural competence may facilitate effective planning. Until recently, nutrition was taught in terms of the "Basic Four," a meal pattern that set the standard for a "good" diet based on the foods and preferences common among the majority in the United States. In the United States, the "Food Guide Pyramid" now acknowledges the possibility of *many* dietary patterns. Grains, legumes, and other plant foods take a prominent place in the Food Guide Pyramid, which can even be used to plan a vegetarian diet. Planning for a special therapeutic diet, such as a diet for a patient newly diagnosed with diabetes mellitus, must be based on an understanding of a person's preferred dietary patterns. These patterns might involve a completely different set of foods from what you might expect,

SOCIOCULTURAL PERSPECTIVES
Cultural Competence in Nursing Care
(continued)

and might involve a very different organization of the day's meals from your own. A culturally competent nurse, working in collaboration with a dietitian, can adapt a therapeutic diet to a patient, rather than forcing the patient to adapt to a whole different dietary pattern.

Another aspect of cultural competence is recognizing the impact of cultural or ethnic differences on interpersonal relationships and communication. The life experiences of minority people of color profoundly affect their relationship with members of the majority population. A lifetime of exposure to large and small acts of discrimination often leaves minority people of color justifiably reluctant to trust others. If you are a member of a minority group, you may need to recognize your own assumptions about the trustworthiness of patients

and coworkers. If you are a member of a majority group, realize that you may need to demonstrate trustworthiness before expecting others to trust you. When dealing with a member of another group, try to examine your own communication patterns from the viewpoint of the other.

As you develop cultural competence, you can be part of a larger effort within your particular health-care institution or agency to make it culturally responsive. You may ask questions about standard policies and procedures and examine them in the light of what you have learned about cultural needs and preferences. Rather than being part of the problem, you may become part of the solution by helping to make the health-care system more culturally sensitive and able to more effectively meet the needs of people of different cultures.

MANAGEMENT

The medical management of diabetes mellitus includes diet, exercise, and the addition of insulin or oral antidiabetic agents as appropriate. To ensure success, the patient must be an active member of the health care team and knowledgeable about all aspects of diabetes and its treatment. No longer is the diabetic patient a passive recipient of health care. He or she must assume responsibility for self-management. It is essential to provide the patient with the knowledge necessary to correlate blood sugars, diet, medications, and exercise to reach the ultimate goal of preventing acute complications and minimizing the effects of long-term degenerative changes.

Diet

The diabetic diet is the cornerstone of treatment for the diabetic patient. However, diet therapy is often ineffective. Lack of adherence to the diet has been identified as the one area of self-management most responsible for poor control of diabetes. To ensure success, it is necessary to individualize the diet to the needs of the patient and to provide adequate teaching to the patient and family or care partners.

The goals of dietary management of diabetes are as follows:

- To have the patient attain and maintain ideal body weight, or at least an improved weight
- To provide adequate nutrition for growth and development in children and in pregnant women
- To achieve blood glucose levels as close to normal as possible
- To prevent acute complications, such as ketoacidosis and hypoglycemia
- To prevent or delay long-term, degenerative complications associated with diabetes mellitus

The most widespread and currently accepted approach to diet therapy is the use of the exchange lists for meal planning created by the American Diabetes Association. This diet is based on the principle that foods within the same exchange list contain about the same amount of calories, carbohydrates, fats, and proteins. Thus, they can be eaten interchangeably. This approach provides flexibility in selecting foods and enhances the patient's ability to stick to the diet.

The number of exchanges a patient can have at each meal are calculated according to the number of prescribed daily calories. Many combinations can be developed. Highlight 28–1 contains sample meal plans using the exchange lists. The timing of meals

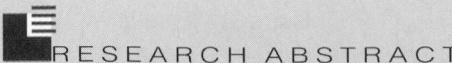

RESEARCH ABSTRACT

How Effective Are Weight-Loss Strategies for People with Type II Diabetes?

Brown SA, Upchurch S, Anding R, et al. Promoting weight loss in type II diabetes. Diabetes Care 1996; 19(6):613.

The potential benefits of weight reduction in obese people with type II diabetes include improved metabolic control and decreased reliance on medications. However, achieving such weight loss is not easy, and several approaches have been tried. To determine which approaches are most effective, Brown and colleagues used meta-analysis to examine the effects of selected weight-loss interventions on weight loss, as well as on a variety of other physiologic outcomes. (Meta-analysis is a research method that uses statistical analysis to integrate the data from a number of independent studies. It allows researchers to determine whether there are trends in research results that support the conclusions of a study.)

For their meta-analysis, Brown and colleagues included 89 studies, published between 1965 and 1994, that in some way tested the effects of weight-loss strategies. Strategies tested were such things as behavioral interventions (education and counseling and behavior modification), diet, exercise, medications, and surgery. The outcomes that were of particular interest to the researchers were weight loss, body mass index, glycosylated hemoglobin levels, fasting blood sugar levels, cholesterol levels, triglyceride levels, blood pressure, and serum insulin levels.

The researchers found that dietary change alone had the most effect on weight loss and metabolic control. Surgery resulted in greater weight loss than did dietary changes, but surgery did not affect metabolic control. The types of diets used in the studies that the researchers reviewed included very-low-calorie diets, the American Diabetes Association reduced-calorie diet, and protein-sparing modified-fast diets.

One thing that surprised the researchers was the small effect on weight loss of an intervention that included diet, behavior therapy, and exercise. They did find that this combination had a significant effect on lowering glycosylated hemoglobin levels and suggest that this in itself is a valuable outcome. They also noted that such studies usually use a comparison group of subjects who also receive some type of standard intervention, and that this makes it harder to show an effect from the experimental intervention.

One value of such a thorough review and synthesis of the literature is the identification of future needs for information. These researchers recommend that, when possible, data collection for weight loss indicators be undertaken over longer periods than just 6 months. With longer periods of data collection, future meta-analyses would be able to determine the long-term effects of interventions on weight loss. Brown and colleagues also encourage future researchers to include better descriptions of their settings and subjects, and to present their data more thoroughly, so that effectiveness can be examined according to such characteristics as ethnicity, education, and socioeconomic background. It may be that some types of interventions for weight loss will work better for particular types of people with type II diabetes.

Questions to Consider

1. Who is responsible for providing for the educational needs of people with diabetes?
2. What type of approaches are used to promote weight loss in obese patients with type 2 diabetes?
3. What type of supervision over time do people receive when they attempt to lose weight using diets such as those examined in the meta-analysis?
4. Does the documentation system for educational and dietary interventions in your clinical setting give future providers enough detail to know what information to reinforce and what information to add?
5. Does your clinical setting support the use of graphs that track people's progress in managing their type 2 diabetes over time? If not, what would a useful tool look like that includes such outcomes as those examined in the meta-analysis?

and snacks is important for patients taking insulin and oral antidiabetic agents in order to maintain stable blood glucose levels and prevent episodes of hypoglycemia and hyperglycemia.

The ADA recommends that 55 to 60% of the total calories consumed be carbohydrate, preferably complex carbohydrate; 15 to 20% protein; and less than 30% fat. The diet should contain less than 10% polyunsaturated fats, less than 10% saturated fats, and only 10 to 15% monounsaturated fats.

The ADA further recommends that people with diabetes limit cholesterol intake to less than 300 mg/d and sodium intake to less than 3 g/d. The ADA exchange lists for meal planning highlight foods that exceed these amounts.

Recent evidence has shown that foods with a

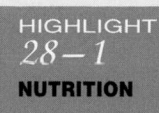 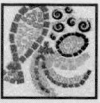

**HIGHLIGHT
28—1
NUTRITION**

Meal-Planning Guidelines for Patients with Diabetes Mellitus

Exchange List	Samples of Equivalent Meals		
BREAKFAST			
1 Fruit	4 oz orange juice	½ banana	½ grapefruit
2 Starch/bread	1 bagel	2 slices toast	1 cup oatmeal
1 Fat	1 tbsp cream cheese	1 slice bacon*	1 tsp butter
1 Milk	8 oz skim milk	8 oz plain nonfat yogurt	8 oz 1% milk
LUNCH			
2 Starch/bread	2 slices bread	1 pita (6 in.)	1 hamburger bun
3 Meat†	½ cup tuna	3 oz ground turkey	3 oz ground beef
1 Vegetable	1 large tomato	1 cup raw vegetables	4 oz vegetable juice
1 Fruit	1 apple	4 oz apple cider	12 cherries
1 Fat	1 tsp salad dressing	1 tsp mayonnaise	1 tsp oil
1 Milk	8 oz skim milk	8 oz lowfat buttermilk	⅔ cup nonfat dry milk
DINNER			
2 Starch/bread	1 cup corn	1 small baked potato	1 cup pasta (cooked)
3 Meat†	3 oz steak	3 oz chicken	3 oz veal cutlet (unbreaded)
2 Vegetable	1 cup raw vegetables *and* ½ cup carrots	1 cup broccoli	½ cup green peppers *and* ½ cup onions
1 Fruit	1¼ cup strawberries	1 peach	1 cup blueberries

---

* 400 mg or more of sodium in two or more exchanges.

† Medium fat meat exchange (7 g protein, 5 g fat, 75 calories).

All foods within each exchange list contain approximately the same amount of carbohydrates, proteins, and fats and therefore can be eaten interchangeably. However, foods from one list or exchange cannot be substituted for foods from another list or exchange. For example, a fruit exchange cannot be substituted for a bread exchange.

---

high soluble fiber content may lower plasma glucose and cholesterol levels. Soluble fibers are found in fruits, legumes, and oats. The ADA exchange lists also highlight foods containing high amounts of fiber.

Although alcohol intake is not recommended, moderate amounts of alcohol may be allowed in the diabetic diet. When alcohol is included in the meal plan, the calories are accounted for by reducing the fat intake (pure alcohol is 7 kcal/g). Alcohol intake in patients who are malnourished or fasting may cause hypoglycemia.

Some foods are considered free foods because they contain less than 20 calories per serving. Examples include sugar-free carbonated drinks, coffee, tea, lettuce, sugar-free gelatin, and 1 tbsp catsup. Seasonings are also free, such as basil, cinnamon, and garlic. Free foods are not restricted and can be eaten in any amount at any time.

Implementation of the diabetic diet requires patient education and often behavior modification as detailed in the nursing process section that appears later in the chapter.

Exercise

Exercise is an important component of diabetes treatment. The benefits include improved insulin sensitivity, potential improvement in glucose tolerance in some patients, promotion of weight loss and attainment of goal body weight, improved cardiovascular status, reduced cholesterol and triglyceride levels, potential reduction in insulin and oral antidiabetic agent requirements, and an improved sense of well-being.

An exercise program should be tailored to meet the patient's individual needs. Factors to consider include the type of diabetes, the patient's age and medical condition, and the presence of long-term degenerative changes. If the patient is taking insulin, consider the type of insulin, the time it is administered, when it reaches its peak, and the injection site used. Insulin is absorbed faster when injected into a site that is exercised. The abdomen, rather than the leg, should be used for an injection site when the patient will be walking or running.

A blood glucose test performed before exercising

lets the patient know whether to eat a snack first. Unless a meal has just been completed, a fruit exchange equal to 15 g of carbohydrate is usually eaten before engaging in moderate exercise. This snack is in addition to food allowed in the regular meal plan. The patient taking antidiabetic medication should always carry a simple carbohydrate snack when exercising and should be prepared to treat hypoglycemia if it occurs. The patient with non-insulin-dependent diabetes mellitus who is not taking insulin or oral antidiabetic agents does not have to eat a snack before exercising.

Exercise should be avoided if blood glucose is higher than 250 mg/dL or when ketones are present in the urine. Exercise at this point raises blood glucose levels by increasing secretion of glucagon and growth hormone, thereby causing the liver to release more glucose.

Because obesity and inactivity are characteristics of the patient with non-insulin-dependent diabetes mellitus, exercise may have a positive effect on controlling hyperglycemia for these patients. Increased physical activity is an important part of any weight reduction program because it increases energy expenditure, increases muscle mass, and decreases body fat. When combined with diet, exercise is an excellent way to attain and maintain ideal or goal body weight.

Exercise may be contraindicated in patients with poor metabolic control and those with active proliferative retinopathy, significant cardiovascular disease, or peripheral neuropathy. Patients with these conditions can exercise only following a thorough medical assessment.

Table 28–4

Categories of Insulin

Category	Onset	Peak Action	Duration
Rapid-acting	½–1 h	2–4 h	5–7 h
Intermediate-acting	2–4 h	8–12 h	18–24 h
Long-acting	4–6 h	18–24 h	>36 h

Table 28–5

Partial List of Insulin Preparations

Category	Insulin	Form	Manufacturer
Rapid-acting	Humulin R	Human	Lilly
	Novolin R	Human	Novo Nordisk
	Velosulin R	Human	Novo Nordisk
	Velosulin R	Pork	Novo Nordisk
	Iletin II R	Pork	Lilly
	Iletin I R	Beef/pork	Lilly
	Purified Pork R	Pork	Novo Nordisk
	Purified Pork S	Pork	Novo Nordisk
	Regular	Pork	Novo Nordisk
	Semilente	Beef	Novo Nordisk
Intermediate-acting	Humulin L	Human	Lilly
	Humulin N	Human	Lilly
	Insulatard NPH	Human	Novo Nordisk
	Novolin L	Human	Novo Nordisk
	Novolin N	Human	Novo Nordisk
	Iletin I Lente	Beef/pork	Lilly
	Iletin I NPH	Beef/pork	Lilly
	NPH	Beef	Novo Nordisk
	Iletin II Lente	Pork	Lilly
	Iletin II NPH	Pork	Lilly
	Insulatard NPH	Pork	Novo Nordisk
	Purified Pork Lente	Pork	Novo Nordisk
	Purified Pork N	Pork	Novo Nordisk
Long-acting	Humulin U	Human	Lilly
	Iletin II PZI	Beef or pork	Lilly
	Purified Beef U	Beef	Novo Nordisk
	Iletin I PZI	Beef/pork	Lilly
	Ultralente	Beef	Novo Nordisk
Mixtures	Mixtard (70% NPH, 30% Regular)	Pork	Novo Nordisk
	Novolin 70/30	Human	Novo Nordisk
	Humulin 70/30	Human	Lilly

Insulin Therapy

INJECTIONS

The beta cells in the pancreatic islets of Langerhans stop producing insulin in patients with insulin-dependent diabetes mellitus. Therefore, these patients must have insulin injections to survive. Insulin can be administered only by injection, because it is a protein and would be destroyed by digestive enzymes if taken orally.

Injectable insulin was originally derived from animal sources by extracting insulin from beef and pork pancreata. Biosynthetic and semisynthetic forms of human insulin are now manufactured and widely prescribed. Human insulin is identical to the insulin produced by the human pancreas and is nearly free of the foreign substances in animal-source insulins. It is, therefore, less likely to stimulate formation of insulin antibodies. Some research has shown that these antibodies may temporarily bind to animal-source insulin and then release it, causing unpredictable blood levels of insulin and poor control of blood glucose. Lipoatrophy at the injection site has also been related to animal insulin impurities.

Insulin is categorized as short- or rapid-acting, intermediate-acting, and long-acting. These categories refer to the following:

- Onset, or when the insulin begins to work
- Peak, or when the insulin provides the maximum effect
- Duration, or the length of time the insulin is active in the body

Table 28–4 summarizes the categories of insulin. Table 28–5 provides a list of insulin preparations and manufacturers.

Insulin is currently available in two concentrations: U-100 and U-500. The most widely used concentration is U-100. U-500 is used in cases of severe insulin resistance. Insulin is measured in United States Pharmacopeia units, which does not refer to volume but to a standard of insulin activity. The concentration refers to the number of units in 1 mL. For example, a vial of U-100 insulin has 100 units in 1 mL. A vial of U-500 insulin has 500 units in 1 mL. Syringes and insulin vials are clearly labeled U-100. Because there is no U-500 syringe, the amount of insulin to administer has to be calculated in milliliters.

The goal of insulin treatment is to mimic the pattern of normal insulin secretion. In the nondiabetic, there is a continuous basal secretion of insulin, with secretion of additional insulin after eating, in response to increased blood glucose levels. Therefore, the type 1 diabetic patient may receive one to several insulin injections each day. Many patients take one or two injections of a mixture of short-acting and intermediate-acting insulins. Some patients inject short-acting insulin before each meal in addition to one long-acting basal dose to control hyperglycemia throughout the day. The Diabetes Control and Complications Trial has shown that three or more insulin injections a day, with dosage based on blood glucose levels, produce better control of blood glucose. This kind of intensive treatment program can delay and prevent long-term degenerative changes associated with diabetes mellitus. Figure 28–2 illustrates several patterns of insulin

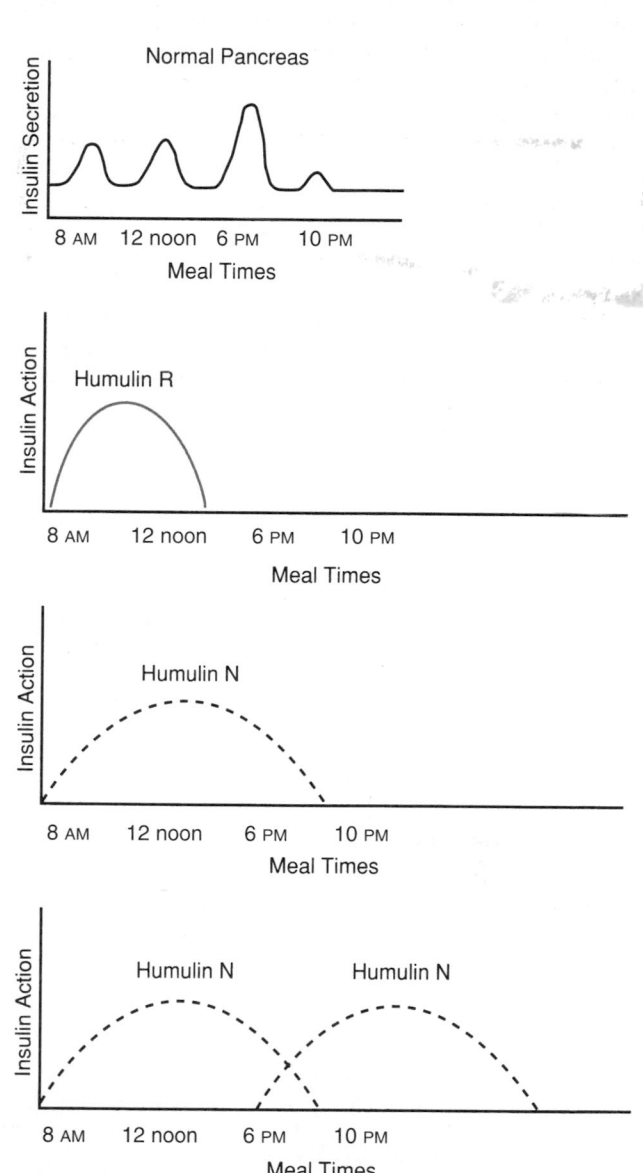

Figure 28–2

Relationship between food intake and the onset, peak, and duration of different patterns of insulin injections and preparations.

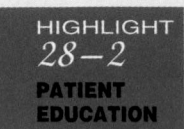 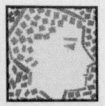

HIGHLIGHT
28–2
PATIENT
EDUCATION

Guidelines for Preparation and Injection of Insulin

Instruct the patient in the following:

Preparation of a Dose of a Single-Action Insulin

1. Gather equipment. Check medication order.
2. Wash hands.
3. If using an intermediate- or long-acting insulin, roll the bottle between your hands to mix it. Do not shake the bottle, because shaking causes bubbles to form. Regular, short-acting insulin does not have to be rolled.
4. Remove metal cap if opening a new bottle. Clean the rubber top with an alcohol swab if previously opened.
5. Draw into the syringe the same amount of air as insulin prescribed, and inject this air into the insulin bottle.
6. While inverting the insulin bottle and keeping the needle tip below the level of insulin, withdraw the prescribed amount of insulin. The syringe should be held vertically at eye level.
7. If air bubbles form in the syringe, tap the barrel of the syringe and move the needle tip above the insulin level so that the air bubbles can be expelled from the syringe and into the air space in the bottle.
8. Double-check to be sure the correct dose of insulin is in the syringe.
9. Remove the needle from the insulin bottle and inject into selected site.

Preparation of a Mixture of Two Insulins with Different Actions (Insulin Mix)

1. Gather equipment. Check medication order.
2. Wash hands.
3. Roll the delayed-acting insulin bottle between your hands to mix it. Do not shake the bottle, because shaking causes bubbles to form. Regular, short-acting insulin does not have to be rolled.
4. Remove metal cap if opening new bottles. Clean the rubber top with an alcohol swab if previously opened.
5. Draw into the syringe the same amount of air as delayed-acting insulin prescribed, and inject this air into the delayed-acting insulin bottle. Withdraw needle empty.
6. Draw into the syringe the same amount of air as short-acting insulin prescribed, and inject this air into the short-acting insulin bottle.
7. While inverting the short-acting insulin bottle and keeping the needle tip below the level of insulin,

withdraw the amount of short-acting insulin prescribed. The syringe should be held at eye level.
8. If air bubbles form in the syringe, tap the barrel of the syringe and move the needle tip above the level of insulin so that the air bubbles can be expelled from the syringe and into the air space in the bottle.
9. Withdraw prescribed amount of short-acting insulin, and remove syringe from bottle.
10. Carefully insert needle into the delayed-acting insulin bottle, and with bottle inverted, pull the plunger down to the total amount of insulin prescribed (short-acting plus delayed-acting = total dose).
11. If an air bubble develops in the syringe while withdrawing the delayed-acting insulin, withdraw the needle, discard the medication and syringe, and start over. This is necessary because in an attempt to expel the air bubble, some of the insulin mixture may inadvertently be expelled also.
12. Withdraw needle and inject into selected site.

Insulin Injection

1. Select the injection site. See Figure 28–3 for sites.
2. Wipe the site with an alcohol swab. Holding the syringe like a pencil, gently pinch a large portion of skin, and insert the needle quickly at a 90-degree angle into subcutaneous tissue. Insert the needle at a 45-degree angle if you have less than an inch of skin when you pinch.
3. Push the plunger down to inject the insulin.
4. Release the skin and withdraw the needle.
5. Press site with alcohol swab but do not massage.

Additional Patient Teaching Instructions

• Store unopened insulin bottles in the refrigerator. Store opened insulin bottles that will be used within 1 month at room temperature of 80°F (26.7°C) or less.
• It is best to bring refrigerated insulin to room temperature before injecting. When cold insulin is injected, absorption rates are delayed because of initial capillary vasoconstriction, and the injection is more painful.
• Do not expose insulin to direct sunlight. Do not freeze insulin.
• Check the expiration date on insulin bottles before purchase. Do not use insulin past the expiration date.
• When traveling, carry insulin and syringes on your person and do not check with baggage. When pre-

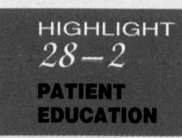 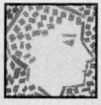

Guidelines for Preparation and Injection of Insulin *(continued)*

paring an insulin mix, always inject air into the intermediate- or long-acting insulin bottle first and then into the regular short-acting insulin bottle. Withdraw the regular insulin first. Do this to avoid contamination of the regular insulin by the intermediate-acting insulin.

• Be sure to remove all air bubbles from the syringe before injecting, because air bubbles take the place of insulin. If air bubbles are injected, you receive less insulin than prescribed.

• When possible, give mixed insulins within 15 minutes after preparation, because after that time, the action of the regular insulin may be blunted.

• Do not inject within 1 inch of the previous injection site. Rotate injection sites to avoid lipodystrophy (lumps or indentations) and to maximize absorption of the insulin. Researchers at the University of Minnesota recommend abandoning site rotation

plans in favor of injecting insulin in the abdomen only for maximum glucose control.

• Do not inject areas that are going to be exercised that day.

• Give insulin injections at the same time each day to ensure continuity of onset, peak, and duration of action.

• When taking less than 50 units of insulin, use low-dose insulin syringes. These syringes hold $\frac{1}{2}$ mL and measure up to 50 units. Each line on the syringe equals one unit of insulin.

• When taking more than 50 units of insulin, use a 1-mL insulin syringe that measures up to 100 units. Each line on the syringe equals two units of insulin.

• Never reuse disposable insulin syringes. Never wipe the needle tip with alcohol before using.

preparations. Highlight 28–2 presents guidelines for preparing and administering insulin injections. Figure 28–3 illustrates sites for insulin injection.

Occasionally, there may be what is known as a "honeymoon" phase or temporary remission in patients with insulin-dependent diabetes mellitus; that is, the beta cells begin to produce insulin again. As endogenous insulin secretion begins, the patient experiences hypoglycemic reactions. Exogenous insulin injections need to be reduced or even eliminated during this temporary remission. The honeymoon

phase is more common in the late teenage years and in young adults and can last from several months to about a year.

OTHER MODES OF INSULIN ADMINISTRATION

Pump

Another method of administering insulin is with a device known as an insulin pump or continuous subcutaneous insulin infusion (CSII). This mode of insulin delivery provides a steady basal dose of in-

Figure 28–3
Insulin injection sites.

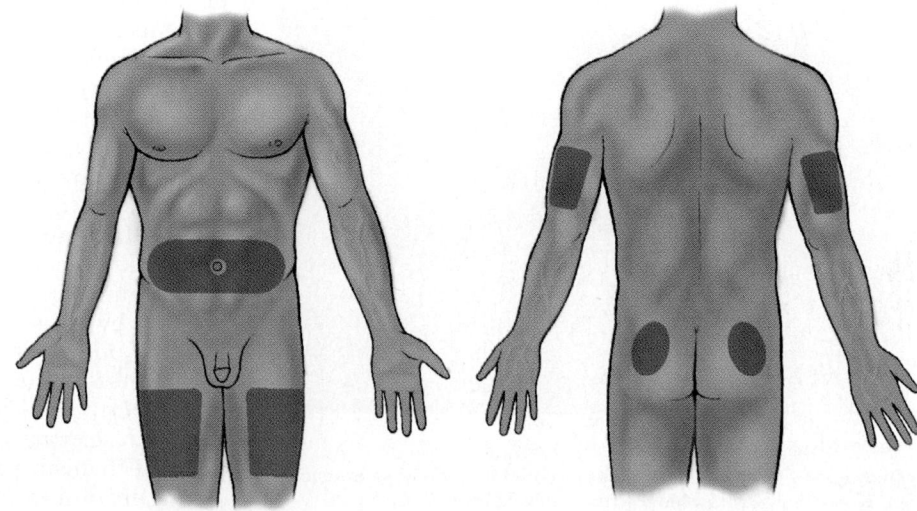

sulin throughout the day and night, as well as a bolus of insulin when food is eaten. The insulin pump is designed to mimic the action of the normal pancreas and replaces insulin injections. It is usually recommended when multiple injections of insulin are not effective in controlling glucose levels.

CSII is called an open-loop infusion system because it does not contain a glucose sensor that automatically adjusts the insulin infusion rate. It is operated by the patient, who must test blood glucose levels to determine the amount of insulin to take. About 40 to 50% of the patient's total daily insulin requirement is administered at the basal rate. The remaining 50 to 60% is given as premeal boluses.

The abdomen is the preferred infusion site because insulin absorption from this area is faster and less affected by exercise than other body sites. However, the upper outer thighs and hips, as well as the arms, can also be used. It can be difficult to deal with tubing and needles in these sites. Needle placement should be in subcutaneous tissue, not muscle. A new site should be chosen at least 1 inch from the previous site each time the infusion set is changed—usually every 48 hours. Tubing is connected to a syringe filled with regular insulin in the pump. The only type of insulin used in a pump is regular insulin. It is slowly pushed automatically from the syringe, thereby providing a basal rate of insulin infusion 24 hours a day. The insulin pump can be programmed to change delivery rates throughout the day. Boluses are given by manual programming before meals.

The insulin pump is the size of a beeper and weighs only a few ounces. It is worn on a belt, in a pocket, or under clothes. The cost of an insulin pump is approximately $4100. Figure 28–4 shows the MiniMed model 507 QR (quick release) insulin pump. The QR is a feature that allows the patient to temporarily disconnect the pump for swimming, showering, or bathing.

Besides providing more effective control of glu-

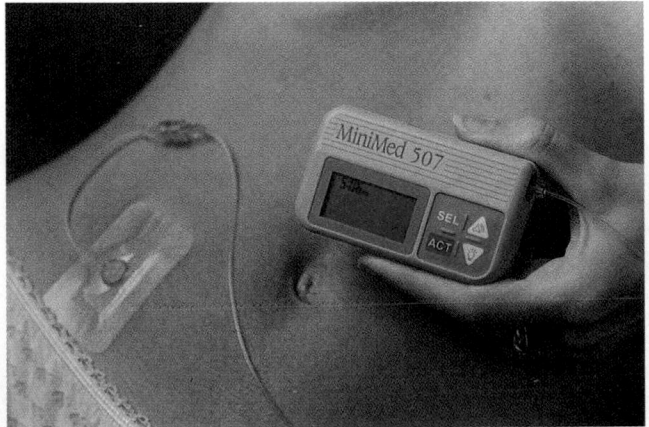

Figure 28–4

MiniMed 507 external insulin pump with Quick-Release Infusion Set. (Courtesy of MiniMed Technologies, Sylmar, CA.)

cose levels, the use of an insulin pump offers greater lifestyle flexibility and convenience. Most patients who need multiple daily injections prefer to use an insulin pump. The selection of candidates is important to ensure a successful outcome. The patient should be mature, have some technical ability, and have the financial resources necessary for this therapy. Pump users must also be able and willing to monitor their blood glucose levels frequently, test their urine for ketones when ill, recognize the warning signs of hypoglycemia and hyperglycemia, and know the techniques of skin and needle care.

Complications associated with the use of an insulin pump include the risk of rapid onset ketoacidosis from technical problems that interfere with insulin delivery. Although ketoacidosis among patients using insulin pumps can be fatal, it is avoidable with proper patient education and self-monitoring of blood glucose, as well as technical improvements and alarm systems in the pump.

Infection at the site of the infusion is a more common complication. Some causes of infection include mechanical irritation from motion of the needle during activity and sensitivity to the needle. To prevent skin infections, the infusion site should be cleaned carefully and allowed to dry before inserting the needle. If the patient has an infection, the infusion set should be removed and discarded. Another infusion site should be used. Patients with infections are treated with oral antibiotics and topical therapies.

Another complication of using the insulin pump is the risk of hypoglycemic episodes and hypoglycemic coma. However, it was shown in the Diabetes Control and Complications Trial that insulin users who try to maintain normal or near-normal blood glucose levels face an increased risk of hypoglycemia no matter what delivery mode they use. These patients should be aware of this possibility and monitor blood glucose levels frequently as a precaution. Because the insulin pump allows programmed reductions in basal insulin delivery during times of decreased insulin need, such as during sleep, use of an insulin pump helps to prevent nocturnal hypoglycemia.

Implantable insulin pumps may soon be available if approved by the Food and Drug Administration. MiniMed Technologies is currently conducting a clinical investigation to demonstrate the safety and efficacy of the MIP-2001, shown in Figure 28–5. This implantable insulin pump is a 5.7-ounce disk-shaped device that automatically releases a constant, preprogrammed amount of insulin into the peritoneal membrane. The pump is refilled about every 3 months by inserting a needle through the skin and into the pump. Because the pump's drug reservoir is maintained at negative pressure, the needle has to be properly seated inside the pump for the vacuum in the reservoir to draw insulin from the syringe. This mechanism prevents the risk of accidentally injecting insulin directly into the patient. Insulin deliv-

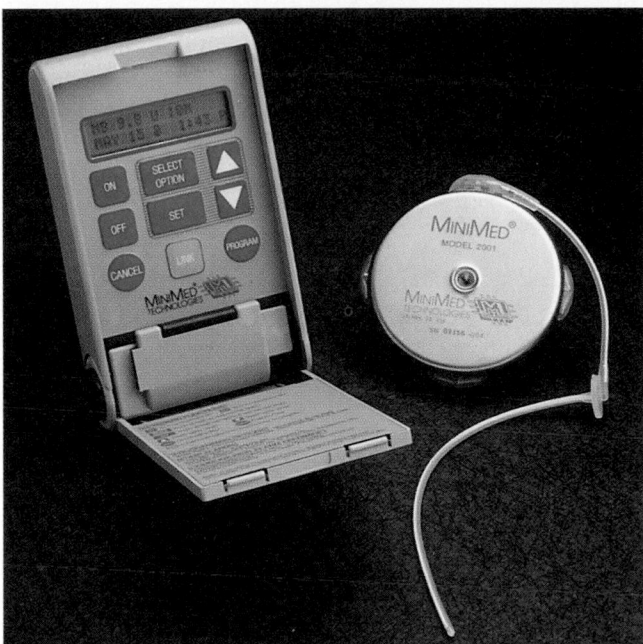

Figure 28–5

MiniMed 2001 implantable insulin pump and hand-held programmer. (Courtesy of MiniMed Technologies, Sylmar, CA.)

ery is controlled by a hand-held external programmer and is customized for each patient by the physician. Patients using an implantable pump must continue to monitor their blood glucose levels four to six times daily. The pump costs about $10,000, excluding physician charges and surgical expenses. The major problem in some patients is blockage of the catheter that delivers insulin.

One goal of current research is to develop a pump that not only infuses insulin but also monitors blood glucose levels, which would be comparable with an artificial pancreas.

Nasal Spray

Research is being conducted on an insulin nasal spray as an alternative insulin delivery route. Insulin nasal spray acts within 10 minutes and lasts for just 1 hour. It could be used to lower blood glucose levels after a meal. The advantage of using insulin nasal spray rather than an injection of short-acting insulin before meals is the lower risk of hypoglycemia developing 3 or 4 hours later.

Oral Antidiabetic Agents

The sulfonylurea oral antidiabetic agents are effective for stable, non-insulin-dependent, nonketotic type 2 diabetics who cannot be treated by diet alone or who are unwilling or unable to take insulin. These agents should not be used in children, insulin-dependent type 1 diabetics, during pregnancy or lactation (because the effects on the fetus and newborn are unknown), or for patients with allergies to sulfonylurea compounds.

Sulfonylureas are effective only in people who have some functioning beta cells and who continue to secrete some endogenous insulin. They stimulate the beta cells to produce more insulin, reduce the accelerated rates of hepatic glucose production in type 2 diabetes, partially reduce the postreceptor defect in cells, and increase the number of cellular insulin receptors. See Table 28–6 for the complete list of sulfonylureas. Highlight 28–3 contains patient education guidelines for administration of sulfonylureas and includes their side effects and drug interactions.

Current Research in the Management of Diabetes

Pancreas transplantation has been performed in thousands of people with diabetes. It significantly improves the quality of life by eliminating the need for insulin injections and normalizing blood glucose levels.

Most transplants are whole organs from cadavers. The donor must be free of pancreatic trauma, pancreatitis, and diabetes and have no history of hepatitis, syphilis, or acquired immunodeficiency

Table 28–6

Characteristics of Oral Antidiabetic Agents

Brand Name	Generic Name	Daily Dosage, mg	Duration, h
1st GENERATION SULFONYLUREAS			
Orinase	Tolbutamide	500–3000	6–12
Diabinese	Chlorpropamide	100–500	up to 60
Dymelor	Acetohexamide	250–1500	12–18
Tolinase	Tolazamide	100–1000	12–24
2nd GENERATION SULFONYLUREAS			
Micronase, Diabeta	Glyburide	1.25–20	16–24
Glucotrol	Glipizide	5–40	12–24
Glynase PresTabs	Micronized glyburide	1.5–12	16–24

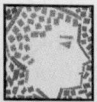

Guidelines for Taking Sulfonylureas

Instruct the patient in the following:

Sulfonylureas or oral antidiabetic agents are not insulin. Insulin is a protein that, if swallowed, would be destroyed by digestion.

Side effects can occur when taking sulfonylureas: Skin rashes in 2% of patients; gastrointestinal disturbances in 5% of patients; and when chlorpropamide is taken with alcohol, 35% of patients experience a disulfiram-like effect.

Hypoglycemic reactions can occur when taking sulfonylureas, especially in the elderly, in malnourished patients, in alcoholics, and in patients with impaired renal or hepatic function. Teach the signs, symptoms, and treatment of these reactions (Table 28–8).

Hypoglycemic reactions can be prolonged and difficult to reverse because of the long duration of action of some of the agents.

Sulfonylureas should be used cautiously in patients with a history of allergy to sulfonamides.

The hypoglycemic action of sulfonylureas is enhanced by sulfonamides, phenylbutazone, anticoagulants, and salicylates. Propranolol can mask the symptoms of hypoglycemia.

Thyroid preparations, corticosteroids, and thiazide diuretics oppose the action of sulfonylureas.

Alcohol may produce a disulfiram-like reaction with any sulfonylurea.

---

syndrome (AIDS). After blood and tissue samples are matched to the recipient, the organ is usually transplanted within 30 hours of harvesting. A sibling who is identical in human leukocyte antigen is considered the ideal living donor because the recipient may not need immunosuppression. The related donor undergoes a glucose tolerance test and C peptide measurement and must be 10 years older than the age at which the recipient developed diabetes. The donor must also be free of islet cell autoantibodies. The success rate for patients with a living related donor is higher than that with a cadaver. However, the use of living donors appears to be limited, because although only the distal half of the pancreas is removed, which alone does not cause diabetes in the donor, abnormal glucose tolerance has developed postoperatively in most human leukocyte antigen–identical donors.

Patients selected as the best candidates for pancreatic transplant are younger, healthier, insulin-dependent diabetics who have brittle diabetes but no severe complications. Diabetic patients who have diabetic nephropathy and whose lives are threatened by renal failure can now receive a simultaneous pancreas and kidney transplant. Candidates for simultaneous pancreas and kidney transplantation are between ages 18 and 55 and free of cardiovascular disease, severe peripheral vascular disease, cancer, or substance abuse problems.

To prevent organ rejection, patients who receive a transplant take life-long oral immunosuppressive medication, such as azathione, cyclosporin (Sandimmune), and steroids. After a 5-year period, 80% of simultaneous pancreas and kidney transplants and 60% of pancreas-only transplants continue to function.

Hyperglycemia is an early symptom of tissue rejection. Therefore, the patient should test blood glucose levels four times a day after discharge from the hospital. Gradually, this can be reduced to once a week. Other symptoms of rejection are tenderness over the graft area, malaise, and fever. Rejection can occur months or years after surgery.

The potential benefits of a successful transplantation are the freedom from insulin injections and the elimination of glucose control issues. In addition, because blood glucose levels are normal, some studies have shown that diabetic neuropathy begins to improve within 2 years and diabetic retinopathy in about 5 years. Serum lipid profiles also show improvement. Even so, many transplant candidates are denied insurance coverage and must use personal resources or seek research funding to cover the cost.

MANAGEMENT DURING ILLNESS

Stress and short-term illness—such as fever, influenza, vomiting, and diarrhea—can lead rapidly to hyperglycemia in the diabetes patient. These conditions increase the need for insulin. The pancreas may be unable to produce sufficient insulin to meet the demand. Stress and illness also increase secretion of the counter-regulatory hormones glucagon, epinephrine, and cortisol, thereby raising blood glucose levels.

The hyperglycemia leads to osmotic diuresis, in which glucose, fluids, and electrolytes are lost. This leads to dehydration, electrolyte depletion, and loss of nutrients. Patients with type 1 diabetes (insulin-dependent diabetes mellitus) rapidly develop ketoacidosis. Patients with type 2 diabetes (non-insulin-dependent diabetes mellitus) are more at risk of developing hyperglycemic hyperosmolar nonketotic syndrome, a life-threatening condition.

During illness, it is important for any patient with diabetes to monitor blood glucose levels every 4 to 6 hours until symptoms of the illness subside. The patient should check urine ketone levels when blood glucose is higher than 250 mg/dL. Fluid intake is increased to minimize the risk of dehydration. Patients who are nauseated or vomiting are advised to take fluids containing glucose and electrolytes, such as regular soda and diluted fruit juices, gelatin, and chicken bouillon. The physician should be notified in the following situations:

- Blood glucose is over 250 mg/dL and ketonuria lasts more than 6 hours
- Signs of dehydration occur (dry mucous membranes, lightheadedness, lethargy, decreased urine output)
- Symptoms of ketoacidosis occur (fruity odor on the breath, abdominal pain, air hunger)
- The patient cannot retain fluids or food for 4 hours
- The illness becomes unmanageable

Patients are instructed never to stop taking insulin when sick. Insulin doses may need to be increased. At times, supplemental injections of insulin are necessary in the patient with insulin-dependent diabetes mellitus. Patients with non-insulin-dependent diabetes mellitus may require insulin injections when acutely ill or if unable to tolerate oral antidiabetic agents.

MANAGEMENT DURING SURGERY

The goal of management during surgery is to prevent hyperglycemia *and* hypoglycemia. Hyperglycemia results from stress and the physiologic effects of surgery. It can lead to ketoacidosis, especially in the patient with type 1 diabetes mellitus. Hypoglycemia, if unrecognized and untreated, can be life-threatening.

Preoperative care includes a complete history, physical examination, and laboratory evaluation to determine the degree of diabetes control. Factors to consider preoperatively are the type of diabetes involved, blood glucose levels, and whether long-term degenerative changes are present. For example, the presence of renal disease can affect the amount of fluids and medications tolerated. Also, if the patient is in poor metabolic control and is losing glucose in the urine, the body uses protein and fat stores for energy. This could prevent a surgical wound from healing properly.

One of three methods is usually used to administer insulin perioperatively:

- Omitting the short-acting insulin and administering one-third to one-half the usual intermediate-acting insulin before surgery
- Adding 10 to 20 units of regular insulin to an intravenous infusion of 1L of 5% dextrose in 0.45% sodium chloride
- Adding 100 units of regular insulin to 500 mL of sodium chloride and piggybacking this to an infusion of 5% dextrose in 0.45% sodium chloride.

The rate of infusion is adjusted according to the blood glucose level, which is monitored every 1 to 2 hours in the perioperative period.

In addition to testing blood glucose levels, the urine is tested for ketones if the blood glucose level is higher than 250 mg/dL.

Patients with type 2 diabetes mellitus who take oral antidiabetic agents may require insulin during and after surgery. Therefore, most oral agents are discontinued about 24 hours before surgery, with the exception of chlorpropamide, which is discontinued 2 to 3 days before surgery. Patients whose disease is controlled by diet alone should be monitored for hyperglycemia because the physiologic stress of surgery may raise blood glucose levels and alter glucose tolerance.

Postoperative care includes maintaining blood glucose levels between 150 and 250 mg/dL to prevent acute complications of hypoglycemia and hyperglycemia. Blood glucose levels are usually measured every 4 to 6 hours. Hypoglycemia can be difficult to identify in the patient recovering from anesthesia, because the usual symptoms may be masked. The patient is also observed for signs of infection, such as inflammatory wound changes or drainage, and elevated temperature. Pain management is important because pain causes release of counter-regulatory hormones that increase the blood glucose level. Patients with diabetic neuropathy are susceptible to developing footdrop and foot ulcerations, so pressure areas are monitored and preventive measures implemented.

EVALUATION OF THERAPY

Blood Glucose Monitoring

Self–blood glucose monitoring is standard practice in managing diabetes. It is the key to attaining and maintaining optimal control of blood glucose levels. Its development has greatly affected the treatment of diabetes. The importance of accuracy in obtaining blood glucose results has led to the development of meters that are simple to use, small, and easy to operate (Fig. 28–6). A meter that measures blood glucose by infrared light is in development, so patients will no longer need to prick a finger for blood.

Before selecting a specific meter, the patient is assessed for the cognitive and psychomotor skills necessary to perform the procedure correctly. Patients with learning difficulties or poor dexterity need a meter that is simple to operate. It is possible to test blood glucose levels by using a reagent strip without a meter. This provides a visual reading based on color changes and gives an approximate blood glucose value. This method cannot be used by patients who are color-blind. Highlight 28–4 presents both patient education guidelines for self-moni-

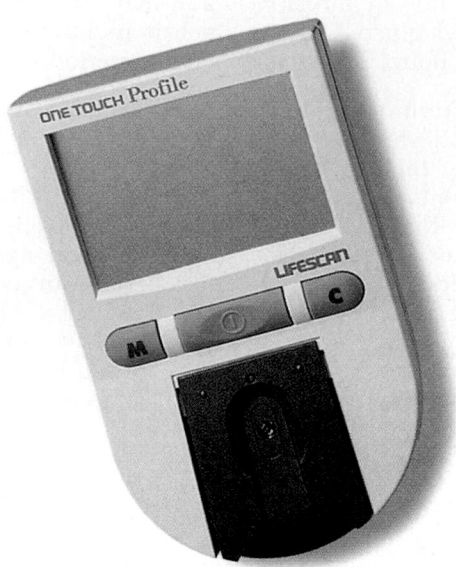

Figure 28–6

LifeScan One Touch Profile diabetes tracking system for home use. (Courtesy of LifeScan, Inc., Milpitas, CA.)

toring blood glucose and factors that can affect test results.

The frequency of testing depends on the patient's state of health and the type of diabetes involved.

The type 1 diabetic patient with fluctuating glucose levels may have to test four to six times a day. The controlled non-insulin-dependent patient can test several times a week. All patients should keep accurate records of the results and report them to the physician regularly.

The major advantage of self-monitoring is the immediate feedback of results, which is important in identifying hypoglycemia and hyperglycemia and in regulating insulin doses. Diabetics who monitor their blood glucose levels are taught to adjust food intake and insulin dose in response to blood glucose levels and to compensate for anticipated changes in physical activity. Self-monitoring allows the diabetic to be an integral member of the health care team and an active participant in his or her own health care.

Disadvantages of self-monitoring include the cost of the meter, testing strips, and lancets if they are not covered by insurance; discomfort caused by piercing the finger; and the potential for infection if good handwashing technique is not followed.

Urine Testing For Glucose

Testing the urine for glucose is no longer considered an accurate measurement of diabetic control because of several disadvantages. First, the blood glucose level must be at least 180 mg/dL, the minimum

---

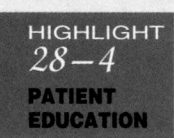 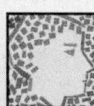

HIGHLIGHT 28–4

PATIENT EDUCATION

Guidelines for Self-Monitoring of Blood Glucose

Instruct the patient in the following:

1. Obtain a large drop of blood from the finger tip or earlobe with a lancet device. Blood flow is enhanced by sticking the side of the finger tip, holding the finger under warm water before sticking, and lowering the hand. To use a reagent strip, place the drop of blood on a fresh reagent strip for the time period specified by the manufacturer. Blot the blood off the strip, and either read the reagent strip visually or insert it into a glucometer. To perform the visual reading, compare the color on the strip to a color chart that comes with the strips. To use a direct-read glucometer, place the drop of blood directly on the meter window.

2. The following factors affect test results:

   • The drop of blood must cover the designated part of the reagent strip or meter window and must be applied as directed by the manufacturer.

   • The timing must be exact according to manufacturer's directions. If the elapsed time is too short, the test results will be lower than they actually are; and if the elapsed time is too long, the test results will be higher than they actually are.

   • The window of the meter must be clean for accurate results.

   • The meter and strips must not be exposed to temperatures higher than 95.4°C (85°F).

   • Reagent strips must not be used after the expiration date.

3. The nurse wears gloves when testing a patient's blood glucose level, but patients do not wear gloves when self-testing.

4. When testing different patients with the same lancet holder device, the nurse changes the lancet and platform between patients. Patients using their own lancet holder device need only change the lancet for each test.

5. Although most meters are calibrated internally when they are manufactured, they can be checked for accuracy with control solutions provided by the manufacturer according to directions.

renal threshold, before the result of the urine glucose test is positive. Further, urine testing cannot detect hypoglycemia, because a negative result shows only that blood glucose is below the renal threshold of 180 mg/dL. Other disadvantages include the lag time between the time glucose is elevated in the blood and when it spills into the urine, variances in individual renal thresholds, false-positive and false-negative results that can occur with certain medications, and the social stigma attached to handling urine.

Urine testing is less expensive than blood testing. For those patients who choose to test their urine, several agents are available. They all contain instructions and have a color chart for reading results. All tests require specific timing for valid results. Each agent has an expiration date. Outdated agents may give inaccurate results and should be discarded.

Urine Testing For Ketones

Urine is tested frequently for ketones in patients with type 1 diabetes mellitus because these patients are prone to ketosis. Patients who test their urine for glucose also test for ketones if the urine glucose level is 1% or higher. Patients who test their blood for glucose are instructed to test their urine for ketones if the blood glucose level is more than 250 mg/dL. In addition, all pregnant women with diabetes are advised to test their urine for ketones daily.

The presence of ketones without an elevated blood glucose level in a pregnant woman indicates starvation ketosis. Starvation ketosis can be caused by inadequate carbohydrate intake by the mother or can result from nocturnal hypoglycemia. If ketones are present, the patient should notify the physician for a change in diet or insulin. The presence of ketones and elevated blood glucose levels during pregnancy significantly increase the risk of fetal morbidity and mortality. Therefore, it is important for the pregnant diabetic patient to test for ketones and glucose, especially in the morning after fasting for the night.

Several agents are available for testing urine for ketones or acetone, which is one type of ketone. Manufacturers' directions should be followed when using these agents. Each agent has an expiration date. Outdated agents may give inaccurate results and should be discarded.

Measurement of Glycosylated Hemoglobin

Measurement of glycosylated hemoglobin, also called hemoglobin A_{1c} (HbA$_{1c}$), can provide an overview of a person's blood glucose levels for the previous 3 months. The red blood cell, of which hemoglobin is a part, has a life span of about 120 days. As glucose enters the blood stream, some attaches or glycosylates to hemoglobin molecules in an irreversible bond. The higher the amount of glucose in the blood stream, the more hemoglobin is glycosylated.

HbA$_{1c}$ levels are not affected by recent food intake, exercise, or stress. The results reveal blood glucose levels during the previous 3 to 4 months, so patients can no longer "cheat" by being especially careful about complying with the diet and taking medication for a few days before visiting the physician. The HbA$_{1c}$ replaces the isolated blood glucose level formerly obtained at office visits to monitor control.

Normal HbA$_{1c}$ levels range from 7 to 11%. However, depending on the method used to measure the components of glycosylated hemoglobin, actual test results vary among laboratories. Good diabetic control is indicated by an HbA$_{1c}$ level of less than 9%. A value of greater than 15% of HbA$_{1c}$ means the patient's diabetes is out of control and the physician should be notified.

Recent studies have identified several factors that can affect the results of the HbA$_{1c}$ test. The results can be lower if the patient has hemolytic anemia, chronic blood loss, or abnormal hemoglobins (S, C, or D). The results can be elevated if the patient has hyperglycemia, thalassemia, or chronic renal failure; is on dialysis; has undergone splenectomy; or has elevated triglyceride or hemoglobin F levels.

ACUTE COMPLICATIONS OF DIABETES MELLITUS

Diabetic Ketoacidosis

Diabetic ketoacidosis is a major, life-threatening complication of diabetes that results from insulin deficiency. It is considered a medical emergency (Nursing Care Guide 28–1.)

Etiology and Pathophysiology
The characteristics of diabetic ketoacidosis are summarized in Table 28–7. The condition is characterized by severe disturbances in protein, fat, and carbohydrate metabolism resulting from a profound insulin deficiency. The levels of the counter-regulatory hormones glucagon, epinephrine, cortisol, and growth hormone are markedly elevated and antagonize the effects of insulin. The patient develops severe hyperglycemia, osmotic diuresis and dehydration, hyperlipidemia, and metabolic acidosis. Electrolyte depletion occurs as ketones are lost in the urine.

Clinical Manifestations
The clinical manifestations of diabetic ketoacidosis usually include hyperglycemia, polyuria, polydipsia, weakness, lethargy, anorexia, nausea, vomiting, blurred vision, headache, muscle aches, and abdominal pain. As hyperglycemia persists, cellular dehydration occurs, which causes sodium and potassium depletion. Dehydration also causes thirst, dry mucous membranes, loss of skin turgor, sunken eyeballs, renal failure, and hypovolemic shock.

The patient in metabolic acidosis has Kussmaul's respirations (deep, rapid breathing), a fruity breath

Text continued on page 1249

Nursing Care Guide 28-1
Patients with Diabetes Mellitus

Assessment Findings:	A 36-year-old single woman is admitted to the hospital with a diagnosis of newly developed type 1 diabetes mellitus. The patient has had polyuria, polydipsia, polyphagia, and a 10 lb weight loss over the previous month. Blood glucose level on admission is 400 mg/dL. The patient is a schoolteacher with little knowledge of diabetes or its management.
Nursing Diagnosis:	Risk for altered health maintenance related to insufficient knowledge of diabetic self-management.

Patient Outcomes	Nursing Interventions	Rationale
Patient verbalizes a basic understanding of the pathophysiology of diabetes mellitus.	Explain the basic pathophysiology of diabetes at the patient's level of understanding. Ask the patient to restate information to validate understanding.	To manage diabetes, the patient must have some understanding of its pathophysiology
Patient demonstrates ability to plan meals using the American Diabetes Association (ADA) exchange lists and stays within prescribed calorie level.	Reinforce diet teaching of ADA exchange lists. Have patient plan sample menus of preferred foods for breakfast, lunch, dinner, and snack within dietary guidelines. Demonstrate how to adjust diet for changes in activity level and illness.	Diet is a primary component in successful self-management of diabetes.
	Provide a copy of the ADA exchange lists.	Written information reinforces learning, clarifies verbal instructions, minimizes the risk of errors, and allows maximum patient control and flexibility.
Patient verbalizes knowledge of prescribed insulin, dosage, and action.	Explain the pharmacokinetics of prescribed insulin preparation and administration schedule.	Insulin is the only antidiabetic agent used to treat type 1 diabetes. The patient must have this information to safely self-administer insulin and minimize the risk of complications.
Patient demonstrates ability to prepare and administer insulin correctly.	Teach the patient how to prepare and administer insulin. Observe the patient performing the procedure daily.	Provides opportunity for repeated feedback to reinforce proper technique and correct errors.
Patient demonstrates ability to test blood glucose and correctly interpret results.	Teach patient to test blood glucose according to manufacturer's instructions. Observe the patient perform the procedure to assess technique, ability to follow instructions, and accuracy of results.	Frequent self-monitoring of blood glucose is the best way to evaluate the diabetic treatment plan. Patient must understand and adhere to the manufacturer's instructions to obtain accurate results. Proper technique in obtaining specimen minimizes the risk of infection.

(continued)

Patients with Diabetes Mellitus (continued)

Patient Outcomes	Nursing Interventions	Rationale
	Provide written information on normal blood glucose values, actions to take when results are abnormal (adjust insulin, modify diet, call physician), and how to adjust for changes in physical activity or illness.	Good diabetic control requires a dynamic balance between diet, insulin, and activity. Adjustment must be made to compensate for changes in any component.
Patient demonstrates ability to test urine for ketones accurately and states when to test.	Teach patient to test urine for ketones according to manufacturer's directions. Observe the patient perform the procedure to evaluate technique and accuracy.	Patient must understand and adhere to the manufacturer's instructions to obtain accurate results.
	Instruct patient to test urine for ketones if blood glucose level is higher than 250 mg/dL or if she is ill or pregnant. Provide written instructions on actions to take if ketones are present in the urine. Reinforce the need to notify physician promptly if ketones are present.	Ketoacidosis indicates incomplete metabolism of body fats. Early detection and treatment minimize the risk of a potentially life-threatening complication. Adjustment in diet or insulin reduces risk of future episodes.
Patient states causes, signs, symptoms, and treatment of hypoglycemia.	*Teach patient the following:* Hypoglycemia is caused by too much insulin, too little food, or a sudden increase in exercise. Signs and symptoms are shaking, sweating, weakness, hunger, dizziness, drowsiness, and confusion. If symptoms occur, take a simple carbohydrate, such as 4 oz fruit juice or regular soda, 2 tsp honey, two lumps of sugar, five or six Life Savers, glucose tablets, or $\frac{1}{2}$ oz of sugar gel icing. Repeat in 10 to 15 minutes if symptoms do not resolve. Follow with a complex carbohydrate and protein snack, such as cheese and crackers and skim milk if the next meal is more than 2 hours away.	Hypoglycemia places the patient at risk for physical injury and irreversible brain damage. It is easily reversed if detected and treated early.
	Teach significant others how to prepare and administer parenteral glucagon if the patient is unconscious.	Glucagon raises blood glucose level by promoting conversion of hepatic glycogen to glucose. *(continued)*

Nursing Care Guide 28–1
Patients with Diabetes Mellitus (continued)

Patient Outcomes	Nursing Interventions	Rationale
Patient states causes, signs, symptoms, and treatment of hyperglycemia and ketoacidosis.	*Teach patient the following:* Hyperglycemia and ketoacidosis are caused by insufficient insulin, too much food, not enough exercise, infection, or stress. Signs and symptoms are unusual thirst, frequent urination, weakness, blurred vision, abdominal pain, nausea and vomiting, and blood glucose level higher than goal range of 70 to 140 mg/dL. If symptoms occur, test blood glucose, take insulin if previously instructed in amount to take, drink fluids, and call physician.	Hyperglycemia and ketoacidosis are acute complications of type 1 diabetes. Early detection and treatment minimize the risk of a life-threatening situation. Maintenance of blood glucose levels below 140 mg/dL slows the progression of long-term degenerative changes of diabetes.
Patient verbalizes understanding of foot-care routine and other hygiene practices to incorporate into lifestyle.	Teach patient daily foot care. Other health care practices include meticulous oral hygiene, a dental appointment every 6 months, annual influenza vaccinations, not smoking, and complete physical examination with evaluation of renal function annually or as recommended by physician. Instruct patient to undergo annual eye examination by an ophthalmologist.	Patients with diabetes are at risk for infection from impaired leukocyte activity. These health care practices minimize the risk of infection and promote early detection of health problems. Diabetic retinopathy is usually the earliest degenerative change of diabetes. Early detection and treatment can minimize impairment of vision.

Evaluation: Compare the patient's status with the expected patient outcomes. If the outcomes are not met, reassess the patient and revise the plan.

Assessment Findings: A 39-year-old man was admitted to the hospital 2 days ago for uncontrolled diabetes mellitus and diabetic ketoacidosis (DKA). He is married, has two young children, and works as a salesman. He travels frequently. The patient says that he has had type 1 diabetes for 10 years, takes one injection of 25 units U-100 Humulin N and 5 units Humulin R insulin every morning and does not bother to monitor his blood glucose levels. He does not follow a diabetic diet. He sees a physician about every 6 months if he is not traveling. At the time of admission, the patient was ill with influenza and his blood glucose level was 800 mg/dL.

Nursing Diagnosis: Ineffective management of therapeutic regimen (individuals) related to lack of understanding of the implications of not following diabetic regimen and difficulty incorporating treatments into personal lifestyle

(continued)

Patients with Diabetes Mellitus (continued)

Patient Outcomes	Nursing Interventions	Rationale
Patient acknowledges insufficient knowledge of diabetic regimen.	Ask the patient how he thinks he developed DKA. Observe verbal and nonverbal cues to identify his readiness to learn. Use feedback and reflection to confirm observations.	Determines patient's level of knowledge and understanding. Teaching is not effective unless patient is ready to learn.
	Review the cause and effect relationship between patient behaviors and control of blood glucose levels.	Accurate information corrects misunderstandings and increases patient's knowledge.
Patient acknowledges noncompliant behavior.	*Determine reason for noncompliance:* Assess patient's and family's cultural and health values.	Compliance involves behavioral changes that are influenced by family, cultural, and individual beliefs about health, susceptibility to disease, and seriousness of disease. Cultural practices may affect the learning process. Verbalization of compliant behaviors ensures that the patient understands what he must do to facilitate change.
	Discuss with patient and family their understanding of the implications of noncompliance.	
	Involve the patient in identifying desired changes in behavior.	
Patient demonstrates willingness to learn about disease and to participate in self-care activities.	*Implement measures to improve compliance:* Explain diabetes at the patient's level of understanding.	An assessment of the patient's learning abilities enables the nurse to develop an individual teaching plan and to facilitate effective teaching and learning. The patient needs to be informed about the disease process and its implications to make informed decisions about the self-care regimen.
	Stress that diabetes is a lifelong, chronic condition and that compliance with the treatment plan is necessary to prevent acute complications and to prevent or delay long-term degenerative changes.	
	Provide complete diabetic teaching to patient and family. Refer to diabetic educator if available.	
	Encourage patient to participate in self-care activities, such as insulin injections, self-monitoring of blood glucose, and selection of foods using diabetic meal plan from the hospital menu.	Participation in self-care activities provides reinforcement of teaching, enhances learning and retention, and increases self-confidence.
Patient verbalizes intent to modify behavior and incorporate diabetic self-management regimen into lifestyle.	Assist patient in identifying ways to incorporate self-management into lifestyle. Provide positive feedback.	Verbalization of intent and commitment facilitates change in behavior. Positive feedback reinforces learning and motivation.

(continued)

Nursing Care Guide 28–1
Patients with Diabetes Mellitus (continued)

Patient Outcomes	Nursing Interventions	Rationale
	Provide written and verbal information on diet plan, medications, activity pattern, symptoms of hyperglycemia and hypoglycemia, what actions to take if they occur, and what to do during periods of illness. Include telephone number of a resource person to answer questions after discharge.	Written information reinforces learning, clarifies verbal instructions, and minimizes the risk of errors. Availability of resource person reduces anxiety.
	Provide information on community resources, diabetic support groups, and diabetic publications. Encourage patient to attend follow-up diabetes education classes. Include patient's spouse in teaching, and encourage family support.	Community resources, support groups, publications, and the involvement of family or significant other provide additional support and information that may reduce anxiety and enhance motivation and compliance.
	Reinforce the benefits of adhering to the prescribed self-management regimen.	Maintenance of blood glucose values below 140 mg/dL slows the progression of the long-term degenerative changes of diabetes.
Patient verbalizes understanding of implications of noncompliance	*Provide information on the pathophysiology of diabetes:* Explain the effects of hypoglycemia and hyperglycemia on body systems. Explain the benefits of new technology to help maintain normal blood glucose levels. Teach patient that he can control diabetes by accepting responsibility for managing his disease.	The basis of self-management is a sound diabetes education program. A patient in control of the disease and able to recognize symptoms is more likely to accept and adhere to the treatment plan.

Evaluation: Compare the patient's status with the expected patient outcomes. If the outcomes are not met, reassess the patient and revise the plan.

Table 28–7
Comparing Diabetic Ketoacidosis and Hyperglycemic Hyperosmolar Nonketotic Syndrome

Diabetic Ketoacidosis	Hyperglycemic Hyperosmolar Nonketotic Syndrome
Usually occurs in type 1 diabetes mellitus	Usually occurs in diagnosed or undiagnosed type 2 diabetes mellitus
Blood glucose level between 300 and 800 mg/dL	Blood glucose level between 600 and 1200 mg/dL, possibly higher
Ketones produced	No ketones produced
Blood pH below 7.35	Blood pH normal
Serum osmolality <350 mOsm/kg	Serum osmolality >350 mOsm/kg

odor from ketones, and nausea and vomiting. Hyperkalemia occurs as potassium moves out of the cell with water in exchange for hydrogen ions. Depression of the central nervous system, and eventually coma, may result from acidosis. The arterial pH is less than 7.35, plasma bicarbonate is less than 15 mEq/L, the blood glucose level is higher than 250 mg/dL, and ketones are present in the blood and urine.

Management

The major goals for treating diabetic ketoacidosis are to correct the hyperglycemia, fluid volume depletion, hyperosmolarity, acidosis, and potassium deficiency. Hyperglycemia is treated with an intravenous infusion of regular insulin in 0.45% normal saline. When the blood glucose level falls to 300 mg/dL, the infusion rate is reduced, and 5% dextrose is added to maintain a blood glucose level of about 250 mg/dL, or until the patient recovers from ketosis.

To correct fluid volume depletion, 1 to 2 L of 0.45% sodium chloride are infused within the first 2 to 3 hours. Intravenous fluids are then administered more slowly, with the rate depending on the state of dehydration. Adequate volume replacement is determined by a systolic blood pressure between 90 and 140 mm Hg, a pulse rate between 60 and 100 beats per minute, and a urine output of at least 30 mL/h.

Patients in ketoacidosis have a serum osmolarity of more than 330 mOsm/L. The normal range for serum osmolarity is 280 to 300 mOsm/L. Treatment consists of hypotonic fluid, usually 0.45% saline. Serum osmolarity is corrected as saline is given to correct hypovolemia. Acidosis is corrected by administration of insulin and fluids. The use of sodium bicarbonate to correct acidosis is avoided because it can precipitate a further drop in serum potassium levels.

Electrolyte imbalance is restored through administration of intravenous potassium. Initially, the potassium level may be normal or high because potassium leaves the cell and enters the plasma as the cells dehydrate. However, as insulin is administered, potassium moves back into the cells and the serum potassium level falls. Twenty to 40 mEq potassium chloride per liter of intravenous fluid is given even if initial serum potassium levels are normal. As diabetic ketoacidosis is resolved, the rate of the potassium infusion is decreased. Potassium level is determined every 2 hours during the first 8 hours of treatment.

Hyperglycemic Hyperosmolar Nonketotic Syndrome

Hyperglycemic hyperosmolar nonketotic syndrome is a life-threatening, emergency situation more common in the elderly type 2 diabetic patient or undiagnosed diabetic patient. Because the initial symptoms of hyperglycemic hyperosmolar nonketotic syndrome can go unnoticed for several weeks, and

they are often confused with other medical conditions, the mortality rate is high. Type 2 diabetics who are most likely to develop hyperglycemic hyperosmolar nonketotic syndrome are elderly patients whose fluid intake is poor and hospitalized patients who are not receiving adequate fluid intake.

Etiology and Pathophysiology

Hyperglycemic hyperosmolar nonketotic syndrome is usually precipitated by an acute illness or infection, fluid loss from osmotic diuresis secondary to hyperglycemia, severe burns, severe diarrhea, hemodialysis, peritoneal dialysis, myocardial infarction, uremia, arterial thrombosis, hypertonic enteral feedings, or pharmacologic agents, such as thiazides, propranolol, phenytoin, and steroids.

Hyperglycemic hyperosmolar nonketotic syndrome is similar to diabetic ketoacidosis, but because it occurs primarily in type 2 diabetics, the lack of insulin is not absolute and lipolysis or fat breakdown does not occur. Therefore, ketones are not produced. However, as a result of the precipitating event, insulin needs increase and the pancreas cannot produce enough insulin for normal metabolism to take place. This results in severe hyperglycemia, with a blood glucose level often higher than 800 mg/dL, and hyperosmolality.

Clinical Manifestations

Hyperglycemic hyperosmolar nonketotic syndrome is evidenced by profound hyperglycemia and dehydration, absence of ketosis, and the presence of neurologic changes ranging from depressed sensorium to coma.

The onset of hyperglycemic hyperosmolar nonketotic syndrome is gradual, with a history of increasing polyuria and polydipsia. These early symptoms are frequently missed, especially in the elderly, which is one reason dehydration is more severe than in diabetic ketoacidosis. The dehydration or loss of fluids also causes electrolyte depletion, hyperosmolality, and hypovolemia.

Patients can also have neurologic signs similar to those of a cerebrovascular accident, which are reversible when the condition subsides. Despite severe hyperglycemia, there are no ketones in the blood or urine. Also, there are fewer complaints of gastrointestinal symptoms than in diabetic ketoacidosis (see Table 28–7).

Management

The primary goals of treatment are to rehydrate the patient to restore fluid volume and to correct electrolyte deficiency. The amount of fluid replacement depends on the level of dehydration and the patient's cardiovascular status. Intravenous fluid replacement is similar to that administered in diabetic ketoacidosis. Blood glucose levels and osmolality decrease as the patient is rehydrated. Elderly patients and those with a previous history of cardiovascular disease are monitored by central venous pressure or Swan-Ganz catheter. Potassium replacement is guided by continuous cardiac monitoring and frequent serum potassium determinations.

Insulin is another important component in the treatment of hyperglycemic hyperosmolar nonketotic syndrome and is given according to the same guidelines as in diabetic ketoacidosis. Blood glucose and electrolyte levels are monitored every 1 to 2 hours until stable.

Hypoglycemia

Acute hypoglycemia occurs when blood glucose levels fall below 50 mg/dL. Hypoglycemia is dangerous because the brain relies solely on glucose for energy. It cannot metabolize fats for energy as the rest of the body can when glucose is not available.

Etiology and Pathophysiology

Hypoglycemia is an acute complication that can occur in patients taking medication for diabetes. The most common causes are too much insulin, inadequate food intake, excessive or prolonged physical activity, and ingestion of alcohol, especially when not eating.

The diabetic patient can have a hypoglycemic insulin reaction from too much insulin if an error is made in preparing the medication, if the insulin is absorbed more rapidly than normal as a result of injection into an extremity that is being exercised, or if the type of insulin is changed from animal-source insulin to human insulin or other highly purified preparation. Hypoglycemia may also develop in patients when blood glucose levels approach normal and insulin requirements decrease.

Hypoglycemia can occur if snacks or meals are late or omitted. All prescribed exchanges of the meal plan have to be eaten on schedule. Hypoglycemia may also occur with delayed or impaired absorption of carbohydrates from gastrointestinal neuropathy.

Physical activity can lower blood glucose levels for as long as 24 hours after exercise. The presence of insulin normally inhibits the production of glucose by the liver. Thus, in the nondiabetic person, endogenous insulin production decreases during exercise, thereby allowing for increased hepatic glucose production. However, the diabetic patient who receives a set amount of exogenous insulin may have a relative excess of insulin, which would inhibit production of glucose by the liver during exercise. Exercise also increases sensitivity of muscle tissue to insulin and promotes increased glucose uptake by muscle to replenish stores of glycogen depleted by exercise. The combination of decreased glucose production by the liver and increased glucose utilization by muscle can lead to hypoglycemia both during and after exercise.

Ingestion of alcohol or ethanol causes hypoglycemia by inhibiting glucose production by the liver (gluconeogenesis). This can occur with as little as 2 or 3 ounces of alcohol on an empty stomach.

Hypoglycemia can also occur when taking propranolol, which can mask the early symptoms of a hypoglycemic reaction; at the onset of menses, when progesterone levels decrease, which decreases insulin requirements; and during the immediate postpartum period, when there is a reduction in placental hormones antagonistic to insulin.

Clinical Manifestations

Hypoglycemia can be classified as mild, moderate, or severe, depending on the patient's symptoms. Although the severity of the hypoglycemic reaction is poorly correlated with blood glucose levels because the exact blood glucose level at which symptoms begin varies from patient to patient, most patients develop symptoms when blood glucose is between 50 and 60 mg/dL.

The patient with mild hypoglycemia exhibits sudden tremors, palpitations, diaphoresis, and hunger—symptoms associated with stimulation of the autonomic nervous system. The patient remains alert and capable of self-treatment, such as ingesting 10 to 15 g of simple carbohydrate (4 to 6 ounces of juice or 6 to 10 Life Savers). After treatment, symptoms subside quickly.

Moderate hypoglycemia impairs central nervous system function. In addition to manifestations of stimulation of the autonomic nervous system, the patient may experience headache, mood changes, irritability, inability to concentrate, confusion, slurred speech, irrational behavior, blurred vision, impaired judgment, and drowsiness. The patient is able to request assistance and may require a second dose of simple carbohydrate to correct the hypoglycemia.

A severe hypoglycemic reaction is one in which the patient needs help from another person for treatment because of severely impaired neurologic function. The patient is unresponsive and may have convulsions. Treatment consists of parenteral glucagon or intravenous glucose.

Management

The major goal for treating hypoglycemia is rapid reversal of the condition by administration of glucose to prevent injury or residual central nervous system damage. It is also important to review principles of self-management with the patient to prevent further hypoglycemic episodes. The production of counter-regulatory hormones assists in recovery from hypoglycemia if glycogen stores are not depleted. An elevated circulating insulin level delays recovery.

Treatment depends on the patient's history, resources, and severity of the hypoglycemic episode. All levels of hypoglycemia in both type 1 and type 2 diabetic persons are treated immediately. Review Table 28–8 for a comparison of the causes, symptoms, and treatment of hypoglycemia and hyperglycemia.

Somogyi Phenomenon

The Somogyi phenomenon is characterized by periods of hypoglycemia followed by rebound hypergly-

Table 28–8

Traits of Hypoglycemia and Hyperglycemia

	Causes	Symptoms	Treatment
Hypoglycemia (insulin shock, insulin reaction)	Too much insulin Excess oral antidiabetic agent Too little food Unusual physical activity	Shaking Sweating Dizziness Anxiety Palpitations Tachycardia Headache Behavioral changes Mental confusion Slurred speech Loss of coordination Drowsiness Coma	Glucose or glycogen Food
Hyperglycemia (diabetic ketoacidosis)	Not enough insulin Insufficient oral antidiabetic agent Eating too much or eating sweets Illness or infection Stress	Polyuria Polydipsia Fatigue Abdominal pain Headache Blurred vision Nausea Vomiting Kussmaul's respiration Fruity breath odor Coma	Insulin Fluids Electrolytes

cemia. Typically, the Somogyi phenomenon occurs during the night, but it can occur any time a hypoglycemic episode occurs. The phenomenon begins with hypoglycemia, followed by oversecretion of counter-regulatory hormones. These hormones stimulate the liver to produce glucose, causing hyperglycemia.

Diagnosing the Somogyi phenomenon may be difficult because the pattern of hypoglycemia followed by rebound hyperglycemia may also be caused by developing insulin resistance. Somogyi phenomenon is suspected in patients whose blood glucose levels fluctuate between hypoglycemia and severe hyperglycemia, those whose blood glucose levels increase despite increasing doses of insulin, and patients who awaken with headaches and complain of restless sleep, nightmares, or enuresis, or who have unexplained nausea and vomiting.

Diagnosis of the Somogyi phenomenon requires measuring blood glucose levels between 2:00 AM and 4:00 AM and again at 7:00 AM. If the blood glucose levels between 2:00 AM and 4:00 AM are below 50 to 60 mg/dL and the 7:00 AM blood glucose level is more than 180 to 200 mg/dL, the Somogyi phenomenon probably occurred.

Treatment for the Somogyi phenomenon is to decrease the evening insulin dose to a level that no longer causes nocturnal hypoglycemia. A bedtime snack is also recommended to counter the duration of the effects of intermediate- and long-acting insulins during the night.

Dawn Phenomenon

The dawn phenomenon is a condition that can occur in some insulin-dependent patients and is characterized by an increase in fasting blood glucose levels between 5:00 AM and 9:00 AM. It is not preceded by an episode of hypoglycemia. A possible cause is the release of growth hormone or cortisol during rapid-eye-movement (REM) sleep in the early morning hours, which increases glucose levels.

Diagnosis requires measuring blood glucose levels at 3:00 AM. If this blood glucose level is normal and the level at 6:00 AM or 7:00 AM is elevated, the dawn phenomenon is suspected.

Treatment consists of delaying the intermediate-acting evening insulin dose until 10:00 PM and eating a bedtime snack. The intermediate-acting insulin would prevent a rise in blood glucose after 3:00 AM.

LONG-TERM DEGENERATIVE CHANGES OF DIABETES MELLITUS

It is important that diabetic patients recognize that they are at risk for developing the long-term, chronic degenerative changes associated with the disease. Although degenerative changes can develop in all patients with diabetes mellitus, research has confirmed that good control of blood glucose levels may delay, or possibly prevent, their onset and can reduce their severity.

Degenerative Vascular Changes

MACROVASCULAR DISEASE

Macrovascular disease, or macroangiopathy, is an atherosclerotic process of large and moderate-size blood vessels that can occur in any person, diabetic or not. However, over the past two decades, research has shown that diabetics face a greater risk of developing these changes at an earlier age. It is now recognized that macrovascular disease is responsible for most of the morbidity and mortality seen in patients with diabetes. Macrovascular disease at least doubles the risk of coronary artery, cerebral vascular, and peripheral vascular disease in these patients. In addition to the usual risk factors of cigarette smoking, hypertension, and elevated cholesterol and triglyceride levels, hyperglycemia is an independent risk factor in the diabetic patient. Research to determine why atherosclerosis occurs more frequently in diabetics continues. There is no conclusive evidence as yet.

People with diabetes should be advised of the increased risk of macrovascular disease and taught to take steps to reduce risk factors associated with its development.

MICROVASCULAR DISEASE

Microvascular disease, or microangiopathy, refers to small-vessel disease that affects the arterioles, venules, and capillaries. It is characterized by thickening of the capillary basement membrane that surrounds the endothelial cells of the capillary, increased capillary permeability, and capillary occlusion. It primarily affects the eyes, kidneys, nervous system, and peripheral circulation. Microangiopathy results in diabetic retinopathy, diabetic nephropathy, and peripheral neuropathy. Guidelines for patient teaching to monitor and minimize the risks associated with microvascular degenerative changes are presented in Highlight 28–5.

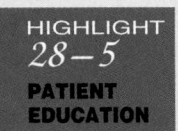 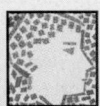

HIGHLIGHT
28–5
PATIENT EDUCATION

Guidelines for Self-Care and Monitoring of Long-Term Degenerative Changes of Diabetes Mellitus

Instruct the patient in the following for diabetic retinopathy:

Have an eye examination annually by an ophthalmologist.

Make an appointment with the ophthalmologist immediately if blurred vision occurs or if there is a change or decrease in vision.

Instruct the patient in the following for diabetic peripheral neuropathy:

Foot-care instructions:

Follow a foot-care routine daily to prevent long-term complications.

Inspect the feet daily for sores, blisters, swelling, redness, and tenderness. Report skin infections or non-healing sores immediately to the physician. Loss of sensation caused by diabetic neuropathy can lead to infection, gangrene, and possible amputation if not detected and treated early.

Wash the feet daily using a mild soap. Pat the feet dry and apply lotion (do not apply lotion between the toes). Use lotion containing lanolin, not petroleum jelly. Test the temperature of the water before submerging the feet to prevent burns. Do not soak the feet.

Wear properly fitting shoes with smooth linings.

Do not walk in bare feet either in the house or outside.

Avoid using a heating pad or hot water bottle on the feet.

Cut the toenails straight and even with the toe itself. If the toenails are thick and hard to cut or if vision is poor, have a physician or podiatrist cut them.

Make an appointment with a podiatrist for treatment of corns, calluses, warts, thickened or rough skin, splinters, or injuries. Do not attempt to treat corns, calluses, or warts with nonprescription preparations or instruments.

Do not cross the legs at the knees or ankles when sitting.

Instruct the patient in the following for diabetic nephropathy:

Renal function is monitored by checking the urine for the presence of protein during physician visits. If overt proteinuria is present, renal function tests are done.

For advanced uremia:

• Follow a protein-restricted diet.
• Monitor blood glucose levels closely, because insulin requirements decrease with uremia and there is an increased likelihood of having a hypoglycemic reaction.

Diabetic Retinopathy

Diabetic retinopathy is characterized by progressive deterioration of the small blood vessels in the retina. It is the leading cause of blindness in the United States and is related to the length of time the patient has had diabetes. After 10 years of having diabetes, 50% of all diabetic patients and 90% of those with poorly controlled blood glucose levels have some form of retinopathy.

There are three stages of diabetic retinopathy. The first and earliest stage is nonproliferative background retinopathy characterized by microaneurysms, which are seen as tiny red dots in the retina. Other changes associated with background retinopathy are the appearance of yellow lipid deposits commonly called hard exudates, small intraretinal hemorrhages that appear as red smudges on the retina, and the presence of macular edema. Blurred central vision caused by the macular edema develops in 10% of diabetic patients and may be the only subjective symptom. Macular edema may progress to loss of central vision in later stages.

The second stage of diabetic retinopathy is preproliferative retinopathy characterized by progression of background retinopathy and further destruction and occlusion of retinal capillaries. The retinal veins become tortuous and bulging, and multiple clustered blot hemorrhages appear, indicating weakened capillary walls. Poor retinal perfusion may stimulate initial growth of abnormal new blood vessels. Areas of retinal ischemia produce soft exudates or cotton-wool spots, which are white, fluffy-looking lesions.

In patients with severe preproliferative retinopathy, there is a 50% chance that the third stage, proliferative retinopathy, will develop within 1 year. This stage is characterized by the growth of networks of new, abnormal blood vessels on the surface of the retina and extending into the vitreous. This growth of new blood vessels is called neovascularization and occurs in response to ischemia in the diseased retina. Light transmission through these areas is diminished.

These new blood vessels are highly brittle and can easily hemorrhage, sometimes filling the vitreous with blood. As the damaged vessels heal and blood is resorbed from the vitreous, fibrous scar tissue forms. The growth of fibrous scar tissue is called fibrous proliferation. As the fibrous tissue contracts, it can place traction on the retina, resulting in retinal detachment. Loss of vision caused by vitreous hemorrhage or retinal detachment can be the patient's first symptom of proliferative retinopathy. Any diabetic patient complaining of spots floating in the field of vision, rapid visual changes, or fogged vision should be referred to an ophthalmologist immediately.

The primary treatment for the early stages of diabetic retinopathy includes normalizing blood glucose levels and blood pressure, both of which are associated with progression of retinopathy. When vision loss becomes a threat, argon laser photocoagulation is performed. In patients with high-risk characteristics of proliferative retinopathy, panretinal photocoagulation is most beneficial. This is a procedure in which 1200 to 1600 laser burns, each measuring 500 μm, are placed throughout the midperipheral retina but not in the macular region. Macular edema is treated by focal argon laser photocoagulation.

Laser photocoagulation is a relatively painless procedure performed on an outpatient basis with anesthetic eye drops. The patient can usually resume activities of daily living the following day, with possible restrictions on heavy lifting. However, the potential side effects are night blindness, decreased visual acuity, decreased peripheral vision, loss of central vision, and, rarely, hemorrhage. Despite its side effects, the benefits of this procedure probably outweigh its risks.

The treatment for vitreous hemorrhage is vitrectomy. In this procedure, both the hemorrhagic area of the vitreous and the fibrous proliferation are removed and replaced with sterile saline. Vitrectomy can improve vision in 50 to 60% of patients treated.

All diabetic patients should undergo eye examination by an ophthalmologist annually, including an intraocular pressure measurement and a dilated pupil fundus examination. Fluorescein angiography is performed to assess retinal vessels and macular edema.

Diabetic Neuropathy

Diabetic neuropathy is the most common complication of diabetes. It occurs in 70% of diabetic patients and is already present in 12% of patients at the time of diagnosis. The incidence and prevalence of neuropathy increase with the patient's age and the severity of hyperglycemia.

Diabetic neuropathy is a group of neurologic complications related to the abnormal metabolism of diabetes that affects the peripheral and autonomic nervous systems. The pathology can be metabolic or vascular and results in a loss of large and small myelin nerve fibers (demyelination), connective tissue proliferation, and thickening of the capillary basement membrane.

A common theory for the pathology of diabetic neuropathy is a disturbance of the pathway of glucose metabolism in nerve tissue during periods of hyperglycemia.

Diabetic neuropathies are classified according to the anatomic distribution of the lesions, type of nerve involvement, degree of vascular involvement, and extent of nerve damage. Diabetic mononeuropathies include nerves chronically exposed to external pressure, such as those affected in carpal tunnel syndrome, extraocular motor paralysis, and footdrop. The symptoms are numbness, tingling, burning, and sudden pain. Medical management includes correction of the nerve entrapment. Pain is treated by splinting, local injections of glucocorticoids, or nerve block. Recovery usually occurs within 3 months. Without treatment, muscle weakness and wasting could result.

Distal symmetric polyneuropathy, also called peripheral neuropathy, is the most common form of diabetic neuropathy. Symptoms include numbness, tingling, burning, dull ache, and cramping that begins in the digits and progresses to the foot and hand. The symptoms are usually worse at night. Eventually, the pain increases. The skin may become so sensitive that the patient cannot tolerate pressure from bed sheets. As the neuropathy progresses, the patient develops muscle weakness, sensory loss, an unbalanced gait, foot ulcers, and loss of fine motor skills. Sensory neuropathy leads to loss of pain and pressure sensation and increases the risk of undetected injury, tissue ischemia, or infection. Medical management includes control of hyperglycemia and medication to relieve pain and allow the patient to sleep at night.

Autonomic neuropathy involves nerves of the small blood vessels, the sweat glands of the skin, the gastrointestinal tract, the genitourinary tract, the cardiovascular system, and the adrenergic system. This type of neuropathy usually occurs in combination with peripheral neuropathy. Symptoms depend on the system involved. Orthostatic hypotension and mild, persistent tachycardia are common manifestations of cardiovascular autonomic neuropathy. When the nerves of the sweat glands are involved, there can be frequent attacks of profuse sweating when eating, and drying and cracking of the skin of the feet. Involvement of the gastrointestinal tract, known as gastroparesis, can cause delayed emptying of the gastric contents, retention and decreased ability to expel gastric contents, nausea, and vomiting of undigested food. Involvement of the small intestine causes watery diarrhea, often at night without warning, followed by constipation. Involvement of the genitourinary tract causes urinary retention, overflow incontinence, and frequent urinary tract infections.

Sexual dysfunction occurs in 50% of male diabetic patients and 35% of the females after 20 years with diabetes. The symptoms in men are impotence, retrograde ejaculation, and inability to maintain an erection. Sexual function may be regained with papaverine injections, vacuum devices, or penile prostheses. Pretreatment counseling of patients and partners is advised. Women have a reduced ability to have an orgasm and experience changes in vaginal lubrication.

Diabetic Nephropathy

Diabetic nephropathy is characterized by proteinuria, hypertension, edema, and renal insufficiency. It occurs in patients who have had type 1 diabetes mellitus for 15 to 20 years. Some 30 to 40% of these patients progress to end-stage renal disease. Patients with type 2 diabetes mellitus develop nephropathy within 5 to 10 years. Three to 5% of these patients progress to end-stage renal disease. In addition, 97% of patients with end-stage renal disease have diabetic retinopathy. Fifty percent are either blind or have significant vision loss. This is known as renal-retinal syndrome.

Pathology and early renal changes develop without clinical signs. Deterioration of renal function is often ongoing for many years before detection. During this time, glomerular changes are taking place: basement membrane thickening, mesangial expansion, and arteriosclerosis of the afferent and efferent blood vessels. The effectiveness of glomerular filtration decreases. Urinary creatinine clearance decreases as the glomerular filtration rate deteriorates. Next, nodular and diffuse lesions form throughout the glomerulus, a condition called Kimmelstiel-Wilson syndrome. These changes occur in insulin-dependent diabetes mellitus and non-insulin-dependent diabetes mellitus patients, but earlier in patients with non-insulin-dependent diabetes mellitus.

The first clinical sign of kidney damage is protein in the urine, which results from increased glomerular capillary permeability caused by thickening of the basement membrane. Proteinuria usually develops within 15 to 20 years after the onset of clinical symptoms of diabetes. Protein can be detected by the dipstick method of testing a single specimen of urine or by testing a 24-hour urine collection. Nephrotic syndrome is diagnosed when the amount of protein excreted exceeds 3.5 g/d. As protein is excreted, plasma albumin concentration falls, leading to protein tissue wasting, sodium and water retention, weight gain, and edema.

Diabetic patients are tested regularly for proteinuria. When it occurs, serum creatinine and urea nitrogen concentrations are also measured. A 24-hour urine test to quantitate the total protein excreted and creatinine clearance may be performed.

Control of blood glucose and hypertension are important factors in slowing the progression of diabetic nephropathy. Normal blood pressure, maintained through the use of diuretics and antihypertensive drugs, decreases the rate at which the glomerular filtration rate declines, reduces proteinuria, and helps prevent cerebrovascular and coronary artery disease.

Renal insufficiency is characterized by proteinuria, hypertension, a glomerular filtration rate below 25 to 30 mL/min (normal is about 125 mL/min), and elevated serum creatinine and blood urea nitrogen levels.

The patient has uremia when the glomerular filtration rate is below 15 mL/min and the serum creatinine level is greater than 4 to 5 mg/dL. The clinical signs at this stage include nausea, vomiting, lethargy, anemia, hypertension, and acidosis. In addition, blood glucose levels fluctuate greatly. Insulin needs decrease as uremia advances, because about 25% of insulin is catabolized by the kidneys.

Medical management includes placing the patient on a protein-restricted diet. Patients with end-stage renal disease require either a kidney transplant or dialysis to forestall death. Patients with diabetic nephropathy are at increased risk for acute renal failure after a radiocontrast procedure, such as intravenous pyelography or computed tomography. Therefore, the patient is well hydrated before the procedure. A minimal amount of dye is given. In addition, intravenous mannitol is commonly administered before the procedure and continued for 24 hours afterward. Serum creatinine concentration is measured daily for 2 to 3 days. It is also important to avoid nephrotoxic drugs and procedures that could lead to infection, such as bladder catheterization, in patients with end-stage renal disease.

❖ SETTINGS, PROVIDERS, AND COLLABORATION FOR CARE

The discovery of insulin and oral antidiabetic agents, along with improved technology and methods of managing diabetes, has enabled people with diabetes to live longer. People who once would have been admitted to the hospital for elevated blood glucose levels are being seen today in outpatient centers or physician's offices. Even newly diagnosed diabetic patients are referred by their physicians to diabetes educators to learn how to manage their disease rather than admitting them to the hospital. They learn how and when to monitor blood glucose levels, prepare and inject insulin, follow exchange lists, recognize and treat hypoglycemia, provide daily foot care, and call the physician.

Many hospitals have developed outpatient programs to keep these patients informed about self-management and self-care practices. People in whom diabetes mellitus is diagnosed are typically treated in outpatient clinics and in the home. Because of the seriousness of the systemic effects of the disease, complications are common. Many diabetics experience frequent hospitalizations for diagnosis and treatment of complications. Depending on the type of complication, many patients need continued care and nursing assistance after discharge.

Because of the chronicity of diabetes, most patients require the assistance of several health professionals to provide the care needed to maintain health, manage complications, or both. The coordinator of the care team may be the case manager, the physician, or the home health nurse. Members of the team may include the following:

- Diabetologist or endocrinologist, who monitors the patient's disease and prescribes appropriate medication for treatment
- Diabetic nurse educator, who teaches the patient and family about the disease, the diet, and how to monitor glucose levels and administer medication
- Dietitian, who assists the patent and family with meal planning and monitoring of the diet plan
- Home health nurse, who assesses the patient's progress, continues the teaching plan of other members of the care team, and administers direct care based on the patient's needs
- Social worker, who helps the family find financial resources and other services in the community
- Psychologist or counselor, who helps the patient and family cope with the effects of a chronic disease and the care needed

Collaboration among these professionals is mandatory to provide treatment, education, and care assistance to the patient and family on a continual or intermittent basis, as needed.

NURSING PROCESS
Diabetes Mellitus

Assessment

Nursing assessment of the patient with diabetes mellitus is based on the type of diabetes the patient has, the duration of the disease, the frequency of acute complications, and the presence of long-term degenerative changes. Assessment includes a complete history and physical assessment, as presented in Table 28–9. The history identifies factors that affect glucose levels, such as dietary and exercise habits, whether the patient takes insulin or oral antidiabetic agents, and the patient's level of knowledge and compliance in managing the disease. The physical assessment confirms physical changes in the multiple body systems affected by diabetes mellitus.

Because diabetes requires self-management, it is important to assess the patient's readiness, willingness, and ability to learn the self-care regimen. Newly diagnosed patients may not be ready to learn yet because of feelings of loss associated with loss of freedom and loss of control over their lives. These feelings indicate a grieving process. The patient may show anxiety, fear, denial, anger, and depression before accepting the disease. Some patients never accept the disease and may fluctuate among these stages throughout life.

Patients who are not newly diagnosed are assessed for assimilation of diabetes management practices into their lifestyle. During your interview, explore aspects of the diabetic treatment plan that have been easy for the patient to assimilate versus those that have been more difficult. For example, the patient who works through the stages of grief and accepts responsibility for self-care by making lifestyle changes, who keeps abreast of new information, and who self-monitors blood glucose levels has coped well. The patient who has not progressed through the grief process and does not take respon-

Table 28–9

Nursing Guidelines for Assessing a Patient with Diabetes Mellitus

Assessment Item	Special Considerations
PATIENT HISTORY	
Duration of diabetes	Ask the patient when the diabetes diagnosis was made.
Reason for admission or appointment	Ask the patient to describe the reason in detail for seeking care.
Patient's diet	Ask the patient to write down from memory everything eaten for the previous 2 days to determine whether patient understands and complies with a previously taught diet.
Insulin therapy	If the patient has been administering insulin at home, observe patient prepare and administer insulin in the hospital. Ask the patient to state the name and dose of the insulin and time taken and to describe its action according to onset, peak, and duration.
Antidiabetic oral agents	If the patient takes oral antidiabetic agents, ask the patient to state the name of the agent. Ask patient whether he or she knows the difference between insulin and oral antidiabetic agents.
Self–blood glucose monitoring	If the patient has been doing this procedure at home, observe while it is performed. Ask the patient to describe how he or she interprets the results.
Knowledge of acute complications	Ask the patient to state the causes, symptoms, and treatment of hypoglycemia, hyperglycemia, and ketoacidosis.
Knowledge of sick-day management	Ask the patient to describe how he or she manages sick days regarding diet and medication. Determine whether patient understands implications of illness, especially infection, nausea and vomiting, and diarrhea.
Foot-care routine	Ask the patient to describe how he or she takes care of the feet. Determine whether patient understands implications of foot-care problems.
Exercise	Determine whether the patient leads a sedentary or active lifestyle and whether he or she understands the effects of exercise on blood glucose levels.
Basic physiology of diabetes	Ask the patient to explain what diabetes is and how it affects the body.
Long-term degenerative changes	Ask the patient to list the long-term changes that can occur with diabetes and how to delay their onset.
Personal history	Find out whether patient lives alone or with others; lifestyle, including occupation, hobbies, and weekend activities; whether patient receives social assistance; and whether there is a family history of diabetes.
Diabetic identification	Ask to see the diabetic identification the patient wears or carries.
PHYSICAL EXAMINATION	
Infections	Assess for the presence or history of *Candida albicans* in the groin, the axillae, and under the breasts, and of vaginal yeast infections in females. Assess for urinary tract infections.
Diabetic dermopathy	Examine the tibial area for the presence of "shin spots," known as diabetic dermopathy, and for necrobiosis, which is characterized by raised reddened lesions with sharply defined borders.
Xanthomas	Examine the elbows and knees for xanthomas, which are yellow fat deposits.
Lipodystrophy	Examine insulin injection sites for the presence of lipodystrophy.
Foot and leg problems	Examine the feet and legs for sores, blisters, reddened areas, or ulcers. Examine the toenails to see whether they are thick and hard to cut. Palpate the dorsalis pedis and posterior tibial pulse. Examine the dorsal part of the foot for hair loss. Palpate ankles for edema.
Physical condition	Assess weight, blood pressure, and pulse. Assess for symptoms of cardiovascular disease—dyspnea, irregular apical or brachial pulse, dependent edema, orthostatic hypotension. Examine hands for sores, burns, or muscle atrophy. Assess for gastrointestinal disturbances, such as diarrhea, especially at night. Assess for impotence or other reproductive problems. Assess for loss of sensation in extremities.

sibility for self-care needs assistance in exploring what has not been accomplished and in developing ways to make these accomplishments a reality.

Assessment also includes determination of the patient's desire and ability to learn. Ask about prior health care experiences the patient has had with diabetes, what the patient wants to learn, the most immediate concern for learning, the patient's level of formal education and reading ability, and the patient's goals. For patient teaching to be successful, the teaching plan must be centered around the patient's needs. For example, if the patient wants to learn how to prepare and administer insulin, the nurse should begin teaching this first. If the patient cannot read, teaching methods must include the use of audio-visuals and discussion rather than printed material.

Assessment of the diabetic patient also includes identifying available support systems, such as the family and significant others. It is advisable to include these persons in the patient teaching process because personal relationships are sometimes affected by the disease.

Nursing assessment of the diabetic patient also includes a physical assessment. Diabetes affects every system in the body. Therefore, the skin, mouth, eyes, and cardiovascular, peripheral vascular, renal, and neurologic systems should be assessed.

Nursing Diagnoses and Planning

Nursing diagnoses and related patient outcomes commonly applicable to patients with diabetes mellitus include the following:

NDx: Anticipatory grieving related to loss of freedom and required changes in lifestyle

Planning: Patient Outcomes
1. Patient verbalizes negative feelings about diabetes, such as anger, fear, and depression.
2. Patient verbalizes questions and concerns.
3. Patient states desire to participate in self-care activities.

NDx: Ineffective individual coping related to realization that diabetes is a chronic condition requiring life-long self-management, medical supervision, and lifestyle changes to prevent long-term degenerative changes

Planning: Patient Outcomes
1. Patient verbalizes perception of disease, benefits of care, and barriers to care.
2. Patient identifies coping patterns and personal strengths to promote effective coping.
3. Patient demonstrates a desire to participate in learning and self-care activities.
4. Patient identifies individual stressors.
5. Patient participates in developing a realistic plan for incorporating changes into lifestyle using appropriate problem-solving techniques.

6. Patient recognizes and uses available support systems.

NDx: Fluid volume deficit related to loss of fluids associated with diarrhea, vomiting, and osmotic diuresis from hyperglycemia

Planning: Patient Outcomes
1. Patient maintains adequate intake of fluids and electrolytes as evidenced by the following:
   Normal skin turgor
   Moist mucous membranes
   Blood pressure and pulse within patient's normal range
   Balanced intake and output
   Urine specific gravity between 1.010 and 1.030
   Normal serum sodium, chloride, magnesium, phosphorus, and potassium levels
   Absence of nausea, vomiting, and diarrhea

NDx: Altered peripheral tissue perfusion related to degenerative vascular changes of diabetes

Planning: Patient Outcomes
1. Patient maintains adequate systemic tissue perfusion as evidenced by the following:
   Blood pressure and pulse within patient's normal range
   Palpable peripheral pulses
   Skin warm and of normal color
   Capillary refill time of less than 3 seconds
   Urine output greater than 30 mL/h
   Verbalization of increased sensation and decreased tingling and numbness in extremities
   Decreased edema in extremities
   Verbalization of increased comfort
   Maintenance of skin integrity

NDx: Risk for injury related to muscle weakness and atrophy, sensory and motor loss secondary to peripheral neuropathy, and symptoms of hypoglycemic insulin reactions

Planning: Patient Outcomes
1. Patient identifies factors that increase the potential for trauma.
2. Patient verbalizes desire to practice measures that prevent trauma.
3. Patient maintains glucose levels below 140 mg/dL, or within target range set by physician, to prevent or delay the onset of degenerative changes.
4. Patient employs measures to prevent onset of hypoglycemic insulin reactions.

NDx: Risk for altered health maintenance related to lack of knowledge of self-care activities

Planning: Patient Outcomes
1. Patient verbalizes a basic understanding of the pathophysiology of diabetes.
2. Patient verbalizes an understanding of prescribed medication, including action, dose, side effects, and schedule of administration.

3. Patient demonstrates the ability to prepare and administer insulin correctly.
4. Patient verbalizes an understanding of the prescribed diet and use of exchange lists.
5. Patient demonstrates the ability to perform blood glucose and urine tests correctly and interpret results.
6. Patient verbalizes the causes, symptoms, and treatment for hypoglycemia and hyperglycemia.
7. Patient verbalizes an understanding of proper foot care routine.
8. Patient describes ways to incorporate the treatment plan into his or her lifestyle.
9. Patient identifies available support systems.

INTERNET CONNECTIONS

Diabetes Mellitus

The National Institute of Diabetes and Digestive and Kidney Diseases of the National Institutes of Health
http://www.niddk.nih.gov/DiabetesDocs.html
This authoritative U.S.-government-sponsored site provides up-to-date information for the public, patients, health educators, and health-care providers about diabetes, as well as links to sites addressing a wide variety of other diseases.

American Diabetes Association
http://www.diabetes.org/
This site provides information for both patients and health professionals. It includes information about professional educational programs and meetings as well as patient-oriented information, including nutritionally appropriate recipes.

Doctor's Guide to Diabetes Information and Resources
http://www.pslgroup.com/DIABETES.htm
Oriented specifically to health professionals, this site provides medical news and alerts, general disease and drug information, discussion groups, and links to other sites.

The Diabetes Homepage
http://www.nd.edu~hhowisen/diabetes.html
A popular site among patients with diabetes, The Diabetes Homepage provides general information about diabetes, travel tips, and personal stories. It also offers information on self-management, diabetes-related organizations, current research, books, and software, including virtual-reality games. This site also provides answers to frequently asked questions, as well as access to chat rooms.

Nursing Interventions and Evaluation

Nursing care of the patient with diabetes mellitus includes maintaining near-normal blood glucose levels, preventing acute complications and long-term degenerative changes, and teaching the patient how to manage the disease at home. Nursing interventions depend on the acuity of the patient's condition, the duration of the disease, the type of diabetes, the reason for admission to the hospital (if hospitalized), the presence of long-term degenerative changes, and the patient's level of knowledge of the disease.

NDx: Anticipatory grieving

An analogy to the stages of the grieving process can be made to the stages the diabetic patient goes through before accepting the disease. First, determine the patient's perception of the disease and its impact on the future. The patient may have misunderstandings about diabetes or may believe myths that need to be corrected. Give the patient time to work through the stages of grief by promoting trust, providing a supportive atmosphere of care and concern, and using therapeutic communication to encourage expression of feelings. The stage of denial can be prolonged, especially because manifestations of illness may not by immediately apparent upon diagnosis. It is possible for a patient to have diabetes for years and have no physical symptoms. It can be difficult for these patients to understand why they must follow a diabetic regimen.

NDx: Ineffective individual coping

Patients unable to cope effectively with diabetes may fear the onset of long-term degenerative changes as well as the changes in lifestyle needed to manage a chronic disease. Signs of poor coping ability are sleep disturbances, fatigue, inability to concentrate, inability to solve problems, and verbalization of inability to cope.

The patient may be anxious about learning new information needed to provide self-care, as well as the ability to incorporate a new routine into daily lives. Nursing interventions to help the patient cope effectively include identifying the patient's strengths and limitations and encouraging the patient to participate in self-care learning activities. Assist the patient in identifying stressors and in using problem-solving techniques.

Patient teaching and allowing the patient to set goals for self-care give the patient a sense of control and help avoid crisis situations. Individualize teaching at the patient's level of understanding, and provide ample opportunities for the patient to verbalize and demonstrate the acquired knowledge and skills. Review strategies for dealing with anxiety-provoking situations by role-playing and visualizing anticipated events.

Arrange a meeting with other diabetic patients who have coped successfully, and encourage the patient to use available support systems to promote successful coping. Provide information on the American Diabetes Association and local community support groups for diabetics. Initiate a social service referral if appropriate.

NDx: Fluid volume deficit

Determine the causative factors leading to hyperglycemia and fluid volume deficit, and the degree of the deficit. Monitor for the clinical manifestations of dehydration, which include decreased or poor skin turgor, dry mucous membranes, thirst, low blood pressure, weak and rapid pulse, and urine output less than intake with a specific gravity higher than 1.030 (not useful if the patient has diabetic nephropathy).

If nausea and vomiting related to ketoacidosis are the causative factors, the metabolic acidosis is treated. Monitor blood glucose levels, administer insulin, maintain a fluid intake of at least 2500 mL/day as tolerated, and administer intravenous fluids and electrolyte replacement as prescribed. Encourage the patient to take slow, deep breaths. Provide oral hygiene after each emesis to reduce nausea and vomiting.

Observe the patient for electrolyte depletion. Report abnormal laboratory results to the physician. When the patient first has a fluid volume deficit, serum potassium levels are normal as potassium leaves the cell. However, potassium levels can fall when insulin is administered and blood glucose levels start to return to normal, because insulin enhances the movement of potassium back into the cells. Hypokalemia can cause cardiac dysrhythmias and death; therefore, it is extremely important to begin potassium replacement within 2 hours after starting insulin. In addition, if the patient is receiving sodium bicarbonate, additional potassium should be given, because bicarbonate can aggravate hypokalemia by promoting movement of potassium back into the cells.

Once the patient is stabilized, discuss the events that led to hyperglycemia and fluid volume deficit to identify actions the patient could take to avoid recurrence.

NDx: Altered peripheral tissue perfusion

Monitor for the manifestations of altered tissue perfusion daily. These include the following:

- Significant decrease in blood pressure
- Resting pulse of more than 100 beats per minute
- Decrease in systolic blood pressure of at least 15 mm Hg with a simultaneous increase in pulse when the patient changes from a lying to a sitting or standing position
- Rapid or labored respirations
- Delayed return of color to feet and lower legs when legs are returned to a dependent position after being elevated for 1 minute
- Dusky red color of lower legs and feet when in a dependent position

- Diminished or absent peripheral pulses
- Capillary refill time of more than 3 seconds
- Urine output of less than 30 mL/h
- Elevated blood urea nitrogen and serum creatinine levels

Consult with the physician to determine the severity of perfusion impairment indicated by these manifestations or if they become more severe.

Nursing interventions also include actions to maintain adequate tissue perfusion. Promote improved circulation in the lower extremities by having the patient perform active foot and leg exercises for 10 minutes every 2 hours. Alternate short periods of slow walking with periods of rest. Instruct the patient to avoid crossing the legs, wearing constricting hose, elevating the knees by the use of a knee gatch or pillows, or standing or sitting for long periods. Because exposure to cold causes vasoconstriction, keep the room warm and provide adequate clothing and blankets. Advise the patient to avoid foods high in fat and cholesterol to slow the progression of atherosclerosis. Discourage cigarette smoking, which causes vasoconstriction. Teach the patient the principles of self-care to prevent and monitor long-term degenerative changes, as well as which signs and symptoms to report to the physician after discharge.

NDx: Risk for injury

The diabetic patient with peripheral neuropathy may be unable to perceive movement or position of the extremities and may also have diminished reflexes, muscle weakness, and atrophy. These patients could injure their extremities and not feel the injury, which can ultimately lead to ulcerations, infection, and amputation. Patient instructions in a daily foot care routine that includes inspection of the feet for sores or reddened areas are summarized in Highlight 28–5.

Nursing interventions also include teaching the patient how to avoid hypoglycemic insulin reactions and how to treat them if they occur. Insulin reactions usually occur suddenly. The symptoms progress rapidly from tremors, shaking, sweating, and dizziness to more severe symptoms of irritability, confusion, impaired judgment, unresponsiveness, unconsciousness, and convulsions. Instruct the diabetic patient to have a simple carbohydrate snack always available to eat if symptoms occur. Delaying the initial treatment of an insulin reaction increases the risk for severe symptoms and the potential for injury to the patient.

NDx: Risk for altered health maintenance

Because diabetes requires lifelong self-care, patient teaching is an integral nursing intervention. After an initial assessment to determine the patient's level of knowledge, develop a teaching plan based on the patient's individual needs (see Nursing Care Guide 28–1).

PALPITATIONS, DIAPHORESIS, PALLOR, AND ANXIETY IN A DIABETIC PATIENT

At 5:30 AM a 34-year-old man with a medical history of type 1 diabetes mellitus was brought to the emergency department by his brother. His clinical manifestations included fever, dehydration, Kussmaul's respirations, and a blood glucose level of 720 mg/dL. He was admitted with a medical diagnosis of diabetic ketoacidosis. Treatment with intravenous (IV) fluids, IV insulin, and electrolyte replacement was initiated and he was transferred to the medical unit.

After the patient was stabilized, my nursing interview and history revealed that he was "depressed" about his recent separation from his wife. He had been sick with the "flu" for the past 3 days but was too busy to seek medical advice early in the course of his illness. Because he was unable to eat, he had skipped his insulin injections for 24 hours before admission for fear of a hypoglycemic reaction.

By 6 PM, his blood glucose levels had fallen to 250 mg/dL. His acidosis was corrected, the IV insulin was reduced, and 5% dextrose was added to the IV fluid. At 8 PM, subcutaneous insulin therapy was initiated and the IV fluid replacement and IV insulin were discontinued. The patient was served dinner, of which he ate about half, and a bedtime snack, which he refused.

When I checked on the patient at midnight, he was sitting up in bed. He said that he had just awakened from a bad dream and that his heart was racing. He appeared anxious and his skin was pale, cool, and clammy.

The patient's signs and symptoms (palpitations, diaphoresis, pallor, and anxiety) represented an acute change in his health status. They could have indicated a number of cardiovascular and metabolic clinical conditions, including parathyroid and thyroid disorders, as well as hypoglycemia. Because these conditions—all potentially dangerous—require different interventions, I continued my assessment.

The patient was alert and responded promptly to my questions. He denied any chest pain, difficulty breathing, or headache. His peripheral pulses were strong. His heart rate was 118 bpm and regular. Respirations were 26 per minute and shallow. Blood pressure was 120/74 mm Hg. Temperature was 38.2°C (100.8°F). I noted some trembling of his hands and increasing anxiety.

Based on his clinical picture, his recent treatment for diabetic ketoacidosis, and his inadequate food intake, I suspected that the patient was having a hypoglycemic reaction. Because hypoglycemia is a life-threatening situation that can quickly deteriorate to loss of consciousness, seizures, coma, and death, I knew I had to respond quickly. I

decided, however, that because the patient was fully alert and responsive, I had time to test his blood glucose level with a blood glucose meter before performing additional nursing actions. The results revealed a blood glucose level of 190 mg/dL. Although my interpretation of his clinical picture did not correlate with this finding, I continued to suspect hypoglycemia (secondary to a rapid drop in the blood glucose level) and therefore immediately implemented the following actions:

1. I summoned another staff member and requested that orange juice and emergency equipment be brought to the bedside.
2. I notified the physician, who ordered a venous blood glucose specimen and serum electrolytes.
3. I gave the patient 4 ounces of orange juice, which he drank.
4. I supported the patient by remaining with him and explaining what was happening to him.
5. I continued to monitor the patient and repeated the fingerstick blood glucose in 10 minutes.
6. I documented my findings and actions.

The patient remained alert and, within minutes, his signs and symptoms began to subside. No further orange juice was offered. Twenty minutes after the episode, his skin was warm and dry and his heart rate had returned to 94 bpm. He said he felt much better. He ate a complex carbohydrate and protein snack. This positive response to treatment confirmed my suspicion of hypoglycemia. Early recognition and appropriate treatment of this medical emergency prevented the possibility of permanent neurologic damage and death.

Think Critically

What actions might have been taken by the nurse if the patient had been difficult to rouse and incoherent at midnight? What interventions would be implemented if a similar scenario occurred at home?

Was the administration of an oral carbohydrate the best action? Should the nurse have postponed the fingerstick until after the patient drank the juice?

What actions should the nurse have taken if the patient did not respond to the orange juice? If the patient had lost consciousness?

How might the hypoglycemic episode in this scenario have been prevented? What additional nursing actions might have been taken?

Why are some patients treated for hypoglycemia before confirmation of this medical condition?

What patient teaching is required to prevent a recurrence of this admission scenario? What assessments and patient needs (in addition to learning needs) must be determined by the nurse?

Compare the patient's status with the expected outcomes. If the outcomes are not met, reassess the patient and revise the plan.

The Elderly: Special Considerations

Seven percent of men and 9% of women over age 65 have diabetes mellitus. The incidence of diabetes increases to 10% of men and 20% of women over age 80. Almost half of elderly diabetic patients can be managed by diet alone; 30% require insulin at some time, and 20 to 25% can be treated with a combination of diet and oral antidiabetic agents.

Glucose tolerance declines with increasing age as blood glucose levels tend to increase. The mean blood glucose level 1 hour after ingesting 50 g of oral glucose in a 75-year-old person is 166 mg/dL, in contrast with 100 mg/dL for a person in the late teens or early twenties. Both the criteria for diagnosing diabetes mellitus and medical management of the disease in the elderly differ from those of younger and middle-aged adult patients. In addition, signs and symptoms of diabetes are often altered or subtle in the elderly. It is important to take these age-related changes into account during screening for diabetes.

Diabetes mellitus in the elderly is diagnosed when the fasting plasma glucose level equals or exceeds 140 mg/dL on more than one occasion, or if—2 hours after ingesting up to 75 g of glucose—the plasma glucose level is higher than 200 mg/dL and one other glucose level is higher than 200 mg/dL during the 2-hour oral glucose tolerance test.

Therapy is focused on avoiding hypoglycemia and symptomatic hyperglycemia. Management is individualized to meet the needs of each patient. The patient's lifestyle and health care needs must be considered. In planning care for the elderly diabetic patient, carefully assess for special needs associated with altered function, such as poor vision, hearing loss, mental changes, and decreased manual dexterity. These factors can affect the person's self-care ability.

Because decreased secretion of counter-regulatory hormones places the elderly diabetic patient at risk for hypoglycemia, the advantage of tight control to delay the onset of long-term degenerative changes is questionable. However, most clinicians agree that the problems associated with cataracts, neuropathy, and infection can be decreased by maintaining blood glucose levels below 200 mg/dL in the elderly.

Initially, diet therapy may be the only treatment tried for the newly diagnosed elderly patient, as long as blood glucose levels are below 300 mg/dL and the person is not hyperosmolar. The diabetic regimen is aimed at imposing minimal restrictions and changes on the person's lifestyle. It is important to emphasize the value of eating nutritious meals regularly. Diet therapy is usually aimed at reducing calories, but older people with diabetes may be consuming too few, rather than too many, calories.

Therefore, consider involving a family member or friend in meal planning to ensure adequate and healthy food intake. Also consider referring the elderly diabetic patient for home-delivered meals or community meal programs. The usual diabetic diet consists of 60 to 70% carbohydrate, 15 to 20% protein, and 20% fat. The patient taking medication for diabetes is cautioned about fasting for religious or other reasons because of the risk of hypoglycemia.

When insulin is the preferred treatment modality, consideration must be given to the person's ability to prepare the insulin accurately, to monitor effects, and to comply with the diet. One or two injections of intermediate-acting insulin or a premixed combination of short-acting and intermediate-acting insulin may be prescribed for use before breakfast and supper. In prescribing insulin, the goal is to keep the patient asymptomatic and the blood glucose levels below 200 mg/dL. Because subcutaneous fat decreases in the elderly, it is most important to rotate injection sites. A syringe magnifier can be obtained for visually impaired diabetics to ensure accuracy in preparing insulin injections.

Oral antidiabetic agents or sulfonylureas are usually effective in patients who have a blood glucose level below 200 mg/dL. Before prescribing, the individual characteristics of these drugs have to be considered, with special attention paid to the needs of each patient. For example, tolazamide has a short half-life, which decreases the risk of hypoglycemia. However, it also has a mild diuretic effect, which may or may not be desirable, depending on such factors as risk for incontinence. Tolbutamide requires two or three daily doses, making compliance a potential problem. The risk of drug interaction is increased if the person takes additional medications, such as salicylates, furosemide, thiazide diuretics, and anticoagulants, which are known to interact with oral antidiabetic agents.

Second-generation sulfonylureas have advantages over first-generation sulfonylureas. Because glipizide is metabolized primarily in the liver, complications resulting from impaired renal function are decreased. Also, hypoglycemia and drug interactions are rare. These drugs are usually taken once a day on an empty stomach, and they are inexpensive.

New technology has made blood glucose testing at home easier. People who have difficulty managing the testing procedure may need assistance from caregivers or may need to use urine testing methods as an alternative. Medicare covers the cost of a blood glucose testing device and testing strips. Homebound patients may qualify for skilled nursing visits through a home-care agency for initial teaching. Encourage the patient to keep a written record of test results. Measurement of glycosylated hemoglobin (HbA_{1c}) several times a year gives an approximation of glucose control. A result of 10% is acceptable for an elderly diabetic patient.

Older adults with diabetes should be encouraged to obtain annual influenza and once-in-a-lifetime pneumonia immunizations. Also, because older people may have difficulty adhering to a regimen of daily foot care, semi-annual podiatric care is recommended. Medicare covers podiatry services for diabetic patients, including home visits for homebound patients. The elderly diabetic patient should be encouraged to wear diabetic identification.

Because proper management of diabetes depends on the patient's ability to learn the self-care routine, patient teaching is an important component of the treatment plan. An assessment of learning needs may be time-consuming, but it is essential in developing effective teaching strategies. The patient is taught whatever information is necessary to live safely with diabetes and maintain optimal wellness and quality of life. Verbal instructions are reinforced with clearly printed or large-type written instruction. Referrals should be considered for home care services and community resources, such as sight centers.

Chapter Review

1. How do insulin requirements change for the diabetic patient during illness? Why does this happen?
2. Describe how you would teach a diabetic patient to prepare and administer insulin.
3. A diabetic patient received a combination of Humulin R and Humulin N at 7:30 AM and had a hypoglycemic episode at 11:00 AM. In determining the cause of the hypoglycemia, what parameters would need to be investigated?
4. Your patient's fasting blood sugar before breakfast is 60 mg/dL. The physician ordered a daily dose of Humulin R 15 units and Humulin N 65 units. What action would you take regarding this order?
5. Your patient states that his fasting blood sugars in the morning are always above 200 mg/dL. He also tells you that, each evening, he takes Humulin N 50 units before dinner. Sometimes when he wakes up in the morning he finds his nightclothes and bed damp from perspiration, and he has a headache. What do you think is occurring? What action should be taken?
6. Describe how you would teach a diabetic patient a foot care routine. Why is it important for a diabetic patient to follow a foot care routine?
7. How would you determine that a newly diagnosed diabetic patient is ready to learn self-care?
8. What would you tell a diabetic patient who claims that his job and lifestyle prevent him from testing blood sugars and following a diet?
9. Describe the causes, symptoms, and treatment of hypoglycemia and hyperglycemia.
10. How does exercise affect blood glucose levels?

Bibliography

American Diabetes Association. Bedside blood glucose monitoring in hospitals. Diabetes Care 1995; 18(1):36.

American Diabetes Association. Gestational diabetes mellitus. Diabetes Care 1995; 18(1):24.

American Diabetes Association. Hospital admission guidelines for diabetes mellitus. Diabetes Care 1995; 18(1):35.

American Diabetes Association. National standards for diabetes self-management education programs. Diabetes Care 1995; 18(1):94.

American Diabetes Association. Nutrition recommendations and principles for people with diabetes mellitus. Diabetes Care 1995; 18(1):16.

American Diabetes Association. Office guide to diagnosis and classification of diabetes mellitus and other categories of glucose intolerance. Diabetes Care 1995; 18(1):4.

American Diabetes Association. Pancreas transplantation for patients with diabetes mellitus. Diabetes Care 1995; 18(1):37.

American Diabetes Association. Screening for diabetes. Diabetes Care 1995; 18(1):5.

American Diabetes Association. Standards of medical care for patients with diabetes mellitus. Diabetes Care 1995; 18(1):8.

American Diabetes Association. Third-party reimbursement for outpatient diabetes education and counseling. Diabetes Care 1995; 18(1):45.

American Diabetes Association. Urine glucose and ketone determinations. Diabetes Care 1995; 18(1):20.

Anderson RM, Fitzgerald JT, Oh MS. The relationship between diabetes-related attitudes and patients' self-reported adherence. Diabetes Educ 1993; 19(4):287.

Anderson S. 7 care tips for managing patients with diabetes. Am J Nurs 1994; 94(9):36.

Cirone N. Diabetes in the elderly. Part I: Unmasking a hidden disorder. Nursing 1996; 26(3):34.

Cirone N. Diabetes in the elderly. Part II: Finding the balance for drug therapy. Nursing 1996; 26(3):40.

Citron M. Why wait? Diabetes Forecast 1996; 49(2):34.

D'Eramo-Melkus G. Type II non-insulin dependent diabetes mellitus. Nurs Clin North Am 1993; 28(1):25.

Davis E, Ward L. Sick-day plan will reduce impact of minor illnesses. Diabetes in the News 1993; 12(1):20.

Deakins DA. Teaching elderly patients about diabetes. Am J Nurs 1994; 94(4):39.

Dinsmoor RS. The newest approaches to preventing diabetes. Diabetes Self-Management 1993; 10(3):6.

Dinsmoor RS. Hypoglycemia without warning. Diabetes Self-Management 1993; 10(2):6.

Doughty R. Beyond randomization: Study participants chart their futures. Living Well with Diabetes 1993; 8(4):10.

Dudley J. Glucose self-monitoring tells you how well you are doing. Diabetes in the News 1994; 13(4):20.

Eliopoulos C. Gerontological nursing. 3rd ed. Philadelphia: JB Lippincott, 1993.

Etzwiler DD. The treatment of diabetes will never be the same. Living Well with Diabetes 1993; 8(4):3.

Expert Committee on the Diagnosis and Classification of Diabetes Mellitus (American Diabetes Association). Report of the Expert Committee on the Diagnosis and Classification of Diabetes Mellitus. Diabetes Care. 1997; 20(7):1183.

Fain JA. National trends in diabetes. Nurs Clin North Am 1993; 28(1):1.

Fishman TD, Freedline AD, Kahn D. Putting the best foot forward. Nursing 1996; 26(1):58.

Funnel MM, Merritt JH. The challenges of diabetes and older adults. Nurs Clin North Am 1993; 28(1):45.

Goetz DR. How you can live with diagnosis of diabetes. Diabetes in the News 1994; 13(4):54.

Hamilton C. As lifestyle changes, so do nutrition needs. Diabetes in the News 1993; 12(1):46.

Hamilton C. Food is the key part of your diabetes control program. Diabetes in the News 1994; 13(4):9.

Hinnen D. Issues in diabetes education. Nurs Clin North Am 1993; 28(1):113.

Hirsch IB, Farkas-Hirsch R. Type 1 diabetes and insulin therapy. Nurs Clin North Am 1993; 28(1):9.

Holten J. The story behind the people behind the numbers. Living Well with Diabetes 1993; 8(4): 6.

Hornsby WG. Exercise keeps your body tuned up and helps control glucose levels. Diabetes in the News 1994; 13(4):15.

Hoyson PM. Oral medications. RN 1995; 58(5):34.

Kendall DM, Robertson RP. Pancreas transplantation in diabetes mellitus. Pract Diabetol 1993; 12(1):14.

Kestel F. Using blood glucose meters: What you and your patient need to know. Part I. Nursing 1993; 23(3):34.

Kestel F. Using blood glucose meters: What you and your patient need to know. Part II. Nursing 1993; 23(4):50.

Kestel F. Using blood glucose meters: What you and your patient need to know. Part III. Nursing 1993; 23(5):51.

Laux L. Visual interpretation of blood glucose test strips. Diabetes Educ 1994; 20(1):41.

Lee ET, Howard BV, Savage PJ, et al. Indian health service provider. INS Primary Care Provider 1995; 20(8):97.

Lorber DL. Complications of diabetes: Eye disease. Pract Diabetol 1993; 12(4):14.

Lorber DL. Complications of diabetes: Kidney disease. Pract Diabetol 1993; 12(1):18.

Lun WS. Use of oral hypoglycemic agents in the elderly. Pract Diabetol 1993; 12(4):10.

Lyon RB, Vinci DM. Nutrition management of insulin-dependent diabetes mellitus in adults: Review by the diabetes care and education dietetic practice group. J Am Diet Assoc 1993; 93(3):309.

Macheca MKK. Diabetic hypoglycemia: Keeping the threat at bay. Am J Nurs 1993; 93(4):26.

Martinez NC. Diabetes and minority populations. Nurs Clin North Am 1993; 28(1):87.

Maser RE, Bussard M, DeCherney DS. Monitoring glucose levels in hospitalized patients with diabetes mellitus. Pract Diabetol 1994; 13(3):7.

Pasmantier RM. Muscle cells' resistance to insulin may start decades before diagnosis of type 11. Diabetes in the News 1993; 12(2):14.

Peragallo-Dittko V. Acute complications. RN 1995; 58(8):36.

Puczynski S. Management of nocturnal hypoglycemia in IDDM. Pract Diabetol 1994; 13(3):2.

Raymond NR, D'Eramo-Melkus G. Non-insulin-dependent diabetes and obesity in the black and Hispanic population: Culturally sensitive management. Diabetes Educ 1993; 19(4):313.

Reising DL. Acute hyperglycemia: Putting a lid on the crisis. Nursing 1995; 25(2):33.

Reising DL. Acute hypoglycemia: Keeping the bottom from falling out. Nursing 1995; 25(2):41.

Rogacz S. Pancreas transplants: Today's cure for diabetes. Living Well with Diabetes 1993; 8(2):14.

Rubin RJ, Altman WM, Mendelson DN. Health care expenditures for people with diabetes mellitus 1992. J Clin Endocrinol Metabol 1994; 78(4):809A.

Scheffler NM. What you need to know and do to care for your feet. Diabetes in the News 1994; 13(4):44.

Schmidt LE, Rost KM, McGill JB, Santiago JV. The relationship between eating patterns and metabolic control in patients with non-insulin-dependent diabetes mellitus (NIDDM). Diabetes Educ 1994; 20(4):317.

Shapiro M, Stegall MD. When insulin isn't enough. RN 1995; 58(7):34.

Simon NR, Frishman WH. Diabetes mellitus in the elderly. Pract Diabetol 1993; 12(1):4.

Strowig SM. Initiation and management of insulin pump therapy. Diabetes Educ 1993; 19(1):50.

Strowig S. Insulin therapy. RN 1995; 58(6):30.

Taxel P, Abourizk NN. Oral agents can play key role in type II diabetes management. Diabetes in the News 1994; 13(4):26.

Thom AL. Nutritional management of diabetes. Nurs Clin North Am 1993; 28(1):97.

Walker EA. Quality assurance for blood glucose monitoring. Nurs Clin North Am 1993; 28(1):61.

Wierenga ME, Hewitt JB. Facilitating diabetes self-management. Diabetes Educ 1994; 20(2):138.

Willis J. Diabetes medical complications. Nursing Times 1995; 91(23):49.

Wilson JP. New diabetes nutrition guidelines. Do you know the score? Nursing 1995; 25(7):65.

Womack RB. Measuring the attitudes and beliefs of American Indian patients with diabetes. Diabetes Educ 1993; 19(3): 205.

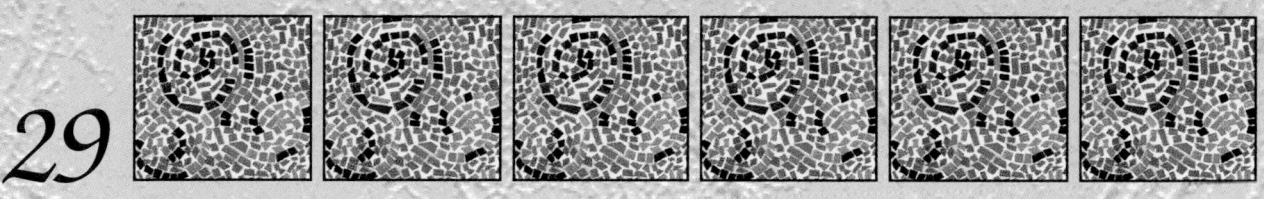

29

Nursing Care of Patients with Other Endocrine Disorders

Study Outcomes

After studying this chapter, you should be able to:

1. Explain the normal anatomy and physiology of the endocrine glands and related structures.
2. Describe the function of the pituitary, adrenal, thyroid, and parathyroid hormones.
3. Describe the etiology, pathophysiology, clinical manifestations, diagnostic procedures, and medical and surgical management of common endocrine disorders.
4. Identify information and physical examination data essential to the assessment of patients with common endocrine disorders.
5. State nursing diagnoses and related expected patient outcomes commonly applicable to patients with endocrine disorders.
6. Describe nursing interventions, with their rationales, commonly applicable to patients with endocrine gland disorders.
7. Explain the basis for evaluation of nursing care provided to patients with common endocrine gland disorders.
8. Identify alternative treatment and care settings for patients with endocrine disorders and the services related to community-based care.
9. Identify special considerations for the elderly patient with altered pituitary, adrenal, thyroid, or parathyroid function.

People who experience endocrine dysfunction are faced with systemic responses that require a plan of holistic care and treatment. Although the primary pathology may be localized to an organ or area, the effects are experienced throughout the body.

Therefore, the nurse must consider the entire person, including all body systems, when planning and implementing care.

Treatment settings vary based on the severity of the disorder, the type of interventions needed, the patient's response to those interventions, and the overall health-care delivery plan. Initial or mild manifestations usually are treated on an outpatient basis in a physician's office or clinic. Severe manifestations or those requiring surgery may involve admission to the hospital. For many patients, treatment happens primarily at home. Support from a visiting nurse and sound education can help the patient recover and adjust to the disorder. No matter where the patient with an endocrine disorder receives care, it is crucial that the patient receive comprehensive, collaborative care.

Pituitary Disorders

The pituitary gland is a vital link in the hypothalamus-pituitary-endocrine system that maintains homeostasis. Pituitary disorders involve a deficiency or excess of one or more of the pituitary hormones. The result is altered function in target organs and tissues throughout the body.

ANTERIOR PITUITARY DISORDERS

Disorders of the anterior lobe of the pituitary gland can cause an alteration in the function of any one or all of the secretory cell types. Altered function of the secretory cells can result in hyposecretion or hypersecretion of one or more anterior pituitary hormones.

Neoplasia

Etiology and Pathophysiology
Pituitary tumors are the most common cause of primary anterior pituitary disorders. Although pituitary tumors can develop at any age, they are most common in adults. They are equally distributed between men and women. Their etiologic factors are unclear.

Pituitary tumors are usually benign, secreting adenomas that arise from one cell type and produce clinical manifestations of hypersecretion of one or two pituitary hormones. Manifestations may also include neurologic signs and symptoms as the expanding pituitary mass presses on adjacent tissues and blood vessels. Pituitary adenomas account for 6 to 18% of all intracranial tumors. Rarely are they malignant.

Clinical Manifestations

Typically, a person with a pituitary adenoma seeks medical attention because of neurologic manifestations.

Neurologic Manifestations

The most common manifestation of pituitary adenoma is headache. It recurs frequently and is unrelated to stress or other apparent physiologic or psychologic factors.

Visual disturbances are the second most common neurologic manifestation. As illustrated in Figure 29–1, expansion of the pituitary mass may press on or displace the optic chiasm and optic nerve. Loss of vision in the lateral portions of both visual fields (bitemporal hemianopia) with no change in visual acuity is the most common visual disturbance.

Other neurologic manifestations are rare but may include vascular disturbances and involvement of the cranial nerves.

Endocrine Manifestations

The most common pituitary adenomas arise from lactotrope and somatotrope cells. They are discussed later in the chapter. Adenomas of corticotrope cells are less common. Those of thyrotrope and gonadotrope cells are rare.

Hypersecretion of a pituitary hormone caused by a secreting adenoma causes increased secretion from the hormone's target gland. For this reason, any person with clinical manifestations of hypersecretion from an endocrine gland controlled by the anterior pituitary must be evaluated for pituitary adenoma.

Diagnosis

Medical diagnosis of a pituitary tumor is based on the patient's history, clinical manifestations, radiologic studies, and determination of serum hormone levels. Pituitary hormone levels are elevated in the presence of a secreting pituitary adenoma. Other possible causes of endocrine dysfunction, such as stress or side effects of medications, must be ruled out before confirming a diagnosis of pituitary tumor.

Management

The primary treatment for pituitary tumor is surgical excision and irradiation. Tumors of lactotrope and somatotrope cells may respond to bromocriptine (Parlodel).

Transsphenoidal Microsurgery

Transsphenoidal microsurgery is the procedure of choice for excision of a pituitary adenoma. It removes the tumor while preserving as much normal pituitary tissue as possible. If the entire pituitary gland is removed by the transsphenoidal approach, the surgery is called a total transsphenoidal hypophysectomy.

In transsphenoidal microsurgery through the mouth, an incision is made at the junction of the gums and upper lip. A surgical microscope is then advanced along the floor of the nasal passage, through the sphenoid sinus, and into the base of the sella turcica (Fig. 29–2). Special microsurgical instruments are used to incise the dura mater and to identify and remove the abnormal tissue. This surgery can also be done through the nose. This may be less traumatic for the patient and may reduce healing time. Destruction of the abnormal tissue by laser is under investigation.

To prevent leakage of cerebrospinal fluid (CSF) after surgery, the dura mater may be patched with a piece of fascia or muscle taken from the leg. The

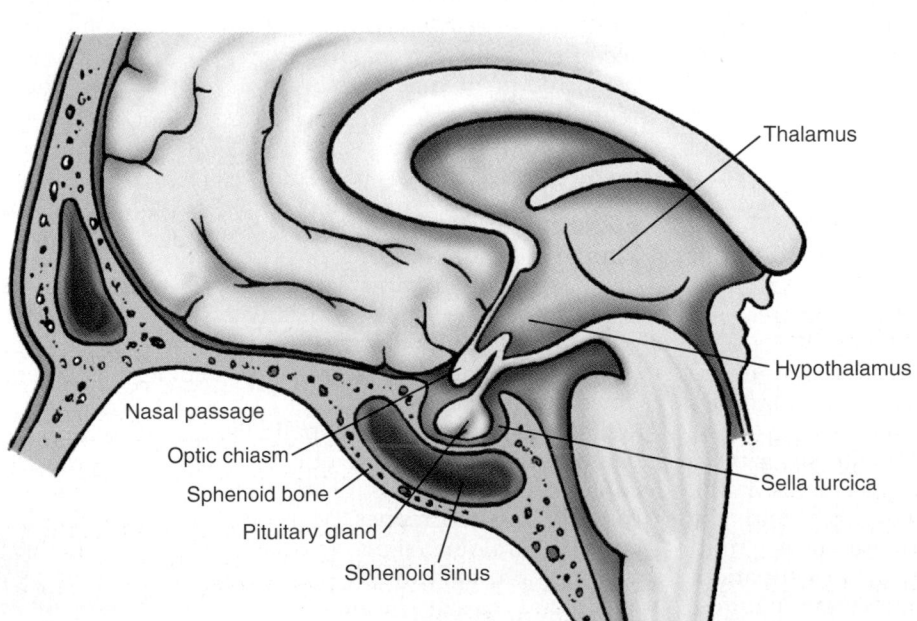

Figure 29–1

Anatomical relationship of the pituitary gland and the optic chiasm.

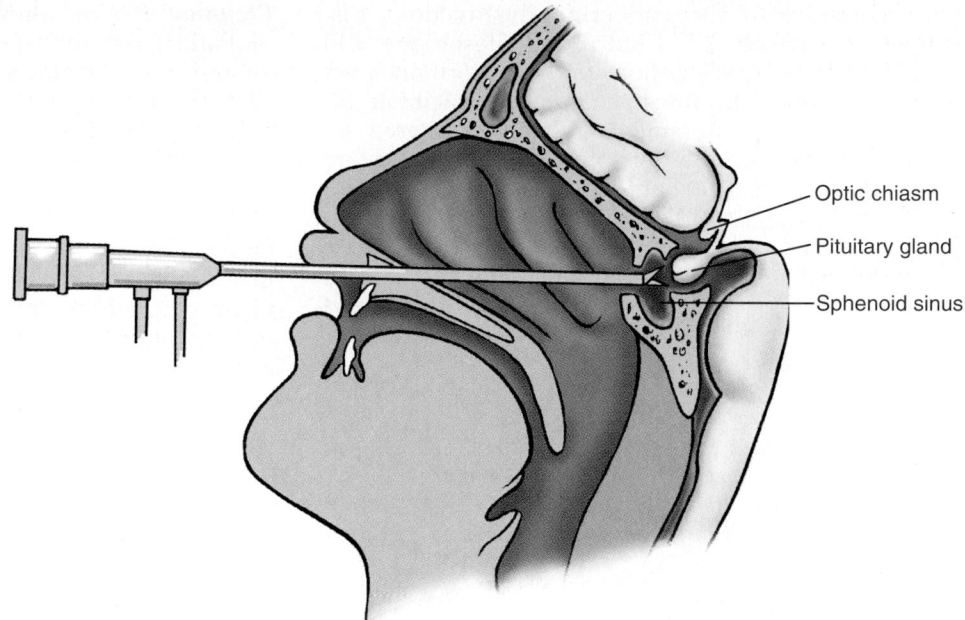

Figure 29–2

Placement of a surgical microscope for transsphenoidal microsurgery.

nose is packed, and a gauze dressing or sling is worn under the nose to absorb drainage and keep the packing in place.

Excision of pituitary adenomas by transsphenoidal microsurgery has a success rate of 70 to 90%. The most common complication is temporary diabetes insipidus (discussed later in this chapter) caused by surgical trauma to the posterior pituitary. Because prophylactic antibiotics are used, meningitis is rare. If a total hypophysectomy is performed, or if normal pituitary tissue is damaged, panhypopituitarism will develop.

The patient will require lifelong hormone replacement therapy because of the absence of adrenocorticotropic hormone, thyrotropin, and the gonadotropins.

Transfrontal Craniotomy

If the pituitary adenoma has spread beyond the sella turcica, a total hypophysectomy is performed using a transfrontal craniotomy approach. Preoperative and postoperative care of a patient undergoing a craniotomy procedure is similar to that of a patient who has undergone transsphenoidal surgery, with specific modifications because the procedure is more invasive.

Irradiation

Treatment of a pituitary adenoma by external radiation is an alternative to surgery in some cases. Successful reduction of tumor size and neurologic manifestations is similar to that achieved through microsurgery. However, reduction in hormone levels is not as rapid. It may take up to 2 years for hormone levels to return to normal.

Stereotactic radiosurgery uses high-energy, pencil-thin beams of external radiation from a linear accelerator to destroy tumor tissue. Its application in the treatment of pituitary tumors is under investigation.

Implantation of radioactive isotopes is seldom performed because of advances in treatment by microsurgery and external radiation, and because of the risk of meningitis and chronic rhinorrhea after the implantation procedure.

NURSING PROCESS
Pituitary Neoplasms

PREOPERATIVE NURSING CARE

Assessment

When obtaining the nursing history, first determine what clinical manifestations are present. If headaches are a problem, ask the patient to describe them and to point to the areas of the head involved. Determine when the headaches first began, how often they occur, what precipitates them, and what relieves them.

If the patient reports visual changes, ask when they first became noticeable. Assess visual acuity and fields even if the patient does not complain of visual disturbance. Because visual changes associated with a pituitary tumor develop very gradually, many people are not aware that their vision has changed.

Assess the patient's knowledge of what might be causing the neurologic symptoms. Remember that neurologic problems are very frightening and apt to be misunderstood.

Assessment of a patient with a suspected pituitary adenoma should include investigation of alterations common to the endocrine dysfunctions discussed in Chapter 27. Clinical manifestations will vary with the specific hormone or hormones affected. Document findings accurately to facilitate diagnosis. Nursing assessments related to altered secretion of specific anterior pituitary hormones are discussed later in this chapter.

While conducting the patient history, allay preoperative and postoperative anxiety. Determine what the patient knows about the surgery, as well as his or her expectations of the postoperative recovery period.

Nursing Diagnoses and Planning

Nursing diagnoses and related expected patient outcomes commonly applicable to patients with a pituitary tumor include the following:

NDx: Risk for trauma related to loss of peripheral vision

Planning: Patient Outcomes
 1. Patient accurately states degree of peripheral vision loss.
 2. Patient identifies safety measures to avoid trauma.
 3. Patient remains free from injury.

NDx: Knowledge deficit: diagnosis and pathophysiology, diagnostic procedures, planned treatment, and expected outcome of treatment

Planning: Patient Outcomes
 1. Patient asks questions and verbalizes concerns.
 2. Patient correctly states diagnosis and is able to verbalize an understanding of the diagnosis.
 3. Patient identifies pressure from pituitary tumor as the cause of neurologic symptoms.
 4. Patient identifies altered secretion from pituitary tumor as the cause of endocrine manifestations.
 5. Patient verbalizes understanding of diagnostic procedures and cooperates in their accurate and timely completion.
 6. Patient identifies planned treatment and the reasons this treatment has been chosen.
 7. Patient verbalizes realistic expectations of treatment.

NDx: Risk for altered cerebral tissue perfusion related to increased intracranial pressure secondary to tumor growth or edema after surgery or irradiation

Planning: Patient Outcomes
 1. Patient remains oriented and alert or easily aroused.
 2. Urine output is less than 100 mL/hour.
 3. Vital signs and neurologic signs remain within normal limits.
 4. Patient avoids activities that increase intracranial pressure (ICP).

NDx: Risk for infection related to surgical incision of the dura mater, oral and nasal mucous membranes, and possibly the leg

Planning: Patient Outcomes
 1. Patient remains afebrile and free from headaches and nuchal rigidity.
 2. Oral and nasal mucous membranes and leg remain free from inflammation, swelling, and purulent drainage.

Nursing Interventions and Evaluation

Nursing care of a patient with a pituitary tumor includes maintaining the patient's safety, monitoring neurologic status, assessing changes in physiologic manifestations of endocrine function, and providing appropriate information and teaching. Changes in vital signs, neurologic signs, and visual fields may indicate growth or regression of the tumor and are reported to the physician promptly.

NDx: Risk for trauma
Assess visual fields and acuity to determine the extent of the loss. Orient the visually impaired patient to the surroundings. Maintain a safe environment to avoid injury. Explain how to use the call bell. Tell the patient to ask for help before getting out of bed if visual impairment is severe.

NDx: Knowledge deficit: diagnosis and pathophysiology, diagnostic procedures, planned treatment, and expected outcome of treatment
Provide ample opportunity for the patient to express thoughts and concerns about the physical changes that he or she is experiencing. Reinforce the physician's explanation of what is causing the symptoms. Use terms the patient can understand. Answer questions and correct any misconceptions about symptoms, diagnosis, and treatment. Refer questions you cannot answer to an appropriate resource.

During the diagnostic phase, assess the patient's ability to understand and cooperate with diagnostic procedures. Provide appropriate instruction and assistance to ensure timely and accurate collection of required specimens.

Discuss the planned procedure with the patient preoperatively. Correct any misconceptions or unrealistic expectations about the surgery or results. Even though excess hormone secretion will cease after surgery, and the patient will feel progressively better, some alterations caused by increased hormone levels may be permanent. These may include excess bone growth or altered cardiac function. Be sure to tell the patient if a piece of fascia or muscle will be removed from the leg. This way, the patient knows to expect a second surgical dressing.

NDx: Risk for altered cerebral tissue perfusion
In your preoperative teaching, tell the patient to avoid sneezing, coughing, bending, vigorous hair brushing, or any activity that could increase ICP after surgery. Increased ICP could lead to CSF leakage. Teach and have the patient practice deep-breathing exercises because they will be used postoperatively to ventilate the lungs and mobilize secretions. Postoperative coughing is prohibited.

Postoperatively, the patient usually feels relatively well, with discomfort similar to a headache. Low doses of narcotic analgesics are prescribed, if needed, for relief. Begin oral fluids as soon as the effects of anesthesia have worn off. Progress the diet as tolerated.

To reduce cerebral edema, elevate the head of the bed 30 degrees at all times. The patient may be positioned on one side or the other. Assess vital signs and neurologic signs to detect any increase in ICP from cerebral edema.

Frequently remind the patient to avoid any activity that may increase ICP. Have the patient take five deep breaths every 30 minutes to prevent pulmonary complications. If the patient becomes nauseated, administer antiemetics promptly because vomiting raises ICP.

Monitor intake and output to detect the onset of diabetes insipidus. Notify the physician promptly if output exceeds 100 mL/hour. Nursing care of the patient who has undergone transsphenoidal microsurgery for excision of a pituitary adenoma is summarized in Nursing Care Guide 29–1.

NDx: Risk for infection
Change the gauze sling or pad under the nose as it becomes soiled to remove a potential site for bacterial growth. Nasal packing is removed after 24 hours by the surgeon. The dura mater usually seals within 72 hours. During this time, assess for CSF leak, which is manifested by frequent swallowing or complaints of a postnasal drip. Test nasal drainage for glucose, which is present in CSF but not in normal nasal secretions. Assess for nuchal rigidity and persistent or severe headache, which warn of meningitis. Administer prophylactic antibiotics as prescribed.

Provide cool mist humidification if prescribed to prevent drying of the oral and nasal mucous membranes. Help the patient with frequent oral hygiene. Use mouthwash, a solution of hydrogen peroxide and saline, or a foam toothette to keep the incision site clean. Do not use a bristle toothbrush because it may injure the tissues. Assess mouth and leg incisions each shift for redness, edema, and inflammation.

Compare the patient's status with the expected outcomes. If the outcomes are not met, reassess the patient and revise the plan.

Hypersecretion of Somatotropin

Etiology and Pathophysiology
Excess secretion of somatotropin (growth hormone) is a rare condition. It can occur at any age, but it appears most commonly between the ages of 10 and 40. There is no clear sex, race, or family predisposition. A secreting benign adenoma of the somatotrope cells is the most common cause of excess somatotropin secretion. Recent studies have identified

excess secretion of growth hormone releasing hormone from the hypothalamus as a possible cause of somatotrope hyperplasia. In rare instances, idiopathic hyperplasia of the somatotrope cells is the cause.

Excess secretion of somatotropin affects all actively growing cells. If it occurs before the epiphyses close, gigantism develops with excess growth of the skeleton and soft tissues. If it occurs after the epiphyses close, acromegaly develops. This disorder is characterized by an increase in connective tissue, cartilage, and soft tissue, and by growth and thickening of the bones in the hands, feet, and face.

Excess somatotropin also alters glucose metabolism by impeding glucose uptake by the cells. This raises blood glucose levels. Somatotropin is therefore called an insulin antagonist. Secondary diabetes mellitus may develop from excess somatotropin secretion. Fat and protein metabolism is also altered, producing elevations in serum lipid levels. Urinary excretion of sodium, potassium, phosphorus, and chloride decreases in the presence of excess somatotropin, thereby increasing serum levels of these electrolytes and promoting fluid retention.

Clinical Manifestations
The onset of clinical manifestations is insidious. Manifestations include the neurologic manifestations of a pituitary tumor, persistent visual disturbances and headaches, and the endocrine manifestations of excess somatotropin secretion.

In acromegaly, changes in appearance occur so slowly that the disease often goes undetected for years. In retrospect, the person may remember a progressive increase in ring, shoe, hat, and glove sizes. A review of old photographs, such as those shown in Figure 29–3, will demonstrate a coarsening of features and thickening and enlargement of the lips. These effects result from increased growth of subcutaneous connective tissue.

Proliferation of cartilage causes enlargement of the ears and nose, increased circumference of the chest, and arthritic changes in the joints of the long bones and spine. Kyphosis is common. Muscle weakness, osteoporosis, and bowing of the long bones develop from altered protein metabolism and hypertrophy of the periosteum. Overgrowth of the maxilla results in prominent zygomatic arches. Mandibular growth produces prognathism (projection of the lower jaw) with wide spaces between the teeth. A forward slanting forehead results from growth of the supraorbital ridges. The hands and feet become wide and spadelike because of the increase in cartilage and radial growth of the bones.

Soft tissue growth is manifested by a deepening or hoarseness of the voice, thickened skin, increased sebum secretion, and enlargement of the tongue and abdominal viscera. Paresthesias may develop from entrapment of nerves by bony or soft tissue overgrowth. Diminished gonad function results in hirsutism, amenorrhea, and infertility in women and in

Patient Care After Transsphenoidal Microsurgery for Excision of a Pituitary Adenoma

Assessment Findings: Six hours after transsphenoidal microsurgery, a patient who was previously alert and oriented is now becoming restless and vague in response to questions. The patient complains of blurred vision but denies headache. Pupils react equally but sluggishly to light. Vital signs are stable.

Nursing Diagnosis: Altered cerebral tissue perfusion related to increased intracranial pressure (ICP) secondary to cerebral edema from surgical trauma

Patient Outcomes	Nursing Interventions	Rationale
Patient remains alert and oriented as evidenced by the following: Is alert or is easily aroused when asleep. Correctly identifies person, place, and a realistic time frame. Responds appropriately to questions.	Elevate head of bed 30 to 45 degrees. Patient may turn side to side. Provide rest periods. Administer prescribed humidified oxygen. Talk with patient while assessing vital signs and neurologic signs.	Elevation promotes venous drainage and reduces cerebral edema. Reduction in external stimuli promotes reduction in cerebral edema. Increases cerebral oxygenation. Deterioration in mental status is a manifestation of increasing cerebral edema.
Patient avoids activities that increase ICP.	Instruct the patient preoperatively and remind him or her postoperatively not to cough, sneeze, bend from the waist, pull or push with arms, hyperflex the neck, or brush hair vigorously. Before discharge, teach the patient to avoid for up to 2 months activities that will increase ICP.	These activities increase ICP. Avoid activities that increase ICP until the sphenoid sinus and sella turcica heal completely.
Patient is free from nausea and vomiting.	Instruct patient to advise nurse at first sign of nausea. Administer prescribed antiemetic promptly.	Vomiting increases ICP.
Patient is alert and oriented, pulse is 60–100 bpm, systolic blood pressure is within 10% of preoperative baseline, respirations are 16–20/min, urine output is less than 100 mL/h, strength in bilateral extremities is equal, and pupils react equally to light.	Monitor vital signs, urine output, and neurologic signs hourly for early signs of increased ICP: restlessness, lethargy, confusion, bradycardia, widening pulse pressure, vague headache, dilated pupils, diplopia, blurred vision, progressive muscle weakness, polyuria. Administer osmotic diuretics, steroids, or anticonvulsants if prescribed.	These manifestations indicate impaired cerebral blood flow, decreased tissue oxygenation, and increased pressure on vital brain centers. Early detection of increased ICP prevents cerebral anoxia and irreversible brain damage. Osmotic diuretics reduce cerebral edema. Steroids reduce inflammation of cerebral tissue. Anticonvulsants prevent seizure activity, which can increase cerebral edema and impair tissue oxygenation.

(continued)

Nursing Care Guide 29–1
Patient Care After Transsphenoidal Microsurgery for Excision of a Pituitary Adenoma (continued)

Evaluation: Compare the patient's status with the expected outcomes. If the outcomes are not met, reassess the patient and revise the plan.

Assessment Findings: Patient has a moderate amount of clear drainage from nasal packing and gauze dressing under the nose.

Nursing Diagnosis: Risk for infection related to surgical incision of the sella turcica and dura mater

Patient Outcomes	Nursing Interventions	Rationale
Patient is free of signs of cerebral spinal fluid (CSF) leak within 72 hours.	Assess for and ask patient about signs of CSF leak: frequent swallowing, sensation of postnasal drip, rapid saturation of gauze pad under nose with clear drainage.	These manifestations indicate leakage of CSF from the sella turcica through the surgical access tract into the posterior nasopharynx. This tract is a possible route for invasion of pathogenic organisms until the dura mater seals. The dura mater should seal within 72 hours.
	Test nasal drainage for glucose with a glucose reagent strip. Alternative assessment for CSF is to examine a drop of nasal drainage on a clean cloth or gauze for a pale yellow halo around the pink serosanguineous drainage.	Differentiates between CSF and serous drainage. Glucose is normally present in CSF but not in serous exudate.
Patient remains afebrile and free of nuchal rigidity.	Change dressing under the nose as it becomes moist or soiled.	Moist dressing provides medium for growth of pathogens.
	Assess for fever, nuchal rigidity, headache every 2–4 hours.	These are manifestations of meningitis.
	Administer prescribed prophylactic antibiotics.	Prevents meningitis.

Evaluation: Compare the patient's status with the expected outcomes. If the outcomes are not met, reassess the patient and revise the plan.

Assessment Findings: Patient has a surgical suture line at the junction of the gums and upper lip. Area is slightly edematous, tender, free from inflammation.

Nursing Diagnosis: Altered oral mucous membrane related to surgical incision and sutures

Patient Outcomes	Nursing Interventions	Rationale
Patient avoids mechanical trauma to suture line.	Instruct patient to use foam toothette and dental floss to remove debris from teeth until suture line heals.	Toothbrush with bristles may irritate suture line and delay healing.

(continued)

Nursing Care Guide 29–1

Patient Care After Transsphenoidal Microsurgery for Excision of a Pituitary Adenoma (continued)

Patient Outcomes	Nursing Interventions	Rationale
Patient rinses oral cavity every 2 hours while awake and after meals until suture line heals in 7–10 days.	Instruct patient to rinse mouth with a solution of equal amounts of hydrogen peroxide and warm water or saline every 2 hours while awake and after meals until suture line heals.	Aids in removal of wound exudate and food particles that can provide a medium for the growth of pathogens and also freshens the mouth.
Patient is free of signs of suture line infection.	Examine suture line and surrounding oral mucous membrane twice a day for increasing edema, tenderness, inflammation, and purulent drainage. Advise physician promptly if signs of infection are present.	Early detection and treatment of localized wound infection minimize the risk of delayed healing and meningitis.
Patient demonstrates ability to use a mirror to examine suture line for signs of infection.	If patient is discharged before suture line heals, teach patient to use a mirror to examine area for symptoms of infection just described.	Promotes independence and safety in management of therapeutic regimen. Demonstration provides opportunity to evaluate learning.
Patient states intent to notify physician if increasing edema, tenderness, inflammation, or purulent drainage occurs.	Instruct patient to notify physician promptly if signs of infection are present.	Ensures early detection and treatment of infection.

Evaluation: Compare the patient's status with the expected outcomes. If the outcomes are not met, reassess the patient and revise the plan.

impotence and sterility in men. Cardiomegaly develops from soft tissue changes in the myocardium and from the increased cardiac workload required by the large body mass. These cardiac changes—compounded by the pathologic effects of elevated blood glucose, lipid, and electrolyte levels—contribute to the development of hypertension, coronary atherosclerosis, and congestive heart failure. These lead to progressive heart failure and premature death.

In gigantism, linear growth progresses steadily until the child or adolescent reaches more than three standard deviations above the mean height for his or her age. Growth is symmetric and proportional. Eventually, the person may exceed 8 or 9 feet in height and 350 lbs in weight. Clinical manifestations related to altered metabolism are similar to those found in acromegaly. Muscle weakness, osteoporosis, and arthritic changes are common. Cardiac hypertrophy develops at an early age and leads to cardiac failure and premature death.

Diagnosis

Medical diagnosis of excess somatotropin secretion is based on history, clinical manifestations, old photographs if available, and elevated serum or plasma growth hormone levels. Blood glucose levels remain elevated above normal for more than 2 hours during an oral glucose tolerance test in the presence of altered glucose metabolism. Radiologic examination of the skull, computed tomographic (CT) scans, and magnetic resonance imaging (MRI) may also be used to visualize the tumor.

The most accurate measurement of excess serum or plasma growth hormone levels is by radioimmunoassay. For accurate results, the patient fasts for 8 to 10 hours and should be free of stress and at complete rest for 30 minutes before specimen collection.

Normal serum or plasma growth hormone levels for adults is less than 10 ng/mL. Levels in children and adolescents may be slightly higher. Persons with somatotrope adenomas may have levels as high as 400 ng/mL.

Management

Medical treatment depends on the severity of the symptoms. Transsphenoidal microsurgery is the treatment of choice to excise the tumor, rapidly re-

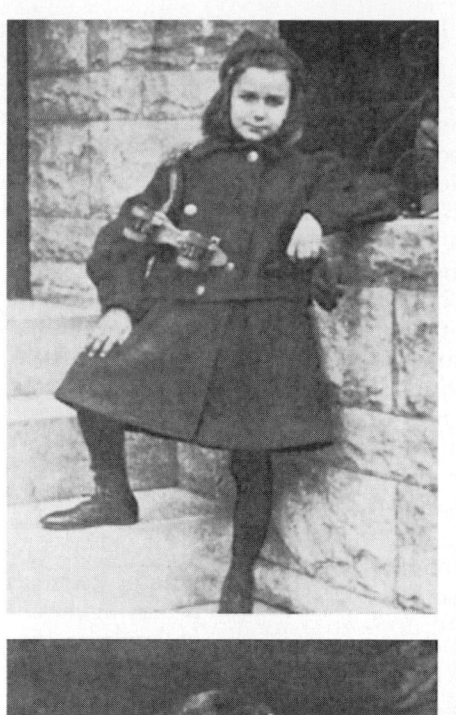
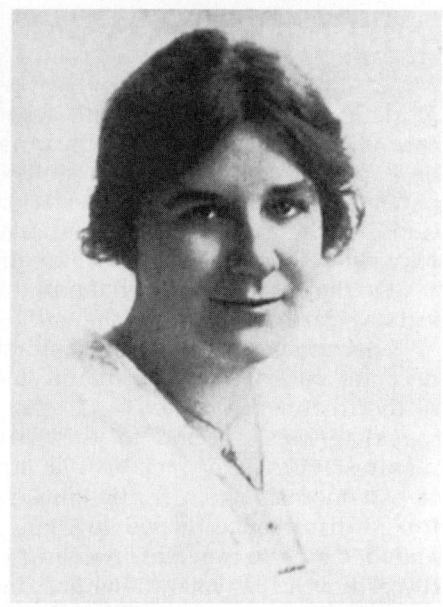
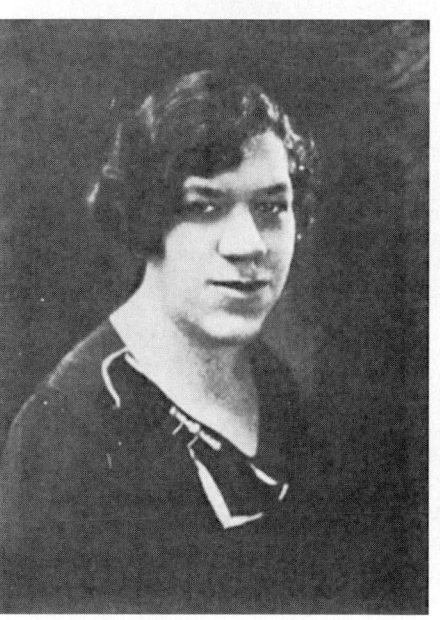
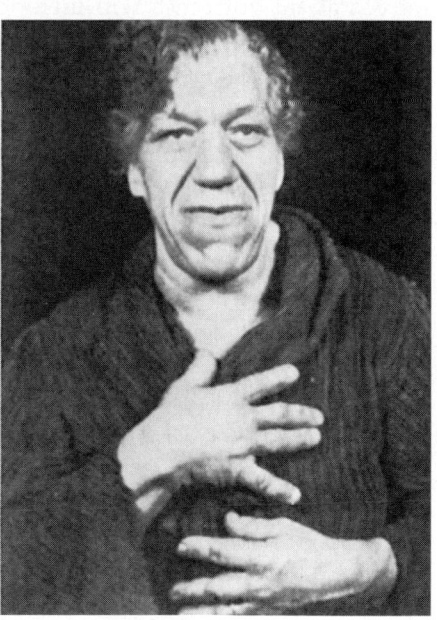

Figure 29–3

A series of photographs that illustrate the progression of acromegaly in a woman from age 9 to 52. (From Mendeloff AI, Smith DE [eds]. Acromegaly, diabetes, hypermetabolism, proteinuria and heart failure. Clin Pathol Conf. Am J Med 1956; 20:133.)

duce somatotropin levels, and preserve normal pituitary function. A transfrontal craniotomy is used if the tumor has extended to surrounding structures and caused optic or cranial nerve damage. External irradiation is effective, but it may take 2 years for hormone levels to decline significantly. The full effect requires 5 to 10 years.

Bromocriptine (Parlodel) suppresses somatotropin secretion in about 2 weeks in cases of acromegaly, and the tumor may shrink somewhat. However, serum growth hormone levels rarely decrease to normal, and the long-term effectiveness of treatment with bromocriptine has not been completely evaluated. Somatostatin is effective in lowering somatotropin secretion. However, it is not practical for long-term use because it has a duration of action of only 5 to 6 hours and inhibits secretion of a number of other hormones.

Early diagnosis and treatment of somatotrope adenomas is important to reduce the severity of permanent alterations that result from excess somatotropin secretion. Features normalize to a degree because of a decrease in soft tissue bulk. And treatment stops the bone and tissue growth, although it does not reverse bone growth that has already occurred. Vascular injury from atherosclerosis, cardiovascular damage, and microvascular changes associated with diabetes are irreversible. Blood glucose levels may return to normal, or secondary diabetes may persist. Prognosis depends on the severity of the alterations that remain after treatment.

NURSING PROCESS GUIDELINES
Acromegaly

Nursing care of a patient with acromegaly combines care of a patient with a pituitary neoplasm and care of a patient with somatotropin excess. Assess the patient for neurologic manifestations of a pituitary tumor and endocrine manifestations of somatotropin hypersecretion. Once medical treatment is planned, assess the patient's understanding of it. Develop a nursing care plan to meet the patient's needs.

The nursing diagnoses and nursing care plan reflect the patient's clinical manifestations, knowledge of the treatment planned, and teaching needs. Nursing diagnoses specific to this patient's endocrine manifestations may include risk for trauma related to osteoporosis and arthritic joint changes, and body image disturbance related to changes in appearance and body characteristics. Nursing diagnoses related to cardiovascular alterations are discussed in Chapter 8. Patient outcomes will include criteria to maintain safety and promote realistic expectations of treatment.

Nursing care includes using side rails for safety and helping the patient ambulate to promote bone recalcification. Position the patient in good alignment when he or she is in bed to prevent deformities and pathologic fractures. Encourage the patient to ask questions about the outcome of treatment. Clarify any misconceptions. Encourage realistic expectations of treatment and allow the patient to vent feelings of anger and grief.

Hypopituitarism

Hyposecretion of any or all of the pituitary hormones may result from a lesion or destructive process in or near the pituitary gland. The most common cause is compression or destruction of pituitary cells by a secreting or nonsecreting adenoma. Other causes of hypopituitarism include iatrogenic factors, postpartum necrosis (Sheehan's syndrome), metastatic lesions, and inflammation secondary to infections of the central nervous system.

Clinical manifestations usually develop slowly and depend on which of the pituitary hormones is deficient. Absence of all pituitary hormones is referred to as panhypopituitarism. It results in hyposecretion at all the target glands. Clinical manifestations include:

  Lethargy
  Fatigue
  Apathy
  Intolerance to cold
  Generalized weakness
  Skin pallor and wrinkling
  Alterations in secondary sex characteristics
  Loss of libido
  Infertility and amenorrhea in women
  Impotence in men
  History of poor health

Diagnosis is based on clinical manifestations and on decreased serum or plasma levels of pituitary or target gland hormones. Treatment involves lifelong replacement therapy with adrenocortical and thyroid hormones. Sex hormones and growth hormone may also be prescribed. Nursing care is similar to that of patients with adrenal cortex and thyroid hypofunction.

❖ Settings, Providers, and Collaboration for Care

The patient with an anterior pituitary disorder may receive care in the hospital or an outpatient setting. If surgery is required, or if the patient is elderly or has other complicating disorders, hospitalization is necessary. After discharge, most patients are seen in a physician's office for follow-up care. If additional nursing care is indicated, referral is made to a home health agency. The home health nurse assesses the patient's recovery, changes dressings, if needed, instructs the patient in further care requirements, and assists the patient and family to cope with the diagnosis.

POSTERIOR PITUITARY DISORDERS

The posterior pituitary (neurohypophysis) stores and secretes antidiuretic hormone (ADH) and oxytocin, which are produced in the hypothalamus. ADH secretion is regulated by osmoreceptors in the hypothalamus, which respond to changes in the osmolality of extracellular fluids. When extracellular fluids become highly concentrated, ADH is released. More water is reabsorbed from the renal tubules, and electrolytes are excreted. As the extracellular fluid becomes more dilute, ADH secretion stops. ADH also has a vasopressive effect; its secretion may be stimulated by severe blood loss or decreased blood pressure.

Disorders of the posterior pituitary are rare and usually secondary to other primary disorders, such as nonendocrine tumors, trauma, and severe infections and inflammatory processes.

Diabetes Insipidus

Etiology and Pathophysiology
Diabetes insipidus is caused by a deficiency in ADH secretion. Primary diabetes insipidus (central or neurogenic diabetes insipidus) is rare. It usually results from a tumor of the hypothalamus or pituitary gland that destroys the portions of the hypothalamus that manufacture or regulate secretion of ADH. Nephrogenic diabetes insipidus is a rare, inherited genetic defect in which the renal tubules do not respond to ADH and water is not resorbed by the kidney.

Secondary diabetes insipidus is a more common

disorder. It develops secondary to head trauma, surgical or irradiation injury, or neoplastic or inflammatory processes that exert pressure on the hypothalamus or hypophysis, or has idiopathic causes. Secondary diabetes insipidus may be temporary or permanent. The permanent version does not develop if the pituitary stalk is intact after total hypophysectomy, because cut axons from the hypothalamus continue to secrete ADH.

In the absence of ADH or failure of the kidneys to respond to ADH, large amounts of fluid and electrolytes are excreted in the urine because the renal tubules do not reabsorb water. As much as 20 L of dilute urine may be excreted daily.

Clinical Manifestations

Polydipsia and polyuria are the classic symptoms of diabetes insipidus. The urine is pale in color, and the specific gravity is less than 1.006. Anorexia and weight loss occur.

If the person cannot drink fluids, severe dehydration, sodium depletion, and vascular collapse develop rapidly.

Diagnosis

Diagnosis is based on clinical manifestations, dehydration tests, and response to vasopressin.

Water-Deprivation Test

The water-deprivation test evaluates the renal tubules' ability to concentrate urine during dehydration. All fluids are withheld for 8 to 12 hours or until 3 to 5% of body weight is lost. Plasma and urine osmolality tests may be done at the beginning and end of the test. The test is positive for diabetes insipidus if the patient continues to excrete large amounts of dilute urine with a low specific gravity.

Nursing implications during the test include frequent assessment of vital signs and clinical manifestations of dehydration and impending hypovolemic shock. The patient will probably need emotional support to cope with the insatiable thirst. Hourly weights are a good indicator of fluid loss. The physician is notified immediately and the test terminated if tachycardia, weight loss of more than 5%, or hypotension develop.

Vasopressin Stimulation Test

The vasopressin stimulation test may be done after a positive water-deprivation test to determine whether the renal tubules' failure to concentrate urine results from renal dysfunction or pituitary diabetes insipidus. A urine specimen is collected for osmolality before and 1 hour after subcutaneous administration of aqueous vasopressin. The vasopressin stimulation test is positive for diabetes insipidus if urine osmolality rises more than 5% after vasopressin administration.

Management

Short-term treatment of diabetes insipidus involves parenteral administration of vasopressin, the phar-macologic form of ADH. This is the treatment of choice for patients with temporary diabetes insipidus resulting from cerebral edema. The pharmacokinetics of antidiuretic hormones are described in Highlight 29–1. Aqueous vasopressin (Pitressin) injection has a short duration of antidiuretic activity and is administered every 6 to 8 hours. Vasopressin tannate has a longer half-life and is administered every 36 to 72 hours.

Desmopressin acetate (DDAVP), a synthetic ADH, is the drug of choice for long-term therapy. DDAVP solution is administered intranasally through a straw once or twice daily. Lypressin (Diapid) nasal spray, another synthetic ADH, must be administered three to four times daily.

Nephrogenic diabetes insipidus is usually controlled with a low-sodium, low-protein diet and thiazide diuretics. This combination promotes water and sodium resorption in the proximal renal tubule and reduces water loss in the distal renal tubule, where ADH is necessary. Protein restriction further reduces water loss by reducing the need for solute excretion.

NURSING PROCESS GUIDELINES
Diabetes Insipidus

Assess for the clinical manifestations of diabetes insipidus in patients who have

> Head trauma
> Cranial surgery or irradiation
> Metastatic lesions to the brain
> A diagnosed pituitary tumor

Monitor vital signs, level of consciousness, urine output, and specific gravity, especially in the unconscious patient who cannot complain of thirst. If urine output exceeds 100 mL/hour for 3 hours with no apparent physiologic cause, notify the physician promptly.

Once diabetes insipidus is diagnosed and therapy implemented, assess and document the patient's response to treatment. If vasopressin tannate is prescribed, warm the vial and shake vigorously to disperse the medication in the oil and to facilitate intramuscular administration. Inject immediately after preparation. If long-term DDAVP or lypressin therapy is required, teach the patient to check the expiration date on the medication, weigh himself or herself daily, and report a 3% weight loss to the physician. Weigh the patient the morning of discharge, calculate 3%, and give this number and the total body weight to the patient to avoid confusion. Include the topics identified in Highlight 29–2 in the teaching plan for a patient with diabetes insipidus who is taking DDAVP. Observe the patient's technique of self-administering the medication to evaluate teaching.

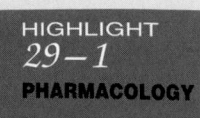 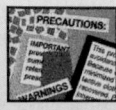

HIGHLIGHT
29—1
PHARMACOLOGY

Antidiuretic Hormones

Definition:

Class of drugs that promote water conservation by increasing reabsorption of water by the distal portion of the renal tubules.

Action:

Reduce urine volume and increase urine concentration and osmolality by increasing renal tubular reabsorption of water. In doses higher than those required for antidiuretic effect, drug also has vasopressor effects.

Uses:

To control the symptoms of neurogenic diabetes insipidus.

Side Effects:

Dose-related. Water intoxication: changes in mental status, confusion, lethargy, headache, weight gain, convulsions, coma. Shortness of breath, heartburn, nausea, abdominal cramps, vulvar pain, rise in blood pressure, angina.

Interactions:

Alcohol, cyclophosphamide, demeclocycline, epinephrine, heparin, and lithium may decrease antidiuretic response. Oral antidiabetic agents, carbamazepine, and clofibrate may increase antidiuretic response.

Nursing Implications:

Take daily weights.

Monitor fluid intake and output and vital signs.

Monitor for side effects: notify physician and withhold dose in the presence of chest pain, dyspnea, decreased level of consciousness, or sudden weight gain.

Geriatric Considerations:

Risk of water intoxication is especially high in the elderly. Monitor cardiovascular status closely.

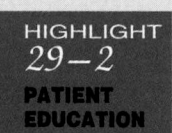 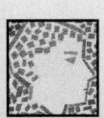

HIGHLIGHT
29—2
PATIENT EDUCATION

Self-Management: Desmopressin Acetate Administration for Diabetes Insipidus

Instruct the patient to:

Expect desmopressin acetate (DDAVP) to reduce frequency and volume of urination and to relieve excessive thirst.

Check expiration date on label. Outdated medication loses its potency rapidly and should be discarded.

Store DDAVP in the refrigerator unless otherwise specified by the manufacturer.

Discard medication and do not use if solution is discolored or if particles are present.

Administer in the evening to control nocturia if a single dose is prescribed.

Monitor pattern of urination. If nocturia or frequent urination during waking hours develops, notify physician. A second morning dose may be prescribed.

Monitor pattern of fluid intake. If frequent thirst develops, notify physician.

Measure dose carefully in calibrated straw.

Inhale high into nasal cavity, not down back of throat.

Weigh daily. Report weight gain of 1 kg (2.2 lbs) in 1 week to physician.

Report to the physician promptly any of the following: feelings of drowsiness, listlessness, headache, shortness of breath, heartburn, nausea, abdominal cramps, vulvar pain, or severe nasal congestion or irritation.

Syndrome of Inappropriate Antidiuretic Hormone

Excess secretion of ADH is a syndrome that develops in critically ill people. The most common cause of the syndrome of inappropriate antidiuretic hormone is secretion of ADH by nonendocrine tumors, especially oat cell carcinoma of the lungs. Other conditions associated with syndrome of inappropriate antidiuretic hormone include severe stress, trauma, cerebral hemorrhage, cranial surgery, central nervous system infections, myxedema, and large doses of radiation and chemotherapy.

In the syndrome of inappropriate antidiuretic hormone, secretion of ADH is not controlled by hypothalamic osmoreceptors and is unrelated to plasma osmolality or extracellular fluid volume. The result is excessive reabsorption of water in the distal renal tubules, leading to expansion of extracellular fluid volume with hemodilution and dilutional hyponatremia.

Assess the patient for clinical manifestations of decreasing urine output with specific gravity of more than 1.030, hyponatremia, weight gain, lethargy, weakness, decreased gastrointestinal motility from hyponatremia, and decreasing level of consciousness progressing to seizures and coma.

The syndrome of inappropriate antidiuretic hormone is best treated by correcting the underlying cause. Fluid restrictions and administration of diuretics, serum albumin, and demeclocycline (Declomycin), a tetracycline that increases free water clearance in the renal tubules, may also be prescribed.

❖ Settings, Providers, and Collaboration for Care

The patient with diabetes insipidus has care managed primarily in the home. It is important for the home health nurse to reinforce the importance of taking medications as ordered and monitoring daily weight.

The patient with the syndrome of inappropriate antidiuretic hormone needs to be closely monitored. The inpatient acute care setting is necessary for assessing and treating conditions that predisposed to the syndrome. The nurse must rely heavily on technical support from team members in the ongoing assessment of laboratory data as well as frequent assessments of changes in activity and level of consciousness.

*A*drenal Disorders

The adrenal glands are located just above each kidney. Each gland has two distinct parts: the cortex and the medulla. These parts differ in function and origin. Thus, different disorders or diseases result from improper function of each part.

ADRENOCORTICAL INSUFFICIENCY: ADDISON'S DISEASE

Etiology and Pathophysiology

Adrenocortical insufficiency is a functional disorder characterized by failure of the adrenal cortex to produce and secrete adrenocortical hormones. Chronic primary adrenocortical insufficiency, or Addison's disease, most commonly results from idiopathic atrophy or destruction of the adrenal cortex by an autoimmune process.

Destruction of the adrenal cortex usually occurs over several years. Addison's disease may occur alone or together with autoimmune-related thyroid disease, insulin-dependent diabetes mellitus, premature gonad failure, and pernicious anemia. Rarely, primary adrenocortical insufficiency results from destruction of the adrenal cortex by tuberculosis or histoplasmosis organisms, metastatic lesions, or surgical removal of both adrenal glands.

Secondary adrenocortical insufficiency is caused by inadequate secretion of adrenocorticotropic hormone (ACTH), either from a pituitary or hypothalamic disorder, or from suppression of adrenal cortex function by exogenous steroid preparations.

The incidence of Addison's disease is about 1 per 100,000 individuals in the United States. It is equally distributed between men and women. It can occur at any age but is uncommon in the elderly. Incidence is higher in people with a history of autoimmune glandular disorders and chronic long-term steroid therapy.

The pathologic changes associated with Addison's disease usually develop after at least 90% of the glandular tissue has been destroyed. They result from increased secretion of ACTH and progressive deficiencies of aldosterone, cortisol, and adrenal androgen.

Aldosterone deficiency results in decreased sodium reabsorption in the distal tubules of the kidneys and increased potassium retention. As sodium is excreted in great amounts in the urine, chloride and water are also excreted. The result of this electrolyte imbalance is depletion of extracellular fluid volume, hyponatremia, hyperkalemia, and mild metabolic alkalosis. As plasma volume decreases, renal perfusion decreases, cardiac output decreases, blood pressure falls, and heart size decreases. Without fluid and sodium replacement, circulatory deterioration leads to peripheral vascular collapse and hypovolemic shock, an often fatal complication referred to as Addison's crisis.

Cortisol deficiency results in the inability to maintain normal blood glucose levels between meals because of impaired gluconeogenesis. Altered metabolism causes muscle weakness, loss of vigor, loss of appetite, inability to withstand even minor stress or illness, and impaired immune response.

In primary adrenocortical deficiency, decreased cortisol secretion also results in loss of the normal negative feedback suppression of ACTH secretion.

Excess ACTH, which is similar in structure to melanocyte-stimulating hormone (MSH), stimulates increased melanocyte formation and increased production of melanin.

Adrenal androgen deficiency has minimal effect on males because testicular androgen production maintains secondary sex characteristics. In females, however, loss of adrenal androgen results in thinning of axillary and pubic hair. Decreased libido and amenorrhea may also occur.

Clinical Manifestations

The onset of symptoms is insidious and occurs over several months. The person becomes profoundly weak and fatigued, with general deterioration in health and physical and mental vigor. Common manifestations include postural hypotension from fluid loss, syncope, muscle weakness, anorexia, nausea, vomiting, abdominal cramps, weight loss, depression, and irritability. The skin develops generalized or patchy hyperpigmentation. In primary adrenocortical insufficiency, the bronze coloration may be especially noticeable on the gums and mucous membranes, skin creases, pressure areas, areolae, and genitalia. Some patients develop vitiligo, patchy areas of decreased pigmentation surrounded by areas of increased pigmentation (Fig. 29–4).

In Addison's crisis, severe hypotension, hypoglycemia, hyponatremia, hyperkalemia, and dehydration lead to profound shock, cardiac dysrhythmias, and death. Hyperpyrexia and severe abdominal and back pain may also occur. Addison's crisis is usually

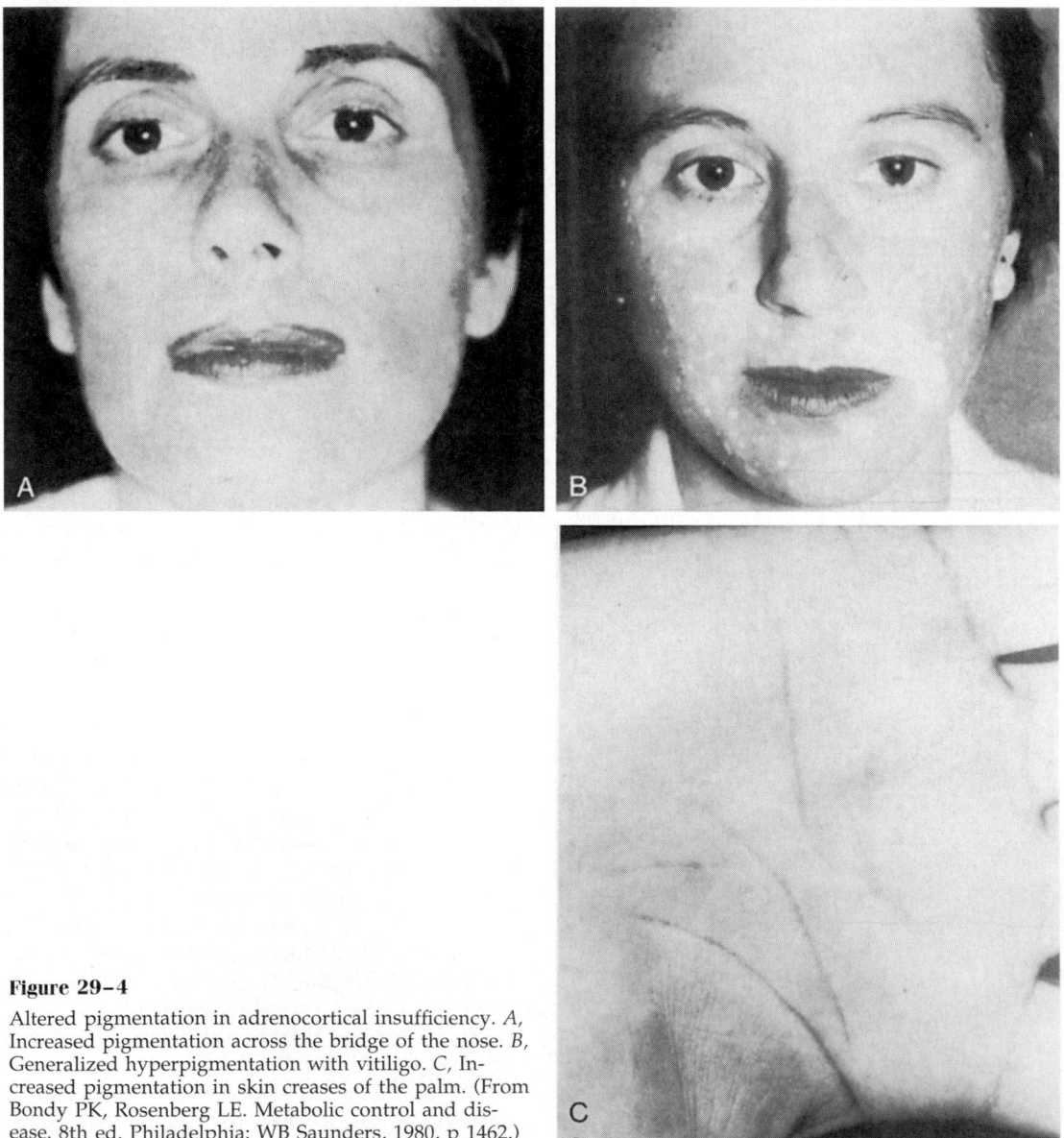

Figure 29–4

Altered pigmentation in adrenocortical insufficiency. *A,* Increased pigmentation across the bridge of the nose. *B,* Generalized hyperpigmentation with vitiligo. *C,* Increased pigmentation in skin creases of the palm. (From Bondy PK, Rosenberg LE. Metabolic control and disease. 8th ed. Philadelphia: WB Saunders, 1980, p 1462.)

Table 29–1

Common Diagnostic Studies of Adrenal Cortex Function*

Study	Purpose and Procedure	Nursing Implications
SERUM STUDIES		

Aldosterone	Assess mineralocorticoid production. Measured in conjunction with 24-hour urine to detect aldosteronism.
	Normal values (upright):
	    Females: 5–30 ng/dL
	    Males: 6–22 ng/dL
		Follow physician's dietary and medication instructions. Unrestricted salt intake is preferred. Record diet and medications on laboratory slip.

Cortisol	Assess cortisol production. Levels normally vary with circadian rhythms, with peak level in early morning.
	Normal values:
	    Morning: 5–25 μg/dL
	    Afternoon: 3–13 μg/dL ($\frac{1}{2}$ of peak level)
	    Evening: $\leq$ peak level
		Specimen may be collected twice on the same day to evaluate circadian effects on cortisol secretion. Minimize stress to avoid artificially elevated levels. Note time collected on laboratory slip.

ACTH	Assess ACTH production. Levels normally vary with circadian rhythms, with peak level in early morning. Immediately place specimens in ice water.
	Normal values:
	    Morning: 20–100 pg/mL
	    Afternoon: 10–40 pg/mL ($\leq$ peak value)
		Implications are the same as for plasma cortisol levels. Single specimen is best collected in early morning. Prepare ice bath before venipuncture.

ACTH stimulation test	Assess response to ACTH in adrenocortical insufficiency. Normally ACTH stimulates increased cortisol production. Baseline serum cortisol laboratory levels are measured. ACTH administered via IV or IM bolus. Serum cortisol levels are drawn 30 and 60 minutes later. Normal values after ACTH: Serum cortisol >20 μg/dL and two to three times baseline	Note on laboratory slip exact time ACTH was administered and specimens were drawn. Check for food restrictions. Instruct patient to avoid strenuous activity on the day before the test.
Dexamethasone suppression test	Assess response to dexamethasone in adrenocortical excess. Normally dexamethasone will suppress cortisol secretion. Baseline morning serum cortisol levels are measured. Oral dexamethasone is administered at bedtime. Serum cortisol levels measured the next morning. Normal values after dexamethasone: Serum cortisol <5 μg/dL	Check physician's orders for drug restrictions. Cortisol levels must be drawn at the same time each day. Note time specimens were drawn and medications on laboratory slip. Instruct patient to avoid strenuous activity the day before the test.

Metyrapone suppression test	Evaluate the pituitary feedback response to differentiate between adrenal hyperplasia and adrenal tumor. Normally metyrapone will block adrenal cortisol synthesis. Baseline cortisol and ACTH levels are measured. Oral metyrapone is administered at midnight. ACTH and cortisol are measured at 8:00 AM.
	Normal values after metyrapone:
	    ACTH: >250 pg/dL
	    Cortisol: <8 μg/dL
		Check physician's orders for drug restrictions. Administer metyrapone with food to prevent gastrointestinal distress. Second specimen must be drawn 8 hours after metyrapone during peak ACTH and cortisol secretion periods. Assess for adrenal insufficiency, which may be induced by metyrapone.

Table continued on following page

Table 29–1

Common Diagnostic Studies of Adrenal Cortex Function* (continued)

Study	Purpose and Procedure	Nursing Implications
URINE STUDIES		

17-Hydroxycorticosteroids (17-OHCS)	Assess urinary levels of glucocorticoid metabolites. 24-hour urine specimen with preservative.
	Normal values:
	  Females: 3–13 mg/24 hr
	  Males: 3–15 mg/24 hr
		Follow standard collection procedures for 24-hour urine specimen. Note start and end time on collection container and patient record. Many drugs affect results; check physician's orders for restrictions. Note medications on laboratory slip.

17-Ketosteroids (17-KS)	Assess androgen metabolites in the urine. 24-hour urine specimen with preservative. Values decrease with age.
	Normal values:
	  Females: 5–15 mg/24 hr
	  Males: 8–25 mg/24 hr
	  >65 yr: 4–8 mg/24 hr
		Implications are the same as for 17-OHCS. Check with laboratory to determine whether specimen must be kept chilled.

Aldosterone	Assess urinary aldosterone levels. Measured in conjunction with plasma aldosterone to detect aldosteronism. 24-hour urine specimen with preservative and kept chilled. Normal values: 35–80 μg/24 hr	Implications are the same as for serum aldosterone. Test results are not affected by patient position, activity, or circadian rhythms.

*Normal values and procedures are guidelines. Contact laboratory performing test for absolute values, interfering substances, specimen preservation, and specific collection procedures.
ACTH, adrenocorticotropic hormone.

precipitated by stress, infection, surgery, salt or fluid loss in hot weather or during exercise, or inadequate replacement or sudden withdrawal of exogenous steroids. It may also be precipitated by illness or stress in people with previously undiagnosed borderline adrenocortical insufficiency.

Diagnosis

Diagnosis of adrenocortical insufficiency is based on identification of low levels of circulating plasma cortisol and low 24-hour urinary 17-hydroxycorticosteroids (17-OHCS) and 17-ketosteroids (17-KS). Plasma ACTH levels are elevated in primary adrenocortical deficiency. In secondary adrenocortical deficiency caused by hyposecretion of ACTH from the pituitary, serum ACTH levels are low, and the ACTH stimulation test causes plasma cortisol values to rise. Table 29–1 identifies common diagnostic studies of adrenal cortex function and their nursing implications. The abnormal responses to these studies that are typical in a patient with Addison's disease appear in Table 29–2.

Additional laboratory studies reveal hyperkalemia, hyponatremia, hypoglycemia, hypochloremia, mild metabolic alkalosis, elevated blood urea nitrogen and serum creatinine levels, eosinophilia, and lymphocytosis.

Management

Treatment of adrenocortical insufficiency includes lifelong hormone replacement. Oral cortisone acetate (Cortone) and hydrocortisone (cortisol, Cortef) are the drugs of choice to replace glucocorticoid activity. The glucocorticoid is administered in divided doses to simulate the body's normal diurnal secretion pattern. The patient takes two-thirds of the total dose on arising in the morning and one-third in the afternoon. It may take as long as 9 months after long-term steroid therapy ends before the hypothalamic-pituitary-adrenal axis can recover enough to respond to acute stress or illness. To prevent Addison's crisis, glucocorticoid dosage may be increased two to three times during periods of stress or illness.

Fludrocortisone acetate (Florinef) is the drug of choice to replace mineralocorticoid activity. It may be prescribed daily to three times a week. To help prevent sodium depletion, the patient follows a diet of unrestricted salt intake. During periods of fluid loss or profuse perspiration, intake of fluid and salt is increased.

Management of acute adrenocortical insufficiency, or Addison's crisis, is a medical emergency. Fluid replacement to reverse hypovolemic shock and steroid replacement are priorities. Hypoglycemia is reversed with parenteral dextrose. Intravenous hydrocortisone is given every 6 hours and isotonic dextrose and saline are infused rapidly. Vital signs and serum electrolyte and blood glucose levels are monitored frequently to evaluate fluid, electrolyte, and blood glucose status. Hyperpyrexia is usually

Table 29–2

Typical Results of Common Diagnostic Studies of Adrenal Cortex Function in Addison's Disease and Cushing's Syndrome*

| Study | Addison's Disease | | Cushing's Syndrome | | |
	Primary Addison's Disease	Pituitary ACTH-Dependent Addison's Disease	Cortisol-Secreting Adrenal Tumor	Pituitary ACTH-Dependent Cushing's Syndrome	Ectopic ACTH-Secreting Tumor
Plasma cortisol	Low	Low	High	High	High
Plasma ACTH	High	Low	High	High	High
17-OHCS	Low	Low	High	High	High
Cortisol response to ACTH stimulation test	None	Normal rise	Marked rise	None	None
Cortisol response to high-dose dexamethasone suppression test			None	Marked drop	None
Cortisol response to metyrapone suppression test			None	Marked rise	Varies

*Data represent typical response, but exceptions are possible on rare occasions.
ACTH, adrenocorticotropic hormone; 17-OHCS, 17-hydroxycorticosteroids.

corrected with reversal of dehydration. If the patient is admitted to an intensive care unit, hemodynamic and cardiac monitoring is employed.

With properly managed hormone-replacement therapy and patient education to minimize the risk of Addison's crisis, a person with chronic adrenocortical insufficiency can expect to live a normal, active life.

❖ Settings, Providers, and Collaboration for Care

Care for the patient in Addison's crisis requires the collaborative efforts of nurse, physician, laboratory technician, pharmacist, respiratory therapist, and dietitian. The patient is admitted to an acute care facility for initial treatment. Continued care for the patient with Addison's disease occurs primarily in the home. Home health nurses collaborate with the physician, patient, and family to plan for management of medications and ongoing health promotion. The patient may also be seen for follow-up care in the physician's office.

NURSING PROCESS
Adrenocortical Insufficiency (Addison's Disease)

Assessment

Obtain a complete nursing history from the patient with diagnosed or suspected chronic adrenocortical insufficiency. Ask specifically about the onset of unusual fatigue, weakness, and lingering minor ill-

nesses. Nonspecific early symptoms are often overlooked by the patient as insignificant or unrelated. Ask about recent or past use of topical, oral, and parenteral adrenocorticosteroid preparations. Obtain baseline weight. Assess vital signs. Check blood pressure and pulse while the patient is lying and standing to identify orthostatic hypotension, which occurs commonly in fluid volume deficit. Determine presymptomatic weight and blood pressure, if documented or known by the patient, and compare with current assessments. Assess mucous membranes and skin turgor for signs of dehydration. Assess for clinical manifestations associated with Addison's disease. Identify the patient's interpretation of clinical manifestations and knowledge of planned diagnostic procedures and treatment to determine teaching needs.

Initial assessment of the patient with acute adrenocortical insufficiency may be limited to a brief history of the current illness, identification of allergies, and determination of hemodynamic status until intravenous fluids and steroids are initiated. Once the patient is stabilized, obtain a complete history and identify the events that precipitated Addison's crisis.

Nursing Diagnoses and Planning

Initial planning may be based on the presence of Addison's crisis. Care then focuses on relieving the crisis and controlling the disease (Nursing Care Guide 29–2). Nursing diagnoses and related expected patient outcomes commonly applicable to pa-

Patients with Acute Adrenocortical Insufficiency: Addison's Crisis

Assessment Findings: Patient with history of chronic adrenocortical insufficiency (Addison's disease) admitted after 24 hours of vomiting and diarrhea. Patient is responsive but lethargic, skin is hot and dry, mucous membranes are dry, temperature is 39.6°C (103.3°F), blood pressure is 90/60 mm Hg, pulse is 110 bpm and thready.

Nursing Diagnosis: Fluid volume deficit related to extracellular sodium and water loss secondary to vomiting, diarrhea, and adrenocortical insufficiency

Patient Outcomes	Nursing Interventions	Rationale
Patient demonstrates adequate extracellular fluid volume by moist mucous membranes, good skin turgor, blood pressure within 10% of normal baseline, pulse 60–100 bpm, urine output > 30 mL/hr, and is alert and responds appropriately.	Administer intravenous hydrocortisone and isotonic dextrose and saline as prescribed.	Provides adrenocorticosteroid hormone, fluid, glucose, and sodium replacement.
	Monitor vital signs, neurologic status, urine output, capillary refill hourly. Monitor pulmonary wedge pressure as appropriate, and electrocardiogram if in intensive care unit. Assess for hyperkalemia, and monitor results of serum electrolyte studies.	Evaluates effectiveness of treatment. Hemodynamic parameters indicate perfusion of vital organs. Hyperkalemia may cause cardiac dysrhythmias.
	Administer antiemetic and antidiarrheal if prescribed.	Prevents further fluid loss.
	Provide oral fluids and high-sodium diet as prescribed when patient is alert.	Maintains adequate fluid and sodium replacement.

Evaluation: Compare the patient's status with the expected outcomes. If the outcomes are not met, reassess the patient and revise the plan.

Assessment Findings: Patient with chronic adrenocortical insufficiency (Addison's disease) is to be discharged after treatment for an episode of Addison's crisis precipitated by gastrointestinal illness.

Nursing Diagnosis: Risk for altered health maintenance related to insufficient knowledge of self-management of chronic adrenocortical insufficiency and lifelong replacement therapy

Patient Outcomes	Nursing Interventions	Rationale
Patient identifies recent gastrointestinal illness as precipitating event of this episode of Addison's crisis.	Review disease process and effect of excess fluid and sodium loss and illness on control of Addison's disease. Discuss probability of recent gastrointestinal illness as precipitating event.	Accurate information corrects misunderstandings and increases patient's knowledge.

(continued)

Nursing Care Guide 29-2
Patients with Acute Adrenocortical Insufficiency: Addison's Crisis (continued)

Patient Outcomes	Nursing Interventions	Rationale
Patient identifies factors that may precipitate Addison's crisis.	Discuss situations that may precipitate Addison's crisis: hot weather, prolonged excessive perspiration, infection, illness, increased stress, injury. Confer with the patient to identify ways to minimize risks.	Knowledge of possible precipitating factors helps prevent or minimize risk of future crises.
Patient states correct actions to take to minimize risk of Addison's crisis or if signs of dehydration develop.	Teach patient and provide in writing the signs of fluid loss. Teach patient to carry prescribed parenteral hydrocortisone and medical alert identification at all times.	Early detection promotes rapid treatment. Written instructions reinforce learning.
	Teach patient, and a caregiver, and observe return demonstration of correct administration of parenteral hydrocortisone. Instruct patient to notify physician during periods of high risk or if signs of fluid loss develop. Teach patient to increase fluid intake, salt intake, and glucocorticoid preparation as prescribed during periods of high risk.	Return demonstration provides opportunity to evaluate learning and correct administration technique. Increased fluid, sodium, and glucocorticoid intake reduces risk of dehydration and crisis episodes.
Patient states intent to keep twice yearly follow-up appointments.	Reinforce importance of twice yearly follow-up by physician.	Evaluates effectiveness of therapeutic regimen.

Evaluation: Compare the patient's status with the expected outcomes. If the outcomes are not met, reassess the patient and revise the plan.

tients with adrenocortical insufficiency (Addison's disease) include the following:

NDx: Risk for fluid volume deficit related to loss of extracellular sodium and water secondary to mineralocorticoid insufficiency

Planning: Patient Outcomes
1. Patient demonstrates adequate extracellular fluid volume as evidenced by the following:
   Stable vital signs within normal limits
   Moist mucous membranes
   Good skin turgor
2. Patient verbalizes understanding of the need for, and intent to take, mineralocorticoid replacement as prescribed.
3. Patient identifies foods and fluids that promote fluid and electrolyte balance.

NDx: Risk for infection related to impaired glucose-regulating mechanisms, impaired immune response, and inability to tolerate stress secondary to glucocorticoid insufficiency

Planning: Patient Outcomes
1. Patient verbalizes understanding of the need for, and intent to take, glucocorticoid replacement as prescribed.
2. Patient identifies foods that maintain blood glucose levels and protein synthesis.
3. Patient remains free from infection.

Nursing Interventions and Evaluation

Nursing care of the patient with adrenocortical insufficiency requires frequent assessment and supportive intervention. This patient faces potentially rapid fluctuations in fluid and electrolyte balance and cardiovascular status, in addition to adrenocortical hormone replacement. Patient education is a primary focus. The patient will need to learn self-management of adrenocortical insufficiency and accept lifelong steroid-replacement therapy to avoid episodes of Addison's crisis. Nursing guidelines for patient education are summarized in Highlight 29–3. In developing a teaching plan, it is important to remember that a patient receiving steroid-replacement therapy to correct a deficiency is much less likely to exhibit side effects than a patient receiving very high doses to suppress an immune or inflammatory response. Highlight 29–4 identifies adrenocorticosteroid preparations.

NDx: Risk for fluid volume deficit

Administer mineralocorticoid replacement as prescribed. Teach the patient the dosage and schedule, expected action, and side effects of the prescribed mineralocorticoid. Monitor vital signs every 4 hours. Assess skin turgor, mucous membranes, and mental status to detect signs of dehydration. Measure intake and output and weigh the patient daily to identify excess fluid loss. Instruct the patient to report increased thirst or light-headedness on standing, which may indicate developing fluid loss. Encourage fluid intake to 3000 mL/day with physician approval.

Administer intravenous fluids, sodium replacement, and antiemetics if prescribed. Consult with the dietitian to provide an unrestricted-salt diet. Help the patient select high-sodium foods from the daily menu. Teach the patient to prevent excess fluid and sodium loss by maintaining adequate salt intake (up to 8 g of sodium daily) and increasing salt intake during hot weather, before strenuous exercise, and in response to fever, vomiting, or diarrhea. Teach the patient about and provide a list of the early signs of dehydration. To prevent Addison's crisis, instruct the patient to notify the physician promptly if these signs occur.

NDx: Risk for infection

Administer glucocorticoid replacement as prescribed. Teach the patient the dosage and schedule, expected action, and side effects of the prescribed glucocorticoid. Place the patient in a quiet room. Be sure that roommates are not infectious. Explain all procedures and answer questions. Keep the environment as free from stress as possible. Encourage communication with the physician and significant others to reduce anxiety. Avoid unnecessary invasive procedures. To minimize the chance of infection, protect the patient from chills, drafts, and exposure to staff and visitors with upper respiratory tract infections. To prevent contamination, use sterile technique when caring for all skin lesions, venipuncture sites, drains, and wounds. Monitor vital signs, examine all open areas, and culture suspicious drainage and wounds for prompt identification and treatment of infections. Encourage rest periods to prevent fatigue.

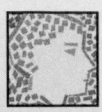

HIGHLIGHT 29–3

PATIENT EDUCATION

Self-Management: Adrenocortical Insufficiency (Addison's Disease)

Instruct the patient to:

Learn about the disease process and the need for lifelong replacement therapy.

Take the prescribed replacement therapy; know the names, doses, routes and times of administration, expected effects, and side effects of each medication.

Recognize the risk of Addison's crisis, conditions that may precipitate crisis, signs and symptoms of impending crisis, and course of action to take.

Notify the physician if unable to ingest or retain food or fluids or if symptoms of crisis develop.

Adjust dosage of prescribed glucocorticoids during illness or increased stress as instructed by the physician.

Carry an emergency syringe of parenteral hydrocortisone at all times and learn how to inject it intramuscularly.

Wear medical alert identification at all times.

Follow a high–complex-carbohydrate, high-protein diet if prescribed.

Maintain high daily sodium intake (up to 8 g), more in hot weather and when diaphoresis is profuse.

Minimize stress and avoid infections and people with infections.

Identify sources of stress, and use relaxation or other techniques to reduce stress.

Avoid fatigue by alternating activity with rest periods.

See physician at least two times a year for follow-up examination and evaluation of treatment regimen.

In consultation with the dietitian and the physician, teach the patient to select a diet high in complex carbohydrates and protein to maintain blood glucose levels and protein synthesis. Help the patient identify sources of emotional stress and methods of dealing effectively with them. Discuss situations and activities that increase the risk of exposure to infectious diseases. Help the patient plan ways to avoid them.

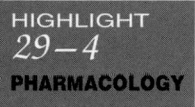 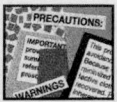

HIGHLIGHT 29–4 PHARMACOLOGY

Adrenocorticosteroids

Definition:

Class of drugs with properties similar to the corticosteroids secreted by the adrenal cortex.

Action:

Mineralocorticoids promote sodium and water retention and potassium excretion by increasing transport through the renal tubular walls. Glucocorticoids promote hepatic gluconeogenesis, alter fat and protein metabolism, and suppress the anti-inflammatory and immune response. In supraphysiologic dosages, both groups of corticosteroids exhibit similar properties.

Uses:

Replacement therapy in adrenocortical insufficiency and for suppression of undesirable inflammatory, immune, or allergic responses.

Side Effects:

Side effects rarely develop with replacement therapy or short-term, high-dose therapy. Among side effects are peptic ulcer, steroid diabetes, delayed wound healing and tissue repair, increased susceptibility to infections, osteoporosis, edema, hypertension, amenorrhea, acne, ecchymoses, hirsutism, cataracts, glaucoma, optic nerve damage, atrophy of the adrenal cortex, a Cushing-like syndrome (fat deposits on the face, trunk, neck, shoulders, wasting of arms and legs), and mood changes. Adrenocorticosteroids are contraindicated in infectious processes because they mask infections.

Interactions:

Antacids decrease absorption. Hyperglycemic effect may necessitate increased doses of antidiabetic agents. Adrenocorticosteroids increase ulcerogenic effects of salicylates. Their use with antibiotics may result in emergence of resistant strains of microorganisms. Amphotericin B and diuretics increase potassium excretion. Barbiturates, phenytoin, and rifampin decrease effect.

Nursing Implications:

Administer oral preparations with food or milk to decrease ulcerogenic effect. Administer parenteral solutions intravenously or by deep intramuscular injection to avoid tissue atrophy. Avoid the deltoid muscle. Do not alter from prescribed dosage or times of administration. Abrupt withdrawal or dosage reduction may precipitate Addison's crisis. Monitor vital signs, intake and output, daily weight, and urine or blood glucose levels. Assess for dependent edema, mood changes, hypernatremia, hypokalemia, altered vision, and infections. Teach the patient the importance of medical supervision, to consult physician before taking any over-the-counter preparations, and to wear medical alert identification.

Geriatric Considerations:

The elderly are more susceptible to the side effects of this class of drugs and often have pre-existing conditions that can be exacerbated by these drugs (eg, cardiovascular disorders, diabetes mellitus). Treatment is usually initiated with lower doses. Monitor closely for fluid retention, electrolyte imbalance, and hyperglycemia.

Compare the patient's status with the expected outcomes. If the outcomes are not met, reassess the patient and revise the plan.

ADRENOCORTICAL EXCESS: CUSHING'S SYNDROME

Etiology and Pathophysiology

Adrenocortical excess (Cushing's syndrome) is a functional disorder characterized by oversecretion of glucocorticoid hormones, primarily cortisol and, to some degree, adrenal androgen. Hyperplasia of the adrenal cortices, especially the zona fasciculata, is the most common cause of adrenocortical excess. This cortical hyperplasia is usually a response to overproduction of ACTH by a benign secreting adenoma of the anterior pituitary or by an ectopic ACTH-secreting tumor. Bronchogenic and small cell carcinomas of the lung and carcinomas of the pancreas or gastrointestinal tract commonly secrete ACTH. Pituitary-dependent Cushing's syndrome, sometimes referred to as Cushing's disease, may occasionally result from oversecretion of corticotropin-releasing hormone (CRH) by the hypothalamus. Another cause of Cushing's syndrome is a cortisol-secreting tumor of the adrenal cortex. A Cushing-like syndrome can also be induced by prolonged administration of high doses of exogenous glucocorticoids.

Cushing's syndrome is fairly rare in the United States, with about 10 cases per million people annually. It most commonly develops between ages 20 and 40. Cushing's syndrome resulting from an adrenal tumor or pituitary hypersecretion is more common in women. Ectopic ACTH-secreting tumors are more common in men.

Most of the physical changes associated with Cushing's syndrome—such as thinning hair, ruddy complexion, and obesity—result from abnormally high levels of cortisol. Increased androgen levels and the mineralocorticoid actions of cortisol also cause some of the alterations.

Unregulated secretion of cortisol causes increased gluconeogenesis and inhibits the ability of insulin to transport glucose into the cells. Elevated cortisol levels accelerate protein catabolism, impair protein synthesis, and increase mobilization of fat from the extremities. Fat deposits increase on the trunk, in the supraclavicular areas, between the shoulders, and, to a lesser degree, on the face. Elevated cortisol levels also impair antibody production and inhibit proliferation of lymphocytes. Susceptibility to peptic ulcers increases because cortisol inhibits gastric mucous production while stimulating gastric acid and pepsin production.

The mineralocorticoid actions of excessive levels of cortisone promote potassium excretion and sodium and water retention. Increased androgen secretion causes masculine-like characteristics in women.

Clinical Manifestations

Cushing's syndrome may develop gradually or rapidly. Early clinical manifestations are muscular weakness and fatigue. In women, alteration in the menstrual cycle is an early symptom. Truncal obesity, "buffalo hump" between the shoulders, and thin extremities are characteristic. The chest and abdomen may become pendulous. Fat deposits and edema combine to give the face a round, moon-shaped appearance. Hyperglycemia produces "steroid diabetes." Protein catabolism leads to weakness, loss of muscle mass, osteoporosis, bone tenderness, and atrophy of the skin. Osteoporosis may result in pathologic fractures and vertebral compression fractures. The skin becomes thin, fragile, and paper-like, with wide purplish striae caused by deterioration of collagen fibers. Hyperpigmentation, similar to that seen in Addison's disease, may develop in persons with secondary Cushing's syndrome caused by excess ACTH secretion. Capillary fragility causes large ecchymotic areas to develop either spontaneously or from minor trauma. The face and neck typically have a ruddy appearance. Decreased protein synthesis impairs healing and response to injury and infec-

tion. Early signs of infection are often suppressed or absent. Rapid mood swings, depression, irritability, euphoria, insomnia, and occasionally psychosis may develop because of the effect of excess cortisol on mental and cognitive functions.

Fluid overload from sodium and water retention may lead to hypertension, edema, cardiac overload, and heart failure. Increased androgen secretion may cause acne, thinning of scalp hair, and decreased libido. In women, oligomenorrhea, amenorrhea, hirsutism, and mild masculinization are common. Figure 29–5 illustrates common clinical manifestations of Cushing's syndrome.

Diagnosis

Diagnosis of Cushing's syndrome is based on the clinical picture and results of laboratory studies. Circulating plasma cortisol levels are several times higher than normal, and the normal diurnal secretion pattern is absent. In 24-hour urine specimens, 17-OHCS and 17-KS levels are elevated. Plasma ACTH level is elevated in pituitary-dependent Cushing's syndrome and in nonpituitary ACTH-secreting tumors but is decreased if a cortisol-secreting adrenal tumor is present. Cortisol response to the dexa-

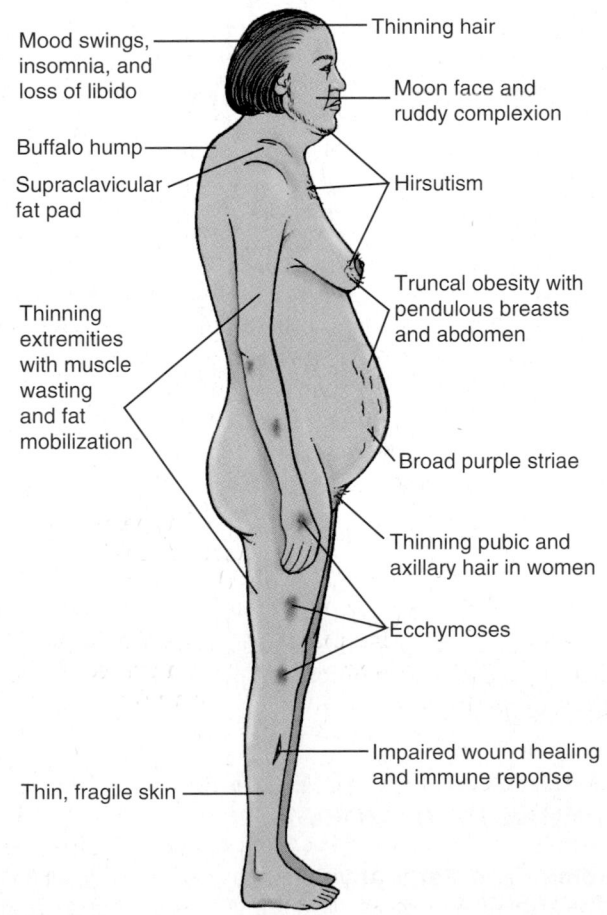

Figure 29–5

Common clinical manifestations of Cushing's syndrome.

methasone and metyrapone suppression tests varies with the cause. Results of common studies of adrenal function in Cushing's syndrome are presented in Table 29–2.

Additional laboratory studies demonstrate hyperglycemia and impaired glucose tolerance, hypokalemia, hypernatremia, hypercalcemia, and leukocytosis. Erythrocytosis, granulocytosis, lymphopenia, and eosinopenia may also be present. Radiologic studies may show osteoporosis, pathologic fractures, collapsed vertebrae, and cardiac hypertrophy.

Radiologic studies, CT scans, MRI, angiography, and studies to diagnose neoplastic disorders help to locate adrenal tumors and identify extra-adrenal sources of ACTH.

Management

The primary goal in managing Cushing's syndrome is to return cortisol levels to normal. Without treatment, half the people with Cushing's syndrome die within 5 years. With treatment, prognosis depends on the severity and duration of the disease at the time of diagnosis, plus the severity of residual cardiovascular effects. The earlier the disorder is diagnosed and treated, the better the prognosis.

Treatment of Cushing's syndrome is determined by the cause. The treatment of choice for pituitary-dependent Cushing's syndrome (Cushing's disease) is transsphenoidal microsurgery to remove the ACTH-secreting tumor while preserving normal pituitary function. Pituitary and adrenal function returns to normal in about 80% of patients with this type of disease. In some women, menses returns and pregnancy is possible. If the pituitary tumor is larger than 1 cm in diameter or has extended beyond the sella turcica, a total transsphenoidal hypophysectomy may be performed. After a total hypophysectomy, the patient requires lifelong replacement of corticosteroids, thyroid hormones, and, in some cases, gonad hormones. Bilateral adrenalectomy, irradiation of the pituitary gland, and administration of adrenal suppressant drugs are alternative treatments if transsphenoidal surgery is contraindicated.

Bilateral or unilateral adrenalectomy is indicated for an adrenal tumor or idiopathic hyperplasia. If a bilateral adrenalectomy is performed, lifelong corticosteroid replacement is required. Ectopic ACTH-secreting tumors respond best if the primary neoplasm is treated. If the neoplasm is inoperable, adrenal suppressant drugs are given. The most commonly used are mitotane (Lysodren), aminoglutethimide (Cytadren), and metyrapone (Metopirone). Mitotane, the most powerful of these drugs, destroys the adrenal zona fasciculata and zona reticularis. Because it has relatively little effect on the zona glomerulosa, patients treated with mitotane become cortisol-deficient but maintain adequate aldosterone secretion. Aminoglutethimide and metyrapone block cortisol synthesis. Nausea and vomiting, central nervous system (CNS) depression, and skin rashes are the most common side effects of adrenal suppressants. Patients are monitored closely for signs of adrenocortical insufficiency during and after treatment of Cushing's syndrome.

If exogenous administration of corticosteroids has resulted in a Cushing-like syndrome, the drug is slowly tapered to the minimal therapeutic level. To reduce the risk of Cushing-like side effects, the corticosteroids required to treat long-term chronic conditions can sometimes be administered on an alternate-day schedule to retain therapeutic effectiveness while maintaining normal ACTH secretion and adrenal responsiveness.

Mineralocorticoid effects of Cushing's syndrome are treated with spironolactone (Aldactone), a mineralocorticoid antagonist.

❖ Settings, Providers, and Collaboration for Care

The patient with Cushing's syndrome is often diagnosed and treated initially in the hospital. However, most ongoing care is delivered on an outpatient basis. The nurse, physician, patient, and family develop a plan of care in the physician's office. Implementation of the plan usually occurs in the home. Primary consideration is given to maintaining a safe environment, fostering rest and return of muscle strength, and giving ongoing health education. Some health teaching is done by the office nurse, but a home health nurse may continue it. A physical therapist may also see the patient at home for evaluation and to provide exercise instructions to improve muscle strength.

NURSING PROCESS
Adrenocortical Excess (Cushing's Syndrome)

Assessment

Obtain a complete nursing history from a patient with diagnosed or suspected adrenocortical excess. Ask specifically about the use of adrenocortical steroid compounds. Obtain weight and measurement of vital signs. Compare these with presymptomatic assessments if documented or known by the patient. Assess for dependent edema, altered skin integrity, and clinical manifestations associated with Cushing's syndrome. Determine the patient's activity level and ability to carry out activities of daily living (ADLs). Identify the patient's interpretation of clinical manifestations, knowledge of planned diagnostic procedures and treatment, and expectations of the outcome of treatment to determine teaching needs.

Nursing Diagnoses and Planning

Nursing diagnoses and related expected patient outcomes commonly applicable to patients with adrenocortical excess (Cushing's syndrome) include the following:

NDx: Risk for infection related to impaired immune response and tissue repair

Planning: Patient Outcomes
1. Patient identifies activities that increase the risk of infection.
2. Patient participates in activities that reduce the risk of infection.
3. Patient remains afebrile and damaged tissue remains free of localized inflammation, edema, and purulent drainage.

NDx: Risk for altered health maintenance related to insufficient knowledge of how disease process alters carbohydrate, protein, and fat metabolism and increases risk of injury as evidenced by hyperglycemia, skin and capillary fragility, muscle weakness, altered center of gravity, osteoporosis, and increased gastric acid and pepsin secretion

Planning: Patient Outcomes
1. Patient verbalizes understanding of the effects of excess cortisol secretion on the body.
2. Patient identifies activities that increase the risk of injury.
3. Patient participates in activities that reduce the risk of injury.
4. Patient remains free of injury.

NDx: Decreased cardiac output related to fluid and electrolyte imbalance

Planning: Patient Outcomes
1. Patient demonstrates adequate cardiac output as evidenced by the following:
   Stable vital signs within normal limits
   Ability to complete self-care activities
   Absence of dependent edema, dyspnea, or orthopnea
   Lungs clear to auscultation
2. Patient identifies and selects low-sodium foods from daily menu choices.
3. Patient demonstrates stable or decreasing weight.

NDx: Body image disturbance related to physical and behavioral changes characteristic of adrenocortical excess

Planning: Patient Outcomes
1. Patient identifies adrenocortical excess as cause of physical and behavioral changes.
2. Patient verbalizes realistic expectations of treatment.
3. Patient verbalizes positive statements about self and future plans.

Nursing Interventions and Evaluation

The focus of nursing care for the patient with adrenocortical excess is to prevent potentially life-threatening infection and injury. Throughout diagnosis and treatment, provide emotional support and information to help the patient and family understand and cope with the physical and mental manifestations of Cushing's disease while developing realistic expectations of treatment.

NDx: Risk for infection
Place the patient in a private room or a room with a noninfectious roommate. To minimize exposure to pathogens, protect the patient from visitors and staff with infectious diseases. Discuss the effect of excess cortisol secretion on the body's immune response and tissue repair. Stress proper hand-washing by staff, the patient, and visitors. Avoid unnecessary invasive procedures. Use sterile technique when caring for all open lesions, venipuncture sites, and drains to prevent contamination. Monitor temperature every 4 hours. Assess all open areas for signs of infection or inflammation. Culture all suspicious drainage and slow-healing wounds.

Monitor the results of white blood cell counts to ensure prompt identification of infection. Signs of inflammation may be masked by excess cortisol. Administer prescribed antibiotics on time to ensure therapeutic blood levels. Encourage the patient to deep breathe and cough every hour while awake. To mobilize respiratory secretions and reduce the risk of pulmonary infection, assist him or her to turn every 2 hours while in bed. Help the patient select a high-protein diet to promote tissue repair.

NDx: Risk for altered health maintenance
Explain the effects of excess cortisol secretion on body systems. Confer with the patient to identify potential sources of trauma, activities that increase the risk of injury, and ways to minimize risk during daily activities. Encourage the patient to take several rest periods during the day to conserve energy. Assist with daily activities as needed, but encourage independence as tolerated to promote self-esteem. Provide a safe, obstacle-free environment. Encourage the patient to wear nonskid shoes to prevent falls. Encourage ambulation and assist as necessary to promote muscle tone and calcium deposition in the bones. Use side rails as appropriate for safety or for self-positioning in bed. Assess skin for redness, breakdown, and ecchymosis. Gently massage bony prominences. Apply skin lubricants at least twice daily to prevent breakdown.

Use a pressure distribution mattress and elbow and heel protectors. Help the patient with position changes every 2 hours while he or she is in bed. Monitor blood glucose levels and administer insulin as prescribed. Unless contraindicated, provide prescribed calorie-restricted, high-protein diet in six small meals a day. Give an antacid or H_2-receptor antagonist, as ordered, to decrease gastric acidity and prevent peptic ulcers. Report gastrointestinal distress, heartburn, and epigastric pain to the physician promptly.

NDx: Decreased cardiac output
Monitor vital signs and apical heart rate and auscultate breath sounds every 4 hours to detect changes in hemodynamic status. Administer prescribed diuretics and antihypertensives. Measure blood pressure daily with the patient lying and sitting or standing to detect orthostatic hypotension. Weigh

the patient daily. Assess for edema. Monitor intake and output to evaluate fluid balance. Assess for signs of hypokalemia and give a potassium supplement if prescribed.

Help the patient select low-sodium and high-potassium foods from the daily menu. Encourage independence in self-care but provide assistance as needed to prevent overexertion. Discontinue all activity in response to tachycardia, dyspnea, fatigue, light-headedness, or change in blood pressure, which signal activity intolerance. Report these symptoms to the physician.

Once a method of treatment is selected, reinforce the physician's explanations, provide opportunity for questions, and correct any misconceptions the patient may have. After surgical excision of an adrenal tumor, a pituitary adenoma, or an ACTH-secreting ectopic neoplasm, the patient is usually in an intensive-care setting for 48 to 72 hours to allow constant monitoring for rapid changes in cardiac function, electrolyte balance, and hemodynamic status caused by the sudden cessation of excess cortisol secretion. Nursing Care Guide 29–3 outlines nursing care of a patient after adrenal surgery.

To prevent Addison's crisis, the physician prescribes parenteral administration of dexamethasone or another glucocorticoid preoperatively, intraoperatively, and postoperatively. Doses become progressively smaller and gradually taper off in the days after surgery. After bilateral adrenalectomy, the patient requires adrenocortical hormone replacement for life, as discussed for the treatment of Addison's disease. Because these patients are at extremely high risk for postoperative infection and delayed wound healing, aggressive pulmonary hygiene, aseptic technique and meticulous wound care are imperative.

If administration of adrenal-suppressant drugs is the selected treatment, teach the patient the name, dose, route of administration, expected therapeutic effects, and side effects. Be sure the patient understands that the desired effects of these drugs may not become apparent for several weeks. Teach and provide in writing the early signs of adrenocortical insufficiency and instruct the patient to notify the physician immediately if they develop. If hormone-replacement therapy is needed for adrenocortical insufficiency, follow the nursing guidelines for teaching self-management (see Highlight 29–3).

NDx: Body image disturbance
Provide factual information about the effect of increased levels of circulating cortisol on the body and mental status to help the patient and family understand changes that have occurred. Encourage the patient to identify and describe feelings about physical changes. Reassure the patient that most physical changes and emotional disturbances resolve with treatment. Help the patient identify relaxation techniques to help control emotions. Maintain a calm, unhurried manner. Explain procedures clearly to promote relaxation and trust. Observe the patient

closely during episodes of emotional instability and depression. Some patients may become dangerous to themselves or others. Request a mental health consultation if appropriate.

Once the treatment method is selected, reinforce the physician's explanations of the treatment and expected outcome. Provide opportunity for discussion and questions to correct any misconceptions the patient may have. Be sure the patient understands what pathologic changes, if any, the physician expects to be residual. Reinforce the need for lifelong follow-up for early detection of recurring or developing adrenocortical insufficiency.

Compare the patient's status with the expected outcomes. If the outcomes are not met, reassess the patient and revise the plan.

PRIMARY ALDOSTERONISM

Etiology and Pathophysiology
Primary aldosteronism is characterized by increased aldosterone secretion. It most commonly results from a benign aldosterone-secreting adenoma of the zona glomerulosa. Bilateral adrenal cortex hyperplasia is the cause in less than 30% of cases. Adrenal carcinoma very rarely causes increased aldosterone secretion. Primary aldosteronism is diagnosed in about 1% of the hypertensive population. It occurs more than twice as often in women as in men and usually develops between ages 30 and 50.

Unregulated hypersecretion of aldosterone results in increased sodium retention in the distal renal tubules, with excess potassium and hydrogen ion excretion and suppression of renin production. As a result of this electrolyte imbalance, increased extracellular fluid volume, hypertension, and hypokalemia develop. Metabolic alkalosis occurs as hydrogen ions are excreted with the potassium. Peripheral edema is either minimal or absent in primary aldosteronism because the proximal renal tubules attempt to compensate for the fluid excess by decreasing sodium reabsorption.

Left ventricular hypertrophy, congestive heart failure, cerebrovascular accidents, and progressive deterioration of renal function and vision result from the pathologic effects of prolonged hypertension.

Clinical Manifestations
Hypertension and hypokalemia are the most significant clinical manifestations of primary aldosteronism. Edema develops only in the presence of congestive heart failure. Hypertension may be mild to severe. Headaches are common and may be accompanied by visual disturbances and orthostatic hypotension. Hypokalemia results in lethargy, fatigue, muscle weakness, cramps, paresthesias, cardiac dysrhythmias, and decreased ability of the kidneys to concentrate urine. Increased urine volume leads to polyuria, nocturia, and polydipsia. Metabolic alkalo-

Nursing Care Guide 29–3
Patient Care After Adrenalectomy for Cushing's Syndrome

Assessment Findings: Patient admitted to surgical intensive care unit from postanesthesia care unit after unilateral adrenalectomy for Cushing's syndrome.

Nursing Diagnosis: Risk for altered systemic tissue perfusion related to fluid loss and electrolyte imbalance secondary to rapid depletion of adrenocortical hormones and risk of postoperative hemorrhage

Patient Outcomes	Nursing Interventions	Rationale
Patient demonstrates adequate extracellular fluid volume by moist mucous membranes, good skin turgor, blood pressure within 10% of normal baseline, pulse 60–100 bpm, urine output > 30 mL/hr, and is alert and responds appropriately.	Administer intravenous hydrocortisone and isotonic dextrose and saline for 24 to 48 hours postoperatively. Administer mineralocorticoid, if prescribed, on the second postoperative day.	Adrenocorticosteroid replacement is necessary to stabilize serum steroid levels during rapid drop in endogenous adrenocortical hormone secretion after surgery. Fluid, glucose, and electrolyte replacement minimizes the risk of Addison's crisis and hypovolemic shock and maintains electrolyte balance.
	Monitor vital signs, neurologic status, urine output, capillary refill hourly. Monitor blood glucose four times daily. Monitor electrocardiogram and pulmonary wedge pressure.	Hemodynamic parameters indicate perfusion of vital organs. Drop in endogenous glucocorticoid secretion places patient at risk for hypoglycemia.
	Examine flank incision and surgical dressings and check under patient frequently for active bleeding. Examine abdomen for hematoma or distension caused by internal bleeding.	Risk of postoperative bleeding is high because adrenal glands and kidneys are highly vascular.
	Provide a noninfectious environment, maintain strict aseptic technique, encourage coughing and deep-breathing, and assist with early ambulation to decrease risk of infection.	Risk of infection is high as a result of suppressed immune response, impaired protein synthesis, and delayed wound healing.
	Administer prescribed analgesics.	Promotes patient comfort, reduces stress, and increases patient participation in postoperative activities that decrease the risk of infection and promote healing.
	After 48 hours, administer prescribed decreasing doses of adrenocortical hormones.	Allows the remaining adrenal gland to gradually resume hormone secretion.
	Monitor for manifestations of adrenocortical deficiency as exogenous hormones are slowly tapered and notify the physician immediately if they develop.	Early detection and treatment prevent or minimize the risk of crisis.

(continued)

Nursing Care Guide 29–3
Patient Care After Adrenalectomy for Cushing's Syndrome (continued)

Patient Outcomes	Nursing Interventions	Rationale
	Provide oral fluids, food, and medications 48 to 72 hours postoperatively as tolerated and discontinue intravenous infusion.	Intravenous access is a potential route of infection.
Evaluation:	Compare the patient's status with the expected outcomes. If the outcomes are not met, reassess the patient and revise the plan.	

sis resulting from hydrogen ion loss correlates to the degree of potassium loss and may result in tetany. Positive Chvostek's (tapping the facial nerve in front of the earlobe elicits spasms of the facial muscle) and Trousseau's (severe carpopedal spasm elicited when a blood pressure cuff is inflated to slightly above the patient's systolic pressure for 1–5 minutes) signs indicate the increased neuromuscular irritability that precedes tetany.

Diagnosis

Diagnosis of primary aldosteronism is based on the presence of hypertension with hypokalemia, low plasma renin levels, and elevated serum and urinary aldosterone levels. Urinary potassium levels exceed 30 mEq/day. Additional laboratory studies demonstrate metabolic alkalosis, hypernatremia, and low urine specific gravity. Impaired glucose tolerance is present in some patients. Mild proteinuria may be present. Renal function studies detect the presence of renal damage.

Radiologic studies, CT scans, MRI, and angiography help to locate adrenal tumors and identify bilateral hyperplasia of the adrenal cortex. Electrocardiograms identify altered electrical conductivity of the myocardium.

Management

The treatment of choice for an aldosterone-secreting adrenal adenoma is unilateral adrenalectomy. Before surgery, hypertension and hypokalemia are corrected by a low-sodium diet, potassium supplements, and administration of spironolactone (Aldactone), an aldosterone antagonist.

Patients with bilateral adrenal hyperplasia are treated medically with spironolactone and a low-sodium, high-potassium diet. Potassium supplements may also be prescribed. If blood pressure remains elevated, other antihypertensive agents and potassium-sparing diuretics may be added.

NURSING PROCESS GUIDELINES
Primary Aldosteronism

Assess for the clinical manifestations of primary aldosteronism in all patients who have hypertension and hypokalemia with no apparent reason for excess potassium loss. Ask specifically about unusual fatigue, muscle weakness, cramps, palpitations, paresthesias, and frequent urination associated with hypokalemia. Monitor vital signs and apical heart rate every 4 hours to assess blood pressure and cardiac rhythm. Measure blood pressure daily with the patient lying and then sitting or standing to detect orthostatic hypotension. Weigh the patient daily. Assess for edema. Monitor intake and output to evaluate fluid balance. Monitor results of serum electrolyte and arterial blood gas studies. Administer potassium supplements and spironolactone as prescribed. Assess and document response to therapy. Assist the patient in the timely completion of diagnostic tests. Explain the rationale for the prescribed low-sodium, high-potassium diet, and help the patient make appropriate choices from the daily menu.

Once the diagnosis is confirmed and a method of treatment selected, reinforce the physician's explanations, provide opportunity for questions, and correct any misconceptions the patient may have. Nursing care after an adrenalectomy was discussed earlier in this chapter. Nursing care after a unilateral adrenalectomy for primary aldosteronism is similar. Because the patient still has one functioning adrenal gland, lifelong steroid replacement therapy is not necessary.

If surgery is contraindicated and lifelong medical treatment is prescribed, teach the patient the name, dose, route and time of administration, expected therapeutic effects, and side effects of prescribed medications. Consult with a dietitian to teach and provide (in writing) a low-sodium, high-potassium diet. Tell the patient to report to the physician unusual weight gain, dependent edema, increasing fatigue, dyspnea, or palpitations. Reinforce the need for lifelong follow-up care for the early detection of altered response to therapy.

PHEOCHROMOCYTOMA

Etiology and Pathophysiology
Pheochromocytomas are the most common pathologic condition associated with the adrenal medulla. They are rare, catecholamine-producing tumors that arise from chromaffin cells of the sympathetic nervous system. These individual or multiple tumors can develop anywhere along the sympathetic nerve chain. More than 90% of these neoplasms occur in the adrenal medulla. The rest develop in extra-adrenal sites along the sympathetic nerve chain in the head or trunk. Extra-adrenal pheochromocytomas are sometimes called paragangliomas.

Pheochromocytomas are characterized by unregulated hypersecretion of catecholamines. They can occur throughout life, but are most common between ages 40 and 60. They are diagnosed in slightly more women than men.

Although the cause of pheochromocytoma is unknown, it is diagnosed most frequently, and at an earlier age, in people with a family history of pheochromocytoma or a history of other endocrine gland neoplasias. It is often associated with hyperparathyroidism, thyroid medullary carcinoma, and multiple endocrine neoplasia (MEN) syndrome. The incidence of multiple tumors increases with a positive family history of pheochromocytoma.

Most pheochromocytomas are benign. They are well-encapsulated, highly vascular tumors that synthesize, store, and secrete catecholamines. Less than 5% are malignant. Malignant tumors metastasize to the bones, liver, lymph nodes, and lungs. Malignant tumors resist radiation and chemotherapy. Survival after diagnosis rarely exceeds 3 years.

Clinical Manifestations
The pathologic changes associated with pheochromocytomas result from heightened physiologic responses to increased levels of circulating catecholamines. Excess secretion may be continuous or paroxysmal and produces cardiovascular and metabolic disturbances that can be fatal if untreated. Overstimulation of α-receptors and β-receptors of the sympathetic nervous system produces increased peripheral vasoconstriction, increased heart rate, increased myocardial contractility and irritability, increased metabolism and oxygen utilization, increased respiratory rate, increased glycogenolysis, decreased peristalsis, stimulation of the sweat and apocrine glands, and pupillary dilatation.

Hypertension is the most significant clinical feature of pheochromocytoma. Most people experience sustained mild to severe hypertension. Many have superimposed paroxysmal episodes of malignant hypertension that reaches 300/180 mm Hg or higher. Malignant hypertensive episodes are caused by intermittent release of large amounts of catecholamines from the tumor. These episodes may be spontaneous or may be precipitated by stress, a change in position, physical activity, or the Valsalva maneuver. They may last from a few minutes to a few hours. Most episodes subside within 40 minutes. As the disease progresses, paroxysmal hypertensive episodes become more frequent.

Hypertension may be accompanied by a pounding headache, tachycardia, palpitations, hyperventilation, dizziness, visual disturbances, nausea, vomiting, and profuse diaphoresis associated with blanching or flushing of the skin. Patients often describe a feeling of impending doom during a hypertensive episode.

Other clinical manifestations include episodes of postural hypotension, abdominal pain, constipation, weakness, fine muscle tremors, hyperreflexia, anxiety, nervousness, insomnia, and increased metabolism and blood glucose levels.

Cardiovascular, pulmonary, and renal problems may develop from sustained hypertension. Congestive heart failure, cerebrovascular accidents, and renal failure are common complications. Death may result from cardiac dysrhythmias, pulmonary edema, or cerebral hemorrhage.

Diagnosis
A diagnosis of pheochromocytoma may be suspected from physical manifestations and a history of periodic or sustained hypertension with no known cause, but a definitive diagnosis cannot be made without laboratory tests.

Catecholamines are almost completely metabolized into inactive waste products, which are excreted and can be measured in the urine. These metabolites are metanephrine, normetanephrine, and vanillylmandelic acid (VMA). One, and usually all, of these substances are increased in pheochromocytoma. Assay of urinary catecholamines and their metabolites can be performed on a single first-voided morning urine specimen as a screening test or on a 24-hour specimen for definitive diagnosis. Proper patient preparation and collection and preservation of the specimen for urinary catecholamines are necessary to ensure an accurate and timely diagnosis. Timed specimens are difficult to collect, so the procedure must be a high priority in the patient's care. Table 29–3 presents guidelines for the collection of a 24-hour urine specimen for catecholamines. The normal values for urinary catecholamines and their metabolites are presented in Table 29–4.

Because of the effects of excessive catecholamine secretion, the patient also exhibits an increased basal metabolic rate and elevated blood glucose levels. Glycosuria and albuminuria may be present. Radiologic studies, CT scans, MRI, and angiography help locate the tumor and identify extra-adrenal sites.

Table 29-3

Nursing Guide to 24-Hour Urine Collection for Urinary Catecholamines

1. Assess the patient's ability to collect the specimen correctly.
2. Advise the patient of the purpose of the test, the length of time required for the test, how to collect the urine, and where to save it.
3. Instruct the patient to void and discard the urine. 24-hour beginning time starts at this point.
4. Provide a specimen container for collection of all urine for the next 24 hours.
5. On the specimen container and patient record, record the exact start time and date, and end time and date.
6. Post a notice in the patient's bathroom and on the patient's record to remind the patient and staff that a 24-hour urine collection is in progress.
7. If any urine is inadvertently discarded, stop the collection and begin a new specimen collection in a new container.
8. At the end of the 24-hour period, instruct the patient to void and add this urine to the specimen container.
9. Many foods and drugs affect urinary catecholamine levels. Restriction of specific substances depends on the evaluation method used. Consult the laboratory to determine which food and drugs must be restricted. Changes in dietary and drug therapies must be ordered by the physician.
10. Explain diet and drug restrictions to the patient.
11. Note any medications administered during specimen collection on the laboratory requisition.
12. Catecholamines and their metabolites are unstable in urine. A preservative, usually hydrochloric acid, may be added to the specimen container, and the container may be kept on ice or refrigerated during collection. The method of specimen preservation depends on the evaluation method used and is determined by the laboratory.

Management

Although less than 0.5% of people with hypertension have pheochromocytoma, it is an important disorder because it is curable with treatment in 90% of

Table 29-4

Urinary Catecholamines and Their Metabolites

Laboratory Test	Normal Values*
Vanillylmandelic acid	<7 mg/24 hr
Epinephrine	0–15 μg/24 hr
Norepinephrine	0–100 μg/24 hr
Metanephrine	0.25–0.8 mg/24 hr

*Normal values are guidelines. Contact laboratory performing test for absolute values.

cases. The treatment of choice is surgical excision of the tumor or tumors. If the tumors are within the adrenal medullae, a unilateral or bilateral adrenalectomy is performed. With removal of both adrenal glands, the sympathetic nervous system takes over the functions of the missing adrenal medullae. Lifelong corticosteroid therapy is required to replace adrenal cortex functions.

Preoperatively, a stimulant-free diet and bedrest with the head of the bed elevated to 45 degrees are prescribed to help reduce blood pressure and prevent hypertensive episodes. Hypertensive crisis is controlled by intravenous administration of phentolamine (Regitine), a rapid-acting alpha-adrenergic blocking agent, followed by oral administration of longer-acting phenoxybenzamine (Dibenzyline) or prazosin (Minipress). Catecholamine-induced cardiac dysrhythmias are treated with propranolol (Inderal) once alpha-adrenergic blockade has been established. These drugs are also administered for 10 days to 2 weeks before surgery to lessen the chance of intraoperative and postoperative complications. Hypovolemic shock caused by rapid relaxation of constricted blood vessels is the most common postoperative complication. Transient hypertensive episodes are common.

In the 10% of patients who are not surgical candidates because of additional medical problems or metastasized malignant pheochromocytomas, symptomatic relief can be obtained by administering phenoxybenzamine, a catecholamine biosynthesis inhibitor. Five-year survival in this group is less than 50%.

❖ Settings, Providers, and Collaboration for Care

The acute-care setting becomes the primary care environment for patients with pheochromocytoma. A multidisciplinary team is needed to address the critical issues of patient care. After discharge, the home health nurse is responsible for assistance with health maintenance.

NURSING PROCESS
Pheochromocytoma

Assessment

Obtain a complete nursing history. Ask specifically about factors that precipitate hypertensive episodes and the manifestations that accompany an episode. Obtain baseline weight, vital signs, and neurologic signs. Assess for clinical manifestations common to pheochromocytoma. Identify the patient's interpretation of clinical manifestations and assess his or her knowledge of planned diagnostic tests and treatment to determine teaching needs.

Postoperatively, the patient is usually in an intensive-care setting for constant nursing observation and monitoring of cardiovascular status.

Nursing Diagnoses and Planning

Nursing diagnoses and related expected patient outcomes commonly applicable to patients with pheochromocytoma include the following:

NDx: Risk for altered systemic tissue perfusion related to rapid fluctuations in cardiovascular status

Planning: Patient Outcomes
1. Patient avoids activities that precipitate hypertensive episodes.
2. Patient notifies nurse immediately about the onset of a hypertensive episode.
3. Patient maintains adequate tissue perfusion preoperatively and postoperatively as evidenced by the following:
   Stable vital signs within normal limits
   Normal neurologic responses
   Urine output more than 30 mL/hr
   Lungs clear to auscultation

NDx: Anxiety related to overstimulation of the nervous system by increased levels of circulating catecholamines

Planning: Patient Outcomes
1. Patient identifies the disease process as the cause of feelings of anxiety.
2. Patient uses relaxation exercises to reduce anxiety levels.

NDx: Altered nutrition: less than body requirements related to increased metabolism, abdominal pain, nausea, vomiting, and/or constipation secondary to prolonged catecholamine hypersecretion

Planning: Patient Outcomes
1. Patient maintains stable weight within recommended norms.
2. Patient defecates soft, formed stool at least every third day.

NDx: Risk for altered health maintenance related to insufficient knowledge of follow-up care

Planning: Patient Outcomes
1. Patient verbalizes understanding of the need for lifelong follow-up care.
2. Patient states intent to advise family members to have screening test for pheochromocytoma.

Nursing Interventions and Evaluation

Nursing care of the patient with pheochromocytoma requires frequent assessment and supportive intervention because of potentially rapid fluctuations in cardiovascular status.

NDx: Risk for altered systemic tissue perfusion
Monitor vital signs and neurologic signs at least every 4 hours, and every 15 minutes during a hypertensive episode. Administer catecholamine-blocking agents as prescribed. Weigh the patient daily. Monitor urine output to detect changes in renal status. Auscultate heart sounds to detect cardiac dysrhythmias and lung sounds to detect congestion and crackles, which may indicate developing pulmonary edema. Keep the head of the bed at 30 to 45 degrees to promote orthostatic reduction of blood pressure and minimize intracranial pressure. Raise side rails to prevent injury from neurologic manifestations or visual disturbances. Prevent chills and provide frequent skin care during profuse diaphoresis. Minimize patient activity as prescribed, and provide a restful environment free of unnecessary stimuli.

Tell the patient to notify a nurse immediately if symptoms of a hypertensive episode develop. Notify the physician at the onset of a hypertensive episode and have phentolamine and emergency cardiac drugs readily available.

Teach the patient to change position slowly and to avoid rapid movements, bearing down, stress, and any activities that precipitated hypertensive episodes in the past. Do not palpate the patient's abdomen because it may stimulate catecholamine release in some people. Post a reminder notice to this effect on the nursing care plan and above the bed. Tell the patient not to smoke and to avoid caffeine because nicotine and caffeine stimulate catecholamine secretion.

Postoperatively, the patient will have a midline or transverse abdominal incision. The first 48 hours after surgery are critical because of unstable blood pressure and the risk of postoperative hemorrhage. The patient is usually in intensive care and requires constant observation and monitoring of cardiovascular status. Administer prescribed intravenous fluids to stabilize blood pressure until the effects of excess catecholamines and preoperative alpha-adrenergic blockers wear off. This takes about 36 hours.

Examine surgical dressings frequently for bleeding. Assess the abdomen for hematoma, which could indicate internal hemorrhage. Large abdominal incisions are very painful. Administer prescribed analgesics to promote comfort, mobility, and participation in breathing exercises. Monitor blood pressure before each dose because many narcotics produce hypotension as a side effect. Monitor urine output hourly for 48 hours after surgery to detect possible kidney damage from surgery or renal failure from profound postoperative shock.

After the immediate postoperative phase, recovery is usually uneventful. The patient is discharged from the hospital once blood pressure readings stabilize and results of a 24-hour urine test for catecholamines and their metabolites are within normal limits. If a bilateral adrenalectomy was performed, the patient will require lifelong replacement therapy with corticosteroids.

NDx: Anxiety
Provide information about the effect of increased levels of circulating catecholamines on the nervous

system. Encourage the patient to identify and describe feelings. Assist the patient in identifying and practicing relaxation techniques that help control anxiety levels. Stay with the patient and provide emotional support during frightening hypertensive episodes. Many patients believe they are going to die. Speak in a calm, reassuring voice, and maintain a calm, unhurried manner to promote relaxation and trust.

NDx: Altered nutrition: less than body requirements

Weigh the patient and compare with normal weight range for people of same sex, height, and body build. Monitor weight at least three times weekly. Monitor blood glucose levels to detect elevation. Provide several small, fiber-rich meals, incorporating the patient's food preferences when nausea is absent. Omit stimulating foods and beverages from the diet. If weight loss is severe, a high-calorie, high-vitamin diet may be prescribed once blood glucose levels are controlled. Administer prescribed stool softeners, laxatives, or enemas to relieve constipation.

NDx: Risk for altered health maintenance

In preparing the patient for discharge, stress the need for lifelong follow-up. The recurrence rate of pheochromocytoma after surgery is about 10%. Teach the patient the symptoms of pheochromocytoma. Tell the patient to report these symptoms to the physician promptly. Periodic 24-hour urine specimens may be collected to measure for catecholamines. Provide the patient with clearly written instructions on the collection procedure (see Table 29–3).

Because there is a familial tendency to develop pheochromocytomas, an important nursing intervention is to advise family members to have a single, first-voided morning urine specimen tested for metanephrines. The specimen for this test is easier and less expensive to collect than a 24-hour specimen, and the test is an accurate screening tool. If results are abnormal, further evaluation for pheochromocytoma is necessary.

Compare the patient's status with the expected outcomes. If the outcomes are not met, reassess the patient and revise the plan.

Thyroid Disorders

Disruptions of thyroid function are among the most commonly diagnosed endocrine disorders. Many are autoimmune disorders. Although the pathophysiology and clinical manifestations of each disorder differ, most result in either increased or decreased hormone production and alter metabolism and cellular function throughout the body. The effect may vary from a subtle change in homeostasis to a life-threatening emergency.

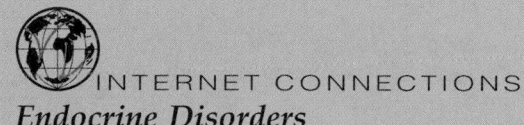

INTERNET CONNECTIONS
Endocrine Disorders

General
The Endocrine Society
http://www.endo-society.org/
This site, oriented toward health-care professionals, provides news and facts, as well as information about publications, scientific meetings, awards and grants, and links to related sites.

Pituitary Disorders
Pituitary Tumor Network Association
http://www.pituitary.com/
This site provides information for health-care professionals as well as patients and their families. General information covers early detection, symptoms, treatments, and resources available to patients with pituitary tumors. Other features include a resource guide for patients, a list of support groups and peer counseling services, a guide to upcoming events, and links to other sites.

Adrenal Disorders
Addison's Disease, National Institute of Diabetes and Digestive and Kidney Diseases
http://www.niddk.nih.gov/AD/AD.html
This encyclopedia-style article provides authoritative information about Addison's disease.

Thyroid Disorders
alt.support thyroid page
http://www.geocities.com/Athens/3626/faqs.html
The site provides answers to frequently asked questions relating to Graves' disease, antithyroid drugs, Hashimoto's thyroiditis, and thyroid function tests.

Health Guides on Thyroid Disease, Thyroid Foundation of Canada
http://www.io.org/~thyroid/English/Guides.html
This site gives access to a series of patient-oriented pamphlets (in English and in French) covering various aspects of thyroid disease.

THYROIDITIS

Thyroiditis is an inflammation of the thyroid gland characterized by enlargement and, often, altered thyroid function. Thyroiditis may be acute, subacute, or chronic. The two most common forms are subacute and chronic.

Acute Thyroiditis

Acute thyroiditis is a rare condition caused by bacterial infection of all or part of the thyroid gland. The patient presents with fever, tenderness on palpation of the thyroid gland, neck pain, swelling, and elevated leukocyte count. Thyroid function is usually normal. Recovery is usually rapid and complete after identification of the causative pathogen and administration of appropriate antibiotics.

Subacute Granulomatous Thyroiditis

The most common form of subacute thyroiditis is granulomatous thyroiditis, also called de Quervain's thyroiditis and giant cell thyroiditis. It is a self-limiting viral infection of the thyroid gland. Although the incidence is not precisely known, it is not considered a rare disease. Subacute thyroiditis is most commonly diagnosed in women between the ages of 30 and 60, usually several weeks after the mumps or an upper respiratory viral infection. Mild cases may be mistakenly diagnosed as pharyngitis.

Subacute granulomatous thyroiditis is characterized by painful enlargement of the thyroid gland with fever, malaise, dysphagia, hoarseness, leukocytosis, and elevated erythrocyte sedimentation rate (ESR). Pain often radiates to the ear, jaw, or occiput and intensifies with movement of the head or swallowing. The skin over the thyroid gland may be warm and red. Signs of hyperthyroidism (nervousness, tachycardia, and palpitations) caused by release of stored thyroid hormone from damaged thyroid follicles are common early in the disease. A subnormal radioactive iodine uptake (RAIU), despite normal or elevated serum thyroxine level, is diagnostic of subacute granulomatous thyroiditis.

Treatment is symptomatic. Aspirin or acetaminophen is prescribed for fever and discomfort. In severe cases, an anti-inflammatory glucocorticoid may be administered. Two to 4 weeks after onset, many patients experience a transient period of hypothyroidism. The benefit of thyroid hormone replacement therapy during this period is inconclusive. Several months are required for complete recovery. To identify the 5 to 10% of patients who develop permanent hypothyroidism from destruction of thyroid follicular epithelial tissue, close medical evaluation during the recovery period is important.

Silent (Painless) Thyroiditis

Silent, or painless, thyroiditis is a recently identified syndrome thought to have an autoimmune etiology. It is characterized by symptoms of hyperthyroidism associated with subnormal radioactive iodine uptake and normal erythrocyte sedimentation rate. There may be slight enlargement, but no tenderness, of the thyroid gland. The hyperthyroid state may last 2 months and be followed by a transient hypothyroid period. Remission is spontaneous, but the syndrome may recur. Propranolol is prescribed if hyperthyroid manifestations are severe.

Chronic Thyroiditis (Hashimoto's Thyroiditis)

The most common form of chronic thyroiditis, Hashimoto's or chronic lymphocytic thyroiditis, is an autoimmune thyroiditis. It occurs at least 10 times more frequently in women than in men and is diagnosed primarily between the ages of 30 and 50. There is often a family history of thyroid disease and other autoimmune disorders. The frequency in people with Down's syndrome or Turner's syndrome is very high.

Hashimoto's thyroiditis is characterized by destructive lymphocytic infiltration and fibrosis of the thyroid tissue. The earliest clinical manifestation is usually a small to moderate enlargement of the thyroid gland called a goiter. The goiter usually develops slowly, is nontender and free of nodules, has a firm to hard, rubbery consistency, and moves freely when the patient swallows. The surface may feel smooth or scalloped. Although a goiter caused by Hashimoto's thyroiditis is usually diffuse and symmetric, some asymmetry of the lobes is not unusual. Rarely, a large goiter compresses adjacent structures, such as the trachea or esophagus, and causes hoarseness or dysphagia. Lymph node enlargement is uncommon. Initially, the patient is euthyroid. If untreated, the goiter gradually increases in size as lymphocytic infiltration and fibrosis of the thyroid tissue progress. The patient develops hypothyroidism as a result of loss of functioning thyroid tissue.

The diagnosis of Hashimoto's thyroiditis is confirmed by demonstration of high titers of circulating antithyroid antibodies in the serum. Clinical and diagnostic manifestations of hypothyroidism help confirm the diagnosis, although results of thyroid function studies may be within normal range if the disease is diagnosed early.

Medical management depends on the size of the goiter and the clinical manifestations present. If the goiter is small and the patient is asymptomatic, no treatment is required. Thyroid hormone therapy is used to treat hypothyroidism and reduce the size of the goiter. Surgery is rare but may be required if thyroid hormone therapy fails to reduce the size of a large unsightly goiter or to relieve pressure symptoms. After surgery, the patient is hypothyroid and requires lifetime maintenance with thyroid hormone replacement. Medical and nursing management of a patient with hypothyroidism and after thyroid surgery is discussed later in this chapter.

FUNCTIONAL DISORDERS

Functional disorders of the thyroid gland are characterized by altered production of thyroid hormone and often are associated with enlargement of the thyroid gland. They are second only to diabetes mellitus among naturally occurring endocrine disorders.

Hypothyroidism

Hypothyroidism is a metabolic disorder usually characterized by a deficiency of the circulating thyroid hormones thyroxine and triiodothyronine. In rare instances, manifestations of hypothyroidism may be caused by an inability of the target tissues to bind with or use available thyroid hormone. Although it can develop in any age group, hypothyroidism is most common after middle age. Hypothyroidism is five times more prevalent in women than in men.

Hypothyroidism that develops during fetal life or infancy and that results in defective physical development and mental retardation is termed *cretinism*. Juvenile hypothyroidism develops during childhood, after the brain is fully developed, but may still cause defective physical development. Early detection and treatment of hypothyroidism in infants and children will prevent mental retardation and promote normal physical development.

Etiology and Pathophysiology

Primary hypothyroidism is a defect in the thyroid gland itself. The gland is unable to produce or release adequate amounts of thyroid hormone. In the adult, primary hypothyroidism most commonly develops in a person with a history of chronic thyroiditis (Hashimoto's thyroiditis), an autoimmune disease in which thyroid tissue is gradually destroyed by thyroid antibodies. Hypothyroidism that is characterized by atrophy of the thyroid gland may be caused by failure of the pituitary gland to secrete thyroid-stimulating hormone, referred to as secondary hypothyroidism, or by failure of the hypothalamus to secrete thyroid-releasing hormone, referred to as tertiary hypothyroidism.

Iatrogenic causes of hypothyroidism include surgical removal or irradiation of the thyroid or pituitary gland and overtreatment of hyperthyroidism with antithyroid agents. Rarely, hypothyroidism may be caused by dietary deficiency of iodine or excess or prolonged ingestion of goitrogens. Goitrogens are drugs and foods that contain thyroid-inhibiting substances that decrease thyroxine production. Although dietary deficiency of iodine is rare in the United States, it is still common in landlocked areas of developing countries. Table 29–5 lists common causes of hypothyroidism.

Pathologic changes associated with hypothyroidism vary with the age of onset of the disorder, its duration before diagnosis, and the severity of the hormone deficiency. The longer and more severe the hormone deficiency, the more profound the changes in physiologic function. In most cases of hypothyroidism, physiologic activities controlled by thyroid

Table 29–5

Causes of Hypothyroidism

Chronic thyroiditis
Pituitary hypofunction
Hypothalamus hypofunction
Iodine deficiency
Idiopathic hypofunction
Neoplasias
Iatrogenic causes:
   Thyroidectomy
   Hypophysectomy
   Irradiation
Drug goitrogens:
   Antithyroid agents
     Propylthiouracil
     Methimazole
   Iodine in large doses
   Lithium carbonate
   Sulfonamides
   Salicylates
Excess ingestion of food goitrogens:
   Plant and animal seafood
   Cabbage and related vegetables
   Turnips
   Rutabaga
   Asparagus
   Spinach
   Soybeans
   Peanuts
   Peas
   Peaches
   Strawberries

hormones slow as the amounts of circulating thyroid hormone decrease. All body processes are affected as basal metabolism and oxygen consumption by the tissues decrease. Personality changes occur as mental processes and responses to stimuli deteriorate. People with severe hypothyroidism develop a generalized accumulation of hydrophilic mucopolysaccharides in interstitial tissues, which causes a thickened, puffy appearance. This mucinous, nonpitting edema is referred to as myxedema, a term often used synonymously with hypothyroidism.

Clinical Manifestations

The clinical manifestations of primary hypothyroidism develop insidiously over a period of months or years as the hormone deficiency worsens. All body systems are affected.

Fatigue, lethargy, and increased somnolence are early symptoms. Decreased metabolism and oxygen consumption are manifested by:

Slowed heart rate
Decreased cardiac output
Decreased blood volume
Decreased pulse pressure
Decreased respiratory rate
Anemia

Subnormal basal temperature
Sensitivity to cold
Impaired wound healing
Easy bruising from capillary fragility
Hypercholesterolemia, with increased risk of coronary atherosclerosis

Anemia combined with decreased cutaneous circulation causes coolness and pallor of the skin. The skin becomes dry, coarse, and inelastic because of decreased secretions from the sweat and sebaceous glands. Hyperkeratosis may develop. Decreased metabolism of carotene results in hypercarotenemia and a yellow tint in the skin. Hair becomes dull, sparse, and brittle. Loss of hair from the temporal third of the eyebrows is a characteristic feature of hypothyroidism. The nails become brittle and grow slowly.

Severe constipation and decreased appetite result from decreased peristalsis. Generalized myxedema results in weight gain and a puffy appearance. Myxedema is also manifested in bagginess around the eyes, puffiness of the face, and swelling of the subclavicular fossae and dorsa of the hands and feet. The typical facial appearance of a person with myxedema is illustrated in Figure 29–6. Numbness and tingling of the hands or feet from pressure around peripheral nerve fibers are common. Thick, slurred speech and hoarseness are caused by myxedema of the tongue and larynx. Aching and stiffness of muscles and joints are common. Muscle movement and reflexes are slow. Women of childbearing age may experience menorrhagia, inability to conceive from failure to ovulate, and loss of libido. Men may develop loss of libido and impotence.

Decreased cerebral blood flow results in headaches, general slowing of mental processes, slowed speech, apathy, and forgetfulness. Syncope, paranoia, or depressive psychoses may develop. Cerebral hypoxia and decreased metabolism may progress to stupor or myxedema coma.

Although myxedema coma is rare, it has a high mortality rate. It is seen most commonly in the elderly and during winter months. Often, it is preceded by exposure to cold, infection, trauma, or use of central nervous system depressants. Myxedema coma may cause death from cerebral hypoxia, bradycardia with severely decreased cardiac output and congestive heart failure, hypothermia, and hypoventilation progressing to respiratory acidosis or failure. Seizures, intestinal ileus, and fecal impaction may also be present in myxedema coma. Deep tendon reflexes are often absent.

Diagnosis

Diagnosis of hypothyroidism is based on the history, clinical manifestations, and identification of low levels of serum T_4, serum T_3, free thyroxine (FT_4), and T_3 resin uptake. In primary hypothyroidism, serum levels of thyroid-stimulating hormone (TSH) are elevated. In hypothyroidism caused by pituitary or hypothalamic dysfunction, TSH levels are lower than normal. Table 29–6 identifies common diagnostic studies of thyroid function and their nursing implications. Abnormal responses to these studies are summarized in Table 29–7.

Management

Treatment of primary hypothyroidism requires lifelong thyroid hormone replacement therapy. Levothyroxine (Synthroid, T_4), a synthetic thyroxine, is the drug of choice. Liothyronine (Cytomel, T_3), liotrix (Thyrolar, T_3/T_4), and desiccated thyroid are alternative thyroid preparations. The dosage of thyroid hormone is individualized to achieve a euthyroid, or normal, hormonal state. The dose is gradually increased from initial to maintenance levels at 1- to 2-week intervals while thyroid function is closely monitored.

Treatment of hypothyroidism secondary to pituitary or hypothalamic dysfunction depends on the nature of the dysfunction. The patient may receive

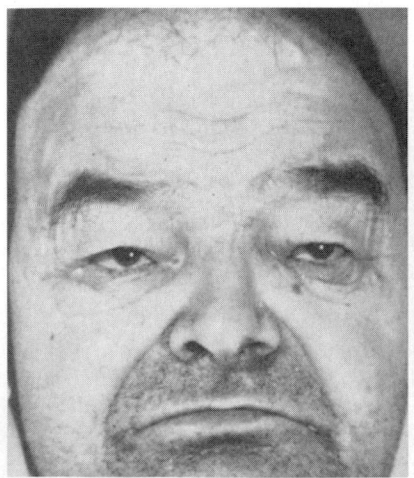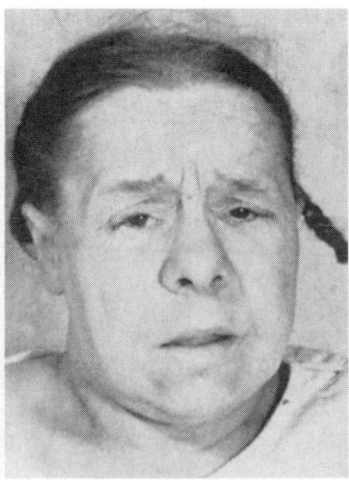

Figure 29–6

Typical facial puffiness and dull expression of patients with myxedema. (From Larsen PR, Ingbar SH. The thyroid gland. In Wilson JD, Foster DW [eds]. Williams textbook of endocrinology. 8th ed. Philadelphia: WB Saunders, 1992, p 451.)

Table 29–6

Common Diagnostic Studies of Thyroid Function*

Study	Purpose and Procedure	Nursing Implications
SERUM STUDIES		
Serum T_4 (total thyroxine)	Assess thyroxine concentration in the blood. Used in conjunction with T_3 to evaluate thyroid function. Normal value: 4.5–13 μg/dL	Levels may be affected by pregnancy, factors that alter the concentration of proteins in the blood, and iodine-containing foods, medications, and contrast media. Note on laboratory requisition the date of diagnostic studies using contrast media and/or use of thyroid or antithyroid medications, goitrogenic medications, or megadoses of mineral supplements containing iodine. Contact laboratory performing test for specific medications that may alter results.
Serum T_3 (total triiodothyronine)	Assess triiodothyronine concentration in the blood. Used in conjunction with T_4 to evaluate thyroid function. Normal value: 70–200 ng/dL	Same as for serum thyroxine.
Free thyroxine (FT_4)	Measurement of the free thyroxine that is unbound to protein in the blood. Not affected by iodine-containing contrast media or medications. Normal value: 0.8–2.4 ng/dL	This test provides a more accurate evaluation of thyroid status in pregnancy and in persons taking medications that alter total thyroxine levels.
Thyroxine-binding globulin (TBG)	Measurement of serum levels of TBG provides an assessment of the thyroxine-binding capacity of the blood. Combined with T_4 to evaluate thyroid function. Normal value: 12–18 μg/dL	Same as for serum thyroxine.
T_3 resin uptake (T_3RU)	Used to indirectly measure the binding of thyroid hormone to TBG in the blood. Radioactive T_3 is added to blood sample to bind with unoccupied sites on TBG. Normal value: 25–35% uptake	Not affected by iodine-containing medications, foods, or contrast media. Other drugs same as for thyroxine.
Thyroid-stimulating hormone (TSH)	Assess circulating levels of TSH secreted by the anterior pituitary gland. Used to differentiate between pituitary dysfunction and primary thyroid dysfunction. Normal value: <10 μIU/mL	Same as for serum thyroxine. This test is also used to diagnose primary hypothyroidism in neonates.

Thyrotropin-releasing hormone (TRH) stimulation test	Assess response of TSH, and sometimes T_3 and T_4, to TRH. Normally TRH stimulates increased TSH production. Baseline TSH level is drawn. TRH bolus is administered intravenously. TSH levels are measured 30 and 60 minutes after TRH is administered. Used to differentiate between hypothyroidism caused by hypothalamic, pituitary, or thyroid dysfunction.
	T_3 and T_4 levels are measured before and 2 hours after TRH administration.
	Normal values after TRH:
	  TSH increases two times baseline with peak at 30 minutes.
	  T_3 and T_4 rise after TRH administration.
		Advise patient of the need for multiple blood samples and of the possibility of transient flushing, nausea, dizziness, and urge to urinate. Monitor for transient effects, and maintain patient safety. Note exact time TRH was administered and specimens drawn on laboratory slip. Same interfering factors as for thyroxine. This test is generally replacing the thyroid-stimulating hormone (TSH) stimulation test.

Table continued on following page

1299

Table 29–6

Common Diagnostic Studies of Thyroid Function* *(continued)*

Study	Purpose and Procedure	Nursing Implications
Antithyroid antibody titer	Detect the presence of thyroid antibodies. Used to differentiate between autoimmune thyroid disorders and toxic thyroid adenoma. Normal value: Titer < 1:100	Antibodies are present in about 10% of healthy persons. Results altered by administration of radioactive iodine within 24 hours of test.
Calcitonin	Assess calcitonin concentration in the blood. Used in the differential diagnosis of cancer of the thyroid gland. Normal values: Men: <19 pg/mL Women: <14 pg/mL	If basal calcitonin is nondiagnostic, additional blood samples are drawn 1 and 5 minutes after a pentagastrin injection.
NUCLEAR MEDICINE STUDIES		

Radioactive iodine (RAI) uptake (^{131}I uptake)(^{123}I uptake)	Measure the rate of iodine uptake by the thyroid gland. A trace dose of RAI is administered orally. The amount of RAI absorbed by the gland is measured at intervals by a gamma counter or scintillation counter placed over the gland. Concurrent 24-hour urine specimen may be collected to assess iodine excretion. Often done in conjunction with thyroid scan.
	Normal values:
	  Absorption by gland:
	    <6% uptake in 2 hr
	    2–25% uptake in 6 hr
	    15–45% uptake in 24 hr
	  24-hour urine:
	    40–80% RAI excreted in 24 hr
		Determine date of last menstrual period in female patients: RAI uptake is never done during pregnancy or lactation. Same interfering factors as for thyroxine. Ask about seafood and iodized salt intake within the previous 2 weeks. Assure the patient that the amount of radioactive iodine used is very small; it is not harmful to the patient and the patient will not be "radioactive." Explain the need for several uptake measurement sessions and the times they are scheduled. Follow standard procedures for patient education and specimen collection if a concurrent 24-hour urine specimen is needed.

Thyroid scan	Similar to an RAI uptake, except that a scintillation detector moves back and forth across the gland to produce a scintigraphic image of iodine concentration and distribution throughout the thyroid gland at specified intervals after administration of radioactive iodine. Determines location, size, shape, and functional activity of the gland. Detects hyperactive "hot spots" and hypoactive "cold spots" within the gland, as well as thyroid tissue outside the gland. Results may be plotted by computed tomography scanner to provide a three-dimensional image. Often done in conjunction with RAI uptake. Normal value: Diffuse tracing with symmetric lobes.	Same as for RAI uptake. Emphasize the need to lie perfectly still without swallowing during the scanning procedure. Each scan usually takes 20 minutes. Be sure that the patient returns to nuclear medicine department at scheduled intervals, usually 6 and 24 hours after RAI intake. Advise physician and/or nuclear medicine department if patient will not be able to cooperate during scanning procedure.

*Normal values and procedures are guidelines. Contact facility performing test for absolute values, interfering substances, patient preparation, and specific procedures.

Table 29–7

Typical Results* of Common Diagnostic Studies of Thyroid Function in Hypothyroidism and Hyperthyroidism

	Hypothyroid Disorders			
	Primary Thyroid Gland Dysfunction	Secondary Dysfunction (Pituitary Dysfunction)	Tertiary Dysfunction (Hypothalamic Dysfunction)	Hyperthyroid Disorders
T_4	Low	Low	Low	High
T_3	Low	Low	Low	High
FT_4	Low	Low	Low	High
T_3RU	Low	Low	Low	High
TSH	High	Low	Low	Normal to low
RAIU	Low	Low	Low	High
Change in $T_4:T_3$ ratio	None	None	None	Increase in T_3 proportionately greater than increase in T_4
TSH response to TRH stimulation test	Normal rise	None	Delayed rise	—
T_3/T_4 response to TRH stimulation test	None	None	Rise	—

* Exceptions are possible in individual cases.

FT_4, free thyroxine; RAIU, radioactive iodine uptake; T_3, triiodothyronine; T_4, thyroxine; TRH, thyrotropin releasing hormone; T_3RU, T_3 resin uptake; TSH, thyroid-stimulating hormone.

temporary thyroid hormone replacement while the underlying disorder is treated, or lifelong replacement if the underlying disorder cannot be corrected.

Hypothyroidism from inadequate iodine intake is corrected with daily iodine supplements. Hypothyroidism caused by excessive ingestion of goitrogens is corrected, if possible, by decreasing or discontinuing the drug or food involved.

Myxedema coma is reversed by intravenous administration of levothyroxine while the patient is treated for shock with intravenous fluids and hydrocortisone. The underlying precipitating factor is identified and treated. Laboratory studies determine the need for intravenous glucose and electrolytes. Oxygen is administered. Mechanical ventilation may be needed to correct hypoventilation and respiratory acidosis. The patient is rewarmed passively to prevent rapid increase in oxygen requirements and shunting of blood from the vital organs to the peripheral circulation. If the patient is unconscious, a nasogastric tube may be inserted to prevent aspiration and gastric distention. Once the patient is stabilized, lifelong thyroid hormone replacement therapy is initiated.

To reduce the severity of permanent effects of physiologic changes associated with prolonged thyroid hormone deficiency, early diagnosis and treatment of hypothyroidism are important. Although treatment reverses most clinical manifestations, cardiovascular changes caused by atherosclerosis and some interstitial myxedema may remain.

With early diagnosis and properly managed hormone replacement therapy, the person with hypothyroidism has an excellent prognosis.

❖ Settings, Providers, and Collaboration for Care

Care for the patient with hypothyroidism can be effectively managed in the home setting. The patient visits the physician's office for regular evaluations of progress. The office nurse or a home health nurse may assess the patient's learning needs and teach the patient about the side effects and therapeutic effects of prescribed medications.

NURSING PROCESS

Hypothyroidism

Assessment

Obtain a complete nursing history from the patient with diagnosed or suspected hypothyroidism. Ask specifically about the onset of early symptoms of unusual fatigue, lethargy, or somnolence. Nonspecific early symptoms are often overlooked by the patient as insignificant or unrelated to the current illness. Allow extra time for the patient to process and respond to questions because mental functions may be slowed.

Obtain baseline vital signs and apical heart rate to determine cardiovascular status. Weigh the patient and compare current weight with the presymptomatic weight, if documented or known by the patient. Note the absence or presence of nonpitting, interstitial myxedema and its distribution. Auscultate for hypoactive bowel sounds. Question the patient and close associates about changes in appearance, behavior, or mental processes. Assess for clinical manifestations associated with hypothyroidism. As each manifestation is identified, ask the patient how long it has been present. Identify the patient's interpretation of clinical manifestations and knowledge of planned diagnostic studies and treatment to determine teaching needs.

Assessment of the patient in myxedema stupor or coma is limited to determination of hemodynamic status until treatment for shock and intravenous administration of thyroid hormone begins. Determine baseline vital signs, neurologic status, and renal function for comparison with later assessments. Obtain a brief history and identification of allergies from a person familiar with the patient if the patient cannot provide information. Complete the history once the patient has been stabilized.

Nursing Diagnoses and Planning

Nursing diagnoses and related expected patient outcomes commonly applicable to patients with hypothyroidism include the following:

NDx: Risk for altered systemic tissue perfusion related to anemia, decreased cardiac output, decreased respirations, and hypothermia secondary to decreased basal metabolism

Planning: Patient Outcomes
1. Patient maintains adequate tissue perfusion as evidenced by:
   Stable vital signs
   Basal temperature higher than 35.5°C (96°F)
   Pulse between 60 and 100 bpm and regular
   Respirations 8 to 16 per minute
   Blood pressure higher than 90/60 mm Hg
   Capillary refill less than 3 seconds
   Alert, oriented to person, place, time
   Urine output more than 30 mL/hour

NDx: Activity intolerance related to fatigue, lethargy, altered sensory perception and muscular responses, slowed mental processes

Planning: Patient Outcomes
1. Patient displays interest in environment.
2. Patient completes daily activities as independently as possible.
3. Patient safety is maintained.

NDx: Constipation related to decreased mobility, decreased gastrointestinal motility, and anorexia

Planning: Patient Outcomes
1. Patient evacuates soft stool at least every 3 days.

NDx: Risk for impaired skin integrity related to loss of elasticity, dryness, and generalized myxedema

Planning: Patient Outcomes
1. Patient's skin remains smooth, supple, and free from breakdown.

NDx: Risk for altered health maintenance related to insufficient knowledge of self-administration of thyroid hormone replacement therapy

Planning: Patient Outcomes
1. Patient verbalizes understanding of the need for, and intent to take, thyroid hormone replacements as prescribed.
2. Patient states name, dose, administration schedule, timetable for expected effects, and adverse and toxic effects of prescribed thyroid hormone.
3. Patient demonstrates ability to monitor radial pulse.
4. Patient states intent to keep follow-up appointments with physician and to notify physician promptly if pulse is less than 60 bpm, higher than 100 bpm, or irregular.

Nursing Interventions and Evaluation

Most patients with hypothyroidism are diagnosed and treated on an outpatient basis. Therefore, nursing care focuses primarily on patient teaching. Patient teaching for self-management is summarized in Nursing Care Guide 29–4. However, because the manifestations of hypothyroidism develop slowly, some patients remain undiagnosed and untreated for several years. These patients require hospitalization to treat severe hypothyroidism or myxedema coma.

NDx: Risk for altered systemic tissue perfusion
Evaluate vital functions and neurologic signs of the hospitalized patient with severe hypothyroidism at least twice daily to identify changes in status and response to treatment. Monitor vital signs, capillary refill, and skin color and temperature to determine changes in cardiovascular status. Auscultate rate, depth, and character of respirations to detect respiratory depression and hypoventilation. Monitor fluid intake and output and daily weights to evaluate fluid balance and renal function. Monitor level of consciousness and orientation to person, place, and time to identify cerebral hypoxia.

Observe the patient's gait, muscle strength, and reflexes to identify slowed neuromuscular responses and impaired coordination. Maintain a warm environment and provide warm blankets, robe, and socks to conserve body temperature and prevent hypothermia. Administer the prescribed thyroid hormone replacement and monitor the patient's response as basal metabolism increases. Highlight 29–5 summarizes the pharmacologic actions, side ef-

Nursing Care Guide 29–4
Patients Learning Self-Management of Hypothyroidism

Assessment Findings:	A 53-year-old woman with a history of progressive slowing of mental processes and lack of energy is diagnosed as having hypothyroidism. Levothyroxine (Synthroid, T_4) has been prescribed.
Nursing Diagnosis:	Risk for altered health maintenance related to insufficient knowledge of self-management of hypothyroidism and lifelong thyroid hormone replacement

Patient Outcomes	Nursing Interventions	Rationale
Patient verbalizes understanding of the physiologic effects of thyroid hormones, the pathologic changes that result from their deficiency, and the rationale for the prescribed treatment.	Reinforce in clear, easily understood terms the physician's explanation of hypothyroidism and its treatment.	Understanding of the disease process and treatment increases patient compliance.
	Allow extra time for patient to understand teaching and to ask questions. Provide repetition and reinforcement as necessary. Reassure patient that slowed thought processes and lack of energy are manifestations of hypothyroidism that will reverse with treatment.	Hypothyroidism slows mental processes. Repetition reinforces learning.
	Provide written instructions.	Written instructions reinforce learning and minimize the risk of errors.
Patient states intent to take levothyroxine daily as prescribed.	Teach patient name, dose, administration schedule, expected action, and side effects of levothyroxine. Stress that thyroid replacement is lifelong and that the patient is not to alter dosage without physician instructions. Advise patient to expect diuresis and increased pulse rate as early responses to treatment.	Legally, all persons must have this information to correctly and safely self-administer medication.
	Instruct patient to take as a single dose, before breakfast.	Food interferes with absorption.
	Teach patient to monitor and record the radial pulse before each dose during the adjustment period, and weekly thereafter. Drug is not taken and the physician is notified promptly if the pulse is higher than 100 bpm or is irregular.	Tachycardia is the earliest sign of overdose of thyroid hormone.
	Instruct patient to advise all physicians treating her that she is taking levothyroxine and to wear MedicAlert identification at all times. Consult with physician before taking over-the-counter preparations.	This will help prevent drug interactions.

(continued)

Nursing Care Guide 29–4
Patients Learning Self-Management of Hypothyroidism (continued)

Patient Outcomes	Nursing Interventions	Rationale
	Consult with physician to determine whether patient is to be instructed to limit ingestion of goitrogens or foods high in iodine.	High iodine intake may alter effectiveness of drug.
	Store drug in light-resistant container in dry location.	Light and moisture cause deterioration of drug.
Patient states intent to keep monthly appointments for evaluation during dosage adjustment and annual appointments thereafter.	Teach patient that effects of levothyroxine are cumulative and require frequent re-evaluation during dosage adjustment. Once a euthyroid state is achieved, annual re-evaluation is necessary to monitor response to therapy and to adjust dosage to meet changing metabolic needs associated with aging.	Evaluates effectiveness of treatment and prevents overdosage or underdosage.
Patient uses energy conservation to complete daily activities.	Teach patient to plan daily activities to allow for frequent rest periods and energy conservation. Example: Plan and complete tasks in one location, rest, begin tasks in another. Remind patient to allow extra time to complete tasks because of slowed mental processes and decreased energy levels. Reassure patient that activity tolerance will increase with treatment.	Euthyroid state will not be attained until several weeks of therapy are completed. Patient will fatigue easily until that time.
	Instruct patient to stop activity and notify the physician if chest pain, palpitations, or tachycardia occurs.	Indicate activity intolerance or possible overdose of levothyroxine.
Patient eats six small meals daily.	Advise patient that six small meals high in protein, carbohydrates, B and C vitamins, and iron will promote optimal nutritional status.	Frequent small meals are better tolerated by individuals with poor appetites than three large meals daily.
	Teach patient to take a few sips of warm liquid 10–15 minutes before eating.	Stimulates peristalsis and improves appetite and digestion.
	Reassure patient that weight loss and increased appetite will occur with treatment.	Indicate increased metabolism.
Patient evacuates soft, formed stool at least once every 3 days.	Determine patient's normal bowel pattern. Discuss the effect hypothyroidism may have on bowel function.	Decreased peristalsis is a manifestation of hypothyroidism and may cause severe constipation.
	Encourage walking or other exercise. Teach patient the importance of fiber and fluids in maintaining normal bowel function throughout life. Provide patient with a list of high-fiber foods.	Exercise stimulates peristalsis and increases abdominal muscle tone. Increased fluids and dietary fiber stimulate peristalsis and soften and provide bulk to the stool to promote bowel evacuation.

(continued)

Nursing Care Guide 29–4

Patients Learning Self-Management of Hypothyroidism (continued)

Patient Outcomes	Nursing Interventions	Rationale
Patient uses skin care products that do not dry or irritate the skin.	Instruct the patient to avoid hot water and soap and to apply moisturizers and creams after bathing.	Soap and hot water dry the skin. Emollients restore moisture and counteract dryness.
Evaluation:	Compare the patient's status with the expected outcomes. If the outcomes are not met, reassess the patient and revise the plan.	

HIGHLIGHT
29–5
PHARMACOLOGY

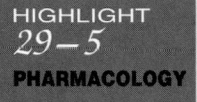 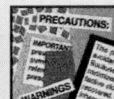

Thyroid Hormone Preparations

Definition:

Class of drugs that increase protein synthesis and stimulate metabolic activity of the cells.

Action:

Exact mechanism of action unknown. By increasing the metabolic activity of the cells, thyroid hormone preparations increase oxygen consumption and energy production; alter carbohydrate, fat, and protein metabolism; and promote growth and maturation of tissues.

Uses:

Replacement therapy in hypothyroid disorders.

Side Effects:

Hypersensitivity reactions (rash, anaphylaxsis) are rare. Side effects appear gradually, primarily result from overdose, and are similar to the manifestations of hyperthyroidism: palpitations, tachycardia, dysrhythmias, elevated pulse pressure, angina pectoris, cardiac failure, headache, tremors, nervousness, insomnia, leg cramps, nausea, diarrhea, anorexia, abdominal cramps, weight loss, heat intolerance, increased basal temperature, sweating, menstrual irregularities.

Interactions:

Cholestyramine and colestipol decrease absorption. Estrogens antagonize action. Thyroid hormone preparations potentiate the effects of anticoagulants, sympathomimetics, and tricyclic antidepressants, and de-

crease effectiveness of antidiabetic agents and digitalis glycosides.

Nursing Implications:

Administer as a single morning dose before eating.

Effects are cumulative.

Monitor changes in pulse, blood pressure, appetite, weight, and activity tolerance.

Withhold dose and notify physician if pulse is higher than 100 beats per minute or if the rhythm is irregular.

Advise patient to expect diuresis and weight loss as the earliest response to therapy.

Stress that replacement therapy is lifelong.

Emphasize need for monthly evaluations during dosage adjustment and annual evaluations once a euthyroid state is achieved.

Store in light-resistant container in dry location.

Consult physician for dietary restrictions; ingestion of iodine and goitrogens may be limited.

Geriatric Considerations:

The elderly are especially susceptible to the metabolic effects of thyroid preparations. Dosage must be increased gradually to avoid cardiovascular and cerebral side effects. Assess for angina due to cardiac overload from increased metabolic demands and for signs of agitation or confusion due to rapid increase in metabolic rate and cerebral perfusion.

fects, and nursing implications of thyroid hormone replacement preparations.

If the patient is in myxedema coma from severe cerebral hypoxia and decreased perfusion, monitor vital signs, pulse pressure, capillary refill, neurologic status, and renal output hourly. Administer oxygen, parenteral fluids and electrolytes, thyroid hormone, and medications to support cardiovascular function as prescribed. Position the patient on one side or the other to prevent aspiration of oral secretions. The patient may require mechanical ventilation to reverse respiratory depression and acidosis. Provide multiple layers of covers and a warm environment to rewarm the patient passively and slowly while preventing surface burns and increased metabolic requirements.

NDx: Activity intolerance

Orient the patient to the surroundings. Explain the call system and ask the patient to demonstrate how to use it. Monitor degree of orientation frequently. Reorient as needed. Explain procedures and requests clearly and slowly. Reinforce them as needed to promote patient understanding and participation. Provide conversation and nonstressful diversional activities to stimulate interest in activities and surroundings. Reassure the patient and family that the current behavior patterns and slowed thought processes are manifestations of hypothyroidism and will reverse with treatment.

Plan care to provide frequent rest periods to conserve energy. To promote self-esteem, allow the patient sufficient time to accomplish activities as independently as possible. Place supplies and personal belongings within easy reach to avoid exertion. Provide help when the patient begins to tire to avoid overexertion while promoting patient participation.

Reassess muscle strength and mobility daily. Encourage ambulation and active range-of-motion exercises to promote muscle strength and flexibility. Tell the patient to call for assistance when getting out of bed. To prevent falls, remove potential hazards from the environment and help with ambulation. Keep the side rails up if needed for patient safety. Check the temperature of bath water to prevent burns. Carefully evaluate the need for and response to sedatives, narcotics, and barbiturates because of hypersensitivity to these drugs of patients with hypothyroidism.

NDx: Constipation

Determine the patient's normal bowel pattern. Monitor for changes in bowel sounds daily. If not contraindicated, provide a diet high in fiber and increase fluid intake by offering fluids hourly to soften the stool and increase bulk. Six small meals daily are better tolerated by patients with a poor appetite and slow digestion. Administer prescribed stool softeners and peristalsis stimulants, such as docusate sodium and casanthranol (Peri-Colace), to promote defecation. Encourage ambulation and activity as tolerated to increase intestinal motility.

NDx: Risk for impaired skin integrity

Assess skin daily for redness or breakdown. Avoid soap. Use oil or lotion in the bath water to prevent dryness. To avoid creating friction, blot the skin dry rather than rubbing it. Massage and lubricate pressure points at least four times daily. Use elbow and heel protectors to prevent breakdown. To promote capillary circulation, help and encourage the patient to ambulate and change position frequently. Provide a diet high in protein, carbohydrates, B and C vitamins, and iron to promote optimal nutrition and provide elements needed for skin maintenance and repair.

NDx: Risk for altered health maintenance

Teach the patient the dosage and schedule, expected therapeutic actions, and side effects of prescribed thyroid hormone replacement preparation (see Highlight 29–5). Advise the patient that diuresis, weight loss, decreasing puffiness, increased pulse rate, increased appetite, and increased activity tolerance are the expected early responses to thyroid hormone replacement. Teach the patient that chest pain, shortness of breath, insomnia, and nervousness are early signs of excess thyroid hormone replacement that must be reported to the physician promptly so that the dosage can be reduced.

Teach the patient how to monitor the radial pulse for 1 full minute and to record the results. Have the patient count the pulse in one wrist while you count it in the other to ensure correct technique. The pulse rate is an important indicator of the body's response to thyroid replacement. It is monitored before each dose during the period of adjustment, and weekly once the patient is euthyroid. The physician is notified promptly if the pulse rate is less than 60 bpm or greater than 100 bpm, or if the rhythm is irregular.

Response to therapy is usually monitored by the physician on a monthly basis until a euthyroid state is achieved, then once yearly. Emphasize that replacement therapy for hypothyroidism is lifelong and that periodic examination to evaluate thyroid function is important. No over-the-counter medications or mineral supplements should be taken without physician approval. Consult with the physician to determine whether the patient should be instructed to limit intake of foods high in iodine, which may alter response to thyroid replacement therapy.

Compare the patient's status with the expected outcomes. If the outcomes are not met, reassess the patient and revise the plan.

Hyperthyroidism

Hyperthyroidism is a disorder of hypermetabolism resulting from exposure of the body tissues to excessive quantities of circulating free thyroxine, triiodothyronine, or both. It is second only to diabetes mellitus among naturally occurring endocrine disorders.

Heredity is a factor in the incidence of hyperthyroidism, and severe emotional or physical stress often precipitates the onset of overt symptoms. Hyperthyroidism is seven to 10 times more common in women and is diagnosed most frequently at puberty, during pregnancy, or between the ages of 30 and 50. In men, it tends to develop after the age of 50 and is more severe.

The most common form of primary hyperthyroidism is Graves' disease. Other causes of hyperthyroid symptoms include toxic nodular goiter, secreting adenoma of the thyroid gland, subacute thyroiditis, pituitary adenoma that secretes excess thyroid-stimulating hormone, overtreatment of hypothyroidism, and thyroid-stimulating medications.

Etiology and Pathophysiology

Primary hyperthyroidism, or Graves' disease, is an autoimmune disorder in which immunoglobulins of the G class (IgG) produce thyroid antibodies similar in action to TSH, but with a stronger and longer-lasting effect. These autoantibodies bind at the TSH receptor sites and stimulate thyroid growth, increased vascularity, and hypersecretion of thyroid hormone. The multiple IgG autoantibodies that have been identified in people with Graves' disease are referred to collectively as thyroid-stimulating immunoglobulins (TSIs).

Graves' disease is a multisystem disorder characterized by hyperthyroidism with diffuse thyroid enlargement and increased vascularity. This thyroid enlargement is called diffuse toxic goiter because it is associated with increased thyroid function. Increased secretion of thyroid hormones produces a sustained hypermetabolic state, with increased oxygen consumption and increased sensitivity and stimulation of the sympathetic nervous system. The physiologic activities of the body triggered by the thyroid hormones increase as the amount of circulating thyroid hormones increases.

About half the people with Graves' disease also develop infiltrative ophthalmopathy, or exophthalmos. About 5 to 10% develop infiltrative dermopathy. Infiltrative ophthalmopathy results from the accumulation of fluid in the fat pads behind the eyeball and inflammatory edema of the extraocular muscles. The increased volume of the orbital content causes the eyeballs to protrude (Fig. 29–7). Infiltrative dermopathy is a raised, hyperpigmented, nonpitting edema of the pretibial area, ankles, and dorsa of the feet that has the appearance of an orange-peel. It is sometimes called pretibial myxedema. An example of severe pretibial myxedema is illustrated in Figure 29–8. The cause of these infiltrative manifestations of Graves' disease is unknown.

Clinical Manifestations

The severity of clinical manifestations in primary hyperthyroidism (Graves' disease) depends on the degree of hormone excess, its duration, how rapidly it developed, and the age of the patient. The disease

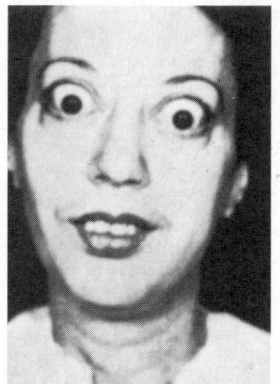

Figure 29–7

Infiltrative ophthalmopathy, or exophthalmos, in a woman with hyperthyroidism. (From Larsen PR, Ingbar SH. The thyroid gland. In Wilson JD, Foster DW [eds]. Williams textbook of endocrinology. 8th ed. Philadelphia: WB Saunders, 1992, p 426.)

usually develops gradually over a period of months or years. In general, the longer the duration of the disease and the more rapid its onset, the more severe the manifestations.

Exaggerated alertness, nervousness, tremulousness, agitation, irritability, insomnia, a feeling of apprehension, and an inability to concentrate are common early symptoms of excess stimulation of the

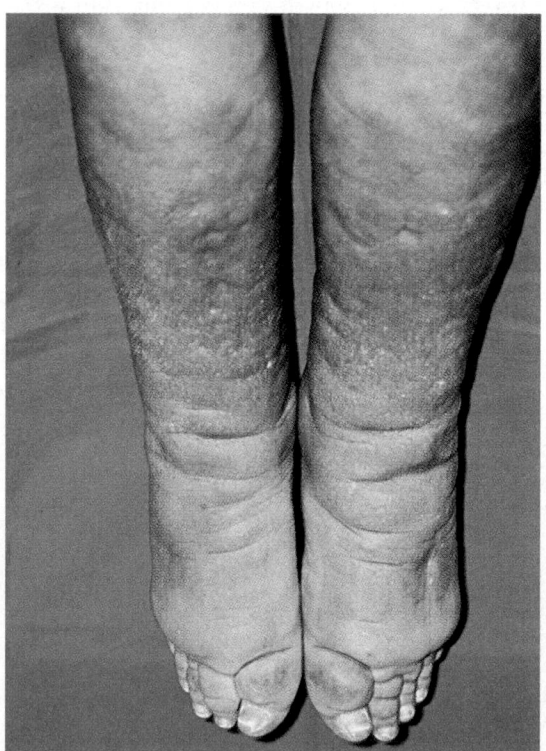

Figure 29–8

Severe pretibial myxedema sometimes present in hyperthyroidism. (From Callen JP, Greer KE, Hood AF, Paller AS, Swinyer LJ. Color atlas of dermatology. Philadelphia: WB Saunders, 1993, p 255.)

sympathetic nervous system. Emotional lability with inappropriate episodes of crying and euphoria may develop. Increased oxygen consumption from hypermetabolism and the need to dissipate excess heat are manifested by tachycardia, palpitations, increased cardiac output, a bounding pulse, increased pulse pressure, systolic hypertension, tachypnea, heat intolerance, diaphoresis, and cutaneous vasodilation. Atrial dysrhythmias may develop. Fatigue, muscle weakness, and muscle wasting result from the production of heat rather than energy during metabolism. Weight loss occurs despite increased appetite.

Sympathetic nervous system stimulation causes fine muscle and tongue tremors, impaired coordination, hyper-reflexia, jerky movement of the eyelids, spasmodic retraction of the eyelids, and a fine tremor of the closed lids. Periorbital edema is common (Fig. 29–9). Photosensitivity, diplopia, and increased lacrimation may develop in conjunction with exophthalmos. The presence of exophthalmos may be masked by the puffiness of periorbital edema.

The skin is warm, moist, smooth, and sometimes flushed. Pruritus may develop. Hard, nonpitting pretibial or ankle edema may be present. The hair is fine, smooth, breaks easily, and does not hold a wave. Hair loss may occur. The nails are soft and easily torn, and the distal nail may separate from the nail bed (onycholysis). Hyperactive bowel sounds, with an increase in the frequency of bowel movements and softening of the stools, is common. Hypercalcemia and osteoporosis from bone demineralization may occur. Women experience decreased libido, changes in the menstrual pattern, and reduced fertility. If conception occurs, spontaneous abortion may result. Men experience decreased libido, impotence, and sometimes gynecomastia.

The thyroid gland may be normal in size or may present as a moderate to massively enlarged diffuse toxic goiter. On palpation, the consistency of the goiter varies from soft to firm and rubbery. It is usually smooth but may feel lobular. A thrill may be felt over a large goiter, and a bruit can often be auscultated.

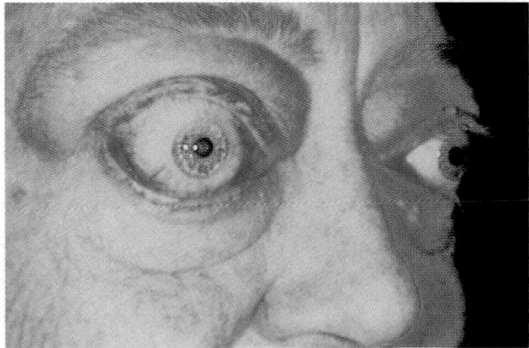

Figure 29–9

Periorbital edema is common in hyperthyroidism. (From Albert DM, Jakobiec FA. Atlas of clinical ophthalmology. Philadelphia: WB Saunders, 1996, p 498.)

Thyrotoxicosis in Graves' disease is a hypermetabolic state characterized by the presence of all the metabolic and neurologic manifestations of hyperthyroidism. Heart failure may develop from prolonged tachycardia and atrial dysrhythmias. The difference between hyperthyroidism and thyrotoxicosis is a matter of degree and severity of symptoms. Sometimes the terms are used interchangeably.

Thyroid storm, or thyroid crisis, is a rare but potentially fatal severe hypermetabolic state characterized by exaggerated clinical manifestations of hyperthyroidism. It may be precipitated by severe stress, infection, surgery, trauma, radioactive iodine therapy, aggressive manipulation of a goiter, or abrupt withdrawal of antithyroid drugs. The clinical manifestations of thyroid storm include fever as high as 41.1°C (106°F), severe tachycardia, profuse diaphoresis, extreme vasodilation, hypotension, atrial fibrillation, hyper-reflexia, abdominal pain, delirium, psychosis, nausea, vomiting, diarrhea, and dehydration rapidly progressing to coma and cardiovascular collapse. Hypokalemia may result from the vomiting and diarrhea.

Diagnosis

Medical diagnosis of hyperthyroidism is based on history, clinical manifestations, and elevated levels of serum T_4, serum T_3, free thyroxine (FT_4), and T_3 resin uptake. In addition, the increase in T_3 is proportionately larger than the increase in T_4, owing, in part, to increased conversion of free circulating T_4 to T_3. Table 29–6 identifies common diagnostic studies to evaluate thyroid function and their nursing implications. Abnormal responses to these studies typical in a patient with hyperthyroidism are summarized in Table 29–7. Identification of elevated antithyroid antibody titers is useful in differentiating between Graves' disease and toxic thyroid adenoma.

Management

Early diagnosis and treatment are important in managing hyperthyroidism. The primary goal is to suppress secretion of thyroid hormones. This is done either with antithyroid preparations or by destroying or removing a portion of the thyroid gland. Choice of treatment is determined jointly by the physician and patient, based on the patient's age, childbearing status, severity of clinical manifestations, and preference. Propranolol, a beta-adrenergic blocking agent, is frequently prescribed during treatment for hyperthyroidism to alleviate the cardiovascular effects of thyroid hormone excess. Dexamethasone may be used as an adjunct in the treatment of thyrotoxicosis. When administered with antithyroid drugs, it inhibits secretion of thyroid hormone and peripheral conversion of T_4 to T_3, rapidly alleviating symptoms.

Mild exophthalmos is primarily treated symptomatically with lubricating methylcellulose eye drops to prevent corneal dryness and ulcerations until the patient achieves a euthyroid state and spontaneous regression occurs. Treatment of severe cases is controversial. Oral glucocorticoid therapy is commonly prescribed for severe or progressing exophthalmos, with extraocular muscle damage or pressure on the optic nerve manifested by changes in visual acuity. Plasmapheresis has been successful in reversing exophthalmos in some patients. Surgical decompression with removal of part of the bony orbit may be necessary to relieve intraorbital pressure and preserve vision. Unfortunately, treatment of hyperthyroidism does not ensure reversal of exophthalmos or complete resolution of its effects.

Antithyroid Drugs

Thioamides are a class of antithyroid drugs that inhibit thyroid hormone synthesis but do not block release of stored hormone. They are used to treat hyperthyroidism in patients who are not candidates for irradiation and as an initial treatment to reduce thyroid gland activity before thyroid surgery or irradiation. Propylthiouracil (PTU) is the drug of choice because it also blocks conversion of circulating T_4 to T_3. Methimazole (Tapazole) is another commonly used thioamide. These drugs are administered in equally divided doses at 8-hour intervals.

Objective manifestations of decreased thyroid function develop in 2 to 3 weeks. Therapy continues for 6 months to several years, with a higher remission rate in patients treated at least 1 year. Long-term remission is achieved in 25 to 30% of patients. Response to therapy is evaluated every 2 to 3 months. The incidence of adverse reactions to thioamides is low. Agranulocytosis is the most serious side effect. Highlight 29–6 summarizes the antithyroid drugs.

Iodine Preparations

In hyperthyroidism, excess iodine temporarily blocks the release of thyroid hormone and reduces the vascularity and size of an enlarged thyroid gland. Iodine is used with antithyroid drugs to rapidly re-

---

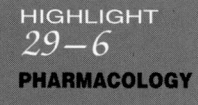 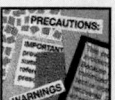

HIGHLIGHT 29–6 PHARMACOLOGY

Thiomide Antithyroid Drugs

Definition:

Class of thiomides that inhibit the synthesis of thyroid hormone but do not inhibit the release of stored hormone.

Action:

Interfere with the binding of iodine with the thyroglobulin molecule, which is necessary for the synthesis of thyroid hormone.

Uses:

Used to treat hyperthyroidism and to reduce thyroid gland activity before thyroid surgery or irradiation.

Side Effects:

Bone marrow depression, agranulocytosis, thrombocytopenia, leukopenia, lymphadenopathy, drowsiness, headache, neuritis, vertigo, paresthesias, nausea, vomiting, dyspepsia, loss of taste, swelling of the salivary glands, jaundice, hepatitis, vasculitis, rash, urticaria, pruritus, hyperpigmentation of the skin, abnormal hair loss, drug fever, lupus-like syndrome, arthralgia, hypothyroidism.

Interactions:

Do not give with other drugs that may cause agranulocytosis. Propylthiouracil potentiates anticoagulants.

Nursing Implications:

Administer in equally divided doses at 8-hour intervals. May be taken with food to lessen gastric distress.

Monitor for signs of response to therapy after 2 to 3 weeks: weight gain, reduced pulse.

Therapy may continue for 6 months to several years.

Monitor for side effects. Instruct patient to notify physician immediately if sore throat, chills, fever, skin rash, swelling of the lymph nodes, bruising, or bleeding develops.

Stress importance of evaluation of therapy and blood studies every 2 to 3 months.

Urge patient not to alter drug regimen or take over-the-counter preparations without consulting physician.

Store in light-resistant container in dry environment.

Avoid use by pregnant women because these drugs cross the placenta.

Avoid use by nursing mothers because these drugs are secreted in breast milk.

Geriatric Considerations:

Agranulocytosis is more likely to develop in the elderly and can develop at any point during therapy.

duce circulating thyroid hormone levels and metabolic activity in hyperthyroid states and before thyroid surgery. The course of therapy is limited to 10 to 14 days because of iodine's temporary effect on hormone release.

Saturated solutions of potassium iodide (SSKI) may be administered to protect the thyroid gland from absorbing radioactivity from the environment after a nuclear power plant accident.

Radioactive Iodine Therapy

Radioactive iodine (^{131}I) is an economical, easily administered agent for treating hyperthyroidism in nonpregnant patients over the age of 30. It is usually administered as a single 4 to 10 mCi dose of oral liquid on an outpatient basis. The patient is instructed to sleep alone for 2 nights, to avoid contact with children, and, because body fluids and wastes will be slightly radioactive for 24 to 48 hours, to flush the toilet two or three times after use. Patients receiving doses larger than 30 mCi (common in the treatment of secreting thyroid adenomas) require hospitalization with appropriate radiation precautions. The radioactive iodine is absorbed and retained by the thyroid gland, where it irradiates and destroys glandular tissue. It produces the ablative effects of surgical removal of thyroid tissue without the potential risks of surgical complications.

Improvement of symptoms begins 2 to 4 weeks after treatment, with maximum effect in about 3 months. Temporary thyroid tenderness just after treatment is common. Hypothyroidism develops in about 10% of patients the first year after treatment, and in 30% of patients within 5 years. These patients take thyroid replacement therapy for life.

Subtotal Thyroidectomy

Surgical removal of up to 90% of the thyroid gland is an alternative method for treating hyperthyroidism in young adults with severe disease or very large goiters, people of childbearing age who are pregnant or who want to become pregnant soon, and people who either do not respond to pharmacologic therapy or have recurrence after pharmacologic treatment. Subtotal thyroidectomy may also be performed as an elected or recommended procedure in persons with simple goiter or thyroid nodules.

Complications of thyroid surgery are rare but can be life-threatening. These include:

- Hemorrhage
- Respiratory obstruction caused by edema of the trachea, larynx, glottis, or surrounding soft tissues
- Laryngeal nerve damage with vocal cord paralysis

Parathyroid injury or accidental removal during the procedure can result in hypocalcemic tetany with respiratory obstruction caused by vocal cord spasm. Postoperative thyroid storm or crisis is very rare. The risk of hemorrhage and thyroid storm is reduced by the administration of antithyroid drugs and iodine before surgery to reduce circulating thyroid hormone levels and the size and vascularity of the thyroid gland.

The use of laser beams guided through fiberoptic scopes to vaporize hypertrophic thyroid tissue is now common in thyroid surgery. The laser surgery requires smaller surgical incisions, causes less trauma to surrounding tissues and residual thyroid tissue, and reduces the risk of hemorrhage and postoperative complications.

❖ Settings, Providers, and Collaboration for Care

For the patient experiencing a thyroid crisis, a multidisciplinary team is necessary to manage care. The patient is hospitalized. However, most patients with hyperthyroidism are diagnosed and treated on an outpatient basis. Therefore, nursing care primarily focuses on patient teaching for self-management. Ongoing care may be effectively provided in the home, under the supervision of the home health nurse. The patient returns to the physician's office for evaluation of progress.

NURSING PROCESS
Hyperthyroidism

Assessment

Obtain a complete nursing history from the patient with diagnosed or suspected hyperthyroidism. Ask specifically about the onset of early symptoms of insomnia, increased alertness and activity despite fatigue, apprehension, agitation, and inability to concentrate. Prompt the patient to think back over at least the past year, because nonspecific early symptoms are often overlooked by the patient as insignificant or unrelated to the current illness.

Obtain baseline vital signs and apical heart rate to identify cardiovascular status. Weigh the patient and compare the current weight with the presymptomatic weight, if it is documented or known by the patient. Note the absence or presence of exophthalmos and hard, nonpitting pretibial edema. Question the patient and close associates about changes in appearance, behavior, or muscle coordination. Auscultate for hyperactive bowel sounds. Test deep tendon reflexes for hyperreflexia. Assess for fine muscle and eyelid tremors and other clinical manifestations associated with hyperthyroidism. If possible, compare current handwriting with a sample 6 months to a year old. A change in handwriting smoothness, and clumsiness in manipulating buttons are signs of fine muscle tremor of the hands. The nurse clinician may examine the thyroid gland to identify size, shape, texture, consistency, tenderness, nodularity, and vascular thrill or bruit. Caution must be taken when examining the thyroid. Minimal manipulation is used to prevent potential precipitation of a thyroid storm. As each manifestation is identified, ask

CLINICAL ❓ THINKING

PARESTHESIAS AFTER THYROIDECTOMY

During breakfast, a 29-year-old female patient who had undergone a subtotal thyroidectomy for Graves' disease 24 hours earlier summoned me as I passed her room. She complained that she was experiencing difficulty setting up her tray and eating due to a tingling sensation and some numbness in her fingers. She also complained of palpitations and shortness of breath. Her postoperative recovery had thus far been uneventful and she had slept well during the night, but she was obviously very anxious and agitated now. I noted some muscle tremors in both hands.

Although postoperative patients may experience numbness and tingling in the extremities secondary to positional pressure exerted during surgery, the presence of this symptom following a thyroidectomy could signal the possibility of hypocalcemia secondary to parathyroid damage. Her other signs and symptoms (palpitations, dyspnea, apprehension, and tremors) supported this possibility but necessitated the consideration of other complications of thyroid surgery as well. These included hemorrhage, acute respiratory obstruction (resulting from edema of the trachea and glottis, pressure from bleeding or hematoma formation, or laryngeal nerve damage), and thyroid storm in addition to the risk of an acute hypocalcemic crisis (tetany).

Further physical assessment was therefore essential for sound clinical decision-making and intervention. The patient's vital signs included a regular pulse rate of 136 bpm, respirations were 30 per minute and moderately labored, her blood pressure had fallen to 94/60 mm Hg and her temperature remained stable at 37.4°C (99.4°F). Mild respiratory stridor was noted, but breath sounds at the base of both lungs were clear. The dressing was dry and intact, a check of the sides and back of the neck and linens was negative. She denied any choking sensation or tightness in the incisional area, and her voice was slightly hoarse.

The absence of fever and hypertension did not support the development of thyroid storm, and although the patient's clinical picture may have heralded the onset of hemorrhage, I continued to suspect hypocalcemia as the cause of this acute change in her health status. I further investigated my suspicion by assessing for Chvostek's and Trousseau's signs. These were both easily elicited, further supporting my suspicion.

Because acute hypocalcemia can lead to tetany, which is a medical emergency and requires prompt intervention to prevent the onset of laryngospasm, cardiac dysrhythmias, and seizures, I immediately took the following actions:

1. I notified the physician.
2. I elevated the head of the bed to a high-Fowler's position.
3. I checked to be sure that an emergency tracheostomy set, suction, oxygen and calcium gluconate were available at the bedside.
4. I started an intravenous line as per hospital protocol.
5. I instituted seizure precautions.
6. I remained with the patient, offered calm reassurance, and explained the complication and its treatment to her.
7. I checked the patient's latest serum calcium and phosphorous levels.
8. I continued to monitor the patient's respiratory, cardiovascular, and neurologic systems.
9. I documented my findings and actions.

The physician ordered STAT serum calcium, magnesium and phosphorous levels, a complete blood count, a 12-lead electrocardiogram (ECG) and IV calcium gluconate, which I administered. The low serum calcium and elevated serum phosphorous levels, the ECG which revealed a prolonged QT interval, and stable hemoglobin and hematocrit valves confirmed my suspicion of hypocalcemia.

The patient remained alert and oriented throughout the treatment, and within 1 hour, normal peripheral sensation returned, her vital signs approached baseline, and she reported feeling more comfortable. Serious consequences were prevented because astute nursing assessments led to the detection and correction of this life-threatening disorder.

Think Critically

If the patient's arterial blood gases had been analyzed at the onset of this scenario, what findings would the nurse have anticipated? What nursing measures might have been implemented if they reflected respiratory alkalosis? Respiratory acidosis?

What additional nursing actions would have been called for if this patient had a history of cardiac disease and was taking digitalis?

Why didn't the nurse initiate oxygen therapy? Was this the best action?

What nursing actions are included in the implementation of seizure precautions? Why?

(continued)

(continued)

If the patient had not responded to treatment and complete airway obstruction had developed, what action should the nurse have anticipated? What similarities and differences would the nursing assessment reveal between the postoperative complications of hypocalcemic crisis thy-roid storm and hemorrhage? What similarities and differences would exist in the nursing actions taken?

What medical regimen can the nurse anticipate if damage to the parathyroid gland was permanent? What teaching must be included in the patient's discharge plan?

the patient how long it has been present. Identify the patient's interpretation of clinical manifestations and knowledge of planned diagnostic studies and treatment to determine teaching needs.

Assessment of the patient in severe thyrotoxicosis or thyroid crisis is limited to determining hemodynamic status until treatment for dehydration, hyperthermia, hypermetabolism, and potential cardiovascular collapse is initiated. Obtain a brief history and identify allergies from a person familiar with the patient if the patient cannot provide information. Determine baseline vital signs, neurologic status, and renal function. Obtain a complete history once the patient is stabilized.

Nursing Diagnoses and Planning

Nursing diagnoses and related expected patient outcomes commonly applicable to patients with hyperthyroidism or Graves' disease include the following:

NDx: Anxiety related to heat intolerance and changes in appearance, behavior, and activity secondary to thyroid hormone excess

Planning: Patient Outcomes
1. Patient verbalizes reduction in anxiety.
2. Patient states effect of excess thyroid hormone production on the body.
3. Patient states understanding of thyroid hormone excess as cause of physical and behavioral changes.

NDx: Risk for altered health maintenance related to insufficient knowledge of self-management of pharmacologic therapy during and after treatment with antithyroid drugs, iodine, or radioactive iodine

Planning: Patient Outcomes
1. Patient states name, dose, administration schedule, timetable for expected effects, and adverse and toxic effects of prescribed medications.
2. Patient demonstrates ability to monitor radial pulse.
3. Patient states realistic expectations of treatment.
4. Patient states intent to keep follow-up appointments with physician.

NDx: Altered nutrition: less than body requirements related to hypermetabolism, hyperactivity, and increased gastrointestinal motility as evidenced by weight loss

Planning: Patient Outcomes
1. Patient states intent to consume a high-calorie, high-protein, high-carbohydrate diet until ideal weight and euthyroid state are attained.
2. Patient states intent to drink up to 4000 mL of fluid daily until euthyroid state is achieved.
3. Patient verbalizes understanding of the need to gradually decrease food and fluid consumption to maintain ideal weight as metabolic rate decreases.

NDx: Risk for trauma related to fatigue, fine muscle tremors, ophthalmic changes, and osteoporosis

Planning: Patient Outcomes
1. Patient verbalizes understanding of the need for frequent rest periods to conserve energy.
2. Patient requests or accepts assistance with activities that require fine motor coordination.
3. Patient demonstrates ability to self-administer prescribed lubricating eye drops.
4. Patient remains free of injury.

NDx: Risk for altered systemic tissue perfusion related to dehydration, hyperthermia, and decreased cardiac output secondary to hypermetabolism and severe thyrotoxicosis or thyroid storm

Planning: Patient Outcomes
1. Patient demonstrates adequate tissue perfusion as evidenced by:
   Basal temperature within normal limits
   Stable vital signs within normal limits
   Normal neurologic responses
   Urine output of more than 30 mL/hour

NDx: Risk for ineffective airway clearance related to tracheolaryngeal obstruction secondary to possible complications of subtotal thyroidectomy: hemorrhage, edema, laryngeal nerve damage, parathyroid gland damage

Planning: Patient Outcomes
1. Patient maintains clear airway as evidenced by:
   Stable vital signs within normal limits
   Respirations regular and unlabored
   Ability to speak and swallow without difficulty

Nursing Interventions and Evaluation

NDx: Anxiety
Provide factual information to the patient and significant others related to the effect of increased levels of circulating thyroid hormones on heat intolerance, appearance, behavior, and activity. Encourage the patient to identify and describe feelings. Help the patient identify relaxation techniques and diversionary activities to help control anxiety while conserving energy. Establish a schedule of activity and rest periods to provide a reassuring routine. Explain procedures in a calm, reassuring voice. Maintain an unhurried manner to promote relaxation and trust. To decrease external stimuli, select roommates carefully and restrict visitors, if necessary. Some patients may require sedation.

The patient with heat intolerance is most comfortable in a cool room with good circulation but free from drafts. Provide lightweight bedding and sleepwear. Frequent hygiene, skin care, and linen changes prevent discomfort and skin breakdown from profuse diaphoresis.

NDx: Risk for altered health maintenance
Teach the patient the name, dose, administration schedule, timetable for expected effects, and side effects of prescribed antithyroid drug, iodine preparation, or radioactive iodine (see Highlight 29–6). Advise the patient taking an iodine preparation to take it after meals, to dilute the solution in a full glass of water or juice to prevent gastric irritation, and to drink it through a straw to avoid discoloring the teeth. Tell the patient to notify the physician promptly about signs of iodine toxicity: metallic taste, stomatitis, coryza, tenderness of the salivary glands, vomiting, bloody diarrhea, and abdominal pain or distention.

To avoid interference with ^{131}I uptake, thioamides and iodine preparations are discontinued 3 to 4 days before radioactive iodine therapy is begun. Instruct the patient to consult the physician before taking any over-the-counter preparations during pharmacologic treatment for hyperthyroidism.

Teach the patient how to monitor the radial pulse for 1 full minute two to three times weekly and record the results. Pulse rate is an important indicator of the body's response to treatment. It should gradually decrease to between 60 and 100 beats per minute. Instruct the patient to notify the physician promptly if the pulse becomes irregular or drops below 60.

Reinforce and clarify the physician's explanations of the expected outcomes of treatment. Encourage the patient to ask questions and verbalize expectations. Inform the physician if the patient expresses unrealistic expectations of treatment so that further discussion and explanation can correct misunderstandings.

The physician monitors response to therapy on a monthly basis until a euthyroid state is achieved, then once or twice yearly. Stress the importance of follow-up thyroid function studies and physical examinations as scheduled. Teach the patient signs of hypothyroidism (which may develop after treatment) and hyperthyroidism (which may signal a recurrence) that should be reported to the physician.

NDx: Altered nutrition: less than body requirements
Weigh the patient or tell the patient to weigh himself or herself two to three times weekly to detect weight gain or loss. Document food intake. Small, frequent, high-calorie, high-protein, high-carbohydrate snacks and supplements may be better tolerated, especially if hyperactivity prevents the patient from sitting down for a meal. The patient may require 4000 to 5000 calories daily to meet metabolic demands. Tell the patient to avoid caffeine, spicy seasonings, and foods high in bulk or fiber, which may further stimulate intestinal motility and decrease absorption of nutrients. Unless contraindicated by cardiac status, encourage fluid intake up to 4000 mL daily to replace excess fluid lost through profuse diaphoresis and frequent stools. Increased production of metabolic wastes also requires large amounts of fluid to promote their dilution and excretion by the kidneys.

As treatment of hyperthyroidism becomes effective and the patient achieves ideal body weight, the patient must decrease food intake to prevent excess weight gain.

NDx: Risk for trauma
Plan care or help the patient plan activities to allow for frequent rest periods and conservation of energy. Monitor physiologic response to activity. Palpitations or increased pulse, systolic blood pressure, or respirations indicate overexertion and the need for reduced activity. Provide a nonstimulating environment, free from hazards. Reassure the patient that fine muscle tremors and difficulty manipulating objects will improve with treatment. Provide assistance as needed with difficult activities to prevent stress, anxiety, and injury. Maintain adequate lighting. Keep the call bell within reach. Provide nonskid slippers or shoes. Help the patient with ambulation as needed to prevent falls.

For the patient with exophthalmos, administer or teach the patient to administer lubricating eye drops to prevent corneal dryness, abrasion, and ulceration.

NDx: Risk for altered systemic tissue perfusion
Monitor vital signs, pulse pressure, capillary refill, neurologic status, and renal output hourly to detect hemodynamic changes in a patient with thyrotoxicosis or thyroid storm. Institute safety measures if the patient is irrational, delirious, or comatose. Apply a hypothermia blanket or ice packs to reduce hyper-

thermia. Propylthiouracil and potassium iodide are administered by mouth or nasogastric tube to rapidly reduce circulating thyroid hormone levels. Propranolol is used to treat cardiac dysrhythmias and reduce sympathetic stimulation. Digoxin, instead of propranolol, is prescribed with cardiac failure. Glucocorticoids and intravenous glucose solutions are administered to treat shock and dehydration and to provide glucose for metabolic requirements. Humidified oxygen is administered to improve tissue oxygenation and meet the high metabolic demands.

NDx: Risk for ineffective airway clearance

The risk of postoperative complications after thyroid surgery is greatly reduced by preoperative preparation. Antithyroid drugs and iodine preparations are administered to reduce levels of circulating thyroid hormone and the size and vascularity of the gland. To prevent tension on the suture line postoperatively, teach the patient to support the head while moving. Discuss the planned procedure with the patient, reinforce and clarify the physician's explanations, and provide an opportunity for the patient to ask questions and verbalize feelings about the surgery and expected outcome.

Postoperatively, apply an ice collar and place the patient in semi-Fowler's position to reduce edema. Administer humidified oxygen and intravenous fluids to meet metabolic requirements and improve tissue perfusion. Examine the dressing and monitor vital signs every 1 to 2 hours for 24 hours, then every 4 hours. To promote optimal respiratory function and mobilization of secretions, encourage early ambulation.

Monitor for and immediately report signs of hemorrhage, including:

- A drop in blood pressure
- A rapid, thready pulse
- Increased tightness of the neck dressing
- Fullness or pressure at the incision site
- A choking sensation or difficulty breathing
- Excessive bloody drainage on the dressing or pillow or behind the neck

Hemorrhage and edema can cause respiratory obstruction by compressing the trachea or larynx. Signs of respiratory obstruction include restlessness, respiratory stridor, crowing on respiration, difficulty swallowing, dyspnea, and cyanosis. If hemorrhage or respiratory distress is suspected, release the edges of the dressing to relieve pressure on internal structures and implement measures for hypovolemic shock. Assist with emergency tracheostomy if necessary to maintain the airway.

Laryngeal nerve damage may result in temporary or permanent loss of voice, paralysis of the vocal cords, or both. Aphonia just after surgery, hoarseness, or a high-pitched voice indicates laryngeal nerve damage. Ask the patient to speak every 2 hours to determine voice quality. If the voice is initially clear and then becomes hoarse, edema may be placing temporary pressure on the nerve. Paralysis of the vocal cords can cause respiratory obstruction and may require a tracheostomy. A tracheostomy tray and suction equipment must be available at the bedside for emergency use.

Acute hypocalcemic tetany is discussed in detail later in this chapter. It can result from damage to, or accidental removal of, the parathyroid glands during thyroid surgery. Notify the physician immediately if the patient is increasingly irritable or has numbness or tingling of the nose, earlobes, toes, fingers, or circumoral areas; muscle twitching; or painful spasms. Assess muscle irritability by eliciting a positive Chvostek or Trousseau sign. If signs of hypocalcemia are present, initiate rebreathing to raise calcium ion levels, institute seizure precautions, and prepare for administration of intravenous calcium chloride or calcium gluconate. Intravenous calcium chloride or calcium gluconate must be available on the unit for emergency use. Tetany can cause respiratory distress from seizures and laryngospasm. A tracheostomy may be required to maintain the airway.

Compare the patient's status with the expected outcomes. If the outcomes are not met, reassess the patient and revise the plan.

Thyroid Hormone Resistance

Thyroid hormone resistance is a recently recognized syndrome characterized by an inability of the target tissues to bind with or use available thyroid hormone. It has a genetic predisposition. The patient presents with manifestations of mild hypothyroidism despite elevated levels of circulating thyroid hormone and normal or elevated levels of TSH. Thyroid enlargement may be present and lead to misdiagnosis. Thyroid hormone resistance is treated by cautious administration of T_3 to overcome hormone resistance. Liothyronine sodium (Cytomel) is commonly prescribed. Some patients respond well to administration of dopamine, a neurotransmitter that also lowers the serum levels of TSH in both euthyroid and hypothyroid persons. Antithyroid drugs and thyroidectomy are contraindicated and will worsen the condition.

STRUCTURAL DISORDERS

A goiter is an enlargement of the thyroid gland not related to inflammation or neoplasia. A diffuse toxic goiter is common in hyperthyroidism, which was discussed earlier in this chapter. People with nontoxic goiters are usually euthyroid. Goiters are more common in women than men.

Simple Nontoxic Goiter

A simple nontoxic goiter is hyperplasia of the thyroid gland that develops in response to the gland's inability to secrete enough thyroid hormone to meet metabolic needs. The enlarged gland compensates for inadequate hormone production and is able to secrete sufficient amounts of thyroid hormone to maintain a euthyroid state.

Simple goiters are more common in young women. They may develop during periods of increased metabolic demands, such as adolescence or pregnancy. Deficiency of dietary iodine is another cause of simple goiter. Because simple nontoxic goiters caused by iodine deficiency are more common in regions far from the seacoast, they often are called endemic goiters.

Clinical manifestations of a simple nontoxic goiter depend on the size of the gland. A large, palpable mass at the base of the neck is the primary manifestation (Fig. 29–10). Displacement or compression of the esophagus or trachea may cause dysphagia, a choking sensation, or respiratory difficulty. A very large goiter may impair venous return from the head, neck, and even the upper limbs. Venous engorgement may lead to dizziness and syncope.

Diagnosis is based on history, clinical manifestations, and the results of thyroid function studies. Once other causes of thyroid enlargement are ruled out, a simple nontoxic goiter is treated by correcting its cause. Temporary thyroid hormone replacement meets metabolic demands while allowing the gland to rest and shrink. Iodine supplements or increased dietary iodine is prescribed for people with iodine deficiency. Foods high in iodine include seafood, seaplants, and iodized salt. Iodine is also used as a dough conditioner in many commercial bread products. Surgery is not recommended but may be needed if the goiter does not shrink sufficiently to relieve obstructive symptoms.

Nodular Goiter

A nodular goiter is similar to a simple goiter, except that the glandular enlargement develops as multiple nodules in women over the age of 40. These multinodular goiters are usually asymptomatic unless they are very large. Occasionally, a nodule may be hyperfunctioning glandular tissue that shows up as a "hot spot" on the thyroid scan and may be associated with symptoms of hyperthyroidism. Treatment varies according to the person's age and clinical manifestations.

NEOPLASIA

Benign thyroid cysts and adenomas are firm, well-encapsulated, noninvasive, slow-growing neoplasms of unknown etiology. Their incidence is higher in people who have received radiation to the head, neck, or chest. Benign neoplasms are usually nonfunctioning and rarely symptomatic. They present as "cold spots" on a thyroid scan. Secreting benign adenomas are very rare and not dependent on TSH to maintain function. Diagnosis of benign neoplasms is

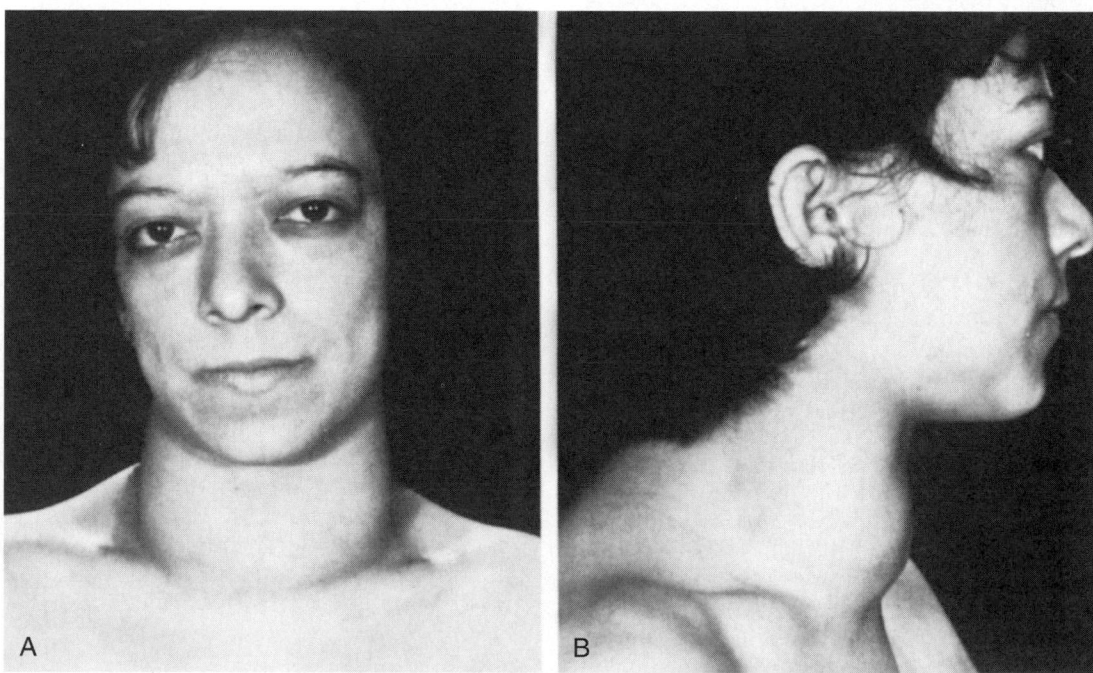

Figure 29–10
Thyroid enlargement due to goiter. Note enlargement at the base of the neck. (From Larsen PR, Ingbar SH. The thyroid gland. In Wilson JD, Foster DW [eds]. Williams textbook of endocrinology. 8th ed. Philadelphia: WB Saunders, 1992, p 425.)

confirmed by needle biopsy. Treatment is conservative, with annual re-evaluation. Functioning adenomas are treated with radioactive iodine or surgery.

It is recommended that individuals perform self-examinations for thyroid cancer. To do this, the individual should look in a mirror with the head tilted back. Swallow a sip of water and observe for any bulges. If a bulge is seen, the thyroid gland should be checked by a physician.

Malignant thyroid neoplasms are rare, destructive, nonsecreting adenocarcinomas that usually develop as a single, firm nodule. Metastasis to the lungs and bones is common. Thyroid cancer occurs with greater frequency in middle-aged women with a history of radiation to the head, neck, or chest. There is a familial tendency. Vocal cord paralysis and hoarseness are common with thyroid carcinoma. Thyroid scan, computed tomography or magnetic resonance imaging, and needle biopsy are used to identify probable malignant lesions.

Subtotal or total thyroidectomy, sometimes followed by radioactive iodine therapy, is the primary treatment. Postoperatively, lifelong thyroid hormone replacement is prescribed to suppress thyroid function and minimize the risk of recurrence. Nursing care related to these treatments is discussed earlier in the chapter.

Papillary carcinoma is the most common form of thyroid cancer. It usually develops as a firm, solitary nodule identified as a "cold spot" on the thyroid scan. It grows slowly and remains confined to the thyroid gland for many years. Prognosis is excellent if the carcinoma is diagnosed and treated before it spreads outside the gland.

Follicular carcinoma is slightly more aggressive than papillary carcinoma, and metastasis is more common. These tumors sometimes retain their ability to synthesize and secrete thyroid hormone. Secreting tumors present as a "hot spot" on the thyroid scan. Secreting follicular tumors respond well to treatment with radioactive iodine.

Medullary carcinoma is a cancer of the parafollicular cells. It is more aggressive than follicular cancer and commonly extends into local lymph nodes and surrounding tissues. Medullary tumors secrete calcitonin. Serum calcitonin levels are used to diagnose the tumor and evaluate the success of treatment. Total thyroidectomy with lymph node dissection is the treatment of choice. Radioactive iodine is not effective. Prognosis is poorer in patients with lymph node involvement.

Undifferentiated carcinoma, also called anaplastic carcinoma, or giant cell or small cell carcinoma, depending on cell structure, is very rare. It rapidly grows into surrounding structures and metastasizes early. Undifferentiated carcinoma is very resistant to treatment, although surgery may be performed to relieve pressure symptoms. Death usually occurs within 6 to 12 months of diagnosis.

Parathyroid Disorders

Functional disorders of the parathyroid glands are characterized by inadequate or excess secretion of parathyroid hormone. Disorders of the parathyroid glands are uncommon but can be life-threatening.

HYPOPARATHYROIDISM

Hypoparathyroidism is an acute or chronic disorder of calcium metabolism. It is caused by inadequate secretion of parathyroid hormone or failure of the target cells to respond to it. The latter condition is called pseudohypoparathyroidism and is an extremely rare genetic disorder.

Etiology and Pathophysiology

The most common causes of hypoparathyroidism are iatrogenic. These include damage to, or accidental removal of, the parathyroids during thyroid gland surgery; irradiation of the neck; and surgical removal of the parathyroids to treat neoplasias or hyperparathyroidism. Rarely, hypoparathyroidism develops after destruction of the thyroid gland with radioactive iodine. In procedures that carry a high risk for damage to the parathyroid glands, parathyroid tissue can be autografted to a muscle of the forearm before the surgery. This practice has been successful in preventing iatrogenic hypoparathyroidism.

Idiopathic hypoparathyroidism is less common and is thought to be a familial autoimmune disorder. Chronic hypomagnesemia, which is frequently associated with alcoholism, malabsorption syndromes, prolonged parenteral nutrition, and administration of cisplatin and aminoglycoside antibiotics, impairs parathyroid hormone release and impairs the response of body tissues to parathyroid hormone. The result is hypocalcemia in the presence of normally functioning parathyroid glands.

Decreased parathyroid hormone activity causes decreased calcium resorption from the bones, decreased intestinal absorption, and decreased reabsorption of calcium in the renal tubules, with increased phosphate retention. Hypocalcemia and hyperphosphatemia result. Decreased concentrations of serum ionized calcium increase neuromuscular excitability. The transmission of neuromuscular impulses speeds up, and repetitive responses to a single stimulus may occur. Spontaneous discharge of neuromuscular fibers occurs in severe hypocalcemia. Calcifications in the optic lens and in the basal ganglia develop in chronic hypocalcemic states.

Clinical Manifestations

The clinical manifestations of hypoparathyroidism are directly related to decreased serum ionized calcium concentration, its severity, rate of fall, and duration. The more rapid the decrease in serum calcium, the more severe the symptoms. Neuromuscular manifestations are most severe in the rapid onset of acute hypocalcemia caused by iatrogenic destruction of, or damage to, the parathyroids.

Early manifestations of acute hypocalcemia include irritability, apprehension, muscle cramps in the extremities and abdomen, and photophobia. Stiffness of the hands and feet and paresthesias characterized by numbness and tingling around the mouth (perioral area), of the nose or earlobes, and in the fingers and toes are common. Positive Chvostek's and Trousseau's signs may be present.

If serum calcium continues to fall, general muscle hypertonia and cramping may progress to hypocalcemic tetany, which is characterized by tonic spasms and sustained contraction of individual muscle groups. Respiratory stridor, crowing on inspiration caused by glottic and laryngeal spasms, bronchospasms, and respiratory arrest may occur as tetany progresses and serum calcium drops below 7 mg/dL. Cardiac dysrhythmias can result from decreased myocardial contractility and atony. Generalized tonic-clonic seizures usually develop if serum calcium drops below 6 mg/dL. Loss of consciousness and incontinence are rarely associated with hypocalcemic convulsions.

Clinical manifestations in chronic hypocalcemia include irritability, lethargy, and personality changes. The skin becomes dry and scaly, with brittle nails and thin, patchy, prematurely gray hair. Premature cataracts develop from lens calcification. Calcification in the basal ganglia may cause brain damage, a Parkinson-like syndrome, psychosis, and seizures. Cardiac dysrhythmias may progress to congestive heart failure.

Diagnosis

Parathyroid hormone levels are determined by radioimmunoassay on a blood specimen taken in the early morning or late evening, when parathyroid hormone secretion is highest. A sample for assessing serum ionized calcium is drawn concurrently. In hypoparathyroidism, the parathyroid hormone level and serum calcium level are low. The serum phosphorus level is elevated. Ectopic calcifications are identified by CT scans of the brain and ophthalmic examination. Cardiac dysrhythmias and a prolonged QT interval are identified by electrocardiography.

Management

Treatment of hypoparathyroidism depends on its severity. Acute hypocalcemic tetany is a medical emergency. It is treated with intravenous calcium gluconate or calcium chloride until serum calcium exceeds 7 mg/dL. Oral calcium and vitamin D therapy is then initiated. Muscle relaxants may also be prescribed if raising the serum calcium level does not control neuromuscular irritability.

Chronic hypoparathyroidism is treated with oral calcium supplements taken with oral vitamin D supplements. Dihydrotachysterol (Hytakerol) and ergocalciferol (formerly called calciferol) are two commonly prescribed vitamin D supplements. A diet high in calcium but low in phosphorus is recommended. The intake of calcium through diet and supplements combined should be about 2 g daily. Aluminum carbonate gel (Basaljel) or aluminum hydroxide gel (Amphojel) may be prescribed to promote phosphorus excretion. In some cases, thiazide diuretics may be effective in promoting calcium reabsorption from the renal tubules.

The goal in treating chronic hypoparathyroidism is to maintain a serum calcium level between 8.5 and 9.5 mg/dL. It requires lifelong treatment and frequent serum calcium determinations to prevent hypercalcemia from excess calcium and vitamin D intake.

NURSING PROCESS
Hypoparathyroidism

Assessment

Obtain a complete nursing history from patients with diagnosed or suspected hypoparathyroidism and from patients at risk for acute hypocalcemia. Patients at risk include:

- Those with diagnosed chronic hypoparathyroidism or low serum calcium or magnesium concentrations
- Those with a history of chronic renal failure, malnutrition, or alcoholism
- Those with a family history of autoimmune endocrine disorders
- Those who have undergone thyroid surgery or radioactive iodine therapy

Assess for clinical manifestations associated with acute and chronic hypoparathyroidism. Obtain baseline vital signs and apical pulse to determine cardiac rhythm. Review laboratory results of serum calcium, ionized calcium, phosphorus, and magnesium values to determine baseline levels. If paresthesias are reported, test for a positive Chvostek or Trousseau sign. Notify the physician immediately if manifestations of impending acute hypocalcemia are present.

Identify the patient's interpretation of the clinical manifestations of the disorder and assess his or her knowledge of planned diagnostic studies and treatment to determine teaching needs.

Nursing Diagnoses and Planning

Nursing diagnoses and related expected patient outcomes commonly applicable to patients with hypoparathyroidism include the following:

NDx: Risk for suffocation and Risk for injury related to increased neuromuscular irritability and tetany secondary to acute hypocalcemia

Planning: Patient Outcomes

1. Patient maintains normal neuromuscular activity and respiratory function as evidenced by:
   Usual mental status
   Regular apical pulse, 60 to 100 bpm
   Negative Chvostek's and Trousseau's signs
   Absence of paresthesias, muscle cramps, tetany, respiratory stridor, convulsions
2. Patient remains free from injury.
3. Patient maintains serum calcium level above 8.5 mg/dL.

NDx: Risk for altered health maintenance related to insufficient knowledge of chronic hypoparathyroidism, treatment regimen, self-management, and follow-up care

Planning: Patient Outcomes

1. Patient verbalizes understanding of the need for, and intent to take, calcium and vitamin D supplements as prescribed.
2. Patient identifies foods that are high in calcium as desirable to include in the daily diet.
3. Patient identifies foods that are high in phosphorus as foods to avoid in the diet.
4. Patient maintains serum calcium level higher than 8.5 mg/dL.
5. Patient states intent to keep follow-up appointments as scheduled.
6. Patient states intent to notify physician promptly if signs of hypocalcemia or hypercalcemia develop.

Nursing Interventions and Evaluation

The nursing priority for the patient with acute or chronic hypoparathyroidism is to prevent manifestations of increased neuromuscular irritability and hypocalcemic tetany by maintaining the serum calcium level above 8.5 mg/dL. If tetany or convulsions occur, airway maintenance is the first concern.

NDx: Risk for suffocation and Risk for injury
Monitor serum calcium levels, vital signs, and apical pulse of patients at risk for acute hypocalcemia. Place a tracheostomy tray and intravenous calcium gluconate at the bedside of postoperative patients after a thyroidectomy, parathyroidectomy, or radical neck surgery. Provide a nonstimulating environment to minimize neuromuscular stimulation.

Monitor neuromuscular irritability and mental status to identify early signs of acute hypocalcemia. Initiate rebreathing in a paper bag or rebreathing mask, notify the physician immediately, and prepare to administer intravenous calcium gluconate if early signs of hypocalcemic tetany develop. Rebreathing decreases exhaled carbon dioxide, raises serum carbonic acid levels, and lowers serum pH. The resulting mild respiratory acidosis temporarily increases serum ionized calcium levels. Monitor for respiratory stridor caused by glottic and laryngeal spasms. A tracheostomy may be necessary to maintain a patent airway if bronchospasms or convulsions occur.

Maintain patient safety if convulsions develop. Nursing care of the patient with acute hypocalcemia is summarized in Nursing Care Guide 29–5.

NDx: Risk for altered health maintenance
Explain the basic concepts of chronic hypoparathyroidism, the function of parathyroid hormone in the body, and the reasons for physical and emotional changes the patient has experienced. Provide an opportunity for the patient to ask questions and verbalize feelings. Reinforce the physician's explanation of the prescribed therapy and clarify any misunderstandings.

Teach the patient the dosage, administration schedule, expected action, and side effects of prescribed calcium and vitamin D supplements. Reinforce the benefit of taking these supplements concurrently, preferably with meals, to enhance calcium absorption. Vitamin D toxicity is a potentially serious complication. Instruct the patient to notify the physician promptly if dry mouth, nausea, vomiting, metallic taste, or constipation develops. Constipation is also a side effect of aluminum carbonate gel and aluminum hydroxide gel. Monitor the number and consistency of stools. Teach the patient to report the early signs of hypocalcemia to the physician promptly. Teach that frequent urination, thirst, slowed mental processes, muscle weakness, and fatigue are early signs of hypercalcemia that must be reported to the physician promptly.

Reinforce the dietitian's explanation of a high-calcium, low-phosphorus diet. Provide a list of foods high in calcium to include in the diet, and a list of foods high in phosphorus to avoid. Although dairy products and canned fish with bones are high in calcium, they are also high in phosphorus and may be restricted. Consult with the physician and dietitian to determine the precise amount of these foods allowed. High phosphorus levels are found in foods rich in protein (meat, poultry, fish, eggs, legumes, nuts). If aluminum carbonate gel (Basaljel) or aluminum hydroxide gel (Amphojel) is prescribed, stress that it is to be taken with a full glass of water or juice immediately after meals to promote excretion of phosphorus. (When used as antacids, these drugs are taken 1 hour after meals.)

Emphasize that treatment of chronic hypoparathyroidism is lifelong and that periodic examination to evaluate response to treatment and to monitor serum ionized calcium levels is necessary to prevent episodes of hypocalcemia or hypercalcemia.

Compare the patient's status with the expected outcomes. If the outcomes are not met, reassess the patient and revise the plan.

HYPERPARATHYROIDISM

Etiology and Pathophysiology

Hyperparathyroidism is a disorder of calcium metabolism caused by excess secretion of parathyroid

Nursing Care Guide 29-5

Patients with Acute Hypoparathyroidism: Hypocalcemic Tetany

Assessment Findings: Twelve hours after a total thyroidectomy, a patient complains of muscle cramps and numbness and tingling of the nose, fingers, and around the mouth. The patient appears anxious. Positive Chvostek's and Trousseau's signs are elicited.

Nursing Diagnosis: Risk for trauma: suffocation related to increased neuromuscular irritability associated with acute hypocalcemia secondary to damage to the parathyroid glands during thyroid surgery

Patient Outcomes	Nursing Interventions	Rationale
Patient notifies nurse immediately if paresthesia develops.	Teach all patients at risk for acute hypocalcemia to notify the nurse immediately of muscle or abdominal cramps, or tingling of the nose, earlobes, fingers, toes, or perioral area.	Detection and treatment of early manifestations of hypocalcemia can prevent acute hypocalcemic crisis.
Patient remains free from injury.	Place tracheostomy tray and intravenous calcium gluconate at the bedside of patients at risk for acute hypocalcemic tetany.	Emergency supplies and medication should be immediately available if needed.
	Monitor apical heart rate and rhythm, or use a cardiac monitor, to identify dysrhythmias caused by low serum calcium levels. Monitor changes in peripheral sensations, mental status, behavior, response to Chvostek's and Trousseau's tests, and neuromuscular irritability at least every 2 hours for 48 hours.	Cardiac dysrhythmias, altered neurologic status, and neuromuscular irritability are manifestations of hypocalcemia.
	Initiate rebreathing, notify the physician, and prepare to administer intravenous calcium gluconate if signs of increased neuromuscular irritability develop.	Rebreathing produces mild respiratory acidosis and temporarily increases serum calcium levels. Intravenous calcium gluconate rapidly restores serum calcium levels.
Patient's respirations remain clear and unlabored.	Assess for respiratory stridor or obstruction caused by hypocalcemic tetany. Be prepared to assist with emergency tracheostomy if they occur. Maintain patent airway and patient safety if seizures develop.	Acute hypocalcemic tetany may cause laryngospasms, bronchospasms, or seizures.
	Monitor parenteral calcium infusion to avoid infiltration. Stop the infusion immediately and notify the physician if infiltration occurs.	Infiltration of calcium may cause tissue necrosis.
	Monitor serum calcium values, vital signs, cardiac rhythm, and patient response during calcium administration.	Evaluates effectiveness of treatment of hypocalcemia and prevents hypercalcemia caused by overtreatment.

Evaluation: Compare the patient's status with the expected outcomes. If the outcomes are not met, reassess the patient and revise the plan.

hormone. It primarily affects people older than 50, and females twice as frequently as males. Incidence increases with advancing age. Hyperparathyroidism is being diagnosed more frequently with the widespread use of multichannel autoanalyzers that include serum calcium evaluation. Some studies performed on people over the age of 50 have found hyperparathyroidism to some degree in as many as 1 man in 1000 and 2 women in 200.

There are several classifications of hyperparathyroidism, each with a different etiology. Of these, primary and secondary hyperparathyroidism are the most common.

Primary hyperparathyroidism is characterized by enlargement of one or more parathyroid glands and increased secretion of parathyroid hormone. Specific etiology is unknown. Single benign adenomas are diagnosed in 85 to 90% of people with primary hyperparathyroidism. Other causes include multiple adenomas and single or multiple gland hyperplasia. Parathyroid cancer, characterized by a serum calcium level over 15 mg/dL, is very rare. The incidence of primary hyperparathyroidism is higher in people with a family history of parathyroid disorders or multiple endocrine neoplasias. Irradiation of the neck or thyroid gland also increases risk.

Secondary hyperparathyroidism is a compensatory response by normal glands to chronic mild hypocalcemia. A sustained increase in the production and secretion of parathyroid hormone results in glandular hyperplasia. Conditions that may precipitate secondary hyperparathyroidism include vitamin D or calcium deficiency, hyperphosphatemia, chronic renal failure, intestinal malabsorption syndromes, rickets, acromegaly, and pseudohypoparathyroidism. Pregnant and lactating women may also experience temporary parathyroid hyperplasia. Secondary hyperparathyroidism usually does not result in hypercalcemia because normal feedback control mechanisms are intact. It is treated by correcting the cause.

Increased parathyroid hormone activity causes increased resorption of calcium from the bones, increased intestinal absorption, and increased reabsorption of calcium in the renal tubules with excess excretion of phosphorus. Hypercalcemia and hypophosphatemia result. Increased concentrations of serum ionized calcium decrease neuromuscular excitability. Transmission of neuromuscular impulses is slowed because of the sedative effect of calcium on nerve fibers. Calcium is deposited in tissues throughout the body. Polyuria and excessive thirst may develop as the body attempts unsuccessfully to excrete excess calcium.

Clinical Manifestations

The clinical manifestations of primary hyperparathyroidism are directly related to increased levels of serum ionized calcium. In its mildest form, and often in secondary hyperparathyroidism, the patient may be asymptomatic or have nonspecific clinical manifestations.

Early symptoms include fatigue, general malaise, lethargy, apathy, and drowsiness. Muscle weakness and atrophy, lack of coordination, activity intolerance, memory lapses, poor concentration, and depression result from slowed impulse transmission.

Abdominal pain, anorexia, nausea, vomiting, and constipation develop from decreased gastrointestinal motility. Gastric secretions increase in response to hypercalcemia. This, plus decreased gastrointestinal motility, increases the risk for peptic ulcers. Acute pancreatitis may develop secondary to sustained hypercalcemia.

Renal calculi, formed by precipitation of calcium in the kidneys, are found in most people with hyperparathyroidism. Renal colic, urinary tract infections, hematuria, and polyuria occur in conjunction with the renal calculi. Metabolic acidosis from impaired renal reabsorption of sodium bicarbonate may develop. Cardiovascular manifestations include bradycardia, dysrhythmias, and calcification of arterial walls. An atrioventricular block may lead to cardiac arrest. Hypertension secondary to renal and cardiovascular involvement is common.

Bone demineralization, caused by the increased subperiosteal calcium resorption that is characteristic in hyperparathyroidism of long duration, is most severe in cortical bone. It causes generalized osteoporosis and weakens the bones. Low back pain, bone pain and tenderness, arthralgia, pathologic fractures, and deformity result. Demineralization around the teeth can also occur. Pseudogout, caused by deposition of calcium crystals in articular cartilage, is a complication of hyperparathyroidism. Anemia, calcifications in the cornea of the eye (band keratopathy), and occipital headache are less common manifestations.

Acute hypercalcemic crisis is a rare, life-threatening complication of hyperparathyroidism. It can also occur with some cancers and after chemotherapy or irradiation because of massive cell destruction. In addition to the clinical manifestations already listed, the patient in hypercalcemic crisis is at high risk for severe dehydration, coma, and cardiac dysrhythmias with cardiac arrest in asystole.

Diagnosis

Diagnosis of primary hyperparathyroidism, especially in mild or asymptomatic people, is based primarily on an elevated serum parathyroid hormone level after the discovery of elevated ionized serum calcium and decreased phosphorus levels, or of elevated 24-hour urinary calcium excretion. An elevated alkaline phosphatase level indicates increased osteoblastic activity of the bones. Radiographic studies may reveal subperiosteal bone resorption, osteoporosis of the skull and other bones, soft-tissue calcification, and renal calculi. Bone densitometry identifies loss of bone mass. Cardiac dysrhythmias, atrioventricular block, widened T wave, and shortened QT intervals are confirmed by electrocardiography.

Management

Early diagnosis and treatment is important in the successful management of primary hyperparathyroidism. The primary goal is to lower serum calcium and prevent complications. Because of the risk of disease progression, surgery is the treatment of choice in most cases. However, for asymptomatic patients with serum calcium levels under 12 mg/dL who have no renal or skeletal manifestations, some physicians favor conservative management with oral phosphate supplements and 4 to 5 L of fluids daily to promote calcium excretion. These patients require frequent follow-up to evaluate treatment and detect hypercalcemia-related complications.

Computed tomography, ultrasonography, magnetic resonance imaging, and arteriography are used commonly to confirm the number and location of parathyroid glands before surgery. In single-gland adenoma, the involved gland is removed. A subtotal parathyroidectomy with removal of three and a half glands is done for multiple-gland hyperplasia. Adequate parathyroid hormone will be secreted by the remaining tissue. Some surgeons remove all identified parathyroid glands and graft a portion of one into a muscle of the forearm. This facilitates later removal if hypercalcemia persists.

Serum ionized calcium levels decrease to near normal levels 24 to 48 hours after surgery. The patient may experience mild symptoms of transient tetany after surgery from the rapid drop in calcium concentration and the rapid absorption of serum calcium by demineralized bone—the "hungry bone syndrome." Once serum calcium and 24-hour urinary calcium excretion have returned to normal, a high-calcium diet and calcium and vitamin D supplements may be prescribed for several months until bone recalcification stabilizes. Prognosis after surgery is good. However, renal damage may be irreversible and bone deformities, if present, will persist.

Hypercalcemic crisis is a medical emergency that can occur any time serum calcium concentration exceeds 12 mg/dL. Intravenous normal saline is rapidly infused to rehydrate the patient and lower serum calcium concentration by expanding fluid volume. Furosemide (Lasix), a loop diuretic; plicamycin (Mithracin), an antibiotic; and calcitonin, a parathyroid hormone antagonist, may also be administered to inhibit bone resorption and promote calcium excretion. The use of intravenous phosphates is limited because of the danger of extraskeletal calcification in patients who are in severely hypercalcemic states. Bisphosphonates have been somewhat effective in inhibiting osteoclastic bone resorption in cases of severe hypercalcemia caused by metastatic bone cancer.

NURSING PROCESS
Hyperparathyroidism
Assessment

Obtain a complete nursing history from the patient with hyperparathyroidism. Assess for clinical manifestations associated with hyperparathyroidism. Ask specifically about the onset of early symptoms of hypercalcemia because nonspecific early symptoms are often overlooked by the patient as insignificant or unrelated to the current illness. Obtain baseline vital signs and apical pulse to determine cardiac rhythm. Identify the patient's interpretation of clinical manifestations and knowledge of the planned diagnostic studies and surgery to determine teaching needs. Assess for changes in neuromuscular and mental status and increased urine output, which may indicate deterioration and impending hypercalcemic crisis. Notify the physician immediately if the patient's condition deteriorates.

Nursing Diagnoses and Planning

Nursing diagnoses and related expected patient outcomes commonly applicable to patients with hyperparathyroidism include the following:

NDx: Risk for fluid volume deficit related to excess urine output secondary to hypercalcemia

Planning: Patient Outcomes
1. Patient consumes 3000 mL of fluid daily.
2. Patient maintains hemodynamic fluid balance as evidenced by:
   Stable weight
   Vital signs within patient's normal range
   Stable neurologic status
   Moist mucous membranes
   Good skin turgor

NDx: Risk for trauma related to impaired neuromuscular function, activity intolerance, and osteoporosis secondary to hypercalcemia

Planning: Patient Outcomes
1. Patient remains free from injury.
2. Patient walks for 15 minutes at least three times daily.
3. Patient verbalizes understanding of the need for, and intent to consume, a high-calcium diet after surgery.

Nursing Interventions and Evaluation

The priorities of care for the patient with hyperparathyroidism are to lower serum calcium levels and prevent renal complications. Care after a subtotal parathyroidectomy is similar to care after a thyroidectomy. Anticipate and assess for signs of mild hypocalcemic tetany caused by the rapid drop in the serum calcium level. Monitor closely for the onset of early signs of acute hypocalcemic tetany, a rare early postoperative complication. Notify the physician if such signs develop.

NDx: Risk for fluid volume deficit

Monitor vital signs, apical pulse, neurologic status, and urine output to detect changes in neuromuscular and cardiac function. Monitor changes in serum calcium determinations. Encourage fluids to 3000 mL daily, unless contraindicated by cardiac status, to maintain hydration, replace fluids lost through excess urine output, and promote excretion of calcium. Record fluid intake and output. Weigh the patient daily to assess fluid loss or gain. Adjust intake accordingly. Closely monitor the patient receiving cardiotonics to detect early signs of toxicity. Hypercalcemia potentiates the effects of cardiotonics. Monitor changes in sensorium to detect decreasing alertness, an early sign of dehydration. Examine mucous membranes and test skin turgor to identify signs of dehydration.

Assess for manifestations of renal colic and renal calculi caused by calcium precipitation in the kidneys. Teach the patient to consume low-calcium, acid-ash foods and fluids (such as cranberry, tomato, and prune juice) to increase urine acidity and promote calcium excretion. Initiate consultation with a dietitian to facilitate patient education. Strain all urine and send excreted calculi for analysis. Test urine daily with a reagent strip to identify hematuria. Encourage mobility to inhibit calcium resorption from the bones. Administer stimulant stool softeners and anti-ulcer medications to counteract the gastrointestinal effects of hypercalcemia.

A patient in hypercalcemic crisis is placed on a cardiac monitor to facilitate early identification of potentially life-threatening cardiac dysrhythmias. Monitor vital signs, central venous pressure, and urine output hourly during high-volume intravenous infusion with normal saline to prevent fluid overload and assess renal function. Administer prescribed medications to lower serum calcium concentrations. Assess for early signs of hypocalcemic tetany to prevent overtreatment of hypercalcemia.

NDx: Risk for trauma

Explain the pathology of hyperparathyroidism and hypercalcemia as the cause for physical and mental alterations. Provide an opportunity for the patient to verbalize feelings and ask questions. Support the patient in maintaining realistic expectations of surgery. Renal damage may not be reversible.

Implement safety measures if mental functions are impaired. Encourage ambulation before and after surgery to diminish muscle atrophy and promote bone recalcification. Maintain an obstacle-free environment to prevent falls. Keep the bed in low position with at least one side rail up. Tell the patient to call for assistance before getting out of bed, and place the call bell within reach. Supervise or assist with ambulation as appropriate. Plan nursing care to allow frequent rest periods to conserve energy.

Teach the patient that a high-calcium diet is important for several months after surgery to maintain adequate serum calcium levels for bone recalcification. Provide a list of foods high in calcium. Review dosage, administration schedule, expected action, and side effects of prescribed calcium supplements. Stress that calcium and vitamin D supplements should be taken together and with meals to enhance absorption. Teach the patient that fatigue, general malaise, lethargy, apathy, and drowsiness are early signs of hypercalcemia, whereas paresthesias, muscle cramps, and irritability are early signs of hypocalcemia. Provide a written list of the signs of calcium imbalance with instructions to notify the physician promptly if they develop. Stress the importance of periodic assessments of serum calcium concentrations to evaluate the effectiveness of surgery.

Compare the patient's status with the expected outcomes. If the outcomes are not met, reassess the patient and revise the plan.

❖ SETTINGS, PROVIDERS, AND COLLABORATION FOR CARE

Care of the patient with hypoparathyroidism or hyperparathyroidism may require the efforts of a variety of health-care professionals in the acute care setting, or care may be delivered in clinics and the home. For the patient experiencing tetany associated with hypoparathyroidism, careful evaluation is needed to manage care. The state of hypercalcemia must also be closely monitored. Thus, the patient diagnosed with tetany or hypercalcemia is usually hospitalized for initial treatment. The prospect of surgical intervention reinforces the importance of the nurse collaborating with a team of health-care providers. Postoperatively, the nurse teaches the patient about continued care (if needed) in the home and sets a follow-up appointment for the patient to be seen at the physician's office. Ongoing care for the patient with hypoparathyroidism or hyperparathyroidism may be effectively provided in the home, under the supervision of the home health nurse.

The Elderly: Special Considerations

Pituitary Disorders in Older Adults

There is no evidence that pituitary disorders are more common in the elderly than in the general population. Indeed, almost all chronic pituitary disorders develop before mid-life. However, because of the complexity of physiologic problems in many older people, manifestations of possible pituitary-related disorders may be falsely attributed to old age, rather than investigated for potentially reversible conditions.

Hypofunction of the thyroid gland and adrenal cortex may result from hypopituitarism caused by altered cerebrovascular blood flow. Deteriorating neurologic function can alter the transmission of, and response to, stimuli to and from the hypothalamus and pituitary gland. In addition, chronic undernutrition has been found to reduce the secretion of hypothalamic and anterior pituitary hormones. Several studies have noted that the older person is able to maintain urine concentration under normal circumstances but cannot alter urine concentration to adjust for fluid excess or deficit. To compensate for decreased renal efficiency in elderly people, the hypothalamic osmoreceptors become more sensitive and ADH secretion increases. This compensatory hypersecretion of ADH is one of the factors in the high incidence of transient syndrome of inappropriate antidiuretic hormone in the elderly after the administration of anesthesia. Impaired renal response also places the elderly person at higher risk for the untoward effects of drugs that may alter ADH activity. Syndrome of inappropriate antidiuretic hormone associated with the administration of sulfonylurea compounds, although rare, occurs almost exclusively in the aged.

Assess all geriatric patients for clinical manifestations of pituitary dysfunction. Evaluate any changes in behavior patterns to rule out the possibility of pituitary neoplasms. Consider any geriatric patient at risk for altered posterior pituitary function caused by anesthesia, response to medications, or fluctuations in extracellular fluid levels. In patient teaching, use large-type and clearly written instructions to reinforce verbal instructions on prescribed medications and self-management. Indicate which side effects necessitate immediate notification of the physician.

Adrenal Disorders in Older Adults

Secretion of ACTH and adrenal hormones diminishes with increased age. Reduced levels of glucocorticoids place the older person at higher risk for hypoglycemia when food intake is decreased or when the person must fast for diagnostic procedures or surgery. Aldosterone secretion is diminished in older adults, placing them at higher risk of excess fluid loss if fluid intake is reduced or if the environment is dry or very warm. It is unclear whether reduced secretion of adrenal sex steroid hormones influences the changes in secondary sex characteristics commonly associated with the aging process.

There is no evidence that adrenal disorders are more common in older adults than in the general population, but tuberculosis in older adults may be associated with Addison's disease. In light of the normal physiologic changes associated with the aging process discussed in Chapter 4, it is apparent that an elderly person with an adrenal disorder may be at higher risk for complications of fluid and elec-

trolyte imbalance than a younger person. Orthostatic hypotension develops more rapidly in an elderly person who experiences a change in blood pressure or fluid balance. Older people receiving long-term glucocorticoid preparations are at higher risk for osteoporosis.

Thyroid Disorders in Older Adults

The major significance of thyroid disorders in the elderly is not in the differences in incidence, manifestations, or complexity of treatment, but in the potential for inaccurate, delayed, or missed diagnosis. Early signs may be incorrectly attributed to manifestations of the aging process. As a person ages, decreasing thyroid gland function is usually compensated for by decreasing metabolic demands and an increase in the proportion of T_3 to T_4. The ratio of T_4 to T_3 is closer to 5:1, compared with 7:1 to 10:1 in younger people.

The incidence of hypothyroidism increases with age, with an estimated prevalence of about 10% among older adults. Early manifestations may be mistaken for a gradual age-related decrease in metabolism. In addition, manifestations of hypothyroidism, such as slowed mentation, decreased cardiac output, and increased sensitivity to cold, may be falsely perceived as age-related changes. Older persons with hypothyroid disorders may have no symptoms except apathy or diminished level of functioning. Diagnosis is based on clinical manifestations and elevated serum TSH levels.

Thyroid hormone replacement should be monitored carefully because the half-life of thyroxine is increased in older adults. Also, older adults may be more susceptible to the metabolic effects of thyroid preparations. Hormone replacement is initiated at a low dose, and increments are made gradually at 4- to 6-week intervals to avoid adverse effects such as agitation, mental changes, and cardiovascular overload. Most older people achieve a euthyroid state at lower than normal dosages.

The most common cause of hyperthyroidism in the elderly is toxic nodular goiter. In contrast to the higher incidence in women younger than age 60, hyperthyroidism occurs equally in elderly men and women. Altered cardiac function is a predominant clinical manifestation. Cardiac disorders, such as atrial fibrillation or congestive heart failure may be caused by hyperthyroidism. Ophthalmic manifestations are less common in older adults. Apathy, lethargy, depression, and anorexia with weight loss and muscle wasting are atypical manifestations that are seen in older people with hyperthyroid disorders. Diagnosis should rely primarily on thyroid function tests rather than on clinical manifestations.

Initial treatment with antithyroid drugs and propranolol followed by radioactive iodine therapy is the treatment of choice in the elderly. A euthyroid state is usually achieved within 6 weeks. Agranulocytosis is an adverse reaction seen in the elderly. It can develop at any time during therapy with anti-thyroid drugs. Instruct the patient to notify the physician immediately if manifestations develop.

Parathyroid Disorders in Older Adults

As discussed earlier in this chapter, the incidence of hyperparathyroidism increases with age. There is no evidence that the incidence of other parathyroid disorders is higher in the elderly than in the general population. However, poor nutrition increases the risk of altered parathyroid function. The chance of misdiagnosis or completely missed diagnosis is higher in older adults because the vague, nonspecific early symptoms of parathyroid disorders may be overlooked as age-associated changes. People with the neurologic alterations of hypocalcemia and hypercalcemia have been misdiagnosed as having Alzheimer's disease or a psychiatric disorder. Parathyroid disorders should be considered as a possibility in older patients who have altered mental or behavioral status in conjunction with nonspecific neuromuscular or gastrointestinal complaints.

Chapter Review

1. How does the action of each of the endocrine glands affect the body?
2. What are the effects of hypersecretions of each of the endocrine glands?
3. What are the effects of hyposecretions of each of the endocrine glands?
4. Which manifestations of endocrine disorders are most critical to the patient's health status?
5. Which nursing diagnoses are appropriate for the patient with an endocrine disorder that affects cardiovascular functioning?
6. What nursing interventions are appropriate for the patient with external feature changes resulting from an endocrine disorder?
7. What pharmacologic therapy is useful for each of the major endocrine disorders?
8. In which treatment settings might nursing care be delivered for the patient with an endocrine disorder?
9. How can life-threatening complications be prevented in patients with severe endocrine disorders?
10. What nursing strategies would you use to bring families (or significant others) of patients with endocrine disorders into active roles on the health-care team?

Bibliography

Abrams AC. Clinical drug therapy: Rationales for nursing practice. 4th ed. Philadelphia: JB Lippincott, 1995.

Aronow WS. The heart and thyroid disease. Clin Geriatr Med 1995; 11(2):219.

Baker KH, Feldman JE. Thyroid cancer: A review. Oncol Nurs Forum 1993; 20(1):95.

Baxter MA. Acromegaly and transsphenoidal hypophysectomy: A case report. AANA J 1994; 62(2):182.

Bilezikian JP. Primary hyperparathyroidism: Another important metabolic bone disease of women. J Womens Health 1994; 3(1):21.

Bland JH. Arthritis symptoms: Is it endocrine disease? Consider ovarian, pancreatic, or parathyroid disease . . . part 2. J Musculoskeletal Med 1994; 11(3):34.

Boulanger BR, Gann DS. Management of the trauma victim with pre-existing endocrine disease. Crit Care Clin 1994; 10(3):537.

Bruton-Maree N, Maree SM. Acute adrenal insufficiency: A case report. CRNA 1993; 4(3):128.

Burke MM, Walsh MB. Regulation: Endocrine, temperature, and infection in gerontologic nursing: Care of the frail elderly. St. Louis: Mosby Year-Book, 1992, pp 167–196.

Carlson L. Aseptic necrosis following transplant. ANNA J 1993; 20(2):185.

Carpenito LJ. Nursing diagnosis: Application to clinical practice. 6th ed. Philadelphia: JB Lippincott, 1995.

Cassel CK, Walsh JR (eds). Geriatric medicine. 3rd ed. New York: Springer-Verlag, 1996.

Cella JH, Watson J. Nurse's manual of laboratory tests. 2nd ed. Philadelphia: FA Davis, 1995.

Coffland FI. Endocrine disorders affecting the cardiovascular system. Crit Care Nurs Clin North Am 1994; 6(4):735.

Cooper JAD, Pappas PG (eds). Cecil review of general internal medicine. 6th ed. Philadelphia: WB Saunders, 1996.

Corsetti A, Buhl B. Managing thyroid storm. Am J Nurs 1994; 94(11):39.

Counsell CM, Gilbert M, Snively C. Challenging diagnosis. Management of the patient with a pituitary tumor resection. DCCN 1996; 15(2):75.

Curtis P, Dworkin H. Nuclear medicine and the thyroid gland: A retrospective review. J Nucl Med Technol 1995; 23(Suppl 4): 8S.

Daniels GH. Thyroid function tests: The pivotal role of sensitive TSH measurements. Consultant 1995; 35(2):209.

Daroff RB, Frishman WH, Lederman RJ, Stewart WC. Beta-blockers: Beyond cardiology. Patient Care 1993; 27(11):47, 52, 54.

DeCoopman J. Breastfeeding after pituitary resection: Support for a theory of autocrine control of milk supply? J Hum Lact 1993; 9(1):35.

DeGroot LJ (ed). Endocrinology. 3rd ed. Philadelphia: WB Saunders, 1994.

Doenges M, Moorhouse M. Nurse's pocket guide: Nursing diagnosis with interventions. 5th ed. Philadelphia: FA Davis, 1996.

Dranov P. Tired? Wired? It could be your thyroid. Am Health 1994; 13(4):90.

Dudek SG. Nutrition handbook for nursing practice. 2nd ed. Philadelphia: JB Lippincott, 1993.

Eliopoulos C. Gerontological nursing. 4th ed. Philadelphia: JB Lippincott, 1996.

Fischbach F. A manual of laboratory diagnostic tests. 5th ed. Philadelphia: JB Lippincott, 1996.

Gambert SR. Hyperthyroidism in the elderly. Clin Geriatr Med 1995; 11(2):181.

Giefer CK, Cassmeyer VL. The syndrome of primary aldosteronism: A case study. Medsurg Nurs 1994; 3(4):277.

Gordon M. Nursing diagnosis: Process and application. 3rd ed. St. Louis: CV Mosby, 1993.

Greenspan FS. Basic and clinical endocrinology. 4th ed. Norwalk, CT: Appleton & Lange, 1994.

Grey AB, Evans MC, Stapleton JP, Reid IR. Body weight and bone mineral density in postmenopausal women with primary hyperparathyroidism. Ann Intern Med 1994; 121(10):745.

Griffith CJ. Nonsteroidal anti-inflammatory drugs: A pharmacologic update. Physician Assist 1994; 18(9):31, 36, 46.

Griffin J, Ojeda S (eds). Textbook of endocrine physiology. 3rd ed. New York: Oxford University Press, 1996.

Guyton AG. Textbook of medical physiology. 9th ed. Philadelphia: WB Saunders, 1995.

Hardy JR. Endocrine therapy in advanced malignancy. Eur J Palliat Care 1995; 2(4):151.

Hart IR. Management decisions in subclinical thyroid disease. Hosp Pract 1995; 30(1):43, 50.

Healy PF. Self-test. Caring for patients with endocrine disorders. Nursing 1995; 25(9):22.

Horowitz M, Wishart JM, Need AG, Morris HA, Nordin BEC. Primary hyperparathyroidism. Clin Geriatr Med 1994; 10(4):757.

Hyperparathyroidism. Harv Womens Health Watch 1996; 3(9):6.

Jankowski CB. Irradiating the thyroid: How to protect yourself and others. Am J Nurs 1996; 96(20):50.

Johnson D. Advanced perioperative nursing: Selected physiological effects of trauma. Semin Periop Nurs 1994; 3(4):185.

Kee JL. Handbook of laboratory and diagnostic tests with nursing implications. 2nd ed. Norwalk, CT: Appleton & Lange, 1994.

Khan JA, Wagner DV, Tiojanco JK, Hoover LA. Combined transconjunctival and external approach for endoscopic orbital apex decompression in Graves' disease. Laryngoscope 1995; 105(2):203.

Kim TS. Primary hyperparathyroidism. Orthop Nurs 1994; 13(3):17.

Kingsbury SJ, Salzman C. Lithium's role in hyperparathyroidism and hypercalcemia. H&CP 1993; 44(11):1047.

Lawler DA. Hormonal response in sepsis. Crit Care Nurs Clin North Am 1994; 6(2):265.

Lehne RA. Pharmacology for nursing care. 2nd ed. Philadelphia: WB Saunders, 1994.

Malseed RT, Harrigan G. Textbook of pharmacology and nursing care: The nursing process. 4th ed. Philadelphia: JB Lippincott, 1995.

Managing thyroid troubles. Health News 1994; 12(1):1.

Maree S, Curll N, Emerson P. Anesthetic management of patients with pheochromocytomas: A report of three cases. CRNA 1993; 4(3):129.

Matteson MA, McConnell ES. Gerontological nursing: Concepts and practice. 2nd ed. Philadelphia: WB Saunders, 1996.

Maugeri D, Russo MS, Carnazzo G, et al. Altered laboratory thyroid parameters indicating hyperthyroidism in elderly subjects. Arch Geront Geriatr 1996; 22(2):145.

McEwen DR. Transsphenoidal adenomectomy. AORN J 1995; 61(2):319.

McMorrow ME. Emergency! Myxedema coma. Am J Nurs 1996; 96(10):55.

Mehta V, Savino JA. Surgical management of the patient with a thyroid disorder. Clin Geriatr Med 1995; 11(2):291.

Miller M, Gold GC. Acute endocrine emergencies. Clin Geriatr Med 1994; 10(1):161.

Moore L. Anesthetic considerations in patients with hyperparathyroidism. CRNA 1993; 4(3):118.

Moore L. Undiagnosed hyperthyroidism. CRNA 1993; 4(3):114.

Morley CT. Case management of the anemic patient: Epoetin alfafocus on osteitis fibrosa. ANNA J 1993; 20(5):604.

Mundy GR. Evaluation and treatment of hypercalcemia. Hosp Pract 1994; 29(6):79.

Nimmagadda U. Anesthesia and the parathyroid gland. Curr Rev Nurse Anesth 1994; 16(21):183, 192.

North American Nursing Diagnosis Association. NANDA nursing diagnoses: Definitions & classifications, 1995–96. St. Louis: NANDA, 1994.

Novak S, Greenwood R. Patterns of urine flow and electrolyte excretion in patients following traumatic brain injury. Clin Rehabil 1995; 9(4):331.

Ouellette RG, D'Agostino EO. Undiagnosed hyperthyroidism. CRNA 1993; 4(3):114.

Perry HM, Miller DK, Morley JE, et al. A preliminary report of vitamin D and calcium metabolism in older African Americans. J A Geriatr Soc 1993; 41(6):612.

Piziak VK, Gilliland PF. Pituitary tumors: Look for early signs and symptoms. Emerg Med 1993; 25(7):124.

Preoperative imaging in hyperparathyroidism. Emerg Med 1995; 27(11):60, 62.

Ram CVS. Secondary hypertension: Workup and correction. Hosp Pract 1994; 29(4):137.

Richuso KM. Commentary on practical points in the care of the patient post-thyroid surgery. AACN Nurs Scan Crit Care 1993; 3(3):24.

Roberts A. Growth hormone and prolactin. Nurs Times 1995; 91(28):29.

Roberts A. Systems of life: The adrenal glands. Nurs Times 1995; 91(45):34.

Roberts A. Systems of life: The adrenal gland 2. Nurs Times 1995; 91(50):31.

Rutecki GW, Whittier FC. Hyponatremia: Cause of hypotonicity directs management. Consultant 1994; 34(5):705, 711.

Shannon MT, Wilson BA. Govoni & Hayes drugs and nursing implications. 8th ed. Norwalk, CT: Appleton & Lange, 1994.

Shuey KM. Heart, lung, and endocrine complications of solid tumors. Semin Oncol Nurs 1994; 10(3):177.

Singer PA, Cooper DS, Levy EG, et al. Treatment guidelines for patients with hyperthyroidism and hypothyroidism. JAMA 1995; 273(10):808.

Smith-Rooker JL, Garrett A, Hodges LC. Case management of the patient with pituitary tumor. Medsurg Nurs 1993; 2(4):265.

Stoffer SS. Addison's disease: How to improve patients' quality of life. Postgrad Med 1993; 93(4):265.

Tagney GC. Commentary on recognition of panic disorder in the emergency department. AACN Nurs Scan Crit Care 1993; 3(1):16.

Taylor K, Schneiderman H. Apathetic hyperthyroidism. Consultant 1993; 33(3):81.

Thyroid disease. Clin Geriatr Med 1995; 11(2):xi, 159.

Tolliss D. Who was Cushing? . . . Harvey Williams Cushing was one of the most prominent and influential neurosurgeons around the turn of the century and is often considered to be one of the fathers of neurosurgery. Nursing Times 1994; 90(39):55.

Ulrich SP, Canale SW, Wendell SA. Nursing care planning guides: A nursing diagnosis approach. 3rd ed. Philadelphia: WB Saunders, 1994.

Vague symptoms may signal thyroid disease. Univ Tex Lifetime Health Lett 1993; 5(10):1.

What's new in drugs. Octreotide enters the market against acromegaly. RN 1996; 59(1):69.

Wojner AW, Graves B. Sterotactic radiosurgery: New practice frontiers for the perioperative nurse. Semin Periop Nurs 1995; 4(3):177.

Wyngaarden JB, Smith LH, Bennett JC (eds). Cecil textbook of medicine. 20th ed. Philadelphia: WB Saunders, 1996.

Young WF. Pheochromocytoma: A brief management guide. Hosp Med 1993; 29(10):67.

Ziomek R. Commentary on endocrine responses to the stress of critical illness. AACN Nurs Scan Crit Care 1993; 3(1):17.

Unit X

Urinary Dysfunction

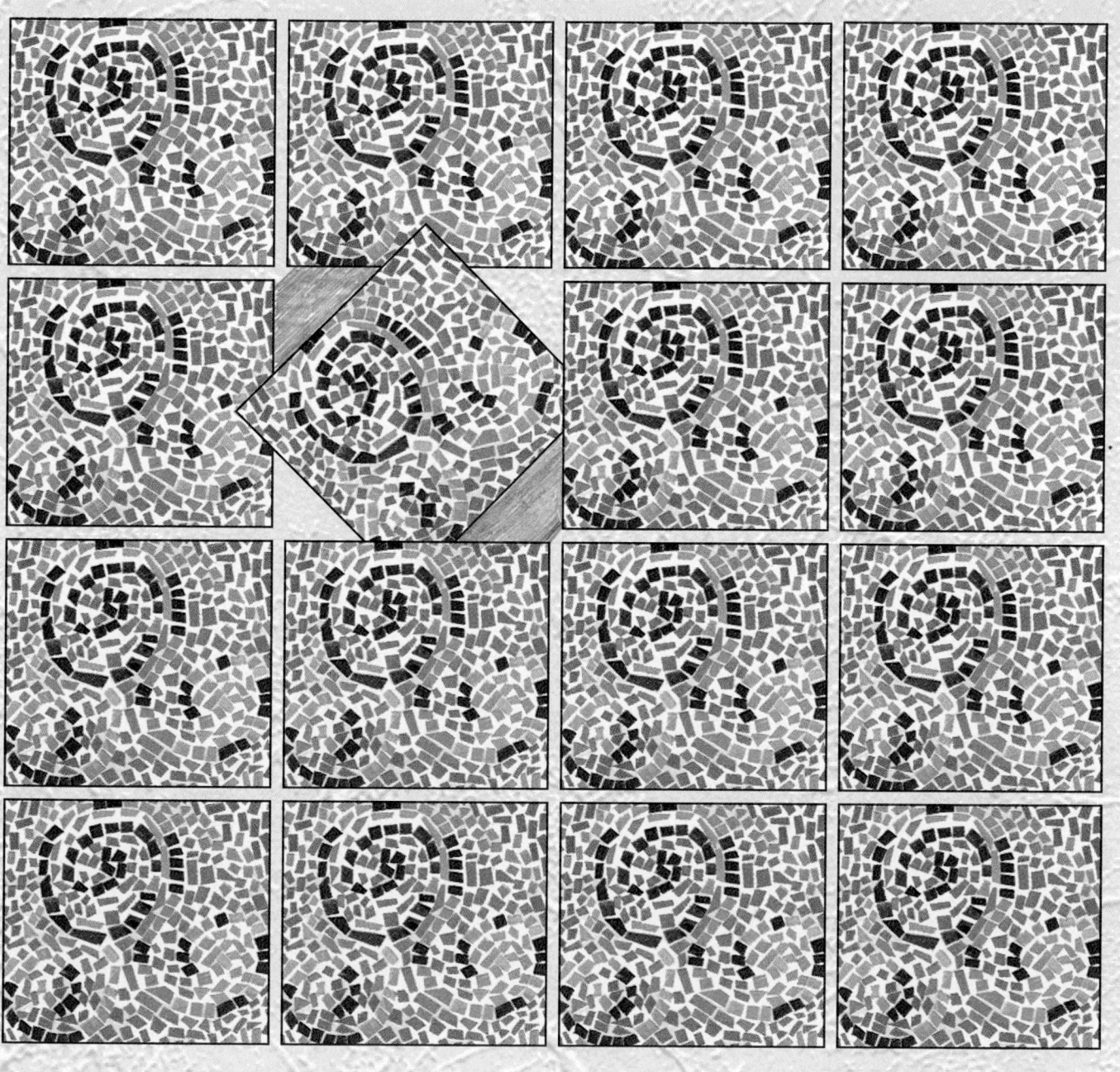

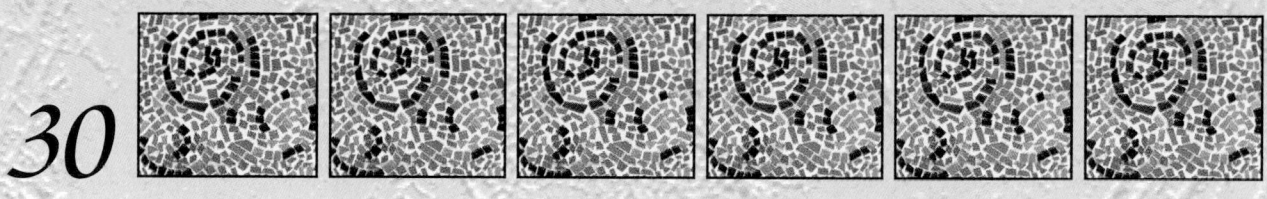

30

Knowledge Base for Patients with Urinary Dysfunction

Study Outcomes

After studying this chapter, you should be able to:

1. Explain the normal anatomy and physiology of the urinary system.
2. Describe common clinical manifestations of urinary tract dysfunction.
3. Identify information and physical examination data essential to the assessment of the urinary system.
4. Identify the most common laboratory and radiologic studies used to diagnose urinary dysfunction.
5. Describe the medical management and surgical procedures commonly used in the treatment of patients with urinary dysfunction.
6. Identify data essential to the assessment of patients undergoing treatment of urinary dysfunction.
7. State the nursing diagnoses and related expected patient outcomes commonly applicable to patients undergoing radiologic and other studies of the urinary tract and treatments of urinary dysfunction.
8. Describe nursing interventions, with their rationales, commonly applicable to patients undergoing radiologic and other studies of the urinary tract and treatments of urinary dysfunction.
9. Explain the basis for evaluation of nursing care provided to patients undergoing treatment of urinary dysfunction.
10. Identify special considerations and resources for the elderly patient with altered urinary function.
11. Identify alternative treatments, care settings, and community-based services for patients with urinary dysfunction.

The urinary system is responsible for maintaining homeostasis by reabsorbing and retaining materials needed by the body, and by filtering and excreting waste materials. Dysfunction in the urinary system has a profound effect on almost all other body systems because function of the urinary tract is critical to the maintenance of overall homeostasis. For example, urinary dysfunction may affect the cardiovascular system, the gastrointestinal system and the accessory organs of digestion, the neurologic system, and even the integumentary system.

Procedures commonly ordered for diagnosis of urinary dysfunction or for treatment of urinary disorders are frequently completed in outpatient facilities such as clinics or freestanding surgical centers. Procedures such as x-rays, scans, dilatations, and cystoscopies may be performed in the physician's office, as well as in the hospital. Nursing care, especially patient education, may vary depending on the setting in which the diagnostic measure or treatment is being completed.

Anatomy and Physiology

The urinary tract consists of the paired kidneys and ureters, the urinary bladder, and the urethra (Fig. 30–1). These structures are essentially the same in both sexes. However, the urethra is longer in the male.

KIDNEYS

The kidneys are paired organs that lie lateral to the vertebral column between the twelfth thoracic (T-12) and the third lumbar (L-3) vertebrae. The kidneys lie in an oblique position. They are found retroperitoneally against the posterior abdominal wall in the right and left upper abdominal quadrants. The average-sized kidney measures approximately 12 to 14 cm ($4\frac{3}{4}$ to $5\frac{1}{2}$ inches) in length, 5 to 7 cm (2 to $2\frac{3}{4}$ inches) in width, and 3 cm ($1\frac{1}{4}$ inches) in thickness. The adult kidney weighs approximately 150 g (5 oz). The left kidney is usually slightly larger than the right, and the position of the liver causes the right kidney to be somewhat lower than the left.

On the medial surface of the kidney there is a concave notch called the hilus. In addition to the ureter, the renal artery, the renal vein, nerves, and lymphatic vessels enter the kidney through the hilus.

The kidneys are enclosed in the thin, fibrous re-

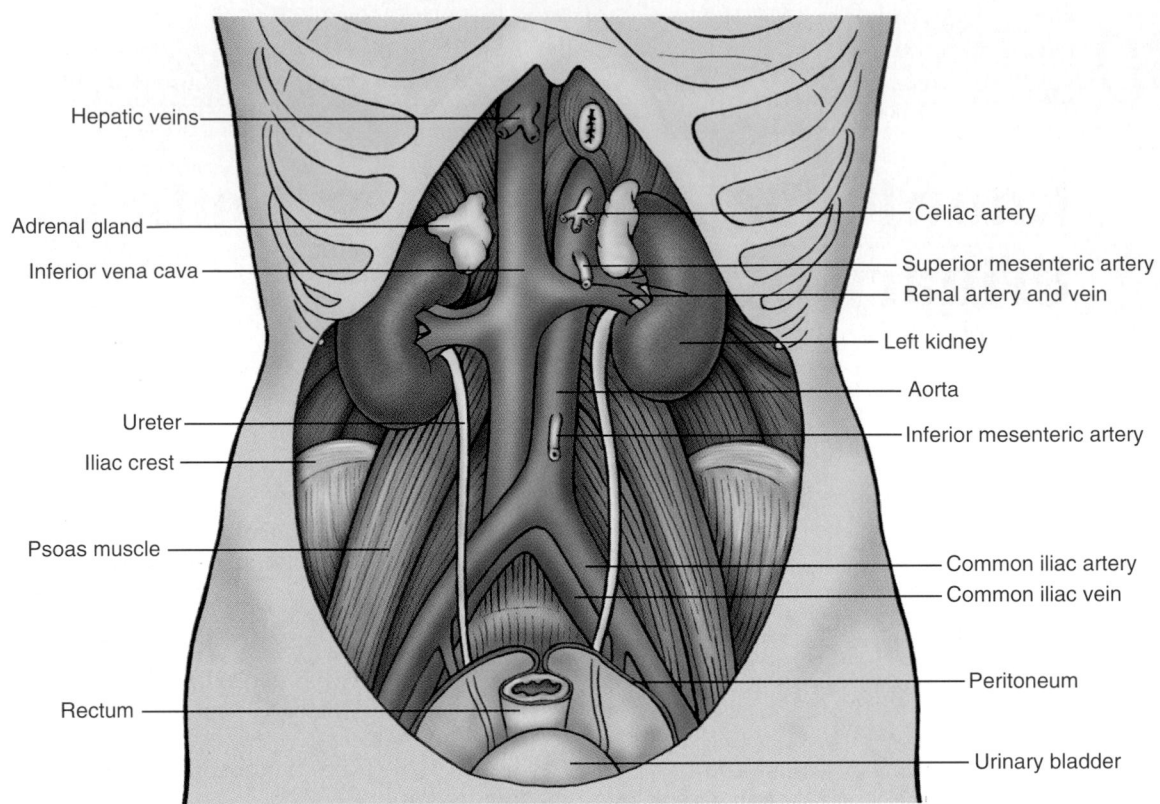

Figure 30–1

The kidneys and related structures.

nal capsule. The capsule is supported by layers of perineal fat and Gerota's fascia. The capsule covers all areas of the kidney except the hilum. The muscles of the back, flank, and abdomen also provide support and protection to the kidneys.

The parenchyma is the functional tissue of the kidney. It consists of the cortex and the medulla (Fig. 30–2). The medulla is below the cortex. The medulla is divided into 10 to 20 triangle-shaped wedges referred to as the renal pyramids. The base of each pyramid faces the cortex. The apex, or renal papilla, faces the center of the kidney. The papillae carry formed urine into the collecting system. The pyramids of the medulla have a somewhat striated appearance, whereas the cortex has a smooth texture.

The cortex extends inward between each of two pyramids, forming the renal columns. The peaks, or apices, of the renal pyramids form a "cup," called a minor calix. Each minor calix joins one or two other minor calices to form a major calix. In each kidney there are approximately eight minor calices and three major calices. The major calices come together at the center of the medulla to form the renal pelvis.

The renal pelvis is a cone-shaped structure that extends from the center of the medulla. It exits the kidney through the hilum and curves downward to

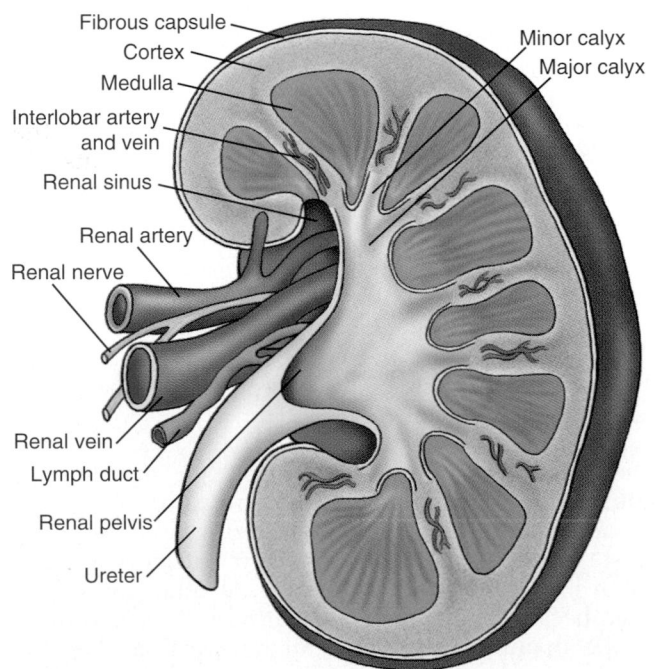

Figure 30–2

The kidney.

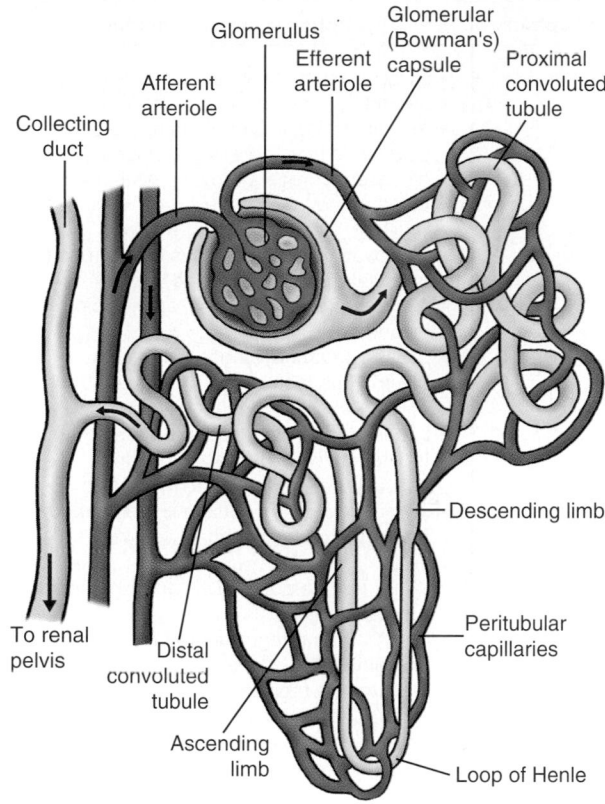

Figure 30–3

The nephron.

form the ureter. The renal pelvis normally holds 5 to 7 mL (approximately $\frac{1}{4}$ ounce) of urine.

The cortex, or outer layer, of the kidney contains the nephrons (Fig. 30–3). The nephron is the functioning unit of the kidney. It contains the glomeruli, which are tufts of capillaries. Blood enters into the glomerulus via the afferent arterioles and exits via the efferent arterioles. The glomerulus is enclosed in Bowman's capsule. Bowman's capsule is the beginning of the tubular system of the nephron. The tubular system consists of the proximal convoluted tubule, the loop of Henle, and the distal convoluted tubules. This structure twists and turns throughout the parenchyma of the kidney. The distal convoluted tubules terminate in one of the many collecting ducts that pass through the papillae and calices, emptying into the renal pelvis.

The renal artery is the major blood supply of the kidneys. The kidneys receive 25% of the total cardiac output. The renal artery arises from the abdominal aorta, branching into the right and left renal arteries. The renal veins empty into the inferior vena cava.

The kidneys have both sympathetic and parasympathetic innervation. Innervation is through the lesser splanchnic nerves.

The overall function of the urinary system can generally be described as the maintenance of the body's internal homeostasis. It accomplishes homeostasis through three mechanisms: glomerular filtration, tubular reabsorption and secretion, and excretion. More specifically, the urinary system performs the following functions:

- Excretes the body's metabolic waste (its primary function)
- Regulates fluid and electrolyte balance
- Helps to maintain acid-base balance
- Assists with calcium metabolism and regulation of blood pressure
- Regulates production of red blood cells

The kidneys selectively reabsorb those essential substances needed to maintain normal body fluid composition and excrete unneeded substances in the form of urine (Fig. 30–4). The kidneys normally filter approximately 180 liters (about 47.5 gallons) of plasma in 25 hours. This translates into approximately 125 mL (about $4\frac{1}{4}$ ounces) per minute. In that time, 1 liter becomes urine and the other 179 liters are reabsorbed, as is two-thirds of the solute, the substances extracted by the kidneys from the plasma. Renal function can be affected by the response of the kidneys to the composition, pressure, and volume of blood flowing through them.

Formation and Excretion of Urine

Glomerulus

The primary function of the kidneys—excretion of metabolic wastes—begins in the glomerulus, also called the capillary tuft. As blood flows through the glomerular capillaries, filtration occurs. Blood plasma flows across the semipermeable membrane of the glomerular tuft, taking smaller molecules with it and leaving larger molecules behind. The substance that moves across the semipermeable membrane into Bowman's capsule is called glomerular filtrate.

The rate at which glomerular filtrate is formed is known as the glomerular filtration rate (GFR). Normally, it is approximately 125 mL (about $4\frac{1}{4}$ ounces) per minute. GFR depends on three factors: the permeability of the glomerular capillary walls, blood pressure, and the effectiveness of filtration. It is also regulated and kept constant by the contraction and relaxation of the afferent and efferent arterioles of the glomerulus. Alterations in any of these factors can significantly alter the GFR.

Creatinine is a metabolic end-product of a substance in skeletal muscle. It is formed and excreted through the glomeruli in constant amounts. Creatinine is not appreciably reabsorbed or secreted by the renal tubules. Thus it is good approximation of the GFR. The creatinine clearance (CrCl) test is

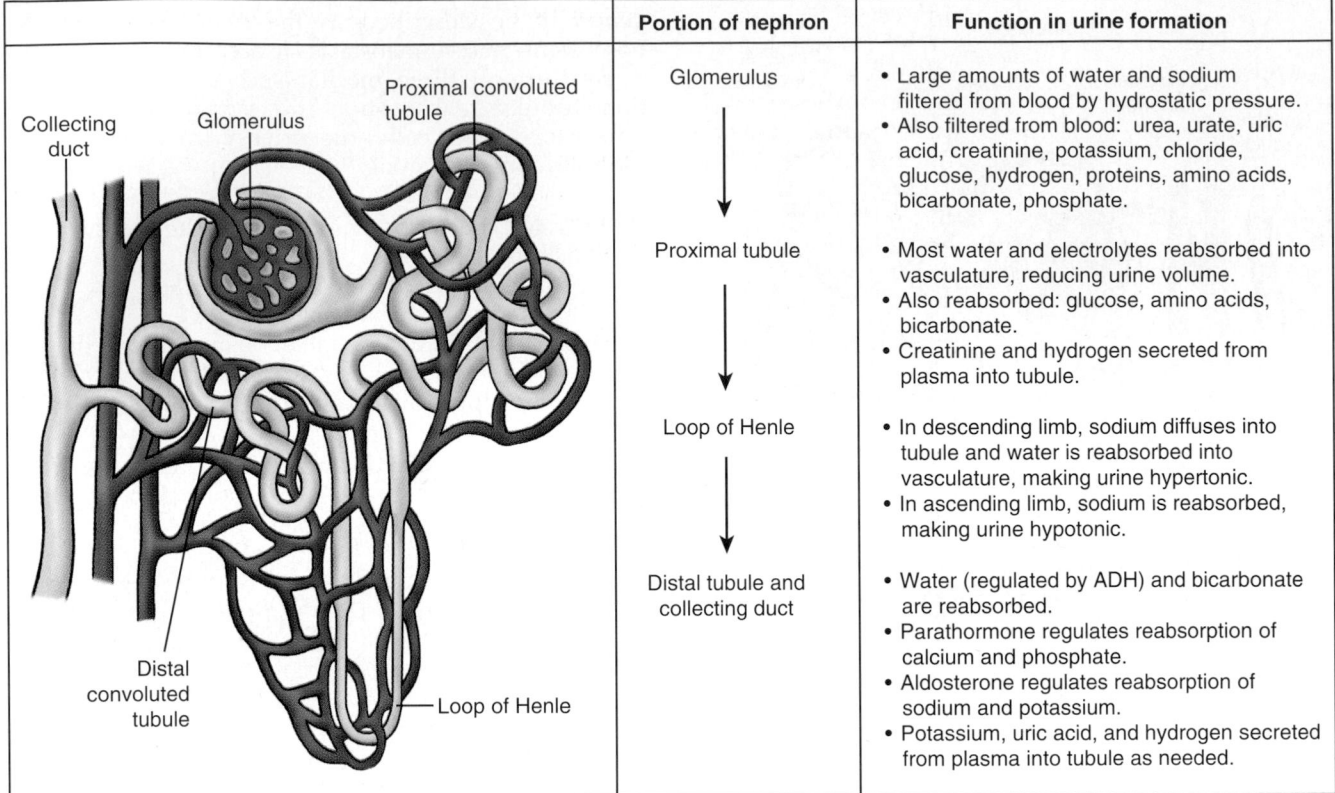

Portion of nephron	Function in urine formation
Glomerulus	• Large amounts of water and sodium filtered from blood by hydrostatic pressure. • Also filtered from blood: urea, urate, uric acid, creatinine, potassium, chloride, glucose, hydrogen, proteins, amino acids, bicarbonate, phosphate.
Proximal tubule	• Most water and electrolytes reabsorbed into vasculature, reducing urine volume. • Also reabsorbed: glucose, amino acids, bicarbonate. • Creatinine and hydrogen secreted from plasma into tubule.
Loop of Henle	• In descending limb, sodium diffuses into tubule and water is reabsorbed into vasculature, making urine hypertonic. • In ascending limb, sodium is reabsorbed, making urine hypotonic.
Distal tubule and collecting duct	• Water (regulated by ADH) and bicarbonate are reabsorbed. • Parathormone regulates reabsorption of calcium and phosphate. • Aldosterone regulates reabsorption of sodium and potassium. • Potassium, uric acid, and hydrogen secreted from plasma into tubule as needed.

Figure 30-4

Normal physiologic function of the nephron in urine formation. ADH, antidiuretic hormone.

therefore used to determine the GFR. The formula for calculating creatinine clearance is as follows:

$$\text{CrCl (GFR)} = \frac{\text{urine creatinine}}{\text{plasma creatinine}} \times \frac{\text{volume of urine}}{\text{minutes of urine collection}}$$

The results are expressed in milliliters per minute, with 90 to 100 mL/min being normal.

Proximal Convoluted Tubule

Glomerular filtration represents only the initial portion of the process of urine formation. After the filtrate is collected in the space within Bowman's capsule, it passes into the proximal convoluted tubule, where reabsorption occurs. Approximately 80% of the water, 50% to 70% of the sodium and chloride, 85% of all electrolytes, and normally 100% of the filtered glucose are reabsorbed here.

Loop of Henle

The filtrate continues through the loop of Henle. The descending portion of this loop is highly permeable to water and moderately permeable to sodium, urea, and other ions. The ascending portion of the loop is slightly permeable to urea and water and actively transports sodium in and out. Approximately 25% of filtrate is reabsorbed through this ascending portion. The medulla of the loop of Henle also produces a high concentration of sodium chloride, which is essential in water homeostasis.

Distal Convoluted Tubule and Collecting Duct

As shown in Figure 30-4, both the distal convoluted tubule and the collecting duct reabsorb and secrete a number of substances. This process changes glomerular filtrate into urine. Urine then flows into the ducts of the renal papillae, into the minor calices, into the major calices, and finally into the renal pelvis. Here the flow of urine is promoted by the intraluminal pressure of the kidney and by peristalsis in the ureters. The urine is transported down the ureter into the bladder.

Regulation of Fluid and Electrolyte Balance

Regulation of fluid and electrolyte balance by the kidneys is achieved through adjustments in filtration, reabsorption, and secretion. If renal blood flow is adequate, the distal tubules of the nephrons control fluid volume by concentrating or diluting urine. If the body is dehydrated, it releases antidiuretic hormone (ADH), which is synthesized by cells of the hypothalamus and stored in the posterior pituitary gland. ADH acts on the distal tubule and collecting ducts to make them permeable to water. Water is then reabsorbed into the blood stream rather than excreted in the urine. If the body is well hydrated or overhydrated, the body does not release ADH, water is not reabsorbed, and water is then excreted in the urine.

Electrolyte balance is influenced by hydrostatic and osmotic pressures. In addition, aldosterone affects sodium and potassium reabsorption. The majority of electrolytes are reabsorbed in the proximal convoluted tubule, and the regulation of electrolytes occurs in the distal convoluted tubule. The distal tubule actively transports sodium and other positive ions in and out. Potassium ions are also secreted into the tubular fluid in the distal tubule and in the collecting duct. Depending on the concentration of the electrolytes in the urine, the tubular cells secrete or further reabsorb electrolytes in the urine. This takes place through diffusion and active transport.

Regulation of Acid-Base Balance

Regulation of acid-base balance (pH) is accomplished by both the lungs and the kidneys. Although the lungs can quickly compensate for mild pH imbalances, the kidneys can compensate for much greater imbalances, though their action is slower than that of the lungs. Because more acids than bases normally enter the blood stream, the kidneys normally excrete more acids than bases to maintain acid-base balance. That is, the kidneys regulate acid-base balance primarily by ridding the blood of excess acid and by conserving base to be reabsorbed into the blood stream. They accomplish this task by secretion of hydrogen ions from the distal tubules into the urine. In response to base excess (alkalosis), the distal tubules do the opposite. They conserve hydrogen ions and excrete bicarbonate into the urine.

Stimulation of Red Blood Cell Production

The renal parenchyma is believed to produce erythropoietin. Erythropoietin stimulates the bone marrow to produce red blood cells. A deficit of erythropoietin therefore causes anemia.

Calcium Metabolism

Active vitamin D is necessary for gastrointestinal absorption of calcium. Active vitamin D also helps regulate calcium deposition in the bone matrix, as well as metabolism of calcium and phosphorus. The active form of vitamin D is 1,25-dihydroxycholecalciferol, and it is the kidney that converts inactive vitamin D to active vitamin D.

Regulation of Blood Pressure

The kidneys help regulate blood pressure through three mechanisms: regulation of plasma volume, the renin-angiotensin-aldosterone system, and prostaglandins.

The kidneys regulate plasma volume by reabsorbing water and by controlling the composition of extracellular fluid.

The renin-angiotensin-aldosterone system plays an important role in the regulation of blood pressure. The release of the hormone renin is caused by a decrease in blood flow, a decrease in serum sodium, or both. Renin is released by the juxtaglomerular apparatus of the nephron. This hormone stimulates the conversion of angiotensinogen to angiotensin I (a mild vasoconstrictor) in the liver. Angiotensinase then converts angiotensin I to angiotensin II in the lungs. Angiotensin II is a powerful vasoconstrictor that also stimulates the release of aldosterone. Aldosterone is a mineralocorticoid that increases the reabsorption of sodium. The increase in sodium increases the amount of water reabsorbed into the blood stream. The increase in water absorbed, together with the vasoconstriction, increases blood pressure.

Prostaglandins are substances produced in the kidney and other tissues. It is believed that they have either vasoconstricting or vasodilating properties that facilitate regulation of glomerular filtration, vascular resistance, and renin production. Research on the role and function of prostaglandins is in progress because their actual mechanism is not completely understood.

URETERS

The ureters are paired, cylindrical, fibromuscular tubes that transport urine by peristalsis from the renal pelvis to the bladder. They are approximately 30 to 33 cm (about 12 to 13 inches) in length and vary in diameter from 1 mm to 1 cm (about $\frac{1}{25}$ to $\frac{3}{8}$ inches). Points of narrowing in the ureters occur at the following sites:

- The ureteropelvic junction
- The point where they enter the bony pelvis as they cross over the iliac vessels
- The ureterovesical junction

There is no true valve or sphincter where the ureters enter the bladder. However, the ureters take an oblique pathway into the bladder. This pathway creates a type of mucosal fold that normally prevents urine from flowing black up the ureters to the kidneys (reflux) during voiding or bladder emptying.

The function of the ureters is to carry urine from

the renal pelvis to the urinary bladder. This task is accomplished through peristaltic contractions of the smooth muscle fibers of the middle layer of the ureters.

BLADDER

The bladder is a hollow, muscular organ that serves as a reservoir for urine (Fig. 30–5). The adult bladder normally has a capacity of 350 to 450 mL (about 12 to 15 ounces). When empty, it lies between the rectum and pubis in the male and in front of the vagina and uterus in the female. When distended, it projects well into the abdomen and can easily be palpated or percussed.

There are three openings (orifices) on the floor of the bladder. One is in the anterior portion, for the urethra. Two are in the posterolateral portion, for the two ureters. The triangular area outlined by these three openings is called the trigone.

The inner lining, or mucosal layer, of the bladder is composed of transitional epithelium. Beneath the mucosa is a submucosal layer made up largely of connective and elastic tissue. Outside the submucosa is the muscular layer, the detrusor muscle. This muscle is a mixture of smooth muscle fibers arranged in a circular, longitudinal, and spiral manner.

The bladder neck, sometimes called the involuntary internal sphincter, is not a true circular sphincter. Rather, it is a thickening formed by the interlaced fibers of the muscular layer of the bladder as they transition into the smoother urethral musculature.

By the process of micturition (voiding, or urination), the bladder is emptied as urine is passed through the urethra and excreted by way of the urinary meatus. Micturition is a highly coordinated and complicated process. However, the normal micturition cycle can be simply separated into two phases: urine storage and bladder emptying. Both phases are controlled and coordinated by the sympathetic, parasympathetic, and central nervous systems.

During urine storage (the filling phase), there is a slow rise in pressure within the bladder, called intravesical pressure. This rise in pressure results from the increasing volume of urine in the bladder. As this pressure increases, stretch receptors in the bladder wall convey afferent impulses through the pelvic nerve to the spinal cord. This action then stimulates the sympathetic efferent nerves, located in spinal cord segments T-11 to L-2. Then, impulses are conveyed back to the bladder and urethra via the hypogastric nerves. The results are the activation of the internal sphincter to maintain continence, and the inhibition of a bladder contraction. The purpose of this inhibition is to allow for more complete bladder filling.

When intravesical pressure reaches a critical point and the bladder is sufficiently distended, nerve impulses are transmitted from the spinal cord to the brain. Although many areas of the brain may be involved in the voiding process, it is the brain stem that is considered to be the actual organizational center for micturition.

Bladder emptying occurs by parasympathetic facilitation and sympathetic inhibition. To initiate voiding, the efferent pelvic nerve, which originates in spinal cord segments S-2 to S-4, stimulates the bladder to contract and permits the bladder neck and urethra to open. At the same time, relaxation of the external urethral sphincter and perineal muscles occurs through inhibition of the pudendal nerve, which also originates in the sacral spinal cord.

Micturition is considered a nerve-mediated event. Thus, any interruption between the sacral spinal cord and the brain stem may result in a disturbance in voiding.

Other factors also contribute to normal micturition. Urine storage requires appropriate bladder sensations during filling, a closed bladder outlet at rest, and the absence of involuntary bladder contractions. Bladder emptying requires a strong and well-maintained bladder contraction, as well as the absence of

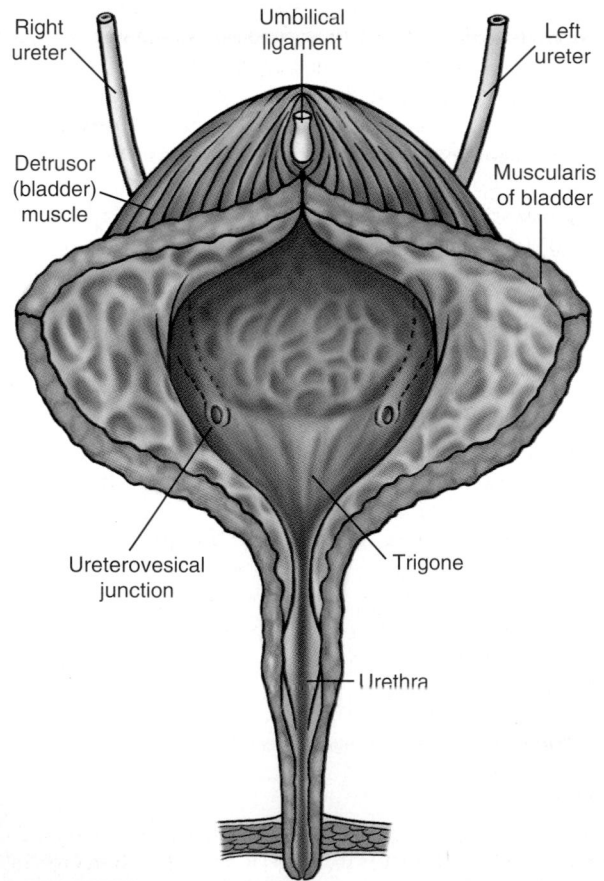

Figure 30–5

The urinary bladder.

Labels: Right ureter, Umbilical ligament, Left ureter, Detrusor (bladder) muscle, Muscularis of bladder, Ureterovesical junction, Trigone, Urethra

anatomic obstruction. Conditions that interfere with these requirements compromise normal voiding.

URETHRA

The urethra is the hollow muscular tube that conveys urine from the bladder to the urinary meatus (opening) for excretion. In women, the urethra is approximately 4 cm (about $1\frac{1}{2}$ inches) in length. It extends from the bladder neck (the involuntary internal sphincter) to the meatus. It is slightly curved and lies beneath the pubis symphysis just in front of the vagina. A voluntary external sphincter surrounds the middle third of the female urethra.

In men, the urethra is approximately 15 cm (about 6 inches) long and is described as being made up of five portions. In descending order they are the prostatic, membranous, bulbous, penile (pendulous), and glandular portions. The prostatic urethra and the membranous urethra are sometimes referred to as the posterior urethra; the bulbous, penile, and glandular portions are referred to as the anterior urethra. As in the female urethra, there is an internal sphincter, and the external sphincter in men surrounds the urethra at the narrowest portion, the membranous urethra.

The urethra serves as a conduit for the elimination of urine from the body. Falling pressure in the urethra causes urine to move from the bladder down into the urethra. The female urethra empties by gravity. The male urethra empties by contraction of the bulbocavernosus muscle.

Clinical Manifestations of Urinary Tract Dysfunction

The elimination of urine is a normal physiologic process that most people take for granted until changes occur that disrupt what are considered normal and usual bladder habits. Because of fear, some people choose to ignore such changes. However, prompt attention to these symptoms is always wise.

DYSFUNCTIONAL VOIDING

Frequency

Urinary frequency is the most common urologic symptom. It refers to an excessive need to urinate. During the daytime, the normal adult usually voids every $3\frac{1}{2}$ to 4 hours, and at night, no more than once. The patient who complains of frequency may be voiding as often as every 1 to 2 hours during the day and night. The many causes of urinary frequency may include the following:

- An increased volume of urine
- Decreased bladder capacity
- Inflammation, with increased sensitivity of the urinary tract
- Pressure from abdominal masses
- Incomplete bladder emptying
- Anxiety

Urgency

Urinary urgency is a sudden and very strong desire to urinate that is difficult to suppress. This symptom suggests an irritation of the bladder, which may be caused by an infection, tumor, or neurologic disease. Often, urinary urgency is triggered by everyday events such as the sound of running water, an abrupt change in position (eg, sitting to standing), and the sensation of warm water on the skin.

Dysuria

Dysuria is painful or difficult urination. It is usually accompanied by frequency and urgency. Together they suggest an inflammation or irritation of the lower urinary tract. The location of the discomfort may be a clue to the cause of dysuria. For instance, pain at the beginning of urination points to a problem in the urethra. Pain during or after urination suggests a problem in the bladder.

Nocturia

Nocturia is night-time urinary frequency. It is generally related to an increase in urine production at night. This symptom may suggest decreased function in the renal parenchyma. However, nocturia often occurs in the absence of any disease. For example, a person who drinks large amounts of fluid in the evening is likely to experience nocturia. Similarly, the diuretic effect of coffee and alcohol, if consumed in the evening, may produce nocturia. Medication-induced nocturia is common in patients who take diuretics for congestive heart failure, especially if the medication is taken in the evening. Additionally, the elderly person who experiences generalized fluid retention during the day will often have nocturia caused by the movement of fluid at rest. Nevertheless, unexplained nocturia is a disturbance that should be investigated if it occurs two or more times each night.

Nocturnal Enuresis

Nocturnal enuresis is the involuntary release of urine during sleep—in other words, bedwetting. This symptom is sometimes confused with nocturia, but the two are distinctly different. The patient with nocturia awakens with the need to urinate and has sufficient time to get to the bathroom. The patient with nocturnal enuresis is unaware of the need to urinate and awakens only after the bed has been wet with urine. Nocturnal enuresis in the adult is highly suggestive of a neurologic disorder.

Hesitancy

Hesitancy is a delay in the start of urination. In men, this symptom may be accompanied by a slow or weak urine stream, an intermittent stream, or postvoid dribbling. Together these symptoms suggest a blockage of the lower urinary tract, which is commonly caused by an enlarged prostate or urethral stricture.

Urinary Retention

Urinary retention is the inability to effectively empty the bladder. Acute urinary retention often occurs postoperatively. However, it may also be medication-induced or the result of injury to the lower back or pelvis. Chronic urinary retention may be related to long-standing obstruction of the lower urinary tract, as well as to neurologic and psychogenic disorders. Most patients who experience urinary retention are completely unable to urinate. Depending on the cause of urinary retention, the urge to void may or may not be present. Urinary retention is also considered to be present if the patient can produce a urinary stream but more than 50 mL of residual urine remains in the bladder.

NURSING PROCESS
Urinary Retention

Assessment

Assess the patient's usual urinary elimination pattern. Ask the patient how often he or she voids and the amount of urine voided. Ask whether the patient has experienced any frequency, urgency, fullness, or discomfort above the symphysis pubis (suprapubic discomfort). Assess the patient for distention by palpating the bladder area and above the symphysis pubis. Check the intake and output record for the past 24 hours. Assess for residual urine by catheterizing the patient immediately after voiding. Measure and record the amount of urine obtained.

Nursing Diagnoses and Planning

The nursing diagnosis and related expected patient outcomes most commonly applicable to patients experiencing urinary retention are as follows:

NDx: Urinary retention related to postoperative complications

Planning: Patient Outcomes
1. Patient voids adequate amounts within reasonable intervals.

2. Patient denies frequency, urgency, fullness, or suprapubic discomfort.
3. Patient is free from visible or palpable bladder distention.
4. Patient has balanced fluid intake and output within 48 hours after surgery.

Nursing Interventions and Evaluation

NDx: Urinary retention
Collect data on the patient's usual urinary elimination patterns. Assess for signs and symptoms of urinary retention, such as complaints of frequency, urgency, fullness, or bladder discomfort. Also assess for bladder distention and small, frequent voidings.

Monitor fluid intake and output. Fluid intake and output should be equal within 48 hours after surgery. In the initial postoperative period, urinary output is expected to decrease as a result of increased blood loss. This blood loss increases the secretion of ADH and aldosterone. Notify the physician if there is no urinary output 6 to 12 hours postoperatively.

Instruct the patient in measures to prevent urinary retention. Teach the patient to void when the urge is felt. Provide privacy. Allow the patient to get up to go to the commode unless contraindicated. Pour warm water over the perineum, run water, or put the patient's hand in warm water. Encourage the patient to try to void every 2 to 3 hours.

Compare the patient's status with the expected outcomes. If the outcomes are not met, reassess the patient and revise the plan.

INCONTINENCE

Incontinence is a symptom, not a disease. It is the involuntary loss of urine, which becomes a social or health problem for the person. Both urologic and neurologic disorders can cause incontinence, but many factors, including aging, can contribute to incontinence. Incontinence is one of the most disruptive disorders of the urinary system. It causes stress for both the patient and the caregiver. It is so embarrassing to many people that they may avoid seeking care. (Because of this embarrassment, it is important to ensure privacy during physical examination and the collection of specimens.) There are five types of urinary incontinence, and the pathophysiology of each is different (Table 30–1).

TOTAL INCONTINENCE. Total incontinence is the constant and involuntary dribbling of urine. It is caused primarily by neurologic disorders, trauma, or anatomic problems.

REFLEX INCONTINENCE. Reflex incontinence is associated with urinary retention. It is caused by a grossly distended bladder that leaks as more urine is produced and as intra-abdominal pressure is exerted on the full bladder. It is common among those who have sustained a spinal cord injury and is seen in autonomic neuropathies and bladder neck obstruction.

CLINICAL ? THINKING

ANURIA AFTER VASCULAR SURGERY

Eight hours after vascular surgery on his leg, a 74-year-old male patient still had not voided. The patient had undergone femoropopliteal bypass grafting for chronic arterial occlusive disease of the lower extremities. (Prior to the surgery, the arterial occlusive disease had progressed so far that the patient was experiencing rest pain in the left leg.) The patient's medical history included the following:

- Angina pectoris treated with sublingual nitroglycerin PRN (as needed)
- Two recent transient ischemic attacks (TIAs)
- Type II diabetes mellitus controlled with diet and an oral sulfonylurea

During report, the nurse on the day shift said that the patient was alert, remained on complete bedrest with the left extended straight, was receiving meperidine (Demerol) intramuscularly with adequate pain control, and had a peripheral intravenous infusing at 100 mL/hour. The nurse also reported that the patient's neurovascular status was satisfactory and that his vital signs were stable.

When I started my shift, I realized that the patient's absence of urinary output over the past 8 hours, despite administration of IV and oral fluids, demanded prompt attention. First, however, I had to try to determine whether the patient's anuria was caused by suppression of urine production in the kidney or by retention of urine in the bladder. I recognized that the possible causes of sudden urinary suppression in a patient with no previous history of renal disease included the following:

- Acute renal failure secondary to a severe hypovolemic and/or hypotensive episode
- Decreased renal perfusion secondary to heart failure and reduced cardiac output
- Renal dysfunction secondary to an adverse reaction to blood or blood products
- Nephrotoxicity from medication

To aid in identifying the problem, I questioned the nurse giving the report about the patient's perioperative course. I also checked the patient's chart for any evidence of the causes of sudden urinary suppression listed above.

The surgery had been performed under spinal anesthesia. The patient had remained entirely free of other complications during the perioperative period. He required no blood transfusions and had no history of nephrotoxic drugs prior to or during his hospitalization. In addition, the patient's post-operative serum creatinine, blood urea nitrogen (BUN), and serum potassium levels were within normal limits. Additional data remained to be gathered during my physical examination of the patient. Nevertheless, the information that I gathered from the patient's chart did not support urinary suppression as the underlying cause of the patient's anuria.

As I entered the patient's room, I therefore reviewed the possible conditions that might cause urinary retention:

- Neurologic disorders
- Obstruction secondary to urethral strictures, urolithiasis, tumors, scarring from chronic urinary tract infections (UTIs), and benign prostatic hypertrophy (BPH)
- The surgical experience, including some preoperative medications and the effects of anesthesia

The patient appeared slightly diaphoretic, anxious, and restless. He complained of pain, a sensation of fullness in the bladder area, and the urge to void.

Physical assessment of the patient revealed the following:

Blood pressure (BP) 146/90 (slightly elevated from his baseline)
Apical pulse—82 beats per minute (bpm) and regular
Respirations—16 per minute and unlabored
Temperature—36.8°C (98.2°F)
Lungs clear to auscultation and percussion
Skin temperature warm, color pink
Peripheral pulses palpated in both lower extremities, and strong in the upper extremities
Capillary refill less than 3 seconds of blanching
No evidence of peripheral edema
Dressing dry and intact

The patient was alert, oriented, and able to follow directions and perform specific tasks.

Inspection and palpation of the bladder revealed a rounded mass above the level of the symphysis pubis, indicative of a distended bladder. Percussion of the suprapubic region produced a dull sound, indicative of a bladder filled with urine. The patient denied any chest pain, flank pain, or tenderness in the region of the costovertebral angle. He denied any history of chronic UTIs, and symptoms such as frequency, hesitancy, or difficulty initiating micturition. He denied having any decrease in the size or force of the urinary stream.

The clinical evidence in favor of adequate cerebral, cardiac, and peripheral perfusion (level of consciousness and cardiovascular stability) sug-

(continued)

CLINICAL ❓ THINKING

(continued)

gested adequate cardiac output and renal perfusion. These findings further supported ruling out urinary suppression as the underlying problem. The possible cardiovascular origin of the patient's restlessness, anxiety, and diaphoresis was likewise ruled out by these findings.

On the other hand, the absence of voided urine—accompanied by bladder distention, complaints of pain in the lower abdomen, elevated blood pressure, diaphoresis, anxiety, and restlessness—prompted me to strongly suspect urinary retention. The patient's history of diabetes mellitus might have contributed to the development of a neurogenic bladder, and subsequent urinary retention. However, the patient's recent surgery and the absence of any history of renal dysfunction, chronic UTIs, and clinical manifestations of BPH led me to believe that the urinary retention was related to his postsurgical status. The patient had numerous risk factors that could have contributed to urinary retention following surgery:

- His age
- The use of spinal anesthesia
- The administration of an anticholinergic preoperative medication
- The vascular nature and site of the surgery
- The patient's immobility and postoperative position
- The use of a narcotic analgesic

These risk factors further supported my suspicion.

I knew that urinary retention is a hazardous condition that can lead to temporary or permanent loss of bladder tone, stasis of urine, and an environment conducive to the development of UTIs. I also realized that it put the patient at risk for urinary tract damage secondary to increased pressure. I therefore instituted the following measures:

1. I placed the patient in semi-Fowler's position and encourage him to exert gentle abdominal pressure with his hand.
2. I provided the patient with privacy; a quiet, relaxed atmosphere; and adequate time to void.
3. I allayed the patient's anxiety and provided reassurance by explaining that this was a common postoperative condition and by maintaining a positive outlook.

4. I instructed the patient in deep-breathing and muscle relaxation techniques.
5. I ran water, flushed the toilet, and placed the patient's hands in warm water.
6. I instituted rest periods for the patient, alternating with additional attempts at urination.
7. I documented my findings and actions.

Despite these interventions, the patient still did not urinate. I therefore called the physician, informed him of my actions and the patient's status, and secured an order for straight urinary catheterization. Catheterization yielded a return of 680 mL of clear, pale yellow urine. These results confirmed my suspicion—that the patient had been experiencing postoperative urinary retention.

The patient expressed relief and voided twice spontaneously during the remainder of my shift. After that, the patient maintained a normal pattern of urinary elimination throughout his hospitalization and recovered uneventfully.

Think Critically

Why is the administration of a diuretic inappropriate for a patient with urinary retention?

What additional measures to promote voiding might the nurse have implemented? What measures were contraindicated for this patient? Why?

A student nurse questioned the use of a straight versus a retention urinary catheter. Why was the straight catheter the better choice?

What nursing responsibilities would be included when catheterizing the patient?

What nursing assessments would the nurse make when decompressing the distended bladder?

For what complications of catheterization would the nurse monitor?

What medications would the nurse anticipate before or in conjunction with catheterization to promote voiding? Why?

What short-term and long-term medical treatment would the nurse have anticipated if the patient's urinary retention had been related to BPH? Calculi?

What nursing actions would be appropriate when anuria is observed in a patient with an indwelling urinary catheter?

URGE INCONTINENCE. Urge incontinence results when the feeling to urinate is so strong and so severe that uncontrolled bladder emptying occurs. This may be due to bladder inflammation from a tumor or infection. However, urge incontinence is more frequently due to uninhibited bladder contractions that are related to neurologic disorders, such as spinal cord injuries.

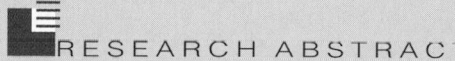

RESEARCH ABSTRACT

What Pads Work Best for Managing Urinary Incontinence in Women?

Baker J, Norton P. Evaluation of absorbent products for women with mild to moderate urinary incontinence. Appl Nurs Res 1996; 9(1):29.

Increasing numbers of women are coping with mild to moderate incontinence resulting from hormonal changes and the loss of pelvic muscle tone. The value of a thorough assessment, and consideration of various interventions, is supported by the recent AHCPR Guidelines on Urinary Incontinence. Nevertheless, the use of absorbent products to control urinary incontinence is widespread. In recognition of this reality, Baker and Norton set out to examine the characteristics of a variety of absorbent products from the viewpoint of the women who choose to use them, either as an initial coping strategy or as a supplement to other interventions.

Over the course of 8 weeks, subjects who ranged in age from 28 to 84 years evaluated 11 different characteristics of eight different absorbent products. To the patients who used them, the five most important characteristics of an absorbent product were:

1. Dryness and confidence
2. Odor control
3. Ability to stay in place
4. Discreetness
5. Comfort

These characteristics were rated most important both before and after the study, although in the post-study survey the rank order changed slightly.

The products that were evaluated included brand-name products marketed for bladder control as well as menstrual pads. Because of the recurrent nature of incontinence and the need for some type of continuous protection, cost was examined for each of the products. The women also rated the products on overall performance.

The top-rated product for overall performance was the Serenity Guard (a moderately expensive product), followed by the Always menstrual pad and the store-brand menstrual pad (the two least expensive products).

Based on the results of the study, the researchers suggested that women who decide to use absorbent products should begin with the least expensive products first and evaluate the capacity of these products to control symptoms. The researchers also encouraged institutions to offer women who experience mild to moderate incontinence a sample pack that includes the full range of products, including menstrual pads and those products marketed specifically for bladder control.

Questions to Consider

1. What types of assessment questions address the urinary elimination patterns of women in your clinical facility?
2. Some women are embarrassed to admit that they have difficulty with bladder control. How can you sensitively address this issue in your assessment?
3. What types of absorbent products are available in your clinical facility?
4. Complete a cost comparison for absorbent products in your community. Be sure to include both discount and retail stores.
5. Over the next week, listen and look for advertising related to absorbent products. Make a list of the product features that are highlighted. How does your list compare with the characteristics rated as most important by the subjects in the study?
6. Locate a copy of the AHCPR Guidelines for Urinary Incontinence in your clinical facility (also available on the AHCPR homepage on the Internet). Examine the recommendations for evaluating the various types of urinary incontinence. Based on these recommendations, what additional information would you provide for women who report symptoms of urge or stress incontinence?

STRESS INCONTINENCE. Stress incontinence is the unexpected loss of small amounts of urine when there is a rapid rise in intra-abdominal pressure, from either coughing, laughing, straining, or physical activity. In most instances, the pelvic muscles supporting the bladder have weakened, and the normal anatomic position of the bladder and urethra has changed. This type of incontinence is most common in women. Causes of stress incontinence include trauma from childbirth and loss of muscle tone secondary to obesity or aging.

FUNCTIONAL INCONTINENCE. Functional incontinence is an involuntary, unpredictable passage of urine. The patient cannot control micturition because of environmental barriers, physical limitations, or disorientation. The patient is unable to reach the bathroom in time to void.

Table 30–1

Classification of Urinary Incontinence

Type	Feature	Cause
Total incontinence	Continuous and unpredictable passage of urine	Injury to the lower urinary tract, sphincter trauma, surgery, or childbirth
Reflex incontinence	Constant urine loss	Neurologic abnormalities such as spinal cord lesions, also drugs, tumors, benign strictures, and prostatic hypertrophy
Urge incontinence	Strong desire to urinate with an uncontrolled emptying	Bladder irritation or reduced bladder capacity after radiation treatment, urinary tract infection, increased urine concentration, the use of caffeine or alcohol, or an enlarged prostate
Stress incontinence	Immediate involuntary loss of urine as a result of an increase in intra-abdominal pressure (coughing, laughing, straining)	Decreased pelvic muscle tone caused by menopause, childbirth, obesity, or surgical procedure interfering with the normal structure
Functional incontinence	Difficulty or inability to reach the toilet in time as a result of environmental barriers, disorientation, and/or physical limitations	Intact lower urinary tract but factors such as immobility, severe cognitive impairment, musculoskeletal impairments, and restricted access to toilets cause the incontinence

NURSING PROCESS
Incontinence

Nursing diagnoses have been identified by North American Nursing Diagnosis Association (NANDA) for each of the five types of incontinence. The nursing care for patients with each of these diagnoses is similar. For purposes of instruction, the following paragraphs describe how to apply the nursing process to the care of a patient with total incontinence.

Assessment

Ask the patient for a detailed voiding history. Questions should relate to time, place, and amount of urine. Ask the patient about awareness of the passage of urine and whether he or she can identify what stimulates voiding. Ask about any past history of urologic or neurologic disease, including dementia. Ask about symptoms of hesitancy, urgency, polyuria (urination in large quantities), dysuria, and nocturia. An accurate history is very important in assessing the incontinent patient. Keep an accurate record of fluid intake and output. Assess the characteristics of the urine. Assess the patient's mental status.

Nursing Diagnoses and Planning

The nursing diagnosis and related expected patient outcomes most commonly applicable to patients with total incontinence are as follows:

NDx: Total incontinence related to independent contraction of detrusor reflex due to trauma or surgery

Planning: Patient Outcomes
1. Patient and significant other demonstrate bladder regimen.
2. Patient's voiding occurs on a planned schedule.
3. Patient's skin is intact.
4. Patient has decrease in episodes of incontinence.
5. Patient and significant other manage bladder elimination.
6. Patient verbalizes feelings of self-worth.

NDx: Ineffective individual coping and Caregiver role strain related to total incontinence of significant other

Planning: Patient Outcomes
1. Patient and caregiver communicate physiologic and emotional needs to each other.
2. Patient and/or caregiver seek outside support services.
3. Patient and/or caregiver identify coping mechanisms to reduce stress.

Nursing Interventions and Evaluation

NDx: Total incontinence
Establish a bladder training program, and assist the patient and significant other in carrying out this program. Set up a schedule for toileting. Ensure that all staff involved know the schedule and adhere to it. The patient may or may not require the placement of an indwelling catheter. Check frequently for incontinence. To prevent skin breakdown, it is essential that the patient remain dry.

Teach the patient and family the bladder regimen, and give support and encouragement. Praise both patient and family for maintenance of the program and for any decrease in episodes of incontinence. Allow the patient and family time to talk about their feelings related to this problem. Answer all questions in terminology the patient can understand.

NDx: Ineffective individual coping and Caregiver role strain

Communicate to the patient and/or caregiver the importance of expressing physical and emotional needs. Teach the patient about support services related to incontinence and related problems, and make available the names, addresses, and phone numbers of these services. Identify, teach, and evaluate the effectiveness of coping mechanisms to reduce stress.

Compare the patient's status with the expected outcomes. If the outcomes are not met, reassess the patient and revise the plan.

PAIN

The most common reason for seeking medical attention for a urologic problem is pain in the urinary tract. The pain may be localized to a specific organ or part, or it may be referred from one area of the urinary tract to another. Generally, pains within the urinary tract originate from distention or inflammation of the system.

RENAL PAIN. Renal pain manifests as a constant and dull ache in the area of the costovertebral angle below the twelfth rib (Fig. 30–6). This type of pain may be sharp or paroxysmal (spasmodic) and may radiate to the lower abdomen and inguinal area. It is important to note that some disorders of the kidney, such as cancer and tuberculosis, are not painful, because of the slow development of these conditions.

URETERAL PAIN. Ureteral pain is colicky and is among the most severe types of pain known. It is caused by sudden obstruction, usually from a calculus, that produces hyperperistalsis and spasm of the ureter. A urinary calculus, or "stone" obstructing the upper ureter produces symptoms similar to those of renal pain, but may also radiate pain to the testis or labia. Pain generated by obstruction of the lower portion of the ureter causes suprapubic discomfort, but may also be felt in the bladder, penis, or urethra.

BLADDER PAIN. Bladder pain due to overdistention causes local discomfort in the suprapubic area. Infection and inflammation of the bladder produce a sharp burning pain that radiates to the distal urethra. This pain intensifies with urination.

NURSING PROCESS
Urinary Tract Pain

Assessment

Assess the characteristics of the pain, including its type, location, duration, severity, frequency, and any precipitating factors. Assess for tenderness or pain with palpation (see Fig. 30–6). Ask what lessens the pain. Observe the patient's reaction to the pain.

Nursing Diagnoses and Planning

The nursing diagnosis and related expected patient outcomes most commonly applicable to patients experiencing urinary tract pain are as follows:

NDx: Pain related to distention or inflammation

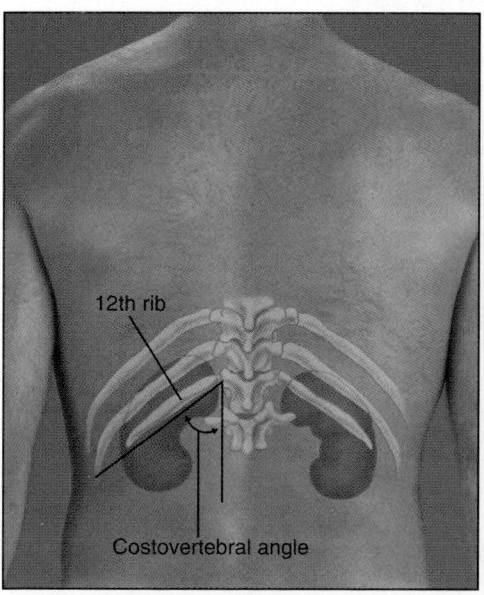
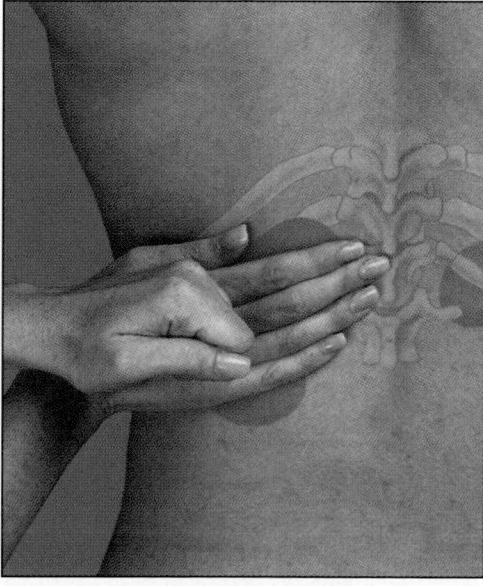

Figure 30–6

Renal pain manifests as a constant, dull ache in the area of the costovertebral angle, below the twelfth rib. Percuss over the costovertebral angle to elicit pain.

12th rib

Costovertebral angle

Planning: Patient Outcomes

1. Patient reports that pain is controlled with analgesics.
2. Patient identifies comfort measures to help relieve pain.
3. Patient uses coping measures such as relaxation techniques to help relieve, lessen, or tolerate pain.

Nursing Interventions and Evaluation

NDx: Pain

Encourage or help the patient to assume comfortable positions and to reposition frequently. Assess when pain is most severe, and encourage or help the patient to rest during those periods. Administer pain medications as ordered prior to activity so that the patient can tolerate the activity better. Teach the patient the use of patient-controlled analgesia if ordered.

Assist the patient in finding alternate methods to alleviate, lessen, or be able to tolerate the pain. Show the patient and family relaxation techniques that may help. Encourage the patient to practice them frequently.

Compare the patient's status with the expected outcomes. If the outcomes are not met, reassess the patient and revise the plan.

CHANGE IN URINE CHARACTERISTICS

Urine color normally ranges from pale yellow to deep gold, depending on its concentration. Significant changes in color may be disease-related. However, an alteration in urine color may also be caused by foods or medications (Table 30–2). Turbidity refers to the clarity of urine. Upon visualization, a normal urine specimen should be clear. A cloudy specimen may indicate urinary tract infection, the cloudiness resulting from the large number of white blood cells in the urine. Benign cloudiness occurs at an alkaline pH and is caused by the precipitation of phosphates in the urine. Benign cloudiness also occurs when a urine specimen has been left standing at room temperature for a long period.

Urine has an odor that at most times is nonspecific. In certain instances, though, the scent of a freshly voided urine specimen may be a clue to an underlying disease. For example, foul-smelling urine is typically associated with a bacterial infection. A strong, pungent odor suggests infection with gram-negative bacteria. The presence of ketone bodies gives urine a sweet, fruity smell. Urine odor that resembles maple syrup or sweaty feet suggests a metabolic disorder.

HEMATURIA

Hematuria, the presence of blood in the urine, is a serious finding that always warrants prompt assessment. This is true whether the blood is grossly visi-

Table 30–2

Causes of Alterations in Urine Color

ALTERATIONS CAUSED BY PATHOLOGIC CONDITIONS

Color	Pathologic Condition
Red	Bleeding in the lower urinary tract
Dark red or smoky gray	Bleeding in the upper urinary tract
Tea colored	Release of myoglobin from severely damaged tissue
Dark yellow	Presence of urobilinogen or bilirubin
Green	Presence of *Pseudomonas* organisms

ALTERATIONS CAUSED BY MEDICATIONS

Color	Medication
Blue to blue-green	Amitriptyline (Elavil)
Brown (in acid urine); yellow-pink (in alkaline urine)	Cascara
Dark urine or amber	Levodopa or methyldopa
Green	Methylene blue
Dark urine	Metronidazole (Flagyl)
Bright yellow	Multiple vitamins (with riboflavin)
Orange-brown, orange-red, or red	Phenazopyridine (Pyridium)
Pink-red in alkaline urine	Phenolphthalein (laxative)
Red, red-brown, or pink	Phenothiazine (Thorazine)
Red, red-brown, or pink	Phenytoin (Dilantin)
Red, orange, or brown	Rifampin

ble or only a microscopic finding. In young adults, trauma, urinary tract infection, and urinary calculi are among the most common causes of hematuria. In middle-aged to elderly patients, hematuria is highly suggestive of a tumor within the urinary tract. Even in this age group, however, infection, calculi, benign prostatic hypertrophy, vascular malformation of the kidney, and medications may also induce bleeding in the urinary tract.

To help pinpoint the site of bleeding, it is important to know *when* blood is observed during urination. Hematuria at the beginning of voiding indicates bleeding of the anterior urethra. Hematuria at the end of the stream suggests bleeding from the posterior urethra, bladder neck, or trigone. Total hematuria—blood throughout the entire urine stream—indicates bleeding within or above the bladder.

When assessing the patient with hematuria, it is helpful to know whether or not pain is associated with the bleeding. Painful hematuria occurs in association with infections or the passage of a calculus. Painless hematuria is more ominous and is considered to be a symptom of a urinary tract neoplasm, unless studies suggest another cause. In addition to noting the presence or absence of pain, it is also important to note the color of the urine. Depending upon the number of red blood cells in the urine, as well as the source and time of bleeding, urine color in the presence of hematuria varies from a light pink to bright red or dark brown.

CHANGE IN URINE VOLUME

There are three types of change in urine volume: anuria, oliguria, and polyuria. Anuria refers to urine output that is 100 mL (about $3\frac{1}{2}$ ounces) or less in a 24-hour period. Oliguria refers to a urine output that is between 100 and 400 mL ($3\frac{1}{2}$ to $13\frac{1}{2}$ ounces) in a 24-hour period. These terms represent varying degrees of decreased urinary output. Both conditions may be the result of acute renal failure, fluid and electrolyte imbalances, bilateral ureteral obstruction, or urethral obstruction.

Polyuria is the excessive secretion of urine, which is generally more than 2500 mL (about $2\frac{1}{2}$ quarts) in a 24-hour period. Common causes of polyuria include a decrease in the concentrating ability of the kidneys, an increase in fluid intake (eg, psychogenic water drinking), diabetes insipidus, diabetes mellitus, and intake of diuretics.

An accurate evaluation of a change in urine volume requires the careful recording of fluid intake and output, as well as astute observations by the nurse. Patient education about the measurement of fluid intake and output is essential to ensure compliance because measurement of intake and output may need to last for several days.

Assessment of the Urinary System

The health history and detailed descriptions of the urinary problems that the patient is experiencing are important components in the diagnosis of urinary system dysfunction. A physical assessment follows the history so that specific problems can be identified and a plan of care established.

HEALTH HISTORY

Ask the patient about the history of the present illness or disorder. Ask what is the patient's chief complaint. Get a detailed description of the complaint. If incontinence is the most significant problem, ask about the time during the day or night it most frequently occurs. Ask whether there is a pre-

cipitating event, and whether fluids were ingested prior to the episode. Ask whether the patient experiences difficulty in urinating, whether burning is present, or whether frequency is a problem. Determine whether the color and consistency of the urine is within normal ranges. Ask whether pain is present during urination. Ask whether a discharge is present with urination or is present around the meatus. Ask the patient to describe the discharge by color and odor. Determine the usual amount of fluids that the patient ingests daily and the approximate amount of output.

Ask the female patient about whether she leaks urine during exercise, coughing, or sneezing. Determine the severity of the problem. Ask the male patient whether he has been circumcised. If not, ask whether his foreskin retracts easily. Also ask the male patient whether he experiences dribbling or nocturnal frequency or has any known prostate problems.

Ask the patient about past medical problems, medications, and previous surgeries. Also ask about the family history of illness. Determine the patient's usual activities of daily living and whether the present condition interferes with the normal daily routine. Complete a brief review of systems, determining whether dysfunctions in any other system might be affecting the urinary system.

Assess the patient's understanding and compliance with health promotion and risk reduction measures related to the health of the system (Highlight 30–1). For example, ask about the amount of fluid the patient drinks in a day, as well as the number of

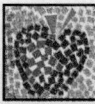

HIGHLIGHT 30–1

HEALTH PROMOTION & RISK REDUCTION

Optimal Urinary System Function

For optimal urinary system function, encourage patients to:

Practice good hygiene habits during and after toileting.

Urinate as urge demands and not deliberately restrain from urinating as needed.

Practice good nutritional habits including drinking plenty of fluids daily (unless medically contraindicated).

Report symptoms of urgency, pain, frequency, nocturia, or hematuria.

Visit a physician annually for a complete physical with a urinalysis if there is any history of urinary dysfunction or if over 50 years of age.

past urinary infections, episodes of bleeding in the urine, and episodes of urinary pain. Carefully document the information obtained.

PHYSICAL EXAMINATION

Begin the examination with a general inspection of the patient. Note the fluid status of the patient by checking skin turgor, looking for signs of edema, and comparing daily fluid intake and output. If edema is present, assess the severity of it. Check the mucous membranes of the mouth. Look for dry, cracked skin and sunken eyes, which may indicate dehydration. Weigh the patient and compare the results with the patient's stated weight. Check the patient's vital signs, noting the blood pressure in particular. Observe the patient's skin color, checking for signs of jaundice.

Check the patient's abdomen for signs of ascites. Note whether the patient seems distended near the symphysis pubis. Wearing gloves, inspect the urethral meatus, looking for redness, deviation, or discharge. Ulcerations in the area may indicate sexually transmitted disease.

Using the stethoscope on the abdomen, auscultate the renal arteries for bruits, which may indicate arterial stenosis or hypertension. Palpate the kidneys and bladder to detect any masses. Have the patient void into a specimen container prior to palpating the bladder. This prevents discomfort from pressure on a full bladder and the urgency to void during the examination and allows for assessment of the urine. Observe the urine for color, consistency, and amount. Ask the patient whether he or she has a feeling of urgency after voiding or whether the bladder does not feel empty. Palpate the kidneys bilaterally, and note any evidence of masses or tenderness. Palpate the bladder, noting its size and the presence of any lumps or tender areas.

Document the findings from the physical examination in detail, using schematics, when appropriate, to describe location. Also note statements from the patient that may explain the findings or present more data about any abnormalities found.

*D*iagnostic Procedures

A variety of diagnostic procedures may be used for patients with problems in the urinary system. Urine studies, such as urinalysis, are important screening and diagnostic procedures for patients with problems outside the urinary system. However, they are even more important for patients with urinary dysfunction. Other tests used to evaluate function of the urinary system include blood studies, radiographic studies, and invasive diagnostic tests such as cystoscopy and biopsy.

URINE STUDIES

Urinalysis

Urinalysis is the simplest and most frequently performed diagnostic procedure. It is an essential component of the urologic evaluation. Macroscopic urinalysis includes assessment of color, turbidity, odor, and specific gravity. It also involves dipstick testing for pH, protein, glucose, ketones, bilirubin, and blood. Microscopic examination of urine sediment is done to detect red and white blood cells, epithelial cells, casts, crystals, bacteria, fungi, and fat globules. Normal urinalysis results are summarized in Table 30–3. The best urine sample for this routine examination is a midstream urine sample—a sample taken from the patient's urine stream about halfway between the beginning and end of urination—from the first or second urination of the morning.

Urine Culture

A urine culture is indicated when symptoms suggest a urinary tract infection. It is performed to identify bacteria infecting the urine so that the proper medication can be selected and treatment initiated. A clear, uncontaminated urine sample is necessary when a culture is to be performed. Once the specimen has been obtained, it should be sent to the laboratory immediately to prevent the overgrowth of bacteria, which may alter the actual bacterial count. If a delay of 20 minutes or longer is anticipated between the collection of the urine and the receipt of the specimen in the laboratory, the sample

Table 30–3

Normal Urinalysis Results

MACROSCOPIC EXAMINATION	
Color	Pale yellow
Turbidity	Clear
Odor	Distinct odor, ammonia-like smell
Specific gravity	1.003–1.030
pH	4.6–8.0
Protein	Negative (qualitative) 10–150 mg/24 hours (quantitative)
Glucose	<250 mg/24 hours
Ketones	Negative
Bilirubin	Negative
MICROSCOPIC EXAMINATION	
Red blood cells	0–5/HPF
White blood cells	0–5/HPF
Casts	1 per every 10–20/LPF
Crystals	None
Bacteria	<1000 colonies/mL

HPF, high-power field; LPF, low-power field.

should be refrigerated. However, refrigeration must not exceed 24 hours.

Urine Cytology

Urine cytology is the microscopic examination of urine to detect the presence of atypical epithelial cells that have been shed from the surface of the urinary tract. This laboratory examination is used as a screening procedure for people at risk of developing cancer within the urinary system. It is also used in the follow-up of people who have had a malignancy within the urinary tract, and it is used to diagnose inflammatory and infectious urinary diseases.

To perform a cytologic evaluation, a minimum of 50 mL of urine is needed. At least three specimens should be collected and examined at different times within a 3-month period. Although the first morning specimen is preferred for urine cytology studies, other types of urine samples may also be used, including a random daytime sample or a catheterized urine sample. Urine samples obtained after bladder irrigation or prostatic massage, as well as those obtained from an ileal conduit or suprapubic aspiration, are also acceptable.

Twenty-Four-Hour Urine Collection

A 24-hour urine collection is considered to be a valid and reliable diagnostic measure for substances excreted in the urine (Table 30–4). This test is commonly performed to measure creatinine and protein excretion in patients with known or suspected renal disease. In patients with a history of urinary calculi, it is used to measure, among other things, calcium and uric acid, which are primary components of urinary calculi.

To collect a 24-hour urine specimen, the patient should be given a container with a tight-fitting lid that holds up to 2 liters. A form or piece of paper on which to make notations is also helpful.

The day and time the collection are to be started are not particularly important. However, for the sake of convenience, the patient should be advised

Table 30–4

Normal Values for a 24-Hour Urine Collection	
Substance	**Value**
Chloride	110–250 mEq
Creatinine clearance	110–150 mL/min for men
	105–132 mL/min for women
Glucose	<250 mg
Potassium	25–100 mEq
Sodium	130–260 mEq
Urea nitrogen	10–15 g

to start the urine collection after rising in the morning and to stay home for the day. If the test is completed while the patient is hospitalized, tell the patient when to start collecting the urine.

On the morning the collection is to begin, the patient should note the exact time of awakening and then immediately void and *discard* the first-voided urine. The patient should collect and save every voiding after this time until the collection period ends. The collection period ends the next morning, exactly 24 hours after it was started, after saving that morning's first-voided urine.

Thorough patient instruction is necessary to ensure that the collection of a 24-hour urine specimen is performed properly. Accurate results depend on the careful documentation of the beginning and end of the collection period as well as the meticulous saving of urine. Remind patients that all urine voided during the collection times must be saved—even urine voided at night. In addition, the container that is being filled with urine should be kept refrigerated, or on ice, while the collection is in progress and until the specimen is delivered to the laboratory. Adherence to this entire procedure is essential because misleading results may be obtained from a specimen improperly collected.

BLOOD STUDIES

Complete Blood Count

For patients with a urinary tract disorder, a complete blood count (CBC) is generally ordered as a screening procedure in the presence of such problems as hematuria and urinary tract infection. The complete blood count values that are of particular interest in these patients are those for hematocrit and hemoglobin (Hct & Hgb, or H & H) and white blood cell count.

Blood Chemistry Studies

Blood chemistry studies are also ordered as screening tests in patients with urinary tract disorders, especially in those with a history of urinary calculi. For patients with renal failure, oliguria, or suspected fluid and electrolyte imbalances, the frequent measurement of serum electrolytes offers a means of assessing the patient's status, as well as the effectiveness of treatment.

Serum Creatinine and Blood Urea Nitrogen

Serum creatinine and blood urea nitrogen (BUN) are two tests commonly used to measure glomerular filtration. They measure the reabsorption of creatinine and urea by the renal tubules.

Creatinine is secreted in very small amounts by the renal tubules, and it is reabsorbed very slowly.

Thus, when a rise in the creatinine occurs, it reflects an actual decrease in glomerular filtration. For this reason, serum creatinine levels are considered a reliable indicator of renal function. The normal adult value for serum creatinine is 0.7 to 1.5 mg/dL. With aging, glomerular filtration tends to decrease, and serum creatinine levels increase. After age 70, a normal creatinine level may be as high as 1.8 mg/dL.

In contrast, urea is rapidly reabsorbed by the renal tubules. Because the level of reabsorption is directly related to the rate of urine flow through the kidneys, a mere slowing of this action quickly produces a measurable increase in urea levels. Although the BUN is a valid test, an increase does not always imply the presence of renal disease. In adults, the normal BUN level is 6 to 23 mg/dL.

NURSING PROCESS GUIDELINES
Blood Studies

Explain that the purpose of the testing is to determine how well the kidneys are excreting wastes. Instruct the patient that there are no food or water restrictions before the test. Because these tests are often routinely ordered, medications that can influence the test results might not have to be withheld prior to the testing, but the physician will consider the impact of these medications when interpreting the test results. If ordered, hold medications that influence the results of these tests (Table 30–5) for 24 hours prior to the test. On the laboratory slip, list any drugs that cannot safely be withheld.

Table 30–5

Medications That Affect Serum Creatinine and Blood Urea Nitrogen (BUN) Levels

Serum Creatinine	BUN
Amphotericin B	Bacitracin
Cefazolin	Cephaloridine
Cephalothin	Gentamicin
Gentamicin	Kanamycin
Kanamycin	Chloramphenicol
Methicillin	Methicillin
Ascorbic acid	Neomycin
Barbiturates	Vancomycin
Lithium carbonate	Methyldopa
Mithramycin	Guanethidine
Methyldopa	Sulfonamides
Phenolsulfonphthalein (PSP)	Propranolol
Sulfobromophthalein	Morphine
Triamterene	Lithium carbonate
	Salicylates
	Hydrochlorothiazide
	Ethacrynic acid
	Furosemide
	Triamterene

Recognize the clinical problems associated with high levels and assess the patient accordingly. An elevated BUN level can indicate dehydration, high protein intake, gastrointestinal bleeding, or prerenal failure. An elevated serum creatinine level indicates acute or chronic renal failure or prolonged shock and can be used with other tests and procedures as a diagnostic tool for many other medical disorders. Check both the BUN and the creatinine levels. If both are elevated, the problem is most likely renal.

RADIOLOGIC STUDIES

Several radiologic studies are used routinely to aid in diagnosing or ruling out disorders of the urinary tract. The studies most commonly performed are outlined in Table 30–6. Also described in this table are several newer studies that are being used with increasing frequency as technology advances. Among them are magnetic resonance imaging (MRI) and various nuclear medicine studies. These studies are very useful for patients who are allergic to the contrast agents used in some diagnostic procedures for disorders of the urinary tract. A decade ago, such allergies would have left physicians no choice but to order extensive invasive testing or steroid preparation. However, these newer technologies are not universally available throughout North America. We will therefore describe the older invasive tests and steroid preparations because they continue to be used in some settings.

The excretory urogram, also called an intravenous urogram or intravenous pyelogram (IVP), remains the mainstay of urologic diagnostic tests. Along with cystoscopy, an excretory urogram is usually ordered for virtually every urologic disorder—from microscopic hematuria to renal cancer. Table 30–6 describes in detail the nursing care of the patient having an excretory urogram.

Patients who have never had radiologic studies using contrast agents may not know that they are allergic to them. An inability to tolerate iodine-containing foods, most often shellfish, is a strong indicator of a allergy to contrast agents. Patients who are allergic may know only that they had a reaction during an x-ray examination performed for an entirely different disorder and thus may not relate it to any urologic tests.

The most severe complication in patients who are allergic to contrast agents is an anaphylactic reaction that causes respiratory and cardiac distress or arrest. Identification of patients at risk before the excretory urogram prevents such a disaster. An excretory urogram can be performed safely even when an allergy to contrast agents exists by administering corticosteroids for 24 hours before, the day of, and for 24 hours after the test, along with an antihistamine (usually diphenhydramine [Benadryl]) 1 hour before the test. For patients with such an allergy, an excretory urogram is scheduled with an anesthesiol-

Text continued on page 1351

Table 30–6

Most Commonly Performed Radiologic and Other Studies of the Urinary Tract

Definition and Description	Clinical Uses	Complications	Nursing Care
KUB (KIDNEYS, URETERS, AND BLADDER)			
A plain radiographic film of the abdomen that visualizes the major organs of the urinary tract	To identify radiopaque stones, large masses, or gross abnormalities of the kidneys, ureters, and bladder Frequently used as an initial diagnostic test for acute flank pain or as follow-up after treatment for stone diseases	None Contraindicated in pregnancy	Physician may order a mild laxative the night before KUB if not done on an emergency basis. Patients may require reassurance about exposure to x-rays.
EXCRETORY UROGRAM (INTRAVENOUS PYELOGRAM [IVP])			
A radiographic study using contrast dye The dye is injected for several minutes intravenously and then observed through a series of films as it passes through the urinary tract. A final film is taken after the patient voids the contrast dye.	Evaluation of the kidneys, ureters, and bladder An IVP identifies the location of stones or masses and aids in diagnosis of congenital anomalies. Renal function can be grossly assessed by the kidney's ability to clear the dye. The postvoid film can identify a significant residual volume.	An unknown allergy to contrast dye may result in severe anaphylactic reaction. In rare cases, use of contrast dye can lead to acute renal failure. Hypersensitivity to contrast dye may result in pruritus, skin flushing, or difficulty breathing.	Question the patient about an allergy sensitivity to contrast dye, iodine, or iodine-containing foods (shellfish). Patients with renal failure, labile diabetes, or myeloma or those in severely dehydrated states should not undergo the test. It is also contraindicated in pregnancy. Patients with a known allergy to contrast dye can usually tolerate the test safely after a steroid preparation. Explain the events that will occur before, during, and after the test. Explain the laxative preparation and dietary restrictions; assist the patient in adhering to the preparation, and evaluate results. (The test preparation usually consists of a routine bowel cleansing preparation given to the patient during the evening before the test. Also a clear liquid diet may be given the day before. NPO [nothing by mouth] status is maintained after midnight the night before the test is done.) After the test, provide nourishment and encourage fluid intake. Monitor intake and output. Observe for symptoms of hypersensitivity reaction. Notify the patient's physician if nausea or vomiting occur; intravenous hydration may be ordered to ensure that the dye is flushed out of the urinary tract completely.

Table continued on following page

Table 30–6

Most Commonly Performed Radiologic and Other Studies of the Urinary Tract *(continued)*

Definition and Description	Clinical Uses	Complications	Nursing Care
RETROGRADE/ANTEGRADE PYELOGRAM			
These procedures are performed in the cystoscopy suite. With the patient under local or regional anesthesia, a cystoscope is inserted (see Cystogram). A ureteral catheter is passed into the ureter, and contrast dye is injected.	Either of these studies may be ordered when IVP has failed to visualize the kidneys or ureters, or in patients with a known allergy to contrast dye. Retrograde pyelography is the least invasive of the two procedures and is preferred for that reason. Antegrade pyelography may be necessary in patients with ureteral abnormalities that prevent passing a ureteral catheter. It is commonly done after percutaneous renal surgery for kidney stones, because a nephrostomy catheter is already in place. Retrograde pyelogram is frequently done before ESWL in patients with radiolucent stones or as part of a follow-up regimen for patients with urologic cancer who are allergic to contrast dye.	Retrograde pyelogram: • Ureteral perforation • Perforation of the renal pelvis • Infection • Urinary retention Antegrade pyelogram: • Renal puncture or damage • Hematuria • Infection • Urinary retention • Perinephric hematoma	Explain the procedure and type of anesthesia to be used. Retrograde pyelography may be done under local anesthesia only; however, both procedures are done under spinal or general anesthesia. Ensure dietary restrictions before the procedure; administer premedications if ordered. After the procedure, monitor vital signs and intake and output, and observe the patient for symptoms of systemic infection secondary to instrumentation. Urine output should be assessed for quantity and for hematuria. Puncture wounds from antegrade pyelography should be dressed, and observed for urine drainage or infection.
CYSTOGRAM			
A radiologic study of the bladder only The patient is catheterized, and contrast dye is instilled through the catheter into the bladder, until the bladder is filled. Several films are taken, then the dye is drained out through the catheter and the catheter is removed. A final film is then taken.	Evaluation of the bladder for gross abnormalities; commonly done after bladder surgery to check for extravasation This study can detect large tumors or diverticula and can identify vesicoureteral reflux. Although not the primary diagnostic test for this, a cystogram can also identify causes of urethral obstruction and some voiding disorders. Also used in trauma patients with suspected bladder injury and in patients with enteritis, diverticulitis, or endometriosis when bladder involvement is suspected	None The amount of contrast dye that extravasates through a small bladder perforation is harmless. Systemic absorption of contrast dye through the bladder wall is rarely enough to cause a reaction in the patient allergic to contrast dye.	Explain the procedure to the patient. There is usually no need for anesthesia or any preparation for a cystogram. Contraindicated in pregnancy Patients who are allergic to contrast dye may receive a steroid preparation.

Table 30–6

Most Commonly Performed Radiologic and Other Studies of the Urinary Tract (continued)

Definition and Description	Clinical Uses	Complications	Nursing Care
VOIDING CYSTOURETHROGRAM			
A radiologic study that captures on film the dynamics of voiding: how the bladder fills and how it empties. A urethral catheter is inserted, and dye is instilled into the bladder until the patient feels an urge to void. The catheter is removed and the patient is asked to void. Films are taken during filling, during voiding, and after voiding.	Evaluation of the lower urinary tract, the urethra, and in some cases, the distal ureters Commonly used as a diagnostic aid for patients with voiding disorders or anomalies when significant vesicoureteral reflux is suspected	Same as for cystogram	Same as for cystogram
ULTRASONOGRAPHY			
Renal ultrasonography: A transducer is passed over the flank or lateral abdomen, depending on the patient's position. Transmission gel is applied to the skin and transducer. Bladder ultrasonography: A transducer is passed over the suprapubic and lower abdominal area.	Renal ultrasonography is used as a diagnostic aid in evaluating the kidneys for congenital anomalies, inflammatory conditions, calcifications, hydronephrosis, renal failure, and masses. Patients with suspicious areas on IVP are sent for ultrasonographic examination to determine whether these areas are cysts or solid masses. Renal ultrasonography is also frequently used to evaluate kidneys after renal transplant. Bladder ultrasonography is sometimes used in evaluating many urologic disorders. A broad categorization would include renal masses, chronic infections, vascular lesions, nephrolithiasis, and other renal diseases, and metastatic evaluations.	None There are no contraindications to ultrasonography.	Explanation of the procedure helps allay fears. Most ultrasonographic studies are painless. Bladder ultrasonography requires a full bladder. As with the other urologic procedures, several of the ultrasonographic studies require exposure of the genitalia and thus can be embarrassing to the patient.
COMPUTED TOMOGRAPHY (CT)			
CT scan may be ordered to study all or part of the urinary tract. A CT scan of the pelvis visualizes the lower structures of the urinary tract. The patient is usually given an oral dose of an iodine-containing preparation prior to the testing. Dur-	CT scans are clinically useful in evaluating many urologic disorders. A broad categorization would include renal masses, chronic infections, vascular lesions, nephrolithiasis, and other renal diseases, and metastatic evaluations.	CT scan has no post-test complications other than a potential delayed hypersensitivity reaction to the contrast material used. Patients with known allergy to contrast dye receive a steroid preparation before any CT scan in which	Assessment for allergy to contrast dye or hypersensitivity to iodine-containing foods should be done on admission. Explain the CT scanner to the patient, including the room and the use of oral and intravenous contrast dye. As with any study,

Table continued on following page

Table 30–6

Most Commonly Performed Radiologic and Other Studies of the Urinary Tract (continued)

Definition and Description	Clinical Uses	Complications	Nursing Care
ing the procedure, the patient lies supine on a table while scans are taken at intervals of 1–2 cm. Some CT scans include intravenous as well as oral injection of contrast medium.		contrast dye will be used. Oral contrast preparations are not absorbed, so alone they are safe. However, the decision to inject contrast dye is often made during the scan; therefore, a steroid preparation is routine for contrast-allergic patients. Hypersensitivity reactions include pruritus, urticaria, skin flushing, and breathing difficulties.	the injection of contrast dye intravenously may cause a flushing or warm feeling. Patients often find it hard to lie still for long periods and find the hard, flat table uncomfortable. After CT scan, monitor intake and output, observe for symptoms of a hypersensitivity reaction, and encourage fluid intake to flush out remaining dye.
MAGNETIC RESONANCE IMAGING (MRI)			
A study based on the reaction of protons and electrons in living tissues to a magnetic field Images are obtained by measuring the energy utilized by the protons and electrons during this reaction to the magnetic field.	Useful in urology for imaging of the retroperitoneum, pelvic area, bladder, and prostate Images can be obtained in three planes: coronal, sagittal, and transverse. Most urologists feel that MRI does not, at this time, replace CT scanning. Continued use of the MRI is necessary. It is quite valuable in patients with an allergy to contrast dye.	Contraindicated in patients with pacemakers Difficult to obtain clear images with the slightest motion, even cardiac, respiratory, or bowel Surgical clips, implants, or any metallic devices within the body will cause artifact. There are no known complications from MRI.	There is usually no preparation for an MRI study. The patient must be sure to remove all jewelry and anything metallic, even credit cards, before entering the MRI area. Describe the procedure and the possibility of feeling claustrophobic during the test. Sedation may be ordered for relaxation.
NUCLEAR MEDICINE STUDIES			
Nuclear medicine studies involve the injection of radioactive tracers into the circulatory system, then following their progression through the various organs using a specialized camera. There are several types of radioactive tracers used, some of the more common being DTPA, DMSA, and Hippuran [131]I.	Nuclear medicine studies are clinically useful in a variety of urologic disorders and in patients in whom the administration of contrast dye is contraindicated, for example: acute or chronic renal failure, evaluation of masses, hydronephrosis and hydroureter, renal transplant evaluation, and trauma. For most urologic disorders, radiography and CT scans are preferred. Bone scans are commonly done as part of a metastatic evaluation. Renal scans are often used to evaluate renal blood flow and function in patients with renal disease.	Contraindicated in pregnancy Hypersensitivity reactions to the radioactive tracers are very rare.	There is no patient preparation for nuclear medicine studies. The radioactive tracer is injected at a specified time before the study, allowing it to concentrate in the desired organ(s). Commercially manufactured kits are available for outpatient use. Intake and output should be monitored after the test, and fluid intake encouraged. In some institutions, patients are placed on radiation precautions for 24 hours. The institution's recommended protocols for disposal of waste products and linen should be followed.

DMSA, dimercaptosuccinic acid; DTPA, diethylene triamine penta-acetic acid; ESWL, extracorporeal shock wave lithotripsy.

ogist present for careful patient monitoring in addition to the steroid preparation.

Patients with chronic diseases known to affect renal function should also receive careful assessment before any diagnostic study using a contrast agent. Elevated BUN and creatinine levels should alert you to possible complications, because compromised renal function makes it difficult for the kidneys to clear the contrast agents. For patients with renal disease, physicians will therefore typically order alternative diagnostic studies that do not involve the use of contrast agents. Such studies include retrograde pyelograms, renal ultrasounds, and nuclear medicine studies.

NURSING PROCESS
Excretory Urogram

Assessment

By far the most important factors to assess in the patient with a urinary tract disorder who is about to undergo radiologic testing are renal function and allergy to contrast agents. Careful questioning during a nursing history can provide valuable information that can prevent dangerous complications.

Assess the patient's knowledge about the procedure, the associated risks, and the potential findings. Ask the patient about fears or anxiety related to the test. Look for nonverbal signs of anxiety, such as the following signs:

- Nervousness
- Increased pulse, respirations, and blood pressure
- Withdrawal from participation in conversations

Note whether the patient asks frequent questions or relates inaccurate information about the procedure.

After the procedure, check the patient's fluid intake and output for several days. Assess the color, consistency, and amount of urine every 8 hours. Check whether the patient is having difficulty voiding or whether he or she is experiencing pain or burning on urination. Consider the results of urinalysis and any other diagnostic tests completed after the procedure.

Nursing Diagnoses and Planning

Nursing diagnoses and related expected patient outcomes most commonly applicable to patients undergoing an excretory urogram include the following:

NDx: Knowledge deficit: nature of the diagnostic test, purpose, preparation, and procedure

Planning: Patient Outcomes
1. Patient verbalizes an understanding of the events that will occur before, during, and after the procedure.
2. Patient identifies allergies or contraindications before the procedure that may predispose to complications.

NDx: Anxiety related to unfamiliar and presumably uncomfortable tests

Planning: Patient Outcomes
1. Patient verbalizes a reduction in anxiety.
2. Patient demonstrates positive problem-solving skills.
3. Patient appears relaxed and less anxious and is resting well.

NDx: Altered urinary elimination related to complications from radiologic procedures

Planning: Patient Outcomes
1. Patient maintains adequate urinary output and fluid intake in the postprocedure period.
2. Patient denies pain or burning on urination after the procedure.

Nursing Interventions and Evaluation

NDx: Knowledge deficit: nature of the diagnostic test, purpose, preparation, and procedure
Identify any allergy to contrast agents or compromised renal function before any study in which contrast agents are used. Explain the procedure to the patient. Provide information about any injections or invasive procedures, the room where the study will be performed, and any unfamiliar machines or equipment. Ask the patient what he or she already understands about the procedure. Reinforce accurate facts and correct any misunderstandings. Explain that the patient will need to drink increased fluids after the test and that his or her urinary output will be closely monitored.

NDx: Anxiety
Acknowledge the patient's anxiety and the perceived threat of the situation. Encourage the expression of feelings of anger, fear, or grief. Orient the patient to the procedure, and explain all activities that will take place in the diagnostic laboratory and afterwards. Allow the family to express feelings and ask questions.

Seek assistance from clergy or significant others if necessary to help allay the patient's anxiety. Answer all questions factually, and provide consistent reinforcement. Encourage questions, self-care, and decision-making as much as possible.

NDx: Altered urinary elimination
After the study, encourage fluid intake and monitor intake and output closely. Provide fluids of choice for the patient to increase the fluid intake. Evaluate the urine for color, consistency, and quantity.

Observe the patient for hypersensitivity reactions after the use of any contrast agents or injectable materials. Pay particular attention to pruritus, rashes, breathing difficulties, generalized edema, or urinary retention.

Compare the patient's status with the expected outcomes. If the outcomes are not met, reassess the patient and revise the plan.

CYSTOSCOPY

Cystoscopy, also called cystourethroscopy, is an examination of the urinary bladder and urethra by direct visualization. Cystoscopy involves the passage of a metal sheath into the urethra. A bridge is connected to the end of the sheath, and through these two parts the examiner passes telescope devices that allow for visual inspection of the bladder and urethra. Any urine in the bladder is first emptied through the sheath. An irrigating solution, usually sterile saline, is allowed to flow by gravity into the bladder. A fiberoptic light connected to a powerful light source is attached to the telescope. Telescopes with two standard lenses are used. These lenses (30-degree and 70-degree) provide direct and wide-angle viewing. The urethra is visualized by looking through one of the telescopes as the sheath is passed through it (Fig. 30–7).

Several types of specimens can be obtained during cystoscopy. Saline washings may be sent for cytologic examination. Biopsy forceps can be passed through the sheath to allow for biopsies of suspicious areas. Bridges with specialized ports allow for the passage of ureteral catheters during cystoscopy. Other specialized instruments can also be used during cystoscopy.

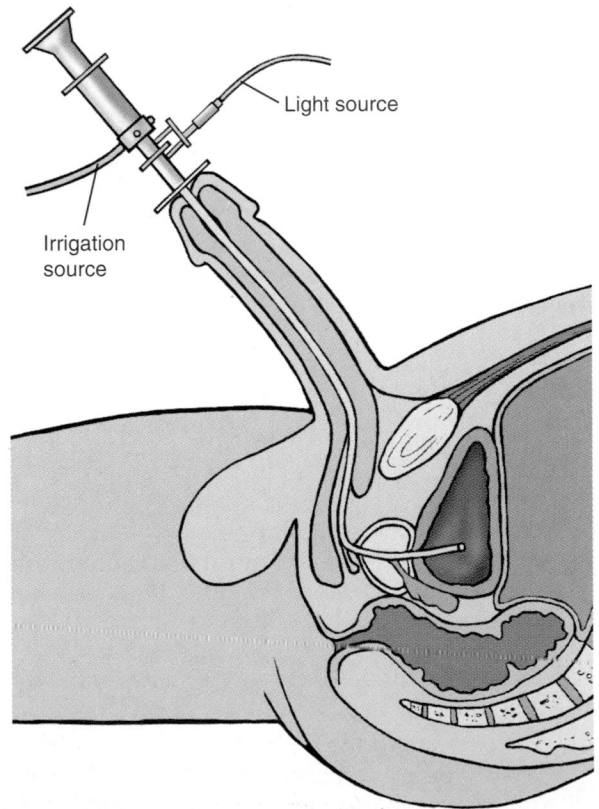

Figure 30–7
Cystoscope in the male bladder.

Routine cystoscopy is performed under local anesthesia. Regional, spinal, or general anesthesia is sometimes used when the patient cannot tolerate local anesthesia, when the physician prefers it, or when multiple biopsies or other painful procedures are anticipated.

Uses

Along with the excretory urogram, cystoscopy is a mainstay of the urologic diagnostic evaluation. No other test can take the place of directly visualizing the interior of the bladder. Cystoscopy is the primary method for diagnosis and follow-up of bladder tumors. It is also an essential part of the diagnostic evaluation for many urologic disorders. Such disorders include prostatism, voiding disorders, fistulas, diverticula, recurrent urinary tract infections, and some congenital anomalies.

Although cystoscopy is used for the evaluation of recurrent urinary tract infections, the presence of an *active* urinary tract infection is a contraindication to cystoscopy. That is because the procedure may spread the infection to other parts of the urinary tract. Significant bladder outlet obstruction from prostatism is considered by some physicians to be a contraindication to outpatient cystoscopy. That is because hematuria, urinary retention, and bladder neck edema are common after any urethral instrumentation. In patients scheduled for cystoscopy, assessment must therefore include questioning about voiding patterns and the results of recent urine cultures.

Complications

Serious complications after simple cystoscopy are very uncommon. Minor complications are possible, and the patient should be advised of symptoms of these complications before leaving for home.

Infection is always a possibility after any urethral instrumentation, including cystoscopy. The patient should therefore be advised to report any fever, persistent burning on urination, or urinary frequency. Hematuria occurs more frequently in men than in women, and after any biopsies. After cystoscopy, the urine may be slightly blood-tinged, but this should clear up within 24 to 48 hours. Gross hematuria with clots may require hospitalization and continuous bladder irrigation. Urinary retention is also more common in men, especially in those with enlarged prostates. If the patient is unable to void after 6 to 8 hours, he should return to the physician's office or to the hospital. Pushing oral fluids copiously can help prevent all these complications.

Serious complications of cystoscopy include urethral, bladder, or ureteral perforation. Fortunately, these complications are rare. Any sudden and severe pain in the lower abdomen during cystoscopy calls for immediate termination of the procedure. Likewise, any sudden change in vital signs requires termination of cystoscopy.

NURSING PROCESS GUIDELINES
Cystoscopy

Review the history and other completed diagnostic studies. Assess the patient's anxiety about the procedure. Cystoscopy provokes great anxiety in some patients, and they will require repeated reassurances and explanations. Evaluate any physical limitations that would prevent the patient from lying in a lithotomy position. Patients with a history of unstable cardiac, neurologic, or psychiatric conditions are not good candidates for cystoscopy under local anesthesia. Communicate these findings to the physician so that alternative or adjunctive measures can be taken.

The nursing diagnoses, related expected patient outcomes, and nursing interventions most commonly applicable to patients undergoing a cystoscopy include those described previously for patients undergoing an excretory urogram. Also see Nursing Care Guide 30–1. The following additional interventions also apply to the care of patients undergoing cystoscopy.

The procedure is often embarrassing to many patients because there is manipulation of the genitalia, and patients may develop increased anxiety prior to the cystoscopy. Explain the necessity of the procedure and exactly what is to be done.

If intravenous sedation or anesthesia (regional, spinal, or general) is to be used during cystoscopy, the patient should receive nothing by mouth (NPO) after midnight prior to the procedure. Teach the patient relaxation methods before the procedure. Most patients can tolerate cystoscopy under local anesthesia when they are well prepared and practice relaxation techniques prior to and during the examination.

After the cystoscopy, monitor fluid intake and output carefully. Encourage increased fluid intake. Notify the physician if the patient does not void within 8 hours or if excessive bleeding or pain is present. Note any hematuria or change in the appearance of the urine. Dysuria and frequency are common for 24 to 48 hours. If an indwelling catheter is present, monitor for patency and measure the output. Document both the color and amount of urine. Administer any ordered pain medication as necessary for discomfort from bladder spasms.

Give the patient written discharge instructions. Review the information verbally in terms that the patient can understand. Also explain to the family any needed home care. Allow time for questions or expression of concerns (see Nursing Care Guide 30–1).

BLADDER BIOPSY

Bladder biopsies may be performed for a number of reasons. Patients with a history of transitional cell carcinoma of the bladder frequently have biopsies of suspicious areas seen on radiographic studies or during cystoscopy. Patients with symptoms indicative of a carcinoma of the bladder, ureter, or renal pelvis may require biopsies of any of these areas. Finally, some infectious conditions or diseases, such as interstitial cystitis, must be diagnosed by pathologic or cytologic evaluation of tissue specimens.

Bladder biopsies are easily performed during cystoscopy, using biopsy forceps to obtain a "cold cup" specimen (a snip of tissue) to send to the pathology laboratory. One or two superficial biopsies can be performed under local anesthesia. More extensive biopsies, often called superficial and deep or random bladder biopsies, are usually performed under regional or general anesthesia.

Specimens of ureteral or renal pelvic tissue can be obtained using any of several instruments passed up the ureter during cystoscopy. For example, small brushes that collect cells and minute pieces of tissue for cytologic evaluation are used to perform brush biopsies. Careful, methodologic specimens can be collected in this manner to determine the origins of suspicious cells found in cytologic studies when no obvious lesions can be found.

When urethral malignancy is suspected, urethral biopsies can be obtained using the same method as for bladder biopsy.

Uses

Bladder biopsies are indicated for diagnosis of transitional cell carcinoma, squamous cell carcinoma, or adenocarcinoma of the bladder. They are also used to diagnose various infectious processes within the bladder wall and interstitial cystitis. Random biopsies of several areas within the bladder mucosa are indicated for staging bladder cancer or for identifying the origin of suspicious or malignant cells found in cytologic studies. Bladder biopsies are always indicated when suspicious areas are seen on cystoscopy. Brush biopsy of the ureter or renal pelvis is indicated when suspicious areas are seen on radiographic studies. Brush biopsy is also indicated when malignant cells are present in a cytologic specimen and no bladder lesions are present. Because transitional cell carcinoma can recur anywhere in the urothelial lining of the urinary tract, such examinations are sometimes necessary as part of a thorough follow-up regimen. (However, periodic excretory urography, cystoscopy, and urinary cytology may suffice in these cases.)

Complications

Patients on anticoagulant therapy or those with known bleeding disorders should not undergo bladder biopsy because hemorrhage may result. If the patient *must* undergo the bladder biopsy, anticoagulants should be discontinued 3 to 5 days before biopsy, when possible. Bladder biopsy should not be performed when an active urinary tract infection is present because sepsis may result.

Nursing Care Guide 30–1
Patients Undergoing Cystoscopy

Preoperative Care

Assessment Findings: Patient presents signs of restlessness, nervousness, increased respiratory rate, and increased heart rate; asks questions about procedures; clenches hands; cries.

Nursing Diagnosis: Anxiety related to fear of procedure, diagnosis, and future treatments or medical management

Patient Outcomes	Nursing Interventions	Rationale
Patient is less anxious as evidenced by smiling; lack of restlessness, crying, or nervousness; and vital signs within normal limits.	Explain the procedure to the patient and family. Describe the preoperative preparation. Allow time for questions and concerns.	An understanding of the procedure may reduce anxiety. Providing time for questions relieves some of the patient's fear of the unknown and allows for correction of misunderstandings.
	Check vital signs, and observe for signs of relaxation in the patient.	Changes in vital signs may indicate reduced anxiety.
Patient verbalizes feeling less anxious.	Teach relaxation techniques. Help the patient find coping strategies that help alleviate the stress and anxiety.	Relaxation exercises promote relief of stress and anxiety.
	Allow time for rest; provide a quiet, comfortable atmosphere.	Rest periods and quiet may promote a reduction in stress and anxiety.

Evaluation: Compare the patient's status with the expected outcomes. If the outcomes are not met, reassess the patient and revise the plan.

Assessment Findings: Patient asks questions about procedure, seems uninformed about preoperative and postprocedure care and treatments; patient and family voice concerns about risks of and necessity for the procedure.

Nursing Diagnosis: Knowledge deficit: nature of procedure and postprocedure care

Patient Outcomes	Nursing Interventions	Rationale
Patient reports accurate information about the procedure, the necessity for it, and the expectations postprocedure.	Be certain the physician has discussed the procedure, risks, complications, and expectations with the patient. Allow the patient to ask questions, and try to expand on the understanding about the procedure for the patient and family.	Having the patient reiterate the information provided allows for an assessment of the patient's understanding of the procedure. Providing time for questions allows for correction of misunderstandings.

(continued)

Nursing Care Guide 30-1
Patients Undergoing Cystoscopy (continued)

Patient Outcomes	Nursing Interventions	Rationale
Patient and family state that they have an understanding of the procedure, the risks, and the postprocedure care needed.	Explain the postprocedure care needed, and tell the patient that the information will be repeated prior to discharge. Include the family in the education sessions. Allow time for questions and concerns. Explain all information in understandable terms.	Providing some information about postprocedure expectations helps relieve anxiety about the postprocedure care needed. Inclusion of the family provides reinforcement for the patient, relieves family anxiety, and gives support to the patient.

Evaluation: Compare the patient's status with the expected outcomes. If the outcomes are not met, reassess the patient and revise the plan.

Postoperative Care

Assessment Findings: Patient is unable to void even with increased fluid intake; patient has difficulty starting stream: patient complains of discomfort with voiding and is able to produce only some dribbling; or patient complains of frequency of urination with small amounts voided each time.

Nursing Diagnosis: Altered urinary elimination related to irritation of urethra secondary to instrumentation

Patient Outcomes	Nursing Interventions	Rationale
Patient resumes normal patterns of urinary elimination with adequate output.	After the procedure, encourage increasd fluid intake (8–10 glasses of water unless contraindicated).	Increased intake of fluids helps restore normal urinary pattern and flushes the system, helping prevent infection.
	Have the patient attempt to void frequently, and measure amount. Ask the patient whether it seems as though the bladder has been emptied.	Frequent voiding prevents accumulation of urine, which may promote bacterial growth or overdistend the bladder.
Patient denies difficulty with urination.	Have the patient report any difficulty with urination. Ask whether there are feelings of burning or irritation. Check the color, consistency, and amount of the urine.	Early assessment for problems may prevent serious complications.

Evaluation: Compare the patient's status with the expected outcomes. If the outcomes are not met, reassess the patient and revise the plan.

Assessment Findings: Patient asks questions about home care and other discharge instructions.

Nursing Diagnosis: Altered health maintenance related to insufficient knowledge about home care

(continued)

Nursing Care Guide 30–1
Patients Undergoing Cystoscopy *(continued)*

Patient Outcomes	Nursing Interventions	Rationale
Patient states accurate information about discharge care, including when to report to the physician.	Give the patient written instructions for self-care after discharge, and have the patient repeat the information. Tell the patient to observe for any change in color or consistency of the urine. Explain that some discomfort may occur from bladder spasms or irritation of the urethra.	Written instructions reinforce the verbal information provided. A reiteration of the instructions allows for an assessment of the patient's understanding of the information. An explanation of the possible complications prepares the patient for them and for early intervention.
	Tell the patient to notify the physician if bleeding, extreme pain, changes in the color or consistency of the urine, or inability to void occurs. Encourage the patient to continue to drink copious amounts of fluid at home to wash out urinary tract.	An explanation of follow-up care needed and when to seek medical assistance may prevent problems. Continued intake of increased amounts of fluids helps flush the urinary system and prevent complications.
Patient and family verbalize an understanding of the instructions given.	Explain all information to the patient's family, and have them repeat the information. Be sure to use terminology that is understandable to them. Allow time for questions.	Including the family reinforces the information and provides support for the patient. Reiteration of the instructions allows for an assessment of the understanding of the information.
Evaluation:	Compare the patient's status with the expected outcomes. If the outcomes are not met, reassess the patient and revise the plan.	

Complications during bladder biopsy include bladder perforation with urinary extravasation, and prolonged bleeding. Biopsies of the ureter or renal pelvis can be complicated by perforation of either of these areas, again with urinary extravasation resulting. Complications after any of these biopsies include persistent bleeding, urinary tract obstruction from edema, sepsis, stricture formation, and formation of scar tissue.

NURSING PROCESS
Bladder Biopsy

Assessment

Assess for bleeding disorders. Check bleeding times preoperatively, and question the patient about excessive bleeding from minor cuts and about frequent bruising. Assess the patient's current medications.

Look especially for the use of nonsteroidal, anti-inflammatory drugs, aspirin or aspirin-containing compounds, and anticoagulants. All of these drugs should be discontinued 3 to 5 days before any biopsies.

Check the results of the urine studies. Recent urine cultures should show no signs of infection. Note the color, consistency, and amount of urine for baseline data to be used in postbiopsy comparisons.

Assess for any physical limitations that would prohibit the patient from lying in a lithotomy position. Assess the patient's understanding of the procedure before teaching is begun. Look for signs of anxiety.

Nursing Diagnoses and Planning

Nursing diagnoses and related expected patient outcomes most commonly applicable to patients undergoing a bladder biopsy include those described previously for patients undergoing an excretory urogram, and the following:

NDx: Pain related to irritation from biopsy site

Planning: Patient Outcomes
1. Patient denies pain or discomfort after the procedure.
2. Patient resumes a normal pattern of urinary elimination after the procedure.

Nursing Interventions and Evaluation

NDx: Pain

After completion of the procedure, monitor the patient's fluid intake and output. Assess the urine for the degree of hematuria. If no Foley catheter is present, the patient should void within 8 hours after the procedure. If a Foley catheter is present, it must remain patent. Continuous or intermittent bladder irrigation may be necessary when significant hematuria is present. Ask the patient about feelings of discomfort, especially when voiding if no catheter is present. Irritation from the biopsies or from the Foley catheter is often uncomfortable enough to warrant medication. Give the prescribed medication as necessary. Belladonna and opium suppositories or anticholinergic drugs may relieve bladder spasms, and a mild pain medication may relieve vague feelings of discomfort.

Compare the patient's status with the expected outcomes. If the outcomes are not met, reassess the patient and revise the plan.

RENAL BIOPSY

Two techniques of renal biopsy are available: needle biopsy and open renal biopsy. Needle biopsy of the kidney, also called closed renal biopsy, is described here. Open renal biopsy, a surgical procedure, is not described in this text.

Needle biopsy of the kidney involves a puncture through the flank into the parenchyma of the lower pole of either kidney. To perform the procedure, the examiner may localize the kidney by ultrasonography or fluoroscopy. Alternatively, the examiner may determine its location simply by locating it in relation to the eleventh or twelfth rib on a recent radiologic study. A local anesthetic (usually 1% lidocaine) is administered through a spinal needle. The placement of the needle in the kidney is determined by its movement during inspiration and expiration (if ultrasonography or fluoroscopy are not used). One of several standard biopsy needles then replaces the spinal needle, and a core of tissue is removed and sent to the pathology laboratory for analysis.

Closed renal biopsy is usually performed in the ultrasound or radiology department of a hospital or, in rare cases, at the patient's bedside.

Uses
Renal biopsy is used to diagnose renal disease. It is also used to evaluate the patient's response to treatment or to evaluate the progression of a previously diagnosed renal disorder. It is much more clinically useful in nephrology than in urology. However, urologists occasionally use closed renal biopsy to aspirate specimens from suspicious areas seen on ultrasonograms or x-rays in order to differentiate between simple cysts and malignancies. In these cases, adjunctive ultrasonography, fluoroscopy, and occasionally computed tomography are used.

Complications
The most common complication of closed renal biopsy is prolonged bleeding in the form of gross hematuria or a perinephric hematoma. Rarely is bleeding severe enough to cause circulatory collapse. However, late hemorrhage occurs in some patients 7 to 10 days after biopsy. Other infrequent complications are arteriovenous aneurysm and inadvertent biopsy of an organ other than the kidney.

Closed renal biopsy is contraindicated in patients with severe hypertension, pyelonephritis, coagulation disorders, and renal tuberculosis. It is also not recommended in patients with a solitary kidney or a kidney in an unusual anatomic position.

NURSING PROCESS
Renal Biopsy

Assessment

Assess all medications that the patient is currently taking. Assess for routine use of aspirin, aspirin-containing compounds, or nonsteroidal anti-inflammatory drugs, and notify the physician of this information. Assess the patient's anxiety level and knowledge about the procedure. This is essential, because patient cooperation is important to the success of the procedure. To assess the patient's level of understanding, ask the patient to explain the information the physician has stated.

After the procedure, assess for signs of bleeding. Check the urinary output for color, and note any drop in blood pressure. Check vital signs for indications of infection (fever) or previously undiagnosed hypertension (elevated blood pressure). Both of these conditions increase the risk of complications after biopsy. Changes in vital signs may also indicate fluid volume deficits caused by bleeding.

Nursing Diagnoses and Planning

Nursing diagnoses and related expected patient outcomes most commonly applicable to patients undergoing renal biopsy include the following:

NDx: Knowledge deficit: nature, purpose, and risks of renal biopsy

Planning: Patient Outcomes
1. Patient verbalizes an understanding of the procedure and the need for cooperation during the procedure.

2. Patient recovers from the procedure without serious complications.
3. Patient tolerates the procedure and adheres to postbiopsy mobility restrictions.

NDx: Risk for fluid volume deficit related to possible bleeding of biopsy site

Planning: Patient Outcomes
1. Patient maintains adequate fluid volume as evidenced by adequate output and lack of signs of bleeding.
2. Patient's vital signs remain within normal ranges for the patient.

Nursing Interventions and Evaluation

NDx: Knowledge deficit: nature, purpose, and risks of renal biopsy
Explain the events that will occur during renal biopsy. Prebiopsy teaching may require several repetitions for the anxious patient. When you can be present during the procedure, describe for the patient what is occurring and help the patient use relaxation techniques.

The patient will be asked to take deep breaths, hold the breath, and lie very still during the procedure. After biopsy, patients often must lie prone for 1 hour, then remain on bedrest for up to 24 hours. If gross hematuria or bleeding from or around the biopsy site persists, bedrest may be ordered for longer periods. Monitor vital signs for several hours after the procedure, and report any significant changes to the physician immediately. Dress the biopsy site with a small dressing or adhesive bandage, and observe frequently for bleeding.

NDx: Risk for fluid volume deficit
Monitor vital signs frequently after biopsy to check for impending shock related to a decrease in fluid volume from bleeding. Check the patient's urine for changes in color. Check the biopsy site for bleeding. Keep a small pressure dressing over the puncture site, and apply digital pressure if you note any bleeding.

Compare the patient's status with the expected outcomes. If the outcomes are not met, reassess the patient and revise the plan.

URODYNAMICS

Urodynamics refers to a series of diagnostic techniques used for the evaluation of voiding disorders. Just as pulmonary function tests study the respiratory system while it is actually functioning, urodynamic procedures study the urinary tract dynamically, while it is actually functioning.

There are various components of urodynamic testing, which incorporate measures of flow, volume, pressure, and electrical response. Used individually or in combination, these measures provide

valuable insight into how the process of micturition is functioning in a particular patient.

The need for urodynamic testing is based in part on findings from the history, physical examination, radiographic investigation, and endoscopic evaluation. The extent of testing required depends on the patient's problem, the urologist's preference for various procedures, and the availability of urodynamic testing equipment.

Without question, simple urodynamic assessment is essential in the evaluation of patients with suspected neurogenic voiding dysfunction. For those with unusual disorders or inconclusive findings from previous studies, sophisticated multichannel studies (or videourodynamics) may be necessary.

At one time urodynamic testing was used solely for the purpose of assessing lower urinary tract function. However, it is now also used to assess the function of the upper urinary tract. Table 30–7 describes the various urodynamic procedures, including their uses, complications, and nursing care.

NURSING PROCESS
Urodynamic Testing

Assessment

Assess the patient for any signs or symptoms that indicate the presence of a urinary tract infection. Check for elevated temperature. Note the results of urine cultures. Check the color and consistency of the urine. If there are signs of a urinary infection, notify the physician. In the presence of urinary tract infection, the testing should be postponed. Irritation of the urinary tract from infection adversely alters test results, and repeated instrumentation in the presence of urinary tract infection could lead to sepsis.

Evaluate the patient's physical condition, because multiple position changes are usually required during the course of the procedure. Check whether the patient can transfer from a bed to a commode with ease. Note whether the patient is able to walk alone or whether assistance is needed. Check whether the patient has the strength to undergo testing at the time it is scheduled. Although urodynamic testing is often performed in patients with impaired mobility, a more complete evaluation can be obtained if the patient feels physically able to cooperate with the testing and is able to move about freely.

Evaluate the patient's mental status, because study results are correlated with the individual's description of sensations during the procedures. If the patient is disoriented, confused, or unable to take instructions, he or she is probably not a candidate for urodynamic testing.

Review the current medications prescribed for the patient to see whether any of them directly alter bladder function. Make note of cholinergic and anticholinergic agents, musculotropic relaxants, polysy-

Table 30-7

Urodynamic Procedures

Definition and Description	Uses	Complications	Nursing Care
URINARY FLOW RATE A measure of the volume of urine expelled from the bladder during a given period of time; it is an assessment of the joint action of the bladder and outlet. Rate is calculated and expressed as mL/sec. It is the easiest, most informative, and only noninvasive urodynamic procedure. Patient is simply required to urinate into a special commode with measuring device attached.	To assess patients with symptoms of outflow obstruction (e.g., BPH, urethral strictures) Before and after any procedure designed to improve urine flow As a screening procedure for those with dysfunctional voiding prior to initiating other invasive urodynamic tests	None	Explain that a full bladder is needed in order to obtain a valid and reliable study. Make sure that the patient understands that this is a test to assess voiding, not defecation; stool interferes with the validity of the test. Instruct the patient to force fluids and delay voiding until time for the test.
CYSTOMETROGRAM (CMG) A measure of bladder pressure (in cm H_2O) during the filling and storage phases of micturition Procedure requires that a catheter be inserted and the bladder slowly filled with water or gas (CO_2) until capacity is reached. Notation is made of amount of fluid or gas infused and of patient's sensations to filling.	To evaluate all types of urinary incontinence; in those with enuresis; for sure or suspected neurogenic voiding dysfunction	A UTI may result from instrumentation of the urethra. Procedure is contraindicated if UTI is present or if patient is experiencing diarrhea.	Fully explain the procedure: Check to see whether the patient is taking any medication that could interfere with results of the tests (cholinergics and anticholinergics have direct effect upon the bladder). Check to see whether patient had a recent negative result on urine culture. After the procedure, an increase in fluid intake helps reduce discomfort felt when voiding and dilutes urine to prevent infection.
ELECTROMYOGRAPHY (EMG) The recording of electrical activity generated by the striated muscles of the external urethral sphincter To establish the recording, two needle, wire, or surface electrodes are strategically placed on the perineum and connected to the urodynamics machine.	To evaluate the coordination of the external urethral sphincter and perineum with detrusor activity during bladder filling and emptying; aids in diagnosing detrusor-sphincter dyssynergia Always performed in conjunction with other urodynamic tests	Some pain may be experienced during the insertion of wire or needle electrodes.	Explain the procedure and assure the patient that it involves only temporary discomfort.

Table continued on following page

Table 30–7

Urodynamic Procedures *(continued)*

Definition and Description	Uses	Complications	Nursing Care
COMBINED MICTURITION STUDY			
The simultaneous recording of urine flow, intravesical pressure, intraabdominal (usually via the rectum) pressure, and sphincter EMG activity during the emptying phase of micturition; requires that the patient be transferred to commode chair following bladder filling (performed during CMG) with monitoring equipment attached	When used in conjunction with CMG, this study offers the clinician the opportunity to evaluate the entire micturition cycle. Helpful in cases of complicated voiding dysfunction to differentiate between outflow obstruction and weak detrusor	Dizziness may occur during the procedure as a result of the change in position.	Same as for previous studies
VIDEOURODYNAMIC STUDY			
The synchronous recording of previously described urodynamic parameters and cystourethrography	Complicated neurologic disease; complicated incontinence; when clinical impression differs from urodynamic findings; unsuccessful therapeutic results from medications or surgery	Same as for previous studies	Same as for previous studies
URETHRAL PRESSURE PROFILE (UPP)			
A study of the pressures along the length of the urethra; requires that a special #8 to #10 French catheter be inserted into the bladder and then pulled back through the urethra at a fixed rate as water or gas is infused	To determine urethral incompetency; to locate areas of increased resistance or obstruction; before and after artificial sphincter implants; in the operating room during surgery for bladder neck reconstruction	Same as for CMG	Same as for previous studies

BPH, benign prostatic hypertrophy; UTI, urinary tract infection.

naptic inhibitors, beta-adrenergic stimulants, and tricyclic antidepressants. Although these drugs are helpful in treating voiding symptoms as well as a variety of other medical problems, they also interfere with urodynamic test results and prevent evaluation of how the urinary tract functions without medication.

Nursing Diagnoses and Planning

Nursing diagnoses and related expected patient outcomes most commonly applicable to patients undergoing urodynamic testing include the following:

NDx: Knowledge deficit: nature of urodynamic testing techniques

Planning: Patient Outcomes
1. Patient verbalizes an understanding of the events that will occur before, during, and after the testing.
2. Patient denies lack of understanding about the testing and verbalizes lack of anxiety about it.

NDx: Risk for infection related to instrumentation of the urinary tract

Planning: Patient Outcomes
1. Patient denies burning or pain on urination, which may be signs of infection.
2. Patient's vital signs are within normal ranges.
3. Patient presents clear urine with no trace of bacteria on urinalysis.

NDx: Altered urinary elimination related to irritation of urethra from catheterization

Planning: Patient Outcomes
1. Patient denies having difficulty voiding.
2. Patient increases fluid intake after the test.
3. Patient's fluid intake and output are adequate.

Nursing Interventions and Evaluation

NDx: Knowledge deficit: nature of urodynamic testing techniques
Explain each urodynamic procedure. However, before proceeding with a detailed description of the tests, call the urodynamic facility to inquire about any special testing techniques that they plan to use. Emphasize to the patient that these studies are neither passed or failed. Rather, they are used to collect information about the patient's voiding pattern.

Prior to testing, dress the patient in a hospital gown only. The limited clothing is necessary because of the amount of equipment that will be attached to the patient during the urodynamic procedures.

Explain to the patient that there will be no premedication given for this test. Although premedicating patients with sedatives or analgesics is common prior to many procedures, it is not done prior to urodynamic testing (unless ordered for a specific reason). These drugs can affect bladder function. And, more importantly, they alter a patient's perception and threaten safety during the procedure.

Tell the patient that after urodynamic testing there may be some perineal discomfort, generally caused by repeated instrumentation. Because of this irritation, the patient may be reluctant to void. Encourage the patient to force fluids for 24 to 36 hours after the studies to increase urine output, stimulate voiding, dilute urine, and flush out bacteria.

NDx: Risk for infection
Because a urinary tract infection can occur after urodynamic testing, instruct the patient to report signs and symptoms of urinary tract infection. These include burning, pain, or discharge with urination. For patients who are prone to developing a urinary tract infection, prophylactic antibiotics may be prescribed. Explain to the patient the frequency, dosage, and side effects of the medication. Encourage increased fluid intake to clear out bacteria.

NDx: Altered urinary elimination
After the study, encourage fluid intake and monitor intake and output closely. Provide the patients with a choice of fluids. Evaluate the urine for color, consistency, and quantity. Check for burning with urination, bloody urine, or pain at the urinary meatus (the opening of the urethra). Provide a bedside urinal or commode if the patient cannot get up to go to the bathroom.

Observe the patient for hypersensitivity reactions after the use of any contrast materials or other injectable materials. Pay particular attention to pruritus, rashes, breathing difficulties, generalized edema, or urinary retention. Tell the patient to report any difficulty in urination or other side effects.

Compare the patient's status with the expected outcomes. If the outcomes are not met, reassess the patient and revise the plan.

Management

NONSURGICAL MANAGEMENT

Nonsurgical management of urinary tract dysfunction involves a combination of treatment modalities. Catheter drainage, medications, self-help measures, and diet therapy are some of the interventions used to assist patients with urinary problems.

Catheter Drainage
The primary purpose of a urinary catheter is to remove urine from the bladder when the patient is incapable of totally emptying the bladder. A catheter may be used in emergency situations or following certain surgical interventions or traumatic injuries. Additionally, a catheter can be used for the following purposes:

- Instilling medication into the bladder
- Diagnostic procedures
- Accurate monitoring of urinary output

In severe cases of urinary incontinence, when other medical problems exist, a catheter is sometimes used to temporarily manage incontinence until a more permanent means of control is established.

Catheters come in a wide variety of shapes and sizes and should be chosen according to the needs of the patient. Pediatric sizes (#10 to #14 French [Fr]) are available for the young adult but are also used in patients with atrophy of the urethral meatus. Large sizes (#25 Fr or greater) are used during bladder irrigation procedures. Coudé-tip catheters are useful in men with enlarged prostates. Mushroom-shaped, or winged, catheters may be used for suprapubic placement or placement as a nephrostomy tube. When a catheter is particularly difficult to insert, a physician may use a stylet or filiform catheter to achieve catheter insertion. Urinary catheters may be made of latex, Silastic, silicone-coated materials, solid silicone, and combinations of these materials.

INDWELLING CATHETERS
Indwelling catheters are used for the continuous drainage of urine from the bladder. They may be employed temporarily after a surgical procedure or they may be required for long-term management of urinary retention. Regardless of their use, all indwelling catheters should be maintained as a sterile,

closed drainage system and should be inserted using strict aseptic technique by qualified personnel.

Use of indwelling catheters can lead to complications, such as inflammation of the urethra, strictures, urinary tract infections, renal and bladder calculi, and hydronephrosis. In men they may be associated with epididymitis and penoscrotal complications. Table 30–8 provides nursing guidelines for the prevention of such side effects.

The presence of an indwelling catheter increases the hospitalized patient's risk of nosocomial infection by 40% to 50%. Patients especially at risk for infection are pregnant women, the elderly, diabetic patients, and those who are immunosuppressed.

Nursing measures such as the application of antimicrobial agents at the urethral meatus have proved ineffective in reducing the risk of catheter-related infections. In fact, these measures may actually *promote* infection by acting as an irritant to the meatal tissue. In addition, repeated washing of the meatus with soap and water may increase the risk of infection. This is due in part to the manipulation of the catheter and in part to the introduction of exogenous bacteria into the bladder. Instillation of antiseptic solutions such as hydrogen peroxide or chlorhexidine into the urinary drainage bag has also proved to be ineffective in reducing catheter-induced urinary tract infections. Routine perineal care during the daily bath is generally sufficient to minimize infection from the indwelling catheter.

In any hospitalized patient with an indwelling catheter, bacteriuria will be present after 24 to 72 hours. Urine cultures are indicated only when symptoms of an upper urinary tract or systemic infection are present. Routine catheter changes—at one time performed to impede bacterial growth— are also not necessary unless the closed drainage system has been broken. Although continuous bladder irrigations may be used after transurethral surgery, routine bladder irrigations are contraindicated. The only exception is that they are used on the express orders of a physician when clots or other residue has blocked catheter drainage.

For patients requiring catheter drainage at home, a low-dose prophylactic antibiotic may be prescribed to control bacterial growth. Some of these patients may also require a routine catheter change or catheter irrigation to prevent occlusion of the catheter from crystals that tend to form on the tip. However, if the tube is patent and draining well, there is really no reason to change or irrigate it. If there is a need to change the catheter, consider decreasing the catheter size if the one removed is larger than a #14 to #16 Fr. Large catheters may irritate the bladder trigone muscle and cause pain. They may also block the paraurethral glands by preventing the natural lubrication from "washing out" the bacteria and debris that has accumulated. In addition, instruct patients about the procedure for transferring the catheter from a drain bag to a urinary leg bag. Advise them to rinse the drain bags overnight at least two or three times each week in a solution of equal parts white vinegar and water, which helps to clean and deodorize them. Provide a teaching checklist for the patient that covers the following subjects:

- The function and anatomical position of the catheter
- Disinfecting the catheter bag
- Emptying the catheter bag
- Fluid intake
- Signs of infection
- Sexual activity
- Anchoring the catheter
- Irrigation (if needed)

SUPRAPUBIC CATHETERS

A suprapubic catheter may be used in place of a urethral catheter when there is urethral injury, prostatic obstruction, or urethral stricture. It is also used after gynecologic surgery and may be used for long-

Table 30–8

Nursing Guidelines for Prevention of Complications of Indwelling Catheters

To minimize the complications associated with indwelling urinary catheters, follow these guidelines:

Use aseptic technique in catheter insertion.

Determine appropriate type and size of catheter before insertion.

Employ a closed drainage system. If irrigations are ordered, all efforts must be made to prevent contamination of the system.

Ensure that drainage bag stays below the level of the bladder at all times.

Remove catheter as soon as possible.

Use aseptic technique when taking urine samples from the aspiration port.

Change catheter only when it becomes obstructed or contaminated; catheters should not be changed on a routine basis.

Empty drainage bags every 8 hours or more often if volume is excessive.

Clean the outlet valve each time, and prevent contact contamination by the measuring container.

Ensure that each catheterized patient has an individualized, labeled measuring container.

Ensure that all catheterized patients maintain adequate hydration; 2 to 3 L/day of water is recommended except in the presence of cardiac insufficiency or renal failure.

Anchor the catheter securely to the leg or lower abdomen by use of tape or catheter strap.

Assess the catheterized patient on a routine basis. Assess fluid intake and output levels patency of the system, color and odor of urine, evidence of sediment, presence/absence of patient discomfort, fever, and hematuria.

Remove catheter by aspirating fluid from the inflation port with a syringe. Because varied amounts of fluid are used to inflate catheter balloons, be sure to check the insertion record before aspiration to determine the amount of fluid used.

term catheterization. Insertion of the catheter may be performed in the patient's bed as opposed to an operating room or cystoscopy room. The catheter is inserted into the bladder using a trocar-cannula device that is inserted directly above the pubic bone. The catheter is held in place either internally, by the design of the catheter, or externally, by a disk or sutures. Initially, the insertion site is cleaned and redressed every day. After healing has occurred, a permanent suprapubic opening should be cleaned and assessed several times per week. At that point a dressing may no longer be necessary. Catheters are changed only if they show evidence of obstruction. Suprapubic catheters should be changed only by qualified personnel. Irrigations may be ordered to maintain patency and should be performed using clean technique.

The catheter must be connected to either a drain bag or a urinary leg bag. Use of the leg bag is beneficial to patients who are ambulatory or who wish to sit in a wheelchair without having a cumbersome drain bag present for everyone to see. One advantage of a suprapubic catheter is that it does not interfere as much with sexual activity as does an indwelling catheter.

INTERMITTENT SELF-CATHETERIZATION

Clean intermittent self-catheterization, also called simply *intermittent self-catheterization*, was reinstituted in the early 1970s as an alternative to indwelling catheterization. The procedure may be used on a long- or short-term basis, depending on the bladder's ability to return to normal function. Paraplegic or quadriplegic patients typically use intermittent self-catheterization and are seldom able to discontinue its use. However, some patients with mildly neurogenic bladders or who have had gynecologic surgery may use this technique for only a few weeks or months.

The theory behind the effectiveness of clean intermittent self-catheterization is the physiologic capacity of the bladder to hold approximately 500 mL. When the amount goes over 500 mL, two problems can occur: (1) blood flow to the bladder is decreased, lowering the defense mechanism of the bladder wall, and (2) bacteria present in the urine multiply rapidly. The longer that contaminated urine is allowed to stay in the bladder, the higher the bacteria count. Consequently, the natural defense mechanism of the bladder wall is decreased as urine volume increases. For this reason, patients should be taught the importance of regular and complete bladder emptying in order to prevent recurrent urinary tract infections.

It is important for the patient to understand the necessity of learning the procedure and that the desired results will not occur without compliance. In order for a self-catheterization program to succeed, the patient must value self-care and be willing to overcome certain fears. Table 30–9 provides nursing guidelines for clean intermittent self-catheterization.

NURSING PROCESS
Indwelling Catheters

Assessment

Review the patient's history and the results of any diagnostic studies completed. Monitor the patient's fluid intake and output. Note conditions that would contraindicate increased fluid intake, such as congestive heart failure or renal failure. Assess the patency of the catheter. Check the color, amount, and odor of the urine. Check vital signs routinely, being alert to an elevated temperature. Check the results of the laboratory data to assess the white blood cell count for indications of infection. Assess patient for chills, back pain, suprapubic pain, and burning with urination.

Nursing Diagnoses and Planning

The nursing diagnosis and related expected patient outcomes most commonly applicable to patients with indwelling catheters are as follows:

NDx: Risk for infection related to catheter and lack of appropriate perineal hygiene

Planning: Patient Outcomes
1. Patient has negative results on urine cultures.
2. Patient remains afebrile.
3. Signs and symptoms of infection, such as burning or pain, cloudy urine, or a discharge, are absent.
4. Patient's white blood cell count is within normal limits.

Nursing Interventions and Evaluation

NDx: Risk for infection
Monitor vital signs every 4 hours, and report temperature elevations. Maintain the patient's fluid intake at 2500 mL or more per day unless contraindicated. Observe the patient's urine for signs and symptoms of urinary tract infection, such as cloudy or very turbid urine. Wash your hands prior to each contact with the patient. Use gloves as necessary. Use aseptic technique when cleansing around the catheter. Maintain the patency of the catheter and tubing. Do not raise the catheter above the level of the bladder, because this allows urine to run back into the bladder. Monitor the results of complete blood cell counts, and report any abnormalities to the physician. Collect cultures as ordered, and note any abnormalities. Teach the patient and family the interventions necessary to prevent infection (see Table 30–8).

Compare the patient's status with the expected outcomes. If the outcomes are not met, reassess the patient and revise the plan.

Medications

Many urologic problems can be treated nonsurgically with a variety of medications, singly or in combinations. The approach to infections of the uri-

Table 30–9

Nursing Guidelines for Clean Intermittent Self-Catheterization (CISC)

Provide all teaching in a private and comfortable environment.

Review the individual's need for the procedure and history.

Individualize the teaching plan based on the assessment of the individual's needs.

Select the appropriate catheter for the individual based on sex, ability to move, individual requirements, and preference.

Explain the procedure.

Describe the basic location of anatomic structures.

Encourage the visualization of anatomic structures.

Utilize a mirror with female patients.

Be aware that the individuals may not know how to view their genital organs and may have many reservations and concerns about their anatomy.

Describe hand-washing techniques necessary prior to insertion.

Explain the need for some individuals to utilize clean gloves, specifically health care professionals and those persons who are immunosuppressed, have genital lesions, or are in long-term care facilities.

Describe the need for a water-soluble lubricant to increase the ease of insertion. (Note that water may be substituted in an emergency situation.)

Demonstrate the insertion procedure with a mannequin, or have the patient view a video on the procedure.

Encourage the patient to become familiar with the equipment.

Clarify any misconceptions and questions.

Assess the individual readiness to perform CISC.

Talk the individual through the procedure, assisting him or her as needed.

For women, explain that insertion is in an upward direction toward the umbilicus. If there is a vaginal prolapse, it may be necessary to perform the procedure in a recumbent position or utilize a vaginal pessary.

For the men, instruct them to hold the penis by the sides, perpendicular to the body, in order to facilitate the passage of the catheter. If there is resistance at the level of the prostate, one can utilize deep breathing or relaxation exercises, or it may require the use of a coudé-tip (bent stiff tip that does not bend against an obstacle) catheter to facilitate the catheterization.

Explain how to perform the Credé maneuver to facilitate complete bladder emptying.

Correct errors, while remembering to encourage and praise the patient's progress.

Explain how to clamp or stop the drainage of urine if it exceeds 500 mL in the first few minutes.

Review the individual's catheterization schedule.

Discuss the need to monitor fluid intake and output.

Describe the importance of assessing the urine output, specifically the color, clarity, amount, and odor.

Emphasize the importance of performing CISC on schedule rather than just when convenient.

Explain how CISC can be performed in public facilities.

Explain alternative means to performing CISC when in a public bathroom. For example, women can perform the CISC while standing up with one foot on the toilet seat to maintain balance, utilizing as clean a technique as possible.

Describe cleansing regimens for the daily care of the catheter. Simple cleansing with soap and water after each use is sufficient; along with soaking the catheter in a solution of half-strength white vinegar and water overnight once per week to clean out exudate and decrease odors.

Discuss the appropriate storage of the catheter in a clean, closed container. Catheters may be stored in any closed container and reused for 4–6 weeks, after which time they are discarded. Catheters with cracks should be discarded.

---

nary tract is either to employ broad-spectrum antibiotics or to use genitourinary-specific antibacterials. In some instances, urinary acidifiers are used to lower the pH of the patient's urine and to control bacterial growth.

Pharmacologic management of dysfunctional voiding is often successful in correcting or improving problems associated with urine storage and bladder emptying. Drugs used to treat these problems act by either blocking, modifying, or mimicking substances that influence lower urinary tract function. These substances include acetylcholine, norepinephrine, histamine, dopamine, the prostaglandins, 5-hydroxytryptamine, and kinins.

For patients with recurrent urolithiasis, medications are prescribed to reduce stone formation. The specific agent used depends on where in the urinary tract the stone was formed as well as its composition.

The goal of drug therapy in acute and chronic renal failure is to maintain fluid and electrolyte balance and ultimately to minimize complications. However, in some situations, drugs are used to prevent or limit the degree of renal failure.

Bladder irrigants are helpful in treating some urologic problems. Irrigants are especially useful for administering medications locally. Using either intermittent or continuous delivery of an irrigant solution permits fluid to flow into and out of the urinary tract without systemic absorption.

Many chemotherapeutic agents used to treat other malignancies are also used to treat urinary carcinomas. One group of chemotherapeutic agents unique to the management of urologic tumors is the intravesical drug category. These drugs are used to treat superficial bladder tumors. These preparations are instilled directly into the bladder through a catheter and offer direct treatment of lesions without the systemic side effects associated with other medications.

For more information on the medications used in the management of urinary disorders, see the discussions of specific disorders in Chapter 31.

Self-Care Measures

Nursing care of patients with urinary problems focuses heavily on teaching patients how to care for themselves. Self-catheterization, discussed previously, is one such self-care measure. Others include Credé voiding, Kegel exercises, bladder drills, and trigger voiding.

CREDÉ OR VALSALVA VOIDING

The purpose of Credé and Valsalva voiding is to aid in the passage of urine out of the bladder. In Credé voiding, a gentle downward massage is applied to the bladder during and after urination. A variation of Credé voiding involves rocking back and forth while sitting on the toilet.

In Valsalva voiding the patient is instructed to bear down as in defecation. However, Valsalva voiding is not recommended for patients with cardiac problems or elderly patients in poor health because this maneuver stimulates the vagus nerve and slows the heart rate.

KEGEL OR PELVIC FLOOR EXERCISES

Kegel exercises (also called pelvic floor exercises) were first developed in the early 1950s for women with simple stress incontinence to help them to control involuntary loss of urine. These exercises are aimed at first identifying and then strengthening the muscles of the pelvic floor. The technique has proved to be effective both for women with stress incontinence and for some men after prostate surgery. Learning the technique is rather simple. For patient instructions, see Highlight 30–2.

For women, a perineometer is used to measure the patient's ability to contract the appropriate muscles. Another way to assess for successful muscle contraction is to insert one gloved finger into the vagina and instruct the patient to tighten as if holding urine back. This also reinforces for the patient which muscles to contract when practicing the procedure.

Although there is some disagreement about how often to practice Kegel exercises, it is usually recommended that the exercises be repeated several times per day. The patient should therefore practice them whenever urination occurs and at other times

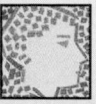

Phase I

Instruct the patient to:

Sit or stand with legs apart.

Pull up the rectum, vagina, and urethra.

Hold the muscles in this position for 4–5 sec.

Repeat the exercises 5 or 6 times, gradually increasing the number of times. (As the muscle strengthens, the individual will be able to do 25 or more exercises at one time.)

Repeat the exercise several times a day, increasing the total number to 200 times.

Exercise while driving, sitting at a desk, or watching television.

Phase II

Instruct the patient to:

Sit on the toilet and start to urinate.

Stop the urine flow by pulling up and tightening the rectum, vagina, and urethra.

Hold this position for 4–5 sec.

Release the muscles and start the stream again.

Repeat the exercise 5 or 6 times with each urination.

throughout the day. Kegel exercises are highly successful when performed on a regular basis. The combination of Kegel exercises and the administration of local or topical estrogen has been helpful for many postmenopausal women with stress incontinence.

BLADDER DRILLS

Bladder drills are also referred to as bladder training. They are designed to help patients regain urinary control through routine scheduling. Bladder drills require the cooperation of both the care provider and the patient. The patient's intake of oral fluids should be up to 2000 to 3000 mL unless otherwise contraindicated. Natural diuretics such as caffeine products and alcohol are to be avoided. The patient is taught to follow a routine voiding pattern, as described in Highlight 30–3. High levels of success are achieved when the plan is individualized, when all participants are motivated in working

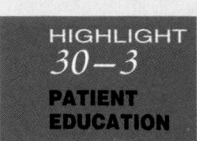
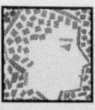

HIGHLIGHT 30–3
PATIENT EDUCATION
Bladder Drills

Instruct the patient to:

Increase oral fluid intake. Encourage the patient to drink up to 200–300 mL of fluids per day unless otherwise medically contraindicated. Tell the patient to avoid natural diuretics such as caffeine products and alcohol.

Establish a voiding pattern. Tell the patient to attempt to urinate every 2 hours, and keep a record of the time and amount. Also note whether the patient was incontinent prior to the voiding time.

Begin the voiding schedule. Start when the patient awakens in the morning. Have the patient void at that time and then every 2 hours throughout the day, extending the time to every 3 to 4 hours at night.

Lengthen the schedule. As the patient is able to halt periods of incontinence, lengthen the time between voidings by 30 minutes until the patient is toileting every 3 to 4 hours throughout the day.

Monitor fluid intake and output. Throughout the process, check the patient's fluid intake and measure the output. Note inadequacies in either measurement.

Reward efforts to comply with the schedule. Give positive reinforcement to the patient for compliance with the routine, and ignore periods of incontinence. The plan needs to be individualized and advanced as the patient progresses.

toward a specific goal, and when the fluid intake and output are considered to be adequate.

TRIGGER VOIDING

For generations, parents trying to toilet-train toddlers have used the simple trigger technique of turning on a water faucet to try to trigger voiding in the child. Likewise, a variety of techniques may be employed to stimulate voiding on cue in patients experiencing difficulty in starting urination. Among the techniques used are the following methods:

- Stroking the inner thighs or abdomen
- Gently pulling on the pubic hair
- Using the Credé method
- Tapping over the symphysis pubis (suprapubic tapping)
- Putting oil of wintergreen in the bedpan of a bedridden client

- Using an alarm clock or timer (enuresis alarm systems)
- Running tap water
- Dipping the hands in warm water
- Pouring warm water over the perineum

Individualized assessment is necessary to determine which trigger mechanism is most effective for each particular patient.

Diet Therapy

Management of the patient with a urinary tract disorder usually includes some dietary modifications. For the patient with chronic renal failure, diet therapy is directed toward control of edema and malnutrition by monitoring intake of protein, sodium, potassium, and water. The objectives of diet therapy for patients with chronic renal failure are described in Highlight 30–4. These objectives are achieved by providing a low-sodium, low-potassium, low-protein, high-carbohydrate diet.

Patients predisposed to urinary calculi may also benefit from a change in diet. The most common

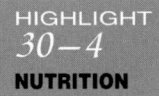
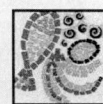

HIGHLIGHT 30–4
NUTRITION
Objectives of Diet Therapy for Patients with Chronic Renal Failure

For the patient with chronic renal failure, diet therapy is directed toward control of edema and malnutrition by monitoring protein, sodium, potassium, and water intake. The overall treatment plan has the following six objectives:

Minimize protein catabolism.

Avoid overhydration or dehydration.

Maintain acid-base balance by correcting or preventing acidosis.

Correct electrolyte depletions and avoid excesses.

Control fluid and electrolyte losses from vomiting and diarrhea.

Maintain nutritional intake and weight appropriate for the patient.

The above objectives are achieved by providing a low-sodium, low-potassium, low-protein, and high-carbohydrate diet. The patient is carefully monitored for problems. Medications are used as adjunct therapy to correct or prevent episodes of vomiting and diarrhea and to maintain acid-base balance.

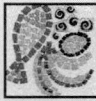

HIGHLIGHT
30-5
NUTRITION

Calcium-Containing Foods

Instruct the patient predisposed to calcium oxalate urinary calculus formation to consult the physician regarding increased intake of calcium-containing foods. The following are calcium-containing foods that can be recommended:

- Dairy products
- Green leafy vegetables
- Whole grains

type of calculus is composed of calcium oxalate. Researchers from Harvard School of Public Health have found that a diet with increased calcium intake was associated with a decreased risk of urinary calculi. A high intake of animal protein has been associated with an increased risk of urinary calculi. Therefore, foods high in calcium may be recommended for patients with urolithiasis (Highlight 30–5). In addition to these dietary restrictions, encourage patients to practice high-volume fluid flushing by drinking up to 3000 to 4000 mL per day (except in the presence of cardiac or renal complications). A high oral fluid intake, followed by bladder emptying every 2 hours, is important regardless of the composition of the patient's urinary stone.

For patients requiring catheterization or those with recurrent urinary tract infections, dietary modifications to acidify the urine are recommended. This is because a lower urinary pH is known to decrease the rate of multiplication of bacteria. Advise these patients to consume foods such as meat, nuts, prunes, plums, cranberries, and whole-grain cereals and breads. On the contrary, these patients should avoid large quantities of milk, fruits, and vegetables because they produce a more alkaline urine. Discourage the intake of caffeine, carbonated beverages, and alcohol. The exception to these restrictions is for patients taking sulfonamides, which require an alkaline urine for maximum effectiveness.

Additional Treatment Options

Urinary continence in women may be assisted by the use of a vaginal ring, pessary, or tampon. These are nonsurgical treatment options that temporarily reposition the bladder and vaginal walls.

Transurethral injection of Teflon for urinary incontinence has been available for more than 20 years but has only recently come to the attention of health care consumers. The 20- to 30-minute procedure creates a bulge in the urethra, thus blocking the leak-

age of the urine. Currently considered experimental, Teflon injections are performed only by specially trained physicians.

SURGICAL MANAGEMENT

One treatment option that is still considered experimental is the implantation of an artificial sphincter for patients with urinary incontinence (Fig. 30–8). This option involves the implantation of a hydraulic pump mechanism that contains a reservoir, a urethral cuff encircling the bladder neck, and a control pump. Inflation of the urethral cuff prevents leakage of urine. Deflation of the cuff by squeezing the control pump implanted in the scrotum in men enables the patient to urinate. The cuff automatically reinflates after urination.

Other surgical interventions for urinary tract disorders are specific to each disorder and thus are discussed with the appropriate problem in Chapter 31.

❖ Settings, Providers, and Collaboration for Care

People with urologic dysfunction may be assessed, diagnosed, and treated in inpatient or outpatient settings, depending on the nature of the tests and the findings. Because of the clinical manifestations of urologic dysfunction, such as severe pain or anuria, some patients may be admitted to a hospital for initial treatment. Once the dysfunction has been diagnosed, acute problems (and surgery) are managed

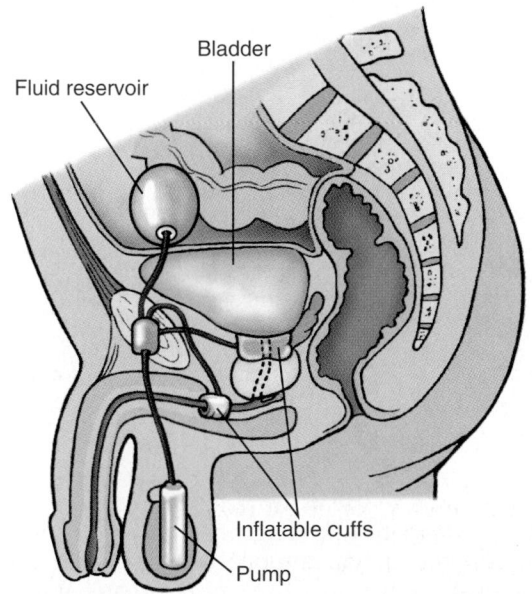

Figure 30–8

Artificial urinary sphincter.

in the hospital. However, once the patient is stable, discharge to the home is likely. If the patient still needs medical intervention, continued visits to the physician's office or to a clinic are likely. In some cases, especially when the patient must have an indwelling catheter for treatment or needs to perform self-intermittent catheterization, a home health nurse visits the patient to assess progress and to provide additional education.

The Elderly: Special Considerations

Common diseases that may produce some form of urinary tract dysfunction in the elderly include dementia, diabetes, neuropathy, Parkinson's disease, and cerebrovascular accident. Urinary incontinence may also be secondary to conditions such as fecal impaction and prostatic hyperplasia. In addition, older adults may develop urinary incontinence secondary to the effects of medications. Drugs that may cause or contribute to incontinence include hypnotics, loop diuretics, adrenergic agents, calcium channel blockers, and drugs containing anticholinergics, such as antidepressants, antihistamines, antipsychotics, and belladonna alkaloids.

In older adults there is a decrease in the muscle tone of the bladder and urethra, which causes the bladder to empty less efficiently. This age-related change may cause urinary retention and a predisposition to urinary infections. Older adults are also at risk of developing urinary incontinence because of the following age-related changes:

- Diminished bladder capacity
- Bladder contractions during filling
- Incomplete bladder emptying
- Urinary urgency and frequency
- Relaxation of the pelvic floor muscles

Additional age-related changes that affect urinary elimination include delayed excretion of water-soluble medications and decreased efficiency of homeostatic mechanisms.

Postmenopausal estrogen depletion leads to weakening of the pelvic floor muscles and atrophy of the vaginal and trigonal tissue. These changes contribute to the increased incidence of urinary incontinence and urinary tract infections in the elderly. Urethral, vaginal, and uterine prolapse are conditions that may occur in older women, producing urinary retention and restricting the flow of urine. The most common problem associated with these conditions is pain during urination. Check to determine whether a discharge is present during urination or is evident around the meatus. Ask the patient to describe the discharge by color and odor. Determine the usual amount of fluids that the patient ingests daily and the approximate amount of urinary output.

Chapter Review

1. Why is the assessment of urine volume in acute renal failure an important nursing function?
2. How can pain within the urinary tract best be assessed?
3. Compare and contrast the importance of a serum creatinine and BUN as diagnostic studies for patients with urinary tract dysfunction.
4. What patient outcomes signal normal urinary elimination following a cystoscopy?
5. What teaching guidelines could you offer to a homebound patient with an indwelling catheter?
6. What are the possible solutions to the prevention of urinary tract infection?
7. Why is nutrition important when planning the care of the patient with chronic renal failure?
8. How do age-related problems affect the care of an elderly patient with a urinary tract disorder?
9. What would happen to the distal tubule and collecting ducts if the ADH were inappropriately secreted?
10. What are the advantages of home health care to a patient with urinary tract dysfunction?

Bibliography

Agency for Health Care Policy and Research. Clinical practice guidelines: Urinary incontinence in adults. AHCPR No. 0038. Rockville, MD: Author, 1992.

Bager M, Woolner B. Primary care for women—assessment and management of genitourinary tract disorders. J Nurse Midwife 1995; 40(2):231.

Bernal H. A model for delivering culture-relevant care in the community. Public Health Nurs 1993; 10(4):228.

Brazier AM, Palmer MH. Collecting clean-catch urine in the nursing home—obtaining the uncontaminated specimen. Geriatr Nurs 1995; 16(5):217.

Burman ME. Health diaries in nursing research and practice. Image J Nurs Sch 1995; 27(2):147.

Colling JC, Owen TR, McCreedy MR. Urine volumes and patterns among incontinent nursing home residents. Geriatr Nurs 1994; 15(4):188.

Criner JA. A nursing management protocol for incontinence. Rehabil Nurs 1994; 19(3):141.

Gill HS. Home care's place within an integrated delivery system. The Journal of Care Management 1995; 1(3):17.

Goldberg J. Preventing kidney stones, a new track. PEN pages. Washington Post Writers Group, 1993.

Helbert JL. Use of home care nursing resources by the elderly. Public Health Nurs 1993; 11(2):104.

Higgins C. Measuring renal function with urea and creatinine tests. Nurs Times 1994; 90(51):35.

Kammerer JK. Case study of the anemic patient: Epoetin alfa—focus on CQI and patient management. ANNA J 1994; 21(5):282.

Kee JL. Laboratory and diagnostic tests with nursing implications. 4th ed. Norwalk, CT: Appleton & Lange, 1995.

Kirkis, EJ. Home health/public health/visiting nurse return to our past. Home Healthc Nurse 1993; 11(5):9.

Kohler-Ockmore J. Catheter concerns. Nurs Times 1993; 89(2):34.

Langley T. Continence: Assessing knowledge. Nurs Times 1994; 90(36):74.

Lowe FC, Brendler CB. Evaluation of the urologic patient: History, physical examination, and urinalysis. In Walsh PC, Retik AB, Stamey TA, Vaughan ED (eds). Campbell's urology. 6th ed, Vol 1. Philadelphia: WB Saunders, 1992, pp 307–331.

Lutumba NA, St-Laurent L, Tanguay C. Urinary incontinence and long-term care. Can Nurse 1995; 91(3):46.

Malone-Rising D. The changing face of long-term care. Nurs Clin North Am 1994; 29(3);417.

McCaffery M. Pain control: Keeping current. Nursing 1994; 24(6): 51.

McDowell BJ. Care of urinary incontinence in the home. Nurse Pract Forum 1994; 5(3):138.

McDowell BJ, Engberg S, Weber E, et al. Successful treatment using behavioral interventions of urinary incontinence in homebound older adults. Geriatr Nurs 1994; 15(6):303.

Miller CA. Medications can cause or treat urinary incontinence. Geriatr Nurs 1995; 16(5):253.

Neary, MA. Community services in the 1990's: Are they meeting the needs of the care givers? J Community Health Nurs 1993; 10(2):105.

Palmer M, Level I: Basic assessment and management of urinary incontinence in nursing homes. Nurse Pract Forum 1994; 5(3): 152.

Penn C, Lekan-Rutledge D, Joers AM, et al. Assessment of urinary incontinence. Journal of Gerontological Nursing 1996; 22 (1):8.

Russell K, Jewell N. Cultural impact of health-care access: Challenges for improving the health of African Americans. J Community Health Nurs 1992; 9(3):161.

Stark JL. Interpreting B.U.N./Creatinine levels. Nursing 1994; 24(9):58.

Thobaben M, Mattingly HJ. Cultural sensitivity: Educating home healthcare nurses to be transcultural nurses. Home Healthc Nurse 1993; 11(4):61.

Warren JW. Catheter associated bacteriuria in long-term care facilities. Infect Control Hosp Epidemiol 1994; 15(8):557.

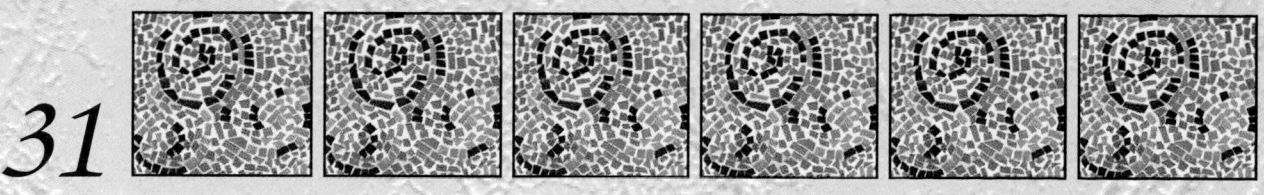

31

Nursing Care of Patients with Urinary Disorders

Study Outcomes

After studying this chapter, you should be able to:

1. Describe common urinary disorders in terms of their etiology, pathophysiology, clinical manifestations, diagnosis, and management.
2. Identify common pharmacologic agents used to treat urinary disorders.
3. Explain the effects of acute and chronic renal failure.
4. Describe the health teaching appropriate for the patient who is at risk for urinary tract infection.
5. Identify physical examination data and other information essential to the assessment of patients with common urinary tract disorders.
6. State nursing diagnoses and related expected patient outcomes commonly applicable to patients with urinary tract disorders.
7. Describe nursing interventions, with their rationales, commonly applicable to patients with urinary tract disorders.
8. Explain the basis for evaluation of nursing care provided to patients with common urinary tract disorders.
9. Identify special considerations for the elderly patient with a urinary tract disorder.
10. Identify alternative treatments, care settings, and community-based services for patients with urinary tract disorders.

Urinary tract disorders are some of the most common health problems in adults. These disorders are not often life-threatening. Nevertheless, morbidity from urinary tract problems is still a threat, especially when the kidney is damaged. The urinary system helps the body to maintain homeostasis through fluid and electrolyte balance. Therefore, disorders of the urinary system have a profound effect on the entire body.

Patients with disorders of the urinary system may be hospitalized for treatment. They may also be treated as outpatients in clinics or even in the home. As hospitals stays become shorter, more patients will be discharged with indwelling catheters and dressings. These patients will need continued treatment in the home or other settings.

*I*nfections and Inflammations

The most common urologic disorders are infections and inflammations. These disorders account for about three-quarters of urologic consultations and almost half of nosocomial infections are urinary tract infections (UTIs).

By definition, an infection exists in the urinary tract when specific microorganisms can be identified through urine culture. To meet the definition of a UTI, there must be more than 10^5 (100,000) organisms per milliliter in a clean-catch urine specimen. Clinicians describe UTIs in relation to the anatomic area involved. For example, cystitis is an infection of the bladder. Urethritis is an infection of the urethra. Pyelonephritis is an infection of the kidney itself.

Most infections and inflammations of the urinary tract are treated in outpatient settings, such as the physician's office. Rarely, however, if a patient has complicating problems or has glomerulonephritis, hospitalization may be necessary.

CYSTITIS

Etiology and Pathophysiology

Cystitis is inflammation of the bladder. It usually results from the invasion of bacteria into the urinary tract. In women, bacteria that enter the urinary tract usually originate from either the rectum or the vagina and ascend upward via the urethra. In men, cystitis is usually the result of another problem in the urinary tract, such as prostatitis or benign prostatic hyperplasia.

Cystitis is more common in women than in men. Up to one-fourth of women experience the problem at least once in their lifetime. This is because of the length of the urethra (2.5 to 4 cm, or 1 to 1.5 inches) and the proximity of the urethral meatus to the vagina and rectum in women. Cystitis can occur following medical procedures involving the urinary tract ("instrumentation"). Or, it can be result from incomplete bladder emptying. Cystitis is also associ-

~~ated with sexual intercourse and pregnancy.~~ In some instances, cystitis develops when bacteria travel to the bladder via the vascular or lymphatic systems from a site elsewhere in the body.

When bacteria enter the bladder, they adhere to and multiply in the bladder's mucosal surface. As the infection intensifies, the surface of the bladder becomes reddened and edematous. Areas of ulceration may also develop. Pain and urinary urgency result when urine comes in contact with the irritated surface of the bladder. This irritation worsens when the bladder becomes even slightly distended with urine.

Clinical Manifestations

The patient with cystitis usually presents with one or more of the following symptoms: dysuria, frequency, urgency, nocturia, nocturnal enuresis, incontinence, urethral pain, low back pain, suprapubic pain, and fever. The patient may also describe episodes of painful straining that are ineffective in producing urine, called tenesmus. Hematuria sometimes occurs in the patient with cystitis. The urine often has a strong odor.

Diagnosis

Although the patient history and presenting symptoms are helpful in making a diagnosis, the urine culture confirms the presence of an infection in the bladder. A urine culture that grows more than 100,000 colonies of bacteria per milliliter of urine documents the existence of an infection. A complete blood count with differential shows an elevated white blood cell count with a "shift to the left." This shift indicates that there is an increase in the number of immature white blood cells, which would be a response to the infection. When the colony count is less than 100,000, additional studies, such as intravenous pyelography and cystoscopy, may be needed. The findings of these studies would then be correlated with other data to make the diagnosis. In patients with cystitis, intravenous pyelography, computed tomography (CT), and ultrasonography may provide evidence of obstruction.

Management

Patients with uncomplicated, acute cystitis are usually treated with an antimicrobial agent. The specific medication to be used is determined by sensitivity testing for the bacteria found growing in the urine. Those most commonly prescribed include ampicillin, amoxicillin, trimethoprim-sulfamethoxazole, and sulfisoxazole. In most instances of acute cystitis, patients are treated for 7 to 10 days. However, some studies suggest that 1-day therapy, or even single-dose therapy, is equally effective in women with acute, uncomplicated cystitis. For patients with chronic recurrent cystitis, antimicrobial therapy may be required for several months. Analgesics, urinary antiseptics, and anticholinergics are also used to treat the pain and bladder spasms that often accompany UTIs. Highlight 31–1 describes measures for prevention of UTIs.

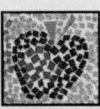

HIGHLIGHT
31–1

HEALTH PROMOTION & RISK REDUCTION

Self-Care for Prevention of Urinary Tract Infections

Instruct the patient to:

Drink 2 to 3 L of fluid daily.

Notify the physician if urgency, frequency, burning, or difficulty in urinating is experienced.

Empty the bladder as soon as the urge is felt.

Clean the perineum from front to back (women only).

Avoid irritating substances such as bubble bath, nylon underwear, and scented toilet paper (women only).

Wear cotton underwear.

Take all of medication, even after symptoms subside, to prevent recurring infections.

Schedule a follow-up visit with the physician to have a repeat urine culture.

~~Empty the bladder following sexual intercourse.~~

NURSING PROCESS
Cystitis

Assessment

Obtain a health history, including a review of the patient's current status and symptoms. Assess for uropenia (diminished urine output), hesitancy, frequency, and dysuria. Ask about voiding patterns. Obtain information about the color and odor of the urine. Ask whether there is any blood or mucus in the urine. Ask the patient to describe any pain or discomfort that has occurred. Because medical treatment most often involves the administration of an antimicrobial agent, also ask the patient about any drug allergies or sensitivities.

Inspect the lower abdomen and the meatus to determine whether tissues are inflamed. Palpate the urinary bladder for distention or pain.

Review the patient's daily hygiene and dietary practices. Discuss activities that may predispose the patient to cystitis. Ask whether symptoms began after sexual intercourse. Check whether the patient frequently takes bubble baths. Note whether the patient wears tight-fitting blue jeans. Ask whether the patient is able to empty the bladder at regular intervals, or whether voiding is often delayed for several hours. The answers to these questions are extremely important and help in developing a teaching plan aimed at preventing recurrence.

Assess the patient's level of knowledge about the disorder and the treatment and care needed. Note the patient's questions and concerns. Invite the family to participate when appropriate. Assess their level of knowledge about the condition.

Nursing Diagnoses and Planning

Nursing diagnoses and related expected patient outcomes most commonly applicable to patients with cystitis include the following:

NDx: Altered urinary elimination related to inflammation and irritation

Planning: Patient Outcomes
1. Patient adheres to established voiding schedule.
2. Patient reports relief of irritating voiding symptoms.
3. Patient resumes normal voiding pattern.

NDx: Pain related to inflammation and irritation

Planning: Patient Outcomes
1. Patient reports comfort and pain relief.
2. Patient is able to void without pain or burning.

NDx: Knowledge deficit: factors that may predispose to cystitis or treatment regimen

Planning: Patient Outcomes
1. Patient lists factors that predispose to cystitis.
2. Patient describes medical and dietary regimen.
3. Patient verbalizes measures to prevent cystitis.

Nursing Interventions and Evaluation

NDx: Altered urinary elimination
Nursing intervention for the patient with cystitis includes measures to alleviate the irritative voiding symptoms. Administer antimicrobial medications as ordered to sterilize the urine. Administer antispasmodics or analgesics as ordered to relieve the accompanying suprapubic discomfort brought on by bladder spasms. Encourage increased fluid intake of up to 3000 mL per day (unless contraindicated for other medical reasons) because dilute urine lessens the irritation to the bladder mucosa.

Often, a patient delays voiding because of the pain and discomfort brought on by urination. Encourage voiding at regular intervals. Frequent bladder emptying decreases intravesical irritation and prevents stasis of urine.

NDx: Pain
Administer analgesics and antispasmodics as ordered. Offer a warm sitz bath to relieve perineal or suprapubic discomfort. Sitz baths may be performed two to three times per day. Encourage the patient to drink 2 to 3 L of fluid per day.

NDx: Knowledge deficit: factors that may predispose to cystitis or treatment regimen
Incorporate information about the dosage and potential side effects of the medication prescribed. Remind the patient to complete the entire course of therapy even though symptoms have subsided. Instruct the patient to drink 2 to 3 L of fluid per day and to obtain adequate rest and nutrition. Review the patient's hygiene practices. Most importantly, teach the patient activities that help to prevent a recurrence of the cystitis. For example, if the patient's bladder infection occurred after sexual intercourse, teach the patient to void immediately after coitus. Similarly, if the patient experiences irritating voiding symptoms after taking a tub bath, encourage showering to prevent the ascent of bacteria into the urinary tract from the bath water. Teach the patient to recognize the symptoms of UTIs and to report these symptoms promptly (see Highlight 31–1). Explain the diagnostic studies completed and the need for any follow-up studies after discharge. Include the family in any of the teaching sessions when applicable.

Compare the patient's status with the expected outcomes. If the outcomes are not met, reassess the patient and revise the plan.

URETHRITIS

Etiology and Pathophysiology
Urethritis is an inflammation of the urethra. The patient presents with signs and symptoms similar to those of cystitis. Urethritis can be acute or chronic.

Urethritis occurs in both men and women. In men the most common cause is gonorrhea. Urethritis is often associated with sexually transmitted disease. Some of the organisms commonly associated with urethritis are *Ureaplasma, Chlamydia,* and *Trichomonas vaginalis.* Urethritis can also be caused by irritants such as soaps, perfumed toilet paper and sanitary napkins, and bubble baths.

Clinical Manifestations
The patient with urethritis presents with burning, frequency, and nocturia. There may be difficulty with urination. Men with urethritis usually have a discharge from the urethral meatus, but women do not. Patients of both sexes often complain of lower abdominal discomfort.

Diagnosis
The diagnosis of urethritis is based on the patient's history and current complaints. Examination of the urine may reveal pus or bacteria. If pyuria (pus in the urine) is found without significant bacteria, the patient should be examined for an infection elsewhere in the urinary tract.

Management
If the urethritis is caused by bacterial invasion, the patient is treated with systemic or topical antibiotics, or both. If it is caused by an irritant, the irritant should be removed. The patient is encouraged to avoid factors that can contribute to the problem. A high fluid intake and sitz baths are also encouraged.

NURSING PROCESS GUIDELINES
Urethritis

The assessment, nursing diagnoses, expected patient outcomes, nursing interventions, and evaluation for patients with urethritis are similar to those described previously for patients with cystitis.

PYELONEPHRITIS

Etiology and Pathophysiology
Pyelonephritis is an infection of the upper urinary tract that produces pain and edema in the kidney, renal pelvis, and surrounding structures. Its onset is usually acute, with symptoms that are often mistaken for those of back strain. ~~It can become chronic, resulting in hypertension and uremia in some patients. Pyelonephritis is the original diagnosis in one-third of patients with renal failure.~~

The most common cause of pyelonephritis is reflux of infected urine from the bladder to the upper urinary tract. However, stasis of urine in the system as a result of obstruction can also lead to pyelonephritis.

Patients at risk of developing pyelonephritis fall into the following categories:

Those who have undergone recent instrumentation of the urinary tract
Those with diabetes mellitus
Those with a history of analgesic abuse
Those with voiding disorders associated with incomplete bladder emptying; elderly patients and pregnant women are also susceptible

The bacteria contaminating the urinary tract in pyelonephritis are usually the normal flora found in feces. Once these microorganisms enter the urinary tract, they adhere to and multiply in uroepithelial tissue. An *Escherichia coli* infection is the most common form of pyelonephritis, although pyelonephritis caused by *Proteus, Pseudomonas, Enterobacter, Klebsiella,* enterococci, *Serratia, Morganella,* and *Staphylococcus* is not uncommon.

Clinical Manifestations
The patient with acute pyelonephritis complains of a persistent ache in the flank or back, cystitis-like symptoms, fever with chills, and general malaise accompanied by nausea, vomiting, and diarrhea. Upon examination, there may be tenderness in the area of the costovertebral angle and an elevated pulse rate, as well as pus, bacteria, and white cell casts in the urine. Patients with chronic pyelonephritis are usually asymptomatic, except for some vague and intermittent flank pain, an occasionally elevated temperature, and evidence of persistent, unresolved bacteriuria.

Diagnosis
The diagnosis of pyelonephritis is based primarily on the patient's history, physical examination, and findings from urinalysis, urine culture, blood count, and radiographic studies. A positive urine culture result and an elevated white blood cell count along with x-ray results that demonstrate changes in the appearance of the kidney and ureter consistent with a long-standing infection confirm the diagnosis.

Management
Once pyelonephritis has been diagnosed, oral or intravenous antibiotic therapy is immediately instituted and continued for at least 2 weeks. For patients with chronic pyelonephritis, intense antibiotic therapy may be required for as long as 6 months to clear the infection. Relief of symptoms includes aspirin for an elevated temperature, antiemetics to control nausea and vomiting, oral or intravenous fluids to prevent dehydration and increase urine output, pain medications and urinary antiseptics to relieve discomfort, and bedrest.

In some cases, surgery is performed to relieve obstruction or eradicate intractable infection. Stones could be removed by performing extracorporeal shock wave lithotripsy, percutaneous ultrasonic pyelolithotomy, or pyelotomy. Nephrectomy could be performed, as a last resort, to eradicate infection. The care of the patient undergoing these procedures is discussed later in this chapter.

NURSING PROCESS
Pyelonephritis

Assessment

Review the patient's health history and medical management. It is important to note whether this is the first occurrence of pyelonephritis. Assess the patient for pain, malaise, fatigue, chills, and fever. Inspect the area of the costovertebral angle for asymmetry or swelling, which would indicate inflammation. Encourage the patient to feel free to talk about the signs and symptoms. Many patients feel embarrassed and anxious about discussing problems of the urinary tract.

Nursing Diagnoses and Planning

Nursing diagnoses and related expected patient outcomes most commonly applicable to patients with pyelonephritis include the following:

NDx: Pain related to inflammation and infection

Planning: Patient Outcomes
1. Patient verbalizes relief from pain.
2. Patient is able to resume usual activities of daily living.

NDx: Activity intolerance related to fatigue

Planning: Patient Outcomes
1. Patient follows a regimen of planned activities and rest periods each day.
2. Patient verbalizes feeling less fatigued and demonstrates signs of increased activity.

3. Patient is able to resume usual activities of daily living.

NDx: Knowledge deficit: nature of the medical diagnosis and treatment regimen

Planning: Patient Outcomes
1. Patient describes cause, effects, and clinical course of pyelonephritis.
2. Patient lists symptoms of pyelonephritis and treatment.
3. Patient states self-care needed to prevent recurrence or complications of pyelonephritis.

NDx: Fear related to the potential development of chronic renal failure

Planning: Patient Outcomes
1. Patient verbalizes fear relating to potential complications of diagnoses.
2. Patient states self-care needed to prevent recurrence or complications of pyelonephritis.

Nursing Interventions and Evaluation

NDx: Pain
Administer analgesics and antiseptics as ordered to relieve pain and discomfort. Administer antiemetics as ordered to alleviate nausea and vomiting. Assist the patient in achieving comfortable positions while on bedrest.

NDx: Activity intolerance
Encourage bedrest during the acute stages. Encourage the patient to do range-of-motion exercises frequently while lying in bed to maintain muscle tone and strength. As symptoms subside, instruct the patient in developing a regimen of activity with frequent rest periods throughout the day.

NDx: Knowledge deficit: nature of the medical diagnosis and treatment regimen
Explain the cause, effects, and clinical course of the disorder to the patient. Allow for questions from the patient at any time. Provide appropriate literature for the patient and family to review.

Alert the patient to signs and symptoms of pyelonephritis that should be attended to when they occur. Teach the patient measures to prevent UTIs. Stress the importance of balancing rest and activity. Instruct the patient to follow a balanced diet with increased fluid intake.

Teach the patient dosage, route, time, frequency, side effects, and toxic effects of any medication prescribed. When the patient suffers from chronic pyelonephritis, stress the importance of compliance with an extended medication regimen. Include the family in any of the teaching sessions when applicable.

NDx: Fear
Encourage the patient to verbalize feelings related to the disease. Discuss the patient's perception of the danger of developing renal failure. Provide information to reduce distortions. Assist the patient in the use of coping skills. Teach the patient measures to prevent the recurrence of pyelonephritis.

Compare the patient's status with the expected outcomes. If the outcomes are not met, reassess the patient and revise the plan.

PERINEPHRIC ABSCESS

Etiology and Pathophysiology
A perinephric abscess is a fluid-filled mass that forms outside the kidney but within its supportive tissue structures. It is associated with chronic upper UTIs, often causes necrosis to surrounding tissues, and usually occurs because of extravasation of infected urine. *E. coli, Pseudomonas,* and *Staphylococcus* are the most common causative organisms.

Clinical Manifestations
Signs and symptoms of a perinephric abscess are similar to those for pyelonephritis. A persistent fever despite the administration of antibiotics for a suspected upper UTI is considered characteristic. Additionally, palpation of a flank mass and observed edema of the skin over the affected area are possible. If the abscess is unusually large, other internal structures, such as the diaphragm and the spine, are displaced. Skin lesions also may erupt over the abscess if the infecting organism is *Staphylococcus.*

Diagnosis
The diagnosis is confirmed by radiologic examination. Ultrasonography or CT of the affected kidney are the procedures of choice. A kidney, ureter, and bladder x-ray examination and excretory urography may also be performed.

Management
Once the abscess has been detected and located, immediate percutaneous drainage is required. Antibiotic therapy is also necessary to prevent sepsis and further extension of the disease. Failure to intervene quickly once the diagnosis is made can result in the death of the patient because of sepsis. In some instances, surgical removal of the abscess and correction of an underlying urinary tract problem are necessary.

NURSING PROCESS GUIDELINES
Perinephric Abscess

The assessment, nursing diagnoses, expected patient outcomes, nursing interventions, and evaluation for patients with a perinephric abscess are similar to those described previously for patients with pyelonephritis. The assessment, nursing diagnoses, expected patient outcomes, nursing interventions, and evaluation for patients undergoing percutaneous drainage of the abscess are similar to those described previously for patients undergoing renal biopsy (see Chap. 30).

GLOMERULONEPHRITIS

Etiology and Pathophysiology

Glomerulonephritis is an inflammation of the kidney that affects the capillary loops in the glomeruli. Its onset is usually secondary to an infection of the upper respiratory tract, most commonly caused by beta-hemolytic streptococci. However, glomerulonephritis can be the result of a primary infection elsewhere in the body and be caused by staphylococci, pneumococci, or a virus (Table 31–1). Glomerulonephritis can occur at any age. It has a higher incidence in men than in women.

Glomerulonephritis is caused by an immunologic reaction. The antigen that initiates the process may be endogenous or exogenous. Endogenous antigens are believed to be already present in the glomerulus or other tissues of the body. Exogenous antigens are from infections occurring in the body. Because of the antigen-antibody response, glomerular injury occurs.

The antigen-antibody complexes are trapped within the glomerulus. This trapping produces an inflammatory response that damages the glomeruli. The glomeruli are unable to filter out the plasma proteins. They are instead spilled into the urine. As the inflammation persists, there is destruction of renal tissue, scarring, and hypertrophy, which impinges on unaffected tubules.

Clinical Manifestations

Patients with glomerulonephritis often present with a sore throat, an elevated temperature, microscopic hematuria, proteinuria, a decreased urinary output, swelling of the face and lower extremities, costovertebral angle tenderness, and flank pain likened to renal colic. As the disease progresses, the patient experiences shortness of breath, lethargy, and anorexia. Signs and symptoms of uremia may become evident. Hypertension often develops. The blood urea nitrogen and serum creatinine levels are elevated.

Diagnosis

The diagnosis of glomerulonephritis is based on findings from the patient's history, physical examination, and urinalysis. A renal biopsy may be performed to confirm the presence of glomerular inflammation.

Management

Glomerulonephritis is a serious condition that could lead to end-stage renal disease if not treated promptly. The goal of medical intervention is to treat the inflammation and accompanying symptoms in order to restore the kidney to normal function. Because the primary infecting organism is often beta-hemolytic streptococci, patients are generally treated with penicillin for 7 to 10 days. Salt restriction may be required to combat the associated edema and hypertension. Bedrest is essential during the acute phase of the disease process and may be necessary for a longer period of time, until renal function has stabilized and proteinuria and hematuria are no longer evident. The usual course of illness is 14 days. The proteinuria and hematuria may last several months. If symptoms do not subside within 2 years, the patient will more than likely be afflicted with chronic glomerulonephritis.

❖ Settings, Providers, and Collaboration for Care

Although the patient may be hospitalized for the diagnosis and early management of glomerulonephritis, most of the treatment is continued in the patient's home with scheduled visits to the physician's office for follow-up care and evaluation. Home health care referral may be necessary for chronic cases or for severe or complicated acute cases.

NURSING PROCESS
Glomerulonephritis

Assessment

Assess the patient with glomerulonephritis by checking the history and laboratory data. Then inquire about any previous infections. Of special interest would be a recent upper respiratory tract infection, skin infection, pericarditis, or lower UTI.

Next, evaluate the current status of the patient. Examine the patient for signs of renal failure, respiratory distress, circulatory congestion, and systemic infection. Also note the patient's nutritional status and current eating habits, the type and location of any pain, the appearance of the urine, and any physical limitations brought on by the associated weakness, lethargy, and fatigue.

Finally, review the laboratory values for quanti-

Table 31–1

Primary and Secondary Causes of Glomerulonephritis

Glomerulonephritis may occur as a primary disease, or it may result from a systemic disease. The following are types of glomerulonephritis that occur as a primary disease:

- Acute glomerulonephritis
- Chronic glomerulonephritis
- Focal glomerular sclerosis
- Idiopathic membranous glomerulonephritis
- Lipoid nephrosis
- Membranoproliferative glomerulonephritis
- Rapidly progressive glomerulonephritis

The following diseases may cause glomerulonephritis:

- Goodpasture's syndrome
- Hemolytic-uremic syndrome
- Henoch-Schönlein syndrome
- Polyarteritis nodosa
- Progressive systemic sclerosis
- Renal failure
- Systemic lupus erythematosus
- Thrombocytopenic purpura
- Wegener's granulomatosis

tative information from the urinalysis, complete blood cell count, and blood chemistry.

Nursing Diagnoses and Planning

Nursing diagnoses and related expected patient outcomes most commonly applicable to patients with glomerulonephritis include the following:

NDx: Activity intolerance related to fatigue, fluid volume excess, and loss of energy

Planning: Patient Outcomes
1. Patient follows a regimen of planned activities and rest period each day.
2. Patient verbalizes feeling less fatigued and demonstrates signs of increased activity.
3. Patient is able to resume usual activities of daily living.

NDx: Fluid volume excess related to decreased glomerular filtration rate

Planning: Patient Outcomes
1. Patient exhibits decreased edema.
2. Signs and symptoms of fluid overload are absent.
3. Patient demonstrates knowledge related to therapeutic regimen to decrease fluid.

NDx: Altered nutrition: less than body requirements related to anorexia, nausea, and vomiting

Planning: Patient Outcomes
1. Patient increases oral intake as evidenced by eating 75% of meals.
2. Patient describes the rationale and procedure for treatment.
3. Patient maintains desired weight.
4. Nausea and vomiting are absent.

Nursing Interventions and Evaluation

NDx: Activity intolerance
Assist the patient in maintenance of bedrest. This is important because there is a direct relationship between physical activity and the presence of proteinuria and hematuria. Even ambulation over a short distance must be restricted until the kidney has had time to heal and there is little or no protein and blood in the urine. Patient education and the encouragement of a caring nurse ensure compliance with this temporary but difficult alteration in the patient's activity level. As symptoms improve, instruct the patient in developing a regimen of activity with frequent rest periods throughout the day.

NDx: Fluid volume excess
Assess the patient frequently for signs and symptoms of fluid overload. Weigh the patient every morning. Monitor fluid intake and output. Instruct the patient in diet that is low in sodium. Assist the patient in coping with any fluid restriction that is ordered. Protect edematous skin from injury. Assess the patient's knowledge of diet and medical regimen. Instruct the patient as needed, including family when necessary.

NDx: Altered nutrition: less than body requirements
Explain to the patient the importance of consuming adequate amounts of nutrients. Monitor intake and output. Weigh the patient daily. Instruct him or her in the prescribed diet. If there is severe edema, hypertension, or oliguria, a low-protein, low-sodium diet with fluid restriction is ordered. Teach the patient to use spices to help improve the taste of food. Plan care so that unpleasant procedures do not take place before meals. Medicate the patient for pain or nausea 30 to 45 minutes before meals as ordered. Provide a pleasant, relaxed atmosphere for meals. Assist the patient in resting or relaxing before meals. Encourage small, frequent feedings. Provide good oral hygiene. Allow the patient to choose food items as much as possible. Encourage support from the family.

Compare the patient's status with the expected outcomes. If the outcomes are not met, reassess the patient and revise the plan.

Obstruction

Urinary tract obstruction can be defined as blockage of the normal glomerular filtrate flow anywhere along the urinary tract. Obstruction of the urinary tract poses serious pathophysiologic consequences for the renal parenchyma in the form of dilatation and thinning of the renal tubules with eventual atrophy of the renal substance itself.

Any disorder that interferes with the peristaltic movement of urine is obstructive. An obstruction can occur at any point in the urinary tract.

Classification systems denoting obstruction vary. One method is to classify obstructions according to congenital or acquired causes. Congenital anomalies are more common in the urinary tract than in any other organ system. These anomalies are generally obstructive. Acquired causes are many and may be found within the urinary tract, invading the tract, or compressing the tract. Other means of classifying obstruction include the duration (acute or chronic), the degree (partial or complete), and the level at which it occurs in the urinary tract (upper or lower).

Pathophysiologic changes secondary to obstruction occur only in those segments of the urinary tract proximal to the obstruction. These changes do not occur throughout the urinary tract all at once. Each portion of the tract tends to protect those parts more proximal to the obstruction. For example, with obstruction of the bladder neck, the bladder undergoes changes, but the ureter is protected until the bladder can no longer compensate.

Initially, obstruction causes back pressure because of stasis of urine in the segment of the urinary tract just above the obstruction. The hydrostatic pressure of the accumulated urine opposes the peristaltic force of the urine flow. In response to the back pressure, the affected segment dilates to accommodate the stagnated urine. In most instances, dilatation stretches the muscle fibers, stimulating hypertrophy. The hypertrophied muscle contracts more strongly in an effort to force urine through the area of obstruction. The affected segment compensates, which means it undergoes changes in order to maintain function.

If obstruction is not relieved, increasing dilatation overstretches the muscle fibers, decreasing muscle tone and the ability to contract. The segment decompensates and is unable to maintain its function of elimination. The area becomes increasingly dilated. The atonic muscle wall may become thinned and weakened. Increased back pressure is transmitted to the next proximal segment in the urinary tract. This cycle of compensation-decompensation occurs in succession to all segments up to the renal pelvis and calices.

Any obstruction of the urinary tract can lead to increased pressure in the renal pelvis and calices, resulting from distention with urine. When the obstruction is in the upper part of the ureter, the resulting distention is known as hydronephrosis. When the obstruction is in the lower part of the ureter, the resulting distention is known as hydroureter (Fig. 31–1). Such pressure can damage the renal parenchyma and interfere with renal function. Renal blood flow may also be compromised. If infection is present, the damage to the kidney could be more severe.

The long-term effects of hydronephrosis and how much function returns after relief of the obstruction are determined by several factors, such as severity (complete or partial obstruction), duration, totality (bilateral or unilateral obstruction), and presence of infection.

Following relief of obstruction, urine output may increase by 3 to 10 times. This response, called postobstructive diuresis, is usually mild and self-limiting but sometimes is severe. This state of markedly excessive, dilute urine output is caused by the impaired ability of renal tubules to concentrate and absorb body fluids and electrolytes (primarily sodium) effectively. This impairment of renal function is secondary to renal damage caused by increased pressure on the tubules as a result of urinary tract obstruction.

Diuresis can be defined as urine output greater than 2000 mL in an 8-hour period. In a broader sense, any urine output above normal (which in adults can range from 700 to 2000 mL) may be considered to be postobstructive diuresis, if only because of its life-threatening potential.

Postobstructive diuresis is characterized by an excessive loss of both water and electrolytes. If judicious treatment is not undertaken in a timely manner, this dramatic polyuria and "salt-losing" may result in rapid depletion of extracellular fluid volume, vascular collapse, and death. Fluid and electrolytes must be replaced appropriately until renal function (concentrating ability) improves.

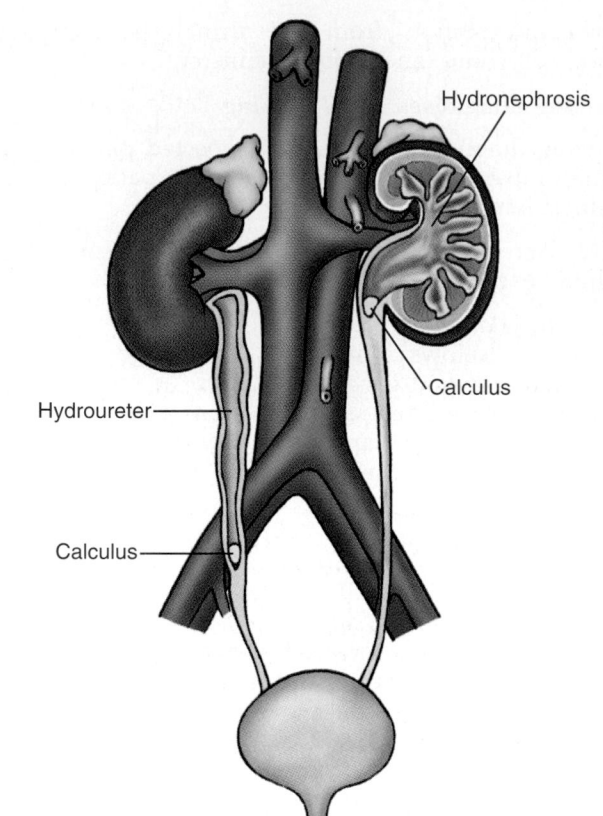

Figure 31–1

Hydronephrosis is caused by obstruction in the upper part of the ureter. Hydroureter is caused by obstruction in the lower part of the ureter.

URINARY CALCULI

Etiology and Pathophysiology

Urinary calculus, or urolithiasis, is the presence of stones in the urinary tract. It is one of the most common urologic problems for adults. About 12% of the population of the United States develops a urinary tract calculus at some time in their lives. For some this may mean a small stone that passes easily and painlessly through the urinary tract. In extreme cases, patients suffer recurrent UTI or loss of renal function from large, obstructing or infected renal stones.

Passing a urinary calculus can be a painful experience. Stones that grow too large to pass spontaneously are treated using a variety of medical and surgical techniques. The recent advent of the use of shock waves to disintegrate stones without the need for surgery has drastically reduced the morbidity formerly associated with this disease. Extracorporeal shock wave lithotripsy is indicated for renal pelvic stones, stones in the renal calices, and stones above the pelvic brim. Extracorporeal shock wave lithotripsy is contraindicated for patients with lower ureteral stones or ureteral obstruction stones that cannot be seen on monitors, patients taking anticoagulants, patients with calcified aortic aneurysms, and patients with atrial fibrillation and ventricular tachycardia or some type of pacemaker.

Approximately 80% of persons with urinary calculus disease are found to have a metabolic or dietary cause for stone formation. In the remaining 20%, diet, fluid intake, and geographic location are thought to be major factors. Generally, persons whose diet includes a high intake of calcium and animal proteins, persons whose fluid intake is chronically low, and persons who live in the Southeast, Southwest, and Northwest United States are at greater risk for urinary calculus formation.

Urinary calculi occur most commonly in the 20- to 50-year-old age group. Stones associated with infection are more common in women. It is believed that stones form when chemicals and other elements commonly found in urine become concentrated and lead to the formation of crystals. The crystals begin to cling together to eventually form a calcification or calculus. The elements that lead to crystal formation may be present in large amounts in the urine as a result of one of many metabolic disorders, diet, or fluid intake.

Most urinary tract stones are formed in the kidney. Ureteral stones are usually renal stones that have moved down the ureter. Bladder stones are common in patients with indwelling urinary drainage tubes or an inability to empty their bladder when voiding.

Clinical Manifestations

Pain is the most common symptom that patients with urinary calculi experience. Renal calculi cause flank pain on the same side as the affected kidney, which may radiate to the groin or the genitalia. Ureteral stones cause pain in the flank and abdominal area, which may also radiate to the genitalia. When the discomfort is dull and aching, the patient may visit the physician's office. Most patients, however, go to the emergency room during an episode of renal or ureteral colic. Cultural and ethnic differences of the patient indicate a wide range of pain threshold perceptions. For example, Asians seldom express emotions that others may consider offensive, and this stoicism may be so extreme that you cannot accurately assess the patient's pain.

Renal colic occurs when the muscular components of the lining of the urinary tract go into spasm in response to irritation from the calculus. Episodes of colic are excruciatingly painful, have a sudden onset, and are often accompanied by severe nausea and vomiting. Large doses of pain medication are often required to give the patient some measure of relief from the pain. Fever and an elevated white blood cell count may be present if the stone has caused an infection.

Diagnosis

Diagnosis of a urinary calculus or calculi is based on the presenting symptoms and on a series of radiographic tests. A plain abdominal film identifies most calculi, although some are composed of elements that are radiolucent. An excretory urogram further outlines the calculus and allows evaluation of its location in the kidney or ureter and any effect the calculus has had on the surrounding tissue. Retrograde pyelogram may be necessary to diagnose renal or ureteral stones in patients with radiolucent stones or in those with an allergy to contrast dye. The urinalysis may show red blood cells, white blood cells, and bacteria.

Management

The treatment for urinary calculus disease depends on the size, number, location, and content of the stone or stones. Eighty to ninety percent of stones that are smaller than 5 mm in diameter pass spontaneously. However, hospitalization may be required to treat the symptoms of colic that may occur as the stone passes. Infection accompanying urinary stones, even if they are smaller than 5 mm, may cause pyelonephritis, requiring antibiotic therapy.

Patients with multiple stones, large impacted stones, or stones that completely obstruct the urinary tract usually require surgical treatment.

Extracorporeal shock wave lithotripsy is now commonly used to treat renal or ureteral calculi. In this procedure, a device called a lithotriptor generates ultrasonic shock waves that shatter the urinary stones. The stone particles then pass through the urinary system and are excreted in the urine. The procedure can be accomplished by partially submerging the patient in warm water (called a "water bath") and sending the shock waves through the water toward the stone. For this method of lithotripsy, the patient must be under anesthesia. A newer method of extracorporeal shock wave lithotripsy is performed without the water bath. In this method, a device is placed on the skin over the stone, and the shock waves are then fired at the stone (Fig. 31–2). There is still some discomfort with this method, so the patient may receive a mild sedative before the procedure.

Surgical interventions are reserved for patients for whom extracorporeal shock wave lithotripsy is

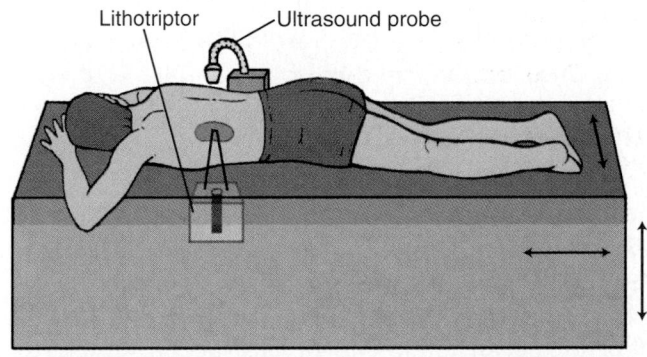

Lithotriptor   Ultrasound probe

Figure 31–2

Extracorporeal shock wave lithotripsy for treatment of urinary tract stones.

contraindicated or would be unsuccessful. A variety of surgical approaches are used, ranging from procedures performed through a small flank incision using flexible ultrasonic instruments (used to break up and remove renal stones) to major surgery, such as nephrolithotomy or nephrectomy.

Lower ureteral or bladder stones are usually removed using instruments that are passed through a cystoscope. Bladder stones that are very large require open surgical removal.

❖ Settings, Providers, and Collaboration for Care

Surgical intervention for urinary calculi is frequently performed on an outpatient basis, unless an extensive procedure is necessary. The patient is admitted to the hospital the morning of the treatment or surgery and remains only until fully recovered from anesthesia. With extracorporeal shock wave lithotripsy, a patient may have a full liquid diet the day before and is given nothing by mouth (NPO status) after midnight. Preoperatively the patient may take a chlorhexidine gluconate shower on the morning of the extracorporeal shock wave lithotripsy and an antiflatulence suppository the night before. Postoperatively the patient will need to force fluids up to 3 to 4 L per day, ambulate, and strain all urine and send urine for fragment analysis. Inform the patient that transportation is needed postoperatively because the patient should not drive for at least 24 hours after the surgery.

The patient is given information related to the required post-treatment care needs before discharge. A follow-up appointment to the physician's office is made. A referral to a home health nurse may be necessary for patients who live alone, are elderly, or have other special care needs.

NURSING PROCESS GUIDELINES
Urinary Calculi

The assessment, nursing diagnoses, expected patient outcomes, nursing interventions, and evaluation for patients with urinary calculi are provided in Nursing Care Guide 31–1 and Highlight 31–2.

UPPER URINARY TRACT OBSTRUCTION

Ureteropelvic Junction Obstruction

Etiology and Pathophysiology

Ureteropelvic junction obstruction is a term that refers to the anatomic site of obstruction. Causes of this type of urinary tract disorder are varied but can usually be attributed to congenital anomalies such as a ureter that has developed abnormally high in the renal pelvis. Inflammation, ischemia, tumors, and calculi are examples of acquired causes of ureteropelvic junction obstruction.

In most cases of ureteropelvic junction obstruction, regardless of the cause, there is hydronephrosis and dilatation of the kidney pelvis and calices. With long-standing obstruction, there is deterioration of renal function. Other pathophysiologic changes can occur but are related to specific causes of the obstruction.

Clinical Manifestations

The patient with ureteropelvic junction obstruction usually describes symptoms of several years' duration. Flank or back pain is the most common symptom. The discomfort felt is usually vague but intensifies with diuresis following an excessive fluid intake. Pyuria, hematuria, and bacteriuria may be present. A flank mass may occasionally be palpable.

Diagnosis

Information from the history and physical examination is correlated with radiographic findings to establish the diagnosis. Excretory urography is performed. Results usually indicate delayed excretion of urine from the affected kidney, as well as variable dilatation of the renal pelvis and calices. Hydronephrosis may also be evident. In some instances, hydration or drug-induced diuresis may accentuate the effects of the obstructive lesion and facilitate diagnosis. Ultrasonography and CT are sometimes performed to document the nonfunctional status of the kidney.

Management

Treatment for ureteropelvic junction obstruction is directed toward restoring renal function, providing relief of symptoms, eliminating infection, and correcting anatomical abnormalities. When renal function has not been compromised, pyeloureteroplasty is the procedure of choice for correcting ureteropelvic junction obstruction. Various surgical techniques are used, but all are focused on restoring normal anatomical structure and function to the kidney. When prolonged and untreated obstruction has resulted in irreversible renal damage, nephrectomy may be indicated.

Ureterovesical Junction Obstruction

The ureterovesical junction is that part of the urinary system where the ureters enter the bladder. Normally, orifices are located on either side of the proximal border of the trigone area.

Etiology and Pathophysiology

The causes of obstruction at the ureterovesical junction are relatively few and are not always clearly defined. Obstruction may occasionally be caused by stricture formation following an operative procedure, or it may be the result of an inflammatory

Nursing Care Guide 31–1
Patients with Renal Calculi

Assessment Findings: Patient complains of severe pain in back and flank area and has fever and increased white blood cell count. Patient is unable to provide self-care as a result of the extreme pain.

Nursing Diagnosis: Pain related to obstruction from renal calculi

Patient Outcomes	Nursing Interventions	Rationale
Patient verbalizes relief of pain or that pain is within tolerable limits.	Investigate complaints of discomfort. Medicate for pain as ordered. Provide comfort measures.	Assessing the patient's pain provides baseline data for later comparisons.
	Encourage patient to practice relaxation exercises.	Relaxation techniques may provide additional relief for the patient.
Patient participates in self-care activities.	Encourage the patient to complete as much self-care as able. Assist the patient when necessary.	Participating in the care may ease some of the emotional stress associated with the condition.
	Medicate for pain before self-care activities.	Medicating the patient before activity may promote more participation from the patient.
	Encourage ambulation and increased fluid intake, as tolerated.	Ambulating and drinking increased amounts of fluids may help pass the calculi, thus eliminating the pain.

Evaluation: Compare the patient's status with the expected outcomes. If the outcomes are not met, reassess the patient and revise the plan.

Assessment Findings: Patient experiences nausea, vomiting, or both and is unable to eat or drink fluids.

Nursing Diagnosis: Altered nutrition: less than body requirements related to nausea and vomiting secondary to extreme pain from renal calculi

Patient Outcomes	Nursing Interventions	Rationale
Patient verbalizes relief of nausea and vomiting.	Evaluate the factor causing the nausea. Administer analgesics and antiemetics as ordered. Monitor the patient's fluid intake and output.	Analgesics relieve the pain that may result in relief of the nausea. Antiemetics relieve the nausea and vomiting.
	Encourage relaxation techniques such as slow, deep breathing. Position the patient for comfort.	Relaxation exercises may provide stress relief and make the patient more comfortable as well as relieve some of the pain.
	Provide small frequent sips of fluids as tolerated.	Replacing fluids slowly may prevent aggravation of the nausea.
	Provide oral hygiene frequently. Encourage the patient to rinse mouth as necessary.	Providing oral hygiene reduces foul odor and taste and prevents increased bacterial growth in the mouth.

(continued)

Nursing Care Guide 31–1
Patients with Renal Calculi (continued)

Evaluation:	Compare the patient's status with the expected outcomes. If the outcomes are not met, reassess the patient and revise the plan.
Assessment Findings:	Patient complains of urgency, bladder fullness, and suprapubic discomfort. The patient's bladder is distended and easily palpable; intake is greater than output, and pain is increasing.
Nursing Diagnosis:	Altered urinary elimination related to obstructed ureter

Patient Outcomes	Nursing Interventions	Rationale
Patient denies feelings of urgency, fullness, or discomfort.	Assess for increasing pain and bladder fullness.	Assessing for bladder distention, discomfort, and dysuria provides a baseline for later comparisons. It also promotes early intervention for problems found.
	Administer analgesics as ordered.	Analgesics may relieve some of the discomfort.
Patient's voiding pattern returns to normal; fluid intake and output are adequate.	Monitor the fluid intake and output, strain all urine, and insert Foley catheter if necessary to relieve pressure. Note the color and consistency of the urine.	Monitoring the fluid intake and output provides for early intervention if problems arise. Straining urine may reveal passage of the calculi.
	Encourage increased fluid intake.	Increased fluids help wash out system and may promote the passage of the calculi.

Evaluation:	Compare the patient's status with the expected outcomes. If the outcomes are not met, reassess the patient and revise the plan.

process precipitated by ureteral instrumentation. More commonly, the cause is secondary to an infective or neoplastic condition or the presence of a stone at the junction. Certain anatomical pathologies can also cause blockage of the flow of urine through the ureterovesical junction. These include ureteroceles, bladder diverticula, and a condition called obstructive megaureter (large or dilated ureter).

Pathophysiologic changes that occur as a result of obstruction at the ureterovesical junction are the same as those that occur with ureteropelvic junction obstruction. Depending on the degree of obstruction, vesicoureteral reflux may also occur.

Clinical Manifestations
The presenting symptoms of ureterovesical junction obstruction are fever, flank pain, and varying degrees of gastrointestinal disturbances. When the blockage is the result of an obstructed megaureter,

adult patients may complain of abdominal pain and hematuria.

Diagnosis
The diagnosis of ureterovesical junction obstruction is based on findings from radiographic studies. Excretory urography, intravenous pyelography, and retrograde pyelography are the procedures most commonly performed.

Management
Treatment of ureterovesical junction obstruction depends on the cause of the problem. In general, obstruction that is the result of an infection, tumor, or urinary calculus is first managed medically. Surgical intervention for these types of problems is considered on an individual basis. When the obstruction is related to presence of a ureterocele, diverticula, or megaureter, surgical removal is usually indicated.

HIGHLIGHT
31–2
NUTRITION

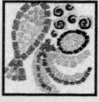

Dietary Needs Related to Type of Calculus

Calculus Type	Dietary Needs
Calcium phosphate	Decrease dairy products to reduce calcium content in urine. Increase meats, eggs, fish, prunes, grapes, and cranberry juice to acidify urine.
Calcium oxalate	Decrease dairy products to reduce calcium content in urine. Decrease colas, coffee, nuts, chocolate, rhubarb, and spinach to decrease oxalate content in urine.
Uric acid	Increase legumes, green vegetables, and fruits (except prunes, grapes, cranberries, and citrus fruits) to increase alkalinity of the urine. Decrease purine sources such as organ meats, gravies, red wines, goose, venison, and seafood.
Struvite (magnesium ammonium phosphate)	Increase eggs, fish, prunes, and cranberries to increase the acidity of the urine. Decrease nuts, poultry, milk, cheese, peas, and corn to decrease phosphate content in the urine.
Cystine	Increase legumes, green vegetables, and fruits (except grapes, prunes, and cranberries) to increase the alkalinity of the urine.

Ureteral Stricture

Etiology and Pathophysiology

A ureteral stricture is an abnormal narrowing of the ureter. Although stricture formation can occur at any point in the ureter, three areas are particularly prone to the development of this abnormality: the ureteropelvic junction, the midureter, and the distal ureter above the ureterovesical junction.

The narrowing of the ureter can sometimes be attributed to congenital malformation or congenital stenosis. More often, this abnormality is acquired as a result of trauma, which can occur with operative procedures or instrumentation of the ureter, the passage or presence of stones within the ureter, or the inadvertent ligation of the ureter. Infections such as renal tuberculosis and retroperitoneal fibrosis can induce ureteral stricture formation. Cancerous tumors and their metastases, radiation therapy, and transplanted kidneys can also be etiologic factors for stricture formation in the ureter. Predisposing factors that have been identified include urinary extravasation, infection, and ischemia to the ureter.

The formation of ureteral strictures is due to a series of fibrotic tissue changes that lead to scar formation and increasing constriction of the ureter. Prolonged constriction decreases the perfusion of the tissues involved, impedes the development of a collateral vascular supply, and interrupts the flow of urine from the kidney to the bladder. As with other types of upper urinary tract obstruction, an untreated ureteral stricture can eventually lead to hydronephrosis and damage of the renal parenchyma.

Clinical Manifestations

Frequently, patients with ureteral strictures are asymptomatic. The stricture may be found during a radiographic examination being performed for another problem. Symptoms include fever, flank pain, gastrointestinal disturbances, and hematuria. Abdominal pain may simulate the pain of appendicitis if the right ureter is obstructed. If the involved kidney is enlarged, it may be palpated or percussed on physical examination. Infection may cause tenderness of the kidney.

Diagnosis

Together with history and physical examination, the diagnosis of ureteral stricture is generally made by excretory urography and retrograde ureteropyelography. These studies often reveal the obstructive lesion, usually with varying degrees of hydronephrosis.

Management

The treatment of a ureteral stricture depends on its location. For a stricture at the ureteropelvic junction, pyeloplasty may be necessary. Midureteral strictures are often treated by surgical excision of the stenotic area, followed by ureteroureterostomy (end-to-end anastomosis of the remaining portions of the ureter). Lower ureteral strictures and ureterovesical junction strictures may be treated by excision of the strictured portion of the ureter, followed by reimplantation of the ureter into the bladder wall. For cases involving extreme hydronephrosis, nephrectomy may be necessary.

Balloon dilatation of ureteral strictures, using a special balloon catheter, has become a popular and successful treatment option for certain situations. The better success rate has been demonstrated with strictures caused by inflammatory processes or those that have been diagnosed on patients who have recently undergone surgery. This technique has not been successful with strictures caused by cancerous tumors, with failed pyeloplasty, or with radiation-induced strictures.

❖ Settings, Providers, and Collaboration for Care

Because patients with upper urinary tract obstructions frequently undergo surgery to correct the problem, hospitalization for a few days is usually necessary. As soon as possible after surgery, the patient is discharged. Follow-up care by both a nurse and a physician may be necessary. Some patients are discharged with catheters, dressings, and other drains still in place. Referral to a home health nurse may be needed to check the patient's status, provide instruction about care needs, and prevent complications after discharge. Additional follow-up usually occurs at the physician's office.

NURSING PROCESS
Upper Urinary Tract Obstruction

PREOPERATIVE NURSING CARE

Assessment

Assess for signs of fever, flank pain, abdominal pain, and gastrointestinal disturbances. Note changes in the patient's voiding pattern as well as any signs of infection. As with any presurgical candidate, the patient's understanding of the condition, the procedure to be performed, and the postoperative routine is evaluated.

Nursing Diagnoses and Planning

Nursing diagnoses and related expected patient outcomes most commonly applicable to the preoperative patient with upper urinary tract obstruction include the following:

NDx: Knowledge deficit: nature of the proposed treatment plan

Planning: Patient Outcomes
1. Patient asks questions that are appropriate and related to presurgical teaching.
2. Patient demonstrates an understanding of the treatment plan.

NDx: Anxiety related to outcome of care and obstruction

Planning: Patient Outcomes
1. Patient verbalizes reasons for anxiety.
2. Patient demonstrates decreased levels of anxiety.
3. Patient demonstrates effective coping skills.

Nursing Interventions and Evaluation

NDx: Knowledge deficit: nature of the proposed treatment plan
Because most upper urinary tract obstructions are treated surgically, preoperative nursing interventions are directed toward preparing the patient for the upcoming surgical procedure. In addition to those activities, which are a part of the routine preoperative case, develop a teaching plan that describes the series of events that will take place. Provide an illustration of the urinary tract to reinforce the physician's explanation of the surgical procedure. This simple visual aid enhances preoperative teaching and helps the patient understand the problem and the proposed treatment plan. Because the patient will return from surgery with multiple drainage tubes, point out locations for drainage tube placement.

NDx: Anxiety
In addition to explaining the preoperative preparation and the surgical intervention to the patient, teach the patient some relaxation techniques. Allow time for the patient to express fears and concerns. Answer all questions as honestly as possible. Seek support from clergy or significant others when appropriate.

Compare the patient's status with the expected outcomes. If the outcomes are not met, reassess the patient and revise the plan.

POSTOPERATIVE NURSING CARE

Assessment

Postoperative assessment of the patient who has undergone surgical correction of an upper urinary tract obstruction includes determination of renal function. Check the patency of urinary drainage tubes, such as a nephrostomy tube or ureteral stent. Inspect the skin surrounding the insertion site of urinary drainage tube. Note any leakage of urine. Observe any urine drainage (whether outside the tube or within the tube) for its color and degree of hematuria. Monitor intake and output. Observe the patient for signs of fluid and electrolyte imbalance.

In addition to evaluating the function of the urinary system, check dressings over the surgical site for excessive or unusual drainage. Continually assess the patient for signs of infection, either of the surgical incision or of the urine and the urinary tract. Assess routine postoperative needs.

Nursing Diagnoses and Planning

Nursing diagnoses and related expected patient outcomes most commonly applicable to postoperative patients with upper urinary tract obstruction include the following:

NDx: Altered urinary elimination related to surgical procedure

Planning: Patient Outcomes
1. Patient's urinary drainage tubes are patent.
2. Patient's urinary output is adequate in relation to intake.

NDx: Risk for infection related to risk of urine stasis within drainage tubes

Planning: Patient Outcomes
1. Patient is free of signs and symptoms of UTI.
2. Patient exhibits normal vital signs and laboratory data.

NDx: Impaired skin integrity related to leakage of urine around drainage tubes

Planning: Patient Outcomes
1. Patient's skin around the drainage tube remains clean and dry and without signs of irritation.
2. Patient's skin around the drainage tube remains intact.

Nursing Interventions and Evaluation

NDx: Altered urinary elimination
Assess urinary drainage for patency. Ensure that urine drains freely. Monitor fluid intake and output. As the patient's mobility increases, ensure that urinary drainage bags are secure and draining freely. Empty bags at regular intervals.

NDx: Risk for infection
Observe for signs and symptoms of a UTI. Note color, consistency, and amount of urine. Monitor vital signs, reporting fever or unexplained tachycardia. Monitor white blood cell count, urinalysis, and urine culture for infection.

NDx: Impaired skin integrity
Keep skin around drainage tubes clean and dry. Reinforce or change dressings as needed. Observe the skin around drainage tubes for redness or breakdown.

Compare the patient's status with the expected outcomes. If the outcomes are not met, reassess the patient and revise the plan.

LOWER URINARY TRACT OBSTRUCTION

Urethral Stricture

Etiology and Pathophysiology
Urethral stricture is defined as a pathologic narrowing of the urethra. It is a problem that is more common in men because of the anatomical structure and length of the urethra. Women do develop urethral strictures, but it is more often a functional obstruction rather than an anatomical obstruction.

Urethral strictures can be congenital or acquired. Chronic infection, sexually transmitted diseases, and trauma to the lower urinary tract or pelvis all are causes of stricture formation. In women, trauma following intercourse, childbirth, vaginal surgery, or chronic urethritis can lead to the development of a urethral stricture. There are also iatrogenic causes of stricture formation. These include manipulation of the lower urinary tract during diagnostic procedures and transurethral surgery as well as the long-term use of indwelling urethral catheters. In some instances, neoplasms, venereal warts, and urethral polyps are underlying causes of urethral stricture formation.

A stricture develops because of the formation of collagen and fibrous tissue at the area of insult within the urethra. This leads to a narrowing and a loss of elasticity of the passageway. Consequently, urine flow out of the bladder is restricted, and dilatation of the system proximal to the strictured area occurs.

Clinical Manifestations
Patients with a urethral stricture usually have obstructive and irritating voiding symptoms. Obstructive symptoms include the following:

Decreased force of the urinary stream (one of the most common complaints)
Hesitancy in initiating the urinary stream
Double voiding (patient voids and then is able to void again within 5 to 10 minutes)
Postvoid dribbling
Interrupted urinary stream
Urinary retention (generally a slowly developing, chronic problem)
Overflow incontinence

Irritating voiding symptoms include dysuria, frequency, nocturia, and urgency and urge incontinence.

Diagnosis
A general and urologic history, coupled with selected diagnostic procedures, confirms the diagnosis of a urethral stricture. Diagnostic studies that are usually performed include urine cultures to identify the presence of any UTI, urine flow studies to measure the amount of decrease in the force of the uri-

nary stream, and radiologic studies, such as voiding cystourethrography and urethrography, to visualize the location and extent of the obstruction.

Management

The goal of treatment is to relieve the obstruction and eradicate any existing infection. The type of treatment selected depends on the location, length, and density of the stricture area.

Mechanical dilatation of strictures is among the most common therapy instituted. It is a nonsurgical procedure that involves the use of urethral sounds (curved metal rods) that graduate in size up to #36 French. A local anesthetic is usually instilled into the urethra before the procedure. The sounds are then passed (starting with the smaller and working up to the larger sizes) into the urethra and through the strictured area to open it to approximately #22 Fr.

Another procedure often performed is internal urethrotomy. This involves an incision of the strictured area under direct visualization through a specially designed endoscope. To prevent recurrence of the stricture after incision, a program of intermittent self-catheterization is sometimes recommended.

Urethroplasty, or surgical repair of the strictured area, is indicated when a previously treated stricture recurs, when dilatation of the area is needed more frequently than every 6 months, when the strictured area is too large for treatment by dilatation or urethrotomy, and when the stricture is the result of severe traumatic urethral injury (eg, severed urethra). Urethroplasty is performed as either a one- or two-stage procedure. In the one-stage operation, the stricture is excised. Anastomosis of remaining urethral ends is carried out. A tissue graft over the anastomosed area may be used. In the two-step procedure, which is thought by some to have the higher success rate, the area of stricture is marsupialized (formation of a pouchlike structure) and allowed to heal. After about 6 months, the tissue is reapproximated to form a new urethra.

The newest treatment alternative for urethral strictures is laser photoradiation. This form of therapy has yielded mixed results. Consequently, its place in the treatment of urethral strictures is still unknown.

Meatal Stenosis

Etiology and Pathophysiology

Stenosis of the external meatus is a problem in both adults and children. Meatal stenosis (or distal urethral stenosis, as the problem is sometimes called in women) can be either congenital or acquired. Congenital meatal stenosis in men is rare but is occasionally associated with hypospadias. In women, congenital distal urethral stenosis is a condition that is problematic in early childhood but that typically disappears after puberty, possibly because of the production of estrogens.

Acquired meatal stenosis is caused by inflammation secondary to an infectious process. In women, it can also result from the trauma of a vaginal delivery.

In men, meatal stenosis is a membranous web of tissue running across the external urinary meatus. In women, a ring of stenosis forms just inside the external urinary meatus. It is the result of collagen and inelastic tissue formation, similar to that which occurs during stricture formation. When meatal stenosis is severe, complete bladder emptying could be compromised. However, the problem primarily affects the quality and control of the urinary stream.

Clinical Manifestations

The signs and symptoms of meatal stenosis are much the same as those described for urethral stricture. In addition, men may describe difficulty directing the urinary stream, which causes urine to spray outside the toilet or urinal. A man may also find it necessary to hold the penis down during voiding. A fine forceful stream, prolonged voiding time, and blood in the urine at the end of voiding (terminal hematuria) are other common complaints.

Diagnosis

To confirm the diagnosis of meatal stenosis, urethral calibration (measurement of the internal diameter of the urethral meatus with special sounds) is usually performed. In some men, this procedure may not be necessary because evidence of meatal stenosis may be visible upon examination of the penis. Additional diagnostic techniques, such as radiographic studies, are usually not performed unless other problems within the urinary system are suspected.

Management

Meatal stenosis can be corrected by dilatation with catheters up to #24 to #26 Fr. This is performed at regular intervals over a specified period of time. To prevent infection during the course of the treatment period, antibiotic therapy is usually initiated.

Surgical intervention such as meatotomy may be performed in men under local anesthesia. This procedure simply involves making an incision through the web of membranous tissue. If surgical intervention is indicated for women with distal urethral stenosis, urethroplasty is performed.

❖ Settings, Providers, and Collaboration for Care

Patients with lower urinary tract obstruction may undergo surgical intervention to correct the disorder. Some types of surgery for urethral stricture or meatal stenosis may necessitate hospitalization for a short period. Others may be performed on an outpatient basis. Follow-up examination in a physician's office is necessary for all types of surgical intervention. A home health nurse may assist the patient with ongoing care necessary after some types of surgery, especially when an indwelling catheter is still in place after discharge. The nurse may also assist the patient in the home with intermittent catheterization for dilatation. The patient may also be taught self-dilatation. Education about infection prevention should take place before discharge but can be reiterated by the home health nurse or physician's office nurse.

NURSING PROCESS
Lower Urinary Tract Obstruction

PREOPERATIVE NURSING CARE

Assessment

Question the patient with lower urinary tract obstruction about the incidence of any previous urinary tract obstructions, UTIs, injuries to the pelvis, or abdominal surgery. Identify all symptoms the patient may be experiencing. Distinguish whether these are truly symptoms. Assess the patient for signs and symptoms of a UTI, such as burning with urination or cloudy urine. Ask whether the patient has a discharge from the urethra.

Nursing Diagnoses and Planning

Nursing diagnoses and related expected patient outcomes most commonly applicable to the preoperative patients with lower urinary tract obstruction include the following:

NDx: Altered urinary elimination related to blockage of the urinary outlet

Planning: Patient Outcomes
  1. Patient voids at regular intervals.
  2. Patient does not strain excessively or use force to empty the bladder.

NDx: Urinary retention related to obstruction of urine flow

Planning: Patient Outcomes
  1. Patient voids at regular intervals.
  2. Patient expresses a sense of complete bladder emptying.

NDx: Risk for infection related to stasis of urine

Planning: Patient Outcomes
  1. Patient is free of signs and symptoms of a UTI.
  2. Patient exhibits normal vital signs and laboratory data.

Nursing Interventions and Evaluation

NDx: Altered urinary elimination
Monitor closely the patient's pattern of urinary elimination. If appropriate, instruct the patient to keep a record of the time and amount of each void. Teach the patient to relax throughout urination rather than trying to strain or force the stream.

NDx: Urinary retention
Monitor the patient's fluid intake and output. Provide adequate fluids. Palpate the bladder for full-

ness. If retention is suspected, obtain an order for catheterization. Catheterize for residual urine.

NDx: Risk for infection
Observe for and document any signs and symptoms of a UTI. Monitor vital signs, reporting fever or unexplained tachycardia. Monitor white blood cell count, urinalysis, and urine culture for infection. Note the color, consistency, and amount of urine. Report any abnormalities.

Compare the patient's status with the expected outcomes. If the outcomes are not met, reassess the patient and revise the plan.

POSTOPERATIVE NURSING CARE

Assessment

The patient who has undergone surgical correction of a lower urinary tract obstruction is likely to have some type of urinary drainage tube, usually an indwelling Foley catheter. Check this tubing to be sure it is draining freely without obstruction. Note the color and quality of the urine passing through the tube.

Bladder spasms are not uncommon when the lower urinary tract has been manipulated. Assess the patient for any pain or discomfort that has resulted from the surgical treatment.

The development of a UTI can also occur following instrumentation of the urethra. Assess the patient for signs and symptoms of an infectious process.

Nursing Diagnoses and Planning

Nursing diagnoses and related expected patient outcomes most commonly applicable to postoperative patients with lower urinary tract obstruction include the following:

NDx: Risk for infection related to instrumentation of the lower urinary tract

Planning: Patient Outcomes
  1. Patient is free of signs and symptoms of a UTI.
  2. Patient exhibits normal vital signs and laboratory data.

NDx: Pain related to bladder spasms

Planning: Patient Outcomes
  1. Patient expresses relief of pain and bladder spasms.
  2. Patient gradually increases activity without discomfort.

Nursing Interventions and Evaluation

NDx: Risk for infection
Observe for and document any signs and symptoms of a UTI. Monitor vital signs, reporting fever or unexplained tachycardia. Monitor white blood cell count, urinalysis, and urine culture for infection. Note the color, consistency, and amount of urine. Report any abnormalities.

NDx: Pain

Any manipulation or instrumentation of the lower urinary tract causes discomfort. Administer analgesics and antispasmodics as necessary to provide the patient with relief of pain or bladder spasms. ~~Limit the patient's activity because too much physical stress can precipitate bladder spasms as well as hematuria.~~

Compare the patient's status with the expected outcomes. If the outcomes are not met, reassess the patient and revise the plan.

Renal Failure

Renal failure or renal insufficiency is the condition of partial or total loss of kidney function. Failure does not occur until there is functional loss of 75% of the kidney's nephrons, the functioning unit of the kidney.

Renal failure may be either acute or chronic, depending on the course of onset. Regardless of the type of failure, the body undergoes significant biochemical changes that, without treatment, result eventually in death. Table 31–2 presents terminology related to renal failure.

ACUTE RENAL FAILURE

Etiology and Pathophysiology

Acute renal failure occurs suddenly and is often reversible. It generally follows ischemic or toxic trauma to the kidney. Recovery from acute renal failure depends on the cause and underlying disease process. If the renal failure is a result of an extensive disease process, the mortality rate is high. Acute renal failure may result from prerenal, renal, or postrenal causes (Fig. 31–3).

Prerenal failure is caused by interference with renal blood flow. The kidney depends on adequate blood flow to maintain function. A decrease in perfusion results in decreased glomerular filtration. Causes of prerenal failure include the following:

- Decreased volume states caused by diarrhea, vomiting, hemorrhage, excessive use of diuretics, burns, and glycosuria
- States that are caused by shifts of volume, such as vasodilation and sepsis
- States of decreased cardiac output, such as congestive heart failure, pericardial tamponade, and acute pulmonary embolus
- States of decreased vascular resistance, such as anesthesia and hepatorenal syndrome
- States of vascular obstruction, such as dissecting aneurysm and bilateral renal artery occlusion

Renal causes are those conditions that cause direct kidney damage or changes. These include nephrotoxic substances, such as aminoglycosides and heavy metals and ischemia. Acute tubular necrosis is the most common renal cause of acute renal failure. Other renal causes include acute glomerulonephritis, trauma, severe muscle exertion, genetic and metabolic disorders, and renal vascular lesions.

Postrenal causes are related to obstruction in the urinary tract from the renal tubules to the urethral meatus. The obstruction can be caused by urethral or bladder cancer, renal calculi, atony of bladder, prostatic hyperplasia or cancer, cervical cancer, postsurgical or traumatic interruption, or retroperitoneal fibrosis.

Acute renal failure is caused by two major mechanisms: (1) ischemic changes to renal cells or (2) renal cell changes as a result of toxic substances. Ischemia may be a result of decreased perfusion leading to the death of renal cells and compromised renal function. Toxic substances decrease renal function by attacking the renal cell membranes and destroying their ability to maintain hemostasis. Some

Table 31–2

Terminology Related to Renal Failure

Term	Definition
Acute renal failure (ARF)	Loss of functional ability of the kidney that is rapid in onset and usually reversible. It may be prerenal, renal, or postrenal in nature.
Acute tubular necrosis (ATN)	Acute renal failure that is renal in nature. The cause is ischemic or toxic injury.
Anuria	Urinary output of less than 100 mL/d.
Azotemia	Buildup of nitrogenous waste products in the blood, specifically blood urea nitrogen and creatinine.
Chronic renal failure (CRF)	Chronic, progressive loss of renal function that is irreversible. Causes of chronic renal failure are numerous.
Metabolic waste products	Byproducts of protein metabolism that are excreted in the urine.
Oliguria	Urinary output of less than 400 mL/d.
Uremia	The clinical manifestations associated with an accumulation of nitrogenous waste products in the blood, typically associated with renal failure.

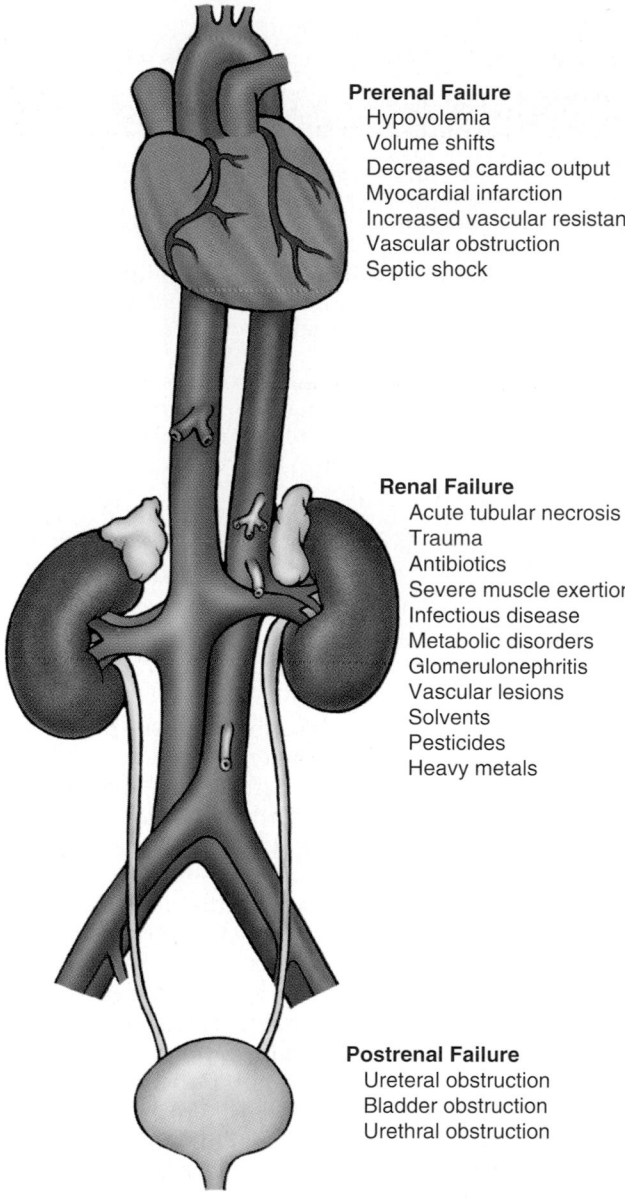

Prerenal Failure
Hypovolemia
Volume shifts
Decreased cardiac output
Myocardial infarction
Increased vascular resistance
Vascular obstruction
Septic shock

Renal Failure
Acute tubular necrosis
Trauma
Antibiotics
Severe muscle exertion
Infectious disease
Metabolic disorders
Glomerulonephritis
Vascular lesions
Solvents
Pesticides
Heavy metals

Postrenal Failure
Ureteral obstruction
Bladder obstruction
Urethral obstruction

Figure 31–3
Causes of the three types of acute renal failure: prerenal, renal, and postrenal.

ronment. The patient may exhibit either oliguria (urine output of less than 400 mL per day) or anuria (urine output of less than 100 mL per day).

Fluid overload is exhibited by edema and hypertension when the intake of fluids exceeds the urinary output and insensible losses. When the overload becomes severe, the signs and symptoms of congestive heart failure and pulmonary edema are present.

Retention of electrolytes and metabolic wastes (such as urea and creatinine) produce a group of symptoms known as uremia. These include nausea, vomiting, drowsiness, fatigue, and shortness of breath. Confusion, convulsions, coma, or gastrointestinal bleeding may also be present.

Pericarditis may result from irritation of the pericardium by the buildup of metabolic wastes. This may be exhibited by fever, development of cardiac friction rub, and pleuritic pain. Cardiac tamponade may develop. This is the accumulation of fluid in the pericardial sac (see Chap. 8). If tamponade has developed, pulsus paradoxus may be present.

The course of renal failure is usually characterized by several phases. The onset phase is the period from the precipitating event to the onset of

medications associated with nephrotoxicity are listed in Table 31–3.

Clinical Manifestations

Symptoms of acute renal failure appear rapidly and result from retention of fluids and metabolic wastes and the inability to regulate electrolytes (Table 31–4). The patient may suffer from acidosis, anemia, fluid and electrolyte imbalances, fluid overload or deficit, gastrointestinal distress, or even uremic encephalopathy. In general, the patient is acutely ill. Biochemical changes occur rapidly and give the person little time to adjust to the altered internal envi-

Table 31–3

Medications Associated with Nephrotoxicity

Drug	Associated Dysfunction
Amphotericin B Kanamycin Bacitracin Tetracycline Rifampin Vancomycin Tobramycin Netromycin Amikacin Streptomycin Cephaloridine Neomycin Cyclosporine Lithium Gentamicin	May cause damage to renal tubules
Probenecid Lithium Heroin	May cause damage to the glomeruli
Penicillin Sulfonamide Acetaminophen Allopurinol	May cause acute nephritis
Some diuretics Opioids Some antihypertensives (injectable)	May cause acute renal failure

Table 31–4

Manifestations of Electrolyte Imbalances in Renal Failure

Electrolyte Imbalance	Manifestations
Hyponatremia (decreased sodium)	Headache, muscle weakness, fatigue, apathy, confusion, coma, postural hypotension, anorexia, nausea, vomiting, abdominal cramping, weight loss
Hypernatremia (increased sodium)	Dry mucous membranes, decreased urinary output, rubbery skin turgor, excitement, tachycardia
Hypokalemia (decreased potassium)	Anorexia, nausea, vomiting, abdominal distention, lethargy, confusion, mental depression, weakness, decreased standing blood pressure, arrhythmias, electrocardiographic changes, thirst, increased urine output
Hyperkalemia (increased potassium)	Nausea, vomiting, diarrhea, irritability, weakness, oliguria, arrhythmias, electrocardiographic changes, sudden death, numbness, tingling
Hypocalcemia (decreased calcium)	Osteoporosis, fractures, tingling, convulsions, muscle spasms, tetany, calcium deposits in tissue, nausea, vomiting, diarrhea, arrhythmias
Hypercalcemia (increased calcium)	Renal calculi, coma, decreased reflexes, lethargy, arrhythmias, muscle fatigue, bone pain, osteoporosis, fractures
Acidosis (decreased bicarbonate)	Headache, malaise, rapid deep respirations, disorientation, stupor, coma, hyperkalemia

symptoms. The oliguric phase occurs from the onset of symptoms, lasting as long as 8 weeks. The longer this phase lasts, the worse the prognosis. The patient is acutely ill during this time. The diuretic phase is marked by a leveling of blood urea nitrogen (BUN) levels and a return to glomerular filtration. The urine output may be greater than 2000 mL per day. Dehydration can occur. The final phase is that of recovery. This phase lasts 3 to 12 months.

Diagnosis

Medical diagnosis is based on symptoms and findings from blood chemistries. These include the following:

Decreased or absent urinary output
Increased levels of BUN, serum creatinine, sodium, potassium, and chloride
Decreased serum calcium, carbon dioxide (bicarbonate), hemoglobin, and hematocrit levels

Management

Medical interventions during the oliguric phase are designed to prevent hyperkalemia, severe acidosis, severe fluid overload and pulmonary edema, infection, convulsions, and pericarditis, which may become life-threatening. Electrolyte imbalances are corrected as soon as possible (Table 31–5).

Drugs used to treat renal failure include cardiotonics, such as digoxin to increase stroke volume, and antihypertensives to reduce the elevated blood pressure. Stool softeners may also be given to prevent constipation and excessive straining. Dietary supplements such as multivitamin preparations may be ordered to maintain optimal nutritional status. Iron supplements are given if anemia is present. When administering any drugs, drug metabolism must be considered, because of the altered metabolism that occurs with renal failure. Fluid must be replaced carefully because fluid overload can easily

Table 31–5

Electrolyte Imbalances in Renal Failure

Electrolyte	Normal Value	Change in Renal Failure	Goal of Treatment
Sodium (Na)	136–145 mEq/L	Increase or decrease	125–145 mEq/L
Potassium (K)	3.5–5 mEq/L	Increase	3–6 mEq/L
CO_2 (bicarbonate)	24–30 mEq/L	Decrease	>15 mEq/L
Calcium (Ca)	9–11 mg/dL	Decrease	9–11 mg/dL
Phosphate (PO_4)	3.0–4.5 mg/dL	Increase	3–5 mg/dL
Albumin	3.5–5.5 g/dL	Decrease	>3.5 g/dL
Urea nitrogen (BUN)	11–23 mg/dL	Increase	<100 mg/dL
Creatinine	0.6–1.2 mg/dL	Increase	<15 mg/dL
Uric acid	2.2–8 mg/dL	Increase	<12 mg/dL

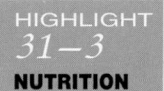 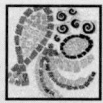

HIGHLIGHT
31–3
NUTRITION

Dietary Restrictions in Acute and Chronic Renal Failure

Rationale for restricted diets in renal failure: To minimize the complications associated with acute and chronic renal failure.

Component	Amounts
Fluid	Sufficient to maintain adequate urine volume, or 700 mL/d plus amount of urine excreted
Protein	0.6–1.0 g/kg of body weight per day; at least 0.35 g/kg/d from high-biologic-value protein to ensure adequate amounts of essential amino acids, adjusted to individual needs
Sodium	500–200 mg/d
Potassium	700–1000 mg/d
Phosphorus and calcium	500–600 mg/d
Carbohydrates	300–400 g/d

occur. The amount of fluid given is usually based on the previous day's output plus an amount to account for the body's insensible loss (400 to 500 mL). The physician determines this amount. Central venous pressure (CVP) monitoring or pulmonary artery monitoring is used to evaluate hemodynamic status.

Dialysis is used to control the buildup of electrolytes, metabolic wastes, and fluids. Hemodialysis is often the preferred method of dialysis in acute renal failure.

Dietary restrictions of protein and potassium are enforced to help reduce the accumulation of electrolytes and metabolic wastes. Fluid and sodium are restricted during the oliguric phase to decrease fluid overload (Highlight 31–3).

During the diuretic phase of acute renal failure, interventions are designed to maintain fluid and electrolyte balance. Interventions vary depending on the excretion of metabolic wastes and electrolytes.

Complete recovery of renal function is slow and requires several days to months. Return of the renal function to normal or near-normal levels is evidenced when the kidney can both conserve and dilute urine and when the serum electrolyte and nonprotein nitrogen levels become normal.

NURSING PROCESS
Acute Renal Failure

Assessment

When acute renal failure has been diagnosed, assess for the following subjective data: voiding patterns, weight gain, nausea, family history of renal disease, recent history of flu-like symptoms, and any medications taken recently, which may give an indication as to the cause of acute renal failure. Obtain the objective data: amount of urine excreted in 24 hours, blood pressure (including postural changes), daily weights, fluid status, peripheral edema, assessment of breath sounds, skin turgor, changes in mental status, and changes in pulse rate and rhythm.

These patients excrete less urine or no urine. The patients may tell you that they have not voided all day. Weight gain indicates fluid retention and is noted especially in the oliguric phase. Assess for nausea, often one of the first signs exhibited with retention of metabolic wastes. Ask about the medication history because it may also be helpful in identifying nephrotoxic substances that have been ingested.

During the oliguric phase, the 24-hour urine output is diminished or absent. During the diuretic phase, output may be greatly increased. Daily weights may increase rapidly during the oliguric phase and decrease during the diuretic phase. Edema, decreased or wet breath sounds, and skin turgor all are signs of fluid status. Observe for changes in mentation, which are symptoms of uremia and electrolyte imbalances. Changes in cardiac rate and rhythm may indicate hyperkalemia or hypokalemia. Electrolyte values and arterial blood gases must be monitored closely (see Table 31–5).

Assess the patient's knowledge level regarding renal failure and the prescribed treatment. Find out whether the patient and family understand the effects of the disease and the treatments used. Assess

▶
■ Clinical Pathway for Acute Renal Failure

Patient Name _____

DRG# _____

Date _____

Expected LOS _____

	Day 1	Day 2	Day 3	Day 4	Day 5
Medication	*Acidosis and/or hyperkalemia:* sodium polystyrene sulfonate (Kayexalate) followed by sorbitol. If potassium >6.5 mEq, give 50% glucose and regular insulin. Sodium bicarb citrate or calcium gluconate. Antihypertensives: hydralazine, methyldopa, propranolol, cardiotonic such as digoxin. *Hyperphosphatemia:* Calcium carbonate or other phosphate binders. Vitamins and minerals (vitamin D, folic acid), stool softener, IV fluids (depends on phase).	Antihypertensive, cardiotonic, diuretic, vitamin and mineral supplement, and stool softener; IV fluids (depends on phase)	Same as Day 2	Antihypertensive	Same as Day 4
Diagnostic Tests	Lytes, BUN, creatinine, Mg²⁺, phosphorus, bicarb, calcium, protein, albumin, lipids, sodium, potassium. Complete blood count with differential. INR (prothrombin time)/activated partial thromboplastin time. Urine for C&S, creatinine, osmolality, lytes, protein, SG, pH. Chest and kidney, ureter, and bladder x-ray. Computed tomography with contrast, renal sonogram, electrocardiogram.	Lytes, BUN, creatinine, Hct and Hgb. Aortorenal angiography. Possible cytoscopy or retrograde pyelography.	Same as Day 2 plus possible renal biopsy.	Lytes, BUN, creatinine, Hgb, Hct, Mg²⁺, phosphorus, albumin, protein.	Serum: BUN, creatinine, lytes. Urine: Urinalysis, lytes, osmolality.
Diet	High-fat and high-carbohydrate, low-protein diet with NA⁺ and K⁺ restriction. Fluid restriction based on lytes. Total parenteral nutrition (only if patient cannot eat).	Same as Day 1.	Same as Day 1.	Same as Day 1.	Same as Day 1.
Activity	Bedrest. ROM every 4 h (when awake). Prevent complications of immobility.	OOB as tolerated, ROM.	OOB as tolerated. Ambulate in room as tolerated.	OOB and ambulate as tolerated.	Same as Day 4.

Treatments/ Nursing Actions	Systems assessment every shift with particular attention to renal: decreased urine volume, frequency, change in color and odor. VS and NS every 4 h. Assess for Chvostek's or Trousseau's sign, neck vein distention, and capillary refill. Monitor medication levels. Assess need to adjust medications (eg, those excreted or metabolized in kidney). Monitor for complications: acidosis, hyperkalemia, hypertension, overload, infection, uremia, ileus, pneumonia, gastrointestinal bleed. Psychosocial assessment. Strict I&O measurement of all body fluid output. Urine SG each void. Daily weight, frequent skin and oral care, water per NC (if needed). Safety precautions, incentive spirometry every 2 h (when awake). Strict aseptic technique for all procedures. Guaiac all stools.	Same as Day 1. Monitor closely for renal failure progression, uremia. Assess need for dialysis (severe acidosis and/or hyperkalemia).	Same as Day 2.	Same as Day 2 with VS and NS every 8 h. Strict I&O, daily weights, skin and mouth care.	Same as Day 4.
Teaching/ Discharge Planning	Orient to hospital and unit. Prepare for diagnostic tests. Provide information about diagnosis. Involve family in care of patient as needed. Review plan of care/clinical pathway with patient and family. Social worker to assess need for social services, health insurance, home environment, need for placement, family support, and financial status.	Continue to provide information regarding diagnosis and diagnostic tests. Explain dialysis if needed. Discharge planning is same as Day 1.	Diet education and fluid restriction. Medication, side effects, time. Importance of rest and gradually increasing activity. Assess ability to perform ADL, home environment, and need for assistive/adaptive devices.	Same as Day 3. Instruct: in signs and symptoms of renal failure, infection. According to identified cause of renal failure, provide prevention or management information. Arrange for outpatient blood and urine tests. Ensure that transportation is available. Verify ability pay for medications and laboratory work. Continue ADL assessment. Refer to home health service.	Review medications, diet laboratory work, fluid and activity restriction. Instruct to do daily weights using same scale. Instruct in signs and symptoms of renal failure, infection. Discharge planning: continue as per Day 4 and arrange to follow-up with physician.

the patient's and family's coping mechanisms. Identify any support systems.

Nursing Diagnoses and Planning

Nursing diagnoses and related expected patient outcomes most commonly applicable to patients with acute renal failure include the following:

NDx: Fluid volume excess related to malfunctioning kidneys

Planning: Patient Outcomes
1. Patient exhibits decreased peripheral, facial, and sacral edema.
2. Patient exhibits systemic signs of fluid overload.
3. Patient relates causative factors and treatments to alleviate overload.
4. Patient has a balanced fluid intake and output.
5. Patient's electrolyte levels are within safe limits.

NDx: Altered nutrition: less than body requirements related to renal failure and dietary restrictions

Planning: Patient Outcomes
1. Patient's weight is within accepted range.
2. Patient verbalizes need for dietary changes.
3. Patient follows prescribed diet.
4. Patient eats 75% of meals.

NDx: Hopelessness related to discomfort secondary to uremia

Planning: Patient Outcomes
1. Patient verbalizes relief of discomforts related to uremia (ie, pruritus, nausea and vomiting, and paresthesia).
2. Patient exhibits relaxed facial expression and body positioning.

Nursing Interventions and Evaluation

NDx: Fluid volume excess
Assess and report signs and symptoms of fluid volume excess, which include significant weight gain, increased blood pressure and pulse, change in mental status, dyspnea, orthopnea, crackles in the lungs, edema, distended neck veins, and elevated CVP. Monitor chest x-ray results. Monitor fluid intake and output. Maintain fluid restrictions as ordered. Restrict sodium intake as ordered. Monitor and document the therapeutic effect and side effects of prescribed medications. Weigh the patient at the same time each day. Alert the physician if signs and symptoms persist or worsen. Prepare the patient and family for dialysis if needed.

NDx: Altered nutrition: less than body requirements
Weigh the patient daily. Assess nutritional status regularly. Document the patient's food intake. Monitor intake and output. Assess the patient for any problems that could be associated with poor intake. These include anorexia, nausea, vomiting, fatigue, and mouth discomfort.

Administer antiemetics as ordered. Encourage the patient to take slow, deep breaths if nauseated.

Provide oral hygiene frequently. Provide small, frequent meals. Ensure that the environment is clean, relaxed, and pleasant. Provide a rest period before meals to minimize fatigue.

Obtain a dietary consultation if needed. Encourage the patient and family to discuss needs with the dietitian. Encourage the family to bring in favorite foods that meet dietary requirements.

NDx: Hopelessness
Assess for nonverbal signs of discomfort. Assess for complaints of nausea, vomiting, pruritus, muscle cramps, or paresthesia. Assist the patient with position changes as needed. Teach relaxation techniques. Administer medications as ordered. (More specific interventions for relieving discomforts can be found in Nursing Care Guide 31–2.)

Patient education is essential in the strict regimen and restrictions that must be employed. Education along with other psychosocial support mechanisms may also help decrease anxiety. Compliance with the medical regimen is essential. Therefore, measures such as therapeutic communication and knowledge of cultural diversities could be instituted to aid in compliance.

Compare the patient's status with the expected outcomes. If the outcomes are not met, reassess the patient and revise the plan.

CHRONIC RENAL FAILURE

Etiology and Pathophysiology
Chronic renal failure is irreversible. It is characterized by progressive reduction of nephrons until the remaining nephrons can no longer maintain the body's internal environment. Owing to the wide variety of causes of chronic renal failure, the early stages of the disease vary. The end-result for the person with renal failure is either uremia and death or treatment by dialysis or transplantation.

The causes of chronic renal failure are numerous. They include chronic glomerulonephritis, acute renal failure, polycystic kidney disease, obstruction, repeated pyelonephritis, and nephrotoxins. Systemic diseases, such as diabetes mellitus, hypertension, lupus erythematosus, polyarteritis, sickle cell disease, and amyloid disease, may also lead to renal failure.

The specific pathophysiologic mechanisms of renal failure depend on the underlying disease process. As nephrons are destroyed, the total glomerular filtration rate falls and clearance is reduced. BUN and serum creatinine levels rise. It is believed that remaining nephrons hypertrophy as a result of increased workload. Glomerular filtration remains effective until 70 to 80% of renal function is lost.

The course of chronic renal failure begins with the stage of diminished renal reserve. Kidney function decreases, but no wastes are accumulated. Early in the disease the kidneys can maintain excretion of solutes or waste products by decreasing water reab-

Text continued on page 1399

Nursing Care Guide 31–2
Patients with Chronic Renal Failure

Assessment Findings:	Patient experiences weight gain, hypertension, tachycardia, dyspnea, crackles in lungs, increasing central venous pressure (CVP), and decreased mentation.
Nursing Diagnosis:	Fluid volume excess related to retention of sodium and water secondary to decreased number of functioning nephrons and decreased glomerular filtration

Patient Outcomes	Nursing Interventions	Rationale
Patient's vital signs are within normal limits, chest is clear, no shortness of breath is apparent, and CVP is appropriate.	Maintain fluid restrictions as ordered. Restrict sodium intake.	Restricting fluids and sodium decreases the workload on the kidneys.
	Monitor vital signs and CVP frequently. Auscultate chest sounds.	Assessment of vital signs allows for early intervention if problems occur.
	Elevate the head of the bed and administer oxygen if needed.	This allows for easier respiratory effort.
Patient presents a decrease in peripheral edema.	Assess signs of edema in extremities. Check for pitting. Look for signs of compromised circulation.	Decreased edema in the periphery indicates a reduction in the fluid volume excess.

Evaluation:	Compare the patient's status with the expected outcomes. If the outcomes are not met, reassess the patient and revise the plan.

Assessment Findings:	Patient experiences muscle cramps, numbness, burning, tingling, and restless leg syndrome (crawling, itching sensation).
Nursing Diagnosis:	Pain related to peripheral neuropathies associated with electrolyte imbalances and nitrogenous waste accumulation

Patient Outcomes	Nursing Interventions	Rationale
Patient denies muscle cramps and paresthesia.	Observe the patient's reaction to discomfort. Explain the cause of the problems.	Understanding the cause of the discomfort may help the patient accept the problem.
	Provide a footboard, and instruct the patient to push feet against the board. Instruct patient to move legs while lying in bed. Keep linens off extremities.	Exercising while in bed helps relieve some of the symptoms of restless leg syndrome.
	Apply cool packs if ordered for comfort. Administer pharmacologic agents as ordered for discomfort.	Cool packs are soothing.
Patient completes activities of daily living without complaints of discomfort.	Assist the patient in completing daily self-care activities as needed. Explain alternative methods for performing tasks, and encourage the patient to do as much as possible.	Helping the patient complete tasks of self-care and encouraging self-participation promotes independence in the patient and prepares the patient for discharge.

(continued)

Nursing Care Guide 31–2
Patients with Chronic Renal Failure (continued)

Patient Outcomes	Nursing Interventions	Rationale
	Teach the patient exercises and relaxation techniques.	Exercises and relaxation techniques may help relieve symptoms of the syndrome.

Evaluation: Compare the patient's status with the expected outcomes. If the outcomes are not met, reassess the patient and revise the plan.

Assessment Findings: Patient scratches and rubs skin continually. Patient complains of severe itching.

Nursing Diagnosis: Impaired skin integrity related to atrophy of sweat glands, accumulation of urate crystals and calcium phosphate crystals on the skin

Patient Outcomes	Nursing Interventions	Rationale
Patient refrains from scratching and rubbing skin.	Assess for pruritus. Tell patient about the effects of continued scratching of the skin.	Assessment of symptoms of pruritus provides for early interventions.
	Apply cool moist packs. Use lotion on the skin as needed.	Cool packs are soothing to the skin. Lotion prevents dryness.
	Discourage frequent bathing. Use mild soaps and tepid water for bathing. Dry skin completely.	Frequent bathing is drying to the skin. Mild soap and water is less irritating.
	Provide diversional activities for the patient.	This takes the patient's mind off the constant feeling of skin irritation.
Patient denies pruritis and presents no evidence of skin irritation.	Monitor the patient for signs of skin breakdown. Look for scratches, signs of infection, reddened areas, and extreme dryness.	Assessing for pruritus and problems associated with it allows for early intervention to prevent skin breakdown.

Evaluation: Compare the patient's status with the expected outcomes. If the outcomes are not met, reassess the patient and revise the plan.

Assessment Findings: Patient is disoriented, experiences poor judgment and reasoning ability. Patient has short attention span, poor memory, irritability, and confusion.

Nursing Diagnosis: Altered thought processes related to accumulation of nitrogenous wastes and electrolyte imbalances

Patient Outcomes	Nursing Interventions	Rationale
Patient verbalizes orientation to time, place, and person.	Check the patient's orientation frequently. Reorient the patient to time, place, and person as needed. Explain to the patient all procedures and equipment used.	Assessing the patient's orientation provides baseline and continual data on the patient's neurologic status. This assists in orienting the patient to the present.
	Decrease external stimuli to a minimum.	Reducing stimuli prevents more confusion for the patient.

Nursing Care Guide 31–2
Patients with Chronic Renal Failure (continued)

Patient Outcomes	Nursing Interventions	Rationale
Patient presents improvement in thought processes.	Assess for alterations in thought processes. Allow time for patient to make decisions. Explain the physiologic basis for the change in mentation to the patient and family. Repeat instructions as needed. Assist the patient in decision-making when appropriate.	Presenting information slowly allows for comprehension by the patient. An understanding of the basis for the disturbances may help the patient and family accept and adjust to the situation. Some assistance in decision-making may be needed because of inability to process information appropriately.

Evaluation: Compare the patient's status with the expected outcomes. If the outcomes are not met, reassess the patient and revise the plan.

Assessment Findings: Patient experiences weakness, fatigue, and decreased endurance. Patient complains of inability to complete activities of daily living.

Nursing Diagnosis: Activity intolerance related to anemia and uremia

Patient Outcomes	Nursing Interventions	Rationale
Patient denies weakness and fatigue.	Assist the patient in identifying activities that result in extreme fatigue. Provide uninterrupted rest periods throughout the day. Teach the patient energy-saving techniques. Help the patient establish goals for increased endurance. Encourage good nutrition habits. Teach the patient to consume foods that are high in iron.	Restricting activities that cause extreme fatigue preserves the patient's energy. Frequent rest is necessary to promote increased energy levels. Using energy-saving techniques reduces the workload on the patient. Good nutrition promotes increased energy.
Patient completes activities of daily living such as self-care practices without complaints of fatigue and weakness.	Assist the patient with self-care as needed. Teach family members how to assist the patient. Have the patient organize the day for maximum activity during periods of maximum strength and energy level. Refer the patient to an exercise therapist for assistance in developing a planned routine of daily exercise.	Assisting the patient with some activities preserves strength. Careful planning for the day may allow for maximum utilization of the patient's abilities. Prescribed exercises may increase strength and endurance.

Evaluation: Compare the patient's status with the expected outcomes. If the outcomes are not met, reassess the patient and revise the plan.

(continued)

Nursing Care Guide 31–2
Patients with Chronic Renal Failure (continued)

Assessment Findings: Patient and family ask questions about the disease process and treatment regimen.

Nursing Diagnosis: Knowledge deficit: nature of disease process and the need for follow-up care and treatment

Patient Outcomes	Nursing Interventions	Rationale
Patient verbalizes an understanding of the disease process, the dietary restrictions, and measures to control problems associated with the disease.	Instruct the patient about the disease process, the dietary implications, and the methods for control of complications associated with the disease. Reinforce fluid and dietary restrictions.	Understanding the disease may promote compliance with the treatment regimen.
	Provide the patient with written instructions and information. Include the patient's family in the education sessions when appropriate.	Written instructions reinforce the verbal information. Including the family provides additional support for the patient.
	Have the patient repeat the information, and correct any misunderstandings. Allow the patient and family to ask questions.	Reiteration of the information allows for correction of misinformation.
Patient demonstrates an ability to weigh himself or herself and to monitor fluid intake and output appropriately.	Teach the patient how to monitor weight and fluid intake and output. Tell the patient to record the results and to present the information to the physician at the follow-up visit.	Recording of the weight and fluid intake and output provides the physician with data about the patient's progress and renal status after discharge.
Patient identifies signs and symptoms that are to be reported to the physician, and verbalizes the need for follow-up care and compliance with treatment plan.	Explain to the patient the signs and symptoms of potential problems that should be reported to the physician, such as weight gain greater than 1 lb/d, uncontrolled nausea and vomiting, increased weakness or confusion, abnormal bleeding, unrelieved itching, skin breakdown, shortness of breath, increased muscle cramping, tremors, or seizures.	Understanding the disease process, the complications, and when to seek assistance may prevent problems for the patient after discharge.
	Explain the importance of follow-up care and compliance with the treatment plan.	Continued medical monitoring of the patient and compliance with the treatment plan are essential to the appropriate management of the disease and prevention of complications.

Evaluation: Compare the patient's status with the expected outcomes. If the outcomes are not met, reassess the patient and revise the plan.

sorption. The ability to concentrate urine is lost. Urinary output increases. These are early signs of chronic renal failure and can cause severe dehydration. The second stage is renal insufficiency. As renal failure progresses, BUN level rises and urinary output decreases. The remaining healthy kidney tissue can no longer compensate. Glomerular filtration rate falls. Metabolic wastes begin to accumulate. The final stage is end-stage renal disease. BUN and serum creatinine levels rise excessively. Homeostasis cannot be maintained, and without dialysis, death occurs.

Clinical Manifestations

The course of chronic renal failure is highly individualized. However, there are common features of the disease process. The manifestations seen are those related to the following:

Imbalance of fluids and electrolytes (see Table 31–4)
Alterations of the body's regulatory mechanisms
Retention of metabolic wastes

Uremia, anemia, and acidosis are always present. Fluid and sodium are either abnormally retained or excreted. Thus, urinary volume may be increased, normal, or decreased. Hypertension is common in chronic renal failure but not always present. The most common cause of a higher blood pressure is an increase in total body water and sodium. No body system remains unaffected by renal failure (Table 31–6).

Diagnosis

Diagnosis of renal failure is based on the history, symptoms, and laboratory studies. The most definitive of these are serum creatinine and creatinine clearance. A rise in serum creatinine level and a fall in creatinine clearance indicate renal failure.

Management

The focus of conservative management is regulation of fluids, electrolytes (see Table 31–5), and metabolic wastes through dietary and volume controls along with medication, treatment of concurrent disorders, and patient comfort. Treatment goals are as follows:

Stabilization of internal environment
Control of fluid and electrolyte imbalances
Absence of infection
Absence of bleeding
Control of blood pressure
Control of concurrent illness
Absence of toxicity of medications that are inadequately excreted
Sufficient nutrient intake to maintain positive nitrogen balance
Control of anorexia and nausea
Control of itching (pruritus)

Fluid and sodium excretion vary significantly from patient to patient. Most patients have a tendency toward hypervolemia because of the inability to excrete sodium and water. Other patients are unable to conserve sodium and water because of an

Table 31–6

Clinical Manifestations of Renal Failure

Body System	Clinical Manifestations	Cause of Manifestations
Cardiovascular	Hypervolemia, hypertension, tachycardia, arrhythmias, congestive heart failure, pericarditis	Increased fluid volume, buildup of metabolic wastes, changes in renin-angiotensin mechanism, chronic hypertension
Hematologic	Anemia, leukocytosis, decreased platelet function, thrombocytopenia	Decreased production of erythropoietin, leading to decreased red blood cell production; decreased red blood cell survival time; decreased platelet activity; loss of blood through bleeding and dialysis
Gastrointestinal	Anorexia, nausea, vomiting, abdominal distention, diarrhea, constipation, bleeding	Buildup of uremic toxins, electrolyte imbalances, changes in platelet activity, conversion of urea to ammonia by saliva
Neurologic	Lethargy, confusion, convulsions, stupor, coma, sleep disturbances, behavioral disturbances, muscle irritability	Uremic toxins, electrolyte imbalances, cerebral swelling caused by fluid shifts
Dermatologic	Pallor, pigmentation, pruritus, ecchymosis, excoriation, uremic frost	Anemia, decreased activity of sweat gland, dry skin, phosphate deposits on skin
Urinary	Decreased urine output, decreased specific gravity, proteinuria, casts and cells in the urine	Damage to the nephron
Skeletal	Osteoporosis, renal rickets, joint pain	Decreased calcium absorption, decreased phosphate excretion

inability to concentrate the urine and therefore tend to be hypovolemic. The desired effect is to maintain the person in a normotensive, normovolemic state.

Virtually every electrolyte and mineral is affected in renal failure. The goal of treatment here is to maintain electrolyte levels within an acceptable limit (see Table 31–5). Control of electrolytes is accomplished through dietary restriction, medication, or both. Because of the chronic nature of the disease, these patients may be able to tolerate electrolyte imbalance without the symptoms experienced by patients without renal disease.

Dietary restrictions can significantly reduce metabolic wastes. Protein restrictions may range from 20 to 80 g per day (see Highlight 31–3). The restriction depends on the ability of the person to excrete wastes from the body. The quality of protein allowed must be high in order to maintain positive nitrogen balance, thus decreasing urea production from muscle wasting. Calories for energy needs are supplied by carbohydrates and fats.

Anemia is present in all renal failure patients owing to multiple causes. Anemia may be treated with iron supplements and folic acid supplementation. The drug epoetin alfa (Epogen) has greatly reduced the problem of anemia. Transfusions are used in cases of severe anemia when the patient is symptomatic.

Gastrointestinal symptoms of these patients range from nausea to gastrointestinal bleeding. Treatment of these manifestations includes administration of antacids and antiemetics, dietary control of nitrogenous wastes, and maintenance of fluid and electrolyte balances.

Hypertension is treated vigorously in this population. A stepwise approach to treatment may be instituted as follows:

Sodium and fluid restriction
Diuretic therapy
Beta blockers
Vasodilators

Sources of infection, such as an indwelling catheter, are avoided. When infection occurs, immediate action is taken to treat the infection.

Patient comfort is promoted. These patients are prone to muscle cramping, pruritus, headaches, ocular irritation, insomnia, and fatigue. Muscle cramping is often associated with sodium depletion. Measures instituted to control the cramping include local heat and massage. Primary treatment is control of the electrolyte imbalance. Pruritus is described as a sensation of deep itching that may be related to the uremic frost or associated with phosphate deposits in the skin. Treatment for pruritus is aimed at decreasing the phosphorus with administration of phosphate binders. Local and systemic agents may be administered to decrease the itching. Ocular irritation is exhibited by burning and watery eyes, thought to be caused by calcium deposits in the conjunctiva. Treatment is aimed at decreasing the

plasma phosphate levels. "Artificial tears" may be used for local comfort. Insomnia and fatigue are related to uremia and possibly psychosocial disturbances. Treatment is designed to decrease metabolic waste buildup and psychosocial support. If necessary, medications are used with caution for sleep. Changes in drug metabolism related to decreased renal function must be considered when administering all medications.

NURSING PROCESS
Chronic Renal Failure

The assessment, nursing diagnoses, expected patient outcomes, nursing interventions, and evaluation for patients with chronic renal failure can be found in Nursing Care Guide 31–2.

DIALYSIS

Dialysis was first utilized in 1960 by means of an artificial kidney with chronic intermittent hemodialysis. When the irreversibility of renal damage was established, treatment was then withdrawn. This practice continues in many countries worldwide where resources are limited.

In 1972 the United States government established legislation to provide payment for the health-care costs of citizens with end-stage renal disease. In the United States, payment for patients with documented end-stage renal disease is provided through Medicare.

Dialysis occurs with the movement of fluids and particles across a semipermeable membrane. This treatment is used to restore fluid and electrolyte balance and acid-base balance and to remove wastes and toxic materials from the body. This treatment is an augmentation of renal function to sustain life in acute and chronic situations.

Dialysis is based on three principles: diffusion, osmosis, and ultrafiltration. Diffusion is the movement of particles across a semipermeable membrane from areas of a higher concentration to those of a lower concentration. Diffusion is used to clear solutes from the body in both hemodialysis and peritoneal dialysis. Osmosis is the passage of solvent (water) across a semipermeable membrane from an area of lesser solute concentration to an area of greater solute concentration. Osmosis is used to remove extra fluid, especially in peritoneal dialysis. Ultrafiltration is the movement of fluid across a semipermeable membrane as a result of an artificially created pressure gradient. Ultrafiltration is more efficient in removing fluids from the body than is osmosis. Ultrafiltration is used to remove excess fluids in hemodialysis. During dialysis, diffusion, osmosis, and ultrafiltration occur simultaneously.

Dialysis of some form is implemented when the following conditions occur:

Unmanageable hyperkalemia
Intractable acidosis
Volume overload
Uremia

There are four main goals of dialysis therapy:

Removal of metabolic waste products
Maintenance of safe concentration of electrolytes
Correction of acid-base imbalance
Removal of excess fluids

These goals can be met through the use of hemodialysis or peritoneal dialysis. The two methods of dialysis vary significantly in procedure, benefits, time required to complete, cost, and appropriateness for the patient. Advantages and disadvantages of hemodialysis and peritoneal dialysis are described in Table 31–7.

Peritoneal Dialysis

Peritoneal dialysis involves the instillation of hypertonic fluid into the peritoneal cavity, where it is allowed to remain for a prescribed period of time before it is drained (Fig. 31–4). Fluids and solutes from the blood stream are transferred through the peritoneum. Solutes, which carry fluids, move from an area of higher concentration in the body to an area of lower concentration in the dialyzing fluid. It is used for both acute and chronic renal failure and can be performed in the hospital or at home.

Peritoneal dialysis offers many advantages to the patient, including the following:

Maintenance of steady state of blood chemistry
Opportunity for patient independence in dialysis therapy
Simplicity of learning procedure
Fewer dietary restrictions
More control over daily life
Safe use in hemodynamically unstable patients

The contraindications for peritoneal dialysis include the following:

Tight abdominal muscles
Diaphragmatic tears
Abdominal drains
Diffuse bowel disease
Respiratory insufficiency
Intra-abdominal cancer
Extensive abdominal adhesions
Infection in the abdomen

Procedure

Access to the peritoneal cavity is gained through placement of a catheter. The physician chooses the

Table 31–7

Some Advantages and Disadvantages of Peritoneal Dialysis and Hemodialysis

	Advantage	Disadvantage
Peritoneal dialysis	Can be used for temporary or permanent dialysis Relatively easy to perform Nonsophisticated equipment needed No vascular access required May be used in either the hospital or home Generally less costly than hemodialysis Patient may be ambulatory (with one type) Can be performed by the patient without assistance in the home Few nutrition restrictions	Takes longer to complete treatment than hemodialysis Slower clearance of toxins Not usable if patient has had recent abdominal surgery or has abdominal wounds Alters the patient's lifestyle Requires abdominal catheter care
Hemodialysis	Can be used for temporary or permanent dialysis Quick removal of toxins More efficient for some patients especially those with complicating disorders (fewer contraindications) May be done in hospital or home Shorter time for treatment needed (3–4 h 3–4 times per week)	Needs a reliable access site, may need a long-term site Needs specially trained personnel in the hospital or assistance at home More costly than peritoneal dialysis Alters the patient's lifestyle Restrictions for diet Requires vascular care The patient is not ambulatory during treatment Has complications such as hemorrhage, air embolus, hemodynamic alterations, and muscle cramping, along with vascular access problems

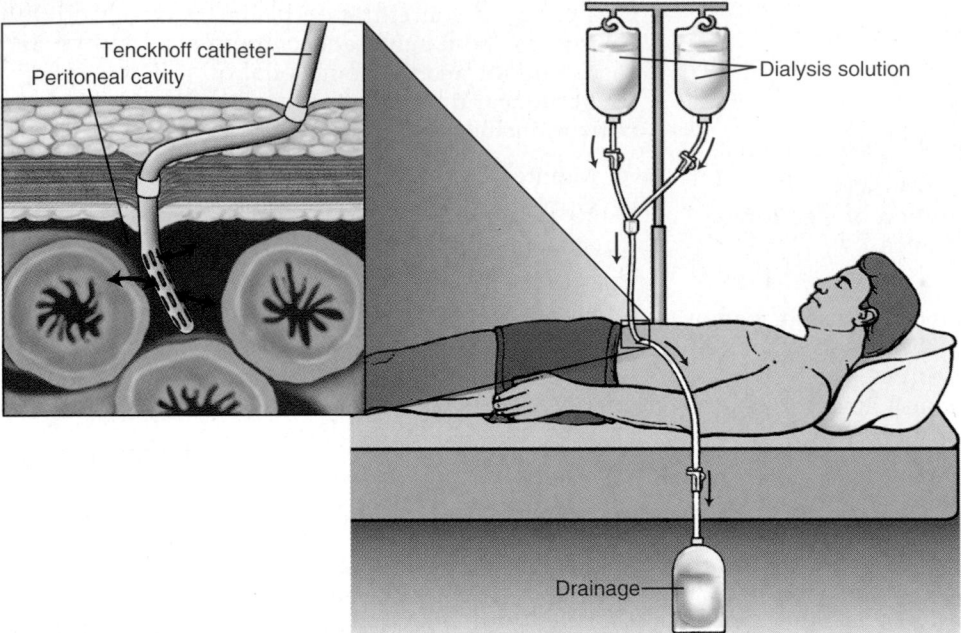

Figure 31–4

Peritoneal dialysis via an implanted abdominal catheter.

appropriate type catheter (Fig. 31–5). If the catheter is to be used for an acutely ill patient, a catheter is placed for each dialysis session. A permanent catheter is inserted for long-term use.

There are several types of peritoneal dialysis. Basically the same principle is used with some modification in the procedure. The types of peritoneal dialysis are as follows:

Intermittent peritoneal dialysis
Continuous ambulatory peritoneal dialysis
Continuous-cycle peritoneal dialysis

Intermittent peritoneal dialysis involves dialyzing for 40 hours per week. The time period is divided into three to seven dialysis runs per week. These usually occur at night. The abdomen remains empty between dialysis runs. The procedure uses a cycling machine.

In continuous ambulatory peritoneal dialysis, dialysate is instilled into the abdomen and left in place 4 to 8 hours. The empty bag is rolled and carried with the patient until it is time to drain the fluid. When it is time for drainage, the bag is unrolled and the fluid is drained by gravity. Continu-

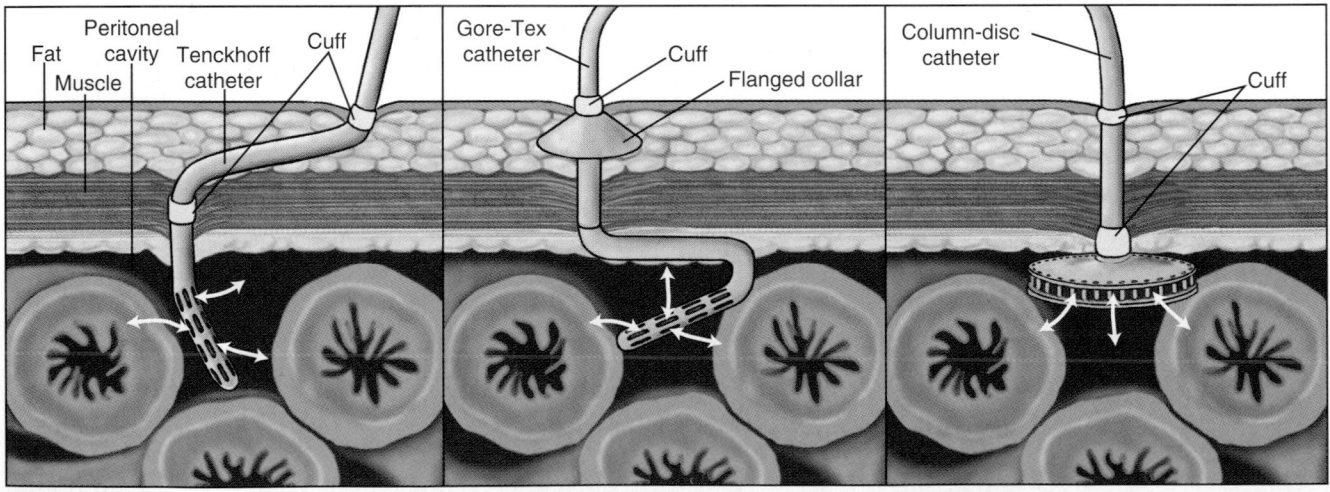

Figure 31–5

Three types of peritoneal dialysis catheters. Tenckhoff's catheter (left) has two Dacron felt cuffs that hold the catheter in place and prevent leakage of the dialysate and bacterial invasion. The use of a subcutaneous tunnel with this type of catheter also helps prevent infection. The Gore-Tex catheter (center) has a Dacron cuff above a flanged collar. The column-disc catheter (right) has cuffs and a large implanted abdominal port.

ous ambulatory peritoneal dialysis requires four exchanges per day on the average. Dialysis is carried out 7 days per week for 24 hours per day for a total of 168 hours per week. This is a manual procedure.

Continuous-cycle peritoneal dialysis is similar to continuous ambulatory peritoneal dialysis in that it is continuous. However, this procedure calls for three cycles to be run via a cycling machine. In the morning, fresh dialysate is instilled into the abdomen and allowed to remain until it is drained just before initiation of the nightly cycles.

Commercial dialysate comes in both 1.5% and 4.26% dextrose, in 2 L bottles or bags. Usual instillation for adults is 2 L per exchange.

Peritoneal dialysis is carried out under strict sterile technique. Mask should always be worn by nurses performing peritoneal dialysis. Povidone-iodine should be used for cleansing the catheter for both connection and disconnection.

Drugs or other substances may be added to the dialysate under sterile technique. These may include potassium, antibiotics, heparin, and insulin, depending on the needs of the patient.

Uses

Peritoneal dialysis may be used in the treatment of both acute and chronic renal failure. Peritoneal dialysis may be chosen if the patient is hemodynamically unstable or cannot tolerate systemic anticoagulation.

Complications

Peritoneal dialysis is considered to be a safe procedure. However, it is not without complications. Among the complications are the following:

> Peritonitis
> Catheter plugging or displacement
> Constipation
> Fluid leakage
> Bowel perforation on catheter insertion
> Bladder perforation on catheter insertion
> Pain
> Hernia
> Electrolyte imbalance
> Fluid imbalance
> Hypoalbuminemia
> Respiratory difficulties

These complications are easily diagnosed and may be resolved with prompt treatment. Careful nursing care and patient education often prevent the development of many of these complications.

NURSING PROCESS
Peritoneal Dialysis

Assessment

Assess fluid and electrolyte status continually. Monitor fluid intake and output. Assess blood pressure and vital signs before, during, and at the completion of dialysis. Monitor and record infusion and drainage of dialysate. Assess for signs of respiratory distress, pain, and discomfort. Assess the patency of the catheter. Assess for any signs of infection. Evaluate the patient's knowledge related to the procedure.

Nursing Diagnoses and Planning

Nursing diagnoses and related expected patient outcomes most commonly applicable to patients undergoing peritoneal dialysis include the following:

NDx: Risk for infection related to peritoneal catheter and dialysis procedure

Planning: Patient Outcomes
1. Patient is free of infection.
2. Patient verbalizes the signs and symptoms of infection.
3. Patient demonstrates sterile technique for bag, tubing, and dressing changes (if performing self-care).

NDx: Risk for fluid volume excess or deficit related to fluid retention or removal

Planning: Patient Outcomes
1. Patient has balanced fluid intake and output, stable weight, and good skin turgor.
2. Patient's vital signs and CVP are within normal limits.
3. Patient's dialysate outflow is greater than or equal to inflow.

NDx: Altered nutrition: less than body requirements related to protein loss in dialysate

Planning: Patient Outcomes
1. Patient has stable weight.
2. Patient has adequate protein intake (1.2 to 1.5 g/kg body weight per day) and a normal serum albumin level (3.5 to 5.5 g/dL).

(Other nursing diagnoses that apply to both peritoneal dialysis and hemodialysis are covered in the section on hemodialysis.)

Nursing Interventions and Evaluation

NDx: Risk for infection
Observe for and report signs and symptoms of peritonitis. These include fever, abdominal pain, cloudy outflow, nausea, and malaise. Maintain sterile technique when changing dialysate bags, connecting and disconnecting the catheter, and performing catheter care (Table 31–8). Maintain sterility of dialysate.

Assess the catheter site for redness, drainage, tenderness, or foul odor. If exudate is present, it should be cultured. Observe for leakage at the site. Continuous leakage can lead to peritonitis.

Instruct the patient in the procedure and the needed care to maintain dialysis at home if needed. Allow the patient and family to ask questions.

NDx: Risk for fluid volume excess or deficit
Observe for and report signs and symptoms of fluid

Table 31–8

Nursing Care Guidelines for Peritoneal Dialysis Catheters

Interventions	Rationale
Use aseptic technique and infection control precautions (handwashing, mask, gloves)	Prevents contamination and risk of infection
Assess the site for erythema, drainage, swelling, or tenderness	Early recognition of infection allows for treatment and prevention of complications
Change dressing and administer site/skin care per physician's orders (iodophor swab solution, sterile occlusive or transparent dressing)	Prevents contamination and potential complications
Instruct patient and family about the signs and symptoms of complications and when to notify the physician or nurse	Early recognition of possible complications and notification facilitates the treatment regimen

overload. These include hypertension, tachycardia, dyspnea, crackles in lungs, distended neck veins, and increased CVP. Record accurately the measurement of inflow and outflow.

Observe for and report signs of outflow problems. Outflow problems may include catheter obstruction by omentum, catheter occlusion by fibrin, and a full colon. For a full colon, administer stool softeners and provide a high-fiber diet. Enemas can be used if necessary. If the catheter is occluded by fibrin, obtain an order to irrigate with heparinized saline. If the omentum obstructs the catheter, turn the patient from side to side, elevate the head of the bed, or apply firm pressure to the abdomen. Notify the physician if outflow problems continue.

Monitor intake and output. Weigh the patient daily. Raise the head of the bed. Drain the dialysate. Notify the physician if respiratory distress occurs.

Assess for signs and symptoms of fluid deficit. These include hypertension, tachycardia, decreased CVP, and poor skin turgor.

NDx: Altered nutrition: less than body requirements
Monitor intake and output. Weigh the patient daily. Provide adequate dietary protein. Consult with the dietitian as necessary. Instruct the patient in proper diet. Provide a list of restricted and encouraged foods with menus. Assist the patient in developing a plan for meals before discharge. Allow the patient and family to ask questions and discuss nutrition options.

Compare the patient's status with the expected outcomes. If the outcomes are not met, reassess the patient and revise the plan.

Hemodialysis

In hemodialysis, blood is removed from a vascular access site. The blood is heparinized, pumped through a dialyzer (Fig. 31–6), and then returned to the patient's circulation. Diffusion and ultrafiltration occur, allowing the blood to be filtered.

Procedure
A hemodialysis system includes a dialyzer, dialysate, vascular access routes, and hemodialysis machine. There are several different designs of dialyzers. The dialyzer has a blood compartment and a dialysate compartment. The two compartments are separated by a semipermeable membrane. The dialysate is an electrolyte solution that can be modified to meet the patient's needs. Toxins and wastes diffuse across the semipermeable membrane from the blood to the dialysate. There are many different models of hemodialysis machines, but their basic function is similar.

Heparin is used for anticoagulation to prevent clots from forming in the dialyzer and tubing. Dosage is based on each patient's individual need. Clotting studies, such as activated partial thromboplastin times and partial thromboplastin time, are performed to monitor the drug's effect. The antidote for heparin is protamine sulfate.

Hemodialysis involves shunting the patient's blood from the body through a dialyzer in which diffusion and ultrafiltration occur and then returning filtered blood to the patient's circulation. Vascu-

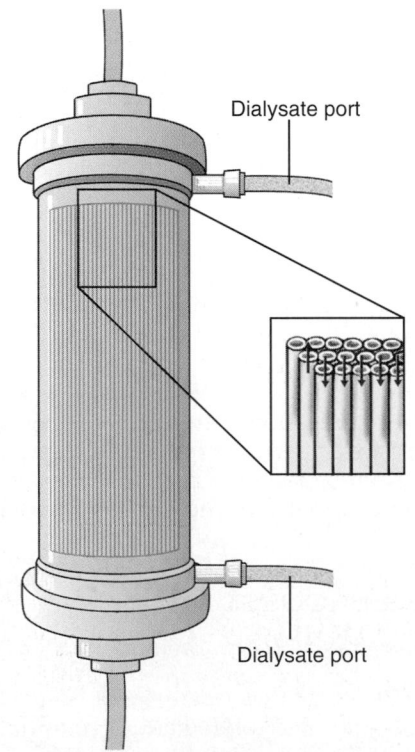

Figure 31–6
One type of dialyzer used in hemodialysis.

Figure 31–7

Sites for creation of an internal arteriovenous fistula. Surgical creation of an arteriovenous anastomosis provides easy access to blood for hemodialysis. This method reduces the risk of infection and makes shunts unnecessary except during hemodialysis.

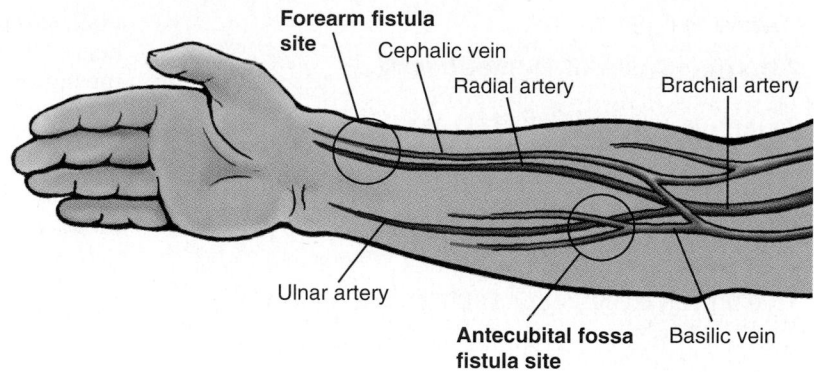

lar access is necessary in order to perform hemodialysis. Several techniques are instituted to establish this access:

> Arteriovenous fistula
> Arteriovenous graft
> External arteriovenous shunt
> Femoral vein catheterization
> Subclavian vein catheterization

The first three are permanent access techniques. The last two are temporary access techniques.

Arteriovenous fistulas are created surgically by joining or anastomosing an artery and a vein. Usually, the surgeon joins the radial artery and cephalic vein to create a forearm fistula. However, the surgeon may sometimes join the ulnar artery and basilic vein to create an antecubital fistula (Fig. 31–7). After surgery, a fistula must mature for 6 to 12 weeks.

Arteriovenous grafts are surgically placed materials that form a bridge between the arterial and venous circulations. Among the materials used are the following:

> Patient's own saphenous vein
> Bovine carotid arteries
> Expanded polytetrafluoroethylene (PTFE or
>   Gore-Tex)

These may be placed in either the arms or the legs. However, the arm is the preferred site.

External arteriovenous shunts are devices made of Silastic-Teflon tubing that is surgically implanted into an adjacent artery and vein. The tubing remains outside the body (Fig. 31–8). An external arteriovenous shunt can be used for 6 to 9 months, which makes it practical for patients with chronic renal failure who are undergoing long-term dialysis.

Use of femoral vein catheters is usually a safe and easy procedure. This involves insertion of two 16-gauge angiocatheters or a specially designed catheter into the femoral vein. These catheters must be removed after each dialysis treatment.

Subclavian vein catheterization involves the placement of a specially designed catheter into the subclavian vein under sterile technique. The advantage of the subclavian catheter is that it can be left in place for repeated use. Care of these types of vascular access is discussed within the context of the nursing process.

Uses

Hemodialysis is usually performed in a hospital or free-standing dialysis clinic. The procedure is usually carried out three times per week. Home dialysis is available for selected patients. Hemodialysis may be used in the treatment of both acute and chronic renal failure.

Complications

The complications of hemodialysis are divided into two categories: (1) those involving the vascular access and (2) those involving the dialysis process (Table 31–9).

Figure 31–8

An external arteriovenous shunt provides access to blood for hemodialysis. The arterial cannula is connected to the dialyzer. Blood returns through the venous cannula. When not connected to the hemodialyzer, the arterial cannula is connected to the venous cannula.

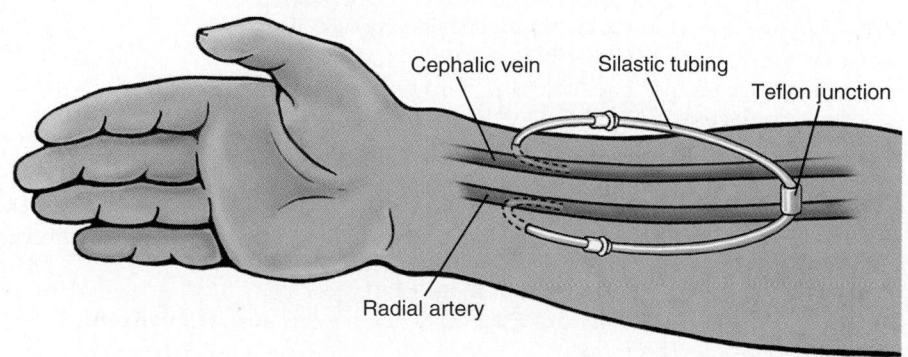

Table 31–9

Complications of Hemodialysis

COMPLICATIONS RELATED TO VASCULAR ACCESS

Clot formation in the graft, fistula, or catheter
Stenosis or narrowing of the anastomosis infection
Aneurysm formation
High-output cardiac failure

COMPLICATIONS RELATED TO THE DIALYSIS PROCEDURE

Hypovolemic shock
Blood loss
Electrolyte imbalance
Air embolus

NURSING PROCESS
Hemodialysis

Assessment

Assessment of the patient undergoing hemodialysis is related to control of fluid and electrolyte balance, prevention of complications, and maintenance of vascular access. Cardiac status is of utmost importance. Assess postural changes of blood pressure, especially at the completion of dialysis. Check all vital signs. Assess heart and lung sounds. Monitor heart rhythm. Assess CVP, if a line is present, and the status of neck veins.

Assess fluid status before and after the procedure. Monitor intake and output. Weigh the patient before and after dialysis. Assess mental status. Mental status changes may indicate disequilibrium dementia or electrolyte imbalance. Monitor electrolyte values.

Check the patency of the vascular access by auscultating for a bruit and palpating for a thrill. The presence of the bruit and thrill indicates an adequate blood flow through the access. Observe and report any numbness, pain, or swelling in the extremity distal to the access. The vascular access is the lifeline of the patient on hemodialysis and must be monitored closely and handled with care. Assessment and care of a vascular access site are summarized in Table 31–10.

Assess the patient's and family's knowledge concerning dialysis, vascular access, and dietary and medical regimen. Assess support systems and the patient's coping mechanisms.

Nursing Diagnoses and Planning

Nursing diagnoses and related expected patient outcomes most commonly applicable to patients undergoing hemodialysis include the following:

Table 31–10

Nursing Care Guidelines for Vascular Access Sites

Type	Interventions	Rationale
Fistula	Inspect needle puncture sites after dialysis. If bleeding occurs, apply pressure to stop bleeding; release pressure to check site every 5–10 min.	Prevents hemorrhaging.
	Do not take blood pressure, perform venipuncture, or draw blood from arm with fistula. Avoid tight clothing or restrictive bands or jewelry. Palpate for thrill and auscultate for bruit every shift. Report absence of thrill or bruit.	Prevents clotting and allows for early intervention at signs of clotting.
	Observe for signs and symptoms of infection. Culture and report any drainage.	Prevents infection and allows for early intervention at signs of infection.
Shunt	Wrap shunt securely with gauze. Tape all connections. Do not use scissors to remove dressings. Keep bulldog or rubber-shod clamp at bedside for use if disconnection occurs. Apply firm pressure at site if shunt pulls out, and notify physician immediately.	Prevents hemorrhaging and disruption of shunt.
	Expose a portion of the loop to check for patency every shift. Palpate for thrill and auscultate for bruit above exit site every shift.	Prevents clotting and allows for early intervention at signs of clotting.
	Use aseptic technique with dressing changes. Observe for signs of infection. Culture any drainage.	Prevents infection and allows for early intervention at signs of infection.

NDx: Risk for fluid volume excess or deficit related to renal failure or fluid removal

Planning: Patient Outcomes
1. Patient has balanced intake and output, stable weight, and good skin turgor.
2. Patient's vital signs and CVP are within normal limits.
3. Patient's dialysate outflow is greater than or equal to inflow.

NDx: Risk for injury related to blood loss from access site

Planning: Patient Outcomes
1. Patient exhibits normal vital signs, normal skin temperature and color, and brisk capillary refill.
2. Patient's access has audible bruit and palpable thrill.

NDx: Risk for infection related to vascular access

Planning: Patient Outcomes
1. Patient is afebrile.
2. Patient's access site is free of erythema, warmth, exudate, swelling, and tenderness.

NDx: Ineffective individual coping related to effects of long-term hemodialysis

Planning: Patient Outcomes
1. Patient expresses a realistic view of the situation and coping resources available.
2. Patient discusses changes in himself or herself and the family as a result of renal failure.
3. Patient verbalizes feelings to health-care professional and family.
4. Patient identifies changes in family roles and processes as a result of renal failure.
5. Patient identifies alternative coping behaviors.

Nursing Interventions and Evaluation

NDx: Risk for fluid volume excess or deficit
Observe for and report signs and symptoms of fluid overload. These include hypertension, tachycardia, dyspnea, crackles in lungs, distended neck veins, and increased CVP. Record accurately the measurement of inflow and outflow.

Observe for and report signs of outflow problems. Outflow problems may include catheter obstruction from kinking or catheter occlusion by fibrin. If the catheter is occluded by fibrin, obtain an order to irrigate with heparinized saline. Notify the physician if outflow problems continue.

Monitor intake and output. Weigh the patient daily. Raise the head of the bed. Notify the physician if respiratory distress occurs. Assess for signs and symptoms of fluid deficit. These include hypertension, tachycardia, decreased CVP, and poor skin turgor.

NDx: Risk for injury
Provide adequate site care (see Table 31–10). Monitor for complications. Report severe or unrelieved pain, numbness, tingling, or swelling of the extremity distal to the access. Observe for symptoms of blood loss. Maintain and monitor equipment.

NDx: Risk for infection
Provide adequate site care. Use aseptic technique when changing dressings. Monitor vital signs. Observe for redness, swelling, warmth, exudate, and tenderness at the site. Culture any drainage. Teach the patient and family to recognize signs and symptoms of infection.

NDx: Ineffective individual coping
It often takes several weeks for the full impact and permanency of dialysis to be realized. The most common psychosocial problems seen are as follows:

Change in body image
Dependence-independence conflict
Difficulty in facing potential death

Relationships with family, relatives, and friends are likely to change. Many patients have much difficulty coping with these changes and problems.

Instruct the patient and family in all areas of the treatment regimen. Allow for questions and verbalization of fears and concerns. Identify the patient's normal patterns of coping. Provide support for decisions made by the patient and family. Accept the patient's reactions to dialysis. Encourage active participation in the patient's care by the patient and the family.

Compare the patient's status with the expected outcomes. If the outcomes are not met, reassess the patient and revise the plan.

❖ Settings, Providers, and Collaboration for Care

Home care teaching for the patient on dialysis must begin as soon as the patient seems receptive. A teaching care plan should be adapted to the patient's needs with follow-up teaching evaluation. Patients should be aware of their special nutritional and medication needs and how to detect changes in kidney function. In addition, an assessment of the family's ability to cope, patient's level of independence, and community resources available is needed.

The primary treatment setting of peritoneal dialysis is the patient's home. Full-service home care programs are available and offer a wide variety of options in the care of dialysis patients. Home care offers the patient greater control over chronic therapy in the best environment, quality dialysis therapy, and less costly modalities. Collaboration between the patient's physician and the dialysis or home health nurse is an ongoing process throughout the treatment period.

The primary outpatient treatment settings for hemodialysis are the free-standing dialysis centers or hospital-based dialysis centers. Home hemodialysis is available but seldom used. The home hemodialysis setting can provide the patient with quality dialysis therapy and control over the therapy, but it is expensive, and many patients and their families feel more secure in the outpatient dialysis center. A home dialysis visiting nurse may be necessary to assist the patient and family with the therapy.

According to the Centers for Disease Control and Prevention (CDC), patients with human immunodeficiency virus (HIV) infection can be treated with either peritoneal dialysis or hemodialysis. HIV-infected patients do not need to be isolated from other patients. CDC guidelines affirm the infection control strategy of Universal Precautions to be used consistently in dialysis centers by all personnel.

RENAL TRANSPLANTATION

Renal transplantation is the surgical transfer of a functioning kidney from one person to another. This is a treatment option for irreversible renal failure. In 1995, approximately 20,000 renal transplantations were performed and approximately 30,000 people were on the waiting lists for transplantation.

Donors for transplantation come from two sources. The first group consists of living-related donors. The other group consists of cadaveric donors. The preferred donor is the living-related donor because genetic matching is closer or even identical. There is a third source of donors that is gaining popularity. This is the living-nonrelated donor. At present some centers are using this source of donors.

The major factors in donor and recipient determination are blood type and histocompatibility typing. Kidneys are not transplanted across blood types. Therefore, if the recipient has type A blood, the donor must have type A blood also. In histocompatibility typing, the human leukocyte antigens are examined. There are three areas that are examined. They are A, B, and DR loci. In living-related donors, an identical match is ideal. However, a half match is acceptable. In cadaveric transplantation, there may be no match at all except the blood type. The matching of donor and recipient varies from center to center. Some use only blood type. Others use human leukocyte antigen–matching in choosing the recipient. The final determining factor in the recipient is called a final cross-match. In this test, the donor's and recipient's blood are mixed and examined for a reaction. If there is a reaction, the recipient and donor are not compatible, and, therefore, the transplantation will not take place.

Cadaveric kidneys may be maintained for as long as 72 hours before transplantation, depending on the preservation method. This allows kidneys to be transported long distances for transplantation.

Donors must meet certain criteria for transplantation. These criteria include the following:

Heart beating
Functioning organs
No history of chronic disease
No history of cancer outside of the central nervous system
Younger than 65 years

Procedure

After removal from the donor, the kidney is preserved on ice or on a perfusion pump. When the donor is cadaveric, multiple organs may be harvested. Because of the preservation of the kidneys, they are the last organs to be harvested. Both kidneys are removed along with the aorta, vena cava, and ureters.

When the donor is living-related, a single kidney is removed through a flank incision. In this nephrectomy procedure, the kidney, renal vein, renal artery, and ureter are removed together. The transplanted kidney is placed in the iliac fossa. Either kidney may be used. Figure 31–9 shows the placement of a transplanted kidney.

The recipient has a hockey-stick incision in either the lower left or right quadrant of the abdomen, depending on the kidney used. The renal artery and vein are attached to the iliac artery and vein. The surgery is performed without entering the peritoneum. Therefore, the patient may eat or drink after recovering from anesthesia.

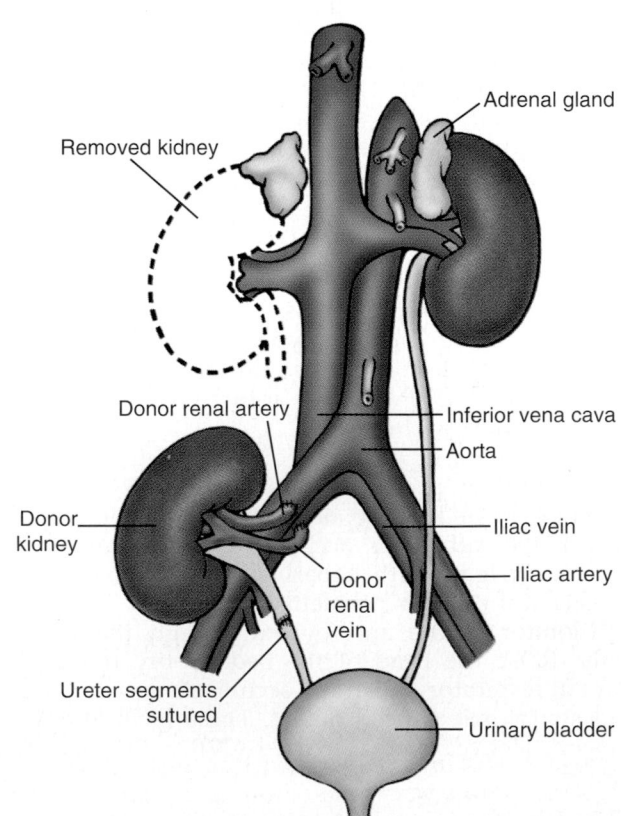

Figure 31–9

Placement of a transplanted kidney.

Depending on the surgeon's preference, the patient returns from the operating room with at least one intravenous line and usually a Foley catheter and some sort of abdominal drain.

In some centers, the patient may go to the intensive care unit for 24 to 48 hours. In other centers, the patient returns to the transplantation floor.

Uses

Renal transplantation is a means of restoring renal function to normal in most patients, thus allowing them to return to a healthy lifestyle. Geriatric patients are not candidates for transplantation, because most centers limit the upper range for receiving a transplant to the age of 55 to 60 years.

Complications

Numerous complications are related to transplantation. These may be grouped into several categories: surgical, medical, and those related to immunosuppression, rejection, or infection.

Surgical complications include vascular problems, such as thrombosis (clotting), stenosis, and leakage. Additional complications include urologic problems, such as obstruction, reflux, fistula, and urine leakage. Other complications include the formation of hematomas, abscesses, and lymphoceles (collections of lymph fluid).

Medical complications include acute tubular necrosis (a form of acute renal failure related to ischemia), fluid overload or dehydration, electrolyte imbalances, hypertension, gastric distress, constipation, and diarrhea.

Rejection is an ever-present danger in transplantation. There are three types of rejection: hyperacute, acute, and chronic. Hyperacute rejection happens immediately, but can usually be avoided by performing the final cross-match. Acute rejection is a treatable form of rejection that generally occurs in the first year after transplantation. Chronic rejection occurs after the first year of transplantation. It is untreatable and generally results in the loss of the graft. See Table 31–11 for signs and symptoms of rejection.

Infection is the plague of all patients taking immunosuppressive medications because these drugs decrease the body's ability to fight off infection. The infections may be bacterial, viral, or fungal. Bacterial infections are the easiest to treat because of the broad spectrum of antibiotics available. The most common fungal infection is caused by yeast and can be treated with amphotericin and, if oral, with clotrimazole (Mycelex). Viral infections can be the most troublesome to transplantation. The most common viral infection is caused by cytomegalovirus. If not detected and treated early, it can eventually result in graft loss or even death of the patient. The other menacing viral infection of the transplant patient is the herpes virus, which can show many forms in the immunosuppressed patient. It can range from simple outbreaks of "fever blisters," to herpes zoster or shingles, to a systemic form that is extremely detri-

Table 31–11

Signs and Symptoms of Transplant Rejection

Acute Rejection (less than 1 year)	Chronic Rejection (more than 1 year)
Weight gain	Gradual decrease in urine output
Edema	Gradual weight gain
Fever	Gradual rise in creatinine level
Increased blood urea nitrogen and serum creatinine levels	Hypertension (new onset)
Increased blood pressure	Proteinuria
Swelling and tenderness at graft site	
Electrolyte imbalances	

mental to the patient's health. Acyclovir (Zovirax) has become instrumental in the treatment of these patients.

The complications related to immunosuppressive medications are varied and range from a marked decrease in white blood cell counts to an increased risk of cancer. All immunosuppressive medications increase the risk of infection.

Immunosuppression

Immunosuppressive medications are given to prevent rejection of the transplanted organ. Five medications are given as therapy immediately after transplantation. These are antilymphocyte globulin, antithymocyte globulin, cyclosporine, steroids, and azathioprine. The type and protocol used for transplant patients varies from center to center. Rejection may be treated with any of these medications mentioned except azathioprine. One other medication used in the treatment of rejection is muromonab-CD3 (OKT3).

Antilymphocyte globulin and antithymocyte globulin act by covering white blood cells, therefore making them less effective. These two medications may be used immediately postoperatively or as a treatment for rejection.

Steroids (prednisone and Solu-Medrol) affect the immune system by decreasing the inflammatory response, sensitivity, and number of some of the white blood cells. These medications are not without side effects. They include increases in blood sugar level, retention of sodium and water, decreased wound healing, stress ulcer formation, mood swings, muscle wasting, steroid acne, and rarely cataracts and degeneration of the weight-bearing joints. Steroids are used for maintenance therapy and treatment of rejection.

Cyclosporine acts directly on T cells to prevent rejection. This medication is extremely expensive. The side effects include toxicity of the kidney and liver, increased hair growth on the face, hypertension, tremors, and rarely seizures.

Azathioprine acts by decreasing white cell activity. Side effects include increased risk of infection and malignancy, hair loss, decrease in number of platelets, nausea, and vomiting.

Muromonab-CD3 (OKT3) is a new treatment for rejection. The major side effect of this medication is pulmonary edema, especially with the first dose. This medication should never be given to a fluid-overloaded patient. Other side effects are fever and malaise.

Obviously, immunosuppressive medications have many disturbing side effects. Therefore, the patient must be educated to expect these. Noncompliance with the medication schedule is often associated with the patient's inability to tolerate the side effects from immunosuppressive drugs as well as afford their high cost.

NURSING PROCESS
Renal Transplantation

Assessment

Assess the patient's vital signs and breath sounds. Record intake and output. Weigh the patient daily. Assess the wound status and graft site. Evaluate the patient's mental and nutritional status. Determine the patient's understanding of the surgery. Check for anxiety or concerns about the procedure. Monitor complete blood cell count, serum electrolytes, and BUN and serum creatinine levels.

Nursing Diagnoses and Planning

Nursing diagnoses and related expected patient outcomes most commonly applicable to patients who have undergone renal transplantation include the following:

NDx: Risk for infection related to immunosuppressive drug therapy

Planning: Patient Outcomes
1. Patient exhibits normal vital signs.
2. Patient is free from redness or purulent drainage at wound site.
3. Patient verbalizes the signs and symptoms of infection.

NDx: Fear related to possibility of rejection

Planning: Patient Outcomes
1. Patient verbalizes specific fears related to transplantation.
2. Patient verbalizes realistic expectations related to transplantation.
3. Patient verbalizes decreased fear.

NDx: Altered health maintenance related to lack of knowledge about signs and symptoms of rejection, side effects of immunosuppressive drugs, and the need to protect the vascular access

Planning: Patient Outcomes
1. Patient verbalizes signs and symptoms of rejection.
2. Patient verbalizes side effects of immunosuppressive drugs.
3. Patient verbalizes importance of protecting vascular access.

Nursing Interventions and Evaluation

NDx: Risk for infection
Monitor the patient's vital signs. Report fever and unexplained tachycardia. Observe for infections in other body systems. Use aseptic technique with all invasive procedures and dressing changes. Instruct the patient in measures to avoid infection (Highlight 31–4).

NDx: Fear
Encourage the patient to verbalize subjective feelings, perceptions of illness, perception of his or her own coping skills, and need for assistance from the nursing staff. Initiate teaching to decrease knowledge deficit. Teach patient what to expect during

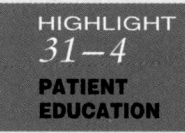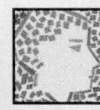

HIGHLIGHT
31–4
PATIENT
EDUCATION

Self-Care for the Renal Transplant Patient

Instruct the patient to:

Recognize and report fever and tachycardia.

Be alert to signs and symptoms of common infections:

Urinary tract infection—cloudy, odorous urine; urinary burning; frequency; and urgency
Upper respiratory tract infection—productive cough with purulent, colored, copius sputum
Otitis media—malaise, earache
Impetigo—inflamed, drainage pustules on skin

Avoid contact with individuals with known infections.

Recognize and report immediately the signs of rejection:
Oliguria
Tenderness over kidney (in iliac fossa)
Sudden weight gain
Fever
Malaise
Increased blood pressure

Protect the vascular access because it may be needed if rejection occurs.

Forbid venipuncture, blood drawing, or blood pressure to be taken in the access extremity.

hospitalization and after discharge. Monitor the level of fear. Encourage the patient to verbalize fear.

NDx: Altered health maintenance

Explain and teach the patient and family about signs and symptoms of infection and rejection and the importance of protecting the vascular access (see Highlight 31–4). Allow the patient and family to ask questions. Give them written instructions and printed literature explaining the postoperative care needed.

Compare the patient's status with the expected outcomes. If the outcomes are not met, reassess the patient and revise the plan.

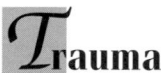 # Trauma

RENAL TRAUMA

Renal trauma is not uncommon and occurs in various blunt or penetrating injuries. In patients with severe multiple trauma, renal injuries are deferred to the priorities of resuscitation and stabilization of vital signs. Severe renal injuries require immediate surgical intervention at the same time that injuries to other vital organs (if present) are treated.

Etiology and Pathophysiology

The usual cause of renal trauma is blunt or penetrating injury to the kidney. Blunt renal trauma occurs more frequently than penetrating trauma. Approximately 60 to 85% of renal trauma cases are blunt trauma injuries. Blunt trauma is caused by direct blows, sports injuries, or rapid deceleration injuries such as motor vehicle accidents or falls from heights. Penetrating renal trauma is caused by stabbing or gunshot wounds.

The kidneys are located in the upper retroperitoneal space, in front of the lower thoracic cage and beneath the liver, spleen, and diaphragm. Under normal circumstances, the kidneys are somewhat mobile. They are surrounded by fat, called Gerota's fascia, and are held in place only by their major blood vessels, which are attached to the aorta and vena cava. The renal capsule is a tough membrane that resists rupture.

Blunt renal trauma occurs when the kidney is violently and suddenly jarred out of its normal position. In the presence of bony fractures, such as lower rib or upper lumbar vertebral fractures, Gerota's fascia and the renal capsule may be penetrated, causing damage to the kidney's internal structure. If the trauma is great enough to rupture the major renal blood vessels, shock quickly occurs and is a life-threatening emergency.

Penetrating renal trauma is frequently associated with other abdominal injuries that require immediate surgical repair. The severity of the trauma to the kidney depends on the location of the entry and exit wounds or the force of the blunt blow to the kidney.

Clinical Manifestations

If the patient is conscious, blunt renal injuries may cause flank or upper abdominal pain. Other possible symptoms include flank or abdominal bruising, masses, or tenderness in the area of trauma. Lower rib fractures or injuries to nearby organs greatly increase the likelihood of renal injuries. Hematuria, either gross or microscopic, is common after renal trauma. The amount of hematuria is not a good indicator of the severity of the injury.

Penetrating renal injury is suspected when an entrance wound is present in the renal area. Symptoms reported by the conscious patient are not specific enough to diagnose renal injury. Because major blood loss and shock are likely when major blood vessels are involved, the patient must be closely monitored. Patients with gunshot wounds are transferred to the operating room, usually immediately after assessment, and after the diagnostic studies can be performed if time permits.

Diagnosis

Classification of renal injury is necessary before treatment decisions are made. The four categories of renal injury are contusion, minor laceration, major laceration, and multiple laceration or shattered kidney.

Diagnostic studies are performed as quickly as possible when renal trauma is evident. Urinalysis involves an evaluation for hematuria as well as the presence of other abnormalities. Hematuria is usually present with renal trauma. However, 10 to 40% of patients with renal trauma do not have hematuria. The amount of hematuria does not correlate with the severity of the trauma. The absence of hematuria does not rule out renal trauma.

When the patient is stable, excretory urography using high doses of contrast material is performed to evaluate the renal injury. Blunt renal injury may be difficult to see on the urogram, and nephrotomography or CT may be necessary. When a kidney cannot be seen at all on a urogram, emergency arteriography or CT is performed if time permits. The number of preoperative diagnostic studies performed depends on the patient's condition. In severely injured patients, diagnosis may be made intraoperatively, and excretory urography is performed with the patient on the operating table.

Management

Conservative treatment is appropriate for most patients with blunt trauma and few patients with penetrating renal trauma. Patients with minor injuries, microhematuria, and normal urography results are discharged on limited activity for a time period. Patients with contusion or minor laceration are admitted and treated with bedrest. Urine evaluations are performed to determine the presence and severity of the hematuria. Antibiotics may be administered.

Most patients recover from these minor injuries without complications. Follow-up after discharge is necessary because late complications, including late bleeding and hypertension, may occur.

For patients with severe blunt renal trauma, and for most patients with penetrating renal trauma, surgical intervention is necessary. Approximately 15% of blunt injuries and 85% of penetrating injuries require exploration and repair. A midline abdominal incision is performed so that abdominal exploration can be performed at the same time. As much functioning kidney as possible is salvaged during the surgical repair. When a shattered kidney or multiple lacerations are present, nephrectomy may be necessary.

The only exception to immediate surgery in severe renal trauma is when the need for nephrectomy is evident in a clinically stable patient. In this case, the nephrectomy can be performed hours or days later.

Follow-up for up to 1 year after the penetrating renal trauma is important to rule out the potential for latent complications of surgical repair, including calcification, areas of nonfunction, and hypertension.

NURSING PROCESS
Renal Trauma

Assessment

Initial assessment of the patient with suspected renal trauma involves assessment of other systems in order of priority. Check the patient's respiratory and cardiovascular status first. Next, complete a neurologic assessment, following that with the assessment of any abdominal or pelvic injuries once the patient is stabilized. Specific renal injuries may not be apparent on assessment. Thus, complete a general abdominal assessment, noting any bruising or penetrating wounds in the flank area. Ask the patient about areas of pain or tenderness. Observe for hematomas or swelling. Blunt injuries are the most difficult to assess and are not usually found without radiologic studies. If a penetrating wound is present, note the location of entrance and exit wounds and amount of bleeding and determine the type of wound (gunshot, stab). Check the urine for gross hematuria.

Nursing Diagnoses and Planning

Nursing diagnoses and related expected patient outcomes most commonly applicable to patients with renal trauma include the following:

NDx: Altered renal tissue perfusion related to hemorrhage from injury

Planning: Patient Outcomes
1. Patient's renal function is adequate, without evidence of bleeding.
2. Patient's vital signs are within normal limits for the patient.

NDx: Pain related to trauma and manipulation during treatment

Planning: Patient Outcomes
1. Patient reports a decrease in pain or that pain is tolerable.
2. Patient rests without interruptions from pain.

NDx: Anxiety related to traumatic event and fear of damage to the kidney

Planning: Patient Outcomes
1. Patient expresses feelings about events that occurred and potential outcomes after treatment.
2. Patient reports decreased anxiety and appears relaxed.

Nursing Interventions and Evaluation

NDx: Altered renal tissue perfusion
During the initial evaluation of the injury in the trauma suite or emergency room, focus nursing interventions on stabilizing the patient. Closely observe the patient for vital sign changes, which may indicate bleeding and impending shock. Note the amount of urine produced hourly. Document the data. Keep the patient on bedrest to prevent further trauma and to aid in healing of minor blunt trauma injuries.

If the patient required surgical intervention, postoperatively monitor the output carefully. Observe for gross hematuria. Check the flank incision for drainage. Take vital signs frequently, watching for changes. Monitor the laboratory data, noting the urinalysis and BUN and serum creatinine levels to assess for renal function. Report an output of less than 30 mL/h to the attending physician.

NDx: Pain
Evaluate the patient's pain tolerance. Give analgesics as prescribed. Position the patient for comfort. Medicate the patient before engaging in care activities. Encourage the patient to practice relaxation exercises.

NDx: Anxiety
Explain all nursing activities to the patient. Allow the patient to participate in care decisions. Let the patient verbalize fears and concerns about the injury and outcomes. Keep the patient informed about the renal status. Help the patient find coping strategies that are effective. Provide periods of rest and quiet as needed.

Compare the patient's status with the expected outcomes. If the outcomes are not met, reassess the patient and revise the plan.

URETERAL TRAUMA

Injuries to the ureter occur far more frequently from penetrating trauma than from blunt trauma. In either case, ureteral trauma is relatively rare, accounting for only a small percentage of injuries seen in trauma. Unfortunately, ureteral injury does not usually manifest itself until several days after the occurrence of the injury.

Etiology and Pathophysiology

The spinal column and large muscles of the back protect the ureters posteriorly. The abdominal wall and contents protect the ureters anteriorly. Because of this protection, only severe blunt trauma (such as falls from extreme heights) can cause ureteral trauma. The type of ureteral injury most frequently sustained during blunt trauma is disruption of the ureter at the ureteropelvic junction.

Penetrating injuries, especially gunshot wounds, account for 95% of ureteral trauma from external causes. A bullet or stab wound can sever or nick the ureter at any point along its course from the kidney to the bladder. Injury to the ureter during difficult abdominal surgeries is much more common than penetrating or blunt causes of ureteral injury.

Clinical Manifestations

No specific symptoms lead to suspicion of ureteral injury. In most cases, the symptoms of ureteral trauma appear several days after the injury. Hematuria is present in most cases of ureteral injury from external causes. As with renal trauma, the amount of hematuria is not a good indicator of the severity of the injury. Penetrating ureteral trauma is suspected when entrance or exit wounds are in the ureteral area. Because most wounds are explored surgically, little time exists for symptomatic evaluation of the patient. Symptoms of a ureteral injury that have been present for several days include fever, flank pain, and infection with generalized abdominal symptoms of pain, tenderness, rigidity and nausea, vomiting, and paralytic ileus.

Diagnosis

Diagnosis of ureteral injury is achieved by radiographic examinations or during surgery. Blunt trauma is usually evaluated with excretory urography. Extravasation of contrast material from the site of the ureteral disruption demonstrates the injury. Penetrating trauma is evaluated by exploratory surgery in most cases. Ureteral trauma is diagnosed at that time by intraoperative urography or intravenously injected indigo carmine, which causes a blue discoloration of the tissue surrounding the site of injury.

Management

Ureteral trauma usually requires surgical repair. The type of surgery depends on which section of the ureter has been injured. Upper ureteral injuries are repaired by pyeloplasty. Lower ureteral injuries are repaired by reimplantation into the bladder. Injuries in the middle of the ureter are corrected by an end-to-end anastomosis. Varying amounts of débridement of surrounding tissue may be necessary after bullet wounds. In most patients, ureteral stents or nephrostomy tubes are used postoperatively to divert urine away from the surgical area. Penrose drains or sumps may also be used.

NURSING PROCESS
Ureteral Trauma

The assessment, nursing diagnoses, expected patient outcomes, nursing interventions, and evaluation for patients with ureteral trauma are similar to those described previously for patients with renal trauma.

BLADDER TRAUMA

The urinary bladder's anatomical location deep in the pelvis usually protects it from injury. Bladder trauma can occur, however, from blunt or penetrating injuries. Penetrating injuries account for only approximately one-fourth of all bladder injuries. The more frequent cause of bladder trauma is blunt injuries that occur in pelvic fractures.

Etiology and Pathophysiology

The type of injury the urinary bladder sustains depends on the amount of urine in the bladder at the time of injury. The empty bladder is more likely not to be injured or to receive less injury than the full bladder. Penetrating trauma is usually due to gunshot wounds or stab wounds. Blunt trauma is classified into three types of injuries: contusion, extraperitoneal, or intraperitoneal. Contusion is not usually a serious injury and does not require surgery. A contusion is often a partial-thickness tear of the bladder wall. Penetration of the bladder wall by a bone fragment during pelvic fracture is an extraperitoneal rupture. Urine leaks out of the bladder into the area directly surrounding the bladder. Intraperitoneal rupture occurs when a severe blow to the lower abdomen causes intolerable strain on a full bladder. In response to the sudden increase in pressure, the full bladder ruptures at its weakest point, the dome, which is located at the top of the bladder. Urine leaks into the peritoneal cavity, around the bowel and nearby organs.

Clinical Manifestations

Most patients with bladder trauma have gross hematuria. Other common symptoms are lower suprapubic or lower abdominal pain. Rectal examination may yield evidence of pelvic hematoma. The patient may report having received a direct blow to the abdomen.

Symptoms of shock are uncommon when the bladder injury is the only injury that the patient sustained. However, additional injuries are frequently present, causing symptoms other than those noted. The multiple trauma patient may suffer from shock and require evaluation of life-threatening injuries initially.

Diagnosis

A plain x-ray of the abdomen is performed initially to observe for pelvic fracture, calcifications, foreign bodies, or bullets. Intravenous urography is performed to rule out ureteral or renal injury and to evaluate the shape of the bladder. The bladder injury may be seen on the urogram, but a cystogram is the best diagnostic tool for diagnosing the extent of the bladder injury. Because this requires catheterization, urethral trauma is first ruled out. Once the catheter is in place, small to large amounts of contrast dye are instilled into the bladder. Small amounts of dye demonstrate injuries at the base of the bladder. Large amounts are instilled to demonstrate injuries to the top of the bladder. In women, a thorough pelvic examination is necessary to detect urethral or vaginal injury in addition to the bladder injury.

Management

Conservative management of minor bladder injuries consists of urinary catheter drainage until the wounds heal. A Foley catheter or suprapubic catheter is used, depending on the location of the injury. The progress of healing is evaluated periodically by cystogram until no contrast dye is extravasated. Small amounts of sterile urine leaking into the area surrounding the bladder are usually not harmful to the patient and are gradually absorbed into the interstitial fluid. Antibiotics may be used during the prolonged catheter therapy to prevent UTIs.

Penetrating wounds are surgically explored and repaired. Surrounding organs and tissue are assessed for damage. The bladder injury is closed with absorbable sutures. A suprapubic catheter is used to divert drainage of urine away from the healing suture line. A large suprapubic tube is used for men. A Foley catheter or a suprapubic tube is used for women, depending on the location of the injury. Penrose drains may be used on either side of the bladder.

Patients with intraperitoneal and extraperitoneal bladder rupture caused by blunt trauma are usually treated with the same type of surgical intervention. Occasionally, in patients with minor ruptures, conservative treatment is used rather than surgery.

NURSING PROCESS
Bladder Trauma

Assessment

Treat the patient with a pelvic fracture as though a bladder injury exists. Evaluate the urine for hematuria. If the patient cannot void, do not catheterize the patient until a urethral injury is ruled out. If the patient is able to void easily, the injury is probably minor. Serious pelvic fractures with bladder injury involve profound blood loss and shock; thus genitourinary assessment may be delayed until the patient is stabilized.

After assessment of vital signs, assess for symptoms of genitourinary injury. Ask the patient about the nature of the trauma sustained and whether a blow to the abdomen occurred. Patients with severe intraperitoneal ruptures may appear to have an "acute abdomen," especially if several hours have

passed since the injury. If the patient reports an inability to void since the injury, bladder rupture is possible.

Nursing Diagnoses and Planning

Nursing diagnoses and related expected patient outcomes most commonly applicable to patients with bladder trauma are similar to those described previously for patients with renal trauma and include the following:

NDx: Urinary retention related to trauma

Planning: Patient Outcomes
1. Patient has an adequate balanced intake and output.
2. Patient resumes normal pattern of voiding after treatment of injury.

NDx: Risk for infection related to disruption of the urinary system

Planning: Patient Outcomes
1. Patient's vital signs remain within normal ranges for the patient.
2. Signs of infection, such as bacteremia, bacteriuria, fever, or dysuria, are absent.

Nursing Interventions and Evaluation

NDx: Urinary retention
Check the catheter drainage for patency. Encourage increased fluid intake if not contraindicated. Administer analgesics and antispasmodics as prescribed to relieve spasms and pain and to prevent interference with urinary output. Monitor the patient's laboratory data. Note hematuria and document the data. After the catheter is removed, encourage the patient to void frequently and measure each voiding. Note the color, consistency, and amount of urine. Use strategies to assist the patient with voiding if there is difficulty.

NDx: Risk for infection
Monitor the patient for symptoms of peritonitis, such as increased abdominal pain, tenderness, fever, and unstable vital signs. Check the incision for signs of infection. Keep drainage from Penrose drains away from the suture line. Assess the urine for cloudiness, sediment, or foul odor. Report any early signs of infection to the attending physician. Keep catheters patent and the drainage system closed. Use aseptic dressing changes when removing and replacing the surgical dressings. Tell the patient to report any untoward symptoms. Review the urinalysis and urine cultures for indications of infection.

Compare the patient's status with the expected outcomes. If the outcomes are not met, reassess the patient and revise the plan.

URETHRAL TRAUMA

Injuries to the urethra are far more common in men than in women and are much more difficult to repair in men. In women, the urethra is entirely internal and somewhat mobile. The male urethra has some nonmobile areas, which are more susceptible to injury than other parts of the urethra. When trauma occurs to these areas, it is difficult to diagnose and correct. Long-term complications are common.

Etiology and Pathophysiology

The urogenital diaphragm is an important anatomical landmark because urethral injuries in men are classified as to whether they occur above it or below it. Anterior urethral injuries occur below the urogenital diaphragm. The anterior portion of the urethra is very mobile. It is injured most frequently from straddle-type injuries such as a fall in which the patient lands sitting or by a direct blow or penetration along the course of the lower urethra.

Posterior urethral injuries occur between the bladder neck and the urogenital diaphragm. The presence of the prostate gland and the numerous ligaments make this portion of the urethra immobile in men. The cause of injuries to the posterior urethra is usually severe blunt trauma such as pelvic fracture.

Anterior and posterior urethral injuries may be either complete or partial. Other causes of urethral injury are self-manipulation injury from a variety of objects or injury during medical instrumentation.

Clinical Manifestations

The presence of blood at the urinary meatus is a sign of urethral injury. The patient may complain of difficulty voiding or may be unable to void at all. Pain is present at the site of injury or throughout the lower abdomen, depending on the extent of the trauma and its cause. Evidence of penile or perineal hematoma is common. Anterior urethral injuries are usually easy to see. The penis may be swollen with blood and urine if the patient has tried to void.

If the urethral injury has been present for several hours or days, symptoms of inflammation and sepsis result. Swelling can involve the penis, scrotum, and perineal area in men and the entire perineal area in women. In complete posterior urethral disruption, a rectal examination yields only the presence of a hematoma because the prostate and bladder are displaced superiorly.

Diagnosis

A plain abdominal x-ray is completed initially to check for pelvic fracture. When blood is present at the urethral meatus, retrograde urethrography is performed. This reveals the site of injury by demonstrating extravasation of contrast dye. If no extravasation is seen, the injury is likely to be either a contusion or a small tear. Urethroscopy may be performed to confirm the diagnosis of minor injuries. Excretory urography and cystography are performed to complete the evaluation when urethral continuity is largely intact.

Management

Urethral contusions with minimal hematuria in a patient who is able to void does not require treatment. Urethral tears without extravasation on urethrogram are treated with a Foley catheter for 7 to 10 days or suprapubic drainage, allowing the injury to heal. Most urethral injuries are treated in this manner.

If surgery is necessary, the type of surgical repair performed depends on the severity of the injury. When serious multiple injuries exist, urinary diversion by placement of a suprapubic cystostomy is performed, and urethral reconstruction is delayed until other injuries can be treated. When only urethral injury exists, particularly a posterior injury, surgical reconstruction is performed immediately. Anterior tears are repaired by suturing the tear or laceration.

NURSING PROCESS GUIDELINES
Urethral Trauma

Ask the patient to describe the injury sustained and the length of time that has passed since it occurred. When serious multiple injuries exist, assess vital systems initially. Once the patient is stable, assess the genitourinary injuries.

In men, assess the external genitalia. Assess the location and type of visible external penetrating wounds. Inspect the penis, scrotum, and perineal area for hematomas or swelling. In inflamed areas, palpation may reveal fluid underneath, the result of extravasation of urine during voiding. Assess the patient for symptoms of infection if significant time has passed since the injury.

In women, check the perineal area for hematomas. Ask whether the patient has difficulty voiding. Note any bloody discharge. Ask about pain or burning during urination.

In all patients, examine the urinary meatus for blood. If blood is present, do not catheterize the patient until further medical examination has occurred. Ask the patient when the last voiding occurred. Send a voided specimen to the laboratory for assessment for hematuria and bacteria.

The nursing diagnoses, related expected patient outcomes, and nursing interventions most commonly applicable to patients with urethral trauma are similar to those described previously for patients with renal or bladder trauma.

❖ SETTINGS, PROVIDERS, AND COLLABORATION FOR CARE

Patients with trauma to the urinary system are frequently seen in the emergency department of the hospital or, at times, in the physician's office. The emergency department physician may complete the first assessment of the patient, but a urologist is usually consulted once the diagnosis of trauma to the urinary system is established. The emergency department nurse implements the initial care as prescribed, before the patient's admission or discharge, depending on the severity of the trauma. Patients may be admitted for surgical repair of the injury. Upon discharge after surgery, the patient may be referred to a home health agency for additional treatment in the home. Follow-up medical treatment takes place at the physician's office. The home health nurse may assess the patient's status and further health-care needs and instruct the patient about dressing changes, pain management, and the care of an indwelling catheter.

Patients seen in the physician's office for initial assessment and treatment usually do not have severe urinary system trauma. They may be diagnosed and treated in the clinic and discharged with instructions for home care. If their trauma is severe, they are referred to the hospital and a urologist for continued treatment.

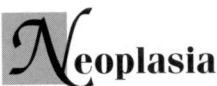
Neoplasia

A neoplasm or tumor is a pathologic overgrowth of tissue, which can be either benign or malignant, solid or cystic, superficial or invasive, as well as primary or metastatic. Many types of tumors can be found in the urinary tract. Eventually, all neoplasia affect its function. This section discusses those tumors that are the most common and that pose the biggest threat to the integrity of the urinary system—primary malignant tumors.

CANCER OF THE KIDNEY

Etiology and Pathophysiology

Malignant tumors of the kidney are the second most common cancers in the urinary tract. (Bladder cancers are more common.) Approximately 45% of patients with the disease die annually. The incidence of kidney cancer is higher (2:1) in men than in women and increases in frequency with age.

The types of malignant tumors generally found in the kidney are as follows:

Renal cell carcinoma (adenocarcinoma of the kidney)
Tumors of the renal collecting system (transitional cell epithelioma)
Wilms' tumor (nephroblastoma)
Sarcoma

Of these, renal cell carcinoma is the most frequently diagnosed tumor and accounts for more than three-quarters of all cases of kidney cancer. It is a disease that causes great concern, yet is challenging to diagnose and treat. Because of the predomi-

nance of renal cell carcinoma over other types of malignant renal tumors, the discussion that follows is specific to this condition.

The cause of renal cell carcinoma is unclear. Research continues in an attempt to identify sources of the disease, as well as groups at risk for developing it. Facts that are known about renal cell carcinoma include the following:

It primarily affects men older than age 40
It is more often seen in urban areas than in rural areas
It is associated with the use of tobacco, especially that used in pipes and cigars

Renal cell carcinoma usually affects only one kidney and apparently originates in the proximal convoluted tubule. The tumor typically grows into the renal medulla but can extend downward to the renal pelvis or out to the renal capsule and perinephric fat. Not uncommon is the extension of the tumor into the renal vein and inferior vena cava. In some instances, a renal cell carcinoma grows large enough to impinge on or invade surrounding muscles and abdominal organs. Enlargement of the affected kidney, as well as hemorrhage and necrosis, is the direct result of tumor growth.

Metastasis of a renal cell carcinoma occurs in about one-fourth of cases. Common sites for metastasis are the lungs, lymph nodes, adrenal gland, liver, opposite kidney, brain, and bone.

Clinical Manifestations

Gross or microscopic hematuria, flank pain, and a palpable flank mass are considered classic symptoms of the presence of a renal cell carcinoma. Ironically, this triad of symptoms is probably present in less than half of patients with the disease. More often, patients with renal cell carcinoma present with symptoms unrelated to the urinary tract. These are usually vague complaints that are common to a number of other conditions. For example, a persistent fever or gastrointestinal disturbances (anorexia, constipation, nausea, or vomiting) may be the first and only symptom in a patient with renal cell carcinoma.

Diagnosis

The diagnosis of renal cell carcinoma is based on radiographic findings. Excretory urography is the study most frequently performed, because it allows for visualization of the kidney's collecting system and permits full assessment of renal contour. Other examinations, such as nephrotomograms, renal sonography, CT, angiography, or magnetic resonance imaging, are used to more specifically define the extent of the tumor or when findings from the intravenous urogram are inconclusive.

Management

Treatment for renal cell carcinoma is immediate surgical removal of the tumor. Radical nephrectomy is usually performed. This procedure is performed through a transabdominal, thoracoabdominal, or extrapleural interspace incision and involves removal of the affected kidney as well as Gerota's fascia, the upper ureter, and at times, the adrenal gland. In some instances, lymph nodes are also excised. When the tumor has invaded the abdomen or vena cava, it is removed and resected as completely as possible.

NURSING PROCESS
Nephrectomy for Cancer of the Kidney

Assessment

In the preoperative period, assess the overall health of the patient with renal cell carcinoma. Because the tumor can affect a number of different abdominal structures and can metastasize to several different locations in the body, a system-by-system approach should be taken to establish the patient's current condition. Note the patient's nutritional status, including eating habits. Check the urinary status, assessing for signs of infection such as fever, discolored urine, or difficulty with urination.

Assess the patient's understanding of the disease process and the treatment plan. Note any misunderstandings.

In the immediate postoperative period, assess the patient's fluid and electrolyte status, because a significant amount of blood is lost during radical nephrectomy. Find out exactly how much blood was lost during the procedure. If replacement fluid was given during surgery, determine the type and amount administered. Assess vital signs, fluid intake and output, hemoglobin and hematocrit results, and urine specific gravity.

Evaluate the patient's respiratory status, because breathing may be compromised as a result of the location and size of the incision necessary for the radical nephrectomy. Respiratory function may also be limited if the patient is experiencing significant discomfort. Assess for pain and the need for analgesia.

Infection is always a threat when the urinary tract has been manipulated or disrupted. Assess for signs and symptoms of infection, noting any temperature elevation, redness at the surgical site, cloudy urine, or discharge.

Assess the patency of any urinary or wound drainage tubes. Note the color and quantity of drainage fluids. Because excessive drainage (sometimes urine) from the surgical site is not uncommon, inspect the area carefully. Note any need for dressing reinforcement or change of dressing.

Once the immediate postoperative period has passed, assess the patient's incision for evidence of wound healing. Evaluate the pattern of bowel elimination. Check the patient for the presence of paresthesia over the surgical site, because peripheral nerves are cut during surgery.

Nursing Diagnoses and Planning

Nursing diagnoses and related expected patient outcomes most commonly applicable to patients undergoing nephrectomy for cancer of the kidney include the following:

NDx: Ineffective breathing pattern related to pain from the surgical site

Planning: Patient Outcomes
1. Patient maintains an effective breathing pattern.
2. Patient coughs, turns, and breathes deeply every 2 hours.
3. Patient's lungs are clear to auscultation.

NDx: Fluid volume deficit related to excessive loss from surgery

Planning: Patient Outcomes
1. Patient's vital signs remain stable.
2. Patient has balanced fluid intake and output.
3. Patient's hemoglobin and hematocrit values remain within normal limits.
4. Patient's blood chemistry levels remain within normal limits.

NDx: Anxiety related to the diagnosis of cancer and the uncertain outcome of treatment

Planning: Patient Outcomes
1. Patient verbalizes fears and concerns related to diagnosis and treatment.
2. Patient asks questions related to fears and concerns.
3. Patient reports decrease in anxiety and appears relaxed.

NDx: Pain related to manipulation during surgery

Planning: Patient Outcomes
1. Patient states that pain is decreased or relieved by analgesia.
2. Patient participates in care without apparent discomfort.
3. Patient is able to rest without interruption from pain.

NDx: Knowledge deficit: nature of surgery and follow-up care

Planning: Patient Outcomes
1. Patient verbalizes the procedure as discussed by the physician and the measures necessary to maintain health of the remaining kidney after discharge.
2. Patient asks questions about follow-up care.
3. Patient reports accurate information about the directions given.

Nursing Interventions and Evaluation

NDx: Ineffective breathing pattern
Auscultate the breath sounds frequently and note any abnormalities. In the postoperative period, respiratory function may be compromised. Check for dyspnea, shallow breathing, or tachypnea. Position

the patient to facilitate maximum respiratory efforts, such as in a semi-Fowler's position. Encourage the patient to cough, deep breathe, and turn frequently, at least every 2 hours. Also encourage the patient to use the incentive spirometer, as instructed, every hour while awake.

NDx: Fluid volume deficit

Postoperative nursing care centers on preventing complications. Check the fluid intake and output carefully, assessing it every 4 hours or more frequently as needed. The immediate postoperative period is the most critical in terms of fluid volume. The electrolyte and fluid balance is labile at this time. Watch for vital sign changes indicating a change in volume status. Check the laboratory data such as the urine specific gravity and the hemoglobin and hematocrit values. Note changes and report them. Increase intravenous fluids as ordered to maintain appropriate output and blood pressure. Measure output hourly and document the results.

NDx: Anxiety

Allow time for the patient to express fears and concerns. Answer all questions as honestly as possible. Seek support from clergy or significant others when appropriate. Include the family in counseling sessions. Allow the patient to make choices about care when appropriate. Explain all procedures before initiating them. Schedule time for the patient to rest as needed. Encourage relaxation exercises.

NDx: Pain

For severe postoperative pain, administer analgesics as prescribed. In addition to relief of pain, this aids in respiratory function by promoting a more effective breathing pattern because the respiratory muscles are not restricted by discomfort. Administer analgesics before treatments and before sleep. Use relaxation techniques to relieve tension, stress, and pain, and position the patient for comfort. Teach the patient how to use patient-controlled analgesia, if ordered.

NDx: Knowledge deficit: nature of surgery and follow-up care

Explain the surgical procedure to the patient, including the postoperative expectations. Describe the equipment that the patient will see postoperatively and the necessity for it. Discuss the discharge plans with both the patient and the family. Include information about the signs and symptoms of wound infection before discharge as well as other complications. Allow time for questions. Caution the patient against lifting heavy objects until allowed by the physician. Encourage the patient to avoid activities that would strain the flank area. Explain interventions to maintain the health of the remaining kidney as described in Highlight 31-5.

Compare the patient's status with the expected outcomes. If the outcomes are not met, reassess the patient and revise the plan.

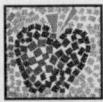

HIGHLIGHT
31-5

HEALTH PROMOTION & RISK REDUCTION

Maintaining the Health of the Remaining Kidney

Instruct the patient to:

Drink at least six to eight glasses of liquid per day.

Void when the urge is felt.

Maintain a program of moderate activity.

Maintain acidity of urine by eating meats, eggs, poultry, fish, grapes, whole grains, and cranberry and prune juice; limit intake of milk and carbonated beverages.

Wipe perineum from front to back (women only).

Keep perineal area clean and dry.

Take prophylactic anti-infectives as prescribed.

Report signs and symptoms of an infection immediately.

Notify physician if a cold or other infection persists for more than 3 days or if unable to maintain fluid intake.

Inform health-care workers of nephrectomy so that measures can be taken to protect kidney.

Avoid activities that could cause trauma to remaining kidney (eg, contact sports, horseback riding).

Consult physician before taking any medications that may be nephrotoxic.

Follow instructions to prevent stone formation if nephrectomy was done for calculi.

Follow instructions for controlling blood pressure if nephrectomy was done because of hypertension.

Data from Ulrich SP, Canale SW, Wendell SA. Nursing care planning guides. 4th ed. Philadelphia: WB Saunders, 1994, pp 531-532.

CANCER OF THE RENAL PELVIS AND URETER

Etiology and Pathophysiology

Primary malignant tumors of the renal pelvis and ureter are extremely rare and account for fewer than 7% of all urinary tract carcinomas. The most common type of tumor found in this part of the urinary tract is transitional cell carcinoma that develops from the uroepithelium. This is also the most common tumor in the bladder. Its incidence is three times greater in men than in women. Chemical carcinogens, phenacetin, cigarette smoking, and chronic infection and inflammation of the upper urinary tract are possible causes of tumor growth. The presence of a transitional cell carcinoma in the renal pelvis or ureter increases the likelihood of the same type of tumor developing in the bladder.

Clinical Manifestations

The most common symptoms in patients with a tumor of the renal pelvis or ureter are hematuria and flank pain. Some patients also present with costovertebral angle tenderness or generalized symptoms, such as weight loss and anorexia. The majority of patients, however, are asymptomatic.

Diagnosis

Tumors of the renal pelvis and ureter are difficult to detect. Therefore, a number of different diagnostic tests are performed to locate the lesion, define its extent, and confirm the diagnosis. Radiologic examination includes one or more of the following: excretory urography, retrograde pyelography, renal ultrasonography, CT, and renal angiography. Ureteroscopy may also be performed in order to directly visualize the area in question. Voided urine samples or brush biopsy specimens may be obtained for cytologic examination. (Refer to Chap. 30 for an explanation of the diagnostic tests.)

Management

Treatment for cancer of the renal pelvis and ureter is surgical removal of the tumor. The actual procedure performed depends on the location and extent of the tumor and may be partial nephrectomy, nephrectomy, or radical nephrectomy.

NURSING PROCESS GUIDELINES
Cancer of the Renal Pelvis and Ureter

The assessment, nursing diagnoses, expected patient outcomes, nursing interventions, and evaluation for patients with cancer of the renal pelvis and ureter are similar to those described previously for patients with cancer of the kidney. When the tumor extends into the bladder, nursing care activities as described for the patient with cancer of the bladder would apply.

CANCER OF THE BLADDER

Etiology and Pathophysiology

Malignant tumors of the bladder are the most common tumors within the urinary system. However, when the entire genitourinary system is considered, prostate tumors are far more prevalent. Almost 50,000 new cases of bladder cancer are diagnosed each year. Five-year survival rates are as excellent for patients who have received treatment of superficial tumors. When tumor growth is extensive, the

5-year survival rate drops to approximately 10 to 50%.

The cause of bladder cancer has been attributed to a number of environmental and occupational health hazards. Among the most common are chemicals used by industrial workers in dyestuff manufacture, rubber manufacture, coal gas production, sewage work, and textile printing. It has been theorized that using cigarettes and artificial sweeteners as well as coffee drinking can increase one's risk of bladder cancer. Patients who have undergone pelvic irradiation, who have a history of chronic infection and inflammation of the urinary tract, who have been treated with cyclophosphamide, or who were born with exstrophy of the bladder (a congenital condition in which the bladder develops outside the abdomen) are also at risk for developing cancer of the bladder.

The incidence of bladder cancer is three times greater in men than in women and affects the Caucasian population twice as often as African-Americans. It is a condition generally seen in patients older than the age of 40.

Three types of tumors are found in the bladder: transitional cell carcinoma, squamous cell carcinoma, and adenocarcinoma. Of these, transitional cell carcinoma is the most common, accounting for approximately 90% of all bladder cancers.

Transitional cell carcinoma develops in the epithelial lining of the bladder. The tumors can appear in many different forms but are generally identified as being papillary or nonpapillary lesions. Papillary tumors are usually superficial lesions that grow outward from the mucosa. Nonpapillary tumors are solid growths that tend to extend deep into the bladder wall and that are more likely to metastasize. Common sites of metastasis are the lymph nodes, liver, lungs, and bone.

Clinical Manifestations

The most common symptom in patients with cancer of the bladder is hematuria. The presence of blood in the urine may be a gross or microscopic finding and can occur with each voiding or intermittently. As was previously mentioned, the amount and severity of hematuria do not correlate with the presence or absence of a disease state. However, it is important to note that in the patient with hematuria, cancer is considered as a valid diagnosis until disproved.

In addition to hematuria, the patient may experience irritative voiding symptoms, such as frequency, urgency, and dysuria. These symptoms are often associated with cancer in situ.

Diagnosis

The medical diagnosis is based on symptoms, history, and diagnostic tests. The goal is to determine the extent of the cancerous lesion in order to classify it according to the stage of penetration or invasiveness into the bladder wall. This differentiation of

Table 31–12

Staging and Treatment of Bladder Cancer

Stage	Description	Treatment
0	Carcinoma in situ Papillary tumor—no invasion	Transurethral resection Intravesical chemotherapy Laser therapy
A	Papillary tumor—lamina propria invasion	Interstitial irradiation Intravesical immunotherapy
B1	Superficial muscle invasion	
B2	Deep muscle invasion	Radical cystectomy and urinary diversion
C	Invasion of perivesical fat	Radiation therapy in inoperable patients
D1	Invasion of contiguous viscera Involvement of pelvic nodes Involvement of juxtaregional nodes	External radiation Systemic chemotherapy
D2	Distant metastases	

bladder tumors helps to delineate the appropriate method of treatment (Table 31–12).

To diagnose cancer of the bladder, voided urine samples are collected for cytologic examination. Radiologic studies, which may include excretory urography or CT, are then performed. Finally, cystourethroscopy is performed and a biopsy taken of the suspect lesion. In many instances, random biopsies of apparently normal tissue are also obtained to help determine the extent of disease.

Management

The type of treatment initiated for cancer of the bladder depends on the form of tumor (papillary versus nonpapillary) and the stages of the disease. A variety of therapies for treatment of bladder cancer exist. These are reviewed here.

Treatment of Papillary or Superficial Bladder Cancer

TRANSURETHRAL RESECTION. Transurethral resection is the initial and most common treatment for superficial bladder cancer. It involves endoscopic removal of the tumors. Assessment of the urinary tract for the recurrence of cancerous lesions is required every 3 to 6 months following tumor resection.

INTRAVESICAL CHEMOTHERAPY. Intravesical chemotherapy allows for high concentrations of chemotherapeutic agents to be instilled directly into the bladder. The advantage to this treatment is that patients avoid toxic side effects that occur with systemic administration of the chemotherapeutic agents. Intravesical chemotherapy is used when superficial bladder cancer is widespread and transurethral resection would not be effective. More frequently, though, it is used as an adjunctive treatment after transurethral resection surgery to decrease the number of tumors and the time between recurrences of the tumors.

LASER THERAPY. The use of lasers to treat superficial bladder tumors is becoming increasingly common. One advantage to this type of treatment is that

multiple tumors can be eradicated without administering anesthesia to the patient. Additionally, blood loss is minimized, trauma to the normal tissue surrounding the tumor is avoided, and tumor spread is prevented by vaporization of the cancerous tissue.

INTERSTITIAL RADIATION. Although external radiation of superficial bladder tumors has not been effective, recent studies from other countries suggest that radium implants are successful in preventing extension and recurrence of the disease.

Treatment of Nonpapillary or Muscle-Invasive Bladder Cancer

SEGMENTAL OR PARTIAL CYSTECTOMY. This procedure may be performed when there is a single, well-defined tumor in the bladder that is not accessible to treatment by transurethral resection. The overall objective is to remove only that portion of the bladder affected by tumor without disrupting or injuring the ureters, bladder neck, or prostate.

INTRAVESICAL IMMUNOTHERAPY. Some urologists have had success in managing, or curing, selected patients with nonpapillary disease by intravesical immunotherapy. The treatment involves the instillation of bacillus Calmette-Guérin into the bladder. A schedule is established in which the instillation of the bacillus Calmette-Guérin is repeated as often as every 5 to 7 days for a 6-week course. At a designated time after the treatments are discontinued, the bladder is rebiopsied. If the tumor has recurred, other treatment options are considered. If there is no evidence of tumor, the patient status is monitored by cystoscopy every 3 months initially, then every 6 months to 1 year.

RADICAL CYSTECTOMY. Radical cystectomy is performed when the bladder cancer is not treatable by conservative measures or when there is recurrence of disease (and the cancer has invaded the muscle wall) following treatment by conservative therapy. In men, radical cystectomy involves removal of the bladder as well as the prostate, seminal vesicles, and proximal urethra. Total urethrectomy is performed if the prostatic urethra is affected by the tumor. In women, the bladder, entire urethra, anterior vaginal wall, uterus, cervix, fallopian tubes, and ovaries are removed. Excision of pelvic lymph nodes is routine in either instance.

Once a radical cystectomy is complete, a means of urinary diversion is created. This procedure is performed at the same time as the cystectomy. The types of urinary diversions most frequently constructed are the ileal conduit, the colon conduit, the cutaneous ureterostomy, and the continent internal ileal reservoir. Ureterosigmoidostomy may also be constructed, but it has many disadvantages and thus is not the surgery of choice in most cases (Fig. 31–10).

RADIATION THERAPY. External radiotherapy is used to treat, and sometimes cure, malignant blad-der tumors in very elderly patients thought to be poor surgical candidates or those who have tumors that are considered to be inoperable. Radiation therapy may also be performed preoperatively to shrink a bladder tumor before cystectomy. In patients with advanced metastatic cancer, it is used as a palliative treatment. The use of interstitial radiation to treat nonpapillary tumors is also promising. For these types of tumors, iridium needles are inserted through an open bladder directly into the tumor. They are left in place for a period of several days, then removed percutaneously.

SYSTEMIC CHEMOTHERAPY. Chemotherapeutic agents such as cisplatin and doxorubicin (Adriamycin) are administered to patients for palliative treatment of nonpapillary bladder tumors. In some instances, patients experience remission of the disease after treatment.

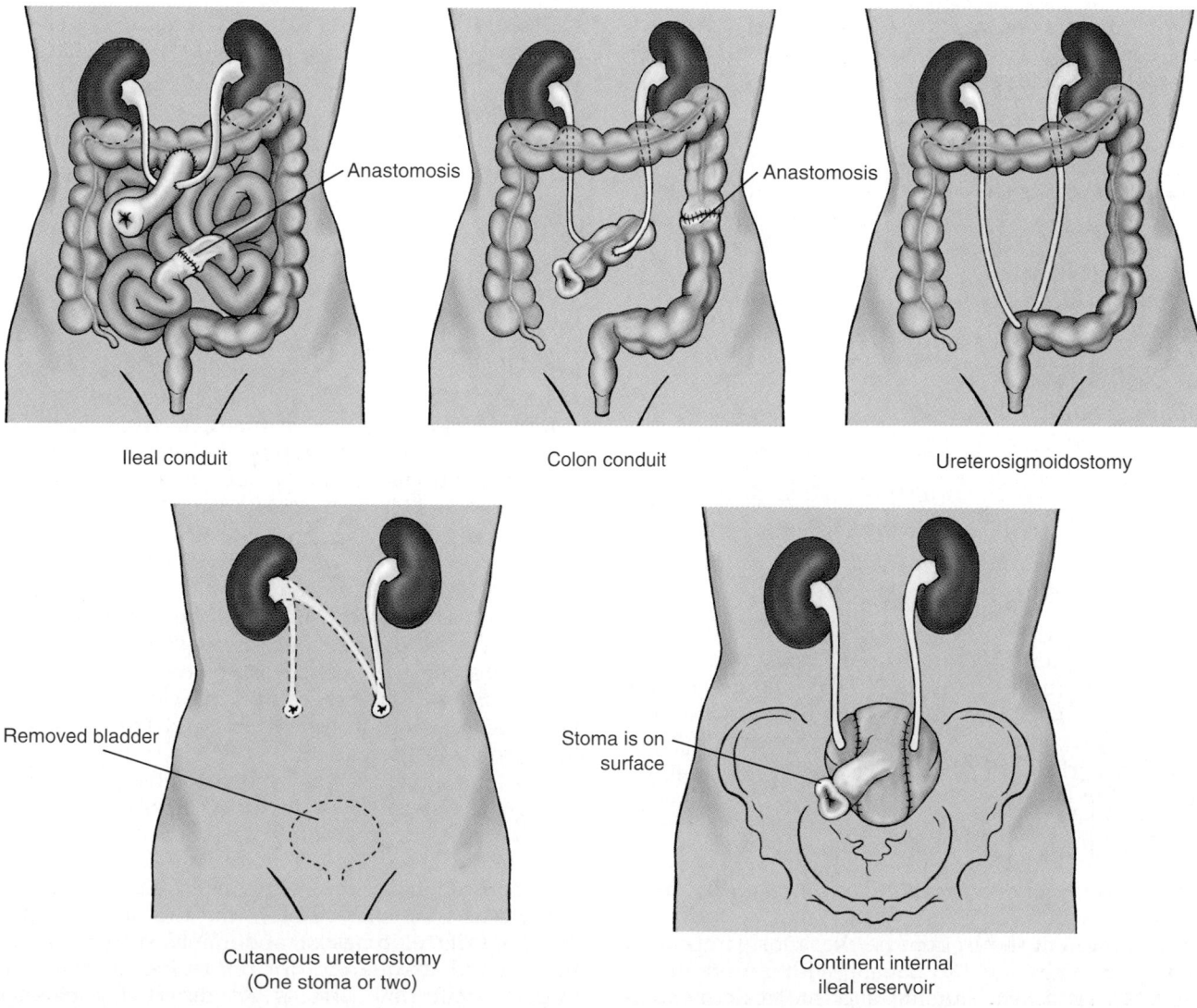

Ileal conduit

Colon conduit

Ureterosigmoidostomy

Cutaneous ureterostomy
(One stoma or two)

Continent internal
ileal reservoir

Figure 31–10

Types of urinary diversion procedures.

NURSING PROCESS
Papillary or Superficial Bladder Tumors

Assessment

Check the patient's history and current findings, focusing on any predisposing or risk factors that may have precipitated the development of a bladder tumor. Evaluate the patient's usual pattern of urinary elimination. Note any irritating or unusual voiding symptoms. Obtain a urine specimen to check for the presence of hematuria. Review laboratory results, noting the urine culture and the presence of bacteria. Explore generalized complaints, such as weight loss, fatigue, anorexia, diarrhea, constipation, or fever. Finally, assess the patient's level of understanding about the disease and the proposed treatment plan. This assessment is applicable in the pretreatment and post-treatment phases for the patient with a papillary or superficial bladder tumor.

Nursing Diagnoses and Planning

Nursing diagnoses and related expected outcomes most commonly applicable to patients with papillary or superficial bladder tumors include the following:

NDx: Altered urinary elimination related to vesical irritation from the presence of bladder tumors

Planning: Patient Outcomes
1. Patient expresses relief of voiding symptoms.
2. Patient's urine has a decrease in blood and an absence of bacteria.
3. Patient voids appropriate amounts of urine.

NDx: Knowledge deficit: nature of the disorder and the treatment plan

Planning: Patient Outcomes
1. Patient asks questions that are appropriate to health teaching.
2. Patient verbalizes an understanding of the disorder and the proposed treatment plan.

Nursing Interventions and Evaluation

NDx: Altered urinary elimination
Offer measures to help the patient relieve irritating voiding symptoms. Warm baths, a routine of timed voiding, or the administration of analgesia may lessen the urinary tract discomfort. Because bleeding is a common problem, obtain urine specimens regularly and perform dipstick checks for hematuria. Encourage fluids unless contraindicated. If an infection is suspected, send a urine specimen to the laboratory for culture.

NDx: Knowledge deficit: nature of the disorder and treatment plan
Because patient education is the most important nursing measure for the patient with cancer of the bladder, explain all nursing and medical interventions to the patient. Provide general information to the patient about the diagnosis, with specific information about the particular type of bladder tumor.

Instruct the patient about the events that are to occur in relation to the treatment plan, specifying all information about the preoperative and postoperative care and guidelines for the patient to follow.

Stress the importance of complying with the long-term treatment plan and follow-up care. Patients often assume that once treatment has been instituted, the tumor is gone forever. However, as many as three-fourths of the patients treated for superficial bladder cancers experience recurrence of the disease at some time. Depending on the physician's preference and the patient's condition, repeat assessment of the urinary tract is performed every 3 to 6 months initially, then every 6 to 12 months, for the rest of the patient's life. Encourage the patient to follow this reassessment schedule.

Compare the patient's status with the expected outcomes. If the outcomes are not met, reassess the patient and revise the plan.

NURSING PROCESS
Nonpapillary or Muscle-Invasive Bladder Cancer

Because radical cystectomy with urinary diversion is the primary method of treatment for patients with these tumors, the application of the nursing process is specific to this type of intervention.

Assessment

Preoperatively, evaluate the patient's overall physical, nutritional, and respiratory status. Ask the patient about usual eating habits. Note the patient's weight in relation to height. Observe for signs of malnutrition. Check for dyspnea, tachypnea, or abnormal breath sounds. Assess the patient's view of sexuality and pattern of sexual activity. This information is valuable in the postoperative period as the patient adjusts to the presence of a stoma. Assess the patient's anxiety in relation to the surgery and to the physical changes that will result from the surgical intervention. Determine the patient's understanding of the disease and the surgical intervention. Determine the patient's ability to cope with the upcoming lifestyle changes. Find out what support systems are available to the patient and who will be at home to assist the patient.

Postoperatively, assess the patient for any respiratory distress, such as difficulty breathing, extreme tachypnea, or wheezing. Note the patient's circulatory status. Assess pulses, color of extremities, heart rate, and blood pressure. Evaluate fluid and electrolyte status frequently. Determine the need for pain relief. As in all types of abdominal surgery, assess the wound frequently for excessive drainage or signs of infection. Assess all drains for patency. Evaluate the color and appearance of the stoma as well as the condition of the surrounding skin. Assess the ostomy appliance every shift and as necessary for placement, leaking around the system, and need for replacement or emptying.

In addition to the assessment of the various physical parameters, assess the patient and family for their reaction to the appearance of the stoma and for their readiness to learn about stoma care. Once past the immediate postoperative period, assess the patient for an understanding of the basics of stoma care as well as the ability to perform the procedure.

Nursing Diagnoses and Planning

Nursing diagnoses and related expected patient outcomes most commonly applicable to patients with nonpapillary or muscle-invasive bladder cancer who are undergoing cystectomy include the following:

NDx: Fluid volume deficit related to the surgical intervention

Planning: Patient Outcomes
1. Patient's fluid intake and output is balanced.
2. Patient's urinary output is 30 mL/h or more.
3. Patient's vital signs are within normal ranges for the patient.

NDx: Impaired skin integrity related to leakage of urine around the stoma

Planning: Patient Outcomes
1. Patient's skin remains intact.
2. Patient's skin remains clean and dry.
3. Patient remains free of infection around stoma.

NDx: Anxiety related to surgical procedure and lifestyle changes

Planning: Patient Outcomes
1. Patient communicates fears and concerns about surgery, body image, and coping with stoma care.
2. Patient identifies relaxation techniques and other coping mechanisms.

NDx: Altered urinary elimination related to the urinary diversion

Planning: Patient Outcomes
1. Patient's urinary output is 30 mL/h or more.
2. Patient's urine is clear, with normal characteristic odor.
3. Patient is able to maintain an appropriate fluid intake and output.

NDx: Body image disturbance related to the urinary stoma

Planning: Patient Outcomes
1. Patient expresses feelings related to the stoma.
2. Patient expresses fears and concerns.
3. Patient asks questions about the care of the stoma.
4. Patient looks at the stoma with the appearance of acceptance.

NDx: Altered health maintenance related to lack of knowledge about the surgical intervention and postoperative stoma care

Planning: Patient Outcomes
1. Patient relates accurate information about the surgical procedure and postoperative expectations.
2. Patient asks questions about the home care necessary.
3. Patient demonstrates appropriate care of the stoma.

Nursing Interventions and Evaluation

NDx: Fluid volume deficit
Monitor the patient's fluid status frequently. Check the fluid intake and output. Document the data. Note any signs of fluid deficit such as changes in vital signs. Monitor the cardiovascular status, checking the patient's blood pressure and pulse rate as per unit protocol. Observe the wound for excessive drainage or signs of hemorrhage. Check drains. Note the amount of drainage. Report any signs of excessive fluid loss, especially hemorrhage. Measure all drainage bag amounts. Document the results.

NDx: Impaired skin integrity
Check the newly created stoma every 2 to 4 hours during the first 24 hours. Note the color, size, and general appearance. Report any excessive bleeding around the stoma. Check the pouch covering the stoma for leakage. Change it as ordered and needed. Cleanse the skin frequently, as prescribed, to prevent excoriation from the drainage. Place a skin barrier around the peristomal skin for protection. Observe for early signs of skin breakdown, such as redness around the stoma or other discoloration or lesions.

NDx: Anxiety
Permit the patient to verbalize feelings about the diagnosis, stoma, and changes in lifestyle and body image. Allow time for questions and concerns from the patient. Refer the patient to clergy or other counseling groups for assistance with the emotional trauma. Invite a member of an ostomy group to visit the patient. Have the patient practice relaxation techniques as frequently as needed to allay anxiety episodes.

NDx: Altered urinary elimination
Check the patient's fluid intake and output frequently, especially in the early postoperative period. Note any extreme imbalances. Report them to the attending physician. Once the patient is able to take oral fluids, encourage increased fluid intake unless otherwise contraindicated. Patients with urinary diversions often restrict fluids to prevent continuous drainage of urine. Explain to the patient the necessity for continuing to take increased oral fluids. The patient may subconsciously dehydrate from continued self-restriction of fluids. Increased fluid intake also assists in infection prevention.

NDx: Body image disturbance

Provide opportunities for the patient to verbalize feelings and concerns about the changes experienced. Before surgery, show the patient examples of the appliances that may be used. Have a member of an ostomy group visit the patient to assist in providing the needed emotional support. Discuss the family's feelings about the surgery and the changes in the patient's physical appearance. Ask the patient what information the physician has provided about sexual activity. (Men will be impotent.) Be accepting of the patient's demonstration of feelings but do not reinforce denial.

NDx: Altered health maintenance

Extensive preoperative teaching, based on the patient's readiness, is necessary to ensure a successful outcome from the surgery. Verify what the physician has explained to the patient and family about the operation. Review these points with the patient. Use illustrations to explain the procedure and the outcome in terms of changes in body image. Help the patient visualize the anatomical structures and identify the location of the incision area and stoma placement. Describe the appearance of the stoma to the patient.

Familiarize the patient with the postoperative equipment and treatments that are to be completed, such as the stoma care, wound care, and intravenous therapy. Explain the need for not allowing the patient to receive anything by mouth (NPO status) and for the use of analgesics.

Because the patient may be admitted to an intensive care unit for the immediate postoperative period, explain the appearance of the unit to the patient. Also explain the equipment and care that will be given in the unit.

Postoperatively, when the patient is stable, begin discharge planning. Consult with an enterostomal therapist for a teaching plan for the patient and family and for continued follow-up care that may be needed. The enterostomal therapist can assist the patient with the transition from hospital care to home care. Several teaching sessions are usually necessary for the patient to understand the stoma care. Refer the patient to an ostomy support group if one is available in the area. This group is extremely helpful in getting the patient to accept the stoma and change in lifestyle necessary to cope with the diagnosis and future. A representative of the group may visit the patient while still in the hospital to assist the patient in understanding the care needed and to give emotional support. A visiting nurse may also provide assistance with the stoma care when needed.

Before discharge, instruct the patient to observe for latent postoperative complications, such as wound infection and obstruction of the stoma. Arrange for a follow-up visit with the physician and the enterostomal therapist to answer questions that may arise after discharge and to evaluate the patient's competency with stoma care.

CANCER OF THE URETHRA

Etiology and Pathophysiology

Primary malignant tumors of the urethra are extremely rare, but they are the only urinary tract carcinomas with a higher incidence in women than in men. The cause of the tumors is unknown, although urethral irritation, urethral polyps, and urethral diverticulum are suggested as possible causes of the disease.

Clinical Manifestations

Clinical manifestations of urethral cancer are nonspecific, making the medical diagnosis difficult.

Diagnosis

The diagnosis is ultimately confirmed by biopsy of suspicious areas within the urethra.

Management

Medical treatment is always surgical removal of the lesion in the urethra.

NURSING PROCESS GUIDELINES
Urethral Cancer

Nursing care of the patient with cancer of the urethra depends on the location and extent of the cancer. Because surgery is the treatment of choice, care is directed at preparing the patient for the surgery and postoperative prevention of complications. If the cancer is extensive, the patient may undergo extensive surgery. In that case, the care is similar to that of the patient with cancer of the bladder with a urinary diversion.

❖ SETTINGS, PROVIDERS, AND COLLABORATION FOR CARE

The patient with urinary tract cancer may be treated and released from the hospital with many care needs that continue into the home setting. Continued treatment may occur in the physician's office, a radiology clinic, or the home. Rehospitalization may also be necessary. The nursing role in alternative care settings can facilitate the care of the patient diagnosed with urinary tract cancer and the family members by determining appropriate community-based resources. A wide range of agencies provide a variety of social and health services through home health care, support groups, referral services, transportation, and other long-term care services. Ongoing communication with the physician, radiologist, oncologist, and home health nurses is necessary and may be coordinated by the case manager.

Cultural factors may affect the patient and family outcomes in the maintenance and restoration of optimal function, especially as the patient moves from the hospital back into a more familiar environment. The nurse should be sensitive to cultural differences

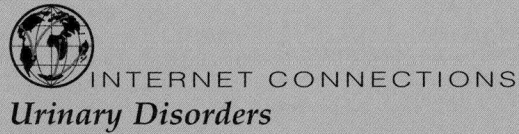

Urinary Disorders

American Association of Kidney Patients
http://cybermart.com/aakpaz/aakp.html
An information resource for patients, including treatment options, education, and links to other sites. In particular, this site provides a link to another site, which offers well-written, frequently asked questions and answers for dialysis patients:
http://cybermart.com/aakpaz/advisory.html

RENALNET
http://ns.gamewood.net//renalnet.html
A resource for health-care professionals in the area of kidney disorders, with such items as news, continuing education resources, professional organizations, and conferences. This site includes information for nursing in the area of kidney disorders as well as other health-care resources and links.

The International Society for Peritoneal Dialysis
http://www.ispd.org/ask.html
A forum for health-care professionals to ask specific questions and receive answers related to peritoneal dialysis.

and incorporate the differences in the care and goals for the client.

Because patients diagnosed with urinary tract cancer may be treated on an outpatient basis at a radiology clinic or even receive chemotherapy in the home, the home health nurse may be needed to assist the client and family as a caregiver or as patient educator. Patients who have been diagnosed with terminal cancer may be referred to a hospice program for continued assistance in the home.

The Elderly: Special Considerations

As discussed in Chapter 30, urinary incontinence is a common problem of older adults, but it is not due solely to age-related changes. Nursing assessment of urinary elimination focuses on the identification of any factors that influence overall urinary elimination or increase the risk of urinary incontinence. Nurses also assess signs and symptoms of urinary incontinence and identify any negative consequences, such as restrictions on activities. The nursing assessment may include the completion of a 2-week baseline voiding diary, completed by the older person or caregiver. This diary includes information about incontinence episodes and precipitating factors, such

as sneezing, coughing, or changing position. Environmental factors related to assistive devices, toilet accessibility, and the presence of caregivers should also be included. A comprehensive assessment may be time-consuming and difficult because many people are reluctant to discuss their bladder habits and problems. The nurse should demonstrate patience, professionalism, and concern for the patient. Use a matter-of-fact approach and direct but open-ended questions.

Nursing care addresses the identified risk factors and is directed toward alleviating incontinence. Measures such as pelvic muscle exercises, discussed in Chapter 30, can be taught. The person with nocturia should be advised to maintain an adequate fluid intake during the day but to limit beverages in the evening. The person should also be advised to leave a night light on near the bathroom as a safety precaution to prevent injury from a fall.

When incontinence cannot be resolved or prevented, nursing goals address the actual and potential negative consequences (eg, social isolation, impaired skin integrity). For the older person experiencing frequency, urgency, or incontinence, time-voiding may be suggested as a means of establishing an accident-free pattern of urinary elimination. Another alternative is to recommend the use of continence products, such as pants liners and special briefs. These items are widely available and can protect against possible embarrassing events.

Because catheterization is one of the leading causes of UTIs, the use of indwelling catheters should be carefully evaluated. For people who have indwelling catheters, the use of aseptic technique is essential when inserting and caring for catheters. It is also important for the person to maintain adequate fluid intake unless contraindicated.

Chapter Review

1. Why is it important to review daily hygiene, activities, and dietary practices in patients with a confirmed diagnosis of cystitis?
2. How does the etiology of glomerulonephritis differ from the etiology of pyelonephritis?
3. How does a decrease in perfusion lead to prerenal failure?
4. What nursing assessments are crucial during the oliguric phase of acute renal failure?
5. What would happen to a patient in the oliguric phase of acute renal failure if fluid and protein intake exceed recommended amounts?
6. Why is the drug epoetin alfa administered to patients with chronic renal failure, and what laboratory work assesses the need for epoetin alfa?

7. What are the advantages of hemodialysis versus peritoneal dialysis for long-term care?
8. How does the inability of the renal tubules to excrete water and sodium affect the fluid volume of a patient with acute renal failure?
9. Why is the monitoring of intake and output and serum electrolytes important in the care of a patient with postobstructive diuresis?
10. What are the advantages of extracorporeal shock wave lithotripsy in the treatment of urinary calculi?
11. How can fluid volume deficit best be assessed in the postoperative patient who has undergone nephrectomy?

Bibliography

Bellomo R, Parkin G, Boyce N. Acute renal failure in the critically ill: Management by continuous veno-venous hemodiafiltration. J Crit Care 1993; 8(3):140.

Bernal H. A model for delivering culture-relevant care: I. The community. Public Health Nurs 1993; 10(4):228.

Blagg CR. The challenge of hemodialysis. Contemporary Dialysis and Nephrology 1993; 14(4):29.

Bove LA. Restoring electrolyte balance—Calcium and phosphorus. RN 1996; 59(3):47.

Bove LA. Restoring electrolyte balance—Sodium and chloride. RN 1996; 5(1):25.

Brundage DJ, Swearengen PA. Chronic renal failure: Evaluation and teaching tool. ANNA-J 1994; 21(5):265.

Bull MJ. Patients' and professionals' perceptions of quality in discharge planning. J Nurs Care Qual 1994; 8(2):47.

Courts NF. Psychosocial interventions for patients receiving hemodialysis. Urol Nurs 1994; 14(3):79.

Davison AM. Continuous therapy for complicated acute renal failure. Nephrology, Dialysis, Transplantation 1994; 9(4):187.

Fitts SS, Guthrie MR. Six-minute walk by people with CRF: Assessment of effort by perceived exertion. Am J Phys Med Rehabil 1995; 74(1):54.

Gillot C. Caring for patients with prostate cancer. Nursing 1994; 24(6):32c.

Hagland M. Making sense of continuous renal replacement therapy. Nurs Times 1994; 90(40):37.

Hall WA, Carty EM. Managing the early discharge experience: Taking control. J Adv Nurs 1993; 18(4):574.

Kammerer JK. Case study of the anemic patient: Epoetin alfa focus on CQI and patient management. ANNA-J 1994; 21(5):282.

Kelly M. Chronic renal failure. AJN 1996; 96(1):36.

Korber KE. Impaired renal function and dietary protein manipulation. Physician Assistant 1994; 18(5):71–73, 76–78, 92–93.

Kutner NG, Lin LS, et al. Continued survival of older hemodialysis patients: Investigation of psychosocial predictors. Am J Kidney Dis 1994; 24(1):42.

Lowenstein AJ, Hoff PS. Discharge planning. A study of nursing staff involvement. J Nurs Adm 1994; 24(4):45.

Marangi AL, Giordano R, et al. Hepatitis B virus infection in chronic uremia: Long term follow up of a two-step integrated protocol of vaccination. Am J Kidney Dis 1994; 23(4):537.

Montemuro M, Martin LS, et al. Participatory control in chronic hospital-based hemodialysis patients. ANNA-J 1994; 21(7):403.

Moss AH. ANNA seeks to collaborate with renal community on guidelines. ANNA-J 1994; 21(7):403.

Mueller V. Quality of life with an ostomy: Building a model for assessment and care. Progressions 1993; 5(1):3.

Neary MA. Community services in the 1990s: Are they meeting the needs of caregivers? J Commun Health Nurs 1993; 10(2):105.

Perez A. Restoring electrolyte balance—Hypokalemia. RN 1995; 58(12):33.

Peterson KJ, Solie CJ. Interpreting lab values in chronic renal insufficiency. AJN 1994; 94(5):56B, 56E, 56H.

Price CA. Acute renal failure, a sequela of sepsis. Crit Care Nurs Clin North Am 1994; 6 (2):359.

Pryor J, Jenkins AD. Use of double-pigtail stents in extracorporeal shock wave lithotripsy. J Urol 1990; 143(3):475.

Rhoads C, Dean J, et al. Comprehensive discharge planning: A hospital-home healthcare partnership. Home Healthcare Nurse 1992; 10(6):13.

Recer P. New test could be breakthrough in treatment of bladder cancer. The Morning News of Northwest Arkansas 1996, February 2, p 6B.

Roy RS. Prostate diseases and treatments. Geriatric Consultant 1993; 10(4):14.

Smith AS. Patient participation in changing behaviors. Home Healthc Nurse 1995; 13(2):45.

Spector RE. Cultural diversity in health and illness. 4th ed. Norwalk, CT: Appleton & Lange, 1996.

Speers AT. A renal jeopardy game. J Nurs Staff Dev 1993; 9(1):41.

Stark J. Acute renal failure in trauma: Current perspectives. Crit Care Nurs Q 1994; 16(4):49.

Thobaben M, Mattingly HJ. Cultural sensitivity: Educating home healthcare nurse to be transcultural nurses. Home Healthc Nurse 1993; 11(4):61.

United Network for Organ Sharing, April 1996. UNOS Research Department Report, Richmond, VA.

Wadhwa NK, Suh H, et al. Peritoneal dialysis with trained home nurses in elderly and disabled end-stage renal disease patients. Adv Periton Dialysis 1993; 9:130.

Warren JW. Catheter associated bacteriuria in long-term care facilities. Infect Cont Hosp Epidemiol 1994; 15(8):557.

Wood JM, Bosley CL. Acute postrenal failure: Reversing the problem. Nursing 1995; 25(3):48.

Unit XI

Immune Dysfunction

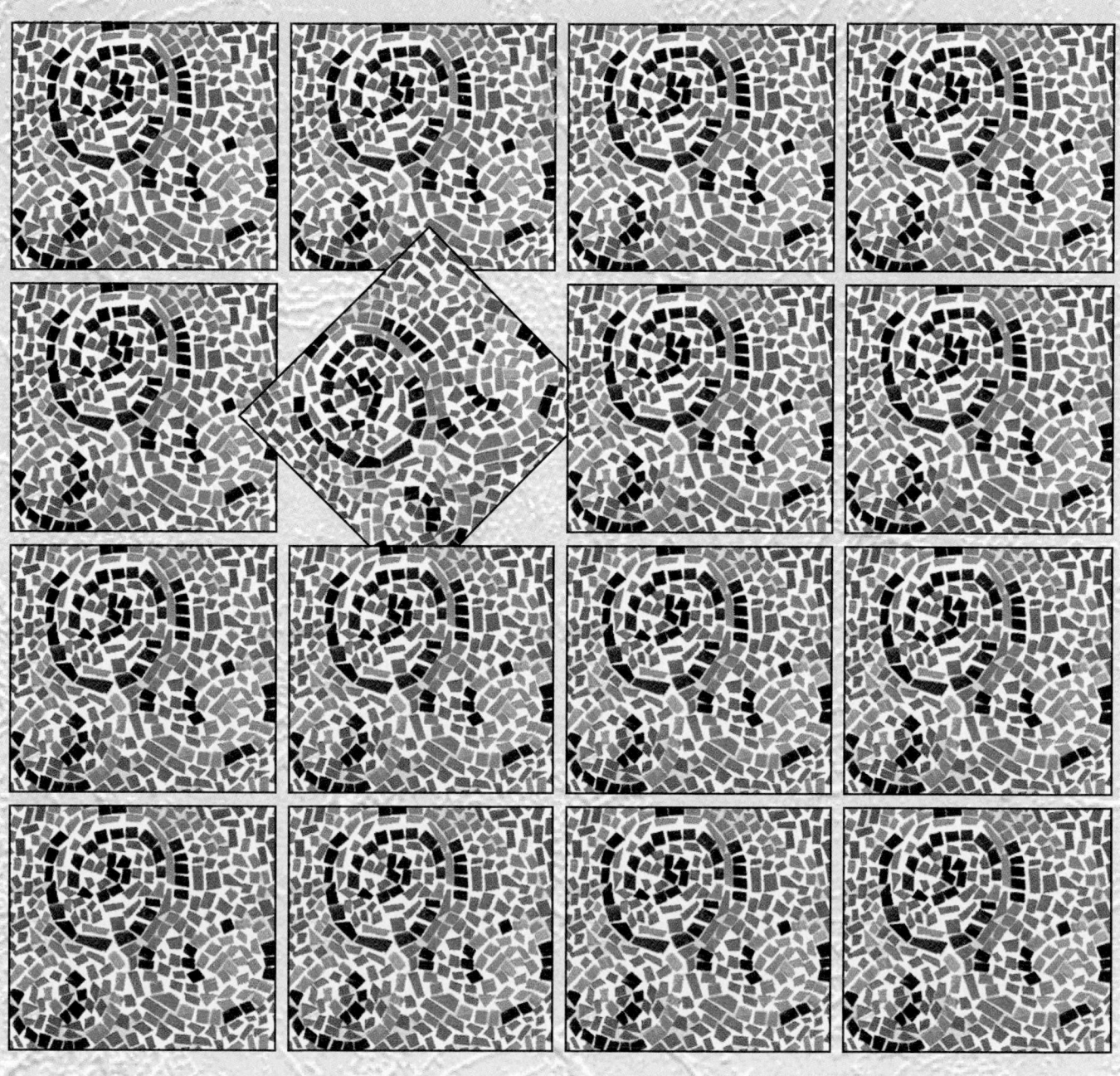

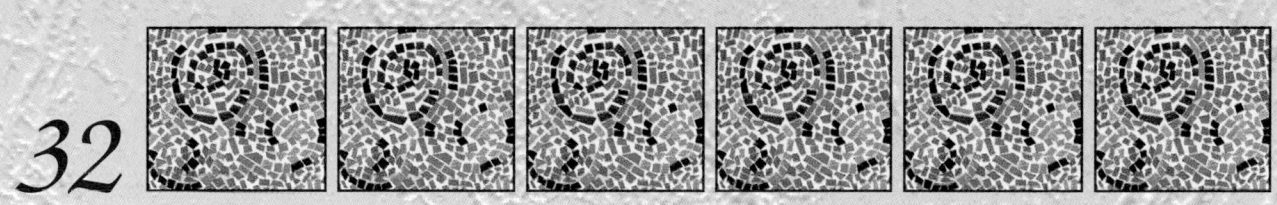

Knowledge Base for Patients with Immune Dysfunction

Study Outcomes

After studying this chapter, you should be able to:

1. Explain the normal anatomy and physiology of the immune system.
2. Discuss immunity and the various types of human immune response.
3. Identify information and physical examination data essential to the assessment of immune status.
4. Describe basic diagnostic tests and modalities of medical management used in the treatment of patients with immune disorders.
5. Describe bone marrow aspiration and bone marrow transplantation.
6. Describe nursing process and related expected patient outcomes commonly applicable to patients undergoing bone marrow aspiration and transplantation.
7. Identify alternative treatment and care settings for patients with immune dysfunction and the services related to community-based care.
8. Identify special considerations for the elderly patient with altered immune function.

The immune system is the body's complex and carefully orchestrated defense mechanism against a host of infectious microbial agents, including viruses, bacteria, fungi, and parasites. Functioning properly, the immune system protects the body through a critically regulated series of cellular interactions that display a wide range of nonspecific and exquisitely specific effects. Nonspecific reactions, also known as innate or natural immunity, result in chronic or acute inflammation. Specific reactions, also known as adaptive or acquired immunity, involve antigen recognition.

These are the two fundamental divisions of the immune system: innate immunity and adaptive immunity. Innate immunity is the first line of defense to stop potential pathogens and infectious agents before they can take hold and cause infection. The adaptive immune system takes over if an organism breaches innate immunity, producing a specific reaction to the infectious agent and usually eliminating the infection.

The immune system has three primary functions: defense, surveillance, and homeostasis (Table 32–1). Defense provides protection against external invaders, primarily microorganisms threatening to gain entry to the body. Surveillance provides protection from internal invaders, such as malignant cells. Homeostasis provides the body with cleanup operations; immune system cells remove dead and damaged cells from all parts of the body.

The ability to carry out these functions depends on four major features of the immune system:

Specificity
Diversity
Memory
Self versus nonself recognition

Specificity refers to the immune system's ability to discriminate among various antigens or molecular invaders. Diversity refers to the extensive number of receptors (estimated at 109 or more) available to recognize different specificities. Memory refers to the immune system's ability to mount a long-lasting reaction to antigens so that, months or even years later, exposure to the antigen results in an accelerated response. Vaccination has capitalized on this ability of the immune system to remember. The final and most basic feature of the immune system is the capacity to distinguish self from nonself. This discrimination is a function of the whole immune system and might be seen as the operational balance. Breakdown of this self-tolerance is thought to be the basic pathologic mechanism of autoimmune diseases (conditions in which the body reacts against itself and causes damage). The ability of the body to react appropriately to self must be as specific as its ability to respond to foreign antigens.

Many of the diagnostic tests and some treatment procedures for immune dysfunction are carried out in clinics and outpatient settings. However, because of the nature of immune dysfunction, protecting the patient from exposure to other infectious processes may require hospitalization during the testing and treatment regimen.

Table 32–1

Functions of the Immune System

Functional Category	Physiologic Effect
Defense	Provides protection against invaders from outside the body, such as microorganisms
Surveillance	Protects the body from internal threats, such as malignant cells
Homeostasis	Maintains the internal environment by removing dead or damaged cells

Anatomy and Physiology

The immune system has no one specific anatomic site. It consists of a complex network of organs and cells dispersed throughout the body. Immune system organs are connected with each other by lymphatic ducts and blood vessels. Several organs, such as the liver and spleen, possess immune functions in addition to their other functions.

Organs that function in the immune system are often called lymphoid organs and are classified as generative (central or primary) and peripheral (or secondary), as shown in Figure 32–1. The two generative lymphoid organs in the human are the thymus and the bone marrow. Lymphocytes arise and mature in these generative organs. Peripheral lymphoid organs include the lymph nodes, spleen, liver, tonsils, and Peyer's patches of the intestine. Peripheral lymph organs filter foreign particles and microorganisms from blood and lymph. They also serve as the location in which mature immune-system cells interact with each other and react with antigens.

GENERATIVE LYMPHOID ORGANS

Thymus Gland

The thymus gland is located in the mediastinal cavity, anterior to and above the heart. The thymus grows from birth to puberty. At puberty, it weighs about 40 g. Undifferentiated stem cells from bone marrow migrate to and enter the thymus gland. In 2 to 3 days, these cells acquire a new function and new surface markers as they mature into T lymphocytes (T cells). Mature T cells enter the blood stream via postcapillary venules of the thymus and then travel to the peripheral lymph organs (Fig. 32–2). T cells are responsible for cell-mediated immunity. The thymus gland also produces multiple hormones (eg,

thymosin) that increase the number of lymphocytes in the peripheral lymphoid organs.

After puberty, the thymus begins to atrophy. In the mature adult, it is a relatively functionless, shriveled mass of fatty tissue. This loss of thymic function is thought to be responsible for some of the immune deficiencies seen in the elderly. As thymic

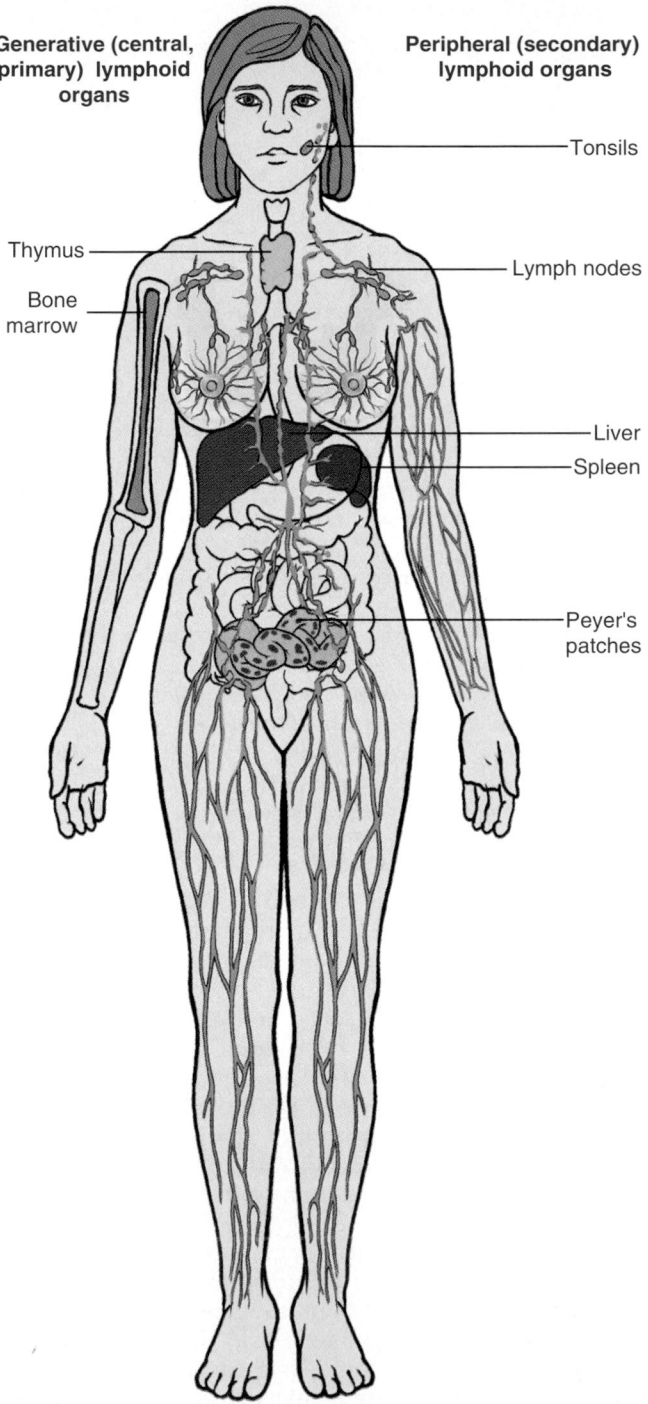

Generative (central, primary) lymphoid organs

Peripheral (secondary) lymphoid organs

Tonsils

Thymus

Bone marrow

Lymph nodes

Liver

Spleen

Peyer's patches

Figure 32–1

Major primary and secondary lymphoid organs and tissues.

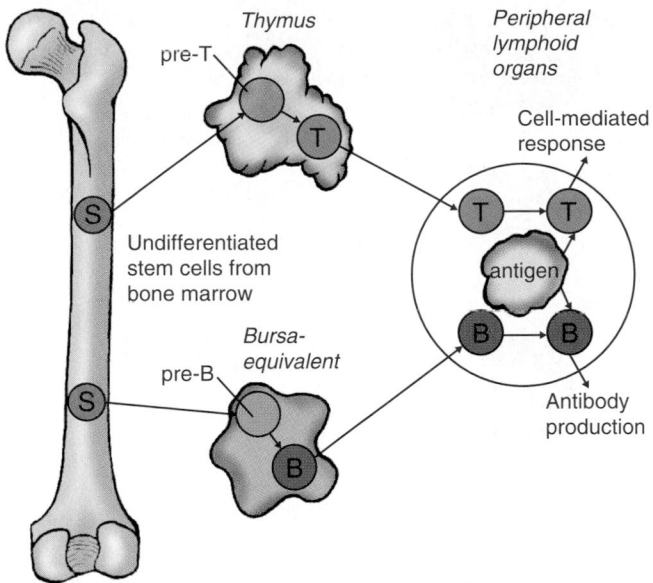

Figure 32-2

Undifferentiated stem cells move from the bone marrow to either the thymus gland or the bursa-equivalent, where they are transformed into T cells or B cells. They then move to one of the secondary lymphoid organs, where they may contact an antigen and become activated.

function decreases with age, the incidence of malignancies and autoimmune disease increases.

Bone Marrow

The bone marrow is the area of the body where undifferentiated stem cells are transformed into mature B lymphocytes (antibody-producing cells). The bone marrow is a highly vascular, sinusoidal tissue dispersed within the bones. If it was merged together, its total weight and volume would be about that of the liver. In the adult, active bone marrow is found in the bones of the ribs, sternum, pelvis, skull, femur, and humerus. Active bone marrow is essential for life.

PERIPHERAL LYMPHOID ORGANS

Lymph Nodes

The lymph nodes and other peripheral lymphoid organs are strategically clustered in areas of the body where contact with external antigens is most likely—that is, around areas of the body exposed to the external environment: the respiratory, gastrointestinal, and genitourinary tracts. In addition, the vascular connections of the liver and spleen make them likely to contact internal antigens. This helps increase the chance that an antigen, whether external or internal, will quickly encounter the active cells of

the immune system and be destroyed before disease occurs.

More than 500 lymph nodes exist in the body, varying from the size of a pinhead to that of a lima bean. Lymph nodes contain lymphocytes, plasma cells, macrophages, granulocytes, and a few erythrocytes. They have several important functions. One is to filter foreign material and other particulate matter from the lymph. Another is to provide a place where immunologically active cells and antigens can come together and interact with each other. As a result of this interaction with antigen, antibody is produced and phagocytic cells are stimulated. These antibodies and phagocytic cells are released into the general circulation via lymph leaving the lymph node. Lymph nodes containing B cells and T cells that have been antigenically stimulated may increase in size and become palpable. Enlarged lymph nodes are an important clinical sign that an immune response is occurring somewhere in the region of the body that drains into the enlarged node.

Lymph nodes are connected by the lymphatic system, which is composed of a network of capillaries, vessels, and ducts. Each lymph node drains a distinct region of the body. This region is determined by the location of the lymphatic vessels that flow to the node. The walls of these lymphatic capillaries and vessels are only one cell thick, so plasma proteins and other substances can be picked up from the interstitial spaces of connective tissues. Capillaries join to form vessels along which the lymph nodes are located. The lymph vessels eventually unite to form the thoracic duct, which joins the venous system at the juncture of the left internal jugular vein and the subclavian vein. Lymph from the right side of the head and neck, the right arm, and the thorax flows to the right lymph duct, which joins the venous system at the juncture of the right subclavian vein and the internal jugular vein. (See Chap. 12 for more information.)

Spleen

The spleen, a peripheral lymphoid organ, has many functions, some of which are immunologic and others of which are separate from the immune system. Many of the spleen's functions depend on its ability to filter blood and store blood cells. The spleen plays a major role in homeostasis by removing worn out or damaged erythrocytes. The spleen is composed of many fine channels that form a meshwork. These channels are lined with phagocytic cells that engulf and destroy materials in the blood passing through the spleen. At birth, the spleen is not completely developed and depends on hormones from the thymus gland to complete its development. Some lymphocytes are produced in the spleen, but most of the active cells come from the bone marrow. The spleen is the largest single collection of lymphocytes and macrophages in the body. Antibodies are also produced here. The spleen is not necessary for life, but its removal is associated with an increased risk of infection, especially if removed before the person reaches age 6.

Tonsils and Peyer's Patches

The tonsils of the oropharynx consist of the palatine tonsils between the palatoglossal and palatopharyngeal arches, the lingual tonsils at the base of the tongue, and the pharyngeal tonsils (also called adenoids) at the back of the pharynx. Tonsils contain collections of lymphocytes and macrophages, as well as memory cells. Peyer's patches are lymphoid nodules in the small intestine where T cells congregate. These organs are most important in the secondary immune response, although they may play a role in the primary immune response as well. These organs may enlarge as they become highly active in the immune response.

Liver

The liver contains a large number of fixed macrophages called Kupffer's cells. These Kupffer's cells help filter blood by phagocytizing microorganisms and other foreign particles passing through the liver.

CELLS OF THE IMMUNE SYSTEM

The cells involved in the immune response are represented in Figure 32–3. The white blood cells, or leukocytes, are responsible for immune functions. There are five kinds of leukocytes: polymorphonuclear leukocytes, monocytes, macrophages, lymphocytes, and plasma cells. Each type of cell has a specialized role in the body's defense system. The polymorphonuclear leukocytes (also called granulocytes) are primarily involved in the acute inflammatory process. Four types of polymorphonuclear leukocytes are neutrophils, eosinophils, mast cells, and basophils.

Neutrophils make up 57 to 67% of the total white blood cell count. These cells can quickly phagocytize large numbers of bacteria and are one of the first lines of defense against infection. The number of neutrophils frequently rises during an infection.

Eosinophils are also phagocytic but respond primarily in allergic reactions, rather than to infection. They work at the site of tissue inflammation to detoxify foreign proteins and antigen-antibody complexes before these substances can damage the body. Normally, eosinophils constitute about 1 to 3% of the total white cell count.

The function of basophils is not entirely clear, but they seem to have a role in mediating inflammatory reactions. Basophils contain large amounts of histamine and secrete heparin. The normal value of basophils is 0 to 0.75% of the total white cell count. A small rise in the number of basophils may occur

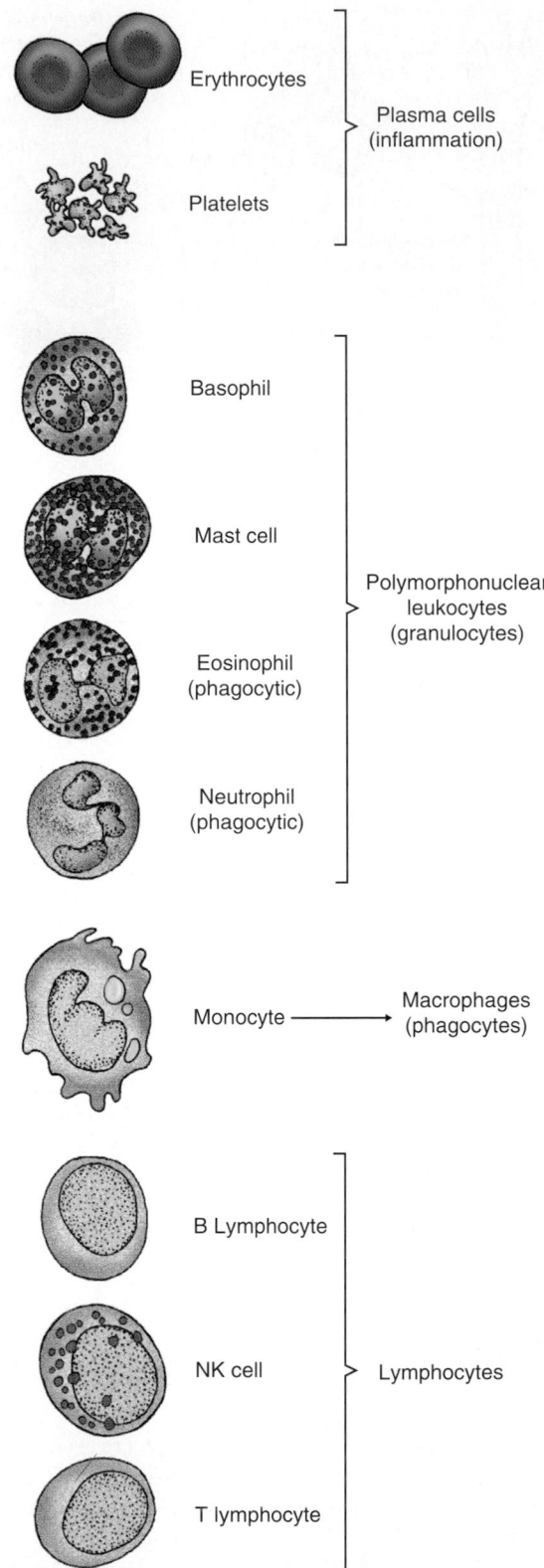

Figure 32–3

Cells involved in the immune response and their precursor origins. NK, natural killer.

in response to stress and chronic inflammation. Mast cells found in the lungs, gastrointestinal tract, and superficial layers of the skin are similar to basophils, except that they are immobile and do not circulate in the blood.

Monocytes and macrophages are two other types of leukocytes. Monocytes are found in blood and normally constitute 3 to 7% of the total white cell count. Monocytes migrate into tissue and become macrophages. Both monocytes and macrophages have great phagocytic ability and can ingest large numbers of microorganisms and other foreign materials. Some macrophages, called fixed macrophages or histiocytes, remain in one place in body tissues and do not travel in the blood. Areas where these fixed macrophages are found include the spleen, Kupffer's cells, pulmonary alveoli, and the gastrointestinal tract. Other monocytes circulate freely in the blood, leaving the blood vessels when needed to localize and contain invaders at the site of an injury.

Lymphocytes and plasma cells are the leukocytes responsible for the specific immune response. Lymphocytes normally make up about 25 to 33% of the total white cell count. There are two types of lymphocytes: T lymphocytes (T cells) and B lymphocytes (B cells). T cells are responsible for cellular immunity; B cells are responsible for humoral immunity (Table 32–2). T cells and B cells have distinct functions but depend on each other for proper functioning. Lymphocytes are the immunologic cells with the important properties of specificity and memory.

T Lymphocytes (T Cells)

T cells are responsible for the cellular, or cell-mediated, response. The cellular response involves tissue reactions that do not require antibodies produced by B cells. Cellular immunity is thought to primarily protect against infection caused by intracellular microorganisms, viruses, and slow-growing bacteria, as well as being responsible for rejection of allografts and malignant cells. T cells normally constitute 80 to 90% of the total circulating lymphocyte population. From the thymus, where they are produced, T cells travel to the peripheral lymphoid organs, take up residence, and carry out their immunologic functions. T-cell functions include the following:

• Mediation of delayed hypersensitivity reactions through release of lymphokines (substances produced by T cells that alter the physiology of other cells)
• Destruction of other cells (cytolytic reactions), such as virus-infected cells and tumor cells
• Regulation of the type and intensity of virtually all aspects of the specific immune response

There are several functionally distinct subsets of T cells. Each T cell has a specific function; these are not multifunctional cells. The subsets of T cells are named for the function they perform. They include helper cells, suppressor cells, cytotoxic (killer) cells, and memory cells (Table 32–3). These cells all function in controlling the specific immune response.

Helper T cells (also called inducer cells, T4 cells, or CD4$^+$32 [because they carry the most CD4 surface molecule] T cells) usually constitute about 60% of the total circulating T cells. Helper T cells interact with B cells to induce antibody production. Some antigens, especially those of low molecular weight, do not induce antibody production by themselves. Most antigens interact with the helper T cells. The helper T cells then induce antibody production by the B cells. Helper T cells also induce other types of T cells and macrophages to become active.

Suppressor T cells (also called T8 cells) inhibit the activities of other T cells and B cells. They turn the immune response off. The usual ratio of helper T cells to suppressor T cells is 2:1. This ratio is

Table 32–2

Classification of Leukocytes

Type of Leukocyte	Role in Immune Function
Polymorphonuclear Leukocytes	Primarily involved in the acute inflammatory response
Neutrophils	Phagocytic cells that are important in defense against infections
Eosinophils	Phagocytic cells that are important in allergic reactions and helminthic infections
Basophils	Release chemical mediators of the allergic reaction
Mast cells	Release chemical mediators of the allergic reaction
Monocytes	Phagocytic cells that attract other cells to the area
Macrophages	Phagocytes that can ingest large numbers of microorganisms
Lymphocytes	Responsible for the specific immune response
T cells	Responsible for cellular immunity
B cells	Responsible for humoral immunity
Natural killer cells	Nonselectively attack unhealthy or abnormal self cells in addition to nonself cells
Plasma cells	Fully differentiated B cells that have been stimulated by an antigen and are actively producing antibodies

Table 32–3

T-Cell Subsets

Type of T Cell	Function
Helper T cells	Stimulate activity of other immunologically active cells
Suppressor T cells	Turn off activity of other immunologically active cells
Cytotoxic (killer) T cells	Killer cells targeted by IgG antibody bound to the cell's surface
Memory T cells	Remember antigen and respond immediately on succeeding exposures to it

reversed in some diseases, such as acquired immunodeficiency syndrome (AIDS).

Cytotoxic (killer) T cells (also called K cells) can kill cells that have been targeted by immunoglobulin G (IgG) antibody bound to the cells' surface. Killer T cells depend on the presence of specific IgG antibody.

Memory T cells are another important subset of T cells. Once T cells have been stimulated by an antigen, some T cells become memory cells. These cells appear in the blood about 5 days after primary exposure to an antigen. They continually travel through the blood to every anatomic site that has a blood supply. This allows the memory T cells to come in contact with the antigen wherever it should enter the body in the future. The next time a memory T cell contacts its specific antigen, it undergoes proliferation and differentiation to effector cell in a matter of hours. These effector cells are then able to stimulate other immune cells to respond to the antigen. The immune response is quickly set into motion.

Natural killer cells, although similar to T cells, are not considered a true T-cell subset. Natural killer cells are cytotoxic to targeted cells. Their action is unique in that prior sensitization to the targeted cell is not necessary and occurs independently of other leukocytes. The cytotoxic action of natural killer cells seems to be most effective against self cells that are either infected by a virus or affected by malignant transformation. Natural killer cells also destroy foreign cells and thus play a role in rejection of grafts and transplanted organs.

B Lymphocytes (B Cells)

B cells are responsible for producing antibodies. The protection that results from these antibodies in blood and body fluids is called humoral immunity. Humoral immunity is important in defending against pyogenic infections and combating the effects of toxins produced by microorganisms. Stem cells are transformed into B cells in the bone mar-

row. Unstimulated B cells are stimulated either directly by an antigen or by lymphokines from a T cell that has recognized an antigen. Once stimulated, the B cell enlarges, divides, and is transformed into plasma cells and memory B cells. The plasma cells actually produce and secrete antibody. Plasma cells are predominantly located in the peripheral lymphoid tissues and are seldom found in peripheral blood. Plasma cells may be found in the peripheral blood in multiple myeloma, scarlet fever, measles, chickenpox, or other severe infection.

B cells are controlled and regulated by the helper and suppressor T cells. The helper T cells turn on or increase antibody production in B cells; suppressor T cells decrease the amount of antibody produced by the B cells. A delicate balance between T-cell subsets and B cells is required to maintain immunologic balance. If this balance is disrupted, disease may result because of too little or too much antibody production.

THE IMMUNE RESPONSE

There are two types of immune responses: nonspecific and specific. They have fairly different functions (Table 32–4). The nonspecific responses are considered the body's first line of defense. They are primarily responsible for defense against outside invaders. Their importance is frequently underestimated. Intact nonspecific responses present a formidable barrier to the microorganisms that are constantly trying to invade the host. Nonspecific responses can differentiate self from nonself, but cannot identify the specific invader. Nonspecific responses are functioning at birth, do not need to be learned, and respond in the same way to all invaders.

The specific immune response is the body's surveillance system that recognizes foreign substances in the body and then selectively eliminates them through a complex series of immunologic responses. The specific immune response, both humoral and

Table 32–4

Differences Between Specific and Nonspecific Immunity

Specific Immunity	Nonspecific Immunity
Second line of defense against infections	First line of defense against infections
Able to identify specific antigens	Unable to identify specific antigens
Reacts differently to different antigens	Reacts the same to all antigens
Response must be learned and developed	Present and functioning at birth

cellular, is initiated when an antigen makes its way past the body's nonspecific defenses and comes in contact with cells of the immune system. This response is highly specific in that it is effective against only the antigen that initiated it.

Nonspecific Immune Response

Nonspecific responses can be grouped into five categories: physical barriers, chemical barriers, interferon, inflammation, and phagocytosis.

PHYSICAL BARRIERS

Physical barriers help keep microorganisms out of the body. Intact skin and mucous membranes are effective at keeping most microorganisms out. Coughing and sneezing help expel microorganisms from the respiratory tract. The action of the cilia lining the respiratory tract also helps remove microorganisms before they can get into the lungs. The flushing action of fluids, such as urine and tears, helps remove microorganisms from their respective body openings.

CHEMICAL BARRIERS

Chemical barriers include various acids and enzymes found in body fluids. Sebaceous secretions contain lactic acid and unsaturated fatty acids, which are active against both bacteria and fungi. Areas of the body with no sebaceous glands, such as between the toes, are common sites of fungal infection. Lysozyme, found in tears, nasal secretions, saliva, and urine, is an enzyme that destroys the cell wall of gram-positive bacteria and, to a lesser extent, gram-negative bacteria. The highly acid pH of the stomach is effective at eliminating most microorganisms present in food and swallowed from the nose and mouth.

INTERFERON

Interferon is a protein produced by macrophages or lymphocytes, often in response to a viral infection. It protects cells that have not yet been infected by the virus by inducing production of another protein in these cells, which in turn inhibits viral replication within them. This action does not appear to be virus-specific. In other words, interferon produced in response to one type of virus protects cells against other types of viruses. However, interferon does appear to be species-specific, in that interferon produced by a rabbit is not effective in a mouse or a human. Interferon also has some immunoregulatory functions, in that it increases production of natural killer cells.

Interferon differs from antibody in several ways. Interferon is produced by several types of cells, whereas antibody is produced only by B lymphocytes. Interferon is effective against a wide variety of viruses; antibody is only effective against the specific virus that stimulated its formation. Interferon works on the host's cells to induce protection, whereas antibody inactivates viruses outside the cells.

Lymphocytes in the spleen, liver, and lungs are important sites of interferon production. Synthesis of interferon begins almost immediately after a virus enters the cell. Blood levels of interferon are detectable in about 2 hours and persist for several days. Virus-neutralizing antibody appears in the blood at about the time that interferon levels are decreasing. Interferon is not constantly present in the blood or body fluids. It is found only immediately after an exposure to a virus.

Currently, there is much research on the therapeutic use of interferon. Interferon is being investigated in the treatment of some malignant diseases, viral infections (especially chronic viral infections, such as hepatitis), and as an aid in reducing the severity of such viral infections as cytomegalovirus in immunosuppressed persons (such as organ transplant recipients).

INFLAMMATION

Inflammation is a complex nonspecific response that occurs when tissue is injured by any means (physical, chemical, anoxia, microorganisms, or their toxins). Inflammation is an attempt by the body to maintain homeostasis and repair the injured tissues. It is a protective response and normally not a harmful reaction. Classic signs of inflammation are redness, swelling, heat, and pain in the area of the injury.

The inflammatory reaction can be divided into three stages. During the first stage, blood vessels in the area of the injury dilate and become more permeable in response to chemical mediators (histamine, serotonin, kinins, and complement proteins) released by the injured cells. This increases the flow of blood and lymph to the injured area and increases the amount of fluid and cells released from the blood vessels. The increased fluid helps dilute and flush out any toxic materials that may be in the area. Neutrophils appear in the area in 30 to 60 minutes. Their prime purpose is to phagocytize (ingest and destroy) any potentially harmful agents, such as microorganisms. In a few hours, lymphocytes and monocytes arrive in the area. The monocytes also phagocytize any harmful agent. These cells all migrate to the area in response to chemotactic factors released by the injured cells. Phagocytosis and exudate formation occur during the second stage. The exudate is composed of fluid and cells that have been drawn to the area. During the third stage, the injured tissue undergoes repair and regeneration (Fig. 32–4).

PHAGOCYTOSIS

Phagocytosis, an important nonspecific immune response, is a process by which a particle is ingested

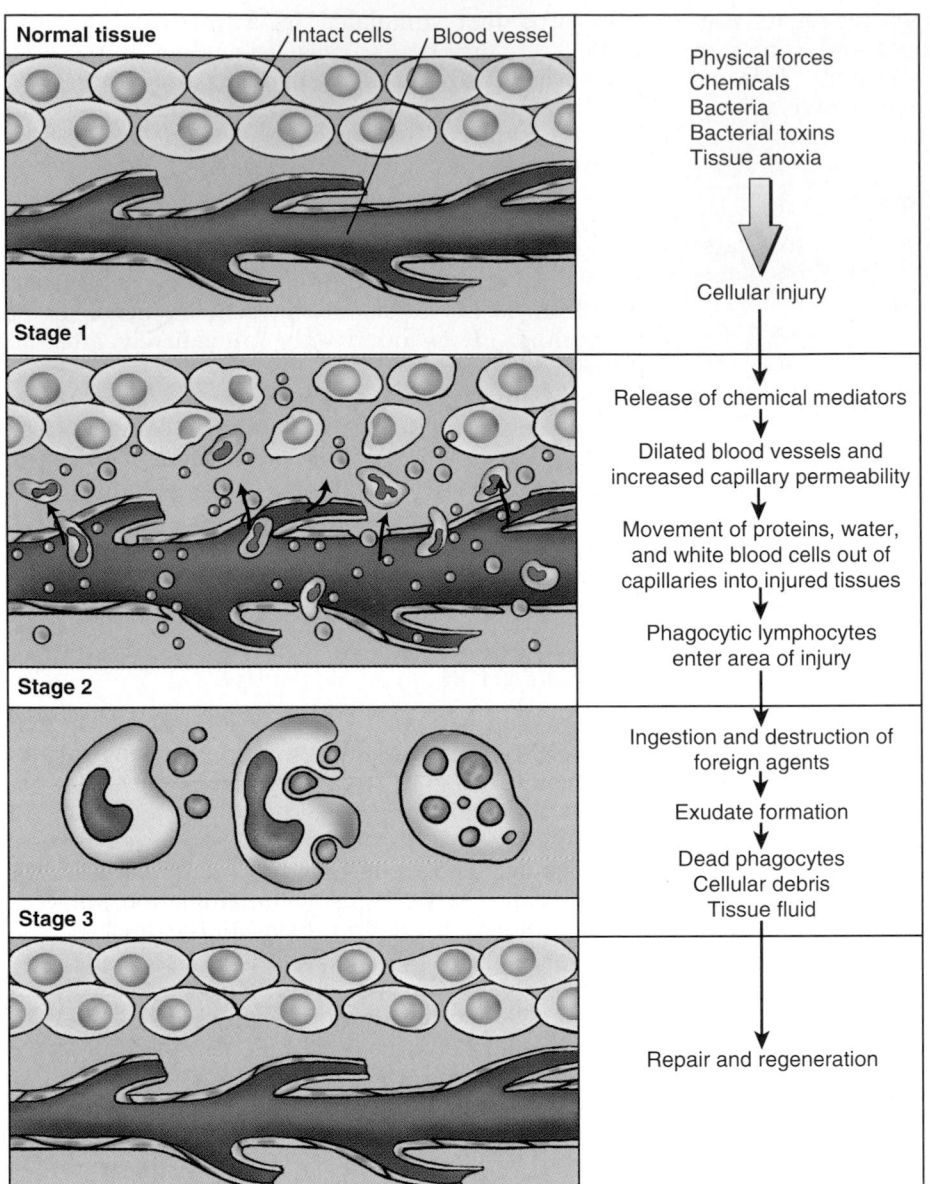

Normal tissue Intact cells Blood vessel

Physical forces
Chemicals
Bacteria
Bacterial toxins
Tissue anoxia

Cellular injury

Stage 1

Release of chemical mediators

Dilated blood vessels and
increased capillary permeability

Movement of proteins, water,
and white blood cells out of
capillaries into injured tissues

Phagocytic lymphocytes
enter area of injury

Stage 2

Ingestion and destruction of
foreign agents

Exudate formation

Dead phagocytes
Cellular debris
Tissue fluid

Stage 3

Repair and regeneration

Figure 32–4
The inflammatory response.

and digested by a cell. Cells with this ability are called phagocytes. Several types of leukocytes have phagocytic abilities, including monocytes, macrophages, neutrophils, and eosinophils. The goal of phagocytosis is to remove foreign substances, such as microorganisms. To accomplish this, the phagocytic cell must travel to the area where the substance is, ingest the substance, and destroy it. Phagocytes are attracted to an area by chemicals called chemotactic factors that are released from bacteria and other host cells, and by components of complement (complement is a series of proteins found in the blood that can destroy bacteria when combined with antigen and antibody). Once a phagocyte encounters a microorganism, it attaches to the surface of the microorganism. The external membrane of the phagocyte then engulfs the organism and encloses it

in a vesicle. This vesicle separates from the rest of the outer membrane and is internalized within the phagocytic cell, at which point it is called a phagosome (Fig. 32–5). Once internalized, most microorganisms are killed by the acid pH, lysozyme from other granules within the phagocyte, a reaction with a superoxide anion (an oxygen molecule that has had an electron removed, making it highly reactive), or most importantly by a reaction with hydrogen peroxide. However, some microorganisms are not killed once they are ingested by a phagocytic cell. *Mycobacterium tuberculosis,* for example, resists intracellular destruction and may survive for long periods of time in macrophages. These viable organisms may spread to other areas of the body via the macrophages and then cause disease where they are deposited when the macrophage finally dies.

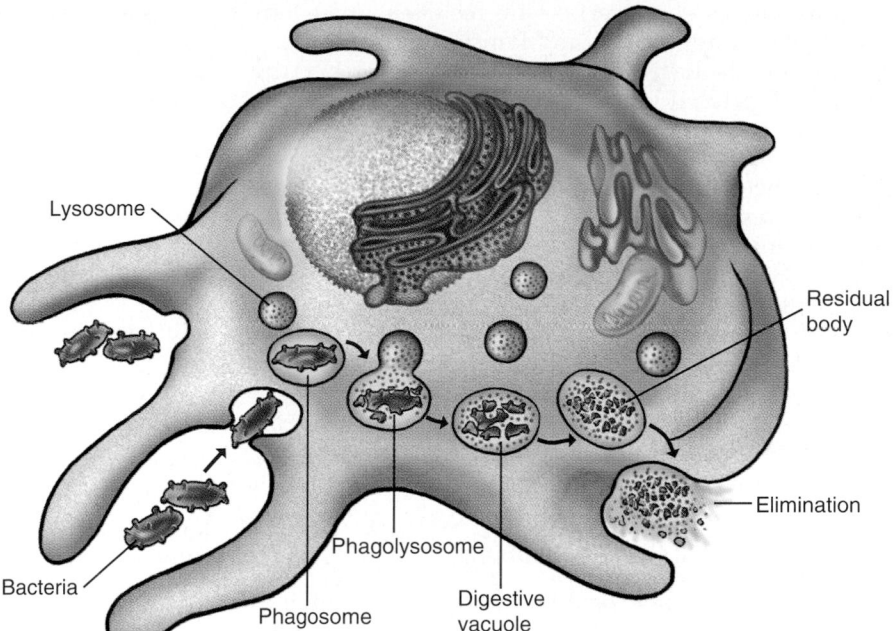

Figure 32–5

Phagocytosis. The ingestion process and intracellular digestion.

Opsonization

Some microorganisms are resistant to phagocytosis, especially those covered by a capsule, such as *Streptococcus pneumoniae* and *Cryptococcus neoformans.* Opsonization helps overcome this barrier to phagocytosis. Opsonization is the coating of the exterior of a microorganism or other foreign particle with a substance that makes the foreign particle more attractive to phagocytes. It is something like putting frosting on a cake to make the cake more attractive and appetizing. Complement protein and antibody are the substances that usually serve as opsonins. Some microorganisms require more opsonization than others. "Rough" strains of bacteria may need only the complement factors, whereas the smooth or encapsulated strains need both the complement factors and antibody before they can be phagocytized.

Defects in Phagocytosis

Defects that may leave the host more susceptible to infections can occur at any step in the phagocytic process. For instance, there may not be enough phagocytic cells in the body (neutropenia). This may be caused by an inherited disorder, such as congenital agranulocytosis or cyclic neutropenia, but is much more common as a result of a neoplastic disease or chemotherapy. Almost any medication has the potential to reduce the number of phagocytic cells, either by direct cytotoxic effect on the cells or indirectly through immunologic mechanisms. Chemotherapeutic agents used to treat malignancies, sulfa drugs, and chloramphenicol are commonly used drugs that reduce phagocyte numbers.

When the number of polymorphonuclear neutrophils drops below 1000/mm³ of blood, the risk of infection rises. This risk of acquiring an infection rises even more if the number of polymorphonuclear neutrophils falls below 500/mm³ of blood. Patients with polymorphonuclear neutrophil numbers lower than 500/mm³ are easily infected by organisms common to all humans, organisms usually maintained at nonthreatening levels. Special precautions to protect the patient from infection may be instituted when the number of polymorphonuclear neutrophils drops to these levels.

Phagocytosis may also be impaired by defects in phagocytic cells' ability to leave the blood vessels or adhere to tissues. Ingestion of large quantities of alcohol and the use of corticosteroids can decrease these abilities, thus impairing the host's phagocytic functions. Defects in the motility of the phagocytes have also been discovered. These defects can be either intrinsic in the cells, as in such rare disorders as Chédiak-Higashi syndrome and juvenile periodontitis, or they may spring from a defect in chemotactic factors. Inactivation or inhibition of chemotactic factors occurs in premature infants and patients with cirrhosis of the liver, Hodgkin's disease, systemic lupus erythematosus, or sarcoidosis.

Opsonization defects can also occur. Splenectomy may cause a defect in the ability to produce the opsonin for *S. pneumoniae.* This may contribute to development of the severe pneumococcal infections to which these patients are prone. Pneumovax (a vaccine for several common strains of *S. pneumoniae*) can help reduce this susceptibility but should be given at least 1 month before splenectomy to be most effective.

The ability of the phagocyte to kill organisms it has ingested may be defective. This is the basic pathologic mechanism in chronic granulomatous disease, which is an inherited disorder that occurs in children and is characterized by recurrent infections of the skin, lungs, bones, and lymph nodes.

Abnormal phagocytosis is usually manifested by recurrent bacterial infections with such organisms as staphylococci, gram-negative enteric bacteria, *Candida*, or *Aspergillus*. Infection may be found in any part of the body but most frequently arises in the skin and respiratory tract. Medical evaluation of patients suspected of having defective phagocytosis involves a complete history and physical examination, complete blood count, bone marrow biopsy, and frequently a number of tests available only at special reference laboratories to evaluate all aspects of phagocytic function. Treatment for defects in phagocytosis is limited. The most important aspect of caring for these patients is early detection and prompt, proper treatment of infections.

Specific Immune Response

The specific immune response can be divided into humoral response, cellular response, and complement. These three immune activities are in response to specific antigens, or unwanted substances.

UNDERSTANDING ANTIGENS

An antigen is a substance that produces a detectable immune response when introduced into a host. Several factors determine whether a substance (usually a molecule) is antigenic. One important factor is the size of the molecule. Usually, molecules with a molecular weight of less than 10,000 are weak antigens or not antigenic at all. Molecules with a molecular weight over 100,000 are usually potent antigens. Small molecules, such as amino acids and monosaccharides, are not antigenic. Large-protein molecules are potent antigens.

A second factor is the chemical complexity of the molecule. Very simple molecules are poor antigens. More chemically complex molecules are more significant antigens. In addition, the host must be genetically able to respond to the substance, and the substance must be administered by the proper route and in an adequate dose. Too much or too little antigen may fail to cause an immune response.

Only a small part of the antigen molecule is responsible for its immunologic activity and actual binding with antibody. This small part, which has the specific structure that makes it a unique antigen, is called the antigenic determinant, or epitope.

Haptens are small molecules that alone are not antigenic but that may bind to another molecule and become antigenic. The antibody produced is specific for an antigenic determinant on the hapten, not on the molecule to which the hapten is bound. Drugs (particularly penicillin) may act as haptens, becoming antigenic when bound to proteins in the body.

HUMORAL IMMUNE RESPONSE

Antibodies, also called immunoglobulins, are specialized proteins. They are formed in response to an antigen and react specifically with that antigen. The function of antibody is to provide a specific and efficient mechanism to protect the body from foreign invaders. B cells are responsible for producing antibodies.

B cells are stimulated either directly by antigen binding with receptors on its surface or indirectly by T cells. Each B cell has a specific receptor site on the surface that reacts only with one specific antigen or a few closely related antigens. In the lymph nodes, antigens that have been phagocytized by macrophages are presented to the B cell on the surface of the macrophage. This mechanism requires far less antigen than is required if the antigen directly stimulates the B cell. Some antigens cannot directly stimulate B cells and require the assistance of T cells to induce antibody production. Once the B cell is stimulated, it enlarges, divides, and transforms into plasma cells. The plasma cells mature and secrete antibody. Each plasma cell produces only one specific type of antibody.

Classes of Antibodies

There are five different classes of human antibodies (Table 32–5). They all have a similar structure, but each has a different role. The basic antibody molecule is composed of four polypeptide chains arranged in a Y shape. There are two heavy chains and two light chains. Each chain has a constant re-

Table 32–5

Properties of Antibody Classes

	IgG	IgA	IgM	IgD	IgE
Percentage of total circulating antibodies	70	21	7	≤0.2	≤0.5
Number of component molecules	1	2	5	1	1
Able to cross the placenta	Yes	No	No	No	No
Able to bind complement	Yes	No	Yes	No	No
Found in body secretions	Unknown	Yes	No	No	No
Has a role in allergic reactions	Yes	Unknown	No	Unknown	Yes

Ig, immunoglobulin.

gion and a variable region. Antigen-binding sites are found in the variable regions (Fig. 32–6).

The major serum antibody is IgG, constituting about 70% of the total circulating antibodies. IgG is antiviral, antibacterial, and effective against toxins. It can move into all body fluids and is the only antibody that crosses the placenta. It has a half-life of about 28 days. (Half-life is the amount of time it takes to metabolize or inactivate half the amount given.)

IgA makes up about 21% of the total circulating antibodies. It is the main antibody found in external secretions, such as tears, saliva, bronchial secretions, and colostrum. It can neutralize viruses and inhibit attachment of bacteria to epithelial surfaces.

IgM is the first antibody produced in response to an antigen. About 7% of the total serum antibodies are of the IgM class. Because of their size, these antibodies are confined to the blood stream.

IgE antibody is present only in minute quantities in the normal human, accounting for only about 0.5% of the total antibody level in the blood. IgE mediates hypersensitivity type I reactions, such as hay fever, asthma, and atopic allergies. The constant region of the IgE molecule binds to the surface of mast cells and basophils. When the appropriate antigen binds to the variable region of the mast cell–bound IgE molecule, the mast cell degranulates, releasing histamine and other chemical substances that play a role in the allergic reaction. Increased levels of IgE can be found in patients infected with intestinal parasites, such as roundworms.

IgD is also normally present only in minute quantities in the blood, constituting about 0.2% of the total circulating antibodies. The immune function of IgD is unknown. It appears to function only on the surface of B cells, where it may have a regulatory role.

Primary and Secondary Responses

The primary antibody response follows the first exposure to an antigen. Detectable levels of antibodies are not present in the serum until about 4 to 10 days after entry of an antigen. During this lag period, the host's defenses are not up to par, and the antigen may have time to produce disease. Antibody levels produced during the primary response are not high, and they do not last for a long time. They peak in 1 to 10 weeks and then drop off to low levels. The first and most abundant antibody produced during the primary response is IgM. It is during the initial exposure to an antigen that long-lived memory B cells are programmed.

The second and succeeding encounters with the same antigen produce the secondary antibody response. This is a faster, more efficient response, which seems to produce better-quality antibodies (Fig. 32–7) than the primary response does. Antibody from the secondary response is detectable within 1 to 2 days after exposure to the antigen and lasts much longer. Plus, antibody titers are much higher than that following the primary response. The most abundant antibody of the secondary response is IgG.

Antibodies work in several different ways to protect the host. They may neutralize or block the action of toxins or other substances produced by microorganisms. The microorganism may be killed by antibodies, or antibodies may block the infective ability of the microorganism. The latter mechanism is especially important in protecting against viruses in the blood stream. Antibodies may also agglutinate microorganisms—that is, cause them to clump and stick together, making it easier for the phagocytic cells to attack the microorganism. Another mechanism used by antibodies is opsonization. This occurs when the antibody alters the surface of the microorganism so that phagocytes are more attracted to it.

CELLULAR IMMUNE RESPONSE

The T cells responsible for cellular immunity are also activated by the presence of an antigen. Lymphokines produced by helper T cells stimulate B cells to produce antibodies. Suppressor T cells produce lymphokines to regulate the immune response so that it does not over-react to an antigen. They inhibit antibody formation. Suppressor T cells are thought to play an important role in tolerance and in autoimmune reactions. Cytotoxic (killer) T cells are stimulated to kill the appropriate foreign cells. This is especially important when the antigen is a tumor cell, a cell grafted from another host, or a virus-infected cell.

COMPLEMENT

Complement is a complex of more than 25 proteins formed in the liver and found in the serum. The complement proteins interact with antigen and anti-

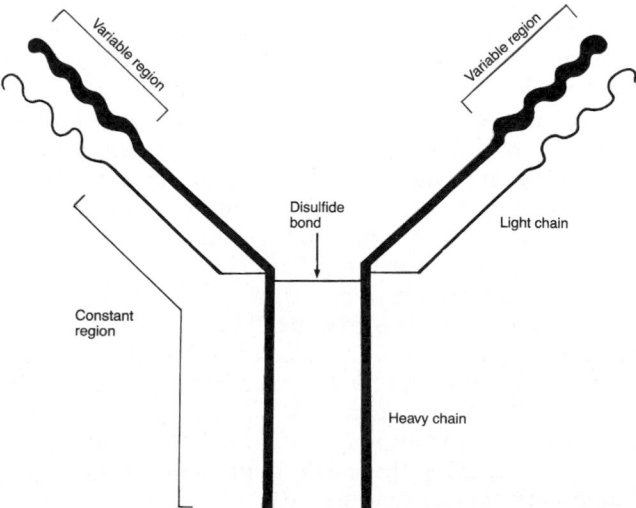

Figure 32–6

The basic antibody molecule is a Y-shaped unit composed of two heavy chains and two light chains. Each chain has a constant region and a variable region that contains the specific antigen-binding site.

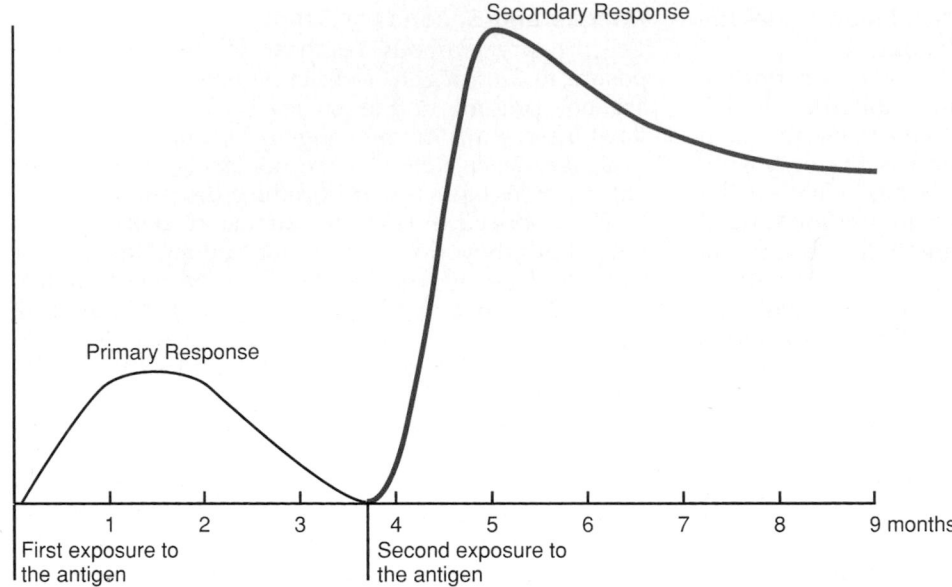

Figure 32–7

Antibody levels of the primary and secondary responses. Levels produced after the first exposure to an antigen are much lower than those produced after succeeding exposures. Antibody production also occurs much sooner after succeeding exposures and lasts much longer.

body in a complex series of reactions that result in lysis of foreign cells, opsonization of foreign cells, and enhancement of the inflammatory and immune reaction (Table 32–6). The cells that are most susceptible to complement-mediated lysis are gram-negative bacteria, white blood cells, and red blood cells. Complement in conjunction with the appropriate antibody is able to neutralize free virus in the blood and therefore is an important defense against viruses and bacteria. Many gram-positive bacteria and fungi resist complement-mediated lysis. There are nine major proteins that make up complement and many minor ones. The nine major proteins are sequentially numbered C1 through C9.

The combination of an antigen with an antibody of the IgG or IgM class is capable of activating C1 and the classic complement pathway. C1 working in conjunction with C2, C3, and C4 acts as the activation unit for the rest of the components. C5 through C9 actually attack the membrane of the antigen and bring about its lysis.

Table 32–6

Results of Complement Activation

Lysis of antigen
Increases phagocytosis
Stimulates T-cell activity
Releases chemotactic factors that draw phagocytic cells
   to the area
Releases histamine and kinins to mediate the inflammatory reaction
Promotes blood clotting
Increases release of white blood cells from the bone marrow
Stimulates antibody formation

The complement system may also be activated by an alternative pathway called the properdin pathway, or amplification loop. Properdin is a serum globulin that, in conjunction with some initiating factors, starts the complement system at the C3 level. This alternative pathway does not require an antigen-antibody reaction to initiate the complement system. Complex antigens, such as polysaccharides, lipopolysaccharides (found in the cell wall of gram-negative bacteria), and glycoproteins (from the capsules of some yeast and bacteria), are capable of activating the alternative pathway.

As a result of the activation of various components of the complement cascade, several biologically active complement split products are produced. These substances are important in mediating the inflammatory process as well as the immune response. The effects of these substances are varied. Several are strong chemotactic agents that attract phagocytic cells to the area to participate in the inflammatory reaction. Some components of complement, in combination with antibody, act as opsonins, helping to increase the effectiveness of phagocytic cells attracted to the area. Other substances promote the release of histamine and kinins, which are important mediators of the inflammatory reaction. Still other substances produced during activation of the complement cascade stimulate B cells to produce antibodies, increase the release of white blood cells from bone marrow, and promote blood clotting. The fibrin network of the blood clot helps prevent the injurious agent from spreading further in the tissues and later, during the healing process, serves as a framework for the new tissue.

Deficiencies of complement components have been reported, but they are rare. These complement deficiencies may leave the patient more susceptible to infections and immune complex disorders or they may have little or no effect on the patient's immune status.

TYPES OF IMMUNITY

Immunity is frequently referred to in terms of the method by which a person came to possess that immunity. When discussed in this way, immunity is described in terms of natural versus acquired immunity.

Natural Resistance

Natural resistance (also called innate or inherited immunity) is that immunity with which a person is born. The nonspecific defense mechanisms (such as chemical and physical barriers) play a role in natural resistance. Some natural resistance is conferred by virtue of species. Some microorganisms are pathogenic for one species but not another. Humans are immune to the microorganisms that cause distemper, dog tapeworm, fowl malaria, and fowl typhoid, but dogs, cats, and birds are not. In contrast, humans are susceptible to the virus that causes mumps, whereas dogs and cats are immune to it. Race also plays a role in natural resistance. When differences in economic and social conditions are taken into account, it appears that African-Americans are more susceptible to tuberculosis than white Americans, but white Americans are more susceptible to diphtheria and influenza than African-Americans. Other factors that play a role in natural resistance are sex, age (the very young and the elderly are more susceptible to infections), and nutritional status (phagocytic cells of a malnourished person are only a third to a tenth as effective as those of a well-nourished person).

Even though natural resistance is often called natural immunity, the term *resistance* is more accurate because much of this phenomenon does not have the precise antigenic specificity that is usually associated with immunity. Natural resistance does not require prior exposure to the antigen and is not a learned response.

Acquired Immunity

Acquired, or adaptive, immunity includes all antigen-specific immunities that a person develops during a lifetime. It develops after exposure to an antigen. Acquired immunity can vary widely from person to person, depending on which antigens they have previously been exposed to. Acquired immunity can be actively acquired or passively acquired (Table 32–7). With actively acquired immunity, the person produces antibodies, sensitized T cells, or both after being exposed to the antigen. Exposure to the antigen may be either natural or artificial. Natural exposure occurs by chance during the course of a person's life and may result in overt infection or

Table 32–7

Acquired Immunity

Acquired immunity can be:
  Actively acquired
    Naturally by actually having the disease
    Artificially by vaccination
  Passively acquired
    Naturally from antibodies (eg, maternal IgG)
    Artificially by injection of antibodies (eg, immune serum globulin)

Ig, immunoglobulin.

subclinical illness. In either case, exposure to the antigen is sufficient to stimulate the immune response. The resulting immunity is called naturally acquired active immunity. Artificially acquired active immunity is developed after the person is purposefully exposed to the antigen in the form of a vaccine or toxoid. Vaccines contain either killed or attenuated (weak but viable organisms) bacteria or viruses. Toxoids are the toxins produced by bacteria that have been altered so that they are no longer toxic but their important antigenic receptor sites remain intact, enabling antibodies to be produced to the antigen-producing toxin.

Passively acquired immunity occurs when the antibodies are produced in one person and then given to another person. These passively acquired antibodies are usually given by injection (eg, immune serum globulin), except in the case of the transfer of maternal antibodies either across the placenta to the fetus or via colostrum and breast milk. When the antibodies are given by injection, it is called artificially acquired passive immunity. The transfer of maternal antibodies to the fetus or newborn infant is called naturally acquired passive immunity. Only IgG antibody crosses the placenta. Colostrum and breast milk contain secretory IgA and IgM. These antibodies are absorbed from the infant's gastrointestinal tract. They also coat it to help prevent intestinal infections.

Although both active and passive immunity provide protection against infections, there are differences between the two. Active immunity lasts much longer and is more effective at preventing subsequent infections than passive immunity. Active immunity lasts for years, as a result of memory T and B lymphocytes, and can be easily reactivated by a booster dose of antigen. Passively received human antibodies have a half-life of about 30 days. Protection from active immunity takes 5 to 14 days to develop after the first exposure to the antigen and 1 to 3 days after subsequent exposures. Passive immunity provides protection immediately.

Artificially acquired active immunity is primarily used prophylactically before exposure to the antigen. Because the incubation period for most infections is less than the time required to develop antibodies, vaccines must be given at least 2 weeks before exposure to the antigen. (An exception is the live measles vaccine, which prevents disease if given less than 48 hours after exposure.) Passively acquired immunity can be used prophylactically if given before an exposure or immediately after an exposure. It may prevent infection from the exposure but does not provide protection for future exposures. Hepatitis B immune globulin and varicella-zoster immune globulin are two preparations used to help prevent disease after exposure to hepatitis B and chickenpox, respectively. Passively acquired immunity is sometimes used therapeutically to help treat an infection that has already been established. It is hoped that these antibodies will be able to decrease the duration and severity of the infection.

Assessment of the Immune System

PATIENT HISTORY

Assessment of the immune system begins with a health history that includes detailed information related to the following:

- Occurrence of infections, neoplastic disease, and autoimmune disorders
- Allergies
- Immunizations
- Condition of nonspecific defenses and factors that can affect them

In regard to infections, obtain information about usual childhood diseases and infections, including the location of infection, date of occurrence, whether any are recurrent, and, if so, how often and what treatment was used. Ask the patient about exposure to tuberculosis, when he or she last underwent a purified protein derivative test or chest x-ray, and what the results were. Question all patients about recent exposure to infections that could currently be in the incubation stage. Obtain information about immunization status and note the type and date of all immunizations.

In regard to malignant disease, ask the patient whether any family members have had cancer and, if so, the type, age at onset, and relationship of the affected person to the patient. (In cases of grandparents and others, note the relationship to the maternal or paternal side of the family.) Also determine whether the patient has ever had a malignancy diagnosed and, if so, the date of diagnosis, type of tumor, and type of treatment. Be sure to find out whether chemotherapy or radiation therapy was received by the patient because of the effects of these treatments on the immune system. Whether or not

the person has had a malignancy, determine the date of the last complete physical, and rectal, breast, and pelvic or prostate examinations. Question the patient about the presence of any symptoms that are warning signs of cancer (see Chap. 34).

Ask about any history of autoimmune disease, such as rheumatoid arthritis, psoriasis, and systemic lupus erythematosus. Also question the patient about allergies and substances known to trigger them, such as pollen, dust, bee stings, contact substances, foods, and medications. Find out what symptoms the patient experiences. Ask about any seasonal variations in occurrence or severity. And inquire about medications or other treatment measures used, and how effective they are.

Question the patient about risk behaviors for sexually transmitted diseases, which can often be present without symptoms. Ask the patient about numbers of sexual partners, whether latex barriers and condoms are used and how often, and whether the patient engages in high-risk behaviors, such as anal intercourse or intravenous drug use. Ask all questions in an open and nonjudgmental way to encourage honesty.

Finally, assess the patient's understanding and compliance with health promotion and risk reduction measures related to immune-system health and functioning of the body's nonspecific defense mechanisms (Highlight 32–1). For example, ask about smoking (how much and for how long), exposure to air pollutants through occupation or living location, stress and coping mechanisms, cough, and skin problems.

PHYSICAL EXAMINATION

On physical examination, observe the patient for signs of infection, such as elevated temperature, chills, or sweating. Examine the entire surface of the body for breaks or lesions of the skin or mucous membranes. Inspect the skin carefully for texture, temperature, color, turgor, and moisture. Dermatitis, urticaria, inflammation, or discharge may indicate an immune disorder. The texture of the skin may change as in scleroderma, where the skin becomes thick, smooth, and shiny. With other disorders, the skin may become dry and scaly. Increased skin temperature may indicate inflammation. Cool skin may suggest circulatory insufficiency, as in Raynaud's disease. Change in color may indicate an underlying immune disorder, such as jaundice in the case of hemolytic anemia, or pallor in the case of asthma.

A wide range of skin lesions may be present, depending on the underlying immune disorder. For example, patients with AIDS may develop Kaposi's sarcoma lesions, which are raised, maculopapular spots ranging from dark pink to bluish-purple. Patients with systemic lupus erythematosus may have a rash across the bridge of the nose and cheeks in a butterfly pattern.

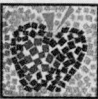

Optimal Immune System Function

Encourage patients to avoid immune-suppressing factors, including:

- Smoking
- Stressors
- Pollution
- Poor nutrition
- B-vitamin deficiency
- Toxic emotions and friendships
- Worry, anxiety
- Being overweight or underweight

Encourage patients to increase immune-enhancing factors, including:

- Proper nutrition
- Moderate exercise
- Relaxation techniques
- Laughter
- Fulfilling work
- Positive relationships
- Constructive channeling of emotions
- Pet therapy
- Aroma therapy
- Weight control
- Massage

Teach patients the importance of:

- Having an annual physical examination
- Reporting unusual fatigue
- Reporting unexplained cough
- Reporting allergies
- Reporting stress responses
- Reporting skin problems

Palpate the anterior and posterior cervical, axillary, and inguinal lymph nodes. If you feel any, note their size, consistency, symmetry, mobility, and tenderness or lack thereof. Tender, inflamed, or fixed lymph nodes warrant further medical assessment. The location helps to identify the possible source of infection by the pattern of node involvement and usual drainage route.

Carefully assess the respiratory system by checking respiratory rate, presence of cough (dry or pro-ductive), and abnormal lung sounds. Special note should be made of cough pattern, presence of sputum, sputum color, the work of breathing, and whether abnormal lung sounds are crackles (rales) or wheezes (rhonchi). Immunosuppressed patients are particularly susceptible to pneumonia and may have tachypnea, cyanosis, and thick yellow or green sputum. They may use accessory muscles to breathe. Allergic patients typically have wheezes, dyspnea, and cough with little sputum production.

The patient's behavior may be an important clue to underlying disease. Because such disorders as systemic lupus erythematosus and AIDS can lead to dementia, assess for signs of cognitive impairment or memory loss. Facial expression is important because facial weakness occurs in myasthenia gravis. Patients with scleroderma may have a characteristic mask-like, nonexpressive look.

Assess the musculoskeletal system for range of motion of all joints and any tenderness or swelling of joints. Check the cardiovascular system for circulatory problems, cardiac dysrhythmias, vasculitis, and anemia. Assess the patient's nutritional status along with age and any functional limitations, such as fatigue and endurance.

Diagnostic Procedures

BONE MARROW ASPIRATION AND BIOPSY

Bone marrow aspiration is performed to obtain a small sample of cells from the bone marrow. Bone marrow biopsy is performed to obtain a core of tissue from the bone marrow so that its structure can be studied. The procedures, which are usually performed at the same time, help diagnose many conditions with hematologic or immunologic abnormalities. A pathologist studies the bone marrow samples to determine the types and number of cells present, the phase of cellular maturation, the presence of any abnormal cells, and information about the iron stores.

A special large-gauge needle with a stylet is used to aspirate a small amount of bone marrow, usually from the iliac crest or the sternum. The skin is prepared with an antiseptic. A local anesthetic is administered at the site of aspiration, first into the skin and then deeper into the periosteum. The large-gauge needle is then inserted through the skin, tissues, and bone into the marrow cavity. The stylet is removed, allowing cells to be aspirated through the needle into a sterile syringe. The biopsy device is then inserted and the biopsy sample taken. The needle is removed and the site dressed with a small sterile dressing. The procedure is not very painful if the skin and periosteum have been properly anesthetized. Most patients feel pressure while the needle is being inserted and then a somewhat painful sensation during actual aspiration of material. Many physicians administer intravenous sedation and analgesia before the procedure, particularly if the client is unusually anxious or fearful. Complications include soreness at the puncture site, bleeding, and infection. The latter two may be life-threatening.

NURSING PROCESS
Bone Marrow Aspiration and Biopsy

Assessment

Assess patients undergoing a bone marrow aspiration for level of anxiety about the test and its results, ability to lie in the required position, knowledge of what to expect, and allergy to the local anesthetic that will be used. Also verify that informed consent has been obtained before the procedure.

Nursing Diagnoses and Planning

Nursing diagnoses and related expected patient outcomes commonly applicable to patients undergoing bone marrow aspiration include the following:

NDx: Knowledge deficit: bone marrow aspiration procedure

Planning: Patient Outcomes
1. Patient states why the test is being performed.
2. Patient states where the test will be performed and what staff members will be involved.
3. Patient describes the usual sensations associated with the procedure.
4. Patient states the approximate length of the procedure.

NDx: Anxiety related to the procedure or its outcome

Planning: Patient Outcomes
1. Patient expresses feelings about the procedure and its outcomes.
2. Patient verbalizes decreased levels of anxiety.
3. Patient attends to directions.

NDx: Pain related to tissue trauma at the site of aspiration

Planning: Patient Outcomes
1. Patient states that pain is manageable or absent.
2. Patient moves about without signs of excessive distress.

NDx: Risk for decreased cardiac output related to blood loss

Planning: Patient Outcomes
1. Evidence of bleeding at the site of aspiration is absent.
2. Vital signs are within the patient's normal limits.

NDx: Risk for infection related to the invasive procedure

Planning: Patient Outcomes
1. Redness and swelling at the site of aspiration are absent.
2. Drainage is absent from the site of aspiration.
3. Patient is afebrile.

NDx: Energy field disturbance related to invasive procedure

Planning: Patient Outcomes
1. Energy field shows no spikes or bulges.
2. Patient expresses harmony of body, mind, and spirit.

Nursing Interventions and Evaluation

NDx: Knowledge deficit: bone marrow aspiration procedure
Explain the procedure to the patient in understandable language. Include the reason for the test, sensations the patient is likely to feel, who will be in the room and what their roles are, what equipment will be used, the position the patient will be in, the fact that the procedure will take 5 to 10 minutes, and how long before results will be known. Be sure to allow time for the patient to ask questions.

NDx: Anxiety
Offer support during the procedure by remaining next to the patient, holding the patient's hand if needed, giving verbal reassurance, and telling the patient what is happening. When the test results come back and the physician has informed the patient of them, provide an opportunity for the patient to express his or her reaction and to ask any additional questions. This support is necessary whether the results were normal or abnormal. Patients need to express feelings of happiness and relief as well as anxiety and sadness.

NDx: Pain
Reassure the patient that discomfort will gradually subside in 24 to 48 hours. Position the patient off the site of aspiration for comfort when in bed, unless otherwise ordered. Administer prescribed analgesics, such as Tylenol, every 4 hours as needed.

NDx: Risk for decreased cardiac output
Monitor the site of aspiration for bleeding. Monitor pulse and blood pressure. If a pressure dressing is in place, as following multiple aspirations for harvest of bone marrow for transplant, leave in place until the day after the procedure.

NDx: Risk for infection
Instruct the patient not to take a bath or shower or otherwise wet the aspiration site for 24 hours. A pressure dressing usually is applied for the first 24 hours. Then the site should be left open to air and kept clean.

Check for temperature elevation and observe the aspiration site for redness, swelling, and foul drainage. If the patient is discharged, stress the importance of reporting these symptoms.

NDx: Energy field disturbance

Invasive procedures, such as bone marrow aspiration or biopsy, can create disturbances in the patient's energy field. These disturbances can be detected as bulges, spikes, or dips by nurses trained in Therapeutic Touch, Reiki, and other practices. Using an energy field practice can smooth and reduce the disturbance.

Having the patient practice what is comforting to him or her is effective as well. Assess what is effective for the patient, such as guided imagery, music therapy, or relaxation techniques and assist the patient in implementing a technique.

Additional Interventions

At least 30 minutes before the procedure, obtain baseline vital signs and administer any premedications (such as a sedative) that have been ordered. Just before the procedure, position the patient with pillows to support the arms, legs, and head as needed. Provide a blanket or other cover for warmth and to maintain the patient's modesty.

Compare the patient's status with the expected outcomes. If the outcomes are not met, reassess the patient and revise the plan.

LABORATORY TESTS

The antigen-antibody reaction is used as the basis of several common laboratory techniques. These techniques use antigen or antibody as a sensitive and highly specific reagent to detect, identify, and quantify proteins and other small molecules (such as drugs) in blood, body fluids, and tissues. These tests can help diagnose specific infections, some forms of cancer, and immune dysfunctions. The tests involve taking a sample of peripheral venous blood or other body fluid (urine, sputum, cerebrospinal fluid) or tissue for laboratory analysis.

Electrophoresis

Electrophoresis is a technique that uses an electric current to separate electrically charged particles in a solution. It is frequently used to separate serum proteins (albumin and the different globulins) so they can be identified and quantified. Electrophoresis is used in diagnosing hypogammaglobulinemia and multiple myeloma. Electrophoresis can also be performed on cerebrospinal fluid and urine.

Radioimmunoassay

Radioimmunoassay is a sensitive and specific laboratory procedure used to detect small amounts of a substance in the blood. The test uses the antibody specific for the antigen in question and a small amount of antigen that has been labeled with a ra-

dioactive material. It is commonly used to detect hormones, proteins, and drugs, such as digoxin, digitoxin, vitamin B_{12}, folic acid, barbiturates, and opiates.

Immunofluorescence

Immunofluorescence is a technique that allows identification of specific antigens. It uses antibodies that have been chemically bound to a fluorescent molecule. The specimen with the unknown antigen is fixed to a glass slide. Then the fluorescent antibody is applied to the specimen. If the antibody is specific for the antigen on the slide, the antibody binds with it and remains on the slide. The slide is examined under a special microscope, and any antibody remaining on the slide will fluoresce. Because it is difficult to accurately quantify the amount of antigen present with this technique, the results are usually given as positive or negative. Immunofluorescence provides relatively rapid results and is used to identify a wide variety of bacteria, viruses, fungi, and protozoa. Specific organisms that can be identified by immunofluorescence include *Candida albicans*, group A streptococci, *Haemophilus influenzae*, herpes virus, influenza virus, *Mycoplasma pneumoniae*, *Neisseria gonorrhoeae*, *Neisseria meningitis*, rabies virus, *Staphylococcus aureus*, and *S. pneumoniae*. This technique can be modified to identify antibody by using fluorescent antigens.

Agglutination

Agglutination refers to the clumping together of microorganisms or other particles. Infection with some organisms causes the body to produce agglutinins (immunoglobulins that cause clumping of the invading organism) specific for that organism. Agglutinins provide a valuable tool to help detect these organisms. The patient's serum is mixed with a suspension of the organisms. If the agglutinin is present in the serum, it causes the organisms to clump together and the result is positive. The serum is then diluted until agglutination no longer occurs. This dilution process determines the titer (quantity of a substance required to react with or to correspond to a given amount of another substance) of the agglutinin. Diseases that may be diagnosed by this method include typhoid fever, tularemia, typhus fever, and undulant fever. Antigens may be attached to small latex particles. If the appropriate agglutinin is present in the serum, these antigen-coated latex particles clump together, allowing the reaction to be seen. Tests for rheumatoid factor, hepatitis B, and some urine pregnancy tests use latex particles.

Complement Fixation Test

Complement fixation is a two-step test usually used to detect a specific antibody. In the first step, the patient's serum is mixed with an identified antigen and a known amount of complement. If the serum contains antibody specific for the antigen, the antibody and antigen react with each other and consume or "fix" the complement in the process. This is an invisible reaction. In the second step, an indicator is added to determine whether complement is still present. If complement is present, the test result is negative, because the patient's serum did not contain antibody specific for the antigen and no reaction took place. If no complement is present, the test result is positive. The test can also be performed to determine whether the patient's serum contains a specific antigen by using a known antibody. The Wassermann test for syphilis is an example of a complement fixation test.

Genetic Testing

Genetic testing is now being performed for many purposes. DNA assays, such as the Southern blot, are used to estimate clonal composition of lymphocyte populations using molecular finger-printing of needle biopsies of lymph nodes. This test requires a blood or tissue specimen containing 25 million leukocytes. DNA finger-printing is a genetic marker used in forensic and clinical applications. Clinical applications include parental testing in disputed paternity cases and monitoring of bone marrow transplant recipients for engraftment when the human leukocyte antigen (HLA) of the marrow donor is identical to that of the recipient.

Allergy Tests

Allergy tests are performed to help determine specific antigens to which the patient is allergic. Four types of allergy tests are available: scratch, prick, intradermal, and radioallergosorbent tests. The scratch, prick, and intradermal tests all involve administration of a small amount of various diluted antigens to the skin and observation for a local reaction, usually redness, swelling, and itching. A rare but possible risk with any of these tests is the development of a generalized allergic reaction or anaphylaxis. The radioallergosorbent test determines the presence of specific IgE antibodies in a blood sample. The results of these tests are used in conjunction with the patient's allergic history to help determine which antigens cause the patient's allergic symptoms.

SCRATCH TESTING

The scratch test is somewhat less sensitive than the other tests, but it is the easiest and safest. More antigens can be tested at one time with the scratch test than with the other methods. Scratch tests are usually performed on the back or forearms. The skin in the area to be used is cleansed with alcohol. Areas that have abnormal or damaged skin should not be used. After the alcohol has dried, small, superficial scratches are made on the skin (Fig. 32–8A). These scratches should not bleed. A drop of a diluted antigen solution is applied to one scratch. Different antigens are applied to multiple scratches. Redness and swelling at a scratch is a positive result. The results are read in 5 to 30 minutes.

PRICK TESTING

The prick test is similar to the scratch test but is a little more sensitive. A drop of antigen is placed on the skin. Then the skin is pricked with a 26-gauge needle through the drop of antigen (Fig. 32–8B). Some redness and swelling at the site is a positive test result. The results are read in 15 to 30 minutes.

INTRADERMAL TESTING

For the intradermal test, a small amount of antigen is injected intradermally (Fig. 32–8C). It is more

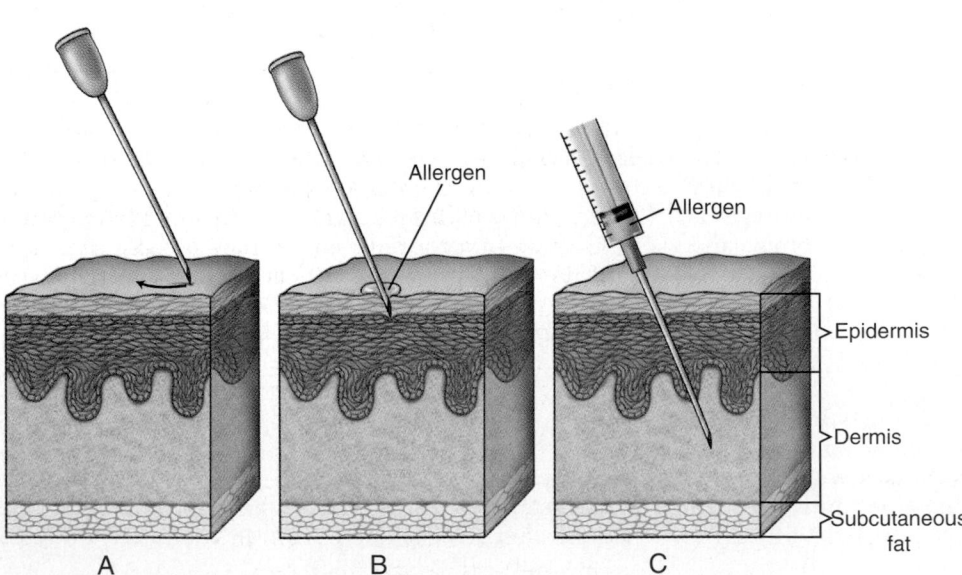

Figure 32–8

Scratch (A), prick (B), and intradermal (C) allergy testing.

painful than the scratch or the prick test. Only a few antigens can be tested at one time, because more space (2 to 3 inches) is needed between each test site. The results are read in 15 to 30 minutes. Some redness and swelling at the site is a positive test result.

RADIOALLERGOSORBENT TESTING

Radioallergosorbent testing determines the presence of allergen-specific IgE antibodies in a blood sample. Radioallergosorbent testing is no more sensitive than the other tests and is more expensive. However, it is useful when the other tests cannot be used, such as when the patient has extensive skin lesions and not enough normal skin area is available. Radioallergosorbent testing is easier for the patient. The only risk is that associated with a simple venipuncture.

NURSING PROCESS GUIDELINES
Allergy Testing

All these allergy tests are most frequently performed as office procedures. In preparation for testing, assess the patient's understanding of the test to be performed and teach accordingly. For the scratch, prick, or intradermal test, check the condition of the skin in the area where the test will be performed. It should be intact and relatively hairless, with some subcutaneous tissue. Assist the patient into a comfortable position that permits easy access to the test site. Thoroughly cleanse the skin in the testing area with alcohol and allow to air dry.

Once the test is done, observe the patient for any reactions. After the appropriate length of time, check the test site. Measure and record the size of the wheal (Fig. 32–9). Upon completion of testing, determine whether the patient understands the results and what follow-up is planned. Do additional teaching about allergies and medications as required.

Patients should be instructed about factors that suppress and enhance immune function (see Highlight 32–1). Encourage the patient to avoid immune-suppressing factors, if possible, and to embrace immune-enhancing behaviors.

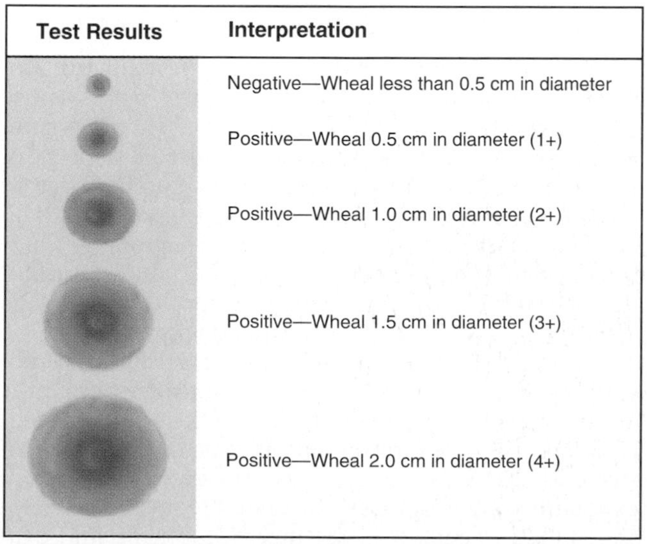

Management

IMMUNIZATIONS

Immunizations have served to increase quality of life and have made some diseases (such as smallpox) a thing of the past. Vaccines containing live antigens are not given to pregnant women because of the theoretical risk to the fetus. Neither are live vaccines given to immunosuppressed persons (those receiving corticosteroids, cancer chemotherapy, radiation therapy, or other immunosuppressive agents) or to persons with a defect in their cellular immunity (such as patients with leukemia, lymphoma, and Hodgkin's disease). Even though the antigen has been weakened during production of the vaccine, it may be able to overcome the incompetent immune system and cause a serious or fatal disease. Some vaccines are produced in eggs and may contain some egg protein. These should not be administered to patients who are allergic to eggs. To maintain maximum effectiveness, vaccines must be stored properly. In fact, vaccine failures have been caused by improper storage.

Vaccination is normally a safe procedure whose benefits far outweigh its risks. In healthy people, multiple antigens can be administered simultaneously and a good response obtained to each antigen. The preferred site for injection of vaccines in adults is the deltoid muscle or the anterolateral thigh because injections in the buttocks may deposit the vaccine in fat tissue, where it is not as effective.

Vaccines are usually thought of as being given in childhood. However, several important vaccines should be given to adults and the elderly. The tetanus-diphtheria vaccine should be given every 10 years to all adults. Many older adults are not adequately protected against tetanus. Influenza and pneumococcal vaccines should be considered for all adults with chronic illness and those over age 65. The hepatitis B vaccine should be considered for adults whose occupation or lifestyle increases the risk of exposure to hepatitis B. A major role for nurses is teaching people the importance of keeping their immunizations up-to-date and the need for other appropriate vaccinations.

Test Results	Interpretation
	Negative—Wheal less than 0.5 cm in diameter
	Positive—Wheal 0.5 cm in diameter (1+)
	Positive—Wheal 1.0 cm in diameter (2+)
	Positive—Wheal 1.5 cm in diameter (3+)
	Positive—Wheal 2.0 cm in diameter (4+)

Figure 32–9

Interpretation of intradermal allergy test results based on the size of the wheal after 15 to 30 minutes.

IMMUNOSUPPRESSIVE THERAPY

Immunosuppression is a reduction or depression in any aspect of the immune system's ability to respond to an antigen. Immunosuppression can be brought about in a number of ways; some have a less severe effect on the immune system than others. Immunosuppressive therapy is used to treat a wide variety of diseases. It is used extensively with most types of organ transplants to help reduce rejection of the transplanted tissue. It is also used for immunologically mediated diseases, such as allergies, rheumatoid arthritis, and vasculitis. Collagen disorders, such as scleroderma, are also frequently treated with immunosuppressives.

Antigen-Specific Immunosuppression

Allergy desensitization is one example of induced immunosuppression that has been used for years. In this method, the antigen that causes the allergy is used to suppress the body's response to it. Small amounts of the antigen are injected into the body in an attempt to prompt the body to produce antibodies of a class other than IgE that are specific to that antigen. Once this occurs, the antigen, on entering the body, reacts with these non-IgE antibodies before it makes its way to the IgE antibodies on the mast cells. This method is not always successful and in some cases may increase hypersensitivity to the antigen.

Another commonly used method of immunosuppression is to administer antibody produced in one person to another person who has been exposed to the antigen specific to that antibody. The antibody binds with the antigen, rendering it nonantigenic before it has a chance to stimulate the immune response in the host. In a sense, the preformed antibody hides the antigen from the immune system. For example, RhoGAM is given to prevent an immune response in Rh-negative persons who have been exposed to Rh-positive blood cells. A woman who is Rh-negative can receive such an exposure during the termination or delivery of a pregnancy. Antibodies in the RhoGAM bind with antigens on the fetal red blood cells and prevent them from stimulating the woman's immune system.

The two methods just discussed are specific and induce immunosuppression only to selected antigens. Other immunosuppressive methods produce a generalized nonspecific immunosuppression to many antigens.

Nonspecific Immunosuppression

ANTILYMPHOCYTE SERUM

Antilymphocyte serum produces a nonspecific immunosuppression. Antilymphocyte serum is produced by injecting animals with human lymphocytes. The animal then produces antibodies against the human lymphocytes. These antibodies are harvested from the animal and purified to make antilymphocyte serum. When antilymphocyte serum is injected into a human, these antibodies destroy the human lymphocytes, causing a transient lymphopenia. Functioning of both T cells and B cells is decreased. Antilymphocyte serum tends to have many unwanted side effects, such as febrile reactions, serum sickness, and sometimes anaphylaxis.

MONOCLONAL ANTIBODIES

Monoclonal antibodies are a new and much more selective variation of antilymphocyte serum. They consist of identical copies of an antibody molecule that reacts with only a single, specific part of the antigenic determinant. Most antigenic determinants have more than one area that stimulates antibody formation, so several antibodies are produced in response to the antigen. A cell that produces the single desired antibody is combined with a continuously replicating cell line. A clone of cells develops that produce only that specific antibody. A monoclonal antibody can be produced to react with almost any antigen.

The use of monoclonal antibodies to detect and treat cancers is under investigation. To detect cancers, a radioisotope is combined with a monoclonal antibody that binds to tumor antigen. This combination is injected into the patient. The patient is then scanned to detect areas where the radioisotope has concentrated. To treat cancers, anticancer drugs or toxins are bound to a monoclonal antibody specific for the tumor. The monoclonal antibody brings the drug directly to the tumor. Monoclonal antibodies have opened many new diagnostic and treatment possibilities. They have also revolutionized laboratory testing procedures and appear to have a promising future.

Pharmacologic Immunosuppression

The most commonly used method of inducing immunosuppression is with drugs. Many drugs cause some degree of immunosuppression, ranging from mild to profound. Drugs do not affect all aspects of the immune response equally. It is much easier to suppress the primary immune response than it is to depress the secondary immune response. Once memory cells have been formed, it is almost impossible to inhibit the immune response. Some drugs affect T cells more than B cells, and vice versa.

The timing of the administration of the immunosuppressant in relation to exposure to the antigen is often critical in determining how effective the agent is. Some immunosuppressant agents, such as corticosteroids and irradiation, must be given just before exposure to the antigen for them to be most effective. Other agents, such as mercaptopurine and azathioprine, must be given immediately after exposure to the antigen for them to be most effective.

Immunosuppressants work either by their effect on T cells and B cells or by their effect on neutrophils and monocytes. The anti-inflammatory properties of a drug can also produce a degree of immunosuppression. The most important agents used to induce immunosuppression are briefly discussed here.

CORTICOSTEROIDS

Corticosteroids are extremely useful immunosuppressants and are used in the treatment of a wide variety of diseases. Corticosteroids affect several parts of the immune system; however, their mechanism of action is not completely understood. A single high dose of corticosteroids causes a prompt reduction in the number of lymphocytes. Both T cells and B cells are affected; however, T cells are more affected than B cells, and helper T4 cells are more affected than suppressor T8 cells. The lymphocytes are not destroyed but are thought to be redistributed and possibly sequestered in the bone marrow. Within 24 hours, the number of lymphocytes returns to normal.

Corticosteroids also impair the ability of the lymphocytes to synthesize antibodies and lymphokines and decrease the number of functioning monocytes and eosinophils. When corticosteroids are given for several days, the amount of antibody present is decreased. Cell-mediated immunity is inhibited by corticosteroids. All these effects leave a patient on corticosteroids more susceptible to infection. Corticosteroids also stabilize mast cells and basophils, inhibiting their ability to release histamine and other chemical mediators of the allergic reaction.

CYTOTOXIC DRUGS

Cytotoxic drugs bring about immunosuppression by killing immunologically competent cells. These agents are able to kill any cell that is replicating. Prior to stimulation by an antigen, the immune cells are in a dormant state. Once stimulated by an antigen, the cells begin to divide and are then susceptible to the cytotoxic drugs. Frequently used cytotoxic drugs are azathioprine (Imuran), cyclophosphamide (Cytoxan), cyclosporine, and methotrexate. Azathioprine is also a potent anti-inflammatory agent. It is frequently used in combination with corticosteroids to help prevent rejection of organ transplants and is used to treat disorders with an autoimmune component.

Cyclophosphamide is a potent immunosuppressant affecting both T cells and B cells. It is used to treat disorders with an autoimmune component and those resulting from an aberrant immune response, such as Wegener's granulomatosis and severe rheumatoid arthritis.

Cyclosporine appears to be highly selective, destroying only helper T cells. It is useful in suppressing rejection of allografts (graft from a genetically different donor of the same species) and is used in many transplant protocols. Methotrexate inhibits humoral and cellular immune responses by inhibiting folate metabolism.

The major side effects of cytotoxic drugs are bone marrow depression, nausea, vomiting, diarrhea, gastrointestinal bleeding, nephrotoxicity, sterility, infection, and an increased risk of cancer.

Radiation

Radiation can decrease the number of lymphocytes in the general circulation and in lymphoid tissues. It also suppresses the function of most immunocompetent cells. Total body radiation and total nodal radiation (administration of radiation to the major lymph node areas) are used as part of transplant protocols.

Surgery

Surgical removal of lymphoid tissue can also induce immunosuppression. Removal of the spleen or thymus gland, especially if performed at an early age, can produce a type of immunosuppression.

NURSING PROCESS GUIDELINES
Immunosuppressive Therapy

Nursing care for patients undergoing immunosuppressive therapy varies with the degree of immunosuppression and the length of time it is expected to persist. Ensure that all patients know why immunosuppression is needed, its expected effect and therapeutic benefit, and side effects or complications that may occur. In cases of antigen-specific immunotherapy, such teaching may constitute the majority of the nursing role. However, when extensive nonspecific immunosuppression is involved, nursing care becomes complex. It includes protection from infection, care required for side effects or complications of the specific therapy used, and care related to any underlying disease.

BONE MARROW TRANSPLANTATION

Bone marrow transplantation is a high-risk procedure performed on patients who have exhausted all other treatment options without success. The object of a bone marrow transplant is to replace defective marrow with healthy marrow from a donor, thereby re-establishing normal marrow function in the recipient.

Types of Bone Marrow Transplantation

There are three types of bone marrow transplant: allogeneic, syngeneic, and autologous.

In an allogeneic transplant, bone marrow is harvested from a HLA-matched donor and infused into the recipient after cytoreduction therapy. A critical difficulty in this type of transplant is the location of a donor who is HLA-compatible and mixed lymphocyte culture–compatible. HLA is found on the surface of all nucleated cells. This antigen can induce an immune response if cells are transplanted into a recipient who does not have the same antigen. HLAs are considered tissue antigens and are different from the ABO antigens on the surface of red blood cells. The immune response that the recipient mounts against these HLAs can cause rejection of the grafted tissue.

An in vitro test for mixed lymphocyte culture is used to help predict the success of the transplant. In this test, peripheral lymphocytes from the donor and the recipient are mixed together in cell culture and observed to determine whether the recipient's lymphocytes are reacting by proliferation to the donor's lymphocytes.

The second type of bone marrow transplant, the syngeneic, is one in which bone marrow is harvested from an identical twin. The advantage of a syngeneic graft over an allogeneic graft is that both donor and recipient are identically HLA-matched, so an immune response based on recognition of foreign cells does not occur.

The third type of transplant is an autologous transplant. There are advantages to this type of transplant, because the donor and the recipient are the same. In an autologous transplant, bone marrow is harvested from the patient when healthy, in remission, or when the bone marrow is microscopically free of malignancy. It is then stored for future use. A disadvantage of autologous transplant is the increased risk of recurrent disease.

Uses

Bone marrow transplantation is an accepted modality of treatment for severe aplastic anemia, acute leukemia, chronic myelogenous leukemia, refractory non-Hodgkin's lymphoma, relapsed Hodgkin's disease, neuroblastoma, severe combined immunodeficiency disorder, and multiple myeloma. Autologous bone marrow transplant is also being used in the treatment of selected solid tumors, including melanoma, refractory sarcoma, and refractory malignancies of the stomach, colon, liver, ovary, and breast.

Harvesting the Transplant

Bone marrow is harvested from the donor via multiple bone marrow aspirations. The goal of the harvest is to obtain a sufficient number of stem cells to re-establish a hematopoietic system in the recipient. To this end, from 600 to 2500 mL of marrow mixed with peripheral blood is obtained from an adult donor, usually from the posterior iliac crest, although the anterior iliac crest and sternum can also be used. Harvesting is performed in the operating room under local or general anesthesia. Once aspi-

rated, the marrow is filtered and heparinized. For allogeneic or syngeneic transplants, the marrow is then taken to the patient for infusion. In autologous transplants, the marrow is frozen until needed. If there is a possibility that malignant cells are present in the marrow, it may be purged before freezing by physical procedures that separate normal from malignant cells based on density, by immunologic procedures involving immunotoxic or monoclonal antibodies, or by chemotherapy.

Patient Preparation

Before starting the transplant procedure, patients are scheduled for a dental examination. Any needed dental work, including fluoride and plaque treatments, is completed. This is to avert the need for dental intervention when the patient's platelet count is low and to decrease the risk of abscesses or gum disease, which can seed infection into the vascular space while the patient is neutropenic. In women, menstruation may be suppressed pharmacologically to prevent menstrual bleeding during the period of thrombocytopenia. Upon admission, most patients undergo insertion of a permanent venous access device, such as a Hickman or Broviac catheter. This makes administration of the many drugs, blood products, and total parenteral nutrition easier for the patient by reducing the number of venipunctures needed. Many of the required blood samples can also be drawn from these lines.

Before the transplant, the patient undergoes a cytoreduction protocol designed to destroy any abnormal cells and suppress the immune system if needed. These protocols typically consist of a combination of chemotherapeutic agents and irradiation. All are immunosuppressive or ablative and leave the patient pancytopenic and at risk for fatal infection or bleeding. Patients are therefore placed on protective isolation. Thrombocytopenic precautions are taken. These protocols also cause severe mucositis, which places the patient at risk for airway obstruction from swelling of the oral pharyngeal tissues, necessitates parenteral nutrition, and may require opiates for pain. Additional side effects include sterility, temporary loss of sexual desire in males secondary to low testosterone levels, amenorrhea in females from decreased estrogen production by the ovary, and hair loss. (Refer to Chap. 34 for a complete discussion of the many other side effects that occur with these modes of treatment.)

Procedure

The transplantation is similar to a blood transfusion. Marrow is infused into the patient's blood stream through a central venous access device. The cells then migrate to bone marrow cavities, where stem cells from the new marrow mature and should begin to function in 10 to 20 days.

Postprocedure Course

Pancytopenia persists for at least the first 3 to 4 weeks after transplantation. Severe immunologic impairment may last as long as a year. During this time, the ratio of helper to suppressor T-cells may be abnormal, T cells may not respond well to antigens, and antibody production is abnormal. Completely normal immune function may not be regained for 12 to 18 months because it takes time for the transplanted immune system to mature and develop normal function.

As a result of the pancytopenia following the transplant, patients remain on protective isolation and receive broad-spectrum prophylactic antibiotics. Thrombocytopenic precautions are observed until the platelet count returns to normal. Because thrombocytopenia lasts weeks to months, repeated transfusions of irradiated platelets may be required. Discharge from the hospital generally occurs about 4 weeks after transplantation.

Complications

Major complications of bone marrow transplantation include infection and bleeding. In fact, viral infections (such as cytomegalovirus pneumonia), fungal infections, hemorrhage, and marrow failure are the chief causes of death in bone marrow transplant patients. These patients are also at risk for veno-occlusive disease of the liver. This complication is apparently related to the amount of chemotherapy and radiation the patient received before transplantation. Veno-occlusive disease is characterized by blocking of the hepatic venules by deposits of collagen and fibrin. This results in obstructed blood flow, liver engorgement, and the development of ascites from "weeping" of sodium- and albumin-rich fluid from the liver's surface. Renal perfusion is also decreased secondary to a decrease in intravascular fluid volume. Clinical manifestations of veno-occlusive disease include weight gain and impaired liver function as indicated by jaundice, increased serum alanine aminotransferase and alkaline phosphatase levels, and coagulation defects. Treatment is supportive and focuses on maintaining intravascular fluid volume to support renal blood flow. Veno-occlusive disease spontaneously resolves in 2 to 3 weeks in about half of those affected.

A complication unique to patients who have received allogeneic transplants is graft-versus-host disease. In graft-versus-host disease, cells of the graft mount an immunologic attack against the cells of the recipient. The effects of graft-versus-host disease primarily affect the skin, liver, gastrointestinal tract, and lymphoid tissues. Skin manifestations range from a mild rash on the palms of the hands, soles of the feet, trunk, and ears to severe desquamation of the skin. Increases in the levels of serum bilirubin, aspartate aminotransferase, and alkaline phosphatase occur as the liver becomes involved and, in severe cases, can lead to liver failure. Involvement of the gastrointestinal tract is characterized by green, watery diarrhea and abdominal cramping that can lead to gastrointestinal bleeding.

About 30% of allogeneic bone marrow transplant patients experience fatal graft-versus-host disease, whereas another 30 to 60% experience a lesser degree of the disease. Once the disease process is under way, there is little effective treatment. In its chronic form, it can be highly debilitating, causing changes in physical appearance and body image.

NURSING PROCESS
Bone Marrow Transplantation

Assessment

Before the transplant, assess how well the patient and significant others understand the underlying disease, the transplant protocol, potential side effects of the protocol, and therapeutic goals of the procedure, as well as the patient's emotional response to the underlying problem and to the scheduled transplant. Patients undergoing bone marrow transplantation must have strong support and a dependable caregiver available.

Assess the patient's physical condition. Give special attention to nutritional status because adequate nutrition is essential to avoid postprocedure complications. Adequate nutrition may be compromised either by the underlying disease or by the chemotherapy and irradiation given before the transplant. Obtain detailed information about the patient's eating patterns and food preferences for use in encouraging nutritional intake following the transplant.

Collect information about the patient's living conditions, financial situation, and available sources of emotional and physical support, because the recovery period is long and ongoing care is required. When the pretransplant chemotherapy and irradiation begin, make ongoing assessments of the patient's physical and psychologic responses to therapy.

Both before and after the transplant, make ongoing observations for signs of inflammation and infection. Monitor temperature frequently at 2- to 4-hour intervals around the clock. Always take the patient's temperature by the same method, either oral or axillary; do not take rectal temperatures. Be sure the thermometer is placed correctly and left for an adequate time. If the patient is taking medications with an antipyretic effect, do not take temperature when the medication is at peak effect; the patient's temperature may appear to be normal because of the medication's effect. Also be aware that even slight temperature elevations are significant and require medical intervention.

Closely observe the patient for nosebleeds, petechiae, conjunctival hemorrhage, and symptoms of cerebral hemorrhage (such as restlessness, confusion, alteration in vital signs, and cardiac dysrhythmias), because bleeding is a potential complication of the procedure. Also check stool and emesis for signs of blood.

Nursing Diagnoses and Planning

Nursing diagnoses and related expected patient outcomes commonly applicable to patients undergoing bone marrow transplantation include the following:

NDx: Altered nutrition: less than body requirements related to mucositis and esophageal ulceration secondary to chemotherapy, radiation, or both

Planning: Patient Outcomes
1. Serum albumin is within normal range.
2. Patient's daily nutritional intake approaches the recommended daily allowance or as prescribed.

NDx: Risk for altered tissue perfusion related to abnormal bleeding secondary to platelet obliteration

Planning: Patient Outcomes
1. Nosebleeds and conjunctival hemorrhages are absent.
2. Signs of cerebral hemorrhage or other internal bleeding are absent.

NDx: Risk for infection related to suppression of the immune system

Planning: Patient Outcomes
1. Skin and mucous membranes are intact.
2. Lungs are clear to auscultation.
3. Monilial or herpetic lesions are absent from the mouth.
4. Vaginal itching and discharge are absent.
5. Patient describes sources of potentially infectious organisms and how to avoid them.
6. Patient remains afebrile.

NDx: Knowledge deficit: transplant protocol, potential side effects, therapeutic goals

Planning: Patient Outcomes
1. Patient describes, in sequence, the major components of his or her treatment plan—for example, chemotherapy, irradiation, duration of transplantation, and postoperative care.
2. Patient describes potential side effects, both long-term and short-term.
3. Patient states why transplantation is being performed and what effect it is expected to have on his or her health status.

NDx: Anxiety related to the procedure and its outcome

Planning: Patient Outcomes
1. Patient discusses concerns about the procedure and its outcomes.
2. Signs of anxiety, such as pacing, trembling, tachycardia, or inability to focus attention, are absent.

NDx: Risk for body image disturbance related to transplant or occurrence of graft-versus-host disease

Planning: Patient Outcomes
1. Patient discusses his or her condition or asks questions about it.

2. Patient makes decisions when asked—for example, what to eat, what to wear, when to get up.
3. Patient maintains social contact with staff, family, and others.

NDx: Risk for diversional activity deficit related to extended length of treatment

Planning: Patient Outcomes
1. Patient pursues some diversional activity, such as reading, watching television, or writing letters.
2. Patient denies that boredom is a problem.

NDx: Risk for altered health maintenance related to insufficient knowledge of self-care after discharge

Planning: Patient Outcomes
1. Patient describes self-care.
2. Patient and significant others verbalize ability and willingness to comply with self-care instructions.
3. Patient identifies person and method of contact in the event of questions or problems.

Other nursing diagnoses and patient outcomes that may apply are related to chemotherapy and irradiation given before the procedure. These are discussed in Chapter 34. Because bone marrow transplantation is in essence the last hope of a dying patient, nursing diagnoses and patient outcomes related to grieving and death, presented in Chapter 3, also apply.

Nursing Interventions and Evaluation

NDx: Altered nutrition: less than body requirements
Administer total parenteral nutrition as ordered. If the patient is not on total parenteral nutrition, give small, frequent meals planned according to the patient's stated food preferences. Offer between-meal supplements as needed. Avoid performing offensive or distressing procedures immediately before meals. Administer antiemetics so that peak action occurs at mealtime. Maintain a calm, relaxed atmosphere at mealtime, and provide companionship when possible.

In most cases, a nutritional assessment should be performed by a dietitian and the resulting recommendations followed regarding how the patient's nutritional needs can best be met. Total parenteral nutrition is usually necessary in the bone marrow transplant patient and should be administered according to hospital procedure.

Weigh the patient daily using the same scale. Record food and fluid intake for periodic calorie counts.

NDx: Risk for altered tissue perfusion
Apply pressure for several minutes to any puncture sites, as from injections or venipunctures, to help lessen the risk of bleeding. Administer blood products as ordered to maintain adequate levels of platelets and red blood cells. As much as possible, avoid

venipunctures and invasive procedures. Obtain platelet count before performing invasive procedures.

NDx: Risk for infection

Place the patient in a private room and help ensure that all personnel wash their hands thoroughly before entering so that the patient is protected from exposure to potentially pathogenic organisms.

Check arrangement of staff assignments so that persons caring for the patient are healthy, free of communicable diseases such as colds and flu, without active herpetic lesions, and not caring for another patient with an infectious process. Screen visitors for communicable diseases. People who are ill are not allowed to visit the patient. However, if a visit is essential to the psychologic well-being of the patient, instruct the visitor in the appropriate precautions.

Live plants and cut flowers are not permitted in the patient's environment because they harbor many bacteria and molds that can be dangerous to the patient during neutropenic episodes. Personnel frequently touch the flowers while admiring, smelling, or moving them. This can contaminate their hands and thus provide a means of spread to the patient.

Provide a low-bacteria diet during neutropenic periods. Also, institute nursing measures to maintain intact nonspecific defense mechanisms, thus decreasing the opportunity for pathogens to enter the body. Measures to prevent damage to the skin are listed in Highlight 32–2.

Promote normal bowel function to avoid possible rectal lacerations, irritation and bleeding, or hemorrhoids from passage of hard stool. Keep stools soft and avoid constipation by increasing bulk in the diet, providing plenty of fluids, encouraging as much exercise as possible, and giving stool softeners, such as docusate (Colace), as needed. Avoid taking rectal temperatures, performing rectal examinations, giving enemas, and doing anything else that may injure the intestinal mucosa.

Perform invasive therapies (such as intravenous catheterization, insertion of nasogastric tubes, and insertion of Foley catheters) only if absolutely necessary. Discontinue them as soon as possible. These therapies are used only for medically indicated reasons, never for the convenience of the staff. Use sterile technique at all times when invasive therapy is necessary.

Encourage the patient to cough and breathe deeply, use an incentive spirometer, maintain good hydration, and get out of bed and walk. Good pulmonary toilet is essential to prevent pulmonary infection.

NDx: Knowledge deficit: transplant protocol, potential side effects, therapeutic goals

Begin teaching during the pretransplantation outpatient phase. Use a bone marrow transplant teaching booklet or other patient education materials such as

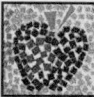

HIGHLIGHT 32–2

HEALTH PROMOTION & RISK REDUCTION

Measures to Prevent Skin Damage After Bone Marrow Transplantation

Turn and position the patient to relieve pressure on the skin areas prone to breakdown.

When moving the patient, take care to avoid shearing forces and abrasions.

Use lotions, bath oil, and skin moisturizers as necessary to prevent dry, chapped skin.

If the patient's skin is delicate, avoid using tape if possible.

Provide good oral hygiene to prevent damage to the mucous membranes.

Use gentle, nontraumatic techniques, such as soft sponges, gauze, or a Water Pik to clean the teeth and gums.

Rinse the mouth frequently with a nonirritating, non–alcohol-based solution such as normal saline from a container that is changed daily.

Keep the lips moist and soft with vitamins A and D ointment or a similar substance.

those available from the National Institutes of Health. Review with the patient information related to the procedure, its therapeutic goals, and its potential side effects. Be alert to any patient comments or behaviors that indicate lack of knowledge. Clarify information, and if necessary, notify the physician of the patient's need for further explanation of the medical treatment.

NDx: Anxiety

Ensure that the patient is kept informed of what to expect during all stages of care. Provide the opportunity for both the patient and significant others to express concerns and ask questions. Involve a psychiatric nurse clinician, social workers, and clergy in patient care early in the hospitalization. Plan care so the patient has private time in which to speak with family members or members of the clergy.

NDx: Risk for body image disturbance

Whenever possible, encourage the patient to make decisions about care, including how to structure the day's activities, what to eat, and what to wear. Encourage the patient to perform as much self-care as possible and to maintain good grooming. Arrange a visit with a former bone marrow transplantation recipient if the patient so desires.

NDx: Risk for diversional activity deficit
Provide appropriate diversional activities, such as prescheduled telephone calls, prescheduled video movie showings, television, books, music, games, hobbies, or puzzles to prevent boredom. Also be sure to spend time with the patient. Consult the occupational or recreational therapist to arrange additional activities for the patient.

NDx: Risk for altered health maintenance
Instruct the patient in self-care after discharge as presented in Highlight 32–3. Include significant oth-

---

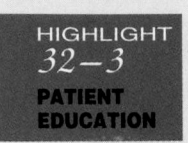 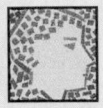

HIGHLIGHT 32–3 PATIENT EDUCATION

Essentials of Self-Care After Bone Marrow Transplantation

Instruct the patient to:

- Expect to tire easily.
- Plan for frequent rest periods or naps.
- Resume pretransplant activities gradually, as tolerance allows.
- Take prophylactic antibiotics as prescribed.
- Monitor for and report nosebleeds, blood in the stool, bleeding gums, hemoptysis, and the appearance of new bruises until platelet count returns to normal.
- Avoid forceful nose blowing until platelet count is normal.
- Use an electric razor until platelet count is normal.
- Avoid contact sports and other activities that risk injury until platelet count is normal.
- Avoid ingestion of irritating or difficult-to-digest foods until platelet count is normal. Then progress to usual diet as tolerated.
- Avoid use of aspirin and aspirin-containing drugs, cough medicines containing guaifenesin, laxatives containing phenolphthalein, and nonsteroidal anti-inflammatory drugs until platelet count is normal.
- Postpone sexual activity until platelet count is at least 50,000.
- Expect vaginal dryness and dyspareunia. Use a vaginal lubricant when intercourse is resumed.
- Monitor for and report signs and symptoms of infection until blood count returns to normal. These include a temperature over 38.4°C (101°F) or persistently over 38°C (100.4°F), shaking chills, sweating, diarrhea lasting more than 2 days, rectal pain, cough, runny nose, shortness of breath, chest discomfort, painful urination, areas of inflammation (redness, swelling, pain), an open sore, or vision change.
- Practice meticulous personal oral and body hygiene. Take a bath or shower daily. Use a mild soap. Take particular care in cleansing underarms and perineal area. Do not share towels or washcloths with others. Use a soft nylon toothbrush and floss daily unless platelet count is below 50,000 or white blood cell count is below 15,000 (1.5). In [that] case, use only soft toothettes.

- Use a mouth rinse of $\frac{1}{2}$ teaspoon of salt and $\frac{1}{2}$ teaspoon of baking soda in 8 ounces of water rather than using commercial mouthwash or hydrogen peroxide, which dry and irritate mucous membranes.
- Avoid crowds and contact with persons known to have a colds or other contagious diseases until blood count returns to normal.
- Walk outdoors regularly.
- Wear sunscreen (SPF 15 or higher) if in direct sun for more than 20 minutes. Sun exposure can aggravate graft-versus-host disease or activate a viral infection.
- Avoid swimming in lakes or crowded pools for at least 6 months.
- Keep the home as free from dust and dirt as possible. Have air conditioning or heating units cleaned before returning home. Use a disinfectant, such as ammonia or bleach, to clean the bathroom fixtures. Wash all dishes in hot water and detergent. Launder bath linens twice a week and bed linens once a week.
- Avoid handling water and soil from flowers and house plants until neutrophil count is sustained at normal levels, because these substances can harbor bacteria.
- Have household cats and dogs treated for parasites and toxoplasmosis before returning home.
- Avoid close contact with all animals. Do not clean cages, litter boxes, aquariums, or the like for 12 to 18 months.
- Monitor for and report signs of graft-versus-host disease. These include rash or itching (especially on the palms of the hands or soles of the feet), frequent liquid bowel movements, clay-colored stool, dark urine, and jaundice.
- Return for weekly blood tests (complete blood count with platelets and differential count) until counts return to normal range.
- Return for biweekly platelet infusions if needed.
- Comply with follow-up schedule of monthly visits to the transplant surgeon, with repeat scans and blood counts for 1 year and every 2 months thereafter.

ers in the teaching, because self-care requirements affect the entire household. Provide all instructions in writing for easy reference. Give clear directions as to whom should be contacted should questions or problems occur.

Compare the patient's status with the expected outcomes. If the outcomes are not met, reassess the patient and revise the plan.

The Elderly: Special Considerations

The immune system is complex. Age-related effects on its structure and function are just beginning to be delineated through research. With advancing age, the cortex of the thymus becomes thinner, and a slow decrease in overall thymic size occurs. Because T cells originate from the thymic cortical cells, these changes suggest that the number of T cells in the peripheral lymphatic tissues declines with age. However, this is difficult to document. No atrophy of the lymph nodes or a decrease in B cells in the blood has been found.

Functionally, it appears that a gradual decrease in immunologic competence occurs during senescence, apparently from defects in aged lymphoid cells. There seems to be some decrease in delayed-type hypersensitivity with aging. Studies in this area suggest that, in senescence, T memory cells can respond to a booster skin test involving an antigen to which the T cells had been exposed at a young age but are unable to react to an antigen seen for the first time because of thymic hypofunction.

In relationship to humoral immunity, numbers of B cells in the peripheral blood and levels of IgM have been found to be unchanged in the aged. However, total serum IgG and IgA levels increase after age 70, suggesting either an enhanced response to antigens or a defect in control of the system. Abnormal regulation of immune function with age is further suggested by an increased incidence of autoantibodies in the aged. This occurs even without associated disease and may result from a loss of tolerance to self-antigens (such as DNA).

In terms of rapid antibody production in the aged in response to antigens, some studies indicate a diminished response and some a normal response. In any case, a response does occur, and thus immunizations have some positive effect. Older clients should be encouraged to undergo annual influenza immunizations and the one-time pneumonia vaccination.

Chapter Review

1. How does specific (or adaptive) immunity differ from nonspecific (or innate)?
2. What role does complement play in inflammation?
3. How does the immune system respond to infection?
4. What role does family history play in immune disorders?
5. What are the differences in sensitivity and specificity of the scratch, prick, and intradermal allergy tests?
6. How does antigen-specific immunosuppression differ from nonspecific immunosuppression?
7. How does immunization use the body's own mechanisms to provide protection?
8. What are possible solutions to the problem of graft-versus-host disease?
9. How do you think a cancer patient would react to a bone marrow biopsy?
10. What is the significance of weight gain in a patient with bone marrow transplant?

Bibliography

Balakrishnan K, Adams LE. The role of the lymphocyte in an immune response. Immunol Invest 1995; 24(1–2):233.

Barnes RMR, Chapel HM. Current practice and future directions in clinical immunology. J R Soc Med 1995; 88(7):395.

Bauer SM. Psychoneuroimmunology and cancer: An integrated review. J Adv Nurs 1994; 19:1114.

Bloodborne infections: A practical guide to OSHA compliance. Arlington, TX: Johnson & Johnson Medical, 1992.

Centers for Disease Control and Prevention. Draft guideline for isolation precautions in hospitals. Fed Reg 1994; 59(214):55552.

Check IJ. Vaccines and immunity assessment: Diagnostic immunology laboratory issues. Clin Immunol Newsl 1994; 14(9):117.

DeLandazuri MO. Immunology research. Clin Sci 1996; 90(3):148.

Dracker RA. Hematopoietic stem cells: Form, method, characteristics. Immunol Invest 1995; 24(1–2):443.

Dobbing EA. Preventing transference of bloodborne pathogens in the workplace: Reducing your risk of contracting HIV/HBV. Point of View 1993; 30(2):8.

Eirik Mollnes T, Harboe M. Recent advances in clinical immunology. Br Med J 1996; 312(7044):1465.

Frank MM, Austen KF, Claman HN, Unanue ER. Samter's immunologic diseases, vol I. Boston: Little Brown, 1995.

Frank MM, Austen KF, Claman HN, Unanue ER. Samter's immunologic diseases, vol II. Boston: Little Brown, 1995.

Gautam AM. Immunology: Why does the human immune system sometimes attack itself? Today's Life Sci 1994; 6(12):28.

Health care workers at risk: An interview with Patricia Wetzel, MD. Asepsis, The Infection Prevention Forum 1995; 17(1):10.

Immunology web links. Immunol Today 1996; 17(2):51.

Important advances in clinical medicine—Allergy and immunology—Epitomes of progress. Connecticut Med 1996; 60(1):21.

Kagnoff MF. Mucosal immunology: New frontiers. Immunol Today 1996; 17(2):57.

Kimball JW. Introduction to immunology. New York: Macmillan, 1990.

Lambert RB, Lambert NK. The effects of humor on secretory immunoglobulin A levels in school-aged children. Pediatr Nurs 1995; 21(1):16.

Lawlor GJ, Fischer TJ, Adelman DC. Manual of allergy and immunology. Boston: Little Brown, 1995.

Michel G, Leverger G, Leblanc T, Nelken B. Allogeneic bone marrow transplantation vs. aggressive post-remission chemotherapy for children with acute myeloid leukemia in first complete remission. Bone Marrow Transplant 1996; 17(2):191.

Norman PS. Clinical aspects of immunology. J Allergy Clin Immunol 1995; 96(1):136.

Putnam FW. Milestones in structural immunology. FASEB J 1995; 9(1):146.

Roitt I, Brostoff J, Male D. Immunology. London: Gower Medical, 1989.

Sissons JGP, Borysiewicz LK, Cohen J. Immunology of infection. Virus Res 1995; 39(2):386.

Stalheim-Smith A, Fitch GK. Understanding human anatomy and physiology. Minneapolis: West Publishing, 1993.

Starzl TE, Murase N, Thomson A, et al. The bidirectional paradigm of transplant immunology. Ann N Y Acad Sci 1996; 770:165.

Stites DP, Abba IT, Parslow TG. Basic & clinical immunology. Norwalk, CT: Appleton & Lange, 1994.

Tizard IR. Immunology—An introduction. Philadelphia: Saunders College Publishing, 1995.

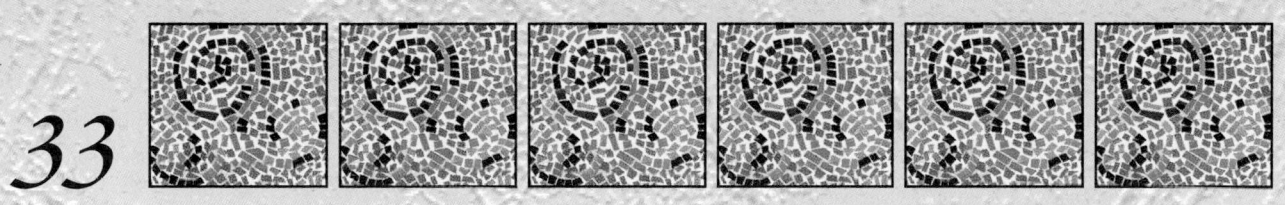

33

Nursing Care of Patients with HIV/AIDS and Other Immune Disorders

Study Outcomes

After studying this chapter, you should be able to:

1. Describe the etiology, pathophysiology, clinical manifestations, diagnostic procedures, and medical management of human immunodeficiency virus (HIV)/acquired immunodeficiency syndrome (AIDS) and other immune disorders.
2. Identify information and physical examination data essential to the assessment of patients with HIV/AIDS and other immune disorders.
3. State nursing diagnoses and related expected patient outcomes commonly applicable to patients with HIV/AIDS and other immune disorders.
4. Describe nursing interventions, with their rationales, commonly applicable to patients with HIV/AIDS and other immune disorders.
5. Explain the basis for evaluation of nursing care provided to patients with HIV/AIDS and other immune disorders.
6. Identify alternative treatment and care settings for patients with HIV/AIDS and other immune disorders, and the services related to community-based care.
7. Identify special considerations for the elderly patient with an immune disorder.

Disorders of the immune system can be categorized as immunodeficiency disorders, hypersensitivity disorders, and autoimmune disorders. In immunodeficiency disorders, the immune system fails to respond in a normal manner. In hypersensitivity disorders, the immune system overreacts, causing tissue damage. In autoimmune disorders, the body reacts immunologically against itself. This chapter presents examples of all three types.

Most immunodeficiency, hypersensitivity, and autoimmune disorders are chronic in nature. During diagnosis and acute episodes, patients may be briefly admitted to a hospital. Much of the follow-up care, however, will be done in an outpatient setting, clinic, or doctor's office. Even care in the terminal stage of acquired immunodeficiency syndrome (AIDS) is being managed by home health agencies and hospice in the patient's home. Often, care and teaching are directed toward helping patients learn to manage these conditions independently. Consequently, involving patients and families in every step of the care process is a critical aspect of providing appropriate nursing care to patients with immune disorders.

*I*mmunodeficiency Disorders

Immunodeficiency refers to a condition in which the immune system fails to produce an adequate response to an antigen. Immunodeficiency may result from a defect or deficiency in B cells (antibody), T cells (cellular), combined B and T cells (antibody and cellular), phagocytes, or complement.

Symptoms of immunodeficiency depend on the immune system components affected and the degree to which their function has been impaired. Symptoms seen with many immunodeficiency diseases include:

- Chronic or frequent infection
- Infection caused by unusual organisms or normal body flora that do not usually cause infection
- Poor response to treatment of the infection
- Chronic diarrhea
- Skin rash
- Abscesses
- Osteomyelitis
- Hepatosplenomegaly
- Failure to grow and thrive

Failure to grow and thrive is known as primary immunodeficiency. Secondary immunodeficiency is acquired later in life as a result of disease or exposure to a toxic agent or other unknown cause.

The ability to diagnose immunodeficiency is expanding as we learn more about the immune system and as laboratory techniques improve.

PRIMARY IMMUNODEFICIENCIES

Primary immunodeficiencies are immunodeficiencies acquired at birth. Stem-cell deficiency, DiGeorge's

1457

syndrome, and agammaglobulinemia are examples of primary immunodeficiencies that are predominantly pediatric problems. Patients with these diseases seldom live to adulthood. The most severe is stem-cell deficiency, also called severe combined immunodeficiency (SCID). This is an inherited trait characterized by absence of both T-cell and B-cell function. DiGeorge's syndrome is known by a lack of thymic development and a subsequent lack of T cells, resulting in impaired cell-mediated immunity. Agammaglobulinemia is an inherited disorder in which there are no B cells or antibodies.

Symptoms of primary immunodeficiencies usually develop very early in life, at about the time protection from maternal antibodies is lost. Treatment consists of aggressive antibiotic therapy for infections and possibly prophylactic antibiotics to help prevent infections. Administration of gamma globulin may be helpful in stem-cell deficiency and agammaglobulinemia. Bone marrow transplants and fetal liver transplants, and fetal thymic transplants may be helpful in treating stem-cell deficiency and DiGeorge's syndrome, respectively.

The most common primary immunodeficiency is selective immunoglobulin A (IgA) deficiency, which affects about 1 in 600 people. Its cause is unknown. It is defined as a serum IgA level of less than 5 mg/dL, with normal or increased levels of the other immunoglobulins and normal T-cell function.

Many patients with selective IgA deficiency have no symptoms and remain relatively healthy. Other patients seem to be more susceptible to respiratory tract and gastrointestinal tract infections. Selective IgA deficiency has also been associated with an increased incidence of allergies and autoimmune disorders. When symptoms do occur, they usually appear by age 10.

Treatment consists of combating infections with the appropriate antibiotics. No safe and effective method is available for replacing the missing IgA. Gamma globulin is not given, because these patients can produce normal amounts of IgG, IgM, IgE, IgD. In addition, their immune system can recognize the injected IgA as foreign and produce antibodies against it. These anti-IgA antibodies then increase the patient's risk of developing a transfusion reaction if blood is ever needed, because anti-IgA antibodies would react with the IgA in the transfused blood. With proper treatment of infections and other associated complications, the prognosis for a normal life span is good.

SECONDARY IMMUNODEFICIENCIES

Etiology and Pathophysiology

Secondary immunodeficiencies are caused by a vast array of diseases and drugs and exhibit a wide range of degree and duration of immunosuppression. In addition to the major immunosuppressant drugs discussed in Chapter 32, many other drugs have the potential to cause immunosuppression as a rare side effect. Some infectious diseases also cause a degree of immunosuppression. These include tuberculosis, leprosy, measles, cytomegalovirus, congenital rubella, and HIV/AIDS. Immunosuppression is also characteristic of malignant disease. It may result from such malignancies as leukemias and lymphomas, which directly involve immune system cells and alter their function. Or it may result from malnutrition and protein depletion frequently associated with malignant diseases. Severe immunosuppression may also result from chemotherapy and radiation therapy used to treat malignant disease.

Patients with severe burns develop some degree of immunosuppression because their integument, a very important defense mechanism, is compromised or destroyed, and antibodies are lost along with the serum in the exudate. Diabetics may have less efficient phagocytic cells, which—combined with high levels of glucose and vascular disease—increases their risk of infection. Alcoholics may experience immunosuppression from the malnutrition and liver damage often associated with the disease. Chronic lung diseases tend to destroy the defense mechanisms of the respiratory tract, leaving the patient more susceptible to respiratory infections. Some degree of immunosuppression may also exist for several weeks after anesthesia and surgery, as well as after trauma, emotional and physical stress, and pregnancy. Chronic drug abuse may also cause some immunosuppression from the effects of impaired nutrition.

Clinical Manifestations

The clinical manifestations in immunodeficiency vary greatly with the degree and duration of immunosuppression. Some patients develop no infections, while others develop one or more fulminating infections. Ultimately, the symptoms depend on what type of infection develops. Many of the more common symptoms are listed in Table 33–1. Infections with opportunistic organisms, such as *Staphylococcus epidermidis* and *Candida albicans*, are much more likely to occur in patients with immunosuppression.

Diagnosis

Diagnosis of secondary immunodeficiency is typically based on the patient's clinical picture and history. Frequent infections, infections with unusual organisms, or minor infections that do not heal are clues that the patient may have an immunodeficiency. Laboratory tests can be done to determine T-cell and B-cell function, as well as levels of antibodies in the blood. Molecular genetic techniques are being used to detect such viruses as Epstein-Barr, HIV, and human T-cell leukemia viruses (HTLV). These techniques can also detect chromosomal deletions or rearrangements that occur in certain malignancies. Skin tests with common antigens can be done to determine whether cell-mediated immunity is intact, although a small percentage of peo-

Table 33–1

Clinical Features in Immunodeficiency

USUALLY PRESENT

Recurrent upper respiratory infections
Severe bacterial infections
Persistent infections with incomplete or no response to therapy

OFTEN PRESENT

Failure to thrive or growth retardation
Infection with unusual organisms
Skin lesions, such as rash, seborrhea, pyoderma, necrotic abscesses, alopecia, eczema, telangiectasia
Recalcitrant thrush
Diarrhea and malabsorption
Persistent sinusitis or mastoiditis
Recurrent bronchitis or pneumonia
Evidence of autoimmunity
Paucity of lymph nodes and tonsils
Hematologic abnormalities: aplastic anemia, hemolytic anemia, neutropenia, and thrombocytopenia

OCCASIONALLY PRESENT

Weight loss, fevers
Chronic conjunctivitis
Lymphadenopathy
Hepatosplenomegaly
Severe viral disease (eg, varicella or herpes simplex)
Arthralgia or arthritis
Chronic encephalitis
Recurrent meningitis
Pyoderma gangrenosa
Adverse reaction to vaccines
Bronchiectasis
Chronic stomatitis or peritonitis

From Lawlor GJ, Fischer TJ, Adelman DC. Manual of allergy and immunology. Boston: Little, Brown, 1995; adapted from Stiehm ER. Immunodeficiency disorders: General considerations. In Stiehm ER (ed). Immunologic disorders in infants and children. 3rd ed. Philadelphia: WB Saunders, 1989.

ple are anergic (having a diminished reactivity to specific antigens).

Management

Specific medical management depends on the underlying cause of the immunodeficiency. If possible, this cause should be eliminated. Infections are treated with antimicrobials effective against the causative organism.

NURSING PROCESS GUIDELINES
Immunodeficiency

Nursing care of the patient with an immunodeficiency depends on the type, degree, and expected duration of the deficiency. For the hospitalized patient, nursing care includes using isolation precautions, checking laboratory test results, and assessing the patient for positive responses to the treatment

plan. If the person is being treated as an outpatient, teach the patient how to minimize the risk of infection. Explain the importance of good personal hygiene, the need to avoid crowds and contact with persons known to be ill, and the need to seek medical care at the first sign of infection rather than attempting self-treatment.

ACQUIRED IMMUNODEFICIENCY SYNDROME

Infection with HIV causes progressive deterioration and dysfunction in cell-mediated immunity. In its most severe manifestation, it results in the disease syndrome known as AIDS. Opportunistic infections that arise during such severe immunosuppression may be fatal. In addition to immune dysfunction, HIV causes slow, progressive wasting disorders— including neurodegeneration—that are commonly fatal in and of themselves.

HIV infection is a pandemic that continues to spread in areas already affected as well as areas apparently unaffected or minimally affected. The epidemiology of HIV infection is becoming increasingly complex over time. With the widespread distribution of risk factors for transmission, and the long infectious period, it is believed that HIV will eventually reach all human communities. The World Health Organization estimated that, in 1995, 12 million people were infected with HIV worldwide. At least 7.5 million were in Africa, 2.2 million were in the Americas, 1.5 million were in Asia and Oceania, and about 0.8 million were in Europe. Of the 12 million, 7.5 million were men and 4.5 million were women.

Etiology and Pathophysiology

The human immunodeficiency virus is an RNA virus in the lentivirus family of nononcogenic, cytopathic retroviruses. HIV has been known by several names. Initially, it was known as lymphadenopathy-associated virus. Then it was called human T-cell lymphotropic virus type III. Then it was called AIDS-related virus. Finally it was named HIV. The virus has two major strains. HIV-1 is very closely related to the primate retrovirus called simian immunodeficiency virus. HIV-2 is clearly associated with immunodeficiency but may be less pathogenic than HIV-1.

Long-term, chronic viral replication leads to progressive and lethal degeneration of the immune system and the central nervous system. Evidence suggests that several factors may modify the host response to HIV, including:

- The route of HIV infection
- The amount of HIV inoculum
- The pathogenic potential of a given HIV strain
- Host genetic factors and certain cofactors, such as other infections and drug use

The primary cells involved in HIV-1 infection are the human T lymphocytes with a particular affinity to the CD4 molecule, and monocyte-macrophages. The CD4+ (T helper) cells appear to be the primary site of viral replication, with a 5-fold to 10-fold higher frequency in lymphoid tissue than in the peripheral blood of HIV-infected people.

HIV-1 Life Cycle

The life cycle of HIV-1 is divided into two phases: establishment of infection and productive infection. Infection is accomplished by a series of virus-cell interactions that include binding of the virus to the cell surface (at the CD4 receptor molecule), fusion, entry of the virus into the cytoplasm, conversion of RNA to DNA, and entry of DNA into the nucleus.

Expression occurs when DNA is transcribed into RNA and viruses are encapsulated and bud through a region of the cell membrane (Fig. 33–1). Figure 33–2 shows an electron micrograph of the budding process schematically represented in Figure 33–1. There is a clear relationship between viral burden and CD4+ T-cell decline, which suggests that HIV infection results directly in cell death. The mecha-

nism is believed to involve accumulation of large amounts of unintegrated viral DNA or mutation of the HIV envelope glycoprotein.

It is unclear why production of new CD4+ T cells cannot replenish the supply. One explanation for the lack of CD4+ T-cell regeneration is that the precursors in the thymus and bone marrow are also infected with HIV.

As mentioned earlier, the primary site of viral replication is the lymph or plasma membrane. Replication within infected macrophages occurs at both the plasma and cytoplasmic membranes. Tissue samples from AIDS patients have also shown virus present in skin, lymph nodes, lungs, spinal cord, and brain. The presence of HIV in these tissues plays a definite role in clinical dysfunction.

Immune Response

The host mounts an anti-HIV immune response almost immediately after infection to neutralize free HIV and eliminate HIV-infected cells. Despite adverse effects on many cellular components of the immune response, the anti-HIV antibody manages to inhibit the infectivity of free HIV or HIV-infected

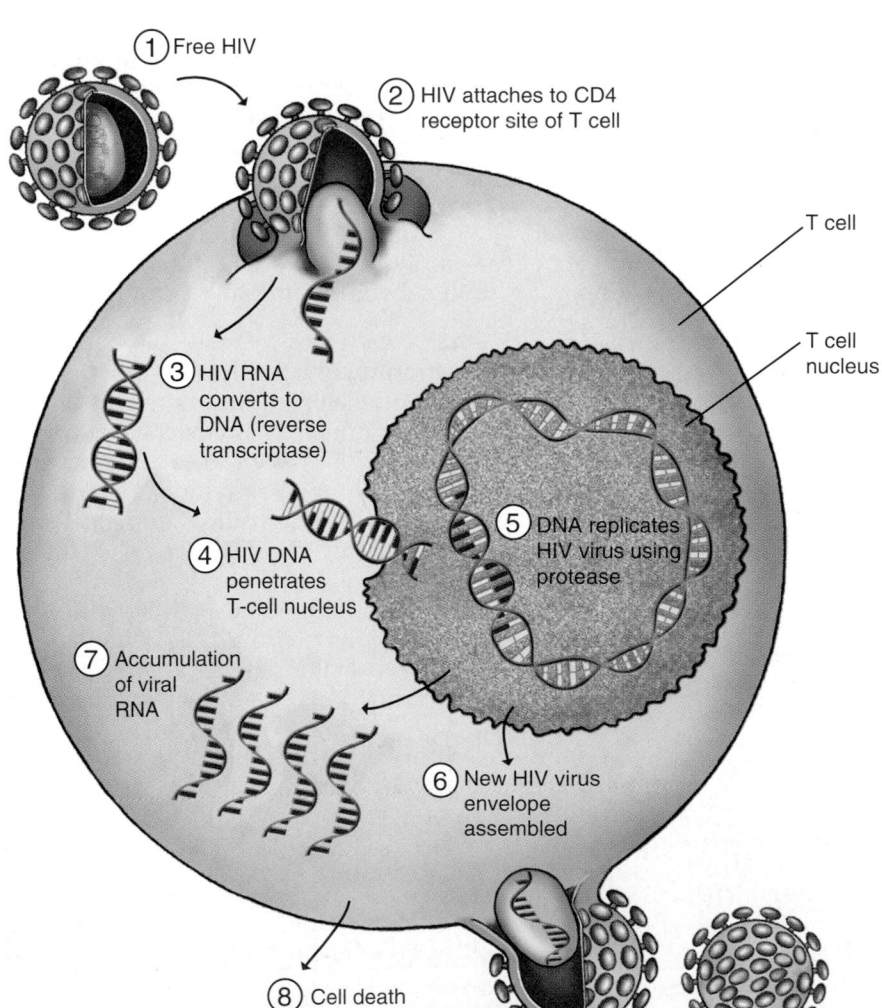

Figure 33–1

Life cycle of human immunodeficiency virus (HIV).

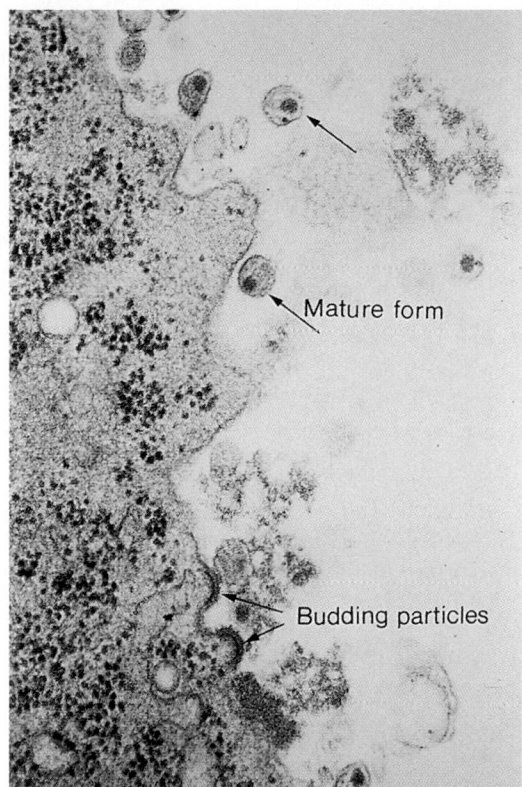

Figure 33-2

Electron micrograph of human immunodeficiency virus (HIV) cultured from a hemophiliac patient. Virus particles range in size from 90 to 120 nm. (Courtesy of Jonathan W.M. Gold, MD.)

cells in acute HIV infection. Similarly, anti-HIV CD8+ lymphocytes, cytotoxic T lymphocytes, natural killer cells, and macrophages clear high numbers of circulating HIV-infected cells. These same antibodies, along with HIV-neutralizing antibodies, are thought to resolve the acute infection and maintain the asymptomatic phase of HIV infection (Fig. 33-3).

No one knows why this highly coordinated, initially effective immune response does not control HIV infection over the long term. The answer probably relates to the ability of HIV to spread by cell-to-cell fusion, use of the CD4 molecule as the HIV receptor, and the ability of HIV to mutate and replicate.

Transmission

HIV is transmitted by exposure to a body fluid containing HIV. Not all persons exposed become infected. The probability of transmission increases with the concentration of HIV and the amount of fluid. Body fluids that have been shown to transmit the virus include blood, semen, cerebrospinal fluid, vaginal secretions, and possibly breast milk. HIV has been isolated from many other body fluids, such as saliva, and urine, but the amount present is not believed to be significant enough to cause infection.

The three major routes of transmission include:

- Sexual contact involving the exchange of body fluids
- Parenteral, by inoculation with infected blood, blood products, or body fluids
- Perinatal, from infected mother to fetus or infant

There is no evidence that HIV is spread during casual contact with an infected person or through air, water, or food. HIV is not transmitted via fomites or insect or animal vectors. HIV cannot move independently. In the United States, transmission of HIV most frequently occurs through sexual activity and intravenous drug use.

Sexual Activity

Transmission of HIV occurs during homosexual and heterosexual activity. It can be transmitted from male to male, male to female, female to male, and, rarely, female to female. At this time, the risk of acquiring HIV from a single sexual encounter with an infected person is not known, although it appears to be less easily transmitted than other sex-

Figure 33-3

Relative levels of immune response to human immunodeficiency virus (HIV) infection.

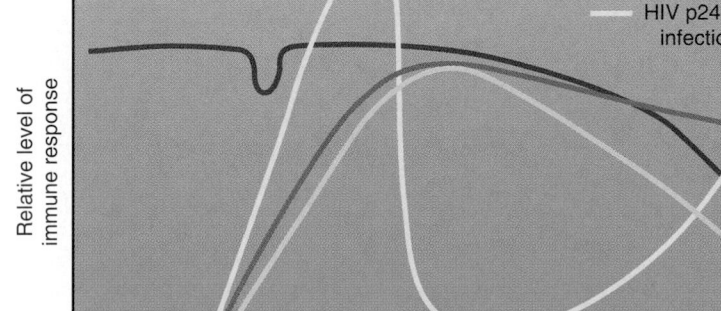

SOCIOCULTURAL PERSPECTIVES

Access to Care
by Janice R. Ellis, PhD, RN

Medical research is providing a greater and greater variety of high-cost, high-tech responses to acute and chronic illness. As these interventions are approved for clinical use, access to them has become an important issue.

In health care, the term *access* refers to a person's ability to receive health care when and where that person needs it. There are three aspects of access to health-care: geographic access, economic access, and cultural access. Let's take a closer look at each, and their effect on patient care.

Geographic access encompasses all of the advantages and disadvantages of the patient's place of residence. One aspect of geographic access is whether the patient can get to the health-care experts and technologies that will best treat a particular health-care problem. For example, cancer care requires not only access to an oncologist but also access to radiation therapy, hospitals with expertise in chemotherapy, and laboratories that can support treatments involving such tasks as the production of monoclonal antibodies. The complexities of providing interdisciplinary treatment, managing adverse responses to new drugs, and balancing the many aspects of care provide a unique challenge in cancer care—a challenge that is often best met in major cancer centers. How does this reality affect the care available to the patient who lives in a rural area and is not able to travel to a specialized center? For the rural patient who *is* able to travel, there is the problem of leaving behind important sources of emotional and social support.

Even within a community, geographic access becomes a concern when transportation options are limited. In larger cities, it may take literally hours to negotiate public transportation to a major care center. For the person who is sick and weak or who must manage small children throughout this process, problems with transportation may prove to be an insurmountable barrier to effective access.

Access to health care also requires the economic resources to pay for care. To pay for health care, most people in the United States rely on health insurance. But there is wide variation in the extent of coverage among different insurance plans. For example, some policies do not provide any coverage for outpatient or ambulatory care. There may also be limits on the types of therapies that will be covered by insurance. As new therapies are developed and approved, they are usually very expensive. For example, an organ transplantation procedure may cost hundreds of thousands of dollars, and maintenance drugs after transplantation add thousands of dollars to this cost each year, perhaps

for life. Although organ transplantation may be an extreme example, even such relatively common interventions as neurosurgery for a brain tumor or glucose monitoring and drug therapy for diabetes require major economic resources.

As third-party payers seek to reduce their costs, they often limit services. These limits pose economic barriers to patients, because the cost of treatment is too great for the patient to pay personally, "out of pocket." Likewise, health insurers may require pre-approval for major care, and they may deny certain claims that do not meet their standards. For example, a treatment that a health-care provider considers the treatment of choice may be deemed "experimental" by a particular insurer, and most insurers will not cover experimental procedures. Who decides what is experimental? The insurer does. The patient may not even be aware of these limitations until the need for such care arises. Then, too late, the patient discovers that the one treatment that may offer a chance of a cure is the one treatment for which an insurer will not pay.

Managed-care companies try to limit costs by controlling the use of services. For example, a patient on a managed-care plan is usually restricted in his or her choice of physicians. Specialty care may be severely curtailed by the requirement that a patient obtain a written referral from a primary care physician to visit a specialist. Some managed-care companies are even limiting the postoperative visits of patients recovering from eye surgery to the ophthalmologist who performed the surgery. Instead, the managed-care company requires the primary care physician to provide postoperative monitoring.

For Americans without health insurance, economic access becomes even more of a problem. Some economic access is provided through Medicaid programs. These programs are designed to provide health care for people receiving public assistance. However, the "working poor," who are not eligible for Medicaid programs, may be caught in the middle. Their employers may not provide health insurance, they are not eligible for Medicaid, and they are certainly unable to pay "out-of-pocket" for health care. As welfare reforms continue to be adopted in the United States, it is clear that many individuals and families will be dropped from public assistance. These individuals and families will often lose all access to health care. Already, advocates for children are expressing concern about how children's health-care needs will be met.

SOCIOCULTURAL PERSPECTIVES

Access to Care

(continued)

Access is also related to a person's feeling accepted and comfortable in the environment where care is provided. When people do not feel that care providers will recognize their uniqueness, and when they feel that their special needs will be disregarded, they may avoid seeking care. Thus, care is not truly accessible for that person. For patients to feel accepted and comfortable, health-care providers must be culturally competent. Cultural competence involves knowledge about cultural differences (such as cultural differences in the expectations of patients) and interpersonal skills in adapting care to these differences.

Cultural competence is very important when caring for people with HIV/AIDS. The population of people who are HIV-positive or who have AIDS includes large numbers of homosexual men, minorities, and those with a history of drug problems. Often, these people already feel marginalized in society, even apart from their HIV status. In health-care environments, they may feel that they cannot discuss their concerns openly—that care providers will respond negatively to them if they disclose the details of their lives.

Likewise, consider the patient from a minority group who finds that all care providers at a particular facility are from the majority group. The patient may feel—perhaps justifiably—that the system will not respond to her unique cultural needs. People whose culture is not the majority culture may encounter care providers who discount their beliefs and life patterns. Situations like these create cultural barriers to access.

The culturally competent caregiver strives to provide health care that reaches out and establishes a bond of trust with all patients. To do this effectively, you will need to continue your education informally as you leave school and begin your practice. This education will take place as you actively engage in relationships with people of various cultures and grow in your understanding of others. An effective relationship of trust provides the access that is essential to positive outcomes.

As a nurse, you will be working with many people who face barriers to their access to health care. If you do not understand how imposing these barriers are and how powerfully they interfere with health care, patients may never receive the care that they so desperately need. You can help to overcome problems of geographic access by creatively helping patients to solve transportation problems, by facilitating effective communication between care providers, and by bringing care to patients who cannot go to the care. You can help to overcome some economic barriers by working with others in the community to establish avenues of economic access. You can help to overcome cultural barriers by committing yourself to the development of the knowledge and skills that will make you a culturally competent nurse.

---

ually transmitted diseases, such as gonorrhea and syphilis.

Certain sexual practices increase the risk of exposure to body fluids and thereby increase the chance of infection. Practices that pose an increased risk of transmission include anal, vaginal, and oral intercourse without the use of a latex barrier. The risk of transmission relates to potential tears in the mucous membrane, which can result in direct viral access to the vascular system. Mucosal damage may not be necessary during anal intercourse because the high rate of fluid absorption in this part of the digestive system may move virus through the mucous membrane. Sexual practices that expose a person to the blood of his or her partner pose an even greater risk of HIV transmission. These include insertion of large objects or fists into the anal or vaginal cavities, and practices that involve the piercing of body parts. The portal of entry in these situations may be a break in the skin or mucous membrane.

Latex barriers—such as gloves, condoms, and vaginal dams—reduce the chance of exposure and thereby reduce the risk of infection. It is important to use latex because HIV may penetrate condoms made from animal skin. Water-soluble lubricants or a spermicide containing nonoxynol-9 should be used with condoms and vaginal barriers. Oil-based lubricants, such as hand lotion, baby oil, or petrolatum jelly (Vaseline), should not be used, because they dissolve latex and cause condoms or gloves to break. High-risk sexual practices, especially anal intercourse, should be discouraged. Limiting the number of sexual partners decreases the number of possible exposures but does not prevent transmission of HIV infection.

Intravenous Drug Use

Transmission by inoculation of infected blood can occur in several ways. The most frequent is through the sharing of blood-contaminated needles and syringes by intravenous drug users. Although the amount of blood present in the needle and syringe may be very small, the frequent, repeated exposure to contaminated blood increases the chance of infection with HIV. Infected intravenous drug users are increasingly infecting their sexual partners who do not use drugs.

Transmission Via Blood Products

HIV can also be transmitted through transfusion of blood or blood products that contain the virus and through organ transplant from an infected donor. Only a small proportion of the patients with AIDS, about 3%, have become infected by this route. Since April 1985, all blood donated in the United States has been screened for antibody to HIV. If antibodies to HIV are present, the blood is not used. Blood donors are also screened for high-risk behaviors for HIV transmission. If a risk activity is reported, blood from that donor is not used. Blood products (such as clotting-factor concentrates) are now being prepared so that the virus, if present, is inactivated. Screening and treating of blood and blood products have almost, but not completely, eliminated this route of transmission.

Perinatal Transmission

Women infected with HIV may pass the virus to their infants during the perinatal period. Although the mechanism of transmission is not known, it may occur by one of the following routes:

- From the maternal circulation to the fetus in utero
- From exposure of the infant to maternal blood and body fluids during labor and delivery
- Possibly through infected breast milk

The risk of transmission from an HIV-infected mother to her child ranges from 20% to 35%. Early use of zidovudine (Retrovir, AZT) by HIV-infected pregnant women has significantly decreased the rate of infection in infants. This provides yet another reason why early diagnosis and intervention are especially important for pregnant women.

Risk to Health-Care Workers

Health-care workers may be exposed to HIV while providing patient care. However, routine care activities do not facilitate transmission. Accidental transmission of HIV can occur if the health-care worker contacts the blood or body fluids of an HIV-infected patient, especially through percutaneous exposure. To minimize the risk of accidental infection, all health-care workers should avoid direct contact with the blood and body fluids of all patients.

The Centers for Disease Control and Prevention (CDC) reconsidered its original infection control guidelines in response to infection of health-care workers by HIV. The result was standard precautions, which encompasses the main components of universal precautions and body substance isolation. In general, standard precautions mandate the use of protective measures when caring for any patient because the secretions of all patients are seen as potentially infectious. Although the precautions were developed specifically to respond to HIV, they are also effective in reducing the risk of exposure to other blood-borne pathogens, such as hepatitis B. They apply to all body fluids and secretions (except sweat), blood, mucous membranes, and non-intact skin.

Standard precautions include personal protective devices and workplace practices. Gloves must be worn whenever contact with blood or body fluids is likely. Hand-washing is performed immediately after removing gloves. Gloves should not be worn outside a patient's room after use. If blood or body fluids are likely to be splashed, spattered, or aerosolized, masks and goggles should be worn to prevent contact with mucous membranes of the eyes, nose, and mouth. Long-sleeved, impermeable gowns must also be worn whenever blood or body fluids could contact the arms or body. When using needles or other sharp items, health-care workers must use extreme care to avoid injuring themselves. Needles should never be bent, broken, or recapped. Needles and other sharps should be discarded immediately in a puncture-resistant container. If a health-care worker is exposed to any body fluid, he or she should immediately wash the area with soap and water. All needle-stick injuries, lacerations, or abrasions with body fluid–contaminated materials or instruments must be reported to the agency's infection control or employee health department. If the contact is deemed a significant exposure, follow-up testing will be instituted. HIV testing should be performed immediately and at 3 months, 6 months, and 1 year. The health-care worker should be counseled concerning risk for contracting HIV, treatment available (antivirals are offered prophylactically), and prevention of possible transmission to sexual partners during the testing period.

Clinical Manifestations

Early in the AIDS epidemic, experts believed the infection included four distinct clinical entities or processes: acute infection, latency, AIDS-related complex, and acquired immunodeficiency syndrome (AIDS). HIV infection is now known to be a single, continuous disease process. However, it is useful to separate the disease into four stages, each with its own intervention implications (Table 33–2). The four stages are acute retroviral infection, asymptomatic HIV disease, symptomatic disease (early and late), and advanced disease. Even though the CDC uses a case definition for AIDS for reporting purposes, the clinical spectrum is more varied and comprehensive care better served through the use of staging.

Acute Retroviral Infection

The acute retroviral syndrome usually begins about 1 to 3 weeks (although it may range from 5 days to 3 months) after initial infection and lasts 1 to 2 weeks. This syndrome appears to be a response to passive HIV replication that occurs in the first few weeks of infection. It is detectable by transient HIV

Table 33–2

HIV Disease: Stages, CD4 T-Cell Values, and Symptoms

Stage	CD4+ T-Cell Count, Cells/mm³	Symptoms
1: Acute retroviral infection	750–1000	Fever, malaise, headache, pharyngitis, erythematous rash
2: Asymptomatic HIV disease	500–750	Diffuse reactive lymphadenopathy, headache
3: Symptomatic HIV disease		
a: Early	<500	Fever, fatigue, night sweats, oral infections, headache, diarrhea
b: Late	<200	Opportunistic infections, cancers, wasting
4: Advanced HIV disease	<50	Cognitive/motor complex, increased mortality

p24 antigenemia. Signs and symptoms include fever, pharyngitis, headache, malaise, and a diffuse cutaneous erythematous rash. Diffuse reactive lymphadenopathy is also quite common, occurring in 75% of cases. Although most of the symptoms are nonspecific and self-limiting, some—especially the lymphadenopathy—may persist throughout the course of HIV disease. Persistent generalized lymphadenopathy (PGL) is defined as the presence of lymph nodes larger than 1 cm in diameter in two or more extrainguinal sites lasting for more than 3 months. Lymphadenopathy does not affect the patient's prognosis and is considered part of "asymptomatic" disease. Headaches may also persist throughout the course of HIV disease and are part of the asymptomatic phase.

It is estimated that the acute syndrome occurs in 90% of cases of HIV infection, but is often misdiagnosed as influenza or infectious mononucleosis from lack of physician awareness and the nonspecific nature of the syndrome. This was especially true in the early years of research on HIV and AIDS, and especially true when the patient was female.

Asymptomatic HIV Disease

The median time from estimated initial infection to the development of symptomatic HIV disease or AIDS is 10 to 11 years (possibly much shorter in infants and children). This is the asymptomatic phase or clinical latency period.

The definition for asymptomatic HIV disease is that no chronic signs or symptoms potentially attributable to HIV infection are present other than diffuse reactive lymphadenopathy or headache. However, an assortment of abnormal laboratory values can be obtained. A combination of anemia, neutropenia, and thrombocytopenia may occur. Chemistry panel abnormalities may occur, such as increased total serum globulin and decreased albumin and cholesterol levels. Transaminase may be elevated with underlying hepatitis.

The immune deficiency caused by HIV infection can be followed by monitoring the circulating CD4+ T-lymphocyte count. The typical normal count of CD4+ is 750 to 1000/mm³. During the asymptomatic phase, the count decreases by about 40 to 80 cells/mm³ per year. This rate of decline, however, may vary widely among individuals and may be altered by antiretroviral therapy. The CD4+ cell count is useful in monitoring the benefits of antiretroviral therapy and the probability of opportunistic infections. Viral load is used for predicting prognosis and is therefore an important marker for developing a medical treatment plan.

Symptomatic HIV Disease

The symptomatic phase of HIV is divided into early and late symptomatic disease. Early symptomatic disease is characterized by a wide array of symptoms ranging from mild to life-threatening. They may be brief and infrequent to persistent and chronic. Symptoms can affect any organ or system in the body and respond well or minimally to therapy. Many of the symptoms continue throughout the remainder of the patient's life. The early symptomatic phase is characterized by a drop in CD4+ T cell count below 500/mm³.

Fever is a common symptom. It may be associated with any number of infections and malignancies but may occur in the absence of any specific disease.

Oral manifestations occur in the great majority of patients in the early symptomatic stage. Among the most common are oral *Candida albicans*, oral hairy leukoplakia, and recurrent herpes simplex lesions.

Night sweats are another common and hallmark symptom of early symptomatic HIV disease. Night sweats are drenching in nature and occur repeatedly over at least a 2-week period. The pathogenesis is poorly understood and may be a reaction to the HIV itself.

Diarrhea may occur at this stage without any specific pathogen identified. Since chronic diarrhea can lead to dehydration and cachexia, it should be treated aggressively.

Patients are considered to have late symptomatic HIV disease as medical problems increase and CD4+ cell counts fall below 200 cells/mm³. At this point, the patient meets the CDC definition for AIDS and should be reported to the CDC unless a previous opportunistic infection already prompted the report. At this stage, the possibility of opportunistic infections increases dramatically and prophylaxis should be instituted if available.

Also at this stage, gastrointestinal disturbance may be caused by any number of enteric pathogens, such as *Giardia lamblia*, *Entamoeba histolytica* (both parasites), and species of *Salmonella*, *Shigella*, and *Campylobacter* (three bacteria). Viruses such as cytomegalovirus (CMV) have been associated with esophageal ulcers, esophagitis, gastritis, isolated intestinal ulcers, terminal ileitis, colitis, hepatitis, pancreatitis, and unexplained wasting. Cryptosporidium (a parasite) is the most widely recognized enteric pathogen in persons with AIDS, causing massive chronic and protracted diarrhea. Fungi, such as *Candida albicans* and *Histoplasma capsulatum* can cause painful lesions as well as gastrointestinal dysfunction. Many other factors may contribute to malnutrition and weight loss, including anorexia, nausea, and metabolic abnormalities. A patient's nutritional status commonly is a more reliable predictor of death than opportunistic infection.

Neurologic problems are common in patients with late symptomatic HIV infection. They produce a wide range of symptoms that involve both the central and peripheral nervous systems. Peripheral neuropathies are an increasingly common problem. They may result from infection of the nervous system with HIV or from opportunistic infections, such as cytomegalovirus infection, toxoplasmosis, cryptococcosis, and tuberculosis. Lymphomas also frequently affect the central nervous system.

The most common neurologic disorder is a nonfocal encephalopathy that is known as HIV-1–associated cognitive/motor complex (formerly known as AIDS dementia complex), which results in cognitive, motor, and behavioral changes. Initially, subtle changes may occur, such as forgetfulness, poor concentration, decreased spontaneity, poor cognitive flexibility, and psychomotor slowing. A flat affect and apathy similar to that seen with depression and anxiety are also common. In the late symptomatic stage, the patient may exhibit an unsteady gait, incoordination, loss of libido, and withdrawal.

Dermatologic manifestations are common in persons with late symptomatic HIV disease. These include varicella, herpes zoster, *Molluscum contagiosum* eczema, seborrheic dermatitis, and folliculitis. Kaposi's sarcoma, a vascular neoplasm, may also occur. The lesions of Kaposi's sarcoma may occur anywhere on the body surface as well as on the oral mucosa and internal organs. Lesions begin as pink, red, or purple nodules or plaques. They are usually firm to palpation and nontender, do not blanch when pressure is applied, and do not itch (Fig. 33–4). Visceral and lymphatic involvement may result in pain if the tumor presses against nerves or organs. The incidence of Kaposi's sarcoma has de-

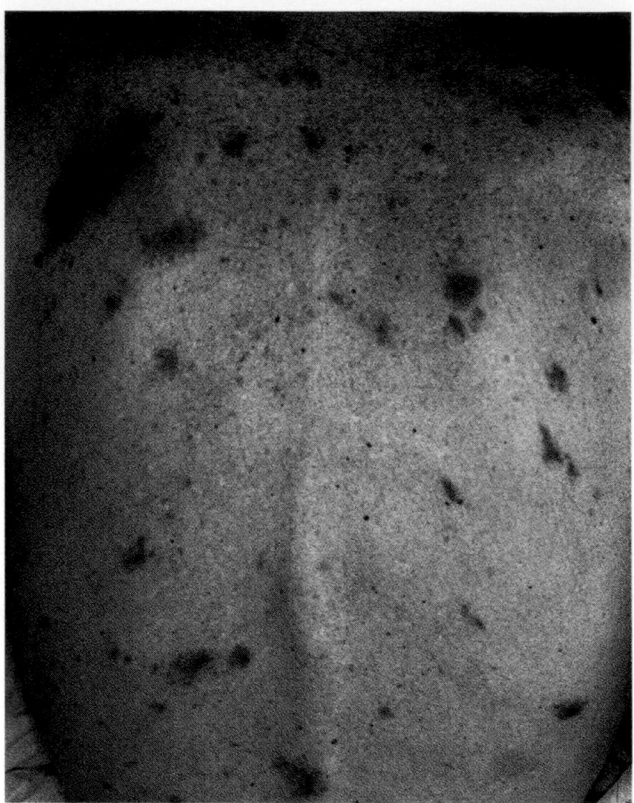

Figure 33–4

Kaposi's sarcoma. (From Callen JP, Greer KE, Hood AF, et al. Color atlas of dermatology. Philadelphia: WB Saunders, 1993, p 220.)

creased from 40% to 14% of all AIDS cases reported to CDC.

The most frequent pulmonary manifestation of AIDS is pneumonia caused by the protozoan *Pneumocystis carinii*. Prophylactic use of trimethoprim/sulfamethoxazole (Bactrim) (pentamidine [Pentam 300] for those allergic to trimethoprim/sulfamethoxazole) has decreased the incidence greatly. Symptoms common to *Pneumocystis carinii* pneumonia include fever, dyspnea, tachypnea, and dry cough. These are sometimes accompanied by chills and chest pain. Lung sounds and chest x-rays may be normal but, more often, they reveal diffuse interstitial infiltrates (Fig. 33–5). Arterial blood gases show a variable degree of hypoxia. A gallium scan may be used in diagnosing *Pneumocystis carinii* pneumonia. Other pulmonary infections that may be seen in persons with AIDS are those caused by cytomegalovirus and *Mycobacterium avium-intracellulare*. Kaposi's sarcoma can also involve the lungs. Other pulmonary conditions that may develop during the late symptomatic stage include *Haemophilus influenzae* infection, pneumococcal pneumonia, streptococcal pneumonia, and reactivated *Mycobacterium tuberculosis*.

Patients with AIDS may develop ophthalmologic problems from opportunistic infection of the eye by

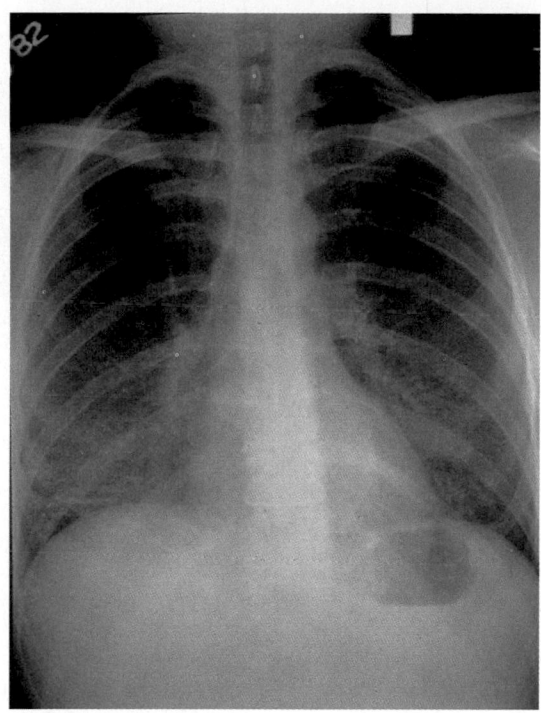

Figure 33-5
Pulmonary pneumocystosis. Chest x-ray shows interstitial infiltrates. (Courtesy of Jonathan W.M. Gold, MD.)

bacterial, fungal, and viral pathogens. Symptoms usually include blurred vision or loss of vision. Cytomegalovirus retinitis is a common problem, especially in advanced disease.

The heart, kidneys, and endocrine glands are less frequently involved in AIDS. A few patients have been found to have myocarditis or pericarditis caused by a variety of infectious agents. Renal involvement has included proteinuria, azotemia, and renal failure. Some patients with invasive cytomegalovirus infection have had adrenal insufficiency requiring supplemental steroid therapy. Others have developed hypercalcemia, suggesting involvement of the parathyroid glands.

In women, there are three important clinical manifestations seen in late symptomatic HIV disease:

Human papillomavirus
Cervical dysplasia and cancer
Vaginal and mucocutaneous *Candida* infection

These conditions may be aggressive, extensive, and difficult to treat. Other manifestations of HIV in women include genital ulcerative disease, cervicitis, and salpingitis. The relationship between HIV disease and pelvic inflammatory disease is being researched as well. The importance of HIV disease in pregnancy must also be considered.

Advanced HIV Disease
Advanced HIV disease occurs when CD4+ cell counts drop below 50 cells/mm³. At this stage, the risk of mortality increases significantly. In advanced disease, serum albumin and cholesterol levels drop, serum globulins rise, and anemia and neutropenia develop. More virulent and persistent opportunistic infections appear and are increasingly resistant to treatment.

Advanced HIV-1 associated cognitive/motor complex symptoms include confusion, vacant staring, disorientation, organic psychosis, seizures, mutism, urinary and fecal incontinence, hemiparesis, paraparesis, blindness, delirium, and coma. The life expectancy at this stage can be as long as 2 years but is frequently shorter.

Diagnosis

The diagnosis of HIV disease is based on a careful medical history and laboratory testing. The HIV test indicates whether antibodies to HIV are present in the person's blood. If the antibody test is positive, it is presumed that the person was infected with HIV at some time in the past, continues to be infected, and is capable of transmitting the virus to others.

When testing for HIV antibodies, two tests are usually done. The first is an enzyme-linked immunosorbent assay. If results of this test for antibodies are repeatedly positive, a confirmatory test for proteins specific to HIV is performed by the Western blot method.

Tests for HIV antibodies can have false-negative and false-positive results. False-negative results occur because there is a gap between infection with the virus and appearance of antibodies (called the window period). For most people, it takes 6 to 8 weeks until antibodies develop (seroconversion), but in some people it may take several months. False-positives can occur for a variety of biologic and technical reasons. For example, an infant younger than 6 months old may have maternal antibodies that cause a positive test result when, in fact, the infant is not infected with HIV.

Serial measures of the level of circulating CD4+ T cells are used to assess disease progression. Levels at or below 500 cells/mm³ usually correlate with early symptomatic disease. Levels lower than 200/mm³ correlate with late symptomatic disease and a worsening prognosis. CD4+ T cell levels also serve as the basis for the CDC classification system for HIV-infected adolescents and adults. The system is based on three ranges of CD4+ T cell counts and three clinical categories, the interface of which produces nine mutually exclusive categories (Table 33-3).

Viral load tests measure the HIV RNA in copies per milliliter. The viral load test is a better predictor for disease progression than CD4 counts. Whereas CD4 counts show where the patient is at the time, the viral load test predicts how quickly the disease will progress. Patients with a viral load of 20,000 have a 1% chance of disease progression in 60 weeks, whereas patients with a viral load of 200,000

Table 33–3

CDC Classifications for HIV Infection

CD4+ T-Cell Categories	Clinical Categories (Definition)		
	A (Asymptomatic; persistent, generalized lymphadenopathy; or acute [primary] HIV infection)	B (Symptomatic but not included in category C)	C (AIDS-indicator conditions included in the surveillance case definition [see Table 33–4])
1 >500/mm³	A1	B1	C1
2 200–499/mm³	A2	B2	C2
3 <200/mm³	A3	B3	C3

AIDS, acquired immunodeficiency syndrome; CDC, Centers for Disease Control and Prevention; HIV, human immunodeficiency virus.

have a 24% chance of disease progression in that time.

The diagnosis of AIDS is made when the patient meets the clinical criteria that have been established by the CDC (Table 33–4). As mentioned earlier, this diagnosis is used mainly for reporting purposes and not for clinical diagnosis or treatment.

Management

There is no known cure for AIDS. Current medical management consists primarily of treating infections and malignancies and administering drugs that inhibit or block HIV replication. Antiretroviral therapy with zidovudine (Retrovir, AZT), didanosine (Videx, ddI), zalcitabine (Hivid, ddC), stavudine (Zerit), and

protease inhibitors (saquinavir [Invirase], ritonavir [Norvir], and indinavir [Crixivan]) are used in various combinations. These drugs block HIV replication by inhibiting HIV reverse transcriptase or by inhibiting the protease enzyme. Newer classes of drugs—such as the protease inhibitors, interleukin 2, and peptide T—are being used to inhibit viral replication.

Treatment given early in the course of HIV infection delays progression to AIDS, but the effectiveness of combination therapy decreases over time. Development of drug resistance is believed to cause the decrease in effectiveness, and combination therapy seems to delay resistance. The introduction of protease inhibitors and nucleoside analogs is show-

Table 33–4

CDC Surveillance Case Definition for AIDS

I. HIV status of patient is unknown or inconclusive
   If laboratory tests for HIV infection were not performed or gave inconclusive results and the patient had no other cause of immunodeficiency listed in IA (see below), a definitive diagnosis of any disease listed in IB (see below) indicates AIDS.
   A. Causes of immunodeficiency that disqualify a disease as an indication of AIDS in the absence of laboratory evidence of HIV infection
      1. The use of high-dose or long-term systemic corticosteroid therapy or other immunosuppressive/cytotoxic therapy within 3 months before the onset of the indicator disease
      2. A diagnosis of any of the following diseases within 3 months after diagnosis of the indicator disease: Hodgkin's disease, non-Hodgkin's lymphoma (other than primary brain lymphoma), lymphocytic leukemia, multiple myeloma, any other cancer of lymphoreticular or histiocytic tissue, or angioimmunoblastic lymphadenopathy
      3. A genetic (congenital) immunodeficiency syndrome or an acquired immunodeficiency syndrome that is atypical of HIV infection, such as one involving hypogammaglobulinemia
   B. Diseases that indicate AIDS (requires definitive diagnosis)
      1. Candidiasis of the esophagus, trachea, bronchi, or lungs
      2. Cryptococcosis, extrapulmonary
      3. Cryptosporidiosis with diarrhea persisting for more than 1 month
      4. Cytomegalovirus disease of an organ other than the liver, spleen, or lymph nodes in a patient older than 1 month

Table 33–4

CDC Surveillance Case Definition for AIDS *(continued)*

5. Herpes simplex virus infection causing a mucocutaneous ulcer that persists longer than 1 month; or herpes simplex virus infection causing bronchitis, pneumonitis, or esophagitis for any duration in a patient older than 1 month
6. Kaposi's sarcoma in a patient younger than 60 years
7. Lymphoid interstitial pneumonia or pulmonary lymphoid hyperplasia (LIP/PLH complex) in a patient younger than 13 years
8. Lymphoma of the brain (primary) affecting a patient younger than 60 years
9. *Mycobacterium avium* complex or *M. kansasii* disease, disseminated (at a site other than or in addition to the lungs, skin, or cervical or hilar lymph nodes)
10. *Pneumocystis carinii* pneumonia
11. Progressive multifocal leukoencephalopathy
12. Toxoplasmosis of the brain in a patient older than 1 month

II. *Patient is HIV positive*
Regardless of the presence of other causes of immunodeficiency (see *IA*, above), in the presence of laboratory evidence of HIV infection, any disease listed in *IB* (see above) or in *IIA* or *IIB* (see below) indicates a diagnosis of AIDS. In addition, beginning in 1993, all HIV-positive adults and adolescents with CD4+ T-cell counts less than 200/mm^3 or with pulmonary tuberculosis, recurrent pneumonia, or invasive cervical carcinoma should also be included in the AIDS case definition.

A. *Diseases that indicate AIDS (requires definitive diagnosis)*
1. Bacterial infections, multiple or recurrent (any combination of at least two within a 2- to 4-year period), of the following types in a patient younger than 13 years: septicemia, pneumonia, meningitis, bone or joint infection, or abscess of an internal organ or body cavity (excluding otitis media or superficial skin or mucosal abscesses) caused by *Haemophilus*, *Streptococcus* (including pneumococcus), or other pyogenic bacteria
2. Coccidioidomycosis, disseminated (at a site other than or in addition to the lungs or cervical or hilar lymph nodes)
3. Histoplasmosis, disseminated (at a site other than or in addition to the lungs or cervical or hilar lymph nodes)
4. HIV encephalopathy
5. HIV wasting syndrome
6. Isosporiasis with diarrhea persisting for more than 1 month
7. Kaposi's sarcoma at any age
8. Lymphoma of the brain (primary) at any age
9. *M. tuberculosis* disease, extrapulmonary (involving at least one site outside the lungs, regardless of whether there is concurrent pulmonary involvement)
10. Mycobacterial disease caused by mycobacteria other than *M. tuberculosis*, disseminated (at a site other than or in addition to the lungs, skin, or cervical or hilar lymph nodes)
11. Non-Hodgkin's lymphoma of B-cell or unknown immunologic phenotype and the following histologic types: small noncleaved lymphoma (Burkitt's or non-Burkitt's) or immunoblastic sarcoma
12. *Salmonella* (nontyphoidal) septicemia, recurrent

B. *Diseases that indicate AIDS (presumptive diagnosis)*
1. Candidiasis of the esophagus
2. Cytomegalovirus retinitis, with loss of vision
3. Kaposi's sarcoma
4. Lymphoid interstitial pneumonia or pulmonary lymphoid hyperplasia (LIP/PLH complex) in a patient younger than 13 years
5. Mycobacterial disease (acid-fast bacilli with species not identified by culture), disseminated (involving at least one site other than or in addition to the lungs, skin, or cervical or hilar lymph nodes)
6. *P. carinii* pneumonia
7. Toxoplasmosis of the brain in a patient older than 1 month.

III. *Patient is HIV negative*
With laboratory test results negative for HIV infection, a diagnosis of AIDS for surveillance purposes is ruled out *unless*

A. *All the other causes of immunodeficiency listed in IA (see above) are excluded; and*
B. *The patient has had either of the following:*
1. *P. carinii* pneumonia diagnosed by a definitive method
2. A definitive diagnosis of any of the other diseases indicative of AIDS listed in *IB* (see above) and a CD4+ helper-inducer T-cell count of less than 400/mm^3

AIDS, acquired immunodeficiency syndrome; CDC, Centers for Disease Control and Prevention; HIV, human immunodeficiency virus.

RESEARCH ABSTRACT

What Factors Influence the Attitudes of Nurses Toward Patients with AIDS?

Baylor RA, McDaniel AM. Nurses' attitudes toward caring for patients with acquired immunodeficiency syndrome. J Prof Nurs 1996; 12(2):99.

In the past decade, the public has come face to face with the reality that we are now in the throes of a worldwide epidemic of acquired immunodeficiency syndrome (AIDS) and of widespread infection with the human immunodeficiency virus (HIV). Nurses encounter people with AIDS in many practice settings. Because of the life-threatening aspects of the disease, and because of its means of transmission, caring for patients with HIV/AIDS can be emotionally charged. The attitudes of nurses toward these patients may be influenced by many characteristics and life experiences.

Baylor and McDaniel therefore sought to discover whether factors such as age, education, and experience influenced the attitudes of nurses toward patients with AIDS. To determine the impact of those factors, they used a motivational theory (the Ajzen-Fishbein Theory of Reasoned Action) as the basis for a survey that was then mailed to 250 registered nurses selected at random. Over 60% ($n = 138$) of the sample responded.

Despite past research that showed that education was related to more positive attitudes toward patients with AIDS, the study conducted by Baylor and McDaniel did not support such a relationship. Also, the researchers found that as years of experience as a nurse increased among the nurses in the sample, attitudes toward homosexuality became less positive. Also, the researchers found that the age of the nurses was not related to any of the attitude scores.

The researchers wondered whether the attitudes of the nurses were related to the amount of actual experience they had in caring for patients with AIDS. They did find such a relationship. The nurses who had more experience in caring for patients with AIDS had more positive attitudes toward health-care use by patients with AIDS and toward homosexuality. However, the researchers did not collect information about the specific types of AIDS-related caregiving experiences that the nurses had. The authors caution against assuming a cause-and-effect relationship between experience with AIDS and positive attitudes toward patients with AIDS. They suggest that the differences in attitude may have been present before the nurses actually worked with people with AIDS.

The researchers are also careful to point out the limits of generalizability. This research sample was drawn from only one midwestern American state, and this factor might have shaped the attitudes of nurses in unique ways.

Questions to Consider

1. What influences in your life have shaped your current attitudes toward caring for people with AIDS?

2. How have your attitudes toward people with AIDS changed over the past few years?

3. How would you rate the attitudes of your classmates toward caring for people with AIDS?

4. Listen to the conversations of nurses in report and on the various clinical units. What differences do you detect in the attitudes of nurses toward people with AIDS and their attitudes toward people with other medical conditions?

5. What classroom and clinical experiences with HIV and AIDS have you had in your nursing program?

6. What opportunities do you have to discuss concerns you may have about caring for people with AIDS?

7. If you know someone with AIDS, how has your relationship with that person shaped your attitudes toward caring for people with AIDS?

ing great promise for extending the lives of patients with HIV disease. New drugs are being introduced each month, and some researchers hope to completely eliminate the virus in the future (Kim et al, 1996).

One of the great challenges in managing HIV is maintaining nutritional status. Gastrointestinal disturbances and muscle wasting are an ongoing problem for many patients. Drugs to increase appetite, such as dronabinol (Marinol), and dietary supplements such as Ensure are commonly prescribed.

Thalidomide has shown promise in preventing wasting but remains controversial for approved use.

Infections are treated early and aggressively because this usually produces a better outcome than delaying treatment until the infection becomes severe. Prophylactic anti-infectives are often given to prevent recurrence of *Pneumocystis carinii* pneumonia, lesions caused by the herpes simplex virus, and candidal infections.

The life expectancy of persons infected with HIV has increased because of our growing knowledge of the disease process, the advent of antiretroviral drugs, and the ability to treat or prevent many of the more common opportunistic infections.

❖ Settings, Providers, and Collaboration for Care

More and more patients are being managed in home care settings with only occasional hospitalization for acute infections or problems. Group homes are commonly available in larger cities to provide assisted living arrangements for persons with HIV who have no other way to live semi-independently. Home health nurses, hospice nurses, and caregivers often work closely alongside family members in caring for persons with HIV. Referrals to other health-care providers may augment the care of the person with HIV.

A social worker or case manager usually becomes the most important person in coordinating services for a person with HIV. The challenge for the case manager is great because the patient's needs may vary from week to week and even day to day. The case manager helps the patient with referrals to social services, food pantries, or support groups. A counselor may be needed to assist with grief and loss issues. The challenge of referrals may be particularly difficult in rural areas, where travel distances are great, public transportation is limited, and many social services available in larger cities do not exist.

Several AIDS-specific services are available through public health agencies but are dwindling in a time of government cost cutting. HOPWA (Housing of Persons with AIDS) is one such service where monies are made available to assist with rental or mortgage payments to prevent persons with AIDS from becoming homeless. State medication programs may be available to help patients pay for a limited number of medications. Federal dollars from the Ryan White Entitlement bill are available for early intervention services. Many of the programs are administered through state and regional health or HIV-related agencies.

Many patients choose complementary therapies—such as vitamins, herbs, or faith healing—in addition to their conventional medical management. It is important to acknowledge the use of complementary therapies and to create a trusting atmosphere in which the patient feels safe in sharing this information. Referrals to reputable caregivers, such as massage therapists, nurses trained in therapeutic touch, or practitioners of biofeedback, may be very helpful to the patient. The nurse can be instrumental in helping the patient sort out legitimate treatment from quackery in order to spend health-care dollars wisely.

Legal and financial advice may be very important early in the course of HIV. Patients should be encouraged to put their legal and financial affairs in order as soon as possible, to prepare a will, to designate medical and legal power of attorney, and to develop advance directives. The nurse can be instrumental in raising these issues and guiding the patient to an attorney familiar with HIV issues.

Hospice is an invaluable resource to help manage patients in the home in the terminal stage of HIV disease. Nurses are available through hospice to provide daily care. Volunteers, chaplains, social workers, and others are commonly available to help with practical, emotional, and spiritual assistance. Medical equipment such as beds, bedside commodes, canes, and walkers can commonly be provided as well.

Although home care may be complex to coordinate, it is usually of great benefit to the patient and loved ones. The experience of caring for someone at home can be a healing and rewarding experience for all those involved.

NURSING PROCESS GUIDELINES
Late Symptomatic and Advanced HIV Disease (AIDS)

Nursing assessment of the patient with AIDS is highly complex because many physical, psychologic, and social issues confront the patient. In addition, the patient's status may change frequently and quickly as new infections and problems develop. Today, many patients are cared for at home with only episodic hospitalizations. Thus, it is important to assess living situation, family support, and other resources available to the patient.

Perform a head-to-toe physical assessment. Obtain a detailed description of current symptoms and their severity. Inspect the patient's skin and mouth for lesions and signs of infection. In the mouth, look specifically for white patches that indicate candidal infection or hairy leukoplakia. Also look for herpes simplex lesions. These are common causes of oral infections in persons with HIV infection. Question the patient about soreness of the mouth, bleeding gums, and difficulty chewing or swallowing.

Ask the patient about weight loss, change in appetite, abdominal pain, and diarrhea. If diarrhea is a problem, ask which remedies have been tried and how effective they were. Assess for signs of dehydration. Also obtain a dietary history to determine the adequacy of the patient's nutritional intake and whether foods being eaten might contribute to hyperactivity of the bowel.

Carefully assess respiratory status, because people with AIDS risk developing respiratory difficulties. Check pulse and respiration, color, and lung sounds. Question the patient about cough, chest pain, and sputum production. If available, review arterial blood gas values or pulse oximetry readings.

Determine the patient's baseline mental status so that changes can be identified. Remember that mental status may change because of the disease itself, opportunistic infections of the central nervous system, metabolic abnormalities caused by other problems, the adverse effects of drugs, or depression. As part of the neurologic assessment, determine the patient's ability to pay attention, to concentrate, and to follow commands. Assess the patient's orientation, reflexes, responses, and gait. Also assess memory, speech, judgment, and mood. Ask family or significant others whether changes have been observed in these parameters.

Assess the patient's emotional status and coping ability. Many patients with HIV infection complain of feeling isolated and alone. These feelings may result from the patient's fear of acknowledging the diagnosis and sharing feelings about it, or from the withdrawal of family, friends, or acquaintances. Keep in mind that—in cases where the patient is homosexual, bisexual, or an intravenous drug user—family and friends may have been unaware of that fact until the time AIDS is diagnosed. This, too, can contribute to withdrawal. Patients infected by a sexual partner may also feel betrayed.

Explore the patient's current ability for self-care,

including (for outpatients) such home management issues as food preparation, shopping, transportation to and from medical facilities, home maintenance, and physical layout of the home. Ask about existing support for psychosocial as well as physical needs from family and friends. Because of the chronic, debilitating nature of HIV disease, assess the family's need for respite care and in-home assistance. Explore the patient's and family's understanding of the disease and its transmission, infections that may develop, available treatment methods, self-care, and available community resources. Infection control guidelines for caring for AIDS patients in the home are listed in Highlight 33–1. These guidelines help protect the caregiver as well as the patient.

Pain and discomfort from a wide variety of causes can be a major problem for the patient with AIDS.

One of the most pervasive and difficult symptoms of HIV disease to manage is an alteration in nutritional status, such as cachexia. Malnutrition and weight loss are a major determinant of the course of

---

HIGHLIGHT
33–1

HEALTH PROMOTION & RISK REDUCTION

Infection-Control Guidelines for Caregivers of People with HIV/AIDS

Wash hands thoroughly with soap and water before and after giving direct care and preparing foods and in between preparing different food items.

Wear latex gloves when handling blood or body fluids. Rubber gloves made for household use should also be worn when cleaning up spilled body fluids. These can be disinfected and reused.

Cover any cuts or broken skin that may come into contact with blood or body fluids with Band-Aids.

When using needles, be very careful to avoid needle sticks. Place used needles in a puncture-proof container (such as a coffee can) immediately after use. Never recap, bend, or break a needle. Keep a puncture-proof container in every room where needles are used and discarded.

Wash the patient's dishes in hot soapy water. Patients with HIV infection do not require separate dishes or eating utensils.

Use typical cleansers for household cleaning. Clean the bathroom regularly with a household disinfectant. Clean up blood spills with a diluted bleach solution (1 part bleach mixed with 10 parts water). Wear gloves for this task. Make a new bleach solution every 24 hours, because old solutions are less effective.

Allow the patient to prepare food for others as long as he or she does not have diarrhea or open lesions on the hands or arms.

Do not share such personal items as a toothbrush or razor with the patient.

Wash clothing and linen in the usual manner with soap or detergent in either hot or cold water. It is not necessary to add bleach to kill the virus.

Prevent exposure of a neutropenic patient to people with active infections.

Protect patients with HIV infection from pathogens found in foods by taking these steps:

- Avoid raw or undercooked meat, poultry, fish, shellfish, or eggs as well as raw (unpasteurized) milk.
- Wash utensils before using them in other foods that are being prepared.
- Do not mix raw foods or their juices with other foods.
- Use a wooden cutting board rather than a plastic one, because plastic ones harbor more bacteria.
- Wash fruit and vegetables thoroughly.

AIDS, acquired immunodeficiency syndrome; HIV, human immunodeficiency virus.

the disease. Because many factors contribute to altered nutrition (such as metabolic disturbances, anorexia, nausea, and diarrhea), nutritional support should be aggressive and a high priority throughout the course of HIV disease. Tips to relieve nausea and vomiting are listed in Highlight 33–2. Oral infections can often contribute to altered nutritional status. Good oral hygiene is important to maintain appetite and ability to eat (Highlight 33–3).

Infections can be complex problems that affect patients with HIV infection. They can cause respiratory distress, gastrointestinal distress, blindness, and mental deterioration. Even a minor infection can be life-threatening. Identifiable infections are treated if therapy is available, and many times prophylaxis is implemented.

Nursing care of HIV-infected patients varies greatly from patient to patient depending on which infections develop and the severity of the disease. A summary of a sample care plan is shown in Nursing

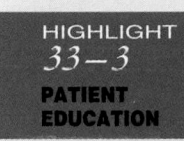 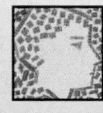

HIGHLIGHT 33–3
PATIENT EDUCATION
Oral Care for the Patient with HIV Infection

Instruct the patient experiencing oral infections or conditions associated with HIV infection to:

Clean the teeth and gums with a soft gauze pad instead of a brush.

Use mouthwash that does not contain alcohol or other astringent agents.

Lubricate the lips.

Avoid irritating foods, such as those that are spicy, contain a lot of acid, are very hot, or are difficult to chew.

Use a local anesthetic, such as viscous lidocaine (Xylocaine), for discomfort.

Obtain treatment for oral infections such as those caused by *Candida* and Herpes simplex virus.

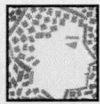

HIGHLIGHT 33–2
PATIENT EDUCATION
Tips to Relieve Nausea in People with AIDS

Take nausea-causing medications after eating rather than before.

Avoid large meals. Instead, eat smaller meals more frequently throughout the day.

Eat slowly and chew foods thoroughly for easy digestion.

Do not drink liquids with meals. Take liquids 1 hour before or after meals.

If nausea is a problem in the morning, eat dry foods—such as cereal, toast, or crackers—before getting up.

Avoid strong smells by eating foods cold or at room temperature.

Avoid sweet, fried, or fatty foods. Eat bland or salty foods.

Suck on ice cubes, mints, or tart candies.

Rest in a chair after eating but do not lie flat for at least 2 hours.

Breathe deeply and slowly when feeling nauseated.

Take antiemetics 30 minutes before meals if nausea persists or is associated with food intake.

Adapted from Beal JA, Martin BM. The clinical management of wasting and malnutrition in HIV/AIDS. AIDS Patient Care 1995; 9(2):70.

Care Guide 33–1. Care becomes increasingly complex as more problems develop and the patient becomes more acutely ill. Much of the patient's care can be provided in an outpatient or home setting, with hospitalization necessary only when serious problems develop that cannot be managed elsewhere. For care at home to be successful, the patient must have needed support services. When possible, involve the family and significant others in daily care. Inform caregivers about changes that should be reported to the patient's health-care providers (Highlight 33–4). Be sure written information is provided as needed, such as for medications, dressing changes, access to the health-care system in an emergency, and so forth.

*H*ypersensitivity Disorders

Hypersensitivity disorders result when the immune system over-reacts to an antigen, causing tissue damage. There are four basic types of hypersensitivity disorders:

- Immediate (Type I) hypersensitivity reactions
- Cytotoxic (Type II) hypersensitivity reactions
- Immune complex (Type III) hypersensitivity reactions
- Cell-mediated (Type IV) hypersensitivity reactions.

(*Text continues on page 1483*)

Nursing Care Guide 33–1
Patients with Late Symptomatic and Advanced HIV Disease (AIDS)

Assessment Findings: Patient asks questions about HIV disease and transmission. Patient expresses uncertainty over clinical course, treatment, and ability to care for self.

Nursing Diagnosis: Risk for altered health maintenance related to lack of knowledge of etiology and transmission of the disease, clinical course, treatment, and self-care

Patient Outcomes	Nursing Interventions	Rationale
Patient explains that AIDS is caused by a virus that weakens the immune system and its ability to fight off infections or prevent development of certain malignancies Patient explains stages of HIV infection. Patient describes types of medical therapy available and their goals.	Explain to the patient what causes the disease, how it affects the body, stages of disease progression, and available treatments, both standard and experimental.	Helps patient cope with an uncertain future.
Patient describes ways HIV is transmitted to others. Patient identifies ways to reduce the risk of spreading the virus to others or acquiring additional sexually transmitted diseases, such as "safer sex" and not sharing needles.	Carefully explain how the disease is transmitted, and instruct the patient on precautions to take to avoid transmitting the disease to others. Include a discussion of safer sexual practices.	Helps patient maintain control, prevent reinfection of self, and infection to others.
	Instruct significant others and people caring for the patient in how to reduce their risk of exposure to the virus (Highlight 33–1).	Prevents infection of caregivers, and helps allay fears.
Patient lists symptoms that require immediate medical evaluation. Patient states where to go for medical evaluation. Patient states name, use, dose, route, frequency, and reportable side effects of all prescribed drugs. Patient describes health habits that promote healthy immune function, including stress reduction, smoking cessation, and good nutrition.	Instruct the patient in self-care. Stress the importance of a nutritious diet, appropriate rest for the management of fatigue, and following orders for prescribed treatments conscientiously.	Promotes sense of self-control.

(continued)

Nursing Care Guide 33–1
Patients with Late Symptomatic and Advanced HIV Disease (AIDS) *(continued)*

Patient Outcomes	Nursing Interventions	Rationale
	Be sure the patient understands basic information about prescribed medications, including the drug name, its intended purpose, the dose, when to take it, how to take it, and any side effects that should be reported.	Helps ensure proper use of medications.
	Instruct the patient on when to seek additional medical attention for symptoms that develop as specified in Highlight 33–4.	Fosters a sense of self-control.

Evaluation: Compare the patient's status with the expected outcomes. If the outcomes are not met, reassess the patient and revise the plan.

Assessment Findings: Patient verbalizes complaints of pain. Patient is restless and moaning or grimacing.

Nursing Diagnosis: Pain related to the effects of HIV infection on various tissues and organs

Patient Outcomes	Nursing Interventions	Rationale
Patient reports decreased pain level.	Assess the character and intensity of pain. Give analgesics as ordered, keeping in mind that they are often more effective when given on a regular schedule than on an as-needed basis.	Medications provide temporary relief of pain by altering perception or decreasing the reception of stimuli.
Patient describes correct use of prescribed analgesics.	Instruct the patient and family in proper use of analgesics.	Correct use of medications ensures better results.
Patient describes nonpharmacologic comfort measures specific to the problem.	Be sure the patient's basic comfort needs are met. These include proper environmental temperature, a comfortable place to lie or sit, ability to reposition frequently, and good personal hygiene.	These measures promote relaxation and enhance pain relief by reducing anxiety.
Patient reports that nonpharmacologic measures result in decreased pain.	Encourage activity as tolerated.	Complementary therapies can be very effective in managing pain and decreasing the need for analgesics.
	Teach and encourage the use of nonpharmacologic complementary pain therapies such as relaxation therapies and cutaneous therapies.	

(continued)

Nursing Care Guide 33–1
Patients with Late Symptomatic and Advanced HIV Disease (AIDS) *(continued)*

Patient Outcomes	Nursing Interventions	Rationale
	Provide guidance and instruction in application of heat and cold massage. Provide guidance and instruction in progressive relaxation, meditation, imaging, and slow rhythmic breathing.	

Evaluation:	Compare the patient's status with the expected outcomes. If the outcomes are not met, reassess the patient and revise the plan.	

Assessment Findings:	Patient's T-cell count is below 200 and patient's self-care practices for hygiene, food handling, and infection control are less than optimal.	
Nursing Diagnosis:	Risk for infection related to immunosuppression and insufficient knowledge to avoid exposure to pathogens	

Patient Outcomes	Nursing Interventions	Rationale
Patient takes anti-infective medications as prescribed.	If patients are on antibiotics or antifungals, instruct them about the name of the drug, purpose, dosage, side effects, and symptoms to report.	Knowledge of medications promotes proper use.
Patient describes methods for hygiene and infection control in home setting.	Instruct the patient and significant others in infection-control practices.	Knowledge of factors that increase risk of reinfection allows modification to reduce the risk.
Patient remains free of infection.	Teach sterile dressing changes and proper care of the device to any patient with a vascular access device.	
	Teach sexually active patients about the dangers of reinfection with HIV. Because the virus mutates, they may become infected with another strain that will exacerbate the current disease. Other sexually transmitted diseases are also a grave threat.	
	Patients should avoid animal droppings.	
	Emphasize the importance of hand-washing to persons with HIV and their caregivers.	Reduces spread of organisms by the hands.

(continued)

Nursing Care Guide 33-1
Patients with Late Symptomatic and Advanced HIV Disease (AIDS) (continued)

Patient Outcomes	Nursing Interventions	Rationale
Patient describes food handling techniques to avoid infection (such as avoiding raw eggs, washing fresh vegetables, and cleaning kitchen surfaces). Patient describes signs and symptoms of infection to report.	Stress the importance of proper food handling. Teach patients to avoid raw seafood, meat, and eggs. Teach patients and families to wash food and food preparation surfaces carefully. Monitor the patient for signs and symptoms of infection. Tell the patient to notify the doctor if they occur (see Highlight 33–4).	Reduces incidence of food poisoning that can be fatal in immunocompromised patients.

Evaluation: Compare the patient's status with the expected outcomes. If the outcomes are not met, reassess the patient and revise the plan.

Assessment Findings: Patient verbalizes complaints of anorexia. Food intake is inadequate for body requirements.

Nursing Diagnosis: Altered nutrition: less than body requirements related to anorexia, gastrointestinal pathogens, nausea, diarrhea, and malabsorption disorders

Patient Outcomes	Nursing Interventions	Rationale
Patient describes prescribed antidiarrheal, antiemetic, and/or appetite stimulant regimen accurately.	Instruct patient on proper use of medication.	Knowledge enhances proper use of medication.
Patient describes signs and symptoms of dehydration and means of treating or preventing its development. Patient lists foods to be avoided because of their irritating or stimulating effect on the gastrointestinal tract. Patient's fluid and electrolyte values are within normal limits. Patient is free of anal or perineal skin irritation from diarrhea.	Monitor the patient's weight, intake and output, calorie counts, and signs of dehydration. Teach the patient to watch for the same signs of problems.	Early assessment may prevent complications.
	Encourage nutritional supplements as tolerated. Significant others should be encouraged to provide appealing and nutritious foods and a dietitian should be consulted as needed.	Prevention of wasting can prolong life. Adequate nutrition has much to do with appetite. Patients with limited appetite must make the most of the food they do eat.

(continued)

Nursing Care Guide 33–1
Patients with Late Symptomatic and Advanced HIV Disease (AIDS) (continued)

Patient Outcomes	Nursing Interventions	Rationale
Patient describes ways to manage nausea and vomiting. Patient remains free of nausea and subsequent weight loss.	Teach patient and family how to reduce nausea and vomiting (see Highlight 33–2).	Involve the patient and family in care and monitoring for problems so early intervention can be instituted.

Evaluation: Compare the patient's status with the expected outcomes. If the outcomes are not met, reassess the patient and revise the plan.

Assessment Findings: Patient complains of soreness in mouth. Mucous membranes are dry and have visible sores or hairy plaques.

Nursing Diagnosis: Altered oral mucous membrane related to *Candida*, herpes simplex, or other infection

Patient Outcomes	Nursing Interventions	Rationale
Number of lesions decreases. Patient chews and swallows soft foods with minimal discomfort. Patient performs mouth care properly.	Provide frequent thorough oral hygiene. Carry out treatments for specific infections as prescribed. Instruct the patient in mouth care as specified in Highlight 33–3.	Infections of the oral mucous membranes can cause great pain and discomfort, and can affect appetite and nutrition. Minimizes pain, discomfort and anorexia. Fosters sense of self-control.

Evaluation: Compare the patient's status with the expected outcomes. If the outcomes are not met, reassess the patient and revise the plan.

Assessment Findings: Patient exhibits signs of confusion and dementia, such as lack of orientation, depression, and changes in reflexes, responses, and gait.

Nursing Diagnosis: Altered thought processes related to underlying disease process, opportunistic infections, or medications

Patient Outcomes	Nursing Interventions	Rationale
Changes in neurologic status are detected promptly and responded to appropriately.	Monitor for changes in thought processes by checking patient orientation, reflexes, responses, and gait. Arrange for prompt medical evaluation if changes occur.	Early intervention can prevent injury and complications.
Patient remains free of injury.	Monitor the patient for suicidal ideation, and refer to a mental health professional if indicated.	Terminally ill patients may become depressed and suicidal.

(continued)

Nursing Care Guide 33–1
Patients with Late Symptomatic and Advanced HIV Disease (AIDS) *(continued)*

Patient Outcomes	Nursing Interventions	Rationale
	Arrange for assistive devices (such as walker, cane, bedside commode, etc.) as needed.	Prevents potential sources of injury.
	Provide additional supervision and assistance with normal activities as needed.	
	Assist the patient and family in identifying potential physical hazards and in providing a safe living environment.	
Patient maintains mental orientation as long as possible.	Keep changes to a minimum.	The patient functions best in an environment that is familiar.
	Establish a daily routine, and be as consistent as possible with staff assignments.	
	Orient the patient as needed.	Maintains orientation as long as possible.
	Avoid giving central nervous system depressant drugs when possible.	
	When giving care, use simple explanations and clear directions given one at a time.	Minimizes distress to patient.

Evaluation: Compare the patient's status with the expected outcomes. If the outcomes are not met, reassess the patient and revise the plan.

Assessment Findings: Patient verbalizes feelings of isolation and awareness that friends and family members are withdrawing. Patient may express feelings of loneliness and missing touch.

Nursing Diagnosis: Social isolation related to stigma, people's fear of contracting the disease, lack of strength, or lack of motivation to maintain normal social activities

Patient Outcomes	Nursing Interventions	Rationale
Patient initiates conversation with professional staff, other patients, or social acquaintances.	Provide the environment and the opportunity for the patient to discuss the diagnosis and his or her reactions to it.	Helps the patient combat the sense of isolation and aloneness.
	Give back rubs, hold the patient's hand, or hug the patient.	Meets the patient's need for touch and encourages others working with the patient to provide appropriate physical contact.

(continued)

Nursing Care Guide 33–1
Patients with Late Symptomatic and Advanced HIV Disease (AIDS) *(continued)*

Patient Outcomes	Nursing Interventions	Rationale
Patient maintains regular contact with family or friends. Patient identifies support persons to rely on in the community. Patient describes available support groups and their meeting times and places. Patient participates in social activities consistent with physical condition.	In line with the patient's ability, encourage social interaction with other patients or with friends or members of a support group in the community. If the patient is bedridden and at home, arrange for contact with an organization that provides volunteer "buddies" or other assistance to persons with HIV infection.	Helps the patient maintain motivation. Prevents social isolation.

Evaluation: Compare the patient's status with the expected outcomes. If the outcomes are not met, reassess the patient and revise the plan.

Assessment Findings: Patient expresses feelings of anxiety, anger, and depression. Patient may withdraw or strike out at those around him.

Nursing Diagnosis: Ineffective individual coping related to an infectious, life-threatening disease with a degree of social stigma

Patient Outcomes	Nursing Interventions	Rationale
Patient verbalizes feelings and concerns.	Provide a nonjudgmental, accepting atmosphere. Involve other support persons such as chaplains, social workers, and psychiatrists.	Allows the patient to express feelings.
Patient identifies sources of support.	Encourage the patient's significant others to stay involved, and provide support and help to them in dealing with their feelings. Refer significant others to support groups and other resources for ongoing help.	Assists family in dealing with grief, helplessness, and other feelings.
	Administer medications to control anxiety and depression as ordered. Be sure the patient and family are knowledgeable about these medications.	Knowledge increases proper use of medications.
Patient discusses feelings about death and dying.	Help the patient deal with uncertainty about dying.	HIV infection is a terminal disease with widely varying trajectories. Provides practical and emotional support.

(continued)

Nursing Care Guide 33–1

Patients with Late Symptomatic and Advanced HIV Disease (AIDS) (continued)

Patient Outcomes	Nursing Interventions	Rationale
Patient prepares for death (makes a will, plans funeral arrangements, gives advance directives for health care).	Put the patient in contact with the local hospice organization. Explore with the patient preparations for death and dying, such as writing a will, making arrangements for power of attorney should the patient become unable to make decisions, making funeral arrangements, and providing advance directives for health care.	Helps patient and family deal with the reality of impending death and feel reassured that patient's wishes are known.
	Support the patient in preparations for death, and if involvement of significant others is desired, support them as well.	Assists patient and family in coping with difficult decisions and feelings.

Evaluation: Compare the patient's status with the expected outcomes. If the outcomes are not met, reassess the patient and revise the plan.

Assessment Findings: The patient is physically weak and unable to perform total self-care. The patient's home setting is less than optimal (for example, the caregiver works or is elderly).

Nursing Diagnosis: Risk for impaired home maintenance management related to incapacitating weakness

Patient Outcomes	Nursing Interventions	Rationale
Patient or caregiver identifies areas of home maintenance in which help is or will be needed.	Conduct early assessment to determine the status of the patient's physical, financial, psychosocial, and home environment to develop and implement the plan of care.	Early intervention can often prevent financial and emotional devastation.
Patient or caregiver identifies sources of assistance in the community.	Begin social service referrals as soon as a patient's HIV status is determined, preferably in the outpatient setting.	Early referrals help patient cope and maintain dignity.

(continued)

Nursing Care Guide 33–1

Patients with Late Symptomatic and Advanced HIV Disease (AIDS) *(continued)*

Patient Outcomes	Nursing Interventions	Rationale
Patient lives at home safely with medical and basic human needs met. Patient uses assistive devices when appropriate.	Refer to community services to help with transportation, meals, shopping, household chores, assistance with medication administration, and financial help.	Relieves many of the burdens associated with caregiving.
	Refer patients to volunteer groups devoted to this kind of help for persons with HIV infection or to hospice organizations or other community resources.	Provides specialized support by people who understand HIV disease.

Evaluation: Compare the patient's status with the expected outcomes. If the outcomes are not met, reassess the patient and revise the plan.

Assessment Findings: Patient and family members question the meaning of suffering and the meaning of existence. Patient and family may express anguish over the moral implications of HIV disease.

Nursing Diagnosis: Spiritual distress related to terminal illness with moral/ethical implications and stigma

Patient Outcomes	Nursing Interventions	Rationale
Patient verbalizes own meaning and belief systems.	Encourage open discussion of spiritual issues without being judgmental.	Allows patient to freely express spiritual concerns.
Patient initiates discussions about spiritual meaning of existence and suffering.	Listen actively. Help the patient find personal beliefs, even if they differ from yours.	Patients do not need routine answers. Instead, they need someone willing to listen, have empathy, and perhaps even struggle with eternal questions, such as "Why me?"
Patient expresses peace about personal belief system.	Assess the patient's need for spiritual comfort and provide whatever seems appropriate, from a chaplain, to a spiritual reading, to discussion, to simply being present.	Patients have a wide range of spiritual needs, not all of which involve conventional religion. It is important to individualize interventions to meet the patient's unique needs.

Evaluation: Compare the patient's status with the expected outcomes. If the outcomes are not met, reassess the patient and revise the plan.

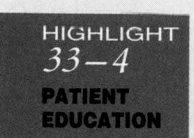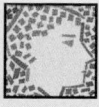

HIGHLIGHT
33–4
PATIENT EDUCATION

Symptoms That Require Immediate Medical Evaluation in the Patient with AIDS

Instruct the patient to seek prompt medical attention for any of the following symptoms:

New cough with or without sputum production

Shortness of breath or dyspnea on exertion

Increased fatigue or malaise

Fever

Night sweats

Headache

Stiff neck

Visual changes, such as floaters, blurred vision, loss of visual field, and sensitivity to light

Change in mental status, such as loss of consciousness or memory, forgetfulness, mood swings, and depression

Development of skin lesions

Pain

New or increased diarrhea, with or without abdominal cramping

Sudden, unintended weight loss

Increased size of painful lymph nodes

The terms hypersensitivity and allergy are often used as synonyms, but they are slightly different variations of the immune response. As the word suggests, hypersensitivity is an over-reaction or inappropriate reaction of the normal immune response to an antigen that results in tissue damage. Allergy or atopy is an altered or unusual reaction to an antigen that causes a deviation from the expected immune response. Hypersensitivity reactions may occur in all people. Allergic reactions occur only in people genetically predisposed to them.

IMMEDIATE HYPERSENSITIVITY REACTIONS (TYPE I)

Immediate hypersensitivity is an immunologic response that occurs within minutes after an antigen combines with the IgE antibody. Allergic reactions are included in this category. The most severe reaction in the group of immediate hypersensitivity re-

actions is anaphylaxis. See Chapter 11 for a discussion of anaphylaxis.

Allergy

Allergic, or atopic, reactions occur in people genetically susceptible to them. About 10% of the population has some type of allergy. Allergic rhinitis, commonly called hay fever, is the most common form of allergy. Less common forms include bronchial asthma, atopic dermatitis, gastrointestinal food allergies, and drug allergies. Examples of specific antigenic substances are given in Table 33–5. Allergy symptoms may start at any age, but most people begin to notice them during childhood.

The pathologic mechanism of allergy is basically the same as that of anaphylaxis, except that the target organs are different. IgE antibody is produced after the first exposure to the antigen. It binds to the mast cells in the target organ (nasal mucosa, bronchi, skin, or gastrointestinal tract). During subsequent exposures, the antigen binds with the mast cell–bound IgE, which triggers the release of chemical mediators.

ALLERGIC RHINITIS

Etiology and Pathophysiology
Allergic rhinitis is a Type I hypersensitivity reaction that occurs in response to inhaled antigens. Pollens, fungal spores, dust, and animal danders are the usual atmospheric allergens. Symptoms are localized to the nasal mucosa and conjunctiva. The etiology of allergic rhinitis is unknown, but there is substantial evidence that genetic factors are involved.

Clinical Manifestations
Typical symptoms of allergic rhinitis include a profuse watery nasal discharge, sneezing, swelling of

Table 33–5

Common Antigenic Substances	
Category of Antigen	**Antigenic Substance**
Drugs	ACTH, anesthetics (local), antibiotics (especially penicillin and cephalosporins), antitoxins, cocaine, dextran, gamma globulin, insulin, iodides, iron, IVP dye, radiographic contrast media, Telepaque, vaccines
Foods	Citrus fruits, eggs, milk, nuts, seafood, strawberries
Insect venom	Bee venom, fire-ant venom, hornet venom, wasp venom

ACTH, adrenocorticotropic hormone; IVP, intravenous pyelography.

the nasal mucosa (which can cause nasal obstruction), and itching of the nose and palate. These symptoms may be accompanied by intense itching and swelling of the conjunctiva, although conjunctivitis may also occur without nasal symptoms. The patient may experience some general malaise, but no fever. The intense sneezing may cause sore muscles in the chest.

Diagnosis

Allergic rhinitis is diagnosed primarily by history and physical findings during an attack. Nasal secretions may be examined for eosinophils, which will be numerous. The number of eosinophils in peripheral blood may be normal or only slightly increased. IgE levels may range from normal to somewhat elevated. To determine specific antigens to which the patient is allergic, skin tests are done as described in Chapter 35.

Management

The ideal treatment of allergic rhinitis is for the patient to avoid the antigen. Unfortunately, this is not always possible, making medical treatment with medication or desensitization necessary to control the allergic response.

Antihistamines are the drugs most useful in treating allergic rhinitis (Highlight 33–5). Antihistamines must be taken regularly to be most effective. However, these drugs have several side effects that tend to limit their use, including their tendency to cause sedation, dry mouth, dizziness, blurred vision, and nausea. Even the highly touted nonsedating antihistamines produce side effects and have not proved as revolutionary as they had been predicted to be.

Systemic corticosteroids are also very effective in controlling the symptoms of allergic rhinitis, but serious side effects limit their usefulness in treating an essentially benign condition. These side effects include increased susceptibility to infection, hypertension, and glaucoma. Given as a nasal spray, corticosteroids and cromolyn sodium can be helpful in controlling allergic rhinitis symptoms with few side effects. There appears to be little, if any, absorption of these drugs from the nasal mucosa.

HIGHLIGHT
33–5
PHARMACOLOGY

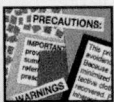

Antihistamines

Definition:

Class of synthetic drugs that inhibit the effects of histamine.

Action:

Attach to the histamine receptor sites on effector cells and thus prevent histamine from occupying them and exerting its effects. Also inhibit acetylcholine by a similar mechanism.

Uses:

Treatment of allergic disorders such as hay fever, urticaria, and drug, food, and cosmetic allergies.

Side Effects:

Dizziness, drowsiness, impaired coordination, inability to concentrate, dry mouth and throat, occasional nausea and vomiting, and insomnia.

Interactions:

Increase the central nervous system (CNS) depressant effect of alcohol, narcotics, hypnotics, analgesics, anesthetics, tranquilizers, reserpine, bromine, and scopolamine. Have an additive effect with anticholinergic drugs, which can result in urinary retention or constipation. Decrease effects of corticosteroids, estradiol, progesterone, and testosterone. Erythromycin and the antifungal agent ketoconazole slow the metabolism of terfenadine (Seldane) and can lead to toxic effects on the heart. Warning signs of a terfenadine reaction are faintness, dizziness, and heart palpitations.

Nursing Implications:

Caution patient against drinking alcoholic beverages or taking other depressant drugs while taking antihistamines, except on specific order of a physician.

Caution patient against driving or performing other dangerous tasks if not completely alert.

Instruct patient to take medication with food or milk if gastrointestinal distress occurs.

Suggest sugarless gum, sour hard candy, or ice chips to relieve dry mouth.

Suggest coffee or tea to combat drowsiness.

Instruct patient to discontinue use of antihistamines 4 days before scheduled allergy testing.

Geriatric Considerations:

Because elderly persons are particularly prone to CNS side effects of antihistamines, interventions to prevent falls or other accidental injuries are essential.

Desensitization is used for patients whose symptoms cannot be controlled with drugs and environmental controls. It is most effective in the treatment of allergies caused by pollen-producing plants. In this form of immunotherapy, the patient is injected with extracts of the pollen or mold spores that produce symptoms. These injections are given weekly in gradually increasing amounts until the maximum dose that the patient can tolerate is reached. Maintenance doses are then given every 2 to 4 weeks. This therapy may be given for 2 to 3 months before the onset of seasonal symptoms, or it may be given throughout the year. In either case, several years are required before the therapy achieves maximal effectiveness.

Desensitization is not a cure; rather, it allows control of symptoms. How it does this is not specifically known, although some suggest that it stimulates production of a new antibody (probably IgG) that prevents the allergen from initiating an allergic response. Because each desensitization injection carries a risk of systemic reaction (such as hives, an asthma attack, or even anaphylactic shock) all injections should be given by a health-care professional prepared to administer epinephrine if needed to counteract a reaction. For this reason too, the patient should be observed for about 20 minutes after the injection. Desensitization is not effective in every patient.

❖ Settings, Providers, and Collaboration for Care

Nearly all treatment of allergic rhinitis is done on an outpatient basis unless the patient has an anaphylactic reaction during the course of desensitization. Clinics or doctor's offices often provide desensitization schedules and provide patient education so the patient can manage symptoms through self-care. Many patients experiment with complementary therapies, such as acupuncture. It is important to help the patient determine if the practitioner is licensed or certified and reputable.

NURSING PROCESS
Allergic Rhinitis

Assessment

Determine what symptoms the patient experiences during an attack. Ask about:

Itching, burning, redness, or swelling of the eyes
Itching, fullness, or popping of the ears
Sneezing
Runny nose
Itchiness of the nose
Mouth breathing
Sore throat
Postnasal drip
Cough
Pain

Dyspnea
Sore chest or abdominal muscles
Dermatitis
Urticaria
Eczema

Obtain information about any family history of allergy, previous testing for or treatment of allergy, and the patient's usual daily environment. Is the patient exposed to dust, chemicals, plants, or animals on a regular basis? Also determine whether symptoms occur year-round or only in a particular season. Ask whether the symptoms are more pronounced at certain times, such as certain times of the year or month, weekdays or weekends, day or night. Ask if they increase during certain weather conditions, such as heat, humidity, cold, or rain. Ask if symptoms occur after certain activities, such as eating specific foods, mowing the lawn, or using perfume, hair spray, or other toiletries. And ask if symptoms correlate with exposure to animals, flowers, tobacco smoke, or paint.

Nursing Diagnoses and Planning

Nursing diagnoses and related expected patient outcomes commonly applicable to patients with allergic rhinitis include the following:

NDx: Risk for altered health maintenance related to lack of knowledge of the disease, environmental control, use of medications, or desensitization therapy

Planning: Patient Outcomes
1. Patient names the antigen(s).
2. Patient briefly explains how the symptoms are produced.
3. Patient describes different treatment options.
4. Patient describes the expected effects of treatment prescribed.
5. Patient lists ways in which exposure to the antigen can be avoided or minimized.
6. Patient describes a specific plan for incorporating the identified measures in his or her lifestyle.
7. Patient names each drug and states the dose, frequency, and route of administration.
8. Patient describes the side effects of each drug.
9. Patient lists things that are contraindicated when taking each drug, such as certain foods, activities, or other medications.

NDx: Pain related to itchy eyes, itchy nose, itchy oral mucous membranes, irritation from nasal secretions, and sore muscles secondary to repeated sneezing

Planning: Patient Outcomes
1. Patient avoids rubbing eyes or nose.
2. Patient describes use of measures to relieve discomfort.
3. Complaints of itchy eyes, nose, or oral mucous membranes are absent.

4. Nasal passages are clear.
5. Patient is free of sneezing.
6. Skin around the nose is free of redness and excoriation.

Nursing Interventions and Evaluation

NDx: Risk for altered health maintenance

Explain the disease process so the patient understands what triggers the symptoms and what happens in the eyes, nose, and throat to cause the symptoms. Explain that allergic rhinitis often occurs only during a particular time of year and that it is not a contagious disease and therefore cannot be given to others.

Help the patient identify ways to avoid the antigen in the environment. These will vary with the antigen involved and the patient's ability and willingness to make changes. If the antigen is an airborne pollen, explore the possibility of an air conditioner to help remove it, so that air inside the house is pollen-free. If the antigen is house dust and dust mites, instruct the patient to "dustproof" the home environment by eliminating furnishings that collect dust, such as drapes, rugs, and overstuffed furniture, by washing all bedding in hot water, using vinyl mattress covers, damp-mopping floors, and dusting with a damp cloth. Urge the patient to wear a dust mask while cleaning. If the allergy involves animal dander, suggest eliminating the use of down quilts or pillows. Also suggest that household pets be bathed frequently or, if necessary, removed from the home (Highlight 33–6).

Teach about prescribed medications. The patient should know the name of each drug, how much to take, when to take it, how to take it, how to use it if it is an inhaler or spray, and common side effects. Warn the patient that antihistamines can cause drowsiness. Also warn the patient not to take alcohol or other over-the-counter drugs with antihistamines because they can potentiate the drug effects.

NDx: Pain

Instruct the patient in measures that can be used to minimize discomfort. Discuss the use of gargles for sore throat and postnasal drip, cold compresses to soothe itchy eyes, and the need to avoid rubbing eyes.

Compare the patient's status with the expected outcomes. If the outcomes are not met, reassess the patient and revise the plan.

CYTOTOXIC HYPERSENSITIVITY REACTIONS (TYPE II)

Cytotoxic reactions produce cell damage. IgG or IgM antibody binds with an antigen on the cell surface. This antigen-antibody combination either triggers the complement cascade, which results in cell damage or cell lysis, or it may act as an opsonin and attract phagocytic cells that cause the damage.

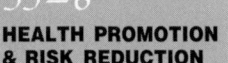 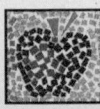

HIGHLIGHT 33–6

HEALTH PROMOTION & RISK REDUCTION

Preventing Allergic Reactions

The following strategies can help minimize the frequency and severity of attacks in patients with allergy, asthma, or both:

Use synthetic pillows.

Eliminate carpets and rugs if possible.

Eliminate curtains. Instead, use blinds or shades.

Avoid fur-bearing animals.

Avoid tobacco smoke.

Use an air filter.

Keep filters on central heating and air conditioning clean. Change them frequently.

Eliminate overstuffed furniture.

Use a vinyl mattress cover.

Use a damp mop and damp dust rag when cleaning.

Wear a dust mask when doing dusty tasks.

Cytotoxic reactions are the basis of several disorders, of which drug-associated hemolytic anemia is one example. In this disorder, a drug bound to the surface of the red blood cells acts as an antigen. Antidrug antibody then binds with the drug on the cell and initiates the complement cascade, which in turn destroys the red blood cells. Common drugs known to cause this reaction are penicillin, quinine, and quinidine.

This type of reaction is also responsible for the hemolysis of incompatible red blood cells after blood transfusion, and for the destruction of such other blood components as platelets, polymorphonuclear leukocytes, and lymphocytes. This reaction, when involving antibodies specific for the basement membrane of the skin, results in the skin blisters and bubbles characteristic of pemphigoid disorders.

IMMUNE COMPLEX HYPERSENSITIVITY REACTIONS (TYPE III)

Immune complex, or Type III, hypersensitivity reactions occur when soluble antigens react with antibodies, usually IgG, and form an immune complex that precipitates in body tissues and in the blood.

Serum sickness is considered the characteristic manifestation of the immune complex hypersensitivity reaction.

Serum Sickness

Etiology and Pathophysiology

Serum sickness was seen frequently in the early part of this century, when antiserum from horses was used to treat diphtheria, tetanus, gas gangrene, and other diseases involving toxins. A toxin was injected into a horse to induce the production of antibodies. Horse serum containing antibodies was then injected into the patient in the hope that the antibodies would inactivate the toxin present in the patient's system. Now serum sickness is induced primarily by drugs (such as penicillin, cephalosporins, sulfonamide, and dextrans) and by antilymphocyte serum.

Several days after injection of the antigen, the body begins to produce antibodies specific for that antigen. These antibodies combine with the antigen, and immune complexes are formed. These immune complexes are deposited in various tissues throughout the body. The complement cascade is activated by these immune complexes. This activation of complement results in tissue damage and inflammation at the site of the immune complexes. This tissue damage and inflammation produce the symptoms of the immune complex hypersensitivity reaction.

Clinical Manifestations

Symptoms of serum sickness develop several days to 3 weeks after initial administration of the antigen. They include:

Fever
Malaise
Rash or hives
Extensive edema of the face, neck, and joints
Arthralgia
Lymphadenopathy
Splenomegaly

These symptoms last for 1 to 2 weeks and then gradually subside. If the patient was previously exposed to the antigen, the symptoms appear within 2 to 5 days because antibodies are produced much more quickly during a secondary immune response.

Diagnosis

Diagnosis of serum sickness is based primarily on the clinical symptoms and history. Laboratory findings include slight leukocytosis, increased erythrocyte sedimentation rate, proteinuria, hematuria, and casts. Electrocardiographic abnormalities are not unusual in serum sickness.

Management

Medical management is directed at relieving symptoms. Antihistamines and analgesics are usually enough to make the patient comfortable. If they do not relieve the patient's symptoms, corticosteroids may be used.

NURSING PROCESS
Serum Sickness

Assessment

Assess the patient's symptoms. Determine their severity and their impact on overall well-being. Observe for hives or rash. Question the patient about itching, and note if the patient is scratching. Also observe for edema and, if present, note the location, extent, and any effect on function. For example, does edema of the face and neck interfere with vision and eye opening? With enunciation? With swallowing? Question the patient about joint pain and note ability to move, walk, and carry out activities of daily living. Take temperature and other vital signs, and assess for enlarged lymph nodes. Assess the patient's knowledge about factors that precipitated the reaction, the expected course of the disease, prescribed treatment, and the need to avoid re-exposure to the antigen.

Nursing Diagnoses and Planning

Nursing diagnoses and related expected outcomes commonly applicable to patients with serum sickness include the following:

NDx: Risk for altered health maintenance related to insufficient knowledge of cause, expected course, prescribed treatment, and need to avoid re-exposure to the antigen

Planning: Patient Outcomes
1. Patient describes what caused the disease.
2. Patient states the expected action and common side effects of prescribed medications.
3. Patient explains the importance of avoiding re-exposure to the antigen.

NDx: Pain related to inflammation and tissue damage

Planning: Patient Outcomes
1. Complaints of joint pain are absent.
2. Patient is able to turn, sit up, walk, and perform activities of daily living.
3. Patient refrains from scratching.
4. Patient reports being comfortable.

Nursing Interventions and Evaluation

NDx: Risk for altered health maintenance
To help the patient understand the disease and its treatment and to avoid re-exposure to the antigen, explain what serum sickness is, what antigen caused the reaction, the 7- to 14-day duration of the disease, the gradual disappearance of the symptoms, and the need in the future to inform all health-care professionals about the reaction. In addition, explain the purpose and expected effects of all treatments and describe the reason for use and common side effects of prescribed medications. If the patient will be responsible for medications and treatments at home, teach dose, route, time, and frequency of

medications as well as the correct method of carrying out any treatments. Advise the patient to obtain a MedicAlert bracelet or necklace to wear at all times.

NDx: Pain

Administer medications and treatments as ordered, and institute palliative nursing measures. Examples include positioning and use of supporting pillows for the patient with arthralgia and cool compresses for the patient with itchy hives.

Compare the patient's status with the expected outcomes. If the outcomes are not met, reassess the patient and revise the plan.

Hypersensitivity Pneumonitides

Etiology and Pathophysiology

The Arthus reaction is another form of immune complex hypersensitivity from which hypersensitivity pneumonitides result. It is a severe localized inflammatory reaction that occurs at the site of repeated injection of a nonirritating but antigenic substance. The Arthus reaction is a model for immune-complex–mediated vascular damage. It is primarily an experimental phenomenon produced by repeatedly immunizing an animal until a high level of antibody has been produced. The antigen is then injected intradermally. The circulating antibody reacts with the antigen, and the immune response produces local tissue damage. The first symptoms are extreme edema and erythema around the injection site. Several hours later the center of the area becomes purplish-black. Over the next few days, tissue in the area necroses. The area heals in 1 to 2 weeks.

The hypersensitivity pneumonitides are human diseases that result from the Arthus reaction mechanism. After repeated exposures to an inhaled antigen, the patient produces antibodies specific to that antigen. Later when the antigen is again inhaled, it reacts with the previously produced antibody, forming antigen-antibody complexes in the interstitial spaces of the lung. These complexes activate the complement cascade, which results in inflammation and tissue damage in the lungs. Farmer's lung, caused by the inhalation of spores from moldy hay, is an example of this type of hypersensitivity pneumonitis. Other types of hypersensitivity pneumonitis and related antigens are listed in Table 33–6.

Clinical Manifestations

Symptoms of hypersensitivity pneumonitis include a dry cough, shortness of breath, fever, chills, myalgia, and malaise. These symptoms develop 4 to 8 hours after exposure and last up to 24 hours. The patient then feels healthy until the next exposure triggers the recurrence of symptoms. Pulmonary function tests and the chest x-rays may be abnormal during the acute attack but are within normal limits in be-

Table 33–6

Types of Hypersensitivity Pneumonitis and Related Antigens

Type of Pneumonitis	Causative Antigen
Bird-breeder's (or pigeon-breeder's) lung	Dry bird excreta
Cheese-worker's lung	Cheese mold or casings
Farmer's lung	Moldy hay
Laundry-worker's lung	Detergent
Malt-worker's lung	Moldy malt or barley
Mushroom-worker's lung	Moldy compost
Painter's lung	Paint
Plastic-worker's lung	Plastic
Wood worker's lung	Moldy wood dust

tween attacks. Chronic disease occurs from low-dose continuous exposure.

Diagnosis

Diagnosis is usually made by a careful and detailed history of the symptoms and physical findings during the actual attack. A test may be done in which the suspected antigen is inhaled and the patient observed to see whether symptoms can be replicated. A careful environmental and occupational history is essential for determining the causative allergen.

Management

The ideal treatment is avoidance of the antigen. When this is not possible, orally administered corticosteroids are used to help control the symptoms. Antihistamines and bronchodilators are not much help in controlling the symptoms of hypersensitivity pneumonitis because histamine and bronchospasm are not the primary cause of symptoms.

❖ Settings, Providers, and Collaboration for Care

Acute cases of hypersensitivity pneumonitis will often be seen in an emergency room setting but can be managed adequately on an outpatient basis. Patient education can assist the patient in seeking outpatient treatment and ultimately avoiding the antigen. A career counselor may be an important referral in helping the patient avoid an antigen present in the occupational setting.

NURSING PROCESS
Hypersensitivity Pneumonitis

Assessment

Obtain a description of the patient's symptoms and their time of onset. Also obtain a history of previous attacks, including when they occurred, how severe they were, how long they lasted, and the type and effectiveness of treatment employed. Take vital signs and note the depth, sound, and effort of respiration, along with the patient's color and any complaints of shortness of breath or chills. Assess the patient's understanding of the disorder, the offending antigen, and treatment. Assess the impact of the disorder on lifestyle.

Nursing Diagnoses and Planning

Nursing diagnoses and related expected patient outcomes commonly applicable to patients with hypersensitivity pneumonitis include the following:

NDx: Risk for altered health maintenance related to insufficient knowledge of cause and treatment of the disorder

Planning: Patient Outcomes
1. Patient describes the relationship of the antigen to the symptoms.
2. Patient states the correct use of prescribed medications.

Nursing Interventions and Evaluation

NDx: Risk for altered health maintenance
Teach the patient about the disease, the correct use of medications prescribed to relieve symptoms, the antigen causing the symptoms, and ways to avoid re-exposure to the antigen. For example, in many cases, the patient may be able to wear a mask when working in the area where the antigen is prevalent. Sometimes a filter on the air-handling system or a different type of system helps eliminate the antigen from the air. Some antigens are so prevalent in the environment that avoidance is not feasible for some patients. In these cases, it may be necessary for the patient to change jobs or lifestyle, or give up a particular hobby to avoid the antigen.

Compare the patient's status with the expected outcomes. If the outcomes are not met, reassess the patient and revise the plan.

CELL-MEDIATED HYPERSENSITIVITY REACTIONS (TYPE IV)

The cell-mediated, or Type IV, hypersensitivity reactions are also called delayed hypersensitivity reactions. These reactions do not depend on antibody or complement, but are mediated by sensitized T cells and the lymphokines they release. When sensitized T cells are stimulated by exposure to antigen, they release lymphokines, one function of which is to initiate the inflammatory reaction and attract phagocytic cells to the area. This type of response takes at least 24 hours to develop. Contact dermatitis is an example of a human disease caused by this mechanism.

Skin Tests

Skin tests to detect delayed hypersensitivity are a valuable diagnostic aid. These tests involve intradermal injection of an antigen. If the patient has been previously exposed to the antigen, erythema and induration (abnormal hardness of the tissue) occur at the injection site in 24 to 48 hours. The induration indicates that cells and plasma have entered the area, and this must be present for the response to be positive.

Skin tests are used to help determine whether the patient has been exposed to a specific disease. An example of such a test is the purified protein derivative (PPD) test used to determine exposure to tuberculosis. A positive skin test indicates only that the patient has at some point been exposed to that antigen. It does not mean that the patient presently has active disease.

Several skin tests can be done at once to determine whether the patient is anergic. Anergy is an impaired or absent delayed hypersensitivity response to an antigen to which the patient has been previously exposed. Anergy to several antigens indicates that the patient's cell-mediated immune responses may be generally impaired. This is not a good prognostic sign because anergic patients are more prone to infection, especially by viruses and fungi.

Graft Rejection

T cells and the cell-mediated immune response are primarily responsible for the rejection of grafted tissues. Graft rejection can be divided into three basic types: hyperacute, acute, and chronic. Hyperacute rejection, characterized by ischemia and necrosis of the graft, occurs within minutes to several hours of transplanting the graft. It may be caused by antibodies present in the recipient that respond to tissue antigens on the donor organ. A subcategory of hyperacute rejection, accelerated rejection, may occur within 2 to 5 days after transplant.

In acute rejection, T cells detect foreign antigens on grafted tissues, become sensitized, and then set the immune response into motion. Phagocytic cells are attracted to the graft by T cell–produced lymphokines. The inner lining of small blood vessels in the graft is damaged. This causes thrombosis of the vessels, resulting in tissue ischemia and eventual death of the graft. The graft may appear to be doing fine for 1 or 2 weeks before signs of acute rejection and failure begin to appear. Rejection usually occurs within 3 months, but could occur a year or more after the transplant. Immunosuppressive drugs are used to decrease or stop rejection of the graft.

Late or chronic rejection of the graft, which occurs months or years after the transplant, appears to result from immune complexes of IgM and complement that form in the blood vessels of the graft.

Table 33–7

Hypersensitivity Reactions and Resulting Disorders

Type of Hypersensitivity	Pathophysiology	Resulting Disorders
Type I Immediate	Antigen combines with IgE, triggering release of chemical mediators from mast cells	Anaphylaxis, allergic rhinitis, asthma
Type II Cytotoxic	IgC or IgM binds with antigen on cell surface, resulting in cell damage	Acute hemolytic transfusion reaction, autoimmune hemolytic anemia
Type III Immune complex	Antigen-antibody complexes are deposited in body tissues and complement is activated, causing tissue damage at the site of antigen-antibody complexes	Serum sickness, vasculitis, hypersensitivity pneumonitis, systemic lupus erythematosus
Type IV Cell-mediated	Sensitized T cells cause cell damage	Graft rejection, tuberculosis, sarcoidosis, leprosy, poison ivy

Immunosuppression does not stop this type of rejection.

The four types of hypersensitivity reactions with their related disorders are reviewed in Table 33–7.

Autoimmune Disorders

Autoimmunity is a condition in which the body reacts immunologically against itself. The body has lost some of its "self-tolerance" and is no longer able to precisely distinguish self from non-self. Autoimmunity may involve T cells, B cells, or both. An autoantibody is one that the body has produced in response to one of its own antigens. The mere presence of an autoantibody does not necessarily mean that an autoimmune disease is present. In fact, more than half of people 70 years old or older have at least one autoantibody.

The exact mechanism by which autoimmunity develops is not completely understood, although it is generally felt that suppressor T cells are important in helping prevent formation of autoantibodies. Several mechanisms for the development of autoantibodies have been proposed:

- A defect in suppressor T cells
- An alteration in a host antigen from a factor, such as a viral disease, that changes the surface of the cell or haptens that bind to the cell
- Exposure to a foreign antigen that is so similar to a self-antigen that the antibody reacts with either one (a cross-reaction)—thought to be the mechanism of rheumatic fever; antibodies formed to beta-hemolytic group A streptococci may cross-react with self-antigens on the heart muscle
- Abnormal stimulation of helper T cells
- Exposure of self-antigens that are usually hidden from the immune system, such as when tissue trauma occurs—specific examples include production of autoantibodies against heart muscle

following a myocardial infarction, against the lens after an eye injury, and against sperm after a vasectomy

A large variety of diseases may have an autoimmune component. They involve all body systems. As a group, autoimmune diseases have several characteristics in common. For example, they occur more frequently in women than in men. Usually, other family members have the disease or detectable autoantibodies. The disease improves with immunosuppressive therapy.

Selected autoimmune disorders are presented here. Others, such as rheumatoid arthritis, are discussed under the body system they affect most.

SYSTEMIC LUPUS ERYTHEMATOSUS

Systemic lupus erythematosus (SLE) is frequently considered the classic autoimmune disease. In SLE, self-tolerance is lost and the immune system attacks the body itself. It is a chronic disorder characterized by alternating periods of exacerbation and remission. It involves most organ systems and occurs most frequently in women of childbearing age.

Etiology and Pathophysiology

The exact etiology of SLE is not yet known, but several factors or triggering mechanisms have been identified. These include genetic predisposition, sex hormones, race, environmental factors (such as ultraviolet radiation, drugs, and chemicals) viruses and infections, pregnancy, fatigue, and physical or emotional stress. It appears that a combination of one or more of these factors, along with a defect in the immune system and possibly a genetic predisposition, are needed for SLE to develop.

The basic dysfunction in SLE is an imbalance in the immune system with depression of T-cell activity and greatly increased antibody production. Antibodies to DNA and RNA are produced, as well as anti-erythrocyte and anti-platelet antibodies. Other immunologic abnormalities found with SLE include decreased amounts of complement, positive rheumatoid factor, and false-positive results in serologic tests for syphilis.

The most important of the immunologic abnormalities in SLE is the presence of antinuclear antibodies in the serum. These antibodies are responsible for the formation of lupus erythematosus cells and immune complexes. Lupus erythematosus cells are polymorphonuclear leukocytes that have ingested immune complexes composed of antinuclear antibodies and complement combined with nuclear material from damaged cells. These lupus erythematosus cells are present in more than 80% of patients with SLE. A Type III hypersensitivity reaction occurs when the immune complexes formed from the antinuclear antibodies, complement, and DNA are deposited in veins and arteries, initiating the inflammatory process in these locations (vasculitis). This vasculitis can cause pain, swelling, and tissue damage in any area of the body.

Clinical Manifestations

SLE is a highly variable disease with no typical presentation. A whole complex of symptoms may develop suddenly, or symptoms may develop slowly, one at a time. Any organ or tissue may be affected at any time. In fact, SLE seems to randomly affect different organs. Symptoms depend on which organs and tissues are involved. Organs commonly affected at one time or another during the course of the disease include joints, skin, pleura, pericardium, heart, kidney, central nervous system, eye, and blood. The course of the disease also varies but generally seems to be most active in the first few years and then to gradually decline.

If SLE can be said to have any typical symptoms, they would include the following:

- Fever and fatigue that tend to occur before and during exacerbations but may be present to some degree all the time
- Migratory joint pain and stiffness
- Skin lesions, particularly an erythematous "butterfly" rash on the face across the bridge of the nose and on the cheeks, composed of discoid (round) or diffuse maculopapular lesions (Fig. 33–6)
- Pleurisy, pericarditis, myocarditis, noninfectious endocarditis, and hypertension
- Glomerulonephritis, renal dysfunction, and renal failure, which are the most serious problems to SLE patients and account for many of the fatalities
- Almost any type of central nervous system pathology, such as impaired cognitive function, psychosis, depression, seizures, peripheral neuropathies, cerebrovascular accidents, and organic brain syndrome
- Anemia, leukopenia, and thrombocytopenia

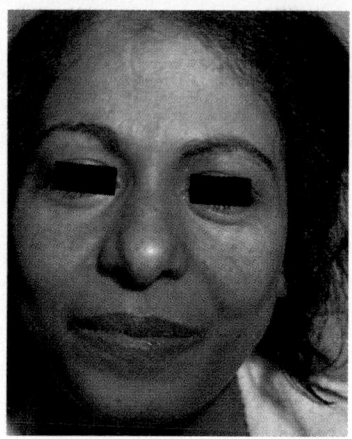

Figure 33–6

Butterfly rash that may accompany systemic lupus erythematosus. (From Lookingbill DP, Marks JG. Principles of dermatology. 2nd ed. Philadelphia: WB Saunders, 1993, p 225.)

- Anorexia, nausea, vomiting, and weight loss
- Hepatomegaly and splenomegaly

Diagnosis

Diagnosis of SLE is based on an evaluation of the patient's history and findings on physical examination. Because of the great variability of symptoms and the lack of conclusive laboratory tests, the diagnosis can be very difficult. Many patients go undiagnosed for years. The presence of 4 of the 11 criteria listed by the American Rheumatism Association in Table 33–8 is sufficient for the diagnosis of SLE.

Specific laboratory tests used in evaluating a patient for SLE include the antinuclear antibody test, the lupus erythematosus cell test, and the anti-DNA test. A positive result on any of these tests suggests SLE but is not conclusive because false-positive and false-negative tests results can occur. Examples of disorders that may test false-positive for SLE include rheumatoid arthritis, scleroderma, carcinoma, tuberculosis, hepatitis, and mononucleosis.

Management

Management of SLE aims to control inflammation and relieve symptoms. It involves ongoing medical care and avoidance of factors that cause exacerbations.

Drug therapy is individualized and depends on the type and severity of present symptoms. During periods of remission, no drug therapy may be required. In mild phases of the disease, aspirin and other nonsteroidal anti-inflammatory drugs are used to relieve pain and control inflammation. When symptoms are not effectively controlled by these drugs, as during periods of acute exacerbation, corticosteroids and immunosuppressants are used. Antimalarial drugs, such as hydroxychloroquine sulfate, are also sometimes used, particularly for patients with severe skin lesions. When all other treatment fails or the patient develops life-threatening complications, cytotoxic drugs may be tried. These are

Table 33–8

American Rheumatism Association Criteria for Diagnosing Systemic Lupus Erythematosus*

Criterion	Definition
Malar rash	Fixed erythema, flat or raised, over the malar eminence, tending to spare the nasolabial folds
Discoid rash	Erythematous raised patches with adherent keratotic scaling and follicular plugging Atrophic scarring may occur in older lesions
Photosensitivity	Skin rash from unusual reaction to sunlight, by patient history or physician observation
Oral ulcers	Oral or nasopharyngeal ulceration, usually painless, observed by a physician
Arthritis	Nonerosive arthritis involving two or more peripheral joints Characterized by tenderness, swelling, or effusion
Serositis	Pleuritis diagnosed by convincing history of pleuritic pain, rub heard by a physician, or evidence of pleural effusion Pericarditis documented by ECG, rub, or evidence of pericardial effusion
Renal disorder	Persistent proteinuria >0.5g daily or >3+ if quantitation not performed Cellular cast (may be red cell, hemoglobin, granular, tubular, or mixed)
Neurologic disorder	Seizures in the absence of offending drugs or known metabolic derangements such as uremia, ketoacidosis, or electrolyte imbalance Psychosis in the absence of offending drugs or known metabolic derangements such as uremia, ketoacidosis, or electrolyte imbalance
Hematologic disorder	Hemolytic anemia with reticulocytosis Leukopenia (<4,000/mm³ total on two or more occasions) Lymphopenia (<15,000/mm³ on two or more occasions) Thrombocytopenia (<100,000/mm³ in the absence of offending drugs)
Immunologic disorder	Positive LE cell preparation Anti-DNA: antibody to native DNA in abnormal titer Anti-SM: presence of antibody to SM nuclear antigen False-positive serologic test for syphilis known to be positive for at least 6 months and confirmed by *Treponema pallidum* immobilization of fluorescent treponemal antibody absorption test
Antinuclear antibody	An abnormal titer of antinuclear antibody by immunofluorescence or an equivalent assay in the absence of drugs known to be associated with "drug-induced lupus" syndrome.

*The presence of at least 4 of these 11 criteria establishes diagnosis.
ECG, electrocardiogram; LE, lupus erythematosus; SM, smooth muscle.

used with great care because of serious side effects, such as an increased risk of infection and renal damage.

❖ Settings, Providers, and Collaboration for Care

During acute exacerbations, patients with SLE may need to be admitted to the hospital to regulate medications and monitor symptoms effectively. During milder phases of the disease or during remission, patients may be managed quite well on an outpatient basis. With good support systems, such as family and support networks, even severely affected patients can be managed at home once medications are regulated.

NURSING PROCESS
Systemic Lupus Erythematosus

Assessment

Obtain a detailed patient history. Determine when the disease began, when it was diagnosed, what symptoms have occurred, what types of treatment have been used, and how effective they have been. Ask what symptoms are currently being experienced, what medications are being taken, and whether the medications are adequately controlling symptoms. Explore the patient's understanding of the disease and its treatment, the effect it has had on the patient's lifestyle and personal and family relationships, and how the patient is coping with this chronic, incurable disease.

Because the effects of SLE are so varied, perform a head-to-toe physical assessment. Assess carefully for any signs of respiratory, circulatory, or renal dysfunction. Take the patient's temperature and observe for any signs of infection, because the patient with neutropenia or who is taking steroids is at increased risk. Observe for skin lesions and alopecia. Do a complete neurologic assessment. Check muscle strength and note joint deformity, stiffness, or pain. Review the patient's usual daily diet, and ask about anorexia, nausea, and vomiting.

Nursing Diagnoses and Planning

Because of the chronic, incurable nature of SLE and its varied effects on different organs and systems, almost all nursing diagnoses are at some time applicable to patients with the disease. Nursing diagnoses and related expected patient outcomes commonly applicable to patients with SLE include the following:

NDx: Pain related to joint inflammation or skin lesions

Planning: Patient Outcomes
 1. Patient reports joint pain or discomfort from skin lesions is relieved.
 2. Patient performs activities of daily living without signs of pain, such as moaning or grimacing.

NDx: Activity intolerance related to fatigue

Planning: Patient Outcomes
 1. Patient describes importance of remaining active while avoiding overexertion and fatigue.
 2. Patient describes how daily activities can be planned to include needed rest periods.

NDx: Risk for infection related to skin lesions, neutropenia, and steroid therapy

Planning: Patient Outcomes
 1. Patient is afebrile.
 2. Signs and symptoms of infection are absent.

NDx: Risk for ineffective individual coping related to the presence of a chronic, incurable disease and the need for lifestyle restrictions

Planning: Patient Outcomes
 1. Patient expresses feelings and fears.
 2. Patient participates in making decisions regarding care.
 3. Patient identifies sources of support.
 4. Patient maintains contact with family and friends.
 5. Patient continues usual participation in social activities.

NDx: Risk for altered health maintenance related to insufficient knowledge of disease, treatment, and self-care

Planning: Patient Outcomes
 1. Patient describes disease process of SLE.
 2. Patient lists factors related to exacerbations.
 3. Patient identifies ways to avoid exacerbating factors.
 4. Patient names prescribed medications and states the purpose of each.
 5. Patient states dosage of each medication and how and when to take it.
 6. Patient lists side effects of medications that need to be reported.

Nursing Interventions and Evaluation

Nursing interventions must be individualized for each patient. They must take into account the patient's knowledge of the disease and treatment, the symptoms the patient is experiencing, the severity of the disease, and the medications that have been prescribed.

NDx: Pain
Administer analgesic and anti-inflammatory drugs as ordered. When muscle or joint pain is severe, maintain bedrest and support affected joints with pillows. During periods of remission, do active or passive range-of-motion exercises to maintain joint mobility and, in the case of active exercise, to maintain muscle strength.

Keep skin lesions clean and dry. Encourage the patient to avoid touching, rubbing, or scratching lesions because these activities increase irritation and the risk of infection. Apply local preparations as ordered to control itching and decrease inflammation.

NDx: Activity intolerance
Help the patient structure daily activities around frequent rest periods to help avoid fatigue and overwork. Caution the patient against inactivity, which can contribute to fatigue, muscle weakness, and joint stiffness. Instruct the patient in self-management of fatigue (Highlight 33–7).

NDx: Risk for infection
Instruct the patient to guard against exposure to infection by staying away from people who have colds, flu, and other infections. Teach the importance of good hygiene, balanced diet, and adequate rest in preventing infection.

In the hospital, monitor the patient's temperature. If elevated, obtain blood, sputum, urine, and other cultures as ordered. Initiate protective isolation if severe neutropenia develops.

NDx: Risk for ineffective individual coping
Allow the patient to express feelings and fears and accept the patient's mood swings. Encourage the patient to make as many decisions about care as possi-

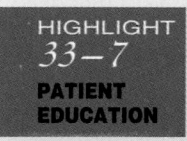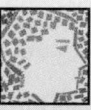

HIGHLIGHT 33–7
PATIENT EDUCATION

Managing Fatigue in Systemic Lupus Erythematosus

To help reduce fatigue, give the patient the following instructions:

Sit whenever possible.

Obtain a handicapped parking permit to conserve energy when shopping.

Avoid hot baths.

Delegate work when possible.

Do not rest for long periods because it promotes joint stiffness.

Schedule moderate low-impact exercise when not fatigued.

Maintain a balanced diet.

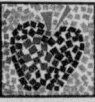

HIGHLIGHT 33–8
HEALTH PROMOTION & RISK REDUCTION

Protecting Against Ultraviolet Light Rays

To help the patient with systemic lupus erythematosus avoid excessive exposure to ultraviolet light, offer the following instructions:

Always wear an effective sunscreen with a high sun protection factor (SPF) rating.

Wear protective clothing (hat with a brim, long sleeves, pants, or long skirt) when outside.

Plan outdoor activities for early morning or late afternoon, when the sun is low in the sky.

Avoid indoor sources of ultraviolet rays, such as fluorescent lights, copy machines, and sunlight filtered through windows.

ble to foster a sense of self-worth and control. Focus the patient on the idea that she or he can learn to cope with the disease rather than be controlled by it.

Help the patient identify available support systems and refer the patient to social services or support groups as needed.

NDx: Risk for altered health maintenance

Teach the patient about SLE, what is known about the cause of the disease, its symptoms, how it is treated, and what course can be expected. Also teach about prescribed medications, including the name of each medication, its use, the dosage, when it is to be taken, and what side effects should be reported. If the patient is taking anti-inflammatory drugs, stress the importance of taking them exactly as prescribed. Abrupt discontinuation of the drug may trigger an exacerbation of symptoms.

Help the patient identify factors that can cause an exacerbation of the disease and ways to avoid them. For example, teach the patient to avoid exposure to ultraviolet light rays (Highlight 33–8). Other exacerbating factors include fatigue and overwork, emotional stress, injuries, and pregnancy.

Compare the patient's status with the expected outcomes. If the outcomes are not met, reassess the patient and revise the plan.

SCLERODERMA

Scleroderma is an autoimmune collagen disorder. It is uncommon and affects women two to three times more frequently than men. Scleroderma occurs in people of all races.

Etiology and Pathophysiology

The etiology of scleroderma is unknown. It occurs in both systemic and localized forms. The two types of the systemic form are diffuse scleroderma (progressive systemic sclerosis, or PSS) and a more localized form of the disease known as the CREST syndrome.

Diffuse scleroderma can progress rapidly and is potentially fatal. It is characterized by diffuse fibrosis in the skin and thickening of the blood vessel walls with narrowing of the lumens and ischemic effects in affected internal organs. The fingers, joints, esophagus, intestine, kidney, and heart are especially affected. Edema and inflammation of the involved tissue result from the ischemic effects and lead to fibrosis and excessive collagen deposits in the tissues.

In contrast to diffuse scleroderma, the CREST syndrome is more localized and more slowly progressive. It is an acronym for the manifestations that occur in the syndrome. These include:

- Calcinosis cutis (calcium deposits on tips of fingers and over bony prominences)
- Raynaud's phenomenon
- Esophageal dysmotility
- Sclerodactyly
- Telangiectasia

Morphea is the most common form of localized scleroderma. It is restricted to the skin and is characterized by asymmetric lesions. The epidermis is normal. The dermis is thickened, with an increased number of fibroblasts and collagen bundles.

Clinical Manifestations

Diffuse scleroderma most often begins with thickening of the skin on the hands or Raynaud's phenomenon. The skin becomes thick, smooth, shiny, and taut. Telangiectases may be prominent, and hyperpigmentation in a speckled light-and-dark pattern may be present. These changes are also common in the face.

The fingers become thick and edematous from ischemic changes caused by the vasospasm of Raynaud's phenomenon. Ischemic ulcers in the fingertips produce characteristic pitted scars (Fig. 33–7).

As the condition progresses, movement of the hands, face, mouth, and chest become limited. Respirations may be impaired, and contractures and atrophy develop. Esophageal stricture and decreased movement may make swallowing difficult.

Renal failure with severe hypertension is a frequent cause of death with systemic scleroderma. Pericarditis, conduction defects, and heart failure are cardiac complications. Pulmonary fibrosis occurs, as does weight loss and malnutrition secondary to esophageal strictures.

Morphea initially presents as one or more areas of purplish induration (Fig. 33–8). Over time, the center of the plaque becomes thick, firm, hairless, and dull white with a lilac-colored active inflammatory border. Inactive lesions are brown or yellow-

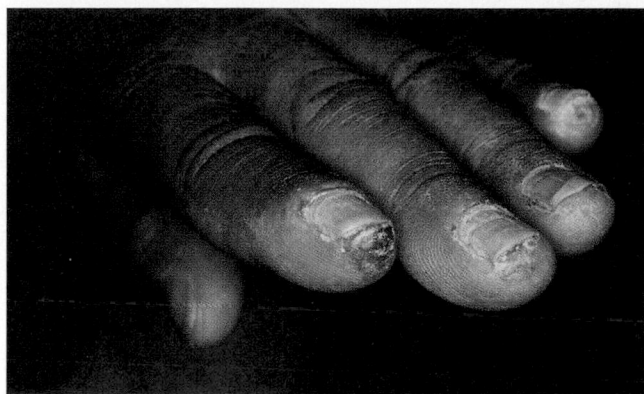

Figure 33–7

Scleroderma with severe Raynaud's phenomenon and ulceration of the fingertips. (From Callen JP, Greer KE, Hood AF, et al. Color atlas of dermatology. Philadelphia: WB Saunders, 1993, p 340.)

brown, and much of the thickening and induration may disappear. Morphea usually occurs on the trunk, although the linear variant is found on the head or extremities. Raynaud's phenomenon is not characteristic of morphea, and the skin does not appear "bound down."

Diagnosis

Both systemic scleroderma and morphea are diagnosed by the presenting lesions. A skin biopsy can confirm a questionable diagnosis.

Laboratory tests used in diagnosing diffuse systemic scleroderma include complete blood count, urinalysis, renal function tests, chest x-rays, antinuclear antibodies, pulmonary function tests, and barium swallow.

Management

Progressive systemic sclerosis resists treatment. Penicillamine (which prevents cross-linking of collagen

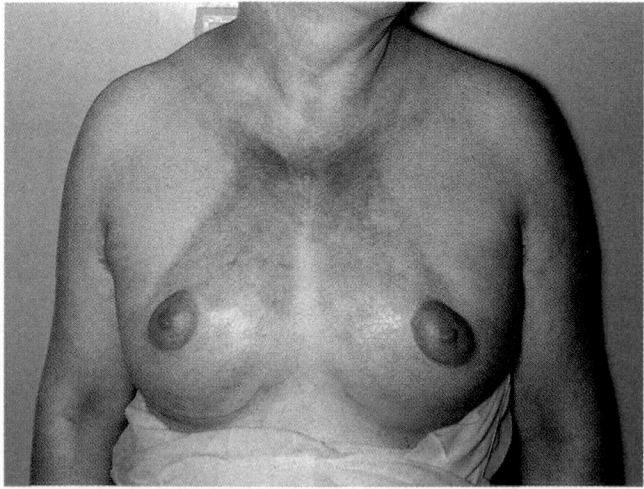

Figure 33–8

Morphea. (From Callen JP, Greer KE, Hood AF, et al. Color atlas of dermatology. Philadelphia: WB Saunders, 1993, p 253.)

fibers), colchicine (which inhibits collagen synthesis), and immunosuppressive drugs (such as prednisone and azathioprine) may be prescribed but usually are ineffective. Salicylates and nonsteroidal anti-inflammatory drugs may relieve musculoskeletal discomfort. Vasodilators may help reduce vasospasm in the hands.

Physical therapy for patients with sclerodactyly prevents flexion contractures. Cold exposure should be avoided; insulated gloves can help prevent vasospasm in the digits.

There is no truly effective treatment for morphea, although topical steroids and occlusion may result in some slight improvement. In most patients, it is a benign disease, and plaques resolve spontaneously.

❖ Settings, Providers, and Collaboration for Care

Nearly all cases of scleroderma and morphea can be managed on an outpatient basis. Physical therapy is prescribed outpatient for ongoing management. Since the disease is normally benign, hospitalization is rarely required. Referral to a physical therapist may be important to prevent contractures. A support group or counseling may also be effective in helping the patient cope with a disease that has no effective treatment.

NURSING PROCESS GUIDELINES
Scleroderma

Because systemic forms of scleroderma can affect many different parts of the body, a complete assessment with emphasis on the skin and other commonly affected organs, such as the esophagus, kidney, and lungs, is necessary. Nursing diagnoses, expected patient outcomes, and nursing interventions are based on the assessment. Depending on the extent of involvement, they will be similar to those for the patient with Raynaud's disease, rheumatoid arthritis, dysphagia, or kidney failure, as well as a chronic skin disease with risk for impaired skin integrity. Assure the patient that most systemic forms of scleroderma progress very slowly. For the patient with a localized form, stress that localized disease rarely progresses to generalized disease. Refer all patients to the Scleroderma Foundation for information and support.

AUTOIMMUNE HEMOLYTIC ANEMIA

Autoimmune hemolytic anemia refers to a variety of disorders characterized by increased destruction of red blood cells associated with the presence of antibodies specific for the red blood cell.

Etiology and Pathophysiology

In more than half the cases, the cause of autoimmune hemolytic anemia is unknown. These are referred to as idiopathic autoimmune hemolytic anemia. In the remaining cases, the cause is secondary to some event, such as a viral illness, a malignant disease, or use of a drug.

Antibodies responsible for this disease, which may be either acute or chronic, are classified as warm or cold depending on the temperature at which they are most active. Warm antibodies are the most common type. They are usually IgG-class antibodies directed at the Rh antigen on the red blood cell. These antibodies are not very active and tend to cause only a very mild anemia. Cold antibodies are most active at a temperature below 37°C (98.6°F). In fact, they are almost inactive at this temperature. They are usually IgM-class antibodies.

Clinical Manifestations

Symptoms vary depending on the extent of the anemia and may include fever, malaise, jaundice, and splenomegaly. The red blood cells are usually normal, but indirect serum bilirubin and urobilinogen levels in urine and stool are often elevated. Patients with cold antibodies experience a hemolytic episode after being chilled.

Diagnosis

The diagnosis of autoimmune hemolytic anemia is usually based on demonstration of immunoglobulins or components of complement on the patient's red blood cells.

Management

If the anemia is secondary to some other disease process, that disease must be treated to resolve the anemia. Blood transfusions are given only if the anemia is life-threatening, because the transfused cells are quickly destroyed. For patients with warm antibodies, corticosteroids are sometimes effective in controlling the hemolysis. For patients with cold antibodies, it is essential to keep them warm to prevent cooling to a temperature at which the antibodies become active. In some cases, particularly those of the idiopathic, warm-antibody type, splenectomy may be done to control the hemolysis.

❖ **Settings, Providers, and Collaboration for Care**

Autoimmune hemolytic anemia often must be treated in the hospital because laboratory studies are critical to proper diagnosis and treatment. Initial monitoring in a hospital is also important in case blood transfusions or surgery is required. Long-term management can be done on an outpatient basis. The patient should be advised to keep in close contact with a primary physician for monitoring of the condition.

NURSING PROCESS GUIDELINES
Autoimmune Hemolytic Anemia

Nursing care of the patient with autoimmune hemolytic anemia combines the care required by any patient with anemia with that required by a patient with the underlying disease. It must be remembered, however, that patients with idiopathic hemolytic anemia are often frustrated by the fact that the cause of their problem is unknown and by the lack of definitive treatment. Thus, it is important to allow the patient as much control as possible over his or her care. Keep the patient well informed about the therapeutic plan, and provide an opportunity for the patient to express feelings and reactions.

CHRONIC FATIGUE SYNDROME

Chronic fatigue syndrome (CFS) or chronic fatigue immune dysfunction syndrome (CFIDS), previously called *yuppie flu* or Epstein-Barr virus syndrome, is a nonfatal disorder characterized by unrelenting fatigue. It occurs almost exclusively in whites, and three-quarters of those affected are women. The syndrome has been diagnosed in persons of all ages, from children to the elderly.

Etiology and Pathophysiology

The etiology of CFS is uncertain. Chronic viral infection, immunoregulatory defect, and depression all have been suggested as possible etiologic agents.

In the late 1980s, CFS was thought to be linked to the Epstein-Barr virus (the main cause of infectious mononucleosis) because several common herpesviruses, including the Epstein-Barr virus, were found in the blood of infected persons. Subsequent research, however, showed that the viruses become reactivated when the immune system is impaired, and it is now believed that Epstein-Barr virus is a result rather than a cause of CFS. Microbiologic studies have been unhelpful thus far. Immunologic studies have also produced inconclusive results and the agent remains a mystery (Jones, 1994).

The role of depression in CFS also continues to be debated. In most cases, a psychiatric disorder is involved. Depression is the most frequent diagnosis, with anxiety and somatization disorder following. Some clinicians believe that depression causes CFS, although nearly one-fourth of patients with CFS have no symptoms of depression or psychiatric disorder. CFS has no simple explanation. It is a complex interaction of trigger factors, immune and possibly cerebral dysfunction, and social attitudes.

In CFS, the function of the immune system is disrupted, and abnormalities in cell-mediated immunity occur. The number of natural killer cells increases, but their cytotoxicity decreases. Production of interleukin-2 increases, and lymphoproliferative responses and production of gamma interferon following an appropriate stimulus decrease. Various abnormalities of peripheral blood lymphocytes have also been found, including an increase in the percentage of suppressor cytotoxic T lymphocytes. None of these findings is unique to CFS, however. In addition to immune system abnormalities, CFS patients have been found to have an abnormally low blood flow to one of the temporal lobes of the brain.

Clinical Manifestations

CFS typically begins with flulike symptoms: recurrent low-grade fever, pharyngitis, night sweats, cervical lymphadenopathy, body aches, and fatigue. Rather than disappearing, as in flu, the symptoms worsen. Persistent overwhelming fatigue or easy fatigability disrupts routines of daily living, and additional symptoms develop, such as muscle weakness, headaches, joint pain, memory loss, insomnia, and problems with vision, balance, and concentration. Physical findings are essentially normal and, because of the differing effect of the disease on various parts of the immune system, patients typically do not suffer from flus, colds, or other common illnesses, but may complain of acne, monilial infection, or shingles. Symptoms persist for an average of 3.5 to 4 years, with many people showing improvement after a year. About 1 in 5 people seem to recover fully, whereas 1 in 20 remain so ill as to be homebound or bedridden.

Diagnosis

CFS is diagnosed based on criteria developed by the CDC (Table 33–9). There is no definitive diagnostic test available.

Management

There is no generally accepted treatment for CFS. Immunoregulatory therapy in the form of high doses of intravenous immunoglobulin G has been reported to effectively reduce symptoms in some patients, but the treatment is costly and the effect of such therapy remains debatable (Lloyd et al, 1990). Supportive therapy and symptomatic treatment is often the only avenue of medical management.

❖ Settings, Providers, and Collaboration for Care

The treatment for CFS is virtually always handled on an outpatient basis. Much of the treatment occurs in a home setting, making the family an important element of treatment as well as an important support system. Patient education is important in helping patients conserve energy and pace activities. A referral to a support group or help-line may assist the patient in coping with a chronic, often debilitating disease that has no accepted treatment.

NURSING PROCESS
Chronic Fatigue Syndrome

Assessment

Obtain a history of the patient's symptoms. Determine what the symptoms are, when they began, and how they have affected the patient's daily function and overall lifestyle. Explore their effects on occupation, role responsibilities, family, and finances.

Nursing Diagnoses and Planning

Nursing diagnoses and related expected patient outcomes commonly applicable to patients with CSF include the following:

NDx: Fatigue related to the pathologic effects of chronic fatigue syndrome

Planning: Patient Outcomes
1. Patient expresses feelings and concerns about the effects of fatigue on his or her life.
2. Patient sets priorities for daily, weekly, and monthly activities.
3. Patient schedules activities and rest periods according to individual tolerance.
4. Patient participates as tolerated in a balance of activities that contribute to physical and psychosocial well-being.

NDx: Risk for altered family processes related to difficulty adjusting to changes in patient, roles, routines, etc.

Planning: Patient Outcomes
1. Family members verbalize feelings about the patient's illness and the resulting changes in patterns of daily living and lifestyle.
2. Family members support the ill person's attempts to cope.
3. Family members maintain a supportive relationship with one another.
4. Family members use available external resources as needed.

Table 33–9

CDC Criteria for Diagnosing Chronic Fatigue Syndrome

Symptoms develop over a few hours to a few days.
- Temperature of 37.5° to 38.6°C (99.5° to 101.5°F) or chills
- Painful cervical or axillary lymphadenopathy
- Unexplained generalized muscle weakness
- Muscle discomfort or pain
- Prolonged (24 hours or more) generalized fatigue after levels of exercise that would have been easily tolerated previously
- Headaches different in type, severity, or pattern from any previously experienced
- Arthralgia without edema or erythema
- Mental disturbances, such as confusion, forgetfulness, irritability, inability to concentrate or reason, painful reaction to bright light, or depression
- Sleep disturbance (too little or too much)

Symptoms persist or recur over at least 6 months.
The persistent fatigue or easy fatigability must be:
- New to the patient (patient has no history of it)
- Unrelieved by bedrest
- Severe enough to decrease the patient's activities by more than half

Other potential causes have been ruled out.

CDC, Centers for Disease Control and Prevention.

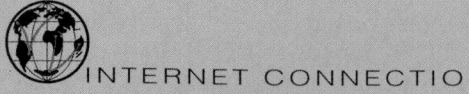

INTERNET CONNECTIONS
HIV/AIDS and Other Immune Disorders

HIV/AIDS
HIV/AIDS Treatment Information Service
http://www.hivatis.org/
This patient-oriented site provides information about U.S. government treatment guidelines for HIV and AIDS. A Public Health Service project, it provides medical news, treatment information, and links to other sources and treatment-related sites.

AIDS Clinical Trials Information Service
http://www.actis.org/
This site provides current information on U.S. government and privately sponsored clinical trials for people with AIDS and HIV infection. Sponsored by the Public Health Service and other U.S. agencies and centers, this site also provide links to a wide variety of research-related U.S. and international sites.

The Red Ribbon Net
http://www.redribbon.net/home.htm
An unusual site offering a wide variety of resources, articles, and information as well as links to government and other sites. This site also provides shopping at the Red Ribbon Mall, participation in the Red Ribbon Coffeehouse, information on biotechnical and pharmaceutical companies, and online classified ads.

Hypersensitivity Disorders
The American Academy of Allergy, Asthma and Immunology
http://www.aaaai.org
An authoritative site that provides information for health professionals including information on professional meetings and societies, scientific information resources, health and medical news, detailed information on pollen and mold counts, and listings of predominant allergens in various areas. This site also provides patient-oriented "tips" brochures relating to asthma and allergies, as well as links to related sites.

Autoimmune Disorders
Lupus Home Page
http://www.hamline.edu/lupus/index.html
An authoritative site sponsored by Hamline University, featuring information on all aspects of lupus as well as links to related sites, medical news, and information on ongoing research.

The Immune Page
http://www.best.com/~immune
This homepage for the Immune Mailing List features information on immune disorders as well as links to related sites. It is designed for patients, families, and health professionals and includes such disorders as chronic fatigue syndrome, candida, lupus, fibromyalgia, Epstein-Barr syndrome, multiple allergies, environmental illness, and chemical sensitivity.

Chronic Fatigue Syndrome/Myalgic Encephalomyelitis
http://www.cais.net/cfs-news
This site provides a tremendous array of U.S. and international references and links to other sources, including news and discussion groups, answers to frequently asked questions for both patients and health professionals, medical news, and information files and resources for health professionals.

Chronic Fatigue Syndrome
http://www.ncf.carleton.ca/ip/social.services/cfseir/ CFSEIR.HP.html
This site provides answers to frequently asked questions, links to related sites, medical news, and resources for emotional support.

NDx: Risk for situational low self esteem related to inability to carry out usual activities and responsibilities secondary to the clinical manifestations of chronic fatigue syndrome

Planning: Patient Outcomes
1. Patient identifies positive aspects of self.
2. Patient expresses optimism about the future.
3. Patient describes ways to maintain a sense of control.

Nursing Interventions and Evaluation

NDx: Fatigue
Focus on helping the patient adapt to the fatigued state. Encourage the patient to express feelings, fears, and concerns about the impact of fatigue on daily activities and lifestyle. Explore with the patient which activities are difficult and the manner and extent to which the fatigue interferes with role activities.

Guide the patient in identifying energy patterns and in scheduling activities in relationship to them. Do this by asking the patient to record fatigue level and activities performed each hour. Provide the patient with directions for recording fatigue, such as use of the Phoben scale of 0 (not tired) to 10 (total exhaustion). Analyze the record with the patient to identify times of peak energy, times of lower energy, and activities that are related to increasing fatigue. Stress careful, consistent planning as the key to living as normal a life as possible. Explain the importance of conserving energy in preparation for active or stressful events, and encourage the patient to plan daily and weekly schedules accordingly. Stress the importance of adequate sleep, naps, and a daily balance of activities that alternates more restful activities with more demanding ones.

Analyze routines and the home environment and make necessary changes to simplify work and conserve energy efficiently. Classify activities as essential or nonessential, and identify those that may be performed by others. Explain that stress depletes energy, and explore with the patient sources of stress in his or her daily life. Help the patient identify how sources of stress might be reduced or eliminated, as well as methods for controlling the effects of stressful situations.

Refer to community resources for household, child care, transportation, or other assistance as needed.

NDx: Risk for altered family processes
Involve family members in planning conferences. Provide accurate information, and encourage questions to promote realistic changes in the family's expectations of the patient. Encourage open discussion of their reactions to the effects of the patient's illness and resulting tensions on the family. Allow expressions of anger and anxiety, and acknowledge these feelings as normal. Explore with the family how role responsibilities in the home can be reorganized to foster family function and decrease stress. Help the family set priorities, and refer to sources of help as needed. Encourage open discussion of secondary gains associated with the sick role, which can contribute to delay in the patient's resumption of the well role.

NDx: Risk for situational low self esteem
Promote expression of feelings. Do this by reflecting the patient's feelings, both positive and negative, and by maintaining an empathetic, nonjudgmental attitude. Help the patient identify positive self-attributes. Recognize and praise positive decisions, activities, and coping strategies. Encourage the patient to structure situations for success through appropriate timing and by allowing adequate time for preparation and rest. Teach cognitive therapy, that is, correction of negative, defeatist thoughts or over-generalizations. Encourage use of relaxation and guided imagery. Inform the patient about sources of support.

Compare the patient's status with the expected outcomes. If the outcomes are not met, reassess the patient and revise the plan.

The Elderly: Special Considerations

Cancer and infection are the two major disorders with increased incidence in the aged. Both are postulated to be due, at least in part, to age-related changes in the immune system.

The "immunologic surveillance" theory holds that malignant cells are marked by antigens identified as foreign by T cells or natural killer cells. The malignant cell carrying the foreign antigen is then destroyed by the T cell in the properly functioning immune system. According to this theory, the increase in cancer seen in the aged results from a decrease in effective surveillance by the immune system. This interpretation is supported by the fact that there is also an increase of cancer in younger persons who are immunosuppressed. However, it is also true that aged persons have had a longer time to be exposed to environmental carcinogens and to acquire mutations in the genes, which also contribute to the risk of cancer.

The increased incidence of infection among geriatric patients results from changes in the immune system, as well as from age-related changes in the body's other defenses. For example, decreased skin turgor, with its associated decreased resistance to friction damage, is a normal effect of aging. Aging also takes its toll on nonspecific defense mechanisms of the respiratory tract. Respiratory muscles weaken and the thoracic cage stiffens. Cilia may have been damaged and their effectiveness decreased by cigarette smoking or other forms of air pollution. Aspiration becomes a problem as the gag and cough reflexes decrease and problems with swallowing develop. These factors may make it difficult for the elderly person to cough and effectively remove foreign matter from the lungs. Thus, they increase susceptibility to influenza and pneumonia.

Changes in the cardiovascular system also contribute to the increasing risk of infection in the elderly. Calcification of the heart valves makes it easier for bacteria to attach and cause endocarditis. The blood supply to peripheral areas of the body may be decreased as cardiac output declines and arterial resistance rises. This leaves peripheral areas of the body more prone to infection and decreases their ability to heal injured tissues.

The gastrointestinal tract becomes more prone to infection as its acidity and motility decrease. Normally, stomach acids destroy most ingested microorganisms. Without this protective acidity, organisms can gain access to the gastrointestinal tract and, because motility has decreased, remain long enough to multiply and cause gastroenteritis and diarrhea.

As renal function decreases, the urinary tract is also more prone to infection. Similarly, structural changes that commonly occur with age, such as urethral stricture and enlargement of the prostate gland, also increase the risk of infection.

Chronic illnesses—such as congestive heart failure, diabetes mellitus, alcoholism, lung disease, and cancer—seem to increase susceptibility to infection. The elderly frequently have one or more of these chronic illnesses, often in addition to other risk factors, such as dehydration and malnutrition.

The geriatric patient with an infection may not exhibit the usual signs and symptoms of infection. Fever is often absent. Many elderly people have a normally low body temperature, and a rise of a degree or more is not identified as an elevation in temperature. Other signs, such as an increase in white blood cell count, cough, pain, and inflammation, may not be present. Often, the only clues that an infection is occurring are subtle changes in behavior, such as a decrease in alertness, fatigue, apathy, irritability, and confusion.

Antibiotics are used to treat the infection in doses adjusted as needed based on age and renal function. In addition, supportive treatment is used to maintain optimal function of all body systems. This is of critical importance because, if present, fever increases the basal metabolic rate, thus increasing the heart rate, respiratory rate, blood pressure, and the need for fluids, oxygen, and energy. This stress may cause the geriatric patient with marginal functioning of body systems to begin to decompensate. For example, cardiac dysrhythmias may develop as a result of the increased demand, and renal function may be impaired. Additional oxygen may be required, especially if the patient has pre-existing lung disease. If the patient is an insulin-dependent diabetic, the need for insulin is increased.

Measures to lower the temperature (antipyretic medications or cooling techniques) are not instituted unless the patient is at risk of delirium, which is likely at a temperature of 40.5°C (105°F) or higher. Temperature is usually not lowered because fever inhibits the growth of pathogens and also provides a clinical indication of the response of the infection to prescribed antibiotics.

Assessment of the aged patient with an infection involves observations specific to the type of infection (eg, if a wound infection, inspect the wound for redness, swelling, and type and amount of drainage; if a respiratory infection, note the presence of cough and type and amount of expectoration, as well as rate, depth, sound, and ease of respirations); observations related to the status of essential body needs and functions; and observation for side effects of the treatments being used.

Take the patient's temperature every 4 hours. Monitor pulse and blood pressure for signs of cardiac dysrhythmias and congestive heart failure, which is a risk during fluid replacement in elderly patients. Monitor respiratory rate and depth, the patient's color, and arterial blood gas values to check for adequate ventilation and oxygenation. Measure and record fluid intake and output to ascertain the patient is not dehydrated and the kidneys are functioning.

NURSING PROCESS GUIDELINES
Infection in the Elderly Patient

Assess nutritional status in terms of the additional demands made by the infection. Observe the patient for side effects of prescribed medications such as mental changes and, if the patient is on bedrest,

monitor for skin breakdown, constipation, confusion, and other effects of immobility.

Because infection can impact on all aspects of the aged person's functioning, many nursing diagnoses and related expected patient outcomes apply. These need to be individualized to the patient based on the circumstances surrounding the patient's infection, the patient's history, present health status, the supporting services available for care, and the patient's response to medical and nursing interventions.

Specific nursing interventions depend on the type and extent of infection and the physician's orders. In all cases, however, provide care in a manner that conserves the patient's energy for fighting the infection while preventing loss of functional ability. To keep the patient oriented, keep a clock, a calendar, and selected personal items near the bedside and use a radio or television to provide sensory stimulation.

If the patient is receiving antibiotic therapy, monitor for diarrhea, which can cause severe fluid and electrolyte imbalance. If diarrhea occurs, notify the physician before administering the next dose. If the patient is taking an aminoglycoside, monitor for hearing loss and for elevated blood urea nitrogen and creatinine levels indicative of nephrotoxicity. Also record fluid intake and output, and ensure adequate hydration.

Specific outcomes depend on the patient, the type of infection, and the nursing diagnosis. Examples might include the following:

Temperature is within patient's normal range.
Lungs are clear on auscultation.
Vital signs are within patient's normal range.
Urinary output is between 1200 and 1500 mL daily.
Skin turgor has elastic recoil.
Blood gas values are within normal range.
Skin and mucous membranes are intact.
Patient is oriented to person, place, and time.

Chapter Review

1. What are the major differences between primary and secondary immunodeficiencies?
2. How does antiretroviral therapy affect the clinical course of a patient with HIV disease?
3. Why is nutritional intervention important when planning care for a patient with late symptomatic HIV disease?
4. How would you manage HIV-1–related cognitive/motor complex (AIDS dementia complex) when caring for a patient with advanced HIV disease?

5. How is the care of a patient with immunosuppressive therapy different from that of a patient with immunodeficiency?
6. Why is respiratory assessment and support important in the patient with allergic rhinitis?
7. What are the similarities and differences between Type I and Type II hypersensitivity disorders?
8. What is the meaning of fatigue when seen in a patient with systemic lupus erythematosus (SLE)?
9. How does depression affect the course of a patient with chronic fatigue syndrome?
10. How does the geriatric patient with an infection differ from a younger adult?

Bibliography

Baker DA. Management of the female HIV-infected patient. AIDS Patient Care 1995; 9(2):78.

Barwick A. Treating systemic lupus erythematosus. Nurs Stand 1993; 7(7):31.

Bauer SM. Psychoneuroimmunology and cancer: An integrated review. J Adv Nurs 1994; 19:1114.

Beal JA, Martin BM. The clinical management of wasting and malnutrition in HIV/AIDS. AIDS Patient Care 1995; 9(2):66.

Bertino LS, Lu LC. The bite of a wolf: Systemic lupus erythematosus. Rehabil Nurs 1993; (18)3:173.

Biagis-Smith J, Coombs VJ, Larson E. HIV infection, exercise, and immune function. IMAGE J Nurs Sch 1994; 26(4):277.

Burmester GR, Daser A, Kanradt T, et al. Immunology of reactive arthritides. Ann Rev Immunol 1995; 13:229.

Centers for Disease Control and Prevention. Draft guideline for isolation precautions in hospitals. Federal Register 1994; 59(214):55552.

Centers for Disease Control and Prevention. The chronic fatigue syndrome [information pamphlet]. Washington, DC: Public Health Service, Department of Health and Human Services, January 1990.

Coler MS. PERC: A nursing syndrome for AIDS. Nurs Diagn 1996; 7(1):19.

Collier AC. Efficacy of combination antiretroviral therapy. Adv Exp Med Biol 1996; 394:355.

Cordell B. Evaluation of a wellness/early intervention/advocacy program for HIV disease. AIDS Patient Care 1995; 9(4):189.

DeVita VT, Hellman S, Rosenberg SA, et al. AIDS: Etiology, diagnosis, treatment, and prevention. 4th ed. Philadelphia: JB Lippincott, 1997.

Dobbing EA. Preventing transference of bloodborne pathogens in the workplace: Reducing your risk of contracting HIV/HBV. Point View 1993; 30(2):8.

Fifth International HIV Conference Proceedings, Vancouver, WA, 1966.

Franco T, Gould DA. Allogeneic bone marrow transplantation. Semin Oncol Nurs 1994; 10(1):3.

Frank MM, Austen KF, Claman HN, Unanue ER. Samter's Immunologic Diseases. Vol I. Boston: Little, Brown, 1995.

Frank MM, Austen KF, Claman HN, Unanue ER. Samter's Immunologic Diseases. Vol II. Boston: Little, Brown, 1995.

Groves DF. "A merry heart doeth good like a medicine..." Holistic Nurs Pract 1991; 5(4):49.

Health care workers at risk: An interview with Patricia Wetzel, MD. Asepsis 1995; 17(1):10.

Hillhouse J, Adler C. Stress, health, and immunity: A review of the literature and implications for the nursing profession. Holistic Nurs Pract 1991; 5(4):22.

Hyde RM. Immunology. Baltimore: Williams & Wilkins, 1995.

Johnson CC. Knowledge of immunology is essential to plan effective nursing for immunocompromised patients. Intensive Crit Care Nurs 1994; 10:121.

Jones CA. These patients truly need our help. RN 1992; 55(10):46.

Jones GA. Is it infectious? J Infect 1994; 28:233.

Kim CU, McGee LR, Krawczyk SH, et al. New series of potent, orally bioavailable, non-peptidic cyclic, sulfones as HIV-1 protease inhibitors. J Med Chem 1996; 39(18):3431.

Lambert RB, Lambert NK. The effects of humor on secretory immunoglobulin A levels in school-aged children. Pediatr Nurs 1995; (21)1:16.

Lange EG, Hertzfield L. Hemolytic transfusion reaction. Nursing 1995; 25(7):33.

Lash AA. Why so many women? Part 1. Systemic lupus erythematosus. MEDSURG Nurs 1993; 2(5):375.

Lash AA. Systemic lupus erythematosus. Part 2. Diagnosis, treatment modalities, and nursing management. MEDSURG Nurs 1993; 2(5):375.

Lawlor GJ, Fischer TJ, Adelman DC. Manual of allergy and immunology. Boston: Little, Brown, 1995.

Lloyd A, Hickie I, Wakefield D, et al. A double-blind, placebo-controlled trial of intravenous immunoglobulin therapy in patients with chronic fatigue syndrome. Am J Med 1990; 89(5):561.

Major C, Li X, Strune G, et al. HIV-1 viral load in progressors vs. non-progressors. 3rd Conference Retro and Opportunistic Infections, January 28–February 1, 1996, p 101.

Montelaro RC, Wigzell H. Vaccines and immunology: Overview. AIDS 1995; 9(Suppl A):S111.

New era makes viral load testing an important tool. AIDS Alert 1996; 11(8):Suppl 1–2.

Nott KH, Vedhara K, Spickett GP. Psychology, immunology, and HIV. Psychoneuroendocrinology 1995; 20(5):451.

Paul WE (ed). Fundamental immunology. 3rd ed. New York: Raven Press, 1994.

Safrit JT, Koup RA. The immunology of primary HIV infection: Which immune responses control HIV replication? Curr Opin Immunol 1995; 7(4):456.

Smith AR, Chang BL. Nursing diagnoses for hospitalized patients with AIDS. Nurs Diagn 1996; 7(1):9.

Thomas PK. The chronic fatigue syndrome: What do we know? Br Med J 1993; 306:1557.

Tizard IR. Immunology: An introduction. Philadelphia: Saunders College Publishing, 1995.

Unquarski PJ. Update on HIV infection. Am J Nurs 1997; 97(1):44.

Williams HF. Integrating the occupational safety and health administration mandates on bloodborne pathogens in the practice setting. J Intravenous Nurs 1995; 18(6 Suppl):s9.

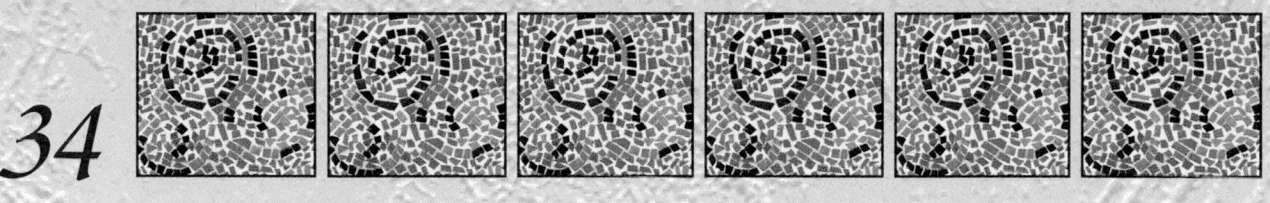

34

Nursing Care of Patients with Oncologic Disorders

Study Outcomes

After studying this chapter, you should be able to:

1. Explain the normal anatomy and physiology of the cell.
2. Describe the etiology, pathophysiology, clinical manifestations, diagnostic procedures, and collaborative management of cancer.
3. Identify information and physical examination data essential to the assessment of patients with cancer.
4. State nursing diagnoses and related expected patient outcomes commonly applicable to patients with cancer.
5. Describe nursing interventions, with their rationales, commonly applicable to patients with cancer.
6. Explain the basis for evaluation of nursing care provided to patients with cancer.
7. Identify alternative treatment and care settings for patients with cancer and the services related to community-based care.
8. Identify special considerations for the elderly patient with cancer.

In the United States, more than 1 million people are diagnosed with cancer each year. Cancer occurs among all age groups, although its incidence is greatest in the elderly. It can affect any body system. Despite the many advances in diagnosis and treatment, many people still consider a diagnosis of cancer to mean suffering and death. Thus, caring for patients with cancer requires an understanding of the normal physiology and pathophysiology of body systems as well as an understanding of the etiology and pathophysiology of malignant tumors, diagnostic and therapeutic measures in current use, and the related nursing care. Because of the psychologic toll of cancer, the nurse also must be sensitive to the needs of both patients and significant others for support. The nurse must be involved in patient and family education regarding care and prevention and knowledgeable about available community resources so that appropriate referrals can be made. Because the trend in cancer care is toward ambulatory services and home care, assessment of patients' support systems, as well as timeliness and comprehen-

siveness of patient and family education, has become a basic tenet of oncology nursing.

Anatomy and Physiology

The cell is the basic unit of all living things. An understanding of its normal structure and function is essential in the study of diseases caused by malignant cells. The human body is composed of more than 75 trillion cells. Most of them reproduce continually to maintain the body's pattern of growth and to replace damaged tissue and dead cells. Figure 34–1 illustrates the major cellular components and describes their function.

Each cell is surrounded by a membrane composed of proteins and lipids. Within the cell are a nucleus and cytoplasm. The nucleus, which is surrounded by a nuclear membrane, contains the cell's genetic controlling material—deoxyribonucleic acid (DNA). Within the nucleus is the nucleolus, which contains additional genetic controlling material—ribonucleic acid (RNA). Cytoplasm surrounds the nucleus and provides a complex microtubule system to transport substances within the cell. Cytoplasm gives the cell its shape and supports all cell structures. Several highly specialized organelles within the cytoplasm perform functions that allow the cell to carry out metabolism, excretion, and reproduction.

The cell cycle describes the life of a cell. It begins at the midpoint of the mitosis, which results in the formation of a particular cell, and ends at the midpoint of the mitosis, which results in that cell dividing into two daughter cells. The cell cycle (Fig. 34–2) is a dynamic process that is divided into five phases: G_1, G_0, S, G_2, and M.

Phase G_1 is a postmitotic period of cell growth characterized by the development of RNA and protein. Cells may leave phase G_1 and enter G_0 or go on to phase S. Phase G_0 is a dormant or resting stage in which the cell performs all normal functions but does not replicate. Phase S, in contrast, is an active period of DNA synthesis that creates two sep-

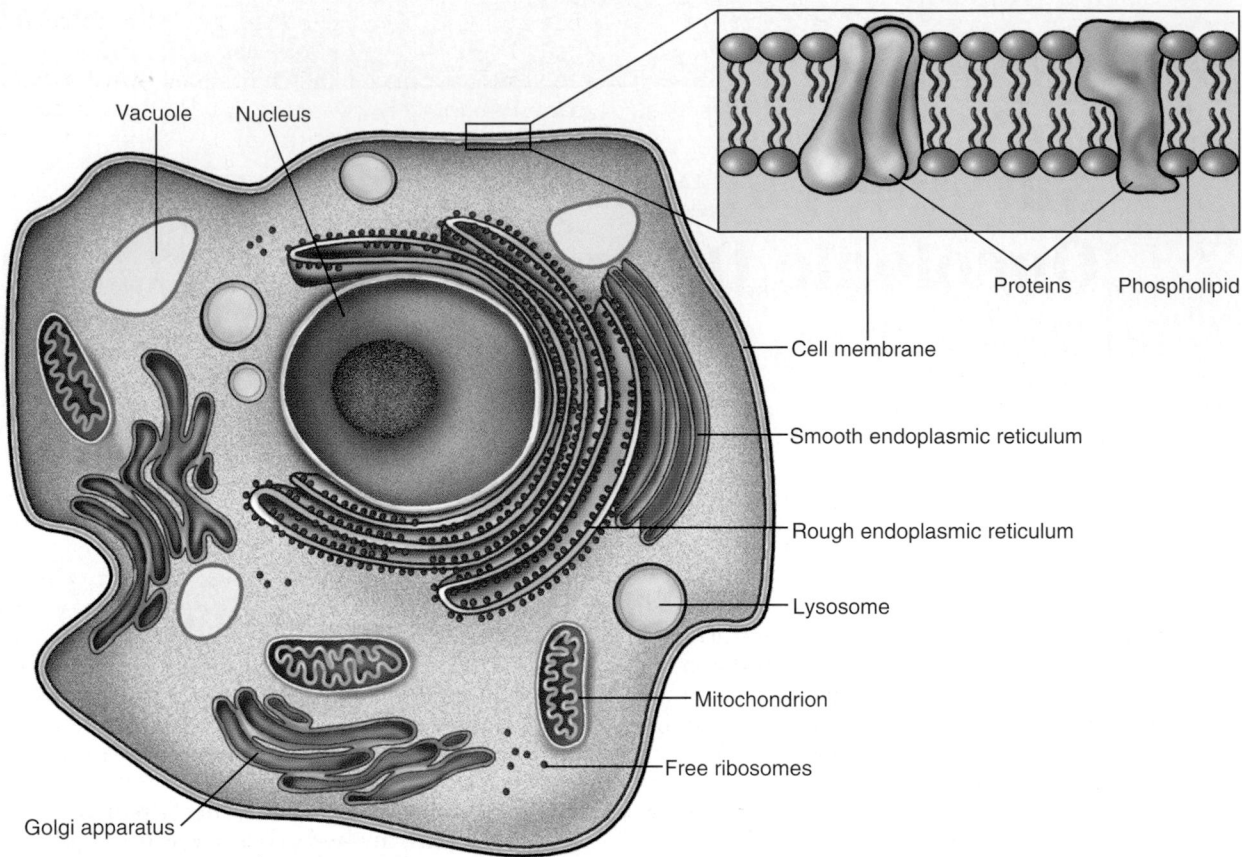

Figure 34–1

Major cellular components. The *cell membrane* controls movement of substances in and out of the cell. Small pores allow passage of small molecules. Other substances move in or out by active transport. The *nucleus* directs and controls all cellular activities by means of the genes, which are located on the chromosomes. The *rough endoplasmic reticulum* has ribosomes on its surface. It synthesizes proteins that combine with fats or carbohydrates. *Smooth endoplasmic reticulum* has no ribosomes on its surface. It is part of the intracellular transport system, with a role in fat metabolism, biotransformation, and calcium storage. *Free ribosomes* synthesize proteins for intracellular enzymes and structures. A *vacuole* is a clear space in the cytoplasm filled with fluid or air. The *Golgi apparatus* concentrates and packages chemical products into secretion granules that float to the cell membrane for excretion into the extracellular fluid. A *lysosome* is an intracellular digestive system capable of breaking down proteins and carbohydrates. It destroys foreign proteins by phagocytosis. A *mitochondrion* manufactures adenosine triphosphate, which supplies the cell with energy.

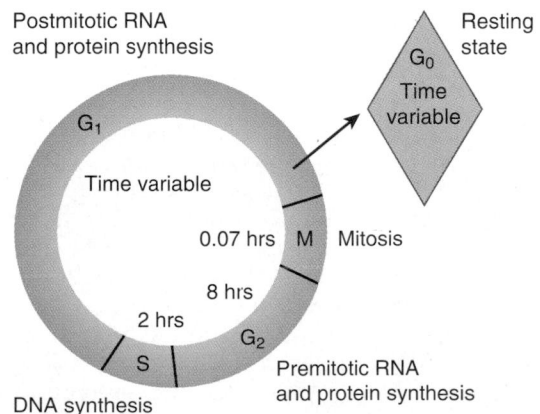

Figure 34–2

The cell cycle.

arate sets of chromosomes in the nucleus. After phase S comes phase G_2, which is a premitotic interval of RNA and protein synthesis similar to G_1. M, or mitosis, is the final phase, during which the cell splits into two daughter cells.

The length of the cell cycle varies from tissue to tissue. It may be as short as 16 hours or extend to 400 hours, as with liver cells. Because the time spent in phases G_2 (8 hours), S (2 hours), and M (0.07 hour) is about the same for all cells, the variability results from different times spent in phases G_1 and G_0. One factor contributing to this variability is that not all cells enter the G_0 phase. The number that do enter G_0 varies, depending on the type of tissue.

Highly differentiated cells, such as neurons, never enter the cell cycle because in the process of developing a highly specialized function they have lost the ability to replicate.

𝒫athophysiology

The term *neoplasm* (new growth) is used to describe a group of cells with an abnormal growth pattern. Neoplasms are classified as either benign or malignant. A benign neoplasm has the following characteristics:

- It is composed of cells that resemble the tissue of origin.
- It is usually encapsulated.
- It grows slowly and by expansion.
- It does not recur or metastasize.
- It does not destroy tissue unless it interferes with blood flow.
- It does not cause systemic symptoms or death unless its location causes it to interfere with vital functions (eg, a brain tumor).

A malignant neoplasm, or cancer, is composed of undifferentiated (immature) cells that have little resemblance to the tissue of origin. The malignant neoplasm tends to grow rapidly, expanding at the periphery and invading and destroying surrounding tissues (Fig. 34–3). It also tends to recur when removed and spreads by way of the blood and lymph to distant areas of the body. It causes systemic manifestations—such as alteration in taste, anorexia, weight loss, and weakness. Ultimately, if not controlled, it causes death.

Malignant cells in epithelial tissue are called *carcinomas*. Malignant cells of connective tissue, muscle, or bone are called *sarcomas*. These are classified as solid tumors because initially they are confined to a specific tissue or organ. Malignant cells of blood are called leukemias; malignant cells of the bone marrow are called myelomas, and those of the lymphatics are called lymphomas. These are classified as hematologic cancers, which are disseminated from their beginning.

When a normal cell undergoes transformation to a malignant cell, a number of changes occur in the cell membrane and intracellular structures. The cell membrane loses its contact inhibition, continuing to grow even when it touches another cell. It develops a strong negative surface charge and does not form intercellular connections. Its antigens may be altered. The number of free ribosomes increases. Protein production changes. More structural proteins, but fewer enzymes, are formed. Proteins normally synthesized only during fetal development appear. The mitochondria are sometimes edematous. Metabolism is altered. It reverts to a simpler pattern usually involving greater use of glucose and more anaerobic pathways. The nucleus of the cell is significantly larger than normal and exhibits abnormal chromosomes and increased amounts of DNA.

Cancer cells also differ from normal cells in that they are anaplastic, that is, primitive, undifferentiated cells that no longer resemble the original cells from which the tumor began (Fig. 34–4). Anaplastic cells replicate much more quickly than normal cells and cannot perform the functions of the tissues from which they are derived. They also do not "age" normally or die "on time."

A tumor's growth rate is described by doubling time. This is the time it takes for the total mass of cells in the tumor to double. The growth rate of a malignant tumor depends on how many cells are actively dividing, cell cycle time, and how many cells are dying. Because many cancer cells seem unable to enter the resting G_0 phase of the cell cycle and simply continue to divide until the blood and nutrient supply is insufficient, there are usually a greater number of malignant cells replicating at any point in time than there would be in normal tissue.

Malignant tumors spread or metastasize through

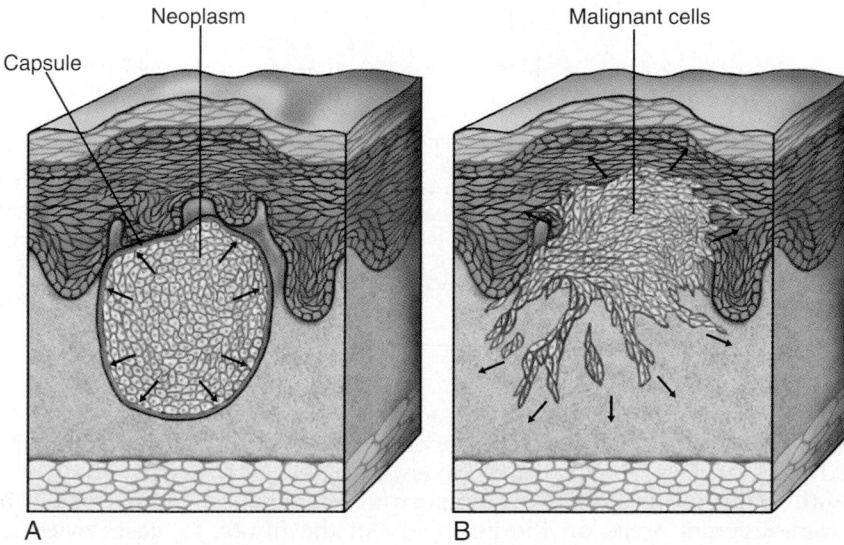

Figure 34–3

A, Benign encapsulated neoplasm. *B,* Malignant neoplasm, showing multiple projections from its periphery into the surrounding tissue.

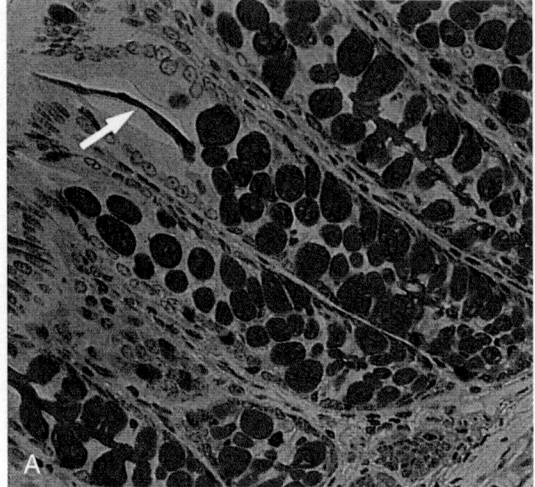
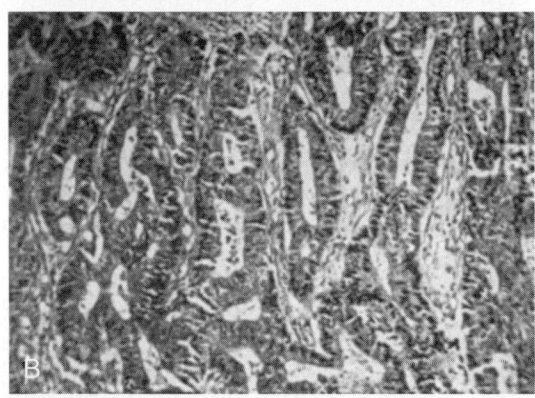
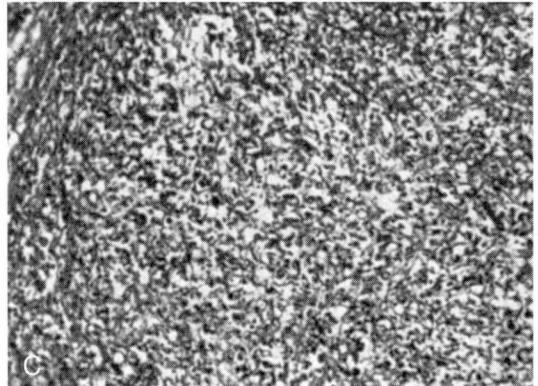

Figure 34–4

A, Photomicrograph of normal colonic tissue. *B,* Photomicrograph of a well-differentiated adenocarcinoma that resembles parent tissue in that glands can be identified. *C,* Photomicrograph of an undifferentiated or anaplastic adenocarcinoma. (*A* from Leeson TS, Leeson CR, Paparo AA. Text/atlas of histology. 2nd ed. Philadelphia: WB Saunders, 1984, p 458; *B* and *C* from Perez-Tamayo R. Mechanisms of disease. Philadelphia: WB Saunders, 1961, p 205.)

both a direct and an indirect process. Direct extension involves the infiltration of malignant cells into adjacent tissues. This occurs in an irregular way, with many projections invading surrounding tissues from different areas on the periphery of the tumor. Depending on the tissues affected, hemorrhage, ul-

ceration, necrosis, or fibrosis can occur. Direct extension can also result in seeding of cancer cells into a body cavity. This occurs when a malignant tumor penetrates into a body cavity and cells drop off and implant on the serosal surface.

Indirect spread involves invasion of vascular or lymphatic channels, in which malignant cells break away from the tumor and travel to distant areas of the body, where they implant and develop into secondary tumors. When spread is by way of the lymphatics, malignant cells first lodge in the lymph nodes that drain the tumor site. They may remain there for some time before again breaking away and traveling to more distant nodes and eventually reaching the thoracic duct and entering the blood stream.

*I*ncidence

Cancer is a general term used to encompass a group of more than 100 malignant disorders. It is second only to heart disease as a cause of human death. Cancer can occur throughout a person's life span. Any organ in the body can be a target for metastasis of malignant cells.

Currently, more than 8 million people in the United States have a history of cancer. More than 5 million have been alive for more than 5 years after diagnosis.

Statistics compiled by the American Cancer Society (ACS) indicate that three of every four families in the United States will experience a family member being diagnosed with an oncologic disorder. One of every three people will be diagnosed with cancer at some time during his or her lifetime. Although the death rate from other diseases over the past 30 years has declined, the death rate from cancer has increased, mostly because of the increased incidence of lung cancer (Fig. 34–5).

GENDER AND AGE

In general, the incidence of cancer is the same in both males and females; however, the age distribution is different. Between ages 20 and 60, the incidence is higher in women. This may reflect the high rates of breast and cervical cancer during these years. After age 60, men have a markedly higher incidence of cancer compared with women.

RACE

Incidence and mortality rates for cancer are generally higher for African-Americans than for white Americans. In 1995, approximately 1,252,000 cancer cases were diagnosed in the United States. About 120,000 of these were among African Americans and

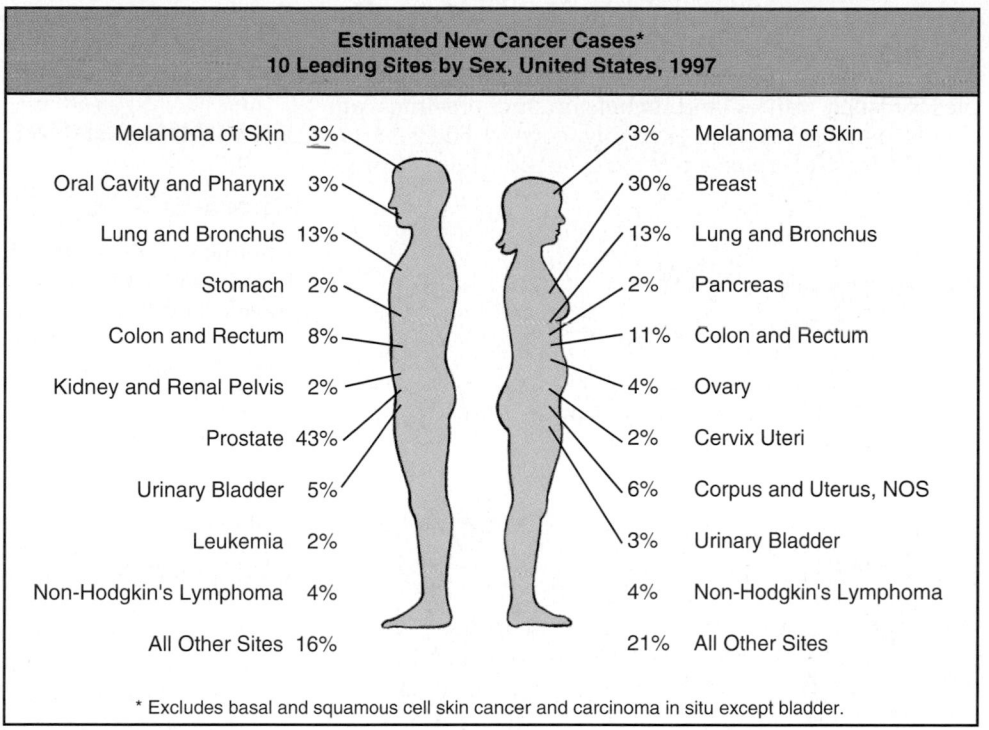

Estimated New Cancer Cases*
10 Leading Sites by Sex, United States, 1997

Male			Female
Melanoma of Skin	3%	3%	Melanoma of Skin
Oral Cavity and Pharynx	3%	30%	Breast
Lung and Bronchus	13%	13%	Lung and Bronchus
Stomach	2%	2%	Pancreas
Colon and Rectum	8%	11%	Colon and Rectum
Kidney and Renal Pelvis	2%	4%	Ovary
Prostate	43%	2%	Cervix Uteri
Urinary Bladder	5%	6%	Corpus and Uterus, NOS
Leukemia	2%	3%	Urinary Bladder
Non-Hodgkin's Lymphoma	4%	4%	Non-Hodgkin's Lymphoma
All Other Sites	16%	21%	All Other Sites

* Excludes basal and squamous cell skin cancer and carcinoma in situ except bladder.

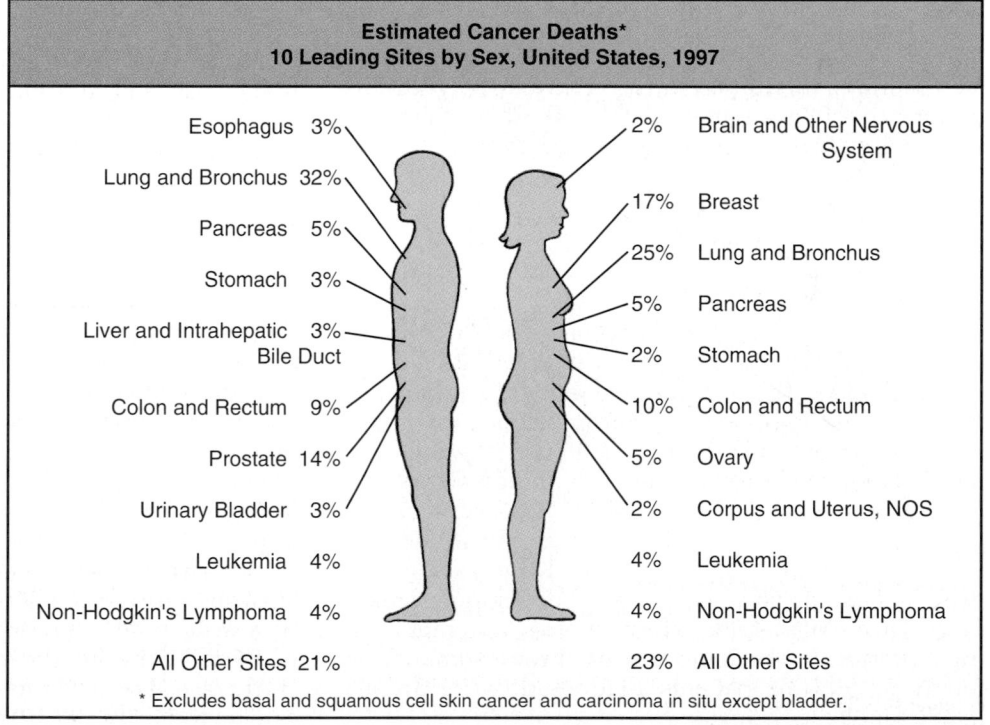

Estimated Cancer Deaths*
10 Leading Sites by Sex, United States, 1997

Male			Female
Esophagus	3%	2%	Brain and Other Nervous System
Lung and Bronchus	32%	17%	Breast
Pancreas	5%	25%	Lung and Bronchus
Stomach	3%	5%	Pancreas
Liver and Intrahepatic Bile Duct	3%	2%	Stomach
Colon and Rectum	9%	10%	Colon and Rectum
Prostate	14%	5%	Ovary
Urinary Bladder	3%	2%	Corpus and Uterus, NOS
Leukemia	4%	4%	Leukemia
Non-Hodgkin's Lymphoma	4%	4%	Non-Hodgkin's Lymphoma
All Other Sites	21%	23%	All Other Sites

* Excludes basal and squamous cell skin cancer and carcinoma in situ except bladder.

Figure 34–5

Estimated cancer incidence and deaths by site and sex. NOS, not otherwise specified. (Redrawn from Parker SL, Tong T, Bolder S, Wingo, PA. Cancer statistics 1997. CA Cancer J Clin 1997; 47[1]:5.)

35,000 among other minority Americans (ACS, 1995). However, these differences may be more reflective of socioeconomic conditions than of any intrinsic racial differences. When social and economic living standards are similar for black and white populations, so are the incidence and death rates from cancer. Incidence and mortality rates for other minority groups, such as Hispanics, are often lower than those for white Americans or African-Americans.

Because cancer risk is strongly associated with lifestyle and behavior, differences in ethnic and cultural groups may sometimes provide clues to factors involved in the development of cancer (see Etiology and Pathophysiology). Cultural values and beliefs can affect attitudes about seeking medical care or following screening guidelines (ACS, 1995). Examples of such values and beliefs include feelings of shame associated with exposing certain body parts and mistrust of people who are outside the cultural group.

GEOGRAPHY

Cancer occurs more frequently in western countries where the life span is estimated to be longer. Exposure to environmental carcinogens may be geographically related.

Etiology

Although the exact etiology of all oncologic disorders is unknown, epidemiologic research has helped to identify risk factors that may influence the development of an oncologic disorder.

The process that causes the uncontrolled and undisciplined growth of cells is thought to involve many steps that may be enhanced by external stimuli. Genetic, environmental, immunologic, and viral factors may individually or as cofactors play an important role in changing normal cells into malignant cells; this process is called carcinogenesis.

GENETIC FACTORS

An important clue to the cause of a malignant disease may actually be hidden in a person's chromosomal characteristics as well as in the tumor itself. The cells of nearly all human malignant tumors and most animal tumors contain chromosomal abnormalities. Evidence exists that people with specific genetic characteristics may have an increased risk of certain cancers.

People with such chromosome disorders as Bloom's, Fanconi's, Down's, and Klinefelter's syndromes have an increased risk of developing leukemia. The Philadelphia chromosomal alteration (a translocation of the long arm of chromosome 22) is found in 90% of patients diagnosed with chronic myelogenous leukemia.

The high incidence of cancer in members of the same family may indicate a genetic predisposition. Cancers of the gastrointestinal tract and thyroid, and retinoblastomas, are known to occur more frequently in patients with a family history of these cancers. Familial cancers may be related to the combined influence of genetics and environment. Cancer of the breast also shows a familial pattern, and mutations of two genes (*BRCA*-1 on chromosome 17 and *BRCA*-2 on chromosome 13) have been identi-

fied in persons with hereditary early-onset breast cancers.

ENVIRONMENTAL FACTORS

Chemicals and Toxic Substances

Chemicals and substances in the environment have been identified as significantly contributing to the development of certain oncologic disorders. Certain chemicals have the ability to alter directly or indirectly the structure of DNA within cells.

Chemical carcinogenesis can be divided into a two-step process of initiation and promotion. A chemical initiator can permanently and irreversibly alter cells. A chemical promoter can temporarily and reversibly alter cells. Carcinogenesis is thought to occur when a cell undergoes a permanent change from a chemical initiator and is then repeatedly exposed to a chemical promoter. This two-step process results in cellular oncogenous transformation.

The high incidence of scrotal cancer seen in chimney sweeps more than 150 years ago was perhaps the first recognition of an occupational cause of cancer. The relationship between soldiers exposed to nitrogen mustard gas during World War I and their subsequent development of cancer was another clue to the dangers of exposure to carcinogenic substances. Many chemical compounds have been shown to produce tumors in animals. Several hundred of these compounds are suspected to be carcinogenic. Most produce cancer in animals and not humans. Examples of agents that exhibit carcinogenic risk to humans include arsenic, asbestos, aromatic amines, benzene, vinyl chloride, and aflatoxins. People may be exposed to chemical carcinogens as part of their lifestyle, occupation, and medical history. Asbestos, a mineral fiber used in insulation, as a fire retardant, and in a number of manufacturing applications, is associated with pleural and abdominal mesothelioma after repeated exposure. Medical therapies that employ certain drugs (eg, hormones, antitumor drugs, and antibiotics) may also cause oncologic disorders.

A variety of federal and state governmental agencies in the United States regulate chemicals proven to be carcinogenic and furnish updated lists of these agents to the public and to people in the workplace. The lists include new information on carcinogenic chemicals in the workplace, in medicinal agents, in foods, and in the environment. In 1986, the U.S. government mandated that employees who are exposed to hazardous substances at work (including carcinogens) be trained by employers in correct handling and use of protective clothing.

It is probably no coincidence that many African-Americans, who have a higher incidence of cancer than do white Americans, have worked in occupations (such as the steel- and tire-making industries) that place them at risk for a variety of cancers (Pottern et al, 1981; Miller & Cooper, 1982; Michaels, 1983; U.S. Department of Health and Human Services, 1986; U.S. Bureau of Census, 1992).

Tobacco

Cigarette smoking is the single most preventable cause of disease and death in the United States. It is estimated that more than 30% of all cancer is related to smoking, including cancers of the lung, mouth, throat, larynx, esophagus, and bladder. Eighty-seven percent of all lung cancer is related to smoking, 90% among men and 79% among women (ACS, 1995). As increasing numbers of women began to smoke, their rate of smoking-related cancers also increased.

The relationship between smoking and cancer is well documented. Risk increases with the length of time and number of cigarettes a person has smoked. In addition, a smoker who also consumes large quantities of alcohol has a substantially increased risk of developing oral cancer. Chemicals that are known tumor promoters and initiators have been detected in both tobacco and cigarette smoke.

Although smoking is a risk factor for all smokers, some racial and ethnic groups have a higher incidence of smoking than others, and this places them at greater risk for the development of cancer. For example, smoking has been identified as a lifestyle risk factor in the following racial or ethnic populations: African-American, Asian/Pacific islanders, Native American Oglala women, and Alaska natives (Olsen & Frank-Stromberg, 1993). Although each patient must be assessed as a unique individual, these statistics are important to keep in mind when assessing members of these groups.

Researchers continue to study the effect of cigarette smoke inhaled by nonsmokers. This "second-hand smoke" is a potent carcinogen and a significant factor in the development of numerous other disorders. Each year, about 3000 nonsmoking adults die of lung cancer from breathing the smoke of other people's cigarettes. The risk of dying of lung cancer is 30% higher for a nonsmoker living with a smoker compared with a nonsmoker living with a nonsmoker (ACS, 1995).

Smoking in the home also jeopardizes the health of family members, especially young children. Several childhood illnesses are associated with exposure to smoke, including respiratory infections and chronic ear infections. The children of parents who smoke compared with children of nonsmoking parents have an increased frequency of chronic cough and other respiratory symptoms. An infant's risk of sudden infant death syndrome (SIDS) has been associated with maternal smoking.

Alcohol

A relationship has been established between consumption of large amounts of alcohol and the subsequent development of cancers of the head, neck, esophagus, and liver, especially when accompanied by smoking cigarettes or chewing tobacco (ACS, 1995). Heavy consumption of beer may increase the risk of colorectal cancer.

When incorporating cultural understanding into practice, it is important to note that, as a group, both African-American (Clark-Tasker, 1993) and Hispanic populations statistically tend to consume more alcohol than the average, perhaps because of social and economic pressures. Although it cannot be assumed that any particular patient may consume excessive alcohol based simply on his or her race or culture, if the health-care professional is aware of these statistical differences he or she may help to identify important ways in which to promote the health of a particular patient (Olsen & Frank-Stromberg, 1993).

Diet

The relationship between dietary intake and cancer is being closely studied. Diet may be responsible for about one-third of oncologic disorders in the United States. Dietary intake may be an environmental promoter and initiator, based on the time periods during which the person is exposed to certain dietary practices. People 40% or more overweight have an increased risk of cancer of the colon, breast, prostate, gallbladder, ovary, and uterus (ACS, 1995).

Dietary fat increases bile secretion, and it is postulated that byproducts of bile salts may act as promoting agents in the development of colon cancer. Fats also affect the endocrine system and increase hormone production, which explains the relationship between high fat intake and hormone-dependent tumors of the breast and prostate.

In animal studies, vitamins A and C, riboflavin, and selenium have been shown to possess a mechanism that appears to have an unexplained ability to protect against the development of cancer. The American Cancer Society suggests a diet that may guard against the development of cancer, which includes fresh vegetables, fruits, and foods that contain high fiber content, vitamins A and C (ACS, 1995).

Statistically, African-Americans have been found to tend to eat more animal fat, less fiber, and fewer fruits and vegetables and to have lower levels of thiamine, riboflavin, vitamins A and C, and iron than white Americans (Hargreaves et al, 1989). The Asian/Pacific islander diet is generally deficient in vitamin A. The Japanese diet tends to be low in vitamin C. Korean and Filipino diets are often high in fat. The diets of the Oklahoma and Alaska Native American tribes lack dietary fiber (Olsen & Frank-Stromberg, 1993). Although assumptions cannot be made about individuals based on these tendencies, creative strategies *may* need to be employed when teaching people of these cultures about cancer prevention.

In areas of the world where salt-cured and

smoked foods are eaten frequently (Asian/Pacific islands, Japan, Alaska), there is a higher incidence of cancer of the esophagus and stomach. Newer methods of food processing and preservation appear to eliminate the cancer-causing byproducts associated with these traditional methods of food treatment (ACS, 1995; Olsen & Frank-Stromberg, 1993).

Radiation

Ionizing and electromagnetic radiation has the ability to interfere with the structure and function of DNA in cells. Radiation is one of the major therapies used to kill cancerous cells. The relationship between the ultraviolet rays of the sun and inducement of skin cancer was documented more than a century ago. People exposed to atomic radiation have a markedly increased risk for breast cancer, leukemia, and lung and thyroid cancer. Radiologists in the early 1900s, before protective methods were employed, had a high incidence of leukemia. Radon, an odorless, colorless gas that is a breakdown product of uranium and can seep into homes from the ground or through the water, is associated with an increased risk of lung cancer.

VIRUSES

The viral etiology theory of cancer suggests that certain viruses have the ability to change the genetic makeup of cells, thus initiating the process of transforming normal cells into malignant cells (oncogenesis). The oncogene (type of gene that can promote the growth of malignant cells) can directly affect cellular DNA. The presence of a virus that can turn on the oncogene may be just one factor in the subsequent development of cancer. Several viruses have been implicated in the development of certain oncologic diseases. Human T-cell leukemia virus (HTLV) is associated with T-cell leukemia and lymphoma. Epstein-Barr virus is associated with Burkitt's lymphoma and tumors of the nasopharynx. Human papillomavirus is associated with cancer of the cervix, as is cytomegalovirus, which is also associated with Kaposi's sarcoma. Other tumors associated with viruses include hairy-cell leukemia, retinoblastoma, and hepatocellular carcinoma (Groenwald et al, 1995).

IMMUNOLOGIC DEFECTS

The body's immunologic system serves as a surveillance mechanism to recognize and destroy foreign agents. The immunologic etiology of cancer purports that this system may play an essential role in regulating the presence of neoplastic cells. When the system fails, tumors are somehow allowed to grow and spread. People with immunologic disorders have a higher risk of developing certain kinds of malignant disorders. This fact is evident in the high incidence

of cancer seen in people with acquired immunodeficiency syndrome (AIDS). People who have received immunosuppressive therapy for neoplastic and non-neoplastic disorders also have an increased incidence of neoplastic diseases.

Immunotherapy holds the hope of enhancing the body's own disease-fighting systems to help control cancer. Biologic response modifiers, such as interferon (a naturally occurring body protein capable of killing cancer cells or stopping their growth) and interleukin-2 (a growth factor that stimulates cells of the immune system to fight cancer), are being studied (ACS, 1995).

PSYCHOSOCIAL FACTORS

Research demonstrates a strong relationship between psychologic stress and the onset and outcome of illness. This seems particularly true after major loss and depression. It is impossible, however, to determine whether a direct cause-effect relationship exists. Research tools cannot measure data of a psychosocial nature.

A group of leukemia and lymphoma patients were studied by Green (1966), who noted a strong relationship between loss of significant others and the subsequent onset of cancer. Not merely major loss, but poor adjustment to loss was reported, resulting in ongoing feelings of helplessness, powerlessness, and depression. LeShan (1966) came to similar conclusions about loss and cancer using interviews and questionnaires in several studies over a 21-year period with about 1000 cancer patients and a cancer-free control group. Another group was studied for 20 years by Engel (1967), who also found that the onset of various illnesses coincided with strong feelings of hopelessness after significant losses. Seeman and Seeman (1983) studied 1000 subjects over a 1-year period and determined that a sense of having personal control in their lives was a crucial factor in maintaining their health status. Those who are engaged in counseling cancer patients also report recurrent, almost universal themes of helplessness and powerlessness with lowered self-esteem. These emotions are a predominant effect if not a contributing causative agent of cancer.

Certain personal attributes have been described as making one "cancer prone." LeShan found in one study (Haber et al, 1987) that 95% of patients with cancer, compared with only 10% without cancer in the control group, exhibited a characteristic profile. This profile describes a person with low self-esteem who sees himself or herself as a victim and harbors resentments that, along with anger and aggression, cannot be expressed. This personality type lacks resiliency, values conformity, and has a narrow range of personal relationships and interests. The person also appears to be dominated by feelings of loss and helplessness. These characteristics existed before the onset of cancer. Once cancer is diagnosed, these patients have a poorer prognosis, with more rapid disease progression. Dysfunctional profiles of their families of origin have also been described.

Conversely, a very different personality profile has been associated with above-average remission rates in cancer (Haber et al, 1987). These people demonstrate a sound sense of self-esteem. They are described as creative, intelligent, successful, confident, vital, open, and flexible. They are the "fighters" who seek, expect, and demand the best possible treatments. They have an internal locus of control. That is, they believe that they can directly affect and control the outcome of their situation and do not feel at the mercy of external controls.

A major danger in emphasizing cancer-prone personality profiles is that patients, especially those prone to self-blame, may feel that their attitude is primarily to blame for the onset, recurrence, or poor course and prognosis of their cancer. The self-guilt this generates increases depression, which in turn negatively affects prognosis, resulting in a cycle of self-fulfilling prophecy. People with significant external locus of control can become more internally controlled. However, this requires significant supportive, long-term counseling to help raise consciousness and self-confidence. Observation of newborns indicates that some people are constitutionally programmed to be more passive. It is unrealistic and unfair to teach such people that the development of a "fighting spirit" is essential to conquer their cancer. In spite of the validity of that "fighting" personality profile, one must use this approach with caution.

Clinical Manifestations

The clinical manifestations of cancer are numerous. Each variant of the disease has unique symptoms and sequence. Manifestations range from vague complaints of unexplained fatigue, weight loss, and elevated body temperature to severe symptoms of pain, inability to function, and life-threatening medical emergencies. Signs and symptoms of some common cancers appear in Table 34–1.

NURSING PROCESS
Cancer Prevention and Screening

Assessment

Cancer screening helps detect cancer at an early stage and helps identify people at high risk. When screening a patient for cancer, assess general health status. Ask about the seven warning signs of cancer:

C Change in bowel or bladder habits
A A sore that does not heal
U Unusual bleeding or discharge
T Thickening or lump in breast or elsewhere
I Indigestion or difficulty swallowing
O Obvious change in wart or mole
N Nagging cough or hoarseness

Assess the patient's knowledge of cancer. Specifically determine the patient's understanding of risk

Table 34–1

Risk Factors and Signs and Symptoms of Common Cancers

Site	Risk Factors	Signs and Symptoms
Lung	Cigarette smoking Exposure to airborne carcinogens Family history	Persistent cough Hemoptysis Recurrent lung infections
Colon	Family or personal history of colon cancer Polyps Inflammatory bowel disease	Bleeding from rectum Blood in stool Change in bowel habits
Breast	Older than age 50	Breast changes: lump, thickening, swelling, dimpling, nipple retraction, nipple discharge, pain, tenderness
Skin	Excessive sun exposure Fair complexion Exposure to carcinogens, such as coal tar, arsenic	Change in size or color of mole Darkly pigmented lesion Ulcerated lesions Lesion that bleeds easily
Cervix	Early sexual activity Multiple sexual partners Genital herpes History of diethylstilbestrol use by mother	Painless bleeding after intercourse or douching (contact bleeding)
Prostate	Older than age 50	Hard, nodular, fixed prostate Difficulty initiating urination Weak stream with dribbling Urinary frequency and urgency Nocturia Urinary retention

factors, self-examination techniques, recommended schedule of screening procedures by health-care professionals, and symptoms to be reported. Explore the patient's current health practices to determine where change is indicated to reduce cancer risk.

Nursing Diagnoses and Planning

Nursing diagnoses and related expected patient outcomes commonly applicable to patients undergoing screening for cancer include the following:

NDx: Risk for altered health maintenance related to insufficient knowledge of risk factors for cancer, signs and symptoms of cancer, self-detection methods, recommended schedule of screening examinations, or risk-reducing behaviors

Planning: Patient Outcomes

1. Patient identifies general factors associated with an increased risk of cancer.
2. Patient describes factors in family history or life-style that predispose to development of cancer.
3. Patient identifies measures that can decrease the risk of cancer.
4. Patient lists the seven warning signs of cancer.
5. Patient performs correctly appropriate self-examinations for detection of cancer.
6. Patient states action to be taken if a warning sign is discovered.
7. Patient states how often screening examinations for particular types of cancer should be done given age, family history, existence of predisposing factors, and so on.

Nursing Interventions and Evaluation

NDx: Risk for altered health maintenance

Review with the patient the common types of cancers and their respective risk factors, signs, and symptoms (see Table 34–1). Discuss health practices that may reduce the risk of cancer (Highlight 34–1), and teach self-examination techniques, such as breast self-examination, skin inspection, or testicular examination. (The details of these examinations are reviewed in related chapters of this book.) Explore with the patient how new health behaviors can be incorporated into his or her lifestyle. Allow ample time for questions and concerns.

Compare the patient's status with the expected outcomes. If the outcomes are not met, reassess the patient and revise the plan.

*D*iagnosis

A complete patient history and physical examination is required to obtain a medical diagnosis. Diagnostic procedures are chosen based on patient symptoms, results of the examination, and the type of cancer suspected. The only definitive way to diagnose can-

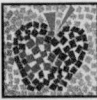

HIGHLIGHT
34–1
HEALTH PROMOTION & RISK REDUCTION

Health Practices That May Reduce Cancer Risk

Eat a diet that includes:

Vegetables and food high in vitamins A and C

High fiber foods: whole grain cereal, fruits, and vegetables

Limit:

Consumption of salt-cured, smoked, and nitrite-cured foods

Fat intake

Alcohol consumption

Avoid:

Smoking

Obesity

Sunlight

Have regular physical examinations

Participate in screening for common types of cancer:

Baseline mammography between ages 35 and 40, every 1 to 2 years between ages 40 and 49, annually after age 50

Monthly breast self-examination after age 20

Annual professional breast examination after age 40, every third year between ages 20 and 40

Monthly testicular self-examination

Annual digital rectal examination for prostate cancer after age 40; prostate-specific antigen level and rectal examination after age 50, earlier if in a high-risk group

Annual test for occult blood in the stool after age 50

Skin inspection

Papanicolaou smear after two negative examination results 1 year apart, every third year between ages 20 (or when sexually active, whichever comes first) and 65

Pelvic examination every third year between ages 20 and 40, annually after age 40

cer is to obtain a specimen of the suspect tissue through biopsy for pathologic study.

Tumors are classified based on their histologic characteristics. The pathologist grades the tissue specimen based on the similarity of tumor cells to normal cells of that tissue as follows:

Grade 1   Well-differentiated (looks like normal cells)
Grade 2   Moderately well-differentiated
Grade 3   Poorly differentiated
Grade 4   Anaplastic

Higher-grade tumors (more immature cells) are considered more malignant and possess a higher likelihood of growth and spread.

STAGING

Cancer staging is a method of identifying the extent of the disease. The TNM staging system is an internationally accepted method for tumor staging. Each anatomic site is classified based on three components: tumor size (T), characteristics of regional lymph nodes and the presence or absence of malignant cells in the lymph nodes (N), and presence or absence of metastatic disease (M).

DIAGNOSTIC PROCEDURES

Blood Tests

Blood tests are scheduled to detect abnormalities. A complete blood count (CBC) is done to review the status of the patient's white blood cells, red blood cells, and platelets. Serum chemicals are monitored to assess the patient's metabolic functions. Serum chemical levels can be elevated by the oncologic process of organ destruction in metastatic cancer. For example, the level of serum alkaline phosphatase, which is produced in the liver and bone, may be elevated if cancer cells are destroying cells of the liver or bone. Other serum chemicals monitored to assess for organ destruction include calcium, aspartate transaminase, and alanine transaminase.

Highly specialized blood tests are done by radioimmunoassay to detect tumor markers. Tumor markers are proteins and hormones produced by certain tumors. These proteins and hormones are usually produced only during fetal development and are called oncofetal proteins and ectopic hormones, respectively. The highly immature nature of cancer cells makes them capable of producing oncofetal proteins and ectopic hormones (hormones produced by organs that do not normally produce them or produced in situations in which they would not normally be produced) that can be measured in the blood. As tumors increase in size, these tumor marker levels increase. As tumor size declines, the levels decrease. An example of an oncofetal protein is carcinoembryonic antigen, which is produced by several tumors of the gastrointestinal tract. It has also been reported in lung, breast, and ovarian tumors. An example of an ectopic hormone is human chorionic gonadotropin (hCG), which is produced by tumors of the testicle, ovary, and pancreas.

Prostate-specific antigen, which increases proportionately to the total mass of the prostate gland, is a tumor marker used in the staging and management of prostate cancer.

Stool Tests

The patient's stool is tested for occult blood. This is an important test for the early detection of colorectal cancer. Before this test, the patient is told not to eat red meat for at least 24 hours. This helps reduce false-positive results. If stool specimen cards are given to the patient for feces sampling over a period of a few days, the patient is instructed to use a disposable glove and place a small smear of the fecal material onto the card. The card is then returned to the health-care provider for testing.

Cytologic Tests

Cytology is the study of the structure and function of cells. Specimens of body fluid may be obtained to detect cancerous cells. Sputum, cervical scrapings, or fluid aspirated from a tumor are examples of tissue specimens examined for cancerous cells.

Sputum cytology is used in the detection of lung cancer. An early morning specimen is usually submitted. For this test, the patient is instructed to rinse the mouth with saline to reduce oral bacteria and food particles in the specimen. The patient then takes several deep breaths and expectorates the sputum into a sterile receptacle. If needed, production of sputum can be assisted by use of a nebulizer to inhale a saline solution. Endotracheal suction can also be used to obtain a sputum specimen.

A Papanicolaou (Pap) test is performed by obtaining a scraping sample of cells from the cervix, endometrium, and vagina. The cells are obtained during an internal examination, and the scraping is transferred to a glass slide. The cells are reviewed by a pathologist and classified based on the presence or absence of abnormal cells. One classification system is as follows:

Class 1   Absence of abnormal cells
Class 2   Suggestive, but inconclusive for malignant cells
Class 3   Presence of malignant cells

The American Cancer Society recommends a Pap test every 3 years for women between ages 20 and 65 who have had two negative tests a year apart and are not in a high-risk group. The American College of Obstetricians and Gynecologists recommends that the test be done yearly. For further discussion of this procedure, see Chapter 40.

Fluid from a suspicious tumor mass may be obtained through an aspiration needle. The fluid from a breast cyst, lymph node, or palpable organ can be examined for the presence of abnormal cells, as can cerebrospinal fluid and washings of cells from the bronchus, esophagus, and stomach.

Patient preparation depends on how and from where the fluid specimen is obtained. The aspiration of fluid from a breast cyst can be performed in an outpatient setting, whereas a cavital washing such as in the case of obtaining bronchial fluid requires that the patient undergo a bronchoscopy and be sedated (see Chap. 14).

Radiographic and Imaging Tests

CHEST X-RAYS

X-rays are a form of electromagnetic radiation that can pass through the body and define internal structures. An x-ray of the chest is obtained to survey the lungs, mediastinum, heart, and thorax by providing a picture of these structures. The x-ray may reveal the location and size of a primary or metastatic chest tumor.

BODY X-RAYS

Radiographic pictures can be obtained to survey the bones and internal organs. These include contrast x-rays of the upper gastrointestinal tract and small bowel studies. Barium is swallowed for the upper gastrointestinal tract examination and given by means of an enema for the small bowel x-ray examination (see Chap. 21).

MAMMOGRAPHY

Mammography is an x-ray examination of the breasts used to detect abnormal breast tissue (see Chap. 42).

TOMOGRAPHY

Tomography uses higher radiation doses than plain x-rays to visualize body structures in linear planes. In this way, sections of the body can be seen without other organs obstructing the field.

FLUOROSCOPY

Fluoroscopy uses higher-than-normal doses of x-ray to visualize an area and ensure accuracy during a procedure, such as a fluoroscopy-guided biopsy.

ULTRASONOGRAPHY

Ultrasonography directs high-frequency sound waves into the body over a specific organ or body part. The sound echoes that are created reveal external features of the organ. Tumor masses can be localized and measured using this non–radiation-producing imaging method. Ultrasonographic pictures are also used to guide the surgeon during a biopsy.

For ultrasonography of the abdomen and pelvis, the patient is required not to urinate for 1 hour before the examination. The patient is also in-structed to drink three to four full glasses of water before the examination. This preparation fills the bladder and helps push the bowel out of the way of the ultrasound waves. In addition, urine in the bladder improves transmission of the ultrasound waves. Before the examination, the patient is instructed to remove clothing and is given a hospital gown. The patient is positioned on a table either face up or face down, depending on the type of examination. An oil or gel is applied over the area to be surveyed. This lubrication prevents air from getting between the sound source and the skin. A transducer that resembles a microphone is passed over the area in different directions. The physician or technician views the results of the sound waves on a monitor, and photographs are taken of the images by a camera attached to the ultrasound equipment.

RADIONUCLIDE SCANNING

A radionuclide is a radioactive material, a small amount of which is given intravenously, carried through the blood stream, and traced in the body using a scanning machine. The resulting radioactivity in the tissue being studied can be increased or decreased relative to normal. Areas of decreased radioactivity, or *cold spots*, represent nonfunctioning tissue whereas areas of increased radioactivity or *hot spots* represent hyperfunctioning tissue. Both hot and cold spots may be associated with tumor growth. Scanning is used to evaluate structures in the brain, bones, liver, gallbladder, lungs, spleen, heart, kidney, pancreas, and thyroid. It begins when the radionuclide is distributed, which can take minutes or hours depending on the material used and the area to be scanned. For example, a liver scan begins about 30 minutes after the injection. A bone scan begins 2 to 3 hours after the injection. The patient is positioned on a table and asked to lie still and possibly change positions during the procedure. Scanning times vary from 15 minutes to 1 hour based on the organ being surveyed.

COMPUTED TOMOGRAPHY

This radiographic procedure produces a detailed, cross-sectional, three-dimensional image using information analyzed by computer and reconstructed as a series of cross-sectional views. A ring encircling the body contains rotating x-ray tubes that survey the body at varying levels. Intravenous or oral contrast material is sometimes used to enhance the computer-produced images of certain organs.

The patient is instructed to drink only clear fluids for the meal preceding the scan. At the time of the scan, the patient, in a hospital gown, is positioned on the table lying face up. The patient is instructed to lie still and told that the table will slowly move through the x-ray scanner and that the sound of gears and motors in the x-ray ring may be heard. The procedure can take as long as 1 hour to complete.

MAGNETIC RESONANCE IMAGING

Magnetic resonance imaging employs magnetic fields and radiofrequency waves analyzed by a computer to produce two- and three-dimensional cross sections of the body. This imaging technique does not expose the patient to any radiation or contrast materials. The patient is placed on a nonmagnetic stretcher that slides into a narrow tunnel-like space in the large magnetic resonance machine. The procedure takes 30 to 90 minutes to complete.

There are no food or fluid restrictions for the examination. The patient is given a gown and asked to remove clothing and metallic objects, such as hairpins, glasses, jewelry, and nonpermanent dentures. Patients with cardiac pacemakers or other metallic implant devices cannot be scanned by this method. A patient history is taken, and the patient is checked with a metal detector before the procedure. The patient is informed that a variety of noises from the machine may be heard during the procedure.

ENDOSCOPY

Endoscopy is the use of fiberoptic instruments to visualize and, in some cases, obtain biopsy samples from inside the body. Through these instruments, physicians can examine the entire gastrointestinal tract, the mediastinum, the bronchial tubes, the bladder, and the abdominal cavity. The specific details of these tests and respective patient preparation and nursing care are detailed in other chapters of this book.

NURSING PROCESS GUIDELINES
Diagnostic Tests for Cancer

Nursing care for patients who undergo radiographic and imaging diagnostic tests involves preparing the patient for the procedure, allaying anxiety, and providing the patient with information related to the test. Explain what the procedure entails, establish a supportive relationship with the patient, and provide time for patient questions. Because these tests have been ordered as part of a diagnostic workup for cancer, be sensitive to the extreme anxiety and apprehension that patients and family may be experiencing. In addition, make sure the patient knows who will convey the results of the tests and when.

NURSING PROCESS
Newly Diagnosed Cancer

Assessment

Assess the patient and family for misunderstandings related to cause, prognosis, or treatment modes of cancer. It is important to correct popular myths, such as the belief that cancer is contagious or that breast cancer can be caused by accidentally hitting the breast. The patient and family should have a realistic view of the prognosis. Cancer is no longer always and immediately fatal, as believed in the past. Rather, some types of cancer respond well to treatment and patients go on to live long, full lives. The patient and family should also understand that there are many different types of treatment, such as surgery, radiation, chemotherapy, and immunotherapy. Explain that the type of treatment selected depends on the type and stage of the disease.

Assess the patient's and family's emotional response to the diagnosis, with particular attention to the patient's readiness to follow through with treatment and make necessary decisions. Also assess the patient's support systems and coping skills. Find out if the patient has a person with whom he or she can share feelings and concerns. Ask about resources available to help the patient carry out the plan of therapy. The latter includes determining such factors as the ability to pay not only for the treatment itself but for help in the home, if needed, and to obtain transportation and assistance to outpatient radiation or chemotherapy treatments and physician visits.

Nursing Diagnoses and Planning

Nursing diagnoses and related expected patient outcomes commonly applicable to patients diagnosed with cancer include the following:

NDx: Risk for ineffective individual coping related to dealing with the diagnosis of cancer and making adjustments in lifestyle necessitated by diagnosis and plan of treatment

Planning: Patient Outcomes
1. Patient openly discusses fears and anxiety.
2. Patient asks questions relevant to the diagnosis, prognosis, and treatment plan.
3. Patient identifies realistic problems.
4. Patient identifies sources of support and how to use them.

NDx: Knowledge deficit: cause, prognosis, type of malignancy, and treatment methods

Planning: Patient Outcomes
1. Patient describes available options, citing the major advantages and disadvantages of each.
2. Patient describes the agreed-upon plan of treatment in terms of time frame, side effects, and expected effect on prognosis.

Nursing Interventions and Evaluation

NDx: Risk for ineffective individual coping
Based on assessment data, plan interventions that encourage coping. Refer the patient and family to community agencies, community resources, and other professionals if indicated. (See Appendix 3.) Many patients benefit from self-help support groups in which people with cancer share their experiences, problems, and concerns.

NDx: Knowledge deficit: cause, prognosis, type of malignancy, and treatment methods
Clarify and reinforce information given to the patient and family by the physician about the disease

and its treatment. Because the emotional stress associated with a diagnosis of cancer can interfere with teaching and learning, provide information in writing and allow opportunities for questions. Repeat information as often as necessary.

Compare the patient's status with the expected outcomes. If the outcomes are not met, reassess the patient's level of understanding and revise the plan.

Cancer Management

The complex nature of oncologic disorders dictates that there is no single treatment. The major treatment modalities of surgery, radiation therapy, and chemotherapy have been used alone and in combination for preventing, controlling, and eliminating cancerous tumors. Immunotherapy is a form of therapy that is being investigated. Treatment selection is based on several individual patient variables, which include the patient's age, type and classification of tumor, stage of disease, response to previous therapies, concomitant medical illnesses, and general health status.

SURGERY

Surgery is the oldest and most frequently used treatment for cancer. Because a definitive diagnosis of cancer requires a biopsy specimen, patients may undergo surgical procedures early in the course of treatment. Surgery has many applications in the treatment of cancer. Surgical procedures are performed for cancer prevention, tissue biopsy, primary tumor removal, disease staging, tumor debulking, hormonal ablation, disease palliation, and reconstruction. (See appropriate chapters for nursing care of the surgical patient and related procedures.)

Preventive Surgery

Preventive surgery involves the surgical removal of premalignant tumors. Many people are predisposed to developing certain tumors for genetic, congenital, or other health reasons. An example is the high incidence of colon cancer in people with multiple colon polyps. For these people, a prophylactic colectomy may be indicated. Men with cryptorchidism (undescended testicles) have a high incidence of cancer of the testicles. The incidence is decreased when surgery to descend the testicles is performed before age 6. Other surgical interventions for cancer prevention include removal of premalignant skin tumors and benign colon polyps.

Biopsy

If a suspicious mass is palpated or revealed by a diagnostic procedure, the definitive method for di-

agnosis is to obtain a biopsy of the mass for examination by a pathologist. Based on the clinical situation, different types of biopsy techniques may be used:

Needle biopsy: Insertion of a needle into a tumor to withdraw fluid or tissue

Incisional biopsy: Removal of a piece of the tumor

Excisional biopsy: Removal of the entire tumor

Closed biopsies: Performed via endoscopy on deep lesions revealed on imaging tests to obtain tissue samples. The surgeon may use the picture from a CT scan to locate a lesion for biopsy.

Tumor Removal

Surgical removal of a malignant tumor may be the only treatment for some tumor types. Early-stage, localized tumors with low incidence of metastasis can be treated by removing the primary tumor. Surgical removal usually includes removal of the tumor mass, part of the surrounding tissue, and the regional lymph nodes.

Staging

Staging surgery reveals the extent of disease spread by sampling regional and distant lymph nodes and sampling and viewing other organs for tumor. An example of tumor staging is the removal of axillary lymph nodes during surgery for breast cancer.

Tumor Debulking

In some cases, cancer surgery involves reducing or debulking the amount of tumor. When the entire tumor cannot be removed, or in cases of widespread metastases, the surgeon removes as much tumor as possible. The remaining tumor is then treated with other therapies, such as radiation and chemotherapy.

Hormonal Ablation

Certain tumor types, such as cancer of the breast and prostate, respond to hormonal manipulation. Removal of hormone-producing organs, such as the ovaries, testicles, or adrenal glands, may be indicated for some patients. In some cases, hormonal ablation is achieved medically through the use of agents that block production of the hormone or its action at target tissues.

Surgical Palliation

Surgery may be indicated in advanced cancer for pain relief or to alleviate organ obstruction. Palliative surgery can improve the quality of a patient's life by relieving physical symptoms caused by the tumor.

Reconstruction and Rehabilitation

Surgical procedures in the area of reconstruction and rehabilitation have improved in the past decade. Major advances in the field of breast and head and neck reconstruction have made it an important component in cancer treatment. Surgical procedures can be used to restore functional losses that may have resulted from previous radiation therapy or surgery.

NURSING PROCESS GUIDELINES
Cancer Surgery

Nursing care of the patient undergoing surgery for cancer does not essentially differ from that given to any surgical patient. However, certain problems and related nursing activities may have greater significance because of the nature of the diagnosis. For example, the psychologic impact of cancer surgery is great. The patient and family may experience a wide range of emotions and reactions to the diagnosis and the need for surgery. In addition, many types of cancer surgery involve change or loss of body function, limitations of mobility, and change in physical appearance, which can be potentially devastating to the patient.

RADIATION

Radiation therapy uses the effects of ionization to damage and kill cancer cells. The exact mechanism is unknown; however, it is believed that as radiation waves are absorbed by cells, energy within the cells increases. This energy releases electrons from atomic orbits, causing the atom to become ionized, a process called ionization, which damages cellular DNA and the cell membrane.

Electromagnetic waves and particle waves are the two types of ionizing radiation. Electromagnetic waves are divided into two types: gamma radiation and roentgen radiation (x-rays). Because of their high energy and penetrating capability, gamma rays are used to treat malignant cells. Gamma rays can be produced from radioactive sources, such as radium or cobalt, or from mechanical sources using electrostatic machines. X-rays are similar to gamma rays but have less energy and are usually produced artificially. X-rays are used in diagnostic procedures rather than for the actual treatment of malignant cells.

Particle radiation uses high-energy beams of atomic particles such as neutrons, protons, and alpha and negative pi mesons to destabilize atoms and cause ionization. The principal difference between each type of particle is the size and charge. Negatively charged particles, such as beta particles, have higher tissue-penetrating power.

Radioactive energy is released during the decay process of radioactive substances, which are also known as radioactive isotopes. The length of time that these isotopes emit radiation is called their active life. The half-life is a measurement of the time it takes for the isotope to lose 50% of its radioactive activity. This time can vary from milliseconds to several days to thousands of years, depending on the element.

The amount of radiation delivered to tissues is measured as the *r*adiation *a*bsorbed *d*ose, known as the rad. The amount of ionizing radiation that has the same biologic effect as 1 rad is called the *r*oentgen *e*quivalent *m*an dose, known as the rem.

Radiation damages rapidly growing cells so they cannot reproduce. A cell is most sensitive to the effects of radiation during the G_2 and mitosis phases of the cell cycle. Some cells lose their ability to reproduce immediately, whereas others may be able to reproduce for only a short time after their initial radiation exposure. In a third group of cells, radiation may cause minor changes within the cell but not enough to destroy the reproductive process. Because both malignant and normal cells can be damaged during radiation therapy, the goal of radiation therapy is to deliver a lethal dose of radiation to the malignant cells while minimizing the amount of radiation to which normal cells are subjected. There is a direct relationship between the presence of molecular oxygen within tissues and the success of radiation on cancer cells. Hypoxic and anoxic cells are more resistant to ionizing radiation. Pharmacologic agents, including chemotherapeutic agents, are being studied for their possible value in increasing cellular oxygen levels and are called radiosensitizers. In addition, agents called radioprotectors that may protect normal tissue from the effects of radiation are being studied.

Radiosensitivity is a measure of susceptibility to radiation-induced damage and cell death. Some tumors are known to be more radiosensitive than others and may be categorized based on the kind of organ tissue that is producing the tumor. Tumors of germinal, epithelial, and skin origin are the most radiosensitive. Radioresistant malignant cells are less sensitive to the effects of ionizing radiation and require extremely high doses of radiation to be destroyed. The amount of radiation required for destruction of radioresistant tumors results in irreversible damage to the normal tissue surrounding the tumor.

Therapeutic Uses of Radiation

Radiation therapy performs many roles in treating early and advanced cancer. Often, it is used as a component of a treatment plan that may include surgery and chemotherapy.

Radiation therapy can eradicate many tumor types. In these cases, the goal of treatment is cure. Radiation may be used to shrink a tumor that is too large to be surgically removed, allowing surgical removal after the radiation is completed. For certain tumors, such as breast cancer, radiation may be administered to regional lymph nodes after the primary tumor has been surgically excised or chemotherapeutically eradicated. Radiation is used for palliative treatment in advanced cancer to provide relief from tumor symptoms such as pain or organ obstruction, to prevent further complications from the tumor, and to treat many oncologic emergencies such as superior vena cava syndrome and spinal cord compression.

Modes of Radiation Therapy

Radiation therapy given by external beam is called teletherapy. When given internally, it is called brachytherapy.

EXTERNAL RADIATION THERAPY

External-beam equipment delivers radiation to a designated area of the body. Dosimetry is the method used to calculate the size of the area or port (section of the body) to be radiated and the amount of radiation necessary based on tumor type, size, and depth. The radiation port is demarcated using a special marking ink on the skin. The markings remain throughout the treatment course, and patients are told not to remove them. Occasionally, small tattoos rather than ink markings are used to demarcate the area.

The radiation is delivered in divided dose increments over a period of several weeks, depending on the amount of radiation required and the size and depth of the tumor. This process of divided doses, called dose fractionation, allows time for normal cellular repair and increased tumor kill. For example, a patient may receive 300 rad daily for 5 days a week over a period of 5 weeks, for a total radiation dose of 6000 rad. The radioactive energy generated is measured in units of electron volts (eV). Some machines deliver low energy levels that are measured in thousands of volts (kiloelectron volts [keV]), also called orthovoltage. Other, more widely used machines, such as the cobalt-60 and the linear accelerator, can deliver greater levels that are measured in millions of volts (MeV), called megavoltage. The cobalt-60 equipment can release as much as 3 MeV, compared with the linear accelerator, which can release as much as 25 MeV. Megavoltage radiation has several advantages over the classic orthovoltage method:

• Deeper tissue penetration
• Less radiation scattered to normal tissues
• Less radiation absorption by bone, resulting in more uniform dosage to the tumor
• Decreased skin toxicity

External-beam radiation therapy is usually performed in an outpatient setting unless the patient's medical condition requires hospitalization.

The patient receives external radiation in a special room that houses the radiation equipment. The patient is positioned on a table (Fig. 34–6), and positioning usually takes longer than the actual radiation treatment. Immobilization devices may be used to prevent movement during treatment. Protective shields may also be placed near the radiation site to protect other body parts from radiation beams. The patient is alone in the room during the treatment; however, the radiation technologist views the patient through a window or video monitor and can communicate with the patient.

INTERNAL RADIATION THERAPY

Brachytherapy is the technique of implanting sealed or unsealed radioactive material adjacent to or within the targeted tumor. Here the tumor is subjected to radioactive activity over a longer period of time as compared with external beam therapy. Sealed isotopes, such as iridium (^{192}Ir) and cesium (^{137}Cs), are contained in tubes, needles, capsules, wires, or seeds. The sealed containers are then placed inside the body cavity. In the treatment of many gynecologic cancers, for example, the source is placed vaginally. In the treatment of pleural effusions, the radioactive material is injected into the pleural space. Interstitial placement of sealed radioactive material involves direct placement of the material into the body tissues, such as the breast, tongue, floor of the mouth, and oropharynx.

Preloading refers to the process of placing containers with the radioactive material already inside.

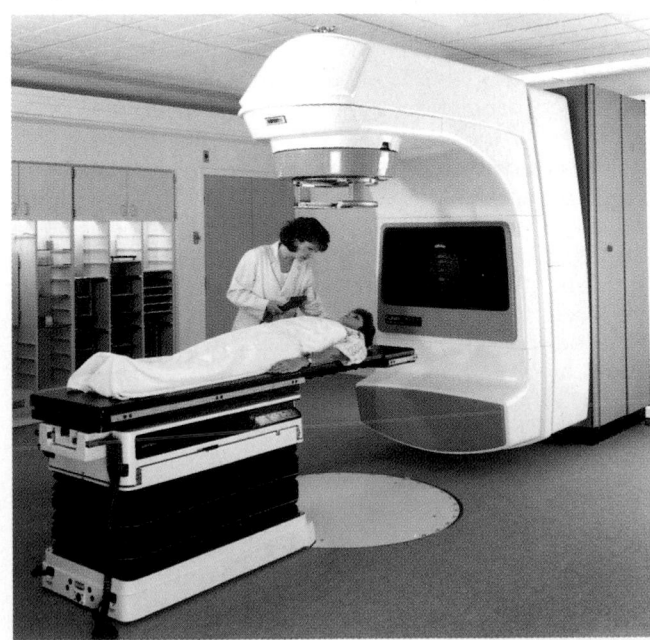

Figure 34–6

A 2300 C/D linear accelerator used for external beam radiation. (Courtesy of Varian Associates, Inc., Palo Alto, CA.)

Afterloading refers to the process of first placing the container within the tissues, and then inserting the radioactive material into the container. Afterloading requires that the needles or tubes be placed into the treatment area and tunneled out of the skin (Fig. 34–7). The procedure is done under local or general anesthesia in the operating room. The radioactive substance is later inserted into the tubes in the patient's hospital room. The patient requires a private room during the procedure, and visitors and staff must limit the amount of time spent in the patient's room. Unsealed isotopes, such as phosphorus (^{32}P) used in the treatment of prostatic cancer and iodine (^{131}I) used in the treatment of thyroid cancer, are administered without a protective container. For unsealed isotopes, the risk of radiation contamination is high. Table 34–2 reviews precautions needed for sealed and unsealed isotopes.

The radioactive implant may remain in place for several days. In some cases, if the amount of radioactivity is small and the half-life of the isotope is very short, the implant remains permanently.

Safety Precautions

The Nuclear Regulatory Commission has developed guidelines for occupational exposure to radiation. Every hospital must have a radiation safety officer responsible for ensuring compliance with standards. Hospital personnel who care for patients receiving radiation are given special dosimetry badges to wear on their clothing. The badges contain film that measures radiation exposure. They are collected monthly and tested for radiation absorption. A permanent record of radiation exposure is kept for all personnel. The results of the dosimetry readings are reviewed regularly by the radiation safety officer. U.S. federal regulations stipulate the maximum permissible annual exposure.

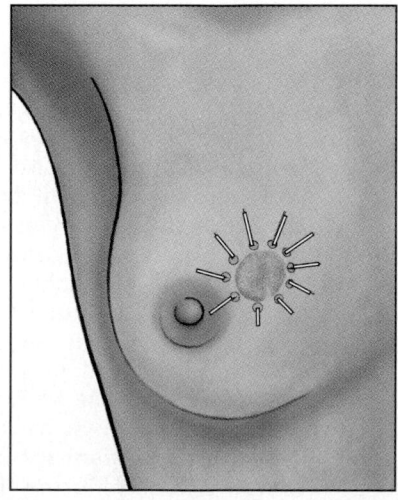

Figure 34–7

Needles in place in the breast, through which iridium seeds in a plastic tube are passed.

Table 34–2

Nursing Precautions for Internal Radiation Therapy
Wear a dosimetry badge.
Keep the telephone number of a radiation safety officer available.
Place a sign on the patient's door: CAUTION, RADIOACTIVE MATERIAL.
Indicate on the patient's chart that radioactive implant is in place.
Provide the patient with a private room and private bath.
Limit visitors. Bar children younger than age 16 and pregnant women.
Instruct visitors to remain at least 6 feet from the radiation source and to stay no longer than 30 minutes.
Place a lead shield at the bedside.
Pregnant nurses should not provide patient care.
Sealed sources require no special treatment of body fluids, excrement, or bed linen.
Place a lead container and long-handled tongs in the patient's room in case the sealed source becomes dislodged.
Additional precautions for unsealed radioactive sources:
Keep the patient in bed.
Serve meals on disposable materials.
Place linen, bandages, trash, and laundry in labeled bags and keep them in the patient's room until disposal.
Wear gloves when handling body fluid samples. Label the samples "radioactive."
Make sure the room is monitored by a radiation safety officer during hospitalization, in case of accidental spill or a dislodged source, and after patient discharge.
Contact the radiation safety officer as needed.

The patient who is receiving external-beam radiation is not radioactive and poses no risk to the hospital staff. Radiation precautions must be followed, however, when caring for a patient with a radioactive implant. Radiation safety is based on three important factors: time, distance, and shielding.

Time spent in the patient's room is limited to a total of 30 minutes per 8 hours. The amount of radiation emitted decreases by the inverse square of the distance from the source. This means that working twice as far from the radiation source reduces the amount of radiation by one fourth (Fig. 34–8). It is important to maintain maximum physical distance from the patient whenever possible. Lead shielding provides some additional protection; however, lead shields and lead aprons have a significant disadvantage. They are cumbersome to use and work with and may actually induce a nurse to remain in the room for longer time periods. The nurse should consistently adhere to principles of time and distance while caring for the patient.

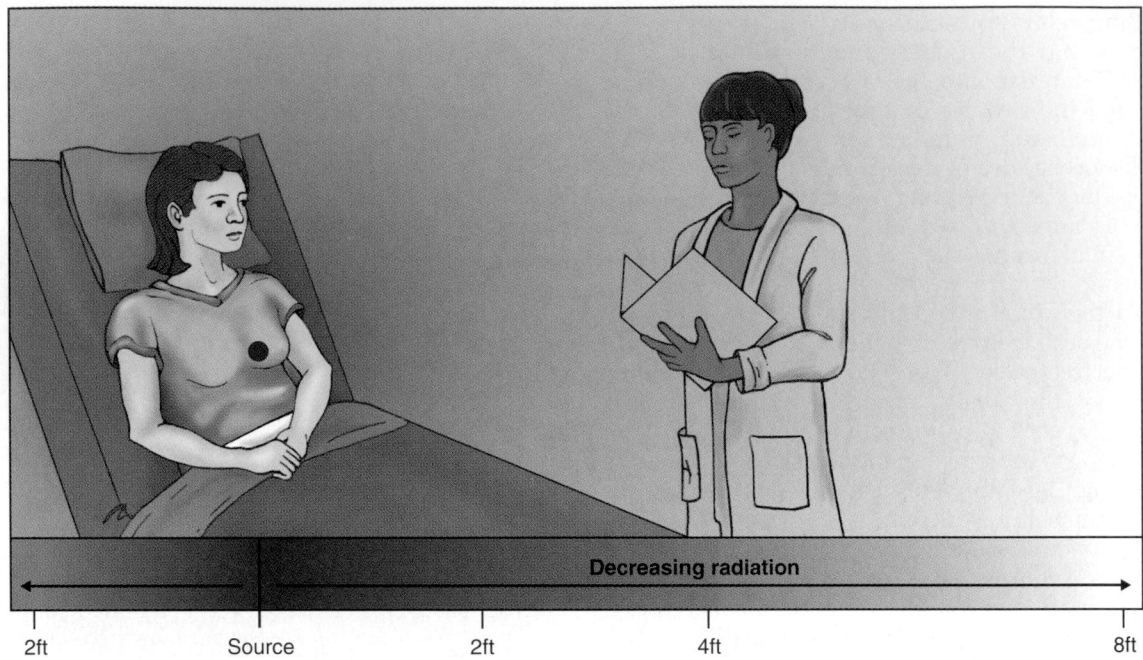

Figure 34–8

Exposure to radioactivity is a function of distance. The nurse nearest the source (the patient) is exposed the most. The nurse at 2 feet receives more than 15 times the radiation that the nurse at 8 feet receives.

Side Effects of Radiation Therapy

During radiation therapy, normal cells are subjected to the ionizing beams. Any tissue near the radiation port can be damaged or destroyed. Side effects of treatment relate to the impact of radiation on normal tissue and depend on the area being treated. Some side effects are acute and temporary. Others develop over time and may be permanent.

SKIN

External radiation must pass through the skin to reach the tumor target. The use of megavoltage therapy has decreased the amount and severity of skin reactions, because here the beams are targeted to become active at greater tissue depth. The most common skin effect is a change in color over the radiation port. The skin may appear tanned or red. A tanning reaction is caused by the increased production of pigment. Reddening of skin color (erythema) is caused by dermal capillary engorgement. Erythema may cause varying degrees of itching over the area. Dry desquamation, which is flaking of the skin, is caused by accumulated dead skin cells. In cases in which basal cells of the skin are destroyed, the dermal level is exposed, which results in the leakage of serum, called moist desquamation.

Skin reactions are usually temporary. However, in cases of severe skin reaction, long-term effects can include scarring, changes in skin texture, and necrosis. Radiation recall is a delayed skin side effect in which the skin of the radiation port becomes irritated after the patient receives certain chemotherapy drugs. Depending on the severity of the recall reaction, vesicles and wet desquamation can develop.

ORAL CAVITY

Radiation can be given through external-beam therapy or interstitial placement of radioactive isotopes to treat tumors of the head and neck region. As the radiation destroys the cancerous cells, healthy cells of the oral cavity are also destroyed. This alters and potentially injures the lining of the oral cavity, the teeth, and the salivary glands.

The rapidly growing cells of the mucous membrane provide a protective lining of cells in the oral cavity. Irritation of the membrane causes an inflammatory response, known as mucositis or stomatitis. Varying degrees of stomatitis can result from injury to the oral mucosa. Severe stomatitis can cause oral pain and infection and can further complicate the patient's nutritional and hydration status. Teeth can be affected indirectly by radiation from periodontal membrane damage and more acidic saliva, which allows an increased amount of oral bacteria. Injury to the salivary glands can decrease saliva production, resulting in a condition known as xerostomia or mouth dryness. Saliva is important for lubricating and cleansing the oral cavity, diluting food, and keeping an alkaline environment, which limits bacterial buildup. Salivary secretions may become thick and difficult to expectorate.

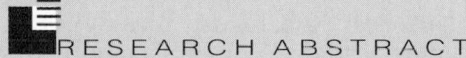

RESEARCH ABSTRACT

What Approaches to Mouth Care Do Nurses Use for Patients Receiving Radiation Therapy to the Head and Neck?

Ganley BJ. Mouth care for the patient undergoing head and neck radiation therapy. A survey of radiation oncology nurses. Oncol Nurs Forum 1996;23(10):1619.

Oral complications from radiation therapy include inflammation, infection, altered function, and discomfort. Management of these complications is varied and not always based on research. Ganley therefore decided to survey the members of the Radiation Special Interest Group of the Oncology Nursing Society regarding their practice patterns for patients receiving radiation therapy to the head and neck. She obtained a 43% response rate to her questionnaire.

Results from Ganley's study indicate that the vast majority of oncology nurses (73%) did not use a standardized tool to assess oral health, even though several tools and scales are available. Most of the nurses in the study (82%) recommended that patients use a soft toothbrush until complications developed. Once complications developed, 55% recommended the use of a soft toothette. Nonabrasive fluoride toothpastes were recommended by 80% of respondents. Salt and baking soda solutions were the most frequently recommended rinsing solutions for patients both before and after the development of complications.

Although Ganley did not set out to establish the most effective method of mouth care during radiation therapy, she did establish that there is a range of practice approaches to the clinical problem, despite general guidelines currently available to clinicians.

Questions to Consider

1. What is the current protocol for assessing and managing oral complications of radiation therapy in your clinical setting?
2. Is there a systematic tool for assessing both objective and subjective dimensions of oral health?
3. What products are available to nurses in your agency to provide oral hygiene?
4. What is the process for obtaining new self-care products in your clinical setting?
5. Are dental consultations a part of the team approach to caring for people undergoing radiation therapy in your clinical setting?

Hypogeusia is the term used to describe an alteration or loss of taste sensation, which is related to the effect of radiation on the patient's taste buds. *Dysgeusia* is the term used to describe the presence of unpleasant tastes sometimes described as metallic. *Ageusia* is the absence of taste sensation.

HEAD

Radiation therapy to the brain can cause cerebral edema. To prevent this, patients are given steroids to combat the inflammatory process.

Patients may also experience nausea and vomiting from the effects of radiation on the brain's chemoreceptor trigger zone. Because hair follicles are destroyed by radiation, patients receiving radiation to the head experience hair loss, called alopecia. Hair may be lost or growth arrested, depending on the amount of radiation received and the hair follicles' response to it. Possible long-term and often delayed side effects include brain cell necrosis and infarction.

CHEST

Primary or metastatic lung tumors can be treated with radiation therapy. Side effects include esophagitis, pneumonitis, and the delayed effect of pulmonary fibrosis. The epithelium of the lungs, trachea, and esophagus can be affected by radiation, resulting in inflammation, infection, and obstruction due to narrowing of these structures. Thus, the patient is at risk for negative effects on hydration and nutritional status and respiratory function.

ABDOMEN

Radiation can damage the rapidly growing cells of the gastrointestinal tract. When the upper abdomen receives radiation, the patient may experience nausea and vomiting. This results from mechanical irritation and inflammation of the cells that line the stomach. When the lower gastrointestinal tract receives radiation, the patient may experience diarrhea and abdominal cramping.

PELVIS

Cancers of the cervix, endometrium, prostate, bladder, and rectum are sometimes treated with radiation therapy by external beam and internal implants. Patients may experience side effects that include diarrhea; cystitis; vaginal, urethral, and rectal stenosis; and sexual dysfunction as a result of bowel, bladder, and gonad irritation.

SEXUAL FUNCTION

Radiation to the pelvis by external-beam or internal implant technique can narrow the vaginal walls, decrease secretion of vaginal lubrication, and inflame and scar vaginal tissue. Patients should be informed of these possible side effects and shown how to use a vaginal dilator or encouraged to continue sexual intercourse as a means to keep the vaginal walls open and flexible. Artificial lubrication can be maintained by commercially available creams and lubricants. Radiation to the pelvis and gonads can cause partial and permanent sterility in males. In females, ovarian function can be eradicated by high levels of radiation. Radiation to the pelvis may cause premature menopause and loss of libido. When possible, the reproductive organs are shielded from radiation. Patients should be informed of the possibility of temporary or permanent sterility. Men should be reminded about the availability of sperm banks.

Sexual function may also be altered by fatigue and weakness, along with the multiple side effects of the disease and treatment.

HEMATOPOIETIC SYSTEM

Radiation can affect production of blood cell components in the bone marrow. Bone marrow is composed of rapidly proliferating cells that include white blood cells, red blood cells, and platelets. Radiation to large areas of the body over bony structures such as the pelvis is most likely to produce bone marrow suppression. The patient's blood cell count should be monitored during treatment and through follow-up. Depression of red blood cells is called anemia. Depression of white blood cells, called leukopenia, can compromise the immune system and render the patient unable to fight infections. Depression of the platelet count, called thrombocytopenia, can increase susceptibility to bleeding.

NURSING PROCESS
Radiation Therapy

Assessment

Assess the patient's understanding of the program of radiation therapy, its goals, and its potential side effects. When external beam therapy is given, assess for changes in skin color, for dry or moist desquamation, and for pain or other discomfort at the radiation sites. For patients receiving radiation to the head and neck region, observe the mouth for signs of inflammation, infection, and ulceration. Also assess and note the patient's dental status. Determine the patient's ability to eat, take fluids, and swallow. Note the consistency of saliva. Question the patient about altered taste.

If the patient is receiving radiation to the chest or back, side effects may mimic the symptoms of the underlying disease. Observe for sore throat, dysphagia, and upper chest pain related to esophagitis, as well as for dyspnea, dry cough, hemoptysis, and elevated body temperature. Also assess the patient's need for supplemental oxygen, cough suppressants, analgesics, and nutritional supplements.

Nursing Diagnoses and Planning

Nursing diagnoses and related expected patient outcomes commonly applicable to patients receiving radiation therapy include the following:

NDx: Risk for altered health maintenance related to insufficient knowledge of treatment, side effects, self-care measures, and required follow-up

Planning: Patient Outcomes
1. Patient describes expected effects of radiation.
2. Patient states the symptoms of side effects most likely to occur given the type of radiation administered.
3. Patient describes the relationship of symptoms to the radiation therapy, noting that specific symptoms will disappear when the radiation therapy is completed.
4. Patient receiving external radiation describes or demonstrates appropriate interventions to control specific side effects.
5. Patient receiving external radiation accurately states symptoms that should be reported to the health-care professional.
6. Patient receiving internal radiation states how the radioactive substance will be placed in the body, where the procedure will be done, and how long the radioactive substance will remain in the body.
7. Patient receiving internal radiation describes the need for a private room, and the influence of time, distance, and shielding on the effects of radiation.
8. Patient receiving internal radiation describes the precautions to be observed.
9. Patient receiving internal radiation describes limitations on movement necessitated by the radiation.
10. Patient having internal radiation identifies self-care activities possible despite the limitation on movement and describes how they will be carried out.

In addition, nursing diagnoses and related expected patient outcomes commonly applicable to patients receiving internal radiation therapy include the following:

NDx: Pain related to the presence of a radiation implant and temporary limitation of movement

Planning: Patient Outcomes
1. Patient accepts analgesics.
2. Patient participates in relaxation exercises.
3. Patient reports lessened discomfort.

Nursing Interventions and Evaluation

NDx: Risk for altered health maintenance

For all patients having radiation therapy, reinforce explanations of the purpose of the radiation, the treatment procedure, and possible side effects. Instruct patients receiving external radiation therapy in self-care and comfort measures (Highlight 34–2). Explain radiation precautions to patients receiving internal radiation therapy and their families before the implant is done (see Table 34–2). After the implant is in place, be sure the patient understands the limitations on movement, as well as what self-care activities are possible and expected.

NDx: Pain

Encourage frequent position changes. Provide an alternating pressure mattress. Support body parts with pillows. Help the patient with relaxation exercises. Provide diversionary activities, such as reading, watching television, and listening to the radio. Administer analgesics and muscle relaxants as needed according to the physician's orders. Pain management is discussed in greater detail later in the chapter.

Compare the patient's status with the expected outcomes. If the outcomes are not met, reassess the patient and revise the plan.

CHEMOTHERAPY

The use of drugs to kill cancer cells has its origin in chemical warfare. After World War I, scientists noted bone marrow suppression in soldiers exposed to nitrogen mustard gas. This led to the hypothesis that the chemical could destroy rapidly growing

---

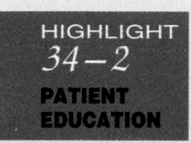 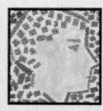

HIGHLIGHT 34–2
PATIENT EDUCATION

Self-Care During External Radiation Therapy

Care of the Skin Affected by Radiation

Instruct the patient to:

Wear loosely fitting clothing.

Gently wash the affected area with a mild soap and pat dry.

Avoid the use of lotion, perfume, and deodorants.

Avoid pressure on the irritated area.

Avoid exposure to the sun.

Avoid swimming in saltwater or chlorinated water.

Avoid applications of heat or cold to irritated areas.

Use a water-soluble lubricant for dry desquamation.

Use either the open or partially open treatment for moist desquamation.

  Open treatment: Keep area clean, dry, uncovered, and exposed to the air.

  Partially open treatment: Keep area clean and covered with a nonadhering dressing. Change dressing *frequently* to keep wound surface clean and dry.

Use cool, moist compresses or water-soluble lubricants for itching.

Take antihistamines and use topical antipruritic lotions as ordered by the physician.

Care of the Mouth Affected by Radiation

Instruct the patient to:

Perform good oral hygiene after eating and at bedtime

using a soft toothbrush, nonabrasive toothpaste, and dental floss.

Increase fluids to at least 2500 mL/d unless otherwise restricted.

Decrease smoking.

Do a daily self-examination of the mouth and report any changes.

Rinse the mouth frequently with mouthwash for xerostomia. Use a mouthwash that does not contain a drying agent such as alcohol.

Breathe through the nose to avoid the drying effect of mouth breathing.

Suck sour, hard candies to help stimulate saliva and create a pleasant taste.

Remove thick oral secretions with a swab, and use an oral gavage bag to irrigate the mouth.

Eat a liquid or blenderized, high-protein diet at room temperature if dysphagia or esophagitis is a problem.

Prevention of Infection

Instruct the patient to:

Wash hands properly.

Keep the fingernails clean and short.

Identify and immediately report any sign of infection, such as fever, severe fatigue, or purulent skin drainage.

cells. During the 1950s, several drugs of the same class were successfully used to shrink lymphatic tumors. By the 1980s, chemotherapy was considered the major intervention to treat and cure more than 12 kinds of tumors, including cancer of the testicle or ovary, Hodgkin's disease, leukemia, and several types of lymphoma. The U.S. government set up an organized system to evaluate new chemotherapeutic drugs under the direction of the National Institutes of Health at the National Cancer Institute. The National Cancer Institute is responsible for overseeing all clinical trials of cancer treatments, including chemotherapy.

Chemotherapeutic drugs are cytotoxic because they disrupt cell development and reproduction. As with radiation, both normal and malignant cells are affected. This is a major limiting factor in the use of chemotherapy. The multiple side effects of chemotherapy range from minor patient discomfort to life-threatening occurrences. This treatment modality has become quite complex as new drugs are developed and new combinations of drugs are formulated and tested. More than 50 different chemotherapeutic agents are used to treat cancer. One or several drugs may be prescribed, depending on the tumor type and stage, previous treatment course, and physical status of the patient.

Chemotherapy can be combined with radiation, surgery, or immunotherapy to treat cancer. It is often used before surgery to shrink large tumors and inhibit microscopic spread of tumor cells. It is also used after the surgical removal of a tumor to similarly inhibit the microscopic spread of tumor cells. This method of chemotherapy, called adjuvant therapy, has been used successfully in the postsurgical treatment of breast, colon, lung, and bone tumors. The treatment goal of chemotherapy can be cure, control, or palliation. Modes of delivery include topical, oral, intravenous, intramuscular, subcutaneous, intrathecal, intra-arterial, intrapleural, and intraperitoneal.

Chemotherapeutic agents are grouped by their activity during the cell cycle. Drugs that affect the cell during certain phases of the cell cycle are considered to be cell cycle specific. Drugs that do not require the cell to be in a specific phase to be effective are called cell cycle nonspecific.

Classification of Chemotherapeutic Agents

Chemotherapeutic agents can be classified into six categories: alkylating agents, antimetabolites, antitumor antibiotics, steroids and hormones, alkaloids, taxanes, and a miscellaneous group. Table 34–3 lists common drugs in each classification.

Alkylating agents interfere with the structure, synthesis, and function of DNA, which results in cell death. They are active in all phases of the cell cycle and are considered cell cycle–nonspecific agents. An exception is the drug cyclophosphamide, whose cellular activity appears to take place in the S

Table 34–3

Classification of Chemotherapeutic Agents

Classification	Chemotherapeutic Agents
Alkylating agents	Cyclophosphamide
	Chlorambucil
	Melphalan
	Busulfan
	Thiotepa
Antimetabolites	Methotrexate
	5-Fluorouracil
	6-Thioguanine
	6-Mercaptopurine
	Cytarabine
Antitumor antibiotics	Doxorubicin
	Daunorubicin
	Dactinomycin
	Mitomycin
Steroids and hormones	Androgens
	Testosterone
	Fluoxymesterone
	Estrogens
	Diethylstilbestrol
	Ethinyl estradiol
	Progestins
	Hydroxyprogesterone
	Medroxyprogesterone
	Megestrol
	Antiestrogens
	Tamoxifen
	Corticosteroids
	Prednisone
	Methylprednisone
	Cortisone
	Dexamethasone
Alkaloids	Vincristine
	Vinblastine
	Podophyllins
	Etoposide
Taxanes	Taxol
	Taxotere
Miscellaneous Agents	L-Asparaginase
	Streptozocin
	Hydroxyurea
	Cisplatin
	Procarbazine

phase. A subclassification in this group includes the nitrosoureas such as carmustine, lomustine, and streptozocin. The action and cytotoxic effects of these drugs resemble those of the alkylating agents; however, they are also effective against cells in the resting phase and can cross the blood-brain barrier. This feature makes them valuable in the treatment of central nervous system tumors.

Antimetabolites interfere with normal biochemical processes that cells need to complete the synthesis of DNA and RNA. These agents are cell cycle specific because their activity takes place during the S phase of the cell cycle. Antimetabolites are more effective against tumors with increased metabolic rates.

Antitumor antibiotics interfere with DNA and RNA synthesis. Their cytotoxic effect results in physical changes to the DNA strands, causing chromosome damage. They are active in all phases of the cell cycle and are considered cell cycle nonspecific.

Hormones and steroids have a wide range of use in cancer treatment. Some tumors require the presence of hormones on their cell surface to grow and have specific areas on the cell membrane where they attach, known as hormone receptors. The antitumor action of hormones depends on the tumor type and the presence of hormonal receptors. Some breast tumors require estrogen for growth. Reducing the availability of estrogen by administering male hormones (such as androgens) or administering antiestrogens (such as tamoxifen) can retard tumor growth. Prostatic cancer requires the presence of androgens to grow and is treated by administering analogues of luteinizing hormone-releasing hormone to inhibit the release of pituitary gonadotropin, antiandrogens to block androgens at target tissues, or estrogen to halt the body's production of the male hormone testosterone. It is also treated by orchiectomy (surgical removal of the testes, which produce testosterone). The complex actions of steroids result in an environment that retards tumor growth. Steroids, such as prednisone, often are combined with other chemotherapeutic agents. They do not suppress bone marrow and, in some cases, can actually stimulate blood cell production.

Plant alkaloids are drugs derived from plants and are cell cycle–specific agents active during the mitosis phase of the cell cycle. They inhibit formation of spindle fibers, thus preventing chromosomes from lining up during the mitosis phase. They also have some activity in the G_2 and S phases, during which they inhibit DNA and protein synthesis. Vincristine and vinblastine, which are derived from the periwinkle plant, are two of the most commonly used alkaloids.

Miscellaneous chemotherapeutic agents are those whose action is not fully understood and whose cytotoxic activity does not fit into the other classifications.

Combination Chemotherapy

Using more than one chemotherapy agent to treat malignant tumors is based on years of research and an increased understanding of the growth, repair, and reproduction of the cancer cell. By combining drugs of different classes, there is an increased chance of being effective at varying times in the cell's reproductive cycle. In many instances, the dosage of one drug used alone would be too high; however, combinations of drugs allow administration of more drugs at lesser dosages. Drugs with varying side effects can be used together.

Chemotherapy combinations have been tested on several tumors. New drug combinations continue to

Table 34–4

Standard Chemotherapy Combinations

Cancer Type	Treatment Combination
Breast cancer	Cyclophosphamide *Methotrexate* *Fluorouracil*
Hodgkin's disease	*Mustard* (nitrogen mustard) *Oncovin* (vincristine) *Prednisone* *Procarbazine*
Ovarian cancer	Doxorubicin Cisplatin
Lymphoma	Doxorubicin Bleomycin Vincristine Dactinomycin

Italicized letters signify how the particular drug combination is referred to in everyday usage (such as the CMF regimen and the MOPP regimen).

be tested. Table 34–4 pairs tumors with their respective standard chemotherapy combinations.

Dosage

The amount of chemotherapy prescribed for a patient is based on several factors, including:

- The type of tumor to be treated
- The patient's history of chemotherapy and radiation therapy
- Bone marrow, kidney, and liver function
- The patient's age
- The patient's physical status
- Concomitant medical illnesses

The dosage of most chemotherapeutic agents is determined by a measurement known as the total body surface area. A special measurement tool called a nomogram calculates the patient's body surface area per square meter (m^2) as a function of the patient's height and weight (Fig. 34–9). For example, if the dosage of doxorubicin is 30 mg/m^2 of body surface area and the patient's body surface area is 1.5 m^2 based on height and weight measurements, the dosage of the drug will be 45 mg.

Treatment Schedules

Chemotherapy is given in time intervals that allow for drug effectiveness and recovery from side effects. For example, in a 28-day treatment cycle, the patient may receive chemotherapy for the first 14 days and no therapy for 14 days. At the end of 28 days, a new cycle begins. The length of time that treatment is prescribed is based on the tumor type, tumor response, and toxicities, along with other factors. Chemotherapy is usually prescribed by a medi-

Body Surface of Adults

Nomogram for determination of body surface from height and mass¹

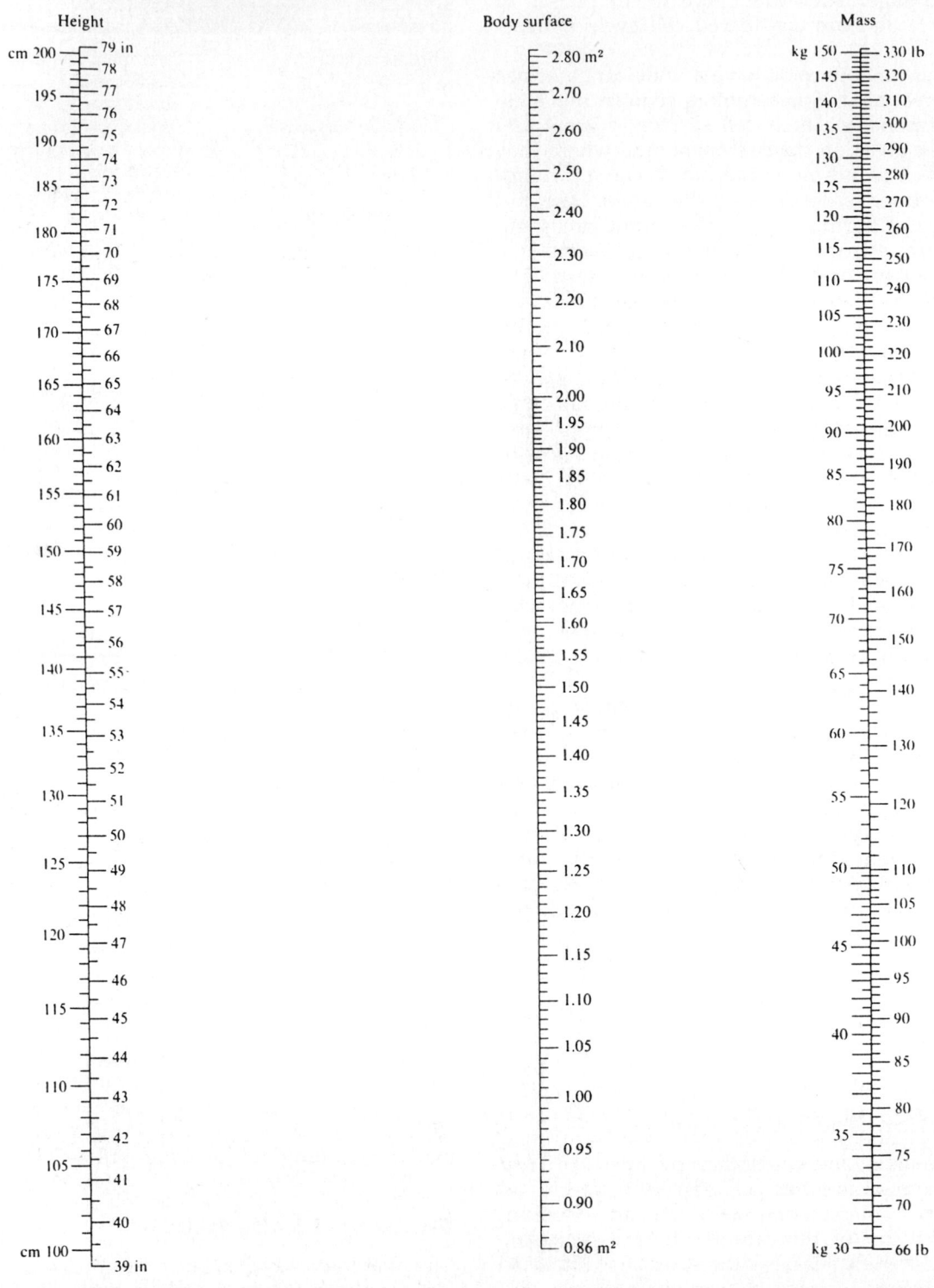

¹ From the formula of Du Bois and Du Bois, *Arch. intern. Med.*, **17**, 863 (1916): $S = M^{0.425} \times H^{0.725} \times 71.84$, or $\log S = \log M \times 0.425 + \log H \times 0.725 + 1.8564$ (*S*: body surface in cm²; *M*: mass in kg; *H*: height in cm).

Figure 34–9

Nomogram to calculate total body surface area for determining chemotherapeutic dose. (From Lentner C [ed]. Geigy scientific tables. 8th ed, Vol 1. Basel, Switzerland: Ciba-Geigy, 1981, p 227.)

cal oncologist, a physician who specializes in the diagnosing and treating of oncologic disorders.

Continuous intravenous infusion of chemotherapy over several hours, days, or weeks is based on the premise that constant exposure of a tumor to small amounts of drugs is effective while less toxic to normal tissues. The use of continuous infusion chemotherapy in gastrointestinal and head and neck tumors is considered standard therapy. Continuous intraperitoneal and intracavital therapy is also being investigated.

Delivery of Chemotherapy

Intravenous use of chemotherapy agents over continuous time intervals and the use of agents that are potentially irritating to veins and surrounding tissues (known as vesicant agents) led to the development of alternative venous access devices. Venous access devices include the central venous catheter, the implantable venous port, and the Ommaya reservoir. Continuous chemotherapy infusion pumps can be portable or implanted under the skin.

CATHETERS

A central venous catheter is surgically placed near the right atrium, is tunneled under the skin of the chest, and exits with an external catheter that is anchored to the skin (Fig. 34–10). The externally placed catheter can be used to obtain blood specimens; to administer chemotherapy or other intravenous medications, blood, and blood products; and for total parenteral nutrition.

Catheters can also be placed intra-arterially and intraperitoneally to administer chemotherapy. Intra-arterial catheters are used when chemotherapy will be delivered directly into an organ, such as the liver. Intraperitoneal catheters are used to bathe the peritoneum with chemotherapy. Chemotherapy can also be instilled into the lungs through an intrapleural catheter.

IMPLANTED VENOUS PORTS

An implanted venous device known as a port is similar to the central venous catheter, except that it has no external catheter (Fig. 34–11). The structure of the port is such that a steel septum with a plastic resealing chamber is implanted under the skin (Fig. 34–12). A special noncoring needle (designed to not pierce the port) is used to access the port. Dressing changes and frequent flushing are not required. The port is flushed by the nurse after treatment or monthly. Patients can be taught to access the port for self-administration of medications and heparinization.

The Ommaya reservoir is a device implanted in the scalp and attached to a catheter threaded into the lateral ventricle for administering chemotherapy to the central nervous system.

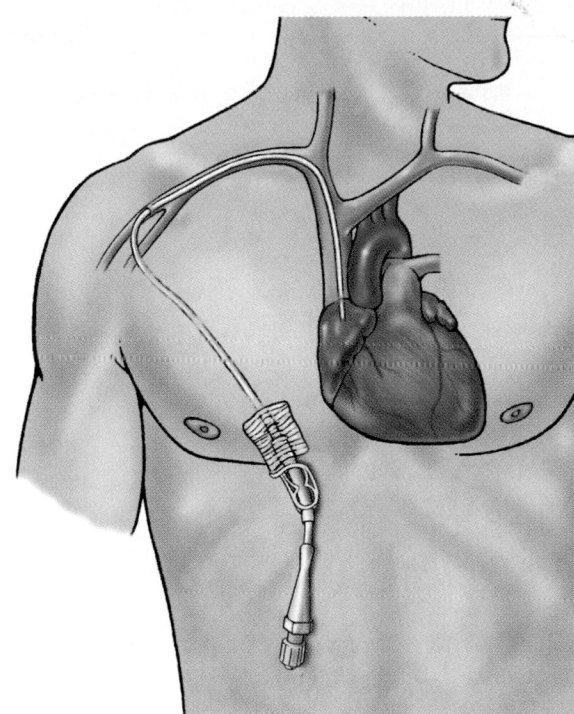

Figure 34–10
Central venous catheter in place.

INFUSION PUMPS

Continuous intravenous administration of chemotherapeutic agents occurs over time intervals that span several hours to several days or weeks. To provide continuous infusion therapy, specialized pumps have been developed. Some are portable and can be attached to a waist belt. The patient can be fully ambulatory and active while receiving continuous chemotherapy (Fig. 34–13). The pump is filled with the chemotherapeutic agent and attached to a central venous line. Some pumps are implanted under the skin and externally filled with the chemotherapeutic agent. The pumps are programmed to deliver small amounts of drug continuously over a given time period.

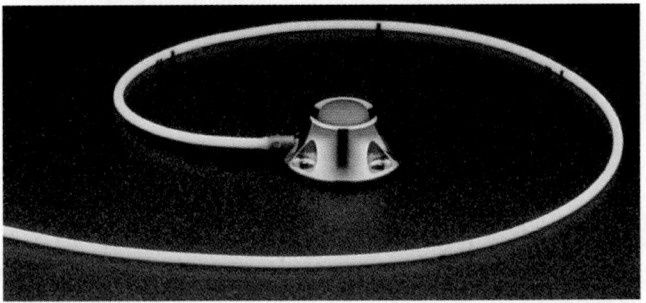

Figure 34–11
Port-A-Cath Low Profile implantable access system. (Courtesy of SIMS Deltec Inc, St. Paul, MN.)

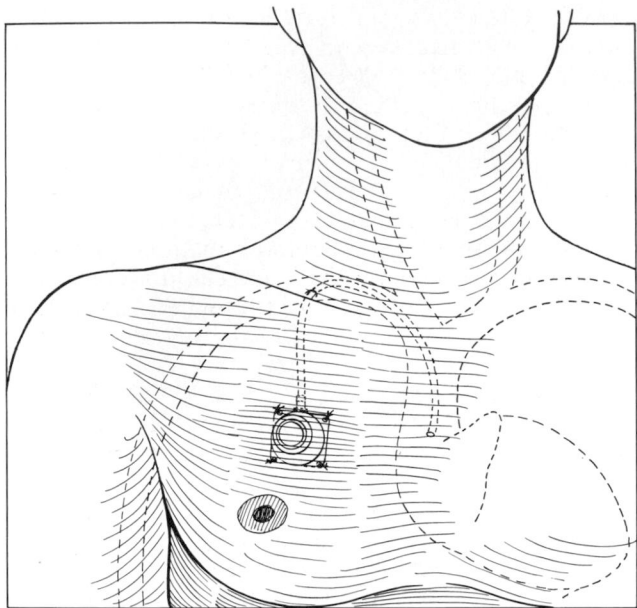

Figure 34–12
Port-A-Cath implantable access system in place in the chest. (Courtesy of SIMS Deltec Inc, St. Paul, MN.)

Safe Handling of Chemotherapeutic Agents

The cytotoxic nature of chemotherapeutic agents requires that personnel who prepare and administer these drugs take precautions to protect themselves

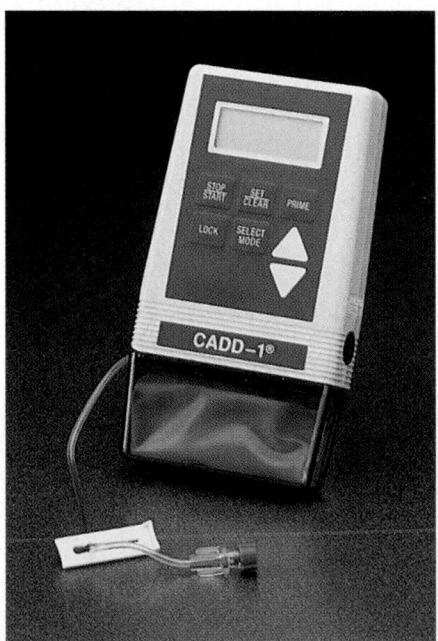

Figure 34–13
Ambulatory infusion pump, which allows continuous intravenous administration of chemotherapy over several hours, days, or weeks without limiting the patient's mobility. (Courtesy of SIMS Deltec Inc, St. Paul, MN.)

from contact with the agents (Table 34–5). Protective gloves, gowns, and masks may be worn to guard against accidental skin contact and airborne fumes. In areas where large volumes of chemotherapy are prepared, a biologic vertical laminar air flow hood is suggested for preparing and administering chemotherapeutic agents.

Side Effects of Chemotherapy

As chemotherapeutic drugs attack malignant tumor cells, normal rapidly growing cells are also temporarily or permanently damaged. Chemotherapeutic agents do not differentiate malignant cells from rapidly growing normal body cells. This results in damage to normal cells, which is manifested as side effects or drug effects similar to those seen with radiation therapy. The side effects can range from minor annoyances to life-threatening toxicities.

GASTROINTESTINAL TOXICITY

The lining of the gastrointestinal tract is composed of rapidly growing cells that are constantly renewed to protect and maintain the integrity of the tract. Any part of the gastrointestinal tract can be affected by chemotherapy, resulting in nausea, vomiting, mucositis, taste alterations, diarrhea, and constipation.

Table 34–5

Precautions for Handling Chemotherapeutic Agents
Wear:
Disposable latex gloves
Mask to cover nose and mouth
Eye protectors, especially if biologic hood is not available
Use:
Biologic air flow hood if mixing chemotherapeutic agents on a regular basis
Soap and water for skin contact
Avoid:
Spills
Aerosolization when drawing up from a vial
Expelling excess drug from syringes into the air
Dispose of:
Needles and syringes in impervious containers
Chemotherapy bottles and tubing as per hospital policy
Body excretions and fluids as per hospital policy
Always:
Read package inserts
Be familiar with the drugs to be administered
Prepare drugs in a quiet area
Wash hands before and after preparation and administration
Review physician's written chemotherapy order
Double-check drug and drug dosage with another colleague before administering

Nausea and Vomiting

Nausea and vomiting are the most common early side effects of chemotherapy. The chemoreceptor trigger zone of the medulla is located near the emetic center and is stimulated by chemicals in the blood. It is believed that this zone in turn stimulates the emetic center. Some drugs, such as cisplatin and the nitrosoureas, cause severe vomiting. Nausea and vomiting may also result from actual irritation of the lining of the gastrointestinal tract.

Several antiemetic drugs are used to minimize nausea and vomiting, with varying results. The antiemetic agents in the phenothiazine class, such as prochlorperazine, are used because they block stimulation of the chemoreceptor trigger zone and the emetic center. Phenothiazines offer only mild relief, and studies indicate that when the more emetic types of chemotherapy (such as the alkylating agents and antimetabolites) are used, effectiveness is minimal.

The antiemetic effects of tetrahydrocannabinol, the active ingredient of marijuana, and nabilone, a synthetic form of tetrahydrocannabinol, have been studied, also with varying results. Most reports suggest that they are more effective for younger patients and that the patient must experience a "high" feeling for the drug to work. It is hypothesized that tetrahydrocannabinol may suppress the chemoreceptor trigger zone.

Metoclopramide, a derivative of the procainamide class of drugs, is an effective antiemetic agent. It blocks the chemoreceptor trigger zone, increases gastrointestinal motility, and causes gastric emptying. In high intravenous doses, metoclopramide is effective against nausea and vomiting. However, extrapyramidal effects may result in patients' experiencing adverse side effects. Antihistamines can be given with the drug to eliminate these side effects.

Antihistamines and steroids have some antiemetic action and are also used to enhance the effectiveness of other antiemetic agents. Anxiolytic drugs, such as lorazepam, have been used alone or with other antiemetics for their amnesic and sedative effect. These agents may also be helpful for anticipatory nausea and vomiting, which occurs before administration of chemotherapy secondary to cognitive associations of nausea and vomiting with chemotherapy.

Advances in the treatment of nausea and vomiting during the past decade have included appreciation of the value of combination antiemetic therapy to both improve efficacy and to decrease toxicity, identification of patient prognostic factors, and the likelihood that certain chemotherapeutic agents will cause nausea and vomiting.

Understanding the physiology of emesis has led to the recognition of serotonin, which activates or binds to 5-hydroxytryptamine receptors on the vagus nerve that send signals to the chemoreceptor trigger zone in the brain. Therefore, serotonin antagonists ondansetron and granisetron have become universal standard agents and are prescribed at times, despite their high cost (Cleri, 1995).

The psychogenic aspects of nausea and vomiting and behavioral interventions continue to be studied. Many patients benefit from relaxation exercises; biofeedback tapes; hypnosis; diversionary activities such as music, reading, or television; desensitization; and mental imaging. Behavioral therapies provide patients with something that they can do to actively participate in their care. Any of these techniques can be used in conjunction with pharmacologic antiemetics.

Anticipatory nausea and vomiting is a learned phenomenon stimulated by something that occurs in association with the true stimulant. Learned stimuli include thoughts, sights, tastes, and odors related to the treatment. Because it is a learned response, anticipatory nausea and vomiting does not occur with the first dose administered. It may, however, increase with each successive cycle of chemotherapy. Vomiting also occurs in association with radiation therapy, obstructions, infections, and intestinal inflammatory diseases.)

The behavioral techniques described earlier are often helpful with anticipatory nausea and vomiting, as are many of the pharmacologic agents also described earlier.

Mucositis

The cytotoxic action of chemotherapy can damage or destroy the cells of the lining of the oral cavity, resulting in varying degrees of mucositis. Mucositis in the oral cavity is also called stomatitis. Mucositis in the esophagus is called esophagitis.

Patients may develop painful oral and esophageal ulcers as the cells of the mucosa are damaged and cellular repair is decreased. Stomatitis and esophagitis can also occur if the patient is immunosuppressed from the disease or treatment or from malnutrition or dehydration. Mucositis can alter the patient's nutritional and hydration status by inhibiting consumption of food and fluids. It also predisposes the patient to infection in the mouth or esophagus. The intensity and degree of inflammation vary, depending on the patient's physical status and the type, dosage, and scheduling of the chemotherapy or radiation therapy prescribed. Severe stomatitis can cause oral pain and infection and can further complicate the patient's nutrition and hydration status.

Patients are usually instructed to rinse their mouth several times a day (before meals and at bedtime, or more frequently) with an alkaline mouthrinse. One useful salt/soda rinse is made up of 1 tsp salt and 1 tsp sodium bicarbonate in 1 quart of water. Patients should avoid hydrogen peroxide rinses except to treat severe forms of plaque not amenable to other forms of treatment, because peroxide mouthrinses dry the mucous membranes. When peroxide mouthrinses are essential, they should be in extremely weak solutions (15 mL hydrogen peroxide to 1 L of water). Alcohol-containing mouthrinses should be avoided because of their potential to irritate the oral mucosa. Oral topical analgesics, antibiotics, antifungal agents, and antiviral pharmacologic agents may be prescribed.

In severe cases of mucositis, analgesics may be necessary. It is not uncommon for patients to be placed on continuous infusion morphine after high doses of chemotherapy. Nutrition can also be a problem when the oral mucosa is seriously compromised. It is often necessary to place patients on hyperalimentation or to use other methods of feeding patients when the oral route is not feasible.

Xerostomia and Taste Alterations

Cytotoxic effects of chemotherapy on the salivary glands can decrease production of saliva, resulting in xerostomia, or mouth dryness. Injury to the taste buds can cause hypogeusia, dysgeusia, or ageusia. These side effects can further compromise the patient's nutrition and hydration status.

Diarrhea

Destruction of the intestinal lining by chemotherapy results in inflammation and inability of the intestine to produce digestive enzymes. Intestinal motility is stimulated, which results in diarrhea. Along with frequent loose bowel movements, patients can also experience abdominal cramping, flatulence, bloating, and irritation of the rectal mucosa. Diarrhea may also be related to the patient's anxieties and fears. The incidence of diarrhea related to chemotherapy is high. It occurs with many of the antimetabolites and antitumor antibiotics. Potential alterations in nutrition and fluid and electrolyte balance result from inadequate digestion and decreased nutrient absorption. Pharmacologic agents that slow intestinal peristalsis, such as diphenoxylate with atropine (Lomotil), may be indicated along with nutritional interventions.

Constipation

Chemotherapy-related constipation is a side effect of the *Vinca* alkaloid drugs. The neurotoxicity of vincristine and vinblastine can cause a decrease in intestinal peristalsis, resulting in constipation. Bowel status must be assessed before and during treatment to avoid constipation and possible paralytic ileus. Older patients are especially susceptible to constipation caused by the *Vinca* alkaloids. Constipation may be further aggravated by a decrease in fluid intake and physical activity. Severe constipation may require manual disimpaction.

SKIN TOXICITY

Skin side effects include hyperpigmentation, photosensitivity, erythematous rashes, radiation recall, alopecia, and chemical tissue infiltration.

Hyperpigmentation of the skin and nail beds is caused by an increased stimulation of the melanin cells in the basal level of the dermis. Skin darkening can be localized in small areas, such as over the veins, or more widespread over the face and trunk. Several agents cause photosensitivity—an acceleration of the tanning process caused by the sun's ultraviolet rays—resulting in marked hyperpigmentation, deeply tanned skin, and severe sunburn. Hyperpigmentation and photosensitivity are known side effects of fluorouracil, methotrexate, and bleomycin.

Erythematous rashes are caused by dilated blood vessels in the skin. These transient rashes sometimes occur after administration of chemotherapy near the injection site or over other areas of the body and may remain for several hours. The rashes are sometimes accompanied by urticaria, skin flaking, and skin dryness. A hypersensitivity reaction to chemotherapy may first be evidenced as a rash and quickly progress to an allergic reaction requiring immediate medical intervention.

Radiation recall is a term used to describe the effect that chemotherapy may have on areas of the skin that have been previously or concomitantly exposed to radiation therapy. This can result in erythema, ulceration, wet desquamation, and permanent hyperpigmentation.

Alopecia can be a devastating side effect because hair is a significant part of a person's self-image. Chemotherapy causes alopecia by damaging rapidly growing and renewing hair follicles. Hair is weakened at the shaft and easily removed from the scalp. The amount of hair lost depends on the drug dosage and treatment duration. Some chemotherapeutic agents do not cause alopecia. Hair loss can range from mild thinning on the scalp to loss of all scalp hair.

Facial and body hair are less frequently affected by chemotherapy because the growth and renewal rate is slower; nevertheless, patients may experience a loss of facial and body hair. Alopecia may cause the scalp to become irritated and sensitive, with flaking of dry skin. Hair loss is almost always temporary. Complete regrowth can be expected after treatment stops. Regrowth time varies, and hair may have a changed color and texture. Hair regrowth is slower in the geriatric population.

Patient preparation must be emphasized as an important component of adaptation to alopecia. Wigs, hairpieces, and hats can be suggested. Scalp hypothermia refers to application of ice to the scalp to decrease blood circulation during chemotherapy administration. This technique has been studied as a means to minimize hair loss. Its use remains controversial on the basis that reducing chemotherapy distribution to the scalp could theoretically create a safe area for cancer cells. Scalp hypothermia is contraindicated in cancers known to spread to the brain and soft tissues of the scalp.

Tissue extravasation is defined as localized tissue damage caused by infiltration of chemotherapy into tissues around the intravenous administration site. Chemotherapeutic drugs that produce tissue damage if they are given directly into the tissues or if they leak out of veins are called vesicants. Venous access devices are used to administer vesicants because they limit the occurrence of tissue infiltration. Vesicant chemotherapeutic agents include

Amsacrine
Nitrogen mustard
Dactinomycin/daunorubicin
Vincristine
Doxorubicin
Epirubicin
Idarubicin
Vinblastine/mitomycin C
Mitomycin C
Vindesine

Irritant chemotherapeutic agents capable of causing tissue irritation if extravasated include cisplatin, carmustine, dacarbazine, etoposide, paclitaxel, plicamycin, streptozocin, and teniposide.

Tissue extravasation can cause local pain, induration, erythema, and necrosis. Medical and nursing interventions for tissue extravasation remain controversial, and institutional protocols vary. Studies report the use of subcutaneously and intravenously administered antidotes at the infiltration site, to attempt to neutralize and inactivate the infiltrated drug or limit tissue absorption. The Oncology Nursing Society recommends the following general interventions for chemotherapy-induced tissue extravasation:

- Stop chemotherapy administration.
- Keep intravenous needle in place and try to aspirate residual chemotherapeutic agent from the intravenous tubing, the needle, and the infiltration site.
- Instill antidote as per hospital protocol and/or physician order (the use of antidotes remains controversial). Antidotes include hydrocortisone, hyaluronidase, and sodium bicarbonate.
- Apply cold or warm compress to area, based on type of agent and hospital policy.
- Elevate arm.
- Observe area at regular intervals.
- Arrange follow-up visit.

Document the following:

- Time and date
- Needle size and type
- Name of chemotherapy agent and approximate amount of drug volume infiltrated
- Drug administration technique and sequence of administration of multiple drugs
- Immediate interventions taken
- Description of infiltration site; photograph site, if possible
- Patient symptoms

HEMATOLOGIC TOXICITY

The action of chemotherapy can directly affect the blood-producing mechanism. Blood components (red blood cells, white blood cells, and platelets) are continually being made by the rapidly growing cells of the bone marrow. The cytotoxic action of chemotherapy inhibits this production. Because red blood cells (erythrocytes) carry oxygen to tissues and carbon dioxide away from tissues, a decrease in their number in circulation causes anemia. The life cycle of red blood cells is about 120 days. They are completely recycled after their death.

White blood cells (leukocytes) are an integral component of the immune system. Decreased production of leukocytes reduces the system's ability to recognize and defend against foreign microorganisms, leading to increased susceptibility to infection. Granulocytes are a type of white blood cell that contains granules on its surface. These granules contain potent chemicals that help destroy foreign bodies. Granulocytes comprise 50 to 70% of the total circulating white blood cell count. Basophils, eosinophils, and neutrophils make up the granulocyte portion of the white blood cell count. About 55 to 60% of bone marrow is devoted to neutrophil production. A normal neutrophil count is 3000 to 6000 cells/mm³. The circulation life is 6 to 10 hours. They are the body's first line of defense against invading organisms. Monocytes are found in the circulation, and macrophages are found mostly in body organs. They are responsible for phagocytosis of invading organisms and dead or damaged cells.

Platelets are blood components that assist with clot formation and blood coagulation. A decrease in the number of platelets in circulation can cause an increased susceptibility to bleeding. Platelets survive for 8 to 10 days in circulation. A normal platelet count is 150,000 to 350,000/mm³.

Peripheral blood cell counts are monitored regularly and are always evaluated before the beginning of a chemotherapy cycle. Based on blood cell count values, therapy is sometimes modified or delayed. Chemotherapy is commonly withheld if the white blood cell count is below 3000/mm³ or if the absolute neutrophil count (ANC) is below 1500/mm³. The ANC is calculated by multiplying the total WBC count by the neutrophils: (Neutrophils + bands) × WBC = ANC. Profound neutropenia (grade 4) is defined as an ANC of less than 500 cells/mm³. The point of lowest blood count (nadir) occurs 7 to 14 days after chemotherapy. Infections from invasion and overgrowth of pathogenic microbes increase in frequency and severity as the ANC decreases. Risk of infection increases when the nadir persists for

Table 34–6

Normal Blood Values

Laboratory Test	Normal Value
Hematocrit	Male: 40–54%
	Female: 37–47%
Hemoglobin	Male: 13.5–18.0 g/dL
	Female: 12.0–16.0 g/dL
White blood cell count	$4.5–13.0 \times 10$
White blood cell dif-ferential count (cal-culated as a per-centage of total white blood cell count)	Segmented neutrophils: 56%
	Bands: 3%
	Eosinophils: 3%
	Basophils: 0.3%
	Lymphocytes: 34%
	Monocytes: 4%
Platelet count	150,000–400,000

more than 7 to 10 days. Normal blood cell count ranges are listed in Table 34–6.

Hematologic toxicity from chemotherapy can result in life-threatening anemia, infection, and bleeding. Hematologic status can also be concomitantly compromised by invasion of the primary tumor into the bone marrow, other hematologic disorders, and malnutrition.

RENAL TOXICITY

Renal toxicity is a less common side effect. Impaired renal function has been documented with such chemotherapeutic agents as cisplatin, methotrexate, and mitomycin C. These drugs are known to be toxic to the renal tubule system and the glomeruli. Renal calculi can form from rapid tumor destruction. Hemorrhagic cystitis caused by bladder irritation is associated with cyclophosphamide.

PULMONARY TOXICITY

Pulmonary toxicity related to chemotherapy is manifested as pulmonary fibrosis and inflammation. It is associated with methotrexate and bleomycin. Bleomycin can cause pulmonary fibrosis, which seems to be related to cumulative doses over 400 units. Geriatric patients may be at increased risk of pulmonary fibrosis related to changes in respiratory muscles and air capacity of the lungs. Pulmonary toxicity is usually irreversible.

NEUROTOXICITY

Sensory and perceptual alterations result from the effects of chemotherapy on nerve conduction fibers. Neurotoxicity is most often associated with the *Vinca* alkaloid agents (vincristine, vinblastine) and is manifested by peripheral neuropathy. Symptoms include the following:

• Lack of body coordination

• Feeling of numbness and tingling in the hands and feet
• Loss of feeling sensation in extremities
• Loss of deep tendon reflexes
• Generalized motor weakness
• In severe cases, atonia of the bowel and bladder

Cisplatin can cause motor and sensory neuropathy, tinnitus, and hearing losses. Procarbazine causes peripheral neuropathy and altered levels of consciousness.

CARDIOTOXICITY

Cardiotoxicity is a major dose-limiting factor for the antitumor antibiotics doxorubicin and daunorubicin. Cardiotoxicity has been documented after patients received a total cumulative dose of these agents ranging from 450 to 550 mg/m² of body surface area. Cardiotoxic effects include dysrhythmia and heart failure.

Other risk factors for cardiotoxicity include increasing age, pre-existing cardiac disease, and a history of radiation therapy to the mediastinum. Patients who receive the anthracycline antitumor antibiotics are closely monitored for signs and symptoms of heart failure.

NURSING PROCESS
Chemotherapy

Assessment

Assess the patient's understanding of the disease and treatment, anxiety level, and coping skills. Also assess the patient's physical and nutritional status. Once therapy begins, do a complete assessment to identify all side effects.

Nursing Diagnoses and Planning

Nursing diagnoses and related expected patient outcomes commonly applicable to patients receiving chemotherapy for cancer include the following:

NDx: Risk for altered health maintenance related to insufficient knowledge of prescribed treatment, side effects, and their management

Planning: Patient Outcomes
1. Patient states what the chemotherapy is expected to accomplish (eg, shrink tumor in preparation for surgery or eliminate cancer cells remaining after surgery).
2. Patient describes schedule of treatments (interval at which treatments are given, when oral chemotherapeutic drugs are to be taken, and so on).
3. Patient describes expected side effects of chemotherapy.
4. Patient accurately describes palliative measures that may be used to help manage side effects.
5. Patient lists symptoms that should be reported to a health-care professional.

CLINICAL ? THINKING

NAUSEA, CHILLS, AND RESTLESSNESS AFTER CHEMOTHERAPY

Twelve days after completing her most recent cycle of chemotherapy, a 51-year-old patient was admitted for a diagnostic evaluation for chronic recurrent urinary tract infections (UTIs). Her initial episode of UTI occurred as a nosocomial infection 6 months earlier, during hospitalization for a modified radical mastectomy for stage III breast cancer. The patient currently reported moderate pain on urination and the presence of blood in her urine. She was scheduled for an intravenous pyelogram and cystoscopy. Treatment with trimethoprim-sulfamethoxazole (Bactrim) and phenazopyridine (Pyridium) would begin after collection of a sterile urine specimen for culture and sensitivity.

On arrival on the unit, the patient had the following baseline vital signs. Her blood pressure was 124/82 mm Hg, her apical pulse was 78 beats per minute and her respirations were 16 per minute and unlabored, and her temperature was 37.6°C (99.8°F). Her skin was warm and dry, her peripheral pulses were readily palpated, and she was alert and oriented.

On her return to the floor after the intravenous pyelogram, I helped the patient into bed and checked her vital signs. Her blood pressure had increased slightly, to 132/84 mm Hg, and her pulse and respirations had increased to 94 beats per minute and 22 per minute. Her breath sounds remained clear. Her temperature had risen to 38°C (100.4°F). She said that she didn't feel "quite right." These findings represented very subtle changes in the patient's condition. Although they did not necessarily indicate a serious change, I suspected that the problem was more than an uncomplicated UTI. I decided to assess and monitor her further.

The patient complained of mild nausea and chills and appeared agitated and restless. Her skin remained warm and dry, her face was flushed, and her peripheral pulses were bounding with adequate capillary refill.

I recognized that the patient's changes in blood pressure, pulse, and respirations might have resulted from pain secondary to the UTI, from stress and anxiety related to the procedure, or from transient hypoxia. However, based on my knowledge and past experiences, the patient's history (neutropenia secondary to chemotherapy treatment and chronic UTIs), and the signs and symptoms I was observing (especially the widening pulse pressure, elevated pulse and respiratory rates, elevated temperature, chills, and bounding peripheral pulses), I

suspected that the patient had developed septicemia and was manifesting the early (hyperdynamic) stage of septic shock.

Although the patient's temperature was below 38.3°C (101°F), I knew that temperature readings vary greatly in the early phase of septic shock. In addition, a temperature of 38°C (100.4°F) in an immunocompromised (neutropenic) patient can be a very significant clinical clue to her condition. Other signs and symptoms may be diminished secondary to an impaired response to bacterial invasion. I rejected the possibility that the patient had developed anaphylactic shock from the intravenous pyelogram. This was based on her absence of clinical manifestations of allergic response, inconsistencies in her blood pressure readings, and her bounding peripheral pulses.

Further questioning revealed that the patient had increasing difficulty in focusing her thoughts. She was mildly disoriented. These changes in level of consciousness strongly supported my suspicion.

Recognizing that septic shock progresses rapidly and commonly causes multiple organ failure and death without prompt and aggressive treatment in patients undergoing chemotherapy, I did not hesitate to implement the following actions:

1. I notified the physician of my suspicion.
2. I placed the patient in high-Fowler's position.
3. I administered oxygen and established an intravenous line as per hospital policy.
4. I stayed with the patient and offered emotional support and brief explanations of her condition and treatment.
5. I continued to monitor the patient's respiratory, cardiovascular, and mental status.
6. I monitored the patient's intake and output.
7. I rechecked for a history of drug allergies.
8. I attached a pulse oximeter.
9. I documented my findings and actions.

The physician ordered a complete blood cell count with white blood cell differential, blood chemistries, blood and urine samples for culture and sensitivity, IV administration of a broad-spectrum antibiotic and fluids, arterial blood gas analysis, a 12-lead electrocardiogram, and a STAT portable chest x-ray. Despite an anticipated low white blood cell count, positive blood and urine cultures and the arterial blood gas analysis results confirmed my suspicion.

The patient's condition stabilized after initiation of therapy. She was transferred to the intensive care unit for continuous monitoring of her response to therapy and the potential onset of com-

(continued)

CLINICAL ? THINKING

(continued)

plications of septic shock, such as acute respiratory distress syndrome, acute renal failure, and disseminated intravascular coagulation. Skilled observations and assessments, identification of early trends, and prompt interventions for this high-risk patient dramatically improved her chance for recovery.

Think Critically

What additional patient cues might have alerted the nurse to early septic shock?

Why did the change in the patient's mental status lend strong support to the nurse's suspicion?

Was placing the patient in high-Fowler's position the best action? Why didn't the nurse place the patient in the "shock" position?

Why does the patient with sepsis who does not demonstrate tachycardia and tachypnea have a poorer prognosis?

What physiologic mechanism underlies the pattern of a widening pulse pressure?

What changes in the patient's urinary output does the nurse anticipate in early septic shock? Late septic shock?

What nursing assessments would have alerted the nurse to the onset of late-stage (hypodynamic) septic shock?

In what ways would nursing actions differ if the patient deteriorated to late-stage septic shock?

The nurse administered an antibiotic after collecting the blood and urine specimens. Why?

What instructions must be included in the discharge teaching about recognizing sepsis at home?

How would the nurse explain the low white blood cell count in the presence of septicemia and septic shock?

What relationship did the nurse recognize between the last chemotherapy treatment and the results of the white blood cell count?

What similarities and differences exist when planning care for patients with cardiogenic, anaphylactic, hypovolemic, and septic shock?

What neutropenic precautions might have been implemented by the nurse? Would it have made a difference to this scenario?

---

6. Patient identifies telephone number at which a health-care professional can be reached.
7. Patient states date and time of next appointment.

Table 34–7 presents other nursing diagnoses that are likely to apply to common side effects, along with expected outcomes and nursing interventions.

Nursing Interventions and Evaluation

Nursing interventions involve preparing the patient and family for chemotherapy and its potential side effects, administering prescribed chemotherapy, monitoring side effects, and teaching comfort and other support measures.

NDx: Risk for altered health maintenance

Using language the patient can understand, explain the action and effects of the chemotherapy to the patient and family. Review the treatment regimen and possible side effects of the drugs, stressing that each person's response is individual, so all of the side effects will not necessarily be experienced. Identify for the patient symptoms that should be immediately reported. Tell the patient how to contact the appropriate health-care professional.

Additional Interventions

Additional interventions depend on the specific body system affected by the chemotherapy. Keep in mind that each patient will experience one, several, or no side effects, based on multiple factors. Always review the chemotherapy treatment plan to evaluate potential common side effects for each patient's treatment. Informed consent must be verified before starting chemotherapy.

When indicated, refer patients and families to other professionals and community programs and agencies. A list of patient resources appears in the Appendix.

Compare the patient's status with the expected outcomes. If the outcomes are not met, reassess the patient and revise the plan.

IMMUNOTHERAPY

Immunotherapy can be defined as treatment with chemical or biological agents intended to help the immune system destroy cancerous cells. The immune system, which is discussed in Chapter 32, possesses protective mechanisms that recognize and defend against foreign matter, such as bacteria, viruses, and tumors. The immunologic approach in the treatment of cancerous cells is predicated on the assumption that certain parts of the immune system

Text continued on page 1544

Table 34-7

Side Effects of Chemotherapy with Related Assessments, Nursing Diagnoses, Expected Patient Outcomes, and Nursing Interventions

Side Effect	Assessment	Nursing Diagnosis	Expected Patient Outcomes	Nursing Interventions
Pulmonary Toxicity Patients with pre-existing pulmonary disease or previous treatment with lung radiation therapy are at risk for pulmonary fibrosis and inflammation.	Obtain pretreatment pulmonary function studies and chest x-ray. Assess for: • Cough • Elevated body temperature • Tachycardia • Dyspnea on exertion • Weakness Auscultate lungs. Obtain vital signs. Ascertain activity status. Check blood gas values.	Risk for ineffective breathing pattern related to inflammation and decreased lung expansion	Lung sounds are normal. Arterial blood gas values are within the patient's normal range.	To alleviate pulmonary fibrosis and inflammation: • Medicate with antibiotics, steroids, and bronchodilators as prescribed. • Adjust patient to comfortable sitting position. • Use respiratory therapy machines. • Administer and monitor effects of oxygen therapy. • Refer to visiting nurse service for home follow-up. • Explain all procedures and interventions. • Monitor cumulative dose of bleomycin.
Cardiotoxicity	Ascertain cardiac history. Check vital signs. Obtain and monitor pretreatment and at intervals: • Electrocardiogram • Echocardiogram • Cardiac scan Observe for signs of heart failure: • Tachycardia • Moist cough • Shortness of breath • Dyspnea on exertion • Distended neck veins • Cardiomegaly • Hepatomegaly • Pedal edema • Orthopnea Ascertain whether patient has previously received radiation therapy. Assess patient's activity level.	Risk for decreased cardiac output related to toxic effects of chemotherapeutic agents on the heart	Signs and symptoms of heart failure are absent.	Teach signs and symptoms of heart failure, and encourage the patient to report all symptoms. Record cumulative doses of doxorubicin and daunorubicin. Monitor and report changes in interval physical assessments and interval cardiac test results to physician.

Table continued on following page

1535

Table 34–7

Side Effects of Chemotherapy with Related Assessments, Nursing Diagnoses, Expected Patient Outcomes, and Nursing Interventions (continued)

Side Effect	Assessment	Nursing Diagnosis	Expected Patient Outcomes	Nursing Interventions
Neurotoxicity	Assess for symptoms of peripheral neuropathy: • Paresthesias of hands and feet • Numbness and tingling sensations of extremities • Muscle pain • Loss of Achilles tendon reflex • Falls, loss of balance • Bone and joint pain • Changes in gait • Bowel and bladder habits Assess effects of neurotoxicity on physical activity.	Risk for injury related to paresthesias, loss of balance, or other symptoms of peripheral neuropathy	Patient remains free of injury.	Explain to the patient that: • Symptoms may be related to chemotherapy. • Reporting of symptoms is important. Instruct the patient to: • Avoid use of heating pads to areas with reduced feeling. • Test bath water temperature to avoid scalding. • Use gloves for washing dishes and gardening, and protect hands when cooking. Assist with and teach range-of-joint-motion exercises. Use foot board if indicated for foot-drop. Use pillows to correct body alignment. Refer patient to visiting nurse service for follow-up care if indicated.
Hematologic Toxicity	Observe for signs and symptoms of infection. Be aware that patients with a low white blood cell count may not exhibit the normal signs of infection, such as productive cough, elevated body temperature, redness of skin, edema, and pain due to the absence of neutrophils. Check the white blood cell count. Obtain vital signs. Inspect all body orifices and skin for infection. Question patient about symptoms of infection. Obtain blood; urine; skin; sputum; and vaginal, rectal, or other cultures as indicated. Obtain history of medication schedule.	Risk for infection related to chemotherapy—induced leukopenia	Patient is afebrile. Signs of specific localized infections are absent. Patient describes measures to reduce the risk of infection.	Implement measures to prevent infection: • Restrict visitors. • Protect the patient from people with known infections. • Provide a private room. • Instruct the patient, family, and visitors in hand-washing technique. • Encourage fluid if not contraindicated by other medical disorders. Suggest a low bacteria diet: • Avoid fresh fruits and vegetables. • Cook all foods. Maintain skin integrity: • Bathe daily with antiseptic soap; include nail care. • Change intravenous tubing every 24 hours. • Avoid injections.

Nursing Diagnosis	Expected Outcomes	Nursing Interventions
(continued from previous page)		Assess fluid intake and output. Assess mental status. • Avoid skin breakdown. • Monitor exit sites of central venous catheters, intravenous lines, or other venous access devices. Prevent respiratory infection: • Encourage ambulation, coughing and deep-breathing, fluid intake. • Avoid smoking. Prevent urinary infections: • Avoid indwelling urinary catheters. • Encourage fluid intake, good hygienic measures after bowel movements. Provide care for skin breakage. Avoid enemas and rectal suppositories. Avoid taking rectal temperatures. Administer antibiotics and antifungal agents as prescribed by physician. Explain to the patient and family how to notify medical personnel if signs of infection appear.
Risk for decreased cardiac output related to bleeding secondary to chemotherapy—induced thrombocytopenia	Signs and symptoms of bleeding are absent. Patient describes self-care measures to decrease the risk of bleeding.	Inspect patient for signs and symptoms of bleeding: • Inspect skin for petechiae, ecchymoses, and hematomas. • Observe neurologic status for changes associated with intracranial bleeding. • Inspect for bleeding into joints. • Measure abdominal girth. • Inspect and test all body secretions and fluids for blood. Check platelet count. Ascertain chemotherapy regimen. Ascertain whether the patient is currently taking steroids or products that contain aspirin. Ascertain whether the patient has experienced: • Hemoptysis • Hematuria • Epistaxis • Wound bleeding • Hematemesis • Melena • Menometrorrhagia Implement measures to prevent and control bleeding: Limit injections and venipunctures. Use small-gauge needles, and apply pressure after all skin punctures. Avoid: • Shaving with straight-edge razor. • Using toothbrush and dental floss. • Straining during bowel movements. • Taking any medication that contains aspirin. • Nasotracheal suctioning. • Vomiting. Eliminate objects in patient's environment that may cause bruising from falls. Suggest: • Mouth care with sponges or gauze • Increased fluid intake and stool softeners, if indicated • Antiemetics, if indicated • For menstruating females: estrogen-progesterone agents can be given to stop menses, if indicated • Soft diet high in fiber and protein

Table continued on following page

Table 34–7

Side Effects of Chemotherapy with Related Assessments, Nursing Diagnoses, Expected Patient Outcomes, and Nursing Interventions (continued)

Side Effect	Assessment	Nursing Diagnosis	Expected Patient Outcomes	Nursing Interventions
Hematologic Toxicity (continued)	Check: • Vital signs. Include blood pressure in reclining, sitting, and standing positions to assess for postural hypotension.			• Limited physical activity • If indicated, pad side rails, prevent falls • Use of humidifier if oxygen therapy is indicated to prevent mucosal drying For nosebleeding: • Place patient in high Fowler's position. • Apply ice packs and pressure to bridge of nose. • Notify physician. Administer and monitor platelet transfusions. Administer antacids and ice water lavages for gastric bleeding if ordered.
	Check hemoglobin, hematocrit. Ask about symptoms of syncope, drowsiness, dyspnea, diaphoresis, and chest pain. Ask about feelings of fatigue. Ascertain ability to carry out usual activities. Review usual schedule and type of activities.	Fatigue related to chemotherapy-induced anemia	Patient identifies a plan for limiting activity and providing frequent rest periods. Patient reports that he or she is able to carry out basic activities of daily living.	Instruct patient to: • Report symptoms. • Limit physical activity. • Plan frequent rest periods. • Take soft diet high in protein, vitamins, and iron. Administer red blood cell transfusion as ordered by physician.
Sexual Dysfunction	Explore questions and concerns related to sexual functioning. Determine current methods of birth control.	Sexual dysfunction related to physiologic and psychologic effects of chemotherapy	Patient describes potential effects of chemotherapy on sexual function. Patient verbalizes concerns about sex role and desirability as a sexual partner. Patient identifies measures supportive of sexual function.	Inform females about: • Possible amenorrhea • Possible onset of early menopause with symptoms of "hot flashes," vaginal dryness, and dyspareunia • Use of birth control methods if premenopausal • Possible dyspareunia related to decreased lubrication of vaginal walls. Use water-soluble lubricant or steroid cream if indicated. • Possible decreased libido related to fatigue and hormonal changes

Toxicity	Assessment	Nursing Diagnosis	Expected Outcomes	Nursing Interventions
				Inform males about: • Possible temporary or permanent sterility • Possible impotence related to therapy, anxiety, and fatigue • Penile prosthesis implantation, if indicated. • Sperm banking before therapy begins, if indicated. Refer patients and partners to appropriate professionals, if indicated. Allow time for discussion of sexual dysfunction. Provide written information about contraception methods.
Skin Toxicity Photosensitivity	Inspect skin for erythema, blisters, and other lesions.	Risk for impaired skin integrity related to sunburn	Skin is intact. Skin is free of erythema and lesions.	Teach patient to: • Avoid the rays of the sun by wearing protective clothing and applying sunscreen (SPF 15) if exposed to the sun. • Report signs and symptoms. • Follow topical medication schedules if ordered. Explain: • Skin reactions are expected and related to the chemotherapy. • Nail growth may be slowed. • Skin changes and vein and nail darkening are usually temporary. Implement measures to assist the patient in adapting to a change in physical appearance.
Alopecia Skin hyperpigmentation	Inspect skin for: • Increased pigmentation • Dark veins near chemotherapy injection sites • Areas of increased pigmentation in mouth and nailbeds • Rashes. Assess: • Patient feelings about hair loss • Patient knowledge related to hair loss.	Risk for body image disturbance related to skin hyperpigmentation and loss of hair	Patient verbalizes acceptance of self with skin and hair changes. Patient identifies positive aspects of self. Patient expresses pleasure at visits from family or friends.	Explain: • Hair loss is almost always temporary (except with high doses of radiotherapy to the scalp). • Timing of hair loss (will start about 14 days after treatment). • Hair sometimes grows back while the patient is still receiving treatment and that it can fall out again. • Hair will start to permanently grow after treatment is withdrawn. • New hair may be different in color and texture. • Facial and body hair can also be affected. • The scalp may become irritated with skin flaking.

Table continued on following page

Table 34-7

Side Effects of Chemotherapy with Related Assessments, Nursing Diagnoses, Expected Patient Outcomes, and Nursing Interventions *(continued)*

Side Effect	Assessment	Nursing Diagnosis	Expected Patient Outcomes	Nursing Interventions

Alopecia
Skin hyperpigmentation *(continued)*
				Suggest:
				• Purchasing a wig or hairpiece before alopecia begins.
				• Cutting long hair to decrease the anxiety associated with losing large amounts of hair.
				• Using a mild shampoo to alleviate scalp irritation.
				• Using hats and scarves.
				• Methods to reduce the rate of hair loss:
				  Limit hair brushing.
				  Avoid using harsh shampoos.
				  Wear a hair net to sleep at night.
				  Review hypothermia technique if indicated and with physician approval.
				Inform the patient that the cost of wigs and hairpieces is covered by most third-party health insurance companies. Local units of the American Cancer Society will lend patients wigs free of charge.

Gastrointestinal Toxicity Nausea and vomiting	Assess: • General appearance • Skin color and turgor. Obtain vital signs: temperature, pulse, respiration, and blood pressure. Determine: • Time, frequency, and amount of emesis • Diet history • Medication schedules. Examine abdomen; auscultate for bowel sounds (intestinal obstruction). Evaluate level of serum electrolytes and chemistries (hypercalcemia, hyponatremia, uremia, dehydration).	Risk for fluid volume deficit related to inadequate fluid intake and excessive fluid loss secondary to nausea and vomiting	Skin turgor is firm. Mucous membranes are moist. Fluid intake approximates output.	Instruct in measures that provide relief: Advise patient to: • Eat salty foods. • Try dry foods such as toast or crackers. • Drink clear, cool liquids. • Eat small portions of low-fat foods. • Report symptoms and severity. • Limit physical activity after meals. Administer antiemetics as prescribed. Suggest taking antiemetics before receiving chemotherapy and using antiemetics in suppository form. Offer support by: • Explaining that nausea and vomiting are expected side effects. • Explaining relaxation techniques.

	Nursing Assessment	Nursing Diagnosis	Expected Outcomes	Nursing Interventions
Stomatitis Xerostomia	Inspect oral cavity for: • Moisture, color, ulceration, inflammation, and fungus • Quality, color, and amount of saliva. Assess for symptoms: pain, dysphagia, inability to open mouth, inability to eat and take fluids, taste changes, voice changes. Observe condition of teeth. Ask about patient-initiated comfort measures. Ask about usual regimen for oral hygiene.	Altered oral mucous membrane related to effects of chemotherapeutic agents on the mucosal cells	Oral mucous membranes are intact. Oral mucous membranes are pink and moist. Patient is able to ingest foods and fluids without oral discomfort.	• Suggesting diversionary activity. • Being available for questions and follow-up. Implement measures to alleviate symptoms: • Encourage and assist with mouth care. • Rinse mouth with alkaline solutions every hour (1 tsp of baking soda in 8 oz of warm water). • Use soft sponge or gauze instead of toothbrush. • Remove thick saliva with gauze; irrigate mouth with salt/soda solution. • Remove dentures for cleaning; keep dentures in place only if comfortable and not causing irritation. • Suggest and evaluate effects of topical analgesics, artificial saliva, and lip lubricant. • Instruct patient to avoid alcohol, smoking, commercial mouthwashes, and hot, spicy, and acidic foods and fluids. Encourage: • Fluids • Ice popsicles • Soft bland diet • Using a straw to sip soups and beverages • Frequent oral irrigation.
Diarrhea	Determine frequency and character of bowel movements. Obtain nutrition history. Obtain height, weight, and vital signs. Assess hydration status: tissue turgor, condition of mucous membranes, and serum electrolyte values. Assess knowledge and symptoms related to diarrhea. Determine: • Patient-initiated measures to control diarrhea. • Previous methods used to control diarrhea.	Diarrhea related to effects of chemotherapeutic agents on the intestinal mucosa	Stool is formed. Stool is evacuated at intervals normal for the individual patient.	Implement measures to control and prevent diarrhea: Avoid: • Bowel-irritating foods • Gas-forming foods • Fatty foods • Lactose- and caffeine-containing products • Smoking Suggest: • Diet low in residue, high in protein and carbohydrates • Small, frequent meals Teach perianal hygiene: • Cleanse with water and mild soap after bowel movement. • Use sitz baths, if indicated.

Table continued on following page

1541

Table 34–7

Side Effects of Chemotherapy with Related Assessments, Nursing Diagnoses, Expected Patient Outcomes, and Nursing Interventions *(continued)*

Side Effect	Assessment	Nursing Diagnosis	Expected Patient Outcomes	Nursing Interventions
Diarrhea *(continued)*				• Apply topical anesthetics to rectal area, if indicated. Administer and monitor the effects of medications to control diarrhea: • Antidiarrheal agents • Antispasmodics • Opiates and opiate substitutes
Constipation	Determine: • Usual bowel habits. • Patient knowledge related to constipation. • Patient symptoms (cramping, pain, abdominal distention). • Schedule of all medications (chemotherapy, *Vinca* alkaloids, narcotics). • Previous medications and interventions used to treat constipation. • Bowel sound patterns.	Constipation related to the effects of chemotherapeutic agents on the bowel	Stool is soft and formed. Stool is evacuated at regular intervals without straining.	Implement measures to prevent and alleviate constipation: Suggest: • Diet high in fiber, roughage, fluid • Drinking warm fluids to stimulate intestinal motility • Increase in physical activity to increase intestinal motility • Using toilet or bedside commode instead of bedpan If patient has history of constipation and will receive *Vinca* alkaloid agents, suggest that all the above start after first chemotherapy dose. Avoid using enemas or suppositories without consulting physician. Administer and monitor the effects of medications prescribed to relieve constipation: • Stool softeners: dioctyl sodium sulfosuccinate, mineral oil • Bulk producers: psyllium, calcium, polycarbophil • Osmotic and saline laxatives: sodium, potassium, and magnesium salts

1542

OTHER ASSESSMENTS AND INTERVENTIONS

Renal toxicity
Renal toxicity is caused by specific chemotherapy agents:
Cisplatin—damage to renal tubules
Methotrexate—renal tubule necrosis with high doses

Cyclophosphamide—hemorrhagic cystitis
Hyperuricemia is due to rapid tumor destruction or tumor lysis in which tumor cells enter the circulatory system and pass through the renal system.

Review renal function studies:
• Serum creatinine
• Creatinine clearance
• Blood urea nitrogen
Review urinalysis.
Check history of renal disease.
Ask about symptoms of dysuria, hematuria (for cyclophosphamide).

• Lactulose is especially effective for constipation caused by *Vinca* alkaloids
• Cathartics: castor oil, senna, cascara, bisacodyl

For cisplatin:
• Hydrate before therapy as per institutional protocol.
• Measure and record urine output.
• Administer diuretics as ordered by physician.
• Monitor renal function regularly.
For methotrexate:
• Hydrate before therapy as per institutional protocol.
• Measure and record urine output.
• Administer sodium bicarbonate to alkalinize urine.
• Monitor urine pH; must be >7 before treatment.
• Monitor renal function regularly.
For cyclophosphamide:
• Hydrate with intravenous therapy.
• Advise increase in oral fluids.
• Institute measures to prevent hyperuricemia.
• Increase oral and intravenous fluids as indicated.
• Alkalinize urine.
• Administer allopurinol (Zyloprim) before and during therapy to break down urates.
• Monitor serum and urine uric acid levels.

can be enhanced to recognize and destroy tumor cells.

Types of Immunotherapy

Historically, immunotherapy has been classified as passive, active, or adaptive. Passive immunotherapy involves administration of antitumor antibodies sensitized to a specific antigen. Active immunotherapy involves use of vaccines prepared from tumor cells to stimulate both cellular and hormonal immunity. Active immunotherapy can be either specific for a certain kind of tumor cell or nonspecific to stimulate general immunity. An example of active nonspecific immunotherapy is the use of bacille Calmette-Guérin (BCG), an extract of tuberculosis bacilli. An example of active specific immunotherapy would involve the use of a vaccine derived from specific tumor cells and given to treat the same tumor.

Adaptive methods involve stimulation of the immune system through administration of chemically treated white blood cells. An example of adaptive immunotherapy is the use of interferons and interleukins. Interferons are a group of proteins naturally produced by the body in response to viral infections and other inducers. Interferons may have clinical value because of their ability to stimulate the immune system and inhibit cell growth. Interleukins are natural substances produced by lymphocytes and monocytes and are being studied for their antitumor properties. Extensive research is being carried out to determine the therapeutic value of interferons and interleukins.

Immunotherapeutic agents are now called biologic response modifiers because they exhibit antitumor effects by mediating the immune response and, in some cases, directly killing tumor cells. Immunotherapeutic agents are divided into categories based on how they affect the tumor and the immune response. The classifications include agents that modulate or stimulate the immune system, agents that kill cancer cells directly, and agents whose action is not yet known. Some immunotherapy agents belong in more than one category. Immunomodulators include interleukins, interferons, and specific and nonspecific vaccines. Immunotherapy is often used in conjunction with other forms of cancer therapy, such as chemotherapy, radiation therapy, and surgery.

Side Effects

The side effects of immunotherapy vary with the type and mode of administration. Intradermal, subcutaneous, and intralesional vaccines can cause localized skin irritation and systemic side effects of elevated body temperature, body chills, diaphoresis, and fatigue. Intravenous administration of immunomodulators has a wider range of systemic side effects, which include elevated body temperature, chills, diaphoresis, fluid retention, nausea, vomiting, and fatigue. Patients receiving investigational forms of immunotherapy are closely monitored for unknown side effects and adverse systemic reactions.

UNCONVENTIONAL THERAPIES

The success of medical research and treatment in eradicating such diseases as polio and smallpox has created a general expectation that there must be a "cure" for cancer. The search for a "miracle" cure for oncologic diseases has led patients to investigate and participate in a wide range of therapies, such as diet programs, vitamin therapies, and unproven and potentially unsafe biologic vaccines. These unproven methods are often costly and, if used instead of generally accepted treatments, can prevent timely treatment and restoration of health.

An example of a psychologic approach to cancer cure that has become quite well known is that developed by the Simontons, a radiation oncologist and psychotherapist team. Their program is based on research suggesting that stress reduces antibody response. Immunoglobulin levels change in response to psychological stimuli, protective "killer cell" lymphocytes become less effective, and proliferation of T lymphocytes declines significantly.

The Simontons, and others, teach patients to use mental imagery and other stress reduction techniques to fortify the immune system against cancer. These techniques are valuable adjuncts to traditional treatment regimens when used with appropriate patients. However, they should never be promoted as a substitute for traditional treatment modalities such as surgery, radiation, and chemotherapy. The Simontons have developed a step-by-step, self-help program for patient and family participation in the treatment of cancer. Their program includes daily practice of progressive relaxation and mental imagery, daily reading assignments to overcome knowledge deficit on cancer, and self-study meditation to strengthen or correct coping behaviors.

The imagery includes visualization of lymphocytes overpowering and destroying cancer cells, tumors shrinking, and improved general health status and well-being.

Patients may request information related to alternative therapies as a means to ensure that they are reviewing all treatment alternatives. Respond to such requests by providing accurate information related to these therapies while listening to and exploring the reasons for seeking unproven methods. If the response is unsatisfactory to the patient, provide referrals to educational materials or other professionals who can provide additional and current information about the health hazards and risks of unproven cancer treatments. Among sources of information are publications of the Food and Drug Administration, the National Cancer Institute, and the American Cancer Society. These agencies have literature that reviews and assesses unproven drugs, substances, and treatment centers.

NURSING PROCESS GUIDELINES
Unconventional Therapies

Be sensitive to the fact that many patients and families who seek unconventional therapy may have exhausted all conventional therapy without regression of disease. A patient's inclination to explore unproven therapies may be founded in desperation and not in reason. Remain objective and present patients with information to help them understand the risks and implications of unproven cancer therapies. Accept the patient's right to choose whatever therapy he or she finds most desirable even if, in your judgment, it is not the correct choice.

Psychosocial Problems of the Patient Receiving Treatment for Cancer

Cancer raises psychosocial problems of varying complexity and severity. Nevertheless, certain themes emerge that are noted and reported by cancer patients with frequent regularity.

ANXIETY AND FEAR

Anxiety and fear are universally experienced with cancer. Patients report that one of the most difficult things they experience is uncertainty. Anxiety induced by that uncertainty promotes a sense of powerlessness and loss of control. Adjustments and changes in role and lifestyle are real and ongoing. Therefore, uncertainty is a constant threat. The degree of anxiety is increased by threatened self-esteem and actual or anticipated loss.

Fear of recurring malignancy, of the effects of chemotherapy, and of metastasis and death are common. Most feared is a lingering and painful death.

THREATS TO SELF-CONCEPT

Disturbance in self-concept results when one is forced to perceive oneself differently. Forced changes in self-concept may result from lowered self-esteem, difference in role performance, or changes in body image. These problems occur frequently in cancer patients. Surgical interventions to remove and, one hopes, cure the cancer, such as a colostomy or ileal conduit, may leave the patient with major changes in body function and image. A laryngectomy requires major adjustments to new communication patterns. An amputation or mastectomy may induce feelings of mutilation. Chronic pain produces feelings of vulnerability and lowers self-confidence. These few examples illustrate the profound abrupt changes in body image and threats to self-esteem that cancer engenders. No wonder many patients feel betrayed by their body when they develop cancer.

Role performance alterations are also common and can lower self-esteem. Effects of surgery and chemotherapy, or of the illness itself, may prevent the breadwinner from working, prevent the homemaker from caring for the household, or make childbearing impossible. Even when the ability to continue at a satisfying job is not cut off, the demands of chemotherapy and the uncertainty of its outcome may prevent a promotion or inhibit challenging assignments.

ALTERED SEXUALITY

Changes in sexual activity may result from alterations in body functions caused by the disease or by surgical treatments, such as excision of the vulva. More common is potential sexual dysfunction from an altered self-concept.

The presence of a stoma or loss of a breast may induce fears of disgust or rejection by the sexual partner. Men may become impotent from changed role performance and dependency. Chemotherapeutic agents and radiation can also induce temporary or permanent sexual dysfunction.

PROFOUND LOSS AND HELPLESSNESS

Feelings of profound loss and helplessness have been identified as major factors that often precede illness. These feelings are also experienced during cancer treatment. Cancer treatments, to be successful, must be intrusive. This can cause fear, anger, and resentment that the patient must willingly submit to "torture." Helplessness to resist the need for mutilating surgery or distressingly toxic chemicals results in profound feelings of powerlessness. Depression commonly results from the sense of loss and may be accompanied by spiritual distress, deep hopelessness, and suicidal thoughts or actions.

Certain losses have profound symbolic meaning. Hair or breast loss for some women is deeply disturbing because both are strongly symbolic of feminine attractiveness.

ISOLATION AND ALIENATION

Isolation commonly occurs in cancer because the disease or treatments produce weakness and difficulty in socializing. Patients are often homebound. Friends may stop visiting from uneasiness, fear of catching cancer, sadness, or embarrassment at not knowing what to say. This raises feelings of alienation in the patient.

Isolation can be self-induced if patients are unwilling to be seen in public because of hair and weight loss or other changes in appearance. The loneliness is compounded if they feel unable to talk freely with loved ones about their feelings and worries. Satisfying jobs are very therapeutic in maintaining a sense of structure in their new "world of turmoil." Continuing to work should be encouraged, even on a part-time basis. Disability leave, when necessary, should be as short-term as possible to reduce feelings of isolation.

FAMILY STRESS

The level of family stress always rises when a member develops cancer. Alterations in family processes cannot be avoided because of changes in routines and schedules. Financial strains occur. Family members must watch helplessly as a loved one suffers and must adapt to changes in the loved one who has cancer.

Family members who have had trouble coping in the past face additional stress. Invariably, the crisis of cancer causes old conflicts to resurface. Unresolved issues or poor relationships can no longer be ignored or left dormant. Superficially healed emotional wounds often are exacerbated and become raw. Cancer, which is a family problem, exposes inadequacies in the family system. The coping styles of patients and their families range from effective to ineffective as the patient adjusts to the diagnosis and required therapies. Coping effectiveness depends on the ability to seek information, to follow-through on treatment, and to talk freely about feelings and concerns, as well as on the availability of an adequate support system.

Type of cancer, extent of the disease, forced changes in body image, age at onset, degree of debilitating symptoms, previous experiences with cancer, and financial means to seek and pay for needed care also have a direct effect on coping abilities.

NURSING PROCESS
Psychosocial Needs of Cancer Patients

The focus of cancer treatment, and its impact on the patient's ability to cope, varies with the prognosis. This focus can be summarized as cure, control, or comfort. Each category of care, as well as the specific type of cancer experienced, presents different psychosocial problems.

CURE. Coping strategies often focus around needed adjustments to body image from curative surgery that causes major body changes. Efforts should be made to reduce anxiety, to ventilate feelings, to maintain a fighting spirit, and to resume a normal lifestyle. Even easily cured types of skin cancer generate fear that must be addressed.

CONTROL. Major adjustments to long-term radiation and chemotherapy result in profound feelings of vulnerability, dependency, and helplessness. Fear, isolation, and threats to self-esteem are common themes. Family stress and knowledge deficit are additional problems frequently noted.

COMFORT. Patients with a terminal prognosis need help to cope and to be spared as much pain, depression, and alienation as possible. A profound sense of loss is often reported, which can lead to hopelessness or spiritual distress as well as grief.

Assessment

When assessing the psychosocial dimension, keep in mind that careful observation and attentive listening to patients and their families provide the basis for identifying reactions and needs. Promote honest communication by expressing empathy and projecting an attitude of calm acceptance. Use clarifying questions to validate perceptions and broad opening questions to permit the patient's priorities to surface. Paraphrase and reflect feelings to mirror reactions and enable the patients to look more clearly at their responses to what they are experiencing.

Remember that sometimes patients cannot identify the nature of their feelings directly and need to initially address them peripherally by discussing and focusing on people or happenings around them. Other times they need to use symbolic language or gestures. Always remember that all behavior has meaning. Rude, petty demands may be expressions of feelings of powerlessness, loss, and anger. Passive compliance may indicate problems of low self-esteem or depression. Compare currently observed coping mechanisms with premorbid behavior patterns through discussion with patients, families, or trusted others.

Identify major strengths and weaknesses as a basis for planning care. These include the ability to relate and communicate effectively with others, to recognize and express feelings, to effectively seek and request help as needed, to make sound decisions, and to follow instructions with consistency.

Assess important resources, such as the quality of medical care, religious faith, supportive family and friends, and adequate finances. Also assess ethnic and cultural influences, previous experience with cancer, other major problems or burdens in life, and, most important, present understanding of the condition and its prognosis.

Nursing Diagnoses and Planning

Nursing diagnoses and related expected patient outcomes commonly applicable to the psychosocial needs of patients undergoing cancer treatment include the following:

NDx: Anxiety related to uncertain outcomes and effects of cancer treatment

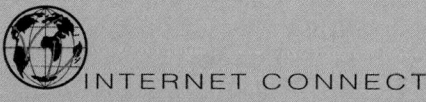

INTERNET CONNECTIONS
Oncologic Disorders

ONCOLINK

http://cancer.med.upenn.edu/

This authoritative site, sponsored by the University of Pennsylvania, provides a vast array of cancer-related information, including disease-oriented menus on specific types of cancer as well as menus oriented toward specific medical specialties. It provides links to support services, global resources, international conferences for health-care professionals, and information about financial issues for patients. It provides links to specific ONCOLINK sites for many types of cancer, some of which are featured in Internet Connections boxes in other chapters of this text.

Oncology Nursing Society Online

http://www.ons.org

This site, sponsored by the Oncology Nursing Society, which has a membership of over 25,000 nurses worldwide, includes e-mail, chat sessions, and forums for oncology nurses. The goal of this site is to provide relevant clinical information for nurses who provide direct care to patients with cancer.

American Cancer Society

http://www.cancer.org/

Information is provided about the American Cancer Society and its programs and events as well as about professional meetings and medical news, lists of cancer-related publications, and links to other resources.

National Cancer Institute

http://www.nci.nih.gov/

A U.S. government–sponsored source of authoritative information includes links to other cancer-related resources.

Netherlands Cancer Institute/Antoni van Leeuwenhoek Hospital

http://www.nki.nl/

This international site provides general information about cancer, including research findings, information on the clinical aspects of cancer, and information on the nursing aspects of cancer. It also provides links to a wide variety of resources.

Planning: Patient Outcomes

1. Patient asks relevant questions.
2. Patient reads information about treatments.
3. Patient expresses anxieties and fears openly to nurse and significant others.
4. Patient uses self-identified effective coping mechanisms to reduce stress.
5. Patient attempts to limit self-identified counterproductive coping mechanisms.
6. Patient sets realistic goals, breaking them down to small, attainable units.
7. Patient focuses on the present, attempting to live "one day at a time."
8. Patient practices progressive relaxation and mental imagery on a daily basis.
9. Patient keeps as active as possible, performing at least a few simple exercises daily and taking brief, daily walks.
10. Patient attends self-help group or keeps scheduled appointments with cancer support counselor.
11. Patient uses problem-solving techniques to reduce fears and uncertainties.

NDx: Body image disturbance related to loss of a body part or to major structural or functional changes (such as stoma, immobility, alopecia, inability to speak)

Planning: Patient Outcomes

1. Patient talks about feelings of loss, crying appropriately.
2. Patient assumes responsibility for care of altered body part.
3. Patient speaks calmly and naturally about new body part, function, or role.
4. Patient states he or she feels comfortable with self.
5. Patient uses effective coping mechanisms to plan rehabilitation.
6. Patient takes steps to secure, adjust, and care for adequate adaptive devices.
7. Patient maintains or resumes social contacts with equanimity.
8. Patient participates in physical activities, relaxation exercises, contact with well-adjusted patients, and other techniques that promote adjustment.
9. Patient plans for future with family and significant others.

NDx: Altered role performance related to inability to

continue working or dependence on others secondary to effects of disease, irradiation, and chemotherapy

Planning: Patient Outcomes
1. Patient talks about feelings regarding role change.
2. Patient describes new role requirements accurately.
3. Patient assertively defines new role with acceptance and satisfaction.

NDx: Sexual dysfunction related to perceived disfigurement and mutilation, loss of role and self-esteem, presence of appliance, fears, or effects of chemotherapy

Planning: Patient Outcomes
1. Patient talks openly and freely to nurse and partner about sexual problems.
2. Patient actively seeks ways to reduce stress and cope with problems, including willingness to participate in sex counseling as needed.
3. Patient discusses alternative techniques for sexual expression with partner.

NDx: Powerlessness related to hospitalization, need to participate in undesirable treatment, or overprotectiveness by family

Planning: Patient Outcomes
1. Patient identifies sense of powerlessness and takes steps to avoid preventable insecurities.
2. Patient assertively expresses legitimate complaints and need for independence and control.
3. Patient actively participates in decision-making.
4. Patient realistically identifies what he or she can continue to do and functions as independently as condition allows.

NDx: Social isolation related to decreased contact with friends or need to stop working

Planning: Patient Outcomes
1. Patient describes feelings of isolation and alienation as common to the cancer experience.
2. Patient shares feelings freely with trusted others.
3. Patient maintains work and social schedule with adaptations for physical disability.

NDx: Altered family processes related to difficulty adjusting to changes in the patient, hospitalization of the patient, disruption of routines, or the financial burden of treatment

Planning: Patient Outcomes
1. Family members verbalize thoughts and feelings about the effects of cancer to each other and with appropriate health-care professionals.
2. Family makes positive affirmations by words and deeds of patient as a valued member.
3. Individual members of family weather crisis without long-term psychological disability or alienation.

4. Family members work together to attack problems and share responsibilities constructively.
5. Family seeks community services and referrals appropriately as needed.

Nursing Interventions and Evaluation

Interventions vary with the prognosis and the treatment focus of cure, control, or comfort.

NDx: Anxiety
Therapeutic communication is the priority intervention in preventing and reducing anxiety. Give the patient information about the anticipated treatment and its effects in clear, simple terms. Stress individual variations of response to chemotherapy and other treatments to avoid suggesting or conditioning the patient to expect unpleasant side effects. Schedule regular opportunities for the patient to discuss and ventilate anxieties and fears in an unhurried, empathetic manner. Avoid false reassurances because they belittle the patient's concerns. Often, encouraging patients to describe anticipated death or other fears in segmented details helps break down and reduce their terror.

Help the patient identify and initiate steps to reduce anxiety. For example, encourage realistic goal setting—small, easily attainable short-term goals for immediate attention and maximum success. Action reduces anxiety, so focus on the "here and now" with small, immediate goals to help reduce the anxiety produced by situations in which one feels helpless. Teach and guide the patient through progressive relaxation techniques because, when muscles are not tense, the person does not feel tense. Total relaxation can result from training in muscle relaxation. Also guide the patient in the use of mental imagery, which may have a positive effect in stimulating and enhancing the body's immune system. Encourage regular daily exercise and activities as valuable means of discharging tensions and dissipating fear and anxiety.

Teach problem-solving techniques, such as assessment, analysis, planning, interventions, and evaluation, as a means of reducing uncertainties that can be resolved. Identify and reinforce patients' strengths to help structure for success. Identify and accept other coping mechanisms (eg, hostility, withdrawal, distraction, or demanding behaviors) as manifestations of stress, while helping the patient to set limits on these behaviors.

Counsel and help patients to structure life and environment to avoid extra stress and to keep unnecessary changes and decisions to a minimum.

Arrange for patients to meet with cancer patients who have had successful outcomes to their treatment to reduce anxiety and promote hope. Encourage or help patients to join a support group, because others who have had similar crises understand the patient's distress and may offer the best help in dealing with it on an ongoing basis. When necessary, administer antianxiety medications as ordered.

NDx: Body image disturbance

To help the patient adjust to altered body parts or function, explain the stages of grief and reassure the patient that grief is a normal reaction to loss of body parts and functions. This helps prevent guilt about the feelings associated with the different stages of grief and promotes self-acceptance. Involve the patient gradually in the care of the altered part to avoid overwhelming him or her. Recognize that the patient's first perception of his or her altered appearance is derived from the response of the nurse, whether it be calm acceptance or revulsion. Because better understanding promotes quality care, identify the patient's areas of concern and his or her symbolic meaning of the lost part or function (eg, mastectomy equals loss of femininity for some women).

Provide reliable resource information about quality wigs, prostheses, or adaptive devices to allow for practical steps to improve the patient's well-being. Arrange fittings for prostheses or use of adaptive devices as soon as possible to avoid development of negative habits, resistance, or apathy.

Discuss social situations that the patient dreads because of altered body parts or function. Role-play these situations with the patient, because rehearsal in a safe setting builds confidence and structures for later success in real situations. Arrange peer visits or involvement with people from self-help groups such as the Ostomy Association, Reach for Recovery, or the Lost Chord Society, because these people understand the patient's situation better than anyone and can teach and motivate most effectively.

Provide information about programs such as the American Cancer Society's "Look Good Feel Better" Program, which has been designed to help cancer patients with creative grooming strategies. It is a 1-day program during which consultants assist with application of make-up, hair care, wig/scarf application, and fashion suggestions. It is available in various sites and information can be obtained from the American Cancer Society.

NDx: Altered role performance

To help the patient adjust to role change without excessive dependency patterns, explore and use the patient's strengths to plan care and rehabilitation. Facilitate honest expression of feelings, which communicates respect and promotes self-esteem and acceptance. Explore with and assist the patient in techniques of biofeedback, behavior modification, hypnosis, imagery, and relaxation, which increase ability to cope with stress and build self-esteem. Encourage as much physical movement as possible to help the patient redefine body space and to build self-confidence.

Be sure to involve the family and patient in planning and problem-solving because patients do not function in isolation. Identify and discuss role changes, role confusion, or role conflicts (eg, breadwinner versus dependent, sick role versus active participant in rehabilitative decisions), so that frustration can be ventilated and areas of confusion corrected. Also identify and discuss stressors that promote role disturbance, such as financial stress, changes in sexual performance, changes in appearance, and changes in physical capabilities. Better understanding promotes acceptance and successful adjustment. Help the patient sort through options and identify ways to structure for success to encourage autonomy and sound decision-making. Explore gender role expectations and needed adaptations for realistic preparation for future demands. Identify family patterns of shielding of or dependency on the patient, because these can promote feelings of inadequacy in the patient.

NDx: Sexual dysfunction

Gently introduce information about the relationship of stress to sexual interest and performance to promote understanding and acknowledgment of the problem. Differentiate between intrapsychic conflicts and organic factors, such as the effects of medication. With the patient's permission, explore the partner's reactions to sexual problems. Identify and discuss myths about cancer and sexual disability to restore hope and confidence. Explore the patient's willingness to discuss alternative techniques to stimulate and satisfy sexual needs (eg, body massage, mutual masturbation, and use of erotic routines and materials as aids to sexual stimulation). Make referrals for counseling or sex therapy as needed. If patients desire to have children, give information about sperm banks for freezing and preserving sperm before surgery or treatments that may cause infertility.

In vitro fertilization and embryo transfer is yet another evolving option for couples who anticipate or are experiencing infertility. The ovaries are continually monitored by periodic ultrasonography to determine the appropriate time for laparoscopic harvest of the ovum. Once ripe follicles are obtained, they are mixed with the partner's semen in a culture dish, which is then incubated for 36 to 40 hours. The resulting embryo is then transferred to the uterus and, if pregnancy occurs, it is established in 2 weeks.

NDx: Powerlessness

To help the patient make decisions and actively participate in planning for the future, begin by respecting the patient's need to grieve the loss of independence, power, and control, as well as body changes and role. Recognize that hospitalization promotes powerlessness. Make all possible efforts to offset that effect. Orient the patient to the hospital environment and personnel to reduce confusion and feelings of being a stranger. Within the confines and demands of the hospital setting, give the patient as much control as possible. Involve the patient in regulation of temperature, lighting, ventilation, television and radio noise, and furniture placement. Encourage decision-making in terms of scheduling. Minimize inconveniences, irritations, and sensory overload because they increase feelings of inadequacy when the patient is helpless to do anything about them.

Avoid reinforcing dependency patterns, which in turn reinforce feelings of powerlessness. Teach the family about factors that promote helplessness (such as overprotecting and isolating the patient) so that members will avoid these destructive tendencies. Also stress that helplessness is a learned response that can be unlearned and replaced with more responsible responses. Make available reference books such as *The American Cancer Society Cancer Book, Coping With Chemotherapy,* or *The Cancer Patient's Handbook* to promote learning and feelings of control. Encourage assertiveness on the part of the patient, and recognize patient demands as coping mechanisms. Respect the patient's legitimate complaints because ignoring them negates all sense of worth and control.

Explore and encourage spiritual supports if the patient finds them useful. Prayer and meditation, scripture readings, attendance at religious services, and chaplains' visits can help patients relate to God's power and reduce their own sense of powerlessness. If expressions of hopelessness and other signs of despair and depression appear, initiate a referral for counseling.

NDx: Social isolation

To promote patient participation in constructive social and diversional activities, encourage the patient to continue working at a satisfactory job as long as possible. When the patient cannot work, help identify ways to increase or maintain meaningful social contacts (such as regularly scheduled telephone calls, tape recordings, visits, or written correspondence) to prevent isolation. Approach significant family members and friends about the importance of continued visits and calls to prevent isolation and alienation. Teach the family to respect the patient's privacy but firmly maintain some social involvement if the patient tends to withdraw. Most often, one-to-one and small-group contacts are less threatening and therefore more acceptable to the patient. If the patient seems religious, visits from a pastor, rabbi, or other spiritual advisor may encourage hope and a sense of receiving God's blessing and presence in their loneliness.

When appropriate, provide specific information or referrals for social involvement because the patient may lack the motivation or energy to seek out and pursue needed information. Consider senior citizen centers, adult education classes, self-help groups, volunteer visitors, and home health aides. If transportation is a problem, provide information on what is available in the community, such as ambulettes and senior citizen vans. Explore diversional activities appropriate to the patient's physical abilities. Make occupational therapy referrals as needed so the patient gains confidence with mastering new small motor skills and is stimulated by new activities.

Empathize with the patient, and validate that feelings of isolation and alienation are a common component of the cancer experience. Encourage the patient to confide and discuss feelings of isolation and alienation openly with significant others. If needed, role-play interactions with significant others to help the patient communicate on a more intimate, meaningful level. Avoid pat phrases and false reassurances and minimization or disrespect of the patient's feelings. This increases the sense of isolation and loneliness. Teach the family to do likewise. Do not lie to a patient; rather, teach the truth in a supportive manner when the patient provides cues that he or she is ready to learn. Take extra time to promote alternative means of significant communication with a patient who has lost speaking ability, to prevent the loneliness, isolation, and alienation characteristic of this disability.

NDx: Altered family processes

To enable the family to maintain mutual support while coping positively with changes caused by cancer and the financial strains of treatment, first recognize that cancer is a family disease. The family's suffering can be as great or greater than that of their loved one because families usually function as integral units. Take time to speak with each family member about his or her own stress. Make referrals as needed to cancer support groups or individual counseling. Because each family member's reactions affect the other members, discuss constructive family coping, including use of humor, respect of individuality, mutual reliance and support, sharing thoughts and feelings, and shared decision-making and planning. These behaviors promote health and well-being. Identify and discuss potentially destructive family coping tendencies, such as denial, separation and withdrawal, exploitation and overdependency, an authoritarian approach to problems, and substance abuse by stressed members as a form of escape. Awareness of these dysfunctional patterns can help resolve them.

Teach families that old problems tend to resurface in times of stress. Make referrals as needed for marriage and individual counseling, family therapy, and substance abuse interventions (Al-Anon, Al-Ateen, Alcoholics Anonymous). Always stress that crises carry potential for positive change and that it is possible to emerge from a crisis as a stronger unit. Avoid giving advice and using appeals to logic because these rarely produce changed behavior. Do provide genuine expressions of empathy to each member. Avoid taking sides in disputes and disagreements because to do so dilutes and negates your influence and ability to help the family as a whole unit. Facilitate freer family communication patterns by clarifying ambiguous messages and identifying destructive patterns to be avoided. Make referrals as needed for financial or other assistance to departments of social services, Medicare, Medicaid, American Cancer Society, hospice, home care agencies, and self-help groups. Remember that the family may not know about these resources.

Cultural Considerations

Oncology nurses are increasingly faced with the frustrations and rewards of working with patients, families, and fellow staff members from cultures different from their own. Culture is not a singular characteristic to be added to a list of items checked off when assessing a patient. Rather, it is the core element on which the cancer experience is constructed.

Seeking the cause and meaning of one's cancer appears to be a universal drive. People, their families, and communities seek an order to the chaos imposed by a cancer diagnosis and direction on how potential suffering should be borne. Each cultural group also has different styles of communication, and both age and gender establish specific parameters for what are considered appropriate topics of discussion and with whom, when, and how such interactions can occur. Culture also prescribes who is appropriate to provide social support and what form this support should take to be considered appropriate and acceptable.

Attitudes toward the side effects of treatment, concepts of body image, sexuality, and the response to pain also vary with cultural norms and expectations about suffering, private behavior, and interactions with authority figures. Perceptions of disability and dependency are also integrated into individual and family identity according to cultural precepts. Even the concept of who constitutes a family and the dynamics that occur within the family differ across cultures. Death, although a universal phenomenon, is experienced in different manners from group to group, and quality of life and spirituality may also be defined in different ways (Kagawa-Singer, 1996).

In providing culturally based care, it is essential that nurses develop a knowledge of the patient's cultural group. This knowledge can be enhanced through observation and openness, which is a gradual process. Patience is also necessary and may present a challenge because of nursing time constraints. However, it is essential to establish a trusting relationship with patients from different cultures. Finally, the nurse is in a key position to facilitate the achievement of goals between patients and all members of the health-care team. The nurse must recognize the practices of the cultural group as being as important as those of the health-care team. If patients see this attitude, they will be more willing to negotiate and comply with recommendations made by the team (Kagawa-Singer, 1996).

The Office of Cancer Communication (OCC) is the organizational component of the National Cancer Institute (NCI) responsible for public education and patient, family, and professional education. One initiative of the OCC is the development of educational programs and materials targeted to underserved and hard-to-reach populations: African-Americans, Hispanics, older Americans, and low-literate people (NCI, 1994).

Complications

PAIN

Pain is a major factor in advanced cancer. The International Association for the Study of Pain has defined pain as "an unpleasant sensory and emotional experience associated with actual or potential tissue damage or described in terms of such damage." The subjective nature of pain is evidenced by the unique psychologic and physiologic responses to pain.

Cancer pain is most often associated with tissue damage and tissue infiltration. As malignant tumors grow within a body part, they stretch normal boundaries of the organ, causing severe pain (Fig. 34–14). As tumors grow and occupy additional space, other organs and structures are affected. Tumor growth and tissue invasion can result in nerve compression, organ and bone invasion, organ obstruction, and organ stretching. Primary or metastatic bone tumors cause pain related to pressure, periosteal irritation, and pathologic fractures. Pain can be experienced as an acute or chronic event. Unrelieved pain can affect a patient's lifestyle, treatment, and ability to cope with his or her disease status.

Physiology of Pain

According to the gate-control theory, pain is a subjective individualized event that represents several interrelated sensory, affective, and personal factors. The gate-control theory demonstrates the relationship between the central nervous system and the peripheral nervous system in the recognition and control of pain. This theory is predicated on the physiologic structure of small, slow-conducting afferent nerve fibers of the peripheral nervous system that merge in the dorsal root of the spinal cord. This area, called the substantia gelatinosa, consists of a layer of cells that cover the spinal cord on both sides and provide a "gate" for pain signals to pass. As pain builds, the fibers of the gate open and pain is experienced. Larger nerve fibers have the capacity to inhibit the transmission of pain and cause the gate to close. Afferent nerve impulses, such as memory, attention, and emotions, can either reduce or enhance the pain because they, too, can stimulate the gate mechanism.

Neurotransmitters are chemicals, such as endor-

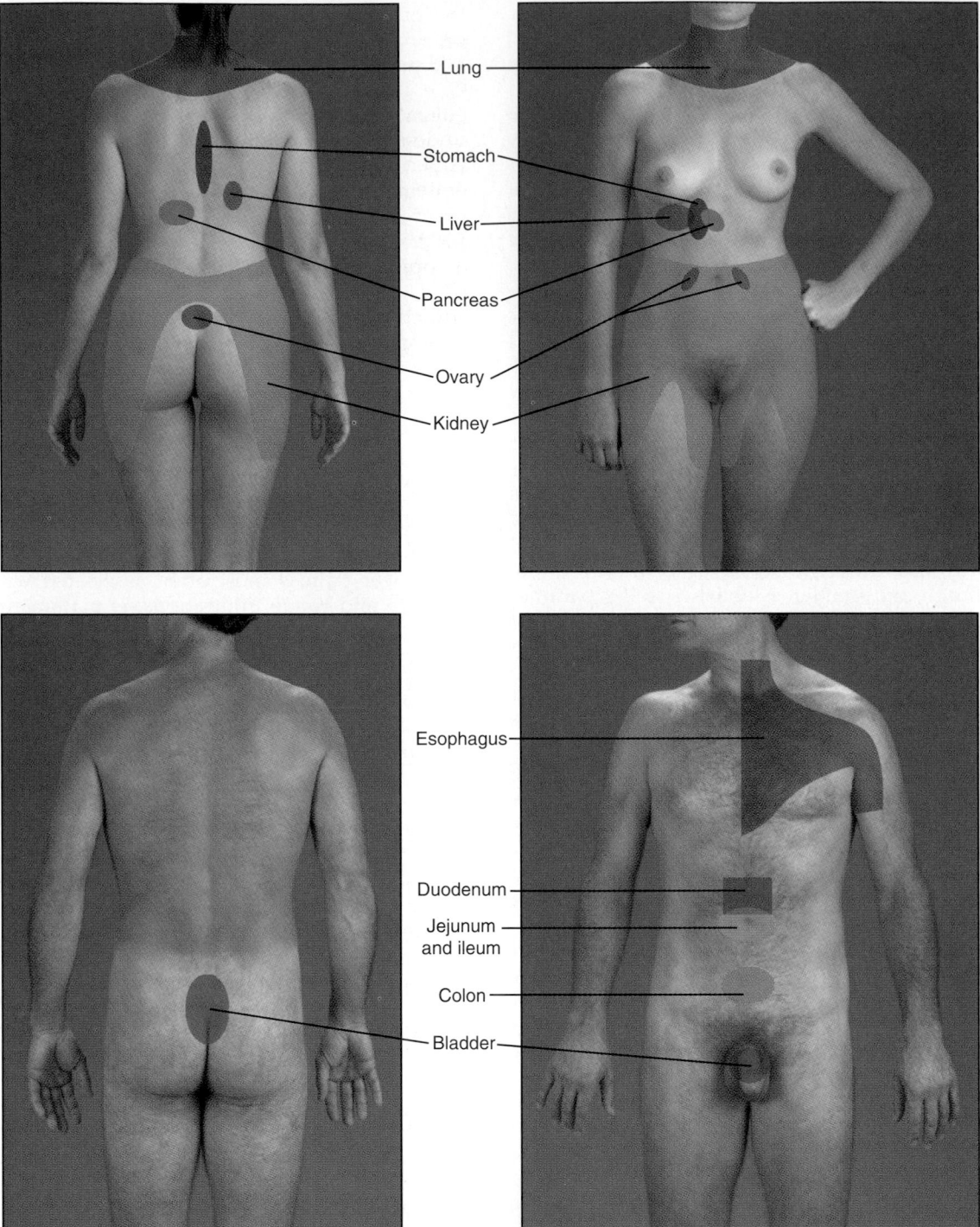

Figure 34-14
Body surface areas where pain is felt from visceral organs that are common cancer sites.

phins and enkephalins, that are produced by the body in response to pain. These chemicals modify and block transmission of pain impulses and function as opiate receptors throughout the nervous system. Drug therapy with narcotics is used to relieve pain through activating opiate receptors in the central and peripheral nervous dystem.

Pain Management

Relief of cancer pain can be achieved for the vast majority of patients. Although the pain may not be completely eliminated, it can be controlled sufficiently to allow the patient to maintain quality of life. To be successful, pain management must be tailored to individual needs, which vary with diagnosis, stage of disease, response to pain, and personal preference. It requires a team approach, with the patient participating as an active member coupled with systematic assessment of pain status at regular intervals.

PHARMACOLOGIC THERAPIES

Pharmacologic therapy is the basic, relatively low risk, inexpensive method of pain control. Analgesics, anti-inflammatory agents, and adjuvant agents (eg, psychotropic drugs and steroids) are used in treating pain, alone or in combination. These agents control pain symptoms with the goal of improving patient comfort. As illustrated in the World Health Organization three-step analgesic ladder, mild to moderate pain is treated with nonopioid drugs, with or without adjuvant agents (Fig. 34–15). An opioid is added if the pain persists or worsens. For continued moderate to severe pain, the potency or dose of the opioid is increased. Because drugs within each category vary in effect, different drugs and doses within each category should be tried before moving the patient to the next step.

Nonopioid analgesics control pain by acting on the peripheral nervous system. They include aspirin, acetaminophen, and nonsteroidal anti-inflammatory agents (NSAIDs), such as ibuprofen. NSAIDs, which are contraindicated for patients with thrombocytopenia, can cause platelet dysfunction and bleeding from impaired blood clotting. They can also cause renal failure, hepatic dysfunction, and gastric ulceration. NSAIDs can interact with other drugs, such as warfarin, digoxin, and oral antidiabetic agents.

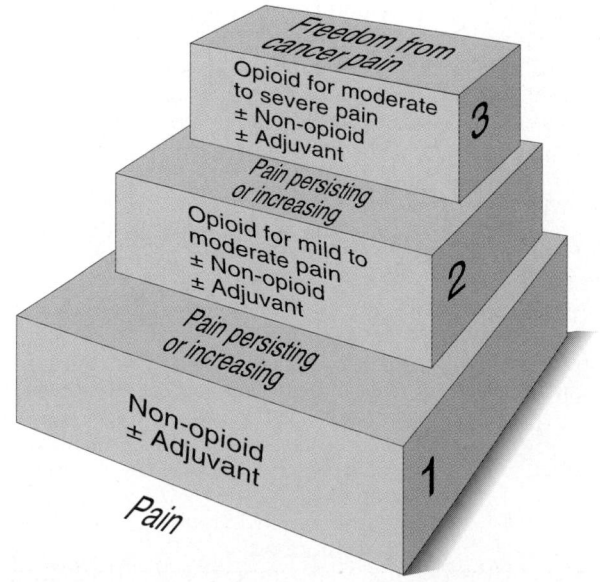

Figure 34–15

The World Health Organization's three-step analgesic ladder. (Reproduced by permission of WHO, from Cancer pain relief. 2nd ed. Geneva: World Health Organization, 1996.)

Opioids control pain by acting on the central nervous system. They include codeine, morphine, oxycodone, hydrocodone, levorphanol, and fentanyl. Side effects from opioids include drowsiness and mental clouding, constipation, nausea and vomiting, drying of the oral mucosa, and respiratory depression. Side effects are managed through dose reduction in conjunction with increased frequency of administration, substitution of another drug, or use of adjuvant agents to counteract them. Long-term use of opioids also induces tolerance and physical dependence, but this is not equivalent to psychological addiction or drug abuse.

Pharmacologic agents can be given by several routes: oral, rectal, transdermal (fentanyl patch), parenteral, and intraspinal (Table 34–8). Oral administration is the route of choice. When this is not possible, the rectal or transdermal route should be tried unless other conditions preclude their use. For example, rectal administration is contraindicated for patients with diarrhea, anorectal lesions, thrombocytopenia, or neutropenia. Transdermal administration is not suited for rapid titration and so is best used for relatively stable pain.

Parenteral administration, indicated when other routes are not possible or are ineffective, can be intravenous or subcutaneous. Intravenous administration provides the most rapid onset of analgesia and may be given in bolus or continuous doses. Because the duration of analgesia after a bolus dose is shorter than with other routes, continuous infusion is a good choice for maintaining a consistent level of analgesia in patients requiring continuous intravenous access for other purposes. When intravenous access is not feasible, subcutaneous opioid infusion is practical in the hospital or the home. Intramuscular administration is avoided because of pain and unreliable absorption.

Patient-controlled analgesia (PCA) is used to help the patient maintain independence and control by matching drug delivery to the need for analgesia. With PCA, the opioid may be administered orally or through a dedicated portable pump to deliver the drug intravenously, subcutaneously, or epidurally (intraspinally). The intraspinal route is considered when patients develop intractable pain in the lower part of the body or when intolerable side effects occur with other routes (USDHHS, 1994).

COGNITIVE-BEHAVIORAL THERAPIES

Cognitive-behavioral therapies provide the patient with a sense of control. They help the patient develop skills needed for coping with pain. They promote patient participation in care. And they can be used in conjunction with pharmacologic therapies. Cognitive-behavioral therapies vary in approach and are intended to decrease tension and increase muscle relaxation. They can potentially assist with pain control while ameliorating nausea and vomiting related to other therapy. Furthermore, they can also

Table 34-8

Advantages and Disadvantages of Selected Pain Therapies

Intervention	Advantages	Disadvantages

Oral analgesics
  Acetaminophen
  Aspirin
  Nonsteroidal anti-inflammatory drugs (NSAIDs)
	Useful for a wide variety of mild to moderate pains.
	Widely available, some over the counter.
	Additive analgesia when combined with opioids and other modalities.
	Can be administered by patient or family.
	Some are inexpensive.
		Ceiling effect to analgesia.
		Side effects, especially gastritis and renal toxicity, can be serious.
		May cause bleeding in severely thrombocytopenic patients.
		Only one NSAID (ketorolac) is available now for parenteral administration.
		Many are expensive.

Oral opioids	Effective for both localized and generalized pain. Ceiling to analgesic effectiveness imposed only by side effects. Multiple drug choices in this class. Sedative and anxiolytic properties useful in some acute treatment settings. Can be administered by patient or family. Some are inexpensive. Long-acting, controlled-release forms available.	Side effects may limit analgesic effectiveness. Prescription of these substances is regulated. Stigma or fears associated with use.
Transdermal opioids (fentanyl)	Long duration of action (48–72 hours) from single patch. Allows use of a strong opioid (fentanyl) in outpatient settings for some patients who have not tolerated morphine and related drugs. Many patients find them easy to use. Provides continuous administration of an opioid without use of needles or pumps. Can be administered by patient or family.	Side effects may not be as quickly reversible as in oral opioid administration. Difficult to modify dosage rapidly. Relatively slow onset of action. Requires additional short-acting medicine for breakthrough pain. Expensive.
Rectal opioids	Relatively easy-to-use alternative route when the oral route is unavailable. Other opioid suppositories available for morphine-intolerant patients. Can be administered by patient or family. Less expensive than subcutaneous or intravenous infusions.	Not widely accepted by patients or families. Side effects may limit analgesic effectiveness. Relatively slow onset of action. Contraindicated if low white blood cell or platelet counts (risks of infection, bleeding).
Subcutaneous infusion	Can provide rapid pain relief without intravenous access. Morphine or hydromorphine are the preferred drugs for this route when administered in the home. When used in patient-controlled analgesia, allows for rapid individual dose titration and provides sense of control for patient.	Only a limited volume of infusate can be administered (eg, 2 to 4 mL/h). Induration, irritation at infusion site may be a complication. Requires skilled nursing and pharmacy support. Often requires expensive drug infusion pump and recurring charges for disposables.
Intravenous infusion	Can provide rapid pain relief. Almost all opioids can be given by this route. Not limited by infusate volumes. When used in patient-controlled analgesia, allows for rapid individual dose titration and provides sense of control for patient.	Infection and infiltration of intravenous lines are potential complications. Requires skilled nursing and pharmacy support. Often requires expensive drug infusion pump and recurring charges for disposables.

Table 34-8

Advantages and Disadvantages of Selected Pain Therapies (continued)

Intervention	Advantages	Disadvantages
Epidural, intrathecal, and intracerebral ventricular routes	Useful for pain that has not responded to less invasive measures. Local anesthetics may be added to spinal opioids and may produce additive analgesia.	Tolerance may occur sooner than with oral or rectal administration. Infection at catheter site can produce meningitis and/or epidural abscess. Pruritus and urinary retention are more common than with oral or parenteral opioid administration. Contraindicated in presence of acute spinal cord compression. Requires special expertise. Requires careful monitoring, especially when therapy begins and when doses are increased. May require expensive drug infusion pump, intervention fees, and recurring charges for disposables.
Regional neurolytic blocks	Effective for pain relief with certain diagnoses (eg, pancreatic cancer). May be useful for movement-related and abdominal visceral pain that is refractory to drug therapy. Can allow dosage (and side effect) reduction of systemic drugs for localized pain.	Risk of postural hypotension, bowel and bladder incontinence, and leg weakness. Procedure is irreversible. Requires special expertise. Expenses for specialized care and operating room costs.
Ablative neurosurgery	May be useful for movement-related lower body pain that is refractory to drug therapy. Fast onset of pain relief. Percutaneous cordotomy can be done under local anesthesia. Can allow dosage (and side effect) reduction of systemic drugs for localized pain.	Six-month duration of pain relief for cordotomy is only 50%. Procedure is irreversible. Requires special expertise. Expensive because of specialized care and operating room costs.

From US Department of Health and Human Services, Public Health Service. Agency for Health Care Policy and Research. Management of cancer pain. AHCPR Publ. 94-0592. Rockville, MD: Author, March 1994.

reduce general anxiety. Some cognitive-behavioral therapies include cognitive distraction and reframing, relaxation therapy and imagery, and biofeedback.

Cognitive Distraction and Reframing

Diversionary activities are used to help redirect pain sensations and perceptions. Diversions used to refocus attention away from the pain may be internal or external. Internal diversions include such activities as counting, praying, or repeating a mantra. External diversions include music, television, reading, rhythmic massage, and use of a visual focal point. In reframing or cognitive reappraisal, the patient monitors himself or herself for negative thoughts and consciously replaces them with positive thoughts or images.

Relaxation Therapy and Imagery

This category includes slow, rhythmic breathing exercises, yoga, meditation, and progressive muscle re-

laxation. Simple relaxation techniques are effective for episodes of brief pain. They can also be used when the patient has difficulty concentrating because of severe pain, anxiety, or fatigue. Advanced relaxation techniques involve hypnosis and guided imagery. These therapies can be learned and self-induced to provide deep relaxation.

Biofeedback

Biofeedback helps with self-regulation of physiologic activities, such as pulse and blood pressure. It can decrease tension and increase muscle relaxation.

PHYSICAL THERAPIES

Physical therapies include cutaneous stimulation, exercise, repositioning, immobilization, and counterstimulation. Types of cutaneous stimulation are application of heat, cold, lotion, massage, pressure, and vibration. Heat can be applied with a hot pack or heating pad, wrapped in a towel to prevent burns. Heat should not be applied over irradiated sites. Heat in the form of ultrasound or diathermy should not be applied over tumor sites.

Cold can be applied for periods of up to 15 minutes using flexible ice packs. Cold provides longer periods of relief than heat but is contraindicated for patients with peripheral vascular disease and for use over irradiated tissue.

Exercise maintains muscle strength and joint mobility. It also provides a sense of well-being. For patients with acute pain, exercise should be self-administered and limited to range of motion. Weight-bearing exercise should be avoided when bone fracture is a risk.

Immobilization may be used to manage acute pain or to stabilize fractures. Joints should be immobilized in a position of function and for as short a time as possible. Repositioning at regular intervals is provided for immobilized patients.

Counterstimulation in the form of transcutaneous electrical nerve stimulation (TENS) or acupuncture can also offer temporary pain relief. Transcutaneous electric nerve stimulation is based on the gate-control theory and is accomplished through a small electrical device powered by a battery pack. It may be worn by the patient and provides electrical stimulation to the skin. The large fibers of the peripheral nervous system are stimulated in an attempt to override pain stimuli and close the gate that controls pain perception (Fig. 34–16).

INVASIVE THERAPIES

Tumor-related pain can be relieved by destroying the causative tumor. This can be accomplished through surgical removal, debulking, or chemotherapy used to shrink the tumor mass. Radiation therapy, directed to localized areas, can be used to treat organ and vessel obstructions and to directly treat bone pain. For pain of widespread bony metastases, one intravenous injection of a beta-particle–emitting agent such as ^{131}I is effective. Nerve blocks and surgical ablation of pain pathways can also be used when other, less-invasive measures are ineffective.

Figure 34–17 presents a flow chart depicting continuing cancer pain management.

NURSING PROCESS
Cancer Pain

Assessment

Assess pain at regular intervals and at the onset of any report of new pain. Keep in mind that the patient's self-report is a critical component of pain assessment but that a patient may be reluctant to report pain because of concerns about derailing treatment of the underlying disease, being a "good" patient, and worries that pain means the disease is worsening.

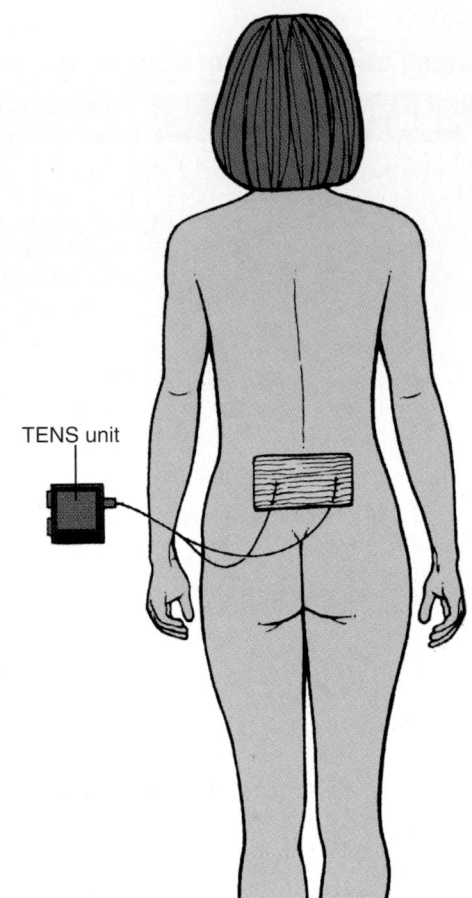

Figure 34–16

Transcutaneous electrical nerve stimulation (TENS) used for relief of low back pain. Electrodes in place on surface of lower back.

As part of the assessment, review the patient's medical history, previous pain history, and previous and present pain control interventions and their outcomes. Obtain information about social networks, and assess mental status and self-care capacity.

Ask the patient to describe the location, onset, duration, character, and intensity of the pain (Fig. 34–18) and to describe any activities that cause an increase in pain and any activities or interventions that alleviate the pain. Specifically ask when the patient has the most and the least pain. During the patient's description of the pain, listen carefully to words used to describe it. Assess how pain affects the patient's physiologic and psychologic well-being.

Nursing Diagnoses and Planning

Nursing diagnoses and related expected patient outcomes commonly applicable to patients with cancer pain include the following:

NDx: Pain related to the malignant process

Planning: Patient Outcomes
1. Patient states names, doses, and time schedule of pharmacologic agents prescribed.

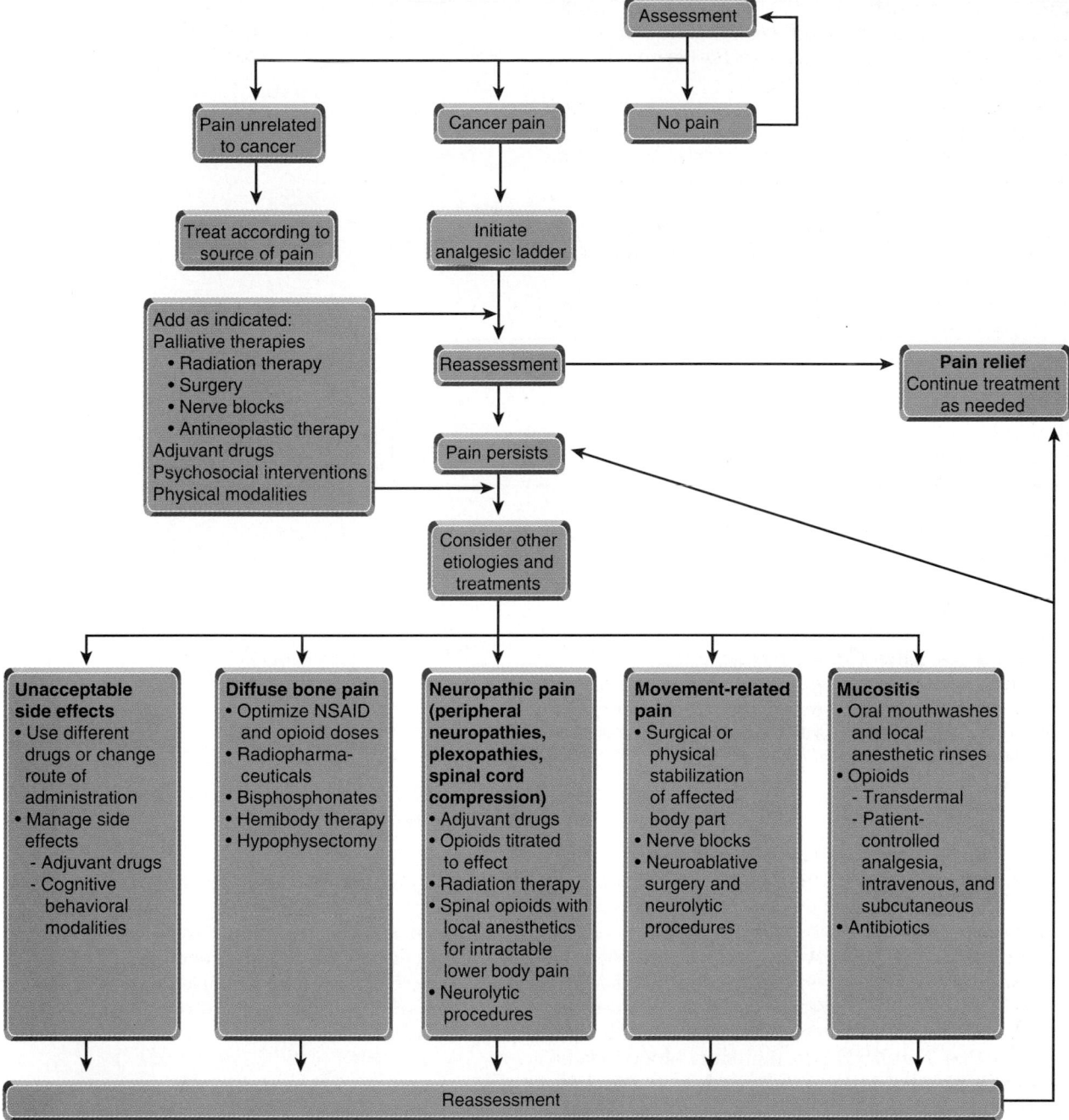

Figure 34–17

Pain management steps for cancer patients. This flow chart helps achieve continuous pain management for patients with cancer pain. (Redrawn from US Department of Health and Human Services, Public Health Service. Agency for Health Care Policy and Research. Management of cancer pain. AHCPR publication 94-0592. Rockville, MD: Author, March 1994.)

2. Patient describes cognitive-behavioral and physical therapies.
3. Patient uses appropriate methods of pain control.
4. Patient reports side effects of pharmacologic agents.
5. Patient describes interventions to alleviate the most common side effects, such as constipation, nausea, and vomiting.
6. Patient reports that pain is controlled or alleviated.

Nursing Interventions and Evaluation

NDx: Pain

Explain in language the patient and family can understand the cause of pain and how the various types of interventions affect the pain experience. Regarding pharmacologic therapy, teach the name of prescribed drugs and the dosage schedule. Also teach about their side effects: what they may include, how to control common ones, and which side

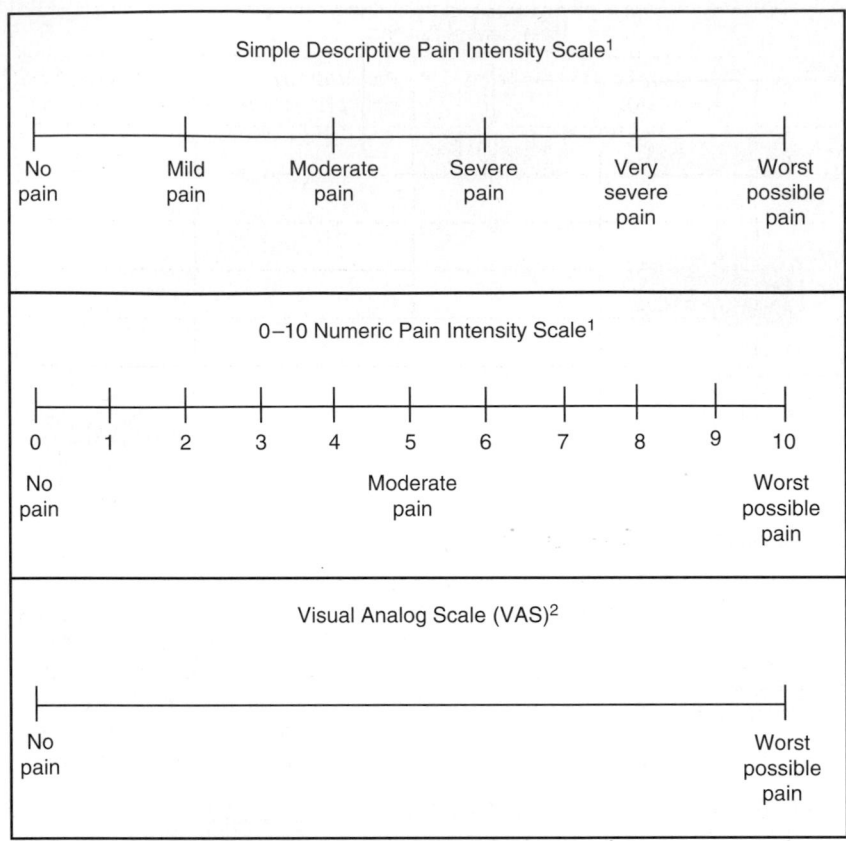

Figure 34–18
Examples of pain intensity scales.

effects should be reported. Recognize that some patients may be reluctant to take pain medication from worries about the side effects, developing tolerance, or becoming addicted. Provide correct information about these concerns and stress the importance of taking medications on a regular schedule. Emphasize that it is easier to prevent pain than to subdue it. Explain that regular doses maintain blood levels of the drug so that drug effectiveness is not lost between doses.

Also instruct the patient and family in the use of behavioral therapies and cutaneous therapies, such as massage, vibration, and the use of heat, cold, lotions, or a TENS device as indicated. Provide the patient and family with a written pain management plan to promote compliance by providing a reference in the event that any part of the plan is forgotten. Encourage the patient to keep a record of pain intensity and its response to pain medications (Fig. 34–19). The patient should assess pain level 1 hour after oral medications and 15 to 30 minutes after parenteral medications.

Collaborate with the physician to manage the effectiveness and side effects of therapy. Initiate consultations or referrals to other professionals as needed. If the patient is not hospitalized, make sure the patient has a follow-up appointment and that the patient and family know how to contact medical personnel in case of an emergency.

Compare the patient's status with the expected outcomes. If the outcomes are not met, reassess the patient and revise the plan.

MALNUTRITION

The nutritional status and well-being of the cancer patient can be affected by several interrelated factors: physical and biological characteristics of the tumor, side effects of cancer treatment, and the patient's dietary intake and emotional state. Loss of appetite and weight loss are common symptoms of advanced cancer. Research suggests that patients who suffer from malnutrition have an inferior prognosis as measured by their response and tolerance to treatment and their length of survival. Nutritional assessment and support should be part of the patient's total treatment plan. Food preferences, past dietary patterns, and physical symptoms caused by the disease process and related therapy should be

Pain Control Record					
Date	Time	Pain intensity (score 0-10)	Medicine I took	Pain intensity 1 hour after taking medicine	What I was doing when I felt pain
11/30/97	3:05 pm	6	2 Tylenol tablets	3	Taking a nap

Figure 34-19

Pain control record for the patient's use. The patient rates pain intensity on a scale of 0 to 10, with 0 being no pain and 10 being the worst pain possible.

considered. The nurse should suggest small frequent meals served in a pleasant environment.

Cachexia

Cachexia is a term used to describe the complex nutritional alterations that result from the disease process, which are further complicated by cancer treatments. Cachexia is characterized by marked anorexia, feeling of abdominal fullness after small amounts of food, marked weight loss (>10% of body weight), and loss of adipose tissue, visceral protein, and skeletal muscle. Cachectic patients complain of fatigue and decreased motor and mental skills. The patient appears physically emaciated from muscle wasting.

The exact cause of cachexia remains unknown, although it has been associated with an imbalanced dietary intake, impaired digestion or absorption, increased use of body nutrients by the tumor, increased metabolic rate, and increased energy expenditure related to the tumor's rapid growth. The treatment of cachexia largely depends on the ability of anticancer therapies to destroy tumors.

The following factors contribute to cachexia.

TUMOR CHARACTERISTICS

Malignant tumors use body nutrients, thereby depriving normal tissues of them. Also, tumors can secrete substances that impair metabolic processes and negatively influence the appetite control center in the hypothalamus. This results in a state of nutrient competition between malignant and normal tissues. Malignant tissues become nourished, leaving the normal tissues to absorb nutrients through catabolism of normal tissues, such as skeletal muscle breakdown, to provide amino acids.

In addition, the physical presence of a tumor mass in the abdomen or gastrointestinal tract can mechanically impair digestion and interrupt the normal feedback system that controls hunger.

CANCER THERAPY

Gastrointestinal side effects associated with radiation therapy and chemotherapy can alter the patient's nutritional status. Nausea, vomiting, taste alterations, mucositis, taste changes, and diarrhea can impair dietary intake. Surgical interventions to treat tumors of the head and neck region and gastrointestinal tract can affect dietary intake and digestion.

PATIENT VARIABLES

Reduced dietary intake may result from the patient's psychologic condition. Anorexia may be a direct consequence of psychologic stress induced by the diagnosis or required therapies. Patients may experience loss of appetite as a consequence of feeling depressed, angry, fearful, anxious, and hopeless.

Nutritional Support

Nutritional assessment and dietary counseling should be part of the patient's total care in all phases of cancer prevention, treatment, and follow-up. Development of a dietary support program should consider the patient's symptoms related to the disease process, treatment side effects, concomitant medical illnesses, and social support networks. Support with oral, enteral, or parenteral nutrition may be indicated.

NURSING PROCESS
Nutrition and Cancer

Assessment

Review the patient's medical history, including type and schedule of treatments and side effects experienced. Determine the patient's knowledge about the effect of cancer and cancer treatments on nutritional status.

Assess current nutritional status by measuring the patient's height and weight, mid-arm muscle circumference, and triceps skinfold to determine external tissue mass. Also review pertinent laboratory data, such as levels of hemoglobin, hematocrit, serum albumin, and blood urea nitrogen. Obtain information on current dietary intake, and calculate the patient's protein, carbohydrate, fat, vitamin, mineral, and fluid needs considering age, activity, and pathology.

Explore the patient's food preferences and patterns of eating. Identify any strategies the patient has initiated to increase dietary intake, and question him or her about their success.

Nursing Diagnoses and Planning

Nursing diagnoses and related expected patient outcomes commonly applicable to patients at risk for nutritional alterations due to cancer are as follows:

NDx: Risk for altered nutrition: less than body requirements related to the malignant disease process and side effects of cancer therapy

Planning: Patient Outcomes
1. Patient describes dietary interventions.
2. Patient maintains weight or limits weight loss.
3. Measurements of serum protein and albumin levels are within normal limits.

4. Measurements of hemoglobin and hematocrit levels are within normal limits.
5. Signs of dehydration are absent.
6. Patient participates in physical activities.

Nursing Interventions and Evaluation

NDx: Risk for altered nutrition: less than body requirements
Discuss aspects of the disease process and treatments that can affect nutritional status with the patient and the family. Teach the basic food groups on the food pyramid and instruct the patient as specified in Highlight 34–3 on ways to improve appetite and meet nutritional needs.

Monitor nutritional status on a regular basis, but always avoid statements that may make the patient feel guilty about anorexia and instruct the family to do the same.

If indicated, consult with the physician regarding enteral and parenteral nutritional supplementation, use of oral liquid supplements, and antiemetic or antidiarrheal medications. Initiate referrals to the dietitian and to community agencies that assist with meal preparation as needed.

Compare the patient's status with the expected outcomes. If the outcomes are not met, reassess the patient and revise the plan.

❖ Settings, Providers, and Collaboration for Care

The complexity of cancer care necessitates a multidisciplinary approach to delivery of services. Among the health-care professionals routinely involved in caring for cancer patients are the following:

* The patient's primary physician
* A medical, surgical, and/or radiation oncologist
* A pathologist
* A radiologist
* An oncology clinical nurse specialist
* A social worker or other psycho-oncology specialist
* Radiation therapists

The primary physician commonly is the first to identify a potential cancer and is responsible for referring the patient to a surgeon or other specialist for definitive diagnosis and beginning treatment. The primary physician also continues to monitor other aspects of the patient's health care throughout the program of cancer treatment.

Within this multidisciplinary team, oncology nurses collaborate with other team members to establish outcomes for patients, provide nursing care as well as education and counseling, coordinate services and continuity of care, serve as a patient advocate, and consult with other professionals as needed to provide optimal care for the patient.

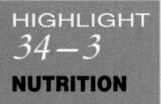 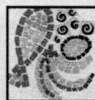

HIGHLIGHT 34–3 NUTRITION

Special Considerations for Patients with Cancer

Instruct patients with cancer to:

Eat small, frequent meals.

Avoid strong-smelling foods.

Increase caloric and nutrient intake:
  Add wine, beer, or milk to soups and sauces.
  Combine ice cream with soda, milk shakes, or yogurt.
  Drink liquid protein supplements.

Increase intake of lean protein.

Serve foods that are cold or room temperature.

Take advantage of times when feeling "well" to prepare food and freeze for later use.

Dine in an environment conducive to eating.

Rinse mouth before eating to wash away bad tastes.

Plan meals that meet fluid and caloric needs.

Keep a food diary.

HOME CARE

Diagnosis and treatment of oncologic disorders often do not include extensive hospitalization. Many patients undergoing radiation therapy, chemotherapy, and immunotherapy may safely be treated and monitored on an ambulatory basis. In addition, patients in the terminal phase of the disease process may wish to remain at home. Home care should be planned during the patient's hospitalization.

Family members and home health-care professionals can provide needed home care. However, family members will require support and instruction in basic patient care skills. The patient should be referred to the hospital's home care department and a referral made to the local visiting nurse service.

Some specialized aspects of cancer care have become routine parts of home care services. Infusion therapy is the most rapidly growing segment within home health services. Venous access devices and infusion pumps have enabled the use of home infusions. Home hyperalimentation and home antibiotic therapy have also become common.

Chemotherapy administration in the home is most common. It is often very cost effective. Patient selection is extremely important because patients and their families must be educated about chemotherapy precautions and when to report problems. Insurance reimbursement must also be verified to avoid undue financial stress. Home care nurses must be well educated in administration procedures, as well as in safety considerations of drug transport, preparation of drugs, spills, patient care, disposal of drugs and supplies, and patient and family education.

Pain management is another segment of cancer care that can be provided in the home. It is important to develop an analgesic regimen that is simple to administer yet provides sufficient pain relief to allow optimal functioning. Patients and family members must be instructed to ensure that pain medications are given on time around the clock and not just as needed. Interventions also must be employed to prevent potential side effects of narcotic regimens (eg, constipation and nausea). An ongoing comprehensive assessment of the patient's pain must also be conducted to note patterns and changes. It is of the utmost importance for the home care nurse to identify and dispel patient and family misconceptions about the use and abuse of narcotics.

In an overall sense, quality assessments in the home care setting are accomplished by examining links between processes of care and patient outcomes (Groenwald et al, 1995).

HOSPICE CARE

For the terminally ill, a familiar environment including family members and friends can be a comforting experience during the final stage of cancer. Hospice care is a philosophy of comprehensive psychologic, physical, and spiritual support for terminally ill patients and their families. Care is provided by interdisciplinary professionals and community volunteers, either in an institution or in the home. The hospice approach, which started in England in the 1960s, is becoming an integral part of terminal care in the United States. Nurses should familiarize patients and their families with hospice services available in their communities.

The hospice nurse must be an experienced practitioner with specialized skill in terminal care. It is essential that the hospice nurse be skilled at working cooperatively and communicating effectively within a multidisciplinary framework.

Other attributes necessary for performing the hospice nurse's role include self-direction and initiative, ability to coordinate care and services provided, leadership within a multidisciplinary team, ability to individualize a plan of care, and ability to foster a relaxed, warm, personal relationship with the patient, family, and other team members (Groenwald et al, 1995).

The Elderly: Special Considerations

The incidence of cancer increases with advancing age. As in the population as a whole, most cancers found in elderly people affect the prostate, the breast, the lung, or the lower gastrointestinal tract. Some cancers, although fewer in number, occur almost exclusively among the aged. These include cancers of the skin, vulva, vagina, urinary bladder, and uterine endometrium. Multiple myeloma and leukemia, especially chronic lymphocytic leukemia, are predominantly diseases of the aged, although not exclusively so.

Etiology and Pathophysiology

The reasons for the relationship between advancing age and the development of malignant disease are not fully understood. At least two factors seem to contribute. The first is defective repair of DNA that has been found in the elderly. Because chromosomes break at all ages—particularly in response to exposure to carcinogens, radiation, and some viruses—it is theorized that the decrease in ability of the elderly to repair DNA causes an accumulation of chromosomal abnormalities that allow uncontrolled cell growth. The second factor is the decreased effectiveness of the immune system in the elderly, particularly in identifying and destroying cells that carry foreign antigens.

Just as the incidence and the occurrence of specific types of cancer differ in the elderly, so do the characteristics of particular tumors. For example, papillary cancer of the thyroid, which is highly treatable in younger women, is very aggressive and highly metastatic in older women. Similarly, malignant melanoma is more aggressive in the elderly, particularly women. In contrast, cancer of the breast has a better prognosis in the elderly because it grows more slowly and tends to metastasize to bone and soft tissue rather than to liver and lungs.

Diagnosis

Early diagnosis is as important in the elderly as in any other age group. Yet in many cases, disease is advanced when the diagnosis is made, because early signs of cancer have been interpreted as normal concomitants of advancing age or symptoms related to coexisting diseases. Any major change in functioning, particularly mental function, should be evaluated as a manifestation of medical conditions such as cancer.

Management

Medical treatment is based on presenting symptoms, the person's overall condition, and the type of malignancy. For example, if the tumor is a very slow-growing one and the patient, because of age or the presence of another severe disease, is unlikely to survive long enough to die of the cancer, palliative treatment may be the choice. In other cases, an all-out program of the most aggressive treatment available may be selected. Whatever the circumstances, however, the patient must have informed input into the decision.

NURSING PROCESS GUIDELINES
The Elderly Patient with Cancer

Stress the importance of cancer screening tests for the elderly at every opportunity. Teach older women how to do monthly breast self-examinations. Because many women do not see a gynecologist after the childbearing years, it is important to stress the value of annual pelvic examinations. Inform older women of the increasing risk of endometrial and vaginal cancer. Explain that, although noticeable symptoms do not occur until the disease is far advanced, diagnosis in an early, most curable stage can be made by pelvic examination. Also stress that any new symptoms should be reported to the health-care provider and not assumed to be "normal aging" or due to an already diagnosed disease.

When caring for an older person who is undergoing diagnostic testing for cancer or who has been diagnosed, be aware that the person may associate cancer with a grim prognosis. This heightens the need for the person to talk about the illness and to receive information, empathy, and support. Because some older adults have developed such long-standing fears that they cannot bring themselves to use the word "cancer," referring only to my "tumor," "growth," "sickness" or even using a nonverbal expression to indicate the problem, be alert to the patient's symbolic terminology and use it rather than forcing a confrontation with fearful words like "cancer" or "malignancy." Quite often, a simple expres-

sion of empathy such as, "It must feel very lonely to be seriously ill," releases a flood of pent-up feelings. Be certain also to correct misconceptions and provide current information based on the patient's emotional readiness to hear. As with younger patients, older patients should be referred for hospice services when appropriate.

Chapter Review

1. What psychosocial and cultural factors could influence a person's willingness and ability to adhere to health practices designed to reduce the risk of cancer?
2. How would you explain to a patient what a class II Pap test result means?
3. What three principles form the basis of radiation safety protocols?
4. What is the general cause of the majority of side effects related to chemotherapy?
5. How does external radiation therapy differ from internal radiation therapy?
6. What is the rationale for each precaution taken when handling chemotherapeutic agents?
7. How are the side effects of chemotherapy similar to and different from the side effects of radiation therapy?
8. What factors contribute to the development of cachexia in the patient with cancer?
9. How do radiation precautions affect the care of a patient receiving internal radiation therapy?
10. Why is nutrition important in caring for a patient with cancer?

Bibliography

Altman GB, Lee CA. Strontium-89 for treatment of painful bone metastasis from prostate cancer. Oncol Nurs Forum 1996; 23(3):523.

American Cancer Society. Cancer facts and figures 1995. New York: Author, 1995.

American Council on Science and Health. What causes human cancer? Reprint of: Update: Is there a cancer epidemic in the United States? Today's OR Nurse 1995; 17(6):28.

American Nurses' Association and the Oncology Nursing Society. Standards of oncology nursing practice. Kansas City, MO: American Nurses' Association, 1987.

Bland KI, Karakousis CP, Copeland EM III (eds). Atlas of surgical oncology. Philadelphia: WB Saunders, 1995.

Burke M. Oncology nursing homecare handbook. Boston: Jones & Bartlett, 1993.

Campbell MK, Pruitt J. Radiation therapy: Protecting your patients' skin. RN 1996; 59(1):46.

Clark JC, McGee RF (eds). Oncology Nursing Society: Core curriculum for oncology nursing. 2nd ed. Philadelphia: WB Saunders, 1992.

Clark-Tasker V. Cancer prevention and early detection in African-Americans. In Frank-Stromberg M, Olsen SJ (eds). Cancer prevention and screening in minorities: Cultural implications for health care providers. St. Louis: CV Mosby, 1993.

Cleri LB. Serotonin antagonists: State of the art management of chemotherapy-induced emesis. In Hubbard SM, Goodman M, Knobf T (eds). Oncology nursing: Patient treatment and support. Philadelphia: JB Lippincott, 1995.

Devita VT. Principles of chemotherapy. In Devita VT, Hellman S, Rosenberg SA (eds). Cancer: Principles and practice of oncology. 4th ed. Philadelphia: JB Lippincott, 1993.

Engel G. A psychological setting of somatic disease: The giving up-given up complex. Proc R Soc Med 1967; 60(6):553.

Eriksson JH. Oncologic nursing. 2nd ed. Springhouse, PA: Springhouse, 1993.

Fernsler JI, Ades TB. Developing strategies for public education in cancer. In McCorkle R, Grant M, Frank-Stromberg M, Baird SB. Cancer nursing: A comprehensive textbook. Philadelphia: WB Saunders, 1996.

Fitch M, Bolster A, Alderson D, et al. Moving toward research-based cancer nursing practice. Can Oncol Nurs J 1995; 5(1):5.

Foley JF, et al (eds). Current therapy in cancer. Philadelphia: WB Saunders, 1994.

Gallagher J. Management of cutaneous symptoms. Semin Oncol Nurs 1995; 11(4):239.

Glynn TJ, Manly MW. How to help your patients stop smoking. NIH Publication No. 95-3064. Bethesda, MD: US Department of Health and Human Services, Public Health Service, National Institutes of Health, September 1995.

Grant M, Ropka ME. Alterations in nutrition. In McCorkle R, Grant M, Frank-Stromberg M, Baird S (eds). Cancer nursing: A comprehensive textbook. Philadelphia: WB Saunders, 1996.

Green WA. The psychosocial setting of the development of leukemia and lymphoma. Ann NY Acad Sci 1966; 125:794.

Groenwald SL, Frogge MH, Goodman M, Yarboro CH (eds). A clinical guide to cancer nursing: A companion to cancer nursing. 3rd ed. Boston: Jones & Bartlett, 1995.

Haber J, et al. Comprehensive psychiatric nursing. New York: McGraw-Hill, 1987.

Hargreaves MK, Baquet C, Gamshadzahi A. Diet, nutritional status, and cancer risk in American blacks. Nutr Cancer 1989; 12:1.

Held JL. Caring for the patient with lung cancer. Nursing 1995; 25(10):34.

Hellman S. Principles of radiation therapy. In Devita VT, Hellman S, Rosenberg SA (eds). Cancer: Principles and practice of oncology. 4th ed. Philadelphia: JB Lippincott, 1993.

Holland JC, Rowland JH (eds). Handbook of psycho-oncology: Psychological care of the patient with cancer. New York: Oxford University Press, 1989.

Holler AI. The American Cancer Society cancer book. Garden City, NY: Doubleday, 1988.

Holmes S. Making sense of radiotherapy: Curative and palliative. Nursing Times 1996; 92(23):32.

Johnson BI, Gross J. Handbook of oncology nursing. 2nd ed. Boston: Jones & Bartlett, 1994.

Kagawa-Singer M. Cultural systems. In McCorkle R, Grant M, Baird SB, Frank-Stromberg M. Cancer nursing: A comprehensive textbook. Philadelphia: WB Saunders, 1996.

Kan MK. Palliation of bone pain in patients with metastatic cancer using strontium-89 (Metastron). Cancer Nurs 1995; 18(4):286.

Lamb MA. Sexuality and sexual functioning. In McCorkle R, Grant M, Baird SB, Frank-Stromberg M. Cancer nursing: A comprehensive textbook. Philadelphia: WB Saunders, 1996.

Lentner C (ed). Geigy scientific tables. 8th ed. Vol. 1. Basel, Switzerland: Ciba-Geigy, 1981.

LeShan L. An emotional life-history pattern associated with neoplastic disease. Ann NY Acad Sci 1966; 125:780.

Lindsey AM, Larson PJ, Dodd MJ, et al. Comorbidity, nutritional intake, social support, weight, and functional status over time in older cancer patients receiving radiotherapy. Cancer Nurs 1994; 17(2):113.

McCorkle R, Grant M, Baird SB, Frank-Stromberg M (eds). Cancer nursing: A comprehensive textbook. 2nd ed. Philadelphia: WB Saunders, 1996.

Michaels D. Occupational cancer in the black population: The health effects of job discrimination. J Natl Black Med Assoc 1983; 75:1014.

Miller W, Cooper R. Rising lung cancer death rates among black men: The importance of occupation and social class. J Natl Black Med Assoc 1982; 74:253.

National Cancer Institute. Chemotherapy and you: A guide to self help during treatment. NIH Publication No. 88-1136. Bethesda, MD: Department of Health and Human Services, 1987.

National Cancer Institute Office of Cancer Communications. Office of the Director Annual Report FY '93. Bethesda, MD: National Cancer Institute, 1994.

National Institute of Health Consensus Development Conference Statement. Oral complications of cancer therapies: Diagnosis, prevention, and treatment. J Am Dent Assoc 1989; 119(1):179.

Olsen SJ, Frank-Stromberg M. Cancer prevention and early detection in ethnically diverse populations. Semin Oncol Nurs 1993; 9(3):198.

Parker SL, Tong T, Bolden S, Wingo, PA. Cancer statistics 1997. CA—Cancer J Clin 1997; 47(1):5.

Pottern LM, Morris LE, Blot WJ, et al. Esophageal cancer among black men in Washington, D.C.: I. Alcohol, tobacco and other risk factors. JNCI 1981; 67:777.

Oncology Nursing Society. Access device guidelines, modules I–III. Pittsburgh: Oncology Nursing Press, 1989–1990.

Oncology Nursing Society. Cancer chemotherapy: Guidelines and recommendations for nursing education and practice. Pittsburgh: Oncology Nursing Press, 1989.

Oncology Nursing Society, Fiscus JA, Hayes NA, Rostad ME, Whedon MA. Safe handling of cytotoxic drugs. Independent study module. Pittsburgh: Oncology Nursing Press, 1989.

Oncology Nursing Society and American Nurses' Association Division of Medical-Surgical Nursing Practice. Outcome standards for cancer nursing practice. Kansas City, MO: American Nurses' Association, 1989.

Otto SE. Advanced concepts in chemotherapy drug delivery: Regional therapy. J Intravenous Nurs 1995; 18(4):170.

Rosenberg S. Principles of surgical oncology. In Devita VT, Hellman S, Rosenberg SA (eds). Cancer: Principles and practice of oncology. 4th ed. Philadelphia: JB Lippincott, 1993.

Sabo CE, Michael SR. The influence of personal massage wtih music on anxiety and side effects associated with chemotherapy. Cancer Nurs 1996; 19(4):283.

Seeman M, Seeman T. Health behavior and personal autonomy: A longitudinal study of the sense of control in illness. J Health Soc Behav 1983; 24(6):144.

Simonton OC, Simonton S. Getting well again. Toronto: Bantam Books, 1980.

Smith SL. Physical exercise as an oncology nursing intervention to enhance quality of life. Oncol Nurs Forum 1996; 23(5):771.

Tenenbaum L (ed). Cancer chemotherapy and biotherapy: A reference guide. 2nd ed. Philadelphia: WB Saunders, 1994.

Thompson SD, Szukiewicz-Nugent JM, Walczak JR. A woman's cancer: When ovarian cancer strikes. Nursing 1996; 26(10):33.

Trichopoulos D, Li FP, Hunter DJ. Causes and prevention: What causes cancer? Sci Am 1996; 275(3):80.

US Bureau of Census: Current population reports, Publication No. 25-1092. Population projections of the United States, by age, sex, race and hispanic origin: 1992–2050. Washington, DC: Government Printing Office, 1992.

US Department of Health and Human Services. Management of cancer pain: Adults. AHCPR Publication No 94-0593. Rockville, MD: Author, March 1994.

US Department of Health and Human Services. Eating hints, recipes and tips for better nutrition during cancer treatment. NIH Publication No. 91-2079. Bethesda, MD: National Institutes of Health, 1990.

US Department of Health and Human Services. Diet, nutrition and cancer prevention: A guide to food choices. NIH Publication No. 87-2878. Bethesda, MD: National Institutes of Health, 1987.

US Department of Health and Human Services. Cancer among blacks and other minorities: Statistical profiles. Bethesda, MD: National Institutes of Health, 1986.

US Department of Health and Human Services. Eating hints, recipes and tips for better nutrition during cancer treatment. NIH Publication No. 81-2079. Bethesda, MD: National Institutes of Health, 1981.

US Department of Health and Human Services, Public Health Service. Agency for Health Care Policy and Research. Management of cancer pain. AHCPR Publication No. 94-0592. Rockville, MD: Author, March 1994.

US Department of Health and Human Services, Public Health Service. Radiation therapy and you: A guide to self-help during treatment. NIH Publication No. 88-2227. Bethesda, MD: National Institutes of Health, 1988.

US Department of Labor, Office of Occupational Medicine, Occupational Safety and Health Administration. Work practice guidelines for personnel dealing with cytotoxic (antineoplastic) drugs. Publication No. 8.1.1., Washington DC: Author, 1986.

Young A, Gilbert J, Sherman M, et al. Intraperitoneal chemotherapy: A prolonged infusion of 5-fluorouracil using a novel carrier solution. Br J Nurs 1996; 5(9):539.

Unit XII

Integumentary Dysfunction

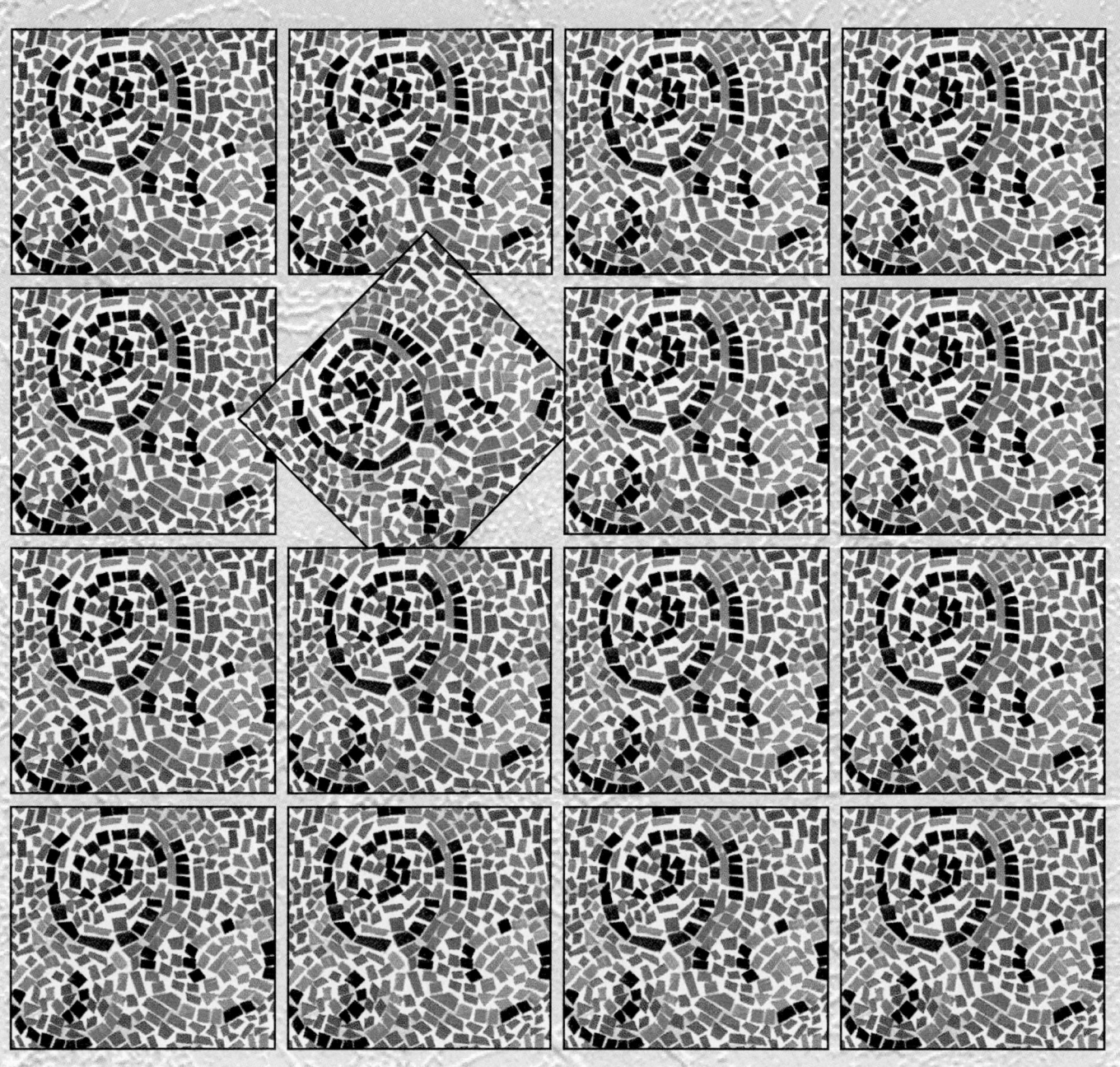

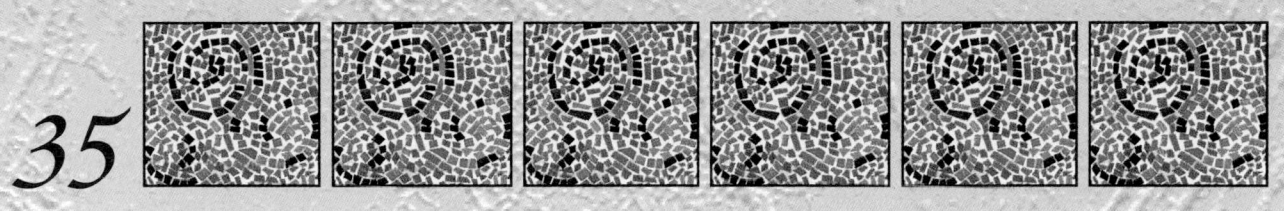

35

Knowledge Base for Patients with Integumentary Dysfunction

Study Outcomes

After studying this chapter, you should be able to:

1. Explain the normal anatomy and physiology of the skin and related structures.
2. Describe common clinical manifestations of skin disease.
3. Identify information and physical examination data essential to the assessment of the skin.
4. Describe basic diagnostic tests and treatment methods used in the management of patients with skin dysfunction.
5. Describe basic surgical procedures and techniques used in the treatment of patients with skin dysfunction.
6. Identify data essential to the assessment of patients undergoing treatment of skin dysfunction.
7. State nursing diagnoses and related expected patient outcomes commonly applicable to patients undergoing treatment of skin dysfunction.
8. Describe nursing interventions, with their rationales, commonly applicable to patients undergoing treatment of skin dysfunction.
9. Explain the basis for evaluation of nursing care provided to patients undergoing treatment of skin dysfunction.
10. Identify alternative treatment and care settings for patients with skin dysfunction, and the services related to community-based care.
11. Identify special considerations for the elderly patient with skin dysfunction.

The skin is the body's largest organ. It accounts for 15% of the body's weight and varies in thickness from 1/50 to 1/4 of an inch. Skin is durable and pliable. It absorbs, reflects, cushions, and limits the effects of environmental factors on the body. It provides a barrier against invasion by microorganisms. It helps regulate temperature, fluid, and electrolytes. It serves as a sense organ for touch, pain, heat, cold, and pressure. Together with the action of ultraviolet light, it provides the body with vitamin D. Last but not least, it serves as the interface between each of us and the world we live in. In a very real sense, we are known by our skin. By building sound knowl-

edge and giving accurate and empathic care, nurses can provide profound relief for patients with skin disorders—disorders that are much more than skin deep.

Anatomy and Physiology

Skin is composed of the epidermis, dermis, subcutaneous fat, and skin appendages, such as the glands and hair follicles (Fig. 35–1).

EPIDERMIS

The epidermis is the outer layer of skin. It is made up of stratified squamous epithelial cells. Ninety-five percent of these are keratinocytes. The other 5% are melanocytes, the pigment cells that produce melanin and give the skin its color. The epidermis is itself composed of five layers:

- Stratum corneum
- Stratum lucidum
- Stratum granulosum
- Stratum spinosum, or prickle-cell layer
- Stratum basale, basal-cell layer, or stratum germinativum

The stratum corneum is the skin's outer layer—its protective barrier. It is made up of many layers of thick or keratinized squamous cells that lack nuclei and cytoplasm. Ten percent of the stratum corneum is water. Lipids that hold water in keratin make up 7 to 9%. Mucous membrane structures, such as the lips and labia, lack stratum corneum. Skin lacking stratum corneum is freely permeable. Minor disruptions of the skin, such as paper cuts, stripping with tape, or extensive hand washing, weaken the barrier.

The stratum lucidum is just below the stratum corneum and is found in thick skin, such as the palms of the hands and soles of the feet.

The basal-cell layer, which is the innermost layer of the epidermis, is the site where new cells are produced to replace those that are sloughed or dam-

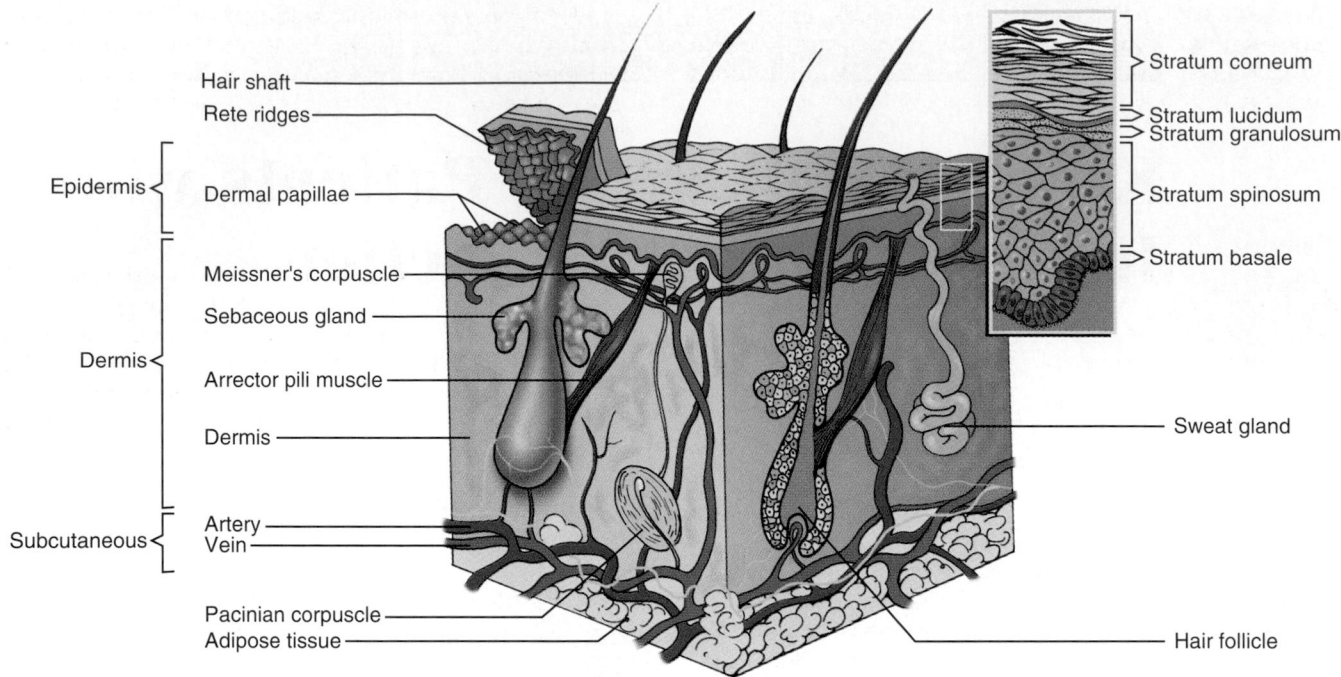

Figure 35-1

Anatomy of the skin.

aged. After being produced, new cells migrate upward and undergo keratinization as they pass through the succeeding layers. Cell migration from the basal layer to the top of the stratum granulosum takes about 2 weeks. These cells form the protective stratum corneum for about another 14 days, after which they reach the surface and are shed.

Basal cells also line the hair follicles and the sweat and sebaceous glands, which are located in the dermis.

The rete ridges anchor the epidermis to the dermis at the dermoepidermal junction.

DERMIS

The dermis is thick and gives bulk to the skin. It is made up of connective tissue, cellular elements, and ground substance. Connective tissues in the form of collagen fibers, elastin fibers, and reticular fibers provide support and give elasticity to the skin.

The cellular elements of the dermis include reticulohistiocytes, myeloid cells, and lymphoid cells. The reticulohistiocytes include:

- Fibroblasts, which are migrating cells that continually break down and re-form collagen fibers and that are important in wound healing
- Histiocytes, which are active in phagocytosis
- Mast cells, which release histamine and heparin when injured and which are increased in itching dermatoses
- Reticulum cells, which may cause increased plasma cells in chronic inflammation

The myeloid cells are the polymorphonuclear leukocytes and eosinophilic leukocytes found especially in allergic dermatoses. Lymphoid cells are found in inflammatory lesions.

Ground substance is gel-like and contains proteins, mucopolysaccharides, soluble collagens, enzymes, immune bodies, metabolites, and other substances. It surrounds the cells of the dermis and contributes to the turgor and suppleness of the skin.

The dermis contains blood vessels that provide nourishment and temperature regulation. The epidermis has no intrinsic blood supply and depends on diffusion from vessels in the papillary dermis for nutrients and oxygen.

In the dermis, two horizontal plexuses, or vascular beds, are interconnected by means of shunts. The deep plexus is in the reticular dermis. The superficial plexus is in the papillary dermis. Increased blood flow in the superficial plexus allows heat loss. Heat is conserved by shunting blood to the deep plexus.

The dermis also contains widespread free nerve endings and receptors, which provide the sensations of touch, temperature, and pain.

SUBCUTANEOUS FAT

The subcutaneous fat is a layer of loose connective tissue containing lipocytes, which are cells that manufacture and store fat. There is a wide variation in individual fat distribution. Some people store enormous quantities of fat, whereas others store little.

Areas of the body such as the eyelids have little. Subcutaneous fat supports the upper skin layers, serves as a caloric reservoir, and insulates the body against heat loss.

GLANDS

The sebaceous, apocrine, and eccrine sweat glands originate in the dermis and extend into the epidermis, opening at or near the surface of the skin. The sebaceous glands are the oil-producing glands of the skin. They secrete sebum, a complex lipoidal mixture that plays a role in vitamin D synthesis. Sebaceous glands are most abundant on the face, scalp, scrotum, and upper trunk. They are absent on the palms and soles.

Apocrine sweat glands, the largest glands of the skin, are found in the axillae, the areolae of the nipples, and the periumbilical, perianal, and genital regions. The apocrine sweat glands begin to function as a result of hormonal influences at puberty. They secrete minute quantities of a sterile, odorless, milky-white fluid that is unnoticed on the skin. Bacterial changes account for distinctive body odors characteristic of the aprocrine glands. The apocrine and sebaceous glands usually have a common excretory path through a hair follicle.

The eccrine sweat glands are distributed over the entire body surface. By secreting sweat through pores of the skin, the eccrine glands provide thermoregulation. The hypothalamus regulates eccrine sweating in response to heat. Emotional stress also produces sweating, especially of the forehead, axillae, palms, and soles. Eccrine sweat glands also excrete lactate ion, urea, ammonia, and sodium chloride in varying quantities.

HAIR

A hair follicle is an invagination of the epidermis, extending at an angle into the dermis. Hair cells form the hair matrix in the bulb. They divide, differentiate, and form a keratinized hair shaft, pushing hair outward at an average rate of 1 cm per month. Melanocytes in the matrix determine hair color.

Tiny, light-colored vellus hairs grow over most body surfaces. Terminal hairs acquire special characteristics at different sites, including the scalp, eyebrow, eyelash, beard, axilla, trunk, extremities, and pubis. Terminal hair, especially scalp hair, contributes to cosmetic appearance and self-image.

Individual hair follicles grow in cycles with an anagen, or growth, phase and telogen, or resting phase. In scalp hair, the anagen phase lasts about 6 years and the telogen phase lasts about 4 months. Normally, 50 to 100 hairs are shed from the scalp each day, with 80 to 90% of scalp hair in the anagen phase and 10 to 20% in the telogen phase. Diffuse hair loss may not be noticed until 50% of the hair is lost.

Testosterone influences hair growth in males and females in curious ways. It stimulates beard growth in males and hair growth in the axillae and groin in both sexes at puberty, yet testosterone also causes scalp baldness.

NAILS

Nails form from a matrix of dividing epidermal cells (keratin). The matrix lies under the proximal nail fold, extending under the nail plate and appearing as the lunula. The nail bed produces keratin, which adheres to the nail plate. Blood vessels in the dermis cause the pink color in the nail bed. The stratum corneum at the proximal nail fold (eponychium) forms the cuticle. The hyponychium lies under the free distal edge of the nail plate, producing stratum corneum, which forms a cuticle at the distal nail bed and plate.

Fingernails grow about 0.1 mm per day. Toenails grow more slowly. Nails range in thickness from 0.3 to 0.65 mm.

Nails reflect local stresses. Persistent occupational trauma thickens them. Nail biting doubles their growth rate.

The specific function of each of these skin components is presented in Table 35–1.

Table 35–1

Functions of Specific Skin Structures

Structure	Function
Epidermis	Barrier
Stratum corneum	Physical
Melanocytes	Light
Langerhans' cells	Immunologic
Dermis	
Connective tissue	Support and elasticity
Cellular elements	Collagen formation; immunologic
Subcutaneous fat	
Connective tissue	Support
Lipocyte	Manufacture and storage of fat energy
Fat	Insulation from cold and trauma
Glands	
Sebaceous gland	Sebum formation
Apocrine gland	Unknown except mammary glands
Eccrine sweat gland	Temperature regulation
Hair	Decorative
Nails	Grasping
Blood vessels	Nourishment, temperature regulation
Nerves	Sensation

Data from Lookingbill DP, Marks JG. Principles of dermatology. 2nd ed. Philadelphia: WB Saunders, 1993.

Clinical Manifestations of Integumentary Dysfunction

ALTERED SKIN COLOR

The normal components of skin color are brown, yellow, red, and blue. *Generalized hyperpigmentation* is the term for an overall increase in the brown component of skin color. Generalized hyperpigmentation resulting from increased production of melanin-stimulating hormone is sometimes seen as a bronzing of the skin in Addison's disease.

Generalized erythroderma is caused by vasodilation of the arterioles and capillaries in the papillary dermis and increased oxyhemoglobin, the red component of skin color. The redness of oxyhemoglobin is more readily apparent in areas such as the lips, where the stratum corneum is absent.

Vasoconstriction decreases capillary blood flow, resulting in a pale or ashen skin color. Pallor is more apparent in the palms, soles, head, and neck areas, where cutaneous arterial flow and capillary perfusion are high.

Cyanosis gives the skin a blue appearance. It occurs when the blood contains 5 g/100 mL or more of reduced hemoglobin. The more brown pigment there is in the skin, the less apparent the reduced hemoglobin or blue color.

ALTERED SKIN TURGOR

Skin turgor is the resiliency of the skin caused by the outward pressure of cells and intercellular fluid. Alteration in skin turgor can be determined by gently pinching the skin. If it does not return to normal position immediately, then skin turgor is decreased. Causes of decreased turgor include dehydration, edema, and normal aging. Skin with decreased turgor is at greater risk for breakdown than skin with normal turgor.

ALTERED SKIN TEMPERATURE

Surface temperature varies over different parts of the body. Normally, skin temperature is between the temperature of the body core (the internal organs) and that of the surrounding environment, or about 35°C (95°F). Body-surface temperature can vary from about 20°C (68°F) to 40°C (104°F) without damage. A local skin temperature of 18°C (65°F) or lower or 45°C (113°F) or higher is associated with pain or injury.

Evaporation of sweat cools the skin. Vasoconstriction can also lower skin temperature, especially in the extremities. Warmer skin temperature can result from heat, stress, and vasodilation.

The actual temperature of the skin is rarely recorded. In most patient-care situations, it is sufficient to document assessment of skin temperature by describing it as warm or cool to touch, by comparing the temperature of symmetric body parts, and by noting whether this temperature is generalized or localized.

ALTERED SKIN SENSATION

Alteration in skin sensation is a subjective assessment of skin integrity. It involves asking the patient how the skin feels. Descriptive terms include itching, burning, pain, decreased sensation, numbness, tingling, and hot or cold. The most common symptom by far in dermatology is itching, or pruritus.

Pruritus results from stimulation of itch receptors located at the junction of the epidermis and the dermis. It can be caused by skin disease or internal disease, or it may be idiopathic. Systemic diseases that can cause pruritus include diabetes mellitus, anemia, and renal, liver, and thyroid disorders. It can also be caused by cancer. In fact, some theories claim that symptoms of itching may precede a malignancy by 2 years. Pruritus can also be due to medications, dry skin, radiation therapy, or contact with perfumes, soaps, wool, and other substances. When the cause is unknown, a medical workup is sometimes performed to rule out internal disease and malignancy.

Pruritus, which is often worse at night, leads to scratching, which in turn can result in redness, excoriations, infection, and changes in pigment. To help reduce these effects, patients with pruritus should keep their fingernails short, wear white cotton gloves, or both.

ALTERED SKIN COMPONENTS: LESIONS

Types of Lesions

MACULE

A macule is a flat lesion characterized by a change in skin color resulting from either a change in the pigment-forming cells (melanocytes) or a change in vascularity. There is no change in the texture of the skin surface (Fig. 35–2). A depigmented lesion appears white because there are no melanocytes. Hypopigmented lesions are lighter than normal skin because of a decreased production of melanin.

Hyperpigmented lesions such as ephelides (freckles) contain fewer melanocytes than adjacent pale skin, but these melanocytes have the capacity to form melanin faster than nonfreckled areas. The hyperpigmentation in a café au lait spot results from

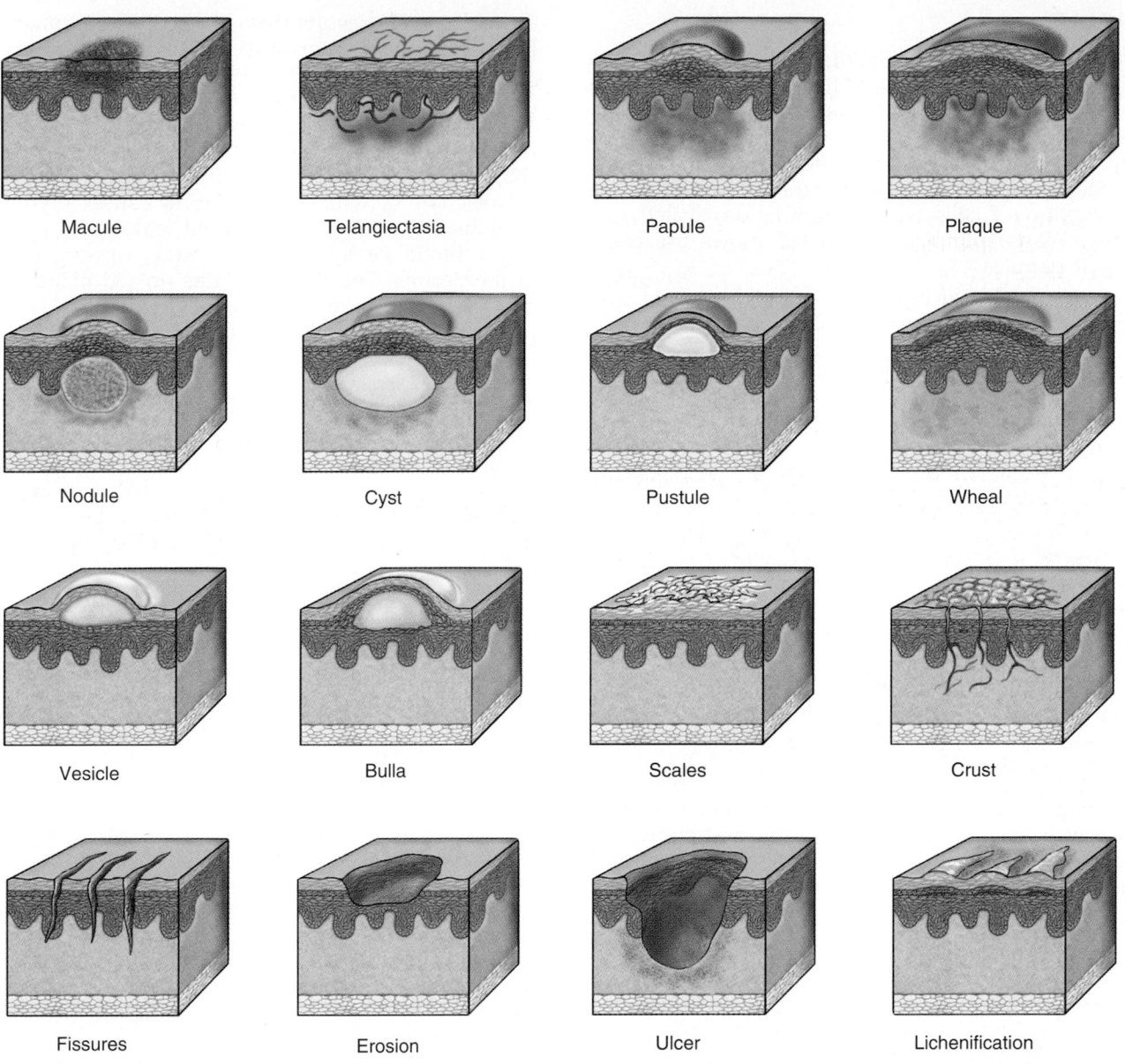

Figure 35-2

Types of skin lesions.

melanocytes lying nearer to the surface of the skin than the basal layer. In the blue hyperpigmentation of a mongolian spot, the melanocytes are deeper than normal, lying within the dermis. The blueness is from the scattering of light as it passes through the dermis and is called the Tyndall phenomenon.

Erythematous macules are flat red lesions caused by a temporary dilatation of capillaries or by a permanent vascular disorder. They blanch with pressure and on diascopy. Drug eruptions and viral exanthems, such as measles, are common causes of transitory capillary dilatation. Capillary hemangiomas are vascular abnormalities that appear as macular patches (nevus flammeus or port-wine stain). Strawberry hemangiomas are superficial,

bright red, rapidly expanding capillary hemangiomas, most of which subsequently undergo complete regression.

Petechiae, purpura, and ecchymoses are skin lesions caused by red blood cells that have extravasated or leaked out into the tissue. These lesions do not blanch with pressure or on diascopy. Size is the distinguishing characteristic of these lesions. Petechiae are pinpoint red lesions that are smaller than purpura. An ecchymosis (black and blue mark) is larger than a purpura.

Telangiectasias are small, permanently dilated blood vessels. They may appear alone or as part of another lesion (see Fig. 35-2). Telangiectasias blanch with pressure and on diascopy.

PAPULE

A papule is a raised palpable lesion less than 1 cm in breadth (see Fig. 35–2). It may involve the epidermis, dermis, or both. Pathophysiologic changes resulting in papular lesions include inflammation, vascular changes, accumulation of epidermal cells in the dermis, thickening of the stratum corneum, and destruction of cells with accumulation of cell remnants. Warts, pimples and raised moles are examples of papules.

PLAQUE

A plaque is a raised lesion that is larger in diameter than a papule but not deeper (see Fig. 35–2). Because they are superficial, plaques are usually considered to be formed by an epidermal process. Plaques occur in disorders such as psoriasis and seborrheic keratosis.

NODULE

A nodule is a raised, solid mass (see Fig. 35–2). It is deeper than a papule and is due to either changes in the epidermis or proliferative events in the dermis. The depth of involvement and palpability are criteria used to differentiate a nodule from a papule.

CYST

A cyst is similar to a nodule, but, instead of being solid, it is filled with liquid or semisolid expressible material (see Fig. 35–2). A sebaceous cyst is filled with material from the sebaceous glands and hair follicles.

TUMOR

A tumor is larger than a nodule and can be benign or malignant. Tumors of the skin are composed of cells having the same origin as the cells that make up the different structures and tissues of normal skin. For example, a basal cell skin tumor originates in the basal cells of the epidermis. A melanoma arises from melanocytes. Some tumors on the skin result from metastases of internal malignancies.

PUSTULE

A pustule is a raised cavity filled with pus, which includes white cells, debris, and microorganisms and their products (see Fig. 35–2). Pustules are usually caused by infection, but some may be sterile. Pustules may arise in hair follicles, resulting in ingrown hairs, or they may arise independently, as is common in acne.

ABSCESS

An abscess is a circumscribed, walled-off cavity filled with pus and serosanguineous fluid. A skin abscess usually results from staphylococcal infection. It can be superficial or deep.

WHEAL

A wheal (hive, urticaria) is a transient, irregularly shaped elevation of the skin. It is caused by a vascular reaction in which vasodilation causes erythema or redness (see Fig. 35–2). Fluid leaks diffusely out of the blood vessels into the tissue, causing edema in the dermis. The fluid contains no red blood cells, and there is no free fluid. Wheals may look like tiny papules or giant erythematous plaques.

VESICLES AND BULLAE

Vesicles and bullae (blisters) are elevated lesions with cavities that contain free fluid (see Fig. 35–2). The cavity wall is usually so thin that it is translucent, allowing the encapsulated fluid to be seen. The fluid flows out when the cavity wall is ruptured. A bulla is larger than a vesicle.

Vesicles or bullae may arise just below the stratum corneum, as in impetigo, or they may arise deeper in the epidermis, such as in the vesicles of contact dermatitis, friction, and dyshidrotic eczema. In bullous pemphigoid, subepidermal vesicles and bullae form at the dermoepidermal junction below the epidermis.

SCALES

Scales are dry, often white areas of thickened stratum corneum associated with hypertrophic disorders that cause increased proliferation of epidermal cells, as seen in psoriasis (see Fig. 35–2). Because of this rapid proliferation, the outer layer of skin contains nuclei and forms scales that remain attached to the skin surface. The fine scales commonly found on erythematous skin are secondary to inflammation.

Ichthyosis is a term that refers to a variety of disorders characterized by dry, rough skin resembling fish scales. There is no preceding redness or inflammation.

CRUSTS

Crusts are formed when fluid reaches the skin's disrupted surface and dries there (see Fig. 35–2). Crust formation may be preceded by the rupture of vesicles, pustules, or bullae or by bleeding. Brown and honey-colored crusts are characteristic of bacterial infection. Dark brown crusts are formed by blood. Crusts are seen in conditions such as eczema and impetigo.

FISSURES, EROSIONS, AND ULCERS

Fissures, erosions, and ulcers leave depressions in the plane of the skin (see Fig. 35-2). A fissure is a thin, linear rent or crack through the epidermis. An erosion is a scraped-out, shallow, open lesion limited to the epidermis, in which part or all of the epidermis is absent. An erosion heals without scarring. An ulcer is typically defined as a deeper, open lesion, devoid of epidermis, extending into the dermis and sometimes into the subcutaneous fat. It should be noted, however, that the Pressure Ulcer Classification System uses the phrase *stage I pressure ulcer* in reference to changes in the epidermis (see Chap. 36).

LICHENIFICATIONS

Lichenifications are palpably thickened areas of epidermis characterized by abnormally prominent skin markings (see Fig. 35–2). Chronic rubbing and scratching, as seen in chronic dermatitis, cause lichenifications.

Shapes of Lesions

Lesions can be described as round, oval or discoid, elongated or tubular, or irregular. There are also ring-shaped lesions that are described as annular. An annular lesion begins to develop in the center of the ring and then spreads to the periphery while healing in the center. These lesions are seen in tinea and impetigo infections (see figures in Chap. 36).

A target or bull's-eye lesion is an annular macule or papule with a purplish or vesicular center. This type of lesion, which occurs in erythema multiforme, is also illustrated in Chapter 36.

An iris lesion resembles the iris of the eye. There are three zones of color change present in concentric rings.

Distribution of Lesions

Lesions can be localized to one area of the body or can be widely distributed. Regional distribution refers to the area of the body affected, such as the groin, scalp, palms, and soles. *Generalized distribution* denotes widespread involvement. *Total* or *universal distribution* denotes entire involvement of the hair, skin, and nails. *Circumscribed distribution* refers to involvement that is sharply limited to a specific area by clean borders.

Other descriptions of distribution patterns include the following: scattered; symmetric; exposed areas; sites of pressure; intertriginous areas or skin surfaces that touch; areas occluded by tight clothing, tape, or dressings; and characteristic sites of specific skin ailments.

Arrangement of Lesions

Lesions can be discrete (separate) or confluent (running together). They may also be grouped or clustered (Fig. 35–3). Lesions described as linear are arranged in a line. Arciform lesions form an arc. Circinate lesions are annular lesions that have grown together to form larger lesions. Polycyclic denotes many circinate lesions. Serpiginous lesions wind like snakes, whereas reticular lesions are net-like, such as a telangiectasia.

Lesions of herpes zoster are described as following the path of a dermatome (the area of skin innervated by a single nerve root). Herpes simplex lesions may be described as grouped, clustered, or herpetiform. Lesions with geographic configurations are sometimes seen in psoriasis.

Evolution of Lesions

A primary lesion develops without any preceding skin change; that is, it is the initial reaction of the skin to the underlying disorder. When a primary lesion changes in character by natural progression of the disorder, scratching, rubbing, or therapeutic intervention, it becomes a secondary lesion. Macules, papules, nodules, vesicles, bullae, pustules, wheals, plaques, and cysts are primary lesions. Scales, crusts, fissures, ulcers, and excoriations are secondary lesions.

Scars

Scars are an alteration in appearance of the skin after repair of an injury with fibrous tissue. In an atrophic, depressed scar, there is too little tissue to fill the healed area completely. Acne is a common cause of atrophic scar formation. Hypertrophic scars, called keloids, contain excess fibrous tissue. They are raised and usually caused by an injury. Keloids are more common among African-Americans. They are treated by surgical excision, intralesional corticosteroid therapy, or radiation.

Atrophy

Skin atrophy results from a loss of subcutaneous tissue. In epidermal atrophy, there is a decrease in the number of epidermal cells, resulting in an alteration of surface appearance. Although the skin may or may not retain its normal skin lines, they are usually absent. Atrophied skin may be bluish and look like wrinkled cigarette paper.

Dermal atrophy results in a clinically detectable depression in the skin caused by a decrease in the papillary or reticular dermal connective tissue. Dermal atrophy is usually caused by inflammation or injury. If dermal atrophy occurs without epidermal atrophy, the skin is normal in color and markings.

Striae commonly result from stretching of the skin, such as during pregnancy or from obesity. The overstretching results in epidermal and dermal atrophy, with a crinkled appearance of the affected skin and blood vessels seen through it.

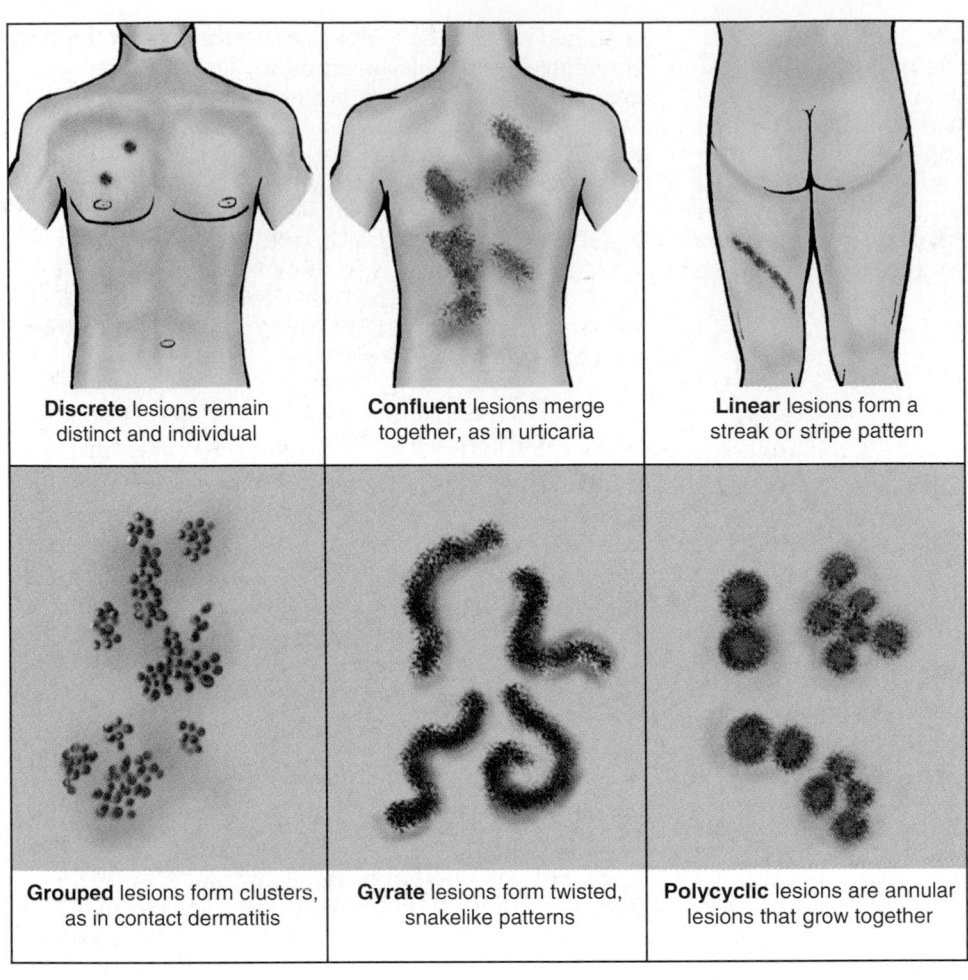

Discrete lesions remain distinct and individual

Confluent lesions merge together, as in urticaria

Linear lesions form a streak or stripe pattern

Grouped lesions form clusters, as in contact dermatitis

Gyrate lesions form twisted, snakelike patterns

Polycyclic lesions are annular lesions that grow together

Figure 35–3

Examples of arrangements or configurations of lesions.

Assessment of the Integumentary System

PATIENT HISTORY

Ask the patient whether he or she is currently experiencing any skin problem. If so, obtain a description. Determine where on the body the problem began and when, and whether it is associated with any other symptoms, such as itching, burning, stinging, numbness, fever, sore throat, nausea, vomiting, or diarrhea. Determine what, if any, treatment measures the patient has used and whether the condition has worsened or improved.

Because factors in both the external and internal environment may contribute to dermatologic disorders, explore any associated with the onset or worsening of the problem, such as exposure to the sun, heat, cold, stress, or menstruation. Take special care to question the patient about recent changes in laundry products, use of hand and body lotions, and use of birth control pills, contraceptive creams, foams, vaginal tablets, vaginal sponges, and condoms.

Explore dietary patterns, and identify any new or rarely eaten foods that have been recently ingested. Review the climates and environments in which the patient has lived and traveled. Explore possible exposure to chemicals, the amount of time spent outdoors exposed to ultraviolet light, and exposure to ionizing radiation therapy.

Question the patient about present and past medical problems, including any known allergies. Identify any prescribed or over-the-counter medication or topical preparation currently used or used in the recent past. Note when any medication use was begun, dosage and frequency of administration, and when the last dose was taken.

Determine whether any member of the patient's family has a history of dermatologic disorders. If so, note the type of problem and the relationship of the affected members to the patient.

Assess the patient's understanding of and compliance with risk reduction and health maintenance

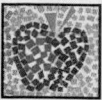

To maintain healthy skin and decrease the risk of skin disease, instruct the patient to:

Drink plenty of water because the integumentary system is about 90% water.

Eat a balanced diet because fruits, vegetables, and fiber provide nutrients essential to the skin.

Exercise to stimulate the flow of nourishing blood and oxygen to the skin, thus creating a healthy glow.

Bathe or shower only once a day and only long enough to clean the body because soap and water can cause skin to become excessively dry.

Use tepid water when washing because it is not as drying as hot water.

Lather gently in circles with your hands and pat the skin dry with a soft towel because scrubbing and rubbing are irritating and can cause skin breakdown.

Apply an emollient every day after bathing to help lock in moisture.

Get enough sleep because fatigue slows circulation and impedes delivery of oxygen and other nutrients to the skin.

Limit exposure of skin to harmful ultraviolet rays by covering up and applying a sunscreen (at least sun protection factor 15) 30 minutes before exposure every day, all year, when going out in the sun. This habit decreases the risk of skin cancer.

Inspect the skin monthly for changes in existing lesions or development of new lesions.

tion. Keep in mind that areas of the skin exposed to the sun are usually deeper in color than nonexposed areas.

If assessing color in a dark-skinned person, increase the light to make the reddish undertone characteristic of healthy dark skin more visible. Remember that erythema of dark skin manifests as a purplish to gray tone. Pallor appears as ashen gray to yellow-brown because of the absence of underlying red tones. The conjunctivae of dark-skinned people are normally yellow, so check the hard palate for evidence of jaundice.

If vascular changes are evident, note location and distribution. Also note their color and size, and palpate for the presence of pulsation. Describe any marks on the skin in terms of location, size, and type of break (tear, erosion, ulcer). Note the amount and color of any drainage. Note any signs of infection. Describe the location and appearance of any rashes, papules, nodules, or other lesions. Note the color, size, shape, and distribution of lesions. Palpate to determine whether lesions are flat or elevated, hard or soft. Use a metric ruler to measure size.

Place the back of your hand on the skin surface to check skin temperature. Describe any local variations in temperature, and note affected areas. When palpating, also note skin texture, mobility, and moisture. Note areas of dry, flaky skin or waterlogged, macerated skin. Observe for edema, which can make the skin appear taut, shiny, and pale. Check skin turgor, and observe for needle tracks, which can indicate substance abuse.

Assess hair and nails. Note the hair color and distribution. Also note whether the hair is thick or thin and shiny or dull. Observe for dandruff, nits, and other hair or scalp alteration. Inspect the nails, noting configuration, color, and consistency. Remember that the angle between the nail and the base should be 160 degrees and that the base of the nails should be firm on palpation.

Throughout the assessment, note the patient's general hygiene. If hygiene appears to be lacking in one or more areas, observe the patient for mobility or other problems that could indicate a self-care deficit.

information related to the care of the skin as presented in Highlight 35–1.

PHYSICAL EXAMINATION

Physical assessment includes examination of the skin on all body surfaces, hair, nails, and mucous membranes. In good light, inspect all areas of the skin and mucous membranes. Observe for color, vascular changes, and breaks or other lesions. Be sure to examine areas between skin folds carefully. If you find local areas of color variation, note the size and loca-

Diagnostic Procedures

Diagnostic procedures that aid in diagnosing skin disorders include direct and microscopic examinations of the lesions (Table 35–2), cultures, biopsies, and patch tests. The nurse wears gloves, uses aseptic technique, or both, when collecting specimens for dermatologic examination. Blood tests, urine tests, and x-rays may be ordered for patients suspected of

Table 35–2

Dermatologic Diagnostic Procedures

Type of Procedure	Description	Uses
DIRECT EXAMINATION		
Wood's light examination	A hand-held, long-wave ultraviolet or black light is used to examine the skin in a darkened room	Accentuates pigment changes in fair-skinned persons Identifies infections characterized by areas of blue-green or red fluorescence when seen under the light
Diascopy	A microscope slide is pressed firmly over a skin lesion so examiner can see whether lesion blanches or stays red	Determines whether a macular or papular lesion results from capillary dilatation (lesion blanches) or from extravasation of blood into tissues (lesion stays red)
MICROSCOPIC EXAMINATION		
Potassium hydroxide (KOH) mount	Scales are scraped from the edge of the lesion onto a slide, treated with KOH, and examined under a microscope for hyphae (fungal filaments) characteristic of fungus infection	Done on scaling lesions to check for fungal infection Results are documented as KOH(−) or KOH(+)
Tzanck test	Fluid from a vesicle is scraped onto a slide, prepared, and examined under a microscope for multinucleated giant cells	Diagnoses herpes viral infections
Oil mount of skin scraping	Skin from a suspicious area is scraped, placed in oil on a slide, and examined under a microscope	Diagnoses scabies by identifying the scabies mite
Darkfield examination	Serous fluid from a suspected chancre or secondary lesion is examined under a microscope for the presence of the spirochete *Treponema pallidum*	Diagnoses active syphilis
Gram's stain	Bacteria are stained with crystal violet, treated, decolorized, and counterstained with a contrasting dye. Bacteria that retain the original violet stain are gram-positive; those that lose the stain but retain the counter-stain are gram-negative.	Diagnoses bacterial infection

having a systemic disorder with dermatologic manifestations.

CULTURES

Fungal, viral, and bacterial cultures confirm and further characterize pathogens. For fungal cultures, skin scrapings are collected from the surface of a lesion. The scrapings are cultured in a fungal media bottle for 1 to 2 weeks. The growth is then examined grossly and microscopically to identify the fungus.

Viral and bacterial cultures are collected from intact bullae, vesicles, and pustules. The lesion is aseptically punctured, and the exudate is swabbed with a culturette for transport to the microbiology laboratory, where it is cultured and examined.

PATCH TEST

The patch test identifies allergens responsible for allergic contact dermatitis. It tests delayed type IV hypersensitivity response to contact allergens. Patch testing is done when the dermatitis persists despite avoidance of likely causative agents and institution of appropriate topical therapy.

The three types of patch test are use, open, and closed. In a use test, the suspected causative agent, such as a cream or cosmetic, is applied to an area of the skin distant from the affected area. This is done twice a day for 5 to 7 days unless a reaction occurs, in which case the test is stopped.

In an open patch test, a suspected allergen is applied to the skin on the inner upper arm once a day for 3 to 5 days.

In a closed patch test, suspected allergens are applied to the skin and covered for 48 hours. Solid materials (such as rubber), topical medications, cosmetics, and the like can be tested in this way. Results of open and closed patch tests are read as described later.

If the allergen evades identification, a standard patch test series can be performed. For this, a kit that contains 20 allergens in nonirritating concentrations packaged in syringe dispensers is used. Each of the allergens to be tested (it may be some or all of the 20) is applied to a patch or other holding device (Fig. 35–4). It is then taped to clear skin, preferably on the patient's upper back, and the perimeter of the test site is outlined with 0.5% gentian violet. The test strips are removed in 48 hours, and an initial reading is done at that time. A second reading is done in 3 to 7 days after application to check for a delayed reaction. Test reactions are read as follows:

+   Weakly positive reaction characterized by erythema, infiltration, and sometimes papules
++   Strongly positive reaction characterized by edema and vesicles
+++ Extremely positive reaction characterized by spreading bullae and ulcers
−   Negative reaction

SKIN BIOPSIES

Skin biopsies are done to obtain skin specimens for microscopic examination and diagnosis of a skin dis-order and to determine the stage of a disease process. Biopsy specimens are obtained from fully developed lesions. Primary lesions are preferred.

Types of Skin Biopsy

The types of biopsies commonly done in dermatology are punch biopsies, shave biopsies, and excision biopsies. The type of biopsy is determined by the physician's preference and by the location and type of lesion. An excision biopsy is done whenever malignant melanoma or deep inflammatory disease is suspected. Shave biopsies are done on raised, superficial lesions other than malignant melanoma. Punch biopsies are appropriate for any superficial lesion, whether inflammatory, bullous, or neoplastic, with the exception of melanoma.

Procedures

Biopsy procedures may be performed in the physician's office or in an ambulatory surgery clinic. In all biopsy procedures, the area around the lesion is cleaned with an appropriate antibacterial agent, and the site is marked with a skin-marking pen. Hair may also be shaved from the area. A 30-gauge needle is used to inject local anesthetic around the site.

PUNCH BIOPSY

To obtain the specimen, a skin punch—which looks like a very-large-bore needle—is pressed into the skin at a 90-degree angle using a rotary motion (Fig. 35–5). The specimen is lifted gently and snipped off at the level of the subcutaneous fat, leaving a smooth, round edge. Hemostasis is achieved with absorbable gelatin sponge (Gelfoam) packing, electrodesiccation, Monsel's solution, or aluminum chloride 35% in isopropyl alcohol 50% applied with a

Figure 35–4

A, Patch test kit. *B*, Patch test applied to the patient's back. (Courtesy of Hermal Pharmaceutical Laboratories, Delmar, NY.)

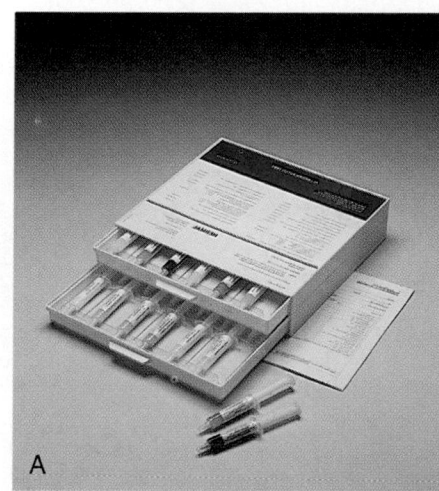
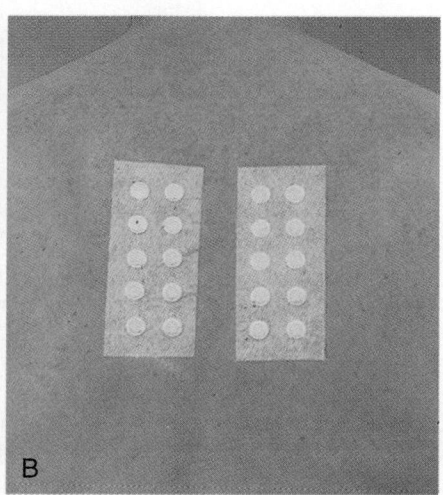

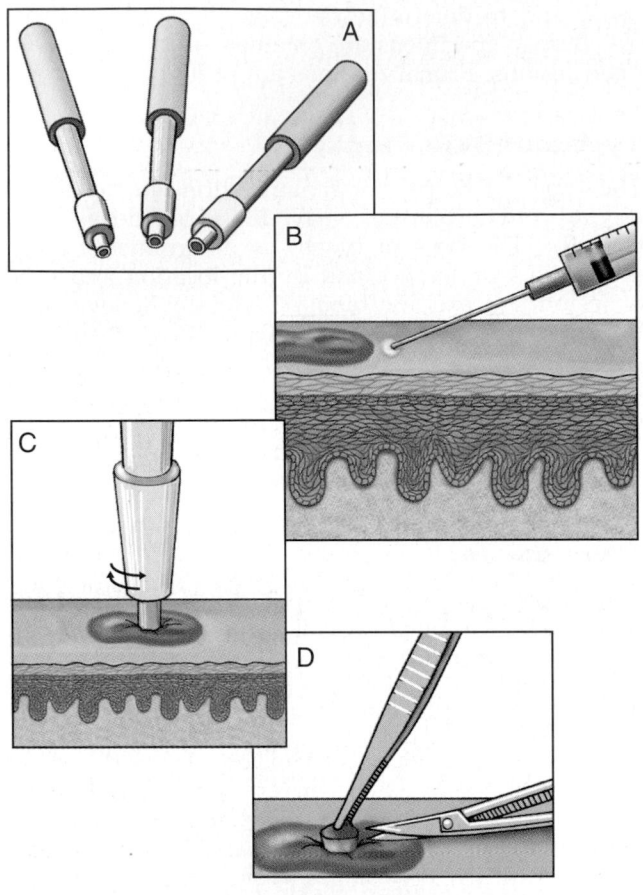

though healing is faster than by secondary intention, the wound margins may not approximate well, depending on the location of the biopsy. On the back, for example, the tissues have limited give.

SHAVE BIOPSY

To obtain a specimen by shave biopsy, a wheal is first raised in the skin by injecting local anesthetic intradermally under the lesion. The lesion is then shaved with a number 15 blade to obtain the specimen.

EXCISION BIOPSY

An excision biopsy is obtained using sterile technique, under local anesthesia by the physician, who uses a scalpel to remove an elliptic section of involved skin (Fig. 35–6). The surgical wound is sutured closed. Absorbable and nonabsorbable sutures are often used for wounds that extend deep into the dermis to facilitate wound closure.

NURSING PROCESS GUIDELINES
Skin Biopsy

Before the procedure, question the patient about allergies to local anesthetics, topical anesthetics, and topical skin preparations. Assess the patient's understanding of the procedure and anxiety level about it. Allow the patient to express concerns and ask questions. Clarify the patient's understanding of the purpose of the biopsy and the procedure involved. Reassure the patient that skin biopsy is a minor procedure, complications are rare, and scarring is minimal. Instruct the patient in self-care, as presented in Highlight 35–2. Make provisions for the patient to obtain biopsy results: make certain he or she knows whether to call, to expect a telephone call, or to return for a follow-up visit. Also explain when and by whom the patient will be informed of the results.

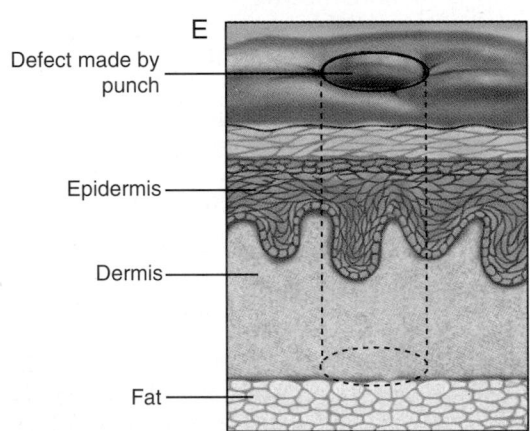

Figure 35–5

Steps of a punch biopsy. *A*, The physician chooses a biopsy tool of appropriate diameter. *B*, Local anesthesia is used to numb the biopsy area. *C*, The physician obtains the biopsy specimen by pressing the biopsy tool into the lesion using a radial motion. *D*, After lifting the specimen with forceps, the physician cuts it at the subcutaneous fat level. *E*, The defect left after punch biopsy can be left open to heal by second intention or, if large, can be sutured.

cotton-tipped applicator. Two to 3 mm punches heal well by secondary intention, leaving a slightly depressed scar that is cosmetically acceptable. Punch-biopsy wounds larger than 3 mm are sutured. Al-

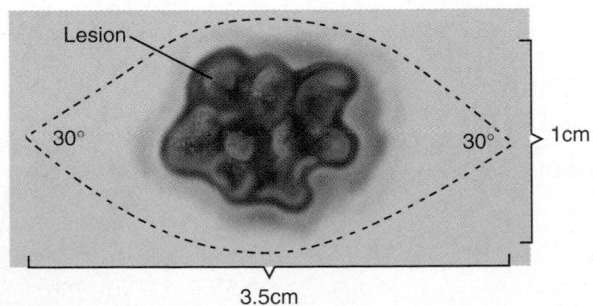

Figure 35–6

An elliptic scalpel excision with a length-to-width ratio of 3.5:1. The apical angles should be 30 degrees.

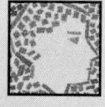

HIGHLIGHT
35–2

PATIENT EDUCATION

Self-Care After Skin Biopsy

Instruct the patient to:

Keep the dressing dry and intact for at least 8 hours.

Leave the site open to air after the initial dressing is removed unless it needs a cover for cosmetic reasons or is located in an area prone to contamination.

Clean the biopsy site once each day with tap water, saline, or a cotton-tipped applicator and hydrogen peroxide after the initial dressing is removed.

Apply topical antibiotic ointment as ordered by the physician.

Report erythema or excessive drainage.

Return for removal of the sutures on *(specify date and time).*

Management

NONSURGICAL MANAGEMENT

Pharmacologic Therapy

Pharmacologic therapy in dermatology may be topical, intralesional, systemic, or a combination of these. Topical administration is the most widely used. Topical preparations deliver medication directly to the involved area of the skin. They are safer than systemic therapy but are often time-consuming, expensive, and aesthetically unpleasant. They may also require a large volume of medication.

Topical medications must be absorbed percutaneously to be effective. Absorption is influenced by the active ingredient, the concentration of the active ingredient, the vehicle or substance that contains the active ingredient, and the condition of the integument to which the topical agent is applied. The active ingredient in a topical preparation is the chemical substance that is responsible for its effects.

VEHICLES USED IN TOPICAL PREPARATIONS

Vehicles used in topical agents are therapeutically inactive substances that contain the active ingredient. The most common vehicles are emollients, creams, ointments, and lotions.

Emollients are skin softeners, such as mineral oil, white petrolatum, lanolin, paraffins, glycerin, and urea. They increase hydration of the stratum corneum by trapping water particles on the skin. Emollients allow scales to fall off the skin by decreasing the binding forces within the horny layers. Emollients are used to treat dry skin, psoriasis, eczema, and pruritus. They can cause folliculitis by occluding hair follicles.

A cream is an oil-in-water emulsion. It is white, nongreasy, and vanishes when rubbed into the skin. Parabens and formaldehyde preservatives are added to creams to prevent the growth of bacteria and fungi. The preservatives can cause allergic-contact dermatitis. Creams are used to treat subacute inflammation. They are usually the preferred vehicle for applying steroids to the face, underarms, and groin.

An ointment is a water-in-oil emulsion. It is greasy and clear. No preservative is required. Ointments provide increased hydration, occlusion, and penetration of the active ingredient. They are the best vehicle to treat thick, hyperkeratotic skin and chronic inflammation associated with dryness, scaling, and lichenification. An ointment is not applied to wet, weepy skin.

A lotion is a liquid suspension. It has a cooling effect on the skin as the water evaporates. Lotions are especially useful in treating hairy areas such as the scalp. A lotion wears off easily. It is not useful as a barrier to promote hydration. Lotions are used to treat wet, weepy skin and acute inflammation with vesiculation.

Other vehicles include gels, powders, and pastes. Table 35–3 presents a summary comparison of the most common topical vehicles and their uses.

ACTIVE INGREDIENTS USED IN TOPICAL PREPARATIONS

Active ingredients used in topical preparations include keratolytics, antiproliferative agents, anti-inflammatory agents, and antifungal, antibacterial, and antiviral agents.

Keratolytics soften and remove the horny layer of the skin. Salicylic acid 2% to 20% is the most commonly used keratolytic agent. Lactic acid is also keratolytic. These agents can be added to any vehicle and combined with other active ingredients. They are used to treat acne, psoriasis, warts, corns, and calluses.

Crude coal tar is an antiproliferative agent that also has antipruritic, astringent, vasoconstrictive, and disinfective properties. It suppresses epidermal deoxyribonucleic acid (DNA) synthesis and enhances ultraviolet B therapy. Crude coal tar is dark in color and smells like tar. It stains clothes and linens and can cause scarring of the skin. Liquid carbonic detergens is a 20% solution of crude coal tar that also stains and scars. Coal tars are used to treat psoriasis, eczemas, and pruritus.

Table 35–3

Comparing Vehicles for Application of Topical Medicine

Vehicle	Description	Use	Advantages	Disadvantages
Lotion	Oil in water (liquid emulsion)	Acute inflammation Wet, weepy skin with vesiculation Hairy areas Scalp	Cooling effect	Wears off easily Not a barrier Does not promote hydration
Cream	Oil in water (semisolid emulsion)	Subacute inflammation Preferred for face, underarms, groin, and hands	Nongreasy	Antibacterial preservatives added May cause contact dermatitis
Ointment	Water in oil	Chronic inflammation Thick, hyperkeratotic skin Dryness, scaling, and lichenification	Provides the most hydration, occlusion, and penetration of active ingredient because it prevents transepidermal water loss	Greasy Cannot be used on wet, weepy skin

Anthralin is a synthetic coal tar used to treat psoriatic plaques. It is an antiproliferative agent that affects mitochondrial DNA. Low concentrations of 0.01 to 0.05% can be applied and left on the skin. High-dose, short-contact anthralin therapy is effective in treating thick plaques. High-dose anthralin is applied in 1 to 3% concentrations to the plaques and removed after 30 minutes to 1 hour.

Anthralin irritates normal skin. Caution must be used to ensure that the medicine is applied only to the area being treated. White petrolatum applied to the normal skin around the plaques before applying anthralin protects uninvolved skin. Anthralin stains clothes and the bathtub. Anthralin treatment is usually administered in inpatient settings or in psoriasis treatment centers, but it can be self-administered at home if the patient understands how to apply the medicine and the implications of staining and damage to normal skin.

TOPICAL AND SYSTEMIC PREPARATIONS

Corticosteroids

Topical corticosteroid preparations are antiproliferative and anti-inflammatory. They provide high therapeutic benefit with little toxicity. However, most potent steroids can cause significant local and systemic side effects. Systemic side effects can occur when a strong preparation of a topical steroid is absorbed into the system through the skin or mucous membrane. Weak topical steroid preparations rarely cause systemic or local side effects. Table 35–4 lists topical steroids in categories by potency.

The vehicle affects the potency of the steroid. The vehicle is selected on the basis of its occlusive property and the presenting condition of the skin. The vehicle is changed as the skin condition progresses from acute to chronic.

Topical corticosteroids are usually applied twice daily. Because the stratum corneum becomes a reservoir for the steroid and continues to release it into the skin after initial application, a thin application provides the same benefit as a thick application.

Topical corticosteroids are absorbed more readily when applied to the mucous membrane, mouth, scrotum, eyelids, and face. Penetration is decreased on the lower arms and legs and dorsa of the hands and feet. The nails, palms, and soles do not readily absorb the drug. The topical steroid must penetrate into the dermis to be effective.

Side effects include skin atrophy, striae, telangiectasias, glaucoma and cataracts when applied around the eyes, and perioral dermatitis (acne eruption around the mouth). Side effects can be avoided

Table 35–4

Topical Corticosteroid Potency

Potency	Proprietary Name	Generic Name
High	Temovate	Clobetasol propionate
	Halog	Halcinonide
	Lidex	Fluocinonide
	Diprosone	Betamethasone dipropionate
	Topicort	Desoximetasone
Medium	Valisone	Betamethasone valerate
	Aristocort	Triamcinolone acetonide
	Kenalog	
	Synalar	Fluocinolone acetonide
	Westcort	Hydrocortisone valerate
Low	Hytone	Hydrocortisone
	Carmol-HC	Hydrocortisone acetate
	Aclovate	Alclometasone

by using no more than 50 g (20 oz) of a potent steroid per week. Cushing's syndrome is rare but has been reported as a side effect of chronic, excessive use of potent topical corticosteroids applied over large areas of skin and usually covered by an occlusive substance such as plastic wrap.

Hydrocortisone cream 0.5% has no side effects and can be purchased over the counter. Hydrocortisone cream 1% is also safe and can also be purchased over the counter.

Intralesional corticosteroid therapy is used to treat keloids and to provide prolonged anti-inflammatory effects in a localized lesion. The corticosteroid is injected into the lesion by the physician with a 30-gauge, half-inch needle or with a pressure jet. The patient may have some pain at the injection site similar to that felt on injection of a local anesthetic by the dentist.

Systemic corticosteroids may be administered orally, intramuscularly, or intravenously for acute dermatitis.

Antibacterials

Systemic antibiotics are used to treat bacterial skin infections. Tetracycline and erythromycin are the most common antibiotics used in dermatology.

Local antibiotics are applied two to four times daily to treat minor local infections or to prevent wound infections. Their efficacy in treating existing infections is questionable.

Chlorhexidine gluconate (Hibiclens) is an antiseptic, antimicrobial skin cleanser with bactericidal activity. It is the preferred anti-infective agent to treat skin infections. It is effective against gram-negative and gram-positive bacteria. Povidone-iodine (Betadine) is also effective against gram-negative and gram-positive bacteria, but local skin sensitivity is more common than with Hibiclens. Neither of these products should be used routinely on wounds that involve more than superficial skin layers.

Hexachlorophene (pHisoHex) is effective against gram-positive bacteria. It has been found to cause neurotoxicity and cannot be applied to mucous membrane or to any open-skin lesions.

Antifungals

Most cutaneous dermatophyte and yeast infections can be treated with topical antifungal agents, such as imidazole carboxamide cream applied twice daily until 2 weeks after the infection is clinically clear. Nystatin and nystatin with corticosteroids (Mycolog) are effective in treating yeast infections but not dermatophytes.

Griseofulvin is a systemic fungistatic antibiotic used to treat dermatophyte infections of the scalp and nails and, sometimes, generalized skin infections. It is administered in daily doses of 500 mg orally for 4 to 6 weeks to treat tinea capitis and 1 g daily for 12 months or more to treat toenail infections. Griseofulvin may cause hematologic, renal, and hepatic toxicity. Periodic blood studies and evaluation of renal and hepatic function are recommended.

Antivirals

Acyclovir is used to treat herpes simplex virus (HSV) infections. It is used primarily for genital herpes infections and for cutaneous HSV infections in immunocompromised patients to decrease healing time, viral shedding, and duration of pain. It may also decrease viral shedding in recurrent HSV infections. Intravenous acyclovir is indicated in the treatment of severe primary herpes simplex, neonatal herpes, and herpes simplex and herpes zoster infections in immunocompromised patients. Oral acyclovir is effective against primary and recurrent HSV infections. Another treatment for herpes zoster is famciclovir (Famvir), which also may reduce the duration of postherpetic neuralgia.

Retinoids

Retinoids are derivatives of vitamin A. They have a direct effect on the growth and differentiation of keratinizing epithelium. Retinoids are used primarily to treat cystic acne and psoriasis.

Isotretinoin (Accutane) is a highly toxic retinoid administered orally to treat severe recalcitrant cystic acne. It inhibits sebaceous gland function and keratinization. A course of therapy consists of 0.5 to 2 mg/kg body weight divided into two doses daily for 15 to 20 weeks.

Isotretinoin is teratogenic. It must not be given to pregnant women because major human fetal abnormalities have been reported. Women are advised not to become pregnant for at least 3 months after discontinuing therapy. Pregnancy tests are required in women of childbearing age before initiating therapy, and birth-control measures should be used during treatment. Other significant adverse effects include intracranial hypertension, corneal opacities, inflammatory bowel disease, hypertriglyceridemia, musculoskeletal symptoms, and cheilitis (dermatitis of the lip). Monthly blood studies are monitored carefully for elevated triglycerides and for positive serum pregnancy. Isotretinoin should be prescribed only by dermatologists. Transient exacerbation of acne sometimes occurs in the early treatment period.

Etretinate (Tegison) is an oral systemic retinoid that is effective in treating pustular, joint, palmar-plantar, and erythrodermic psoriasis. Studies in Europe have shown it to be effective in combination with psoralen plus ultraviolet A (PUVA) treatments for plaque psoriasis. Etretinate is teratogenic and hepatotoxic. No safe time has been established for pregnancy after discontinuing use of the drug.

Tretinoin (Retin-A) is a topical retinoid used to treat acne vulgaris and comedones (blackheads). It is available as a cream, gel, or solution. Tretinoin stimulates mitotic activity and increases turnover of follicular epithelial cells, causing extrusion of comedones. It is applied once daily at bedtime. Patients may experience a temporary exacerbation of their condition because of the action of the medication on deep, unseen lesions. Inform patients that erythema and desquamation (peeling) are expected during the first 1 to 3 weeks of therapy. Patients should stay out of sunlight or use a sun protection factor (SPF) 15 sunscreen during treatment because of increased sensitivity to ultraviolet rays.

Antimetabolites

Antimetabolites inhibit DNA synthesis in cells and are used as antiproliferative agents in treating dermatologic conditions. Methotrexate is used to treat psoriasis. It is usually given by mouth in three divided doses over 2 days weekly or given weekly by intramuscular injection. Laboratory studies to determine the effect of methotrexate on lymphocytes and renal and liver function are done frequently during the course of treatment. Liver biopsies are also done before initiating treatment and periodically while undergoing treatment. The patient must abstain from alcohol to prevent liver damage.

Fluorouracil is an antimetabolite used to treat multiple actinic keratosis and superficial basal-cell carcinoma. It is available in a cream or solution. Clinically apparent lesions and subclinical lesions undergo selective inflammatory response during treatment. Normal skin does not become inflamed as a result of application of topical fluorouracil. The inflammatory response progresses through stages of erythema, vesiculation, erosion, ulceration, and necrosis if the medication is continued. A course of therapy for actinic keratosis is usually 2 to 4 weeks or until the response reaches the erythema stage. The arms may require 6 to 8 weeks of treatment.

The patient is closely monitored to assess when an adequate response is achieved. Gloves are worn to apply fluorouracil, and caution is used when applying it around the eyes, nose, and mouth.

Antihistamines

Hydroxyzine hydrochloride (Atarax) is a systemic antihistamine used to treat pruritus. As much as 25 to 50 mg by mouth four times daily is administered to treat severe itching. The patient can take another dose during the night if he or she becomes uncomfortable. Precautions must be taken so the patient is not oversedated. The patient should not take the medicine during the day if driving or working.

Hydroxyzine hydrochloride and diphenhydramine hydrochloride (Benadryl) are prescribed for histamine-mediated allergic skin disorders, such as urticaria. Diphenhydramine is not as effective as hydroxyzine in treating pruritus.

Sun Sensitizers

Methoxsalen, a psoralen derivative, is used to increase skin sensitivity to ultraviolet A (UVA) light in the treatment of cutaneous T-cell lymphoma, vitiligo, and psoriasis. It can be taken systemically, applied topically, or added to bath water. The systemic approach requires 30 to 60 mg doses of the medication to be ingested 2 hours before PUVA therapy. Oral methoxsalen is prescribed according to the pa-

tient's body weight (0.6 mg / kg). The most common side effects after ingestion are nausea, vomiting, and diarrhea. Ginger may be helpful in limiting these symptoms.

If applied topically, methoxsalen is applied only to affected areas 20 minutes before UVA exposure. Care must be taken to avoid healthy skin to minimize risk of hyperpigmentation and phototoxicity.

Bath water delivery of methoxsalen is not considered the best approach since it requires more patient time and effort. The bath is prepared by dissolving 50 mg of medication in 50 mL of near-boiling water and adding it to 100 L of tepid bath water. The patient then bathes the entire body except head and scalp for 10 minutes, towel dries, and then exposes himself or herself to UVA 10 minutes later. These time intervals must be kept constant because they influence the patient's photosensitivity. Varying them may result in a phototoxic reaction even though the appropriate dose of light was administered.

Patients taking oral methoxsalen are instructed to wear UVA-blocking glasses indoors and outdoors for 24 hours after ingesting the medication and to avoid sun exposure. UVA-protective goggles must also be worn by patients who take psoralen baths and take etretinate.

Psoralen is sometimes used to treat vitiligo in natural sunlight.

Sunscreens

Sunscreens block out the sun's burning ultraviolet rays and allow the skin to tan gradually. They are applied to sun-exposed areas of the skin at least 30 minutes before going outdoors and reapplied after swimming or heavy perspiration. The ratio between the amount of sun exposure needed to cause redness with a sunscreen and the amount needed without a sunscreen is the sun protection factor (SPF). SPF is always listed on the sunscreen bottle. The Skin Cancer Foundation grants its seal of acceptance to products of SPF 15, which meet the criteria to aid in the prevention of sun-induced damage to the skin. SPF 15 is appropriate for all skin types. Table 35–5 lists the sun-reactive skin types used in dermatology practice.

Because both UVA and UVB rays are harmful and directly related to the development of skin cancer, patients must be instructed to read labels and use a sunscreen that protects against both types of radiation. Because of erosion of the ozone layer and the resultant increase in UVC radiation, sunscreens protecting against UVC as well as UVA and UVB rays will be available in the near future.

Topical Treatments

Water is one of the most important therapeutic agents in dermatology. Dry skin is due to a lack of water in the stratum corneum. The keratinocytes in the stratum corneum are capable of absorbing vast amounts of water.

Table 35–5

Classification of Sun-Reactive Skin Types Used in Dermatology Practice

Type*	Description
I	Always burn, never tan (often have red hair, blue eyes; of Irish ancestry)
II	Always burn, sometimes tan (blonde, brunette; blue or brown eyes)
III	Always tan, rarely burn
IV	Always tan, never burn (Mediterranean)
V	Asian
VI	Black

*To assess skin type, ask patients if they burned or tanned as a child on the first day they spent outdoors in the sun each summer.

BATHS

Therapeutic baths are soothing, antipruritic, cleansing, relaxing, hydrating, débriding, and anti-inflammatory. Topical medicines and ultraviolet therapies penetrate the skin more deeply if the skin is hydrated and débrided before treatment.

To hydrate the skin, the patient soaks in plain, warm water of approximately 35° to 39°C (96°–103°F) for 20 minutes once or twice daily. The entire body, up to the neck, is immersed. Underarms, groin, and feet can be washed with soap and water at the end of the bath. After the bath, the skin is patted dry. An ointment, such as white petrolatum, is applied to damp skin to hold the water in the skin.

A similar procedure is used to débride scaling skin. After 20 to 30 minutes in the bath, the patient uses a soft cloth to gently débride the buildup of scales. The water temperature may be as high as 39°C (103°F) for patients with psoriasis.

Cool-water baths are antipruritic. The same procedure is followed for antipruritic baths as for hydrating baths. For patients with acute dermatitis, the water temperature should be 35°C (96°F).

Crude coal tar baths are antieczematous and antipruritic and increase photosensitivity. Two capfuls are added to 6 to 8 inches of bath water or as prescribed.

Starch baths and Aveeno Colloidal Oatmeal are soothing and antipruritic for generalized itching, dry skin, winter itching, and urticaria.

Bath oils may relieve itching and dryness. They should not be added to the bath water but rather applied to the skin after bathing to minimize the risk of falls from slipping in the tub.

WET DRESSINGS

Wet dressings are prescribed to treat acute inflammation, oozing, crusting, and itching. They may be prescribed for psoriasis, eczematous dermatitis, and sunburn.

Water is the most important agent used in wet dressings. Active ingredients used in wet dressings include potassium permanganate, Burow's solution, and silver nitrate. Gauze pads, wraparound gauze, cotton sheets torn into smaller sizes, towels, or old T-shirts can be used to apply wet dressings. The fabric is soaked in water or other prescribed agent and then applied to the skin for 15 to 30 minutes. An occlusive wrap is never applied over a wet dressing. Special masks, gloves, and cotton socks to treat the face, hands, and feet can be purchased or improvised.

OCCLUSIVE DRESSINGS

Occlusive dressings may be prescribed to enhance the action of keratolytics and, occasionally, other topical preparations. An occlusive dressing, such as plastic wrap, placed over a topical preparation can enhance penetration of the medication 10 to 100 times. Although deeper penetration of the topical preparation is usually beneficial to the patient, occlusive dressings increase the risk of skin irritation and toxic side effects. This is especially true with topical corticosteroids. Occlusive dressings also interfere with heat exchange and increase the risk of infection and folliculitis. Occlusive dressings should be used only with an order from a dermatologist. The patient and the skin condition are frequently monitored for adverse side effects of therapy.

SCALP TREATMENTS

Keratolytic agents are applied to the scalp to débride the scales of psoriasis. The scalp is hydrated under running water for a few minutes before applying the keratolytic agent. Salicylic acid 2% (Baker's P&S) is an over-the-counter preparation that is keratolytic. It can be applied to the scalp to débride scales. Salicylic acid 2% to 10% is also available in an oil base. The oil softens the scales, and the salicylic acid loosens them. The scales can then be gently débrided by being lifted with a soft-tooth comb. This procedure can be repeated for a severe, neglected buildup of scales in psoriasis.

Corticosteroids are applied in a lotion base to erythematous psoriatic lesions on the scalp. Corticosteroids are also indicated in treating eczematous dermatitis and seborrheic dermatitis of the scalp.

Radiation Therapy

IONIZING RADIATION

Ionizing radiation therapy is effective in treating basal-cell and squamous-cell skin cancer. However, it is time-consuming and requires multiple visits over a period of 1 to 2 months. Radiation therapy is a good alternative to surgery for patients unable or unwilling to undergo a surgical procedure and for lesions located in anatomic sites that are difficult to treat surgically. It should not be used in children because of increased risk of future skin cancer from the radiation. The side effects of radiation therapy are discussed in Chapter 34.

Total-body electron-beam radiation is effective in treating the skin lesions of mycosis fungoides. Electron-beam therapy uses electrons instead of photons. The electrons have limited penetration through the skin, so internal organ damage is avoided.

ULTRAVIOLET RADIATION

Ultraviolet radiation is effective in treating psoriasis, eczema, uremic pruritus, vitiligo, and mycosis fungoides. Its primary use is the treatment of psoriasis.

Artificial light sources have been developed that emit ultraviolet radiation in the UVB middle-wave spectrum and in the UVA long-wave spectrum. These bulbs are arranged in ultraviolet phototherapy cabinets with 12 to 60 bulbs per cabinet. An ultraviolet cabinet may have UVB bulbs, UVA bulbs, or both.

UVB treatment may be combined with tar, anthralin, white petrolatum, steroid therapy, or a combination of these. A nurse or specially trained phototherapist administers the treatment. The patient wears UVB-blocking goggles during the treatment and keeps the eyes closed. The eyelids do not provide adequate protection from the UVB rays. The patient stands nude in the cabinet and is treated with gradually increasing doses of UVB radiation. Treatments range from a minimum of 10 millijoules (mJ) to a maximum of 999 mJ, with a 10 to 20% increase determined by the patient's response to treatment. Treatments are administered daily or three times weekly until improvement is noted. The nurse inspects the patient before each treatment for untoward reactions such as sunburn, itching, or for a skin flare. Sunburn-sensitive areas can be covered during treatment, and no treatment is given to sunburned areas. Many patients see improvements after 8 to 10 treatments, with remission of as long as 18 months.

PUVA consists of exposure to long-range UVA rays 2 hours after administration of psoralen, a photosensitizing drug. UVA rays promote tanning and are the type of rays used in commercial tanning booths. In a tanning booth, however, patients would not achieve a therapeutic dose because no photosensitizing drug is administered to increase UVA penetration into the skin.

PUVA treatments, like UVB treatments, are administered according to established protocols, with gradual increments at each treatment until the patient shows improvement. When the patient achieves an acceptable clearing of lesions (80–100%), the number of treatments is tapered to achieve a monthly maintenance schedule. PUVA therapy has improved the quality of life for many psoriasis patients over the past 10 years.

Patients must wear wraparound UVA-blocking glasses indoors and outdoors during daylight hours for 24 to 48 hours after psoralen ingestion to prevent cataract formation. Wraparound UVA-blocking goggles are also worn during the treatment. Patients who have received PUVA therapy are at increased risk for skin malignancies in sun-exposed areas and are instructed to have periodic skin examinations. Other risks associated with PUVA treatment include itching, pain, blistering sunburn, freckles over the entire body, and hyperpigmentation or total-body tan.

When administering ultraviolet light therapy, consideration is given to the patient's skin type (see Table 35–5). Caution and a conservative approach are used in administering ultraviolet therapy to patients with type I and type II skin, who are at higher risk for skin cancer.

SURGICAL MANAGEMENT

Common surgical procedures in dermatology are the ellipsoidal scalpel excision described previously, curettage and desiccation, cryosurgery, and Mohs' micrographic surgery.

Dermatologic Surgical Procedures

CURETTAGE AND DESICCATION

Curettage and desiccation is the most common procedure used for the removal of early basal cell and squamous cell skin cancers. It is also a valuable treatment for destroying the lesions of Bowen's disease, actinic keratosis, skin tags, seborrheic keratosis, nevi, and hemangiomas.

Procedure

Curettage consists of using a sharp curet to remove material from the skin lesion for a biopsy. Curettage is followed by desiccation (electrosurgery or surgical diathermy), which coagulates and destroys tissue with electric current. Electrocoagulation controls bleeding by creating instant dehydration, which generates heat in the tissue adjacent to the needle point. Cellular fluids evaporate, blanching the area. Tissue destruction results from the conversion of electric energy emitted by an electrode into heat in a warm body.

The type and location of a lesion are more important than its size in determining the suitability of curettage and desiccation for removal. Local anesthesia is infiltrated around and under the lesions to be removed. No dressing is required for small lesions. The physician may prescribe topical antibiotics and dressings for larger wounds.

Postoperative Course

Healing usually takes 1 to 3 weeks by granulation. A crust forms and sloughs in 7 to 10 days. If the lesion was large, two or three successive crusts may form and slough off. Premature removal of the crust should be prevented. Areas with good blood supply and abundant subcutaneous fat heal most rapidly.

The cure rate of primary early small basal-cell and squamous-cell skin cancers with this procedure is excellent (about 96%). The procedure is simple and convenient and leaves a cosmetically acceptable scar in most sites.

CRYOSURGERY

Cryosurgery uses liquid nitrogen to destroy warts, actinic keratosis, seborrheic keratosis, and benign lentigo.

Procedure

Liquid nitrogen ($-195.6°C$ [$-384°F$]) is applied to the lesion with either a cotton swab or a cryospray gun. An ice ball develops at the site of freezing. A blister forms within 24 hours and dries in several days. Then, the skin with the lesion peels off. Cryosurgery does not require local anesthesia. If needed, the procedure may be repeated at 2- to 3-week intervals until the lesion disappears.

Postoperative Course

Immediately after cryosurgery, the operative area swells and, within hours, develops redness, throbbing, and mild pain. This is usually followed in 24 to 48 hours by development of a blister filled with clear or blood-tinged fluid. The site oozes for several days, after which the swelling begins to decrease. A scab forms in 7 to 10 days and falls off in 3 to 4 weeks. Healing time is longer for lesions on the neck, trunk, and extremities. Complications are rare, and the cosmetic result is excellent.

HIGHLIGHT
35–3
PATIENT EDUCATION   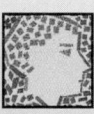 **Self-Care After Dermatologic Cryosurgery**

Instruct the patient to:

Take two acetaminophen tablets every 4 to 6 hours, apply warm soaks for 10 to 15 minutes every 2 to 3 hours, or both, to relieve discomfort.

Expect the area to swell. In 1 to 2 days, a blister filled with clear or blood-tinged fluid will develop.

Keep the affected area elevated to decrease swelling. Support an affected arm on pillows, prop an affected leg on a chair, or sleep in a semi-upright position with three or four pillows supporting the back.

Avoid breaking the blister.

Keep the affected area clean by washing with mild soap and water or cleansing with cotton or gauze and hydrogen peroxide. Apply a thin film of antibiotic ointment if ordered and cover with an adhesive bandage, nonadherent gauze, or other dressing.

Report fever or increasing redness around the affected area because it could indicate infection.

Return for a follow-up appointment on *(specify date and time)*.

NURSING PROCESS GUIDELINES
Cryosurgery

Confirm the patient's understanding of the procedure. Question the patient about any history of cryoglobulinemia, cold urticaria, or other inability to tolerate the procedure. When the procedure is completed, instruct the patient in self-care, as presented in Highlight 35–3.

MOHS' MICROGRAPHIC SURGERY

Mohs' micrographic surgery is used to treat recurrent basal-cell epithelioma, primary and recurrent squamous-cell skin cancer, morphea (fibrosing, sclerosing), basal-cell epithelioma, and basal-cell epitheliomas on the face and other sites. It is associated with a 99% cure rate for primary and recurrent skin cancer; and it minimizes damage to healthy tissue.

Procedure

After the area is prepared and anesthetized, the lesion is removed in thin horizontal layers along a grid pattern so that the exact location of each can be pinpointed on the wound. Following removal of each layer, the wound is covered with a dressing, and the patient waits while the specimen is prepared for microscopic examination. The undersurface and borders are examined. If malignant cells are still present, another layer of tissue is removed but only in the area of cancer involvement seen under the microscope. The process is repeated until a cancer-free plane is reached. The surgery is usually completed in a few hours but can take more than 1 day.

Wound closure varies with the extent and location of surgery. Flap or graft procedures may be done for large wounds. A smaller wound is sutured or allowed to granulate.

Postoperative Course

The postoperative course varies with the extent of the wound and the type of closure. Small wounds are simply kept clean and dry. Large wounds with grafts require care, as described later in this chapter.

LASER SURGERY

The carbon dioxide (CO_2) laser is used in dermatology for removal of warts, scars, and selected types of skin cancer.

The CO_2 laser beam is absorbed by water and hence by body cells, most of which are composed of about 85% water. When the CO_2 laser beam is absorbed by intracellular water, it causes the water to boil. This, in turn, causes the cells to swell and burst, releasing water vapor, carbon, and cell fragments. Put another way, the CO_2 laser vaporizes tissues instantly. It does no damage to surrounding structures and has a maximum penetration depth of 0.1 mm.

Port-wine stains, telangiectasias, and cherry angiomas are treated with the pulsed dye laser, which penetrates 1 mm. It is selective for hemoglobin and pigmented tissue and can coagulate surface vessels precisely and safely.

The argon laser, which penetrates up to 6 mm, is used in dermatology to treat deep cavernous hemangiomas. It passes through water and is absorbed in tissue protein, resulting in deep coagulation.

Laser surgery has no associated restrictions for elderly patients or pregnant women. Because laser wavelengths are non-ionizing forms of radiation, laser light does not accumulate or cause cellular changes. Laser treatment has not been found to cause cancer.

Procedure

Local anesthesia is used for most laser procedures. Some procedures are performed after the operative area is numbed with ice.

Postoperative Course

After CO_2 laser surgery, the wound is cleaned with 3% hydrogen peroxide, and antibiotic ointment and a dry dressing are applied. Discomfort, usually treated effectively with non-narcotic analgesics or topical lidocaine, may occur 3 to 5 days postoperatively. Reepithelialization of the wound begins at the periphery and proceeds centrally, taking anywhere from 1 to 2 months depending on size and location. During the first 1 to 3 weeks of this process, as blood vessels regrow, spontaneous bleeding may occur. This is usually controlled easily by direct pressure.

The postoperative course after other types of laser surgery varies with the specific laser. For example, after surgery with a laser, that does not create an open wound, healing can occur in as few as 2 days. After tattoo removal, a scar similar to a burn scar remains.

NURSING PROCESS GUIDELINES
Dermatologic Laser Surgery

Be sure to assess the patient's expectations of the outcomes of surgery. If the patient has unrealistic expectations, alert the surgeon and provide additional information and discussion. Keep in mind that comprehensive preoperative teaching is essential for promoting patient compliance with safety procedures and preventing undue anxiety. Prepare the patient for expected sights and sounds. Clearly explain the need to wear protective goggles, the need to remain still, and the reason for the DANGER signs posted on the doors.

After the procedure, instruct the patient in self-care, as presented in Highlight 35–4.

Closure of Skin Wounds

Skin wounds can be closed in a variety of ways: simple side-to-side approximation, granulation, skin grafting, or use of skin flaps. The method of closure used varies with the size, type, and location of the wound, as well as the patient's general condition.

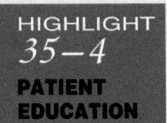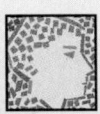

HIGHLIGHT 35–4
PATIENT EDUCATION

Self-Care After Dermatologic Carbon Dioxide Laser Surgery

Instruct the patient who has had a carbon dioxide laser procedure to:

Leave the initial pressure dressing in place for 24 hours.

Keep the site dry for 48 hours.

Clean the wound with hydrogen peroxide, and apply a thin layer of antibiotic ointment three times a day beginning 48 hours after surgery.

Keep the wound covered with a dry, sterile dressing, or cover only when the potential for exposure to contaminants exists, as directed by the physician's preference.

Take non-narcotic analgesics and apply 5% lidocaine ointment as directed for discomfort, which may occur 3 to 7 days postoperatively.

Accept as a normal occurrence spontaneous bleeding from the healing site for 1 to 3 weeks after surgery.

Apply direct pressure to control minor, spontaneous bleeding.

Recognize that clear, yellow drainage is normal and not a sign of infection.

Protect the wound from friction, which may cause blister formation until healing is complete in several months.

Inspect the healed area regularly to ensure early detection of recurrence.

SIDE-TO-SIDE APPROXIMATION

Suturing the edges of a wound together is the simplest method of closing a skin wound. The result is best when the wound is elliptic in shape, the edges of the wound are perpendicular, and the skin lines were followed in making the incision. An elliptic excision is illustrated in Figure 35–6.

Wounds closed by side-to-side approximation are dressed with adhesive bandages or gauze dressings. The patient is instructed to keep the wound dry for 24 hours and to return to the clinic if problems arise with bleeding, purulent drainage, or excessive pain. Acetaminophen is recommended for pain. Suture removal depends on the site and wound tension. Facial sutures are usually removed in 5 to 7 days.

GRANULATION

A wound is sometimes allowed to granulate in from the edges and heal by secondary intention. Healing by secondary intention is slower. Reliance on granulation depends on the size and anatomical location of the wound and patient preference.

SKIN FLAPS

A flap is tissue raised from one area of the body and transferred either to an adjacent area with its blood supply intact or to a distant site where the blood supply is re-established. The indications for flaps include the following:

- Replacing full-thickness tissue loss
- Covering densely scarred areas that have a compromised blood supply
- Covering exposed tendon, bone, or nerve
- Providing protection for delicate structures (such as vascular grafts in the groin)
- Providing coverage to reduce infection until final surgery can be performed

Flaps can be classified according to blood supply, location of donor tissue in relation to the defect, or anatomic composition. Flaps based on blood supply are classified as random-pattern or axial-pattern flaps. Random-pattern flaps consist of skin and subcutaneous tissue supplied with blood from random vessels. Axial-pattern flaps have a known arterial and venous blood supply.

Flaps based on location of the donor tissue in relation to the defect are described as local or distant. Local flaps are created from tissue adjacent to the defect. Distant flaps are designed in one area of the body and transferred to a defect in another area. Free flaps are a type of distant flap that are completely detached from the donor site and moved into a defect where a new blood supply is created by attaching vessels in the flap to vessels in the defect (Fig. 35–7).

Flaps based on anatomic composition are classified as skin, muscle, bone, fascia, omentum, or com-

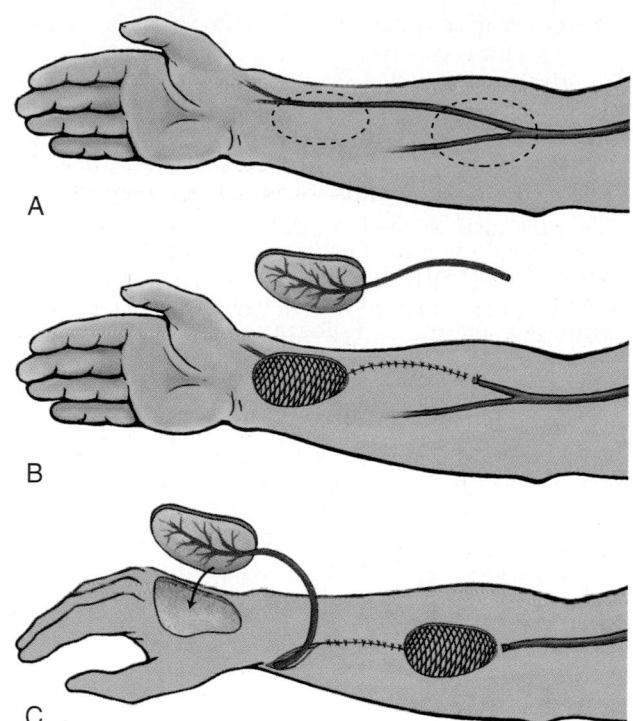

Figure 35–7

A, Possible donor sites for a flap to cover a defect on the back of the patient's hand. *B,* A free flap from the selected donor site. *C,* Flap with blood supply intact, ready to cover the defect. In *B* and *C,* the crosshatching indicates skin grafting of donor site. (Adapted from McCarthy JG [ed]. Plastic surgery. Vol. 1: General principles. Philadelphia: WB Saunders, 1990, p 297.)

posite grafts. A musculocutaneous flap is composed of skin and the underlying muscle.

The word *pedicle* is sometimes used to describe the tissue that houses the blood supply for a flap. In the past, flaps were transferred with long pedicles to cover defects. For example, the nose was reconstructed with tissue from the underside of the arm. A long pedicle flap was raised and the tissue sutured to the nose. Thus, the patient had the arm attached to the nose until a blood supply was re-established from local vessels. Today, the pedicle is seldom visible. It is tunneled through other tissues. For example, to reconstruct the breast, a surgeon may use a flap from the abdomen or back. The pedicle supplying blood to the tissue is located in the abdomen or axilla. It is imperative to understand where the blood supply is coming from for a flap, because no amount of pressure can be applied to the flap without risking necrosis of the tissues. Free flaps do not have a pedicle, because the surgeon has created a new blood supply for the tissues.

SKIN GRAFTS

Skin grafting transplants skin that has been totally detached from its blood supply in a donor site to a recipient site. This is done to cover defects that result from skin loss caused by trauma, burns, or excision of a cutaneous malignancy.

For a graft to "take"—attach and revascularize to the "bed" or recipient site—it must have a good blood supply and the grafted tissue must be immobilized. Shearing of the graft from the bed destroys any ingrowth of capillaries. Both the bed and the graft must also be free of infection.

Types of Skin Grafts by Source

Skin grafts are classified according to source as autografts, homografts (allografts), and heterografts (xenografts).

An autograft is skin transferred from a donor site to a recipient site on the same person. The donor site is the area of healthy, intact skin on the body from which the graft is taken. Although grafts are thin, the donor site is an open wound. Donor sites heal in about 2 weeks and can be used over and over. Only an autograft can supply permanent skin coverage.

A homograft, or allograft, is skin transplanted from one person to another. Most homografts come from cadavers because no advantages have been found in the use of living donors. Homografts usually remain attached for 3 to 10 weeks before sloughing off.

A heterograft, or xenograft, is skin transferred from an animal to a human. Heterografts are used to limit fluid loss, control temperature, decrease the risk of infection, and stimulate epithelialization. Most heterografts are porcine (pig skin). Because it is a foreign protein, the heterograft does not grow and is sloughed off in 3 to 7 days. A heterograft is replaced on a regular basis until the wound is healed or autografting is complete.

Because homografts and heterografts provide only temporary emergency cover for burns or other trauma, they are referred to as biologic dressings.

Types of Skin Grafts by Thickness

Skin grafts consist of epidermis and varying thicknesses of dermis (Fig. 35–8). Thus, they are divided into full-thickness and split-thickness grafts, depending on the number of skin layers taken from the donor site. The type of skin graft used is determined by the location and size of the defect and the desired cosmetic and functional result.

Full-thickness skin grafts are used to repair defects extending into the subcutaneous tissue, especially when the skin loss is on the face. Donor sites for full-thickness grafts include the retroauricular area, supraclavicular area, eyelids, abdomen, and thigh. The donor site is selected to best match skin color, texture, and hair growth on the recipient area. Because all skin layers are removed, donor sites must be sutured closed or covered with split-thickness skin grafts.

A full-thickness graft has less tendency to contract or to become hyperpigmented postoperatively and is functionally superior to a split-thickness graft in that it is more resistant to trauma.

Split-thickness skin grafts are used to cover large

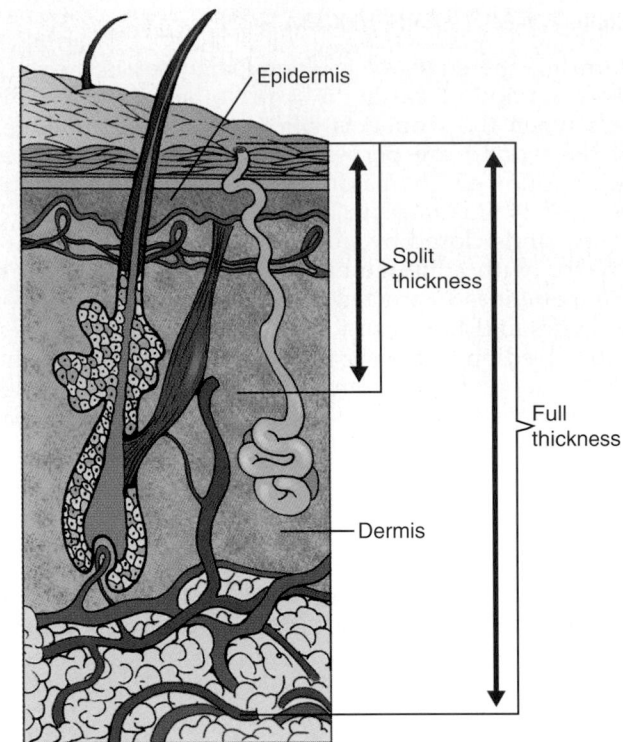

Figure 35–8

Cross-section of skin showing the depth of split-thickness and full-thickness grafts.

areas of denuded skin from burns and other trauma. Closure of wounds after excision of large, pigmented nevi or burn scars may also require a split-thickness skin graft. In some instances, a primary defect is covered with a flap and the secondary defect is covered with a split-thickness skin graft. The split-thickness graft revascularizes more rapidly and requires shorter immobilization to survive than a full-thickness skin graft. However, it is less resistant to trauma, tends to contract, lacks sensation, has impaired sweating ability, and has a poor cosmetic appearance. The anterior thigh is the most common donor site for split-thickness skin grafts.

Mesh grafts are thin split-thickness grafts with many tiny slits cut into the graft. The slits allow the graft to be stretched or expanded in two directions to 1.5 to 9 times its original size. Mesh grafts are used to cover extensive wounds or irregular surfaces, such as the ankle, that could not have otherwise been covered because of a lack of available donor sites (Fig. 35–9). Once the graft takes, epidermal cells grow into the spaces until the interstices have completely filled in. Use of a mesh graft also allows rapid closure of the wound and decreases the risk of infection. The graft can be held in place with sutures, staples, sterile tape, or dressings.

Autografting Procedure

A donor site is selected on the basis of the following:

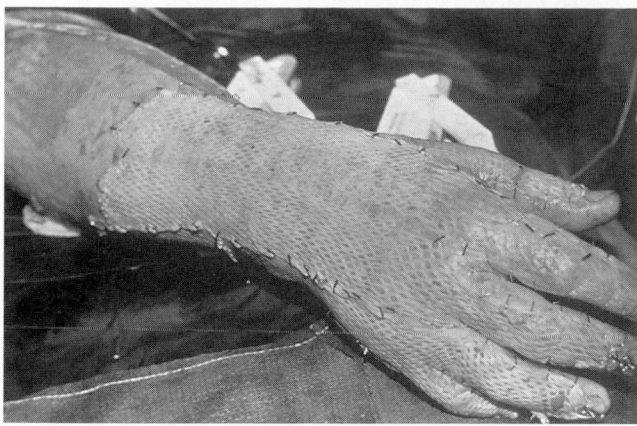

Figure 35–9

Mesh graft used to cover an extensive defect of the upper extremity.

- Healthy condition of the skin
- Match to the recipient site in terms of color, texture, and hair growth
- Inconspicuousness of its location

The graft is removed from the donor site with a dermatome or razor blade. It is then prepared and fitted to the recipient site, where it may or may not be sutured into place. Because a dry graft will lift off the wound or curl at the edges and will not take, the completed graft is usually covered with petrolatum-impregnated dressings and wrapped in several layers of roller gauze such as Kerlix to protect it and

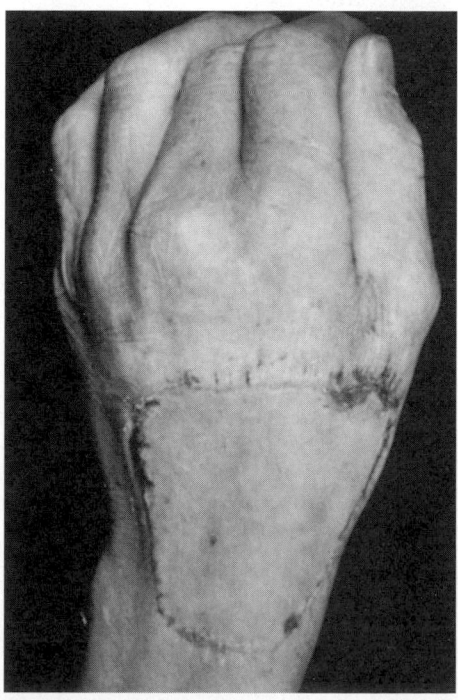

Figure 35–10

Typical appearance of a skin graft at 5 days, when "take" has been completed. (From Peacock EE. Wound repair. 3rd ed. Philadelphia: WB Saunders, 1984, p 223.)

to keep it from drying out. Depending on location, the graft site may also be splinted to keep adjacent joints from moving and dislodging the graft.

The donor site, which heals by re-epithelialization, may be covered with a transparent dressing for moist healing or with a single layer of nonadherent gauze for dry healing. Both types of dressing are covered with a pressure dressing for 24 to 48 hours to control bleeding.

Postgrafting Course

The surgeon performs the first dressing change of the graft site about 3 days after the grafting procedure. By this time, a successful graft, or a "take," appears pink and is attached to the bed of the wound. If the graft was meshed, the interstices show beginning signs of new epithelial cell growth (Fig. 35–10). Revascularization is indicated by pinkness of the graft.

NURSING PROCESS
Autografting

Assessment

Assess the condition of the dressings covering the graft site. Check that they are intact, and observe for purulent drainage or foul odor, which can indicate infection. Check peripheral circulation. Inspect any splints for proper application and placement. During dressing changes, assess the graft for adherence to the bed. Look for signs of epithelialization, vascularization, and new granulation. Be alert also for signs of infection, including redness of the skin surrounding the graft site. Inspect the donor site for signs of both healing and infection.

Assess the patient's compliance with instructions about care of the graft and donor sites, including maintaining immobility, preventing pressure on the sites, and keeping sites free from contamination.

Assess the patient's general physical and psychologic response to the procedure. Keep in mind that immobility can affect all body systems and that patients undergoing grafting are coping not simply with the stress of the procedure itself but with the stress of the trauma or disease that necessitated grafting. Thus, it is critical to assess the patient's anxiety level, coping skills, and sources of support.

Nursing Diagnoses and Planning

Nursing diagnoses and related expected patient outcomes commonly applicable to patients who have had skin grafting include the following:

NDx: Risk for infection related to multiple routes of possible invasion by microorganisms secondary to breaks in the skin

Planning: Patient Outcomes

1. Spreading erythema around the graft is absent.
2. Purulent drainage is absent.
3. Foul odor from the graft site is absent.

NDx: Risk for altered peripheral tissue perfusion (graft) related to trauma to the graft site

Planning: Patient Outcomes

1. Patient observes precautions, such as keeping the part elevated and free from pressure, designed to protect the graft.
2. Graft remains in close contact with its bed.
3. Graft is pink.

NDx: Pain related to surgical trauma at newly created donor sites

Planning: Patient Outcomes

1. Patient accepts medication and other comfort measures for pain.
2. Patient sleeps.
3. Patient states that pain is manageable or relieved.

NDx: Risk for altered health maintenance related to insufficient knowledge of self-care of grafts and protection of new skin

Planning: Patient Outcomes

1. Patient describes self-care measures.
2. Patient demonstrates care of the graft.
3. Patient verbalizes willingness and ability to perform required self-care.

When grafts or flaps are necessary because of extensive traumatic wounds or disfiguring surgery for cancer, many additional nursing diagnoses are likely to apply.

Nursing Interventions and Evaluation

NDx: Risk for infection
Use strict aseptic technique during graft care until the graft has taken. Wear cap, mask, gown, and sterile gloves. After the initial dressing change by the surgeon, remove dressings, gently clean the graft, and reapply dressings according to the surgeon's orders.

NDx: Risk for altered peripheral tissue perfusion
Maintain the patient on bed rest. Elevate the graft site to promote drainage from the area, thereby decreasing the risk of rupturing fragile new capillaries in the graft by increased intravascular pressure. Do not disturb the dressing, and take precautions to ensure that the dressing is not moved.

Position the patient off the graft and donor sites, and prevent any movement at these sites. Use prescribed splints to immobilize joints adjacent to the graft.

Use a bed cradle or other device to prevent sheets from lying on the graft or donor sites. If the patient has been undergoing physical therapy and tank or tubbing treatments before grafting, such therapy is discontinued until ordered resumed by the physician. It is resumed as soon as possible to maintain joint function and mobility.

NDx: Pain
Administer prescribed analgesics as needed. Remember that new donor sites are more painful than graft sites. Enhance the effect of analgesics by maintaining a restful atmosphere; offering comfort measures such as a back rub, washing the patient's mouth, face, and hands; and providing distraction, such as light music, if desired by the patient. Do not change the patient's position for comfort unless it can be done without moving or putting pressure on the graft site.

NDx: Risk for altered health maintenance
Instruct the patient on care of the graft and in protection of the new skin as it grows (Highlight 35–5).

Additional Interventions
Protect the selected donor site from injury and infection before surgery, if the site is known.

Compare the patient's status with the expected outcomes. If the outcomes are not met, reassess the patient and revise the plan.

Plastic Surgery Procedures

Plastic or reconstructive surgery is done to reconstruct defects from congenital or acquired disorders or to improve appearance or function. It can involve

---

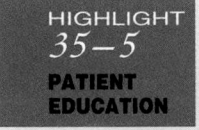 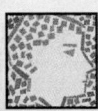

HIGHLIGHT
35–5

PATIENT EDUCATION

Self-Care of Grafts and Protection of New Skin

Instruct the patient to:

Wear pressure garments as directed over recipient site.

Elevate involved extremities.

Wear layers of clothing as needed to prevent cold injury.

Massage graft and donor sites with lanolin or cocoa butter to soften the skin, decrease itching, and increase circulation. Do this at least once a day for 2 to 18 months once the area is healed in 2 to 3 weeks.

Avoid exposure of the graft sites to sunlight, heat, or other potential sources of trauma. Because there is a loss of feeling in the area, risk of injury is increased.

Avoid exposure of the donor site to sunlight because the new skin has increased sensitivity.

Return for a follow-up visit on *(specify date and time)*.

Table 35–6

Common Plastic Surgery Procedures

Procedure	Description	Postoperative Course
Blepharoplasty	Correction of saggy, baggy, wrinkled eyelids by removing excess skin and fat Usually done as same-day surgery under local anesthesia	Iced compresses to reduce swelling and discoloration Topical antibiotics may be applied to sutures Sutures removed in 3 to 7 days
Rhytidoplasty/rhytidectomy (facelift)	Removal of facial wrinkles by separating skin from muscle, pulling it up and back, and removing excess Usually done as same-day surgery under local anesthesia	Rest for 24 hours with head elevated and neck straight (not flexed) to promote circulation and decrease edema and risk of bleeding Dressings removed in 3 to 5 days, face cleaned of crusted drainage, and topical antibiotic applied Swelling and bruising resolve over several weeks Effect not permanent
Liposuction	Removal of diet-resistant fat from such areas as neck, chin, abdomen, thighs, buttocks, and flanks to improve body contour A small cannula is inserted under the skin and moved back and forth as suction is applied to remove fat	Compression garment or tape is kept in place for 7 to 10 days Anticoagulants are contraindicated because of bleeding risk Change in body contour may not be apparent for 2 to 4 months because of edema

bone, muscles, cartilage, and nerves as well as skin. Plastic surgery performed primarily for aesthetic effect is often referred to as cosmetic surgery. Information about commonly performed plastic surgery procedures is presented in Table 35–6.

NURSING PROCESS GUIDELINES
Rhytidoplasty or Liposuction

Basic nursing care for a patient undergoing rhytidoplasty or liposuction is the same as for anyone undergoing a minor surgical procedure. Instructions for self-care at home following rhytidoplasty or liposuction are found in Highlights 35–6 and 35–7.

❖ Settings, Providers, and Collaboration for Care

Most dermatologic problems are associated with a negligible mortality rate and are more annoying than disabling. As a result, along with those treated by a dermatologist, many of these problems are self-treated or treated by the patient's primary physician as part of a general practice. Almost all dermatologic problems are managed in ambulatory care settings, such as physician offices or clinics. Exceptions to this include patients with major infections, dis-

eases that require aggressive steroids and other supporting therapy (such as pemphigus), or severe burns, and those undergoing extensive reconstructive or plastic procedures.

Because many dermatologic disorders are cyclic and chronic in nature, continuity of care is essential in supporting the patient in complying with therapy and coping with his or her disease. All caregivers need to understand the patient's lifestyle and life demands and how these affect the disease and its treatment. Caregivers also need to use the same methods and must all work toward the same goals. Collaboration of caregivers across settings and time is the means by which such continuity of care can be achieved.

The Elderly: Special Considerations

Skin changes throughout life are associated with aging, heredity, lifestyle, and environmental factors. As people age, the epidermis becomes thinner and has less water content. This results in dry skin. The activity of the sebaceous and apocrine glands decreases, which adds to the dry skin problem.

The dermis becomes less flexible and loses elasticity. Some of the fatty cushion is lost. These changes cause wrinkles and increased susceptibility to tear injuries. Fingernails and toenails become thicker and brittle. Additional details about age-related changes of the skin, hair, and nails are dis-

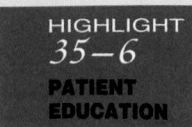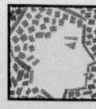

HIGHLIGHT 35–6
PATIENT EDUCATION
Self-Care After Rhytidoplasty

Instruct the patient to:

Rest for 48 hours and then gradually resume activities.

Avoid taking aspirin.

Avoid lifting and bending for 10 days because these actions encourage edema and bleeding.

Keep the head elevated when in bed, and avoid flexing the neck to prevent impaired circulation to the face.

Expect tightness in the face, and take non-narcotic analgesics as directed for discomfort.

Ingest liquids through a straw, progressing to a soft diet and then a regular diet when able to chew comfortably.

Shampoo hair when all sutures have been removed.

Use hair blow-dryer on warm only, because ears remain numb for some time and can be burned.

Expect face to appear swollen and bruised for several weeks.

Report signs of infection immediately: redness, increased pain, warmth, purulent drainage, fever, and chills.

Return for follow-up visit on *(specify date and time).*

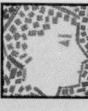

HIGHLIGHT 35–7
PATIENT EDUCATION
Self-Care After Liposuction

Instruct the patient to:

Rest for 12 hours and then gradually resume activities.

Remove the compression garment or tape in 7 to 10 days as directed by the surgeon.

Apply ice packs to affected area to reduce swelling.

Take nonaspirin pain relievers for discomfort.

Avoid consumption of alcohol and aspirin.

Return for follow-up visit and suture removal in 5 to 7 days.

Use discretion in eating to avoid weight gain.

---

cussed in Chapter 4. Blood vessels become more fragile with aging, resulting in ecchymosis and petechiae from minimal trauma. Common lesions that appear on the aging skin are described in Chapter 36.

Benign clinical features on sun-exposed areas include actinic keratosis, telangiectasia, open comedones, solar lentigines, and follicular cysts. Wrinkles, freckles, irregular pigmentation, and loss of elasticity also result from the cumulative effects of sun exposure. Skin changes associated with sun exposure can be minimized by protecting the skin throughout life. Measures to protect the skin include avoiding sunlight exposure between 10 AM and 3 PM, wearing protective clothing and hats, and using sunscreens of at least SPF 15.

Skin changes associated with smoking include lines or wrinkles on the face radiating at right angles from the upper and lower lips and corners of the eyes. There may be deep lines on the cheeks or numerous shallow lines on the cheeks and lower jaw. Facial features develop a subtle gauntness with a prominence of bony contours. "Smoker's face" has a leathery, worn, and rugged appearance.

Chapter Review

1. How does hemoglobin level affect the potential for cyanosis?
2. How does a nodule differ from a papule?
3. What do fissures, erosions, and ulcers have in common?
4. What questions would you ask a patient who arrives at the clinic because of a "rash"?
5. When assessing an African-American patient, you note a yellow tinge to the conjunctiva. What is the likely meaning of this observation?
6. How would you interpret a ++ reaction to a patch test?
7. What laboratory values would you expect to monitor monthly in a patient taking isotretinoin and why?
8. What are the similarities and differences between lotions and creams?
9. What self-care instructions must be given to patients receiving PUVA therapy?
10. Why is a dependent position contraindicated for an extremity with a new skin graft?

Bibliography

Arndt K, LeBoit P, Robinson J, Wintroub BU. Cutaneous medicine and surgery: An integrated program in dermatology. Philadelphia: WB Saunders, 1996.

Bacon P. Nutrition and skin care. Commun Nurse 1995; 1(7):34.

Baker T. Surgical rejuvenation of the face. St. Louis: Mosby–Year Book, 1993.

Barker MO. Sunscreens. Dermatol Nurs 1995; 7(4):247.

Bergmann K, Johannsen L. Liposuction: A surgical intervention to improve body contour. Dermatol Nurs 1994: 6(4):239.

Callen JP, Greer K, Hood A, et al. Color atlas of dermatology. Philadelphia: WB Saunders, 1993.

Drake LA, Dinehart SM, Goltz RW, et al. Guidelines of care for Mohs' micrographic surgery: American Academy of Dermatology. J Am Acad Dermatol 1995; 33(2, Pt 1):271.

Elbaz J. Liposuction and plastic surgery of the abdomen. Edinburgh: Churchill Livingstone, 1993.

Elson M (ed). Evaluation and treatment of the aging face. New York: Springer-Verlag, 1995.

Fosko S, Stecher J. The role of home health nursing: A dermatologic case study. Dermatol Nurs 1995; 7(3):185.

Grevey SC, Zax RH, McCall MW. Melanoma and Mohs' micrographic surgery. Adv Dermatol 1995; 10:175.

Haas AA. Wound healing. Dermatol Nurs 1995; 7(1):26.

Habif TP. Clinical dermatology. 3rd ed. St. Louis: Mosby–Year Book, 1996.

Hamra S. Composite rhytidectomy. St. Louis: Quality Medical Publishers, 1993.

Ho C, Nguyen Q, Lowe NJ, et al. Laser resurfacing in pigmented skin. Dermatol Surg 1995; 21:1035.

Lejour M. Vertical mammaplasty and liposuction. St. Louis: Quality Medical Publishers, 1994.

Lookingbill DP, Marks JG. Principles of dermatology. Philadelphia: WB Saunders, 1993.

Lynch PJ. Dermatology. 3rd ed. Baltimore: Williams & Wilkins, 1994.

Maksud DP, Anderson RC. Psychological dimensions of aesthetic surgery: Essentials for nurses. Plast Surg Nurs 1995; 15(3):137.

Matarasso A. Superficial suction lipectomy: Something old, something new, something borrowed. . . . Ann Plast Surg 1995; 34(3):268.

McConnell EA. Clinical do's and don'ts: Administering intradermal injections. Nursing 1996; 26(2):18.

Motley RJ. The technique of micrographic surgery for excising skin tumours. J Wound Care 1995; 4(8):380.

Murphy GF, Herzberg AJ. Atlas of dermatopathology. Philadelphia: WB Saunders, 1996.

Nicol N, Fenske N. Photodamage: Causes, clinical manifestations, and prevention. Dermatol Nurs 1993; 5(4):263.

Pitman GH. Liposuction. Dermatol Surg 1995; 21(5):441.

Psillakis J (ed). Deep face-lifting techniques. New York: Thieme Medical, 1994.

Ratner D, Grande D. Mohs' micrographic surgery: An overview. Dermatol Nurs 1994; 6(4):269.

Ruane-Morris M, Thompson G, Lawton S. Community liaison in dermatology. Prof Nurse 1995; 10(11):687.

Rumsfield J. Sunscreens: What you and your patients should know. Dermatol Nurs 1990; 2(3):139.

Sallavanti RA. Protecting your eyes in the laser operating room. Todays OR Nurse 1995; 17(4):23.

Schnur PL, Weinzweig J. A second look at the second-look technique in face lifts. Plast Reconstr Surg 1995; 96(7):1724.

Strzyzewski NM. The cycle of perioperative nursing care for plastic surgery patients. Plast Surg Nurs 1995; 15(2):78, 88.

Swartz S, Sheretz E. The technique of patch testing: Role of the office staff. Dermatol Nurs 1993; 5(2):133.

Talbot L, Curtis C. The challenges of assessing skin indicators in people of color. Home Healthcare Nurse 1996; 14(3):167.

Whyte A. Pre and postoperative evaluation of patients undergoing cutaneous surgery. Dermatol Nurs 1994; 6(4):248.

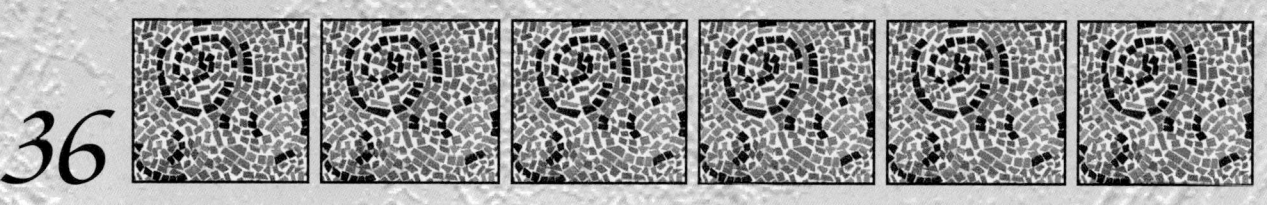

36

Nursing Care of Patients with Integumentary Disorders

Study Outcomes

After studying this chapter, you should be able to:

1. Describe the etiology, pathophysiology, clinical manifestations, diagnostic procedures, and management of common skin disorders.
2. Identify information and physical examination data essential to the assessment of patients with common skin disorders.
3. State nursing diagnoses and related expected patient outcomes commonly applicable to patients with skin disorders.
4. Describe nursing interventions, with their rationales, commonly applicable to patients with skin disorders.
5. Explain the basis for evaluation of nursing care provided to patients with common skin disorders.
6. Identify alternative treatment and care settings for patients with common skin disorders and state the services related to community-based care.
7. Identify special considerations for the elderly patient with a skin disorder.

Skin disorders are a major cause of disability, disfigurement, and discomfort. Nearly everyone suffers from some type of skin disorder at some point. It may be localized or disseminated, asymptomatic or accompanied by severely distressing symptoms. It may be infectious or caused by exposure to sunlight, an allergen, or an irritant. For many disorders, the cause is unknown. Skin changes also accompany a variety of systemic disorders and often are the first manifestation of the underlying problem. Because many skin disorders are chronic and can be disfiguring, patients require not only sound physical care but also consistent encouragement and emotional support.

*I*nfections

Most pathogenic organisms that cause skin infections reach the skin by an external route. The stratum corneum usually provides a barrier to invading organisms. When this barrier is altered and invading organisms enter, the body's secondary immunologic barrier localizes the infection and prevents systemic invasion. Most people recover completely from acute infectious skin ailments. However, some suffer from chronic skin infections. These can result from poor hygiene, chronic irritation that alters the physical barrier, or an immunologic defect.

BACTERIAL INFECTIONS

Common bacterial infections of the skin include folliculitis (Fig. 36–1), furuncle, carbuncle, abscess, impetigo (Fig. 36–2), cellulitis (Fig. 36–3), erysipelas, and paronychia. The etiology, pathophysiology, clinical manifestations, diagnosis, and management of each of these infections appear in Table 36–1.

NURSING PROCESS
Bacterial Skin Infection

Assessment

When assessing a patient with a bacterial skin infection, obtain a complete history, including duration of the lesions and personal and family history of similar lesions. Ask about associated subjective symptoms, such as tenderness or pruritus. Determine whether trauma or insect bites preceded the inflammation. Review personal hygiene practices. Note the brand names of cleaning and cosmetic agents.

Examine the patient to assess and document objective symptoms: the types of lesions present, the extent of involvement of the primary disorder, and the presence of secondary infection. Note the appearance of lesions and their number, configuration, and distribution. Mark them on a body outline to aid in tracking the course of the disorder.

Determine the patient's understanding of and emotional response to the disease process and the prescribed treatment. Also assess understanding of factors that may contribute to the disease process, such as poor hygiene, tight-fitting clothing, fiber

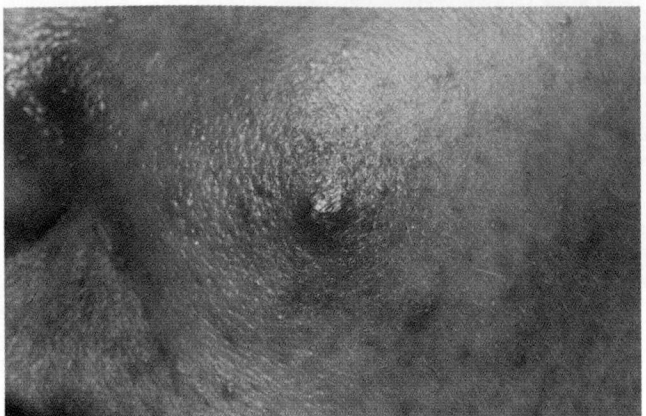

Figure 36-1

Folliculitis. (From Murphy GF, Herzberg AJ. Atlas of dermatopathology. Philadelphia: WB Saunders, 1996, p. 102.)

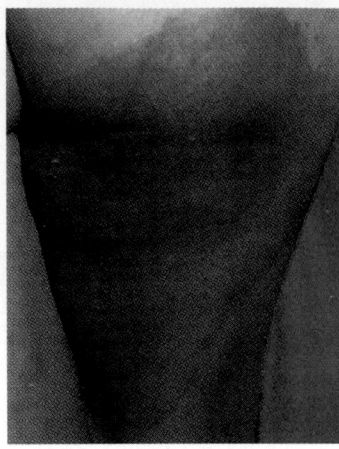

Figure 36-3

Deep red, swollen, tender area characteristic of cellulitis. (From Lookingbill DP, Marks JG. Principles of dermatology. 2nd ed. Philadelphia: WB Saunders, 1993, p. 232.)

content of clothing, trauma to the skin, maceration caused by obesity, and use of occlusive cosmetics.

Assess the patient's physical, psychologic, and financial ability to comply with prescribed hygiene and other self-care treatments. If needed, assess whether significant others or community resources are available to help with self-care.

Nursing Diagnoses and Planning

Nursing diagnoses and related expected patient outcomes commonly applicable to patients with a bacterial skin infection include the following:

NDx: Impaired skin integrity related to the presence of lesions

Planning: Patient Outcomes
1. Skin lesions clear.

NDx: Risk for infection related to spread

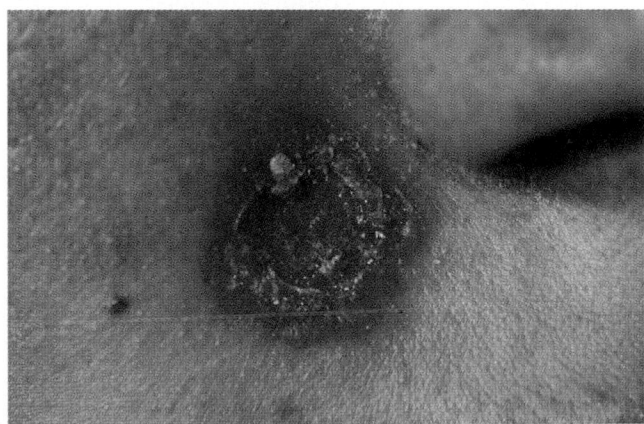

Figure 36-2

Vesicular impetigo characterized by a thick, honey-yellow adherent crust covering the eroded surface. (From Murphy GF, Herzberg AJ. Atlas of dermatopathology. Philadelphia: WB Saunders, 1996, p. 98.)

Planning: Patient Outcomes
1. Patient describes measures to reduce the risk of spread.
2. Infection remains localized.

NDx: Risk for altered health maintenance related to insufficient knowledge of prevention of and early intervention for recurrence

Planning: Patient Outcomes
1. Patient describes measures to reduce risk of recurrence.
2. Patient has no recurrences.
3. Patient identifies signs of recurrence and the importance of early treatment.

Nursing Interventions and Evaluation

NDx: Impaired skin integrity

Instruct the patient to apply warm, moist compresses for 20 minutes three times daily to increase circulation and hasten healing. Urge the patient to use astringent compresses made with aluminum acetate (Burow's) solution to promote drying. Stress the importance of allowing the area to dry thoroughly between compresses by wearing loose-fitting, porous clothing and by proper positioning to allow air circulation to the area.

NDx: Risk for infection

Instruct the patient in self-administration of prescribed systemic and topical antibiotics. Also instruct him or her in self-care to prevent the spread of infection, as presented in Highlight 36-1. Stress the need to avoid scratching as an important deterrent to spread. In an institutional setting, follow isolation precautions to limit the spread of organisms to other patients.

Advise the patient to notify the physician immediately of any increase in redness, tenderness, odor, or drainage, or if the infection is not significantly better in 2 or 3 days.

Table 36–1

Common Bacterial Infections of the Skin

Infection	Etiology and Pathophysiology	Clinical Manifestations	Diagnosis and Management
Folliculitis	Superficial infection of the hair follicle usually caused by *Staphylococcus aureus*. Predisposing factors include open wounds, maceration, dirt, friction, tight-fitting clothing, occlusive cosmetics, and ointments. Bacteria enter through hair follicle and infect epidermal lining, resulting in pustule formation. May spread to new areas through inoculation by the fingernails.	Single or multiple papules and pustules with central hair (see Fig. 36–1).	*Diagnosis:* Based on clinical appearance. Culture may confirm presence of *S. aureus.* *Management:* Daily cleaning with chlorhexidine gluconate (Hibiclens) or povidone-iodine (Betadine) for several weeks. If extensive, systemic antibiotics (such as erythromycin or dicloxacillin) for 7–10 days.
Furuncle (boil)	Deep folliculitis usually caused by *S. aureus.* Predisposing factors include repeated irritation, pressure, friction, heavy perspiration.	Small, red, elevated, tender nodule.	*Diagnosis:* Based on clinical appearance. Exudate may be cultured to identify causative organism. *Management:* Hot, wet compresses qid. Incision and drainage for painful lesions. Should not be squeezed because this can force pathogens deeper into the tissues. Systemic antibiotics and topical antiseptic agents are used for furunculosis. In chronic cases, antibiotic ointment may be applied to the nares once daily as prophylaxis.
Carbuncle	Large pus-filled mass in the dermis that drains purulent exudate through several points on the surface. Forms when furuncles develop in adjoining hair follicles and coalesce. Occur most often where the skin is thick and inelastic, such as the back of the neck and buttocks.	Painful, red, swollen area with multiple pustules. Fever and malaise are common. Leukocytosis may occur.	*Diagnosis:* Based on clinical appearance and bacterial culture. *Management:* Immobilization of the affected area and systemic antibiotic therapy. Carbuncles are never manipulated or incised to avoid spreading the infection.
Abscess	Similar to a furuncle except it usually results from traumatic inoculation of bacteria through a puncture wound, laceration, or surgical incision.	Tender red nodules that enlarge and become increasingly painful. Regional lymph node involvement is common.	*Diagnosis:* Based on clinical appearance. Exudate may be cultured to identify causative organism. *Management:* Hot, wet compresses qid. Incision and drainage for painful lesions. Should not be squeezed because this can force pathogens deeper into the tissues. Systemic antibiotics and topical antiseptic agents are used. In chronic cases, antibiotic ointment may be applied to the nares once daily as prophylaxis.

(continued)

Table 36–1

Common Bacterial Infections of the Skin *(continued)*

Infection	Etiology and Pathophysiology	Clinical Manifestations	Diagnosis and Management
Impetigo	Superficial skin infection caused by *S. aureus* or group A streptococci. Pustules form as part of the inflammatory response. When they break, crusted lesions form. Healing occurs without scarring.	Honey-colored crusts on an erythematous base. Areas beneath the crusts are glistening, weeping, and eroded. Usually occurs on the face (see Fig. 36–2).	*Diagnosis:* Based on appearance. A culture may be obtained from a weeping erosion after the crust is removed. *Management:* Oral antibiotics, usually erythromycin or dicloxacillin for 7–10 days. Crusts removed by gentle scrubbing with chlorhexidine. Antiseptic ointment is applied. If caused by *Streptococcus*, patient is monitored for glomerulonephritis.
Cellulitis	Deep infection of the skin and subcutaneous tissue usually caused by group A streptococci or *S. aureus*. Bacteria enter the dermis through a break in the skin or by means of the bloodstream. Inflammation results and spreads horizontally through the tissues. Impaired lymphatic circulation secondary to the infection or from lymph node resection or radiation therapy predisposes to recurrent episodes.	Involved area is warm, red, swollen and painful. Systemic symptoms include fever, malaise, chills, leukocytosis with a left shift, and a slightly elevated sedimentation rate. Occurs most often in the lower legs (see Fig. 36–3).	*Diagnosis:* Based on clinical appearance and laboratory findings. *Management:* Bedrest and elevation of the affected area. Parenteral antibiotics for severe cases; oral antibiotics for mild cases. Resolves in about 2 weeks with treatment. Long-term prophylactic antibiotics may be given for recurrent episodes.
Erysipelas	Acute inflammatory form of cellulitis with significant lymphatic involvement. Usually caused by *S. aureus*. As infection spreads, vesicles and bullae may form over a large area. May cause subcutaneous abscess and widespread infection.	Red, hot, shiny, indurated, tender area of skin with a sharp advancing border and streaking (red lines along lymphatic vessels in the direction of the lymph nodes). Most common on the lower legs, face, and ears.	*Diagnosis:* Based on clinical appearance and laboratory findings. *Management:* Bedrest and elevation of the affected area. Parenteral antibiotics for severe cases, oral antibiotics for mild cases. Resolves in about 2 weeks with treatment. Long-term prophylactic antibiotics may be given for recurrent episodes.
Paronychia	Acute or chronic infection of the nail fold usually caused by *S. aureus*. Acute form usually results from trauma. Chronic form occurs when hands are repeatedly exposed to moisture.	*Acute:* sudden edema, redness, and throbbing pain, most often in second or third finger. *Chronic:* Mild swelling, tenderness, redness involving all or several fingers.	*Diagnosis:* Culture may be done to identify the causative organism. *Management:* For acute form, incision and drainage with systemic antibiotics. For chronic form, keep hands dry and apply topical thymol solution until cuticle regrows.

NDx: Risk for altered health maintenance
Instruct the patient to shower and shampoo daily with an antibacterial soap to eliminate the causative pathogen from the skin. Review the medical prescription and instructions for prophylactic antibiotic therapy. Teach the patient to avoid contributing factors, such as bath or hair oils, occlusive cosmetics, laundry softeners, tight-fitting clothing, and obesity.

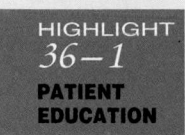 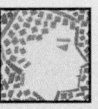

HIGHLIGHT 36–1
PATIENT EDUCATION
Preventing the Spread of Bacterial Skin Infections

Instruct the patient to:

Refrain from squeezing or otherwise manipulating skin lesions because this can rupture the wall of tissue formed in the body's effort to localize the infection.

Wash hands thoroughly before and after treating the infected area.

Clean surrounding skin with an antibacterial soap.

Apply a thin layer of any ordered antibiotic ointment to the surrounding skin.

Wash all clothing and linens that come in contact with the lesion in hot, soapy water after each use.

Keep wounds covered with a dry dressing after incision and drainage.

Dispose of soiled dressings by wrapping in paper and burning, if possible.

Avoid scratching lesions.

Avoid sharing towels or other linens.

Teach the patient how to recognize early recurrence of infection, and stress the importance of seeking immediate treatment.

Additional Interventions
Instruct the patient about immobilizing affected areas and limits on activity. Stress the importance of good nutrition to promote healing. Refer for home care if the patient needs frequent evaluation or does not have the knowledge or ability to manage the condition at home.

Compare the patient's status with the expected outcomes. If the outcomes are not met, reassess the patient and revise the plan.

Necrotizing Fasciitis

Necrotizing fasciitis is a Group A streptococcal infection of the fascia and adjacent tissues. It is called a "flesh-eating disease" because of the rapid, massive tissue destruction that it causes.

Etiology and Pathophysiology
The Group A streptococcal infection responsible for necrotizing fasciitis usually develops following a traumatic injury that causes a break in the skin. The injury need not be large; it may simply be a small cut. Factors that place individuals at particular risk

for this infection include diabetes mellitus, obesity, arteriosclerosis, alcoholism, and intravenous drug abuse. Necrotizing fasciitis occasionally occurs postoperatively in apparently healthy individuals and, in a few cases, in healthy individuals without any history of traumatic injury.

The tissue destruction of necrotizing fasciitis is due to toxins secreted by the infecting organism in the tissue beneath the skin. These toxins contain enzymes that break down protein. Necrosis progresses from the superficial fascia to the subcutaneous fat, which contains nerves, arteries, and veins, and may even extend to the muscle and epidermis. As this destruction progresses, gas accumulates in the muscle and a characteristic odor becomes apparent on the fourth or fifth day of infection.

Clinical Manifestations
Necrotizing fasciitis has an acute onset. Initially the skin around the wound appears red and shiny. Pain, often described as heavy, is much more severe than would be expected based on the appearance of the wound. A low-grade fever (38°–38.5°C [100.4°–101.3°F]), tachycardia greater than 120 beats per minutes, mild leukocytosis, and hematocrit of less than 36% are other findings. As the infection progresses, the erythema spreads and severe edema develops. The skin in the affected area becomes bluish-purple, and blisters filled with yellow fluid appear. "Dishwater" pus, which is a foul-smelling watery fluid resulting from the necrosis of fat and other tissue, develops. Numbness replaces severe pain as nerves in the subcutaneous tissue are destroyed. Creatinine phosphokinase becomes elevated secondary to muscle necrosis, and septic shock may ensue.

Diagnosis
Necrotizing fasciitis is diagnosed based on clinical presentation. Culture and Gram stain of necrotic tissue demonstrate Group A streptococci. Gas in the tissue is seen on radiographs as a feathery pattern.

Management
Management is aimed at preventing progression of the infection and development of septic shock. Surgical débridement of all necrotic tissue is done and antibiotic therapy instituted. Broad-spectrum antibiotics are used because multiple bacteria are typically found in the wound. The drug of choice is penicillin, up to 40 million units IV. For patients allergic to penicillin, metronidazole (Flagyl), clindamycin phosphate (Cleocin), an aminoglycoside, or a combination of these is used. If surgical débridement is not possible, hyperbaric therapy in addition to antibiotic treatment may be tried. Fluids, electrolytes, colloids, and blood products are given as needed to stabilize hemodynamic status, since extracellular fluid may accumulate in the interstitium. If septic shock develops, management is as described in Chapter 11.

NURSING PROCESS GUIDELINES
Necrotizing Fasciitis

Maintain the patient on strict contact precautions because Group A streptococcal infection is highly contagious. Medicate for pain. Because pain is so severe, arrange for PCA if appropriate for the patient. Since necrotizing fasciitis is a rapidly progressing disease (1 inch of flesh per hour can be destroyed), mark and date the area of erythema or necrosis with a skin marker every 2 hours. Monitor for signs of developing shock: check for drop in systolic blood pressure, tachycardia, weak peripheral pulses, urinary output decreased to less than 30 mL per hour, and capillary refill longer than 3 seconds. Also monitor for an allergic reaction to antibiotics. Change dressings on débrided wounds every 4 hours and as necessary using strict sterile technique. Usually a wet to dry dressing containing hydrogen peroxide or saline and an antibiotic is ordered. Mark the size of the wound and note odor, amount of drainage, and appearance of surrounding skin at each dressing change. Immediately report increased drainage odor, wound extension, or bleeding. Provide nutrition as ordered with calories up to twice the normal requirement. Initially, parenteral hyperalimentation or tube feedings are usual with oral foods and fluids resumed when tolerated. Psychologic support for both the patient and the family is critical, given the serious and often fatal nature of this disease.

FUNGAL INFECTIONS

Fungal infections are classified as dermatophyte (tinea) and nondermatophyte (yeast) infections.

Dermatophyte Infections

Etiology and Pathophysiology
Dermatophytes cause superficial fungal infections of the skin and its appendages. These dermatophytes produce keratinase, an enzyme that breaks down keratin. They live only on dead keratin, the main constituent of the hair, nails, and outer horny layer of the skin. Dermatophyte infections, referred to in lay language as ringworm, are classified according to the area of the body involved (Table 36–2).

The source of the infecting organism may be another person, an animal, or soil. Dermatophytes that grow only on humans are called anthropophilic; those that grow on animals, zoophilic; and those that live in the soil, geophilic. Zoophilic and geophilic dermatophytes may infect humans. Dermatophyte infections are most often spread by direct contact, although spread through fomites, such as combs and bed linens, also occurs. Factors that increase susceptibility to dermatophyte infection include a warm, humid environment and a break in the stratum corneum.

When infected by a dermatophyte, the stratum corneum becomes thickened and infiltrated with fungal hyphae (threadlike elements of the mycelium of the fungus). There may be inflammation in the dermis. Slow-growing dermatophytes affect only the stratum corneum, with no dermal inflammation. Zoophilic dermatophytes cause more skin inflammation than anthropophilic dermatophytes. Dermatophyte infections do not invade beyond the epidermis because they depend on keratin and because human serum is fungistatic.

Clinical Manifestations
A major characteristic of a tinea infection is its active border. This border is red, scaly, and slightly elevated. It surrounds a central area that usually is paler in color than adjacent nonaffected skin. This characteristic appearance is the reason tinea is commonly known as ringworm.

Table 36–2 describes clinical manifestations by site of infection on the body. Figure 36–4 illustrates two types of dermatophyte infection.

Diagnosis
Diagnosis is based on the clinical presentation and the finding of hyphae on a potassium hydroxide (KOH) preparation. KOH positivity is diagnostic of a fungal infection.

Table 36–2

Classification of Dermatophyte Infections by Site and Clinical Manifestations

Infection	Site	Clinical Manifestations
Tinea capitis	Scalp	Noninflammatory tinea capitis: scaling area with broken hair shafts Inflammatory tinea capitis: plaques, pustules, lymphadenopathy, possible scarring, and possible permanent hair loss
Tinea corporis	Body, arms, legs	Elevated, scaling, erythematous, serpiginous border with central clearing
Tinea cruris	Groin	Sharply demarcated area with elevated, scaling, serpiginous borders
Tinea pedis	Feet	Interdigital maceration or diffuse scaling on soles and sides of feet or vesicles and pustules on instep
Tinea manuum	Hand	Dry, scaling hyperkeratotic lesions, usually on only one palm
Tinea unguium (onychomycosis)	Nails	Separation from the nail bed with debris under the nail

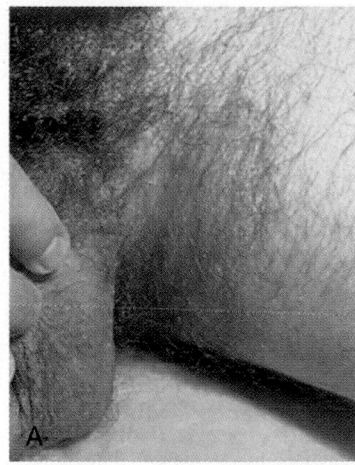

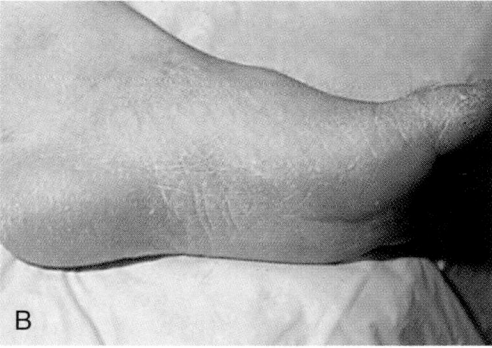

Figure 36-4

A, Tinea cruris. Note sharply marginated scaling border. *B*, Chronic tinea pedis. Note diffuse plantar scaling in moccasin distribution. (From Lookingbill DP, Marks JG. Principles of dermatology. 2nd ed. Philadelphia: WB Saunders, 1993, pp. 145–146.)

Management

Topical agents are prescribed for most tinea infections. The imidazole creams are antifungal agents that can be applied twice daily for 1 to 2 weeks after cleaning the area with soap and water. If the area is severely inflamed, with vesicles or bullae, wet soaks may be used. Four to 6 weeks of treatment, perhaps more, may be required. Systemic antifungal agents, such as griseofulvin, are prescribed for widespread fungal disease, tinea capitis, and tinea unguium (onychomycosis).

NURSING PROCESS
Dermatophyte Infection

ASSESSMENT

Inspect the involved areas. Note the appearance, number, and location of lesions. Ask about associated symptoms, such as itching. Have the patient describe when and how the lesions developed. Ask about at-home treatment, including use of over-the-counter preparations. Determine whether any household member or other contact person has a similar infection and whether the patient has pets or has recently been exposed to other animals. When the affected area is the groin or the foot, explore the type and frequency of athletic activity.

Nursing Diagnoses and Planning

Nursing diagnoses and related expected patient outcomes commonly applicable to patients with a dermatophyte infection include the following:

NDx: Impaired skin integrity related to open lesions secondary to dermatophyte infection

Planning: Patient Outcomes
1. Patient describes or demonstrates prescribed therapeutic measures.
2. Lesions heal.

NDx: Risk for altered health maintenance related to insufficient knowledge of prevention of spread and recurrence of tinea infection

Planning: Patient Outcomes
1. Patient lists basic precautions to be taken to prevent spread to others.
2. Patient describes preventive measures.

Nursing Interventions and Evaluation

NDx: Impaired skin integrity
Explain the importance of keeping the area clean, dry, and free from irritation. Instruct the patient to use a clean washcloth and towel daily and to pat the skin dry thoroughly, paying particular attention to skin-fold areas. Encourage exposure of the affected areas to air as often as possible. Instruct the patient to apply the prescribed topical agent twice daily until the skin is clear and then for 2 weeks more. Stress that it may take 4 to 6 weeks, possibly longer, for the lesions to clear. Caution the patient against becoming discouraged and stopping the treatment.

NDx: Risk for altered health maintenance
To prevent spread of the infection, instruct the patient to wash his or her hands thoroughly after touching the affected area. Tell the patient to avoid tight-fitting clothing that chafes or occludes the area. Clothes should be absorbent (cotton) rather than synthetic. Powders should not be allowed to cake in skin folds. Teach the patient measures to prevent recurrence (Highlight 36–2).

Additional Interventions
If itching is a problem, suggest application of cool compresses. Suggest sitz baths for tinea cruris. Provide instruction on how to protect family and other contacts from the infection.

Compare the patient's status with the expected outcomes. If the outcomes are not met, reassess the patient and revise the plan.

Nondermatophyte Infections

Infections caused by nondermatophytes, or yeast fungal infections, include candidiasis and tinea versicolor.

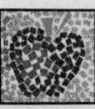

Preventing Recurrence of Dermatophyte Infections

Instruct the patient to take the following measures to keep skin clean and dry:

Bathe daily, preferably after activities causing exertion and sweating.

Dry skin thoroughly, paying particular attention to intertriginous and interdigital areas.

Apply talc or antifungal powder once a day if needed to control moisture.

Place cotton wads between toes at night if needed to absorb moisture and to prevent maceration.

Avoid tight-fitting clothing, which decreases air circulation and creates a warm, moist environment.

Wear cotton underwear and socks to promote air circulation and absorption of moisture.

Change clothes frequently.

Launder clothing and linens in hot water.

Avoid wearing a wet bathing suit for a prolonged period.

Wear leather sandals or other footwear that allows air circulation over the feet.

Avoid wearing the same shoes 2 days in a row.

Avoid plastic shoes, sneakers, or other footwear that hold moisture.

Avoid sharing combs, brushes, hats, clothing, or personal linens.

CANDIDIASIS

Candidiasis (moniliasis) is an inflammatory reaction caused by *Candida albicans* infection in the epidermis.

Etiology and Pathophysiology

C. albicans is present normally on the skin and in the gastrointestinal tract, mouth, and vagina. When it penetrates and colonizes the surface of the skin or mucous membrane, it becomes pathogenic. Factors that predispose to candidiasis include pregnancy, use of oral contraceptives, diabetes, antibiotic or topical corticosteroid therapy, and depression of cell-mediated immunity, as in acquired immunodeficiency syndrome (AIDS) or chemotherapy. The elderly and patients with cancer, particularly leukemia, appear to be at increased risk.

C. albicans penetrates only the outer layers of the skin or mucous membrane. The toxins it releases cause an acute inflammatory response. The primary lesion is a pustule whose contents spread under the stratum corneum and peel it away.

Clinical Manifestations

The infected skin area appears glistening, fiery red, or moist pink and may be surrounded by erythematous papules, a border fringe of white scale, and satellite pustules, which are so called because they are outside the area of opposing skin surfaces (Fig. 36–5). The patient has severe itching and burning.

Skin-fold areas are affected most often because they provide the warm, moist environment that yeast need to grow. These include the perianal area, groin, toe webs, and areas under pendulous breasts or between abdominal folds. Candidiasis affecting these areas is referred to as *Candida* intertrigo. In acute oral candidiasis (thrush), the mucosa typically is red and sore, with a white, creamy exudate or adherent white plaques, although a variety of presentations can occur. The tongue is almost always involved. In addition, candidiasis can cause chronic paronychia (nail infection).

Diagnosis

Candidiasis is diagnosed based on the presenting symptoms and a KOH preparation that shows hyphae. A Wood's lamp may also be used to visualize fungal spores, which show blue-green on the skin under the light.

Management

Most intertriginous candidal infections are treated with topical agents, including the imidazole derivatives and nystatin. They are applied sparingly twice daily.

NURSING PROCESS GUIDELINES
Candidiasis

The assessment, nursing diagnoses, expected patient outcomes, nursing interventions, and evaluation for

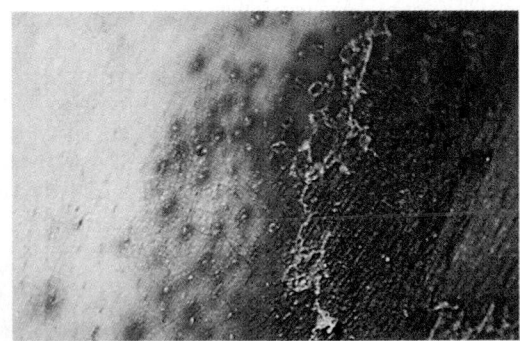

Figure 36–5

Candidiasis. Beefy red erythema with satellite papules and pustules. Note fringe of scale at edges of lesion. (From Lookingbill DP, Marks JG. Principles of dermatology. 2nd ed. Philadelphia: WB Saunders, 1993, p. 199.)

patients with candidiasis are similar to those described previously for patients with a dermatophyte infection, with several additional considerations. Assess carefully for factors that decrease host resistance, because candidiasis usually is an opportunistic infection. These factors include immunosuppressive drug therapy, antibiotic therapy, diabetes, cancer, and nutritional problems. If the patient with candidiasis has limited mobility, position him or her to maintain good air circulation to the affected and at-risk areas. For example, place a pillow between the patient's knees or under each arm to support them away from the chest walls and allow air circulation to the axillae.

TINEA VERSICOLOR

Tinea versicolor is a common, chronic disorder that causes hypopigmentation or loss of skin color. It is seen worldwide but is most common in hot, tropical climates. Tinea versicolor is not known to be contagious.

Etiology and Pathophysiology
The term *tinea* is a misnomer because tinea versicolor is a nondermatophyte infection. It is caused by the yeast *Pityrosporum orbiculare*, which is part of the normal skin flora. It occurs in greatest numbers in areas of sebaceous glands. Factors that may predispose to infection include high heat and humidity, malnutrition, burns, corticosteroid therapy, pregnancy, and oral contraception.

The spores of the yeast proliferate in the outer layers of the stratum corneum. Infection occurs when the spores are transformed to hyphae, which penetrate deeper in the stratum corneum, resulting in thickening and scaling of the stratum corneum. It is not known whether hypopigmentation occurs from thickened infected stratum corneum, which may block out ultraviolet (UV) rays, or whether it results from enzymes acting on surface lipids, thus inhibiting the enzyme responsible for melanin production.

Clinical Manifestations
The lesions of tinea versicolor are macular and vary in size, shape, and color. Typically, they begin as multiple small, round macules that enlarge radially to become confluent patches. They may cover the upper trunk, lower abdomen, and proximal portions of the extremities. After sun exposure, the infected skin does not tan.

Diagnosis
Tinea versicolor is diagnosed based on clinical presentation and the finding of hyphae on a KOH preparation.

Management
Tinea versicolor is treated primarily for cosmetic reasons. Antifungal creams are effective, but the lesion recurs as soon as treatment is stopped. If the infection is widespread, it is more economical to treat with selenium sulfide shampoo.

Oral ketaconazole eliminates lesions for 6 to 9 months. However, the drug carries the risk of hepatotoxicity.

NURSING PROCESS GUIDELINES
Tinea Versicolor

Assess the patient's knowledge of the skin condition. Determine how long the lesions have been present. Examine the entire skin to determine the extent of the lesions. Ask the patient whether any past treatments have been successful or unsuccessful. Determine the patient's ability and interest in self-management of this skin condition.

Explain that, although tinea versicolor is caused by a fungus, it is not contagious and can be controlled. Teach the patient how to use selenium sulfide shampoo and apply antifungal creams as follows:

- Apply selenium sulfide shampoo to the trunk, arms, and thighs in the shower. Leave it on for 10 minutes and then rinse it off. Do this three nights in a row, then weekly, then every 2 to 3 weeks as needed to maintain control.
- Apply antifungal cream in a thin layer to the affected skin areas. Because the entire trunk may be affected, explain that the cream may be applied using the palms of the hands and downward strokes. Inform the patient that applicators to reach the back can be purchased in drug stores specializing in skin-care products.

If oral ketaconazole is prescribed, be sure to explore and document any history of liver disease and alcohol use because the drug can be hepatotoxic. Explain that it may take several months for hypopigmented areas to clear.

VIRAL INFECTIONS

Viral infections of the skin are caused by papovavirus, poxvirus, and herpesvirus.

Warts

One of the most common skin ailments, warts (or verrucae) are benign epidermal neoplasms. They occur most commonly between ages 12 and 16.

Etiology and Pathophysiology
Warts are caused by infection with human papillomavirus (HPV). HPV is a subgroup of deoxyribonucleic acid (DNA)–containing papovaviruses that replicates in the epidermis. The altered DNA stimulates epidermal thickening and hyperkeratosis. Different HPV strains are responsible for different types of lesions.

Warts are transmitted by touch. Plantar warts are usually transmitted between young adults using common showers. Numerous warts may develop around a single primary wart through autoinoculation. Warts are commonly found on the hands secondary to nail biting or other trauma.

Clinical Manifestations

Warts are characterized by epidermal thickening and hyperkeratosis (Fig. 36–6). They interrupt normal skin lines and may have small red dots from thrombosed capillaries or small black dots, hemosiderin, on their surfaces. The clinical manifestations of the different types of warts and their most common locations are listed in Table 36–3.

Diagnosis

Most warts are diagnosed by appearance. They undergo biopsy only if there is suspicion of squamous cell cancer. Darkfield examination and serology tests may be done if the lesions are suspected to be condylomata lata associated with secondary syphilis. HPV has not been cultured, and HPV typing is experimental at this time.

Management

Medical treatment involves destruction of the infected keratinocytes and is about 80% effective. Although two-thirds of all warts disappear in 2 years without treatment, their unsightly appearance and awkward locations prompt many people to seek treatment. Painless plantar warts are often best left to resolve spontaneously rather than subjecting the patient to a prolonged program of treatment.

Cryosurgery is the most common method of treatment (see Chap. 35), but chemical destruction (keratolytic therapy) is preferred in children and patients with numerous warts. For chemical destruction, the lesion is first soaked in water, then salicylic

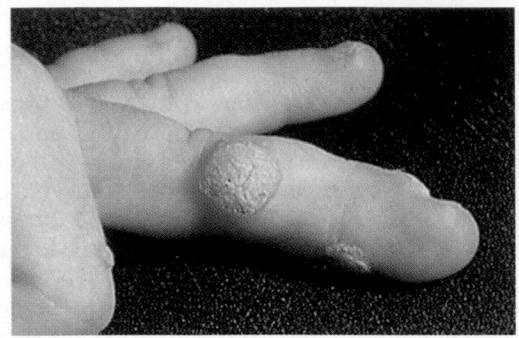

Figure 36–6

Warts. (From Lookingbill DP, Marks JG. Principles of dermatology. 2nd ed. Philadelphia: WB Saunders, 1993, p. 67.)

acid and lactic acid in varying strengths in flexible collodion are applied to the wart. The area is covered with tape for 6 to 8 hours. The tape is removed and the dead tissue rubbed off with an emery board or pumice stone. This treatment can be repeated once or twice daily. The acid solution is caustic to normal skin.

Podophyllin 25% in benzoin tincture is a cytotoxic agent used to treat condylomata acuminata (genital warts) in moist areas. It is applied carefully to the lesion during an outpatient visit and washed off by the patient in 6 to 8 hours. Treatment is repeated weekly in the clinic or office until warts are resolved. Severe systemic reactions can occur from absorption of podophyllin, including renal toxicity, polyneuritis, and shock. It is not used during pregnancy. The patient may use podofilox (Condylox) at home to treat condylomata acuminata.

Cantharidin is a vesicant or blistering agent applied to the wart after paring with a scalpel. The wart is then occluded for 24 hours or until it starts

Table 36–3

Clinical Manifestations, Common Locations, and Treatment of Warts

Type	Appearance	Common Locations	Treatments
Common (verruca vulgaris)	Flesh-colored or brownish gray scaling, vegetative papule or nodule	Hands	Cryosurgery Curettage and desiccation Cantharidin
Plantar	Solitary, grouped, or mosaic scaling papules	Feet	Chemical destruction (salicylic acid and lactic acid in flexible collodion)
Flat	Flesh colored or tan, soft, 1–3 mm	Face, neck, and sometimes forearms and hands	Cryosurgery Tretinoin (Retin-A)
Filiform	Soft, finger-like growth	Face and neck	Curettage and desiccation Cryosurgery
Condyloma acuminatum (moist)	Soft, vegetative	Mucocutaneous skin in anogenital area	Cryosurgery Podophyllin 25% in benzoin tincture 5-Fluorouracil Laser surgery

to hurt. The blister crusts and falls off in 7 to 14 days. The wart is retreated if necessary.

Desiccation followed by curettage of dead tissue is most effective for common and filiform warts (see Chap. 35). Tretinoin has been found useful in treating flat warts. Recalcitrant warts have been treated intradermally with topical 5-fluorouracil and bleomycin. Laser surgery is used to treat condylomata acuminata extending into the vagina and may be used to treat other types of warts after all other treatment methods have failed.

There are no vaccines to treat warts, and biologic treatments are not recommended to induce immune responses.

NURSING PROCESS GUIDELINES
Warts

When caring for a patient with warts, note the number, appearance, and location of the warts. Ask whether the warts tend to be rubbed or irritated during daily activities and whether they cause discomfort or pain because of their location. Determine when they appeared and whether any measures have been used to treat them. Additional assessments, as well as nursing diagnoses, expected outcomes, and nursing interventions, relate to the selected mode of treatment. When chemical destruction is selected, carefully instruct the patient in the correct application of the topical medication. Also provide written instructions and tell the patient to follow only these because package-insert directions vary. Caution the patient against letting the medication come in contact with the normal skin surrounding the warts. Also caution against treating the warts more often than prescribed because marked irritation can result.

Molluscum Contagiosum

Molluscum contagiosum is a DNA viral infection of the epidermis. It occurs most often among children and among persons infected with human immunodeficiency virus (HIV). In fact, molluscum on the face may be an initial warning sign of HIV infection.

Etiology and Pathophysiology
Molluscum contagiosum is caused by a DNA poxvirus that infects the epidermis. The virus replicates in the cytoplasm of a keratin cell, resulting in proliferation of the epidermis and in eosinophilic cytoplasmic inclusion bodies.

Molluscum is spread by autoinoculation, scratching, or touching a lesion. Venereal transmission occurs in sexually active persons.

Clinical Manifestations
The lesion of molluscum contagiosum appears as a flesh-colored, dome-shaped papule with a cheesy core. In children, the lesions appear on the face,

trunk, and extremities. In sexually active persons, they are most common on the genitalia.

Diagnosis
Diagnosis is based on clinical observation. It can be confirmed with Wright's stain.

Management
Curettage and cryosurgery are reliable methods of treatment. Spontaneous remission commonly occurs within 6 to 9 months.

NURSING PROCESS GUIDELINES
Molluscum Contagiosum

The assessment, nursing diagnoses, expected patient outcomes, nursing interventions, and evaluation for patients with molluscum contagiosum vary with the treatment mode selected. See Chapter 6 for specific information on the care of patients undergoing curettage or cryosurgery.

Herpes Simplex

Herpes simplex virus (HSV) is one of the most common viruses found in humans. Although most of the adult population has been infected with HSV, not all infected people have experienced a clinically active eruption.

There are two types of herpes simplex virus: HSV-1 and HSV-2. HSV 1 typically is associated with oral infections, such as fever blisters or cold scores (Fig. 36–7). HSV 2 typically is associated with genital infections. HSV-1 genital infections and HSV-2 oral infections do occur and are in fact increasing in frequency. HSV-1 may also infect the eye (herpes keratitis) and the brain (herpes encephalitis).

See Chapters 22 and 43 for a discussion of the etiology, pathophysiology, clinical manifestations, medical diagnosis, and treatment of HSV-1 and HSV-2, respectively.

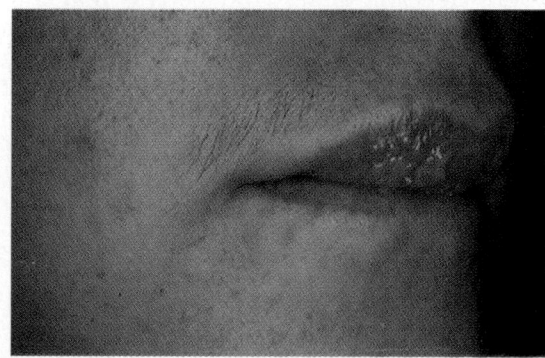

Figure 36–7

Herpes simplex on the upper lip. Early lesion appears as a localized swelling that subsequently reveals itself to be a group of vesicles. (From Hurwitz S. Clinical pediatric dermatology: A textbook of skin disorders of childhood and adolescence. 2nd ed. Philadelphia: WB Saunders, 1993, p. 321.)

NURSING PROCESS GUIDELINES
Herpes Simplex Virus Type 1 Oral Infection

See Chapter 22 for the assessment, nursing diagnoses, expected outcomes, nursing interventions, and evaluation commonly applicable to patients with genital and oral infections. Be sure to explain to patients with herpes simplex of the lip that the lesion can be spread by kissing, by orogenital sexual contact, or by any contact of the lesion with impaired skin (eg, the patient's own finger with a paper cut, macerated skin from excessive hand-washing).

Because the virus can be shed even when lesions are not apparent, protect yourself and others by routinely wearing gloves when performing oral or tracheal suctioning, oral care, or perineal care. When coming into direct contact with herpetic lesions or secretions, wear gown and gloves, and wash your hands carefully on completing care.

See Chapter 43 for discussion of the care of the patient with genital herpes.

Herpes Zoster

Herpes zoster (shingles) is a viral infection usually affecting the skin of a single dermatome. It occurs in 10% to 20% of the population (Habif, 1996). Its incidence has increased among the elderly and the immunosuppressed. It is equally common in men and women.

Etiology and Pathophysiology

Herpes zoster results from activation of the latent varicella-zoster virus in persons who have had varicella (chickenpox) or by exposure to the varicella virus in persons with no immunity to it.

The varicella-zoster virus enters the cutaneous nerves during an episode of chickenpox and travels to the dorsal root ganglia, where it becomes latent. It later reactivates, replicates, and travels back down the sensory nerve to the skin. The epidermis becomes inflamed, and bullae and multinucleated giant cells develop, along with perivascular inflammation in the dermis. Factors associated with reactivation of the virus include advancing age, immunosuppression, fatigue, emotional upset, and radiation therapy.

Clinical Manifestations

Herpes zoster lesions appear as grouped vesicles in a linear pattern on an erythematous base (Fig. 36–8). They follow the course of a peripheral sensory nerve, are usually unilateral, and do not cross the midline. Although individual lesions crust and drop off in about 10 days, one episode may produce continuous eruptions over a prolonged period.

Severe itching, burning, and pain occur 4 or 5 days before the eruption. Fever, headache, and malaise may also precede the eruption by several days. Lymphadenopathy may be present as well. These symptoms gradually subside as the eruption ap-

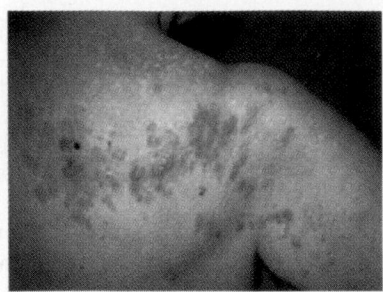

Figure 36–8

Herpes zoster affecting a single dermatome. Vesicles are grouped and vary in size. (From Lookingbill DP, Marks JG. Principles of dermatology. 2nd ed. Philadelphia: WB Saunders, 1993, p. 166.)

pears. The course of herpes zoster can be long and drawn out over a year. It can be exasperating and demoralizing for the patient. Secondary infection is also a concern.

For elderly and immunosuppressed patients, herpes zoster infection can be very serious. One-third of patients older than 60 years infected with herpes zoster acquire postherpetic neuralgia (pain persisting in a dermatome for months or years after the eruption has resolved). This pain is often severe, accentuated by tactile stimuli, and exhausting.

Disseminated zoster occurs only in patients with severe immunosuppression. It occurs 5 to 7 days after the initial eruption. Symptoms include fever, malaise, and generalized vesicular eruptions. The liver, lungs, and central nervous system may be involved.

Diagnosis

Characteristic lesions distributed along the dermatome are diagnostic for herpes zoster infection.

Management

Treatment of localized herpes zoster lesions includes cool compresses, Burow's compresses, and acetaminophen with codeine for pain. In patients over age 65 or who are immunosuppressed, oral acyclovir can help reduce viral shedding time and the risk of postherpetic neuralgia. Disseminated zoster is treated with intravenous acyclovir, which reduces pain and stops dissemination and vesicle formation.

NURSING PROCESS
Herpes Zoster

Assessment

Inspect the affected area. Note the appearance and distribution of lesions. Question the patient about when the lesions developed. Ask about associated pain, itching, headache, and malaise. Check for elevated temperature. Because the incidence of herpes zoster is increased in immunosuppressed people, review the patient's medical history and current health status. Also explore the patient's stress and fatigue levels because these factors are also implicated in reactivation of the varicella virus. Assess for signs of secondary infection.

Nursing Diagnoses and Planning

Nursing diagnoses and related expected patient outcomes commonly applicable to patients with herpes zoster include the following:

NDx: Impaired skin integrity related to presence of lesions secondary to herpes zoster infection

Planning: Patient Outcomes
1. Patient explains or demonstrates skin-care regimen.
2. Lesions heal without secondary infection.

NDx: Pain related to inflammation secondary to herpes zoster infection

Planning: Patient Outcomes
1. Patient uses a variety of pain-control techniques.
2. Patient reports increased comfort.

NDx: Risk for ineffective individual coping related to prolonged, severe discomfort and change in appearance

Planning: Patient Outcomes
1. Patient verbalizes concerns about the herpes zoster infection and its symptoms.
2. Patient identifies plans for coping with the effects of the herpes zoster infection.
3. Patient expresses confidence in ability to cope with the herpes zoster infection.

Nursing Interventions and Evaluation

Adhere to standard precautions for nonimmunocompromised patients with localized herpes zoster. Use airborne and contact precautions for all patients with disseminated herpes zoster and for immunocompromised patients with localized disease. Maintain these precautions until all lesions are crusted. Instruct patients about precautions at home. Stress the importance of avoiding contact with pregnant women to avoid transmitting the disease to the mother and fetus.

Adhere to airborne precautions for exposed susceptible patients beginning 10 days after exposure and continuing through 21 days after the last exposure or up to 28 days if varicella zoster immune globulin (VZIG) was given (CDC Special Communication, 1996.)

NDx: Impaired skin integrity
Keep the affected area clean, dry, and free from irritation. Wash with mild soap and warm water. Rinse and pat dry thoroughly. If a dressing is used, change it frequently, making sure it does not rub or irritate the lesions. Review with the patient the importance of adequate rest and good nutrition, including the need for vitamin C, to the healing process.

Instruct the patient to avoid scratching the lesions to avert further tissue damage and to decrease the risk of secondary infection. Tell the patient to notify the physician if purulent drainage, fever, or severe malaise develops.

NDx: Pain
Acknowledge that the pain and itch can be excruciating, and reassure the patient that a variety of pain-control methods can be used to provide relief.

Administer or teach self-administration of prescribed analgesics and antipruritics. Explain the importance of taking the medication at bedtime because the pain and itching tend to be worse at night. Because pain and itch are not always satisfactorily relieved with medication, encourage the use of showers and cool compresses if approved by the physician. Also guide the patient in the use of such pain-control techniques as progressive relaxation, imaging, and distraction.

Help the patient select clothing that is loose and soft, so it does not trigger pain through tactile stimulation of the affected area. If needed, plan for a bed cradle to decrease the pressure of bed linens.

NDx: Risk for ineffective individual coping
Recognize that patients with herpes zoster are at risk for ineffective individual coping for a variety of reasons, including prolonged severe pain, lack of adequate rest and sleep because of the pain, interference with usual activities, inability to dress in the usual style because of the need for loose clothing, and disfigurement, particularly when the face is affected. Encourage the patient to verbalize concerns and feelings, and acknowledge their validity. When necessary, correct any misinformation. Guide the patient in realistically assessing the problems and in identifying methods of coping and sources of support.

Compare the patient's status with the expected outcomes. If the outcomes are not met, reassess the patient and revise the plan.

*I*nflammations

ECZEMATOUS DERMATITIS

Eczematous dermatitis (eczema) is a common superficial skin inflammation characterized by itching, erythema, and edema of the involved area. Papules, vesicles, crusts, scales, and fissures also may develop.

Nonspecific Eczematous Dermatitis

Etiology and Pathophysiology

Nonspecific eczematous dermatitis is an idiopathic self-perpetuating epidermal eruption. It can be acute or chronic, localized or generalized. Statistics reflect

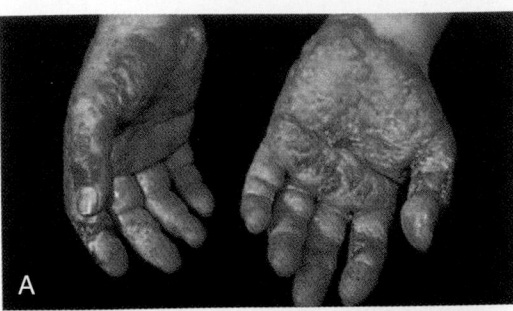
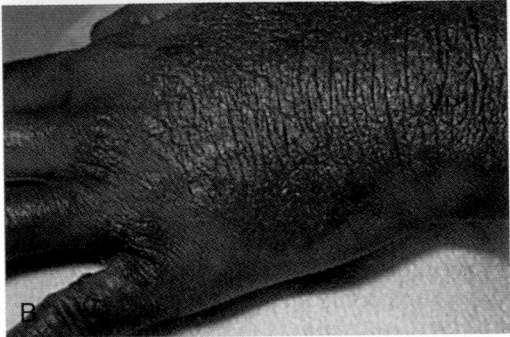

Figure 36-9

A, Acute nonspecific eczematous dermatitis. Note vesicles affecting the epidermis and erythema affecting the dermis. *B,* Chronic nonspecific eczematous dermatitis. Note lichenified, scaled areas affecting the epidermis and erythema affecting the dermis. (From Lookingbill DP, Marks JG. Principles of dermatology. 2nd ed. Philadelphia: WB Saunders, 1993, p. 122.)

a greater incidence of eczema in people who have allergies.

In this disorder, a papulovesicular eruption develops with intense itching. Scratching results in histamine release, which causes more itching and worsens the dermatitis. In chronic eczematous eruptions, the epidermis becomes hyperkeratotic or thickened. Perivascular inflammation is present in both acute and chronic eczema.

Clinical Manifestations

Severe itching that interferes with sleep and activities of daily living is characteristic of nonspecific eczematous dermatitis. Acute presenting symptoms include vesicles, weeping, and crusted patches. Oozing papules are the presenting lesions in subacute eczema. Chronic eczema is characterized by lichenified, scaling plaques. Secondary lesions seen in eczemas are crusts, scales, and fissures. An indistinct border between normal and eczematous skin is characteristic. Figure 36-9 illustrates acute and chronic nonspecific eczema.

Idiopathic eczemas that have been classified by presenting lesions, common sites, and possible causes are identified in Table 36-4.

Diagnosis

Presenting lesions, Tzanck's preparation, KOH, and Gram's stain differentiate acute eczematous dermatitis from contact dermatitis, herpes, fungal infection, and impetigo. History, KOH, patch tests, and skin biopsy help differentiate chronic eczematous dermatitis from contact dermatitis, psoriasis, drug eruption, and fungal infection.

Management

Eczematous dermatitis is treated with topical or intralesional corticosteroids. Oral prednisone in tapered doses may be given for acute and subacute eczema. Because eczema is a chronic disease and long-term steroid use is associated with severe side effects, systemic steroid therapy is used only when absolutely necessary.

The glucocorticoid triamcinolone, 40 mg intramuscularly, can be given for acute eczema. It can help for up to 4 weeks. Erythromycin and dicloxacillin are antibiotics prescribed for secondary bacterial infections.

Wet dressings and baths soothe the skin, reduce inflammation, and remove crusts and scales. Antihistamines are prescribed for itching, especially at bedtime.

Table 36-4

Idiopathic Eczemas Classified by Presenting Lesion, Site, and Contributing Factors

Idiopathic Eczema	Possible Contributing Factors	Presenting Lesion	Site
Dyshidrotic	Excessive hand-washing "Housewives' eczema"	Deep-seated vesicles Tapioca-like appearance	Palms, soles, sides of fingers
Autosensitization (intradermal eruption)	Hypersensitivity reaction to substance produced by acute dermatitis of hands or feet	Subacute dermatitis	Face, neck, arms, and thighs
Xerotic ("winter's itch")	Low humidity, dry skin	Dry, fissured skin	Trunk, extremities, especially lower legs
Nummular	Biopsychosocial factors	Oval patches with crusted papulovesicles Coinlike appearance	Trunk, extremities

NURSING PROCESS
Eczema

Assessment

Assess the patient's knowledge of the condition. Determine the onset, duration, and previous treatments, including self-remedies and over-the-counter drugs. Assess the extent of the lesions and the discomfort caused by itching. Also assess the impact of the condition on the patient's self-esteem and lifestyle.

Nursing Diagnoses and Planning

Nursing diagnoses and related expected patient outcomes commonly applicable to patients with nonspecific eczematous dermatitis include the following:

NDx: Impaired skin integrity related to presence of acute or chronic eruption

Planning: Patient Outcomes
1. Eruption clears.
2. Frequency and severity of recurrences decrease.

NDx: Risk for body image disturbance related to presence of skin lesions

Planning: Patient Outcomes
1. Patient verbalizes positive, realistic perception of self.
2. Patient expresses confidence in own coping ability.
3. Patient participates in social activities.

Nursing Interventions and Evaluation

NDx: Impaired skin integrity
Instruct the patient in self-administration of prescribed steroid therapy. Also instruct in the application of wet dressings and the use of therapeutic moisturizing baths. Explain the importance of taking antihistamines, especially at bedtime, to prevent unintentional scratching, which perpetuates the eczema. Encourage cool baths and the use of skin moisturizers, such as petrolatum, to decrease itching and dryness during waking hours. Stress that seeking immediate treatment for acute eczema and control of the itch–scratch cycle is essential to the control and prevention of chronic eczema.

NDx: Risk for body image disturbance
Encourage the patient to express feelings about the eczema and its impact on personal appearance. Be alert for behaviors or verbalizations indicating negative feelings about self. Explore with the patient how to use clothing to conceal affected areas and to enhance overall appearance.

Compare the patient's status with the expected outcomes. If the outcomes are not met, reassess the patient and revise the plan.

Contact Dermatitis

Contact dermatitis is a common inflammatory skin ailment caused by an external agent. Statistics show that contact dermatitis causes more than 50% of occupational illnesses, excluding injuries. It accounts for 25% of lost work time and costs millions of dollars each year.

There are two types of contact dermatitis—irritant contact dermatitis and allergic contact dermatitis.

Etiology and Pathophysiology
Irritant dermatitis is caused by substances that are toxic to the skin, such as acids, alkalis, solvents, and detergents.

Allergic contact dermatitis is a tissue inflammation caused by an immunologic reaction to chemicals such as plants, rubber, metals, and medicines. The most common causes of allergic contact dermatitis are listed in Table 36–5.

Irritant dermatitis is an inflammatory skin reaction to a toxic substance. It usually occurs within a few hours after contact but may develop after days of multiple exposure to a weaker irritant.

Table 36–5

Common Causes of Allergic Contact Dermatitis

Allergy	Source	Cross-Sensitivity
Rhus (plant)	Poison ivy, poison oak, poison sumac	Cashews, mangoes, lacquer trees, ginkgo trees, smoke of burning plants
Paraphenylenediamine	Hair dye	Aso and aniline dyes, benzocaine, procaine, hydrochlorothiazide, sulfonamides
Nickel	Garters, jewelry, earrings (including hypoallergenic)	
Rubber	Clothing, footgear, dress shields, gloves, breast pads, condoms, contraceptive diaphragms, eyelash curlers	
Ethylenediamine	Triamcinolone (Mycolog) cream, dyes, insecticides, rubber accelerators, synthetic waxes, resins	Aminophylline, paraphenylenediamine

Allergic contact dermatitis is caused by a cell-mediated, type IV immunologic reaction. The sensitization phase occurs when a chemical on the skin combines with an epidermal protein. A hapten-protein complex is formed, and the antigen stimulates T lymphocytes to produce effector memory and suppressor lymphocytes in the lymph nodes. This phase takes 7 days. On re-exposure to the antigen, the elicitation phase occurs, resulting in the inflammation of allergic contact dermatitis. The allergic response is later suppressed by the suppressor T cells.

Contact dermatitis, like other eczematous dermatitis conditions, is characterized by perivascular inflammation of the dermis, with vesicle formation and spongiosis (intercellular edema of the spongy layer of the skin) in the epidermis.

Clinical Manifestations

Clinical manifestations of irritant contact dermatitis include vesicles, fluid-filled papules, and lichenified plaques with sharp margins. Contact with the irritant may precede the eruption by hours or days.

In allergic contact dermatitis, the eruption occurs 1 to 4 days after exposure to the allergen. A vesicular, papular eruption occurs in the area of contact. The configuration varies. Linear streaks of papulovesicles are characteristic for contact dermatitis caused by poison ivy or other plants (Fig. 36–10).

Diagnosis

There is no standard method for diagnosing irritant contact dermatitis. Patch testing is done for allergic contact dermatitis (see Chap. 35).

Management

Acute, severe, and generalized contact dermatitis is treated with a 10-day course of systemic steroids and baths or wet dressings. If a secondary infection occurs, it is treated with systemic antibiotics because topical antibiotics can aggravate contact dermatitis.

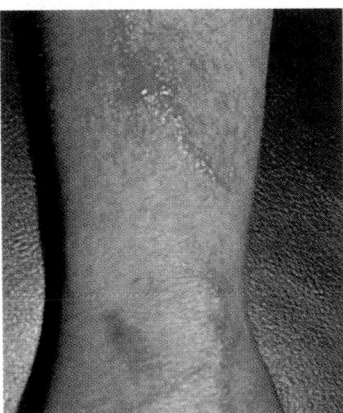

Figure 36–10

Linear streaks of papulovesicles characteristic of contact dermatitis caused by poison ivy or other plants. (From Lookingbill DP, Marks JG. Principles of dermatology. 2nd ed. Philadelphia: WB Saunders, 1993, p. 124.)

Topical steroids and systemic antihistamines are prescribed for less severe cases. Acute contact dermatitis subsides within 3 weeks.

Chronic eczematous dermatitis develops with repeated exposure to the irritant or allergen. It is treated as chronic eczema.

NURSING PROCESS
Contact Dermatitis

Assessment

Obtain a patient and family history of skin disease. Ask the patient about recent use of prescribed and over-the-counter oral and topical medications and preparations. Include medications the patient is preparing for use by someone else.

Obtain a work history. Does the patient handle chemicals? Is the work environment hot and humid or very dry? Obtain a home and recreation history.

Document the location, course, and appearance of the lesions. Determine what the patient has used to treat the condition.

Nursing Diagnoses and Planning

Nursing diagnoses and related expected patient outcomes commonly applicable to patients with contact dermatitis include the following:

NDx: Risk for altered health maintenance related to insufficient knowledge of the cause and prevention of contact dermatitis

Planning: Patient Outcomes
1. Patient identifies causative factors.
2. Patient describes ways to avoid causative factors.

Nursing Interventions and Evaluation

NDx: Risk for altered health maintenance
Explain that avoiding the causative irritant or allergen is the best way to prevent recurrence. Teach about sources of the irritant or allergen and cross-sensitivities to allergies (see Table 36–5). Explain that allergens may be transmitted by the hands or possibly by pets that have picked up allergens on their coats. Acknowledge that avoidance of the causative factor may be difficult and in some cases may require changes in lifestyle and occupation. Explore with the patient what changes may be necessary and how they might be instituted. Explain that protective clothing rarely helps. Advise the patient to avoid factors that increase sensitivity, such as perspiration and tight-fitting clothing.

For nickel dermatitis, instruct the patient to purchase a kit to test jewelry for nickel. Any jewelry that tests positive for nickel can be covered with four coats of clear nail polish and is then safe to wear.

Additional Interventions
Help the physician and the patient identify etiologic factors by history and patch testing. Teach the pa-

tient how to use prescribed topical therapies to treat contact dermatitis. These can include wet dressings of cool water; aluminum acetate solution; soothing, tepid baths; and colloidal oatmeal (Aveeno) baths.

Teach the patient to use topical steroids by applying a thin layer using aseptic technique and only to affected areas. Warn against applying the medication more often than directed.

Compare the patient's status with the expected outcomes. If the outcomes are not met, reassess the patient and revise the plan.

Seborrheic Dermatitis

Etiology and Pathophysiology
Seborrheic dermatitis is a common, chronic inflammatory condition that affects hairy areas of the body. It is characterized by hyperkeratosis in the epidermis and perivascular inflammation in the dermis. Its cause is unknown.

Clinical Manifestations
Seborrheic dermatitis occurs in hairy regions that contain many sebaceous glands. These areas include the scalp, eyebrows, eyelids, nasolabial folds, ears, chest, and intertriginous areas (axilla, groin, buttocks, inframammary folds). The patches and plaques of seborrhea are bilateral, symmetric, and erythematous, with indistinct borders and greasy, yellowish scales (Fig. 36–11).

Dandruff, a mild form of seborrheic dermatitis, presents as fine, white scales with no erythema.

Diagnosis
The diagnosis of seborrheic dermatitis is based on clinical presentation.

Management
Treatment of seborrheic dermatitis consists of shampoos that contain any of the following keratolytic ingredients: sulfur, salicylic acid, coal tar, selenium sulfide, or zinc pyrithione. These preparations remove scales and soften the horny layer.

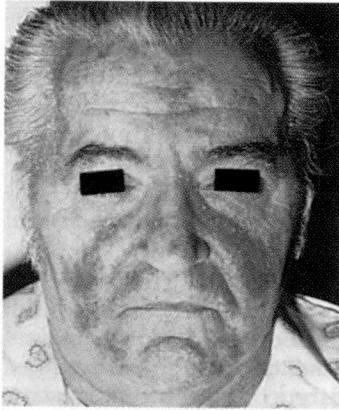

Figure 36–11

Seborrheic dermatitis. (From Lookingbill DP, Marks JG. Principles of dermatology. 2nd ed. Philadelphia: WB Saunders, 1993, p. 130.)

Topical steroid lotion is applied to hairy areas that are highly inflamed or that do not respond to treatment. Hydrocortisone 1% cream can be used to control seborrhea in nonhairy areas. High-potency steroid creams are contraindicated because, although they are initially effective, recurrent episodes of seborrheic dermatitis cease to respond and the treated skin develops atrophic changes.

NURSING PROCESS GUIDELINES
Seborrheic Dermatitis

Assess the extent, onset, and duration of the seborrhea. Instruct the patient to wash his or her hair with an antiseborrheic shampoo, leave it on the scalp for 5 minutes, and rinse it out. Also instruct the patient to apply hydrocortisone 1% lotion sparingly to the involved area of the scalp at bedtime. If areas of the face are affected, instruct the patient to apply a thin layer of hydrocortisone 1% cream to the face twice daily as ordered by the physician. Remind the patient that a corticosteroid cream is readily absorbed on the face and that a thin layer provides the same therapeutic effect as a thick layer. Advise the patient to discontinue the hydrocortisone when the condition clears and to reapply at the first sign of recurrence.

Stasis Dermatitis

Stasis dermatitis is an eczematous eruption of the lower legs. The lower leg above the medial malleolus is the most common site.

Etiology and Pathophysiology
Stasis dermatitis is a complication of peripheral vascular disease. Venous incompetence causes increased hydrostatic pressure, swelling, and edema. Capillary proliferation and extravasation of red blood cells and vascular fluid cause inflammatory eczematous dermatitis. Skin changes are similar to those seen in chronic, nonspecific dermatitis.

Clinical Manifestations
The clinical manifestations of stasis dermatitis are edema, brown pigmentation, dull erythema, petechiae, thickened skin, scaling, and weeping of the skin (Fig. 36–12). Varicose veins may be present. Peripheral pulses are present. Dusky erythema precedes ulceration.

Diagnosis
The diagnosis of stasis dermatitis is made clinically. Cellulitis, contact dermatitis with a recent history of topical medication, fungal infection, and arterial disease may have to be ruled out.

Management
Medical treatment consists of support hose or restrictive boots to prevent venous stasis and edema.

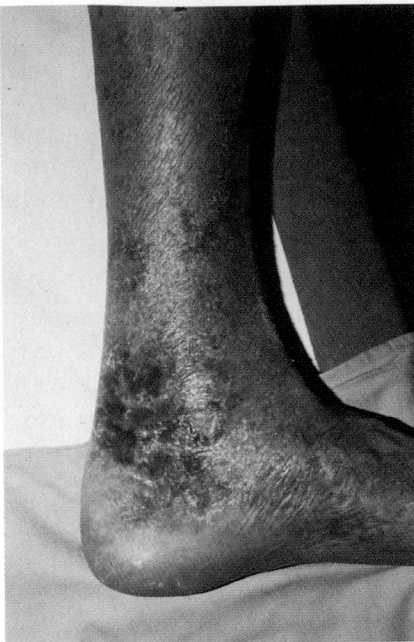

Figure 36–12

Bilateral stasis dermatitis. Note brawny, indurated edema of the ankle. (From Murphy GF, Herzberg AJ. Atlas of dermatopathology. Philadelphia: WB Saunders, 1996, p. 265.)

Standing for long periods is discouraged. Weight reduction is necessary if the patient is obese. Frequent rest periods with leg elevation promote venous return. Wet dressings are applied to the skin if oozing or crusting is present. Topical steroids may also be prescribed.

If ulceration occurs, antiseptic cleansing is important to prevent infection. Antibiotics are not helpful in the healing process unless cellulitis is present. Topical antibiotics are contraindicated because they can cause contact dermatitis from the compromised epidermal barrier. Skin grafts may be required for deep ulcers.

NURSING PROCESS GUIDELINES
Stasis Dermatitis

The assessment, nursing diagnoses, expected patient outcomes, nursing interventions, and evaluation for patients with stasis dermatitis are similar to those described for patients with peripheral vascular disease and to those concerning symptomatic relief for patients with eczematous dermatitis. If grafting is necessary because of ulceration, provide nursing care as described in Chapter 35.

DRUG ERUPTIONS

Drug eruptions are the most common cause of generalized erythematous eruptions.

Etiology and Pathophysiology

Drug eruptions are usually caused by new drugs started within 1 week of the eruption. Three common types are morbilliform eruption (generalized, measles-like erythema), acute urticaria, and erythema multiforme (a skin and mucous-membrane reaction characterized by the sudden onset of an erythematous eruption of which the characteristic lesion is the bull's eye or target lesion). Toxic epidermal necrolysis is a rare reaction in which the epidermis peels away from the dermis. The involved area resembles a severe burn and, if large, may be life-threatening.

Clinical Manifestations

The most common drug-related reaction is a generalized, itchy, maculopapular, bright red morbilliform eruption with confluent lesions over large areas (Fig. 36–13).

The hives of acute urticaria are erythematous plaques with pale centers and red borders. They may be confluent and have a geographic configuration. Distribution may be generalized or localized on specific areas of the body. Individual hives last less than 24 hours, but new hives may continue to develop after the initial eruption. There is severe itching.

Target lesions are diagnostic for erythema multiforme. Three zones of color must be present in the lesions to diagnose erythema multiforme. The lesions have a central, dark area surrounded by pale edema, with a peripheral rim of erythema. The distribution is often symmetric and is frequently found on the palms and soles.

Diagnosis

Patient history of recent new drug use and clinical manifestations help to diagnose a drug reaction. The only skin test helpful in diagnosing a drug reaction is a penicillin test for immediate hypersensitivity reaction in hives.

Management

Use of the offending drug should be discontinued. If the patient is taking several drugs and the offender

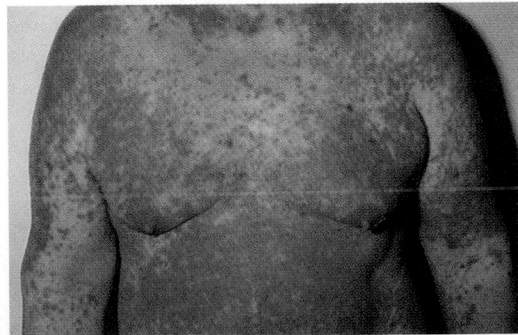

Figure 36–13

Generalized symmetric erythematous rash caused by an allergic drug reaction. (From Lookingbill DP, Marks JG Jr. Principles of dermatology. 2nd ed. Philadelphia: WB Saunders, 1993, p. 218.)

Table 36–6

Drugs Commonly Associated with Allergic Skin Reactions

Drug	Reaction Rate (Per 100 Recipients)
Trimethoprim-sulfa-methoxazole (Septra, Bactrim)	5.9
Ampicillin	5.2
Semisynthetic penicillins	3.6
Blood, whole human	3.5
Blood platelets	2.8
Erythromycin	2.3
Sulfisoxazole	1.7
Penicillin G	1.6
Gentamicin sulfate	1.6
Cephalosporins	1.3
Quinidine	1.2

Data from Arndt KA, Jick H. Rates of cutaneous reactions to drugs: A report from the Boston Collaborative Drug Surveillance Program. JAMA 1976; 235:918.

is not apparent, the number of drugs administered should be reduced to a minimum. Possible offenders should be changed to alternatives if feasible. Table 36–6 lists drugs that frequently cause dermatologic drug eruptions.

Symptomatic treatment may include:

- Antihistamines
- Soothing baths
- Cool, wet dressings
- Antipruritic lotions, such as calamine
- Body lotions with menthol
- Topical steroids

Systemic steroids are rarely required, but severe reactions may necessitate hospitalization and intravenous steroid therapy. Patients with hives should not take aspirin or salicylates, which may exacerbate the condition.

NURSING PROCESS GUIDELINES
Drug Eruption

Assess extent and characteristics of the eruption. Ask the patient whether any new drugs or over-the-counter preparations have been taken 7 to 10 days before eruption. Specifically ask about acetylsalicylic acid, penicillin, and other antibiotics, which frequently cause drug eruptions.

When a drug eruption is suspected, withhold the possible offender and notify the physician. Advise outpatients to discontinue use of the drug and to see or call the physician when a drug eruption is suspected.

Once a drug eruption is diagnosed and the causative agent is identified, instruct the patient in methods of symptomatic relief as prescribed, and explain that the drug eruption may worsen over the next few days before it improves. Total clearing may take 1 to 2 weeks. Also explain the importance of alerting health care providers and pharmacists to the allergy and carrying medical alert information at all times. This is critical because a patient with a history of an urticarial drug reaction is at risk for anaphylaxis if the offending drug is taken again.

ACNE

Acne is a skin disorder of multifactorial origin that affects the sebaceous glands.

Acne Vulgaris

Acne vulgaris is the most common skin disease seen by dermatologists. It can affect people of all ages but is most common among adolescents. In one survey, 85% of high school students indicated that they had acne. Although acne vulgaris is more prevalent and usually more severe in males, in females it may continue into the third and fourth decades of life.

Etiology and Pathophysiology

Etiologic factors associated with acne vulgaris include androgenic hormone stimulation, which causes increased sebum production by the sebaceous glands, obstruction of the sebaceous glands caused by keratinous impaction, and proliferation of anaerobic bacteria. The contents of the dilated sebaceous unit extravasate into the dermis, causing inflammation and comedo formation (Fig. 36–14).

Clinical Manifestations

The open comedo consists of a dilated pore filled with black keratinous material (blackhead). The closed comedo is a small, skin-colored, dome-shaped papule (whitehead). These lesions are not inflamed.

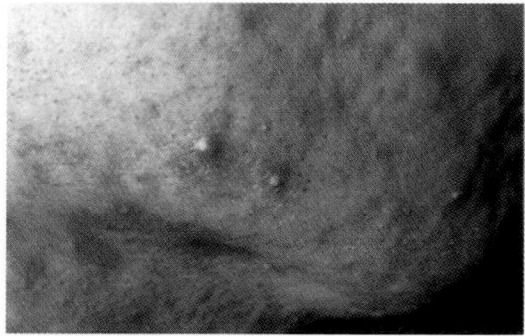

Figure 36–14

Acne. (From Lookingbill DP, Marks JG. Principles of dermatology. 2nd ed. Philadelphia: WB Saunders, 1993, p. 191.)

The inflammatory lesions are papules, pustules, nodules, and cysts, often surrounded by erythema. The face and upper trunk are the most common sites for comedones and the inflammatory lesions of acne vulgaris. Cystic acne is characterized by suppurated nodules and by large deep cysts that commonly cause permanent scarring.

Diagnosis

Diagnosis of acne vulgaris is made clinically by the appearance of the lesions.

Management

Treatment of acne includes the following:

- Topical keratolytic agents, such as benzoyl peroxide
- Topical comedolytic agents, such as tretinoin (Retin-A)
- Topical antibiotics, such as clindamycin (Cleocin T)
- Systemic antibiotics, such as tetracycline and erythromycin
- Systemic retinoids for severe recalcitrant acne

NURSING PROCESS
Acne Vulgaris

Assessment

Determine the patient's concept of the severity of his or her acne condition, and assess the psychosocial response to it. Keep in mind that acne occurs most often in teenage years, when self-consciousness is greatest. Individual psychosocial responses vary greatly. Assess the actual extent of the acne, presence or absence of excoriations, and tissue damage.

Question the patient about over-the-counter preparations or other remedies that have been used to treat the acne and the degree of success of these remedies.

Obtain a history of any other possibly related diseases, such as endocrine disorders, medicines the patient may be taking that can cause steroid-induced acne (eg, corticosteroids), and use of cosmetics that might aggravate acne, especially in late-onset acne in women. Assess the patient's interest in treatment and ability to comply with the prescribed regimen.

The nurse working in a dermatologist's office or with a dermatologist in a clinic setting is also responsible for follow-up assessments on the effectiveness of treatments, patient compliance, and psychosocial effects of the disease and treatment.

Nursing Diagnoses and Planning

Nursing diagnoses and related expected patient outcomes commonly applicable to patients with acne vulgaris include the following:

NDx: Risk for body image disturbance related to the presence of lesions

Planning: Patient Outcomes
1. Patient verbalizes positive feelings about self.
2. Patient expresses confidence in ability to treat and control the acne.

NDx: Risk for altered health maintenance related to insufficient knowledge of the cause and treatment of acne vulgaris

Planning: Patient Outcomes
1. Patient lists basic principles of skin care.
2. Patient explains prescribed medical treatment, including the name, frequency, method of use, and precautions related to prescribed medications.
3. Patient explains importance of consistent daily treatment.

Nursing Interventions and Evaluation

NDx: Risk for body image disturbance
Encourage the patient to express feelings about the acne and its impact. Monitor the patient for expression of negative feelings about his or her body. Be alert to behaviors or verbalizations indicating feelings of powerlessness, fear of negative reactions or rejection by others, or unwillingness to look at or touch affected skin areas.

Listen to the patient's complaints, and avoid giving soothing advice that minimizes the seriousness of the acne. Offer encouragement about the patient's ability to control the condition.

Dispel myths about acne (eg, that it is caused by ingestion of sweet or greasy foods, uncleanliness, masturbation, or sexual activity). Stress that it is caused largely by factors beyond individual control, such as heredity and large sebaceous glands.

NDx: Risk for altered health maintenance
Instruct the patient in the basic principles of skin care. Caution the patient to avoid overdrying the skin with soaps and cleansers, which may exacerbate the condition. Recommend washing the face with a mild soap twice a day to remove surface oil. If an oily feeling is a problem, recommend a mild abrasive soap or a drying agent. Advise the patient to keep hair off the face and to shampoo daily if necessary. Stress the importance of not touching affected areas and not picking or squeezing the lesions.

Instruct the patient in the prescribed medical treatment and associated precautions (Table 36–7). Explore with the patient how he or she will incorporate the prescribed regimen into daily activities. Stress that improvement requires consistent daily treatment and that it will be 4 to 6 weeks before obvious improvement can be seen. Encourage a healthy diet, which can reduce the severity of the condition. Explain that, although stress or ingestion of chocolate and fatty foods may worsen the condition in some people, no etiologic connection has been proved.

Table 36–7

Topical and Systemic Medications for Acne Vulgaris

Medication	Action	Administration	Patient Teaching
TOPICAL PREPARATIONS			
Benzoyl peroxide	Antibacterial and keratolytic agent decreases inflammatory lesions Decreases sebum production Promotes breakdown of comedo plugs	Lotion, cream, or gel applied to affected area once a day initially May go to 4 times daily as tolerance permits	Available over the counter and by prescription Redness and scaling may occur when first used Avoid contact with eyes, mouth, mucous membrane, denuded skin areas
Tretinoin (vitamin A acid)	Speeds turnover of epithelial cells, forcing out comedones and suppressing formation of new plugs Enhances penetration of other antiacne drugs	Cream, gel, or liquid applied at bedtime after skin is washed, toweled dry, and left to dry further for 15–30 min	Do not use if pregnant Stop use of abrasive soaps or keratolytics before using tretinoin May cause blistering, peeling, crusting, burning, or edema Do not apply to open areas or to areas of sunburn or windburn Avoid contact with eyes, nose, and mouth
Antibiotics (erythromycin, tetracycline, clindamycin)	Suppresses growth of *Propionibacterium acnes* Decreases skin surface free fatty-acid levels Decreases comedones, pustules, papules	Apply thin layer to clean, dry skin	No systemic side effects
SYSTEMIC PREPARATIONS			
Antibiotics (tetracycline, erythromycin)	Anti-infective agents used in moderate to severe inflammatory acne characterized by pustules, abscesses, scarring	Small doses given over months to years	Take tetracycline 2 hr before meals Stop if pregnancy occurs to avoid potential altered tooth formation in the fetus as result of effect of tetracycline on calcium metabolism Potential side effects include photosensitivity, nausea, diarrhea, and vaginitis
Isotretinoin (vitamin A derivative)	Decreases sebum production, inflammation, keratinization, and secondarily the number of *P. acnes* Used for severe, recalcitrant acne	0.5–1 mg/kg/day in 2 divided doses for 15–20 wk	Teratogenic, causing hydrocephalus, microcephalus, cleft palate, facial and external ear deformities, and cardiovascular defects Pregnancy test done and contraception begun 1 mo before therapy Contraception continued until 4–8 wk after treatment ends Cheilitis, dryness or itching of the skin, nose, and mouth, and nosebleeds are almost universal side effects Blood triglycerides are measured before and during treatment to check for evaluation Supplementary vitamin A and alcohol should be avoided

Additional Interventions

Re-evaluate the patient on return visits. If there is no improvement in 2 months, the physician should re-evaluate the patient for more intensive treatment.

Compare the patient's status with the expected outcomes. If the outcomes are not met, reassess the patient and revise the plan.

Acne Rosacea

Acne rosacea is a chronic inflammatory disorder of adulthood that affects the blood vessels and pilosebaceous units of the face. It is most common in women between the ages of 30 and 50 years. Acne rosacea is most severe in men and increases in severity if untreated.

Etiology and Pathophysiology

Acne rosacea is a fairly common disorder of unknown etiology. It is characterized by intrafollicular pustules in the epidermis and telangiectasia with perivascular inflammation. Sun exposure, spicy foods, alcohol, and caffeine have been suggested as causes of the vascular component of rosacea.

Clinical Manifestations

Acne rosacea begins as an erythematous eruption over the nose and central part of the face called a butterfly distribution (Fig. 36–15). Papules and pustules develop. Telangiectasias are also present.

Diagnosis

Diagnosis of acne rosacea is based on clinical appearance.

Management

Metronidazole 0.75% topical gel (MetroGel) is used to treat the inflammatory papules, pustules, and erythema of acne rosacea. It is applied twice daily to the affected area, with improvement typically seen in 3 weeks. Pustules and papules can also be treated

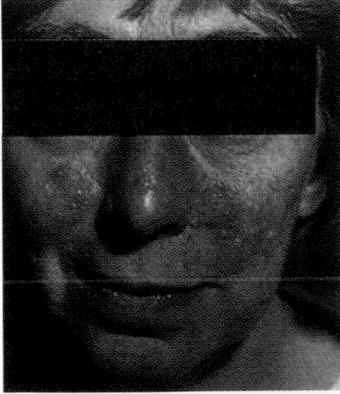

Figure 36–15

Severe rosacea. Note the butterfly distribution of acne-like pustules over the nose and cheeks. (From Lookingbill DP, Marks JG. Principles of dermatology. 2nd ed. Philadelphia: WB Saunders, 1993, p. 194.)

with oral antibiotics. Hydrocortisone 1% cream can be used to help decrease erythema. The condition may recur once treatment is discontinued.

NURSING PROCESS GUIDELINES
Acne Rosacea

Explore the patient's lifestyle to check for factors that might contribute to the acne rosacea. Inquire specifically about exposure to the sun, ingestion of spicy foods, and alcohol and caffeine intake.

Advise the patient that antibiotics may be needed for months or years to treat rosacea and to prevent recurrences and complications. Explain that most people show improvement within weeks after starting the antibiotics, although the telangiectasias persist.

Teach the patient using metronidazole gel to wash the affected area thoroughly before applying the medication. The patient should apply a thin film twice a day. After applying the medication, the patient also can apply cosmetics, if desired.

PSORIASIS

Psoriasis is a chronic hereditary disorder with a wide variation in severity and distribution of skin lesions. Its course is unpredictable and marked by remissions and exacerbations. It occurs equally among males and females and is more frequent among light-skinned races. Psoriasis affects 1.5 to 2.0% of the population in Western countries and has a low incidence among West Africans, American Indians, and Asians. It can occur at any age. The average age of onset is in the late twenties, particularly in women. Psoriasis can be economically, socially, psychologically, and physically disabling.

Etiology and Pathophysiology

The multifactorial genetic and environmental stimuli responsible for the clinical expression of psoriasis are unclear. About one-third of affected people have a positive family history for psoriasis. About 80% of identical twins are affected concurrently. Among environmental factors that appear to trigger its expression are the following:

- Skin injury, such as from surgery or sunburn
- Infections, such as a cold, sinusitis, or sore throat
- Hormonal changes
- Stress
- Drugs, such as lithium, beta-blockers, systemic corticosteroids, indomethacin, and antimalarials
- Alcohol
- Smoking
- Obesity

The normal epidermis has a cell turnover rate of 28 days. The psoriatic cell turnover rate can be as fast as 4 days. This results in hyperkeratosis, acan-

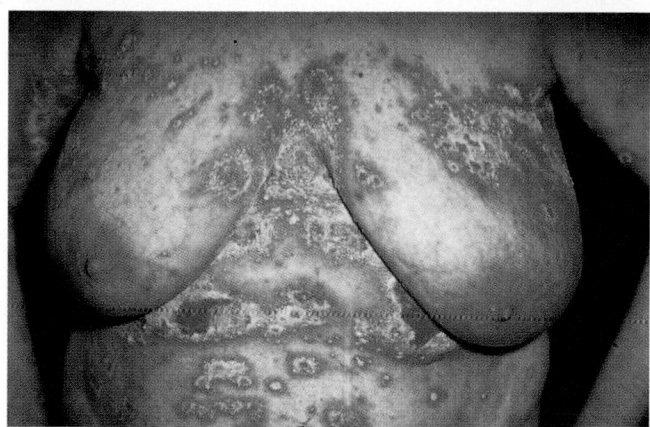

Figure 36–16

Psoriasis. (Courtesy of Columbia-Presbyterian Dermatology Associates, New York, NY.)

thosis (increased thickness of the prickle cell layer) with elongated rete pegs, infiltration by neutrophils, and an accumulation of scales. Perivascular inflammation develops in the dermis.

Clinical Manifestations

A psoriasis lesion is an erythematous plaque with a sharp, well-defined border and silvery white scales. If the scale is removed, the lesion may bleed because of the proximity of dilated blood vessels to the surface. Lesions are usually symmetric and may be few in number, or they may cover the total surface of a part (Fig. 36–16).

The most common sites of psoriasis are the elbows, knees, scalp, and lumbosacral skin, but it can occur on all skin surfaces. It affects the nails in 30% of patients. Pitting of the nails is the classic nail change in psoriasis, especially in patients with concomitant arthritis. Other nail changes are yellowish discoloration, onycholysis (separation of the nail from the bed), thickening, grooving, splitting, and subungual hyperkeratosis. Often associated with severe nail involvement is mutilating psoriatic arthritis involving the interphalangeal joints of the hands and feet, the sacroiliac, hip, and cervical areas. The skin lesions and arthritis may occur together, or the arthritis may precede the onset of psoriasis.

Table 36–8 presents the various types of psoriasis.

Table 36–8

Types of Psoriasis

Type	Lesions	Characteristics	Sites
Plaque (nummular, common)	Round, oval plaques that may be small or very large and confluent, serpiginous, or geographic Silvery white scales present on plaques in untreated psoriasis		Elbows, knees, scalp, trunk
Inverse	Red, sharply defined Less scaling because of maceration	May be exclusively inverse or appear with plaque psoriasis	Intertriginous folds of axillae, inguinal, intergluteal, and perianal skin
Guttate	Small, droplike psoriasis lesions with minimal scaling	Appears abruptly, often after streptococcal infections	Trunk and proximal extremities
Palmar	Hyperkeratosis and thick scales on the palms and fingers	May result from trauma to the area Often occurs with elbow and knee lesions	Volar surfaces of fingers and palms
Erythrodermic (exfoliative)	Generalized redness Little scaling	Can result from overaggressive treatment, such as tar and ultraviolet light Requires cautious, nonirritating treatment and hospitalization	Generalized
Acute generalized pustular psoriasis (von Zumbusch's)	Skin becomes red and tender Tiny pustules appear at edges of lesions and coalesce to form lakes of pus	Plaque psoriasis irritated by drugs, pregnancy, or infections If patient is very ill, hospitalization is necessary Loss of fluid, albumin, and heat	Generalized

Diagnosis

Psoriasis is diagnosed by the characteristic lesions. Uncharacteristic lesions and lesions that do not respond to treatment undergo biopsy.

Management

The goal of medical management is to decrease epidermal proliferation and dermal inflammation. Treatment includes application of emollients, keratolytics, coal tar, anthralin, and topical steroids. Phototherapy (ultraviolet B light, or UVB) and photochemotherapy (psoralen ultraviolet light, or PUVA) are treatments for generalized and difficult cases of psoriasis. Retinoids, antimetabolites, and occasionally systemic steroids are used for severe, acute, and recalcitrant psoriasis. Refer to Chapter 35 for a discussion of pharmacologic therapy and topical treatment, including UV radiation.

Patients with pustular von Zumbusch's psoriasis or erythroderma require hospitalization, rest, and conservative skin care. They must be observed for heart failure, pulmonary embolus, exhaustion, pneumonia, and sepsis.

NURSING PROCESS
Psoriasis

Assessment

Obtain a history of the current condition. Ask when it began, what area of the body was first affected, how it progressed, whether there were any identifiable precipitating factors, what treatments have been used, and whether they were effective. Question the patient about any family history of psoriasis, noting age of onset in family members and a description of the course of the disease, including remissions and exacerbations.

Inspect the skin. Examine all areas for involvement, including scalp, ears, trunk, groin, buttocks, perianal area, arms, legs, intertriginous areas under the arms and breasts, hands, feet, and nails.

Compare the actual extent of the psoriasis with the patient's perception. Question the patient about associated symptoms, such as fever and pruritus. Remember that some patients with psoriasis do not itch, whereas others will be scratching during the interview.

Explore the psychosocial impact of the disease on the patient. Ask the patient to describe how the condition affects his or her comfort, lifestyle, body image, employment, and social relationships.

Assess for factors that make some treatment plans unrealistic for individual patients. For example, some patients may be unable or unwilling to apply corticosteroids or tar preparations three times daily. In particular, patients in frequent contact with the public may be unwilling to apply tar preparations that will cause them to smell like tar.

Nursing Diagnoses and Planning

Nursing diagnoses and related expected patient outcomes commonly applicable to patients with psoriasis include the following:

NDx: Impaired skin integrity related to skin lesions secondary to psoriasis

Planning: Patient Outcomes
1. Patient performs skin care correctly.
2. Skin lesions clear.

NDx: Pain related to itching

Planning: Patient Outcomes
1. Patient lists basic self-care measures to reduce or control pruritus.
2. Patient states that pruritus is relieved or controlled.

NDx: Risk for body image disturbance related to unsightly or extensive psoriatic lesions with dry, flaky scales

Planning: Patient Outcomes
1. Patient verbalizes positive feelings about self.
2. Patient maintains good grooming.
3. Patient interacts with staff members, family, and friends.

NDx: Risk for ineffective individual coping related to presence of a chronic disease and the demands of the treatment regimen

Planning: Patient Outcomes
1. Patient identifies potential precipitating factors.
2. Patient discusses ways to avoid precipitating stressors.
3. Patient describes available support sources.
4. Patient expresses confidence in ability to cope.

Nursing Interventions and Evaluation

NDx: Impaired skin integrity

Teach the patient with psoriasis about the disease. Advise the patient to avoid factors that may aggravate psoriasis, such as obesity, consumption of alcoholic beverages, sunburn, trauma to the skin, scratching, dry skin, stress, infection, and shaving with a razor.

Instruct the patient in the prescribed therapy. Provide verbal and written instructions on the sequence of therapy, application of therapeutic agents, and the frequency of treatment.

Teach the patient to use topical steroids sparingly for acute lesions and to use an emollient on nonacute lesions. Review the side effects (skin atrophy, striae, telangiectasia) of aggressive topical steroid therapy. Explain that side effects are insidious and can be irreversible, but they usually occur only with long-term therapy.

Instruct the patient in self-administration of prescribed tar therapy and over-the-counter topical preparations as discussed in Chapter 35. Encourage patients with extensive psoriasis to make treatment a priority.

When therapeutic baths are ordered, instruct the patient to use a circular motion and to gently rub lesions to remove loose scales and to pat, not rub, the skin dry. When UV light treatments are ordered, instruct the patient to report any burning or tenderness of the skin, which can indicate overexposure. Also explain the use of sunscreens and how to shield sunburned areas.

Teach the patient with a history of extensive psoriasis to seek treatment during the early signs of exacerbation of the condition.

NDx: Pain

Instruct the patient in measures to reduce the discomfort of pruritus (Highlight 36–3).

NDx: Risk for body image disturbance

Be sensitive to the patient's feelings about appearance. Encourage verbalization about them. Take care to avoid any inadvertent expressions of distaste when treating the affected areas. Use touch as appropriate to indicate acceptance. Stress that the disease is not contagious and that the skin returns to normal with effective treatment. Encourage good grooming, interaction with others, and participation in self-care.

NDx: Risk for ineffective individual coping

Provide encouragement and emotional support. Psoriasis is a chronic, frustrating condition for the patient to deal with because of frequent exacerbations and remissions. Foster verbalization of concerns and feelings, which may involve anger, revulsion, inadequacy, powerlessness, anxiety, and depression. Guide the patient toward a realistic view of the problem, acknowledging its negative aspects but also focusing on treatment and control. Discuss the role of stress and emotional factors in flare-ups of the disease, and explore with the patient ways to minimize stress. Stress-reducing measures to be considered include a program of physical exercise, relaxation therapy, and counseling.

Provide the patient with information about community support services for psoriasis patients. Tell the patient about nurse-managed psoriasis day-care treatment centers, which are found in major metropolitan areas in the United States, Canada, and Europe. These centers provide acute care for exacerbations of psoriasis, patient education, follow-up, and maintenance of chronic psoriasis. Support services of dietitians, social workers, psychiatrists, psychologists, podiatrists, and self-help groups are offered at some centers. The centers are usually affiliated with a university medical center dermatology program or owned and operated by a board-certified dermatologist. Registered nurses usually manage the patient care as ordered by the physician.

Nursing care in these centers includes PUVA, UVB, combination PUVA and UVB, full day-care treatment programs, hand and foot UV treatments, hot quartz-lamp therapy, Goekerman treatment (tar and UV), modified Goekerman treatments, Ingram treatments (anthralin and UV), administration of and follow-up for patients on chemotherapy, and a great deal of encouragement.

Also inform the patient about voluntary psoriasis organizations, such as the Psoriasis Foundation in Portland, Oregon, and the Psoriasis Research Institute at Stanford University, Stanford, California. These organizations publish newsletters that have practical information for patients. Information on the disease process and new products and letters from psoriasis patients are commonly found in these newsletters.

Compare the patient's status with the expected outcomes. If the outcomes are not met, reassess the patient and revise the plan.

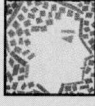

HIGHLIGHT
36–3
PATIENT EDUCATION

Reducing Pruritus Caused by Psoriasis

Instruct the patient to:

Avoid scratching itchy areas because this creates the scratch–itch cycle and can cause excoriation.

Use a room humidifier for moisture if the environment is dry.

Use warm, not hot, water for bathing.

Avoid use of strong soaps.

Lubricate the skin with petrolatum when it is free of topical therapeutic agents.

Take antihistamines as prescribed.

Structural Disorders

BULLOUS DISEASES

Pemphigus Vulgaris

Pemphigus vulgaris is the most common and severe form of pemphigus. It is characterized by flaccid, easily ruptured bullae that develop on apparently normal skin and mucous membranes. Pemphigus vulgaris usually occurs during middle or old age, with an equal incidence in men and women. It occurs among all races and ethnic groups. There may

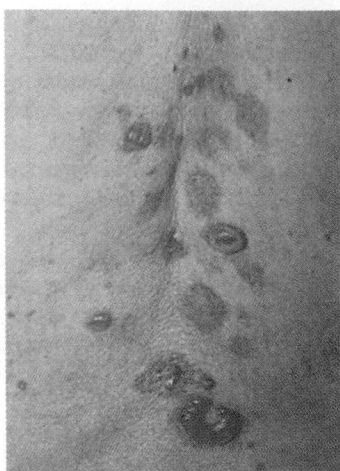

Figure 36–17

Flaccid bullae of pemphigus vulgaris forming on noninflamed skin. (From Lookingbill DP, Marks JG. Principles of dermatology. 2nd ed. Philadelphia: WB Saunders, 1993, p. 172.)

be increased prevalence in persons of Jewish descent (Moschella & Hurley, 1985).

Etiology and Pathophysiology

Pemphigus vulgaris is a serious chronic or acute autoimmune disease. The bullae of pemphigus vulgaris are intradermal. They form below the basal layer of the skin and result from a loss of cohesion between epidermal cells. Little inflammation is associated with the condition unless ruptured bullae become infected.

Clinical Manifestations

The flaccid bullae usually develop on noninflamed skin (Fig. 36–17). As they rupture, they leave large, denuded, bleeding, weeping, crusted erosions. Although bullae can develop anywhere on the body, the oral mucosa is often the initial site, with the scalp, face, chest, axillae, groin, and umbilicus the next most often affected sites. The bullae extend laterally when pressure is applied (Nikolsky's sign).

Diagnosis

A skin biopsy is performed for direct immunofluorescent studies of the perilesional skin to detect characteristic changes, such as the presence of immunoglobulin G (IgG) in the epidermal intercellular space. Serum antibody studies may demonstrate the presence of IgG pemphigus antibody.

Management

The goal of medical treatment is to administer enough steroids, alone or in combination with a cytotoxic agent (eg, azathioprine, cyclophosphamide, or methotrexate), to suppress the clinical manifestations of the disease. Gold is another treatment for pemphigus.

The patient is hospitalized and monitored closely while high doses of intravenous corticosteroids are administered to control acute pemphigus. As the condition begins to resolve and new blisters stop forming (and Nikolsky's sign disappears), oral corticosteroid therapy is begun and the dosage gradually reduced.

The patient can be weaned off all medicine when there are no clinical manifestations or pemphigus antibodies present in the serum. The patient is followed closely, and treatment resumes if symptoms return or if pemphigus antibody appears in the serum.

Wet dressings for 15 minutes, four times daily, help to remove debris from the lesions and prevent infection. Potent topical fluorinated steroids can be prescribed for localized occurrences.

Systemic corticosteroids prevent death from bronchopneumonia, metabolic changes, exhaustion, septicemia, and renal failure. Today, the major cause of death is from complications of long-term corticosteroid therapy (Habif, 1996).

NURSING PROCESS GUIDELINES
Pemphigus Vulgaris

The assessment, nursing diagnoses, expected patient outcomes, nursing interventions, and evaluation for patients with pemphigus vulgaris are a combination of those for patients with a chronic, life-threatening disease, those for patients with open skin lesions, and those for patients whose treatment involves steroids and cytotoxic agents.

Bullous Pemphigoid

The blisters of bullous pemphigoid arise from erythematous or urticarial plaque. It has been reported in all age groups but occurs mainly in people more than 60 years of age. Although the disease is serious because it occurs in the elderly, the mortality rate is low.

Etiology and Pathophysiology

Bullous pemphigoid is another autoimmune disease. The blister in bullous pemphigoid forms below the epidermis at the dermoepidermal junction. Perivascular inflammation develops in the dermis.

Clinical Manifestations

Localized bullous pemphigoid is most common on the lower extremities. Other sites include the groin, axillae, and other flexural areas. The bullae are large and tense (Fig. 36–18). They do not extend laterally when pressure is applied. Healing usually occurs without scarring if no infection develops.

Diagnosis

Biopsy specimens for direct and indirect immunofluorescence reveal a linear band of IgG and complement when the blister forms.

Management

The disease may subside spontaneously within months or years. Localized pemphigoid can be

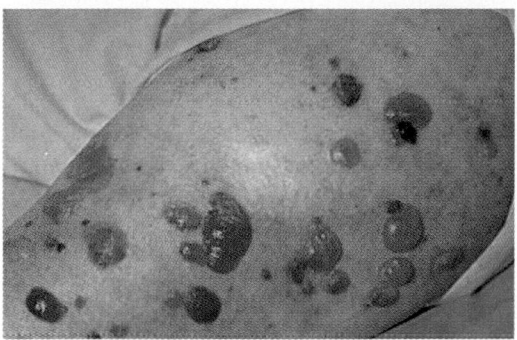

Figure 36–18
Tense blisters of bullous pemphigoid. (From Lookingbill DP, Marks JG. Principles of dermatology. 2nd ed. Philadelphia: WB Saunders, 1993, p. 173.)

treated with wet dressings and potent topical fluorinated steroids. Widespread bullae require treatment with systemic steroids and immunosuppressive agents.

NURSING PROCESS GUIDELINES
Bullous Pemphigoid

The assessment, nursing diagnoses, expected patient outcomes, nursing interventions, and evaluation for patients with bullous pemphigoid are similar to those described for patients with any chronic disease characterized by skin lesions. Because bullous pemphigoid is common in the elderly, pay particular attention to the patient's ability to perform the prescribed treatments and to obtain needed supplies. Support the patient's spirits by emphasizing that bullous pemphigoid is usually not fatal and that it may spontaneously subside.

STINGS

Hymenoptera stings cause about 30 deaths each year in the United States. Hymenoptera include honeybees, bumblebees, wasps, hornets, yellow jackets, mud daubers, and fire ants.

Etiology and Pathophysiology
The venoms of the Hymenoptera are a mixture of allergens and active amines and peptides. Any component of the venom may cause an allergic reaction. Cross-sensitization to Hymenoptera venom may occur. A person's reaction to a Hymenoptera sting is a combination of local and systemic effects of the peptides and amines in the venom and individual hypersensitivity to allergens in the venom.

Clinical Manifestations
Reactions to Hymenoptera venom may be immediate or delayed (after 2 hours). Immediate nonallergic reactions are characterized by local edema, erythema, pain, and itching. These subside within a few

hours. Multiple stings may cause malaise, nausea, and fever, and can be fatal. Patients with hypersensitivity have more severe and prolonged local reactions. They also may experience generalized urticaria and pruritus, severe bronchospasm, and laryngeal edema, leading to shock and death. Such anaphylactic reactions usually occur within 10 to 30 minutes after the sting.

The sting of fire ants produces a cluster of cutaneous lesions. Two hemorrhagic puncta at the site of attachment are surrounded by a circle of pustules from multiple stings. Immediate pain usually subsides quickly and a 2 to 10 mm wheal forms. A vesicle forms in about 4 hours. After 24 hours, the lesion becomes a pustule on an erythematous base.

Diagnosis
Patients usually are aware of having been stung by a bee or ant. The reaction is diagnosed by the symptoms. The most sensitive test for Hymenoptera allergy is the venom test, but it is still imperfect.

Management
The honeybee is the only stinging insect that leaves the stinger in the skin. It is removed carefully by scraping with a flat blade to avoid breaking or squeezing the venom sac and spreading the venom. Treatment for mild, local reactions includes ice, elevation, and antihistamines. For a delayed local reaction after 24 hours, systemic steroids may be prescribed for 5 days. There is no effective treatment for the local reaction to a fire ant sting except to keep it clean to prevent secondary infection.

To protect against anaphylaxis in the allergic person, epinephrine (0.1–0.5 mL of 1 : 1000 solution) is given subcutaneously and repeated every 5 to 15 minutes as needed. Airway maintenance and administration of intravenous fluids, vasopressors, and oxygen are emergency measures instituted if anaphylaxis occurs.

Hyposensitization (venom immunotherapy) is conducted on patients with a history of severe systemic reaction and a positive venom skin test.

NURSING PROCESS
Insect Sting

Assessment

Determine the number of stings, their location, the time of occurrence, and whether the causative insect is known. Keep in mind that multiple stings and stings on the head and neck have the most serious potential and that anaphylactic reactions usually occur within 10 to 30 minutes after a sting.

Determine whether the patient has a known allergy to Hymenoptera. Ask about any previous stings and the reaction to them.

Assess for both systemic and local reactions. Observe for signs of respiratory distress and question about nausea. Inspect the area of the sting for edema and erythema. Question the patient about pain and itch, especially of the soles of the feet and the palms of the hands.

Nursing Diagnoses and Planning

Nursing diagnoses and related expected patient outcomes commonly applicable to patients with an insect sting include the following:

NDx: Risk for ineffective breathing pattern related to bronchoconstriction and laryngeal edema

Planning: Patient Outcomes
1. Respiratory rate and depth are within normal limits.
2. Respirations are easy and silent.
3. Cyanosis is absent.

NDx: Risk for altered health maintenance related to insufficient knowledge of prevention of stings and self-care measures for persons allergic to Hymenoptera venom

Planning: Patient Outcomes
1. Patient lists ways to limit exposure to Hymenoptera.
2. Allergic patient explains importance of carrying MedicAlert identification and a bee-sting kit.
3. Allergic patient states protocol to be followed in the event of a bee sting.
4. Allergic patient describes importance of discussing hyposensitization therapy with the physician.

Nursing Interventions and Evaluation

NDx: Risk for ineffective breathing pattern
Administer epinephrine as ordered to protect the allergic patient from anaphylaxis. Hasten absorption of the epinephrine by massaging the injection site to increase circulation. Monitor respiratory and cardiovascular status. If anaphylaxis occurs, maintain an airway, administer oxygen and intravenous fluids, and support cardiovascular status as discussed in Chapter 33.

NDx: Risk for altered health maintenance
Instruct the patient allergic to Hymenoptera venom in self-care (Highlight 36–4).

Compare the patient's status with the expected outcomes. If the outcomes are not met, reassess the patient and revise the plan.

Pressure Ulcers

A pressure ulcer is "any lesion caused by unrelieved pressure resulting in damage of underlying tissue" (AHCPR Clinical Practice Guideline No. 15, 1994). Depending on stage, pressure ulcers can range from nonblanchable erythema of intact skin to full-thickness skin loss with extensive destruction of underlying muscle and bone. Terms formerly used to de-

---

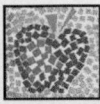

HIGHLIGHT
36–4

HEALTH PROMOTION & RISK REDUCTION

Instructions for Patients Allergic to Hymenoptera Stings

Instruct the patient to:

Carry MedicAlert identification indicating allergy to Hymenoptera at all times.

Keep accessible at all times a commercially available bee-sting kit containing a tourniquet, syringe, epinephrine, and antihistamine tablets. In the event of a sting:

- Inject self with epinephrine immediately.
- If stung by a honeybee, scrape the site swiftly with the fingernail to remove the stinger.
- If stung on an extremity, apply a tourniquet above the sting.
- Clean the area of the sting with soap and water.
- Apply ice to the area of the sting.
- Proceed to the nearest health care facility.

Explore the need for hyposensitization therapy with the physician.

Decrease exposure to bees by:

- Avoiding feeding areas, such as flower gardens, orchards, areas of clover, garbage cans, picnic sites, and other areas with food refuse.
- Wearing shoes outdoors because yellowjackets and fire ants are found in the ground.
- Wearing dark colors when outside because bees are attracted to bright colors.
- Avoiding use of perfumes and scented soaps, deodorants, or hair sprays when going outside because these attract bees.
- Remaining still if a bee is buzzing around because movement increases the risk of being stung.
- Keeping home area free of bees by keeping garbage cans covered, eliminating decorative fruit trees such as crabapple, and having nests or hives removed by an exterminator.
- Shaking out clothing and linens that have been line-dried outdoors before using them.

---

scribe these lesions include *decubitus ulcers, ischemic ulcers, pressure sores,* and *bed sores.*

The reported incidence of pressure ulcers ranges from 3 to 20%. For example, a survey of nursing home admissions showed an incidence of 15 to 20% (Bryant, 1992), whereas a survey of 177 acute care hospitals with a total census of 31,530 showed an incidence of 11.1% (Meehan, 1994). In studies involving age, pressure ulcers have been found to occur most often among the frail elderly. In studies involving ethnicity and race, the highest incidence of pressure ulcers has been found among white people, but the highest percentage of stage IV (most extensive damage) ulcers has been found among dark-skinned or African-American persons.

Pressure ulcers diminish the quality of life for those affected and are of high cost to the health care system because of nursing requirements, expensive treatment methods, and increased length of stay. For these reasons, the Agency for Health Care Policy and Research (AHCPR) selected pressure ulcers as a topic on which to develop clinical practice guidelines for use by physicians and other health care practitioners. Clinical Practice Guideline No. 3: *Pressure Ulcers in Adults: Prediction and Prevention* (AHCPR, 1992) recommends strategies for identifying at-risk persons, implementing preventive measures, and treating early stage I ulcers. This document was followed by Clinical Practice Guideline No. 15: *Treatment of Pressure Ulcers* (AHCPR, 1994). These guidelines form the basis of the discussion that follows.

Etiology and Pathophysiology

Unrelieved pressure is the major cause of pressure ulcers: The greater the pressure and the longer it lasts, the more likely a pressure ulcer is to develop. This is because body tissues require an adequate supply of oxygen and nutrients and removal of carbon dioxide and other waste products of metabolism to remain viable and healthy. Maintaining adequate blood flow through the capillaries is essential to meeting these requirements. When external pressure on the tissues exceeds 32 mm Hg (the capillary closing pressure), the network of capillaries collapses and the supply of oxygen and nutrients to the cells, as well as removal of metabolic waste products, is interrupted. This results in tissue ischemia and, if unrelieved, in tissue death or necrosis.

Areas most prone to pressure that exceeds the capillary closing pressure are those close to a bone, where soft tissue becomes compressed between the underlying source of pressure and the bone. In the supine position, these areas include the sacrum, heels, elbows, scapulae, spine, and the back of the head. For example, the mean pressure exerted on a heel resting on a hospital mattress is 85 mm Hg (plus or minus 20 mm Hg) (Macklebust, 1986). This is 53 mm Hg higher than the capillary closing pressure. In the side-lying position, susceptible areas are the malleoli, the medial and lateral condyles of the greater trochanter, the ribs, the acromion process, and the ear.

A second major factor capable of causing pressure ulcers is shear, a condition in which the skin remains stationary while the underlying tissue shifts, causing angulation and thrombosis of the involved blood vessels and leading to tissue anoxia. Shear occurs when the head of the bed is elevated more than 30 degrees because gravity pulls the body downward while the resistance of the bed surface tends to hold the body in place. In recognition of the role of both pressure and shear in the development of pressure ulcers, the term *presshear* has been suggested as an accurate descriptive term (Yarkony, 1994).

In addition to the primary role of presshear in the etiology of pressure ulcers, several other external and internal factors contribute to their development. Friction, the force created when two contacting surfaces move across each other, as when a patient is moved up in bed, removes the outer surface of the skin and thus contributes to skin loss. Moisture on the skin—whether from perspiration, leaking gastrostomy tubes, fistulas, incontinence, or other sources—increases the presshear effect, makes the skin more permeable to irritating substances, and increases the likelihood of colonization by microorganisms.

Internal factors that contribute to pressure ulcer development include the following:

- Relative immobility, such as when the patient is bed or wheelchair bound, is unable to ambulate without help, or has trouble repositioning, as with spinal cord injury, contractures, or altered level of consciousness
- Impaired sensory perception, also found in spinal cord injury and altered level of consciousness
- Diabetes
- Malnutrition
- Anemia
- Advanced age
- Elevated temperature (above 39°C [102.2°F])
- Compromised immune status
- Chemotherapy or steroid therapy

See Table 36–9 for the relationship of these factors to the development of pressure ulcers.

Clinical Manifestations

Decreased blood flow to the skin causes it to blanch and lose its normal red tones. This occurs in both dark and light-skinned people, but it may be more difficult to detect in dark-skinned people. After a period of decreased blood flow or tissue ischemia, hyperemia occurs. Normal reactive hyperemia presents as a localized area of redness that blanches when the fingertips are pressed against it. It lasts less than 1 hour after pressure is relieved. Normal reactive hyperemia is a compensatory mechanism in which local vasodilation increases blood flow, thus providing the oxygen and nutrients needed to make up the metabolic deficit that developed during the period of ischemia. It is an effective protective mechanism, provided the period of ischemia is not long enough to cause tissue damage.

A second type of reactive hyperemia is abnormal. It persists for more than an hour. With abnormal hyperemia, the skin area appears bright pink to red from excessive vasodilation. Induration (localized edema under the skin) is present. The area does not blanch. This indicates that tissue damage has

Table 36–9

Internal Risk Factors for Pressure Ulcer Development

Factor	Relationship to Pressure Ulcer Development
Impaired sensory perception	Person does not feel discomfort from pressure and thus does not unconsciously act to turn or report.
Malnutrition	Cells require nutrients to remain viable. In malnutrition, essential nutrients are deficient, resulting in impaired cellular function, susceptibility to tissue breakdown, and impaired healing.
	Decreased serum albumin is related to the susceptibility to ulcer formation and to the severity of the ulcer.
	Decreased zinc, vitamin A, and vitamin C impair wound healing because they are necessary for the synthesis of collagen.
Cachexia	Decreased adipose tissue means less protection from pressure over bony prominences.
Obesity	Adipose tissue is poorly vascularized and therefore more susceptible to ischemia.
Anemia	In anemia, less hemoglobin is available to transport oxygen to the impaired tissues, and oxygen is essential to tissue viability.
Diabetes	Circulatory changes associated with diabetes lead to hypoxia and impaired leukocyte function thus increasing the risk of pressure ulcers and impairing their healing.
	Diabetic neuropathy predisposes to trauma and therefore to pressure ulcer development.
Spinal cord injury	Pressure from impaired mobility, insensitivity to ischemia, and hypoxemia from the loss of vasomotor control below the level of the lesion contribute to the development of pressure ulcers.
Steroid therapy/immuno-suppressant therapy	Steroids and immunosuppressants suppress inflammation, which is the first step in wound healing.
Advanced age	Changes in the elderly include decreased epidermal turnover, increased skin fragility, increased dryness, reduced microvasculature, decreased cellular immunity, reduced pain perception, and lessened ability to verbalize discomfort, all of which either predispose to pressure ulcers or inhibit healing.
Edema	Edema impairs circulation and, therefore, the delivery of oxygen and nutrients to the involved tissue.
Fever/infection	Elevated temperature increases metabolic rate, thereby increasing the need for oxygen. This makes already-hypoxic tissue more susceptible to ischemia.
Incontinence	Increases exposure of skin to moisture and irritating substances, thereby increasing risk of maceration or excoriation.

occurred and, according to AHCPR guidelines, represents a stage I pressure ulcer (Fig. 36–19). A stage I pressure ulcer causes discomfort, such as tingling or burning, and may be superficial or a sign of deeper tissue damage. A stage II ulcer is characterized by a partial-thickness skin loss that involves the epidermis, dermis, or both. It appears as an abrasion, blister, or shallow crater. A stage III ulcer involves full-thickness skin loss with damage or necrosis of subcutaneous tissue that may extend down to the underlying fascia. It appears as a deep crater with or without undermining of adjacent tissue. A stage IV ulcer involves full-thickness skin loss with extensive destruction, necrosis, or damage to muscle, bone, or supporting structures. Undermining and sinus tracts may also be present.

Stage II, III, and IV pressure ulcers always contain bacteria because there is a break in the skin surface. When the number of bacteria is sufficient to cause clinical infection, foul-smelling drainage appears. In the absence of infection, there may be a continuous loss of serum from large ulcers, which depletes body protein needed for healing.

Diagnosis

Pressure ulcers are diagnosed based on history and observation and are staged as described above. For accurate staging, the bed of the ulcer must be observed. This means that any eschar must be removed before a pressure ulcer is staged (Fig. 36–20). Pressure ulcers should never be reverse-staged. In other words, a stage III pressure ulcer does not become a stage II. Rather, it is a granulating stage III or a healed stage III pressure ulcer.

Soft-tissue infection associated with pressure ulcers is diagnosed by culture of fluid obtained by needle aspiration or culture of tissue from ulcer biopsy. Swab cultures are not used because they detect only surface organisms.

Management

A complete history is obtained and physical examination done because effective management requires that the ulcer be assessed within the context of the patient's overall physical, psychologic, and social health.

Nutritional management is an essential aspect of

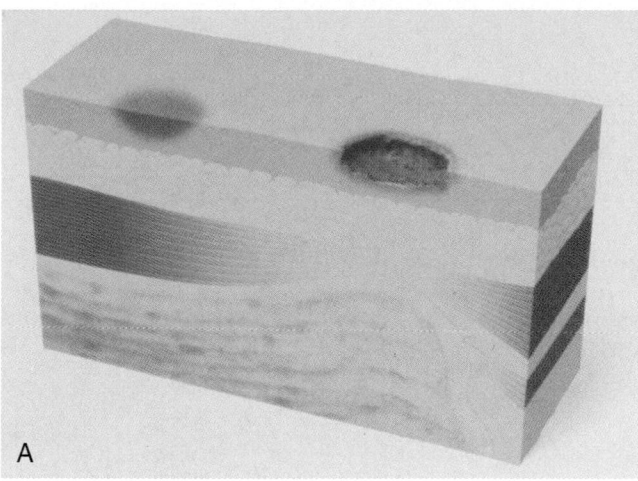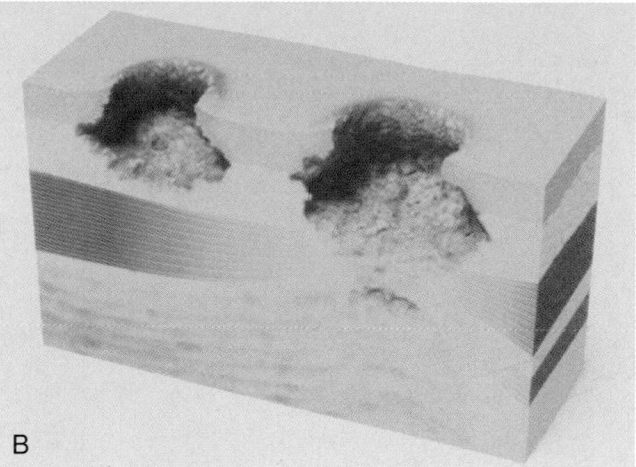

Figure 36–19

A, Stage I and II (partial thickness) pressure ulcers. A Stage I ulcer is known by nonblanchable erythema of intact skin. A stage II ulcer presents as a superficial abrasion, blister, or shallow crater involving the epidermis and possibly the dermis. *B,* Stage III and IV (full-thickness) pressure ulcers. A Stage III ulcer may extend down to but not through the underlying fascia. A deep crater, it may or may not undermine adjacent tissue. A Stage IV ulcer involves extensive tissue destruction, necrosis, or damage to muscle, bone, or supporting structures. (Courtesy of Coloplast Corporation, Skin Care Division, North Mankato, MN.)

care for all patients with pressure ulcers because an adequate supply of nutrients is needed to support the healing process. If the patient's oral intake does not supply needed nutrients, dietary supplements are prescribed. If the diet remains inadequate, nutritional support is used to place the patient in positive nitrogen balance. This support usually takes the form of tube feedings that contain 30 to 35 kal/kg/day and 1.25 to 1.5 protein/kg/day. Vitamin and mineral supplements are given if deficiencies are suspected or confirmed.

A second focus of management is the pressure ulcer itself. This varies with its stage and condition. In cases in which moist, devitalized tissue supportive of bacterial growth is present, management begins with débridement or removal of this tissue to create an environment conducive to healing. In the case of heel ulcers with dry eschar, débridement is used only if edema, erythema, fluctuance, or drainage is present. The various methods of débridement

in current use are identified and described in Table 36–10. To clean pressure ulcers with thick exudate, whirlpool therapy may be used.

Topical antibiotics effective against gram-negative, gram-positive, and anaerobic organisms may be used on clean pressure ulcers that are producing

Table 36–10

Methods of Pressure Ulcer Débridement

Method	Description
Sharp	Scalpel, scissors, or other sharp instrument is used to remove dead tissue.
	Effective for areas of thick, adherent eschar.
	Used when débridement is urgent, as with advancing cellulitis or sepsis.
	Clean, dry dressings are used to cover the wound for 8–24 hours after débridement. Then moist dressings are used.
Mechanical	Wet to dry dressings, hydrotherapy, wound irrigation, and dextranomers are used to remove dead tissue.
Enzymatic	Topical débridement agents (e.g., Collagenase, Travase, Elase) are applied to the surface of devitalized tissue.
	If area of necrosis is hard, crosshatching is necessary to allow enzyme penetration.
Autolytic débridement	Ulcer is covered with synthetic dressings that allow dead tissue to be digested by enzymes normally found in wound drainage.
	Not appropriate for infected wounds.

![Pressure ulcer with eschar labeled STAGE III with ESCHAR]

Figure 36–20

Pressure ulcer with eschar.

Table 36–11

The Braden Scale for Predicting Pressure Ulcer Risk

Patient's Name				Evaluator's Name	Date of Assessment	Score*			

SENSORY PERCEPTION
Ability to respond meaningfully to pressure-related discomfort

1. **COMPLETELY LIMITED:** Unresponsive (does not moan, flinch, or grasp) to painful stimuli, owing to diminished level of consciousness or sedation,
OR
limited ability to feel pain over most of body surface.

2. **VERY LIMITED:** Responds only to painful stimuli. Cannot communicate discomfort except by moaning or restlessness,
OR
has a sensory impairment which limits the ability to feel pain or discomfort over 1/2 of body.

3. **SLIGHTLY LIMITED:** Responds to verbal commands but cannot always communicate discomfort or need to be turned,
OR
has some sensory impairment, which limits ability to feel pain or discomfort in 1 or 2 extremities.

4. **NO IMPAIRMENT:** Responds to verbal commands. Has no sensory deficit that would limit ability to feel or voice pain or discomfort.

MOISTURE
Degree to which skin is exposed to moisture

1. **CONSTANTLY MOIST:** Skin is kept moist almost constantly by perspiration, urine, etc. Dampness is detected every time patient is moved or turned.

2. **MOIST:** Skin is often but not always moist. Linen must be changed at least once a shift.

3. **OCCASIONALLY MOIST:** Skin is occasionally moist, requiring an extra linen change approximately once a day.

4. **RARELY MOIST:** Skin is usually dry; linen requires changing only at routine intervals.

ACTIVITY
Degree of physical activity

1. **BEDFAST:** Confined to bed.

2. **CHAIRFAST:** Ability to walk severely limited or nonexistent. Cannot bear own weight or must be assisted into chair or wheelchair.

3. **WALKS OCCASIONALLY:** Walks occasionally during day but for very short distances, with or without assistance. Spends most of each shift in bed or chair.

4. **WALKS FREQUENTLY:** Walks outside the room at least twice a day and inside room at least once every 2 hours during waking hours.

MOBILITY
Ability to change and control body position

1. **COMPLETELY IMMOBILE:** Does not make even slight changes in body or extremity position without assistance.

2. **VERY LIMITED:** Makes occasional slight changes in body or extremity position but unable to make frequent or significant changes independently.

3. **SLIGHTLY LIMITED:** Makes frequent though slight changes in body or extremity position independently.

4. **NO LIMITATIONS:** Makes major and frequent changes in position without assistance.

	1. VERY POOR:	2. PROBABLY INADEQUATE:	3. ADEQUATE:	4. EXCELLENT:
NUTRITION Usual food intake pattern	Never eats a complete meal. Rarely eats more than one-third of any food offered. Eats 2 servings or less of protein (meat or dairy products) per day. Takes fluids poorly. Does not take a liquid dietary supplement, OR is NPO or maintained on clear liquids or IV for more than 5 days.	Rarely eats a complete meal and generally eats only about half of any food offered. Protein intake includes only 3 servings of meat or dairy products per day. Occasionally will take a dietary supplement, OR receives less than optimal amount of liquid diet or tube feeding.	Eats more than half of most meals. Eats a total of 4 servings of protein (meat, dairy products) each day. Occasionally refuses a meal, but usually takes a supplement if offered, OR is on a tube feeding or TPN regimen, which probably meets most of nutritional needs.	Eats most of every meal. Never refuses a meal. Usually eats a total of 4 or more servings of meat and dairy products. Occasionally eats between meals. Does not require supplementation.
	1. PROBLEM:	2. POTENTIAL PROBLEM:	3. NO APPARENT PROBLEM:	
FRICTION AND SHEAR	Requires moderate to maximal assistance in moving. Complete lifting without sliding against sheets is impossible. Frequently slides down in bed or chair, requiring frequent repositioning with maximum assistance. Spasticity, contractures, or agitation leads to almost constant friction.	Moves feebly or requires minimal assistance. During a move, skin probably slides to some extent against sheets, chair, restraints, or other devices. Maintains relatively good position in chair or bed most of the time but occasionally slides down.	Moves in bed and in chair independently and has sufficient muscle strength to lift up completely during move. Maintains good position in bed or chair at all times.	

Total score

*16, minimum risk; 13–14, moderate risk; 12 or less, high risk; NPO, nothing by mouth; IV, intravenously; TPN, total parenteral nutrition. Copyright 1988 by Barbara Braden and Nancy Bergstrom.

exudate or failing to show signs of healing after 2 to 4 weeks. These agents include silver sulfadiazine and triple-antibiotic therapy. Systemic antibiotics must be given when bacteremia, sepsis, advancing cellulitis, or osteomyelitis is present.

In selected cases, operative procedures are used to repair pressure ulcers, including direct closure, skin grafting, skin flaps, musculocutaneous flaps, or free flaps. Electrical stimulation (electrotherapy) can be used for stage II, III, and IV pressure ulcers unresponsive to therapy.

❖ Settings, Providers, and Collaboration for Care

Patients at risk for or with pressure ulcers are found in all health-care settings as well as in the home. Thus, preventive care must be given in all settings. Treatment of existing ulcers can also be delivered in any setting except for cases treated with operative procedures or complicated by sepsis or other extensive infection that requires admission to an acute care facility. In all settings, effective treatment requires collaboration among physicians, nurses, dieticians, physical therapists, and direct caregivers.

NURSING PROCESS
Pressure Ulcers

Assessment

Perform a baseline assessment to identify the normal character of the patient's skin, the presence of existing pressure ulcers, potential areas of pressure ulcer development, and the patient's overall risk for developing pressure ulcers. Assess the skin in good light, ideally either natural or fluorescent. Ensure a comfortable room temperature to avoid environmentally induced flushing, pallor, or cyanosis.

Note the general appearance of the skin. Is it thin, transparent, wrinkled, lacking in turgor? Is it dry or moist to the touch? What is its color tone? Are there areas of discoloration? If a pressure ulcer exists, note the following:

- Stage
- Color
- Size in centimeters (length, width, and depth)
- Presence of undermining
- Sinus tracts, or tunneling
- Location
- Presence of exudate (including amount, color, consistency, and odor)
- Necrotic tissue
- Granulation tissue and epithelialization
- Condition of the skin around the ulcer

Be certain to determine how long the patient has had the pressure ulcer and whether it is painful.

In assessing for areas of potential pressure ulcer formation, inspect the skin over bony prominences carefully. Observe for erythema. If hyperemia is present, distinguish between abnormal hyperemia and normal reactive hyperemia, in which the area has suffered a period of ischemia without tissue damage. Palpate the area to check for increased temperature, which can indicate inflammation. Also check for edema, which makes the tissue feel spongy. Note if there is little subcutaneous tissue since, without its padding effect, these areas are more susceptible to pressure. Also note obesity. Adipose tissue has a limited vascular supply and thus is itself at increased risk for pressure damage. Observe for abrasions from shear or friction, and for excoriation from prolonged exposure to moisture from incontinence, drainage, or perspiration. Carefully assess skin exposed to casts, traction, drainage tubes, or other appliances that may exert excessive pressure.

Determine the patient's overall risk for pressure ulcers by reviewing the history for risk factors (see Table 36–9). In addition, use a risk-identification tool, such as the Braden scale, which provides a risk score for individual patients and which has been shown to be sensitive and reliable (Table 36–11).

After your baseline assessment, perform continuing assessments at scheduled intervals. Reassess at-risk skin areas at least once a day, with any change in physical status, and at the time of discharge. Reassess existing pressure ulcers weekly because the treatment plan will require revision if the ulcer worsens. Also perform a nutritional assessment at least every 3 months if the patient cannot eat by mouth or has had an involuntary weight change or other indication of risk for malnutrition. Figure 36–21 presents a sample nutritional assessment for patients with pressure ulcers. Assess patients with infected pressure ulcers for signs of sepsis, including unexplained fever, tachycardia, hypotension, and a deteriorating mental status.

Assess the patient's and the family's understanding of the risks, prevention, and treatment of pressure ulcers. Assess the abilities, goals, values, and lifestyle of the patient and the caregiver, because any plan of care must be consistent with these if it is to be successful.

Nursing Diagnoses and Planning

Nursing diagnoses and related expected patient outcomes commonly applicable to patients with pressure ulcers include the following:

NDx: Risk for impaired tissue integrity related to the effects of presshear, moisture, nutritional deficiency

Planning: Patient Outcomes
1. Patient or caregiver describes interventions to prevent pressure ulcers.
2. Patient or caregiver demonstrates a moving and positioning routine that reduces pressure, shear, and friction.
3. Patient ingests a diet containing adequate amounts of nutrients needed to maintain skin integrity.
4. Skin remains intact.

Patient Name: _____ Date: _____ Time: _____

To be filled out for all patients at risk on initial evaluation and every 12 weeks thereafter, as indicated. Trends will document the efficacy of nutritional support therapy.

Protein Compartments

Somatic:

Current Weight (kg)   _____
Previous Weight (kg)   _____ (_____date)
Percent Change in Weight   _____

Height (cm)   _____
Height/Weight   _____
Current Body Mass Index (BMI)   _____ [wt/(ht)^2]
Previous BMI   _____ (_____date)
Percent Change in BMI   _____

Visceral:

Serum Albumin   _____
        (Normal ≥ 3.5 mg/dL)
Total Lymphocyte Count (TLC)   _____ (optional)
        (White Blood Cell count x percent Lymphocytes/100)

        Guide to TLC:

        • Immune competence   ≥1,800 mm^3
        • Immunity partly impaired <1,800 but ≥ 900 mm^3
        • Anergy   < 900 mm^3

State of Hydration

24-Hour Intake _____mL 24-Hour Output _____mL

Note: Thirst, tongue dryness in non-mouth-breathers, and tenting of cervical skin may indicate dehydration. Jugular vein distention may indicate overhydration.

Estimated Nutritional Requirement

Estimated Nonprotein Calories (NPC)_____/kg   Estimated Protein _____ (g/kg)
Actual NPC   _____/kg   Actual Protein   _____ (g/kg)

Recommendations/Plan

1.
2.
3.
4.

Figure 36–21

Nutritional assessment of a patient with a pressure ulcer. (Redrawn from Bergstrom N, Bennett MA, Carlson CE, et al. Pressure ulcer treatment. Clinical Practice Guideline. Quick Reference Guide for Clinicians, No. 15. Rockville, MD: U.S. Department of Health and Human Services, Public Health Service, Agency for Health Care Policy and Research. AHCPR Pub. No. 95-0653. Dec. 1994.)

NDx: Impaired tissue integrity related to the effects of presshear, moisture, nutritional deficiency

Planning: Patient Outcomes
1. Patient or caregiver demonstrates a moving and positioning routine that reduces pressure, shear and friction.
2. Patient ingests a diet containing adequate amounts of nutrients needed to maintain skin integrity.
3. Size of pressure ulcer decreases.
4. Amount of drainage decreases.
5. Pressure ulcer is free of infection.

Nursing Interventions and Evaluation

NDx: Risk for impaired tissue integrity
Protect skin from mechanical and chemical trauma. Begin with hygiene designed to maintain skin health. Clean at-risk skin areas regularly with warm water. Wash gently, pat thoroughly dry, and apply lubricant. Avoid unnecessary friction when washing and drying because it can abrade the epidermis. Also avoid use of soap and alcohol-based solutions because they are drying and leave a residue that supports bacterial growth. Clean areas exposed to drainage, urine, or fecal matter immediately. If a

water-repellant ointment is used to protect the skin from drainage or incontinence, clean it off completely at regular intervals because it can support bacterial growth and lead to skin maceration.

Protect the skin from pressure by ensuring that the patient's position is changed at regular intervals to redistribute body weight, thereby altering the areas under pressure and preventing prolonged decreased blood flow. Small changes in position or the movement of a small pillow or foam pad from under one bony prominence to another should occur every 15 minutes. In addition, the bedridden patient should be turned around the clock on an individualized schedule based on skin condition. Intervals should not exceed 1.5 to 2 hours. For example, a patient who has had a cerebrovascular accident should not lie on the paralyzed side for more than 20 minutes. To provide maximum pressure relief, rotate the patient through six positions: dorsal, prone, right- and left-side lying, and right and left Sims'. The Sims' positions protect against trochanteric pressure and, if pillows are used to maintain the legs in a nearly parallel position, can also help to prevent contractures. At each position change, check the skin for warm or reddened areas. If present, position the patient off these sites. To promote adherence to a turning schedule, post it prominently at the bedside. Include a turning clock or chart showing at which hour the patient should be in which position.

To protect specific areas from pressure, use a bridging technique with pillows supporting the body above and below a bony prominence, thus raising the bony area off the mattress.

If the lower leg is placed on a pillow to keep the heel off the mattress, be sure to provide support and avoid pressure under the knee because it can impede blood flow. To further relieve pressure on the feet and legs, use a pillow or footboard to support the weight of the bedding.

Patients who are chair bound need similar care. Teach the patient to shift position every 15 minutes and to raise off the chair for a few seconds every 30 minutes to relieve pressure over the ischial tuberosities. Remind or help the patient to do this as necessary. All patients confined to a wheelchair should use a cushion custom-designed to the patient's individual pattern of pressure distribution in the sitting position.

Use specialized equipment for bedridden and chair-bound patients if their conditions warrant it. Examples include the following:

- Polyurethane foam mattress, which places more of the body's supporting surface in contact with the mattress and thus more evenly distributes pressure
- Gel-type flotation pad that gives with weight
- Alternating-pressure mattress that, through alternate inflation and deflation of areas of the mat-

tress, shifts pressure from one area of the body to another at regular intervals
- Water bed that floats the body, thereby distributing pressure evenly over its entire supporting surface

Do not use rings or donuts since they impede circulation to the area they are trying to protect. To further relieve pressure and promote circulation, help patients with range-of-motion exercises and ambulation, if possible.

Protect the patient from shear by keeping the head of the bed flat or elevated less than 30 degrees. When higher elevation is required, as for meals, keep the patient from sliding by using a well-padded foot board. Lower the head of the bed again as soon as possible. To protect the patient from shear and friction, use a pull sheet to lift the patient to minimize rubbing of the patient's body against the sheets when being moved. Do not drag the patient to reposition. Use a small amount of cornstarch on the lower bed sheet to allow the skin to slide when the patient moves. Provide a trapeze to help the patient to lift his or her buttocks off the bed when repositioning. Use foam or sheepskin booties to protect the heels from rubbing when the patient moves, but check them often to be sure they have not slipped off and that the strap is not constricting circulation.

Protect the patient's skin from moisture by controlling temperature to reduce perspiration. Keep all clothing and linen dry. Avoid placing plastic-backed pads directly under the patient because they hold moisture against the skin rather than drawing it away. They also cause sweating. Use moisture barrier ointments, condom-type drainage, retracted penis pouches connected to straight drainage, and fecal incontinence pouches to protect skin from contact with drainage, urine, or feces.

To promote early identification of developing pressure ulcers, teach the caregiver or patient to monitor skin condition. If the patient is self-monitoring, instruct him or her in the use of a mirror to ensure that all at-risk areas can be inspected.

NDx: Impaired tissue integrity

Eliminate all pressure from the area of an existing pressure ulcer by adapting the pressure-relief measures described earlier to the needs of the individual patient. Do not allow a patient to sit or lie on an existing pressure ulcer for even a few minutes because it impairs healing.

Clean pressure ulcers at the time of first treatment and at every dressing change thereafter. Proper cleaning helps prevent bacterial colonization from progressing to infection and enhances wound healing by removing necrotic tissue, exudate, and metabolic waste. To be effective, a cleaning method must clean without mechanically or chemically damaging the healing wound bed. Therefore, do not use skin cleaners or antiseptics on pressure ulcers because they are irritating and cytotoxic. Use a nonirritating solution, such as normal saline, and apply minimal mechanical force if using gauze or sponges to avoid damaging granulation tissue and increasing the depth of the wound.

To clean areas of undermining and tunneling, use an angiocatheter and 250 to 500 mL of normal saline to irrigate the debris from the wound. Warm normal saline to body temperature for patient comfort and to encourage wound healing. Use of an angiocatheter is recommended because 4 to 15 pounds per square inch (psi) of pressure is needed to clean a wound. Less pressure does not clean effectively, and higher pressure traumatizes the bed and may drive bacteria deeper into the tissue. An angiocatheter delivers 8 psi, whereas the traditional bulb syringe delivers only 2 psi.

Cover the pressure ulcer with a dressing selected to promote healing given the characteristics of the ulcer. Stage I pressure ulcers, in which the skin is intact, may be covered with a film dressing to protect against shear. For noninfected ulcers in which the skin is broken, use a dressing that maintains a moist wound surface because this stimulates re-epithelialization, as shown in Figure 36–22 (Bryant, 1992). An occlusive film or hydrocolloid dressing, which can be left in place up to a week provided the seal remains intact, accomplishes this and also prevents bacterial contamination. For draining pressure ulcers, select a dressing that will absorb exudate. For noninfected ulcers, a composite dressing with an occlusive cover may be used. For infected pressure ulcers, always use a nonocclusive dressing. When dressing large ulcers, fill dead space (areas of tissue destruction under intact skin surfaces) loosely. Avoid overpacking, which can increase damage by increasing pressure.

In caring for a pressure ulcer, infection control is essential. Protect against cross-contamination through careful hand washing and use of contact precautions in addition to standard precautions. Keep dressing supplies separate for each patient and store them to protect against accidental environmental contamination. Wear clean gloves and use clean dressings when caring for pressure ulcers. Always treat the most contaminated area—the one closest to the anus—last. Be sure to take out only the number of dressings needed. Never return unused dressings to the pack, and never remove additional dressings from the pack unless you have removed your gloves and washed your hands. Place all soiled dressings in a securely fastened plastic bag. If the patient is being cared for at home, instruct the caregiver in proper aseptic technique and obtain a return demonstration.

Because healing is impossible in the absence of adequate nutrition and hydration, collaborate with the physician, dietician, direct caregiver, and patient to design interventions to achieve this goal.

Additional Interventions

If the patient has pain from the pressure ulcer or its treatment, eliminate contributing factors by repositioning the patient, covering the ulcer, or adjusting the support surfaces. Provide analgesia as needed such as before débridement, cleaning, and dressing changes.

Compare the patient's status with the expected outcomes. If the outcomes are not met, reassess the patient and revise the plan.

Neoplasia

Neoplasms of the skin are very common. Most people have one or more types during their lifetime. In addition to being classified as benign or malignant, neoplasms of the skin are further categorized according to the skin structure from which they arise: epidermal lesions, dermal and subcutaneous lesions, and pigmented lesions.

Pigmented lesions are derived from the pigment-forming cells, the dendritic melanocytes in the epi-

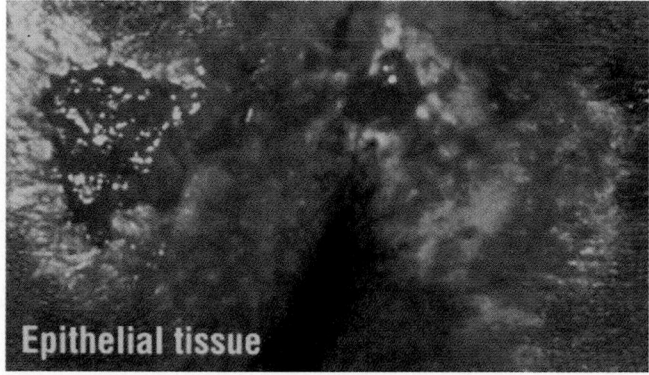
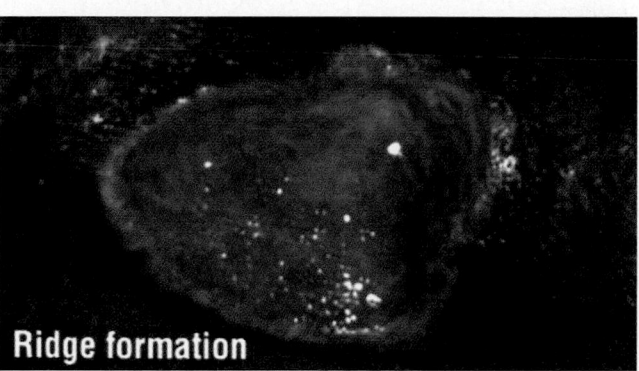

Figure 36–22

A, New tissue growth at the edges of a pressure ulcer. *B*, Ridge formation at the edge of a pressure ulcer. (Courtesy of Kathi Thimsen-Whitaker, RN, MSN, CETN.)

Table 36–12

Benign Neoplasms of the Skin

Type	Description
EPIDERMAL	
Skin tags	Soft, flesh-colored 1–10 mm pedunculated papules of unknown cause
	Occur most often on neck, eyelids, axilla, and inframammary areas of adults more than 50 years of age
	Removed with scissors or frozen nitrogen if irritated or cosmetically unacceptable
	Specimen sent for pathologic examination if necrotic, crusted, or otherwise suspicious looking
Seborrheic keratosis	Flesh-colored, tan, brown, and black, round or oval 2 mm to 2 cm papules or plaques that appear greasy and pasted to the skin
	Develop in middle age or later and most frequently occur on head, neck, trunk, and extremities
	May resemble pigmented basal cell epithelioma, malignant melanoma, or actinic keratosis
	An excisional or shave biopsy is performed for diagnosis
	If irritated or cosmetically unacceptable, may be removed by liquid nitrogen, curettage and desiccation, or excision
Corns	Painful area of hyperkeratosis (overgrowth of horny layer) appearing as a whitish gray or yellowish brown with a translucent core and normal skin lines
	Caused by pressure from poor-fitting shoes or skeletal deformity
	Treated by use of proper-fitting footwear, orthotic devices, rings or pads to reduce mechanical trauma, paring down by a podiatrist, or surgical correction of any underlying deformity
Epidermal cyst	Sebaceous cyst whose wall is lined with keratin-secreting epithelial cells and which is connected to the skin surface by a narrow channel, the opening of which may be imperceptible or blocked with keratin plug
	Presents as round, smooth, protruding movable mass common on face, back, or base of ears, chest, or back
	May remain small or grow until rupturing into dermis, initiating inflammatory response
	Inflamed cysts may require incision and drainage
	Large cysts can be excised for comfort and appearance
DERMAL AND SUBCUTANEOUS NEOPLASMS	
Cherry (senile) hemangioma	Proliferation of blood vessels in the dermis presenting as multiple red to purple raised flat or dome-shaped papules on the trunk that bleed slightly with trauma
	Commonly occur after age 30
	Can be removed by scissor excision or curettage and desiccation
Xanthoma	Accumulation of lipid-laden histiocytes in the dermis associated with chronic hyperlipoproteinemia (persistent elevated serum cholesterol or triglycerides)
	Xanthelasma known by yellowish plaques on the eyelids
	Eruptive xanthoma known by crops of yellow papules on erythematous base found on buttocks and extensor aspects of elbows and knees that clear when serum triglyceride levels return to normal
	Tuberous xanthoma known by plaquelike or nodular lipid deposit on elbows and knees
	Tendenous xanthomas known by hard nodules on the tendons, usually the Achilles or the extensor tendons of the finger
	Xanthomas can be excised if a problem cosmetically or otherwise
	May recur unless the hyperlipoproteinemia is controlled
Neurofibroma	Collection of neural fibers in the dermis caused by overgrowth of cells from neural crest
	Presents as soft, skin-colored papules or nodules that invaginate into skin on compression (buttonhole sign)
	Neurofibromatosis (von Recklinghausen's disease or elephant man disease)
	Characterized by multiple lesions, café au lait spots, axillary freckles, and disfiguring skeletal and central nervous system involvement
	Inherited as autosomal dominant trait
Dermatofibroma	Area of dermal fibrosis, usually on legs, that presents most often as a solitary, firm, slightly elevated lesion ranging in color from light tan to dark brown
	Dimpling sign is characteristic of the lesion (pinching the lesion results in a dimple)
	Enlarging or atypically covered lesions can undergo biopsy; otherwise, treatment is unnecessary
	Common in women
Keloid	Excessive proliferation of scar tissue in response to trauma
	Presents as shiny, firm, protuberant mass with irregular border extending beyond area of original trauma
	Excessive proliferation of scar tissue in response to trauma
	Presents as shiny, firm, protuberant mass with irregular border extending beyond area of original trauma

Table 36–12

Benign Neoplasms of the Skin *(continued)*

Type	Description
Keloid *(continued)*	Pink in light-skinned persons and dark brown in dark-skinned people
	Occurs most often on earlobes, shoulders, upper chest, and back in dark-skinned persons
	Best treatment is prevention (e.g., avoiding surgery or other trauma)
	Intralesional steroid injections over months may decrease size
	Laser and radiation therapy also used with some success
Lipoma	Subcutaneous fat tumor of unknown cause that presents as 1–10 cm soft, elevated mass under normal skin on the trunk, neck, or upper extremities
	Most common in women aged 40–50 yr
	Excision biopsy sometimes performed to rule out malignancy; otherwise, no treatment needed

PIGMENTED LESIONS

Type	Description
Ephelis (freckle)	Irregularly shaped 1–6 mm discrete brown macule caused by increased melanin production in basal layer
	Develops during childhood on sun-exposed skin and darkens with ultraviolet exposure
Lentigo	Brown-black macule caused by increased number of melanocytes and resultant increased melanin
	Actinic lentigo (liver spot) has indistinct border, occurs in sun-exposed areas, and develops in later life
	Can be removed with liquid nitrogen or bleached with hydroquinone if cosmetically unacceptable. Porcelana is a 2% preparation available over the counter
Melasma	Symmetric, macular hyperpigmented lesions on the cheeks and forehead with a well-defined border
	Occurs in women secondary to sunlight exposure, pregnancy (known as chloasma), and use of oral contraceptives
	Lesions fade slowly when precipitating factor is eliminated or may be bleached with hydroquinone
	Sunscreens with sun protection factor 15 may aid in prevention
Pigmented nevi (moles)	Benign tumors composed of nevus cells, which are derived from melanocytes
	Most people have 30–40 nevi
	Biopsy performed if changes occur in color, size, or border; if there is bleeding, crusting, or persistent itching; or if a new mole occurs after age 40 yr
	Repeatedly irritated or unsightly nevi can be removed by shave, punch, or excisional biopsy
	All are sent for pathologic examination regardless of clinical appearance

PREMALIGNANT LESIONS

Type	Description
Actinic keratosis (senile or solar keratosis)	Most common precancerous lesion
	Excessive exposure to ultraviolet rays results in atypical keratinocytes and hyperkeratosis of epidermis and chronic inflammation in dermis
	Lesions are well-defined, round, or irregularly shaped red to brownish to grayish papules covered by dry adherent scale that feels like sandpaper
	Occurs most often on face, ears, neck, and dorsal hand or forearm
	Surrounding skin is often dry, leathery, and wrinkled, with freckles and other signs of chronic sun exposure
	Treatment consists of removal by liquid nitrogen, curettage and electrodesiccation, or simple excision, especially if malignant change is suspected
	Multiple lesions are treated with 5-fluorouracil (Efudex)
	Without treatment, lesions enlarge and 25% develop into squamous cell carcinoma
	Occurs more often in women than in men
Bowen's lesion	Intraepidermal squamous cell carcinoma or cancer in situ found in older, light-skinned men
	Risk factors include exposure to environmental chemical carcinogens and chronic sunlight exposure
	Lesion is a well-defined erythematous eczematous plaque covered with yellow to yellow-brown crust
	Diagnosis is by means of punch biopsy, and treatment is surgical excision
	Periodic follow-up skin evaluation is required
Cutaneous horn	Hard keratotic protrusion developing from normal skin
	Horns are removed and examined because base of horn may have squamous cell cancer
Leukoplakia	White plaque on the mucous membrane of mouth or vagina
Dysplastic nevus	Flat atypical nevus about 10 mm in diameter with irregular border and palpable dermal component
	In dysplastic nevus syndrome, 10–100 or more nevi occur on all areas of the body—scalp, axilla, trunk, groin
	Diagnosed by biopsy and treated by removal or monthly self-examination, examination by physician every 3–6 mo, and medical photography to detect change

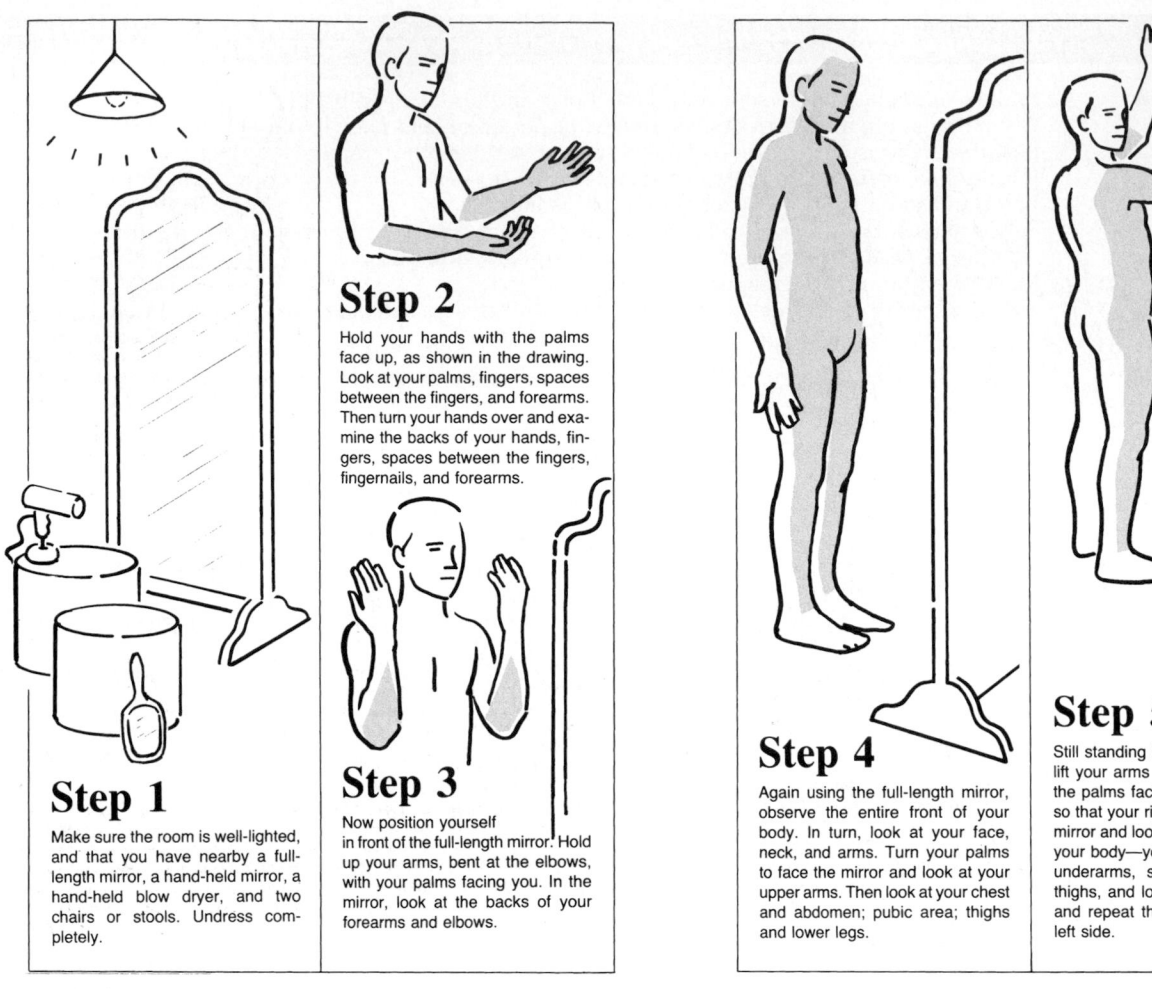

Step 1

Make sure the room is well-lighted, and that you have nearby a full-length mirror, a hand-held mirror, a hand-held blow dryer, and two chairs or stools. Undress completely.

Step 2

Hold your hands with the palms face up, as shown in the drawing. Look at your palms, fingers, spaces between the fingers, and forearms. Then turn your hands over and examine the backs of your hands, fingers, spaces between the fingers, fingernails, and forearms.

Step 3

Now position yourself in front of the full-length mirror. Hold up your arms, bent at the elbows, with your palms facing you. In the mirror, look at the backs of your forearms and elbows.

Step 4

Again using the full-length mirror, observe the entire front of your body. In turn, look at your face, neck, and arms. Turn your palms to face the mirror and look at your upper arms. Then look at your chest and abdomen; pubic area; thighs and lower legs.

Step 5

Still standing in front of the mirror, lift your arms over your head with the palms facing each other. Turn so that your right side is facing the mirror and look at the entire side of your body—your hands and arms, underarms, sides of your trunk, thighs, and lower legs. Then turn, and repeat the process with your left side.

Figure 36–23

Technique for self-examination of the skin. (Courtesy of the American Cancer Society.)

dermis, and the nevus cells arranged in nests in the dermis. Some lesions are further identified as premalignant because of their high incidence of transformation into a malignant tumor.

BENIGN NEOPLASMS

Most cutaneous neoplasms are benign. Information on common benign neoplasms of the skin is presented in Table 36–12.

NURSING PROCESS
Benign Skin Neoplasm

Assessment

Assess the lesion, noting and documenting its location, size, color, symmetry, and border characteristics. Observe for crusting, bleeding, and areas of erosion.

Determine when the lesion first appeared. Ask the patient to describe any changes the lesion has

undergone. Specifically, ask whether the lesion has changed in size. Is it larger? Is it smaller? Has it changed in depth? Has there been any bleeding, crusting, or ulceration? Has there been a color change? Is it darker? Is it lighter? Does it itch? Is it painful?

Question the patient about previous similar lesions, history of sun exposure, exposure to occupational hazards, and any coexisting medical problems.

Assess the patient's psychologic response to the skin lesion. Be alert for signs of anxiety over possible malignancy. Also be attuned to indications of undue embarrassment, fear of others' reactions, fear of rejection, or negative feelings about the body.

Nursing Diagnoses and Planning

Nursing diagnoses and related expected patient outcomes commonly applicable to patients with a benign neoplasm of the skin include the following:

NDx: Anxiety related to procedures to be done and the perceived possibility of skin cancer

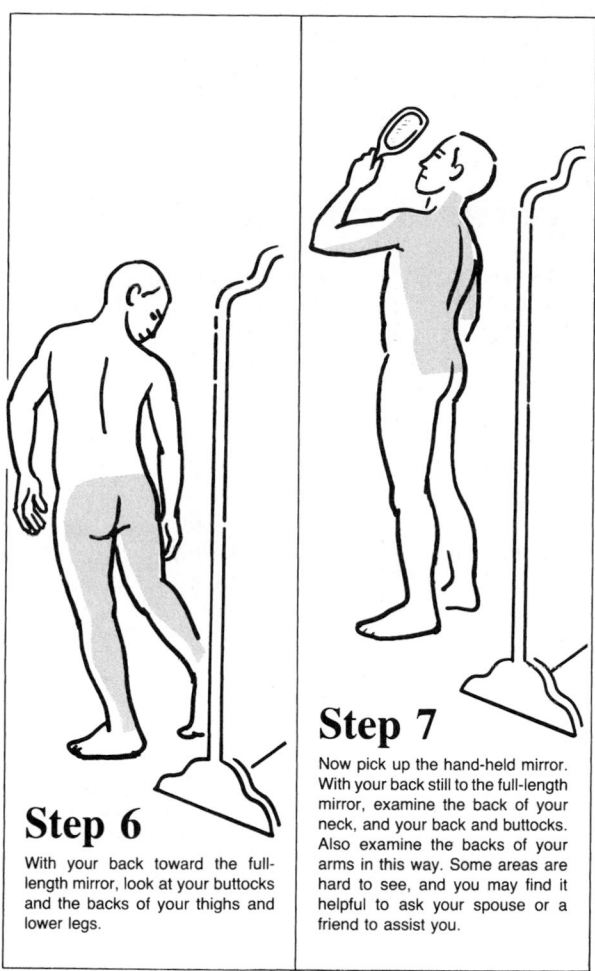

Step 6

With your back toward the full-length mirror, look at your buttocks and the backs of your thighs and lower legs.

Step 7

Now pick up the hand-held mirror. With your back still to the full-length mirror, examine the back of your neck, and your back and buttocks. Also examine the backs of your arms in this way. Some areas are hard to see, and you may find it helpful to ask your spouse or a friend to assist you.

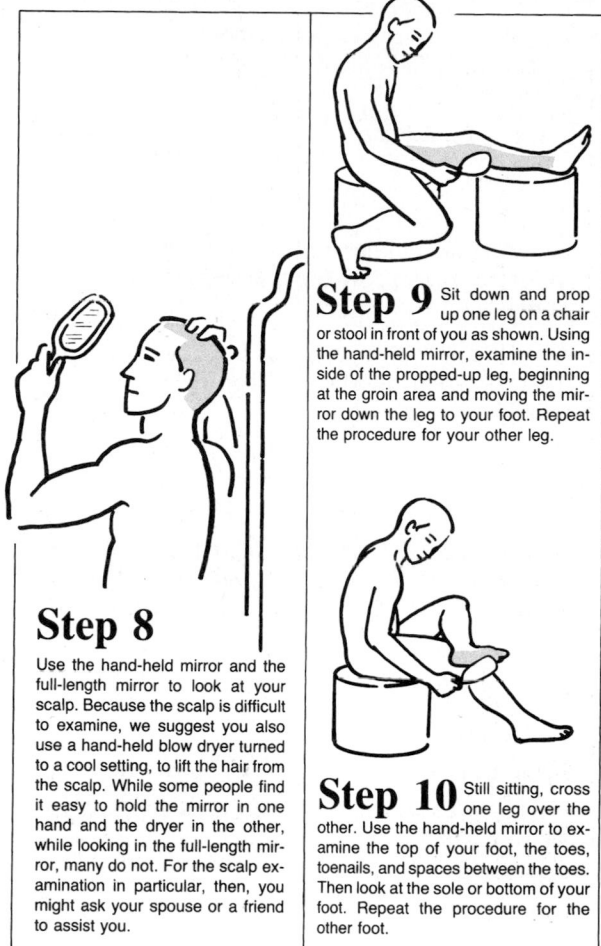

Step 9 Sit down and prop up one leg on a chair or stool in front of you as shown. Using the hand-held mirror, examine the inside of the propped-up leg, beginning at the groin area and moving the mirror down the leg to your foot. Repeat the procedure for your other leg.

Step 8

Use the hand-held mirror and the full-length mirror to look at your scalp. Because the scalp is difficult to examine, we suggest you also use a hand-held blow dryer turned to a cool setting, to lift the hair from the scalp. While some people find it easy to hold the mirror in one hand and the dryer in the other, while looking in the full-length mirror, many do not. For the scalp examination in particular, then, you might ask your spouse or a friend to assist you.

Step 10 Still sitting, cross one leg over the other. Use the hand-held mirror to examine the top of your foot, the toes, toenails, and spaces between the toes. Then look at the sole or bottom of your foot. Repeat the procedure for the other foot.

Figure 36–23 *(continued)*

Planning: Patient Outcomes
1. Patient verbalizes concerns about procedures to be done.
2. Patient discusses fear of malignancy.
3. Patient states that anxiety is reduced.

NDx: Risk for altered health maintenance related to insufficient knowledge of follow-up care, self-examination of the skin, changes in lesion to be reported to physician

Planning: Patient Outcomes
1. Patient states instructions for follow-up self-care.
2. Patient describes technique of skin self-examination.
3. Patient identifies ways to decrease the risk of benign lesions becoming malignant lesions.
4. Patient lists changes in lesions to be reported to the physician.

NDx: Risk for body image disturbance related to presence of cosmetically unacceptable lesions

Planning: Patient Outcomes
1. Patient identifies ways in which lesions can be camouflaged.

2. Patient realistically discusses the effect of the lesion on appearance.
3. Patient verbalizes positive feelings about self.

Nursing Interventions and Evaluation

NDx: Anxiety
Support the patient during diagnostic and surgical procedures by reinforcing the physician's explanation of the purpose and protocol of the procedures. Answer the patient's questions and correct any misconceptions. If a biopsy has been done, inform the patient of when and from whom he or she will receive a pathology report.

NDx: Risk for altered health maintenance
Instruct the patient in self-examination of the skin (Fig. 36–23). Explain why and how often it should be performed. Teach measures to decrease the risk of skin cancer as well as the early warning signs of a nevus transforming into a malignant melanoma (Highlight 36–5). Use the ABCD acronym:

Asymmetry
Border irregularity
Change in color, surface, or sensation in a mole
Diameter more than 6 mm

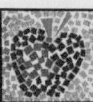

HIGHLIGHT 36–5
HEALTH PROMOTION & RISK REDUCTION
Preventing and Detecting Skin Cancer

Instruct the patient to take the following measures to minimize exposure to ultraviolet radiation:

Avoid being out in the sun between 10 AM and 3 PM, when ultraviolet radiation light is most intense.

Start with short (15–20 minutes) exposures in early morning or late afternoon when sun exposure cannot be avoided.

Apply a sunscreen with 15 or higher sun protection factor (SPF) every day all year when out in the sun if light complexioned or if skin burns easily.

Reapply even water-resistant sunscreens after swimming, strenuous exercise, or prolonged sunbathing.

Apply a lip balm with an SPF of 15 or higher.

Wear protective clothing such as a hat and long sleeves when out in the sun.

Remember that ultraviolet rays penetrate clouds.

Avoid use of tanning lamps or commercial tanning booths.

Instruct the patient to monitor skin changes as follows:

Perform monthly self-evaluation of skin. Pair with breast self-examination or testicular self-examination when possible.

Return for professional follow-up every 3 months for a year and then every 6 months for life after a skin cancer is removed.

Report changes in color, shape, size, occurrence of crusting, scaling, itching, bleeding, and redness or swelling of skin around an existing lesion.

Report development of any new lesions.

Stress the importance of seeing a dermatologist for evaluation and biopsy if any signs of malignancy occur.

After diagnostic and surgical procedures, instruct the patient in the importance of follow-up care. Provide the patient with written instructions for wound care, use of topical or systemic medications, and time, date, and place of follow-up visit.

NDx: Risk for body image disturbance
Explore the patient's perception of the effect of the lesion on his or her appearance. Provide a realistic perspective when necessary. Discuss cosmetic camouflage for lesions on exposed areas of the body.

Compare the patient's status with the expected outcomes. If the outcomes are not met, reassess the patient and revise the plan.

MALIGNANT NEOPLASMS

Basal cell epithelioma, squamous cell carcinoma, and malignant melanoma are the three types of skin cancer. They each arise from the epidermis.

Basal Cell Epithelioma

Basal cell epithelioma (BCE) is probably the most common of all human cancers. It is most common in blue-eyed men over age 40 years with blond or red hair and fair skin. BCE is rare in dark-skinned people and Asians. BCE rarely if ever metastasizes, but it is locally invasive and can destroy all the tissue, cartilage, and bone in the area.

Etiology and Pathophysiology
BCE usually develops in sun-exposed areas of the skin. The longer the sun exposure, the higher the risk. These areas include the face, scalp, neck, forearms, hands, and back. Arsenic in drinking water, ionizing radiation, burn scars, and vaccinations may also increase the risk of developing BCE.

BCE contains cells that resemble the elongated, palisaded basal cells of the epidermis. The epidermis becomes thickened. The invasive buds and lobules of basaloid cells spread through the dermis.

Clinical Manifestations
BCEs present in many different sizes and forms. A pearly, translucent border and telangiectasias (dilated blood vessels) are highly characteristic. The tumor may show no signs of tissue invasion for years or may be rapidly destructive.

A noduloulcerative BCE, the most common form, has a central ulceration and pearly, nodular border (Fig. 36–24). The nodule may have a gelatinous appearance. It begins as a small, waxy nodule, often with a few small telangiectasias on its surface. The lesion increases slowly in size and undergoes central ulceration. It is commonly found on the face.

A pigmented BCE differs from the noduloulcerative type only in its irregular brown pigmentation.

A morphea-like, fibrosing, or sclerosing BCE is a slightly elevated, firm, yellowish plaque with an ill-defined border often extending beyond what is clinically apparent. The skin remains intact for many years before ulceration occurs. It usually appears on the head and neck.

A superficial BCE looks different from the other types and is less aggressive. Superficial BCEs vary in size and can be multiple. They resemble eczematous or psoriatic lesions but have a pearly, rolled border. Superficial BCEs occur predominantly on the trunk.

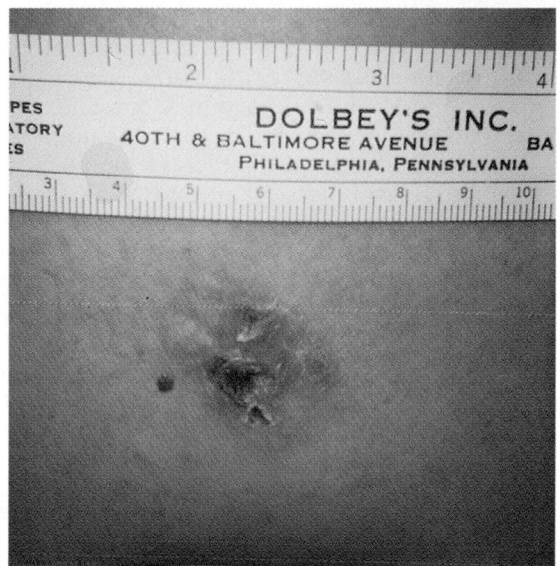

Figure 36–24

Basal-cell carcinoma. Note the translucent nodule. (Courtesy of Columbia-Presbyterian Dermatology Associates, New York, NY.)

Diagnosis

Diagnosis of BCE is based on histologic examination of shave, punch, or excisional biopsies.

Management

Curettage and desiccation is the most common method of treating BCEs. It is 96% to 100% effective in appropriate lesions. The lesions best treated by curettage and desiccation are in areas of increased subcutaneous fat, such as the cheek, forehead, and trunk. This method is not recommended for lesions larger than 2 cm, those over bone or cartilage, tumors bordering mucosa or eyelids, or morphea-like BCEs.

Surgical excision has a high cure rate in the same locations amenable to treatment with curettage and desiccation. The resulting tissue defect is similar, but healing time is shorter.

Mohs' micrographic surgery is done in cases of recurrent BCE, sclerosing BCE, and tumors in the nasolabial fold. It is usually performed only on malignancies affecting the head, neck, or hands, where the best cosmetic outcome is needed.

Radiation therapy is noninvasive, less painful to the debilitated patient, and as effective as other methods while leaving about the same tissue defect. Multiple radiation therapy sessions are required, and the patient is at risk for radiation osteosis and chondritis when exposure is over bone or cartilage, especially in the naso-orbital areas.

The skill of the surgeon is more important than the method of treatment in determining the cure rate for BCE.

Squamous Cell Carcinoma

Squamous cell carcinoma (SCC) is the second most common skin cancer. It occurs more frequently in men around the age 60 years. SCC is more likely to metastasize than BCE, especially in lymphatic drainage areas, such as the neck, ears, or nose. However, statistical figures for metastasis are not high. If it does metastasize, it can be fatal.

Etiology and Pathophysiology

SCC has a tendency to arise on skin damaged by the sun or other radiation. It often arises from pre-existing lesions, including actinic keratosis, radiation dermatitis, Bowen's lesions, keratoacanthoma, cutaneous horns, scars, burn scars, vaccinations, ulcers, and draining sinuses.

DNA, ribonucleic acid (RNA), and proteins in the skin are altered by exposure to various carcinogens. These include UV radiation, x-rays, coal tar, and arsenic. Alteration in the genetic code and cell structure results in epidermal hyperkeratosis and atypical keratinocytes. An invasive tumor and inflammation develop in the dermis.

Clinical Manifestations

Change from a precancerous lesion is often heralded by induration of the lesion and surrounding inflammatory changes. In early stages, SCC may appear to be a thickened actinic keratosis. Arising from normal skin, it appears as a solitary, slowly enlarging nodule with an indurated base. The nodule is firm and develops a central crust that ultimately ulcerates (Fig. 36–25).

SSC may clinically resemble a BCE, but it tends to enlarge more rapidly and usually is firmer, with greater induration and inflammation.

Diagnosis

Diagnosis of SSC is confirmed by biopsy and histologic examination.

Management

Treatment for SSC typically involves surgical excision. Elderly or debilitated patients who cannot tolerate a surgical procedure may undergo radiation therapy. Mohs' micrographic surgery may be the treatment of choice for difficult or recurrent lesions or lesions without well-defined borders.

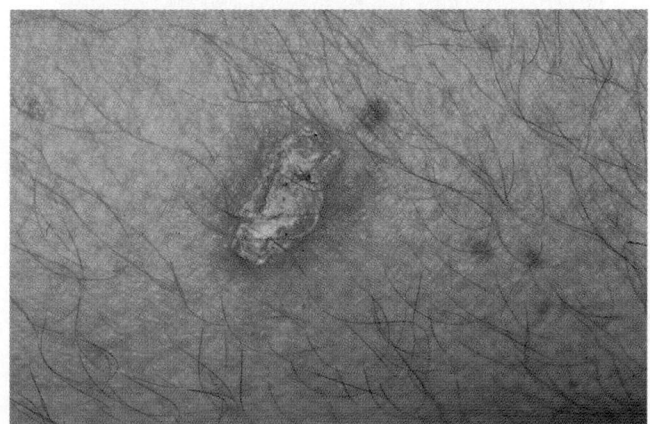

Figure 36–25

Squamous-cell carcinoma. (Courtesy of Columbia-Presbyterian Dermatology Associates, New York, NY.)

Cutaneous Malignant Melanoma

Cutaneous malignant melanoma, or malignant melanoma, is a neoplasm of pigment-forming cells (melanocytes). Although it is the least common form of skin cancer, it is the most common fatal illness seen by dermatologists. The disease is not life-threatening when recognized and treated early.

The incidence of malignant melanoma has been increasing steadily. It occurs most frequently in white men.

Etiology and Pathophysiology

Exposure to environmental carcinogens, recurrent sunburn, sun exposure, and immunosuppression are believed to be the primary etiologic factors in malignant melanoma. Hereditary tendencies and periods of increased hormonal activity may also be factors.

Atypical pigmented melanoma cells are seen in the epidermis. There are various-sized nests of atypical melanoma cells in the dermis.

Malignant melanoma can metastasize. It requires more aggressive treatment than SCC and BCE. If malignant melanoma is diagnosed early, the patient can be cured.

Clinical Manifestations

Positive signs of malignant melanoma, in order of significance, include a lesion with variegated color, irregular border, and irregular surface (Fig. 36–26).

The variegated colors include shades of blue, white, and red in a brown or black lesion. Bluish black, bluish red, or bluish gray melanomas may be uniform in color.

Diagnosis

The only method of diagnosing cutaneous malignant melanoma is biopsy of the lesion. Diagnosis is established by an excisional biopsy with a 2 to 4 mm margin. Incisional biopsy is done on a large lesion. If the lesion is confirmed to be a malignant melanoma, more extensive surgery is done.

After diagnosis of a primary melanoma, a clinical staging workup is completed that includes chest x-ray, complete blood count, blood chemistry, and liver-function tests. Liver, brain, and bone scans do not detect metastases in asymptomatic patients but are performed as base studies for later comparison.

Clinically, Stage I melanomas are localized, Stage II melanomas have regional node disease, and Stage III melanomas are disseminated. Patients with stage II and III melanomas usually die within 10 years of diagnosis. The best prognosis is with melanomas less than 1.7 mm thick.

Management

Wide excision with a 2 to 3 cm margin on all sides is the treatment for stage I melanoma. A wide excision includes removal of skin, fat, and muscle and leaves a large defect that typically requires grafting.

Patients with stage II melanomas and clinically abnormal regional lymph nodes should have excision of the primary tumor, as with stage I, and radical regional lymph node dissection.

Systemic interferon is used for stage III melanoma. Regional hyperthermic limb perfusion is considered as an alternative to radical amputation for recurrent melanoma with intransigent metastases in an extremity.

NURSING PROCESS
Skin Cancer

Assessment

Perform a complete skin assessment, and note the size, location, appearance, and duration of the lesion for which treatment is being sought. Assess the skin for additional lesions. Question the patient about any concurrent physical problems. Assess the patient's emotional response to the problem as well as his or her understanding of it. Be alert for signs of anxiety out of proportion to the diagnosis.

After medical treatment, make assessments required by the type of treatment used. For example, after a wide excision for malignant melanoma done under general anesthesia, make postoperative assessments as described in Chapter 6.

Nursing Diagnoses and Planning

Nursing diagnoses and related expected patient outcomes commonly applicable to patients with skin cancer include the following:

NDx: Anxiety related to treatment, cosmetic result of treatment, prognosis, recurrence

Planning: Patient Outcomes
1. Patient verbalizes concerns.
2. Patient realistically describes expected cosmetic result of treatment and prognosis.
3. Signs of undue anxiety are absent.

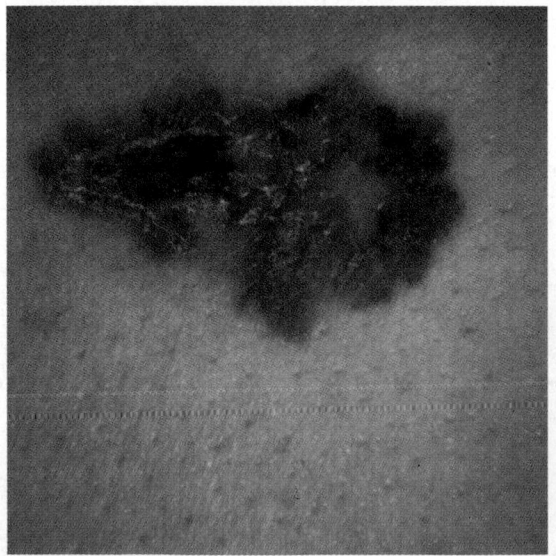

Figure 36–26

Malignant melanoma—an irregular lesion with varying pigmentation and early central thickening. (Courtesy of Columbia-Presbyterian Dermatology Associates, New York, NY.)

INTERNET CONNECTIONS
Integumentary Disorders

General
American Academy of Dermatology
http://www.aad.org/
This authoritative site provides a great deal of information oriented to both patients and health professionals. It provides links to patient information and support groups as well as health-care news and resources.

Psoriasis
National Psoriasis Foundation
http://www.psoriasis.org/
This site also offers information for patients and health professionals. It presents the NPF On-Line Psoriasis Information Resource and provides answers to frequently asked questions, general information, photographs and descriptions of psoriasis, therapy information, case histories with descriptions and photographs, and current research, in addition to related sites worldwide.

Skin Cancer
ONCOLINK/Skin Cancer
http://www.oncolink.upenn.edu/disease/skin1/
Part of the ONCOLINK network, this informative site describes a wide variety of skin cancer types and provides links to an exhaustive list of related resources.

An Introduction to Skin Cancer and Related Topics
http://www.maui.net/~southsky/introto.html
This patient-oriented site focuses on prevention of skin cancer and descriptions of melanoma and related topics. It provides information on environmental factors, types of skin cancer, skin protection, and the effects of ultraviolet light, as well as answers to frequently asked questions.

NDx: Risk for altered health maintenance related to insufficient knowledge of follow-up care for prevention and early detection of recurrence

Planning: Patient Outcomes

1. Patient identifies ways to decrease risk of skin cancer.
2. Patient explains the procedure for and importance of monthly skin self-examination.
3. Patient lists skin changes to be reported to the physician.
4. Patient explains need for follow-up care.

NDx: Impaired skin integrity related to removal of a skin cancer

Planning: Patient Outcomes

1. Patient describes wound care as ordered by the physician.
2. Wound heals without excessive scarring or infection.

Nursing Interventions and Evaluation

NDx: Anxiety
Encourage the patient to ask questions and express concerns and feelings about the disease, treatment, and prognosis. Allay unnecessary anxiety by clarifying and reinforcing information provided by the physician as needed. Acknowledge anxiety as normal. Provide emotional support by listening, being understanding, and providing encouragement. Because recurrence is a major source of anxiety, emphasize the high rate of cure. For patients with basal-cell carcinoma or SCC, stress that metastasis is rare. Reassure patients with stage I or II malignant melanoma that the prognosis for cure is excellent with early removal.

NDx: Risk for altered health maintenance
Instruct the patient in follow-up care needed for prevention and early detection of recurrence (See Highlight 36–5).

NDx: Impaired skin integrity
Instruct the patient in wound care. Keep in mind that instructions vary with the type of surgery performed and with the physician's preference. For example, cleaning of the wound with hydrogen peroxide, application of a topical antibiotic as prophylaxis against infection, and use of a dressing to protect against trauma and contamination may be ordered. Be sure the patient knows what solution, medication, and types of dressing to use, how often to use them, and how to care for the wound aseptically. Have the patient demonstrate wound care when possible.

Provide specific instructions as needed based on the location and extent of the wound. For example, for surgery around the mouth, tell the patient to drink with a straw and to avoid unnecessary movement from chewing and talking. Instruct patients who have had excision and suturing of the thigh to avoid running, jumping, and other activities that could strain the suture line and disrupt healing. If wide excision with grafting is performed for malignant melanoma, provide instructions on wound care, as discussed in Chapter 35.

Additional Interventions
When a diagnosis of malignant melanoma is first suspected, reinforce to the patient that biopsy and excision are urgent.

Compare the patient's status with the expected outcomes. If the outcomes are not met, reassess the patient and revise the plan.

The Elderly: Special Considerations

Skin disorders are one of the most common complaints of older adults. As in any age group, the disorder may be limited to the skin or may be a manifestation of systemic disease. The most common skin lesions found in the elderly are keratoses and basal cell and squamous cell carcinomas, all of which are associated to some degree with long-term exposure to sunlight. Seborrheic dermatitis is also common in the elderly. It is characterized by scaling and erythema, and it occurs primarily on the eyebrows, forehead, and nasolabial fold. It is more severe and resistant to treatment in people who are immunosuppressed or who have Parkinson's disease.

Xerosis (dry skin) is by far the most common of all skin problems in the elderly, affecting most people over age 75 years to some degree. It is characterized by pruritus and dry, scaly skin. Dry skin results from decreased sebum production and is worsened by exposure to cold, dry weather, and by the use of soaps and other drying agents. Treatment of xerosis involves bathing only once or twice a week, avoiding deodorant soaps, and using emollients, such as Keri or Eucerin. Antihistamines should be used with caution because of the high risk for adverse effects in older adults.

Fungal infections may occur because warm, moist areas between skin folds provide good conditions for fungal growth. These conditions are associated with obesity, impaired mobility, and inadequate cleaning and drying of skin-fold areas, such as the groin, axilla, perineum, and under the breasts. The elderly are also at risk for pressure sores and drug-related skin reactions.

Systemic diseases frequently associated with skin disorders in the elderly include neurologic and vascular disorders; gout, diabetes, and other metabolic disturbances; and cancer in organs other than the skin.

Chapter Review

1. What is the relationship between lymphatic impairment and cellulitis?
2. What is the meaning of a worsened drug eruption 24 hours after the offending agent has been discontinued?
3. Why is it essential to effective management that you assess the patient's perception of the importance of an acne condition?
4. What are possible solutions to the problem of pruritus in a patient with eczema?
5. What factors might contribute to noncompliance with tar preparation therapy prescribed for a patient with psoriasis?
6. What evidence supports the therapeutic effect of antihistamines when used in the management of patients with psoriasis?
7. Why is a nutritional assessment important in the care of a patient with a pressure ulcer?
8. How is the care of a patient at risk for pressure ulcer development similar to that of a patient with a pressure ulcer?
9. How is the care of a patient with a squamous cell carcinoma likely to differ from that of a patient with a malignant melanoma?
10. What assessments are necessary prior to teaching an elderly patient about self-examination of the skin?

Bibliography

Agency for Health Care Policy and Research, U.S. Department of Health and Human Services, Publication No. 92-0047, Pressure ulcers in adults: Patient guide, prediction and prevention clinical practice guideline, No. 3, Rockville, MD: Author, 1994.

Agency for Health Care Policy and Research, U.S. Department of Health and Human Services, Publication No. 92-0048, Preventing pressure ulcers: Consumer version, No. 3, Rockville, MD: Author, 1992.

Agency for Health Care Policy and Research, U.S. Department of Health and Human Services, Publication No. 95-0050, Pressure ulcers in adults: Prediction and prevention, Quick Reference Guide for Clinicians, No. 3, Rockville, MD: Author, 1992.

Agency for Health Care Policy and Research, U.S. Department of Health and Human Services, Publication No. 92-0654, Treating pressure sores: Consumer version, No. 15, Rockville, MD: Author, 1994.

Arndt KA. Manual of dermatologic therapeutics. 4th ed. Boston: Little, Brown, 1994.

Arndt K, Robinson J, LeBoit P, Wintroub BU. Cutaneous medicine and surgery: An integrated program in dermatology. Philadelphia: WB Saunders, 1996.

Barker M. Sunscreens. Dermatol Nurs 1995; 7(Aug):247.

Bergfeld WF. The evaluation and management of acne: Economic considerations. J Am Acad Dermatol 1995; 32(5, Pt 3):S52.

Bergstrom N, Braden B. A prospective study of bed sore risk among institutional elderly. J Am Geriatr Soc 1992; 40:747.

Berson DS, Shalita AR. The treatment of acne: The role of combination therapies. J Am Acad Dermatol 1995; 32(5, Pt 3):S31.

Bielan B. What's your assessment: Allergic contact dermatitis. Dermatol Nurs 1995; 7(6):352.

Bielan B. What's your assessment: Herpes zoster. Dermatol Nurs 1993; 5(2):122.

Beilan B. What's your assessment: Skin tags. Dermatol Nurs 1996; 8(1):58.

Beilan B. What's your assessment: Tinea corporis. Dermatol Nurs 1994; 6(5):94.

Black P. Acne vulgaris. Prof Nurse 1995; 11(3):181.

Breslow RA, Bergstrom N. Nutritional prediction of pressure ulcers. J Am Diet Assoc 1994; 94(11):1301.

Breslow RA, Hallfrish J, Goldberg AP. Malnutrition in tube-fed nursing home patients with pressure sores. J Parenter Enter Nutrition 1991; 15:663.

Bryant RA: Acute and chronic wounds: Nursing management. St. Louis: Mosby-Year Book, 1992.

Bryant RA: Wound management. J ET Nurs 1992; 19(2):66.

Callen JP, Greer K, Hood A, et al. Color atlas of dermatology. Philadelphia: WB Saunders, 1993.

Camisa C. Treatment of severe psoriasis with systemic drugs. Dermatol Nurs 1995; 7(Apr):107.

Canning S, Kurban A. Laser treatment of cutaneous malignancies. Dermatol Nurs 1993; 5(6):447.

Colburn L. Pressure ulcer prevention for the hospice patient: Strategies for care to increase comfort. Am J Hosp Care 1987; 4(2):22.

Converse J. Reconstructive plastic surgery. Philadelphia: WB Saunders, 1990.

Cress RD, Holly EA, Ahn DK. Cutaneous melanoma in women. V. Characteristics of those who tan and those who burn when exposed to the summer sun. Epidemiology 1995; 6(5):538.

Crewe RA. Problems of rubber ring nursing customs and a clinical survey of alternative cushions for ill patients. Care Sci Pract 1987; 5(2):22.

Degreef H. International Committee on Wound Management: Wound management and quality of life in the elderly. Ostomy Wound Manage 1994; 40(3):96.

De Keyser G, Dejaeger E, De Meyst H, Evers GCM. Pressure-reducing effects of heel protectors. Adv Wound Care 1994; 7(4):30.

Farber EM. Therapeutic perspectives in psoriasis. Int J Dermatol 1995; 34(7):456.

Fawzy NW. A psychoeducational nursing intervention to enhance coping and affective state in newly diagnosed malignant melanoma patients. Cancer Nurs 1995; 18(6):427.

Fitzpatrick TB, Eisen AZ, Wolff K, et al. Dermatology in general medicine. 4th ed. New York: McGraw-Hill, 1993.

Fleming ID, Amonette R, Monaghan T, Fleming MD. Principles of management of basal and squamous cell carcinoma of the skin. Cancer 1995; 75:699.

Fosko S, Stecher J. The role of home health nursing: A dermatologic case study. Dermatol Nurs 1995; 7(June):185.

Frankel E. Continuing education forum: Psoriasis. J Am Acad Nurse Pract 1995; 7(May):237.

Galloway G, Lawson G. Photochemotherapy (PUVA) protocol. Dermatol Nurs 1995; 7(Dec):348.

Gilleaudeau P, McClelland P. Cyclosporine: A new therapeutic option for severe, recalcitrant psoriasis. Dermatol Nurs 1994; 6(6):395.

Gloster HM, Brodland DG. The epidemiology of skin cancer. Dermatol Surg 1996; 22(3):217.

Grevey SC, Zax RH, McCall MW. Melanoma and Moh's micrographic surgery. Adv Dermatol 1995; 10:175.

Grizzard D. Understanding the pathophysiology of psoriasis: A nursing perspective. Dermatol Nurs 1991; 3(5):305.

Habif TP. Clinical dermatology. 3rd ed. St. Louis: CV Mosby, 1996.

Hanan K, Scheele L. Albumin v weight as a predictor of nutritional status and pressure sore development. Ostomy Wound Manage 1991; 9(Mar/Apr):22.

Ho C, Nguyen Q, Lowe NJ, et al. Laser resurfacing in pigmented skin. Dermatol Surg 1995; 21(12):1035.

Howard R, Frieden IJ. Tinea capitis: New perspectives on an old disease. Semin Dermatol 1995; 14(1):2.

Hunter JAA. Clinical dermatology. 2nd ed. Cambridge, MA: Blackwell Science, 1995.

Janniger CK, Schwartz RA. Seborrheic dermatitis. Am Fam Physician 1995; 52:149, 159.

Kaminester L. The many guises of psoriasis. Emerg Med 1993; 25(May):26.

Kligman AM. Acne vulgaris: Tricks and treatments. Part 1: Cutis 1995; 56(5):141.

Kligman AM. Acne vulgaris: Tricks and treatments. Part II: The benzoyl peroxide saga. Cutis 1995; 56(5):260.

Knight D, Scott H. Contracture and pressure necrosis. Ostomy Wound Manage 1990; 26(Jan/Feb):60.

Koo J. The psychosocial impact of acne patients' perceptions. J Am Acad Dermatol 1995; 32(5, Pt 3):S26.

Kosiak FJ, Kubiosk WG, Olson M, et al. Evaluation of pressure as a factor in ischial ulcers. Arch Phys Med Rehabil 1958; 39:623.

Kottke FJ. The effects of limitation of activity upon the human body. JAMA 1966; 196:117.

Kovacs SO, Hruza LL. Superficial fungal infections: Getting rid of lesions that don't want to go away. Postgrad Med 1995; 98(6):61.

Layton A. Acne: Assessment and treatment. Commun Nurse 1995; 1(7):36.

Lebwohl M, Abel E, Zanolli M, et al. Topical therapy for psoriasis. Int J Dermatol 1995; 34(10):673.

Leyden JJ. New understandings of the pathogenesis of acne. J Am Acad Dermatol 1995; 32(5, Pt 3):S15.

Lookingbill DP, Marks JG. Principles of dermatology. 2nd ed. Philadelphia: WB Saunders, 1993.

Lowe NJ, Lowe PS, Wasiowich E. Psoriasis ambulatory treatment centers: United States experience. Dermatol Nurs 1992; 4(Apr):126.

Macklebust J: Using wound care products to promote a healing environment. Crit Care Nurs Clin North Am 1996; 8(2):141.

Macklebust J, Margolis D: The businessization of health care [editorial; comment]. Adv Wound Care 1996; 9(6):6.

Macklebust J, Margolis D: The need for collaboration in wound care [editorial]. Adv Wound Care 1996; 9(1):4.

Macklebust J, Margolis D: Pressure ulcers: The great insult [editorial]. Adv Wound Care 1996; 9(2):4.

Macklebust J, Sieggreen MY: Attacking all fronts: How to conquer pressure ulcers. Nursing 1996; 26(12):34.

Maksud D, Anderson R. Psychological dimensions of aesthetic surgery: Essentials for nurses. Plastic Surg Nurs 1995; 15(Fall):137.

Margolis DJ, Lewis VI. A literature assessment of the use of miscellaneous topical agents, growth factors, and skin equivalents for the treatment of pressure ulcers. Dermatol Surg 1995; 21(2):145.

Matarasso A. Superficial suction lipectomy: Something old, something new, something borrowed. . . . Ann Plast Surg 1995; 34(Mar):268.

McHenry PM, Williams HC, Bingham EA. Management of atopic eczema. BMJ 1995; 310(6983):843.

Mead M. Psoriasis and skin. Pract Nurse 1995; 10(6):406.

Meehan M. National pressure ulcer prevalence survey. Adv Wound Care 1994; 7(3):27.

Moschella S, Hurley HJ. Dermatology. 3rd Ed. Philadelphia: WB Saunders, 1992.

Meusch R, Lillis PJ. Liposuction: The tumescent technique. Dermatol Nurs 1991; 3(4):255.

Murphy GF, Herzberg AJ. Atlas of dermatopathology. Philadelphia: WB Saunders, 1996.

National Pressure Ulcer Advisory Council. Pressure ulcers: Incidence, economics, risk assessment. Consensus Development Conference Statement. West Dundee, IL:S-N Publications, 1989.

Parker T, Zitelli J. Malignant melanoma. Dermatol Surg 1996; 22(3):234.

Payling KJ. Skin cancer. Prof Nurse 1995; 11(3):175.

Pitman G. Liposuction. Dermatol Surg 1995; 21(May):441.

Pocock DG, Legere-Strunt L. What's your diagnosis? . . . Basal cell and squamous cell carcinoma. Consultant 1995; 35(Jan):83, 87.

Richards C. The effects of psoriasis and its treatment. Part 1. Nurs Times 1995; 91(21):38.

Richards C. Topical and systemic treatment of psoriasis. Part 2. Nurs Times 1995; 91(25):38.

Rodeheaver G, Baharestani MM, Brabec ME, et al. Wound healing and wound management: Focus on debridement . . . an interdisciplinary round table [corrected]. Adv Wound Care 1994; 7(1):22. Published erratum appears in Adv Wound Care 1994; 7(3):4.

Ruane-Morris M, Thompson G, Lawton S. Community liaison in dermatology. Prof Nurse 1995; 10(11):687.

Rumsfield J. Sunscreens: What you and your patients should know. Dermatol Nurs 1990; 2(3):139.

Ruth-Sahd LA, Pirrung M. The infection that eats patients alive . . . necrotizing fasciitis. RN 1997; 60(3):28.

Schnur P, Weinzweig J. A second look at the second-look technique in face lifts. Plast Reconstr Surg 1995; 96(Dec):1724.

Schwartz RA, Janniger CK. Tinea capitis. Cutis 1995; 55(1):29.

Sieggreen MY, Macklebust J: Managing leg ulcers. Nursing 1996; 26(12):41.

Shelk JL. Phototherapy: A nursing overview. Dermatol Nurs 1991; 3(6):401.

Silva-Lizama E. Tinea versicolor. Int J Dermatol 1995; 34(9):611.

Special Communication. Guideline for isolation precautions in hospitals. Part I. Evolution of isolation practices. Part II. Recommendations for isolation precautions in hospitals. The Hospital Infection Control Practices Committee, Centers for Disease Control and Prevention, Public Health Service, US Department of Health and Human Services. Am J Infect Control 1996; 24:24.

Stiller MJ. A management update on psoriasis. Hosp Med 1994; 30(Jan):28.

Strzyzewski N. The cycle of perioperative nursing care for plastic surgery patients. Plast Surg Nurs 1995; 15(Summer):78.

Swanson J, Dibble S. Genital herpes: Clinical features, sources of information, recurrences and treatment in young adults. Dermatol Nurs 1993; 5(5):365.

Thompson G. Treating psoriasis. Commun Nurse 1995; 1(7):31.

Venables J. The management and treatment of eczema. Nurs Stand 1995; 9(44):25.

Voelker R. Making sense of a group A *Streptococcus* scare. JAMA 1994; 272(3):190.

Yarkony G. Pressure ulcers: A review. Arch Phys Med Rehabil 1994; 75(8):908.

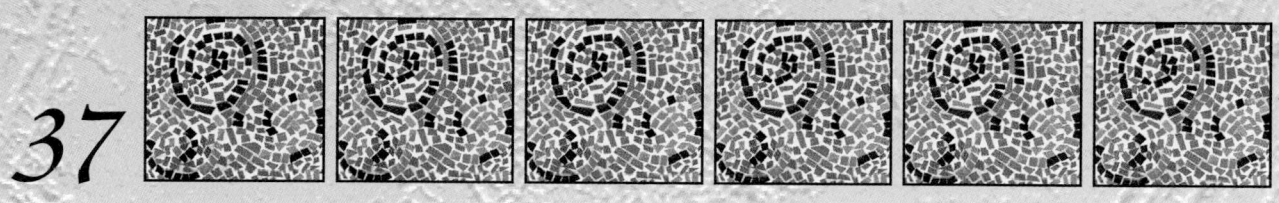

37

Nursing Care of Patients with Burns

Study Outcomes

After studying this chapter, you should be able to:

1. Describe the etiology, pathophysiology, clinical manifestations, diagnostic procedures, and medical-surgical management of thermal, chemical, and electrical burn injuries.
2. Identify information and physical examination data essential to the assessment of patients with burn injuries.
3. State nursing diagnoses and related expected patient outcomes commonly applicable to patients with burn injuries.
4. Describe nursing interventions, with their rationales, commonly applicable during the immediate, emergent, acute, and rehabilitation phases of burn care.
5. Explain the basis for evaluation of nursing care to patients with burn injuries.
6. Identify special considerations for the pregnant patient with burn injuries.
7. Identify alternative treatment and care settings for patients with burn injuries and the services related to community-based care.
8. Identify special considerations for the elderly patient with burn injuries.

Each year, more than 2.5 million Americans sustain a burn injury. Some 100,000 of them require hospitalization, and 6000 eventually die from their injuries.

A burn can be one of the most devastating injuries that can occur to the human body. It can affect almost every organ system and is one of the most severe injuries the body can endure and still survive.

In addition to physical injury, the burn survivor may also endure psychologic, social, and economic problems. The survivor may suffer loss of home, loss of employment, and possibly loss of family members. Some burn survivors have been the victims of crime. A major burn injury affects not only the injured person, but everyone associated with that person.

A team approach is absolutely essential for successful care of the burn patient. The burn team consists of surgeons, internists, nurses, physical and occupational therapists, social workers, nutritionists, psychiatrists, skin bank personnel, epidemiologists, various technicians, and clergy. This team not only must work together but must communicate continually. Frequent team conferences are required to allow all members of the team to formulate a care plan. One goal of the team is to keep the family and, when possible, the patient aware of the plan of care. The nurse coordinates the team because, usually, it is the nurse who spends the most time at the patient's bedside. Burn patients are one of nursing's toughest challenges as well as one of its greatest rewards.

During the initial phases of burn injuries, especially when the injury is severe, the patient may be treated in a special burn center or burn unit in an acute care institution. During the rehabilitation phase of the treatment, care may still be delivered in the hospital setting or in another specialized rehabilitation center. For minor burns, or for some patients during the rehabilitation phase, care may be delivered in an outpatient setting of the hospital, in a clinic, or even in the home. Referrals are made to community nursing services whenever possible and families are taught to do wound care so patients can be cared for in their home.

Assessment of the Burn Injury

As discussed in Chapter 35, the skin has many functions, including the following:

- It protects against infection.
- It prevents loss of body fluids.
- It helps regulate body temperature.
- It acts as an excretory organ.
- It produces vitamin D.
- It contributes to individual identity.

Depending on the depth and size of the burn injury, these functions will be either altered or eliminated. Although all skin functions are important, loss of the first three from a major burn injury must be addressed immediately to prevent the patient's death.

HISTORY OF THE BURN INJURY

A brief history of the cause and circumstances of the injury is critical in managing the burn patient appropriately. To calculate the patient's fluid requirements, for example, it is important to know when the injury occurred. If possible, determine whether the patient was injured in an enclosed space. This information alerts burn center personnel to the possibility of inhalation injury and acute airway obstruction. Enclosed areas—such as tunnels, tanks, and furnace rooms—reduce the patient's access to fresh air, leading to pulmonary injury, carbon monoxide (CO) poisoning, and asphyxiation.

Determine how the injury occurred. Water heater explosions, propane gas explosions, and other explosions that cause burn injuries commonly throw the patient some distance and may result in internal injuries and fractures. If the patient has a chemical burn, it is helpful to know what type of agent caused it. It is also helpful to know whether the patient lost consciousness.

Also try to determine whether the patient has any chronic illnesses, such as diabetes mellitus, hypertension, substance abuse problems, or cardiac, pulmonary, or renal disease. Try to find out if the patient takes any medications, has allergies or sensitivities, or needs tetanus immunization.

FACTORS FOR DETERMINING BURN SEVERITY

To classify the severity of a burn injury, many factors must be considered, including the depth of the burn, size of the burned area, part of the body

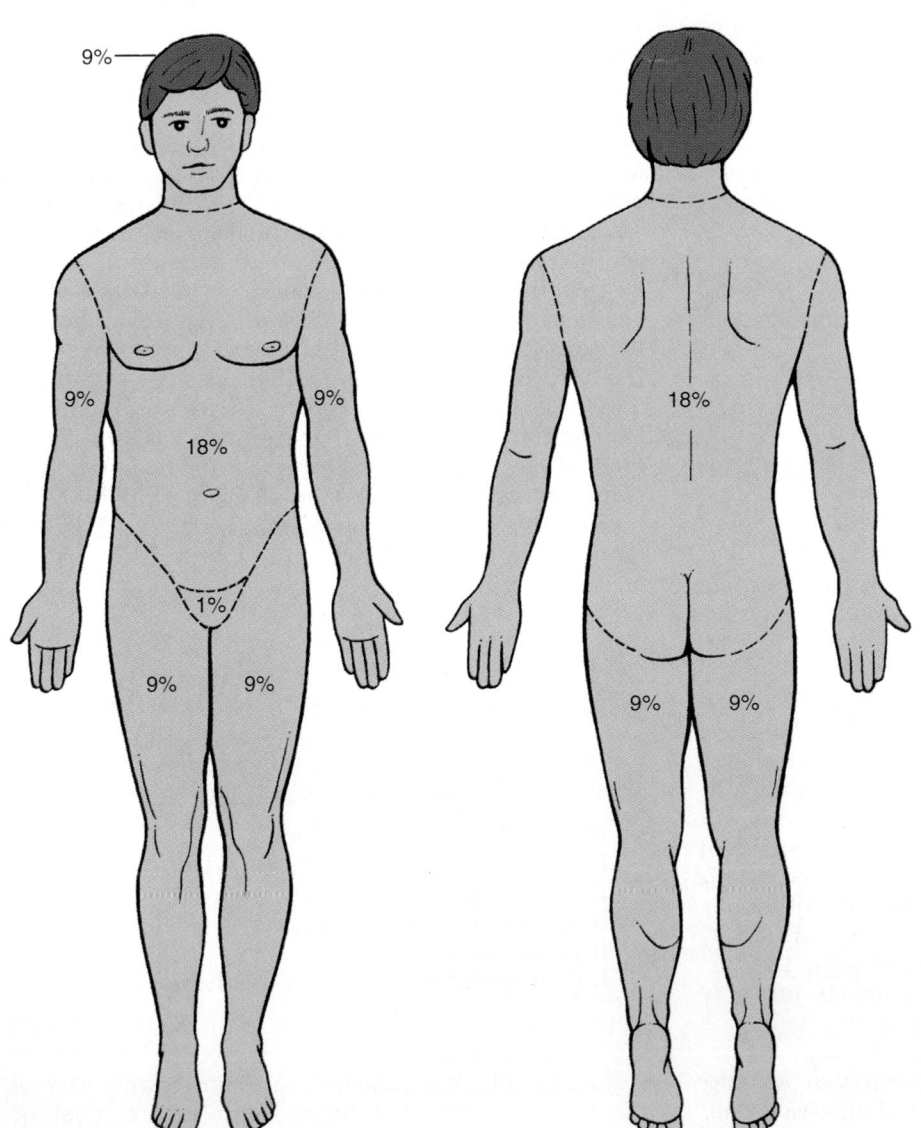

Figure 37–1

The rule of nines is used to estimate the size of a burned area. In this method, each body part is assigned a percentage that relates to the number nine, as shown in the illustration. Added together, all parts equal 100%. By observing the size and location of a burn, and assigning the appropriate body percentage shown, the examiner can roughly determine what percentage of the patient's body has been burned.

burned, age of the patient, medical history, and additional injuries acquired at the time of the incident.

Burn Area

The size of the burn is expressed as the percentage of total body surface area (TBSA). The quickest and easiest method of estimating the size of the area burned is called the *rule of nines* (Fig. 37–1). The rule of nines is a good method for rapid assessment at the scene of an injury or in the emergency department. It does not, however, provide the accurate calculation of percentages necessary for intensive in-hospital care.

The Lund and Browder chart is another method of estimating TBSA burned. This method accounts for the changes in body proportion that occur with age. Its greater accuracy can help determine the exact fluid replacement requirements after a burn injury. Figure 37–2 illustrates a commonly used version of the Lund and Browder method modified by Berkow.

Body Part Affected

The part of the body burned is an important factor in determining the severity of the injury. Certain areas of the body present serious potential complications. Burns that involve the face, neck, and chest are associated with a greater possibility of pulmonary complications. Burns of the hands, feet, or joints require intense physical and occupational re-habilitation. Burns of the perineum have a high rate of infection. Because of the high incidence of complications, any burn involving the hands, face, eyes, ears, feet, or perineum is considered a major burn injury, regardless of the burn's size.

Burn Depth

Determining the depth of a burn identifies which skin layers have been damaged or destroyed and provides the burn team with important information in developing treatment plans for the patient.

The severity of damage to the innermost layer of the epidermis, the stratum germinativum or basal cell layer, has significant impact on burn care. This layer is the site where new cells are produced to replace destroyed or damaged cells. Basal cells are also found in the dermis lining the hair follicles and the sweat and sebaceous glands. It is the presence of adequate numbers of basal cells that determines whether a burn wound heals spontaneously by regenerating new skin or whether it requires skin grafting to heal.

New technology is being developed to aid professional staff in determining the depth of a burn. A laser Doppler flowmeter is being used in some burn centers to measure wound perfusion and predict wound outcomes. Accuracy in early prediction of burn depth aids the team in making management decisions sooner and potentially decreasing hospitalization time.

Burn depth, as summarized in Table 37–1, is

Table 37–1

Types of Burn Injuries

Classification	Skin Layers Damaged	Clinical Manifestations	Sensation	Healing Time	Result
Superficial (first-degree)	Epidermis	Pink to red No blisters or bullae Skin dry Minimal edema	Painful for short duration	3–5 days	No scarring
Partial-thickness (second-degree)	Entire epidermis, partial dermis	Red to ivory-white Blisters and bullae Wet, glistening surface Edema formation Slow blanching and capillary refill	Very painful	14–28 days	Scarring varies
Full-thickness (third-degree)	Entire epidermis, entire dermis, and sometimes fat, muscle, bone	White, black, cherry-red, tan Thrombosed vessels No blister formation Dry, leathery surface No elasticity Massive edema	Painless	No healing potential	Scarring

Body Area	0-1 Years	1-4 Years	5-9 Years	10-14 Years	15 Years	Adult
Head	19	17	13	11	9	7
Neck	2	2	2	2	2	2
Ant. Trunk	13	13	13	13	13	13
Post. Trunk	13	13	13	13	13	13
R. Buttock	2.5	2.5	2.5	2.5	2.5	2.5
L. Buttock	2.5	2.5	2.5	2.5	2.5	2.5
Genitalia	1	1	1	1	1	1
R. U. Arm	4	4	4	4	4	4
L. U. Arm	4	4	4	4	4	4
R. L. Arm	3	3	3	3	3	3
L. L. Arm	3	3	3	3	3	3
R. Hand	2.5	2.5	2.5	2.5	2.5	2.5
L. Hand	2.5	2.5	2.5	2.5	2.5	2.5
R. Thigh	5.5	6.5	8	8.5	9	9.5
L. Thigh	5.5	6.5	8	8.5	9	9.5
R. L. Leg	5	5	5.5	6	6.5	7
L. L. Leg	5	5	5.5	6	6.5	7
R. Foot	3.5	3.5	3.5	3.5	3.5	3.5
L. Foot	3.5	3.5	3.5	3.5	3.5	3.5

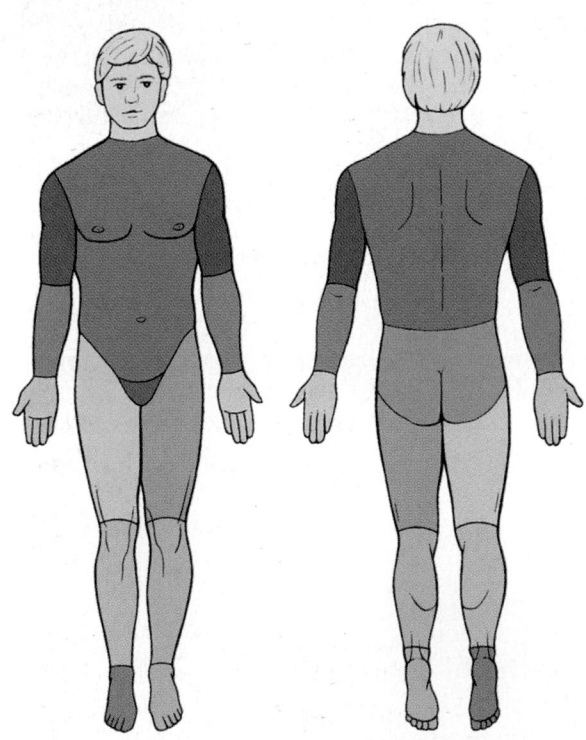

Figure 37–2

Berkow's adaptation of Lund and Browder's method of calculating the percentage of total body surface area (TBSA) burned. This method accounts for age-related changes in body proportion.

classified as either partial thickness or full thickness. Partial-thickness injuries are subdivided into superficial injuries or deep injuries.

SUPERFICIAL AND PARTIAL-THICKNESS BURNS

Superficial Burns

Superficial burn injuries (previously called first-de-gree burns) are commonly caused by brief contact with a hot object, low-voltage electricity, a spatter scald, or, most commonly, ultraviolet light (sunburn). They involve only the epidermis of the skin; therefore, skin functions are minimally affected.

These burn wounds are typically pink to red in color, with a dry surface, no vesicles, and no or minimal edema. They are painful, blanch with pressure, and have quick capillary refill. The burn area may blister and peel after 24 hours. Superficial partial-thickness burns heal spontaneously, without scarring, in 3 to 5 days. An example of a superficial partial-thickness burn can be seen in Figure 37–3A.

Partial-Thickness Burns

Partial-thickness burn injuries (previously called second-degree burns) are caused by more prolonged contact with hot objects, hot liquids, or chemicals. These burns involve all of the epidermis and part of the dermis but do not destroy the sweat glands, hair follicles, or basal cells lining them.

Partial-thickness burns are red, mottled, or white in color. Fluid-filled surface vesicles or bullae form rapidly and may or may not be intact on the patient's arrival at the hospital. An important characteristic is that these burns are wet and glistening. Hairs present in the wound will remain firmly in place if pulled. The patient usually experiences a great deal of pain from a deep partial-thickness burn because of the damaged nerve endings. Blanching and capillary refill will occur but not as

rapidly as with the more superficial injury. Edema is present and varies from moderate to severe. An example of a deep partial-thickness burn can be seen in Figure 37–3B.

In the care of partial-thickness burns, it is important to prevent conversion of the wound to a full-thickness injury from further trauma, infection, poor tissue perfusion, or prolonged pressure. Partial-thickness burns can heal spontaneously by regeneration from the basal cells. However, to minimize functional loss and scarring, the burn team may opt to graft wounds that will take more than 2 to 3 weeks to heal. In some patients, original skin color may not return because melanocytes have been destroyed. These cells are located primarily in the deepest layer of the epidermis and produce the melanin that determines skin pigmentation.

FULL-THICKNESS BURNS

A full-thickness burn injury (previously called third-degree burn), as seen in Figure 37–3C, involves de-

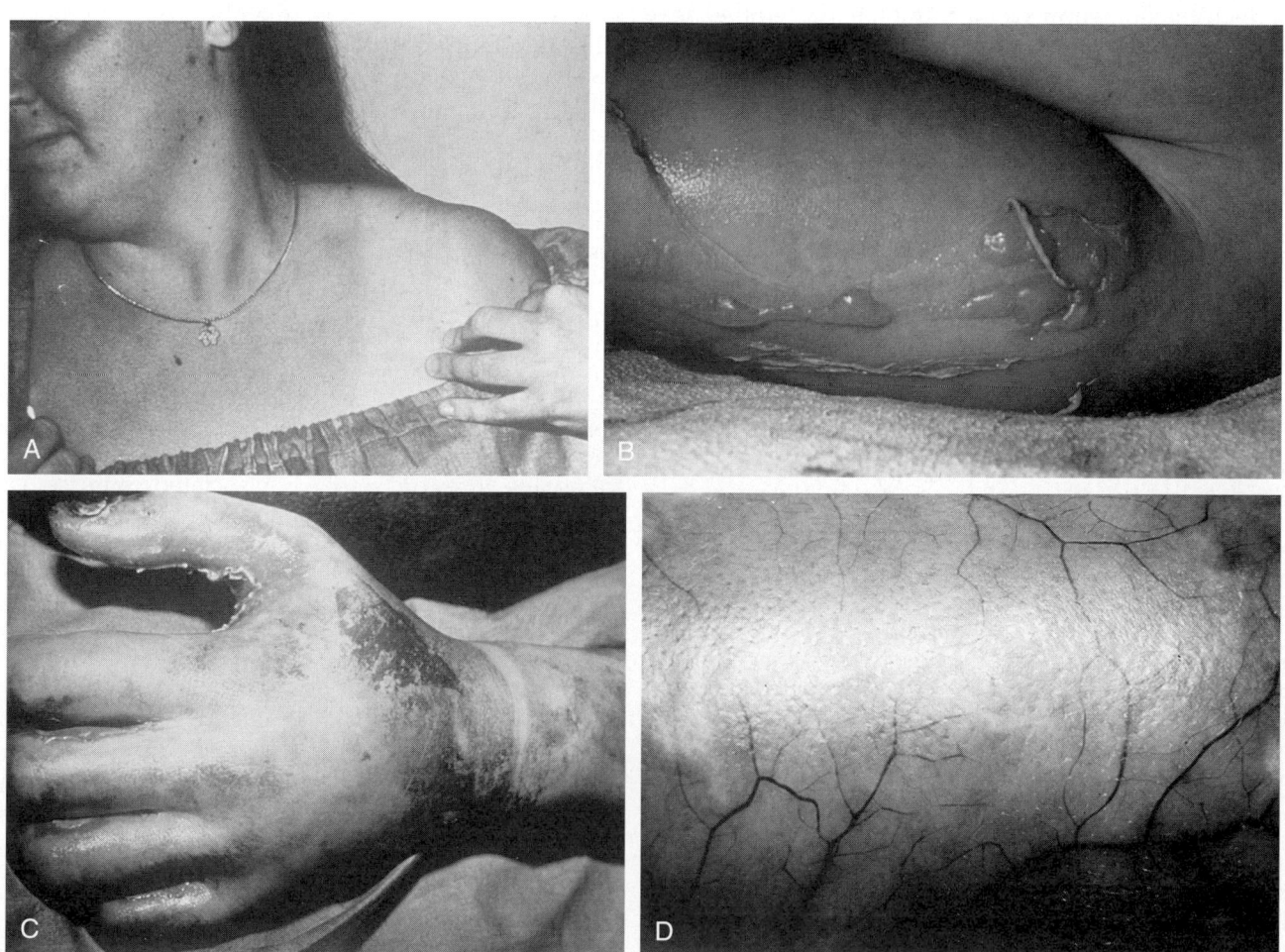

Figure 37–3

A, Sunburn is the most common example of a superficial partial-thickness burn injury. *B,* Glistening wet surface, thick peeling skin, and fluid-filled vesicles typical of a deep partial-thickness burn injury. *C,* Dry, leathery-white, taut skin and severe edema in a full-thickness burn injury. *D,* Thrombosed vessels with hemolyzed blood seen beneath the surface of a full-thickness burn injury. Note the taut skin from severe edema.

struction of the epidermis and dermis. These injuries are commonly caused by prolonged contact with flames, electricity, chemicals, hot liquids (immersion), and hot objects. Brief contact with high-voltage electricity can also cause a full-thickness burn injury.

A full-thickness burn injury may be black, waxy white, cherry-red, or tan. It is leathery, dry, and hard. The capillary bed is destroyed, and thrombosed vessels may sometimes be seen within the wound (see Fig. 37–3D). Blanching does not occur. Any hairs remaining in the wound can be pulled out easily. Although full-thickness burns are painless from nerve destruction, any surrounding areas of partial-thickness burn injury will still be very painful. Surface edema may not appear as severe in a full-thickness burn as with a partial-thickness burn because loss of the skin's elasticity does not allow for expansion. However, it is important to remember that edema develops in the deeper tissues. Increased pressure on blood vessels and internal structures can cause serious problems.

Because the epidermis, dermis, and basal cells are destroyed, spontaneous healing will not occur by re-epithelialization from within. If the wound is the size of a half dollar or smaller, doctors may elect to allow the wound to cover itself through contractions of wound margins. This will leave a small scar and is commonly referred to as allowing the wound to "scar in." Larger wounds must receive skin grafts to heal.

It should be noted that initial assessment of the depth of a burn injury is not always accurate. It may take 2 to 3 days for the full extent of the injury to become apparent. In addition, extensive burns usually present with several depths of tissue injury. It is therefore important to consider the history and cause of the burn injury when initially assessing the patient and determining treatment.

Burn Agent

Burns are classified as thermal (heat, hot liquids, radiation), chemical, and electrical. The depth of the injury caused by hot liquids depends on the temperature of the liquid and the length of exposure. Typically, oil burns are deeper because oil reaches higher temperatures and adheres to the skin, lengthening exposure time.

Management of chemical and electrical burns is complicated by the nature of the agent causing the burn. Chemical burns continue to destroy tissue until adequately irrigated with water to dilute the chemical. Electrical burns cause extensive injury to internal organs, muscles, nerves, and blood vessels. These internal injuries are difficult to assess at the time of the initial injury, yet may greatly complicate care. Some may take months or years to become apparent. In addition, electrical arcing may cause clothing to ignite, resulting in a thermal burn in addition to the electrical injury. A complete history

of the circumstances of the injury helps the burn team to anticipate problems.

Age of the Patient

The child under age 10 and the adult over age 50 with a burn injury are considered at high risk during treatment. The dermis of young and elderly patients is thinner, allowing a deeper burn from exposure to the heat source. Diminished blood supply to the skin in the elderly lengthens healing time, while a weaker immune response increases the risk of infection. Recovery of the elderly patient may be further complicated by pre-existing health problems that compromise cardiovascular, respiratory, and nutritional status and increase the risk of complications. Because of higher mortality, any burn to a person in these age groups is considered a potentially serious burn injury and should be evaluated in an emergency department.

Medical History

It is extremely important to obtain a medical history from the patient, a family member, or a significant other. Pre-existing conditions (such as cardiovascular disease, diabetes, seizure disorder) may be exacerbated by a burn injury and may complicate the patient's recovery. Allergies should be prominently noted in the patient record and posted on the front of the chart, on the medication record, and in the nursing care plan. Tetanus immunization status should also be noted.

Associated Injuries

Many patients suffer other injuries in addition to the burn injury. These occur most often when the patient is involved in a motor-vehicle accident, an explosion, or when the victim jumps from a building to escape fire or smoke. Associated injuries can range from minor to life-threatening and can include internal injuries, lacerations, fractures, spinal cord injury, and head trauma. Any additional injury will further complicate the patient's recovery.

CRITERIA FOR TRANSPORT TO A BURN CENTER

The following list includes the injuries that the American Burn Association has identified as those for which the patient should be transported to a burn center after initial assessment and treatment at an emergency department:

- Partial-thickness and full-thickness burns of 10% or more of the body surface in patients younger than 10 years or older than 50 years
- Partial-thickness and full-thickness burns of more than 20% of the body surface in other age groups

- Full-thickness burns of more than 5% of the body surface area in any age group
- Partial-thickness and full-thickness burns that involve the face, hands, feet, genitalia, perineum, or major joints
- Electrical burns, including lightning injury
- Chemical burns
- Inhalation injury with burn injury
- Full-thickness circumferential burns of the extremity and chest
- Lesser burns in patients with pre-existing medical problems that could complicate management
- Associated injuries or pregnancy

When trauma-related injuries pose a greater immediate risk than the burn injury, the patient may be treated in a trauma center until stable before being transferred to a burn center. This decision is made by the trauma physician in consultation with the regional burn center.

Care of the Burn Injury

Care of the patient with a burn injury is determined in part by the time elapsed since the injury occurred. Burn care includes four phases: the immediate phase, at the scene of the injury; the emergent phase, during the first 48 to 72 hours; the acute phase, which begins with reabsorption of interstitial fluid (at the end of the emergent period) and ends with wound closure; and the rehabilitation phase.

Although for clarity of presentation each of the phases of burn care is discussed individually, it is important to remember that, to provide continuity of care, many aspects of patient care overlap the phases. For example, wound care, which is presented as a primary focus of the acute phase, begins with immediate care at the scene and continues through the rehabilitation phase. Rehabilitation, discussed as the final phase of burn care, begins on first contact with health care professionals and continues through all phases of burn care. Nursing Care Guide 37–1 illustrates this necessary overlap of patient care among the four phases.

IMMEDIATE PHASE

The priority of immediate care at the scene, as summarized in Table 37–2, is to stop the burning process, prevent further injury, and maintain vital functions until the ambulance arrives with monitoring and life-support equipment. The nurse at the scene must first determine the safest access to the victim. Next, the victim must be moved to a safe area before treating. Successful treatment cannot be given in a smoke-filled area, nor can the nurse be of help if he or she is overcome from inhaling smoke or injured by falling debris.

Stop the Burning Process

The first step in treating the victim is to stop the burning process to halt the penetration of heat to deeper tissue, causing greater damage. First, remove the heat source. If the victim is still on fire, roll him or her immediately on the ground or smother the flames in a blanket. If skin is warm to the touch, cool it with water. Clothes should be removed and the patient transported to the hospital covered in a clean dry sheet or blanket. Loss of skin leaves the body unable to regulate temperature. Thus, the victim is at high risk for hypothermia if the burn covers more than 10% TBSA.

If the injury resulted from a chemical, use caution in approaching the scene to prevent contact with the chemical, particularly when the accident involved a spill or explosion. All persons who touch the patient should first put on a double set of rubber gloves to prevent contact with any chemical on the patient's skin or clothing. Protective clothing and eye covering are also desirable. Do not waste time in determining the correct neutralizing agent. The priority is to remove any chemical in contact with the patient. First, rapidly remove the patient's garments, which will retain the chemical agent. Next, brush any chemical in powdered or visible form from the skin. Flush the skin with large amounts of water for at least 15 to 30 minutes to dilute and wash away the chemical. Use a shower or hose if available. Flush chemical burns of the eyes from the inner canthus, next to the nose, toward the outer canthus to avoid washing the chemical from one eye into the other. Remove contact lenses, and continue eye irrigation throughout transport to the hospital.

It is extremely important that anyone assisting at the scene of an electrical burn take precautions in approaching the victim to prevent becoming a second victim. Make sure the electrical current has been turned off or removed before touching the victim. Use a long pole made of dry wood or dry rubber to remove the victim from the electrical source if the current cannot be turned off. Cardiopulmonary resuscitation (CPR) may be needed if the victim has no pulse. Many victims of electrical injury respond quickly to cardiopulmonary resuscitation and can be resuscitated.

Maintain a Patent Airway

Proper airway management is imperative. Assess the victim's breathing. The airway must be open and free of debris. Establish a patent airway, if needed, by using the chin lift maneuver. If the victim is not breathing, perform rescue breathing.

Treat Life-Threatening Injuries

Very often, these victims have life-threatening injuries in addition to the burn injury. Associated inju-

Text continued on page 1655

Nursing Care Guide 37-1
Patients with Thermal Burn Injuries

Assessment Findings: Patient is 1 hour post–thermal burn injury of the anterior torso, neck, chin, and upper arms. Fire occurred in the patient's small bedroom. Patient is alert and oriented. Nasal hairs are singed, external nares blistered. Oral mucous membranes are pink, moist. Breath sounds: clear and unlabored; respiratory rate: 16, regular and unlabored.

Nursing Diagnosis: Risk for ineffective airway clearance related to possible upper airway edema secondary to inhalation of superheated air

Patient Outcomes	Nursing Interventions	Rationale
Patient maintains patent airway with regular, unlabored respirations between 12 and 20 per minute.	Identify body surface areas burned. Determine the circumstances of the burn injury.	Risk of upper airway injury is greater in burns of the face, neck, or upper chest and if the fire occurred in a confined space.
	Examine the patient for singed nasal hairs; soot on the tongue, pharynx, or in the sputum; redness or blistering of the lips, face, or buccal mucosa.	These manifestations indicate possible upper airway burn injury.
	Auscultate breath sounds, and assess rate, depth, rhythm of respirations, level of consciousness, and voice quality at least hourly.	Edema narrows respiratory passages, causing frequent cough, wheezing, crackles (rales), stridor, or hoarseness. Restlessness, increasing respiratory rate, altered respiratory depth, irregular respiratory rhythm, and decreasing level of consciousness (LOC) indicate impaired respiratory function.
	Elevate the head of the bed.	Elevation promotes venous drainage to reduce edema and promotes chest expansion and diaphragmatic excursion to ease breathing.
	Provide humidified oxygen.	Prevents drying of respiratory tissues and improves oxygenation.
	Administer intravenous narcotic analgesics as needed and before wound care.	Pain increases anxiety and oxygen requirements.
	Encourage position changes, deep breathing, coughing, and use of incentive spirometer.	Prevents stasis of secretions and promotes respiratory function.
	Monitor arterial blood gases.	An increasing partial pressure of carbon dioxide ($PaCO_2$) and a decreasing partial pressure of oxygen (PaO_2) indicate respiratory compromise.
	Notify physician promptly of any indication of deteriorating respiratory status.	Intubation may be necessary to maintain patent airway. Early intervention prevents further deterioration in status and the risk of hypoxia.

(continued)

Nursing Care Guide 37–1
Patients with Thermal Burn Injuries (continued)

Evaluation:	Compare the patient's status with the expected outcomes. If the outcomes are not met, reassess the patient and revise the plan.
Assessment Findings:	Patient is 2 hours–thermal burn injury with partial-thickness burns over 40% of total body surface area (TBSA). Burned areas are edematous and blistered, with open areas weeping serous fluid. Patient is lethargic, urine output is 25 mL/hour via indwelling urinary catheter, blood pressure (BP) is 90/60, pulse rate is 100 beats per minute (bpm), central venous pressure (CVP) is 5 cm of water (H_2O), intravenous (IV) lactated Ringer's solution infusing 600 mL/hour via large-bore IV catheter. Patient is to receive 9600 mL of IV fluid resuscitation over 24 hours from time of the burn injury.
Nursing Diagnosis:	Risk for fluid volume deficit related to inadequate replacement of fluids lost through evaporation from the burn wound and fluid shift into interstitial spaces

Patient Outcomes	Nursing Interventions	Rationale

Patient maintains adequate hydration as evidenced by:
  Being mentally alert
  Urine output > 30 mL/hour
  BP > 90/60
  Heart rate 60–100 bpm
  CVP 4–15 mm H_2O
Moist mucous membranes
Capillary refill < 3 seconds
	Weigh patient and obtain vital signs on admission. Monitor vital signs, LOC, CVP, urine output, and capillary refill at least hourly.	Changes in these parameters indicate the adequacy of fluid resuscitation. Hypovolemia is indicated by decreasing LOC, urine output < 30 mL/hour, BP < 90/60, heart rate > 100 bpm, dry mucous membranes, delayed capillary refill.

	Maintain IV infusion for fluid resuscitation. Calculate flow rate to ensure that 50% of the total fluid volume prescribed for the initial 24-hour period from the time of the injury will infuse over the first 8 hours. The remaining 50% infuses over the next 16 hours. Assess infusion sites hourly.	Infusion of large volumes of fluids and electrolytes is necessary to maintain perfusion of vital organs and tissues during the emergent period when fluids shift into interstitial spaces and are lost through the burn wound.
	Auscultate breath sounds hourly. Notify physician immediately if dyspnea, orthopnea, crackles (rales), cough, or pink, frothy sputum develops.	Fluid overload from too rapid fluid infusion may cause pulmonary edema.

Evaluation:	Compare the patient's status with the expected outcomes. If the outcomes are not met, reassess the patient and revise the plan.
Assessment Findings:	Patient with burn injury is restless, moans when touched, complains of pain. Patient states pain is intolerable.
Nursing Diagnosis:	Pain related to burn injury

(continued)

Nursing Care Guide 37–1
Patients with Thermal Burn Injuries (continued)

Patient Outcomes	Nursing Interventions	Rationale
Patient states pain is within tolerable limits	Administer intravenous morphine or other narcotic analgesic in small, frequent doses or continuous infusion during the emergent phase and fluid mobilization in the acute phase.	Subcutaneous or intramuscular medication is poorly absorbed during the emergent and fluid mobilization phases because of fluid imbalances. Small, frequent doses or continuous infusion provides better pain management.
	Administer bolus dose of analgesic before wound care.	Minimizes pain during painful procedures and reduces fear of the procedure.
	Monitor respirations, LOC.	Narcotics are a central nervous system (CNS) depressant.
	Assist patient to assume comfortable position within limits of injury. Provide emotional support and comfort measures. Encourage distraction and relaxation exercises. Allow patient to assist with wound care.	These measures promote relaxation and enhance pain relief by reducing anxiety. Patient participation provides a sense of control.

Evaluation: Compare the patient's status with the expected outcomes. If the outcomes are not met, reassess the patient and revise the plan.

Assessment Findings: Patient has partial- and full-thickness burn wounds.

Nursing Diagnosis: Risk for infection related to open burn wounds, suppressed immune response

Patient Outcomes	Nursing Interventions	Rationale
Patient remains free from infection as evidenced by: 1. Absence of fever 2. Daily increase in wound granulation and healing 3. Wound free of increasing edema, foul odor, purulent drainage 4. <100,000 bacteria per gram of wound tissue	Maintain good hand-washing technique for all persons entering patient's room. Use aseptic technique, and wear cap, mask, gown, and sterile gloves during wound care. Change gloves between wounds.	Minimizes risk of wound contamination and cross-contamination between wounds.
	Cleanse wounds one to two times daily or as prescribed.	Cleansing removes exudates, eschar, and necrotic tissue, which inhibit healing and provide a medium for the growth of microorganisms.

(continued)

Nursing Care Guide 37–1
Patients with Thermal Burn Injuries (continued)

Patient Outcomes	Nursing Interventions	Rationale
	Assess wounds after cleansing for signs of healing or infection. Small blood vessels, bleeding, shiny-pink granulation tissue indicate healing. Four odor, purulent drainage, expanding redness, or edema indicates infection. Notify physician if wound is not healing or if signs of infection are present.	Infection is the most common cause of death in the acute phase of burn care. Wounds that fail to heal may be infected. Burn wounds with manifestations of surface infection must undergo biopsy for tissue culture to diagnose infection because surface colonization is common but does not necessarily indicate tissue infection.
	Gently apply topical agent and cover with gauze dressings as prescribed. Be sure dressings do not constrict blood flow.	Antimicrobial topical agents minimize risk of infection. Gentle handling of the wound prevents disruption of fragile granulation tissue and new blood vessels.
	Provide care of graft and donor sites as discussed in Chapter 35.	Proper care prevents disruption of the graft, which will inhibit wound healing and closure. Donor sites are a new wound and potential site for infection.
	Maintain a warm environment and minimize patient exposure during wound care.	Prevents hypothermia.
Patient demonstrates correct wound care technique before discharge.	Teach patient how to cleanse and re-dress open wounds, as presented in Highlight 37–1.	Correct wound care technique minimizes the risk of infection and promotes healing.
Patient verbalizes care of newly healed skin.	Teach patient to take precautions to prevent trauma to newly healed skin and to protect it from exposure to ultraviolet light and hot objects.	Newly healed skin is fragile and sensitive to ultraviolet light and heat.
	Teach patient to massage emollient moisturizers into skin.	Restores moisture and suppleness, stimulates circulation, and reduces flaking and itching.
Patient puts on pressure garment correctly and verbalizes intent to wear it at least 23 hours a day.	Teach patient the purpose of pressure garment. Stress that it must be worn at least 23 hours a day to be effective.	Pressure garments minimize the risk of hypertrophic scarring if worn at least 23 hours daily.
	Be sure the patient has two garments before discharge. Review garment care as presented in Highlight 37–1.	Garment must be washed and air-dried daily.

Evaluation: Compare the patient's status with the expected outcomes. If the outcomes are not met, reassess the patient and revise the plan.

(continued)

Nursing Care Guide 37–1
Patients with Thermal Burn Injuries (continued)

Assessment Findings: Family preparing to visit loved one 8 hours post–thermal burn injury of 60% of TBSA. Patient is intubated; severe edema has distorted physical features and has closed eyes. Bulky dressings cover most burned areas.

Nursing Diagnosis: Anxiety related to appearance of loved one, unknown outcome of treatment

Patient Outcomes	Nursing Interventions	Rationale
Family is prepared for the appearance of the patient.	Discuss the patient's appearance with the family before they see the patient.	Preparation for what they will see will lessen the shock.
	Explain the need for the endotracheal tube and how it is helping the patient. Explain why the patient's features are distorted.	Understanding what they see will lessen their anxiety.
	Encourage family to speak to the patient and touch unburned areas. Assure them that the patient can still hear and understand.	Communication and touch can provide emotional support for patient and family.
Family asks questions and verbalizes concerns.	Encourage questions and expression of thoughts and concerns both before and after visits.	Provides emotional support and opportunity for family to express concerns.
	Offer pastoral services to family and patient.	Demonstrates concern for spiritual needs.
Family verbalizes understanding that the outcome of treatment is uncertain because of the severity of the burn injury.	Answer questions honestly in terms the family can understand. Reinforce the physician's explanations of the desired outcome and prognosis of treatment. Do not give false assurances. Refer questions you cannot answer to appropriate resources.	Accurate information provides assurance that everything possible is being done for the patient.

Evaluation: Compare the patient's status with the expected outcomes. If the outcomes are not met, reassess the patient and revise the plan.

Assessment Findings: Patient is 54 hours post–thermal burn injury of 40% of TBSA. Urine output has been >100 mL/hour for 2 hours.

Nursing Diagnosis: Risk for fluid volume excess related to mobilization of fluids from interstitial spaces into the intravascular circulation

(continued)

Nursing Care Guide 37–1
Patients with Thermal Burn Injuries (continued)

Patient Outcomes	Nursing Interventions	Rationale

Patient maintains fluid balance as evidenced by the following:
Urine output 30–100 mL/hour
  BP > 90/60 but < 140/90
  Heart rate 60–100 bpm
  Regular rhythm
  CVP > 4 but < 15 mm H$_2$O
  Lungs clear to auscultation
  Body weight within 5% of preinjury weight
	Assess for respiratory distress, auscultate breath sounds, monitor urine output and vital signs at least hourly. Weigh patient daily. Compare with patient's baseline values.
	Monitor electrolyte levels.
	Auscultate heart and bowel sounds.
	Maintain intravenous infusion.
	Offer oral fluids if bowel sounds are present and patient is free of nausea and able to drink.
		Diuresis, with corresponding loss in body weight, is an expected manifestation of fluid mobilization. The rapid shift of fluid into the vascular circulation may result in left ventricular failure or pulmonary edema.
		Diuresis may cause rapid shift in serum electrolytes.
		Fluid intake will prevent dehydration.

Evalution: Compare the patient's status with the expected outcomes. If the outcomes are not met, reassess the patient and revise the plan.

ries occur when the victim is burned in an accident (such as airplane or motor vehicle), an explosion, or a fall or jump from a burning building. Assess circulatory status and perform cardiopulmonary resuscitation if needed. Apply direct pressure to control bleeding. Maintain body and spinal alignment to stabilize skeletal injuries.

Maintain Peripheral Circulation

Remove rings, bracelets, necklaces, ankle bracelets, anything that is potentially constrictive. As edema develops, these objects will compress the blood vessels and impair circulation to the distal portion of the extremity. Assess the status of distal circulation, checking for pulses, cyanosis, impaired capillary refill, paresthesias, and deep-tissue pain.

EMERGENT PHASE

The emergent phase, sometimes referred to as the fluid resuscitation stage, is the first 2 to 3 days after a burn injury. The focus of medical and nursing management during this phase of burn care is identification and treatment of life-threatening alterations in respiratory function, fluid and electrolyte balance, and peripheral vascular circulation. Although pain management and intensive care of the burn wound itself begin in the emergent period, they are primary focuses of the acute period and are discussed in detail later.

Respiratory Function

Respiratory failure is a major cause of death from a burn injury in the emergent phase. As many as 60 to 70% of the patients who die in a burn center have an inhalation injury.

As illustrated in Table 37–3, several types of airway problems may develop in burn patients depending on the circumstances of the burn accident. Many patients with severe respiratory involvement from a burn injury die before reaching the hospital. Death from respiratory compromise during the early post-burn period can be attributed to:

- Inhalation of carbon monoxide, smoke, or noxious chemicals
- Acute airway obstruction caused by inhalation of superheated air
- Pulmonary complications caused by decreased vital capacity

CARBON MONOXIDE POISONING

Carbon monoxide is a colorless, odorless, and tasteless gas that is nonirritating to the mucous membranes. It is produced by the incomplete combustion of carbon-containing materials. Carbon monoxide poisoning is most likely to occur when a fire occurs in an enclosed space.

Pathophysiology

Carbon monoxide has an affinity for hemoglobin that is 200 times stronger than that of oxygen. When

Table 37-2

Priorities of Care at the Scene of a Thermal Burn Injury

Priority	Intervention
PRIMARY SURVEY AND MANAGEMENT	

Assess scene safety	Do not attempt to treat unless:
	   Patient has been removed from smoke-filled or unsafe area
	   Double gloves have been applied if chemicals were involved
	   Electric current has been turned off, or patient has been moved from the current with nonconductive tools

Stop the burning process	Roll the victim, smother the flames, or douse with water Remove clothing that does not stick Flush burn with cool-to-tepid water
Manage airway distress	Assess respiratory status Maintain patent airway Perform rescue breathing
Treat associated life-threatening injuries	Assess circulatory status Perform CPR, if needed Assess for bleeding Apply direct pressure to control bleeding Maintain cervical alignment
Maintain peripheral circulation	Remove rings, bracelets, anklets, and so on Open shirts, pants, skirts; remove belts
Maintain body temperature	Cover victim with a clean sheet and blankets
Initiate fluid resuscitation, if possible	Start an intravenous line with a large-bore needle. Administer Ringer's lactate solution at 500 mL/h (for patients older than 15 years of age)
SECONDARY SURVEY AND MANAGEMENT	
Maintain airway	Assist ventilation Closely monitor for the need to intubate

Assess level of consciousness	Determine the patient's level of consciousness using the AVPU method:
	  A = alert
	  V = responds to verbal stimuli
	  P = responds only to painful stimuli
	  U = unresponsive

Identify associated injuries	Stabilize fractures Cover open wounds with dressings

Obtain patient history	Determine characteristics of injury:
	  Cause of burn
	  Possibility of inhalation:
	    Fire in an enclosed space
	    Patient unconscious
	  Chemicals involved
	  Time of injury
	Obtain patient-related factors:
	  Age, illnesses, medications, allergies, etc

Monitor patient	Monitor vital signs and ventilatory status

CPR, cardiopulmonary resuscitation.

carbon monoxide is introduced into the blood stream, it binds with hemoglobin and forms carboxyhemoglobin by displacing oxygen molecules. Hypoxemia results from decreased oxygen transport to the tissues. Even when low levels of carbon monoxide are present, blood levels of carboxyhemoglobin are elevated.

Clinical Manifestations

The severity of the clinical manifestations of carbon monoxide poisoning directly correlates with the concentration of carbon monoxide present in the blood. Cerebral hypoxia is the earliest consequence of carbon monoxide poisoning. Symptoms include intense headache, restlessness, impaired judgment, slowed thought processes, irritability, confusion, and slight breathlessness. Visual acuity may be impaired. Although the skin color may be either pale or cyanotic, it often has a pink flush caused by vasodilation in response to tissue hypoxia. A unique indicator of carbon monoxide poisoning is a cherry-red appearance of the mucous membranes.

Table 37–3

Respiratory Alterations Associated with Thermal Burn Injuries

Type of Injury	Cause	Clinical Manifestations	Management	Nursing Implications
Carbon monoxide poisoning	Mild exposure (10–20% COHb)	Headache Decreased visual acuity Possible breathlessness Irritability	Inhalation of 100% oxygen Monitor arterial blood gases Monitor COHb level	Administer 100% oxygen Observe patient color Monitor arterial blood gases Monitor COHb levels Monitor vital signs
	Moderate exposure (20–40% COHb)	Decreased blood pressure Increased pulse Cheyne-Stokes respirations Dilated pupils Confusion Headache Irritability Vertigo Nausea and vomiting Decreased visual acuity Reddish skin color	Same Intubation may be needed for ventilation	Same as above
	Major exposure (40–60% COHb)	Dysrhythmias Seizures Coma	Same as above	Same as above
	Extreme exposure (>60% COHb)	Usually, respiratory arrest and death	Same as above	Same as above
Inhalation injury above the glottis	Inhalation of super-heated air	*Early:* Soot on tongue, pharynx, or sputum Singed nasal hairs Dry, red buccal mucosa Burns on face, neck, upper chest *Late:* Dyspnea Coughing Wheezing Hoarseness Inability to control secretions	Early intubation Mechanical respiratory support Baseline arterial blood gases Baseline chest x-ray examination	Administer prescribed oxygen Observe for increased cough and hoarseness Auscultate lung fields Observe lung expansion Monitor vital signs Monitor arterial blood gases
Inhalation injury below the glottis	Inhalation of smoke and chemicals of combustion	Fever Dyspnea Wheezing Rales Decreased tidal volume Poor gas exchange Productive cough	Administration of oxygen Intubation, if required Baseline arterial blood gases Baseline chest x-ray examination	Administer prescribed oxygen Suction hourly Monitor vital signs and oxygen saturation Monitor arterial blood gases Turn patient every 1–2 h
Restrictive disease	Mechanical impairment of vital capacity	Anxiety Restlessness Decreased level of consciousness Labored breathing	Administration of oxygen Intubation, if required Baseline arterial blood gases Baseline chest x-ray examination	Administer prescribed oxygen Monitor vital signs Monitor arterial blood gas results and oxygen saturation

COHb, carboxyhemoglobin.

Later symptoms include drowsiness or stupor, vertigo, muscular rigidity of the jaw, convulsions, dilated pupils, respiratory stridor, and a rapid, bounding pulse. A carboxyhemoglobin level of 50% or greater is usually associated with loss of consciousness, coma, or death.

INHALATION INJURY ABOVE THE GLOTTIS

Inhalation injury is seen more commonly above the glottis than below it. It is usually caused by inhalation of superheated air (>149°C [300°F]), but may also be caused by steam inhalation, aspiration of scalding liquids, and explosions. These inhalation injuries result in a thermal burn and edema of the tissues of the upper airway. Acute airway obstruction usually occurs within the first 30 minutes to 48 hours after the burn.

Pathophysiology

Thermal damage to tissues of the respiratory tract is usually confined to the upper airway because the lower airway is protected from heat by the tremendous ability of the tracheobronchial tract to cool airborne particles. As the damaged tissue in the upper airway becomes edematous, the airway narrows and eventually closes.

Clinical Manifestations

Upper respiratory tract injury should be suspected if the patient was in a confined space during the fire. Acute airway obstruction can be prevented if a thorough history is obtained and accurate observations made that allow early detection and intervention. The patient is usually able to breathe until final obstruction occurs. However, early intubation, when the edema is minimal, is indicated if upper airway injury is suspected.

Early manifestations of upper respiratory tract injury include soot on the tongue, pharynx, or in sputum; singed nasal hairs; a burn involving the face, neck, or upper chest; and a dry, red buccal mucosa.

Late signs include dyspnea, use of accessory muscles, coughing, wheezing, inability to cough up secretions, a change in the voice, and increasing hoarseness. If any of the late signs are noted, the patient must be intubated immediately.

INHALATION INJURY BELOW THE GLOTTIS

Smoke contains many noxious and potentially toxic chemicals in addition to carbon monoxide. These chemicals result from combustion of various substances and can cause damage to the lower respiratory tract and pulmonary tissue when inhaled.

Pathophysiology

Inhalation of smoke and noxious chemicals damages the mucosa lining the alveoli and lower respiratory passages, causing inflammation, edema, and increased secretions from the inflamed mucosa. Edema inhibits oxygen and carbon dioxide exchange, and progressive hypoxia develops. Pulmonary edema or bronchiolitis with subsequent atelectasis, pneumonia, and adult respiratory distress syndrome are common.

Clinical Manifestations

Symptoms of damage from inhalation of noxious or toxic substances may not occur for several days after the burn injury. The symptoms include fever, dyspnea, wheezing, crackles (rales), decreased tidal volume, poor gas exchange, productive cough, pleuritic pain, and densities on chest x-ray examinations. When obtaining the history from a burn patient or fire department personnel, it is important to determine whether burning chemicals were involved in the fire.

RESTRICTIVE LUNG DISEASE

Patients with massive chest wall edema or circumferential chest burns have decreased vital capacity and increased pulmonary resistance, known as restrictive lung disease. The etiology and pathophysiology of restrictive disease are poorly understood. They are, however, associated with increased risk of pulmonary complications, such as atelectasis and pneumonia.

Clinical manifestations of restrictive disease include increasing anxiety and restlessness followed by decreasing level of consciousness, shallow and rapid respiration, and cyanosis.

ASSESSING RESPIRATORY FUNCTION

Medical diagnosis of carbon monoxide poisoning is based on the patient's history, clinical manifestations, and laboratory determination of carboxyhemoglobin levels and arterial blood gases. Pulse oximetry is used as an adjunct. However, because the oximeter is not sensitive to the presence of carbon monoxide–bound hemoglobin but only indicates the saturation of oxygen-bound hemoglobin, oximetry does not eliminate the need for arterial carbon monoxide measurements. A carboxyhemoglobin level of more than 20% is considered toxic. It is important to determine whether the patient received oxygen during transport to the hospital. This will allow estimation of carboxyhemoglobin levels at the scene, and if the patient is at high risk for carbon monoxide poisoning.

Arterial blood gases (ABGs) are measured on admission for any patient with

- Burns of the upper chest, neck, and face
- Evidence of burns of the upper airway
- Suspected exposure to superheated air
- Risk of inhalation of noxious fumes
- History of a chronic respiratory disorder

Initial values are used as a baseline to compare with repeat arterial blood gas determinations every 4 to 6 hours to monitor the patient's respiratory function. An increasing partial pressure of carbon dioxide ($PaCO_2$) and a decreasing partial pressure of oxygen

(PaO$_2$) indicate impending airway obstruction or respiratory failure from inhalation injury or restrictive disease.

Diagnosis of acute airway obstruction is based on the patient's history, clinical manifestations, and arterial blood gas values or on direct visualization of the respiratory passages with a fiberoptic bronchoscope. Depending on the severity of the upper airway injury, the patient may be either prophylactically intubated or re-examined by bronchoscope every 4 to 6 hours for the first 24 to 36 hours.

Diagnosis of lower airway injury is based on the patient's history of inhalation of noxious chemicals and clinical manifestations and examination with the fiberoptic bronchoscope. A sophisticated method of diagnosing lower airway injury is the xenon-133 lung scan. This costly procedure requires transport to the nuclear medicine department. A chest x-ray is usually done at the patient's bedside. This provides the physicians with a baseline for comparing pulmonary changes later in the patient's course of treatment.

MANAGING RESPIRATORY FUNCTION

The medical treatment of alterations in respiratory function associated with thermal burn injuries depends on the type and severity of the respiratory dysfunction. All patients are treated with humidified oxygen and aggressive pulmonary hygiene, as discussed in Chapter 14. Those with carbon monoxide poisoning receive inhalation of 100% oxygen to shorten the half-life of the carbon monoxide molecules and to increase the oxygen saturation of the blood. Hyperbaric oxygen treatment may be considered as a means of administering high concentrations of oxygen and shortening the half-life of the carbon monoxide molecules even more.

Respiratory status and arterial blood gas results are monitored frequently. The patient is intubated at the first indication of deteriorating respiratory status. Patients with confirmed upper airway injury may be intubated prophylactically. Early intubation prevents the risk of hypoxia and is less traumatic to the tissues if performed before edema becomes severe. If the patient is intubated for upper airway obstruction with no lower airway pulmonary involvement, mechanical ventilation is rarely necessary. Intubation is usually necessary only until the edema resolves in 2 or 3 days. Care of the intubated patient and the patient with altered respiratory function is discussed in detail in Unit 4.

NURSING PROCESS
Altered Respiratory Function After Burn Injury

Assessment

Obtain as accurate a description as possible of the circumstances surrounding the incident. Determine the cause of the burn injury (thermal, chemical, or electrical) and whether there was exposure to smoke, superheated air, or noxious chemicals to determine the risk of respiratory involvement. Ask where the patient was found and whether he or she was in an enclosed space. Determine whether the patient was unconscious. Unless the patient also has head trauma, loss of consciousness indicates probable hypoxia from inhalation of carbon monoxide, smoke, or noxious chemicals. Ask whether the patient stopped breathing at any time prior to arrival at the hospital and if so, for how long.

Assess for flushed skin, pallor, cyanosis, and cherry-red mucous membranes. These signs indicate carbon monoxide poisoning but may be difficult to see on a dark-skinned person or a patient who has been burned. Observe for burns of the face, neck, and upper chest. Burns in these areas increase the possibility of respiratory injury. Assess for soot on the tongue, on the pharynx, or in the sputum and for the presence of singed nasal hairs, which indicate possible inhalation injury.

Use arterial blood gas analysis and pulse oximetry to determine the patient's oxygen saturation. Assess vital signs and voice quality to provide a baseline for early detection of altered respiratory function. Observe the patient's breathing pattern, rate, and depth for difficulty in breathing and use of accessory muscles. Auscultate for wheezes, stridor, or crackles (rales), which indicate upper airway edema or accumulation of secretions. Breath sounds may be distant or difficult to hear if the thorax is edematous from burns. Assess for general signs of hypoxia. Agitation, restlessness, and anxiety are early signs of hypoxia. Hoarseness, change in voice quality, persistent cough, and decreasing level of orientation or consciousness are late signs of upper airway edema and hypoxia.

Nursing Diagnoses and Planning

Nursing diagnoses and related expected patient outcomes commonly applicable to patients with altered respiratory function after a major burn injury include the following:

NDx: Impaired gas exchange related to carbon monoxide poisoning secondary to smoke inhalation

Planning: Patient Outcomes
1. Respiratory pattern is regular and unlabored.
2. Arterial blood gas results are acceptable.

NDx: Risk for ineffective airway clearance related to airway edema secondary to inhalation of superheated air, smoke, or noxious chemicals

Planning: Patient Outcomes
1. Patient is alert and oriented.
2. Patient's respirations remain clear and unlabored, more than 12 and fewer than 20 per minute.
3. Patient speaks without hoarseness or persistent cough.

Nursing Interventions and Evaluation

The primary goal for nursing care of a patient with respiratory dysfunction after a burn injury is to ensure that the patient maintains adequate ventilation and oxygenation.

NDx: Impaired gas exchange

Encourage deep breathing and administer 100% humidified oxygen to displace the carbon monoxide, which binds with hemoglobin in the blood stream. Observe for decreasing level of consciousness and inability to follow simple commands, which indicate cerebral hypoxia. Monitor laboratory results of carboxyhemoglobin levels and arterial blood gases. Decreasing levels of carboxyhemoglobin are a reliable indicator of the effectiveness of treatment. Limit patient activity to decrease oxygen requirements.

NDx: Risk for ineffective airway clearance

Administer humidified oxygen to increase oxygen saturation and tissue oxygenation. Elevate the head of the bed, if not contraindicated by associated injuries, to ease diaphragmatic excursion, promote venous drainage, and reduce edema. Encourage coughing and deep breathing. Turn the patient hourly to promote lung expansion and to prevent stasis of secretions. Patients with an inhalation injury have copious secretions. Suction as necessary to maintain patent airway, but avoid unnecessary suctioning because it can increase edema. Talk to the patient frequently. Explain procedures and treatments to allay anxiety, decrease oxygen requirements, and encourage verbalization of concerns.

Monitor respiratory status and auscultate breath sounds at least hourly to detect deterioration in condition. Note the rate and rhythm of respirations and the use of accessory muscles. Monitor the quality of the patient's voice every hour by asking a question that requires a brief, multiple-word answer to detect laryngeal edema. Report deterioration in arterial blood gas values, pulse oximeter saturation, increasing restlessness, anxiety, respiratory stridor, wheezes, crackles, frequent cough, hoarseness, or decreasing level of consciousness to the physician immediately and prepare for intubation.

Compare the patient's status with the expected outcomes. If the outcomes are not met, reassess the patient and revise the plan.

Hypovolemia and Electrolyte Imbalance

Severe hypovolemia and electrolyte imbalance, commonly referred to as burn shock, occur after a major burn injury because large volumes of plasma and proteins are lost through the burn wound and shift from the vascular system into the interstitial spaces, where they cause severe edema. Burn shock differs from hemorrhagic shock in that the blood volume lost is plasma, not whole blood. Although the plasma is effectively removed from the intravascular circulation, much of it remains in the body to be reabsorbed or remobilized in 3 to 14 days. Despite these differences, the physiologic effects of burn shock and hemorrhagic shock are the same.

Pathophysiology

Several factors contribute to the fluid shift from intravascular to interstitial spaces, which leads to edema and burn shock:

- Capillaries at the site of the burn injury, and to a lesser extent throughout the body, become more permeable and leak large amounts of water, electrolytes, albumin, and globulin into the interstitial spaces.
- Histamine is released from the damaged cells, causing vasodilation and engorgement. This, in turn, increases hydrostatic pressure in the vessels, pushing more fluid from the highly permeable vessels and into the interstitial spaces.
- Large protein molecules leak through the permeable capillaries into the interstitial spaces. These molecules, which normally pull fluid into the intravascular circulation, now pull it into the interstitial spaces.
- The lymphatic system, which normally drains excess interstitial fluid and returns it to the general circulation, becomes overwhelmed by the amount of interstitial edema. In addition, because the lymphatic vessels have very thin walls, they are the first to be compressed by burn wound edema, further inhibiting their ability to drain fluid.

The decreased volume of circulating intravascular fluid results in decreased venous return, decreased cardiac output, and decreased perfusion and function of vital organs, especially the brain, kidney, and heart. Hypovolemia and decreased cardiac output may cause myocardial hypoxemia and further compromise cardiac function. Decreased perfusion results in tissue hypoxia and anaerobic metabolism with the production of lactic acid. The release of catecholamines in response to trauma and stress alters glucose metabolism, promoting the breakdown of glycogen stores in the liver to create glucose. Acid end-products and lactic acid accumulate in the blood because decreased renal perfusion impairs renal function. Metabolic acidosis results.

Along with this massive fluid shift and hypovolemia, electrolyte imbalance occurs with a major burn injury. Aldosterone, which promotes sodium and water reabsorption in the renal tubules, is secreted in response to reduced circulating intravascular fluid. The retained sodium quickly accumulates in the interstitial spaces as fluid continues to shift out of the vascular system. Additionally, the sodium pump fails; normally it pumps sodium out of the cell in exchange for potassium. Sodium accumulates within the cells of the tissues, bringing water with it, as potassium is released. Additional potassium is released into the intravascular spaces from tissue cells and hemolysis of red blood cells damaged by the burn. Urinary excretion of potassium is impaired because of decreased renal perfusion and function. As a result of these processes, serum sodium levels decrease as serum potassium levels increase. The physiologic events that cause hypovolemia and electrolyte imbalance after a major burn injury are illustrated in Figure 37–4.

After the first 16 to 24 hours, the hydrostatic pressure in the interstitial spaces begins to resist the flow of fluid out of the capillaries. Normal capillary membrane permeability is gradually restored and fluid loss slows. Edema continues to increase, but more slowly, until approximately 48 hours after injury, at which time it stabilizes and then begins to decrease. Diuresis begins at about 3 days.

Clinical Manifestations

The clinical manifestations of burn shock include those common in hypovolemic shock: dehydration, decreased urine output, hematuria, hypotension,

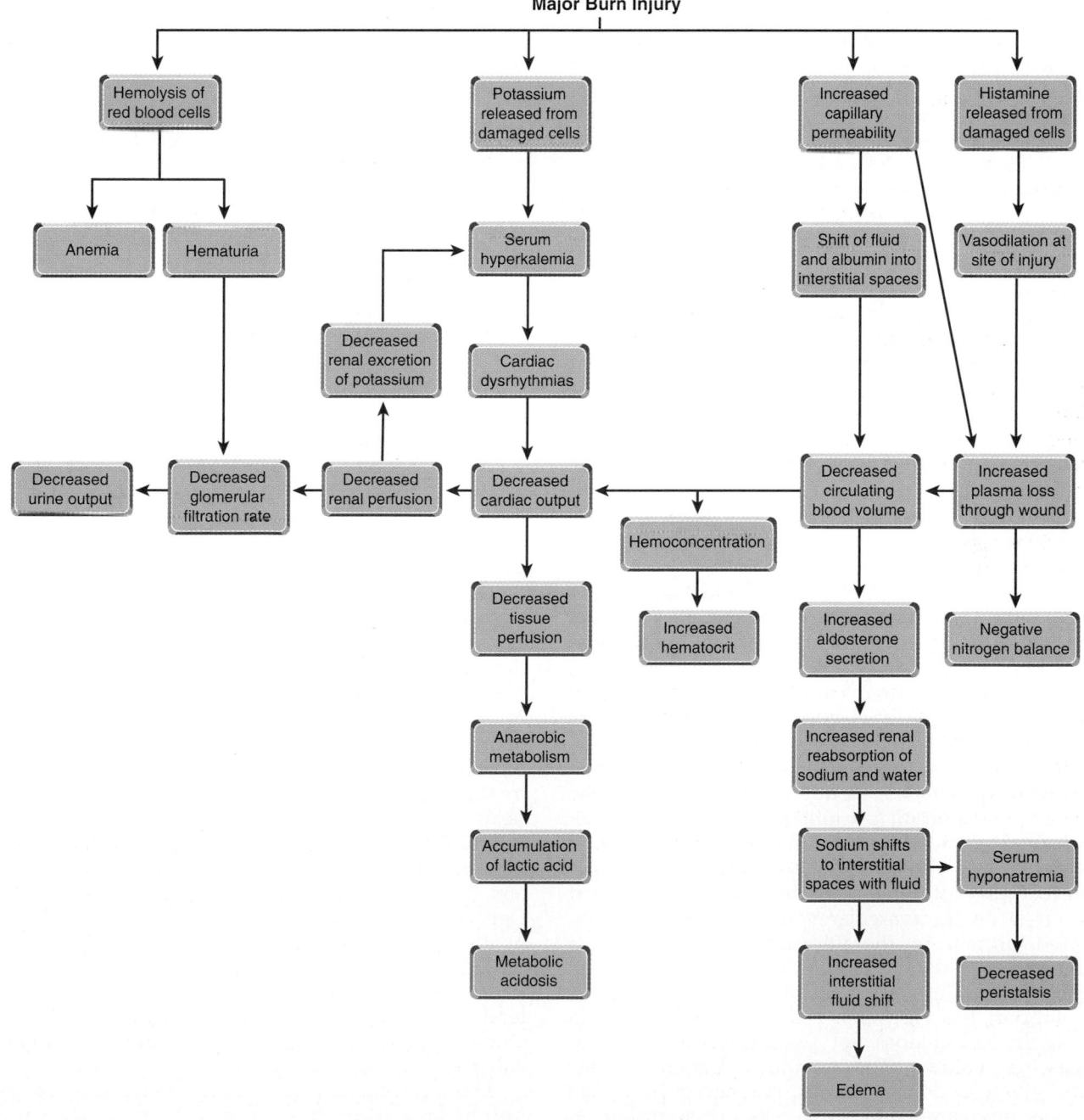

Figure 37–4

Physiologic events that lead to hypovolemia, electrolyte imbalance, and metabolic acidosis following a major burn injury.

tachycardia, weak pulse, decreased central venous pressure, decreased cardiac output, decreased pulmonary artery wedge pressure, decreasing level of consciousness, and dry mucous membranes. Cardiac dysrhythmias may result from the hyperkalemia and decreased peristalsis from the hyponatremia.

Diagnosis

Medical diagnosis is based on the clinical manifestations and the results of laboratory studies. These studies include serum electrolytes and proteins, serum and urine osmolality, urine specific gravity, hematocrit, blood urea nitrogen (BUN), and arterial blood gas analysis. Results will show increasing serum and urine osmolality, increased specific gravity, increased hematocrit, hyponatremia, hyperkalemia, hypoproteinemia, elevated blood urea nitrogen, and metabolic acidosis. The patient is in negative nitrogen balance because of excess tissue catabolism and protein loss through the burn.

Management

Treatment of hypovolemia and electrolyte imbalances associated with burn shock is an immediate priority if rapid deterioration and death are to be prevented. Adequate fluid replacement in burn shock is so vital that it is commonly referred to as fluid resuscitation. To maintain cardiac output, perfusion of vital organs, and renal function, the patient must receive fluids in volumes adequate to replace fluids lost through the burn wound and interstitial edema. Generally, burns of more than 20% of TBSA require parenteral fluid resuscitation.

The goal of fluid resuscitation is to replace fluid lost through injured tissue and sequestered in the interstitial spaces in a manner that closely approximates the amount and type of fluid lost, as well as the speed of the loss. A few studies indicate that the entire fluid loss may occur within 12 to 18 hours after the burn, but most indicate continued fluid loss for as long as 36 to 48 hours.

Because of increased capillary permeability and the need to replace electrolytes, Ringer's lactate (crystalloid fluid) is the choice for the fluid resuscitation. Colloids (human plasma protein fraction [Plasmanate], salt-poor albumin) are not used for the first 24 hours because capillaries continue to leak until about 30 to 36 hours after the burn. Because infused colloids will also leak into the tissues, it is believed that colloid replacement will have little if any effect on intravascular volume. In addition, increased protein in the interstitial spaces exerts a pulling force, which tends to increase interstitial edema by pulling water with it. Many burn specialists support the view that colloid administration in this early period does not significantly increase intravascular volume. The amount of Ringer's lactate to be given is determined by Advanced Burn Life Support guidelines and varies slightly according to whether the patient is an adult or a child. The adult formula, based on the age, weight, and TBSA burned, is as follows: 2 to 4 mL Ringer's lactate × kg body weight × percentage burn, administered in the first 24 hours.

The rate of fluid administration is calculated from the time the burn injury occurred. Half of the calculated volume is replaced in the first 8 hours from the time of injury. Capillary permeability and intravascular loss are the greatest during this time. The remaining fluid is administered over the next 16 hours.

It is important to remember that the fluid replacement formula is only a guide. In the face of obvious hypovolemia or hypervolemia, the infusion rate must be adjusted regardless of what requirements have been calculated. In some specific cases it can be predicted that the calculated replacement will be insufficient to meet the patient's resuscitation needs. Examples include:

- Pulmonary injury, in which great fluid losses occur in the lungs secondary to increased alveolar capillary permeability, which is not measured in the TBSA burned and therefore not considered in the formulas
- Electrical burns, in which internal injury cannot be accurately measured
- Patients in whom resuscitation is delayed
- Patients burned while intoxicated

The usual causes for over-resuscitation are overestimation of burn percentage and overly aggressive fluid replacement in the field.

After the first 24 hours, the fluid lost is free water, an electrolyte-free solution that is lost as evaporative water loss through the burn wound. Evaporative loss, which is normally 10 mL/kg a day, may increase to 2.5 to 12 L a day and must be replaced. Capillary permeability gradually returns toward normal by the end of the second postburn day. Colloids can be effective at this time to keep the amount of fluid administered to a minimum. The fluid therapy of choice, for adults, after the first 24 hours postburn is to infuse 0.3 to 0.5 mL × kg body weight × percentage TBSA burn of a colloid-containing fluid in addition to enough electrolyte-free fluid to maintain adequate urinary output and a serum sodium of 140 mEq/L.

Monitoring serum sodium is an important tool in determining whether the patient is hypernatremic and dehydrated or hyponatremic and overhydrated. Depending on the severity of the burn and the patient's gastrointestinal status, parenteral fluid replacement may no longer be required after 48 hours. Patients with small burns may never require parenteral replacement if they can tolerate adequate amounts of electrolyte solutions and nutritionally balanced fluids by mouth.

Diuretics are avoided in the early postburn period because the decreased urine output results from hypovolemia, which would be further aggravated by increasing the amount of fluid excreted.

NURSING PROCESS
Hypovolemia and Electrolyte Imbalance After Major Burn Injury

Assessment

Obtain baseline vital signs and weight on admission for later comparison and evaluation of fluid replacement. Obtain an accurate baseline weight. Ask the patient, significant other, emergency personnel, or transferring agency what time the burn injury occurred. Examine the patient to locate all burned areas. Assist in determining the size of the injury by using the agency's chart to calculate TBSA burned. Data regarding accurate weight, time of the injury, and TBSA burned are essential in calculating the amount of fluid to be administered during fluid resuscitation.

Assess the patient's level of consciousness. Talk to the patient to determine awareness of person, place, and time. Level of consciousness and orientation are indicators of cerebral perfusion. Be sure someone has told the patient where he or she is and what has happened. Many patients are not initially aware of exactly what has occurred or what hospital they have been taken to, especially if the burn center is not in a local facility.

Auscultate bowel sounds and obtain specimens for baseline serum chemistries (sodium [Na], potassium [K], chloride [Cl], bicarbonate [HCO$_3$], blood urea nitrogen, glucose) and arterial blood gases for later comparison and evaluation of electrolyte and acid-base balance.

Nursing Diagnoses and Planning

Nursing diagnoses and related expected patient outcomes commonly applicable to patients with hypovolemia and electrolyte imbalance after a major burn injury include the following:

NDx: Risk for fluid volume deficit related to inadequate replacement of fluids lost through evaporation from the burn wound and fluid shift into interstitial spaces

Planning: Patient Outcomes
1. Patient is alert and oriented.
2. Patient maintains adequate hydration as evidenced by the following:
   Heart rate regular and more than 60 but fewer than 110 beats per minute (bpm)
   Blood pressure stable and higher than 90/60
   Urine output more than 30 mL per hour
   Central venous pressure 4 to 12 mm of water
   Capillary refill less than 3 seconds
   Moist mucous membranes
3. Patient's weight increases by 15 to 20%.
4. Patient has bowel sounds and is free of nausea.

Nursing Interventions and Evaluation

The primary goal of the nursing care of a patient with hypovolemia and electrolyte imbalance after a major burn injury is to minimize burn shock by providing adequate fluid resuscitation and electrolyte replacement. Determination of the adequacy of fluid resuscitation is based on the premise that adequate fluid replacement ensures perfusion and function of vital organs.

NDx: Risk for fluid volume deficit
Establish intravenous access as soon as possible using a 16- to 18-gauge IV catheter to facilitate rapid fluid infusion. Multiple IV catheters may be necessary. Administer and document fluid replacement to make sure the patient receives prescribed fluids in the appropriate time frame. Monitor intravenous administration and infusion sites at least hourly to detect altered flow rate, leakage, or infiltration. The risk of problems with parenteral infusions is greater with rapid infusion of high volumes of fluid. Auscultate breath sounds hourly to detect crackles, which may indicate pulmonary edema and fluid overload from rapid fluid infusion. Report inability to maintain prescribed flow rate or any infusion-related problems to the physician immediately.

Insert an indwelling urinary catheter with a low-volume graduate to measure urine output accurately. Monitor heart rate, blood pressure, capillary refill, level of consciousness, and urine output hourly to evaluate the adequacy of fluid replacement and perfusion of vital organs. Tachycardia may be present even with adequate fluid resuscitation because of trauma, pain, and anxiety. Heart rate should return to normal range within 18 to 24 hours. Blood pressure should be within low-normal limits for the patient by history and age. Capillary refill of less than 3 seconds and a clear sensorium indicate adequate peripheral and cerebral perfusion. Urine output greater than 30 mL/hour in adults (or 0.5 mL/kg/hour) indicates adequate renal perfusion. A central venous catheter may be inserted for more accurate hourly measurement of hemodynamic status and fluid balance. Occasionally, a Swan-Ganz catheter is inserted to monitor cardiac output and pulmonary wedge pressure. It is not uncommon for initial central pressures and cardiac output to be low and then return to normal range in 18 to 24 hours. Care of the patient with a central line is discussed in Chapter 8.

Weigh the patient at the same time daily with the same scale and the same amount of clothing to monitor fluid balance. Accuracy is improved if the patient can be weighed without dressings or topical creams covering the burn wounds. Note on the flow sheet or chart whether dressings were removed. An increase in body weight of 15 to 20% is expected with successful fluid resuscitation.

Auscultate the abdomen every 4 hours to determine the presence of bowel sounds. Hyponatremia and poor bowel perfusion may cause hypoperistalsis. The presence of bowel sounds and the absence of nausea indicate good bowel perfusion and adequate serum sodium levels. Attach the patient to a cardiac monitor to detect dysrhythmias caused by hyperkalemia. Review serum electrolyte and arterial blood gas values daily to monitor electrolyte balance and metabolic acidosis.

Compare the patient's status with the expected outcomes. If the outcomes are not met, reassess the patient and revise the plan.

Circumferential Burns

Impaired peripheral circulation and compromised respiratory movement may occur with a full-thickness burn that involves the entire circumference of a limb or the thorax.

Pathophysiology

In a full-thickness burn injury, elastin is destroyed and tissues cannot expand to accommodate increasing edema. The wound becomes covered by eschar—a dry, tight, inelastic covering that forms from dead tissue and wound exudate. If eschar forms around the circumference of a limb, it acts as a tourniquet, compressing lymphatic vessels and impairing arterial blood flow and venous return. Circulation may be so compromised that the viability of the limb is impaired. If the circumferential burn involves the upper torso, chest expansion for respiration may be impaired.

Clinical Manifestations

The clinical manifestations of impaired peripheral circulation caused by a circumferential burn of an extremity include cyanosis distal to the burn wound, loss of the distal pulse measured by Doppler ultrasound, delayed capillary refill, and paresthesias or decreased sensation. The clinical manifestations of compromised respiratory function resulting from a circumferential burn of the torso are decreased tidal volume and respiratory excursion with increasing signs of respiratory distress and hypoxia.

Diagnosis

A medical diagnosis of impaired peripheral circulation or respiratory compromise caused by circumferential burn is based on the clinical manifestations. Hypoxia is confirmed by decreasing oxygen saturation on pulse oximetry or arterial blood gases.

Management

Treatment for circulatory impairment in an extremity or restriction of chest expansion is an escharotomy, a shallow incision made through the eschar with a scalpel or electrocautery. The incision is made lengthwise, only along the lateral and medial aspects of the extremity and never inside the fingers. Hand and finger escharotomies do not improve local circulation but do increase the risk of loss of function. If escharotomies are performed on the torso, incisions along the anterior axillary lines are made and joined by transverse incisions. An escharotomy immediately releases pressure on underlying tissues to restore blood flow to the extremity or to allow expansion of the chest.

An escharotomy is performed at the bedside. Because it involves only the dead eschar in a full-thickness burn injury, no analgesia other than what the patient is already receiving is required. The incision is usually covered by the same topical agent used on the patient's burn wounds. An escharotomy can be seen in Figure 37–5.

NURSING PROCESS
Circumferential Burns

Assessment

Assess the depth of the wound to identify possible areas of full-thickness injury and eschar formation. Assess pulses, color, temperature, sensation, and capillary refill in extremities with circumferential full-thickness burns immediately on admission to determine baseline neurovascular status. Use a Doppler ultrasound instrument to assess nonpalpable pulses. To assess capillary refill, press on the skin or nailbed distal to the injury and note how long it takes for the color to return. Color should return in less than 3 seconds.

If the circumferential injury involves the torso, assess respiratory status and chest expansion with each respiration. Auscultate breath sounds. The patient should be able to fully expand the chest with each respiration. Breath sounds should be present in all lobes.

Nursing Diagnoses and Planning

Nursing diagnoses and related expected patient outcomes commonly applicable to patients with circumferential burns include the following:

NDx: Risk for peripheral neurovascular dysfunction related to edema and circulatory impairment secondary to circumferential full-thickness burn injury of the extremity

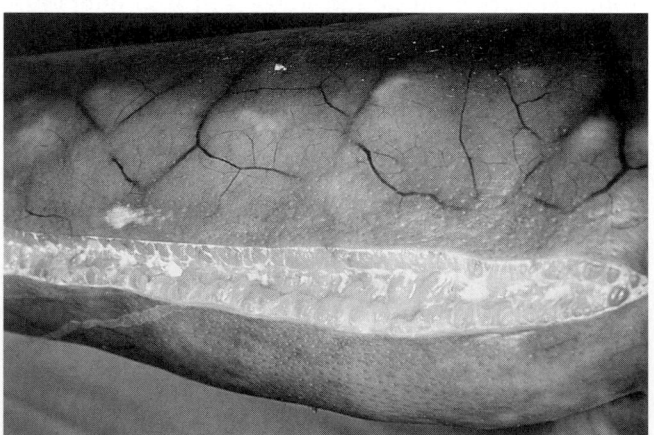

Figure 37–5

Escharotomy into the dead tissue of a full-thickness burn helps relieve pressure from edema on underlying deep tissues and blood vessels.

Planning: Patient Outcomes
1. Patient maintains peripheral circulation distal to circumferential full-thickness burn injury as evidenced by the following:
   Distal pulses present
   Normal sensation distal to the injury
   Capillary refill less than 3 seconds

NDx: Risk for ineffective breathing pattern related to impaired chest expansion secondary to circumferential full-thickness burn injury of the torso

Planning: Patient Outcomes
1. Patient is able to expand chest fully with each respiration.
2. Patient breathes with regular, unlabored respirations.

Nursing Interventions and Evaluation

The primary goal of nursing care of a patient with circumferential burns is to maintain adequate peripheral circulation and adequate chest expansion.

NDx: Risk for peripheral neurovascular dysfunction
Remove all clothing and rings, necklaces, bracelets, anklets, and any other jewelry or item that could occlude peripheral circulation with edema formation. Elevate burned extremities above the level of the heart to promote venous return and to minimize edema.

Monitor neurovascular status of extremities and digits distal to circumferential full-thickness burns at least hourly to ensure early detection of impaired peripheral circulation. Report inability to obtain pulse by Doppler ultrasound, cyanotic or pale skin or nailbeds, cool temperature, loss of sensation or paresthesias, or capillary refill longer than 3 seconds to the physician immediately.

Prepare the patient for an escharotomy by reinforcing the surgeon's explanation of how and why the procedure is performed. Provide reassurance that the procedure is painless. Obtain signed consent. Assemble sterile supplies for the procedure: scalpel, gauze sponges, drapes, gloves, and waterproof covering to protect the bed. Assist during the escharotomy, and apply prescribed antibacterial agent over the incisions to prevent infection.

Continue to assess the extremities distal to the escharotomy hourly for circulatory impairment. In some cases, the escharotomy requires revision.

NDx: Risk for ineffective breathing pattern
Monitor respiratory status of the patient with a circumferential full-thickness burn of the thorax at least hourly to ensure early detection of compromised respiratory function. Chest expansion and breath sounds should remain equal bilaterally. Monitor oxygen saturation with pulse oximeter. Pulse oximetry cannot be used if all digits and both ear lobes have full-thickness burns. Review arterial blood gas results for decreasing oxygen saturation and increasing carbon dioxide levels. Report increas-

ing anxiety or restlessness, dyspnea, labored or shallow respirations, absent or diminished breath sounds, unequal chest expansion, deterioration of arterial blood gases, or increased pressure alarming on the ventilator to the physician immediately. If necessary, prepare the patient for escharotomy as described previously. Continue to monitor respiratory status and chest expansion hourly after torso escharotomy to ensure adequate respiratory function.

Compare the patient's status with the expected outcomes. If the outcomes are not met, reassess the patient and revise the plan.

ACUTE PHASE

The acute phase of burn care immediately follows the emergent phase. It is sometimes referred to as the postemergent phase, the fluid mobilization phase, or the diuretic phase.

The acute phase begins with reabsorption of fluid from the interstitial spaces and its mobilization into the intravascular circulation. It continues until the wound is closed either by spontaneous healing or by successful skin grafts. During the acute phase, the focus of the health team is fluid and electrolyte balance, pain management, care of the wound to prevent infection, meeting metabolic requirements, and supporting the patient and family's psychologic adjustment. Rehabilitation and physical therapy continue through acute care.

Fluid Mobilization and Electrolyte Imbalance

Pathophysiology
After the first 24 hours, the hydrostatic pressure in the interstitial spaces begins to resist the flow of fluid out of the capillaries and the capillaries begin to return to their preburn function. Edema continues to increase, but more slowly, until approximately 48 hours after injury, at which time it stabilizes and then begins to decrease.

As capillary permeability decreases, the leakage of large protein molecules and fluid into the interstitial spaces stops. Slowly at first and then more rapidly, fluid is pulled out of the tissues and into the intravascular system. As edema decreases, the lymphatic system is able to drain excess interstitial fluid and return it to the general circulation. The increased volume of intravascular fluid results in increased venous return, increased cardiac output, and increased perfusion and function of vital organs. During fluid mobilization, as large volumes of fluid are reabsorbed back into the circulation, the patient is at risk for rapid onset of left ventricular failure and pulmonary edema from fluid overload.

With improved systemic perfusion and fluid mobilization, the cellular sodium pump resumes normal function, pumping sodium out of the cell in

HEMORRHAGE AFTER SEVERE BURN INJURY

On the morning after her admission to the burn unit, I was assigned to care for a 47-year-old woman who had been burned in an accidental house fire. While attempting to extinguish a fire in the broiler, the right sleeve of the patient's robe caught fire. Hearing her screams, her 20-year-old son immediately helped her to the kitchen floor, where he rolled her in towels and extinguished the flames. He then extinguished the fire in the broiler and called for an ambulance.

The patient was taken to the emergency department (ED) of a community hospital for evaluation and stabilization. She was then transported via ambulance to the regional burn center.

Despite the proximity of her burns to the respiratory tract, the patient demonstrated no evidence of inhalation injury. The kitchen was large and a sliding glass door was open at the time of the incident. The patient had not experienced any loss of consciousness, dyspnea, hoarseness, and carbonaceous sputum. She had no symptoms of increased carboxyhemoglobin levels, such as headache, nausea, vomiting, or cherry-red skin. She was free from trauma and injuries associated with the accident. She had been in excellent health before this incident, with no history of illness, hospitalization, or allergies.

The patient was admitted to the burn unit with mixed deep partial-thickness and full-thickness burns of her anterior chest, neck, chin, right and left hands, circumferential burns of her right arm below the elbow, and burns of the anterior aspect of the right arm above the elbow.

Her clothing and jewelry had been removed at the community hospital, and she was covered with a sterile sheet and blanket for transport. The extent of the burn injury had been assessed and fluid requirements were calculated according to the Parkland formula. Fluid resuscitation had been initiated in the ED and an indwelling urinary catheter inserted. It drained about 40 mL per hour during transport. Oxygen therapy had been initiated and the patient was medicated with morphine sulphate intravenously.

Upon arrival to the burn unit, the patient's airway, breathing, and circulation were thoroughly assessed again. Her respirations were 22 per minute and unlabored. Apical pulse was 102 and regular. Blood pressure was 130/80. Temperature was 37.2°C (99°F). She was alert and oriented to person, place and time. She was anxious and cooperative.

A central venous line was substituted for the peripheral intravenous line. A nasogastric tube was inserted and connected to intermittent low suction. Bloods were drawn for a complete blood count (CBC), serum electrolytes, serum glucose, blood urea nitrogen (BUN), creatinine, clotting studies, and carboxyhemoglobin. A chest x-ray, arterial blood gases (ABGs), 12-lead electrocardiogram (ECG), urinalysis, and pulse oximetry were ordered. The patient was scheduled for a fiberoptic bronchoscopy, was given a tetanus toxoid booster, and was started on a regimen of histamine antagonist and antacid therapy. Aggressive fluid resuscitation, oxygen therapy, and pain management with IV morphine sulphate in small doses were continued. The burn wounds were cleaned, débrided, and treated with silver sulfadiazine.

The patient greeted me with a series of questions about her hospitalization and course of treatment. She was alert and oriented, and stated that the medication was adequately controlling her pain. I proceeded to perform a thorough physical assessment, beginning once again with her respiratory status. Although she continued to show no evidence of inhalation injury, I knew that respiratory difficulties could still develop. Her respirations were 20 per minute, unlabored and regular. Despite the chest burns, she had no restriction of respiratory excursion. Chest movements were equal bilaterally. There was no use of the accessory muscles of respiration, and breath sounds were clear on auscultation. Her blood pressure was 128/76, and her apical pulse was 92 and regular.

Examination of her peripheral circulation in the lower extremities revealed strong, bilateral pedal pulses, capillary refill of less than 3 seconds, and skin that was pink and warm to the touch. Radial pulses were weak to palpation, but evident with the use of a Doppler ultrasound stethoscope. Capillary refill was 3 seconds in both hands. Both arms and hands were edematous. The patient denied paresthesias and demonstrated no limitation of range of motion (ROM). Following this assessment, I elevated both her arms on pillows to facilitate venous return.

Her abdomen was soft with hyperactive bowel sounds auscultated in all four quadrants. The nasogastric tube set to low intermittent suction was draining small amounts of brownish fluid. A litmus test of the gastrointestinal aspirate confirmed that the patient was within the desired range of alkalinity. Urinary output remained between 40 and 50 mL per hour, and showed no evidence of a burgundy color and myoglobinuria.

When I returned 1 hour later, the patient complained of numbness and tingling in her right

CLINICAL ? THINKING

(continued)

hand. I could no longer palpate the radial pulse, nor could I locate it with the Doppler ultrasound. Capillary refill was about 5 seconds and she had limited ability to move her fingers. Assessment findings of the left hand showed no significant changes in the past hour.

Knowing that a circumferential burn could act as a tourniquet and occlude arterial circulation as fluid shifted and accumulated in the interstitial tissue, I recognized that these findings in the patient's right arm represented a dangerous change in her clinical condition. The ensuing neurologic disturbance and tissue ischemia could threaten the viability of the extremity and required emergency intervention. I immediately notified the physician and assisted with an escharotomy, performed at the bedside, to re-establish adequate peripheral circulation. The patient tolerated the procedure well, and adequate circulation to the extremity was restored.

I cared for the patient again on day three of her hospitalization, during which time she remained stable and progressed as anticipated by the clinical pathway for patients with burns. That evening, as I prepared to perform my final assessment of the patient and an evaluation of the outcomes of her nursing and medical therapy, I noted that she was somewhat agitated and restless, and that her face appeared flushed. Upon closer inspection of her face and skin, I observed numerous small areas of petechiae on her face, shoulders, and lower extremities. I also noted a large ecchymotic area on her left arm at the site where the blood pressure cuff usually encircled her arm. These new developments in the patient's clinical picture indicated a tendency to bleed and warranted further investigation.

Her vital signs remained stable, with a slight rise in her pulse rate to 108 beats per minute (bpm). She had no evidence of an increased respiratory effort. I decided to report my findings to the physician, who said he would check the patient shortly. When I returned, I noticed that the dressing over the IV site was saturated with serosanguineous drainage. The IV site continued to ooze when I removed the dressing.

Although petechiae and ecchymosis can be related to a number of blood dyscrasias (such as thrombocytopenia) this additional symptom of bleeding without a known hemorrhagic disease, hepatic disorder, or anticoagulant therapy led me to suspect that the patient was experiencing disseminated intravascular coagulation (DIC). The possibility of DIC, a clotting and bleeding disorder

that often occurs secondary to a serious underlying medical condition, was supported by the patient's history of recent burns with its widespread tissue damage and necrosis. The patient denied any personal or family history of bleeding disorders, and was not taking any medication that might otherwise account for the bleeding.

Despite the patient's stable blood pressure, the presence of restlessness and tachycardia were consistent with the presence of some bleeding. Knowing that orthostatic hypotension can precede an actual drop in blood pressure secondary to bleeding, I checked the patient's blood pressure in the lying and sitting positions and found greater than a 10-mm Hg difference in the systolic readings. This represented some degree of hypovolemia, and although hypovolemia in a burn patient often occurs secondary to fluid shifts and inadequate fluid resuscitation, the patient had already been successfully and uneventfully resuscitated. Also, bleeding and hemorrhage related to trauma were unlikely in this case.

To identify additional sites of bleeding, I continued my assessment and decided to check the nasogastric aspirate for blood to determine if there was any gastrointestinal bleeding. The results were positive for occult blood. Although a patient with a burn is at high risk for bleeding from a Curling's ulcer, hemorrhagic gastritis, or both, the patient's treatment with histamine antagonists and antacids greatly reduced the likelihood that this was the source of the bleeding. Instead, this finding further supported the likelihood of DIC.

To check for thrombosis in the extremities, I evaluated the peripheral circulation in her legs and found that they were cool to the touch with evidence of mottling and cyanosis. I eliminated shock and hypovolemia as the underlying reason for this inadequate peripheral circulation based on the patient's blood pressure. This finding very strongly supported my suspicion. As I explained to the patient that she required immediate medical attention, she began to bleed from the nose. Bleeding from various unrelated sites, in conjunction with acrocyanosis, left little doubt in my mind about the patient's condition.

Because DIC is a life-threatening condition that can lead to widespread vascular occlusion with extensive organ damage, hemorrhage, shock, coma, and death, I implemented the following nursing measures at once:

1. I called for assistance and asked the nurse who responded to notify the physician at once.

(continued)

CLINICAL ❓ THINKING

(continued)

2. I sat the patient up and instructed her to apply gentle pressure to her nares.

3. I applied a pressure dressing to the IV site.

4. I continued to monitor the patient's vital signs and neurologic status for signs of continued bleeding or thrombosis.

5. I checked the patient for additional signs of bleeding, such as hematomas and hematuria.

6. I checked the patient for changes in the extent of petechiae and ecchymosis.

7. I monitored the patient for additional gastrointestinal bleeding.

8. I monitored the patient for renal failure, pulmonary embolism, adult respiratory distress syndrome (ARDS), and intracranial hemorrhage or thrombosis.

9. I continued to monitor the patient for acrocyanosis.

10. I initiated safety measures and bleeding precautions to prevent injury and further bleeding.

11. I explained what was happening to the patient, answered her questions, and provided emotional support.

12. I documented my findings and actions.

The physician arrived and ordered a CBC with platelet count, prothrombin time (PT), partial thromboplastin time (PTT), fibrinogen level, fibrinogen degradation product (FDP) test and D-dimer assay, and type and cross-match for blood products.

The results of the laboratory tests confirmed the suspicion of DIC. The patient's treatment was directed at stopping the bleeding by replacing platelets and coagulation factors, and at supportive treatment of the underlying burns. The patient was transfused with platelets and fresh frozen plasma, and stopped bleeding within 48 hours.

Although the patient faced a lengthy rehabilitation from the burns as well as the possibility of new complications, the nurse's competent care and prompt and comprehensive treatment improved the patient's chance for survival. Early recognition of two emergency situations by the nurse saved both the patient's life and her limb.

Think Critically

Did the patient meet the American Burn Association's criteria for transfer to a burn facility? Why? Why not?

According to the rule of nines, about what percentage of the patient's total body surface area would the nurse have documented as burned?

How does the loss of consciousness during the fire increase the chances for inhalation injuries?

How might this scenario have differed if the patient had experienced inhalation injuries? An electrical burn?

What nursing assessments should be made while the burn patient is receiving narcotic analgesics? When might they be contraindicated?

The patient asks the nurse, "How serious are my burn injuries?" What would be the nurse's best response?

The patient's son expresses concern regarding his mother's psychologic adjustment and ability to cope with possible scarring, and the possible limitation of function. What would be the nurse's best response?

How does the role of the home health nurse fit in with the interdisciplinary approach of the entire burn team?

Should the nurse have checked the patient's hematocrit (Hct) levels to support the suspicion of DIC? Would this finding lend accurate support? Why? Why not?

Were frequent blood pressure checks utilizing the ecchymotic area, following the discovery of the ecchymosis, the best action by the nurse? Why? Why not? What were the options?

What additional assessments might the nurse have made to further support the suspicion of DIC?

The nurse anticipated the possible inclusion of heparin in the patient's treatment regimen for DIC. Why might this paradoxical treatment be utilized? Why is it controversial?

What assessments would the nurse make to determine whether the patient had developed acute tubular necrosis (ATN) secondary to impaired tissue perfusion and organ necrosis? Could the nurse differentiate renal failure secondary to hypovolemia and inadequate fluid resuscitation from renal failure secondary to thrombosis? If yes, how? If not, why not?

Could the nurse differentiate decreased peripheral perfusion of an extremity related to a circumferential burn from that related to thrombosis secondary to DIC? If yes, how? If not, why not?

Table 37–4

Comparison of Fluid and Electrolyte (F&E) Shift in Emergent and Diuretic Phases

F&E Characteristic	Emergent Phase	Acute (Diuretic) Phase
Capillary permeability	Increases	Returns to normal
Interstitial edema	Increases	Decreases
Intracellular sodium	Increases	Decreases
Intracellular potassium	Decreases	Increases
Extracellular sodium	Decreases	Increases
Extracellular potassium	Increases	Decreases
Vasodilation	Increases	Decreases
Cardiac output	Decreases	Increases
Venous return	Decreases	Increases

exchange for potassium. Fluid leaves the cells with the sodium, decreasing intracellular edema. A comparison of the fluid and electrolyte shifts in burn shock in the emergent phase and fluid mobilization in the acute phase is presented in Table 37–4.

Clinical Manifestations
The earliest clinical manifestation of the onset of fluid remobilization in the acute phase is a rapid increase in urine output. The blood pressure and heart rate return to the patient's normal limits as the central venous pressure, cardiac output, and pulmonary artery wedge pressure increase.

Management
Fluid loss in the acute phase is vastly reduced and results mainly from evaporative loss of free water through the burned skin. The larger the size of the burn wound, the greater the evaporative loss. This fluid is primarily replaced with 5% dextrose in water to maintain fluid balance, urine output, and a serum sodium of 140 mEq/L. In addition, colloids are administered to replace protein loss and to pull fluid from the interstitial space back into the vascular system. Fluid replacement in the acute phase is at a much slower rate, and lesser volume, than in the emergent phase.

NURSING PROCESS
Fluid Mobilization After a Major Burn Injury

Fluid mobilization in the acute phase of burn care represents a continuation of care as the patient experiences a physiologic shift from a state of circulatory hypovolemia to a state of potential fluid overload. With fluid mobilization, the focus of care changes from treating hypovolemia to replacing evaporative fluid loss and maintaining electrolyte balance. Nurs-

ing care during fluid mobilization is similar to, and a continuation of, the care of the burn patient presented in the emergent phase (see Nursing Care Guide 37–1).

Assessment
The initial indication of fluid mobilization is an increase in urine output to greater than 50 mL/hour. Document the precise time of increased urine output, and notify the physician so the infusion rate of parenteral fluids can be decreased.

Nursing Diagnoses and Planning
Nursing diagnoses and related expected patient outcomes commonly applicable to patients with fluid mobilization after a burn injury include the following:

NDx: Risk for fluid volume excess related to over-replacement of fluids lost through evaporation from the burn wound or mobilization of fluids from the interstitial spaces into the circulatory system

Planning: Patient Outcomes
1. Patient remains free of manifestations of fluid overload as evidenced by:
   Heart rate regular and more than 60 but fewer than 100 beats per minute
   Blood pressure stable and higher than 90/60 but lower than 140/90
   Respirations clear and unlabored
   Central venous pressure 4 to 12 mm H_2O
   Capillary refill less than 3 seconds
   Moist mucous membranes
2. Patient's urine output is more than 30 mL/hour but less than 100 mL/hour after initial diuresis.
3. Patient's weight is within 5% of preburn weight after diuresis.
4. Patient has bowel sounds and is free of nausea.

Nursing Interventions and Evaluations

NDx: Risk for fluid volume excess
Monitor parenteral infusions hourly to ensure correct rate of flow and to prevent fluid overload. Continue to auscultate bowel sounds every 4 hours to detect hypoperistalsis or paralytic ileus caused by dilutional hyponatremia. The intravenous infusion may be discontinued or changed to a saline (heparin) lock if bowel sounds are present and the patient is free of nausea and able to ingest adequate amounts of fluids.

Urine measurement can usually be decreased to every 4 hours for 24 hours when output is greater than 50 mL/hour for 4 consecutive hours. Expect output to be greater than 100 mL/hour during initial diuresis. Be sure the urine-collection container can hold the increased urine volume. The indwelling urinary catheter may be removed if the patient is able to use the bedpan or urinal without contaminating the burn wound. Urine specific gravity decreases as the urine becomes more dilute. Diuresis is complete when urine specific gravity returns to normal and output is less than 100 mL/hour for 4 hours.

Continue hourly measurements of hemodynamic parameters until diuresis is complete. Vital signs, central venous pressure, and pulmonary artery wedge pressures should remain within normal limits. An increase in heart rate or peripheral or central blood pressure or a change in heart rhythm may indicate left ventricular failure. Continue electrocardiogram monitoring for early detection of cardiac dysrhythmias caused by rapid shift in serum potassium levels. Review results of electrolyte studies to evaluate electrolyte balance.

Observe for increased restlessness, anxiety, or dyspnea, and auscultate breath sounds for crackles (rales) and wheezes, which indicate pulmonary edema from fluid overload. Elevate the head of the bed to promote pulmonary venous drainage and to ease diaphragmatic excursion if not contraindicated by the location of injuries. Because of the generalized interstitial edema, assessment of dependent edema and distended neck veins is not clinically useful in detecting fluid overload in the burn patient.

Report deterioration in the patient's circulatory or respiratory status to the physician immediately. Continue to weigh the patient daily to monitor fluid balance. Expect rapid weight loss during diuresis. Fluid replacement is successful if the patient is within 5% of preburn weight at the end of diuresis.

Compare the patient's status with the expected outcomes. If the outcomes are not met, reassess the patient and revise the plan.

Pain Management

Burn patients are in pain 24 hours a day because of unprotected nerve endings until the wound heals or is grafted. Wound care and physical therapy add to the already intense pain. Burn patients may undergo repeated surgical procedures during hospitalization and after discharge. Often the surgeries will follow each other in rapid succession. After these procedures, the patient usually experiences a temporary increase in pain and discomfort.

Narcotic analgesics are used for pain management. Intravenous morphine sulfate administered in frequent, small doses or by continuous low-dose infusion or patient-controlled analgesia, combined with a bolus dose before painful procedures, is most effective for pain management during the emergent phase and fluid remobilization. Oral, subcutaneous, and intramuscular routes are contraindicated at this time because of poor absorption. When fluid balance is stabilized, oral narcotic agents can be used. The addition of psychotropic agents and the use of guided imagery, hypnosis, and relaxation techniques may increase the effectiveness of pain control for some patients. Inhalation of a preset mixture of oxygen and nitrous oxide just before highly painful procedures is being evaluated as part of pain management.

NURSING PROCESS
Pain After a Burn Injury
Assessment

Assess the need for pain medication. Burn injuries are extremely painful and remain so until grafting is completed or until the wound closes spontaneously. Pain is intensified by movement and wound care procedures. The patient may verbalize pain or demonstrate pain by facial grimacing, refusal to move, stiffness, guarding, or refusing treatments. Anorexia, dilated pupils, elevated blood pressure, and increased pulse or respiratory rate may also indicate pain. Ask the patient to identify the location and type of pain to confirm that the patient's wounds, treatments, or associated injuries are the cause of the pain.

Nursing Diagnoses and Planning

Nursing diagnoses and related expected patient outcomes commonly applicable to patients with pain after a burn injury include the following:

NDx: Pain related to open burn wounds, treatments, and dressing changes

Planning: Patient Outcomes
1. Patient expresses relief from analgesics and is adequately medicated to tolerate painful procedures.
2. Pain from open burn wounds decreases in intensity as healing occurs.
3. Patient talks about, participates in, and tolerates wound care.

Nursing Interventions and Evaluations

Pain assessment and management are critical to the recovery of the burn patient. Almost every procedure and intervention, whose goal is to promote wound healing, causes pain. People have different degrees of tolerance and response to pain; therefore, administration of analgesics must be adjusted for each patient. General nursing interventions in pain management are discussed in detail in the care of the postoperative patient in Chapter 6.

NDx: Pain
Administer narcotic analgesics as needed. Monitor the patient's response to determine the need for additional medication or increased or decreased dosage. Administer intravenous narcotic analgesic 5 minutes before dressing changes, débridement, and other painful procedures to allow enough time for the medication to take effect.

Acknowledge the patient's pain and fear of procedures that increase pain. Assure the patient that feelings of fear, anger, hostility, and frustration are normal. Explain the cause of the pain and the goals of pain management to correct misconceptions and fears of drug addiction. Explain procedures, and allow the patient to make decisions and participate in his or her care as much as possible. Encourage verbalization, keep the patient informed, and give the patient a degree of control to reduce anxiety and fear and promote pain management by reducing feelings of helplessness. Explore with the patient the use of distraction, deep breathing, and other relaxation techniques to reduce anxiety and enhance pain relief.

Compare the patient's status with the expected outcomes. If the outcomes are not met, reassess the patient and revise the plan.

Wound Care

Although wound care begins at the scene of the injury and continues throughout the emergent, acute, and rehabilitation periods, it is a primary focus of the acute period. The two most common methods of wound care are the open method and the closed method. Table 37–5 summarizes their characteristics, advantages, and disadvantages. The goals of wound care are to:

- Minimize wound and systemic infection.
- Prevent conversion of a partial-thickness wound to a full-thickness wound.
- Débride the injury to remove all dead tissue and prepare healthy granulation tissue for grafting.

- Complete wound closure as soon as possible, using grafts when necessary.
- Minimize scar and contracture formation to maximize appearance and function.

Although no burn wound is sterile, it is important to keep the wound as clean and free from microorganisms as possible. Risk of burn wound infection is high for two reasons. First, the body's primary line of defense, the skin, is extensively damaged, disrupting natural protection against invasion. Second, the body's immune system is suppressed after a major burn injury. The patient's normal flora, as well as nosocomial bacteria from the hospital environment, becomes a source of infection. The most common organisms in burn wound infection are *Pseudomonas, Klebsiella, Streptococcus, Staphylococcus aureus,* and other strains of *Staphylococcus.*

Protein exudate in the burn wound provides an ideal medium for microorganism growth. Wound infection places the patient at risk for systemic sepsis. As the infectious process destroys healthy tissue, necrosis deepens the wound, and a partial-thickness burn can convert to a full-thickness burn wound. An infected wound will not heal.

The surface of most burn wounds is contaminated by a small number of organisms. This is referred to as colonization of the wound and is not considered a wound infection. Wound infection occurs when microorganisms have penetrated the surface of the wound and invaded the eschar or underlying viable tissue. Because of the eschar covering the wound, colonization of the surface of the wound, and the body's inflammatory response to

Table 37–5

Comparison of Open and Closed Methods of Wound Care

Method	Description	Advantages	Disadvantages
Open	Wounds covered with topical agent Gauze dressings not used	Wound easily visualized and assessed Avoids dark, warm, moist environment conducive to growth of microorganisms Wound care takes less time	Topical antibacterial agent is easily rubbed off onto equipment or falls onto the floor, becoming cleaning problem, safety hazard, and source of cross-contamination. Must be reapplied frequently to maintain wound coverage and provide a barrier against infection
Closed	Wounds covered with topical agent and gauze dressing	Wound always covered, providing a constant barrier against infection Topical agent does not contaminate equipment or fall onto the floor	Dressings provide dark, warm, moist environment conducive to growth of microorganisms Visual assessment of the wound is difficult Dressings become stuck to wound if not enough agent applied or if too much time elapsed, making it difficult to remove, thus causing bleeding, increased pain, and damage to healing skin

the injury, an infected burn wound may be difficult to identify by inspection. Increasing localized edema, increasing redness and warmth along the wound edges, purulent drainage, or foul odor when dressings are removed indicates infection. Figure 37–6 illustrates the difference in appearance between a clean, noninfected wound and an infected wound.

Penetration of the surface of the wound by microorganisms is determined by biopsy. A small piece of eschar or tissue is excised, microscopically examined, and cultured for determination of the types of organisms present, the number per gram of tissue, and the antibiotics to which the organisms are sensitive. Once bacteria exceed 100,000 per gram of tissue with invasion of subadjacent unburned tissue, the wound is defined as infected. A topical or systemic antibiotic to which the pathogen is sensitive is prescribed, and the wound is evaluated for débridement.

Sepsis from burn wound infection is the leading cause of death in the acute period of burn care. It may occur at any time until the wounds are completely closed. Clinical manifestations of sepsis include anorexia, malaise, headache, confusion, elevated or subnormal temperature, chills, increased pulse and respirations, decreased blood pressure, and decreased urine output. Blood cultures confirm septicemia. Wound, urine, and all invasive access sites may be cultured to identify the primary source of infection. Broad-spectrum intravenous antibiotics effective against gram-negative bacteria are started immediately. Once sensitivity studies are complete, antibiotic therapy and the topical agent may be changed to increase effectiveness against the identified microorganism. The patient may require aggressive supportive interventions to prevent or to treat septic shock.

DÉBRIDEMENT

On admission to the hospital or burn unit, the burn wound is cleansed, and all loose and nonviable tissue is removed or débrided. Once the wound is initially débrided, the depth of the burn is reassessed. Débridement may be necessary many more times throughout the healing process to remove wound exudate and necrotic tissue that could be a perfect medium for bacterial growth. The need for extensive nursing débridement has largely been eliminated by early excision and grafting of the burn wounds. Rarely is it necessary to wait for eschar separation and tissue granulation before placing a skin graft on the burn wound.

Enzymatic débridement uses a commercially prepared enzyme agent (such as Travase), which is applied to the eschar and covered with sterile gauze dressings. The enzyme breaks down the eschar, speeds natural separation, and makes mechanical removal easier. The use of these agents is controversial because of variations in effectiveness and possible degradation of viable tissue.

Wound débridement is a painful procedure and should be preceded by appropriate pain medication.

HYDROTHERAPY

Hydrotherapy is the use of water to clean burn wounds. This can be done by submerging patients in hydrotherapy tubs, using shower table devices, or having patients wash their own wounds in a regular shower. The type of hydrotherapy and wound cleansing depend on the patient's wound care needs and level of independence.

Hydrotherapy tanks allow for the soaking of wounds and gentle débridement of nonviable tissue. This method is cumbersome for dependent patients

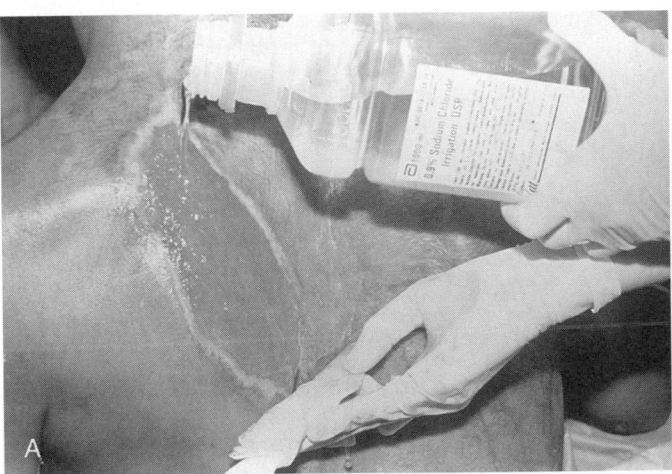
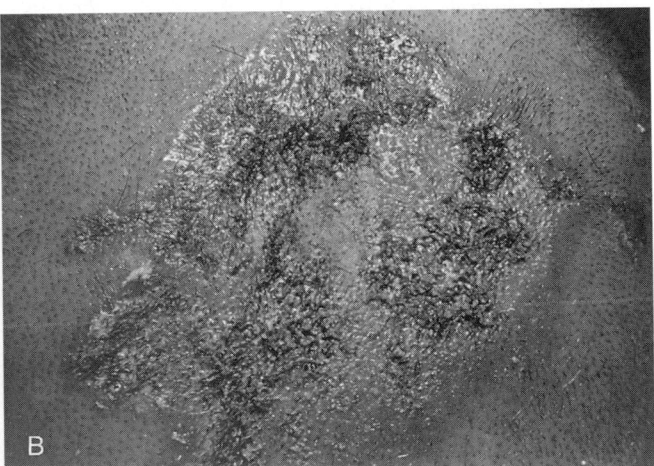

Figure 37–6

A, A clean, uninfected burn wound with new tissue growth around the edges. *B,* An infected burn wound with black necrotic tissue in the bed of the wound.

and significantly limits access to patients during wound care procedures.

Shower tables and patients showering independently allow for easy accessibility for care and visualization of wounds. This method may also decrease possible cross-contamination caused by submerging all wounds in the same water. Hypothermia can be a problem with showering if precautions are not taken. Both methods are currently in use, and preferences for each vary among burn centers.

TOPICAL AGENTS

Many topical agents are available for use in burn care. They provide a physical barrier against the invasion of microorganisms and inhibit the growth of microorganisms in the wound and eschar. Each agent has its advantages and disadvantages. The three most widely used agents are silver sulfadiazine, mafenide acetate (Sulfamylon), and silver nitrate. The pharmacokinetics and nursing implications of topical agents commonly used in burn wound care are described in Table 37–6.

TETANUS PROPHYLAXIS

Tetanus toxoid is administered as soon as possible in burn injuries in which dead tissue is present and in those associated with penetrating injuries. Patients receive a tetanus booster if already immunized against tetanus but with more than 5 years elapsed since the last booster. Patients who have never been immunized against tetanus should receive hyperimmune human tetanus globulin as well as the tetanus immunization series.

GRAFTING PROCEDURES

As discussed in Chapter 35 and summarized in Table 37–7, there are three common types of skin grafts by source: homograft, heterograft, and autograft. Application of a graft slows evaporative loss through the wound, reduces pain, and reduces the risk of infection.

Homografts and heterografts are used as a temporary biologic dressing either to protect the wound bed while small adherent bits of eschar separate or to provide temporary wound coverage until the bed is ready to accept a permanent graft. Figure 37–7 shows the use of porcine heterografts as a temporary biologic dressing on the bed of a full-thickness burn injury.

Autografts are used in burn wound care to permanently cover a full-thickness burn, which is incapable of regenerating skin, or deep partial-thickness burns that will require more than 3 weeks to heal. Split-thickness skin grafts and mesh grafts are most commonly used. Solid sheets of split-thickness grafts are preferred for closing wounds on the face be-

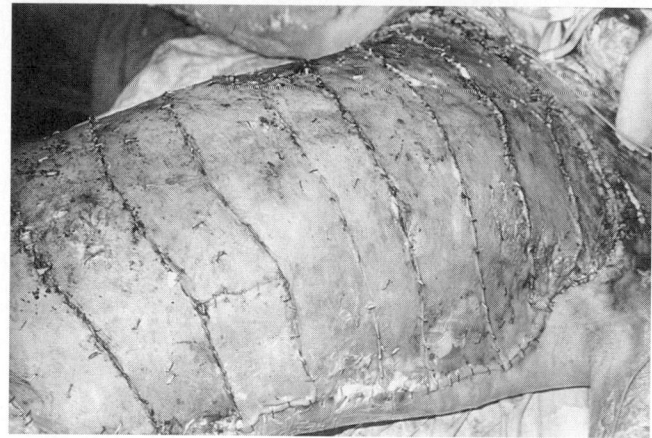

Figure 37–7

Solid sheets of porcine heterograft used to temporarily cover a full-thickness burn wound of the anterior torso.

cause scarring is minimal. It is important that the patient understand that the grafted skin will retain properties of the area of the body from which it was grafted.

Once a graft is applied, it is covered with petrolatum-impregnated dressings or dressings soaked in topical antimicrobial solutions and then wrapped in a bulky gauze dressing to protect it from trauma and to keep it from drying out. A dry graft will lift off the wound or curl up at the edges and will not take (adhere and grow on the wound). The graft site may also be splinted to keep adjacent joints from moving and dislodging the graft.

The first dressing change is done approximately 3 to 5 days after the grafting procedure. By this time, a successful autograft will be pink and appear as though it is attached to the bed of the wound. If the graft was meshed, the interstices usually show signs of new epithelial cell growth in 5 to 7 days. The interstices will continue to fill in until the spaces disappear completely. The meshed appearance of the skin may eventually disappear. Figure 37–8 shows a successful mesh graft, with new epithelial cell growth beginning to fill in the interstitial spaces.

The donor sites for skin grafts heal in about 3 weeks and can be reused. Although donor sites heal quickly, each one is a new open wound in an immunocompromised patient and increases the burn patient's morbidity risk. As illustrated in Figure 37–9, a donor site has the wet appearance of a deep partial-thickness burn wound and can be as painful. An infected donor site can become a full-thickness wound and place the patient at risk for sepsis. Because blood and serum are lost through the donor site, its area is added to the TBSA of open wounds when calculating the patient's fluid and nutritional requirements.

Table 37–6

Commonly Used Topical Agents

Agent	Description	Action	Advantages	Disadvantages	Nursing Implications
Silver sulfadiazine	White, soluble cream	Broad-spectrum antimicrobial sulfonamide effective against gram-negative and gram-positive bacteria and yeast	Soothing to wound Easily applied Does not affect acid-base balance Dressings not required	May not penetrate eschar completely Transient leukopenia may occur in first 4 days Gram-negative bacilli may become resistant after prolonged use	Clean wound to remove old cream and loose necrotic tissue. Use sterile glove, tongue blade, or gauze pad to aseptically apply $\frac{1}{16}$-inch thick layer 2–3 times daily. Apply additional cream between scheduled applications to areas rubbed off.
Mafenide acetate (Sulfamylon)	Thick, white, water-soluble cream	Broad-spectrum bacteriostatic sulfonamide agent effective against many gram-negative and gram-positive organisms and certain anaerobes	Excellent penetration of eschar Not inactivated by pus or serum or affected by pH changes	May cause burning or stinging on application Inhibits carbonic anhydrase, resulting in alkaline urine and metabolic acidosis Leukopenia may occur. Hypersensitivity reactions may occur as late as 10–14 days after use.	Application is the same as for silver sulfadiazine. Dressings are optional.
Silver nitrate	0.5% aqueous solution	Wide-spectrum bactericidal agent	Painless on application High degree of effectiveness Prevents cross-contamination of burn wounds	Poor penetration of eschar, allowing subeschar infection and sepsis Caustic to skin if allowed to dry Heat loss through wet dressings Joint mobility may be impaired Hyponatremia and hypochloremia possible Time consuming, messy dressings	Apply bulky dressings soaked in silver nitrate solution. Re-wet dressings at least every 2 hours using a bulb syringe or catheters embedded in the dressing. Apply petrolatum to unburned skin bordering burn to prevent skin staining. Silver nitrate is most commonly used in patients with neutropenic reaction to silver sulfadiazine.
Bacitracin	Ointment	Minimal antibiotic effect	Painless on application Prevents drying of wound Keeps eschar soft	No major antibiotic effect	Apply to clean wound twice daily. Cover with petrolatum gauze and bandage. Bacitracin is used for small burns and facial burns.

Table 37–7

Comparing Graft Types

	Heterograft	Homograft	Autograft Sheet	Autograft Meshed 1.5:1	Autograft Meshed 3:1	Allograft
Biologic dressing	Yes	Yes	Yes	Yes	Yes	Yes
Permanent	No	No	Yes	Yes	Yes	Yes
Cosmetic results	N/A	N/A	Superior	Moderate	Poor	Good*
Maximal skin coverage	Yes	Yes	Poor	Moderate	Superior	*
Source	Pig	Cadaver	Patient	Patient	Patient	Cadaver
Fragility	N/A	N/A	Minimal	Moderate	Maximal	*

*This technique is still in the research phase.
N/A, not applicable.

Lack of available donor sites in a massive burn injury presents a major problem in burn care. Recently there has been development of an epidermal skin equivalent grown from full-thickness skin biopsies. These biopsies are processed, grown in culture dishes and after about 3 weeks produce small patches of skin suitable for use in wound closure. There are different types of products available. Some are just epithelial cells and others are joined to an allograft dermal structure. So far this treatment's efficacy remains controversial because the quality of the new skin is poor, the actual take of the graft is 10 to 30%, and the cost is very high. All agree however, that this type of therapy holds great promise for the future but still warrants more study and development.

NURSING PROCESS
Burn Wound Care

Assessment

Assess burn wounds for signs of healing or infection. A clean wound is free of redness, edema, and purulent or foul-smelling drainage and is the same temperature to the touch as other parts of the body. A partial-thickness wound heals by re-epithelialization as skin buds and new patches of epithelial cells develop. Healthy granulation tissue in a full-thickness wound is moist and pink to red in color and looks like fleshy bumps or masses emerging from the bed and edges of the wound. Granulation tissue indicates adequate revascularization of the wound bed and readiness to receive a graft. Figure 37–10

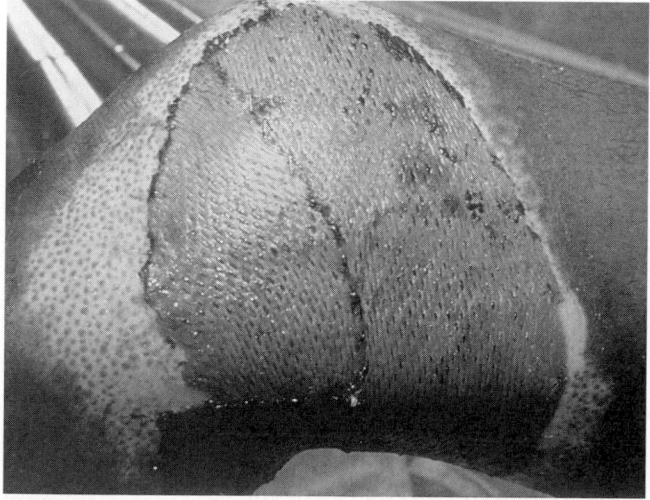

Figure 37–8
Successful mesh graft with new epithelial cell growth in the interstitial spaces.

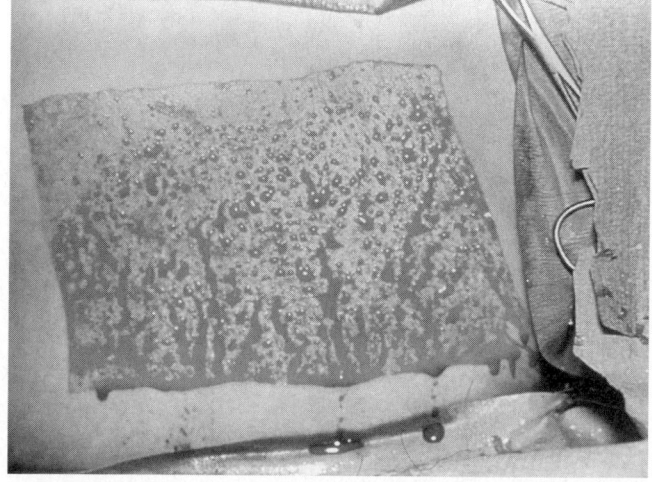

Figure 37–9
A newly harvested donor site has the wet appearance of a deep partial-thickness burn wound.

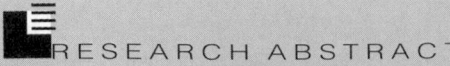

RESEARCH ABSTRACT

Can a 19th-Century Dressing Promote Skin Graft Healing in the 1990s?

Sanford S, Gore D. Unna's boot dressings facilitate outpatient skin grafting of hands. J Burn Care Rehab 1996; 17(4);323.

Burn injuries can have a great impact on a person's self-care ability and work productivity. Promoting maximum healing and return of function is therefore a major goal during recovery and rehabilitation from burn injuries to the hands.

Skin grafting is a common surgical intervention for such injuries. However, potential complications during recovery from skin grafting include infection, graft rejection, and formation of scar tissue. Good follow-up care after grafting is therefore crucial. In an effort to develop a burn care dressing for the hands that could be managed in home environments, Sanford and Gore conducted a small trial using Unna's boot dressings and splinting.

Unna's boot dressings were orginally developed in the late 1880s to treat venous ulcers. Traditionally, they were constructed of gauze soaked in a mixture of zinc oxide, calamine, glycerin, and gelatin wrapped around the extremity and covered with an elastic bandage. They offered moist protection with compression to the site of the wound (Barr, 1996).

In this study, a splint was added to the "boot" once the wound was dressed. Donor sites were covered with calcium alginate gauze for protection and pain relief. Patients were discharged after their immediate postoperative recovery (4–6 hours). They received prescriptions for antibiotics and analgesics at home. Clinic visits were scheduled for the second and fifth postoperative day to assess for signs of healing and complications. During these visits patients were also instructed in range-of-motion exercises.

Sanford and Gore limited their sample to people who suffered from burn injuries to the distal arm and whose home environments would allow sufficient assistance with self-care during the immediate discharge period. Twelve people participated in the study. The results of the study included a 95 to 100% "take" on all graft sites and no infection in the graft sites. Range of motion improved for all but two of the patients studied. Continued outpatient rehabilitation was needed for all subjects.

The researchers say that this approach to managing burns of the hand, and graft sites, may be a cost-effective and clinically acceptable method. Given the limitations of their selected sample, generalizations to all burn-injured patients cannot be made. However, for a selected group of patients with limited burn injuries, supportive home environments, and supportive facilities, the approach seems feasible.

Reference

Barr D. The Unna's boot as a treatment for venous ulcers. Nurse Practitioner 1996; 21(7):55.

Questions to Consider

1. What innovations in burn care management are used in your clinical facilities?

2. How are patients and families prepared to manage wounds in their home environments?

3. What criteria would you use to determine whether a person's home environment would allow him or her to manage a wound effectively?

4. When an Unna's boot is used to treat a burn injury, the wound is completely covered. How would you instruct a patient and family to monitor for signs of complications?

5. What outpatient systems are in place in the clinical facilities in your area to help people manage their burn injuries in the home environment?

illustrates the appearance of healthy epithelial and granulation tissue.

After a grafting procedure, examine the dressings to ensure that they are intact, that peripheral circulation is adequate, and that splints are properly applied. Assess dressings over donor sites for bleeding and excessive drainage.

Nursing Diagnoses and Planning

Nursing diagnoses and related expected patient outcomes commonly applicable to patients being treated for burn wound injuries include the following:

NDx: Risk for infection related to burn wounds, donor site wounds, and multiple routes of possible invasion by microorganisms

Planning: Patient Outcomes

1. Patient's débrided wounds show daily evidence of healing by increased granulation tissue or reduced area or depth.

2. Patient remains free from infection as evidenced by the following:
   Patient is afebrile.
   Skin around wounds is the same temperature as other parts of the body.

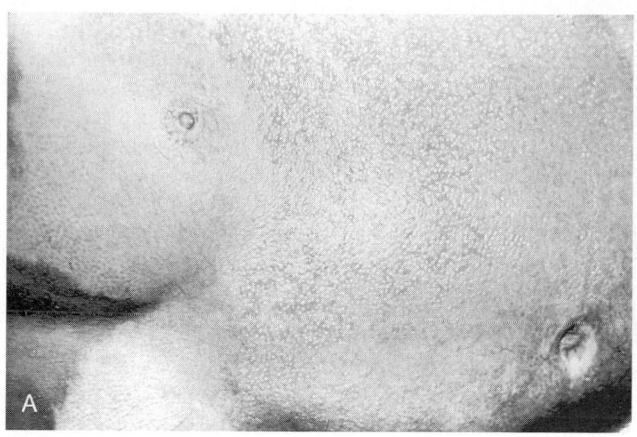 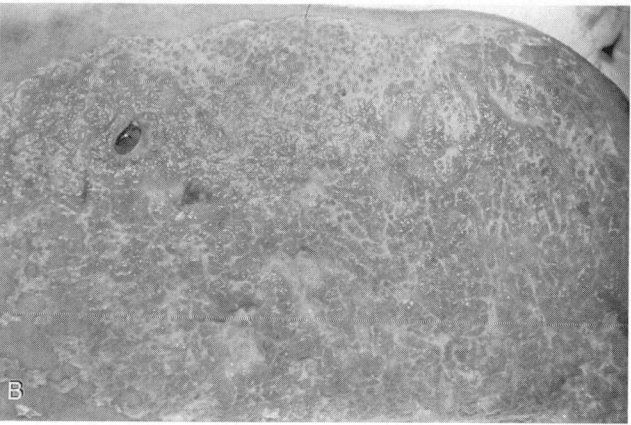

Figure 37–10

A, Skin buds and patches of epithelial tissue growing in a partial-thickness burn wound. *B*, Fleshy masses of granulation tissue growing in the bed of a full-thickness burn wound.

Wounds are free of increasing edema or redness, foul odor, purulent drainage.

There are fewer than 100,000 bacteria per gram of wound tissue.

NDx: Impaired physical mobility related to pain from burn wounds and donor sites.

Planning: Patient Outcomes

1. Patient expresses relief of pain to tolerable level.
2. Patient maintains function and mobility of all joints.

Nursing Interventions and Evaluation

The focus of the nursing care of a patient with burn wound injuries is to keep the wounds, grafts, and donor sites clean and free from infection to maximize comfort, minimize scarring, and promote graft adherence and new skin growth.

NDx: Risk for infection

Wash hands before and after all patient contact. Improper hand-washing is the biggest cause of nosocomial infections. A single room with equipment used only for the patient, and with specialized air flow and filtration system, further reduces the risk of cross-contamination.

Use aseptic technique, and wear a mask, gown, and sterile gloves during wound care to prevent contamination. Remove all of the topical agent and dressings from the wound, cleanse the wound, and re-dress daily or as prescribed to minimize growth of microorganisms. Keep the wound covered at all times with a topical agent to promote healing and provide a physical barrier against invasion by microorganisms. Wounds should not be uncovered for longer than necessary during wound care to minimize invasion of bacteria. Bulky dressings provide protection from trauma, which can delay healing.

Examine the wound with each dressing change for signs of healing or infection. Failure to heal is often the earliest sign of infection. Monitor vital signs every 4 hours to detect systemic signs of sepsis. Continue to observe all burn wounds and graft and donor sites at least daily until all wounds have closed.

Use aseptic technique in caring for all catheters, infusion sites, and invasive monitoring devices. Any access site is a potential route of entry for pathogens into the body.

Notify the physician immediately of any manifestations of wound infection or sepsis to ensure rapid treatment. Obtain specimens for culture and sensitivity to facilitate diagnosis. Administer the first dose of parenteral antibiotic as soon as possible to minimize the risk of septicemia. Do not delay the initiation of antibiotic therapy to collect all specimens if they cannot be immediately obtained because pathogens will continue to grow. Document any antibiotic administered before specimen collection on the laboratory requisition.

Once all wounds and donor sites have healed, the risk of wound infection is eliminated. Nursing interventions to promote adherence and growth of skin grafts and the care of donor sites are presented in Chapter 35.

NDx: Impaired physical mobility

Consult with the physician and physical and occupational therapists to determine whether splints will be applied after grafting. Splints immobilize joints adjacent to the grafts to prevent skin movement, which could dislodge the grafts. Discuss the use and benefits of the splints with the patient and family. Advise them to expect bulky dressings that may further limit movement. They should expect pain from the donor sites. Knowledge of anticipated sensations reduces fear of the unknown. Understanding of postoperative procedures and restrictions promotes participation and compliance, which promote healing.

After surgery, administer prescribed analgesics as needed. New donor sites are as painful as partial-thickness burn injuries, inhibiting the patient's desire and ability to move. Assure the patient that donor site pain will decrease as it heals. Re-epithelialization occurs more rapidly in donor sites covered with occlusive dressings than with fine-mesh gauze. Table 37–8 compares healing time and characteristics of three commonly used donor-site dressings.

Maintain the patient on bedrest if necessary to immobilize the grafted area. Examine splints frequently to ensure that they are secure and correctly positioned. Elevate the limb to reduce edema. Monitor temperature, pulses, and capillary refill distal to the splint to confirm adequate peripheral circulation. Position the patient off the graft and donor sites to reduce pain and to promote blood flow and healing. Use a bed cradle or other device to prevent sheets from lying on the graft or donor sites. Air cushion beds may be used to improve air flow to the donor sites to keep them drier. Discontinue physical therapy to involved limbs for 3 to 5 days to prevent dislodging the graft. The surgeon will resume physical therapy as soon as possible to maintain joint function and mobility. If possible, continue exercises to noninvolved joints throughout the postoperative period to maintain muscle tone and joint flexibility.

Compare the patient's status with the expected outcomes. If the outcomes are not met, reassess the patient and revise the plan.

Metabolic Needs

The body's metabolic needs remain at near-normal levels during fluid resuscitation in the emergent period after a burn injury. Then, in direct proportion to the extent of the burn injury, the metabolic rate rises rapidly and continues to rise until it peaks between the sixth and tenth days after the burn. Metabolic requirements during the acute period can increase 15 to 100% as the metabolic rate rises. After peaking, metabolism slowly decreases until it returns to near-normal levels with closure of the wound.

Pathophysiology

The metabolic response to a burn injury can be attributed to many factors. Most significant of these are hypermetabolism, to compensate for heat loss, and severe protein wasting.

A major burn injury destroys the skin's ability to conserve heat and regulate body temperature. As large amounts of fluid evaporate through the open wound, body heat is lost. Use of wet silver nitrate dressings and hydrotherapy may accelerate heat loss. The basal metabolic rate rises to compensate for the heat loss. High caloric intake is necessary to provide fuel to meet hypermetabolic requirements and prevent catabolism of body tissues for energy.

Protein wasting results from the loss of protein in wound exudate and the catabolism of skeletal muscle to meet metabolic needs. Protein loss through wound exudate is maximum in the early postburn period and then gradually decreases until wound closure. Protein is used for tissue repair and wound healing and may be oxidized as fuel to replace heat loss. In the absence of adequate protein intake to replace protein losses and to meet metabolic needs, the body breaks down muscle tissue.

Protein loss and muscle wasting also contribute to excess nitrogen loss. The burn patient may lose 30 g of nitrogen a day as opposed to 6 to 7 g of nitrogen lost daily by postsurgical patients. This loss results in a severe negative nitrogen balance, which further impairs the body's ability to repair tissue.

Failure to maintain sufficient caloric and protein intake to meet metabolic needs could result in weight loss, decreased resistance to infection, im-

Table 37–8

Comparison of Donor Site Care			
Variable	**Duoderm**	**Biobrane**	**Fine Mesh Gauze**
Healing time	7–10 days	10–14 days	12–16 days
Mobility	Moderate	Moderate	Poor
Risk of conversion to deeper wounds	Minimal	Moderate	Significant
Pain management	Minimal to no pain	Moderate pain	Severe pain
Special considerations	Wound becomes exudative. Reinforce dressing for moderate leakage. Replace if only exudate causes nonadherence.	Pressure dressing is applied to Biobrane for the first 24 h to promote adherence. As donor site heals, if pockets of bloody or serous drainage form, the Biobrane is trimmed at that spot.	Heat lamps may be used over donor sites for the first 24 h to dry sites. As the donor site heals, the fine mesh gauze is trimmed. If donor site becomes "soupy," the fine mesh gauze is trimmed and an antimicrobial agent is applied.

paired wound healing, and loss of body tissues. The burn patient could lose as much as 1 kg of body mass a day. Weight loss for a patient with a 40% TBSA burn could be as much as 20% of the patient's preburn weight.

Clinical Manifestations

Current body weight compared with the preburn weight is the most reliable factor in determining nutritional status. In addition to weight loss, signs of malnutrition include sunken and dull eyes, dry lips, sparse and brittle hair, pale and swollen tongue, inflamed gums, and a distended abdomen. A low serum albumin level confirms a decrease in body proteins and the need for increasing protein in the patient's diet.

Management

An extensive nutritional evaluation and close monitoring by the nutritionist and the nurse is essential for proper nutrition for the burn patient. Several formulas have been developed to calculate approximate caloric need. One of the more widely used is the Curreri formula:

(25 kcal × kg preburn weight)
+ (40 kcal × % TBSA burned)

Daily calorie requirements can exceed 5000 in patients with major burn injuries.

Patients with a burn of less than 20% TBSA without complications receive a high-protein, high-calorie diet with multivitamin supplements. Patients with larger burns or complications usually require enteral feedings. Parenteral hyperalimentation (intravenous infusion of amino acid, fat, and dextrose solutions) may be required only by patients who have severe complications or persistent paralytic ileus.

Paralytic ileus and acute stress (Curling's) ulcer are the most common gastrointestinal complications in the burn patient. Paralytic ileus is more common. It usually develops in the emergent or early acute period of recovery. Causative factors include hyponatremia, hypovolemia, and stress. Sepsis may also be a contributing factor. Paralytic ileus is detected by the absence of bowel sounds. It is usually treated by withholding food and oral fluids until gastrointestinal function returns. Nasogastric intubation for gastric decompression may be necessary.

The exact cause of Curling's ulcer is not known. Physical and psychologic stress, caused by the initial injury and later by surgical procedures or sepsis, and the release of massive amounts of histamine from damaged tissues appear to be major factors. Other contributing factors include elevated steroid, epinephrine, and norepinephrine levels caused by stress; decreased gastroduodenal blood flow caused by shock; slowed peristalsis resulting from hyponatremia; and changes in the gastric mucosa caused by hypovolemia.

Early enteral feedings and prophylactic use of antacids or histamine blockers begun during the emergent period and continued into the acute period have greatly reduced the incidence of Curling's ulcer in the burn patient. Chapter 22 presents a detailed discussion of the diagnosis and medical and nursing management of acute stress (Curling's) ulcer.

NURSING PROCESS
Increased Metabolic Needs After Burn Injury

Assessment

Weigh the patient on admission to establish a baseline for comparison with later weights. If significant fluid resuscitation has already occurred, question the patient, family, or friends to determine preburn weight. Determine food allergies, preferences, eating habits, and cultural and religious influences. Auscultate the patient's abdomen for bowel sounds, which indicate the presence of peristalsis.

Nursing Diagnoses and Planning

Nursing diagnoses and related expected patient outcomes commonly applicable to patients with increased metabolic needs after a burn injury include the following:

NDx: Altered nutrition: less than body requirements related to hypermetabolism and protein wasting as manifested by weight loss

Planning: Patient Outcomes
1. Patient consumes an adequate amount of food to meet calculated nutritional requirements.
2. Patient weight loss is less than 10% of preburn weight.

Nursing Interventions and Evaluation

The goal of nursing care of a patient with increased metabolic needs after a burn injury is to assist the patient to meet increased nutritional requirements necessary to prevent body wasting during wound healing and tissue repair.

NDx: Altered nutrition: less than body requirements
Weigh the patient at the same time daily with the same scale and the same amount of clothing to monitor weight loss. Accuracy is improved if the patient can be weighed without dressings or topical creams covering the burn wounds. Note on the flow sheet or chart whether dressings were removed.

Maintain a warm environment to reduce heat loss. Use radiant warmers, heat-reflecting blankets, or regular blankets to maintain the patient's body temperature between 37° and 38°C (98.6° and 100.4°F). Reducing heat loss reduces metabolic caloric requirements. Monitor the patient's temperature, and adjust the warming devices accordingly.

Beginning enteral feedings within the first 24 to 48 hours postburn has been shown to decrease the incidence of post-traumatic ileus and preserve the integrity of the bowel mucosa. If started slowly and gradually increased, this method is usually well tolerated by the patient. Oral feedings are started as soon as the patient is able to tolerate them without nausea. As oral feedings increase, enteral feedings can be decreased so that the patient's total nutritional needs are maintained.

Review the approximate nutritional requirements calculated by the dietitian or physician. Consult with the dietitian, physician, and patient to formulate a plan to meet the patient's nutritional needs. Review nutritional needs with the patient to increase understanding and cooperation. Stress that adequate nutrition is necessary for burn wounds to heal properly. The ability to eat regular food is psychologically important to most people. Six or more small meals are better tolerated than three large meals. Provide nutritional supplements and snacks to meet high-calorie, high-protein requirements. Encourage significant others to bring food to the patient from home. Avoid unpleasant procedures, sights, or odors immediately before and at mealtime to provide an environment conducive to eating. Encourage oral hygiene before meals to freshen the mouth. Assist the patient to sit up or assume a comfortable position for meals if not contraindicated. Assist with eating if necessary, but allow the patient as much independence as possible to restore self-image.

Maintain daily calorie count to monitor nutritional intake. Assess lab values for serum albumin, total protein, and vitamin levels. Document the amount of all food and fluid ingested, and submit totals to the dietitian daily for calculation.

Monitor the patient's energy level daily, and observe for manifestations of deterioration in nutritional status. Report sunken, dull eyes; dry, cracked lips or mucous membranes; sparse, brittle hair; pale, swollen tongue; inflamed gums; distended abdomen; or impaired wound healing to the physician for re-evaluation of nutritional intake.

Compare the patient's status with the expected outcomes. If the outcomes are not met, reassess the patient and revise the plan.

Psychosocial Needs

The adult patient with a major burn injury presents with many psychosocial needs. The implications of the injury involve not just the patient but also family, close friends, associates, and employer. In addition to sustaining a life-threatening injury, the patient may have family members or friends who were injured or who perished in the fire. It is not uncommon for the survivors of an accident to feel guilty that they survived when others did not. The individual must deal with the reality that he or she may not survive. These patients are aware not only of their own condition but also of patients around them who do or do not survive. If intubation is required, the patient will be unable to speak until the endotracheal tube is removed and may not be able to write because of burns of the hands. At a time when anxiety is highest, the individual is unable to ask questions, communicate, or make needs easily known.

The burn patient may also be anxious about the survival of family or friends who were also injured. If several members of the same household are injured, they may be hospitalized in different agencies. It is not uncommon for patients to be hospitalized in burn centers that are long distances from home and loved ones. In addition, the home and all possessions may have been lost.

Patients who have sustained burns of the head, face, neck, or hands may be concerned about the possibility of permanent disfigurement or disability. It is important to realize that patients who have sustained burns over less visible parts of their bodies will also be concerned about scars and disfigurement. The patient may fear rejection by family, friends, loved ones, and strangers because of appearance or because of limitations in ability to function.

The patient may resent or be ashamed of dependency on others during hospitalization and may fear the possibility of still being dependent on, or a burden to, others after discharge. Long convalescence, financial hardship, and possible permanent deformities may force the postponement or cancellation of previous plans for the future.

The cost of extended hospital and outpatient care is often a major concern to patients, especially those who have no medical insurance or whose insurance does not cover all expenses. Although most patients are discharged once their wounds heal, extended convalescence, rehabilitation, and further surgery will continue for many months or years. During this time, the patient may not be able to work, resulting in further financial hardship. The injury may prevent return to previous employment, increasing concern over future employment and long-term financial responsibilities.

Because the psychosocial needs of the burn patient can be so involved, it is important that the burn team include mental health specialists, social workers, and clergy. These specialists provide psychosocial support, which is needed by the patient, family, loved ones, and other members of the burn team. Therapeutic support may include discussions with the patient and loved ones, medications to reduce anxiety, hypnosis, and biofeedback training. Many burn centers include mental health specialists as part of their staff support.

NURSING PROCESS
Psychosocial Needs After Burn Injury

Assessment

Assess psychosocial needs during conversations and therapeutic interactions with the patient, family, and visitors. Determine the circumstances of the accident, other persons injured or killed, and their relationship with the patient. Ask the patient to identify ways he or she has coped with stressful situations in the past. Observe nonverbal cues of emotional status, and encourage the patient to verbalize feelings. Decreased compliance with therapies, persistent hostility or anger, decreased appetite, poor sleep patterns at night, poor eye contact, refusal to look at self, a monotone or sharp voice, refusal to discuss care or injuries, conflict with family or staff, refusal to see visitors, denial of having any worries or concerns, or any marked change in the patient's outlook or behavior pattern may indicate need for aggressive psychologic support.

Nursing Diagnoses and Planning

A burn injury may affect any aspect of an individual's life and emotional health. Because similar burn injuries affect individuals differently, all psychosocial nursing diagnoses are potentially applicable. Nursing diagnoses and related expected patient outcomes commonly applicable to patients with psychosocial needs after a burn injury include the following:

NDx: Post-trauma response related to major burn injury as evidenced by recurrent nightmares, sleep-pattern disturbances, survival guilt, angry outbursts

Planning: Patient Outcomes
1. Patient acknowledges the impact of the circumstances of the burn injury on self.
2. Patient talks about the event.
3. Patient verbalizes fear, anger, guilt.
4. Patient reports lessening of frequency of re-experiencing the event.
5. Patient sleeps through the night.

NDx: Body image disturbance related to change in appearance, fear of loss of ability to function independently and to fulfill role performance because of burn injuries

Planning: Patient Outcomes
1. Patient grieves and expresses feelings of loss.
2. Patient verbalizes realistic perceptions of appearance.
3. Patient states realistic expectations of long-term ability to function independently and to fulfill role expectations.
4. Patient expresses desire to be discharged.

Nursing Interventions and Evaluation

The goal of nursing care of the patient with psychosocial needs after a burn injury is to assist the patient to cope with the short- and long-term effects of the injuries, hospitalization, treatment, and convalescence.

NDx: Post-trauma response
Provide continuity of nursing care so the patient can develop a positive relationship with primary caregivers. Share information at multidiciplinary conference to determine which member of the health team,

clergy, or family can offer the best support for the patient at any given time during recovery.

Spend time talking with the patient when no painful procedures are being performed to provide an opportunity to express feelings and ask questions. Be an active, nonjudgmental listener. Talking about a traumatic event can often help the person come to terms with it. As discussed in Chapter 3, expect the patient to respond to the accident and subsequent injury and losses with denial, shock, anger, guilt, and depression. Assure the patient these feelings are normal after a traumatic event and loss. Assist the patient to understand what happened and the reality of personal involvement. Stay with a patient who has awakened from a nightmare to provide reassurance of safety and to lessen anxiety.

NDx: Body image disturbance
Prepare the patient and visitors for the patient's appearance, especially if facial burns and edema are present. Preparation for what they will see lessens the shock. Explain that edema severely alters initial appearance. Encourage the patient with burns of the head, face, and neck to look in a mirror once the edema has receded. Often the imagined image is worse than reality. Encourage the patient to discuss anticipated results of healing, reconstructive surgery, and rehabilitation with the health team so long-term expectations are realistic. Reassure the patient that the appearance of suture lines of sheet grafts and interstices of mesh grafts usually normalize over time.

Encourage visits by family and friends to prevent feelings of rejection and social isolation. Encourage the patient to leave the sheltered environment of the burn unit for brief excursions to hospital corridors, the cafeteria, or hospital grounds to prepare for the reaction of strangers to the burn scars.

Encourage full participation in the planned program of rehabilitation and wound care to promote full recovery and to minimize the risk of long-term disability. Answer questions honestly. Do not give false reassurances. Refer questions you cannot answer to appropriate resources. Explain procedures, and prepare the patient for anticipated events and sensations to reduce feelings of powerlessness. Give choices when possible to provide a sense control and increase self-esteem. Consult with the patient, family, and health team to develop a plan to provide emotional and financial support for the patient and family throughout hospitalization and postdischarge rehabilitation.

Compare the patient's status with the expected outcomes. If the outcomes are not met, reassess the patient and revise the plan.

REHABILITATION PHASE

Rehabilitation is a process of treatment and education through physical and occupational therapy that enables the patient to restore and maintain maxi-

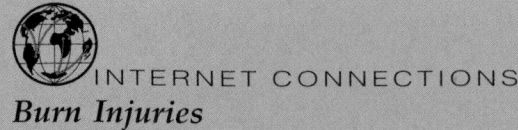

INTERNET CONNECTIONS
Burn Injuries

Burn Center of the University of Washington at Harborview Medical Center
http://weber.u.washington.edu/~engrav/index.html#BC
This site provides information about the University of Washington model for burn rehabilitation and plastic surgery, as well as patient information.

British Columbia Burn Network Society
http://www.vanserve.org/proinfo.html
This site provides detailed information for health professionals related to burn assessment, management, and rehabilitation.

mum function of injured body parts and to achieve maximum independence in activities of daily living. Rehabilitation begins on admission to the hospital or burn unit, continues throughout the healing process and discharge, and culminates in the individual's return to maximum function in society.

In conjunction with nursing and medical management, the goal of rehabilitation is to promote optimum wound healing with minimum contracture and scar formation. While physicians and nurses stabilize the patient in the emergent period, physical and occupational therapists develop care plans to prevent cosmetic and functional deformities that would leave the patient physically impaired or require needless surgery to correct. These initial plans are revised as the patient's physical condition and wound status change throughout the acute period and into the rehabilitation phase. Therapy sessions are scheduled at least daily and may ultimately include retraining in activities of daily living or job rehabilitation to adapt to loss of function or limb loss. Burn patients usually require long-term rehabilitation, and therapy continues on an outpatient basis after discharge.

Contractures

As burn wounds heal, scar tissue forms. As the healing process continues, connective fibers in the scar tissue contract or shorten. Contraction of scar tissue over a joint can cause deformity and loss of function and mobility of the joint.

Contractures and joint deformities are prevented by exercise, positioning, and splinting throughout the healing process. All patients with deep partial- or full-thickness burns of the joints and burns of the

hands, feet, or neck require physical therapy. Early excision and grafting allow earlier resumption of exercises and help minimize contracture formation and loss of function. Therapy begins with range-of-motion exercises to prevent contractures and then progresses to strengthening exercises and activities of daily living to maintain function. If involved joints are unable to be exercised because of associated injury or recent grafting, splints are applied to maintain functional anatomic position of the joints. Splints may be worn at night throughout the healing process to prevent flexion contractures as scar tissue contracts. If contractures do form, surgical release is required to return function to the joint.

Hypertrophic Scarring

Deep burn wounds initially appear flat and pink as they heal. In some patients with deep partial- or full-thickness burns, excess collagen deposits form in the scar tissue. In these cases, approximately a month after initial healing, the skin becomes raised, is very firm, and lacks moisture. Hyperactive collagen formation continues for about 1 year before growth slows, and the scarred skin again becomes supple.

Elastic pressure garments prevent or reduce hypertrophic scarring. Pressure garments, such as those shown in Figure 37–11, are custom-made to conform to body areas burned. By exerting constant uniform pressure over the healed wound, they minimize the proliferation of scar tissue. Pressure garments are applied after the burn wounds have healed or have been grafted, are removed only to bathe, and are worn until the scar matures and softens, which takes approximately 1 year. To be effective, they must be worn at least 23 hours a day and refitted frequently to maintain pressure. Emollients are used in conjunction with pressure garments to soften the skin.

Cosmetic surgery to excise hypertrophic scar tissue cannot be performed for 18 months to 2 years after the initial closure of the wound. Continued hyperactive growth of the scar tissue during this time would result in unsatisfactory cosmetic results.

NURSING PROCESS
Rehabilitation After Burn Injury

Assessment

Assess the severity and location of burn injuries to identify patients at risk for contractures and hypertrophic scarring. Patients with full-thickness or deep partial-thickness burns around joints and on the hands, feet, or neck are at high risk for contractures. Examine old scars and determine the healing pattern of old wounds to identify persons at risk for hypertrophic scarring. Hypertrophic scarring occurs more frequently in individuals of African and Mediterra-

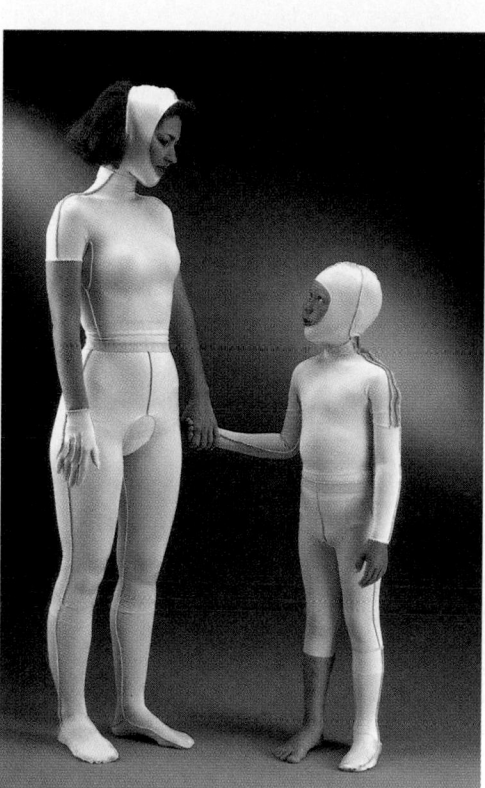

Figure 37–11

Models wearing Jobskin interim care garments. Pressure garments have been proved effective in managing hypertrophic scarring. (Courtesy of Beiersdorf-Jobst, Inc, Charlotte, NC.)

nean ancestry. Question the patient and family about specific home- and work-related mobility and dexterity requirements.

Nursing Diagnoses and Planning

Nursing diagnoses and related expected patient outcomes commonly applicable to patients requiring rehabilitation after a burn injury include the following:

NDx: Risk for impaired physical mobility related to contractures

Planning: Patient Outcomes
1. Patient performs active and passive range-of-motion exercises as prescribed.
2. Patient remains free of contractures.
3. Patient performs activities of daily living independently.

NDx: Risk for altered health maintenance related to insufficient knowledge of physical therapy exercises, use of pressure garments, self-management of grafts and burn scars

Planning: Patient Outcomes
1. Patient demonstrates ability to perform wound care.
2. Patient performs active and passive range-of-motion exercises at home as prescribed.

3. Patient wears pressure garment at least 23 hours a day.
4. Patient remains free of contractures and hypertrophic scarring.
5. Patient resumes social and employment activities.

Nursing Interventions and Evaluation

The goal of nursing care of the patient requiring rehabilitation after a burn injury is to assist the patient to maintain mobility and function of involved joints and limbs and to minimize scarring.

NDx: Risk for impaired physical mobility
Consult with the patient, family, physicians, and therapists to develop a plan for rehabilitation. Reinforce the therapists' explanation of the purpose of splints and exercises. Active patient participation in the planning stages and understanding of the benefits of physical therapy increase compliance and give the patient a sense of control over a stressful situation.

Always keep burned skin surfaces separated by gauze dressings to prevent adhesions and contractures. Unless contraindicated by multiple burned areas or associated injuries, position the patient as described in Table 37–9 to reduce the risk of contracture formation. Position per physician's orders if contraindications to standard positions are present. Apply splints to burned joints at night or as prescribed to prevent flexion contractures. Assess circulation distal to the splints every 2 hours to ensure tissue perfusion.

Administer prescribed analgesic before physical therapy sessions to minimize pain and to maximize compliance. Resume physical therapy to immobilized joints as soon as possible after grafting procedures to minimize the risk of contractures. Encourage, assist, and remind the patient to perform prescribed independent exercises as often as possible between therapy sessions to maintain joint mobility. Document how often the patient does independent exercises and how much assistance is needed. Early, active exercise reduces the risk of contractures and increases strength. Ambulate the patient as soon as possible to promote strength and inhibit bone decalcification.

NDx: Risk for altered health maintenance
Many patients are discharged before burn wounds are completely healed. Teach the patient and a caregiver how to cleanse the wound, reapply topical agent, and re-dress the wound to promote healing and to minimize the risk of infection. A hand-held shower can be used for cleansing the wound. Observe the patient or caregiver performing wound care to evaluate learning, and answer questions on technique. Review, and provide in writing, the signs of infection and instructions on what to do if they occur.

Newly healed skin burns easily and is sensitive to ultraviolet light, yet until nerve regeneration occurs, it is hyposensitive to heat, cold, and touch.

Table 37–9

Nursing Interventions to Prevent Contractures

Area Burned	Nursing Interventions
Anterior neck	Hyperextend the neck. Place a rolled towel under the back of the neck, or position the patient at the top of one mattress with the head hanging over and resting on a second mattress underneath. Do not use a pillow under the head at any time.
Posterior neck	Flex the neck. Use no pillow or only a small pillow under the head, and encourage frequent side-to-side and turning motion.
Ears	Do not use a pillow. Place gauze between auricle and head to prevent adhesions.
Upper chest and anterior shoulder	Place a rolled or folded towel parallel to the spine between the scapulae with arms on mattress. Do not use a pillow under the head.
Axilla	Extend arm up over head.
Antecubital fossa, popliteal fossa	Maintain elbow or knee in extension. Hyperextend knee by pressing it into the mattress several times a day.
Hand, ankle, foot	Splint in anatomical position, with digits separated by gauze.
Groin	Maintain hip in extension. If possible, avoid elevating head of bed and hyperextend hip several times a day by placing the patient in a prone position. Place gauze between burned surfaces of the genitalia.

Teach the patient to use a thermometer or an area of unburned skin to test the temperature of water before use to prevent scalding. Instruct the patient to remain out of the sun for at least 1 year, to use sunscreen, and to always wear a hat to prevent sunburn. Newly healed skin is fragile and must be protected from friction and trauma. Examine the skin daily to detect injury or blisters from splints or pressure garments. As new epithelial cells grow, grafts and donor sites flake and itch. Teach the patient to massage in an emollient moisturizer daily to soften the skin, to relieve itching, and to increase circulation. Lotions, lanolin, and cocoa butter are commonly used.

Reinforce the therapist's instructions to the patient in the purpose, use, and care of splints and pressure garments for the prevention of contractures and hypertrophic scarring. Schedule a time when the patient is rested and relatively free of pain to be measured for prescribed pressure garments. Observe the patient or caregiver in the application and removal of splints and pressure garments to ensure proper usage. Review, and provide in writing, time of application and removal and care instructions. The patient needs two pressure garments so a clean one can be put on each day after bathing. Instruct the patient to wash the soiled one in a nondetergent, nondeodorant mild soap, such as Ivory Snow, to rinse well, and to hang the garment to dry. Reinforce the need to wear the pressure garment at least 23 hours a day to achieve desired results. Patient education for self-management after a burn injury is summarized in Highlight 37–1.

Compare the patient's status with the expected outcomes. If the outcomes are not met, reassess the patient and revise the plan.

Care of the Patient with a Chemical Burn Injury

More than 25,000 products on the market today are capable of resulting in a chemical burn injury. These products, available for home, industrial, agricultural, and military use, are the cause of more than 3000 deaths a year in the United States. It is estimated that more than 60,000 people require medical attention for chemical injuries annually.

Chemicals are broadly classified as acids, alkalis, and vesicants. They are more precisely grouped by their local and systemic actions, as summarized in Table 37–10.

In general, chemical agents do not "burn" or destroy tissue by heat. Instead, they destroy cellular protein by coagulation, a solidification of the protein into a gelatinous mass. Incomplete removal or inadequate dilution of the chemical can cause further tissue damage by residual chemicals.

Body tissues can be damaged by chemical agents on skin contact and penetration, ingestion, and inhalation. The extent of tissue damage depends on several factors. The greater the quantity of chemical agent that comes in contact with the tissues, the stronger or more concentrated the agent, and the longer the duration of contact, the more severe the damage. An agent that rapidly penetrates to underlying tissues can cause extensive deep injury. Some chemical agents not only cause contact tissue dam-

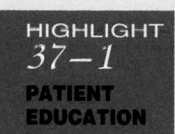 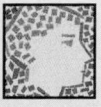

HIGHLIGHT 37–1

PATIENT EDUCATION

Discharge Instructions for Burn Care

Instruct the patient to perform the following:

Wound Care

Wash hands before and after wound care.

Wash the wound gently once a day with a mild, non-detergent, nondeodorant soap (eg, Ivory) to remove all old topical preparation and wound drainage. The wound may be cleansed in the shower.

Apply a thin layer of prescribed antibacterial cream or ointment and cover with dressing.

Examine wound and surrounding area for redness, swelling, purulent drainage, warmth, or foul odor. Report any of these observations to physician immediately.

Return for follow-up appointment on *(specify date)*.

Use and Care of Pressure Garments

Wear pressure garments at least 23 hours a day. Remove only for shower or bath.

Examine skin under garment for blisters or irritation. If found, call for an appointment and do not wear the garment until seen by the physician.

Wash the garment in a mild nondetergent, nondeodorant soap (eg, Ivory Snow) and hang to air-dry.

Care of Newly Healed Skin

Take precautions to avoid bumps, bruises, or trauma to the fragile newly healed skin.

Rub emollient moisturizer (eg, Lubriderm, Nivea, lano-lin, cocoa butter) into the new skin several times a day.

Apply moisturizer under pressure garment as a protective emollient.

Test the temperature of kitchen, bath, or shower water with a thermometer or an area of nonburned skin to prevent scalds.

Always apply sunscreen with a minimum sun protection factor (SPF) of 15 before leaving the house, and cover healed skin with loose-fitting clothing, hat, socks, or gloves to prevent sunburn. Pressure garments alone do not protect the skin from ultraviolet light. Always wear clothing over the garments. Skin must be protected for a minimum of 1 year.

Wear loose-fitting cotton clothes to prevent rubbing of the skin. Do not wear belts or other constricting items over newly healed skin.

Proper Diet and Exercise

Eat foods rich in protein and high in calories.

Weigh yourself at least twice a week.

Report any weight loss to the physician.

After skin has healed, continue to weigh yourself once a week and maintain even weight to prevent pressure garments from becoming too loose.

Perform prescribed exercises to increase joint mobility and muscle strength.

Walk each day and climb stairs a few times a day to improve health and stamina.

---

age but also are toxins that can cause systemic effects or poisoning.

Clinical Manifestations

Clinical manifestations of chemical burns depend on the area of contact. A chemical skin burn will have the same appearance as any burn of the same depth. Full-thickness chemical burns are often red, yellow, or brown in color. Contact with the eyes can produce initial tearing, blepharospasm, inflammation of the conjunctiva and sclera, and an uncontrollable urge to rub the eyes. Ingestion of a chemical results in esophageal, tracheobronchial, or gastric injuries as well as the risk of systemic poisoning and death.

Inhalation of toxic gases or powdered chemicals can cause burns of the upper respiratory tract, respiratory distress, and the risk of systemic poisoning from absorption through respiratory mucosa.

Determination of the depth of the burn and TBSA involved is often difficult. Chemical burns initially appear less severe than they actually are. Additional tissue destruction as a result of continued chemical penetration into deeper tissues may occur for 72 hours after the initial contact. These expanded areas of tissue destruction often appear as yellow-brown or mildly discolored marks rather than burns. An untreated chemical burn is illustrated in Figure 37–12.

Table 37–10

Classification of Chemical Agents

Classification	Effect on Tissue	Systemic Effect	Method of Neutralization	Examples	Products Commonly Found in
Oxidizing agents	Blisters, ulcerations	Diarrhea, gastrointestinal bleeding, seizures, death	Water	Sodium hypochloride Chromic acid Potassium permanganate	Clorox Metal cleaners Disinfectants
Reducing agents	Eschar formation		Water	Nitric acid Hydrochloric acid Alkyl mercuric acid	Industry Metal cleaning
Corrosive agents	Rapidly penetrate Thick eschar	Central nervous system depression, hypotension, pulmonary, edema, hepatic necrosis, nephrotoxicity, death	Brush off powder first Ethyl alcohol or cooking oil followed by copious water 1% copper sulfate/water Water	Phenols White phosphorus Dichromate salts Sodium metals Lye Calcium oxide Lime	Sanitizers, plastic Explosives, insecticides Cleaning agents Drain cleaners Portland cement Agriculture
Protoplasmic poisons	Eschar formation Local vasoconstriction	Hepatic necrosis, nephrotoxicity, binds calcium Bone decalcification	Water Water/intravenous calcium Water/subcutaneous calcium	Picric acid Tannic acid Sulfosalicylic acid Acetic acid Formic acid Oxalic acid Hydrofluoric acid	Industry Glass etching
Desiccants	Produce excessive heat; cause severe cell dehydration		Water	Sulfuric acid Muriatic acid	
Vesicants	Blisters, edema Ischemic and anoxic necrosis		Water	Cantharides Dimethyl sulfoxide Dichlorodiethyl sulfide (mustard gas) Chlorovinyldichloroarsine	Veterinary uses Military uses

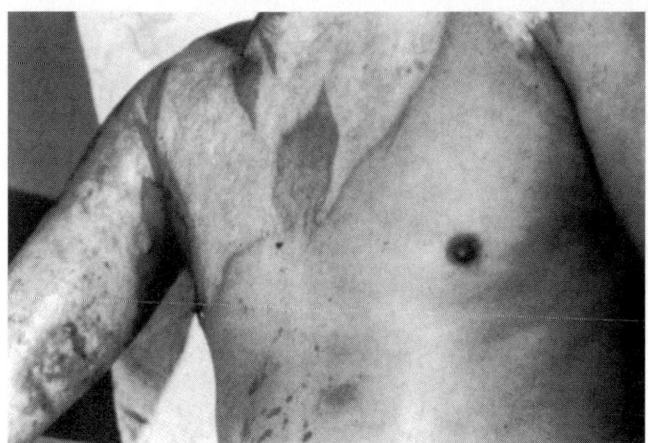

Figure 37–12

Skin discoloration characteristic of a chemical burn injury. (From Artz CP, Moncrief JA, Pruitt BA [eds]. Burns: A team approach. Philadelphia: WB Saunders, 1979, p 365.)

Management

Rapid intervention is of prime importance to limit tissue destruction in a chemical injury. Flushing the wound with copious amounts of water cannot be overemphasized. Water has been shown to dilute and physically remove the agent, decrease the rate of chemical reaction, decrease inflammatory reaction by decreasing tissue metabolism, reduce hygroscopic action, and restore wound pH levels toward normal in chemical injuries caused by some concentrated acids and alkalis. The use of copious amounts of water also dissipates the heat that is produced when some chemical agents are mixed with water.

Irrigation of chemical eye injuries continues with normal saline for up to 48 hours to minimize the risk of permanent damage and vision loss. The ophthalmologist may apply a Morgan lens to the eye to facilitate continuous irrigation. Ophthalmic steroid, antibiotic, and anesthetic preparations reduce inflammation and scarring, prevent infection, and increase patient comfort.

Some chemical injuries require further treatment after irrigation and dilution to completely neutralize the agent and to stop tissue destruction. Neutralizing agents for each classification of chemical are included in Table 37–10.

Any patient who has ingested chemicals is evaluated for esophageal and gastric injuries by esophagoscopy within 12 hours of admission. Systemic steroids and antibiotics reduce inflammation, scarring, and infection. Reconstructive surgery or a temporary or permanent gastrostomy for feeding may be required in cases of extensive esophageal damage. Psychiatric evaluation to determine immediate risk to self and others is required if the ingestion of chemicals was a suicide attempt. Suicidal patients are monitored continuously to prevent additional attempts and require long-term psychiatric follow-up.

The extent of respiratory injury after inhalation of chemical agents is evaluated by bronchoscopy. Injury to the trachea and bronchi has also been reported after ingestion of chemicals. Treatment with steroids, antibiotics, bronchodilators, and intubation and ventilator support is implemented as needed.

Fluid resuscitation and wound care in chemical injuries are similar to methods used for other burn injuries. However, because of the difficulty in initially determining the full extent and depth of the injury, standard fluid resuscitation calculation is used only as a guideline. Closely monitor the patient for signs of inadequate fluid resuscitation to prevent hypovolemic shock and acute tubular necrosis.

NURSING PROCESS GUIDELINES
Chemical Burn Injury

Nursing care of patients with chemical burn injuries is similar to that described earlier in this chapter for patients with burn injuries. The goals of the nursing care plan for patients with chemical burn injuries are to assist the patient to limit tissue destruction, avoid or minimize burn shock, keep the wounds clean and free from infection, maximize comfort, meet nutritional needs, maintain mobility and function, minimize scarring, provide psychosocial support, and maintain vision if the eyes are involved.

Identify the area of contact, type of chemical agent, method and duration of contact, and treatment administered at the scene of the accident. Specifically ask whether any of the agent came in contact with the eyes or was swallowed or inhaled. If possible, obtain the container of the agent to ensure accurate identification. The label of many chemical containers gives information on treatment for exposure and ingestion and how to neutralize the agent.

Examine the involved area and surrounding tissue to determine the severity of damage. Remember that because chemical penetration and tissue destruction continue for as long as 72 hours, initial assessment may not reflect the final severity of the injury. Monitor the wound every hour during the irrigation and then every 4 hours after the irrigation. Changes in skin color, additional skin loss, or blistering indicate an increase in the extent or depth of injury.

If the chemical was ingested, monitor for manifestations of gastrointestinal damage and respiratory involvement from aspiration. If the chemical or its fumes were inhaled, auscultate lung sounds and monitor for manifestations of respiratory injury. Report difficulty swallowing, vomiting, and signs of respiratory distress to the physician immediately. Administer enteral or gastrostomy feedings to meet nutritional needs if the patient is receiving nothing by mouth.

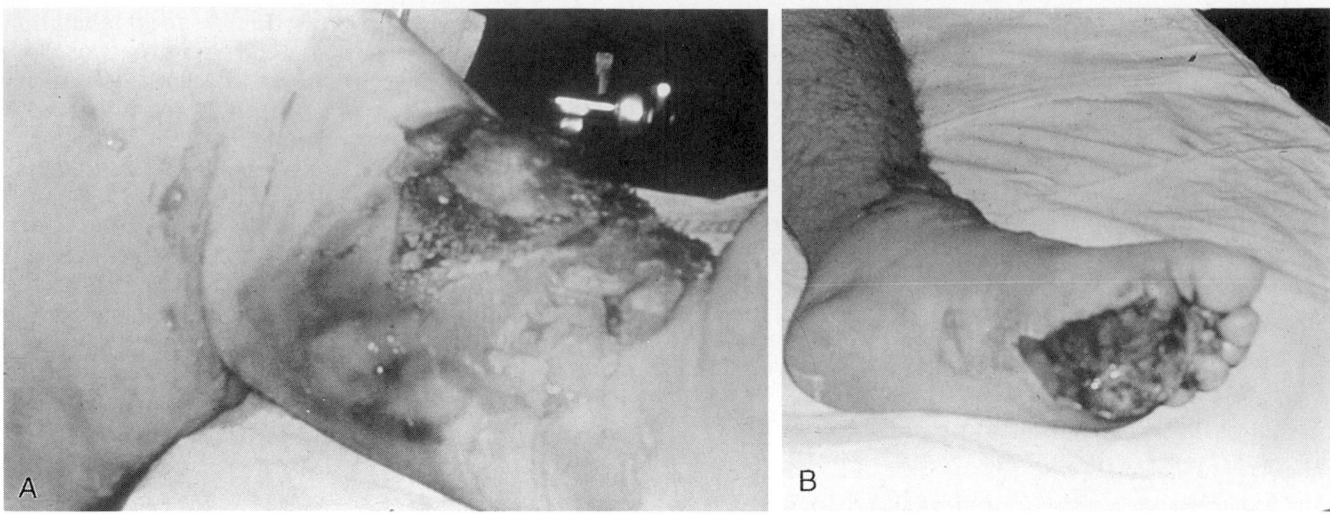

Figure 37–13

Electrical burn injury. The entrance wound (*A*) is typically charred and resembles a full-thickness burn wound. The exit wound (*B*) appears as though something exploded out of it.

Care of the Patient with an Electrical Burn Injury

More than 1000 deaths in the United States each year result from electrical shock. More than 90% of the deaths from high voltage injuries occur in males between ages 20 and 34. Even nonfatal electrical injuries can cause extensive deep muscle, bone, and tissue damage along the path of the electrical current as it flows through the body. The stronger the current and the longer the contact, the more severe the internal damage. High-voltage current and lightning can generate temperatures in body tissues as high as 2500°C (4500°F). Different body tissues vary in their resistance to the flow of current. More dense tissues have greater resistance. The slower passage of the current generates more heat and tissue damage.

Clinical Manifestations

An entrance–exit wound is the most common visible characteristic of an electrical burn injury. An entrance wound is created at the point of contact as the current enters the body. It has a charred appearance and resembles a full-thickness thermal burn injury. An entrance wound is usually located on an extremity, the most common point of contact with the electrical source. The exit wound, or point at which the current leaves the body, may be located anywhere on the body. It has dry, open edges and looks as though something exploded out through it. Figure 37–13 illustrates the appearance of entrance and exit wounds. Electrical current may enter and exit the patient more than once, resulting in multiple sets of entrance and exit wounds, as shown in Figure 37–14. If contact with an electrical flash ignites

clothing, the patient may suffer a thermal burn injury as well as an electrical injury.

If the current crosses the heart, cardiac dysrhythmias can occur, including premature atrial and ventricular beats, ventricular fibrillation, and cardiac standstill. Fractures may result from sudden, forceful contraction of muscles stimulated by the passage of electric current. Decortication of bone may be caused by the force of the current. Extensive deep bone, muscle, and tissue necrosis may require amputation. Paralysis may result from permanent nerve damage.

Acute tubular necrosis may develop from obstruction of the renal tubules by hemoglobin released from damaged red blood cells and by myoglobin released from damaged muscle tissue. Although acute tubular necrosis occurs in full-thick-

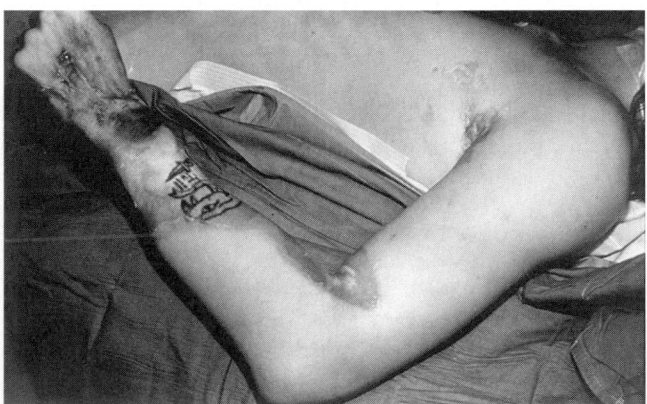

Figure 37–14

Multiple entrance and exit wounds formed as electric current exited and re-entered the body.

ness thermal burns, it is much more common in electrical injury because of extensive muscle damage. The risk of acute tubular necrosis is highest in patients with myoglobinuria or hematuria, signs that the by-products of muscle damage and hemocoagulation are being excreted in the urine.

Late complications of electrical injury may not be apparent for months after the initial injury. These include cataracts, meningitis, progressive spinal cord damage, motor dysfunction, pain syndromes, bacterial endocarditis, and osteomyelitis.

Management

If the patient is in ventricular fibrillation or cardiac standstill, cardiopulmonary resuscitation is initiated at the scene of the accident and continued during transport to the hospital. Advanced cardiac life-support measures, including defibrillation, are implemented on admission to the hospital or as soon as trained personnel are available at the scene.

Patients with a history of loss of consciousness or cardiac arrest in the field, or with documented cardiac dysrhythmias, should have cardiac monitoring for at least 24 hours after admission.

Fluid Replacement

Patients with electrical injuries caused by brief contact with low-voltage electricity can usually be resuscitated with the volume calculated for standard fluid replacement. High-voltage or prolonged-contact electrical injuries, however, involve extensive internal damage along the path of the electric current. Although surface wounds may appear small, the patient requires large-volume fluid resuscitation to replace the rapid loss of fluids into damaged internal tissues and to prevent acute tubular necrosis. Standard fluid-replacement calculation based on TBSA is used only as a rough guideline for fluid resuscitation because the internal tissue destruction is much greater than visible surface injuries. The adequacy of fluid resuscitation is determined by the criteria for successful fluid resuscitation presented earlier in this chapter.

Intravenous mannitol may be administered to promote excretion of myoglobins and to decrease the chance of acute tubular necrosis. To avoid dehydrating a hypovolemic patient, mannitol is administered only if hematuria is present and urine output is greater than 50 mL/hour. Sodium bicarbonate is administered if metabolic acidosis results from the myoglobinemia and altered renal function.

Wound Management

Low-voltage and brief-contact injuries with minimal internal damage are treated similarly to thermal burns with a topical antibacterial agent. The wound is allowed to slough and heal by granulation or may be excised and grafted. To assess the extent of muscle damage and the possible need for amputation in high-voltage injuries, deep incisions to the muscle fascia, called fasciotomies, are made near the entrance of the wound. The exposed tissues are examined for damage and necrosis. If the tissues are viable, the fasciotomy may be extended along the muscle to relieve pressure from edema within the muscle compartment, thereby preventing further tissue damage from impaired circulation. If the fasciotomy reveals extensively damaged or necrotic muscle, the wound is surgically débrided and grafted. If tissue damage is too extensive for revitalization, the limb is amputated. High-voltage electrical injuries may also result in the loss of internal organs.

The patient with a major electrical injury requires intensive rehabilitation because of extensive tissue, muscle, and skeletal damage. Even if amputation of a limb is not required, the damaged nerves and muscles require retraining and exercise. If a limb is amputated, prosthetic devices and training in their use are needed.

NURSING PROCESS GUIDELINES
Electrical Burn Injury

Nursing care of patients with electrical burn injuries is similar to that described earlier in this chapter for patients with burn injuries. The goals of the nursing care plan for patients with electrical burn injuries are to assist the patient to salvage viable tissue, avoid or minimize burn shock, keep the wounds clean and free from infection, maximize comfort, meet nutritional needs, maintain mobility and function, minimize scarring, provide psychosocial support, and adapt to limb loss and use of a prosthesis if amputation was necessary.

Question the patient or persons accompanying the patient to determine the type of current, voltage, amperage, and duration of contact. Determine whether the patient lost consciousness, had a cardiac arrest, or was defibrillated before arrival at the hospital. Examine the entire body for entrance and exit wounds because the current can re-enter the body after exiting. Assess the size and depth of external burn injuries. Determine the presence of associated injuries such as thermal burns, lacerations, and fractures. Obtain baseline electrocardiogram readings and cardiac enzyme levels to evaluate cardiac muscle damage or conduction disorders.

Administer parenteral fluid resuscitation to minimize burn shock and the risk of acute tubular necrosis. Monitor the patient hourly to evaluate fluid replacement. The risk of hypovolemia is high in electrical injuries because the extent of internal tissue damage cannot be accurately determined. If hematuria or myoglobinuria are present, increase the rate of parenteral fluid administration to maintain urine output at 75 to 100 mL/hour until the urine clears. The physician may also order 44 to 50 mEq of sodium bicarbonate per liter of lactated Ringer's solution to produce an alkaline urine and to reverse metabolic acidosis. Myoglobin and hemoglobin are more readily excreted in an alkaline urine. Mannitol is administered to aid in the prevention of tubular necrosis if the urine does not clear.

Prepare the patient for fasciotomy and wound débridement, reinforcing the physician's explanation of the procedure and its purpose. If amputation is necessary, reinforce the physician's explanation of the need for it, and provide emotional support while preparing the patient for surgery. Care of a patient after a fasciotomy, amputation, or other orthopedic injury that may be associated with an electrical burn injury is described in Unit 6.

Monitor the patient daily for peripheral and central nervous system damage. The extent of nerve damage may slowly progress for an extended period of time after the initial injury, and early manifestations may be masked by associated tissue injury. Teach the patient, and provide in writing, the manifestations of the long-term complications of electrical injury to aid in early detection and treatment. Explain that they often are not apparent for months after the injury.

Care of the Pregnant Patient After Burn Injury

The possibility of pregnancy in any woman of childbearing age must be considered and is a complication in burn management. A pregnant woman with TBSA burns of 60% or more or who has suffered an inhalation injury is at high risk for loss of that pregnancy.

As with all burn patients, airway stabilization and management are the first and most important concerns. Hypoxia is not tolerated by the fetus and will cause premature labor or abortion, or both.

Constant fetal monitoring is important, particularly in the second or third trimester, to determine fetal distress. Early consultation with both an obstetrician and a burn center physician is imperative.

Delayed or inadequate fluid resuscitation may also cause premature labor or loss of the pregnancy, or both. Response to fluid resuscitation must be closely monitored because fluid needs may exceed calculated amounts. Electrolyte disturbances, alterations in clotting factors, and depletion of fibrinogen and platelets are common complications in pregnant burn patients.

Pregnant patients require that there be no delay in assessment, management, and consultation to ensure viability of the fetus. Transfer to a burn center is recommended.

The Elderly: Special Considerations

Older people are at an increased risk both for getting burned and for experiencing delayed recovery and complications after a burn injury. Diminished vision may affect perception and cause injuries while working around stoves, heaters, open flames, and hot water. If visual impairment interferes with reading labels, the older person is at increased risk for a chemical injury. Older people with disorders that affect their memory may leave the stove on, forget about lighted cigarettes, or have difficulty using the phone to call for help. Decreased tactile sensitivity may lead to burns from bathing in hot water or from using a heating pad. Decreased mobility may prevent rapid evacuation once a fire starts.

An older person with burn injuries may be a victim of abuse or self-neglect. Examine the patient's entire body for wounds, and bruises. Question the patient, family members, and caregivers to determine how the injury occurred. Consult with other members of the health team if the injury does not fit the explanation of the incident, if conflicting explanations are given, or if the explanation of the incident keeps changing. Report incidents of abuse or neglect to the proper authorities.

Older people are considered to be at high risk after even a minor burn injury. Pruitt showed a 75% mortality rate for patients older than 60 years with a burn as small as 25 to 30% TBSA. Many factors increase mortality in the elderly. Because of the aging process, the skin is thinner, less elastic, and has less subcutaneous fat. This increases the susceptibility of the patient to a deeper burn injury because the muscle tissues and bone are closer to the body surface. Dehydration and nutritional deficiencies slow wound healing and increase the risk of infection.

Pre-existing disorders affect the person's ability to survive a burn injury, and chronic diseases of the heart, lungs, kidney, and liver are more common in older adults. Impaired function of these vital organs is a significant factor in the high mortality rate. Older patients may have concurrent diseases, such as diabetes, respiratory disorders, and cardiovascular diseases that complicate their recovery from the burn injury.

Special care must be taken in the fluid resuscitation of the geriatric patient because of decreased ability to adjust rapidly to fluctuations in circulating fluid volume. Older patients are likely to experience pulmonary edema and cardiac failure during fluid resuscitation. Even with careful management, some research has shown that approximately 15% of older adult patients die within the first 5 days after burn injuries from either over–fluid resuscitation or under–fluid resuscitation.

Monitor vital signs, urine output, and cardiac status for signs of cardiac failure. Ambulate the elderly patient as soon as possible, and provide frequent pulmonary hygiene to minimize the risk of circulatory and respiratory complications.

A major concern in burn wound management is delayed eschar separation in a full-thickness injury as a result of decreased peripheral blood flow common in the elderly. Delayed separation increases susceptibility to infection and slows wound healing.

Impaired blood flow also delays revascularization and the growth of granulation tissue. Skin grafting may be delayed, and the risk of graft failure is greater. Handle all burned areas gently to prevent further trauma. Maintain meticulous aseptic wound care to prevent infection and to promote wound closure.

Finally, older patients, especially those who have lost their home and possessions in a fire, may become seriously depressed. Disruption of their living situation and the loss of irreplaceable possessions may present a monumental coping challenge. The resources of the entire burn team should be used to support the patient in this crisis. The patient may benefit from an evaluation for antidepressant medications along with counseling and problem-solving approaches to help the person develop effective coping strategies. Successful treatment of the geriatric burn patient is one of the most difficult challenges in all of burn care.

Chapter Review

1. Why is it important to get an accurate weight on a burn patient on admission to the hospital?
2. Calculate the fluid resuscitation requirements for a 38% burn.
3. What are the criteria that warrant a burn patient being transferred to a Burn Center?
4. List the symptoms of smoke inhalation.
5. Why do burn patients need a high-calorie, high-protein diet?
6. How are contractures of the extremities prevented in burn patients?
7. What is the purpose of pressure garments for burn patients?
8. Why is it important to rinse the skin of a chemical burn patient with copious amounts of fluid?
9. Why might an electrical burn patient have myoglobin urea?
10. What are some of the special considerations when caring for a geriatric burn patient?

Bibliography

Atiles L, Mileski W, Purdue G, et al. Laser Doppler flowmetry in burn wounds. J Burn Care Rehabil 1995; 16:388.

Baby P, Subramanian N. Management of mass burns casualty in a government hospital—a nurse's angle. Nurs J India 1994; 85(10):237.

Bingham HG, Hudson D, Popp J. A retrospective review of the burn intensive care unit admissions for a year. J Burn Care Rehabil 1995; 16(1):56.

Bolinger B. Burn care in the home. J WOCN 1995; 22(3):122.

Carpenito LJ. Nursing diagnosis: Application to clinical practice. 6th ed. Philadelphia: JB Lippincott, 1995.

Clarke R. Caring for burns patients. Community Nurse 1996; 1(12):14.

Clark WR. Smoke inhalation: Diagnosis and treatment. World J Surg 1992; 16:24.

Dattolo J, Trout S, Connolly ML. Nursing forum. Home health care and burn care: An educational and economical program. J Burn Care Rehabil 1996; 17(2):182.

Doenges ME, Moorhouse MF. Nurse's pocket guide: Nursing diagnoses with interventions. 4th ed. Philadelphia: FA Davis, 1993.

Edwards K. Burns. Nurs Stand 1995; 10(7):36.

Eliopoulos C. Gerontological nursing. 3rd ed. Philadelphia: JB Lippincott, 1993.

Everett JJ. Pain assessment from patients with burns and their nurses. J Burn Care Rehabil 1994; 15(2):194.

Faldmo L, Kravitz M. Management of acute burns and burn shock resuscitation. AACN Clin Iss Crit Care Nurs 1993; 4(2):351.

Fishbach F. A manual of laboratory and diagnostic tests. 5th ed. Philadelphia: JB Lippincott, 1995.

Gibran NS, Heimbach DM. Pharmacokinetics of antibiotics in patients with thermal injury. Infect Med 1993; 10(3):45.

Goodwin CW. Metabolism and nutrition in the thermally injured patient. Critical Care 1995; 1:97.

Gordon M. Nursing diagnosis: Process and application. 3rd ed. St. Louis: Mosby Year-Book, 1994.

Greenfield E, Jordan B. Advances in burn wound care. Crit Care Nurs Clin North Am 1996; 8(2):203.

Hansbrough W, Dore C, Hansbrough JF. Management of skin grafted burn wounds with xeroform and layers of dry coarse-mesh gauze dressings results in excellent graft take and minimal nursing time. J Burn Care Rehab 1995; 16(5):331.

Hunt JL, Purdue GF. The elderly burn patient. Am J Surg 1992; 164(5):472.

Kirkpatrick JJR, Curtis B, Naylor IL. Back to the future for wound care? The influences of Padua on wound management in Renaissance Europe. Wound Repair Regeneration 1996; 4(3):326.

Kuehn CN. Management of a self-immolation victim: A nursing challenge in burn care. Crit Care Nurs Clin North Am 1994; 6(4):863.

Nebraska Burn Institute, St. Elizabeth Community Health Center, Lincoln Medical Educational Foundation. Pre-hospital advanced burn life support course manual. Lincoln, NE: Nebraska Burn Institute, 1991.

North American Nursing Diagnosis Association. NANDA nursing diagnoses: Definitions and classification 1997–1998. Philadelphia: Author, 1996.

Orr J, Hain T. Burn wound management: An overview. Prof Nurse 1994; 10(3):153.

Richard R, Miller SF. Emergent and resuscitative phases of burn patient care: Rehabilitation considerations. Top Emerg Med 1995; 17(1):70.

Ronk LL. Surgical patients with multiantibiotic-resistant bacteria. AORN J 1995; 61(6):1023.

Ruppert SD, Kernicki JG, Dolan JT. Dolan's critical care nursing: Clinical management through the nursing process. 2nd ed. Philadelphia: FA Davis, 1996.

Shannon MT, Wilson BA, Stang CL. Govoni and Hayes drugs and nursing implications. 8th ed. Norwalk, CT: Appleton & Lange, 1995.

Sutherland S. Nursing forum: Procedural burn pain intensity under conditions of varying physical control by the patient. J Burn Care Rehabil 1996; 17(5):457.

Warden GD. Burn shock resuscitation. World J Surg 1992; 16:16.

Unit XIII

Reproductive Dysfunction

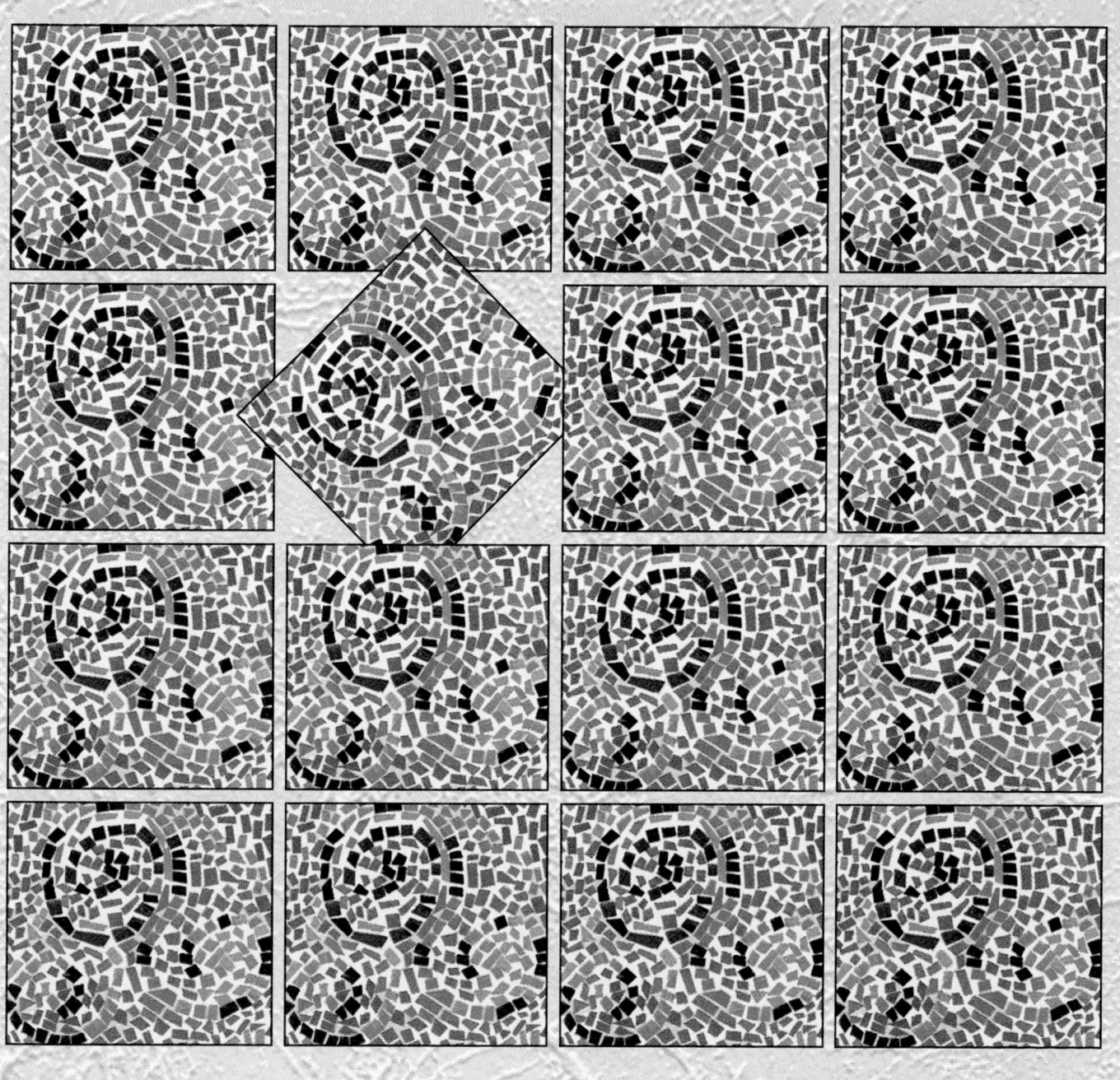

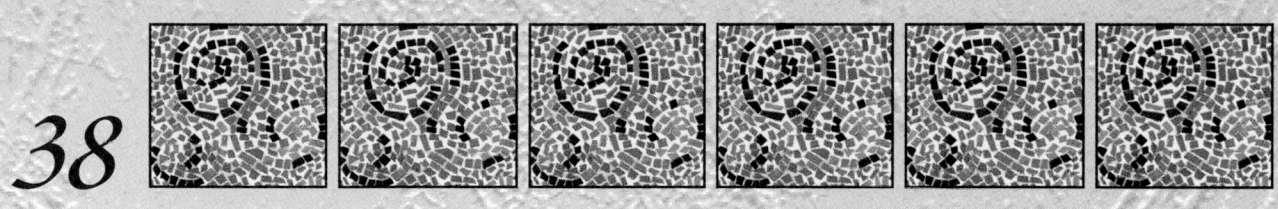

38

Knowledge Base for Men with Reproductive Dysfunction

Study Outcomes

After studying this chapter, you should be able to:

1. Explain the normal anatomy and physiology of the male reproductive system.
2. Describe common clinical manifestations of male reproductive system dysfunction.
3. Identify information and physical examination data essential to the assessment of male reproductive status.
4. Describe basic diagnostic tests and treatment modalities used in the collaborative management of patients with male reproductive system disorders.
5. Describe basic surgical procedures used in the treatment of patients with male reproductive system disorders.
6. Identify data essential to the assessment of patients undergoing treatment of male reproductive system disorders.
7. State nursing diagnoses and related expected patient outcomes commonly applicable to patients undergoing treatment of male reproductive system disorders.
8. Describe nursing interventions, with their rationales, commonly applicable to patients undergoing treatment of male reproductive system disorders.
9. Explain the basis for evaluation of nursing care provided to patients undergoing treatment of male reproductive system disorders.
10. Identify alternative treatment and care settings for men with reproductive disorders and the services related to community-based care.
11. Identify special considerations for the elderly patient with altered male reproductive system function.

In preparation for study of the nursing care of men with reproductive disorders, this chapter begins by reviewing the anatomy and physiology of the male reproductive system. This is followed by discussions of the clinical manifestations common to male reproductive disorders, assessment of the system, and diagnostic tests and basic surgical interventions used in treating these disorders.

Patients with common male reproductive disorders receive care in a variety of settings, such as physicians' offices, ambulatory care centers, acute inpatient facilities, and long-term care institutions. The chapter closes with a discussion of special considerations in caring for the elderly.

Anatomy and Physiology

The male reproductive system is composed of internal and external genitalia (Fig. 38–1). The external genitalia consist of the penis and the scrotum. The internal genitalia are the testes, seminiferous tubules, interstitial cells, epididymis, vas deferens, seminal vesicles, ejaculatory ducts, prostate gland, bulbourethral glands (Cowper's glands), urethra, and spermatic cords.

EXTERNAL GENITALIA

Penis

The penis is attached to the pubic area in front of the scrotum. It functions as the organ for both copulation (sexual intercourse) and urination. The shaft of the penis is composed of three cylindric masses of erectile tissue. Two of these cylinders that form the penis, the corpora cavernosa, are arranged laterally and the third, the corpus spongiosum, forms the ventral surface of the penis. The urethra runs through the middle of the penis, creating a common passageway for both urine and seminal fluid.

At the distal end of the penis, the corpus spongiosum expands to form a slightly bulging structure called the glans penis, which terminates in a longitudinal slit at the external meatus. The glans penis is richly endowed with nerve fibers and is extremely sensitive to tactile stimulation. The skin covering the penis is hairless and loosely adherent to the underlying tissues. At the neck of the penis the skin is folded doubly, covering the glans to form a loose, retractable casing called the *prepuce*, or *foreskin*. Under the prepuce and in the neck of the penis are small glands that produce a cheeselike substance called *smegma*, a secretion with no known function.

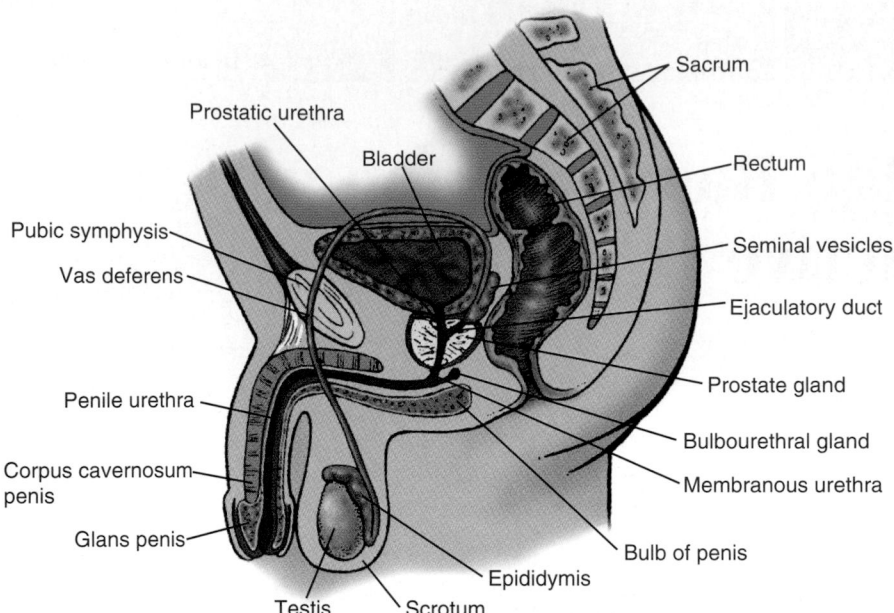

Figure 38–1

The male reproductive system: internal and external genitalia.

Scrotum

The scrotum is a skin-covered pouch suspended from the perineal region that covers, protects, and regulates the temperature of the testes. It is divided by a septum into two sacs, each of which contains and supports one testis together with its connecting tube, the epididymis, and the lower part of the spermatic cord.

The scrotum consists of a thin layer of skin arranged in folds, known as *rugae*, and an incomplete layer of smooth-muscle fibers called the *dartos muscle*. This muscle contracts when the body is cold, causing the testes to be drawn upward against the perineum. In hot weather, the scrotum relaxes and allows the testes to hang more freely away from the body. These changes in the scrotum are important thermoregulators because spermatogenesis is adversely affected by temperature extremes. The skin covering the scrotum is darker in color than that of the rest of the body and, at puberty, the scrotum becomes sparsely covered with hair. Because of the rugae, the skin of the scrotum has the potential for great distention, as when edema develops within the scrotal sac.

INTERNAL GENITALIA

Testes

The testes are the gonads, or reproductive glands, of the male and therefore are the counterpart of the female's ovaries. They have the dual function of producing sperm and the male hormone, testosterone. The testes are small, ovoid glands, usually of equal size, with the left one hanging lower than the right in the scrotal sac. During fetal development, the testes are located in the abdominal cavity behind the peritoneum. About 2 months before birth, the testes descend into the scrotum and are held in position by the spermatic cords. If the testes fail to descend, the condition is known as *cryptorchidism*.

In the internal structure of the testes, two components are important: the seminiferous tubules and the interstitial cells. The seminiferous tubules are a series of long, convoluted, threadlike structures packed densely into the testes, which eventually converge into a collection of excretory ducts. Sperm are produced in the seminiferous tubules and are then stored in the corresponding epididymis and vas deferens.

Sperm are produced at the rate of about 300 million each day and, once ejaculated, have a life expectancy of about 48 hours in the female reproductive tract. Spermatogenesis continues throughout the male life cycle, although it diminishes with advancing age.

The *interstitial cells*, also called *Leydig's cells*, are scattered in clusters in the connective tissue lying between the seminiferous tubules. These cells carry out the second function of the testes: production of the male sex hormone, testosterone. Interstitial cells are located close to the blood vessels in the testes and secrete this hormone directly into the blood stream.

Secretion of testosterone is governed by gonadotropin-releasing hormone (GnRH) from the hypothalamus, which stimulates the anterior pituitary to secrete interstitial cell–stimulating hormone. Interstitial cell–stimulating hormone in turn stimulates hyperplasia of the interstitial cells of the testes and the production of testosterone. The secretion of testosterone subsequently inhibits the secretion of interstitial cell–stimulating hormone and luteinizing hormone–releasing hormone. This negative feedback mechanism controls the rate at which testosterone is produced. Secretion of testosterone results in the enlargement of the penis, scrotum, and testes; the maturation of sperm; and the appearance of secondary sex characteristics. Testosterone continues to be secreted throughout most of the remainder of life but gradually decreases in amount beginning at about 50 years at age.

Epididymis

The epididymis is a long tube about 6 m (20 ft) in length, coiled into a comma-shaped structure, adhering to the top and side of each testis. Each epididymis is divided into a head, a central body, and a tapered portion that is continuous with the vas deferens, called the *tail*. The epididymis begins the first portion of the paired male genital duct system in which sperm mature and are then propelled from the testes toward the urethra during ejaculation.

Vas Deferens

The vas deferens is a tubular structure that connects the epididymis with the ejaculatory duct. Sperm are stored in the vas deferens without losing their fertility for periods ranging from several hours to as long as 42 days depending on the degree of sexual activity. The vas deferens has thick muscular walls and can be palpated in the scrotal sac as a smooth, movable cord. The muscular layers of the vas help propel the sperm through the duct system. The vas deferens from each testis ascends from the scrotum and passes through the inguinal canal and into the pelvic cavity. Here it extends over the top and down the posterior surface of the urinary bladder, narrows to a tip, and joins the duct of the seminal vesicle to form the ejaculatory duct.

Seminal Vesicles

The seminal vesicles are two convoluted membranous pouches located along the lower part of the posterior surface of the bladder directly in front of the rectum. The seminal vesicles secrete a slightly alkaline fluid containing large amounts of fructose. This secretion, which is a component of semen, helps to protect and nourish the sperm and activates their motility. Normal secretory activity of the seminal vesicles depends on adequate levels of testosterone. Each seminal vesicle joins with the corresponding vas deferens to form an ejaculatory duct.

Ejaculatory Ducts

The ejaculatory ducts are two short tubes that pass through the prostate gland to empty the semen-containing sperm into the urethra.

Prostate Gland

The prostate gland in the adult is an encapsulated, three-lobed structure the size and shape of a chestnut. It is located at the base of the urinary bladder, behind the symphysis pubis, and close to the rectal wall (see Fig. 38–1). The initial 2 to 3 cm (0.8–1.1 in) of the urethra pass through a small hole in the center of the prostate gland.

Internally, the prostate is partly glandular and partly muscular. The glandular tissue secretes a thin, milky alkaline fluid into excretory ducts that open into the prostatic portion of the urethra. During ejaculation, the muscle fibers of the prostate contract and eject the prostatic secretion into the urethra, thus adding it to the semen. The alkalinity of this secretion helps protect the sperm from acid present in the male urethra and female vagina and thus increases sperm motility.

Because the prostate gland is anterior to the rectal wall, it is easily palpable by rectal examination, thus facilitating early diagnosis of prostatic problems, such as infections and enlargements. Because of the anatomic relationship of the prostate to the urethra, many prostatic problems cause urinary symptoms.

Cowper's Glands

Cowper's glands (bulbourethral glands) are two small, pea-sized structures located on either side of the urethra inferior to the prostate. During sexual arousal, these glands secrete a small amount of clear alkaline fluid into the urethra. This appears as a droplet at the tip of the penis before ejaculation occurs. Like the secretions of the seminal vesicles and prostate gland, this secretion neutralizes the acidic environment of the male urethra and the female vagina.

Urethra

The urethra, the terminal duct of the male reproductive system, serves as the pathway for eliminating urine and semen. It measures about 20 cm (8 in) in length and is divided into prostatic, membranous, and penile parts. Although the urethra is the passageway out of the body for both urine and semen, excretion of these fluids never occurs simultaneously. The nervous reflexes involved in the expulsion of semen (ejaculation) automatically inhibit urination.

Spermatic Cords

The spermatic cords are two cylindric structures from which each testis is suspended in the scrotal sac. The cords extend from the inguinal rings to the testes and enclose the vas deferens, blood vessels, lymphatic vessels, nerves, and muscle fibers. When these muscle fibers contract, the spermatic cord shortens and pulls the attached testis upward within the scrotal sac.

SEMEN

Semen, or seminal fluid, is a milky, viscid fluid with a pH of about 7.5. It contains about 120 million sperm per milliliter as well as secretions from the epididymides, seminal vesicles, prostate gland, and bulbourethral glands. These secretions combine to create optimal conditions for the survival and function of the sperm.

MALE SEXUAL RESPONSE

Male sexual response requires a coordinated series of physiologic events that results in erection and ejaculation. Erection is the enlargement and hardening of the penis in response to physical or psychological stimulus. Ejaculation is the expulsion of semen from the urethra to the outside. Afferent input from physical or psychologic stimuli are transmitted by the pudendal nerve and pass up the spinal cord for integration in the cerebrum. Efferent nerve fibers then transmit the impulses to the sacral portion of the parasympathetic nervous system, resulting in arteriolar dilatation in the penis and filling of the venous sinusoids in the corpora cavernosa and corpus spongiosum with blood. As this erectile tissue fills with blood, venous outflow is impaired and the penis becomes hard and elongated, facilitating its penetration into the vagina during sexual intercourse. The penis is returned to its nonerectile state through the stimulation of the sympathetic nerve fibers, which results in constriction of the penile arterioles, a reduction of the inflow of blood, and increase in venous drainage.

Erection can also occur without cerebral cortical control by way of a spinal cord reflex mechanism integrated in the sacral area of the cord. In response to tactile stimulation of the penis, scrotum, inner aspects of the thigh, or the anal epithelium, a neural signal is transmitted via the pudendal nerve to an erector center in the sacral portion of the spinal cord. This center then sends out impulses by way of parasympathetic nerves, causing a redirection of blood flow to the cavernous spaces in the penis, which results in an erection. This reflex mechanism is particularly evident in the patient whose spinal cord has been severed.

The response time for an erection varies. It can be very short, occurring within a few seconds of stimulation, or it can take significantly longer. Advancing age, intake of alcohol, fatigue, and stress may increase the time for an erection to be produced.

Erection is experienced on numerous occasions by practically all males from birth to old age both during sleep and while awake. During the sexually active years, a male may report three to four erections at night.

Erections that are nonsexual in nature occur with tension of the perineal muscles, as when lifting a heavy object or straining during defecation. They can also result from irritation of the glans penis, inflammation of the other genital organs, or a full bladder.

Ejaculation is the expulsion of semen from the urethra to the outside. When the level of sexual stimulation becomes extremely intense, the reflex centers in the lumbar section of the spinal cord send impulses by way of sympathetic nerves to the genital organs. These impulses cause peristaltic contractions of the ducts in the testes, epididymides, and vas deferens that propel sperm into the urethra (emission). Simultaneously, rhythmic contractions of the seminal vesicles and prostate gland expel semen and prostatic fluid into the urethra as well. The ejaculatory act itself occurs when impulses reaching the pudendal nerves stimulate the skeletal muscles at the base of the penis, causing forceful expulsion of the semen to the exterior. During ejaculation, the internal sphincter of the neck of the urinary bladder is tightly closed so that sperm cannot enter the bladder, nor can urine be eliminated. The average amount of semen ejaculated during the sexual act is 2.5 to 5 mL.

After ejaculation and orgasm occur, the male enters the refractory period. During this phase, regardless of the type and intensity of sexual stimulation, he will not respond. He cannot achieve a full erection and ejaculation. The length of the refractory period varies among men; for some it may last only a few minutes, whereas others may remain refractory for as long as 24 hours. During the refractory period, detumescence occurs, and the penis returns to the nonerectile state.

Clinical Manifestations of Male Reproductive Dysfunction

SEXUAL DYSFUNCTION

There are three major manifestations of sexual dysfunction in men: erectile dysfunction or impotence, premature ejaculation, and retrograde ejaculation.

Erectile dysfunction or impotence is the persistent inability to obtain or maintain penile erection suitable for vaginal penetration and completion of intercourse. Untreated impotence may result in infertility. Premature ejaculation, a common sexual problem, refers to the expulsion of semen shortly after the onset of sexual excitement or before orgasm of the sexual partner. In retrograde ejaculation the semen is discharged in a reverse direction from the posterior urethra into the bladder. The retrograde deposition of semen into the bladder produces a functional state of infertility. See Table 38–1 for a summary of causes and management of each dysfunction.

The diagnosis and treatment of sexual dysfunction in men is a specialty field. Refer to appropriate books for specific information on this subject. When caring for such patients, be aware of the sensitive nature of the topic and the need for privacy.

PAIN

Pain is one of the most common clinical manifestations for which men with reproductive system dysfunction seek medical attention. Pain may result from an infectious process, a neoplasm, or a structural abnormality. Its type and location vary with its cause. For example, perineal pain and dysuria (burning on urination) occur with prostatitis, whereas pain in the inguinal and lower abdominal areas is characteristic of epididymitis.

URINARY RETENTION

Urinary retention is the inability to empty the bladder adequately with each voiding. This occurs in reproductive tract disorders that obstruct the passage of urine through the urethra. It is a common clinical manifestation of benign hypertrophy of the prostate gland and of advanced carcinoma of the prostate. Urinary retention is signaled by frequency of urination, difficulty initiating the urine stream, a weak urine stream, and dribbling.

Table 38–1

Causes and Management of Impotence, Premature Ejaculation, and Retrograde Ejaculation

Sexual Dysfunction	Causes	Management
Impotence	Psychogenic 　Anxiety 　Depression Endocrine 　Diabetes mellitus 　Hypogonadism Neurologic 　Multiple sclerosis 　Spinal cord injury Vascular 　Hypertension Pharmacologic 　Alcohol 　Propranolol 　Cimetidine Surgical 　Radical prostatectomy 　Partial penectomy Metabolic 　Renal failure 　Cirrhosis	Sex therapy for patient and partner *Three treatment options for organic impotence:* Medications: 　Oral-Yocon (Yohimbine) PO 　Testosterone injections every 2 to 4 weeks 　Self-injection of drug: 　　combination papaverine 　　hydrochloride, 　　phentolamine mesylate, and 　　prostaglandin E_1 into penis for neurogenic 　　impotence Vacuum erection device Surgical penile prosthesis
Premature ejaculation	Psychogenic 　Guilt or fear about sex 　Anxiety 　Ambivalence toward women	Sex therapy for patient and partner
Retrograde ejaculation	Transurethral resection of prostate Diabetes mellitus Spinal cord injury Guanethidine monosulfate (Ismelin)	Limited treatment Imipramine (Tofranil) 25 mg three times daily PO 　or pseudoephedrine (Allerid) 60 mg three times 　daily PO

*PO, orally.

Assessment of the Male Reproductive System

PATIENT HISTORY

When obtaining a history from a man with reproductive dysfunction, be aware that he may be anxious and embarrassed by the nature of the questions and the examination. Use tact and skill in gathering information. Provide a quiet, private environment and be open, supportive, and nonjudgmental in attitude and approach. This is essential because, without privacy, sufficient time for patient-nurse interaction, and a professional manner, nursing assessments and interventions are likely to be incomplete, incorrect, or ineffective. Patients are unlikely to respond comfortably or completely to questions about sexual ability and presence of a penile discharge or to verbalize concerns about the effects of a surgical procedure on sexual function if other patients can hear the conversation or if the interaction is interrupted by other staff.

Be sure to communicate with the patient at a level he can understand. Keep questions simple and clear. Do not assume that the patient knows the biologic terms for reproductive organs or that he can describe the functions of these organs. In attempting to elicit information about a specific dysfunction, use simple but correct terminology. Avoid terms that may be unfamiliar to the patient because he may be embarrassed to ask their meaning and thus give incorrect information.

Begin the history with nonthreatening, relatively neutral questions to give the patient time to become comfortable with you. Ask if he has children, and if so, ask about their number and ages, and review his medical history. Explore the type, date, and treatment of any previous genitourinary problems. Determine whether he is currently taking any over-the-counter medications, prescription medications, or herbal remedies. Note the drug name, dose, route, frequency, reason for use, and effectiveness. Determine the date of his last genital and rectal examination and the frequency of self-examination of the testes. Ask whether he is circumcised. Review sexual status. Include age of first intercourse, current frequency of intercourse, problems with intercourse (either erectile or ejaculatory), sexual satisfaction, and type of birth control. If the patient is over age 50, inquire about the occurrence of symptoms of male menopause, such as insomnia, impaired ability to concentrate, and listlessness.

Explore current symptoms. Ask about pain or discomfort, determining its location, type, and relationship to intercourse, defecation, or voiding. Inquire about changes in defecation pattern. Ask about any penile discharge, with attention to color (white, yellow, green, clear, bloody), consistency (thin, thick), odor (none, sweet, foul), amount, and time of onset. Inquire about the presence of penile or scrotal edema and of penile, scrotal, or inguinal masses. Because urinary symptoms often accompany reproductive disorders, collect information about dysuria, hesitancy, frequency, straining to urinate, nocturia, decreased force of the urinary stream, and dribbling or incontinence. This information may be collected through both interview and a self-scoring patient questionnaire, such as the American Urological Association (AUA) symptom index (Table 38–2). This scoring system is recommended by the Agency for Health Care Policy and Research (AHCPR) for use when initially assessing a patient who has symptoms of benign prostatic hyperplasia (BPH). The system results in a score indicative of whether symptoms are mild (0–7), moderate (8–19), or severe (20–35).

PELVIC EXAMINATION

The male pelvic examination is an organized assessment of the structural condition of the reproductive organs. It includes inspection and palpation of the external genitalia (penis and scrotum) and inguinal and femoral areas, and palpation of the prostate gland. Male pelvic examinations are usually performed either by a physician or a nurse practitioner.

Patient Preparation

Tell the patient what to expect and how the examination will proceed. In preparation for the examination, ask the patient to urinate unless he has a urethral discharge. This prevents discomfort and urgency when the prostate gland is palpated. Ask the patient to stand and drop his pants and shorts below his knees for the examination. If the patient cannot stand, help him remove his pants and shorts and help him onto the examining table. Drape him in the supine position with knees slightly flexed.

Examination Procedure

To minimize the risk of transmitting pathogens, employ standard precautions. Wearing clean gloves, begin the examination with assessment of the external genitalia. Note the amount and distribution of pubic hair and inspect the base of the hairs for nits or lice. Inspect the anterior and posterior surfaces of the penis for edema, erythema, masses, ulcerations, or other abnormalities.

If the patient is not circumcised, retract or have the patient retract the prepuce (foreskin) to expose the glans. Note any accumulation of smegma beneath it. Assess the glans for ulcers, scars, or other lesions, as well as for signs of inflammation or infection. Note the position of the urethral meatus and examine it for any sign of discharge. If the foreskin has been retracted, return it to its original position and proceed to palpate the entire shaft of the penis for tenderness, masses, and induration.

Examine the contour of the scrotum for lumps

Table 38–2

American Urological Association Symptom Index

Have the patient answer the following questions.

1. Over the past month, how often have you had a sensation of not emptying your bladder completely after you finished urinating?
2. Over the past month, how often have you had to urinate again fewer than 2 hours after you finished urinating?
3. Over the past month, how often have you found you stopped and started again several times when you urinated?
4. Over the past month, how often have you found it difficult to postpone urination?
5. Over the past month, how often have you had a weak urinary stream?
6. Over the past month, how often have you had to push or strain to begin urination?
7. Over the past month, how many times did you most typically get up to urinate from the time you went to bed at night until the time you got up in the morning?

AUA SYMPTOM SCORE (Circle one number on each line)

	Not at all	Fewer than 1 time in 5	Less than half the time	About half the time	More than half the time	Almost always
1.	0	1	2	3	4	5
2.	0	1	2	3	4	5
3.	0	1	2	3	4	5
4.	0	1	2	3	4	5
5.	0	1	2	3	4	5
6.	0	1	2	3	4	5
7.	0	1	2	3	4	5
	(never)	(once)	(twice)	(3 times)	(4 times)	(5 times or more)

Sum of 7 circled numbers (AUA Symptom Score) _____

Results:	0–7	Mild BPH
	8–19	Moderate BPH
	20–35	Severe BPH

From Barry MJ, Fowler FJ Jr, O'Leary MP, et al. The American Urological Association Symptom Index for benign prostate hyperplasia. J Urol 1992; 148:1549.

and edema. Remember that the left side of the scrotum normally hangs about 0.5 inches (1.27 cm) lower than the right. Inspect the scrotal skin for erythema, excoriations, ulcers or other lesions, gross deviations in coloration, and the presence of large or distended scrotal veins. Next, palpate the contents of the right and left compartments of the scrotal sac. Note the size, shape, and relative position of the testes, epididymes, and spermatic cords. Normally, the testes are freely movable. Gently squeezing them produces a dull, aching sensation that radiates to the lower abdomen. No nodules or swellings should be evident.

If you find an abnormal scrotal mass, note its size, shape, location, movability, consistency, and tenderness, and proceed to evaluate the area further by transillumination. This is done in a darkened room by placing a flashlight head flat against the affected side of the scrotum and observing for the transmission of light as a red glow. A red glow indicates the presence of serous fluid, which transmits light, as opposed to a swelling or mass containing blood or tissue, neither of which transmits light.

Examine femoral and inguinal areas with the patient in supine and standing positions. Ask the patient to bear down to help visualize a femoral hernia, if present. Check the area for bulges, edema, tenderness, and palpable lymph nodes. Next, palpate the right and left inguinal canals with the right and left index fingers, respectively, by gently invagi-

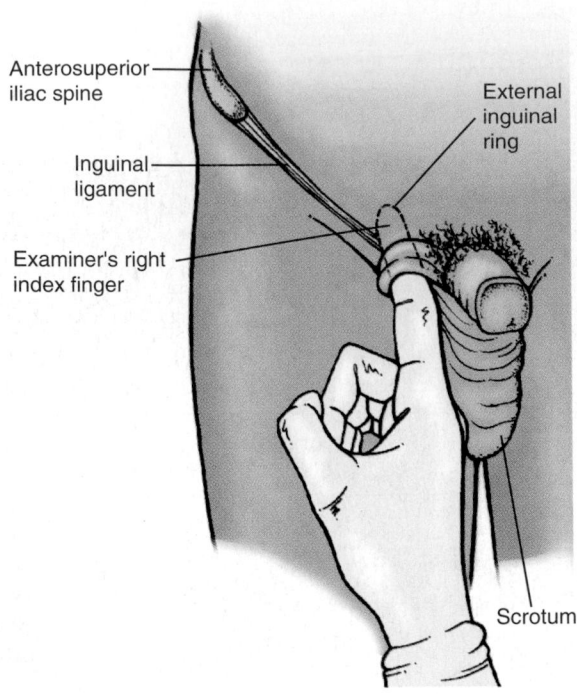

Figure 38–2
Palpating for inguinal hernia at the right inguinal ring.

nating the loose scrotal skin to allow the finger tip to press against the inguinal ring (Fig. 38–2). Instruct the patient to strain down or cough while you feel for a bulge of tissue against the finger tip, which indicates a hernia.

Before proceeding to the examination of the prostate gland tell the patient that his penis may become erect from prostate stimulation. Explain that,

if this does occur, it is an involuntary reflex response that does not indicate sexual arousal.

Perform a digital rectal examination to examine the prostate gland. With the patient in a side-lying position or standing with his back to you and bent over with flexed elbows and upper chest on the examining table, insert a gloved, lubricated index finger into the rectum and evaluate the size and consistency of the prostate gland (Fig. 38–3). The normal prostate is 3.8 cm (1.5 in) long 5 cm (2 in) wide, nontender, and feels smooth and rubbery. The seminal vesicles are usually not palpable unless infected or inflamed.

On conclusion of the examination, check the penis for discharge, which may appear after prostatic manipulation. If discharge is present, a drop may be collected and sent for microscopic analysis (prostatic fluid smear). Cleanse the rectal area of any lubricant and help the patient to a comfortable position.

During the course of the reproductive system as-

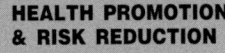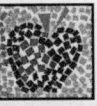

HIGHLIGHT
38–1

HEALTH PROMOTION
& RISK REDUCTION

Optimal Male
Reproductive Function

To maintain a healthy reproductive system and decrease the risk of disease, instruct male patients to:

Maintain good penile hygiene

- Retract the foreskin if uncircumsized.
- Wash the penis from the tip down to the base using soap and warm water.
- Rinse the penis well since soap residue supports bacterial growth and can be irritating to the skin and mucous membrane.
- Dry the penis thoroughly because moisture can lead to maceration, which supports bacterial growth.
- Pull the foreskin back down over the glans.

Have an annual digital rectal examination beginning at age 40.

Perform testicular self-examination monthly.

Seek medical attention promptly if any of the following problems develop:

- Perianal, inguinal, or scrotal pain
- Scrotal swelling
- Dysuria
- Frequency of urination
- Nocturia
- Difficulty initiating voiding
- Erectile dysfunction

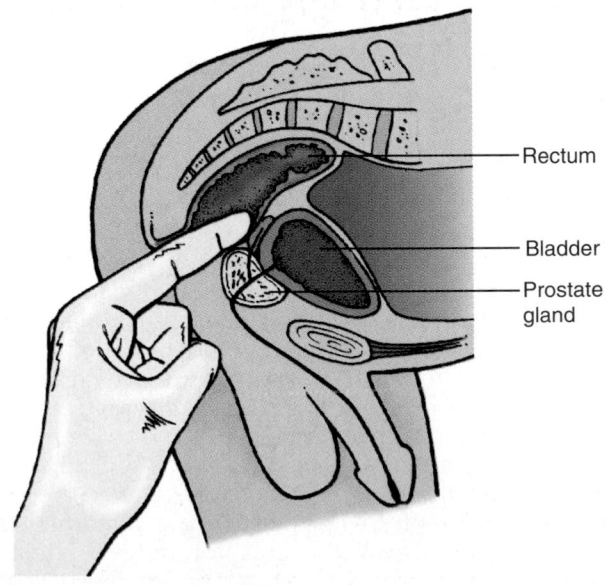

Figure 38–3
Palpating the prostate gland by digital rectal examination.

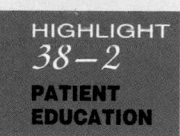 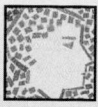

HIGHLIGHT
38–2
PATIENT
EDUCATION   **Testicular Self-Examination**

Before explaining how to perform testicular self-examination, give the patient the following information:

The most common symptom of testicular cancer is a small pea-sized mass on the front or side of the testicle.

Testicular cancer is highly curable, particularly when treated early in its development.

Because a small mass can be felt on testicular self-examination before any other symptoms develop, testicular self-examination allows early detection and treatment, and increases the chances of cure.

Perform testicular self-examination once a month after a warm bath or shower, because the heat relaxes the scrotal skin and makes it easier to feel anything unusual.

Then instruct the patient in the testicular self-examination procedure:

Stand naked in front of a mirror. Look for any swelling on the skin of the scrotum.

Examine each testicle gently with both hands. The index and middle fingers should be placed underneath the testicle while the thumbs are placed on the top, as shown in Figure 38–5. Roll the testicle gently between the thumbs and fingers. One testicle may be larger than the other.

Find the epididymis (a cordlike structure on the top and back of the testicle that stores and transports the sperm). Be sure you don't confuse the epididymis with an abnormal lump.

Feel for a small lump, about the size of a pea, on the front or the side of the testicle. These lumps are usually painless.

Contact the doctor immediately if you find a lump.

Adapted from National Cancer Institute. Testicular self-examination. (National Institutes of Health Publication No. 92-2636.) Washington, DC: U.S. Department of Health and Human Services, Public Health Service, 1992.

sessment, assess the patient's understanding of, and compliance with, health promotion and risk reduction information related to the care of the reproductive system (Highlight 38–1). Also determine whether the patient knows the importance of, and how to perform, a testicular self-inspection (Highlight 38–2 and Fig. 38–4).

Diagnostic Procedures

SEMEN ANALYSIS

Semen analysis is a microscopic examination of ejaculated sperm. It reveals information about the concentration, density, motility, and morphology of sperm and is done when an infertility problem is suspected. The test is repeated at least once, because sperm concentration can vary daily. Semen analysis is also performed 6 weeks after vasectomy to verify that no sperm are present and that sterilization was successful.

The patient collects the semen specimen after a prescribed period of sexual abstinence, at least 2 or 3 days. Preferably, a fresh specimen is obtained by

masturbation while in the physician's office. A less satisfactory specimen can be obtained by the patient at home after masturbation or coitus interruptus. If the specimen cannot be collected by either method because of religious reasons, use of a plastic condom is suggested. Ordinary rubber condoms are not acceptable because spermicides (powders and lubricants) are used in their manufacture. The 2 to 6 mL specimen is placed in a clean, wide-mouthed plastic

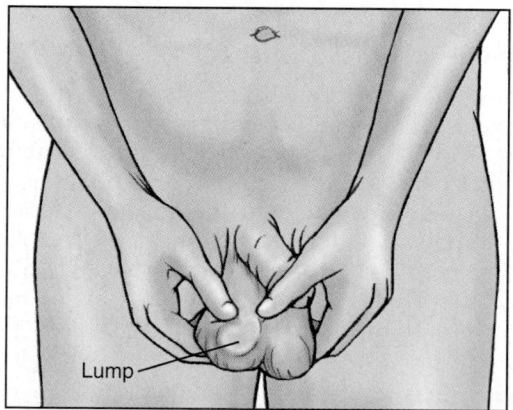

Figure 38–4

Position of hands for testicular self-examination.

container supplied by the physician. It must be kept at room temperature and delivered to the laboratory within 1 hour to ensure accurate results. Date and time of ejaculation, as well as other identifying information, are noted on the container. Instruct the patient on when and how to obtain test results.

LABORATORY STUDIES (BLOOD)

Blood tests used to help diagnose male reproductive disorders include prostate-specific antigen (PSA), prostatic acid phosphatase, alkaline phosphatase, alpha-fetoprotein, human chorionic gonadotropin, testosterone, serum follicle-stimulating hormone, and luteinizing hormone.

Prostate-Specific Antigen

PSA is an organ-specific marker that is elevated in BPH and prostate cancer. Increased levels can also be seen with prostatic inflammation and following prostatic manipulation or instrumentation. It is used as an annual screening test for prostate cancer and to detect residual and recurrent cancer after therapy. The most commonly used measurement is the monoclonal antibody test, which has a 4 mg/mL upper limit of normal. Studies show that PSA level alone has a low sensitivity and specificity for differentiating between organ-confined prostate cancer and BPH (Djavan & Roehrborn, 1994). The use of the PSA PS density, PSA velocity or rate of change, and age-specific reference ranges is currently the most promising attempt to improve the value of PSA levels as a prostate cancer marker. Studies show that monitoring PSA velocity (rate of change) for a consistent, defined increase over time may be the test's most practical value. The Mayo Clinic recommends that African-American men and men with family histories of prostate cancer begin screening examinations with digital rectal examination and PSA at age 40 (Cupp & Osterling, 1993). The American Cancer Society recommends an annual PSA level for most men at age 50.

Prostatic Acid Phosphatase

Prostatic acid phosphatase is an isoenzyme of acid phosphatase. Normal prostatic tissue has a concentration of acid phosphatase 100 times greater than other tissues. Serum activity of the prostatic isoenzyme is greatly elevated in metastatic cancer of the prostate that has extended beyond the prostatic capsule. Prostatic acid phosphatase is used as a tumor marker for prostate cancer. It also can be used to monitor the course of the disease.

Alkaline Phosphatase

Alkaline phosphatase is an enzyme found primarily in bone, liver, and biliary ducts. It is a tumor marker and is elevated in patients with metastatic bone lesions of the prostate.

Alpha-Fetoprotein

Alpha-fetoprotein is a tumor marker that is elevated in patients with testicular malignancies (non-seminomatous). The test is usually done before and after orchiectomy (removal of the testis). Persistent elevated alpha-fetoprotein levels after orchiectomy suggest metastatic spread of the tumor.

Human Chorionic Gonadotropin

Human chorionic gonadotropin is a tumor marker sometimes found in patients with testicular cancer. If human chorionic gonadotropin is present, the test is repeated after orchiectomy. Persistent elevation suggests metastatic spread of the tumor.

Testosterone

Testosterone is the major male hormone secreted by the testes. Testosterone measurements are useful in assessing hypogonadism, erectile dysfunction or impotence, and cryptorchidism. Both total and free testosterone are decreased in hypogonadism.

Serum Follicle-Stimulating Hormone and Serum Luteinizing Hormone

Follicle-stimulating hormone produces spermatogenesis and luteinizing hormone stimulates secretion of androgens. Measurements of these hormones are helpful in the differential diagnosis of hypogonadism and infertility in men.

SEQUENTIAL BACTERIOLOGIC LOCALIZATION CULTURES

Sequential bacteriologic localization cultures are done on sequence-segmented voided specimens of urethral discharge, midstream urine, and expressed prostatic fluid. They are used along with fluid smears to diagnose chronic bacterial prostatitis and nonbacterial prostatitis or to rule out prostatodynia (a condition with symptoms of prostatitis but without evidence of prostate inflammation). Sequential bacterial localization cultures are not usually done if acute bacterial prostatitis is suspected, because prostatic massage could lead to bacteremia.

The procedure for collecting the specimens requires that the patient be cooperative, well hydrated, and have a full bladder. The procedure must be carefully explained and executed to ensure accurate results, as follows:

- Obtain four wide-mouthed sterile containers in which to collect the specimens.

- Wearing a glove, thoroughly cleanse the urinary meatus and glans with a disinfectant. (If the patient is not circumcised, first retract the foreskin and leave it retracted until all specimens are collected.)
- Instruct the patient to void 10 mL of urine into the first sterile container and stop. This is a sample of urethral discharge.
- Instruct the patient to void up to 200 mL of urine into a clean urinal and stop. This urine is discarded.
- Instruct the patient to void 10 mL of urine into a second sterile container and stop. This is the midstream specimen.
- Instruct the patient to bend over, then insert a gloved finger into the rectum, and massage the prostate gland. Massage the gland until drops of prostatic fluid appear at the urinary meatus. Collect them in the third sterile container.
- Instruct the patient to void 10 mL of urine into the fourth sterile container.
- Label all specimens carefully.

Culture and sensitivity must be performed on these specimens within 4 hours of collection to ensure accuracy.

In chronic bacterial prostatitis, more than 10 white blood cells appear in a high-power field in the expressed prostatic fluid and the third voided specimen. In addition, the bacterial count of the specific infecting organism is greater in the expressed prostate secretions and the postmassage urine specimen than in the first two urine samples. In nonbacterial prostatitis, the expressed prostate secretions and postmassage urine specimen contain more than 10 white blood cells per high power field and cultures of urine and prostatic fluid are negative for bacterial growth. In prostatodynia, the expressed prostate fluid sample is normal and all cultures are negative.

VISUALIZATION TECHNIQUES

Urethrocystoscopy

Urethrocystoscopy (cystoscopy and panendoscopy) is a direct visualization of the bladder and urethra. It can demonstrate prostate enlargement, obstruction of the urethra and bladder neck, bladder stones, trabeculation, and diverticula.

Guidelines issued by the AHCPR do not recommend urethrocystoscopy as a means of determining the need for treatment in BPH. The test is recommended for men with prostatism (any abnormal condition of the prostate resulting in obstructed urine flow) who have a history of hematuria, bladder cancer, or lower urinary tract surgery, especially transurethral resection of the prostate. To help the surgeon determine the most appropriate technical approach, urethrocystoscopy is an optional test in men with moderate to severe symptoms who have

chosen (or require) surgical or other invasive therapy.

Ultrasonography

Scrotal ultrasonographic studies are done to diagnose scrotal pathology and structural abnormalities. These studies can confirm the presence of scrotal abscesses, tumor, hydrocele, spermatocele, scrotal hernia, torsion and associated testicular infarction, and chronic epididymitis.

Prostatic ultrasonography is used as an adjunct to digital rectal examination of the prostate. Transrectal ultrasonography allows for the most accurate estimation of prostate size and shape and helps detect areas of the prostate that may be suspicious for cancer. Transrectal ultrasonography is useful in detecting tumor at an early stage by revealing differences in tissue density. The term "echogenicity" refers to the pattern of echoes created by the tissues of the organ being examined (Greene, et al, 1992). The normal ultrasound pattern of the parenchyma in the peripheral zone of the prostate is called *isoechoic*. Relative to this, other areas are either less echogenic (darker, or hypoechoic) or more echogenic (lighter, or hyperechoic). Compared with normal tissue, cancerous tissue is usually hypoechoic.

Transrectal ultrasonography increases the accuracy of directing biopsies to hypoechoic areas. Preparation of the patient for the procedure includes administering a Fleet enema or bisacodyl suppository to remove feces or barium from the rectal area to ensure clear imaging.

BIOPSIES

Prostate Biopsy

There are three common types of prostate biopsy: transperineal using a core needle, transrectal using a core needle, and transrectal fine-needle aspiration biopsy. Figure 38–5 and Table 38–3 compare the three types.

NURSING PROCESS GUIDELINES
Prostate Biopsy

Biopsy of the prostate gland may be performed in a variety of care settings, such as the physician's office, a same-day surgical suite, or a hospital ultrasonography department. The majority of patients are not admitted before or after the biopsy unless there is a coexisting medical problem or a complication develops. As with any biopsy, but especially one involving an internal organ, be sure the patient understands the reason for the biopsy and knows what to expect regarding the procedure and postprocedure care.

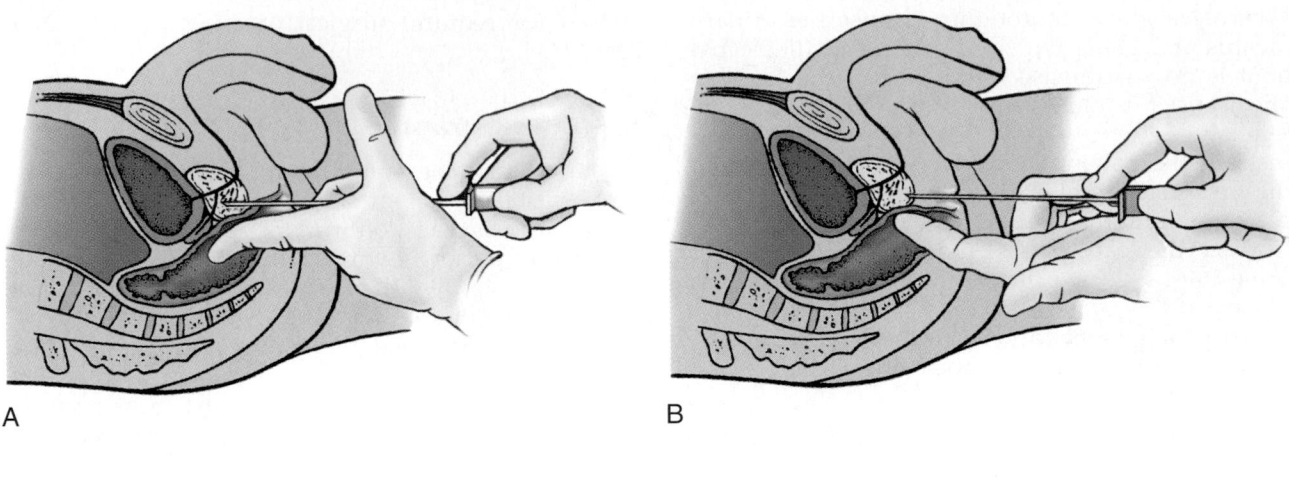

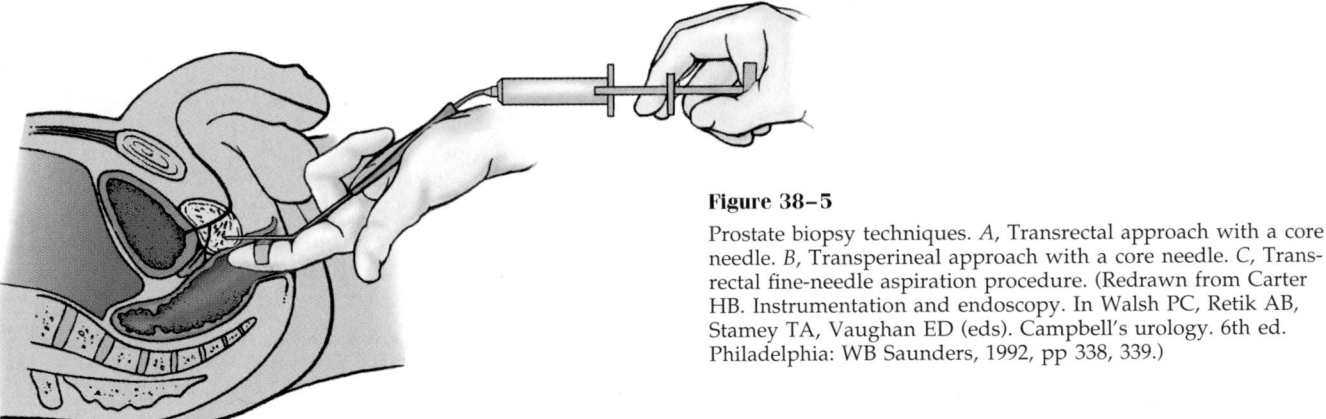

Figure 38–5

Prostate biopsy techniques. *A*, Transrectal approach with a core needle. *B*, Transperineal approach with a core needle. *C*, Transrectal fine-needle aspiration procedure. (Redrawn from Carter HB. Instrumentation and endoscopy. In Walsh PC, Retik AB, Stamey TA, Vaughan ED (eds). Campbell's urology. 6th ed. Philadelphia: WB Saunders, 1992, pp 338, 339.)

Address any concerns verbalized by the patient and check that any prebiopsy instructions, such as for an enema or antibiotics, have been followed. After the biopsy, instruct the patient to avoid exercise or heavy exertion for 4 hours but otherwise to resume normal activities and diet. Instruct him to take any prescribed antibiotics as directed. Urge him to report promptly any bleeding from the biopsy site, chills, a temperature higher than 38.3°C (101°F), difficulty urinating, or excessive pain. Tell the patient he may see blood in his urine for days to weeks, in his semen for months, and—with a transrectal biopsy—after bowel movements for days. Also tell the patient that ejaculation may be uncomfortable for weeks.

If the transperineal approach is used, suggest taking sitz baths for 1 to 2 days for comfort and cleanliness. Instruct the patient to avoid all unnecessary touching near the biopsy site. Inform all patients that the physician will contact them about the biopsy results. Explain that, if the biopsy is negative for cancer, follow-up visits to the physician are necessary to monitor any changes in PSA level and the prostate gland.

Penile Biopsy

Penile biopsy is performed to confirm a suspected diagnosis of carcinoma of the penis. The biopsy can be obtained either by percutaneous fine-needle aspiration or tissue excision.

NURSING PROCESS GUIDELINES
Penile Biopsy

As with any biopsy, make sure the patient understands the reason for the biopsy and knows what to expect about the procedure and its aftercare. Allay anxiety, and support the patient's ability to cope. The latter is particularly important for the patient having a penile biopsy because many men have advanced disease by the time they first seek medical attention. It is estimated that 15 to 50% of men delay seeking medical care for more than a year after the appearance of signs and symptoms because of personal neglect, embarrassment, fear, denial, guilt, or ignorance.

Table 38–3

Comparison of Three Types of Prostatic Biopsy

Type	Description	Advantages	Disadvantages
Transrectal core needle	Core needle (18 gauge) attached to a biopsy gun is inserted into the rectum along the palmar surface of index finger of one hand. Core needle is advanced to the prostatic area to be biopsied. Tissue samples are obtained and withdrawn into biopsy gun. The patient is instructed to take a broad spectrum antibiotic, such as ciprofloxacin (Cipro) before and after the procedure. This procedure may be performed with or without rectal ultrasonography.	No anesthesia required Sepsis and bleeding unusual Patient discomfort likened to that of digital rectal examination	Antibiotics required before and after procedure Fleet enema required before procedure Expensive if performed with rectal ultrasonography
Transperineal core needle	The prostatic area to be biopsied is located rectally with the index finger. With the other hand, the perineum is locally anesthetized. The core needle (attached to a biopsy gun) is inserted through the perineum into the prostate, and tissue samples are obtained. This procedure may be performed with or without rectal ultrasonography.	No periprocedural antibiotics are required Risk of bleeding and sepsis are minimal	Expensive if performed with rectal ultrasonography No longer the preferred method of biopsying the prostate
Transrectal fine-needle aspiration	A 23-gauge needle attached to an aspiration syringe is inserted into the rectum, guided by a gloved index finger, to the suspicious area. Suction is then applied to the syringe and the prostatic aspirate is suctioned into the needle. Suction is then released and the needle containing the prostatic aspirate is removed. This procedure may be performed with or without rectal ultrasonography.	No anesthesia, antibiotics, or enema required Provides cytopathologist with cellular material Minimal complications	Expensive if performed with rectal ultrasonography

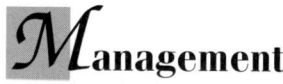anagement

SURGICAL MANAGEMENT

Surgery for the patient with dysfunction of the male reproductive system is performed to diagnose and treat prostatic abnormalities, congenital defects affecting fertility, chronic prostatitis, benign and malignant diseases of the reproductive organs, and for permanent contraception (sterilization). Surgical procedures used in the treatment of male reproductive disorders are summarized in Table 38–4.

Preoperative Preparation
Preoperative preparation begins with consideration of patient's age, general health status, and the presence of coexisting medical problems in view of the proposed surgery. Overall patient status is assessed, with particular attention to cardiopulmonary, hepatic, and renal/urologic function. In young patients with dysfunction of the reproductive system, endo-

crine function may also be studied. In patients having prostatic surgery, renal and urologic functions are evaluated. This evaluation usually includes assessing blood urea nitrogen, serum creatinine, and urine. Assessment of prothrombin time, partial thromboplastin time, and bleeding time is ordered if the proposed surgery carries a significant risk of bleeding. Any clotting defects are corrected before surgery. Medical clearance before surgery is essential in elderly patients with significant heart disease, hypertension, anemia, renal disease, or diabetes mellitus.

Fluid, electrolyte, and acid-base balance are assessed preoperatively to provide a baseline for postoperative comparison. In the elderly hypertensive patient with significant longstanding prostatic obstruction and urinary retention, the bladder is decompressed gradually before surgery. Even with gradual bladder decompression, some decrease in renal function and change in blood pressure may occur. If dehydration is present, the patient must be hydrated carefully with appropriate electrolyte replacements.

Table 38-4

Surgical Procedures Used to Treat Reproductive Disorders in Men*

Surgical Procedure	Description	Setting	Length of Stay†
Circumcision	Excision of the prepuce from the penis	Ambulatory surgical unit	Up to 23 hours
Vasectomy	Transection of a portion of each vas deferens	Ambulatory surgical unit	Up to 23 hours
Orchiopexy	Surgical placement of an undescended testicle into scrotal sac	Ambulatory surgical unit	Up to 23 hours
Orchiectomy	Excision of one or both testicles	Ambulatory surgical unit	Unilateral: Up to 23 hours Bilateral: 1–2 days
Hydrocelectomy	Excision of hydrocele (cystic mass filled with clear fluid that forms around a testicle)	Ambulatory surgical unit	Up to 23 hours
Spermatocelectomy	Excision of spermatocele (cystic mass filled with milky fluid that forms at the upper pole of the testicle)	Ambulatory surgical unit	Up to 23 hours
Prostatectomy	Excision of part or all of the prostate	Acute-care operating room	Transurethral resection: 1–2 days Radical prostatectomy: 4–6 days
Penectomy	Excision of part or all of the penis	Partial: Ambulatory surgical unit Total: Acute-care operating room	Partial: Up to 23 hours Total: 1–2 days
Retroperitoneal lymphadenectomy	Excision of iliac and lumbar lymph nodes in testicular carcinoma (teratocarcinoma, embryonal carcinoma, teratoma)	Acute-care operating room	4–6 days
Iliac lymphadenectomy	Excision of iliac lymph nodes in radical retropubic prostatectomy	Acute-care operating room	4–6 days

*Note: Follow-up care should include specific instructions for wound care, observation of surgical site for bleeding or infection, any voiding difficulty, pain medication, antibiotic therapy, and appointment for first postoperative visit.
†May be adjusted for age, complications, and medical diagnosis.

Any infection in the patient's genitourinary system must be identified and treated with antibiotic therapy before surgery. Additional antibiotics may be given intramuscularly or intravenously a few hours before surgery to ensure effective blood levels during urethral catheterization or surgical manipulation. It is not uncommon for urinary tract infection to recur after surgery.

Mechanical bowel preparation in the form of preoperative enemas may be ordered to prevent postoperative straining, which can induce postoperative bleeding, especially after prostatic surgery. Skin preparation includes mechanical cleansing of the skin preoperatively and shaving the skin area from the nipples to mid-thigh, depending on the extent of the procedure. In many cases, both of these procedures are done in the operating room just before the operative procedure.

Complications

There are many potential postoperative complications of surgery on the male reproductive system. These are summarized in Table 38–5. The risk of complications is particularly high in the confused elderly, who may inadvertently remove drainage tubes and, in the process, traumatize the surgical site, induce bleeding, and contaminate the wound. The risk is intensified because the tubes usually have to be replaced, which requires further manipulation of the area.

VASECTOMY

Vasectomy is the transection of a portion of each vas deferens. It is used primarily as a method of sterilization to control male fertility. It also may be done

Table 38-5

Complications of Surgery on the Male Reproductive System

Complications	Risk Factors
Hemorrhagic shock	Prostate surgery, because the gland is highly vascular
Urinary tract infection	Instrumentation of the urinary system
	Use of catheters, collection bags, bladder irrigations
Wound infection	Perineal prostatectomy, because of the proximity of the incision to the rectum
Respiratory problems	Old age
	Smoking
	Presence of other respiratory disease
Deep thrombophlebitis	Use of lithotomy position, which increases pressure on the popliteal veins during surgery
	Handling of major vessels and resulting inflammation, as in prostatic surgery and pelvic and retroperitoneal lymphadenectomy
	Old age, with its predisposition to venous stasis, immobility, and slower postoperative recovery
Fluid and electrolyte imbalance	Transurethral prostatectomy, because use of hypotonic solution during the procedure predisposes to hyponatremia
Bladder distention, which can lead to damage to the suture line	Obstruction of urinary drainage tubes by clots, mucus, tissue particles
Altered voiding: retention or incontinence	Urethral trauma
Altered sexual function	Surgical trauma varies from minor, such as temporary retrograde ejaculation, to impotence and infertility, as in radical resective procedures

to prevent epididymo-orchitis in the older patient who is undergoing a prostatectomy.

Contraindications

Vasectomy is contraindicated for men who are psychologically unstable or mentally incompetent, for anyone anxious about the procedure because of religious convictions, and for men whose partner disagrees about having the procedure performed.

Patient Preparation

Before a decision is made to perform the surgery, at least one interview is conducted between the surgeon and the patient, preferably accompanied by the spouse or partner. At this time, an informed consent is signed that explains the procedure, its risks, alternative contraceptive methods, and vasectomy reversal with current success rate.

Vasectomy is a minor surgical procedure and is usually performed in an ambulatory surgical unit or in the physician's office. A semen analysis may be done preoperatively to provide a baseline against which to judge the disappearance of sperm after vasectomy. Because vasectomy is done under local anesthesia, food and fluids are not usually withheld. The patient is usually instructed to take a shower and may be asked to shave his scrotum before surgery.

Procedure

Vasectomy may be done in a variety of ways using local anesthesia. One common procedure involves cutting and ligating the vas deferens on both sides (Fig. 38-6).

Postoperative Course

Vasectomy does not result in immediate infertility because viable sperm are found in the ampulla of the vas postoperatively. About 10 to 15 ejaculations after vasectomy are required to clear the sperm from the ductal system. The patient usually becomes aspermatic within 3 months. This is confirmed by semen analysis.

Complications

Complications are infrequent and, when they occur, usually minor. They include wound infection, scrotal hematoma, scrotal abscess, epididymitis, sperm granuloma, and spontaneous reanastomosis of the vas.

NURSING PROCESS GUIDELINES
Vasectomy

Assess the patient's understanding of the extent of the procedure and the facts on reversibility. Also assess his perception of its effect on masculinity and sexual performance. Provide additional information and clarify misconceptions as needed. After the procedure, instruct the patient in self-care (Highlight 38-3).

PROSTATECTOMY

Prostatectomy refers to the partial or total removal of the prostate gland. In a simple prostatectomy,

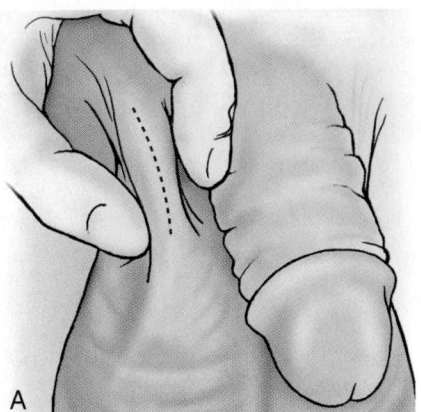

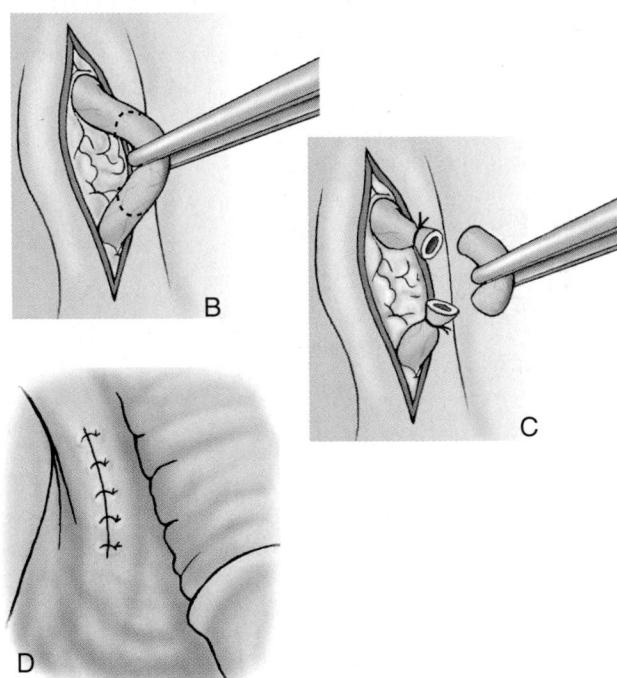

Figure 38–6

A, Longitudinal incision of the scrotum for vasectomy. *B,* Vas deferens exposed. *C,* Small segment of each vas deferens is removed and severed ends are ligated with a suture. *D,* Appearance of scrotal wound after closure.

only the enlarged portion of the gland is removed. In a total prostatectomy, the entire gland and its capsule are excised. A more extensive procedure is the radical prostatectomy, which involves removal of the entire prostate, its capsule, the seminal vesicles, a cuff of the bladder neck, and sometimes pelvic lymph nodes.

An alternative to simple prostatectomy for patients with a small (30 g or less of resected weight) prostate gland is transurethral incision of the prostate. This is an outpatient endoscopic surgical procedure in which an instrument passed through the urethra is used to make one or two cuts in the prostate gland and its capsule, thereby reducing constriction of the urethra.

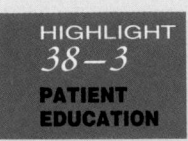 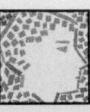

HIGHLIGHT
38–3
PATIENT EDUCATION

Discharge Instructions After Vasectomy

Instruct the patient to do the following:

Change the gauze dressing when stained. Remove the dressing when skin stops oozing.

Apply an ice pack to the scrotum for 12 hours for swelling, alternating 30 minutes on and 1 hour off.

Take sitz baths and acetaminophen, unless contraindicated (per directions on label), for discomfort.

Resume usual activity in 24 hours, but avoid strenuous activity and heavy lifting for 1 week.

Wear a scrotal support for 2 days.

Abstain from sexual intercourse for 3 days.

Use an alternative method of contraception until your physician reports that sperm are no longer found in the semen.

Report bleeding, drainage, fever, or persistent scrotal pain to the physician.

Return for a checkup on *(specify date and time).*

There are four standard surgical approaches to prostatectomy: transurethral resection of the prostate, suprapubic or transvesical prostatectomy, retropubic prostatectomy, and perineal prostatectomy (Fig. 38–7).

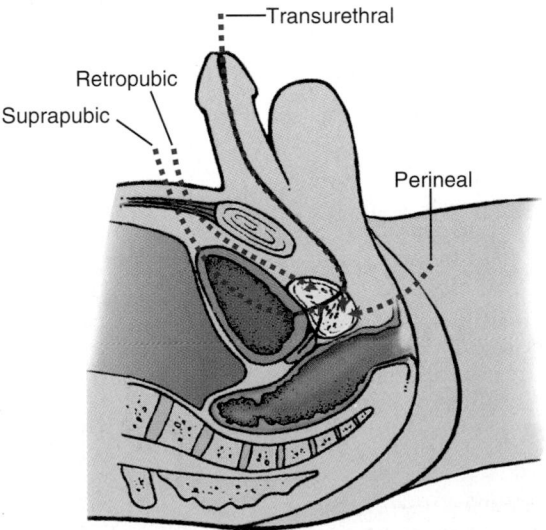

Figure 38–7

Four surgical approaches to prostatectomy.

TRANSURETHRAL PROSTATECTOMY. Transurethral resection of the prostate is the most commonly performed simple prostatectomy procedure. It is performed on 90 to 95% of men undergoing prostatectomy in the United States (Kendall, 1994). It is used to treat symptomatic BPH when the prostate is only moderately enlarged and occasionally is used for patients with malignancy who are poor surgical risks. It is an endoscopic procedure preferably done under local anesthesia using a cystoscope and a resectoscope inserted into the urethra to scrape out the enlarged portion of the gland. To keep the operative area clear, a nonelectrolyte irrigating solution (glycine) is continuously run into the bladder to flush away removed tissue. On completion of the procedure, a large (22 to 24) three-way Foley catheter with a 30 mL balloon is inserted for urinary drainage.

The major advantage of this procedure is that there is no external incision. One disadvantage is that the prostate tissue can regrow because it is not completely removed. There is also the risk of postoperative bladder neck scarring and urethral stricture.

SUPRAPUBIC (TRANSVESICAL) PROSTATECTOMY. In a suprapubic prostatectomy, an incision is made into the lower abdomen and the bladder is opened. The prostate is then removed, working from inside the bladder. A urethral catheter and a suprapubic catheter are both inserted for urinary drainage, and a surgical drain is placed in the abdominal wound. This approach is used when the prostate is too large for a transurethral resection of the prostate and in cases when coexisting bladder problems, such as calculi, need to be treated.

RETROPUBIC PROSTATECTOMY. In a simple retropubic prostatectomy, a low abdominal incision is made, the bladder retracted, and an incision made into the anterior prostatic capsule, through which the gland is removed. A urethral catheter is inserted for urinary drainage, and drains are placed in the abdominal wound. This procedure is done when the prostate is too large for a transurethral resection of the prostate, when cancerous tissue is to be removed, and when the lithotomy position is contraindicated for the patient.

A major advantage of a retropubic prostatectomy is that bleeding is easily controlled because of direct access to the surgical site.

PERINEAL PROSTATECTOMY. In a perineal prostatectomy, the prostate is removed through an incision made in the perineum between the scrotum and the rectum. It is done under spinal or general anesthesia, with the patient in an exaggerated lithotomy position (with the thighs flexed back almost against the trunk). A urethral catheter is inserted to empty the bladder, and a drain is placed in the perineal wound.

A perineal prostatectomy is done when the prostate is too large for a transurethral resection of the prostate and in situations in which abdominal surgery is contraindicated. This procedure is rarely done. It is short but has the disadvantages of potential rectal injury, increased risk of thrombophlebitis because of the patient's position, and the surgeon's inability to reach pelvic lymph nodes for a staging lymphadenectomy if a malignancy is found at surgery. The risk for infection is also greater in perineal prostatectomy because of the location of the incision.

Radical prostatectomy is used as a curative procedure for prostatic cancer. It may be done by either a retropubic or a perineal approach, although the former is often preferred because of the accessibility of the pelvic lymph nodes.

Contraindications

Prostatectomy is contraindicated in the presence of significant sepsis or bladder infection and in patients with an unstabilized medical problem, such as heart disease, marked pulmonary disease, and diabetes mellitus. It is also contraindicated immediately after relief of severe urinary retention because the expected diuresis can result in hyponatremia, which should be corrected before surgery.

Preoperative Preparation

Informed consent is essential before surgery. The possibilities of bleeding, urinary tract infection, incontinence, stricture, sexual dysfunction, and retrograde ejaculation must be explained to the patient. If vasectomy is also planned, this should be noted on the consent form.

Patients are instructed not to take aspirin or any nonsteroidal anti-inflammatory drug for one week before surgery because of the increased risk of bleeding associated with their use. The evening before surgery, patients scheduled for a transurethral, suprapubic, or retropubic prostatectomy have a Fleet enema or soapsuds enema according to the physician's preference. Before a perineal prostatectomy, patients have enemas until clear to decrease the risk of infection. In some cases, stool softeners are also ordered preoperatively. All patients remain on nothing-by-mouth (NPO) status after midnight. Skin preparation is done immediately before surgery. The area from the umbilicus to mid-thigh is shaved and prepared before suprapubic and retropubic prostatectomy. Scrotal, perineal, and perianal areas are also prepared before perineal prostatectomy. There may or may not be a skin preparation for a transurethral resection of the prostate, depending on the surgeon's preference.

Postoperative Course

The postoperative course varies with the type of prostatectomy performed. After a TURP, intravenous fluids are given and then discontinued if clear fluids are taken and tolerated well. The patient is rapidly progressed to a regular diet. A three-way Foley urethral catheter is in place initially and may be attached to a continuous bladder-irrigation system. Such a system allows a constant flow of sterile solution, usually normal saline, into the bladder to prevent blockage of the catheter with clots or pieces of tissue debris. Continuous bladder irrigations are usually stopped when bladder drainage has been pink-tinged and clot-free for 24 hours. After a suprapubic prostatectomy, the patient is maintained on NPO status and on intravenous fluids until peristalsis returns.

Time and sequence of removal of the urethral catheter are variable. If a cystostomy tube is in place, the urethral catheter may be removed after 24 hours and the suprapubic catheter left in place. The suprapubic catheter can then be clamped for periods of time to determine whether the patient can void. Once adequate voiding is established, the suprapubic catheter is removed.

The patient who has had a simple retropubic prostatectomy will also be on NPO status and receiving intravenous fluids. He may also have a nasogastric tube attached to low suction in place until peristalsis returns. The urethral catheter is removed in about 3 to 5 days, and the wound drain is advanced and then withdrawn if there is no leakage of urine.

The course after perineal prostatectomy is similar to that after a transurethral resection of the prostate, except that the urethral catheter remains in place until the urine is clear, an average of 12 days.

With all types of prostatectomy, ambulation begins early. Long periods of sitting are discouraged because the increased intra-abdominal pressure caused by the position can precipitate bleeding.

Bladder spasms are normal after any prostatectomy. They occur most frequently after transurethral and suprapubic procedures and are treated with belladonna and opium (B&O) rectal suppositories and/or other oral analgesics or antispasmodics such as oxybutynin chloride (Ditropan).

Complications

Complications of prostatectomy include bleeding, urinary tract infection, inability to void after the catheter is removed, dribbling, voiding in small amounts, urinary incontinence, urethral scarring, transurethral resection syndrome, thrombophlebitis, and foot drop.

Bleeding is a particular risk after transurethral resection of the prostate because the prostate gland is very vascular and the pressure of irrigating solution used during the procedure can temporarily prevent venous bleeding and obscure the need for hemostasis. To treat postoperative venous bleeding, some surgeons increase pressure in the balloon of the Foley catheter and put traction on the catheter to increase pressure in the prostatic fossa. The catheter is taped to the patient's thigh in the position of traction and released within a few hours (usually 2 to 4) to prevent tissue ischemia and necrosis.

Urinary elimination problems can occur after all simple prostatectomy procedures and are usually caused by surgical trauma to the bladder neck and urethral sphincter. In the radical prostatectomy patient, urinary incontinence may develop after removal of the Foley catheter. This may be from bladder neck contracture, urinary tract inflammation, or disruption of the urethrovesical anastomosis.

Postoperative urinary incontinence occurs in about 1% of patients who have undergone transurethral resection of the prostate and in 0.5% of patients after an open simple prostatectomy (USDHHS, 1994, Pub No. 94-0582). The incidence of urinary incontinence after radical retropubic prostatectomy has been reduced, with rates of 2 to 8% being reported (Goluboff et al, 1995). It is believed that use of Walsh's nerve-sparing surgical technique and the direct anastomosis of the bladder mucosa to the urethral mucosa, as part of the procedure, have contributed to the improvement of postoperative urinary continence.

In the prostatectomy patient experiencing urinary incontinence, return to a normal urinary pattern is usually gradual, with partial control regained in days or weeks, and full control sometimes taking 3 months to 1 year. In a small percentage of these patients, urinary incontinence continues beyond 1 year. Placement of an artificial urinary sphincter may then be considered.

Cystitis, often combined with urethritis and pyelonephritis and caused by a gram-negative organism, can result in dysuria and pyuria. The catheter, which predisposes to infection, is removed as soon as possible.

Transurethral resection syndrome is a hypervolemic dilutional hyponatremia that can occur after transurethral resection of the prostate, especially in patients with large (over 50 g) prostate glands and lengthy (longer than 1.5 hours) operating times. It is caused by increased absorption of nonelectrolyte irrigating fluid (glycine 1.5%) used during surgery into the vascular compartment through open venous sinuses or perforations in the prostatic capsule. With the decreased sodium and ensuing fluid and electrolyte imbalance, the patient may show signs of cerebral edema and increased intracranial pressure, such as increased blood pressure, bradycardia, confusion, disorientation, muscle twitching, visual disturbances, nausea, and vomiting. These symptoms may not result entirely from hypervolemia and hyponatremia but may be due in part to ammonia intoxication related to metabolism of glycine (Kendall, 1994).

Management includes intravenous fluids given at keep-open rate and administration of diuretics. In some patients with more severe symptoms, 200 to 300 mL of 3 to 5% IV hypertonic saline also may be required. Prophylactically, some urologists induce diuresis with furosemide (Lasix) at the time of anesthetic induction.

Thrombophlebitis, a potentially serious complication, may develop in any patient but is a special risk in those with a history of thrombophlebitis and in older, obese men with venous insufficiency. Venous stasis during surgery, dehydration, and pressure on veins from the operating table's leg straps may contribute to development of this complication. Foot drop may also occur from pressure on the peroneal nerve by the stirrups or from improper positioning on the operating table.

After transurethral resection of the prostate and suprapubic and retropubic procedures, sexual dysfunction in the form of retrograde ejaculation is common. Retrograde ejaculation (flow of semen back into the bladder rather than out through the urethra) occurs because the bladder neck has been opened, and the sperm takes the path of least resistance. After perineal and radical prostatectomy, impotency can occur from injury to the pelvic nerve plexus, which provides autonomic innervation to the corpora cavernosa.

Table 38-6 summarizes the different types of prostatectomy and their similarities and differences.

NURSING PROCESS
Simple Prostatectomy

PREOPERATIVE NURSING CARE

Nursing care for the patient scheduled for a simple prostatectomy is similar to that for any preoperative patient (see Chap. 6). Assess the patient's level of anxiety and provide appropriate verbal and nonverbal nursing interventions. Review the patient's knowledge of the surgical procedure (reason for and extent and type of surgery). Explain the expected outcome of surgery and perioperative routines.

POSTOPERATIVE NURSING CARE
Assessment
Assess the patient's physiologic stabilization. Monitor vital signs, oxygen saturation via pulse oximetry, central venous pressure if applicable, laboratory data, and true urine output (total output for a given period of time minus the amount of normal saline irrigant instilled continuously via a three-way indwelling urinary catheter). Assess the patency of the urethral catheter frequently, checking for the following signs of obstruction: increase in bladder spasms or pain, absence of urine and normal saline irrigant outflow from the indwelling urinary catheter, and distention of the lower abdomen on palpation. Observe the color of urinary output from the urethral and/or suprapubic catheters.

Assess postoperative hematocrit, hemoglobin, and serum electrolytes and report changes promptly. Check the abdominal or perineal dressings for bleeding every 15 minutes for 2 hours, then every hour for 8 hours, or more frequently as indicated. Observe the wound (present after all types of prostatectomies other than transurethral resection of the prostate and transurethral incision of the prostate) for color and amount of drainage. Also observe for bloody drainage at the penile meatus at the junction of the catheter and penis. This can be due to an obstruction of the catheter, which causes bloody urine to be expelled around it. If the catheter is patent and this bloody drainage occurs in small to moderate amounts, it is of no concern. If it increases significantly, report this to the physician.

Observe all patients, especially the elderly, with coexisting medical problems for complications related to these medical problems and for signs of hemorrhagic shock and gram-negative sepsis. As the postoperative period progresses, observe the patient for development of complications previously described.

Nursing Diagnoses and Planning

Nursing diagnoses and related expected patient outcomes commonly applicable to patients who have had a simple prostatectomy include the following:

NDx: Risk for urinary retention related to obstruction of urinary drainage tubes and/or removal of part of the bladder neck and prostatic urethra

Planning: Patient Outcomes
1. Urinary drainage tubes are patent and draining.
2. Bladder distention is absent.
3. After catheter removal and depending on the type and extent of prostatectomy, patient voids continently in amounts more than 90 to 120 mL per voiding, within 8 hours of catheter removal or has a postvoiding residual urine volume of less than 50 mL.

NDx: Risk for fluid volume excess related to dilutional hyponatremia secondary to absorption of irrigating fluid during transurethral resection of the prostate

Planning: Patient Outcomes
1. Patient is free of agitation and confusion.
2. Pulse oximetry is within normal limits for patient's age and condition.
3. Blood pressure and pulse are stable within patient's normal range.
4. Serum sodium and potassium levels and serum osmolarity are within normal limits.

NDx: Pain related to surgical tissue trauma and bladder spasms

Planning: Patient Outcomes
1. Patient states that discomfort is lessened or relieved.
2. Patient moves more freely in bed and ambulates more easily when out of bed.

NDx: Risk for infection related to instrumentation of the bladder or presence of an incision and urinary drainage apparatus

Planning: Patient Outcomes
1. Wounds, if present, are free of erythema, drainage, and induration.
2. Urine is clear.
3. Urine cultures are negative.
4. Patient drinks 2.5 L of fluid daily.

Table 38–6

Comparison of Different Types of Prostate Surgery

	Simple Transurethral Resection	Simple Transvesical (Suprapubic) Resection	Simple Retropubic Resection	Radical Retropubic Resection	Simple Perineal Resection	Radical Perineal Resection
INDICATION FOR SURGERY	Moderate enlargement of the prostate	Large obstructing prostate and coexisting bladder problems (stones, diverticula) that are surgically treatable	Large obstructing prostate high in pelvic cavity, no coexisting bladder disease	Large early-stage prostatic cancer	Large obstructing prostate low in pelvic cavity	Large early-stage prostatic cancer
PRESENCE AND LOCATION OF INCISION	None; prostate removed via urethra	Low horizontal abdominal incision (above symphysis pubis), then through bladder wall to prostate	Horizontal incision above symphysis pubis (bladder not entered)	Vertical midline incision from umbilicus to pubis	An inverted U-shaped incision between scrotum and rectum	A larger inverted U-shaped incision between scrotum and rectum
TISSUE REMOVED	Enlarged prostatic chips via resectoscope	Enlarged portion of the prostate gland is enucleated; prostatic capsule remains in place	Enlarged portion of prostate gland is enucleated; prostatic capsule remains in place	Entire prostate gland, including prostatic capsule, prostatic urethra and seminal vesicles, are removed; if frozen section of lymph nodes is positive, iliac lymphadenectomy is performed	Enlarged prostate gland	Entire prostate gland, including prostatic capsule, prostatic urethra, and seminal vesicles, are removed
TYPE OF URINARY DRAINAGE	Three-way urethral Foley catheter with 30 mL balloon, constant bladder irrigation	Three-way urethral Foley catheter with 30 mL balloon, constant bladder irrigation Suprapubic cystotomy tube	Three-way urethral Foley catheter with 30 mL balloon, constant bladder irrigation	Three-way urethral Foley catheter with 30 mL balloon, constant bladder irrigation, occasionally a suprapubic tube	Two- or three-way urethral Foley catheter with 30 mL balloon	Two- or three-way urethral Foley catheter with 30 mL balloon

DRESSINGS AND DRAINS, EXPECTED WOUND DRAINAGE	None	Abdominal dressing including Penrose drain outside bladder to drain accumulated urine and blood; suprapubic cystotomy tube, if used, may drain bloody urine	Abdominal dressing including Penrose drains in retropubic space to drain accumulated urine and blood	Abdominal dressing with Penrose or Hemovac/Jackson-Pratt to drain accumulated urine and blood; if used, a suprapubic cystotomy tube may drain blood-tinged urine	Perineal dressing with Penrose drain may drain serosanguineous drainage (urine may be present first few days)	Perineal dressing with Penrose drain may drain serosanguineous drainage (urine may be present first few days)
PRESENCE AND FREQUENCY OF BLADDER SPASMS	Yes, frequently	Yes, frequently	Yes, but infrequently	Yes, but infrequently	Yes, but infrequently	Yes, but infrequently
TYPE OF VOIDING COMPLICATIONS AFTER REMOVAL OF URETHRAL CATHETER	Inability to void, voiding in small amounts, dribbling, urgency, incontinence, dysuria may occur	Inability to void, voiding in small amounts, dribbling, urgency, incontinence, dysuria may occur	Inability to void, voiding in small amounts, dribbling, urgency, incontinence, dysuria may occur	Inability to void, voiding in small amounts, dribbling, urgency, incontinence, dysuria may occur; in addition, urinary incontinence may persist for 6 months postoperatively	Inability to void, voiding in small amounts, dribbling, urgency, incontinence, dysuria may occur	Inability to void, voiding in small amounts, dribbling, urgency, incontinence, dysuria may occur; in addition, urinary incontinence may persist for 6 months postoperatively
PRESENCE OF SEXUAL DYSFUNCTION	Minor changes in sexual function, temporary retrograde ejaculation possible	Minor changes in sexual function, temporary retrograde ejaculation possible	Minor changes in sexual function, temporary retrograde ejaculation possible	Major changes in sexual function, sexual impotence, and sterility	Major changes in sexual function, sexual impotence, and sterility	Major changes in sexual function, sexual impotence, and sterility

CLINICAL ❓THINKING

RESTLESSNESS AND PAIN AFTER PROSTATECTOMY

A 71-year-old patient returned to the surgical unit after having a radical retropubic prostatectomy for prostate cancer. For the first 10 hours, he remained stable and rested quietly. He had an intravenous infusion of D_5/Ringer's lactate solution running at 100 mL/h, a nasogastric tube to low suction, a three-way indwelling urethral catheter with continuous bladder irrigation with normal saline, a patient-controlled analgesia (PCA) pump with meperidine (Demerol) and was receiving prophylactic antibiotic therapy.

On my 11 PM rounds, I found the patient to be slightly anxious and restless. He complained of pain and reported a constant urge to bear down and void. I explained that these sensations were a common adverse effect of the surgery, encouraged him not to bear down, reviewed the instructions regarding his PCA, checked the doctor's order, and administered an antispasmodic to alleviate his discomfort. An assessment of his vital signs revealed that his blood pressure was 120/90 mm Hg (a change from the previous reading 120/80 mm Hg). He had a regular, apical pulse rate of 94, a respiratory rate of 20 per minute, and a temperature of 38°C (100.4°F).

I noted that his pulse and respiratory rates were slightly increased from previous recordings, which could have resulted from the patient's pain, elevated temperature, or both. His skin was warm, dry, and pale. All peripheral pulses were palpable, and capillary refill was within normal limits. His urinary drainage was reddish with a few clots. A small amount of serosanguineous drainage appeared on his low abdominal dressing. He remained alert and oriented.

Although the patient's vital signs remained within normal limits, I noted and documented the decreased pulse pressure and slight increase in the pulse and respiratory rates. There was no obvious cause for alarm. However, because the changes could be early indications of an unfavorable change, I decided to monitor the patient closely.

When I returned to check on the patient 20 minutes later, I noted a disturbing change in his condition. He was sitting up in bed, pulling on his urinary catheter, and appeared irritable. He was pale and diaphoretic, his extremities were cool and clammy, and his mucous membranes were dry. His blood pressure had fallen to 86/62 mm Hg, apical pulse rate was 130 and regular, respirations were 28 per minute and shallow, and temperature remained 38°C. His peripheral pulses were diminished, and capillary refill was greater than 3 sec-

onds. No adventitious breath sounds were auscultated, and, although his verbal responses were vague, he denied any chest discomfort or leg pain.

I recognized that the patient's clinical manifestations could represent a number of life-threatening conditions. The absence of chest pain argued against an acute myocardial infarction. Although the patient was at high risk for pulmonary embolism, the absence of adventitious lung sounds and leg pain helped me to eliminate that possibility.

Similarly, the absence of a temperature greater than 38.3°C (101°F), the narrowing pulse pressure, and the absence of any evidence of allergy (such as skin rash, pruritis, or urticaria) argued against septic shock and anaphylactic shock as possible underlying causes.

The patient's drop in blood pressure could possibly have been related to the meperidine, have represented orthostatic hypotension, or have been a vasovagal response to pain. However, the patient's current surgical history of prostatectomy with its high risk for postoperative hemorrhage, his severe bladder spasms (which might have initiated bleeding), the pattern of his vital signs (decreasing blood pressure, narrowing pulse pressure, tachycardia, and tachypnea), and his deteriorating mental status led me to suspect that the patient was bleeding from disruption of the vessels at the surgical site.

A quick check of the dressing showed no evidence of bleeding. However, the urinary drainage was becoming increasingly bright red. This further supported my suspicion of hypovolemic shock secondary to hemorrhage.

The bright red color of the bloody urinary drainage indicated arterial rather than venous bleeding. I knew the patient's prognosis would be poor unless I acted quickly because hypovolemic shock can progress rapidly to acute respiratory distress syndrome, disseminated intravascular coagulation, acute renal failure, cardiopulmonary arrest, and death. Because there was little time to spare if the patient was to survive, I immediately implemented the following actions:

1. I called for assistance and asked another staff nurse to notify the surgeon and to gather emergency equipment.
2. I placed the patient in a supine position with his legs elevated.
3. I increased the infusion rate of the IV and the rate of flow of the continuous bladder irrigation.
4. I administered oxygen and established another IV with a large-bore catheter as per hospital policy.

CLINICAL ❓ THINKING

(continued)

5. I covered the patient with a light blanket.
6. I remained with the patient, offered emotional support, and calmly provided a clear explanation of his condition and the procedures initiated.
7. I continued to monitor his airway, respiratory, cardiovascular, and mental status.
8. I monitored his intake and output.
9. I attached a cardiac monitor and pulse oximeter.
10. I documented my findings and actions.

Upon his arrival, the physician confirmed my suspicion of hemorrhagic shock and ordered STAT blood specimens for a complete blood count, hemoglobin and hematocrit, electrolytes, prothrombin time, partial thromboplastin time, creatinine and blood urea nitrogen levels, type and cross-match; arterial blood gas analysis; a 12-lead electrocardiogram; and IV fluids, which I administered.

The patient's vital signs stabilized following administration of 1 L of Ringer's lactate solution and 1 U of whole blood. He then returned to the operating room for identification and repair of the source of bleeding.

Recognition of the classic signs of hypovolemic shock, and knowledge of how to deal with the crisis, helped to reverse the course of this potentially devastating event and saved the patient's life.

Think Critically

Should the nurse in this scenario have intervened earlier in this chain of events? What early clues might have signaled an impending crisis?

Could hypovolemic shock have been prevented altogether?

What nursing actions would have been different if this patient was experiencing septic shock? Anaphylactic shock?

What early evidence of a sympathetic nervous system compensatory response to hypovolemia did the nurse note? What is the physiologic mechanism for this response?

What action should the nurse have taken if placing the patient in a supine position increased his dyspnea?

What is the rationale for not placing the patient's head below the level of the heart?

Why did the nurse cover the patient with a light blanket?

What was the nurse's rationale for increasing the rate of flow of the continuous bladder irrigation?

What actions should the nurse have taken if the patient's condition had deteriorated to a more advanced stage of shock before the physician arrived?

What was the rationale for administering Ringer's lactate solution? Whole blood?

What assessments should the nurse make following rapid administration of volume-expanding fluids and whole blood?

What contraindications of fluid resuscitation should the nurse be aware of?

What changes in the results of the patient's arterial blood gas analysis would the nurse anticipate? Why?

What changes in the patient's hemoglobin and hematocrit would the nurse anticipate? Why?

What assessments would the nurse make to monitor for hypoperfusion of the kidneys?

The patient said, "What's happening to me? Am I going to die?" What is the nurse's best response?

What two priority nursing diagnoses will the nurse include in the patient's nursing care plan following this scenario?

NDx: Risk for injury related to accidents secondary to impairments and/or related to inadvertent removal of urinary drainage tubes or dressings

Planning: Patient Outcomes
1. Patient avoids falls or other accidents.
2. Patient's urinary drainage tubes and dressings remain intact and in place.

NDx: Risk for impaired tissue integrity related to irritation of abdominal or perineal skin by drainage from a suprapubic, retropubic, or perineal incision

Planning: Patient Outcomes
1. Skin and suture line are intact.
2. Skin surrounding suture line is free of erythema.

NDx: Risk for constipation related to change in oral intake, immobility, and fear of pain or disruption of the suture line

Planning: Patient Outcomes
1. Patient ingests 2.5 L of fluid daily (if not medically contraindicated).

2. Patient eats foods allowed that promote regular bowel function.
3. Patient ambulates progressively while hospitalized.
4. Patient's first bowel movement after surgery occurs without straining.

NDx: Risk for sexual dysfunction related to prostatectomy

Planning: Patient Outcomes
1. Patient describes the degree of sexual dysfunction expected with the specific type of prostatectomy to be performed as described by the urologist/surgeon.
2. Patient verbalizes belief that, in time, satisfying sexual relationships can be resumed.

NDx: Risk for altered health maintenance related to insufficient knowledge of postprocedure self-care

Planning: Patient Outcomes
1. Patient lists signs and symptoms to be reported.
2. Patient describes limitations on activity and sexual intercourse and states date of return to work.
3. Patient describes measures to prevent constipation and staining.
4. Patient states reason for use and directions for each discharge medication.
5. Patient states the date of his follow-up visit.

Nursing Interventions and Evaluation

NDx: Risk for urinary retention
To keep urinary drainage catheters patent and free of obstruction, maintain the flow of the normal saline irrigant at the prescribed rate or the rate needed to keep the urine pink-tinged to clear. Empty the urinary drainage bags frequently, especially if the irrigant is running at a rapid rate. Remind the patient about the urinary drainage tube, and instruct him not to lie on it. Check the position of the catheter anchored with tape or a leg band to the patient's inner thigh to prevent tension on the catheter. Check the drainage tube frequently for kinking. Keep the tubing in a straight line from the bed down to the collection bag to ensure proper drainage. Clip or pin the tube to the bed sheet to prevent looping or coiling below the bed and undue tension on the catheter. Position the drainage bag on the same side to which the patient is turned while in bed to ensure proper gravity drainage.

If the patient has significant bladder spasms and there is no urinary/irrigant outflow to the drainage bag, irrigate the urinary catheter by hand if so ordered. Use strict sterile technique, sterile gloves, fresh sterile equipment, and solution as ordered, usually 30 to 60 mL of normal saline. Record amounts of solution instilled and returned on the intake and output sheet, because the amount instilled must be subtracted from the amount returned to determine true urine output.

Do not speed up the irrigant in an attempt to dislodge the obstruction if there is no urinary outflow because this may force the clot to become more deeply seated in the eye of the urethral catheter. This further compounds the obstruction and contributes to an overdistended bladder, bleeding, and an increase in bladder spasms. It may even require replacement of the catheter, which can cause further tissue trauma and raise the risk of sepsis.

When ordered, remove the catheter early in the day, preferably before breakfast, and give the patient 8 to 10 hours to void in sufficient quantity with each voiding (usually 90 to 120 mL per voiding). Do post-void residual catheterization as ordered to check for retention. Bladder ultrasonography may be used to assess for retention.

Tell the patient what to expect during and after the catheter removal. Give the patient a urinal, and instruct him to urinate into it at the first urge to void. Ask him to inform you each time he voids so that you can measure the urine and note its color and character. Maintain careful intake and output records for the 8 to 10 hours immediately after removal of the catheter. During this time, encourage the patient to drink at least one liter of fluid, unless medically contraindicated, so that a sufficient volume of fluid is ingested in the trial voiding period. This amount of fluid may be modified if IV fluids are being provided. A burning sensation while voiding is common during the first 24 hours after removal of the catheter. This high fluid intake dilutes the urine and reduces discomfort. Suggest that the patient ambulate in the room or within reach of a urinal to avoid any potentially embarrassing urgency incontinence.

Promote voiding by reassuring the anxious patient and providing privacy. Depending on the individual patient, encourage perineal (Kegel) exercises, give a warm bath, provide a warmed urinal, run water, or place 5 to 10 mL of spirits of peppermint in the urinal to stimulate voiding. Be supportive to the patient who is unable to void or develops urinary retention and must be recatheterized. Statements like, "I know this must be uncomfortable and difficult for you" let the patient know you are concerned about him and empathize with him.

NDx: Risk for fluid volume excess
Monitor the patient for increasing restlessness, confusion, and muscular twitching, and notify the physician if they occur. Also monitor vital signs. Report any significant elevation in blood pressure or drop in pulse rate. Monitor serum electrolyte values and report abnormal results, especially serum sodium levels below the normal range. If transurethral resection syndrome with dyspnea and pulmonary congestion develops, assist the patient into a sitting position to facilitate breathing and administer oxygen. Slow the rate of intravenous administration to keep-open rate to avoid further fluid overload. Use a calm approach, and reassure the patient to decrease the anxiety accompanying this change in condition. With severe symptoms of transurethral resection

syndrome, IV hypertonic saline solution, usually 250 to 500 mL of 3 to 5% sodium chloride, and osmotic diuretics may be given. After administration of the hypertonic intravenous solution and diuretics, record the patient's intake and output and daily weight.

NDx: Pain
Encourage the use of patient-controlled analgesia if in place, or medicate the patient as ordered. For incisional pain, give analgesics. For bladder spasms, give analgesics, antispasmodics, or both. If belladonna and opium rectal suppositories are ordered for bladder spasms, insert them carefully to avoid traumatizing the operative site.

To further relieve bladder spasms, keep the catheter patent and draining, and make sure there is no inadvertent tension on it. Also keep the patient well hydrated.

Support the effect of medication with physical and psychological comfort measures. Change dressings if needed, give back rubs, and position the patient comfortably. Maintain a quiet, restful environment, and encourage slow, deep breathing and other relaxation techniques. Pain management is crucial during the first 48 hours after prostatectomy. The elderly patient in pain may become increasingly restless and may injure himself when attempting to get out of bed to "go to the bathroom" in an attempt to relieve the discomfort of bladder spasms.

NDx: Risk for infection
Wash hands carefully before and after caring for the patient. Maintain standard precautions by wearing clean gloves for perineal care and catheter care. Use strict sterile technique during dressing changes and when irrigating urethral or suprapubic catheters by hand. Maintain the sterility of the normal saline irrigant and equipment, and label the irrigant with date and time. Discard any irrigating solution that is older than 24 hours. Keep the penile meatus and catheter junction clean and free of bloody drainage. To do this, wrap a sterile abdominal pad loosely around the penis at the penile catheter junction after catheter care. Hold it in place with a strip of adhesive tape on the outside of the abdominal pad, and change as necessary. Encourage oral fluid intake to 2.5 L in 24 hours unless medically contraindicated. Monitor for and report signs of infection, such as elevated temperature, chills, change in type and consistency of wound drainage, and incisional pain. Administer ordered antibiotics on time.

NDx: Risk for injury
To prevent the patient from falling out of bed or inadvertently removing urinary drainage tubes, observe the patient, his dressings, and urinary drainage tubes every 15 minutes initially and then with decreasing frequency on the basis of patient need and condition. Tape the urethral catheter to the patient's inner thigh to prevent inadvertent tension on the catheter and resulting bladder trauma. Place the

call light near the patient and encourage him to use it to call for help. Instruct him to move slowly and carefully in bed to avoid dislodging the tube. Remind him not to get out of bed without assistance until directed to do so. Keep the bed in low position with side rails up.

When the patient is allowed out of bed, move and secure the urinary drainage tubes and bags well ahead of any movement by the patient from bed to chair or when returning to bed. This is a crucial time, when inadvertent removal of catheters can occur because of a sudden movement by the patient in an attempt to help, or from failure of the nurse to carefully place urinary drainage bags and normal saline irrigant ahead of him. Verbally cue and guide the patient carefully when any movement is attempted. Inadvertent removal of the catheter(s) may mean that the patient has to return to the operating room for replacement of suprapubic or urethral catheters.

NDx: Risk for impaired tissue integrity
After suprapubic prostatectomy, serosanguineous drainage and urine may leak out around the suprapubic catheter. Cleanse the skin around the suprapubic catheter and incision with an antibacterial agent such as a povidone-iodine preparation (Betadine). Apply a dry, sterile dressing. Change the dressing frequently to prevent skin maceration. Hold the dressing in place with Montgomery straps to help prevent skin breakdown from frequent application and removal of adhesive tape that could occur with dressing changes. This is very important for elderly patients, whose skin is particularly sensitive to mechanical injury.

After perineal prostatectomy, change the perineal dressing as often as needed to keep the skin dry, clean, and free of fecal contamination. If ordered, give sitz baths for cleanliness and comfort.

NDx: Risk for constipation
Encourage the patient to drink 2 L of fluid per day while hospitalized unless medically contraindicated. When diet permits, encourage him to eat fresh fruits, vegetables, whole-grain products (bread, cereals), and bran. Ambulate the patient progressively and consistently. Administer a stool softener or laxative as prescribed. Record the occurrence of the patient's first bowel movement, which is usually within 3 days of resuming oral food and fluids.

NDx: Risk for sexual dysfunction
Include the significant other in discussions of sexuality. Be sure the patient knows and understands the degree of dysfunction he can expect on the basis of the extent of the procedure performed. Establish a climate that makes him feel comfortable asking questions related to sexuality. If questions about sexuality were included in preoperative teaching and were addressed, postoperative discussion will be easier. Ask, "Do you have any questions for the doctor or me about how this surgery might affect

your sex life?" Answer those questions simply to reaffirm and clarify information given to the patient by the physician. Before discharge, remind the patient about any postoperative restrictions on his sexual activity, as recommended by the physician. Instruct the patient to report cloudy urine, which is associated with retrograde ejaculation, once sexual activity is resumed. If impotence is anticipated, provide emotional support for the patient and significant other. Refer for sexual counseling if indicated.

NDx: Risk for altered health maintenance

Teach the patient appropriate self-care measures (Highlight 38–4). Initiate a referral to a home health-care agency if necessary.

Additional Interventions

For 48 to 72 hours after surgery, avoid all rectal treatments (except belladonna and opium suppositories) to prevent injury to the prostatic surgical site. If urinary incontinence persists at discharge, on the basis of a discussion with the physician, reassure the patient that as healing occurs his ability to void more continently will improve. Discuss the use of Kegel exercises to help regain urinary continence. In cases of severe incontinence, a Cunningham clamp may be ordered for the patient to wear. (See Chap. 39 for more information.)

Compare the patient's status with the expected outcomes. If the outcomes are not met, reassess the patient and revise the plan.

PENILE IMPLANTS

A penile implant is a prosthetic device inserted into the corpora cavernosa to restore erectile potency. Penile prostheses may also be used as adjunct therapy for some patients with a neurogenic bladder to facilitate either intermittent self-catheterization or to maintain the placement of an external urinary drainage device (condom catheter).

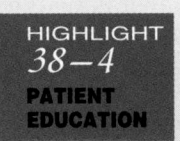 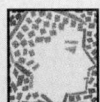

HIGHLIGHT 38–4

PATIENT EDUCATION

Discharge Instructions After Prostatectomy

Before explaining discharge instructions after prostatectomy, give the patient the following information:

Bloody urine is common just after surgery. Small pieces of tissue or blood clots can be passed during urination for up to 2 weeks after surgery.

Strenuous exercise and sports activities such as tennis, golf, swimming, and lifting objects heavier than 20 lbs must be avoided for 6 weeks. These activities can stimulate bleeding.

Absence from sexual intercourse is recommended for a minimum of 3 weeks. Check with the physician before resuming this activity.

Showering rather than bathing in a tub is recommended. To limit dilation of pelvic blood vessels, also avoid hot-tubs.

Driving a car and sitting for long periods of time in a car are restricted for at least 3 weeks. Check with the physician before attempting either activity.

Most patients can return to work in 4 to 6 weeks, depending on the type and extent of prostatectomy performed and the nature of the work.

Then give the patient these instructions:

Keep readily available the name and phone number of the urologist and surgeon.

Promptly report abrupt episodes of frank bleeding to the physician.

Report signs of urinary tract infection, including fever higher than 37.6°C (99.8°F), chills, painful urination, back or side pain (flank area), and general malaise.

Report increases in bloody urine not cleared by drinking fluids (up to 32 oz in 30 minutes) that last for a few hours or one to two voidings.

Notify physician if urinary stream decreases or if urinating becomes difficult.

Take medications, especially antibiotics if prescribed, on time as ordered.

Avoid straining at stool because this can initiate bleeding.

Maintain a high daily intake of nonalcoholic fluids (2 to 2.5 L/day) to ensure soft, regular bowel movements, to limit clot formation, and to prevent infection.

Include fresh vegetables, fruits, whole-grain products (such as shredded wheat), and bran in a well-balanced diet.

Report signs of constipation early to the physician. Avoid use of enemas and suppositories because they can stimulate bleeding. A mild laxative or stool softener may be used.

Return for a follow-up visit on *(specify date and time).*

Contraindications

Any patient undergoing this procedure must have a general state of health good enough to undergo the surgery safely. For example, conditions such as unstable coronary artery disease, thrombocytopenia, or prostate enlargement would make the patient an unsatisfactory candidate for penile implant surgery. In addition, any urinary tract infection must be corrected before insertion of the prosthesis.

Patient Preparation

To determine the appropriateness of implanting a penile prosthesis, the patient's response to any nonsurgical treatment (such as hormone or sex therapy) is reviewed. In addition, the patient and partner must be psychologically and intellectually able to cope with the prosthesis. Once the decision is made that the patient is a suitable candidate for the implant, he and his partner are usually involved in selecting the type of prosthesis to be inserted.

The patient is informed that the erection achieved with the implant will probably not be exactly like that achieved naturally. He is also told that, if his production of sperm has not been affected by the cause of the impotency, he can father a child.

Because infection is a common postoperative complication, prophylactic intravenous antibiotic therapy, usually with an aminoglycoside such as gentamicin, is started preoperatively. Skin preparation includes a shower with an antibacterial cleansing solution, such as 2% povidone-iodine, the night before and the morning of surgery. It also includes a surgical shave of the genital area, which is done in the operating room.

Because implantation of a penile prosthesis is usually performed under general anesthesia, instructions are given not to eat or drink anything for 8 to 10 hours before the operation.

Types of Prostheses

There are two basic types of prostheses: an inflatable prosthesis and a noninflatable or solid rod prosthesis. The inflatable prosthesis has three components: two hollow silicone cylinders with a fluid reservoir

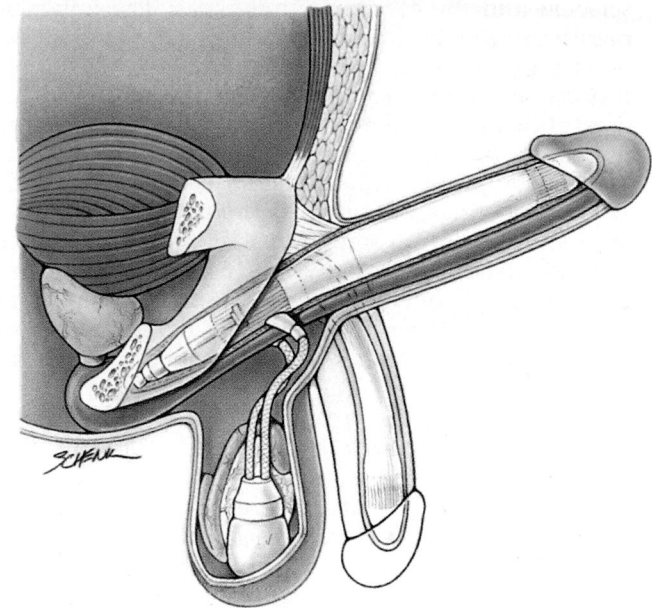

Figure 38–8

Penis in flaccid and erect positions with an inflatable penile prosthesis in place. (Courtesy of American Medical Systems, Inc., Minnetonka, Minnesota. Medical illustration by Michael Schenk.)

and a pump bulb, all connected by kink-resistant tubing (Fig. 38–8). The prosthesis is activated by compressing the pump, which is implanted in one of the scrotal sacs. Fluid from the reservoir located in the retropubic space beside the bladder is then transferred to the cylinders in the penis, causing them to inflate, thus simulating a normal erection in size and appearance. In the noninflatable prosthesis, two silicone rods are implanted into the penis, resulting in a permanent erectile state. The major advantages and disadvantages for the inflatable and noninflatable penile prostheses are listed in Table 38–7.

Procedure

The surgical technique for implanting the penile prosthesis varies depending on the type of device

Table 38–7

Advantages and Disadvantages of Inflatable and Noninflatable Penile Prostheses

Type of Implant	Advantages	Disadvantages
Inflatable	More natural-appearing erection	Higher mechanical failure
	Duration of erection regulated by patient	Insertion time longer
	Does not cause penile erosion	More expensive
	Cytoscopic examinations can be performed easily	Manual dexterity required for activating the prosthesis
Noninflatable	No mechanical parts to malfunction	Penis is always in an erect or semi-erect position
	Insertion time shorter	Erection less rigid than normal
	Less expensive	Problem with concealment
		May interfere with future cystoscopic surgery
		May erode through the penis

selected and the surgeon's preference. The inflatable prosthesis can be inserted either by the suprapubic or upper scrotal approach. Because the scrotal approach allows better access for implanting the cylinders and fluid-filled reservoir, as well as for inserting the pump bulb, this technique is often used. In placing the pump in the scrotal sac, some consideration may be given to whether the patient is right- or left-handed. For example, if the patient is right-handed, the right scrotal sac is usually used. When the three components are connected, the implant is checked for proper inflation and deflation. Before surgery is completed, a Jackson-Pratt drain may be inserted for 24 hours.

The noninflatable prosthesis can also be inserted through the scrotal or suprapubic approach. This procedure usually takes about 30 minutes compared with the 60- to 90-minute operating time for implanting the inflatable prosthesis.

Because some edema is likely to form around the urethra with all types of implants, a Foley catheter is usually inserted before the patient leaves the operating room. The catheter is left in place for the first 24 hours.

Postoperative Course

Antibiotic therapy is continued postoperatively. After discharge from the hospital, the patient is maintained on an oral broad-spectrum antibiotic for about 2 weeks. Moderate pain in the genital area, which may also be referred to the lower abdomen, is expected for the first 24 to 48 hours postoperatively. Pain can usually be controlled with meperidine hydrochloride (Demerol HCL) 75 to 100 mg intramuscularly every 4 to 6 hours as needed, or a similar narcotic analgesic for the first 24 hours and then oxycodone hydrochloride and acetaminophen (Percocet), one to two tablets, every 4 hours as needed. Ice pack applications are usually ordered for the operative area during the first 24 hours to control pain and edema.

Edema and ecchymosis of the penis and scrotum are typical postoperatively and may continue for 7 to 10 days, especially with the inflatable prosthesis. Pain medication is used as ordered during this time. Voiding is not usually a problem after the Foley catheter is removed. Blood loss is usually minimal for all types of implants. If a Jackson-Pratt drain or similar wound drainage system was inserted, as in the case of the patient with an inflatable prosthesis, up to 30 mL of serosanguineous drainage for the first 24 hours is considered within normal limits.

Before discharge from the hospital, the patient with the inflatable implant is taught to locate the pump and apply gentle traction to maintain its position in the most dependent portion of the scrotal sac.

At discharge, all drains have been removed and the patient is usually able to take a shower or bath. He may also be instructed to take sitz baths for 20 minutes four to five times a day for penile and scrotal comfort. If any sutures are in place, they are removed about 1 week after returning home. Sexual activity can usually be resumed in 6 to 8 weeks, depending on the type of prosthesis inserted and whether or not any complications have occurred.

Complications

Postoperative complications for inflatable and noninflatable prostheses are similar and include infection and urinary retention. In addition to these complications, the patient with an inflatable prosthesis may experience a rupture or leak of the cylinders and reservoir. The pump could malfunction or cause an erosion of the scrotum. Or a scrotal hematoma may form.

Specific complications associated with the various noninflatable types are usually limited to device failure and extrusion or perforation of the cylinders through the urethra or skin of the penis.

NURSING PROCESS
Implantation of a Penile Prosthesis

PREOPERATIVE NURSING CARE

Nursing care for the patient scheduled for implantation of a penile prosthesis is similar to that for any preoperative patient, as described in Chapter 6.

POSTOPERATIVE NURSING CARE

Assessment

Assess the patient's physiologic status by taking vital signs, observing Foley catheter and wound drainage for color and amount, monitoring any intravenous fluid intake, and checking the site for signs of infection and inflammation. Assess for signs of complications specific to the surgery, such as hemorrhage, infection, and penile erosion. Also observe for development of any problem that may be associated with the effects of having general anesthesia, as described in Chapter 6. Assess for pain. Determine its type, location, and intensity. Observe for swelling in the operative area and surrounding tissue. With removal of the Foley catheter, determine the patient's ability to initiate urination and empty his bladder. Throughout the postoperative period, assess the patient's emotional state and his reactions to the change in the body image.

Nursing Diagnoses and Planning

Nursing diagnoses and related expected patient outcomes commonly applicable to patients who have undergone implantation of a penile prosthesis include the following:

NDx: Pain related to surgical trauma

Planning: Patient Outcomes
1. Patient asks for and accepts pain medication.
2. Patient keeps ice pack applications in place as ordered.

3. Patient states he has less discomfort in the penile and scrotal areas.
4. Patient moves more easily.

NDx: Risk for infection related to presence of a surgical wound

Planning: Patient Outcomes

1. Patient's temperature is within normal limits.
2. Wound drainage is free of pus and foul odor.

NDx: Risk for body image disturbance related to penile surgery

Planning: Patient Outcomes

1. Patient looks at penis and scrotum.
2. Patient is willing to discuss the prosthesis and its care.
3. Patient assumes self-care activities.

NDx: Risk for urinary retention related to swelling around the urethra

Planning: Patient Outcomes

1. Patient voids continently, 90 to 120 mL per voiding, within 8 hours after the Foley catheter is removed.
2. Complaints of urgency, dysuria, bladder fullness, or suprapubic discomfort are absent.
3. Urinary bladder is free of distention.

NDx: Risk for altered health maintenance related to insufficient knowledge of self-care activities after discharge

Planning: Patient Outcomes

1. Patient lists signs and symptoms that should be reported to the physician.
2. Patient describes restrictions on activity.
3. Patient describes care of the wound.
4. Patient states the name of prescribed antibiotic, expected effects, and the dose, route, and frequency of administration.
5. Patient states when he may resume sexual intercourse.
6. Patient describes when he should inflate and deflate the prosthesis (if applicable).
7. Patient demonstrates the method of repositioning the pump in the scrotal sac (if applicable).
8. Patient states the date of his follow-up visit.

Nursing Interventions and Evaluation

NDx: Pain

Remind the patient that medication has been ordered for his pain. Give analgesics according to the physician's order. Apply ice packs to the penile and scrotal areas as ordered to ease discomfort and minimize edema formation. Avoid tissue ischemia by applying the ice packs for 30 minutes and then removing them for 1 hour to allow the tissues of the penis and scrotum to recover. Repeat this schedule for the time period ordered. Provide an egg-crate pad or flotation pad for the patient to sit on when he is in a chair, or when his bed is in high Fowler's position, to minimize pressure on the penis and scrotum. Use a bed cradle to keep the weight of the bed linens off the patient's penis.

NDx: Risk for infection

Instruct and assist the patient as needed to cleanse the perineal area after each bowel movement to avoid fecal contamination of the wound. Also change linen and the dressing if it is soiled with urine, because moisture increases the chance of infection.

If a Jackson-Pratt or similar wound drainage system is in place, ensure that the tube is free of kinks and is properly secured to the patient's dressing. Maintain the patency of the wound drainage system because accumulated blood and body fluid provide a good medium for growth of microorganisms.

After the Foley catheter is removed, encourage the patient to wash his hands thoroughly before each voiding to decrease the risk of wound contamination with pathogens. Administer antibiotics as ordered for prophylaxis and monitor for side effects.

NDx: Risk for body image disturbance

Remind the patient with an inflatable prosthesis that his penis will have a normal appearance once the swelling has subsided. In the case of the noninflatable implant, remind the patient that, even after the edema disappears, his penis will always be in an erect or semierect state depending on the type of prosthesis. Reassure him, however, that the prosthesis can be concealed by wearing the correct clothing. For example, explain to the patient with the rigid type of implant that wearing snug-fitting jockey shorts, with his penis placed up against his abdomen, and loose trousers will help conceal his semierect penis.

Provide for privacy when carrying out any intervention that requires exposure of the patient's genital area (such as Foley catheter care or emptying the wound drainage system). Suggest that the patient look at his penis during dressing changes. Also encourage him to maintain his personal appearance by shaving, wearing his own pajamas, and combing his hair. Urge the patient to discuss any negative feelings he may have with his sexual partner. Assist in the patient's and partner's adjustment to the image change by listening, facilitating their expressions of concern, and responding clearly to their questions.

NDx: Risk for urinary retention

Allow the patient to stand to void for optimal relaxation of the external urinary sphincter and perineal muscles. Provide for adequate fluid intake to facilitate the desire to void. Encourage voiding within 2 to 3 hours after catheter removal and, if voiding occurs, note the color of the urine. Measure and record the amount. If less than 50 mL is voided, suspect urinary retention with overflow, and notify the physician.

If the patient cannot void after 8 hours, review his fluid intake for this time period, and palpate the suprapubic area for bladder distention. Inform the

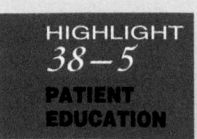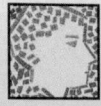

HIGHLIGHT 38–5
PATIENT EDUCATION

Discharge Instructions After Penile Implant Surgery

Instruct the patient to:

Clean the wound daily by washing gently with soap and warm water. Use sitz baths if ordered.

Take prescribed antibiotics on time and until gone.

Avoid strenuous physical activity, such as jogging, lifting, or contact sports, for about 3 weeks while a fibrous sheath is forming around the cylinders.

If you have an inflatable prosthesis, practice inflating and deflating it daily for 2 weeks when directed to do so. This promotes formation of fibrous tissue around the implant.

Promptly report any breakdown of skin around the implant, persistent or intensified penile pain, and—if the prosthesis is inflatable—inability to pull the pump to the lowest part of the scrotum, scrotal pain, drainage from the penis or scrotum, and fever higher than 37.7°C (100°F).

Return for a follow-up visit on *(specify date and time)*.

physician that the patient has not voided. A decision as to whether he needs to be catheterized immediately will depend on the presence of discomfort, bladder distention, and amount of fluid intake. If the patient is not catheterized, measures to promote urination should continue to be implemented, such as standing to void and running water in the sink.

NDx: Risk for altered health maintenance
Instruct the patient in appropriate self-care after discharge (Highlight 38–5).

Compare the patient's status with the expected outcomes. If the outcomes are not met, reassess the patient and revise the plan.

❖ Settings, Providers, and Collaboration for Care

The patient with a problem of the male reproductive system may receive care in a variety of settings depending on the complexity of the disorder. In a managed-care setting, the primary physician or nurse practitioner is often the first to note a problem and is responsible for referring the patient to either a urologist or a general surgeon for definitive diag-

nosis and treatment. The location of diagnostic testing varies with the type of study ordered. For example, sequential bacteriologic localization cultures are usually obtained in the urologist's office or urology clinic, whereas a urethrocystoscopy is often performed in an ambulatory surgical unit.

Surgery of the male reproductive system is carried out in an outpatient unit of a hospital, a freestanding surgical center, or in an operating room of an acute care facility. Where the surgery is performed is dependent on a number of factors, including the diagnosis, extent of surgery planned, degree of risk involved, and the presence of coexisting medical problems.

In many surgical procedures of the male reproductive system, the patient is admitted and discharged the day of surgery (see Table 38–4). Regardless of the length of stay for the patient, most patients report to the surgical unit the day of surgery. The preoperative assessment is usually performed within a week of the planned procedure. This assessment requires the collaborative effort of a variety of health-care team members, such as the anesthesiologist or nurse anesthetist, the nurse, and the laboratory technician, to ensure the patient's safe, uneventful postoperative recovery. The nurse, as part of this multidisciplinary team, completes a nursing assessment and implements a teaching plan. On the day of surgery, the nurse reviews the patient's record and collaborates with the other members of the team as needed.

Before discharge, the nurse assesses the patient's need for any home health-care services. Such services may include one or more visits from a community health nurse, home health aide, or an infusion therapist. In the home, the nurse is usually the primary collaborator, coordinating all the home health care that the patient is receiving.

Depending on the nature of the problem, the patient may also require a referral to a sex therapist or counselor, to a nutritionist, to a support group, or to community services such as the Cancer Society or Meals on Wheels.

The Elderly: Special Considerations

Beginning at about age 50, the male reproductive system begins to undergo age-related changes. There is a very gradual reduction in production of testosterone and sperm. The size and firmness of the testes diminish because of a degenerative process within the seminiferous tubules and a decrease in the number of interstitial cells. Despite these changes, however, a man's ability to procreate continues, although fertilization of an ovum is less frequent because of fewer viable sperm.

Other organs of the male reproductive system also change with advancing age. The elasticity of the skin surrounding the scrotum decreases considerably. This leads to increased relaxation, folding, and sagging of the scrotal tissue and reduced scrotal vasocongestion in response to sexual tensions.

At about age 50, the prostate gland undergoes atrophic changes with an increase in connective tissue, collagen, and smooth muscle fibers, and a decrease in its vascular supply. Prostatic secretions may become calcified (Mikkelsen, 1995). Prostatic enlargement is found in three-fourths of men age 65 and older. The exact cause of this benign prostate enlargement remains unclear.

With aging, the penis becomes smaller and its tissue and blood vessels undergo hardening and lose elasticity. Because an erection depends on blood supply to the penis, vascular sclerosis results in decreased speed and firmness of erection. Thus, as a normal effect of aging, an occasional inability to have an erection may occur. If a consistent impotent state develops in the older male, it is usually secondary to chronic illness such as diabetes mellitus or hypertension or to drug therapy.

No event analogous to menopause occurs in the male reproductive system; that is, there is no specific point in time when the male becomes unable to reproduce. Nonetheless, some middle-aged men experience symptoms typically associated with menopause and are said to have male climacteric syndrome. These symptoms include insomnia, irritability, listlessness, impaired ability to concentrate, depression, and fatigue. Although in some cases a relationship between male climacteric syndrome and a consistently low (less than 300 ng) serum testosterone level has been found, it appears that psychologic factors play a significant role in its development.

There are many potential psychological contributing factors. Prime among them are changes in sexual response cycle. Decreasing speed of erection and the difficulty some men have in maintaining an erection can lead to disturbing fears of reduced sexual performance. In fact, it appears that previously monogamous men may engage in extramarital affairs seeking to reaffirm their virility at this time. Added to this is career crisis, which many men experience simultaneously. They may be excluded from promotions, feel they are seen as inflexible and out of step, and realize that their career goals may never be attained. This can cause feelings of failure and may lead to depression and further a weakened self-esteem.

Management of male climacteric syndrome focuses primarily on psychosocial support (Levy, 1994) with a possible referral for psychotherapy, if needed. Although hypogonadism affects less than 4% of the older male population, androgen therapy may be prescribed if its decrease is suspected as the cause of male climacteric syndrome. In these cases, replacement therapy—such as testosterone enanthate or testosterone cypionate, 50 to 400 mg intramuscularly every 2 to 4 weeks—may be ordered. With this treatment, remission of symptoms should occur within 2 to 3 months. The use of testosterone therapy is contraindicated in patients with coronary artery, liver, or renal disease, and in those with an enlarged prostate gland or prostatic cancer.

Chapter Review

1. Why is it important to ask the male patient to void before he undergoes a pelvic examination?
2. What is the meaning of an elevated PSA in the patient with prostate cancer?
3. What evidence supports the therapeutic effect of applying ice packs to the scrotum as part of the postoperative nursing care for the patient with an inflatable penile implant?
4. How do you think a patient would react if informed that he must have his prostate gland removed?
5. What is the meaning of a significant elevation in blood pressure, decreased pulse rate, confusion, and muscle twitching when seen in a patient in the early postoperative period after transurethral resection of the prostate?
6. What are some nursing interventions for the patient who has undergone transurethral resection of the prostate and who has a nursing diagnosis of risk for urinary retention related to Foley catheter removal?
7. Why are long periods of sitting contraindicated for a patient recovering from a prostatectomy?
8. What evidence supports the therapeutic effect of administering a bellodonna and opium suppository as part of the nursing care plan for the patient who has undergone transurethral resection of the prostate?
9. How is the postoperative nursing care of the patient with a simple retropubic prostatectomy different from that of the patient recovering from a transurethral resection of the prostate?
10. Why is the confused elderly patient at increased risk for postoperative complications when surgery is performed on the male reproductive system?

Bibliography

Ackerman MD, Montague DK, Morganstern S. Impotence: Help for erectile dysfunction. Patient Care 1994; 28(5):22.

Beers M. Male hypogonadism and impotence. In Abrams W et al (eds). The Merck manual of geriatrics. 2nd ed. Whitehouse Station, NJ: Merck & Co, 1995, p 839.

Bruskewitz R, Wasson J. Disorders of the lower genitourinary tract: Bladder, prostate, and testicles. In Abrams W et al (eds).

The Merck manual of geriatrics. 2nd ed. Whitehouse Station, NJ: Merck & Co, 1995, p 785.

Carpenito LJ. Handbook of nursing diagnosis. 6th ed. Philadelphia, JB Lippincott, 1995.

Carpenito LJ. Nursing diagnosis: Application to clinical practice. 6th ed. Philadelphia: JB Lippincott, 1995.

Carter HB. Instrumentation and endoscopy. In Walsh PC, Retik AB, Stamey TA, Vaughan ED (eds). Campbell's urology. 6th ed. Philadelphia: WB Saunders, 1992, p 331.

Cohen S, Gittes RRS. Patient assessment: Examination of the male genitalia. Am J Nurs 1979; 74(4):694, 711.

Cupp MR, Osterling JE. Prostate-specific antigen, digital rectal examination and transrectal ultrasonography: Their roles in diagnosing early prostate cancer. Mayo Clin Proceeds 1993; 68(3):297.

Djavan B, Roehrborn CG. Prostate specific antigen: When to measure it. How to interpret results. Consultant 1994; 34(6):909.

Eliopoulos C. Gerontological nursing. 3rd ed. Philadelphia, JB Lippincott, 1993.

Eliopoulos C. Manual of gerontologic nursing. St. Louis: Mosby–Year Book, 1995.

Fishbach FT. A manual of laboratory diagnostic tests. 5th ed. Philadelphia: JB Lippincott, 1995.

Goldstein M. Surgery of male infertility and other scrotal disorders. In Walsh PC, Retik AB, Stamey TA, Vaughan ED (eds). Campbell's urology. 6th ed. Philadelphia: WB Saunders, 1992, p 3114.

Goluboff ET, Chang DT, Olsson CA, Kaplan SA. Urodynamics and the etiology of post-prostatectomy urinary incontinence: The initial Columbia experience. J Urol 1995; 153(3Pt2):1034.

Gray M, Dobkin K. Genitourinary system. In Thompson JL et al (eds). Clinical nursing. 3rd ed. St. Louis: CV Mosby, 1993, p 957.

Greene D, Shabsigh R, Scardino P. Urologic ultrasonography. In Walsh PC, Retik AB, Stamey TA, Vaughan ED (eds). Campbell's urology. 6th ed. Philadelphia: WB Saunders, 1992, p 342.

Guyton AC, Hall J. Textbook of medical physiology. 9th ed. Philadelphia, WB Saunders, 1996.

Johnson B. Sexuality and aging. In Stanley M, Beare PG. Gerontological nursing. Philadelphia: FA Davis, 1995, p 426.

Kendal AR. Treatment of benign prostate hyperplasia. In Seidman EJ, Hanno PM (eds). Current urologic therapy. 3rd ed. Philadelphia: WB Saunders, 1994, 370–374.

Levy J. Sexuality and aging. In Hazzard WR, et al (eds). Principles of geriatric medicine and gerontology. 3rd ed. New York: McGraw-Hill, 1994, pp 115–122.

Lowe FC, Brendler CB. Evaluation of the urologic patient: History, physical examination, and urinalysis. In Walsh PC, Retik AB, Stamey TA, Vaughan ED (eds). Campbell's urology. 6th ed. Philadelphia: WB Saunders, 1992, p 307.

Lue TF. Physiology of erection and pathophysiology of impotence. In Walsh PC, Retik AB, Stamey TA, Vaughan ED (eds). Campbell's urology. 6th ed. Philadelphia: WB Saunders, 1992, p 709.

Matsumoto A. The testis. In Bennett JC, Plum F (eds). Cecil textbook of medicine. 20th ed. Philadelphia: WB Saunders, 1996, p 1325.

Mebust WK. Transurethral surgery. In Walsh PC, Retik AB, Stamey TA, Vaughan ED (eds). Campbell's urology. 6th ed. Philadelphia: WB Saunders, 1992, p 2900.

Meacham R, Murray M. Reproductive function in the aging male. Urol Clin North Am 1994; 21(August):549.

Mikkelsen D. Structure and function of the male genitourinary system. In Copstead LE (ed). Perspectives on pathophysiology. Philadelphia: WB Saunders, 1995, p 612.

National Cancer Institute. Testicular self-examination. (National Institutes of Health Publication No. 92-2636.) Washington, DC: U.S. Department of Health and Human Services, 1992.

O'Keefe M, Hunt DK. Assessment and treatment of impotence. Med Clin North Am 1995; 79(2):415.

Pagana K, Pagana TJ. Mosby's diagnostic and laboratory test reference. 2nd ed. St. Louis: Mosby–Year Book, 1995.

Paulson DF. Perineal prostatectomy. In Walsh PC, Retik AB, Stamey TA, Vaughan ED (eds). Campbell's urology. 6th ed. Philadelphia: WB Saunders, 1992, pp. 2887–2899.

Presti JC, Stoller ML, Carroll PR. Urology. In Tierney LM, McPhee SJ, Papadakis MA (eds). Current medical diagnosis and treatment 1997. 36th ed. Stamford, CT: Appleton and Lange, 1997, pp 854–891.

Seeley T, Stephens T, Tate P. Anatomy and physiology. 3rd ed. St. Louis: Mosby–Year Book 1995.

Sigman M, Howards SS. Male infertility. In Walsh, PC, Retik AB, Stamey TA, Vaughan ED (eds). Campbell's urology. 6th ed. Philadelphia: WB Saunders, 1992, p 661.

Stamey TA, McNeal JE. Adenocarcinoma of the prostate. In Walsh PC, Retik AB, Stamey TA, Vaughan ED (eds). Campbell's urology. 6th ed. Philadelphia: WB Saunders, 1992, p 1159.

Stamm W, Turch M. Urinary tract infections and pyelonephritis. In Isselbacher K et al (eds). Harrison's principles of internal medicine. 13th ed. New York: McGraw-Hill, 1994, p 548.

Steinberg G, Brendler CB. Diseases of the prostate. In Bennett JC, Plum F (eds). Cecil textbook of medicine. 20th ed. Philadelphia: WB Saunders, 1996, p 1341.

Stewart S. Structure and function of the male genitourinary system. In Porth CM (ed). Pathophysiology. 4th ed. Philadelphia: JB Lippincott, 1994, p 727.

Stutzman RE, Walsh PC. Suprapubic and retropubic prostatectomy. In Walsh PC, Retik AB, Stamey TA, Vaughan ED (eds.) Campbell's urology. 6th ed. Philadelphia: WB Saunders, 1992, p 2851.

U.S. Department of Health and Human Services. Clinical Practice Guidelines. Benign prostatic hyperplasia: Diagnosis and treatment. Pub No. 94-0582. Rockville, MD: Public Health Service, 1994.

U.S. Department of Health and Human Services. Patient Guide: Treating your enlarged prostate: Pub No. 94-0584. Rockville, MD: Public Health Service, 1994.

Walsh PC. Radical retropubic prostatectomy. In Walsh PC, Retik AB, Stamey TA, Vaughan ED (eds). Campbell's urology. 6th ed. Philadelphia: WB Saunders, 1992, p 2865.

Watson J, Jaffe M. Nurse's manual of laboratory and diagnostic tests. 2nd ed. Philadelphia: F.A. Davis, 1995.

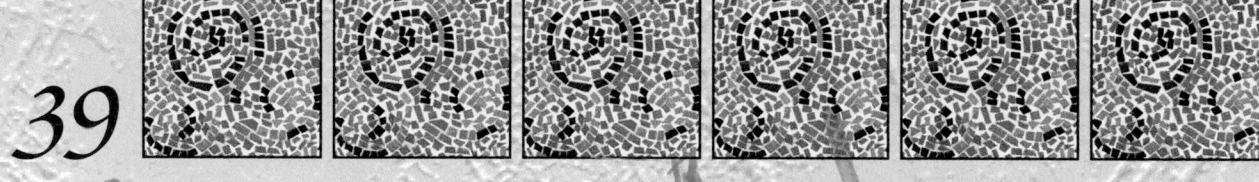

Nursing Care of Men with Reproductive Disorders

Study Outcomes

After studying this chapter, you should be able to:

1. Describe the etiology, pathophysiology, clinical manifestations, diagnostic procedures, and management of common disorders of the male reproductive system.
2. Identify information and physical examination data essential to the assessment of men with common reproductive disorders.
3. State nursing diagnoses and related expected patient outcomes commonly applicable to men with reproductive disorders.
4. Describe nursing interventions, with their rationales, commonly applicable to men with common reproductive disorders.
5. Explain the basis for evaluation of nursing care provided to men with common reproductive disorders.
6. Identify alternative treatment and care settings for men with reproductive disorders and the services related to community-based care.
7. Identify special considerations for the elderly man with a reproductive disorder.

The male reproductive system can be affected by a wide variety of disorders, acute and chronic. They range in severity from minor to life-threatening. Regardless of the prognosis, however, each of the disorders has the potential to exert a profound effect on the patient because of its relationship to sexuality and reproductive capacity. Thus, sensitivity to the psychosocial dimension of patient care is particularly critical when caring for men with reproductive disorders.

Men with disorders of the reproductive system receive care in a variety of settings depending on the severity of the condition. These settings might include the physician's office, an ambulatory surgical site, acute inpatient hospitalization, and long-term and home health care.

*I*nfections and Inflammations

BALANOPOSTHITIS

Balanoposthitis refers to the coexistence of two inflammatory conditions: balanitis and posthitis. Balanitis is an acute or chronic inflammation of the glans penis. Posthitis is an inflammatory process involving the prepuce (foreskin).

Etiology and Pathophysiology

Inflammation of the glans penis and prepuce is usually caused by the combined factors of accumulating smegma, glandular secretions, desquamating cells, and the invasion of a microorganism under the foreskin. Infecting organisms include *Streptococcus*, *Staphylococcus*, coliform bacillus, and those that are sexually transmitted (eg, *Candida albicans*, chlamydia, and the herpes simplex virus).

In some cases, balanoposthitis may be a manifestation of a pre-existing disease, such as diabetes mellitus, or a complication associated with the use of a Foley catheter or external condom catheter.

A major factor in the development of balanoposthitis is poor personal hygiene in the uncircumcised male who fails to retract his foreskin regularly. The warm, moist environment of the space between the glans and foreskin (preputial sac) provides a good culture medium for growth of microorganisms.

Clinical Manifestations

Symptoms of balanoposthitis usually begin within 2 to 3 days after exposure to the infecting organism. Initially, the patient complains of itching and soreness of the glans and prepuce. These symptoms are followed by pain, discharge, local edema, difficulty retracting the foreskin, redness, and a burning sensation when voiding. As the condition progresses, superficial ulcers form on the surface of the glans. Systemic effects, such as fever and malaise, may also develop. If the infection remains untreated, the edema increases, the primary ulcer continues to erode penile tissue, and new ulcers extend up the shaft of the penis. Finally, the entire penis and sometimes the scrotum can become gangrenous and necrotic.

Diagnosis

The diagnosis is based on inspection and palpation of the penis. A culture and a Gram stain of the drainage can identify the infecting organism.

Management

Medical treatment of balanoposthitis depends on the cause. If the culture report is positive, oral antibiotic therapy appropriate for the infecting organism is ordered. In the presence of candidiasis or another fungal infection, an antifungal agent such as nystatin ointment (Mycostatin) or powder is prescribed. An analgesic, such as acetaminophen (Tylenol) or a combination of oxycodone hydrochloride and acetaminophen (Percocet), may be ordered to control pain.

Local therapy for balanoposthitis includes retracting the foreskin (if possible), cleansing the glans with mild or antibacterial soap and water, returning the foreskin over the glans, and applying warm water or saline soaks. The frequency and duration of this treatment depend on the severity of the infection.

If the foreskin cannot be retracted, a warm saline irrigation of the subpreputial area may be ordered. If the infection is severe, a dorsal slit may be made in the foreskin. After the infection has resolved, a circumcision may be recommended to prevent a recurrence.

NURSING PROCESS
Balanoposthitis

Assessment

Ask the patient about symptoms experienced, their duration, and any self-care measures used. Also determine the patient's genital hygiene and sexual practices, including the time of last sexual contact. Inspect the penis for irritation, redness, edema, discharge, and ulceration. If a Foley catheter or external catheter is in place, question its continued use.

Nursing Diagnoses and Planning

Nursing diagnoses and related expected patient outcomes commonly applicable to patients with balanoposthitis include the following:

NDx: Pain related to inflammation of the penis

Planning: Patient Outcomes
1. Patient reports that itching, pain, and soreness have decreased or disappeared.
2. Patient voids without discomfort.

NDx: Risk for altered health maintenance related to insufficient knowledge of prescribed treatment and prevention of recurrence

Planning: Patient Outcomes
1. Patient describes or demonstrates the procedure for applying warm soaks to his penis.
2. Patient states the name, expected effects, dose, route, and frequency of the prescribed medication.
3. Patient describes the role of proper penile hygiene in preventing a recurrence.
4. Patient demonstrates proper cleaning of the penis.
5. Patient states the frequency with which the penis should be cleaned.

Nursing Interventions and Evaluation

NDx: Pain
Wearing examination gloves, assist or instruct the patient in retracting his foreskin and cleaning the glans. Using soap and warm water, clean the glans from the tip down the penile shaft to avoid spreading the infection up the urethra, rinse well, and return the foreskin to its original position. After cleaning, apply warm soaks (gauze pads or a clean face cloth soaked in warm water or saline) for 20 minutes. Change the soaks frequently during this time to maintain constant warmth and achieve vasodilation, increased local circulation, and relief of inflammation. On completion of the soaks, dry the penis thoroughly because moisture can macerate the skin, which predisposes to growth of pathogens. Do not reapply an external condom catheter until the infection resolves. Administer or instruct the patient in the use of analgesics as ordered.

NDx: Risk for altered health maintenance
Briefly explain the action of the prescribed antibiotic or anti-infective medication. Review with the patient its dose, frequency, and side effects. If the route of administration is topical, such as with an ointment or a powder, be sure to describe or demonstrate the correct application. If possible, ask the patient to give a return demonstration.

Instruct the patient in daily penile hygiene to prevent a recurrence, as specified in Highlight 39–1. Some patients, especially the elderly, may need a referral to a community health agency for visiting nurse and home health aide services.

Compare the patient's status with the expected outcomes. If the outcomes are not met, reassess the patient and revise the plan.

EPIDIDYMITIS

Epididymitis is an inflammation or infection of the epididymis. It is the most common of all intrascrotal problems. It affects an estimated 600,000 men in the United States each year.

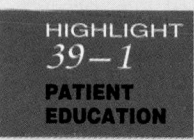 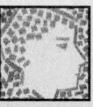

HIGHLIGHT
39—1
**PATIENT
EDUCATION**

Preventing Recurrent Balanoposthitis

Instruct the patient to clean the penis daily as follows:

Retract the foreskin.

Wash the penis from the tip to the base using soap and warm water.

Rinse the penis well because soap residue supports bacterial growth and can irritate the skin.

Dry the penis thoroughly because moisture can lead to maceration, which also supports bacterial growth.

Pull the foreskin back down over the glans.

Etiology and Pathophysiology

Epididymitis, which is usually unilateral, is most often caused by an infection originating in either the prostate gland or the urinary tract that spreads to the prostate via the vas deferens. Because urinary tract infection commonly occurs after urologic procedures such as catheterization and cystoscopy, epididymitis is considered a complication of these procedures. Infecting organisms include *Streptococcus, Staphylococcus, Escherichia coli*, and *Pseudomonas*. In sexually active men, *Chlamydia trachomatis* and *Neisseria gonorrhoeae* are common causes of epididymitis. Epididymitis caused by the cytomegalovirus has been seen in immunocompromised patients after renal transplantation. In addition, a traumatic type of epididymitis may occur 3 to 4 weeks after a difficult vasectomy. Occasionally, epididymitis develops from an infection elsewhere in the body, such as pneumococcal pneumonia or tuberculosis. In these cases, the infecting organism reaches the epididymis via the lymphatic vessels or blood.

In the acute phase of epididymitis, inflammation and swelling usually begin in the tail (cauda epididymis) and then extend to involve the rest of the epididymis. The entire scrotal sac containing the infected epididymis becomes a single, erythematous, painful mass often accompanied by the formation of a hydrocele (a collection of clear fluid in the tunica vaginalis). Acute epididymitis may become somewhat chronic, continuing for several weeks and possibly resulting in peritubular fibrosis and occlusion of the epididymis. Often, however, the infection resolves and the epididymis returns to normal after several months.

Complications of epididymitis include orchitis, which is most common, abscess formation, hydro-

cele, and sterility. Sterility is more likely to occur with chronic bilateral epididymitis. Recurrence tends to occur when the underlying disease process (eg, recurrent urinary tract infection) remains unresolved.

Clinical Manifestations

Symptoms of epididymitis include severe pain and tenderness in the groin and scrotum on the affected side, nausea, vomiting, and fever. To avoid pressure on the groin and scrotum, the patient usually walks with a characteristic "duck waddle." He may also have symptoms of urinary tract infection, including dysuria, frequency, pyuria, and urgency.

Diagnosis

The diagnosis is based on physical findings and laboratory analyses. On inspection, the scrotum is red and edematous. The epididymis feels thickened and enlarged when palpated. The white blood cell count is usually elevated to between 20,000 and 30,000. Cultures of urine and urethral and prostatic secretions help to identify a causative organism.

If torsion of the spermatic cord (twisting of the cord) is suspected, a Doppler ultrasound study of the scrotum is done. Good blood flow to the scrotum rules out torsion.

Management

Management of epididymitis includes bedrest, usually for 3 to 5 days, elevation of the scrotum, application of ice packs, analgesics, antipyretics, antiemetics, and nonsteroidal anti-inflammatory agents. Pending the results of Gram's stains and cultures, a broad-spectrum oral antibiotic, such as tetracycline or ciprofloxacin, is prescribed. In severe cases, combination intravenous antibiotics (eg, ampicillin and gentamicin) may be necessary. Antibiotic therapy is adjusted as needed when sensitivity studies are complete. If epididymitis becomes chronic, long-term low-dose trimethoprim and sulfamethoxazole may be prescribed.

External heat is usually not prescribed because of its possible adverse effect on spermatogenesis. An epididymectomy (removal of the epididymis) may be performed if the infection is refractory to antibiotic therapy or recurs.

See Chapter 43 for the management of patients with a sexually transmitted disease caused by *N. gonorrhoeae* or *C. trachomatis*.

NURSING PROCESS
Epididymitis

Assessment

Ask the patient about the onset, degree, and duration of scrotal pain. Also ask about symptoms indicative of a urinary tract infection, such as frequency and burning on urination. Inspect the scrotal area for heat, redness, and edema. Observe the patient's gait for the characteristic duck waddle. Obtain an oral or tympanic temperature.

Once the diagnosis is made, assess the patient's understanding of the infection and its cause, expected course, and treatment. Explore his concerns and feelings about the diagnosis and its effects on sexual function.

Nursing Diagnoses and Planning

Nursing diagnoses and related expected patient outcomes commonly applicable to patients with epididymitis include the following:

NDx: Pain (scrotal) related to the inflammatory/infectious process

Planning: Patient Outcomes

1. Patient states that pain is diminished or absent.
2. Patient can move in bed and walk without discomfort.

NDx: Hyperthermia related to infection

Planning: Patient Outcomes

1. Patient's temperature is reduced or returned to normal range.
2. Patient's daily fluid intake is at least 3000 mL (unless contraindicated).
3. Oral mucous membranes are moist.

NDx: Fear related to possible development of sterility as a complication

Planning: Patient Outcomes

1. Patient discusses his concerns that he may become sterile.
2. Patient asks questions about his chances of becoming sterile.
3. Patient describes the importance of preventing recurrences of epididymitis.

NDx: Risk for altered health maintenance related to insufficient knowledge of cause of infection, treatment, self-care activities, and prevention of a recurrence

Planning: Patient Outcomes

1. Patient states the cause of his infection.
2. Patient describes local treatments, including their frequency and rationale.
3. Patient explains antibiotic therapy, including the dose, frequency, and side effects.
4. Patient maintains scrotal elevation at all times.
5. Patient describes self-care activities.
6. Patient describes measures to prevent recurrences.

Nursing Interventions and Evaluation

NDx: Pain

Administer or instruct the patient on the use of the analgesic according to the physician's order. Inform the patient that he should ask for the medication or take it when he begins to experience discomfort. Explain that the drug's effectiveness in controlling pain is greatest when it is given early in the pain cycle. Because vomiting can increase the patient's

Table 39–1

How to Build a Bellevue Bridge

Wash and thoroughly dry the patient's upper thighs, groin, penis, and scrotum.

Shave the anterior upper thighs.

Apply a skin preparation such as tincture of benzoin to shaved areas.

Apply one strip of wide (3 to 6 in.), nonallergenic tape under the scrotum and on both thighs.

Apply a second strip of tape, of the same length and width, adhesive side down, on top of the first strip.

Place several 4 × 3 in. gauze sponges under the scrotum and resting on the adhesive strips. If the scrotum is very edematous, a folded, smooth towel may be used in place of the gauze sponges.

local and general discomfort, give or instruct the patient on the use of an antiemetic that is prescribed for nausea.

Elevate the scrotum to promote drainage of fluid and relief of edema and its associated discomfort. While the patient is on bedrest, elevate the scrotum by applying a Bellevue bridge as described in Table 39–1 and depicted in Figure 39–1. An alternative method of elevating the scrotum is to place a rolled towel under it while the patient is on bedrest. However, this is usually only a temporary measure, because the towel is not supported with tape and can easily be displaced with any movement. When the patient is out of bed, instruct him to wear an athletic or scrotal support until the edema subsides.

Instruct the patient in applying ice packs—using a commercial cold pack, ice bag, or examination glove filled with ice—to the scrotum as ordered to reduce edema and discomfort. Emphasize the importance of covering the cold pack with a towel to absorb moisture and prevent skin maceration. Also explain the need to remove the pack after 30 minutes to avoid tissue ischemia and to leave it off for 1 hour to allow the scrotal tissue to recover. Remind

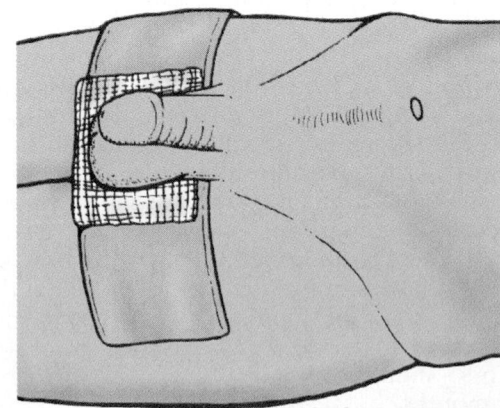

Figure 39–1

Bellevue bridge.

the patient to repeat this schedule for the time period ordered.

NDx: Hyperthermia

Instruct the patient to take his temperature every 4 hours and to take antipyretics as prescribed. Acetaminophen (Tylenol), 650 mg orally every 4 hours, is commonly prescribed for an oral temperature of 38.3°C (101°F) or higher. Cool bed baths may be suggested to help reduce temperature by promoting convection and evaporation. Instructions should also include drinking at least 3 L of fluids daily (unless contraindicated) to replace fluid lost through diaphoresis and increased metabolism.

Instruct the patient to brush his teeth, gargle, and rinse with non-drying mouthwash at least four times daily to help restore moisture to the oral mucous membranes. Also apply petroleum jelly to prevent the lips from drying and cracking. If bed linen and clothing become damp from diaphoresis, explain the need to change them to promote comfort and heat loss.

NDx: Fear

Encourage the patient to ask questions and verbalize any concerns about the effect of the infection on his fertility. Clarify any misconceptions. For example, some men worry that the infection will cause erectile dysfunction. Inform the patient that sterility is usually a complication of bilateral epididymitis and may develop with recurrences of the infection. Stress the importance of preventing this recurrence.

If infertility is suspected as a complication, referral to a sex therapist or counselor may be necessary.

NDx: Risk for altered health maintenance

Explain the cause of epididymitis using a simple anatomic illustration of the reproductive system to facilitate understanding. Explain the need for bedrest, the use of cold packs and scrotal support to prevent further edema and relieve discomfort, and the reason for antibiotic therapy. If the patient requires hospitalization, stress the importance of taking the medication after discharge, if ordered. Review dose, frequency, and side effects to be reported. If the epididymitis is caused by an organism transmitted through sexual contact, advise the patient to avoid sexual intercourse until the partner or partners have been examined and treated, if needed, to decrease the risk of reinfection.

Provide information on measures to prevent the recurrence of epididymitis. These measures include maintaining a daily fluid intake of at least 3000 mL, emptying the bladder frequently, and, if epididymitis is associated with prostatitis, engaging in sexual activity or masturbation to provide periodic release of prostate secretions. Emphasize that, regardless of the cause, early diagnosis and treatment of any infection of the genitourinary tract are essential.

Compare the patient's status with the expected outcomes. If the outcomes are not met, reassess the patient and revise the plan.

ORCHITIS

Orchitis is an acute infection or inflammation of one or both of the testes.

Etiology and Pathophysiology

Orchitis rarely occurs as a primary infection. Most often orchitis results from ascending infection from the epididymis (epididymo-orchitis). Occasionally it results from spread through the blood or lymphatic vessels, from another part of the body. An example of the latter is infection secondary to mumps.

Occasionally, orchitis follows trauma to the scrotal area or develops after a vasectomy or other genitourinary surgery. This traumatic or granulomatous orchitis is considered to be an infectious process resulting from a lowered resistance of the injured tissue to bacteria.

In cases of epididymo-orchitis, the testis is tense, swollen, and bluish, with many punctate hemorrhages on the surface and multiple foci of necrosis. This process progresses occasionally to suppuration involving the whole testis and then abscess formation. It is usually associated with an acute hydrocele, which may become a pyocele (collection of pus in the tunica vaginalis) if the abscess ruptures. Secondary atrophy and sterility from fibrosis and destruction of the tubules and ductal system are frequent sequelae if both testes are involved.

The onset of mumps orchitis usually occurs 4 to 6 days after the appearance of parotitis (inflammation of the parotid glands) and, in approximately 70% of the cases, is unilateral. Some degree of atrophy and reduced spermatogenesis develop in the involved testis in about half of affected men. In cases of bilateral orchitis with significant testicular atrophy, sterility usually occurs.

Clinical Manifestations

The signs and symptoms of bacterial and mumps orchitis are generally the same. Both begin with a high temperature, chills, and sudden pain in the involved testis that radiates to the inguinal area, often accompanied by nausea and vomiting. After 48 hours, the testis is usually hot, red, tender, and obviously swollen. The scrotal skin may also be red and edematous.

Clinical manifestations of traumatic orchitis vary widely. Some men experience the symptoms just described. Others may complain only of painless intrascrotal edema of several weeks' duration.

Diagnosis

The diagnosis is based primarily on the patient's presenting signs and symptoms, related history, and visual inspection of the area. Palpation of the testis is usually not possible because of its extreme tenderness. It may be difficult to differentiate granulomatous orchitis from a testicular tumor on the basis of physical findings. If a testicular tumor is suspected, the testis is removed and a histologic examination is done to establish a diagnosis. A biopsy of the involved testis is not done because of the great danger of metastatic spread if a malignant neoplasm is present.

Management

Treatment of bacterial orchitis is essentially the same as for epididymitis. To decrease inflammation of the testis and the accompanying edema, bedrest, scrotal elevation, and cold applications are usually ordered. Antibiotic therapy is prescribed according to the specific etiologic organism. Analgesics, antiemetics, antipyretics, and nonsteroidal anti-inflammatory agents are also ordered as needed. If a concomitant hydrocele occurs, fluid may be aspirated to provide symptomatic relief by reducing pressure on the testis. If an abscess develops, an orchiectomy is performed.

Management of mumps orchitis is similar to that of bacterial orchitis. Comfort measures include bedrest, elevation of the scrotum, and cold applications. Occasionally, administration of large doses of a corticosteroid may reduce the pain, but the local findings and clinical course remain unchanged.

In cases of severe mumps orchitis with extensive edema, incision and drainage of the hydrocele may be done to reduce pressure in the tunica. If done within the first 48 hours of acute swelling, it appears that this not only relieves symptoms but also markedly reduces subsequent testicular atrophy.

Because gamma globulin administered in the early stages of parotitis has been reported to decrease the incidence of orchitis, it is given to any postpubertal male who is exposed to mumps and who has neither had the disease nor received the mumps vaccine as a child.

NURSING PROCESS
Orchitis

Assessment

Assessment of the patient with orchitis is similar to that of the patient with epididymitis. Obtain information about the pain, including its onset, location, and intensity. Examine the scrotum for heat, redness, and edema. Take an oral or tympanic temperature.

Ask the patient if he had mumps or if he received the mumps vaccine as a child. If he has not had mumps or the vaccine, determine whether he has been exposed to the disease within the past 3 weeks.

Once the diagnosis is established, assess his understanding of the disease and its treatment, as well as his concerns and feelings about it. Determine how he views its effect on subsequent sexual function.

Nursing Diagnoses and Planning

Nursing diagnoses and related expected patient outcomes commonly applicable to patients with orchitis include those discussed under the care of the patient with epididymitis and, if incision and drainage of the scrotum has been performed, the following:

NDx: Risk for infection related to incision and drainage of the scrotum

Planning: Patient Outcomes
1. The wound is clean.
2. Purulent drainage is absent.

Nursing Interventions and Evaluation

Nursing interventions related to the nursing diagnoses of pain, hyperthermia, fear, and altered health maintenance deficit are similar to those described previously for the care of the patient with epididymitis.

NDx: Risk for infection
If incision and drainage of a hydrocele is performed, a scrotal dressing is usually applied to absorb any fluid that may drain after the procedure. Since short-term hospitalization is usually all that is required for the procedure, the patient or significant other is instructed on wound care before discharge from the same-day surgical day care setting. Explain that the dressing should be changed when wet with drainage because a moist dressing facilitates bacterial contamination of the wound by capillary action. Further, tell the patient that a dressing saturated with drainage also places him at risk for scrotal skin breakdown.

Instructions include how to remove the dressing and the need to observe the wound for redness and for drainage, noting the color, consistency, and amount. Demonstrate gentle cleansing of the wound with sterile water or saline, and explain the importance of removing any drainage, which may serve as a source of irritation if left on the scrotal surface.

Finally, explain how to apply a scrotal support to provide elevation and secure the dressing.

Additional Interventions
Explain the use of corticosteroid therapy, if prescribed. Give instruction on the dose, frequency, and side effects and regarding the importance of taking this medication with milk or food.

For the patient who does not have active immunity against mumps, stress the importance of promptly seeking medical care if exposure occurs. Be sure that the patient understands that he has a 25% chance of acquiring mumps orchitis with exposure. Explain that gamma globulin is usually given at the time of exposure and, although it may not prevent him from acquiring mumps, the disease is likely to be less severe and there is a reduced risk for complications, including sterility.

Compare the patient's status with the expected outcomes. If the outcomes are not met, reassess the patient and revise the plan.

PROSTATITIS

Prostatitis is an inflammation of the prostate gland. Prostatic inflammations are common and are classified as acute bacterial, chronic bacterial, nonbacterial, and prostatodynia.

Etiology and Pathophysiology

Acute bacterial prostatitis is usually caused either by an ascending urethral infection or by bacterial invasion (usually gram-negative) via the blood or lymph.

Chronic bacterial prostatitis may follow an episode of acute bacterial prostatitis or result from prostatic enlargement and obstruction.

Nonbacterial prostatitis is the most common type. It is usually found in young, sexually active men and typically occurs after an episode of nonspecific urethritis.

Prostatodynia refers to the presence of symptoms of prostatitis without physical findings. The etiology of this prostate condition is unknown, but some data indicate that pelvic and perineal muscle spasm and abnormal spasm of the urethral sphincter during voiding contribute to symptomatology.

Further information on the causes and pathophysiology of prostatitis is presented in Table 39–2.

Clinical Manifestations

Symptoms of all types of prostatitis include urgency and frequency of urination, nocturia, dysuria, and dull pain in the perineal and rectal areas. With acute and chronic bacterial prostatitis, urethral discharge, myalgia, and arthralgia also occur. Chills and fever are also prominent manifestations of acute, bacterial disease. Painful ejaculation may occur with nonbacterial prostatitis.

Diagnosis

The diagnosis of acute bacterial prostatitis is based on presenting symptoms, digital rectal examination, and urine cultures of two clean voided urine specimens (first voided and mid-stream).

In acute bacterial prostatitis, the prostate is warm, tender, and swollen on palpation. Pyuria is found on urinalysis. The infecting organism can usually be cultured from the urine. Prostatic fluid studies are not done because massage of the prostate, which is required to obtain the specimen, is painful and could cause bacteremia.

Pus cells in the prostatic fluid smear in a sequential bacteriologic localization study are characteristic of chronic bacterial prostatitis.

The diagnosis of nonbacterial prostatitis is sup-

Table 39–2

Etiology and Pathophysiology of Prostatitis

Type of Prostatitis	Etiology	Pathophysiology
Acute bacterial	*Escherichia coli* (most common), *Klebsiella, Proteus, Streptococcus, Staphylococcus, Pseudomonas, Mycobacterium tuberculosis* Usually caused by ascending urethral infection Often associated with urethral instrumentation or catheterization	Diffuse inflammation with edema and hyperemia involving part or all of the prostate May progress to abscess formation or hemorrhage Complications: Epididymo-orchitis, septicemia, urinary retention
Chronic bacterial	Sequela of acute bacterial prostatitis Complication of prostatic enlargement and obstruction	Inflammatory reaction is less marked and more focal than in acute bacterial prostatitis May progress to fibrosis, scarring, contraction of the vesical neck, and prostatic calculi Complication: Epididymitis
Nonbacterial	Cause: unknown Often occurs in young, sexually active men after an episode of nonspecific urethritis Suggested causes include allergic or autoimmune response, sexually transmitted *Chlamydia* or other unknown pathogen	Similar to chronic bacterial prostatitis In addition, increased number of leukocytes and macrophages containing fat in the prostatic secretions
Prostatodynia	Cause: Unknown May be associated with inadequate relaxation of the perineal muscles May be psychogenic	No abnormal findings

ported by increased numbers of leukocytes in prostatic secretions and postmassage urine in the presence of negative cultures. In prostatodynia, the diagnosis is usually based on clinical manifestations and on a negative sequential bacteriologic localization study.

Management

Management varies with the type of prostatitis. The basic treatment for acute bacterial prostatitis is one co-trimoxazole double-strength (Bactrim) twice daily for 30 days unless the results of culture and sensitivity support a change in antibiotic. Also used are fluoroquinolone agents, such as ciprofloxacin hydrochloride, which have been shown to be highly effective in treating acute bacterial prostatitis. In severe cases, combination IV antibiotics, such as gentamicin and ampicillin, may be necessary. In addition, analgesics, nonsteroidal anti-inflammatory agents, antipyretics, anticholinergics (eg, oxybutynin chloride) to relieve urinary symptoms, stool softeners, sitz baths, and sexual abstinence are prescribed.

Chronic bacterial prostatitis is also treated with co-trimoxazole double-strength (Bactrim), taken twice daily for 4 to 16 weeks, as the drug of choice. If symptoms persist, co-trimoxazole single-strength or nitrofurantoin (Furadantin), 100 mg daily, is prescribed on a long-term basis along with regular prostatic massage to release necrotic cells, bacteria, and other debris. If these measures are not effective, prostatectomy may be necessary.

Nonbacterial prostatitis is difficult to treat because the cause is unknown. A trial course with an antibiotic (eg, erythromycin or tetracycline) may be given in case a nonidentified, susceptible organism is involved. Otherwise, treatment consists of controlling symptoms with oxybutynin chloride, nonsteroidal anti-inflammatory agents such as indomethacin or ibuprofen, stool softeners, and sitz baths for comfort. Normal sexual activity is encouraged.

The aim of treatment of prostatodynia is relaxation of the perineal muscles. Thus, an alpha-blocking agent (eg, prazosin) or a muscle relaxant (eg, diazepam) may be prescribed to relax the perineal muscles. Stool softeners and warm sitz baths may be prescribed for comfort. Despite these symptomatic therapies, the patient should be informed that symptoms may reappear.

NURSING PROCESS
Prostatitis

Assessment

Obtain a pertinent history and determine the current status of the patient's symptoms. In particular, ask about the location and intensity of pain, the presence of urethral discharge, and voiding symptoms such as dysuria, frequency, and nocturia.

Take an oral or tympanic temperature. Rectal temperatures are contraindicated because of the lo-

cation of the infection. Review relevant laboratory data, including the white blood cell count and reports of urine and prostatic fluid analyses.

If the patient's history reveals recurrent prostatitis, determine which medications and comfort measures he has used in the past.

Assess the patient's ability to handle discomfort and his emotional reaction to the illness. Determine whether the patient has concerns about sexual and reproductive functions.

Also determine the patient's understanding of his problem, its cause (if known), the therapeutic plan, and prevention of recurrences.

Nursing Diagnoses and Planning

Nursing diagnoses and related expected patient outcomes commonly applicable to patients with prostatitis include the following:

NDx: Pain related to the inflammatory response

Planning: Patient Outcomes
1. Patient states that pain intensity has decreased or that pain is gone.
2. Patient appears to be comfortable, as indicated by factors such as a relaxed body posture and blood pressure and pulse that are within normal limits.
3. Patient reports that specific urinary symptoms have decreased or disappeared.

NDx: Anxiety related to the outcome of disease and the possible impact on sexual functioning

Planning: Patient Outcomes
1. Patient states that he feels less anxious and is more relaxed.
2. Patient engages in diversional activities.
3. Patient readily expresses his concerns.

NDx: Risk for altered health maintenance related to insufficient knowledge of treatment plan, prevention of a recurrence if possible, and self-care activities for control of symptoms

Planning: Patient Outcomes
1. Patient discusses the plan of care, including bedrest, if ordered, drug therapy, frequency of the medication, side effects to report, and comfort measures.
2. Patient discusses the need for possible restriction of certain foods and fluids.
3. Patient describes measures to prevent a recurrence, such as compliance with prescribed drug therapy, drinking at least 3000 mL of fluid daily, and promptly seeking medical attention if symptoms of urinary tract infection occur.

Nursing Interventions and Evaluation

NDx: Pain
For the patient hospitalized with acute bacterial prostatitis, administer prescribed analgesics according to the physician's order and the patient's need. If a nonsteroidal anti-inflammatory drug (eg, ibupro-

fen or indomethacin) is also ordered, be sure that the medication is taken with meals or milk to avoid gastric irritation.

Administer anticholinergic drugs as ordered for discomfort associated with voiding. Monitor the patient's response, and observe for side effects, such as dry mouth, thirst, blurred vision, tachycardia, and urinary retention.

Give or provide instructions on the use of sitz baths if ordered for control of pain and spasm. Also administer prescribed stool softeners to avoid straining at stool, which may increase the pain. Encourage the patient to drink six to eight large glasses of water or other fluid daily to help keep the feces soft and to help dilute the urine so that it will not exacerbate any bladder or urethral irritation.

NDx: Anxiety

Provide time for expression of concerns and feelings. Reassure the patient that sexual and reproductive functions are not impaired. In the case of acute bacterial prostatitis for which sexual abstinence is ordered, explain that this restriction is in effect only until the inflammation is resolved. For the patient with prostatitis other than the acute bacterial type, encourage sexual intercourse to provide periodic emptying of the prostate. If a sexual partner is not available, suggest masturbation.

In the case of prostatitis that cannot be resolved, explain that the condition is not communicable and is not associated with an increased incidence of cancer.

NDx: Risk for altered health maintenance

Provide information about antibiotic and other therapy. Depending on the type of prostatitis, explain that therapy is intended either to eliminate the infecting organism or to control symptoms.

If co-trimoxazole is ordered, reinforce the need to drink at least eight full glasses of liquid daily. Explain that the drug is excreted primarily through the kidneys and that adequate urine production is essential to avoid crystals forming within the urinary tract.

Because co-trimoxazole or another antimicrobial agent is usually ordered for at least 30 days, emphasize the importance of taking the medication at the prescribed time and for the length of time prescribed.

If the patient has prostatodynia and will be taking an alpha-blocking drug, explain why the drug has been ordered and the effect it may have on blood pressure. To avoid postural hypotension, tell the patient to rise slowly when changing from a lying to a sitting position. If he becomes lightheaded, he should lie down. Also, instruct the patient to notify the physician if palpitations, dizziness, or headache occurs.

Inform the patient with chronic bacterial prostatitis that periodic gentle prostate massage may be performed by the physician to release pus cells and bacteria that may be present.

Advise about the need for restricting certain fluids and foods if they are associated with increased symptoms. For example, alcohol, caffeinated beverages, and foods containing hot spices may exacerbate symptoms by increasing prostate secretions. To prevent pressure on the inflamed prostate, explain the importance of avoiding constipation by drinking 8 to 10 glasses of fluid daily and including high-fiber foods in the diet, such as fruit, vegetables, and grain products.

To prevent a recurrence of bacterial prostatitis, stress the need for fluid intake of at least 3 L daily. Explain that this decreases the risk of urinary tract infection and the reappearance of prostatitis.

Finally, tell the patient to contact the physician if symptoms of acute bacterial prostatitis reappear. If the patient has chronic bacterial prostatitis, nonbacterial prostatitis, or prostatodynia, he should contact the physician if symptoms worsen.

Additional Interventions

When bedrest is prescribed, the patient will need help with hygiene, toileting, and diversional activities. To facilitate compliance with the bedrest order, explain that the purpose of remaining in bed is to decrease swelling and pain in and around the prostate. If the patient is treated at home, referral to a community health agency for visiting nurse supervision and home health aide assistance may be needed.

Compare the patient's status with the expected outcomes. If the outcomes are not met, reassess the patient and revise the plan.

❖ SETTINGS, PROVIDERS, AND COLLABORATION FOR CARE

Men with infections or inflammatory conditions of the reproduction system usually receive care either in the physician's office or an ambulatory care setting. In severe cases of acute bacterial prostatitis or acute epididymitis that require IV antibiotic therapy, acute inpatient hospitalization is ordered. As the patient responds, antibiotic therapy may continue in a long-term care facility or at home with the use of a home infusion therapy service. For the patient with balanoposthitis, referral to a visiting nurse may be necessary to assess compliance with any treatment prescribed. For the elderly patient, daily home health aide services may also be needed to assist with penile hygiene.

*S*tructural Disorders

PHIMOSIS

Phimosis is a disorder in which the foreskin (prepuce) cannot be retracted over the glans penis (Fig. 39-2).

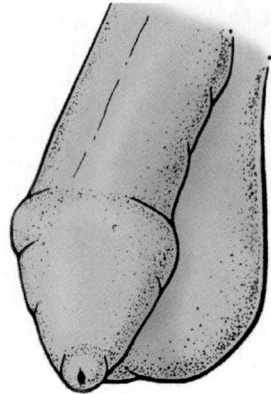

Figure 39-2

Phimosis. The foreskin contracts over the tip of the meatus, resulting in a narrowed opening.

Etiology and Pathophysiology

Phimosis may be congenital or acquired. It develops in children when the foreskin fails to separate from the glans. In the adult, it develops as a complication of recurrent infection of the glans and foreskin (balanoposthitis). Fibrosis and scar formation make the foreskin tight and inelastic. Complications of phimosis include constriction of the penile blood vessels and stenosis of the meatus.

Clinical Manifestations

In addition to a nonretractable foreskin, signs and symptoms of infection may develop, such as swelling, redness, purulent discharge, and pain. Erections may be painful. If stenosis of the urinary meatus develops, the patient will experience decreased urinary flow, dysuria, and straining to void.

Diagnosis

The diagnosis of phimosis is based on the patient's complaints and on inspection of the penis.

Management

When phimosis obstructs urination, a dorsal slit of the foreskin may be necessary as an emergency measure. A meatotomy (see Chap. 31) may also be needed. Antibiotics and warm soaks are ordered for balanoposthitis. After obstruction and infection have been resolved, circumcision is usually recommended to prevent a recurrence.

In the adult, circumcision is usually performed under regional (spinal) anesthesia. The outer and inner surfaces of the foreskin are incised; any adhesions are dissected away; and the appropriate amount of foreskin is excised. Absorbable sutures are used to approximate the two surfaces of the foreskin (Fig. 39-3). A nonadherent dressing, such as petrolatum (Vaseline) gauze, is then applied.

Complications of circumcision include bleeding, temporary hyperesthesia of the glans (increased sensation), urinary retention, infection, and formation of a subcutaneous hematoma.

Preoperative Preparation

Although circumcision usually involves only local anesthesia, food and fluids may be withheld beginning about 6 hours before surgery to allow the use of general anesthesia if necessary. A preoperative antianxiety agent, such as diazepam (Valium), may be prescribed, or conscious sedation with midazolam may be used. The penile area is usually shaved in the operating room.

Postoperative Course

The patient's length of stay in the hospital after a circumcision is short. The patient is usually discharged on the same day that the surgery is performed.

Pain is usually managed with oxycodone hydrochloride and acetaminophen (Percocet) and then acetaminophen as the intensity diminishes. The application of ice packs to the penile area may be ordered for 24 hours to decrease edema and discomfort.

A dry dressing may cover the petrolatum gauze and may need to be changed with each voiding. A warm tub bath may be ordered for cleansing the penile wound on the second or third day postoperatively. Sexual intercourse is usually permitted 1 week after surgery.

NURSING PROCESS
Circumcision

PREOPERATIVE NURSING CARE

Provide basic preoperative care as described in Chapter 6. Be sensitive to the patient's need for privacy, and be sure that he knows his penis will be edematous for several days after surgery.

POSTOPERATIVE NURSING CARE

Assessment

After circumcision, make standard postoperative assessments, with special attention to observing the dressing for bleeding. If there is no dressing, ob-

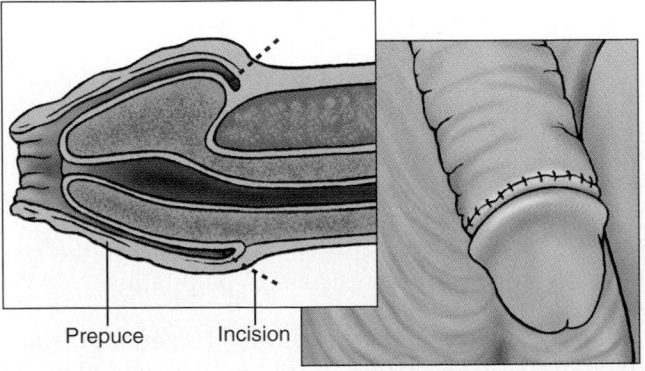

Prepuce   Incision

Figure 39-3

Surgical procedure for circumcision.

serve the penis for edema, bleeding, and development of a hematoma. Assess for the presence and degree of pain. Monitor urinary output closely, especially the first voiding, to ensure a patent urethra.

Nursing Diagnoses and Planning

Nursing diagnoses and related expected patient outcomes commonly applicable to patients who have had a circumcision include the following:

NDx: Pain (penile) related to surgery

Planning: Patient Outcomes
1. Patient uses ice pack applications as directed.
2. Patient reports that pain is decreased or gone.
3. Patient appears comfortable; he does not grimace or groan.

NDx: Risk for urinary retention related to edema of the meatus

Planning: Patient Outcomes
1. Patient voids at least 200 mL of urine within 8 hours after surgery.
2. Urine stream is normal in force and size.

NDx: Risk for infection related to penile surgery

Planning: Patient Outcomes
1. Foul-smelling or purulent drainage is absent.
2. Temperature is within normal limits.

NDx: Risk for altered health maintenance related to insufficient knowledge of discharge self-care activities

Planning: Patient Outcomes
1. Patient describes proper wound care.
2. Patient describes the signs of a developing infection or subcutaneous hematoma.
3. Patient states when sexual intercourse may be resumed.

Nursing Interventions and Evaluation

NDx: Pain
Instruct the patient on the use of analgesics as prescribed and ice packs to the penis if ordered. Caution the patient to avoid touching the glans, because this can increase his pain and contaminate the wound.

NDx: Risk for urinary retention
To facilitate resumption of a normal voiding pattern, encourage fluids and make them available on the bedside table. Leave the urinal within easy reach. Tell the patient to notify a nurse before the first voiding so that output can be measured and patency of the meatus validated. If the patient needs to stand up to void, provide assistance as necessary. If the patient has not voided within 8 hours after surgery, inform the physician. Catheterization may be necessary to relieve the urinary retention.

NDx: Risk for infection
Before discharge, demonstrate removal and reapplication of petrolatum gauze and outer dressing, as appropriate. Explain the importance of changing the dressing when moist and observing the penile wound for redness and purulent drainage. Instruct the patient to wash his hands thoroughly before handling the penis for urination and to avoid touching the operative area except for dressing changes.

NDx: Risk for altered health maintenance
Instruct the patient in self-care activities after discharge (Highlight 39–2).

Compare the patient's status with the expected outcomes. If the outcomes are not met, reassess the patient and revise the plan.

PARAPHIMOSIS

Paraphimosis is a condition in which the uncircumcised foreskin is retracted over the glans penis and cannot be easily returned to its normal position.

Etiology and Pathophysiology
The cause of paraphimosis is usually chronic balanoposthitis. The accumulation of scar tissue under the foreskin inhibits its flexibility so that, when retracted, it cannot be easily pulled down over the glans. The retracted foreskin quickly develops into a

---

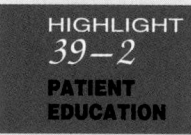 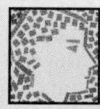

HIGHLIGHT 39–2
PATIENT EDUCATION

Discharge Instructions After Circumcision

Instruct the patient to do the following:

Wash hands well before changing the dressing.

Touch the glans gently because it may be very sensitive.

Apply ice packs as ordered.

Reapply the petrolatum jelly (Vaseline) dressing for the length of time ordered.

Observe for discharge or hematoma formation, and, if present, notify the physician immediately.

Take a warm tub bath on the second or third day to clean the penile area.

Remind the patient of the following:

Edema of the penis will disappear within a few days.

Sexual intercourse may be resumed in 1 week.

Sutures are absorbable.

Return for follow-up care on *(specify date and time)*.

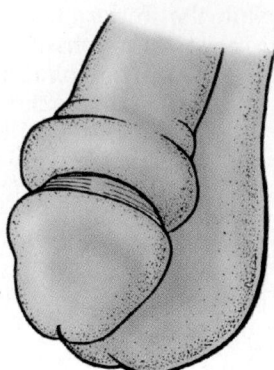

Figure 39–4
Paraphimosis.

constricting ring around the glans, with subsequent venous occlusion and possible arterial obstruction.

Paraphimosis may also occur after urethral instrumentation if the foreskin is retracted and left in that position. Complications of paraphimosis include urethral obstruction and gangrene of the glans.

Clinical Manifestations

When a constricted foreskin is allowed to remain in a retracted position, penile edema develops, accompanied by severe pain (Fig. 39–4). If the obstruction is not relieved as soon as it is observed, the glans becomes bluish from impaired blood supply.

Diagnosis

The diagnosis is based on inspection of the penis and on palpation of the foreskin for the constricting ring.

Management

Manual reduction is the treatment of choice for paraphimosis. Before it is attempted, the penis may be elevated and cool compresses applied to decrease some of the edema. An analgesic, such as intramuscular meperidine hydrochloride (Demerol), may be prescribed before the procedure because reduction usually is painful. After application of 4% lidocaine ointment for local anesthesia, the penis is squeezed in a gloved hand for 5 minutes to try to reduce the size of the glans. The glans penis is then pushed back while the foreskin is pulled down over it. If this is unsuccessful, emergency surgery is necessary. A dorsal slit into the constricting ring of the foreskin is made to prevent necrosis of the glans. To prevent a recurrence, circumcision may be recommended.

NURSING PROCESS
Paraphimosis

Assessment

Inspect the glans penis, and note any bluish color or edema. Palpate for a constricting ring. Assess for pain, and ask the patient when he last voided. Ask the patient about any decrease in the size or force of the urinary stream. Elicit any history of infection of the foreskin and glans as well as a description of usual hygienic care of the penis.

Nursing Diagnoses and Planning

Nursing diagnoses and related expected patient outcomes commonly applicable to patients with paraphimosis include the following:

NDx: Pain (penile) related to a constricted, retracted foreskin

Planning: Patient Outcomes
1. Patient reports that pain or soreness has decreased.
2. Patient describes the use of comfort measures for residual soreness.

NDx: Risk for altered health maintenance related to insufficient knowledge of hygienic care of the penis

Planning: Patient Outcomes
1. Patient describes the correct technique for cleaning the glans penis.
2. Patient verbally indicates his intention to perform daily penile hygiene.
3. Patient describes the importance of preventing infections of the glans and foreskin.

NDx: Risk for urinary retention related to penile edema

Planning: Patient Outcomes
1. Patient's urinary stream is of normal size and force.
2. Patient is free of bladder distention after voiding.

Nursing Interventions and Evaluation

NDx: Pain
Administer a narcotic analgesic, if ordered, before manual reduction. This is typically needed when treatment has been delayed and manual reduction will probably not be easy.

For residual soreness after reduction, instruct the patient to elevate the penis and to apply cool compresses to help reduce the remaining edema. If the physician orders a non-narcotic analgesic, such as acetaminophen, review its correct use.

NDx: Risk for altered health maintenance
If circumcision is not performed, teach the patient to cleanse the glans (see Highlight 39–1). Emphasize the importance of complying with this routine to prevent balanoposthitis or a recurrence of paraphimosis.

NDx: Risk for urinary retention
After reduction of the foreskin, ask the patient to void. Help him to stand and use the toilet rather than the urinal, if possible, because it is more comfortable and will facilitate voiding, especially if the glans is still painful and edematous.

Compare the patient's status with the expected outcomes. If the outcomes are not met, reassess the patient and revise the plan.

CRYPTORCHIDISM

Cryptorchidism is the failure of one or both of the testes to descend into the scrotum shortly before birth. A cryptorchid testis is usually located in one of three sites: intra-abdominal, within the inguinal canal, or just external to the canal.

Etiology and Pathophysiology

The cause of cryptorchidism is unclear but may be related either to an abnormality in the hypothalamic-pituitary-testicular axis resulting in deficient circulating testosterone or to structural problems such as a short spermatic cord occurring during fetal development. Some evidence suggests that sons of mothers who have taken diethystilbestrol (DES) may be born with undescended testes. It occurs in 30% of premature male newborns and in less than 3% of full-term males. In most of these cases, the testes descend spontaneously during the first year, resulting in an 0.8% incidence of true cryptorchidism.

Complications of cryptorchidism include infertility, testicular cancer, and torsion of the testis. The undescended testis is also commonly associated with an inguinal hernia on the affected side.

Infertility occurs because spermatogenesis depends on the cooler temperature found in the scrotum. Failure of the testes to descend results in a progressive decrease in sperm production until it ceases completely when puberty is complete.

All males with bilateral cryptorchidism whose testes were not positioned in the scrotum before age 2 (and more than 60% of those treated before this age) are infertile. Infertility also occurs in up to 30% of males with unilateral cryptorchidism, even when surgically corrected, suggesting that the opposite testis is congenitally abnormal.

Cancer occurs 10 to 50 times more often in a cryptorchid testis than in a normal testis, accounting for approximately 10% of all testicular tumors. Males at greatest risk include those with untreated cryptorchidism and those treated at puberty or after. Seminoma is the type of malignant tumor most likely to develop.

Torsion of the undescended testis (twisting of the spermatic cord that suspends the testis) may develop because of excessive mobility of the testis. Because torsion interrupts the blood supply to the testis, surgery must be performed quickly to maintain testicular function.

Clinical Manifestations

The major clinical manifestation of cryptorchidism is the absence of one or both of the testes from the scrotal sac. This is associated with atrophy of the scrotum on the affected side.

Diagnosis

The diagnosis of cryptorchidism is made easily by inspecting and palpating the scrotum. If the undescended testis cannot be palpated in the inguinal canal, tests such as ultrasonography, computed tomographic (CT) scan, and testicular venography can be done to locate it within the body. If it is not located by one of these methods, a laparoscopy or surgical exploration may be necessary.

Management

Treatment of cryptorchidism depends on the age of the patient when the diagnosis is made. If the testis has not descended by 1 year of age, human chorionic gonadotropin or gonadotropin-releasing hormone may be given to try to stimulate descent. If this is not successful by 2 years of age, surgical placement of the testis in the scrotum (orchiopexy) is done to avoid testicular degeneration, which occurs after this age.

If cryptorchidism remains undetected or untreated until adulthood, the treatment is orchiopexy, which is done primarily to provide cosmetic enhancement and to facilitate early detection of a testicular malignancy.

The surgical approach for orchiopexy can vary with the location of the cryptorchid testis but most often involves an inguinal incision on the affected side to free the spermatic cord of any adhesions and to repair the associated hernia. This is followed by an incision at the top of the scrotum on the opposite side and the creation of a subdartos pouch. The testis is then mobilized, brought down, and implanted in the pouch with a traction suture holding it in place. The incision is closed with absorbable sutures, and Steri-Strips are applied as the dressing. An alternative to orchiopexy is orchiectomy (removal of the testis). This is done if a malignancy is suspected or if the testis is found to be atrophied.

NURSING PROCESS GUIDELINES
Orchiopexy

Nursing care of the patient having an orchiopexy is similar to that of the patient having a testicular biopsy, an inguinal herniorrhaphy, or an orchiectomy. After surgery, elevate the scrotum on a Bellevue bridge while the patient is in bed to limit edema and discomfort. Apply an athletic support for ambulation. Give medication, such as meperidine hydrochloride or oxycodone hydrochloride, as ordered for postoperative pain. Instruct the patient in self-care after discharge (Highlight 39–3).

Before and after surgery, carefully assess the patient's emotional state. Depending on the circumstances, there may be a great deal of anger that the condition was not diagnosed and treated earlier and that the patient is now infertile. In addition, the patient experiences the stress of surgery and the in-

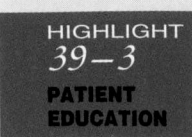
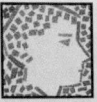

HIGHLIGHT 39–3
PATIENT EDUCATION
Discharge Instructions After Orchiopexy

Instruct the patient to do the following:

Take pain medication as prescribed.

Dry the groin and scrotal areas gently after bathing or showering to avoid disrupting the incision. (Tell the patient not to worry if the Steri-Strips fall off in a few days. This is expected and will not disrupt wound healing).

Wear an athletic support to elevate the scrotum and promote comfort.

Avoid strenuous physical activity and heavy lifting for 6 weeks or until otherwise instructed.

Avoid driving for 2 weeks.

Report immediately any redness, increased tenderness, or drainage from either the inguinal or scrotal incisions.

Perform a monthly testicular self-examination because the risk of testicular cancer is increased in cyptorchidism, even when surgically treated.

Return for a follow-up appointment on *(specify day and time)*.

creased risk of cancer. Refer the patient to a mental health professional or support group as needed.

❖ SETTINGS, PROVIDERS, AND COLLABORATION FOR CARE

The man with a structural disorder of the reproductive system may receive care in a variety of settings. The patient with paraphimosis usually receives care in the physician's office or an ambulatory care setting. If the condition develops while the patient is hospitalized or confined to a long-term-care facility, treatment may be provided at the bedside. Orchiopexy and circumcision are usually performed in an ambulatory surgical day care setting with the patient discharged the day of surgery. Referral to a home health care agency or visiting nurse service for wound care may be needed.

PRIAPISM

Priapism is a prolonged, uncontrolled penile erection that is not associated with tactile stimulation or sexual desire.

Etiology and Pathophysiology

Priapism can result from conditions such as sickle-cell anemia, leukemia, multiple sclerosis, and local and metastatic tumors encroaching on the penile veins. Priapism has been noted to develop after intracavernal injection of vasodilator drugs for treatment of impotence and has also been associated with the use of certain drugs, including the phenothiazines, hydralazine, prazosin, heparin, alcohol, and marijuana. In most cases, however, its cause is unknown.

In priapism, penile enlargement is prolonged because obstruction prevents blood from flowing from the corpora cavernosa. This venous congestion within the corpora cavernosa results in thrombosis and fibrosis, which can lead to impotence, urinary retention, and penile necrosis.

Clinical Manifestations

With priapism, the penis is very large and hard, and the patient has severe, constant penile pain. If arterial circulation is impaired, the penis may also be cold and pale from ischemia. Priapism is often present for hours or days before the patient seeks treatment.

Diagnosis

The diagnosis of priapism is based on the presenting symptoms and the patient's associated medical history.

Management

Because of the risk of impotence and penile necrosis, priapism is viewed as a urologic emergency. Immediate treatment usually includes analgesia, prostatic massage, sedation, and local cold applications to try to reduce penile congestion. If the patient cannot void and the bladder is distended, a urethral catheter is inserted. If the obstruction is such that this is not possible, suprapubic drainage is instituted. Hydration therapy may be ordered. This is true especially if the patient has sickle-cell disease because dehydration may lead to more sickling, further compromising venous outflow from the corpora cavernosa. Needle aspiration of the cavernosa for clots and blood, followed by intracavernosal injection of an alpha-adrenergic drug (eg, epinephrine or phenylephrine), may be performed for decompression and detumescence.

In cases in which a cause is identified, the underlying condition is treated in an attempt to reverse priapism. For example, if priapism is drug-induced, the medication is promptly discontinued. When priapism results from intracavernosal injection of vasodilator drugs, administration of an alpha-adrenergic drug into the corpora cavernosa will usually return the penis to the nonerectile state. If priapism is due to a metastatic process, chemotherapy or irradiation may be used. To decrease the risk of impotence, surgery is performed if priapism does not subside within 48 hours of onset. The procedure with the greatest success rate creates a venous fistula to shunt blood from both corpora cavernosa to the corpus spongiosum. This is quickly performed with a biopsy needle or a narrow knife blade under local anesthesia. If impotence develops as a complication, a penile implant may be recommended.

❖ Settings, Providers, and Collaboration for Care

Patients with priapism may receive initial care in the urologist's office, outpatient clinic, or emergency room. If surgery is needed, the procedure is usually performed in an ambulatory surgical setting with the patient being discharged the same day. Referral to the visiting nurse service for a next-day visit may be needed to assess for penile pain and edema and difficulty voiding. When priapism develops secondary to a serious underlying cause, such as sickle-cell anemia or a metastatic tumor, the patient may be required to be admitted to the hospital.

NURSING PROCESS
Priapism

Assessment

Ask the patient how long his penis has been in a continuous erectile state. Also ask about the presence and severity of pain. Assess for early signs of ischemia, and note the color and temperature of the penis. Determine when the patient last urinated and whether he noticed any change in the amount or force of the stream. If urinary retention is suspected, palpate the suprapubic area for bladder distention.

As the medical plan of care is implemented, assess the patient's understanding of it and the expected outcomes. If surgery is planned, determine the patient's understanding of the purpose and nature of the procedure.

Nursing Diagnoses and Planning

Nursing diagnoses and related expected patient outcomes commonly applicable to patients with priapism include the following:

NDx: Pain (penile) related to circulatory changes in the penis

Planning: Patient Outcomes
1. Patient reports that pain is diminished.
2. Patient appears more comfortable; he does not grimace or moan and is less restless.
3. Patient's blood pressure, pulse, and respiration are within his normal range.

NDx: Risk for urinary retention related to urethral obstruction

Planning: Patient Outcomes
1. Patient initiates voiding on need, with output of at least 120 mL.
2. Bladder distention is absent.

NDx: Risk for sexual dysfunction related to vascular changes in the penis

Planning: Patient Outcomes
1. Patient expresses his concerns about the effect that priapism may have on subsequent sexual function.
2. Patient discusses his concerns and prognosis with his sexual partner.
3. Patient lists alternative methods of sexual expression.
4. Patient describes the role of a penile implant in treating impotence.

Nursing Interventions and Evaluation

NDx: Pain
Administer prescribed analgesics and sedatives promptly. If analgesics are ordered as needed (PRN), give the medications before the pain becomes severe and difficult to control. Before discharge, give the patient instructions about any analgesic that has been prescribed.

Apply and instruct the patient on the application of cold packs to the penis, if ordered. They control edema and can decrease pain perception according to the gate control theory. Enhance the effectiveness of analgesic and sedative medications by maintaining a calm, quiet environment, maintaining general physical comfort, and guiding the patient in controlled breathing exercises.

NDx: Risk for urinary retention
Facilitate voiding by helping the patient to a standing position, providing privacy, offering fluids, and using the power of suggestion (eg, running water in the sink or pouring warm water over the hands or genital area). Record the time and amount of voiding. Report to the physician signs of urinary retention, such as a palpable bladder or voiding of small amounts.

NDx: Risk for sexual dysfunction
Provide time for the patient to ask questions and express his concerns about future sexual performance. If the patient sought treatment immediately, stress that the incidence of impotence is greatly diminished when priapism is resolved within 24 hours of onset. If he delayed seeking treatment and impotence is suspected, discuss alternate methods of sexual expression such as touching, closeness, and orogenital stimulation. Provide information on the use of a penile implant as a method of treating impotence. Encourage discussion with his sexual partner, if available, and refer to a sex therapist if needed.

Compare the patient's status with expected outcomes. If the outcomes are not met, reassess the patient and revise the plan.

HYDROCELE

A hydrocele is an abnormal collection of fluid within the layers of the tunica vaginalis, which surrounds the testis (Fig. 39–5). It may be unilateral or bilateral and may occur in an infant or adult.

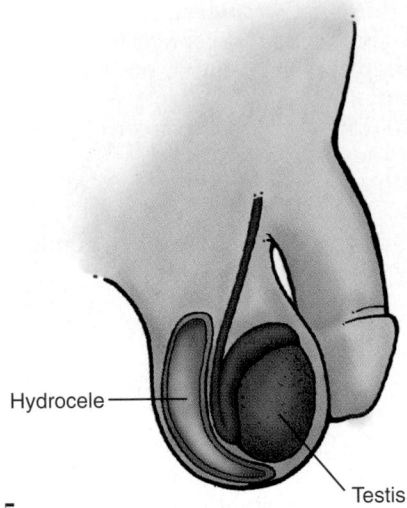

Hydrocele ——

—— Testis

Figure 39–5
Hydrocele.

Etiology and Pathophysiology

A hydrocele in the adult can occur secondary to epididymo-orchitis, scrotal trauma, testicular neoplasm, or hypoalbuminemia. In most cases, however, it is idiopathic.

Normally, the space between the two layers of the tunica vaginalis contains only 1 to 3 mL of clear, serous fluid. Formation and reabsorption occurs constantly. A hydrocele occurs either from increased production or from decreased reabsorption of this fluid. The size of the hydrocele depends on the extent of the imbalance between production and reabsorption. A large hydrocele can impair physical and sexual activity and may compromise the blood supply to the testis, leading to testicular atrophy.

Characteristics of the fluid in the hydrocele sac vary depending on its cause. For example, fluid related to a testicular neoplasm is usually clear yellow, whereas fluid associated with infection may be cloudy and contain bacteria.

Clinical Manifestations

Painless swelling of the scrotum is the classic sign of hydrocele, except when caused by an infection.

Diagnosis

The diagnosis of a hydrocele is based on the patient's history, physical examination, and transillumination or ultrasonography of the scrotum.

Management

Treatment is usually unnecessary for small hydroceles that cause no discomfort. Treatment may also be unnecessary for some large hydroceles, because they may spontaneously disappear as the underlying condition is resolved.

When treatment is required because of size and discomfort, the most conservative approach is to aspirate the fluid. A sclerosing drug, such as 5% tetracycline, may then be injected into the scrotal sac.

Because some hydroceles recur, this treatment may need to be repeated every few months. In some cases, a hydrocelectomy may be indicated.

Hydrocelectomy is the excision of the fluid-filled sac in the tunica vaginalis. In the adult, it is usually done under regional anesthesia. IV conscious sedation with midazolam may also be used. An anterolateral scrotal incision is made on the affected side. The sac is then opened and drained through the incision. Excess tunica is excised; the edges of the remaining tunica are sutured together; and the incision is closed with absorbable sutures. A Penrose drain, which is usually removed in 48 hours, may be placed in the scrotal sac and brought out through a stab wound in the most dependent portion of the scrotum. A compression-type dressing secured with a scrotal support is applied to help control postoperative edema.

Complications of hydrocelectomy include hematoma formation and wound infection. The hydrocele may occasionally recur.

❖ Settings, Providers, and Collaboration for Care

Hydrocelectomy is usually performed in an ambulatory surgical day care setting, and the patient is discharged on the day of surgery. If the patient needs help with wound care after discharge, a referral to the local visiting nurse may be necessary.

NURSING PROCESS
Hydrocelectomy

PREOPERATIVE NURSING CARE

Nursing care of the patient scheduled for a hydrocelectomy includes all the basic assessments and interventions for any patient undergoing surgery. If a knowledge deficit or anxiety state exists, provide information as needed. Give the patient ample opportunity to explain his concerns.

POSTOPERATIVE NURSING CARE

Assessment

Make standard postoperative assessments as discussed in Chapter 6. Also determine the degree of scrotal edema, and note the color and amount of any wound drainage.

Nursing Diagnoses and Planning

Nursing diagnoses and related expected patient outcomes commonly applicable to patients having a hydrocelectomy include the following:

NDx: Pain (scrotal) related to surgery and associated edema

Planning: Patient Outcomes
1. Patient requests medication for pain control as needed.

2. Patient maintains scrotal elevation.
3. Patient maintains cold pack applications as directed.
4. Patient reports that the pain has decreased or disappeared.

NDx: Risk for altered health maintenance related to insufficient knowledge of self-care after discharge

Planning: Patient Outcomes
1. Patient describes the procedure for applying cold packs to the scrotum.
2. Patient describes or demonstrates changing of the scrotal wound dressing.
3. Patient states reasons for keeping the scrotum elevated.
4. Patient lists symptoms to be reported that indicate a wound complication (fever, increased local pain and tenderness, purulent drainage, localized swelling, bleeding).

Nursing Interventions and Evaluation

NDx: Pain
Administer an analgesic or instruct the patient in its use according to the physician's order. Apply ice packs to the scrotum as ordered to control postoperative swelling and pain.

Maintain elevation of the scrotum by ensuring that the scrotal support applied in the operating room is in place. Replace the support if soiled. Inform the patient that use of the scrotal support helps to decrease or minimize postoperative edema and discomfort.

NDx: Risk for altered health maintenance
The length of hospital stay after a hydrocelectomy is usually less than 23 hours. Therefore, preparing the patient for self-care after discharge is important. Give careful instructions to help the patient take care of the wound and detect potential complications (Highlight 39–4).

Compare the patient's status with expected outcomes. If the outcomes are not met, reassess the patient and revise the plan.

VARICOCELE

A varicocele is a cluster of dilated veins of the pampiniform plexus, a network of veins originating from the spermatic veins, which supply the testes (Fig. 39–6).

Etiology and Pathophysiology
A varicocele occurs predominantly between the ages of 15 and 40. It is usually considered to be idiopathic, although a defect in the valves of the internal spermatic veins has been suggested as a possible cause. Although varicoceles can develop bilaterally, the left side is more commonly affected, probably because the left spermatic vein is under greater back pressure than the right spermatic vein.

A varicocele is commonly associated with infer-

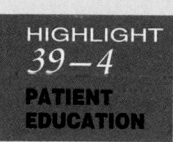
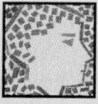

HIGHLIGHT 39–4
PATIENT EDUCATION

Discharge Instructions After Hydrocelectomy

Instruct the patient to:

Apply ice packs to the scrotum as directed.

Wash hands before changing dressing.

Remove the soiled dressing and cleanse the wound gently with soap and water.

Observe for purulent or bloody discharge or localized swelling and notify the physician if necessary.

Reapply a clean scrotal support.

Keep the scrotum elevated until edema has resolved.

Remind the patient of the following:

Scrotal edema will disappear in 2 to 4 weeks.

Sutures are absorbable.

Avoid sexual intercourse and strenuous physical activity until directed by the physician.

If a drain is in place, it will be removed by the physician.

Return for follow-up care on *(specify date and time).*

tility, although the reason is not clear. One widely accepted explanation is that venous enlargement increases the temperature in the scrotum, thus impairing sperm production and motility.

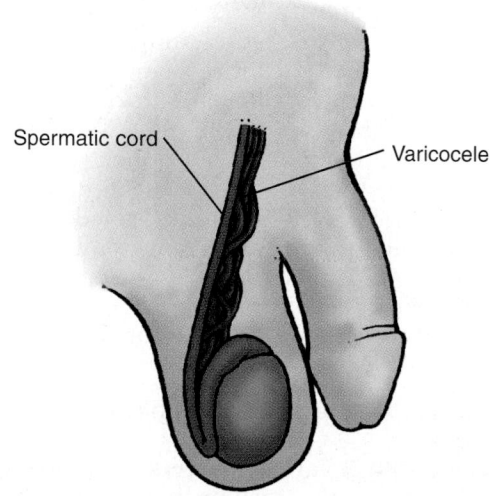

Spermatic cord

Varicocele

Figure 39–6
Varicocele.

In men older than 40 years of age, development of a left varicocele is usually secondary to a left renal tumor. Development of a right varicocele suggests an obstructing abdominal mass because the right spermatic vein inserts into the inferior vena cava.

Clinical Manifestations

For many men, infertility is the only symptom. Others may complain of a feeling of heaviness or a dull ache in the scrotum on the affected side.

Diagnosis

On physical examination, dilated, tortuous veins posterior to and above the affected testis may be palpated with the patient in an upright position. The varicocele usually disappears when the patient lies down. In addition, when the patient performs a Valsalva maneuver, a rush of blood can be felt in the scrotum. A Doppler ultrasonogram or a venogram may be required to confirm the diagnosis. In cases of a suspected underlying malignancy, a CT scan or other similar tests may be ordered.

Management

Discomfort can often be relieved merely by wearing a scrotal support. In some cases, embolization (occlusion of the internal spermatic vein on the affected side, using a balloon-tipped catheter, coil, or sclerosing agent) of the varicocele may be performed at the time of venography. If this is not effective, or if infertility continues, a varicocelectomy is done.

There are three surgical approaches to varicocelectomy: inguinal or upper scrotal, retroperitoneal, and laparoscopic. With each approach, the spermatic vein, its branches, or both are ligated and venous collateral circulation is assumed by the deep pelvic venous system.

In the inguinal and retroperitoneal approaches, a varicocelectomy is usually done under local anesthesia. The incision is closed with either Dacron sutures or skin staples and is covered with a sterile dressing. A laparoscopic varicocelectomy is performed under general anesthesia. The patient is admitted to an ambulatory surgical setting and is discharged on the day of surgery. The three small incisions are usually closed with absorbable sutures, Steri-Strips, and covered with a sterile dressing. With each approach, a scrotal support is applied to decrease edema.

When a varicocelectomy is performed on infertile men, semen quality improves considerably. Impregnation occurs in 35 to 50% of the cases reported.

Complications of a varicocelectomy are rare and include wound infection and the formation of a hydrocele.

❖ Settings, Providers, and Collaboration for Care

The patient with a varicocele usually receives initial care in the urologist's office or in a urology ambulatory care setting. If surgery is needed, it is done in an ambulatory surgical day care unit and the patient is discharged on the day of surgery. A referral to a visiting nurse service for one postoperative home visit may be made for wound care and assessment of compliance with the discharge plan of care.

NURSING PROCESS GUIDELINES
Varicocelectomy

Nursing care of the patient having a varicocelectomy is the same as that for the patient having a hydrocelectomy, with one additional consideration. If the patient is undergoing a varicocelectomy because of an associated infertility problem, he is likely to be highly anxious about its outcome. Preoperatively, determine the patient's understanding of the effects of varicocelectomy on fertility. Be sure that he understands that restoration of fertility cannot be guaranteed. The result may not be known for several months. Provide time for him to express his concerns and his hopes.

The patient usually goes home 4 to 6 hours after the surgery. Before discharge, give instructions about the prescribed analgesic, wound care, and development of possible complications. Instruct him to remain at home for about 5 days, to avoid driving for 7 days, to avoid strenuous physical activity for 3 weeks, and to return for a follow-up visit and suture removal, if needed, in 1 week. Also instruct the patient to follow the physician's guidelines for resumption of sexual activity.

Neoplasia

CANCER OF THE PENIS

Etiology and Pathophysiology

Penile carcinoma accounts for less than 17% of all malignancies among men in the United States (Schellhammer, 1994). The incidence of penile carcinoma varies greatly with hygienic standards and cultural religious practices. Neonatal circumcision dramatically reduces the occurrence of penile carcinoma. Among uncircumcised Africans and Asians, penile carcinoma accounts for 10 to 20% of male malignancies. Carcinoma may also arise from the scarred penile shaft skin after mutilating circumcision (Schellhammer, 1994). The incidence of penile cancer is extremely low in Israel and Moslem countries that practice neonatal circumcision.

The precise cause of penile cancer is not known. However, in uncircumcised men with phimosis and poor personal hygiene, the chronic presence and irritation of smegma may contribute to its development. Viral infection may have some influence on carcinoma. A three- to eightfold increase in the incidence of cervical carcinoma among sexual partners

Table 39–3

TNM Classification of Penile Carcinoma

Primary Tumor (T)

Tx	Primary tumor cannot be assessed
T0	No evidence of primary tumors
TIS	Carcinoma in situ
Ta	Noninvasive verrucous carcinoma
T1	Tumor invades subepithelial connective tissue
T2	Tumor invades corpus spongiosum or cavernosum
T3	Tumor invades the urethra or prostate
T4	Tumor invades other adjacent structures

Regional Lymph Nodes (N)

Nx	Regional lymph nodes cannot be assessed
N0	No regional lymph node metastasis
N1	Metastasis in a single superficial inguinal lymph node
N2	Metastasis in multiple or bilateral superficial inguinal lymph nodes
N3	Metastasis in deep inguinal or pelvic lymph node(s), unilateral or bilateral

Distant Metastasis (M)

Mx	Presence of distant metastasis cannot be assessed
M0	No distant metastasis
M1	Distant metastasis

Used with permission of the American Joint Committee on Cancer. The original source for this material is the AJCC Manual for staging of cancer, 4th edition (1992) published by JB Lippincott Company, Philadelphia.

of patients with penile carcinoma has been documented and may relate to infection with the herpesvirus. Penile carcinoma has also been associated with the sexually transmitted human papilloma virus.

Clinical Manifestations

Carcinoma of the penis presents initially as a small lesion. Most occur on the glans or inner surface of the foreskin. In time, the lesion may extend to involve the entire glans, shaft, and corpora. At the time of initial diagnosis, 40 to 80% of patients with invasive carcinoma have palpable adenopathy. About half of this adenopathy is secondary to metastasis and half to an inflammatory reaction.

Penile cancer is progressive and typically causes death for untreated patients within 2 years (Schellhammer, 1994). Thus, early detection is essential. However, many patients delay seeking medical attention because of embarrassment, denial, failure to detect the lesion under a phimotic foreskin, fear, guilt, or ignorance (Lasater, 1992).

Diagnosis

A biopsy is done to identify the malignant histology and the depth of invasion. It is critical to mapping out therapy. A biopsy may be done as a separate procedure or may be done at the time of surgery, with confirmation of tumor by frozen section followed by immediate surgical excision by partial or total penectomy.

The largest majority (95%) of penile tumors are low-grade squamous cell carcinomas. Evidence shows that high-grade tumors are frequently associated with regional nodal metastases (Schellhammer, 1994).

The Tumor, Nodes, and Metastases (TNM) staging system best describes the depth of invasion with penile cancer (Table 39–3). In many cases, it replaces the Jackson system, which may be inadequate in revealing the depth of neoplastic invasion (Table 39–4). Currently, both classifications may be used when staging penile carcinoma (Schellhammer, 1994).

A potential serum tumor marker antigen, TA-4, becomes significantly elevated as the disease progresses (Lasater, 1992). It can serve as an index of the patient's response to treatment.

Management

Management of penile cancer is tailored to the individual patient, taking into consideration the stage of the disease, coexisting medical problems, and the patient's preference. Therapeutic options include:

- Circumcision
- Excision of the lesion
- Mohs' micrographic surgery, which is surgical removal of skin cancer by excising the tissue in thin layers with tissue mapping and microscopic examination of frozen horizontal tissue sections
- Cryosurgery
- Carbon dioxide and neodymium:yttrium-aluminum-garnet lasers
- External radiation therapy
- Topical 5-fluorouracil–based cream
- Partial penectomy

Table 39–4

Jackson Classification for Clinical Staging of Carcinoma of the Penis

Stage	Extent of Disease
I	Tumor confined to the glans or the prepuce or both
II	Tumor extends onto the shaft of the penis
III	Tumor with inguinal metastases that are operable
IV	Tumor involving adjacent structures or tumor associated with inoperable inguinal or distant metastases

- Total penectomy with perineal urethrostomy
- Chemotherapy
- Inguinal lymphadenectomy
- Hemipelvectomy or hemicorporectomy in certain carefully selected patients

Controversy exists about the timing and extent of surgery in the presence of inguinal metastases. It is recommended that lymphadenectomy (inguinal/pelvic) be performed if the patient has clinically palpable inguinal nodes. This follows treatment of the primary lesion and a course of antibiotics to resolve the extensive lymphadenopathy that is present from either infection or metastases (Schellhammer, 1994). Complications of phlebitis, pulmonary embolism, wound infection, and lymphedema can occur after lymphadenectomy. Improved preoperative and post-operative care and improved surgical techniques and procedures have lessened the occurrence of these complications.

Penectomy

There are two types of penectomy: partial and total. Partial penectomy is performed if the lesion is located on the distal shaft of the penis or is limited to the glans. In a partial penectomy, with the patient in a lithotomy position, a tourniquet is applied around the penis. The tumor area is demarcated, and an incision is made that amputates the corpora cavernosa, corpus spongiosum, and urethra. The remaining urethra and retracted skin flaps are sutured into a penile stump, which allows the patient to void in a normal, upright position and is serviceable for some sexual function. An indwelling catheter may be inserted at the time of surgery and left in place for 24 to 48 hours.

Total penectomy is performed for penile cancer when the lesion involves the proximal penile shaft such that a functional penile stump cannot be created. For this procedure, also done with the patient in a lithotomy position, an incision is made from the pubis down and around the penis into the perineum. The roots of the corpora cavernosa are identified; the urethra is isolated; and the penis is amputated. Next, the urethra is brought out through the perineum, creating a perineal urethrostomy, which allows for voiding in a sitting position. A urethral catheter is inserted into the bladder through the perineal urethrostomy; an incisional drain is placed in the wound; and a compression dressing is applied to prevent scrotal edema (Fig. 39–7).

For some patients, phallic reconstruction using microneurovascular tissue transfers is possible after a total penectomy.

Preoperative Preparation

Any infection in the tissue of the penis is treated with antibiotics and resolved before surgery is scheduled, because infection is associated with an increased risk of postoperative hemorrhage, tissue sloughing, and necrosis. The penile lesion is cleansed and, if extensive, is kept covered with a

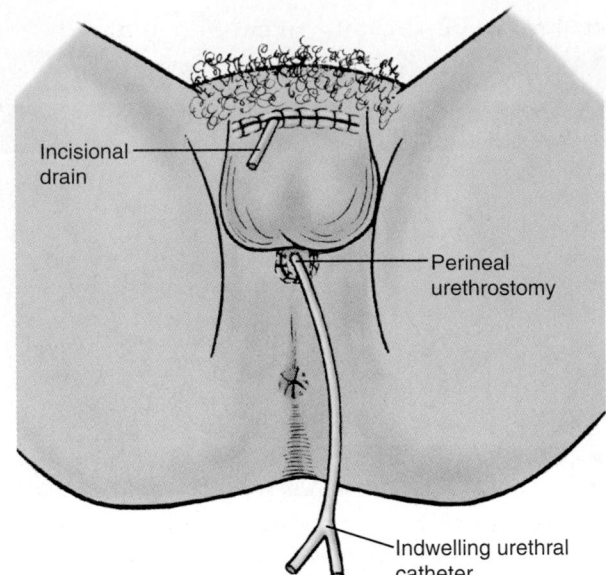

Figure 39–7

Total penectomy: incision, drain, and perineal urethrostomy.

dry, sterile dressing to prevent contamination. A preoperative shave from the umbilicus to the mid-thigh may be done. If an inguinal/pelvic node dissection is planned, cleansing enemas, antiembolic stockings, and antibiotics may be ordered.

Postoperative Course

After a penectomy, compression dressings are kept in place for 36 to 48 hours and are reinforced as needed. When a total penectomy is done, the dressings are held firmly in place by a scrotal support. Drainage is expected and should be serosanguineous, not frankly bloody.

After inguinal/pelvic node dissection, percutaneous closed-catheter suction is in place in the wound to prevent accumulation of drainage. The patient is on bedrest with the legs elevated until shortly before discharge. The patient is maintained on low-dose heparin or warfarin sodium (Coumadin) therapy during this time. The patient may be discharged with instructions to continue antibiotic therapy. Appropriate referrals to a visiting nurse service for home care services should take place before discharge. Follow-up instructions should include the date and the time of the first postoperative visit. At follow-up visits after a total penectomy and perineal urethrostomy, the patient is checked carefully for signs of urethral stenosis and infection. If urethral stenosis occurs, dilatation of the urethra may be necessary. This procedure can be done in the physician's office.

❖ Settings, Providers, and Collaboration for Care

Patients with penile cancer usually receive initial care in the physician's office or ambulatory care unit. In some cases, a biopsy may be done at this visit; in other cases, the patient is admitted to the hospital for biopsy, staging, and tumor excision.

If a total penectomy is performed and a perineal urethrostomy is established, collaboration with an enterostomal nurse therapist is essential and postsurgical care may continue on a subacute or transitional care unit. If the patient is discharged directly home from the acute care setting, referral to a visiting nurse service for assessment of home care management and wound care is a priority. The assistance of a home health aide may also be needed.

For patients with a noninvasive carcinoma biopsied in an outpatient setting, subsequent treatment may be in a radiation facility or an ambulatory surgical unit for laser therapy. For patients receiving IV chemotherapy for lymph node metastasis, treatment may be administered in an ambulatory or inpatient oncology unit or in the oncologist's office.

NURSING PROCESS
Penectomy

PREOPERATIVE NURSING CARE

Preoperative care varies somewhat according to the stage of the disease and the extent of the scheduled surgery. Basic assessments, nursing diagnoses, expected patient outcomes, and nursing interventions for any preoperative cancer patient apply. In addition, be alert for anticipatory grieving, particularly in the patient scheduled for a total penectomy, with its concomitant loss of the capacity for normal urination and sexual intercourse.

POSTOPERATIVE NURSING CARE

Assessment

Assess the return to physiologic stabilization as for any postsurgical patient. Take vital signs. Check the dressing for drainage. Check the urinary catheter for patency. Note the amount and color of urinary output.

If an inguinal/pelvic node dissection has been done, measure drainage from the wound suction, and note its appearance. Observe for swelling in the lower extremities, which indicates lymphedema. Assess for signs of thrombophlebitis. These include swelling, pain, and redness in the calf and a positive Homans' sign. Check the wound for edema, redness, skin sloughing, and other signs of infection, which are likely to occur from 4 to 12 days after surgery. If the patient is discharged within this time, instruct him to observe for and promptly report any of these complications.

Because penectomy is radical, disfiguring surgery, carefully assess the patient's psychological response. Observe for signs of sadness, such as sighing, and for avoidance behaviors, such as anger or withdrawal. Be aware of the patient's need to grieve, and determine his stage of grieving. Assess

for problems related to the grieving process, such as difficulty eating and sleeping. Assess the patient's interest and willingness to participate in self-care and his outlook toward the future. Assess interaction with significant others. In terms of his interaction with his sexual partner, assess his willingness to discuss the surgery, to demonstrate affection, and to plan for the future.

Nursing Diagnoses and Planning

Nursing diagnoses and related expected patient outcomes commonly applicable to patients who have had surgery for cancer of the penis include those related to pain, anxiety, and knowledge deficit: postoperative course, plan of continued care, and self-care after discharge. Additional nursing diagnoses and related expected patient outcomes particularly applicable to patients who have had a total penectomy include the following:

NDx: Body image disturbance related to loss of sexual and urinary functions of the penis

Planning: Patient Outcomes
1. Patient looks at the operative site.
2. Patient sits to void.
3. Patient wipes front to back after voiding and defecating.
4. Patient verbalizes acceptance of change in urinary and sexual functions.
5. Patient refers to himself in positive masculine terms.

NDx: Sexual dysfunction related to loss of the penis

Planning: Patient Outcomes
1. Patient identifies alternative methods of sexual expression.
2. Patient discusses concerns about the loss of ability to have intercourse and desirability as a sexual partner with his partner.

NDx: Risk for powerlessness related to the diagnosis of cancer and the effects of penectomy

Planning: Patient Outcomes
1. Patient identifies the areas over which he has control.
2. Patient makes choices regarding care.
3. Patient participates in self-care.
4. Patient participates, with his significant other, in decision-making about family concerns.

Nursing Interventions and Evaluation

NDx: Body image disturbance
Convey caring, acceptance, and perception of the patient as masculine. Avoid any facial expressions or comments that could be interpreted by the patient as indicating revulsion, pity, or perceived loss of masculinity. Provide the patient with privacy during care and during conversations about his treatment. Be especially sensitive to the patient's need for privacy when the catheter is removed and he first has to sit to void. Collaborate with the enter-

ostomal therapist as needed, especially about problems with the urethrostomy.

NDx: Sexual dysfunction

Encourage the patient to express his feelings and concerns and to share them with his sexual partner. Encourage physical expressions of affection, and provide privacy for visits between the patient and his partner. Refer the patient and his partner to a clinical specialist, professional sex therapist, or other resource as indicated.

NDx: Risk for powerlessness

Keep the call bell within reach. Make frequent, brief visits to the patient's room to prevent him from feeling alone and helpless.

Make the patient aware of areas of his care over which he has control by discussing needs with the patient and asking for his preferences in how to meet them. Provide him with as many choices as possible about his daily schedule, his activities, and his treatments. Encourage independence in self-care activities when the patient is able.

Assist the patient in identifying areas outside of his immediate illness and care over which he has control. As health permits, encourage him to keep informed of household events and to participate in related discussions and decision-making.

These interventions are particularly important because feelings of powerlessness are common among the elderly admitted to an acute-care health facility for any reason. Because cancer of the penis is most often diagnosed in men older than 60 years, these patients are already at risk for powerlessness before this radical surgery.

Compare the patient's status with expected outcomes. If the outcomes are not met, reassess the patient and revise the plan.

CANCER OF THE TESTIS

Testicular carcinoma represents about 1 to 2% of all malignancies in males (3000 to 4000 new cases annually in the United States) but is the most common solid tumor in men between the ages of 20 and 40 (Seidmon, 1994). It is particularly prevalent among Caucasians. With advances in chemotherapy, radiotherapy, diagnostic techniques, and surgical skills, the survival rate for testicular tumors exceeds 90%, making it the most curable cancer in all age groups (Seidmon, 1994).

Etiology and Pathophysiology

The exact cause of the various testicular malignancies is unknown. However, there is evidence to suggest that cryptorchidism, age, environmental factors, maternal treatment with DES during pregnancy, mumps orchitis, and trauma all increase the risk of the disease.

Of all primary testicular cancers, 90 to 95% arise from the germ cell epithelium of the testis and are classified as either seminomas or nonseminomas. Seminomas are the most common of all testicular malignancies. They grow slowly; they are usually localized (confined to the testicles and retroperitoneal lymph nodes); and they have a good prognosis. Nonseminomas tend to be invasive and metastasize quickly via the lymphatic system or the blood. Nonseminomatous testicular tumors include three types: embryonal carcinoma, teratoma, and choriocarcinoma.

Clinical Manifestations

Early testicular cancer is asymptomatic except for a painless, hardened area or lump on the testis found during testicular self-examination or during a routine physical examination. In some cases, the lump is not noticed until a dull ache, pain, or heavy feeling develops in the lower abdominal, inguinal, or scrotal area. If associated infection, necrosis, or hemorrhage develops within the tumor, acute testicular pain occurs. In some patients, presenting symptoms are from metastasis. These symptoms include a neck mass (supraclavicular), respiratory symptoms, gastrointestinal disturbances, a palpable abdominal mass, bone pain, central and peripheral nervous system manifestations, lower extremity edema, anorexia, and weight loss.

Diagnosis

Testicular tumors can be palpated on bimanual examination of the scrotal contents and will not transilluminate when a light is placed behind the scrotum. A malignancy is confirmed by frozen section done with the patient under anesthesia and prepared for an inguinal radical orchiectomy. A biopsy is never done as an isolated procedure to confirm testicular cancer because of the risk of precipitating metastasis.

Before confirmation and orchiectomy, serum levels of the tumor markers beta-subunit human chorionic gonadotropin and alpha-fetoprotein are obtained. These are measured again after orchiectomy and periodically thereafter to check the effectiveness of treatment. Persistent elevation of one or more of these markers indicates a residual tumor. In addition, nonspecific markers—such as lactic dehydrogenase and Regan isoenzyme of alkaline phosphatase—can be useful in following the patient's response to therapy (Pontes, 1994).

After an orchiectomy, diagnostic studies are done to determine the clinical stage of the disease and to plan further treatment. Diagnostic tests used for staging purposes include:

- CT or magnetic resonance imaging (MRI) scan of the chest, abdomen, and pelvis
- Intravenous pyelogram
- Scrotal ultrasound

On the basis of the results of these tests, the extent of testicular cancer is pathologically and clinically staged.

Table 39–5

TNM Classification System for Testicular Tumors

Primary Tumor (T)

Tx	Unknown
T0	No evidence of primary tumors
T1	Tumor confined to the testis
T2	Tumor beyond the tunica albuginea
T3	Involvement of rete testis or epididymis
T4a	Invasion of the cord
T4b	Invasion of the scrotum

Regional Lymph Nodes (N)

N1	Microscopic node involvement
N2	Multiple node involvement
N3	Extranodal extension (resectable)
N4	Unresectable nodes or incomplete resection

Distant Metastasis (M)

M0	No evidence of metastasis
M1	Metastatic disease

The TNM classification system for testicular tumors best describes the depth of invasion with testicular carcinoma (Table 39–5). Its use has increased with the advent of surveillance protocols and identification of prognostic factors associated with the primary tumor (Pontes, 1994). In the past, most classifications were based on pathologic findings because patients underwent retroperitoneal lymph node dissection (Table 39–6). Currently either or both classifications may be cited in staging testicular carcinoma (Seidmon, 1994).

Management

The initial treatment of cancer of the testis is inguinal radical orchiectomy done at the time of biopsy. Subsequent treatment is based on the type of tumor, presence of tumor markers, and clinical stage of the disease. Treatment has progressed to the point at which radiotherapy alone or limited chemotherapy combined with a modified retroperitoneal lymph node dissection has led to decreased morbidity and improved quality of life for these patients (Seidmon, 1994).

Seminomas are treated by inguinal radical orchiectomy and may be followed by postoperative external beam radiation to the lymph drainage areas of the testes. For more extensive disease, multidrug chemotherapy using a combination of various agents—cisplatin, etoposide, actinomycin D, cyclophosphamide, doxorubicin, bleomycin, and vinblastine—may be given before or after radiation. Lymphadenectomy is rarely employed because seminomas are highly radiosensitive.

Nonseminomatous testicular tumors (NSTTs) are usually treated by radical orchiectomy, retroperitoneal lymphadenectomy, chemotherapy, or a combination. In patients with advanced NSTT, a tendency has developed in recent years to treat patients aggressively with high-dose chemotherapy and bone marrow autotransplant as the second line of therapy if the initial chemotherapy fails (Pontes, 1994). However, this approach is considered investigational in some areas of the United States. All patients with testicular cancer, regardless of the type or stage, require careful follow-up with a CT scan (chest, abdominal, and pelvic scans), assessment of tumor markers, and monthly physical examinations for the first 2 years after diagnosis. Frequency of follow-up may then be decreased because most recurrences appear within the first 24 months, although some late relapses do occur.

Inguinal Orchiectomy

In an inguinal radical orchiectomy, the testis, tunica vaginalis, and all except a stump of the spermatic cord are removed. The inguinal canal is explored for metastasis through an incision high in the groin. A gel-filled testicular prosthesis may be inserted for cosmetic effect before the wound is closed with metal staples or silk sutures.

Retroperitoneal Lymph Node Dissection

Retroperitoneal lymph node dissection involves bilateral removal of lymph nodes and channels in the iliac and lumbar regions using either a transabdominal or thoracoabdominal approach. Retroperitoneal lymph node dissection may be used to treat stage I and II nonseminomatous testicular tumors. The amount of surgical dissection depends on the clinical stage. The status of lymph nodes can be determined by a CT scan or by MRI or both. With the increased effectiveness of systemic chemotherapy, questions of submitting all patients with negative metastatic workups to prophylactic lymphadenectomy are being evaluated (Pontes, 1994). After an orchiectomy, surveillance protocols with well-defined criteria for entry have shown the feasibility of this conservative approach for patients with selected

Table 39–6

Pathologic and Clinical Staging of Testicular Carcinoma

Stage	Definition
Stage A (I)	Tumor confined to the testis
Stage B1 (IIa)	Few nodes in the retroperitoneum usually detected at the time of node dissection
Stage B2 (IIb)	Nodes greater than 2 to 6 cm
Stage B3 (IIc)	Nodes greater than 6 cm
Stage C (III)	Spread above the diaphragm, especially to the lungs or involving abdominal solid organs

stage I and stage II nonseminoma. If retroperitoneal lymph node dissection is indicated, surgical approaches that preserve ejaculatory function (modified nerve-sparing retroperitoneal lymph node dissection) can be performed. If a relapse occurs after retroperitoneal lymph node dissection, chemotherapy can be instituted.

PATIENT PREPARATION. Preoperative orders are reviewed with the patient at his preoperative nursing screening visit. Mechanical bowel preparation begins 3 to 4 days before surgery to decrease the risk of postoperative paralytic ileus. Instruct the patient to take ordered laxatives, enemas, and a low-residue diet, which is changed to clear liquids 24 hours before the operation. Instruct the patient to have nothing by mouth (NPO) after midnight.

Coughing, deep breathing, and the use of an incentive spirometer are reviewed as prophylaxis against pulmonary complications. Tell the patient that he will be encouraged to move around while in bed and to flex his ankles and legs. Reassure him that pain medication will be available.

Skin preparation usually consists of a shower with an antimicrobial soap the evening before surgery. A shave from the chest to the midthigh is usually done at the time of surgery. Central and arterial lines may be inserted preoperatively.

Cryopreservation of semen for sperm banking may also be done preoperatively if desired by the patient. This may be chosen because retrograde ejaculation, which produces functional sterility, may develop from surgical damage to the sympathetic nerves that control propulsion of semen into the urethra. The nurse reinforces the information given by the surgeon about the extent of surgery and gives the patient appropriate reassurance to the patient, family, and significant others.

PROCEDURE. Retroperitoneal lymph node dissection is a major operative procedure that lasts 3 to 6 hours, sometimes longer, and involves either a transabdominal or a thoracoabdominal approach. In the transabdominal approach, a midline incision is made from the xiphoid process to the symphysis pubis. With a thoracoabdominal approach, the right 10th rib is resected; the pleura are entered; and chest tubes are inserted. The incision extends from the chest down to the lower abdomen.

POSTOPERATIVE COURSE. Management of patients who have not received chemotherapy before retroperitoneal lymph node dissection is the same as that of patients who have had abdominal surgery. Postchemotherapy patients with retroperitoneal lymph node dissection are usually taken to the critical care unit (Brock, 1993). The patient must maintain NPO status and has a nasogastric tube in place attached to low suction until peristalsis returns. It is not uncommon for patients to develop postoperative ileus, which relates to the extent of the surgical dissection. IV fluids and electrolytes are given to replace those lost as a result of surgery and gastric suction. In patients with postchemotherapy retro-

peritoneal lymph node dissection, fluid management can be difficult. This is thought to be due in part to pulmonary toxicity if bleomycin was used (Brock, 1993). Fluids may be restricted and urinary output monitored very carefully. Initially the patient may receive colloid IV solutions of human plasma protein fraction or salt-poor albumin to prevent fluid overload. Crystalloid fluid (Ringer's lactate solution) is then ordered to maintain fluid balance. Pulmonary function is monitored very carefully. The patient is observed carefully for the complication of noncardiogenic pulmonary edema. A Foley catheter is kept in place to monitor urinary output.

The patient is usually ambulated on the first postoperative day and discharged within 5 to 6 days.

COMPLICATIONS. Complications of retroperitoneal lymph node dissection include atelectasis, paralytic ileus, wound infection, and wound dehiscence.

❖ Settings, Providers, and Collaboration for Care

Patients with testicular cancer usually begin their care in the physician's office or an ambulatory care setting. Once surgery is planned, the patient is admitted to the hospital, and the patient's length of stay is dependent on the stage of the disease and the extent of the surgical procedure. As part of the discharge plan, a subacute or transitional care unit may be recommended to allow the patient to continue his convalescence in a supervised setting before returning home. If the patient is discharged directly home from the acute care setting, referral to a visiting nurse service may be indicated to monitor the patient's progress and provide wound care.

NURSING PROCESS
Inguinal Orchiectomy

PREOPERATIVE NURSING CARE

Preoperative care of the patient scheduled for an inguinal orchiectomy requires that the nurse have an in-depth database about the man with a testicular malignancy. Basic assessments, nursing diagnoses, expected patient outcomes, and nursing interventions that relate to any preoperative patient with cancer apply. Note any symptoms that may indicate metastatic spread. In addition, be aware of the wide-ranging implications that a diagnosis of testicular cancer has for the patient, significant other, and family. It affects virtually every area of life, including social, economic, psychological, sexual, and reproductive function. Fertility issues should be discussed if the patient and significant other are interested in having children. In some cases, sperm banking may be an option. This is done before radiation, chemotherapy, or retroperitoneal lymph node dissection to prevent harvesting mutagenic sperm.

Once the testicular tumor has been analyzed and

a treatment plan is established, provide information and the realistic reassurance necessary.

POSTOPERATIVE NURSING CARE

Assessment

Assess the patient's physiologic response to surgery. Monitor the patient's vital signs, and observe for bleeding and scrotal edema. Assess the degree and location of pain. Note the time and amount of first voiding, because catheterization may be necessary if adequate voiding is not established within 8 to 10 hours.

In the postoperative period, assess the patient's emotional response to the surgery. Does he fear that the orchiectomy has resulted in demasculinization? If a testicular implant was not inserted, is he concerned about the appearance of the empty scrotal sac?

If further diagnostic testing and additional treatments are necessary, determine the patient's level of understanding of these procedures.

Nursing Diagnoses and Planning

Nursing diagnoses and related expected patient outcomes commonly applicable to patients who have undergone an inguinal orchiectomy include the following:

NDx: Pain (inguinal and scrotal) related to surgical trauma and accompanying edema of the scrotum

Planning: Patient Outcomes
1. Patient requests pain medication.
2. Patient reports that pain is decreased or no longer present.
3. Patient moves in bed and ambulates without major discomfort.

NDx: Risk for body image disturbance related to removal of the testis

Planning: Patient Outcomes
1. Patient describes realistically the effects of the surgery on his appearance and function.
2. Patient verbalizes feelings about himself in relationship to the removal of the testis.
3. Patient looks at the incision.
4. Patient expresses feelings of self-worth and sexual adequacy.
5. Patient resumes self-care activities.

NDx: Risk for altered health maintenance related to insufficient knowledge of diagnosis, plan of further treatment, postdischarge care, and testicular self-examination

Planning: Patient Outcomes
1. Patient describes the plan of further treatment.
2. Patient describes and demonstrates care of the wound.
3. Patient states the signs and symptoms of wound complications that should be reported.

4. Patient describes the importance of monthly testicular self-examination as a means of early detection of cancer in the remaining testis.
5. Patient demonstrates testicular self-examination.
6. Patient states the date and time of the first postoperative follow-up visit and the importance of keeping the frequent (monthly) subsequent appointments.

Nursing Interventions and Evaluation

NDx: Pain
Administer analgesics according to the physician's order and the patient's need. Support their effectiveness with comfort measures to promote skeletal muscle relaxation. Splint the incision by placing a pillow over it whenever the patient coughs, deep-breathes, turns, or moves.

Because scrotal swelling usually accompanies an orchiectomy and contributes to the patient's discomfort, keep the scrotum elevated through the application of a Bellevue bridge or the use of an athletic support. Apply ice packs to the scrotal area as ordered.

NDx: Risk for body image disturbance
Encourage the patient to express how he thinks about and views himself as a result of the surgery. During wound care, describe the appearance of the wound, and allow the patient to see it if he desires. If a testicular prosthesis was not inserted at the time of the orchiectomy and the patient expresses concerns about the appearance of the empty scrotal sac, encourage him to discuss an implant with his physician. Clarify the physician's explanation about the effects of surgery and any further treatment on the patient's sexual function.

Provide a quiet environment for the patient and his partner or significant other to share their feelings about the impact of the surgery on their relationship. Give information, and recommend community resources such as the American Cancer Society (ACS), Make Today Count, or a local mental health center for support after discharge.

Encourage independence in self-care activities as soon as possible.

NDx: Risk for altered health maintenance
Reinforce the physician's explanation of the type of cancer found, the extent of the disease, and plans for future treatment.

If a dressing continues to be required at the time of discharge, explain the care of the wound, and ask the patient to demonstrate it. Instruct the patient to report immediately any signs of wound complications such as increased erythema, bloody or purulent drainage, wound dehiscence, or fever.

Stress the importance of monthly testicular self-examination, because a malignant tumor can develop in the remaining testis, and instruct the patient in the technique if needed.

Provide information regarding the date and time of the first follow-up visit.

Compare the patient's status with expected outcomes. If the outcomes are not met, reassess the patient and revise the plan.

NURSING PROCESS GUIDELINES
Retroperitoneal Lymph Node Dissection

Preoperative and postoperative nursing care for the patient undergoing retroperitoneal lymph node dissection is similar to that described for any patient with cancer who is having major surgery (see Chaps. 6 and 34). If the thoracoabdominal approach is used, nursing care described for the patient having chest surgery also applies (see Chap. 14).

Be sensitive to the fact that cancer of the testis primarily affects young men and often occurs when they are trying to establish and maintain families. Encourage the patient by telling him that advancements in chemotherapy, radiotherapy, diagnostic techniques, and modified nerve-sparing retroperitoneal lymph node dissection have raised the survival rate above 90%. This makes testicular cancer the most curable cancer in all age groups (Seidmon, 1994).

Because retrograde ejaculation may accompany extensive bilateral retroperitoneal lymph node dissection, there is a risk of sterility, and this may be overwhelming to the patient and his partner if an extensive lymph node dissection is planned. In some cases, the patient may feel that he cannot continue an intimate relationship because of his sterility. Be sure to assess the patient's coping strategies, and help him to use them during this period of adjustment. Encourage the patient to discuss his feelings and concerns with his partner. Remind the patient that his ability to have an erection and experience orgasm has not been affected.

Be aware that there may also be a grief reaction over the perceived loss of reproductive function and the possibility of premature death. Allow time for the patient to progress through the stages of grieving. Reassure the patient that his feelings related to the loss are expected responses to the diagnosis of cancer and changes experienced. Be empathic about the loss, and offer a realistic but hopeful approach based on the long-term survival rate after retroperitoneal lymph node dissection. Provide information about local mental health counseling services and support groups for continued assistance in working through the grief after discharge from the hospital.

BENIGN PROSTATIC HYPERPLASIA

Etiology and Pathophysiology

Benign prostatic hyperplasia (BPH) is an overgrowth of cells in the prostate gland. This increase in the number of cells, with its concomitant enlargement of the gland, appears to be a normal part of aging. Its

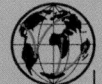

INTERNET CONNECTIONS
Disorders of the Male Reproductive System

General
Health Answers/Men's Health
http://healthanswers.com/health_answers/
search_get_answer/forums/menhealth/index.htm
This authoritative site provides information on a wide variety of issues and disorders related to the male reproductive system.

Disorders of the Prostate
The Prostatitis Home Page
http://www.prostate.org/
This page, sponsored by the Prostatitis Foundation, provides information for patients and for health-care professionals. It includes answers to frequently asked questions, information on treatment options, and links to other sites, including a site for the Prostatitis Foundation.

American Prostate Society
http://www.ameripros.org/
This site provides statistics on prostate cancer.

exact cause, however, is not known. The fact that it occurs only in aging men with normal testicular function suggests that hormones play an important part in its development. Nutritional, metabolic, neoplastic, arteriosclerotic, and inflammatory processes may also contribute.

BPH usually occurs in the form of nodules in the lateral or middle lobes of the prostate. These nodules almost always develop in the inner portion of the gland. As they grow, they compress the normal prostatic tissue toward its outer surface. This creates a so-called surgical capsule around the nodule (a structural difference between the nodule and the normal prostatic tissue), which allows the nodule to be surgically removed or enucleated without removing the entire gland. In addition to compressing normal prostatic tissue outward, nodular enlargement can impinge on the lateral walls of the urethra and reduce its diameter to a slit. This narrowing increases resistance to the outward flow of urine and results in hypertrophy of the detrusor muscles of the bladder in an attempt to compensate. This in turn leads to the formation of trabeculae (fibromuscular bands or cords) and bladder diverticula, which predispose to infection and development of bladder calculi from retention of urine in these spaces. Ureters may dilate because of the increased voiding pressure. Even the kidneys may become distended, with resultant renal insufficiency.

Clinical Manifestations

Many men with BPH have no clinical symptoms. When they do occur, the classic symptoms are frequency of urination, nocturia, difficulty starting and stopping the urine stream, a weak stream, overflow dribbling, and a feeling of being unable to completely empty the bladder. If cystitis develops secondary to the stasis of retained urine in the bladder, dysuria, urgency, and hematuria occur. As urethral obstruction becomes complete, symptoms of acute urinary retention also appear.

If prostatic enlargement and urethral obstruction develop very slowly, the patient may not report symptoms. The problem may be discovered on routine examination, at which time the patient may already have significant renal insufficiency and related secondary anemia as well as hypertension.

Diagnosis

In the initial evaluation of the patient with prostatism, the Agency for Health Care Policy and Research (AHCPR) recommends the following:

- A detailed medical history including a focus on the urinary tract and co-existing medical problems
- A physical examination that includes a digital rectal examination
- A focused neurologic examination
- Urinalysis (to rule out renal insufficiency)
- Test of prostate-specific antigen levels

The patient should also be asked to complete the American Urological Association (AUA) Symptom Index (see Chap. 38) to help quantify symptom severity.

The diagnosis of BPH is based on a history and palpation of a smooth, firm, elastic enlargement of the prostate gland on digital rectal examination. The examiner may also observe the patient's voiding to confirm a decrease in the size or force of the urinary stream.

Management

Treatments for BPH delineated in the AHCPR Clinical Practice Guidelines include watchful waiting, alpha-blocker therapy, finasteride therapy, balloon dilatation, transurethral incision of the prostate, transurethral resection of the prostate, and open prostatectomy. The treatment selected for a specific patient is based on the severity of the symptoms, degree of prostatic involvement, and presence of complications.

Watchful waiting is a strategy of management in which the patient is monitored by his physician but receives no active intervention for BPH. Patients are usually instructed in self-care behaviors designed to manage the problem. These behaviors include:

- Engaging in regular prostatic massage and sexual intercourse to help decrease prostatic congestion
- Limiting the amount of fluids, especially alcohol, taken at any one time to avoid distending the bladder and making voiding difficult
- Urinating at the first urge
- Avoiding drugs that can precipitate urinary retention, such as anticholinergics, antidepressants, decongestants, and tranquilizers

Alpha-blocker therapy is a treatment using any of the α_1-adrenergic receptor blockers, including doxazosin, prazosin, and terazosin. These medications inhibit alpha-adrenergic mediated contraction of prostatic smooth muscle. This muscle relaxation decreases straining on urination and facilitates bladder emptying. Response to treatment with alpha blockers occurs within weeks to a few months. Side effects of these drugs include tiredness, orthostatic hypotension, dizziness, and headaches.

Finasteride therapy is treatment with the drug finasteride (Proscar). Finasteride is an inhibitor of the enzyme 5-alpha reductase, which converts testosterone to dehydrotestosterone, a powerful androgen responsible for the development of the prostate gland. When the action of this enzyme is inhibited, conversion of testosterone into dihydrotestosterone is impaired; levels of dihydrotestosterone drop; and the prostate gland decreases in size in most men. This response can take 6 months to occur and is not always associated with a decrease in symptoms of urinary obstruction. Side effects of finasteride therapy include decreased volume of ejaculate and, in a few men, reduced sexual urge and difficulty with erection.

Balloon dilatation is a procedure in which a catheter with a balloon at the end is inserted through the urethra and into the prostatic urethra. The balloon is then inflated to stretch the urethra where it is narrowed by the prostate.

Transurethral incision of the prostate is an endoscopic surgical procedure limited to patients with smaller prostates (30 g or less of resected weight) in which an instrument is passed through the urethra to make one or two cuts in the prostate and prostatic capsule, thus reducing constriction of the urethra. This procedure can be done on an outpatient basis.

Transurethral resection of the prostate is the surgical removal of the prostate's inner portion by endoscopic approach through the urethra, with no external skin incision. This is the most common active treatment for symptomatic BPH and usually requires a 1- to 3-day hospital stay.

Open prostatectomy involves surgical removal (enucleation) of the inner portion of the prostate via a suprapubic or retropubic incision in the lower abdominal area. Perineal prostatectomies are rarely done. Open prostatectomy requires a longer hospital stay. See Chapter 38 for discussion of these procedures.

Watchful waiting is recommended for patients with an AUA Symptom Index of 7 or less. For patients with moderate to severe symptoms (8 or above) information about the benefits and risks of the various treatments should be given as a basis for decision-making on the part of the patient. This information should include a clear statement about the range of uncertainty associated with the benefits and risks of each treatment option. One source of this information is the pamphlet entitled *Patient Guide: Treating Your Enlarged Prostate,* which is available from the AHCPR.

AHCPR guidelines recommend surgery for patients with refractory urinary retention who have failed at least one attempt at catheter removal and for those who have recurrent urinary tract infections, recurrent gross hematuria, bladder stones, or renal insufficiency clearly caused by BPH.

Several new treatment modalities for BPH are being investigated for their risks and benefits, including laser prostatectomy, hyperthermia, thermal therapy, prostatic stents, and hormonal manipulation.

In a laser prostatectomy, specially designed laser fibers are introduced into the prostatic urethra under direct vision by means of either a cystoscope or transurethral ultrasound imaging. The energy delivered by the laser fibers results in prostatic tissue vaporization and ablation. Evidence from short-term, noncontrolled trials suggests that laser prostatectomy produces significant symptom score improvement (AHCPR, 1994).

Hyperthermia and thermal therapy of the prostate (transrectal or transurethral) utilize electromagnetic waves with a frequency greater than 200 MHz (microwaves) to induce heating and presumably tissue damage. To destroy normal tissue, a temperature in excess of 45°C (113°F) is probably required. The use of temperature above 45°C is referred to as thermal therapy (thermotherapy). Use of temperatures from 40 to 44°C (104–111.2°F) is referred to as hyperthermia (AHCPR, 1994).

Prostatic stents are stainless-steel, biologically inert devices that can be placed into the prostatic urethra under either endoscopic or fluoroscopic control. When expanded in the prostatic urethra, they partially relieve obstruction from the surrounding prostatic tissue. Over a period of a few weeks to a few months, the stents are covered with normal transitional cell epithelium. Stents can be used in extremely poor-risk patients who do not respond to drug therapy or to intermittent catheterization.

❖ Settings, Providers, and Collaboration for Care

The patient with BPH usually begins his care in the physician's office or in an ambulatory care unit. In the event that acute urinary obstruction develops, the patient may seek treatment in a hospital emergency room. If surgery is planned, the patient is usually admitted to the hospital on the day of surgery with a 1- to 3-day inpatient postoperative recovery period allowed. Since BPH primarily affects

the elderly, further convalescence may be necessary in a subacute or transitional care unit before the patient returns home. Once he is discharged to home, home health care services from a visiting nurse service may be necessary. In some cases, the patient may need long-term care placement.

NURSING PROCESS GUIDELINES
Prostatectomy

See Chapter 38 for a discussion of the nursing care of patients undergoing all types of prostatectomy. Also see the Clinical Pathway for the patient undergoing a transurethral resection of the prostate.

CANCER OF THE PROSTATE

Cancer of the prostate occurs primarily in men older than 50 years of age. Its highest incidence is in men approximately 70 years of age; more than 80% of cases occur in men over 65 years of age (Stewart, 1994). Prostate cancer is the second leading cause of cancer deaths among men, after lung cancer. According to ACS estimates, about 317,000 men will be diagnosed with prostate cancer in 1996 in the United States. Some 41,100 will die of it. Cancer of the prostate is more frequent in African-Americans than in other ethnic groups.

Etiology and Pathophysiology

The cause of prostate cancer is unknown, although hormones are generally believed to play a role. Genetic, viral, environmental, and dietary factors may also be involved. Familial clustering of the disease has been observed, but no genetic markers have been described (Stewart, 1994). Viruses, such as cytomegalovirus and type 2 herpesvirus, are seen more frequently in cancerous prostatic tissue. A higher incidence of prostate cancer has been observed among men who have prolonged occupational exposure to cadmium through welding, alkaline battery production, or electroplating. Men with other work-related exposures include farmers, typesetters, ship fitters, and those involved in horticulture (Stewart, 1994). Dietary research has shown that a low-fat diet slowed tumor growth in laboratory animals that had harbored human cancers. Diets high in fruits and vegetables, especially tomatoes, have shown an inverse association with prostate cancer. Carotenoids and retinoids may be protective (Greco and Kulowiak, 1994).

The most common form of prostatic cancer is adenocarcinoma. The histologic grade of the carcinoma, as determined by features such as nuclear morphology, cell size, and glandular differentiation, is an important prognostic factor (Garnick, 1995). There is no universally accepted grading system, but most grading systems refer to well differentiated, moderately differentiated, and poorly differentiated.

Patient Name: _____

DRG#: 336 _____

Date: _____

LOS: 48 hr (PO#2) _____

	Day 1	Day 2 (PO#1)	Day 3 (PO#2)
Medication	Colace (stool softener) started on the day before surgery and continued postoperatively IV-Abx Eg ANCEF—one dose before surgery After surgery—B&O suppository or Ditropan for bladder spasms. Demerol (2 doses) for unrelieved bladder spasms.	Colace Ditropan or B&O suppository for bladder spasms while the catheter is in place Antibiotic PO (eg, Cipro) q 6 h	Colace Ditropan for unrelieved bladder spasms PO antibiotic q 6 h
Diagnostic Tests	Preadmission CBC, creatinine, PT, PTT bleeding time, urinalysis, ECG, chest x-ray	HCT and Hgb may be ordered if the blood loss is significant. Electrolytes if imbalance suspected.	
Diet	NPO 6–8 hours before surgery Postoperatively: when fully awake clear liquids to diet as tolerated	Diet as tolerated.	Diet as tolerated.
Activity	Bedrest	Ambulate with assistance. Sitting limited to 15-minute intervals.	Ambulate independently. Sitting limited to 15-minute intervals.
Treatments/Nursing Actions	Use a three-way Foley catheter, usually with continuous N/S bladder irrigation. Maintain traction on catheter if ordered (traction usually removed in 6 hours). Manual bladder irrigation PRN—eg, if the urine flow stops, hand irrigate. Instruct the patient to report any voiding or dribbling around the catheter. Monitor the color of the urine: It should be pink to clear. Continuous irrigation may need to be increased if urine changes from pink to red with clots. I & O: force fluids, unless contraindicated. Monitor vital signs as ordered. Position the catheter bag on the side to which the patient is turned. Keep the catheter tubing in a straight line from the bed to the drainage bag. Keep the Foley anchored to the leg. Instruct the patient on the use of relaxation techniques for pain.	Assess vital signs and lung sounds. The Foley is removed in 24 hours—instruct the patient to void when the urge is present. Allow the patient to stand to void. Measure each voiding. Report any voiding less than 50 mL. Check for bladder distention if voiding small amounts. Assess the color of the urine. Report bright red blood or clots in the urine. The IV is usually discontinued. I & O: force fluids—2–3 L unless contraindicated.	Assess vital signs and lung sounds. Check color of urine, report bright red blood or clots. Measure each voiding—report voiding less than 50 mL Check for bladder distention if voiding small amounts. I&O Force fluids to 2–3 L unless contraindicated. The patient is discharged if voiding adequately with no bleeding and no infection.
Teaching/Discharge Planning	Before surgery, assess the patient's understanding of the procedure as instructed by MD and clarify misunderstandings. Explain the need for a Foley catheter, irrigation, frequency of vital signs, bedrest, and management of discomfort. Instruct re: turning, coughing, deep breathing, use of incentive spirometer if ordered. Postoperatively, continue to reinforce preoperative teaching.	Reinforce preoperative teaching. Stress need for 2–3 L fluid per day. Explain reason for limiting sitting to 15-minute intervals.	Instruct the patient not to strain while having a BM; continue use of a stool softener. Avoiding sitting for long periods. Stress the need for 2–3 L of fluids per day. Instruct the patient to avoid heavy lifting and sexual activity for 6 weeks. Teach the patient to use Kegel exercises to regain urinary control. Reinforce follow-up care with MD. Notify MD if fever or blood in urine occurs. Review any discharge medications (eg, Colace, Cipro) with the patient. Stress the need for an annual prostate examination. The frail elderly may need discharge to a nursing home or subacute unit for convalescence.

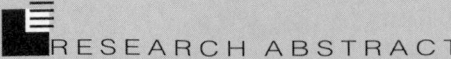

RESEARCH ABSTRACT

Does Education Improve Prostate Cancer Awareness in African-American Men?

Collins, M. Increasing prostate cancer awareness in African American Men. Oncology Nursing Forum 1997; 24(1):91.

Prostate cancer is a major health problem for all men in the United States. According to the U.S. Department of Health and Human Services, however, the mortality rate for African-American men is almost two and a half times the rate for white men. Delayed diagnosis is believed to be a major factor in the difference in mortality rates.

Because of the incidence of prostate cancer, the American Cancer Society and the National Cancer Institute recommend a digital rectal examination for all men after the age of 40 years. In an effort to increase awareness of the need for screening for prostate cancer among African-American men, Collins tested an educational intervention on knowledge outcomes in a convenience sample of African-American men. Collins recruited 75 African-American subjects from a variety of community settings and asked them to complete pre-intervention and post-intervention questionnaires designed to measure knowledge about prostate cancer. Collins developed the questionnaire from American Cancer Society materials, and she used a panel of expert nurses to review the test for content validity. No reliability measures were obtained.

Collins then used group scores to look for trends. She noticed an increase in knowledge overall from pre-test to post-test. However, statements relating to prostate cancer's being the second leading cause of cancer death in men and to urinary frequency as an early warning sign continued to be the most frequently missed items.

No hypothesis testing was performed to examine whether setting made a difference in the results. Since some of the subjects were recruited at a prostate cancer screening conducted in a local church, they may have had some knowledge about prostate cancer that motivated their participation. Interactions with the physician during the screening may also have reinforced some concepts. The lack of such interaction by other subjects may have resulted in lower scores.

Culturally sensitive educational strategies may be more effective than current strategies in reaching high-risk populations. Development of such strategies is currently under way.

Questions to Consider

1. How often are health risk screenings offered in your community?
2. Are culturally sensitive messages included in advertising for these health risk screenings?
3. Do you include health promotion and risk reduction information during illness-related encounters with patients?
4. What reasons do patients give for not obtaining routine screenings for such problems as prostate cancer?

In the Gleason grading system, the primary neoplasm is scored on a scale of 2 to 10 (2 to 4, well differentiated; 5 to 7, moderately differentiated; and 8 to 10, poorly differentiated). Well-differentiated tumors suggest a favorable prognosis, whereas poorly differentiated tumors usually suggest more advanced disease (Garnick, 1995).

Clinical Manifestations

Most patients with early prostatic cancer are asymptomatic. In these cases, the tumor is found when the prostate is palpated via a digital rectal examination during a routine physical examination or occasionally during surgery for BPH. Less commonly, patients present with symptoms of bladder outlet obstruction as seen in BPH: difficulty initiating the urinary stream, decrease in size and force of the stream, involuntary release of urine, and, in some cases, acute urinary retention. Prostate cancer can present on digital rectal examination as a discrete nodule or diffuse induration of the prostate. Because

symptoms usually do not occur until late in the disease, metastases to the lymph nodes, bone, lung, and liver can be seen. Central nervous system involvement usually comes after bone involvement. The patient may complain of low back pain, pathologic fractures, bone pain, unexplained weight loss, anemia, shortness of breath, enlarged lymph nodes, lymphedema, or neurologic symptoms.

Diagnosis

The digital rectal examination, assessment of prostate-specific antigen levels, and transrectal ultrasonography are commonly used methods for detecting prostatic cancer.

The ACS and the AUA recommend that men have a digital rectal examination beginning at age 40 as part of a regular annual physical examination. Beginning at age 50, they recommend both an assessment of prostate-specific antigen levels and a digital rectal examination in that order. For men at high risk (African-American, family history of pros-

Table 39–7

Recommendations for Age-Specific Prostate-Specific Antigen Reference Ranges

Age	Reference Range (ng/ml)
40–49	0.0–2.5
50–59	0.0–3.5
60–69	0.0–4.5
70–79	0.0–6.5

tate cancer), the ACS advocates an annual assessment of prostate-specific antigen levels and digital rectal examination before age 50. The National Cancer Institute (NCI), on the other hand, does not support this annual screening protocol.

Studies to resolve the controversy are under way. Age-specific reference ranges of prostate-specific antigen levels are also being used to more selectively evaluate patients for prostate cancer (Table 39–7). The age-specific reference ranges are a refinement of the previously accepted normal range of 0 to 4 ng/mL (Garnick, 1995).

If results of either the prostate-specific antigen assessment or digital rectal examination are abnormal, transrectal ultrasonography is ordered. With transrectal ultrasonography, the adenocarcinoma appears as hypoechoic densities in the peripheral zone of the prostate (see Chap. 38). The diagnosis of prostate cancer is confirmed by transperineal or transrectal biopsy, usually performed with transrectal ultrasonography. The tumor is assigned a grade based on the level of differentiation.

After the diagnosis is confirmed, a staging workup is ordered to determine whether the cancer is confined to the prostate or has metastasized. A pelvic CT or MRI scan is commonly used to assess for lymph node involvement. If the pelvic lymph nodes are suspicious, a biopsy of at least one of the nodes may be done to determine the pathologic stage of the disease, since the presence of positive lymph nodes influences the treatment plan. A chest x-ray or chest CT scan is usually done to assess for metastatic spread to the chest. A bone scan is done because bones are a frequent site of early metastatic prostate cancer disease. A baseline prostate-specific antigen level is obtained unless already done during screening. A serum prostatic acid phosphatase may also be obtained.

Prostate-specific antigen and serum prostatic acid phosphatase are useful as tumor markers in the staging and management of prostatic cancers. Prostate-specific antigen levels are used to monitor the effectiveness of treatment as well as to detect tumor progression or recurrence. Prostate-specific antigen can be used in this way because it is produced by both normal and malignant prostatic ductal epithe-

lial cells, and its amount increases proportionately to total prostate mass. Serum prostatic acid phosphatase titers are elevated in patients with prostatic cancer because acid phosphatase, which is produced by the acinar cells, is absorbed into the circulation rather than secreted into the seminal fluid and kept in the prostate. This makes measurement of serum prostatic acid phosphatase a useful biochemical test for monitoring the progression or regression of prostatic cancer. The results of these tumor marker studies are used to determine the tentative, or clinical, stage of the disease (Garnick, 1995).

Several staging systems, including the TNM system, are currently used to identify the clinical spread of the disease. However, the most widely accepted system divides prostate cancer into Stages A to D2, as presented in Table 39–8 (Garnick, 1995).

Management

Treatment for cancer of the prostate depends on several factors, including the stage of the tumor and the age and health of the patient. Treatment modalities include surgery, radiation therapy, hormone therapy (androgen deprivation), and in some cases chemotherapy in Stage D disease following relapse after hormonal therapy.

Radical prostatectomy is the primary method of treatment for localized prostatic cancer (A_2 and B_1 stages) in an otherwise healthy male who has an additional life expectancy of at least 10 years. Using either the perineal or retropubic approach, a radical prostatectomy involves the removal of the entire prostate gland and capsule, as well as the ampulla, vas deferens, seminal vesicles, adjacent lymph nodes, and a cuff of the bladder neck.

Table 39–8

Staging of Prostate Cancer

A	No clinical indication of disease
A1	Focal, usually well-differentiated tumor
A2	Diffuse, usually poorly differentiated tumor
B	Tumor confined to the prostate
B1	Small, discrete nodule in one lobe of the gland
B2	Large nodule, multiple nodules, or multiple areas of tumor involvement
C	Tumor localized to tissues surrounding the prostate gland
C1	Tumor of less than 70 g that has extended outside the prostatic capsule and involves the seminal vesicles
C2	Tumor of more than 70 g that has extended outside the prostatic capsule and involves the seminal vesicles
D0	Tumor that has metastasized
D1	Metastasis to the pelvic lymph nodes and/or ureteral obstruction with hydronephrosis
D2	Metastasis to bone, soft tissue, other organs, or distant lymph nodes

Impotence, some degree of urinary incontinence, and significant blood loss are traditional side effects of radical prostatectomy. However, recent modifications in the technique of radical prostatectomy developed by Walsh allow bleeding to be controlled and autonomic innervation to the corpora cavernosa preserved so that erectile function is maintained in many men younger than 60 years of age. The Walsh technique, which also involves a mucosa-to-mucosa ureterovesical anastomosis, maintains urinary continence in many patients. The decision to use the Walsh technique depends on preoperative and intra-operative findings regarding the spread of the tumor (Held et al, 1994).

Other potential complications of prostatectomy are bladder neck contracture, thrombophlebitis, pulmonary embolus, rectal injury, and urinary infection.

When urinary incontinence, a potential complication of both simple and radical prostatectomy, occurs, an artificial urinary sphincter may be implanted in patients with the manual dexterity and the mental and emotional ability to operate the device. Artificial urinary sphincters are implantable, fluid-filled, solid silicone devices used to treat urinary incontinence. The prosthesis consists of three components: a cuff, a control pump, and a pressure-regulating balloon attached to each other with kink-resistant tubing. The pump is placed in the scrotum, and the fluid-filled reservoir is placed in the abdomen. When the patient squeezes the pump, fluid leaves the urethral cuff and flows into the reservoir, thus allowing the patient to empty his bladder (Fig. 39–8). Complications associated with this surgery include infection, hematoma, urethral erosion, and pump malfunction. The overall continence rate after this surgery is approximately 91% (Light, 1994). A wait of at least 6 months to 1 year before implantation of this device is recommended since this length of time is needed for many patients to achieve continence using noninvasive techniques, such as Kegel exercises, scheduled voiding, and pharmacologic interventions, such as oxybutynin (Ditropan).

The injection of a periurethral bulking agent is another option for treating prostatectomy-associated incontinence caused by urethral sphincter insufficiency. Injection of materials such as polytetrafluoroethylene (PTFE) or GAX-collagen (Contingen) into the periurethral area can increase urethral compression. These injections are done via cystoscopy. This treatment, which is not as successful in patients who have undergone pelvic radiation therapy as in those who have not, has a cure or improvement rate of about 32% (AHCPR, 1992).

Radiation therapy is used in patients with localized disease (Stages A and B), patients who are poor surgical risks regardless of stage, and patients who refuse surgery. In some cases, radiation therapy may be prescribed as adjuvant therapy after a radical prostatectomy to decrease the likelihood of tumor recurrence. It is delivered by external beam or by internal interstitial implantation of radioactive seeds. For some patients, a combination of external and internal radiation therapy may be used to provide a higher dose of radiation with fewer side effects.

External beam radiation therapy is chosen more often for larger lesions. Advances in radiation therapy have allowed the delivery of larger doses to more precisely defined anatomic areas. Computer modeling is utilized to precisely outline and deliver doses while minimally affecting surrounding normal tissues. Complications of external radiation include gastrointestinal and genitourinary symptoms and sexual impotence.

A variety of radioactive isotopes have been used for internal interstitial radiation therapy. This modality entails surgical implantation, guided by transrectal ultrasonography, of radioactive seeds containing iodine-125, gold-198, or iridium-191. Complications or side effects of internal radiation depend on the dose and source used and its placement in relation to anatomic structures. The choice of isotope depends on the stage of disease, use of concurrent therapy, and length of placement of the implant (Held et al, 1994). Although most implants are permanent, iridium-191 is removed after 24 to 72 hours. See Chapter 34 for a detailed discussion of the care of patients undergoing radiation therapy.

Radiation therapy is also used palliatively to control pain associated with bone metastases. External beam therapy may be used to debulk specific areas of metastasis, thus eliminating some of the cause of the pain. If pain relief is not achieved with the maximum dose of external radiation, or when pain results from widespread bony metastases, an IV injec-

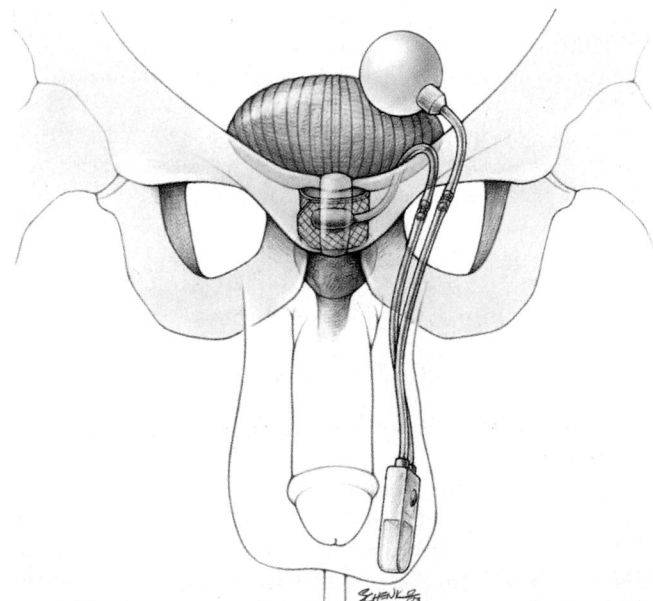

Figure 39–8

Artificial urinary sphincter. (Courtesy of American Medical Systems, Inc, Minnetonka, MN. Medical illustration by Michael Schenk.)

tion of a beta particle–emitting agent, such as strontium-89, may be given.

Hormone therapy (androgen deprivation) is a mode of treatment for prostatic cancer, usually for Stage D1 or D2. The goal of hormone therapy is to limit the amount of circulating androgens because prostate cells depend on androgen for cellular maintenance. Androgen is produced in the testicles and the adrenal glands. Deprivation of androgen can often lead to regression of disease and improvement of symptoms. Methods of achieving deprivation of androgen include surgical castration (bilateral orchiectomy), administration of exogenous estrogens, use of analogues of luteinizing hormone–releasing hormone (LHRH) that inhibit the release of pituitary gonadotropins, and use of antiandrogens that block the androgens at target tissues.

Bilateral orchiectomy (removal of both testes), commonly performed for palliation of metastatic disease, reduces testosterone levels by 90% and usually produces almost immediate pain relief. For some patients, however, this treatment option is psychologically unacceptable.

Administration of estrogens, such as DES, inhibits the release of LHRH from the hypothalamus, thus decreasing the release of follicle-stimulating hormone and luteinizing hormone from the anterior pituitary. This decreases the signal that causes testosterone production by the testes. DES is usually safe in dosages of 3 mg/day or less in men with no pre-existing cardiovascular disease. A problem with this treatment is gynecomastia and the risk of significant long-term cardiovascular side effects.

LHRH analogues such as leuprolide acetate (LUPRON) and goserelin acetate (Zoladex) can have an estrogen-like effect and can be effective in the management of prostate cancer. Leuprolide acetate is injected intramuscularly once a month or every third month depending on the preparation. Goserelin acetate is implanted subcutaneously in the abdomen for continuous release over 28 days. These drugs have fewer cardiovascular complications than DES. Antiandrogens—such as flutamide (Eulexin), megestrol (Megace), and bicalutamide (Casodex)—interfere with the action of androgen in prostatic cancer cells.

Combined androgen blockade therapy utilizing combinations of LHRH analogues and antiandrogens has been useful in achieving total androgen blockade. Many experts think that the combination of an LHRH analogue (eg, leuprolide) with an antiandrogen (eg, flutamide) represents the best therapy for newly diagnosed metastatic prostate cancer (Garnick, 1995). Patients receiving combined androgen blockade therapy appear to have better clinical responses, with lower levels of acid phosphatase and less pain.

Systemic chemotherapy may be used once hormonal therapy is no longer effective, although fewer than 10% of patients usually respond. The following drugs are used alone or in combinations: cyclophosphamide (Cytoxan), cisplatin (Platinol), estramustine (EMCYT), 5-fluorouracil, and suramin (Bayer 205). In terminal phases of prostatic cancer, high doses of prednisone (40 to 60 mg/day) can produce short periods of subjective improvement, characterized by euphoria and relief of bone pain (Garnick, 1995).

An experimental procedure showing promising results in treating localized prostate cancer is percutaneous prostate cryosurgery. It involves application of subfreezing temperatures to the tumor. Unlike a radical prostatectomy, prostatic cryosurgery involves no major abdominal incision. In addition, there is less bleeding and pain, and the patient appears to be at lower risk for incontinence and impotence than after conventional prostate surgery. Also, cryosurgery of the prostate can be performed in about 2 hours instead of 5 hours for a radical prostatectomy.

The patient having prostate cryosurgery is admitted to the hospital on the day of surgery and is usually discharged in 24 to 48 hours. To decrease the risk of postoperative infection, the patient is instructed to take cleansing enemas on the evening before surgery and prophylactic antibiotics, such as ciprofloxacin (Cipro), on the day before surgery. With the use of general or epidural anesthesia, a suprapubic bladder catheter is inserted, as well as a urethral warming device to protect the urethra from the freezing process. Using a transrectal ultrasonographic probe, three to five cryoprobes containing liquid nitrogen are inserted into the prostate gland through small puncture wounds in the perineum. When the tumor is located, the liquid nitrogen's temperature is reduced to subfreezing and the cancer cells are destroyed. Complications of this procedure are bleeding, urinary incontinence, urethrorectal fistula, urethrocutaneous fistula, and prostatic abscess.

Postoperatively the patient is monitored closely for hematuria, scrotal edema, sepsis, and bladder spasm. If spasms occur, belladonna and opium suppositories may be prescribed.

The suprapubic catheter remains in place until urethral edema secondary to the freezing process has subsided, usually about 2 weeks.

Also under experimental study is the use of prostate cancer vaccines to stimulate the body's immune system to produce its own defense against prostate tumors. This work is in its early stages and, to date, has been tried on very ill patients who have not responded to other treatment.

❖ **Settings, Providers, and Collaboration for Care**

The patient with prostate cancer usually receives care in a variety of settings depending on a number of factors, including the stage of the disease when diagnosed, the patient's age, and his general health status. Before a plan of care can be developed, a prostatic biopsy of the suspicious area is done, usually with the aid of ultrasonography. This procedure may be performed in the physician's office, an ambulatory care setting, or medical imaging facility.

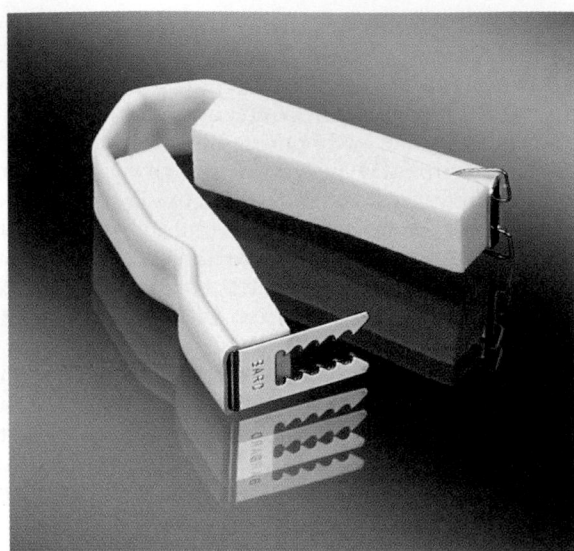

Figure 39–9

Cunningham clamp for urinary incontinence. (Courtesy of Bard Medical Division, C.R. Bard, Inc, Covington, GA.)

When the extent of the disease is determined, treatment settings may include acute inpatient hospitalization for surgery, post-hospital recovery on a subacute or transitional care unit, and home health care services. In advanced disease, or if a patient is considered a poor surgical risk, he may be referred to a radiotherapy unit for palliative care. If IV chemotherapy is planned, treatment may be administered in an ambulatory or inpatient oncology unit or in the physician's office. For the patient in the terminal stage of the disease, hospice care either at home or in a long-term care facility may be recommended.

NURSING PROCESS GUIDELINES
Prostate Cancer

Nursing care of the patient with cancer of the prostate varies according to the extent of disease, the type of treatment selected, and whether the patient is newly diagnosed or admitted for progression of the disease, a recurrence, or terminal care. Assessments, nursing diagnoses, expected patient outcomes, and nursing interventions applicable to patients with various stages of cancer who are undergoing radiation or chemotherapy are presented in Chapter 34. Nursing care of the patient undergoing a radical prostatectomy involves aspects of care for the patient having a simple prostatectomy for BPH through an abdominal or perineal approach (see Chap. 38), with several considerations. Radical prostatectomy is more extensive surgery than simple prostatectomy, thus greater preoperative teaching and support are necessary at the patient's preoperative visit. A somewhat longer postoperative recovery period may occur in the hospital. The patient and family need to be involved in discharge planning for continuity of care and management of problems as they occur. They may need referrals to appropriate community resources. Information resources from the ACS and the NCI for coping with cancer can be given to the patient.

If incontinence occurs postoperatively, instruct the patient to perform perineal (Kegel) exercises (contract the perineal muscles as if stopping and starting the urinary stream during voiding, and tighten and relax the buttocks) to improve urinary and rectal sphincter tone. For urinary incontinence, also instruct the patient to limit oral fluids during the evening to decrease incontinence at night and to avoid alcoholic beverages and caffeine because of their diuretic effect.

If intermittent catheterization, insertion of an indwelling catheter, or use of an external condom catheter attached to a drainage bag is ordered for persistent incontinence in significant amounts, instruct the patient and the family in the appropriate care. If a Cunningham clamp (Fig. 39–9)—an adjustable, lightweight, foam-lined, molded clamp that fits over the penis behind the glans—is ordered, instruct the patient and the family in its use, as specified in Highlight 39–5.

If fecal incontinence is a problem, instruct the patient in perineal exercises as described previously to improve rectal sphincter tone. Also review the prescribed bowel regimen, and stress the importance of strict adherence to the regimen if fecal incontinence is to be controlled.

If the patient is in the terminal phase of cancer of the prostate, management of pain is especially im-

---

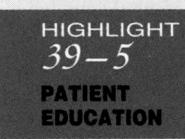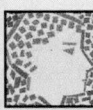

HIGHLIGHT 39–5

PATIENT EDUCATION

Using a Cunningham Clamp

Instruct the patient to:

Wash, dry, and powder the penis before applying the clamp.

Apply the clamp horizontally on the penis behind the glans.

Remove the clamp, and allow the bladder to empty at least every 4 hours to avoid bladder infection.

Inspect the penis for skin irritation and edema each time the clamp is removed.

Alternate use of the clamp with an external condom catheter if skin irritation occurs.

Secure the clamp on a looser notch if mild to moderate penile edema occurs; discontinue use of the clamp if severe edema develops.

portant. If there are localized areas of bone pain, radiotherapy to these sites is possible. Larger areas may be treated with half body or even total body radiation for pain control (Stein, 1994). Long-acting analgesics such as morphine sulfate (MS-Contin), transdermal fentanyl (Duragesic) may be needed to control pain. The patient may need blood transfusions to treat anemia. Urinary retention, renal obstruction, and hematuria may also present challenging problems.

If impotence occurs as a result of surgery, encourage the patient to discuss his reactions and feelings and to share them with his spouse or significant other. If the patient is concerned about and interested in the ability to have sexual intercourse, encourage him to discuss the possibility of a penile implant with the physician. Refer the patient to a sex therapist or counselor if appropriate.

Men often express concern about their male identity. Psychosocial and sexual implications related to the treatment of prostate cancer must be addressed early by medical and nursing staff. One of the most important messages for the patient to hear is that these concerns are reasonable and can be discussed. If the patient is on testosterone-depleting hormonal therapy, it may be helpful to explain that hormonal changes do not affect the personality of an adult (Ofman, 1993). For men who have an orchiectomy, testicular implants are available to help maintain a masculine identity and body image.

The Elderly: Special Considerations

Cancer of the prostate, BPH, and cancer of the penis are disorders found in older men. For each, early diagnosis and treatment offer the best prognosis. To achieve this, health teaching is essential. Because cancer of the prostate is initially asymptomatic, except for a hardened area on the gland itself, teach older men the importance of an annual physical examination that includes rectal palpation of the prostate. Also alert them to symptoms of BPH, such as urinary frequency, a weak stream, and difficulty starting the stream. Stress the importance of seeking medical care as soon as symptoms begin. If the disease progresses, the bladder neck may become obstructed, causing urinary retention and increasing the risk of infection in the bladder and adjacent structures.

With regard to cancer of the penis, explain that it first appears as a pimple, a warty growth, or a hardened or reddened area; if treated early, it is almost 100% curable. Instruct men to inspect the penis routinely for lesions, and have any suspicious areas promptly examined by a physician.

Common causes of problems with sexual function in the older man include medications, chronic disease, and disorders of the reproductive tract itself. Problems such as anemia, diabetes, and malnutrition can decrease libido. In other cases, however, sexual activity is diminished indirectly, through fear of the effects of sexual activity on an existing health problem, such as heart disease. Many drugs can also adversely affect sexual function. These include alcohol, reserpine, and chlorpromazine, all of which can weaken erection and delay ejaculation.

It is important to stress to older men the importance of routine physical examinations. Such examinations allow chronic diseases to be identified and treated early in their course and help to prevent, limit, or reverse negative effects. In addition, inform patients that medications may alter sexual function, and encourage them to discuss the problem with their physician. If medication-related problems develop, the problem may be eliminated by a change in medication or a reduction of the dose. Keep in mind that older men, like older women, sometimes believe that interest in sexual activity and concern about the sexual organs is only for younger people. Thus, they may be reluctant to seek care or they may accept changes in sexual function as effects of age rather than as potential disorders that can and should be treated. Be alert to these feelings, and present information designed to correct such misconceptions in an open but sensitive manner.

Chapter Review

1. How do you think a patient would react if informed that his testes needed to be removed?
2. Why should the uncircumcised male be instructed on the importance of daily penile hygiene?
3. What evidence supports the therapeutic effect of applying a Bellevue bridge for the patient with epididymitis?
4. How can the effectiveness of applying ice packs to the scrotum in the patient with orchitis or epididymitis be evaluated?
5. How will the patient with a total penectomy urinate?
6. What is the meaning of an alpha-fetoprotein measurement greater than 30 ng/mL in a patient 1 year after treatment for cancer of the testes?
7. How can the effectiveness of finasteride be evaluated when caring for a patient with BPH who has been taking this medication for 6 months?
8. What is the meaning of an elevated serum alkaline phosphatase level in the patient with a history of prostate cancer?
9. Why might an older man delay seeking treatment for a disorder affecting the reproductive system?
10. What are some possible solutions to the problem of urinary incontinence in the patient who is recovering from a radical prostatectomy?

Bibliography

American Cancer Society. Cancer facts and figures 1995. Atlanta: Author, 1995.

Badlani G. Balanitis and balanoposthitis. In Seidmon EJ, Hanno PM (eds). Current urologic therapy. 3rd ed. Philadelphia: WB Saunders, 1994, pp 453–454.

Bakemeyer C, Schmall HJ. Treatment of testicular cancer and the development of secondary malignancies. J Clin Oncol 1995; 3: 283.

Ball T. Epididymitis and orchitis. In Seidmon EJ, Hanno PM (eds). Current urologic therapy. 3rd ed. Philadelphia: WB Saunders, 1994, pp 485–489.

Berger RE. Sexually transmitted diseases: The classic diseases. In Walsh PC, Retik AB, Stamey TA, Vaughan ED (eds). Campbell's urology. 6th ed. Philadelphia: WB Saunders, 1992, pp 823–846.

Brenner ZR, Krenzer, ME. 1995 Update on cryosurgical ablation for prostate cancer. Am J Nurs 1995; 4:44.

Brock D, Fox S, Gosling G, et al. Testicular cancer. Semin Oncol Nurs 1993; 9(4):224.

Brock G. Priapism. In Seidmon EJ, Hanno PM (eds). Current urologic therapy. 3rd ed. Philadelphia: WB Saunders, 1994, pp 439–441.

Burke M, Walsh M. Gerontologic nursing: Care of the frail elderly. St. Louis: CV Mosby, 1992.

Bruskewitz R. Disorders of the lower genitourinary tract: Bladder, prostate, and testicles. In Abrams W, Beers M, Berkow R, et al (eds). The Merck manual of geriatrics. 2nd ed. Whitehouse Station: Merck Research Laboratories, 1995, pp 785–795.

Carapella J. Radical prostatectomy: A case study. J Post Anesthesia Nurs 1994; 9(6):366.

Carpenito LJ. Nursing care plans and documentation. 2nd ed. Philadelphia: JB Lippincott, 1995.

Carpenito LJ. Handbook of nursing diagnosis. 6th ed. Philadelphia: JB Lippincott, 1995.

Carpenito LJ. Nursing diagnosis: Application to clinical practice. 6th ed. Philadelphia: JB Lippincott, 1995.

Criste G, Gray D, Gallo B. Prostatitis: A review of diagnosis and management. Nurse Pract 1994; 19(7):32, 37.

Davis DA, Cohen PR. Balanitis. J Urol 1995; 153(2):424.

Devine CJ, Jordan GH, Schlossberg SM. Surgery of the penis and urethra. In Walsh PC, Retik AB, Stamey TA, Vaughan ED (eds). Campbell's urology. 6th ed. Philadelphia: WB Saunders, 1992, pp 2957–3032.

Djavan B, Roehborn C. Prostate-specific antigen: When to measure it, how to interpret results. Consultant 1994; 34(6):909.

Dugan JA, Bostwick DG, Myers RP, et al. The definition and preoperative prediction of clinically insignificant prostate cancer. JAMA 1996; 275(4):288.

Eliopoulos C. Gerontological nursing. 3rd ed. Philadelphia: JB Lippincott, 1993.

Eliopoulos C. Manual of gerontological nursing. St. Louis: CV Mosby, 1995.

Garnick M. Prostate cancer. In Dale D, Federman D (eds). Scientific American Medicine. New York: Scientific American, 1995, pp 1–11.

Garnick M. Testicular cancer and other trophoblastic diseases. In Isselbacher K, Braunwald E, Wilson J, et al (eds). Harrison's principles of internal medicine. 13th ed. New York: McGraw-Hill, 1994, pp 1858–1862.

Giger J, Davidhizar R (eds). Transcultural nursing. 2nd ed. St. Louis: CV Mosby, 1995.

Gomella LG. Paratesticular tumors and masses. In Seidmon EJ, Hanno PM (eds). Current urologic therapy. 3rd ed. Philadelphia: WB Saunders, 1994, pp 500–503.

Greco K, Kulowiak L. Prostate cancer prevention: Risk reduction through life-style, diet, and chemoprevention. Oncol Nurs Forum 1994; 21(9):1504.

Greifzu S, Tiedemann D. Prostate cancer: The pros and cons of treatment. RN 1995; 58(6):22.

Hanno P. Carcinoma of the prostate, Stage C. In Seidmon EJ, Hanno P (eds). Current urologic therapy. 3rd ed. Philadelphia: WB Saunders, 1994, pp 384–386.

Held J, Osborne DM, Volpe H, Waldman AR, et al. Cancer of the prostate: Treatment and nursing implications. Oncol Nurs Forum 1994; 21(9):1517.

Howards SS. Surgery of the scrotum and testis in childhood. In Walsh PC, Gittes RF, Perlmutter AD, Stamey TA (eds). Campbell's urology. 6th ed. Philadelphia: WB Saunders, 1992, pp 1939–1950.

Kedia K. Testicular malignancy after orchiopexy. In Seidmon EJ, Hanno PM (eds). Current urologic therapy. 3rd ed. Philadelphia: WB Saunders, 1994, pp 497–500.

Kendall AR. Treatment of benign prostate hyperplasia. In Seidmon EJ, Hanno PM (eds). Current urologic therapy. 3rd ed. Philadelphia: WB Saunders, 1994, pp 370–376.

Lasater SJ. 1992 Cancer of penis: Perioperative interventions. AORN J 1992; 56(1):19.

Lehne R. Pharmacology for nursing care. 2nd ed. Philadelphia: WB Saunders, 1994.

Light JK. Treatment of urinary incontinence in the male. In Seidman EJ, Hanno PM (eds). Current urologic therapy. 2nd ed. Philadelphia: WB Saunders, 1994, pp 317–318.

Lynch PH. Cutaneous diseases of the external genitalia. In Walsh PC, Retik AB, Stamey TA, Vaughan ED (eds). Campbell's urology. 6th ed. Philadelphia: WB Saunders, 1992, pp 861–882.

Meares EM. Prostatitis and related disorders. In Walsh PC, Retik AB, Stamey TA, Vaughan ED (eds). Campbell's urology. 6th ed. Philadelphia: WB Saunders, 1992, pp 807–822.

Mebust WK. Transurethral surgery. In Walsh PC, Retik AB, Stamey TA, Vaughan ED (eds). Campbell's urology. 6th ed. Philadelphia: WB Saunders, 1992, pp 2900–2922.

Meeker MH, Rothrock JC. Alexander's care of the patient in surgery. 10th ed. St. Louis: CV Mosby, 1995.

Mikkelsen, D. Alterations in structure and function of the male genitourinary system. In Copstead LE (ed). Perspectives on pathophysiology. Philadelphia: WB Saunders, 1995, pp 635–647.

Moore S, Kuhrik M, Shea L, Kuhrik N. Nerve-sparing prostatectomy. Am J Nurs 1992; 4:59.

Ofman U. Psychosocial and sexual implications of genitourinary cancers. Semin Oncol Nurs 1993; 9(4):286.

Osterling JE. Adenocarcinoma of the prostate: Clinical stages B_0, B_1, and B_2. In Seidmon EJ, Hanno PM (eds). Current urologic therapy. 3rd ed. Philadelphia: WB Saunders, 1994, pp 380–384.

Pontari MA. Phimosis and paraphimosis. In Seidmon EJ, Hanno PM (eds). Current urologic therapy. 3rd ed. Philadelphia: WB Saunders, 1994, pp 455–456.

Pontes J. Nonseminomatous testicular tumors. In Seidmon EJ, Hanno PM (eds). Current urologic therapy. 3rd ed. Philadelphia: WB Saunders, 1994, pp 493–495.

Rajfer J. Congenital anomalies of the testis. In Walsh PC, Retik AB, Stamey TA, Vaughan ED (eds). Campbell's urology. 6th ed. Philadelphia: WB Saunders, 1992, pp 1543–1562.

Rajfer J. The testis and epididymis: Congenital disorders. In Seidmon EJ, Hanno P (eds). Current urologic therapy. 3rd ed. Philadelphia: WB Saunders, 1994, pp 477–480.

Rauscher J, MacLeod S. Laparoscopic vein ligation. AORN J 1993; 57(3):664.

Razanauzskas M, Hoebler L. Treating prostate cancer with cryosurgery. Nursing 1994; 24(11):66–68.

Redman J. Circumcision. In Seidmon EJ, Hanno PM (eds). Current urologic therapy. 3rd ed. Philadelphia: WB Saunders, 1994, pp 526–528.

Richie JP. Neoplasms of the testis. In Walsh PC, Retik AB, Stamey TA, Vaughan ED (eds). Campbell's urology. 6th ed. Philadelphia: WB Saunders, 1992, pp 1222–1263.

Roberts RG. Benign prostate hyperplasia. Consultant 1994; 34(7): 1077.

Sagalowsky A, Wilson J. Hyperplasia and carcinoma of the prostate. In Isselbacher K, Braunwald E, Wilson J, et al (eds). Harrison's principles of internal medicine. 13th ed. New York: McGraw-Hill, 1994, pp 1862–1865.

Sarna L. Cancer in the elderly. In Stanley M, Beare P (eds). Gerontologic nursing. Philadelphia: FA Davis, 1995, pp 323–337.

Schellhammer P. Carcinoma of the penis. In Seidmon EJ, Hanno PM (eds). Current urologic therapy. 3rd ed. Philadelphia: WB Saunders, 1994, pp 458–464.

Schellhammer P, Jordan G, Schlossberg S. Tumors of the penis. In Walsh PC, Retik AB, Stamey TA, Vaughan ED (eds). Campbell's urology. 6th ed. Philadelphia: WB Saunders, 1992, pp 1264–1298.

Seidmon EJ. Percutaneous cryosurgery of the prostate using transrectal ultrasound guidance. In Seidmon EJ, Hanno PM (eds). Current urologic therapy. 3rd ed. Philadelphia: WB Saunders, 1994, pp 396–398.

Seidmon EJ. Seminoma. In Seidmon EJ, Hanno PM (eds). Current urologic therapy, 3rd ed. Philadelphia: WB Saunders, 1994, pp 489–493.

Shortliffe LD. Prostatitis. In Seidmon EJ, Hanno PM (eds). Current urologic therapy. 3rd ed. Philadelphia: WB Saunders, 1994, pp 365–370.

Smith JA. Carcinoma of the prostate: Stages A_1 and A_2. In Seidmon EJ, Hanno PM (eds). Current urologic therapy. 3rd ed. Philadelphia: WB Saunders, 1994, pp 377–379.

Stamey TA, McNeal JE. Adenocarcinoma of the prostate. In Walsh PC, Retik AB, Stamey TA, Vaughan ED (eds). Campbell's urology. 6th ed. Philadelphia: WB Saunders, 1992, pp 1159–1221.

Stamm W. Urinary tract infections and pyelonephritis. In Isselbacher K, Braunwald E, Wilson J, et al (eds). Harrison's principles of internal medicine. 13th ed. New York: McGraw-Hill, 1994, pp 548–554.

Stanley M, Beare P (eds). Gerontologic nursing. Philadelphia: FA Davis, 1995.

Stein B. Carcinoma of the prostate: Stage D. In Seidmon EJ, Hanno P (eds). Current urologic therapy. 3rd ed. Philadelphia: WB Saunders, 1994, pp 386–389.

Steinberg G, Brendler C. Diseases of the prostate. In Bennett JC, Plum F (eds). Cecil textbook of medicine. 20th ed. Philadelphia: WB Saunders, 1996, pp 1351–1355.

Stewart S. Structure and function of the male genitourinary system. In Porth CM. Pathophysiology: Concepts of altered health states. 4th ed. Philadelphia: JB Lippincott, 1994, pp 727–743.

Stone N. Varicocele. In Seidmon EJ, Hanno PM (eds). Current urologic therapy. 3rd ed. Philadelphia: WB Saunders, 1994, pp 512–516.

US Department of Health and Human Services, 1994, Agency for Health Care Policy and Research. Clinical Practice Guidelines. Benign prostatic hyperplasia: Diagnosis and treatment. Pub No. 94-0582. Rockville, MD: Public Health Service.

US Department of Health and Human Services, 1994. Patient guide: Treating your enlarged prostate: Pub No. 94-0584. Rockville, MD: Public Health Service.

US Department of Health and Human Services, 1992, Agency for Health Care Policy and Research. Clinical Practice Guidelines. Urinary incontinence in adults. Pub No. 92-0038. Rockville, MD: Public Health Service.

Waldman AR, Osborne D. Screening for prostate cancer. Oncol Nurs Forum 1994; 21(9):1512.

Walsh PC. Benign prostatic hyperplasia. In Walsh PC, Retik AB, Stamey TA, Vaughan ED (eds). Campbell's urology. 6th ed. Philadelphia: WB Saunders, 1992, pp 1007–1027.

Walsh PC. Radical retropubic prostatectomy. In Walsh PC, Retik AB, Stamey TA, Vaughan ED (eds). Campbell's urology. 6th ed. Philadelphia: WB Saunders, 1992, pp 2865–2886.

Wasson JH, Albertsen P. Prostate disease, an emergency only for the patient. Emerg Med 1995; 27(7):20.

Zderic SA. Hydrocele and spermatocele. In Seidmon EJ, Hanno PM (eds). Current urologic therapy. 3rd ed. Philadelphia: WB Saunders, 1994, pp 483–485.

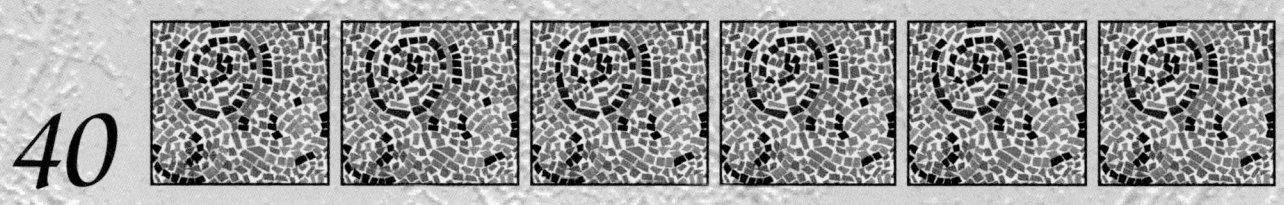

40

Knowledge Base for Women with Reproductive Dysfunction

Study Outcomes

After studying this chapter, you should be able to:

1. Explain the normal anatomy and physiology of the female reproductive system.
2. Describe common clinical manifestations of reproductive system dysfunction.
3. Identify information and physical examination data essential to the assessment of reproductive system status.
4. Describe basic diagnostic tests and treatment modalities used in the collaborative management of women with reproductive system disorders.
5. Describe basic surgical procedures used in the treatment of women with reproductive system disorders.
6. Identify data essential to the assessment of women undergoing treatment of reproductive system disorders.
7. State nursing diagnoses and related expected patient outcomes commonly applicable to women undergoing treatment of reproductive system disorders.
8. Describe nursing interventions, with their rationales, commonly applicable to women undergoing treatment of reproductive system disorders.
9. Explain the basis for evaluation of nursing care provided to women undergoing treatment of reproductive system disorders.
10. Identify alternative treatment and care settings for women with reproductive dysfunction, and the services related to community-based care.
11. Identify special considerations for the elderly woman with altered function of the reproductive system.

A clear understanding of normal reproductive structure and function throughout the life span is essential to effective nursing care of women with gynecologic problems. In addition, the nurse needs strong therapeutic communication skills and sensitivity to women's needs and feelings within their particular cultural contexts.

Despite the openness of society in regard to some aspects of reproduction and sex, many women experience embarrassment and are reluctant to seek health care for prevention and treatment of problems in these areas. New outpatient settings, such as women's health clinics, are responding to the in-crease in the number of women with health concerns related to midlife transitions, sexuality, and domestic violence.

Anatomy and Physiology

The female reproductive system consists of internal genitalia and external genitalia and is regulated by a complex system of hormones. The external genitalia, or vulva, include the mons veneris or mons pubis, labia majora, labia minora, clitoris, fourchette, vestibule, Skene's glands (located within the urethral meatus), Bartholin's glands, hymen, introitus, and perineum (Fig. 40–1).

The internal genitalia include the vagina, uterus, fallopian tubes, and ovaries (Fig. 40–2).

EXTERNAL GENITALIA

The mons pubis is a soft mound of adipose tissue located in front of the symphysis pubis. After puberty, the mons pubis is covered with coarse hair.

The labia majora are two longitudinal folds of adipose tissue that begin at the mons pubis and continue downward and backward on each side of the vaginal opening, or introitus, until they meet at the midline of the perineum. Their outer surfaces are covered with pigmented skin. Coarse hair, which protects the internal structures, and apocrine sweat glands develop during puberty. The inner surfaces of the labia majora are smooth and hairless.

The labia minora are two smaller folds of tissue that lie within the labia majora. They are smooth and hairless but contain large numbers of sebaceous glands. The labia minora extend downward from the clitoris, which is a small mass of erectile tissue located under the prepuce just beneath the pubic arch, to the fourchette, which is a ridge of tissue just below the vaginal opening. The clitoris is highly sensitive tissue and plays a role in female sexual response during intercourse.

The vestibule is the flat, boat-shaped area be-

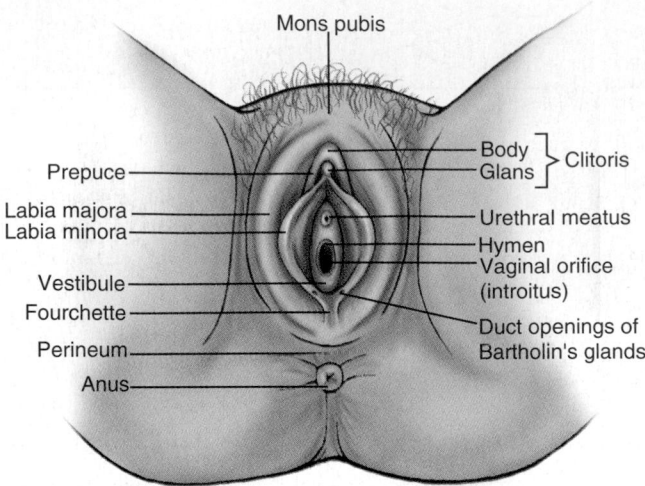

Figure 40–1

Female external genitalia.

tween the labia minora. The vestibule contains the urethral meatus and the opening of the ducts of Skene's glands, which are lateral and posterior to the meatus. It also contains the introitus and the openings of Bartholin's glands, which are posterior and slightly lateral to it.

The hymen is a fold of mucous membrane that partially covers the vaginal opening. The hymen is commonly broken in the adult as a result of sexual intercourse, strenuous exercise, tampon use, or related activities.

The perineum is the area between the vagina and the anus. It consists of muscles, fascia, and skin.

INTERNAL GENITALIA

Vagina

The vagina is a muscular tubelike organ lined with mucous membrane. It has horizontal rugae, or folds, that give it great elasticity. The vagina is located between the urethra and bladder to the anterior and the rectum to the posterior. The vagina connects the uterus to the vulva. It accommodates the penis during intercourse and serves as a passageway for delivery of a baby and for discharge of uterine secretions and menstrual flow.

The vagina is about 3.5 inches (9 cm) in length and is directed upward and back from the introitus toward the coccyx. Its distal end is cuplike in shape and is referred to as the fornix. The cervix of the uterus projects into the fornix and creates a blind pouch on all sides. Thus, there is the posterior fornix, the anterior fornix, and the lateral fornices.

The cells lining the vagina are rich in glycogen. This glycogen is broken down into lactic acid by lactose-fermenting bacteria that are normally found in the vagina. The lactic acid lowers the pH of the

vagina and thus creates an environment that inhibits growth of pathogenic bacteria.

Uterus

The uterus is a hollow, thick-walled muscular organ shaped like an inverted pear. It is the site of menstruation, implantation of the fertilized ovum, fetal development, and the muscular contractions of labor.

The uterus has two main divisions: the body and the cervix. The body, or corpus, is the upper portion of the uterus. The top, domelike portion of the body is the fundus. The angle marking the opening of the fallopian tubes on each side is called the cornu. The isthmus is the constricted portion of the uterus that lies between the body and the cervix, or lower, narrow portion of the uterus, which opens into the vagina.

The uterine cavity is triangular and lined with endometrium. It joins the cervical canal at the internal os. The external os marks the opening of the cervical canal into the vagina.

The uterus is located in the pelvis, with the cervix at almost a right angle to the vagina. The bladder is in front of and below the uterus, and the rectum is below and behind it. The peritoneum is reflected from the abdominal wall over the outer surface of the uterus. This creates a space between the bladder and the vagina (uterovesical pouch) and between the vagina and the rectum. This latter space is the cul-de-sac of Douglas and is the lowest point in the pelvic cavity. Through this cul-de-sac, the peritoneal cavity can be entered through the posterior vaginal wall with little risk of damaging pelvic structures (Fig. 40–3).

The position of the uterus in the pelvic cavity is maintained by a series of ligaments (Fig. 40–4). It is

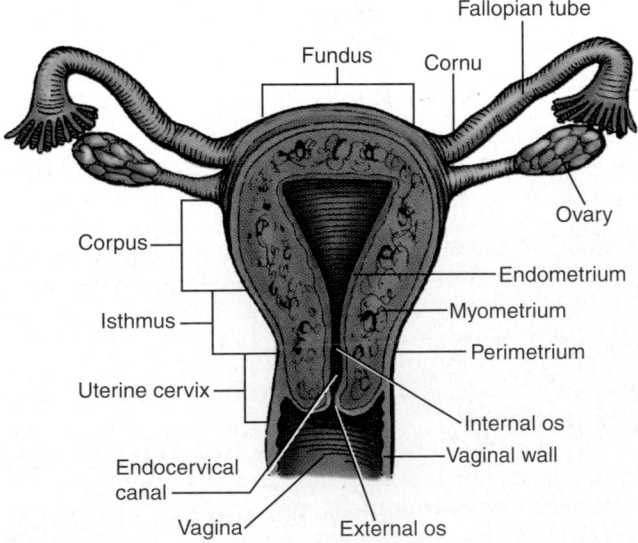

Figure 40–2

Female internal genitalia.

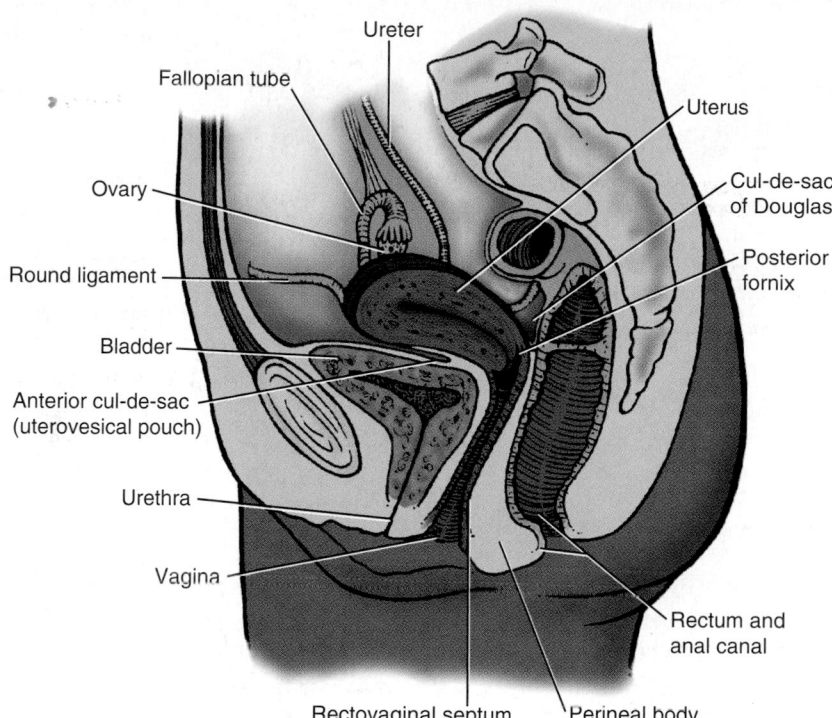

Figure 40-3

Lateral view of the female internal genitalia.

attached to either side of the pelvic cavity by double sheets of peritoneum called the broad ligaments. The cardinal ligaments lie in the base of the broad ligaments and are the primary supports of the uterus. The uterosacral ligaments arise from the sides of the cervix and attach to the sacrum. The round ligaments attach to the uterus just below the entrance of the fallopian tubes and pass within the broad ligament to the pelvic wall, ending in the labia majora.

This system of support allows some movement of the uterine body, so the uterus can deviate from its usual anteverted, slightly anteflexed position and may be in midposition or retroverted.

Fallopian Tubes

The fallopian or uterine tubes transport ova from the ovaries to the uterus and are the usual site of fertilization of the ovum by a sperm. They are about 10 cm long and are located between the folds of the broad ligaments. The portion of the tube nearest to the uterus is the isthmus. The middle portion is the ampulla, and the distal funnel-shaped section is the infundibulum. The infundibulum is surrounded by long, slender, finger-like projections called fimbriae (Fig. 40-5). Wavelike movements of the fimbriae serve to attract the mature ovum released from the ovary at ovulation into the tube for possible fertilization and transport to the uterus.

The mucosal lining of the tube is contiguous with that of the uterus, the vagina, and the peritoneum. Thus, infection of any of these organs can spread to the peritoneum and cause peritonitis.

Ovaries

The ovaries are two organs the size and shape of almonds. One ovary is located in the broad ligament on each side of the uterus below and behind the

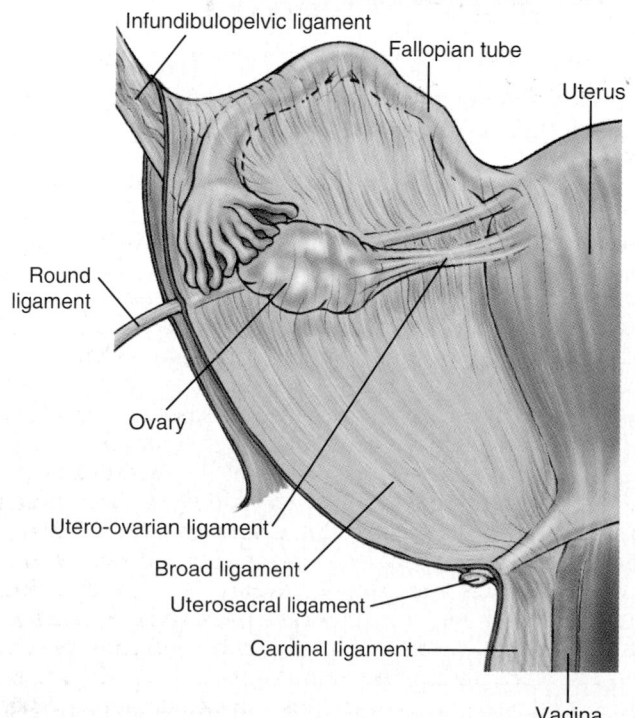

Figure 40-4

Uterine ligaments.

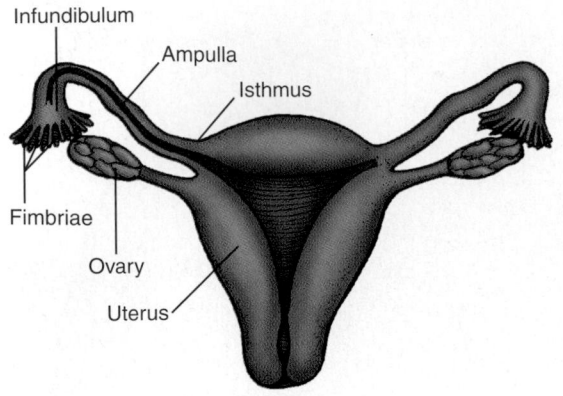

Figure 40–5

Parts of the fallopian tube and their relationship to the ovary and the uterus.

fallopian tube. Like the uterus, ovaries are held in place by a series of ligaments. The utero-ovarian ligament attaches the ovary to the uterus. The infundibulopelvic ligament attaches the ovary to the side wall of the pelvis.

The ovaries' function is to produce and discharge ova. They also secrete the female sex hormones estrogen and progesterone. These are necessary for the development and maintenance of female reproductive structures and secondary sex characteristics and play an essential role in the menstrual cycle and pregnancy.

FEMALE HORMONAL CYCLE

The female hormonal cycle is a periodic recurrent series of changes involving the hypothalamus, anterior pituitary gland, uterus, and ovaries. The purpose of the cycle is to prepare the body for pregnancy through the release of a single mature ovum and to prepare the uterus for implantation. The cycle is initiated at puberty, and its onset is indicated by menarche. Menarche is the first menstruation, or periodic uterine bleeding, associated with shedding of the endometrium. The average age of menarche in the United States is 12.5 years. The first day of menstruation is counted as the first day of the cycle. The average length of the cycle is 28 days, although in normal females it can vary between 20 and 45 days.

The frequency of the cycle can be affected by physical and emotional factors, including illness, fatigue, weight fluctuation, excessive exercise, eating disorders, stress, anxiety, medications, and change in environment. The cycle is divided into four phases: the proliferative phase, the secretory phase, the ischemic phase, and the menstrual phase. The menstrual phase is the time of the menstrual flow. The proliferative phase is from the end of menstruation to ovulation. The secretory phase is from ovulation to 3 days before onset of the next menses. The ischemic phase is these last 3 days.

These phases are named for the changes occurring in the endometrium. However, related changes are occurring simultaneously in the hypothalamus, anterior pituitary gland, ovary, and cervix.

Proliferative Phase

Immature oocytes are present in each ovary at birth. Each oocyte is surrounded by a protective sac of cells and is called a primordial follicle. Under the influence of gonadotropin releasing hormone from the hypothalamus, the anterior pituitary secretes follicle-stimulating hormone and luteinizing hormone. Follicle-stimulating hormone initiates the growth of several primordial follicles. One of these takes precedence and continues to develop under the influence of both follicle-stimulating hormone and luteinizing hormone, while the others regress. The cells of this follicle produce a clear fluid that contains increasing amounts of estrogen as growth progresses. This maturing follicle moves to the surface of the ovary, where it appears as a blister-like structure called a graafian follicle. At this time, estrogen levels peak and the luteinizing hormone level surges. This surge is believed to trigger ovulation, in which the graafian follicle ruptures and releases the mature ovum.

Estrogen produced by the follicle during its development stimulates rapid growth of the endometrium. The thickness of the endometrium increases eightfold as a result of increased cells and progressive growth of the endometrial glands and vascular system. Thus, while an ovum is maturing in the ovary, the lining of the uterus is beginning to be prepared for implantation.

In response to increasing levels of estrogen, the cells of the cervical mucosa enlarge and increase secretion of mucus. The pH becomes more alkaline, shifting from about 7.0 to 7.5. The mucus becomes copious in amount and is thin, clear, and watery. These changes facilitate the passage of sperm into the body of the uterus. By the time of ovulation, cervical mucus assumes a full, fernlike pattern when allowed to dry (Fig. 40–6).

Secretory Phase

After ovulation, the ruptured follicle remaining on the surface of the ovary becomes the corpus luteum. This change occurs primarily in response to luteinizing hormone from the anterior pituitary. The cells of the corpus luteum, or yellow body, produce progesterone, which increases in amount throughout the secretory phase. Estrogen is also produced, but not in pre-ovulation amounts. In the uterus, stimulation by increasing levels of progesterone causes the endometrial glands to dilate, become more tortuous,

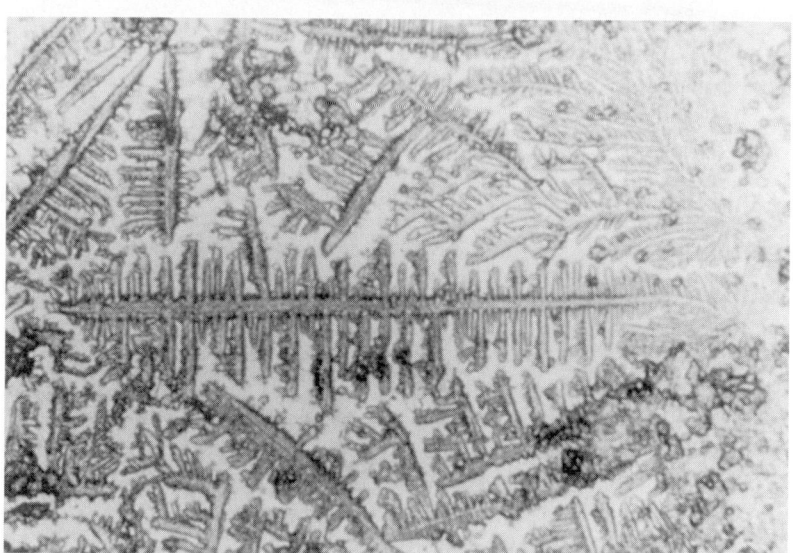

Figure 40-6

Photomicrograph of fernlike pattern of dried cervical mucus at ovulation. (From Edwards RG, Brody SA. Principles and practice of assisted human reproduction. Philadelphia: WB Saunders, 1995, p 190.)

and begin to secrete small quantities of endometrial fluid. Cellular deposits of lipid and glycogen increase; the endometrium becomes edematous; and the vascularity becomes more prominent. These changes result in a highly secretory endometrium containing large amounts of stored nutrients needed to sustain a fertilized ovum. If fertilization and implantation occur, the endometrium develops further under the continuing stimulation of progesterone. If fertilization of the ovum does not occur, the ischemic phase begins.

Ischemic Phase

During the ischemic phase, the corpus luteum degenerates, and levels of estrogen and progesterone fall. With the withdrawal of progesterone, arteries constrict, causing the endometrium to become pale, shrunken, and anemic. This leads to areas of necrosis in the endometrium. Subsequently, blood leaks into the tissues, and small necrotic patches of endometrium break off.

Menstrual Phase

The menstrual phase is the time during which the menstrual flow occurs. The menstrual discharge is composed of blood, cervical and vaginal secretions, mucus, and shreds of endometrium. It does not normally contain clots. The discharge, which is dark red and has a characteristic odor, differs from one woman to another in duration and amount. The average duration is 5 days, although anywhere from 2 to 8 days is within normal range. The amount may be scant, moderate, or heavy, with blood loss varying between 30 and 150 mL.

The female hormonal cycle is presented diagrammatically in Figure 40–7.

FEMALE SEXUAL RESPONSE

Normal sexual functioning is considered within the context of a relationship and involves mutual satisfaction without harm to either partner (Bachmann & Ayers, 1995). Communication between partners is a major factor in healthy sexual functioning.

Female sexual response occurs in four phases: excitement, plateau, orgasmic, and resolution. During each phase, identifiable changes occur in both external and internal genitalia. Individual sexual responsiveness can be affected by illness, use of medications, and other medical-surgical interventions.

In the excitement phase, psychological and physical stimulation causes the genitalia to increase in size and change in color from vasocongestion. Shortly thereafter, vaginal secretions are evident. This phase lasts from minutes to hours.

The plateau phase is brief, lasting from 30 seconds to 3 minutes. A sexual flush appears on the skin of the upper body. The genitalia continue to enlarge. Strong uterine contractions begin late in this phase.

In the orgasmic phase the physiologic tension built up during the previous phases is released and repeated involuntary vaginal contractions occur and uterine contractions continue.

During the resolution phase, which can last from minutes to several hours, the genitalia resume their previous size and positioning. Restimulation of external genitalia can result in additional orgasmic phases.

MENOPAUSE

Menopause is a normal physiologic transition and does not mean the end of an active sexual life. The World Health Organization defines menopause as

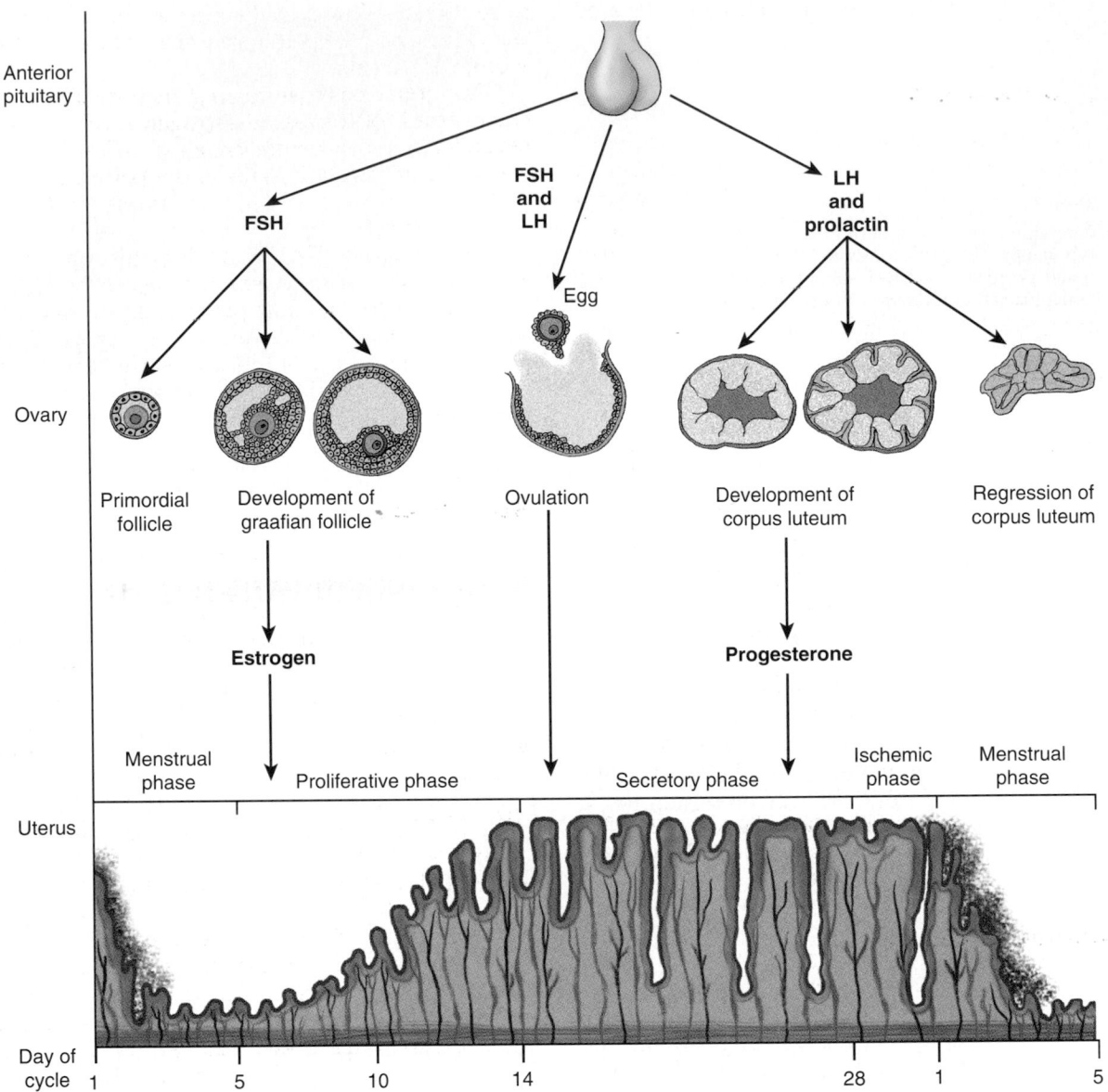

Anterior
pituitary

FSH
and
LH

LH
and
prolactin

FSH

Egg

Ovary

Primordial
follicle

Development of
graafian follicle

Ovulation

Development of
corpus luteum

Regression of
corpus luteum

Estrogen

Progesterone

Menstrual
phase

Proliferative phase

Secretory phase

Ischemic
phase

Menstrual
phase

Uterus

Day of
cycle 1 5 10 14 28 1 5

Figure 40-7

Female hormonal cycle.

the permanent cessation of menstruation resulting from the loss of ovarian follicular activity (1981). The menstrual flow becomes smaller in amount. Menses become less frequent, then irregular, and finally cease. Ovulation usually ends before the last menses. Perimenopause is the period just before, during, and after menopause. The average age of menopause for women in the U.S. is approximately 50 years of age, but individual onset varies widely. When menopause occurs before the age of 45, it is called premature menopause.

As more women enter the perimenopause, the perception of the changes shifts from a pathologic to a developmental perspective. More and more women are seeing the perimenopausal period as an expected developmental transition in life. With in-

creased life expectancy, women will spend more time in the postmenopausal period that in previous generations. The nurse can help women identify how to make the transition in a positive health-promoting way through teaching, counseling, and support.

The changes experienced during menopause occur as the ovaries become less sensitive to pituitary gonadotropins. This results in diminished ovarian estrogen. No progesterone is produced after the last ovulatory cycle. Estrogen, however, continues to be produced in small quantities by the adrenal glands and the ovaries even after the final menses. The amount of estrogen is not sufficient to block output of pituitary gonadotropins through a negative feedback loop, so the level of follicle-stimulating hormone rises with menopause and remains elevated thereafter.

Physical Changes

Many physical changes are initiated at the time of menopause. Most result from the aging process in general and are not the direct result of diminished estrogen. Pubic hair begins to thin and turn gray and may ultimately disappear. The vulval structures begin to atrophy. The labia become thin as their fatty tissue is resorbed and become pale as the deep pigmentation is lost. The cervix shrinks and retracts. The ovaries atrophy, becoming white, wrinkled, and no longer able to be palpated. The fallopian tubes, uterus, and vagina also decrease in size. In addition, the vagina becomes less elastic as the rugae disappear and the mucosa thins. Vaginal secretions decrease in amount and in acidity, thus predisposing to dyspareunia (painful sexual intercourse) and vaginal infection. The pelvic fascia and musculature atrophy, and pelvic support is lost, leading in some cases to urinary stress incontinence. Breasts gradually lose their firmness as fatty deposits are resorbed.

The skin becomes wrinkled as a loss of protein and subcutaneous tissue occurs. Bone loss accelerates as estrogen decreases, and osteoporosis (thin, porous bone) with its associated risk of fractures can ensue, particularly if combined with low body weight, lack of physical exercise, chronic low calcium intake, or excessive intake of caffeine and alcohol.

Psychosocial Effects

Each woman responds to the transitional changes of menopause in a unique way. The ending of the monthly pattern of menstruation is a significant change infused with individual meaning. This may be a time for reflection on the previous years of womanhood. The loss of the reproductive feature of one's feminine identity may be grieved with the same range of emotions as other significant losses (Wear & Nixon, 1994).

Menopause can mean the beginning of freedom to enjoy one's sexuality without concern about pregnancy and contraception. It also means freedom from menstruation, which can have particular importance for women with a history of premenstrual and menstrual discomfort or heavy bleeding. However, menopause marks the end of the ability to bear children. This can create a sense of loss in many women, but it is frequently more marked in women who have never had children. This sense of loss can also be exaggerated in women who devoted most of their time and effort to their children and developed few meaningful outside interests. Thus, when the last child leaves home for school, work, or marriage, life may seem empty and without purpose. Often adding to the loss at this time in life is the developing dependency, sickness, or death of a woman's parents.

Emotional changes during menopause are not a direct result of decreased estrogen levels but may be secondary to concurrent changes in levels of neurotransmitters, alterations in sleep patterns, and general social expectations for an unpleasant response to menopause.

Menopause is also an undeniable sign of aging. This can raise anxiety and feelings of being less attractive and less feminine, especially in U.S. society, with its focus on the desirability of youth. Some women believe that it indicates the end of sexual activity or a satisfying sexual relationship. Still other women have a great fear of an accidental pregnancy and a "change-of-life baby."

Symptoms

Some women experience no unpleasant symptoms during menopause. Some have mild discomforts. Some have significant distress. Symptoms that may occur include hot flushes (also called hot flashes), sleep pattern disturbances, weakness, fatigue, dizzy spells, palpitations, anxiety, depression, negative mood changes, headaches, weight gain, vaginal dryness resulting in dyspareunia (painful intercourse), and decreased libido. Of these, only the hot flushes and vaginal dryness have been shown to occur directly in response to a drop in estrogen level.

It is believed that the drop in estrogen level affects the temperature-regulating center in the hypothalamus, resulting in an increased sensitivity to heat. This, in turn, leads to a hot flush, which is a vasomotor disturbance that occurs as the body attempts to cool itself. Hot flushes usually start on the head, neck, and chest and may progress to include other parts of the body. Profuse sweating usually follows the pattern of flushing. Hot flushes may occur anywhere from once a week to as often as 20 to 30 times daily and last from a few minutes to 30 minutes. They can be triggered by anything that affects body temperature, such as a warm room, warm food, alcohol, or an emotional upset. Their unexpected occurrence in social situations is a source of embarrassment for some women.

Insomnia is also believed to be an effect of decreased estrogen level, although this has not been proved. It is true, however, that hot flushes occurring at night can interfere with normal sleeping, causing headaches and feelings of fatigue, nervousness, and depression that are associated with sleep deprivation.

Atrophy of the lower urinary tract structures, possibly aggravated by lowered estrogen levels, can cause dysuria and urinary urge incontinence. Some degree of hirsutism occurs in many women as the moderating effect of estrogen decreases and the influence of androgen increases.

Management

Historically, the medical community has approached treatment of menopause from a narrow, physiologic perspective. As the number of women experiencing perimenopause increases, there is an increased demand for a more holistic approach to this period of transition.

Hormone replacement therapy, which involves a combination of estrogen and progesterone, or estrogen replacement therapy alone effectively reduces menopausal symptoms of hot flushes, vaginal dryness, and sleep disturbances. Long-term therapy also significantly decreases postmenopausal bone loss and the related risk of hip and vertebral fractures (McKeon, 1994). In addition, replacement therapy improves blood lipid levels by decreasing low-density lipoproteins and increasing high-density lipoproteins and appears to protect postmenopausal women against heart attacks and strokes (Lobo & Speroff, 1994). As a result, hormone replacement therapy is now frequently recommended for women even in the absence of distressing menopausal symptoms, particularly those at risk for osteoporosis. For maximum effectiveness in preventing osteoporosis, replacement is maintained for life because bone loss accelerates as soon as the estrogen replacement therapy is discontinued.

Hormone replacement therapy may be cyclical or continuous low-dose conjugated estrogen alone for a woman who has no uterus. Or it may be a cyclical or continuous regimen of estrogen and progesterone

---

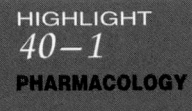

HIGHLIGHT
40-1
PHARMACOLOGY

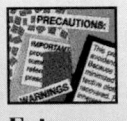

Estrogens

Definition:

Female sex hormones secreted by the ovarian follicles and placenta and in smaller amounts by the adrenal cortex and male testis.

Action:

Promote development of the vagina, uterus, fallopian tubes, breasts, and secondary sex characteristics as well as closure of long bone epiphyses. Stimulate the proliferative phase of the uterine cycle and changes in reproductive organs during pregnancy. Also lower blood cholesterol level and promote retention of sodium and water.

Uses:

Replacement therapy to treat menopausal symptoms, both naturally occurring and following oophorectomy; atrophic vaginitis; secondary amenorrhea; and in the palliative treatment of inoperable cancer of the prostate and breast in males and inoperable cancer of the breast in postmenopausal females. Also used for contraception in combination with progestogen.

Side Effects:

Breakthrough bleeding, changes in menstrual flow; dysmenorrhea; amenorrhea; vaginal discharge; cervical erosion; monilial vaginitis; enlargement, tenderness, and secretion of the breasts; headache; dizziness; chorea; libido changes; depression; thrombophlebitis and embolism; hypertension; edema; nausea; vomiting; abdominal cramps; bloating; diarrhea; constipation; appetite and weight changes; jaundice; hyperglycemia; hypercalcemia; acne; oily skin; hirsutism or alopecia; leg cramps; and intolerance to contact lenses. Gynecomastia, testicular atrophy, and impotence also occur in men.

Interactions:

None that are clinically significant.

Nursing Implications:

Give the package insert to the patient and review the information before the first dose, as required by Food and Drug Administration regulation.

Instruct the patient to immediately report chest pain; shortness of breath; pain, numbness, or stiffness in the legs or buttocks; abdominal pain; severe headache; visual changes; vaginal bleeding or discharge; breast lumps; edema of the extremities; jaundice; dark urine; or light stool.

Teach breast self-examination.

Explain to women on cyclic therapy for menopausal symptoms that ovulation has not occurred and that they are not able to get pregnant despite the fact that vaginal bleeding occurs during the week they do not take the drug.

Explain to male patients that gynecomastia and impotence may occur when the drug is taken for a long time. Reassure them that these effects will disappear when the drug is discontinued.

Note the type, amount, and duration of estrogen therapy.

for women who need to protect the endometrium from the risk of cancer (Highlight 40–1). Dosages are individualized to provide relief of symptoms and minimize risk of side effects.

Potential side effects of the cyclical regimen include breast tenderness, fluid retention, weight gain, headache, and nausea. In addition, most women who have not had hysterectomies develop withdrawal bleeding at the end of each 25-day medication cycle. This resembles menstruation but, since no ovulation has occurred, the woman is not fertile. Such withdrawal bleeding is a major factor in noncompliance with hormone replacement therapy. Continuous regimens are gaining popularity because they avoid monthly withdrawal bleeding after an initial period of unpredictable bleeding. Breast tenderness is also reduced with this regimen.

At current low doses, estrogen replacement therapy and hormone replacement therapy no longer carry an increased risk of endometrial cancer. Women with a history of abnormal bleeding may still be candidates for therapy but should be followed with endometrial biopsies (Hargrove & Eisenberg, 1995). Whether current hormone replacement therapy is associated with an increased risk of breast cancer remains a debated issue. Although many studies indicate that it is not associated with any increased risk of breast cancer and may in fact offer some protection, others show an increased risk (Speroff et al, 1994). The Women's Health Initiative, funded by the National Institutes of Health, is conducting long-term clinical trials to examine the risk of breast cancer in women receiving hormone replacement therapy. Recommendations are due in the year 2002 (Institute of Medicine, 1993).

Hormone replacement therapy is contraindicated in women with:

- A history of breast, endometrial, or other tumors whose growth may be responsive to estrogen
- Recurrent vascular thrombosis
- Liver disease
- Abnormal genital bleeding
- A current pregnancy

It is used with caution in women who:

- Were exposed at birth to diethylstilbestrol (DES)
- Are obese
- Have thrombophlebitis, diabetes, migraine headaches, depression, seizure disorder, or kidney or gallbladder disease who may experience worsening of their symptoms

❖ Settings, Providers, and Collaboration for Care

With the aging of the baby boomers, the number of women entering perimenopause is increasing rapidly. As in earlier developmental stages, this group places new demands for services on the health care system. The developmental nature of menopause makes it a natural focus for informal women's groups as they seek information for self-care in managing menopausal changes.

Most women do not seek care for menopausal symptoms from traditional health care providers or settings. Instead they rely on informal social networks and popular sources of information to navigate the multidimensional changes experienced during menopause. Nurses, who are primarily women, can be excellent sources of information for women through contact with naturally occurring groups, such as those found in churches, communities, and workplaces.

Clinics focused exclusively on women's health, with an emphasis on prevention and self-care, provide an alternative to traditional crisis-oriented settings. Advanced practice nurses are often the primary care providers in such settings. They are able to renegotiate the nurse-patient relationship to allow for more of a partnership, with a recognition of the varied experiences of women who demand choice among options rather than one treatment approach for everyone. As a time of transition, menopause is an opportunity to explore lifestyle changes that could improve a woman's overall health.

NURSING PROCESS
Menopause
Assessment

Use open-ended questions to gain a sense of the woman's current experience of transitional changes. Include such questions as "How are you adjusting to menopause?" and "Which symptoms create the most difficulty for you?" If not reported, be sure to ask about vasomotor symptoms, bleeding patterns, genitourinary symptoms, emotional changes, discomforts, and sexual changes. Assess the patient's understanding of the physiology of menopause. Determine her understanding of the relationship of menopause to osteoporosis and cardiovascular disease, and preventive estrogen replacement therapy. Ask about her fears and concerns. Assess her overall lifestyle, especially her diet, exercise and coping patterns, and her social support network. Convey an empathic attitude throughout the interview.

Nursing Diagnoses and Planning

Nursing diagnoses and related expected patient outcomes commonly applicable to menopausal women include the following:

NDx: Risk for altered health maintenance related to insufficient knowledge of menopause and related self-care

Planning: Patient Outcomes
1. Patient defines menopause.
2. Patient identifies personal changes attributable to endocrine changes.

3. Patient discusses effects of menopause on personal lifestyle realistically and without misconceptions.
4. Patient states cause, duration, and significance of common menopausal symptoms.
5. Patient describes the value of diet, exercise, and stress management strategies in minimizing symptoms in the menopausal and postmenopausal woman.
6. Patient identifies the importance of annual pelvic examinations.
7. Patient for whom hormone replacement therapy is prescribed describes expected benefits, side effects, contraindications, and administration regimen.

8. If appropriate, patient describes her continued need for birth-control measures.
9. Patient states importance of reporting any postmenopausal bleeding or staining to the clinician.

NDx: Anxiety related to the physical and psychologic changes of menopause

Planning: Patient Outcomes
1. Patient discusses menopause freely, without misconceptions or mannerisms that indicate anxiety.
2. Patient reports reduced feelings of anxiety and symptoms associated with anxiety.
3. Patient expresses confidence in her ability to effectively maintain family, work, and social roles.

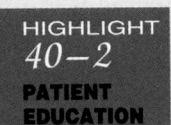 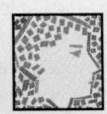

HIGHLIGHT 40–2

PATIENT EDUCATION

Basic Health Practices for the Menopausal Woman

Give the menopausal woman the following instructions.

Diet: Eat a variety of foods. Keep fat intake at no more than 30% of the diet. Eat five servings a day of fruits and vegetables, especially those high in calcium (green, leafy vegetables).

Exercise: Engage in regular weight-bearing exercise (such as walking) to prevent osteoporosis and promote cardiovascular fitness. Select activities that you find enjoyable. Exercise at least three times weekly for 30 minutes each time. Three 10-minute exercise sessions each day can also be beneficial.

Stress: Develop skills in relaxation therapy. Use positive self-talk and humor.

Sleep: Establish a regular schedule for sleep and activity. Avoid stimulants.

Support: Identify, develop, and use social support networks, such as friends, relatives, and women's groups. Plan activities with older women who have successfully navigated the transition of menopause.

Additional information for the menopausal woman.

Use a reliable method of birth control for at least 1 year after menopause.

Institute measures to minimize the effects of hot flushes.
  Reduce intake of stimulants, alcohol, and spicy foods.
  Consider use of vitamin E and B-complex supplements.

Maintain a cool work and home environment.
Wear layered clothing of natural fibers.
During a hot flush, visualize and seek a cool, breezy location. Sip a cool drink.
When bathing, use lukewarm water.

Manage urinary symptoms.
  Drink 6 to 8 glasses of water daily.
  Empty your bladder before and after sexual intercourse.
  Perform Kegel exercises (see Highlight 40–3).

Manage symptoms of vaginal dryness.
  Spend more time in foreplay to gain maximum lubrication.
  Communicate the need for more time to your partner.
  Consider the use of water-soluble lubricant if intercourse is painful.
  Make time for pleasurable, noncoital interaction with your partner.

Perform self-examination of your breasts and vulva.

Have a mammogram yearly after age 50.

Consider bibliotherapy with popular books that may encourage self-reflection and help you navigate the changes of menopause in health-promoting ways.

Perform a mid-life review and examine the meaning of losing reproductive function.

Explore any negative cultural messages surrounding menopause that could interfere with self-acceptance. Identify positive female role models from your social network for the next stage of life. Develop latent interests and satisfying leisure activities that enhance self-esteem.

Nursing Interventions and Evaluation

NDx: Risk for altered health maintenance

Discuss menopause and its associated physical changes with the woman. Also discuss its effects on reproduction and sex and symptoms that may normally occur, their significance, and their treatment. Emphasize that not all women develop all symptoms. If the woman experiences discomfort from hot flushes and perspiration, suggest relief measures (Highlight 40–2).

Structure this discussion so that the woman is at ease and actively contributes information and ideas. Use open-ended questions to elicit beliefs and feelings about current or potential menopausal changes. From the woman's responses, identify any misconceptions and correct them.

Instruct the woman in basic health practices essential to the well-being of the menopausal woman. Provide information about hormone replacement therapy so that she can make an informed choice. Explain the benefits of estrogen in reducing hot flushes and vaginal dryness and in preventing osteoporosis and cardiovascular disease. Emphasize that, with combination therapy, the risk of endometrial cancer is no longer increased. Discuss concerns about the possible risk for breast cancer. If hormone replacement therapy is prescribed, review the medication schedule and help the woman develop a plan for ensuring consistent self-administration. Review educational materials provided with hormone therapy prescriptions.

NDx: Anxiety

When taking care of an anxious menopausal patient, allow her to express her feelings and concerns about menopause, aging, and personal goals. Provide information and correct misconceptions as described earlier. Encourage her to consider friends who have passed menopause and who are still leading active, involved lives. Encourage regular exercise to reduce stress, control weight, and maintain cardiovascular fitness.

Compare the patient's status with the expected outcomes. If the outcomes are not met, reassess the patient and revise the plan.

Clinical Manifestations of Female Reproductive Dysfunction

AMENORRHEA

Amenorrhea is the absence of menstruation. It is classified as primary, secondary, or physiologic. Physiologic amenorrhea is a normal developmental state. It refers to the absence of menses before puberty, during pregnancy and lactation, and after menopause. Primary and secondary amenorrhea are

symptoms of underlying pathology. In primary amenorrhea, the menarche has never occurred. Secondary amenorrhea is the absence of menstruation for 6 months after regular cycles have been established (Webb, 1995).

The possible causes of primary and secondary amenorrhea are multiple. They include lesions at every level of reproductive system control and function, as well as disorders of supporting body systems. Primary or secondary amenorrhea may result from:

- Hypothalamic or pituitary disorders
- Ovarian lesions
- Congenital defects involving the uterus, vagina, or hymen
- Removal of the uterus or both ovaries
- Thyroid, pancreatic, or adrenal dysfunctions
- Cirrhosis, nephritis, or other chronic illness
- Psychogenic disorders, such as anorexia nervosa or bulimia

Temporary secondary amenorrhea may occur as the result of emotional stress, strenuous exercise, low body weight, severe illness, or drugs such as the phenothiazines. It can also occur for up to 6 months or longer after a woman stops taking oral contraceptives.

ABNORMAL UTERINE BLEEDING

There are a variety of patterns of abnormal uterine bleeding. Oligomenorrhea is infrequent or scant episodes of bleeding. Polymenorrhea is frequent but regular episodes of bleeding. Menorrhagia is bleeding that occurs at regular intervals but is excessive in both amount and duration. Metrorrhagia is bleeding that occurs at irregular times and is not excessive. Menometrorrhagia is excessive and prolonged bleeding occurring frequently and irregularly.

The cause of abnormal uterine bleeding may be endocrine or organic. Organic causes include disorders of pregnancy, diseases of the pelvic organs, and disorders of other body systems, such as blood dyscrasias and hypertension. Most often, bleeding related to organic causes is associated with an ovulatory cycle, whereas bleeding related to an endocrine problem is associated with an anovulatory cycle.

Menorrhagia occurring at puberty is most often caused by low estrogen and results in failure of the endometrium to proliferate normally. However, bleeding and clotting disorders are also possible causes, as is adenocarcinoma, which can occur in young women whose mothers took diethylstilbestrol during pregnancy.

In older premenopausal women, menorrhagia is associated with ovarian tumors, submucous fibroid tumors of the uterus, infection of the endometrium, polyps, and pelvic inflammatory disease.

Metrorrhagia is most often caused by a pregnancy-related disorder, such as ectopic pregnancy, threatened abortion, or hydatidiform mole. It is also frequently iatrogenic from the administration of exogenous hormones such as estrogen, androgens, or corticosteroids. Bleeding unrelated to the menstrual cycle may indicate cancer of the cervix or cancer of the endometrium. In fact, a perimenopausal or postmenopausal woman with metrorrhagia is considered to have a malignancy until proven otherwise.

Abnormal uterine bleeding can also be caused by intrauterine devices, ruptured ovarian cysts, and drugs such as phenothiazines, anticoagulants, anticholinergic agents, thiazide diuretics, and digitalis.

LEUKORRHEA

The term *leukorrhea* refers to any vaginal discharge other than blood. It may result from excessive production of normal secretions that moisten the mucous membrane of the reproductive tract, or it may be an abnormal exudate from a pathologic lesion.

Normal secretions include the thick, viscous mucus produced by Bartholin's glands, which lubricates the introitus and the membranes of the vulva. This increases with sexual arousal and may be described as a vaginal discharge, because most women cannot identify the actual source of secretion.

The vagina does not contain secretory glands. It is moistened by clear mucus produced by the cervical glands in varying amounts during the sexual cycle. These cervical glands become hyperactive as a result of hyperemia or endocrine factors and are the chief sources of leukorrhea.

Leukorrhea is also a symptom of vaginal or cervical infection. With vaginal infections, the discharge is mucopurulent or purulent and is commonly accompanied by pruritus. With cervical infections, the discharge may be moderate to copious, purulent, and possibly foul smelling.

Normal uterine secretions do not cause a vaginal discharge. However, uterine polyps and benign and malignant uterine tumors can cause a leukorrheal discharge, especially when they are infected or necrotic. Vascular or endocrine changes can also alter uterine secretion so that leukorrhea may result.

DYSMENORRHEA

Dysmenorrhea is cyclic pain associated with menstruation. It may be primary or secondary.

Primary Dysmenorrhea

In primary dysmenorrhea, no pathology of the reproductive organs or pelvis accounts for the pain. It occurs with an ovulatory cycle. Its onset is just before or at the same time as the onset of the menstrual flow. It lasts from a few hours to 1 or 2 days. Usually, the pain is worst as the flow begins and decreases as the flow becomes established. It is a sharp, sometimes colicky pain located in the lower abdomen with radiation to the lower back, groin, or thighs. Sometimes, it is described as a dull, intense ache and may be accompanied by headache, nausea, anorexia, bloating, diarrhea, faintness, or fatigue.

Primary dysmenorrhea occasionally occurs with the first menses but more often begins 6 to 12 months after menarche. This is because primary dysmenorrhea occurs only with cycles in which ovulation occurs, and the first cycles after menarche are frequently anovulatory.

Primary dysmenorrhea is associated with excessive uterine contractility, both in baseline uterine tone and in strength of contractions. Recent research indicates that abnormally high levels of endometrial prostaglandins are responsible for the high contractility of the uterus as well as for other symptoms accompanying the pain.

Other factors that relate to the incidence and severity of primary dysmenorrhea are poor posture, poor hygiene, a sedentary lifestyle, nulliparity, constitutional illness, and fear or lack of knowledge of normal reproductive function.

Treatment depends on the severity of the problem. For many women, the pain is relieved by nonprescription prostaglandin inhibitors, particularly ibuprofen, along with rest, hot fluids, heat to the lower abdomen, manual pressure on the abdomen, effleurage, mild exercise (eg, walking or swimming), or similar conservative measures. Effectiveness increases if treatment begins when dysmenorrhea begins, rather than waiting until it is well established.

When basic treatments are not effective, oral contraceptives may be prescribed. Hormonal contraceptive therapy is effective because primary dysmenorrhea occurs with ovulatory cycles and this therapy inhibits ovulation. If this therapy is contraindicated, prostaglandin inhibitors (nonsteroidal anti-inflammatory drugs [NSAIDs] such as naproxen, indomethacin, mefenamic acid) may be prescribed. These drugs, which are taken as soon as the menses begins, usually provide relief. They act by inhibiting synthesis of prostaglandins, thus preventing the high prostaglandin levels that cause uterine, gastrointestinal, and vascular smooth muscle spasm. All these drugs have side effects, such as dizziness, headache, nausea, and diarrhea. However, they are generally mild and tolerable, particularly when taken with food. Because fatal anaphylaxis has been reported, NSAIDs are contraindicated for women with a history of allergy to aspirin or any NSAID.

NURSING PROCESS
Primary Dysmenorrhea

Assessment

Ask the woman to describe the type, degree, time of onset, and duration of pain experienced, as well as any symptoms (eg, nausea, diarrhea, and headache) that accompany the pain. Determine the woman's perception of dysmenorrhea, including its cause and its meaning for reproductive function. Obtain information about relief measures that the woman has tried, how they are used, and how effective they are. Note the presence of physical factors—such as poor posture, poor hygiene, and lack of exercise—that contribute to dysmenorrhea. Assess the woman's knowledge of and attitude toward menstruation.

Nursing Diagnoses and Planning

Nursing diagnoses and related expected patient outcomes commonly applicable to women with primary dysmenorrhea include the following:

NDx: Pain related to abdominal cramps secondary to menstruation

Planning: Patient Outcomes
1. Patient describes or demonstrates the use of nonpharmacologic comfort measures.
2. Patient identifies prescribed medications, listing the name, dose, frequency, indications for use, and possible side effects.
3. Patient reports pain relief at follow-up visit.

NDx: Risk for altered health maintenance related to insufficient knowledge of menstruation or self-care measures to help decrease or prevent future dysmenorrhea

Planning: Patient Outcomes
1. Patient describes menstruation and its effects without misconceptions.
2. Patient explains the relationship of good posture, exercise, good hygiene, and balanced diet to prevention of dysmenorrhea.
3. Patient states the importance of avoiding fatigue and constipation just before menses.

Nursing Interventions and Evaluation

NDx: Pain
Provide information on the optimal timing and use of relief measures employed by the woman if assessment data indicate its need. Also give information about available relief measures, other than those already used, that may help to control symptoms. If medications are ordered, review the name, dose, frequency, indications for use, and possible side effects with the woman. Make certain that the woman understands that prostaglandin inhibitors act to prevent cramping, not to suppress pain, and thus are most effective when taken at the earliest sign of pain.

NDx: Risk for altered health maintenance
Encourage a positive attitude toward menstruation by providing relevant facts and allowing the woman to discuss her feelings and experiences. Explain the value of regular exercise, good posture, balanced diet, and good hygiene in preventing dysmenorrhea.

Advise the woman to do waist-bending exercises before the onset of menstruation. Have her avoid constipation, which creates additional abdominal pressure, and the stress of fatigue at this time.

Compare the patient's status with the expected outcomes. If the outcomes are not met, reassess the patient and revise the plan.

Secondary Dysmenorrhea

In secondary dysmenorrhea, demonstrated pelvic disease is the source of the pain. This pain may begin 1 to 2 days before the onset of menstruation and can last for the duration of menses. Women may undergo several diagnostic tests, such as ultrasonography and laparoscopy, to determine the cause of secondary dysmenorrhea. Treatment is directed at the underlying cause. Disorders that can cause secondary dysmenorrhea include endometriosis, stenosis of the cervical os, endometrial polyp, fibroid tumor of the uterus, chronic pelvic inflammatory disease, endometrial hyperplasia, and endometrial cancer.

INTERMENSTRUAL PAIN

Intermenstrual pain, or mittelschmerz, is pain that occurs at about the middle of the hormonal cycle. It lasts from a few hours to a few days and varies from slight discomfort to severe pain. In some cases, it is followed by brownish spotting or by bleeding from the ruptured follicle similar to a scant menstrual flow. When macroscopic bleeding is not evident, microscopic examination of vaginal discharge demonstrates the presence of red blood cells.

Intermenstrual pain is believed to be related to ovulation. The nature of the relationship is uncertain. It has been suggested that the pain results from swelling of the ovary as the graafian follicle matures (Speroff et al, 1994).

Assessment of the Female Reproductive System

When assessing reproductive status, consider the intimate nature of the parts and functions affected. Be aware that, despite the increasing openness about sexuality in our society, discussion of reproductive structure and functioning is a source of embarrassment to many women. Provide privacy and adequate time for uninterrupted conversation. Establish a trust relationship and use communication that is nonjudgmental, open, and respectful of cultural differences. Start with the least intimate assessment questions first. Without privacy, sufficient time for communication, and a professional manner, nursing assessments are likely to be incomplete, incorrect, and ineffective. Women are unlikely to answer questions about vaginal discharge, pain on intercourse, or sexual satisfaction completely and comfortably, or ask questions such as "How long do I have to wait to have intercourse after I get home?" if there are other patients present or if the conversation is interrupted by other hospital personnel speaking to the nurse.

Never assume that a patient knows the correct terms for body parts or that she can name or describe body functions. The nurse may be comfortable talking about menses, leukorrhea, or dyspareunia, but the patient may not understand the terms. Further, the patient may feel that she should understand and be embarrassed to ask their meaning. This can block communication and result in an incorrect or incomplete database.

PATIENT HISTORY

Because symptoms related to menstruation are the most important in the diagnosis of gynecologic disorders, the history usually begins with complete information about the woman's menstrual status, including:

* Age of menarche
* Frequency, duration, and amount of flow (how many pads or tampons soaked per day).
* Characteristics of the discharge, such as color, odor, and presence or absence of clots
* Date of the last menstrual period (LMP); if the woman is not sure, obtain an estimated date
* Whether she uses tampons, pads, or both, because tampon use is linked to dysmenorrhea, vaginal infection, and toxic shock syndrome
* Whether any menstrual periods have been missed

Inquire about mittelschmerz (midcycle pain) and dysmenorrhea, including time of onset, duration, type of discomfort, severity of discomfort, and effective and ineffective remedies. Ask about premenstrual symptoms, such as depression, headaches, anxiety, breast tenderness, and fluid retention. Also inquire about intermenstrual bleeding. Try to establish the amount of bleeding. If the patient reports a few drops, it is considered staining. If she reports the equivalent of 5 or 6 mL, it is called spotting. Estimate bleeding based on the knowledge that one regular sanitary pad or tampon holds 25 to 50 mL of blood. Ask the patient about the appearance of the blood and its relationship to intercourse (or other contact) or pain. If the woman is middle-aged or older, determine the age of menopause or the presence of menopausal symptoms. Regardless of age, obtain the date of the last Papanicolaou (Pap) test and the type, date, and treatment of any past gynecologic problems. Also determine the frequency of breast self-examination and the date of the last mammogram.

Review the woman's sexual and obstetric status. Include the age of first intercourse, sexual orientation, number and type of sexual partners, current frequency of intercourse with and without contraception, type of contraception used, type of protection against STDs used, sexual satisfaction, and sexual difficulties. Ask whether menses is or has been affected by contraceptives used. Obtain the number and description of pregnancies and labors, and the number of spontaneous or induced abortions. Also determine the frequency and type of sexually transmitted diseases and gynecologic surgeries. Inquire whether there is any possibility that the woman may be pregnant at present.

Ask about symptoms, such as breast changes. Note their type and relationship to menses. Ask about pain. Note its type, location, and relationship to menses, sexual intercourse, urination, defecation, or insertion of a tampon. Ask about vaginal discharge. Note its time of onset, duration, amount, color (clear, white, yellow, brown), consistency (thin, thick, cottage cheese–like), odor (none, sweet, fishy), and association with irritation or itching.

Because urinary symptoms are frequent manifestations of gynecologic disorders, also note the presence or absence of urinary frequency, urgency, pain, incontinence, nocturia, or hematuria. For similar reasons, note constipation, tenesmus, diarrhea, or other gastrointestinal symptoms.

Assess for a history of sexual abuse or domestic violence by including such questions as "Have you ever had sex against your will?" and "Do you feel safe in your current relationship?" In such circumstances, the woman may benefit from a compassionate listener who explores options with her for ensuring her safety. Discuss referral sources for psychological support and legal assistance. Additional time may be needed to support her through the pelvic examination.

Assess the woman's understanding of and compliance with health promotion and risk reduction information related to the care of the female reproductive system (Highlight 40–3).

PELVIC EXAMINATION

A pelvic examination is an organized assessment of the structural condition of the reproductive organs. It includes inspection of the external genitalia, cervix, and vagina; evaluation of vaginal and perineal muscle tone; and palpation of the internal genital organs.

Patient Preparation

In preparation, ask the patient to urinate. This allows an easier, more comfortable examination and eliminates changes in the position of the pelvic organs from distention of the urinary bladder. Clothing is then removed from the waist down, and the patient is positioned and draped in a lithotomy or

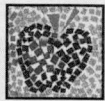

HIGHLIGHT
40—3

HEALTH PROMOTION & RISK REDUCTION

Optimal Female Reproductive Function

To help women in reproductive years achieve optimum health status, reduce risk, and promote early detection of reproductive system disease, take advantage of each health-related encounter to highlight health promotion and risk reduction activities as follows.

Discuss the importance of a routine physical examination (including breast and pelvic examination) by a health care provider every 1 to 3 years. Encourage the woman to ask questions during the examination and request a mirror during the pelvic examination so that she can visualize her own cervix. Refer to clinics and other screening opportunities in the community that may be free or low cost if her insurance coverage is inadequate.

Stress the value of a Papanicolaou (Pap) test to detect cervical neoplasms or premalignant lesions. After two negative smears, 1 year apart, the Pap test should be obtained at least every 3 years once a woman is sexually active, or age 20, whichever comes first. Women older than 65 years of age with previously normal Pap tests do not need to continue routine testing.

Recommend that the patient obtain a baseline mammogram by age 40, every 1 to 2 years between ages 40 and 49, and every year after age 50.

Strongly encourage the woman to promptly report any postmenopausal bleeding to a health care provider to rule out the possibility of endometrial cancer.

Assess the patient's current smoking status. If the woman smokes, advise her to quit. Highlight benefits based on concurrent risk factors. If the woman is interested in quitting, encourage her to set a quit date within 2 weeks. Offer self-help materials and referrals to community support groups. Encourage the use of a nicotine patch. Schedule a follow-up call or visit. If the woman is an ex-smoker, support her continued nonsmoking status.

Assess the patient's current exercise pattern. Encourage the woman to plan regular weight-bearing exercise to prevent osteoporosis and promote cardiovascular fitness. Activities should be enjoyable and performed at least three times weekly, preferably most days, for 30 minutes.

Teach the woman to practice safer sex. Mention that the safest sex is abstinence or self-masturbation. Urge her to determine her human immunodeficiency virus status, and that of her partner. Encourage her to remain in a monogamous relationship. Recommend barrier protection in the form of condoms and spermicide. Tell her to avoid anal intercourse because of trauma to mucous membranes. Also tell her to avoid high-risk behaviors, including multiple partners, intravenous drug use with needle sharing, and unprotected oral and genital sex.

Teach the woman to perform monthly self-examinations of the breasts (see Chap. 42) and vulva to become familiar with normal body changes related to endocrine cycles. For self-vulvar examination, use a simple diagram to help the woman to identify structures. Tell her to locate a hand mirror, bath towel, and flashlight and to follow these instructions. Place the bath towel on the closed commode or edge of tub. Sit comfortably with thighs spread apart. Hold the mirror with the non-dominant hand so that the vulva can be visualized. As an alternative, squat down and put the mirror on the floor below the vulva. Examine the external genitalia for signs of redness, swelling, irritation, skin breakdown, changes in skin color, presence of lesions, and vaginal drainage.

Teach the woman to perform Kegel or pelvic floor exercises to increase the tone of pelvic floor muscles for maintaining optimum genitourinary functioning. Tell her to learn to contract the pubococcygeal (PC) muscle by stopping and starting the urine stream when going to the bathroom. To manually check the strength of the PC muscle, insert two clean fingers into the vagina and tighten the muscle around the fingers. The contraction should isolate this muscle while keeping abdominal, gluteal, and thigh muscles relaxed. Tell her to contract the PC muscle and hold it for several seconds. Tell her to relax and repeat the exercise several times. Once the Kegel exercise is learned, instruct her to perform it frequently throughout the day.

Suggest that the woman read books that offer positive approaches to self-care, and encourage use of community resources that focus on women's health issues.

---

dorsal recumbent position on the examining table. If the patient cannot assume either of these positions, Sims' position may be used. In many states it is mandatory that a female chaperone be present during the examination. This person can also provide emotional support for the woman.

Examination Procedure

The examiner wears clean gloves for the examination, which begins with assessment of the external genitalia. This includes inspection for any structural abnormalities, such as alterations in the size and contour of the labia, distribution of pubic hair, or enlargement or atrophy of the clitoris. The presence of parasites, skin lesions (eg, rashes or ulcerations, tumors, signs of irritation, or change in pigmentation) is noted. The possibility of sexual abuse should be considered if there are any signs of trauma. Also noted is the presence or absence of the hymen, as well as discharge or other signs of infection in Bartholin's glands, Skene's glands, the urinary meatus, and the vagina. With increasing cultural diversity of the population, practitioners may see women who have experienced genital mutilation in the form of female circumcision during childhood. The appearance of the vulva can be markedly altered and make speculum examination of these women difficult if not impossible.

Second, a speculum examination is performed. A medium or possibly large speculum is usually used for multiparous patients, and a small speculum is used for elderly or nulliparous patients. The aim is to have the best possible visualization without discomfort to the patient. The speculum produces a sensation of pressure in the vagina but does not usually cause discomfort. Instructing the patient to bear down opens the introitus and relaxes the perineal muscles (Fig. 40–8).

The cervix is visualized and inspected for color, contour, position, shape, and patency of the external os, presence of polyps, erosions (red areas), and discharge. At this time, the examiner may offer to use a mirror so that the woman can see what her cervix looks like. If any cytopathologic smears or cervical cultures are indicated, they are obtained at this time. As the speculum is inserted and withdrawn, the vaginal mucosa is assessed. Color and consistency as well as the presence of rugae, ulcers, masses, and discharge are noted.

Next, one or more well-lubricated fingers are inserted into the vagina and the degree of muscle tone is evaluated. The patient is then asked to bear down

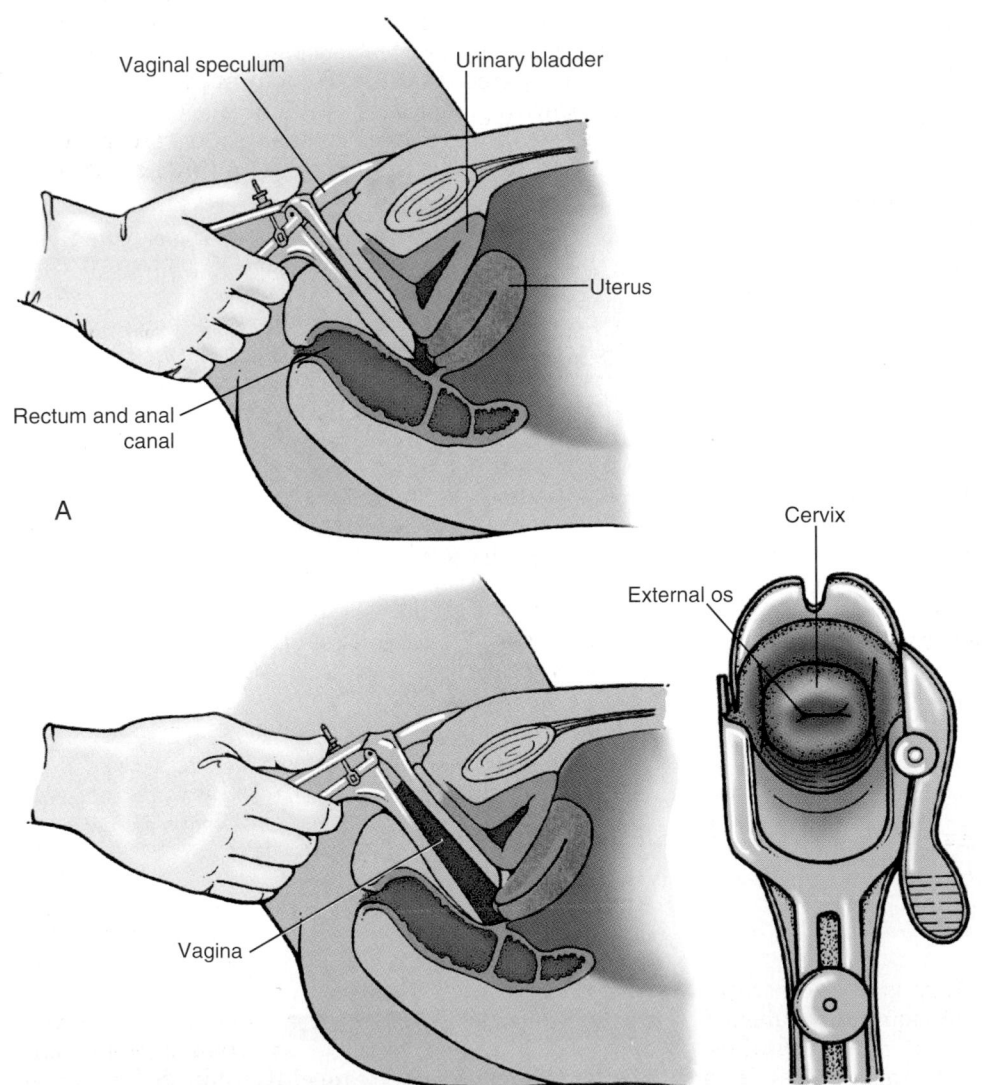

A

B

C

Figure 40–8

Speculum examination of the cervix. *A*, Insertion of a speculum. *B*, Open speculum within the vagina. *C*, Examiner's view of the cervix through an open speculum.

so that the effect of increased intra-abdominal pressure on the position of the bladder, uterus, and rectum can be noted.

Examination of the internal genitalia starts with palpation of the cervix. It is assessed for size, shape, consistency, relationship to the vagina, and mobility. The occurrence of bleeding as a result of the digital contact (friability) is also noted because this is a common indication of a polyp or malignancy. This is followed by a bimanual examination, which allows assessment of the other internal organs and the pelvic supports. One or two fingers of one hand are inserted into the vagina while the other hand is placed on the lower abdomen just above the symphysis pubis. By compressing the abdominal wall with the fingers of both hands, the pelvic contents may be palpated. This is most accurate when the abdominal wall is thin and soft and the patient is relaxed and cooperative. Ask the patient to take slow, deep breaths and relax the abdominal muscles as much as possible. The examination begins with determination of the size, contour, position, and mobility of the uterus. Finally, the lateral aspects of the pelvis are examined. Before menopause, the ovaries can readily be felt and are slightly tender to palpation. Any enlargement as well as mobility or fixation is noted. Normal fallopian tubes are not usually palpable. In the presence of pathology, a tube may be felt as a definite, fixed mass adherent to the ovary.

A rectovaginal examination may be done to confirm the position of the uterus or to further assess the ovaries and tubes (adnexa). A stool sample for occult blood may also be obtained at this time.

Upon conclusion of the examination any excess lubricant or secretions are wiped from the vulva, and the patient is helped to a sitting position. To avoid postural hypotension and the possibility of falling, women, particularly the elderly, should remain sitting for a brief interval before being helped to the standing position.

Throughout the examination, be sure to tell the patient what to expect. For example, tell her to expect a feeling of pressure in the vagina when the speculum is inserted. Tell her that she may feel some tenderness when the bimanual examination is done. If a rectovaginal examination will be done, inform the patient beforehand.

Diagnostic Procedures

PAPANICOLAOU TEST

A Pap test as used in gynecology is a microscopic examination of a smear of exfoliated cells obtained from the vaginal vault, outer cervix, and cervical os. It detects abnormal cells and is primarily used as a screening device for cancer of the cervix. It may also be used to detect infection or to evaluate the hormonal status of a woman who has an infertility problem or who is taking estrogen.

When a Pap smear is obtained, the patient assumes the dorsal recumbent or lithotomy position as for a pelvic examination, and a warmed speculum, which may be rinsed in saline but not lubricated, is inserted. Lubricant is contraindicated because it may prevent accurate interpretation of the test results. For the same reason, the gloves worn by the examiner should not be powdered.

The cellular samples are collected using a specially designed wooden or plastic spatula and a rubber-tipped vaginal pipette, a saline-moistened, cotton-tipped applicator, or a brush like a pipe cleaner called a cytobrush (Fig. 40–9). Material from the posterior vaginal fornix is collected with the blunt end of the spatula. The other end is then used to scrape cells from the entire circumference of the cervix. Finally, the pipette, applicator, or cytobrush is inserted into the external os to collect cells from the endocervix. The samples are immediately smeared on glass slides, each of which is carefully labeled as to source and immediately fixed by either dipping in 95% alcohol or spraying with a commercially prepared solution. This prevents drying and accompanying cellular distortion.

Results are reported to the health care provider using the Bethesda System with information about:

- Adequacy of the specimen
- General category of the specimen (normal, benign changes, or epithelial cell abnormality)
- Descriptive diagnoses (eg, atypical squamous cells of undetermined significance [ASCUS], low-grade squamous intraepithelial lesion [LSIL], high-grade squamous intraepithelial lesion [HSIL], or glandular cell)

Since the Pap test is a screening test, positive (abnormal) findings indicate the need for further tissue studies obtained through biopsy or operation (Warner & Parsons, 1996).

The Pap test is 90 to 95% accurate on positive reports and 95 to 98% accurate on negative reports. In most cases of false-negative results, the cause is an inadequate sample or improper fixation.

To maximize accuracy, the smear should not be obtained during menses because the menstrual discharge makes evaluation of the smear difficult. Tub baths, douches, and intercourse should be avoided for 48 hours before the test. After cauterization of the cervix, cellular distortion is present for 6 weeks, therefore smears are not obtained during this time. After radiation treatments, the interval is longer. Smears are not done for 1 month after use of intravaginal creams and medications because these cause intense cellular exfoliation.

The Pap test is usually a painless procedure that allows evaluation of a wider area than a biopsy and does not remove viable tissue. It produces little or no trauma or inflammation, although some spotting after the procedure can occur and is considered normal.

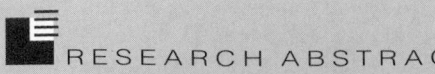

RESEARCH ABSTRACT

How Can Nurses Develop Teaching Materials to Prepare Women for the Experience of Gynecologic Procedures?

Nugent LS, Clark R. Colposcopy: Sensory information for client education. JOGNN 1996; 25(3):225.

Past research suggests that people who receive sensory information about upcoming procedures experience less distress. Because so many procedures related to women's health are performed on an outpatient basis, there is a need to develop brief but useful informational materials to prepare women for what to expect. Nugent and Clark therefore created a model for developing patient informational materials for procedures that was based on the actual sensory experience of women who have undergone a particular procedure. Their model involved four stages: standardizing the procedure, discovering the experience, validating the experience, and writing the message. They used these stages to develop a script for women undergoing a colposcopy procedure in an outpatient setting. Subjects for their study were 60 women aged 17 to 69 years.

The researchers first observed current practice in performing colposcopies to develop a standardized description of the procedure. During the second stage, the researchers asked half of the subjects to describe what sensations they experienced ("felt, heard, saw, smelled, or tasted") during the colposcopy. The researchers made a list of the common sensations and asked the other women in the study if they agreed with the descriptions of the sensations at various points in the procedure. With this additional feedback, the researchers finalized a script to be used in the future for women undergoing the procedure. This script included the vocabulary identified by the women who had participated in the study. The focus of the script was on describing probable sensations, such as temperature ("The vinegar will feel cool") and momentary discomforts ("You will feel a pinch as the biopsy is being taken"), that the woman would feel. The focus was also on pertinent actions of the clinician, such as when instruments would be inserted and removed ("Now I will remove the speculum").

The researchers suggest that future research examine the effects of scripted sensory preparation on such outcomes as anxiety and adherence to follow-up appointments. They also recommend testing various methods of presenting sensory information (spoken, videotaped, and written).

Questions to Consider

1. Listen to the types of information nurses in your clinical facility use to prepare people for procedures. Notice whether the information includes sensory detail. Following the procedure, ask people what information was most helpful to them.
2. How well are people in your clinical facility prepared for procedures?
3. Who is responsible for providing information about procedures to patients? Do they use verbal explanations or supplemental audiovisual materials?
4. Although extensive sensory information may be helpful to many people, what cues would you listen and look for to know whether someone was not interested in so much detail?
5. What sources of information might you use to develop a script to prepare women for other gynecologic procedures?
6. Think back to times when you have undergone a procedure. What types of information were you given? What was most helpful? What was least helpful?

"Do-it-yourself" Pap tests are now available. A woman using one of these tests obtains her own smear and mails it to a laboratory for interpretation. When women are identified who have followed or who plan to follow this procedure, instruct them as to the correct method of obtaining the smear. Also stress that this is not a substitute for a pelvic examination in which the sexual organs are inspected and palpated for abnormalities.

SCHILLER TEST

The Schiller test is used primarily after positive Pap test results to identify areas of the cervix or vagina that should be biopsied. It is a simple test in which an iodine solution is applied to the epithelium of the cervix and the vagina. Because these epithelial cells are normally rich in glycogen and readily pick up iodine, they become a deep mahogany color. Cancerous epithelium, in contrast, does not contain glycogen and does not pick up iodine or change color. Thus, epithelium with malignant changes appears as a glistening light area.

COLPOSCOPY

Colposcopy is the procedure in which the cervix is visualized and magnified in a bright light for the

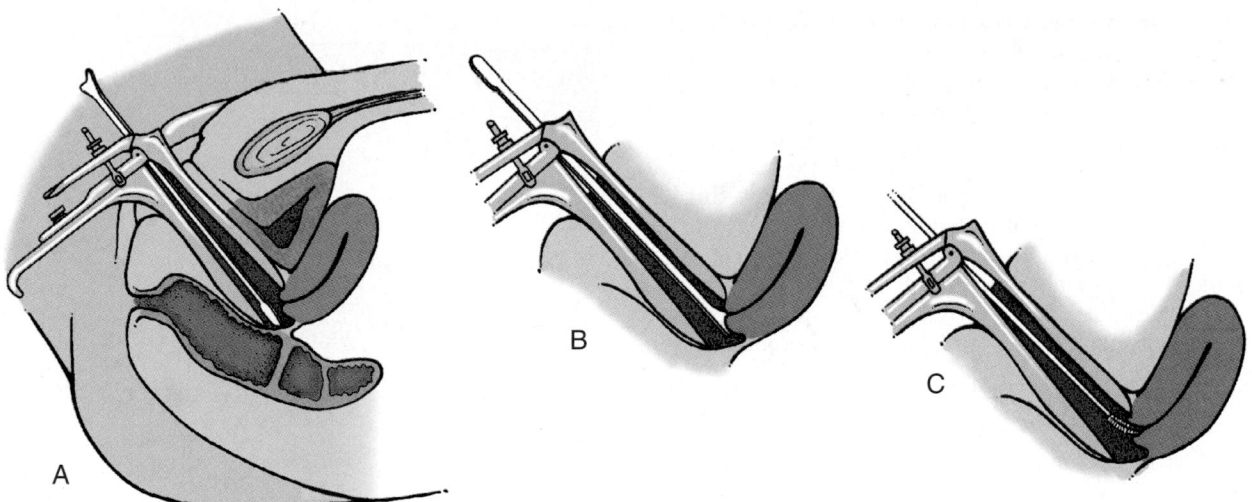

Figure 40–9

Method of obtaining a specimen for a Pap test. *A*, Blunt end of an Ayre spatula used to scrape the specimen from the posterior fornix. *B*, Most pointed tip of the bifid end of an Ayre spatula inserted into the cervical os and rotated 360 degrees to obtain a specimen from the squamocolumnar junction. *C*, Cytobrush inserted into cervical os and rotated 360 degrees to collect a specimen from the endocervix. A glass pipette or cotton swab may also be used.

purpose of identifying areas of abnormality. The instrument used is the colposcope, which is a low-power microscope. This procedure is done when Pap tests indicate persistent atypical or pathologic changes.

It is a simple procedure and takes no longer than the usual inspection of the cervix. Its major advantage is that areas where suspect cells originate can be identified to help to assess their size and severity, as well as selection of optimal biopsy sites. The disadvantage of colposcopy is that only the outer areas of the cervix can be studied. Provision of information regarding the physical sensations of the procedure may be helpful in preparing the patient for the experience (Nugent & Clark, 1996).

CERVICAL BIOPSY

A cervical biopsy is done when a Pap test result is abnormal or when a cervical lesion is seen with or without a colposcopy or a Schiller test. The purpose of the biopsy is to diagnose or rule out a malignancy. It can also serve as a basis for treatment by determining the exact histopathology of the lesion. Because there are few nerve fibers in the cervix, usually little or no anesthesia is needed for a simple biopsy. However, if the procedure involves dilatation of the cervix, anesthesia is required because the endocervix contains numerous nerve fibers.

Cervical biopsies are usually performed 1 week after the end of the menstrual period. This timing decreases the amount of bleeding from the procedure by avoiding the increased vascularity of the cervix that occurs before and after the menses.

Punch Biopsy

The simplest and most frequent type of cervical biopsy is a punch biopsy. This is an outpatient procedure. No anesthesia is needed, and there is only momentary discomfort as the punch biopsy forceps are used to remove a small piece of tissue from the area of the cervical lesion. In cases in which a specific area cannot be pinpointed, a multiple punch biopsy may be done.

There is minimal bleeding with punch biopsies, and it is easily controlled with pressure, application of silver nitrate solution, or electric cautery. If electric cautery is used, there is an unpleasant odor from the burning tissue and some discomfort is felt. A foul-smelling, gray-green discharge begins on or about the fourth day after the procedure and continues for up to 3 weeks.

Excision Biopsy

A second type of biopsy is an excision biopsy. In this type, a cervical lesion with adjacent normal tissue is removed with a scalpel. The excised area is larger than with a punch biopsy. There is more bleeding, and sutures may be required. This is an outpatient procedure. Local anesthesia may be used.

Cone Biopsy

A third type of biopsy is a conization of the cervix, or cone biopsy. This biopsy is done when the location of a lesion cannot be pinpointed, when a lesion involves a large area or extends into the cervical canal, or when smear results are positive but biopsy results are negative.

Cone biopsy is an inpatient or outpatient procedure in which a scalpel or laser is used to remove a cone-shaped piece of tissue from the central cervix (Fig. 40–10). The size and shape of the cone vary with the size and shape of the lesion. The procedure is done under either local or general anesthesia. Sutures may be used to prevent bleeding postoperatively.

Unless absolutely necessary, conization is generally not performed on women who desire to bear children because it can lead to incompetence of the cervix or infertility.

After conization, the next two or three menses may be heavy and prolonged, and a dark brown premenstrual discharge may occur. This is considered normal, and no therapy is indicated. Complications of cone biopsy include hemorrhage, infection, and, less frequently, cervical stenosis. If hemorrhage occurs, it is controlled by a vaginal pack retained for 24 to 48 hours. Cauterization may be required if other measures fail. Infection is treated with antibiotics, and stenosis is treated with dilatation.

"Hot" conization, which uses electrocautery, is performed as a therapeutic measure in women with chronic cervicitis that has extended into the deep tissues of the cervix. Tissue removed in this procedure cannot be used for diagnostic purposes because the cautery chars the tissue and prevents pathologic examination.

NURSING PROCESS GUIDELINES
Cervical Biopsy

Provide emotional support and allay anxiety. Allow time and opportunity for the patient to verbalize her

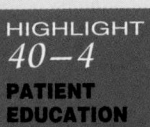 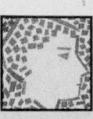

HIGHLIGHT
40–4
PATIENT EDUCATION

Discharge Instructions After Cervical Biopsy

Instruct the patient to:

Rest for 24 hours after the procedure. Avoid heavy lifting or any strenuous exercise or activity.

Call the physician or go to the clinic or hospital if bleeding in excess of a normal menstrual period occurs.

Avoid having intercourse or douching until the time specified by the physician.

Use pads rather than tampons until the physician advises otherwise.

Note: If vaginal packing is in place, do not remove it until instructed to do so by the physician. Usually vaginal packing is left in place for 8 to 24 hours.

concerns. Tell her the type and amount of discomfort that accompanies the procedure, as well as expected effects on the menstrual cycle, such as the occurrence of two or three heavy, prolonged menstrual periods after conization. Also inform the patient when, and by whom, she will be told the results of the biopsy. Provision of emotional support is particularly important when the biopsy is being done to rule out or diagnose malignancy.

Explain postbiopsy instructions to the patient before discharge (Highlight 40–4). Also be certain that the patient knows the date and time as well as the importance of scheduled follow-up visits.

After the procedure, assess the patient's physiologic stabilization by checking the amount of vaginal bleeding and measuring vital signs until stable. If a general anesthetic was given, make the usual postoperative assessments as discussed in Chapter 6.

ENDOMETRIAL CYTOLOGY

Endometrial cytology is done to screen for uterine cancer. The specimen is obtained by aspiration of endometrial secretions, cells, or lavage fluid through a cannula inserted into the uterine cavity via the cervical os. Mild, temporary cramping may accompany this procedure.

This test is of greatest importance to women older than age 50 because this is when endometrial cancer is most likely to occur. It is used in addition to the Pap test because cells rarely exfoliate from the endometrium during the early stages of a malignancy and thus would not be found in a Pap test.

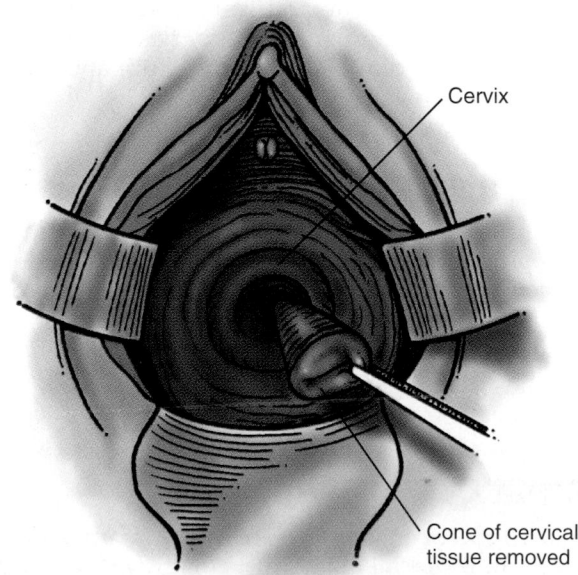

Cervix

Cone of cervical tissue removed

Figure 40–10
Cone biopsy.

ENDOMETRIAL BIOPSY

An endometrial biopsy may be used to diagnose endometrial cancer or to assess the endometrium for the effects of progesterone in women seeking treatment for infertility. It is not used as a routine screening test but is reserved for women with unexplained postmenopausal bleeding (Warner & Parsons, 1996).

The biopsy specimen is most often obtained by use of an aspirating curet attached to some form of negative pressure, although a nonaspirating curet or punch biopsy forceps may be used. To minimize the pain of the procedure, a prostaglandin synthetase inhibitor may be given orally 20 minutes before the procedure. If malignant cells are being looked for, specimens are obtained from several sites in the uterine cavity. This is typically done with a hysteroscopy.

HYSTEROSCOPY

Hysteroscopy is a procedure that allows direct visualization of the intrauterine cavity and is particularly useful in evaluating abnormal uterine bleeding. The procedure is contraindicated by pregnancy, suspected or diagnosed cancer of the cervix, pelvic inflammatory disease, or a history of recent uterine perforation. The procedure is done on either an inpatient or outpatient basis (Siegler, 1995). An instrument called a hysteroscope, which is equipped with a light source, is inserted through the cervix into the uterus and then the endometrial cavity is distended with carbon dioxide or dextran solution. The inside of the uterus can then be checked for polyps, submucous myomas, or adhesions.

Hysteroscopy may be done with paracervical block anesthesia or, if a flexible scope is used, without anesthesia. Physical preparation and positioning is the same as for a pelvic examination; however, unlike a routine pelvic examination, moderate cramping is likely to occur. This discomfort can be reduced by pre-procedure preparation about what to expect and by the presence of a supportive person, as is allowed when the procedure is done in an office setting (Prather & Wolfe, 1995). Hysteroscopy usually allows adequate visualization of the endometrium within 10 minutes. Photographs can be taken; biopsies can be obtained; or intrauterine devices or small polyps can be removed. Future uses for office hysteroscopy may include endometrial ablation, in which lasers are used to eliminate the lining of the uterus, and transcervical sterilization, in which tubal ligation is done through the cervix (Garry, 1995; Goldrath, 1995).

Post-procedure care includes assessing for rare complications of uterine perforation, bleeding, bradycardia, and pulmonary embolism. Vital signs should be monitored for at least 10 minutes. Referred shoulder pain is possible from irritation of the phrenic nerve. If severe, briefly place the woman in Trendelenburg position. Discharge instructions include the use of over-the-counter analgesics for pain, observation for signs of infection, and abstinence from intercourse and use of vaginal products for 2 weeks (Prather & Wolfe, 1995).

HYSTEROSALPINGOGRAPHY

Hysterosalpingography is an x-ray and fluoroscopic procedure in which a contrast medium is used to visualize the size, shape, position, and structure of the uterus and fallopian tubes. It can demonstrate pathology, such as malformation of the uterus and tubes, and the presence of intrauterine tumors or tubal adhesions that may cause infertility in some women. With the patient in the lithotomy position, a cannula is inserted through the vagina and into the cervical canal. A contrast substance, such as Ethiodol or Conray, is injected into the uterine cavity, and x-rays are taken as the cavity is filled and the substance moves through the tubes.

To prevent ascending infection, a pre-procedure antibiotic may be administered 2 hours before the test and continued if tubal dilatation is detected (Orr & Shingleton, 1994). During this test, which takes about 30 minutes, the patient may have uterine cramping and a transient sensation of dizziness. After the test, a vaginal discharge, which is sometimes bloody, may occur for 1 to 2 days.

The procedure is not done during the week before, during, or after menstruation. It is also not done when there is a recent or current episode of abnormal uterine bleeding, active infection of the reproductive tract, or severe cardiorespiratory disease.

ULTRASONOGRAPHY

Ultrasonography can be used to produce an image of the pelvic organs. In this procedure, intermittent high-frequency sound waves are projected toward the pelvis, and the pattern of the sound waves is recorded as they bounce back after hitting tissues of different densities. This procedure can locate pelvic masses. It reveals their size, position, and relationship to normal pelvic structures, and it identifies their internal composition (eg, solid or cystic).

Ultrasonography is used in planning the operative approach to pelvic tumors, planning and evaluating radiation therapy for pelvic malignancies, diagnosing extrauterine pregnancy, monitoring fetal growth, and determining the position of a "lost" contraceptive intrauterine device. It is also used in the diagnosis of other pathologic disorders, such as ovarian cysts and endometriosis.

Vaginal ultrasound is particularly effective in evaluating the need for endometrial biopsy to detect changes in a postmenopausal woman with a history of abnormal bleeding who is on hormone replacement therapy (Hargrove & Eisenberg, 1995; Warner & Parsons, 1996).

Management

NONSURGICAL MANAGEMENT

Pharmacologic therapy is the primary form of non-surgical intervention used to treat gynecologic disorders. Hormone therapy is used to treat disorders of the menstrual cycle and disorders such as atrophic vaginitis and endometriosis. Antineoplastic agents are used for treatment and palliation of many gynecologic cancers. Anti-infective agents are used to treat infectious disorders ranging from simple vaginitis to life-threatening toxic shock syndrome.

SURGICAL MANAGEMENT

Gynecologic surgery is performed to restore normal anatomy, remove abnormal tissue, or provide relief from distressing symptoms. Surgery is used to diagnose and treat the following:

- Menstrual abnormalities
- Congenital defects affecting fertility or sexual identity
- Chronic pelvic inflammatory disease or endometriosis
- Malignant diseases of the reproductive organs
- Traumatic injuries to the reproductive organs or supporting structures
- Therapeutic or incomplete spontaneous abortion

Table 40–1 summarizes gynecologic surgical procedures other than those discussed in depth here.

Preoperative Preparation

As for any surgery, the physician assesses the patient's overall status, with particular attention to pulmonary, myocardial, renal, and hepatic function. The physician checks for existing health problems other than that for which the surgery is being done and also evaluates drugs currently being taken by the patient.

Nutritional status, fluid-electrolyte status, and acid-base balances are assessed preoperatively to provide a baseline for postoperative evaluation and intervention. This is critical to the care of aged patients, patients who were recently pregnant, those taking oral contraceptives or diuretics, and those on special diets. All of these patients are susceptible to postoperative fluid and electrolyte imbalance.

To decrease the risk of postoperative infection, any vulvitis, vaginitis, or cervicitis is treated before the patient's admission for surgery. It is particularly important to identify and treat monilial infections, because monilial sepsis has a relatively high mortality rate. Women at risk for monilial sepsis include the elderly, the debilitated, those on long-term anti-

Table 40–1

Surgical Procedures Used to Treat Specific Gynecologic Disorders

Procedure	Description
Oophorectomy	Removal of an ovary
Salpingectomy	Removal of a fallopian tube
Myomectomy	Removal of a tumor of the uterine musculature
Colporrhaphy	Plastic repair of the vagina
Anterior	Repair of relaxed anterior vaginal wall to correct a cystocele
Posterior	Repair of relaxed posterior vaginal wall to correct a rectocele
Vaginectomy	Removal of the vagina
Vulvectomy	Removal of the vulva
Simple	Excision of vulva with wide skin margin
Radical (Wertheim's operation)	Excision of vulva with deep lymph node dissection
Total pelvic exenteration	Removal of uterus, fallopian tubes, ovaries, cervix, part of the vagina, and bladder; urinary diversion performed and a bowel resection with colostomy
Anterior pelvic exenteration	Total pelvic exenteration minus the bowel resection and colostomy
Posterior pelvic exenteration	Total pelvic exenteration minus the cystectomy and urinary diversion
Ovarian cystectomy	Removal of a cyst from an ovary
Bartholin's marsupialization	Creation of a channel for drainage from a Bartholin cyst by opening the gland and suturing the edges to the vaginal wall

biotic therapy, and those on immunosuppressive or corticosteroid therapy.

The patient is checked for urinary tract infection and treated, if necessary, because flare-ups of existing infection are likely after surgery as a result of catheterization and dissection in the area of the bladder.

To decrease the risk of blood loss, surgery is usually scheduled 1 week after the patient's last menstrual period.

For menopausal or postmenopausal women, estrogen suppositories may be ordered to aid proliferation of the vaginal epithelium and thus facilitate healing. These vaginal suppositories are given once a day for 3 to 4 weeks before surgery.

In addition to the routine scrub of the operative area, douches may be ordered to cleanse the vagina of mucus and epithelial debris. If hair removal is desired, it is done by the surgeon using clippers just before performing the incision. This helps to prevent infection.

If it is a major procedure, the intestine is also prepared. Anti-infective therapy, such as neomycin sulfate and erythromycin base on the day before surgery, is given to decrease bacteria in the intestine. The patient is given a low-residue diet for 3 days preoperatively and an enema on the evening before surgery to empty the rectum. As an alternative, GoLYTELY taken orally over 3 hours the day before surgery may be ordered.

Systemic antibiotics may be administered just before surgery if major wound contamination is expected, especially for vaginal and abdominal hysterectomies.

Patients are instructed to avoid coitus for 1 week before surgery.

Patients who smoke are advised to quit in preparation for anesthesia and to consider long-term cessation. At a minimum, they should refrain from smoking 12 to 24 hours before surgery.

Complications of Gynecologic Surgery

A major risk associated with gynecologic surgery is the development of a postoperative thromboembolism, which results from the effects of anesthesia, immobility, and soft tissue damage.

Predisposing factors include obesity, age older than 40 years, recent use of oral contraceptives, history of thrombus formation, and presence of malignant disease. Preventive measures include intraoperative and postoperative external pneumatic compression stockings, early movement and ambulation, elevation of the foot of the bed to 20 degrees, adequate hydration to maintain the fluidity of the blood, prophylactic anticoagulant therapy, and routine postoperative examination of the calf for early recognition of deep vein thrombosis (Copeland, 1993).

Infection is a second major postoperative complication. Wound infection is common because of vaginal pathogens and the closeness of the anus to the operative site. At particular risk are women who:

- Are obese or malnourished
- Have pre-existing sepsis, diabetes, or malignancy
- Are undergoing an operation that involves an opening between the vagina and the pelvis

Infection may also occur in the urinary tract and in the chest. Catheterization increases the risk of urinary tract infection. Smoking increases the risk of chest infection.

Prevention includes preoperative showering with an anti-infective soap, preoperative antibiotic infusions, bowel preparation, incentive spirometry, and meticulous intraoperative aseptic techniques.

A third complication is hemorrhage, which may occur early or late. Early hemorrhage may result from incomplete hemostasis, loosening of a ligature on a major blood vessel, or perforation. It may also be a reactive hemorrhage from severed vessels that did not bleed during surgery because of hypotension. Late hemorrhage, which occurs several days after the operation, results from suture dissolution or infection. Regardless of type, measures to control bleeding are initiated, and blood is replaced when necessary. Other complications are accidental injury to the bladder, ureter, or rectum, because of their close proximity to the operative site; intestinal obstruction; and wound dehiscence.

Depression and sexual dysfunction occur in some women after gynecologic surgery. Depression may be related to the perceived loss of an important organ or of an important function, or it may be a reaction to the total stress of the preoperative symptoms, the surgery, and the recovery period. Sexual dysfunction may occur secondary to depression or as a result of physical damage to the reproductive tract or atrophy of the vagina, which occurs after removal of the ovaries. It may also be due to the lack of an understanding partner. Empathic emotional support during all phases can help to identify the patient's concerns.

Common Gynecologic Surgical Procedures

LAPAROSCOPY

Laparoscopy is a procedure in which the internal organs of the pelvis are visualized and examined. This is done with a laparoscope that is inserted through an incision in the abdominal wall. It is used for both diagnostic and therapeutic purposes (Fig. 40–11).

Uses

As a diagnostic technique, it is used to evaluate chronic pelvic pain, a palpable abdominal mass, or a history of infertility. It allows identification of endometriosis, pelvic inflammatory disease, ectopic pregnancy, ovarian neoplasms, and signs of abdominal malignancy or metastasis. It can be used to obtain biopsies and also to determine patency or blockage of the fallopian tubes.

As a therapeutic procedure, the principal use of laparoscopy is for tubal sterilization. It may also be used for procedures such as removal of peritubal adhesions, ablation of endometrioma, removal of intrauterine devices that have perforated through the uterine wall, and aspiration of ova for in vitro fertilization.

CLINICAL ? THINKING

ABDOMINAL PAIN AND MOIST DRESSINGS AFTER HYSTERECTOMY

As I approached the patient for a routine check of vital signs, she exclaimed, "I'm so glad you're here, I couldn't reach the call bell." The patient, a 40-year-old obese woman with a medical history of insulin-dependent diabetes mellitus, had undergone a total abdominal hysterectomy for extensive uterine fibroids 5 days earlier. Her postoperative course had been complicated by the development of a wound infection that was currently being treated with antibiotic therapy. The patient was sitting in a chair and appeared pale, mildly diaphoretic, and quite anxious. She reported that she had just vomited and was now experiencing abdominal pain. She was clutching her abdomen and said that the abdominal dressing felt moist.

I decided to help the patient back to bed before I assessed her clinical condition further. I recognized that her abdominal pain could be related to many factors, including incisional pain, infection, abdominal distention, a distended bladder, constipation, muscle spasm, a tight dressing, or a reaction to the antibiotic. It could also indicate dehiscence of the surgical wound and evisceration of the abdominal contents through the wound, which was what I suspected.

Although the patient did not report a feeling that something had popped or given way, her history of obesity and diabetes, along with the current disruption of the wound healing process secondary to infection, were factors that placed her at high risk for this complication. The facts that her incision was a vertical abdominal one, that the episode was precipitated by a sudden strain and increased intra-abdominal pressure related to vomiting, and that she felt a sudden increase in moisture (hemorrhage and increased purulent drainage were unlikely) supported my suspicion.

I recognized that the patient's clinical picture could be ominous and required further investigation. My suspicion was confirmed when I inspected the dressing and noted that it was saturated with serosanguineous drainage. I removed the dressing and found that the wound edges had separated and a loop of intestine protruded through the wound. Although not immediately life-threatening, wound evisceration is a medical/surgical emergency that can be complicated by shock, peritonitis, septicemia, and compromised blood supply and necrosis of the abdominal viscera. Therefore, I quickly implemented the following actions:

1. I called for help.

2. I asked another staff nurse to bring the necessary supplies to the bedside and to notify the physician immediately.
3. I placed the patient in a low-Fowler's position with her knees slightly flexed.
4. I assessed the viscera for signs of ischemia.
5. I placed sterile dressings, soaked in warm sterile normal saline solution, loosely over the exposed viscera.
6. I instructed the patient to lie still.
7. I monitored the patient's vital signs for evidence of shock.
8. I reassured the patient and provided support by explaining what had happened and the reasons for my actions.
9. I started an intravenous line as per hospital protocol.
10. I kept the patient on nothing-by-mouth (NPO) status and anticipated insertion of a nasogastric tube.
11. I kept the dressing moist until the doctor arrived.
12. I documented my findings and actions.

After the physician arrived, the patient was prepared for surgery. I checked for the surgical consent, notified the operating room staff, and administered preoperative medications as ordered.

The patient returned to the unit after débridement and closure of the wound and recovered uneventfully. Sound clinical decisions and appropriate nursing actions prevented the development of serious complications and possibly eventual death.

Think Critically

Should the nurse have assessed the patient's vital signs sooner?

What was the rationale for positioning the patient in this manner? For starting the IV? For maintaining the patient NPO? For anticipating a nasogastric tube?

What was the rationale for placing warm saline-soaked sterile dressings over the wound?

Why didn't the nurse attempt to reinsert the viscera into the abdominal cavity?

How did each risk factor contribute to the development of this complication?

Could the nurse in this scenario have foreseen or prevented this complication of surgery? What nursing actions might have been implemented?

What is the physiologic basis for shock associated with wound evisceration?

What additional nursing actions should have been implemented if the patient had been in shock?

Patient Preparation

Laparoscopy may be performed in either an inpatient or outpatient setting. The patient takes nothing by mouth (NPO) from midnight before the procedure. Bowel cleansing and abdominal skin preparation are done at the discretion of the physician. A short-acting general anesthetic is used most often because little sedation is required and the patient is awake, alert, and, if an outpatient, is able to go home within 2 hours. Local or regional anesthesia may also be used, but more sedation is required and the recovery period is longer.

Procedure

The patient's bladder is emptied, and then an incision is made into the lower rim of the umbilicus. The abdomen is insufflated with carbon dioxide or nitrous oxide to distend it and separate the organs. The patient is placed in Trendelenburg position so that the gas displaces the bowel up and out of the pelvis.

In a one-incision technique, a laparoscope with an electric cautery forceps is then inserted. In a two-incision technique, another incision is made below the umbilicus but above the symphysis pubis, and a second instrument needed for the procedure is inserted. When the procedure is completed, as much gas as possible is expelled from the abdomen, and sutures or clips are used to close the incisions. Healing occurs without a noticeable scar.

Contraindications

Previous surgery, abdominal adhesions, or obesity makes visualization difficult and may result in an unsatisfactory procedure. The procedure cannot be used for women with cardiovascular, respiratory, or other disorders that prevent the use of the Trendelenburg position or abdominal insufflation.

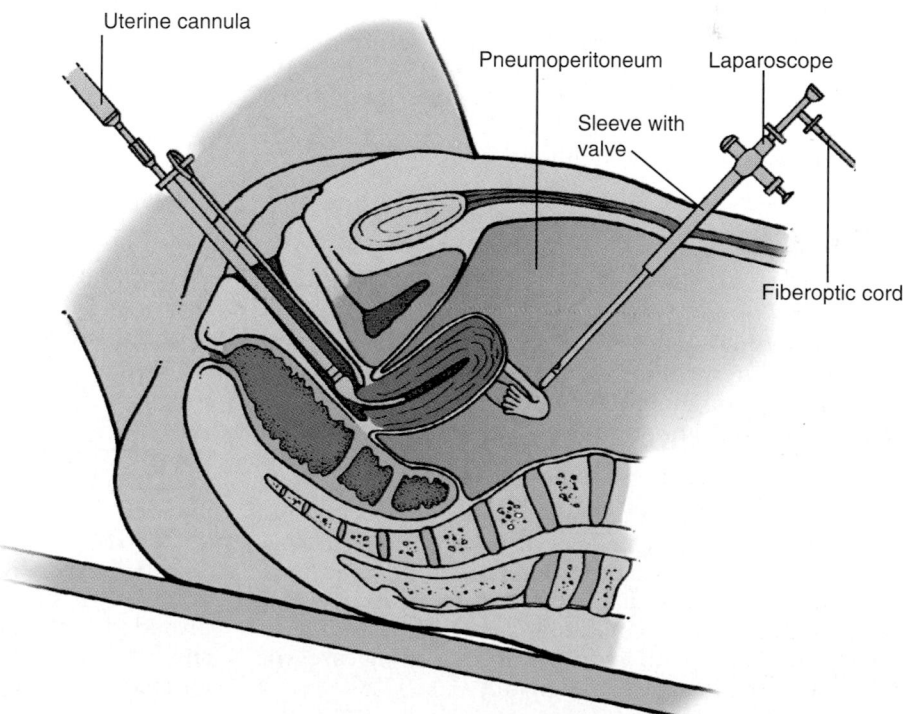

Figure 40–11

Laparoscopy.

Complications

The most serious complication of laparoscopy is intestinal burns when diathermy (electrical current to coagulate tissue) is used. Burns can cause necrosis and perforation of the bowel and consequently peritonitis. Other possible complications include embolism secondary to the insufflation, infection, and—rarely—bleeding, which requires a laparotomy.

NURSING PROCESS GUIDELINES

Laparoscopy

If the patient is having a local anesthetic, obtain baseline vital signs. Tell her that the procedure usually takes less than 1 hour. Tell the patient that, once the anesthesia is given, she may feel some pressure but will not feel pain. Finally, tell the patient that she will be placed in a tilted position with her head somewhat lower than her feet.

After the procedure, monitor physiologic stabilization. Take vital signs every 15 minutes for 1 hour, or until the patient is stable. Allow the patient activity as tolerated, and give fluids and a light snack if she is not nauseated. Monitor the patient for discomfort. Referred shoulder pain and chest soreness from irritation of a branch of the phrenic nerve are common after insufflation. A sore throat is common if the patient was intubated. Keep the patient supine or in low Fowler's position to reduce the pressure of intra-abdominal gas on the diaphragm. Give analgesics (usually aspirin or aspirin substitutes) as ordered to relieve the chest and shoulder discomfort. Tell the patient to resume a regular diet. Give the patient warm saline gargles to relieve the sore throat if general anesthesia was used. Explain to the patient that these symptoms are normal and that the medication, position change, and gargle will provide relief. Reassure the patient that these symptoms should disappear in a few days. Instruct the patient in self-care as needed (Highlight 40–5).

CRYOSURGERY

Cryosurgery is a technique in which tissue is destroyed by exposure to extreme cold. A probe, usually containing liquid nitrogen, is used to produce subfreezing temperatures that cause necrosis and subsequent sloughing of tissue from cellular dehydration and disruption of the cell membrane.

Uses

This local freezing technique is used to treat chronic cervicitis, endocervicitis, cervical erosions, cervical polyps, and benign leukoplakia. It is also used as a preventive measure to remove tissue when dysplasia, a precancerous condition, is evident and as a palliative measure to reduce tumor size in cases of inoperable or recurrent malignancy.

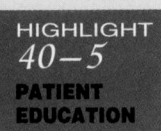 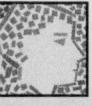

HIGHLIGHT 40–5
PATIENT EDUCATION

Discharge Instructions After Laparoscopy

Instruct the patient to:

Take analgesics as ordered for relief of chest and shoulder discomfort.

Gargle with warm water and salt for relief of sore throat.

Avoid heavy lifting for 1 week.

Resume intercourse when comfortable to do so.

Report oral temperature higher than 37.7°C (100°F) and any redness, swelling, or drainage from the wound.

Patient Preparation

Cryosurgery is an ambulatory procedure performed in an office or clinic setting. No anesthesia is usually required. It is done 1 week after the end of the menstrual period. This prevents destruction of a possible early pregnancy and allows the active phase of cervical regeneration, which takes place after menses, to occur. Premedication with an NSAID can reduce cramping from the procedure.

Procedure

The patient is placed in lithotomy position, and a medium or large speculum is inserted. The patient is then instructed not to move. This is to prevent the probe from accidentally touching and damaging normal tissues. The probe is placed on areas to be treated for 1 to 3 minutes and, upon completion, a perineal pad is applied.

Postoperative Course

After the procedure, a profuse watery discharge occurs. On about the fourth day, it contains cellular debris and may have an odor. The discharge lasts from 2 to 4 weeks. Because the cervix is left friable, some physicians instruct their patients to avoid sexual intercourse, swimming, and the use of tampons for 2 weeks after the procedure. Showers are recommended, but a bath may be used if the tub is well scrubbed.

An intravaginal antibiotic cream, such as Triple Sulfa or Furacin, may be prescribed to aid healing, provided that the patient does not have acute cervicitis or perimetritis. For these women, oral antibiotics are prescribed for 1 week.

Complications

Possible complications of the procedure include occasional spotting, cervical stenosis, infection, and damage to normal tissue through accidental touching with the probe.

NURSING PROCESS GUIDELINES
Cryosurgery

When caring for patients having cryosurgery, intervene to decrease anxiety and promote patient compliance with postoperative instructions. Before the procedure, assess the patient's knowledge of the procedure, awareness of the reason for which it is being performed, and understanding of the discomfort involved. Before discharge, review with the patient characteristics of the vaginal discharge to be expected and instructions about bathing, swimming, use of tampons, and sexual intercourse.

ELECTROCAUTERY

To cauterize is to burn. In electrocautery, an instrument consisting of a holder and a wire is heated by a current of electricity. This is used to burn abnormal tissue in cases of cervical dysplasia or venereal warts. The burned cells exfoliate and new, healthy tissue is regenerated. The treatment may have to be repeated because the abnormality sometimes recurs. Electrocautery is usually an outpatient or office procedure.

When electrocautery is used to treat cervical dysplasia, the patient is placed in the lithotomy position and a vaginal speculum is inserted. Little or no anesthesia is required because electrocauterization does not cause specific pain, although it may cause uterine cramping. There is an unpleasant odor and a foul-smelling, gray-green discharge that begins on or about the fourth day and continues for up to 3 weeks.

LASER SURGERY

Laser surgery is used in many ways in gynecologic practice. It can be used for cervical conization, tubal ligation, excision of polyps, precancerous lesions, and vulvar carcinoma. When combined with hysteroscopy, it can also be used for intrauterine endometrial ablation in the treatment of menorrhagia. To accomplish endometrial ablation, the woman is sedated and given general, spinal, or local anesthesia. Her uterus is kept continuously distended by a gravity infusion of sterile normal saline. The physician directs the laser via the hysteroscope to the endometrial surfaces. The resultant adhesions prevent future bleeding. The procedure is done in less than 1 hour (Goldrath, 1995).

NURSING PROCESS GUIDELINES
Gynecologic Laser Surgery

The assessment, nursing diagnoses, expected patient outcomes, nursing interventions, and evaluation of patients having laser surgery for a gynecologic problem include those for patients having surgery (see Chap. 6), as well as those that relate to the specific gynecologic disorder for which the patient is being treated. Instruct all women in basic self-care after gynecologic laser surgery (Highlight 40–6).

DILATATION AND CURETTAGE

Dilatation and curettage (D&C) is a common operative procedure in which the cervix is dilated and the entire uterine endometrium is scraped out.

Uses

A D&C has both diagnostic and therapeutic uses. As a diagnostic tool, it allows evaluation of the contour

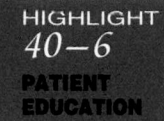
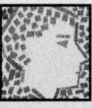

HIGHLIGHT 40–6
PATIENT EDUCATION

Self-Care After Gynecologic Laser Surgery

Instruct the patient to:

Apply ice pack to the perineum immediately after surgery to prevent swelling.

Keep a condom filled with cotton and topical antibiotic in the vagina for 24 hours after extensive vaginal surgery to keep the vaginal walls from adhering to each other, if directed to do so by the physician.

Take over-the-counter analgesics as directed to relieve abdominal cramping, which can last up to 36 hours.

Take sitz baths for comfort after bowel movements or whenever needed.

Dry the perineal area thoroughly after sitz baths by gently patting or using a hand-held blow dryer on its lowest setting.

Facilitate urination if necessary by squirting warm water over the vulva or voiding in the sitz bath.

Take stool softeners as directed to ease constipation and painful defecation, which can occur for up to 14 days after vulvar or perianal laser treatments.

Consult the physician before resuming sexual intercourse.

Return for a checkup on *(specify date and time).*

of the uterine cavity and cytopathologic examination of the endometrium. It is used to diagnose uterine malignancies and may be performed when there is unexplained, irregular uterine bleeding to determine whether its cause is a hormonal dysfunction or a cancer. Because tissue is obtained from all areas of the uterus, missed diagnoses of malignancies are infrequent.

As a therapeutic tool, it is used to control abnormal uterine bleeding, relieve dysmenorrhea, empty the uterus after an incomplete abortion, or perform an abortion.

With increased use of vaginal ultrasonography, endometrial biopsy techniques, and hysteroscopy, the use of D&C is declining.

Patient Preparation

Before a D&C, the patient must have medical clearance for anesthesia and surgery, and remains on NPO status after midnight on the day of the operation. A perineal shave or clipping, an enema, or a douche may be ordered by the surgeon preoperatively, but this is currently the exception rather than the rule.

Procedure

The procedure is usually done under general anesthesia. However, it can also be done using local anesthesia with the patient mildly sedated. The patient is placed in lithotomy position; the perineum and vagina are prepared with povidone-iodine (Betadine); and a bimanual examination is done to determine the position of the uterus. A speculum is inserted to allow access to the cervix. The size of the uterine cavity is assessed by insertion of an instrument called a sound. Metal dilators of increasing size are then used to gradually open the cervix for passage of the curet and for the tissues to be removed from the uterus (Fig. 40–12). When dilatation is accomplished, the endometrium is removed either by scraping with a curet or by the application of suction. When the latter is done, it is called a suction curettage. All material removed is sent to the laboratory for cytopathologic examination.

Postoperative Course

Postoperatively, vaginal bleeding occurs, and it may contain a few small clots. The bleeding progressively

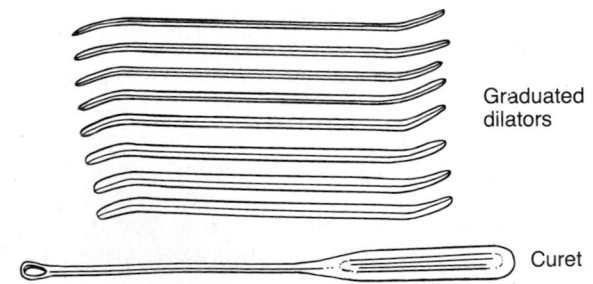

Figure 40–12
Graduated dilators and curet.

decreases in amount and becomes darker. It usually ends in a few days but may continue as spotting for up to 8 weeks if the D&C is performed after a spontaneous abortion. A recurrence of bright red bleeding or the development of a foul odor from the discharge is abnormal.

Abdominal cramping may occur during the first few postoperative days. This is treated with mild analgesics, such as aspirin, NSAIDs, or codeine sulfate. Use of a heating pad or hot-water bottle on the abdomen may also help. Continuous, sharp abdominal pain that is not relieved by medication is abnormal.

The patient is allowed diet and activity as tolerated after her recovery from anesthesia. If the procedure was performed on an outpatient basis, she will be ready to return home in about 8 hours.

The procedure is contraindicated by pregnancy or the presence of an acute infection. Hemorrhage that occurs 7 to 14 days after the procedure is the most common complication.

NURSING PROCESS
Dilatation and Curettage

PREOPERATIVE NURSING CARE

Preoperatively, prepare the patient for the procedure by clarifying the patient's understanding of what is to be done, and ensure that the physician's orders for preoperative diet and skin preparations are carried out. If the D&C is done as an outpatient procedure, be sure that the patient or the patient's significant other understands and is capable of carrying out preparations to be done at home.

POSTOPERATIVE NURSING CARE

Assessment

Assess physiologic stabilization by checking the patient's vital signs and monitoring vaginal bleeding. Check the patient's vital signs every 15 minutes until stable and then as indicated by the patient's condition. Monitor vaginal bleeding by keeping a pad count and by noting the degree of saturation.

After the first postoperative hour, perineal pads should not require changing more than once per hour for the remainder of the first postoperative day. About 60 mL of blood are needed to saturate a pad. Bleeding is excessive when pads are changed every hour and more than one pad is saturated during an 8-hour interval.

Take the patient's temperature every 4 hours. Notify the physician if it is higher than 37.7°C (100°F) orally. Note all fluid intake and the time and amount of voiding. Assess the patient for physical discomfort and for her emotional reaction to the procedure.

Nursing Diagnoses and Planning

Nursing diagnoses and related expected patient outcomes commonly applicable to women who have had a D&C include the following:

NDx: Pain related to abdominal cramping

Planning: Patient Outcomes
1. Patient reports that pain is minimal or absent.
2. Patient appears free of pain (eg, she does not hold her abdomen or draw up her legs).

NDx: Risk for altered health maintenance related to insufficient knowledge of discharge instructions

Planning: Patient Outcomes
1. Patient explains discharge instructions accurately.
2. Patient states the need for and time of any follow-up appointment.

Nursing Interventions and Evaluation

NDx: Pain
Administer analgesics or apply heat to the abdomen according to physician's orders. Assure the patient that abdominal cramping after a D&C is normal, and help her perform relaxation exercises.

NDx: Risk for altered health maintenance
Explain the normal recovery process following a D&C, and instruct the woman in self-care (Highlight 40–7). Be sure the woman knows the reason for and time of any follow-up appointment needed.

Compare the patient's status with the expected outcomes. If the outcomes are not met, reassess the patient and revise the plan.

BILATERAL TUBAL LIGATION

Bilateral tubal ligation (BTL) is a surgical sterilization procedure for women in which the fallopian tubes are cut, cauterized, or clipped to prevent passage of a mature ovum to the uterus. The procedure is most often done through the abdomen via a mini-laparotomy incision or laparoscopic approach. This elective procedure is often done during the immediate postpartum period or as part of a planned cesarean section.

Postoperative discomfort is minimal. When the patient has fully recovered from the anesthesia and her vital signs are stable, she may be discharged from the hospital.

Bleeding and infection are possible complications. For this reason, women are instructed to report redness, swelling, or drainage at the site of the incision; an oral temperature higher than 37.7°C (100°F); bleeding more than 12 hours after the procedure; or fainting.

The patient should rest for 24 to 48 hours after the procedure. She should avoid heavy lifting for 1 week. After laparoscopy, sexual intercourse may be resumed when the woman feels comfortable enough to do so. Tubal ligation should be considered a permanent form of sterilization.

HYSTERECTOMY

Hysterectomy is an operation in which the uterus is removed. In a total hysterectomy, or panhysterectomy, the entire uterus including the cervix is excised, and its several supporting ligaments are then reattached to the vaginal cuff to maintain normal vaginal depth.

When the ovaries are also removed, the procedure is a hysterectomy with bilateral oophorectomy (Fig. 40–13). When the fallopian tubes are also removed, the procedure is a hysterectomy with a bilateral salpingo-oophorectomy (BSO). The latter operation is done in many cases of pelvic malignancy. It may also be done for a benign disorder, depending on the philosophy of the physician and specific patient characteristics. Some surgeons believe that the adnexa (ovaries and fallopian tubes) should be removed at the time of hysterectomy as prophylaxis against cancer of the ovary, which is insidious in its development and is therefore often not discovered until an advanced stage. Others believe that the risk of ovarian cancer is not sufficient to warrant an oophorectomy, because the role of the aging ovary in preventing skeletal or cardiovascular disease is not certain. In all cases, the patient's age, general health, and emotional status are considered, and the woman herself is included in the decision-making process.

In a radical hysterectomy, the entire uterus, the nearby supporting (parametrial) tissues, and the uppermost part of the vagina are removed. A pelvic lymphadenectomy (removal of the pelvic lymph nodes) is frequently done in connection with a radical hysterectomy.

After a hysterectomy, a woman no longer menstruates and cannot become pregnant. When a bilat-

---

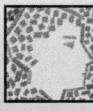

HIGHLIGHT 40–7

PATIENT EDUCATION

Discharge Instructions After Dilatation and Curettage

Instruct patient to:

Avoid strenuous exercise and heavy work. Gradually increase overall activity, and return to a full routine in 2 weeks.

Avoid tampons and douches for 1 week.

Avoid sexual intercourse for 2 weeks or until all bleeding stops.

Report signs and symptoms of infection: pain, fever, chills, or foul-smelling discharge.

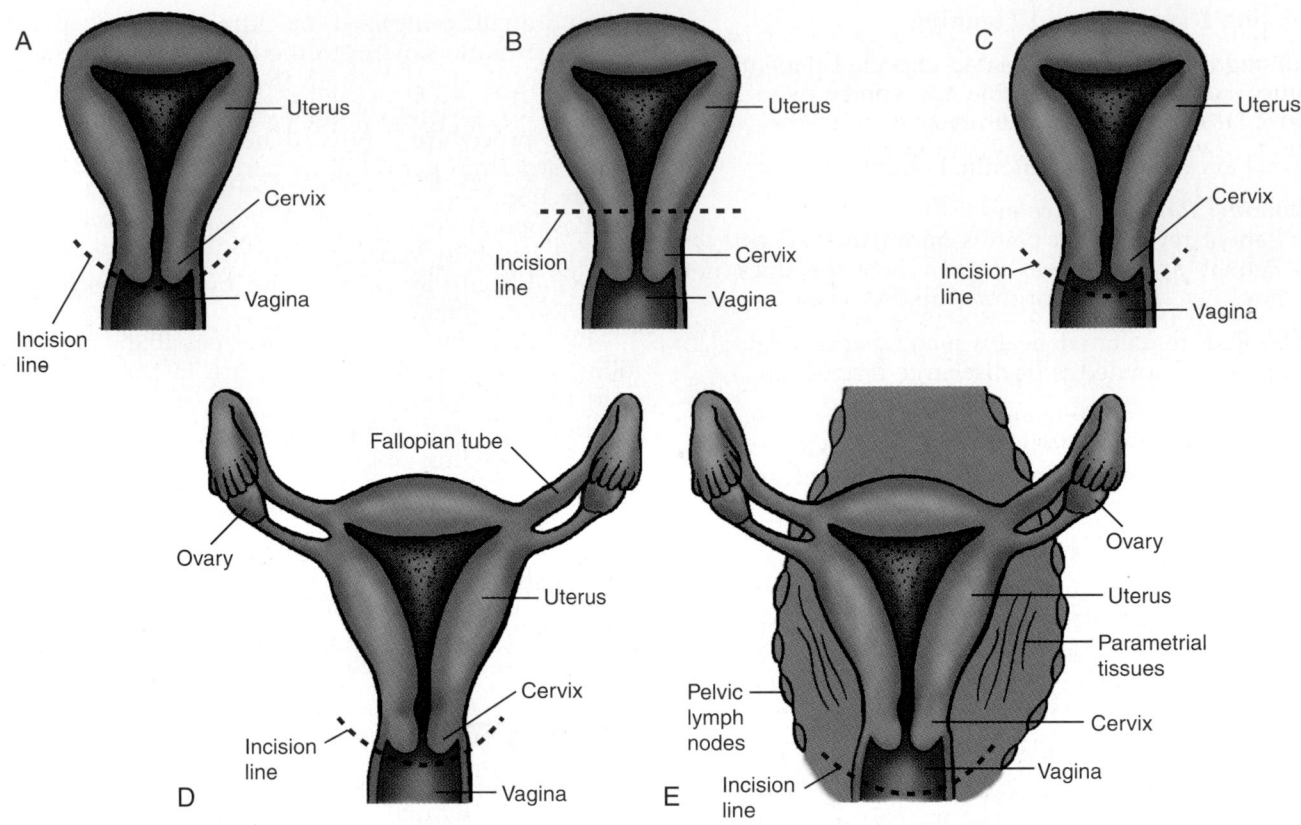

Figure 40–13

Types of hysterectomy. *A*, Total hysterectomy. *B*, Subtotal hysterectomy. *C*, Total hysterectomy with vaginal cuff excision. *D*, Total hysterectomy with bilateral salpingo-oophorectomy. *E*, Radical hysterectomy with pelvic lymphadenectomy.

eral oophorectomy is also done, menopause occurs because the ovaries, the source of estrogen and progesterone, have been removed. This is a surgical or induced menopause. Its symptoms are the same as those of natural menopause, although they may be more severe because of the abrupt decrease in hormone levels.

Hysterectomy may be performed by either the abdominal or vaginal route.

Abdominal Hysterectomy
Abdominal hysterectomy is the more frequent approach. It is performed when gynecologic cancer is suspected or when the uterus is in a fixed position or contains large myomatous (fibroid) tumors. It is also used when there are ovarian lesions, when the adnexa are to be removed in addition to the uterus, and when the woman has had multiple pelvic operations. This approach allows for full inspection of the abdominal cavity. A total abdominal hysterectomy with bilateral salpingo-oophorectomy (removal of ovaries and fallopian tubes) is abbreviated TAH&BSO.

Vaginal Hysterectomy
The vaginal route is used when a vaginal repair is being done along with the hysterectomy. It may also be used when the uterus is being removed because

of small myomata (tumors/fibroids of the uterine muscle), for recurrent uterine bleeding from endocrine imbalance, or for prolapse. The major advantages of this procedure are that it can be done quickly, requires relatively light anesthesia, and has minimal postoperative discomfort. However, it is associated with an increased chance of postoperative infection and other complications, particularly in women younger than age 35 (because of the great vascularity of the pelvis) and in women older than age 60 (because of the normal changes occurring with aging). Women who are 18 to 50 years of age with no concurrent medical problems and adequate support at home may be able to have the procedure done on an outpatient basis (Bran et al, 1995).

Preoperative Preparation
Preoperative preparation for a hysterectomy is the same as for any other vaginal or abdominal surgery. To minimize respiratory complications, women who smoke are counseled to stop smoking a minimum of 12 to 24 hours before surgery. If possible, they should consider cessation 8 weeks before surgery. If abdominal or vaginal hair is a concern, clippers may be used on the morning of surgery or in the operating suite just before performing the incision to prevent infection. A preoperative shower using antiseptic soap, vaginal douche, enema, or all three may be

ordered according to the surgeon's preference. Antibiotics may be given prophylactically 6 to 8 hours before surgery, during surgery, and for several doses after surgery. Preoperative concerns about psychosexual functioning are addressed.

Postoperative Course

Postoperatively, the patient has a perineal pad in place if a vaginal hysterectomy was done, and a perineal pad and abdominal dressing if an abdominal approach was used. If a radical hysterectomy was done, catheters connected to a closed suction drain, though not recommended, are sometimes used to draw excess fluid from the area of surgery (Orr & Shingleton, 1994). The catheters are inserted below the incision and kept in place until there is only scant drainage, usually for 3 to 5 days.

An intravenous fluid line is maintained until adequate amounts of fluid are taken orally and tolerated well. The patient's diet is then advanced as tolerated. Because abdominal hysterectomy involves movement of the bladder, most women have urethral catheter drainage for 1 to 2 days postoperatively.

The patient is ambulatory in 24 hours and has her abdominal sutures or staples removed on day 5.

If a vaginal hysterectomy is done, and a vaginal pack is used to control bleeding, it is usually removed in 24 to 48 hours. Abdominal cramping may occur occasionally, and there may be no sensation in the vagina for several months. Suture removal is unnecessary because the sutures are typically resorbable.

Hormone replacement therapy is usually prescribed for women after a hysterectomy and bilateral oophorectomy, provided that the woman does not have a carcinoma of the breast, a reproductive system disorder that may be stimulated by it, or other contraindication (eg, a history of thrombophlebitis). When ordered, hormone replacement therapy is primarily a prophylaxis against osteoporosis, with possible protection against future cardiac disease.

Complications

Postoperative complications of a hysterectomy include hemorrhage; hematoma; infection; thrombophlebitis; nerve injury; and pulmonary, bowel, and bladder problems. Complications occur more frequently in women who are elderly or obese or who have a concurrent problem, such as diabetes, emphysema, or a cardiovascular disorder.

Hemorrhage after an abdominal hysterectomy may be abdominal or vaginal. After a vaginal hysterectomy, it may be vaginal or intraperitoneal. It may occur early or late. Hemorrhage that occurs in the immediate 24-hour postoperative period is usually caused by inadequate hemostasis during surgery. This may be slight and self-limited or it may be massive. Vaginal bleeding may be controlled with a vaginal pack or a vaginal suture. If it is not

controlled or if bleeding is abdominal, a laparotomy to ligate the bleeding vessels is required. Such women then are at risk for additional complications, such as disseminated intravascular coagulation.

Late bleeding occurs 10 to 14 days postoperatively and probably results from resorption of sutures. Most often, it is slight vaginal bleeding easily controlled by a vaginal pack. Occasionally, it may be profuse and require surgery to control it.

Urinary complications are retention, infection, and fistula formation. Retention of urine in the bladder is a very common occurrence, particularly after vaginal hysterectomy with an anterior repair (see Chap. 41). It can result from the bladder being temporarily atonic from anesthesia and analgesia, trauma to the bladder's nerve supply, or edema at the junction of the urethra and bladder. When retention occurs, a Foley catheter is inserted for about 5 days. The catheter is then removed, and the patient is catheterized for residual urine after voiding. If there is more than 100 mL of residual urine, the Foley catheter is reinserted and the cycle is begun again. To avoid this problem, a suprapubic tube may be inserted at the time of operation to provide for urinary drainage. The suprapubic tube is clamped after 5 days, and most patients void spontaneously at that time.

Cystitis is also a frequent postoperative complication among patients with indwelling catheters and, therefore, is common after a vaginal hysterectomy and repair. It is treated with antibiotics chosen by urine culture and sensitivity. Occasionally, pyelonephritis occurs, with its high temperature, chills, and flank pain. As with cystitis, antibiotics are prescribed by urine culture and sensitivity. If there is no response to the medication, a pyelogram is done to rule out operative damage to the urinary tract.

Rarely, a fistula may occur as a result of damage to the ureter or bladder. Persons at greatest risk for fistula development are those having a radical hysterectomy (excision of uterus and supporting tissue, adnexa, upper vagina, and pelvic lymph nodes), especially if radiation therapy preceded surgery.

Bowel complications occur almost exclusively after an abdominal hysterectomy, especially when large tumors are involved. Paralytic ileus results from nerve trauma associated with handling the viscera. It is characterized by extreme abdominal distention, nausea, and vomiting. There are no bowel sounds, and there is no crampy colicky pain. Treatment consists of insertion of a nasogastric tube or restriction of food and fluids until bowel sounds are normal, the administration of a bowel stimulant, and enemas.

Mechanical obstruction from the formation of adhesions is a second bowel complication. Symptoms include nausea, vomiting, abdominal distention, crampy colicky pain, and high-pitched bowel sounds. It is treated initially with insertion of a nasogastric tube and intravenous fluids. If improvement does not ensue, a laparotomy is necessary.

■■■■■■▶
■
■ Clinical Pathway for Total Abdominal Hysterectomy

Patient Name _____   Date _____

DRG# _____   Expected LOS 4 _____

	Day 1	Day 2 (PO#1)	Day 3 (PO#2)	Day 4 (PO#3)
Medication	• Prophylactic antibiotics • Endocarditis protocol • IV fluids per anesthesia	• Pain medication (IV, IM, PCA, or epidural) to maintain pain at a tolerable level • Stop IV fluids when PCA discontinued and tolerating PO fluids • Change to IM/PO medication	• PO pain medication	• Continue PO medication at home as needed
Diagnostic Tests	• Hematology panel • Type and screen • HCG if patient is at risk • P4 if on diuretic • ECG, CXR per anesthesia	• Hematology panel in AM		
Diet	• NPO per anesthesia	• Clear liquids • Increase to regular diet as tolerated	• Regular diet with emphasis on balance of food groups • Avoid foods that are constipating	
Activity	• Ad lib preoperatively	• Dangle, then stand at bedside within 6 to 12 hours of return to the floor • Ambulate in hall with assistance tid • May shower	• Ambulate ad lib	
Treatments/ Nursing Actions	• DVT protocol if ordered • Bowel prep or douche per order • Postoperative recovery protocol	• Assess pain level and follow pain management protocol • Assess bowel sounds • Assess dressing q8h • Assess vaginal bleeding q8h • Discontinue Foley and assess for adequate voiding within 6 h • Urinary retention protocol if unable to void adequately • Turn, cough, and deep breathe q2h • Assess need for an incentive spirometer • Assess intake and output • Assess for phlebitis	• Assess bowel sounds • Assess wound q8h • Assess vaginal bleeding • MD to remove dressing 24 to 48 hours after arrival on floor • Wound management and staple removal per MD order • Assess intake and output	
Teaching/ Discharge Planning	• Review plan of care • Teach how to cough and deep breathe • Teach use of an incentive spirometer	• Teach importance of increased activity level • Teach to change vaginal pad every 4 hours and to report excessive bleeding • Support emotional adjustment to loss of uterus	Home care instruction: • Pain medication • List of open pharmacies • Wound care • Return visit • Activity • Diet and fluids • Consider referral to home care nurse if functional status needs assistance	

(continued)

■■■■■■▶
■
■ **Clinical Pathway for Total Abdominal Hysterectomy** *(continued)*

Patient Name _____   Date _____

DRG# _____   Expected LOS 4 _____

	Day 1	**Day 2 (PO#1)**	**Day 3 (PO#2)**	**Day 4 (PO#3)**
Target Goals	Postoperative: • Able to report pain level • Stable vital signs • Clear breath sounds • Moves all extremities • Urine output > 30 mL/h • Dressing dry and intact • Vaginal bleeding is not excessive (<1 saturated pad per 8h)	• Vaginal bleeding diminishes (<1 saturated pad per 8h) • Able to void spontaneously 6 to 8 h after Foley discontinued • Bladder not distended • Pain 0–2 on a 10-point pain scale • Incision intact without redness or drainage • Steady gait with assistance • Lab results WNL or abnormal addressed by MD • No sign of phlebitis • Verbalizes feelings regarding loss of uterus	• Verbalizes DC instructions and plan for follow-up care, information regarding HRT • Free of signs of infection (T <38° C) • Minimal vaginal bleeding • Blood count stable • Able to void q3–4h • Bladder nondistended • Pain 0–2 on 10-point pain scale • Nausea controlled • Diet tolerated • Steady gait unassisted • Normal bowel sounds and status	

Pulmonary complications occur most often in patients who smoke and those with pre-existing respiratory diseases, such as chronic bronchitis, asthma, and emphysema. Usually, these patients are treated for several days preoperatively with prophylactic antibiotics and aerosol treatments. Despite this, pneumonitis and atelectasis from a mucous plug, which must be removed by bronchoscopy, may occur.

Circulatory complications from trauma to the deep veins of the thigh or pelvis include thromboembolism and thrombophlebitis occurring 1 week or more after surgery. Obese, diabetic, or cachectic patients are those most likely to develop thromboembolic complications, and they are sometimes given anticoagulants preoperatively.

Obese and diabetic patients are also most likely to develop an incisional infection after an abdominal hysterectomy. If infection does occur, it is treated with local heat, antibiotics, and drainage of any abscesses that form.

Other potential complications are evisceration, hematoma, and nerve injury. Patients at risk for evisceration are diabetics, the obese, the very thin, and those with respiratory problems or malignant disease treated with radiation. Signs of impending evisceration are low-grade fever and increasing serosanguineous discharge from the incision.

Hematoma is a delayed complication occurring with both abdominal and vaginal procedures. Its incidence is highest in young women with an abundant blood supply to the pelvic organs. The more extensive the surgery, the more likely a hematoma is to occur. Signs of hematoma are increased temperature and decreased hematocrit. Occasionally, a hematoma may be palpated in the lower pelvis.

Injury to the femoral nerve may result from prolonged pressure during the operation. Symptoms are numbness, paresthesia, and weakness of the thigh. This is a transient phenomenon. No medical treatment is usually necessary.

NURSING PROCESS
Hysterectomy

PREOPERATIVE NURSING CARE

Nursing care for the patient scheduled for a hysterectomy is similar to that for any preoperative patient (see Chap. 6), with the following considerations. It is particularly important to assess the patient's understanding of the procedure and its effects and to provide clarification as needed because of the many common misconceptions regarding hysterectomy. Among these misconceptions are that a hysterectomy causes loss of sexual function, loss of attractiveness to men, obesity, hirsutism, premature aging, or senility. It is also a common misconception that removal of the cervix results in a decrease in length of the vagina and a loss of sexual satisfaction.

POSTOPERATIVE NURSING CARE

Assessment

Assess physiologic stabilization by monitoring vital signs and checking for bleeding. Check the patient's vital signs every 15 minutes until stable and then with decreasing frequency as indicated by the patient's condition.

Check the abdominal dressing and perineal pad for bleeding every 15 minutes for 2 hours, every hour for 8 hours, and then every shift. A moderate amount of serosanguineous drainage normally occurs.

Occlusive surgical dressings on the abdomen should be left undisturbed for 48 hours unless contamination occurs. Once changed, assess the wound for redness, edema, and drainage. Note whether the suture line is approximated.

After a hysterectomy, pain in the area of the incision is expected. Assess the severity of the patient's pain, and note to what extent the pain interferes with coughing, deep breathing, and moving.

Assess adequacy of urinary elimination by checking for bladder distention, measuring fluid intake and output, and catheterizing for residual urine. Keep in mind that a decrease in output or low back pain may indicate accidental ligation of a ureter during surgery.

If the patient has an indwelling catheter postoperatively, measure output every 8 hours and check the drainage system for improper position, kinks, or accidental compression by the side rail, which can impede drainage. After removal of the catheter, continue to measure output for 2 or 3 days. Also, palpate the bladder for distention, and, if ordered, catheterize the patient for residual urine. If the residual is more than 100 mL, notify the physician. Patients who do not have an indwelling catheter after surgery should empty the bladder within the first 8 hours postoperatively.

Assess gastrointestinal function because, after a hysterectomy, all patients have decreased peristalsis secondary to the effects of anesthesia, handling of the bowel during surgery, and pain medication. Listen for bowel sounds and observe for abdominal distention, belching, and passage of flatus. Ask the patient about gas pains. Note the size, color, and consistency of bowel movements.

Because thrombophlebitis is a common postoperative complication of hysterectomy, observe for signs and symptoms of developing phlebitis, such as pain, redness, heat in the calf, and a positive Homans' sign.

Because hysterectomy involves loss of a body part and, in the premenopausal woman, loss of the capacity for childbearing, be sure to assess the patient's psychological response to the surgery. Crying spells or transient feelings of sadness or depression are not unusual, but verbalization of negative feelings about the effect of the surgery on her, fear of other people's reactions, and preoccupation with loss of the uterus can indicate a disturbance in self-concept and difficulty coping.

Because of the organs involved, also assess the patient for indications of sexual dysfunction. These include behavior that seeks reassurance of femininity and desirability and a verbal statement of an actual or expected problem with sexual desire, performance, or satisfaction.

Nursing Diagnoses and Planning

Nursing diagnoses and related expected patient outcomes commonly applicable to patients who have had a hysterectomy include the following:

NDx: Pain related to tissue trauma secondary to surgical excision of the uterus

Planning: Patient Outcomes
1. Patient reports that pain is relieved.
2. Nonverbal signs of pain, such as grimacing or guarding, are absent.
3. Patient splints the incision when coughing or moving.
4. Patient gets out of bed, sits, and ambulates without undue discomfort.
5. Patient uses personal methods of coping with pain.
6. Patient performs relaxation exercises.

NDx: Impaired physical mobility related to postoperative abdominal and pelvic discomfort

Planning: Patient Outcomes
1. Patient effectively helps herself sit up and get out of bed when allowed to do so.
2. Patient ambulates in the room when the physician's orders allow.

NDx: Risk for ineffective airway clearance related to shallow respirations and ineffective coughing

Planning: Patient Outcomes
1. Respirations are of normal depth.
2. Secretions are expectorated.
3. Breath sounds are clear.

NDx: Risk for altered peripheral tissue perfusion related to immobility

Planning: Patient Outcomes
1. Calves are free of heat, redness, and swelling.
2. Homans' sign is negative.
3. Symptoms of pulmonary embolism are absent: respirations are of normal rate and depth, and the patient is free of cyanosis, chest pain, and hemoptysis.

NDx: Risk for altered sexuality patterns related to removal of the uterus

Planning: Patient Outcomes
1. Patient describes personal impact of the loss of her uterus.

2. Patient identifies common misconceptions regarding the effect of hysterectomy on libido and sexual enjoyment.
3. Patient discusses sexual concerns with her partner.
4. Patient reports attainment of satisfying sexual functioning.

NDx: Risk for altered health maintenance related to insufficient knowledge of discharge instructions

Planning: Patient Outcomes
1. Patient describes limitations on activity.
2. Patient lists symptoms to be reported.
3. Patient describes possible emotional reactions.
4. Patient states the date and time of the follow-up visit.

Nursing Interventions and Evaluation

NDx: Pain
Administer narcotic analgesic and sedative drugs liberally according to physician's orders during the first 2 postoperative days because pain is most severe during this time. Use patient-controlled analgesia systems if available, or give at scheduled times to prevent anticipatory pain. By the third day, the patient is usually more comfortable, and medications can be decreased in strength and frequency. Use independent nursing measures to relieve pain, such as maintenance of a comfortable environment, position changes, and backrubs throughout the postoperative period because they enhance the effect of analgesics as well as decrease the need for them. Also teach and assist the patient with relaxation exercises.

If the patient's discomfort is primarily from gas in the bowel, apply heat to the abdomen and encourage ambulation and use of a rocking chair. A rectal tube may also be ordered. For discomfort on coughing or moving, premedicate and teach the patient to splint the incision and to use the method of getting up and sitting down as described later.

NDx: Impaired physical mobility
Encourage early ambulation because it promotes circulation, muscle tone, lung expansion, and bowel function. After an uncomplicated hysterectomy, the patient should be ambulatory within 24 hours. A longer period of bedrest is required when the operative procedure is more extensive or when the patient has coexistent health problems.

Instruct the patient in getting out of bed with the least strain and discomfort to facilitate ambulation. Elevate the head of the bed, and instruct her to do the following:

1. Turn on her side, facing the side of the bed she will get out of
2. Bend her knees as if she were sitting in a chair
3. Put her feet over the edge of the bed
4. Push up on her elbow
5. Sit up straight

If the patient complains of perineal discomfort on sitting down, instruct her to pull the buttocks together before lowering herself onto the chair. Gradually encourage her to ambulate in her room and then in the corridor as tolerated.

NDx: Risk for ineffective airway clearance
Medicate the patient as needed for pain, because pain can lead to shallow respirations. Place the patient in semi-Fowler's position or flat with pillows under her shoulders to encourage chest expansion. Keep clothing and bedding loose so that the chest is not constricted. Instruct the patient to cough and deep breathe every 2 hours for at least 24 hours after surgery, and encourage expectoration of any secretions. Encourage use of an incentive spirometer if ordered. If the patient had an abdominal hysterectomy, support the incision by splinting the abdomen with a pillow or folded blanket to facilitate effective coughing and deep breathing.

NDx: Risk for altered peripheral tissue perfusion
Monitor for factors that predispose to venous stasis and hence to thrombus formation. Check to see that there is no undue pressure or obstruction in the popliteal area. Instruct the patient to avoid keeping legs and thighs in a flexed position, because this impedes venous return. Keep the legs extended and uncrossed. To further aid in preventing thrombophlebitis, lower the head of the bed to the flat position every 2 hours until the patient is ambulatory to prevent stasis of blood in the pelvic veins. Elevate the foot of the bed 20 degrees to facilitate venous return. Teach the patient to change position and dorsiflex her feet 20 to 25 times every hour while awake until she is ambulatory. Apply antiembolic or pneumatic compression stockings as ordered to support venous return. If the patient has varicose veins, intermittent elevation of the legs for 2- or 3-hour periods may be ordered to prevent venous stasis.

NDx: Risk for altered sexuality patterns
Review normal sexual function and related structures, and describe the effects of the hysterectomy on them. Identify common misconceptions regarding the effect of a hysterectomy on sexual function and enjoyment, and present the correct facts related to each. Refer to Highlight 40–2 if the woman is started on hormone replacement therapy. Throughout the discussion, encourage the woman to share the meaning of losing her uterus or ovaries or what she has heard or thinks and also to ask any questions that she may have. Encourage the woman to share concerns about future sexual activity with her partner, and provide time and privacy for such discussion. With the woman's permission, offer to answer her partner's questions and provide written educational materials.

NDx: Risk for altered health maintenance
Instruct the woman in self-care after discharge as specified in Highlight 40–8. Also be certain that the

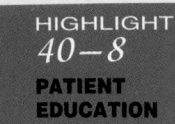
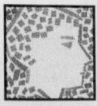

HIGHLIGHT 40-8
PATIENT EDUCATION
Discharge Instructions After Hysterectomy

Instruct the patient to:

Report any bleeding, other vaginal discharge, or temperature elevation to the health care professional.

Avoid tub baths for 2 to 3 weeks.

Avoid activities that increase pelvic congestion for several months. These include sitting for long periods of time, jogging, fast walking, horseback riding, and douching.

Be prepared for feelings of weakness and fatigue.

Avoid strenuous activities such as heavy lifting and vacuum cleaning for 6 to 8 weeks.

Avoid sexual intercourse for 3 weeks after vaginal hysterectomy and for 6 weeks after an abdominal hysterectomy.

Remember that after an abdominal hysterectomy, abdominal soreness and a feeling that the vagina is narrow and short may occur during intercourse for 3 to 4 weeks.

Recognize that periods of emotional lability and feelings of depression and sadness are normal.

Return for a follow-up appointment on *(specify date and time).*

woman knows when to return for her follow-up appointment and the importance of it.

Compare the patient's status with the expected outcomes. If the outcomes are not met, reassess the patient and revise the plan.

VAGINAL PACKING

The vagina may be packed with gauze to provide pressure to control postoperative bleeding or to hold a prolapsed uterus in place within the vagina to decrease edema and aid healing of ulcerated areas before corrective surgery. See Chapter 41 for a discussion of uterine prolapse.

Insertion of a vaginal packing is a sterile procedure that requires good lighting and good exposure of the vagina. The patient empties her bladder and is assisted into a left Sims' or dorsal recumbent position. The vulva is cleansed. If the pack is to control bleeding, a speculum is inserted, and any free blood or clots are swabbed from the vagina. Gauze is then packed firmly into the posterior fornix, the anterior

fornix, and then the remainder of the vagina. If the pack is being used to support a prolapsed uterus, the organ is manually positioned and then the packing is inserted. A T-binder is used to hold the pack in place.

The amount of packing used is recorded in the patient's chart. It is usually removed in 8 to 48 hours.

NURSING PROCESS GUIDELINES
Vaginal Packing

If the purpose of the pack is to control bleeding, inspect the vaginal area to assess continuing blood loss. Monitor voiding for as long as the packing is in place, because the pressure of the packing can impinge on the bladder neck.

The Elderly: Special Considerations

In the geriatric patient, changes initiated at menopause have become marked. The pubic hair is thin and gray or, in some cases, absent. The labia are pale and thin, possibly wrinkled. The ovaries are atrophied and are no longer able to be palpated on pelvic examination. The fallopian tubes, uterus, and vagina have decreased in size. Pelvic support is weak from atrophy of the pelvic fascia and muscles. The vaginal mucosa is thin and the rugae have disappeared, leaving the vagina less elastic. Vaginal secretions are decreased and less acidic.

Although a Pap test may not be deemed necessary for women older than 65 years of age whose previous smears have never showed an abnormality, an annual pelvic examination is needed to ensure early detection of other diseases of the reproductive system that affect the older woman. A small or medium speculum is used for the pelvic examination. Help the patient to get on and off the examining table as needed, and help her to assume the lithotomy position. At the time of examination, the patient is carefully assessed for signs of vaginitis because thinning of the vaginal epithelium and changing pH in the vagina predispose to infection. If appropriate to her lifestyle, determine whether dyspareunia is a problem and recommend the use of a vaginal lubricant to replace normal secretions.

Chapter Review

1. What type of anticipatory guidance should be provided to women during the perimenopausal period?
2. What information is necessary to help a woman decide whether hormone replacement therapy is the best option for her?

3. What are the advantages and disadvantages of the various schedules for hormone replacement therapy?

4. How do the various types of abnormal uterine bleeding differ from one another?

5. What information should be given to a woman before a pelvic examination?

6. What are the major examinations used in the screening and diagnosis of women for reproductive system disorders?

7. What are the advantages and disadvantages of laparoscopy and laser surgery in the treatment of women with reproductive system disorders?

8. What subjective data are essential in planning care for women undergoing surgical intervention for disorders of the reproductive system?

9. What are the key concepts that you would discuss with a patient in preparation for discharge after an abdominal hysterectomy?

10. How might care need to be adapted for a woman from a nondominant culture during an assessment of the reproductive system?

11. What are the most common complaints related to the reproductive system that motivate women to seek health care?

12. How would you prepare a woman for an invasive diagnostic procedure related to the reproductive system?

Bibliography

American Geriatrics Society, Task Force on Older Women's Health. Older women's health. J Am Geriatr Soc 1993; 41:680.

Appleby J. Management of the abnormal Papanicolaou smear. Med Clin North Am 1995; 79(2):345.

Bachmann GA. Sexual function in the perimenopause. Obstet Gynecol Clin North Am 1993; 20(2):379.

Bachmann GA, Ayers CA. Psychosexual gynecology. Med Clin North Am 1995; 79(6):1299.

Bailey C. Education for home-care providers. J Obstet Gynecol Neonatal Nurs 1994; 23(8):714.

Barnhart KT, Freeman EW, Sondheimer SJ. A clinician's guide to the premenstrual syndrome. Med Clin North Am 1995; 79(6):1457.

Berek JS, Adashi EY, Hillard PA: Novack's gynecology. 12th ed. Baltimore: Williams & Wilkins, 1996.

Berek J, Hacker NF. Practical gynecologic oncology. Baltimore: Williams & Wilkins, 1994.

Bernhard LA, Sheppard L. Health, symptoms, self-care, and dyadic adjustment in menopausal women. J Obstet Gynecol Neonatal Nurs 1993; 22(5):456.

Blackledge GRP, Jordan JA, Shingleton HM (eds). Textbook of gynecologic oncology. Philadelphia: WB Saunders, 1991.

Bosarge PM. Hormone therapy: The woman's decision. Contemp Nurse Pract 1995; 1(4)Supplement:3.

Bran DF, Spellman JR, Summit RL. Outpatient vaginal hysterectomy as a new trend in gynecology. AORN J 1995; 62(5):810.

Brocklehurst JC (ed). Textbook of geriatric medicine and gerontology. 4th ed. New York: Churchill Livingstone, 1992.

Bump RC, Gurt WG, Fantl JA, Wyman JF. Assessment of Kegel pelvic muscle exercise performance after brief verbal instruction. Am J Obstet Gynecol 1991; 165(2):322.

Burgel BJ. Occupational health: Nursing in the workplace. Nurs Clin North Am 1994; 29(3):431.

Calle EE, Flanders WD, Thun MJ, Martin LM. Demographic predictors of mammography and Pap smear screening in US women. Am J Public Health 1993; 83(1):53.

Carpenito LJ. Nursing diagnosis: Application to clinical practice. Philadelphia: JB Lippincott, 1995.

Cassey MZ, Savalle-Dunn J. Sketching the future: Trends influencing nursing informatics. J Obstet Gynecol Neonatal Nurs 1994; 23(2):175.

Chikotas N, Dempster J. Secondary amenorrhea. J Am Acad Nurse Pract 1995; 7(9):453.

Christian A. The relationship between women's symptoms of endometriosis and self-esteem. J Obstet Gynecol Neonatal Nurs 1993; 22(4):370.

Cook MJ. Perimenopause: An opportunity for health promotion. J Obstet Gynecol Neonatal Nurs 1993; 22(3):223.

Copeland LJ (ed). Textbook of gynecology. Philadelphia: WB Saunders, 1993.

Covington C, Collins JE. Back to the future of women's health and perinatal nursing in the 21st Century. J Obstet Gynecol Neonatal Nurs 1994; 23(2):183.

Cunningham FG, MacDonald PC, Gant NF, et al. Williams Obstetrics. 19th ed. Norwalk, CT: Appleton & Lange, 1993.

Dickson GL. Fifty-something: A phenomenological study of the experience of menopause. In Munhall PL (ed). In women's experience. New York: National League for Nursing, 1994.

Eliopoulos C. Gerontological nursing. 3rd ed. New York: Harper & Row, 1993.

Freda MC. Childbearing, reproductive control, aging women, and health care: The projected ethical debates. J Obstet Gynecol Neonatal Nurs 1994; 23(2):144.

Freeman SB. Menopause without HRT: Complementary therapies. Contemp Nurse Pract 1995; 1(1):40.

Fromm LM, McCarty T, Dorin M, Harrington DJ. Psychosocial aspects of gynecology. In Copeland LJ (ed). Textbook of gynecology. Philadelphia: WB Saunders, 1993.

Funke BL, Nicholson ME. Factors affecting patient compliance among women with abnormal Pap smears. Patient Educ Counseling 1993; (20):5.

Garry R. Good practice with endometrial ablation. Obstet Gynecol 1995; 86(1):144.

Goldrath MH. Hysteroscopic endometrial ablation. Obstet Gynecol Clin North Am 1995; 22(3):559.

Greendale GA, Judd HL. The menopause: Health implications and clinical management. J Am Geriatr Soc 1993; 41(4):426.

Greer G. The change: Women, aging and menopause. New York: Knopf, 1992.

Gries-Griffin J. Abnormal Pap test results. Adv Nurse Pract 1995; 3(7):16.

Guyton AC. Textbook of medical physiology. 9th ed. Philadelphia: WB Saunders, 1996.

Hammond CB. Women's concerns with hormone replacement therapy: Compliance issues. Fertil Steril 1994; 62(Suppl 2)(6):157S.

Hargrove JT, Eisenberg E. Menopause. Med Clin North Am 1995; 79(6):1337.

Hulka BS. Links between hormone replacement therapy and neoplasia. Fertil Steril 1994; 62(Suppl 2)(6):168S.

Institute of Medicine (US) Committee to review the NIH Women's Health Initiative. An assessment of the NIH Women's Health Initiative. Washington, DC: National Academy Press, 1993.

LeBoeuf FJ, Carter SG. Discomforts of the perimenopause. J Obstet Gynecol Neonatal Nurs 1996; 25(2):173.

Lee KA, Lentz JM, Taylor DL, et al. Fatigues as a response to environmental demands in women's lives. Image: J Nurs Sch 1994; 26(2):149.

Lewis JA, Bernstein J. Women's health: A relational perspective across the life cycle. Boston: Jones and Bartlett Publishers, 1996.

Lightfoot-Klein H. Prisoners of ritual: An odyssey into female genital circumcision in Africa. New York: Harrington Park Press, 1989.

Lobo RA, Speroff L. International consensus conference on post-menopausal hormone therapy and the cardiovascular system. Fertil Steril 1994; 62(Suppl 2)(6):176S.

Lovejoy NC. Precancerous and cancerous cervical lesions: The multicultural "male" risk factor. Oncol Nurs Forum 1994; 21(3):497.

Lowdermilk DL. Home care of the patient with gynecological cancer. J Obstet Gynecol Neonatal Nurs 1995; 24(2):157.

Lynch MA, Ferri RS. Health needs of lesbian women and gay men. Clinician Rev 1996; 7(1):85.

Matteo S (ed). American women in the nineties: Today's critical issues. Boston: Northeastern University Press, 1993.

Mayer DK, Linscott E. Information for women: Management of menopausal symptoms. Oncol Nurs Forum 1995; 22(10):1567.

McCloskey JC, Bulechek GM (eds). Nursing interventions classification (NIC). 2nd ed. St. Louis: Mosby-Year Book, 1996.

McDonald TW. Hysterectomy: Indications, types, and alternatives. In Copeland LJ (ed). Textbook of gynecology. Philadelphia: WB Saunders, 1993.

McKeon VA. Hormone replacement therapy: Evaluating the risks and benefits. J Obstet Gynecol Neonatal Nurs 1994; 23(8):647.

Messing MJ, Gallup DG. Carcinoma of the vulva in young women. Obstet Gynecol 1995; 86(1):51.

Mezrow G. Dysmenorrhea. In Mishell DR, Brenner PF (eds). Management of common problems in obstetrics and gynecology. 3rd ed. Boston: Blackwell Scientific Publications, 1994.

Miller MA. Culture, spirituality, and women's health. J Obstet Gynecol Neonatal Nurs 1995; 24(3):257.

Mishell DR, Brenner PF (eds). Management of common problems in obstetrics and gynecology. 3rd ed. Boston: Blackwell Scientific Publications, 1994.

Munhall PL (ed). In women's experience. New York: National League for Nursing, 1994.

NAACOG, the Organization for Obstetric, Gynecologic, and Neonatal Nursing. NAACOG Standards for the nursing care of women and newborns. 4th ed. Washington, DC: Author, 1991.

Nance TA. Intercultural communication: Finding common ground. J Obstet Gynecol Neonatal Nurs 1995; 24(3):249.

Neufeld KR, Degner LF, Dick JAM. A nursing intervention strategy to foster patient involvement in treatment decisions. Oncol Nurs Forum 1993; 20(4):631.

Newman M, Hudson PO. Solution-oriented therapy techniques for women's health nurses. J Obstet Gynecol Neonatal Nurs 1994; 23(1):15.

Northrup C. Women's bodies, women's wisdom: Creating physical and emotional health and healing. New York: Bantam Books, 1994.

Nugent LS, Clark CR. Colposcopy: Sensory information for client education. J Obstet Gynecol Neonatal Nurs 1996; 25(3):225.

Oestreich S. A closer look at hormone replacement therapy. Adv Nurse Pract 1995; 3(1):10.

Orr JW, Shingleton HM. Complications of gynecologic surgery: Prevention, recognition, and management. Philadelphia: JB Lippincott, 1994.

Pate RR, et al. Physical activity and public health: A recommendation from the Centers for Disease Control and Prevention and the American College of Sports Medicine. JAMA 1995; 273(5):402.

Poorman SG. Human sexuality and the nursing process. Norwalk, CT: Appleton & Lange, 1988.

Prather C, Wolfe A. The nurse's role in office hysteroscopy. J Obstet Gynecol Neonatal Nurs 1995; 24(9):813.

Pullen C, Edwards JB, Lenz CL, Alley N. A comprehensive primary health care delivery model. J Prof Nurs 1994; 10(4):201.

Quillian JP, Dempster JS. Domestic violence. J Am Acad Nurse Pract 1995; 7(7):351.

Ravnikar VA. Diet, exercise, and lifestyle in preparation for menopause. Obstet Gynecol Clin North Am 1993; 20(2):365.

Robinson KD, Kimmel EA, Yasko JM. Reaching out to the African-American community through innovative strategies. Oncol Nurs Forum 1995; 22(9):1383.

Runowicz CD, Goldberg GL, Smith HO. Cancer screening for women older than 40 years of age. Obstet Gynecol Clin North Am 1993; 20(2):391.

Russell DJ. The pelvic mass: Diagnosis and management. Med Clin North Am 1995; 79(6):1481.

Sand G. Is it hot in here or is it me? New York: Harper Collins, 1993.

Sheehy G. Menopause: The silent passage. New York: Simon & Schuster, 1993.

Siegler AM. Office hysteroscopy. Obstet Gynecol Clin North Am 1995; 22(3):457.

Smith MK. Implementing annual cancer screening for elderly women. J Gerontol Nurs 1995; 21(7):12.

Spector RE. Cultural concepts of women's health and health-promoting behaviors. J Obstet Gynecol Neonatal Nurs 1995; 24(3):241.

Speroff L, Glass RH, Kase NG. Clinical gynecologic endocrinology and infertility. 5th ed. Baltimore: Williams & Wilkins, 1994.

Star WL, Lommel LL, Shannon MT (eds). Women's primary health: Protocols for practice. Washington, DC: American Nurses Publishing, 1995.

Taylor D. Perimenopausal symptoms and hormone therapy. In Star WL, Lommel LL, Shannon MT (eds). Women's primary health: Protocols for practice. Washington, DC: American Nurses Publishing, 1995.

Thompson JD, Rock J. The Linde's operative gynecology. 7th ed. Philadelphia: JB Lippincott, 1992.

Tortolero-Luna G, Mitchell MG, Rhodes-Morris HE. Epidemiology and screening of ovarian cancer. Obstet Gynecol Clin North Am 1994; 21(1):1.

U.S. Task Force on Preventive Services. Clinician's handbook of preventive services. Washington, DC: US Dept. of Health and Human Services, 1994.

Warner EA, Parsons AK. Screening and early diagnosis of gynecologic cancers. Med Clin North Am 1996; 80(1):45.

Wathen PI, Henderson MC, Witz CA. Abnormal uterine bleeding. Med Clin North Am 1995; 79(2):329.

Wear D, Nixon LL. Literary anatomies: Women's bodies and health in literature. Albany, NY: State University of New York, 1994.

Webb TS. Evaluation and management of amenorrhea. Adv Nurse Pract 1995; 3(6):28.

White JE, Begg L, Fishman NW, et al. Increasing cervical cancer screening among minority elderly. J Gerontol Nurs 1993; 19(5):28.

Wilcox LS, Mosher WD. Factors associated with obtaining health screening among women of reproductive age. Public Health Rep 1993; 108(1):76.

Williamson ML. Sexual adjustment after hysterectomy. J Obstet Gynecol Neonatal Nurs 1992; 21(1):42.

Willson JR. Obstetrics and gynecology. 9th ed. St. Louis: CV Mosby, 1991.

Womeodu RJ, Bailey JE. Barriers to cancer screening. Med Clin North Am 1996; 80(1):115.

Wood SH, Ransom VJ. The 1990s: A decade for change in women's health care policy. J Obstet Gynecol Neonatal Nurs 1994; 23(2):139.

World Health Organization. Research on the menopause (Technical Report, Series 670). Geneva, Switzerland: Author, 1981.

Youngkin EQ. Estrogen replacement therapy and the estraderm transdermal system. Nurse Pract 1990; 15(5):19.

Youngkin EQ, Davis MS. Women's health: A primary care clinical guide. Norwalk, CT: Appleton & Lange, 1994.

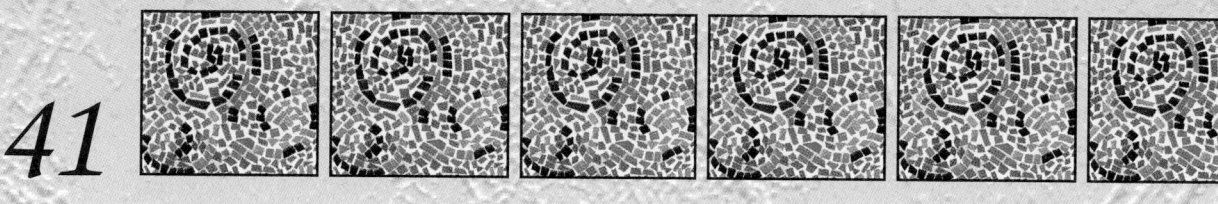

41

Nursing Care of Women with Reproductive Disorders

Study Outcomes

After studying this chapter, you should be able to:

1. Describe the etiology, pathophysiology, clinical manifestations, diagnostic procedures, and management of common disorders of the female reproductive system.
2. Identify information and physical examination data essential to the assessment of women with common reproductive system disorders.
3. State nursing diagnoses and related expected patient outcomes commonly applicable to women with reproductive system disorders.
4. Describe nursing interventions, with their rationales, commonly applicable to women with reproductive system disorders.
5. Explain the basis for evaluation of nursing care provided to women with common reproductive system disorders.
6. Identify alternative treatment and care settings for women with reproductive disorders and the services related to community-based care.
7. Identify special considerations for the elderly woman with a reproductive system disorder.

The female reproductive system can be affected by a wide variety of disorders, including inflammations, infections, functional and structural abnormalities, and neoplastic processes. Most of these disorders are not life-threatening but, nonetheless, can have a profound effect on physical comfort, self-esteem, and the capacity for sexually satisfying relationships.

Care for women's health concerns is offered along a continuum of settings, including community-based health promotion services, outpatient treatment of medical-surgical disorders, inpatient acute-care support following major surgical interventions, home care follow-up for recuperation, and hospice services for palliative care. Nurses work collaboratively to identify the most appropriate setting for women to achieve positive health outcomes.

The consumer movement offers new opportunities for women to consider themselves partners with the health-care team in meeting their needs for information to maintain optimum health, especially as it relates to the reproductive system. Coordination between settings is especially important for conditions that require frequent monitoring, lifestyle adjustments, or both.

Infections and Inflammations

VULVITIS

Etiology and Pathophysiology

Vulvitis, or inflammation of the vulva, may be a manifestation of a systemic disease, an extension of vaginitis, or a local disorder. The skin of the vulva is subject to all the inflammatory disorders that can affect any other skin area. However, it is particularly prone to inflammation from mechanical or chemical irritation because of its anatomical location. Many factors are potential sources of irritation, including:

- Tight-fitting clothing
- Exposure to urine, fecal matter, vaginal discharges, and secretions of vulvar glands
- Exposure to external irritants, such as bath and laundry soap, feminine hygiene sprays and powders, spermicides, and vaginal lubricants containing propylene glycol

Clinical Manifestations

Pruritus is the classic symptom of vulvitis. In addition, there is usually a burning sensation that worsens with urination or defecation. The vulvar tissues appear red and swollen. If the patient has scratched in trying to relieve the itch, abrasions and areas of secondary infection may be present. If the vulvitis is an extension of a vaginitis, a vaginal discharge may be present.

Diagnosis

A detailed history focusing on medical risk factors, personal hygiene, and psychogenic factors is obtained to identify potential causal factors. A complete physical evaluation is done to check for any systemic disorder, such as diabetes, that may be the cause of the vulvitis. A pelvic examination is done, and vaginal smears or cultures are obtained to determine whether a source of infection is present in the vagina.

Management

Medical management depends on the cause of the vulvitis. Along with topical and/or systemic therapy for the underlying problem (when one is identified), local measures are prescribed to relieve symptoms. Most cases can be managed in an outpatient setting.

NURSING PROCESS
Vulvitis

Assessment

The assessment of a patient with vulvitis includes the history and current status of her symptoms. It also includes a review of medical risk factors, stress-related factors, and personal habits that can potentially contribute to the inflammatory process. And it includes an inspection of the area.

Obtain information about the patient's symptoms, including local and systemic symptoms experienced, their duration, factors that can be related to their onset or exacerbation, relief measures used, and the effectiveness of these measures. Explore the patient's patterns of sexual activity. Ask about perineal hygiene and use of perfumed soaps, powders, or other cosmetic products that may irritate tissues or cause an allergic reaction. Ask about the type of undergarments usually worn. Determine the patient's perception of the cause and significance of the problem, and use it later as a guide in planning health teaching.

Inspect the vulvar area for irritation, scratch marks, such parasites as *Phthirus pubis* (pubic lice or "crabs"), and discharge.

Nursing Diagnoses and Planning

Nursing diagnoses and related expected patient outcomes commonly applicable to patients with vulvitis include the following:

NDx: Pain related to pruritus

Planning: Patient Outcomes
1. Patient reports that pruritus is relieved.
2. Vulvar tissue is free of erythema and edema.

NDx: Risk for altered health maintenance related to insufficient knowledge of measures to aid in preventing recurrence of vulvitis

Planning: Patient Outcomes
1. Patient lists materials and types of clothing that predispose to inflammation of the vulva.
2. Patient lists types of cleansing and hygienic products that can cause an allergic reaction.
3. Patient describes proper techniques of cleansing the vulva, explaining how each helps to prevent vulvitis.

4. Patient describes proper technique for self-examination of the vulva.

Nursing Interventions and Evaluation

NDx: Pain
Assist or instruct the patient in the use of comfort measures, such as sitz baths, cool or warm compresses possibly with Burow's solution (dilute solution of aluminum acetate and acetic acid), topical steroid ointments or creams, and oral antihistamines for severe pruritus.

NDx: Risk for altered health maintenance
Instruct the patient as specified in Highlight 41–1 to help her avoid recurrence of the vulvitis.

Compare the patient's status with the expected outcomes. If the outcomes are not met, reassess the patient and revise the plan.

VAGINITIS

Vaginitis is an inflammation of the vagina. It is a common, often recurrent, gynecologic disorder that in most cases is not serious but is very uncomfortable and annoying.

Etiology and Pathophysiology
Vaginitis results from mechanical irritation of the vagina, as from:

- Tampons, sexual intercourse, or a pessary (device inserted in the vagina to support the uterus)
- Chemical irritation, as from douche solutions, contraceptive creams, soaps, or vaginal deodorants
- Fecal contamination
- Infestation with parasites, such as pinworms
- An infectious process caused by sexually transmitted organisms

Infections of the vagina are also caused by nonsexually transmitted organisms, such as *Streptococcus*, *Staphylococcus*, and *Escherichia coli*.

Factors that predispose to the development of vaginitis are those that cause an overall decrease in body defenses and those that specifically alter the vaginal defenses. They include malnutrition, stress, systemic disease (such as diabetes or immune disorders), broad-spectrum antibiotic therapy, pregnancy, postmenopausal thinning of the vaginal epithelium, allergies, oral contraceptives, contraceptive sponges, excessive douching, tampons, inadequate personal hygiene, tight-fitting undergarments, and excessive sucrose and lactose in the diet. Sexual activity without the use of condoms and sexual activity with multiple sexual partners also predispose to vaginitis by increasing the risk of exposure to causative organisms.

Clinical Manifestations
Leukorrhea is the most common symptom of vaginitis, regardless of cause. The amount, color, consist-

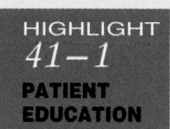 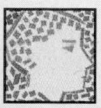

HIGHLIGHT 41–1
PATIENT EDUCATION

Preventing Vulvitis

Teach the patient about the following:

Cleaning the Vulva

Do not use soap between the labia: Odors are on the pubic hair, not on the skin, and rinsing is sufficient to remove secretions.

Rinse the vulva thoroughly after washing because soap residue supports bacterial growth and is irritating to the skin. Be particularly careful to rinse and dry the vulvar area completely when taking a shower.

Keeping the Vulva Dry

Moisture can cause maceration of the skin and is conducive to bacterial growth. Frequently change perineal pads used during menstruation or used because of stress incontinence or a vaginal discharge.

Select clothing that allows for adequate air circulation.

- Avoid tight-fitting pantyhose, pantsuits, and slacks.
- Wear 100% cotton underpants or, as a second choice, those with a cotton crotch.
- Do not wear underpants to bed.
- Wear knee-high or thigh-high stockings whenever possible.

- Wear pantyhose with a cotton crotch, and never wear them under slacks.

Protecting the Vulva from Irritation

Do not scratch the vulvar area.

Avoid clothing that rubs against the area.

Do not wear synthetic fibers and colored fabrics in direct contact with the vulva because they retain warmth and moisture and may cause an allergic reaction.

Avoid strong and excessive amounts of laundry soaps, fabric softeners, talcum powder, perfumed soaps, scented or colored toilet paper, and deodorant sprays, which can also cause allergic reactions that produce itching, rashes, and irritation.

Presoak underpants in one-half strength bleach for 20 minutes and then wash on a hot laundry cycle or boil underpants for 20 minutes and then launder as usual to kill yeast that may be harbored in the garments (Kaufman, 1994).

Use cornstarch if needed to keep the area dry and prevent irritation of adjacent skin surfaces.

---

ency, and odor of the discharge vary with the specific causative agent (Table 41–1). Vulvar pruritus and burning are also associated with most cases of vaginitis.

Diagnosis
A pelvic examination is done to inspect the vaginal mucosa and rule out the presence of a foreign body. With vaginitis, the mucosa generally appears erythematous and congested. A vaginal smear or culture is taken to identify a specific infective organism. A clean-catch urinalysis may be necessary to distinguish between cystitis or urethritis and vaginitis.

Management
If the vaginitis is from a foreign body or chemical irritant, the basic treatment is to remove or eliminate the offending agent. If an infectious process is involved, anti-infectives specific to the causative agent are administered. Heat in the form of sitz baths, soaks, or perineal irrigations may be used to increase circulation and promote comfort and healing. Tea (regular, not herbal) baths are particularly soothing. These baths, whose active ingredient is

Table 41–1

Characteristics of Vaginal Discharge Associated with Different Types of Vaginitis

Cause of Vaginitis	Characteristic Discharge
Mechanical irritation (such as from wearing tampons or a pessary)	Serosanguineous or purulent Possible foul odor
Chemical irritation (such as from douche solutions, feminine hygiene products, or contraceptive sponges)	Moderate to copious With or without odor White, gray, or yellow
Infectious process	
Gardnerella vaginalis	Greater than normal amount Gray-white with fishy odor
Candida albicans	Scant white Cottage cheese–like
Trichomonas vaginalis	Copious Sometimes frothy Yellow-green

tannic acid, are prepared using two to three tea bags per bath.

❖ SETTINGS, PROVIDERS, AND COLLABORATION FOR CARE

Prevention, detection, and treatment of most gynecologic infections in women of reproductive age can be accomplished by advanced practice nurses. These nurses work in office partnerships with family practice physicians and specialists in obstetrics and gynecology. They are also employed as staff in both public and private women's clinics.

NURSING PROCESS
Vaginitis
Assessment

Collect information about the symptoms experienced, their duration, comfort measures used, and the effectiveness of these measures. Ask about any use of over-the-counter medications for vaginal infections. Determine the color, consistency, amount, and odor of vaginal discharge. Also determine whether this is an isolated episode of vaginitis or a recurrence. Identify factors contributing to development of the problem, as well as possible routes of spread, by obtaining information about hygiene and sexual practices, including the time of the last sexual contact, method of birth control used, duration of relationship with the sexual partner, and whether safer sex is practiced (eg, find out whether a condom was used, and if the patient is in a monogamous relationship).

Explore the patient's understanding of normal vaginal defenses and the development and spread of infection. Assess the impact of the infection on the patient's self-esteem and sexual relationships.

Nursing Diagnoses and Planning

Nursing diagnoses and related expected patient outcomes commonly applicable to patients with vaginitis include the following:

NDx: Pain related to pruritus and inflammation

Planning: Patient Outcomes
1. Patient states that itching and burning have decreased.
2. Patient reports voiding without discomfort.

NDx: Risk for altered health maintenance related to insufficient knowledge of prevention of spread and recurrence of vaginitis, normal variations in vaginal secretions

Planning: Patient Outcomes
1. Patient describes personal hygienic habits that decrease the risk of vaginitis.
2. Patient verbalizes need for abstinence or her

partner's use of a condom until the infection has cleared, and partner's need for concurrent treatment.
3. Patient describes normal variations in vaginal discharge.

Nursing Interventions and Evaluation
NDx: Pain
Prepare the patient for discomfort that may occur during the pelvic examination as a result of inflamed vaginal tissues, even though a small speculum is used. Tell her that a small amount of bleeding may occur after the examination. Provide a perineal pad. If a clean-catch urine specimen is needed, give clear, detailed instructions. A urine specimen that has contacted the vulva can lead to misdiagnosis of cystitis or urethritis.

Explain the use of prescribed drugs and other therapeutic measures. Demonstrate the use of vaginal applicators and the correct insertion of vaginal creams or suppositories.

If douches are ordered, review the procedure with the patient and instruct her to douche before inserting vaginal medication, not after. Emphasize that she is not to douche during menses. Stress the importance of not scratching the vulvovaginal area, because this can lead to secondary infection.

NDx: Risk for altered health maintenance
Instruct the patient as specified in Highlight 41–2 to help her prevent spread of infection to her sexual partner, prevent recurrence of the problem, and understand normal variations in vaginal discharge so that the need for further treatment can be more easily identified.

Compare the patient's status with the expected outcomes. If the outcomes are not met, reassess the patient and revise the plan.

ATROPHIC VAGINITIS

Atrophic vaginitis, a disorder affecting postmenopausal women, is a superficial inflammation of the thin, vaginal epithelium.

Etiology and Pathophysiology
As estrogen levels drop after menopause, the vaginal epithelium becomes thin, the number of lactobacilli in the vagina decreases, and vaginal pH increases. These changes make the vagina more susceptible to irritation and invasion by aerobic gram-positive or gram-negative organisms.

Clinical Manifestations
Atrophic vaginitis produces a thin, watery, usually yellow, slight to moderate vaginal discharge. The patient has a burning sensation in the vaginal area. Sexual intercourse is painful. Itching and foul odor do not occur.

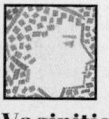

HIGHLIGHT
41–2
PATIENT EDUCATION   **Vaginitis**

Teach the patient about the following:

Prevention of Spread

Abstain from intercourse until the infection resolves. If abstinence is not feasible, have partner use a condom. Encourage partner to obtain concurrent treatment if needed.

Personal Hygiene Measures to Decrease Risk of Recurrence

Wipe the perineal area from front to back to avoid spreading organisms from the anal area to the vaginal and urethral area.

Void before and after intercourse to flush bacteria from the urethrovaginal area.

Avoid douches unless medically ordered, because douches can change the pH of the vagina and encourage the growth of pathogens.

Avoid use of tampons or use them intermittently with pads.

Normal Variations in Vaginal Discharge

The normal amount of vaginal discharge is 1 to 3 tsp.

Vaginal discharge is milky just before and after the menses and becomes thick mucus at ovulation.

Diagnosis

The diagnosis is based on the patient's history, the appearance of the vaginal epithelium, and such diagnostic tests as Papanicolaou (Pap) smears, culture, and vaginal microscopic examination. The vaginal epithelium is diffusely red, and superficial hemorrhagic areas may be seen. This is in stark contrast to the normal pallor of the atrophic epithelium found in the postmenopausal patient.

Management

Estrogen administered two to three times weekly in the form of vaginal cream or suppository thickens the vaginal epithelium and provides prompt relief. To prevent recurrence, estrogen therapy must be continued. Systemic therapy may be substituted in an attempt to have the long-term benefits of more reliable serum levels.

Warm douches of a weak acid solution, such as 15 mL ($\frac{1}{2}$ oz) of acetic acid (vinegar) to 1 L of water cleanse the vagina, lower its pH, and exert a soothing effect on the inflamed tissues.

NURSING PROCESS GUIDELINES
Atrophic Vaginitis

Nursing care is planned to enable the patient to carry out self-care activities effective in providing relief from symptoms and preventing a recurrence.

Instruct the patient on the use of vinegar douches and instillation of the estrogen preparation, if ordered. If the use of the applicator is painful, suggest use of a water-based product, such as K-Y jelly, for lubrication or application of the cream with a finger until the soreness lessens. If estrogen therapy is not prescribed, the patient may use other water-soluble lubricants during intercourse. Instruct the patient about the need for careful hand-washing before and after vaginal treatments.

TOXIC SHOCK SYNDROME

Etiology and Pathophysiology

Toxic shock syndrome is a rare but acute illness caused by one or more toxins produced by the bacterium *Staphylococcus aureus*. Although it can occur after any staphylococcal infection, its incidence is greatest among young, menstruating women who are using tampons, particularly the superabsorbent, rayon type. The tampons, which can hold a large amount of menstrual blood and are left in place for an extended length of time, provide an excellent environment for staphylococcus multiplication. The organisms are then believed to enter the blood stream through lesions in the vaginal mucosa. The Centers for Disease Control and Prevention has developed a case definition of toxic shock syndrome and currently tracks its incidence.

Clinical Manifestations

Toxic shock syndrome usually begins with the sudden onset of a fever of 38.9°C (102°F) or higher accompanied by headache, vomiting, diarrhea, muscle aches, weakness, and fatigue. Shock ensues, and signs of impaired cardiopulmonary, hepatic, and renal function are evident. The patient becomes hypotensive, and respiratory distress from pulmonary edema may develop. Bilirubin and creatine kinase levels rise. Urinary output decreases, blood urea nitrogen level increases, and the patient becomes disoriented. Mucous membranes and conjunctivae may become hyperemic, and an erythematous macular skin eruption may develop. This rash, which may appear first on the body or on the palms of the hands, fingers, soles of the feet, and toes, desquamates in 7 to 10 days.

Complications of toxic shock syndrome include disseminated intravascular coagulation, acute tubular necrosis, and pulmonary edema.

Diagnosis

The diagnosis of toxic shock syndrome is suggested by the rapid onset of characteristic symptoms in otherwise healthy, menstruating females. The presence of skin desquamation and five of the clinical findings confirms the diagnosis. Blood cultures may show the presence of *S. aureus*.

Management

Initial care for a woman with toxic shock syndrome usually takes place in an intensive care unit, so that frequent multisystem assessment and support is available. If a localized source of infection (such as a tampon) is identified, it is removed. Antibiotic therapy for *S. aureus* is given. Life support interventions to counteract the massive vascular response may be necessary. Intubation and ventilation may be required to maintain adequate respiration. Careful monitoring of neurological and renal function are also instituted.

NURSING PROCESS GUIDELINES
Toxic Shock Syndrome

Nursing care varies with the specific effects of the disease. Interventions may include shock management, neurological monitoring, ventilation assistance, parenteral medication administration, and invasive hemodynamic monitoring. As the patient recovers, health teaching is provided as needed (Highlight 41–3). See Chapter 11 for an in-depth discussion of shock management.

*F*unctional Disorders

PREMENSTRUAL SYNDROME

Premenstrual syndrome is a cyclic phenomenon characterized by an individualized yet basically consistent pattern of symptoms that occur between ovulation and menses, and regress or disappear during menstruation.

Premenstrual syndrome affects women of all races, cultures, and socioeconomic levels. Its incidence increases with age and parity. The onset of premenstrual syndrome frequently follows puberty, pregnancy, periods of amenorrhea from oral contraceptives or excessive weight loss, tubal ligation, ovarian surgery, or hysterectomy. Premenstrual syndrome is also more common among women who have had spontaneous abortions (miscarriages), toxemia, postpartum depression, or an adverse reaction to oral contraceptives.

Etiology and Pathophysiology

The cause of premenstrual syndrome is unknown, although many theories have been set forth and are

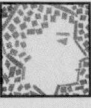

HIGHLIGHT 41–3 PATIENT EDUCATION

Preventing Toxic Shock Syndrome

Instruct the patient to:

Wash hands thoroughly before handling tampons.

Use regular or slender tampons instead of super-absorbent tampons, because the superabsorbent type predispose to development of toxic shock syndrome.

Change tampons after bowel movements.

Change tampons every 1 to 4 hours.

Use a pad, not a tampon, at night.

Insert and remove tampons carefully to avoid abrasions to the vaginal mucosa, which can serve as entry points for pathogenic bacteria. Use a water-based product such as K-Y Jelly for lubrication if needed. Avoid tampons with rough edges because they can damage the lining of the vagina.

Use pads rather than tampons if you have a history of toxic shock syndrome.

currently under study. Suggested causes include estrogen-progesterone imbalance, in which estrogen is in relative excess compared with progesterone, altered serotonin levels, prostaglandin interactions, and individual responses to stress (Barnhart et al, 1995).

Stress and the associated endocrine changes may also play a factor in the psychophysiologic responses of women during the premenstrual phase (Star et al, 1995).

Clinical Manifestations

The symptoms of premenstrual syndrome are nonspecific and vary from person to person. Symptoms that occur as part of premenstrual syndrome are presented in Table 41–2.

Symptoms, which can occur for 1 to 2 days or for 2 weeks, disappear or regress with the onset of menstruation and can vary in severity from month to month.

Diagnosis

The diagnosis of premenstrual syndrome is based on the timing and cyclic nature of the patient's symptoms. The symptoms must occur in the premenstrual period during consecutive cycles and disappear with the onset of the menstrual flow. For this to be evaluated, a record is needed of symptoms experienced

Table 41–2

Clinical Manifestations of Premenstrual Syndrome

PHYSICAL SYMPTOMS

Gastrointestinal	Nausea, abdominal bloating, abdominal cramping, anorexia, bulimia, cravings, exacerbation of hemorrhoids
Reproductive	Breast swelling, tenderness, pain; change in sex drive (may be either increased or decreased to absent)
	(Note: Patients with premenstrual syndrome generally do not have dysmenorrhea; they do ovulate and are able to conceive and carry a fetus to term)
Urologic	Frequency of urination, dysuria
Neurologic	Sensitivity to noise, touch, smell; lack of coordination, slurred speech, visual difficulties such as difficulty focusing, tearing, or dry eyes; fainting; dizziness; headaches; numbness and tingling in hands; insomnia; seizures
Dermatologic	Acne, hives, styes, rashes
Respiratory	Asthma
Cardiovascular	"Pounding of the heart," cardiac dysrhythmias
Musculoskeletal	Back pain, joint pain, muscle ache, stiff neck
Systemic	Fatigue, lethargy, weight gain, infections
EMOTIONAL SYMPTOMS	Anger, anxiety, crying, irritability, feelings of depression, poor self-concept, tension, paranoia, violence, suicidal thoughts, withdrawal

Acute symptoms such as headaches, panic attacks, seizures, and depression often occur after long periods (5 waking hours or 13 sleeping hours) without eating.

and their time of occurrence in relationship to the menstrual cycle. This type of record is called a menstrual log, calendar, or chart and is kept by the patient on a daily basis for 1 to 4 months.

The diagnosis is made after thorough history, physical examination, and relevant diagnostic tests have ruled out any other medical or psychiatric disorder, such as thyroid dysfunction or depression.

Management

Medical management is basically symptomatic because the cause of premenstrual syndrome is unclear. Medications with the best evidence of controlling the most distressing symptoms include antidepressants (particularly serotonin uptake inhibitors), anxiolytics, and ovulation suppressors. A medical oophorectomy using a gonadotropin-releasing hormone agonist has also shown some effectiveness in relieving severe symptoms (Barnhart et al, 1995). Some clinicians have tried diuretics, prostaglandin inhibitors, oral contraceptives, antifungal therapy, and vitamin therapy, though none of these therapies are approved for such use. Hormone therapy in the form of progesterone has also been used but is not currently approved by the Food and Drug Administration (Star et al, 1995).

Stress reduction, aerobic exercises that increase beta-endorphin levels, and the dietary changes described in Highlight 41–4 are usually recommended before medications are prescribed, because most medications have not proved to be effective and may be associated with adverse effects.

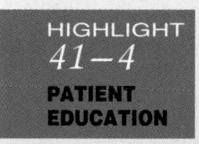 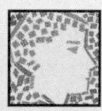

HIGHLIGHT 41–4

PATIENT EDUCATION

Relieving Premenstrual Syndrome

Instruct the patient to:

Obtain adequate sleep and take naps as needed. Fatigue magnifies the symptoms of premenstrual syndrome.

Use relaxation techniques to induce sleep if needed.

Get regular physical exercise. Exercise induces sleep and decreases premenstrual stress.

Eat a well-balanced diet.

Eat six small meals each day to maintain a consistent blood sugar level.

Avoid strict dieting for 7 to 10 days before menstruation.

If a vitamin or mineral supplement is needed, take moderate doses. Avoid megadoses, which can be harmful.

Use a log to track and evaluate the effect of prescribed medication on individual symptom patterns.

NURSING PROCESS
Premenstrual Syndrome

Assessment

Assess the status of the patient's symptoms. What are they? When do they occur in relationship to the menstrual cycle? This information is best obtained by use of a menstrual log. Explain the need for the log, help the patient design a log suited to her needs, and teach her to fill it out. Figure 41–1 depicts types of logs used by different patients.

Determine what measures the patient has used to try to obtain relief and the effect of each. Also determine the patient's lifestyle, including patterns of exercise and nutrition, stressful factors, coping methods, and interpersonal relationships and support systems, because PMS impacts on all areas of the patient's life and is affected by so many factors.

Nursing Diagnoses and Planning

Nursing diagnoses and related expected patient outcomes commonly applicable to patients with premenstrual syndrome include the following:

NDx: Risk for ineffective individual coping related to a cyclic disease with highly variable symptoms and no single cure

Planning: Patient Outcomes
1. Patient identifies the disease as real and describes it in general terms.
2. Patient demonstrates from her menstrual log what her symptom pattern is and how it fits the criteria for premenstrual syndrome.
3. Patient describes role of stress in precipitating or aggravating symptoms of premenstrual syndrome.
4. Patient identifies sources of stress in her daily life and appropriate ways to manage them.
5. Family members or significant others state willingness to support the patient and participate in health-teaching program.

NDx: Risk for altered health maintenance related to insufficient knowledge of effective self-care measures and prescribed medications

Planning: Patient Outcomes
1. Patient states the need for adequate rest and exercise, and the rationale for it.
2. Patient plans a daily diet incorporating recommended diet modifications.
3. Patient identifies common misconceptions regarding effective treatment measures that may be suggested.
4. Patient states the name of prescribed medications, expected effects, and the dose, route, and frequency of administration.
5. Patient describes adverse reactions that should be reported to the health professional.

Nursing Interventions and Evaluation

NDx: Risk for ineffective individual coping
Provide health teaching about the disease process to the patient, emphasizing that the symptoms are not imagined and that her symptom pattern may differ from others with the same disorder. Encourage faithful use of the symptom log for at least two cycles to help identify individual patterns and responses. Use the patient's menstrual log to clarify its cyclic nature.

Explain the importance of avoiding stress during the premenstrual interval when symptoms are present. Assist the patient with anxiety reduction. Help her identify sources of stress in her life and appropriate methods of stress management, such as autogenic training, calming techniques, and simple relaxation therapy. Explore with the patient the feasibility of planning known stressful activities at a time when she is symptom free.

Facilitate support system enhancement to bolster the patient's coping ability. Include significant others in health teaching. Suggest participation in premenstrual syndrome support groups, and tell the patient how to contact one in her geographic area.

NDx: Risk for altered health maintenance
Instruct the patient as specified in Highlights 41–4 and 41–5 to help her make changes in lifestyle and diet to decrease the impact of premenstrual syndrome. If indicated, teach the patient about prescribed medications. Describe their expected effects, method of administration, and adverse reactions to be reported. Encourage the patient to continue self-monitoring her symptoms during therapy to evaluate its effectiveness.

Compare the patient's status with the expected outcomes. If the outcomes are not met, reassess the patient and revise the plan.

ENDOMETRIOSIS

Endometriosis is a condition in which tissue similar to the endometrium of the uterus occurs in other locations, outside the uterus. The most common of these ectopic locations are the ovary and the cul-de-sac of Douglas, although the pelvic ligaments, pelvic peritoneum, vulvar perineum, ureters, bladder, or cecum may also be involved (Fig. 41–2). The disease, which seems to be increasing in incidence, occurs primarily among 30- to 40-year-old nulliparous women of upper socioeconomic classes. A familial tendency has been reported, principally in sisters but also between mothers and daughters. Endometriosis is rare among African-American women, women who give birth at a young age, and women who have had many children.

Etiology and Pathophysiology
The cause of endometriosis is not known, although

Day of Month	Jan	Feb	Mar	Apr	May	June	July	Aug	Sept	Oct	Nov	Dec
1												
2												
3												

A

Symptom being charted: _____   Rating Scale: Mild=1

Moderate=2

Severe=3

Day of Month	Jan	Feb	Mar	Apr	May	June	July	Aug	Sept	Oct	Nov	Dec
1												
2												
3												

B

Symptoms ⟶

Month and Day	Insomnia	Bloating	Nausea	Headache	Irritability	Menstruation
11/1						
11/2						
11/3						

C

Figure 41–1

Examples of menstrual logs. For all charts, the patient writes "M" in the blocks for the dates that menses occurs. *A*, Basic chart used to show relationship of symptoms to the menstrual cycle. Each day the patient records symptoms experienced in the block for that date. *B*, Type of chart used when the severity of a given symptom is being charted over a cycle. Where indicated at the top of the form, the patient fills in the name of the symptom being charted. Each day the patient rates her experience of the symptom (see rating scale at top of form) and writes the rating score in the block corresponding to that date. This is particularly useful when it is not clear that a symptom occurs only premenstrually. *C*, This type of chart is used when the patient has many symptoms and it is difficult to distinguish which are related to the menstrual cycle. Each day the patient places a check mark in the box corresponding to the date and the symptoms experienced. This type of chart can also be used to rate the severity of each symptom by substituting a rating score, as in Chart B, for the check mark. Note: If the time of ovulation is not known, as with long or irregular cycles or after a hysterectomy, the patient keeps a chart of basal body temperature as well as of symptoms. (Adapted from *Self-Help for Premenstrual Syndrome* by Dr. Michelle Harrison. Copyright © 1982, 1985 by Michelle Harrison. Adapted by permission of Random House, Inc.)

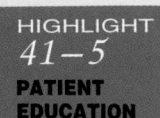
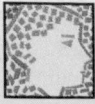

HIGHLIGHT
41–5

PATIENT EDUCATION

Special Considerations for Patients with Premenstrual Syndrome

Instruct the patient with PMS to do the following:

Eat small amounts of fruits, vegetables, and foods high in protein and complex carbohydrates frequently, to prevent hypoglycemia and decrease cravings for sweets.

Include in the daily diet foods high in vitamin B_6 and magnesium, such as leafy green vegetables, legumes, whole grains, and cereals.

Avoid alcohol, caffeine, artificial sweeteners, and tobacco, which can contribute to anxiety, irritability, and insomnia.

Avoid excessive sodium for 7 to 9 days before menstruation to decrease fluid retention, which

causes breast tenderness, bloating, and weight gain. (This means that foods high in sodium as well as hidden sources of sodium, such as some frozen food preservatives and water passing through a water-softening system, must be identified.)

Include in the daily diet 1 tbsp or more of a food high in linoleic acid and vitamin E, such as corn oil or safflower oil.

Drink 8 to 10 glasses of water daily.

Avoid megadoses of vitamins because they have toxic effects and no known advantage over a well-balanced diet.

there are many theories. The most prominent suggests that endometriosis results from small bits of uterine endometrial tissue being propelled upward through the fallopian tubes into the pelvic cavity rather than downward through the cervix and vagina during menstruation. Another theory is that primitive cells, present in the abdominal cavity from the time of fetal development, mature into endometrial cells under the hormonal changes of puberty. A

third is that endometrial cells from the uterus are carried by the blood or lymph to secondary sites.

The condition presents in the affected areas as multiple cystic nodules lined with ectopic endometrial tissue. This tissue undergoes proliferative and secretory changes in response to estrogen and progesterone just as the uterine endometrium does. When the menses begins, in response to decreased circulating levels of these hormones, the ectopic tis-

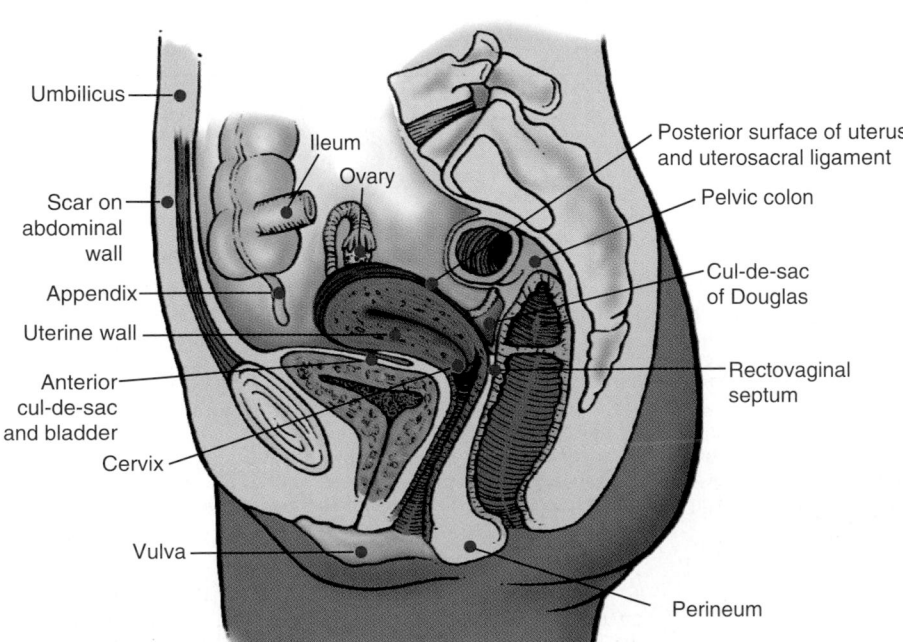

Figure 41–2

Common locations for endometriosis.

sue also sloughs and bleeds. This bleeding gives the lesions their brown or blue-black color. It also causes an inflammatory reaction, which eventually results in the formation of adhesions. These adhesions may be so extensive that the pelvic organs become fused together and immobile.

When endometrial cysts occur on the ovary, they are often referred to as "chocolate" cysts because of their color and the brown fluid found within them.

Because the ectopic tissue is hormone dependent, the disease is active as long as the ovaries are functioning. Remissions usually occur during pregnancy and with the onset of menopause.

Clinical Manifestations

There is no specific pattern of symptoms characteristic of endometriosis. Symptoms vary with the location of the endometrial tissue. Similarly, there is no relationship between the severity of symptoms and the severity of the disease process. Patients with massive endometriosis may have few symptoms, whereas patients with minor lesions may have severe symptoms.

The symptom most frequently associated with endometriosis is dysmenorrhea. It is distinctive in that it typically begins 2 to 3 days before menses, becomes progressively worse during menstruation, and may persist for several days thereafter. This pattern of pain is thought to reflect hormone-mediated changes in the ectopic tissue, plus the associated pressure and inflammation. The pain may be located low in the abdomen, deep in the pelvis, or in the rectal or sacrococcygeal areas.

Deep dyspareunia (painful intercourse) is another symptom of endometriosis. It occurs if the uterosacral ligaments are involved. The patient may complain of dysuria if the bladder is affected, or constipation and pain on defecation if the rectal wall is affected.

Infertility is another concurrent finding with endometriosis. In fact, infertility is commonly the problem that brings the patient to a health-care professional. The mechanism by which endometriosis causes infertility is unknown. It has been suggested that prostaglandins released from the ectopic endometrial tissue interfere with normal ovum release, tubal mobility, uterine relaxation, or steroidogenesis. Regardless of the underlying cause, treatment of endometriosis may result in a subsequent pregnancy in many cases. Delayed childbearing may play a role in the development of endometriosis and subsequent infertility.

Diagnosis

Diagnosis of endometriosis is considered based on history and palpation of characteristic masses on bimanual examination. Laparoscopy with or without a biopsy may be done to confirm the diagnosis.

Management

Medical management of endometriosis depends on the severity of symptoms and the age and lifestyle of the patient. When symptoms are minimal, nonsteroidal anti-inflammatory drugs may be effective. Over-the-counter ibuprofen preparations, such as Advil or Nuprin, are tried first. If they fail to provide relief, such drugs as naproxen (Anaprox, Naprosyn) and prescription ibuprofen (Motrin) may be ordered. If the patient wishes to have a child, a pregnancy can provide relief from symptoms. This relief can be extended if the patient breast-feeds the infant.

In cases where a child is desired but infertility accompanies the endometriosis, conservative hormone therapy or surgical intervention is used.

Hormone Replacement Therapy

Types of hormone therapy used to treat endometriosis include oral contraceptive therapy, progestogen therapy, synthetic androgens, and gonadotropin-releasing hormone agonists.

Low-dose combination oral contraceptives or progestogen therapy may be used to induce a pseudopregnancy state (Highlight 41–6). This inhibits ovulation and menstruation, resulting in endometrial atrophy. Treatment lasts about 9 months and is effective in relieving pain. It also provides relief from infertility in about 40% of patients. A disadvantage of treatment is that uncomfortable symptoms of early pregnancy may develop, such as breast tenderness, nausea, vomiting, and fatigue.

Synthetic androgen therapy with danazol may also be tried. A pseudomenopause is induced by inhibiting follicle-stimulating hormone and luteinizing hormone, suppressing ovulation and ovarian activity, and preventing proliferation of the uterine and ectopic endometrium. The dosage is 200 to 400 mg of danazol given twice daily for 4 to 6 months at a time. Pain relief occurs in almost all patients. Conception occurs in about half.

Disadvantages of this treatment include high cost, tendency of symptoms to recur when the drug is discontinued, unknown long-term effects, and the occurrence of such side effects as hot flushes, hirsutism, weight gain, decreased vaginal secretions, and decreased breast size.

Gonadotropin-releasing hormone agonists are also used to decrease serum estradiol levels with eventual reduction in luteinizing hormone and follicle-stimulating hormone levels. This group of drugs is given intramuscularly or by nasal spray. Side effects include those of decreased estrogen. Advantages of this group of drugs include less severe masculinizing side effects than danazol.

Surgical Intervention

When surgical therapy is selected for the patient who desires a pregnancy, the aim is to remove all ectopic endometrial tissue and return the pelvis to as normal a condition as possible. This is usually done through a laparoscope with the use of laser or cautery techniques. Laser surgery leaves two to five "Band-Aid" ($\frac{1}{4}$ to $\frac{1}{2}$ inch) incisions and allows the patient to go home the same day and resume her

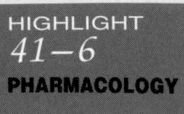
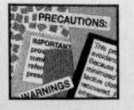

HIGHLIGHT 41–6 PHARMACOLOGY

Progesterones

Definition:

This is a class of drugs composed of the natural female hormone progesterone and its synthetic derivatives. Large amounts of progesterone are secreted by the corpus luteum during the menstrual cycle and by the placenta during pregnancy. Small amounts are secreted by the mature follicle before ovulation and by the adrenal cortex.

Action:

Progesterone is responsible for the secretory phase of the endometrium during the menstrual cycle. It also relaxes the uterine muscle, promotes development of the breast, and maintains the endometrium during pregnancy. Its metabolic effects include protein catabolism and retention of sodium and water.

Uses:

Treatment of dysfunctional uterine bleeding, amenorrhea, and dysmenorrhea. Some are also used to shrink endometrial carcinomas, to treat endometriosis, and as oral contraceptives.

Side Effects:

Breakthrough bleeding, dysmenorrhea, amenorrhea, monilial vaginitis, breast enlargement and tenderness, fluid retention, hypertension, thromboembolic disease, dizziness, migraine, depression, hyperglycemia, cholestatic jaundice, rash, and photosensitivity.

Interactions:

None of clinical significance.

Nursing Implications:

In accord with U.S. Food and Drug Administration regulations, be sure that patient has the package insert, which explains possible side effects. Review this information with the patient before the first dose is given. Instruct the patient to report visual changes, migraine, or other unusual symptoms immediately.

Give oil solution deep intramuscularly, and rotate injection sites.

---

usual routine within a week. Pretreatment with one of the gonadotropin-releasing hormone agents may help decrease the size of lesions.

When pregnancy is not desired and other options have not relieved symptoms, a total hysterectomy with bilateral salpingo-oophorectomy is the most effective treatment. However, if the patient is relatively young, an ovary may be spared and, in many cases, control of symptoms is obtained.

NURSING PROCESS GUIDELINES
Endometriosis

Assess the patient's understanding of the health problem. Does she have any misconceptions about its cause or outcomes? Some people believe endometriosis is caused by using tampons or that it develops into a malignancy.

As the therapeutic plan is instituted, assess the patient's understanding of it and its expected outcomes. For example, if the patient is having surgery, assess her understanding of preoperative preparation and the postoperative course.

Instruct the patient in methods of pain relief, including use of prescribed medications, application of heat to the abdomen through the use of a heating pad or hot water bottle, and abdominal massage. These interventions help to "gate" or block pain at the spinal cord by stimulating the large peripheral nerves of the abdomen. Encourage use of distraction to further enhance "gating."

Use exercise promotion to aid in limiting discomfort through a decrease in prostaglandins and increase in beta-endorphins (Star et al, 1995).

If infertility is not a concern, explain the role of pregnancy and breastfeeding in stopping the progression of the disease and in providing relief of symptoms.

Provide sexual counseling to help the woman and her partner consider alternative means of sexual expression, such as touching and mutual masturbation, until sexual intercourse is not painful.

Help the patient understand the plan of treatment and its expected effect. For example, if the patient is placed on hormone therapy, explain the planned duration of therapy; the dose, time, and frequency of medication; and its effects. Discuss the effect of menstruation and the possibility of pregnancy. Prepare her for side effects, such as the breast tenderness and nausea, that can occur with progestogens and the hot flushes and decreased

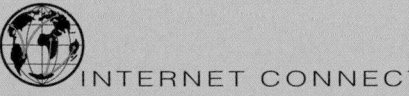

vaginal secretions that may accompany antigonadotropic drugs.

Use coping enhancement to help the patient identify and use new skills to manage feelings of anxiety, such as simple relaxation. Refer to the Endometriosis Association for additional consumer information about endometriosis. Suggest participation in a local support group if available.

Structural Disorders

DISORDERS CAUSED BY WEAKENED PELVIC SUPPORTS

The main organs of the pelvis are the bladder and upper urethra to the anterior, the vagina and the uterus in the middle, and the rectum and sigmoid colon to the posterior. These organs are maintained in their correct positions by the pelvic diaphragm, which is composed of the levator ani muscle, the

pelvic fascia, and the pelvic ligaments. Weakening of any of these supporting structures can result in genital prolapse, which is the abnormal descent of one or more of the pelvic viscera (Fig. 41–3).

Terms used to describe specific forms of genital prolapse are as follows:

Cystocele: Protrusion of the urinary bladder into the vagina through the anterior vaginal wall.
Rectocele: Protrusion of the rectum into the vagina through the lower, posterior vaginal wall.
Urethrocele: Protrusion of the urethra into the vagina through the anterior vaginal wall.
Enterocele: Protrusion of the intestinal wall into the vagina through the posterior vaginal wall.
Uterine prolapse: Downward displacement of the uterus into the vaginal canal.
  First degree: Cervix is between the level of the ischial spines and the vaginal introitus.
  Second degree: Cervix protrudes through the introitus.

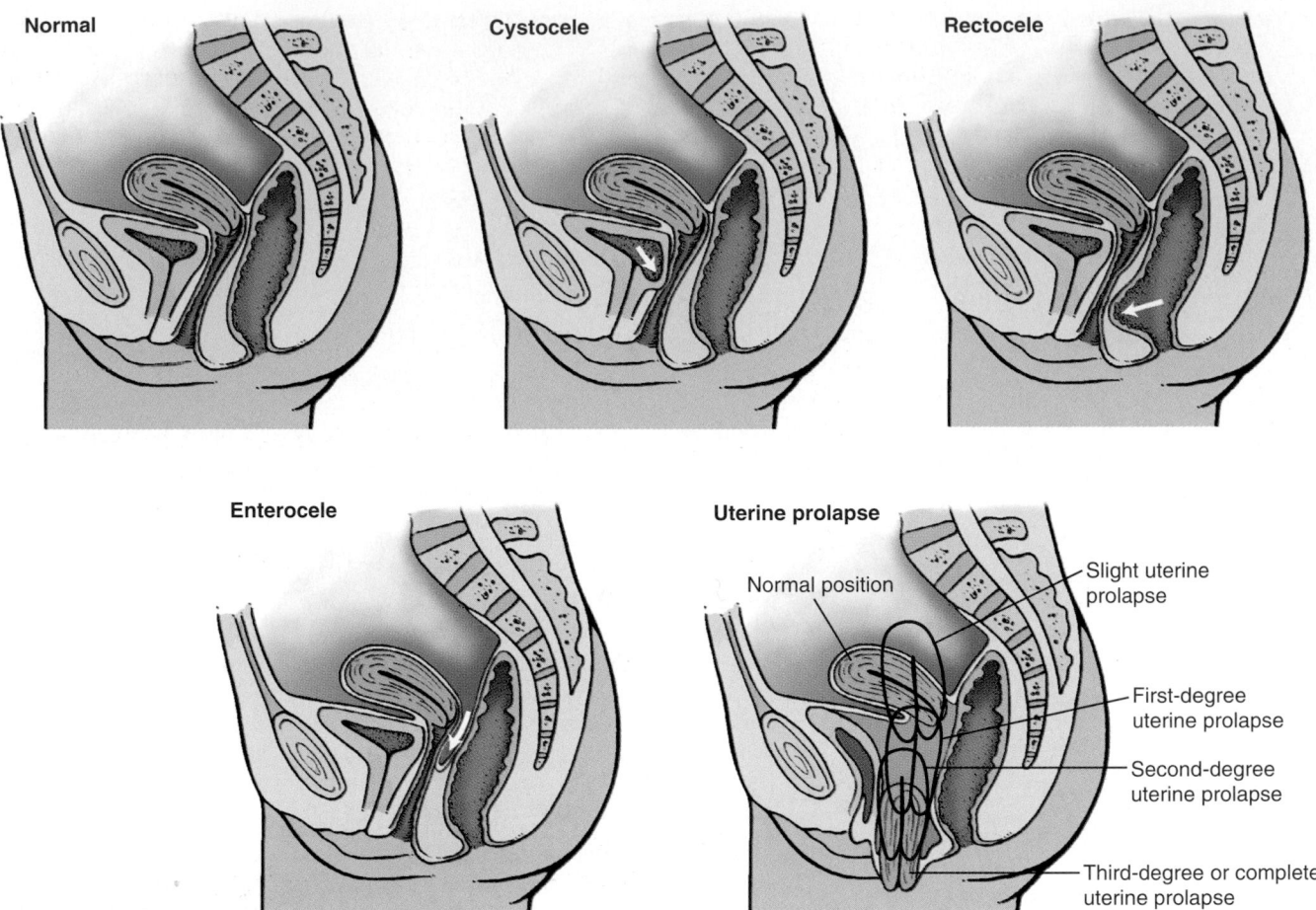

Figure 41–3

Types of genital prolapse.

Third degree (complete prolapse): The cervix and the entire body of the uterus have passed through the introitus, and the vagina is inverted.

Colpocele: Protrusion of a fold of vaginal mucosa outside the vaginal orifice.

Sometimes, the term *pelvic relaxation* is used to refer collectively to all these displacements of the pelvic organs.

Etiology and Pathophysiology

Although congenital incompetence of the pelvic support system occasionally occurs, the primary cause of weakened pelvic support is damage as a result of childbirth. This is further aggravated by weakening of the pelvic diaphragm and loss of elasticity and strength of the fascia that normally occur with aging, by the lack of estrogen after menopause, and by any condition that increases intra-abdominal pressure. Such conditions include chronic coughing associated with smoking or bronchitis, constipation, heavy lifting, obesity, pregnancy, large tumors, and ascites.

Clinical Manifestations

The patient with a weakened pelvic support and a genital prolapse has one or more of the following signs and symptoms:

- A lump protruding from the vagina. Typically the lump is painless and has been slowly increasing in size for months or even years. It is usually worse on standing or straining, and disappears when the patient lies down or presses on it. The patient may say she feels like she is sitting on a ball.

- Discomfort. A dragging sensation may be felt in the lower abdomen, or a feeling of pressure and heaviness may be felt in the vaginal area. This is often described as a feeling that everything inside is dropping out. The patient may also have a low backache (lumbosacral pain), especially after she has been standing for a length of time. This is caused by stretching of the supporting ligaments of the pelvis and the related peritoneum.

- Difficult defecation. With a rectocele, constipation results from overstretching and forward pouching of the rectum. The patient may have to press on the rectocele from inside the vagina to defecate. Hemorrhoids are commonly present.

- Disturbances of micturition. Difficulty emptying the bladder can be caused by a cystocele. The patient may have to press on the cystocele from within the vagina to empty her bladder. If the bladder is not emptied, residual urine in the prolapsed bladder can lead to chronic cystitis with its symptoms of frequency and dysuria. Stress incontinence, which is the escape of urine on coughing, laughing, or other muscular effort, may also occur from a change in the urethrovesical angle created by a cystocele or urethrocele. With a urethrocele, postvoiding incontinence may occur. This is the escape of urine on sitting down after voiding.
- Dyspareunia. Pain on intercourse may result from a change in the relationship of the pelvic organs to the vagina. In other cases, intercourse may simply be unsatisfactory as a result of vaginal relaxation.

There is no definite relationship between the severity of the patient's symptoms and the severity of the problem of pelvic relaxation.

Diagnosis

Diagnosis of genital prolapse is based on the patient's history and the findings of the physical examination.

Vaginal relaxation often can be identified by simple inspection. The vaginal orifice has a gaping appearance, and the anterior and posterior walls of the vagina are separated. Diagnosis is confirmed by placing the examining fingers into the vagina and asking the patient to bear down. With vaginal relaxation, no muscular resistance around the lower vagina is felt.

Uterine prolapse is also visible on inspection. The degree of prolapse is determined by asking the patient to bear down as the speculum is withdrawn toward the vaginal orifice.

Cystocele and rectocele can sometimes also be seen on inspection. More often, however, they recede when the patient is lying in a flat position. In this case, diagnosis is made by asking the patient to bear down or strain and observing the cystocele or rectocele come into view.

On physical examination, a urethrocele shows as a marked bulging just below the urethral orifice. Urethrography or urethroscopy may be used to confirm the diagnosis.

An enterocele is diagnosed by asking the patient to bear down during a rectovaginal examination. If an enterocele is present, a loop of small bowel will enter the sac and separate the examining fingers in the rectum and vagina, respectively.

Management

Nonsurgical measures are used when the patient cannot withstand surgery or when the severity of her symptoms does not warrant surgery. In most cases, medical management of genital prolapse resulting from weakness in the pelvic support system is surgery. The decision for treatment is based on the severity of the patient's symptoms. In most cases, surgery is elective. It is required only for a third-degree uterine prolapse, which produces chafing, ulceration, and bleeding from exposure of the displaced uterus to the external environment and to friction from clothing.

Pelvic Floor Exercises

Pelvic floor exercises may be prescribed for patients not in need of surgery but in whom relief of symptoms is desired. As might be expected, these are more effective in early-stage than in late-stage pelvic relaxation. They are most successful as a preventive measure done before childbirth. Highlight 41–7 describes two exercises effective in toning the pubococcygeal musculature: Kegel exercises and the elevator exercise.

Surgical Intervention

The treatment of choice for genital prolapse is a

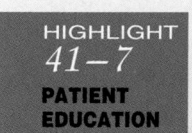 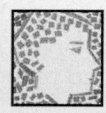

HIGHLIGHT
41–7
PATIENT
EDUCATION   **Pelvic Floor Exercises**

Instruct the patient as follows:

Kegel Exercises

Isolate the pelvic floor muscles for contraction while keeping the abdominal, gluteal, and thigh muscles relaxed. This can be learned during a vaginal examination or through the use of biofeedback equipment. As an alternative, it can be learned by starting and stopping the urine stream to check for isolation of the pelvic floor muscles, although this is not recommended on a routine basis.

Contract the perineal muscles tightly for a count of 3 to 10 seconds.

Relax for the same amount of time, then repeat the contraction.

Repeat the exercises up to 100 times per day (Star et al, 1995).

Elevator Exercise

Contract the perineal muscles gradually in steps. To do this, visualize the vaginal canal as an elevator shaft and stop at four or five "floors" on the way to the top (maximum contraction) and on the way down (complete relaxation).

vaginal hysterectomy with an anterior or posterior colporrhaphy (or both), or colpoperineorrhaphy. Vaginal hysterectomy was discussed in Chapter 40. An anterior colporrhaphy corrects a cystocele. It involves plication (stitching folds in the wall of an organ to reduce its size) of the endopelvic fascia and removal of excess anterior vaginal wall. This commonly results in some narrowing and shortening of the vagina but does not interfere with vaginal function.

A posterior colporrhaphy, which corrects a rectocele, is essentially the same procedure but on the posterior vaginal wall. Posterior repairs are a major cause of vulvar and vaginal stenosis and resulting dyspareunia. Postoperative stenosis can be minimized by the use of dilators and lubricants and the resumption of coitus 6 weeks after surgery. Nonetheless, posterior repairs are not done in adolescent girls and young women unless there is a major relaxation because, even if the size of the vagina is adequate for sexual function after recovery from surgery, dyspareunia may occur after menopause because of normal vaginal atrophy.

When both anterior and posterior colporrhaphies are done, the procedure is referred to as an *AP repair.*

If there is damage to the pelvic floor, a colpoperineorrhaphy is done. In this procedure, the muscles of the pelvic floor are repaired along with tightening of the vaginal walls.

Repairs of pelvic relaxations are not done until after the patient has given birth to the desired number of children, because any repair would be disrupted by a vaginal delivery. The surgery is also not performed until the patient is medically prepared. This includes healing of ulcerations that may be present if the vagina or uterus is completely prolapsed. To facilitate healing, the patient may be placed on bedrest, estrogen may be prescribed, and a vaginal pack may be inserted. The vaginal pack, which may be soaked in glycerin, can interfere with voiding by pressing on the urethrovesical angle. If this occurs, an indwelling catheter is inserted.

NURSING PROCESS
Posterior Colporrhaphy

PREOPERATIVE NURSING CARE

The assessment, nursing diagnoses, expected patient outcomes, nursing interventions, and evaluation for the patient scheduled for a posterior colporrhaphy are similar to those for any preoperative patient, as discussed in Chapter 6. Be sure to assess for recent use of birth control pills, because this predisposes to fluid and electrolyte imbalance postoperatively. A bowel preparation and a cleansing douche on the morning of surgery are components of the usual preoperative routine.

POSTOPERATIVE NURSING CARE
Assessment

Postoperatively, assess the patient's physiologic stabilization. Monitor vital signs, and observe the patient for bleeding. Assess the level of her pain using a standardized tool. Also assess for signs of pulmonary complications and developing thrombophlebitis. If an indwelling catheter is in place, as is usual for 24 to 48 hours, assess the adequacy of urinary elimination by monitoring output.

Nursing Diagnoses and Planning

Nursing diagnoses and related expected patient outcomes commonly applicable to patients who have had a posterior colporrhaphy include the following:

NDx: Risk for infection related to the presence of a vaginal suture line

Planning: Patient Outcomes
1. Foul-smelling or purulent vaginal drainage is absent.
2. Temperature is normal.
3. Leukocytosis is absent.

NDx: Risk for impaired tissue integrity related to pull on the vaginal suture line

Planning: Patient Outcomes
1. Patient maintains position as directed to prevent stress on the suture line.
2. Patient defecates without straining.

NDx: Pain related to tissue trauma

Planning: Patient Outcomes
1. Patient turns and sits up without excessive discomfort.
2. Patient becomes increasingly active.
3. Patient reports that discomfort has decreased.

NDx: Risk for altered health maintenance related to insufficient knowledge of postdischarge self-care activities

Planning: Patient Outcomes
1. Patient describes postdischarge self-care activities.

Nursing Interventions and Evaluation

Institute standard postoperative care, as discussed in Chapter 6. Provide care as described next to meet the specific needs of the patient who has had a posterior colporrhaphy.

NDx: Risk for infection
Begin measures to support healing and prevent infection immediately. Give sterile perineal care twice a day and after each use of the bedpan or toilet. Sterile cotton balls may be used to cleanse the area with a solution, such as normal saline or benzalkonium chloride, or the solution may simply be poured over the perineum while the patient is positioned on a fracture pan. In either case, gently but

thoroughly pat the area dry to avoid creating a dark, warm, moist area conducive to bacterial growth. Occasionally, use of a heat lamp may be ordered for 15 to 20 minutes after perineal care to dry the area and increase circulation needed for healing.

Administer sterile douches as ordered to cleanse the incisional area within the vagina and to facilitate healing. Some surgeons order small douches of normal saline twice a day starting on the first postoperative day. Others leave the suture line undisturbed and order douches beginning 5 to 10 days postoperatively.

NDx: Risk for impaired tissue integrity
Keep the patient either flat or in low Fowler's position to prevent pressure on the suture line, which would impede healing. Implement physician's orders related to diet and medications to control gastrointestinal function. Orders usually call for a liquid diet and paregoric to inhibit bowel function for 5 days and mineral oil on the fifth postoperative evening, followed by an oil retention enema the next day. This facilitates defecation without straining.

NDx: Pain
Give analgesics according to physician's orders. Ice packs may be applied for perineal discomfort. A rubber glove filled with chipped ice fits comfortably to the area. Cover the ice pack and position it so that its weight is on the bed and not on the patient. Apply analgesic ointments as ordered for relief.

Instruct the patient to pinch her buttocks together before sitting down. This decreases pressure on the operative area and reduces discomfort.

After the sutures are removed, sitz baths may ease perineal discomfort.

Ndx: Risk for altered health maintenance
Instruct the patient on self-care after discharge (Highlight 41–8).

Compare the patient's status with the expected outcomes. If the outcomes are not met, reassess the patient and revise the plan.

NURSING PROCESS GUIDELINES
Anterior Colporrhaphy

The assessment, nursing diagnoses, expected patient outcomes, nursing interventions, and evaluation for patients having an anterior colporrhaphy are similar to those described previously for patients having a posterior colporrhaphy, with the following exception.

Because the anterior rather than the posterior wall of the vagina is the operative site, cleansing of the bowel preoperatively is not necessary. Laxatives, a clear-liquid diet, and soapsuds enema are not necessary, so only a cleansing douche as ordered by the surgeon is given on the morning of surgery.

Postoperatively, the patient ambulates within 12 to 24 hours and progresses to a regular diet as soon as tolerated. Mineral oil is usually ordered to prevent straining at stool, which puts stress on the suture line by increasing intra-abdominal pressure.

Usually, the patient has an indwelling catheter for 4 days because, if more than 100 mL of urine accumulates in the bladder, the pressure can disrupt the repair. If the patient does not have an indwelling catheter, she should be asked to void every 4 hours. Inability to void or pain in the area of the bladder should be reported to the physician. If this occurs, insertion of a catheter is usually ordered. Insertion can be difficult postoperatively because of swelling and distortion of the urethral meatus. Asking the patient to take a slow, deep breath can assist in locating the opening.

RETRODISPLACEMENT OF THE UTERUS

Normally, the position of the uterus is one of anteflexion and anteversion. Anteflexion refers to the forward tilt of the entire uterus, which causes the fundus to point toward the symphysis pubis and the cervix to point downward and backward toward the sacrum (Fig. 41–4). Anteversion refers to the near right angle between the cervix and the vagina.

Retrodisplacement of the uterus refers to a backward displacement. If the fundus of the uterus bends backward on the cervix, it is called retroflexion (Fig. 41–5A). If the entire uterus is tipped backward so that the fundus no longer points forward, it is called retroversion (Fig. 41–5B).

Etiology and Pathophysiology
Primary retrodisplacement has no known cause and may be congenital. Secondary or acquired retrodisplacement may result from injury during childbirth, mechanical displacement by a tumor or distended

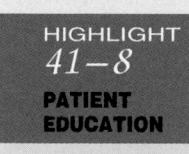
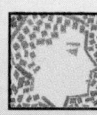

HIGHLIGHT
41–8

PATIENT EDUCATION

Self-Care After Posterior Colporrhaphy

Instruct the patient to:

Take a douche and a tub bath each day until your follow-up visit.

Avoid sexual intercourse until after the follow-up visit.

Take a laxative each night to avoid straining during defecation and the related stress on the suture line.

Avoid jarring activities and prolonged periods of walking or sitting for 6 weeks.

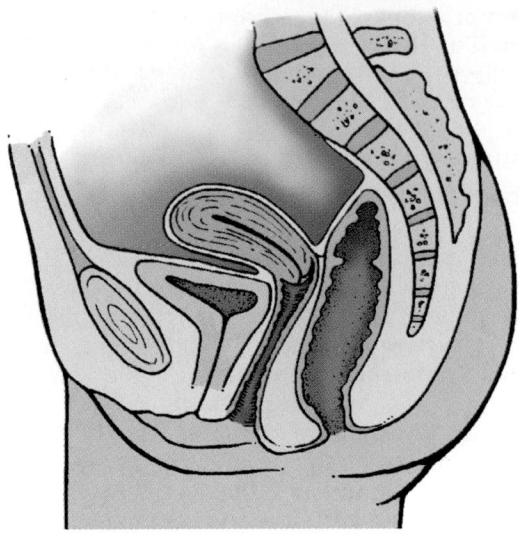

Figure 41–4
Normal uterine position.

bladder, or adnexal disease, such as endometriosis or another inflammatory disorder.

Clinical Manifestations

Symptoms that may be associated with retrodisplacement are dysmenorrhea, low backache, dyspareunia, and a feeling of pelvic pressure. In acquired cases, infertility may also be present. Many patients have no symptoms, even with severe retrodisplacement.

Diagnosis

Diagnosis of a uterine retrodisplacement is based on pelvic examination. The cervix is seen to point to the symphysis pubis rather than to the sacrum, and the fundus is palpated posteriorly rather than in its normal anterior position.

Management

In cases of acquired retrodisplacement of the uterus, medical management is directed at treating the underlying problem. When a treatable underlying disease is not identified, and the uterus is freely mobile and able to be directed into normal position on a bimanual pelvic examination, no management may be needed. If intervention is required, postural therapy or a pessary may be prescribed.

With postural therapy, the patient assumes the knee-chest position three or four times per day for 5 minutes at a time. In this position, air distends the vagina, and the uterus falls forward (Fig. 41–6). This provides symptomatic relief for some patients, particularly those with a postpartum retrodisplacement.

Treatment with a pessary involves insertion of a Hodge pessary to maintain the uterus in its correct position. This pessary works by putting tension on the posterior fornix. It is inserted in an office setting and left in place for 2 to 3 months. During this time, follow-up visits are scheduled to ascertain that the pessary is in fact holding the uterus in the correct position.

NURSING PROCESS GUIDELINES
Retrodisplacement of the Uterus

Explain the relationship of poor posture and improper lifting to back pain because many patients believe that any low back pain is caused by the womb being out of place. Teach principles of correct body mechanics.

Teach the patient to assume the knee-chest position if postural therapy is ordered. Reinforce that this should be done for 5 minutes three or four times every day.

If a pessary is ordered, instruct the patient to report any difficulty with urination, vaginal bleeding or other drainage, and any foul vaginal odor. Make sure the patient knows when to return for a follow-up examination.

If the uterus is mobile and dyspareunia is the only symptom, sexual counseling can probably solve the problem. Explain that because the uterus and ovaries move upward as sexual excitement increases, symptom relief can be obtained by heightening sexual arousal through foreplay before intercourse.

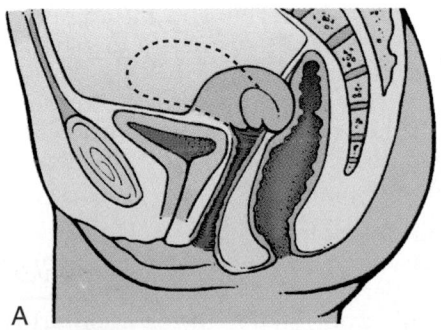

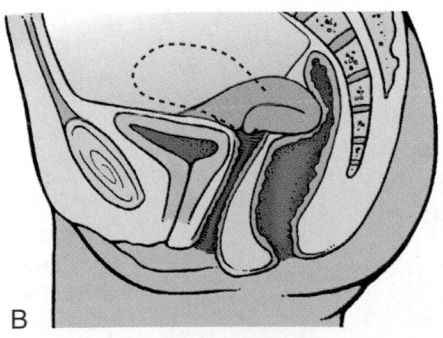

Figure 41–5
Retrodisplacement of the uterus: *A*, Retroflexion; *B*, retroversion.

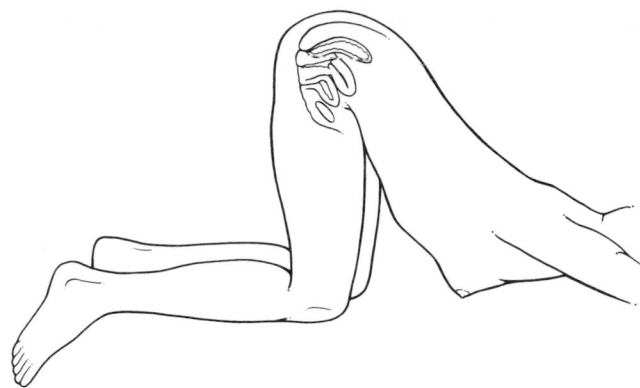

Figure 41-6

In the knee-chest position, the uterus and pelvic organs migrate forward.

GENITAL FISTULAS

A genital fistula is an abnormal opening between the vagina or the uterus and either some part of the urinary tract, some part of the intestinal tract, or both (Fig. 41-7).

Etiology and Pathophysiology

In the past, genital fistulas were common because of trauma during labor and delivery. Today, genital fistulas occur primarily from injury during a radical hysterectomy or secondary to tissue necrosis and sloughing from radiation therapy. In some cases, fistulas may result from the destruction of tissue by

malignant tumors or chronic disorders (such as Crohn's disease) or ulceration from a foreign body (such as a pessary). Rarely women undergoing a simple hysterectomy or an anterior vaginal repair may develop a fistula secondary to trauma or as the result of poor healing.

The most common type of vaginal-intestinal fistula is a rectovaginal fistula (Fig. 41-8). Fistulas involving the sigmoid colon or small intestine also occur. The latter result from malignant disease, pelvic or intestinal operations, or other medical conditions such as Crohn's disease.

Clinical Manifestations

If a vaginal-intestinal fistula is tiny, the only sign may be occasional foul-smelling leukorrhea or an occasional passage of gas or fecal matter from the vagina. In fact, this may occur only when the patient's stool is abnormally loose. With large fistulas, the signs become more prominent, to the point at which there may be constant fecal drainage through the vagina. Irritation of the vagina, vulva, and perineum develops, and an offensive odor is present. Infection may occur in the surrounding tissues.

Diagnosis

Passage of feces through the vagina is evidence of a vaginal-intestinal fistula. The exact location of the fistula in the intestinal tract is identified by sigmoidoscopy or a barium enema.

Management

Very small vaginal-intestinal fistulas in otherwise healthy women may close spontaneously in 1 to 3

Figure 41-7

Types of genitourinary fistulas. *A*, Vesicovaginal (bladder to vagina). *B*, Vesicouterine (bladder to uterus). *C*, Urethrovaginal (urethra to vagina). *D*, Ureterovaginal (ureter to vagina). Fistulas range in size from tiny and difficult to locate to large, disfiguring the base of the bladder. The primary symptom of a genitourinary fistula is leakage of urine into the vagina, which can be a source of embarrassment for the woman. The fistula may be seen during a vaginal examination with the patient in the knee-chest position and confirmed by an intravenous pyelogram. If healing does not occur in 6 months, surgical closure is used.

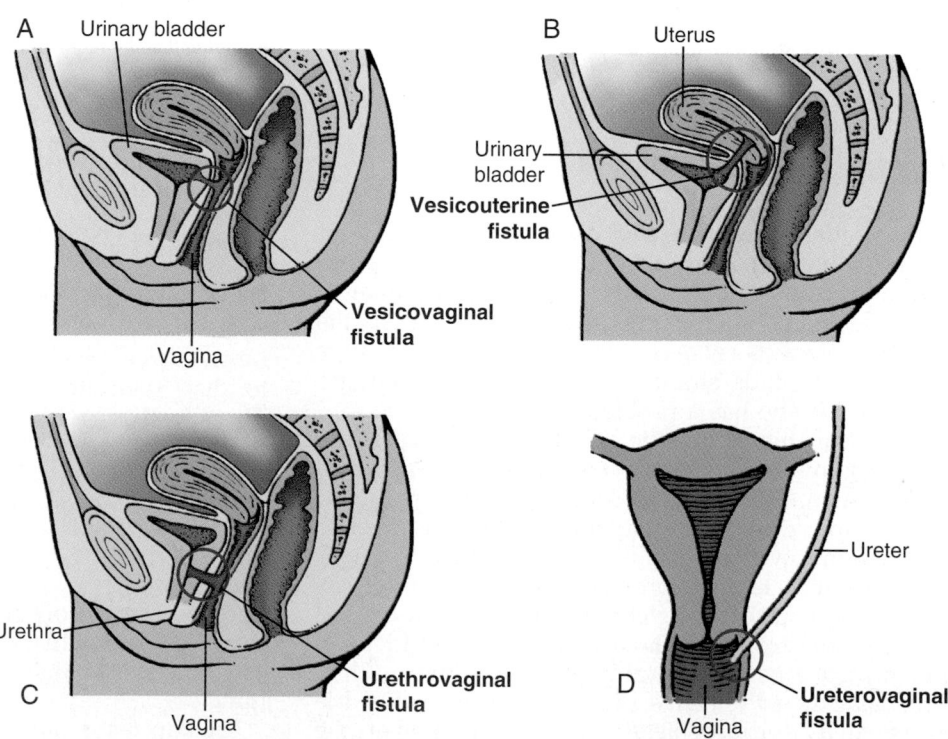

A Urinary bladder
Vesicovaginal fistula
Vagina

B Uterus
Urinary bladder
Vesicouterine fistula

C Urethra
Urethrovaginal fistula
Vagina

D Ureter
Vagina
Ureterovaginal fistula

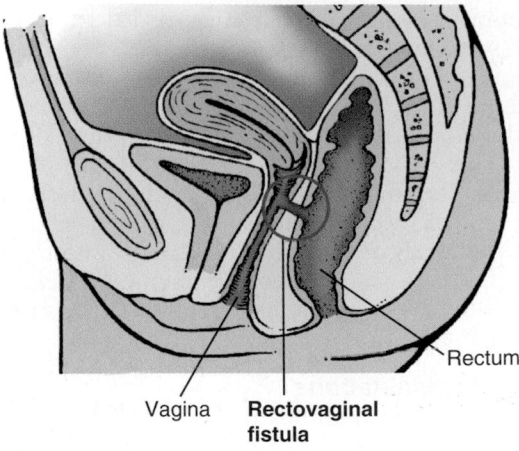

Figure 41-8
Rectovaginal fistula.

months. Larger fistulas require surgical repair. This is best done 4 to 6 months after injury, when edema and inflammation have subsided. Repair of a rectovaginal fistula is done vaginally. For fistulas involving other parts of the intestinal tract, abdominal surgery is necessary. In patients with tissues around the fistula that are badly infected, a temporary colostomy (see Chap. 21) may be performed above the level of the fistula to allow healing of the area before a repair is attempted.

Palliative measures, such as douches and enemas, are prescribed during the interval before surgery. Measures are also taken to improve the general health status of the patient. Antibiotic therapy may be prescribed to treat or prevent infection.

Just before surgery, routine preoperative care is given, including standard bowel preparation.

NURSING PROCESS GUIDELINES
Vaginal-Intestinal Fistula

If the patient has had the fistula for a period of time, explore her methods of dealing with the problem. Determine how often she cleanses the area, what cleansing solution is used, and whether she douches or takes enemas. Also determine what type of protective pads she uses, how often she changes them, and if she has a problem with odor.

Question her about the effects of the fistula and its symptoms on personal lifestyle. Assess for problems in sexual, family, and social relationships.

Care for or teach the patient or other caregiver to treat the involved areas as follows. Cleanse the perineal area and change protective pads or undergarments frequently to prevent skin breakdown caused by irritation from fistula drainage. Use mild soap and water, rinse thoroughly, and dry thoroughly. According to physician's orders, pour a weakly basic (such as sodium bicarbonate) solution over the vulva to neutralize pH and reduce tissue irritation if

drainage from the fistula is acidic. If drainage from the fistula is basic, a weakly acidic (such as acetic acid) solution is recommended. Apply vitamin-based ointments to provide a protective film to prevent irritating drainage from coming into direct contact with the skin.

If ordered, give douches to cleanse and soothe vaginal mucous membranes. Always give gently because too much pressure can force fluid back through the fistula tract.

If the fistula is rectovaginal, administer enemas as ordered to decrease the feces available to escape through the fistula. This helps control leakage, odor, and irritation of skin and mucous membranes. Use a soft, rubber enema tube, and direct it toward the side of the rectum opposite the fistula. Be sure to insert the tube beyond the level of the fistula to prevent the enema fluid from simply draining into the vagina.

Neoplasia

POLYPS

Polyps are tumors that have stalks or pedicles. They are common in vascular organs and bleed easily. In the female reproductive system, two common types of polyps are cervical polyps and endometrial polyps.

Cervical Polyps

Etiology and Pathophysiology
Cervical polyps, which may be single or multiple, develop when an area of the mucosa in the cervical canal proliferates. They are usually small and appear as bright red, spongy tissue protruding out of the cervical canal on a pedicle into the vagina. The tip of the polyp is often ulcerated. Cervical polyps rarely undergo malignant change.

Clinical Manifestations
Small cervical polyps usually do not cause symptoms. Large cervical polyps cause bleeding similar to that associated with early cancer of the cervix. This bleeding, which results from the vascularity of the polyp, is usually scant, although hemorrhage can occur during menstruation. It may be intermenstrual bleeding or contact bleeding that occurs after coitus, douching, or a vaginal examination.

Diagnosis
Large cervical polyps can be felt by the examining finger during palpation of the cervix. Smaller polyps can be seen on inspection through a bivalve speculum.

A Pap test is always done at the time of diagnosis because finding a polyp proves neither that it is the cause of the symptom nor that it is the only pathology present.

Management

Polyps associated with symptoms are usually removed. This can often be done by simply twisting the pedicle off and cauterizing the point of attachment to the uterine wall. If multiple polyps are present, the cervical canal is dilated and cauterized. Lasers are increasingly used to remove polyps. Recurrence is fairly common.

Endometrial Polyps

Etiology and Pathophysiology

Endometrial polyps are composed of functional or nonfunctional endometrial tissue. When the tissue of the polyp is functional, it changes in response to hormones as does the general uterine mucosa. When it is nonfunctional or immature, it does not respond to hormonal stimulation.

Endometrial polyps may be single or multiple and vary in size from small to large enough to fill the uterine cavity. Endometrial polyps are extremely unlikely to undergo malignant change. However, during the menopausal and postmenopausal years, there is an increased incidence of uterine cancer in females who also have endometrial polyps.

Clinical Manifestations

Many endometrial polyps are asymptomatic unless they are large enough to protrude through the cervical canal and have become ulcerated. When this occurs, moderate metrorrhagia results. If the blood supply through the pedicle of the polyp is impeded, necrosis with bleeding and a foul-smelling discharge can occur.

Diagnosis

Many endometrial polyps are discovered accidentally during a dilatation and curettage or after a hysterectomy. Large, protruding polyps can be seen during a pelvic examination.

Management

Large, symptomatic polyps are surgically removed. With the patient under anesthesia, the cervix is dilated and the polyp removed at its base. A curettage is then performed to identify and remove any other small polyps that might be present.

NURSING PROCESS GUIDELINES
Cervical or Endometrial Polyps

Fear is common among women who have any type of neoplasm. This fear may be exaggerated in the patient with a cervical or endometrial polyp because her first symptom may have been spotting similar to that publicly identified as a first sign of cervical cancer. It is important, therefore, to assess the patient's understanding and emotional acceptance of the polyp as a benign growth. If a knowledge deficit or anxiety state exists, provide information and give the patient opportunity to express her concerns. Printed materials indicating the benign nature of polyps are sometimes an effective aid in allaying anxiety.

Teach patients with these polyps about the need for routine gynecologic examinations even after menopause, because endometrial cancer does occur more often in women with a history of endometrial polyps.

LEIOMYOMAS

Leiomyomas (also called myomas, fibromas, and fibroids) are benign, smooth-muscle tumors found in the wall of the uterus. Leiomyomas are the most common tumor of the female reproductive tract. It is estimated that one of five women older than 35 years has them. They occur most frequently in African-American women and in nulliparous women.

Etiology and Pathophysiology

The exact cause of leiomyomas is unknown, but their development seems to be linked to excess estrogen relative to progesterone. This type of imbalance occurs if the level of progesterone is normal but the level of estrogen is increased or if the level of estrogen is normal but the level of progesterone is decreased.

Leiomyomas develop slowly during the reproductive years except during pregnancy, when their growth is accelerated. They atrophy after menopause. They vary in size from that of a small seed to that of a grapefruit. They are firm, round, or oval. They tend to be multiple. Depending on location, they are classified as

• Intramural (in the middle of the uterine wall surrounded by myometrium)
• Submucous (just under the endometrium)
• Subserosal (on the outer surface of the uterus just under the serosal covering

Figure 41–9 depicts these leiomyomas.

As intramural leiomyomas grow, the size of the uterus increases and the inner wall becomes nodular in contour and consistency.

Submucous leiomyomas may grow a pedicle and occasionally can be seen protruding from the cervix and, more rarely, from the vagina. As they grow, they begin to fill the uterine cavity and can eventually touch the opposite wall and distort the shape of the cavity.

Subserous tumors tend to be pedunculated and large. They are called intraligamentary if they grow out between the folds of the broad ligament.

Most often, leiomyomas occur in the body of the uterus, although they can occur in the cervix.

Clinical Manifestations

In many cases, leiomyomas, even multiple large

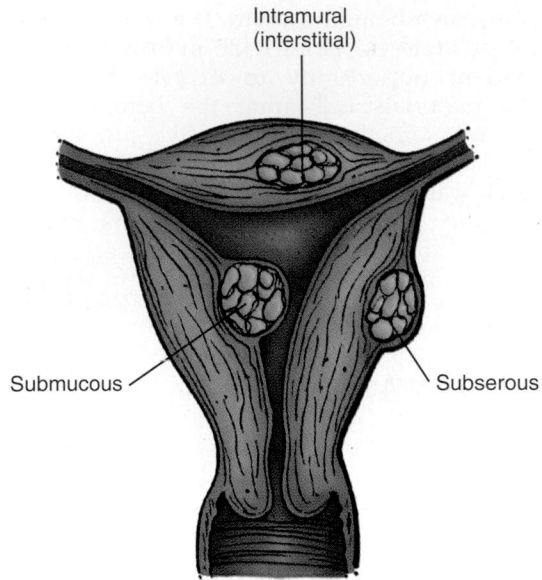

Figure 41–9
Types of leiomyomas.

ones, cause no symptoms. When symptoms do occur, the onset is usually between ages 40 and 45. They are related to the size and location of the tumors. Symptoms are not present until a fibroid is the size of a softball or grapefruit.

Excessive, prolonged menstruation is the most common symptom of intramural and submucous tumors because of an increase in endometrial surface. In some cases, blood loss is sufficient to cause anemia and its symptoms of fatigue, weakness, and lethargy.

Symptoms from large tumors and from subserosal tumors that grow outward from the uterus rather than into the uterine cavity are caused by pressure on adjacent pelvic organs. If pressure is exerted on the rectum, constipation and pain on defecation occur. With pressure on the bladder, the patient may have frequency of urination and dysuria. If the urethra is compressed, retention and hydroureter can occur.

Large tumors of any type can cause a sensation of low abdominal pressure or "bearing down," dysmenorrhea, backache, and weight gain. There may also be a palpable abdominal mass and general enlargement of the abdomen. Large tumors in the body of the uterus can cause spontaneous abortions and, if they grow into the openings of the fallopian tubes, can cause sterility.

If a leiomyoma is pedunculated and the pedicle twists, the resultant interference with blood supply causes severe pain, nausea, and vomiting.

Diagnosis

Leiomyomas are suspected when the patient has a history of characteristic symptoms and one or more nodular outgrowths can be felt on the uterus during a bimanual pelvic examination. Sonograms, diagnostic curettage, and hysterograms may be used to confirm the diagnosis and to rule out pregnancy and other disorders.

Management

Medical management varies depending on the severity of the symptoms, the age of the patient, her desire for childbearing, the location and size of the tumor, and the presence of complications.

If the patient is close to menopause and the leiomyomas have not caused the uterus to enlarge to simulate a 12-week or more gestation, the patient is observed every 3 to 6 months and, provided no rapid increase in size occurs, the leiomyomas are left to undergo normal postmenopausal atrophy. If a rapid increase in size occurs, definitive treatment is needed to rule out the possibility of carcinoma.

If the patient is not menopausal and does not desire to have a child or the leiomyomas are so large that a successful pregnancy is unlikely and bleeding is severe, a hysterectomy is the treatment of choice. When relief of symptoms and subsequent childbearing is the aim, a myomectomy is performed. This procedure, in which the tumors are excised, is always preceded by a diagnostic curettage to rule out any other cause of the presenting symptoms, such as adenocarcinoma. A disadvantage of the procedure is the risk that the tumors may recur.

NURSING PROCESS GUIDELINES
Leiomyomas

The assessment, nursing diagnoses, expected patient outcomes, nursing interventions, and evaluation for patients with a leiomyoma are similar to those described in Chapter 40 for patients having a hysterectomy. In addition, if surgery is scheduled because the tumors suddenly increase in size, the patient may be very fearful that she has cancer. If so, provide opportunities for her to express feelings and concerns, and reinforce facts as needed.

If a myomectomy is done on a patient who is premenopausal and desirous of having a child, give support in the form of information on successful pregnancy after myomectomy.

BENIGN OVARIAN TUMORS

Etiology and Pathophysiology

Ovarian tumors are classified as non-neoplastic or neoplastic.

Non-neoplastic Tumors
Non-neoplastic tumors are physiologic in origin. In other words, they are enlargements of normal ovar-

ian structures. Two common types are follicle cysts and corpus luteal cysts.

Follicle cysts develop in a graafian follicle that has not ruptured or that has ruptured but quickly resealed. These very common cysts tend to be multiple, small, and self-limited. They are filled with serous fluid, which is rich in estrogen. This may delay the onset of menstruation or cause a prolonged menses. Because the fluid is resorbed and the cyst disappears in 4 to 8 weeks, the symptoms occur for only one or two cycles, and no treatment is usually necessary.

Corpus luteal cysts occur when the corpus luteum does not degenerate but keeps on growing and producing progesterone. This delays the onset of menses or causes prolonged spotting or pain. Like follicular cysts, corpus luteal cysts rarely persist beyond one or two menstrual cycles, and treatment is usually unnecessary.

Neoplastic Tumors

Neoplastic tumors are new growths that develop from the tissues of the ovary. One of the most common benign ovarian tumors is the dermoid cyst that arises from germ cells and contains a thick, yellow sebaceous substance along with rudiments of other tissues, such as teeth, hair, bone, brain, and eyes. They are slow-growing tumors and occur most often in women between ages 18 and 35.

Clinical Manifestations

Small ovarian tumors usually do not cause symptoms. When symptoms do occur, they are related to pressure from the tumor on surrounding organs. Common symptoms include a nagging or pulling sensation in the pelvis, a feeling of pelvic pressure, dyspareunia, constipation, painful defecation, urinary frequency, backache, and, with large tumors, an increase in the size of the abdomen. If the tumor is hormone producing, menstrual irregularities or masculinization may occur. If a cyst ruptures, signs and symptoms associated with any acute abdominal emergency such as ruptured appendix or a ruptured ectopic pregnancy are seen.

Diagnosis

Eighty percent of all benign ovarian tumors are discovered by palpation during a routine pelvic examination. Because diagnosis of an ovarian tumor can be difficult, laparoscopy may be used to confirm it.

Management

The size of the tumor determines the medical intervention. A small tumor (less than 5 cm) in a woman of childbearing age who does not have any symptoms is monitored for one to two menstrual cycles to determine whether it will regress like a physiologic cyst, remain the same, or continue to enlarge. If it enlarges, then surgery is performed. If the tumor is benign and there is healthy ovarian tissue, a cystectomy is performed. Oophorectomy is done if the tumor involves all of the ovarian tissue.

Tumors greater than 5 cm in size and tumors in women older than 40 years are always treated surgically because of the increased incidence of malignancy in these cases.

NURSING PROCESS GUIDELINES
Benign Ovarian Tumor

Nursing care of the patient with a benign ovarian tumor depends on the type of tumor and the plan of medical treatment. If a diagnostic laparoscopy is done, nursing care is provided as described in Chapter 40. If a cystectomy is performed, basic nursing care is that required by any patient having abdominal surgery.

A particular nursing concern related to the patient with a benign ovarian tumor is the patient's understanding of the disorder and its symptoms. Nursing assessments and interventions are planned to ascertain that the patient understands that the tumor is harmless, that it does not have a malignant potential, and that it does not indicate infertility.

When the problem is a physiologic cyst that delays onset of menstruation, assess the patient's emotional response and design interventions accordingly. In some cases, the patient may be highly anxious because she believes she is pregnant. In other cases, she may be devastated to find she is not pregnant and needs reassurance that the cyst does not mean she is sterile. Be sure to provide time and opportunity for her to express her concerns.

MALIGNANT NEOPLASMS

Cancer of the Vulva

VULVAR CARCINOMA IN SITU

Vulvar carcinoma in situ is a neoplasm in which histologic changes are present in the vulvar epidermis but do not affect the adjacent tissue layers.

In the past, vulvar carcinoma in situ was a disease affecting primarily 50- to 60-year-old women. In recent years, however, incidence among younger women has been increasing so that, today, the average age of onset is between 30 and 40 years of age.

Etiology and Pathophysiology

The cause of vulvar carcinoma in situ is unknown, although a high degree of association with sexually transmitted diseases, particularly exposure to human papillomavirus, has been reported.

Clinical Manifestations

The two primary symptoms of vulvar carcinoma in situ are pruritus and a surface lesion. Pruritus occurs in about half of all affected women and often occurs for some time before any other finding.

Surface lesions vary greatly in appearance. They may be white, like leukoplakia; red; pink; or mahogany. They may be eczematous, dry or moist, and are often raised (papular).

Diagnosis

Diagnosis depends on careful inspection of the vulva using a bright light, magnifying glass, and vinegar or other staining technique with subsequent colposcopic examination. Any suspicious areas should undergo biopsy. About half of all cases of vulvar carcinoma in situ are discovered during routine screening examinations.

Management

Single lesions are treated by wide, local excision or laser beam therapy. The affected area as well as a border of disease-free tissue is excised, and the wound is sutured. If healing is uncomplicated, no scar or defect results because of the elasticity of the tissues involved. Fluorouracil cream 5% may also be used but does not have as high response rates (National Cancer Institute, 1996d).

If lesions are multiple, treatment may be a partial, total, or skinning vulvectomy. A partial vulvectomy is designed to remove affected tissue while retaining as much normal tissue as possible. Often the clitoris, prepuce, or frenulum can be spared and hence sexual sensation preserved.

In a total vulvectomy, all of the structures of the vulva are removed.

In a skinning vulvectomy, the vulvar skin is excised and replaced with a split-thickness graft from the buttocks or inner thigh. The purpose of this procedure is to replace the skin at risk. Its major advantage is that the subcutaneous vulvar tissue is not disturbed; therefore, there is little functional or cosmetic defect.

A disadvantage to the skinning vulvectomy is that 6 to 7 days of bedrest are required while the graft is adhering. For this reason, it is not the procedure of choice for nonsexually active elderly patients or those otherwise at risk for complications of immobility.

Lifetime follow-up is necessary for all patients. A checkup is done every 3 to 6 months for the first 2 years and annually thereafter provided there is no sign of recurrence.

INVASIVE CANCER OF THE VULVA

Invasive carcinoma of the vulva is an uncommon disorder that occurs most frequently in women age 65 and older. It is often associated with condylomata acuminata (vulvar warts), but no direct cause and effect relationship has been identified. Other possible risk factors are syphilis, smoking, and diabetes.

Currently, the incidence of invasive cancer of the vulva is increasing, possibly because more women are living to the age at which the disease tends to occur. It is found among the poor in all areas of the world.

Etiology and Pathophysiology

Because the vulva is covered with skin, all the types of cancer that can occur on other areas of the skin can occur on the vulva. The most common type of vulvar malignancy is squamous cell carcinoma. This seems to begin as a small area of epithelial thickening that develops into a small nodule that may ulcerate, become infected, or develop into a small, warty or cauliflower-like growth. Most often, it begins on the labia majora and is well localized and demarcated. It tends to extend slowly. Metastasis occurs late and is via the lymph, affecting first the superficial inguinal lymph nodes and then the deep femoral nodes. Eventually liver, lungs, and other internal organs are involved. If local recurrence occurs, it is usually close to the site of the primary lesion and within 2 years after initial treatment.

Carcinoma of the vulva is staged according to the size of the tumor, location of the primary tumor, lymph node involvement, and presence or absence of distant metastases.

Clinical Manifestations

Like vulvar carcinoma in situ, the primary symptoms of cancer of the vulva are long-term pruritus and the presence of a lump or small nodule that may break down and ulcerate. Slight soreness progressing to pain occurs as the disease progresses. If the growth ulcerates and becomes infected, bleeding and a foul-smelling discharge may also be present.

Diagnosis

A positive diagnosis is based on the results of a biopsy.

Management

Basic treatment of invasive vulvar cancer is radical vulvectomy and inguinal lymphadenectomy. Pelvic lymphadenectomy is also done if metastasis is found in the inguinal lymph nodes. It is not done if the inguinal lymph nodes are negative because metastasis is not found in the pelvic nodes unless it is also present in the inguinal lymph nodes. Because of the increase in morbidity associated with pelvic lymphadenectomy, radiation rather than excision may be the treatment, especially in elderly or medically ill patients.

In a radical vulvectomy, tissue is excised from the anus to just above the symphysis pubis. This includes the mons pubis, the terminal section of the urethra and the vagina, and parts of the round ligaments and saphenous veins. In an inguinal lymphadenectomy, the groin is incised and the lymph nodes are dissected and removed.

Preoperative Preparation

To decrease the likelihood of wound infection postoperatively, the skin of the lower abdomen, groin, and upper thighs as well as the vulva may be scrubbed with a detergent germicide each day for several days before surgery. Antibiotics may be ordered prophylactically and continued into the postoperative period. Heparin may also be given preoperatively as prophylaxis against thrombus formation and is often continued for 5 days postoperatively. Enemas, a cleansing douche, and a shower using an antibacterial soap are given the night before surgery. An abdominal perineal shave may be done in the operating room just before making the incision. Because good nutritional status is needed for wound healing, hyperalimentation may be started 4 to 6 days before surgery if the patient is malnourished. If palpable lymph nodes are present in the groin, a computed tomographic scan is also done preoperatively. In some protocols for advanced-stage vulvar cancer, a preoperative course of radiation with or without chemotherapy (5-fluorouracil with or without cisplatin) is used.

Postoperative Course

Postoperatively, the patient has a vulvar wound and a wound in each groin from the inguinal node dissection. Depending on the surgeon's preference, these wounds may be left uncovered, covered with a light dressing, or covered with a pressure dressing to decrease the amount of serum and blood that collects in the wound.

Some patients may have a Hemovac or drainage catheter attached to suction inserted through a stab wound in each inguinal area to prevent accumulation of blood or serum, which could lead to disruption of the wound. This drainage is usually maintained for about 5 days.

Fluids are given intravenously for 48 to 72 hours. The patient then progresses from clear fluids to a full low-residue diet. A low-residue diet is given to prevent pressure on the suture line associated with straining on defecation.

To prevent urethral stenosis and contamination of the wound with urine, a Foley catheter is in place for up to 4 or 5 days after surgery.

The patient is ambulated as soon as possible, usually on the first postoperative day. Sutures are removed in 2 to 3 weeks. Sexual activity can be resumed when healing is complete, usually in about 3 months.

Complications

Wound breakdown from necrosis of the tissue edges at the suture line is the most frequent complication of radical vulvectomy. It occurs in about half the women who undergo this procedure.

The patient is also at risk for thrombosis in the deep leg veins and therefore for the development of a pulmonary embolism. Leg edema is a long-term complication if there is insufficient development of collateral vascular channels after removal of the saphenous vein.

A decrease in sexual satisfaction may occur after a radical vulvectomy. However, there are many women who maintain the ability to reach orgasm.

Other potential complications include stress incontinence, cystocele, and rectocele. Patients who present with advanced disease or have a recurrence following radical vulvectomy may be candidates for pelvic exenteration (complete removal of pelvic structures) surgery following radiation treatment.

❖ SETTINGS, PROVIDERS AND COLLABORATION FOR CARE

With the pressures of cost-containment limiting the amount of time spent in acute-care settings, women with gynecologic cancer receive more of their care in alternative settings, such as the home and outpatient treatment settings. Care that can be effectively delivered in these settings includes postoperative rest, wound management, ostomy care and teaching, intravenous therapy (analgesia, antibiotics, chemotherapy), and symptom palliation. Outpatient radiation therapy with home care support is also effective and can reduce hospitalization costs. In addition to cost containment, advantages of home care include reduced exposure to pathogens, ready access of social support, more uninterrupted time for rest, and reduced family stress (Lowdermilk, 1995). Coordination among providers in the various settings is needed for appropriate placement and design of care.

NURSING PROCESS
Radical Vulvectomy and Inguinal Lymphadenectomy

PREOPERATIVE NURSING CARE

The assessment, nursing diagnoses, expected patient outcomes, nursing interventions, and evaluation for a patient scheduled for radical vulvectomy and inguinal lymphadenectomy are similar to those for any patient scheduled for major surgery (see Chap. 6), with several considerations.

Carefully assess the condition of the skin and the patient's available strength to assist in positioning herself in bed because the patient's mobility is limited in the days just after surgery.

Also assess nutritional status and determine dietary patterns and food preferences, because a good nutritional intake is necessary postoperatively if the large wound is to heal. Determine the patient's usual pattern of bowel elimination because both diarrhea and constipation must be avoided until the wound heals.

POSTOPERATIVE NURSING CARE

Assessment

After a radical vulvectomy, assessments are those required by any patient who has had an extensive surgical procedure. Take vital signs and check the groin dressing for bleeding every 15 minutes initially. Assess the level of pain. Measure urinary output. Observe drainage from the wound for color and amount. Monitor intravenous fluid intake. Observe the site for signs of infiltration or inflammation. Be alert to any signs of cardiopulmonary or renal dysfunction, because these systems are often compromised in the older person.

As the postoperative period progresses, continue to observe the wound edges for signs of necrosis. When oral intake is re-established, assess the patient's tolerance of it as well as her bowel function because both constipation and diarrhea must be avoided to protect the suture line. With removal of the Foley catheter, assess the patient's ability to initiate urination and empty the bladder. Also note any difficulty with the direction of the urinary stream.

Carefully observe the skin over bony prominences for signs of developing pressure ulcers. Check calves for redness, edema, heat, and pain, which could indicate thrombosis.

Throughout the postoperative period, also assess the patient's emotional state. Note the patient's willingness to talk about the surgery and to look at the wound. Observe nonverbal reactions to these activities.

Nursing Diagnoses and Planning

Nursing diagnoses and related expected patient outcomes commonly applicable to patients who have had a radical vulvectomy include the following:

NDx: Pain related to surgery and thick, taut sutures

Planning: Patient Outcomes
1. Patient states she has less perineal discomfort.
2. Patient moves more easily.
3. Patient defecates and, after the catheter is removed, urinates without signs of undue discomfort.

NDx: Risk for impaired tissue integrity related to pull on and disruption of the suture line

Planning: Patient Outcomes
1. Suture line is intact.
2. Patient maintains a low Fowler's or side-lying position.
3. Patient uses trapeze to move.
4. Patient defecates without straining.

NDx: Risk for infection related to contamination of large vulvar wound

Planning: Patient Outcomes
1. Wound is clean.
2. Purulent drainage is absent.

NDx: Urinary retention related to inability to relax the perineum

Planning: Patient Outcomes
1. Patient initiates voiding on need.
2. Patient empties bladder completely.

NDx: Risk for ineffective airway clearance related to shallow breathing and ineffective coughing

Planning: Patient Outcomes
1. Respirations are quiet and easy.
2. Lungs are clear to auscultation.

NDx: Risk for altered peripheral tissue perfusion related to obstruction of venous flow

Planning: Patient Outcomes
1. Calves are free of redness, pain, edema, and heat.

NDx: Body image disturbance related to the loss of external genitalia and large area of scar tissue

Planning: Patient Outcomes
1. Patient looks at the operative site.
2. Patient asks about care at home and resumption of normal activities.
3. Patient expresses pleasure at visits from significant others.
4. Patient demonstrates interest in grooming and appearance.

NDx: Risk for sexual dysfunction related to loss of external genitalia

Planning: Patient Outcomes
1. Patient asks questions regarding future sexual function.
2. Patient discusses sexual function with her mate.
3. Patient discusses alternate patterns of sexual satisfaction.

NDx: Diversional activity deficit related to long, uncomfortable recovery period

Planning: Patient Outcomes
1. Patient participates in meaningful diversional activities.
2. Patient denies excessive boredom.

NDx: Risk for altered health maintenance related to insufficient knowledge of discharge instructions

Planning: Patient Outcomes
1. Patient lists signs and symptoms that should be reported to the health-care professional.
2. Patient accurately describes measures to prevent leg edema.
3. Patient describes and demonstrates care of the wound.
4. Patient states the date of her follow-up appointment.

Nursing Interventions and Evaluation

NDx: Pain
Because of the location of the surgical wound, the extent of the tissue removed, and the thick, taut sutures needed to hold the wound edges together, pain is a major problem in the groin and perineal area. Consider use of patient-controlled analgesia during the initial postoperative period. Thereafter, administer a milder analgesic as ordered to provide relief. Usually, some analgesic is required until the sutures are removed.

NDx: Risk for impaired tissue integrity
Maintain the patient in a low Fowler's or side-lying position to prevent pull on the suture line and possible disruption. Place a pillow to support her lum-

bar area and a pillow between her legs for maximum comfort. With the patient in a side-lying position, bend the upper leg and support it with a pillow in a slightly forward position. Use an over-the-bed trapeze bar to allow the patient to move herself while controlling the amount of pull on the suture line.

Use a bed cradle to keep the pressure of bed covers away from the operative area.

Prevent constipation because it can cause straining during defecation and pressure on the suture line. Progress the patient from clear fluids to a low-residue diet when gastrointestinal function returns, and give stool softeners as ordered.

NDx: Risk for infection
Keep the wound clean and dry to prevent infection and wound breakdown, which can delay healing for as long as 6 months.

Cleanse the wound by applying a sterile solution of normal saline to the area twice a day using an aseptic syringe or a Water Pik machine. Dry the area with a hair dryer. Sitz baths may be given after the sutures are removed, although reinfection is always a risk.

Change dressings frequently because there is a great deal of drainage from this type of wound, and moisture increases the risk of infection. In addition, uncover the wound and leave it exposed to the air at frequent intervals to allow drying and decrease maceration of the tissues.

Give perineal care after each bowel movement and after each voiding once the Foley catheter is removed. This not only reduces the risk of infection, but the warm solution on the perineal area is soothing and stimulates healing.

Because feces can contaminate the wound, also take care to avoid diarrhea.

NDx: Urinary retention
After the Foley catheter is removed (in 2 to 3 weeks), the patient may have difficulty voiding because of an inability to relax the perineum. When she does void, the stream of urine may be deflected to one side and hit her leg. If the urethral meatus has been adequately positioned and anchored during surgery, this effect simply results from edema and will disappear as healing occurs. In the meantime, instruct the patient to stand when voiding to alleviate the problem.

NDx: Risk for ineffective airway clearance
Teach the patient to cough and deep-breathe every 2 hours to help prevent respiratory complications.

NDx: Risk for altered peripheral tissue perfusion
Monitor use of pneumatic compression stockings or apply antiembolic stockings to prevent thrombus formation. Equip the patient's bed with a footboard, and teach her to do leg exercises every hour while awake and in bed. Change her position frequently. Never use the knee gatch because this produces stasis in the perineal area.

When the patient is ambulatory, instruct her to avoid sitting or standing in one position for a long period of time.

NDx: Body image disturbance
An integral part of the postoperative nursing care of the patient with a radical vulvectomy is the continued provision of psychologic support begun during the preoperative period.

The patient may grieve over the permanent change in her body as a result of loss of pubic hair, loss of other parts of the vulva, or the scar tissue that forms. She may no longer feel feminine, sexually attractive to her partner, or sexually adequate. This grief may be manifested by crying, introspection, withdrawal, or depression. Accept the patient's moods, and allow her to vent her feelings and ask questions. Help the family to understand and accept the patient's behavior.

NDx: Risk for sexual dysfunction
Provide opportunities for the patient to discuss her sexual concerns. Discuss the use of water-soluble lubricants to replace lubrication normally provided by the glands of the vulva as well as methods of attaining sexual satisfaction despite loss of the clitoris.

NDx: Diversional activity deficit
Because the recovery period is long and uncomfortable, the patient can easily become discouraged. To combat this, plan diversional activities on the basis of her stated interests.

NDx: Risk for altered health maintenance
Because healing is not always complete at the time of discharge from the hospital, instruct the patient in self-care (Highlight 41–9). Initiate a referral to a home-care agency if needed.

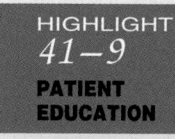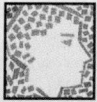

HIGHLIGHT
_41–9_
PATIENT EDUCATION

Discharge Instructions After Radical Vulvectomy

Instruct the patient to:

Clean the wound according to the surgeon's instructions.

Wear support stockings and elevate the legs at frequent intervals to prevent leg edema.

Report bleeding, foul discharge, persistent leg edema, fever, and calf redness, edema, or pain.

Maintain communication with significant other and use social support systems during the recovery period.

Return for checkup on (specify date and time).

Additional Interventions

Use a pressure-reducing device (air, water, foam, or gel) to distribute the patient's weight evenly to make her more comfortable and help prevent skin breakdown (USDHHS, 1992).

If a strong perineal odor exists, as often happens, perform perineal care more frequently and dispose of soiled dressings promptly. Ventilate the room well, and use deodorizers as needed because patients tend to be very sensitive to odors.

Take care not to dislodge the Foley catheter during the 2 to 3 weeks that it is in place because edema in the vulvar area makes it very difficult and painful to reinsert. Pay careful attention to asepsis to prevent urinary tract infection, which is a particular risk because of the extended time the catheter is in place.

Compare the patient's status with expected outcomes. If the outcomes are not met, reassess the patient and revise the plan.

Cancer of the Cervix

Cancer of the cervix is the most common cancer of the female reproductive system. Peak rate of carcinoma in situ is between 20 and 30 years of age. Rates for invasive cervical cancer rise rapidly for African-American women after age 25. Women over age 65 who have not been routinely screened also have high rates of invasive cervical cancer. Increased efforts to screen older poor women, especially African-American women, are needed (National Cancer Institute, 1996b).

Etiology and Pathophysiology

The cause of cancer of the cervix is unknown, but many high-risk factors have been identified. The most important is the human papillomavirus, especially types 16 and 18. Other risk factors include:

• Never having been screened for cervical cancer
• Early age of first sexual intercourse (less than 17 years)
• Early age of first pregnancy
• Multiparity
• History of multiple sexual partners
• History of herpes simplex virus 2 or other sexually transmitted diseases
• Positive human immunodeficiency virus (HIV) status
• African, Mexican, or Native American ethnic background
• Low socioeconomic status
• Cigarette smoking (active and passive)
• Long-term use of oral contraceptives (National Cancer Institute, 1995b).

Ninety percent of all cervical cancers are squamous cell carcinomas. They have a gradual onset, originating with a precursor lesion called dysplasia. These preinvasive abnormalities are referred to as cervical intraepithelial neoplasia (CIN) and are graded as follows:

CIN I: Mild dysplasia (noninvasive, low-grade squamous intraepithelial lesion)
CIN II: Moderate dysplasia (invasive, high-grade squamous intraepithelial lesion)
CIN III: Severe dysplasia (carcinoma in situ, invasive, high-grade squamous intraepithelial lesion)

Dysplasias may regress to normal tissue, may simply persist, or may progress to become invasive carcinoma. The more severe the dysplasia, the more likely it is that an invasive change will occur. HIV-positive women are more likely to have invasive carcinoma (National Cancer Institute, 1995b).

Research is currently ongoing to develop a vaccine to prevent infection from human papillomaviruses, which can lead to the development of cervical cancer (Suzich et al, 1995).

The main routes of spread of cancer of the cervix are into the vaginal mucosa, the myometrium of the uterus, the lymph nodes around the cervix, and by direct extension into other structures of the pelvis, such as the bladder, rectum, and pelvic wall. Distant metastases can occur through the lymphatic or circulatory system, although a predilection to spread within the pelvis seems to exist.

The second form of cervical cancer is adenocarcinoma. This develops in the mucus-producing glands of the cervix. It does not have an identified precursor state. It can be present within the cervix for an extended length of time before detection. It is often recurrent. The method of spread and the treatment are similar to that of squamous carcinoma.

Clinical Manifestations

The first symptom of cancer of the cervix is a thin, watery, blood-tinged vaginal discharge, which in most cases is not even noticed by the patient. Later, the classic symptom of intermittent, painless bleeding between periods develops. This bleeding, which is referred to as contact bleeding because it occurs after sexual intercourse, douching, or other contact, is the symptom usually responsible for the patient seeking health care. If treatment is not begun, the bleeding becomes heavier, more frequent, and of longer duration as the tumor increases in size. The amount and duration of the menses also increase so that, ultimately, the bleeding is continuous.

Late symptoms are related either to spread of the disease within the pelvis or to metastasis to distant organs. Pain referred to the flank or leg occurs if the disease affects the ureters, pelvic wall, or sciatic nerve. Dysuria and hematuria occur if the disease spreads to the bladder. Rectal bleeding occurs if the rectum has been invaded. Extensive spread to the pelvic wall, with blockage of the lymphatic and venous channels, causes edema in the lower extremities. Massive hemorrhage and uremia occur before death.

Diagnosis

Early diagnosis of cervical cancer is of critical importance because it is almost always curable in early stages and almost impossible to cure in late stages. Screening of all at-risk women by a cervical Pap test allows detection of precursor dysplasia or early malignant disease. All women are considered to be at risk for cervical cancer as soon as they either become sexually active or reach 18 to 20 years of age. Their first Pap test should be done at this time.

At one time, it was recommended that the test be repeated on an annual basis. Some clinicians now believe, however, that annual screening is necessary only if the patient is at high risk for cervical cancer based on the risk factors discussed previously. If the patient is not in a high-risk group and results of two initial Pap tests performed 1 year apart are normal, these clinicians believe that the test needs to be done only every 3 years until age 65. Other clinicians continue to believe that all women should have an annual Pap test, especially in view of the false-negative rate, which has been estimated as high as 30%. Women older than age 65 whose Pap test results have always been normal are not considered at risk for the disease, and screening is no longer necessary.

If a Pap test has abnormal results, a repeat test and a colposcopic examination of the cervix are done. Any suspicious-appearing areas undergo biopsy or, if no suspicious areas are seen but results of the repeat Pap test are abnormal, a cold cone biopsy is done, especially if the transformational zone is not visualized.

Diagnosis of cancer of the cervix is based on characteristics of the biopsy specimen.

Management

The plan of medical management for a patient with cervical cancer depends on the stage of the disease (Table 41–3) and the patient's age, desire for childbearing, and general health status.

The usual treatment of carcinoma in situ is either cervical conization, carbon dioxide laser destruction, or hysterectomy. Conization is done when a wide area of normal tissue surrounds the excised malignancy and the patient is young and desires to have children. Laser destruction allows for a controlled eradication of the affected area but it is expensive (Ulmer, 1994). If childbearing is not a concern and the patient is premenopausal, a simple hysterectomy with the ovaries left intact may be done because metastasis from the cervix to the ovary is rare.

A new treatment for CIN is the loop electrosurgical excision procedure, which can be performed under local anesthesia in an outpatient setting. The excision is accomplished when electricity passes through a wire loop positioned on the tissue suspected of pathology.

Invasive cancer of the cervix is usually treated with surgery. If the cancer is Stage I or Stage IIA, and if the patient is young and wishes to maintain

Table 41–3

Staging of Cervical Cancer

Stage	Characteristics
0	Confined to the epithelium (carcinoma in situ)
I	Confined to the cervix
A	Microinvasive cancer
B	Invasive cancer
II	Extends beyond the cervix but does not involve the pelvic wall or lower third of the vagina
A	Involves vagina but not the parametrium
B	Involves the parametrium
III	Extends to lower third of the vagina and may or may not involve the pelvic wall or parametrium; hydronephrosis or a nonfunctioning kidney; no cancer-free space between tumor and pelvic wall on rectal examination
A	Involves lower third of the vagina but not the pelvic wall
B	Involves pelvic wall or parametrium; hydronephrosis or nonfunctioning kidney
IV	Extends beyond the true pelvis or involves the bladder or rectal mucosa
A	Involves adjacent organs
B	Involves distant organs

ovarian function, a radical hysterectomy with pelvic lymph node dissection may be done. See Chapter 40 for a description of a radical hysterectomy (Wertheim's operation) and the related nursing care.

Invasive cancer of the cervix may be treated by either radiation or surgery, or a combination of both.

Pelvic Exenteration

Pelvic exenteration is a radical surgical procedure done most often for advanced or recurrent cancer of the cervix. It is performed only if the cancer is limited to the pelvis and therefore a possibility of cure exists. The patient cannot be elderly or obese and must be able physically to withstand the extensive procedure and psychologically cope with the long recovery period and the changes in body function that result.

There are three types of pelvic exenteration. In a total exenteration, all of the pelvic organs are removed. In women, this includes the vagina, uterus, fallopian tubes, ovaries, bladder, distal ureters, rectum, distal sigmoid colon, internal iliac artery and vein, lymph nodes, and the entire pelvic floor. To allow for bowel function and urinary elimination, a colostomy and an ileal or sigmoid conduit are also performed. An opening is left through the perineum to allow for drainage, which occurs for up to a year after surgery.

In an anterior pelvic exenteration, all of the pelvic structures are removed except the bowel. In a posterior pelvic exenteration, all the pelvic structures are removed except the urinary bladder.

PREOPERATIVE PREPARATION. Before surgery, extensive diagnostic testing is done to rule out metastases beyond the pelvis. If no metastases are found, preparation for the surgical procedure is begun.

Physical preparation includes laxatives, enemas, and antibiotic therapy for 4 to 5 days before surgery. These measures, along with a low-residue diet that is changed to clear liquids 48 hours preoperatively, are designed to empty and disinfect the bowel. Twenty-four to 48 hours preoperatively, a long intestinal tube is passed through the nose into the ileum (see Chap. 21). On the day before surgery, the sites for stoma placement are marked on the abdomen. That evening, an abdominal perineal shave is done. If the patient has poor veins, a subclavian catheter may be inserted.

POSTOPERATIVE COURSE. The patient is usually in an intensive care unit for 3 to 4 days after surgery because of the high risk of shock, cardiac abnormalities, and renal failure. The intestinal tube is kept in place and attached to low suction and the patient is kept on a nothing by mouth (NPO) order until peristalsis returns, usually in 4 to 6 days. When signs of bowel function return, the tube is clamped and clear fluids are given. If no distention occurs, the diet is advanced as tolerated.

The patient receives IV fluids to maintain hydration and replace electrolytes lost as a result of the surgery and the intestinal tube. Albumin is given to decrease edema (IV albumin pulls fluid into the vascular space by osmosis) and to aid in replacing protein that is lost during the first 2 weeks postoperatively.

Respiratory therapy and measures to prevent circulatory complications begin just after surgery. The patient is ambulated within 24 to 48 hours. Care related to the colostomy and ileal conduit is instituted (see Chaps. 21 and 31).

Vaginal intercourse is not possible after this operation unless a plastic surgery procedure is later done to construct an artificial vagina.

NURSING PROCESS GUIDELINES
Pelvic Exenteration

Preoperative and postoperative assessments, nursing diagnoses, expected patient outcomes, nursing interventions, and evaluations for patients undergoing pelvic exenteration are similar to those described previously for patients having a colostomy, a urinary diversion, and a radical hysterectomy with bilateral salpingo-oophorectomy. Several additional interventions also apply.

Keep in mind that pelvic exenteration is a radical procedure done because of extensive underlying pathology. It results in significantly greater changes in body appearance and function than any one of these procedures alone and therefore causes greater physical and psychological stress. It is essential to assess the coping skills of the patient and her significant other. Help her to identify support systems and use them during her period of adjustment. Consideration of a referral for psychological support for the couple should be made before surgery.

Recognize that the patient often experiences an initial period of dependency, followed by a grief reaction over the mutilation of her body. As with any grief reaction, the first stage is shock and disbelief. The patient may deny the body changes and refuse to look at the surgical wounds. As she begins to realize the loss is real, the patient may become depressed and withdrawn or may be angry and hostile. Finally, she begins to participate in care and move toward independence. Progression through these stages is not unidirectional; rather, fluctuations between responses is common. Be alert to mood changes, and be accepting of them.

The patient's sexual adjustment may need additional time and support. Arrange private time for the patient to be alone with her partner. Provide counseling in alternative methods of sexual gratification if desired, because vaginal intercourse is no longer possible.

Radiation Therapy
Irradiation used in the treatment of cancer of the cervix is in the form of internal (intracavitary) therapy, external beam radiation therapy, or both. Intracavitary radiation therapy may be used alone to treat early, small, microinvasive carcinomas of the cervix. A combination of intracavitary radiation therapy and external beam irradiation to the pelvic lymph nodes is the initial treatment of all invasive cervical carcinomas beyond Stage IIA. External beam irradiation may be administered to shrink a very large tumor before the use of intracavitary radiation. In cases where the tumor has invaded the pelvic walls, external beam irradiation is used primarily for its palliative effects. If metastasis to the bone has occurred, radiation therapy is used to decrease the pain.

EXTERNAL BEAM RADIATION THERAPY. External beam radiation therapy and the related nursing care are discussed in Chapter 34.

INTRACAVITARY RADIATION THERAPY. Internal, or intracavitary, radiation is used to irradiate malignant cells in the cervix and the endometrial cavity. The procedure involves insertion of a radiation source, usually cesium, into the vagina and endometrial cavity by means of a specially designed applicator that holds it in place. Intracavitary radiation therapy is well suited for the treatment of cervical lesions because the accessibility of the cervix and the cervical canal allows the radiation source to be placed close to the lesion and a high dose of radiation to be delivered to it. Also, normal cervical and

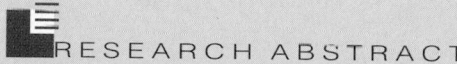

RESEARCH ABSTRACT

What Side Effects of Internal Radiation Therapy Are Most Common?

Fieler VK. Side effects and quality of life in patients receiving high-dose rate brachytherapy. Oncol Nurs Forum 1997; 24(3):545.

Radiation therapy is one intervention used to treat gynecologic cancers. The dose of radiation can be delivered by internal or external methods. *Brachytherapy* is the term used to describe internal methods of delivery of radiation therapy.

Fieler was interested in exploring the relationship between side effects from brachytherapy and perceived quality of life. Her research built on previous studies indicating that patients placed high value on information while undergoing radiation treatment.

Fieler used the Medical Outcome Study (MOS) Short Form Health Survey, a tool with established reliability and validity, to measure the perceived quality of life of her subjects. She also developed two Side Effect Checklists based on the literature, one for the nine subjects in her study undergoing bronchial radiation therapy and one for the 18 subjects undergoing gynecologic radiation therapy.

Fieler asked the patients to self-administer the questionnaires, then analyzed the results for the two groups. The women who received treatment for gynecologic cancers reported fatigue, diarrhea, urinary frequency, and urinary burning as the most frequently experienced side effects. Urinary frequency received the highest severity ratings at three of the six data collection points, including a peak severity at 3 months after treatment. Since the frequency and severity ratings for several of the side effects continued at 3 months after treatment, Fieler suggested that future studies follow patients for a long period.

Scores on the quality-of-life measure did not change significantly over the data collection points, even though the purpose of brachytherapy for some subjects—especially those with bronchial brachytherapy sites—was designed as palliation.

Fieler notes that her research supports previous work on the side effects experienced by people undergoing external beam radiation, although urinary side effects were reported more frequently in her sample.

Fieler suggests that knowledge learned from subjects who undergo brachytherapy can be used to help prepare future patients for what to expect. Such information also helps researchers identify the need for interventions that address the most important patient problems. The National Institute for Nursing Research currently funds studies on symptom management, and studies on the management of brachytherapy-related symptoms might be good candidates for such funding.

Questions to Consider

1. Which of the following types of radiation therapy are available to women in your area: low-dose external beam, low-dose internal beam (brachytherapy), high-dose afterloading?
2. What types of questions do women ask about their anticipated exposure to radiation therapy?
3. In your experience, how common are the side effects reported by the subjects in Fieler's study?
4. What self-care measures do women use to cope with the fatigue of cancer and radiation therapy?
5. What indicators or assessment tools do you use to assess the quality of life of your patients?

---

vaginal tissue is particularly well able to withstand the effects of radiation. This allows administration of a higher dose before adverse effects on normal tissue occur.

PATIENT PREPARATION. Because distention of the bowel or using a bedpan for a bowel movement can change the position of the radiation source relative to adjacent tissues, in preparation for intracavitary radiation therapy, the patient is placed on a low-residue diet and given a cleansing enema. A cleansing douche is also given. An anesthesia workup is done, the patient is placed on NPO status after midnight, and she is premedicated and prepared for transport to the operating room the next morning.

PROCEDURE. Most intracavitary radiation in the United States is given by means of an afterloading device. When such a device is used, the patient is examined under anesthesia in the operating room. The applicator is inserted and held in place with vaginal packing. When the patient has emerged from the anesthesia, an x-ray is taken to verify placement of the applicator. The patient is then returned to her room, where the radiation source is inserted.

This type of system allows strict control of the radiation received by the patient and minimizes radiation exposure of other health-team members through limited, strategic contact with the patient.

A Foley catheter is inserted before the applicator. Catheter drainage is necessary to prevent distention of the bladder and movement of tissues closer to the radiation core.

POSTPROCEDURE COURSE. After insertion, the radiation source remains in place for 48 to 72 hours. During this time, the patient is maintained on strict bedrest. Intravenous fluids are given until oral fluids are tolerated to prevent dehydration, which can easily occur from loss of fluid secondary to the destruction of tissue at the site of irradiation. The patient is progressed to a low-residue diet and anticholinergics (such as diphenoxylate hydrochloride and atropine [Lomotil]), 2 mg four times daily, are given to prevent diarrhea. Antiemetics, such as prochlorperazine maleate (Compazine), are given for nausea, sedatives for sleep, and mild narcotic analgesics for pain.

After removal of the radiation source and the applicator, the patient is given a soapsuds enema and a douche. She is allowed out of bed, returned to a regular diet, and discharged the following day.

COMPLICATIONS. Patients having intracavitary radiation therapy may acquire radiation sickness, with nausea, vomiting, diarrhea, malaise, and fever. (See Chap. 34 for a complete discussion.) Other complications that may occur include cystitis, proctitis, vesicovaginal fistula, ureterovaginal fistula, phlebitis, hemorrhage, chronic radiation enteritis, and burning perineum syndrome (Miaskowski, 1996).

NURSING PROCESS
Intracavitary Radiation Therapy

PREOPERATIVE NURSING CARE

The assessment, nursing diagnoses, expected patient outcomes, nursing interventions, and evaluation for patients scheduled for intracavitary radiation therapy are similar to those for other preoperative patients, with several considerations.

Carefully assess the patient's ability to withstand the limitations imposed by the procedure, and identify appropriate support activities. For example, does she dread 3 days in a private room with limited interpersonal contacts? If so, what diversional activities does she prefer? What is the condition of her skin? Are more than usual measures indicated if she is to complete 2 to 3 days of bedrest without skin breakdown?

Describe what the patient should expect after insertion of the radioactive implant. Prepare her for the indwelling catheter, strict bedrest, and low-residue diet. Give a careful explanation of the lead shield and the limited staff and visitor contact, and assure her that, nonetheless, she will have close supervision.

Explain that nausea, uterine cramping, and foul-smelling vaginal drainage are expected and that medications will be given to make her comfortable.

POSTOPERATIVE NURSING CARE

Assessment

After insertion of the radiation source, assess the patient's vital signs every 4 hours. It is not unusual for temperature to rise above 37.7°C (100°F) on the first evening after insertion as part of the body's response to tissue destruction.

Check for the presence and amount of vaginal bleeding because hemorrhage is a potential complication of the therapy. Determine the amount of discomfort from vaginal cramping and limited mobility, and the effectiveness of medications in providing relief.

Observe the skin over pressure areas for signs of impending breakdown. Especially assess the skin of the buttocks and perineum for erythema, a possible precursor of desquamation.

Monitor for signs of cystitis, proctitis, phlebitis, dehydration, and radiation sickness because all can occur as complications of intracavitary radiation therapy.

Assess how well the patient is coping with the experience. Is she manifesting signs of anxiety, frustration, or depression?

Nursing Diagnoses and Planning

Nursing diagnoses and related expected patient outcomes commonly applicable to patients undergoing intracavitary radiation therapy for cancer of the cervix include the following:

NDx: Risk for injury related to accidental movement of radiation source

Planning: Patient Outcomes
1. Patient stays in flat, dorsal position.
2. Bladder distention is absent.

NDx: Pain related to uterine contractions and limited movement

Planning: Patient Outcomes
1. Patient appears comfortable. She does not grimace, moan, clench fist, or hold abdomen.
2. Patient states that she has less cramping.

NDx: Risk for fluid volume deficit related to abnormal fluid loss secondary to tissue destruction at the site of irradiation

Planning: Patient Outcomes
1. Patient has a fluid intake of at least 3000 mL/day.
2. Mucous membranes are moist.
3. Skin turgor is elastic.

NDx: Risk for altered health maintenance related to insufficient knowledge of discharge instructions

Planning: Patient Outcomes
1. Patient describes and demonstrates douche pro-

cedure, indicating when and how it is to be done, what solution is to be used, and how the equipment is to be cleaned.

2. Patient states when sexual intercourse can be resumed.
3. Patient lists symptoms to be reported.
4. Patient states date and time of follow-up appointment.

Nursing Interventions and Evaluation

Protection of the nurse, visitors, and other hospital personnel from excessive exposure to radiation is an essential part of nursing care for the patient receiving intracavitary radiation. Place the patient in a private room, preferably at the end of a corridor where there is little traffic, and place signs on the door indicating that radiation is in use. If a private room is absolutely not available, the patient may be placed in a semiprivate room provided the other patient is postmenopausal or has had a bilateral oophorectomy.

Do not allow pregnant nurses, pregnant visitors, or persons younger than 18 years in the patient's room. Plan to work as far from the radiation source as possible and to keep the lead shield between you and the radiation source at all times.

Spend time on the day of admission orienting the patient to the call system, radio, television, and general hospital routines. Also teach exercises to be done during the days of the treatment to help eliminate the need for reteaching when the radiation source is in place and time spent at the bedside must be limited.

Always be well organized so that quality care can be given in the least possible amount of time. Remember that urine, feces, soiled linens, dressings, and the like are not radioactive. (See Chap. 34 for additional discussion of precautions related to radiation.)

NDx: Risk for injury

Maintain the patient on absolute bedrest in the dorsal position after insertion to prevent movement of the radiation source. Elevate the head of the bed to a maximum of 10 to 15 degrees for comfort. Avoid turning the patient on her side. If turning is absolutely necessary, place a pillow between her knees and, with her body in straight alignment, roll her like a log.

Use a fracture pan if the patient needs to have a bowel movement despite the cleansing enema, low-residue diet, and anticholinergic drugs.

NDx: Pain

Give narcotics as ordered at regular intervals for uterine contractions, which result from the presence of the applicator in the dilated cervical canal. Administer antiemetics as ordered for nausea. Encourage relaxation exercises and use of distraction.

NDx: Risk for fluid volume deficit

Determine what fluids appeal to the patient, and make them accessible. Encourage her to drink at least 3000 mL/day to prevent dehydration from fluid loss at the site because of tissue destruction by the radiation. Fluid also relieves bladder irritation. Record intake and output.

NDx: Risk for altered health maintenance

Instruct the patient in self-care after discharge (Highlight 41–10).

Additional Interventions

Bathe the patient's upper body, and give a partial back rub to provide comfort and improve circulation to the skin. Do not bathe below her waist unless she is soiled.

Use a pressure-reducing surface (air, foam, water, or gel) to help prevent pressure ulcers. Provide a footboard, and instruct the patient to perform foot and leg exercises every hour while awake to

---

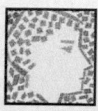

**HIGHLIGHT
41–10

PATIENT
EDUCATION**

Discharge Instructions After Intracavitary Radiation for Cancer of the Cervix

Explain to the patient the following information:

Expect some vaginal bleeding for 1 to 3 months after irradiation.

Foul-smelling vaginal discharge will occur for some time.

Douches are to be taken according to physician's order. (Specify the solution to be used and the frequency with which douching should be done. Demonstrate proper technique for performing the procedure and for cleaning the equipment. Request a return demonstration).

Use emollient cream to ease pruritus.

Sexual intercourse may be resumed in 7 to 10 days, depending on the condition of the cervix and the vagina. Intercourse may be difficult because radiation therapy can cause vaginal atrophy.

Instruct the patient to:

Report any persistent sexual difficulties because vaginal dilatation may be required.

Report persistent rectal irritation.

Return for a follow-up appointment on *(specify date and time)*.

stimulate venous return. Encourage range-of-motion exercises for the arms.

Compare the patient's status with expected outcomes. If the outcomes are not met, reassess the patient and revise the plan.

Chemotherapy

Chemotherapy is usually not effective in the treatment of cancer of the cervix. This is partly because most of these cancers are squamous cell adenomas, which are typically unresponsive to chemotherapy, and partly because the malignancies being treated are in an area that was previously irradiated and therefore lacks sufficient blood supply to deliver chemotherapeutic agents to the area in the concentration needed for an effect.

When chemotherapy is used, it consists of drugs such as hydroxyurea used in combination with radiation treatment. Clinical trials with such drugs as cisplatin and ifosfamide are underway, especially for patients with Stage IV disease. Fluorouracil and mitomycin may be tried for patients with recurrent disease. (See Chap. 34 for a discussion of the principles of chemotherapy and the nursing care of patients receiving it.)

Cancer of the Uterus

Adenocarcinoma of the endometrium is the most common gynecologic cancer in the United States. The number of women with endometrial cancer has been increasing since the 1960s. Factors that are thought to account for this increased incidence include better detection, an increase in the number of women living to the time of life when the disease is most likely to occur, and the use of estrogen (without progesterone) replacement therapy after menopause.

The highest incidence of cancer of the uterine body occurs in postmenopausal women. It is more likely to occur in women who are obese, nulliparous, diabetic, or who had a late menopause.

Etiology and Pathophysiology

Most malignant tumors affecting the body of the uterus are adenocarcinomas (carcinoma involving the glandular tissue), which are believed to develop from areas of hyperplastic endometrium. This hyperplasia is an overgrowth of endometrial glands and stroma. It is thought to result from prolonged, persistent estrogen stimulation such as occurs from successive anovulatory menstrual cycles or exogenous estrogen therapy. Hyperplasia does not always result in adenocarcinoma, but when it does, the change occurs over a period of 5 years or more.

Adenocarcinoma of the uterus is staged according to the areas involved and the histologic type of the tumor. The stages are as follows:

Stage I: Cancer is confined to the body of the uterus. This stage is further subdivided into G1, highly differentiated; G2, differentiated with some solid areas; and G3, completely undifferentiated or predominantly solid.

Stage II: Cancer involves both the body of the uterus and the cervix.

Stage III: Cancer extends outside the uterine body but not outside the true pelvis. The bladder and rectum are not affected.

Stage IV: Cancer involves the bladder or rectum or extends outside the true pelvis.

Uterine adenocarcinoma is a slow-growing tumor. Prognosis is best when the tumor is limited to the body of the uterus and is highly differentiated (Stage I, G1). The prognosis worsens with involvement of the cervix (Stage II), loss of differentiation (G2 and G3), and deep invasion of the myometrium.

Metastases to the pelvic lymph nodes are common. They are seen in about 11% of patients with Stage I disease and 36% of those with Stage II.

Clinical Manifestations

Abnormal uterine bleeding is the primary indicator of endometrial cancer. This is most often postmenopausal bleeding because the greatest incidence of the disease is in women over age 50. The bleeding is sometimes profuse and may be accompanied by lower abdominal cramping and expulsion of clots. Premenopausal women usually have prolonged heavy periods and intermenstrual bleeding, which is usually painless.

Diagnosis

An endometrial biopsy, which is 90% accurate and can be done on an outpatient basis, is commonly used to diagnose endometrial cancer (Warner & Parsons, 1996). Pap tests are not reliable in diagnosing endometrial carcinoma because tumor cells are not shed until late in the disease. Staging (0–IV) is done to determine the best treatment regimen.

Management

The basic treatment of uterine cancer is total abdominal hysterectomy and bilateral salpingo-oophorectomy. In addition, preoperative or postoperative radiation therapy is frequently used. This may be in the form of vaginal radium implants or external beam irradiation to the whole pelvis. Depending on the extent of the disease, radical hysterectomy or pelvic lymphadenectomy, or both, may be done. Chemotherapy in the form of doxorubicin and cisplatin, alone or in combination, may be used as an adjunct to surgery and radiation therapy. When the malignancy is extensive (Stages III and IV), hormone therapy in the form of large doses of a progestin may be given. Hormone therapy is continued for as long as the patient shows an objective, positive response. Tamoxifen has been used for patients who do not respond to progestins (National Cancer Institute, 1995f).

NURSING PROCESS GUIDELINES
Uterine Cancer

Nursing care of patients with cancer of the uterine body is similar to that described previously for patients with a diagnosis of any type of malignancy. Additional nursing considerations relate to the plan of medical treatment. When surgery is done, the principles of nursing care for a patient having a hysterectomy with a bilateral salpingo-oophorectomy apply. If internal or external radiation therapy is used, then the principles of nursing care for a patient undergoing this treatment modality apply.

Because cancer of the uterine body occurs most often in older women, consider two items specifically when assessing the patient and planning her care. First, if she has not had routine gynecologic examinations since her last child was born or since menopause occurred, she may blame herself for her diagnosis. Second, older women in our society are erroneously perceived as asexual. As a result, they tend to hesitate to raise issues relating to sexual function because they fear the reaction of other people. To ensure that the patient receives the information she needs, open the topic to discussion and thus acknowledge to the patient that sexual concerns are normal and appropriate.

Cancer of the Ovary

Cancer of the ovary is an insidious disease with a poor prognosis because symptoms do not occur until the cancer is well advanced. Although it can occur at any age, the greatest incidence is between ages 50 and 59.

Etiology and Pathophysiology
The cause of ovarian cancer is not known, although hormonal stimulation, environmental factors, and familial tendencies are all considered possible factors in its development. Factors that appear to decrease the risk of ovarian cancer include use of oral contraceptives, childbearing, breastfeeding, history of a tubal ligation or hysterectomy, and a low-fat diet (National Cancer Institute, 1996c). A definite relationship between the risks for ovarian cancer and a woman's lifetime number of ovulations has been documented, along with a strong association between a high number of ovulations and a mutated tumor suppressor gene called p53, which is a factor in about two-thirds of all ovarian cancers (Schildkraut et al, 1997). Thus, it appears that factors such as pregnancy, use of oral contraceptives, and breast feeding, which suppress ovulation, decrease the risk of ovarian cancer by decreasing the risk for mutation of gene p53. There appears to be some etiologic relationship between ovarian cancer and breast cancer because breast cancer is three to four times more likely to develop in women who have ovarian cancer than in other women.

Ovarian cancers spread easily throughout the peritoneal cavity. Spread is said to be local when it involves the fallopian tubes, uterus, or broad ligament. Spread is termed regional when it involves the pelvic peritoneum, bladder, sigmoid colon, rectum, or pelvic side wall. It is called abdominal when it involves the omentum, bowel, liver, or diaphragm. Spread out of the abdomen to areas such as the lungs or bone is uncommon.

Clinical Manifestations
Unfortunately, ovarian cancer rarely causes symptoms until there has been extensive growth of the tumor. When symptoms do occur, they result primarily from the pressure of the tumor on other pelvic organs and are similar to the symptoms that occur with benign neoplasms.

Symptoms include a feeling of pelvic pressure or heaviness, vague abdominal discomfort, dyspepsia, bloating, constipation, urinary frequency, dyspareunia, and an increase in the size of the abdomen. In late stages of the disease, weight loss is evident and symptoms arise that are related to organs affected by metastasis.

Diagnosis
There is no method in use to screen for and diagnose ovarian cancer in its early stages. Transvaginal ultrasonography, color Doppler studies, and the serum tumor marker CA-125 have been considered along with the Pap smear for ovarian cancer but they are not economically feasible for use as screening tests at this time.

A presumptive diagnosis of ovarian cancer is made when a hard, fixed, firm mass is palpated in the area of the ovary during a pelvic examination. In postmenopausal women, whose ovaries are normally atrophied, palpation of the ovary itself leads to a suspicion of ovarian cancer.

Laboratory tests, x-rays, and laparoscopy are used to rule out other pelvic diseases but not to diagnose cancer of the ovary. Diagnosis is confirmed and the stage of disease determined by exploratory laparotomy and examination of tissue specimens by a pathologist. The latter includes examination of ascitic fluid or, if none is encountered, examination of peritoneal washings.

Management
Total abdominal hysterectomy with bilateral salpingo-oophorectomy with or without omentectomy is the basic treatment for early ovarian cancer. Both ovaries are removed because of the frequency of bilateral tumors. The uterus is removed because the serosa and endometrium are common sites of metastasis. If the disease is advanced (not localized), as much tumor as possible is also removed (debulking). Consideration for preservation of childbearing capacity may be given to women with early Stage I disease (NIH Consensus Development Panel, 1995).

Postoperatively, some form of systemic chemotherapy (cisplatin and cyclophosphamide) or radiation (intraperitoneal ^{32}P or abdominal/pelvic irradiation) is usually prescribed, depending on the stage of the disease. Early Stage I disease does not require additional treatment. (See Chap. 34 for a discussion of chemotherapy.)

Patients with Stage III disease who complete a course of chemotherapy, have a negative CT scan, and have no clinical symptoms of disease may have a "second-look" procedure done to determine whether they have a possible cure or whether there is asymptomatic disease still present that requires the continuation of chemotherapy. In these cases, a laparoscopy is done first. If tumor is seen, obviously therapy must continue. If disease is not seen, a laparotomy is performed to allow more thorough examination.

Recurrent ovarian cancer resistant to cisplatin may be treated with paclitaxel (NIH Consensus Development Panel, 1995). Intraperitoneal administration of chemotherapy agents, such as paclitaxel, is under investigation as adjuvant therapy.

Because of the lack of a strong standard approach to the treatment of ovarian cancer, patients are often encouraged to participate in clinical trials of new protocols (National Cancer Institute, 1995c).

NURSING PROCESS GUIDELINES
Ovarian Cancer

Nursing care of patients with ovarian cancer is similar to that described previously for patients with other types of cancer and to that described previously for patients having a hysterectomy with bilateral salpingo-oophorectomy. Several additional interventions also apply.

Because patients with cancer of the ovary have an increased chance of acquiring cancer of the breast, counsel on the need for monthly breast self-examination and the importance of an annual mammogram. If needed, teach the method of breast self-examination, and obtain a return demonstration.

When caring for a patient having a second-look procedure, expect the patient to be highly anxious. Provide her the opportunity to verbalize her worries. If the procedure discloses further malignancy, allow the patient to ventilate her feelings about the recurrence of the cancer and offer support to her significant others.

The Elderly: Special Considerations

Reproductive disorders of aging women may be classified into two groups:

1. Those that, for unknown reasons, occur almost exclusively in older women.
2. Those that can occur at any age but for which age-related factors increase the risk.

Disorders in group 1 include cancer of the ovary, uterus, and vulva. Cancer of the ovary, which tends to occur in women who have not been pregnant, has the highest mortality of any cancer of the female reproductive system. Its poor prognosis relates to the fact that there are no symptoms until very late in the disease, so diagnosis is often delayed.

Cancer of the uterus, whose first symptom is vaginal bleeding, is most common in women who are obese, nulliparous, diabetic, or who have a history of anovulation, amenorrhea, or late menopause.

Vulvar carcinoma appears first as simply pruritus or as a small lesion on the vulvar skin. More than half the time, this cancer is diagnosed on a routine screening examination.

Disorders for which age-related factors increase risk include vaginitis and symptomatic weakened pelvic supports.

Thinning of the vaginal epithelium, which results from decreased estrogen after menopause, increases the risk of vaginitis. Adding to this is the fact that systemic diseases (such as diabetes) that predispose to vaginitis are more often present in the aged.

Symptomatic weakened pelvic supports tend to be a problem in aging women because the initial damage caused by childbirth is worsened by weakening of the pelvic diaphragm and loss of elasticity and strength of fascia, which occurs with age.

Morbidity and mortality from these disorders could be dramatically reduced by early diagnosis and treatment. Unfortunately, many women do not have routine gynecologic examinations after menopause. One reason for this is a lack of knowledge. Some older women are simply not aware that there are serious reproductive disorders that occur late in life and that can be diagnosed early only by a gynecologic examination.

A second reason is the prevalent view in our society that all sexually related activities or concerns are taboo for the aging woman. This misconception can generate feelings of embarrassment and guilt, making the woman reluctant to seek medical care.

The implications for nursing are clear. Teach women the importance of obtaining routine gynecologic examinations throughout life. Also teach the importance of obtaining immediate medical care for symptoms such as bleeding, vaginal discharge, and dyspareunia or pelvic pain.

Correct the perception of older women as being without sexual desires or needs. Treat older women seeking care for a reproductive tract disorder in a sensitive, serious manner.

Chapter Review

1. What information would you include in a teaching plan for women with inflammation of the external genitalia?
2. How are menstrual logs used in diag-

nosing and managing premenstrual syndrome?

3. What information will a woman receiving hormone therapy for endometriosis need to know?

4. What instructions would help a woman understand and practice pelvic floor exercises?

5. What nursing interventions would assist a woman with a genitourinary fistula to cope with her symptoms while awaiting spontaneous healing?

6. What nursing interventions are used to prevent physiologic complications of a radical vulvectomy?

7. What are the major treatment differences between carcinoma in situ and invasive cancer of the cervix?

8. What are the advantages and disadvantages to providing home care for women after gynecologic surgery?

9. What psychosocial considerations are important in caring for a woman having a pelvic exenteration?

10. What social stereotypes might prevent older women from receiving comprehensive care for disorders related to the reproductive organs?

Bibliography

Barnhart KT, Freeman EW, Sandheimer SJ. A clinician's guide to the premenstrual syndrome. Med Clin N Am 1995; 79(6):1457.

Berek J. Practical gynecologic oncology. Baltimore: Williams & Wilkins, 1994.

Bran DF, Spellman JR, Summitt RL. Outpatient vaginal hysterectomy as a new trend in gynecology. AORN Journal 1995; 62(5):810.

Carpenito LJ. Nursing diagnosis: Application to clinical practice. 4th ed. Philadelphia: JB Lippincott, 1995.

Cartwright-Alcarese F. Addressing sexual dysfunction following radiation therapy for a gynecologic malignancy. Oncol Nurs Forum 1995; 22(8):1227.

Chikotas N, Dempster J. Secondary amenorrhea. J Am Acad Nurse Pract 1995; 7(9):453.

Creehan PA. Toxic shock syndrome: An opportunity for nursing intervention. JOGNN 1995; 24(6):557.

Eisenhauer LA. A typology of nursing therapeutics. Image J Nurs Sch 1994; 26(4):261.

Galindo D, Kaiser FE. Sexual health after 60. Patient Care 1995; 29(7):25.

Garry R. Good practice with endometrial ablation. Obstet & Gynecol 1995; 86(1):144.

Gurfolino V, Dumas L. Hospice nursing: The concept of palliative care. Nurs Clin North Am 1994; 29(3):533.

Guyton AC. Textbook of medical physiology. 9th ed. Philadelphia: WB Saunders, 1996.

Jones HW, Wentz GS (eds). Novak's textbook of gynecology. 11th ed. Baltimore: Williams & Wilkins, 1988.

Kaufman RH, Friedrich EG, Gardner HL (eds). Benign diseases of the vulva and vagina. 4th ed. Chicago: Year Book Medical Publishers, 1994.

Kornblith AB, Thaler HT, Wong G, et al. Quality of life of women with ovarian cancer. Gynecol Oncol 1995; 59:231.

Kuhns-Hastings J. Management of female incontinence with Kegel exercises. AAOHN J 1988; 36(2):78.

Lowdermilk, DL. Home care of the patient with gynecologic cancer. JOGNN 1995; 24(2):157.

Lubkin LM. Chronic illness: Impact and interventions. 3rd ed. Boston: Jones and Bartlett Publishers, 1995.

Mastrangelo R. Taming the beast known as PMS. Adv Nurse Pract 1994; 2(10):11.

McCloskey JC, Bulechek GM (eds). Nursing interventions classification (NIC). 2nd ed. St. Louis: Mosby Year-Book, 1996.

Miaskowski C. Special needs related to the pain and discomfort of patients with gynecological cancer. JOGNN 1996; 25(2):181.

Miller B, Morris M, Levenback C, et al. Pelvic exenteration for primary and recurrent vulvar cancer. Gynecol Oncol 1995; 58:202.

Mishell DR, Brenner PF (eds). Management of common problems in obstetrics and gynecology. 3rd ed. Boston: Blackwell Scientific Publications, 1994.

NAACOG, the Organization for Obstetric, Gynecologic, and Neonatal Nursing. NAACOG Standards for the nursing care of women and newborns. 4th ed. Washington, DC: Author 1991.

National Cancer Institute. Cervical cancer 208/00103. PDQ Treatment Statements for Physicians. Available [gopher:/gopher.nih.gov:70/00/clin/cancernet/pdqinfo/soa/Cervical%20cancer_Physician], 1996a.

National Cancer Institute. Paclitaxel 208/02424. PDQ Drug Information Statement. Available [gopher://gopher.nih.gov:70/00/clin/cancernet/pdqinfo/drugs/Paclitaxel], 1995a.

National Cancer Institute. Prevention of cervical cancer 208/04734. PDQ Screening/Prevention Statements. Available [gopher://gopher.nih.gov:70/00/clin/cancernet/pdqinfo/screening/Prevention%20of%20cervical%20cancer], 1995b.

National Cancer Institute. Prevention of ovarian cancer 208/05375. PDQ Supportive Care/Screening/Prevention Information. Available [gopher://gopher.nih.gov:70/00/clin/cancernet/pdqinfo/screening/Prevention%20of%20ovarian%20cancer], 1995c.

National Cancer Institute. Screening for cervical cancer 208/04728. PDQ Supportive Care/Screening/Prevention Information. Available [gopher://gopher.nih.gov:70/00/clin/cancernet/pdqinfo/screening/Screening%20for%20cervical%20cancer], 1996b.

National Cancer Institute. Screening for ovarian cancer 208/05145. PDQ Supportive Care/Screening/Prevention Information. Available [gopher://gopher.nih.gov:70/00/clin/cancernet/pdqinfo/screening/Screening%20for%20ovarian%20cancer], 1995d.

National Cancer Institute. Treatment for ovarian epithelial cancer 208/00950. PDQ Treatment Statements for Physicians. Available [gopher://gopher.nih.gov:70/00/clin/cancernet/pdqinfo/soa/Ovarian%20epithelial%20cancer_Physician], 1996c.

National Cancer Institute. Treatment of endometrial cancer 208/01176. PDQ Treatment Statements for Physicians. Available [gopher://gopher.nih.gov:70/00/clin/cancernet/pdqinfo/soa/Endometrial%20cancer_Physician], 1995e.

National Cancer Institute. Treatment of uterine sarcoma 208/03371. PDQ Treatment Statements for Physicians. Available [gopher://gopher.nih.gov:70/00/clin/cancernet/pdqinfo/soa/Uterine%20sarcoma_Physician], 1995f.

National Cancer Institute. Vulvar cancer 208/01038. PDQ Treatment Statements for Physicians. Available [gopher:/gopher.nih.gov:70/00/clin/cancernet/pdqinfo/soa/Vulvar%20cancer_Physician], 1996d.

Neufeld KR, Degner LF, Dick JAM. A nursing intervention strategy to foster patient involvement in treatment decisions. Oncol Nurs Forum 1993; 20(4):631.

NIH Consensus Development Panel. Ovarian cancer: Screening, treatment, and follow-up. JAMA 1995; 273(6):491.

Orr JW, Shingleton HM. Complications of gynecologic surgery: Prevention, recognition, and management. Philadelphia: JB Lippincott, 1994.

Schildkraut JM, Bastos E, Berchuck A. Relationship between lifetime ovulatory cycles and over-expression for mutant p53 in epithelial ovarian cancer. J Natl Cancer Inst 1997; 89(13):932.

Star WL, Lommel LL, Shannon MT. (eds) Women's primary health protocols for practice. Washington, DC: American Nurses Publishing, 1995.

Suzich JA, Ghim SJ, Palmer-Hill FJ, et al. Systemic immunization with papillomavirus L1 protein completely prevents development of viral mucosal papillomas. Proc Natl Acad Sci U S A 1995; 92(25):11553.

Thompson JD, Rock J. Te Linde's operative gynecology. 7th ed. Philadelphia: JB Lippincott, 1992.

Ulmer BC. Cervical intraepithelial neoplasia. AORN J 1994; 59(4): 851.

U.S. Department of Health and Human Services, Public Health Service, Agency for Health Care Policy and Research. Management of cancer pain. Rockville, MD, 1994. (AHCPR Pub. No. 94-0592).

U.S. Department of Health and Human Services, Public Health Service, Agency for Health Care Policy and Research. Pressure ulcers in adults: Prediction and prevention. Rockville, MD, 1992. (AHCPR Pub. No. 92-0047).

Warner EA, Parsons AK. Screening and early diagnoses of gynecologic cancers. Med Clin N Am 1996; 80(1):45.

Willson JR. Obstetrics and Gynecology. 9th ed. St. Louis: CV Mosby, 1991.

Zivnuska J. Endometriosis: An overview of diagnosis and treatment. Adv Nurse Pract 1995; 3(1):15.

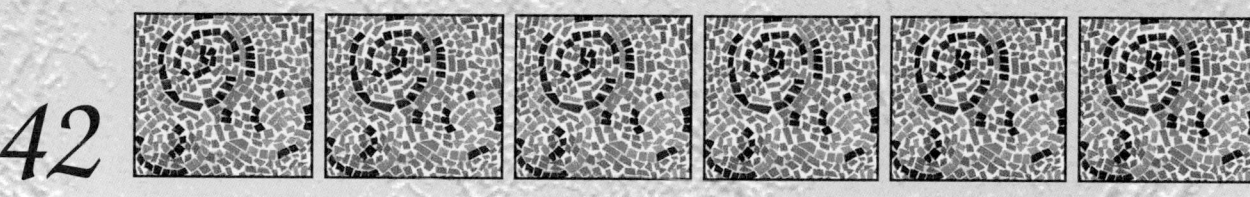

Nursing Care of Patients with Breast Disorders

Study Outcomes

After studying this chapter, you should be able to:

1. Explain the normal anatomy and physiology of the breast.
2. Identify information and physical examination data essential to the assessment of the breast.
3. Describe basic diagnostic tests used in the management of breast disorders.
4. Describe the etiology, pathophysiology, clinical manifestations, diagnostic procedures, and collaborative management of common breast disorders.
5. Identify information and physical examination data essential to the assessment of patients with common breast disorders.
6. State nursing diagnoses and related expected patient outcomes commonly applicable to patients with breast disorders.
7. Describe nursing interventions, with their rationales, commonly applicable to patients with breast disorders.
8. Explain the basis for evaluation of nursing care provided to patients with common breast disorders.
9. Identify alternative treatment and care settings for patients with breast disorders and the services related to community-based care.
10. Identify special considerations for the elderly patient with a breast disorder.

Breast-related concerns represent one of the most common reasons for women to seek health care. This is due in part to the many media campaigns designed to heighten awareness of the increasing incidence of breast cancer in the United States and of the positive relationship between early detection and cure. Unfortunately, this heightened awareness is often accompanied by heightened anxiety. Thus, the nursing care of any woman presenting with a breast concern requires sensitivity to her anxieties and fears. It also requires individualized health teaching to place the patient's concerns in proper perspective while encouraging her to continue practicing positive health-seeking behaviors.

Social and economic changes have dramatically altered the health-care delivery system in the United States. Thus, patients with breast disorders now seek care in a variety of delivery settings, and a greater variety of health-care professionals may become involved with their care. With early hospital discharge and much patient care being delivered in outpatient and home-care settings, patients and their families may move quickly from one setting to another. These changes present new challenges to the nurse to provide continuity of care for women undergoing treatment.

Anatomy and Physiology

EXTERNAL ANATOMY

The breasts are paired specialized glands shaped like cones. They are situated on the anterior chest from the second or third rib to the sixth or seventh rib and extend from the sternal edge to the midaxillary line (Fig. 42–1). Two-thirds of the breast lies over the pectoralis major muscle. The remaining one-third lies over the serratus muscle. The nipple is located centrally and is surrounded by the areola.

The breasts are generally symmetric; however, it is not unusual to observe slight differences in size and shape. The skin that covers the breasts is identical to the skin on the rest of the body. The skin of the nipple and areola is deeply pigmented.

For purposes of description, each breast is divided into four quadrants: upper outer quadrant (UOQ), upper inner quadrant (UIQ), lower outer quadrant (LOQ), and lower inner quadrant (LIQ), as shown in Figure 42–2. The quadrants are delimited by imaginary lines that cross at the nipple. The vertical line extends from the 12 o'clock position to the 6 o'clock position, and the horizontal line extends from the 3 o'clock position to the 9 o'clock position. The "tail" of the breast reaches into the axilla.

INTERNAL ANATOMY

The breast is made up of three types of tissue: glandular tissue, fibrous tissue, and fat (Fig. 42–3). The

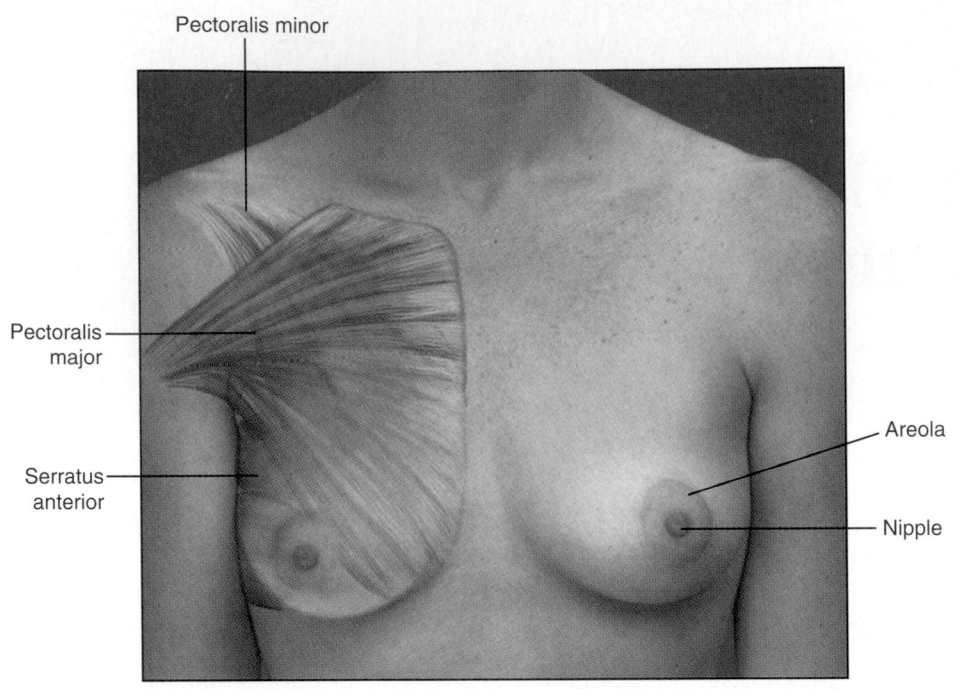

Figure 42–1

Position of breasts on chest wall.

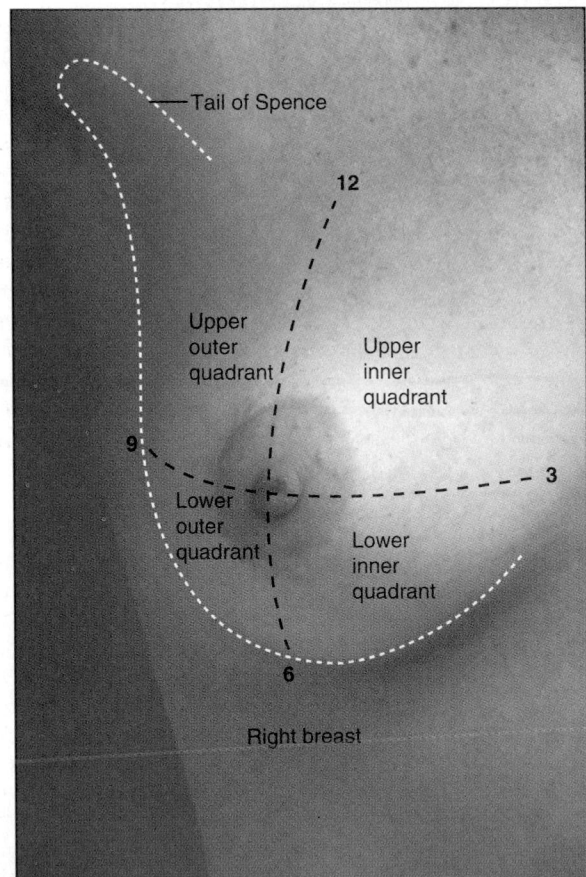

Figure 42–2

Four quadrants of the breast, including the upper outer quadrant, lower outer quadrant, and lower inner quadrant, and upper inner quadrant, and tail of Spence.

proportions of these tissues vary based on a number of factors, including age, stage of the reproductive cycle, and nutritional status of the person. Glandular tissue forms 12 to 20 lobes which branch into 50 to 60 lobules. The lobes are arranged in a circular pattern and are lined with milk-producing structures called acini. Each lobule ends in a duct called a lactiferous sinus. During lactation, the breast's complex ductal system secretes colostrum and milk to the surface of the nipple through contraction of smooth muscle. The glandular tissue is supported by fibrous tissue. This fibrous tissue includes ligaments

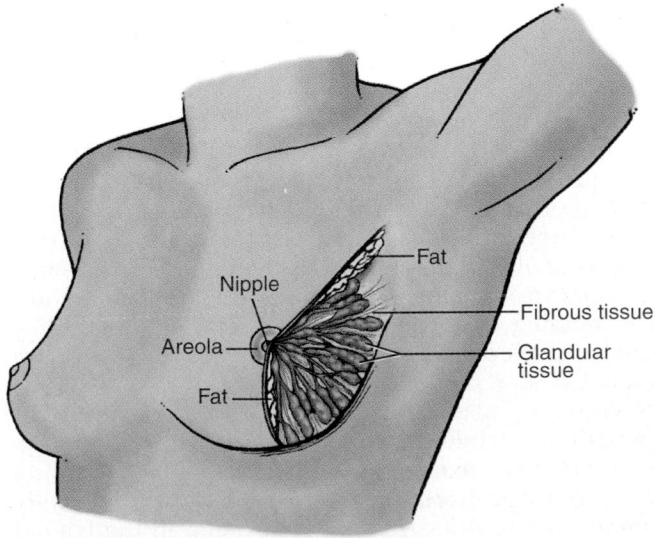

Figure 42–3

Anatomy of a normal breast.

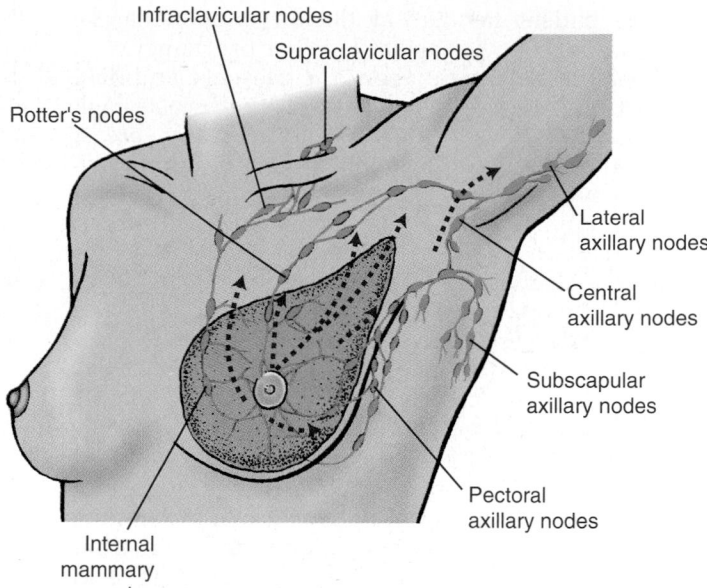

Figure 42–4
Lymphatic drainage of the breast.

called Cooper's ligaments, which are connected to the skin and chest wall underneath the breast. The fibrous tissue has the ability to elongate and increase in volume as the breast grows, especially in response to pregnancy and lactation. The third and most predominant tissue of the breast is fat. Fat cells can be found throughout the breast and serve to cushion the glandular and fibrous tissue.

The venous and lymphatic systems of the breast work together to protect the organ from bacteria, viruses, and such foreign tissue as tumor cells. Blood reaches the breast through the internal mammary artery. The lymphatic vessels have multiple draining pathways throughout the breast (Fig. 42–4). The majority of lymph nodes are in the axillary region. These include the pectoral, subscapular, lateral, and central axillary lymph nodes. The axillary lymph nodes and internal mammary nodes under the sternum drain into the infraclavicular and then into the supraclavicular lymph nodes.

PHYSIOLOGY

The growth and development of the female breast is a dynamic, continuous process that begins during intrauterine life, progresses through puberty and adulthood, and regresses after menopause. The hormonal system, along with factors of heredity, aging, and nutrition, is responsible for the growth and development of the breast. The onset of puberty stimulates the ductile tissue to produce the basic structures of the adult breast. Normal breast development also requires the production of prolactin and growth hormone by the anterior pituitary gland.

During the menstrual cycle, the internal structures of the breast may be affected by fluctuating concentrations of estrogen and progesterone. This can result in increased breast tenderness, heaviness, nodularity, and mild pain before and during menstruation.

The breast of the older woman changes based on individual physiology and the termination of ovarian function after menopause. This leads to structural changes in the breast known as involution. Glandular tissue undergoes significant reduction, with an increase in fat deposits and connective tissue. As the tissue atrophies, the breasts may lose their elasticity, resulting in sagging, smaller, and less dense breasts. The breasts begin to look and feel different as the lobular and alveolar structures decrease. In the aged adult, only small areas of tissue remain, surrounded by hard, fibrous connective tissue. These normal breast adaptations may mimic breast cancer in some older women and should certainly be differentiated from other suspicious lesions.

*A*ssessment of the Breast

PATIENT HISTORY

When assessing the breasts, start by asking about any family history of breast disease. Note the type of disorder and the relationship of the affected persons to the patient. Obtain information about any personal history of breast disease. Note the type of problem, dates of occurrence, treatment, and outcome. Determine the date and result of the patient's last mammogram and the time of the last breast self-examination. Obtain the date of the last menstrual period to determine the place in the menstrual cycle.

Ask the patient her age at the onset of menarche and, if applicable, her age at her first pregnancy.

Question the patient about the presence and date of onset of any current problems in the breasts. Ask the patient whether she has noticed any breast lumps. If so, note the location, when the lump was first discovered, and whether any changes occur in the lump in relationship to menses. Inquire about the occurrence of breast tenderness, discharge, or swelling. Ask the patient whether she is breast-feeding. Ask the patient whether she has noticed any axillary tenderness, lumps, or rash.

PHYSICAL EXAMINATION

Examination of the breasts includes inspection and palpation of each breast, nipple, and axillary region. Conduct the examination in a comfortable environment. Make sure the room is warm, private, and quiet. Ask the patient to remove her clothing from the waist up and provide her with a cover that opens in the front. Tell the patient what the procedure will entail and establish a supportive relationship. Begin the examination with the patient in a sitting position with arms at her sides. Inspect the breasts for size, symmetry, contour, skin color and texture, venous patterns, and lesions. Note any asymmetry, swelling, rashes, scars, ulcerations, lesions, dimpling, lumps, or unusual surface phenomena. Inspect the areola for shape, color, hair, and masses. Observe the nipples and note their size, shape, and symmetry and the direction in which they point. Also observe for retraction, rashes, skin changes, and discharge. Inspect axillae for hair distribution, cleanliness, discoloration, bulging, retraction, edema, observable masses, rashes, and ulcerations. Inspect the breasts with the patient in the following positions: (1) seated with arms at sides, (2) seated with arms over head, (3) seated with arms pressed against hips, and (4) seated and leaning forward from the waist (Fig. 42–5).

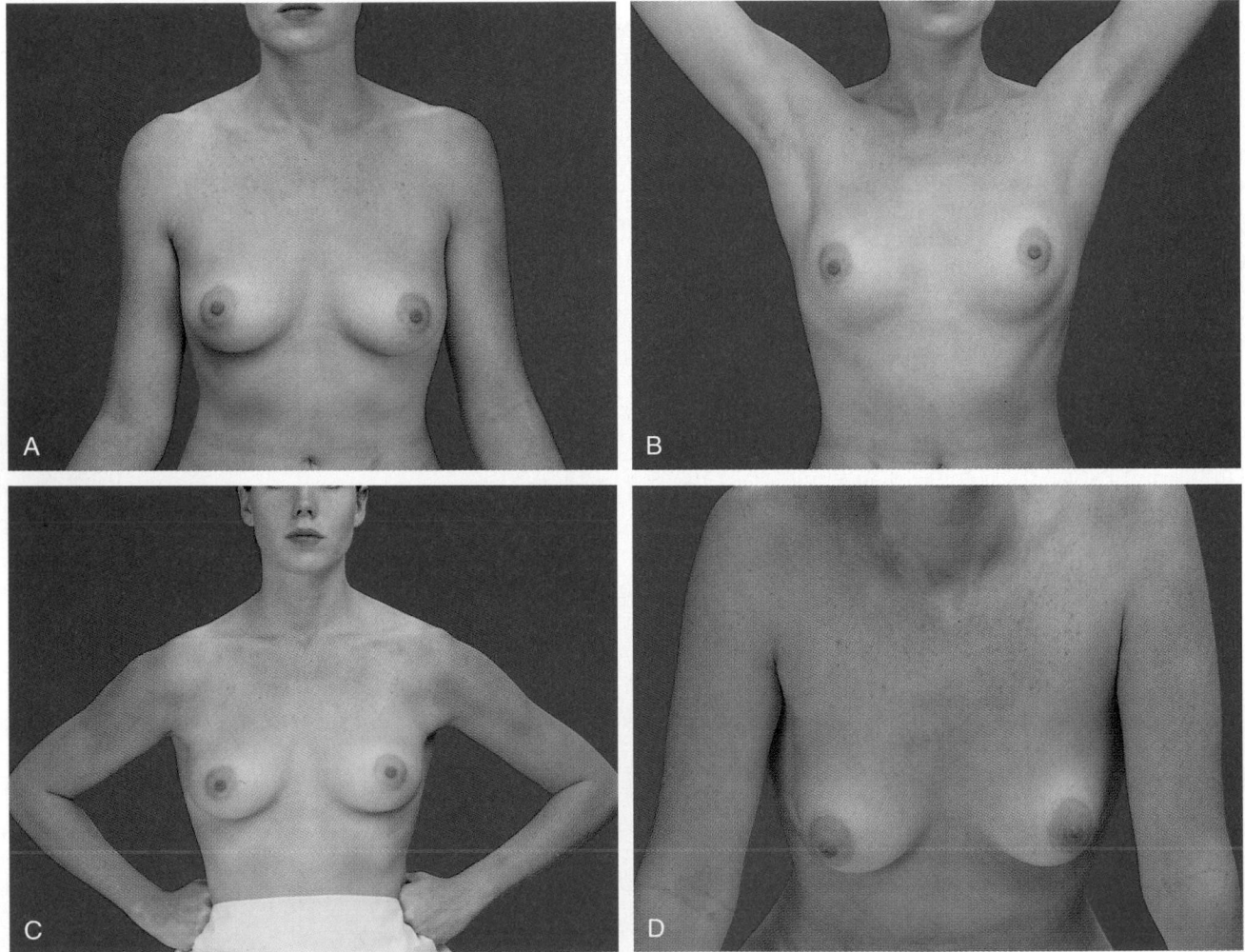

Figure 42–5
Patient positions during examination of the breast. Note the distribution of breast tissue in the different positions. *A,* Patient position at start of breast examination: sitting with arms at sides. *B,* "Arms over the head" position. *C,* Patient with arms lowered and hands pressed against hips. *D,* Forward leaning position, typically used for patient with large, pendulous breasts.

With the patient still in a sitting position, hands at her sides, systematically palpate each breast and axilla, noting masses, consistency, tenderness, and lymph nodes. Use the pads of your fingers in a firm, circular motion, feeling the tissue under the skin of the breasts. There are different patterns that can be followed when palpating the breasts. These include spiral, spokes of a wheel, vertical lines, and horizontal lines (Fig. 42–6). No one pattern is best; but do use the same technique every time and always be certain to examine each quadrant, the tail of the breast, and the axillary region. Compare the breasts with each other. If the patient states that she has noticed a problem in one breast, begin by palpating the other breast to establish a baseline. Try to find the lump without the patient's pointing to it and then verify the position with the patient after palpating the breasts.

Finally, ask the patient to lie on her back on the examining table. Ask her to put her hand behind her head on the side you are palpating. This position helps to spread the breasts out, so that deeper abnormalities can be detected through palpation. If you feel one or more lumps, describe the size, num-ber, consistency, shape, boundaries, mobility, tender-ness, and location. Take a few extra minutes during your examination to have the patient demonstrate how she does her breast self-examination. This will allow you an opportunity to review her technique and reinforce with her the rationale for self-exami-nation.

Assessment of the breast area of the male patient is conducted in the same way as the assessment of the breasts of a female patient.

The breasts of a pregnant or lactating patient are firm, hard, enlarged, and tender and have increased vascularity. The areolae are darker in color. The nip-ples have a discharge in the last trimester of preg-nancy and during lactation.

The breasts of an aging patient have decreased subcutaneous fat and loss of elasticity. Therefore, they have more wrinkles and are flattened and drooping. They feel stringy and nodular. The axillae have decreased hair and increased concavity.

After the breasts have been examined, record findings from the history and physical examination. An example of a recording is: "Patient reports find-ing a small mass in the left breast 5 days ago. In-

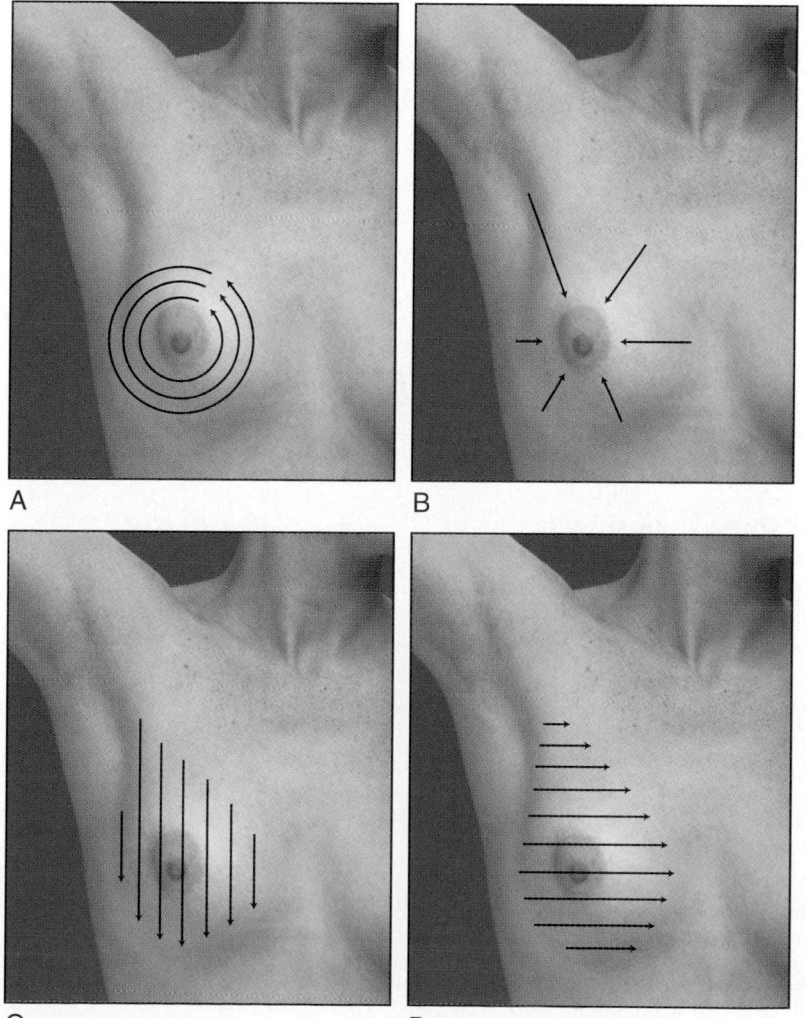

Figure 42–6

Different patterns used in palpation of the breasts. *A*, spiral; *B*, spokes of a wheel; *C*, vertical lines; and *D*, horizontal lines.

How To Do Breast Self-Examination

Do breast self-examination (BSE) every month. Become familiar with how your breasts usually look and feel. Do BSE to find any change from what is normal for you.

If you still menstruate, the best time to do BSE is 2 or 3 days after your period ends. These are the days when your breasts are least likely to be tender or swollen.

If you no longer menstruate, pick a certain day–such as the first day of each month–to remind yourself to do BSE.

If you are taking hormones, talk with your doctor about when to do BSE.

Here's what you should do to check for changes in your breasts.

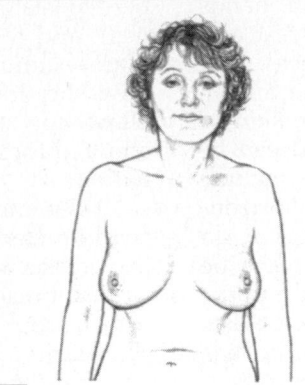

1 Stand in front of a mirror that is large enough for you to see your breasts clearly. Check each breast for anything unusual. Check the skin for puckering, dimpling, or scaliness. Look for a discharge from the nipples.

Do steps 2 and 3 to check for any change in the shape or contour of your breasts. As you do these steps, you should feel your chest muscles tighten.

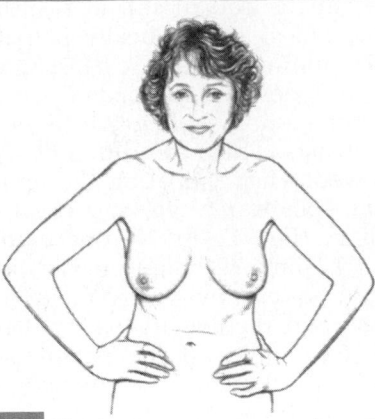

3 Next, press your hands firmly on your hips and bend slightly toward the mirror as you pull your shoulders and elbows forward.

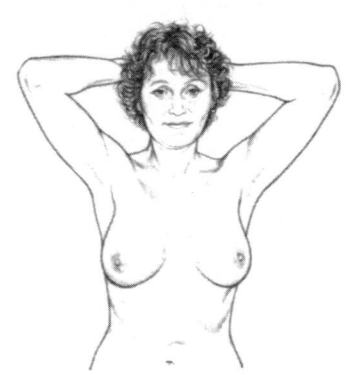

2 Watching closely in the mirror, clasp your hands behind your head and press your hands forward.

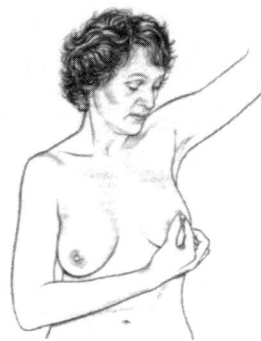

4 Gently squeeze each nipple and look for a discharge.

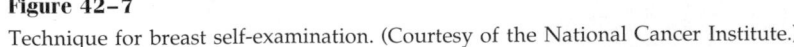

Figure 42–7

Technique for breast self-examination. (Courtesy of the National Cancer Institute.)

spection of the breasts reveals symmetric, small breasts. Palpated one 2 cm, round, hard, mobile, nontender nodule in the LUOQ 3 cm from the nipple at 2 o'clock. No axillary nodes palpated. The patient was referred to a physician." Also include a diagram of the anterior chest indicating where the nodule was palpated.

BREAST SELF-EXAMINATION

Breast self-examination is a procedure that involves systematic monthly self-examination (observation and palpation) of the breasts and underarm areas. Breast self-examination allows a woman to become familiar with the structure of her own breasts so

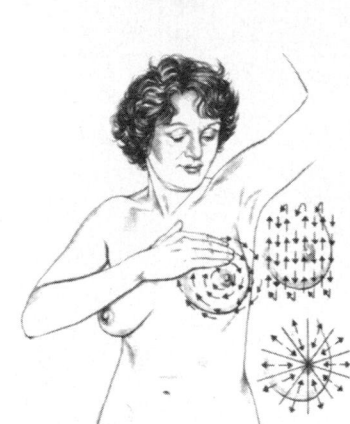

5 Raise one arm. Use the pads of the fingers of your other hand to check the breast and the surrounding area–firmly, carefully, and thoroughly. Some women like to use lotion or powder to help their fingers glide easily over the skin. Feel for any unusual lump or mass under the skin.

Feel the tissue by pressing your fingers in small, overlapping areas about the size of a dime. To be sure you cover your whole breast, take your time and follow a definite pattern: lines, circles, or wedges.

Some research suggests that many women do BSE more thoroughly when they use a pattern of up-and-down lines or strips. Other women feel more comfortable with another pattern. The important thing is to cover the whole breast and to pay special attention to the area between the breast and the underarm, including the underarm itself. Check the area above the breast, up to the collarbone and all the way over to your shoulder.

Lines: Start in the underarm area and move your fingers downward little by little until they are below the breast. Then move your fingers slightly toward the middle and slowly move back up. Go up and down until you cover the whole area.

Circles: Beginning at the outer edge of your breast, move your fingers slowly around the whole breast in a circle. Move around the breast in smaller and smaller circles, gradually working toward the nipple. Don't forget to check the underarm and upper chest areas, too.

Wedges: Starting at the outer edge of the breast, move your fingers toward the nipple and back to the edge. Check your whole breast, covering one small wedge-shaped section at a time. Be sure to check the underarm area and the upper chest.

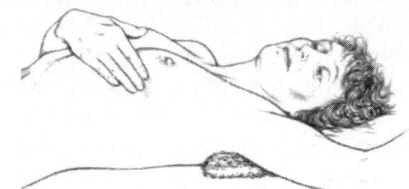

6 It's important to repeat step 5 while you are lying down. Lie flat on your back, with one arm over your head and a pillow or folded towel under the opposite shoulder. This position flattens the breast and makes it easier to check. Check each breast and the area around it very carefully using one of the patterns described above.

7 Some women repeat step 5 in the shower. Your fingers will glide easily over soapy skin, so you can concentrate on feeling for changes underneath.

If you notice a lump, a discharge, or any other change during the month–whether or not it is during BSE–contact your doctor.

Figure 42–7 *Continued*

that she will be able to recognize external and internal changes.

About 90% of all breast masses are found by women themselves. Because treatment of breast cancer at an early stage is much more successful than treatment at later stages, the importance of early detection through self-examination cannot be over-emphasized. All women should be taught breast self-examination and should practice it monthly. The National Cancer Institute recommends the breast self-examination technique shown in Figure 42–7.

When teaching breast self-examination, stress that the procedure should be done each month 2 or 3 days after the completion of menstruation, or at the same time each month for those who are not menstruating. Explain that this simple procedure allows detection of early changes in the structure of the breasts. Also mention that only about 10 to 15% of all breast masses are malignant and that 90% of cancers confined to the breast are curable. Reassure the patient that firm palpation of the breast does not damage breast tissue. Stress that breast self-examination is not a substitute for mammography or breast examination by a clinician. Use teaching aids, such as simulated breast models and videos, that are available through breast health clinics and community agencies. After teaching breast self-examination, ask for a return demonstration. Provide written patient education materials for the woman to take home. Some patients may need you to help them develop an individualized reminder system if they think they may not remember to perform breast self-examination. Be certain that the woman understands that any changes found in the breast should be reported to the physician.

In teaching breast self-examination to the elderly, use written material with large print and speak slowly and clearly. Discuss normal changes that occur in the breasts with age, as well as the continuing importance of self-examination. Keep in mind that many physiologic factors can decrease the incidence and effectiveness of self-examination in older women. Diminished eyesight from glaucoma or cataracts may interfere with the woman's ability to see breast changes. Joint changes that affect range of motion in the upper extremities may limit the ability to palpate. Decreased peripheral sensation also may prevent effective breast self-examination. If any of these factors are present, the breast examination should be done by a nurse or a physician on a monthly basis, or the nurse should work with the woman to adapt BSE practice to her special needs.

*D*iagnostic Procedures

RADIOLOGIC EXAMINATIONS

Mammography

Mammography is an x-ray examination of the breast. It is used to survey the status of breast tissue by providing a picture of the internal structure of the breast (Fig. 42–8). Mammography complements a physical examination of the breast because it can reveal breast masses that are too small or too deep to be palpated manually. Mammography can detect a tumor that otherwise would not be felt for a few years. In addition, mammography allows comparison of current breast status with that shown on previous films so that changes, such as the increased 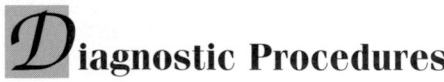 of a mass, can be identified.

 ̇tain a mammogram, the x-ray technician

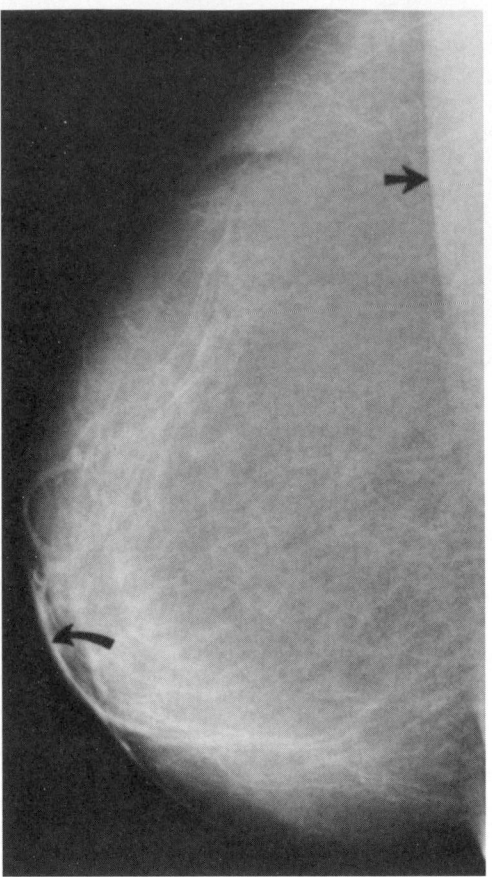

Figure 42–8

A normal mammogram. The curved arrow shows the nipple in profile. The straight arrow shows the pectoralis major muscle. (From Putman CE, Ravin CE. Textbook of diagnostic imaging. 2nd ed. Philadelphia: WB Saunders, 1994, p 2101.)

compresses the breast to be examined between two plastic plates and takes vertical and horizontal pictures. In certain instances, contrast mammography (ductography, galactography) can be performed to determine the presence of duct ectasia, intraductal papilloma, obstruction, or filling defects. In contrast mammography, radiopaque dye is introduced into a mammary duct via its nipple orifice and a mammogram is taken of the breast.

A mammogram should be scheduled in the middle of the menstrual cycle so that the breasts are not too sensitive and can be flattened as much as possible for the procedure.

Some physicians recommend that women refrain from consuming chocolate and caffeine a month before and salt a week before a mammogram to reduce water retention and swelling of the breasts. Women should be instructed to avoid application of powders, creams, or deodorant on the day of the mammogram because the chemical residue from these preparations can interfere with optimal visualization.

Women who have silicone breast implants need an x-ray technician and physician who know how to position the breasts and read the results because a clear mammogram is difficult to obtain when silicone implants are present.

Mammography has created controversy because it exposes the breasts to radiation. Although the amount of radiation exposure is small, the cumulative effect of several mammograms may expose the breasts to radiation-induced breast cancer. However, it is estimated that a woman would be at only a slightly higher risk for breast cancer if she had more than 20 mammograms during her lifetime.

In light of the controversy over the value of mammography versus the risk of radiation, the National Cancer Institute recommends an annual mammography screening only for women over 50 years of age; women over 40 who have a family history of breast cancer; and women over 35 who have had breast cancer.

The American Cancer Society, however, recommends that annual mammography screening begin at age 40.

In addition, a professional breast examination is recommended every 3 years for women 20 to 40 years of age, and every year after age 40.

Xeromammography

Xeromammography provides an x-ray image of the breast that is photoelectrically recorded on paper rather than film. It reveals increased circulation around the tumor site. The radiation exposure is less than with the standard mammographic technique. Xeromammography is becoming increasingly popular because the greater detail produced by the high contrast is easier to read and can be more accurate than mammography in certain instances.

Thermography

Thermography is a procedure that operates on the theory that all objects give off heat and that some of the heat emitted by the body is infrared radiation. With the aid of special instruments, thermography takes a picture of these infrared emissions, which vary depending on the temperature of the source from which they come. It is thought that cancerous masses generate more heat than their surrounding tissue because of increased circulation; thus, a thermogram may provide an indication of the possible location of a cancerous lesion. This tool is not widely used as a screening technique and is not as accurate as mammography in finding small, deep cancers within the breast.

Diaphanography

Diaphanography is a technique that involves shining a light through the breast to illuminate its interior. Different types of tissue transmit and scatter light in different directions. These differences in light trans-

mission are detected by infrared-sensitive cameras and are viewed on a television screen. Currently this technique is still not able to detect the small lesions that appear on a mammogram. However, diaphanography is being refined and evaluated for future potential because it offers the distinct advantage of using a means of scanning other than radiation.

Ultrasonography

If a questionable area is detected on a mammogram or on physical examination, an ultrasonogram can be obtained to study the area further. High-frequency sound waves in the form of ultrasonic echoes are recorded as they strike tissues of different densities and an image of the organs or tissue is made. Therefore, ultrasonography can be used to differentiate a breast cyst from a tumor. This test is sometimes called sonography.

BREAST BIOPSY

If a suspicious mass appears on any of the diagnostic tests or if a breast lump is palpated and thought to be cancerous, a biopsy is done for definitive diagnosis.

Breast biopsy methods include fine-needle, wide-needle, and surgical biopsy. A needle biopsy involves the insertion of a needle into a breast mass to remove fluid or tissue. A fine-needle biopsy, or aspiration biopsy, is the procedure used when a mass is suspected of containing fluid. A sac collapses after the fluid is removed. A wide-needle biopsy is a procedure used to obtain a small piece of tissue from a breast mass. Needle biopsies are performed with the use of local anesthetics and can be done in an outpatient setting. The fluid and tissue that are in the needle and syringe are sent to the laboratory for analysis. If the needle biopsy shows cancer cells, a surgical biopsy is performed to remove tissue for examination. In addition, any suspicious lumps that are too small or are inaccessible to aspiration also undergo surgical biopsy. One type of surgical biopsy is an excisional biopsy, also called a lumpectomy, in which the entire mass is removed.

To locate suspicious but nonpalpable areas of breast tissue before excisional biopsy, a needle wire localization procedure may be performed. About 1 to 2 hours before the breast biopsy, the radiologist inserts a thin, hollow-core localizer needle into the breast under mammographic, sonographic, or stereotactic visualization. Local anesthesia is used. A mammogram is then taken to confirm the correct placement of the needle at the area of suspected abnormality. Then, a flexible hook wire 0.01 inches in diameter is inserted through the needle. The needle is removed, leaving the hook wire in place. A final mammogram confirms the location of the wire. The patient proceeds to surgery with the hook wire in place. The surgeon, guided by the hook wire and mammograms, surgically removes the wire and the surrounding abnormality.

A second type of biopsy is an incisional biopsy, which involves removal of only a piece of the mass. Surgical biopsies typically are outpatient procedures performed under local or general anesthesia. Sutures are used to close the wound, and a sterile dressing is applied to the incision.

The biopsy specimen is sent to a pathology laboratory, where it can be examined as a frozen section or as a permanent section. A frozen section is a sample of tissue that is immediately frozen so that it can be quickly prepared for microscopic review. This can be done within a few minutes, while the patient is still in the operating room. A permanent section of the biopsy tissue involves several steps in preparation for microscopic review. This procedure is more reliable but takes about 24 hours to complete.

When the biopsied tissue is malignant, hormone receptor assays are performed. The cancer cells are tested to determine whether they are estrogen or progesterone receptors. They are examined to ascertain whether these hormones promote the growth of cancer. Results of hormone receptor status will be reported as either positive or negative. These results, along with tumor size, staging, and grading, help in determining the future course of treatment for the patient.

NURSING PROCESS
Breast Biopsy

Assessment

Assess the woman's understanding of the breast biopsy: why it is done, what will happen during the procedure, and what will happen if the breast biopsy reveals a malignancy. Also assess the patient's anxiety level. Review the patient's history and ob-

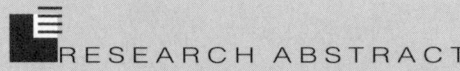

RESEARCH ABSTRACT
How Can Nurses Best Help Women and Their Partners Facing a Breast Biopsy?

Northouse LL, Tocco KM, West P. Coping with breast biopsy: How healthcare professionals can help women and their husbands. Oncol Nurs Forum 1997; 24(3):473.

Although most breast lumps are not malignant, the period between discovery of a lump and biopsy of a suspicious lesion is usually very stressful for women and their partners. Northouse, Tocco, and West therefore set out to discover the following about women and their husbands facing breast biopsy:

- The types of information they received prior to biopsy
- The perceived level of concern of the woman and her husband
- The type of help preferred by the woman and her husband

The subjects selected by Northouse and colleagues for this study were participants in a larger study on psychosocial adjustment. Of those participating in the larger study, 73% of the women and 65% of the men agreed to participate in the smaller study.

The researchers were particularly interested in the experience of the husbands of women awaiting breast biopsy, because the literature addressing their needs or their role in supporting the woman undergoing breast biopsy was very sparse.

For this study, the researchers selected a semistructured interview that included questions about information, concerns, and possible support from health-care providers. The interviews took place in the homes of the participants 1 week before the scheduled biopsy.

The information that the subjects reported having received before the biopsy was grouped into the following categories:

Definitely cancer (2%)
Suspicious (5%)
Needs further assessment (56%)
Probably not cancer (36%)
No comment (1%)

The researchers express concern that even 2% of the women were told that they definitely had cancer prior to the biopsy. The researchers observe that these women may have experienced unwarranted distress, since cancer cannot be diagnosed definitively without biopsy.

Using a five-point scale, the researchers also asked the participants to rate their level of concern about the impending biopsy. A level of 1 indicated "no concern," and a level of 5 indicated that the participants were "very concerned." Of the women studied, 38% rated their concern a 5, and 14% rated it a 4, meaning that slightly more than half of the women rated their concern on the high end of the scale. Husbands reported even higher concern scores, with 53% rating their level of concern a 5 and 22% rating it a 4.

(continued)

serve the patient for any factors that have implications for care before, during, or after the procedure.

Nursing Diagnoses and Planning

Nursing diagnoses and related expected patient outcomes commonly applicable to patients undergoing a breast biopsy include the following:

NDx: Anxiety related to the procedure and its outcomes

Planning: Patient Outcomes
1. Patient attends to questions and directions.
2. Patient verbalizes concerns, feelings, and fears about the breast biopsy.
3. Patient states that anxiety is reduced.
4. Patient participates actively in decisions regarding her treatments.

NDx: Risk for altered health maintenance related to insufficient knowledge of biopsy procedure and follow-up care

Planning: Patient Outcomes
1. Patient describes the preparation for the procedure, expected discomfort, and the expected postprocedure course.
2. Patient states the purpose of the biopsy.
3. Patient states how and when she will be made aware of the results.
4. Patient describes treatment options.
5. Patient states follow-up care requirements.

Nursing Interventions and Evaluation

NDx: Anxiety
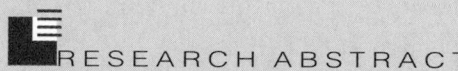
Allow time and opportunity for the patient to verbalize her feelings and concerns about the breast biopsy. This is especially important because the emotional trauma stemming from a diagnosis of malignancy may be overwhelming. Be prepared to deal with a wide variety of patient reactions, ranging from quiet acceptance to anger, tears, or denial. Be particularly sensitive to the support needs of the

---

![L] RESEARCH ABSTRACT

How Can Nurses Best Help Women and Their Partners Facing a Breast Biopsy? (Continued)

The women's suggestions for how health-care professionals could help were grouped into the following categories:

- Provide more information or education (32%)
- Shorten the time between discovery and results of the biopsy (29%)
- Provide support and reassurance (28%)
- Approach the woman with a positive, respectful attitude (9%)
- Involve family in all discussions (2%)

Women in the sample recommended that the information shared at this time be easy to understand and that someone be available to answer questions. Shortening the time before the actual biopsy would show respect for the woman and her partner. Tracking this outcome would be an objective way of measuring responsiveness to patient concerns.

The suggestions of husbands for ways in which health-care providers could help were grouped into slightly different categories:

- Nothing needed (59%)
- Provide more information (21%)
- Help the husband support the woman (8%)
- Shorten the time between discovery and results of the biopsy (7%)
- Improve attitude (3%)
- Offer support (2%)

It is interesting that even though the husbands expressed higher levels of concern than did the women themselves, they had fewer suggestions for help from professionals.

Nurses are in a good position to act as patient advocates. The results of this study indicate that women and their partners appreciate educational and interpersonal interventions during the time surrounding a breast biopsy.

Questions to Consider

1. What involvement do professional nurses have with women facing breast biopsies and their partners?
2. How long does it currently take to schedule a breast biopsy in your community?
3. Is breast self-examination incorporated in the teaching for women at your clinical facility? If not, what community resources for teaching breast self-examination are available?
4. How, when, and by whom are women told the results of their breast biopsies? Are nurses involved?
5. With the pressure on nurses to be more efficient, a patient may feel that she or he is treated more like a number than a person. What can you do to convey genuine concern to a woman and her partner during a brief encounter such as during the time before a breast biopsy is performed?

patient's spouse or significant other. Remember that when family supports are insufficient or when the patient is alone, the role of the nurse can become pivotal in ensuring the patient's emotional well-being. Allowing patients to be involved in making decisions on the type of surgery should result in less anxiety postoperatively.

NDx: Risk for altered health maintenance

Before the biopsy, review its purpose with the patient. If local anesthesia will be used, explain that during the procedure she will feel slight pressure on the breast but will not feel pain. Reassure the patient that the physical recovery from a breast biopsy is typically easy and without complications. Explain that there may be some pain at the incision site and that mild analgesics are usually prescribed. Tell the patient that a small dressing will cover the incision site and will remain in place for 2 to 3 days. Instruct the patient to check the dressing and report any bleeding to the physician. Tell the patient that she may be required to wear a surgical bra for 2 to 3 days postoperatively to provide gentle pressure to the surgical site. This garment, usually applied in the operating room or in the recovery room, will help reduce swelling and provide breast support. Also instruct the patient to take prescribed analgesics for pain or discomfort. Be certain to inform the patient when and by whom she will be told the results of the biopsy. Ensure that the patient knows the date and time of any required follow-up visit, as well as the importance of such appointments. This is especially critical if a diagnosis of breast cancer has been made. Explain that there is time to reflect treatment options or obtain another opinion if desired, but that the decision on a plan of intervention should not be delayed.

Additional Interventions

After the procedure, monitor the patient for physiologic stabilization. Take vital signs and check the amount of bleeding at the dressing site. If general anesthesia has been used, make the usual postoperative assessments, as discussed in Chapter 6.

Compare the patient's status with the expected outcomes. If the outcomes are not met, reassess the patient and revise the plan.

*I*nfections and Inflammations

MASTITIS

Mastitis is inflammation of the soft tissue of the breast that generally, but not exclusively, occurs at the beginning or end of lactation.

Etiology and Pathophysiology

The most common causative agent of mastitis is *Staphylococcus aureus*. The infecting organism may enter the breast through a lactiferous duct or a nipple fissure, via a periductal lymphatic, or by hematogenous spread. Predisposing factors are poor drainage of a duct with milk stasis and lowered maternal defenses. An increased risk for mastitis is present when the supply of breast milk greatly exceeds the demand for it and when abrupt weaning of the infant occurs.

Clinical Manifestations

Classic local symptoms of mastitis are tenderness, redness, and heat in one area of the breast. Systemic symptoms are flulike and include fever, malaise, generalized muscle aching, and nausea or vomiting.

Diagnosis

Diagnosis is based on physical examination of the breast. A culture of breast milk may be obtained from a lactating patient.

Management

In most cases, no intervention is needed other than warm soaks and analgesics for comfort. To drain the breast and combat milk stasis, breast-feeding is continued. If symptoms of mastitis are present longer than 24 hours, antibiotics are usually prescribed. Dicloxacillin and the cephalosporins are the most commonly recommended antibiotics. Most clinicians consider both these drugs to be safe during breast-feeding.

Complications

Breast abscess is the most frequent complication of mastitis. A breast abscess appears as a localized indurated area just below the surface of warm, tender skin. It is treated with incision and drainage. Breast-feeding may have to be stopped if an incision and drainage is performed.

NURSING PROCESS GUIDELINES
Mastitis

Explain to the patient what mastitis is and what causes it. Instruct the patient in the use of warm compresses covered with a dry cloth, a warm towel wrapped in plastic wrap, or a hot water bottle placed on the breast. Tell the patient to force fluids, especially fresh fruit juice and water, and explain the importance of taking antibiotics as directed. Stress the importance of continuing to breast-feed, and reinforce the following breast-feeding technique:

- Continue nursing to empty the breast
- Keep the baby's chin close to the sore area
- Make certain to empty the affected breast

Explain that if nursing is not possible, milk should be pumped or manually expressed because there is an increased risk of abscess if nursing is abruptly stopped. Instruct the patient to nurse frequently for shorter periods and to break the suction by inserting a finger into the corner of the baby's mouth before removing the baby from the breast. Explain that the use of a nursing support brassiere while sleeping as well as during the day increases comfort. Also stress the importance of adequate rest. Suggest that the patient keep the breasts soft by massaging the nipples while in a hot shower or bath to help milk flow. Caution against the use of ointment or cream on the nipples because this may clog the nipple. Tell the patient to seek help early if symptoms recur. Consult a lactation consultant in your institution if one is available and refer the patient to the La Leche League, a breast-feeding organization that offers counseling, peer support groups, and practical advice.

MAMMARY DUCT ECTASIA

Mammary duct ectasia is inflammation and dilatation of the breast ducts.

Etiology and Pathophysiology
Mammary duct ectasia occurs when the breast ducts beneath the nipple become dilated and fill with cellular and fatty debris. This deposited debris produces a gray to greenish sticky discharge at the nipple. Ductal ectasia occurs in women between 35 and 50 years of age.

Clinical Manifestations
The patient presents with a sticky gray to greenish discharge from the nipple and may complain of burning and itching at the nipple. In its early stages, the disease is painless. However, as it progresses, the patient may develop a drawing pain around the nipple and areola. As the inflammation progresses, an infection or abscess may develop.

Diagnosis
Diagnosis is based on patient symptoms and physical examination of the breast.

Management
Medical intervention is based on the extent of the disease process, patient complaints, and patient history. Early ductal ectasia may be treated with warm compresses and antibiotics. More advanced ductal ectasia, if accompanied by abscess and nipple retraction, may require removal of the involved duct as well as antibiotic therapy.

NURSING PROCESS GUIDELINES
Mammary Duct Ectasia

Nursing care of patients with mammary duct ectasia is directed primarily at providing information to increase understanding of the breast disorder, providing emotional support, and allaying the patient's anxiety.

Structural Disorders

GYNECOMASTIA

Gynecomastia is the unusual growth of breast tissue in males (Fig. 42–9).

Etiology and Pathophysiology
Gynecomastia is thought to occur in response to a disturbance in the normal ratio of male to female hormones. Enlargement of male breast tissue may result from normal physiologic development, pathologic conditions, or obesity. It also may occur as a side effect of certain medications.

Gynecomastia may be present for a short period of time in young males aged 12 to 17. This transient state is thought to be a normal part of the young male growth cycle. Gynecomastia is also associated with several diseases, including hypogonadism, Klinefelter's syndrome, tumors of the lung, testicular tumors, tuberculosis, liver failure, and hyperthyroidism. Medications that can cause gynecomastia include hormone therapy with estrogens and androgens, reserpine, phenothiazine, methyldopa, meprobamate, ergotamine, hydroxyzine, marijuana, digitalis, isoniazid, and sertraline. There may be a relationship between gynecomastia and the development of male breast cancer, but that relationship is limited. About 12 to 40% of men with breast cancer have a history of gynecomastia.

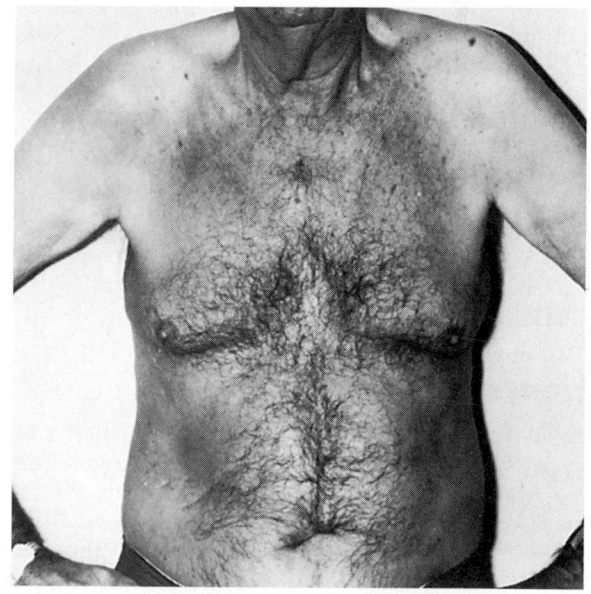

Figure 42–9

Gynecomastia. (From Bland KI, Copeland EM III. The breast: Comprehensive management of benign and malignant diseases. Philadelphia: WB Saunders, 1991, p 149.)

Clinical Manifestations

The primary clinical manifestation in gynecomastia is unilateral or bilateral painful or tender breast enlargement.

Diagnosis

Diagnosis includes a complete physical examination to check for other abnormalities—such as testicular masses—and to assess the development of the genitals. The breasts are examined for masses, and a complete drug history is obtained. Endocrine studies, liver function studies, and tests are done to rule out other systemic disorders.

Management

In general, gynecomastia requires no special therapy except treatment of the underlying cause, as appropriate. If the gynecomastia is thought to be drug induced, the drug may be discontinued or changed. In some cases, the patient may request that surgery be employed to reduce the size of the breasts, to alleviate tenderness or for cosmetic reasons.

NURSING PROCESS GUIDELINES
Gynecomastia

Nursing care of the patient with gynecomastia focuses on providing the patient with information about the causes of gynecomastia and assisting the patient with the prescribed medical treatment. For patients who are having their breasts surgically removed, nursing care is similar to that for the female patient undergoing a mastectomy. When caring for these patients, be certain to consider the sensitive nature of gynecomastia. The patient may be self-conscious about having a "female" body shape, along with having to undergo a "female" surgical procedure.

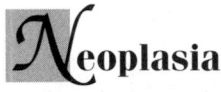eoplasia

BENIGN BREAST DISEASE

Fibrocystic Breast Disease

Fibrocystic breast disease (FBD)—also called mammary dysplasia, fibrocystic mastopathy, and chronic cystic mastopathy—is a benign condition affecting at least one of two premenopausal women. FBD is characterized by a palpable irregularity of the breast accompanied by pain and tenderness. It is most prominent just before menstruation.

The incidence of FBD peaks at about age 40 and is greater in nulliparous women than in those who have had children. FBD is also more common in women with an early menarche, late menopause, or a history of anovulatory cycles.

Etiology and Pathophysiology

The precise cause of FBD is unknown; however, it is generally believed that estrogen with its proliferative effects unopposed by progesterone plays a significant role. This view is supported by the fact that the use of oral contraceptives, which provide a balance of estrogen and progesterone, is associated with a lowered incidence of FBD. Estrogen replacement therapy, on the other hand, is associated with an increasing incidence of FBD with continued use.

Ingestion of methylxanthines, a closely related group of alkaloids including caffeine, theobromine, and theophylline, has also been considered as a contributing factor in the development of FBD. Methylxanthines have been postulated to act as competitive inhibitors of the enzyme that catalyzes hydrolysis of cyclic adenosine monophosphate (cAMP), thus prolonging cAMP activity, which stimulates fibrocystic changes in the breast. This view is supported by the finding that the level of cAMP is significantly increased in women with FBD as compared with women free of breast disease. However, subsequent studies have not all supported these findings.

FBD is characterized by a variety of histopathologic changes, which include cyst formation, stromal fibrosis, and epithelial proliferation. In women with FBD, breast tissue does not completely return to its basal state following menses. Rather some dilatory changes persist. This ultimately leads to permanent ductal dilatation and the formation of cysts. Fibrosis, which most often occurs in the upper outer quadrant of the breast, also contributes to the process of cyst formation because it obstructs the ducts and causes retention of alveolar secretions. These changes have not been found to predispose to malignancy, although they can complicate the detection of malignancy.

The breast discomfort that is associated with FBD occurs as a result of nerve irritation secondary to edema, nerve compression secondary to stromal fibrosis, and an inflammatory response.

Clinical Manifestations

Breast pain, frequently described as an aching fullness, is the most common symptom of FBD. Often, it is bilateral and may occur initially in the upper outer quadrant. Discomfort begins about a week before menses and then decreases with the onset of menstruation.

As the condition progresses, discomfort increases in both severity and duration. The breasts also become granular and tender. Firm masses that increase in size premenstrually may be palpated. These masses are located most often in the upper outer quadrant and may be bilateral in a mirror image.

They are typically well demarcated and freely moveable.

Diagnosis

The diagnosis of FBD is suggested by the patient's age and history in combination with the findings on physical examination. Diffuse bilateral nodularity with cyclic fluctuation in size and related discomfort are key findings supporting the diagnosis of FBD as opposed to a malignancy. Mammography showing a dense pattern with microcalcifications is also typical of FBD. Any persistent mass is biopsied because direct examination of tissue is the only certain method of differentiating a benign from a malignant process.

Management

Management of FBD is directed at preventing progression of the disease and providing symptomatic relief. Many types of treatment have been tried but no one is clearly preferred.

Hormone therapy designed to protect the breast tissue from stimulation by unopposed estrogen is the most common pharmacologic treatment. Danazol (Danocrine), which inhibits anterior pituitary production of follicle-stimulating hormone and luteinizing hormone and thus suppresses ovarian estrogen production, reduces or eliminates symptoms of FBD. Pain relief is reported within 2 to 3 months of treatment, and decreased nodularity in 3 to 6 months. Danazol is expensive, however, and causes such dose-related side effects as weight gain, menstrual irregularities, acne, and sometimes hirsutism and deepening of the voice. Low-dose estrogen and progesterone, which suppress ovarian production of estrogen while providing a balance of extrinsic estrogen and progesterone, also provide symptomatic relief in some women, as can progestins, which correct the estrogen-to-progestin ratio of luteal insufficiency.

A simpler form of therapy and one that is recommended as the initial treatment in women with diffuse fibrocystic changes is decaffeination (reduction or elimination of caffeine from the diet). Advantages of decaffeination are that it is inexpensive and has no side effects or other risks. Effectiveness of this treatment is evaluated in 2 to 4 months.

In women with a persistent dominant cyst, aspiration is commonly indicated, and the aspirate is sent for cytopathologic analysis. If aspiration is not successful, if there is a residual mass after aspiration, or if the cyst recurs, excision may be recommended.

Other measures that have been tried with some success include vitamin therapy in the form of vitamin A, vitamin E, or vitamin B complex and diuretics, which relieve fluid engorgement. Women have also reported relief with dietary supplementation with essential fatty acids, elimination of dietary salt, avoidance of cigarette smoking, and reduction of stress. Many of these factors are currently under investigation.

NURSING PROCESS
Fibrocystic Breast Disease

Assessment

Begin assessment of the patient with fibrocystic breast disease with a history that includes information relevant to her risk status for breast cancer. Determine when she last had a mammogram, the date of her last breast examination by a health-care professional, and whether she practices BSE. Ask about the results of these examinations. Obtain a description of her current symptoms, including when they began and their severity, duration, and relationship to the menstrual cycle. Explore relief measures that have been tried and the effectiveness of these measures. Inspect and palpate the breasts as described previously. Note and describe any discharge, areas of irregularity or tenderness, or other abnormality. Assess the woman's anxiety level and her understanding of the problem. Also assess her knowledge of BSE, which is an important part of follow-up care.

Nursing Diagnoses and Planning

Nursing diagnoses and related expected patient outcomes most commonly applicable to patients with FBD include the following:

NDx: Pain related to swelling and nerve irritation secondary to fibrocystic changes

Planning: Patient Outcomes
1. Patient describes self-care measures for relief of discomfort associated with FBD.
2. Patient reports decreased breast discomfort.

NDx: Anxiety related to the cause and prognosis of FBD and its relationship to cancer

Planning: Patient Outcomes
1. Patient expresses her feelings and concerns about FBD.
2. Patient realistically describes the relationship between FBD and her risk of breast cancer.

NDx: Risk for altered health maintenance related to insufficient knowledge of prescribed medical treatment and required follow-up care

Planning: Patient Outcomes
1. Patient describes the purpose, name, dose, route, frequency, and common side effects of any prescribed pharmacological therapy.
2. Patient describes any planned aspiration or excision procedure.
3. Patient states importance and schedule of follow-up care: BSE, mammography, professional breast examinations.

Nursing Interventions and Evaluation

NDx: Pain
Instruct the patient in self-care measures to alleviate the discomfort associated with FBD, as presented in

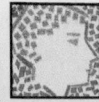

HIGHLIGHT 42–1
PATIENT EDUCATION

Self-Care Measures for Relief of Discomfort Associated with Fibrocystic Breast Disease

Instruct the patient to:

Wear a well-padded support brassiere to decrease tension on ligaments and the inflammatory response such tension triggers.

Avoid sleeping in the prone position, which puts pressure on the breasts.

Apply ice or heat to the breasts for temporary relief of pain.

Limit dietary ingestion of caffeine by avoiding regular coffee, tea, colas, and chocolate.

Limit dietary salt during the week before menstruation to help limit premenstrual swelling.

Take mild analgesics as needed for discomfort during the week prior to menstruation.

Take steps to avoid and limit stress, which, either through a neuroendocrine response or increased awareness of symptoms, appears to exacerbate fibrocystic breast disease.

Highlight 42–1. Discuss the therapeutic value of each. Explain that discomfort is usually reduced after menopause.

NDx: Anxiety

Approach the patient with empathy and tact. Encourage the woman to express her feelings and concerns and to ask questions about the disease, its prognosis, and its treatment. Correct any identified misconceptions or areas of misinformation. Interpret for the patient her risk of cancer. Keep in mind that for many years women with FBD were considered to have an increased risk of cancer and women may still assume that this is true. Explain that, in fact, women with FBD constitute a minority of those with breast cancer. Acknowledge that identification of a suspicious mass can be more difficult in the presence of FBD, but reassure the patient about the effectiveness of BSE, professional breast examinations, and mammograms in the early identification of malignant lesions.

NDx: Risk for altered health maintenance

If pharmacologic therapy is prescribed, teach the patient its purpose as well as the name, dose, route, frequency, and common side effects of prescribed drugs. If aspiration or excision is planned, describe the planned procedure and its purpose to the patient. Review needed follow-up care, describing both its purpose and importance.

Teach BSE, as described previously. Obtain a return demonstration and provide written instructions for the patient to review as needed. Also provide the patient with a written schedule of follow-up care.

Compare the patient's status with the expected outcomes. If the outcomes are not met, reassess the patient and revise the plan.

Fibroadenoma

Fibroadenomas are benign tumors of the breast. The tumors are round, firm, encapsulated, movable, and nontender.

Etiology and Pathophysiology

Fibroadenomas are solid benign breast tumors that are usually composed of fibrous or glandular tissue. They may be multiple and can occur bilaterally. Fibroadenomas occur most often in women between 20 and 40 years of age. They are more common in African-American women than in white women.

Clinical Manifestations

Fibroadenomas are painless, movable breast masses with well-defined borders. The size of the fibroadenoma is not affected by the menstrual cycle.

Diagnosis

Diagnosis includes examination of both breasts and regional lymph nodes. A mammography may be done to visualize and localize the mass. The only way to distinguish a benign fibroadenoma from a malignant tumor is to biopsy the mass.

Management

The usual medical treatment of choice is excision. The breast tissue is sent to a pathologist for examination for malignant cells.

NURSING PROCESS GUIDELINES
Excision of a Fibroadenoma

The assessment, nursing diagnoses, expected patient outcomes, nursing interventions, and evaluation for patients undergoing excision of a fibroadenoma are similar to those described previously for patients undergoing breast biopsy.

Intraductal Papilloma

Intraductal papilloma is a small benign tumor that grows in the lining of the breast ducts near the nipple.

Etiology and Pathophysiology

Intraductal papilloma is most common in women between 45 and 50 years of age. It is typically found as a solitary tumor. Usually it is not precancerous.

Clinical Manifestations

The primary symptom of intraductal papilloma is bleeding from the nipple. This results from irritation of the lining of the breast duct by the tumor. This irritation causes the lining of the breast duct to bleed, and the blood empties at the nipple. The discharge is spontaneous, and the disease is usually unilateral.

Diagnosis

Diagnosis is based on patient symptoms and physical examination of the breasts and regional lymph nodes.

Management

Surgical removal of the involved breast duct is the usual medical treatment. If multiple intraductal papillomas exist, the entire duct system may be removed.

NURSING PROCESS GUIDELINES
Excision of an Intraductal Papilloma

The assessment, nursing diagnoses, expected patient outcomes, nursing interventions, and evaluation for patients undergoing excision of an intraductal papilloma are similar to those described previously for patients undergoing breast biopsy.

CANCER OF THE BREAST

Despite major advances in diagnosis and treatment, breast cancer is still the most common form of cancer among American women, second only to lung cancer as the leading cause of cancer death. It is estimated that one in eight women will be diagnosed with breast cancer during her lifetime. Of those diagnosed, one in four will die of breast cancer. In 1997, 181,600 new cases were expected to be diagnosed, and an estimated 43,900 women were expected to die of the disease (Parker et al, 1997). These statistics are slightly lower than those for 1996.

In the United States, breast cancer is more common in white women than in African-American women; however, among women under the age of 45, African-American women are more likely to develop breast cancer than white women. Rising incidence rates may be a reflection of early detection methods but may also be related to changes in diet, lifestyles, and environmental exposures. The incidence of breast cancer increases as women age. About 77% of women with newly diagnosed breast cancer are over 50 years of age.

Breast cancer does occur in men. However, male breast cancer is rare, accounting for less than 1% of all breast cancers.

Etiology and Pathophysiology

The exact cause of breast cancer is unknown, but many risk factors appear to influence its develop-

Table 42-1

Risk Factors for Cancer of the Breast

Gender:	99% in women
Age:	Incidence increases with age. About 80% of women diagnosed are over 35 years of age.
Family history of breast cancer:	History of breast cancer in both mother and sister or mother and maternal grandmother, especially if it developed before menopause or bilaterally. Recent research has shown that defective genes can be linked to breast cancer.
Personal history of breast cancer:	A previous diagnosis of breast cancer in one breast increases the chance of breast cancer occurring in the remaining breast.
Reproductive history:	Reproductive factors that may influence the development of breast cancer are early menarche, late menopause, nulliparity, or first birth after age 30.
Obesity:	Risk increases when weight is 20% above average for height and age.

ment and clinical course (Table 42-1). The major risk factors include increasing age, first-degree relatives diagnosed with breast cancer, and a previous personal history of breast cancer. Hormones, particularly estrogen, have also been linked to development of breast cancer and are the subject of current investigation. At present, it is generally believed that estrogens do not cause breast cancer but that they facilitate the subsequent growth of the malignant breast tumor. Short courses of postmenopausal estrogen replacement therapy do not appear to increase breast cancer risk, but long-term therapy may be a risk. Use of oral contraceptives in general is not associated with increased risk, but prolonged use before the first pregnancy may pose a risk. Some evidence also suggests a link between dietary fat intake, alcohol consumption, and breast cancer. However, the precise relationship remains unclear.

A variety of genetic mutations associated with cancer have also been identified. Of greatest import for breast cancer is the isolation of the genes *BRCA*-1, on chromosome 17, and *BRCA*-2, on chromosome 13. Mutations in these genes are thought to account for the majority of hereditary, early-onset breast cancers.

At present, testing for *BRCA*-1 and *BRCA*-2 is done only in the research setting. The tests are labor intensive and expensive. Interpretation of the results is technically difficult, resulting in an unknown rate of false-negative findings, in which the test shows no genetic alteration when one may be present. Persons who undergo testing for *BRCA*-1 and *BRCA*-2 genetic mutation must receive counseling to help them understand the personal and social ramifications of genetic testing. These include the psychologic issues of survivor guilt, transmitter guilt, privacy, family coercion for testing in children, the right not to know, prenatal testing, and personal identity issues as well as the social issues of insurability, employability, and confidentiality. At this time, persons with a familial history of breast cancer who wish to be tested for *BRCA*-1 and *BRCA*-2 genetic mutations must be referred to a testing center by their family physicians.

The physiology of breast cancer resembles that of other cancers. It is an uncontrolled growth of cells within the breast tissue. These cells have the unique ability to metastasize locally, regionally, and systemically. They can break away from the main tumor and travel through the lymphatic system and blood stream to other sites. The most common sites of metastases are the lungs, bone, and liver.

Malignant cells usually originate in the epithelial tissues of the breast and are considered carcinomas. The large majority arise in the ductal system and are known as ductal carcinoma. The minority arise in the lobular system and are known as lobular carcinoma. Less than 1% of breast cancers originate in the nonepithelial connective tissue of the breast. These tumors are classified as sarcomas of the breast. The growth of cancerous cells within the breast ducts beneath the nipple is known as Paget's disease.

The upper outer quadrant is the most common site of breast cancer. About half of all breast cancers are found in the upper outer quadrant and the "tail" of the breasts. The next most prevalent site of breast cancer is around the nipple, at about 20%. The inner quadrants show the least incidence of tumors.

Breast tumor cells are also classified by pathologists as noninvasive or invasive. Noninvasive tumor cells are confined to the duct in which they originated and are thus called carcinoma in situ. Invasive tumor cells, which constitute more than 90% of all breast cancers, have broken through the duct walls and have encroached upon other tissues of the breast.

Each case of breast cancer exhibits unique characteristics that may ultimately affect the patient's prognosis. These include tumor size and pathologic classification, estrogen receptor activity of the tumor, lymph node status, and the presence or absence of distant metastases.

Clinical Manifestations

The primary clinical manifestation of breast cancer is the appearance of an abnormal mass of tissue in the breast. Although an appreciable number of tumors are detected by mammography and the clinical examination, many women find their own breast tumors. The mass is typically firm, dense, singular, and irregular in shape. Associated symptoms may include skin dimpling, nipple retraction, enlargement of the breast, changes in the texture or color of the skin of the breast or nipple, peau d'orange skin, increase in vascularity of the breast, discharge from the nipple, and pain or tenderness in the breast, nipple, or axilla (Fig. 42–10). The regional lymph nodes of the axilla may be palpable as a result of tumor spread or as part of the immune system's response to the breast tumor. In more advanced disease, the infraclavicular and supraclavicular lymph nodes may also be enlarged and palpable.

Diagnosis

The diagnosis of breast cancer requires a complete history and physical examination of the patient. Careful breast inspection and palpation are performed to identify the breast tumor. Mammography and other low-voltage radiography tests are used to visualize the mass, locate small nonpalpable tumors, or aid in differentiating benign from malignant tumors. The only definitive way to differentiate between a benign and malignant breast tumor is to obtain a specimen of suspect breast tissue through biopsy for pathologic study.

Staging of breast cancer is a method of identifying the extent of the disease. Clinical and pathologic staging classifies the size of the primary breast tumor (T), the presence or absence of tumor in the regional lymph nodes (N), and the presence or absence of distant organ metastases (M). This staging method is known as the TNM classification (Table 42–2). It is used by physicians to categorize breast cancer into Stage I, Stage II, Stage III, and Stage IV (Table 42–3). Ninety percent of patients with newly diagnosed breast cancer are in the early stages, Stages I and II, which means that the cancer is limited to the breast and axillary lymph nodes, and there is a very good chance for complete recovery. For example, a woman whose breast tumor is smaller than 2 cm, whose axillary lymph nodes have been proven to be free of tumor, and who is free of metastatic spread would be described as having Stage I breast cancer. This woman's chance of cure would be excellent after her primary tumor was removed. In contrast, a woman with Stage IV disease would have metastatic disease in other organs, and less chance of disease control and recovery. Each successive stage carries with it a poorer prognosis.

Breast tumors are also classified by hormonal activity. The biopsy tissue of the tumor is always studied for hormonal receptors because the growth of some breast tumors can be stimulated by estrogen and progesterone. A tumor's estrogen activity is classified as estrogen receptor positive or negative (ER+, ER−). More than half of all breast cancers are diagnosed as estrogen receptor positive. Studies have shown that women with estrogen receptor–positive tumors have a greater chance of remaining disease free and that, if metastatic disease should occur, they can be treated with hormonal manipulation.

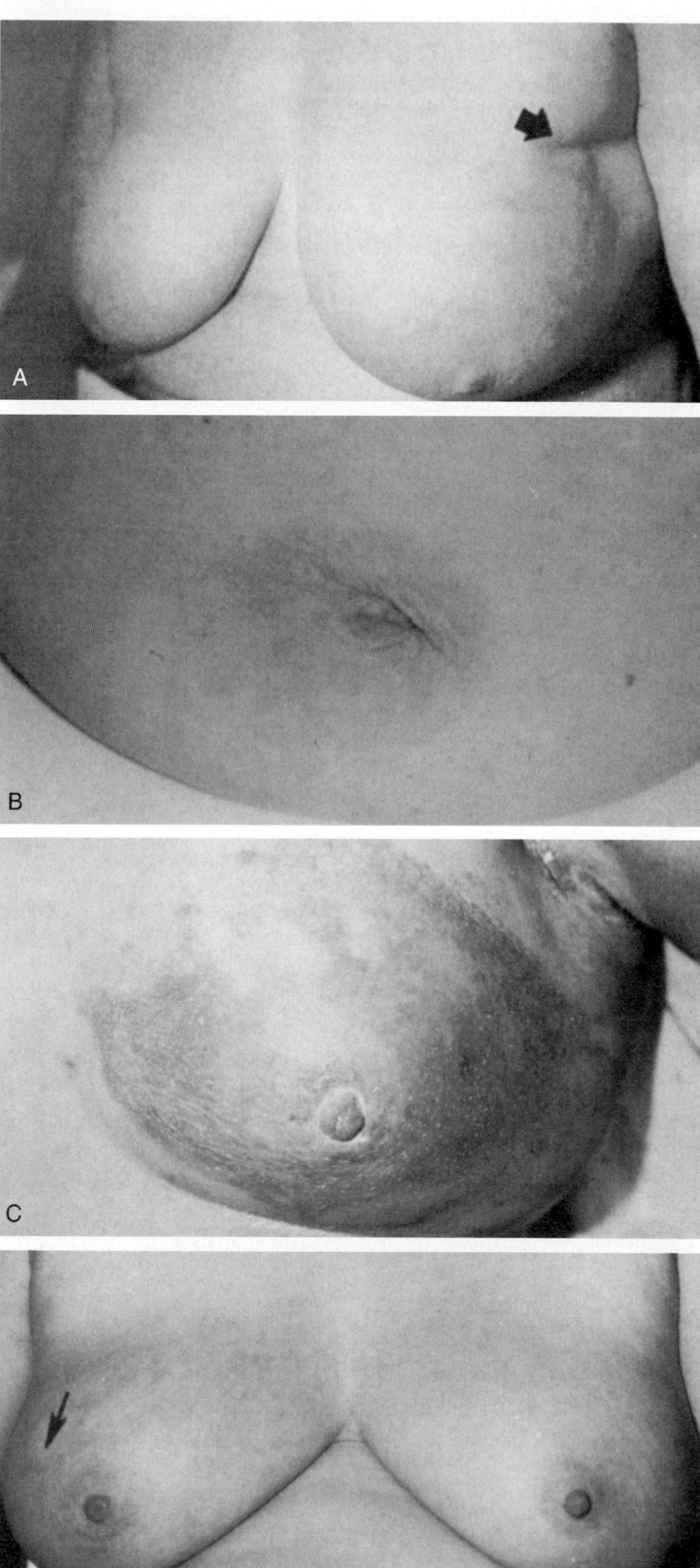

Figure 42–10

Breast changes associated with breast cancer. *A*, Dimpling. *B*, Nipple retraction. *C*, Peau d'orange skin, which resembles the skin of an orange. It is thick and hard with prominent pores as a result of blocked lymphatic drainage. *D*, Increased venous prominence.

Table 42-2

American Joint Committee on Cancer TNM Classification of Breast Cancer

PRIMARY TUMOR (T)

T0	No evidence of primary tumor
T1	<2 cm
T2	>2<5 cm
T3	>5 cm
T4	Any size with direct extension to the chest wall or skin
TX	Tumor cannot be assessed

NODES (N)

N0	No regional lymph node metastasis
N1	Metastasis to movable ipsilateral axillary lymph node or nodes
N2	Metastasis to ipsilateral axillary node or nodes fixed to one another or to other structures
N3	Metastasis to ipsilateral internal mammary node or nodes
NX	Nodes cannot be assessed

METASTASIS (M)

M0	No distant metastasis
M1	Distant metastasis present
MX	Metastasis cannot be assessed

Management

Management is based largely on the stage of the disease. Because a large majority of women have one or several identified risk factors that influence the development of breast cancer, the single most important means to control the disease rests with early detection through BSE and mammography, since breast cancer that has not spread to the lymph nodes has an excellent chance of being cured.

Once a tumor has been located, the patient is examined to detect palpable lymph nodes or possible spread to other areas of the body. Based on patient history and symptoms, further tests may be ordered, including chest x-ray examination, bone scan, and blood studies to determine whether metastatic disease is present.

The treatment of breast cancer may involve surgery, chemotherapy, hormonal therapy, or radiation therapy. Local treatment for breast cancer consists of surgery alone or surgery followed by radiation therapy aimed at treating the breast tissue itself. Chemotherapy and hormonal therapy are what are called systemic treatments because they target the rest of the body. Often two or more therapies are combined in the patient's treatment plan.

Surgical Intervention

The primary treatment of breast cancer is surgical removal and pathologic study of the tumor. The excised tumor is measured, classified pathologically, and tested for hormone receptors.

Currently, there are several surgical options that are used to treat breast cancer: These include modi-

fied radical mastectomy as well as breast conservation procedures (Table 42-4). After a positive biopsy is obtained, the surgeon discusses these options with the patient. The type of surgical intervention selected is based on the patient's clinical status, risk factors, the location and size of the tumor, the clinical stage of the disease, and the patient's preference.

MODIFIED RADICAL MASTECTOMY. The modified radical mastectomy involves removal of the entire breast, skin, and axillary lymph nodes but preserves the major pectoral muscles. As opposed to a radical mastectomy, which involves removal of the breast, skin, axillary nodes, and underlying muscle, the modified radical mastectomy results in a more cosmetically acceptable chest wall and leaves the patient with more strength in her arm and shoulder. The modified radical mastectomy also allows for easier breast reconstruction. Studies have shown no difference in survival between patients treated with modified radical mastectomy and those treated with radical mastectomy. As a result, radical mastectomy is rarely done today. In studies that have compared early-stage breast cancer patients treated by modified radical mastectomy and those treated by breast-conserving surgery and radiation, no significant difference has been found in survival rates.

PATIENT PREPARATION. The patient remains on NPO (nothing by mouth) status from midnight preceding the day of surgery, and an intravenous fluid line is started before surgery. Skin preparation may include a shower or bath and a local scrub with an antiseptic solution. About an hour before surgery, the patient is asked to void and, if applicable, to remove dentures, contact lenses, nail polish, and jewelry. Vital signs are taken and recorded. Side rails are raised after administration of the prescribed preoperative medication.

PROCEDURE. As previously stated, in a modified radical mastectomy, the entire breast, skin, and axillary lymph nodes are removed, but the major muscles of the chest are left intact (see illustration in Table 42-4). A wound drainage catheter is inserted through a stab wound under the axilla to prevent accumulation of blood or serum under the incision and to promote wound healing. A large pressure

Table 42-3

Breast Cancer Staging Based on TNM Classification

Stage	Tumor Size (T)	Nodes (N)	Metastasis (M)
Stage I	T1	N0	M0
Stage II	T2	N0, N1	M0
Stage III	T3	N0, N1	M0
	T1	N2	M0
	T2	N3	M0
Stage IV	T4	N0, N1, N2, N3	M1

Table 42–4

Surgical Interventions for Breast Cancer

Procedure	Description	Diagram
Lumpectomy or tylectomy	Removal of the breast tumor and small amounts of surrounding tissue	
Partial mastectomy or segmental resection	Removal of the tumor plus approximately 2 to 3 cm of surrounding tissue	
Quadrantectomy	Removal of a quadrant of the breast with the tumor, and fascia covering the greater pectoral muscle.	
Local regional treatment	Removal of the tumor with the surrounding tissue and axillary lymph nodes	

Table continued on following page

Table 42—4

Surgical Interventions for Breast Cancer (Continued)

Procedure	Description	Diagram
Total mastectomy	Removal of the entire breast, with the pectoral muscles and axillary lymph nodes left intact	
Modified radical mastectomy	Removal of the entire breast, skin, and axillary lymph nodes. The pectoral muscles are left intact.	Pectoralis minor muscle
Radical mastectomy	Removal of the entire breast, skin, pectoralis major muscle, pectoralis minor muscle, and axillary lymph nodes	Pectoralis minor muscle — Pectoralis major muscle

dressing is applied to the chest wall. Breast reconstruction can be performed at the same time a mastectomy is done, especially if the patient has already received chemotherapy for a previous breast tumor.

POSTOPERATIVE COURSE. Oral fluids with progression to a regular diet are resumed when the patient has recovered from anesthesia. Intravenous therapy is maintained until the patient is physiologically stable and able to tolerate adequate amounts of oral fluid. Activity is gradually resumed once the patient is alert, and simple exercises that do not stress the suture line are started to promote circulation and prevent limitation of movement of the arm and shoulder. Examples of these exercises are squeezing a ball and flexing the elbow on the affected side.

The wound drainage catheter remains in place for 1 to 4 days, depending on the amount of drainage collected. It is removed by the physician when fluid collection is less than 100 mL in a 24-hour period. The surgical dressing is usually removed and the incision checked for healing after the first 24 hours. By the fifth postoperative day, some of the surgical sutures and clips may be removed. Managed-care regulations require that most patients be discharged within 1 to 2 days of their surgery, with sutures, dressings, and drains intact. Teaching and discharge planning must focus on preparing patients to manage their care at home. Well-planned follow-up care is essential for this patient population.

COMPLICATIONS. Possible complications after a modified radical mastectomy include fluid accumulation under the incision, lymphedema, infection, bleeding, limited range of motion of the arm and shoulder, and problems with psychologic adjustment.

NURSING PROCESS
Modified Radical Mastectomy

PREOPERATIVE NURSING CARE

Assessment

Obtain a complete health history from the patient. Include information about the onset and course of the present illness, past illnesses and surgeries, and psychologic, sociologic, and family history. Examine the breasts. Note the size and location of any palpable mass, discharge from the nipple, dimpling of the skin, areas of ulceration, deviation of the direction of the nipple, or any other abnormality. Determine the patient's understanding of the disease process, plan of treatment including the surgery, and the expected prognosis. Assess the patient's anxiety level and level of coping. Assess the patient's support systems.

Nursing Diagnoses and Planning

Nursing diagnoses and related expected patient outcomes commonly applicable to patients who are scheduled for a modified radical mastectomy include the following:

NDx: Knowledge deficit: mastectomy procedure, perioperative routines, breast reconstruction option

Planning: Patient Outcomes
1. Patient states the rationale for the mastectomy.
2. Patient describes the planned mastectomy procedure, including the postoperative appearance of the chest and axilla.
3. Patient decribes preoperative and postoperative activities.
4. Patient describes surgical breast reconstruction as a possibility now or at a later date.

NDx: Anxiety related to the diagnosis of breast cancer and the scheduled surgery

Planning: Patient Outcomes
1. Patient verbalizes her concerns.
2. Patient attends to information and directions.
3. Patient participates in the decision-making process.
4. Physiologic and behavioral signs of severe anxiety are absent.

Nursing Interventions and Evaluation

NDx: Knowledge deficit: mastectomy procedure, perioperative routines, breast reconstruction option
Review with the patient information provided by the surgeon about the mastectomy procedure to be done. Be sure the patient has a realistic expectation of the postoperative appearance of the chest and the axilla. If the patient had previous experience with someone who had a radical mastectomy, stress that the modified technique avoids the chest and axillary disfigurement of the early procedure, so clothes with lower necklines may be worn. Also stress that more strength is left in the arm because the major chest muscles remain intact and that there is less chance of lymphedema in the arm on the affected side because fewer lymphatic vessels are severed. Encourage the patient to ask questions, and clarify information as needed.

If immediate breast reconstruction is planned, assess the patient's understanding of the procedure and the expected physical result. (Refer to the section on breast reconstruction later in this chapter.) Describe perioperative routines. Make sure the patient understands that a wound drainage system and a large pressure dressing will be in place postoperatively on the affected side. The patient may also be required to wear a surgical bra postoperatively to keep the dressings in place.

Explain that the hand and arm on the mastectomy side will be elevated on pillows to facilitate fluid drainage and inhibit swelling. Also explain that pain and tightness over the chest wall and pain in the upper back, shoulder, and arm are expected but that analgesics will be ordered to maintain comfort. Demonstrate deep-breathing and coughing exercises, and inform the patient that these exercises will be started in the recovery room and repeated every hour during the initial postoperative period. Demonstrate exercises for the affected shoulder and arm. Obtain a return demonstration of all exercises before surgery.

NDx: Anxiety
People differ in their ability to deal with anxiety. Allow time for the patient who wants to verbalize her feelings and concerns about the diagnosis and treatment of breast cancer. Seek out a breast cancer specialist in the institution who may be available to speak with your patient before surgery or involve the patient in a presurgical orientation. Respect the right of privacy for the patient who does not wish to talk about these issues. Advise the patient of such support programs as Reach to Recovery because she may relate better to someone who has already been through the treatment process. Give the patient educational materials she can consult when she is ready.

Include the patient and family in the planning of care. Encourage the patient to make decisions and to participate in self-care measures.

Compare the patient's status with the expected

outcomes. If the outcomes are not met, reassess the patient and revise the plan.

POSTOPERATIVE NURSING CARE

Assessment

Assess the patient's return to physiologic stability. Check vital signs and inspect the dressing and sheets under the patient for bleeding. Check the wound drainage system and note the color and amount of drainage. Check the intravenous infusion and inspect the site of insertion for signs of infiltration or phlebitis. Assess for pain and assess the mobility of the affected arm. Inspect the affected arm for signs of infection, including redness, warmth, and edema. Assess the level of stress and anxiety the patient and family are experiencing by observing and listening to both nonverbal and verbal communication.

Nursing Diagnoses and Planning

Nursing diagnoses and related expected patient outcomes most commonly applicable to patients who have had a modified radical mastectomy include the following:

NDx: Pain related to surgical trauma of the anterior chest

Planning: Patient Outcomes
1. Patient takes pain medication as needed.
2. Patient utilizes nonpharmacologic methods of pain management.
3. Patient reports reduced pain.

NDx: Risk for infection related to vascular and lymphatic alteration from surgery

Planning: Patient Outcomes
1. Patient explains the need to protect the affected arm from trauma.
2. Patient lists precautions to be taken to protect the affected arm.
3. Patient verbalizes understanding of aseptic technique in caring for dressing, drains, and incision at home.

NDx: Risk for impaired physical mobility related to breast surgery

---

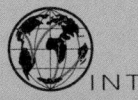

INTERNET CONNECTIONS
Breast Disorders

ONCOLINK/Breast Disease
http://cancer.med.upenn.edu/disease/breast/
This authoritative site, part of ONCOLINK, provides current medical news, links to CancerNet references from the National Cancer Institute, and links to related web sites. It also provides information about the psychosocial aspects of breast cancer. Also included is information about the causes of breast cancer; recommendations for screening, diagnosis, treatment, and prevention; and related topics.

Breast Cancer Roundtable/Breast Cancer References
http://www.seas.gwu.edu/student/tlooms/MGT243/health_professionals.html
This site provides information for health professionals, including professional references, resources, statistics, research findings, course lists, discussions, and papers.

American Cancer Society Professional Education and Development Program for Breast Cancer
http://nysernet.org/bcic/acs2/pro.ed/index.html
This site offers links to an extensive list of articles for health professionals.

Patient's Guide to Breast Cancer/Beth Israel Health Care System of New York
http://www.wp.com/bicbs/gtoc.html
This extremely detailed, patient-oriented site provides information on a wide variety of topics related to breast cancer, including breast self-examination, treatment options, and breast reconstruction.

American Cancer Society Breast Cancer Network
http://www.cancer.org/bcn.html
This authoritative site provides extensive patient-oriented information.

Doctor's Guide to Breast Cancer Information and Resources
http://www.pslgroup.com/BREASTCANCER.HTM
An authoritative site oriented especially to health-care professionals, this site provides information about a wide variety of subjects related to breast cancer. It also provides access to discussion groups, news groups, and support groups. It also addresses common questions that patients ask after diagnosis, as well as frequently asked questions about breast changes.

Planning: Patient Outcomes
1. Patient states the rationale for exercising the affected arm.
2. Patient demonstrates range-of-motion exercises.
3. Patient plans progressive exercise regimen 3 to 5 times a day.
4. Patient lists activities of daily living that enhance arm and shoulder movement.

NDx: Risk for fluid volume excess (local) related to impaired lymph flow in the affected arm

Planning: Patient Outcomes
1. Patient identifies factors that may contribute to the development of lymphedema.
2. Patient lists signs and symptoms of lymphedema.
3. Patient describes precautions to be taken to decrease the risk of lymphedema.
4. Patient performs exercises of affected arm and shoulder 3 to 5 times a day.

NDx: Risk for body image disturbance related to the loss of the breast

Planning: Patient Outcomes
1. Patient verbalizes feelings, concerns, and questions about change in body image.
2. Patient views incision, if able, before discharge.
3. Patient is receptive to information about prostheses.
4. Patient expresses positive feelings about self.

NDx: Risk for sexual dysfunction related to the loss of the breast

Planning: Patient Outcomes
1. Patient asks questions about sexual activity.
2. Patient verbalizes feelings about the effect of the mastectomy on her relationship with her sexual partner.

NDx: Risk for altered health maintenance related to insufficient knowledge of postoperative and postdischarge self-care

Planning: Patient Outcomes
1. Patient states precautions to be taken for operative side.
2. Patient demonstrates correct method of BSE.
3. Patient states time and date of follow-up visit.
4. Patient resumes family and social roles.

NDx: Risk for ineffective individual coping and risk for ineffective family coping related to perceived changes in lifestyle, self-concept, and living with a cancer diagnosis.

Planning: Patient Outcomes
1. Patient and family express fears and concerns regarding changes in lifestyle.
2. Patient and family verbalize perceptions of the effects of living with a diagnosis of cancer.
3. Patient and family identify positive coping strategies.

Nursing Interventions and Evaluation

NDx: Pain

Monitor the extent of the patient's pain and give prescribed narcotic analgesics as needed. Use a pain rating scale to get an accurate assessment of the patient's perception of her pain. Expect the patient to experience incisional pain on the first postoperative day. Reassure the patient during the initial period after surgery that the severity of the incisional pain will decrease to soreness by the second or third postoperative day. In addition to administering analgesics, institute other comfort measures, such as repositioning, rubbing the patient's back, and applying heat as ordered to the upper back, shoulder, and upper arm. Guide the patient in the use of relaxation techniques and provide diversionary activities according to her preference.

NDx: Risk for infection

Explain to the patient that the removal of lymph nodes in the axillary region makes the arm more prone to infection. Instruct her to protect the affected arm and hand from injury as described in Highlight 42–2. Place a sign near the patient's bed and on her Kardex to communicate to hospital personnel that the affected arm cannot be used for drawing blood, taking blood pressure, or administering intravenous fluids. Teach her signs and symptoms of infection and instruct her to report any abnormalities to her health-care provider.

NDx: Risk for impaired physical mobility

Start passive range-of-motion exercises of the arm and shoulder on the affected side, and provide a soft ball for the patient to squeeze as soon as possible postoperatively. Instruct the patient to begin active range-of-motion exercises gradually and to begin to use the affected arm and shoulder to care for herself as soon as the drain is removed and permission is obtained from the physician. Passive and active range-of-motion exercises are critically important because they assist in easing arm and shoulder tension, promote joint movement, re-establish elasticity to the chest wall muscles, prevent further movement limitations, and aid in re-establishing arm and shoulder strength. When explaining their importance to the patient, stress that exercising will help her regain activity and strength in her affected arm and shoulder and can reduce stiffness and pain in her neck and back.

Teach the patient appropriate range-of-motion exercises such as those used in the Reach to Recovery program (Highlight 42–3 and Fig. 42–11). Instruct her to gradually increase the exercises and to continue to exercise 3 to 5 times per day at home until full range of joint motion of the arm and shoulder is regained. Suggest that she integrate the exercises into her usual self-care and housework (Table 42–5). Caution her to avoid exercising beyond the point of discomfort and to avoid heavy lifting. Also provide the patient with information

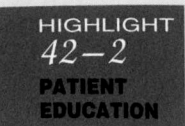 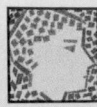

HIGHLIGHT 42-2 PATIENT EDUCATION

Hand and Arm Precautions After Modified Radical Mastectomy

Instruct the patient to:

Avoid

- Burns while cooking or smoking
- Sunburns
- Injections, vaccinations, drawing of blood samples, and blood pressure measurements on the affected arm when possible
- Nicks and scratches
- Cutting cuticles and nails
- Touching hot or cold objects
- Elastic cuffs on blouses and sleepwear

Always

- Carry heavy packages or handbags on the other arm.
- Wash cuts promptly with soap and water, apply an antibacterial medication, and monitor for redness, soreness, or other signs of infection.
- Wear watches and jewelry loosely on the affected arm.
- Wear protective gloves when gardening and when using strong detergents.
- Use a thimble when sewing.
- Use lotion on cuticles, push cuticles back with a soft cloth, and file nails.
- Use mitt-type potholder when cooking.
- Use an electric razor for underarm shaving.
- Report signs of swelling, redness, and pain in affected arm.

about community organizations—such as the American Cancer Society and the YWCA—that sponsor postmastectomy exercise programs. Instruct the patient to report any changes, such as numbness, tingling, or weakness in the affected arm.

NDx: Risk for fluid volume excess (local)

Explain to the patient that lymphedema is an abnormal accumulation of lymphatic fluid that can occur in the arm on the affected side from severing of lymphatic and blood vessels. The extent of lymphedema ranges from mild to severe and may occur any time after surgery. Stress that there is much less risk of lymphedema after a modified radical mastectomy than after a radical mastectomy. Caution the patient not to overdo arm exercises because lymphedema can be the result of or can be exacerbated by

strenuous activity of the arm and shoulder. Explain that lymphedema can also be caused by infection or injury and that the hand and arm precautions outlined in Highlight 42-2 can help prevent this.

If lymphedema occurs, teach the patient to facilitate venous return by elevating the arm to 45 degrees abduction and 60 to 90 degrees flexion. If needed, tell her that a custom-fitted elastic arm sleeve can be used to assist venous return. In severe cases, explain that a pneumatic massage sleeve can be used to drain lymphatic fluid from the arm. Instruct the patient in a low-salt diet and the use of diuretics if prescribed. Referrals to physical therapists who work with lymphedema patients can also be very beneficial. It is the responsibility of the nurse to ensure that each mastectomy patient has received proper education in the rehabilitative measures specific to her surgery to reduce the incidence of lymphedema.

NDx: Risk for body image disturbance

Discuss the meaning of the loss to the patient and encourage her to talk about her feelings. Reassure her that it is normal to be concerned about changes in appearance and the reactions of others after loss of a breast. Acknowledge and accept feelings of loss, grief, or fear of rejection. Encourage the patient to look at the incision. If the patient hesitates to look at it, describe it to her. Continue to provide opportunities for her to see it, but do not force her do so. Consider encouraging the patient and her partner to look at the wound together to promote shared feelings and support. Remember that after the initial emotional reaction, most patients adapt smoothly to the diagnosis and view the surgery as life-saving.

Provide the patient with information about obtaining a breast prosthesis. Explain that a temporary lightweight prosthesis can be used once the dressing is removed. If desired, a soft gauze pad may be used to cover the healing incision and protect it from contact with the prosthesis. Inform the patient that a permanent prosthesis may be worn in about 2 months, after the incision is healed. This prosthesis is an artificial breast mound usually made of molded silicone or foam. Stress that there are many styles and shapes available and that the prostheses are similar to natural breast tissue in weight, shape, and texture. Suggest that the patient wear a blouse and sweater to judge the symmetry when she is being fitted for the form, which fits inside a pocket sewn into a brassiere and swimwear.

Inform the patient that there are advanced-practice nurses and stores with employees that specialize in fitting women with breast prostheses. These specially trained people often go to the patient's home to fit her with a prosthesis. Locate information about these services by looking under "Surgical Appliances and Supplies" in the yellow pages. Explain that prostheses may cost from $50 to $200, but that most health insurance plans reimburse the cost fully or partially.

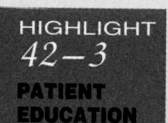 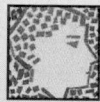

HIGHLIGHT 42–3

PATIENT EDUCATION

Postmastectomy Exercises

Instruct the patient to:

Perform exercises with the affected arm and shoulder once given permission from the physician.

- "Climb the wall": Face and move close to the wall. Put fingers on the wall at the same level as the shoulder, and gradually "walk" up the wall with the fingers (Fig. 42–11*A*).
- Using a rope hung over a bed trapeze or over the door, pull down and up on each side alternately. Reach as high as possible. Allow some discomfort but not a lot of pain (Fig. 42–11*B*).
- Tie a rope to the doorknob and hold it. Start with hand at shoulder height, and then raise the hand. Put the other hand on the hip to help balance (Fig. 42–11*C*).
- Hold a rubber ball in the affected hand and squeeze it (Fig. 42–11*D*).
- Hold a rubber ball with an elastic band in the affected hand. Hold the hand up at the shoulder level, and throw the ball down and then catch the ball when it comes back up to the hand (Fig. 42–11*E*).
- Using a rope 3 feet long, hold one end in the affected hand over the shoulder, and hold the other end in the other hand behind the back at the waist. Move the affected hand over the head and back (Fig. 42–11*F*).

Use both arms whenever possible, to take the mind off the affected arm, to have something to compare it with, and to give balance.

Move arms smoothly, slowly, and gradually using sweeping or swinging movements. Facilitate this by standing in front of a mirror while doing exercises or by doing them to music.

Use the other arm in the beginning to help the affected arm to perform the exercises or to start the exercises.

Breast reconstruction is an alternate way for the patient to regain her breast shape. Provide the patient with information about the various procedures available. Explain that when breast reconstruction is not performed immediately following a mastectomy, the mastectomy site must be fully healed before subsequent reconstruction can be done. This usually takes 3 to 6 months; encourage the patient to speak to women who have had breast reconstruction. If she is interested, The Reach to Recovery program of the American Cancer Society can provide this referral.

NDx: Risk for sexual dysfunction
Recognize the role the breast plays in a woman's sexuality and that the patient may feel that her femininity and role as a sexual partner have been lessened. Respect the individual nature of each patient's response to breast surgery. Remain supportive and nonjudgmental while encouraging the woman to verbalize her concerns and fears. Encourage discussion about sexual activity, and handle it in a sensitive and open manner. Make certain the patient understands that sexual intercourse may be resumed as soon as she wishes, although alternate coital positions may be necessary to avoid pressure on the healing incision. When possible, determine the concerns and feelings of the patient's sexual partner, and provide information and the opportunity to vent as needed. Support sharing of feelings between the patient and her partner.

NDx: Risk for altered health maintenance
Instruct the patient to avoid the use of ointments and creams on the incision and the use of antiperspirant in the affected axilla. Stress the importance of promptly reporting any changes in the incisional area or adjacent axilla or any pain, redness, or swelling in the affected arm. Explain that the patient may experience numbness or altered skin sensation in the axilla and in the area surrounding the incision. Tell the patient that some women experience "phantom breast sensations" for a short period of time postoperatively (eg, a woman may experience sensory phenomena seemingly originating in the missing breast or nipple).

Teach or review breast self-examination and instruct the patient to immediately report any changes in the remaining breast. Provide the patient with information on community agencies and programs that provide support, information, or other assistance to patients with breast cancer (see Appendix).

NDx: Risk for ineffective individual coping and Risk for ineffective family coping
It is important to recognize that receiving a diagnosis of cancer and undergoing surgical treatment and, perhaps, additional adjuvant therapy can seriously challenge the ability of the patient and her family to cope with the situation. Encourage the patient and family members to verbalize their fears concerning the cancer diagnosis, especially of disease recur-

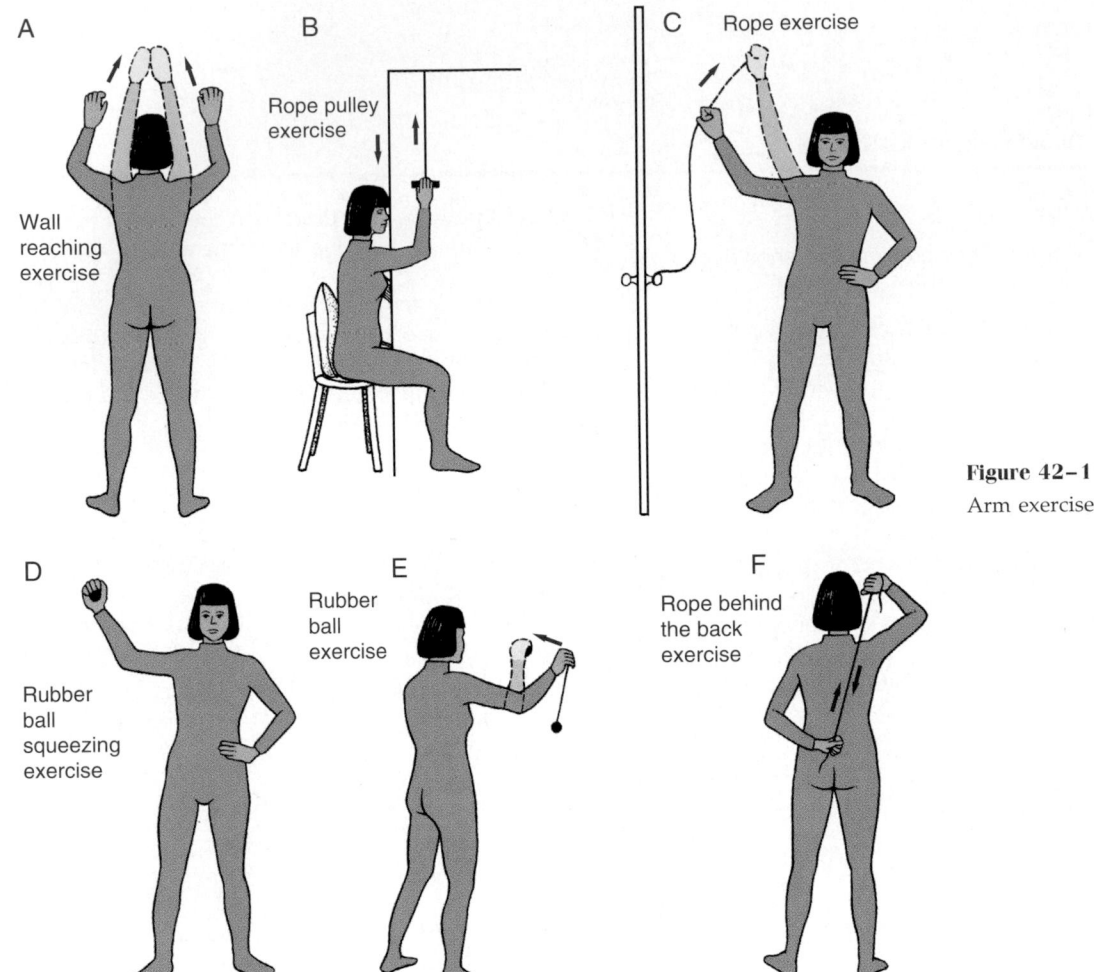

A

Wall reaching exercise

B

Rope pulley exercise

C

Rope exercise

D

Rubber ball squeezing exercise

E

Rubber ball exercise

F

Rope behind the back exercise

Figure 42–11

Arm exercises for mastectomy patients.

rence. Discuss with the patient and family their concerns about lifestyle changes. Determine how the patient and family have coped in the past with major life crises. Help them to identify successful coping

strategies. Provide referrals for family counseling if needed.

Compare the patient's status with the expected outcomes. If the outcomes are not met, reassess the patient and revise the plan.

LUMPECTOMY. Lumpectomy is a breast-preserving procedure performed with axillary lymph node dissection. It is an option when there are no metastases and the breast tumor is well defined, is less than 5 cm in diameter, and does not involve the nipple. Patients who choose this surgical option will be given a course of postoperative radiation therapy. Clinical trials have shown that lumpectomy with axillary node dissection, followed by adjuvant radiation therapy, is as effective as mastectomy for treating early-stage breast cancer.

PATIENT PREPARATION. The physical preparation of the patient scheduled for a lumpectomy is similar to that of the patient scheduled for a modified radical mastectomy.

PROCEDURE. The tumor is excised along with a small amount of surrounding normal tissue. Then, a separate incision at the axilla is made and the axillary lymph node dissection is performed. The lymph

Table 42–5

Activities of Daily Living to Enhance Arm and Shoulder Exercises

Housework

Mop floors
Vacuum
Sweep with a broom
Knead dough
Wash windows
Raise and lower
    windows
Hang clothes on a line
Weed a garden
Cook/stir
Make a bed

Self-Care

Fasten a brassiere
Wash and dry the back
Pull a zipper
Button
Comb and brush hair

Crafts and Sports

Weave
Knit/crochet
Sew
Type
Play golf
Paint
Swim

■ Clinical Pathway for Modified Radical Mastectomy or Lumpectomy with Axillary Node Dissection

Patient Name _____

Date _____

DRG# _____

Expected LOS   48–72 h _____

	Day 1 (Day of Surgery)	Day 2 (PO #1)	Day 3 (PO #2)	Day 4 (PO #3)
Medication	Prophylactic antibiotics IV fluids per anesthesiologist Parenteral pain medications	Pain medication (IV, IM, PCA, PO) D/C IV when tolerating PO intake	PO pain medication	Continued PO pain medication at home prn
Diagnostic Tests		Oncology consult Blood work as needed	Bone scan	
Diet	NPO for surgery Clear liquids postop	Clear liquids Advance to regular diet as tolerated	Regular diet	Resume normal diet at home
Activity		OOB Ambulating	OOB Ambulating Arm exercises as tolerated	Progress to normal activity level and arm exercises at home as tolerated
Treatments/Nursing Actions	PACU: Monitor airway, VS, drainage, incision Elevate arm and institute arm precautions	Monitor VS, drainage, and incision Elevate arm and maintain arm precautions Offer emotional support	Assess drainage, dressing, and incision Elevate arm and maintain arm precautions Offer emotional support	Discharge to home with dressing and temporary drain
Teaching/Discharge Planning		Reach to Recovery referral Assess need for visiting nurse	Teach drain care, incision care, and dressing care Discuss prostheses and community support groups	Provide discharge instructions, emphasizing followup appointments and need to perform BSE

Derived from Sciartelli CH. Using a clinical pathway approach to document patient teaching for breast cancer surgical procedures. Oncol Nurs Forum 1995; 22(1):131.

nodes are removed and all tissue sent to the pathology laboratory. A closed self-suction drain is inserted in the wound, which is covered with a light gauze dressing. The procedure is usually done under general anesthesia and takes 1 to 2 hours.

If a lumpectomy has already been done for diagnosis, axillary lymph node dissection is performed as a second procedure once the diagnosis of cancer is confirmed and the patient selects this option as opposed to a modified radical mastectomy. These procedures are commonly performed in a day-surgery setting.

POSTOPERATIVE COURSE. Oral fluids with progression to a regular diet are resumed when the patient has recovered from the anesthesia. The intravenous line started at the time of surgery is discontinued as soon as the patient tolerates oral intake. Activity is also gradually resumed once the patient is alert. Initial pain from the axillary dissection typically changes to soreness and tightness after the first 24 hours. When drainage from the wound has tapered off, the drain is removed, usually the second

postoperative day. The incision heals in about 2 weeks, and then adjuvant radiation therapy is given to the patient.

COMPLICATIONS. Dissection of the axillary lymph nodes may block the flow of lymph, creating a risk of lymphedema. This risk is greatest in the 6 weeks after surgery, before collateral lymph circulation has developed.

NURSING PROCESS

Lumpectomy and Axillary Node Dissection for Breast Cancer

The nursing care of the patient undergoing lumpectomy for breast cancer is presented in Nursing Care Guide 42–1.

PREVENTIVE SURGERY. Some women desire and some physicians recommend bilateral mastectomies for women who have multiple risk factors for breast

Text continued on page 1874

Nursing Care Guide 42–1
Patients Undergoing Lumpectomy and Axillary Node Dissection for Cancer of the Breast

Preoperative Care

Assessment Findings: Patient has no experience with lumpectomy and axillary node dissection. Patient asks questions about the procedure, perioperative events, and follow-up care.

Nursing Diagnosis: Knowledge deficit: lumpectomy procedure, perioperative events, follow-up care

Patient Outcomes	Nursing Interventions	Rationale
Patient describes lumpectomy within the framework of the overall treatment plan.	Review the physician's plan of care with the patient. Include a description of what lumpectomy involves, as well as the plan for subsequent radiation and/or chemotherapy.	Patients under stress often misinterpret or do not hear information. Reviewing information improves understanding of the procedure and plan of care and contributes to informed consent.
Patient describes perioperative routines.	Describe general perioperative routines.	Prepares the patient for perioperative events, thus involving the patient in the plan of care, promoting cooperation, and decreasing the risk of anxiety over routine measures.

Evaluation: Compare the patient's status with the expected outcomes. If the outcomes are not met, reassess the patient and revise the plan.

Assessment Findings: Patient states, "I'm so worried I don't know what to do. I hope I made the right choice when I chose the lumpectomy. Maybe it would have been better to have everything removed so there would be less chance the cancer will come back. People with cancer have horrible deaths and I don't want to die." Patient also states, "I hope I won't look deformed after this operation."

Nursing Diagnosis: Anxiety related to possibility of prolonged illness, pain, and death; concern that selecting lumpectomy as the method of treatment was the best choice; concern about postoperative appearance

Patient Outcomes	Nursing Interventions	Rationale
Patient expresses concerns freely.	Allow verbalization of concerns	Verbalizing concerns to another provides perspective, allows for correction of misconceptions, and permits a supportive relationship.
Patient expresses comfort with her decision to have a lumpectomy.	Stress that lumpectomy with radiation is as effective as mastectomy for early-stage cancer according to available studies.	Provides positive facts that help build the patient's confidence in her treatment decision.

(continued)

Nursing Care Guide 42-1

Patients Undergoing Lumpectomy and Axillary Node Dissection for Cancer of the Breast (continued)

Patient Outcomes	Nursing Interventions	Rationale
Patient describes expected postoperative appearance of the breast and axilla realistically.	Explain to patient that lumpectomy is not recommended by a surgeon unless the breast is large enough to prevent subsequent deformity.	Provides the patient with positive facts to counteract anxiety over postoperative appearance.
Signs of severe anxiety are absent.	Remind the patient that remission in early-stage cancer is the rule.	Provides positive facts on which to focus and base hope for a successful surgical outcome.

Evaluation: Compare the patient's status with the expected outcomes. If the outcomes are not met, reassess the patient and revise the plan.

Postoperative Care

Assessment Findings: Patient complains of pain in the area of the surgery.

Nursing Diagnosis: Pain related to tissue trauma secondary to surgical dissection of the breast and axilla

Patient Outcomes	Nursing Interventions	Rationale
Patient reports that pain is controlled. Behavioral signs of severe pain are absent.	Administer parenteral analgesics for pain in the immediate postoperative period.	Parenteral analgesics provide prompt pain relief, thus promoting rest and facilitating the healing process.
	Administer prescribed oral analgesics as needed, beginning 8 to 12 hours postoperatively.	Provides pain control, promoting rest and facilitating healing and movement.
	Assist the patient into a comfortable position with support for the affected arm.	Position of comfort promotes rest. The affected area is supported to prevent pull on traumatized tissues and stress on suture lines.

Evaluation: Compare the patient's status with the expected outcomes. If the outcomes are not met, reassess the patient and revise the plan.

Assessment Findings: Postoperative patient has had an excision of a breast mass and an axillary node dissection.

Nursing Diagnosis: Impaired tissue integrity related to surgery of the breast and axilla

(continued)

Nursing Care Guide 42–1

Patients Undergoing Lumpectomy and Axillary Node Dissection for Cancer of the Breast (continued)

Patient Outcomes	Nursing Interventions	Rationale
Wound drainage changes from bright red to serosanguineous within 12 hours after surgery. Drainage gradually tapers off, ending in 46 to 72 hours.	Check amount and color of wound drainage. Expect drainage to be bright red initially and to change to serosanguineous after about 12 hours. Tell the patient to expect an initial volume of about 75 mL per 8 hours, gradually tapering to 0 after 48 to 72. If done as a same-day procedure, instruct patient on how to empty drain and dress wound.	Increase in amount or reversion to a brighter red color indicates bleeding.
Incision remains intact.	Caution the patient about stretching her arm or performing any painful activities. Tell the patient a brassiere may be worn if desired for support.	Tension on the suture line can cause disruption and hemorrhage because the breast is highly vascular. Support brassieres maintain the breasts in an upright position. Large breasts are pendulous and may strain the suture line.

Evaluation: Compare the patient's status with the expected outcomes. If the outcomes are not met, reassess the patient and revise the plan.

Assessment Findings: Patient has a break in the skin from the surgical incision and has had an axillary lymph node dissection.

Nursing Diagnosis: Risk for infection related to presence of an incision and alteration of the lymphatic system on the affected side

Patient Outcomes	Nursing Interventions	Rationale
Wound remains free of infection, as evidenced by absence of redness, warmth, swelling, and drainage.	Instruct the patient to keep the suture line dry and dressings intact according to surgeon's directions. Instruct the patient to observe the suture line daily for redness, warmth, swelling, or drainage, and report to surgeon if present.	Decreases the spread of microorganisms into the incisional area. Evaluates wound for signs of infection, allowing early medical intervention should infection occur.
Patient lists precautions to be taken to protect the affected arm.	Instruct the patient to protect the affected arm from infection as described in Highlight 42–2.	Patient is at risk for infection due to the effects of surgery on the lymphatic system

Evaluation: Compare the patient's status with the expected outcomes. If the outcomes are not met, reassess the patient and revise the plan.

(continued)

Nursing Care Guide 42–1

Patients Undergoing Lumpectomy and Axillary Node Dissection for Cancer of the Breast (continued)

Assessment Findings: Patient has had axillary lymph nodes removed, resulting in a temporary obstruction to lymph flow.

Nursing Diagnosis: Risk for fluid volume excess (local) related to impaired lymph flow in the affected arm

Patient Outcomes	Nursing Interventions	Rationale
Affected arm and hand are free of edema.	Elevate affected arm on a pillow.	Allows gravity to assist in the removal of excess fluid from affected area.
	Monitor for circulatory impairment. Compare affected arm with nonaffected arm. Check for paleness and edema. Palpate radial pulse. Check temperature of arm. Check capillary refill time.	Evaluates circulation in the affected arm and allows prompt medical intervention if impairment occurs.
Patient describes precautions to be taken.	Instruct the patient to gradually increase exercises but to avoid strenuous activity of the arm and shoulder as well as injury or infection in the arm and hand (see Highlight 42–2).	Strenuous activities, injury, and infection can contribute to lymphedema.

Evaluation: Compare the patient's status with the expected outcomes. If the outcomes are not met, reassess the patient and revise the plan.

Assessment Findings: Patient complains of discomfort and a feeling of tightness in the area of the incision.

Nursing Diagnosis: Risk for impaired physical mobility related to discomfort on moving the affected arm

Patient Outcomes	Nursing Interventions	Rationale
Patient performs range-of-motion exercises as directed.	Instruct the patient in range-of-motion exercises when permitted by surgeon.	Promotes joint mobility and tone and strength of muscles of affected arm and shoulder.
Patient states importance of not going beyond the point of "hurt" when exercising.	Caution the patient not to continue any exercise movement past the point of "hurt."	Pain can be a warning sign indicating tissue damage.

Evaluation: Compare the patient's status with the expected outcomes. If the outcomes are not met, reassess the patient and revise the plan.

(continued)

Nursing Care Guide 42–1
*Patients Undergoing Lumpectomy and Axillary Node Dissection
for Cancer of the Breast* (continued)

Additional Assessments and Interventions

Assess for signs of body image disturbance and concerns about sexual activity. Encourage the patient to discuss her concerns frankly with her spouse or sexual partner. Reassure the patient that touching the breasts during lovemaking does not cause injury or the recurrence of cancer.

Provide the patient with information about community resources available to help women deal with their diagnosis and treatment (see Appendix).

Teach or review the importance of and the technique of monthly breast self-examination. Emphasize to the patient how the lumpectomy may have changed the feel or contour of the breast.

Review the plan for follow-up care with the patient. Make certain she knows where and when to report for her next appointment.

---

cancer. These include women who have a strong family history of breast cancer, have had many biopsies, or have breasts that are very hard to examine. This is not a widely used procedure, and a second opinion should always be obtained before prophylactic mastectomies are performed.

Chemotherapy

Several types of chemotherapeutic drugs are used to treat breast cancer. Combinations of chemotherapeutic drugs are common because

- different types of drugs can destroy cancer cells in different stages of the cell cycle
- if a single drug is used, there is more chance of the tumor becoming resistant to the antineoplastic agent
- if a combination of drugs is used, dosages and side effects are less than if a single drug is used alone.

The most frequently used combinations are cyclophosphamide (Cytoxan), methotrexate, and fluorouracil (CMF) and cyclophosphamide (Cytoxan), doxorubicin (Adriamycin), and fluorouracil (CAF). Cyclophosphamide is an alkylating agent; 5-fluorouracil and methotrexate are antimetabolites; doxorubicin is an antitumor antibiotic. Alkylating agents interfere with DNA replication. Antimetabolites interfere with the enzymes needed for the synthesis of RNA and DNA.

Chemotherapy may be used to treat both early and advanced disease. The specific drugs chosen and length of treatment vary according to type of disease. Currently, the anti-cancer agent paclitaxel (Taxol) is widely used to treat a variety of metastatic diseases, including advanced breast cancer. Also used to treat metastatic disease is high-dose chemo-

therapy, in which the maximal safe dosage of a drug is given in conjunction with a bone marrow transplant, peripheral stem cell transplant, or hematopoietic growth factors to stimulate bone marrow recovery.

The side effects of chemotherapy depend on the drugs used and the patient's reaction to the drugs. Refer to Chapter 34 for a discussion of the side effects of chemotherapy.

Hormonal therapy is a specific form of therapy that slows the growth of neoplastic tissue by changing the hormonal balance. Hormone receptor status is important in deciding whether hormonal therapy is indicated. A tumor that is estrogen receptor positive suggests that the tumor cells may grow more rapidly in the presence of estrogen. To prevent estrogen from entering these cells and stimulating growth, an antiestrogen is administered. Tamoxifen is the agent most commonly prescribed. Hormones can be used alone or in combination with other chemotherapeutic drugs.

When chemotherapy is used in conjunction with radiotherapy or surgery, it is called adjuvant chemotherapy. Adjuvant chemotherapy is given after removal of early-stage breast tumors to prevent recurrence and metastasis from microscopic spread. Adjuvant chemotherapy is usually given for a set amount of time, which may be as short as 6 months or as long as 24 months. Currently, premenopausal women with positive axillary lymph nodes receive adjuvant chemotherapy after surgery. Postmenopausal women with positive lymph nodes and estrogen receptor positive tumors receive oral hormonal therapy, such as tamoxifen.

In the past, adjuvant therapy was not recommended for patients with negative lymph nodes. Because of the high recurrence rate (about 30%) in this group, the National Cancer Institute now recommends that adjuvant chemotherapy should be considered for these patients.

Chemotherapy is also used to treat patients with advanced breast cancer. Patients who experience symptoms of metastatic disease, such as pain and organ dysfunction, receive chemotherapy combinations designed to control tumor cells that have already spread to other body organs. A remission is attained when tumor growth is halted and the size of the tumor decreases. In these cases, chemotherapeutic drugs are given for an indefinite period of time and, if the tumor progresses, another combination of chemotherapy agents may be tried.

Refer to Chapter 34 for a discussion of nursing care applicable to patients receiving chemotherapy.

Radiation Therapy

Radiation therapy is given by external beam or by implanting radioactive material into the breast tissue. It is used to treat both localized and advanced breast cancer. Radiation may be used after limited breast surgery, such as a lumpectomy with axillary node dissection, to decrease the chance of recurrence at the operative site and in the regional lymph nodes. For advanced local disease, radiation is used to shrink large breast tumors to an operable size so that they can be removed. In patients with metastatic breast cancer, radiation is used as a palliative method to locally control tumor cells that have spread to other body parts.

External radiation is usually given on an outpatient basis for about 5 weeks, and an additional "boost" of radiation is given 2 weeks later. The radiation boost is accomplished through additional external beam radiation or by the use of internal iridium implants, which deliver radiation in a concentrated form to the breast tissue. Radiation implants require hospitalization. Small plastic tubes are threaded through the breast (see Fig. 34-7) in the operating room with the patient under general or local anesthesia. Radioactive seeds, usually iridium, are introduced into the tubes. The number and placement of the tubes depend on the size and location of the breast tumor. The tubes are kept in place for 45 to 60 hours, and the patient is confined to a private hospital room. Small amounts of radiation are emitted from the radiation implants. For this reason, the amount of time spent in the patient's room by visitors and hospital staff is limited.

Radiation may be used in combination with surgery or chemotherapy, or both. Refer to Chapter 34 for a discussion of nursing care applicable to patients receiving radiation therapy.

❖ Settings, Providers, and Collaboration for Care

The care of patients with breast cancer presents a complex challenge for caregivers that requires a multidisciplinary approach to delivery of services. The health-care professionals routinely involved in caring for patients with breast cancer include the following:

- The patient's primary physician
- A medical, surgical, and/or radiation oncologist
- A pathologist
- A radiologist
- An oncology clinical nurse specialist
- A social worker or other psycho-oncology specialist
- Radiation therapists

The primary physician often initially identifies a suspicious breast lump and is responsible for referring the patient to a breast surgeon for definitive diagnosis and beginning treatment. The primary physician continues to monitor other aspects of the patient's health care throughout the program of breast cancer treatment.

As an integral part of this multidisciplinary team, nurses collaborate with other team members to establish outcomes for patients and provide direct nursing care as well as education and counseling. Nurses also coordinate services and continuity of care, provide patient advocacy and support, and consult with other health-care professionals as needed to maximize care to patients.

Plastic Surgery Procedures

Many women, for a variety of reasons, wish to alter the size and shape of their breasts through plastic surgery. The procedure, known as mammoplasty, can be used to increase or decrease breast size, tighten breast tissue, or reconstruct a missing breast. Mammoplasty is usually performed under general anesthesia and, based on the extent of alteration desired, may require several procedures over a period of months.

BREAST RECONSTRUCTION

Breast reconstruction, also known as reconstructive mammoplasty, is a surgical procedure that creates a natural-looking breast shape. This is achieved either by insertion of an implant under the skin and muscles of the chest wall in the area of a mastectomy, or by transference of skin, fat, and muscle from another part of the body to the mastectomy site (autogenous tissue transfer). Breast reconstruction can be performed immediately following a mastectomy. If breast reconstruction is to be delayed, then the procedure is performed after the mastectomy site has fully healed, usually in 3 to 6 months. If the patient must undergo chemotherapy or radiation, reconstruction is delayed until the completion of this adjuvant therapy. The timing of the procedure must be decided in close consultation with the patient, the plastic surgeon, and the oncologist.

To increase symmetry of the reconstructed and the natural breast, breast reduction, breast augmentation, or mastopexy may be performed on the natural breast. The need for such alteration is most likely in women over the age of 40.

The result of reconstruction, with or without alterations of the other breast, is not an exact duplication of the natural breast, but for some patients reconstruction is more desirable than using a prosthesis. In all cases, it is important that the patient and plastic surgeon set realistic goals for the outcome of the breast reconstruction. The results of the reconstruction should be judged against those expectations. With current advances in autogenous breast reconstruction techniques, the actual results of reconstruction often exceed patients' expectations.

Procedures

SIMPLE IMPLANT RECONSTRUCTION

The breast implant is a sealed sac containing a fluid such as saline or silicone gel. The implant is custom fitted to match the remaining breast or, in the case of bilateral reconstruction, the woman and her plastic surgeon select the implant size and shape.

The breast implant considered safest for use today is filled with saline. Silicone gel implants have been restricted for use on a research basis and explicitly for breast reconstruction by the U.S. Food and Drug Administration (FDA) because of associated risks. These risks include local tissue reactions if silicone leaks from the implant or if the implant ruptures, less than optimal mammogram interpretation because of the presence of the implant or local tissue reaction, the potential for an autoimmune reaction, and the possible carcinogenicity of the implant itself. All women receiving silicone implants must sign a consent form that outlines the risks, and they must agree to participate in FDA-approved clinical studies to evaluate the safety and effectiveness of the implants.

In simple implant reconstruction, the surgeon uses the mastectomy scar and makes a small incision. The implant is inserted in a pocket created under the pectoralis muscle (Fig. 42–12). This method is chosen if the woman's pectoral muscles have been preserved and there is a sufficient amount of skin remaining on the chest wall. A variation of this procedure involves placing the implant between the skin and the muscle.

In another procedure, a tissue expander is used to stretch the operative site to accommodate an implant. A deflated sac is placed in the site in the upper chest. A small amount of saline is injected into the sac via a subcutaneous filling port at weekly intervals until the desired size is attained and the overlying skin is sufficiently stretched. In a few months, when the expander has reached the desired size, another surgery is performed in which the expander is removed and a permanent implant is inserted.

AUTOGENOUS TISSUE TRANSFER

In autogenous tissue transfer, the surgeon transfers a flap of skin, fat, and muscle, along with its intact blood supply (known as *pedicled* tissue), to the mastectomy site and creates a breast mound. The two most common donor sites of this pedicled myocutaneous flap are the transverse rectus abdominis muscle (TRAM flap) and the latissimus dorsi muscle (LD flap).

In rectus abdominis reconstruction, the surgeon harvests the flap from the donor site of the lower abdominal area and tunnels it subcutaneously to the site of the mastectomy, where the breast mound is then fashioned. The TRAM flap provides enough skin and fat to form the breast without the need of an implant (Fig. 42–13).

In latissimus dorsi reconstruction, the surgeon tunnels the myocutaneous flap obtained from the donor site of the upper posterior back to the mastectomy site. Because the LD flap usually has insufficient bulk, an implant is needed to supply the volume of the breast mound (Fig. 42–14).

When lower abdominal tissue is unavailable, a free-flap procedure may be performed. Flaps from

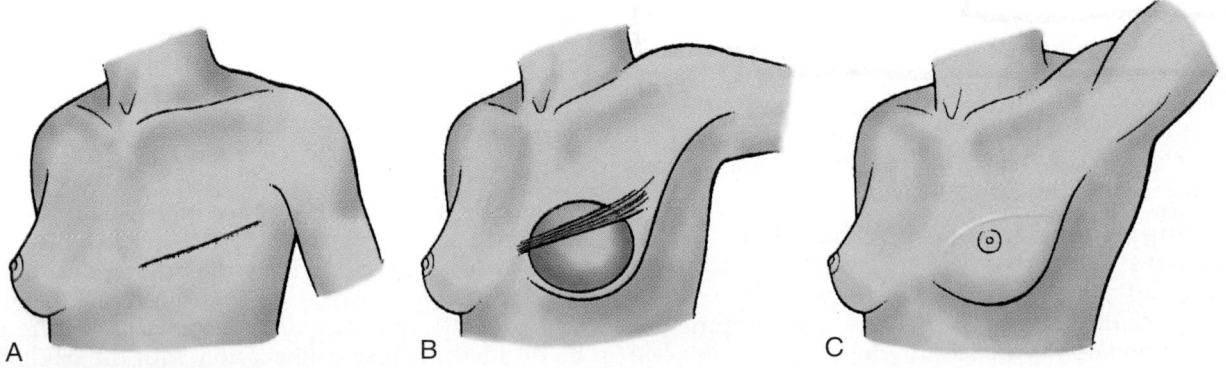

Figure 42–12

Simple breast reconstruction. *A,* Appearance of chest before reconstruction. *B,* Appearance of chest with implant in place. *C,* Appearance of chest with nipple and areola reconstructed.

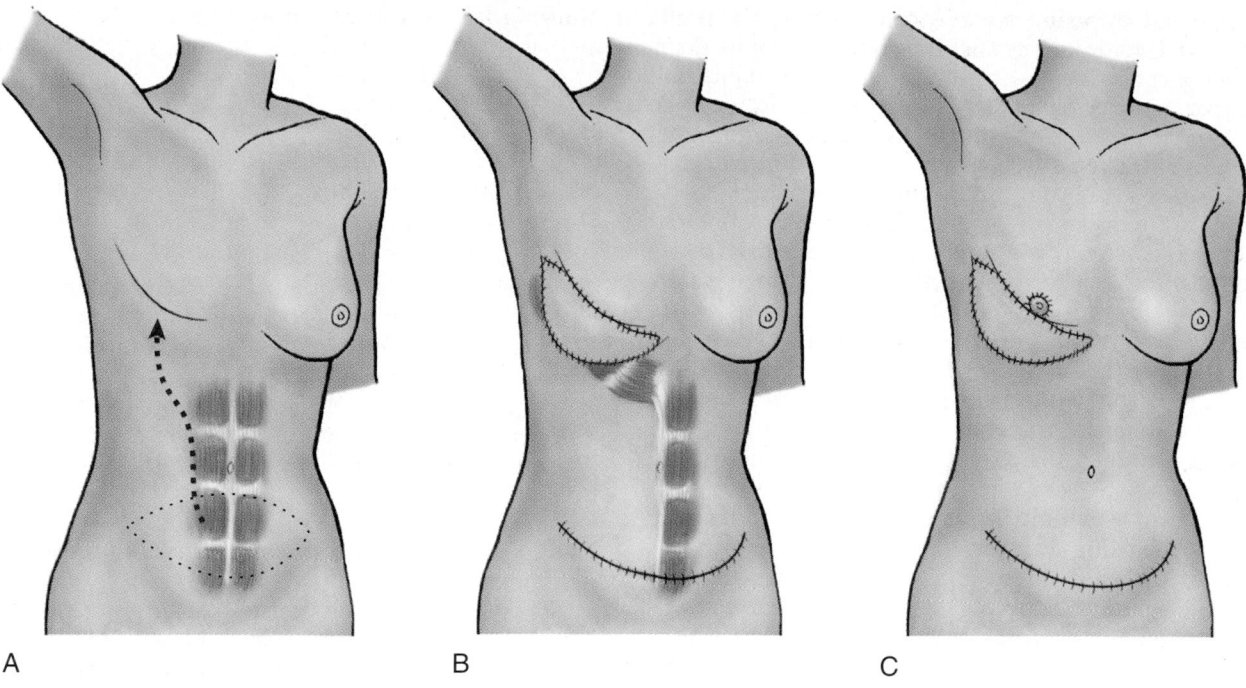

Figure 42-13

In transverse rectus abdominis muscle (TRAM) flap reconstruction, the surgeon creates a flap of muscle and skin from the lower abdomen (*A*), then tunnels this flap up through the upper abdomen to the chest wall (*B*). The postoperative result is shown in *C*.

the gluteal, lateral thigh, or peri-iliac areas can be used to create the breast mound. In the free-flap procedure, microsurgical techniques are used to an-astamose blood vessels, thus re-establishing blood

supply to the reconstructed breast. In both pedicled and free-flap procedures, a significant scar is left at the patient's donor site.

In all procedures, the nipple and areola may also

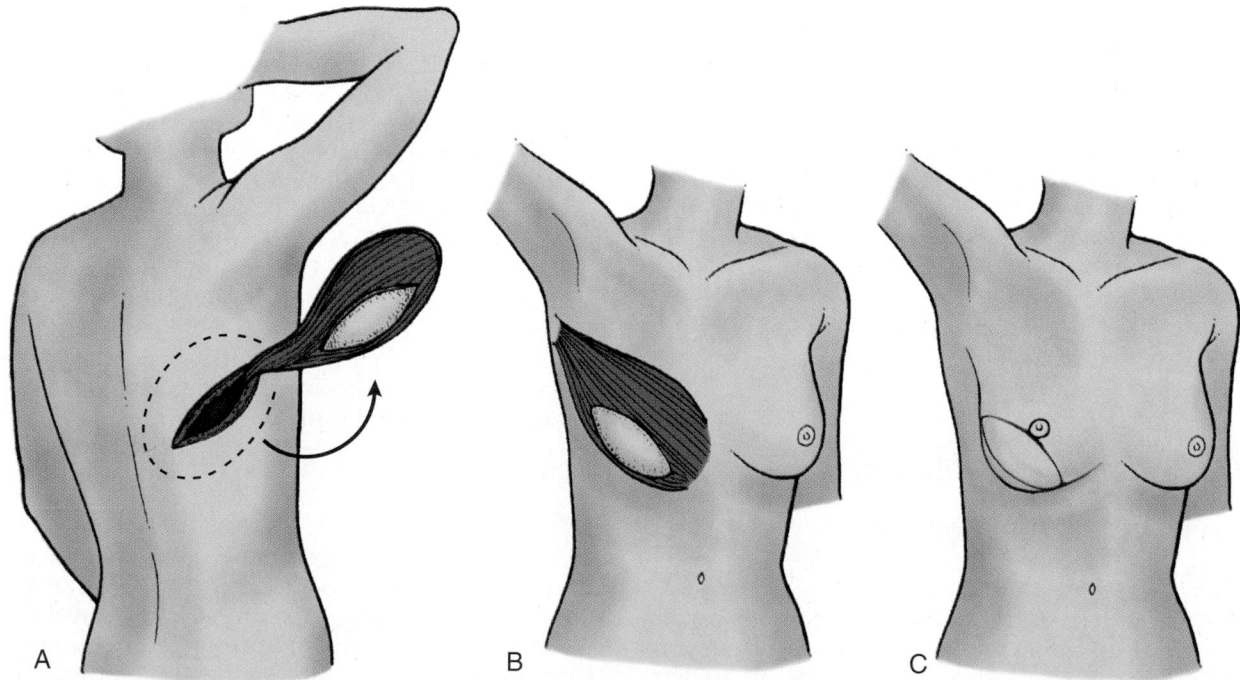

Figure 42-14

Latissimus dorsi (LD) flap procedure. *A*, Latissimus dorsi muscle and skin flap raised on the patient's back. *B*, Flap tunneled under the skin from the back to the anterior chest to create the contour of a breast. *C*, Appearance when reconstruction is complete.

be recreated by using some of the nipple and areola from the remaining breast (known as nipple sharing) or grafting tissue from the toe, thigh, labia minora, or earlobe. The reconstructed breast, areola, and nipple are, for the most part, insensate. Breast reconstruction usually requires two or more surgical procedures, depending on the desired outcome.

The numerous issues and concerns that created controversy over the timing of reconstruction in relation to the mastectomy have been shown to be groundless by current research. In an extensive review of the literature, Corral and Mustoe (1996) concluded that there is no evidence that immediate breast reconstruction causes a delay in detecting cancer recurrence or in any way interferes with the patient's prognosis. Immediate breast reconstruction was shown to lessen the psychologic trauma associated with mastectomy. It was not shown to cause a delay in initiating adjuvant chemotherapy, nor did it cause an increase in postoperative complications in women who underwent adjuvant chemotherapy. Thus, while the issue of immediate versus delayed reconstruction continues to be debated in practice, research results support the benefits of immediate reconstruction for the patient (Corral & Mustoe, 1996).

Complications

The common complications of reconstructive surgery are bleeding and infection at the implant site, insufficient blood circulation at the graft site, and formation of fibrous scar tissue around the implant. If an infection develops, antibiotics are prescribed, and the implant may have to be removed until the infection subsides. Insufficient blood supply to the skin and muscle graft can result in tissue necrosis. If this occurs, the implant must be removed. Fibrous tissue formation occurring around the implant results from the body's reaction to its presence. In about 10% of cases, the fibrous capsule causes the implant to feel hard, and the woman may experience pain. The capsule can be removed by massaging the area or through surgical intervention. The surgeon may instruct the patient to massage the implant postoperatively for 3 to 6 months to prevent capsule formation, soften the implant, and give it a more natural contour.

NURSING PROCESS
Breast Reconstruction Surgery

PREOPERATIVE NURSING CARE

Assessment

Assess the patient's understanding of the reconstruction procedure, the expected physical result, and its possible side effects. Also assess level of anxiety, because even though breast reconstruction is an elective procedure, patients may still be highly anxious over the prospect of anesthesia and further surgery.

Nursing Diagnoses and Planning

The nursing diagnoses and related expected patient outcomes commonly applicable to patients scheduled for breast reconstruction surgery include the following:

NDx: Knowledge deficit: reconstruction procedure and outcome

Planning: Patient Outcomes
1. Patient states reason for selecting reconstructive surgery over other prosthetic options.
2. Patient verbalizes realistic expectations of treatment.
3. Patient describes the preparation for the procedure, expected discomfort, and expected postoperative course.

Nursing Interventions and Evaluation

NDx: Knowledge deficit: reconstruction procedure and outcome
Encourage the patient who is considering breast reconstruction surgery to thoroughly explore all prosthetic options and to realistically appraise the outcomes of the surgery. Explain that the reconstruction is basically designed to provide a normal appearance when the patient is dressed, without the need for an external prosthesis. It will not necessarily duplicate the remaining breast. Stress that it is important to maintain realistic expectations of the outcome of reconstruction. Show pictures of breast reconstruction to the patient. Suggest talking with other women who have completed breast reconstruction by contacting the local American Cancer Society or Reconstruction Education for National Understanding (RENU) for peer support and information.

Inform the patient of the cost and time commitment involved with the multiple-step procedure of breast reconstruction. Review the schedule for procedures and make certain the patient understands that it may take 3 to 6 months before the optimal result of the surgery is evident. Allow time for the patient to ask questions, verbalize concerns, and express the outcome that she desires from breast reconstruction.

When the decision is made to have breast reconstruction surgery, provide basic preoperative teaching as discussed in Chapter 6.

Compare the patient's status with the expected outcomes. If the outcomes are not met, reassess the patient and revise the plan.

POSTOPERATIVE NURSING CARE

Assessment

Assess the patient's return to physiologic stabilization. Check the temperature of the skin flap and observe for blanching, duskiness, and decreased capillary refill, which are indicators of impaired perfusion. Report a temperature drop or mottling immediately. Observe the incisional area for redness, drainage, and other indicators of infection. Check the function of drainage devices and report drainage that exceeds 50 mL/hour.

Nursing Diagnoses and Planning

Nursing diagnoses and related expected patient outcomes commonly applicable to patients who have had breast reconstruction surgery include the following:

NDx: Pain related to surgical trauma to the anterior chest

Planning: Patient Outcomes
1. Patient reports that pain is relieved or controlled.
2. Patient moves freely without signs of excessive discomfort.

NDx: Risk for altered breast tissue perfusion related to pressure on blood vessels or chilling

Planning: Patient Outcomes
1. Breast is free of pressure from weight, tight dressings, and the like.
2. Patient denies feeling chilled.

NDx: Risk for altered health maintenance related to insufficient knowledge of self-care after discharge

Planning: Patient Outcomes
1. Patient describes appropriate self-care.
2. Patient expresses willingness and ability to carry out self-care instructions.

Nursing Interventions and Evaluation

NDx: Pain
Monitor the extent of the patient's pain and administer pain medication as ordered and needed. By the second postoperative day, medications can be decreased in strength and given less frequently. Use nursing measures, such as position changes and back rubs, to both decrease the pain and enhance the effect of analgesics. Teach and encourage the use of relaxation techniques. Encourage the patient to employ measures (such as diversionary activities) that have successfully decreased pain in the past.

NDx: Risk for altered breast tissue perfusion
Position the patient on her back or the nonoperative side to avoid pressure on the breast mound, which could impair circulation and lead to tissue necrosis. Also avoid pressure from dressings, clothing, or other sources. To avoid decreases in surface circulation, keep the patient from getting chilled.

NDx: Risk for altered health maintenance
Instruct the patient in self-care after discharge as presented in Highlight 42–4.

Compare the patient's status with the expected outcomes. If the outcomes are not met, reassess the patient and revise the plan.

AUGMENTATION MAMMOPLASTY

Augmentation mammoplasty is a procedure in which breasts are enlarged by inserting implants filled with a fluid substance between the breast tissue and the chest wall. A tight bandage is applied after the procedure to anchor the implant.

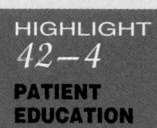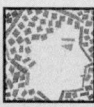

HIGHLIGHT 42–4

PATIENT EDUCATION

Self-Care After Breast Reconstruction Surgery

Instruct the patient to:

Avoid trauma to the breast mound.

- Sleep on the side or back.
- Refrain from wearing a brassiere for 4 to 6 weeks.
- Avoid lifting arms above shoulder level for 4 to 6 weeks.
- Avoid lifting more than 5 lbs for 4 to 6 weeks.
- Limit pressure on the breast during sexual activity.
- Avoid contact sports.

Perform monthly breast self-examination for early detection of recurrence of breast cancer in the unaffected breast and in the axillary regions of both breasts.

Report signs of infection, fluid accumulation, skin changes, bleeding, or contracture of the breast to the surgeon.

Return for a check-up on *(specify date and time)*.

The use of implants for breast augmentation has been sharply restricted by the U.S. FDA, and all implant recipients must sign a specific and lengthy informed consent form that covers the short- and long-term risks of implants and must agree to be listed in a national registry and participate in clinical studies.

NURSING PROCESS GUIDELINES
Augmentation Mammoplasty

The assessment, nursing diagnoses, expected patient outcomes, nursing interventions, and evaluation for patients undergoing augmentation mammoplasty are similar to those described previously for patients undergoing breast reconstruction surgery.

REDUCTION MAMMOPLASTY

Reduction mammoplasty is a procedure that reduces the size of the breast by surgically removing breast tissue and relocating the nipple and areola. This procedure may be necessitated by very large breasts that cause back and shoulder pain or cause brassiere straps to cut the shoulders. Based on the extent of the reduction, multiple incisions may be made in different locations on the breast. Drainage catheters are inserted, and a dressing is applied. There may be a loss of breast function after breast reduction.

DERMAL MASTOPEXY

Dermal mastopexy is a procedure in which excess breast skin and fat are removed in an attempt to uplift sagging breasts. The nipple and the areola are relocated.

NURSING PROCESS GUIDELINES
Reduction Mammoplasty or Dermal Mastopexy

The assessment, nursing diagnoses, expected patient outcomes, nursing interventions, and evaluation for patients undergoing reduction mammoplasty or dermal mastopexy are similar to those described previously for patients undergoing mastectomy, with the following additional considerations. Anxiety is common even though the procedure is elective. There is also a risk for body image disturbance because, although improved cosmetic appearance is a goal, change in and loss of a body part are involved. Nursing needs differ from those of the mastectomy patient in that the patient undergoing reduction mammoplasty or dermal mastopexy is not faced with an underlying life-threatening disease that may recur.

The Elderly: Special Considerations

Breast cancer is the most common breast disease of older women. Because its incidence increases with age, routine breast examinations and other screening measures are essential to early detection. Thus, information related to self-examination and professional breast examination and the patient's last mammogram should be obtained as part of every woman's history. Further, every plan of care must include interventions designed to promote the regular use of screening techniques.

Older women should be taught to practice breast self-examination unless a physical or psychologic disorder is present that makes this inappropriate. If breast self-examination is not possible, then monthly breast examinations by a health-care professional or other person should be considered. When teaching breast self-examination or performing breast examination on an older woman, consider the possibility that nipple retraction, which can be a sign of an underlying tumor, may also be an age-related change. To differentiate between the two, exert gentle pressure around the nipple and watch for nipple eversion, or teach the patient to do so. If the nipple everts, the cause of the retraction is age-related.

Breast problems are relatively rare among older

men. Breast cancer can occur, so patients should be taught to observe for and to report any breast changes. Gynecomastia also occurs among older men and can result from cirrhosis, thyroid disease, testicular tumors, bronchogenic carcinoma, or such drugs as spironolactone.

Chapter Review

1. What are the implications of a family history of breast cancer for an individual patient?
2. What is the meaning of dimpling noted during a breast examination?
3. Why is regular breast self-examination important?
4. How does a sonogram differ from a mammogram?
5. What are the similarities and differences between a benign and a malignant breast tumor?
6. How is the care of a patient with breast cancer similar to the care of a patient with any cancer?
7. How is the care of a patient undergoing lumpectomy and lymph node dissection different from the care of a patient undergoing modified radical mastectomy?
8. What would happen to a patient who has had an axillary node dissection if the arm on the affected side were accidentally injured?
9. What instructions should be given to a patient being discharged with a Jackson-Pratt drain in place after same-day surgery for axillary node dissection?
10. What are the advantages and disadvantages of immediate reconstructive surgery for a patient who has had a mastectomy?

Bibliography

American Cancer Society. Breast cancer facts and figures, 1996. Atlanta, GA: Author, 1996.

American Cancer Society. Breast cancer management: Part 1. CA Cancer J Clin 1995; 45(4):2.

American Cancer Society. Breast cancer management: Part 2. CA Cancer J Clin 1995; 45(5):2.

American Cancer Society. Standards for breast-conservation treatment. CA Cancer J Clin 1992; 42(3).

American Cancer Society. Cancer facts and figures, 1997. New York: Author, 1997.

American Joint Committee on Cancer. Manual for staging of cancer. 3rd ed. Philadelphia: JB Lippincott, 1988.

Armsden G, Lewis F. Behavioral adjustment and self-esteem of school age children of women with breast cancer. Oncol Nurs Forum 1994; 21(1):39.

Bandyk E, Gilmore M. Perceived concerns of pregnant women with breast cancer treated with chemotherapy. Oncol Nurs Forum 1995; 22(6):975.

Baron R, Walsh A. Nine facts everyone should know about breast cancer. Am J Nurs 1995; 95(7):29.

Benedict S, Williams RD, Baron PL. The effect of benign breast biopsy on subsequent breast cancer detection practices. Oncol Nurs Forum 1994; 9:(21):1467.

Bilodeau B, Degner L. Information needs, sources of information, and decisional roles in women with breast cancer. Oncol Nurs Forum 1996; 23(4):691.

Bruning N. Breast implants: Everything you need to know. Alameda, CA: Hunter House, 1992.

Bryla C. The relationship between stress and the development of breast cancer: A literature review. Oncol Nurs Forum 1996; 23(3):441.

Bullough B, Hindi-Alexander M, Fetouh S. Methylxanthines and fibrocystic breast disease. Nurse Pract 1990; 15(3):36.

Burnett C, Steakley C, Tefft M. Barriers to breast and cervical cancer screening in underserved women of the District of Columbia. Oncol Nurs Forum 1995; 22(10):1551.

Champion VL. Results of a nurse-delivered intervention on proficiency and nodule detection with breast self-examination. Oncol Nurs Forum 1995; (22)5:819.

Coleman E, Coon S, Thompson P, Lemon S, Depuy R. Impact of silicone implants on the lives of women with breast cancer. Oncol Nurs Forum 1995; 22(10):1493.

Corral C, Mustoe T. Controversy in breast reconstruction. Surg Clin North Am 1996; 76(2):309.

Crabbe W. The tamoxifen controversy. Oncol Nurs Forum 1996; 23(5):761.

Crockford E, Holloway I, Walker J. Nurses' perceptions of patients' feelings about breast surgery. J Adv Nurs 1993; 18: 1710.

Dest V, Fisher S. Breast cancer: Dreaded diagnosis, complicated care. RN 1994; 57(6):49.

DiFronzo L, O'Connell T. Breast cancer in pregnancy and lactation. Surg Clin North Am 1996; 76(2):267.

Donegan W, Redlich P. Breast cancer in men. Surg Clin of North Am 1996; 76(2):343.

Douglass M, Bartolucci A, Waterbor J, Sirles A. Breast cancer early detection: Differences between African-American and white women's health beliefs and detection practices. Oncol Nurs Forum 1995; 22(5):835.

Drugay M. Battling breast cancer in older women: Where do we stand? Geriatr Nurs 1992; Sept/Oct: 240.

Eberlein T, Crespo L, Smith B, Hergrueter C, Douville L, Eriksson E. Prospective evaluation of immediate reconstruction after mastectomy. Ann Surg 1996; 218(1):29.

Elkowitz A, Colen S, Slavin S, Seibert J, et al. Various methods of breast reconstruction after mastectomy: An economic comparison. Plast Reconstr Surg 1993; 92(1):77.

Elliot L, Eskenazi L, Beegle P, Podres P, Drazan L. Immediate TRAM flap reconstruction: 128 consecutive cases. Plast Reconstr Surg 1993; 92(2):217.

Ferrans CE. Quality of life through the eyes of survivors of breast cancer. Oncol Nurs Forum 1994; (21)10:1645.

Giardino E, Wolf Z. Symptoms: Evidence and experience. Holistic Nurs Pract 1993; 7(2):1.

Gould K, Gates ML, Miakowski C. Breast cancer prevention: A summary of the chemoprevention trial with tamoxifen. Oncol Nurs Forum 1994; 21(5):835. [Published erratum appears in Oncol Nurs Forum 1995; 22(4):615.]

Gould K, Gates ML, Miakowski C. Breast cancer prevention: A summary of the chemoprevention trial with tamoxifen. Oncol Nurs Forum 1994; 21(5):835.

Granda C. Nursing management of patients with lymphedema associated with breast cancer therapy. Cancer Nurs 1994; 17: 229.

Harrison-Woermke DE, Graydon JE. Perceived informational needs of breast cancer patients receiving radiation therapy after excisional biopsy and axillary node dissection. Cancer Nurs 1993; 16(6):449.

Hassey-Dow K. Contemporary issues in breast cancer. Boston: Jones and Bartlett, 1996.

Helzlsouer KJ. Epidemiology, early detection, and prevention of breast cancer. Curr Opin Oncol 1993; 5:955.

Hidalgo D. Are breast prostheses safe for use in reconstruction? Yes. Important Adv Oncol 1993; p 179.

Hughes K. Decision making by patients with breast cancer: The role of information in treatment selection. Oncol Nurs Forum 1993; 20(4):623.

Hughes K. Psychosocial and functional status of breast cancer patients. Cancer Nurs 1993; 16(3):222.

Jarvis C. Physical examination and health assessment. 2nd ed. Philadelphia: WB Saunders, 1996.

Jatoi I, Baum M. American and European recommendations for screening mammography in younger women: A cultural divide? Br Med J 1993; 307:1481.

Kelly P, Winslow E. Needle wire localization for nonpalpable breast lesions: Sensations, anxiety levels, and informational needs. Oncol Nurs Forum 1996; 23(4):639.

Leasia S, Monahan F. A practical guide to health assessment. Philadelphia: WB Saunders, 1997.

Lewis F, Deal L. Balancing our lives: A study of the married couple's experience with breast cancer recurrence. Oncol Nurs Forum 1995; 22(6):943.

Long E. Breast cancer in African-American women. Cancer Nurs 1993; 16(1):1.

Marshburn J, et al. Mass mammography screening: Using an information system to track participation and identify target populations. Cancer Pract 1994; 2(2):146.

McCorkle R, Grant M, Baird S, Frank-Stromborg M. Cancer nursing: A comprehensive textbook. 2nd ed. Philadelphia: WB Saunders, 1996.

Miaskowski C, Dibble S. The problem of pain in outpatients with breast cancer. Oncol Nurs Forum 1995; 22(5):791.

Miki Y, Swensen J, Shattuck-Eidens D, et al. A strong candidate for the breast and ovarian cancer susceptibility gene BRCA1. Science 1994; 266:66.

Miller LT. Lymphedema: Unlocking the doors to successful treatment. Innov Oncol Nurs 1994; 10:57.

Mock V. Body image in women treated for breast cancer. Nurs Res 1993; 42(3):153.

Nielsen B, Miakowski C, Dibble SL. Pain with mammography: Fact or fiction? Oncol Nurs Forum 1993; 20:639.

Osteen RT. Selection of patients for breast cancer surgery. Cancer 1994; 74:366.

Page D. The woman at high risk for breast cancer. Surg Clin North Am 1996; 76(2):221.

Parker SL, Tong T, Bolden S, Wingo PA. Cancer statistics, 1997. CA Cancer J Clin 1997; 47(1):5.

Peters CR. Augmentation mammoplasty. Plast Surg Nurs 1990; 10(1):25.

Powell DE, Stelling CB. The diagnosis and detection of breast disease. St. Louis, MO: Mosby-Year Book, 1994.

Radford D, Zehnbauer B. Inherited breast cancer. Surg Clin North Am 1996; 76(2):205.

Reifsnider E. Educating women about benign breast disease. AAOHN J 1990; 38(3):121.

Rimes K. Mammography: Role of the occupational health nurse. AAOHN J 1993; 41(12):592.

Rutledge DN. Factors related to women's practice of breast self-examination. Nurs Res 1987; 36(2):117.

Schain WS, D'Angelo TM, Dunn ME, et al. Mastectomy versus conservative surgery and radiation therapy: Psychological consequences. Cancer 1994; 73:1221.

Schrover L. The impact of breast cancer on sexuality, body image, and intimate relationships. CA Cancer J Clin 1991; 41(2): 112.

Sciartelli C. Using a clinical pathway approach to document patient teaching for breast cancer surgical procedures. Oncol Nurs Forum 1995; 22(1):131.

Sensiba ME, Stewart DS. Relationship of perceived barriers to breast self-examination in women of varying ages and levels of education. Oncol Nurs Forum 1995; (22)8:1265.

Shapiro CL, Henderson IC. Adjuvant therapy of breast cancer. Hematol Oncol Clin North Am 1994; 8:213.

Stevenson T, Goldstein J. TRAM flap breast reconstruction and contralateral reduction or mastopexy. Plast Reconstr Surg 1993; 92(2):228.

Stombler RE. Breast implants and the FDA: Past, present, and future. Plast Surg Nurs 1993; 13(4):185.

The FDA's regulation of silicone breast implants. Washington, DC: U.S. Government Printing Office, 1993.

Thomas DB. Breast cancer in men. Epidemiol Rev 1993; 15(1):220.

Varricchio CG, Johnson KA. The use of tamoxifen in the prevention and treatment of breast cancer. In Hubbard SM, Greene PE, Knobf MT (eds). Current issues in cancer nursing practice updates. Vol 2. Philadelphia: JB Lippincott, 1993.

Wilkins E, August D, Chang A, Smith D. Immediate, bilateral transverse rectus abdominis musculocutaneous (TRAM) flap reconstruction after mastectomy. Am Surg 1993; 59(8):519.

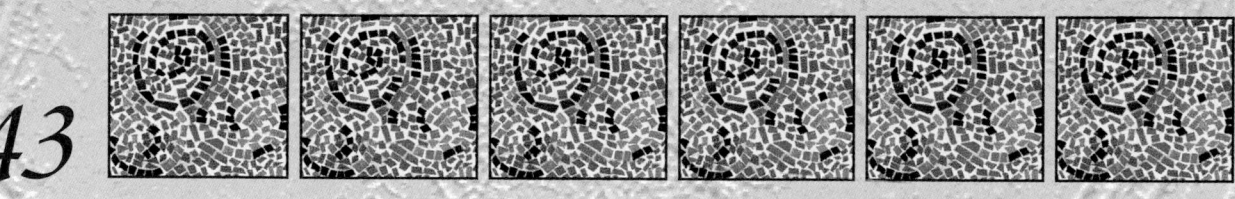

43

Nursing Care of Patients with Sexually Transmitted Diseases

Study Outcomes

After studying this chapter, you should be able to:

1. Describe the etiology, pathophysiology, clinical manifestations, diagnostic procedures, and collaborative management of common sexually transmitted diseases.
2. Identify information and physical examination data essential to the assessment of patients with common sexually transmitted diseases.
3. State nursing diagnoses and related expected patient outcomes commonly applicable to patients with sexually transmitted diseases.
4. Describe nursing interventions, with their rationales, commonly applicable to patients with sexually transmitted diseases.
5. Identify alternative treatment and care settings for patients with sexually transmitted diseases and the services related to community-based care.
6. Explain the basis for evaluation of nursing care provided to patients with common sexually transmitted diseases.

Sexually transmitted diseases (STDs) are caused by organisms transmitted through sexual contact: genital-genital, oral-genital, oral-anal, or genital-anal. These reportable diseases, which are most prevalent among teenagers and young adults, constitute a major public health problem. The number of infected people is increasing, as is the number of people with multiple coexisting STDs. The incidence continues to rise even though the acquired immunodeficiency syndrome (AIDS) epidemic has increased public awareness of the need for measures to prevent transmission of sexually transmitted diseases. (AIDS is discussed in Chap. 33.) Sequelae of STDs include infertility, ectopic pregnancy, perinatal infection, even death.

All sexually active adults are at risk for STDs. For this reason, all health-care facilities play an important role in their prevention and control. Traditionally, STD clinics have been considered the primary treatment facility for people at risk or who have contracted an STD. However, other settings—such as family planning clinics, emergency depart-

ments, young-adult clinics, and private doctor's offices—also care for these patients. An effective plan of care requires a multidisciplinary team. This team, on which the nurse plays a critical role, integrates four necessary components: education, detection, treatment, and prevention of further transmission.

Reporting STDs is necessary for adequate disease control. In addition to assisting local health authorities in identifying and treating sexual partners, reporting also provides data for compilation of STD trends and statistics. All states require that syphilis, gonorrhea, and AIDS be reported. The nurse should be familiar with individual state requirements for other STDs. The local health department can serve as a resource for additional information.

Sexually Transmitted Vaginitis

Vaginal infections are among the most common gynecologic problems seen in adult women. The three most common types of vaginal infections are vulvovaginal candidiasis, trichomoniasis, and nonspecific vaginitis, more correctly identified as *Gardnerella vaginalis* vaginitis (Table 43–1).

Vaginal fluid is composed of multiple elements, including water, electrolytes, epithelial cells, microbial organisms, fatty acids, carbohydrates, and proteins. Vaginal fluid is clear, milky, or cloudy, depending on the hormonal fluctuation of estrogen and progesterone. A large number of microorganisms normally inhabit vaginal fluid. Common organisms include lactobacilli, corynebacteria, streptococci, *Staphylococcus epidermidis*, and *G. vaginalis*. Although potentially pathogenic microbial organisms may be recovered from the vagina at any given time, they do not necessarily indicate infection. The complex milieu of the vaginal flora maintains a balance that normally suppresses the overgrowth of pathogens.

Several factors influence the quantity and quality of organisms in vaginal fluid. During the reproduc-

Table 43–1

Common Types of Sexually Transmitted Vaginitis

Infection	Clinical Manifestations	Medical Treatment	Transmission	Comments
Candidiasis	Severe vulvovaginal itching White, curdlike, nonodorous vaginal discharge (in some cases discharge may be normal) Edema, redness, excoriation of vulva and perineum Burning, pain, dyspareunia	*Antifungal agents:* vaginal tablets or creams *Clotrimazole:* 100 mg tablets or 1% cream BID for 7 days *Miconazole:* 100 mg tablets or 2% cream BID for 7 days *Butaconazole:* 2% cream for 3 days *Terconazole:* 0.4% cream for 7 days	Role of sexual transmission limited and less important than in other sexually transmitted diseases	Factors that promote growth of *Candida* infections include: Pregnancy Oral contraceptives Antibiotics Diabetes Corticosteroids Immunosuppression Menstruation
Gardnerella vaginalis vaginitis	Frequently malodorous vaginal discharge Fishy odor Thin, grayish white, nonirritating discharge	*Metronidazole:* 500 mg PO bid for 7 days	May be sexually transmitted	*G. vaginalis* and anaerobic bacteria act synergistically to produce infection Usually mild Does not cause inflammation Males do not require treatment
Trichomoniasis	Profuse, malodorous, uncomfortable vaginal discharge White to greenish gray watery discharge (may appear frothy) Dysuria Pruritus	*Metronidazole:* single dose, 2g PO or 250 mg PO tid for 10 days	Sexually transmitted Abstain from sexual intercourse during active infection or use condom Prevention: condom	Treat sex partners concurrently 70% can be diagnosed on Papanicolaou test

bid, twice daily; PO, orally; tid, three times daily.

tive years, the pH of the vagina is normally acidic (pH 4.0–4.5). Maintenance of this low vaginal pH depends on adequate levels of estrogen, glucose, and glycogen, as well as the presence of lactobacilli. Estrogen increases the glycogen content of the epithelial cells of the vaginal wall. Vaginal epithelial cells, lactobacilli, and other microorganisms use glycogen and glucose for metabolism, making it less available for the growth of harmful organisms. More important, they produce lactic acid as a product of metabolism. Lactic acid maintains the low vaginal pH. When the balance of the normal vaginal environment is altered, the vaginal pH becomes more alkalotic, providing an environment conducive to the overgrowth of potentially pathogenic organisms. Variables that may alter vaginal pH include pregnancy, diabetes, douching, and use of soaps, feminine hygiene sprays, and deodorant menstrual pads or tampons.

VULVOVAGINAL CANDIDIASIS

Etiology and Pathophysiology

Fungal infections account for 20 to 30% of vaginal infections. *Candida albicans* causes 80 to 90% of these vaginal fungal infections. Small numbers of *C. albicans* commonly inhabit the vagina in asymptomatic women. Infection is associated with an alteration in the normal vaginal microbial environment and decreased host resistance rather than contagious spread.

The role of sexual transmission in the epidemiology of candidiasis is not completely understood. However, it is thought to be less substantial than in other STDs. Most cases of genital candidiasis in men can be traced to an infected female sexual partner. However, the role of male transmission to women is not clear. In addition, fungal infections are not associated with the presence of other STDs. These factors suggest that sexual contact plays a limited role in the transmission of genital *Candida*.

C. albicans primarily affects women during their menstruating years; it rarely occurs before menarche or after menopause. The effects of estrogen, including the presence of glycogen stores in the epithelium, support the growth of *Candida*. Overgrowth of vaginal *Candida* and subsequent infection are associated with a number of host and epidemiologic factors. Pregnancy, oral contraceptives, menstruation, antibiotics and corticosteroids, diabetes, and immunosuppression have all been identified as predisposing factors to the development of candidiasis.

Candidiasis is twice as common in pregnant women as it is in nonpregnant women. The incidence increases as the pregnancy advances. Ten percent of candidal infections seen during pregnancy occur during the first trimester, whereas 36 to 55% occur in the third trimester. In addition, cure rates are lower and recurrence rates higher during pregnancy. The increase in the occurrence and severity of candidal infections in pregnancy is usually attributed to depressed cellular immunity and the increase in vaginal glycogen stores commonly seen during pregnancy. The same mechanism (increased availability of glucose and glycogen) has been suggested as the explanation for the reported increased incidence of vulvovaginal candidiasis in diabetic women and oral contraceptive users. Recurrent episodes of vulvovaginal candidiasis may be the first manifestation of diabetes.

Incidence of vulvovaginal candidiasis increases with systemic antibiotic use, particularly antibiotics active against lactobacilli, such as the penicillins, cephalosporins, and tetracyclines. It is hypothesized that antibiotics alter vaginal flora by decreasing the numbers of lactobacilli, thus elevating the pH and providing glycogen to promote growth of *C. albicans*. Some authorities suggest that patients with a history of candidal infections who are taking systemic antibiotics known to be active against lactobacilli should also receive concomitant antifungal therapy.

Clinical Manifestations

The most common symptom of genital candidiasis is severe vulvovaginal itching. Pruritus may be accompanied by external dysuria related to urine passing over the infected vulva. Vaginal discharge is typically thick and white. It has no odor and resembles cottage cheese. It may appear as white, adherent plaques on the surface of the vaginal wall. In many cases, however, vaginal discharge appears normal.

Other signs and symptoms of vulvovaginal candidal infection include vulvar edema, erythema, and perineal fissures and excoriation, reflecting the effects of frequent scratching. In men, the most common manifestation is balanitis, which is an inflammation of the glans penis. Symptoms include erythema, glazed-skin appearance, and mild desquamation or crusting.

Diagnosis

Diagnosis is based on clinical manifestations and is confirmed by microscopic examination of vaginal fluid for hyphae or pseudohyphae. If results of microscopic examination are normal, cultures may be taken to verify the diagnosis. A new 2-minute slide latex agglutination test may also be used for diagnosis.

Management

Local application of antimycotic agents is the treatment of choice for genital candidiasis. Imidazole derivatives are often used. They include miconazole, clotrimazole, triconazole, econazole, and butaconazole. These medications are broad-spectrum antimycotics with high cure rates. Miconazole (Monistat 7) and clotrimazole (Lotrimin) can be purchased without a prescription. Triazoles, such as the topical agent terconazole (Terazol) and the oral medication fluconazole (Diflucan), may be prescribed, particularly for recurrent candidiasis. For additional information on the pharmacologic treatment of candidiasis, see Table 43–1.

TRICHOMONIASIS

Etiology and Pathophysiology

Trichomoniasis is one of the most common sexually transmitted urogenital infections. About 2.5 million cases are diagnosed yearly in the United States. It is caused by *Trichomonas vaginalis*, a single-cell flagellated protozoan. *T. vaginalis* is frequently found in coexistence with other sexually transmitted pathogens. For example, 40% of women with gonorrhea also have trichomoniasis. Usually, it is difficult to isolate in men. Some studies indicate that exposed men are unaffected or that trichomoniasis is a self-limiting, typically benign disease in men.

Clinical Manifestations

Trichomoniasis is characterized by a profuse, malodorous, often uncomfortable vaginal discharge that may be associated with mild dysuria. The discharge is homogeneous, greenish gray, and watery, and often appears purulent or frothy (Fig. 43–1). The vaginal and cervical epithelia may appear reddened and inflamed. On colposcopic examination, pinpoint hemorrhagic spots may be apparent on the cervix, giving it a strawberry appearance characteristic of trichomoniasis. Asymptomatic infection also occurs, and some estimate that it may be as high as 50% of infected women. In men, *T. vaginalis* is present in the lower urinary tract and may cause prostatitis (infection of the prostate gland) in a few cases. More typically, men are asymptomatic carriers.

Diagnosis

Diagnosis of trichomoniasis is usually made on the basis of clinical symptoms and a wet-mount microscopic examination of vaginal fluid that demonstrates the presence of motile *Trichomonas* organisms. *Trichomonas* is occasionally seen on Papanicolaou

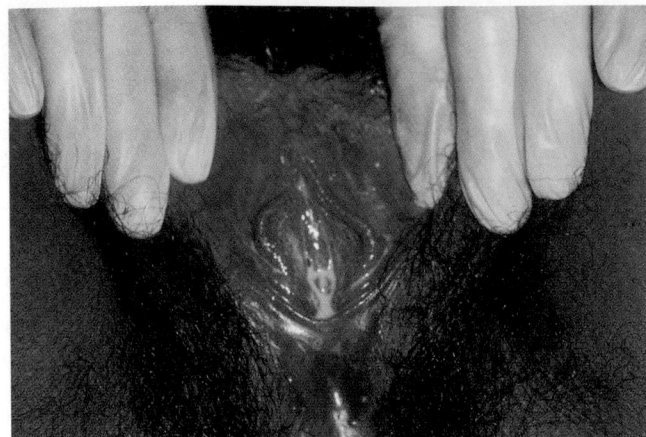

Figure 43–1

Trichomoniasis vaginal discharge. The discharge is profuse and watery and appears purulent. (Courtesy of Leonard Wolf, MD, New York, NY.)

(Pap) tests. If wet-mount smear fails to demonstrate the organism in the presence of clinical symptoms, cultures are recommended.

Management

Metronidazole (Flagyl) is the only consistently effective drug used to treat trichomoniasis. A single dose, 2 g orally, is recommended because it is more likely to guarantee compliance, is inexpensive, and has the same cure rate as an extended regimen (500 mg two times a day for 7 days). Simultaneous treatment of the patient's sexual partners is recommended to decrease the incidence of reinfection.

Gardnerella vaginalis VAGINITIS

Etiology and Pathophysiology

In the past, all vaginal infections not attributable to candidiasis, trichomoniasis, or gonorrhea were labeled nonspecific vaginitis, reflecting the unknown cause of the infection. In 1954, Gardner and Dukes identified *Haemophilus vaginalis* as the causative organism. Now called *G. vaginalis*, these small gram-negative bacteria are present in at least 95% of women with symptoms of nonspecific vaginitis.

As indicated previously, *G. vaginalis* is a frequent constituent of normal vaginal discharge, occurring in 40% of asymptomatic women. It is hypothesized that *G. vaginalis* infection occurs from a complex alteration in the vaginal flora that promotes an increase in *G. vaginalis* as well as anaerobic bacteria that act synergistically to produce symptoms associated with nonspecific vaginitis.

Similar to candidiasis, the role of sexual transmission in the epidemiology of *G. vaginalis* is questionable and not well understood. *G. vaginalis* is more prevalent in the male partners of infected women. Ninety percent of men in sexual contact with infected women are positive for *G. vaginalis*. Men usually do not require treatment except to pre-

vent recurrences in their female partners. The incidence of *G. vaginalis* infection is positively correlated with the following risk factors in women: parity (number of pregnancies), number of sexual partners, use of an intrauterine device, and the presence of cervical infections.

Clinical Manifestations

G. vaginalis is generally not considered a severe infection. Vaginal leukocytes are not greatly increased, and the vaginal epithelium is not greatly inflamed. The primary clinical manifestation is a slightly increased malodorous vaginal discharge. The discharge is usually nonirritating, thin, homogeneous, adherent, and grayish white. It emits a characteristic fishy odor, particularly after sexual intercourse. If symptoms occur in men, they are similar to those associated with nongonococcal urethritis—a slight watery urethral discharge with or without dysuria.

Diagnosis

Clinical diagnosis of *G. vaginalis* infection is based on the presence of three of four signs:

- Characteristic homogeneous vaginal discharge
- pH of vaginal fluid greater than 4.7
- Release of foul, fishy odor when vaginal fluid is mixed with 10% potassium hydroxide (whiff test)
- Presence of "clue cells" on microscopic examination of vaginal fluid (clue cells are vaginal epithelial cells that appear granular because of bacteria on the cell surface)

Management

Metronidazole (Flagyl), 500 mg twice daily for 7 days, is the most effective therapeutic agent in the treatment of nonspecific vaginitis. It is active against anaerobic bacteria as well as *G. vaginalis*. The cure rate is 85%. If alcohol is ingested during therapy with this drug, it produces nausea and vomiting. Metronidazole is contraindicated in the first trimester of pregnancy. Clindamycin vaginal cream 2%, one applicator intravaginally half strength for 7 days, is recommended as alternative treatment. During the second and third trimesters, oral metronidazole may be used.

NURSING PROCESS
Vaginitis

Assessment

A thorough history is the most important part of the nursing assessment of the woman with a vaginal infection. Question the patient about signs and symptoms of vaginitis (vaginal discharge, pruritus, dysuria). Analyze each symptom according to its onset, duration, character, and relieving and aggravating factors. Ask the patient to describe the color, consistency, amount, and odor of the vaginal discharge. Determine whether this is an initial or recurrent infection. Question the patient about previous vaginal infections and her history of other STDs.

Table 43–2

Assessment of Patients with Sexually Transmitted Diseases

Assessment Area	Topics to Address
General considerations	Perform assessment in an environment that provides for patient confidentiality, privacy, and psychologic and physical comfort
	Ask open-ended questions using language and terms familiar to the patient
	Communicate a warm, empathetic, nonjudgmental attitude.
Health history	Chief complaint
	History of current illness, including the following details about signs and symptoms: onset, initial or recurrent, precipitating factors, duration, frequency, character, location, relieving and aggravating factors
	Health history, including medical conditions, previous surgeries, treatments and therapies, and allergies
	Sexual history
	Reproductive and gynecologic history, including:
	Triad (age at onset, frequency, duration of menses)
	Pain or abnormal bleeding during or between periods or during sexual intercourse
	Fertility/infertility
	Number and outcomes of pregnancies, miscarriages, abortions
	Infections during pregnancy
	Gynecologic conditions
	Infections of the genitourinary tract (such as vaginitis, cervicitis, pelvic inflammatory disease, urethritis)
	Endometriosis
	Tumors, cysts: benign, malignant
	Contraceptive practices
	Health maintenance
	Hygiene practices
	Frequency of Papanicolaou tests, gynecologic examinations
	Medications taken (prescription and over the counter), including drug name, dose, reason for use, side effects, last dose taken, and effectiveness
	Health maintenance activities, including personal hygiene practices, activities of daily living, health promotion activities (diet, exercise, sleep), and frequency of physician or clinic visits
Communication status	Orientation
	Language spoken
	Ability to communicate ideas
	Ability to understand verbal communication of others
	Ability to cooperate in plan of care
Educational status	Learning needs (eg, disease process, mode of transmission, prevention)
	Educational level
	Ability to learn new information
	Readiness to learn, including emotional readiness and motivation
	Preferred methods of learning
Psychosocial assessment	Age
	Marital status
	Employment history
	Financial status
	Recent travel
	Family members, significant others
	Availability of support
	Emotional response to illness
	Current or anticipated response of significant others to illness
	Current or anticipated effect of illness on social activities, interpersonal relationships, sexual identity, self-esteem, lifestyle
	Ability and motivation to comply with treatment regimens

Table continued on following page

Table 43–2

Assessment of Patients with Sexually Transmitted Diseases *(continued)*

Assessment Area	Topics to Address

Physical assessment	Observe for clinical manifestations of sexually transmitted diseases throughout assessment:
	  Use inspection and palpation as the primary methods of assessment for sexually transmitted diseases.
	  Wear gloves to inspect the mouth, genitals, perineum, and anus, and to palpate lesions.
	  Perform examination for sexually transmitted diseases in a warm, well-lighted room.
	  Provide the patient with a gown, and use a drape to protect patient's privacy and to cover areas not under examination.
	Assess for systemic symptoms:
	  Obtain vital signs, apical and radial pulses, respiratory rate and rhythm, blood pressure, and temperature.
	Assess the patient's mouth and throat:
	  Inspect the oral cavity, tongue, lips, gingiva, and palpate for lesions, sores, or signs of infection.
	Assess the patient's skin:
	  Note color, texture, temperature, vascularity, and moisture. Inspect for lesions. If present, note the type (vesicles, papules, macules, pustules, buboes, ulcers), size, shape, configuration, location, and distribution.
	  Note signs of inflammation, including edema, erythema, induration, and exudate (color, amount, odor, consistency).
	  Note signs of pruritus, such as scratches and excoriation. Observe for scabies burrows.
	  Palpate lesions for consistency (soft, firm), mobility, and tenderness.
	  Inspect body and pubic hair for evidence of lice or nits.
	Examine the genitalia and anus (examine men in a supine or standing position; examine women in the lithotomy position):
	  Inspect the genitalia, perineum, and anus for lesions, signs of inflammation, and pruritus.
	  Palpate lesions when necessary for consistency and presence or absence of pain.
	  Inspect the vaginal introitus and labia in women and urethral meatus and anus in men and women for signs of discharge and inflammation. Note the color, consistency, amount, and odor of any vaginal, urethral, or rectal discharge.
	  Palpate the inguinal lymph nodes for enlargement or tenderness.

Assess the patient's knowledge of normal vaginal function and discharge. Review her health status and personal hygienic practices. Of particular interest are practices that may predispose her to infection or exacerbate an existing infection, such as frequent douching with solutions that may adversely alter the normal vaginal pH and practices that increase warmth, moisture, and trauma to the vagina. Question the patient about the presence of factors known to promote candidiasis, such as antibiotic and oral contraceptive use, diabetes, pregnancy, and other immunosuppressive conditions or medications.

Obtain an obstetric, gynecologic, and sexual history. Assess the patient's emotional response to the presence of a vaginal infection. Be sure to provide an environment that is private, supportive, and nonthreatening. Also ensure that no biases and assumptions affect the interview. Disclosure of sexuality issues, including lesbian and gay issues, can be a problem if the interviewer is not aware of personal biases or feels uncomfortable and uninformed about varied sexual practices. Many women are anxious, especially if they view the cause of their condition as unknown or as a sign of venereal disease. Others are reluctant to discuss their symptoms or to provide the necessary historic data because of fear or embarrassment. Thus, it is essential to be reassuring, empathetic, and nonjudgmental.

Physical examination includes inspection of the external genitalia and vaginal opening for discharge, odor, or signs of inflammation (eg, redness, swelling, or excoriation). This is followed by a vaginal and cervical examination performed by a physician or a nurse using a speculum.

See Table 43–2 for a summary of assessment data relevant to patients with STDs.

Nursing Diagnoses and Planning

Nursing diagnoses and related expected patient outcomes commonly applicable to patients with sexually transmitted vaginitis include the following:

NDx: Pain related to the inflammatory process

Planning: Patient Outcomes

1. Patient reports using measures recommended to reduce discomfort and using medication as prescribed.
2. Patient states that itching and burning have been relieved.
3. Edema, redness, and excoriation of the vaginal epithelium and external genitalia have disappeared.

NDx: Risk for altered health maintenance related to insufficient knowledge of normal vaginal function, personal hygiene, disease process, or sexual mode of transmission

Planning: Patient Outcomes

1. Patient accurately describes normal vaginal functioning and the characteristics of normal vaginal discharge.
2. Patient identifies three factors that may alter normal vaginal physiology and predispose to infection.
3. Patient identifies three health practices that decrease the risk of vaginal infection.
4. Patient states the cause and symptoms of specific vaginal infections.
5. Patient describes the role of sexual contact in transmission of specific vaginal infections.
6. Patient describes methods for preventing transmission of infection.

NDx: Anxiety related to cause of vaginitis and concerns about physical and lifestyle effects

Planning: Patient Outcomes

1. Patient discusses her concerns about vaginal infection and its potential effects.
2. Patient reports feeling less anxious about the vaginal infection and its outcome.
3. Patient's behavior suggests reduced anxiety (relaxed posture, absence of nervous mannerisms).

Nursing Care Guide 43–1 presents additional nursing diagnoses and patient outcomes that may apply to patients with sexually transmitted vaginitis or any other STD.

Nursing Interventions and Evaluation

NDx: Pain

Review the medication treatment plan with the patient, including the name, dose, route, and times the medication is to be taken. Caution the patient to use all the medication as prescribed and not just until the symptoms have abated. Verify that the patient knows how to insert vaginal creams and suppositories as prescribed.

Recommend the use of cool compresses, sitz baths, and loose cotton undergarments to reduce discomfort until the medication takes effect, usually 1 or 2 days.

NDx: Risk for altered health maintenance

Using simple, nontechnical language, teach the patient about normal vaginal flora, vaginal pH, and the constituents of normal vaginal discharge. Include a discussion of factors that may alter normal vaginal physiology (eg, pregnancy, medications, menstruation). Once the diagnosis is made, review the cause, symptoms, and treatment of the patient's specific infection. Present basic facts about the mode of transmission, treatment, and prevention of the infection (Highlight 43–1).

NDx: Anxiety

Provide an opportunity for the patient to express her concerns about having acquired a vaginal infection. Give particular attention to correcting any myths or misconceptions the patient may have about vaginal discharge and the nature of vaginal infections. Present the information tactfully and sensitively in a quiet, private, nonthreatening environment. Emphasize the positive aspects of the diagnosis—that effective treatment is available and that no long-term effects occur. Be sure to inform the patient of the possibility of sexual transmission of the causative organisms.

Compare the patient's status with the expected outcomes. If the outcomes are not met, reassess the patient and revise the plan.

*G*enital Herpes

Etiology and Pathophysiology

The herpes simplex viruses (HSVs) are one of a group of four herpesviruses known to infect humans. There are two HSVs—herpes simplex virus 1 (HSV-1) and herpes simplex virus 2 (HSV-2). Although clinically indistinguishable, the two viruses have different biologic properties. The molecular composition, growth patterns in cultures, and antibodies they elicit are different. Clinically, both can cause recurrent vesicles and blisters anywhere on the body, although each has a predilection for specific sites.

HSV-1 is most frequently associated with lesions occurring above the waist. Examples of herpes infections commonly produced by HSV-1 are herpes labialis, otherwise known as the common cold sore or fever blister; herpes gingivostomatitis, an infection of the oral cavity and gums; and herpes keratitis, an infection of the eye. Infections attributable to HSV-2 generally occur below the waist. Genital herpes is a primary example.

Both HSVs are capable of producing infections at alternate sites. It is estimated that HSV-1 produces about 15% of genital infections. Changes in sexual practices and mores, including an increase in

Text continued on page 1900

Nursing Care Guide 43–1

Patients with Sexually Transmitted Diseases

Assessment Findings: Patient complains of pain and pruritus in genital area and burning on urination.

Nursing Diagnosis: Pain related to the inflammatory process

Patient Outcomes	Nursing Interventions	Rationale
Patient states that pain or pruritus is diminished or absent. Patient's nonverbal behavior indicates physical comfort (relaxed posture, facial expression, movements). Patient is able to carry out normal daily activities.	Help the patient reduce or eliminate pain or pruritus: Explain the cause of the patient's pain and pruritus. Help the patient identify factors that precipitate or contribute to pain and pruritus. Common factors include the following: • Physical and environmental factors: pressure, friction, warmth, moisture or dryness, scratching, manipulation, daily activities, time of day • Psychosocial factors: anxiety, fear, fatigue, lack of diversional activities Help the patient identify and use strategies for relieving pain or pruritus. Instruct the patient in proper self-administration of oral or topical medications to relieve pain or pruritus. • Caution patient to use analgesics before pain is severe. • Instruct patient to use applicator, gauze, or gloves when applying topical medications to infected areas. • Review dosage, schedule, and side effects of medications. Instruct patient in alternative techniques for management of pain and pruritus: Explore the patient's previous pain experiences and methods for alleviating pain. Determine the patient's prior knowledge and willingness to use alternative strategies for management of pain and pruritus.	Knowledge of causative factors reduces psychologic stress, reducing pain. Recognition of precipitating factors allows patient to avoid behavior that causes pain or pruritus. Correct use of medication ensures better results. Methods that have been previously successful in relieving pain and pruritus are likely to continue to be successful.

(continued)

Nursing Care Guide 43–1
Patients with Sexually Transmitted Diseases (continued)

Patient Outcomes	Nursing Interventions	Rationale
	Provide guidance and instruction in the following:	
	• Cutaneous stimulation (application of heat and cold massage)	Gates pain.
	• Distraction (plan daily activities, use breathing techniques, engage in recreational activities)	Distraction and relaxation succeed by lowering the patient's perception of pain.
	• Relaxation (progressive relaxation, meditation; slow, rhythmic breathing; imaging)	
	Advise patient to avoid excessive warmth, moisture, or dryness (wear loose clothing and cotton undergarments, avoid overdressing, avoid activities that cause pressure or friction at site), use mild soap, blot skin dry.	Reduces stimulation of nerve endings and irritation of local tissues.
	Administer medication to relieve pain and pruritus.	Medications provide temporary relief of pain and pruritus by altering perception or decreasing the reception of stimuli.
	Tell patient to ask for medication before symptoms are severe.	
	Respond to patient's request for medication within acceptable time limits.	
	Monitor effectiveness of medication.	

Evaluation: Compare the patient's status with the expected outcomes. If the outcomes are not met, reassess the patient and revise the plan.

Assessment Findings: Patient has a sexually transmitted infection caused by an infectious organism capable of infecting other unaffected sites.

Nursing Diagnosis: Risk for infection (secondary) related to bacterial contamination

Patient Outcomes	Nursing Interventions	Rationale
Signs of secondary infection—inflammation and purulent discharge unrelated to primary infection—are absent.	Prevent secondary infection and spread of disease to unaffected sites by:	
Patient carries out recommended hygienic practices.	Helping patient maintain adequate hygiene.	
Infection remains confined to original or commonly encountered genital sites.	Teaching women to wipe the perineal/rectal area from front to back after voiding or defecating and blotting skin dry to avoid spreading organisms and infected discharge from	Wiping from front to back prevents organisms from moving from dirty areas to clean. Blotting reduces transfer of organisms from one area to another.

(continued)

Nursing Care Guide 43–1

Patients with Sexually Transmitted Diseases *(continued)*

Patient Outcomes	Nursing Interventions	Rationale
	affected to unaffected areas. Rinsing with a peri-bottle filled with lukewarm water may be helpful in maintaining perineal hygiene.	Use of the peri-bottle allows water to flush organisms from the area.
	Douching is usually not recommended but may be indicated for voluminous or malodorous vaginal discharge. Consult with physician before advising patient.	Douching modifies the normal acidic pH of the vagina and can eliminate normal vaginal flora, which provide a self-cleaning property to the vagina.
	Recommend daily baths or showers using mild soap and lukewarm water.	Showers and baths help to remove organisms from the body surface.
	Instruct patient to avoid excessive warmth and moisture; keep room cool; wear cotton underwear; avoid constrictive clothing, pantyhose, and overdressing.	Warm, moist environments are excellent media for the growth of microorganisms.
	Explain importance of not manipulating or touching lesions or secretions. Many STDs can be spread by autoinoculation. Hands are a source of infective organisms.	Reduces the spread of the organisms by the hands.
	Advise frequent changes in undergarments and sanitary pads when secretions or vaginal discharge is present to decrease accumulation and potential spread of secretions.	Frequent changes remove organisms that can be spread over the skin surface.
	Recommend sitz baths with lukewarm water for cleanliness and comfort. Caution against too frequent soaking, which may cause skin maceration.	Warm water flushes organisms from the body surface. Warmth also brings white blood cells to the area, which help fight infection.
Patient performs wound- and skin-care techniques as instructed.	Instruct patient in proper technique of wound irrigation, if ordered, using normal saline, sterile water, hydrogen peroxide, or antiseptic.	Wound irrigation may be indicated for extensive tissue damage resulting from ruptured abscesses, draining sinuses, or fistulas since it removes secretions and debris from the area to allow healing to occur.
	Instruct patient in use of heat lamp if ordered to increase circulation to the affected area or to dry lesions.	Heat reduces moisture, making the environment less conducive to organism growth. Heat also causes vasodilaton, which in-

(continued)

Patients with Sexually Transmitted Diseases (continued)

Patient Outcomes	Nursing Interventions	Rationale
		creases the presence of white blood cells to fight infection and red blood cells and protein for healing.
	Prevent further injury:	
	Advise against scratching (see interventions for pruritus).	Scratching the area can cause irritation and excoriation of the skin.
	Caution against self-medication with over-the-counter drugs or previously used medication unless recommended by physician.	May cause tissue irritation or alter effect of prescribed medications.
	Advise patient to maintain adequate nutrition and fluid intake.	Adequate hydration decreases risk of urinary tract infections because good urinary output flushes organisms quickly out of the urinary system. Protein and vitamins are needed for tissue repair.

Evaluation:	Compare the patient's status with the expected outcomes. If the outcomes are not met, reassess the patient and revise the plan.
Assessment Findings:	Patient states he or she "will try" to follow the treatment regimen but his or her sexual partner "isn't going to like it." Patient asks "Is this really necessary? I think you people like to make a big deal out of nothing."
Nursing Diagnosis:	Risk for noncompliance with prescribed treatment and palliative measures related to sexual lifestyle and behaviors, lack of knowledge regarding rationale for following treatment regimen and using preventive measures, anger and hostility, or unsatisfactory relationship with caregivers

Patient Outcomes	Nursing Interventions	Rationale
Follow-up tests of cure are negative.	Determine patient's ability and willingness to comply with treatment regimen. Remember that successful therapy depends on patient compliance. Potential noncompliers include individuals who are: • Unable to follow directions • Unable to comprehend verbal or written instructions because of intellectual deficits, inability to read, language barriers • Hostile, uncooperative, and unmotivated	Recognition of reasons for noncompliance assists in the formulation of interventions likely to be successful.

(continued)

Nursing Care Guide 43–1

Patients with Sexually Transmitted Diseases (continued)

Patient Outcomes	Nursing Interventions	Rationale
	• Distrustful of health-care professionals • Uninformed about the reasons for taking medicatons as prescribed (Note: Selection of the type of medication and route of administration is influenced by the health-care professional's perception of the patient's potential compliance. A single-dose parenteral medication may be indicated rather an an oral regimen for potential noncompliers.)	
Patient is able to state the action, dosage, schedule, and potential side effects of prescribed medication. Patient reports taking medications as prescribed.	Provide instruction in self-administration of medication: Relate and explain the action, dosage, schedule, and possible side effects of prescribed medications.	The patient must understand expected behaviors to self-administer medication correctly.
	Assist the patient in planning how to incorporate taking medications into daily routine. Suggest ways the patient can remember to take medications (eg, always before or after meals; place medications in a convenient, visible place).	Problem-solving with the medication schedule assists the patient with compliance.
	Provide written instructions, including name and telephone number of person to contact if questions arise or if side effects develop.	Questions often arise during the actual experience of self-administration. Having a resource available provides access to needed information and promotes compliance.
	Advise patients on how to manage omission of one or more doses.	Provides information about appropriate reaction to a common problem so that blood levels of medication can be maintained.
Patient states the rationale for following the prescribed regimen.	Explain the rationale for following the prescribed treatment regimen by instructing the patient in the following: • Medications must be taken at the prescribed intervals for the recommended number of days to effect a cure and to avoid complications, long-term sequelae, and transmission to others.	Provides the patient with information that promotes compliance.

(continued)

Patients with Sexually Transmitted Diseases (continued)

Patient Outcomes	Nursing Interventions	Rationale
	• Resolution of symptoms before completion of the treatment course does not indicate a cure; continue taking medications. • One or more follow-up visits to test for cure may be necessary. Some organisms may be resistant to the prescribed medicine.	
Patient returns for follow-up visit.	Set a date and time for a follow-up visit that is convenient for the patient. Provide an opportunity for the patient to ask questions and express concerns.	By absolving the patient of the responsibility of scheduling a revisit, the likelihood of compliance is increased. Clarifies misinformation and reduces patient anxiety.
Patient reports complying with recommendations for preventing transmission to others during treatment period.	To prevent transmission to others: • Advise patient to abstain from sexual intercourse until completion of treatment or follow-up test of cure. • Recommend use of condoms if patient appears unlikely to comply. • Inform patient of potential effects on sexual partners. Long-term sequelae, adverse effects, and complications from STDs are more common in women and include pelvic inflammatory disease, infertility, and poor pregnancy and perinatal outcomes.	Semen and vaginal secretions contain infective material for an undetermined period of time during treatment. Provides a barrier to reduce the possibility of transmission of organisms. Provides rationale to promote patient compliance.

Evaluation: Compare the patient's status with the expected outcomes. If the outcomes are not met, reassess the patient and revise the plan.

Assessment Findings: Sexual partner will not come for treatment. Patient expresses doubt about need for preventive measures, stating "If you're going to get it, you're going to get it."

Nursing Diagnosis: Risk for infection (reinfection) related to insufficient knowledge of the disease, its mode of transmission, and prevention; failure to comply with treatment and recommended preventive measures; resumption of sexual relations with untreated partners

Patient Outcomes:	Nursing Interventions	Rationale
Patient states the rationale for altering personal behaviors that increase the risk of infection.	Help the patient prevent reinfection and incorporate preventive techniques into sexual lifestyle.	Modifications of sexual lifestyle can prevent reinfection.

(continued)

Nursing Care Guide 43–1
Patients with Sexually Transmitted Diseases (continued)

Patient Outcomes:	Nursing Interventions	Rationale
Patient identifies factors that increase the risk of infection.	Collaborate with patient to identify factors that increase risk of infection. High-risk factors include the following: • Multiple sex partners • Sex with anonymous partners • Sex with prostitutes (male or female) • Unprotected sexual intercourse • Sex with partners who have multiple partners	Knowledge of factors that increase the risk of infection allows modifications to reduce the risk.
Patient describes preventive behaviors and health practices for reducing the risk of reinfection or infection with other STDs. Patient states intention to use preventive measures and recommended health practices or to change high-risk behaviors. Symptoms of reinfection are absent at follow-up visit.	Recommend the following behaviors or measures to reduce the risk of reinfection: • Use condoms when engaging in genital or anal intercourse. Condoms are the primary preventive measure for reducing the risk of exposure to STD. • Know your partner: Avoid sex with multiple partners, anonymous partners, and prostitutes. • Observe the genitals of prospective sexual partners for signs of STD. • Avoid sex with partners who manifest signs and symptoms of STDs. • Urinate after sex, and wash genitals.	Condoms form a barrier against transmission of infective material. Limiting sexual contact to known partners reduces risk of reinfection Evidence of infection may be present, alerting the patient to the risk of reinfection. Decreases the risk of reinfection. Urine has a flushing action, which helps to remove organisms. Washing the genitals removes surface organisms.
Patient seeks treatment at first sign of STD.	• Obtain medical assistance at the first sign of STD. • Complete the recommended treatment course • Avoid sex with previously exposed untreated partners. • Assist the patient in identifying preventive measures that are realistic and acceptable given his or her values and lifestyle.	Early medical intervention is beneficial to the patient and reduces the spread of the disease to sexual partners. Incomplete treatment may lead to redevelopment of the infection and to the development of antibiotic-resistant organisms. Prevents re-exposure from infected sexual partner. Realistic and acceptable preventive methods are more likely to be included in the patient's sexual lifestyle.

(continued)

Nursing Care Guide 43–1
Patients with Sexually Transmitted Diseases (continued)

Patient Outcomes	Nursing Interventions	Rationale
	• Communicate a nonjudgmental, objective, and supportive attitude. • Recognize and accept that a person's sexual values and practices may be different from one's own. • Discuss alternatives with the patient.	Accepting behaviors by the nurse promote nurse-patient communication. Rejection of the patient's sexual values and practices interferes with communication and patient learning. Provides and clarifies information to allow the patient to modify potentially infective behavior.

Evaluation: Compare the patient's status with the expected outcomes. If the outcomes are not met, reassess the patient and revise the plan.

Assessment Findings: Patient has a history of an STD but states "I know nothing about this disease" and "I don't know how I could have gotten this."

Nursing Diagnosis: Knowledge deficit: sexual structure and functioning, disease process (eg, etiology, risk factors, incubation and period of infectivity, clinical course, long-term sequelae, and complications), modes of transmission, preventive measures, potential effects on sexual partners, rationale for informing sexual contacts and rationale for following treatment regimen as prescribed

Patient Outcomes	Nursing Interventions	Rationale
Patient states the cause, symptoms, clinical course, and mode of transmission of disease. Patient describes health practices for reducing the risk of infection and transmission. Patient describes potential adverse effects and long-term sequelae of untreated disease for self and others. Patient states the rationale for following recommended treatment regimens and health practices.	Provide health teaching when indicated. Determine the patient's • Prior knowledge • Learning level • Motivation • Readiness • Ability to incorporate new information • Emotional status • Preferred learning methods	Provides information when deficits exist. This information guides the teaching-learning situation.
	Postpone health teaching except for essential information if the patient's emotional status interferes with ability to learn.	States of high emotion can interfere with the patient's ability to take in information.
Patient asks questions derived from a knowledge of the disease process.	Provide instruction in the following, as necessary: • Sexual structure and functioning • Disease process • Mode of transmission • Preventive measures • Treatment	Information is essential to appropriate changes in behavior.

(continued)

Nursing Care Guide 43–1
Patients with Sexually Transmitted Diseases (continued)

Patient Outcomes	Nursing Interventions	Rationale
	• Complications and long-term sequelae	
	• Possible effects on sexual partners	
	Use visual aids (photographs, illustrations, and films when available) to augment instruction.	Multisensory teaching methods increase learning.
	Encourage questions and comments. Solicit feedback. Use return demonstration.	Active involvement of the learner makes learning more effective.
	Provide adequate time for teaching.	A hurried approach can be a block to learning.
	Furnish the patient with written literature as well as verbal instruction to reinforce learning and provide a reference for home use.	Reinforces teaching and allows review of material at a later time.
	Use language and terms familiar to the patient.	For communication to be effective, language must be understood by the listener.

Evaluation:	Compare the patient's status with the expected outcomes. If the outcomes are not met, reassess the patient and revise the plan.

Assessment Findings:	Patient appears tense and is trembling. Patient states, "This can't have happened to me. My boyfriend will leave me. I don't want to name people, and I wanted to have children someday."
Nursing Diagnosis:	Anxiety related to nature and location of symptoms; potential response of significant others to the diagnosis; identification and notification of sexual contacts; potential complications and long-term sequelae and misinformation about STD.

Patient Outcomes	Nursing Interventions	Rationale
Patient reports feeling less anxious. Patient's nonverbal behavior indicates decreased anxiety (relaxed facial expression, absence of nervous gestures, or other overt signs of anxiety). Patient asks appropriate questions. Patient is able to retain new information	Offer reassurance and comfort.	Reassurance and comfort are empathic behaviors that reduce anxiety.
	Validate and demonstrate to the patient that you understand his or her feelings.	Encourages patient to share feelings and thus receive support by allaying fears of being perceived negatively.

(continued)

Nursing Care Guide 43–1

Patients with Sexually Transmitted Diseases (continued)

Patient Outcomes	Nursing Interventions	Rationale
	Allow patient to express his or her feeling within limits (eg, crying, anger, frustration).	Reduces internal tension.
	Assist patient in identifying causes of anxiety.	Recognition of causative factors can help with interventions to reduce anxiety.
	Correct misconceptions.	Misconceptions can lead to unnecessary anxiety.
	Provide information when knowledge deficit contributes to anxiety.	Understanding based on knowledge helps to reduce fear of the unknown.
	Collaborate with patient to develop strategies for reducing anxiety. For example, help patient decide how to inform significant others; develop self-care plan to reduce symptoms; provide name and telephone number of person to contact if problems arise or anxiety increases.	By developing a "plan of attack," a sense of control develops and anxiety is reduced.
	Assist patient to view STD from a realistic perspective by emphasizing the following:	Provides the patient with positive facts on which to focus and base hope for a successful outcome.
	• Early treatment prevents complications and serious sequelae in most cases.	
	• STDs are the same as other infections except for the mode of transmission.	Provides information that may make the diagnosis more acceptable to the patient.
	• Acquisition of STD does not indicate sexual promiscuity, uncleanliness, and so on.	Addresses common misconceptions and provides information that can reduce anxiety.

Evaluation: Compare the patient's status with the expected outcomes. If the outcomes are not met, reassess the patient and revise the plan.

Assessment Findings: Patient states "I can't get close to anybody again. I couldn't stand going through this again, and I couldn't take thinking I gave this to anyone else. Who would want me anyhow?"

Nursing Diagnosis: Risk for sexual dysfunction related to fear of transmission to others, lack of knowledge of sexual structure and function, painful intercourse, change in body image, and guilt or embarrassment

Patient Outcomes	Nursing Interventions	Rationale
Patient plans to resume sexual activity after successful treatment.	Correct misinformation about sexual functioning or STD, if indicated.	Correct information reduces anxiety about the diagnosis, which can interfere with sexual functioning.

(continued)

Nursing Care Guide 43–1
Patients with Sexually Transmitted Diseases (continued)

Patient Outcomes	Nursing Interventions	Rationale
Patient plans to incorporate measures for preventing exposure to STDs in future sexual relationships.	Review methods for preventing acquisition of STDs.	Accurate information about disease transmission can reduce anxiety about recurrence.
	Assure patient that disease cannot be transmitted after adequate treatment and test of cure unless reinfection occurs.	Provides the patient with positive facts on which to focus.
Patient states knowledge of STD has decreased fear of transmitting infection to others.	Assist patient in identifying methods for preventing transmission if cure is unavailable (ie, herpes).	Reduces anxiety about the risk of transmission, which can inhibit sexual function.
Patient reports ability to engage in satisfactory sexual relationships at follow-up visits.	Assist patient in planning to implement recommended changes in sexual or social lifestyle.	Help in planning initiates the process and allows for enchange of ideas, which increases the likelihood of arriving at a realistic plan with which the patient will comply.

Evaluation: Compare the patient's status with the expected outcomes. If the outcomes are not met, reassess the patient and revise the plan.

oral sex, may account for the increased occurrence of HSV-1 and HSV-2 at opposite sites. HSV-1 genital infections are less likely to recur than HSV-2. Also, there is evidence that exposure to HSV-1 as a child offers some protection against severe outbreaks of HSV-2 later in life.

Transmission
HSV is transmitted by direct skin-to-skin contact with an infected lesion or infected secretions. The virus enters the body through small breaks in the skin or through susceptible mucosal surfaces, such as the oropharynx, cervix, or conjunctivae. HSV is readily inactivated both at room temperature and by drying. Transmission by aerosolization or inanimate objects is unusual and rare.

Genital herpes is transmitted by sexual contact, either genital or oral-genital. Autoinoculation—transfer of virus from one site to another on the infected person's body—can also occur. Patients should be taught to wash their hands immediately after manipulation of or contact with an infected lesion or secretions.

In asymptomatic viral shedding, the virus is present on skin, on mucosal surfaces, or in secretions, but lesions or other clinical symptoms are absent. Although this has been documented, the frequency of asymptomatic viral shedding and its role in transmission is not currently known. It is believed to be small, however.

Recurrence
After initial exposure, herpesviruses have the ability to remain in the body in a latent state and cause recurrent disease. Much of the psychologic distress experienced by patients with HSV genital infections is attributable to the problem of recurrence. Unlike other infectious diseases that are communicable only for a limited time, herpes is infectious during each episode of recurrence. Consequently, the opportunity for transmission is greatly increased. Person A can give it to person B during an initial infection and to persons C, D, and E during subsequent recurrences.

The biologic mechanism by which latency is established is not fully understood. It is known that the site of latency is the sensory nerve root ganglia located outside the central nervous system. During initial infection, the virus ascends the peripheral sensory nerves at the site of infection and establishes residency in the sensory nerve root ganglia, where it remains latent until circumstances cause it to reactivate. HSV can remain latent for years. It is not known why some people are infected and never manifest symptoms of the disease, whereas others have frequent outbreaks. The patient's immunologic

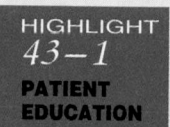
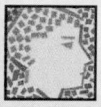

HIGHLIGHT
43–1
PATIENT EDUCATION

Sexually Transmitted Vaginal Infections

Explain the following to the patient:

Most vaginal infections are primarily transmitted through sexual contact.

- Trichomoniasis is a sexually transmitted disease. Nonsexual transmission by means of fomites, such as wet towels, soap dishes, and the backwash from toilets is a possible but infrequent occurrence.
- *Gardnerella vaginalis* may be transmitted by sexual contact. Transmission by fomites is considered possible.
- The designation of candidiasis as a sexually transmitted disease is controversial. Predisposing factors that alter the normal vaginal flora, increase the vaginal pH, or alter the immune response must be present for infection to occur. Sexual transmission of candidiasis is possible because men may harbor and transmit the fungus.

Sexual partners may need to be treated depending on the type of vaginitis and likelihood of the man carrying the organism.

- Treatment of partners is recommended for trichomoniasis, especially if the infection is recurrent.

- Partners of women with candidal infections are usually not treated unless the woman's infection is chronic or recurrent and the man also has symptoms of infection.
- If treatment is recommended, both partners should be treated simultaneously to avoid reinfection.

The full dose of medication should be taken as prescribed.

- All medications ordered must be taken even if symptoms disappear.
- Alcohol should be avoided for 48 to 72 hours after treatment with metronidazole, which is the treatment of choice for both trichomoniasis and *G. vaginalis* vaginitis.

Patients with chronic or recurrent candidal infections should seek treatment at the first sign of infection. Prophylactic antifungal medications may be recommended during antibiotic or immunosuppressive therapy.

---

status definitely plays a significant role. The size of the initial viral inoculum may play a role as well.

Clinical Manifestations

The clinical manifestations of genital herpes vary greatly depending on whether the patient is experiencing a primary, an initial, or a recurrent infection. A true primary infection represents the patient's first exposure to HSV. A primary infection can be verified by the absence of antibodies to HSV on serologic testing during the acute phase of the disease.

An initial infection is also the patient's first clinical manifestation of the disease. However, serologic testing is positive for HSV antibodies, indicating previous asymptomatic acquisition of HSV. Prior exposure to HSV-1 or HSV-2 seems to have an ameliorating effect on initial outbreaks, which tend to be milder than primary HSV genital infections.

In recurrent genital herpes, the patient has had at least one prior outbreak and has high antibody levels.

Primary Genital Herpes

The incubation period for primary genital herpes ranges from 2 to 20 days. In most cases, symptoms begin about 1 week after sexual contact. Initially, the lesions are multiple and small (1–2 mm) and appear as papules on a reddened base. They may be preceded by local irritation and a sensation of burning, tingling, or discomfort. The papules soon become fluid-filled vesicles or pustules that rupture and form shallow, wet, painful ulcers. Ultimately, the ulcers either re-epithelialize or crust over and heal without scarring. Pain, itching, dysuria, vaginal and urethral discharge, and enlarged lymph nodes are the major local symptoms. Itching is associated with vesicular formation and pain with ulcers.

Local symptoms are accompanied by a systemic viremia in 40% of men and 70% of women during primary episodes. Fever, headache, malaise, muscle pain, and back stiffness are frequent systemic symptoms that peak 4 or 5 days after the onset of lesions and resolve within 7 to 10 days. Local symptoms usually resolve in 20 days.

The severity of primary genital herpes varies with the location and number of lesions. In men, lesions appear anywhere on the glans, prepuce, or shaft of the penis. Herpetic urethritis may occur. Usually, symptoms of primary herpes are more severe in women than men.

In women, herpes lesions may appear on the vulva (predominantly the labia minora and fourchette), vagina, cervix, perineum, and buttocks (Fig. 43–2). These lesions usually last about 10 to 20 days. The major site of infection is the cervix. Ninety percent of women experiencing a primary episode of genital herpes have concomitant HSV cervicitis. Additional lesions may appear at other sites, but the cervix is always involved during primary herpes. If the cervix is the only site, vaginal discharge may be the only symptom. Consequently, the infection may remain undiagnosed.

For some women, the number and location of the lesions cause such severe pain that it is impossible to walk or sit. The pain is associated with pressure on the lesions. Severe local symptoms resulting in an inability to urinate may require that the patient be hospitalized for treatment. Complications of primary genital herpes include aseptic meningitis and disseminated infection. Disseminated skin and mucous membrane infections and infections of the internal organs are rare in patients with a normal immune response but may be seen in immunocompromised patients, such as those undergoing bone marrow transplantation and those with AIDS.

Recurrent Genital Herpes

The average number of recurrences is three or four in the first year after a primary episode of herpes. The frequency, duration, and severity of recurrences

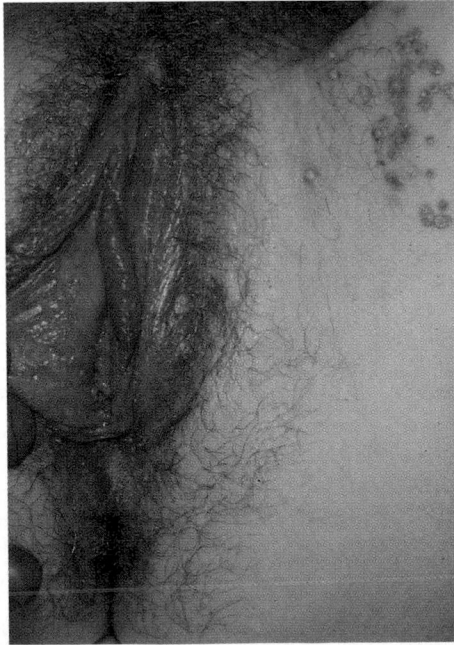

Figure 43–2

Genital herpes lesion located on the vulva and inner thigh of a female patient. Lesions begin as papules and progress to fluid-filled vesicles that rupture to form ulcers. (Courtesy of Leonard Wolf, MD, New York, NY.)

tend to decrease over time. Eighty percent of HSV-2 and 50% of HSV-1 genital infections recur within the first year after a primary infection. Some primary infections never recur.

In contrast to primary herpes, the signs and symptoms of recurrent disease are localized to the genital area and are milder and of shorter duration. Systemic symptoms are not present. About half the people with recurrent genital herpes experience symptoms before lesions appear. Prodromal symptoms include paresthesias (tingling, burning, "pins and needles"), itching, redness, and discomfort at the site. These may be present at any time from 30 minutes to 48 hours before lesions appear. Occasionally, patients complain of sacral neuralgia (sharp, shooting pains in the legs, hips, or buttocks) 1 to 5 days before onset of lesions. Characteristic local symptoms—pain, itching, and burning on urination—recur less frequently in men and are milder in women than during first-time infection.

The main sites of recurrence are the penis and vulva. In contrast to primary infections, lesions are unilateral and, in women, infection of the cervix is infrequent. Cervical infection cannot be ruled out without cultures, but only 5 to 15% of recurrent infections involve the cervix. The average duration of recurrent symptoms and viral shedding is 4 or 5 days. Complete healing occurs in 10 days.

Anecdotal evidence suggests that certain predisposing factors can trigger or precipitate an outbreak of recurrent herpes. The following are frequently identified predisposing factors:

* Heat (both fever and an external elevation in temperature)
* Intercourse, which may cause friction or trauma to the site
* Stress
* Anxiety
* Emotional upset
* Menstruation
* Ovulation

Genital Herpes and Pregnancy

The effects of genital herpes on pregnancy and in the newborn are of major concern to patients and health-care workers. Neonatal herpes is a severe disease with high mortality and morbidity rates and incapacitating long-term effects.

The potential effects of genital herpes on pregnancy relate to whether the infection is primary or recurrent. Primary infection during pregnancy is associated with more severe, harmful effects. Before 20 weeks of gestation, primary infection results in a threefold increase in the incidence of spontaneous abortion. Primary infection in the third trimester is associated with an increase in preterm labor. There are currently no data to indicate an increased incidence of congenital anomalies in infants born to mothers with primary or recurrent genital herpes.

The most serious and frequent problem encountered in pregnancy is the transmission of herpes infection to the neonate during vaginal delivery. Although neonatal infection is rare (1 in 7500 births, or about 400–500 cases yearly), the effects can be devastating. Symptomatic HSV infection of the newborn may appear during the first month after birth. Symptoms may vary. A local infection of the eyes, skin, or mucous membranes may occur. About 70% of affected infants have skin lesions. Seventy percent of affected infants acquire disseminated visceral infections. Of these, 83% die if untreated, and 60% of survivors have serious neurologic sequelae. With treatment, the mortality rate decreases but the morbidity rate and long-term sequelae appear to remain the same.

Risk of a newborn acquiring herpes during vaginal delivery varies with the number of viruses in the vaginal canal and the duration of the second stage of labor. Forty percent of infants born vaginally to mothers with positive cultures for herpes at the time of delivery are infected with neonatal herpes.

Unfortunately, at least half of infants with neonatal herpes are born to mothers who did not exhibit signs or symptoms of herpes at delivery. Shedding of the virus without symptoms appears to be an important source of infection at birth.

Until recently, management of pregnant patients with a history of recurrent genital herpes infection included weekly cultures beginning the 32nd to 36th week of pregnancy. However, major studies now indicate that antepartum cultures do not predict status at the time of delivery. It is therefore recommended that weekly cultures be abandoned and vaginal delivery be allowed if there is no evidence of genital herpetic lesions during labor. Cesarean section is recommended for women with lesions at the time of onset of labor or time of membrane rupture.

If the patient had positive cultures during the previous week or had clinical evidence of infection, a cesarean section is recommended. Infants exposed to HSV at birth during inadvertent vaginal delivery should be observed closely for 1 month for signs of HSV infection.

Genital Herpes and Cervical Cancer

Evidence has accumulated during the past two decades suggesting a possible relationship between HSV-2 genital infections and the development of cervical cancer. Some studies indicate a higher incidence of cervical dysplasia, which is an alteration in the size, shape, or organization of cells, and cervical cancer among women with a history of HSV-2. Herpes tends to infect the same area where cervical cancer frequently develops. There is also evidence that HSV-2 can cause malignant transformation of cells.

Epidemiologically, HSV genital infections are increasing among the adolescent population. Cervical cancer is more common in women who were sexually active before the age of 17 years. Some researchers have suggested that HSV-2 infections in adolescence may initiate or contribute to a chain of events that culminates in cervical cancer many years later. None of the evidence demonstrates a cause-and-effect relationship.

Diagnosis

Most cases of genital herpes are diagnosed clinically. The appearance of characteristic lesions and a thorough patient history strongly suggest the diagnosis. Virus isolation by tissue culture is the definitive test for HSV infection. HSV appears on tissue culture in 1 to 4 days; however, the laboratory may hold the culture for 7 to 10 days to confirm a negative result.

In situations in which a more rapid diagnosis is needed, detection by cytology—microscopic examination of cells for changes typical of viral infection—may be useful. Cytology results can be available in 15 minutes. Tzanck's and Pap tests are commonly used for cytologic studies. Cytologic results are falsely negative in 40% of cases of cervical HSV shedding. Tzanck's smears for vulvar skin lesions are 90% to 95% accurate.

Management

Currently, no treatment completely or permanently eradicates genital herpes. The antiviral agent acyclovir is an effective medication for treatment of primary genital herpes. Intravenous administration (5 mg/kg every 8 hours for 5 to 7 days) significantly decreases viral shedding, shortens the signs and symptoms of the disease, and accelerates healing of primary herpes and mucocutaneous infection in immunocompromised patients by as many as 10 days.

Oral acyclovir is slightly less effective, and topical acyclovir is the least effective route of administration. Either may be prescribed to treat primary or recurrent disease. Acyclovir may decrease viral shedding in recurrent disease but does not appear to otherwise significantly affect the duration of symptoms. Continued oral administration of acyclovir does suppress recurrences and may be recommended for selected patients. However, the safety of daily, long-term use of acyclovir has not been established. When the medication is discontinued, recurrences resume.

Clearly, the goal is to find a treatment that eradicates latent virus and prevents recurrences, as well as a safe vaccine to prevent initial infection. Other antiviral agents and treatments have been proposed, but so far none have proved effective.

Semiannual Pap tests are recommended for women with a history of genital herpes. In addition, both men and women should avoid sexual contact while lesions are present to prevent transmission. Table 43–3 outlines the clinical course and treatment of genital herpes.

NURSING PROCESS
Genital Herpes

Nurses working in all types of health-care settings are likely to encounter patients with genital herpes. A knowledge of the disease process, clinical manifestations, modes of transmission, and current therapies is essential to providing care for these patients.

The psychologic and emotional distress experienced by patients with herpes may pose a greater problem than the actual physical symptoms. In addition to the social stigma of having contracted a venereal disease, patients must cope with the knowledge that they have a recurrent disease, manifested by genital lesions, which can be transmitted to current and future sexual partners. Of concern to

Table 43–3

Clinical Course and Treatment of Genital Herpes

Factor	Primary Infection	Recurrent Infection

Mode of transmission	Direct contact with herpes lesion or infected secretions
	Virus enters through break in skin or through mucous membrane
	Transmitted primarily through sexual contact
	May be transmitted to infant during vaginal delivery
		Reactivation of previously acquired herpes simplex virus
		Factors that may precipitate recurrent infection include:
		  Exposure to heat (fever or external temperature)
		  Mensturation
		  Sexual intercourse
		  Stress, anxiety

Incubation	2–20 days	Unknown

Signs and symptoms	Local:
	  Genital lesions (begin as papules, progress to fluid-filled vesicles that rupture to form ulcers)
	  Pain
	  Pruritus
	  Dysuria
	  Vaginal and urethral discharge
	  Enlarged lymph nodes
	Systemic:
	  Symptoms of viremia:
	    Fever
	    Malaise
	    Headache
	    Muscle pain
	    Back stiffness
		Local:
		  Genital lesions (fewer and more localized than primary infection)
		  Pain, pruritus, and dysuria are milder in recurrent infections and may be absent in males
		
		Systemic:
		  None
		  Prodromal (occurring just before appearance of lesions:
		    Paresthesias
		    Pruritus
		    Redness
		    Discomfort

Duration of symptoms	Local: 8–30 days Systemic: 7–10 days	Local: 4–10 days Prodromal: 0.5–48 hr before appearance of lesions

Medical treatment	*Acyclovir* (Zovirax sterile powder, IV)
	  Indication: For initial or recurrent infections in immunocompromised patients, and for severe initial clinical episodes in patients not immunocompromised
	  Dosage: 5 mg/kg over 1 hour every 8 hr for 5–7 days
	Zovirax capsules (PO)
	  Dosage: 200 mg PO every 4 hr when awake for total of five capsules daily for 10 days
	Zovirax 5% ointment (topical)
	  Dosage: Cover all lesions every 3 hr or six times daily for 7 days (5-inch ribbon of ointment covers 4 square inches of surface area)
		Zovirax capsules
		  Indication: Intermittent therapy for recurrent infection
		  Dosage: 200 mg every 4 hr; total of five capsules daily for 5 days (begin medication at earliest prodromal sign)
		  Indication: Chronic suppressive therapy for recurrent disease
		  Dosage: 200 mg tid up to 6 months (may require up to five capsules per day to suppress disease)
		Zovirax sterile powder (IV)
		  See under primary infection
		Zovirax 5% ointment
		  See under primary infection

IV, intravenous; PO, orally; tid, three times daily.

women is the association of genital herpes with cervical cancer and the potential effect of the disease on the method of delivery and health of future offspring. These complex emotional and social problems may generate feelings of anxiety, fear, and depression. The nurse needs to be prepared to provide education, counseling, and emotional support.

Assessment

Assessment begins with a thorough history and physical examination of the lesions. Throughout the assessment process, observe and inquire about the patient's emotional and social response to the disease. Educational needs are identified by assessing the patient's knowledge about the disease, current health practices, and lifestyle.

Carry out the nursing assessment in a physical environment that provides both privacy and good lighting and that promotes the patient's psychologic and physical comfort.

Patients may be reluctant to provide information about their disease and response to it. The perception of herpes as socially unacceptable and the intimate nature of the mode of transmission often inhibit open, honest communication. It is important to communicate an empathetic, accepting, and nonjudgmental attitude. Use open-ended questions designed to encourage verbalization whenever possible.

Initially determine whether the infection is primary or recurrent, and ascertain the onset, duration, frequency, and severity of local and systemic symptoms (if applicable). Question the patient about factors that aggravate or relieve the symptoms and about current therapies used. In cases of recurrent herpes, help the patient identify factors that may precipitate outbreaks.

Obtain a sexual history, including frequency of sexual relations, number of partners, and mode of sexual contacts. Question the patient about a history of other sexually transmitted diseases. Obtain an obstetric and gynecologic history from female patients. Of particular importance are the frequency of Pap tests and current methods of contraception.

To assess the impact of herpes on the patient's emotional and social wellbeing, question the patient about the effects of herpes on his or her interpersonal relationships, lifestyle, sexual identity, and self-esteem.

Potential emotional reactions to herpes include shock, anger, depression, and withdrawal. Disbelief and denial are common initial reactions. "How could it happen to me?" and "Herpes happens to other people" are feelings frequently communicated by patients on learning the diagnosis. Shock is often followed by anger. For example, a patient may express anger at herself for having contracted the infection, at her partner for "having given it to me," and at health-care professionals for their inability to provide a cure. A pattern of emotional stress, depression, and withdrawal, frequently referred to as the "herpes syndrome," may develop.

Patients may experience sadness either at the loss of sexual freedom and identity or about the change in body image and personal health. Lowering of self-esteem and guilt for having contracted an STD are common. Fear of rejection or fear of transmitting the disease in future relationships may cause the patient to withdraw from social contacts. The stress experienced by patients exhibiting severe emotional responses to herpes may, in fact, precipitate more frequent recurrences.

During the assessment interview, observe and actively listen for cues to the patient's emotional response to herpes. Some questions that may help the patient begin to communicate his or her feelings include the following:

> "Whom have you told about your diagnosis?"
> "How has herpes affected your sexual relationships, social activities, and lifestyle?"
> "What do you find most difficult about having herpes?"

Some patients will appear, or verbally indicate that they are, depressed. Assess these patients for signs and symptoms of clinical depression.

Nursing Diagnoses and Planning

Nursing diagnoses and related expected patient outcomes commonly applicable to patients with genital herpes include the following:

NDx: Pain related to the inflammatory process and irritation of the genital vesicles

Planning: Patient Outcomes
1. Patient reports that itching and burning are controlled by medication.
2. Patient voids without pain or burning.

NDx: Risk for infection (secondary) related to impairment of skin integrity

Planning: Patient Outcomes
1. Lesions are free of purulent drainage.
2. Tissues surrounding the lesions are free of edema.
3. Patient's temperature is normal.
4. Palpable lymph nodes are absent.

NDx: Risk for altered health maintenance related to insufficient knowledge of disease process and prevention of transmission

Planning: Patient Outcomes
1. Patient states cause and mode of herpes transmission.
2. Patient describes progress of primary and recurrent herpes, including signs and symptoms of prodromal and acute phases of infection.
3. Patient states methods and measures for preventing transmission to others.
4. Patient describes possible complications of herpes.

NDx: Anxiety related to the diagnosis of herpes and its potential physical and lifestyle effects.

Planning: Patient Outcomes

1. Patient verbalizes concerns about herpes and its effects.
2. Patient accurately describes effects of genital herpes on sexual activity and reproductive capacity.
3. Patient states knowledge of the disease and measures for preventing transmission have decreased his or her fear of transmitting the infection to others.
4. Behavioral signs of anxiety are absent.

NDx: Risk for ineffective individual coping related to diagnosis of a chronic STD and its potential effects.

Planning: Patient Outcomes

1. Patient describes changes in health habits and lifestyle that may decrease recurrence.
2. Patient lists factors that may precipitate recurrent infection.
3. Patient informs significant others or sexual partners about genital herpes.
4. Patient participates in social relationships and activities.
5. Patient asks questions and requests additional information about herpes.
6. Patient joins herpes support group.
7. Patient reports viewing the infection as a minor inconvenience.
8. Symptoms of depression are absent.

Nursing Interventions and Evaluation

NDx: Pain

Recommend self-care and health-management techniques for symptomatic relief during active infection (Highlight 43–2).

NDx: Risk for infection

Instruct the patient to avoid touching or scratching the lesions because this can result in infection of the area with a new organism introduced from the hands and can spread the herpes infection to other parts of the body by autoinoculation. Stress the importance of performing meticulous perineal hygiene and wearing clean, loose undergarments.

NDx: Risk for altered health maintenance

Teaching and counseling of the patient with genital herpes are based on the assessment of the patient's learning needs, emotional status, and whether the infection is primary or recurrent. The patient's emotional status can affect readiness to learn. Newly diagnosed patients are often emotionally upset and anxious. They require time to assimilate the knowledge that they have herpes before they can begin to absorb information that will ultimately help them cope with the disease. Consequently, initial instruction of patients with primary herpes is often limited

---

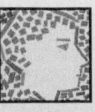

HIGHLIGHT 43–2

PATIENT EDUCATION

Symptomatic Relief of Genital Herpes

Recommend the following self-care measures for symptomatic relief during active infection with genital herpes:

Keep the lesions and adjacent areas clean and dry.

Avoid the use of lubricants and creams, which may prolong healing time and contribute to secondary infection.

Wear loose clothing and cotton underwear to decrease pressure and irritation on the lesions and to promote drying.

Apply drying agents such as Campho-Phenique for relief of pain and itch.

Use soaks and compresses to promote drying and comfort (cool, wet compresses for itching, sitz baths for local pain and discomfort).

Take aspirin or acetaminophen as per directions for pain.

---

to basic information about the disease, mode of transmission, and therapy.

As the patient indicates greater readiness to learn, provide additional information about the cause and mode of transmission as well as differences among primary, initial, and recurrent infections and possible complications. Supplement verbal instruction with written information to which the patient can later refer because patients experiencing high levels of anxiety may not remember much of what was taught.

Correct any misconceptions or myths the patient may have about herpes. Use common, unemotional terms familiar to the patient to assist him or her in viewing the disease in a realistic perspective. It may be helpful to explain that genital herpes lesions are the same skin lesions as the cold sore frequently seen on the lips or face. Also tell the patient that much research is being done to develop a treatment to eradicate the disease permanently.

Avoid terms such as *incurable* when discussing the diagnosis with the patient because the goal is to provide information without increasing anxiety. Emphasize the fact that recurrent outbreaks, if they occur, become less frequent and, in most cases, ultimately cease over time.

Instruct the patient on measures to prevent transmission and complications (Highlight 43–3).

NDx: Anxiety

Encourage the patient to verbalize feelings and concerns about the diagnosis and its potential effects on health and lifestyle. Provide an opportunity for the patient to talk in a nonthreatening environment that provides privacy.

While listening to the patient, pay particular attention to any clues that anxiety is due, at least in part, to lack of information, misconceptions, or unrealistic expectations about the disease and its effects. Provide accurate information using nontechnical and unemotional language. Acknowledge the patient's anxiety while providing practical, factual information that will assist the patient in developing a realistic perspective on the problem and ability to cope with it.

NDx: Risk for ineffective individual coping

Counseling includes interventions to assist the patient in coping with the psychologic and social ramifications of the disease. Identify strategies for self-management that help the patient gain a sense of control and confidence in his or her ability to cope with the disease.

The potential for recurrent, unpredictable outbreaks of infection is a major area of difficulty for herpes patients. Review with the patient the relationship of physical and psychologic stress to recurrent outbreaks. Identify personal and environmental factors—such as an elevation in either the internal or external temperature, stress, anxiety, menstruation, and sexual intercourse—that may precipitate outbreaks. Review specific techniques for reducing stress, such as relaxation techniques, exercise, yoga, and imaging. Emphasize the importance of maintaining a healthy lifestyle. Describe the role of diet, exercise, and adequate rest in maintaining an optimal immune response and possibly decreasing outbreaks.

Explore with the patient the need to inform others about the disease. It is generally recommended that patients inform prospective sex partners, whom they plan to see over time, relatively early in the relationship. Help the patient identify ways of telling others by making specific suggestions. Advise the patient to introduce the topic in a calm, direct, nonthreatening manner that does not frighten the other person. Suggest introductory statements such as "Do you know what cold sores are?" or "Have you heard of herpes?" as opposed to "There's something I think you should know." Advise the patient to assume that the person does not know much about herpes and to talk about the facts and how to prevent transmission. It is also helpful if the patient

---

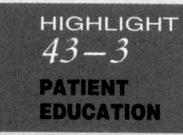 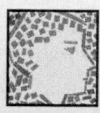

HIGHLIGHT 43–3

PATIENT EDUCATION

Preventing Transmission and Complications of Genital Herpes

To enable the patient to prevent transmission of genital herpes:

Explain to the patient the following:

- The herpesvirus is transmitted by direct skin-to-skin or mucous membrane contact with one or more herpes lesions or infected secretions.
- Sexual contact is the most frequent mode of transmission.
- Infection may be spread by contamination of the hands to other sites.
- Contact with grossly contaminated objects is a possible but rare mode of transmission.

Instruct the patient to do the following:

- Avoid touching the lesions.
- Wash hands thoroughly if lesions are inadvertently touched.
- Inspect the genital area frequently to detect recurrent lesions early.

- Abstain from sexual intercourse when the prodromal signs and symptoms appear and continue until the lesions are no longer present.
- Consider the use of condoms between outbreaks. (It is not known whether the infection can be transmitted during asymptomatic periods. Condoms are not sufficient protection during active herpes because the virus is smaller than the pores of the condom, and it is not known whether the virus can penetrate the condom and in what numbers.)

To assist the female patient in avoiding obstetric complications of genital herpes:

Advise the patient to do the following:

- Inform her gynecologist/obstetrician of her herpes history.
- Obtain a Papanicolaou test every 6 months.

Explain to pregnant patients that a cesarean section is performed if there is active infection at the time of delivery.

can talk about herpes as a fairly insignificant problem that can be dealt with relatively easily.

If you are comfortable with role-playing, offer to play the role of another person to allow the patient to practice telling a prospective partner. Another technique is for the patient to practice telling others by first telling a trusted friend or relative.

Inform the patient about resources available to persons with genital herpes. A quarterly publication called "The Helper" from the National Herpes Research Center of the American Social Health Association contains articles on the latest scientific research as well as ways of coping with herpes. The same organization sponsors support groups for herpes patients that are located throughout the United States. Self-help groups provide information, emotional support, and group identification. Members learn that they are not alone and that others have similar feelings and problems. The group offers an opportunity to work through problems and to learn from the experiences of others. Local chapters of "Help" can be located through the telephone book or through the National Herpes Resource Center.

Compare the patient's status with the expected outcomes. If the outcomes are not met, reassess the patient and revise the plan.

Gonorrhea

Gonorrhea is a sexually transmitted infection caused by *Neisseria gonorrhoeae*, a gram-negative bacterium that has a predilection for certain types of epithelial tissue commonly found in the urogenital tract.

Each year, about 1 million cases of gonorrhea are reported in the United States. In addition, it is estimated that 1 to 1.5 million cases go unreported.

Similar to other STDs, gonorrhea is most prevalent in the teenage and young-adult age groups. The incidence increases in the late teens and early 20s and declines with advancing age. Although the overall rate of gonorrhea has remained relatively constant during the past few years, there have been increases and decreases within specific demographic groups. For example, reported cases of gonorrhea in females, particularly during the teenage years, dramatically increased during the past two decades.

This increase in reported rates of gonorrhea in females, particularly in the younger age groups, may reflect several factors, including better recognition and diagnosis in females and changes in sexual mores and practices, especially earlier and more frequent sexual activity.

On the basis of statistics from reported cases in the United States, demographic risk factors for gonorrhea include low socioeconomic status, nonwhite race, urban residence, unmarried status, multiple sexual partners, early onset of sexual activity, male homosexuality, and history of gonorrhea. Many of these risk factors may influence, at least in part, the reporting of gonorrhea. The demographic groups just identified are more likely to attend public health clinics. Such clinics are more compliant with case reporting than private clinics and physicians who cater to a more affluent segment of the population.

Etiology and Pathophysiology

Initially, the *N. gonorrhoeae* bacterium attaches to the mucous membranes of structures in the lower urogenital tract, such as the urethra, Bartholin's glands, and cervix. Within 24 to 48 hours, the organism invades the mucosal epithelium. *N. gonorrhoeae* causes a vigorous leukocyte response, which leads to the development of a purulent discharge.

Gonorrhea is transmitted from one infected person to another through close body contact. Sexual contact is the most common mode of transmission. Transmission by inanimate objects or close nonsexual personal contact is possible but extremely rare, with the exception of vertical transmission from mother to infant during the birthing process.

Clinical Manifestations

Gonorrhea has a broad range of clinical manifestations, including asymptomatic, symptomatic, and complicated infection at several different sites.

In men, gonorrhea presents most often as an acute urethritis. The major symptoms are a profuse, purulent white or yellowish urethral discharge, accompanied by meatal inflammation and discomfort on urination (Fig. 43–3). Initially, the exudate may be scant and mucoid. Within 24 hours, however, it is usually purulent and relatively abundant. The incubation period ranges from 1 to 14 days, but the onset of symptoms usually occurs 3 to 7 days after sexual contact with an infected partner.

About one-quarter of men exhibit only scant, minimally purulent discharge that may be apparent

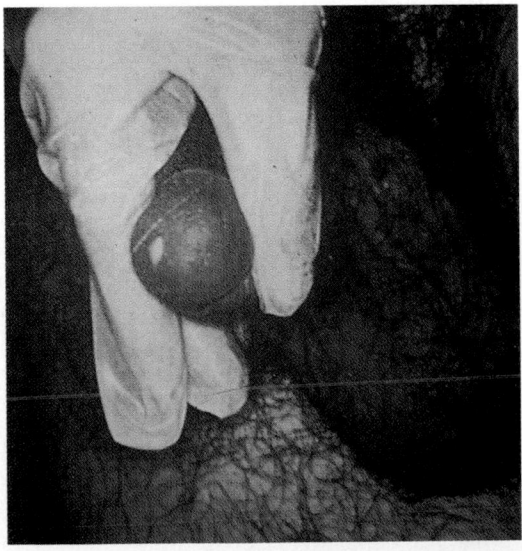

Figure 43–3
Gonococcal urethritis. Note the white, purulent discharge at the meatus. (Courtesy of New York City Health Department.)

exclusively in the morning. In a few infected men, signs and symptoms of urethritis never develop. Complications in men are rare and relatively minor.

In women, the infection is frequently asymptomatic, or the signs and symptoms are so inconsequential that they remain unnoticed.

The primary site of infection in women is the cervix. Colonization of the urinary tract with *N. gonorrhoeae* also occurs in most infected women. Other sites of initial infection may include the periurethral Skene glands and Bartholin glands. Although the incubation period is more variable in women, most who experience symptoms do so within 10 days of exposure and usually within 2 to 5 days.

Urinary frequency, dysuria, and purulent vaginal discharge are the three most common presenting symptoms. On physical examination, signs of cervical inflammation—including mucopurulent cervical discharge, erythema, friability, and tenderness on cervical palpation—are common findings. Apart from pelvic inflammatory disease, which refers to a range of inflammatory disorders of the upper female genital tract including endometritis, salpingitis, tubo-ovarian abscess, and pelvic peritonitis, abscess of a Bartholin gland is the most common complication of gonorrhea in women.

Anorectal infection occurs in about 35 to 50% of women and homosexual men with gonorrhea. In men, infection results from anal intercourse. In women, anorectal infection probably results from contamination of the perineum with discharge originating at the infected cervix. Symptoms range from minor anal itching and mucopurulent discharge to severe rectal pain, bleeding, and constipation.

If gonococci invade the bloodstream, disseminated gonococcal infection may follow. Whether or not systemic infection occurs is influenced by the strain of the infecting gonococcal organism and the person's immunologic status.

Disseminated gonococcal infection is more common in women than men because women are more likely to have untreated gonococcal infections. Clinical manifestations include signs and symptoms commonly seen in bacterial infections (eg, fever, malaise, anorexia, leukocytosis). Skin lesions are the most common manifestation. Usually they appear on the distal extremities as erythematous macules that progress to form pustules. Tenosynovitis (inflammation of the tendon sheaths), septic arthritis, and polyarthralgias are also common clinical manifestations. Fortunately, disseminated gonococcal infection responds well to antibiotic therapy.

Gonococcal pelvic inflammatory disease is the most common and serious complication of gonorrheal infection in women. In 10 to 20%, the initial urogenital infection spreads to the upper genital tract. It is theorized that the gonococci ascend the genital tract during menstruation and are disseminated either to the uterus, where a transient endometritis may occur, or directly to the fallopian tubes. The tubes become reddened and edematous and contain a purulent exudate. The exudate may drip from the ends of the tubes, causing pelvic peritonitis and subsequent pelvic adhesions.

The clinical manifestations of pelvic inflammatory disease vary. Symptoms usually do not occur until during or just after the next menstrual period. The symptoms of acute pelvic inflammatory disease include fever, shaking chills, anorexia, malaise, vaginal discharge, abdominal discomfort, and occasional nausea.

The most common clinical manifestations are fever and bilateral lower abdominal pain. Some patients have a history of abnormal vaginal bleeding and prolonged menstruation before symptoms. Pelvic peritonitis may be manifested by direct and rebound lower abdominal tenderness and muscle guarding. Pelvic examination may reveal mucopurulent cervicitis and urethral discharge. Manipulation of the cervix causes marked discomfort.

Long-term sequelae include tubo-ovarian abscess, ectopic pregnancy, and infertility from intra-abdominal adhesions, with chronic pelvic pain and menstrual irregularities. Management of pelvic inflammatory disease includes prompt administration of antimicrobial therapy, monitoring, and follow-up for complications. The sooner appropriate antibiotic therapy is initiated, the less chance there is of permanent damage to the reproductive tract.

Diagnosis

Because the symptoms of gonorrhea are similar to those of other STDs, clinical diagnosis must be confirmed by laboratory tests. Microscopic examination of stained smears of urethral exudate and subsequent identification of polymorphonuclear leukocytes and the typical gram-negative intracellular diplococci are considered sufficient for diagnosis of gonococcal urethritis in men. Gram's stains are unreliable in women. Cervical cultures are the preferred method and detect 80 to 90% of cervical infections.

Management

Components of management include the following:

- Identification of the sites of infection
- Selection of an effective antimicrobial regimen
- Identification, diagnosis, and treatment of sexual contacts
- Repeated cultures or smears 4 to 7 days after treatment to verify cure

Many antibiotics have proved effective in treating gonorrhea, including the penicillins, tetracyclines, and cephalosporins. Severity of disease, site of infection, expense, patient compliance, and toxicity are all factors considered in the selection of an antimicrobial regimen. For uncomplicated disease, a single parenteral treatment with ceftriaxone is recommended. Single-dose therapy is inexpensive and eliminates patient compliance as a factor in treatment. Doxycycline is also given for possible coinfection with *Chlamydia trachomatis*.

Other recommended regimens include cefixime,

ciprofloxacin, and ofloxacin given orally as a single dose.

In cases of complicated disease (those involving disseminated infection and pelvic inflammatory disease), hospitalization is frequently recommended, especially if the woman is a nulligravida. Regimens include intravenous ceftriaxone followed by oral cefixime or ciprofloxacin. For pelvic inflammatory disease, combination antibiotic therapy is recommended because of the complex nature of the disease, high failure rates, and significant long-term sequelae. Medications should be effective against *N. gonorrhoeae*, *C. trachomatis*, and anaerobic bacteria, all of which have been implicated in pelvic inflammatory disease. Table 43–4 presents common treatment regimens for gonorrhea.

NURSING PROCESS
Gonorrhea

Nurses may encounter patients with gonorrhea under a variety of circumstances. Men seek treatment because the symptoms are usually obvious and uncomfortable. However, at least half of female patients experience few if any symptoms associated with lower genital tract gonococcal infections. Although gonorrhea is diagnosed during routine gynecologic examinations in some women, usually by Pap tests, many remain unaware of the infection. Consequently, many women do not seek health care until they have symptoms of pelvic inflammatory disease.

Nurses working with high-risk female patients in various settings (eg, clinics for treating STDs, family planning clinics, inpatient obstetric and gynecologic services) can play an important role in case finding and prevention. A thorough history and a high degree of suspicion are necessary to identify cases of gonorrhea in asymptomatic female patients.

Assessment

Obtain social, sexual, obstetric, and gynecologic histories, as well as a general health history. Explore the patient's lifestyle and attitudes toward health by asking such questions as the following:

"Do you consider yourself a healthy person?"
"What do you do to protect yourself from disease?"
"How do you stay healthy?"

Note the presence of high-risk factors, such as lower socioeconomic class, early onset of sexual activity, frequent sexual contact with numerous sexual partners, and history of gonorrhea or other STD.

Question the patient about his or her preferred method of contraception. Barrier methods, such as condoms and diaphragms, are recommended because they decrease transmission of gonorrhea. Oral contraceptives are also associated with decreased incidence of the disease, whereas intrauterine devices are related to an increase in the incidence of both urogenital infections and pelvic inflammatory disease.

Question the patient about the occurrence of symptoms associated with complicated and uncomplicated gonococcal infections. A review of symptoms, past and present, is the key to patient assessment and case finding.

If the patient responds affirmatively to having one or more of the symptoms under review, analyze the symptom further. For example, if the patient reports an abnormal discharge, ask about the onset, duration, color, odor, amount, and consistency of the discharge. Analyze complaints of pain according to location, onset, duration, frequency, and aggravating and relieving factors. Also ask the patient to describe the pain. Find out, for example, whether the pain is dull, sharp, stabbing, or gnawing.

Perform a physical assessment guided by the patient's history and symptoms. For example, inspect discharge, and inspect and palpate the site of pain.

Assess also the patient's learning needs and ability to understand and absorb new information. Assess the patient's knowledge about transmission, prevention, signs and symptoms, complications, and long-term sequelae of gonorrhea. Educational background, prior knowledge, level of anxiety, and motivation can all affect the patient's ability to learn. Consider each of these factors in determining when and how to communicate information about the disease to the patient.

Assess the patient's emotional response to a confirmed or possible diagnosis of gonorrhea. Some patients may express anger, fear, or denial. Others may be cavalier or unconcerned about the diagnosis and its implications. Actively listen to and observe the patient for clues to his or her psychologic response to the disease. Validate impressions by asking open-ended questions designed to convey empathy and understanding as well as provide and obtain information. Responses to questions such as "Has there been or do you anticipate a change in your sexual relations because of gonorrhea?" can provide information about both emotional and social effects of the disease on the patient.

Be sure to communicate a nonjudgmental attitude and a sense of caring throughout the assessment interview.

Nursing Diagnoses and Planning

Nursing diagnoses and related expected patient outcomes commonly applicable to patients with gonorrhea include the following:

NDx: Pain related to inflammation of the urogenital tract and irritation from vaginal discharge

Planning: Patient Outcomes
1. Patient keeps genital area clean and dry.
2. Patient describes hygienic measures to be used after elimination to avoid spreading infective discharge.

Table 43–4

Treatment Regimens for Gonorrhea, Syphilis, and Chlamydial Infection

Infection	Medication	Recommended Dosage	Special Considerations
Gonorrhea, uncomplicated	Ceftriaxone	125 mg IM in a single dose	Drug of choice for uncomplicated gonorrhea Divided dose given at two sites (4.8 ml/injection) Moderately painful injection Single-dose treatment is recommended for noncompliant patients Effective for pharyngeal and rectal gonorrhea and incubating syphilis Recommended for treating gonorrhea in homosexual men Probenecid decreases renal excretion of penicillin; increases serum levels
	Cefixime	400 mg PO in a single dose	Easiest treatment to administer and most acceptable to patients
	Ciprofloxin	500 mg PO in a single dose	Contraindicated for pregnant or nursing women and for those ≤17 years of age
	Combination therapy: Single dose ceftriaxone *or* cefixime *or* ciprofloxacin plus doxycycline	125 mg IM *or* 400 mg PO *or* 500 mg PO 100 mg two times daily for 7 days	
Disseminated gonococcal infection	Ceftriaxone followed by cefixime	1 mg IM or IV every 24 hr until improvement; 400 mg PO two times a day for 7 days	IV medications for hospitalized patients
Gonococcal PID Outpatient	Cefoxitin plus probenecid in a single dose *or* ceftriaxone concurrently with doxycycline *or* oflaxacin concurrently with clindamycin	2 g IM 1 g PO *or* 250 IM 100 mg PO twice daily for 7 days *or* 400 mg PO twice daily for 14 days 450 mg PO four times a day	Cefoxitin and probenecid recommended when *Neisseria gonorrhoeae* is most likely causative organism Ceftriaxone and doxycycline recommended when *Chlamydia trachomatis* is most likely causative organism; may also be prescribed for gonoccal PID
Inpatient	Cefoxitin *or* cefotetan *plus* doxycycline	2 g IV every 6 hr *or* 2 g IV every 12 hr *plus* 100 mg IV four times daily until improvement, followed by 100 mg PO two times a day for 14 days	Regimen should be continued for at least 48 hr after patient shows improvement

Table continued on following page

Table 43–4

Treatment Regimens for Gonorrhea, Syphilis, and Chlamydial Infection (continued)

Infection	Medication	Recommended Dosage	Special Considerations
Patients with multiple episodes of PID; possible pelvic abscess	Cefoxitin *plus* doxycycline *plus* clindamycin	2 g IV every 6–8 hr for 10 days *plus* 100 mg IM or PO every 12 hrs *plus* 900 mg IV every 8 hr	Triple antibiotic therapy when causative organism unknown or more than one organism suspected; effective for gonorrheal, chlamydial, and anaerobic infections
Chlamydial infection	Doxycycline *or* azithromycin	100 mg PO twice daily for 7 days *or* 1 g PO in a single dose	Successful treatment for gonorrhea as well as chlamydial infection Recommended for patients who cannot tolerate tetracycline and for pregnant patients
PID	See gonococcal PID		
Syphilis Duration less than 1 y	Benzathine penicillin G	2.4 million units IM	Divide dose into 1.2 million units into each buttock Medication of choice for treatment of primary and secondary syphilis of less than 1 yr duration and for contacts of these patients
	Doxycycline	100 mg PO twice daily for 15 days	Use when penicillin is contraindicated (i.e., penicillin allergy)
Duration more than 1 y	Benzathine penicillin G *or* doxycycline *or* erythromycin *or* aqueous procaine penicillin	2.4 million units once per week for 3 wk *or* 100 mg PO twice daily for 30 days *or* 500 g PO four times daily for 30 days *or* 600,000 units IM daily for 15 days	Medication of choice for syphilis of more than 1 yr duration Recommended for penicillin-allergic patients; may cause gastrointestinal disturbance Recommended for penicillin-allergic pregnant patients Impractical for outpatient therapy
Pregnant patient with penicillin allergy	Penicillin regimen appropriate for the patient's stage of syphilis		There are no proven alternatives to penicillin. Desensitization will be required, and skin testing may be helpful
Neurosyphilis	Crystalline penicillin G *followed by* benzathine penicillin G *or* aqueous procaine penicillin G *plus* probenecid	2 to 4 million units IV every 4 hours for at least 10 days *followed by* 2.4 million units IM weekly for 3 wk *or* 2.4 million units IM daily for 15 days *plus* 500 mg PO four times daily for 10 days	More intensive therapy may be recommended for neurosyphilis as a result of treatment failures with standard treatment of syphilis of more than 1 yr duration

IM, intramuscular; PO, orally; PPNG, penicillinase-producing *Neisseria gonorrhoeae*; IV, intravenous; PID, pelvic inflammatory disease.

3. Patient reports experiencing less discomfort.
4. Patient is free of discomfort on urination.
5. Vaginal or urethral discharge is absent or decreased.

NDx: Risk for altered health maintenance related to insufficient knowledge of disease process, prevention of transmission, potential complications, and long-term sequelae

Planning: Patient Outcomes

1. Patient states the cause, symptoms, complications, and mode of transmission of gonorrhea.
2. Patient describes health practices to reduce the risk of reinfection and transmission.

NDx: Anxiety related to possible long-term sequelae, perceived threat to self-concept, naming sexual contacts

Planning: Patient Outcomes

1. Patient's behavior indicates decreased anxiety (eg, relaxed position, free of nervousness and irritability).
2. Patient asks appropriate questions.
3. Patient reports feeling calm and in control.

NDx: Risk for ineffective management of therapeutic regimen (individuals) related to prescribed health practices, naming of sexual contacts

Planning: Patient Outcomes

1. Patient states reasons for following the therapeutic regimen.
2. Patient reports taking medication as prescribed.
3. Patient returns for follow-up and test of cure.
4. Repeat cultures and tests are negative.
5. Patient expresses intent to use prophylactic measures during future sexual activity.
6. Patient provides names of sexual contacts.

Nursing Interventions and Evaluation

NDx: Pain

Advise the patient to keep the external genitalia clean and dry and to avoid scratching. Caution patients, especially women, to be careful not to spread infected discharge to the urethral meatus or the rectum, particularly after voiding or defecation and during menstruation.

NDx: Risk for altered health maintenance

Teach the patient about the disease process, potential complications, and preventive measures to help ensure compliance with treatment and to prevent reinfection and transmission.

Select teaching strategies based on the patient's prior knowledge, level of anxiety, and ability to learn as well as available materials. With some patients, it may be necessary to review basic anatomy and physiology of the reproductive and urinary tracts. Photographs are often helpful in communicating this information. Films, videotapes, and slides, if available, are also effective, especially when teaching adolescents and young adults. Be sure to use terminology the patient can understand. Avoid complex explanations and the provision of more information than the patient needs or is ready to learn.

If the patient is experiencing moderate to severe anxiety or demonstrates lack of motivation to learn, little learning will occur. In both cases, it may be necessary to limit the amount of information to essentials, such as methods for preventing reinfection and the importance of compliance and follow-up.

Written materials that the patient can take home are helpful adjuncts to teaching, especially when the patient is overly anxious.

Review the cause, symptoms, and mode of transmission of gonorrhea with the patient. Emphasize the importance of abstaining from sexual contact until negative cultures are obtained at a follow-up visit. Explain that a test of cure is necessary to ensure successful treatment because some strains of gonorrhea are resistant to specific antibiotics. Explain that the use of condoms during sexual intercourse reduces the risk of reinfection.

Inform the patient about potential complications and long-term sequelae, especially in untreated or inadequately treated gonorrhea. Inform women that they are at increased risk for disseminated gonococcal infection and pelvic inflammatory disease, which can cause infertility. Also inform men of this fact to promote compliance in treatment, reporting of sexual contacts, and use of preventive measures.

NDx: Anxiety

When possible, help the male or female patient to identify the cause of anxiety. Information can then be provided to address issues or misconceptions presented by the patient.

A nonjudgmental, empathic attitude is essential to effective counseling of patients with STDs, especially gonorrhea, which is often associated in the public's mind with sexual promiscuity. Be sensitive to the difficulty many patients experience accepting the diagnosis and providing names of sexual partners. Encourage the patient to talk about his or her anxiety. Acknowledge the patient's realistic concerns, and provide reassurance when appropriate.

NDx: Risk for ineffective management of therapeutic regimen (individuals)

Recognize that the patient's lifestyle, socioeconomic status, and cultural background may be different from your own. A sincere and caring attitude is essential to gaining the patient's trust. Ask open-ended questions to determine the patient's attitude toward sexual relationships, health care, and health-care professionals. Provide information to correct misconceptions and to promote compliance with the treatment regimen and recommended health practices.

Many patients may be afraid or hesitant to identify contacts. An understanding of the disease process and potential harm of undiagnosed infections may help the patient resolve this ambivalence and resistance to naming contacts. Emphasize that, although sexual partners (especially women) may have no symptoms early in the disease, complications can develop later or reinfect the patient.

Review the incubation period with the patient to determine which sex partners need evaluation and possible treatment. In the case of uncomplicated lower urogenital tract infection, the patient's sexual contacts during the 4 weeks preceding the onset of symptoms are contacted. In cases of disseminated gonococcal infection and pelvic inflammatory disease, the patient's sexual partners during the preceding 3 months are contacted.

Additional Interventions

Hypersensitivity reactions are the most frequent adverse effect to cephalosporins. Because of structural similarities between penicillins and cephalosporins, patients allergic to one type of drug may experience cross-reactivity with the other. The incidence of cross-reactivity in clinical practice is low: only about 5 to 10% of penicillin-allergic patients experience an allergic reaction to a cephalosporin. Cephalosporins may be used for patients with mild penicillin allergy. However, cephalosporins should not be given to patients with a history of severe allergic reaction because of the potential for fatal anaphylaxis.

Also advise the patient to avoid exposure to direct or artificial sunlight during doxycycline therapy because a phototoxic reaction (exaggerated sunburn) may develop as a result of the medication. Doxycycline should not be administered together with calcium supplements, milk products, iron supplements, magnesium-containing laxatives, and most antacids. Doxycycline is contraindicated in pregnant or nursing women.

Emphasize the importance of taking all medication for the prescribed time interval. Although the symptoms may subside or even disappear during the course of therapy, a complete cure cannot be ensured unless the regimen is followed and the patient returns for repeat tests or cultures 4 to 7 days after treatment. Instruct the patient to refrain from sexual intercourse until negative cultures are obtained on follow-up examination.

Compare the patient's status with the expected outcomes. If the outcomes are not met, reassess the patient and revise the plan.

Syphilis

Syphilis is an STD caused by the spirochete *Treponema pallidum*. The disease is most widespread in urban areas, particularly on the East, West, and Gulf Coasts among lower socioeconomic groups and cocaine users. The course of the disease is remarkably variable and prolonged. In untreated patients, 30 to 40 years may elapse between initial infection and the appearance of severe, late clinical manifestations. Its clinical course occurs in four stages:

1. The primary syphilis stage is characterized by the development of a painless chancre, usually genital, about 3 weeks after initial exposure. Chancres may be accompanied by nontender, regional lymphadenopathy.
2. The secondary syphilis stage occurs 6 to 8 weeks after the onset of primary infection. The most common symptoms are skin or mucous membrane lesions. Influenza-like symptoms usually accompany the skin lesions. Symptoms of secondary syphilis resolve 2 to 10 weeks after onset with or without treatment.
3. The latent stage of syphilis is detectable only by a positive serologic test. There are no apparent clinical manifestations. Some patients never progress beyond latent syphilis.
4. Tertiary or late-stage syphilis occurs in about one-third of untreated patients. Tertiary syphilis may affect almost any body system and produce serious complications and sequelae, including permanent disability and death.

Modern diagnostic tests, effective treatments, and public education have greatly reduced the incidence of all stages of syphilis. Manifestations of late syphilis are especially rare today. Currently, the primary public health concern is finding, treating, and preventing early syphilis, although awareness of the late manifestations remains necessary to ensure accurate diagnosis and treatment.

Etiology and Pathophysiology

The causative agent, *T. pallidum*, is a spiral-shaped organism that enters the body through intact mucous membranes or a break in the skin. Transmission of *T. pallidum* occurs primarily during sexual relations through direct contact with a syphilitic lesion or its exudate. If the exudate is secreted into body fluids—such as saliva, semen, or vaginal discharge—contact with the infected fluids can transmit the disease as well.

It appears that exposure to relatively few *T. pallidum* organisms can produce the disease. Because the spirochete enters the blood stream soon after initial exposure, contact with contaminated blood is another potential mode of transmission. *T. pallidum* can also be spread transplacentally from an infected mother to her fetus as early as the ninth week of gestation.

T. pallidum does not live outside the human body for any appreciable time. Therefore, transmission by objects such as towels, toilet seats, and drinking glasses is a highly improbable, rare occurrence.

Once *T. pallidum* invades the skin, it attaches to, but does not appear to penetrate, human cells. During the incubation period, *T. pallidum* stimulates both cell-mediated and humoral immunity. Lymphocytes and macrophages are present locally. Antitreponemal antibody is present in the serum of 70 to 80% of patients with a primary lesion.

During the primary stage, it may appear that the infection is contained and limited to the localized chancre lesion. However, the infection has in fact begun to spread through the circulation and, if untreated, ultimately produces the systemic symptoms characteristic of secondary syphilis.

The appearance of secondary syphilis despite evidence of an active immune response to the infection is an example of the complexity of the host's response to this disease. The period of latency after secondary syphilis symptoms resolve indicates that, eventually, the host suppresses the infection so that no clinical manifestations are apparent. However, one-third of untreated patients acquire tertiary syphilis as many as 20 to 30 years later. The persistence of *T. pallidum*, in the presence of an immune response, over a prolonged period in many patients has led to speculation that syphilis suppresses certain and as yet unidentified aspects of the immune response.

Clinical Manifestations

Primary Syphilis

The classic symptom of primary syphilis is the development of a painless, genital ulcer at the site of entry. The chancre sore appears about 3 weeks after sexual contact with an infectious person. Typically, it begins as a reddened macule and progresses to a papule that erodes to produce a round to oval, well-defined ulcer with raised borders. The chancre is usually painless unless secondary infection occurs. Untreated, it heals in 3 to 6 weeks. In men, the most common genital sites are the coronal sulcus, glans penis, and prepuce (Fig. 43–4). In women, frequent sites are the labia, vulva, and cervix. Cervical lesions are often missed because of the lack of apparent symptoms. Lesions may also occur on extragenital sites. The most common extragenital site is the perianal region (Fig. 43–5). Other common sites include the mouth, tongue, breasts, and fingers. Although the chancre of primary syphilis usually occurs as a single lesion, multiple lesions are possible. Atypical lesions at unusual sites are becoming more common, a fact that is attributed to changes in sexual practices. As a general rule, any genital or extragenital

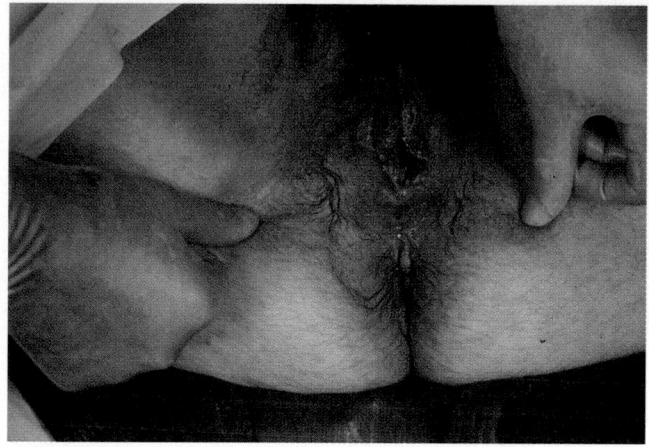

Figure 43–5

Primary chancre in female patient located on posterior fourchette and perineum. (Courtesy of Leonard Wolf, MD, New York, NY.)

ulcer should be considered potentially syphilitic until proved otherwise.

Secondary Syphilis

If the patient is not treated during the incubation period or the primary stage, symptoms of secondary syphilis develop about 6 to 8 weeks after the chancre's initial appearance. Symptoms of secondary syphilis are multiple and varied and can affect almost any organ of the body. Systemic influenza-like symptoms commonly occur, such as malaise, fever, headache, sore throat, anorexia, and arthralgia. Generalized, nontender lymphadenopathy is present.

Generalized skin rashes are the most frequently encountered clinical manifestation of secondary syphilis. Cutaneous eruptions often appear as well-demarcated, copper-colored macules on the palms and soles, although they may appear anywhere on the body (Fig. 43–6). Papulosquamous rashes—small, scaly, reddened elevations—are the most common cutaneous lesions associated with secondary syphilis. The mucous membranes of the mouth may be involved, with the appearance of white erosions called mucous patches.

Lesions may also take the form of flat-topped, wartlike papules called condylomata lata (Fig. 43–7). Syphilis is often referred to as the "great imitator" because of the variety of the skin lesions seen in secondary syphilis, which may mimic and are often confused with other dermatologic conditions. Patchy hair loss may also occur in association with skin lesions and affect the eyebrows and beard as well. With or without treatment, cutaneous symptoms usually heal in 2 to 10 weeks. Other less common symptoms of secondary syphilis include bursitis, arthritis, periostitis, hepatitis, and nephrotic syndrome as a result of immune complex deposition.

Latent Syphilis

Latent syphilis begins with the resolution of secondary signs and symptoms and ends when and if the

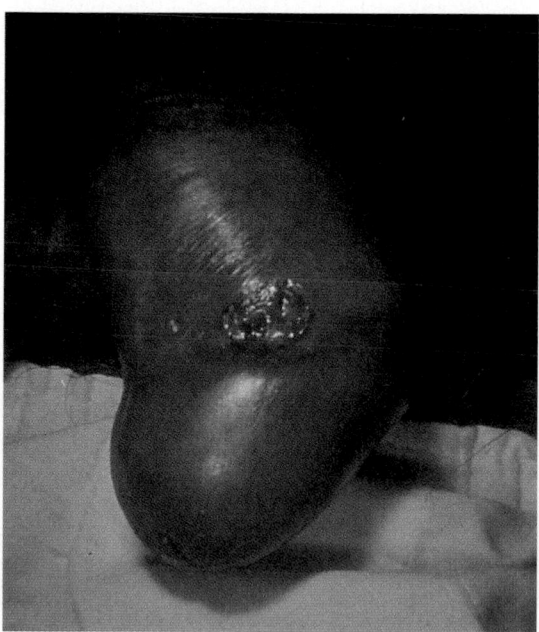

Figure 43–4

Penile chancre typical of primary syphilis. (Courtesy of New York City Health Department.)

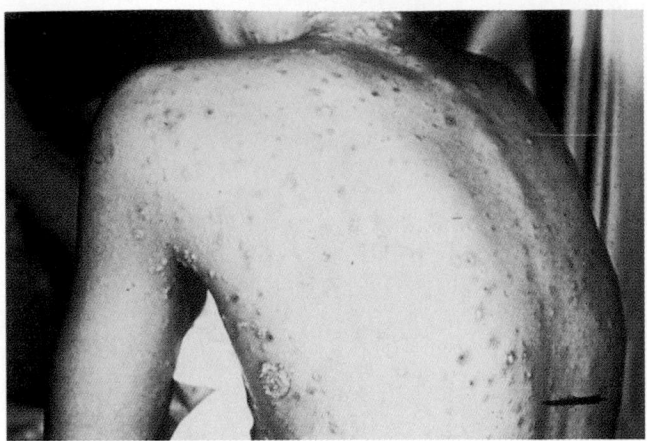

Figure 43–6

Generalized skin rash seen in secondary syphilis. (Courtesy of the New York City Health Department).

clinical manifestations of tertiary syphilis develop. Latent syphilis is defined as the stage at which there are positive serologic test results or a history of syphilis but no current clinical manifestations. The latent period is divided into early and late latency. Early latency refers to syphilis of less than 1 year's duration. During early latency, the patient may experience relapses of the mucocutaneous symptoms experienced during the second stage. In early latency, the patient is still capable of transmitting the disease. Late latent syphilis is infection of greater than 1 year's duration. Relapses do not occur, and the patient is no longer considered infectious, except when donating blood or giving birth, when the infection may pass to the fetus.

Tertiary (Late) Syphilis

Tertiary syphilis is rarely seen today because the disease is usually diagnosed and treated during the primary and secondary stages. In the past, the major morbidity and mortality associated with syphilis were from the variable expression of tertiary syphilis in the skin, bones, central nervous system, and viscera, particularly the heart and great vessels.

Cutaneous and osseous manifestations were previously the most common signs of tertiary syphilis. The typical lesion, the gumma, is a granulomatous infection that begins as a nodule that breaks down to form an ulcer. Gummas can cause slow destruction of tissue and fibrosis, which may impair functioning of affected structures. Gummas may appear on any tissue or organ, although the skin and bone are the primary sites. Gummas respond well to antibiotic therapy.

Cardiovascular symptoms develop in 10% of patients with late syphilis, 30 to 40 years after initial exposure. Aortitis is the most prominent symptom and may result in aortic valve insufficiency and heart failure.

Neurosyphilis is less common, affecting 8% of untreated patients, 2 to 30 years after initial infec-

tion. Neurosyphilis may produce a variety of syndromes, including syphilitic meningitis, paresis, and tabes dorsalis (a degeneration of the dorsal column of the spinal cord).

Diagnosis

Because of the diversity of clinical manifestations in each of the stages and its similarity to other conditions, syphilis can be absolutely diagnosed only by laboratory tests. The darkfield microscopic examination and serologic tests are the most common diagnostic tools.

To perform a darkfield examination, serous exudate from a moist lesion is examined microscopically for the presence of *T. pallidum* using a dark field to highlight the organisms. This test is the most specific and only absolute method for diagnosing syphilis. However, the patient must have skin lesions for this test to be performed. It is the method of choice for diagnosing primary syphilis. It is also effective for diagnosing secondary, early latent, relapsing, and congenital syphilis, each of which is manifested by skin lesions. The test is not reliable for late latent or tertiary syphilis. Local health departments often supply darkfield microscopy as a service.

There are two types of serologic tests: treponemal and nontreponemal. They differ in the antigens they use and the types of antibodies that are measured. Nontreponemal tests are relatively inexpensive and easy to do. The Venereal Disease Research Laboratory (VDRL) test and the rapid plasma reagin card test are currently the most widely used nontreponemal tests. Nontreponemal tests are used to determine the presence of reagin in the patient's se-

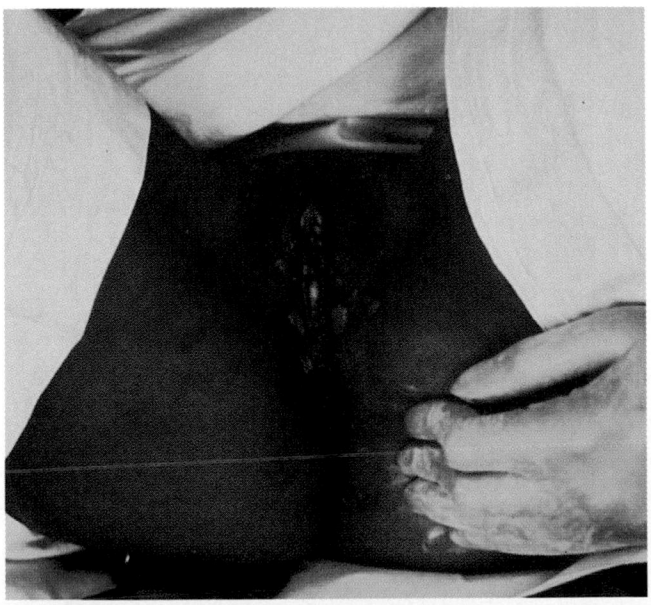

Figure 43–7

Condylomata lata. Wartlike papules may be seen as clinical manifestations of secondary syphilis. (Courtesy of Leonard Wolf, MD, New York, NY.)

rum. Reagin is a heterogeneous group of antibodies that combine with a specific antigen. The test is not specific for syphilis, and at least 1% of the general population have false-positive test results. A false-positive result can occur after an acute illness or immunization and during pregnancy. Chronic false-positive results most often occur with chronic infections, autoimmune diseases, and narcotic addiction.

Because it takes 1 to 3 weeks after the appearance of a chancre in primary syphilis for the patient's serum to become antibody-positive, nontreponemal tests may also indicate false-negative results during the incubation period and early primary stage. If the test is negative in the presence of symptoms of primary syphilis (a chancre), it should be repeated in 2 weeks. Nontreponemal tests are 100% accurate in secondary syphilis and 70% accurate in tertiary syphilis. Nontreponemal tests are most frequently used for premarital and prenatal screening. For positive test results without symptoms, the VDRL is repeated and, if it remains positive, the treponemal test described next is performed. Nontreponemal tests may be used to evaluate the patient's response to treatment through serial measurement of antibody titers.

Treponemal tests are more specific than nontreponemal tests because they are designed to detect antibodies specific for *Treponema*. The standard treponemal test used today is the fluorescent treponemal antibody-absorption (FTA-ABS) test. Because it is technically more difficult and expensive to perform, the FTA-ABS is usually reserved to verify other tests. The FTA-ABS is highly sensitive in all stages of syphilis.

Management

Parenteral penicillin G is the drug of choice for treating all stages of syphilis. Treatment regimens with penicillin G or an appropriate substitute are based on the length of illness and type of syphilis. Patients should be examined clinically and serologically at 3 and 6 months to determine if adequate treatment has occurred. All patients with syphilis should be tested for human immunodeficiency virus (HIV). In areas where HIV is prevalent, patients with primary syphilis should be retested for HIV after 3 months. Patients who demonstrate neurologic or ophthalmic disease should be fully evaluated for neurosyphilis and syphilitic eye disease. Since there are no proven alternatives to penicillin, pregnant women allergic to penicillin should be treated with penicillin after desensitization. See Table 43–4 for treatment regimens for syphilis.

NURSING PROCESS
Syphilis

The availability of simple screening tests, an inexpensive cure, and increased public awareness have contributed to a rapid decline in the incidence of syphilis since the mid-1940s. Once the premier venereal disease, syphilis is now less common than herpes, gonorrhea, and chlamydia. However, the incidence of syphilis is still considered significant. Nurses working in STD centers, inner-city hospitals, and clinics are especially likely to encounter patients with syphilis. All nurses have a responsibility to be informed about the clinical manifestations and course of this disease. It is particularly important for nurses to recognize the signs and symptoms of early syphilis so that the potentially severe complications of tertiary and congenital syphilis can be avoided.

Assessment

Early in the assessment interview, question the patient about his or her reason for seeking health care. Some patients seek treatment because they have symptoms. Others are referred as a result of positive serologic test results or as the sexual contacts of diagnosed patients. In all situations, be sure to project a nonjudgmental, supportive, and caring attitude. Often patients are not aware that they have contracted syphilis. Initial responses to the diagnosis range from shock and denial to hostility or apathy. Ensure the patient's confidentiality and privacy throughout the assessment process.

Question the patient about his or her sexual history and lifestyle, history of other STDs, and past and present symptoms.

Because the symptoms of primary syphilis are mild and may go unnoticed, and symptoms of secondary syphilis are often confused with or attributed to other causes, ask both specific and open-ended questions to help the patient to remember and describe symptoms. Examples of questions that may be asked to obtain information about the patient's symptoms include the following:

> "Have you ever had a painless canker or ulcer sore anywhere on your body, particularly in your mouth or on your genitals?"
> "Have you had any skin rashes? If so, when did the rash occur? Where was it located? What did it look like?"
> "Did you experience any influenza-like symptoms with the rash?"
> "Did you treat the rash? If so, how?"

It is sometimes helpful to use photographs of typical syphilitic skin lesions to help the patient recognize and identify previous skin rashes.

Obtain a psychosocial history that includes the patient's education and employment history, marital status, home environment, and relationship with significant others. The reaction of significant others, the availability of support systems, and the patient's lifestyle all influence the patient's response to the diagnosis, compliance with treatment, and willingness to identify sexual contacts.

Thoroughly examine the patient's skin in a private well-lighted room. Assess the skin for macules, papules, vesicles, nodules, erosions, and ulcers. Note the location, size, distribution, and symmetry of any lesions. Question the patient about changes in the lesions, such as redness, swelling, and exudate. Wear gloves to palpate the lesions for consistency (soft, firm, or indurated) and pain or tenderness. Examine the patient's mouth for ulcers or white mucous patches on the tongue, gingiva (gums), or palate. When appropriate, examine the external genitalia, including the suprapubic and perianal areas, as well as the penis and scrotum in men and the vulva and perineum in women. In women, note any vaginal discharge. Because many patients present with more than one STD, also assess the patient for symptoms of others.

Throughout the process, assess the patient's knowledge of syphilis, including the mode of transmission, clinical manifestations, congenital, and long-term effects.

Nursing Diagnoses and Planning

Nursing diagnoses and related expected patient outcomes commonly applicable to patients with syphilis include the following:

NDx: Risk for altered health maintenance related to insufficient knowledge of cause, signs, symptoms, clinical course, and mode of transmission of syphilis

Planning: Patient Outcomes
1. Patient states the cause of syphilis.
2. Patient describes signs, symptoms, and clinical course of syphilis in adults.
3. Patient describes potential effects of congenital syphilis.
4. Patient identifies the primary mode of transmission.

NDx: Risk for ineffective management of therapeutic regimen (individuals) related to lack of knowledge, lifestyle, distrust of health professionals

Planning: Patient Outcomes
1. Patient lists potential long-term effects of untreated or inadequately treated syphilis.
2. Patient describes the recommended treatment regimen.
3. Patient takes medications as prescribed.
4. Patient returns for follow-up visits.
5. Serologic tests for cure are negative.

NDx: Risk for infection (reinfection) related to sexual practices and lifestyle

Planning: Patient Outcomes
1. Patient describes the rationale for abstaining from sexual relations with former partners until they are examined and treated.
2. Patient identifies at least three ways to prevent reinfection.

NDx: Anxiety related to concerns about personal health status, possible transmission to others, social stigma of having contracted an STD, identification of sexual partners.

Planning: Patient Outcomes
1. Patient reports feeling less anxiety.
2. Nonverbal behaviors indicate that the patient is less anxious (eg, posture and facial expression are relaxed, voice is calm).
3. Patient retains information.
4. Patient provides names of sexual partners for contact tracing by health agency.
5. Patient refers sexual partners within specific time frames.

Nursing Interventions and Evaluation

NDx: Risk for altered health maintenance
The primary nursing intervention for patients with syphilis is education. Patient education helps to ensure compliance with treatment and follow-up as well as cooperation in identifying partners. Instruct the patient in the cause, transmission, and clinical course of syphilis. Explain the incubation periods for primary and secondary syphilis to help the patient identify time periods when sexual partners may have been exposed to the disease. Instruct the patient in the three modes of transmission of syphilis.

Inform patients about the risk of congenital syphilis. Describe the effects, which include skin and mucous membrane lesions and involvement of the bone and central nervous system. Explain that infants of female patients who have syphilis or who contract syphilis during pregnancy are at greatest risk. Inform the patient that the earlier in pregnancy treatment is begun, the lower the risk to the fetus. If the patient is pregnant, provide an opportunity for her to express her concerns and anxieties in a supportive atmosphere. Offer appropriate reassurances concerning the health of the fetus.

NDx: Risk for ineffective management of therapeutic regimen (individuals)
Explain the treatment plan and rationale to the patient in detail. Review the dosage, schedule, and side effects of prescribed medications (see Table 43–4). Emphasize the importance of taking oral medications at the recommended times for the prescribed number of days. Provide the name and telephone number of someone to call if the patient has any questions or experiences any side effects during treatment. Be sure to inform the patient with early syphilis of the possibility of a Jarisch-Herxheimer reaction after the first treatment with parenteral benzathine penicillin G. This reaction is believed to be caused by the release of large amounts of antigenic material after initial treatment. It is characterized by influenza-like symptoms that appear 2 to 6 hours after injection and last about 6 hours.

If applicable to the individual patient, explain that longer treatment times are required for both oral and parenteral medications when a person has had syphilis for more than a year. Inform the patient about the long-term effects of untreated or inadequately treated syphilis. Explain that the lack of current symptoms does not indicate a cure. Stress the importance of returning for follow-up care to

SOCIOCULTURAL PERSPECTIVES

The Impact of Changes in Family Structure on Health Care

by Janice R. Ellis, PhD, RN

Family structures have undergone rapid change and transformation during the past 25 years. What people consider family can vary from the dyad of husband and wife, to the nuclear family of parents and children, to the extended family of grandparents, parents, aunts, uncles, and children. Couples and groups of unrelated people who live in a family relationship with one another may consider themselves to be families. Families may include gay and lesbian couples and their biologic or adopted children, single adults or teens with children, and grandparents raising children. Children in a family may be birth children, adopted children, stepchildren, or foster children.

Our legal definitions of family, and the health-care policies that result from these definitions, may not take all of these relationships into account. Yet to ignore or discount them is to ignore an essential aspect of a person's life and support system. Let's look at some of the implications of these family changes for nursing care.

When a patient has a serious or life-threatening illness, we often make assumptions about who should be allowed to visit, who should have information, and who should be consulted about problems. If we act based on assumptions about family and relationships, we may shut out the most important people from someone's life at a time of crisis. Remember, a competent adult has the right to decide who should and who should not be included in the circle of information and concern.

Therefore, nurses have a responsibility to ask the patient who should be included in this circle of concern and ensure that these preferences are put in writing for the entire health-care team. When a patient asks that a person not legally related be a part of the decision-making processes, written directives are essential to ensure that those desires can be legally carried out regardless of the circumstances. Although nurses should not give legal advice, they can help patients understand that they have options and choices and that these include designating a decision maker. Within a health-care agency, policies should be in place to help direct nurses in effective actions to support these patient choices. If those policies do not exist, nurses can act as catalysts to begin the process of developing effective policies.

Another area in which changes in family structure pose a challenge to nurses is in planning for visitors. Some units have policies that provide much more liberal visiting hours and privileges to family members than to others. Health-care institutions limit visitors in this way to provide rest for patients and to ensure that needed care can be accomplished. However, they *allow* visits by certain significant support people because these visits have a positive effect on anxiety, ability to rest, and even recovery. Who constitutes family in this instance is not a legal decision but rather one in which staff members apply policy and make decisions. As a nurse, you must be sure that you do not mistakenly shut out people who are important to patients just because your own experience does not regard them as family. "Family," in this instance, must be viewed from the patient's viewpoint, not the institution's.

Other assumptions about family are also a problem. If your own experience with family is that family is supportive and caring, you may make the assumption that this is true for all patients. However, family relationships are broken by many different kinds of problems. The presence of some families, far from providing support, may be detrimental to the patient's wellbeing. Some families have histories that include excessive anger, abuse, rejection, or other serious problems in relationships. The patient may need to be free *not* to have family involved in care and to be able to ask that the staff support this choice. This demands skillful communication from the nurse to meet the patient's needs and not increase the alienation within the family.

Sexually transmitted diseases pose a particular challenge in assisting people both in protecting themselves and in obtaining appropriate care. In the United States, most states have public-health policies that include follow-up of sexually transmitted diseases. If we do not understand that people have a wide variety of lifestyles and relationships, we may fail to ask appropriate questions or may ask questions in such a way that the patient is unwilling to be honest. Questions posed in ways that reveal underlying assumptions on the part of the health professional are unlikely to result in effective communication.

Working with teens who are sexually active presents a particular challenge in this regard. While teens may be legally emancipated in terms of seeking care, they may be dependent on family in regard to paying for and accessing care. When teens present for care for a sexually transmitted disease, they may be very fearful of the reactions of parents. Teens are sometimes in rebellion and reject families who could be helpful to them. Others come from families that are abusive and rejecting of *them*, where no help or support will be available. Helping teens to sort out their options, providing nonjudgmental answers to concerns, and ensuring that teens do not become alienated from essential health-care resources all require that the nurse set aside personal views and assumptions about families and actively listen to what patients have to say.

determine the effectiveness of treatment to avoid the long-term effects of this disease.

The patient is usually instructed to return in 1 week. During this time, advise the patient to abstain from sexual relations to avoid transmitting the disease. Caution the patient to avoid sex with previous or current partners until they have been examined, to decrease the risk of reinfection.

Remember that the quality of the nurse-patient interaction also affects compliance. Effective communication skills and a nonjudgmental attitude are essential for working with the patient with syphilis. Promote compliance and follow-up by being objective and empathic and by projecting interest in the patient's wellbeing. Provide information and instructions in terminology the patient can understand, with ample time for the patient to ask questions and express concerns.

NDx: Risk for infection

Advise the patient to avoid sex with former partners until they have been evaluated and treated to prevent reinfection. For both heterosexual and homosexual patients, recommend the use of condoms as a means of preventing future exposure to syphilis and other STDs. Remember that although many patients object to using condoms on a regular basis, they can often be convinced to use them when engaging in high-risk sexual encounters, such as sex with anonymous partners or prostitutes. Help the patient identify methods or behaviors for avoiding future bouts with STDs. Examples include observing the genitals of prospective sexual partners, refraining from sex with partners who have signs or symptoms of STDs, and seeking health care at the first sign of a possible infection. The most effective interventions for helping the patient change behavior to prevent reinfection and transmission are patient education and development of a therapeutic nurse-patient relationship.

NDx: Anxiety

Provide opportunity for the patient to express his or her concerns about having contracted syphilis and fear of transmitting the disease to others. Assure the patient that syphilis is curable provided that the treatment regimen is adhered to and the patient returns for follow-up testing.

Explain the importance of cooperation in naming sexual partners. Allow the patient time to verbalize anxiety about this, but reinforce its necessity and ultimate benefit to those named. Once named, sexual partners are contacted in one of two ways. Traditionally, health-care personnel contact the partner and the patient's confidentiality is maintained. More recently, selected patients are encouraged to refer sexual contacts for evaluation themselves. The first method offers greater assurance of follow-up with sexual partners. The second method is less costly and promotes assumption of responsibility on the part of the patient.

Because of the importance of early treatment, the traditional method of contact tracing is more frequently used in cases of syphilis. However, if the patient is offered the opportunity to refer sexual contacts, explain that he or she must comply within specified time limits or the health agency will contact the sexual partners. Assist the patient who chooses self-referral to decide how to present the information to the partners. Consider role playing as a helpful technique to this end. Do not offer the option of self-referral to the patient who is disinterested or has poor communication skills.

Compare the patient's status with the expected outcomes. If the outcomes are not met, reassess the patient and revise the plan.

Chlamydia trachomatis

Infections caused by *C. trachomatis* are the most prevalent of the STDs. Depending on the population studied, *C. trachomatis* is five to ten times more common than gonorrhea. An estimated 3 to 4 million Americans contract a chlamydial infection each year.

C. trachomatis produces a broad spectrum of diseases and complications. In developing countries, *C. trachomatis* causes a chronic infectious disease of the conjunctiva and cornea known as trachoma. Trachoma is the leading cause of preventable blindness in the world. Chlamydiae have long been known as the causative organism of lymphogranuloma venereum, an STD found mainly in the tropics that affects the lymph organs in the genital area. However, only recently has *C. trachomatis* been recognized as the causative agent in a number of other genital tract infections previously considered to be of unknown origin.

C. trachomatis is a primary causative agent in nongonococcal and postgonococcal urethritis in men. It produces half of the estimated 500,000 cases of epididymitis, inflammation of the cordlike structure on the posterior border of the testis in which sperm is stored.

In women, chlamydia has been implicated as one of the major causes of cervicitis and pelvic inflammatory disease. Consequently, *C. trachomatis* infections play a significant role in the increasing incidence of ectopic pregnancy and infertility, both potential long-term sequelae of pelvic inflammatory disease. *C. trachomatis* in pregnancy is associated with postpartum endometritis in the mother and eye infections and pneumonia in the newborn.

The diversity of the diseases produced by *C. trachomatis* is explained by the fact that there are 15 strains of this bacterium. The strains can be roughly divided into three groups: those that cause trachoma and other adult eye infections, those that cause lymphogranuloma venereum, and those that cause genital tract infections.

In industrialized western society, *C. trachomatis* is almost exclusively a sexually transmitted disease. Populations at risk for chlamydial infections are the same as those at risk for other STDs. *C. trachomatis* is more common in adolescents and 20- to 25-year-old heterosexuals who have multiple partners, lower socioeconomic status, and gonococcal infections. Other risk factors include gender and ethnicity, with infection being more common in African-American women.

Etiology and Pathophysiology

C. trachomatis microorganisms are unique. Classified as bacteria, they also share properties with viruses. Considered obligatory intracellular parasites, *C. trachomatis* organisms take over and use the energy system of living cells to meet their own energy needs and to replicate. *C. trachomatis* has a predilection for columnar and transitional cell epithelia, such as those found in the reproductive tract. The organism can remain latent for a prolonged period within the cell. Replication progresses slowly because of its dependence on the cell's energy system. The incubation of *C. trachomatis* is 1 to 2 weeks after exposure; infection may be asymptomatic, however.

Clinical Manifestations

In men, *C. trachomatis* causes urethritis, which is characterized by a white or mucoid urethral discharge that may be intermittent or occur only in the morning. In some cases, dysuria and urethral itching may also occur.

In women, the most common site for *C. trachomatis* genital infections is the cervix. Although most women with positive culture results for *C. trachomatis* of the cervix have no symptoms, at least one-third have local signs of infection. A mucopurulent cervical discharge that appears yellow to green when viewed on a cotton swab is the most frequent symptom. This may or may not be accompanied by cervical erosion, an area on the cervix that is edematous, congested, and friable. Clinical recognition of chlamydial cervicitis requires a high degree of suspicion and thorough examination of the cervix. Cervical infection, especially asymptomatic infection, provides a reservoir for potential transmission of *C. trachomatis* to male sexual partners and neonates.

In pregnancy, there is 60 to 70% risk of neonatal infection if the mother has a *C. trachomatis* infection of the cervix at the time of delivery. Infants acquire the infection through contact with the infected cervicovaginal secretions. The primary sites of infection are the conjunctiva and respiratory tract.

C. trachomatis is also a major cause of pelvic inflammatory disease, with the primary site of infection being the fallopian tubes and infertility and ectopic pregnancy being the two most common serious sequelae. The exact number of cases of infertility and ectopic pregnancy attributable to *C. trachomatis* remains unknown. However, on the basis of the number of suspected cases of chlamydial salpingitis, it appears to be considerable.

Chlamydia also appears to be an important cause of acute urethral syndrome in women. This syndrome is characterized by dysuria, frequency, and the absence of bacteriuria.

Diagnosis

Until recently, tissue culturing was the only method available for making a definitive diagnosis of chlamydial infections of the genital tract. Although this test is sensitive and specific, it is also complex and expensive and requires a 6- to 7-day wait for definitive results.

Another test for diagnosing chlamydia, the direct-slide monoclonal antibody test, is now available and seems to be as specific and sensitive as culturing. The main advantages of this test are its lower cost, rapid results (total processing takes 30–40 minutes), and relative simplicity.

Other tests, such as cytologic examination of stained smears (the Pap test) and serology, are either unreliable or have little value as diagnostic aids.

Screening for chlamydial infection is recommended for the following groups:

- Patients who come to sexually transmitted disease clinics
- People with chlamydia-associated syndromes
- Sex partners of patients with chlamydial genitourinary infections
- Pregnant patients at high risk (adolescents and unmarried women or married women with a history of STD or multiple partners)

Management

Doxycyline and azithromycin are highly effective antibiotics for treating *C. trachomatis* infections. Sulfisoxazole is approved but has inferior efficacy to the other regimens.

The following treatment regimens are recommended for all confirmed chlamydial urogenital tract infections and for chlamydia-associated syndromes (eg, mucopurulent cervicitis and nongonococcal urethritis) because the causative agent is chlamydia in more than half the cases:

> *Doxycycline*: 100 mg by mouth twice a day for 7 days
> *Azithromycin*: 1 g by mouth in a single dose
> *Erythromycin base:* 500 mg by mouth four times a day for 7 days is recommended for patients who cannot tolerate doxycycline or when use of doxycycline is contraindicated, as in pregnancy

Chlamydia is often found in association with gonorrhea infections. When gonorrhea is also present, treatment should be initiated that is effective against both organisms (see Table 43–4).

Sex partners of patients with urogenital tract chlamydial infections should be evaluated for STD and treated with one of the regimens previously listed.

NURSING PROCESS
Chlamydia trachomatis *Infection*

Assessment

Nursing assessment of the patient with confirmed or suspected chlamydial genital tract infection begins with a thorough history and analysis of symptoms. The health history includes a comprehensive sexual and social history. This information helps identify patients at risk for infection and reinfection with *C. trachomatis* and also provides information about the patient's educational needs.

Question the patient about his or her age, socio-economic status, and sexual lifestyle. Ask about the number of sexual partners because this is considered the most significant predictor of risk for chlamydial infection. Also obtain information about the patient's contraceptive preferences, history of infection with other STDs or chlamydia-associated syndromes (such as pelvic inflammatory disease in women or nongonococcal urethritis in men), and possible infection in current sexual partners.

Because symptoms of lower genital tract infections in women are often absent or so mild that they go unnoticed, many women seen for an initial evaluation do so because their partners received a diag-nosis of nongonococcal urethritis. Thus, the nursing assessment must focus on symptoms to rule out vaginitis and other STDs, as well as to identify the subtle symptoms of chlamydial infection.

Question the patient about vaginal discharge. Note the character of the discharge (amount, color, odor, consistency) and onset, duration, and presence of associated symptoms, such as pain, itching, and skin changes. Also question the patient about factors that aggravate or alleviate symptoms, such as sexual intercourse, menses, or temperature changes. The typical discharge of chlamydia-associated cervical infections is mucoid, clear to amber in color, and varies from scant to profuse. The discharge is not associated with pain or itching, except in patients with concurrent urinary tract infection indicated by frequency, urgency, and dysuria.

Because of the frequently mild or asymptomatic nature of chlamydial cervicitis, women often do not seek health care until the infection has spread to the upper genital tract. Therefore, the nursing assessment also focuses on symptoms of pelvic inflammatory disease, which is often less acute when caused by chlamydia as opposed to gonorrhea.

Question the patient about lower abdominal pain, metrorrhagia (bleeding between periods), and dyspareunia. Also assess for systemic symptoms, such as fever, malaise, nausea, and vomiting even though these are less common with chlamydial infections than with other pelvic infections. Be sure to determine onset and duration of symptoms in sequence with menstruation. The onset of these symptoms immediately after menstruation is more indicative of pelvic inflammatory disease, a progressive infectious process that occurs primarily from chlamydia or gonorrhea and less often with other bacterial organisms.

Men usually present with more observable and characteristic symptoms. Question male patients about white or mucoid urethral discharge that may be intermittent or occur only in the morning. Also ask about dysuria and urethral itching.

Assess the patient's knowledge of the disease process, mode of transmission, and associated syndromes throughout the history taking and physical examination. Examples of specific questions that may be asked to assist in assessing the patient's learning needs include the following:

> "How is chlamydial infection spread from one person to another?"
> "What factors in your sexual lifestyle do you think increase your risk of contracting the infection?"
> "How can you prevent reinfection?"
> "Do you know the possible complications of this infection for yourself, your partner, and your future children?"

Assess also the psychologic response of the patient diagnosed with a chlamydial infection. Responses can range from disinterest to severe anxiety. Varia-

---

INTERNET CONNECTIONS
Sexually Transmitted Diseases

The Johns Hopkins University School of Medicine STD Research Group
http://www.med.jhu.edu/jhustd/frame3.htm
Sponsored by a research group at The Johns Hopkins University School of Medicine, this site provides links to a wide variety of sites related to sexually transmitted diseases. Among the topics addressed are research, "safe sex," behavioral medicine, public health, patient education, HIV/AIDS, gonorrhea, chlamydia, syphilis, trichomonas, herpes, and genital warts.

American Social Health Association
http://sunsite.unc.edu/ASHA/
This site provides answers to frequently asked questions, as well as news releases, surveys, and links to related sites.

1993 STD Treatment Guidelines (CDC)
http://wonder.cdc.gov/rchtml/Convert/STD/Title3301.html
This U.S. government–sponsored site provides information about prevention and treatment of a wide variety of sexually transmitted diseases.

bles include the interpersonal relationships with sexual partners, the severity of symptoms, and the presence of complications or associated syndromes. Women with pelvic inflammatory disease may display anger, denial, or depression related to potential adverse effects on fertility. Patients involved in monogamous relationships may express anger at their partners and question their commitment. As for patients with other STDs, communicate a nonjudgmental, empathetic attitude and sensitivity to the patient's feelings and concerns.

Nursing Diagnoses and Planning

Nursing diagnoses and related expected patient outcomes commonly applicable to patients with chlamydial infections include the following:

NDx: Risk for altered health maintenance related to insufficient knowledge of disease process, transmission, and prevention of chlamydial infections

Planning: Patient Outcomes
1. Patient lists the symptoms and potential complications of chlamydial infections.
2. Patient asks pertinent questions derived from knowledge of the disease process.
3. Patient describes methods for reducing the risk of transmission and reinfection.

NDx: Risk for infection (reinfection) related to sexual lifestyle, lack of knowledge about the mode of transmission or prevention

Planning: Patient Outcomes
1. Patient lists factors that increase the risk of infection.
2. Patient describes the rationale for altering personal behaviors that increase the risk of infection and transmission.
3. Patient describes plans to use a barrier method of contraception.
4. Recurrence of infection is absent.

NDx: Risk for ineffective management of therapeutic regimen (individuals) related to lack of knowledge about the importance of following treatment regimens and behavioral recommendations

Planning: Patient Outcomes
1. Patient states the dosage, schedule, and side effects of prescribed medications.
2. Patient states the rationale for taking medications as prescribed.
3. Patient reports taking medications as prescribed.
4. Patient indicates intention to abstain from sexual intercourse or to use condoms until treatment is completed.

NDx: Anxiety related to potential complications and long-term sequelae for self or sexual partners

Planning: Patient Outcomes
1. Patient verbalizes decreased anxiety.
2. Nonverbal behavior indicates that anxiety is within normal limits (relaxed posture; absence of

hand wringing, crying, shaking; relaxed facial expression).
3. Patient retains information.
4. Patient states that he or she will inform sexual contacts.
5. Sexual contacts present for evaluation.
6. Patient states accurate and realistic expectations for prognosis after treatment.
7. Patient describes measures for preventing reinfection.

Nursing Interventions and Evaluation

NDx: Risk for altered health maintenance
Instruct the patient in the disease process—symptoms, mode of transmission, and complications. Emphasize the significance of asymptomatic infection and the importance of seeking treatment immediately at the first sign of infection to reduce complications and long-term sequelae. It is particularly important for men to understand the potential for serious complications in untreated female partners. Review methods for preventing infection.

NDx: Risk for infection
Help the patient identify factors in his or her sexual lifestyle that increase the risk of reinfection. Recommend use of barrier methods of contraception, such as the diaphragm and the condom. The condom is especially effective in preventing chlamydial infection. If appropriate, suggest a reduction in the number of sexual partners as a means of decreasing the risk of chlamydial infection or infection with other STDs. Variables affecting compliance with these recommendations include the patient's values and the role of the patient's current sexual lifestyle in his or her identity and self-esteem.

NDx: Risk for ineffective management of therapeutic regimen (individuals)
Instruct the patient in the purpose, dosage, scheduling, and side effects of prescribed medications. Emphasize the importance of taking prescribed medications on time and in the recommended dosage for the entire treatment interval to achieve a cure. Otherwise, the patient may stop taking the medications as soon as the symptoms abate. In addition, advise the patient to abstain from sexual intercourse until the treatment is completed and sexual partners have been examined or treated. If the patient indicates that he or she cannot comply, recommend use of a condom during the course of treatment. Caution the patient to seek treatment immediately if symptoms recur.

NDx: Anxiety
Encourage the patient to verbalize his or her concerns and feelings about contracting an STD. With women especially, help the patient view the infection in a realistic perspective. Stress that, once diagnosed, chlamydia is an easily treated infection with a 95% cure rate and that pelvic inflammatory disease is unlikely with timely treatment of lower geni-

RESEARCH ABSTRACT

What Factors Influence Condom Use in Divorced and Separated Women?

Marion LN, Cox CL. Condom use and fertility among divorced and separated women. Nursing Research 1996; 45(2):110.

The time surrounding a woman's separation and divorce constitutes a high-risk period for contracting sexually transmitted diseases or becoming pregnant. Marion and Cox were therefore interested in exploring condom use among these women.

The researchers used the Interaction Model of Client Health Behavior (IMCHB) as a guide to select variables that might influence whether or not a woman used condoms during sexual encounters during this period. The model includes clusters of variables related to the client, interaction between the client and health-care professionals, and health outcomes. The researchers were most interested in those variables that might be modified through nursing interventions. For this study, Marion and Cox therefore selected instruments related to the subject's intrinsic motivation, cognitive appraisal, and affective response to condom use.

The researchers grouped the subjects as fertile or infertile based on the self-reported use of contraceptive methods other than use of a condom. Alarmingly high numbers of the women in both groups did not use condoms. More than 75% reported that they had not used condoms during their most recent intercourse. The researchers note, however, that women in the fertile group reported more frequent condom use. Factors that influenced the use of condoms in the fertile group included past use of condoms, perceived partner influence, partner acceptance of condom use, and feelings toward condom use.

The variables measured did not help the research-ers understand as much about condom use among the *infertile* women in the sample. For that group, factors influencing condom use included the length of the relationship, partner acceptance of condom use, the number of children at home, and a sense of competence in the use of condoms.

Based on these findings, Marion and Cox suggest that nurses impress upon women who are experiencing separation and divorce the risks of contracting a sexually transmitted disease if they do not use condoms. Additional information on how to use condoms effectively, as well as actual guided practice on a model, may be helpful. Women need to know the importance of protection against *disease* as well as protection against pregnancy. The researchers also encourage nurses to include the partners of divorced or separated women in discussions related to sexual health.

Questions to Consider

1. What questions do you routinely ask patients about sexuality?
2. What information about effective use of condoms should be shared with women who are experiencing separation and divorce?
3. What can you do to persuade women to consider use of barrier methods of protection in addition to birth control methods such as oral contraceptives?
4. What advantages and disadvantages would there be to interviewing and educating partners together about their shared sexual health?

tal tract infection. For the patient with pelvic inflammatory disease, point out that infertility related to this condition has decreased from 75% to 20% during the past 20 years because early treatment and improved surgical interventions have decreased the risk of permanent tubal damage. If the patient is pregnant, explain that the risk of transmission to the fetus occurs only at delivery. Reassure the patient that treatment during pregnancy and compliance with recommended preventive measures virtually eliminate this risk. When possible, provide the patient with written literature to reinforce information communicated during patient teaching and counseling. Suggest a follow-up visit for the patient whose verbalizations and behavior indicate excessive anger, anxiety, or potential for depression.

Additional Interventions
Encourage the patient to refer sex partners for evaluation and possible treatment.

Compare the patient's status with the expected outcomes. If the outcomes are not met, reassess the patient and revise the plan.

Nongonococcal Urethritis

Nongonococcal urethritis is an inflammation of the urethra in the absence of infection with *N. gonorrhoeae*. The incidence of this STD is 2.5 times greater than gonococcal urethritis. Most cases of nongonococcal urethritis are caused by *C. trachomatis* and

Ureaplasma urealyticum. By convention, the diagnosis of nongonococcal urethritis is restricted to men, although *C. trachomatis* can produce a urethral syndrome in women as well.

The prevalence of sexually transmitted urethritis, both gonococcal and nongonococcal, has increased significantly in the United States, England, and Sweden during the past 30 years. Although recent statistics indicate that the incidence of nongonococcal urethritis has reached a plateau, the number of cases continues to rise. Nongonococcal urethritis accounts for more than half the cases of urethritis reported by STD clinics and 80 to 90% of cases of urethritis seen at campus health services. Nongonococcal urethritis is most frequently diagnosed in heterosexual men aged 20 to 24 years.

Etiology and Pathophysiology

C. trachomatis is the major cause of nongonococcal urethritis. It can be isolated from the urethras of 50% of men with nongonococcal urethritis, about 20% of men with gonococcal urethritis, and 0 to 5% of men without urethritis. *C. trachomatis* has been identified as the most frequent cause of postgonococcal urethritis. Postgonococcal urethritis occurs shortly after curative therapy for gonorrhea. Because gonorrhea has a shorter incubation period (2–7 days) than chlamydial urethritis (2–3 weeks), men infected with both organisms first present and are diagnosed and treated for gonorrhea. Nearly all men simultaneously infected with both organisms and treated with penicillin go on to develop postgonococcal urethritis because *C. trachomatis* is unaffected by penicillin.

Between 10 and 40% of nongonococcal urethritis infections are thought to result from *U. urealyticum,* one of two mycoplasmas known to infect men. The causal relationship between urethritis and *U. urealyticum* is not as clear-cut as that between *C. trachomatis* and nongonococcal urethritis. *U. urealyticum* is not always pathogenic. It can be isolated from the urethras of sexually active men who do not have urethritis as well as from those who do.

Why *U. urealyticum* produces disease in some men and not others is unknown. It has been suggested that only one or several of the 14 serotypes of *U. urealyticum* are capable of causing disease. Another explanation could be the difference in host response to the organism. Considering the frequently benign nature of the organism, treatment is not indicated for men with culture results positive for *U. urealyticum* unless there are clinical symptoms. In contrast, asymptomatic chlamydial nongonococcal urethritis is treated.

About 20 to 30% of nongonococcal urethritis infections are not caused by *C. trachomatis* or *U. urealyticum.* A variety of organisms have been suggested or proved to be etiologically related to nongonococcal urethritis, including *Trichomonas vaginitis, Gardnerella vaginalis, Candida albicans,* and herpes simplex.

Clinical Manifestations

The characteristic clinical manifestation of nongonococcal urethritis is urethral discharge. The urethral discharge associated with nongonococcal urethritis is usually white or mucoid and may be present only in the morning or may cause intermittent staining. A more profuse, purulent discharge suggests gonococcal urethritis. Dysuria and urethral itching are also common. The manifestations of nongonococcal urethritis are frequently mild. Asymptomatic pyuria is common. More severe symptoms (frequency, urgency, hematuria, and inguinal adenopathy) suggest another or concurrent genital infection.

Diagnosis

Diagnosis of nongonococcal urethritis is based on evidence of urethritis—either clinical symptoms or laboratory demonstration of polymorphonuclear leukocytes on Gram's staining of a urethral smear in the absence of gonorrhea. Laboratory facilities for isolating *C. trachomatis* and *U. urealyticum* are not always available. New and easier techniques for identification of these two organisms are being introduced.

Management

Response of nongonococcal urethritis to medications is variable because the causative organism is usually not identified. In 30 to 40% of cases, infection recurs within 6 weeks of treatment. Poor success may be partially attributable to lack of compliance with the treatment regimen or reinfection from an untreated or new sexual partner. Identification and treatment of sexual contacts, especially in cases of chlamydial infection, is necessary to keep partners from reinfecting each other or spreading the disease. Failure rates are lowest for chlamydia, higher for *U. urealyticum,* and highest for nongonococcal urethritis of unknown origin.

The recommended initial treatment regimen is erythromycin base, 500 mg orally four times daily for 7 days. This is usually effective for chlamydial nongonococcal urethritis, less so for *U. urealyticum,* and successfully treats gonorrhea. It is important for the patient to abstain from sexual intercourse during treatment.

NURSING PROCESS GUIDELINES
Nongonococcal Urethritis

The assessment, nursing diagnoses, expected patient outcomes, nursing interventions, and evaluation for patients with nongonococcal urethritis are similar to those described for patients with *C. trachomatis.* Additional considerations include the variable response of nongonococcal urethritis to medication and the high likelihood of recurrence. These factors can negatively affect compliance and can precipitate a heightened emotional response with related inappropriate or ineffective coping behavior.

Condylomata Acuminata

Condylomata acuminata are warts that appear in the anogenital area and that are caused by infection with human papillomavirus (HPV). Until recently, condylomata acuminata were considered to be minor, relatively inconsequential lesions of more psychologic than physical significance. However, the increasing incidence of anogenital warts and their relationship to genital cancer has led to an increased focus on this STD. Anogenital warts are most commonly caused by HPV types 6 or 11 and are not considered to have malignant potential. Other types—16, 18, and 31—have been strongly associated with genital neoplasia.

Similar to other STDs, genital warts are most frequently seen in the young (aged 16–25 years), sexually active population. Previously diagnosed more frequently in men, genital warts now appear to be at least as common in women. It is estimated that about 2% of women of childbearing age have flat condylomata infections of the cervix. At least 70% of these lesions are subclinical and commonly undiagnosed.

Etiology and Pathophysiology

There are more than 20 subtypes of the HPV. Several have been identified as the etiologic agents in common skin warts, whereas others have been associated with the occurrence of genital warts.

Genital warts are transmitted by direct skin-to-skin contact, primarily through sexual activity. Nonsexual transmission is also possible. Infection by autoinoculation and exposure during birth has been documented.

The virus infects the nuclei of epithelial cells, transforming the cells and causing them to proliferate. Cell-mediated immunity seems to play an important role in both the ultimate severity and recovery from the infection. People with modest depressions in cell-mediated immunity are more susceptible to HPV infection and are less likely to respond well to therapy or to have the warts regress spontaneously. Genital warts are more likely to appear and are more severe during pregnancy, when cell-mediated immunity is reduced.

The incubation period, from time of exposure to the appearance of lesions, is long and highly variable. The average incubation period is 3 months, with a range of 3 weeks to 8 months. In men, lesions can appear anywhere on the penis. The coronal sulcus on the inner aspect of the prepuce is often the initial site of appearance. Penile warts are more common among uncircumcised men.

Clinical Manifestations

There are several varieties of genital warts. The classic venereal wart is a raised, irregular, fissured papule. It is usually pinkish and taller than it is wide, with finger-like projections that give it a pointed appearance (Fig. 43–8).

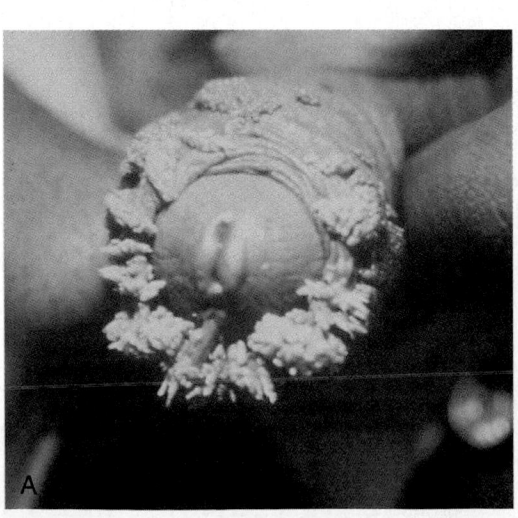
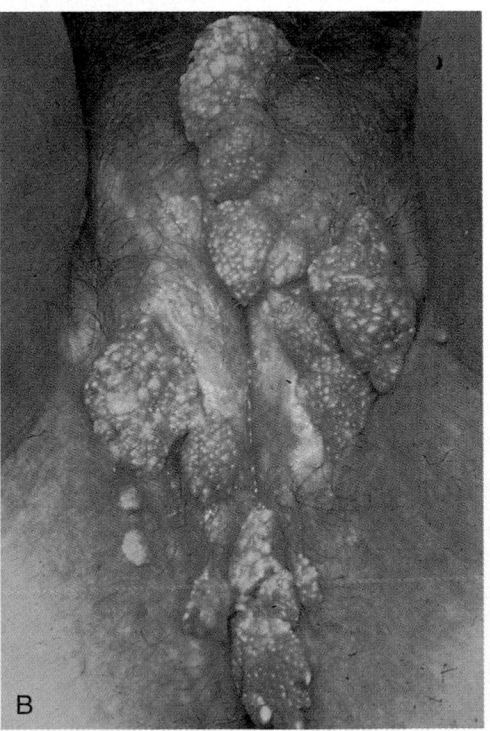

Figure 43–8

A, Extensive condylomata acuminata of the penis. *B*, Condylomata acuminata in a female patient. (Courtesy of the New York City Health Department.)

Condylomata may also be flat. Flat condylomata can occur in great numbers and are the type most frequently seen in the cervix, although they can also be on the vagina or on other mucosal surfaces as well as the skin. Flat condylomata are difficult to see with the naked eye, usually do not cause symptoms, and consequently often remain undiagnosed.

Giant condylomata acuminata are larger, rounded, soft papules or nodules with a strawberry-like surface. Although rare, these warts have a higher incidence of complications.

In women, the initial site is commonly the posterior vaginal introitus and adjacent labia. Lesions may spread to other parts of the vulva, perineum, and anus. Anal warts are more commonly seen in women and homosexual men. Another nongenital site is the mouth.

Genital warts are usually multiple and may coalesce to form larger masses. When venereal warts occur around the vaginal, urethral, and rectal orifices, internal spread is a possible complication. Common symptoms of intraurethral involvement are urethral bleeding, discharge, and dysuria. About half of women with lesions on the vaginal introitus have cervical involvement. Seventy percent of patients with perineal lesions have anal condylomata.

In addition to causing psychologic distress and embarrassment, complications from large genital warts include a tendency toward ulceration with bleeding and secondary infection. Major complications are rare but documented. In men, giant condylomata may grow relentlessly and destroy genital structures. In women, malignant transformation to cervical in situ squamous cell carcinoma and vulvovaginal carcinoma has been suggested but remains unproved.

Although vulvovaginal warts often enlarge during pregnancy, it is usual for them to regress after delivery. Most infants are unaffected, but occasional transmission of the virus does occur. In infants, lesions appear primarily on the genitals, larynx, and trachea. To avoid this problem, it is suggested that as many warts as possible be removed before delivery.

Diagnosis

Diagnosis of condyloma acuminata in the urogenital area or anal and rectal areas is based on the appearance of the lesion. Recognition of cervical lesions may require colposcopic examination.

Management

Podophyllin, a cytotoxic agent, is the treatment of choice for classic venereal warts. Podophyllin is applied topically to all surfaces of the wart, with care being taken to avoid normal skin surfaces. Podophyllin cannot be used during pregnancy or for cervical or oral warts. Local side effects include pain and a burning sensation at the site. Treatment is repeated every 7 days for up to 4 weeks or until the lesions resolve. No more than 0.5 to 1 mL of podophyllin is applied at any one time. Severe systemic side effects, although rare, have been reported and include neuropathy, hepatotoxicity, and granulocytopenia.

Trichloroacetic and dichloroacetic acids are used to treat flat warts on the external genitalia. Again, avoidance of surrounding skin is important, because application causes instant, nonreversible tissue destruction. As with podophyllin, warts are retreated weekly.

Cryosurgery, another common treatment, takes place in the physician's office with a cotton-tipped applicator dipped in nitrous oxide or liquid nitrogen. It causes a local burning sensation. Cryosurgery is very effective against keratotic (horny, elevated) warts and can also be used on classic and flat warts. Retreatment three or four times at weekly intervals is usually necessary. Because of pain, only five to seven warts can be treated at one time.

Electrocautery provides the same results, but local anesthesia is necessary. This is the treatment of choice for large numbers of lesions. It is sometimes necessary to admit the patient and use general anesthesia for multiple lesions. Postoperatively, the treated area resembles a burn.

Surgical excision may be necessary for the larger, giant condylomata. This procedure ensures complete removal while also furnishing specimens for histologic examination.

Alternative treatments, such as application of 5-fluorouracil (5-FU) cream and carbon dioxide (CO_2) laser destruction, have gained in popularity. 5-FU is recommended for treatment of mucous membrane warts, such as those located on the urinary meatus or intra-anal canal. 5-FU cannot be used on the epidermis of genital organs or in pregnant women. The mild to moderate pain associated with application on mucous membranes is controlled with 5% lidocaine ointment or analgesics. The efficacy of 5-FU is comparable to podophyllin and trichloroacetic acid.

Destruction of warts by vaporization with a CO_2 laser is recommended by some physicians for treatment of flat warts. The effectiveness of this therapy is about the same as that of other cryodestructive techniques. However, recurrence rates are expected to be lower because the procedure is done under colposcopy, which detects small subclinical lesions. Also, a small amount of normal tissue surrounding the lesion that may harbor the virus is treated. After therapy, antibacterial cream and a gauze dressing are applied to treated areas. Subsequently, the cream is reapplied and the dressing changed twice daily. Patients are instructed to keep the area clean and dry. Sitz baths are recommended for anal warts. Patients return for follow-up 3 to 6 weeks after treatment.

Untreated, most warts resolve spontaneously within 1 to 2 years. Concern for an effective treatment reflects the possible association with genital cancer, the increasing incidence of genital warts, and the psychologic effects of infection.

Research is currently under way to develop a vaccine to prevent infection from human papillomaviruses, which are related to the development of cervical cancer (Suzich et al, 1995).

NURSING PROCESS GUIDELINES
Genital Warts

Depending on the patient and the location, number, and size of genital warts, any of the nursing diagnoses, expected patient outcomes, and nursing interventions presented in Nursing Care Guide 43–1 may apply.

In almost all cases, risk for altered health maintenance related to insufficient knowledge of increased risk for genital malignancy will be a pertinent nursing diagnosis. Patients should be instructed in the importance of annual gynecologic examinations to ensure early detection should a malignancy develop.

Pediculosis Pubis

Phthirus pubis, also called the crab louse, is one of three species of sucking lice known to infect humans. The others are *Pediculus humanus*—the body louse—and *Pediculus humanus capitis*—the head louse. Pediculosis pubis, infestation with pubic lice, is considered to be an STD because the primary mode of transmission is through sexual contact. Approximately 3 million cases of lice infestation are treated in the United States each year. Pubic lice and head lice account for most of these cases.

Etiology and Pathophysiology
Pubic lice are minute (about 1 mm), crablike in appearance, and light in color. They live outside the human body, on skin surfaces, attached to the body hair. Pubic lice have six legs each, with a hooklike claw and opposing thumb that allows them to hold onto hair (Fig. 43–9).

Lice depend on human blood for survival. They obtain blood with their mouths through a piercelike wound made in the skin surface. The life span of an adult female louse is 20 to 30 days. During this time, the female lays about 50 eggs, called nits. Nits are glued to and are visible on the hair. After an incubation period of 5 to 10 days, the eggs hatch. The life span of the pubic louse is influenced by the temperature, humidity, and availability of blood. Lice do not survive off the host without access to blood for more than 24 hours. The optimal temperature for their survival is (87°F) 30.5°C. If the host is febrile or overheated by exercise, lice leave the body.

Although the pubic region is the main site of infestation, the axillae, eyebrows, eyelids, and even mustaches may also be affected. Lice are primarily transmitted from one person to another through intimate body contact. Less frequently, lice can be spread by fomites, such as infested clothing, linens, and toilet seats. As with other STDs, single, young people between the ages of 15 and 25 years are the population at highest risk for pubic lice infestation.

Clinical Manifestations
The primary symptom of lice infestation is pruritus. The scratching elicited by pruritus can cause local erythema, irritation, and inflammation. After prolonged periods of infestation, some people have an apparent immunity and do not manifest the pruritus associated with lice.

Diagnosis
Diagnosis is based on the history, symptoms, and demonstration of lice or nits on the hair follicles.

Management
Lice infestation is totally curable without long-term effects. Topical application of Kwell—a 1% gamma benzene hexachloride preparation available as a lo-

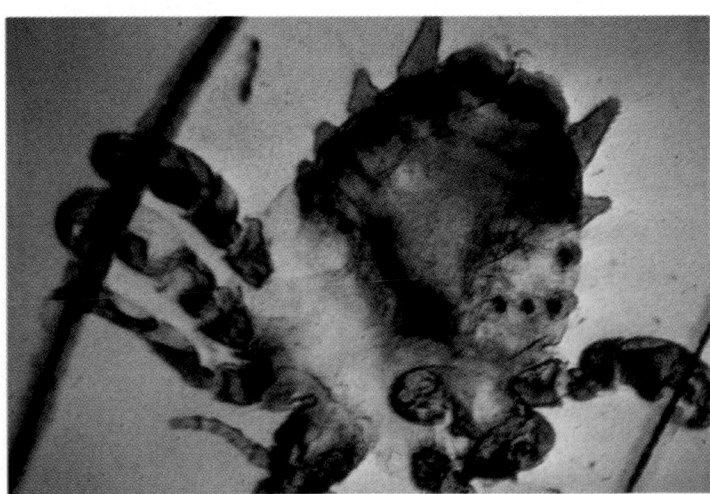

Figure 43–9

Pubic louse 1 mm in length. Note the crablike appearance and hooklike claw at end of each leg. (Courtesy of the New York City Health Department.)

tion, shampoo, or cream—is the most frequently used pediculicide. Infestation of the eyebrows or eyelids is treated with an occlusive application of petroleum jelly (Vaseline).

An antipruritic or anti-inflammatory medication such as hydrocortisone cream may be recommended for itching.

Patients with pubic lice are also evaluated for the presence of other STDs.

NURSING PROCESS
Pediculosis Pubis

Assessment

Assess the patient's understanding of the ways in which pubic lice are transmitted from one person to another, the use of the pediculicide and any other prescribed medications, treatment of contaminated clothing and household goods, and the need for evaluation and possible treatment of other household members and sexual partners.

Nursing Diagnoses and Planning

Nursing diagnoses and related expected patient outcomes commonly applicable to patients with pediculosis pubis include the following:

NDx: Risk for altered health maintenance related to insufficient knowledge of transmission and treatment of pediculosis pubis

Planning: Patient outcomes
1. Patient states correct use of pediculicide and any other prescribed medications.
2. Patient describes treatment of household objects necessary to effectively eliminate pubic lice infesting them.
3. Patient explains need for evaluation and treatment of sexual contacts and other household members.

Nursing Interventions and Evaluation

NDx: Risk for altered health maintenance
Briefly describe the life cycle of the pubic louse. Explain that, although sexual contact is the primary mode of transmission, pubic lice can also be spread by fomites, such as linens and toilet seats. Instruct the patient in the treatment of pubic lice, as specified in Highlight 43–4.

Compare the patient's status with the expected outcomes. If the outcomes are not met, reassess the patient and revise the plan.

$\mathcal{S}$cabies

Scabies is caused by *Sarcoptes scabiei*, which are small, parasitic mites that produce intense itching

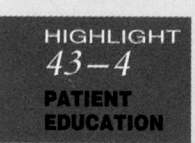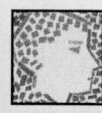

HIGHLIGHT 43–4 PATIENT EDUCATION

Treatment of Pediculosis Pubis

Instruct the patient with pediculosis pubis to do the following:

Use Kwell as follows (in the unusual cases in which an alternative pediculicide is ordered, provide instructions in accord with the package insert):

- Apply Kwell to affected areas for 8 hours, and then wash off thoroughly by showering.
- Avoid contact of Kwell with eyes and mucous membranes.
- Do not use Kwell if pregnant or lactating or on infants and small children.
- Do not apply Kwell to severely excoriated skin.
- Follow directions carefully. Do not overuse, apply incorrectly, or fail to remove after specified time because mild toxic effects on the nervous system can occur.

Rid home of pubic lice as follows:

- Dry clean or wash contaminated clothing and linen with detergent and hot water.
- Treat upholstery and carpets with specially formulated sprays if needed.

Prevent spread and reinfection by encouraging or obtaining evaluation and treatment of sexual contacts and all household members.

Inform the patient that itching may continue for several days after effective treatment, and teach the use of antipruritic or anti-inflammatory drugs if prescribed.

and skin lesions in humans. Scabies has worldwide distribution. Traditionally, scabies appeared to be associated with poverty, poor hygiene, and sexual promiscuity. Today it is recognized that scabies is not limited to social class. Scabies is transmitted primarily through close personal contact with an infected person.

Etiology and Pathophysiology
The scabies mite penetrates the superficial layers of the skin and produces linelike burrows associated with itching, discomfort, and rash. The life span of the adult female mite is 30 days, during which time

she lays two or three eggs per day. Young mites reach maturity in 10 days.

In sexually active young adult people, sexual contact is the most likely mode of transmission. However, scabies can also be transmitted through contact with contaminated clothing, bed linen, and other personal articles. Nonsexual spread within households is a common mode of transmission.

Clinical Manifestations

After a relatively long incubation period, patients present with a chief complaint of a pruritic, papular rash. The itching is either exclusively nocturnal or increases at night. The symptoms frequently appear initially on the webs and sides of the fingers. Wrist and elbow surfaces, the axillae, waistline, genitalia, buttocks, backs of the knees, and toes are common sites. At most sites, a small, papular rash is visible. The rash may appear erythematous and excoriated from scratching. Burrows are not always evident. When they do appear, they can usually be seen on the finger webs, wrists, elbows, or penis. The burrows look like small, dark lines that cross the normal skin lines.

Diagnosis

Scabies resembles other pruritic dermatologic conditions. Definitive diagnosis is based on the presence of the mite, its eggs, or its feces. Skin scrapings or biopsy samples from the papules or burrows are microscopically examined for evidence of the mite. Because these can be difficult to find, diagnosis is frequently based on the history and characteristic appearance and distribution of the lesions.

Management

Topical lindane (Kwell) cream or lotion, a 1% gamma benzene hydrochloride preparation, is the most common treatment for scabies. The cream or lotion is thinly applied to the entire body from the neck down, with special attention paid to the hands and feet. The application remains on the body for 8 to 12 hours, after which it is showered off. Repeated treatments, should they become necessary because of reinfestation or resistance, are limited to two additional applications at 1-week intervals.

Sexual contacts and household members of patients with scabies are evaluated and treated if necessary. Some experts recommend treating contacts with or without clinical manifestations of the disease, because the incubation period may be as long as 2 months.

NURSING PROCESS GUIDELINES
Scabies

The assessment, nursing diagnoses, expected patient outcomes, nursing interventions, and evaluation for patients with scabies are similar to those described for patients with pediculosis pubis.

Chapter Review

1. How is the care of a patient with trichomonas similar to that of a patient with *Gardnerella vaginalis* vaginitis?
2. Why is follow-up important when planning care for a patient with syphilis?
3. What is the significance of herpes simplex virus when seen in a patient who is pregnant?
4. Why is partner identification important when planning care for a patient infected with *Chlamydia*?
5. What would happen to a patient with gonorrhea if left untreated?
6. How can the effectiveness of treatment be evaluated when caring for a patient with syphilis?
7. What is the advantage of azithromycin versus doxycycline for a patient diagnosed with chlamydial infection?
8. What is the meaning of a single, well-circumscribed, nontender genital lesion seen when caring for a patient in the clinic?
9. How is the detection of chlamydial infection in a male patient different from that in a female patient?
10. Why is an annual Pap test important when planning care for a patient with condylomata acuminata?

Bibliography

Augenbraun MH. Sexually transmitted diseases in HIV-infected persons. Infect Dis Clin North Am 1994; 8(2):439.

Ault KA, Faro S. Pelvic inflammatory disease: Current diagnostic criteria and treatment guidelines. Postgrad Med 1993; 93(2): 85.

Biswas M. Bacterial vaginosis. Clin Obstet Gynecol 1993; 36:166.

Blackwell-Weinrich A. Update: Sexually transmitted diseases. Childbirth Instr 1993; 3(3):18, 38.

Bolan G, Fontenot C, Hook E, McCormak W. Syphilis: Are you missing it? Patient Care 1993; 27(16):126.

Centers for Disease Control. Sexually transmitted diseases treatment guidelines. MMWR 1993; 42(RR-14).

Centers for Disease Control and Prevention. Fluoroquinolone resistance in *Neisseria gonorrhoeae*—Colorado and Washington, 1995. MMWR 1995; 44:761.

Clottey C, Dallabetta G. Sexually transmitted diseases and human immunodeficiency virus: Epidemiologic synergy? Infect Dis Clin North Am 1993; 7(4):753.

Dempster JS. Continuing education forum. STDs: A contemporary epidemic. J Am Acad Nurse Pract 1995; 7(3):133.

Drugs for sexually transmitted diseases. Med Lett Drugs Ther 1994; 36:1.

Faro S. Review of vaginitis. Infect Dis Obstet Gynecol 1993; 1:153.

Genc M, Mardh P-A. A cost-effectiveness analysis of screening and treatment for *Chlamydia trachomatis* infection in asymptomatic women. Ann Intern Med 1996; 124:1.

Gibbs R, Sweet R. Evaluating and treating obstetric and gynecologic infections. Califon, NJ: Gardiner-Caldwell Syner Med, 1995.

Grady WR, Tanfer K. Condom breakage and slippage among men in the United States. Fam Plann Perspect 1994; 26:107.

Graves A, Gardner WA. Pathogenicity of trichomonas vaginalis. Clin Obstet Gynecol 1993; 36:145.

Greenaway C, Ronald A. Three common causes of genital ulcer disease. Med North Am 1994; 17(4):253.

Hansfield HH. Recent developments in STDs: I. Bacterial diseases. Hosp Pract 1992; 26(7):47.

Hatcher RA, Stewart F, Trussell J, et al. Contraceptive technology. 16th ed. New York: Irvington Publishers, 1994.

Heine P, McGregor JA. Trichomonas vaginalis: A reemerging pathogen. Clin Obstet Gynecol 1993; 36:137.

Hillis SD. PID prevention: Clinical and societal stakes. Hosp Practice 1994; 29(4):121.

Holmes M, Safyer S, Bickell N, Vermund S, Hanff P, Phillips R. Chlamydia cervical infection in jailed women. Am J Public Health 1993; 83(4):551.

Hutchinson CM, Hook EW, Shepherd M, et al. Altered clinical presentation of early syphilis in patients with human immunodeficiency virus infection. Ann Intern Med 1994; 121:94.

Krieger JN. Trichomoniasis in men: Old issues and new data. Sex Transm Dis 1995; 22:83.

Larsen B. Vaginal flora in health and disease. Clin Obstet Gynecol 1993; 36:107.

Lehne R. Pharmacology for nursing care. Philadelphia: WB Saunders, 1994.

Magid D, Douglas JM, Schwartz JS. Doxycycline compared with azithromycin for treating women with genital *Chlamydia trachomatis* infections: An incremental cost-effectiveness analysis. Ann Intern Med 1996; 124:389.

Martin DH, Mroczkowski TF. Dermatologic manifestations of sexually transmitted diseases other than HIV. Infect Dis Clin North Am 1994; 8(3):533.

McCance DJ. Human papillomaviruses. Infect Dis Clin North Am 1994; 8(4):751.

McCormack WM. Pelvic inflammatory disease. N Engl J Med 1994; 330:115.

McHugh DR. Syphilis: An old disease with modern health concerns. Nurse Pract Forum 1996; 7(1):34.

Melnick SL, Burke GL, Perkins LL, et al. Sexually transmitted diseases among young heterosexual urban adults. Public Health Rep 1993; 108(6):673.

Moran JS, Levine WC. Drugs of choice for the treatment of uncomplicated gonococcal infections. Clin Infect Dis 1995; 20(Suppl 1):S47.

Pastorek J. Prevention of hepatitis B: What the obstetrician/gynecologist can do. Female Patient 1994; 19(Suppl):29.

Poymer T. Diagnosing and treating warts and verrucas. Commun Nurse 1995; 1:2.

Roberts SJ, Sorensen L. Lesbian health care: A review and recommendations for health promotion in primary care settings. Nurse Pract 1995; 6:42.

Rosenberg MJ. Sexually transmitted diseases: What women should know for the '90s. Natl Womens Health Rep 1993; 15(2):1.

Schuler KA. Commentary on syphilis: A review and update of the "new" infection of the '90s. ENAS Nurs Scan Emerg Care 1993; 3(1):2.

Smotkin D. Human papillomavirus infection of the vagina. Clin Obstet Gynecol 1993; 36:188.

Steinberg LJ, Cibley LJ, Rice P. Genital warts: Diagnosis, treatment and counseling for the patient. In Remington JS, Swartz MN (eds). Current clinical topics in infectious diseases. Boston: Blackwell Scientific Publications, 1993.

Stergachis A, Scholes D, Heidrich FE, et al. Selective screening for Chlamydia trachomatic infection in a primary care population of women. Am J Epidemiol 1993; 138(3):143.

Stevens PE. Structural and interpersonal impact of heterosexual assumptions on lesbian health care clients. Nurs Res 1995; 44(1):25.

Stevens PE. Lesbians' health-related experiences of care and noncare. West J Nurs Res 1994; 16(6):639.

Suzich JA, Ghim SG, Palmer-Hill FJ, et al. Systemic immunization with papillomavirus L1 protein completely prevents development of viral mucosal papillomas. Proc Natl Acad Sci U S A 1995; 92(25):11553.

Tagg PI. Patient education. Chlamydia: What you should know. Nurse Pract 1996; 21(2):133.

Taylor-Robinson D. The history and role of mycoplasmagenitalium in sexually transmitted diseases. Genitourin Med 1995; 71:1.

Thomas DL, Quinn TC. Serologic testing for sexually transmitted diseases. Infect Dis Clin North Am 1993; 7(4):793.

Tomberlin MG, Holtom PD, Owens JL, et al. Evaluation of neurosyphilis in human immunodeficiency virus–infected individuals. Clin Infect Dis 1994; 18:288.

Toomey KE, Moran JS, Rafferty MP, Beckett GA. Epidemiological considerations of sexually transmitted diseases in underserved populations. Infect Dis Clin North Am 1993; 7(4):739.

Weber JT, Johnson RE. New treatments for *Chlamydia trachomatis* genital infection. Clin Infect Dis 1995; 20(Suppl 1):S66.

Weinstock H, Dean D, Bolan G. *Chlamydia trachomatis* infections. Infect Dis Clin North Am 1994; 8(4):797.

Witkin SS. Immunology of the vagina. Clin Obstet Gynecol 1993; 36:122.

Unit XIV

Eye and Ear Dysfunction

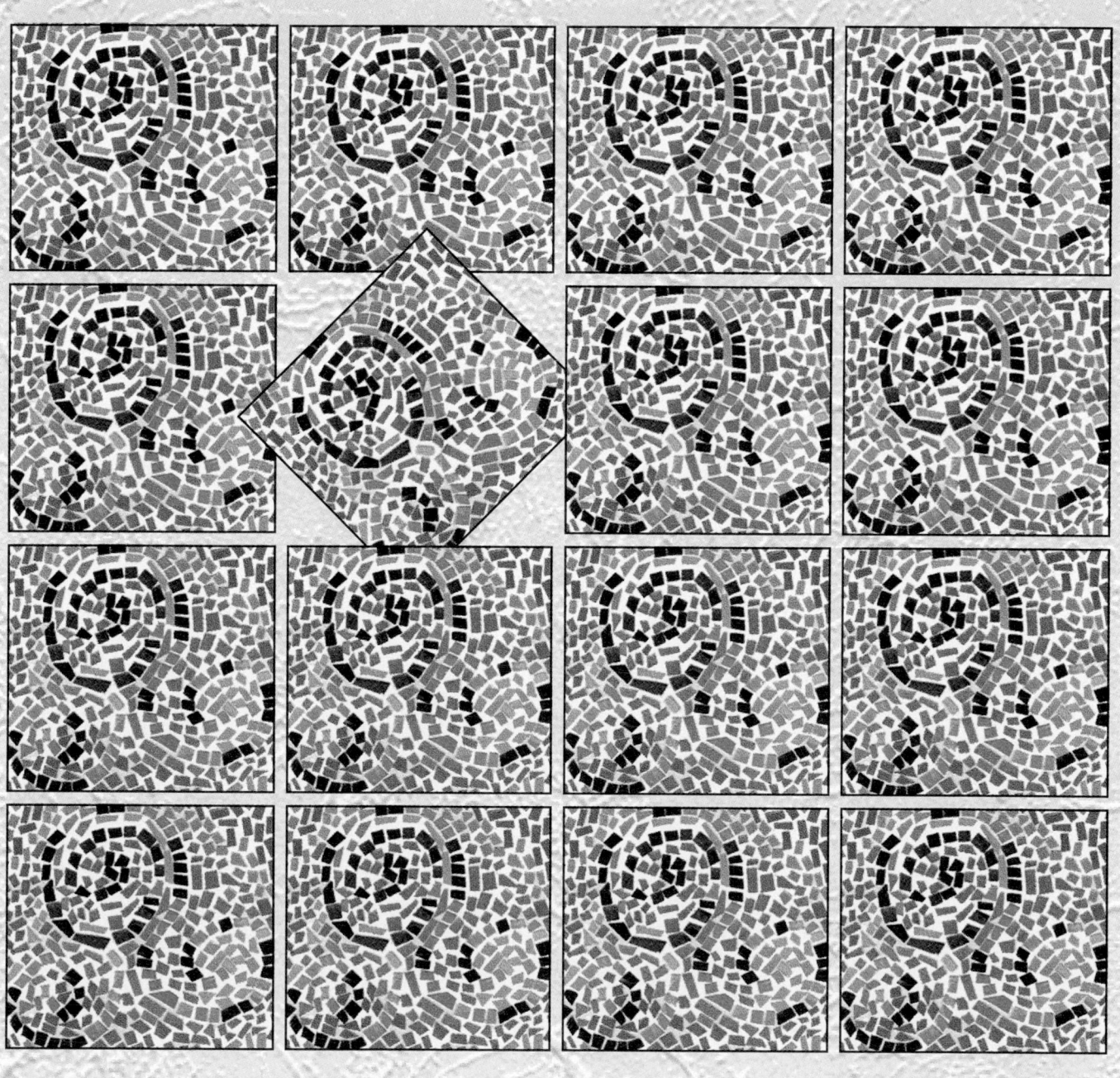

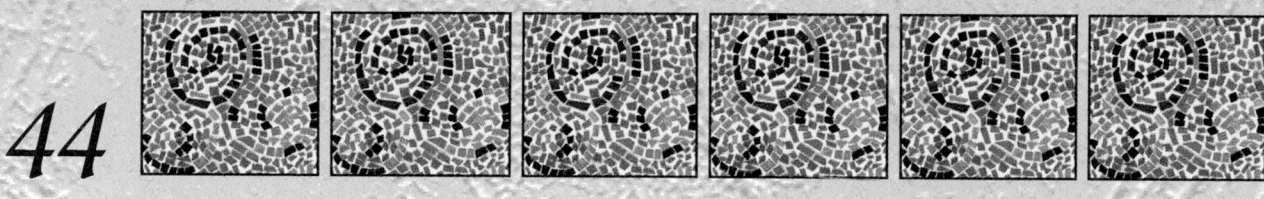

44

Knowledge Base for Patients with Eye Dysfunction

Study Outcomes

After studying this chapter, you should be able to:

1. Explain the normal anatomy and physiology of the eye.
2. Describe common clinical manifestations of eye dysfunction.
3. Identify information and physical examination data essential to the assessment of the eye.
4. Describe basic diagnostic tests and modalities of management used in the treatment of patients with eye disorders.
5. Describe basic ocular surgery.
6. Identify data essential to the assessment of patients undergoing treatment of eye disorders.
7. State nursing diagnoses and related expected patient outcomes commonly applicable to patients undergoing treatment of eye disorders.
8. Describe nursing interventions, with their rationales, commonly applicable to patients undergoing treatment of eye disorders.
9. Explain the basis for evaluation of nursing care provided to patients undergoing treatment of eye disorders.
10. Identify alternative treatment and care settings for patients with eye dysfunction and the services related to community-based care.
11. Identify special considerations for the elderly patient with altered ocular function.

For many Americans, fear of blindness is second only to fear of cancer. Coupled with the steady aging of the American population, this fear has helped to make vision preservation and appropriate eye care a major, growing health concern. This has resulted in a rapidly expanding body of knowledge and a wealth of technologic advances related to the diagnosis and treatment of eye disease. As a nurse, you may be called upon to assist in the diagnosis and treatment of patients with ocular disorders. To do so accurately requires a thorough understanding of ocular anatomy and physiology, pathophysiology, ocular nursing care measures, and patient responses to sometimes distressing disorders.

Anatomy and Physiology

PROTECTIVE STRUCTURES OF THE EYE

The eyeball, also known as the globe, is cradled and protected in a bony cup called the orbit positioned anteriorly in the skull. Accessory structures, including the eyebrows, eyelids, eyelashes, and lacrimal apparatus, also help to protect the eye. The eyebrows help to protect the eye from direct rays of light, as well as from perspiration or other foreign matter that may fall from the brow or forehead. The eyelashes help screen the eye from dust and other foreign particles.

The upper and lower eyelids, or palpebrae, cover the eyeball from the medial canthus to the lateral canthus. They spread lubricating solutions over the globe, protect the eyes from excessive light and foreign objects, cover the eyes during sleep, and keep them moist by preventing evaporation of secretions.

The band of connective tissue that gives form to the eyelids is called the tarsal plate. Embedded in it are the meibomian glands, whose ducts open onto the margin of each eyelid. These modified sebaceous glands secrete an oily substance that helps prevent the lids from adhering to each other. The eyelids are lined with a mucous membrane called the palpebral conjunctiva. This membrane continues into the bulbar conjunctiva, which covers the sclera, the visible white portion of the eye.

The lacrimal apparatus consists of the structures involved in the production and drainage of tears (Fig. 44–1). Tears are produced by the lacrimal gland, which is located in the upper, outer aspect of each orbit. The tears empty through the excretory lacrimal ducts onto the conjunctiva of the upper lid and are spread across the eyeball by blinking. They then enter the lacrimal puncta, which are two small openings located in the inner canthus of each upper and lower eyelid. They then pass into the lacrimal canals, the lacrimal sac, the nasolacrimal duct, and

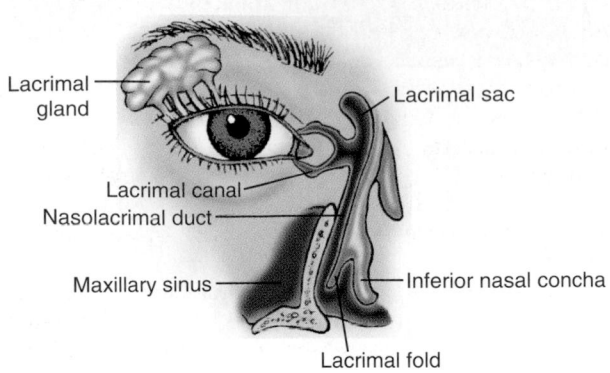

Figure 44–1

The lacrimal apparatus.

finally into the inferior meatus of the turbinate bone of the nose.

Tears contain water, salts, mucus, a bactericidal enzyme called lysozyme, as well as other chemical substances. Tears clean, lubricate, and moisten the eyeball. They wash the surface of the eye constantly, increasing dramatically when the eye is exposed to an irritating substance or the emotional stimulus of the parasympathetic nervous system.

MUSCLES CONTROLLING THE EYE

The muscles that control the eye are of two types: those external to the eyeball and those internal to the eyeball. The six external muscles are attached to the outside of the eyeball and to the bones of the orbit. They are voluntary, skeletal muscles that func-

tion to move the eyeball under the control of cranial nerves III, IV, and VI.

The upper eyelid is raised by the levator palpebrae superioris muscle, which is under the control of cranial nerve III and the sympathetic nervous system. The lid is closed by the orbicularis oculi muscle, which is controlled by cranial nerve VII.

The iris and ciliary muscles work inside the eyeball. They are controlled through the complex neural network involving the optic nerve (cranial nerve II) and oculomotor nerve (cranial nerve III). The iris and ciliary muscles are smooth, involuntary muscles that regulate the size of the pupil and control the shape of the lens during the process of accommodation (focusing the eye).

EYEBALL STRUCTURE

The eyeball is spherical and composed of three distinct layers, or coats, that surround two fluid-filled cavities (Fig. 44–2). The three layers are the external fibrous coat, the middle vascular coat, and the internal nervous coat. The two cavities are the posterior cavity filled with vitreous humor and the anterior cavity filled with aqueous humor.

External Coat

The external fibrous coat, which gives the eyeball its shape, has two distinct parts: the cornea and the sclera. The cornea, which covers the iris, is transparent and avascular. The remainder of the external coat is the opaque sclera, part of which is seen as the white of the eye. This visible portion of the sclera is covered with the bulbar conjunctiva, whose

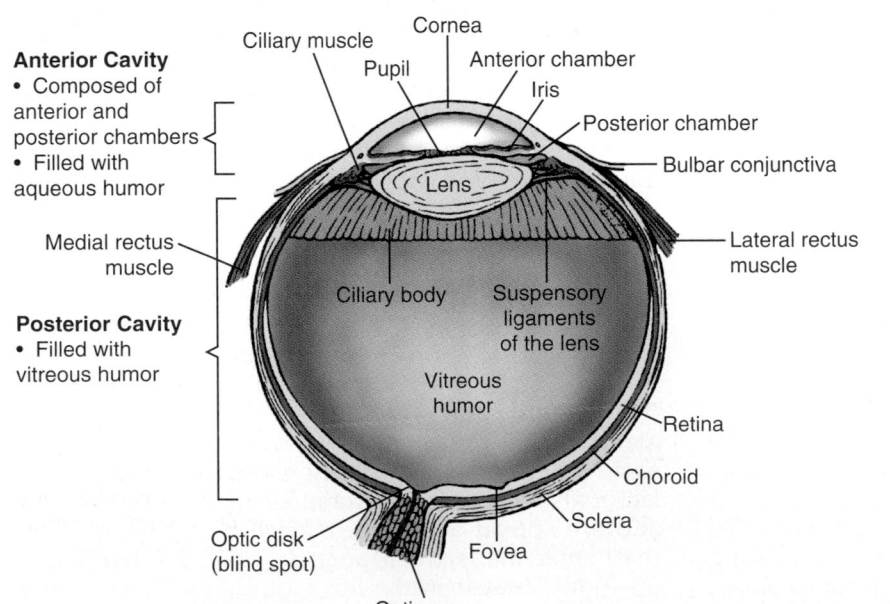

Figure 44–2

Structure of the eyeball.

epithelium is continuous with the layer of epithelium covering the outer surface of the cornea.

Middle Coat

The middle vascular coat is composed of three parts that together are referred to as the uveal tract. They are the iris, the ciliary body, and the choroid.

The iris is the colored area of the eye. Its muscles contract and relax, changing the size of the opening in the center, which is the pupil. By this action the iris regulates the amount of light entering the eye and contributes to a clear visual image.

Around the outer edge of the iris, the middle coat becomes the ciliary body, which is composed of the ciliary muscle and the ciliary processes. The ciliary muscle alters the shape of the lens as needed to focus light rays from near or distant objects on the retina. The ciliary processes produce aqueous humor.

The choroid is the most posterior portion of the middle coat. It is a deeply pigmented, highly vascular membrane that lines most of the sclera. It absorbs light rays to prevent reflection within the eyeball and, through its blood supply, nourishes the retina.

Inner Coat

The inner or neural coat is the retina. It covers the choroid and is found only in the back of the eye. The retina forms the visual image. It consists of an outer pigmented layer, which stores vitamin A needed to produce the photopigment rhodopsin, and an inner neural layer. Rods and cones, which are the photoreceptors, are found in the neural layer and are the visual receptors that develop generator potentials. Cones, stimulated only by bright light, are responsible for color vision and visual acuity. Rods allow for vision in dim light and are responsible for perception of different shades of dark and light, shapes, and movement. Rods are located in the peripheral retina. Cones are concentrated in the fovea, the center of a small avascular area called the macula lutea or yellow spot, which is responsible for sharpest vision.

From the photoreceptor cells containing the rods and cones, sensory information is relayed via the bipolar neurons to the ganglion cells of the retina. The axons of the ganglion cells exit the retina as the optic nerve in the area known as the optic disk or "blind spot" because of the absence of any photoreceptors.

The optic disk consists of distensible tissue and can expand beyond its normal 1.5 mm diameter if capillary pressure increases. The optic disk is lighter in color than the other parts of the retina and contains a characteristic "physiologic cup" at its center, which occupies nearly one-third of the disk.

INNER STRUCTURE OF THE GLOBE

There are two main cavities within the eyeball: the anterior cavity and the posterior cavity. The anterior cavity has anterior and posterior chambers, separated by the iris. The anterior cavity is filled with aqueous humor, the fluid responsible for maintaining intraocular pressure. Aqueous humor is secreted by the choroid plexuses of the ciliary processes into the posterior chamber at the rate of 2 to 5 mm^3/minute. It then flows through the pupil into the anterior chamber through a trabecular meshwork and ultimately to the canal of Schlemm, a venous sinus found at the junction of the sclera and the cornea, from which it drains into the blood (Fig. 44–3). An automatic feedback regulatory system works to maintain normal intraocular pressure between 12 and 20 mm Hg.

The posterior cavity, between the lens and the retina, is filled with vitreous humor. This is a relatively stable gelatinous mass that allows substances to diffuse through it but has little flow of fluid. The mass of the vitreous-filled posterior chamber gives support to the posterior cavity and keeps the retina in place.

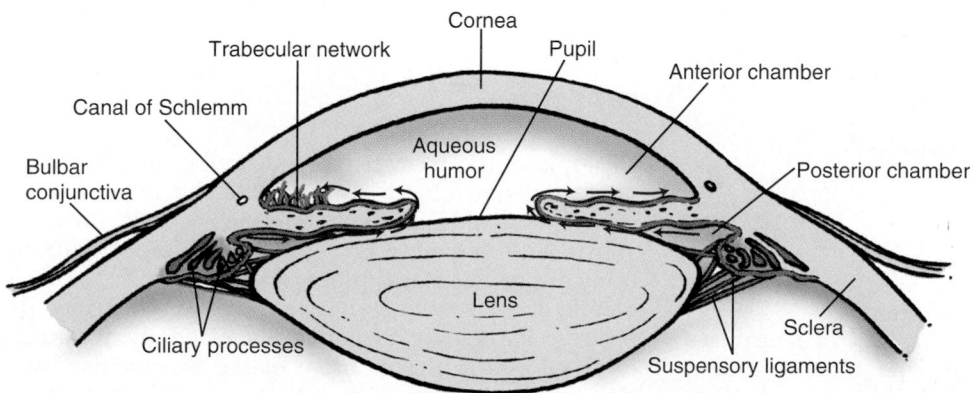

Figure 44–3

Circulation of aqueous humor. Produced by the choroid plexuses of the ciliary processes, it enters the posterior chamber, flows through the pupil, fills the anterior chamber, and flows peripherally through the trabecular meshwork into the canal of Schlemm and ultimately into the venous system.

The crystalline lens that separates the anterior and posterior cavities is a transparent, colorless, biconvex structure. It is enclosed in a clear capsule and held in place by suspensory ligaments. The lens refracts, or bends, light rays entering the eye so that they converge on the retina to form images. In a process called accommodation, the lens changes its shape and hence its refractive ability to adjust for vision at varying distances.

NORMAL VISION AND THE VISUAL PATHWAYS

Ideally, light rays from objects in the visual field entering the eye are refracted by the cornea, the aqueous humor, the lens, and the vitreous humor so that they fall directly on the retina and produce a clear image. Light rays from objects in the nasal half of the visual field of each eye fall on the temporal half of the retina and vice versa. Similarly, light rays from objects in the superior portion of the visual field fall on the inferior portion of the retina. The result is a retinal image that is upside down and reversed right to left.

Stimulation of the retina by light rays initiates the breakdown of photopigments in the photoreceptor neurons and leads to development of generator potentials and, ultimately, nervous impulses. These nervous impulses travel along the axons of the ganglion cells while maintaining their spatial relationships to one another and come together to exit the eye as the optic nerve. At the optic chiasm, nerve fibers from the nasal or medial portion of the retina cross to the opposite side. The fibers then continue with the uncrossed temporal fibers as the right or left optic tract to the geniculate nucleus of the thalamus. Here they synapse with third-order neurons, which conduct the impulses to the visual area of the right and left occipital lobe, respectively (Fig. 44–4). Thus, the left optic tract receives impulses only from the left side of the retina, and the right optic tract receives fibers only from the right side of the retina. As a result, visual stimuli from the left side of the visual fields are interpreted in the right occipital lobe, and visual stimuli from the right side of the visual fields by the left occipital lobe.

Clinical Manifestations of Eye Dysfunction

BLURRED VISION

Vision is blurred or misty from a lack of sharpness or detail in the visual image. The most common cause of gradual blurring is a refractive error that prevents light rays from converging directly on the

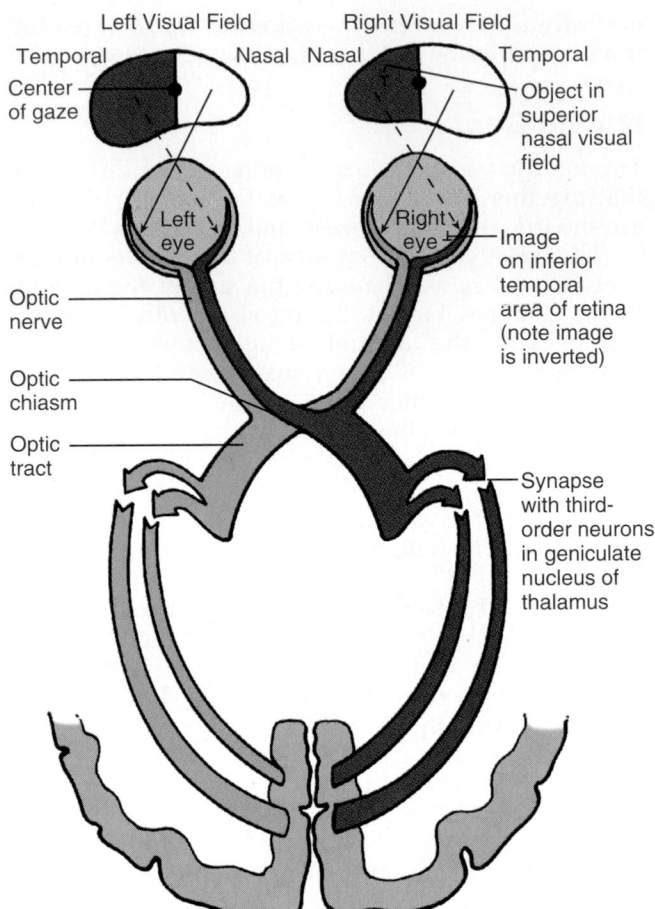

Figure 44–4
Visual pathways.

retina. Other problems originating in the eye that can cause blurred vision are tear film abnormalities, foreign bodies, inflammation of ocular structures, cataract (opacity of the lens), and glaucoma (disease characterized by increased intraocular pressure that results in optic nerve atrophy and blindness). Systemic diseases that can cause blurred vision include diabetes mellitus, hypertension, and kidney diseases. It can also be caused by tobacco and drugs, such as alpha blockers, phenothiazines, and sulfonamides.

DIPLOPIA

Diplopia is the term used to describe double vision, or seeing one object as two. It is horizontal if the images are side by side and vertical if they are above and below each other. In some situations, transient horizontal diplopia can be a normal physiologic event that just happens to be noted by the patient. Pathologic diplopia is caused by weakness or paralysis of one or more of the extraocular muscles that can result from a transient ischemic attack, thyroid eye disease, myasthenia gravis, trauma, or such drugs as alcohol, imipramine, diazepam (Valium), lidocaine (Xylocaine), and nitrofurantoin (Macrodantin).

PHOTOPSIA

Photopsia is the subjective appearance of flashing light or sparks in the visual field. This occurrence is sometimes a forewarning of retinal detachment.

FLOATERS

Floaters are minute particles in the vitreous seen by the patient as stringy, wriggling moving spots or black specks in the visual field. They occur because the particles cast a shadow on the retina. They are common in nearsighted people and in the aged. They tend to be most noticed when the person is tired or worried. Most floaters have no clinical significance, although the presence of many floaters can be a symptom of retinal detachment.

SCOTOMATA

Scotomata are absolute, or fixed, nonmoving blind spots in the visual field. They suggest retinal or neurologic lesions. They may also occur as dose-dependent reactions to drugs, such as isoniazid (INH), streptomycin, and sulfonamides.

PHOTOPHOBIA

Photophobia is an unusual intolerance to light that may or may not reflect a pathologic state. Photophobia differs from photosensitivity, which is an increased reactivity of the skin and other tissues to ultraviolet light.

The causes of photophobia are varied. It occurs in albino people because lack of pigment in the choroid does not protect it sufficiently from light. It also occurs in people whose occupations involve exposure to constant bright sunlight, snow dazzle, constant darkness, furnace heat, or fine, close work. It is also associated with disorders of the anterior segment structures, such as acute conjunctivitis, the presence of foreign bodies (including contact lenses) on the cornea, keratitis, corneal abrasion, and acute iritis. It is a primary symptom of nonocular conditions, such as migraine headaches, meningitis, and Rocky Mountain spotted fever. It also occurs as an idiosyncratic effect of drugs, such as atropine and other cholinergic blockers, chloroquine and other antimalarial drugs, monamine oxidase (MAO) inhibitors, rabies vaccines, and the drugs vidarabine (Vira-A) and idoxuridine, which are used to treat ocular herpes simplex.

PAIN

Areas of the eye sensitive to pain are the lid margins, lacrimal apparatus, cornea, and the uveal tract. The lens and retina are insensitive to pain because they have no sensory innervation.

Eye pain takes many forms and has many causes. Aching is associated with fatigue and muscle imbalance. A specific example is asthenopia, or eyestrain. This results from long, intensive use of the eyes in the presence of uncorrected refractive error. Pain in the lid margins is caused by stretching and inflammation and is usually mild to moderate. The cornea is richly supplied with sensory nerve fibers. An ulceration causes stabbing moderate to severe pain. The pain is localized and aggravated by eye movement. Moderate to severe pain also accompanies contact with chemical irritants, uveitis, and herpes zoster infections. Severe, deep-pressure pain in the eye or eyebrow area is characteristic of increased intraocular pressure.

LOSS OF VISION

Loss of the ability to see may be gradual or sudden in onset, permanent or temporary, and may involve all or part of the visual field (Table 44–1). Loss of vision may result directly from ocular or orbit dysfunction, from neurologic or systemic disorders, from trauma, or from drugs.

Sudden vision loss is associated with retinal detachment, vitreous hemorrhage, and occlusion of the central retinal artery or vein. Slow central loss is associated with nuclear cataract and macular degeneration. Slow peripheral loss is characteristic of open-angle glaucoma.

*A*ssessment of the Eye

PATIENT HISTORY

Begin the history by asking the patient for general information about eye status. Ask questions such as the following:

- How is your vision?
- When were your eyes last examined?
- Do you wear eyeglasses or contact lenses? If yes, for what reason? Nearsightedness? Farsightedness? Other? For how long have you worn glasses? When was your lens prescription last changed?
- Have you noted any changes in vision, such as double vision, blurriness, spots before your eyes?
- Have you noted any other eye symptoms, such as redness, soreness, burning, swelling of the lids or around the eye, itching, excessive tearing, ex-

Table 44–1

Visual Field Defects

TERMINOLOGY

Anopia: absence of vision
Hemianopia: blindness in half the visual field in one or both eyes
Homonymous: referring to the same side (right or left) of the visual field
Quadrantic: referring to one quadrant of the visual field

Visual Defect	Description of the Defect	Illustration
Left anopia	Total blindness on the left side	
Binasal hemianopia	Blindness on the nasal side of both visual fields	
Bitemporal hemianopia	Blindness on the temporal side of both visual fields	
Right homonymous hemianopia	Blindness in the right side of each visual field	
Altitudinal hemianopia	Blindness in the upper or lower half of each visual field	
Homonymous left lower quadrantic hemianopia	Blindness in the lower left quadrant of each visual field	

cessive dryness, or discharge or "sleep" from the eye?

Obtain additional clarifying information about any reported changes in vision or other symptoms. Determine time and speed of onset, whether both eyes were affected equally, relationship of the problem to close work or to distance vision, any identifiable precipitating circumstances, any associated systemic symptoms, any treatment instituted, and the response to treatment. If the patient reports spots before the eyes, ask whether they are fixed or moving. If blurred vision or loss of vision is reported, determine whether the entire visual field is involved or whether a particular central or peripheral area is involved.

Ask the patient about any previous eye disorders, noting type, date of occurrence, and treatment. After this, obtain a general medical history, giving particular attention to known allergies, chronic systemic diseases (such as diabetes and hypertension) that can affect the eye, and use of medication. Specifically ask about cardiac or pulmonary diseases, because certain ophthalmic medications have cardiac and respiratory side effects. Inquire about any family history of diabetes and eye disorders, especially myopia, strabismus, glaucoma, and blindness.

Explore occupational risks by asking about the type of work normally done, the type of lighting used, and any exposure to industrial hazards. Question the patient about recreational activities, because fast-moving racquetballs and tennis balls are potential sources of eye trauma.

Assess the patient's understanding of and compliance with information related to preventive care of the eyes (Highlight 44–1).

PHYSICAL EXAMINATION

Visual Acuity

Visual acuity refers to the sharpness or distinctness of images seen by the eye. Because acuity is primarily a function of the cones, which are concentrated in the central area of the retina, tests of visual acuity are basically tests of central vision. These tests compare what a patient can see at a specified distance with what persons with normal eyes have been found to see at the same distance.

Tests of visual acuity typically use a Snellen chart, which is placed at eye level 20 feet (6 meters) away from the patient. This chart consists of letters

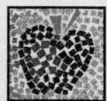

Preventive Care of the Eyes

Keep the eyes clean.

- Keep the hands away from the eyes.
- When necessary to touch the eye, wash hands thoroughly first.
- When cleaning the eye area, move from the inner canthus to the outer.
- Remove old makeup thoroughly.
- Avoid transfer of microorganisms from one eye to the other by never using the same section of washcloth, tissue, and the like to clean both eyes.
- Never share eye makeup with another person.
- Discard old eye makeup, especially mascara, which can serve as a medium for bacterial growth.

Use good, well-placed lighting for all tasks.

Rest eyes at intervals during periods of close work by looking off into the distance or walking around for a few minutes.

Protect eyes from irritation and trauma.

- Wear safety glasses to protect against occupational hazards and when using equipment in the home that can throw off dust, wood shavings, pieces of metal, and so on.

- Use protective eyewear when participating in recreational activities such as tennis or racquetball, where blunt trauma from high-speed balls is a risk.
- Wear dark glasses or other shading device to protect the eyes from bright sunshine, sun lamps, and excessive glare.
- Cover the eyes when using hair spray, and aim other aerosols carefully to avoid contact with the eyes.
- Use ammonia and other household chemicals with irritating fumes only in well-ventilated areas.

Protect eyes from exposure to blood and body fluids by wearing goggles during periods of exposure.

Have an eye examination every 5 years in early adulthood, every 2 years after age 35, and more often if you have, or there is a family history of, diabetes or glaucoma.

Obtain an eye examination immediately if there is a change in vision, eye pain, photophobia, pupil or iris abnormality, nodule, or persistent watering or discharge.

---

in lines that are printed in progressively smaller type from the top to the bottom of the chart. Alongside each line, the distance in feet from which persons with normal vision can read the line is noted.

To test distance vision, position the patient 20 feet from the Snellen chart in good light. Test the eyes individually, right eye first, by covering the other without pressing on the eyeball. Have the patient read aloud down the chart to the smallest line where letters are clear enough to read. Record the visual acuity as the patient's distance from the chart (in this case 20 feet) over the number at the end of the smallest line he or she can read. Thus, a visual acuity of 20/60 means that the patient can see at 20 feet what a person with normal vision (20/20) can see at 60 feet. If the patient misreads some of the letters in the smallest line, subtract the number of missed letters from the overall visual acuity. For example, if the patient missed 2 letters on the 20/60 line, visual acuity would be recorded as $20/60^{-2}$. If the patient missed three letters, visual acuity would be recorded as $20/60^{-3}$.

If the patient wears corrective lenses, test acuity first without the lenses and note "sc" (sine correctio, without correction) next to the result. Repeat the test with corrective lenses, and record "cc" (cum correctio, with correction) next to the result. Normal acuity for distance vision is 20/20. Best corrected visual acuity of less than 20/200 in the better eye or a visual field of less than 20 degrees is defined as legal blindness.

Use an eye chart with rows of numbers or E's pointing in varying directions for patients unable to identify letters. If the patient cannot see any letters, try holding up fingers to see if the patient can count them. Do one eye at a time. Document the result of this test as "Counts fingers at (specify number) feet." For a patient to be classified as having finger-counting acuity, he or she must have identified 50% or more finger presentations correctly.

Test patients who fail a finger-counting test for ability to perceive hand motion. Ask the patient to cover the left eye, then wave your hand in one direction (up-down or left-right). Classify the patient as having hand motion acuity if he or she correctly determines the direction of movement in 50% or more of the presentations. Document the results as "Hand motion at (specify number) feet." Repeat for the other eye.

If a patient fails the hand motion test, proceed to test for light perception. Turn off all room lights. Ask the patient to cover the left eye. Direct a bright light into the exposed right eye at random intervals, turning the light off in between. Ask the patient to report when light is seen. Classify the patient as having light-perception acuity if the patient correctly identifies 50% of the presentations. Repeat for the other eye.

Near-vision acuity is tested if the patient is older than 40 or complains of difficulty with reading or the like. A Jaeger chart, which consists of a series of letters or numbers, is used. It is held 14 inches in front of the face, and the patient is asked to read the smallest characters possible, using reading glasses if worn. Vision is recorded as J1 through J12, with J1, or the ability to read the smallest characters, being normal.

In situations in which eye charts cannot be used, a working estimate of the patient's vision can be obtained using any printed material.

Outer Eye Structures

Begin examination of the outer structures of the eye by noting the position of the eyelids in relationship to the globes. Keep in mind that, normally, no sclera is visible above the iris. Observe the lids for abnormalities, such as ptosis (drooping), retraction, edema, erythema, incomplete closure, and the presence of any lesions. Observe the condition and direction of the lashes, being certain to note whether they are crusted or brushing the globe. If any lesions are present, note location, size, shape, and characteristics.

Inspect the conjunctiva and sclera. Do this by separating the lids between the index finger and the thumb and asking the patient to look up, down, and to each side (Fig. 44–5A). Note any deviation from

the normal smooth white of the sclera (the sclera of people with black skin may normally have a slight yellow cast) as well as the presence of bulging, inflammation, or nodules. Also note the vascular pattern. Inspect the palpebral conjunctiva of the lower eyelid, which is normally a pale, glistening pink, by asking the patient to look up and gently using the thumb to evert the lid (Fig. 44–5B).

Check the clarity of the cornea. Shine a light obliquely onto each eye and observe for cloudiness and opacities.

Inspect each iris. Note shape, color, clarity, and any unusual markings. Be certain to compare the color of the two because, although variation is normal in a small segment of the population, it can also indicate blood in the anterior chamber (hyphema), uveal infection, tumor, or a retained foreign body.

Observe the size and shape of each pupil. Note any abnormal dilation or constriction, as well as any deviation from the normal round, uniform shape. Test the pupillary response to light and accommodation. To test the reaction to light, ask the patient to look into the distance, and then moving from the side to the center, shine a bright light on the pupil of each eye in turn. Observe for the direct response, that is, pupillary constriction in the eye into which the light was shone. Also observe for the consensual response, which is constriction of the pupil of the opposite eye. Repeat for the other eye. Compare the responses of both eyes in amount and speed of constriction and subsequent dilation.

Test for accommodation or the "near reaction" by holding your finger or similar object 4 to 6 inches (10 to 15 cm) from the patient's nose. Ask the patient to look at a distant object behind you and then quickly look at the finger. Observe for pupillary constriction and convergence (the medial movement of both eyes), which normally occur when looking at something near.

Record normal pupillary findings as PERRLA, which stands for *pupils equal, round, reactive to light and accommodation.*

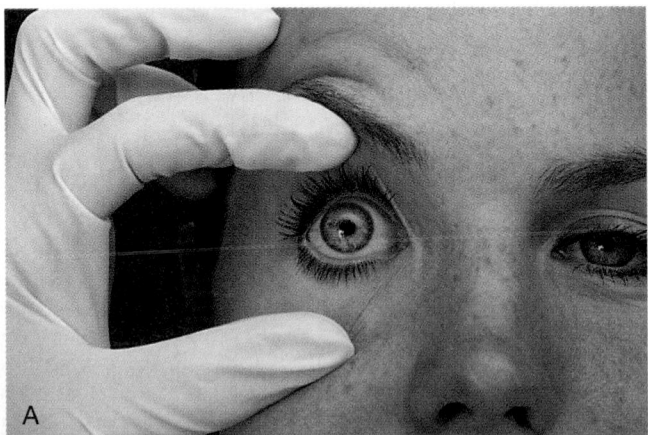 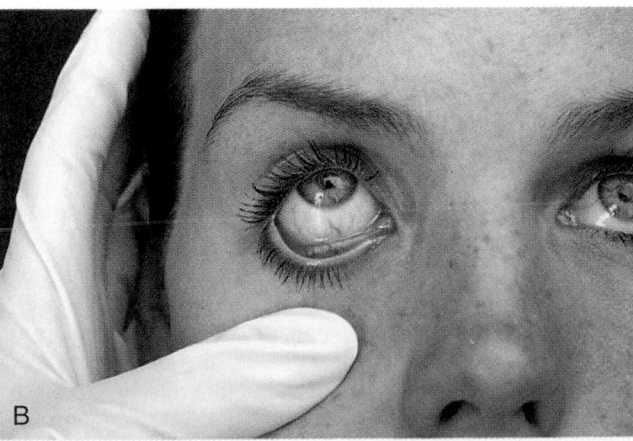

Figure 44–5

A, Examination of the sclera. *B,* Examination of the palpebral conjunctiva of the lower lid.

Extraocular Muscles

The six extraocular eye muscles function to produce a parallel gaze and coordinated movement of the two eyes. Check for parallel gaze by shining a light into the patient's eyes while instructing the patient to look at the light source. Note the location of the light reflection on the corneas. The reflections should be on or just medial to the center of the pupil if the eyes are in parallel alignment.

Assess movement of the eyes by having the patient follow a finger as it is moved through the six cardinal positions of gaze (Fig. 44–6). Instruct the patient to hold the head still and follow the finger with the eyes. Hold the finger about 12 inches in front of the patient, and slowly move it through the fields, first horizontally, then diagonally through the oblique fields, and finally straight up and down.

Throughout the test, observe for parallel eye movement. As the gaze moves from up to down, observe the iris, which should be slightly overlapped by the upper eyelid at all times. Observe also for nystagmus (involuntary, rhythmic, or twitching eye movement), which may occur normally at the end point of any gaze but is otherwise abnormal.

To complete examination of the extraocular muscles, ask the patient to follow your finger as it moves in toward the bridge of the nose. Observe for convergence of the eyes, which is normally sustained to within 5 to 8 cm.

Visual Fields

The most elementary form of visual field testing is the confrontation test. This is a simple test that provides a rough measure of peripheral vision. Begin by facing the patient, positioning yourself so that your face is level with and in front of the patient's face. Instruct the patient to cover the right eye and with the left eye look directly into your right eye. Close or cover your left eye. This position enables you and the patient to have approximately the same visual field. Slowly bring a raised finger or other small object from the periphery of the right side into the field of vision. Be certain to hold it at arm's length midway between yourself and the patient. Ask the patient to say "Now" when the object comes into sight. Compare the time that the patient sees the object with when you see it. Provided your visual fields are normal, both you and the patient should see it at the same time.

Repeat this procedure moving from the left periphery into the field of vision, from above into the field of vision, and from below into the field of vision. Repeat for the opposite eye. Document normal findings as "Visual fields full to confrontation." Retest any areas of discrepancy. Document areas of deficit according to this model: "Unable to detect (specify number) cm object upper outer quadrant of visual field O.D." O.D. refers to the right eye; O.S. refers to the left eye.

More precise examination of the visual fields requires sophisticated mechanical and computerized testing of peripheral vision.

Color Vision

Color vision is not routinely tested. When it is indicated, as for a driver's license, a job requiring color discrimination, or by a patient's history of difficulty in discriminating color, test using a set of plates or cards on which numbers in primary colors are superimposed on a background of multi-toned dots.

Show the plates to the patient one at a time and ask him or her what is seen. Record the test results as a fraction, with the number of figures correctly identified as the numerator and the total number of plates presented as the denominator. A person with a color vision defect will be unable to identify all of the figures correctly. Color vision defects may be hereditary or may be the result of drug toxicity, nutritional deficiency, or disease of the optic nerve or fovea.

Figure 44–6
Cardinal fields of gaze.

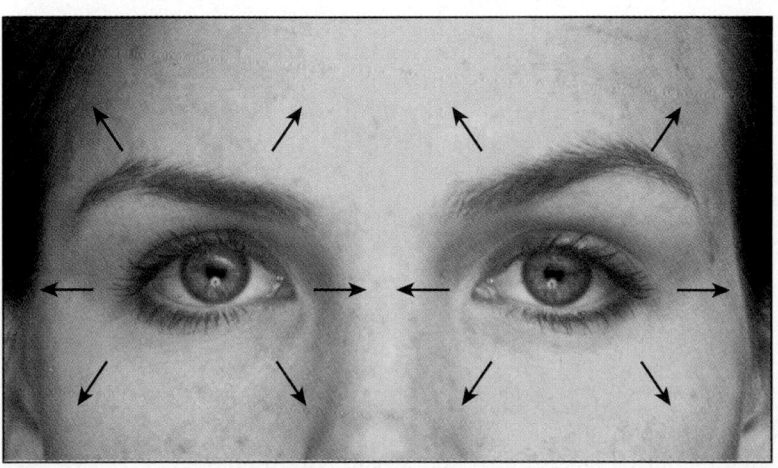

Ocular Fundus

The ocular fundus is composed of the retina, optic disk, macula, and retinal vessels. It can be visualized with an ophthalmoscope, an instrument containing a light source, viewing aperture, and a series of lenses attached to a disk that can be rotated with the index finger without interrupting the examination. These lenses vary in their ability to converge or diverge light. The lens of zero diopters is clear glass and does not affect the light rays passing through it. Plus diopter lenses, indicated on the ophthalmoscope by black numbers, have a progressively shorter focus and are needed to examine farsighted eyes. Negative diopter lenses, indicated by red numbers, have a progressively longer focus and are used for nearsighted eyes unless corrective contact lenses are in place. The lens needed for an examination depends on the type and severity of refractive error in both the eye of the patient and the eye of the examiner.

Ophthalmoscopy is done in a darkened room. To examine the patient's right eye, hold the ophthalmoscope set at zero diopters in your right hand and use your right eye. Repeat this procedure to examine the patient's left eye, remembering to use your left eye.

Stand about 15 inches away and slightly to the side of the patient's line of vision. Place the ophthalmoscope firmly under the medial aspect of your orbit, and shine the light beam on the pupil of the eye to be examined. Looking through the ophthalmoscope, note the appearance of the red reflex, which is an orange-red glow in the pupil, and observe for any opacities interrupting it. Focusing on the red reflex, move your head and the ophthalmoscope forward as a unit until it is almost touching the patient's eyelashes. Rotate the lens disk to focus on the retina, which should now be in view.

Systematically inspect the retina for hemorrhage, exudate, or areas of altered color. Begin by identifying the optic disk, which appears as a yellow-orange to creamy pink round or oval area upon which the blood vessels of the retina converge. If the disk is not immediately evident, locate it by following a blood vessel in the direction in which it enlarges and has branches joining it. When the disk is located, note size, shape, and the clarity of its margins, keeping in mind that the nasal side is sometimes blurred. Also note its color, because dark congestion is associated with papillitis, and a pale or white disk may reflect glaucoma or optic atrophy. Examine the physiologic cup, noting its normal central depression and the emerging retinal vessels. Identify both the arterioles, which are normally light red and have a bright reflection, and the veins, which are dark red, without reflection. Veins are one-quarter to one-third larger in diameter than the arterioles. Observe for abnormal branching, fullness, contour, and integrity. Proceed to examine the periphery of the retina, and end with examination of the macula, which is sensitive to light. Locate the macula, which is an avascular area without margins

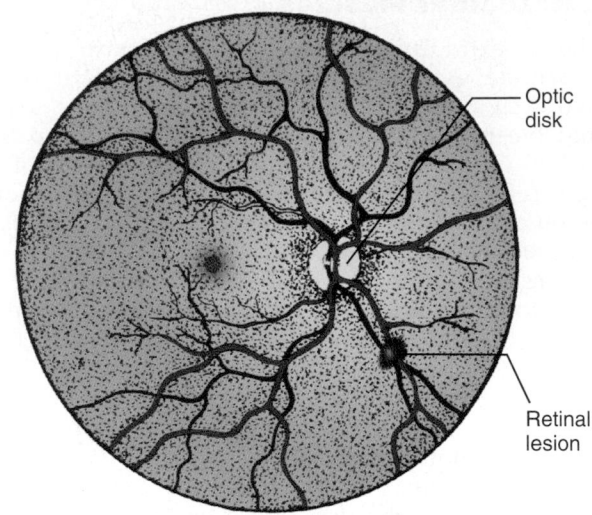

Figure 44–7

The retinal lesion pictured here would be described as 5 o'clock, one disk diameter from the disk, and less than one-quarter disk diameter in size.

temporal to the optic disk, by asking the patient to look directly at the light.

Describe the position of any retinal lesions by referring to location on an imaginary clock face and distance from the optic disk measured in disk diameters (Fig. 44–7).

*D*iagnostic Procedures

MEASUREMENT OF INTRAOCULAR PRESSURE

Tonometry is the measurement of intraocular pressure based on the amount of corneal indentation produced by a given weight or force. The instrument used for this measurement is the tonometer. Normal intraocular pressure is 12 to 20 mm Hg.

The most accurate measurement of intraocular pressure is by applanation tonometry. In this procedure, the cornea is anesthetized with a fluorescein anesthetic solution. Then the Goldmann or applanation tonometer (Fig. 44–8) is brought into contact with the cornea with the patient sitting at the slit lamp or without the slit lamp if a miniaturized, hand-held tonometer is used.

Testing may also be done with a noncontact tonometer. A puff of air is directed at the patient's cornea and provides a digital readout of intraocular pressure based on the resultant deflection of the cornea. This method is fast, simple, and nonpainful. The patient looks straight ahead as an air puff is directed at each eye in turn. A loud "whoosh" is heard as each air puff is released, and a slight momentary pressure on the eye is felt.

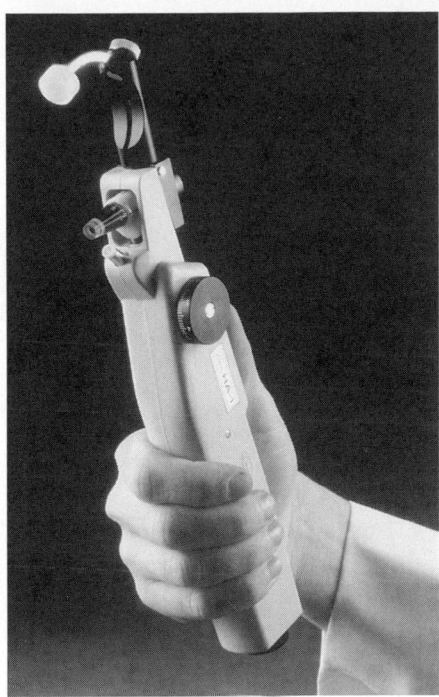

Figure 44–8

An applanation tonometer. (Courtesy of Kowa Optimed, Torrance, CA.)

Another inexpensive but relatively reliable type of indentation tonometry is done with the Schiøtz tonometer. With the patient lying down, anesthetic drops are instilled in the eyes. The foot of the tonometer is then placed on the cornea, and the amount of indentation caused by the weight of the instrument is indicated on the tonometer scale. The scale reading and weight used are then correlated on a chart to determine actual intraocular pressure.

SLIT-LAMP EXAMINATION

A slit-lamp biomicroscope is an instrument that projects a high-intensity beam of light through a narrow slit. Used in a darkened room, the examiner shines the light on a segment of the patient's eye. Then, by looking through a magnifying lens, the examiner can view the conjunctiva, lens, vitreous humor, iris, and cornea.

TOPICAL FLUORESCEIN STAINING

Fluorescein dye is used to detect foreign bodies as well as corneal ulcers or abrasions. The dye is instilled into the conjunctival sac in drop form or by impregnated strips and is spread over the anterior surface of the eye by blinking. The result is that corneal abrasions appear green, foreign bodies have a green ring around them, and conjunctival ulcers appear yellow-orange.

Topical administration creates few adverse ef-fects. Care must be taken, however, to avoid contact with soft contact lenses because they can be stained by the dye. When using fluorescein from a multidose bottle, take extreme care to avoid contaminating the dropper tip. Once the bottle is contaminated, microorganisms can multiply and be transmitted from one patient to another. Cases of *Pseudomonas* corneal ulcers have been reported following use of contaminated solutions of fluorescein.

GONIOSCOPY

Gonioscopy is an examination of the angle of the anterior chamber of the eye. The examiner places a special contact lens similar to a jeweler's loupe over the anesthetized cornea. It is used to determine whether the iridocorneal angle is open or closed in patients with known or suspected glaucoma.

FLUORESCEIN ANGIOGRAPHY

Fluorescein angiography is a contrast study used in conjunction with fundus photography to evaluate the vessels and structures of the internal eye.

Procedure
The patient is screened for allergy to the contrast medium, and the pupil of the eye being tested is dilated. A 5% or 10% sodium fluorescein solution is injected into the antecubital vein, and a fundus camera is used to photograph the sequential phases of retinal circulation (Fig. 44–9). Because the healthy vessel wall is impermeable to the fluorescein dye, diseased vessels are readily identified by their characteristic leakage pattern. Within 24 hours, the dye begins to be excreted by the kidneys. This produces a green-tinged or bright yellow urine that may persist for as long as 48 hours after the procedure. In light-skinned persons, skin discoloration may also occur for 6 to 12 hours.

Complications
Some patients experience a sensation of heat and flushing immediately after injection of the dye. Others develop nausea, vomiting, fainting, or minor allergic reactions. In rare cases, severe reactions may occur, such as bronchospasm, anaphylaxis, convulsions, or cardiac arrest (Bartlett et al, 1992). Therefore, personnel involved in caring for patients having fluorescein angiography testing must have access to emergency equipment and be knowledgeable in its use.

ULTRASONOGRAPHY

Ocular ultrasonography uses high-frequency sound waves to detect tumors and other abnormalities not visible with direct assessment. It is particularly useful in cases of retinal disorders, tumors, vitreous hemorrhage, and dense cataracts.

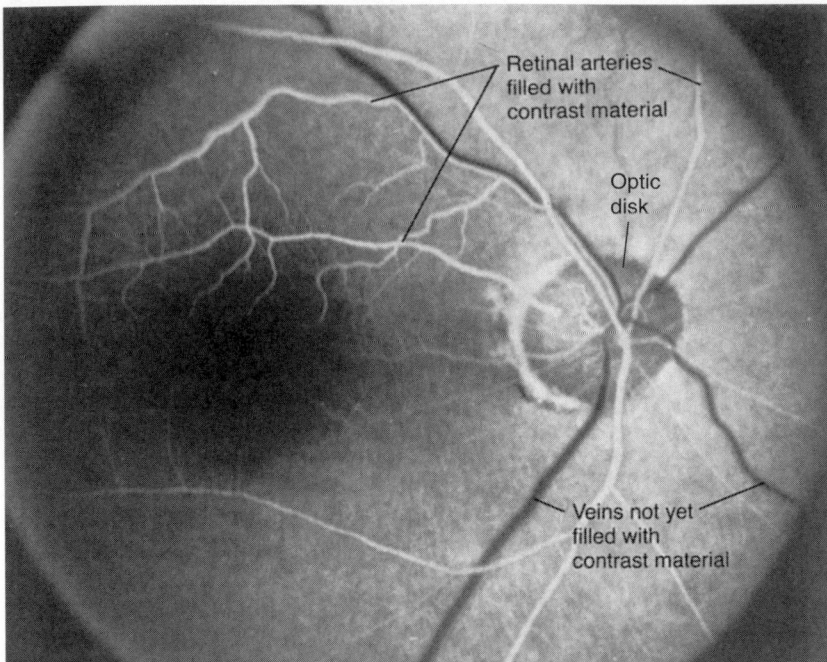

Figure 44–9
Retinal circulation as seen with fluorescein angiography. Arteries fill with contrast material first, veins several seconds later. Note that the veins are slightly wider than the arteries and that both veins and arteries converge at the optic disk. (From Brown MM. Retinal vascular disorders: Nursing and medical implications. Nurs Clin North Am 1981; 16(3):419.)

A small transducer is placed in contact with the eyeball to generate sound waves. The waves spread through the eye as vibrations and ultimately are recorded on a screen. The eye being tested remains open throughout the procedure, and the patient may be asked to change his or her gaze.

COMPUTED TOMOGRAPHY

The computed tomographic (CT) scan of the ocular orbit provides a three-dimensional view of the size, position, and relationships of ocular and adjacent structures. The scan may be done with or without contrast dye and allows accurate diagnosis of orbit pathology, including lesions, fractures, and visual problems. The only potential complication is an allergic response to the contrast medium, if used.

MAGNETIC RESONANCE IMAGING

Magnetic resonance imaging (MRI) is a noninvasive test that uses a strong magnetic field to create images of the eye and orbit. It provides better definition of tissues and fluids in the eye than computed tomography does, but it cannot be used in patients with pacemakers, metallic implants, or foreign bodies that may be dislodged by the magnetic field. It is also contraindicated for pregnant patients.

ELECTRORETINOGRAPHY

Electroretinography (ERG) is a test of the function of rods and cones. In this test, the pupil is dilated and a topical anesthetic applied. A sequence of lights at various intensities and intervals is flashed and the electrical response of the retina recorded via an electrode placed on the cornea with a contact lens. This test is used to diagnose retinal disease and to evaluate the potential for vision in an eye with a dense opacity.

VISUAL EVOKED POTENTIALS

Tests of visual evoked potentials assess the integrity of the visual pathways from the optic nerve to the occipital cortex. Changes in electrical activity in the occipital cortex in response to stimulation of the retina with light are monitored via electrodes placed on the scalp and analyzed by computer. The result is a measurable electrical wave that deviates from normal in the presence of optic nerve dysfunction or demyelinating disease.

*M*anagement

PHARMACOLOGIC THERAPY

The majority of drugs used to treat disorders of the eye are administered topically either in solution or ointment form. Some are used solely for an external effect; others must penetrate the eye to be effective. Many classes of drugs are used in ophthalmic treatment because of the variety of disease processes that can affect the eye.

Understanding Ophthalmic Medications

The eye, especially the cornea and the conjunctiva, is highly sensitive to pain. Thus, anesthetics are used to allow complete eye examination, to measure intraocular pressure by other than a noncontact approach, to remove foreign bodies, and to prevent pain during treatments or surgical procedures. Topical preparations, which produce anesthesia in about 30 seconds, can cause transient stinging, burning, redness, and photophobia. They also interfere with epithelial healing and therefore are not applied repeatedly for painful irritations. Prolonged use can result in keratitis and corneal opacity.

Anti-infective drugs used to treat eye infections include antibacterial, antiviral, and antifungal agents. They may be given systemically, injected beneath the conjunctiva, injected into the vitreous, or applied topically as drops or ointment. Frequent or prolonged use of antibiotics is contraindicated because of the risk of hypersensitivity reactions, which include stinging, burning, itching, urticaria, edema, and dermatitis, as well as the risk of secondary infection.

Corticosteroids suppress hyperemia, photophobia, pain, and the cellular effects of inflammation. They are used to treat inflammations caused by irritation or allergy. These anti-inflammatory agents are not used to treat infections or abrasions because they inhibit normal defense mechanisms. Corticosteroids cause transient stinging or itching on instillation. They may also cause decreased visual acuity, visual field defects, cataracts, glaucoma, and optic nerve damage.

Nonsteroidal anti-inflammatory agents include flurbiprofen (Ocufen), which inhibits production of prostaglandins, diclofenac sodium (Voltaren), and ketorolac tromethamine (Acular).

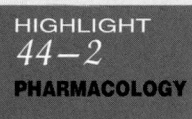 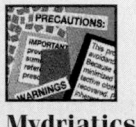

HIGHLIGHT
44–2
PHARMACOLOGY

Mydriatics

Definition:

Drugs that dilate the pupil. Two classes are sympathomimetics (adrenergics) and anticholinergics (cholinergic blocking agents), also called cycloplegics (drugs that paralyze the ciliary muscle).

Action:

Sympathomimetic mydriatics dilate the pupil by stimulating the radial muscle fibers of the iris. They also constrict ocular blood vessels, decrease the formation of aqueous humor, and increase its outflow.

Anticholinergic mydriatics dilate the pupil by paralyzing the circular muscles of the iris and prevent accommodation by paralysis of the ciliary body.

Uses:

Sympathomimetic mydriatics are used to dilate the pupil for examination of the fundus, control bleeding or dilate the pupil for surgery, maintain postoperative mydriasis, shrink blood vessels and lessen injection in conjunctivitis and uveitis, and decrease congestion and irritation due to hay fever, colds, eye strain, and other irritants.

Anticholinergic mydriatics are used for accurate measurement of refractive error and in the treatment of inflammatory conditions of the uvea.

Side Effects:

Stinging upon instillation, photophobia, local irritant or allergic reactions. Sympathomimetics can also cause headache, rebound miosis, and with long use, pigmentation of the lids, conjunctiva, or cornea. Rare systemic reactions include hypertension, tachycardia, dysrhythmias, anxiety, sweating, and trembling. Anticholinergics can also cause increased intraocular pressure and systemic effects, including dry mouth and skin, flushing, headache, tachycardia, fever, abdominal distention, urinary retention, restlessness, ataxia, and confusion.

Interactions:

Only the sympathomimetic drug phenylephrine has significant interactions with other drugs. Phenylephrine increases the pressor effects of guanethidine and the monoamine oxidase inhibitors; levodopa decreases the mydriatic effect of phenylephrine.

Nursing Implications:

Instill the drops and teach the patient to instill the drops as described in Table 44–2. Instruct the patient to compress the area of the lacrimal sac for 1 minute after instillation to prevent systemic absorption. Explain to patients that the pupil will be large and the eye sensitive to light. Suggest the use of dark glasses.

When cycloplegic drugs are used, inform the patient that blurred vision is expected and that driving and use of machinery or household appliances such as meat slicers should be avoided. Tell the patient to discontinue use of the drug if eye pain occurs.

Autonomic drugs include both sympathetic and parasympathetic agents. In the eye, sympathetic stimulation causes pupil dilation (mydriasis), lessens tone in the ciliary muscle, and increases intraocular tension. Parasympathetic stimulation causes pupillary constriction (miosis), increases tone in the ciliary muscle, and decreases intraocular pressure by increasing the outflow of aqueous humor.

Drugs that dilate the pupil are called mydriatics (Highlight 44–2), and those that constrict the pupil are miotics (Highlight 44–3). Drugs that paralyze the ciliary muscle and dilate the pupil are cycloplegic mydriatics.

Carbonic anhydrase inhibitors, which lower intraocular pressure by decreasing production of aqueous humor, are used in managing acute attacks of angle-closure glaucoma and as adjunctive treatment for chronic open-angle glaucoma. The side effects of these drugs are numerous and often severe. They include fever, skin eruptions, gastrointestinal symptoms, drowsiness, fatigue, malaise, depression, renal calculi, and aplastic anemia.

Beta-adrenergic blocking agents, which lower intraocular pressure when applied topically as eye drops, are used to treat glaucoma. The precise mode of action of these drugs is unknown, but they are thought to reduce formation of aqueous humor and to slightly increase its outflow. Because some systemic absorption occurs, these drugs should not be used in patients with heart block or pulmonary disease because they can cause severe cardiac and respiratory reactions. Beta blockers do not constrict the pupil. The usual dosage is twice daily. Beta blockers include timolol (Timoptic), levobunolol (Betagan), betaxolol (Betoptic) and carteolol (Ocupress). Some side effects of this class of medications are ocular irritation, bradycardia, hypotension, and dyspnea.

Lubricants—such as zinc sulfate, petrolatum, and artificial tears—are used for temporary relief of minor eye irritation. They are also used by contact lens wearers, those with artificial eyes, and persons with dry eyes caused by a normal, age-related decrease in tear production.

The osmotic agents glycerin, mannitol, isosorbide, and urea, which shift fluid from the anterior chamber to the plasma, are used in selected situations when intraocular pressure must be quickly reduced. Because they are potent diuretics with systemic effects, rapid changes in fluid and electrolyte balance can occur. Thus, patients with cardiac, renal, or hepatic disease must be closely monitored for heart failure and pulmonary edema.

Administering Ophthalmic Medications

Most ophthalmic drugs are topically administered as drops or ointments. Although ointments are more

---

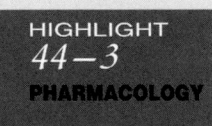 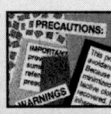

HIGHLIGHT 44–3 PHARMACOLOGY

Miotics

Definition:

Cholinergic drugs (direct-acting or anti-cholinesterase agents) that constrict the pupil.

Action:

Constrict the pupil by stimulating contraction of the sphincter muscle of the iris.

Uses:

Treat glaucoma by improving the outflow of aqueous humor from the anterior chamber and decreasing intraocular pressure. Manage accommodative esotropia (turning inward of the eye with accommodation).

Side Effects:

Blurred vision; photosensitivity; eye, brow, and lid pain; cataract formation. In dark-skinned people, reversible loss of eyelid skin color from hypersensitivity. Potential systemic effects include abdominal cramps, diarrhea, increased salivation, bronchial constriction, and pulmonary edema.

Interactions:

Virtually all miotics have significant interactions either with one another or with other drugs. Refer to the package insert or to a pharmacology text for interactions of any miotic before administering the drug or doing patient teaching.

Nursing Implications:

Instill the drops and teach the patient to instill the drops as described in Table 44–2. Instruct the patient to compress the area of the lacrimal sac for 1 minute after instillation to decrease the risk of systemic absorption. Tell the patient that blurred vision is expected, and warn against driving, using machines, and so on. Suggest instilling the medication at bedtime if possible to avoid difficulties with blurred vision. Suggest the use of dark glasses if the eyes are sensitive to light.

stable than drops and provide longer contact with the eye, they cause blurred vision and are more likely to precipitate a hypersensitivity reaction. An alternative method of administration now in use for the administration of pilocarpine (a cholinergic drug used to constrict the pupil and thus lower intraocular pressure in patients with glaucoma) is a drug-diffusion system known as Ocusert. This system is about the size of a hard contact lens and is placed in the upper or lower cul-de-sac (Fig. 44–10). It consists of a central reservoir that releases drug through membranes at a constant, controlled rate. Advantages of this type of administration are that it provides slower release with better control of intraocular pressure, lowers the needed dosage, and lessens toxicity. Disadvantages are that it is more expensive, can cause conjunctival irritation, and may become dislodged during sleep.

Ophthalmic drops and ointments are instilled as outlined in Table 44–2.

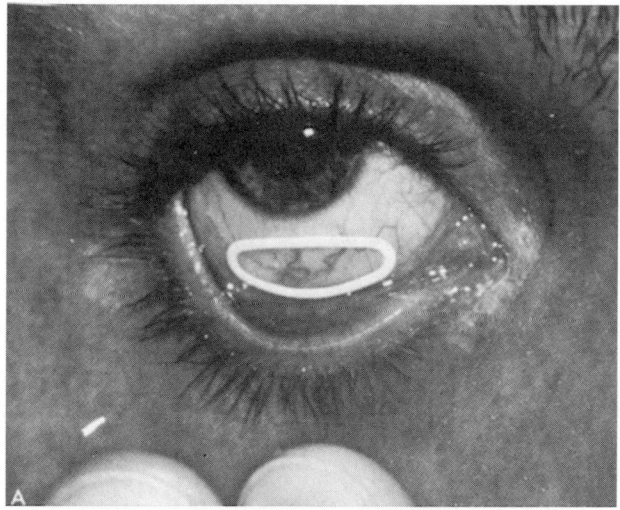

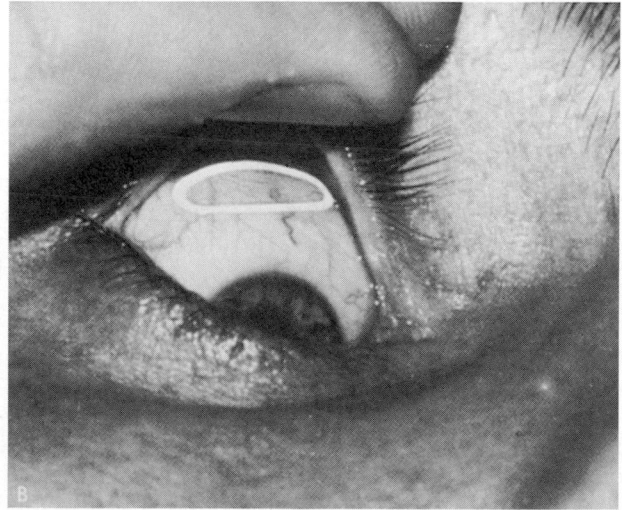

Figure 44–10

Ocusert-Pilo. *A*, In the lower cul-de-sac. *B*, In the upper cul-de-sac. (From Jeglum EL. Ocular therapeutics. Nurs Clin North Am 1981; 16(3):456.)

Table 44–2

How To Instill Ophthalmic Drops and Ointments

INSTILLATION OF OPHTHALMIC DROPS

1. Wash hands to reduce surface microorganisms.
2. Explain the procedure to the patient to decrease anxiety and promote cooperation.
3. Put on gloves if there are secretions in the patient's eye(s) to protect self from contamination.
4. Check name, strength, and expiration date of medication to ensure correct administration of medication free of chemical and physical changes due to age.
5. Ask the patient to open the eyes, tilt the head backward, and look up to position the head for instillation.
6. Retract lower lid downward against the cheekbone or grasp skin of lower lid between thumb and index finger and pull forward to create a pocket-shaped area for drug placement.
7. Hold the medication bottle with the eyedropper tip down like a pencil to provide optimal control of the bottle.
8. Place the wrist of the hand holding the bottle on the patient's cheek to bring bottle close to the eye without touching the eye or eyelashes, which could contaminate the medication and could injure the eye.
9. Squeeze the bottle gently to allow one drop to fall into the pocket between the lower lid and the globe.
10. Release the lower eyelid slowly because quick release may cause medication to splash into the puncta and drain.
11. Tell the patient to gently close the eyelid to distribute the medication. Warn the patient not to squeeze the eyelid shut, because squeezing tends to force medication into the nasal lacrimal system, thus decreasing its absorption.
12. Wait 5 minutes before instilling another drop to promote maximum drug absorption.
13. Wash hands.
14. Record.

INSTILLATION OF OPHTHALMIC OINTMENTS

1–6. Perform steps 1 through 6 as for Instillation of Ophthalmic Drops.
7. Hold ointment tube like a pencil near **but not touching** the eye or eyelashes to avoid contamination of the medication and injury to the eye.
8. Squeeze a thin ribbon of ointment from the inner to the outer canthus along the lining of the sac.
9. Release the lower eyelid slowly because quick release may remove ointment from the pocket.
10. Ask the patient to gently close the eyes to distribute the ointment.
11. Advise the patient that the ointment may cause blurred vision, which creates a potential for injury.
12. Wash hands.
13. Record.

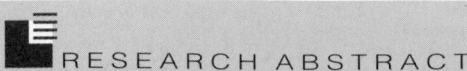

RESEARCH ABSTRACT

What Do Patients Think of Outpatient Eye Surgery?

Mei-Lin L. A telephone survey of day-surgery eye patients. J Adv Nurs 1997; 25:355.

It is now common for ophthalmic surgical procedures to be performed in outpatient settings. But what do patients think of outpatient eye surgery?

To begin to answer that question, Mei-Lin conducted a telephone survey of a random sample of patients who had undergone outpatient eye surgery in one outpatient setting in England. The patients were eligible for same-day surgery if they could take care of themselves and if there was support for them after surgery.

To conduct her research, Mei-Lin developed an interview instrument with questions about the person's experience at three different time periods. Almost 80% of the subjects were over 70 years old. Just over 84% of them had undergone cataract surgery.

The majority of patients rated their overall satisfaction as excellent (>55%) or satisfactory (>39%). They also gave excellent ratings to the care that they received on the day of surgery (>76%). Areas needing attention included

- Decreasing waiting time during the preoperative period
- Providing better pain relief
- Providing a warmer environment on the day of surgery
- Improving retention of information presented both preoperatively and postoperatively

The researcher suggests that her findings were valuable in helping the outpatient facility that she studied in its efforts to improve services. Nevertheless, the economic pressures to deliver services at lower costs will likely continue, and information such as that obtained in this study can be a valuable indicator of the quality of outpatient services. The researcher also notes several limitations of the study, including small sample size, possible interference from the researcher's involvement, and reliability problems with the survey instrument.

Questions to Consider

1. What types of procedures are routinely offered in outpatient settings in your area?
2. What criteria are used to select patients as candidates for surgery in these settings?
3. How do same-day surgery facilities in your area prepare patients for procedures and postoperative care?
4. Recovery from eye procedures may require a time of limited vision. What arrangements are made by the same-day surgery facilities in your area to ensure the safety of patients once they leave?
5. What issues might patients in the same-day surgical facilities in your area identify as needing improvement?
6. How would you adapt your patient teaching strategies to accommodate more limited contact with patients in such settings?

SURGICAL INTERVENTIONS

Ocular Surgery

When the situation allows, eye surgery is preferably done under local anesthesia because the recovery time is faster and because any risk of postanesthesia vomiting is eliminated. Vomiting increases intraocular pressure, which can lead to bleeding and strain on sutures. The risk of accidental external trauma to the affected eye by a patient who becomes restless during recovery from general anesthesia is also eliminated.

Preoperative preparation includes instillation of antibiotic drops, usually beginning 24 hours before surgery. Once the patient has arrived at the unit or preoperative holding area, mydriatic agents are administered at specified intervals to dilate the pupil. In many cases, a sedative or tranquilizing agent may be administered. Other preparations may include facial wash with antiseptic soap and hair shampoo the evening before surgery, NPO (nothing by mouth) status from midnight before surgery, facial shave on the day of surgery for male patients, and insertion of an intravenous line or heparin lock.

Further preparation of the eye is carried out in the operating room. The eyelids, lid margins, eyebrows, and surrounding skin are then cleansed with an antimicrobial solution, and the eye is irrigated with normal saline.

At the end of the surgery, antibiotics are injected subconjunctivally, and an antibiotic-steroid ointment is instilled.

Postoperatively, the operated eye is usually covered with an eye patch on top of which a rigid eye shield may be placed to protect the eye from accidental trauma, particularly at night. Activities that increase intraocular pressure should be avoided, such as bending over from the waist, lifting 25 pounds or more, straining at bowel movements, and coughing. In rare cases, reading and watching television are prohibited to limit rapid eye movement. Patients are usually allowed to get up to go to the bathroom immediately on return from surgery and to take short walks accompanied by a nurse until their stable gait returns. Surgery usually is performed in a day-surgery setting, where the patient is discharged several hours after the operation to recuperate at home. In selected cases, such as when surgery is being performed on the patient's only eye, overnight hospitalization may be suggested.

NURSING PROCESS
Ocular Surgery

PREOPERATIVE NURSING CARE

Assess the patient's understanding of his or her eye disorder, what the surgery is designed to accomplish, and what to expect before, during, and after surgery. Pay particular attention to understanding of the intraoperative experience if local anesthesia is to be used.

Assess the patient's reaction to the scheduled surgery. Because vision is so important to our appreciation of the world around us and to everyday function, reactions can vary from unrealistic expectations regarding return of normal vision to acute anxiety over possible loss of vision.

Assess the patient's current visual status to identify safety precautions and personal assistance the patient may need. Assess functional vision in the eye not scheduled for surgery to determine postoperative needs if the operated eye is patched.

Review the patient's general health status. Obtain information about any chronic diseases and their management. Determine whether the patient has hay fever or other allergies that can cause sneezing or coughing and therefore increase pressure within the eye, which can disrupt sutures or alignment of tissues. Ask what, if any, medications are routinely taken or used (including eye drops used for other conditions) and on what schedule. If the patient will be spending time in the hospital or clinic, ask whether the patient is on a special diet and what, if any, treatments are routinely required.

Review and clarify the information given to the patient in the clinic or ophthalmologist's office at the time the surgery was scheduled. Be sure the patient understands the expected outcome of the surgery and knows when it will be done and how long it will take.

Review postoperative care with the patient, and include the family or significant other if possible. Explain that quick movements, coughing, bending over from the waist, and rubbing the eyes should be avoided. Tell the patient whether to expect an eye patch and, depending on the surgery, remind the patient that improved vision may not be noticed immediately after surgery.

To avoid creating undue anxiety and to help place the patient at ease, approach the patient with limited vision from the unaffected or least affected side. Also be sure to identify yourself as you enter speaking range.

To promote safety, keep the call bell and any visual aids used by the patient within reach at all times. Find out activities for which the patient needs assistance, and help as needed. Place all small objects, such as wastebaskets and foot stools, safely outside the patient's walking area. If furniture or equipment is moved, return it to its original position so the environment remains obstacle-free and familiar to the patient.

Administer the ordered preoperative medications on time so that the eye is ready for surgery. Observe for pupil dilation after administration of mydriatic agents. Keep in mind that dark eyes take longer to dilate than light eyes. If expected dilation does not occur, notify the physician, because a larger dose may be needed. Be sure the patient voids just before leaving for the operating room because a full bladder can make the patient restless during the surgery.

POSTOPERATIVE NURSING CARE

Assessment

Assess the patient's return to physiologic stability. Take vital signs according to agency protocol, guided by the patient's condition. Observe for any drainage, and assess for type and amount of discomfort. Check for nausea, which occasionally occurs from preoperative sedation, so that immediate action can be taken to prevent potential vomiting with its resulting increase in intraocular pressure.

Observe for compliance with position and activity restrictions. Be alert to signs of excessive compliance, that is, the patient who stays rigidly in one position. This behavior can indicate unusual discomfort or severe anxiety.

Throughout the postoperative period, make ongoing assessments of the patient's need for safety measures and assistance with personal activities, as well as assessments related to any coexisting chronic disease.

Nursing Diagnoses and Planning

Nursing diagnoses and related expected patient outcomes commonly applicable to patients who have had eye surgery include the following:

NDx: Risk for infection related to surgical interruption of the intact ocular surface

Planning: Patient Outcomes
1. Patient is afebrile.
2. Ocular redness is absent.
3. Purulent discharge is absent.
4. Severe pain is absent.

NDx: Risk for trauma: tissue related to pressure on suture line

Planning: Patient Outcomes

1. Patient verbalizes importance of not disturbing integrity of suture line.
2. Patient rests and sleeps on back or unoperated side.
3. Patient avoids activities known to increase intraocular pressure.
4. Patient wears eye shield as instructed.

NDx: Risk for impaired home maintenance management related to activity restrictions imposed by eye surgery

Planning: Patient Outcomes

1. Patient performs own activities of daily living within constraints of activity restrictions.
2. Patient identifies plan for meeting activities of daily living if unable to do so independently.

NDx: Risk for altered health maintenance related to insufficient knowledge of postoperative self-care activities

Planning: Patient Outcomes

1. Patient instills eye drops aseptically.
2. Patient identifies purpose of medications.
3. Patient states frequency of medications.
4. Patient correctly applies eye shield.
5. Patient describes activity restrictions.
6. Patient lists symptoms to be reported to the health-care provider.
7. Patient returns for scheduled follow-up visit.

Nursing Interventions and Evaluation

NDx: Risk for infection

Instruct the patient to wash both hands immediately before and after touching the eye. Teach the patient to administer any prescribed eye drops without contaminating the dropper tip (see Table 44–2).

Because reduction in visual acuity is an early sign of postoperative infection, advise the patient to check the vision every day. Instruct the patient to do this by looking at the same object, using only the eye that had the surgery.

Tell the patient to expect some crusty drainage on the eyelid or eyelashes. If a fever develops, pain increases, ocular redness increases, or the amount of drainage increases or becomes purulent, notify the ophthalmologist immediately.

NDx: Risk for trauma

Position the patient on the unaffected side or back to prevent pressure on the suture line. Remember that ophthalmic suture material is finer than a human hair. While it promotes adequate closure of tissue, excessive pressure on the suture line should be avoided. Because suture lines can also have tension placed on them by increased intraocular pressure, advise the patient to avoid activities known to increase it. These include bending over at the waist, straining at stool, lifting heavy objects, vigorous

nose blowing, and coughing. If an eye shield is prescribed, apply it properly and teach the patient how to apply it and when to wear it (Table 44–3, Fig. 44–11). Eye shields are usually worn while sleeping or resting, when outside, and when engaged in activities in which the eye could be injured.

NDx: Risk for impaired home maintenance management

Patients cannot drive after surgery until given clearance by the physician. Help establish a transportation plan for return from the surgery center and for follow-up care appointments.

Also help the patient establish a plan for modifying the home environment. For example, suggest placing needed articles at counter height to avoid use of low-level cabinets. Use of these lower cabinets would involve bending.

Patients may feel fatigued the first few days after surgery. If time permits, encourage the patient to prepare a few meals ahead and store them in the refrigerator or freezer.

Advise the patient to develop a mechanism for alerting a friend or neighbor that emergency assistance is needed. Have the patient place a list of emergency numbers near each telephone in the

---

Table 44–3

How To Clean the Eye and Apply an Eye Shield

CLEANING THE EYE

1. Obtain needed equipment: cotton balls, irrigating solution, small plastic bag.
2. Wash hands to prevent contamination of the eye.
3. Tell patient to close the eye to prevent injury.
4. Moisten cotton ball with irrigating solution.
5. Put on gloves to create a barrier against contact with secretions.
6. Using the moistened cotton ball to soften secretions, wipe from medial to lateral canthus one time. This moves secretions from a clean to a dirty area.
7. Dispose of cotton ball in plastic bag to limit exposure of others to secretions.
8. Repeat as needed.
9. Seal plastic bag to limit exposure of others to secretions.

APPLYING AN EYE SHIELD

1. Wash hands to prevent contamination of the eye.
2. Wipe patient's forehead and cheek with skin preparation to reduce skin irritation by creating a surface for tape to adhere.
3. Ask patient to close both eyes to relax the eyelids.
4. Apply patch or shield over closed eye, exerting slight pressure against the eyelid (see Fig. 44–11A).
5. Cover the patch or shield with pieces of overlapping tape to ensure even pressure against the eye (see Fig. 44–11B).
6. Apply tape from cheek to middle of forehead (see Fig. 44–11C).

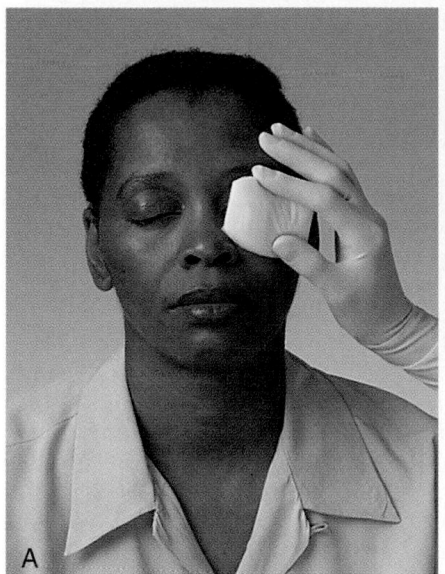
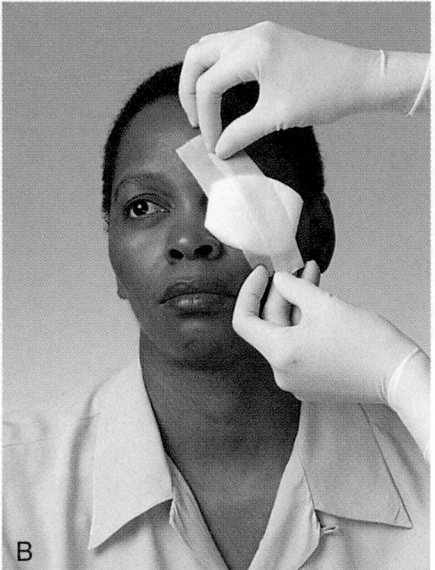
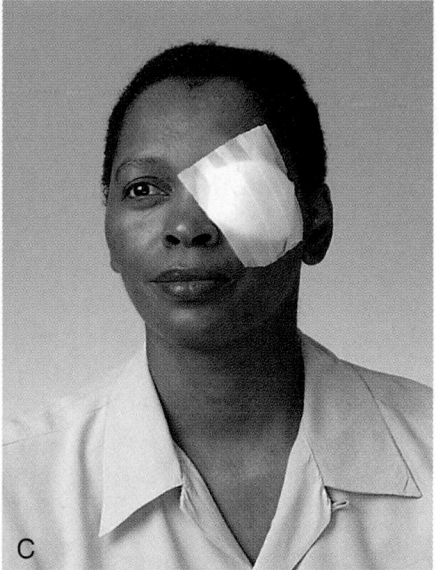

Figure 44-11

Application of an eye patch. *A*, Patch applied over closed eyelid. Note finger placement to avoid pressure on globe. *B*, Overlapping tape applied from cheek to forehead. *C*, Correctly applied patch. Note that cheek is pulled slightly upward.

house. If help is needed, having the numbers nearby speeds the process, and the patient does not need to rely on memory.

If activity restrictions imposed by surgery will create difficulty for the patient at home, assist with finding a source of home care. Temporary nursing agencies can provide in-home assistance with activities of daily living, including personal care and meal preparation. Determine whether these care-related expenses are covered by the patient's insurance plan, or whether she or he is able and willing to pay the cost as an out-of-pocket expense. Collaborate with a social worker as needed.

NDx: Risk for altered health maintenance

Often, patients are discharged with one or more types of eye drops. Make sure the patient knows the name and purpose of each medication, how often to use it, and in which eye. If medications have different frequencies of administration, alert the patient to this fact, and provide a written chart describing how often each is to be used. Teach the patient to instill the eye drops (see Table 44–2), and obtain a return demonstration to evaluate his or her technique. If the patient needs assistance with instilling eye drops, help identify who will instill them and train the caregiver as needed. Provide instruction in additional aspects of self-care as needed (Highlight 44–4).

Additional Interventions

Reassure the patient that some mild pain or pressure in the eye is normal. Encourage use of prescribed pain medication as needed. Report development of acute pain or severe pressure to the physician because these can indicate hemorrhage or other complications.

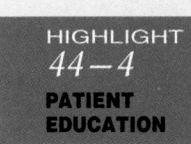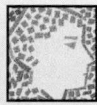

HIGHLIGHT 44–4
PATIENT EDUCATION

Discharge Instructions After Eye Surgery

Instruct the patient to:

Use strict aseptic technique when caring for the eye.

Change eye dressing and keep eye shield in place as per the physician's orders.

Use eye medication as directed. (Be certain that the patient knows the name, dose, route, frequency, and expected effect of all medications and can correctly instill topical ophthalmic preparations.)

Avoid activities that increase intraocular pressure: sudden, jarring movements; bending; coughing; sneezing; forceful nose blowing; and sexual intercourse.

Avoid straining at stool: drink at least 2000 mL of fluid daily (unless contraindicated), eat a high-fiber diet, and take stool softeners as ordered.

Wear dark glasses for photophobia.

Avoid use of eye makeup until otherwise instructed.

Report any increased pain, decreased vision, or purulent drainage.

Return for a follow-up visit on *(specify date)*.

If both eyes are patched, intervene to prevent sensory deprivation and a sense of social isolation. Investigate how much and what type of sensory stimulation the patient prefers. Play a radio, encourage visitors, arrange for a family member, friend, or volunteer to read to the patient, or the like. When interacting with the patient, provide sensory-related information. Describe the weather or make a comment about the time of day.

Compare the patient's status with the expected outcomes. If the outcomes are not met, reassess the patient and revise the plan.

Corneal Transplant

A corneal transplant, also known as a keratoplasty, is the surgical removal of a patient's cornea and replacement of it with a donor cornea.

Uses

Corneal transplants are done when a patient's vision is impaired because the cornea is clouded and opaque as a result of trauma, degeneration, or infection.

Donor Cornea

The cornea to be transplanted comes from a donor who died of an acute disease or accident and was free of infection and disease. Preferably, the donor is a young adult so that the cornea has a large number of endothelial cells. This increases the success rate of the transplant.

When a donor dies, the eyes are closed, and gauze pads wet with saline are placed over them along with a small ice pack. Within 2 to 4 hours, the eyes are enucleated. The cornea is usually transplanted within 24 to 48 hours, but technologic developments in preservation solutions make transplants possible up to 7 days after procurement. Corneas can also be frozen, dehydrated, or refrigerated for later transplantation.

Patient Preparation

Antibiotic eye drops are given preoperatively to reduce the chance of infection, and pilocarpine hydrochloride or another miotic is administered to flatten and elongate the iris. An oral sedative such as diazepam (Valium) may also be ordered.

Corneal transplant surgery does not usually require blood or tissue typing, because the cornea is avascular. It does not need its own blood or lymph supply because it receives nutrition externally from tears and internally from the aqueous humor.

In selected cases, a "tissue-matched" corneal transplant may be performed. Patients undergoing this procedure usually have rejected a previous corneal transplant.

Procedure

Corneal transplant surgery is usually performed under local anesthesia on an outpatient basis, or with an overnight hospital stay. It is done using general anesthesia if the patient cannot remain motionless, as with coexisting Parkinson's disease. Anesthesia is also used if medical problems, such as respiratory disease, prevent the patient from lying flat and breathing because, under general anesthesia, the patient can receive ventilation assistance from a ventilator.

Corneal transplantation is performed under the operating room microscope. The patient's cornea is measured to determine what size the graft should be. Next, the donor tissue is measured. Using an instrument that resembles a tiny cookie cutter, the predetermined size button of cornea is cut from the donor tissue. Once the donor tissue is ready, the same instrument is used to excise the diseased corneal tissue from the patient. The whole cornea is not removed. Rather, the central area through which light rays pass en route to the retina is removed.

The carefully measured donor button is then placed in the exact spot where the diseased cornea was removed, and the new and clear corneal tissue is carefully sutured in place. Subconjunctival injections of antibiotics are administered, and an antibiotic ointment is instilled. The eye is carefully closed, and an eye patch and shield are applied and secured with tape.

Postoperative Course

The eye patch and shield remain in place until the next morning, when they are removed by the surgeon. Diet and activity are resumed based on the patient's tolerance. Because the cornea is avascular, healing is very slow, and recovery of vision after corneal transplant surgery is not as rapid as after cataract surgery.

Complications

Rejection may occur after a corneal transplant, although the rate is relatively low because the cornea has neither a blood nor a lymph supply. When rejection does occur, the transplanted cornea becomes opaque. Episodes of rejection are treated with steroids, but a repeat keratoplasty may be required.

NURSING PROCESS GUIDELINES
Corneal Transplant

Nursing care of patients having corneal transplant surgery is similar to the nursing care of patients having any type of eye surgery, with the following considerations.

Corneal transplant surgery happens in a semi-urgent manner. When the patient, in consultation with the ophthalmologist, decides he or she wants and needs a corneal transplant, the person's name is placed on a waiting list. When tissue becomes available, the patient is notified by the ophthalmologist. Therefore, patients may not have much time to prepare psychologically for the upcoming surgery. Also stressful for some patients is the tissue donation and the fact that someone had to die to make the tissue available for transplantation. Thus, patients may be glad they are getting a second chance at sight, but may also feel sadness for someone else's loss.

If possible, offer the patient the opportunity to speak with another patient who has had corneal transplant surgery. These volunteers have a unique view of the procedure and how it has affected their lives. Eye Banks Association of America (E.B.A.A.) has a volunteer organization called the Ambassadors for Corneal Transplant. The local tissue bank may be able to supply a list of area representatives.

Remind the patient that recovery of vision following corneal transplant surgery is not as rapid as following cataract surgery, so that he or she is not discouraged when the patch is removed and the visual acuity is not a perfect 20/20. Reinforce the fact that the visual acuity the first day may not be an indicator of final visual outcome.

Postoperatively, instruct the patient in self-care as needed (Highlight 44–5).

Enucleation

Enucleation is the removal of the eyeball. It is done primarily in cases where trauma, severe glaucoma or infection have led to a blind, intractably painful eye not responsive to retrobulbar injection of alcohol for pain relief. Enucleation is also used in the treatment of malignant neoplasms of the eye or orbit, although other forms of treatment are becoming available to help preserve appearance and function (see Chap. 45).

When an enucleation is performed, the eye muscles are severed, the optic nerve is cut a short distance from where it exits the eye, and the globe is removed intact. A small round ball is inserted into the socket and covered with conjunctiva. A small cap, called a conformer, is placed between the lids to promote healing. It sometimes falls out on its own 1 or 2 weeks after the operation. Once healed, the socket is similar in appearance to the mucous membrane of the mouth.

A variation on this procedure is evisceration, in which the cornea and intraocular contents including the retina are removed. A ball of silicone or hydroxyapatite (sea coral) is inserted into the scleral shell, which is then sutured closed under the conjunctiva. Final appearance of the socket is similar to that following enucleation but, after healing occurs, a prosthesis with a tiny peg on the underside is

---

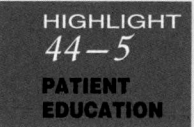 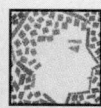

HIGHLIGHT 44–5
PATIENT EDUCATION

Self-Care After Corneal Transplant

Instruct the patient to:

Avoid restricted activities:

- Do not drive until given specific clearance by the ophthalmologist.
- Do not shower or wash hair unless shampooing can be done from behind, as in a beauty salon, so that no soapy or dirty water can come in contact with the eye.
- Do not lie on the operative side.
- Do not bend over from the waist because this increases intraocular pressure.
- Do not lift or carry more than 25 lb.
- Do not have sexual intercourse for 1 week after surgery.

Engage in unrestricted activities as desired: ride in a car, watch television, read, play cards, do close work, climb steps, take sponge or tub baths, carry less than 25 lb.

Instill prescribed antibiotic and steroid eye drops as directed in Table 44–2. Be certain to wait at least 5 minutes between different drops to promote maximum absorption.

Check vision daily in the eye that has had the corneal transplant.

Report any reduction in visual acuity immediately to the ophthalmologist because this is an early sign of infection and/or rejection.

Wear an eye shield at night to prevent rubbing or bumping the eye during sleep. Also wear the shield when engaging in activities such as playing with children or pets that might cause accidental injury.

Apply the eye shield as described in Table 44–3.

Expect some white or yellow-white drainage that appears as dry crustings on the eyelids or eyelashes and is most noticeable in the morning or after sleeping.

Remove the drainage as directed in Table 44–3. Notify the ophthalmologist if the drainage increases, has a foul odor, or is a color other than white or yellow-white.

Expect mild itching.

Report eye pain not relieved by acetaminophen (Tylenol) or accompanied by nausea or fever; seeing spots before the eyes; seeing bright flashes of light or a curtain coming in from the side or obstructing part of the visual field; or any change in visual acuity.

Return for follow-up care the day after surgery and then as scheduled.

fitted into a hole in the ball and, thus, the prosthesis can move in tandem with the unaffected eye by means of the still-attached extraocular muscles (Kostick & Linberg, 1995).

NURSING PROCESS GUIDELINES
Enucleation

Recognize that different patients will react differently to this disfiguring surgery. Those already blind and in severe pain are likely to have feelings of relief mixed with some anxiety about appearance. Symptom-free patients with a malignancy are likely to be highly anxious and very distressed from the diagnosis of cancer as well as the loss of vision and surgical disfigurement. Allow all patients the opportunity to verbalize feelings and acknowledge all patients' need to grieve the loss of the eye. Stress that grieving is normal and that grief work is a process that takes time to complete. Reassure the patient that ocular prostheses can make cosmetic appearance close to normal. Explain that prostheses are usually custom-designed and painted, and are fitted about 4 to 6 weeks after surgery. Show the patient a picture of a person with an ocular prosthesis to demonstrate this point. If the patient is concerned about appearance before the prosthesis is fitted, suggest wearing sunglasses. Provide an opportunity for

---

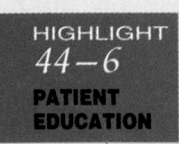 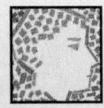

HIGHLIGHT
44–6
PATIENT EDUCATION

Removal, Care, and Insertion of an Ocular Prosthesis

Instruct the patient in the removal, care, and insertion of an ocular prosthesis as described here.

Removal of an Ocular Prosthesis

1. Gather equipment: container with lid.
2. Wash hands to reduce surface microorganisms.
3. Sit up and flex chin slightly for easy removal.
4. Place hand against cheek, palm side up (Fig. 44–12A) to create a platform for the prosthesis to rest on when removed.
5. Pull lower lid slightly down and (Fig. 44–12B) toward ear to extend surface area for easy prosthesis removal.
6. Allow prosthesis to slide out onto fingers and then grasp (Fig. 44–12C).
7. Exert gentle pull if needed.
8. Place prosthesis in container and cover for protection.

Care of an Ocular Prosthesis

1. Gather equipment: clean container with lid, mild soap, towel, and container.
2. Wash hands to reduce surface microorganisms.
3. Drape area with cloth or towel to act as a cushion for the prosthesis should it be dropped.
4. Close sink drain to prevent loss of prosthesis.
5. Rinse prosthesis with tepid tap water to remove secretions.
6. Put prosthesis in palm of nondominant hand for cleaning.
7. Rub small amount of mild soap over prosthesis with finger pad to reduce surface tension and ease removal of secretions.
8. Use tepid water to rinse soap residue from prosthesis because extreme temperatures can shatter prosthesis.
9. Check prosthesis for surface deposits or scratches, which can irritate lids.
10. Place prosthesis in container cushioned with a gauze pad for safe storage.

Insertion of an Ocular Prosthesis

1. Wash hands to reduce surface microorganisms.
2. Drape towel over work area to protect prosthesis should it be dropped.
3. Take prosthesis from container and rinse with tepid water.
4. Raise upper lid against eyebrow using nondominant hand (Fig 44–12E) to fully expose socket.
5. Place prosthesis between thumb and forefinger of dominant hand with the notched end of prosthesis closest to nose.
6. Slide the prosthesis under the upper lid until most of iris is covered (Fig. 44–12F).
7. Slowly release upper eyelid.
8. Retract lower lid down toward cheek until bottom edge of prosthesis slips underneath it (Fig. 44–12G) to permit entrance of bottom edge of prosthesis into socket itself.
9. Release hands slowly.

Note: When the nurse is removing, cleaning, or inserting an ocular prosthesis for a patient, the procedure is explained to reduce anxiety and promote cooperation; nonsterile gloves are worn to create a barrier against contact with secretions; and the prosthesis is stored in a container labeled with the patient's name.

meeting another person who has had an enucleation if the patient so desires.

Instruct the patient with an enucleation on extra precautions to take to minimize the potential for injury to the remaining eye (see Highlight 44–1). Stress the importance of protective eyewear and keep in mind that some patients may be encouraged to wear eyeglasses, even if no visual correction is needed in the seeing eye, because the clear lenses provide added protection against flying debris, dust, and dirt.

Initiate a referral to a home-care agency for assistance with removing, cleaning, and inserting the prosthesis (Highlight 44–6 and Fig. 44–12).

Laser Therapy

The argon laser is used as a noninvasive, outpatient treatment for such problems as flat tears in the retina, proliferative vascular diseases such as diabetic retinopathy, sickle cell anemia hemoglobinopathy, age-related macular degeneration (ARMD), and glaucoma. During the procedure, the patient sits with the head stabilized in the slit-lamp frame. The pupil is dilated with topical cycloplegics, and anesthetic drops are instilled. A Goldmann lens is then placed on the cornea and the laser treatment administered. The eye is irrigated to remove the viscous lens lubricant, and an eye patch is applied according

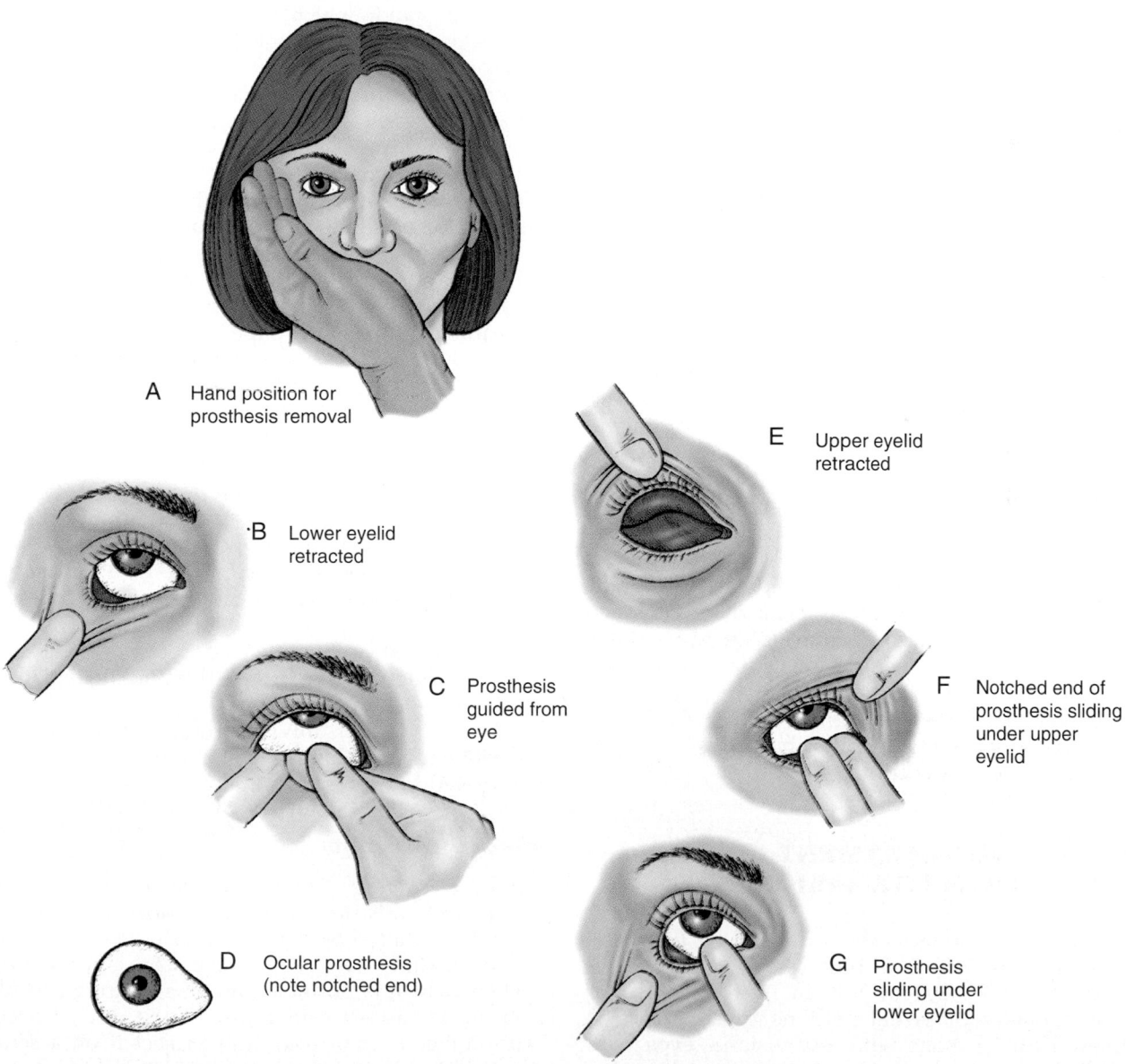

A Hand position for prosthesis removal

B Lower eyelid retracted

C Prosthesis guided from eye

D Ocular prosthesis (note notched end)

E Upper eyelid retracted

F Notched end of prosthesis sliding under upper eyelid

G Prosthesis sliding under lower eyelid

Figure 44–12

Removal (*A through C*) and insertion (*E through G*) of an ocular prosthesis (*D*).

to the preference of the physician. Most patients have no restrictions on activity following the procedure.

The Nd:YAG laser, a photo disrupter laser, is used to lyse vitreous strands or to open the posterior capsule. The procedure is similar to the one just described, except that a Peyman lens is used to lyse vitreous strands, and neither anesthetic nor lens is required for opening the posterior capsule.

Lasers should always be used in a closed room and aimed away from the doorway. On the outside of the door should be a sign indicating that a laser is in use. Persons in the room with the patient during laser therapy should wear protective eyewear specifically designed for the type of laser in use. The number of persons in the room should be restricted to limit the number who could be injured should the laser be misdirected or deflected.

NURSING PROCESS GUIDELINES
Laser Therapy for an Eye Disorder

Before the procedure, obtain baseline vital signs and intraocular pressure and assess and document visual acuity.

Describe to the patient what will be seen and heard during the procedure. Explain that staff members will be wearing protective eyewear. Describe the bright light of the laser and the clicking of the machine as each laser spot is delivered. Reassure the patient that most people do not feel anything because a local or topical anesthetic is used. Stress the importance of focusing on the object placed in the line of vision as directed and not looking elsewhere without consulting the ophthalmologist.

Advise the patient of the potential for corneal injury until the anesthetic wears off. Caution the patient not to rub or bump the eye.

If a short course of topical steroids, such as prednisolone acetate (Pred Mild), is prescribed to reduce the inflammation that sometimes accompanies laser therapy, instruct the patient on how, when, and why to use the drops.

Remember that before the patient leaves the facility, intraocular pressure must be rechecked to be sure no increase has occurred.

SUPPORTIVE TREATMENT FOR THE PATIENT WITH LOW VISION

Low vision (legal blindness) is defined by the Internal Revenue Service as a best corrected central visual acuity of 20/200 or less in the better eye or widest diameter of visual field no greater than 20 degrees. Thus, persons with low vision—even with the help of corrective eyeglasses or contact lenses—have difficulty reading newspaper type, a sign on a bus, labels on canned goods, or recognizing friends in the street. In adults, low vision is commonly associated with macular degeneration, glaucoma, diabetic retinopathy, or cataracts.

Supportive care focuses on enhancing remaining vision to maintain maximum function and quality of life. This is accomplished through the use of optical and nonoptical vision aids and modifications in the home and work environment.

Optical Aids

The simplest types of optical aid are hand-held nonprescription magnifying glasses. Of these, the small half-dollar–size lens is most effective in that it gives the clearest image. It works well for reading small areas of fine print, such as price tags and entries in telephone books. It can easily be carried in the pocket or on a cord around the neck. Magnifiers on a circular stand, which can be easily moved across the page, are convenient and useful for reading newspapers and books.

Available prescription aids include telescopes, prisms, and microscopes. Hand-held monocular telescopes with prescription lenses designed to boost vision in the better eye can be used for seeing street signs and looking for traffic. They can be focused and can be easily carried or worn around the neck. Another type of telescope is a jeweler's loupe, which can be clipped to the top rim of glasses and used for such tasks as seeing where to sign a document or reading numbers on paper currency. A full-diameter telescope set in an eyeglass frame is also available. This can be worn only when sitting still but is valuable for such activities as watching television or attending a play.

A bioptic telescope mounted in the top part of regular eyeglasses can provide acuity of distance vision while the lower lens provides normal distance judgment. In some states, persons with low vision can obtain a driver's license if use of a bioptic telescope can provide a visual acuity meeting the state's standards.

Prisms that are pressed onto eyeglasses can be used to widen a constricted peripheral field of vision.

For near vision only, microscopic spectacles can be obtained with high-power magnifying lenses incorporated into prescription eyeglasses.

Electronic Aids

An ever-growing number of electronic vision enhancement aids are available. Most of these are magnifiers that project print onto a screen enlarged up to 60 times its original size. One such enlarger system, which is portable and small enough to fit in a briefcase, uses a camera about the size of a cigarette lighter to scan print and project it on a screen. Another is designed to enlarge and project print onto a screen as it is typed, enabling a low-vision person to proofread and make corrections.

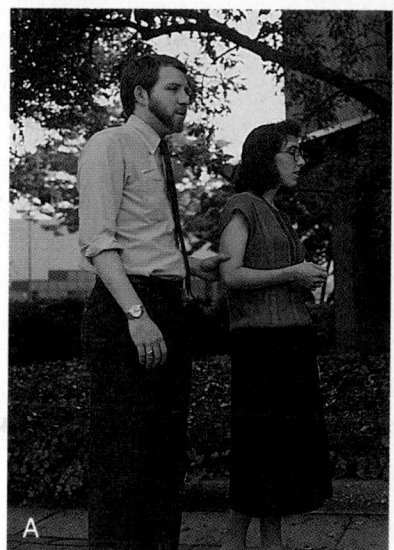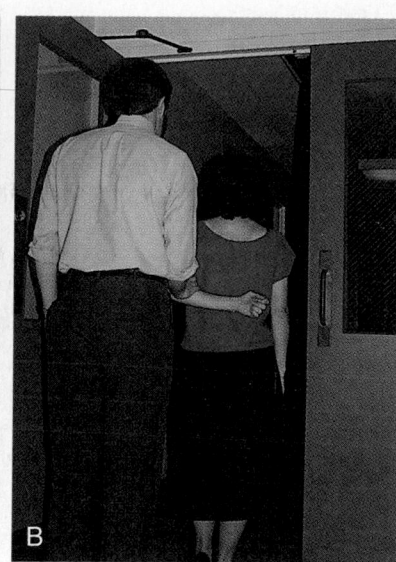

Figure 44–13

A, When escorting a visually disabled person, allow him or her to grasp your upper arm as shown. *B,* When approaching a narrow passage, bring your arm behind your back to alert the visually disabled person. (Courtesy of Cleveland Society for the Blind.)

Also available are devices called optical-to-tactile converters. These devices produce a raised outline of printed letters on a "tactile screen" by adjusting the levels of tiny rods. The letters are then read by touch. A more complex device is the Reading Machine, which uses a computer and a voice synthesizer to read printed materials aloud.

Nonoptical Accessory Aids

Many nonoptical aids can be used to enhance the ability of low-vision patients to perform routine activities. For example, to facilitate reading, a clear sheet of yellow plastic can be placed over the page to decrease glare and make print darker. A small pointer can be used to direct focus to one word at a time. Large-print materials, such as the *New York Times* or *Reader's Digest* large-print editions and the Doubleday Large Print Home Library, increase access to news, best sellers, and how-to information.

To help low-vision patients write checks or fill out other documents, an overlay can be made of dark plastic or construction paper with spaces cut out that correspond to areas that need to be filled in. Similarly, dials with enlarged or raised markings are available for stoves, and there are push-button telephones with extra-large, raised, palpable numbers.

Not all aids are needed by or work well for all people. A major factor that influences their selection is the person's specific goals. Some people want to see street signs. Others want to read a menu. Still others want to be able to type. Another factor is the person's physical capability. Can the person hold a large magnifying glass or support the frame of a telescopic aid on the nose? Yet another factor is the person's acceptance of the aid, since some aids have

a rather unusual appearance. Because many optical aids are not covered by insurance, cost is yet another factor.

Some clinics that specialize in caring for people with low vision facilitate the selection process by lending the patient aids for trial use. Others have simulated environments, such as kitchens and offices, where the patient can learn to use a particular aid.

For persons whose visual impairment exceeds that which can be accommodated by these aids, other types of support are available.

Braille is a system of raised dots representing letters and numbers that are identified or "read" by the fingers. This system is taught by agencies for the blind and other educational institutions. A large variety of materials are available in braille, including books, magazines, playing cards, medical equipment, and various household goods.

To facilitate mobility, patients can use the traditional white cane with a red tip. Another option is the newer laser cane, which can locate obstacles and changes in terrain from up to 20 feet away. Some patients use a guide dog to help navigate and travel. These aids have the secondary purpose of identifying people who may need assistance. When helping a visually disabled person to ambulate, offer your arm for the person to grasp (Fig. 44–13). Table 44–4 offers more guidelines for helping a visually disabled person.

❖ Settings, Providers, and Collaboration for Care

Patients with ophthalmic problems can receive care in a variety of settings. As outpatients, they are examined in physicians' offices, outpatient clinics, and

Table 44–4

Helping a Visually Disabled Person

- Ask if the person would like assistance. If it is needed, most will appreciate the offer. It is better to offer than not.
- When entering a room, announce your presence. State the reason for the visit. Let the person know when you are leaving.
- If speaking to a visually disabled person when others are present, refer to all persons by name. That way, the person knows for whom the greeting is meant. Visually disabled people cannot tell when you are looking at them.
- Avoid pointing, nodding, or shrugging gestures, and terms such as "over there." Remember that visually disabled people are comfortable with language such as "look," "see," and "blind."
- When speaking with a visually disabled person, use a normal, conversational tone. Visually disabled people are not necessarily hearing impaired. Do not shout.
- If a visually disabled person travels with a guide dog, resist the temptation to call or pet the animal, unless given permission. Remember that the animal is there to enhance the safety of the visually disabled person. Any distraction can jeopardize the person's safety.
- When escorting a visually disabled person, allow him or her to grasp your upper arm as demonstrated in Figure 44–13A. Stay one step ahead, and alert the person to changes in terrain and obstacles in the path. If walking near a curb, walk next to the curb. If approaching a narrow passage, bring your arm behind the back. This change alerts the visually disabled person to the narrow door opening (Fig. 44–13B).
- Orient any visually disabled person to the environment before leaving him or her alone. Use one piece of furniture in the room as a reference point, and give directions from it. For example, "There is a chair directly in front of you. To its left is a table." Allow the visually disabled person to put his or her hand on the back of the chair. This action provides reassurance as to its location. Remove hazards, such as throw rugs, footstools, and wastebaskets, because the person might trip in an unfamiliar environment.
- When helping a visually disabled person into a car, check the seat and guide the person's hand onto the door handle. The person will be able to finish the process. If the person travels with a guide dog, allow him or her to settle the dog into the car.
- Describe the table setting and any food in detail. Use the hours of the clock as a guide. For example: "There is roast beef at 6 o'clock. The potatoes are at 3 o'clock. A glass of milk is located just above the spoon."
- When handing money to a visually disabled person, announce its denomination. Most visually disabled people have a system for sorting money.
- Once the person has placed an object, do not move it unless consent is given. Visually disabled persons cannot find things if they are moved.

Adapted with permission from When you meet a blind person. Cleveland, OH: Cleveland Sight Center of the Cleveland Society for the Blind, 1989.

specialty walk-in centers. If patients require surgery, it can be performed in a general hospital, a free-standing surgicenter or a specialty center. Today, most ophthalmic procedures can be done on an ambulatory basis.

A variety of ophthalmic providers may be enlisted to care for patients with ocular dysfunction. In addition to nurses, these providers include ophthalmologists, optometrists, opticians, ophthalmic medical personnel, ophthalmic surgical assistants, certified orthoptists, ophthalmic photographers, ocularists, and ultrasonographers.

An ophthalmologist is a licensed physician who specializes in the diagnosis and treatment of diseases of the eye and the visual system. The ophthalmologist has 3 or more years of specialized medical training and clinical experience in eye care. This is the only ophthalmic provider who can deliver total eye care (medical and surgical as well as contact lenses and other vision services) and also diagnose other medical disorders.

Optometrists are licensed individuals who have not attended medical school but are educated to examine the eyes and determine if visual problems exist. They assess visual acuity and prescribe corrective spectacles, contact lenses, and exercises. Opticians make lenses, frames, and other optical devices and/or contact lenses upon prescription. They determine the lens form best suited to the wearer's needs and also adjust, replace, and repair lenses, frames, and other ophthalmic devices.

Ophthalmic medical personnel include three levels of providers: ophthalmic assistant, ophthalmic technician, and ophthalmic technologist. These providers—who represent the basic, intermediate, and highest levels of qualification respectively—are not licensed or certified as independent practitioners. They function as assistants to the ophthalmologists with whom they work. Their assigned responsibilities may include history-taking and administration of various ophthalmic tests. They do not generate medical or surgical diagnoses, or prescriptions.

Orthoptists are certified by the American Orthoptic Council and assist ophthalmologists in assessing and caring for people with disorders of ocular movement. Orthoptists may also direct patients in ocular exercises.

Ophthalmic photographers and ultrasonographers assist in diagnosing eye disorders. Ophthalmic photographers are specially trained to take pictures of both the anterior and posterior chambers of the eye. Ophthalmic ultrasonographers use high-frequency sound waves that are reflected by the ocular tissues to visualize internal structures of the eye and orbit on a screen. Ocularists are technicians who make ophthalmic prostheses (artificial eyes).

Through patient and family teaching, nurses play a major role in the prevention of visual impairment and blindness. Nurses also provide direct care to patients with ophthalmic disorders. To fulfill these roles effectively, nurses must collaborate with the various ophthalmic care providers and must coordinate care delivered through a variety of settings.

The Elderly: Special Considerations

As a person ages, changes occur in accessory structures of the eye, in structures of the eyeball itself, and in vision.

The skin in the orbital area darkens slightly and crow's feet develop at the periphery of the outer canthus as a person ages. Muscle tone and elasticity in the eyelids diminish, and this may lead to drooping of the upper lids and pouches under the lower lid. Xanthelasma, a collection of benign yellow nodules of lipid deposits, is common on the medial aspects of both the upper and the lower lids, especially in people with hypercholesterolemia.

An opaque white or gray ring may be seen around the iris. This is called arcus senilis and results from hyaline degeneration or lipid deposits in the cornea. The pupil becomes progressively smaller, a condition known as senile miosis. The lens yellows, becomes less transparent, and loses elasticity. Vitreous floaters are common. Retinal blood vessels appear slightly narrowed and irregular. The optic disk shrinks in diameter. If macular degeneration, a common disease of older adulthood, occurs, the macula will be broken or thinned.

As the pupil becomes smaller, less light reaches the retina so that up to three times as much light is needed for routine activities. At the same time, increasing opacity of the lens scatters light rays and increases the person's sensitivity to glare. Inelasticity of the lens causes loss of accommodation. As a consequence of these changes, older adults experience difficulty seeing near objects (presbyopia).

As the lens yellows with age, color vision changes. Discrimination of low tone colors, such as blues, greens, and violets, becomes difficult. Other age-related vision changes include narrowed peripheral vision and increased time needed to adapt to darkness.

Chapter Review

1. What are the similarities and differences between the aqueous humor and the vitreous humor?
2. What is the mechanism by which visual stimuli from the left side of the visual fields are interpreted by the right side of the brain and vice versa?
3. How do scotomata differ from floaters?
4. What types of visual acuity testing are done on patients unable to read an eye chart?
5. What tests and findings are implied by the documentation of PERRLA on a patient's record?
6. How does the direct response of the pupil to light differ from the consensual response?
7. How would you help a patient who must avoid actions that increase intraocular pressure plan for self care?
8. How would wearing an eye shield affect a patient's ability to carry out usual daily activities?
9. How would the specific plan of care for a patient having a corneal transplant differ from a general plan of care for patients having eye surgery?
10. What instructions for self care should be given to a patient following ocular laser therapy?

Bibliography

Albert DM. Source book of ophthalmology. Cambridge, MA: Blackwell Scientific, 1995.

Albert DM, Jakobeic FA. Principles and practice of ophthalmology. Philadelphia: WB Saunders, 1994.

Bankes JL. Clinical ophthalmology: A text and colour atlas. 3rd ed. Edinburgh: Churchill Livingstone, 1994.

Bartlett J, Ghormley N, Jaanus S, et al. Ophthalmic drug facts. St. Louis: Facts & Comparisons, 1992.

Booth B. Information nurses need to tell patients about glaucoma. Nurs Times 1994; 90(May 11–17):39.

Carr L, Talley D. Complications of anterior segment laser procedures. Optom Clin 1995; 4:33.

Crick RP, Khaw P. Textbook of clinical ophthalmology. 2nd ed. River Edge, NJ: World Scientific, 1995.

Dornic D. Ophthalmic pocket companion. 4th ed. Woburn, MA: Butterworth-Heinemann, 1995.

Farkas P. Integrating disposable or planned replacement lenses into contact lens practice. Optom Clin 1994; 4:61.

Fishbaugh J. Focus. Nursing care of the patient with cornea graft rejection. Insight 1995; 20(4):34.

Fishbaugh J. Observations of subspecialties. Retina: indocyanine green (ICG) angiography. Insight 1994; 19(3):30.

Fraunfelder FT, Roy FH. Current ocular therapy 4. Philadelphia: WB Saunders, 1995.

Hunt L. Complications of indirect laser photocoagulation. Insight 1994; 19(Dec):24.

Irvin SM. Identification of potential problems for elderly outpatients after preoperative medication: A case study. J Post Anesth Nurs 1995; 10(Jun):159.

Jalkh AE, Celorio JM. Atlas of fluorescein angiography. Philadelphia: WB Saunders, 1993.

Kanski J. Clinical ophthalmology: A systematic approach. 3rd ed. Woburn, MA: Butterworth-Heinemann, 1994.

Kelly M. Consequences of visual impairment on leisure activities of the elderly. Geriatr Nurs 1995; 16(Nov–Dec):273.

Kostick D, Linberg J. Evisceration with hydroxyapatite implant. Ophthalmology 1995; 102(10):1542.

Medical Economics Staff. Physicians' desk reference for ophthalmology. 25th ed. Montvale, NJ: Medical Economics, 1996.

Murray PI, Fielder AR. Pocket book of ophthalmology. Woburn, MA: Butterworth-Heinemann, 1996.

Newell F. Ophthalmology: Principles and concepts. 8th ed. St. Louis: Mosby-Year Book, 1996.

Lindquist TD, Lindstrom RL. Ophthalmic surgery update #4. St. Louis: Mosby-Year Book, 1996.

Pavan-Langston D (ed). Manual of ocular diagnosis and therapy. Boston: Little, Brown, 1996.

Peralta L, Adame H. Corneal transplant: A new lease on life. Semin Perioper Nurs 1995; 4(Oct):227.

Perry JC. Care of the ophthalmic patient. 2nd ed. San Diego: Singular Publishing, 1995.

Ready R. Commentary on sports-related eye trauma. ENAs Nurs Scan Emerg Care 1994; 4(Mar–Apr):10.

Rosenthal BP, Cole RG. Functional assessment of low vision. St. Louis: Mosby-Year Book, 1995.

Sandler RL. Glaucoma. Am J Nurs 1995; 95(3):34.

Small RG. The clinical handbook of ophthalmology. London: Parthenon, 1994.

Tasman W, Jaeger EA (eds). The Wills Eye Hospital atlas of clinical ophthalmology. Philadelphia: Lippincott-Raven, 1995.

Taylor RH. Key topics in ophthalmology. Philadelphia: Coronet Books, 1995.

Vaughan D, Asbury T, Riordan-Eva P. General ophthalmology. 4th ed. Los Angeles: Lange, 1995.

Year book of opthalmology. St. Louis: Mosby-Year Book, 1996.

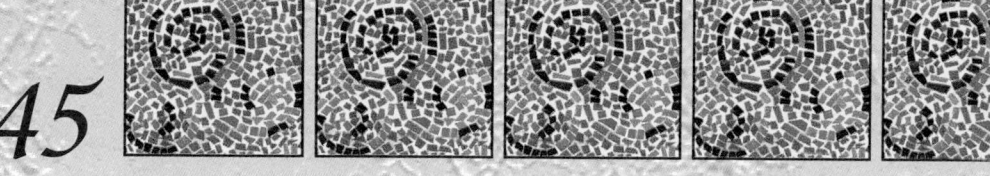

45

Nursing Care of Patients with Eye Disorders

Study Outcomes

After studying this chapter, you should be able to:

1. Describe the etiology, pathophysiology, clinical manifestations, diagnostic procedures, and medical management of common eye disorders.
2. Identify information and physical examination data essential to the assessment of patients with common eye disorders.
3. State nursing diagnoses and related expected patient outcomes commonly applicable to patients with eye disorders.
4. Describe nursing interventions, with their rationales, commonly applicable to patients with eye disorders.
5. Explain the basis for evaluation of nursing care provided to patients with common eye disorders.
6. Identify special considerations for the elderly patient with an eye disorder.

Ophthalmic disorders and ocular manifestations of systemic disease can occur suddenly or evolve over time. Regardless of onset, any threat to a patient's vision is accompanied by the common experience of fear—fear of losing vision or being unable to regain it. To care for these patients appropriately, the nurse needs sensitivity and empathy in addition to sound clinical understanding.

*I*nfections and Inflammations

CONJUNCTIVITIS

Etiology and Pathophysiology

An inflammation or infection of the conjunctiva is called conjunctivitis. The bulbar conjunctiva, which covers the eyeball and is partially exposed to the environment, is prone to inflammation from allergens and irritants, as well as infection from bacteria and viruses. The palpebral conjunctiva, which lines the eyelids, is susceptible to infection because of its close proximity to the eyelashes.

Allergic conjunctivitis occurs after repeated exposure to such allergens as pollen and grass, or from such irritants as smoke and chemicals. When such an irritant is encountered by a previously exposed patient, histamine and other inflammatory mediators are released. Histamine-sensitive blood vessels are stimulated, and vasodilation occurs. These blood vessels can leak fluid, causing tissue edema. Allergic conjunctivitis may be seasonal in occurrence.

Bacterial conjunctivitis results most often from gram-positive or gram-negative bacteria, such as *Pneumococcus*, *Staphylococcus*, *Neisseria gonorrhoeae*, and *Streptococcus*. Bacterial conjunctivitis is also referred to as pink eye, and is highly communicable. It usually begins in one eye but may be transmitted to the other eye by accidental contamination.

Clinical Manifestations

Common symptoms of conjunctivitis include itching, burning, photophobia, and the sensation of a foreign body in the eye. Ptosis, exudation or drainage, hyperemia (increased prominence of conjunctival blood vessels), and chemosis (conjunctival edema) may be evident. The texture of the conjunctiva becomes uneven and irregular, with follicles and exudate noted (Fig. 45–1).

Specific types of conjunctivitis have key characteristics. In allergic conjunctivitis, itching is the primary symptom. It is accompanied by a smooth conjunctiva, tearing, and bilateral redness. Bacterial conjunctivitis, on the other hand, presents with marked hyperemia, mild conjunctival edema, and epiphora (persistent overflow of tears). Discharge is initially watery but progresses to a purulent state.

Diagnosis

A complete history is obtained to check for recent exposure to bacteria, viruses, or allergens. Swabs or scrapings of the conjunctiva and cornea may be taken to assist in identifying a causative organism.

Management

Management depends on the cause of the conjunctivitis. Allergic conjunctivitis is treated by topical instillation of various ophthalmic eye drops. These include corticosteroid eye drops such as prednisolone

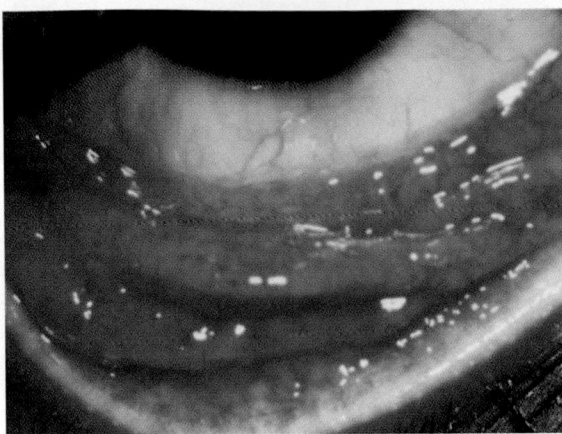

Figure 45–1

Adult follicular conjunctivitis with a mucopurulent discharge. (From Albert DM, Jakobiec FA [eds]. Atlas of clinical ophthalmology. Philadelphia: WB Saunders, 1996, p 62.)

acetate (Econopred Plus), vasoconstrictors for short-term use, and such antiallergy drugs as sodium cromoglycate (cromolyn sodium) and levocarbastine (Livostin), an H_1 antagonist that inhibits release of histamine.

Bacterial conjunctivitis is treated with antibiotics appropriate for the organism. Patients are started on a broad-spectrum antibiotic as soon as cultures are taken. Once the microorganism is identified, the antibiotic is changed if needed.

NURSING PROCESS
Conjunctivitis

Assessment

The assessment of a patient with conjunctivitis begins with a detailed history. Carefully note complaints of itchy, watery eyes, foreign body sensation, photophobia, drainage, or a change in vision. Ask the patient about use of contact lenses and lens solutions. Also ask about sensitivity to pollen, dust, feathers, foods, materials, cosmetics, and drugs. Note any systemic disease, such as asthma or sexually transmitted disease. Have the patient document any recent exposure to such irritants as smoke, tobacco, or noxious chemicals. Ask about previous episodes of similar symptoms and, if acknowledged, whether they are seasonal. Inquire about recent travel to dry climates and places with poor hygiene. Determine whether the patient uses cosmetics or borrows them from others.

After taking the history, examine the patient's eyes. Test visual acuity. Note whether the patient squints or tries to keep the eyes closed because of photophobia. Observe for drainage in the eyes or on the eyelashes. Note the amount, color, and character (clear, white, purulent, ropelike, or patchy). Check eyelid position, keeping in mind that the upper eyelid should rest at the superior limbus, where the cornea and sclera meet. Inspect the bulbar conjunc-

tiva for abnormally prominent blood vessels, a pink overcast to the sclera, as is common in pink eye, and edema. Remember that the bulbar conjunctiva is normally smooth and flat. Expose the palpebral conjunctiva by gently pulling the eyelid down against the cheekbone. Look for deviations from its normal flat, smooth, pale-pink appearance. For example, it may be beefy red with an irregular, or cobblestone, texture.

Nursing Diagnoses and Planning

Nursing diagnoses and related expected patient outcomes commonly applicable to the patient with conjunctivitis include the following:

NDx: Pain related to the inflammatory process

Planning: Patient Outcomes
1. Patient denies photophobia.
2. Patient reports relief of pain and itching.

NDx: Risk for altered health maintenance related to insufficient knowledge of cause, prevention of recurrence, spread of conjunctivitis

Planning: Patient Outcomes
1. Patient lists causes of conjunctivitis.
2. Patient describes measures to prevent recurrence.
3. Patient describes measures to prevent spread of bacterial conjunctivitis.

Nursing Interventions and Evaluation

NDx: Pain
Instruct the patient in the use of comfort measures to reduce pain and itching. These include cool compresses and refrigerating eye drop medications, so the medication is cool when instilled.

Instruct the patient to reduce the effects of photophobia by wearing sunglasses or a wide-brimmed hat, and using window shades. To prevent rubbing the eye, assist the patient to identify a substitute activity, such as scratching the cheek. Urge the patient to perform the substitute activity in response to an overwhelming urge to rub the eye.

Encourage the patient to avoid perfumed soaps and makeup because these contain chemicals that may cause itching. Provide information on available hypoallergenic soaps and cosmetics.

NDx: Risk for altered health maintenance
Explain the causes of conjunctivitis to the patient. Instruct the patient in how to prevent transmission and recurrence of the conjunctivitis (Highlight 45–1).

Compare the patient's status with the expected outcomes. If the outcomes are not met, reassess the patient and revise the plan.

KERATITIS

Etiology and Pathophysiology

Keratitis is an inflammation or infection of the cornea. If a microorganism is involved, it may also be referred to as a corneal ulcer. Keratitis can be caused by exposure to the environment or by such microor-

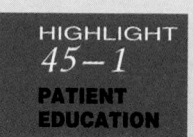
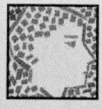

ganisms as bacteria, fungi, viruses, and amoebae. Exposure keratitis can develop when the eye fails to close completely, such as after a cerebrovascular accident or in cases of Bell's palsy or exophthalmos. Because of incomplete closure, the cornea obtains insufficient moisture and develops multiple small areas of breakdown in the epithelium.

Microbial infection can occur when corneal integrity is disturbed by trauma, surgery, or injury from chemicals or mechanical forces. If microorganisms invade only the superficial layers of the cornea, complete healing is possible. However, if infection spreads deep into the stroma and endothelium, scar tissue may form. If extensive scarring results, a corneal transplant may be necessary to restore clarity.

Herpes simplex keratitis, caused by herpes simplex virus 1, is a major cause of corneal ulceration. This form of keratitis is normally self-limiting, but in the immunocompromised patient, such as the person receiving radiation or chemotherapy, it can invade the stroma and cause opacities.

Clinical Manifestations

Clinical manifestations vary with the causative factor. A dry, scratchy, foreign-body sensation develops with exposure keratitis. Exposed areas of the conjunctiva are red and swollen, with small erosions on the lower third to half of the cornea. Symptoms of bacterial keratitis include epiphora, reduced visual acuity, photophobia, iridescent vision, and, fre-

quently, a mucopurulent discharge. Ocular pain and hypopyon (a collection of purulent material in the anterior chamber) may also be present.

Diagnosis

A history of any recent ocular injury, surgery, abrasions, or exposure to viruses is obtained, and baseline visual acuity is assessed. Scrapings of observable lesions or corneal swabs of drainage are obtained and cultured. Slit-lamp examination is done after a topical dye, such as fluorescein, is instilled to highlight areas of nonintact corneal epithelium.

Management

Management depends on the specific cause of the keratitis or ulcer. Exposure keratitis is treated with an ocular lubricant ointment (HypoTears ointment, Lacri-Lube S.O.P., Refresh P.M.) composed of petrolatum, lanolin, and mineral oil. These products melt and are spread by the tear film over the external eye and thus decrease ocular dryness. If ocular lubrication is still insufficient, an eye patch may be applied to help the eyelid protect the cornea. Soft contact lenses may be tried to protect the eye and to decrease the irritative force of the eyelid against the cornea. If these measures are insufficient, the eyelid may be sutured closed.

Microbial keratitis is treated with an anti-infective to which the microorganism is sensitive. For patients with known or suspected cases of bacterial keratitis, broad-spectrum antibiotics, such as fortified cefazolin (Ancef), tobramycin (Tobrex), or gentamicin (Genoptic), are prescribed until the exact causative organism is determined.

Severity of the ulcer determines the frequency of eye drop instillation and location of patient care. The presence of large or deep corneal ulcers requires one or two eye drops to be administered on an hourly schedule, with each eye drop's instillation time evenly spaced. For instance, if fortified cefazolin (Ancef) and gentamicin (Genoptic) are each ordered every hour, one is administered on the hour and the other on the half-hour.

Herpes simplex virus 1 infections are treated with antiviral agents such as idoxuridine (Stoxil), vidarabine (Vira-A), trifluridine (Viroptic), and acyclovir (Zovirax). Corticosteroids must be avoided because their immunosuppressive ability enhances activity of the virus and places the patient at risk for secondary infection.

NURSING PROCESS
Keratitis

Assessment

Begin assessment of a patient with known or suspected keratitis or corneal ulcer with a detailed history. Ask what led the patient to seek treatment (a red or painful eye, a severe foreign-body feeling, drainage, or something else). Determine when the problem started, whether it has gotten worse, and what treatments have been tried, such as over-the-counter eye drops or ointments. Inquire about other problems, such as photophobia, epiphora, change in vision, and ocular drainage. Do not limit the discussion to eye problems because viral keratitis can cause skin eruptions, severe pain, and flulike symptoms. Have the patient describe pain on a scale of 1 to 10, because the level of pain experienced may be disproportionate to symptoms demonstrated. If the patient wears contact lenses, ask about lens-care practices. Use of homemade saline or hydrogen peroxide lens cleaning solutions may be contributing factors in the development of *Acanthamoeba* keratitis.

Carefully explore any travel to developing countries or areas where contact with contaminated water may have occurred. Also note any recent ocular injury, trauma, or minor abrasion. Remember that patients may try to downplay or deny an injury, thinking it too minor to mention.

Review medications the patient is currently using, and note the use of oral or topical steroids.

Assess visual acuity and ask whether any recent changes have been noticed. Note the amount and color of any drainage present.

Nursing Diagnoses and Planning

Nursing diagnoses and related expected patient outcomes commonly applicable to patients with keratitis or a corneal ulcer include the following:

NDx: Sensory/perceptual alterations (visual) related to impaired corneal transparency

Planning: Patient Outcomes
1. Patient demonstrates techniques to maximize use of existing vision.
2. Patient reports improved visual acuity.

NDx: Sleep pattern disturbance related to need for frequent eye drops

Planning: Patient Outcomes
1. Patient rests and sleeps when possible given constraints of treatment.
2. Patient is oriented to time, place, and person.
3. Patient is cooperative.
4. Patient denies irritability.

NDx: Risk for injury related to impaired ability to process sensory information from the environment and presence in an unfamiliar location

Planning: Patient Outcomes
1. Patient avoids falls.
2. Patient avoids injury to eye, self, or others.

NDx: Pain related to corneal nerve fiber irritation

Planning: Patient Outcomes
1. Patient states that pain-control measures have reduced or eliminated pain.
2. Patient reports that pain is at a manageable level.

Nursing Interventions and Evaluation

Since the best treatment for keratitis is prevention, identify and closely monitor patients at risk for exposure keratitis such as those on ventilators, those who are comatose, those with exophthalmos, and those who have had a cerebrovascular accident. Instill ocular lubricant ointments as ordered, at least every 8 hours. If necessary, apply an eye patch over the closed eyelid. See Chapter 44 for more information about these procedures.

To reduce the chance of microbial spread, administer and store fortified eye drops at the patient's bedside. Keep the medications on ice to maintain their pharmacologic properties. Enclosing the bottle of eye drops in a resealable plastic bag in a basin of ice works well.

If patients are to receive the same eye drops in each eye, such as timolol maleate (Timoptic), use separate bottles, clearly labeled O.S. (oculus sinister) for the left eye and O.D. (oculus dexter) for the right eye. This separation decreases the chance of microbial spread from the infected eye to the other eye.

NDx: Sensory/perceptual alterations (visual)
Determine the patient's existing visual acuity. Find out what activities the patient believes he or she is having difficulty performing. Adjust the environment to facilitate patient independence. If glare is a problem, promote the use of indirect lighting and the wearing of hats or sunglasses. Try to maintain a consistent location for the patient's belongings.

If the patient has difficulty with reading, encourage the use of large-print materials and audiovisual programs. Remember that eye ointments may affect the clarity of vision, further reducing acuity.

NDx: Sleep pattern disturbance
Medical treatment of keratitis frequently involves administering one to several kinds of eye drops to patients, each on their own hourly basis. This treatment pattern prevents a normal sleep cycle and may produce a state of acute confusion. Allow the patient as much rest as possible, given the treatment plan, by providing a calm, restful environment, drawing the drapes, dimming the lights, playing quiet music, and maintaining a quiet room.

Allow the patient as many uninterrupted sleep cycles as possible. Group together required care activities, such as measuring vital signs and performing activities of daily living. Be alert for indications of sleep deprivation, such as irritability, short attention span, limited short-term memory, and forgetfulness. Reassure the patient that these symptoms are normal and temporary. Recognize that he or she may be very concerned about not being a "good patient." Try to allay those concerns. Set up designated rest periods. Post a note on the door, and act as the patient's advocate. Permit the patient to be disturbed only for emergency measures or for those situations he or she has indicated.

NDx: Risk for injury

When patients whose vision is already limited by the effects of inflammation are admitted to a hospital, a complete orientation to the environment is essential. Find out what the patient can see and what needs to be pointed out. Help the patient find objects in the room. Move low objects (such as wastebaskets and footstools), rolling equipment (such as a sphygmomanometer), and small objects (such as telephone cords) out of the room's commonly traveled paths. Avoid giving straws to patients with reduced vision. Their visual limitations can alter depth perception, which makes hand-eye coordination difficult. The patient could easily poke his or her eye while attempting to drink through a straw. Allow the patient to unpack, so he or she knows where personal articles have been placed. Keep them in the designated place. Be sure to illuminate corners of the patient's room, avoiding shadows where small objects can hide. (See Chap. 44 for additional guidelines for helping a visually disabled person.)

NDx: Pain

Pain associated with keratitis can range from absent to severe. Have the patient rate the pain on a scale of 1 to 10 to obtain a baseline. Note whether the patient shields the eyes from the light. If pain is accompanied by photophobia, reduce room lighting to a minimum. Use indirect lighting to provide adequate illumination for safety. Encourage the use of window shades, sunglasses, and hats.

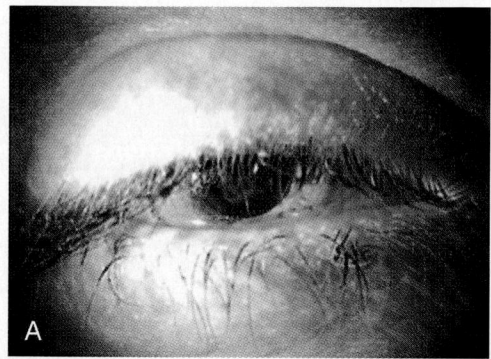

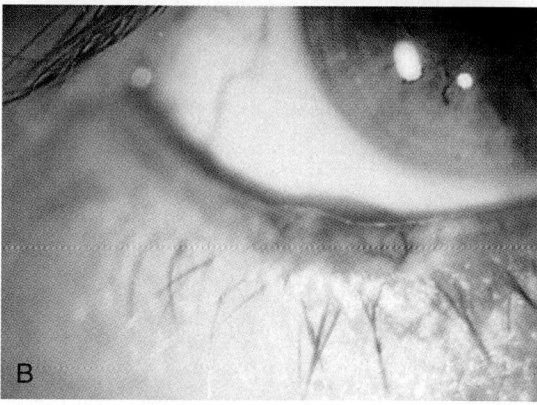

Figure 45–2

A, Blepharitis. Note heavy crusting and scales at the base of the eyelashes, along with swelling and patchy redness. *B*, Chalazion involving multiple meibomian glands. (From Albert DM, Jakobiec FA [eds]. Atlas of clinical ophthalmology. Philadelphia: WB Saunders, 1996, pp 48, 49.)

Table 45–1

Application of an Ocular Compress

1. Wash hands to prevent contamination of the eye, and put on gloves to create a barrier if secretions are present.
2. Explain the procedure to the patient to decrease anxiety and to promote cooperation.
3. Fold a clean washcloth into quarters to fit the ocular area and to provide clean surfaces for four applications.
4. Dampen the washcloth with running water that feels warm on the inner wrist to provide warmth to the eye without causing injury. The sensitivity of the wrist is equal to that of the globe.*
5. Tell the patient to close the eye so the cornea is not irritated by the washcloth.
6. Hold the washcloth in place until it cools (approximately 2 to 4 minutes).
7. Repeat Steps 3 to 5 for three more applications using a separate quarter of the washcloth each time to decrease the risk of microorganism spread.

*If cool compresses are desired, change water temperature and follow same procedure.

Administer ordered analgesics as needed. A typical order would be for acetaminophen or acetaminophen with codeine. Oral analgesics usually provide adequate analgesia. Initiate nonpharmacologic interventions, such as distraction with music, television, visitors, a cool cloth to the forehead, or warm compresses to the inflamed facial lesions (Table 45–1). Be sure to monitor the patient's pain rating after intervention.

Compare the patient's status with the expected outcomes. If the outcomes are not met, reassess the patient and revise the plan.

OTHER INFECTIONS AND INFLAMMATIONS

Other inflammations and infections of the eye are blepharitis, hordeolum, chalazion, dacryocystitis, and endophthalmitis. Blepharitis and chalazion are pictured in Figure 45–2. The etiology, pathophysiology, diagnosis, management, and nursing care related to all these infections are presented in Table 45–2. Self-care for patients with blepharitis, hordeolum, and chalazion is presented in Highlight 45–2.

Table 45–2

Selected Infections and Inflammations of the Eye

Etiology and Pathophysiology	Clinical Manifestations	Diagnosis and Management	Nursing Process Guidelines
BLEPHARITIS: CHRONIC INFLAMMATION OF THE EYELID			
Staphylococcal type is often transmitted by sharing contaminated makeup, especially mascara. Seborrheic type, in which oily scales develop at the margins of the eyelids, is associated with seborrhea of scalp, ears, and eyebrows.	Extremely itchy, red, swollen eyelid Scales (dry in staphylococcal, oily in seborrheic) Small ulcerations at the lid-lash margin Areas of eyelash loss	Diagnosis based on history and examination Treatment includes warm, moist compresses to promote drainage, followed by gentle scrubbing of lid-lash margin with small amount of baby shampoo to loosen and remove scales. Antibiotic ointment may be ordered to prevent secondary infection of conjunctiva and neighboring structures.	Obtain a history of the problem and question about the use of perfumed soaps, makeup, or other products that might be irritating to the external eye. Instruct the patient in self-care at home.
HORDEOLUM: INFECTION OF GLANDS AT THE LID-LASH MARGIN			
Usually caused by *Staphylococcus* If untreated, cellulitis may develop.	Sharp or dull pain, accompanied by a small, red, tender area at the eyelid margin on the external lid or a tiny, beady area on the inside of the lid	Diagnosis based on history and examination Treatment includes warm, moist compresses to promote drainage, followed by gentle scrubbing of the lid-lash margin with a small amount of baby shampoo to loosen and remove scales. Antibiotic ointment may be ordered to prevent secondary infection of the conjunctiva and neighboring structures. Acetaminophen may be ordered for pain. Preventive program of eyelid hygiene is indicated for recurrent hordeola.	Obtain a history of the problem and question about the use of perfumed soaps, makeup, or other products that might be irritating to the external eye. Instruct the patient in self-care at home.
CHALAZION: CHRONIC INFLAMMATION OF A MEIBOMIAN GLAND			
Most common on the inner (conjunctival) side of the eyelid Starts as acute inflammation and progresses to a localized elevation	Red, swollen eyelid Full, scratchy feeling Photophobia Excessive tearing Eye fatigue When fully developed, no signs of inflammation	Diagnosis based on history and examination Treatment includes warm compresses and eyelid scrubs. If recurrent or visually unappealing, may be excised as a minor office procedure	Obtain a history of the problem and question about the use of perfumed soaps, makeup, or other products that might be irritating to the external eye. Instruct the patient in self-care at home.

Table 45–2

Selected Infections and Inflammations of the Eye (continued)

Etiology and Pathophysiology	Clinical Manifestations	Diagnosis and Management	Nursing Process Guidelines
DACRYOCYSTITIS: INFECTION OF THE NASOLACRIMAL SAC OR DUCT			
Common causes of acute form are *Staphylococcus aureus* and beta-hemolytic *Streptococcus*. Common causes of chronic form are *Candida albicans* and *Streptococcus pneumoniae*.	Raised, warm, red area near medial canthus. Purulent material may exude through the puncta when pressure is applied to the canthus.	Diagnosis based on history and examination. Treatment includes warm, moist compresses followed by nasolacrimal massage. If persistent or recurrent, antibiotics are prescribed. If obstruction of the duct or nose is the underlying problem, surgery may be needed.	Instruct the patient to: Wash hands before touching eyes. Wipe secretions from medial to lateral canthus and discard tissues carefully to prevent spread of microorganisms. Promote drainage of secretions by applying compresses and performing nasal puncta massage. To do so, close eyes, depress medial canthus with index finger to create pressure in nasolacrimal system, hold 3 to 5 seconds, and release to create milking action that reduces obstruction. Repeat several times. Instill eye drops by placing index finger over medial canthus and pressing gently while eye drops are instilled. Hold for several minutes to prevent medication from flowing out.
ENDOPHTHALMITIS: INFECTION OR INFLAMMATION OF THE INTERNAL EYE			
Infection occurs as a result of microbial invasion secondary to traumatic wound, surgical procedure. Transmission via blood stream is associated with sharing of needles used for intravenous drug abuse.	Progressive decrease in visual acuity. Ocular redness. Severe, throbbing eye pain. May be corneal edema, decreased red reflex, and purulent drainage on lids or in anterior chamber	Diagnosis includes cultures of specimens from anterior chamber and external eye. Treatment includes topical, subconjunctival, and intravenous broad-spectrum antibiotics. In some cases, it also includes intravitreal antibiotics.	Recognize that any patient reporting a sudden change in visual acuity requires an immediate, detailed, accurate assessment because sight is at risk. Use direct questions to assess type and severity of symptoms and their onset. Be sure to ask about recent surgery, the possibility of a foreign body, and use of street drugs and shared needles. Observe exposed arms for needle marks or tracks. Test visual acuity and compare with baseline records, if available. Check for red reflex, observe for redness of conjunctiva, compare pupils, and check corneal clarity. Help patient identify factors that worsen pain, such as bright light, and modify environment accordingly. Give analgesics as prescribed.

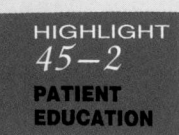 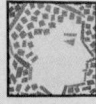

HIGHLIGHT 45–2
PATIENT EDUCATION

Preventing and Treating Blepharitis, Hordeolum, and Chalazion

Instruct the patient to:

Wash hands before touching eyes.

Apply warm, moist compresses for 15 minutes four times per day, as described in Table 45–1.

Perform eyelid scrubs after compress application:

- Rub baby shampoo in a horizontal motion over closed eyelids at the eyelid/eyelash line using a finger tip or cotton swab.
- Gaze downward when scrubbing the upper eyelid and upward when scrubbing the lower eyelid.

Instill prescribed antibiotic ointment, as described in Chapter 44.

Avoid driving if ointment makes vision blurry.

Wear sunglasses or hats with wide brims to reduce photophobia.

Take acetaminophen as directed for pain caused by hordeolum.

Avoid scratching or rubbing the eye to prevent further irritation or spread of infection.

Avoid attempting to burst a hordeolum.

Notify ophthalmologist if eye becomes red or if purulent drainage occurs.

Avoid sharing washcloths or towels with other family members.

Remove makeup daily.

Avoid sharing cosmetics.

Avoid use of perfumed soap or other chemical irritants.

Structural Disorders

REFRACTIVE ERRORS

Etiology and Pathophysiology

The axial length of the eye and its refractive power combine to focus images clearly on the retina (emmetropia). Myopia, or nearsightedness, is caused either by an increase in the length of the eye or by a refractive ability greater than necessary for the length of the eye. In myopia, images focus before reaching the retina, causing the image to appear unfocused (Fig. 45–3).

Hyperopia, or farsightedness, is just the opposite. A short eye length, or a refractive ability weaker than necessary for the length of the eye, may cause the image to be focused behind the retina. Again, the image appears unfocused.

Astigmatism is caused by a variation in the corneal curvature. Light rays arriving from different directions are not focused equally. Images fall distorted on the retina.

Presbyopia occurs normally with the aging process. The lens and the fibers holding it in place become less flexible with age and lose their ability to make the adjustments necessary to focus near images on the retina. As a result, images are focused behind the retina.

Aphakia means absence of a lens. It is the state that occurs after surgical removal of the lens. Because the adjustments in the shape of the lens focus images on the retina, its absence drastically alters the patient's near vision. Images are focused well behind the retina.

Clinical Manifestations

Patients with a refractive error may have vague complaints, such as visual fatigue, discomfort, or headache. They may notice themselves, or others may notice them, rubbing their eyes or squinting.

Diagnosis

Baseline visual acuity is measured, and, through a process called refraction, refractive error is diagnosed. The patient looks at a Snellen chart located in the distance while lenses of varying diopters (measures of power) are placed in front of the eye. The patient is asked to state when the images or pictures are clearest.

Management

Because the anteroposterior length of the eye cannot be adjusted, refractive errors must be treated by changing the focusing ability. This is most often accomplished by the use of lenses. In myopia, the eye's focusing ability is too great for its length. A concave, or "minus" diopter, lens is used to reduce the focusing ability. Strength of a concave lens would be expressed as −3.00 diopters, or minus three diopters.

A "plus" diopter, or convex, lens adds focusing power to the eye. Plus diopter lenses are used to treat hyperopia. For example, a convex lens might be expressed at +2.50 diopters.

Presbyopia is also treated with a convex lens. Presbyopic correction is "added" to the patient's usual lenses. Patients not needing distance correction can wear special eyeglasses just for close work, or near vision.

Astigmatism is corrected with a lens of one-sided curvature. When this lens is used, the focusing ability of the cornea in different planes is adjusted.

Glasses are the easiest and least expensive method of lens correction. They are easy to adapt to

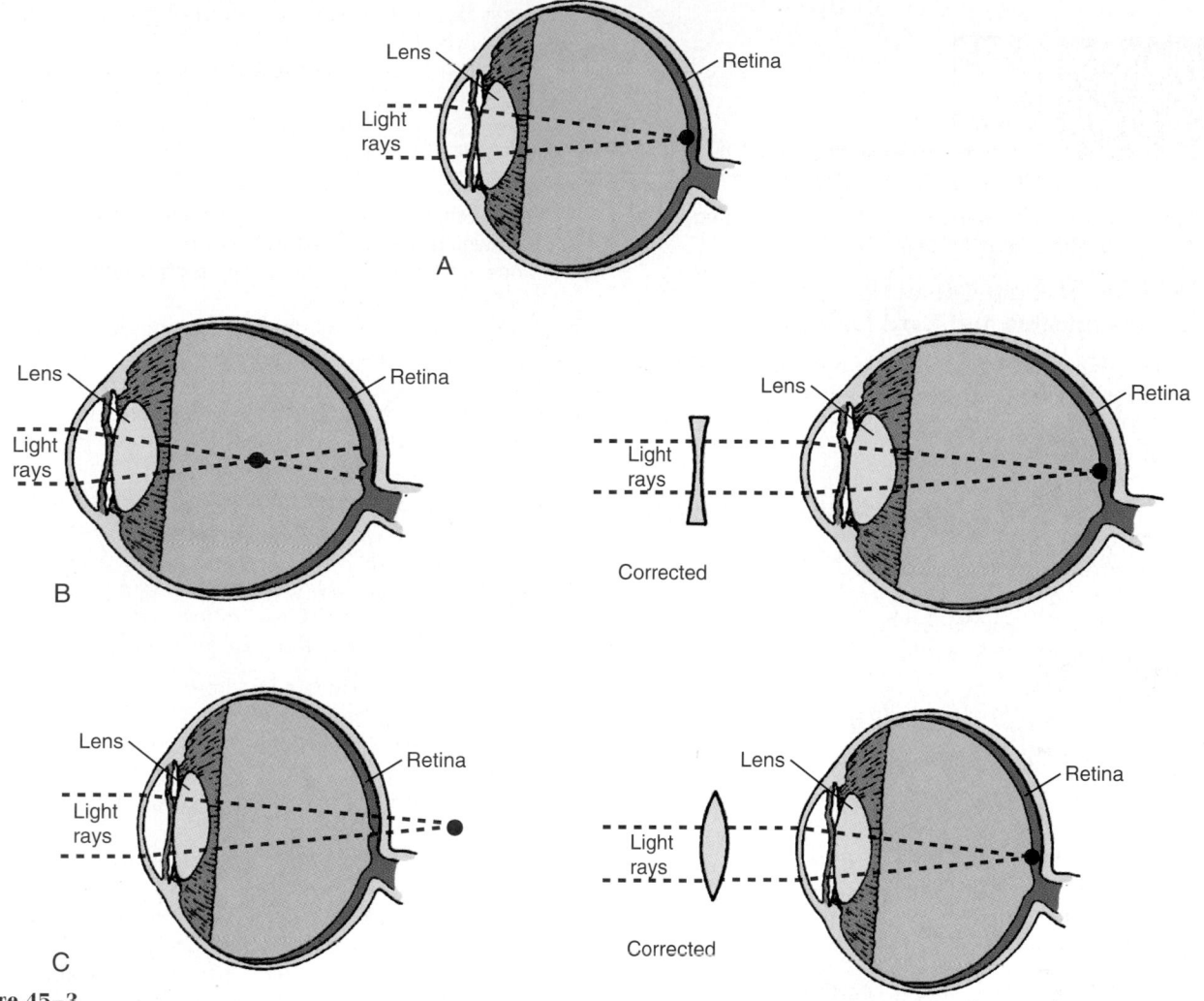

Figure 45–3

A, Emmetropia. Light rays are focused directly on the retina, resulting in a clear visual image. *B*, In myopia, light rays are focused anterior to the retina. A concave lens moves the focus back onto the retina and results in a clear image. *C*, In hyperopia, light rays are focused posterior to the retina. A convex lens moves the focus forward so that light rays focus directly on the retina.

using; however, they alter a person's body image and make objects in the peripheral vision seem out of focus compared with those viewed through the eyeglasses. A second method is the use of contact lenses, which are made of durable plastic and float on the tear film in front of the cornea. With blinking, tears are forced under the edges of the contact lens. The tears float debris away from the contact lens and provide moisture to the cornea.

Contact lenses come in three forms: hard, gas permeable, and soft. The term "rigid" contact lens refers to both hard and gas permeable. There are specially shaped contact lenses for persons with astigmatism.

Rigid contact lenses are smaller than soft lenses. They fit over a portion of the cornea and provide better correction for astigmatism. However, some patients experience dry eyes or corneal warping while wearing a rigid contact lens. Warping is less a problem with gas-permeable lenses than with hard

lenses because the former permit more oxygen to reach the cornea. The removal, cleaning, and insertion of rigid contact lenses are discussed in Highlight 45–3.

Soft contact lenses are made of a less rigid plastic. They fit over the entire cornea and can be worn for a longer period of time than hard lenses because the cornea receives more oxygen and nutrients through them. On the negative side, soft contact lenses can absorb medications. They can be damaged easily because of their thin, "plastic-wrap" consistency. And they create difficulty for the patient with astigmatism because this lens type does not correct it as well as rigid lenses. A specific type of soft lens, called a toric lens, is specifically designed to correct astigmatism. However, these lenses are more expensive and require careful fitting.

Soft contact lenses can be worn on a daily-wear or extended-wear basis. Extended-wear lenses are thinner than daily-wear lenses to enhance corneal

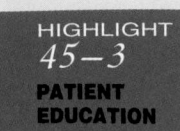
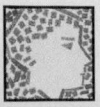

Removal, Cleaning, and Insertion of Contact Lenses

Instruct the patient in the removal, cleaning, and insertion of contact lenses as described here.

Removal of Rigid Contact Lenses (Gas-Permeable and Hard Lenses)

1. Wash hands to reduce microorganisms and decrease risk of cross-contamination.
2. Fill lens case two-thirds full with soaking solution to keep lens moist.
3. Look forward and flex chin slightly.
4. Drape towel on surface below head to catch lens if dropped.
5. Open eyes widely to increase exposed area and facilitate lens removal.
6. To remove right lens: Place right hand against right cheek to catch the lens when it is released from the eye.
7. Use left hand to pull eyelid up and outward toward left ear.
8. Blink to release the lens from the cornea into your right hand.
9. Clean lens (following list).
10. Place lens in storage case.
11. Repeat steps 5–8 to remove left lens, placing left hand against left cheek.
12. Label case with name to prevent loss.

Cleaning of Rigid Contact Lenses

1. Wash hands to reduce microorganisms and decrease risk of cross-contamination.

2. Lay cloth on flat surface to create a work area onto which lens can fall if dropped.
3. Close sink drain to prevent lens from accidentally washing down the drain.
4. Place lens in palm of hand open side up so there is a "bowl" in which to place the cleaning solution.
5. Place two drops of cleaning solution on the lens.
6. Use finger pad to rub solution smoothly over both sides of the lens to loosen debris. Do not use fingernail because it can damage lens.
7. Hold lens by edge and rinse with soaking solution.
8. Examine lens for cleanliness and nicks by holding it up to the light.
9. Repeat procedure for opposite lens.

Insertion of Rigid Contact Lenses

1. Wash hands to reduce microorganisms and reduce the risk of cross-contamination.
2. Moisten index finger of nondominant hand with wetting solution to provide a platform for the lens.
3. Moisten both surfaces of the lens with wetting solution for comfort on insertion.
4. Position lens with convex side facing finger tip on dominant hand index finger.
5. Look straight ahead, bending chin slightly to position the eye to receive the lens.
6. Retract the lower lid against the orbital rim with the middle finger of the nondominant hand.
7. Retract upper lid against bony margin of the brow to maximize corneal exposure.

(continued)

---

oxygenation. They can be worn 24 hours a day for several days without removal. They must be removed at least weekly and thoroughly cleaned. Although promoting ease of wear, these lenses can harbor microorganisms, predisposing the patient to the development of a serious eye infection. See Highlight 45–3 for instructions on the removal, cleaning, and insertion of contact lenses. Contact lenses must be disinfected using a chemical or heat method. The type of disinfection is ordered by the prescribing practitioner.

Also available and growing in popularity are disposable contact lenses. These lenses are designed to be worn for a 1- to 2-week period and discarded. They have the advantages of easy use, decreased maintenance, and enhanced cleanliness.

Indications for contact lens wear include uncomfortable fit of eyeglasses on the nose because of their weight; cosmetic appearance; need for clear peripheral vision because of occupation or leisure pursuits; monocular aphakia; and significant difference between the refractive errors of the left eye (O.S.) and the right eye (O.D.).

Contact lens wear should not be taken lightly. Complications of contact lens wear include corneal abrasions that can lead to corneal ulcers; corneal edema from insufficient oxygen reaching the cornea or from lens overwear; and giant papillary cell conjunctivitis, a sensitivity reaction seen in patients who are long-term contact lens users. Symptoms of this latter condition disappear when lenses are not worn for a while.

Contact lenses should not be worn by patients with impaired corneal sensitivity, those with a lack of manual dexterity, or those who are unable or not motivated to adhere to a lens-care protocol. Contact lenses should not be worn by those who work in a dusty, dry, or smoky environment.

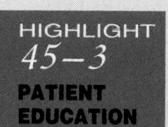
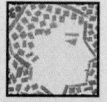

HIGHLIGHT
45—3
PATIENT EDUCATION

Removal, Cleaning, and Insertion of Contact Lenses *(continued)*

8. Bring the finger holding the lens toward the cornea to bring lens in contact with the ocular surface.
9. Allow eyelids to close by slowly releasing the lower lid and then the upper lid. Avoid quick release of lids, which can break lens contact with the eye.
10. Do not move until the tear film has centered the lens on the cornea and vision is clear to decrease the risk of losing the lens if it has been blinked from the eye.
11. Repeat for other eye.

Removal of Soft Contact Lenses

1. Wash hands to reduce microorganisms and decrease risk of cross-contamination.
2. Fill lens case with 0.9% saline solution to prevent damage to the lens from dehydration.
3. Gaze upward to expose area for lens removal.
4. Use dominant hand middle finger to retract lower lid down against the cheek bone.
5. Use finger of dominant hand to slide lens onto sclera, which is less sensitive than the cornea.
6. Secure the lens between the thumb and index finger of the dominant hand and remove.
7. Place lens in saline-filled lens case.
8. Repeat for other eye if needed.
9. Label case with name to prevent loss.

Cleaning of Soft Contact Lenses

1. Wash hands to reduce microorganisms and decrease risk of cross-contamination.

2. Place lens in palm of hand open side up so there is a "bowl" in which to place the cleaning solution.
3. Place several drops of cleaning solution on the lens.
4. Spread cleaning solution gently and smoothly over both surfaces of the lens to loosen debris and avoid tearing the lens.
5. Hold lens by its edge and rinse with 0.9% saline solution.
6. Inspect lens for cleanliness and damage by holding it up to the light.
7. Repeat for opposite lens.

Insertion of Soft Contact Lenses

1. Wash hands to reduce microorganisms and decrease the risk of cross-contamination.
2. Remove lens from storage case using finger pad, not the fingertip, to avoid damaging the lens.
3. Place lens on index finger pad of dominant hand.
4. Look forward and flex chin slightly.
5. Use middle finger of nondominant hand to retract lower lid against cheek to expose area for lens insertion while avoiding pressure against globe.
6. Retract upper lid against eyebrow using index finger of nondominant hand.
7. Gaze slightly upward.
8. Carry lens up toward the eye, and place lens on sclera below or on the cornea.
9. Release eyelids slowly.
10. Close eyelids gently to allow lens to center.

Refractive errors can also be treated by surgical alteration of the shape of the cornea. Radial keratotomy corrects myopia by making incisions in the cornea with a scalpel to flatten it. Photorefractive keratectomy is a procedure that uses a laser to reshape the curve of the cornea by removing microscopic layers of corneal tissue. Both of these outpatient procedures are designed to eliminate or reduce the need for glasses or contact lenses in moderately nearsighted people with healthy eyes, a stable refractive error, and no more than mild astigmatism. Following surgery, the eye may be patched for 24 hours for protection. Eye discomfort is expected, particularly in the first 72 hours, and sensitivity to light and glare and a foreign-body sensation may persist for a few weeks.

Visual improvement is not immediately noticeable, taking from 3 to 6 months to reach its maximum. Ophthalmic drops to control pain and prevent

infection will be used several times daily for up to 6 months.

Potential complications of these procedures include:

- A corneal haze that occurs in all patients temporarily, but may persist and impair vision
- Infection, which can lead to corneal scarring and impaired vision
- Astigmatism or farsightedness, from overcorrection
- Persistent sensitivity to glare and the perception of halos around lights
- Increased intraocular pressure, from ophthalmic medications
- Insufficient correction, which may require use of corrective lenses or additional surgery

Because of these risks, one eye is done first and the second 3 or more months later.

NURSING PROCESS GUIDELINES
Correction of Refractive Error

Help the patient match his or her need for visual correction, motivation, manual dexterity, and lifestyle with the appropriate method of visual rehabilitation. Identify the factor most important to the patient: appearance, cost, or ease of use, as well as any limitations from pre-existing medical problems.

CONTACT LENSES

If contact lenses are considered, explore the patient's ability to meet not only the initial cost but the cost of lens-care products. If selected, instruct the patient to remove, clean, and insert the lenses, as presented in Highlight 45–3.

Remind the patient not to exceed the established wearing schedule, and advise him or her to remove daily-wear contact lenses before napping or sleeping. Reinforce the importance of proper lens cleaning and of washing hands immediately before and after caring for contact lenses. Stress the importance of notifying the contact lens professional if red, puffy, or watery eyes, purulent drainage, or eye pain develops.

RADIAL KERATOTOMY OR PHOTOREFRACTIVE KERATECTOMY

Make sure the patient has a ride home after the procedure because vision will not be clear. Instruct the patient to:

*   Use eye drops and return for follow-up visits as directed.
*   Take a few days off from work.
*   Avoid touching or bumping the eye.
*   Wear sunglasses when in bright light, because the eye will be sensitive to light until it heals.
*   Avoid swimming or sitting in a whirlpool or hot tub.
*   Avoid activities that carry a risk of accidental injury to the eye, such as ball games.
*   Avoid wearing eye makeup.

Stress the importance of not driving until vision clears and notifying the physician if pain increases 24 hours or more after surgery, if blurred vision worsens, if drainage develops, or if redness intensifies.

ENTROPION AND ECTROPION

Etiology and Pathophysiology
Inward turning of the eyelid is called entropion. Outward turning of the eyelid is called ectropion (Fig. 45–4). Entropion occurs as a result of the aging process, chronic inflammation, or scarring disorders, such as trachoma. This change in eyelid direction may allow the eyelashes to deviate inward, brushing against the cornea and causing severe pain.

Ectropion is caused by relaxation of the orbicu-

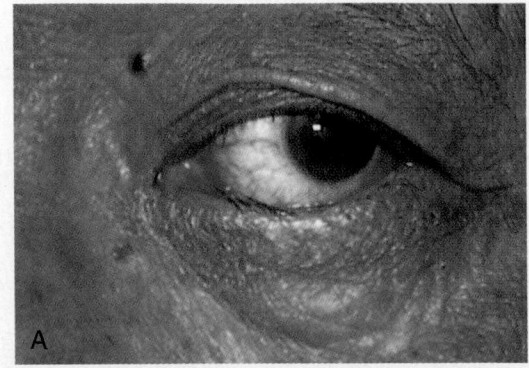

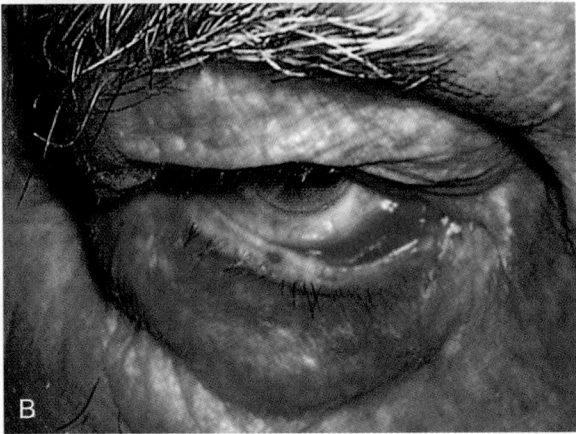

Figure 45–4

A, Entropion. Note how lashes of the inwardly turned lower lid can rub against the globe, potentially causing corneal damage. *B,* Ectropion of lower lid. (From Albert DM, Jakobiec FA [eds]. Atlas of clinical ophthalmology. Philadelphia: WB Saunders, 1996, p 374.)

laris oculi or by seventh nerve palsy. It is usually bilateral and occurs with aging, but may also be congenital. Failure to correct the eyelid position can cause skin excoriation and corneal ulceration.

Clinical Manifestations
Patients with entropion complain of a "foreign-body" sensation that has developed gradually. On inspection, the eyelid is seen to be inwardly deviated. Tearing and conjunctival injection may be present. A corneal ulcer may be noted.

With ectropion, patients complain of epiphora accompanying the corneal irritation from dry, scratchy eyes. The eyes feel dry despite the tearing because the tears cannot wash correctly over the cornea to keep it moist because of the outward deviation of the lower eyelid. Instead of draining toward the medial canthus, tears splash down onto the cheek, causing local irritation. This irritation is caused by the enzyme lysozyme, which is found in tears. If corneal drying has caused exposure keratitis, multiple dotlike areas are noted.

Diagnosis
Diagnosis is based on history and physical examination.

Management

Entropion is treated on a temporary basis by taping the lower eyelid down and laterally with a small adhesive tape strip. On a more permanent basis, a minor surgical procedure can be performed to shorten the eyelid horizontally.

The goal of ectropion treatment is to keep the cornea moist. Lubricating eye drops and ointments are used to protect the cornea. Acetaminophen (Tylenol) or acetaminophen with codeine (Tylenol with Codeine) may be ordered for pain. Surgery may be done to invert the puncta into its normal position.

NURSING PROCESS GUIDELINES
Entropion or Ectropion

Instruct the patient to instill ocular lubricants, drops, and ointments as ordered to keep the cornea moist and thus decrease pain resulting from ocular drying or irritation. Encourage the use of nonpharmacologic measures, such as increasing hydration, increasing the moisture content of the room, and patching the eye in the closed position.

Encourage the patient to use a gentle, fragrance-free soap for cleaning the ocular area because perfumes and colors found in soaps may irritate the area and cause further drying. Remind the patient to rinse the area well to remove soap residue, and to dry gently.

CATARACTS

A cataract is an opacity of the crystalline lens of the eye (Fig. 45–5). Although one eye is often affected first, most cataracts ultimately become bilateral, with proportional visual loss in both eyes.

Etiology and Pathophysiology

The most common type of cataract is that associated with old age. Normally, the lens, which is composed of 65% water and 35% minerals, is clear and avascular. However, as people age, lens fibers, which continue to be produced, become more densely packed and can reduce transparency. The lens also becomes yellow with age. This yellowing causes some colors—such as blue, green, and violet—to appear gray. Some evidence of cataracts can be seen in most patients older than 70 years.

Cataracts can also occur when the integrity of the lens capsule is disturbed by trauma. Fluid enters the lens, and an opacification can quickly develop. Still other causes of cataract formation include toxicity to chemicals and medications such as corticosteroids, nutritional deficits, or exposure to high-voltage electricity or radiation. Cataracts progress more rapidly in diabetics than in nondiabetics.

Clinical Manifestations

A gradual, painless blurring of central distance vision is the chief clinical manifestation of a cataract

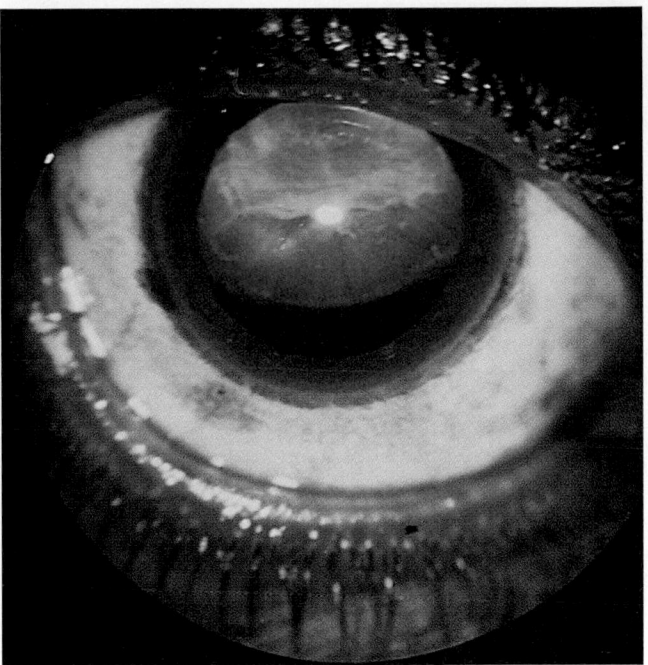

Figure 45–5

In senile cataract, the crystalline lens becomes progressively gray and opaque. (From Jarvis C. Physical examination and health assessment. 2nd ed. Philadelphia: WB Saunders, 1996, p 347.)

(Fig. 45–6). Additional symptoms may include glare spots, ghostly images, double vision from light rays being split by the opacity and falling in two places in the retina, a need for more light for reading or near work, headaches, and irritability. These symptoms may develop rapidly over several months or may arise over several years.

Diagnosis

An advanced cataract can be seen as a white discoloration immediately behind the pupil when the eye is obliquely illuminated. Less advanced cataracts are identified by ophthalmoscopic examination and slit-lamp biomicroscopy. As part of the examination, visual acuity is measured carefully in both eyes, and a test of the patient's ability to handle glare is done.

If cataract extraction with insertion of an intraocular lens (IOL) is planned, A-scan ultrasonographic measurements and keratometry are performed to determine the focusing power needed.

Management

The only method of curing vision loss as a result of cataracts is surgical removal. However, surgery is not required for every patient. The decision to remove cataracts, and when to do so, depends on changes in the cataracts over time in relationship to the patient's age, health status, visual loss, and impact on activities of daily living. Usually, cataract extraction is indicated when visual loss significantly interferes with the patient's usual activities; when

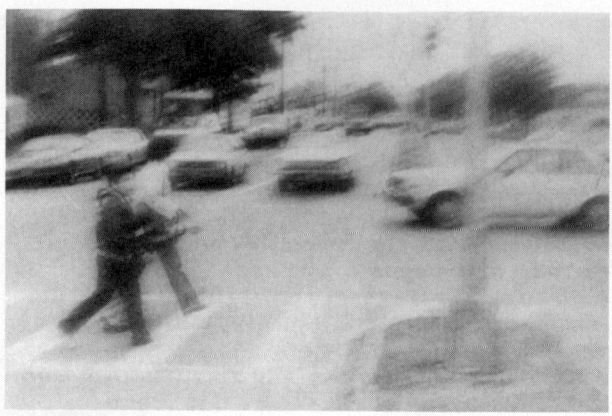

Figure 45–6

Images as seen by a patient with a cataract. (Permission to use this photograph has been granted by the American Foundation for the Blind, 15 West 16th Street, New York, NY 10011.)

vision in the better eye is less than 20/50 or when there is a need for visualization or treatment of structures in the posterior chamber of the eye.

Cataract surgery is usually performed under local anesthesia as ambulatory surgery. An overnight stay in the hospital is needed only if complications arise, if surgery is being performed on the patient's only seeing eye, or if the patient requires monitoring of a pre-existing medical problem. If both eyes are affected, the more opaque cataract is removed first and the second about a month later.

Cataract extraction leaves the patient aphakic (without a lens) and requires lens replacement by an IOL implant, contact lenses, or cataract glasses. Of the three, IOL implant is rapidly becoming the preferred method of lens replacement by both patients and surgeons. The IOL is invisible, permanent, and cannot be felt. It also affords the best postextraction visual correction.

Cataract glasses are the least desirable form of lens replacement. They allow good central vision but restrict peripheral vision and cause objects to appear about 30% larger than reality. As a result, objects look closer than they are and straight lines look curved. Further, because the brain cannot fuse images of very different sizes, if the lenses have not been removed from both eyes, the patient has double vision unless only one eye is focused. These visual field distortions result in difficulty walking, reaching for things, pouring liquids, and, of course, driving until the patient adjusts to them, which takes at least 4 to 8 weeks.

Contact lenses may be used by persons who are nonallergic and who have the dexterity needed to handle the required daily care for removal, cleaning, and replacement. Contact lenses are preferred over cataract glasses because of the improved image size (objects appear only 8% to 10% larger) and peripheral vision they offer. In addition, double vision

does not occur even if only one crystalline lens is removed.

Patient Preparation for Cataract Surgery
Before the start of surgery, the periorbital area is injected with local anesthetic. The area is cleansed with an antiseptic scrubbing solution and then sterile drapes are placed.

Procedure
There are two types of cataract surgery: extracapsular and intracapsular. In extracapsular cataract extraction (ECCE), a small incision is made at the corneoscleral limbus under the operating room microscope. The eye is entered through the anterior chamber, and the anterior lens capsule is removed. The nucleus is then removed either by gentle pressure applied to the eye or by phacoemulsification, a procedure in which high-frequency sound waves delivered through an ultrasonic needle inserted into the lens are used to break the cataract into fine pieces. Phacoemulsification is increasingly used because a smaller incision is required, activity restrictions are needed for a shorter period, and healing time is reduced. With both extracapsular cataract extraction techniques, the retained lens material is then irrigated from the eye and aspirated through an instrument. The posterior lens capsule is left in place to protect the retina and to create a supportive structure for the lens implant. If a lens is to be implanted, it is usually placed in the posterior chamber, behind the iris, and in front of the posterior lens capsule.

Intracapsular cataract extraction surgery is an older and less frequently performed technique in which a freezing probe is introduced into the eye and affixed to the lens. The lens is then removed intact, so no posterior capsule remains. If an IOL is to be implanted, it is placed in the anterior chamber, between the cornea and the iris, or sutured in the posterior chamber. This method leaves the retina and vitreous less protected.

After extraction by either procedure, the eye is sutured closed with material finer than a human hair. An antibiotic is injected subconjunctivally, an ophthalmic antibiotic ointment is instilled, and an eye patch is applied over the patient's closed eyelid. A metal shield is taped in place over the eye patch.

Complications
Complications that can occur with or after cataract surgery include cystoid macular edema (CME), vitreous loss, expulsive hemorrhage, postoperative inflammation or infection, retinal detachment, glaucoma, or endophthalmitis. Over several weeks to months, the posterior capsule can also become opaque, causing the patient to say the cataract has returned. This late opacification is treated with a laser to create a small opening through which light rays can reach the retina.

NURSING PROCESS
Cataract Surgery

PREOPERATIVE NURSING CARE

Nursing care of the patient scheduled for cataract surgery is similar to that described for any patient having ocular surgery (see Chap. 44), with several considerations. Ask about the use of nonsteroidal and anti-inflammatory drugs, such as ibuprofen (Motrin) or aspirin, because these can affect platelet function, creating a potential for increased bleeding during surgery. Because many cataract surgery patients live alone, it is important to obtain information about the patient's social support systems. Ask who, if anyone, will be available to assist with eye drop instillation, application of the eye shield, and transportation for follow-up care visits.

Review preoperative instructions with the patient, caregiver, or both, and, having ascertained the patient's ability to read, provide a written copy to be taken home because anxious persons may forget information. Use off-white paper to reduce glare and large-print, high-contrast letters to make reading easier. Provide a telephone number for the patient to call if questions arise.

POSTOPERATIVE NURSING CARE

Assessment

Assess the patient's return to physiologic stability. As per established institutional protocol but guided by the patient's condition, check vital signs and evaluate the dressing for evidence of bleeding.

Nursing Diagnoses and Planning

Nursing diagnoses and related expected patient outcomes commonly applicable to patients who have had cataract extraction surgery include the following:

NDx: Risk for injury: ocular trauma and fall related to altered depth perception, effects of medication, and presence in an unfamiliar environment

Planning: Patient Outcomes
1. Patient's eye heals without evidence of trauma.
2. Patient avoids injury.

NDx: Pain related to surgical manipulation of tissue and use of suture material

Planning: Patient Outcomes
1. Patient differentiates expected discomfort from pain.
2. Patient refrains from rubbing.

NDx: Risk for impaired home maintenance management related to activity restrictions imposed by surgery

Planning: Patient Outcomes
1. Patient identifies home modifications necessary to coincide with activity restrictions.

2. Patient plans and prepares meals ahead.
3. Patient arranges transportation to market, follow-up care, and other locations as needed.

NDx: Risk for altered health maintenance related to insufficient knowledge of application of eye shield, eyelid hygiene, administration of medications, activity restrictions, and plans for follow-up care

Planning: Patient Outcomes
1. Patient correctly applies eye shield.
2. Patient correctly cleanses eyelid.
3. Patient states name, purpose, and schedule of administration for medications.
4. Patient identifies signs and symptoms of complications to report.
5. Patient describes activity restrictions.
6. Patient describes plans for follow-up care.

Nursing Interventions and Evaluation

NDx: Risk for injury
Patching one eye after surgery alters depth perception. As a result, patients perceive distances to be different than they are and objects in places where they are not. Tell the patient to hold on to handrails whenever available and to use adaptive equipment, such as a walker or cane, if he or she usually does so. Stress the importance of not reaching for objects, such as door frames, backs of chairs, and other furniture for support because these objects may not be where they appear, possibly causing the patient to lose balance and fall. Falling can rupture the stitches, which opens the wound, and can potentially cause a loss of vision. In addition, patients may also have received medications that they are not used to, such as diazepam (Valium) or midazolam (Versed). Because this can alter the patient's gait, stress the need for caution when ambulating.

Orient the patient to the surroundings. Make sure the patient knows the location of the call light, bathroom, small objects on the floor, and the side rails. Remove small objects from traveled paths if possible.

Help the patient identify and arrange for removal of hazards in the home environment. Examples of such hazards include rugs, dog dishes, and footstools.

Encourage the patient to wear the eye shield as directed. This shield protects the eye during times when risk of an injury is increased, such as when ambulating during the night. The shield also protects the eye from accidental injury caused by rubbing the eye during sleep.

NDx: Pain
Tell the patient to use a cool cloth on the forehead and to elevate the head slightly when in bed to promote comfort. Also instruct the patient to take acetaminophen (Tylenol) as ordered and needed. Because pain is unusual after cataract surgery, stress the importance of notifying the ophthalmologist im-

mediately if pain occurs that is unrelieved by acetaminophen (Tylenol) or is accompanied by nausea. The latter is associated with increased intraocular pressure (IOP).

Explain that mild itching is normal and is caused by the presence of the suture rubbing against the conjunctiva. Suggest refrigerating the eye drops to provide a cool, comfortable sensation when the drop is instilled, provided refrigerating the medication will not significantly alter its chemical or pharmacologic properties.

NDx: Risk for impaired home maintenance management

Immediately after surgery, patients usually cannot bend from the waist, lift more than 20 to 25 pounds, or drive. The length of time these restrictions are needed varies somewhat on the basis of the exact surgical procedure performed, size of the incision, patient condition, and presence of complications. Promote compliance with these restrictions by helping the patient develop a plan for adapting the home environment. Do this before surgery, if possible. Encourage the patient to cook a few meals ahead, so they only need reheating. Advise placing pots, pans, and objects from low cupboards at counter height so that bending is unnecessary to access lower cupboards. Suggest placing pet dishes on a low stool or box, and instruct the patient to sit on a chair and lean forward to fill the dish.

Driving is not permitted immediately after surgery because an eye patch and shield are covering the operative eye. Help the patient establish a transportation plan for marketing, errands, and follow-up care. Refer to community senior citizen programs or agencies that may provide assistance.

NDx: Risk for altered health maintenance

Teach the patient to remove crusty drainage from the eyelid and to apply an eye shield. (See Chap. 44 for more information.)

Review the purpose of each medication. When they are discharged, patients frequently have two different eye drops prescribed: an antibiotic such as gentamicin (Genoptic) to prevent infection, and a steroid such as prednisolone acetate (Pred Mild). Sometimes patients are advised to use a combination eye drop composed of an antibiotic and a steroid, such as prednisolone acetate and gentamicin sulfate (Pred-G).

If medications are in a suspension (eg, prednisolone acetate [Pred Mild]), reinforce the critical importance of vigorously shaking the bottle of eye drops while slowly counting to a minimum of 25. This shaking is necessary to distribute the medication in the solution. Check that the patient knows how to instill the eye drops, and observe the patient's technique. Remind the patient to close the eye gently and keep it closed for at least 3 minutes after instilling the medication to reduce the likelihood of washing the medication into the nasolacrimal system with blinking.

There are times when patients are discharged and ordered to take several eye drops. For example, the patient using timolol maleate (Timoptic) to control his or her glaucoma will continue to use the drop in the operated eye, unless specifically advised otherwise. If more than one drop is to be instilled into the same eye on the same schedule, instruct the patient to wait a minimum of 5 minutes between drops to promote maximum absorption of the drops.

Teach the patient signs and symptoms of complications. Stress the importance of promptly reporting pain not relieved by acetaminophen (Tylenol), spots or bright flashes of light in the visual field, a curtain that obscures part of the visual field, or a reduction in visual acuity.

Compare the patient's status with the expected outcomes. If the outcomes are not met, reassess the patient and revise the plan.

GLAUCOMA

Glaucoma is a cluster of related disorders, with increased IOP as the common element. It is the second major cause of blindness in the United States and the primary cause of blindness in African-Americans. Of the 2 million people who have glaucoma, about half are unaware that they have it (American Academy of Ophthalmology, Quality of Care Committee, Glaucoma Panel, 1989). This lack of awareness is due to the asymptomatic nature of the disease's early course: Vision is lost gradually and without pain. Thus, glaucoma is often referred to as the "sneak thief" of sight.

Glaucoma is found more commonly in patients with a family history of glaucoma, diabetes, severe myopia, hypertension, or retinal detachment.

Etiology and Pathophysiology

Normal IOP is 10 to 21 mm Hg. The increased IOP in glaucoma results from an imbalance between production of aqueous humor and its outflow from the eye. In glaucoma, aqueous humor is drained from the eye more slowly than it is produced. Drainage is through the anterior chamber angle, trabecular meshwork, and into the canal of Schlemm, where it enters a series of capillaries that absorb it into the systemic circulation. Increased IOP causes ischemia and atrophy of the optic disk, and peripheral vision is lost. There is some variance in the patient's susceptibility to ocular damage from increased IOP, however. At the same IOP, one patient may have extensive peripheral sight loss and another minimal evidence of damage.

There are two classifications of glaucoma: primary and secondary. Primary glaucoma refers to those cases in which glaucoma is the main problem. It did not result from something else. Secondary glaucoma occurs as a sequela of another problem, such as a tumor, surgery, or recurrent ocular inflammation.

Glaucoma is also differentiated by the appearance of the anterior chamber angle. In angle-closure glaucoma, the iris slides forward, closing off the normally open angle. Angle-closure glaucoma is also referred to as narrow-angle or acute glaucoma (Fig. 45–7). If the angle remains open, it is referred to as open-angle glaucoma.

Clinical Manifestations

Patients with primary open-angle glaucoma are largely asymptomatic, which is why they can experience severe vision loss before the problem is detected (Fig. 45–8). With progression, vague symptoms such as foggy vision or a reduced near-vision acuity (accommodation) can occur. Patients may complain of headaches or achy pains behind the eye.

On examination, the optic disk may appear pale or gray with the size and depth of the physiologic cup increased. Palpation of the globe over the closed eyelid may reveal an increased firmness, a crude estimation of IOP.

Angle-closure glaucoma patients present with a very different clinical picture. They look sick and complain of a sudden onset of severe unilateral ocular pain, which may radiate to the forehead. These patients may report nausea and vomiting and seeing halos around lights. On slit-lamp examination, the sclera is frequently seen to be injected (red), and the cornea looks steamy (as if looking through a steam-

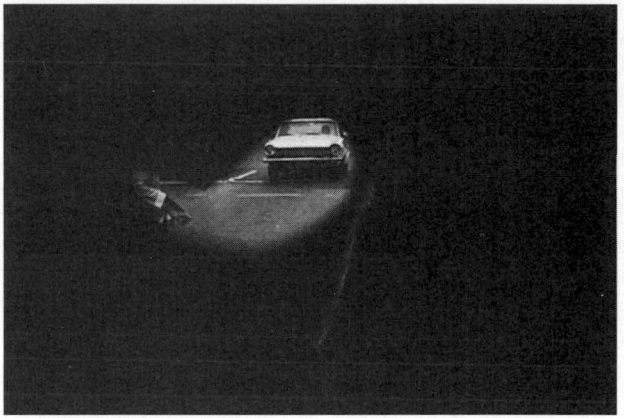

Figure 45–8

Image seen by a patient with advanced glaucoma. Note small center island of vision. (Permission to use this photograph has been granted by the American Foundation for the Blind, 15 West 16th Street, New York, NY 10011.)

filled room). The pupil is usually mid-size to slightly dilated and slow to react to light. It may not be equal in size when compared with the other eye.

Diagnosis

Diagnosis of glaucoma is based on history and physical findings. The fundus is examined with the direct ophthalmoscope. A tonometer is used to measure IOP, which is greater than 21 mm Hg in the majority of patients with glaucoma. Gonioscopy, a procedure in which a special contact lens is placed over the anesthetized cornea, is done to visualize the anterior chamber and its angles. A visual field test is performed to investigate and document areas of vision loss, and fundus photographs are taken of the optic disk to provide baseline data for use in future comparisons.

Management

Once glaucoma is diagnosed, the goal of treatment is to reduce IOP to a level tolerated by the eye without damage. For primary open-angle glaucoma, eye drops supplemented with oral carbonic anhydrase inhibitors as needed are used initially. Topical eye drops control IOP by either enhancing outflow or reducing the production of aqueous humor. Oral carbonic anhydrase inhibitors are used to reduce production of aqueous humor. These drugs can cause a number of very unpleasant and annoying side effects. Pilocarpine hydrochloride (Pilocar) causes burning and itching. It can cause local skin irritation and abdominal cramps as well as induced myopia. Timolol maleate (Timoptic) can cause bronchospasm in patients with reactive airway disease. The beta-blocker effect reduces the body's ability to respond to periods of decreased myocardial contractility. Severe respiratory and cardiac reactions have also been seen. This drug must be used with caution in diabetic patients because it masks signs and symptoms of hypoglycemia. Echothiophate iodide

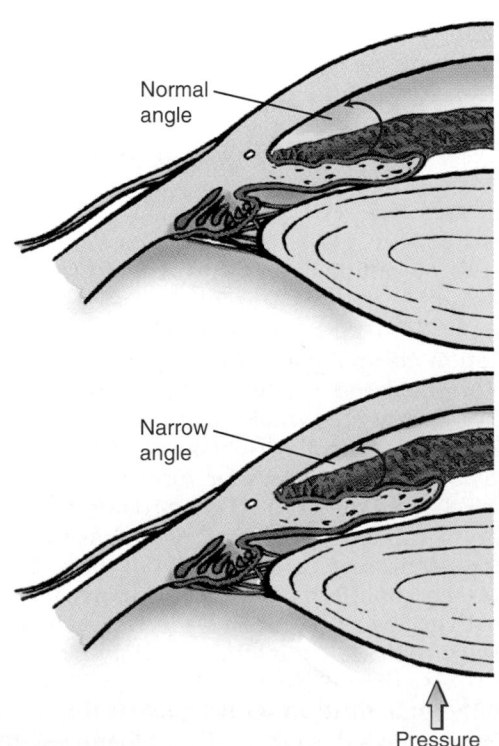

Figure 45–7

Normal angle versus a narrow angle caused when the iris slides forward, as in acute glaucoma.

(Phospholine Iodide) can be associated with stinging and burning on instillation as well as brow ache, headache, and the formation of iris cysts. Because it can also lead to the formation of cataracts, this drug should be used only in aphakic patients. Acetazolamide (Diamox) can cause anorexia, vomiting, constipation, weight loss, renal calculi, nervousness, tremors, ataxia, and paresthesia. The number and variety of side effects can make staying on the prescribed medications a problem for the patient.

Angle-closure glaucoma is treated by topical agents and oral or intravenous hyperosmotics to rapidly bring down IOP. Oral hyperosmotics such as glycerin (Osmoglyn) or isosorbide (Ismotic) can cause serious side effects, such as nausea, vomiting, severe headache, confusion, disorientation, pulmonary edema, and subarachnoid hemorrhage. These agents should be administered over ice and consumed over a 20- to 30-minute period. Patients must be observed closely for development of side effects. Intravenous hyperosmotics are usually administered to hospitalized patients.

If pharmacologic treatments for primary open-angle glaucoma are insufficient, argon laser trabeculoplasty is performed. A slit-lamp mounted laser is used to create a series of laser burns in the trabecular meshwork. As the area scars, contraction causes tightening of the trabecular meshwork fibers. The drainage channels are pulled open, which enhances outflow of aqueous and lowers IOP in about 85% of patients. This procedure is performed on an outpatient basis, either at the ophthalmologist's office or hospital. Over time, the effectiveness of argon laser trabeculoplasty is reduced. Medications may need to be resumed or continued for this reason.

Angle-closure glaucoma patients also benefit from laser procedures. After topical or local anesthesia, the laser is used to create a hole in the peripheral iris. This new hole creates an alternate pathway for aqueous humor to drain from the posterior chamber into the anterior chamber and then through the trabecular meshwork. Once IOP is reduced in the eye experiencing angle-closure glaucoma, some patients may undergo a preventive laser iridotomy in the other eye.

With either laser trabeculoplasty or iridotomy, a brief rise in IOP can occur. To combat this rise, which can further damage the optic nerve, apraclonidine hydrochloride (Iopidine) is used. However, it can cause bradycardia, vasovagal attacks, chest heaviness, and nausea. Because of the potential cardiovascular side effects, vital signs are taken before and after each dose, and emergency equipment is kept nearby.

Intraocular surgery is done when pharmacologic or laser therapy fail to keep IOP at a level the eye can tolerate. Surgical procedures either create an alternate pathway for the drainage of aqueous humor or destroy structures responsible for the production of aqueous humor. Procedures aimed at reducing aqueous production are called cyclodestructive procedures. A freezing force is delivered to the ciliary body area through the sclera, causing destruction of the site of aqueous production.

In glaucoma filtering surgery, a channel connecting the anterior chamber and the subconjunctival space is created. The aqueous humor moves up through this channel to collect under the conjunctiva. From here, it is absorbed into the systemic circulation and IOP is lowered in a controlled manner.

In glaucoma shunting procedures, an implanted reservoir and connecting tube are used to facilitate movement of aqueous humor from the anterior chamber to the reservoir. The aqueous humor forms a bubble over the reservoir and under the conjunctiva, where it is absorbed into systemic circulation. Thus, obstructions in the trabecular meshwork that prevented aqueous outflow are bypassed.

Complications of glaucoma filtering and shunting surgery include hypotonia resulting from excessive reduction in IOP, scar tissue formation, obstruction of the shunt, and progression of cataracts.

A peripheral iridectomy is performed for the treatment of angle-closure glaucoma when a laser iridotomy is not effective or is not an option. A small, wedge-shaped section of the peripheral iris is removed, creating a new channel for aqueous humor to follow when flowing from the posterior to the anterior chamber.

NURSING PROCESS
Glaucoma

Assessment

Begin the assessment by asking why the patient presented for treatment. Keep in mind that symptoms of glaucoma are vague and undefined, so listen carefully and do not minimize them. Explore specific symptoms, such as headaches, pain behind the eye or radiating to the forehead, and frequent changes of eyeglasses. Also note complaints that could indicate angle-closure glaucoma: seeing halos around lights, reduced visual acuity, nausea, and vomiting.

Question the patient about a personal or family history of glaucoma, diabetes, hypertension, or myopia, and determine whether these are associated with the development of glaucoma. Also ask about any previous ocular trauma or surgery.

Inquire about other medical problems. Carefully note any cardiac or respiratory diseases, because they may contraindicate the use of beta blockers. Question about allergies to medications, especially preservatives, because many glaucoma patients receive eye drops that contain a variety of preservatives.

Ask the patient to describe a usual day to obtain information needed to help the patient establish a manageable treatment plan for eye drop instillation.

Observe the patient's general appearance while obtaining the history. Does the patient appear fatigued? Does the patient have signs of dehydration that can result from nausea and vomiting associated with increased IOP?

Check visual acuity. Compare the right eye with the left eye. Ask the patient how current vision compares with how well he or she usually sees. Be sure to document this information for medical and legal purposes.

Carefully observe the pupils, noting their size and shape. Remember that patients using certain glaucoma medications, such as pilocarpine hydrochloride (Pilocar), will have small pupils (referred to as miotic), whereas the pupils of the patient with angle-closure glaucoma may be asymmetric, with the affected eye slightly dilated and slow to react.

If the patient has previously been diagnosed with glaucoma, assess his or her knowledge of the disease and its treatment. Identify all medications the patient uses or takes as well as their frequency. Compare this list with prescribed medications and their frequency. Clarify any differences between prescribed and actual use.

Nursing Diagnoses and Planning

Nursing diagnoses and related expected patient outcomes commonly applicable to patients with glaucoma include the following:

NDx: Risk for injury related to peripheral vision loss

Planning: Patient Outcomes
1. Patient describes how to use existing vision to promote safety.
2. Patient avoids self-injury.

NDx: Pain related to increased intraocular pressure

Planning: Patient Outcomes
1. Patient associates pain with increased IOP.
2. Patient describes level of pain as tolerable.
3. Patient states pharmacologic interventions are effective.
4. Patient uses nonpharmacologic interventions for effective pain relief.

NDx: Risk for ineffective management of therapeutic regimen (individuals) related to side effects of medications, specifics of treatment regimen, and patient-identified reasons

Planning: Patient Outcomes
1. Patient describes importance of treatment regimen.
2. Patient creates a treatment schedule with which she or he is able to comply.
3. Patient follows treatment regimen.

Nursing Interventions and Evaluation

NDx: Risk for injury
Explain the type of vision loss associated with glaucoma to enable the patient to plan effective safety measures. Stress that because peripheral vision loss accompanies glaucoma, there is a risk of stumbling over obstacles off to the side as a result of not see-ing them. Tell the patient to remove small articles from frequently traveled paths. Also explain that an object may suddenly appear in the field of vision.

Orient the patient to any new environment, from the examining room to the operating room. Help the patient settle into the room, but permit him or her to place personal objects. This helps the patient to remember the location of belongings and also allows the patient to place the objects in locations appropriate for his or her needs. Do not move objects without consent.

Avoid approaching the patient from the periphery. Instead, always approach from the front. If the doorway is not within the patient's line of sight, call out a greeting when entering the room. These actions avoid startling the patient and decrease the potential for injury.

Several glaucoma medications cause miosis. The small pupil changes size very slowly when adapting to dim lighting. Explain this slowed adaptation to the patient. Caution the patient to move slowly and to use available security measures, such as handrails, when adapting to dim lighting.

NDx: Pain
Patients with angle-closure glaucoma are frequently in moderate to severe pain. Note the patient's position when entering the room. Frequently, the eye pain or headache is so severe that the patient is holding the head. To promote pain relief, provide an atmosphere of comfort. Ask whether dim lighting helps ease the pain or makes it worse, and adjust lighting accordingly. Provide cool compresses for the patient's forehead. Administer analgesics, such as meperidine (Demerol), as ordered for intense pain. Keep in mind the route of choice is intramuscular because the patient may have nausea and onset of action is rapid. Monitor the patient's level of comfort before, during, and after interventions, and adjust accordingly.

Stress to the patient that ocular pain will be relieved once the IOP is reduced. Begin interventions to lower IOP as soon as possible.

NDx: Risk for ineffective management of therapeutic regimen (individuals)
Primary open-angle glaucoma is an incurable disease. Once started on medications, the patient will probably require them for an extended period. Help the patient understand that these treatments attempt to prevent loss of vision. Nothing can restore vision lost from glaucoma.

Unfortunately, side effects from glaucoma medications are common. Alert the glaucoma patient to them. Advise him or her to contact the nurse or ophthalmologist as soon as they occur. Reinforce the importance of not stopping the drug if side effects occur. If side effects do occur and the decision is to keep the patient on the medication, work with the patient to minimize side effects.

Side effects are not the only reason for noncompliance. Other reasons include cost, availability, and specific treatment schedule. When a variance between the treatment regimen and how the patient is actually practicing is observed, discuss those observations with the patient. The patient may have misinterpreted the instructions about the regimen or may have deviated for a reason. Remember that only the patient can say why the variance exists. Any successful treatment regimen must be negotiated with and agreed to by the patient.

If the problem is cost, explore resources available to the patient. State or federal assistance may be available, or local civic groups may provide a small source of funding. Refer the patient to a local social service agency to investigate sources of aid.

If the problem is scheduling difficulties, work with the patient to determine what is creating the difficulty. Is the problem one of needing to use a medication four times daily, but the patient only remembers it or only has help available two times daily? If so, check whether the patient can be changed to a regimen that requires use only twice daily.

If the problem is a memory error, help the patient develop a reminder mechanism. Checklists showing when each dose is due can be posted on the refrigerator or in another patient-determined location. When the patient administers the drops or takes the pill, the dose is checked off. If such a list is used, have the patient bring it to follow-up visits. Review the checkoff list with the patient, and monitor compliance at the same time.

Other strategies for dealing with noncompliance related to memory error include involving family or friends as a reminder checkup and placing medications in visible strategic locations. If the problem is remembering a midday dose, the medication can be tossed into the brown-bag lunch. When the bag is opened, the patient sees the bottle and remembers the dose.

Perhaps the problem of noncompliance is one of transportation difficulties. Patients cannot use medications they do not have. In these cases, examine available resources for transportation. Investigate the possibility of transferring the prescription to a pharmacy closer to the patient's home or near a location to which he or she frequently travels. Encourage the patient to look in the yellow pages to find out whether a neighborhood pharmacy offers delivery. Call local agencies, churches, or civic clubs, such as the Lions Club, that might transport the patient to the pharmacy or deliver the medication to the patient.

Whatever the cause, remember that no plan for reducing noncompliance can be successful unless it involves the patient. The nurse's role is to generate ideas and suggestions. Goals can be achieved only when the patient supports the idea.

Compare the patient's status with the expected outcomes. If the outcomes are not met, reassess the patient and revise the plan.

NURSING PROCESS GUIDELINES
Laser Therapy for Glaucoma

Nursing care for patients having laser therapy for glaucoma is similar to that described for patients having laser therapy for any disorder of the eye. (See Chap. 44.) For the patient with glaucoma, be sure to measure and record IOP on arrival for therapy and to check both IOP and vital signs before and after administering apraclonidine hydrochloride (Iopidine).

RETINAL HOLES, TEARS, AND DETACHMENTS

Etiology and Pathophysiology

A retinal detachment is a separation of the retina from the underlying choroid. The retina is physically attached to the choroid in only two places: posteriorly at the optic nerve and anteriorly at the ciliary body. The remaining retinal areas are held against the choroid by pressure from the vitreous. Thus, a retinal detachment can result from any factor that causes the retina to be pushed or pulled from the choroid. Such factors include hemorrhage, tumor, collection of exudate behind the retina caused by an inflammatory process (such as uveitis), or forward pull by the vitreous as a result of traction from newly formed blood vessels in it, as in diabetic neovascularization. However, the most common cause of retinal detachment is a hole or tear in the retina, which allows vitreous to gradually seep between and separate it from the choroid (Fig. 45–9). Such holes or tears may be due to trauma or to age-related degeneration of the retina. They occur most commonly at the outer edges of the retina where it is the thinnest.

Retinal detachments subsequently occur in the second eye in about one of five people.

Clinical Manifestations

The most common indication of a retinal hole, tear, or detachment is a painless change in vision. Patients complain of suddenly seeing flashes of bright lights (photopsia), a shower of spots before their eyes, or the sensation of a curtain being pulled down over part of their vision (Fig. 45–10). Some patients experience no awareness of the problem until the macular area is involved.

Light flashes are usually the result of traction on the retina. As the retina is pulled away, small capillaries break and release red blood cells and fragments into the vitreous. These fragments and cells cast a shadow on the retina, creating the perception of spots.

Diagnosis

The diagnosis of a retinal hole, tear, or detachment is made on the basis of the patient's history and the

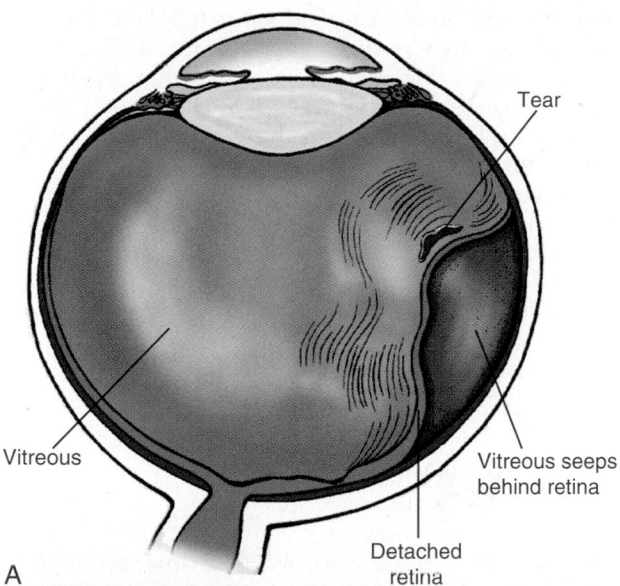

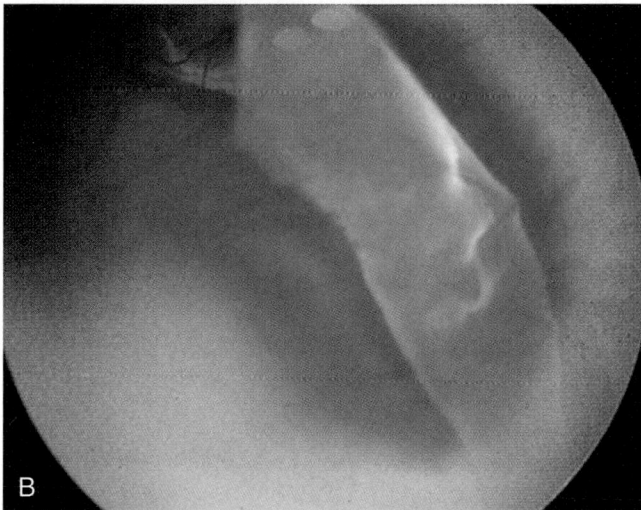

Figure 45–9

A, Illustration of a retinal detachment. B, Fundus photograph of a very large retinal tear with a rolled posterior border. (B, from Albert DM, Jakobiec FA [eds]. Atlas of clinical ophthalmology. Philadelphia: WB Saunders, 1996, p 244.)

ocular examination. When the retina is examined, small holes or tears can be seen. Tears are usually shaped like an arrowhead or a horseshoe. If a detachment is present, a hole or tear may be noted in close proximity. Areas of retinal detachment appear as gray inward bulges that may contain ripples or folds that jiggle with eye movement.

The detached area of the retina appears gray because it obstructs the view of the normal pink-orange color of the underlying choroid. The retina itself is transparent.

Management

The goal of treating retinal holes and tears is to prevent a retinal detachment. Small holes located in the periphery are often left untreated when the patient can be closely monitored for an increase in hole size.

Tears in the retina are treated with photocoagulation, cryotherapy, or diathermy. The goal of each procedure is to induce an inflammatory response between the retina and the underlying pigment epithelium and choroid to seal the edges of the tear.

Photocoagulation uses laser light focused on the pigment epithelium to coagulate it to the overlying retina. With cryotherapy, a supercooled probe is placed on the conjunctiva over the borders of the hole or tear. This freezes the area, creating an inflammatory response while not disturbing nearby ocular structures. Diathermy uses energy from a high-frequency current sufficient to cause tissue coagulation. It is also applied to the external eye overlying the retinal tear or hole.

Surgery is necessary to repair areas of retinal detachment because spontaneous reattachment is rare. The usual procedure is called a scleral buckle.

Scleral buckling is designed to repair the retinal detachment by indenting the sclera, forcing the choroid to come into closer contact with the retina. It is usually an inpatient procedure performed under general anesthesia. The conjunctiva is retracted to expose the sclera, through which microsurgical instruments, such as cutters and sources of light, are inserted. Using these instruments, wrinkles and folds in the retina are flattened, enabling the retina to assume its normal smooth position. Adhesions or traction bands between the retina and vitreous are cut and removed if needed. A vitrectomy is performed if needed to remove blood and other particles in the vitreous.

Once the retina is back in place and any subretinal fluid drained, the endolaser may be used to promote reattachment. Use of the laser creates intense heat, which seals the edges and creates an inflam-

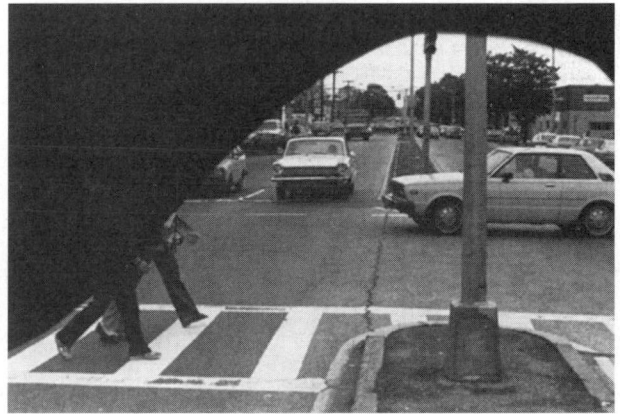

Figure 45–10

Example of visual defect seen by a patient with a retinal detachment. (Permission to use this photograph has been granted by the American Foundation for the Blind, 15 West 16th Street, New York, NY 10011.)

matory response. Silicone bands or implants, also known as a buckle, are placed to encircle the sclera or cover the area of the retinal tear to promote reattachment (Fig. 45–11). These implants help maintain the retina in contact with the choroid.

If needed, silicone oil or a gas, such as perfluoropropane or sulfur hexafluoride, is injected to help keep the retina in contact with the choroid. Because of its lower specific gravity, the gas or oil floats up against the retina and holds it in place.

When the procedure is completed, a subconjunctival injection of antibiotic is administered and topical antibiotic ointment instilled. An eye patch and shield are taped in place over the closed eyelid.

Complications of retinal detachment repair include infection, failure of the detachment to reattach, and increased IOP.

NURSING PROCESS
Surgery for Retinal Detachment

PREOPERATIVE NURSING CARE

Nursing care for the patient scheduled for surgery for a retinal detachment is similar to that for any patient having eye surgery, as described in Chapter 44, with several considerations. Be sure to determine when the patient last had anything to eat or drink, because the need for surgery can develop without warning. Instruct the patient in any preoperative activity restrictions, because rest in a specific position may be required to reduce stress on the area of detachment. This restriction is seen most frequently when the macula is intact but threatened by the location of the detachment. If the macula is severely threatened, total eye rest may be needed. Patients on

total eye rest may not read or watch television because these two activities cause rapid eye movements. Rarely, bilateral eye patches may be used to further ensure total eye rest. If these are needed, provide auditory or other nonvisual types of sensory stimulation.

Retinal detachment surgery may take several hours, depending on the nature, location, and complexity of the detachment. Inform the family or significant other of this information, so they will not become unduly anxious about how long the patient is in surgery. Tell the patient that he or she may feel stiff and sore for 1 or 2 days after surgery if it is a long procedure.

POSTOPERATIVE NURSING CARE

Assessment

The care of the patient after retinal detachment surgery is similar to that of any patient receiving general anesthesia. Assess the patient's return to physiologic stability. Monitor respiratory and cardiovascular status. Check vital signs in accordance with institutional policy and guided by the patient's condition. Observe the eye patch and shield for evidence of drainage. Assess for nausea, which sometimes results from the anesthetic agents as well as from manipulation of the eye during the procedure. Auscultate bowel sounds because diet can be resumed when they return and nausea is absent.

Once the initial eye patch is removed, the patient is started on cycloplegic agents, such as atropine or cyclopentolate (Cyclogyl), to dilate the pupil and rest the muscles of accommodation. Antibiotic and steroid eye drops, such as gentamicin (Genoptic) and prednisolone acetate (Pred Mild), respectively, or an antibiotic/steroid combination, such as prednisolone acetate and gentamicin (Pred-G) eye drops, will be ordered. Be sure to assess the patient's ability to instill these drops.

Nursing Diagnoses and Planning

Nursing diagnoses and related expected patient outcomes commonly applicable to patients who have had surgery for a retinal detachment include the following:

NDx: Risk for self care deficit related to positioning and activity restrictions required after surgery

Planning: Patient Outcomes
1. Patient describes how to manage personal care needs while maintaining activity restrictions.

NDx: Risk for injury: fall related to presence in an unfamiliar environment

Planning: Patient Outcomes
1. Patient avoids falling.
2. Retina remains reattached.

NDx: Pain related to surgical manipulation of tissue

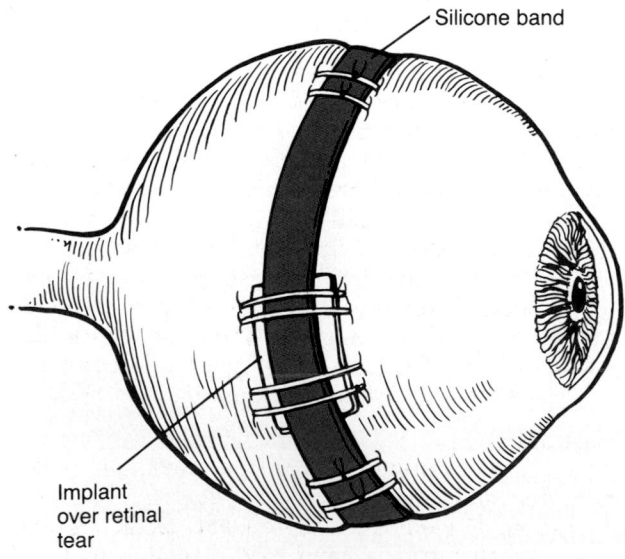

Silicone band

Implant over retinal tear

Figure 45–11
Scleral buckle for the treatment of retinal detachment.

Planning: Patient Outcomes
1. Patient reports pain is relieved or reduced to a manageable level.
2. Behavioral signs of severe pain are absent.

Nursing Interventions and Evaluation

NDx: Risk for self care deficit

When gas or oil is used to promote retinal reattachment, extreme care must be taken to keep the gas or oil bubble positioned against the repaired area of the retina. Maintain the patient in the position specified by the ophthalmologist. Usually, the patient's head will be parallel to the floor and turned to the side. Instruct the patient to lie on the abdomen and turn the head to the correct side. Place pillows for comfort and for support of the arms and lower back. Because the same position—head parallel to floor—must be maintained when the patient is out of bed or sitting up, instruct him or her to walk with the head down and turned to the appropriate side. Advise the patient to use the overbed table to rest the turned head. Monitor these activity restrictions, which must be maintained until the gas bubble absorbs, which may take 4 to 8 days.

Discuss how the patient can continue these restrictions while still meeting personal care needs. For example, to bathe, a basin of water can be placed on the bed next to the patient, or the patient can bathe at the sink as long as the head is kept flexed at the neck, thus parallel to the floor, and turned to the correct side.

The patient must also get used to eating with food in the lap or alongside. Encourage eating easy, hand-held foods. Provide assistance with tray set-up and item selection if necessary.

If the patient is going home with these restrictions, review the home situation and assist the patient in identifying self-care measures that comply with the restrictions.

Discuss how household chores, such as cooking or washing dishes, can be performed while maintaining these restrictions. As needed, explore community resources available, such as Meals on Wheels or home-care assistance.

NDx: Risk for injury

Make sure the patient has been oriented to the environment. Keep doors completely opened or closed. Place furniture and other items outside of the traffic flow areas of the room. Keep the call light within easy reach. Also place other needed articles within sight and reach. Because depth perception may be impaired, elevate the side rails at the head of the bed. Advise the patient to call for assistance with ambulation.

NDx: Pain

A significant amount of tissue manipulation occurs during scleral buckling surgery. Monitor the patient's level of pain. As necessary and prescribed, administer acetaminophen with codeine (Tylenol with Codeine) or other analgesic. If the pain is severe, or the patient is nauseated, administer intramuscular injections of prescribed analgesics. Initiate appropriate nonpharmacologic interventions, such as quiet music or conversation. Once the initial eye patch has been removed, place cool compresses over the closed eyelid for relief of discomfort from edema of the conjunctiva and sclera.

Compare the patient's status with the expected outcomes. If the outcomes are not met, reassess the patient and revise the plan.

Degenerative Disorders

MACULAR DEGENERATION

The macula is responsible for processing finely detailed vision used for recognizing faces and street signs, reading a label, threading a needle, and writing a check. It is 100 times more sensitive to detail than the peripheral retina.

Age-related macular degeneration (AMD) is the leading cause of irreversible vision loss in persons older than 65 years.

Etiology and Pathophysiology

AMD is a progressive form of permanent vision loss, the cause of which is unknown. In the atrophic form, the macula thins and functions poorly. In the exudative form, new and fragile blood vessels grow beneath the macula from the underlying choroid (a process called subretinal neovascularization). Blood and serous fluid leak out, causing the macula to bubble up and detail vision to be lost. The longer these vessels continue to grow, leak, and bleed, the greater the degree of detail vision lost.

AMD can occur bilaterally or unilaterally. In most cases of bilateral AMD, the disease progresses at different rates in each eye.

Clinical Manifestations

In the initial stages of AMD, the patient may notice blurry vision when reading or have no difficulty with near vision, yet experience trouble reading distant objects such as street signs. Because the macula is no longer smooth and flat, objects may look bent, crooked, or distorted. Straight lines look irregular. Patients may notice that sizes, shapes, and colors of objects look different when viewed with each eye. Patients may also complain about seeing a fixed gray spot just off the center of vision and compare it with the after-effect of a flash bulb (Fig. 45–12).

Diagnosis

The retina is examined for drusen, the small, yellow-white deposits frequently associated with macular degeneration, as well as for blisters and blood vessels.

An Amsler grid, a hand-held card that looks like graph paper with a dot in the center, is used to detect the presence of metamorphopsia, which is the

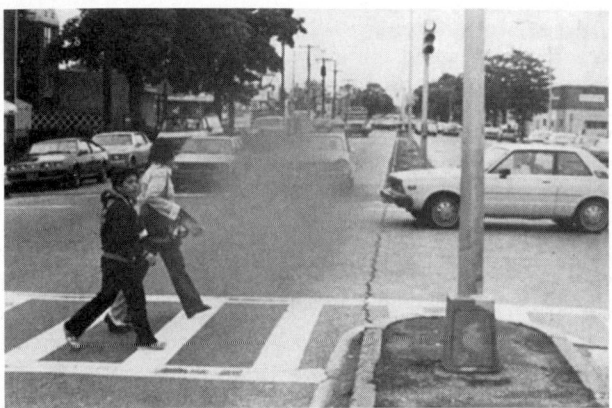

Figure 45–12

Image seen by patient with macular degeneration. (Permission to use this photograph has been granted by the American Foundation for the Blind, 15 West 16th Street, New York, NY 10011.)

distortion of straight lines. The patient with AMD frequently sees areas of distortion in the straight lines. The patient with AMD may also note that areas on the grid are dark or missing.

Fluorescein angiography may be used to check the retinal vasculature and determine whether blood vessel leakage is present. The photographs taken during this angiography provide important baseline data.

Management

Unfortunately, there is no medical, surgical, or laser treatment for atrophic AMD. The patient whose only symptom is drusen is given an Amsler grid and instructed to check vision daily. In exudative macular degeneration, when abnormal blood vessels are present and detected early, laser therapy can be used. Laser therapy seals the blood vessels, stopping their progression, leaking, and bleeding. However, while sealing the leaking blood vessels, small nearby areas of the retina are destroyed. As a result, the gray spot seen previously becomes a black scotoma, or blind spot.

It is not always possible or in the patient's best interest to perform laser therapy. It depends on the amount of blood present, the general health of the macula, and the location of the abnormal blood vessels. It is important for the patient to know that vision usually does not improve after laser therapy but that distortion is lessened or eliminated.

NURSING PROCESS GUIDELINES
Macular Degeneration

Determine when the patient noticed the change in acuity and under what conditions the reduced acuity is noted, such as in dim light, when tired, or when reading. Review the patient's and family's medical history because age, female sex, smoking,

and a family history of macular degeneration place the patient at a greater risk for developing AMD.

Explore how the change in vision has affected lifestyle. Ask whether there are things he or she is no longer able to do or has increased difficulty doing. Measure distance and near visual acuity. Be sure the patient wears reading glasses if used.

Use a quiet, simple approach when teaching the patient newly diagnosed with AMD. Remember that the diagnosis can alter the patient's lifestyle dramatically and permanently. Expect many questions, but be aware that the patient is often too afraid of the answers to ask them.

Advise the patient that macular degeneration is a permanent form of vision loss, but total vision loss and blindness occur very rarely. Review the normal anatomy of the eye and vision, using models as needed. Review the pathology of AMD, using the analogy of tree roots bubbling up the sidewalk as appropriate.

Provide the patient with written, large-print

INTERNET CONNECTIONS
Eye Disorders

American Academy of Ophthalmology/Eye Diseases and Conditions
http://www.eyenet.org/public/faqs/faqs.html
A patient-oriented site providing answers to frequently asked questions in the areas of eye diseases, eye health, and eye safety, as well as links to many other sites. Conditions covered include cataracts, glaucoma, low vision, and macular degeneration.

National Eye Institute
http://www.nei.nih.gov/
This U.S. government–sponsored site provides general information, publications, information about clinical studies, and related resources.

Frequently Asked Questions: Glaucoma
http://www.web-xpress.com/athens/glaucoma.html
A patient-oriented list of frequently asked questions that, as of spring 1997, was still under development. It discusses various types of glaucoma and their diagnosis and treatment.

Macular Degeneration Foundation
http://www.eyesight.org/
This extensive site provides a newsletter, links to related resources, and answers to frequently asked questions about eye disease.

handouts to take home. To improve the contrast between the letters on the page and the paper, thus making reading easier, send the patient home with a yellow transparent cover sheet, which can be inexpensively made from a yellow, transparent report cover.

Review and demonstrate use of the Amsler grid. Have the patient practice using it, and obtain a return demonstration in its use before he or she leaves. Instruct the patient to check both eyes each day while wearing his or her reading glasses. Also have the patient use one object in the living area, such as a clock or door frame, to check vision each day. Stress the importance of notifying the ophthalmologist whenever new or larger areas of distortion are noted.

Assist the patient to identify ways in which existing vision can be maximized. Ways can vary from changing light bulbs to using optical scanners. Determine what help the patient wants and what will be used as opposed to what the caregiver believes should be used.

Encourage the use of incandescent light because glare can be visually handicapping for these patients. Fluorescent lighting causes more glare. Instruct the patient to use a 75-watt to 100-watt light bulb and to position the light source so the light rays fall directly down onto the page. In the early stages of AMD, these changes might be all that is needed.

Refer the patient with significant vision loss to a local low-vision specialist for evaluation and recommendation of additional visual resources, such as magnifiers, hand-held or eyeglass-mounted telescopes, and optical scanners.

No one knows the stressors of living with macular degeneration the way another macular degeneration patient does. Ask the patient if he or she would find it helpful to speak with other patients. If acceptable to the patient, make a referral to the local support group. The services of a clinical nurse specialist, psychologist, or mental health professional may be available through the local center or community agency that services the visually handicapped.

Sometimes job changes are required. Refer to state agencies, such as the Bureau for Vocational Rehabilitation, for assistance with retraining.

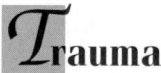

Trauma

CONTUSIONS, ABRASIONS, LACERATIONS, AND PENETRATING INJURIES

Etiology and Pathophysiology

Contusions result from the impact of a blunt object, such as a baseball bat or racquetball. Such impact causes an immediate and significant rise in IOP, which results in tearing and bleeding of susceptible tissues and major arterioles in the angle. Rupture of the globe can occur, as well as subconjunctival hemorrhage (called hyphema). Severe blunt injuries can even dislocate the lens. The incidence of this type of injury is increasing because of the popularity of such sports as tennis, racquetball, and soccer.

A corneal abrasion occurs when the epithelium is removed by a scratching or irritating force. Common causes of corneal abrasions include foreign bodies, eyelashes, dust, and dirt. Abrasions can also occur from natural objects, such as tree branches, grass blades forced out at high speeds from lawn mowers or weed removers, and from contact lens overwear and excessive exposure to sunlight. After abrasion, the cornea usually regenerates in 24 to 48 hours without scarring.

Lacerations, caused by sharp objects such as scissors, a fishhook, animal or human teeth, or glass fragments can affect any part of the external eye. The most common sites of lacerations are the eyelid and cornea. Corneal lacerations can be serious because ocular contents can prolapse through the corneal laceration. Deep corneal lacerations can heal with a scar. If the scar significantly affects vision, a corneal transplant may be necessary (see Chap. 44).

High-speed particles, such as BBs, metal, bullets, rock pellets, and flying glass projectiles are able to penetrate the eye. Objects can become embedded in the eye after a fall onto a sharp object, such as a tree branch or a pair of scissors. Rupture of the eye can result. Once inside the eye, the foreign body can create an ocular inflammation or infection.

Clinical Manifestations

Patients experiencing a contusion, or black eye, usually relate a history of recent trauma to the area. Visual acuity usually is not affected. Edema of the eyelids, periorbital edema, and a hyphema are frequently seen. Photophobia or diplopia may occur.

Abrasions create a "foreign-body" sensation in the eye, often accompanied by tearing and photophobia. Visual acuity may be reduced if the cornea is involved. Vertical scratches may be seen on the cornea if particulate matter has lodged under the eyelid, because the foreign body is scraped across the cornea during each blink.

Patients with a laceration of the eye or eyelid usually report a history of being struck by an object. An irregular cut of the eyelid or the surface of the eye may be visible. Because the eyelid is very vascular, the amount of bleeding may seem out of proportion compared with the severity of the laceration. Pieces of the eyelid may be missing.

Most penetrating injuries cause a marked loss of vision. However, injuries from small particles traveling at a significant speed may produce only mild pain and blurring of vision. Other signs of penetrating injuries include an irregular pupil, vitreous hemorrhage, laceration of the conjunctiva or cornea, and hyphema.

Some patients present for treatment with the object still protruding from the eye. Extreme care must be taken not to disturb this object because it may be holding ocular contents in place.

Diagnosis

The diagnosis is based on a careful patient history and examination. Visual acuity is examined before conducting any part of the examination to document the patient's visual status, for medical and legal reasons, before care is administered. Near and distance vision are tested.

If a foreign body is suspected, the upper eyelid is everted and the bulbar and palpebral conjunctiva examined with a slit lamp. Fluorescein is used to highlight areas of corneal abrasion. This dye, when viewed with a blue filter, colors any abraded area a vivid and easily detected green.

The cornea, sclera, iris, and lens are examined with the slit lamp or direct ophthalmoscope for evidence of an entrance wound. X-rays and computed tomographic (CT) scans of the eye and orbit can be used to locate objects and fragments. Ultrasonography may also be used to determine the location of the intraocular foreign body in relationship to ocular structures. Magnetic resonance imaging (MRI) may also be used if a nonmetal foreign body is suspected.

Management

Contusions usually require ice to reduce swelling. If the force caused bleeding into the anterior chamber (hyphema), the patient is placed on bedrest because rebleeding in the first few days is possible. Patients with a hyphema may receive aminocaproic acid (Amicar) to prevent further bleeding. Patients with hyphema should sleep and rest with the head elevated, so the blood will settle to the lower anterior chamber and away from the visual pathway. IOP is monitored because blood in the anterior chamber can potentially obstruct the trabecular meshwork and prevent drainage of aqueous humor.

Corneal abrasions are treated by removing the cause, when possible. For example, a foreign body on the conjunctiva is irrigated away. An ophthalmic antibiotic, such as gentamicin (Gentacidin), is then instilled. The eye is patched closed for 24 hours, the usual healing and regenerating time necessary for the corneal epithelium.

Lacerations usually require stitches. If the laceration does not involve the edge of the eyelid, a simple closure is possible. Lacerations involving the cornea must be treated as an ocular emergency because the laceration creates an opening through which microorganisms can directly enter the eye and ocular contents can prolapse. These lacerations are repaired under the operating room microscope. Once repaired, an ophthalmic antibiotic, such as gentamicin (Gentacidin) ointment, is instilled and an eye patch and shield applied. Visual acuity is carefully monitored over the next few days. Deep corneal lacerations may heal with a scar.

A foreign body may or may not be removed, depending on its composition and location in the eye. Foreign bodies made of metals such as iron and copper must be removed because these metals are toxic to ocular tissues. Materials such as porcelain and glass are well tolerated by the eye and might not need to be removed. The exact surgical procedure depends on the location of the object. Special equipment, such as metal locators and magnets, may be used.

NURSING PROCESS
Ocular Trauma

Assessment

When obtaining a history from a patient with a known or suspected ocular injury, provide for patient comfort. If photophobia is present, dim the room lights. If tearing is a problem, provide adequate tissues. Unless the problem is obvious, such as a bleeding eyelid or an object protruding from the eye, ask the patient why he or she is seeking care. Ask when it began or happened and what he or she was doing at that time. If an injury is described, ask about the circumstances and the first aid, if any, that was given on the scene. Find out what materials the patient was working with, such as metal or glass. Ask whether the patient takes any medications, especially anticoagulants or aspirin. Also determine when the patient last had a tetanus shot and whether he or she has any allergies. If surgery may be necessary, ask when food and fluids were last consumed.

Obtain a baseline acuity for near and distance vision. Examine the external eye. Are any foreign bodies present? Are the eyelids intact? If sections of the eyelid are missing, ask the patient or family if they know where the missing fragments are. In many cases, these segments can be reattached. Observe the external eye for ecchymosis.

Observe for signs and symptoms of anxiety, because patients with ocular trauma are worried about their vision and whether any permanent damage has been done.

Nursing Diagnoses and Planning

Nursing diagnoses and related expected patient outcomes commonly applicable to patients with ocular trauma include the following:

NDx: Pain related to irritation of the corneal nerve fibers

Planning: Patient Outcomes
1. Patient participates in the examination without indication of excessive pain.
2. Patient reports intensity of symptoms to be manageable.

NDx: Anxiety related to possible loss of vision or failure to regain vision

Planning: Patient Outcomes
1. Patient reports anxiety level is manageable.
2. Behavioral signs of severe anxiety are absent.

NDx: Risk for altered health maintenance related to insufficient knowledge of prevention of future ocular injuries

Planning: Patient Outcomes
1. Patient lists common causes of ocular trauma.
2. Patient identifies measures to use in the prevention of ocular trauma.

Nursing Interventions and Evaluation

NDx: Pain

Because of the large number of nerve fibers in the cornea, abrasions can be extremely painful. The pain can actually be so severe that it disables the patient. Immediately promote comfort by dimming the lights of the examination room. Once the diagnosis of a corneal abrasion has been made, instill a drop of topical anesthetic, such as proparacaine (Ophthetic), as ordered. Keep in mind, however, that repeated use of topical anesthetics retards healing. Apply an eye patch for overnight wear. Patch the eyelid in the closed position to prevent it from rubbing against the abrasion with blinking.

Administer oral analgesics, such as acetaminophen (Tylenol), as ordered for severe pain. Keep the lights dimmed, provide quiet conversation or distraction, and apply a cool cloth over the closed eyelids for brief periods to further promote comfort.

These measures to reduce pain and photophobia should also be effective in reducing tearing, which is usually a reflex mechanism.

NDx: Anxiety

Expect the patient to be anxious over the possibility of short-term or permanent vision loss. Acknowledge this anxiety, as well as anticipatory grief, as normal reactions. Listen supportively. Reassure the patient that measures to save vision are being taken. Also be sure to keep the patient and family informed of what is happening. Ask the patient about measures that would provide comfort, such as the presence of a cleric or friend. Remind the patient that, after trauma, vision may take a while to return to baseline. Help the patient recognize the improvement when it occurs.

NDx: Risk for altered health maintenance

Most eye injuries are preventable. Instruct the patient that abrasions from tree branches and high-speed grass particles can be prevented by wearing sunglasses or safety glasses. The same is true for abrasions caused by high-speed metal particles.

Encourage the patient to use protective eyewear when participating in sports, especially high-speed sports, such as racquetball and tennis. Encourage local racquet clubs to discourage play unless participants are wearing appropriate protective eyewear. Warn cross-country skiers and hikers about the potential for injury while participating in these activi-

ties. Remind the patient that excessive exposure to sunlight, such as falling asleep in the sun, can cause severe corneal damage. Caution the patient who wears contact lenses against excessive wear. Review a reasonable wearing schedule with the patient, as well as its rationale.

Discuss safe handling of sharp objects in the home, school, work place, and other high-risk areas. Stress that persons not familiar with the sharp object should be supervised in its use.

Additional Interventions

Guilt frequently is experienced by others involved in the trauma, such as the hockey player who shot the puck that injured the patient, or the fellow racquetball player who hit the ball that struck the patient in the eye. If these people are present, be aware of this need and help them deal with their feelings of guilt.

Compare the patient's status with the expected outcomes. If the outcomes are not met, reassess the patient and revise the plan.

CHEMICAL BURNS

Etiology and Pathophysiology

Chemicals can come into contact with the eye or eyelids in many forms and from a variety of sources, such as steam, molten metal, hot ashes, strong acids (battery acid), and alkalis (lye, lime). Because of the devastating effects on the eye, contact with chemicals is an ocular emergency.

The extent of damage depends on the exact chemical involved, duration of time between exposure and institution of first aid, degree of penetration into the eye, and definitive treatment in an emergency care setting.

For example, when acids come in contact with the eye, direct damage of the tissue results. However, the acids form a cover of coagulated tissue that protects ocular structures from further penetration of the chemical. Alkaline chemicals, on the other hand, can cause both immediate and delayed changes because they are able to penetrate deeply into tissues and cause damage long after initial exposure.

Because of its anatomical position, the cornea is typically affected by chemical burns. Perforation and scarring of the cornea are common. Entropion of the eyelids can also result. Intraocular structures can be affected, such as the lens and trabecular meshwork, leading to the development of cataracts and glaucoma.

Clinical Manifestations

A patient with a chemical burn relates a history of something splashing into the face. The pain is intense, and the patient may be unable to open the eyes.

First- and second-degree burns of the periorbital area may be present as a result of irritation by the chemicals. The conjunctiva may be red, ischemic, or

Table 45–3

Emergency Treatment for Chemical Burns of the Eye

1. Flush affected eye immediately with a large amount of clean water or irrigating solution for 10 minutes to shorten chemical contact with ocular tissues.
2. Hold patient's hands away from face if necessary because of the normal protective response to cover eyes with hands, an action that limits access to the eye.
3. Hold eyelids open widely during procedure because a larger area can be flushed.
4. Quickly check visual acuity to provide baseline information for medical and legal reasons.
5. Obtain a sample of the chemical involved. Send it and its container with the injured person to the hospital or emergency care center to help identify the specific substance.
6. Get the patient to the hospital or emergency care center.
7. Tell someone to alert the hospital or emergency care center that patient is en route to enable the facility to have equipment ready on the patient's arrival.

absent. All or part of the corneal epithelium may be absent. Total anesthesia of the cornea is possible, as well as a corneal haze, which can make evaluation of the internal eye difficult or impossible. In some cases, the cornea turns totally white.

Diagnosis

The diagnosis of a chemical burn is based on history and ocular examination. No assessment is conducted or history obtained, however, until after ocular irrigation has begun.

Management

Treatment of a chemical burn should begin at the site of exposure. Copious irrigation with water or saline should be conducted even before transport to the emergency care center (Table 45–3). If the patient is unable to hold the eyelids open—a normal response—someone should provide assistance. If no facilities exist for irrigating the eye, the patient is instructed to hold the eyes open under a running shower. A sink filled with water, into which the patient submerges the head, will also work. The patient must be reminded to keep the eyes open to adequately flush the area.

Table 45–4

Irrigation of the Eye

1. Obtain the following necessary equipment:
   0.9% saline (1-L bag)
   Macrodrip IV tubing
   IV pole or other suspension device
   Topical anesthetic drops (proparacaine [Ophthaine])
   Eyelid speculum or irrigating contact lens
   Gloves (unsterile)
   pH paper
   Towels
   Collection container
2. Simultaneously obtain history as tubing or contact lens is being flushed with saline solution because time is of the essence.
   Determine the following:
   Time of injury
   Type of chemical or irritant
   First aid given on site
   Allergy to -caine drugs
3. Briefly describe procedure to patient to promote cooperation and to decrease anxiety.
4. Assess visual acuity for medical and legal reasons before starting treatment.
5. Put on gloves to reduce potential for exposure to chemicals.
6. Assess pH by dabbing paper in cul-de-sac to determine nature of chemical and help plan treatment.
7. Instill proparacaine (Ophthaine) prn or per protocol to enhance comfort by anesthetizing the external eye.
8. Turn the patient onto the affected side so drainage flows away from the unaffected eye.
9. Place irrigating contact lens or eyelid speculum to spread eyelids because normal reflex is to close eyes. Avoid using contact lens if particulate matter is suspected, because it could be ground into cornea.
10. Direct irrigating solution from the medial to the lateral canthus to flush surface without recontamination.
11. Monitor the patient's level of comfort throughout, and instill anesthetic drops as necessary.
12. Reassure the patient throughout procedure to reduce feeling of anxiety.
13. Irrigate both eyes simultaneously if both are affected to reduce chemical contact time with eye tissue.

IV, intravenous; prn, as occasion requires.

On arrival at the emergency care center, the eyes are again irrigated copiously with 0.9% saline. Ophthalmic anesthetic drops, such as proparacaine (Ophthaine), are instilled periodically for patient comfort. The irrigations are continued until the pH is approximately 7.0.

Once the irrigations are complete, an eye drop program to combat ocular inflammation is begun. Antiglaucoma agents and pupillary dilation drugs are used. A short-term course of steroid drops may be used, but long-term administration may contribute to problems with corneal healing.

Because patients are usually admitted to the hospital, IOP and indications of healing can be closely monitored. Recovery from a chemical burn is a long process, and there is great uncertainty about return of vision. Some patients fail to recover much vision. In cases of severe chemical burns affecting the cornea, a transplant may be required, but success is limited after this type of injury.

NURSING PROCESS GUIDELINES
Chemical Ocular Burn

Nursing care of the patient with a chemical ocular burn is similar to that of the patient with mechanical trauma, with several specific considerations.

When assessing a patient with a known or suspected chemical burn, be sure to begin the irrigation first (Table 45–4).

Question the patient about allergies. If no allergy to drugs of the -caine family exists, instill a drop of proparacaine (Ophthaine) to anesthetize the external eye. During irrigation, periodically assess the patient's level of comfort, and administer additional drops of proparacaine as necessary.

Find out when the exposure to the chemical occurred, the name and type of chemical, whether a sample of the chemical can be obtained, and the emergency care that was administered at the scene. Also determine whether contact lenses were being worn at the time of exposure, because they will need to be removed. Use strict aseptic technique because the potential for infection exists from disruption of the intact surface of the eye.

Be sensitive to the patient's high level of anxiety. Almost constant reassurance and positive reinforcement are necessary throughout the assessment, diagnosis, intervention, and evaluation processes. Answer questions honestly yet hopefully. Be aware that grieving for loss of vision will occur.

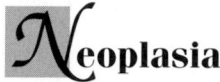 eoplasia

Both benign and malignant tumors can affect the structures of the eye. Malignant tumors can arise in the retina or the uveal tract, or may be due to metastasis from another site in the body. The most common primary malignancy of the eye is choroidal melanoma, with about 1500 cases diagnosed in the United States each year. Choroidal melanoma is almost always unilateral and is more common among white people. It is spread easily because of the rich blood supply of the choroid, and is frequently found in asymptomatic patients who present with a different ophthalmic complaint. Treatment consists of local excision and radiation, radioactive plaque therapy, in which a plaque containing seeds of radioactive isotope is sutured to the sclera overlying the tumor, or enucleation of the globe (see Chap. 44).

The Elderly: Special Considerations

Many of the patients seen with ocular disorders are older adults. Cataracts occur commonly, and loss of muscle tone and tissue elasticity can contribute to development of an ectropion.

Older adults may have chronic conditions, such as dementia or cardiovascular disorders, that cause fatigue or mental changes. These two factors may complicate assessment and treatment because ophthalmic assessments require a great deal of patient participation. The nurse must be sensitive to detecting problems that may interfere with assessment or treatment and adapt communication techniques to the needs of the older adult. For example, if the person has difficulty responding to questions, it may be appropriate to involve a family member or caregiver in the interview. Also, if several tests are required, the patient may appreciate a break between them. If hearing problems interfere with communication, the nurse must be careful to phrase questions appropriately to assist the older adult in providing accurate information. Questions may need to be rephrased if a vague or questioning expression is noted.

Geriatric ophthalmic patients must receive care that is based on complete knowledge of their medical history. For example, nonspecific beta blockers, such as timolol maleate (Timoptic), can cause shortness of breath and trigger episodes of heart failure in patients with respiratory or cardiac problems. Certain drugs must be used with caution in the older adult. For example, acetazolamide (Diamox) can cause mental changes.

With aging, pupil reactivity slows. Many ophthalmic drugs used to treat glaucoma can cause miosis. The small pupil and prolonged reactivity may interfere with the person's ability to move safely from bright to dim environments, and vice versa.

Careful attention must also be directed to a treatment regimen that the older adult can manage. For example, an older adult who has arthritis or orthopedic problems may require special adaptation for comfort during surgery. When planning care, ask whether the older adult can see the fine print on the label of the eye drop bottle and whether the patient with arthritic hands can instill the required eye drops. Keep the medication regimen as simple as possible by asking the physician if longer-acting eye drops can be used to decrease the frequency of administration.

As patients age, color sensitivity to blues, greens, and violets decreases. Care must be exercised when incorporating visual cues into the treatment process as reminders for patients. Many eye drops come in bottles with colored tops. The nurse must assess whether the patient can determine the color of the top before providing visual cues such as "use one drop from the green-topped bottle three times a day."

Chapter Review

1. Which types of pathophysiologic changes in the eye cause pain, and which do not?
2. Why is information about sexually transmitted diseases an essential part of the history for a patient complaining of conjunctivitis?
3. What kinds of questions need to be asked a patient with a hordeolum to determine if he or she is able to comply with the treatment regimen?
4. How do such factors as physical status, mental status, and lifestyle affect a person's suitability for the various types of refractive correction available?
5. How does the vision loss associated with glaucoma differ from the vision loss associated with cataracts?
6. What patient characteristics would support a decision that cataract surgery is needed, and which would not?
7. How do patients with open-angle glaucoma and angle-closure glaucoma differ in their clinical manifestations, medical treatment, and nursing care needs?
8. What difference in history of visual loss would be expected between a patient with open-angle glaucoma and a patient with a retinal detachment?
9. What adaptations to the standard hospital admission process would be required by a patient with advanced macular degeneration?
10. How can a nurse help a patient cope with a new diagnosis of macular degeneration?

Bibliography

Albert D, Jakobiec F (eds). Principles and practice of ophthalmology: Clinical practice. Philadelphia: WB Saunders, 1994.

Albert DM. Source book of ophthalmology. Cambridge, MA: Blackwell Scientific, 1995.

Bankes JL. Clinical ophthalmology: A text and colour atlas. 3rd ed. Edinburgh: Churchill Livingstone, 1994.

Booth B. Information nurses need to tell patients about glaucoma. Nurs Times 1994; 90(May 11–17):39.

Brady BA. Macular degeneration: Helping your patient cope. Nursing 1995; 25(June):62.

Caramella F. Silicone oil as a vitreous substitute in vitreoretinal surgery. J Ophthalmic Nurs Technol 1994; 13(Sept–Oct):241.

Carr L, Talley D. Complications of anterior segment laser procedures. Optom Clin 1995; 4(4):33.

Crick RP, Khaw P. Textbook of clinical ophthalmology. 2nd ed. River Edge, NJ: World Scientific, 1995.

Dornic D. Ophthalmic pocket companion. 4th ed. Woburn, MA: Butterworth-Heinemann, 1995.

Farkas P. Integrating disposable or planned replacement lenses into contact lens practice. Optom Clinics 1994; 4(1):61.

Fishbaugh J. Focus. Nursing care of the patient with cornea graft rejection. Insight 1995; 20(Dec):34.

Fishbaugh J. Observations of subspecialties. Retina: indocyanine green (ICG) angiography. Insight 1994; 19(Oct):30.

Fleming JB. Laser therapy and angle-closure glaucoma. Optom Clin 1995; 4(4):97.

Gaffney MM, Kelly MP. What is this entity? . . . lattice degeneration of the retina. J Ophthalmic Nurs Technol 1995; 14(Mar–Apr):89.

Glynn-Milley C, Mackay J. Home care for the postoperative cataract patient. Insight 1995; 20(4):21.

Hunt L. Complications of indirect laser photocoagulation. Insight 1994; 19(Dec):24.

Irvin SM. Identification of potential problems for elderly outpatients after preoperative medication: A case study. J Post Anesth Nurs 1995; 10(June):159.

Kanski JJ. Clinical ophthalmology: A systematic approach. 3rd ed. Woburn, MA: Butterworth-Heinemann, 1994.

Kelly M. Consequences of visual impairment on leisure activities of the elderly. Geriatr Nurs 1995; 16(Nov–Dec):273.

Kostick D, Linberg J. Evisceration with hydroxyapatite implant. Ophthalmology 1995; 102(10):1542.

Kowalski CK. Cataracts at any age. Home Healthc Nurse 1994; 12(Mar–Apr):43.

Kulick M, Hoffman C. Nutrition supplement usage recommendation by eye care specialists for macular degeneration of the eye: A statewide survey of Michigan. Top Clin Nutr 1995; 10(Sept):67.

Lindquist TD, Lindstrom RL. Ophthalmic surgery update #4. St. Louis: Mosby-Year Book, 1996.

Medical Economics Staff. Physicians' desk reference for ophthalmology. 24th ed. Oradell, NJ: Medical Economics, 1995.

Meissner J. Caring for patients with glaucoma. Nursing 1995; 25(Jan):56.

Monshizadeh R, Haimovici R. Advances in vitreoretinal surgery: Macular hole repair and perfluorocarbon liquids. J Ophth Nurs Technol 1995; 14(Sept–Oct):220.

Murill CA, et al. Primary care of the cataract patient. Stamford, CT: Appleton & Lange, 1994.

Murray PI, Fielder AR. Pocket book of ophthalmology. Woburn, MA: Butterworth-Heinemann, 1996.

Newell F. Ophthalmology: Principles and concepts. 8th ed. St. Louis: CV Mosby, 1996.

Pavan-Langston D (ed). Manual of ocular diagnosis and therapy. Boston: Little, Brown, 1996.

Peralta L, Adame H. Corneal transplant: A new lease on life. Semin Perioper Nurs 1995; 4(Oct):227.

Perry JP. Care of the ophthalmic patient. 2nd ed. San Diego, CA: Singular Publishing, 1995.

Ralph J, Otero C, Hammond B. Operation cataract. Nurs Stand 1995; 9(34):18.

Ready R. Commentary on sports related eye trauma. ENAs Nurs Scan Emerg Care 1994; 4(Mar–Apr):10.

Rosenthal BP, Cole RG. Functional assessment of low vision. St. Louis: Mosby-Year Book, 1995.

Sandler R. Clinical snapshot: Glaucoma. Am J Nurs 1995; 95(Mar):34.

Sandler RL. Glaucoma. Am J Nurs 1995; 95(Mar):34.

Shields JA, Shields CL. Intraocular tumors: A text and atlas. Philadelphia: WB Saunders, 1992.

Sighted: Foods for better vision. Tufts Univ Diet Nutr Lett 1995; 12(Jan):1.

Sivalingam E. Glaucoma: An overview. J Ophthalmic Nurs Technol 1996; 15(1):15.

Small RG. The clinical handbook of ophthalmology. London: Parthenon, 1994.

Spires R. Contact laser transscleral cyclophotocoagulation in the treatment of glaucoma. J Ophthalmic Nurs Technol 1995; 14(Jul–Aug):154.

Spires R. Glaucoma filtration surgery and the shell tamponade technique. J Ophthalmic Nurs Technol 1994; 13(Jan–Feb):17.

Spires R. Traumatic hyphema. J Ophthalmic Nurs Technol 1995; 14(Jan–Feb):21.

Talley D. Laser therapy for open angle glaucoma. Optom Clin 1995; 4:85.

Tasman W, Jaeger EA (eds). The Wills Eye Hospital atlas of clinical ophthalmology. Philadelphia: Lippincott-Raven, 1995.

Taylor RH. Key topics in ophthalmology. Philadelphia: Coronet Books, 1995.

Vaughan D, Asbury T, Riordan-Eva P. General ophthalmology. 4th ed. Los Angeles: Lange, 1995.

White T. Aqueous shunt implant surgery for refractory glaucoma. J Ophthalmic Nurs Technol 1996; 15(Jan–Feb):7.

Woods D. Idiopathic macular hole. J Ophthalmic Nurs Technol 1995; 14(Mar–Apr):57.

Year book of ophthalmology. St. Louis: Mosby-Year Book, 1996.

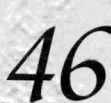
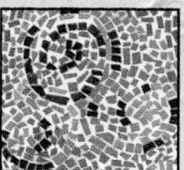
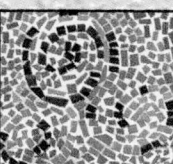
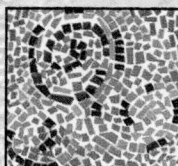
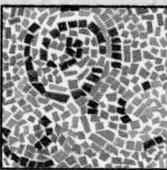
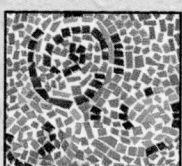
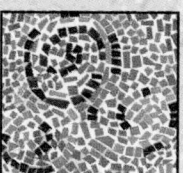

46

Knowledge Base for Patients with Ear Dysfunction

Study Outcomes

After studying this chapter, you should be able to:

1. Explain the normal anatomy and physiology of the ear.
2. Describe common clinical manifestations of ear dysfunction.
3. Identify information and physical examination data essential to the assessment of the ear.
4. Describe basic diagnostic tests and treatments used in the collaborative management of patients with ear disorders.
5. Describe basic surgical procedures used in the treatment of patients with ear disorders.
6. Identify data essential to the assessment of patients undergoing treatment of ear disorders.
7. State nursing diagnoses and related expected patient outcomes commonly applicable to patients undergoing treatment of ear disorders.
8. Describe nursing interventions, with their rationales, commonly applicable to patients undergoing treatment of ear disorders.
9. Explain the basis for evaluation of nursing care provided to patients undergoing treatment of ear disorders.
10. Identify alternative treatment and care settings for patients with ear dysfunction and the services related to community-based care.
11. Identify special considerations for the elderly patient with altered function of the ear.

The ear is a complex organ whose function is a major determinant of the quality of a person's life experience. As the organ of hearing, the ear facilitates communication and provides important information about the environment—such as the sound of oncoming traffic, sirens, and cries of warning—all of which can be critical to safety and well being. The ear's vestibular system functions together with other body systems to maintain balance and equilibrium, also critical to a sense of safety and well-being.

This chapter presents an overview of the anatomy and physiology of the ear, followed by a discussion of clinical manifestations common to ear disorders, assessment of the ear, and related diagnostic measures. Finally, it reviews otologic surgical procedures and specific considerations basic to caring for an elderly person who has an ear disorder.

Anatomy and Physiology

The ear is a complex structure that consists of three parts: the external ear, the middle ear, and the inner ear (Fig. 46–1). The temporal bones of the skull house the ears and protect important structures, including the internal auditory canal, seventh and eighth cranial nerves, labyrinth, and cochlea.

EXTERNAL EAR

The external ear includes the auricle (pinna) and the external auditory meatus (ear canal). The auricle projects from the side of the head and is composed primarily of cartilage, which gives shape to the ear. The lobule (earlobe) contains adipose and subcutaneous tissue. The external auditory canal is a tube-shaped passage about 2.5 cm in length that extends inward medially, proximally, and downward in adults. The canal is lined with skin and contains hair and cerumen (wax)-producing glands.

The external ear is separated from the middle ear by the tympanic membrane (eardrum) located at the proximal end of the external auditory canal. Sound waves are collected and focused by the auricle and travel within the canal, impinging on the tympanic membrane, causing it to vibrate. This vibration sets the ossicles (bones) of the middle ear into motion.

MIDDLE EAR

The middle-ear space, also referred to as the tympanic cavity, is a small, irregular, air-filled cavity within the petrous section of the temporal bone. It is separated from the inner ear by a thin, bony wall and two membrane-covered openings—the oval and

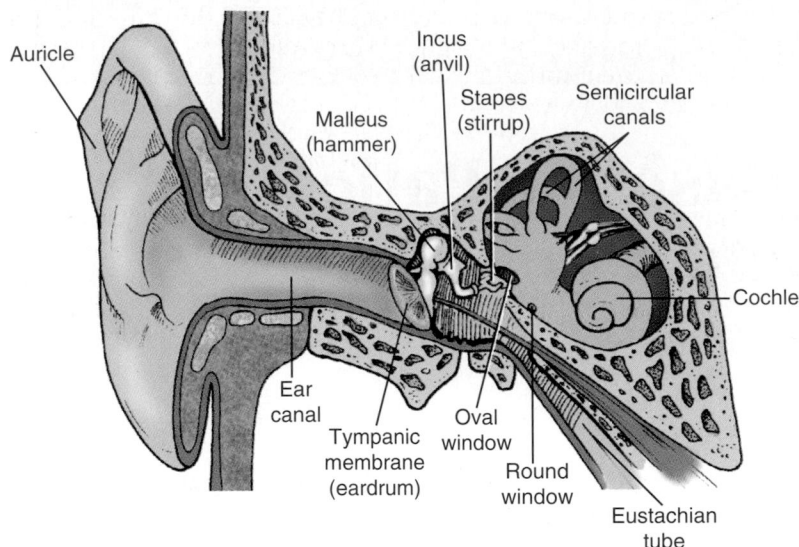

Figure 46–1

Anatomical structure of the ear. The tympanic membrane separates the external ear from the middle ear. The middle ear is separated from the inner ear by a thin, bony wall and two membrane-covered openings—the oval and round windows.

round windows. Anteriorly, the middle ear communicates with the eustachian tube, which forms a channel between the middle ear and the nasopharynx. This connection allows air to enter the middle-ear space, which equalizes the pressure on both sides of the tympanic membrane. Eustachian tube dysfunction can lead to various middle ear disorders. Posteriorly, there is an opening into the mastoid antrum, which communicates with the mastoid air cells.

The three ossicles within the middle ear are the smallest bones in the body. These tiny bones connect the tympanic membrane to the oval window. The malleus (hammer) is the most lateral ossicle (closest to the outside of the head) and attaches to the tympanic membrane at the umbo. The malleus is attached to the incus (anvil), which in turn is connected to the stapes (stirrup) at a ball-and-socket joint called the incudostapedial joint. These connections, or articulations, and the two tendons within the middle ear, the tensor tympani tendon and the stapedius tendon, modify movement of the ossicles in response to displacement by sound waves, thereby protecting the ear from damage by very loud sounds.

When sound waves enter the ear canal, they set the tympanic membrane in motion. These vibrations, amplified by the ossicles, which function as a system of levers, are transmitted through the oval window to the fluid-filled structures of the inner ear.

INNER EAR

The inner ear (labyrinth) is the most complex and important portion of the auditory system. Within it are found the structures necessary for both hearing and balance. The inner ear is a closed, fluid-filled space located within the petrous portion of the temporal bone. The structures that make up the inner ear are as follows:

- The vestibule, which houses the utricle and saccule
- The semicircular canals, which respond to movements of the head in three planes
- The cochlea, which contains the organ of hearing

The bony portion, known as the osseous labyrinth, contains the membranous labyrinth. Perilymphatic fluid, a plasma filtrate, fills the space between the bony labyrinth and the membranous labyrinth. Endolymphatic fluid, similar to both cerebrospinal fluid and perilymphatic fluid, fills the membranous labyrinth. Abnormal communications of these fluids with other parts of the ear or changes in amounts of fluid within these spaces are thought to cause some symptoms associated with various inner ear disorders. The vestibule lies posterior to the cochlea and anterior to the semicircular canals. Within the vestibule, two fluid-filled sacs, the utricle and saccule, which are oriented at 90 degrees to each other, respond to slow head movements, straight-ahead movements, and gravity through a complex relationship of polarization and depolarization of the cell membranes of the cilia contained within. Impulses result from this depolarization and are sent along the vestibular nerve to the brain to interpret environmental stimuli and help the brain alter body position or eye movement to maintain equilibrium.

The semicircular canals also aid in the body and brain response to changes in direction of head movement. These three canals—the anterior, posterior, and lateral (horizontal) semicircular canals—lie in planes at right angles to each other. They can respond to changes of head movement in all three planes and provide information to the cerebellum by means of cranial nerve VIII to correct for change in direction or movement. Movement of the fluid within these canals causes a sensation of dizziness or vertigo, which may be associated with motion sickness or other vestibular disorders.

The cochlea is a bony, tubelike structure coiled like a snail shell, which contains the organ of hearing—known as the organ of Corti. The cochlea is also filled with perilymphatic fluid. The volume of this fluid is equal to about two drops of water. The oval and round windows are where the middle ear interfaces with the inner ear. The oval window is filled by the footplate of the stapes and is the opening where sound vibrations enter the inner ear and move the fluid in the cochlea. The round window provides an exit for sound waves from the inner ear. The organ of Corti contains receptor cells in the form of cilia, or hair cells. These specialized hair cells respond to various frequencies of sound, and their response is transformed into an electrical impulse that is sent along the cochlear nerve to the brain, where it is interpreted as sound.

PROCESS OF HEARING

Hearing involves the collection, amplification, transformation, and interpretation of sound waves. Sound waves set particles of air in motion, which enter the external auditory meatus (canal) and in turn displace the eardrum or tympanic membrane. This movement of the eardrum vibrates the ossicles (malleus, incus, and stapes). The function of the ossicles is to amplify the force of sound 15 to 20 times and to transmit sound to the cochlea by displacement of the stapes footplate in the oval window. This displacement sets the perilymphatic fluid in motion, which then stimulates the receptor hair cells in the cochlea's organ of Corti. These signals are transformed from vibratory energy into electrical impulses by the hair cells and then sent as electrical impulses to the brain to be interpreted as sound.

*C*linical Manifestations of Ear Dysfunction

HEARING LOSS

The major clinical manifestation of ear disorders is loss of hearing. This occurs for a wide variety of reasons and is classified as conductive, sensorineural, or mixed.

Conductive Hearing Loss

Conductive hearing loss results from any condition that interferes with normal transmission of sound waves from the external or middle ear to the inner ear. Causes of conductive hearing loss are varied and numerous. Foreign bodies in the external ear, excessive wax buildup, or bony growths of the ear canal can contribute to conductive loss associated with the external ear. Causes of conductive hearing loss associated with the middle ear include upper respiratory tract infections, allergies, eustachian tube dysfunction, middle-ear infections and effusions, growths (benign or malignant), and any condition that affects ossicular function (eg, otosclerosis or traumatic disruption). In addition, congenital defects, hereditary disorders, and complications of ear surgery may result in conductive hearing loss.

Sensorineural Hearing Loss

Sensorineural hearing loss results from damage within the inner ear or to the neural pathway that communicates with the brain. This type of hearing loss can be temporary, fluctuating, or permanent. Its onset may be sudden or gradual. Sudden sensorineural hearing loss may develop from viral infection. Initially, it may be quite profound, but it usually returns to normal. Certain infectious diseases (mumps, measles, meningitis) may cause sensorineural hearing loss.

Ototoxic drugs (Table 46–1) can cause sensorineural hearing loss and can also affect the vestibular portion of the inner ear, causing vertigo in addition to hearing loss. Other causes of sensorineural hearing loss include Meniere's disease, noise trauma, tumors of the auditory nerve, hereditary factors, congenital defects, and long-term noise exposure. Presbycusis, the progressive sensorineural hearing loss associated with the process of aging, is the most common type of sensorineural hearing loss.

Table 46–1

Drugs Toxic to the Inner Ear
Alkylating agents used in chemotherapy, such as cisplatin
Aminoglycosides
Gentamicin
Kanamycin sulfate
Neomycin sulfate
Streptomycin sulfate
Tobramycin sulfate
Antiarrhythmics
Quinidine
Anti-infectives
Vancomycin
Erythromycin (intravenous only)
Antimalarials
Chloroquine hydrochloride
Quinine sulfate
Diuretics
Ethacrynic acid
Furosemide
Aspirin

Mixed Hearing Loss

Mixed hearing loss is the term used to refer to cases in which hearing loss has both conductive and sensorineural components.

Severity of Hearing Loss

Hearing loss is further categorized by severity. Persons with a mild to moderate hearing loss (15–50 dB hearing loss) are referred to as hearing-impaired. (Decibels [dB] are a measure of the loudness, or intensity, of sound.) Severe hearing loss is defined as 50 to 80 dB of hearing loss. People suffering from a hearing loss of greater than 80 dB in both ears are said to have a profound hearing loss or may be referred to as "deaf" (Fig. 46–2).

OTALGIA

Otalgia is ear pain. It can be associated with conductive hearing loss, especially if caused by infection, trauma, or pressure disturbances associated with eustachian tube dysfunction. Ear pain may affect one or both ears and may be constant or intermittent. It can range in severity from mild fullness or pressure in the ear to excruciating throbbing, pounding, and pressure pain.

Many patients report otalgia that is unrelated to the ears but instead is a result of temporomandibu-

lar joint (TMJ) syndrome, in which the articulation of the mandible causes referred pain to the nearby ear. In addition, patients with head and neck tumors may present for medical examination because of the referred otalgia associated with the growth of the tumor.

OTORRHEA

Otorrhea is drainage from the ear. It may be clear, bloody, serosanguineous, or purulent. Skull fractures and other trauma may result in clear, watery otorrhea, which indicates a cerebrospinal fluid (CSF) leak. Bloody otorrhea may suggest hemorrhage alone or hemorrhage and CSF combined. Infections of the external and middle ear can produce a purulent otorrhea, which may be thick, yellow, foul smelling, and, in some cases, bloody. Tumors may produce bloody or serosanguineous drainage.

TINNITUS

Tinnitus is a subjective sensation of buzzing, ringing, or other types of noise heard in one or both ears. It may be constant or intermittent and varies in severity. Tinnitus is frequently associated with most types of sensorineural hearing loss. It may also be a symptom of other types of ear disorders, such as chronic ear infection or labyrinthitis, or may be a symptom of systemic disease, such as hypertension, arteriosclerosis, anemia, hypothyroidism, or drug toxicity.

VERTIGO

Vertigo is different from dizziness, although the terms are often (and incorrectly) used interchangeably. Dizziness is a sensation of imbalance, unsteadiness, or faintness. It is sometimes associated with giddiness, weakness, confusion, and blurred or double vision. It can be mild or severe, with abrupt or gradual onset. It may be aggravated by standing up too quickly and alleviated by rest. Dizziness may occur secondary to anemia, cardiac dysrhythmias, carotid sinus hypersensitivity, anxiety disorder, orthostatic hypotension, transient ischemic attack, drug therapy, and whiplash.

Vertigo is a sensation of revolving in space or of the surroundings revolving around oneself. It is often associated with nausea, vomiting, nystagmus, staggering gait, and tinnitus or hearing loss. These symptoms can occur together or separately. True vertigo may have its origins in the inner ear (labyrinthitis, vestibular neuritis, perilymph fistula, Meniere's disease). It may indicate the presence of a tumor of the acoustic nerve or the posterior fossa, or it may result from head trauma or ototoxicity secondary to drug therapy (Fig. 46–3). Vertigo can also be

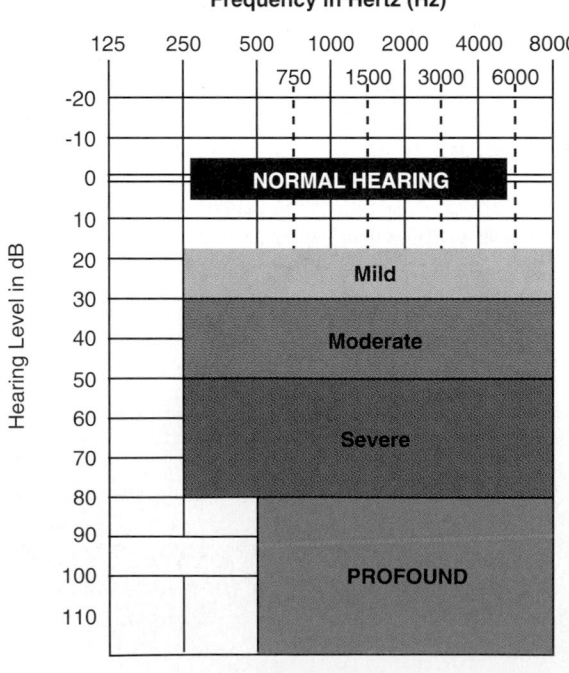

Frequency in Hertz (Hz)

Figure 46–2

Audiogram outlining the ranges for classification of hearing loss. (Redrawn from Lilly LF. Cochlear implants: The second generation. Periop Nurs Q 1986; 2[3]:10, with permission of Aspen Publishers, Inc, © 1986.)

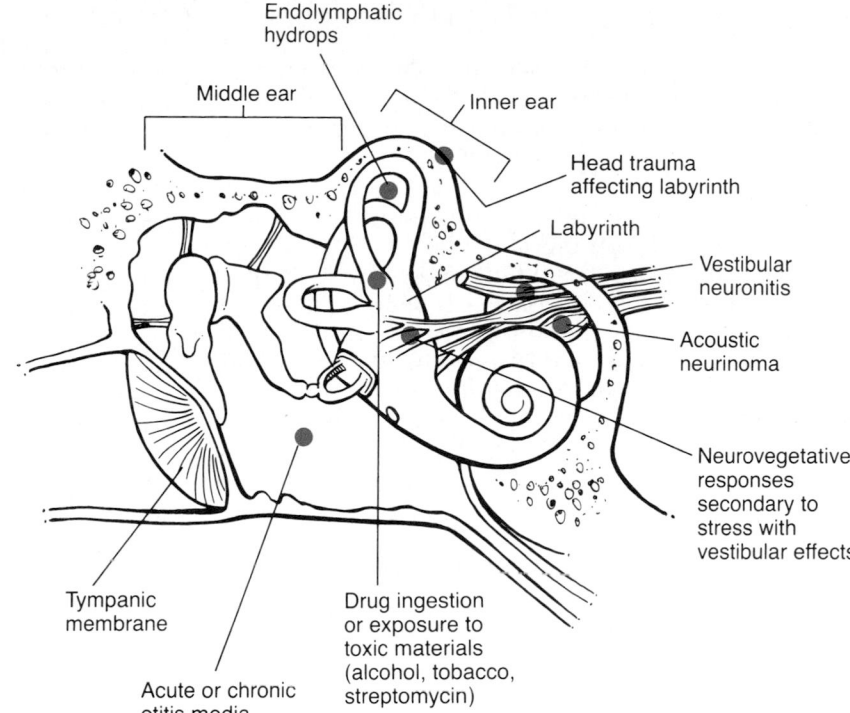

Figure 46–3
Common locations and types of pathologic changes causing vertigo.

precipitated by positional head changes, as in benign paroxysmal positional vertigo. Drugs used to treat vertigo are listed in Table 46–2.

*A*ssessment of the Ear and Hearing

PATIENT HISTORY

Systematically question the patient about the primary symptoms of ear disorders: hearing loss, otalgia (ear pain), drainage, tinnitus, and vertigo. Obtain the following information.

If the patient has hearing loss, determine whether onset was sudden or gradual. If gradual, determine the period over which the patient or fam-

ily thinks it developed. Ask the patient or family about any event precipitating or associated with the hearing loss. Determine whether the hearing loss is unilateral or bilateral. Also determine its severity and how it is manifested. Can the patient hear a watch ticking next to the ear? Can the patient hear the telephone ringing in the same room? Are one-on-one conversations muffled? Can the patient hear environmental sounds, such as traffic or sirens? Ask about interventions that the patient uses to compensate for the loss, such as a hearing aid, lip reading, relying on the better ear for hearing, and so on.

If the patient has ear pain or discomfort, determine whether its onset was sudden or gradual. Also investigate pain characteristics, including:

- Type or severity of pain (throbbing, feeling of fullness, dull ache, sharp, stabbing pain)
- Changes in the quality of pain (sharp, throbbing pain may subside suddenly after rupture of the

Table 46–2

Drugs Used to Treat Vertigo

Drug	Classification	Indication for Use	Route of Administration
Dimenhydrinate (Dramamine)	Antihistamine	Mild vertigo	PO, IM, rectal suppository
Meclizine hydrochloride (Antivert)	Antihistamine	Mild vertigo	PO
Promethazine (Phenergan)	Antiemetic	Severe vertigo	PO, IM, rectal suppository
Diazepam (Valium)	Tranquilizer	Severe vertigo	PO, IM, IV

IM, intramuscularly; IV, intravenously; PO, orally.

tympanic membrane in an acute infectious process)

- Precipitating factors (worse when chewing or yawning, TMJ syndrome)
- Location (can it be reproduced by pulling on the auricle or palpating the TMJ?)

Ask about measures the patient has used to alleviate the pain (eg, heat, soft diet).

If the patient has ear drainage, determine its type and onset. Sudden purulent drainage associated with decreased pain may indicate spontaneous rupture of the tympanic membrane. Also determine duration, location, amount (copious, clear drainage after head trauma may signal a skull fracture), color, consistency, precipitating factors (eg, upper respiratory tract infection or a blow to the head), and associated factors (eg, skin irritation, canal itching, fever, pain).

If the patient has tinnitus, determine its onset, whether it is bilateral or unilateral, and its severity, duration, quality (high or low pitched, roaring, humming, or hissing), and precipitating factors (exposure to extremely loud noise, possible proximity to noise out of hearing range, such as ultrasonic alarms).

If the patient has vertigo, determine its onset and duration, whether it is intermittent or constant, its quality and severity, associated symptoms (eg, nausea, vomiting, ataxia), precipitating factors if noted, and the type and effectiveness of relief measures used.

Allow the patient to use his or her own words to describe all symptoms instead of forcing a choice from a set of adjectives presented to the patient. This provides a more accurate characterization of the symptoms. Assess the patient's understanding of any previously diagnosed chronic ear disorder. If a hearing aid or other assistive device is used, determine the patient's perception of its effectiveness and the consistency of its use. Assess the patient's knowledge of and ability to care for the aid, and note any complaints about it or other assistive devices.

Obtain a complete medical history, because some ear disorders result from childhood disease. Note early childhood diseases, such as mumps and measles, and explore any history of allergies. Establish dates and frequency of past ear problems, noting type of problem (eg, infection, perforation, drainage, pain) and location. Investigate the patient's drug history. Question about the use of drugs associated with hearing loss, tinnitus, or loss of equilibrium. Also ask about chronic use of aspirin or other salicylates, because they can cause tinnitus that resolves after discontinuing drug therapy. Question the patient about recent head trauma or other injury. Also obtain a surgical history, noting ear surgery, tonsillectomy, and adenoidectomy.

Review the patient's familial history to check for hearing or ear disorders, and obtain an occupational history to document long-term exposure to noise associated with work environments. Because recent research suggests that long-term exposure to loud music—either through personal headset stereos or as a member of an audience—can result in permanent hearing loss, question the patient about amount and frequency of exposure to these factors.

As part of the history, assess the patient's understanding of and compliance with activities that promote otologic health and help reduce the risk of otologic disease (Highlight 46–1).

PHYSICAL EXAMINATION

Examine the auricles and surrounding tissues for deformity, nodules, or other lesions. Observe the postauricular and auricular area for drainage. Check for redness, warmth, or swelling, and for pain on palpation or pulling of the auricle. Also assess for tenderness when pressure is exerted on the tragus, the cartilaginous projection anterior to the ear canal opening. The function of the seventh cranial nerve (facial nerve) should be assessed by observing for symmetry of facial movements while the patient smiles, puffs the cheeks, closes the eyes, and raises the eyebrows.

Next, use an otoscope to visualize the external canal and tympanic membrane directly. Tip the patient's head away from you and toward the side of the unexamined ear. Pull the auricle up and back to straighten the entrance to the canal, and insert the speculum of the otoscope. Advance it slowly and gently in accordance with patient comfort. Observe the ear canal for redness, swelling (sometimes determined by the size of the speculum that can be comfortably introduced), wax accumulation, discharge, or foreign body. Assess the eardrum for bulging, retraction, perforation, and scarring. Note color, luster, presence or absence of the light reflex, and

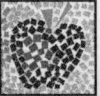

HIGHLIGHT 46–1

HEALTH PROMOTION & RISK REDUCTION

Preventive Care of the Ears

Instruct the patient in preventive care of the ears as follows:

Avoid using cotton-tipped applicators or other objects to clean ears.

Protect ears from excessive noise exposure; use care with personal headsets and so forth.

Seek medical attention promptly for any problems relating to the ear, such as drainage, pain, or decreased hearing.

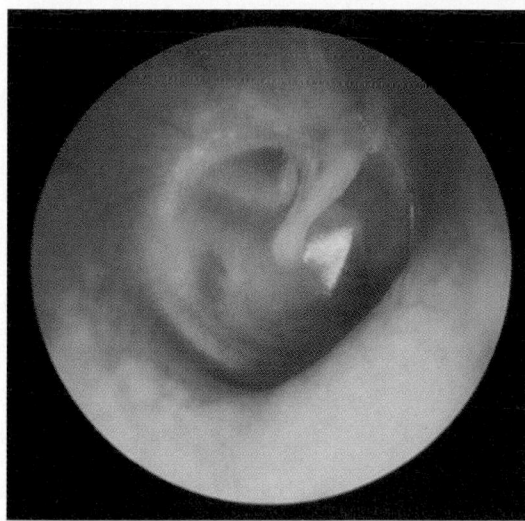

Figure 46–4

Right tympanic membrane. Note the umbo, the handle of the malleus, and the cone of light. (From Bluestone CD, Klein JO. Otitis media in infants and children. 2nd ed. Philadelphia: WB Saunders, 1995.)

thickness. Normally, the eardrum is pearly gray, translucent, and shaped like a concave disk. A light reflex should be present. The light reflex appears as a cone of light reflected from the light of the otoscope and, in a normal examination, appears at the 5-o'clock position in the right ear and 7-o'clock position in the left ear (Fig. 46–4). The malleus handle normally can be seen through the tympanic membrane.

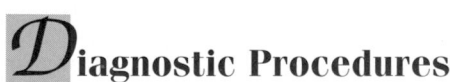iagnostic Procedures

PNEUMATOSCOPY

Pneumatoscopy tests the ability of the eardrum to respond to changes in air pressure introduced into the ear canal and the middle ear. A pneumatic otoscope is used to introduce air into the ear and to assess mobility of the tympanic membrane. The air causes the tympanic membrane to move in and out if it is intact. The membrane does not move if a perforation is present (because the air simply passes through the opening) or if there is fluid in the middle ear space.

TUNING FORK TESTS

A tuning fork is a small metal instrument that consists of a stem and two prongs tuned to a specific frequency. Holding the stem and striking one prong against a solid object creates a sound of that frequency. Tuning fork tests are used to differentiate

between conductive and sensorineural hearing loss. They can be helpful in evaluating the severity of hearing loss and the need to refer for more extensive audiometric testing.

WEBER'S TEST

Weber's test helps distinguish conductive from sensorineural hearing loss. It uses bone conduction of sound waves produced by a vibrating tuning fork to determine whether sound is lateralized (referred to one side). The stem of the vibrating tuning fork (a low-frequency fork of 256 or 512 Hz) is placed on the midline of the skull at the forehead or on the two front teeth of the maxilla. The patient is then asked to indicate in which ear the tone is heard by pointing to the ear. A patient with a unilateral conductive hearing loss hears the tone more loudly in the affected ear because background noise is blocked by the conductive defect and bone conduction is enhanced. A patient with a unilateral sensorineural hearing loss hears the tone more loudly in the unaffected ear. Patients with normal hearing or equal amounts of hearing loss bilaterally perceive sound as heard in the midline.

RINNE TEST

The Rinne test compares hearing ability by air and bone conduction. The vibrating stem of the tuning fork is first placed on the mastoid process (behind the auricle), and then moved quickly to about 5 cm (2 inches) lateral to the opening of the external auditory canal. The patient then indicates whether the tone sounds louder with the fork behind or in front of the ear. Patients with normal hearing or sensorineural hearing loss perceive the tone as louder in front of the ear (sound heard by air conduction). Patients with conductive hearing loss perceive the sound as louder behind the ear (sound heard by bone conduction).

AUDIOMETRIC TESTING

Audiometry is the measurement of the sensivity of hearing to various frequencies of sound. Some of the types of audiometry include pure tone audiometry, speech audiometry, impedance audiometry, acoustic reflex testing, and electric response audiometry (Table 46–3). In general, these tests are performed by an audiologist, who provides test results and interpretation to the referring individual.

VESTIBULAR TESTS

BALANCE, GAIT, AND PAST-POINTING TESTS

Balance, gait, and past-pointing tests are used to assess vestibular function and help identify the area of any vestibular lesion. In the Romberg test, the

Table 46–3

Basic Audiometric Tests

Test	Function
Pure-tone audiometry	This test is the standard measure of hearing acuity. To test air conduction, pure tones within the range of 250–8000 Hz are presented at varying intensities to one ear at a time through earphones, beginning with the better-hearing ear. The patient signals when a sound is heard (even if very faint) by raising a hand or pushing a button. For bone-conduction testing, tones are delivered through a bone vibrator placed against the forehead or mastoid process rather than an earphone. Masking noise is presented to the untested ear by an earphone to prevent it from participating in the test of the opposite ear. Results are recorded on an audiogram.
Speech audiometry	
Speech-reception threshold	This test determines the lowest intensity at which the patient can hear and correctly repeat 50% of a list of two-syllable words presented through earphones. The result usually corresponds closely to the air-conduction threshold.
Speech discrimination	A list of 50 monosyllabic words is presented through earphones to the patient. The score indicates the percentage of words that the patient can hear and repeat correctly.

patient is asked to stand with feet together, arms out in front, and eyes closed for 20 seconds. Slight swaying is normal, but loss of balance is not. Another test of balance is to ask the patient to stand alternately on one foot and then the other foot with eyes closed and arms at the sides. Again, slight swaying is normal, but the patient should be able to maintain balance on each foot for at least 5 seconds. For gait evaluation, the patient is instructed to walk backward and forward heel to toe, first with the eyes open and then with them closed. Patients with no abnormality can perform both maneuvers successfully.

For the past-pointing test, the patient is seated facing the examiner, who holds out an index finger at the level of the patient's shoulder. The patient is requested to touch the examiner's finger with the right index finger and then close the eyes, lower the arm, and touch the examiner's finger again. The examination is repeated for the left side. The examiner observes and notes the degree and direction of past-pointing. The findings are normal when the patient can touch the examiner's finger with eyes open or closed.

ELECTRONYSTAGMOGRAPHY

Electronystagmography is a method of measuring and recording eye movement by detecting and recording changes in background electrical activity produced by eye motion. This measurement is based on the corneoretinal potential. The results are used to evaluate interactions between the vestibular system and muscles controlling eye movement—the vestibulo-ocular reflex. This test is used to diagnose vestibular dysfunction and is important in assessing causes of dizziness, vertigo, and tinnitus. It can suggest the presence and location of central or peripheral lesions.

CALORIC TEST

The caloric test is also a test of vestibular function and is performed routinely as part of electronystagmography. In this study, the ear is stimulated alternately with warm (44°C, 111.2°F) and cold (30°C, 86°F). This can be done by irrigating the ear with water or by using testing equipment that consists of water- or air-filled tubing, which is inserted in the ear canal. A normal person responds to warm or cold stimulation with nystagmus (an involuntary jerking movement of the eye). Warm stimulation produces nystagmus toward the side of instillation, whereas cold stimulation produces nystagmus in the opposite direction. Vestibular lesions are suggested in people who show no nystagmus with caloric testing, or when nystagmus velocity or frequency is decreased.

Caloric testing with water instilled in the ear canal is contraindicated in patients with a tympanic membrane perforation. Otoscopy is performed before beginning the test to examine for this possibility and to evaluate for any obstruction to instillation, particularly (and most commonly) cerumen.

*M*anagement

Treatment of patients with disorders of the ear depends on the particular disease or disorder, its cause, severity of symptoms, and resulting impairment.

PHARMACOLOGIC THERAPY

Many ear disorders can be treated effectively with medications. Antibiotics can control most infectious processes. Antihistamines can reduce the allergic reactions and swelling that affect eustachian tube function. Diazepam and related drugs are used to control the symptoms of dizziness and vertigo, although they do not correct the disease process. Diuretics and a low-salt diet are prescribed to help control symptoms of Meniere's disease.

VESTIBULAR REHABILITATION

The use of vestibular rehabilitation in managing vestibular disorders has increased greatly in recent years. When the vestibular system is affected adversely, the body attempts to compensate or counteract this problem. It has been shown that inactivity slows the rate and degree of this physiologic attempt to make up for the problem.

The aim of this therapy is to promote compensation by actively using the vestibular system through a series of exercises and strategies. In other words, patients are taught repetitive maneuvers that actually cause dizziness. The more actively the patient uses the vestibular system, the greater the degree of compensation for the balance disorder. A physical therapist is consulted to provide vestibular rehabilitation.

SURGICAL INTERVENTIONS

Ear surgery can be performed to replace or restore structure and function, correct deformities, remove diseased tissues or growths, or relieve symptoms that incapacitate the patient. Extensive ear surgery generally requires a postauricular incision, whereas other procedures can be performed endaurally (through the canal).

Complications of Ear Surgery

Complications of ear surgery are rare, but risks include hearing loss, vestibular dysfunction, infection, and temporary or permanent facial nerve paralysis. Temporary facial paralysis may result from swelling around the nerve or manipulation during surgery. Because of this risk, facial nerve function should be assessed and documented before surgery. Potential complications also include anxiety and depression. These are most likely to develop if the patient has unrealistic expectations for the surgical outcome or timetable for improvement.

Common Surgical Procedures Performed on the Ear

TYMPANOPLASTY AND MYRINGOPLASTY

Tympanoplasty refers to a variety of reconstructive procedures performed on deformed or diseased portions of the middle ear. It is performed to eradicate disease in the middle ear and to preserve or improve hearing by repairing or replacing some or all of the conductive mechanisms. The types of tympanoplasty are shown in Figure 46–5. Extensive tympanoplastic procedures may use fascia, cartilage, perichondrium, bone, prostheses, or any combination of these to repair or replace structures damaged in the middle ear. Tympanoplastic procedures are performed in an outpatient setting.

Myringoplasty is a simple repair of a perforated eardrum. To repair a perforation of the tympanic membrane, graft material (usually harvested from temporalis fascia, a vein from the back of the hand, or occasionally skin) is placed just medial or lateral to the perforated eardrum. The graft may be held in place by absorbable gelatin film (Gelfilm) or absorbable gelatin sponge (Gelfoam) soaked in saline or an otic preparation. The external canal may be packed with sterile strip gauze, gelatin sponge, or an expanding wick made of cellulose. A mastoid dressing is usually applied for 24 hours.

NURSING PROCESS
Tympanoplasty

PREOPERATIVE NURSING CARE

Nursing care of the patient scheduled for a tympanoplasty is similar to that for any preoperative patient, as discussed in Chapter 6, with several considerations. Be sure the patient understands that hearing improvement usually is not apparent until 6 weeks after surgery. Realistic expectations for outcomes and a timetable for improvement can help avoid postoperative anxiety and depression. Discuss postoperative restrictions and potential physical and sensory alterations with the patient before surgery.

POSTOPERATIVE NURSING CARE

Assessment

Assess the patient's comfort level and the need for physical safety measures. Determine the patient's ability to hear and understand instructions, because edema, ear packing, and the outer dressing may all impair hearing in the operative ear.

Assess the patient for severe vertigo or dizziness, which can indicate a surgical complication. Also observe for excessive bleeding and inability to wrinkle the forehead, close the eyes, or smile symmetrically, which can indicate facial nerve trauma. On follow-up contact with the patient, assess for signs of sec-

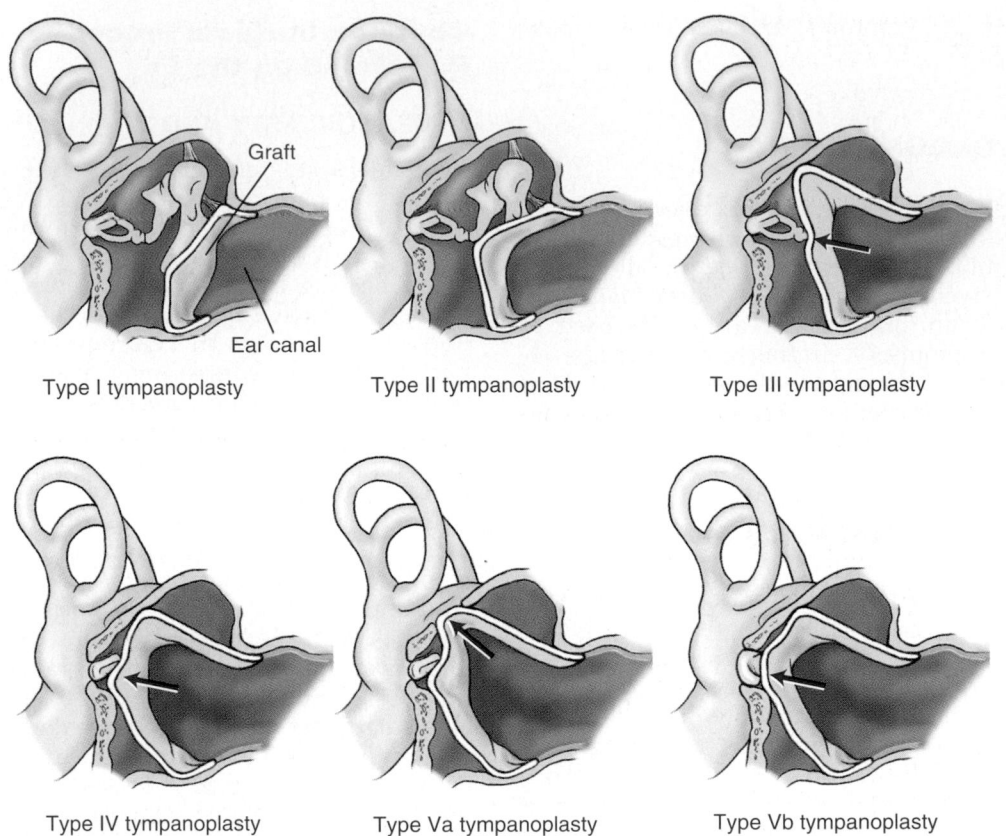

Type I tympanoplasty

Type II tympanoplasty

Type III tympanoplasty

Type IV tympanoplasty

Type Va tympanoplasty

Type Vb tympanoplasty

Figure 46–5

Types of tympanoplasty. In type I, the graft rests on the malleus and the middle ear space, and the structures are essentially normal. This is different from types II to V, in which there is progressive loss of middle ear structure. (Modified from Paparella MM, Shumrick DA, Gluckman JL, Meyerhoff WL. Otolaryngology. 3rd ed. Vol 2: Otology and neuro-otology. Philadelphia: WB Saunders, 1991, p 1416.)

ondary infection, such as fever, headache, or increased ear pain. Report any of these symptoms immediately.

Nursing Diagnoses and Planning

Nursing diagnoses and related expected patient outcomes commonly applicable to patients who have had a tympanoplasty include the following:

NDx: Sensory/perceptual alterations (kinesthetic) related to vertigo or dizziness secondary to surgical manipulation of the ear

Planning: Patient Outcomes

1. Patient takes medications as ordered for vertigo, dizziness, or unsteadiness.
2. Patient initiates movements slowly, avoiding actions or movements that precipitate or worsen vertigo or dizziness.
3. Patient reports that vertigo or dizziness is relieved.

NDx: Impaired verbal communication related to decreased hearing secondary to edema, ear packing, and the surgical dressing

Planning: Patient Outcomes

1. Effective communication is maintained between the patient and others.
2. Patient directs staff, family, and others in effective alternative communication techniques (eg, directing others to speak into the unaffected ear, writing messages).

NDx: Pain related to surgical trauma to the ear

Planning: Patient Outcomes

1. Patient uses noninvasive pain-control techniques, such as positioning.
2. Patient takes medications as ordered for pain.
3. Patient verbalizes relief of discomfort.

NDx: Risk for injury related to vertigo, dizziness, or unsteadiness

Planning: Patient Outcomes

1. Patient requests assistance when ambulating and getting in and out of bed when dizziness or vertigo is present.
2. Patient moves into different positions slowly to minimize or prevent vertigo or dizziness.
3. Patient remains free of injury.

NDx: Risk for infection related to surgical disruption of the body's first line of defense

Planning: Patient Outcomes
1. No increase in ear pain occurs.
2. Purulent drainage and foul odor from the ear are absent.
3. Incision line is clean and approximated.
4. Patient is afebrile.

NDx: Risk for altered health maintenance related to insufficient knowledge of self-care after tympanoplasty

Planning: Patient Outcomes
1. Patient describes self-care of the ear after surgery.
2. Patient lists activities to be avoided or altered during the postoperative period.
3. Patient explains prescribed medication regimen.
4. Patient identifies symptoms to be reported.
5. Patient states the reason for and date of follow-up visit.

Nursing Interventions and Evaluation

NDx: Sensory/perceptual alterations (kinesthetic)
Encourage the patient to take medication for vertigo or nausea as needed. Vomiting should be avoided if possible, to prevent dislodgement of grafts. Stress that vertigo and nausea are not abnormal after ear surgery. Maintain a dimmed, quiet environment. Avoid sudden movements of the patient's bed or chair. Instruct the patient to initiate movements slowly, particularly sitting or standing up. Avoid any activities that precipitate or exacerbate vertigo or dizziness.

NDx: Impaired verbal communication
If the patient's ability to hear is significantly altered by the surgery, direct all communication to the unaffected ear. Speak directly into the unaffected ear from a few inches away using a normal tone of voice. Use touch, gestures, or the written word in extreme situations to ensure accurate communication. Leave written instructions at the bedside if appropriate. Encourage the patient to inform others when they cannot be heard and to direct them in ways of enhancing communication.

NDx: Pain
Administer medications for pain as needed, in accordance with the physician's orders, and explain their expected effect. Maintain a calm environment. Make the patient comfortable within the limits of the positioning restrictions. Severe pain is rare after tympanoplasties, but individual differences in pain tolerance do exist. Severe pain may indicate a surgical complication.

NDx: Risk for injury
Keep the head of the bed elevated and the side rails up at all times. Assist the patient in and out of bed and with ambulation. Ensure that the call light is within reach.

NDx: Risk for infection
Use strict aseptic technique when caring for the ear. Do not remove the initial ear dressing, but reinforce as needed. Administer antibiotics as ordered. Monitor vital signs, especially temperature.

NDx: Risk for altered health maintenance
Instruct the patient in self-care at home, as specified in Highlight 46–2.

Compare the patient's status with the expected outcomes. If the outcomes are not met, reassess the patient and revise the plan.

MYRINGOTOMY

Myringotomy is a procedure in which an incision is made into the tympanic membrane to relieve pres-

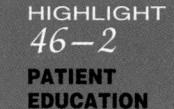 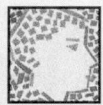

HIGHLIGHT 46–2
PATIENT EDUCATION

Discharge Instructions After Tympanoplasty

Instruct the patient to do the following:

Wash hands thoroughly before caring for the ear.

Keep water out of the ear canal for at least 3 weeks. Place a cottonball in the ear canal, and apply petrolatum ointment over the cotton to form a seal when shampooing the hair.

Avoid coughing, sneezing, and nose blowing. If necessary, coughing and sneezing should be done with the mouth open. Accumulated nasal secretions should be gently drawn back and expectorated through the mouth.

Avoid heavy lifting, straining, or vigorous activity for at least 3 weeks.

Avoid constant or prolonged use of ear cotton. A cottonball can be inserted for short periods to collect drainage (while sleeping) or for exposure to excessive dust or dirt.

Expect reddish brown to brown ear drainage, which usually becomes clear and disappears within a week or two.

Do not swim until given permission from the surgeon.

Avoid air travel until cleared by the surgeon.

Take antibiotics as prescribed for entire course of medication.

Report any increase in pain, development of fever, redness of areas surrounding the ear, or purulent drainage.

sure behind the eardrum and to promote drainage of purulent or serous fluid from the middle ear.

Uses

Myringotomy is usually performed when medical treatment, such as antibiotic and decongestant therapy, has failed to resolve eustachian tube blockage associated with serous otitis media. It is also indicated in the case of a painful, bulging tympanic membrane, which can occur with acute suppurative otitis media.

Procedure

A myringotomy is performed with local anesthetic as an outpatient procedure. A single incision is made into the posterior-inferior portion of the eardrum. Fluid is removed from the middle ear by suction. In some cases, a tympanostomy tube is inserted through the opening in the tympanic membrane to ventilate the middle ear and equalize the pressure between the external and the middle ear (Fig. 46–6). If no tube is inserted, the incision heals rapidly and usually without incident. If the tube is left in place, it slowly pushes its way out of the eardrum over a period of months and the eardrum heals.

NURSING PROCESS GUIDELINES
Myringotomy

Assess for ear drainage; if present, note the amount and color. A small amount of brownish or reddish brown drainage is normal for 24 to 48 hours though it may be too scant to be noticeable. Excessive drain-

age, especially clear fluid, should be reported immediately.

Instruct the patient in the importance of not getting water into the ear until the myringotomy incision is healed or the tube is extruded from the ear. This is best documented by physical examination at a follow-up visit. Encourage the patient to use cotton with petroleum jelly or earplugs when showering or shampooing. Stress that swimming or diving must be avoided unless specially designed earplugs are used.

MASTOIDECTOMY

Mastoidectomy is the excision of a part of the mastoid process of the temporal bone. Infection of the mastoid process is usually the result of chronic otitis media. Depending on the extent of the excision, the procedure is classified as a simple, radical, or modified radical mastoidectomy.

Uses

Mastoidectomy is done to eradicate infection, gain access to the middle or inner ear, or remove a cholesteatoma. A cholesteatoma is a sac that fills with sebaceous material and degenerated skin. It develops from an ingrowth of squamous epithelium of the external ear canal into the middle ear through a tympanic membrane perforation. A cholesteatoma is a complication of chronic otitis media and is potentially dangerous because of its capacity to destroy bone. If left untreated, a cholesteatoma may result in otologic or intracranial complications. Complications include facial paralysis, dizziness, and brain abscesses.

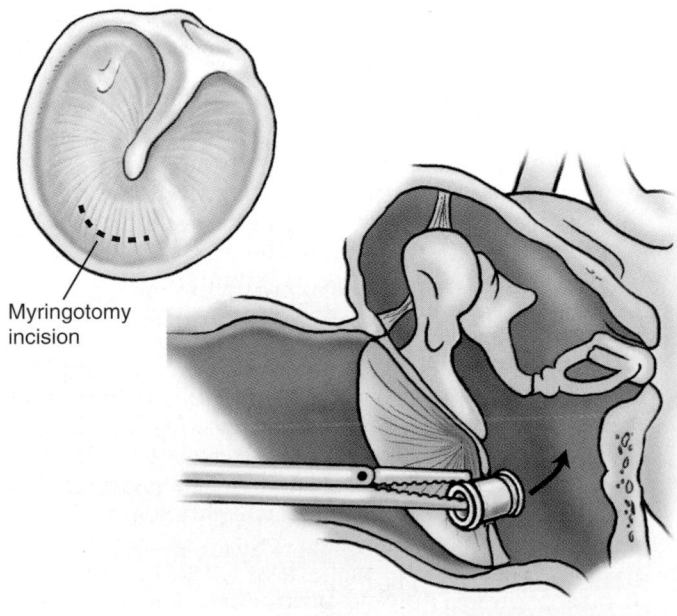

Myringotomy incision

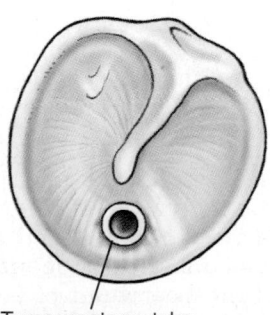

Tympanostomy tube

Figure 46–6

Myringotomy with insertion of a tympanostomy tube.

Figure 46-7

Types of mastoidectomy incision. *A*, Postauricular approach. *B*, Endaural approach. (After Goycoolea MV, Paparella MM, Nissen RL. Atlas of otologic surgery. Philadelphia: WB Saunders, 1989, pp 131, 134.)

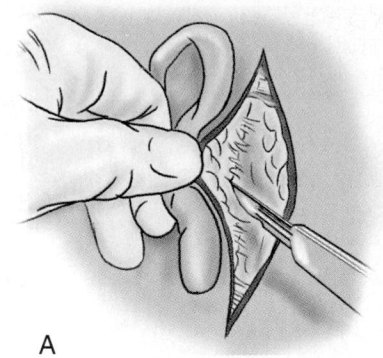

A

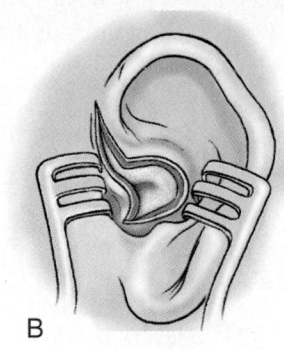

B

Procedure

Mastoidectomy is most often performed as an inpatient procedure under general anesthesia and may be done through a postauricular or an endaural incision (Fig. 46-7).

In a simple mastoidectomy, all accessible air cells in the mastoid process are removed. In a radical mastoidectomy, the wall of the external auditory canal, the tympanic membrane, and most of the middle ear structures are removed, and the opening to the eustachian tube is plugged. In a modified radical mastoidectomy, the mastoid air cells and posterior canal wall are removed, but the tympanic membrane and ossicles are saved. A drain may be inserted in the inferior part of the incision, and a mastoid dressing is applied.

Postoperative Course

The patient is assisted out of bed on the evening of surgery and is discharged in 24 to 48 hours. Dizziness may necessitate assistance with ambulating. Sutures, the outer ear packing, and bulky dressing are removed on about the sixth postoperative day. Unrestricted activities can be resumed in about 3 weeks.

Potential complications of a mastoidectomy include wound infection, bleeding, and facial nerve injury. These are not common but do occur more often after mastoidectomy than after tympanoplasty alone.

NURSING PROCESS GUIDELINES
Mastoidectomy

Assess the patient's return to physiologic stabilization after the procedure. Monitor vital signs, and inspect the dressing for bleeding or drainage. Assess for signs of facial nerve injury because the facial nerve (cranial nerve VII) passes through the internal auditory canal and exits through the mastoid process. Observe for signs of facial paralysis, such as drooling, sagging of the side of the face or mouth, or inability to close the eyelid on the operative side. Ask the patient to smile, wrinkle the forehead, and

pucker the mouth as if to whistle. Also assess for pain, dizziness, and nausea. Keep the head of the bed elevated at least 30 degrees, and instruct the patient to lie on the unaffected side. Reinforce the dressing as needed, and immediately report excessive bleeding to the surgeon. Administer antibiotics as ordered. Give oral fluids, progressing to a regular diet as tolerated. Instruct the patient in self-care after discharge. Discharge instructions are the same as for the patient who has undergone tympanostomy (see Highlight 46-2).

COCHLEAR IMPLANTATION

A cochlear implant (Fig. 46-8) is an auditory prosthesis that provides sound awareness for patients with profound sensorineural hearing impairments from damage or loss of hair cells in the organ of Corti. The implant bypasses this damaged hair-cell population and directly stimulates the auditory nerve. This helps people identify environmental sounds (eg, the telephone and doorbell) and improves communication ability by providing the patient with auditory cues that assist in lip reading. Cochlear implants have been especially successful in patients who became deaf after learning to speak. In some patients, use of the telephone has become possible. The internal component of the prosthesis includes one or more electrodes, which are implanted into or onto the cochlea, and a receiver (usually a coil), which is surgically implanted behind the top of the auricle and transmits the electrical signal to the electrode. These internal components are implanted under general anesthesia through a postauricular incision.

The external components of a cochlear implant consist of a small microphone with an ear hook that is worn over the ear and is connected by a thin cord to a speech processor (about the size of a deck of cards) and to a transmitter coil with a magnet that holds it in place over the receiver stimulator. These are put in place when the wound has healed adequately, usually in 10 to 15 days. Once the device is in place, sound is picked up by the microphone and sent to the processor, where it is broken down and

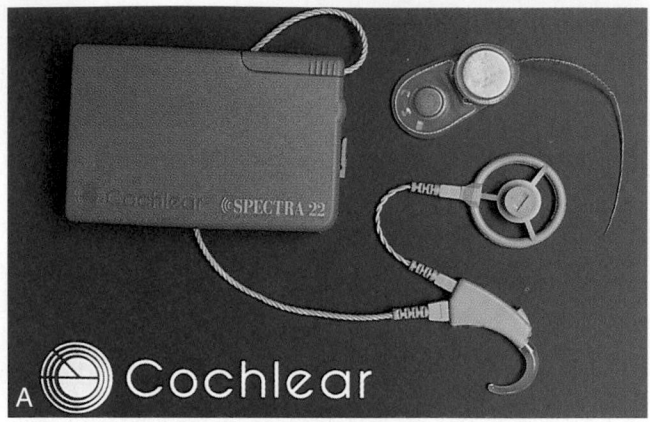

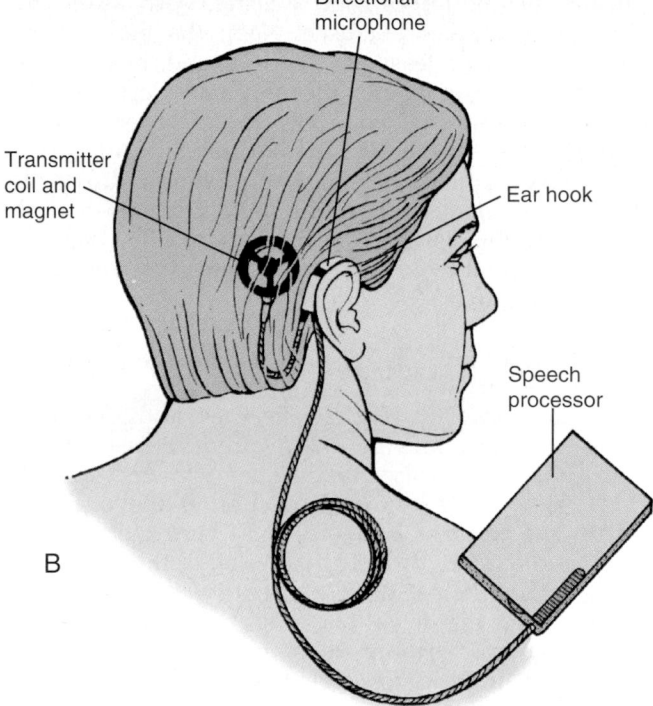

Figure 46–8

Cochlear implant. *A,* The Nucleus 22-channel cochlear implant. *B,* Patient with the prosthesis in place. The magnet holds the transmitter coil in place over the internal coil. The patient's hair usually conceals these components as well as the directional microphone and ear hook. The programmable speech processor to which the signals are sent is carried in the patient's shirt pocket. (*A* courtesy of Cochlear Corporation, Englewood, CO.)

packaged. This converted sound information is then transferred to the external device, which fits over the internal coil (receiver). The sound is further processed and sent along the electrodes to the cochlea. The electrical signal is picked up by any surviving nerve fibers and sent to the auditory center of the brain. No change in the patient's hearing occurs until this time.

NURSING PROCESS GUIDELINES
Cochlear Implant

Nursing assessments and interventions for patients undergoing cochlear implantation are similar to those for patients undergoing a mastoidectomy. The following additional considerations apply to the care of patients having a cochlear implant.

Maximum participation of the patient in the care-planning process is essential. Achieving this is a challenge because of the patient's communication disability. Many of these patients do not know sign language (neither do their nurses), and although some have outstanding lip-reading capabilities, others have lived a life of isolation since the onset of their profound deafness. A consensus on communication strategies to be used should be established well before the perioperative period.

It is vitally important that the patient's expectations for the surgical outcome be realistic. It is often difficult to dissuade patients from the expectation that sound perception will return to the predeafened state, and postsurgical depression can be profound in patients who have not accepted the limitations of cochlear implantations. Make sure the patient understands what types of sound will be perceived and that no change in hearing will occur until the rehabilitation program begins at least 1 month after surgery. Once the implant is activated, patients receive sound information that helps them interpret these sounds as speech. These sounds are sometimes described as the sound one hears when blowing on a comb covered with paper. Patients receive timing information (How long does the word or syllable last?) and some inflection instruction (Does the word or sentence end like a question or a statement?). When this information is combined with lip-reading, patients can usually understand the subject being discussed.

❖ Settings, Providers, and Collaboration for Care

Patients with ear disorders are seen and treated primarily in the outpatient setting, usually physician offices or hospital clinics. When surgical intervention is indicated, the type of procedure dictates whether hospitalization is required. Many surgical procedures allow the patient to be discharged the same day, although some necessitate a hospital stay of varying length. Some disorders (such as infection or cerebrospinal fluid leak) may also be treated in the inpatient hospital setting. Treatment of ear disorders involves several types of health care professionals—nurses, physicians, audiologists, and physical therapists.

Audiologists perform routine hearing tests as well as other more specialized tests. These include impedance audiometry, electronystagmography, and auditory brainstem response. Audiologists fit patients for hearing aids and provide in-depth patient education about caring for and using them. Candidates for cochlear implantations undergo extensive testing and counseling by audiologists preoperatively. Most of the rehabilitation after a cochlear implantation is also performed by audiologists as the patient learns to use the device to achieve maximum hearing potential.

Physical therapists with specialized training are consulted to provide vestibular rehabilitation for patients with balance disorders. The physical therapist instructs the patient on vestibular exercises and provides needed follow-up on their use.

The nurse plays an integral role in coordinating the care of these patients. The nurse interacts with all members of the health care team, providing patient information as needed. The nurse also plays a critical role in patient education, reinforcing instructions, and providing independent teaching.

The Elderly: Special Considerations

The external ear undergoes relatively minor changes with age. The lobes elongate slightly, and the auricle enlarges a little. Age-related changes of the external ear canal include production of a higher concentration of keratin, the growth of longer and thicker hair, and thinning and drying of the skin lining the canal. These changes predispose the older adult to a buildup of cerumen. An age-related diminution in sweat gland activity further increases the potential for cerumen accumulation by making the wax drier.

Age-related changes of the middle ear include diminished resiliency of the tympanic membrane, calcification and hardening of the ossicles, and weakening and stiffening of the muscles and ligaments. These changes can interfere with conduction of sound waves.

In the inner ear of elderly people, neurons diminish and endolymph, hair cells, and blood supply decrease. The basilar membrane is less flexible, and the spiral ganglion and arterial blood supply undergo degenerative changes. The auditory nerve is affected by narrowing of the auditory meatus. Central processing systems in the brain also degenerate.

As a consequence of these age-related changes, older adults experience presbycusis. This is a diminished ability to hear high-pitched sounds, especially in the presence of background noise. In practical terms, older adults have more difficulty hearing sibilant consonants, such as *ch, f, g, s, sh, t, th,* and *z.* With high-pitched sounds filtered out, words become distorted and jumbled, and sentences become incoherent. Nursing care of older adults with presbycusis is discussed in Chapter 47.

Chapter Review

1. How does the functional status of the ear affect quality of life?
2. How is sound transformed and interpreted as the spoken word?
3. What are the similarities and differences between sensorineural and conductive hearing loss?
4. How does dizziness differ from vertigo?
5. Why is establishing a communication method preoperatively important in the care of a patient undergoing otologic surgery?
6. How is the care of a patient undergoing a tympanoplasty similar to that of a patient undergoing a mastoidectomy?
7. What types of disease processes can produce otorrhea?
8. Why is safety an important consideration when planning care for a patient who has undergone ear surgery?
9. What methods may be used to facilitate communication with a hearing-impaired patient after surgery?
10. Why is it important to question a patient about drug regimens when obtaining a health history?

Bibliography

Ballenger J. Snow J (eds). Otorhinolaryngology: Head and neck surgery. 15th ed. Baltimore: Williams & Wilkins, 1996.

Bates B. A guide to physical examination. 6th ed. Philadelphia: JB Lippincott, 1994.

Bingham B. Atlas of clinical otolaryngology. St. Louis: Mosby-Year Book, 1992.

Boettcher FA, Gratton MA, Schmiedt RA. Effects of noise and age on the auditory system. Occup Med 1995; 10(3):577.

Brackmann DE, Shelton C, Arriaga M (eds). Otologic surgery. Philadelphia: WB Saunders, 1994.

Bull PD. Lecture notes on diseases of the ear, nose and throat. 8th ed. Cambridge, MA: Blackwell Scientific Publications, 1996.

Carpenito LJ. Nursing diagnosis application to clinical practice. 6th ed. Philadelphia: JB Lippincott, 1995.

Cummings CW, Frederickson JM, Harker LA, et al. Otolaryngology–head and neck surgery. 2nd ed. St. Louis: Mosby-Year Book, 1993.

Davidson TK. Clinical manual of otolaryngology. 2nd ed. New York: McGraw-Hill, 1992.

DeSouza C, Goycoolea KV, Ruah CB. Textbook of the ear, nose and throat. London: Sangam, 1995.

Gasaway DC. Hearing protection devices compendium 1995. Occup Health Saf 1995; 64(10):125, 133, 138.

Girardi M, Konrad H. Management of benign paroxysmal positional vertigo. ORL Head Neck Nurs 1996; 14(2):25.

Glasscock ME, Shambaugh GE Jr (eds). Surgery of the ear. 4th ed. Philadelphia: WB Saunders, 1990.

Hawke M, Martin RL. A photographic study of the normal and diseased ear. Hear J 1995; 48(6):29, 34.

Hawke M, McCombe A. Diseases of the ear: A pocket atlas. Ontario: Manticore Communications, 1995.

Haybach PJ. Tuning in to ototoxicity. Nursing 1993; 23(6):34.

Hughes GB, Pensak ML. Clinical otology. 2nd ed. New York: Thieme, 1997.

Jarvis C. Physical examination and health assessment. 2nd ed. Philadelphia: WB Saunders, 1996.

Johnson A, Nylen PR. Effects of industrial solvents on hearing. Occup Med 1995; 10(3):623.

Pollock KJ. Meniere's disease: A review of the problem. ORL Head Neck Nurs 1995; 13(2):10.

Roland PS, Meyerhoff ML, Marple BF. Hearing loss. New York: Thieme, 1997.

Rybak LP. Ototoxicity. Otolaryngol Clin North Am 1993; 26(3):30.

Schuknecht HF. Pathology of the ear. 2nd ed. Philadelphia: Lea & Febiger, 1993.

Schuller D, Schleuning AJ (eds). De Weese and Saunders' otolaryngology: Head and neck surgery. St. Louis: Mosby-Year Book, 1994.

Sigler BA, Schuring LT. Ear, nose and throat disorders. St. Louis: CV Mosby, 1993.

Silverstein H, Wolfson RJ, Rosenberg S. Diagnosis and management of hearing loss. Clin Symp 1992; 44(3):2.

Stafford N. ENT. Edinburgh: Churchill Livingstone, 1994.

Yost WA. Fundamentals of hearing: An introduction. 3rd ed. San Diego: Academic Press, 1994.

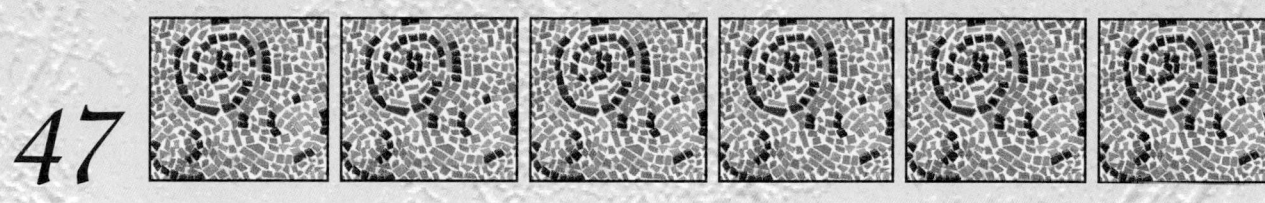

47

Nursing Care of Patients with Ear Disorders

Study Outcomes

After studying this chapter, you should be able to:

1. Describe the etiology, pathophysiology, clinical manifestations, diagnostic procedures, and management of common ear disorders.
2. Identify information and physical examination data essential to the assessment of patients with common ear disorders.
3. State nursing diagnoses and related expected patient outcomes commonly applicable to patients with ear disorders.
4. Describe nursing interventions, with their rationales, commonly applicable to patients with ear disorders.
5. Explain the basis for evaluation of nursing care provided to patients with common ear disorders.
6. Identify alternative treatment and care settings for patients with ear disorders and the services related to community-based care.
7. Identify special considerations for the elderly patient with an ear disorder.

Ear disorders affect adults of all ages and can be acute or chronic in nature. They range in severity from infections that resolve without residual effects to disorders that cause significant incapacitation. Examples of the latter are otosclerosis, which alters ear structure and causes hearing loss, and Meniere's disease, which affects balance and is characterized by recurrent episodes of vertigo and progressive nerve deafness. Treatment varies with the type and severity of the disorder and may involve supportive measures, pharmacologic therapy, or surgery.

*I*nfections and Inflammations

EXTERNAL EAR INFECTIONS

Infections of the external ear include furunculosis, bacterial otitis, and otomycosis. A furuncle, or boil, is a localized suppurative inflammation of the skin and underlying tissues of the outer ear. External otitis involves the skin of the auricle or the outer ear canal. It is one of the most common types of ear infection and may be an acute or chronic disorder. Otomycosis is a fungal infection of the external ear canal and is especially common in warm, damp climates.

Etiology and Pathophysiology

Infections of the external ear may be localized, as in the case of a furuncle, or generalized, involving the entire canal. A furuncle is caused by a bacterium, usually *Staphylococcus aureus*, that enters through hair follicles or sweat glands. A suppurative inflammation ensues, and pus and a local core of dead tissue are discharged. Local skin irritation predisposes to the development of furuncles.

Generalized external otitis may result from swimming in contaminated water. Bacteria—such as *Pseudomonas aeruginosa*, *Escherichia coli*, *Proteus vulgaris*, and *S. aureus*—are among the causative pathogens. Allergic people may acquire external otitis from irritants, such as hair dye or hair spray. The irritant causes the person to scratch the skin around the ear, thus allowing pathogens access through the excoriated area. Another predisposing factor to development of external otitis is trauma that results from cleaning the ear canal with objects such as cotton swabs and bobby pins.

Clinical Manifestations

Furuncles usually cause severe pain that may be associated with tinnitus and hearing loss in the affected ear. The extent of hearing loss relates to the amount of swelling in the ear canal. Fever, headache, and enlarged cervical lymph nodes may also occur.

Pain, possibly excruciating, is a common symptom of generalized external otitis. It is caused by inflammation and swelling of the skin of the auricle and external ear canal. The discomfort is increased by chewing, opening the mouth, or touching the auricle. The external canal may appear red and edematous. A purulent, foul-smelling, sticky, yellow otorrhea may be present. Other symptoms include itching and hearing loss, which develop if the external canal becomes swollen or filled with purulent material. Low-grade fever and headache may also occur.

With otomycosis, itching may be an intense symptom. Pain and a stinging sensation may also be felt in the external auditory canal.

Diagnosis

External ear infections are diagnosed primarily by physical examination. A history of the problem differentiates chronic external otitis from the acute condition. Otoscopy, when possible, reveals a red, swollen external ear canal. Culture and sensitivity of purulent material may be performed to identify the causative pathogens.

Management

Early administration of topical antibiotics is usually effective in treating furuncles. However, incision of the furuncle may be necessary in some cases. This is followed by application of warm, moist dressings to enhance drainage and relieve discomfort.

Management of external otitis depends on its cause. Treatment is directed toward alleviating the infectious process and accompanying symptoms. A combination of topical and systemic medications, commonly antibiotics and corticosteroids, is usually effective in treating generalized external otitis. Treatment may require hospitalization and intravenous antibiotic administration if severe cellulitis has developed. To reduce the pain associated with generalized acute external otitis, codeine, propoxyphene napsylate (Darvocet), aspirin, or acetaminophen may be ordered. Heat therapy to the infected area may also be recommended to relieve discomfort.

For chronic external otitis, treatment involves cleaning the infected ear canal by suction to remove the accumulated debris. Antibiotic ointments or ear drops are usually effective in treating the infectious process. These may be applied to the ear canal via a cotton wick inserted in the canal by the physician. These topical treatments may require multiple outpatient visits for cleansing and packing changes until the condition is under control. Analgesics can be prescribed for the relief of mild pain.

Otomycosis may be treated with antibiotics. The infected area may also be cleaned with a dilute solution of aluminum acetate and acetic acid known as Burow's solution. There are also a variety of antifungal agents that may be used depending on the physician's preference. The most important principle in managing the infection is frequent and regular cleaning of the canal. Ear drops containing antifungal agents are administered after cleaning.

NURSING PROCESS GUIDELINES
External Ear Infection

Obtain information about the patient's history and symptoms. Inspect the affected ear for redness, swelling, or discharge. Determine whether the pa-

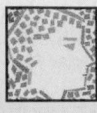

HIGHLIGHT 47–1

PATIENT EDUCATION

Preventing External Otitis

Instruct the patient to:

Avoid cleaning the ears with cotton swabs, bobby pins, match sticks, or other small, hard objects that can damage tissue.

Avoid getting water in the ears by wearing ear plugs or cotton smeared with petrolatum ointment when showering, washing hair, or swimming.

Avoid cosmetic products, such as hair dyes and hair sprays, that cause irritation or itching.

---

tient has recently used cosmetic products, such as hair dyes or sprays, which may have contributed to the inflammation. Also determine if the patient had been swimming before the onset of symptoms.

Review information related to prescribed drug or heat therapy with the patient, caregiver, or both. Reassure the patient that any hearing loss attributed to the infection is temporary, and normal hearing should return when the infection resolves. If tinnitus is a problem, suggest soft background music to mask it. Tell the patient how to prevent recurrence (Highlight 47–1).

MIDDLE-EAR INFECTIONS

Otitis media is a general term used to refer to middle-ear infections caused by bacteria or, less frequently, by viruses. Otitis media may occur secondary to pneumonia, influenza, measles, mumps, or scarlet fever. Common infections in this category include acute, serous, or chronic otitis media and mastoiditis (Table 47–1).

NURSING PROCESS GUIDELINES
Otitis Media or Mastoiditis

Assess for the signs and symptoms of middle ear or mastoid infection and obtain pertinent health history data for patients in whom there is a suspicion of serous otitis media. Include questions about allergies and recent altitude changes, as in diving, flying, or driving in the mountains. In acute otitis media, otoscopy may reveal a red, bulging eardrum (Fig. 47–1).

Review with the patient the name, purpose, dose, frequency and route of prescribed medications. In the case of antibiotics, stress the importance of taking all the medication prescribed. Instruct patients

Table 47–1

Middle Ear Infections

Disorder	Etiology and Pathophysiology	Clinical Manifestations	Management
Acute otitis media	Microorganisms enter the middle ear from the nasopharynx via the eustachian tube and establish infectious process Occurs most commonly in infancy and childhood If untreated, perforation of eardrum may result	Throbbing pain and feeling of fullness in affected ear Fever Headache Nausea Vomiting Vertigo Conductive hearing loss A red, bulging ear drum (see Fig. 47–1) with a visible fluid level or a perforated eardrum with fluid in the canal.	Antibiotic therapy for 10 days In severe cases, myringotomy for drainage may be necessary Antihistamine if allergies are a contributing factor
Chronic otitis media	Untreated or repeated attacks of acute otitis media If not resolved, may lead to tympanic membrane perforation, ossicle destruction, and conductive hearing loss	Thick, purulent, persistent or recurrent discharge Gradual hearing loss Occasional pain, nausea, and vertigo.	Cleaning of ear canal and removal of infectious material from the middle ear by suction followed by topical antibiotics If severe, systemic broad-spectrum antibiotics Tympanoplasty if middle-ear structures are damaged
Serous otitis media	Incomplete resolution of acute otitis media Allergic reaction Any obstruction of the eustachian tube leads to the accumulation of noninfectious fluid in the middle ear space.	Conductive hearing loss, pressure, and tinnitus in affected ear Absence of pain and fever Possibly a retracted eardrum with a visible fluid level	Systemic sympathomimetic amines for vasoconstriction (to improve eustachian tube function) Drainage of middle ear by aspiration of fluid or insertion of a tympanostomy tube Correction of underlying problem
Mastoiditis	Extension of middle ear infection results in formation of infectious fluid or pus that fills air cells of the mastoid If untreated, may progress to brain abscess, meningitis, facial paralysis or suppurative labyrinthitis	Pain Tinnitus Otorrhea Hearing loss Also redness, swelling and tenderness in the area of the mastoid process	Intensive parenteral antibiotic therapy beginning with penicillin and adjusted PRN based on culture and sensitivity studies Myringotomy and tubes also performed Mastoidectomy may be indicated in patients who do not respond to antibiotic therapy and tubes

with serous otitis media in self-care (Highlight 47–2).

LABYRINTHITIS

Labyrinthitis is an inflammation of the labyrinth of the inner ear. It can be caused by bacterial infection or, most commonly, by viral infection.

Etiology and Pathophysiology

Purulent (bacterial) labyrinthitis is extremely rare in the adult population but may accompany or be sec-

ondary to acute or chronic otitis media. It may also be secondary to purulent meningitis if pathogens gain access to the subarachnoid space via the cochlear aqueduct. Viral labyrinthitis is associated with upper respiratory tract infection and may be responsible for the nonconductive hearing loss that follows chickenpox and other viral infections.

Clinical Manifestations

Labyrinthitis is characterized by profound sensorineural hearing loss, severe vertigo, and loss of equilibrium. It may also be accompanied by tinnitus. The sensorineural hearing loss associated with puru-

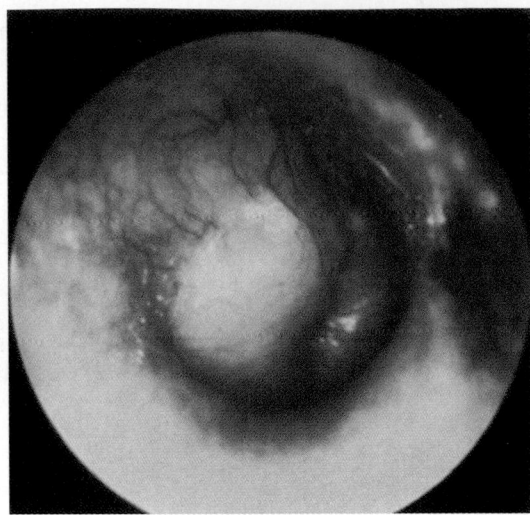

Figure 47–1

Bulging right eardrum with fluid or pus behind it as seen in acute otitis media. (From Bluestone CD, Klein JO. Otitis media in infants and children. 2nd ed. Philadelphia: WB Saunders, 1995.)

lent labyrinthitis is almost always permanent. Viral labyrinthitis is also associated with profound sensorineural hearing loss, but some or all of the hearing may be recovered after the acute phase. Vertigo, although incapacitating during the acute episode, gradually subsides. Other symptoms of labyrinthitis, whether purulent or viral, may include fever, chills, nausea, vomiting, and purulent otorrhea.

Diagnosis

Medical diagnosis is based on clinical presentation and history of otitis media, upper respiratory tract infection, or other viral infection. Audiometric test-

ing may be done to document hearing loss. Vestibular testing may be performed to evaluate impairment of vestibular function.

Management

Vestibular suppressants, such as diazepam, are prescribed and the patient is maintained on bedrest to control vertigo. The patient diagnosed with bacterial labyrinthitis is hospitalized and started on high-dose intravenous antibiotic therapy. Intravenous fluids may be ordered to supplement oral intake, thus preventing dehydration in cases of severe nausea and vomiting. Vestibular rehabilitation may be recommended to improve compensation for disequilibrium. If symptoms do not respond to medical treatment, a labyrinthectomy or vestibular nerve section may be necessary.

NURSING PROCESS GUIDELINES
Labyrinthitis

Assess the patient's physical condition. Pay particular attention to symptoms associated with vertigo and the need for safety precautions because of imbalance. Assess the extent of hearing loss in relation to the patient's ability to communicate and understand instructions and explanations.

To control vertigo, instruct the patient to take medication before symptoms become severe and to avoid sudden position changes, such as from lying to sitting to standing. Also help the patient identify and avoid stimuli that may exacerbate vertigo, such as fluorescent lights. Reassure the patient that vertigo, nausea, and vomiting will gradually subside as the infection resolves.

If patients have adequate hearing in the opposite ear, expect that they will have only minor difficulty in adjusting to the hearing loss. However, if there is already a significant loss in the unaffected ear, a distinct impairment in the ability to communicate and understand may be noticed. Help the patient to instruct others in communication-enhancement techniques, such as face-to-face communication, use of gestures, and speaking close to the less-affected ear. If these techniques are not helpful, encourage the use of written materials to convey information. Help the patient to understand and accept the possibility that the hearing loss may be permanent.

*S*tructural Disorders

PERFORATION OF THE TYMPANIC MEMBRANE

Etiology and Pathophysiology

A tympanic perforation is a hole or tear in the eardrum. It most often results from infection or trauma, such as puncture with a foreign object, skull frac-

---

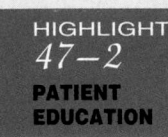 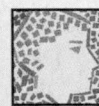

HIGHLIGHT 47–2 PATIENT EDUCATION

Serous Otitis Media

Instruct the patient to:

Perform the Valsalva maneuver to inflate the eustachian tube unless medically contraindicated. To do this, pinch the nostrils together and vigorously blow the nose several times daily to help open the eustachian tube and permit air to enter the middle ear.

Take decongestants and antihistamines as prescribed by the physician.

Avoid exposure to known allergens.

Seek prompt medical treatment if nasopharyngeal infection recurs, or allergic symptoms persist, to prevent development of chronic serous otitis media.

ture, or sudden increase in air pressure, as may occur in an explosion.

Clinical Manifestations

Clinical manifestations of a perforated tympanic membrane are pain and discharge (blood or middle-ear fluid) from the affected ear. When the perforation results from infection, pain is worse before the tympanic membrane perforates. After perforation the release of built-up pressure usually results in a significant reduction in pain. If the perforation results from trauma, the pain exists at the moment of perforation but does not usually persist.

Diagnosis

Earache and bleeding from the ear, possibly accompanied by some hearing loss, suggest perforation if the patient has a recent history of trauma. The diagnosis can be confirmed by otoscopy (Fig. 47–2).

Management

Tympanic membrane perforations often heal spontaneously. Prophylactic antibiotics may be prescribed to prevent infection. A tympanoplasty may be required if the perforation does not heal within 6 months of the traumatic event. A persistent conductive hearing loss may indicate a disruption of the ossicles, which necessitates surgical exploration and repair of the middle ear. Chronic perforations secondary to repeated middle ear infection have less chance of healing spontaneously and will probably require surgical repair.

NURSING PROCESS GUIDELINES
Perforated Tympanic Membrane

Question the patient about pain, tinnitus, vertigo, and hearing loss. Examine the ear for bleeding and

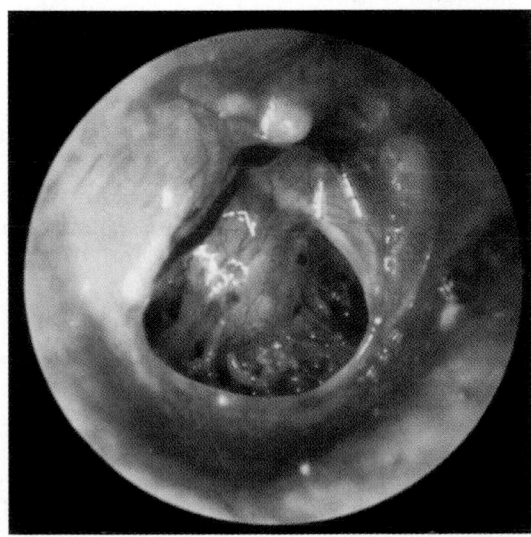

Figure 47–2
Large "dry" central perforation of the right tympanic membrane. (From Bluestone CD, Klein JO. Otitis media in infants and children. 2nd ed. Philadelphia: WB Saunders, 1995.)

drainage. If trauma has occurred recently, keep in mind that clear drainage may indicate a skull fracture with cerebrospinal fluid draining through the perforated eardrum.

Stress the importance of adhering to the prescribed regimen of antibiotics. Explain the importance of keeping the ear canal dry during the healing process. Instruct the patient to avoid swimming. The ear should be protected by placing a cotton ball with petrolatum jelly applied over it to form a seal when the patient is showering or shampooing. Remind the patient that vigorous nose blowing during the recovery period can disrupt the healing process.

Teach the patient to identify signs of infection, such as fever, pain, drainage, and warmth of the ear or canal. Stress the need to seek prompt medical treatment should these occur.

OTOSCLEROSIS

Etiology and Pathophysiology

Otosclerosis is an overgrowth of spongy bone around the oval window and stapes footplate that prevents movement of the stapes in the oval window. This results in a conductive hearing loss because sound cannot be transmitted from the oval window to the cochlea. The cause of otosclerosis is unknown. The condition usually appears in early adulthood and exhibits a familial tendency. It is more common in women and may be exacerbated by pregnancy.

Clinical Manifestations

Otosclerosis is characterized by a progressive, conductive hearing loss. Sometimes a mixed hearing loss is noted in cases of longstanding otosclerosis. Both ears may be affected to varying degrees. Tinnitus may be an accompanying symptom.

Diagnosis

Progressive hearing loss without a history of middle-ear infections suggests otosclerosis. Diagnosis can be confirmed through audiometric testing.

Management

There is no cure for otosclerosis or known treatment or prevention. Some physicians advocate the use of oral fluoride to slow the progression of sensorineural hearing loss in patients with mixed hearing loss. Fluoride does not stop the progression of conductive hearing loss and is not a substitute for stapes replacement surgery. A hearing aid may be prescribed to help the patient's hearing to some degree, but the treatment of choice in most cases is stapes replacement surgery.

Stapedectomy is a microsurgical procedure in which the stapes suprastructure is removed and replaced with a prosthesis. This prosthesis is usually made of stainless steel, polyethylene, or some other synthetic material (Fig. 47–3).

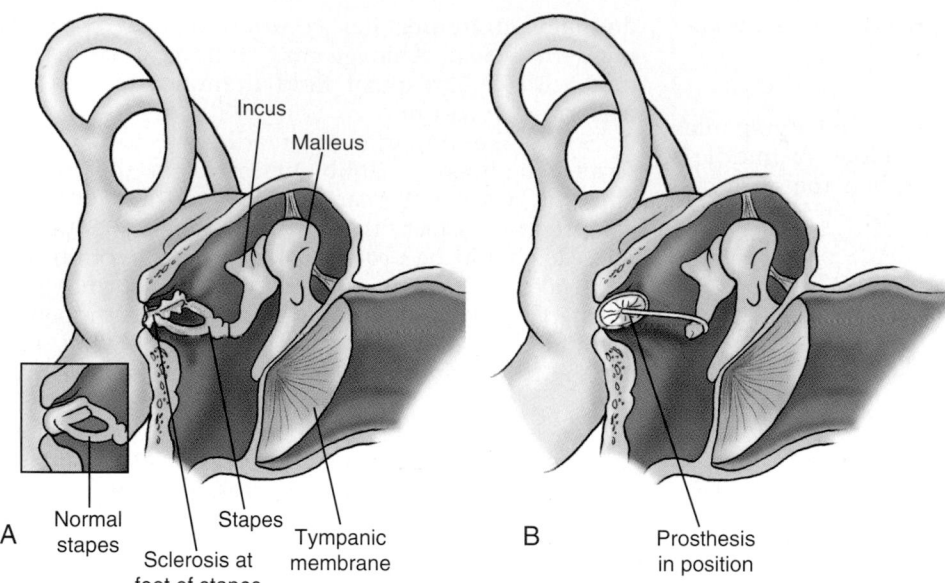

A
Normal stapes
Incus
Malleus
Stapes
Tympanic membrane
Sclerosis at foot of stapes

B
Prosthesis in position

Figure 47–3
Diagram of the middle ear showing (A) sclerosis at the foot of the stapes and (B) a prosthesis in place after stapedectomy.

Procedure

Stapes replacement surgery is usually performed under local anesthesia so the patient can report the effect on hearing, as well as the occurrence of vertigo or other symptoms during the procedure. The entire procedure is performed through the ear canal. Access to the middle-ear space is gained by rolling back the tympanic membrane. The joint between the incus and stapes is separated. The suprastructure of the stapes is carefully removed, and a fenestra (hole) is made in the footplate of the stapes with the Argon laser. The prosthesis is then positioned between the incus and the fenestra and crimped to the incus. The patient is asked to repeat words or numbers to test improvement in hearing, which is usually immediate. The ear canal is packed lightly with an absorbable gelatin sponge (Gelfoam) and usually left without a dressing.

Postoperative Course

Discharge is usually the day of surgery unless the patient suffers intractable dizziness or vomiting, in which case overnight hospitalization is required. Patients are usually kept on bedrest for several hours after surgery, and then gradual activity is initiated. There are usually fewer problems with vertigo and nausea after the laser stapedotomy procedure than with non-laser stapedectomy. The patient is seen about 1 week postoperatively in the physician's office, at which time any undissolved ear packing may be removed.

The improved hearing that the patient may have noted at the time of the operation usually decreases immediately after surgery because of the ear packing and tissue edema. Hearing returns over the next 2 to 6 weeks with removal of the packing and resolution of surgical edema.

Complications

The most frequent complication of stapedectomy is postoperative vertigo. This is quite common and usually resolves slowly.

Other complications that can occur include hearing loss, infection, displacement of the newly placed prosthesis, taste disturbance, mouth dryness, perilymph fistula, and temporary or permanent facial paralysis.

NURSING PROCESS GUIDELINES
Stapedectomy

Assess the patient for discomfort or dizziness, and observe the operative ear. Keep in mind that there is generally minimal pain and drainage after surgery. Ask the patient to smile, close the eyes, puff the cheeks, and bare the teeth to check seventh cranial (facial) nerve function.

Administer medications as prescribed for dizziness or vertigo. Remind the patient to move slowly to avoid precipitating or worsening vertigo and to ask for assistance with ambulation. Instruct the patient in self-care measures (Highlight 47–3). Be sure the patient knows when and where to return for follow-up care.

MENIERE'S DISEASE

Meniere's disease is a recurrent and usually progressive disorder of the inner ear that affects hearing and the vestibular system.

Etiology and Pathophysiology

The cause of Meniere's disease is not known, but it

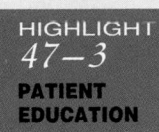 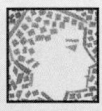

HIGHLIGHT 47–3

PATIENT EDUCATION

Discharge Instructions After Stapedectomy

To prevent infection, instruct the patient to:

Wash hands with soap and water before caring for the ear.

Keep water out of the ear canal for at least 3 weeks. To shampoo hair or shower, place a cottonball in the ear canal and apply petrolatum ointment over the cotton to form a seal.

Avoid swimming for 6 weeks.

Prevent displacement of the prosthesis from pressure changes in the ear by following these instructions:

    Avoid nose blowing when possible. Nasal secretions should be drawn back and expectorated through the mouth.

    Avoid coughing and sneezing. If necessary, cough or sneeze with mouth open.

    Avoid exposure to upper respiratory tract infections.

    Avoid bending and lifting heavy objects and other strenuous activities for at least 3 weeks.

Avoid air travel for 4 weeks or as specified by surgeon.

Identify complications early and report any of the following symptoms

    Sudden hearing loss

    Fever

    Severe persistent vertigo or dizziness

Additional information for the stapedectomy patient:

Periods of vertigo or dizziness may occur for several days. Take precautions to prevent falls.

Hearing may improve or fade at times during the first 3 weeks. It is normal to experience cracking and popping of the ear, and sound like your head is "in a barrel."

A nerve for taste passes through the ear, and it is not unusual for taste sensation to be altered slightly for several weeks or months after surgery.

---

is thought to affect the vestibular system by metabolically altering the labyrinthine fluid, causing the membranous labyrinth to dilate with endolymph (Sigler & Schuring, 1993).

Clinical Manifestations

Meniere's disease is characterized by recurrent attacks of severe vertigo, fluctuating sensorineural hearing loss, and tinnitus. Often only one ear is affected, although 20 to 30% of patients have bilateral involvement. Onset of the disease is sudden and usually occurs between ages 20 and 60.

Patients may describe a vague feeling of pressure or fullness in the ear at the beginning of an attack. Tinnitus and vertigo ensue, and sometimes are severe enough to incapacitate the patient. These symptoms may be accompanied by headache, diaphoresis, nystagmus, and imbalance. In the acute stage of an attack, any abrupt motion of the head or eyes may precipitate nausea and vomiting. Vertigo lasts for several hours or days but gradually subsides and is absent between attacks. Tinnitus and hearing impairment, however, remain.

Diagnosis

Meniere's disease is diagnosed primarily from the patient's history and presenting symptoms. Audiometric testing often reveals a decrease in speech discrimination and a sensorineural hearing loss. Caloric testing and electronystagmography are performed to document nystagmus characteristic of Meniere's disease. Radiography, computed tomography, and brain stem–evoked response audiometry are performed to rule out acoustic neuromas or other types of brain lesions.

Management

During an acute attack of Meniere's disease, medical management is directed toward the relief of symptoms. Vestibular suppressants, such as meclizine (Antivert) and diazepam (Valium), are given to control vertigo. Prochlorperazine (Compazine) or other antiemetics may be prescribed for nausea. In addition, mild sedatives or tranquilizers may be prescribed.

Dietary restrictions have been suggested as advantageous in the treatment of Meniere's disease. These include a low-sodium diet and decreased fluid intake to control fluid retention in the endolymphatic system, as well as restrictions on caffeine and alcohol. Diuretics are ordered as part of the treatment and may create the need for potassium supplements to replace potassium lost through diuresis.

Surgical treatment is a last resort for patients with unilateral Meniere's disease and intractable or incapacitating vertigo. Endolymphatic shunts, which channel fluid from the inner ear into the subarachnoid space or the mastoid, help equalize fluid pressures within the inner ear. In vestibular neurectomy, the section of the eighth cranial (acoustic) nerve that controls balance is transected. This procedure is usually effective in relieving vertigo but carries the risk of hearing loss if the acoustical portion of the nerve is damaged. Cryosurgery to produce a fistula in the inner ear for fluid drainage also effectively relieves vertigo in some patients. Labyrinthectomy cures vertigo but causes irreversible hearing loss and alteration in balance.

NURSING PROCESS
Meniere's Disease

Assessment

Obtain information about the onset, duration, severity, and frequency of attacks. Explore the type of vertigo experienced. Many patients describe a feeling of being pulled to the ground, which is commonly referred to as a drop attack. Determine whether the vertigo leads to nausea and vomiting. Help the patient identify any precipitating event or forewarning of the attack.

Inquire about associated symptoms, such as ringing or roaring in the ears, ataxia, and a sudden, noticeable change in hearing. Subjectively assess the extent of the hearing loss. Although it is not always possible in the acute phase of the attack, make an effort to obtain psychosocial data, such as occupation, family role, and community activities to assess the possible effects of this chronic disease on the patient and the family.

Nursing Diagnoses and Planning

Nursing diagnoses and related expected patient outcomes commonly applicable to patients with Meniere's disease include the following:

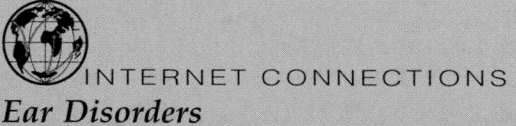

INTERNET CONNECTIONS
Ear Disorders

American Academy of Otolaryngology
http://www.entnet.org/
This authoritative site provides health tips and information for patients, medical news, a members-only section, and links to other sites.

National Institute on Deafness and Other Communication Disorders/ Meniere's Disease
http://www.nih.gov/nidcd/meniere.htm
An encyclopedia-style article providing information about causes, symptoms, diagnosis, and treatment of Meniere's disease. Current research is also briefly discussed.

NDx: Risk for altered health maintenance related to insufficient knowledge of disease, treatment, and self-care

Planning: Patient Outcomes
1. Patient describes condition and symptoms accurately.
2. Patient lists signs and symptoms of an impending attack, stating what is to be done when these occur.
3. Patient describes measures to reduce severity of attacks and to protect self from injury.

Nursing Interventions and Evaluation

NDx: Risk for altered health maintenance
Explain the disease process to the patient and the family or significant others. Instruct the patient and family in self-care. Begin by helping the patient identify warning signs of attacks and measures to protect self from harm. Review interventions to reduce the severity of attacks. Instruct the patient to take medications as prescribed when an attack begins and to lie down on the unaffected side in a darkened, quiet room, avoiding sudden movements and activities, including reading.

To help prevent attacks, instruct the patient to avoid noisy places and exposure to loud music, television, and other sound in the home. Instruct the patient to avoid exposure to bright light by suggesting that low-wattage light bulbs be used in the home, curtains or blinds be kept closed, dark glasses be worn outside or in bright light, and car windows be tinted to the extent legally permitted. Instruct the patient to refrain from sudden, jerky movements and to avoid actions, such as bending over or twisting the head, that predispose to vertigo. Encourage the patient to move slowly, to bend at the knees, and to turn the whole body rather than just the head.

Urge the patient to avoid or limit use of nicotine, caffeine, and decongestant medications, all of which cause vasoconstriction. This may decrease circulation to the inner ear and interfere with fluid absorption, thus increasing the risk of an attack. Reinforce the importance of compliance with the low-salt diet. If a patient experiences constant tinnitus, suggest using a white-noise machine to mask it. Instruct the patient to take measures to avoid fatigue and minimize stress.

There is often a great deal of anxiety associated with Meniere's disease because the patient never knows when an attack will occur. Acknowledge this fact, and refer the family and patient to support groups to help the patient learn to cope with the long-term effects of the disease process. Information on the Meniere's network of self-help groups and related services can be obtained from The Ear Foundation.

Compare the patient's status with the expected outcomes. If the outcomes are not met, reassess the patient and revise the plan.

The Elderly: Special Considerations

About half of community-living older people and up to 96% of older people residing in nursing homes have hearing loss. Hearing impairment is more likely in men, people of lower economic status, and people exposed to prolonged job-related or recreational noise. The probability of hearing impairment also increases with a family history of otosclerosis, and it is greater in white populations than in nonwhite populations. Diabetes and vascular disorders, such as hypertension and arteriosclerosis, are particular problems that affect the elderly and predispose them to hearing impairments. The delayed excretion of ototoxic drugs, often prescribed or taken by the elderly, may also contribute to irreversible hearing loss. (See Chap. 46 for more information about ototoxic drugs.)

PRESBYCUSIS

Etiology and Pathophysiology

Presbycusis is a progressive sensorineural hearing loss that occurs as a part of the aging process. It results from the loss of hair cells in the cochlea that function to stimulate the organ of Corti. Among the elderly, there is considerable variation in the degree of hearing loss and impairment. Therefore, age alone does not determine the impact and consequences of presbycusis.

Clinical Manifestations

Presbycusis actually begins in youth. Characteristically, hearing acuity for the highest frequencies (18,000 to 20,000 Hz) is lost first. This loss is not noticeable until the frequencies coincide with the range of tones found in speech.

Diagnosis

Diagnosis of presbycusis is based primarily on the patient's history (frequently as given by the family). Often, the patient is unaware of the severity of the hearing impairment, whereas family members are acutely aware of it. Audiometric testing documents the degree and severity of the hearing loss.

Management

In most cases, a hearing aid is the best means of enhancing communication for patients with presbycusis. A variety of hearing aids are available to match the varied hearing losses of the hearing-impaired population. An audiologist should be consulted to match the appropriate aid with the patient's hearing loss.

NURSING PROCESS
Presbycusis

Assessment

Assess the degree of hearing loss. Question the patient or family member about the onset and duration of the hearing loss. Hearing loss associated with aging is insidious, and onset and duration may be difficult to identify. Question the patient about additional symptoms—such as pain, tinnitus, dizziness, or nausea—to rule out another disease process as the cause of the hearing loss. Obtain a thorough history of illnesses, including a medication history. Include any familial history of ear disease or other contributing factors.

Assess the patient's overall physical condition. Investigate coping techniques that the patient or the family may have used to deal with the hearing loss. Lip-reading is rare in patients with this type of hearing loss, but patients do unconsciously rely on seeing the face of the speaker to get more information from the spoken word. Many times the patient already has a hearing aid but does not use it. Try to discover the reasons for nonuse. For some aging patients, the mechanics of battery changes in these small devices are too difficult if they also have impaired vision.

Attempt to assess the psychological response to the hearing disorder. Has the patient accepted the existence of the disability? How has he or she reacted or adjusted to the disability? Assess and document the patient's social support system.

Assess the patient's motivation to use a hearing aid, because one of the major impediments to improving hearing in the elderly is resistance to using the device. Patients often do not want to admit the need for the device or may reject it for cosmetic reasons. Many patients have difficulty adjusting to life with a hearing aid and instead withdraw from social situations, thereby removing the need for the aid. It is important to determine the patient's financial resources as well. Hearing aids represent a significant investment and usually are not covered by insurance.

Nursing Diagnoses and Planning

Nursing diagnoses and related expected patient outcomes commonly applicable to patients with presbycusis include the following:

NDx: Impaired verbal communication related to hearing loss

Planning: Patient Outcomes
1. Patient asks others to speak toward the better hearing ear when applicable.
2. Patient instructs others in ways of increasing effective communication. For example, in cases of severe hearing impairment, the speaker should speak in a normal tone of voice 2 or 3 inches from the patient's ear. In less severe cases, the speaker should maintain face-to-face communication with the patient.
3. Patient instructs others to communicate in writing when necessary

NDx: Risk for injury related to alteration in perception of auditory stimuli

Planning: Patient Outcomes

1. Patient identifies precautions to be taken to avoid physical injury as a result of hearing loss.
2. When necessary, patient describes environmental modifications to provide a safe environment. For example, severely hearing-impaired people may need assistive devices to alert them to a telephone ringing or a smoke alarm.
3. Patient remains free of injury.

NDx: Risk for social isolation related to impaired communication

Planning: Patient Outcomes

1. Patient maintains social contact with staff, family, and significant others.
2. Patient participates in routine recreational activities.

NDx: Noncompliance related to purchase or use of hearing aid

Planning: Patient Outcomes

1. Patient discusses benefits and disadvantages of proposed hearing aid.
2. Patient demonstrates ability to maintain and use hearing aid.
3. Patient discusses financial considerations in obtaining hearing aid.

NDx: Risk for altered health maintenance related to insufficient knowledge of community resources for the hearing impaired

Planning: Patient Outcomes

1. Patient lists specific community resources that deal with hearing-impaired people.
2. Patient uses applicable resources.
3. Patient discusses financial resources available for assistance in purchase of hearing aid.

Nursing Interventions and Evaluation

NDx: Impaired verbal communication

Provide a quiet, private, and calm environment for the patient. Devote full attention to the communication process. Face the patient directly when speaking. Speak slowly and clearly. Do not exaggerate lip movements. Use normal conversational tones. In cases of severe hearing impairment, gestures or written communication may be necessary. Encourage the family to help in the communication effort because they may have an effective system in place already.

NDx: Risk for injury

Provide for the physical safety of the hospitalized patient. Reinforce safety and patient-care instructions, and evaluate the patient's understanding of them. Educate the patient on assistive listening devices to reduce the risk of injury at home.

NDx: Risk for social isolation

In an acute care setting, provide a room for the patient close to the nursing station. This will help the patient better maintain visual contact with care providers and reduce isolation. Encourage recreational activities and, if possible, organize a support group of other patients with similar hearing disability. On discharge, provide the patient with a list of local senior citizen organizations.

NDx: Noncompliance

Encourage the patient who may benefit from the use of a hearing aid to consult an audiologist for fitting with the most appropriate hearing aid. Help the patient understand the benefits and drawbacks of the hearing aid. If the patient already has a hearing aid, explore reasons for its nonuse and help to identify ways to eliminate or cope with these barriers.

NDx: Risk for altered health maintenance

Provide information regarding community resources for the hearing impaired.

Compare the patient's status with the expected outcomes. If the outcomes are not met, reassess the patient and revise the plan.

Chapter Review

1. What is the most important principle in the medical management of the patient with external otitis?
2. How do the symptoms of external otitis differ from those of otitis media?
3. How is the care of a patient with mastoiditis similar to the care of a patient with acute otitis media?
4. Why are safety precautions important when caring for a patient with labyrinthitis?
5. How does getting water in the ear affect the patient with a perforated tympanic membrane?
6. Why is stapes replacement surgery always done under local anesthesia?
7. What does the inability to close the eye tightly mean in a patient who has just undergone a stapedectomy?
8. What are possible solutions to the problem of vertigo in a patient with Meniere's disease?
9. How would the effectiveness of a low-salt diet for a patient with Meniere's disease be assessed?
10. What environmental factors may contribute to the incidence of hearing loss in the elderly?

Bibliography

Ballenger JJ. Diseases of the nose, throat, ear, head and neck. Philadelphia: Lea & Febiger, 1992.

Ballenger J, Snow J (eds). Otorhinolaryngology: Head and neck surgery. 15th ed. Baltimore: Williams & Wilkins, 1996.

Bates B. A guide to physical examination. 6th ed. Philadelphia: JB Lippincott, 1994.

Bingham B. Atlas of clinical otolaryngology. St Louis: Mosby-Year Book, 1992.

Brackmann DE, Shelton C, Arriaga M (eds). Otologic surgery. Philadelphia: WB Saunders, 1994.

Bull PD. Lecture notes on diseases of the ear, nose and throat. 8th ed. Cambridge, MA: Blackwell Scientific Publications, 1996.

Carpenito LJ. Nursing diagnosis application to clinical practice. 5th ed. Philadelphia: JB Lippincott, 1993.

Davidson TK. Clinical manual of otolaryngology. 2nd ed. New York: McGraw-Hill, 1992.

DeSouza C, Goycoolea KV, Ruah CB. Textbook of the ear, nose and throat. London: Sangam, 1995.

Girardi M, Konrad H. Management of benign paroxysmal positional vertigo. ORL Head Neck Nurs 1996; 14(2):25.

Glasscock ME, Shambaugh GE (eds). Surgery of the ear. 4th ed. Philadelphia: WB Saunders, 1990.

Hawke M, Martin RL. A photographic study of the normal and diseased ear. HEAR J 1995; 48(6):29, 34.

Hawke M, McCombe A. Diseases of the ear: A pocket atlas. Ontario: Manticore Communications, 1995.

Haybach PJ. Tuning in to ototoxicity. Nursing 1993; 23(6):34.

Hughes GB, Pensak ML. Clinical otology. 2nd ed. New York: Thieme, 1997.

Jarvis C. Physical examination and health assessment. 2nd ed. Philadelphia: WB Saunders, 1996.

Meyerhoff W, Rice D. Otolaryngology: Head and neck surgery. Philadelphia: WB Saunders, 1992.

Otolaryngology: Head and neck surgery. 2nd ed. St Louis: Mosby-Year Book, 1993.

Pollock KJ. Meniere's disease: A review of the problem. ORL Head Neck Nurs 1995; 13(2):10.

Roland PS, Meyerhoff ML, Marple BF. Hearing loss. New York: Thieme, 1997.

Rybak LP. Ototoxicity. Philadelphia: WB Saunders, 1997.

Schuknecht HF. Pathology of the ear. 2nd ed. Philadelphia: Lea & Febiger, 1993.

Schuller D, Schleuning AJ (eds). DeWeese and Saunders' otolaryngology: Head and neck surgery. St. Louis: Mosby-Year Book, 1994.

Sigler BA, Schuring LT. Ear, nose and throat disorders. St Louis: Mosby-Year Book, 1993.

Silverstein H, et al. Diagnosis and management of hearing loss. Clin Symp 1992; 44(3):2.

Stafford N. ENT. Edinburgh: Churchill Livingstone, 1994.

Yost WA. Fundamentals of hearing: An introduction. 3rd ed. San Diego: Academic Press, 1994.

$\mathcal{A}$ppendix 1

Reference Values for Laboratory Tests

Reference values for laboratory tests serve as important guides in evaluating laboratory data on individual patients. They should not be considered equivalent to normal, however, because there is no sharp dividing line between normal and abnormal values, and the transition from a clearly normal to a clearly abnormal value as a result of a pathologic process is gradual.

The following tables present reference values for commonly performed laboratory tests. These values are given in conventional units as well as in SI (Système International d'Unités) units because the United States is the only industrialized nation that has not adopted the International System of Units.

Because laboratory techniques may differ, values in the tables may differ from those of other laboratories and textbooks, as well as from values given in specific chapters in this text.

Reference Values for Hematology

	Conventional Units	SI Units
Acid hemolysis (Ham test)	No hemolysis	No hemolysis
Alkaline phosphatase, leukocyte	Total score 14–100	Total score 14–100
Cell counts		
Erythrocytes		
Males	4.6–6.2 million/mm^3	4.6–6.2 × 10^{12}/L
Females	4.2–5.4 million/mm^3	4.2–5.4 × 10^{12}/L
Children (varies with age)	4.5–5.1 million/mm^3	4.5–5.1 × 10^{12}/L
Leukocytes, total	4500–11,000/mm^3	4.5–11.0 × 10^9/L
Leukocytes, differential counts*		
Myelocytes	0%	0/L
Band neutrophils	3–5%	150–400 × 10^6/L
Segmented neutrophils	54–62%	3000–5800 × 10^6/L
Lymphocytes	25–33%	1500–3000 × 10^6/L
Monocytes	3–7%	300–500 × 10^6/L
Eosinophils	1–3%	50–250 × 10^6/L
Basophils	0–1%	15–50 × 10^6/L
Platelets	150,000–400,000/mm^3	150–400 × 10^9/L
Reticulocytes	25,000–75,000/mm^3 (0.5–1.5% of erythrocytes)	25–75 × 10^9/L
Coagulation tests		
Bleeding time (template)	2.75–8.0 min	2.75–8.0 min
Coagulation time (glass tube)	5–15 min	5–15 min
D-Dimer	<0.5 μg/mL	<0.5 mg/L
Factor VIII and other coagulation factors	50–150% of normal	0.5–1.5 of normal
Fibrin split products (Thrombo-Welco test)	<10 μg/mL	<10 mg/L
Fibrinogen	200–400 mg/dL	2.0–4.0 g/L
Partial thromboplastin time (PTT)	20–35 sec	20–35 sec
Prothrombin time (PT)	12.0–14.0 sec	12.0–14.0 sec
Coombs' test		
Direct	Negative	Negative
Indirect	Negative	Negative

Table continued on following page

Reference Values for Hematology *Continued*

	Conventional Units	SI Units
Corpuscular values of erythrocytes		
Mean corpuscular hemoglobin (MCH)	26–34 pg/cell	26–34 pg/cell
Mean corpuscular volume (MCV)	80–96 μm^3	80–96 fL
Mean corpuscular hemoglobin concentration (MCHC)	32–36 g/dL	320–360 g/L
Erythrocyte sedimentation rate (ESR)		
Wintrobe		
Males	0–5 mm/h	0–5 mm/h
Females	0–15 mm/h	0–15 mm/h
Westergren		
Males	0–15 mm/h	0–15 mm/h
Females	0–20 mm/h	0–20 mm/h
Haptoglobin	20–165 mg/dL	0.20–1.65 g/L
Hematocrit		
Males	40–54 mL/dL	0.40–0.54
Females	37–47 mL/dL	0.37–0.47
Newborns	49–54 mL/dL	0.49–0.54
Children (varies with age)	35–49 mL/dL	0.35–0.49
Hemoglobin		
Males	13.0–18.0 g/dL	8.1–11.2 mmol/L
Females	12.0–16.0 g/dL	7.4–9.9 mmol/L
Newborns	16.5–19.5 g/dL	10.2–12.1 mmol/L
Children (varies with age)	11.2–16.5 g/dL	7.0–10.2 mmol/L
Hemoglobin, fetal	<1.0% of total	<0.01 of total
Hemoglobin A_{1c}	3–5% of total	0.03–0.05 of total
Hemoglobin A_2	1.5–3.0% of total	0.015–0.03 of total
Hemoglobin, plasma	0.0–5.0 mg/dL	0.0–3.2 $\mu mol/L$
Methemoglobin	30–130 mg/dL	19–80 $\mu mol/L$

Conventional units are percentages; SI units are absolute counts.

Reference Values* for Blood, Serum, and Plasma

	Conventional Units	SI Units
Acetoacetate plus acetone		
Qualitative	Negative	Negative
Quantitative	0.3–2.0 mg/dL	30–200 $\mu mol/L$
Acid phosphatase, serum (Thymolphthalein monophosphate substrate)	0.1–0.6 U/L	0.1–0.6 U/L
ACTH (see Corticotropin)		
Alanine aminotransferase (ALT, SGPT), serum	1–45 U/L	1–45 U/L
Albumin, serum	3.3–5.2 g/dL	33–52 g/L
Aldolase, serum	0.0–7.0 U/L	0.0–7.0 U/L
Aldosterone, plasma		
Standing	5–30 ng/dL	140–830 pmol/L
Recumbent	3–10 ng/dL	80–275 pmol/L
Alkaline phosphatase (ALP), serum		
Adult	35–150 U/L	35–150 U/L
Adolescent	100–500 U/L	100–500 U/L
Child	100–350 U/L	100–350 U/L
Ammonia nitrogen, plasma	10–50 $\mu mol/L$	10–50 $\mu mol/L$
Amylase, serum	25–125 U/L	25–125 U/L
Anion gap, serum, calculated	8–16 mEq/L	8–16 mmol/L
Ascorbic acid, blood	0.4–1.5 mg/dL	23–85 $\mu mol/L$
Aspartate aminotransferase (AST, SGOT), serum	1–36 U/L	1–36 U/L
Base excess, arterial blood, calculated	0 ± 2 mEq/L	0 ± 2 mmol/L
β-Carotene, serum	60–260 $\mu g/dL$	1.1–8.6 $\mu mol/L$

Reference Values* for Blood, Serum, and Plasma *Continued*

	Conventional Units	SI Units
Bicarbonate		
Venous plasma	23–29 mEq/L	23–29 mmol/L
Arterial blood	21–27 mEq/L	21–27 mmol/L
Bile acids, serum	0.3–3.0 mg/dL	0.8–7.6 µmol/L
Bilirubin, serum		
Conjugated	0.1–0.4 mg/dL	1.7–6.8 µmol/L
Total	0.3–1.1 mg/dL	5.1–19.0 µmol/L
Calcium, serum	8.4–10.6 mg/dL	2.10–2.65 mmol/L
Calcium, ionized, serum	4.25–5.25 mg/dL	1.05–1.30 mmol/L
Carbon dioxide, total, serum or plasma	24–31 mEq/L	24–31 mmol/L
Carbon dioxide tension (PCO_2), blood	35–45 mmHg	35–45 mmHg
Ceruloplasmin, serum	23–44 mg/dL	230–440 mg/L
Chloride, serum or plasma	96–106 mEq/L	96–106 mmol/L
Cholesterol, serum or EDTA plasma		
Desirable range	<200 mg/dL	<5.20 mmol/L
LDL cholesterol	60–180 mg/dL	1.55–4.65 mmol/L
HDL cholesterol	30–80 mg/dL	0.80–2.05 mmol/L
Copper	70–140 µg/dL	11–22 µmol/L
Corticotropin (ACTH), plasma, 8 AM	10–80 pg/mL	2–18 pmol/L
Cortisol, plasma		
8:00 AM	6–23 µg/dL	170–630 nmol/L
4:00 PM	3–15 µg/dL	80–410 nmol/L
10:00 PM	<50% of 8:00 AM value	<50% of 8:00 AM value
Creatine, serum		
Males	0.2–0.5 mg/dL	15–40 µmol/L
Females	0.3–0.9 mg/dL	25–70 µmol/L
Creatine kinase (CK), serum		
Males	55–170 U/L	55–170 U/L
Females	30–135 U/L	30–135 U/L
Creatine kinase MB isoenzyme, serum	<5% of total CK activity	<5% of total CK activity
	<5% ng/mL by immunoassay	<5% ng/mL by immunoassay
Creatinine, serum	0.6–1.2 mg/dL	50–110 µmol/L
Estradiol-17β, adult		
Males	10–65 pg/mL	35–240 pmol/L
Females		
Follicular phase	30–100 pg/mL	110–370 pmol/L
Ovulatory phase	200–400 pg/mL	730–1470 pmol/L
Luteal phase	50–140 pg/mL	180–510 pmol/L
Ferritin, serum	20–200 ng/mL	20–200 µg/L
Fibrinogen, plasma	200–400 mg/dL	2.0–4.0 g/L
Folate, serum erythrocytes	2.0–9.0 ng/mL	4.5–20.4 nmol/L
	170–700 ng/mL	385–1590 nmol/L
Follicle-stimulating hormone (FSH), plasma		
Males	4–25 mU/mL	4–25 U/L
Females, premenopausal	4–30 mU/mL	4–30 U/L
Females, postmenopausal	40–250 mU/mL	40–250 U/L
γ-Glutamyltransferase (GGT), serum	5–40 U/L	5–40 U/L
Gastrin, fasting, serum	0–110 pg/mL	0–110 mg/L
Glucose, fasting, plasma or serum	70–115 mg/dL	3.9–6.4 nmol/L
Growth hormone (hGH), plasma, adult, fasting	0–6 ng/mL	0–6 µg/L
Haptoglobin, serum	20–165 mg/dL	0.20–1.65 g/L
Immunoglobulins, serum (see Reference Values for Immunologic Procedures)		
Insulin, fasting, plasma	5–25 µU/mL	36–179 pmol/L
Iron, serum	75–175 µg/dL	13–31 µmol/L
Iron binding capacity, serum		
Total	250–410 µg/dL	45–73 µmol/L
Saturation	20–55%	0.20–0.55

Table continued on following page

Reference Values* for Blood, Serum, and Plasma *Continued*

	Conventional Units	SI Units
Lactate		
Venous whole blood	5.0–20.0 mg/dL	0.6–2.2 mmol/L
Arterial whole blood	5.0–15.0 mg/dL	0.6–1.7 mmol/L
Lactate dehydrogenase (LDH), serum	110–220 U/L	110–220 U/L
Lipase, serum	10–140 U/L	10–140 U/L
Lutropin (LH), serum		
Males	1–9 U/L	1–9 U/L
Females		
Follicular phase	2–10 U/L	2–10 U/L
Midcycle peak	15–65 U/L	15–65 U/L
Luteal phase	1–12 U/L	1–12 U/L
Postmenopausal	12–65 U/L	12–65 U/L
Magnesium, serum	1.3–2.1 mg/dL	0.65–1.05 mmol/L
Osmolality	275–295 mOsm/kg water	275–295 mOsm/kg water
Oxygen, blood, arterial, room air		
Partial pressure (PaO_2)	80–100 mm Hg	80–100 mm Hg
Saturation (SaO_2)	95–98%	95–98%
pH, arterial blood	7.35–7.45	7.35–7.45
Phosphate, inorganic, serum		
Adult	3.0–4.5 mg/dL	1.0–1.5 mmol/L
Child	4.0–7.0 mg/dL	1.3–2.3 mmol/L
Potassium		
Serum	3.5–5.0 mEq/L	3.5–5.0 mmol/L
Plasma	3.5–4.5 mEq/L	3.5–4.5 mmol/L
Progesterone, serum, adult		
Males	0.0–0.4 ng/mL	0.0–1.3 mmol/L
Females		
Follicular phase	0.1–1.5 ng/mL	0.3–4.8 mmol/L
Luteal phase	2.5–28.0 ng/mL	8.0–89.0 mmol/L
Prolactin, serum		
Males	1.0–15.0 ng/mL	1.0–15.0 μg/L
Females	1.0–20.0 ng/mL	1.0–20.0 μg/L
Protein, serum, electrophoresis		
Total	6.0–8.0 g/dL	60–80 g/L
Albumin	3.5–5.5 g/dL	35–55 g/L
Globulins		
Alpha$_1$	0.2–0.4 g/dL	2.0–4.0 g/L
Alpha$_2$	0.5–0.9 g/dL	5.0–9.0 g/L
Beta	0.6–1.1 g/dL	6.0–11.0 g/L
Gamma	0.7–1.7 g/dL	7.0–17.0 g/L
Pyruvate, blood	0.3–0.9 mg/dL	0.03–0.10 mmol/L
Rheumatoid factor	0.0–30.0 IU/mL	0.0–30.0 kIU/L
Sodium, serum or plasma	135–145 mEq/L	135–145 mmol/L
Testosterone, plasma		
Males, adult	300–1200 ng/dL	10.4–41.6 nmol/L
Females, adult	20–75 ng/dL	0.7–2.6 nmol/L
Pregnant females	40–200 ng/dL	1.4–6.9 nmol/L
Thyroglobulin	3–42 ng/mL	3–42 μg/L
Thyrotropin (hTSH), serum	0.4–4.8 μIU/mL	0.4–4.8 mIU/L
Thyrotropin-releasing hormone (TRH)	5–60 pg/mL	5–60 ng/L
Thyroxine (FT_4), free, serum	0.9–2.1 ng/dL	12–27 pmol/L
Thyroxine (T_4), serum	4.5–12.0 μg/dL	58–154 nmol/L
Thyroxine-binding globulin (TBG)	15.0–34.0 μg/mL	15.0–34.0 mg/L
Transferrin	250–430 mg/dL	2.5–4.3 g/L
Triglycerides, serum, after 12-hour fast	40–150 mg/dL	0.4–1.5 g/L
Triiodothyronine (T_3), serum	70–190 ng/dL	1.1–2.9 nmol/L
Triiodothyronine uptake, resin (T_3RU)	25–38%	0.25–0.38
Urate		
Males	2.5–8.0 mg/dL	150–480 μmol/L
Females	2.2–7.0 mg/dL	130–420 μmol/L
Urea, serum or plasma	24–49 mg/dL	4.0–8.2 nmol/L

Reference Values* for Blood, Serum, and Plasma *Continued*

	Conventional Units	SI Units
Urea nitrogen, serum or plasma	11–23 mg/dL	8.0–16.4 nmol/L
Viscosity, serum	1.4–1.8 × water	1.4–1.8 × water
Vitamin A, serum	20–80 µg/dL	0.70–2.80 µmol/L
Vitamin B$_{12}$, serum	180–900 pg/mL	133–664 pmol/L

* Reference values may vary depending on the method and sample source used.

Reference Values for Therapeutic Drug Monitoring (Serum)

	Therapeutic Range	Toxic Concentrations	Proprietary Names
ANALGESICS			
Acetaminophen	10–20 µg/mL	>250 µg/mL	Tylenol Datril
Salicylate	100–250 µg/mL	>300 µg/mL	Aspirin Bufferin
ANTIBIOTICS			
Amikacin	25–30 µg/mL	Peak >35 µg/mL Trough >10 µg/mL	Amikin
Chloramphenicol	10–20 µg/mL	>25 µg/mL	Chloromycetin
Gentamicin	5–10 µg/mL	Peak >10 µg/mL Trough >2 µg/mL	Garamycin
Tobramycin	5–10 µg/mL	Peak >10 µg/mL Trough >2 µg/mL	Nebcin
Vancomycin	5–10 µg/mL	Peak >40 µg/mL Trough >10 µg/mL	Vancocin
ANTICONVULSANTS			
Carbamazepine	5–12 µg/mL	>15 µg/mL	Tegretol
Ethosuximide	40–100 µg/mL	>150 µg/mL	Zarontin
Phenobarbital	15–40 µg/mL	40–100 ng/mL (varies widely)	Luminal
Phenytoin	10–20 µg/mL	>20 µg/mL	Dilantin
Primidone	5–12 µg/mL	>15 µg/mL	Mysoline
Valproic acid	50–100 µg/mL	>100 µg/mL	Depakene
ANTINEOPLASTICS AND IMMUNOSUPPRESSIVES			
Cyclosporine	50–400 ng/mL	>400 ng/mL	Sandimmune
Methotrexate, high dose, 48-hour	Variable	>1 µmol/L 48 hr after dose	Mexate Folex
Tacrolimus (FK-506), whole blood	3–10 µg/L	>15 µg/L	Prograf
BRONCHODILATORS AND RESPIRATORY STIMULANTS			
Caffeine	3–15 ng/mL	>30 ng/mL	
Theophylline (Aminophylline)	10–20 µg/mL	>20 µg/mL	Elixophyllin Quibron
CARDIOVASCULAR DRUGS			
Amiodarone (Obtain specimen more than 8 h after last dose)	1.0–2.0 µg/mL	>2.0 µg/mL	Cordarone
Digitoxin (Obtain specimen 12–24 h after last dose)	15–25 ng/mL	>35 ng/mL	Crystodigin
Digoxin (Obtain specimen more than 6 h after last dose)	0.8–2.0 ng/mL	>2.4 ng/mL	Lanoxin
Disopyramide	2–5 µg/mL	>7 µg/mL	Norpace
Flecainide	0.2–1.0 ng/mL	>1 ng/mL	Tambocor
Lidocaine	1.5–5.0 µg/mL	>6 µg/mL	Xylocaine

Table continued on following page

Reference Values for Therapeutic Drug Monitoring (Serum) *Continued*

	Therapeutic Range	Toxic Concentrations	Proprietary Names
Mexiletine	0.7–2.0 ng/mL	>2 ng/mL	Mexitil
Procainamide	4–10 μg/mL	>12 μg/mL	Pronestyl
Procainamide plus NAPA	8–30 μg/mL	>30 μg/mL	
Propranolol	50–100 ng/mL	Variable	Inderal
Quinidine	2–5 μg/mL	>6 μg/mL	Cardioquin
			Quinaglute
Tocainide	4–10 ng/mL	>10 ng/mL	Tonocard
PSYCHOPHARMACOLOGIC DRUGS			
Amitriptyline	120–150 ng/mL	>500 ng/mL	Elavil
Bupropion	25–100 ng/mL	Not applicable	Triavil
			Wellbutrin
Desipramine	150–300 ng/mL	>500 ng/mL	Norpramin
			Pertofrane
			Tofranil
Imipramine	125–250 ng/mL	>400 ng/mL	Janimine
Lithium	0.6–1.5 mEq/L	>1.5 mEq/L	Lithobid
(Obtain specimen 12 h after last dose)			
Nortriptyline	50–150 ng/mL	>500 ng/mL	Aventyl
			Pamelor

Reference Values for Urine

	Conventional Units	SI Units
Acetone and acetoacetate, qualitative	Negative	Negative
Albumin		
Qualitative	Negative	Negative
Quantitative	10–100 mg/24 h	0.15–1.5 μmol/d
Aldosterone	3–20 μg/24 h	8.3–55 nmol/d
δ-Aminolevulinic acid (δ-ALA)	1.3–7.0 mg/24 h	10–53 μmol/d
Amylase	<17 U/h	<17 U/h
Amylase/creatinine clearance ratio	0.01–0.04	0.01–0.04
Bilirubin, qualitative	Negative	Negative
Calcium (regular diet)	<250 mg/24 h	<6.3 nmol/d
Catecholamines		
Epinephrine	<10 μg/24 h	<55 nmol/d
Norepinephrine	<100 μg/24 h	<590 nmol/d
Total free catecholamines	4–126 μg/24 h	24–745 nmol/d
Total metanephrines	0.1–1.6 mg/24 h	0.5–8.1 μmol/d
Chloride (varies with intake)	110–250 mEq/24 h	110–250 mmol/d
Copper	0–50 μg/24 h	0.0–0.80 μmol/d
Cortisol, free	10–100 μg/24 h	27.6–276 nmol/d
Creatine		
Males	0–40 mg/24 h	0.0–0.30 mmol/d
Females	0–80 mg/24 h	0.0–0.60 mmol/d
Creatinine	15–25 mg/kg/24 h	0.13–0.22 mmol/kg/d
Creatinine clearance (endogenous)		
Males	110–150 mL/min/1.73m²	110–150 mL/min/1.73m²
Females	105–132 mL/min/1.73m²	105–132 mL/min/1.73m²
Cystine or cysteine	Negative	Negative
Dehydroepiandrosterone		
Males	0.2–2.0 mg/24 h	0.7–6.9 μmol/d
Females	0.2–1.8 mg/24 h	0.7–6.2 μmol/d
Estrogens, total		
Males	4–25 μg/24 h	14–90 nmol/d
Females	5–100 μg/24 h	18–360 nmol/d
Glucose (as reducing substance)	<250 mg/24 h	<250 mg/d

Reference Values for Urine *Continued*

	Conventional Units	SI Units
Hemoglobin and myoglobin, qualitative	Negative	Negative
Homogentisic acid, qualitative	Negative	Negative
17-Hydroxycorticosteroids		
Males	3–9 mg/24 h	8.3–25 μmol/d
Females	2–8 mg/24 h	5.5–22 μmol/d
5-Hydroxyindoleacetic acid		
Qualitative	Negative	Negative
Quantitative	2–6 mg/24 h	10–31 μmol/d
17-Ketogenic steroids		
Males	5–23 mg/24 h	17–80 μmol/d
Females	3–15 mg/24 h	10–52 μmol/d
17-Ketosteroids		
Males	8–22 mg/24 h	28–76 μmol/d
Females	6–15 mg/24 h	21–52 μmol/d
Magnesium	6–10 mEq/24 h	3–5 mmol/d
Metanephrines	0.05–1.2 ng/mg creatinine	0.03–0.70 mmol/mmol creatinine
Osmolality	38–1400 mOsm/kg water	38–1400 mOsm/kg water
pH	4.6–8.0	4.6–8.0
Phenylpyruvic acid, qualitative	Negative	Negative
Phosphate	0.4–1.3 g/24 h	13–42 mmol/d
Porphobilinogen		
Qualitative	Negative	Negative
Quantitative	<2 mg/24 h	<9 μmol/d
Porphyrins		
Coproporphyrin	50–250 μg/24 h	77–380 nmol/d
Uroporphyrin	10–30 μg/24 h	12–36 nmol/d
Potassium	25–125 mEq/24 h	25–125 mmol/d
Pregnanediol		
Males	0.0–1.9 mg/24 h	0.0–6.0 μmol/d
Females		
Proliferative phase	0.0–2.6 mg/24 h	0.0–8.0 μmol/d
Luteal phase	2.6–10.6 mg/24 h	8–33 μmol/d
Postmenopausal	0.2–1.0 mg/24 h	0.6–3.1 μmol/d
Pregnanetriol	0.0–2.5 mg/24 h	0.0–7.4 μmol/d
Protein, total		
Qualitative	Negative	Negative
Quantitative	10–150 mg/24 h	10–150 mg/d
Protein/creatinine ratio	<0.2	<0.2
Sodium (regular diet)	60–260 mEq/24 h	60–260 mmol/d
Specific gravity		
Random specimen	1.003–1.030	1.003–1.030
24-hour collection	1.015–1.025	1.015–1.025
Urate (regular diet)	250–750 mg/24 h	1.5–4.4 mmol/d
Urobilinogen	0.5–4.0 mg/24 h	0.6–6.8 μmol/d
Vanillylmandelic acid (VMA)	1.0–8.0 mg/24 h	5–40 μmol/d

Reference Values for Toxic Substances

	Conventional Units	SI Units
Arsenic, urine	<130 μg/24 hr	<1.7 μmol/d
Bromides, serum, inorganic	<100 mg/dL	<10 mmol/L
Toxic symptoms	140–1000 mg/dL	14–100 mmol/L
Carboxyhemoglobin, blood	% Saturation	Saturation
Urban environment	<5%	<0.05
Smokers	<12%	<0.12
Symptoms		
Headache	>15%	>0.15

Table continued on following page

Reference Values for Toxic Substances *Continued*

	Conventional Units	SI Units
Nausea and vomiting	>25%	>0.25
Potentially lethal	>50%	>0.50
Ethanol, blood	<0.05 mg/dL <0.005%	<1.0 mmol/L
Intoxication	>100 mg/dL >0.1%	>22 mmol/L
Marked intoxication	300–400 mg/dL 0.3–0.4%	65–87 mmol/L
Alcoholic stupor	400–500 mg/dL 0.4–0.5%	87–109 mmol/L
Coma	>500 mg/dL >0.5%	>109 mmol/L
Lead, blood		
Adults	<25 μg/dL	<1.2 μmol/L
Children	<15 μg/dL	<0.7 μmol/L
Lead, urine	<80 μg/24 hr	<0.4 μmol/d
Mercury, urine	<30 μg/24 hr	<150 nmol/d

Reference Values for Cerebrospinal Fluid

	Conventional Units	SI Units
Cells	<5/mm³; all mononuclear	<5 × 10⁶/L, all mononuclear
Glucose	50–75 mg/dL (20 mg/dL less than in serum)	2.8–4.2 mmol/L (1.1 mmol less than in serum)
IgG		
Children under 14	<8% of total protein	<0.08% of total protein
Adults	<14% of total protein	<0.14% of total protein
IgG index $\left(\dfrac{\text{CSF/serum IgG ratio}}{\text{CSF/ serum albumin ratio}}\right)$	0.3–0.6	0.3–0.6
Oligoclonal banding on electrophoresis	Absent	Absent
Pressure, opening	70–180 mmH₂O	70–180 mmH₂O
Protein, total	15–45 mg/dL	150–450 mg/L
Protein electrophoresis	Albumin predominant	Albumin predominant

Reference Values for Tests of Gastrointestinal Function

	Conventional Units		Conventional Units
Bentiromide	6-hour urinary arylamine excretion greater than 57% excludes pancreatic insufficiency	Maximum (after histamine or pentagastrin)	
β-Carotene, serum	60–250 ng/dL	Males	9.0–48.0 mmol/h
Fecal fat estimation		Females	6.0–31.0 mmol/h
Qualitative	No fat globules seen by high-power microscope	Ratio: basal/maximum	
		Males	0.0–0.31
Quantitative	<6 g/24 h (>95% coefficient of fat absorption)	Females	0.0–0.29
		Secretin test, pancreatic fluid	
Gastric acid output		Volume	>1.8 mL/kg/h
Basal		Bicarbonate	>80 mEq/L
Males	0.0–10.5 mmol/h		
Females	0.0–5.6 mmol/h	D-Xylose absorption test, urine	>20% of ingested dose excreted in 5 h

Reference Values for Immunologic Procedures

	Conventional Units	SI Units
Complement, serum		
C3	85–175 mg/dL	0.85–1.75 g/L
C4	15–45 mg/dL	150–450 mg/L
Total hemolytic (CH_{50})	150–250 U/mL	150–250 U/mL
Immunoglobulins, serum, adult		
IgG	640–1350 mg/dL	6.4–13.5 g/L
IgA	70–310 mg/dL	0.70–3.1 g/L
IgM	90–350 mg/dL	0.90–3.5 g/L
IgD	0.0–6.0 mg/dL	0.0–60 mg/L
IgE	0.0–430 ng/dL	0.0–430 μg/L

LYMPHOCYTE SUBSETS, WHOLE BLOOD, HEPARINIZED

Antigen	Cell Type	Percentage	Absolute
CD3	Total T cells	56–77	860–1880
CD19	Total B cells	7–17	140–370
CD3 and CD4	Helper-inducer cells	32–54	550–1190
CD3 and CD8	Suppressor-cytotoxic cells	24–37	430–1060
CD3 and DR	Activated T cells	5–14	70–310
CD2	E rosette T cells	73–87	1040–2160
CD16 and CD56	Natural killer (NK) cells	8–22	130–500

Helper/suppressor ratio: 0.8–1.8.

Reference Values for Semen

	Conventional Units	SI Units
Volume	2–5 mL	2–5 mL
Liquefaction	Complete in 15 min	Complete in 15 min
pH	7.2–8.0	7.2–8.0
Leukocytes	Occasional or absent	Occasional or absent
Spermatozoa		
Count	60–150 × 10^6/mL	60–150 × 10^6/mL
Motility	>80% motile	>0.80 motile
Morphology	80–90% normal forms	>0.80–0.90 normal forms
Fructose	>150 mg/dL	>8.33 mmol/L

Tables from Rakel RE (ed). Conn's current therapy 1997. Philadelphia: WB Saunders, 1997.

$\mathcal{A}$ppendix 2

Common Abbreviations

a	before	BPH	benign prostatic hypertrophy
aa	of each	bpm	beats per minute
ABG	arterial blood gas	B.R.P.	bathroom privileges
ac	before meals	BS	bowel sounds
ACH	acetylcholine	BUN	blood urea nitrogen
ACT	activated clotting time	Bx	biopsy
ACTH	adrenocorticotropic hormone		
ADH	antidiuretic hormone	c	with
ADL	activities of daily living	CA	cancer
ad lib	as desired	Ca^{2+}	calcium
AFP	alpha-fetoprotein	CABG	coronary artery bypass graft
A/G ratio	albumin-globulin ratio	CAD	coronary artery disease
AHCPR	Agency for Health Care Policy and Research	CAPD	continuous ambulatory peritoneal dialysis
AHG	antihemophilic globulin	CAT	computerized axial tomography
AIDS	acquired immunodeficiency syndrome	CBC	complete blood count
ALG	antilymphocyte globulin	CC	chief complaint
ALL	acute lymphocytic leukemia	CCK	cholecystokinin
ALS	amyotrophic lateral sclerosis	CCPD	continuous cycle peritoneal dialysis
ALT	alanine aminotransferase	CCT	crude coal tar
AML	acute myelocytic leukemia	C&D	curettage and desiccation
ANA	antinuclear antibody	CDC	Centers for Disease Control and Prevention
AP	anteroposterior		
APTT	activated partial thromboplastin time	CF	circumflex artery
A/R pulse	apical/radial pulse	CFS	chronic fatigue syndrome
ARDS	adult respiratory distress syndrome	CHF	congestive heart failure
ASCVD	arteriosclerotic cardiovascular disease	CK	creatine kinase
ASHD	arteriosclerotic heart disease	Cl^-	chloride
AST	aspartate aminotransferase	CLL	chronic lymphocytic leukemia
ATG	antithymocyte globulin	CML	chronic myelocytic leukemia
ATN	acute tubular necrosis	CMV	cytomegalovirus
ATP	adenosine triphosphate	CNS	central nervous system
AV	atrioventricular	c/o	complained of
AVM	arteriovenous malformation	CO	cardiac output
AVR	aortic valve replacement	CO_2	carbon dioxide
		COP	Cytoxan, Oncovin, prednisone
BaE	barium enema	COPD	chronic obstructive pulmonary disease
BCE	basal cell epithelioma	COPP	Cytoxan, Oncovin, prednisone, procarbazine
bid	twice daily		
BK	below knee	CPK	creatine phosphokinase
BMR	basal metabolism rate	CPR	cardiopulmonary resuscitation
BP	blood pressure	CRF	chronic renal failure

CS	complete stroke
C&S	culture and sensitivities
CSF	cerebrospinal fluid
CT	computed tomography
CVA	cerebrovascular accident
CVA	costovertebral angle
CVD	cardiovascular disease
CVP	central venous pressure
Cx	cervix
Cysto	cystoscopy
D/C	discontinue
D&C	dilation and curettage
DIC	disseminated intravascular coagulation
Diff	differential white blood cell count
DJD	degenerative joint disease
DM	diabetes mellitus
DNA	deoxyribonucleic acid
DOA	dead on arrival
DOE	dyspnea on exertion
DPT	diphtheria, pertussis, tetanus toxoid
DRTBC	drug-resistant tuberculosis
Dx	diagnosis
EBV	Epstein-Barr virus
ECF	extracellular fluid
ECFVD	extracellular fluid volume deficit
ECFVE	extracellular fluid volume excess
ECG (EKG)	electrocardiogram
EEG	electroencephalogram
EENT	eye, ear, nose, and throat
EMG	electromyogram
ENT	ear, nose, and throat
ESR	erythrocyte sedimentation rate
ESRD	end-stage renal disease
FBS	fasting blood sugar
FFP	fresh frozen plasma
FH	family history
FSF	fibrin stabilizing factor
FUO	fever of unknown origin
FWB	full weight bearing
Fx	fracture
GEST	graded exercise stress test
GFR	glomerular filtration rate
GI	gastrointestinal
G6PD	glucose-6-phosphate dehydrogenase
gtt	drops
GTT	glucose tolerance test
GU	genitourinary
HAV	hepatitis A virus
HBV	hepatitis B virus
HCO_3	bicarbonate ion
H_2CO_3	carbonic acid
Hct	hematocrit
HCVD	hypertensive cardiovascular disease
HDL	high-density lipoproteins
HF	heart failure

Hg	mercury
Hgb	hemoglobin
HLA	human leukocyte globulin
HMO	health maintenance organization
HNP	herniated nucleus pulposus
HPI	history of present illness
H_2PO_4	hydrogen phosphate ion
HPV	human papillomavirus
h	hour
h.s.	at bedtime
HSV	herpes simplex virus
HTN	hypertension
hx	history
IABP	intra-aortic balloon pump
ICF	intracellular fluid volume
ICP	intracranial pressure
ICS	intercostal space
ICU	intensive care unit
I&D	incision and drainage
IDDM	insulin-dependent diabetes mellitus
IHSS	idiopathic hypertrophic subaortic stenosis
IM	intramuscular
IMB	intermenstrual bleeding
I&O	intake and output
IPD	intermittent peritoneal dialysis
IPPB	intermittent positive pressure breathing
ISG	immune serum globulin
ITP	idiopathic thrombocytopenic purpura
IV	intravenous
IVC	intravenous cholangiogram
IVP	intravenous pyelogram
JVD	jugular vein distention
K^+	potassium
kg	kilogram
KOH	potassium hydroxide
KUB	kidney, ureter, bladder
L	liter
LAP	leukocyte alkaline phosphatase
LBP	low back pain
LCA	left coronary artery
LCD	liquid carbonic detergents
LDH	lactate dehydrogenase
LDL	low-density lipoproteins
LE	lupus erythematosus
LE prep	lupus erythematosus prep
LLL	left lower lobe
LLQ	left lower quadrant
LMP	last menstrual period
LOC	level of consciousness
LP	lumbar puncture
LVEDP	left ventricular end-diastolic pressure
L&W	living and well
lytes	electrolytes

m	murmur		PEEP	positive end-expiratory pressure
MCH	mean corpuscular hemoglobin		PERRLA	pupils equal, round, reactive to light and accommodation
MCHC	mean corpuscular hemoglobin concentration		PFT	pulmonary function test
MCV	mean corpuscular volume		PGL	persistent generalized lymphadenopathy
MD	muscular dystrophy		PH	past history
mEq	milliequivalent		PI	present illness
MG	myasthenia gravis		Plt	platelet
Mg^{2+}	magnesium		PMI	point of maximal impulse
MI	myocardial infarction		PMNs	polymorphonuclear leukocytes
mm Hg	millimeters of mercury		PMP	past menstrual period
MOPP	mechlorethamine (Mustargen), vincristine (Oncovin), procarbazine, prednisone		PND	paroxysmal nocturnal dyspnea
			PNS	peripheral nervous system
			PO	by mouth
mOsm	milliosmole		POD	postoperative day
MRI	magnetic resonance imaging		PPD	purified protein derivative
MS	multiple sclerosis		PRN	according to necessity
MVR	mitral valve replacement		pro time	prothrombin time
			PS	progressive stroke
Na^+	sodium		PSA	prostate-specific antigen
NAD	no acute distress		PSRO	Professional Standards Review Organization
$NaHCO_3$	sodium bicarbonate			
NH_3	ammonia		PT	prothrombin time
NIDDM	non-insulin-dependent diabetes mellitus		P.T.	physical therapy
NPH	neutral protamine Hagedorn (insulin)		PTA	percutaneous transluminal angioplasty
NPN	nonprotein nitrogen		PTA	plasma thromboplastin antecedent
NPO	nothing by mouth		PTA	prior to admission
NVD	neck vein distention		PTCA	percutaneous transluminal coronary angioplasty
NWB	non-weight-bearing			
			PTFE	polytetrafluoroethylene
O_2	oxygen		PTH	parathyroid hormone
OBS	organic brain syndrome		PTT	partial thromboplastin time
OD	overdose		PUVA	psoralen plus ultraviolet A
O.D.	right eye		PVC	premature ventricular contraction
OOB	out of bed		PVD	peripheral vascular disease
O.R.	operating room		PWB	partial weight bearing
ORIF	open reduction internal fixation		PWP	pulmonary wedge pressure
O.S.	left eye			
O.T.	occupational therapy		qd	every day
O.U.	both eyes		qh	every hour
			qhs	at bedtime
P	after		qid	four times a day
PA	posteroanterior		qns	quantity not sufficient
PA	pulmonary artery		qod	every other day
P&A	percussion and auscultation		qoh	every other hour
PAC	premature atrial contraction		qs	as much as necessary
$Paco_2$	partial pressure of arterial CO_2			
PACU	postanesthesia care unit		RBC	red blood cells
PAEDP	pulmonary artery end-diastolic pressure		RCA	right coronary artery
Pao_2	partial pressure of arterial oxygen		RDA	recommended dietary allowance
Pap	Papanicolaou smear		RIND	reversible ischemic neurologic deficit
PAP	prostatic acid phosphatase		RLL	right lower lobe
PAP	pulmonary artery pressure		RLQ	right lower quadrant
PBI	protein-bound iodine		R/O	rule out
p.c.	after meals		ROS	review of symptoms
PCA	patient-controlled analgesia		RSR	regular sinus rhythm
PCP	*Pneumocystis carinii* pneumonia		Rx	treatment
PCWP	pulmonary capillary wedge pressure			

s̄	without
SA	sinoatrial
SAH	subarachnoid hemorrhage
SBE	subacute bacterial endocarditis
sc	subcutaneous
SCC	squamous cell carcinoma
SCID	severe combined immunodeficiency
sed rate	sedimentation rate
SIADH	syndrome of inappropriate antidiuretic hormone
SLE	systemic lupus erythematosus
SOB	short of breath
s.o.s.	administer once if necessary
S/P	status post (occurred in past)
SPF	sun protection factor
SR	systems review
SSE	soapsuds enema
stat	at once
STD	sexually transmitted disease
STS	serologic test for syphilis
T_3	triiodothyronine
T_4	thyroxine
tab	tablet
TBC	tuberculosis
TBG	thyroxine-binding globulin
TEN	toxic epidermal necrolysis
TENS	transcutaneous electrical nerve stimulator
THA	total hip arthroplasty
THR	total hip replacement
TIA	transient ischemic attack
TIBC	total iron-binding capacity
tid	three times a day
TP	total protein
t-PA	tissue plasminogen activator
TPN	total parenteral nutrition
TSP	total serum protein
TSS	toxic shock syndrome
TURP	transurethral prostatic resection
Tx	traction
ung	ointment
URI	upper respiratory infection
US	ultrasound
UTI	urinary tract infection
UV	ultraviolet
UVA	ultraviolet A
UVB	ultraviolet B
UVJ	ureterovesical junction
VC	vital capacity
VDRL	Veneral Disease Research Laboratories test
VLDL	very-low-density lipoprotein
VNA	Visiting Nurse Association
VS	vital signs
VSS	vital signs stable
wa	while awake
WBC	white blood count
WNL	within normal limits

$\mathcal{A}$ppendix 3

Resources

GENERAL RESOURCES

Academy of Medical-Surgical Nurses
East Holly Avenue
Box 56
Pitman, NJ 08071
609-256-2323

Agency for Health Care Policy and Research
Publications Clearinghouse
P.O. Box 8547
Silver Spring, MD 20907
800-358-9295
301-495-3453
InstantFax service: 301-594-2800
Internet: http://www.ahcpr.gov/
e-mail: info@po5.ahcpr.gov

American Cancer Society
1599 Clifton Road NE
Atlanta, GA 30392
404-320-3333
800-ACS-2345 (800-227-2345)
Internet: http://www.cancer.org

American Nurses' Association
600 Maryland Avenue SW
Suite 100 West
Washington, DC 20024
800-274-4ANA

Centers for Disease Control and Prevention
Department of Health and Human Services
U.S. Public Health Service
Atlanta, GA 30333
404-639-3534
Internet: http://www.cdc.gov
e-mail: netinfo@cdcl.cdc.gov

National Cancer Institute
Cancer Information Service
9000 Rockville Pike
Bethesda, MD 20892
1-800-4-CANCER
Internet: http://www.nci.nih.gov

National Wellness Institute
1045 Clark Street, Suite 210
PO Box 827
Stevens Point, WI 54481-0827
715-342-2969

North American Nursing Diagnosis Association (NANDA)
1211 Locust Street
Philadelphia, PA 19107
800-647-9002

UNIT 1. KNOWLEDGE BASE FOR MEDICAL-SURGICAL NURSING

Death, Dying, and Bereavement

Choice in Dying, Inc.
200 Varick Street
New York, NY 10014-4810
800-989-9455

Foundation for Hospice and Home Care
National Association for Home Care
228 7th Street SE
Washington, DC 20003
202-547-7424
Fax: 202-547-3540

The Hastings Center
Institute of Society, Ethics and the Life Sciences
255 Elm Road
Briarcliff Manor, NY 10510
914-762-8500

Hemlock Society, USA
P.O. Box 11830
Eugene, OR 97440-4030
541-342-5748

Hospice Association of America
519 C Street NE
Washington, DC 20002
202-546-4759

Hospice Educational Institute
190 Westbrook Road
Essex, CT 06426
800-331-1620
Fax: 860-767-2746

National Hospice Organization
1901 N. Moore Street
Arlington, VA 22209
800-658-8898
703-243-5900

Thanatology Foundation
161 Ft Washington Avenue
New York, NY 10032
212-928-2066

United Network for Organ Sharing
100 Boulder Pkwy Suite 500
P.O. Box 137700
Richmond, VA 23225
800-24-DONOR

Aging

Administration on Aging
330 Independence Avenue SW, Suite 4760
Washington, DC 20201
202-619-0556
Internet: http://www.aoa.dhhs.gov/

Aging Network Services
4400 East-West Highway, Suite 907
Bethesda, MD 20814
301-657-4329

Alliance for Aging Research
2021 K Street NW, Suite 305
Washington, DC 20006
Internet: http://www.alz.org/pubpol

American Society on Aging
833 Market Street, Suite 516
San Francisco, CA 94130
415-974-9600

National Council on the Aging, Inc.
409 Third Street SW, Suite 200
Washington, DC 20024
202-479-1200

National Gerontological Association
7250 Parkway Drive, Suite 510
Hanover, MD 21076
800-723-0560

The National Institute on Aging Information Center
PO Box 8057
Gaithersburg, MD 20870-8057

Surgery

Association of Operating Room Nurses
2170 South Parker Road, Suite 300
Denver, CO 80231
303-755-6300

UNIT II. CARDIOVASCULAR DYSFUNCTION

American Heart Association National Center
7320 Greenville Avenue
Dallas, TX 75231
800-242-8715
214-373-6300
Internet: http://www.amhrt.org/
e-mail: inquire@amhrt.org

American Red Cross
430 17th Street
Washington, DC 20006
202-737-8300
Internet: http://www.crossnet.org/

Heart Information Center
National Heart, Lung, and Blood Institute
US Public Health Service
9000 Rockville Pike
Building 31, Room 4A21
Bethesda, MD 20892
301-251-1222

Mended Hearts
American Heart Association
7320 Greenville Avenue
Dallas, TX 75231
800-242-8715
214-373-6300
Internet: http://www.amhrt.org/
e-mail: inquire@amhrt.org

National Heart Savers Association
9140 W. Dodge Road
Omaha, NE 68114
402-398-1993

Society for Vascular Nursing
309 Winter Street
Norwood, MA 02062
617-762-3630

UNIT III. HEMATOLOGIC DYSFUNCTION

American Association of Blood Banks
8101 Glenbrook Road
Bethesda, MD 20814
301-907-6977

Cooley's Anemia Foundation
105 East 22nd Street, Room 911
New York, NY 10010
800-221-3571

Leukemia Society of America
733 Third Avenue
New York, NY 10017
212-573-8484
800-955-4LSA
Internet: http://www.kumc.edu/gec/s

National Association for Sickle Cell Disease
3345 Wilshire Blvd, Suite 1106
Los Angeles, CA 90010
800-421-8453
Internet: http://www.access.bridgenet.org/center/local/sickle.html

National Hemophilia Foundation
110 Greene Street, Suite 303
New York, NY 10012
212-219-8180
Internet: http://www.stepstn.com/nord/org/

UNIT IV. RESPIRATORY DYSFUNCTION

American Academy of Allergy, Asthma, and Immunology
611 East Wells Street
Milwaukee, WI 53202
800-822-2762
Internet: http://www.execpc.com/~edi/aaaai.html

American Academy of Otolaryngology–Head and
Neck Surgery
One Prince Street
Alexandria, VA 22314
703-836-4444

American Lung Association
1740 Broadway
New York, NY 10019
212-315-8700
800-LUNG-USA

American Thoracic Society, Section on Nursing
1740 Broadway
New York, NY 10019
212-315-8700

Asthma and Allergy Foundation of America
11125 15th Street NW, Suite 502
Washington, DC 20005
800-7-ASTHMA

Asthma Care Association of America
PO Box 568
Spring Valley Road
Ossining, NY 10562
914-762-2110

Canadian Lung Association
75 Alberta, Suite 908
Ottawa, Ontario, Canada K1P 5E7
613-237-1208

International Association of Laryngectomees
1599 Clifton Road NE
Atlanta, GA 30329
404-329-7651

Lung Disease Hotline
National Jewish Medical and Research Center for
Immunology and Respiratory Medicine
1400 Jackson Street
Denver, CO 80206
800-222-LUNG
303-398-1477

National Association for Medical Equipment Services
625 Slaters Lane, Suite 200
Alexandria, VA 22314-1171
703-836-6263
Fax: 703-836-6730

National Asthma Education Program
11225 15th Street NW, Suite 502
Washington, DC 20005
202-466-7643

Respiratory Nursing Society
5700 Old Orchard Road, First Floor
Skokie, IL 60077
847-965-8673

Society of Otorhinolaryngology and Head/Neck Nurses
116 Canal Street, Suite A
New Smyrna Beach, FL 32068
904-428-1695

UNIT V. NEUROLOGIC DYSFUNCTION

Alzheimer's Disease and Related Disorders Association
919 N. Michigan Avenue, Suite 100
Chicago, IL 60611
800-272-3900

Alzheimer's Disease Education and Referral Center
ADEAR Center
PO Box 8250
Silver Spring, MD 20907-8250
800-438-4380
Fax: 301-495-3334

American Association of Neuroscience Nurses
224 North Des Plaines
Suite 601
Chicago, IL 60661
312-993-0043
Internet: http://www.prairienet.org/aann/homepage.html
e-mail: AssnNeuro@aol.com

American Association of Spinal Cord Injury Nurses
75-20 Astoria Blvd.
Jackson Heights, NY 11370
718-803-3782

American Brain Tumor Association
3725 North Talman Avenue
Chicago, IL 60618
Internet: http://www.neurosurgery.mgh.harvard.edu/abta/

American Parkinson Disease Association
116 John Street
New York, NY 10038
800-223-2732

American Society for Parenteral and Enteral Nutrition
8630 Fenton Street, Suite 412
Silver Spring, MD 20910
301-587-6215
Internet: http://www.peakcom.com/clinnutr.org/

American Speech/Language/Hearing Association
10801 Rockville Pike
Rockville, MD 20852
800-638-8255

Amyotrophic Lateral Sclerosis Association
21021 Ventura Boulevard, Suite 321
Woodland Hills, CA 91364-2206
818-340-7500
800-782-4747
Fax: 818-340-2060
Internet: http://www.kumc.edu/gec/s

Epilepsy Foundation of America
4351 Garden City Drive
Landover, MD 20785
800-332-1000
Internet: http://www.swcp.com/..djf/

Guillain-Barré International Foundation
P.O. Box 262
Wynnewood, PA 19096
610-667-0131

Hereditary Disease Foundation
1427 7th Street, Suite 2
Santa Monica, CA 90401

Huntington's Disease Foundation of America
140 West 22nd Street, 6th Floor
New York, NY 10011
800-345-4372
Internet: http://www.lib.uchicago.e

Muscular Dystrophy Association
3561 East Sunrise Drive
Tucson, AZ 85718
602-529-2000
Internet: http://www.aztec.asu.edu/cirs

Myasthenia Gravis Foundation
53 West Jackson Boulevard, Suite 909
Chicago, IL 60604
800-541-5454
Internet: http://www.med.unc.edu/mg

National Amyotrophic Lateral Sclerosis Foundation
185 Madison Avenue
New York, NY 10019
800-782-4747

National Head Injury Foundation
1140 Connecticut Avenue NW, Suite 812
Washington, DC 20036
800-444-6443
Internet: http://www.ncats.newaygo.mi.u

National Institute of Neurological Disorders and Stroke
National Institutes of Health
Bethesda, MD 20892
301-496-4000
Internet: http://www.nih.gov/ninds/nindseeo.htm

National MS Society
733 3rd Avenue, 6th floor
New York, NY 10017
800-624-8236
Internet: http://www.nmss.org
e-mail: info@nmss.org

National Parkinson Foundation
1501 NW Ninth Avenue
Miami, FL 33136
800-443-7022
Internet: http://www.parkinson.org/

National Spasmodic Torticollis Association, Inc.
P.O. Box 873
Royal Oak, MI 48068

National Spinal Cord Injury Association
600 West Cummings Park, Suite 2000
Woburn, MA 01801
617-935-2722
Members and those with spinal cord injuries: 800-962-9629
Internet: http://www.spinalcord.org/

Parkinson's Disease Foundation
William Black Medical Research Building
Columbia University Medical Center
640 West 168th Street
New York, NY 10032

800-327-4545
Internet: http://www.parkinsons-foundation.org/

The Stroke Foundation
898 Park Avenue
New York, NY 10021
800-367-1990
Internet: http://www.hsf.ca/research/index.html

Tourette Syndrome Association
42-40 Bell Boulevard
Bayside, NY 11361
800-327-0717
Internet: http://www.amda.ab.ca/mpinfo/pcinfo/agency35.html

UNIT VI. MUSCULOSKELETAL DYSFUNCTION

Arthritis Foundation
P.O. Box 19000
Atlanta, GA 30326
404-872-7100
800-542-0295
Internet: http://www.arthritis.org
e-mail: help@arthritis.org

National Amputation Foundation
12-45 150th Street
Whitestone, NY 11357
212-767-0596

National Arthritis/Musculoskeletal and Skin Diseases
Information Clearinghouse
9000 Rockville Pike
Bethesda, MD 20892
800-283-7800

National Association of Orthopaedic Nurses
East Holly Avenue
Box 56
Pitman, NJ 08071
609-256-2310

National Osteoporosis Foundation
1150 17th Street NW
Washington, DC 20036
202-223-2226
Internet: http://www.nof.org/

UNIT VII. GASTROINTESTINAL DYSFUNCTION

Crohn's and Colitis Foundation of America
444 Park Avenue South
New York, NY 10016-7374
800-343-3637
Internet: http://www.amda.ab.ca/mpinfo/pcinfo/directory/agency24.html

Nutrition Screening Initiative
2626 Pennsylvania Avenue NW, Suite 301
Washington, DC 20037
202-625-1662

Society of Gastrointestinal Nurses and Associates
1070 Sibley Tower
Rochester, NY 14604
716-546-7241

United Ostomy Association
19772 MacArthur Blvd., Suite 200
Irvine, CA 92612-2405
Internet: http://www.uoa.org/

Wound Ostomy and Continence Nurses Society
2755 Bristol Street, Suite 110
Costa Mesa, CA 92606
712-476-0268

UNIT VIII. HEPATIC DYSFUNCTION

Alcoholics Anonymous
PO Box 549
Grand Central Station
New York, NY 10163
212-870-3400
Fax: 212-870-3003

American Liver Foundation
1425 Pompton Avenue
Cedar Grove, NJ 07009
800-223-0179

National Clearinghouse for Alcohol and Drug Information
11426 Rockville Pike, Suite 200
Rockville, MD 20852-3007
800-729-6686
TDD: 800-487-4889
Fax: 301-468-6433

National Council on Alcoholism and Drug
Dependence, Inc.
12 W. 21st Street
New York, NY 10010
800-NCA-CALL

UNIT IX. ENDOCRINE DYSFUNCTION

American Association of Diabetic Educators
500 North Michigan Avenue, Suite 1400
Chicago, IL 60611
312-661-1700

American Diabetes Association
1660 Duke Street
Alexandria, VA 22314
800-232-3472
Internet: http://www.diabetes.org

UNIT X. URINARY DYSFUNCTION

American Nephrology Nurses' Association
East Holly Avenue
Box 56
Pitman, NJ 08071
609-256-2320

The Bladder Health Council
American Foundation for Urologic Disease
1120 N. Charles Street
Baltimore, MD 21201
800-242-2383

HIP (Help for Incontinent People)
P. O. Box 544
Union, SC 29379
800-BLADDER

The Simon Foundation for Continence
P. O. Box 835
Wilmette, IL 60091
Patient information: 800-23-SIMON
Professional information: 708-864-3913

UNIT XI. IMMUNE DYSFUNCTION

HIV/AIDS

AIDS Action Council
1875 Connecticut Avenue, Suite 700
Washington, DC 20009
202-986-1300
Internet: http://www.thebody.com/

AIDS Hotline for the Hearing Impaired
800-243-7889

American Foundation for AIDS Research
733 3rd Avenue, 12th Floor
New York, NY 10017
212-682-7440

Centers for Disease Control and Prevention
Department of Health and Human Services
US Public Health Service
Atlanta, GA 30333
404-639-3534
AIDS statistics: 404-332-4570
Internet: http://www.cdc.gov
e-mail: netinfo@cdcl.cdc.gov

Housing of Persons with AIDS (HOPWA)
TDH HIV Division
1100 49th Street
Austin, TX 78756
(512) 490-2520

National AIDS Hotline
800-342-AIDS

National AIDS Information Clearinghouse
800-458-5231

National Association of People with AIDS
1413 K Street NW
Washington, DC 20005
202-898-0414
Fax: 202-898-0435

Spanish AIDS Hotline
800-344-7432

Cancer

American Cancer Society
1599 Clifton Road NE
Atlanta, GA 30392
404-320-3333
800-ACS-2345 (800-227-2345)
Internet: http://www.cancer.org

American Chronic Pain Association
PO Box 850
Rocklin, CA 95677
916-632-0922

Canadian Cancer Society
National Office
10 Alcorn Avenue, Suite 200
Toronto, Ontario, Canada M4V 1E4
416-961-7223

Cancer Care, Inc.
1180 Avenue of the Americas
New York, NY 10036
800-813-HOPE

CancerNet
NCI International Cancer Information Center
Building 82, Room 123
Bethesda, MD 20892
301-496-4907
Internet:
    http://biomed.nus.sg:80/Cancer/welcome.html
    gopher://gopher.nih.gov/11/clin/cancernet
e-mail: cancernet@icicb.nci.nih.gov

Cancer Nursing

Raven Press
1185 Avenue of the Americas
New York, NY 10003
212-930-9500

Chemocare
231 North Avenue West
Westfield, NJ 07090
800-55-CHEMO

International Association for the Study of Pain
909 NE 43rd Street, Suite 306
Seattle, WA 98105-6020
206-547-6409

Leukemia Society of America
733 Third Avenue
New York, NY 10017
212-573-8484
800-955-4LSA
Internet: http://www.kumc.edu/gec/s

National Cancer Institute
Cancer Information Service
Office of Cancer Communications
Bethesda, MD 20205
1-800-4-CANCER

National Cancer Institute Information Associates Program
9300 Old Georgetown Road
Bethesda, MD 20814-1519
800-624-7890
301-496-7600

National Institutes of Health
Office of Clinical Center Communications
Building 10, Room 1C255
9000 Rockville Pike
Bethesda, MD 20892
301-496-4000

Oncology Nursing Forum

The Oncology Nursing Press
501 Holiday Drive
Pittsburgh, PA 15220
412-921-7373

Oncology Nursing Society
501 Holiday Drive
Pittsburgh, PA 15220
412-921-7373
Internet: http://www.nauticom.net/www/onsmain/
e-mail: member@nauticom.net

Seminars in Oncology Nursing

WB Saunders Company
Periodicals Order Fulfillment
6277 Sea Harbor Drive
Orlando, FL 32887-4800
800-654-2452
Fax: 407-363-9661

The Susan G. Komen Breast Cancer Foundation
5005 LBJ Freeway, Suite 370
Dallas, TX 75244
800-IMAWARE

United Cancer Council
1803 N. Meridian Street
Indianapolis, IN 46202
317-879-4100

United Ostomy Association
19772 MacArthur Blvd., Suite 200
Irvine, CA 92612-2405
Internet: http://www.uoa.org./

Other Immune Dysfunction

American Academy of Allergy, Asthma, and Immunology
800-822-2762
Internet: http://execpc.com/~edi/aaaai.html

Asthma and Allergy Foundation of America
11125 15th Street NW, Suite 502
Washington, DC 20005
800-7-ASTHMA

Chronic Fatigue and Immune Dysfunction Syndrome
Association
P.O. Box 220398
Charlotte, NC 28222-0398
704-362-CFID
800-442-3437
Internet: http://www.ybi.com/cfids/

Chronic Fatigue Immune Dysfunction Syndrome Society
P.O. Box 230108
Portland, OR 97223
503-684-5261

Lupus Foundation of America
4 Research Place, Suite 180
Rockville, MD 20850
301-670-9292
Internet: http://www.lupus.org/lupu

National CFS Association
3521 Broadway, Suite 222
Kansas City, MO 64111
816-931-4777

Scleroderma International Foundation
1725 York Avenue, #29F
New York, NY 10128
212-427-7040

United Scleroderma Foundation
PO Box 399
Watsonville, CA 95077
800-722-4673
408-728-2202
Internet: http://www.social.com/hea

UNIT XII. INTEGUMENTARY DYSFUNCTION

American Academy of Facial Plastic and
Reconstructive Surgery
110 Vermont Avenue NW, Suite 220
Washington, DC 20005
202-842-4500

American Burn Association
c/o Cleon W. Goodwin, MD
Secretary, American Burn Association
New York Hospital–Cornell Medical Center
525 East 68th Street, Room L-706
New York, NY 10021
800-548-BURN

American Society of Plastic and Reconstructive
Surgical Nurses
East Holly Avenue
Box 56
Pitman, NJ 08071
609-256-2340

Burn Awareness Coalition
PO Box 17840
Encino, CA 91416
818-994-4661

Burn Foundation
1128 Walnut Street
Philadelphia, PA 19107
215-629-9200
Internet: http://www.ot.com/burn_prevention/

Burn Institute
3702 Ruffin Road, #101
San Diego, CA 92123-1812
619-541-2277

Burn Prevention Foundation
5000 Tilghman Street, Suite 110
Allentown, PA 18104
610-481-9810
Internet: http://www.ot.com/burn_prevention/fact_sheets

Dermatology Nurses Association
East Holly Avenue
Box 56
Pitman, NJ 08071
609-256-2330

Emergency Nurses Association
216 Higgins Road
Park Ridge, IL 60068
708-698-9400

National Institute for Burn Medicine
909 E. Ann Street
Ann Arbor, MI 48104
313-769-9000

Psoriasis Foundation
6600 Southwest 92nd Avenue, Suite 300
Portland, OR 97223
503-244-7404
Fax: 503-245-0626

Wound, Ostomy, and Continence Nurses
2755 Bristol Street, Suite 110
Costa Mesa, CA 92626
714-476-0268

UNIT XIII. REPRODUCTIVE DYSFUNCTION

Alta Bates-Herrick Breast Cancer Risk Counseling
2001 Dwight Way
Berkeley, CA 94704
510-204-4286

Association of Women's Health, Obstetric, and
Neonatal Nurses
700 14th Street NW
Washington, DC 20005
202-662-1600

CanSurmount
American Cancer Society
1599 Clifton Road NE
Atlanta, GA 30392
404-320-3333
800-ACS-2345 (800-227-2345)
Internet: http://www.cancer.org

ENCORE
National YWCA
Health Promotion Department
726 Broadway
New York, NY 10003
212-475-5990

Endometriosis Association
8585 North 76th Place
Milwaukee, WI 53223
800-992-3636
414-355-2200
Internet: http://www.ivf.com/endoassn.ktml

National Herpes Hotline
Herpes Resource Center
13827 Research Triangle Park
Raleigh, NC 27709
800-230-6039

I Can Cope
American Cancer Society
1599 Clifton Road NE
Atlanta, GA 30392
404-320-3333
800-ACS-2345 (800-227-2345)
Internet: http://www.cancer.org

Impotence Anonymous
119 South Ruth Street
Maryville, TN 37802
615-926-7025

La Leche League International
1400 N. Meacham Road
Schaumburg, IL 60173
1-800-LALECHE
847-519-7730

Look Good, Feel Better
American Cancer Society
1599 Clifton Road NE
Atlanta, GA 30392
404-320-3333
800-ACS-2345 (800-227-2345)
Internet: http://www.cancer.org

Make Today Count
1235 East Cherokee
Springfield, MA 65804
800-432-2273

National Alliance of Breast Cancer Organizations
9 East 37th Street, 10th Floor
New York, NY 10016
800-719-9154
212-719-0154

National Breast Cancer Coalition
1707 L Street
Washington, DC 20036
202-296-7477
Fax: 202-265-6854

National Sexually Transmitted Disease Hotline
800-227-8922

National Women's Health Network
514 10th Street NW, Suite 400
Washington, DC 20004
202-628-7814

Prostatitis Foundation
2029 Ireland Grove Rd.
Bloomington, IL 61704
309-664-6222

Reach to Recovery
American Cancer Society
1599 Clifton Road NE
Atlanta, GA 30392
404-320-3333
800-ACS-2345 (800-227-2345)
Internet: http://www.cancer.org

RESOLVE
PO Box 474
Belmont, MA 02178
617-484-2424

Sexuality Information and Education Council of the
United States (SIECUS)

Publication Department
130 W. 42nd Street, Suite 350
New York, NY 10036-7802
212-819-9770

Us Too International
930 North York Road, Suite 50
Hinsdale, IL 60521
630-323-1002

Y-Me: National Breast Cancer Hotline
800-221-2141

UNIT XIV. EYE AND EAR DYSFUNCTION

Eye Dysfunction

American Council of the Blind
1155 15th Street NW, Suite 720
Washington, DC 20005
202-467-5081
Fax: 202-467-5085

American Foundation for the Blind
11 Penn Plaza, Suite 300
New York, NY 10001
212-502-7600

American Society of Ophthalmic Registered Nurses
655 Beach Street
PO Box 193030
San Francisco, CA 94119
415-561-8513

Canadian National Institute for the Blind
1929 Bayview Avenue
Toronto, Ontario, Canada M4G 3E8
416-486-2500

Eye Bank Associations of America
1001 Connecticut Avenue NW, Suite 601
Washington, DC 20036
202-775-4999

Lighthouse National Center for Education
111 East 59th Street
New York, NY 10022
800-334-5497

National Association for the Visually Handicapped
22 West 21st Street
New York, NY 10010
212-889-3141

Recording for the Blind and Dyslexic
20 Roszel Road
Princeton, NJ 08540
800-221-4792
609-452-0606

Ear Dysfunction

Acoustic Neuroma Association
PO Box 398
Carlisle, PA 17013
717-249-4783

Alexander Graham Bell Association for the Deaf, Inc.
3417 Volta Place NW
Washington, DC 20007
202-337-5220

American Academy of Audiology
1735 N. Lynn Street
Arlington, VA 22209
703-610-9022

American Speech-Language-Hearing Association
10801 Rockville Pike, Dept. AP
Rockville, MD 20852
301-897-5700

American Tinnitus Association
PO Box 5
Portland, OR 97207
503-248-9985

Better Hearing Institute
PO Box 1848
Washington, DC 20013
800-EAR-WELL

Canadian Hard of Hearing Association
2435 Holly Lane, Suite 205
Ottawa, Ontario, Canada K1V 7P2
800-263-8068
613-526-1584
Fax: 613-526-4718
TTY: 613-526-2692

Deafness Research Foundation
55 E. 34th Street
New York, NY 10016
212-768-1181

Ear Foundation
Baptist Hospital
Nashville, TN 37236
800-545-HEAR

International Hearing Dog, Inc.
5901 E. 89th Avenue
Henderson, CO 80640
303-287-3277

International Hearing Society
20361 Middlebelt Road
Livonia, MI 48512
800-521-5247

National Association of the Deaf
814 Thayer Avenue
Silver Spring, MD 20910
301-587-1788

National Institute on Deafness and Other
Communication Disorders
National Institutes of Health
Building 31, Room 3C35
9000 Rockville Pike
Bethesda, MD 20892
301-907-7653

Self-Help for Hard of Hearing People
7910 Woodmont Avenue, Suite 1200
Bethesda, MD 20814
301-657-2248

Vestibular Disorders Association
PO Box 4467
Portland, OR 97208
503-229-7705

*I*ndex

Note: Page numbers in *italics* indicate illustrations. Page numbers followed by t indicate tables; those followed by c indicate nursing care guides; those followed by d indicate other display materials.

A

Abbreviations, 2033–2036
ABCD mnemonic, for skin cancer, 1635–1636
Abdomen, acute, assessment in, 1119d–1121d
  auscultation of, 968
  examination of, 968–969
  palpation of, 192, 969
  percussion of, 192, 968–969
Abdominal adhesions, 148t
Abdominal angina, in elderly, 1106
Abdominal aortic aneurysm, *367*, 367–370
  case study of, 368d–369d
  clinical manifestations of, 367, 368d
  diagnosis of, 367–368
  etiology and pathophysiology of, 367
  management of, 368–370
  risk factors for, 370
  rupture of, 368d–369d, 370
Abdominal distention, gas and, 961
Abdominal incisions, 993–995, 994t–995t
Abdominal pain, 964, 964t, 965. See also *Pain.*
  characteristics of, 965
  in appendicitis, 1065, *1065*
  in Crohn's disease, 1067, 1069
  in diverticular disease, 1082, 1083
  in elderly, 1015
  in peritonitis, 1062, 1063
  in ulcerative colitis, 1070
  sources of, 965t
Abdominal perineal resection, 1101–1106
  complications in, 1102
  patient preparation for, 1101
  postoperative care in, 1103–1106
  postoperative course in, 1101–1102
  preoperative care in, 1103
  procedure for, 1101, *1102*
Abdominal rigidity, in peritonitis, 969
Abdominal surgery, paralytic ileus after, 1075–1077
Abducens nerve, 723t
Ablative neurosurgery, 1555t
ABO blood group, 432–433, *434*
Abrasion, corneal, 1987–1989
  fluorescein staining of, 1945
  scalp, 816–817
Abscess, anorectal, 1071–1074, *1072*
  brain, 770–773
    nursing process in, 771–773
    prevention of, in head injury, 821–822
    sinusitis and, 602
  breast, 1852

Abscess *(Continued)*
  liver, 1179
  lumbar, appendicitis and, 1064t
  lung, 647–648
  pancreatic, fistula formation and, 1124–1126, *1125*
  pelvic, appendicitis and, 1064t
  perinephric, 1375
  peritonsillar, 607–608
  skin, *1571*, 1572
  soft tissue, 1595–1599, 1598t, 1599d
  subphrenic, appendicitis and, 1064t
Absence seizures, 796t
Absolute granulocyte count, 444
Absolute neutrophil count (ANC), 131
Abuse, spouse, 19
Acceptance, in bereavement, 37
  in death and dying, 33–34
Accessory nerve, 724t
Accident prevention. See *Safety measures.*
Accutane (isotretinoin), 1581
ACE inhibitors, 213, 214d
  for heart failure, 275
  for myocardial infarction, 297
Acebutolol (Sectral), 377t
Acetaminophen (Tylenol), 893d, 1553, 1554t
  hepatotoxicity of, 1178t
Acetazolamide (Diamox), for glaucoma, 1980
Acetohexamide (Dymelor), 1239, 1239t, 1240d
Acetylcholine, 713, 726
  in muscle contraction, 840
  in myasthenia gravis, 782, *782*
Acetylcholinesterase, 713
Acetylsalicylic acid. See *Aspirin.*
Achalasia, *1044*, 1044–1046, 1046d
Acid burns. See *Chemical burns.*
Acid treatment, for genital warts, 1027
Acid-base balance, buffer systems in, 103, 104t
  disturbances of, 102–113. See also *Acidosis; Alkalosis.*
  in arterial blood, 540, 540t, 542, 543, 544t
  renal mechanisms of, *103*, 103–104, 104t, 543, 1333
  respiratory control of, 103, *103*, 104t, 543
Acidophilic adenoma, 828–832, 831t
Acidosis, metabolic, 104–106, 105t
  compensated, 543
  hypoxemia and, 530
  in acute renal failure, 1390t
  in burns, 1660, *1661*

Acidosis *(Continued)*
  in diabetes, 1227. See also *Diabetic ketoacidosis.*
  in ileostomy client, 1013, 1014d
  in shock, 406, 407
  respiratory, 108t, 108–111, 543
  hypercarbia and, 530
  in acute renal failure, 1390t
Acne rosacea, 1616, *1616*
Acne vulgaris, *1613*, 1613–1616, 1615t
  retinoids for, 1581–1582, 1615t
Acoustic nerve, 723t
  in Menière's disease, 829
Acoustic neuroma, 828–832, 831t
Acquired hypoprothrombinemia, 517
Acquired immunity, 1429, 1430, 1441t, 1441–1442
Acquired immunodeficiency syndrome (AIDS), 19–20. See also *Human immunodeficiency virus (HIV) infection.*
  CDC criteria for, 1468, 1468t–1469t
  resources for, 2041
Acromegaly, 1269–1274, *1273*
ACTH, 1205t
  measurement of, 1279t
  secretion of, 1214, *1215*
ACTH stimulation test, 1279t, 1280
ACTH-secreting tumors, Cushing's syndrome and, 1285, 1286, 1287
Actinic keratosis, 1633t
Action potential, 712, 713
  of cardiac cell, 169, *170*, 171
Activase (alteplase), 217, *218*
  for myocardial infarction, 295, 296d
Activated partial thromboplastin time, 443t, 448
Activities of daily living. See also *Self-care.*
  assistance with, 18–19
  in myasthenia gravis, 784
  in stroke, 812–813
  postmastectomy, 1868t
  self-help devices for, 884
Activity. See also *Exercise.*
  after spinal surgery, 764–765
  in Parkinson's disease, 788, 789d
  metabolic equivalents for, 298
  postoperative, 153–154
Activity intolerance. See *Exercise; Fatigue; Rest.*
Acupuncture, 1556
Acute abdomen, assessment in, 1119d–1121d
Acute bacterial prostatitis, 1733t, 1733–1735

Acute bronchitis, 639–641, 640d

Acute cholecystitis, liver abscess in, 1179

Acute gastritis, 1023–1025

Acute generalized pustular psoriasis, 1616–1619, 1617t

Acute hemolytic transfusion reaction, 462, 483, 488–489

Acute lymphocytic leukemia, 493, 494t. See also *Leukemia*.

Acute myelocytic leukemia, 493, 494t. See also *Leukemia*.

Acute necrotizing ulcerative gingivitis, 1017–1019, 1018t

Acute pancreatitis, 1118–1122
case study of, 1119d–1121d
in elderly, 1131
pancreatic fistula and, 1124–1126, *1125*

Acute renal failure, 1388–1394. See also *Renal failure, acute*.

Acute sinusitis, 602–603

Acute tubular necrosis, definition of, 1388t
in electrical injury, 1688–1689

Acute urethral syndrome, chlamydia and, 1921

Acute viral rhinitis, 600, 600d

Acyclovir (Zovirax), for genital herpes, 1903, 1904t
for herpes simplex virus infection, 1581

Adaptive immunity, 1429, 1430, 1441t, 1441–1442

Addison's crisis, after adrenalectomy, 1289
clinical manifestations of, 1278–1280
management of, 1280–1281
nursing care guide for, 1282c–1283c

Addison's disease, 1277–1285
assessment in, 1281
clinical manifestations of, *1278*, 1278–1280
diagnosis of, 1279t–1281t, 1280
etiology of, 1277
in elderly, 1323
management of, 1280–1281, 1284d
nursing care guide for, 1282c–1283c
nursing diagnoses and planning in, 1281–1283
nursing interventions in, 1281–1285
pathophysiology of, 1277–1278
self-care in, 1282c–1283c, 1284d

Adenocarcinoma. See also *Cancer*.
of cervix, 1830. See also *Cervical cancer*.
of kidney, 1416–1418
of lung, 695–696
of prostate, 1754–1755. See also *Prostate cancer*.
of uterus, 1836–1837

Adenocard. See *Adenosine (Adenocard)*.

Adenohypophysis, disorders of, 1265–1274
hormones of, 1205t
structure and function of, 1208, *1208*, 1209–1210

Adenoma, acidophilic, 828–832, 831t
adrenal, Cushing's syndrome and, 1286
pheochromocytoma as, 1292–1295
primary aldosteronism and, 1289–1292
chromophilic, 828–832, 831t
chromophobe, 828–832, 831t
hepatic, 1194
parathyroid, 1320
pituitary, 828–832, 831t, 1265–1269, *1266*, *1267*, 1270c–1272c
Cushing's syndrome and, 1285, 1287
hyperthyroidism and, 1307

Adenoma (Continued)
somatotropin hypersecretion and, 1269–1274
surgery for, 1266–1269, *1267*, 1270c–1272c
in Cushing's disease, 1287
thyroid, 1315
zona glomerulosa, primary aldosteronism and, 1289–1292

Adenosine (Adenocard), for dysrhythmias, 215–216, 216d
for paroxysmal atrial tachycardia, 245
in cardiopulmonary resuscitation, 263, 263t

Adenosine triphosphate, in muscle movement, 842

Adhesions, abdominal, 148t
intestinal, 1074, *1074*, 1084–1093

Adhesive skin traction, 859–860. See also *Traction*.

Adjuvant chemotherapy, 1874

Adolescents, gynecomastia in, 1853–1854
sexually transmitted diseases in, 1919d. See also *Sexually transmitted diseases (STDs)*.

Adrenal(s), structure and function of, 1206t, 1213–1216, *1214*, *1215*, 1216t

Adrenal adenoma. See *Adrenal tumors*.

Adrenal androgen deficiency, in adrenocortical insufficiency, 1277

Adrenal cortex, hormones of, 1206t, 1214–1215, *1215*
structure and function of, 1206t, 1213–1215, *1214*
failure of, in Addison's disease, 1277

Adrenal cortical hyperplasia, primary aldosteronism and, 1289–1292

Adrenal disorders, 1277–1295
diagnostic tests for, 1279t–1280t, 1281t
in elderly, 1323
Internet connections for, 1295d

Adrenal hormones, 1206t, 1214–1215, *1215*, 1216t

Adrenal medulla, 1206t, *1214*, 1215–1216
hormones of, 1206t, 1215–1216, 1216t

Adrenal suppressant drugs, for Cushing's syndrome, 1287, 1289

Adrenal tumors, Cushing's syndrome and, 1286
pheochromocytoma as, 1292–1295
primary aldosteronism and, 1289–1292

Adrenalectomy, Addison's crisis after, 1289
adrenocortical insufficiency after, 1289
for Cushing's syndrome, 1287
for pheochromocytoma, 1293
nursing care guide for, 1290c–1291c
postoperative care in, 1289

Adrenalin (epinephrine), cardiac effects of, 405t
for anaphylaxis, 418
for cardiogenic shock, 413
for Hymenoptera stings, 1621, 1622
in cardiopulmonary resuscitation, 263, 263t

Adrenocortical excess, 1285–1289. See also *Cushing's syndrome*.

Adrenocortical insufficiency, 1277–1285. See also *Addison's disease*.
in elderly, 1323
postoperative, 1289

Adrenocorticotropic hormone. See *ACTH*.

Adult day health centers, 22

Adult respiratory distress syndrome (ARDS), 686–688

Advance directives, 42–43

Advanced cardiac life support, 262. See also *Cardiopulmonary resuscitation (CPR)*.

Adventitious breath sounds, 537
in heart failure, 270–271, 277

Advil (ibuprofen), 893d

Adynamic ileus. See *Paralytic ileus*.

Afferent neurons, 711, *712*

African-Americans, asthma in, 659
cancer incidence in, 1506–1507, 1508
cyanosis in, 182
diabetes in, 1226, 1227
glucose-6-phosphatase deficiency in, 488, 488d
hypertension in, 372–373
pallor in, 182
prostate cancer in, patient teaching for, 1756d
risk factors for, 373t
sickle-cell anemia in, *484*, 484–487, 485d, 486t, 487d

Afterload, 403–404
cardiac output and, 172–173

Agammaglobulinemia, 1458

Age spots, 58, *58*

Agency for Health Care Policy and Research, Clinical Practice Guidelines of, 7–8

Age-related macular degeneration, 1985–1987, *1986*

Age-related memory impairment, 63

Ageusia, in chemotherapy, 1530
in radiation therapy, 1521

Agglutination, diagnostic, 1445
in immune response, 1439

Agglutinin, 1445

Aging. See also *Elderly*.
cognitive function and, 63
normal changes of, 49–69
coping strategies for, 50t
physiologic changes of, 51–69
cardiovascular, 64–65
cognitive, 63
endocrine, 68–69
gastrointestinal, 65–66
in body composition, 51
integumentary, 10–11, *58*
musculoskeletal, 66–67, *67*
neurologic, 67–68
pharmacokinetics and, 52–58, 53d, 54t, 55d–57d
reproductive, 68
respiratory, 65
sensory, 60–63
thermoregulatory, 59–60
urinary, 66
psychosocial aspects of, 49–51, 50t
resources for, 2038
sleep and, 63–64

Agitation, postoperative, 150

Agranulocytes, 429, *430*

Agranulocytosis, 491–493

AIDS. See *Acquired immunodeficiency syndrome (AIDS)*.

AIDS dementia complex, 1466, 1478c–1479c

Air embolism, in total parenteral nutrition, 988

Air splints, 883–884

Airway(s), artificial, 559–567. See also *Endotracheal intubation; Tracheostomy*.

Airway(s) (Continued)
in coma, 728
lower, 525, 525–526
nasopharyngeal, 559, 560
oropharyngeal, 559, 560
upper, 524, 525
Airway burns, 1657t, 1658
Airway management. See also Endotracheal intubation; Mechanical ventilation.
in amyotrophic lateral sclerosis, 777
in anesthesia, 139, 140, 140
in burns, in emergent phase, 1658–1660
in immediate phase, 1649, 1650c–1651c, 1656t
in Guillain-Barré syndrome, 774
in hypocalcemia, 1318, 1319c
in increased intracranial pressure, 734
in intermaxillary fixation, 1048, 1049d
in oral surgery, 1051
in pneumonia, 645
in respiratory acidosis, 110
in seizures, 800
in stroke, 809
in supraglottic laryngectomy, 619c–623c
in tetany, 1318, 1319c
in total laryngectomy, 629–630
in tracheostomy, 566–567, 624d–625d
in unconsciousness, 727, 728
postoperative, 145, 146t, 151
in pneumonectomy, 702c
in thyroidectomy, 1314
Airway obstruction, atelectasis and, 680, 680
in tracheostomy, 566–567, 624d–625d
Airway resistance, 528
Alanine aminotransferase, assessment of, 1161t, 1162
Albumin, 428
for portal hypertension, 1144
serum, geriatric pharmacokinetics and, 54
in hepatic disorders, 1161t, 1163–1164
transfusion of, 456. See also Transfusion(s).
Albuterol, for asthma, 661, 662t
Alcohol use/abuse, acne rosacea and, 1616, 1616
acute pancreatitis and, 1118, 1122, 1122d
as surgical risk factor, 122–123
cancer and, 1509
chronic pancreatitis and, 1122, 1124
fatty liver and, 1137
folic acid deficiency in, 479
hepatocellular carcinoma and, 1195
in diabetes, 1233
hypoglycemia and, 1250
nutritional deficiencies in, 1139t, 1153
premature atrial contractions and, 243–244, 244
premature junctional contractions and, 247
Alcoholic cirrhosis, 1180–1193, 1181t. See also Cirrhosis.
Aldactazide, 377t
Aldactone (spironolactone), 377t
for heart disease, 216, 217d, 218d
for portal hypertension, 1144, 1144d
for primary aldosteronism, 1291
Aldomet (methyldopa), 378t, 380t
Aldosterone, 1206t
deficiency of, in adrenocortical insufficiency, 1277
in blood pressure regulation, 1333

Aldosterone (Continued)
in heart failure, 270
secretion of, 1214, 1215
serum, measurement of, 1279t
urine, measurement of, 1280t
Aldosteronism, 1289–1292
Aldrete's Postanesthetic Recovery Score, 144t, 157, 157t
Alendronate (Fosamax), for osteoporosis, 905, 906d
Alienation, in cancer, 1545–1546, 1550
Alkali burns. See Chemical burns.
Alkaline phosphatase, assessment of, 1161t, 1162
in prostate cancer, 1704
Alkaline reflux gastritis, postgastrectomy, 998t
Alkalosis, metabolic, 106–108, 107t
compensated, 543
in primary aldosteronism, 1289–1291
respiratory, 111t, 111–112, 543
hypocarbia and, 530
Alkeran (melphalan), for multiple myeloma, 511
Alkylating agents, 1524, 1524t
Allergens, common, 1483t
skin tests for, 1489
Allergic conjunctivitis, 1963–1964, 1965d
Allergic contact dermatitis, 1609t, 1609–1611, 1610
Allergic rhinitis, 601, 1483–1486
antihistamines for, 575
nasal polyps and, 611, 611
Allergy(ies), 1483–1486, 1490t. See also Hypersensitivity.
anaphylaxis in, 417t, 417–418, 420. See also Anaphylaxis/anaphylactic shock.
as immediate hypersensitivity reaction, 1483–1486, 1490t
asthma and, 659, 661
desensitization for, 1448, 1485
drug, 1483t, 1612, 1612–1613, 1613t
food, 1483t
insect venom, 1483t, 1622
Internet connections for, 1498d
patch test for, 1576–1577, 1577
prevention of, 1486d
skin tests for, 1489
to contrast media, 201, 1346
transfusion-related, 457, 458, 459c–461c, 461–462, 483, 488–489, 1486
vs. hypersensitivity, 1483
Allergy tests, 1446, 1446–1447
Allerid (pseudoephedrine), for retrograde ejaculation, 1699
Allograft, skin, 1588–1590
for burns, 1673–1678, 1675, 1675t
Allopurinol (Zyloprim), for gout, 900, 900d
Alopecia, chemotherapy and, 1530, 1539t
Alpha 2, assessment of, 1161t, 1162
Alpha-adrenergic blocking agents, 213, 213d
for benign prostatic hyperplasia, 1753
Alpha-fetoprotein, in liver cancer, 1162t, 1164
in prostate cancer, 1704
Alteplase (Activase), 217, 218
for myocardial infarction, 295, 296d
Altered health maintenance, risk for. See Patient teaching.
Alternative therapies, for cancer, 1544–1545
Altitudinal hemianopia, 1940t

Aluminum carbonate gel (Basaljel), for hypoparathyroidism, 1317, 1318
Aluminum hydroxide gel (Amphojel), for hypoparathyroidism, 1317, 1318
Alveoli, 526, 526–527
Alzheimer's disease, 765–766, 790–792, 791t
Internet connections for, 779d
Amantadine (Symmetrel), for influenza, 649
Amaurosis fugax, 361
Ambulation, after stroke, 809, 812
postoperative, in hysterectomy, 1799
safety measures for, 944
Ambulatory aids, 878–881, 880
for visually impaired, 1959, 1960d
Ambulatory care nurse, 26–27
Ambulatory health care, settings for, 21–22
Ambulatory surgery, 115–116, 156t, 156–158, 157t
facilities for, 22
Amebiasis, liver abscess in, 1179
metronidazole for, 1179, 1180d
Amenorrhea, 1775
ovarian cyst and, 1825
American Association of Occupational Health Nurses (AAOHN), 28
American Nurses' Association (ANA), certification by, 5t, 6
Standards of Clinical Nursing Practice of, 6–7, 7t
American Urologic Association symptom index, 1700, 1701t
Amiloride (Midamor), 377t
Amino acids, hepatic utilization of, 1137
Aminocaproic acid, 516d
Aminoglutethimide (Cytadren), for Cushing's syndrome, 1287
Aminoglycosides, in elderly, 54t
Aminosalicylic acid, for tuberculosis, 653, 654t
Aminotransferase (AST), in heart disease, 209, 209
Ammonia, blood, in hepatic disorders, 1162t, 1164
hepatic breakdown of, 1137
Amphiarthrodial joints, 841, 842, 842t
Amphojel (aluminum hydroxide gel), for hypoparathyroidism, 1317, 1318
Amplification loop, 1440
Amputation, 868–878
clinical pathway for, 875d–876d
for osteosarcoma, 938, 939c–942c
guillotine, 872
in peripheral vascular disease, 346
levels of, 868–872, 873
neuroma formation and, 873
nursing care guide for, 939c–942c
nursing process in, 873–878, 939c–942c
phantom limb sensation in, 872
postoperative care in, 874–878, 875d–876d, 878d
preoperative care in, 873–874
prostheses for, 881–884, 882–884
stump care in, 875d–876d, 877, 878d, 879
traumatic, 930–932
Amrinone (Inocor), cardiac effects of, 405t
for cardiogenic shock, 413
for heart failure, 274
Amsler grid, 1985–1986, 1987
Amylase, pancreatic, 956, 957, 958t
in acute pancreatitis, 1118

Amylase *(Continued)*
 salivary, 951, 958t
Amyotrophic lateral sclerosis (ALS), 775–777
Anabolism, 1224t
Anal. See also under *Anorectal; Anus.*
Anal examination, 969
Anal fissure, 1073t
Anal packing, 1074
Anal sphincters, 956
Analgesia. See also *Pain; Pain management.*
 in elderly, 54t
 patient-controlled, 152, *152,* 847, 1553
 postoperative, 152–153
Analgesics, 1553, *1553*
 advantages and disadvantages of, 1554t
 narcotic, 1553, *1553,* 1554t–1555t
 for burns, 1670
 in elderly, 54t
 infusion pump for, 152, *152*
 postoperative, 152–153
 preoperative, 127–128
 routes of administration for, 1554t–1555t
 nonopioid, 1553, *1553*
 route of administration for, 1553, 1554t–1555t
Anaphylaxis/anaphylactic shock, 417t, 417–419, 420. See also *Shock.*
 case study of, 418–419
 contrast media and, 1346
 Hymenoptera stings and, 1621–1622, 1622d
 prevention of, 422d
 transfusion-related, 462
Anatomical dead space, 526, 528
Androgen, 1206t
Androgen deficiency, in adrenocortical insufficiency, 1277
Androgen deprivation, for prostate cancer, 1759
Anectine (succinylcholine), 141t
Anemia, 467–489
 aplastic, 479–482
 assessment in, 468–469
 chemotherapy and, 1531–1532, 1536t–1538t
 clinical manifestations of, 468
 definition of, 467
 diagnosis of, 468
 hemolytic, 468, 482–489
 autoimmune, 488–489, 1495–1496
 drug-associated, 1486
 Heinz body test for, 443t, 449
 transfusion reaction and, 462, 483, 488–489, 1486
 hemorrhagic, 467, 470–472, 473c–475c
 hypoproliferative, 467, 472–482
 in glucose-6-phosphatase deficiency, 488, 488d
 in radiation therapy, 1522
 in renal failure, 1400
 in thalassemia, 487–488
 iron deficiency, 470d, 472–476
 macrocytic, 468
 Schilling test for, 451
 management of, 468
 microcytic hypochromic, 468
 normocytic normochromic, 468
 nursing process in, 469–470
 of folic acid deficiency, 479
 pernicious, 476–479
 in chronic gastritis, 1025, *1025*
 Schilling test for, 451, 478

Anemia *(Continued)*
 vs. folic acid deficiency, 479
 sickle-cell, 484–487
 leg ulcers in, 437, 484, 487, 487d
 test for, 443t, 448–449
Anergy, 1489
Anesthesia, 136–142
 assessment for, 127
 general, 137–142
 complications of, 140–142
 hypothermia in, 140
 inhalation, 139, 139t
 intravenous, 140, 141t
 stages of, 137–139
 malignant hyperthermia and, 142
 preoperative medications for, 127–128
 recovery from, 143–149
 regional, 137, 138t
 topical, ocular, 1947
Anesthesiologist, 135
Aneurysm(s), 365–372
 abdominal aortic, *367,* 367–370. See also *Abdominal aortic aneurysm.*
 assessment for, 371–372
 berry, 367
 cerebral, sites of, *815*
 subarachnoid hemorrhage and, 814–816, *815*
 types of, 814, *815*
 classification of, 366, *366*
 definition of, 365
 dissecting, *366,* 366–367
 etiology of, 366–367
 false, 366, *366*
 femoral, 371–372
 fusiform, 366, *366,* 367, *371*
 location of, *367*
 nursing interventions for, 372
 pathophysiology of, 366–367
 peripheral arterial, 371
 rupture of, 367, 368d–369d, 370–371
 saccular, 366, *366,* 367
 subarachnoid hemorrhage and, 814–816, *815*
 thoracic aortic, *367,* 370–371
 true, 366, *366*
 types of, 814, *815*
Anger, in bereavement, 36–37
 in death and dying, 32
Angina, abdominal, in elderly, 1106
Angina pectoris, 175, 175t, 285–291
 assessment in, 188, 287–288
 clinical manifestations of, 286
 coronary artery bypass grafting for, *289,* 289–292, 290d, 291d
 coronary stents for, 292, *293*
 diagnosis of, 286
 drug therapy for, 286–289
 etiology of, 285–286
 in elderly, 318–319
 laser angioplasty for, 293
 management of, 286–287, 289–293
 settings and providers for, 293
 nursing diagnoses and planning in, 287–288
 nursing interventions for, 288–289
 pathophysiology of, 285–286
 percutaneous transluminal coronary angioplasty for, 292, *292*
 Prinzmetal's, 286
 stable, 286
 unstable, 286
 variant, 286
Angioblastoma, 828–832, 831t

Angiography, cardiac, 200–202, *202*
 cerebral, 750–752, *751*
 fluorescein, ocular, 1945, *1946*
 in arterial insufficiency, 339t
 in musculoskeletal disorders, 850t
 in subarachnoid hemorrhage, 815–816
 in venous insufficiency, 340t
 nursing care in, 342t
 pulmonary, 548
Angioma, 828–832, 831t
Angioplasty, 344–346, 345d
 laser, 344
 coronary artery, 293
 percutaneous transluminal, 343–344
 percutaneous transluminal coronary, *292,* 292–293
 for coronary artery disease, 292, *292*
 for myocardial infarction, 295
Angiotensin, in blood pressure regulation, 1333
 vasoconstriction and, 329t
Angiotensin II, 173
Angiotensin-converting enzyme (ACE) inhibitors, 213, 214d
 for heart failure, 275
 for myocardial infarction, 297
Angle-closure glaucoma, 1979–1982
Anisoylated plasminogen streptokinase activator complex (APSAC), for myocardial infarction, 295, 296d
Anistreplase, for myocardial infarction, 295, 296d
Ankle dorsiflexion, 747
Ankle plantar flexion, 747
Ankle sprains, 913–914
Ankylosing spondylitis, 898–899
Annular lesions, 1573
Annuloplasty, 310, *310.* See also *Cardiac valvular disease, surgery for.*
Anogenital warts, 1603–1605, 1604t, *1926,* 1926–1928
Anopia, 1940t
Anorectal. See also under *Anal; Anus.*
Anorectal abscess, 1071–1074, *1072*
Anorectal fistula, 1071, *1072,* 1073t
Anorectal infection, in gonorrhea, 1909
Anorexia, 958–959
 in chronic pancreatitis, 1123, 1124
 in elderly, in heart disease, 318–319
 in hematologic disorders, 518
 in hepatic disorders, 1139t, 1153–1154, 1154t, 1156c
 in elderly, 1166
 in HIV infection, 1470, 1472–1473, 1473d, 1477c–1478c
Anoxia, 529
Antacids, 967d, 1021d
 for acute gastritis, 1024
 for elderly, 1015
 for esophagitis, 1021d
 for hiatus hernia, 1042, 1043d
 for peptic ulcer disease, 1027–1028
 hypermagnesemia and, 101
 patient teaching for, 1043
 side effects of, 1022d, 1023
Antegrade pyelography, 1348t
Anterior cerebral artery, 716, *717*
 stenosis of, 807t
Anterior chamber, 1937, *1937*
Anterior colporrhaphy, 1818, 1819
Anterior cord syndrome, 824t
Anterior cruciate ligament injuries, 914
Anterior pelvic exenteration, 1786t
Anterior spinal artery, 716

Anterior spinothalamic tract, 722
Anterolateral thoracotomy incision, 580
Anthralin, 1580
Antiagglutination, 433, *434*
Antiagglutinin, 433
Antiandrogens, for prostate cancer, 1759
Antianxiety agents, in elderly, 54t
Antiarrhythmics, 215–216, 216d
  for myocardial infarction, 297
  in elderly, 54t
Antibiotics. See also specific drugs.
  antitumor, 1524, 1524t
  for acne, 1615t
  for Crohn's disease, 1067
  for cystitis, 1372
  for elderly, 1500
  for gonorrhea, 1909–1910, 1911t–1912t
  for *H. pylori* infection, 1028
  for infective endocarditis, 234, 235d
  for liver abscess, 1179, 1180d
  for necrotizing fasciitis, 1599
  for pneumonia, 643t, 644d
  for pressure ulcers, 1625–1626
  for prostatitis, 1734, 1735
  for pyelonephritis, 1374
  for skin infections, 1581
  for syphilis, 1912t, 1917
  nephrotoxic, 1389t
  ocular, 1947
  prophylactic, for infective endocarditis, 234
    in cardiac valvular disease, 234–235, 310, 316
    in hypertrophic cardiomyopathy, 306
    in sickle-cell anemia, 485
  topical, 1581
  vaginal candidiasis and, 1885
Antibody(ies), 428–429, 1438t, 1438–1439, *1439*. See also *Immunoglobulin(s).*
  cold, in autoimmune hemolytic anemia, 1496
  functions of, 1439
  monoclonal, 1448
  production of, 1438, 1439, *1440*
    B cells in, 1434
  structure of, 1438–1439, *1439*
  vs. interferon, 1435
  warm, in autoimmune hemolytic anemia, 1496
Antibody response, primary, 1439, *1440*
  secondary, 1439, *1440*
Antibody tests, for HIV infection, 1467
Antibody-antigen interactions, 1438, 1439, *1440*
  complement activation and, 1440t, 1440–1441
Anticholinergics, for achalasia, 1045
  for asthma, 661, 662t
  for Parkinson's disease, 787
  preoperative, 128
Anticholinesterases, for myasthenia gravis, 783, 783d
Anticipatory grieving, 34–36, 37
  in spinal cord injury, 826–827
Anticoagulants, 344d, 385t
  acquired hypoprothrombinemia and, 517
  drug interactions with, 386t
  for myocardial infarction, 297
  for peripheral vascular disease, 345t
  for pulmonary embolism, 682
  for stroke, 807
  for venous thrombosis, 385t, 385–386, 386t

Anticoagulants (*Continued*)
  for prophylaxis, 682
  in elderly, 54t
  in hemodialysis, 1404
  International Normalized Ratio for, 447–448
  postoperative, in cardiac valvular surgery, 316
    in colectomy, 1001d
  prothrombin time in, 447
  therapeutic monitoring for, 208–209
Anticoagulation factors, 432
Anticonvulsants, 796, 797d–798d
  for increased intracranial pressure, 732
Antidiabetic agents, 1239, 1239t, 1240d
  for elderly, 1261, 1323
Antidiarrheal drugs, 964, 964d
Antidiuretic hormone (ADH), 1205t
  deficiency of, in diabetes insipidus, 1274–1275, 1276d
  in fluid balance, 1333
  in heart failure, 270
  inappropriate secretion of, 83, 83t, 1277
    hyponatremia and, 91, 92
    in elderly, 1323
    in lung cancer, 696, 697, 698, 699d
  production of, 1209
Antiemetics, for chemotherapy, 1529
  preoperative, 128
Antifungal agents, for dermatophytoses, 1601
  for skin infections, 1581
  for vaginal candidiasis, 1884t, 1885
  ocular, 1947
Antigen(s), in specific immunity, 1434–1435
  prostate-specific, 1704
    in screening, 1757, 1757t
    in staging and management, 1757
Antigen-antibody interactions, 1438, 1439, *1440*
  complement activation and, 1440t, 1440–1441
Antigenic determinant, 1438
Antihemophilic factor, 456, 517d
Antihistamines, 1484c
  for allergic rhinitis, 128, 1484
  for chemotherapy-related nausea and vomiting, 1529
  for pruritus, 1582
  preoperative, 128
Antihypertensives, 375–376, 377t–380t, 379d
  diuretics as, 216, 217d, 218d
  for hypertensive crisis, 380t
  for thoracic aortic aneurysm, 371
  in elderly, 54t
  noncompliance with, 375–376, 383–384
Anti-inflammatory agents. See also *Nonsteroidal anti-inflammatory drugs (NSAIDs).*
  for asthma, 661, 662t
  in elderly, 54t
Antilipemics, 216–217, 218d, 287
Antilymphocyte globulin, for transplant immunosuppression, 1409
Antilymphocyte serum, 1448
  serum sickness and, 1487–1488
Antimetabolites, 1524, 1524t
  for skin infections, 1582
Antimicrobials. See *Antibiotics; Antifungal agents; Antiviral agents.*
Antinuclear antibodies, in systemic lupus erythematosus, 1491, 1492t

Antiplatelet agents, for peripheral vascular disease, 345t
Antipruritics, for jaundice-related pruritus, 1140, 1141d
Antiretrovirals, for HIV infection, 1468
Antithrombin, 432
Antithymocyte globulin, for transplant immunosuppression, 1409
Antithyroid antibody titer, 1300t
Antithyroid drugs, for hyperthyroidism, 1308, 1309, 1309t, 1314
Antituberculosis drugs, 653–655, 654t–655t
Antitumor antibiotics, 1524, 1524t
Antitussives, 575, 575d
Antiviral agents, for herpes simplex encephalitis, 770
  for skin infections, 1581
  ocular, 1947
Antrum, gastric, 952, *952*
Anturane (sulfinpyrazone), for gout, 900, 900d
Anuria, 1343
  definition of, 1388t
  in acute renal failure, 1389
Anus, 956. See also under *Anal; Anorectal.*
  examination of, 969
Anvil, 1996, *1996*, 1997
Anxiety, after cardiac arrest, 265c
  catecholamine hypersecretion and, 1295
  chest pain in, 175
  dyspnea and, 110–111
  hyperventilation and, 530
  in angina, 288
  in breast biopsy, 1851–1852
  in cancer, 1545, 1548
  in dysrhythmias, 255
  in genital herpes, 1907
  in leukemia, 500c–501c, 503
  in myocardial infarction, 300
  in sexually transmitted diseases, 1898c–1899c
  preoperative, 130
    in cardiac surgery, 220, 223–224
    in colostomy surgery, 1006
    in lumpectomy, 1870d–1871d
    in mastectomy, 1863–1864
  tension headache and, 800
Anxiolytics, in elderly, 54t
Aorta, *164, 167, 168*
Aortic aneurysm, abdominal, *367,* 367–370. See also *Abdominal aortic aneurysm.*
  thoracic, *367,* 370–371
Aortic occlusion, 363–365
Aortic stenosis, effort syncope in, 176
Aortic valve, *164, 167, 167, 168,* 171
Aortic valve regurgitation, 308. See also *Cardiac valvular disease.*
Aortic valve stenosis, 307–308. See also *Cardiac valvular disease.*
Aortofemoral graft, 364–365
Aortoiliac graft, *364,* 364–365
AP-1, assessment of, 1161t, 1162
Aphakia, 1970
Aphasia, 738–739
  in stroke, 814
Aphthous ulcers, 1017–1019, 1018t
Apical impulse, palpation of, 191
Aplastic anemia, 479–482
Apocrine glands, *1568,* 1569, 1569t
Appendectomy, 1065–1066, 1066d
Appendicitis, 1063–1066
  in elderly, 1106–1107
  Internet connections for, 1068d
Appetite, loss of. See *Anorexia.*

Applanation tonometry, 1944–1945, *1945*

Appliances, colostomy, *1008*, 1008–1009

Apraclonidine (Iopidine), for glaucoma, 1980

Apresoline (hydralazine), 213, 378t, 380t

APSAC, for myocardial infarction, 295, 296d

Aqueous humor, 1937, *1937*

Arachnoid, 714, *716*

Arachnoid villi, 718

Arciform lesions, 1573

Arcus senilis, 1961

ARDS (adult respiratory distress syndrome), 686–688

Arfonad (trimethaphan), 380t

Argon laser trabeculoplasty, for glaucoma, 1980

Arm, prosthetic, 882, *882, 883*

Arm casts, 854t. See also *Cast(s).*

Arm drift, 747

Arm exercises, after mastectomy, 1865–1866, 1867d, *1868*, 1868t
after pneumonectomy, 583, 586

Arousal, 726

Arrhythmia(s). See also *Dysrhythmia(s).*
sinus, 178, 242, *243*

Arterial blood gas(es), in adult respiratory distress syndrome, 686–687
in pulmonary embolism, 681–682
partial pressure of, 540

Arterial blood gas analysis, 539–544
acid-base balance and, 542–543, 544t
bicarbonate in, 540, 540t
blood specimens for, 442, 543
carbon dioxide diffusion in, 540
carbon dioxide transport in, 542–543
in metabolic acidosis, 104–105
in metabolic alkalosis, 107
in respiratory acidosis, 109
in respiratory alkalosis, 111
in shock, 407t
interpretation in, 540–543, 544t
normal values in, 540t
oxygen diffusion in, 540
oxygen transport in, 540
oxyhemoglobin dissociation curve in, 540–542, *541*
$PaCO_2$ in, 540, 540t, 542–543
PaO_2 in, 540, 540t, 541–542
parameters in, 540, 540t
pH in, 540, 540t, 543, 544t
physiologic basis of, 540t, 540–543
procedures in, 543–544
SaO_2 in, 540, 540t, 541–542
uses of, 540

Arterial blood pH, 540, 540t, 543, 544t
oxygen transport and, 542
$PaCO_2$ and, 542–543
SaO_2 and, 542

Arterial blood specimen, 442, 543

Arterial bypass grafts, 344–346
in chronic arterial occlusive disease, *364,* 364–365, *365*
postoperative care in, 347–348
preoperative care in, 346–347

Arterial dilators, 212d, 213

Arterial disorders, 351–372. See also *Peripheral vascular disease.*
assessment in, 337–339
diagnosis in, 339t, 339–340, 341c, 342t
in atherosclerosis, 361–364
in elderly, 397–398
in thromboangiitis obliterans, 351–354

Arterial disorders *(Continued)*
management of, nonsurgical, 342–344
surgical, 344–348
pain in, 332–334
skin changes in, 334t, 334–337

Arterial embolism, 357–361

Arterial puncture, 442, 543
in total parenteral nutrition, 987

Arterial thromboembolism, 357–361
in peripheral arterial aneurysm, 371, 372

Arterial ulcerations, pain in, 333–334, 334t, 335

Arteries, diameter of, blood flow and, 328
elastic recoil of, blood flow and, 328
structure and function of, 324, *324, 326*

Arteriography. See *Angiography.*

Arterioles, 324, *324, 328*
diameter of, blood flow and, 328

Arteriosclerosis. See *Atherosclerosis.*

Arteriosclerosis obliterans, 363–365

Arteriovenous anastomoses, 325

Arteriovenous fistula, for hemodialysis, 1405, *1405,* 1406

Arteriovenous graft, for hemodialysis, 1405, 1406

Arteriovenous malformation, subarachnoid hemorrhage and, 814–816, *815*

Arteriovenous shunt, for hemodialysis, 1405, *1405,* 1406

Arthritis, 890–898
degenerative, 897–898
Lyme, 901–902, 902d
post-streptococcal, 237
psoriatic, 1617
rheumatoid, 890–897. See also *Rheumatoid arthritis.*

Arthritis Foundation, 896

Arthrocentesis, 851t

Arthrodesis, for rheumatoid arthritis, 892

Arthrogram, 850t

Arthroplasty, 867–868, *868,* 869c–872c

Arthroscopy, 851t

Arthus reaction, 1488

Artificial airways, 559–567
in coma, 728

Artificial larynx, 618, *627*

Artificial limbs, 881–884, *882–884*

Artificial pacemakers, external, 259, *259*
internal, 256–259, *257, 258*

Artificial respiration, in cardiopulmonary resuscitation, 262, 264t

Asbestosis, 688, 689–691

Ascending reticular activating system, 726

Aschoff's nodules, 236–237

Ascites, 1139t, 1141–1149, 1155c–1156c
assessment in, 1145–1146
clinical manifestations of, 1143
definition of, 1142
Denver shunt for, 1145
diuretics for, 1144, 1144d
in cirrhosis, 1181–1182, 1182t, 1190c–1191c
LeVeen shunt for, 1144–1145, *1146*
low-sodium diet for, 1143d, 1144
management of, 1143d, 1144d, 1144–1145, 1145t, *1146*
nursing diagnoses and planning in, 1146–1147
nursing interventions in, 1147–1149
paracentesis for, 1144, 1145d, 1145t
pathophysiology of, 1141–1143, *1142*

Ascites *(Continued)*
sodium-restricted diet for, 1143d, 1144

Asepsis, surgical, 143

Aseptic meningitis, 769
nursing process in, 771–773

Aspartate aminotransferase, assessment of, 1160–1162, 1161t

Aspiration, bone marrow, 451, 1443–1445
fluid, for cancer diagnosis, 1513–1514
tracheopulmonary, in amyotrophic lateral sclerosis, 777
in enteral nutrition, 984
in esophageal balloon tamponade, 1187, 1191c–1192c, 1193
in myasthenia gravis, 785
in prosthetic intubation, 1055, 1058
in supraglottic laryngectomy, 618, 622c–623c, 624d–625d
postoperative, 146t
prevention of, 647
in stroke, 809

Aspiration pneumonia, 647

Aspirin, 893d, 1553, 1554t. See also *Nonsteroidal anti-inflammatory drugs (NSAIDs).*
for coronary artery disease, 284
for myocardial infarction, 295, 297
for venous thrombosis prophylaxis, 682
gastritis and, 1024
hepatotoxicity of, 1178t
in thrombosis prevention, 432d

Assessment, in nursing process, 8

Assisted suicide, 41, 42b

Assistive devices, 878–881, 884
ambulatory, 878–881, *880*
visual, 1958–1959, *1959,* 1960d

Association of Operating Room Nurses (AORN), 116, 117t

AST (aminotransferase), in heart disease, 209, *209*

Asterixis, in hepatic encephalopathy, 1150

Asthenopia, 1939

Asthma, 659–668
allergens and, 659
assessment in, 664
bronchospasm in, 659
clinical manifestations of, 660
cough variant, 660
diagnosis of, 660–661
drug therapy for, 659, 661–664, 662t–663t
drugs to be avoided in, 667t
patient teaching for, 665–667
etiology of, 659–660
exercise in, 667–668
incidence of, 659
Internet connections for, 665d
management of, *661,* 661–664
step-care approach in, 661, 662t–663t
nursing diagnoses and planning in, 664
nursing interventions in, 664–668
pathophysiology of, 659–660, *660*
peak flow meter in, 663, *663*
severity of, 659, 660
management and, 661, 662t–663t
status asthmaticus in, 660
stress management in, 665

Astigmatism, 1970–1974

Astrocytes, 712, *713*

Astrocytoma, 828–832, 831t

Atelectasis, 679–681, *680*
postoperative, 146t, 996
pulmonary contusion and, 695

Atenolol (Tenormin), 214, 377t

Atherosclerosis, 280, 360–363. See also *Coronary artery disease.*
  abdominal aortic aneurysm in, 367, 370d
  angina pectoris in, 175, 175t, 188, 285–291
  assessment in, 354, 362
  chronic arterial occlusive disease and, 363–365
  clinical manifestations of, 360–361
  etiology of, 360
  hypertension and, 338t, 373, 373t, 375
  in diabetes, 1252
  management of, 361
  nursing diagnoses and planning in, 354–355, 362
  nursing interventions in, 355, 362–363
  pathogenesis of, 360
  peripheral arterial aneurysms and, 370
  peripheral vascular disease in, 331–348. See also *Peripheral vascular disease.*
  risk reduction for, 363d
  thoracic aortic aneurysm in, 370
Atherosclerotic plaque, *282, 283*
  in myocardial infarction, 293
Athlete's foot, 1600t, 1600–1601, *1601*
Atopy. See *Allergy(ies).*
Atrial diastole, 165, *166,* 171, 191
Atrial diastolic gallop, 180
Atrial dysrhythmias, 243–247
Atrial fib-flutter, 246
Atrial fibrillation, 178, *246,* 246–247
Atrial flutter, *245,* 245–246
Atrial kick, 165, 171, 246
Atrial natriuretic hormone, 173
  in heart failure, 270
Atrial systole, 165, *166,* 171, 191
Atrial tachycardia, paroxysmal, *244,* 244–245
Atrioventricular groove, 165, 168
Atrioventricular heart block, *251–253,* 251–255
  first-degree, 251, *251*
  second-degree, 251–253, *252*
  third-degree, *253,* 253–255
Atrioventricular node, 169–171, *170*
Atrioventricular valves, *164, 167, 167, 168,* 171
Atrium, 165–167, *166*
Atrophic rhinitis, 601
Atrophic vaginitis, 1806–1807
Atrophy, of skin, 1573
Atropine, for dysrhythmias, 216, 216d
  in cardiopulmonary resuscitation, 263, 263t
Atrovent (ipratropium bromide), for asthma, 661, 662t
Audiologist, 2008–2009
Audiometric testing, 2001, 2002t
Auditory nerve, 723t
Augmentation mammoplasty, 1879
Auricle, 1995, *1996*
Auscultation, of abdomen, 968
  of chest, 191, *536,* 536–537
    for heart sounds, 191
    for lung sounds, 192, *536,* 536–537
Autoantibodies, IgG, hyperthyroidism and, 1307
  in type 1 diabetes, 1226
  production of, 1490
Autografts, cardiac valve, 313
  skin, 1588–1590
    for burns, 1673–1678, *1675,* 1675t
Autoimmune disorders, 1490–1500

Autoimmune disorders *(Continued)*
  autoimmune hemolytic anemia as, 1495–1496
  chronic fatigue syndrome as, 1496–1500
  common characteristics of, 1490
  Internet connections for, 1498d
  rheumatoid arthritis as. See *Rheumatoid arthritis.*
  scleroderma as, 1494–1495, *1495*
  systemic lupus erythematosus as, 1490–1494
Autoimmune hemolytic anemia, 1495–1496
  transfusion reaction and, 462, 483, 488–489, 1486
Autoimmunity, in type 1 diabetes, 1226
Autonomic dysreflexia, 823, 825, 826
Autonomic nervous system, anatomy and physiology of, 725–726, 726t
Autonomic neuropathy, diabetic, 1252d, 1254
Autosensitization eczema, 1608t
Autotransfusion, 453. See also *Transfusion(s).*
  in hypovolemic shock, 410
  nursing care guide for, 454c–455c
Avascular necrosis, 935
Aveeno Colloidal Oatmeal, 1583
Axillary lymph node(s), *435, 1843, 1843.* See also *Lymph nodes.*
  in breast cancer, 1858, 1860t
Axillary lymph node dissection, 1862d
  in lumpectomy, 1868–1874, 1871c–1873c
  in modified radical mastectomy, 1860–1868, 1869d
Axillobifemoral graft, *364,* 364–365
Axons, in nerve regeneration, 827, *827*
  myelinated, 712
Azathioprine, for immunosuppression, 1410, 1449
Azithromycin, for chlamydia, 1912t, 1921
Azotemia, definition of, 1388t

B
B cell(s), *429, 430,* 445t, *1432,* 1433, 1433t, 1434
  formation of, 1431, *1431*
  humoral immunity and, 1434
  in antibody production, 1438
  interaction of with T cells, 1434
Bacillus Calmette-Guérin, for bladder cancer, 1420
Bacitracin, for burns, 1674t
Back injuries, disc herniation and, 793–795, *794,* 794t
  prevention of, 795d
Back pain, 911–913
Back school, 912
Bacterial conjunctivitis, 1963–1964, *1964,* 1965d
Bacterial endocarditis, 233–236, 235d, 236d
Bacterial keratitis, 1965–1967
Bacterial meningitis, 767–769
  nursing process in, 771–773
Bacterial orchitis, 1731–1732
Bacterial prostatitis, 1733t, 1733–1735
  sequential bacteriologic localization cultures for, 1704–1705
Bacteriuria, with catheterization, 1362
Bactrim (co-trimoxazole), for prostatitis, 1734, 1735
Balance, assessment of, 2001–2002

Balance *(Continued)*
  impairment of, 1998–1999, *1999,* 1999t. See also *Dizziness; Vertigo.*
  inner ear in, 1996
  tests of, 2001–2002
Balanitis, candidal, 1885
Balanoposthitis, 1727–1728, 1729d
  paraphimosis and, 1737–1739
  phimosis and, 1735–1736
Balloon dilatation, esophageal, for achalasia, *1044,* 1045
  urethral, for benign prostatic hyperplasia, 1753
Balloon tamponade, for esophageal varices, 1186–1188, *1187,* 1191c–1192c, 1193
Balloon valvuloplasty, 311. See also *Cardiac valvular disease, surgery in.*
Band neutrophils, 445t
Bandaging. See also *Dressings.*
  for strains, 913
  in skin traction, 859–860, *860*
  stump, 875d–876d, 877, 878d, *879*
Barbiturates, for increased intracranial pressure, 732
  for seizures, 796, 797d–798d
  in anesthesia, 141t
Bargaining, in bereavement, 37
  in death and dying, 32
Barium enema, 971
Barium swallow, *970,* 970–971
Baroreceptors, 173
Barrel chest, 534, *534*
Bartholin's glands, 1766, *1766*
Bartholin's marsupialization, 1786t
Basal cell, 1567, *1568, 1568*
Basal cell epithelioma, 1636–1637, *1637,* 1638–1639
Basal ganglia, 719–720
Basaljel (aluminum carbonate gel), for hypoparathyroidism, 1317, 1318
Basic life support, in cardiac arrest, 261
Basilar artery, 714–715, *717*
Basilar skull fracture, 818, *818*
Basophils, 429, *429, 430,* 445t, *1432,* 1432–1433, 1433t
Bath oils, 1583
Baths, therapeutic, 1583
  for psoriasis, 1618, 1619
  for vaginitis, 1805–1806
Battle's sign, 818
BB, in heart disease, *209,* 209–210
Beck's triad, 317
Beclomethasone, for asthma, 661, 662t, 663t
Bed rest. See also *Immobility; Rest.*
  in disc herniation, 794–795
  in glomerulonephritis, 1376, 1377
  in heart failure, 275, 279
  in hematologic disorders, 452
  in myocardial infarction, 295–296
  in rheumatoid arthritis, 895
  in thromboembolic disease, 385, 387
  pulmonary embolism and, 681
  skin care in, 279–280
Bed sores. See *Pressure ulcers.*
Bedwetting, 1335–1336
Bee stings, 1621–1622, 1622d
Behavioral changes, in stroke, 808
Bellevue bridge, *1730,* 1730d
Bell's palsy, 829t–830t
Bence-Jones proteins, 511
Bendroflumethiazide (Naturetin), 377t
Benemid (probenecid), for gout, 900, 900d
Benign neoplasm, 1505, *1505*

Benign prostatic hyperplasia, 1752–1754
American Urologic Association symptom index for, 1700, 1701t
in elderly, 1761
prostatectomy for. See *Prostatectomy.*
prostate-specific antigen in, 1704
urinary hesitancy in, 1336
Benign senescent forgetfulness, 63
Benzathine penicillin, for syphilis, 1912t, 1917
Benzodiazepines, for seizures, 796, 797d–798d
preoperative, 128
Benzoyl peroxide, for acne, 1615t
Benzthiazide (Exna), 377t
Bereavement, 36–39. See also *Grief.*
dysfunctional grief in, 39–40
in stigmatized or violent death, 37–38
in sudden death, 38–39
stages of, 36–37
Berry aneurysm, 367
Beta blockers, 377t, 379d, 576d
for angina, 286, 287–289
for dysrhythmias, 215, 216d
for glaucoma, 1947
for heart disease, 214–215
for myocardial infarction, 297
Beta-adrenergic agonists, for asthma, 661, 662t–663t
for heart failure, 274–275
Betadine (povidone-iodine), 1581
Betapace (sotalol), for dysrhythmias, 215, 216d
Betaseron (interferon beta-16), for multiple sclerosis, 779
Bicarbonate, arterial blood, 540, 540t
fluid distribution of, 85
for ileostomy client, 1013, 1014d
in acid-base balance, 102, 102–103
Bigeminal pulse, 179, 179
Bile, 957
hepatic production of, 1137t, 1137–1138
Bile acid sequestrants, for jaundice-related pruritus, 1140, 1141d
Bile acids, oral, for gallstones, 1110–1111
Bile drainage, in cholecystectomy, 1114, 1114, 1115, 1117
discharge instructions for, 1117d
in liver transplant, 1197
Bile ducts, x-ray studies of, 972
Bile salts, 957
functions of, 1138
Bileaflet valve, 312, 313
Biliary cirrhosis, 1181t, 1181–1193. See also *Cirrhosis.*
Bilirubin, 957
measurement of, 1161t, 1163
metabolism of, 1138, 1138
assessment of, 1161t, 1163
unconjugated, 1138
urine, 1161t, 1164
Bilirubin conjugation, hepatic, 1137t, 1137–1138
Biliverdin, 1138
Billroth I procedure, 996, 996–997
for peptic ulcers, 1028
Billroth II procedure, 996, 996–997
for peptic ulcers, 1028, 1028
Bimanual examination, pelvic, 1781
Binasal hemianopia, 1940t
Biofeedback, in pain management, 1555
Biologic dressings, for burns, 1673, 1673, 1675t

Biologic response modifiers, for cancer, 1544
Biologic tissue valves, 313, 313
Biopsy, bladder, 1353–1357
bone marrow, 451, 1443–1445
breast, 1849–1852, 1850d–1851d
brush, 1353
cervical, 1783–1784, 1784, 1784d
endometrial, 1785
excision, 1578, 1578, 1579d
for cancer, 1516
liver, 1164, 1165t
lung, 552
lymph node, 451
of burns, 1672
of melanoma, 1638
penile, 1706
pleural, in tuberculosis, 652
prostate, 1705–1706, 1706, 1707t
punch, 1577–1578, 1578
renal, 1357–1358
shave, 1578, 1579d
skin, 1577–1578, 1578, 1579d
for melanoma, 1638
Bioptic telescope, 1958
Biot's breathing, 532, 533
Birth control pills. See *Oral contraceptives.*
Bishydroxycoumarin (coumarin), 385t
Bismuth subsalicylate (Pepto-Bismol), for *H. pylori* infection, 1028
Bitemporal hemianopia, 1940t
Bites, insect, hypersensitivity to, 1483t, 1621–1622, 1622d
Black eye, 1987–1989
Black lung disease, 688–691
Blackheads, 1613, 1613–1614
Bladder, biopsy of, 1353–1357
cancer of, 1419–1424
assessment in, 1422–1423
biopsy for, 1353–1357
clinical manifestations of, 1419
diagnosis of, 1419–1420
etiology of, 1419
nursing diagnoses and planning in, 1422, 1423
nursing interventions in, 1422, 1423–1424
pathogenesis of, 1419
staging of, 1420t
treatment of, 1420t, 1420–1421, 1421
catheterization of. See *Urinary catheterization.*
emptying of, 1334–1335. See also *Voiding.*
inflammation of, 1371–1373
neurogenic, 823, 825, 826
catheterization of, 1361–1363
in multiple sclerosis, 780, 781
pain in, 1341–1342
prolapse of, 1815–1819, 1816
structure and function of, 1334, 1334–1335
traumatic injuries of, 1413–1414, 1415–1416
Bladder distention, in autonomic dysreflexia, 823, 825, 826
postoperative, 154–155
Bladder drills, 1365–1366, 1366d
Bladder irrigation, 1362, 1364
in prostatectomy, 1711–1712
Bladder spasms, after prostatectomy, 1712, 1715t, 1718, 1719
Bladder training, 1365–1366, 1366d

Bleeding. See also *Hemorrhage.*
abnormal uterine, history in, 1778
anemia and, 467, 470–472
from esophageal varices, 1183–1189
balloon tamponade for, 1186–1188, 1187
drug therapy for, 1183–1186
nursing process for, 1189–1193, 1191c–1192c
sclerotherapy for, 1186
surgery for, 1188, 1189
from hemorrhoids, 1096
gastrointestinal, 964–968, 966d. See also *Gastrointestinal bleeding.*
hemothorax and, 694
in acquired hypoprothrombinemia, 517
in anticoagulation, 386
in bone marrow transplant, 1451
in disseminated intravascular coagulation, 517–518
in diverticular disease, 1082
in hematologic disorders, 436–437
in hemophilia, 516–517
in hepatic disorders, 1149
in hepatic trauma, 1194
in leukemia, 494, 504d
in peptic ulcer disease, 1029, 1029, 1030d–1031d
in polycythemia vera, 489, 490
joint, 436–437, 438, 516
nasal, 610–611
in nasal fracture, 612
postoperative, 615c
postoperative, 149
in hysterectomy, 1795
in prostatectomy, 1709t, 1712, 1713, 1716d–1717d
in tonsillectomy, 607
rectal, in colorectal cancer, 1100
under cast, 855
uterine, 1775–1776
history in, 1778
in cervical cancer, 1830
in uterine cancer, 1836
Bleeding disorders, 513–515
self-care in, 482d
Bleeding time, 443t, 448
Blepharitis, 1967, 1968t, 1970d
Blepharoplasty, 1591t
Blind spot, pathologic, 1939
physiologic, 1936, 1937
Blindness. See *Vision impairment.*
Blistering disorders, 1619–1621
Bloating, 961
Blocadren. See *Timolol.*
Blood, characteristics of, 427–428
coagulation of, 429–432, 431. See also *Coagulation.*
color of, 427
components of, 428, 428–429
cross-matching of, 434
formed elements of, 428, 429, 429
functions of, 427
hepatic filtration of, 1138
hepatic storage of, 1139
in urine, 1342–1343. See also *Hematuria.*
in vomitus, 960, 966
assessment for, 1184d–1186d
from esophageal varices, 1183, 1184d–1186d
menstrual, 1769
pH of, 428
viscosity of, 328–329, 428

Blood ammonia, in hepatic disorders, 1162t, 1164
Blood cells, formation of, 429, *430*
   nutrients for, 441d
   types of, *428, 429, 429*
Blood filtration, hepatic, 1137t, 1138
Blood flow, autoregulation of, 329
   blood viscosity and, 328
   control of, 405
     humoral, 329, 329t
     local, 329
     neural, 329
   elastic recoil and, 328
   factors affecting, 328–329
   laminar, 328
   turbulent, 328
   vessel diameter and, 328
Blood glucose monitoring, in diabetes, 1241–1242, *1242*, 1242d, 1244c–1245c
   in elderly, 1261
Blood groups, 432–433, *434*
Blood pressure. See also *Hypertension; Hypotension.*
   age-related changes in, 64–65
   diastolic, 177
   electrolytes and, 100d
   in heart disease, 177–178
   intraarterial monitoring of, 206–207
   measurement of, 190
   normal values for, 177
   regulation of, 173, 177
     renal, 1333
   systolic, 177
Blood specimens, arterial, 442, 543
   collection of, 442, 543
   venous, 442, 545
Blood studies, in heart disease, 207–210
   in hematologic disorders. See *Blood tests.*
   in musculoskeletal disorders, 851t
   in respiratory disorders, 539–545, 540t, *541*
   in urinary tract disorders, 1345–1346, 1346t
   preoperative, 125t
   reference values for, 2023–2027
   specimen collection for, 442, 543
Blood tests, 442–451, 443t, 445t–447t
   activated partial thromboplastin time, 443t, 448
   bleeding time, 443t, 448
   blood samples for, 442
   clotting factor assays, 448
   coagulation, 443t, 447t, 447–448
   complete blood count, 442–447, 443t, 1532t
   direct Coombs' test, 443t, 449, 450t
   erythrocyte fragility test, 443t, 449
   erythrocyte sedimentation rate, 443t, 449
   Heinz body test, 443t, 449
   hematocrit, 443t, 444, 1532t
   hemoglobin, 443t, 444, 1532t
   hemoglobin electrophoresis, 448
   Ivy bleeding time, 443t, 448
   leukocyte alkaline phosphatase stain, 443t, 449
   nursing process for, 450–451
   partial thromboplastin time, 443t, 448
   platelet aggregation, 443t, 447
   platelet count, 443t, 446–447, 1532t
   prothrombin time, 443t, 447–448
   red blood cell count, 443t, 444

Blood tests *(Continued)*
   red blood cell indices, 446, 446t
   reference values for, 1532t, 2023–2024
   reticulocyte count, 443t, 449
   serum folic acid, 443t, 450
   serum iron, 443t, 449–450
   sickle-cell test, 443t, 448–449
   specimen collection for, 442, 543
   stained red cell examination, 443t, 446
   total iron-binding capacity, 443t, 450
   white blood cell count, 442–444, 443t, 1532t
     differential, 443t, 444, 445t, 1532t
Blood transfusions. See *Transfusion(s).*
Blood types, 432–433
Blood urea nitrogen, drugs affecting, 1346t
   in heart disease, 208
   in urinary tract disorders, 1345, 1346
Blood vessels. See also under *Arterial; Vascular; Venous.*
   capacitance, 325
   diameter of, blood flow and, 328
   elastic recoil of, blood flow and, 328
   resistance, 328
   structure and function of, 323–328, *324–328*
Blood volume, 427
Blood-brain barrier, 717–718
Blood-forming organs, 433
   diagnostic tests for, 451–452
Blue toe syndrome, 371
Blurred vision, 1938
Body cast, 853–858, 855t. See also *Cast(s).*
   cast syndrome and, 856, 858
Body composition, age-related changes in, 51
   drug therapy and, 52–54
Body fat, 1568–1569, 1569t
   age-related changes in, 51
   liposuction of, 1591t, 1592d
Body image, after amputation, 876–877, 943
   after chest surgery, 586, 594c–595c
   after mastectomy, 1866–1867
   after oral surgery, 1052
   after orchiectomy, 1751
   after penectomy, 1747–1748
   after radical neck dissection, 636c
   after radical vulvectomy, 1829
   after total laryngectomy, 630
   in burns, 1680, 1681
   in cancer, 1545, 1549
   in elderly, 58
   in jaundice, 1141
   postoperative, 155
   with colostomy, 1010, 1105
   with ocular prosthesis, 1956–1957
   with penile implant, 1723
   with urostomy, 1424
Body preoccupation, 32
Body transcendence, 32
Body water, 75–76, *76*. See also under *Fluid.*
Body weight, age-related changes in, 51
   fluid component of, *76*
   reduction of. See *Weight loss.*
Boil, 1595–1599, 1598t, 1599d
Bone, avascular necrosis of, 935
   blood supply of, 839
   cancellous, 838, *838*
   classification of, 839
   cortical, 838, *838*

Bone *(Continued)*
   deformities of, in hematologic disorders, 438
   flat, 839
   formation of, 838–839
   infection of, 887–890
     posttraumatic, 934
   innervation of, 839
   irregular, 839
   long, 839, *840*
   metastases to, 943
   microscopic anatomy of, 837–838, *838*
   Paget's disease of, 908
   pain in, 846–847
     in hematologic disorders, 438
   remodeling of, 840
   repair of, 839–840
   short, 839
   structure and function of, 837–838, *838*
   tuberculosis of, 889–890
   types of, 837
Bone cells, 838
Bone cyst, 935–938, 936t
Bone demineralization, in hyperparathyroidism, 1320
Bone densitometry, 905
Bone grafts, for fracture nonunion, 934
Bone lesions, in multiple myeloma, 511, 512
Bone loss, age-related, 904. See also *Osteoporosis.*
   in Paget's disease, 908
Bone marrow, B cell production in, 1431, *1431*
   blood cell production in, 429, 433, 837
   hypertrophy of, in hematologic disorders, 441
   red, 839
   yellow, 839
Bone marrow aspiration and biopsy, 451, 1443–1445
Bone marrow failure, aplastic anemia and, 479–482
Bone marrow transplantation, 1449–1455
   allogeneic, 1450
   assessment in, 1451
   autologous, 1450
   complications of, 1451
   course in, 1450–1451
   for aplastic anemia, 480
   graft-versus-host disease in, 1451
   hepatic veno-occlusive disease in, 1451
   marrow harvesting in, 1450
   nursing diagnoses and planning in, 1452
   nursing interventions in, 1452–1455, 1453d, 1454d
   opportunistic infections in, 1451, 1453, 1454d
   patient preparation for, 1450
   procedure for, 1450
   self-care in, 1454d, 1454–1455
   syngeneic, 1450
   types of, 1449–1450
   uses of, 1450
Bone scan, in musculoskeletal disorders, 850t
Bone tumors, benign, 935–938, 936t
   classification of, 935
   malignant, 936t, 938–943
   metastatic, 943
Bouchard's nodes, 897
Bounding pulse, 178–179, *179*

Bowel cleansing, in hepatic encephalopathy, 1150
  preoperative. See *Bowel preparation.*
Bowel distention, in autonomic dysreflexia, 823, 825, 826
Bowel history, 961, 968
Bowel incontinence. See *Fecal incontinence.*
Bowel movements. See also *Constipation; Diarrhea.*
  after ileostomy, 1012–1013, 1014, 1014d, 1015
  in colorectal cancer, 1100
  in elderly, 1015
  in heart failure, 278
  patterns of, 961
Bowel obstruction, postoperative, 148t
Bowel preparation, for abdominal perineal resection, 1101
  for diagnostic studies, 971, 975
  for gynecologic surgery, 1787
  for intestinal resection, 1000
  for prostatectomy, 1711
  preoperative, 124, 971
Bowen's lesions, 1633t
Bowman's capsule, 1331, *1331*
Boyle's law, 527–528
Braces, 881
Brachytherapy, 1518–1519, *1519.* See also *Radiation therapy.*
  for breast cancer, *1519,* 1875
  for prostate cancer, 1758
Braden Scale, for pressure ulcers, 1626t–1627t, 1628
Bradycardia, 178
  external pacing for, 259
  sinus, 240–241, *241*
Bradykinesia, 739–740
  in Parkinson's disease, 787, *787*
Bradykinin, in shock, 407
  vasodilation and, 329t
Bradypnea, 532, *533*
Braille, 1959
Brain. See also under *Cerebral.*
  age-related changes in, 68, 765–766
  arterial blood supply of, 714–716, *717*
  circulation in, 714–715, *717*
  computed tomography of, 749
  concussion of, 819
    nursing process in, 821–822
  contusion of, 819
    nursing process in, 821–822
  hematoma of, 819–820
  magnetic resonance imaging of, 749, *750*
  positron emission tomography of, 749
  protective coverings for, 713–714, *715*
  structure and function of, *718–720,* 718–721
  venous drainage of, 716
Brain abscess, 770–773
  nursing process in, 771–773
  prevention of, in head injury, 821–822
  sinusitis and, 602
Brain death, 41, 745
  organ donation and, 46
Brain injury, closed, 818–819, *819*
  hematoma in, 819–820, *820*
    in elderly, 832
  management of, 819
    settings and providers for, 821
  nursing process in, 821–822
  penetrating, 819
  stress ulcers in, 1033
Brain stem, 720–721

Brain surgery, 757–761. See also *Intracranial surgery.*
Brain tumors, 828–832, 831t
  in increased intracranial pressure, 730, 730t
  surgery for, 757–761. See also *Intracranial surgery.*
Brainstem auditory evoked potentials, 757
Brainstem dysfunction, decerebrate posturing in, 733, *734*
BRCA-1, in breast cancer, 1857–1858
BRCA-2, in breast cancer, 1857–1858
Breast, abscess of, 1852
  after menopause, 1843
  age-related changes in, 1843, 1845, 1880
  benign tumors of, 1856–1857
  biopsy of, 1849–1852, 1850d–1851d
  development of, 1843
  fibroadenomas of, 1856
  fibrocystic disease of, 1854–1856, 1956d
  in lactation, 1842, 1845
  in menstrual cycle, 1843
  in pregnancy, 1845
  inflammation of, 1852–1853
  intraductal papilloma of, 1856–1857
  involution of, 1843
  male, enlargement of, *1853,* 1853–1854, 1880
  palpation of, 1845, *1845*
  physical examination of, *1844,* 1844–1848, *1845*
  pigeon, 534, *534*
  plastic surgery of, 1875–1880
    augmentation, 1879
    dermal mastopexy, 1880
    reconstructive, 1875–1879, *1876–1877,* 1879d
    reduction, 1879–1880
  quadrants of, 1841, *1842*
  self-examination of, *1846–1847,* 1846–1848
  structure and function of, 1841–1843, *1842, 1843*
Breast cancer, 1857–1880
  biopsy for, 1849–1852, 1850d–1851d
  chemotherapy for, 1874–1875
  clinical manifestations of, 1511t, 1858, *1859*
  diagnosis of, 1858
    breast self-examination in, *1846–1847,* 1846–1848
    diaphanography in, 1849
    mammography in, *1848,* 1848–1849
    thermography in, 1849
    ultrasonography in, 1849
    xeromammography in, 1849
  estrogen and, 1773, 1857, 1858
  etiology of, 1857–1858
  genetic factors in, 1508, 1857–1858
  hormonal therapy for, 1874
  in elderly, 1880
  incidence of, 1857
  Internet connections for, 1864d
  male, gynecomastia and, 1853
  management of, 1860–1875
    setting and providers for, 1875
  nodal metastasis in, 1858, 1860t
  ovarian cancer and, 1837
  pathophysiology of, 1857–1858
  radiation therapy for, *1519,* 1875
  risk factors for, 1511t, 1857, 1857t
  staging of, 1858, 1860t
  surgery for, 1860–1874
    in locoregional treatment, *1861*

Breast cancer *(Continued)*
  lumpectomy in, 1868–1874, 1869d–1874d
  mastectomy in, 1860–1868, *1861–1862,* 1869d. See also *Mastectomy.*
  preventive, 1869–1874
  procedures in, *1861–1862*
  reconstructive, 1875–1879, *1876–1877,* 1879d
Breast disorders, 1843–1880
  assessment in, 1843–1848
  diagnosis in, biopsy in, 1849–1852, 1850d–1851d
  diaphanography in, 1849
  mammography in, *1848,* 1848–1849
  thermography in, 1849
  ultrasonography in, 1849
  xeromammography in, 1849
  infectious and inflammatory, 1852–1853
  neoplastic. See *Breast cancer.*
  physical examination in, *1844,* 1844–1848, *1845*
  structural, 1853–1854
Breast implants, in augmentation mammoplasty, 1879
  in reconstructive surgery, *1876–1877,* 1876–1879, 1879d
  mammography of, 1848–1849
Breast prosthesis, 1866
Breast reconstruction, 1867, 1875–1879, *1876–1877*
Breast-feeding, breast changes in, 1842, 1845
  mastitis in, 1852–1853
Breath odor, 968
Breath sounds, 536–537
  adventitious, 537
  in heart failure, 270–271, 277
Breathing. See also *Respiration.*
  Biot's, 532, *533*
  diaphragmatic, 130, 553
    in chronic obstructive pulmonary disease, 676, *676*
  mechanics of, 528
  pursed-lip, 130, 553
    in chronic obstructive pulmonary disease, 676
  work of, 528
Breathing exercises, 552–553
  postoperative, 130, *130*
    after lobectomy, 589c
    after pneumonectomy, 582–583, 585–586
Bretylium, for ventricular tachycardia, 250
  in cardiopulmonary resuscitation, 263, 263t
Briggs' adapter, 555t
Broad ligaments, 1767, *1767*
Broca's aphasia, 738–739, 814
Broca's area, 719, *738*
Bromocriptine (Parlodel), for somatotropin hypersecretion, 1273
Bronchial breath sounds, 537
Bronchial toilet. See *Chest physiotherapy.*
Bronchiectasis, 679, *679.* See also *Chronic obstructive pulmonary disease (COPD).*
Bronchioles, 526, *526*
Bronchitis, acute, 639–641, 640d
  chronic, 668–669. See also *Chronic obstructive pulmonary disease (COPD).*
Bronchoalveolar carcinoma, 696
Bronchodilators, 575, 576d
  for asthma, 661, 662t–663t

Bronchodilators (Continued)
  for chronic obstructive pulmonary disease, 671, 673t
  nebulized, 675, *675*
Bronchophony, 537
Bronchoscopy, *439*, 548–550
Bronchospasm, in asthma, 659
Bronchovesicular breath sounds, 537
Bronchus, *525*, 525–526
  in asthma, 660, *660*
Brook's ileostomy, 1011
Broviac catheter, in total parenteral nutrition, 990–993
Brown-Séquard syndrome, 743, *743*, 824t
Brudzinski's sign, 768, *768*
Bruising, in fractures, 916
Brunner's glands, 956
Brush biopsy, 1353
Buck's traction, 859, *860*
Buddhism, beliefs and practices of, in death and dying, 35t
Buerger-Allen exercises, 352, 353, 353d
Buerger's disease, 351–354, 353d
  Raynaud's phenomenon and, 356
Buffer systems, 103, 104t
Bulbar conjunctiva, *1936*, 1936–1937, *1937*
Bulbourethral glands, 1697
Bullae, *1571*, 1572
Bullet wounds, cardiac, 317
  of brain, 819
  of kidney, 1411–1412
  of liver, 1194
  of spinal cord, 823
  of ureter, 1412–1413
Bullous disorders, 1619–1621
Bullous pemphigoid, 1620–1621, *1621*
Bull's-eye lesion, 1573
Bumetanide (Bumex), 377t
BUN, in heart disease, 208
Bunion, *910*, 910–911
Burn center, transfer to, criteria for, 1648–1649
Burn shock, 1660–1664, *1661*
Burns, 1643–1691
  agents of, 1648
  assessment of, 1643–1649
  associated injuries in, 1648
  biopsy of, 1672
  burn center transfer for, 1648–1649
  carbon monoxide poisoning in, 1655–1660, 1657t
  case study of, 1666d–1668d
  chemical, 1648, 1684–1687
    agents in, 1684, 1686t
    clinical manifestations of, 1685, *1687*
    decontamination measures in, 1649
    esophageal, 1047t
    incidence of, 1684–1685
    management of, 1687
    nursing interventions for, 1687
    of eye, 1649, 1687, 1989–1991, 1990t
    tissue damage in, 1684–1685
  circumferential, 1664–1665
    of chest, 1658
  clean, 1672, *1672*, 1675
  compartment syndrome and, 932–933
  contractures in, 1682–1684, 1684t
  Curling's ulcer in, 1033, 1679
  débridement of, 1672
  depth of, 1645–1648, *1647*
  disseminated intravascular coagulation in, 1666d–1668d
  diuretic phase of, 1665–1670

Burns (Continued)
  dressings for, 1671, *1671*, 1673
    biologic, 1673, *1673*, 1675t
  electrical, 1648, *1688*, 1688–1690
    first aid in, 1649
  electrolyte imbalance in, 1660–1664, *1661*, 1665–1670
  epidermal skin equivalent for, 1675
  eschar formation in, 1664
  esophageal, 1687
  family stress in, 1653c
  fluid management in, 1651c, 1654c–1655c, 1656t, 1662–1664, 1669–1670
  fluid shift in, 1665–1670
  full-thickness, *1647*, 1647–1648
  grafts for, 1587–1590, *1588, 1589, 1673,* 1673–1678, *1675*, 1675t
  healed, skin care for, 1683–1684
  healing of, 1675–1676, *1677*
  hemorrhage in, 1666d–1668d
  history in, 1644, 1656t
  hydrotherapy for, 1672–1673
  hypertrophic scarring of, 1682–1684
  hypovolemia in, 1660–1664, *1661*
  in children, 1648
  in elderly, 1648, 1690–1691
  in pregnancy, 1690
  infection of, 1671–1672, *1672*
    prevention of, 1652c–1653c, 1671, 1677
  inhalation injury in, 1657t, 1658
  Internet connections for, 1682d
  location of, 1645
  management of, 1649–1691
    acute-phase, 1665–1681
    airway management in, 1649, 1650c–1651c, 1656t
    emergent-phase, 1655–1665
    immediate-phase, 1649–1655, 1656t
    respiratory dysfunction in, 1655–1660
    stopping burning process in, 1649, 1656t
    treatment of life-threatening injuries in, 1649–1655
  medical history and, 1648
  metabolic needs in, 1678–1680
  nursing care guide for, 1650c–1655c
  nutrition in, 1678–1680
  pain in, 1651c–1652c, 1670–1671
  paralytic ileus in, 1679
  partial-thickness, 1647, *1647*
  patient age and, 1648
  physical therapy for, 1682, 1684t
  pressure garments for, 1682, *1683*, 1684, 1685d
  psychosocial needs in, 1680–1681
  rehabilitation in, 1681–1684
  respiratory dysfunction in, assessment of, 1658–1659, 1664
    management of, 1659–1660, 1664–1665
  restrictive lung disease and, 1658, 1664–1665
  self-care in, 1683–1684, 1685d
  severity of, 1644–1648
  size of, *1644*, 1645, *1646*
  stress ulcers in, 1033
  superficial, 1646–1647, *1647*
  tetanus prophylaxis for, 1673
  thermal, 1648
  topical agents for, 1673, 1674t
  urine output in, 1669–1670
  wound care in, 1652c–1653c, 1671–1678
    assessment in, 1675–1676

Burns (Continued)
  nursing diagnoses and planning in, 1676–1677
  nursing interventions in, 1677–1678
  open vs. closed methods of, 1671t
  patient teaching for, 1684, 1685d
Burping, 961
Bursitis, 902
Butaconazole, for vaginal candidiasis, 1884t, 1885
Butterfly rash, in systemic lupus erythematosus, 1491, *1491*, 1492t

C

C (parafollicular) cells, 1211, 1212
Cachexia, cancer, 1559
Caffeine, fibrocystic breast disease and, 1854, 1855
  palpitations and, 176–177
  premature atrial contractions and, 243–244, *244*
  premature junctional contractions and, 247
Caged-ball valve, 312, *312*
Calan (verapamil), 213, 215d, 378t
  for dysrhythmias, 215, 216d
  for heart disease, 213, 215d
  for hypertrophic cardiomyopathy, 306
Calcitonin, 1212
  assays of, 1300t
  for Paget's disease, 908
  parathyroid hormone and, 1213
Calcium, cardiac function and, 208
  deficiency of. See *Hypocalcemia.*
  dietary, daily requirement for, 95
    sources of, 904d, 1367d
    urinary calculi and, 1367, 1367d, 1379
  excess of. See *Hypercalcemia.*
  fluid distribution of, *85*
  ionized, 95
  magnesium and, 95
  normal values for, 95
  parathyroid hormone and, 1213
  phosphorus and, 95, 1213
  renal metabolism of, 1333
  supplemental, 96, 97, 903d
    for elderly women, 67
    for hypoparathyroidism, 1317
    for osteoporosis, 905
    in osteomalacia, 903, 903d, 904
    intravenous, 97
  vitamin D and, 1213
Calcium channel blockers, 213–214, 215d
  for angina, 286–289
  in elderly, 54t
Calcium chloride, for hypocalcemia, 96, 97
Calcium gluconate, for hypocalcemia, 96, 97
Calcium imbalances. See *Hypercalcemia; Hypocalcemia.*
Calcium oxalate calculi. See *Urinary calculi.*
Calcium phosphate calculi. See *Urinary calculi.*
Calcium score, 200
Calculi, biliary. See *Gallstones.*
  diet and, 1383t
  urinary. See *Urinary calculi.*
Callus, bone, 839
Caloric test, 2002
Campylobacter jejuni, Guillain-Barré syndrome and, 773
Canal of Schlemm, 1937, *1937*

Canaliculi, bile, 1136, *1136*
Cancellous bone, 838, *838*
Cancer, 1503–1562. See also specific sites and types.
　anaplastic cells in, 1505, *1506*
　anxiety in, 1545, 1548
　bladder, 1419–1424
　　biopsy for, 1353–1357
　body imaging in, 1545, 1549
　bone, 936t, 938–943
　bone metastases in, 943
　brain, 828–832, 831t
　cachexia in, 1559
　carcinoma, 1505
　cardiac, 317–318
　cell cycle and, 1503–1504, *1504*
　cervical, 1829–1836
　chemicals and, 1508–1509
　chemotherapy for, 1523–1534. See also *Chemotherapy.*
　classification of, 1505
　clinical manifestations of, 1511t
　colorectal, 1100–1106, *1101*
　complications in, 1551–1562
　cultural factors in, 1506–1508, 1509, 1551
　diagnosis of, 1512–1516
　　biopsy in, 1516
　　blood tests in, 1513
　　cytologic tests in, 1513–1514
　　imaging studies in, 1514–1515
　　radiography in, 1514–1515
　　stool tests in, 1513
　endometrial, 1836–1837
　　in elderly, 1838
　environmental factors in, 1508–1510
　esophageal, 1053–1058
　etiology of, 1508–1511
　family stress in, 1546, 1550–1551
　gastric, 1058–1059
　　gastrectomy for, *996*, 996–1000
　gender and, 1506, *1507*
　genetic factors in, 1508
　geographic factors in, 1508
　gynecologic, 1825–1838
　　in elderly, 1838
　helplessness in, 1545, 1549–1550
　hematologic, 493–1512
　hepatic, 1195–1196
　　alpha-fetoprotein in, 1162t, 1164
　　portal hypertension in, 1141–1149
　home care in, 1561
　hospice care in, 1561
　immunologic defects and, 1510
　immunologic surveillance theory and, 1499
　immunotherapy for, 1510, 1534–1546
　in elderly, 1499, 1561–1562
　incidence of, 1503, 1506–1508, *1507*
　Internet connections for, 1547d
　isolation in, 1545–1546, 1550
　laryngeal, 616–637
　loss in, 1545, 1549–1550
　lung, 695–698, 699d, 700c–707c
　management of, settings and providers for, 1560–1561
　mediastinal, 698
　metastasis in, 943, 1505–1506
　monoclonal antibodies for, 1448
　newly diagnosed, nursing care in, 1515–1516
　nutrition in, 1558–1560, 1560d
　occupational factors in, 1508–1509
　ocular, 1991

Cancer *(Continued)*
　of renal pelvis, 1418–1419
　oral, 1049–1053
　ovarian, 1837–1838
　　in elderly, 1838
　pain in, 1551–1558
　　assessment in, 1556
　　body surface sites of, *1552*
　　home care for, 1561
　　management of, 1552–1556, *1557.* See also *Pain management.*
　　nursing diagnoses and planning in, 1556–1557
　　nursing interventions in, 1557–1558
　　palliative treatment for, surgical, 1516
　pancreatic, 1126–1131
　　Internet connections for, 1113d
　pathophysiology of, 1505–1506
　penile, 1744–1748, 1745t
　powerlessness in, 1545, 1549–1550
　prevention of, surgery for, 1516
　prostate, 1754–1761
　psychosocial factors in, 1510–1511
　psychosocial problems in, 1545–1551
　　assessment of, 1546
　　nursing diagnoses and planning in, 1546–1548
　　nursing interventions in, 1548–1551
　race and, 1506–1508
　radiation therapy for, 1517–1523. See also *Radiation therapy.*
　renal cell, 1416–1418
　resources for, 2041–2042
　risk factors for, 1509–1510, 1511t
　risk reduction for, 1512d
　sarcoma, 1505
　screening for, 1511–1512, 1512d
　self-concept disturbance in, 1545, 1549
　seven warning signs of, 1511
　sexual dysfunction in, 1545, 1549
　skin, 1636–1639
　sociocultural factors in, 1506–1508
　solid tumors in, 1505
　spread of, 1505–1506
　staging of, 1513
　　surgery for, 1516
　surgery for, 1516–1517
　syndrome of inappropriate antidiuretic hormone in, 697
　testicular, 1748–1752
　　cryptorchidism and, 1739
　　human chorionic gonadotropin in, 1704
　toxins and, 1508–1509
　tumor doubling time in, 1505–1506
　unconventional therapies for, 1544–1545
　ureteral, 1418–1419
　urethral, 1424–1425
　uterine, 1836–1837
　　in elderly, 1838
　viral infections and, 1510
　vulvar, 1825–1830
Cancer nursing, resources for, 2042
Candidiasis, cutaneous, *1602*, 1602–1603
　oral, 1017–1019, 1019t, 1602
　　in HIV infection, 1465
　vaginal, 1804–1806, 1805t, 1884t, 1884–1885
　　in HIV infection, 1467
　　nursing care in, 1886–1889
　　patient teaching in, 1901d
Canes, 880
　for blind, 1959
Canker sores, 1017–1019, 1018t

Cantharidin, for warts, 1604–1605
Cantor tube, *977*, 978
Capillaries, 324, 325, *328*
　diameter of, blood flow and, 328
　elastic recoil of, blood flow and, 328
　lymphatic, 329–331, *330, 331,* 1431
Capillary hemangioma, 1571
Capillary refill, abnormal, in heart disease, 181
Capitance vessels, 325
Capreomycin, for tuberculosis, 653, 654t
Capsule of Glisson, 1135
Captopril (Capoten), 213, 214d, 378t
Carafate (sucralfate), 1022d
　for peptic ulcers, 1028
Carbamazepine, for seizures, 796, 797d–798d
Carbohydrate deficiency, clinical manifestations of, 1077t
Carbohydrate metabolism, hepatic, 1136–1137, 1137t
　in diabetics vs. nondiabetics, *1225*
　in hepatic disorders, 1162t
　insulin in, 1223–1224
Carbon dioxide, arterial, decreased, 530
　increased, 530
　arterial blood pH and, 542, 543, 544t
　oxygen transport and, 542
　partial pressure of, 540, 540t
　transport of, 542–543
Carbon dioxide diffusion, 540, 540t
Carbon dioxide laser. See *Laser surgery.*
Carbon dioxide narcosis, 108–109
　in emphysema, 670–671
Carbon monoxide poisoning, 1655–1660, 1657t
Carbonic acid, in acid-base balance, *102,* 102–103
Carbonic anhydrase inhibitors, for glaucoma, 1947, 1979–1980
Carbuncle, 1595–1599, 1598t, 1599d
Carcinogens, alcohol as, 1509
　chemical, 1508–1509
　dietary, 1509–1510
　radiation as, 1510
　tobacco as, 1509
　viruses as, 1510
Carcinoma, 1505
Cardene (nicardipine), 213, 215d
Cardia, 952, *952*
Cardiac. See also under *Cardiovascular; Heart.*
Cardiac angiography, 200–202, *202*
Cardiac arrest, 261–264, 263t
　cardiopulmonary resuscitation in, 261–263, 262t–264t
　drugs for, 263t
　family needs in, 263–264
　survival in, nursing care guide for, 265c–268c
Cardiac catheterization, 200–202, *201,* 201t
　angiography in, 200–202, *201*
　complications of, 201–202, 205d
　discharge instructions for, 201d, 205d
　indications for, 200
　left-sided, 200
　nursing care guide for, 203c–205c
　patient preparation for, 201, 203d–204d
　postprocedure care for, 201d, 201–202, 204d–205d
　right-sided, 200
Cardiac cell, depolarization and repolarization of, 169, *170,* 171
Cardiac circulation, 163, 165–167, *166*

Cardiac cirrhosis, 1198
Cardiac compression, in cardiopulmonary resuscitation, 262, 264t
Cardiac conduction system, 169–171, 170
surgery of, 261
Cardiac contractility, 172, 404
Cardiac cough, 174, 270
Cardiac cycle, 171
heart sounds and, 179–181, 180
Cardiac dysfunction. See *Heart disease.*
Cardiac dysrhythmias. See *Dysrhythmia(s).*
Cardiac enzymes, 209, 209
in myocardial infarction, 294
Cardiac function, 163–231
age-related changes in, 64–65
anatomic aspects of, 163–173
as surgical risk factor, 121
electrolytes and, 208
in chronic obstructive pulmonary disease, 668, 669t
in elderly, 230–231
in hypercalcemia, 97, 98–99
in hypermagnesemia, 100
in hypomagnesemia, 100
in metabolic acidosis, 104, 106
in surgical patient, 121
postoperative, monitoring of, 145–149
post-transplant, 228–229
Cardiac glycosides, 211d, 211–212
Cardiac index, 402, 402t
in cardiogenic shock, 413
Cardiac isoenzymes, 209, 209–210, 210
Cardiac life support. See also *Cardiopulmonary resuscitation (CPR).*
advanced, 262
basic, 261
Cardiac output, 402, 402t
afterload and, 403, 403–404
contractility and, 404
decreased, after cardiac arrest, 265c–266c, 267c–268c
after cardiac surgery, 222
after cardiac valvular surgery, 314, 315
fatigue and, 182
hyperkalemia and, 89, 90
hypokalemia and, 86, 88
in dysrhythmias, 255
in heart failure, 268, 271, 278
in hyperkalemia, 90
in hypokalemia, 88
in metabolic acidosis, 106
in myocardial infarction, 302
in respiratory acidosis, 110
in shock, 406, 407, 408, 420, 421
monitoring of, 207
normal values for, 172
oxygen transport and, 542
regulation of, 172, 172
definition of, 172
determinants of, 402–403, 403
drug effects on, 405t
heart rate and, 402–403, 403
in anesthesia, 140–141
normal values for, 402t
oxygen delivery and, 405
preload and, 403, 403
stroke volume and, 402, 403
Cardiac rehabilitation, 229–230, 289
Cardiac septum, 165, 166
Cardiac surgery, 217–229
cardiopulmonary bypass, 220–221, 221
complications of, 222, 222t
conduction system, 261

Cardiac surgery (*Continued*)
coronary artery bypass grafting, 289, 289–292, 290d, 291d, 295
for heart failure, 275
indications for, 218–219
intra-aortic balloon counterpulsation, 229
nursing care in, postoperative, 225–227
preoperative, 222–225, 224t
postoperative management in, 221–222, 225–227
preoperative preparation for, 219–220, 222–225
rehabilitation after, 229–230
technique of, 219
temporary pacing in, 258–259
transplant, 227–229, 228
types of, 219t
valve-replacement, 234
valvular, 234, 310, 310–313, 312–314. See also *Cardiac valvular disease, surgery in.*
Cardiac tamponade, 317
in pericardial effusion, 239, 240
Cardiac transplantation, 227–229, 228
Cardiac trauma, 316–317
Cardiac tumors, 317–318
Cardiac valves, 164, 167, 167, 168, 171
disorders of, murmurs in, 181
heart sounds and, 179–181, 180
Cardiac valvular disease, 306–317
antibiotic prophylaxis in, 234–235, 310
aortic stenosis in, 307–308
aortic valve regurgitation in, 308
care settings and providers for, 313–314
classification of, 306–307
infective endocarditis and, 233–236
mitral valve prolapse in, 309–310
mitral valve regurgitation in, 309
mitral valve stenosis in, 308–309
mixed, 307
regurgitation in, 307, 307
rheumatic, 236–237. See also *Rheumatic heart disease.*
stenosis in, 306–307, 307
surgery in, 234, 310–317
care settings and providers for, 313–314, 316–317
postoperative care in, 313–317
valve replacement, 234, 311–317, 312t, 312–314
valvuloplasty in, 310, 310–311
Cardinal ligaments, 1767, 1767
Cardiogenic pulmonary edema, 270, 280, 281d–282d
Cardiogenic shock, 411, 411–413, 412t, 419–420. See also *Shock.*
Cardiomyopathy, 303–306
causes of, 303
dilated, 303–305, 304
hypertrophic, 304, 305–306
idiopathic, 303
nonsurgical management of, 306
obliterative, 306
restrictive, 304, 306
transplant for, 227–229, 228
Cardiopulmonary bypass, 220–221, 221
complications of, 222, 222t
postoperative care in, 221–222, 225–227, 226t
Cardiopulmonary resuscitation (CPR), ABCs of, 262, 264t
crash cart for, 262, 262t

Cardiopulmonary resuscitation (CPR) (*Continued*)
Do Not Resuscitate (DNR) orders and, 43–46, 45
drugs for, 263t
duration of, 263
equipment for, 262t
family needs in, 263–264
in cardiac arrest, 261–264, 262t–264t
Cardiotoxicity, of chemotherapy, 1532, 1535t
Cardiovascular assessment, 187–192
Cardiovascular disorders, in chronic renal failure, 1399t
resources for, 2038
Cardiovascular function, age-related changes in, 64–65, 230–231
as surgical risk factor, 121
in anesthesia, 140–141
in hypertension, 374, 374–375
in hyponatremia, 91
in surgical patient, 121
regulation of, 172–173
Cardioversion, 259–260, 261d
Cardioverter-defibrillator, implanted, 260, 261d
Cardizem (diltiazem), 378t
for dysrhythmias, 215, 216d
for heart disease, 213, 215d
Carotid artery, 714–715, 716
Doppler studies of, 749–750, 751
Carotid artery hemorrhage, in radical neck dissection, 634c–635c
Carotid artery stenosis, 751
Carotid endarterectomy, for stroke, 808
Carotid massage, 176
Carotid pulse, 178
palpation of, 178
Carotid sinus pressure, for paroxysmal atrial tachycardia, 245
Carpal tunnel syndrome, 909, 909–910
Raynaud's phenomenon and, 356
Cartilage, 842–843
knee, tears of, 914
Case management, 21
Cast(s), 853–858
application of, 853
compartment syndrome and, 857, 932–933
complications of, 853–857
discharge instructions for, 857d, 858
drainage in, 856
nursing interventions for, 856–858, 919–924, 920c–923c
removal of, 853
types of, 854t–855t
Cast cutter, 853
Cast syndrome, 856, 858
Catabolism, 1224t
Catapres (clonidine), 378t
Cataract glasses, 1976
Cataracts, 60, 1975, 1975–1978, 1976
Catecholamines, endogenous, adrenal secretion of, 1215–1216, 1216
hypersecretion of, from pheochromocytoma, 1292
urinary, assays of, 1292, 1293t
exogenous, for heart disease, 214
Cathartics, after upper GI series, 970, 971
Catheter(s), Broviac, in total parenteral nutrition, 990–993
chemotherapy, 1527, 1527
femoral vein, for hemodialysis, 1405, 1406

Catheter(s) *(Continued)*
  Hickman, in total parenteral nutrition, 993
  in peritoneal dialysis, 1401–1402, *1402*
    care of, 1404d
    obstruction of, 1404
  peripherally inserted central, in total parenteral nutrition, 987
  subclavian vein, for hemodialysis, 1405, 1406
  urinary, 1361
  ventricular, in intracranial pressure monitoring, 731, *731*
Catheter infection, in total parenteral nutrition, 987
  prevention of, 989
Catheterization, cardiac, 200–202, *201,* 201t
  nursing care guide for, 203c–205c
  for meatal stenosis, 1386
  in total parenteral nutrition, 987, 989
    in home care, 990–993
  in transtracheal oxygen administration, 557, 557–558, 558d
  pulmonary artery, 403, *404*
  urinary. See *Urinary catheterization.*
Cauda equina, 722
Cauda equina lesion, sensory impairment in, *743*
Caudal block, 137, 138t. See also *Anesthesia.*
Caustics, ingestion of, 1687
Cavitary malignant abscess, of lung, 647
Cavitation, tubercular, 650, *650*
CD4+ cells, in HIV infection
  in acute retroviral stage, 1465t
  in advanced stage, 1465t, 1467
  in asymptomatic stage, 1465, 1465t
  in diagnosis, 1467, 1468t
  in symptomatic stage, 1465t, 1465–1466
Cecum, structure and function of, 956
Cefixime, for gonorrhea, 1909–1910, 1911t, 1914
Cefotetan, for gonorrhea, 1909–1910, 1911t, 1914
Cefoxitin, for gonorrhea, 1909–1910, 1911t, 1914
Ceftriaxone, for gonorrhea, 1909–1910, 1911t, 1914
Celestin tube, 1055
Celiac sprue, *1078,* 1078–1079
  malabsorption in, 1077t, 1077–1078
Cell(s), cancer, 1505–1506, *1506*
  structure of, 1503, *1504*
Cell cycle, 1503–1504, *1504*
Cell-mediated (Type IV) hypersensitivity reaction, 1489–1490, 1490t
Cellular immunity, 1433–1434, 1434t, 1439
Cellulitis, 1595–1599, *1596,* 1598t, 1599d
Central cord lesions, sensory impairment in, *743*
Central cord syndrome, 824t
Central line, in total parenteral nutrition, 987
  care of, 989, *990*
  infection of, 987, 989
Central nervous system, anatomy and physiology of, 718–722, *718–722*
  gray matter of, 712
  white matter of, 712
Central venous catheter, for chemotherapy, 1527, *1527*
Central venous pressure, 402t, 403

Central venous pressure monitoring, 202
  for cardiac output, 207
Cephalosporins, for gonorrhea, 1909–1910, 1911t, 1912t, 1914
Cerebellar ataxia, in multiple sclerosis, 780
Cerebellum, 721
Cerebral aneurysms, sites of, *815*
  subarachnoid hemorrhage and, 814–816, *815*
  types of, 814, *815*
Cerebral angiography, 750–752, *751*
Cerebral arteries, 716, *717*
Cerebral circulation, 714–715, *717*
Cerebral concussion, 819
  management of, setting and providers for, 821
  nursing process in, 821–822
Cerebral contusion, 819
  nursing process in, 821–822
Cerebral cortex, motor, 719, *720*
  sensory, 719, *720*
Cerebral death, 41, 745
  organ donation and, 46
Cerebral edema, 82
Cerebral function, age-related changes in, 68
Cerebral hematoma, 819–820, 821
Cerebral hemispheres, 718, 719, *719, 720*
Cerebral hemorrhage, cerebrovascular accident and, 804, *805.* See also *Cerebrovascular accident (CVA).*
  subarachnoid, 814–816, *815*
Cerebral hypoxia, 530
  in carbon monoxide poisoning, 1656
Cerebral perfusion pressure, 731
Cerebral venous sinuses, 716
Cerebrospinal fluid (CSF), 718
  analysis of, 754t
    in bacterial meningitis, 769
    in brain abscess, 771
    specimen collection for, 753–754, 755c–756c, 757
  circulation of, *717,* 718
  drainage of, from ear, 1998, 2000
    in increased intracranial pressure, 733
    ventricular shunt for, 802–804, *803*
  formation of, 718
  in increased intracranial pressure, 730, 730t
  postoperative leakage of, in brain surgery, 761
  in spinal surgery, 762
  reference values for, 2030
Cerebrovascular accident (CVA), 804–814
  Alzheimer's disease and, 790, 791d, 792
  assessment in, 808
  behavioral changes in, 808
  case study of, 810d–812d
  classification of, 806t
  clinical manifestations of, 806–807, *807,* 807t
  completed, 806t
  diagnosis of, 807
  embolic, 804, *805*
  etiology of, 804–805
  gastrointestinal bleeding in, 966d
  hemorrhagic, 805, *805*
  in elderly, 832
  language impairment in, 807t, 808, 814
  management of, 807–808
  motor impairment in, 808, 809–813
  nursing diagnoses and planning in, 808–809
  nursing interventions in, 809–814

Cerebrovascular accident (CVA) *(Continued)*
  pathophysiology of, 804–805
  progressive, 806t
  reversible ischemic neurologic deficit and, 806t
  right vs. left hemispheric involvement in, 807, *807*
  risk factors for, 805–806, 806d
  sensory impairment in, 808, 813
  thrombotic, 804
  transient ischemic attack and, 806t
  unilateral neglect in, 813
Cerebrum, 718, *719*
Certification, 5–6, 6t
  in medical-surgical nursing, 5t, 5–6
Certified registered nurse anesthetist, 135
Cervical biopsy, 1783–1784, *1784,* 1784d
Cervical cancer, 1830–1836
  adenocarcinoma, 1830
  chemotherapy for, 1836
  clinical manifestations of, 1511t, 1830
  diagnosis of, 1831
  etiology of, 1830
  genital herpes and, 1903
  in HIV infection, 1467
  management of, 1831–1836
  metastasis in, 1830
  Papanicolaou test for, 1513, 1779d, 1781–1782, *1783,* 1831
  pathophysiology of, 1830
  pelvic exenteration for, 1831–1832
  radiation therapy for, 1832–1836
  risk factors for, 1511t
  squamous cell, 1830
Cervical conization, for cancer, 1831
Cervical dysplasia, cryosurgery for, 1790–1791
  electrocautery for, 1791
  in HIV infection, 1467
Cervical intraepithelial neoplasia, 1830
Cervical laminectomy, 761–765, 763d. See also *Spinal surgery.*
Cervical lymph nodes, *435.* See also *Lymph nodes.*
  removal of, in radical neck dissection, 631–637, 634c–637c
Cervical mucus, ferning of, 1768, *1769*
Cervical polyps, 1822–1823
Cervical spine, 715. See also under *Spinal; Spine.*
  disc herniation in, 792–795, *793,* 793t, 794d
  injury of, 822–827. See also *Spinal cord injury.*
  traction of, 824, 826, 861, *861.* See also *Traction.*
Cervical tongs, 824
Cervicitis, chlamydial, 1920, 1921. See also *Chlamydia trachomatis infection.*
  discharge in, 1776
  gonococcal, 1909. See also *Gonorrhea.*
  herpetic, 1902
Cervix, speculum examination of, 1780, *1780*
  structure and function of, 1766, *1766*
Chalazion, 1968t, 1970d
Chancre, in syphilis, 1915, *1915*
Chemical burns, 1648, 1684–1687. See also *Burns.*
  agents in, 1684, 1686t
  clinical manifestations of, 1685, *1687*
  esophageal, 1047t
  incidence of, 1684–1685

Chemical burns (Continued)
  management of, 1687
  nursing interventions for, 1687
  of eye, 1649, 1687, 1989–1991, 1990t
  tissue damage in, 1684–1685
Chemical carcinogenesis, 1508–1509
Chemoreceptor trigger zone, 960
Chemotactic factors, 1436
Chemotherapy, 1420, 1421
  adjuvant, 1874
  assessment in, 1532, 1535t–1543t
  cardiotoxicity of, 1532, 1535t
  case study of, 1533d–1534d
  catheters for, 1527, 1527
  combination, 1525, 1525t
  continuous infusion, 1527
  delivery of, 1527, 1527, 1528
  dosage of, 1525, 1526
  drugs for, classification of, 1524t, 1524–
    1525
  for brain tumors, 830
  for breast cancer, 1874–1875
  for cervical cancer, 1836
  for hematologic disorders, 464
  for hepatic cancer, 1195
  for Hodgkin's disease, 505
  for leukemia, 494t, 495
  for lung cancer, 696–697
  for multiple myeloma, 511
  for non-Hodgkin's lymphoma, 508, 508t
  for ovarian cancer, 1837–1838
  for pancreatic cancer, 1128
  for polycythemia vera, 489–491
  for prostate cancer, 1759
  for testicular cancer, 1749
  for uterine cancer, 1836
  gastrointestinal toxicity of, 1528–1530,
    1540t–1542t
  hematologic toxicity of, 1531–1532,
    1536t–1538t
  home administration of, 1561
  implanted ports for, 1527, 1527, 1528
  infusion pump for, 1195, 1527, 1528
  intravesical, 1365
    for bladder cancer, 1420
  neurotoxicity of, 1532, 1536t
  neutropenia in, 1437
  nursing diagnoses and planning in,
    1532–1534, 1535t–1543t
  nursing interventions in, 1534, 1535t–
    1543t
  principles of, 1523–1524
  pulmonary toxicity of, 1532, 1535t
  renal toxicity of, 1532, 1543t
  safety precautions for, 1528, 1528t
  sexual dysfunction and, 1538t–1539t
  side effects of, 1528–1532, 1535t–1543t
  skin toxicity of, 1530–1531, 1539t–1540t
  tissue extravasation and, 1531
  treatment schedules for, 1525–1527
Chenodeoxycholic acid, for gallstones,
  1110–1111
Chenodiol, for gallstones, 1110–1111
Cherry hemangioma, 1632t
Chest. See also under Thoracic; Thorax.
  anatomic landmarks of, 181, 190–191
  auscultation of, 191, 536, 536–537
  barrel, 534, 534
  burns of, restrictive lung disease and,
    1658, 1664–1665
  drainage of, 575–580. See also Chest tube
    drainage.
  excursion of, 535
  funnel, 534, 534

Chest (Continued)
  lines of, 533
  palpation of, 181, 190–191, 534–535
  percussion of, diagnostic, 192, 535, 535–
    536, 536
    therapeutic, 553–555
  pigeon, 534, 534
Chest compression, in cardiopulmonary
    resuscitation, 262, 264t
  postoperative, 585–586
Chest films, 547, 547–548
  for lung cancer, 1514
  in cardiac assessment, 192–193
  in emphysema, 671
  in tuberculosis, 652
  portable, 193
  preoperative, 126t
Chest pain, after cardiac arrest, 266c–267c
  assessment of, 188
  cardiac, 175, 175t, 188, 285–289. See also
    Angina pectoris.
  in infective endocarditis, 235–236
  in myocardial infarction, 294, 295, 296,
    300
  in pericarditis, 238, 239
  in pleuritis, 658
  noncardiac, 175
Chest physiotherapy, 552–556, 587
  after lobectomy, 589c
  after pneumonectomy, 582–583, 585–586
  breathing exercises in, 130, 552–553
  in chronic obstructive pulmonary dis-
    ease, 672, 675–676
  in mechanical ventilation, 571
  in unconscious client, 728
  percussion in, 553–555
  postural drainage in, 553, 554
  vibration in, 555–556
Chest trauma, 690–695
  flail chest in, 691, 691–692
  hemothorax in, 694
  pneumothorax in, 692–693, 693, 694
  pulmonary contusion in, 695
  rib fractures in, 690–691
  subcutaneous emphysema in, 695
Chest tube drainage, 575–580
  assessment in, 577–578
  equipment for, 576–577, 577d
  extubation in, 579
    accidental, 578–579
  for empyema, 658
  for hemothorax, 694
  for pneumothorax, 694
  Heimlich valve in, 579–580
  indications for, 575
  nursing diagnoses and planning in, 578
  nursing guide for, 590c
  nursing interventions in, 578–579
  pneumothorax in, 577, 578, 579
  postoperative, 580
    in cardiac surgery, 222, 225
    in lobectomy, 590c
  water-seal system in, 576–577, 577
Chest wall, abnormalities of, 534, 534
  inspection of, 534, 534
Cheyne-Stokes respirations, 532, 533, 730
Chief cells, 952
Children, burns in, 1648
  second-hand smoke effects on, 1509
Chlamydia trachomatis infection, 1920–1924
  assessment in, 1922–1923
  cervicitis and, 1920, 1921
  clinical manifestations of, 1921
  diagnosis of, 1921

Chlamydia trachomatis infection (Continued)
  epididymitis in, 1728–1730
  etiology of, 1921
  in pregnancy, 1920
  incidence of, 1920
  management of, 1921
  nongonococcal urethritis and, 1920,
    1921, 1924–1925
  nursing diagnoses and planning in, 1923
  nursing interventions in, 1922–1924
  ocular, 1920
  pathophysiology of, 1921
  pelvic inflammatory disease and, 1920,
    1921, 1923–1924
  risk factors for, 1921
  transmission of, 1920–1921
Chlorhexidine gluconate (Hibiclens), 1581
Chloride, cardiac function and, 208
Chlorothiazide (Diuril), 377t
Chlorothiazide diuretics, hepatic encepha-
    lopathy and, 1150
Chlorpromazine (Thorazine), hepatotoxic-
    ity of, 1178t, 1179
Chlorpropamide (Diabinese), 1239, 1239t,
    1240d
Chlorthalidone (Hygroton), 377t
Chocolate cyst, 1813
Cholangiocellular carcinoma, 1195
Cholangiography, 972
Cholangiopancreatography, in mechanical
    lithotripsy, 1111
Cholangitic cirrhosis, 1181, 1181t. See also
    Cirrhosis.
Cholecystectomy, 1113–1118
  laparoscopic, 1113–1114
  open, complications of, 1115
    conventional, 1114–1118, 1115d
    discharge instructions in, 1117d
    laser, 1115
    postoperative care in, 1116–1118
    postoperative course in, 1114–1115
    preoperative care in, 1116
    procedure for, 1114
    settings and providers for, 1115
  patient preparation for, 1113
Cholecystitis, 1109–1118
  acute, liver abscess in, 1179
  diagnosis of, 1109–1110
  etiology of, 1109
  in elderly, 1131
  incidence of, 1109
  Internet connections for, 1113d
  management of, 1110–1118
  pathophysiology of, 1109
  surgery for, 1113–1118
Cholecystogram, oral, 971–972
Cholecystojejunostomy, 1127, 1127
Cholecystokinin, 952, 953t, 957
Cholecystotomy, 1113
Choledocholithotomy, 1113
Choledochostomy, 1113
Cholelithiasis, 1109–1118
  diagnosis of, 1109–1110
  dissolution therapy for, 1110–1113, 1115
  etiology of, 1109
  in elderly, 1131
  incidence of, 1109
  Internet connections for, 1113d
  management of, 1110–1118
  pathophysiology of, 1109
  prevention of, 1110d
  surgery for, 1113–1118
Cholesteatoma, excision of, 2006–2007,
  2007

Cholesterol, elevated, coronary artery disease and, 280–285
  drug therapy for, 216–217, 218d
  heart disease and, 186, 210, 280–285
  vascular disease and, 338t
  functions of, 1137
  in hepatic disorders, 1164
  serum, normal values for, 337
  total, in hepatic disorders, 1162t, 1164
Cholesterol esters, in hepatic disorders, 1162t, 1164
Cholestyramine (Questran), 343d
  for jaundice-related pruritus, 1141d
Cholinergic crisis, 782–783
Cholinesterase inhibitors, for myasthenia gravis, 783, 783d
Chondrosarcoma, 935–938, 936t
Chordoplasty, 311. See also *Cardiac valvular disease, surgery in.*
Chorea, 740
Choroid, *1936, 1937*
Choroidal melanoma, 1991
Christianity, beliefs and practices of, in death and dying, 35t
Chromaffin cells, 1215
Chromophilic adenoma, 828–832, 831t
Chromophobe adenoma, 828–832, 831t
Chronic arterial occlusive disease, 363–365
Chronic bacterial prostatitis, 1733t, 1733–1735
  sequential bacteriologic localization cultures for, 1704–1705
Chronic bronchitis, 668–669, *669,* 669t, 671–678. See also *Chronic obstructive pulmonary disease (COPD).*
  clinical manifestations of, 669t
  etiology of, 668–669
  vs. emphysema, 669t
Chronic constrictive pericarditis, 239
Chronic cystic mastopathy, 1854–1856, 1956d
Chronic fatigue syndrome, 1496–1500
Chronic gastritis, 1025
Chronic gingivitis, 1017–1019, 1018t
Chronic hepatitis, 1171, 1171t
  active, 1175
  persistent, 1174–1175
Chronic illness, in elderly, costs of, 62d–63d
Chronic lymphocytic leukemia, 493–494, 494t. See also *Leukemia.*
  nursing care guide for, 497c–502c
Chronic myelocytic leukemia, 494, 494t. See also *Leukemia.*
Chronic nonbacterial prostatitis, sequential bacteriologic localization cultures for, 1704–1705
Chronic obstructive pulmonary disease (COPD), 668–678
  assessment in, 673–674
  breathing techniques for, 672, 675–676
  bronchiectasis in, 679, *679*
  chronic bronchitis in, 668–669, *669,* 669t
  clinical manifestations of, 668, 669, *669,* 669t, 670–671, *671*
  emphysema in, 669t, 669–671, *670, 671*
  energy conservation in, 676–677, *677*
  etiology of, 668
  exercise in, 672, 676–677
  infection in, prevention of, 671d
  management of, 671–673, 672d, *673*
    settings and providers for, 673, *674*
  mechanical ventilation in, 672d

Chronic obstructive pulmonary disease (COPD) *(Continued)*
  nebulized drugs for, 675, *675*
  nursing diagnoses and planning in, 674–675
  nursing interventions in, 675–678
  nutrition in, 668, 669, 678d
  oxygen therapy for, 672, 675
  pathophysiology of, 668
  pulmonary function studies in, 669, 671, 674
  pulmonary hypertension in, 685–686
  pulmonary rehabilitation for, 673, *674*
  respiratory acidosis in, 108–111
  respiratory infections in, 671d, 678d
Chronic osteomyelitis, 889–890
Chronic pancreatitis, 1122–1124
  in elderly, 1131
Chronic renal failure, 1394–1400. See also *Renal failure, chronic.*
Chronic rhinitis, 601
  turbinate hypertrophy and, 611
Chronic sinusitis, 603–604
Chronic subdural hematoma, 820
Chronic thyroiditis, 1296
  hypothyroidism and, 1296, 1297
Chronic venous insufficiency, 388–394, 389–395
  pathogenesis of, 389
  varicose veins and, 386, 389–390, 391c–392c
  venous stasis ulcers and, 332, 333–334, 335, 386, 390–395
  venous thrombosis and, 386
Chvostek's sign, in hypocalcemia, 96, *96*
  in metabolic alkalosis, 111
  in respiratory alkalosis, 111
Chyme, in small intestine, 956
  in stomach, 952, 953, 954, *954*
Chymotrypsin, 956, 957, 958t
Cigarette smoking. See *Smoking.*
Cilia, 526
Ciliary body, *1936, 1937*
Ciliary muscles, 1936
Cimetidine (Tagamet), 1022d
  for peptic ulcers, 1024, 1028
Ciprofloxacin, for gonorrhea, 1909–1910, 1911t, 1914
Circinate lesions, 1573
Circle of Willis, 716, *717*
Circulating nurse, 135, 143
Circulation. See also *Blood flow.*
  cardiac, 163, 165–167, *166*
  cerebral, 714–715, *717*
  cerebrospinal fluid, *717,* 718
  control of, humoral, 173
    intrinsic, 172–173
    neural, 173
  enterohepatic, 1138
  factors affecting, 328–329
  peripheral, control of, 405
  systemic, *324.* See also under *Vascular.*
Circulatory overload, transfusion-related, 462
Circumcision, 1708t
  for phimosis, *1736,* 1736–1737, 1737d
Circumflex artery, *164, 168,* 168–169
Cirrhosis, 1137, 1180–1193
  alcohol and, 1153
  ascites in, 1181–1182, 1182t, 1190c–1191c
  bleeding in, 1183–1189, 1184d–1186d, 1191c–1192c
  cardiac, 1198

Cirrhosis *(Continued)*
  chronic active hepatitis and, 1175
  clinical manifestations of, 1181t, 1181–1182, 1182t
  complications of, 1183–1189
  diagnosis of, 1182–1183
  esophageal varices in, 1181, *1182.* See also *Esophageal varices.*
    management of, 1183–1189
  etiology of, 1180–1181
  hepatocellular carcinoma and, 1195
  in elderly, 1198
  Laënnec's, 1180–1181, 1181t
  management of, 1183
  nursing care guide for, 1190c–1193c
  pathophysiology of, 1180–1181
  portal hypertension in, 1141–1149
  postnecrotic, 1181, 1181t
  primary biliary, 1181, 1181t
Cisternal puncture, 754
Cisterns, 718
CK (creatine kinase), in heart disease, *209,* 209–210, *210*
  in myocardial infarction, 294
CK-BB, in heart disease, *209,* 209–210
  in myocardial infarction, 294
CK-MB, in heart disease, *209,* 209–210
  in myocardial infarction, 294
CK-MM, in heart disease, *209,* 209–210
  in myocardial infarction, 294
Clapping, 553–555
Claudication, intermittent, 332, 333
Clean intermittent self-catheterization, 1363, 1364t
Client. See under *Patient.*
Clindamycin, for *Gardnerella vaginalis* vaginitis, 1886
  for pelvic inflammatory disease, 1912t
Clinical nurse specialist, 5, 27–28
  certification of, 5t, 5–6
Clinical pathway, 12
  for acute renal failure, 1392d
  for coronary artery bypass graft, 290d
  for endoscopy, 116d
  for hysterectomy, 1796d–1797d
  for modified radical mastectomy, 1869d
  for pneumonia, 644d
  for spinal surgery, 763d
  for transurethral resection of prostate, 1755d
Clinical Practice Guidelines, 7–8
Clitoris, 1765, *1766*
Clonazepam, for seizures, 796, 797d–798d
Clonidine (Catapres), 378t
Close chest compression, in cardiopulmonary resuscitation, 262, 264t
Closed pneumothorax, 692–693, *693,* 694
Closed thoracotomy, 580t
Clotrimazole, for vaginal candidiasis, 1884t, 1885
Clotting. See *Coagulation.*
Clubbing, of fingers, 182, 534, *535*
  in heart disease, 182
Cluster headaches, 800. See also *Headache.*
CO_2 laser. See *Laser surgery.*
CO_2 narcosis, 108–109
Coagulation, 429–432, *431*
  clot formation in, 429, *431*
  disseminated intravascular, 517–518
  drug effects on, 448t
Coagulation disorders, 515–518
  chemotherapy and, 1531, 1536t–1538t
  in hepatic disorders, 1149

Coagulation factors, *431*, 432, 433t
  assays for, 448
  transfusion of, 456–457. See also *Transfusion(s)*.
Coagulation tests, 443t, 447–448
  in liver disease, 1162t, 1164
  preoperative, 125t
  reference values for, 2023–2024
Coal tars, 1579, 1583
  for psoriasis, 1579, 1583, 1618, 1619
Coal workers' pneumoconiosis, 688–691
Coccyx, *715*
Cochlea, *1996*, 1997
Cochlear implant, 2007–2008, *2008*
Cochlear nerve, 723t
Code cart, 262, 262t
Coffee-ground vomitus, 960, 966
  assessment for, 1184d–1186d
Cognitive distraction, in pain management, 1555
Cognitive function, age-related changes in, 63, 765–766
  assessment of, 746
    in elderly, 63
    in hepatic disorders, 1160
  in acute renal failure, 1396c–1397c
  in head injury, 822
  in heart disease, 185
  in hepatic disorders, 1160
  in HIV infection, 1466, 1478c–1479c
  in hypernatremia, 93, 94
  in metabolic acidosis, 104, 105, 106
  in metabolic alkalosis, 107, 108
  in respiratory acidosis, 109
Cognitive screening, in head injury, 817d
Cognitive-behavioral therapies, for pain management, 1553–1555
Colchicine, for gout, 900, 900d
Cold, vasoconstriction and, in Raynaud's disease, 355–356
Cold antibodies, in autoimmune hemolytic anemia, 1496
Cold application, in epididymitis, 1730
  in musculoskeletal disorders, 850–853
  in pain management, 1556
  in rheumatoid arthritis, 892
Cold chemical cardioplegic solutions, 220
Cold sores, 1017–1019, 1018t, *1605*, 1605–1606
Cold stimulation test, in arterial insufficiency, 339t
Colds, 600, 600d
  in elderly, 632
Colectomy, colostomy for. See *Colostomy*.
  for cancer, 1101–1106
  malabsorption in, 1077t, 1077–1078
  with ileostomy. See also *Ileostomy*.
    for ulcerative colitis, 1011–1015, 1071, *1071*
Colestipol hydrochloride (Colestid), for jaundice-related pruritus, 1141d
Colles' fracture, 927–930
Colloids. See also *Fluid management*.
  for hypovolemic shock, 410
  in fluid resuscitation, for burns, 1662
Colon. See also under *Intestinal; Rectal*.
  polyps of, 1098–1100, *1099*
  structure and function of, 956–957
  x-ray studies of, 971
Colon conduit, 1421, *1421*
Colonic resection, 1000–1015
  clinical pathway for, 1001d

Colonic resection (*Continued*)
  colostomy in, 1003–1011, *1004, 1005*. See also *Colostomy*.
  patient preparation for, 1000
  postoperative care in, 1002–1003
  postoperative course in, 1001–1002
  preoperative care in, 1002
  procedure for, 1001
  uses of, 1000
Colonoscopy, 974–975, 976d
Color vision, 1937
  assessment of, 1943
  in elderly, 1992
Colorectal cancer, 1100–1106
  abdominal perineal resection of, 1101–1106, *1102*
  clinical manifestations of, 1511t
  colostomy for, 1003–1011
  diagnosis of, 1101
  etiology of, 1100
  ileostomy for, 1011–1015. See also *Ileostomy*.
  incidence of, 1100
  management of, 1101–1106
    settings and providers for, 1102
  metastases in, 1100
  pathophysiology of, 1100
  polyps and, 1098
  prevention of, 969, 1100d
  risk factors for, 1100, 1511t
  stool test for, 1513
  ulcerative colitis and, 1070
Colostomy, 1003–1011
  complications of, 1005, *1005*
  diet for, 1090c–1091c
  double-barrel, 1004, *1004*
  end, 1004, *1004*
  equipment for, *1008*, 1008–1009
  fecal output from, 1003, 1004–1005
  in abdominal perineal resection, 1101, 1105
  loop, 1004, *1004*
  patient preparation for, 1004
  patient teaching for, 1006–1007, 1010–1011, 1092c–1093c
  permanent, 1003–1004
  postoperative care in, 1007–1011
  postoperative course in, 1004–1005
  preoperative care in, 1005–1007
  procedure for, 1004
  self-care in, 1006–1007, 1009–1011, 1092c–1093c
  stoma care in, 1009–1010, 1086c–1087c, 1092c–1093c
  temporary, 1003, 1083, 1085c–1093c
  types of, 1003, *1004*
  uses of, 1003–1011
Colpocele, *1816*, 1816–1819
Colporrhaphy, 1786t
  anterior, 1818, 1819
  posterior, 1818–1819, 1819d
Colposcopy, 1782d, 1782–1783
  patient teaching for, 1782d
Column-disc catheter, for peritoneal dialysis, *1402*
Coma, 726t, 726–730, 727t
  airway management in, 727, 728
  assessment in, 727
  brain death in, 745
  clinical manifestations of, 726t, 726–727
  constipation in, 729–730
  diagnosis of, 727
  etiology of, 726

Coma (*Continued*)
  exercises in, 729
  Glasgow Coma Scale for, 727, 727t
  hepatic, 1149–1153
  in heart disease, 184
  incontinence in, 729
  management of, 727
  myxedema, 1298, 1301, 1302, 1306
  nursing diagnoses and planning in, 727–728
  nursing interventions in, 728–730
  nutrition in, 728–729
  pathophysiology of, 726–727
  personal care in, 729
  positioning in, 729
  skin care in, 728
  terminology for, 726t, 726–727
Comatose, 726t
Combined micturition study, 1360t
Comedo, *1613*, 1613–1614
Comminuted fracture, 818, *917*
Commissurotomy, 310–311. See also *Cardiac valvular disease, surgery in*.
Common bile duct, 1136, *1136*
  x-ray studies of, 972
Common cold, 600, 600d
  in elderly, 632
Communication, cultural aspects of, 1231d
  in aphasia, 738–739, 814
  in hearing loss, 2019, 2020
  in laryngitis, 609, 610
  in Parkinson's disease, 790
  intermaxillary fixation and, 1048
  supraglottic laryngectomy and, 621c–622c
  total laryngectomy and, 618–626, *626–628*
  tracheostomy and, 567
  with non-native English speakers, 666d–667d
Compact osteoma, 935–938, 936t
Compartment syndrome, 932–933
  in burns, 1664–1665
  in casted limb, 857, 932–933
Complement, 1439–1441, 1440t
  deficiencies of, 1440–1441
Complement fixation test, 1445–1446
Complementary therapies, in HIV infection, 1471
Complete blood count (CBC), 442–447, 443t, 445t, 446t
  in cancer, 1513
  in cystitis, 1372
  in urinary tract disorders, 1345
  preoperative, 125t
  reference values for, 1532t, 2023–2024
  with differential, in heart disease, 208
Complex partial seizures, 796t
Compound fracture, 916, *917*
Compression fracture, 823, *823, 917*
  vertebral, *917*
Compression injuries, of peripheral nerves, 828
  of spinal cord, 823, *823, 917*
Compression stockings, application of, 389d
  for varicose veins, 390
  for venous thrombosis, 388
Computed tomography, electron beam, in heart disease, 199–200
  gastrointestinal, 976
  hepatic, 1163t

Computed tomography (*Continued*)
  in cancer diagnosis, 1514
  in hematologic disorders, 452
  in musculoskeletal disorders, 850t
  in neurologic disorders, 749
  ocular, 1946
  of liver abscess, 1179
  of urinary tract, 1349t–1350t
  preoperative, 126t
Computers. See *Internet connections.*
Concussion, 819
  management of, settings and providers
    for, 821
  nursing process in, 821–822
Condoms, HIV transmission and, 1463
  use of by divorced/separated women,
    1924d
Conductive hearing loss, 743, 1997. See
    also *Hearing loss.*
  in otosclerosis, 2015–2016
Condylomata acuminata, 1603–1605, 1604t,
    1926–1928
Condylomata lata, in syphilis, 1915, *1916*
Cone biopsy, cervical, 1783–1784, *1784*
Cones, retinal, 1937
  electroretinography of, 1946
Confrontation test, 1943
Confusion, in Alzheimer's disease, 790,
    791d, 792
  in dementia, 832
  in head injury, 821
  in HIV infection, 1466, 1478c–1479c
Congenital heart disease. See also *Heart
    disease.*
  antibiotic prophylaxis in, 234–235
  infective endocarditis and, 233–236
Congenital syphilis, 1918
Congestive heart failure. See *Heart disease;
    Heart failure.*
Conization, cervical, for cancer, 1831
Conjunctiva, bulbar, *1936*, 1936–1937, *1937*
  examination of, 1942, *1942*
  palpebral, 1935–1936, *1936*
Conjunctivitis, 1963–1964, *1964*, 1965d
Consciousness. See also *Mental status.*
  altered, 726t, 726–730, 727t. See also
    Coma.
    assessment in, 727
    clinical manifestations of, 726t, 726–
      727
    diagnosis of, 727
    etiology of, 726
    Glasgow Coma Scale for, 727, 727t
    in heart disease, 184
    in increased intracranial pressure, 730
    management of, 727
    nursing diagnoses and planning in,
      727–728
    nursing interventions in, 728–730
    pathophysiology of, 726–727
    terminology for, 726t, 726–727
  arousal and, 726
  characteristics of, 727
  components of, 726
  content of, 726
  definition of, 726
  level of, in shock, 407t, 408
  range of, 726t
Consent, for surgery, 117–118
Conservation laryngectomy, nursing care
    guide for, 619c–623c
Constipation, 961–963
  after barium enema, 971
  after prostatectomy, 1719

Constipation (*Continued*)
  after upper GI series, 970, 971
  antacids and, 1022d, 1023
  chemotherapy and, 1530, 1542t
  hypercalcemia and, 97, 98
  hypokalemia and, 86, 88
  in colorectal cancer, 1100
  in diverticular disease, 1082–1083
  in elderly, 72c, 1015
  in enteral nutrition, 984
  in hypothyroidism, 1298, 1304c, 1306
  in spinal cord injury, 823, 825, 826
  in stroke, 813
  in unconscious client, 729–730
  laxatives for, 962d
Contact bleeding, in cervical cancer, 1830
Contact dermatitis, 1609t, 1609–1611, *1610*
Contact lenses, 1971–1972, 1972d–1973d,
    1974
  for cataract, 1976
Contact notification, in gonorrhea, 1913–
    1914
  in syphilis, 1917, 1920
Contact precautions, for hepatitis, 1176,
    1177
Contact solvents, for gallstones, 1111
Continent ileostomy, 1012, *1013*
Continent internal ileal reservoir, cutane-
    ous, 1421, *1421*
Contingen (GAX-collagen), for urinary in-
    continence, 1758
Continuous passive motion device, 868,
    914
Continuous positive airway pressure, 569.
    See also *Mechanical ventilation.*
Contraception, in divorced/separated
    women, 1924d
Contractility, 404
Contracture(s), Dupuytren's, 909–910
  in burns, 1682–1684, 1684t
  in rheumatoid arthritis, 895
  posttraumatic, 933–934
  prevention of, in unconscious client, 729
Contrast media, allergy to, 201, 1346–1351
Contrecoup injury, 819, *819*
Contusion, 913
  bladder, 1413–1414
  cerebral, 819
    nursing process in, 821–822
  ocular, 1987–1989
  peripheral nerve, 828
  pulmonary, 695
  renal, 1411–1412
  scalp, 816–817
  urethral, 1414–1415
Conus medullaris, 721, 722
Convulsions. See *Seizure(s).*
Cooper-Rand electronic speech aid, 620,
    627
Cooper's ligaments, 1843
COPD. See *Chronic obstructive pulmonary
    disease (COPD).*
Coping, in genital herpes, 1907–1908
  in multiple sclerosis, 781
  with psychosocial aspects of aging, 49–
    51, 50t
Corgard (nadolol), 214, 377t
  for bleeding esophageal varices, 1183–
    1186
Cornea, *1936*, 1936–1937, *1937*
  examination of, 1942
  laser surgery for, for refractive errors,
    1973, 1974
Corneal abrasion, 1987–1989

Corneal lacerations, 1987–1989
Corneal lesions, fluorescein staining of,
    1945
Corneal transplant, 1954–1955
Corneal ulcer, 1965–1967
Corns, 1632t
Coronary angiography, 200–202, *202*
Coronary artery(ies), *164*, 167–169, *168*
Coronary artery bypass graft (CABG), for
    coronary artery disease, *289*, 290d,
    291d, 291–292
  for myocardial infarction, 295
  minimally invasive, 291
Coronary artery disease, 280–285. See also
    Heart disease.
  angina pectoris and, 175, 175t, 188, 283,
    285–291. See also *Angina pectoris.*
  atherosclerotic plaque in, *282*, 283. See
    also *Atherosclerosis.*
  calcium score in, 200
  clinical manifestations of, 283–284
  coronary artery bypass grafting for, *289,
    289–292, 290d, 291d*
  coronary stents for, 292, *293*
  diagnosis of, 283
  electron beam computed tomography in,
    199–200
  etiology of, 282–283
  in females, 280–281
  laser angioplasty for, 293
  magnetic resonance imaging in, 199
  management of, 284
    settings and providers for, 293
  myocardial infarction and, 283, 293–303.
    See also *Myocardial infarction.*
  nursing interventions in, 284–285
  pathophysiology of, *282*, 283
  percutaneous transluminal coronary an-
    gioplasty for, 292, *292*
  prevention of, 282, 285d
  progression of, 283
  risk factors for, 184–187, 283
  reduction of, 282, 284–285, 285d
Coronary sinus, *168*, 169
Coronary stents, 292–293, *293*
Coronary veins, *164*, *168*, 169
Corpus callosum, 719
Corpus cavernosum, 1695, *1696*
Corpus luteal cysts, 1825
Corpus luteum, 1768, 1769
Corpus spongiosum, 1695
Corrosives, burns from, 1686t. See also
    Chemical burns.
Cortef. See *Hydrocortisone (Cortef).*
Cortex, visual, 719, *720*
Cortical bone, 838, *838*
Cortical death, 41
Corticospinal tract, 722
Corticosteroids, endogenous, adrenal syn-
    thesis of, 1213–1214
  for asthma, 661, 662t–663t, 663, 665
  for canker sores, 1018t
  for chemotherapy-related nausea and
    vomiting, 1529
  for chronic obstructive pulmonary dis-
    ease, 671–672
  for contrast media allergy, 1346–1351
  for Crohn's disease, 1067
  for increased intracranial pressure,
    732
  for ocular disorders, 1947
  for pemphigus vulgaris, 1620
  for purpura, 514
  for rheumatic heart disease, 237

Corticosteroids *(Continued)*
for skin disorders, 1580–1581
for transplant immunosuppression, 1409
in chemotherapy, 1524t, 1525
in immunosuppression, 1449
intralesional, 1581
metered-dose inhaler for, *661,* 661–663
topical, 1580t, 1580–1581
for psoriasis, 1618
for seborrheic dermatitis, 1611
Corticosterone, 1206t
Corticotropin-releasing hormone, 1209t
Cortisol, endogenous, 1206, 1215
deficiency of, in adrenocortical insufficiency, 1277
in glucose metabolism, 1224
measurement of, 1279t
exogenous. See *Hydrocortisone (Cortef).*
Cortisone (Cortone), 1206t
for Addison's disease, 1280
Coryza, 600, 600d
in elderly, 632
Cosmetic surgery, breast, for augmentation, 1879
for reduction, 1879–1880
facial, 1590–1591, 1591t, 1592d
for burns, 1682
Costal angle, 523
Costovertebral angle pain, 1341, *1341*
Co-trimoxazole (Bactrim), for prostatitis, 1734, 1735
Cough, 528–529
antitussives for, 575, 575d
assessment of, 531
cardiac, 174, 270
chronic, 529
dry, 529
expectorants for, 575
in asthma, 660
in bronchiectasis, 679
in chronic bronchitis, 668, 669, 669t
in chronic obstructive pulmonary disease, 668, 669, 669t
in influenza, 649
in orthopnea, 270
in tuberculosis, 651
mucolytics for, 575
paroxysmal, 529
postoperative, 585
incision splinting for, 582, *583,* 585, 586
nursing care guide for, 591c–592c
Cough variant asthma, 660
Coughing exercises, 130, *131*
Coumadin. See *Warfarin (Coumadin).*
Coumarin, 385t
for venous thrombosis, 385t, 385–386, 386t
Counterpulsation, intra-aortic balloon, 229, *414*
for cardiogenic shock, 413
Counterstimulation, in pain management, 1556
Coup injury, 819, *819*
Cowper's glands, *1696,* 1697
CPR. See *Cardiopulmonary resuscitation (CPR).*
Crabs, *1928,* 1928–1929
Crackles, 192, 537
in heart failure, 270–271, 277
Cramps, in hypocalcemia, 1318, 1319c
in renal failure, 1395d, 1400
Cranial nerves, 722, 723t–724t

Craniopharyngioma, 828–832, 831t
Cranioplasty, 758. See also *Intracranial surgery.*
for fractures, 818
Craniotomy, 758, *758.* See also *Intracranial surgery.*
transfrontal, for pituitary adenoma, 1267–1269
Cranium, 713, *715*
Crash cart, 262, 262t
Creams, 1579, 1580t
Creatine kinase (CK), in heart disease, *209,* 209–210, *210*
in myocardial infarction, 294
Creatinine, 1331
serum, in heart disease, 208
in urinary tract disorders, 1345–1346
Creatinine clearance (CrCl) test, 1331–1332
Credé voiding, 1365
Crepitation, 537
Crepitus, 916
CREST syndrome, 1494–1495
Cretinism, 1297
Critical path, 12
Crohn's disease, *1066,* 1066–1069
anorectal abscess in, 1071–1074, *1072*
in elderly, 1106
Internet connections for, 1068d
malabsorption in, 1077t, 1077–1078
vs. ulcerative colitis, 1072t
Cromolyn (Intal), for asthma, 661, 662t, 663t
Crude coal tars, 1579, 1583
for psoriasis, 1579, 1583, 1618, 1619
Crusts, *1571,* 1572
Crutches, *880,* 880–881
Crutchfield tongs, 861, *861*
Cryoprecipitate, transfusion of, 456–457. See also *Transfusion(s).*
Cryosurgery, for genital warts, 1027
for prostate cancer, 1759
for retinal tears, 1983
for skin disorders, 1585, 1585d
for warts, 1604, 1604t
gynecologic, 1790–1791
Cryptogenic cirrhosis, 1181, 1181t. See also *Cirrhosis.*
Cryptorchidism, 1696, 1739–1740
orchiopexy for, 1739–1740, 1740d
Cryptosporidiosis, in HIV infection, 1466
Crypts of Lieberkühn, 956
Crystalloids. See also under *Fluid.*
for hypovolemic shock, 411
in fluid resuscitation, for burns, 1662
Cul-de-sac of Douglas, 1766, *1767*
Cullen's sign, in acute pancreatitis, 1118
Cultural assessment, 13
Cultural competence, in nursing care, 1230d–1231d
Cultural issues, 12–14. See also *Racial/ethnic groups.*
in cancer, 1506–1508, 1509, 1551
in communication, 1231d
in diabetes, 1227
in diet, 1230d
in immunity, 1441
in Laënnec's cirrhosis, 1180
in pain tolerance, 1379
in preoperative management, 128
Culture, definition of, 12
Cultures, sequential bacteriologic localization, 1704–1705
skin, 1576
throat, 604, 605, *605,* 606

Cultures *(Continued)*
urine, 1344–1345
in cystitis, 1372
sequential bacteriologic localization, 1704–1705
Cunningham clamp, for urinary incontinence, 1760, 1760d
Cupping, 553–555
Curettage and desiccation, for basal cell epithelioma, 1637
for skin disorders, 1584–1585
Curling's ulcer, 1033, 1679
bleeding from, 966d
in burns, 1679
postoperative, 148t
Cushing's disease, 1285–1286
Cushing's syndrome, 1281t, 1285–1289, *1286*
adrenalectomy for, 1287, 1290c–1291c
in elderly, 1323
pituitary-dependent, 1285–1286
Cushing's ulcer, 1033
Cutaneous horn, 1633t
Cutaneous malignant melanoma, *1638,* 1638–1639. See also *Skin cancer.*
self-examination for, *1634–1635,* 1635–1636
warning signs of, 1635–1636
Cutaneous T-cell lymphoma, PUVA therapy for, 1582
Cutaneous ureterostomy, 1421, *1421*
Cyanosis, 181–182, 334, 434, 529–530
in dark-skinned clients, 532
in hematologic disorders, 434
skin color in, 1570
Cyanotic heart disease, 181–182
Cyclophosphamide (Cytoxan), for immunosuppression, 1449
for multiple myeloma, 511
for non-Hodgkin's lymphoma, 508
Cycloserine, for tuberculosis, 653, 654t
Cyclosporine, for immunosuppression, 1197d, 1409–1410, 1449
Cyst(s), *1571,* 1572
bone, 935–938, 936t
corpus luteal, 1825
dermoid, 1825
epidermal, 1632t
follicle, 1825
in fibrocystic breast disease, 1854–1855
ovarian, 1824–1825
chocolate, 1813
pilonidal, 1073t
sebaceous, 1572
thyroid, 1315
Cystectomy, for bladder cancer, 1420–1421
Cystic acne, 1614
Cystic bile ducts, 1136, *1136*
x-ray studies of, 972
Cystine calculi. See *Urinary calculi.*
Cystitis, 1371–1373
after hysterectomy, 1795
after prostatectomy, 1709t, 1712
Cystocele, 1815–1819, *1816*
anterior colporrhaphy for, 1818
Cystogram, 1348t
Cystometrogram (CMG), 1359t
Cystoscopy, *1352,* 1352–1353, 1354c–1356c
Cystourethrogram, voiding, 1349t
Cytadren (aminoglutethimide), for Cushing's syndrome, 1287
Cytology, endometrial, 1784
Cytomegalovirus infection, in HIV infection, 1466, 1467

Cytomel (liothyronine), for hypothyroidism, 1298, 1305t
Cytoplasm, 1503, *1504*
Cytotoxic drugs, for immunosuppression, 1449
Cytotoxic (Type II) hypersensitivity reaction, 1486, 1490t
Cytotoxic T cells, 1434, 1434t, 1439
Cytoxan (cyclophosphamide). See *Cyclophosphamide (Cytoxan).*

D

Dacryocystitis, 1969t
Danazol (Danocrine), for endometriosis, 1813
  for fibrocystic breast disease, 1854
Dandruff, 1611
Darkfield examination, for *T. pallidum,* 1916
Dartos muscle, 1696
Data collection, 8
Dawn phenomenon, 1251
Day care, adult, 22
Day surgery, 115–116, 156t, 156–158, 157t
  facilities for, 22
Daypro (oxaprozin), 893d
DDAVP (desmopressin acetate), for diabetes insipidus, 1275, 1276d
De Quervain's thyroiditis, 1296
Deafness. See *Hearing loss.*
Death and dying, 31–46
  advance directives in, 42–43
  anticipatory grieving in, 34–36, 37
  as developmental stage, 32
  assisted suicide in, 41, 42b
  bereavement and, 36–39. See also *Grief.*
  brain death in, 41, 745
  Do Not Resuscitate (DNR) orders in, 43–45, *45*
  hospice care in, 23
    in cancer, 1561
    in HIV infection, 1471
  in AIDS, 1472, 1473, 1480c–1481c, 1482c
  in cancer, 1561
  legal definition of, 41
  nursing process in, 34–36
  organ donation and, 45–46
  personal awareness of, 31–32
  religious beliefs and practices in, 35t, 40–41
  resources for, 2037–2038
  spiritual aspects of, 34, 40–41
  stages of, 32–33
  stigmatized, 37–38
  sudden, 38–39
  violent, 37–38
Débridement, of burns, 1672
  of pressure ulcers, 1625, 1625t
  of scale, 1583
Decadron (dexamethasone), for hyperthyroidism, 1308
  for increased intracranial pressure, 732
Decaffeination, for fibrocystic breast disease, 1855
Decerebrate posturing, 733, *734*
Decongestants, 574d, 575
Decorticate posturing, 733, *734*
Decubitus ulcers, 1622–1631. See also *Pressure ulcers.*
Deep venous thrombophlebitis/thrombosis, 384–388. See also *Thrombosis.*
Deep-breathing exercises, postoperative, 130, *130*

Defecation, 957
  aids to, 963
  bleeding on, from hemorrhoids, 1096
  in heart failure, 278
Defibrillation, 260, 261d
  in cardiac arrest, 262
Defined enteral formulas, 981
Degenerative joint disease, 897–898
  nonsteroidal anti-inflammatory drugs for, 893d
Deglutition, 951. See also *Swallowing.*
Dehiscence, wound, postoperative, 147t, 153
Dehydration, as surgical risk factor, 121
  hypernatremia and, 93–94
  hyperosmolar, 75–79, 77t
  in diabetic ketoacidosis, 1243, 1249
  in elderly, 112–113
  in hyperglycemic hyperosmolar nonketotic syndrome, 1249
  in intestinal obstruction, 1074, 1075
  management of. See *Fluid management.*
Delirium, 726t
  in elderly, 832
Delta agent, 1170–1171, 1171t
Demeclocycline, for syndrome of inappropriate antidiuretic hormone, 697
Dementia, Alzheimer's, 790–792, 791t
  in HIV infection, 1466, 1478c–1479c
  senile, 765–766, 832
Demyelination, in multiple sclerosis, 778, *778*
Denial, in bereavement, 36
  in colostomy client, 1010
  in death and dying, 32
Dental examination, 968
Dental hygiene. See also *Oral care.*
  in bone marrow transplant, 1454d
Dentures, in elderly, 1059
Denver shunt, for ascites, 1145
Deoxycorticosterone, 1206t
Depakote (divalproex), for seizures, 796, 797d–798d
Depolarization, membrane, 169, *170,* 171, 712–713, *714*
Depression, after gynecologic surgery, 1787
  in bereavement, 37
  in chronic fatigue syndrome, 1496
  in death and dying, 32–33
Dermal atrophy, 1573
Dermal mastopexy, 1880
Dermatitis, contact, 1609–1611, *1610*
  eczematous, 1607–1612
  seborrheic, 1611, *1611*
  stasis, 332, 333–334, 334t, 335, 390–395, 1611–1612, *1612*
    in homeless persons, 394–395
    pain in, 332, 333–334
    venous thrombosis and, 386
Dermatofibroma, 1632t
Dermatologic disorders. See *Skin disorders.*
Dermatomes, *724, 725*
Dermatophyte infections, 1600t, 1600–1601, *1601*
  in elderly, 1630
Dermis, 1568, *1568,* 1569t
Dermoid cyst, 1825
Desensitization, for allergic rhinitis, 1485
  for allergies, 1448, 1485
Desflurane (Suprane), 139, 139t
Desiccants, burns from, 1686t. See also *Chemical burns.*

Desmopressin acetate (DDAVP), for diabetes insipidus, 1275, 1276d
Developmental tasks, of elderly, 32
Dexamethasone (Decadron), for hyperthyroidism, 1308
  for increased intracranial pressure, 732
Dexamethasone suppression test, 1279t
Dextrose in water. See *Intravenous infusion.*
Diabeta (glyburide), 1239, 1239t, 1240d
Diabetes insipidus, 1274–1275, 1276d
Diabetes mellitus, 1223–1262
  alcohol in, 1233
    hypoglycemia and, 1250
  anticipatory grieving in, 1258
  assessment in, 1255–1257, 1256t
  atherosclerosis in, 1252
  blood glucose monitoring in, 1241–1242, *1242,* 1242d, 1244c–1245c
    in elderly, 1261
  chronic arterial occlusive disease and, 363–365
  classification of, 1227–1228
  clinical manifestations of, 1228–1229
  complications of, acute, 1243–1251
    long-term, 1251–1255
    prevention/delay of, 1226, 1235
    self-care for, 1252d
  coping in, 1258–1259
  cultural factors in, 1227
  dawn phenomenon in, 1251
  diagnosis of, 1229, 1229t
  diet in, 1231–1233, 1232d, 1233t, 1244c
    in elderly, 1261
  economic impact of, 1226
  etiology of, 1226
  exercise in, 1233–1234
    hypoglycemia and, 1250
  fasting blood sugar in, 1229
  fluid management in, 1259
  foot care in, 1252d
  genetic factors in, 1226
  gestational, 1228
    diagnostic criteria for, 1229t
    starvation ketosis in, 1243
    urinary testing for ketones in, 1243
  glucose control in, importance of, 1226
  glucose intolerance and, 1228
  glycosylated hemoglobin in, 1243
  heart disease and, 186
  history in, 1255, 1256t
  hyperglycemia in, 1241, 1246c, 1249–1250, 1251t. See also *Diabetic ketoacidosis.*
    in dawn phenomenon, 1251
    in Somogyi phenomenon, 1250–1251
    management of, 1249
    monitoring for, 1241–1243, *1242,* 1242d
    pathogenesis of, 1227
  hyperglycemic hyperosmolar nonketotic syndrome in, 1248t, 1249–1250
  hypoglycemia in, 1241, 1244c, 1245c, 1250, 1251t
    in Somogyi phenomenon, 1250–1251
    insulin pump and, 1238
    monitoring for, 1241–1243, *1242,* 1242d
  hypotension in, 1259
  in elderly, 68, 1261–1262
  incidence of, 1226
  insulin for, 1235–1240, 1244c
    administration of, by injection, 1236d–1237d, *1237,* 1244c
      by pump, 1237–1239, *1238, 1239*

Diabetes metillus *(Continued)*
  frequency of, *1235*, 1235–1237
    intranasal, 1239
    oral, 1239, 1239t, 1240d, 1261
  concentrations of, 1235
  for elderly, 1261
  patient teaching for, 1236d–1237d
  types of, 1234t, 1235
Internet connections for, 1258d
management of, 1224, 1230–1243
  current research in, 1239–1240
  during illness, 1240–1241
  during surgery, 1241
  evaluation in, 1241–1243
  honeymoon phase in, 1237
  noncompliance in, 1246c–1248c,
    1260d
  nursing care guide for, 1244c–1246c
  settings and providers for, 1255
nursing care guide for, 1244c–1248c
nursing diagnoses in, 1257–1258
nursing interventions in, 1258–1261
oral antidiabetic agents for, 1239, 1239t,
  1240d
  in elderly, 1261
oral glucose tolerance test in, 1229
pancreatic transplant for, 1239–1240
pathophysiology of, 1226–1227
patient teaching in, 1242d, 1244c–1248c
peripheral vascular disease in, 331–348.
  See also *Peripheral vascular disease.*
physical examination in, 1255, 1256t
physiologic response to food ingestion
  in, *1225*, 1227
risk factors for, 1226, 1228
self-care in, 1230–1243, 1258–1259
  in elderly, 1261–1262
  nursing care guide for, 1244c–1246c
somatotropin hypersecretion and, 1269
Somogyi phenomenon in, 1250–1251
sulfonylureas for, 1239, 1239t, 1240d
  in elderly, 1261
terminology of, 1224t
type 1, 1227, 1228t
  as autoimmune disease, 1226
type 2, 1227, 1228t
  weight loss in, 1232d
urine tests in, for glucose, 1242–1243
  for ketones, 1243, 1245c
vaginal candidiasis in, 1885
vascular complications in, 338t, 1252d,
  1252–1255
Diabetic ketoacidosis, 1226, 1228, 1243–
  1249, 1248t
  clinical manifestations of, 1243–1249
  etiology of, 1243
  hypokalemia in, 1249
  management of, 1249
  nursing care guide for, 1246c–1248c
  pathogenesis of, 1227
  pathophysiology of, 1243
  vs. hyperglycemic hyperosmolar nonke-
    totic syndrome, 1248t
  with insulin pump, 1238
Diabetic nephropathy, 1252d, 1254–1255
Diabetic neuropathy, 1252d, 1253–1254
Diabetic retinopathy, 1252d, 1253
Diabinese (chlorpropamide), 1239, 1239t,
  1240d
Diagnosis-related groups (DRGs), 20
Diagnostic procedures, preoperative, 123–
  124, 125t–127t, 130
  in elderly, 158
Dialysis, 1400–1408

Dialysis *(Continued)*
  care settings and providers for, 1407–
    1408
  goals of, 1401
  hemodialysis, 1404–1408. See also *Hemo-
    dialysis.*
  indications for, 1400–1401
  peritoneal, 1401–1404. See also *Peritoneal
    dialysis.*
  principles of, 1400
Diamox (acetazolamide), for glaucoma,
  1980
Diaphanography, breast, 1849
Diaphragm, thoracic, 524, *525*
  excursion of, 536
  urogenital, 1415
Diaphragma sellae, 714
Diaphragmatic breathing, 130, 553
  in chronic obstructive pulmonary dis-
    ease, 676, *676*
Diapid (lypressin), for diabetes insipidus,
  1275
Diarrhea, 963–964
  antacids and, 1022d, 1023
  chemotherapy and, 1530, 1541t–1542t
  drugs for, 964, 964d
  hyperkalemia and, 89, 90
  hyponatremia and, 91, 92, 93
  in colorectal cancer, 1100
  in Crohn's disease, 1067, 1069
  in enteral nutrition, 984
  in HIV infection, 1465, 1477c
  in ileostomy client, 1013, 1014d
  in ulcerative colitis, 1070
Diarthrodial joints, *841*, 842, 842t
Diastole, ventricular, 165, *166*, 171, 191
Diastolic blood pressure, 177
Diastolic murmurs, 181
Diathermy, for retinal tears, 1983
Diazepam (Valium), hepatotoxicity of,
  1178t, 1179
Diazoxide (Hyperstat), 213, 378t, 380t
Dichloroacetic acid, for genital warts, 1027
Diclofenac (Voltaren), 893d
Dicumarol (bishydroxycoumarin), 385t
Diencephalon, 720
Diet. See also *Nutrition.*
  cancer and, 1509–1510, 1512d
  colorectal cancer and, 1100, 1100d
  colostomy, 1010
  cultural aspects of, 1230d
  diabetic, 1231–1233, 1232d, 1233t
    in elderly, 1261
  diverticular disease and, 1082
  gastric cancer and, 1058, 1058d
  gluten-free, 1078–1079, 1080d
  high-calcium, 97
    urinary calculi and, 1367, 1367d, 1379
  high-fat, 184d
  high-phosphorus, 1318
  high-potassium, 183d
  high-protein, 472d
    in fluid volume excess, 80
  high-sodium, 93, 184d
  high-vitamin, 472d
  ileostomy, 1014d
  in acute pancreatitis, 1122, 1122d
  in acute renal failure, 1391, 1391d, 1394
  in atherosclerosis prevention, 363d
  in chronic gastritis, 1025
  in chronic pancreatitis, 1123, 1124
  in chronic renal failure, 1391d, 1400
  in colostomy, 1090c–1091c
  in constipation, 963

Diet *(Continued)*
  in Crohn's disease, 1067, 1069, 1069d
  in diarrhea, 964
  in diverticular disease, 1083, 1084d
  in edema, 177
  in elderly, 52, 53d
    oral problems and, 65–66
  in esophageal cancer, 1058
  in esophagitis, 1020, 1023
  in fibrocystic breast disease, 1854, 1855
  in fluid volume excess, 80, 81
  in glomerulonephritis, 1377
  in gout, 901, 901d
  in heart disease, 183d–185d, 184–185,
    210
  in heart failure, 275, 276d, 279
  in hematologic disorders, 440–441, 441d
  in hepatic disease, 1153–1154
  in hiatus hernia, 1041, 1042–1043,
    1044d
  in Hodgkin's disease, 506–507
  in hypercalcemia, 98, 99
  in hyperkalemia, 90
  in hypermagnesemia, 101–102
  in hypernatremia, 94
  in hypertension, 382d, 382–383
  in hypocalcemia, 96, 97
  in hypokalemia, 88
  in hypomagnesemia, 100, 101
  in hyponatremia, 93
  in hypoparathyroidism, 1318
  in hypothyroidism, 1298, 1304c, 1306,
    1313
  in iron deficiency anemia, 470d, 476
  in lactase deficiency, 1080, 1081, 1081d
  in Meniere's disease, 2017
  in myocardial infarction, 297
  in osteomalacia, 903d, 904d
  in osteoporosis, 906, 907
  in peptic ulcer disease, 1027, 1032
  in pharyngitis, 606d
  in premenstrual syndrome, 1809d
  in prostatitis, 1735
  in supraglottic laryngectomy, 623c
  in urinary tract disorders, 1366d, 1366–
    1367, 1367d
  in vomiting, 960
  intermaxillary fixation and, 1048–1049,
    1049d
  low-fat, 284, 285d
  low-potassium, 90
  low-protein, 1151d
    in hepatic encephalopathy, 1150,
      1151d
  low-sodium, 184d, 382d, 1143d
    in heart failure, 275, 276d, 279
    in hypernatremia, 94
    in portal hypertension, 1143d, 1144
  magnesium sources in, 101
  postgastrectomy, 998t, 1000, 1039–1040
  postoperative, 155
    in cholecystectomy, 1114
    in oral surgery, 1052
  potassium sources in, 84, 183d
  preoperative, 124
  prostate cancer and, 1754
  urinary calculi and, 1367, 1367d, 1378,
    1379, 1383d
  vegetarian, vitamin B$_{12}$ deficiency and,
    478
Diet history, 968
Diethylstilbestrol (DES), for prostate cancer, 1759
  testicular cancer and, 1748

Dietitian, qualifications and responsibilities of, 24t

Differential white cell count, 443t, 444, 445t

Diffuse scleroderma, 1494–1495

Diffuse toxic goiter, in hypothyroidism, 1307

Diffusion, 1224t
facilitated, 1223, 1224t

Diflusinal (Dolobid), 893d

DiGeorge syndrome, 1457–1458

Digestion, age-related changes in, 65, 1015
gastric, 952–954, 954
mastication in, 951

Digestive enzymes, gastric, 952–953, 953t, 958t
intestinal, 958t
pancreatic, 957–958, 958t
salivary, 951, 958t

Digital rectal examination, prostate palpation in, 1702, 1702, 1756–1757

Digital subtraction angiography, in arterial insufficiency, 339t

Digital subtraction venography, in venous insufficiency, 340t

Digitalis, for heart failure, 274, 278
in elderly, 54t
palpitations and, 176–177

Digitalis toxicity, heart block and, 251–253, 254d
hypomagnesemia and, 101
in myocarditis, 238
toxicity of, 274

Digits, clubbing of, 182, 534, 535
in heart disease, 182

Digoxin (Lanoxin), 211d, 211–212
for fluid volume excess, 79–80
for heart failure, 274, 278
toxicity of, 274

Dilantin (phenytoin), for increased intracranial pressure, 732
for seizures, 796, 797d–798d

Dilatation and curettage, 1791–1793, 1793d

Dilated cardiomyopathy, 303–305, 304, 306

Diltiazem (Cardizem), 378t
for dysrhythmias, 215, 216d
for heart disease, 213, 215d

Diphenylhydantoin, for seizures, 796, 797d–798d

Diplopia, 742, 1938

Direct antiglobulin test, 443t, 449, 450t

Direct Coombs' test, 443t, 449, 450t

Disc, intervertebral, 714, 715
herniation of, 752, 752, 792–795, 793, 793t, 794d
pain in, 911–913
straight-leg-raise test for, 912
surgery for, 673d, 761–767, 763d

Discharge, from postanesthesia care unit, 143–144, 144t
in ambulatory surgery, 157t, 157–158

Discharge planner, 26

Discharge planning, 155, 156d. See also *Patient teaching.*
postoperative, 129d, 131–133, 155, 156d

Dislocations, 915–916

Dissecting aneurysm, 366, 366–367, 367

Disseminated intravascular coagulation (DIC), 517–518
in burns, 1666d–1668d

Distal convoluted tubules, 1331, 1331
in urine formation, 1332, 1332

Distal splenorenal shunt, for esophageal varices, 1188, 1189

Distal symmetric polyneuropathy, diabetic, 1252d, 1254

Distributive shock, 413–422, 420. See also *Shock.*

Disuse syndromes, 843–846

Diulo (metolazone), 377t

Diuresis, in burns, 1666–1670
postobstructive, 1378

Diuretics, 79, 216, 217d, 218d, 377t
for heart disease, 216, 217d, 275
for hypernatremia, 94
for portal hypertension, 1144, 1144d
in elderly, 54t
loop, 377t
osmotic, 732d
for increased intracranial pressure, 731–732
patient teaching for, 218d
potassium-sparing, 79, 377t
potassium-wasting, 79
self-management for, 1144d
thiazide, 377t
hepatic encephalopathy and, 1150
hypercalcemia and, 97, 98

Diuril (chlorothiazide), 377t

Divalproex (Depakote), for seizures, 796, 797d–798d

Diverticular disease, 1081, 1081–1084, 1082
in elderly, 1106
temporary colostomy for, 1085c–1093c

Diverticulitis, 1081, 1081–1084, 1082

Diverticulosis, 1081, 1081–1084, 1082

Dizziness, 1996–1997, 1998
diagnosis of, 2001–2002

DNA assays, 1446

Do Not Resuscitate (DNR) order, 43–45, 45

Dobutamine (Dobutrex), cardiac effects of, 405t
for cardiogenic shock, 413
for heart disease, 214, 274–275

Dolobid (diflusinal), 893d

Domestic violence, 19

Dopamine (Intropin), cardiac effects of, 405t
for cardiogenic shock, 214
for heart disease, 214, 274–275
in cardiopulmonary resuscitation, 263, 263t
in Parkinson's disease, 787

Doppler treadmill test, in arterial insufficiency, 339t

Doppler ultrasound, carotid, 749–750, 751
in arterial insufficiency, 339t
in distal pulse recording, 335, 337, 339
in venous insufficiency, 340t

Dorsal position, 135, 136

Double vision, 742, 1938

Double voiding, 1385

Double-barrel colostomy, 1004, 1004

Douching, for atrophic vaginitis, 1806
for infectious vaginitis, 1806, 1892c

Dowager's hump, 67, 67, 905, 905

Doxazosin, for benign prostatic hyperplasia, 1753

Doxycycline, for chlamydia, 1912t, 1921
for gonorrhea, 1909–1910, 1911t, 1914
for pelvic inflammatory disease, 1912t

Drain bag, for urine, 1362, 1363

Drainage, bile, in cholecystectomy, 1114, 1114, 1116, 1117, 1117d
in liver transplant, 1197
cast, 856

Drainage *(Continued)*
cerebrospinal fluid, in increased intracranial pressure, 733
chest, 575–580. See also *Chest tube drainage.*
from ear, 1998
assessment of, 2000
gastrointestinal, intubation for, 976–978, 977
in casts, 855
in cholecystectomy, 1114, 1114, 1116, 1117
discharge instructions for, 1117d
in liver transplant, 1197
in prostatectomy, 1715t
of anorectal abscess, 1072–1074
of liver abscess, 1179
of pancreatic fistula, 1125, 1126
postural, 553, 554
percussion in, 553–555
vibration in, 555–556
urinary. See *Urinary catheterization.*

Draping, surgical, 136

Dressings. See also *Bandaging.*
central line, care of, 989, 990
for burns, 1671, 1671, 1673
biologic, 1673, 1673, 1675t
Unna's boot as, 1676d
for prostatectomy, 1715t
for skin grafts, 1673, 1676d
gastrostomy, 986
occlusive, 1583
patient teaching for, 155
stump, 874, 875d–876d, 877, 878d, 879
wet, 1583

Drooling, after oral surgery, 1053

Drops. See *Ear drops; Eye drops.*

Drug eruptions, 1612, 1612–1613, 1613t

Drug therapy. See also specific drugs.
agranulocytosis and, 491–493
aplastic anemia and, 480t
blood urea nitrogen in, 1346t
coagulation delay in, 448t
dosage in, nomogram for, 1525, 1526
effects of, on direct Coombs' test, 450t
erythematous eruptions in, 1612, 1612–1613, 1613t
feeding tube administration in, 986
for cancer. See *Chemotherapy.*
for ear disorders, 2003
for respiratory disorders, 574d–576d, 574–575
for urinary tract disorders, 1363–1365
hemolytic anemia in, 1486
hepatotoxicity in, 1177, 1178t
hypersensitivity in, 1483t
in elderly, 52–58
compliance with, 54–58, 55d, 56d–57d
costs of, 62d–63d
nursing care guide for, 56c–57c
nutrition and, 51–52
pharmacokinetics and, 52–54, 54t
neutropenia in, 1437
ototoxicity in, 1997, 1997t
pharmacokinetics in, age-related changes in, 52–58, 53d, 54t, 55d–57d
preanesthesia, 127–128, 133
preoperative, 127–128, 133
reference values for, 2027–2028
renal toxicity in, 1389t
routine, perioperative care and, 122
serum creatinine in, 1346t
serum sickness in, 1487–1488
topical, 1579–1581

Drug therapy *(Continued)*
   active ingredients in, 1579–1581
   occlusive dressings for, 1583
   vehicles for, 1579, 1580t
  urine color changes in, 1342t
Drug-induced hepatitis, 1177t, 1177–1179,
   1178t
  in elderly, 1198
Drusen, in macular degeneration, 1985,
   1986
Dry cough, 529
Dry eye, ectropion and, 1974
Dry mouth, chemotherapy and, 1530,
   1541t
  in radiation therapy, 1520
Dry skin, 1608t
  in elderly, 58–59
Dullness, 536
  abdominal, 968–969
Dumping syndrome, postgastrectomy,
   998t, 1000
Duodenal ulcers, 1025–1033. See also *Peptic ulcers.*
Duodenum, *955,* 955–956
  structure and function of, 956–957, *958*
Dupuytren's contracture, 909–910
Dura mater, 714, *716*
Durable power of attorney for health care,
   42–43, *44*
Dural tear, in skull fracture, 818
Dural venous sinuses, 716
Dyazide, 377t
Dymelor (acetohexamide), 1239, 1239t,
   1240d
Dynamic cardiomyoplasty, 276, 305
Dyrenium (triamterene), 377t
Dysfunctional grieving, 39–40
Dysgeusia, in chemotherapy, 1530
  in radiation therapy, 1521
Dyshidrotic eczema, 1608t
Dyskinesia, 740
Dysmenorrhea, 1776–1777
  endometriosis and, 1813
  uterine retrodisplacement and, 1820
Dyspareunia, endometriosis and, 1813
  genital prolapse and, 1817
  postmenopausal, 1771, 1800
  uterine retrodisplacement and, 1820
Dysphagia, diet in, 606d
  hypomagnesemia and, 101
  in achalasia, 1044, 1045
  in elderly, 1059
  in oral cancer, 1054
  in peritonsillar abscess, 607
  in pharyngitis, 604, 605
  in supraglottic laryngectomy, 622c–623c
  in tonsillitis, 606, 606d
  self-management of, 1046d
Dysplastic nevus, 1633t
Dyspnea, 529
  anxiety and, 110–111
  assessment of, 188, 531
  in ascites, 1143, 1155c
  in asthma, 660
  in chronic obstructive pulmonary disease, 668
  in elderly, 65
  in emphysema, 670
  in heart disease, 174–175, 270, 277, 278
  in hematologic disorders, 433–436
  in occupational lung diseases, 688
  in respiratory acidosis, 110
  paroxysmal nocturnal, 174, 270
  positional, 174

Dyspnea on exertion, 174
Dysrhythmia(s), 240–261. See also specific
   types.
  after cardiac valvular disease, 315
  after pneumonectomy, 584
  anxiety in, 255
  artificial pacemakers for, 256–259
   external, 259, *259*
   internal, 256–259, *257, 258*
  assessment in, 255
  atrial, 243–247
  atrioventricular heart block as, *251–253,*
   251–255
  cardiac conduction surgery for, 260–
   261
  cardiogenic shock in, 412
  cardioversion for, 259–260
  care settings for, 261
  decreased cardiac output in, 255
  defibrillation for, 260
  digitalis and, 274
  digoxin and, 212
  drug therapy for, 215–216, 216d
  electrocardiography in, *194,* 194–197,
   195, 196t. See also *Electrocardiography (ECG).*
  electrophysiologic studies in, 197
  hyperkalemia and, 87, 89, 90
  hypokalemia and, 86, 88
  implantable cardioverter-defibrillator for,
   260, 261d
  in cardiac arrest, 261
  in electrical injury, 1688, 1689
  in hypomagnesemia, 100
  in myocardial infarction, 296–297
  in myocarditis, 238
  junctional, 247–248
  management of, 253
  nursing diagnoses and planning in, 255
  nursing interventions and evaluation in,
   255–256
  patient teaching in, 255–256
  postoperative, 221, 225
  potassium imbalance and, 208
  sinus, 178, 240–242, *241–243*
  Stokes-Adams syndrome in, 176
  ventricular, 248–251
Dystonia, 740
Dysuria, 1335
  in cystitis, 1372, 1373
  in menopause, 1771

E

Ear, age-related changes in, 2009
  drainage from, 1998
   assessment of, 2000
  examination of, 2000–2001, *2001*
   in elderly, 60–61
  external, age-related changes in, 2009
   infections of, 2011–2012, 2012d
   structure and function of, 1995, *1996*
  inner, age-related changes in, 2009
   infection of, 2013–2014
   structure and function of, 1996, *1996*
  middle, age-related changes in, 2009
   infection of, 2012–2013, 2013t, *2014*
    brain abscess and, 771
    myringotomy for, 2005–2006, *2006*
   structure and function of, 1995–1996,
    1996
  noise in, 820, 1998
   assessment of, 2000

Ear *(Continued)*
  pain in, 1998
   assessment of, 1999–2000
  structure and function of, 1995–1997,
   1996
Ear disorders, assessment in, 1999–2001
  diagnosis of, 2001–2002, 2002t
  drug therapy for, 2003
  history in, 1999–2000
  in elderly, 2009
  infectious and inflammatory, 2011–2014
  management of, 2002–2003
   settings and providers for, 2008–2009
  resources for, 2044–2045
  risk reduction for, 2000d
  surgery for, 2003–2008
  surgery in, complications of, 2003
  vestibular rehabilitation in, 2003
Ear drops, 2012
Eardrum, 1995, *1996,* 1997
  examination of, 2000–2001, *2001*
  perforation of, 2014–2015, *2015*
  surgical repair of, 2003–2005, *2004*
Ecchymosis, 1571
  in fractures, 916
Eccrine glands, *1568,* 1569, 1569t
ECG. See also *Electrocardiography (ECG).*
ECG gating, 199
Echocardiography, 199, *199*
Echothiophate iodine (Phospholine Iodide),
   for glaucoma, 1979–1980
Economic factors, in chronic illness, in elderly, 62d–63d
  in health care access, 18
  in surgery, 119–120
Ectopic beats, 297
Ectopic pregnancy, chlamydial salpingitis
   and, 1921
Ectropion, *1974,* 1974–1975
Eczema, of aging, 49–51, 50t
  of cancer, 1545–1551
  of surgery, 119, 120d
  PUVA therapy for, 1582, 1584
Eczematous dermatitis, 1607–1612
  nonspecific, 1607–1609, *1608,* 1608t
Edecrin (ethacrynic acid), 377t, 380t
Edema, 79–81, *80*
  cerebral, 82
  diuretics for, 216, 217d, 218d
  in acute renal failure, 1389–1390, 1395c
  in burns, 1660–1661, *1661,* 1664–1665
  in heart disease, 177, 189, 277
   in elderly, 318
  in hypothyroidism, 1297, 1298, *1298,*
   1307, *1307,* 1308, *1308*
  in lymphedema, 396–397
  in venous insufficiency, 334t
  of casted parts, 853
  periorbital, in hypothyroidism, 1308,
   1308
  pitting, 80, *80,* 177
   in third-space shift, 82
  pulmonary, after pneumonectomy, 584
   cardiogenic, 270, 280, 281d–282d
   in heart failure, 270
   noncardiogenic, 686–688
Edrophonium (Tensilon IV), in myasthenic
   vs. cholinergic crisis, 783
Edrophonium test, for myasthenia gravis,
   783
Education, nursing, 3–5
Efferent neurons, 711–712, *712*
Effort syncope, 176
Ego differentiation, 32

Ego preoccupation, 32
Ego transcendence, 32
Egophony, 537
Ejaculation, 1698
   premature, 1698–1699, 1699t
   retrograde, 1699, 1699t
      after prostatectomy, 1709t, 1713, 1715t, 1719–1720
      after retroperitoneal lymphadenectomy, 1752
Ejaculatory ducts, structure and function of, *1696*, 1697
Ejection click, 180–181
Elastic cartilage, 843
Elastic compression stockings, application of, 389d
   for varicose veins, 390
   for venous thrombosis, 388
Elastic pressure garments, for burns, 1682, *1683*, 1684, 1685d
Elastic recoil, vascular, 328
Elastic wrap, for strains, 913
   for stump, *879*
Elbow, bursitis of, 902
   tennis, 902
Elderly, 49–74. See also *Aging.*
   abdominal pain in, 1015
   adrenal disorders in, 1323
   anorexia in, in heart disease, 318–319
      in hematologic disorders, 518
   antacids for, 1015, 1021d
   assessment of, 69–74
      history taking in, 69
      nursing care guide for, 70d–74d
      physical examination in, 69
   atrophic vaginitis in, 1806–1807
   benign prostatic hyperplasia in, 1752–1754, 1761. See also *Benign prostatic hyperplasia.*
   beta blockers in, 379t
   body composition in, 51
      drug therapy and, 52–54
   bowel movements in, 1015
   breast cancer in, 1880
   breast disorders in, 1880
   bullous pemphigoid in, 1620–1621, *1621*
   burns in, 1648, 1690–1691
   cancer in, 1499, 1561–1562
   cardiovascular function in, 64–65, 397–398
   cataracts in, *1975*, 1975–1978, *1976*
   cerebrovascular accident in, 832
   chronic illness in, costs of, 62d–63d
   cirrhosis in, 1198
   constipation in, 1015
   day care for, 22
   dehydration in, 112
   delirium in, 832
   dementia in, 832
   dentures in, 1059
   developmental tasks of, 32
   diabetes in, 1261–1262
   drug therapy in, 52–58, 53d, 54t, 55d–57d
      compliance with, 54–58, 55d, 56d–57d
      costs of, 62d–63d
      nursing care guide for, 56d–57d
      nutrition and, 51–52
      pharmacokinetics and, 52–54, 54t
   dysphagia in, 1059
   ear disorders in, 2009
   endocrine function in, 68–69, 1218–1219
   esophageal disorders in, 1059
   exercise for, 65

Elderly *(Continued)*
   eye disorders in, 1991–1992
   fever in, 318
   fluid management in, 112
   gallstones in, 1131
   gastrointestinal function in, 65–66, 1015
      lower tract, 1106–1107
      upper tract, 1059–1060
   growing population of, 49
   gynecomastia in, 1880
   hair in, 59
   health care spending on, 18–29
   health needs of, 18–19
   health promotion for, 14t, 14–15
   hearing in, 60–61, 766, 1997, 2019–2020
   heart disease in, 230–231, 318–319
   hematologic disorders in, 464–465, 519
   hepatic disorders in, 1165–1166, 1198
   hepatitis B vaccine for, 1175d
   hepatitis in, 1198
   herpes zoster in, 1606–1607
   home assessment for, 944
   hypercalcemia in, 1324
   hyperkalemia in, 112
   hypertension in, 230
   hypocalcemia in, 1324
   hyponatremia in, 112–113
   immune disorders in, 1499–1500
   infection in, 1499–1500
   influenza in, 650
   intestinal ischemia in, 1106
   joint disorders in, 67, 884–885
   kyphosis in, 67, *67*
   macular degeneration in, 1985–1987, *1986*
   memory loss in, 63, 765–766, 790, 791d, 792
   mental processes in, 63
   musculoskeletal function in, 66–67, *67*, 884–885, 943–944
   nails in, 59
   neurologic function in, 67–68, 765–766, 766
   nonsteroidal anti-inflammatory drugs in, 893d
   nutrition in, gastrointestinal function and, 65–66
   ocular disorders in, 1961
   orthostatic hypotension in, 64–65, 71c
   osteoporosis in, 67, 71c
   pancreatic disease in, 1131
   parathyroid disorders in, 1324
   penile cancer in, 1761
   peptic ulcer disease in, 1059–1060
   peripheral vascular disease in, 348
   pets for, 50
   pituitary disorders in, 1322–1323
   pneumonia in, 707
   postherpetic neuralgia in, 1606–1607
   powerlessness in, 73c–74c
   prostate cancer in, 1761
   reproductive function in, 68, 1761–1762
      in females, 1800, 1838
      in males, 1724–1725
   resources for, 2038
   respiratory function in, 65, 587, 632, 698–707
   safety measures for, 70c–72c
   self-esteem in, 58
   sexuality of, 68, 1761
   shock in, 422
   skin in, 10–11, *58*, 1591–1592, 1630
   sleep in, 63–64, 766

Elderly *(Continued)*
   smell in, 61
   stress response in, 1218
   subdural hematoma in, 832
   surgery in, 158–159
   tactile sensation in, 61–63, 766
   taste in, 61
   thermoregulation in, 59–60
   thyroid disorders in, 1323–1324
   traction in, 885
   tuberculosis in, 707
   urethral prolapse in, 1368
   urinary function in, 66
   urinary incontinence in, 1425
   urinary tract disorders in, 1368, 1425
   uterine prolapse in, 1368
   vaginal prolapse in, 1368
   vascular disorders in, 397–398
   vision in, 60, 71c, 766
   voiding in, 65–66, 1425
   water intoxication in, 112–113
   wellness strategies for, 69d
   xerosis in, 1630
Electrical bone stimulator, 934–935
Electrical injury, 1648, *1688*, 1688–1690. See also *Burns.*
   first aid in, 1649
   peripheral nerve, 828
Electrocardiographic gating, 199
Electrocardiography (ECG), 193–197
   ambulatory, 197
   in atrial fibrillation, 246, *246*
   in atrial flutter, 245, *245*
   in atrioventricular heart block, 251, *251–253*, 252, 253, 254d
   in exercise stress testing, 195–197
   in junctional escape rhythm, *247*, 247–248
   in myocardial infarction, 294, 295, 296–297
   in pacemaker evaluation, 257, *258*, 259
   in paroxysmal atrial tachycardia, 244
   in premature atrial contractions, *243*
   in premature ventricular contractions, 248, *248*
   in pulmonary embolism, 682
   in sinus arrhythmia, *243*
   in sinus bradycardia, *241*
   in sinus tachycardia, *242*
   in ventricular fibrillation, *250*
   in ventricular tachycardia, 249, *249*
   interpretation in, *194*, 195, *195*, 196t
   preoperative, 125t
   signal-averaged, 195
   tracings on, 193–195, *194*, *195*
   waveforms on, 193, *194*
Electrocautery, for genital warts, 1027
   gynecologic, 1791
Electroencephalography (EEG), 754–757
   in seizure disorders, 796
Electrolyte(s), blood pressure and, 100d
   measurement of, in heart disease, 208
   preoperative, 125t
Electrolyte balance, renal mechanisms of, 1332–1333
Electrolyte imbalance, 84–102
   after ileostomy, 1013, 1014d
   as surgical risk factor, 121
   hypercalcemia as, 97–99. See also *Hypercalcemia.*
   hyperkalemia as, 89–91. See also *Hyperkalemia.*
   hypermagnesemia as, 101–102. See also *Hypermagnesemia.*

Electrolyte imbalance *(Continued)*
hypernatremia as, 93–94. See also *Hypernatremia.*
hypocalcemia as, 94–97. See also *Hypocalcemia.*
hypokalemia as, 84–89. See also *Hypokalemia.*
hypomagnesemia as, 99–101. See also *Hypomagnesemia.*
hyponatremia as, 91–93. See also *Hyponatremia.*
in acute renal failure, 1389, 1390t, 1395
in burns, 1660–1664, *1661,* 1665–1670
in chronic renal failure, 1390t, 1399–1400
in elderly, 112–113
in intestinal obstruction, 1074, 1075
Electromyography (EMG), 757, 852t
in urinary tract assessment, 1359t
Electron beam computed tomography, cardiac, 199–200
Electronic aid, for visually impaired, 1958–1959
Electronystagmography, 2002
Electrophoresis, 1445
serum protein, in hepatic disorders, 1161t, 1163–1164
Electrophysiologic studies, 197
Electroretinography, 1946
Elimination, preoperative, 124
Embolectomy, 346
for pulmonary embolism, 682–683
Embolic stroke, 804, *805.* See also *Cerebrovascular accident (CVA).*
Embolism, air, in total parenteral nutrition, 988
arterial, 357–361
in peripheral arterial aneurysm, 371, 372
definition of, 357
fat, 933
mesenteric, intestinal ischemia and, in elderly, 1106
pathogenesis of, 384
pulmonary, 386, 681–685. See also *Pulmonary embolism.*
Embolization, of varicocele, 1744
Emergency care, settings for, 21–22
Emergency surgery, 118
Emesis. See also *Vomiting.*
coffee-ground, assessment for, 1184d–1186d
Emetic agents, 960
Emmetropia, 1970, *1971*
Emollients, 1579
Emotional disturbances, in chronic fatigue syndrome, 1496, 1499
in HIV infection, 1472, 1479c–1481c
in hyperthyroidism, 1307–1308
in premenstrual syndrome, 1809t
Emphysema, 669t, 669–678, *670, 671.* See also *Chronic obstructive pulmonary disease (COPD).*
centrilobar, 670, *670*
clinical manifestations of, 669t, 670–671, *671*
diagnosis of, 671
etiology of, 670
panlobar, 670, *670*
pathophysiology of, 670
pneumothorax in, 692
subcutaneous, 695
vs. chronic bronchitis, 669t

Employment. See also under *Occupational.*
in chronic obstructive pulmonary disease, 678
Empyema, 657–658
sinus, 602
Enalapril (Vasotec), 213, 214d, 378t
Encephalitis, 769–770
nursing process in, 771–773
Encephalopathy, hepatic, 1149–1153
in cirrhosis, 1182t
Enchondroma, 935–938, 936t
End colostomy, 1004, *1004*
Endarterectomy, 346
Endocardial isolation, 261
Endocardial resection, 261
Endocarditis, infective, 233–236, 235d, 236d
Endocardium, 164–165
Endochondral ossification, 839
Endocrine disorders, assessment in, 1217–1218, 1218t
clinical manifestations of, 1218t
history in, 1217
hypersecretion in, primary, 1216–1217
secondary, 1217
hyposecretion in, primary, 1216–1217
secondary, 1217
in elderly, 1218–1219, 1322–1324
inability to use hormone in, 1217
Internet connections for, 1295d
nursing process in, 1217–1218
patient teaching in, 1217–1218, 1218d
prevention of, 1217, 1219d
resources for, 2041
treatment of, settings and providers for, 1218
Endocrine dysfunction, primary, 1216–1217
secondary, 1217
Endocrine function, age-related changes in, 68–69
as surgical risk factor, 122
Endocrine system, assessment of, 1217–1218, 1218t
in vascular control, 173
structure and function of, 1203–1216, *1204,* 1205t–1207t
Endocrine therapy, for breast cancer, 1874
for endometriosis, 1813, 1814d
for fibrocystic breast disease, 1854
for prostate cancer, 1759
Endocrine tumors, mediastinal, 698
End-of-life issues. See *Death and dying.*
Endolymphatic fluid, 1996
Endometrial biopsy, 1785
Endometrial cancer, 1836–1837
in elderly, 1838
Endometrial cytology, 1784
Endometrial hyperplasia, cancer and, 1836
Endometrial polyps, 1823
Endometriosis, 1810–1815
clinical manifestations of, 1813
diagnosis of, 1813
etiology of, 1810–1812
Internet connections for, 1815d
management of, 1813–1814, 1814d
nursing care in, 1814–1815
pathophysiology of, *1812,* 1812–1813
sites of, *1812*
Endometrium, in female hormonal cycle, 1768, 1769
Endophthalmitis, 1969t
Endoscopic polypectomy, colonic, 1099

Endoscopic retrograde cholangiography, 972
Endoscopic retrograde cholangiopancreatography, in mechanical lithotripsy, 1111
Endoscopic sclerotherapy, for esophageal varices, 1186
Endoscopic surgery, 119
Endoscopy, clinical pathway for, 116d
in cancer diagnosis, 1515
in gastrointestinal disorders, *973, 973–975, 974, 975d, 976d*
in respiratory disorders, 548–550
Endosteum, 839
Endotracheal intubation, 559–564. See also *Airway management.*
cuff care in, 562d
cuff inflation and deflation in, 562–563
equipment for, 559–560, *560*
extubation in, 563–564
for anesthesia, *26,* 137
in coma, 728
in inhalation injury, 1659
in unconscious client, 728
nursing process in, 561–563
nutrition in, 563d
oronasal care in, 563
suctioning in, 728
tube insertion in, 561
tubes for, 559–560, *560, 561, 564*
Enduron (methyclothiazide), 377t
Enema. See also *Bowel preparation.*
barium, 971
for rectovaginal fistula, 1822
lactulose, for hepatic encephalopathy, 1150, 1152d
neomycin, for hepatic encephalopathy, 1150
preoperative, 124, 971
Energy conservation, in chronic obstructive pulmonary disease, 676–677, *677,* 678d
Energy field disturbance, in bone marrow aspiration and biopsy, 1445
Enflurane (Ethrane), 139, 139t
Enteral nutrition, 980–986. See also *Nutrition.*
aspiration in, 984
pneumonia and, 647
assessment in, 984
at home, 986
bolus feedings in, 981
constipation in, 984
continuous, 981
dehydration in, 984
delivery systems for, *983,* 983–984
diarrhea in, 984
feeding administration sets in, 983, *983*
feeding pumps in, 983–984, *984*
feeding tubes in, 983
formulas for, 981, 985
dilution of, 984
in unconscious client, 728
intermittent feedings in, 981
medication administration in, 986
methods of delivery in, 981
nursing diagnoses and planning in, 984–985
nursing interventions in, 985–986
overhydration in, 984
rate of administration in, 984, *985*
routes of delivery in, 981t, 981–983
skin care in, 985, 986
tube flushing in, 985–986

Enteral nutrition *(Continued)*
tube maintenance in, 984–985
tube malposition in, 984
types of, 980–981, 981t
uses of, 980
Enterocele, 1815–1819, *1816*
Enteroendocrine cells, 952
Enterohepatic circulation, 1138
Enterokinase, 958
Enterostomal therapist, 1424
Entropion, *1974*, 1974–1975
Enucleation, 1955–1957, *1957*
Enuresis. See also *Urinary incontinence.*
nocturnal, 1335
Enzymatic débridement, of burns, 1672
Enzymes, cardiac, 209, *209*
hepatic, age-related decrease in, 1165–1166
assessment of, 1160–1161, 1161t
pancreatic. See *Pancreatic enzymes.*
Eosinophils, 429, *429*, *430*, 445t, 1432, *1432*, 1433t
in phagocytosis, 1436
Ependymal cells, 712, *713*
Ependymoma, 828–832, 831t
Ephelis, 1633t
Epicardium, 164–165
Epidermal atrophy, 1573
Epidermal cyst, 1632t
Epidermal skin equivalent, for burns, 1675
Epidermis, 1567–1568, *1568*, 1569t
Epididymis, structure and function of, *1696*, 1697
Epididymitis, 1728–1731, *1730*
chlamydial, 1920. See also Chlamydia trachomatis *infection.*
Epididymo-orchitis, 1731–1732
Epidural analgesia, 1555t
Epidural anesthesia, 137, 138t. See also *Anesthesia.*
Epidural hematoma, 819–820, *820*
management of, 820
settings and providers for, 821
nursing process in, 821–822
Epidural sensor, in intracranial pressure monitoring, 731, *731*
Epidural space, 714
Epiglottis, *524*, 525, *609*
Epilepsy, 795–800. See also *Seizure(s); Seizure disorders.*
Internet connections for, 779d
Epinephrine, 1206t, 1215–1216, 1216t
as vasoconstrictor, 173
blood flow and, 329, 329t
hypersecretion of, from pheochromocytoma, 1292
in glucose metabolism, 1224
urinary assays of, 1293t
Epinephrine (Adrenalin), cardiac effects of, 405t
for anaphylaxis, 418
for cardiogenic shock, 413
for Hymenoptera stings, 1621, 1622
in cardiopulmonary resuscitation, 263, 263t
Epistaxis, 610–611
in nasal fracture, 612
postoperative, 615c
Epitope, 1438
Epoetin alfa (Procrit), 469, 470d
Epstein-Barr virus syndrome, 1496–1497
Equilibrium, assessment of, 2001–2002
disturbances of. See *Dizziness; Vertigo.*
inner ear in, 1996

Erectile dysfunction, 1698–1699, 1699t
after prostatectomy, 1709t, 1713, 1715t, 1719–1720, 1761
in diabetes, 1254
in elderly, 1725, 1761
intracavernosal injection for, priapism and, 1740–1741
penile implant for, 1720–1724, *1721*, 1721t, 1724d
Erectile function, 1698
Erection, prolonged, 1740–1741
in autonomic dysreflexia, 823
Erikson, Erik, 32
Erosion, *1571*, 1572–1573
Eructation, 961
Erysipelas, 1595–1599, 1598t, 1599d
Erythema. See also *Rash.*
chemotherapy and, 1530
Erythema multiforme, 1612
Erythematous macules, 1571
Erythrocyte(s), 429, *429*, *430*
abnormalities of, 447t
disorders of, 467–491
in inflammation, 1432
phagocytosis of, 1138
production of, kidneys in, 1333
sickled, test for, 443t, 448–449
staining of, 446
Erythrocyte count, 443t, 444
Erythrocyte fragility test, 443t, 449
Erythrocyte sedimentation rate (ESR), 443t, 449
in heart disease, 208
in myocardial infarction, 294
Erythroderma, generalized, 1570
Erythrodermic psoriasis, 1616–1619, 1617t
Erythromycin, for acute gingivitis, 1018t
for chlamydia, 1912t, 1921
for nongonococcal urethritis, 1925
for syphilis, 1912t
hepatotoxicity of, 1178t
Erythropoiesis, 429, *430*
Erythropoietin, renal production of, 1333
Eschar, burn, formation of, 1664
pressure ulcer, 1624, *1625*
Escharotomy, 1664, *1664*, 1665
Esidrix. See *Hydrochlorothiazide.*
Esophageal balloon tamponade, 1186–1188, *1187*, 1191c–1192c, 1193
Esophageal burns, 1687
Esophageal bypass, 1054
postoperative care in, 1057–1058
preoperative care in, 1055–1057
Esophageal cancer, 1053–1058
clinical manifestations of, 1054
diagnosis of, 1054
etiology of, 1053
Internet connections for, 1056d
pathophysiology of, 1053–1054
surgery for, 1054, 1055–1058
postoperative care in, 1057–1058
preoperative care in, 1055–1057
Esophageal dilatation, for achalasia, *1044*, 1045
Esophageal disorders, in elderly, 1059
Esophageal myectomy, for achalasia, 1045–1046
Esophageal speech, 618, *626*
Esophageal varices, 1183–1189
bleeding in, balloon tamponade for, 1186–1188, *1187*, 1191c–1192c, 1193
case study of, 1184d–1186d
drug therapy for, 1183–1186
sclerotherapy for, 1186

Esophageal varices *(Continued)*
surgery for, *1188*, 1189
in cirrhosis, 1181, 1181t, *1182*, 1183–1193
in portal hypertension, 1142
management of, 1183–1189
nursing care guide for, 1191c–1192c
nursing process in, 1189–1193
Esophagitis, 1019–1023
chemotherapy and, 1529, 1541t
reflux, hiatus hernia and, 1041, 1043
Esophagogastroduodenoscopy, *973*, 973–975, *974*, 975d
Esophagogastrostomy, 1054
postoperative care in, 1057–1058
preoperative care in, 1055–1057
Esophagoscopy, in hepatic disorders, 1163t
Esophagostomy feeding, 981t. See also *Gastrointestinal intubation.*
Esophagus, chemical burns of, 1047t
drug-induced injury of, 1047t
foreign body in, 1047t
perforation of, 1047t
structure and function of, 951–952, *952*
Estrogen, 1206t, 1207t
breast cancer and, 1857, 1858
in menopause, 1770
Estrogen therapy, after hysterectomy, 1795
for endometriosis, 1813
for fibrocystic breast disease, 1855
for menopause, 1772d, 1772–1773
for osteoporosis, 905
for prostate cancer, 1759
topical, for atrophic vaginitis, 1806
Ethacrynic acid (Edecrin), 377t, 380t
Ethambutol, for tuberculosis, 653, 653t, 654t
Ethical issues, Do Not Resuscitate (DNR) orders, 43–45, *45*
euthanasia, 41, 42b
Ethionamide, for tuberculosis, 653, 654t
Ethmoidal sinus, *601*
infection of, 601–604
Ethnic groups. See *Racial/ethnic groups.*
Ethon (methyclothiazide), 377t
Ethosuximide (Zarontin), for seizures, 796, 797d–798d
Ethrane (enflurane), 139, 139t
Ethylenediamine dermatitis, 1609t, 1609–1611
Etretinate (Tegison), 1581
Eustachian tube, 525, 1996, *1996*
inflation of, 2014d
Euthanasia, 41, 42b
Evaluation, in nursing process, 11–12
Evisceration
ocular, 1955–1956
postoperative, 147t, 153
in hysterectomy, 1788d–1789d, 1797
Evoked potential studies, 757
Ewing's sarcoma, 935–938, 936t
Exchange diet, diabetic, 1231–1233, 1233t
Excision biopsy, 1578, *1578*, 1579d
Excretory urogram, 1346, 1347t, 1351
Exercise, cardiac benefits of, 284–285
for elderly, 65
heart disease and, 187
in asthma, 667–668
in chronic obstructive pulmonary disease (COPD), 672, 676
in diabetes, 1233–1234
hypoglycemia and, 1250
in hematologic disorders, 452
in myocardial infarction, 297–298
in pain management, 1556

Exercise *(Continued)*
  in peripheral vascular disease, 333, 336,
      338d, 343
  in rheumatoid arthritis, 895
  in traction, 862
  in venous thrombosis, 387
  intermittent claudication and, 332, 333
  ischemic pain and, 332, 333
  metabolic equivalents for, 298
  osteoporosis and, 905, 906, 907d
  postoperative, 131, *132,* 151, 153–154
      after spinal surgery, 764–765
  talk test for, 284–285
Exercise stress testing, 195–197, 286
  in myocardial infarction, 298
  submaximal, 298
Exercises, breathing, 130, *130,* 552–553
      after lobectomy, 589c
      after pneumectomy, 582–583, 585–586
  Buerger-Allen, 352, 353, 353d
  coughing, 130, *131*
  leg, postoperative, 131, *132,* 151, 153
  neck, after radical neck dissection, 632,
      633, 637c
  pelvic floor (Kegel), 1365, 1365d, 1779d,
      1817, 1817d
  postmastectomy, 1865–1866, 1867d,
      1868, 1868t
  range-of-motion, in rheumatoid arthritis,
      895
    in unconscious client, 729
  shoulder, in stroke, 809
    postoperative, after mastectomy,
        1865–1866, 1867d, *1868,* 1868t
      after thoracostomy, 583, 586, 593c,
          701c, 705c
Exna (benzthiazide), 377t
Exophthalmos, in hyperthyroidism, 1307,
    1307, 1308
  treatment of, 1308–1309
Expected outcomes, in nursing process, 9
Expectorants, 575
Expiratory reserve volume, 537, *538,* 539t
Exposure keratitis, 1965
Expressive aphasia, 738–739, 814
External ear, 1995, *1996.* See also under
    Ear.
  age-related changes in, 2009
  infections of, 2011–2012, 2012d
External fixation devices, *863,* 863–865,
    922c–923c
Extracapsular cataract extraction, 1976
Extracellular fluid, 75, *76*
Extracellular fluid volume deficit, 75–79,
    77t
  from third-space shift, 81t, 81–82
Extracellular fluid volume excess, 79–81,
    80
Extracellular third-space volume shift, 81t,
    81–82
Extracorporeal shock wave lithotripsy, for
    gallstones, 1111–1113, *1112,* 1115
  for urinary calculi, 1378, *1379,* 1379–
      1380
Extraocular muscles, 1936, *1936*
  examination of, 1943
  weakness of, in myasthenia gravis, 782,
      784
Extrapyramidal tract, 722
Extubation, endotracheal, 563–564
  gastrointestinal, 980
Eye. See also under *Ocular; Ophthalmic.*
  abnormalities of, in hypertension, 375,
      376

Eye *(Continued)*
  in renal failure, 1400
  age-related changes in, 1961
  black, 1987–1989
  C. trachomatis infection of, 1920
  chemical burns of, 1649, 1687, 1989–
      1991, 1990t. See also *Chemical burns.*
  contusion of, 1987–1989
  dry, ectropion and, 1974
  examination of, 1940–1944
    in elderly, 60
  foreign bodies in, 1987–1989
    fluorescein staining of, 1945
  irrigation of, 1990t, 1990–1991
    for chemical burns, 1649, 1687
  muscles of, 1936, *1936*
    examination of, 1943
  pain in, 1939
  prosthetic, 1955–1956, 1956d, *1957*
  protective structures of, 1935–1938,
      1936–1938
  removal of, 1955–1957, *1957*
  structure and function of, 1935–1938,
      1936–1938
  tumors of, 1991
  ultrasonography of, 1945–1946, 1960
Eye care, in unconscious client, 729
Eye chart, 1940–1941
Eye disorders, assessment in, 1939–1944
  clinical manifestations of, 1938–1939
  degenerative, 1985–1987
  diagnosis of, 1944–1946
    computed tomography in, 1946
    electroretinography in, 1946
    fluorescein angiography in, 1945, *1946*
    fluorescein staining in, 1945
    gonioscopy in, 1945
    magnetic resonance imaging in, 1946
    slit-lamp examination in, 1945
    tonometry in, 1944–1945, *1945*
    ultrasonography in, 1945–1946
    visual evoked potentials in, 1946
  drugs for, 1946–1949
    administration of, 1948–1949, *1949,*
        1949t, 1953
    in elderly, 1991–1992
    types of, 1946–1948
  history in, 1939–1940
  in elderly, 1961, 1991–1992
  in HIV infection, 1466–1467
  in hypertension, 375, 376
  in renal failure, 1400
  infectious and inflammatory, 1963–1967,
      1968t–1969t, 1970d
  Internet connections for, 1986
  management of, 1946–1961
    settings and providers for, 1959–1961
  neoplastic, 1991
  physical examination in, 1940–1944
  prevention of, 1941d
  resources for, 2044
  structural, 1970–1985
  surgery for, 1950–1958
    anesthesia for, 1950
    laser, 1957–1958
    outpatient, 1950d
    patient preparation for, 1950
    postoperative care in, 1951–1954
    postoperative course in, 1950–1951
    preoperative care in, 1951
  traumatic, 1987–1991
Eye drops, administration of, 1948–1949,
    1949, 1949t, 1953
  after cataract surgery, 1978

Eye patch, *1953*
  safety measures for, 1977
Eye rest, 1984
Eye shield, 1952t
Eyeball, 1935, *1936*
  external coat of, 1936–1937
  inner coat of, 1937
  middle coat of, 1937
  removal of, 1955–1957
  rupture of, 1987–1989
  structure of, external, *1936,* 1936–1937
    internal, *1937,* 1937–1938
Eyebrow, 1935, *1936*
Eyeglasses, 1970–1971
  cataract, 1976
Eyelashes, examination of, 1942
Eyelid, 1935, *1936*
  eversion of, *1974,* 1974–1975
  examination of, 1942
  inversion of, *1974,* 1974–1975
  laceration of, 1987–1989
  movement of, 1936
Eyestrain, 1939

F

F waves, 246, *246*
Facelift, 1591t, 1592d
Facial cancer, self-examination for, 1053d
Facial edema, in hypothyroidism, 1297,
    1298, *1298*
Facial nerve, 723t
  examination of, 2000
  paralysis of, 829t–830t
    after ear surgery, 2003
Facilitated diffusion, 1223, 1224t
Factor IX concentrate, 456–457, 517, 517d
Factor VIII concentrate, 456, 517
Fainting, in heart disease, 176
Falciform ligament, 1135, *1136*
Fallopian tubes, structure and function of,
    1767, *1768*
False aneurysm, 366, *366*
Falx cerebelli, 714
Falx cerebri, 714
Familial polyposis, 1098
Family concerns, in Alzheimer's disease,
    792
  in burns, 1653c, 1680–1681
  in cancer, 1546, 1550–1551
  in cardiac arrest, 263–264
  in cardiopulmonary resuscitation, 263–
      264
  in head injury, 822
  in hip fractures, 925d
  in increased intracranial pressure, 737–
      738
  in lung cancer, 705c–706c
Family structure, changes in, 1919d
Famotidine, 1022d
Farsightedness, 1970–1974, *1971*
Fascia, 840
Fasciitis, necrotizing, 1599–1600
Fasciotomy, for electrical burns, 1689, 1690
Fasting blood sugar test, 1229
Fat, dietary, deficiency of, 1077t
  in total parenteral nutrition, 990
  restriction of, 284, 285d
  subcutaneous, 1568–1569, 1569t
    age-related changes in, 51
    liposuction of, 1591t, 1592d
Fat embolism, 933
Fat metabolism, bile salts in, 1138

Fat metabolism *(Continued)*
  in diabetics vs. nondiabetics, *1225*
  insulin in, 1223–1224
Fatigue, immobility and, 844–845
  in acute renal failure, 1397c
  in anemia, 468, 469–470
  in angina, 289
  in chronic fatigue syndrome, 1496–1497,
    1498–1499
  in heart disease, 182, 279
  in hematologic disorders, 433–436
  in hepatitis, 1173, 1177
  in Hodgkin's disease, 507
  in hypothyroidism, 1297–1298, 1304c,
    1306
  in infective endocarditis, 235, 236
  in leukemia, 497c, 503
  in multiple sclerosis, 781
  in myasthenia gravis, 782, 785
  in polycythemia vera, 490
  in respiratory acidosis, 110
  in systemic lupus erythematosus, 1493,
    1493d
  management of, 182
Fat-restricted diet, 284, 285d
Fatty liver, 1137, 1180–1193, 1181t. See
    also *Cirrhosis.*
  alcohol and, 1153
Fatty stool, in chronic pancreatitis, 1123,
    1124
  in gluten-induced enteropathy, 1078
  in liver disease, 1138, 1153
  in malabsorption, 1077
Fear. See also *Anxiety.*
  in cancer, 1545, 1548
Fecal impaction, 961
Fecal incontinence, 1760
  in unconscious client, 729
  with colostomy, 1008
Fecal output, from colostomy, 1003, 1004–
    1005
  from ileostomy, 1012–1013, 1014, 1015
Fecal retention, in autonomic dysreflexia,
    823, 825, 826
Fecal urobilinogen, 451, 1161t, 1164
Feeding, after oral surgery, 1052
  in esophageal cancer, 1055, 1058
  tube, 980–986. See also *Enteral nutrition.*
Feeding pumps, 983–984, *984*
Feeding tubes, *977,* 981t, 981–984, *983.* See
    also *Enteral nutrition.*
Feet. See *Foot.*
Feldene (piroxicam), 893d
Female hormonal cycle, 1768–1769, *1770*
  ischemic phase of, 1769, *1770*
  menstrual phase of, 1769, *1770*
  proliferative phase of, 1768, *1770*
  secretory phase of, 1768–1769, *1770*
Female sexual response, 1769
Femoral aneurysm, 371–372
Femoral artery occlusion, 363–365
Femoral head, avascular necrosis of, 935
  fractures of, 885, 924–927
Femoral hernia, 1093–1096, *1094*
  examination for, 1701
Femoral vein catheter, for hemodialysis,
    1405, 1406
Femoral vein thrombectomy, 386
Femoropopliteal graft, 364–365, *365*
Fentanyl (Sublimaze), for anesthesia, 141t
  transdermal, 1554t
Ferrous dumarate, for iron deficiency ane-
    mia, 470d, 476, 477d

Ferrous gluconate, for iron deficiency ane-
    mia, 470d, 476, 477d
Ferrous sulfate, for iron deficiency anemia,
    470d, 476, 477d
Fetor hepaticus, 1150
Fever, after intestinal resection, 1003
  in elderly, 318, 1500
  in HIV infection, 1465
  in septic shock, 421
  postoperative, 148t
Fever blisters, 1017–1019, 1018t, *1605,*
    1605–1606
Fiber, dietary, diverticular disease and,
    1082
  for constipation, 963
Fiberoptic surgery, 119
Fibrillary waves, 246, *246*
Fibrin clot, formation of, 429, *431*
Fibroadenoma, of breast, 1856
Fibrocartilage, 843
Fibrocystic breast disease, 1854–1856,
    1956d
Fibroids, uterine, 1823–1824, *1824*
Fibromas, uterine, 1823–1824, *1824*
Fibrosarcoma, 935–938, 936t
Fight or flight response, 173
Filgrastim (Neupogen), for agranulocyto-
    sis, 491, 492d
Filiform warts, 1603–1605, 1604t
Filter, vena cava, 386
Fimbriae, 1767, *1768*
Financial factors, in chronic illness, in el-
    derly, 62d–63d
  in health care access, 18
  in surgery, 119–120
Finasteride (Proscar), for benign prostatic
    hyperplasia, 1753
Finger(s), clubbing of, 182, 534, *535*
  in heart disease, 182
Finger counting test, 1941
Fingernail. See *Nail(s).*
FIO$_2$, in oxygen therapy, 555t
Fire ant stings, 1621–1622, 1622d
Fissure, *1571,* 1572
  anal, 1073t
Fistula, anorectal, 1071, *1072,* 1073t
  arteriovenous, for hemodialysis, 1405,
    1405, 1406
  genital, *1821,* 1821–1822
    after hysterectomy, 1795
  pancreatic, 1124–1126, *1125*
Fixed split, 179, *180*
Flaccid muscle, 840
Flagyl. See *Metronidazole (Flagyl).*
Flaps, skin, 1587, *1587*
Flat bones, 839
Flat warts, 1603–1605, 1604t
Flatfoot, 910–911
Flatness, on percussion, 536
Flatus, 961
Flesh-eating disease, 1599–1600
Floaters, 1039
Fludrocortisone (Florinef), for Addison's
    disease, 1280
Fluid, cation and anion distribution in, *85*
  extracellular, 75, *76*
  intracellular, 75, *76*
Fluid aspiration, for cancer diagnosis,
    1513–1514
Fluid balance, renal mechanisms of, 1331,
    1332–1333
Fluid imbalance, 75–84. See also under
    Fluid volume.

Fluid imbalance *(Continued)*
  after ileostomy, 1013
  extracellular fluid volume deficit as, 75–
    79, 77t
  extracellular fluid volume excess as, 79–
    81
  extracellular third-space shift as, 81t, 81–
    82
  in acute renal failure, 1389–1390, 1395c
  in chronic renal failure, 1399–1400
  in elderly, 112
  in hemodialysis, 1404
  in peritoneal dialysis, 1403–1404
  intracellular fluid volume excess as, 82–
    84, 83t, *83t*
Fluid intake, in elderly, 66
Fluid loss, in diarrhea, 963
Fluid management. See also *Intravenous in-
    fusion; Transfusion(s).*
  in acute renal failure, 1390–1391, 1391d,
    1392d, 1394, 1395c
  in Addison's disease, 1282c, 1284
  in adult respiratory distress syndrome,
    687
  in ascites, 1147, 1148, 1155d–1156d
  in asthma, 663
  in burns, 1651c, 1654c–1655c, 1656t,
    1662–1664, 1669–1670
  in chronic renal failure, 1391d, 1399–
    1400
  in constipation, 963
  in cystitis, 1373
  in dehydration, 77–78
  in diabetic ketoacidosis, 1249
  in edema, 177
  in elderly, 112
  in electrical injury, 1689–1690
  in enteral nutrition, 984
  in fluid volume excess, 81
  in gastrointestinal bleeding, 966
  in gastrointestinal intubation, 979
  in heart failure, 279
  in hemorrhagic anemia, 471
  in hypercalcemic crisis, 1321, 1322
  in hyperglycemic hyperosmolar nonke-
    totic syndrome, 1249–1250
  in hyperparathyroidism, 1321, 1322
  in hyponatremia, 92–93
  in hypovolemic shock, 410–411, 420, 421
  in ileostomy, 1014d
  in increased intracranial pressure, 736–
    737
  in intracellular fluid volume excess, 83–
    84
  in lung cancer, 697
  in metabolic acidosis, 106
  in metabolic alkalosis, 107, 108
  in neurogenic shock, 417, 420, 421
  in peritoneal dialysis, 1404
  in pneumonia, 643, 646
  in portal hypertension, 1144
  in prostatectomy, 1718–1719
  in prostatitis, 1735
  in septic shock, 415, 420, 421
  in third-space shift, 82
  in transurethral resection syndrome,
    1713
  in vomiting, 960
  postoperative, 145–149, 151
    in cardiac surgery, 222, 226, 227
  preoperative, 124
Fluid overload, 79–81, *80*
Fluid resuscitation, in burns, 1662

Fluid shift, in burns, 1660–1661, *1661,* 1666–1670
Fluid volume deficit, as surgical risk factor, 121
  extracellular, 75–79, 77t
  from third-space shift, 81t, 81–82
  in diabetic ketoacidosis, 1243, 1249
  in elderly, 112–113
  in hyperglycemic hyperosmolar nonketotic syndrome, 1249
Fluid volume excess, as surgical risk factor, 121
  extracellular, 79–81, *80*
  in heart disease, 279
  intracellular, 82–84, 83t, *83t*
Fluorescein angiography, ocular, 1945, *1946*
Fluorescein staining, ocular, 1945
Fluorescent treponemal antibody-absorption (FTA-ABS) test, 1917
Fluoroscopy, cardiac, 193
  chest, 547–548
  in cancer diagnosis, 1514
5-Fluorouracil, for genital warts, 1027
  for skin infections, 1582
Fluothane (halothane), 139, 139t
Flutter waves, 246, *246*
Folic acid antagonists, 450t
Folic acid deficiency, 450, 450t, 479
  anemia of, 450, 450t, 479
  clinical manifestations of, 1077t
Follicle, 1569
  of oocyte, 1768
Follicle-stimulating hormone, 1205t
  in ovulation, 1768
  measurement of, in males, 1704
Follicle-stimulating hormone–releasing hormone, 1209t
Follicular thyroid cancer, 1316
Folliculitis, 1595–1599, *1596,* 1597t, 1599d
Food. See also *Diet; Nutrition.*
  calcium content of, 904d
  goitrogenic, 1297, 1297t
  high-calcium, 1318, 1367d
  high-potassium, 183d
  high-protein, 472d
  high-sodium, 184d
  high-vitamin, 472d
  hypersensitivity to, 1483t
  low-sodium, 184d
  physiologic response to, in diabetics vs. nondiabetics, *1225,* 1227
  purine content of, 901, 901d
Foot, disorders of, 910–911
  flat, 910–911
  fungal infections of, 1600t, 1600–1601, *1601*
  prosthetic, 882–884, *883*
Foot care, in diabetes, 1252d
  in vascular disorders, 336–337, 355, 355d
Forane (isoflurane), 139, 139t
Forced expiratory volume, 539t
Forced vital capacity, 539t
Forearm prosthesis, 882, *882,* 883
Foreign body, esophageal, 1047t
  intraocular, 1987–1989
    fluorescein staining of, 1945
Foreign language speakers, communication with, 666d–667d
Foreskin, 1695
  constricting, 1737–1739, *1738*
  inflammation of, 1727–1728

Foreskin (*Continued*)
  nonretractable, 1735–1737, *1736*
Formulas, enteral, 981, 985
  dilution of, 981
Fosamax (alendronate), for osteoporosis, 905, 906d
Fourchette, 1765, *1766*
Four-point gait, 881
Fracture(s), 916–930
  assessment in, 919
  casts for, 853–858, 854t, 855t. See also *Cast(s).*
  clinical manifestations of, 916–918
  closed, 916
  Colles', 927–930
  comminuted, 818, *917*
  compartment syndrome and, 932–933
  compound, 916, *917*
  compression, 823, *823,* *917*
  delayed union of, 934
  depressed, *818,* *917*
  diagnosis of, 918
  etiology of, 916
  external fixation devices for, *863,* 863–865, 922c–923c
  fat embolism and, 933
  greenstick, *917*
  hip, 885, *917,* 924–927, 925d, 926d, 928d–929d
  immobilization of, 918
  in elderly, 924–930
    of hip, 885, *917,* 924–927, 925d, 926d, 928d–929d
    of wrist, 927–930
  in Paget's disease, 908
  internal fixation devices for, *865,* 865–867, 867d
  longitudinal, *917*
  malunion of, 934
  management of, 918–919
  mandibular, *1046,* 1046–1049, 1049d
  nasal, 612
  nonunion of, 934–935
  nursing diagnoses and planning in, 919
  nursing interventions in, 919–924
  organ injuries in, 916–918
  pathologic, in multiple myeloma, 512
    in osteoporosis, 905, 906
  pathophysiology of, 916
  pelvic, bladder injury in, 1413–1414
    urethral injuries in, 1415
  reduction of, 918
    closed, 918
    open, 918, 920c–923c
  repair of, 839–840
  rib, 690–691
    flail chest and, *691,* 691–692
  simple oblique, *917*
  simple transverse, *917*
  skull, 817–818, *818*
    management of, 818
      settings and providers for, 821
      nursing process in, 821–822
  soft tissue injuries in, 916
  spiral, *917*
  traction for, 858–863
  types of, *917*
  wrist, 927–930
Frank-Starling law, 172, 403, *403*
Frank-Starling mechanism, 269
Freckle, 1633t
Free thyroxine (FT$_4$) assay, 1299t, 1301t
Fremitus, tactile, 535

Fresh frozen plasma, 455–456. See also *Transfusion(s).*
Friction rub, 537
  in pleuritis, 658
  pericardial, 181
Frontal lobe, 719, *719*
Frontal sinus, *601*
  infection of, 601–604
  palpation of, *602*
Frozen red cell transfusion, 453. See also *Transfusion(s).*
Fulminant hepatitits, 1176
Functional incontinence, 1338, 1340t, 1340–1341
Functional residual capacity, 537–538, *538,* 539t
Fundus, gastric, 952, *952*
Fungal infections, of skin, 1600t, 1600–1603, *1601,* 1601d, *1602*
  in elderly, 1630
Fungal osteomyelitis, 889–890
Funnel chest, 534, *534*
Furadantin (nitrofurantoin), for prostatitis, 1734
Furosemide (Lasix), 79, 377t
  for heart disease, 216, 217d, 218d
  for hypertension, 377t, 380t
Furuncles, 1595–1599, 1598t, 1599d, 2011–2012
Fusiform aneurysm, 366, *366,* 367, *371*

G

G_0 phase, of cell cycle, 1503, 1504, *1504*
G_1 phase, of cell cycle, 1503, 1504, *1504*
G_2 phase, of cell cycle, 1503, 1504, *1504*
Gait, assessment of, 747, 848–849, 2001–2002
  crutch, *880,* 880–881
Gallbladder, structure and function of, 957, *958*
  ultrasonography of, 976
  x-ray studies of, 971–972
Gallbladder disease, 1109–1118
  diagnosis of, 1109–1110
  etiology of, 1109
  in elderly, 1131
  incidence of, 1109
  Internet connections for, 1113d
  management of, 1110–1118
  pathophysiology of, 1109
  surgery for, 1113–1118
Gallium scan, in musculoskeletal disorders, 850t
Gallstones, 1109–1118
  dissolution therapy for, 1110–1113, 1115
  in elderly, 1131
  Internet connections for, 1113d
  location of, *1110*
  prevention of, 1110d
  surgery for, 1113–1118
Gamma globulins, 428
Gamma glutamyl transpeptidase, assessment of, 1161t, 1162
Ganglia, 712, 909–910
Gangrene, 334t, 335
  gas, 934
  pain in, 333–334
Gardnerella vaginalis vaginitis, 1804–1806, 1805t
  nursing care in, 1886–1889
  patient teaching in, 1901d

Gas, intestinal, 961
Gas exchange, 528
Gas gangrene, 934
Gas pains, postoperative, 155
Gas transport, 528
Gastrectomy, *996*, 996–1000
  complications of, 998t
  patient preparation for, 997
  postoperative care in, 999–1000
  postoperative course in, 997
  preoperative care in, 997–999
  subtotal, 996, *996*
    for peptic ulcer disease, 1028–1029,
      1034c–1041c
    nursing care guide for, 1034c–1041c
  total, 996, *996*
Gastric acid hypersecretion, antacids for,
    967d, 1021d
  histamine₂-receptor antagonists for,
    1022d
  stress ulcers and, 1033
Gastric analysis, 969–970
Gastric cancer, 1058–1059
  gastrectomy for, *996*, 996–1000
  H. pylori and, 1025, 1026
  Internet connections for, 1056d
Gastric decompression, intubation for,
    976–978, *977*
Gastric dilation, postgastrectomy, 998t
Gastric glands, 952
Gastric inhibitory peptide, 952, 953t
Gastric juice, 952, 953, 953t, 958t
Gastric lavage, for bleeding, 967
  for bleeding esophageal varices,
    1183
  for sputum collection, 546–547
Gastric motility, 954
Gastric pull-up, postoperative care in,
    1057–1058
  preoperative care in, 1055–1057
Gastric secretions, 952–953, 953t
Gastric ulcers, 1025–1033. See also *Peptic
    ulcers.*
  stress, 1033, 1679
    bleeding from, 966d
    in burns, 1679
    postoperative, 148t
Gastric washing. See *Gastric lavage.*
Gastrin, 952, 953, 953t
Gastritis, acute, 1023–1025
  alkaline reflux, postgastrectomy, 998t
  chronic, 1025
Gastrocolic reflex, 957
Gastroduodenal reflex, 957
Gastroesophageal reflux, 1019–1023
  hiatus hernia and, 1041, 1043
  with tube prosthesis, 1055
Gastrointestinal bleeding, 964–968,
    966d
  acute, 965
  chronic, 965
  clinical manifestations of, 965–966
  drug therapy for, 967, 967d
  etiology of, 965
  from stress ulcers, 966d
  gastric lavage for, 967
  in cirrhosis, 1183, 1184d–1186d
  in stroke patients, 966d
  lower, 965
  management of, 966–968, 967d
  pathogenesis of, 965
  persistent, 965
  recurrent, 965
  upper, 965

Gastrointestinal disorders, anorexia in,
    958–959
  bleeding in, 964–968, 966d
  clinical manifestations of, 958–968
  constipation in, 961–963
  diagnosis of, 969–976
    barium enema in, 971
    cholangiogram in, 972
    colonoscopy in, 974–975, 976d
    computed tomography in, 976
    endoscopy in, *973*, 973–975, *974*,
      975d
    esophagogastroduodenoscopy in, *973*,
      973–975, *974*, 975d
    gastric analysis in, 969–970
    magnetic resonance imaging in, 976
    oral cholecystogram in, 971–972
    ultrasonography in, 975–976
    upper gastrointestinal series in, *970*,
      970–971
  diarrhea in, 963–964, 964d
  history in, 968
  in chronic renal failure, 1399t, 1400
  in elderly, 1015
  in HIV infection, 1465, 1466, 1473c,
    1477c–1478c
  in radiation therapy, 1521
  intestinal gas in, 961
  lower tract, 1061–1107
    functional, 1074–1081
    in elderly, 1106–1107
    infectious and inflammatory, 1061–
      1074
    Internet connections for, 1068d
    neoplastic, 1098–1106
    structural, 1081–1098
  management of, 976–1015
  nausea in, 959–961
  pain in, 964, 964t
  physical examination in, 968–969
  prevention of, 969d
  resources for, 2040–2041
  risk factors for, reduction of, 969d
  upper tract, 1017–1060
    in elderly, 1059–1060
    infectious and inflammatory, 1017–
      1025
    Internet connections for, 1056d
    neoplastic, 1049–1059
    structural and functional, 1025–1046
    traumatic, 1046–1049, 1047t
  vomiting in, 959–961
Gastrointestinal function, age-related
    changes in, 65–66, 1015, 1106
  in heart disease, 183d–185d, 183–185
  in hematologic disorders, 441
  postoperative, 155
  reference values for, 2030
Gastrointestinal intubation, 976–980
  extubation in, 980
  for decompression and drainage, 976–
    978
  for feeding. See *Enteral nutrition.*
  nursing process in, 979–980
  procedure for, 978–980
  tubes for, 976–978, *977*
Gastrointestinal obstruction, in peptic ulcer
    disease, 1029
Gastrointestinal surgery, 993–1015
  atelectasis in, 996
  complications of, 996
  ileus in, 996
  incisions in, 993–995, 994t–995t
  infection in, 996

Gastrointestinal surgery *(Continued)*
  urinary retention in, 996
  wound dehiscence in, 996
Gastrointestinal toxicity, in chemotherapy,
    1528–1530, 1540t–1542t
Gastrointestinal tract, anatomy and physi-
    ology of, 949–958, *950*
  tissue layers of, 949–950
Gastrostomy, percutaneous endoscopic,
    982, 982–983
  ostomy care in, 986
  surgical, 982
Gastrostomy feeding, 980–986, 981t, *982*.
    See also *Enteral nutrition.*
  aspiration in, pneumonia and, 647
  in esophageal cancer, 1055
  in unconscious client, 728
Gate-control theory, of pain, 1551
Gated heart studies, 198
GAX-collagen (Contingen), for urinary in-
    continence, 1758
Gaze, assessment of, 1943, *1943*
  cardinal positions of, 1943, *1943*
Gemfibrozil (Lopid), 216–217, 218d
General anesthesia, 137–142. See also *An-
    esthesia.*
Generalized tonic-clonic seizures, 796t
Genetic testing, 1446
Genital fistulas, *1821*, 1821–1822
  after hysterectomy, 1795
Genital herpes. See *Herpes genitalis.*
Genital prolapse, 1815–1819, *1816*
Genital warts, 1603–1605, 1604t, *1926*,
    1926–1928
Genitalia, female, 1765–1768
  age-related changes in, 1771
  examination of, 1779–1781, *1780*
    in elderly, 1800
  external, 1765–1766, *1766*
  internal, 1766–1768, *1766–1768*
  male, age-related changes in, 1724–1725,
    1761–1762
  examination of, 1699t, 1700–1703
  external, 1695–1696, *1696*
  internal, *1696*, 1696–1698
Genitourinary disorders, in radiation ther-
    apy, 1521
Genitourinary fistulas, *1821*, 1821–1822
  after hysterectomy, 1795
Genitourinary function, age-related
    changes in, 68
Geographic access, to health care, 1462d
Geriatric patients. See *Elderly.*
Geriatrics, 49
Gerontology, 49
Gestational diabetes, 1228
  diagnostic criteria for, 1229t
  starvation ketosis in, 1243
  urinary testing for ketones in, 1243
Ghon's complex, 650
Ghon's lesion, 650
Giant cell thyroiditis, 1296
Giant cell tumor of bone, 935–938, 936t
Gigantism, 1272–1274
Gingiva, examination of, 968
Gingival hyperplasia, anticonvulsants and,
    799
Gingivitis, 1017–1019, 1018t
Glans penis, inflammation of, 1727–1728
Glasgow Coma Scale, 727, 727t
Glasses, 1970–1971
  cataract, 1976
Glaucoma, 1978–1982
  beta-blockers for, 1947

Glaucoma (Continued)
  carbonic anhydrase inhibitors for, 1947
  diagnosis of, goniometry in, 1945
    tonometry in, 1944–1945, 1945
  Internet connections for, 1986
  pilocarpine for, administration of, 1949,
    1949
Glioblastoma, 828–832, 831t
Gliomas, 828–832, 831t
Glipizide (Glucotrol), 1239, 1239t, 1240d
Global aphasia, 738–739, 814
Globe, 1935, 1936
  external coat of, 1936–1937
  inner coat of, 1937
  middle coat of, 1937
  removal of, 1955–1957
  rupture of, 1987–1989
  structure of, external, 1936, 1936–1937
    internal, 1937, 1937–1938
Globulin(s), 428
  serum, in hepatic disorders, 1161t, 1163–
    1164
Glomerular filtrate, 1331
Glomerular filtration, 1331–1332, 1332
Glomerular filtration rate (GFR), 1331–
  1332
Glomeruli, renal, 1331, 1331
Glomerulonephritis, 1376t, 1376–1377
Glossectomy, for cancer, 1050–1053
Glossitis, in pernicious anemia, 1025,
  1025
Glossopharyngeal nerve, 723t
Glossopharyngeal neuralgia, 829t–830t
Gloves, 1464
Glucagon, 1207t, 1224
  for hypoglycemia, 1245c–1246c
Glucocorticoids, 1206t, 1214–1215, 1215
  exogenous, for Addison's disease, 1280
Gluconeogenesis, 1224t
Glucose, blood levels of, diabetic monitor-
    ing of, 1241–1242, 1242, 1242d,
    1244c–1245c
  in heart disease, 208
  hormonal regulation of, 1223–1226
  renal threshold for, 1227
  serum, in hepatic disorders, 1162t
  urine, diabetic monitoring of, 1242–1243
Glucose imbalance. See also Hyperglycemia;
  Hypoglycemia.
  in total parenteral nutrition, 987–988,
    992d–993d
Glucose intolerance, 1228
  diagnostic criteria for, 1229t
  heart disease and, 186
  in elderly, 68
  in liver disease, 1137
Glucose metabolism, age-related changes
    in, 1261
  counter-regulatory hormones in, 1224
  glucocorticoids in, 1214, 1215
  hepatic, 1137–1138
  in diabetics vs. nondiabetics, 1225
  insulin in, 1223, 1224, 1225
  regulation of, 1223–1226
Glucose monitoring, in diabetes, 1241–
    1243, 1242, 1242d, 1244c–1245c
Glucose-6-phosphatase deficiency, 488,
    488d
  Heinz body test for, 443t, 449
Glucotrol (glipizide), 1239, 1239t, 1240d
Gluten-free diet, 1078–1079, 1080d
Gluten-induced enteropathy, 1078, 1078–
  1079
  malabsorption in, 1077t, 1077–1078

Glyburide (Glynase, Micronase), 1239,
  1239t, 1240d
Glycerin (Osmoglyn), for glaucoma, 1980
Glycogen, 1224t
Glycogenesis, 1223, 1224t
Glycogenolysis, 1223, 1224t
  hepatic, 1137–1138
Glycosylated hemoglobin, 1243
  in diabetes, 1243
Glynase Pres Tabs (micronized glyburide),
  1239, 1239t, 1240d
Goiter, diffuse toxic, in hypothyroidism,
  1307
  in Hashimoto's thyroiditis, 1296
  nodular, 1315
  simple nontoxic, 1314–1315, 1315
Goitrogens, 1297, 1297t
Goldmann tonometer, 1944–1945, 1945
GoLYTELY, 971
Gonadotropic hormones, 1205t
Gonadotropin-releasing hormone, 1209t
  in testosterone secretion, 1696
Gonadotropin-releasing hormone agonists,
  for endometriosis, 1813, 1814
Goniometer, 848
Gonioscopy, 1945, 1979
Gonococcal urethritis, 1908, 1908–1909. See
  also Gonorrhea.
Gonorrhea, 1908–1914
  assessment in, 1910
  clinical manifestations of, 1908, 1908–
    1909
  diagnosis of, 1909
  epididymitis in, 1728–1730
  etiology of, 1908
  incidence of, 1908
  management of, 1909–1910, 1911t–1912t
  nursing diagnoses and planning in,
    1910–1913
  nursing interventions in, 1913–1914
  pathophysiology of, 1908
  postgonococcal urethritis and, 1925
  transmission of, 1908
Gore-Tex catheter, for peritoneal dialysis,
  1402
Goserelin acetate (Zoladex), for prostate
  cancer, 1759
Gout, 899, 899–901, 900d
  in leukemia, 495, 496
Gowns, 1464
Graafian follicle, 1768
Graduated elastic compression hose, appli-
    cation of, 389d
  for varicose veins, 390
  for venous thrombosis, 388
Graft(s), arterial bypass, 344–346
  in chronic arterial occlusive disease,
    364, 364–365, 365
  postoperative care in, 347–348
  preoperative care in, 346–347
  arteriovenous, for hemodialysis, 1405,
    1406
  bone, for fracture nonunion, 934
  coronary artery bypass, 289, 290d, 291d,
    291–292
  skin, 1587–1590, 1588, 1589, 1673–1678.
    See also Skin grafts.
    dressings for, 1673, 1676d
    splints for, 1677
    Unna's boot for, 1676d
  tympanic membrane, 2003, 2004
Graft rejection, 1489
Graft-versus-host disease, in bone marrow
  transplant, 1451

Grand mal seizures, 796t
Granulation, 1587
Granulocyte, 429, 430, 444, 1432, 1433,
  1433t
Granulocyte transfusion, 456. See also
  Transfusion(s).
Granulomatous thyroiditis, 1296
Graves' disease, 1307–1314. See also Hypothyroidism.
Grey matter, 712
Gridiron incision, 995t
Grief, 36–39. See also Bereavement.
  anticipatory, 34–35, 37
  dysfunctional, 39–40
    in amputation, 877, 941c
  in elderly, 51
  in male infertility, 1752
  in pelvic exenteration, 1832
  in spinal cord injury, 826–827
  stages of, 32–33, 36–37
  stigmatized or violent death and, 37–38
  sudden death and, 38–39
Griseofulvin, 1581
Ground substance, 1568
Growth hormone, hypersecretion of, 1269
  in glucose metabolism, 1224
  reference values for, 1272
Growth hormone–inhibiting hormone,
  1209t
Growth hormone–releasing hormone,
  1209t
Guanabenz (Wytensin), 378t
Guanadrel (Hylorel), 378t
Guanethidine (Ismelin), 378t
Guide dogs, 1960d
Guillain-Barré syndrome, 773–775
Guillotine amputation, 872
Gumma, in syphilis, 1916
Gums, examination of, 968
  hyperplastic, anticonvulsants and, 799
  inflammation of, 1017–1019, 1018t
Gunshot wounds, cardiac, 317
  cerebral, 819
  hepatic, 1194
  renal, 1411–1412
  spinal cord, 823
  ureteral, 1412–1413
Guttate psoriasis, 1616–1619, 1617t
Gynecologic cancer, 1825–1838
  in elderly, 1838
  Internet connections for, 1815d
Gynecologic disorders. See also Reproduc-
    tive disorders, female.
  assessment in, 1777–1785
  diagnosis of, 1781–1785
  drug therapy for, 1786
  history in, 1778
  in elderly, 1800, 1838
  in HIV infection, 1467
  management of, 1786–1800
    pharmacologic, 1786
    surgical, 1786–1800. See also Gyneco-
      logic surgery.
  risk reduction for, 1779d
Gynecologic examination, 1778–1781,
  1780
  in elderly, 1800
  patient preparation for, 1778–1779
  procedure for, 1779–1781, 1780
Gynecologic history, 1887t
Gynecologic surgery, 1786–1800
  complications of, 1787
  laparoscopic, 1787–1790
  patient preparation for, 1786–1787

Gynecologic surgery *(Continued)*
　types of, 1786t
　uses of, 1786
Gynecomastia, *1853*, 1853–1854
　in elderly, 1880
Gyrate lesions, *1574*
Gyrus, 718

H

HACEK organisms, 234
Haemophilus influenzae pneumonia, 641
Hair, age-related changes in, 59
　examination of, 1575
　structure of, 1569
　terminal, 1569
　vellus, 1569
Hair follicle, 1569
Hair loss, age-related, 59
　chemotherapy and, 1530, 1539t
　in radiation therapy, 1521
Hair removal, preoperative, 124
Half-life, 1517
Hallux valgus, *910*, 910–911
Halo device, 824, 826, 861, *861*
Halothane (Fluothane), 139, 139t
Hammer, 1996, *1996*, 1997
Hammer toe, *910*, 910–911
Hand, prosthetic, 882, *882*, *883*
Hand and arm precautions, in mastectomy, 1865, 1866d
Hand grip, 747
Hand motion test, 1941–1942
Hashimoto's thyroiditis, 1296, 1297
Haustral churning, 956–957
HAV-Ab/IgG, 1174t
HAV-Ab/IgM, 1173, 1174t
Haversian canals, 838, *838*
Havrix, 1174
Hay fever, 601, 1483–1486
HB$_c$Ab, 1173, 1174t
HB$_e$Ag, 1173, 1174t
HB$_e$Ag, 1173, 1174t
HB$_s$Ab, 1173, 1174t
HB$_s$Ag, 1173, 1174t
HCV-Ab, 1174t
Head injury, 816–822
　assessment in, 821
　brain injury in, 818–819
　cognitive screening in, 817d
　complications of, 819–820
　etiology of, 816
　hematoma in, 819–820
　　in elderly, 832
　management of, settings and providers
　　for, 820–821
　nursing diagnoses and planning in, 821
　nursing interventions in, 821–822
　rehabilitation in, 820–822
　scalp injury in, 816–817
　skull fractures in, 817–818, *818*
　stress ulcers in, 1033
Headache, 800–802
　brain tumors and, 828
　clinical manifestations of, 800
　cluster, 800
　diagnosis of, 800
　in hyponatremia, 92, 93
　in increased intracranial pressure, 733
　in subarachnoid hemorrhage, 814–815
　management of, 800–801
　migraine, 800
　nursing process in, 801–802
　pituitary adenoma and, 1266

Headache *(Continued)*
　spinal, epidural anesthesia and, 137
　　lumbar puncture and, 754
　tension, 800
Health beliefs and practices, cultural aspects of, 13
　religion and, 1230d
Health care, access to, 1462d–1463d
　cost controls for, 20–21
　nonhospital, increase in, 17–21
　　practice roles in, 26–29
　　practice settings for, 21–29
Health care costs, increase in, 18
Health care providers, HIV infection in, 1464
　radiation exposure of, 1519, 1519t, *1520*
　tuberculosis prevention in, 652–653
Health care reform, 6
Health insurance, 18
　health care access and, 1462d
Health maintenance. See *Patient teaching.*
Health maintenance organizations (HMOs), 20
Health promotion, 14t, 14–15
Health-care proxy, 42–43, *44*
Healthy People 2000, 14t, 14–15
Hearing, age-related changes in, 60–61
　assessment of, 2001–2002, 2002t
　　audiologist in, 2008–2009
　　audiometry in, 2001, 2002t
　　Rinne test in, 2001
　　tuning fork tests in, 2001
　　Weber's test in, 2001
　physiology of, 1995–1997
Hearing aids, for presbycusis, 2019, 2020
Hearing loss, 743–744, 1997–1998. See also
　Ear disorders.
　age-related, 60–61, 766, 1997, 2009,
　　2019–2020
　assessment in, 1999–2000
　conductive, 743, 1997
　drugs and, 1997, 1997t
　in Meniere's disease, 2017–2019
　in otosclerosis, 2015–2016
　Internet connections for, 2018
　mixed, 1998
　nursing process in, 743–744
　postoperative, 2003, 2005
　resources for, 2044–2045
　sensorineural, 743, 1997–1998
　　cochlear implant for, 2007–2008, *2008*
　　in labyrinthitis, 2013–2014
　　tinnitus and, 1998
　severity of, 1998, *1998*
　tympanoplasty for, 2003–2005, *2004*
Hearing tests. See *Hearing, assessment of.*
Heart. See also under *Cardiac; Cardiovascular.*
　age-related changes in, 64–65
　anatomy and physiology of, 163–167,
　　164–167
　blood flow in, 163, 165–167, *166*
　chambers of, 165–167, *166*
　examination of, 190–192
　function of, 163
　left dominant, 169
　position of, 163, *165*
　pumping action of, 165–167, *166*
　right dominant, 168
　traumatic injuries of, 317
　tumors of, 318
　vasculature of, *164*, 167–169, *168*
Heart attack. See *Myocardial infarction.*
Heart block, *251–253*, 251–255

Heart block *(Continued)*
　digitalis toxicity and, 254
　first-degree, 251, *251*, 254d
　second-degree, 251–253, *252*
　third-degree (complete), *253*, 253–255
Heart disease, 233–319. See also *Heart failure.*
　age and, 185–186
　angina pectoris in, 175, 175t, 188, 285–
　　291
　antibiotic prophylaxis in, 234–235, 237
　assessment in, 187–192
　capillary refill in, 181
　cardiogenic shock in, 411–413
　cardiomyopathy as, 303–306
　chest pain in, 175, 175t
　clinical manifestations of, 174–185
　clubbing in, 182
　congenital, infective endocarditis and,
　　233–236
　congestive heart failure as, 264–280
　coronary artery disease as, 280–285
　cyanotic, 181–182
　diabetes mellitus and, 186
　diagnosis of, 192–210, 230
　　blood studies in, 207–210
　　cardiac catheterization in, 200–202,
　　　203d–205d
　　echocardiography in, 198, *199*
　　electrocardiography in, 193–197, *194,*
　　　195, 196t
　　electron beam computed tomography
　　　in, 199–200
　　electrophysiologic studies in, 197
　　exercise stress testing in, 195–197
　　fluoroscopy in, 193
　　gated heart studies in, 198
　　hemodynamic monitoring in, 202–207
　　magnetic resonance imaging in, 199
　　positron emission tomography in, 198
　　radionuclide imaging in, 197–198
　　x-ray studies in, 192–193
　diet in, 183d–185d, 184–185, 210, 284,
　　285d
　dyspnea in, 174–175
　dysrhythmias in, 240–261. See also *Dys-*
　　rhythmia(s).
　edema in, 177
　exercise and, 187, 284–285, 285d
　family history of, 185
　fatigue in, 182
　functional classification of, 312t
　gastrointestinal dysfunction in, 183–184
　glucose intolerance and, 186
　heart sounds in, 179–181, *180*
　hyperkalemia and, 89, 90
　hyperlipidemia and, 186
　hypertensive, 177–178, 186, *374*, 374–375
　hypokalemia and, 86, 87, 88
　hypotension in, 177–178
　in acromegaly, 1272
　in acute renal failure, 1389
　in elderly, 230–231, 318–319
　infectious/inflammatory, 233–240
　intra-aortic balloon counterpulsation in,
　　229
　knowledge base for, 174–231
　lipoproteins and, 186, 209
　management of, care settings for, 230
　　drug therapy in, 211d–218d, 211–217
　　　in elderly, 230–231
　　　preoperative modification of, 219–
　　　　220
　　health-care providers in, 230

Heart disease *(Continued)*
nonsurgical, 210–217
risk factor reduction in, 210–211
surgical, 217–229. See also *Cardiac surgery.*
multiple role expectations and, 187
murmurs in, 181
myocardial infarction and, 293–303
neck vein distention in, 181
neoplastic, 318
neurologic dysfunction in, 183–184
nursing care in, 233–319
obesity and, 186, 210
oral contraceptives and, 187, 210–211
pallor in, 182
palpitations in, 176–177
patient history in, 187–192
pericardial friction rub in, 181
physical examination in, 189–192
prevention of, 189d, 282, 284, 285d
diet in, 284, 285d
exercise in, 284, 285d
pulmonary edema in, 270, 280
pulse alterations in, 178–179
rehabilitation in, 229–230
renal dysfunction in, 182–183
rheumatic, 236–237
antibiotic prophylaxis in, 234–235, 237
infective endocarditis and, 233–236
pericarditis in, 238–239
risk factors for, 184–187, 283
reduction of, 210–211, 282, 284–285, 285d
screening for, 230
sex and, 186
smoking and, 186–187, 210, 211, 285
stress and, 187, 210, 285
syncope in, 176
transplantation in, 227–229, *228*
type A personality and, 187
valvular, 306–317. See also *Cardiac valvular disease.*
antibiotic prophylaxis in, 234–235
infective endocarditis and, 233–236
rheumatic heart disease and, 236–237
ventricular assist device in, 229
Heart failure, 264–280
acute vs. chronic, 270
after cardiac valvular disease, 314, 315, 316
assessment in, 276–277
atrial natriuretic hormone in, 270
bed rest in, 279
clinical manifestations of, 270–271
compensatory mechanisms in, 268, *269,* 269–270
definition of, 268
diagnosis of, 271–272, 273d
diastolic, 269
diet in, 275, 276d
diuretics for, 216, 217d, 218d
drug therapy for, 272–276, 273d
dyspnea in, 174–175, 270, 277, 278
edema in, 79, 177, 189, 277
etiology of, 268–270
fluid management in, 279
high-output, 268
in chronic obstructive pulmonary disease, 678
in hypertension, *374,* 374–375
increased heart rate in, 269
left-sided, 270–271, *271*
low cardiac output syndrome in, 271, 277

Heart failure *(Continued)*
low-output, 268
management of, 271–276
settings and providers for, 276
nursing diagnoses and planning in, 277–280
nursing interventions in, 273d, 278–280
orthopnea in, 270, 277
oxygen therapy in, 279
patient teaching in, 273d, 279
renin-angiotensin system in, 270
respiratory dysfunction in, 174–175, 270, 277, 278
rest in, 275
right-sided, 270, 271, *272*
surgery for, 275–276
systolic, 269
vasoconstriction in, 270
ventricular dilatation in, 269–270
ventricular hypertrophy in, 269
Heart murmurs, 181
auscultation of, 191
in aortic regurgitation, 308
in aortic stenosis, 307–308
in mitral prolapse, 309
in mitral regurgitation, 309
in mitral stenosis, 309
Heart rate, 402–403
abnormal. See *Bradycardia; Tachycardia.*
assessment of, 178–179
cardiac output and, 402, *403*
increased, in heart failure, 269
normal values for, 178
on electrocardiogram, 195, *195,* 196t. See also *Electrocardiography (ECG).*
Heart sounds, abnormal, 179–181, *180*
auscultation of, 191
Heart transplant, 227–229, *228*
Heart valves, abnormalities of. See *Cardiac valvular disease.*
prosthetic, 312–313, *312–314*
Heartburn, in esophagitis, 1020
in hiatus hernia, 1041, 1043
Heart-lung machine, 220–221, *221*
Heat application, in musculoskeletal disorders, 850–853
in pain management, 1555–1556
in rheumatoid arthritis, 892
Heat intolerance, in hyperthyroidism, 1308, 1313
Heberden's nodes, 897
Heimlich Microtrach system, in transtracheal oxygen administration, *557,* 557–558, 558d
Heimlich valve, 579–580
Heinz body test, 443t, 449
Helicobacter pylori, chronic gastritis and, 1025
peptic ulcer disease and, 1026, 1027
Helper T cells, 1433, 1434t, 1439
Helplessness, cancer and, 1510, 1545, 1549–1550
Hemangioma, 828–832, 831t, 935–938, 936t, 1194
capillary, 1571
cherry (senile), 1632t
strawberry, 1571
Hemarthrosis, 436–437, 438, 517
Hematemesis, 960, 966
assessment for, 1184d–1186d
from esophageal varices, 1183, 1184d–1186d
Hematocrit, 443t, 444
normal values for, 1532t

Hematologic abnormalities, as surgical risk factor, 122
in HIV infection, 1465
Hematologic cancer, 1505
Hematologic disorder(s), agranulocytosis as, 491–493
anemia as, 467–489
assessment in, 442
bed rest in, 453
bleeding in, 436–437
bone and joint deformities in, 438
bone marrow transplantation in, 464
chemotherapy in, 464
clinical manifestations of, 433–441
coagulation disorders as, 515–518
diagnosis of, 442–452
blood tests in, 442–447, 443t, 445t–447t
bone marrow biopsy in, 451
coagulation tests in, 443t, 447–448
computed tomography in, 452
lymph node biopsy in, 451
magnetic resonance imaging in, 452
nuclear resonance imaging in, 452
ultrasonography in, 451–452
dyspnea in, 433–436
exercise in, 453
fatigue in, 433–436
gastrointestinal dysfunction in, 441
Hodgkin's disease as, 503–507
immunodepression in, 438–440
in chronic renal failure, 1399t, 1400
in elderly, 464–465, 519
in radiation therapy, 1522
infections in, 438–440
infectious mononucleosis as, 512–513
Internet connections for, 506d
jaundice in, 440
joint bleeding in, 436–437, 438
leukemia as, 493–504
management of, 452–465
nonsurgical, 452–463
surgical, 453–465
multiple myeloma as, 508–512
non-Hodgkin's lymphoma as, 507–508
nutrition in, 440–441, 441d, 453
oral lesions in, 437–438, 439, 439d
oxygen therapy in, 453
patient teaching in, 442d
polycythemias as, 489–491
protective isolation in, 453
pruritus in, 440
purpuras as, 513–515
radiation therapy in, 464
resources for, 2038
self-care in, 482d
splenectomy in, 462–464
transfusions in, 453–463. See also *Transfusion(s).*
ulcerative lesions in, 437–438
weakness in, 434, 436
Hematologic system, anatomy and physiology of, 427–433
assessment in, 442
components of, 427
Hematologic toxicity, of chemotherapy, 1531–1532, 1536t–1538t
Hematology, reference values for, 2023–2024
Hematoma(s), after hysterectomy, 1797
epidural, 819–820, *820*
management of, 820
settings and providers for, 821
nursing process for, 821

Hematoma(s) (Continued)
intrahepatic, 1194
management of, settings and providers for, 821
postoperative, 147t
subdural, 819–820, 820
in elderly, 832
management of, 820
settings and providers for, 821
nursing process for, 821
Hematopoiesis, 429, 430
organs of, 433, 837
Hematuria, after cystoscopy, 1352
after renal biopsy, 1357, 1358
in renal cancer, 1416
in renal trauma, 1411
in ureteral trauma, 1413
Hemianalgesia, 743–744
Hemianopia, 1940t
in stroke, 813
Hemodialysis, 1404–1408
advantages and disadvantages of, 1401t
assessment in, 1406
care settings and providers for, 1407–1408
complications of, 1405, 1406t
dialyzers for, 1404, 1404
goals of, 1401
heparin in, 1404
indications for, 1400–1401
nursing diagnoses and planning in, 1406–1407
nursing interventions in, 1407
principles of, 1400
procedure for, 1404–1405, 1405
vascular access in, 1405, 1405, 1406
Hemodynamic monitoring, 202–207
cardiac output in, 207
central venous pressure in, 202, 403
intraarterial blood pressure in, 206–207
pulmonary artery pressure in, 200, 202–206, 206, 207
pulmonary artery wedge pressure in, 403, 404
pulmonary vascular resistance in, 404
systemic vascular resistance in, 404
Hemodynamic resistance, 328
Hemodynamics, 402–405
normal values for, 402t
terminology for, 402t
Hemoglobin, 429
glycosylated, in diabetes, 1243
in red cell indices, 446, 446t
normal values for, 1532t
reduced, 427
Hemoglobin A₁c, in diabetes, 1243
Hemoglobin count, 443t, 444
Hemoglobin electrophoresis, 448
Hemoglobin S, 484, 484
Hemoglobin S test, 443t, 448–449
Hemoglobin saturation percentage (SaO₂), 540, 540t, 541–542
measurement of, 544–545, 546
Hemolytic anemia, 468, 482–489
autoimmune, 488–489, 1495–1496
transfusion reaction and, 462, 483, 488–489, 1486
drug-associated, 1486
Heinz body test for, 443t, 449
Hemolytic jaundice, 1140
Hemolytic transfusion reaction, 462
case study of, 483
Hemophilia, 515, 515–517
antihemophilic factor for, 456

Hemophilia (Continued)
clotting factors for, 456–457
cryoprecipitate for, 456–457
Hemorrhage. See also Bleeding.
assessment in, 410t
classification of, 409–410, 410t
in acquired hypoprothrombinemia, 517
in burns, 1666d–1668d
in disseminated intravascular coagulation, 517–518
in hematologic disorders, 436–437
in hemophilia, 516–517
in leukemia, 494
in peptic ulcer disease, 1029, 1029
intracranial, cerebrovascular accident and, 804, 805. See also Cerebrovascular accident (CVA).
nasal, in nasal fracture, 612
postoperative, 615c
postoperative, in gastrectomy, 998t
in gynecologic surgery, 1787
in hysterectomy, 1795
in prostatectomy, 1709t, 1712, 1716d–1717d
in tonsillectomy, 607
subarachnoid, 814–816, 815
subconjunctival, 1987–1989
under cast, 855
vitreous, in diabetes, 1253
Hemorrhagic anemia, 467, 470–472. See also Anemia.
nursing care guide for, 473c–475c
Hemorrhagic disorders, 513–515
Hemorrhagic shock, 409–410, 410t. See also Shock.
Hemorrhoidectomy, 1097–1098, 1098d
Hemorrhoids, 1096, 1096–1098
Hemostasis, in bleeding disorders, 516d, 516–517
in epistaxis, 610, 611
Hemostatic agents, 516d
Hemothorax, 694
in chest tube drainage, 577
in total parenteral nutrition, 987, 988
Heparin, 385t
acquired hypoprothrombinemia and, 517
endogenous, 432
for pulmonary embolism, 682
for stroke, 807
for venous thrombosis, 385, 385t, 682
for prophylaxis, 682
in hemodialysis, 1404
therapeutic monitoring for, 208–209
Hepatic. See also Liver.
Hepatic abscess, 1179
Hepatic adenoma, 1194
Hepatic artery, 1135, 1136
Hepatic artery infusion, in chemotherapy, 1195
Hepatic carcinoma, 1194, 1195–1196
alpha-fetoprotein in, 1162t, 1164
portal hypertension in, 1141–1149
Hepatic cirrhosis. See Cirrhosis.
Hepatic disorders, 1169–1198
altered protein metabolism in, 1137
anorexia in, 1139t, 1153–1154, 1154t, 1156c
ascites in, 1139t, 1141–1149, 1155c–1156c
assessment in, 1154–1160
blood studies in, 1160–1164, 1161t
clinical manifestations of, 1139t, 1139–1154
clotting disorders in, 1149
computed tomography in, 1163t

Hepatic disorders (Continued)
diagnostic studies in, 1160–1165
nursing process in, 1164–1165
diet in, 1153–1154
encephalopathy in, 1139t, 1149–1153, 1157c–1158c
endoscopy in, 1163t
esophagoscopy in, 1163t
glucose intolerance in, 1137
history in, 1154–1158
hyperammonemia in, 1137
hypoglycemia in, 1137
in elderly, 1165–1166, 1198
infectious and inflammatory, 1169–1179
Internet connections for, 1176
jaundice in, 1139t, 1139–1141, 1156c–1157c
liver biopsy in, 1164, 1165t
liver enzyme studies in, 1160–1161, 1161t
liver scan in, 1163t
liver transplant for, 1196–1198
magnetic resonance imaging in, 1163t
neoplastic, 1194–1196
nutritional deficiencies in, 1139t, 1153–1154, 1154t, 1156c
peritoneoscopy in, 1163t
physical examination in, 1158–1160
prevention of, 1159c
resources for, 2041
skin care in, 1156c–1157c
steatorrhea in, 1138
structural, 1180–1193
traumatic, 1193–1194
ultrasonography in, 1163t
varicose veins in, 389
Hepatic ducts, 1136, 1136
x-ray studies of, 972
Hepatic encephalopathy, 1139t, 1149–1153, 1157c–1158c
in cirrhosis, 1182t, 1192c–1193c
Hepatic enzymes, age-related decrease in, 1165–1166
assessment of, 1160–1161, 1161t
Hepatic function, 1136–1139
age-related changes in, 1165–1166
as cardiac risk factor, 122
assessment of, 1154–1160
in shock, 408
Hepatic function(s), bile production and bilirubin conjugation as, 1137t, 1137–1138
blood filtration as, 1137t, 1138
carbohydrate metabolism as, 1136–1137, 1137t
detoxification as, 1137t, 1138–1139
lipid metabolism as, 1137, 1137t
protein metabolism as, 1137, 1137t
storage, 1137t, 1139
Hepatic lobules, 1135, 1136
Hepatic metabolism, assessment of, 1162t
Hepatic toxins, 1177t, 1177–1178
Hepatic transplant, 1196–1198
Hepatic tremor, 1150
Hepatic vein, 1135, 1136
Hepatitis, 1169–1179
drug-induced, 1177t, 1177–1179, 1178t
in elderly, 1198
Internet connections for, 1176
postnecrotic cirrhosis and, 1181
toxic, 1177t, 1177–1179, 1178t
viral, 1169–1177
assessment in, 1176
chronic, 1171, 1171t, 1174–1175

Hepatitis *(Continued)*
   clinical manifestations of, 1172, 1173t
   complications of, 1174–1176
   diagnosis of, 1172–1173, 1173t, 1174t
   etiology of, 1169–1172, 1171t
   fulminant, 1176
   icteric phase of, 1172, 1173t
   immunization for, 1173–1174, 1175d
   incubation period for, 1172
   infection precautions for, 1176
   jaundice in, 1172, 1173t
   management of, 1174
     settings and providers for, 1176
   markers of, 1173, 1174t
   nursing diagnoses and planning in, 1176
   nursing interventions in, 1177
   pathophysiology of, 1169–1172, 1171t
   posticteric phase of, 1172, 1173t
   post-transfusion, 1171, 1171t
   preicteric phase of, 1172, 1173t
   prevention of, 1173–1174, 1175d, 1176, 1177
   recurrence of, 1174–1175
Hepatitis A, prevention of, 1159c
Hepatitis A virus, 1169, 1170t
Hepatitis B, immunization for, 1159c, 1447
   prevention of, 1159c
Hepatitis B vaccine, 1174
   for elderly, 1175d
Hepatitis B virus, 1169–1170, 1170t
Hepatitis C, immunization for, 1159c
Hepatitis C virus, 1170t, 1171
Hepatitis D virus, 1170t, 1170–1171
Hepatitis E virus, 1171t, 1172
Hepatitis G virus, 1171–1172
Hepatocellular carcinoma, 1194, 1195–1196
   alpha-fetoprotein in, 1162t, 1164
   portal hypertension in, 1141–1149
Hepatocellular jaundice, 1140
Hepatocytes, 1135
   necrosis of, in hepatitis, 1169
Hepatomegaly, in heart disease, 184
   in heart failure, 271
   in hematologic disorders, 441
   in infectious mononucleosis, 513
Hepatotoxic drugs, 1177, 1178t
Hereditary spherocytosis, 482–484
Hernia, femoral, 1093–1096, *1094*
   examination for, 1701
   hiatus, 1033–1044
   inguinal, 1093–1096, *1094*
     examination for, 1701, *1702*
   intestinal, 1093–1096, *1094*
     incarcerated, 1094
     strangulated, 1094
Herniorrhaphy, 1094–1096, 1096d
Herpes genitalis, 1889–1908
   assessment in, 1905
   cervical cancer and, 1903
   clinical manifestations of, 1900–1903
   coping in, 1907–1908
   course of, 1904t
   diagnosis of, 1903
   etiology and pathophysiology of, 1889–1900
   in pregnancy, 1902–1903
   latent infection in, 1900–1901
   management of, 1903, 1904t
   nursing diagnoses and planning in, 1905–1906
   nursing interventions in, 1906–1908
   patient teaching in, 1906, 1906d, 1907d
   prevention of, 1906, 1907d

Herpes genitalis *(Continued)*
   primary infection in, 1900–1903, 1904t
   recurrent, 1900–1901, 1902, 1904t
   self-care in, 1906d, 1906–1907
   support groups for, 1907–1908
   transmission of, 1900
Herpes labialis, 1017–1019, 1018t, *1605*, 1605–1606
Herpes simplex encephalitis, 770
   nursing process in, 771–773
Herpes simplex keratitis, 1965–1967
Herpes simplex virus, type 1, 1605, 1889–1900
   type 2, 1605, 1889–1900
Herpes simplex virus infection, 1605–1606
   acyclovir for, 1581
   genital, 1889–1908. See also *Herpes genitalis.*
   lesion arrangement in, 1573
   neonatal, 1902–1903
   of lip, 1017–1019, 1018t, *1605*, 1605–1606
Herpes zoster, *1606*, 1606–1607
Heterograft, skin, 1588–1590
   for burns, 1673–1678, *1675*, 1675t
Hexachlorophene (pHisoHex), 1581
Hiatus hernia, 1033–1044, *1042*
   in elderly, 1059
Hibiclens (chlorhexidine gluconate), 1581
Hiccups, postoperative, 149t
Hickman catheter, in total parenteral nutrition, 993
High-calcium diet, urinary calculi and, 1367, 1367d, 1378
High-density lipoproteins (HDL), heart disease and, 186, 209
High-fiber diet, in diverticular disease, 1083, 1084d
High-protein diet, in fluid volume excess, 80
Hilus, renal, 1329
Hinduism, beliefs and practices of, in death and dying, 35t
Hip fractures, 885, 924–927
   case study of, 928d–929d
   clinical pathway for, 926d
   home care in, 925d, 927
Hip replacement, 867–868, *868*, 869c–872c
Hip spica cast, *855*. See also *Cast(s).*
Hispanics. See also *Racial/ethnic groups.*
Histamine, gastric secretion of, 952, 953t
   vasodilation and, 329t
Histamine H$_2$-receptor antagonists, 1022d
   for acute gastritis, 1024
   for peptic ulcers, 1024
History, diet, 968
   gynecologic, 1887t
   reproductive, 1887t
   sexual, female, 1778
     male, 1700
History taking, 8
HIV. See *Human immunodeficiency virus (HIV); Human immunodeficiency virus (HIV) infection.*
HIV-1–associated cognitive/motor complex, 1466, 1478c–1479c
Hives, drug-related, 1612
Hoarseness, in laryngitis, 608–610, *609*
Hodge pessary, for uterine retrodisplacement, 1820
Hodgkin's disease, 503t, 503–507
   nursing care guide for, 509c–511c
Holding area, 133
Holistic health paradigm, 13
Holter monitor, 197

Homan's sign, 384, 683
Home, modifications in, for allergies, 1486, 1486d
Home assessment, for elderly, 944
Home care, 22–23
   enteral nutrition in, 986
   for allergies, 1486, 1486d
   for amyotrophic lateral sclerosis, 776
   for cancer, 1561
   for hip fractures, 925d, 927
   for HIV infection, 1471
   for neurologic disorders, 765
   for respiratory disorders, 587
   for rheumatoid arthritis, 894
   for stroke, 808
   for tuberculosis, preventive measures in, 656d
   mechanical ventilation in, 572d–573d
   Medicare coverage for, 27t
   total parenteral nutrition in, *990*, 990–993, 991d–993d
   transtracheal oxygen therapy in, *557*, 557–559, 558d
Home care aides, supervision of, 26
Home health aide, qualifications and responsibilities of, 24t
Home health nurse, 27
Home maintenance, after cataract surgery, 1978
Homeless persons, self-care planning for, 394–395
Homelessness, 19
Homografts, cardiac valve, 313
   skin, 1588–1590
     for burns, 1673–1678, *1675*, 1675t
Homonymous hemianopia, 1940t
Hopelessness, cancer and, 1510–1511
   in amyotrophic lateral sclerosis, 777
Hordeolum, 1968t, 1970d
Hormone(s), adrenal, 1214–1216, *1215*
   age-related changes in, 68–69
   blood flow and, 329, 329t
   hypersecretion of, 1216–1217
   hyposecretion of, 1217
   hypothalamic, 1208–1209, 1209t
   in chemotherapy, 1524t, 1525
   negative feedback control of, 1204, 1208, *1208*, 1210, *1210*
   parathyroid, 1212–1213, *1213*
   pituitary, 1209–1210, 1210t
   regulation of, 1204, 1208, *1208*, 1210, *1210*
   thyroid, *1211*, 1211–1212, 1212t
   tropic, 1209
Hormone receptors, 1203–1204
   cell membrane, 1203–1204, *1208*
   intracellular, 1204, *1208*
Hormone replacement therapy, after hysterectomy, 1795
   for endometriosis, 1813, 1814d
   for menopause, 1772d, 1772–1773
Hormone therapy, for breast cancer, 1874
   for endometriosis, 1813, 1814d
   for fibrocystic breast disease, 1854, 1855
   for osteoporosis, 905
   for prostate cancer, 1759
   topical, for atrophic vaginitis, 1806
Horner's syndrome, 824t
Hornet stings, 1621–1622, 1622d
Hose, compression, 388, 389d, 390
Hospice care, 23
   in cancer, 1561
   in HIV infection, 1471
Hospice nurse, 27

Hospital-acquired pneumonia, 641. See also *Pneumonia.*
  case study of, 928d–929d
  prevention of, 642d
Hospitals, shift away from, 17–21
Hot flashes, 1771
Housemaid's knee, 902
Huffing, postoperative, 585
Human chorionic gonadotropin, in testicular cancer, 1704
Human immunodeficiency virus (HIV), host response to, 1459–1461, *1461*
  life cycle of, 1460, *1460, 1461*
  pain management in, 1475c–1476c
  transmission of, 1461–1464
Human immunodeficiency virus (HIV) infection, 19–20, 1459–1473. See also *Acquired immunodeficiency syndrome (AIDS).*
  acute retroviral infection in, 1464–1465, 1465t
  antibody tests for, 1467
  assessment in, 1471–1472
  asymptomatic, 1465, 1465t
  CD4+ cells in, 1460, 1465, 1465t
    disease progression and, 1465t, 1465–1466, 1467
    in diagnosis, 1467, 1468t
  CDC classification of, 1468t
  clinical manifestations of, 1465–1467
    requiring immediate evaluation, 1483d
  complementary therapies in, 1471
  diagnosis of, 1467
  drug therapy for, 1469–1470
  emotional aspects of, 1472, 1479c–1481c
  etiology of, 1459
  gastrointestinal disorders in, 1465, 1466, 1473c, 1477c–1478c
  gynecologic complications in, 1467
  HIV-1–associated cognitive/motor complex in, 1466, 1478c–1479c
  immune response in, 1460–1461, *1461*
  in health care workers, prevention of, 1464, 1472d
  incidence of, 1459
  Internet connections for, 1498d
  latent, 1465, 1465t
  life expectancy in, 1470–1471
  lymphadenopathy in, 1465
  management of, settings and providers in, 1471
  molluscum contagiosum in, 1605
  neurologic complications in, 1466, 1478c–1479c
  nurses' attitudes toward, 1470d
  nursing care in, 1471–1473, 1474c–1482c
  nutrition in, 1470, 1472–1473, 1477c–1478c
  ocular complications in, 1466–1467
  opportunistic infections in, 1466, 1467, 1470, 1476c–1477c
    prevention of, 1464, 1472d, 1476c–1477c
  oral care in, 1465, 1473d, 1478c
  oral lesions in, 1465, 1473d
  pathophysiology of, 1459–1461, *1460, 1461*
  resources for, 2041
  respiratory complications in, 1466, *1467*
  risk reduction for, 1464, 1472d
  self-care in, 1472, 1474c–1475c
  skin lesions in, 1466, *1466*
  social isolation in, 1472, 1479c–1480c
  social services for, 1471

Human immunodeficiency virus (HIV) infection *(Continued)*
  stages of, 1464–1467, 1465t
  symptomatic, 1465t, 1465–1467
  syphilis and, 1917
  transmission of, 1461–1464
  tuberculosis in, 650, 652, 654
  viral load tests for, 1467–1468
Human papillomavirus, condylomata acuminata and, 1926
Human papillomavirus infection, cervical cancer and, 1830
  in HIV infection, 1467
  warts and, 1603
Humoral immunity, 1434
Hungry bone syndrome, 1321
Hyaline cartilage, 842, 843
Hydralazine (Apresoline), 213, 378t, 380t
Hydrocele, 1741–1743, *1742*
Hydrocelectomy, 1708t, 1742–1743, 1743d
Hydrocephalus, 802–804, *803*
Hydrochlorothiazide, 377t
  for heart disease, 216, 217d, 218d
Hydrocortisone (Cortef), 1215
  for Addison's disease, 1280
  for asthma, 661, 662t, 663t
  for seborrheic dermatitis, 1611
HydroDIURIL. See *Hydrochlorothiazide.*
Hydroflumethiazide (Saluron), 377t
Hydrogen breath test, 1080
Hydrogen ion concentration, *102,* 102–103. See also *pH.*
Hydronephrosis, 1378, *1378*
  in ureteropelvic junction obstruction, 1380
Hydrostatic pulmonary edema, 270, 280
Hydrotherapy, for burns, 1672–1673
Hydrothorax, in total parenteral nutrition, 987, 988
Hydroureter, 1378, *1378*
17-Hydroxycorticosteroids, measurement of, 1280t
Hygiene, in unconscious client, 729
  oral. See *Oral care.*
    penile, 1702, 1728, 1729d
    pulmonary. See *Pulmonary hygiene.*
    vulvovaginal, patient teaching for, 1805d, 1807d
Hygroton (chlorthalidone), 377t
Hylorel (guanadrel), 378t
Hymen, 1766, *1766*
Hymenoptera stings, 1621–1622, 1622d
Hyperalimentation. See *Total parenteral nutrition.*
Hyperammonemia, bowel cleansing for, 1150, 1151d
  hepatic encephalopathy and, 1149–1150, 1157c–1158c
  in liver disease, 1137
Hyperbilirubinemia, in anemia, 469
Hypercalcemia, 94, 97–99
  clinical manifestations of, 98, 1318
  diagnosis of, 98
  etiology of, 97
  hypomagnesemia and, 99
  iatrogenic, in hypoparathyroidism, 1318
  in acute renal failure, 1390t
  in elderly, 1324
  in hyperparathyroidism, 1320
  in multiple myeloma, 508, 512
  management of, 99
  pathophysiology of, 97
Hypercalcemic crisis, 98, 1320
  treatment of, 1321, 1322

Hypercapnia, 530, 542
  in chronic obstructive pulmonary disease, 668, 669t, 675
  in mechanical ventilation, 570
  in respiratory acidosis, 109
Hypercholesterolemia. See also *Hyperlipidemia.*
  definition of, 284
  xanthelasma in, 1961
Hypercortisolism, 1285–1289. See also *Cushing's disease.*
  in elderly, 1323
Hyperemia, reactive, 1623–1624, *1628*
Hypereosinophilic syndrome, obliterative cardiomyopathy in, 306
Hyperextension injuries, of spinal cord, 822–823, *823,* 824t
Hyperflexion injuries, of spinal cord, 822, *822,* 824t
Hyperglycemia, 1224–1225
  diabetic, 1241, 1246c, 1249–1250, 1251t. See also *Diabetic ketoacidosis.*
  in dawn phenomenon, 1251
  in Somogyi phenomenon, 1250–1251
  management of, 1249
  monitoring for, 1241–1243, *1242,* 1242d
  pathogenesis of, 1227
  in enteral nutrition, 984
  in total parenteral nutrition, 987, 992d–993d
  lipolysis and, 1224–1225
Hyperglycemic hyperosmolar nonketotic syndrome, 1248t, 1249–1250
Hyperkalemia, 84, 89–91
  cardiac function and, 208
  in acute renal failure, 1390t
  in burn shock, 1660–1661
  in elderly, 112
  in metabolic acidosis, 104, 105
Hyperlipidemia, coronary artery disease and, 280–285
  definition of, 284
  drug therapy for, 216–217, 218d, 284
  heart disease and, 186, 210
  vascular disease and, 338t
Hypermagnesemia, 99, 101–102
Hypernatremia, 91, 93–94
  in acute renal failure, 1390t
  in burn shock, 1662
Hyperopia, 1970–1974, *1971*
  assessment for, 1941–1942
  contact lenses for, 1971–1972, 1972d–1973d, 1974
  in elderly, 60, 1961
Hyperosmolar fluid volume deficit, 75–79, 77t
Hyperosmolar nonketotic syndrome, in total parenteral nutrition, 992d–993d
Hyperosmotics, for glaucoma, 1980
Hyperparathyroidism, 1318–1322
  assessment in, 1321
  clinical manifestations of, 1320
  diagnosis of, 1320–1321
  etiology of, 1318–1319
  in elderly, 1324
  nursing diagnoses and planning in, 1321
  nursing interventions in, 1321–1322
  pathophysiology of, 1319
  primary, 1320
  secondary, 1320
Hyperpigmentation, chemotherapy and, 1530, 1539t–1540t
  generalized, 1570

Hyperpigmentation (Continued)
  in Addison's disease, 1278, *1278*
  in Cushing's syndrome, 1286
  of lesions, 1570–1571
Hyperpituitarism, acromegaly and, 1269–1274, *1273*
  gigantism and, 1272–1274
  in elderly, 1322–1323
  pituitary adenoma and, 1265–1269, *1267, 1270c–1272c*
Hyperpnea, 532
Hyperresonance, on percussion, 536
Hypersensitive carotid sinus syncope, 176
Hypersensitivity, anaphylaxis in, 417t, 417–418
  anergy in, 1489
  vs. allergy, 1483
Hypersensitivity disorders, 1473–1490. See also *Allergy(ies)*.
  Internet connections for, 1498d
Hypersensitivity pneumonitis, 1488t, 1488–1489
Hypersensitivity reactions, cell-mediated (Type IV), 1489–1490, 1490t
  cytotoxic (Type II), 1486, 1490t
  immediate (Type I), 1483–1486, 1490t
  immune complex (Type III), 1486–1489, 1490t
  skin tests for, 1489
Hypersplenism, 463
  splenectomy for, 463–464
Hyperstat (diazoxide), 213, 378t, 380t
Hypertension, 372–384
  abdominal aortic aneurysm and, 367, 370d
  assessment in, 376–381
  atherosclerosis and, 338t, 373, 373t, 375
  clinical definition of, 64
  clinical manifestations of, 375
  complications in, 376
  definition of, 177
  diagnosis of, 375
  diastolic, 177
  diet in, 382d, 382–383
  electrolytes and, 100d
  etiology and pathophysiology of, *373*, 373t, 373–375, *374*
  heart disease and, 177–178, 186, *374*, 374–375
  hypertensive crisis in, 376, 380t
  in autonomic dysreflexia, 825
  in chronic renal failure, 1399, 1399t, 1400
  in diabetic nephropathy, 1254–1255
  in elderly, 64, 230
  in heart disease, 177–178
  in primary aldosteronism, 1289, 1291
  incidence of, 372–373
  Internet connections for, 361d
  intracranial, 730–738. See also *Increased intracranial pressure (ICP)*.
  intraocular. See *Intraocular pressure, increased*.
  malignant, 373, 375
    pheochromocytoma and, 1292, 1294
  management of, 375–376, 376t–380t, 379d
    behavior modification in, 383d, 384
    noncompliance in, 375–376, 383d, 384
    settings and providers for, 376
    stepped-care guidelines for, 382d
  nursing diagnoses and planning in, 381
  nursing interventions for, 381–384
  pheochromocytoma and, 1292, 1294

Hypertension (Continued)
  portal, 1139t, 1141–1149. See also *Portal hypertension*.
  postoperative, in cardiac surgery, 222
  primary, 373
    benign, 373
  pulmonary, 685–686
    in chronic obstructive pulmonary disease, 668
  secondary, 373
  stages of, 372t
  systolic, 177, 372
  target organ effects in, 374, *374*
  vascular disease and, 338t, 373, 373t
Hypertensive crisis, 376, 380t
Hyperthermia, for benign prostatic hyperplasia, 1754
  in hyperthyroidism, 1308, 1313, 1314
  malignant, 142
Hyperthyroidism, 1306–1314
  case study of, 1311d–1312d
  clinical manifestations of, *1307*, 1307–1308, *1308*
  etiology of, 1307
  in elderly, 1323
  nursing diagnoses and planning in, 1312
  nursing interventions in, 1312–1314
  pathophysiology of, 1307
Hypertonic fluid volume deficit, 75–79, 77t
Hypertrophic cardiomyopathy, *304*, 305–306
Hyperuricemia, in gout, 899
Hyperventilation, 532, *533*, 542
  for increased intracranial pressure, 732
  hypocapnia and, 542
  hypocarbia and, 530
  in increased intracranial pressure, 734
  respiratory alkalosis and, 111, 543
Hypervolemia, after prostatectomy, 1713, 1718–1719
  as surgical risk factor, 121
  from extracellular fluid volume excess, 79–81, *80*
  from intracellular fluid volume excess, 82–84, 83t, *83t*
  from third-space shift, 81t, 81–82
  management of. See *Fluid management*.
  transfusion-related, 462
Hyphema, 1987–1989
Hypoalbuminemia, in portal hypertension, 1142
Hypocalcemia, 94–97
  clinical manifestations of, 95–96, 1077t, 1316, 1317
  etiology of, 95
  hypomagnesemia and, 99
  hypoparathyroidism and, 1316–1318
  in acute renal failure, 1390t
  in elderly, 1324
  management of, 96, 1317
  nursing interventions in, 96–97, 1318
  pathophysiology of, 95
  postgastrectomy, 998t
  tetany in. See *Tetany*.
Hypocapnia, 530, 542
  in mechanical ventilation, 570
Hypochloremia, in metabolic alkalosis, 107
Hypogeusia, in chemotherapy, 1530
  in radiation therapy, 1521
Hypoglossal nerve, 724t
Hypoglycemia, diabetic, 1241, 1245c, 1250, 1251t
  in Somogyi phenomenon, 1250–1251

Hypoglycemia (Continued)
  monitoring for, 1241–1243, *1242*, 1242d
    with insulin pump, 1238
  in insulin reaction, 1250, 1259
  in liver disease, 1137
  in total parenteral nutrition, 987–988
  postprandial, postgastrectomy, 998t
Hypoglycemics, oral, in elderly, 54t
Hypokalemia, 84–89
  cardiac function and, 208
  clinical manifestations of, 86, 1077t
  diagnosis of, 86
  etiology of, 84–85
  hepatic encephalopathy and, 1150
  in acute renal failure, 1390t
  in diabetic ketoacidosis, 1249, 1259
  in primary aldosteronism, 1289, 1291
  management of, 86, 87d, 88d
  metabolic alkalosis and, 106
  nursing process in, 86–89
  pathophysiology of, 84–85
  vitamin B_{12} therapy and, 478
  with hypomagnesemia, 86
Hypolipemic drugs, 343d
Hypomagnesemia, 99–101
  clinical manifestations of, 1077t
  hypoparathyroidism and, 1316
  with hypokalemia, 86
Hyponatremia, 91–93
  after prostatectomy, 1712
  clinical manifestations of, 1077t
  in acute renal failure, 1390t
  in burn shock, 1660–1661, 1662
  in elderly, 112–113
Hypoparathyroidism, 1316–1318, 1322
  hypocalcemia and, 95, 1316–1318, 1319c
  in elderly, 1324
  nursing care guide for, 1319c
Hypophosphatemia, clinical manifestations of, 1077t
  in hyperparathyroidism, 1320
Hypophysis. See *Pituitary* entries.
Hypopigmentation, in tinea versicolor, 1603
Hypopituitarism, 1274
  in elderly, 1322–1323
Hypoproliferative anemia, 467, 472–482. See also *Anemia*.
Hypoprothrombinemia, acquired, 517
Hypospadias, meatal stenosis and, 1386
Hypotension, causes of, 178
  definition of, 177
  in diabetes, 1259
  in elderly, 64–65, 71c
  in fluid volume deficit, 77, 78
  in heart disease, 177–178
  in shock, 406, 407t
  orthostatic (postural), 178
    in elderly, 64–65, 71c
    injury prevention in, 71c
  postoperative, in cardiac surgery, 222
Hypothalamic disorders, hypothyroidism in, 1297, 1298–1301, 1301t
Hypothalamic hormones, 1206t, 1208, *1208*, 1208–1209, 1209t
Hypothalamus, 720
  negative feedback control by, 1208, *1208*, 1210, *1210*
  structure and function of, 1205t, *1208*, 1208–1209, 1209t
Hypothermia, after cardiopulmonary bypass, 221, 225, 227

Hypothermia *(Continued)*
  for increased intracranial pressure, 733,
    736
  in anesthesia, 140
  scalp, in chemotherapy, 1530
Hypothyroidism, 1297–1306
  assessment in, 1301, 1310–1312
  clinical manifestations of, 1297–1298,
    1298
  cretinism and, 1297
  diagnosis of, 1298, 1299t–1301t
  etiology of, 1297, 1297t
  granulomatous hyperthyroidism and,
    1296
  Hashimoto's thyroiditis and, 1296, 1297
  iatrogenic, 1297
  in elderly, 1323
  juvenile, 1297
  management of, 1298–1301
  nursing care guide for, 1303c–1305c
  nursing diagnoses and planning in, 1302
  nursing interventions in, 1302–1306
  pathogenesis of, 1297
  secondary, 1297, 1301t
  tertiary, 1297, 1301t
Hypoventilation, 532, *533*
  hypercapnia and, 542
  metabolic alkalosis and, 107, 108
  respiratory acidosis and, 108, 109, 110,
    543
Hypovolemia, 75–79, 77t, 79–81, *80*
  absolute, 408
  as surgical risk factor, 121
  from extracellular fluid deficit, 75–79,
    77t
  from third-space shift, 81t, 81–82
  hypernatremia and, 93–94
  in burns, 1660–1664, *1661*
  in electrical injury, 1689–1690
  in intestinal obstruction, 1074, 1075
  relative, 408
Hypovolemic shock, 408t, 408–411, *409*,
    419. See also *Shock.*
  in musculoskeletal injuries, 932
Hypoxemia, 529–530
  clinical manifestations of, 1147
  cyanosis and, 181–182
  in chronic obstructive pulmonary dis-
    ease, 668, 675
  in respiratory acidosis, 108, 109, 110
  oxygenation failure and, 531
Hypoxia, 529–530
  cerebral, 530
    in carbon monoxide poisoning, 1656
  in mechanical ventilation, 570
Hysterectomy, 1793–1800
  abdominal, 1794
  clinical pathway for, 1796d–1797d
  complications of, 1795–1797
  for cancer, 1831
  for endometriosis, 1814
  for genital prolapse, 1818
  for leiomyomas, 1824
  for ovarian cancer, 1837
  for uterine cancer, 1836
  genital fistulas after, 1795, *1821*, 1821–
    1822
  patient teaching for, postoperative,
    1799–1800, 1800d
    preoperative, 1797
  postoperative care in, 1798–1800
  postoperative course in, 1795
  preoperative care in, 1797
  preoperative preparation for, 1794–1795

Hysterectomy *(Continued)*
  radical, 1793, *1794*
  total, 1793, *1794*
  types of, 1793–1794, *1794*
  vaginal, 1794
  vaginal packing in, 1800
  with bilateral oophorectomy, 1793–1794,
    1794
  with bilateral salpingo-oophorectomy,
    1793, *1794*
Hysterosalpingography, 1785
Hysteroscopy, 1785

I

Ibuprofen (Motrin), 893d
Ichthyosis, 1572
ICP. See *Increased intracranial pressure
  (ICP).*
Icterus. See *Jaundice.*
Idiopathic hemolytic anemia, 1495–1496
Idiopathic postmenopausal osteoporosis,
  905
Idiopathic thrombocytopenic purpura,
  513–515
I:E ratio, in chronic obstructive pulmonary
  disease (COPD), 675–676
IgA, 1438t, 1439
  deficiency of, 1458
IgD, 1438t, 1439
IgE, 1438t, 1439
  in allergic reaction, 1483
IgG, 1438t, 1439
IgG autoantibodies, hyperthyroidism and,
  1307
IgM, 1438t, 1439
Ileal conduit, 1421, *1421*
Ileal pouch–anal canal anastomosis, 1012,
  1012
Ileocecal valve, 956
Ileostomy, 1011–1015
  Brook's, 1011
  complications of, 1013, 1014d
  continent, 1012, *1013*
  end, 1011
  fecal output from, 1012–1013, 1015
  loop, 1011–1012
  patient preparation for, 1011
  postoperative care for, 1014–1015
  postoperative course in, 1012–1013
  preoperative care for, 1013–1014
  procedure for, 1011–1012, *1012*
  self-care in, 1014d
  uses of, 1011
Ileum, *955*, 955–956
Ileus, mechanical, 1074–1075, *1075*
  paralytic. See *Paralytic ileus.*
Iliac artery occlusion, 363–365
Iliac lymphadenectomy, 1708t
Ilosone. See *Erythromycin.*
Imagery, in pain management, 1555
Imipramine (Tofranil), for retrograde ejaculation, 1699
Immediate (Type I) hypersensitivity, 1483–
  1486, 1490t
Immobility, 843–846
  assessment in, 843–844
  cast therapy and, 858
  in musculoskeletal disorders, 843–846
  in rheumatoid arthritis, 895
  in traction, 862
  infection prevention in, 845
  nursing diagnoses and planning in, 844
  nursing interventions in, 844–846

Immobility *(Continued)*
  self-care in, 845–846
  skin care in, 845
  traction and, 858–863
Immobilization, in pain management, 1556
  in spinal cord injury, 824, 825, 826
  of fractures, 918
Immobilizer, knee, *914*, 916
Immune complex (Type III) hypersensitivity reaction, 1486–1489, 1490t
Immune disorders. See also *Autoimmune
  disorders.*
  defective opsonization in, 1437
  defective phagocytosis in, 1437–1438
  diagnosis of, 1443–1447
    agglutination in, 1445
    allergy testing in, *1446*, 1446–1447
    bone marrow aspiration and biopsy
      in, 1443–1445
    complement fixation test in, 1445–
      1446
    electrophoresis in, 1445
    genetic testing in, 1446
    immunofluorescence in, 1445
    laboratory tests in, 1445–1447
    radioimmunoassay in, 1445
  history in, 1442
  hypersensitivity. See *Allergy(ies); Hyper-
    sensitivity.*
  immunodeficiency, 1457–1482. See also
    Immunodeficiency disorders.
  in elderly, 1455, 1499–1500
  Internet connections for, 1498d
  management of, 1447–1455
  physical examination in, 1442–1443
  resources for, 2041–2043
  risk reduction for, 1443d
Immune hemolytic anemia, 488–489
  transfusion reaction and, 462, 483, 488–
    489
Immune response, age-related changes in,
  1455
  cellular, 1433–1434, 1434t, 1439
  nonspecific, 1434, 1434t, 1435–1438
    chemical barriers in, 1435
    inflammation in, 1435, *1436*
    interferon in, 1435
    opsonization in, 1437, 1439
      defects in, 1437
    phagocytosis in, 1435–1437, *1437*
      defects in, 1437–1438
    physical barriers in, 1435
  specific, 1434t, 1434–1435, 1438–1441
    antibodies in, 1438t, 1438–1439
    antigens in, 1438
    cellular, 1439
    complement in, 1439–1441, 1440t
    humoral, 1438–1439
    primary, 1439, *1440*
    secondary, 1439, *1440*
Immune serum globulin, for hepatitis A,
  1173–1174
  for hepatitis B, 1174
  transfusion of, 457. See also *Transfu-
    sion(s).*
Immune system, 1429–1445
  age-related changes in, 1455
  cells of, *1432*, 1432–1433, 1433t
  defensive functions of, 1429, 1430t
  diversity in, 1429
  health promotion for, 1443d
  homeostatic functions of, 1429, 1430t
  memory in, 1429
  self vs. nonself recognition in, 1429

Immune system *(Continued)*
  specificity in, 1429
  structure and function of, *1430,* 1430t,
    1430–1442
  surveillance functions of, 1429, 1430t
Immunity, acquired (adaptive), 1429, 1430,
    1441t, 1441–1442
  active, 1441
  cellular, 1433–1434, 1434t, 1439
  humoral, 1434
  innate, 1429, 1441t, 1441–1442
  nonspecific, 1434, 1434t
  passive, 1441
  types of, 1441–1442
Immunization, 1447
  artificially acquired active immunity
    and, 1441
  hepatitis A, 1159c, 1173–1174, 1175d
  hepatitis B, 1159c, 1174, 1175d
  influenza, 646, 649
  pneumococcal, 646
Immunodeficiency. See also *Immune disor-
    ders.*
  definition of, 1457
  primary, 1457–1458
  secondary, 1458–1459
  severe combined, 1458
Immunodeficiency disorders, 1457–1482
  clinical manifestations of, 1457, 1458,
    1459t
  diagnosis of, 1458–1459
  etiology of, 1458
  management of, 1459
  nursing care in, 1459
  pathophysiology of, 1458
Immunodepression, in hematologic disor-
    ders, 438–440
Immunofluorescence, 1445
Immunoglobulin(s), 428–429, 1438t, 1438–
    1439, *1439.* See also *Antibody(ies).*
Immunoglobulin A, deficiency of, 1458
Immunoglobulin E, in allergic reaction,
    1483
Immunologic disorders. See *Immune disor-
    ders.*
Immunologic function, in surgical patient,
    121
Immunologic procedures, reference values
    for, 2031
Immunologic surveillance theory, 1499
Immunosuppression, 1448–1449. See also
    Immune disorders; Immunodeficiency.
  antigen-specific, 1448
  disseminated zoster in, 1606
  in burns, 1458
  in cancer, 1458
  in HIV infection, 1460, 1465–1466
  in systemic disease, 1458
  opportunistic infections and, 1409, 1458,
    1459t
  therapeutic, antilymphocyte serum in,
    1448
    corticosteroids in, 1449
    cytotoxic drugs in, 1449
    for aplastic anemia, 480
    in heart transplant, 228–229
    in transplantation, 1409–1410
      cyclosporine for, 1197d
    infections and, 1409
    monoclonal antibodies in, 1448
    nonspecific, 1448
    pharmacologic, 1448–1449
    radiation in, 1449
    surgery in, 1449

Immunotherapy, for cancer, 1510
  intravesical, for bladder cancer, 1420
Impedance plethysmography, 340t
Impetigo, 1595–1599, *1596,* 1598t, 1599d
Implanted ports, for chemotherapy, 1527,
    1527, 1528
Implementation, in nursing process, 11–
    12
Impotence, 1698–1699, 1699t
  after prostatectomy, 1709t, 1713, 1715t,
    1719–1720, 1761
  in diabetes, 1254
  in elderly, 1725, 1761
  intracavernosal injection for, priapism
    and, 1740–1741
  penile implant for, 1720–1724, *1721,*
    1721t, 1724d
Incarcerated hernia, 1094
Incentive spirometry, 130–131, *131,* 538–
    539
Incision(s), abdominal, 993–995, 994t–
    995t
  splinting of, 130, *131*
    post-thoracotomy, 582, *583,* 585, 586
  suturing of, 1586–1587, *1587*
  thoracotomy, 580
Incision and drainage, of anorectal abscess,
    1072–1074
Incontinence, fecal, in colostomy client,
    1008–1009
  in unconscious client, 729
  stress, Kegel exercises for, 1365, 1365d
  urinary, 1336–1341, 1340t. See also *Uri-
    nary incontinence.*
Incontinence pads, 1339d
Increased intracranial pressure (ICP), 730–
    738
  assessment in, 733
  case study of, 735d–737d
  clinical manifestations of, 730
  diagnosis of, 730–731, *731*
  drug therapy for, 731–732, 732d
  etiology of, 730, 730t
  hydrocephalus and, 802–804, *803*
  hyperventilation in, 733, 734
  hypothermia in, 733, 736
  in intracranial hematoma, 820
  management of, 731–733
  nursing diagnoses and planning in, 733–
    734
  nursing interventions in, 734–738
  papilledema in, 828–829
  pathophysiology of, 730
  postoperative, 759, 761
    in transsphenoidal microsurgery,
      1268–1269, 1270c–1271c
  supportive measures in, 732–733
  surgery for, 733
Increased intraocular pressure, drug ther-
    apy for, 1947
  in glaucoma, 1978–1979
Incus, 1996, *1996,* 1997
Indapamide (Lozol), 377t
Inderal. See *Propranolol.*
Indomethacin, 893d
Indwelling catheters, 1361–1362, 1363
Infants, hepatitis B infection in, 1170
Infarction, pulmonary, abscess and, 647
Infection(s), bone, posttraumatic, 934
  cardiac, 233–240
  catheter, 1362, 1363
    in total parenteral nutrition, 987, 989
    prevention of, 987
  in agranulocytosis, 491, 492, 493

Infection(s) *(Continued)*
  in elderly, 1499–1500
  in hematologic disorders, 438–440
  in internal fixation, 865, 867
  in leukemia, 495, 497c–498c, 504d
  opportunistic, immunosuppression and,
    1409, 1458, 1459t
    in bone marrow transplant, 1451,
      1453, 1454d
    in HIV infection, 1466, 1467, 1470,
      1476c–1477c
      prevention of, 1464, 1472d, 1476c–
        1477c
  postoperative, in gynecologic surgery,
    1787
  prevention of, 1464, 1472d, 1476c–1477c
    after adrenalectomy, 1289
    in Addison's disease, 1284
    in radiation therapy, 1523d
    in sickle-cell anemia, 485
    patient teaching for, 440d
    standard precautions for, 439t
  shunt, 804
  surgical, prevention of, 143
  transfusion-related, 457, 458
  wound, postoperative, 147t, 153
Infectious mononucleosis, 512–513
Infective endocarditis, 233–236, 235d,
    236d
Inferior vena cava, filter in, 386
  in hepatic circulation, 1135–1136
Infertility, after retroperitoneal lymphade-
    nectomy, 1752
  chlamydial salpingitis and, 1921
  cryptorchidism and, 1739
  endometriosis and, 1813
  orchitis and, 1731
  varicocele and, 1743
Infiltrative dermopathy, in hyperthyroid-
    ism, 1307, *1307*
Infiltrative ophthalmopathy, in hyperthy-
    roidism, 1307, *1307,* 1308
  treatment of, 1308–1309
Inflammatory bowel disease, 1066–1071
  anorectal abscess in, 1071–1074, *1072*
  Crohn's disease in, 1066–1069
  ileostomy for, 1011–1015
  in elderly, 1106
  Internet connections for, 1068d
  ulcerative colitis in, 1069–1071
Inflammatory response, 1435, *1436*
  phagocytosis in, 1435–1437, *1436, 1437*
  defects in, 1437–1438
  plasma cells in, 1432, *1432,* 1433, 1433t
Influenza, 648–650
  immunization for, 646, 649, 1447
Information sources, 2037–2045
Informed consent, for surgery, 117–118
Infratentorial surgery, 757, 759t. See also
    Intracranial surgery.
Infundibulopelvic ligaments, 1768
Infusion pump, for chemotherapy, 1527,
    1528
  for narcotic analgesics, 152, *152*
Inguinal hernia, 1093–1096, *1094*
  examination for, 1701, *1702*
Inguinal lymph nodes, *435.* See also *Lymph
    nodes.*
Inguinal lymphadenectomy, in radical vul-
    vectomy, 1826–1830, 1829d
Inguinal orchiectomy, 1708t, 1749, 1750–
    1752
Inhalation anesthetics, I25, 139t. See also
    Anesthesia.

Inhalation injury, subglottic, 1657t, 1658
  supraglottic, 1657t, 1658
Inherited immunity, 1429, 1441t, 1441–
  1442
Injection, insulin, 1236d–1237d, *1237*
  nerve injury in, 827
Injuries. See *Trauma.*
Injury prevention. See *Safety measures.*
Innate immunity, 1429, 1430, 1441t, 1441–
  1442
Inner ear. See also under *Ear.*
  age-related changes in, 2009
  infection of, 2013–2014
  structure and function of, *1996*, 1996–
    1997
Inocor (amrinone), cardiac effects of, 405t
  for cardiogenic shock, 413
  for heart failure, 274
Inotropic agents, for heart failure, 272–274
Inotropy, 404
Insect stings, hypersensitivity to, 1483t,
  1621–1622, 1622d
Insomnia, in elderly, 64
  in menopause, 1771
Inspiratory capacity, 537–538, *538*, 539t
Inspiratory reserve volume, 537, *538*, 539t
Inspiratory-expiratory control, in chronic
    obstructive pulmonary disease
    (COPD), 675–676
Insulin, endogenous, 1206t, 1223–1224
  absence of, 1224–1225
  in carbohydrate metabolism, 1223–
    1224
  in fat metabolism, 1224
  in protein metabolism, 1224
  secretion of, 1224
  exogenous, administration of, by injec-
      tion, 1236d–1237d, *1237*
    by pump, 1237–1239, *1238*, *1239*
    frequency of, *1235*, 1235–1237
    intranasal, 1239
    oral, 1239, 1239t, 1240d
    patient teaching for, 1236d–1237d
  concentrations of, 1235
  for elderly, 1261
  in illness, 1240–1241
  in surgery, 1241
  preparation of, 1236d
  types of, 1234t, 1235
  for diabetic hyperglycemia, 1249
Insulin antagonists, 1224
Insulin mix, preparation of, 1236d
Insulin pump, 1237–1239, *1238*, *1239*
Insulin reaction, hypoglycemia in, 1250,
  1259
Insulin resistance, in type 2 diabetes, 1227,
  1228t
Insulin-dependent diabetes (type 1), 1227,
  1228t. See also *Diabetes mellitus.*
Insulin-requiring diabetes (type 2), 1227,
  1228t. See also *Diabetes mellitus.*
Intal (cromolyn), for asthma, 661, 662t,
  663t
Integumentary disorders. See also under
  Skin.
  Internet connections for, 1639d
  resources for, 2043
Intercostal spaces, 523
Interferon(s), exogenous, 1435
    for cancer, 1544
  in nonspecific immune response, 1435
Interferon beta-16 (Betaseron), for multiple
  sclerosis, 779
Interleukins, for cancer, 1544

Intermaxillary fixation, *1046*, 1046–1049,
  1049d
Intermittent calf compression, 682, *682*
Intermittent claudication, 332, *332*, 333–
  334
Intermittent positive-pressure breathing,
    567–568. See also *Mechanical ventila-
    tion.*
Intermittent self-catheterization, 1363,
  1364t
Intermittent skin traction, 860
Internal carotid artery, 714–715, *717*
  stenosis of, 807t
Internal fixation devices, *865*, 865–867,
  867d
  for hip fractures, 924, 926d, 928d–929d
Internal urethrotomy, 1386
  nursing care in, 1387–1388
International Normalized Ratio, 447–448
Internet connections, for Alzheimer's dis-
    ease, 779d
  for autoimmune disorders, 1498d
  for breast cancer, 1864d
  for burns, 1682d
  for cancer, 1547d
  for cardiac disorders, 287d
  for diabetes, 1258d
  for ear disorders, 2018
  for endocrine disorders, 1295d
  for endometriosis, 1815d
  for eye disorders, 1986
  for gallbladder disease, 1113d
  for glaucoma, 1986
  for gynecologic cancers, 1815d
  for hearing loss, 2018
  for hematologic disorders, 506d
  for hepatic disorders, 1176
  for human immunodeficiency virus
      (HIV) infection, 1498d
  for hypersensitivity disorders, 1498d
  for leukemia, 506d
  for lower gastrointestinal disorders,
    1068d
  for lower respiratory disorders, 665d
  for macular degeneration, 1986
  for male reproductive disorders, 1752d
  for Meniere's disease, 2018
  for multiple sclerosis, 779d
  for pancreatic cancer, 1113d
  for prostate disorders, 1752d
  for rheumatoid arthritis, 896d
  for seizure disorders, 779d
  for sexually transmitted diseases, 1922d
  for skin disorders, 1639d
  for upper gastrointestinal disorders,
    1056d
  for vascular disorders, 361d
Interstitial cells, testicular, 1696
Interstitium, 527
Intertrigo, *Candidiasis*, 1602
  fungal, in elderly, 1630
Interventricular groove, 165, 168
Intervertebral disc, 714, *715*
  herniation of, *752*, 792–795, *793*, 793t,
    794d
  pain in, 911–913
  straight-leg-raise test for, 912
  surgery for, 761–767, 763d
Intestinal adhesions, 1074, *1074*, 1084–1093
Intestinal decompression, in mechanical ileus, 1075
  in paralytic ileus, 1076
Intestinal gas, 961
Intestinal gastrin, 953, 953t

Intestinal hernias, 1093–1096, *1094*
Intestinal intubation, for adhesions, 1084
Intestinal ischemia, in elderly, 1106
Intestinal juice, 956, 958t
Intestinal obstruction, mechanical, 1074–
  1075
Intestinal resection, 1000–1015
  clinical pathway for, 1001d
  colostomy in, 1003–1011, *1004*, *1005*. See
    also *Colostomy.*
  ileostomy in, 1011–1015
  malabsorption in, 1077t, 1077–1078
  patient preparation for, 1000
  postoperative care in, 1002–1003, 1007–
    1011
  postoperative course in, 1001–1002
  preoperative care in, 1002
  procedure for, 1001
  uses of, 1000
Intestinal tube, for adhesions, 1084
Intestinal villi, *955*, 956
Intestinal volvulus, 1074, *1074*
Intra-aortic balloon counterpulsation, 229,
  414
  for cardiogenic shock, 413
Intra-arterial blood pressure monitoring,
  206, 206–207
Intracapsular cataract extraction, 1976
Intracavernosal injection, priapism and,
  1740–1741
Intracavitary radiation therapy, for cervical
    cancer, 1832–1836
  side effects of, 1833d, 1834
Intracellular fluid, 75, *76*
Intracellular fluid volume excess, 82–84,
  83t, *83t*
Intracerebral ventricular analgesia, 1555t
Intracranial hemorrhage, cerebrovascular
    accident and, 804, *805*. See also *Cere-
    brovascular accident (CVA).*
  subarachnoid, 814–816, *815*
Intracranial hypertension. See *Increased intracranial pressure (ICP).*
Intracranial pressure, increased, 730–738.
    See also *Increased intracranial pressure
    (ICP).*
  monitoring of, 730–731, *731*
  normal values for, 730
Intracranial surgery, 757–761
  complications of, 759
  for brain tumors, 829–830
  for seizures, 796
  infratentorial, 757, 759t
  nursing interventions in, 759–761
  patient preparation for, 758
  postoperative care in, 760–761
  postprocedure course in, 758–759
  preoperative care in, 759–760
  procedure for, 758, *758*
  stereotaxic, 830
  supratentorial, 757, 759t
  uses of, 758
Intradermal testing, *1446*, 1446–1447,
  1447
Intraductal papilloma, of breast, 1856–
  1857
Intramembranous ossification, 838–839
Intraocular foreign body, 1987–1989
  fluorescein staining of, 1945
Intraocular lens implant, after cataract extraction, 1976–1978
Intraocular pressure, increased, drug ther-
    apy for, 1947
  in glaucoma, 1978–1979

Intraocular pressure *(Continued)*
    normal values for, 1978
    measurement of, 1944–1945, *1945*
Intraoperative management, 134–143. See
    also *Surgery.*
    nursing activities in, 117t
Intraoperative period, elderly in, 159
    nursing process in, 142–143
Intrathecal analgesia, 1555t
Intravenous anesthetics, 140, 141t. See also
    Anesthesia.
Intravenous cholangiogram, 972
Intravenous drug abuse, HIV transmission
    and, 1463–1464
Intravenous hyperalimentation. See *Total
    parenteral nutrition.*
Intravenous infusion, for dehydration, 77–
    78
    in third-space shift, 82
    intracellular fluid volume excess and, 82,
    84
Intravenous opioids, 1554t
Intravenous pyelogram, 1346, 1347t, 1351
Intravenous urogram, 1346, 1347t, 1351
Intravesical chemotherapy, for bladder
    cancer, 1420
Intravesical immunotherapy, for bladder
    cancer, 1420
Intrinsic factor deficiency, in chronic gas-
    tritis, 1025
    pernicious anemia and, 476–479
    Schilling test for, 443t, 451, 478
Intropin (dopamine). See *Dopamine (Intro-
    pin).*
Intubation, chest. See *Chest tube drainage.*
    endotracheal, 559–564. See also *Endotra-
    cheal intubation.*
    gastrointestinal, 976–980
    intestinal, for adhesions, 1084
    nasogastric. See *Nasogastric intubation.*
Intussusception, 1074, *1074*
Inverse psoriasis, 1616–1619, 1617t
Iodine, deficiency of, goiter and, 1315
    dietary intake of, 1211
    for hyperthyroidism, 1309–1310, 1313
Iodine-131, for hyperthyroidism, 1309–
    1310, 1313
Iodine-131 uptake, 1300t
Iodipine (apraclonidine), for glaucoma,
    1980
Ipratropium bromide (Atrovent), for
    asthma, 661, 662t
Iris, *1936,* 1937
    examination of, 1942
    muscles of, 1936
Iris lesion, 1573
Iron, serum, assay for, 443t, 449–450
Iron deficiency, clinical manifestations of,
    1077t
    postgastrectomy, 998t
Iron deficiency anemia, 470d, 472–476,
    477d
Iron supplements, for iron deficiency ane-
    mia, 470d, 476, 477d
Irreducible hernia, 1094
Irrigation, bladder, 1362, 1364
    in prostatectomy, 1711–1712
    of chemical burns, 1649, 1687
    of eye, 1990t, 1990–1991
        for chemical burns, 1649, 1687
    of gastrointestinal tube, 980
    of pressure ulcers, 1630–1631
    perineal, in abdominal perineal resec-
        tion, 1105

Irritant contact dermatitis, 1609–1611, *1610*
Ischemia. See also *Venous insufficiency.*
    in atherosclerosis, 361
    myocardial, 175
        angina pectoris and, 175, 175t, 188,
            283, 285–291
        pain in, 331–334, 362
Ischemic neuropathy, 332, 333–334
Ischemic ulcers, 1622–1631. See also *Pres-
    sure ulcers.*
Islam, beliefs and practices of, in death
    and dying, 35t
Ismelin (guanethidine), 378t
Ismotic (isosorbide), 212d, 212–213
    for glaucoma, 1980
Isoenzymes, cardiac, *209,* 209–210, *210*
Isoflurane (Forane), 139, 139t
Isolation, hearing loss and, 2020
    in cancer, 1545–1546, 1550
    in hematologic disorders, 452
    in HIV infection, 1472, 1479c–1480c
    in tuberculosis, 652
    negative pressure room for, 652
Isometric contraction, 841
Isoniazid (INH), for tuberculosis, 653, 653t,
    654t
    for prevention, 655, 655t
    hepatotoxicity of, 1178, 1178t
Iso-osmolar extracellular fluid volume ex-
    cess, 79–81
Iso-osmolar fluid volume deficit, 75–79,
    77t
Isoptin (verapamil), 378t
Isosorbide (Ismotic), 212d, 212–213
    for glaucoma, 1980
Isotonic contraction, 841
Isotretinoin (Accutane), 1581
    for acne, 1615t
Itching. See *Pruritus.*
Ivy bleeding time, 443t, 448

J

Jackknife position, 135, *136*
    lateral, 135, *136*
Jaeger chart, 1942
Jarisch-Herxheimer reaction, 1918
Jaundice, body image and, 1177
    hemolytic, 1140
    hepatocellular, 1140
    in elderly, 1166
    in hematologic disorders, 440
    in hepatic disorders, 1139t, 1139–1141,
        1156d–1157d
    in hepatitis, 1172, 1173t, 1177
    in pancreatic cancer, 1127
    liver abscess and, 1179
    obstructive, 1140
Jaw, fracture of, *1046,* 1046–1049, 1049d
Jejunostomy feeding, 981t, 983. See also
    Gastrointestinal intubation.
    ostomy care in, 986
Jejunum, *955,* 955–956
Jeweler's loupe, 1958
Joint(s), degenerative disease of, 897–898
    dislocations of, 915–916
    range of motion of, assessment of, 848t
    sprains of, 913–914
    subluxations of, 915–916
    types of, *841,* 842, 842t
Joint bleeding, 436–437, 438, 517
Joint contractures, Dupuytren's, 909–910
    in burns, 1682–1684, 1684t
    in rheumatoid arthritis, 895

Joint contractures *(Continued)*
    posttraumatic, 933–934
    prevention of, in unconscious client, 729
Joint deformities, in hematologic disorders,
    438
    in rheumatoid arthritis, 891, *891*
Joint disorders, in elderly, 67, 884–885
    in Lyme disease, 901
    total joint replacement for, 867–868, *868,*
        869c–872c
Joint fusion, for rheumatoid arthritis, 892
Joint pain, 846–847
    in sickle-cell anemia, 46d, 485, 486
Joint stiffness, in arthritis, 891, 892, 897–
    898
    posttraumatic, 933–934
Judaism, beliefs and practices of, in death
    and dying, 35t
Jugular venous distention, 181, 192, *192*
    in heart failure, 271
Junctional dysrhythmias, 247–248
Junctional escape beats, 247
Junctional escape rhythm, 247, *247*
Junctional pacemaker, 171
Juvenile diabetes (type 1), 1227, 1228t. See
    also *Diabetes mellitus.*

K

Kanamycin, for tuberculosis, 653, 654t
Kaposi's sarcoma, in HIV infection, 1466,
    1466
Kegel exercises, 1365, 1365d, 1779d, 1817,
    1817d
Keloid, 1632t–1633t
Keratinocytes, 1567
Keratitis, 1964–1967
Keratolytics, 1579
    for scalp, 1583
    for warts, 1604
Keratoplasty, 1954–1955, 1955d
Keratosis, actinic, 1633t
    seborrheic, 1632t
Kernig's sign, 768, *768*
Ketoacidosis, diabetic. See *Diabetic ketoaci-
    dosis.*
Ketoconazole, for tinea versicolor, 1603
Ketones, urine tests for, 1243, 1245c
Ketorolac (Toradol), 893d
Ketosis, 1137
    starvation, 1243
17-Ketosteroids, measurement of, 1280t
Kidney(s). See also under *Renal.*
    age-related changes in, 66
    biopsy of, 1357–1358
    blood supply of, 1331
    cancer of, 1416–1418
    excretory functions of, 1331, *1332*
    glomerular filtration in, 1331–1332, *1332*
    in acid-base balance, *103,* 103–104, 104t,
        543, 1333
    in blood pressure regulation, 1333
    in calcium metabolism, 1333
    in fluid and electrolyte balance, 1331,
        1332–1333
    in red cell production, 1333
    in vitamin D activation, 1333
    innervation of, 1331
    shattered, 1411–1412
    structure and function, 1329–1333,
        1330–1332
    transplantation of, *1408,* 1408–1411,
        1409t, 1410d
    tubular reabsorption in, 1331, *1332*

Kidney, ureter, bladder film, 1347t
Kidney stones. See *Urinary calculi.*
Killer T cells, 1434, 1434t, 1439
Kirschner wires, 860
Knee, bursitis of, 902
    cartilaginous injuries of, 914
    housemaid's, 902
    ligamentous injuries of, 913–914
    sprains of, 913–914
Knee immobilizer, *914,* 916
Knee lift, 747
Knee replacement, 867–868, 869c–872c
Knee-chest position, for uterine retrodis-
    placement, 1820, *1821*
Kock pouch, 1012, *1013*
Kübler-Ross, Elisabeth, 32, 33
Kupffer's cells, *1136,* 1138
Kussmaul's respirations, 532, *533*
    in diabetic ketoacidosis, 1227, 1243
    in metabolic acidosis, 104, 105
Kwell (lindane), for pubic lice, 1928–1929,
    1929d, 1930
Kyphosis, 534, *534*
    assessment for, 848
    in elderly, 67, *67*
    in osteomalacia, 903
    osteoporosis and, 905, *905*

L

Labetalol (Normodyne), 378t
Labia majora, 1765, *1766*
Labia minora, 1765, *1766*
Laboratory tests, reference values for,
    2023–2031
Labyrinth, *1996,* 1996–1997
Labyrinthitis, 2013–2014
Laceration, closure of, 1586–1587
    corneal, 1987–1989
    eyelid, 1987–1989
    hepatic, 1194
    renal, 1411–1412
    scalp, 816–817
    urethral, 1414–1415
Lacrimal apparatus, 1935–1936, *1936*
LactAid, 1080
Lactase, 958
Lactase deficiency, 1079–1081
    in gluten-induced enteropathy, 1078
Lactate dehydrogenase (LDH), assessment
    of, 1161t, 1162
    in heart disease, 209, *209,* 210, *210*
    in myocardial infarction, 294
Lactation, breast in, 1842, 1845
    mastitis in, 1852–1853
Lactic acid, for warts, 1604
Lactulose, for hepatic encephalopathy,
    1150, 1152d
Lacunae, osseous, 838, *838*
Laënnec's cirrhosis, 1180–1193, 1181t. See
    also *Cirrhosis.*
Laminectomy. See also *Spinal surgery.*
    cervical, 761–765, 763d
Language assessment, 738–739, 746–747
Language deficits, 738–739
    in stroke, 807t, 808, 814
Lanoxin. See *Digoxin (Lanoxin).*
Laparoscopic cholecystectomy, 1114–1118
    complications of, 1115
    discharge instructions in, 1117d
    postoperative care in, 1116–1118
    postoperative course in, 1114–1115
    preoperative care in, 1116
    procedure for, 1114
    settings and providers for, 1115

Laparoscopy, 1787–1790
    complications of, 1790
    contraindications to, 1789
    nursing care in, 1790, 1790d
    patient preparation for, 1789
    procedure for, 1789, *1789*
    uses of, 1787
Laparotomy, incisions in, 994t–995t
Large intestine. See *Colon.*
Laryngeal nerve injury, in thyroidectomy,
    1314
Laryngectomee, communication with, 620–
    626, *626–628*
Laryngectomy, case study of, 624–625
    conservation (supraglottic), 617–622
        nursing care guide for, 619c–623c
        radical neck dissection in, *631,* 631–
            637, 633c–636c
    critical thinking exercise for, 624–625
    partial, 617
    radical neck dissection in, *631,* 631–637,
        634c–637c
    total, 618–637
        assessment in, postoperative, 628
            preoperative, 627–628
        care settings and providers for, 632
        communication after, 618–626, *626–*
            628
        nursing diagnoses and planning in,
            postoperative, 629
            preoperative, 627–628
        nursing interventions in, postopera-
            tive, 629–631
            preoperative, 628
        patient teaching in, 630, 631d, 632
        permanent tracheostomy in, 618,
            618
        postoperative care in, 628–631, 637
        preoperative care in, 626–628
Laryngectomy tube, 618
    changing of, 630
Laryngitis, 608–610, *609*
Laryngopharynx, *524,* 525, 951
Laryngoscopy, 550
Larynx, *524,* 525
    artificial, 618, *627*
    cancer of, 616–637
        clinical manifestations of, 617
        diagnosis of, 617
        etiology of, 616–617
        laryngectomy for, 617–637. See also
            Laryngectomy.
        management of, 617–637
        pathophysiology of, 616–617
        risk factors for, 616–617, 617d
    injuries of, 612–616
    structure of, *609*
Laser angioplasty, coronary artery, 293
Laser cholecystectomy, 1115
Laser photocoagulation, for diabetic reti-
    nopathy, 1253
    for retinal tears, 1983
Laser prostatectomy, 1754
Laser surgery, corneal, for refractive er-
    rors, 1973, *1974*
    for bladder cancer, 1420
    for cancer, 1831
    for endometriosis, 1813–1814
    for genital warts, 1027
    for glaucoma, 1980
    for hypothyroidism, 1310
    for macular degeneration, 1986
    for retinal detachment, 1983–1984
    for skin disorders, 1586, 1586d
    gynecologic, 1791, 1791d

Laser surgery *(Continued)*
    ocular, 1957–1958
    palliative, for esophageal cancer, 1055
Laser thermal angioplasty, 344
Laser trabeculoplasty, for glaucoma, 1980
Lasix (furosemide), 79, 377t
    for heart disease, 216, 217d, 218d
    for hypertension, 377t, 380t
Lateral cord syndrome, 824t
Lateral spinothalamic tract, 721
Latissimus dorsi muscle flap, in breast re-
    construction, 1876–1879, *1877,* 1879d
Lavacuator tube, *977*
Lavage, gastric, for bleeding, 967
    for bleeding esophageal varices, 1183
    for sputum collection, 546–547
Laxatives, 962d
    hypermagnesemia and, 101
LD flap, in breast reconstruction, 1876–
    1879, *1877,* 1879d
Leaflet repair, 311. See also *Cardiac valvular*
    disease, surgery in.
Left bundle branch, 171
Left coronary artery, *164, 168,* 168–169
Left ventricular afterload, 172
Leg, prosthetic, 882–884, *883, 884*
Leg bag, for urine, 1362, 1363
Leg casts, 854t. See also *Cast(s).*
Leg exercises, postoperative, 131, *132,* 151,
    153
Leg ulcers. See also *Venous stasis ulcers.*
    in sickle-cell anemia, 437, 484, 487, 487d
Legal issue(s), advance directives as, 12–
    13, *43, 44*
    brain death as, 41
    Do Not Resuscitate (DNR) orders as,
        43–45, *45*
    in surgery, 117–118
    informed consent as, 117–118
    medical durable power of attorney as,
        42–43, *44*
Legally blind, supportive treatment for,
    1958–1959, *1959,* 1960d
Legionella pneumophila pneumonia, 641
Leiomyomas, 1823–1824, *1824*
Lens, contact, 1971–1972, 1972d–1973d,
    1974
    crystalline, *1937, 1938*
        absence of, 1970
        age-related changes in, 1961
    intraocular, after cataract extraction,
        1976–1978
Lentigo, 1633t
Leukemia, 493–503
    acute lymphocytic, 493, 494t
    acute myelocytic, 493, 494t
    assessment in, 495–496
    cellular changes in, 494t
    chronic lymphocytic, 493–494, 494t
        nursing care guide for, 497c–502c
    chronic myelocytic, 494, 494t
    clinical manifestations of, 494t, 494–495
    diagnosis of, 495
    Internet connections for, 506d
    management of, 494t, 495
    nursing diagnoses and planning in, 496
    nursing interventions in, 496–504, 497c–
        502c
    prognosis in, 494t
    self-care in, 503, 504d
Leukocyte(s), 429, *429, 430.* See also *White*
    blood cell count.
    disorders of, 491–513
    polymorphonuclear, 1432, *1432*
    types of, *1432,* 1432–1433, 1433t

Leukocyte alkaline phosphatase stain, 443t, 449
Leukocytosis, 429, 442
  chemotherapy and, 1531, 1536t–1538t
  in myocardial infarction, 294
Leukopenia, 429, 444
  in agranulocytosis, 491–493
  in radiation therapy, 1522
Leukoplakia, 1049, *1050*, 1633t
Leukorrhea, 1776
  in vaginitis, 1776, 1804–1805, 1805t
Leukotriene modifiers, for asthma, 661
Leuprolide acetate (LU-PRON), for prostate cancer, 1759
Levator palpebrae superioris muscle, 1936
LeVeen shunt, for portal hypertension, 1144–1145, *1146*
Levin tube, 977, *977*
Levodopa, for Parkinson's disease, 787
Levophed (norepinephrine), cardiac effects of, 405t
Levothyroxine (Synthroid), for hypothyroidism, 1298, 1303c–1304c, 1305t
Leydig's cells, 1696
Lice, pubic, *1928*, 1928–1929
Lichenification, *1571*, 1573
Lidocaine (Xylocaine), for dysrhythmias, 215, 216d
  for myocardial infarction, 297
  for premature ventricular contractions, 249
  in cardiopulmonary resuscitation, 263, 263t
Lifestyle changes. See also *Patient teaching; Self-care.*
  after myocardial infarction, 299d
  for heart disease prevention, 284–285, 285d
  in hypertension, 382d, 383d, 383–384
  in peptic ulcer disease, 1032–1033
Ligaments, 842
  injuries of, 913–914
  ovarian, 1768
  uterine, 1766–1767, *1767*
Light reflex, tympanic membrane, 2001, *2001*
Light-touch perception, assessment of, 748
Limb prostheses, 881–884, *882–884*
Limb-girdle dystrophy, 785–786
Lindane (Kwell), for pubic lice, 1928–1929, 1929d, 1930
Linear lesions, 1573, *1574*
Linton tube, for esophageal varices, 1187–1188
Liothyronine (Cytomel), for hypothyroidism, 1298, 1305t
Liotrix (Thyrolar), for hypothyroidism, 1298, 1305t
Lip, cancer of, 1049–1053. See also *Oral cancer.*
  examination of, 968
  herpes simplex infection of, 1017–1019, 1018t, *1605*, 1605–1606
Lipase, intestinal, 958t
  pancreatic, 956, 957, 958t
Lipid metabolism, hepatic, 1137, 1137t
Lipids. See also *Hyperlipidemia.*
  in total parenteral nutrition, 990
  serum, in heart disease, 209
Lipogenesis, 1224, 1224t
Lipolysis, 1224t, 1224–1225
Lipoma, 1633t
Lipoproteins, heart disease and, 186, 209
Liposuction, 1591t, 1592d

Lisinopril (Prinivil), 213, 214d
Lithotomy position, 135, *136*
Lithotripsy, extracorporeal shock wave, 1378, *1379*, 1379–1380
  for gallstones, 1111–1113, *1112*, 1115
  mechanical, for gallstones, 1111, 1115
Liver. See also under *Hepatic.*
  abscess of, 1179
  biopsy of, 1164, 1165t
  blood formation in, 433
  blood supply of, 1135–1136, *1136*
  cancer of, 1195–1196
    alpha-fetoprotein in, 1162t, 1164
    portal hypertension in, 1141–1149
  fatty, 1137, 1180–1193, 1181t. See also *Cirrhosis.*
    alcohol and, 1153
  immunologic functions of, 1432
  in bile production and bilirubin conjugation, 1137t, 1137–1138
  in blood filtration, 1137t, 1138
  in carbohydrate metabolism, 1136–1137, 1137t
  in detoxification, 1137t, 1138–1139
  in lipid metabolism, 1137, 1137t
  in protein metabolism, 1137, 1137t
  lobes of, 1135, *1136*
  palpation of, 192, 969, 1159, *1160*
  percussion of, 1159, *1160*
  storage functions of, 1137t, 1139
  structure and function of, 957, *958*, 1135–1139
  traumatic injuries of, 1193–1194
  tumors of, benign, 1194
    malignant, 1195–1196
  ultrasonography of, 976
  veno-occlusive disease of, bone marrow transplant and, 1451
Liver flap, 1150
Liver function, age-related changes in, 1165–1166
  in heart failure, 271
Liver scan, 1163t
Liver spots, 58, *58*
Liver transplant, 1196–1198
Living will, 42–43, *43*
Lobectomy, 580t, 586–587
  complications of, 581
  incisions in, 580
  nursing care guide for, 588d–596d
  patient preparation for, 580–581
Local anesthesia, 137, 138t. See also *Anesthesia.*
Locus of control, 1511
Long arm cast, 854t. See also *Cast(s).*
Long bones, 839, *840*
Long leg cast, 854t. See also *Cast(s).*
Long-term care facilities, rehabilitation in, 23
Long-term care services, 23
Loniten (minoxidil), 213, 378t
Loop colostomy, 1004, *1004*
Loop diuretics, 377t. See also *Diuretics.*
Loop electrosurgical excision procedure, for cervical cancer, 1831
Loop of Henle, 1331, *1331*
  in urine formation, 1332, *1332*
Looser's zones, 903
Lopid (gemfibrozil), 216–217, 218d
Lopressor (metoprolol), 377t
  for dysrhythmias, 215, 216d
  for heart disease, 214
Lordosis, assessment for, 848
Loss, in cancer, 1510, 1545, 1549–1550
Lotions, 1579, 1580t

Lou Gehrig's disease, 775–777
Lovastatin (Mevacor), 216–217, 218d, 343d
Low back pain, 911–913
Low cardiac output syndrome, 271, 277
Low vision, supportive treatment for, 1958–1959, *1959*, 1960d
Low-density lipoproteins (LDL), heart disease and, 186, 209
Lower esophageal sphincter, 951, *952*
Lower extremity prostheses, 882–884, *883*, *884*
Lower gastrointestinal endoscopy, 974–975, 976d
Lower midline incision, 994t
Lower motor neuron disease, 739, 740t
Lower motor neurons, 722
Lower paramedian (rectus) incision, 994t
Low-fat diet, 284, 285d
Low-potassium diet, 90
Low-protein diet, 1151d
  in hepatic encephalopathy, 1150, 1151d
  in renal failure, 1391d, 1400
Low-sodium diet, 184d, 382d, 1143d
  in fluid volume excess, 80, 81
  in heart failure, 275, 276d, 279
  in hypernatremia, 94
  in hypertension, 382d
  in portal hypertension, 1143d, 1144
Lozol (indapamide), 377t
Lubricants, ocular, 1947
Lumbar abscess, appendicitis and, 1064t
Lumbar puncture, 753–754, 755c–756c, 757
  in bacterial meningitis, 769
  in increased intracranial pressure, 731
  in subarachnoid hemorrhage, 815
Lumbar spine, 715. See also under *Spinal; Spine.*
Lumbar sympathetic block, in arterial insufficiency, 339t
Luminal (phenobarbital), for seizures, 796, 797d–798d
  hepatotoxicity of, 1178t, 1179
Lumpectomy, *1861*, 1868–1874, 1869d–1874d
  clinical pathway for, 1869d
  complications of, 1869
  nursing care guide for, 1870c–1874c
  patient preparation for, 1868
  postoperative course in, 1869
  procedure for, 1868–1869
Lund and Brower chart, 1645, *1646*
Lung(s), abscess of, 647–648
  age-related changes in, 65, 587
  auscultation of, 192, *536*, 536–537
  biopsy of, 552
  contusion of, 695
  elastic recoil of, 527
  structure and function of, 524, *525*
Lung cancer, 695–698, 699d, 700c–707c
  adenocarcinoma, 696
  assessment in, 697
  chemotherapy for, 696–697
  chest x-ray for, 1514
  clinical manifestations of, 696, 1511t
  diagnosis of, 696
  etiology of, 695
  Internet connections for, 665d
  large-cell, 696
  management of, 696–697, 699d
  metastasis in, 696
  nursing diagnoses and planning in, 697
  nursing interventions in, 697
  nutrition in, 699d
  oat-cell, 696
  pathophysiology of, 695–696

Lung cancer (*Continued*)
  radiation therapy for, 696, 1521
  risk factors for, 1511t
  self-care in, 698, 699d
  small-cell, 696
  sputum cytology in, 1513
  squamous cell, 695–696
  surgery for, 696, 700c–707c
    nursing care guide for, 700c–707c. See
      also *Pneumonectomy.*
  syndrome of inappropriate antidiuretic
      hormone in, 696, 697, 698, 699d
  types of, 695
Lung capacities, 538, *538*, 539t
Lung disease. See also *Respiratory disorder(s).*
  occupational, 688–690
  restrictive, burns and, 1658
Lung receptors, 528
Lung scans, 548
Lung sounds, adventitious, 537
    in heart failure, 270–271, 277
Lung volume reduction surgery, for em-
    physema, 672–673
Lung volumes, 538, *538*, 539t
LU-PRON (leuprolide acetate), for prostate
    cancer, 1759
Lupus erythematosus, systemic. See *Sys-
    temic lupus erythematosus.*
Lupus erythematosus cells, 1491
Luteinizing hormone, 1205t
  in female hormonal cycle, 1768
  measurement of, in males, 1704
Luteinizing hormone–releasing hormone,
    1209t
Lyme disease, 901–902, 902d
Lymph, characteristics of, 331
  circulation of, 329–331, *330, 331*, 1431
Lymph nodes, 331
  axillary. See *Axillary lymph node(s).*
  biopsy of, 451
  cervical, *435*
    removal of, in radical neck dissection,
      631–637, 634c–637c
  enlarged, in HIV infection, 1465
  functions of, 433
  palpable, *435*
  palpation of, 1443
  structure and function of, 1431
Lymphadenectomy, axillary, 1862d
    in lumpectomy, 1868–1874, 1871c–
      1873c
    in modified radical mastectomy, 1860–
      1868, 1869d
  iliac, 1708t
  in radical neck dissection, 631–637,
      633c–636c
  inguinal, in radical vulvectomy, 1826–
      1830, 1829d
  pelvic, in radical vulvectomy, 1826–
      1830, 1829d
  retroperitoneal, 1708t, 1749–1750, 1752
Lymphadenitis, 396
Lymphadenopathy, *435*
  in HIV infection, 1465
Lymphangitis, 396
Lymphatic disorders, 395–397
Lymphatic drainage, of breast, 1843, *1843*
Lymphatic system, structure and function
    of, 329–331, *332, 333*, 1431
Lymphedema, 396–397
  postmastectomy, 1866, 1866d
Lymphocyte(s), *429, 430*, 445t, *1432*, 1433,
    1433t. See also *B cell(s); T cell(s).*
  formation of, 1430–1431, *1431*

Lymphocytic thyroiditis, 1296
Lymphoid cells, dermal, 1568
Lymphoid organs, generative, 1430–1431
  peripheral, *1431*, 1431–1432
Lymphokines, 1439
Lymphoma, cutaneous T-cell, PUVA ther-
    apy for, 1582
  Hodgkin's, 503–507, 504t
  non-Hodgkin's, 507t, 507–508
  nursing care guide for, 509c–511c
Lypressin (Diapid), for diabetes insipidus,
    1275
Lysodren (mitotane), for Cushing's syn-
    drome, 1287
Lysozymes, in nonspecific immune re-
    sponse, 1435, 1436

M

M phase, of cell cycle, 1504, *1504*
Macroangiopathy, diabetic, 1252, 1252d
Macrocytic anemia, Schilling test for, 451
Macronodular cirrhosis, 1181, 1181t
Macrophages, *1432, 1433*, 1433t
  in phagocytosis, 1436
Macula, examination of, 1944, *1944*
Macular degeneration, 1961, 1985–1987,
    1986
  Internet connections for, 1986
Macule, 1570–1571, *1571*
Mafenide acetate (Sulfamylon), for burns,
    1674t
Magnesium, calcium and, 95
  cardiac function and, 208
  daily requirement for, 99
  deficiency of, 99–101. See also *Hypomag-
    nesemia.*
  excess of, 99, 101–102
  fluid distribution of, *85*
  normal values for, 99
  sources of, 101
  supplemental, 100, 101
    for hypertension, 100d
Magnesium sulfate, for hypomagnesemia,
    100, 101
  in cardiopulmonary resuscitation, 263,
    263t
Magnesium tolerance test, 100
Magnetic resonance imaging, cardiac,
    199
  gastrointestinal, 976
  hepatic, 1163t
  in cancer, 1515
  in hematologic disorders, 452
  in musculoskeletal disorders, 851t
  in neurologic disorders, 749, *750*
  ocular, 1946
  of urinary tract, 1350t
  preoperative, 126t
Magnifiers, 1958
Malabsorption, after ileostomy, 1013
Malabsorption syndromes, 1077t, 1077–
    1078
  in elderly, 1106
Malar rash, in systemic lupus erythemato-
    sus, 1491, *1491*, 1492t
Male climacteric syndrome, 1725
Malignant fibrous histiocytoma, 935–938,
    936t
Malignant hypertension, 373, 375. See also
    Hypertension.
  pheochromocytoma and, 1292, 1294
Malignant hyperthermia, 142

Malignant melanoma, *1638*, 1638–1639.
    See also *Skin cancer.*
  choroidal, 1991
  self-examination for, *1634–1635*, 1635–
    1636
  warning signs of, 1635–1636
Malignant neoplasm, 1505, *1505*. See also
    Cancer.
Malleus, 1996, *1996*, 1997
Malnutrition, as surgical risk factor, 120–
    121
  clinical manifestations of, 1077t
  in alcoholism, 1139t, 1153
  in cancer, 1558–1560, 1560d
  in hepatic disorders, 1139t, 1153–1154,
    1154t
  in malabsorption syndrome, 1077t,
    1077–1078
  postgastrectomy, 998t
Maltase, 958
Mammary duct ectasia, 1853
Mammary dysplasia, 1854–1856, 1956d
Mammography, *1848*, 1848–1849
Mammoplasty, augmentation, 1879
  reconstructive, 1875–1879, *1876–1877*,
    1879d
  reduction, 1879–1880
Managed care, 6, 20–21
  access to care and, 1462d–1463d
Managed care organizations, 20
Mandibular fracture, *1046*, 1046–1049,
    1049d
Mandibulectomy, for cancer, 1050–1053
Mannitol (Osmitrol), 732d
  for increased intracranial pressure, 732
Mantoux test, 652
Manual heart compression, in cardiopul-
    monary resuscitation, 262, 264t
Marie-Strümpell disease, 898–899
Marijuana, for chemotherapy-related nau-
    sea and vomiting, 1529
Masks, oxygen, 555t
MAST suit, 411
Mastectomy, 1860–1868, 1869d
  modified radical, 1860–1868, *1862*
    breast prosthesis for, 1866
    clinical pathway for, 1869d
    complications of, 1863
    hand and arm precautions in, 1865,
      1866d
    lymphedema after, 1866, 1866d
    patient preparation for, 1860
    postoperative care in, 1864–1868
    postoperative course in, 1862–1863
    preoperative care in, 1863–1864
    procedure for, 1860–1862, *1861*
    range-of-motion exercises for, 1865–
      1866, 1867d, *1868*
  partial, *1861*
  radical, *1862*
  reconstructive surgery after, 1867, 1875–
    1879, *1876–1877*
  total, *1862*
Mastication, 951
Mastitis, 1852–1853
Mastoidectomy, 2006–2008, *2008*
Mastoiditis, 2012–2013, 2013t
  brain abscess and, 771
Mastopexy, dermal, 1880
Maxillary sinus, *601*
  infection of, 601–604
  palpation of, 602
Maximal voluntary ventilation, 539t
Maximum expiratory flow rate, 539t

Maximum midexpiratory flow, 539t
MB, in heart disease, 209, 209–210
McBurney's point, tenderness over, in appendicitis, 1065, 1065
Mean corpuscular hemoglobin (MCH), 446, 446t
Mean corpuscular hemoglobin concentration (MCHC), 446, 446t
Mean corpuscular volume (MCV), 446, 446t
Meatal stenosis, 1386–1388
Mechanical ileus, 1074, 1074–1075
Mechanical lithotripsy, for gallstones, 1111, 1115
Mechanical ventilation, 567–574. See also Airway management.
 assessment in, 570
 assist, 569
 assist-control, 569
 at home, 572d–573d
 continuous positive airway pressure, 569
 control, 569
 fighting the ventilator in, 571
 in adult respiratory distress syndrome, 687
 in chronic obstructive pulmonary disease, 672d
 in flail chest, 691, 692
 intermittent positive-pressure breathing in, 567–568
 modes of, 569–570
 negative-pressure ventilators in, 568t, 568–569
 nursing diagnoses and planning in, 570–571
 nursing interventions in, 571
 nutrition in, 563d
 positive end-expiratory pressure, 569
 positive-pressure ventilators in, 568t, 568–569
 pressure support, 569
  in mechanical ventilation, 569
 pressure-cycled, 568t, 569
 respiratory alkalosis in, 111
 safety measures for, 570
 sighs in, 570
 synchronized intermittent mandatory, 569
  in weaning, 574
 time-cycled, 568t, 569
 volume-cycled, 568t, 569
 weaning in, 571–574
Median nerve compression, in carpal tunnel syndrome, 909–910
Median sternotomy incision, 580
Mediastinal shift, after pneumonectomy, 584, 703c
Mediastinal tumors, 698
Mediastinoscopy, 550
Mediastinum, 164
Medicaid, 18
Medical antishock trousers, 411
Medical power of attorney, 42–43, 44
Medical-surgical nurse, certification of, 5t, 5–6
 generalist, 4
 specialist, 3, 4
Medical-surgical nursing. See also Nursing.
 certification in, 5t, 5–6
 Clinical Practice Guidelines for, 7–8
 culturally sensitive, 12–14
 definition of, 3
 demographic changes affecting, 18–20
 future of, 29

Medical-surgical nursing (Continued)
 health care reform and, 6
 nature of, 3
 nonhospital settings for, 17–29
  reasons for, 17–21
  types of, 21–29
 nursing process in, 8–12
 preparation for, 3–5
 scope of, 3
 settings for, 17–29
 societal changes and, 6
 specialties in, 3
 spiritual aspects of, 13–14
 standards of practice for, 6–7, 7t
 trends in, 6
Medicare, cost controls for, 20
 diagnosis-related groups and, 20
 for home care, 27t
Medulla oblongata, 721
Medullary thyroid cancer, 1316
Medulloblastoma, 828–832, 831t
Megaureter, obstructive, ureterovesical junction obstruction and, 1382
Meibomian glands, 1935–1936, 1936
Melanocytes, 1567, 1569t
 in hyperpigmented lesions, 1570–1571
Melanocyte-stimulating hormone, 1205t
Melanocyte-stimulating hormone–inhibiting hormone, 1209t
Melanocyte-stimulating hormone–releasing hormone, 1209t
Melanoma, 1638, 1638–1639. See also Skin cancer.
 choroidal, 1991
 self-examination for, 1634–1635, 1635–1636
 warning signs of, 1635–1636
Melasma, 1633t
Melatonin, 1204–1208, 1207t
Melphalan (Alkeran), for multiple myeloma, 511
Membrane depolarization, 169, 170, 171, 712–713, 714
Membrane polarization, 712–713, 714
Membrane potential, 712, 714
Membranous labyrinth, 1996
Memory, assessment of, 746
 immunologic, 1430
 impairment of, age-related, 765–766
  in Alzheimer's disease, 765–766, 790, 791d, 792
Memory B cells, 1434
Memory T cells, 1434, 1434t
Menarche, onset of, 1768
Meniere's disease, 829t–830t, 1998–1999. See also Vertigo.
Meningeal irritation, signs of, 768, 768
Meninges, 714, 716
Meningioma, 828–832, 831t
Meningitis, 767–769
 bacterial, 768–769
 nursing process in, 768, 771–773
 prevention of, in head injury, 821–822
 viral, 768–769
Meningococcal meningitis, 768
 nursing process in, 768, 771–773
Meniscal tears, 914
Menometrorrhagia, 1775–1776
Menopause, 1769–1775
 assessment in, 1773
 heart disease and, 280–281
 hormonal changes in, 1770–1771
 hormone replacement therapy for, 1772d, 1772–1773

Menopause (Continued)
 management of, 1772d, 1772–1773
 nursing diagnoses and planning in, 1773–1774
 nursing interventions in, 1774
 osteoporosis and, 905
 physical changes in, 1771
 premature, 1769
 psychosocial effects of, 1771
 self-care in, 1774d, 1775
 surgical, 1794, 1795. See also Hysterectomy.
 symptoms of, 1771
Menorrhagia, 1775–1776
Menstrual cycle, 1768–1769, 1770
 ischemic phase of, 1769, 1770
 menstrual phase of, 1769, 1770
 proliferative phase of, 1768, 1770
 secretory phase of, 1768–1769, 1770
Menstrual log, 1808–1809, 1810, 1811
Menstruation, absence of, 1775
 cessation of, 1769–1770. See also Menopause.
 onset of, 1768
 painful, 1776–1777
 premenstrual syndrome and, 1807–1810, 1809d, 1809t
 tampon use in, toxic shock syndrome and, 1807–1808, 1808d
Mental processes, age-related changes in, 63
Mental status. See also under Cognitive.
 age-related changes in, 63, 765–766, 766
 in acute renal failure, 1396c–1397c
 in head injury, 822
 in heart disease, 185
 in hypernatremia, 93, 94
 in metabolic acidosis, 104, 105, 106
 in metabolic alkalosis, 107, 108
 in respiratory acidosis, 109
Mental status examination, 746
 in hepatic disorders, 1160
Mercaptans, 1149
Mesenteric vascular disease, intestinal ischemia and, in elderly, 1106
Mesh graft, 1588, 1589
 for burns, 1673–1678, 1675
Mesodermal tumors, mediastinal, 698
Mestinon (pyridostigmine), for myasthenia gravis, 783, 783d, 785
Metabolic acidosis, 104–106, 105t
 compensated, 543
 hypoxemia and, 530
 in acute renal failure, 1390t
 in burns, 1660, 1661
 in diabetes, 1227. See also Diabetic ketoacidosis.
 in ileostomy client, 1013, 1014d
 in shock, 406, 407
Metabolic alkalosis, 106–108, 107t
 compensated, 543
 in primary aldosteronism, 1289–1291
Metabolic autoregulation, of blood flow, 329
Metabolic equivalents, 298
Metabolic waste products, definition of, 1388t
Metabolism, in diabetics vs. nondiabetics, 1225
Metahydrin (trichlormethiazide), 377t
Metanephrine, hypersecretion of, from pheochromocytoma, 1292
 urinary assays of, 1293t
Metarterioles, 324

Metastasis, 1505–1506

Metered-dose inhaler, *661*, 661–663

Methimazole (Tapazole), for hyperthyroidism, 1309, 1309t

Methotrexate, for skin infections, 1582

Methoxsalen, in PUVA therapy, 1582

Methyclothiazide (Ethon), 377t

Methyl tert-butyl ether (MTBE), for gallstones, 1111

Methyldopa (Aldomet), 378t, 380t

Methylxanthines, 576d

　fibrocystic breast disease and, 1854

Metoclopramide, for chemotherapy-related nausea and vomiting, 1529

Metolazone (Zaroxolyn), 377t

Metopirone. See *Metyrapone (Metopirone)*.

Metoprolol (Lopressor), 214, 377t

　for dysrhythmias, 215, 216d

Metronidazole (Flagyl), 1180d

　for acne rosacea, 1616

　for *Gardnerella vaginalis* vaginitis, 1884t, 1886

　for liver abscess, 1179, 1180d

　for trichomoniasis, 1884t, 1886

　for vaginal candidiasis, 1884t, 1885

Metrorrhagia, 1775–1776

Metyrapone (Metopirone), for Cushing's syndrome, 1287

Metyrapone suppression test, 1279t

Mevacor (lovastatin), 216–217, 218d, 343d

Miconazole, for vaginal candidiasis, 1884t, 1885

Microangiopathy, diabetic, 1252d, 1252–1255

Microbial keratitis, 1965–1967

Microcirculation, 325, *328*

Microdiskectomy, 762

Microglia, 712, *713*

Micronase (glyburide), 1239, 1239t, 1240d

Microvilli, intestinal, *955, 956*

Micturition. See *Voiding*.

Midamor (amiloride), 377t

Midbrain, 720

Middle cerebral artery, 716, *717*

　stenosis of, 807t

Middle ear. See also under *Ear*.

　age-related changes in, 2009

　infection of, 2012–2013, 2013t, *2014*

　　brain abscess and, 771

　　myringotomy for, 2005–2006, *2006*

　structure and function of, 1995–1996, *1996*

Midstream urine sample, 1344

Midsystolic click, 181

Migraine headaches, 800. See also *Headache*.

Miliary tuberculosis, 650

Miller-Abbott tube, *977, 978*

　for adhesions, 1084

Milrinone (Primacor), for heart failure, 274

Milroy's disease, 396–397

Mineralocorticoids, 1206t, 1214, *1215*

Minerals, hepatic storage of, 1139

Minimally invasive coronary artery bypass graft, 291

Minipress (prazosin), 213, 213d, 378t

　for benign prostatic hyperplasia, 1753

Minnesota tube, for esophageal varices, 1187–1188

Minors, consent of, 118

Minoxidil (Loniten), 213, 378t

Minute ventilation, 539t

Miosis, senile, 1961

Miotics, 1947, 1947d

Mitosis, 1504, *1504*

Mitotane (Lysodren), for Cushing's syndrome, 1287

Mitral valve, *164*, 167, *167, 168*, 171

Mitral valve prolapse, 309–310. See also *Cardiac valvular disease*.

Mitral valve regurgitation, 309. See also *Cardiac valvular disease*.

Mitral valve stenosis, 308–309. See also *Cardiac valvular disease*.

Mittelschmerz, 1777

MM, in heart disease, 209, 209–210

Mobile clinics, 21

Mobility, with casts, 858

Mobility aids, for visually impaired, 1959, 1960d

Mobility impairment, 843–846. See also *Immobility*.

Mobitz block, type I, 251–252, *252*

　type II, *252*, 252–253

Modified Fowler position, 135, *136*

Modified radical mastectomy, 1860–1868, 1869d. See also *Mastectomy*.

Mohs' micrographic surgery, 1585

　for basal cell epithelioma, 1637

　for squamous cell carcinoma, 1637

Mole, 1633t

Molluscum contagiosum, 1605

Mongolian spot, 1571

Moniliasis. See *Candidiasis*.

Monoclonal antibodies, 1448

Monoctanoin, for gallstones, 1111

Monocular telescope, 1958

Monocytes, *429, 430*, 445t, *1432, 1433*, 1433t

　in phagocytosis, 1436

Mononuclear cells, 429

Mononucleosis, 512–513

Mons pubis, 1765, *1766*

Morphea, 1494–1495, *1495*

Morphine. See also *Narcotics, analgesic*.

　for myocardial infarction, 296

　infusion pump for, 152, *152*

Morton's neuroma, 910–911

Motor aphasia, 738–739, 814

Motor assessment, mobility assessment in, 843–844

Motor cortex, 719, *720*

Motor neuron, 711, *712*

Motor neuron disease, 739, 740t

Motor system assessment, 747

Motor system dysfunction, 739–742, 740t

　in stroke, 808, 809–813

Motrin (ibuprofen), 893d

Mourning. See *Bereavement; Grief*.

Mouth. See under *Oral*.

Movement, energy for, 842

　physiology of, 841–842

Mucociliary escalator, 526

Mucolytics, 575

Mucosa, gastrointestinal, 950

　duodenal, 956

　gastric, 952

　oral, 951

Mucositis, chemotherapy and, 1529–1530, 1541t

　in radiation therapy, 1520

Mucous cells, 952

Mud dauber stings, 1621–1622, 1622d

MUGA scan, 198

Multicultural nursing care, 12–14

Multidisciplinary team, 24t–25t

Multiple myeloma, 508–512, 935–938, 936t

Multiple sclerosis (MS), 777–781

　clinical manifestations of, 778–779

　demyelination in, 778, *778*

　diagnosis of, 779

　etiology of, 777

　Internet connections for, 779d

　management of, 779–780

　　settings and providers for, 780

　pathophysiology of, 777–778, *778*

Mumps orchitis, 1731–1732

Murmurs, 181

　auscultation of, 191

　in aortic regurgitation, 308

　in aortic stenosis, 307–308

　in mitral prolapse, 309

　in mitral regurgitation, 309

　in mitral stenosis, 309

Muromonab-CD3, for transplant immunosuppression, 1410

Muscle(s). See also under *Neuromuscular*.

　extraocular, 1936, *1936*

　　examination of, 1943

　　weakness of, in myasthenia gravis, 782, 784

　flaccid, 840

　skeletal, structure and function of, 840–842

Muscle contraction, 840–841

Muscle contraction headaches, 800. See also *Headache*.

Muscle contusions, 913

Muscle cramps, in hypocalcemia, 1318, 1319c

　in renal failure, 1395d, 1400

Muscle pain, 846–847

Muscle relaxants, 846d

Muscle rigidity, in Parkinson's disease, 787, *787*

Muscle spasticity, 840

　in multiple sclerosis, 780

Muscle strains, 913

Muscle strength, assessment of, 747, 747t, 848

Muscle tone, 840

　assessment of, 747

Muscle wasting, in burns, 1678

Muscle weakness. See *Weakness*.

Muscular dystrophy, limb-girdle, 785–786

Muscularis, gastrointestinal, 950

Musculoskeletal assessment, 847–849

　for elderly, 884

　neurovascular assessment in, 849

　　in cast therapy, 857

　　in traction, 862

　patient history in, 847

　physical examination in, 848–849

Musculoskeletal disorders, activity intolerance in, 844–845

　amputation in, 868–878

　assessment of, 847–849

　assistive and supportive devices in, 878–881

　clinical manifestations of, 843–847

　cold application in, 850–853

　diagnostic procedures in, 850t–852t

　external fixation devices for, *863*, 863–865

　heat application in, 850–853

　impaired mobility in, 843–846

　in elderly, 884–885, 943–944

　in hyperparathyroidism, 1320

　infectious and inflammatory, 887–902

Musculoskeletal disorders (Continued)
  malignant hyperthermia and, 142
  management of, 849–885
  neoplastic, 935–943
  pain in, 846–847
  patient history in, 847
  physical examination in, 847–849
  resources for, 2040
  self-help devices for, 884
  structural, 902–913
  surgery for, 863–878
  total joint replacement in, 867–868, 868, 869c–872c
  traumatic. See Musculoskeletal injuries.
Musculoskeletal function, age-related changes in, 66–67, 67
Musculoskeletal injuries, 913–935
  avascular necrosis in, 935
  compartment syndrome in, 932–933
  complications of, 932–935
  contractures in, 933–934
  delayed healing in, 934–935
  fat embolism in, 933
  infection in, 934
  joint stiffness in, 933–934
  major, 915–935
  minor, 913–915
  pathologic ossification in, 935
  shock in, 932
Musculoskeletal system, age-related changes in, 943–944
  anatomy and physiology of, 837–843, 838, 840, 841
Myasthenia gravis, 782, 782–785
Myasthenic crisis, 782, 783
Mycobacterium tuberculosis, 650
  sputum studies for, 652
Mycoplasma pneumoniae pneumonia, 641
Mycosis fungoides, PUVA therapy for, 1582, 1584
Mycotic osteomyelitis, 889–890
Mydriatics, 1946d, 1947
Myelin, 712
Myelography, 752, 752–753
Myeloid cells, dermal, 1568
Myeloma, 508–512, 935–938, 936t
Myocardial depressant factor, in shock, 407
Myocardial infarction, 175, 293–303
  analgesia in, 296
  aspirin for, 295
  assessment in, 298–300
  cardiac enzyme/isoenzyme levels in, 209, 209–210, 210
  cardiac monitoring in, 296–297
  cardiogenic shock in, 411–413
  clinical manifestations of, 294
  complications of, 295
  coronary artery disease and, 280–285
  definition of, 293
  diagnosis of, 294
  diet in, 297
  drug therapy for, 297
  etiology of, 293
  exercise in, 297–298
  location of, 293–294
  management of, 295–298
    settings and providers for, 298
  nursing diagnoses and planning for, 299
  nursing interventions for, 299–300
  oxygen therapy for, 296, 302
  pain in, 294, 295, 296, 300
  pathophysiology of, 293–294

Myocardial infarction (Continued)
  prevention of, 282, 284, 285d
    diet in, 284, 285d
    drugs in, 284
    exercise in, 284–285, 285d
  radioisotope scanning in, 198
  recovery from, nurses' knowledge of, 301d
  self-care after, 299d
  silent, 294
  surgery for, 295
  thrombolytics for, 217, 218, 295, 296d, 297
Myocardial ischemia, 175
  angina pectoris in, 175, 175t, 188, 283, 285–291
  thrombolytics for, 217, 218
Myocarditis, 237–238
  rheumatic, 236–237
Myocardium, 164–165
  impulse conduction over, 169, 170, 171
Myofibrils, 840
Myomas, uterine, 1823–1824, 1824
Myomectomy, 1786t, 1824
Myopia, 1970–1974, 1971
  assessment for, 1941–1942
  contact lenses for, 1971–1972, 1972d–1973d, 1974
  photorefractive keratectomy for, 1973, 1974
  radial keratotomy for, 1973, 1974
Myositis ossificans, 935
Myringoplasty, 2003–2005, 2004
Myringotomy, 2005–2006, 2006
Mysoline (primidone), for seizures, 796, 797d–798d
Myxedema, 1297, 1298, 1298. See also Hypothyroidism.
  pretibial, in hyperthyroidism, 1307
Myxedema coma, 1298, 1301, 1302, 1306
Myxomatous degeneration, 309

N
Nabilone, for chemotherapy-related nausea and vomiting, 1529
Nadolol (Corgard), 214, 377t
  for bleeding esophageal varices, 1183–1186
Nail(s), age-related changes in, 59
  bacterial infection of, 1598t
  candidiasis of, 1602
  clubbing of, 182, 534, 535
  examination of, 1575
  fungal infection of, 1600t, 1600–1601
  in psoriasis, 1617
  orthopedic, 865–867
  structure and function of, 1569, 1569t
Napping, by elderly, 64
Naproxen (Naprosyn), 893d
Naqua (trichlormethiazide), 377t
Narcotics, abuse of. See Substance abuse.
  analgesic, 1553, 1553, 1554t–1555t
    for burns, 1670
    in elderly, 54t
    infusion pump for, 152, 152
    postoperative, 152–153
    preoperative, 127–128
    routes of administration for, 1554t–1555t
  anesthetic, 141t
Nasal bleeding, 610–611

Nasal bleeding (Continued)
  in nasal fracture, 612
  postoperative, 615c
Nasal cannula, 555t
Nasal cavity, 524, 525
Nasal decongestants, 574d, 575
Nasal discharge, in rhinitis, 600–601
  in sinusitis, 601–602
Nasal drip pad, 604
Nasal fracture, 612
Nasal obstruction, 611–612
Nasal packing, 604, 614c
Nasal polyps, 611, 611
Nasal secretions, assessment of, 531
  excessive, 529
Nasal septum, deviated, 611–612, 612
Nasal spray, insulin, 1239
Nasal surgery, cosmetic, 610–611
  for deviated septum, 610–611
  for polyps, 611, 611
  nursing care guide for, 613c–616c
  reconstructive, 1591t
Nasal turbinates, hypertrophic, 611
Nasoenteric tubes, 983
Nasogastric feeding, 982. See also Enteral nutrition; Nutrition.
  aspiration in, pneumonia and, 647
  in unconscious client, 728
Nasogastric intubation, 976–980. See also Gastrointestinal intubation.
  for intestinal decompression, in mechanical ileus, 1075
  in paralytic ileus, 1076
  in intestinal resection, 1000, 1001, 1002
Nasointestinal feeding, 981t, 982. See also Gastrointestinal intubation.
Nasopharyngeal airway, 559, 560
Nasopharynx, 524, 525, 951
Nasotracheal tube, 559, 560. See also Endotracheal intubation.
National Advisory Council on Nursing Education and Practice (NACNEP), 29
National Amputation Foundation, 878
National health promotion, 14t, 14–15
National Hemophilia Foundation, 517
Native Americans. See also Racial/ethnic groups.
  diabetes in, 1227
Natural killer cells, 1432, 1433, 1433t, 1434
Natural resistance, 1441
Naturetin (bendroflumethiazide), 377t
Nausea, 959–961
  chemotherapy and, 1529, 1540t
  in HIV infection, management of, 1473d, 1478c
  in radiation therapy, 1521
  in renal colic, 1379, 1381c
Nd:YAG laser. See Laser surgery.
Nearsightedness, 1970–1974, 1971
Nebulized drugs, for chronic obstructive pulmonary disease, 675, 675
Neck. See also under Cervical.
  stiff, in disc herniation, 793
  in meningitis, 768, 768
Neck exercises, after radical neck dissection, 632, 633, 636c
Neck vein distention, assessment of, 192, 192
  in heart disease, 181
Necrotizing fasciitis, 1599–1600
Nedocromil, for asthma, 661, 662t, 663t
Needle biopsy, renal, 1357–1358

Needles, safety precautions for, 1464, 1472d
Negative feedback control, of hormones, 1208, *1208*, 1210, *1210*
Negative pressure room, 652
Neisseria gonorrhoeae, 1908. See also *Gonorrhea*.
Nembutal (sodium pentothal), for increased intracranial pressure, 732
Neomycin, 1151d
Neomycin enema, for hepatic encephalopathy, 1150, 1151d
Neonatal herpes, 1902–1903
Neonatal syphilis, 1918
Neonate, HIV transmission to, 1464
Neoplasm, benign, 1505, *1505*
    malignant, 1505, *1505*. See also *Cancer*.
Neostigmine (Prostigmin), for myasthenia gravis, 783, 783d
Neostigmine test, for myasthenia gravis, 783
Nephrectomy, for cancer, 1415–1418, 1418d
Nephritis. See *Glomerulonephritis; Pyelonephritis*.
Nephroblastoma, 1416–1418
Nephrogenic diabetes insipidus, 1274–1275
Nephron, 1331, *1331*
    in urine formation, 1332, *1332*
Nephropathy, diabetic, 1252d, 1254–1255
Nephrotic syndrome, in diabetes, 1255
Nephrotoxic drugs, 1389t
Nerve(s), peripheral, regeneration of, 712
Nerve blocks, 137, 138t. See also *Anesthesia*.
Nerve cells. See *Neuroglia; Neuron(s)*.
Nerve conduction studies, 757
Nerve deafness, 743
Nerve impulse transmission, 712–713
Nerve root compression, 793t
Nervous system, autonomic, anatomy and physiology of, 725–726, 726t
    cells of, 711–712, 712, 713
    central, 718–722, *718–722*. See also *Brain; Spinal cord*.
    nerve impulse transmission in, 712–713, *714*
    parasympathetic, in vascular control, 173
    peripheral, anatomy and physiology of, 722–725, *724*
    sympathetic, in vascular control, 173
Neupogen (filgrastim), for agranulocytosis, 491, 492d
Neuralgia, glossopharyngeal, 829t–830t
    trigeminal, 829t–830t
Neurofibroma, 1632t
Neurogenic bladder, 823, 825, 826
    catheterization of, 1361–1363
    in multiple sclerosis, 780, 781
Neurogenic shock, 416–417, 420. See also *Shock*.
Neurogenic tumors, mediastinal, 698
Neuroglia, 712, *713*
Neurohypophysis, 1208, *1208*, 1209–1210
    disorders of, 1274–1282
    hormones of, 1205t
Neurologic assessment, 745–748
    after spinal surgery, 762, 763d
    cranial nerve examination in, 723t–724t
    health history in, 745
    in head injury, 821
    in HIV infection, 1472
    in increased intracranial pressure, 733

Neurologic assessment (*Continued*)
    in stroke, 808
    in subarachnoid hemorrhage, 816
    mental status examination in, 746
    motor function assessment in, 747, 747t
    physical examination in, 745–746
    postoperative, 760
        in cardiac surgery, 225
    quick, 748, 748t
    reflex assessment in, 748
    sensory function assessment in, 747–748
    speech and language assessment in, 746–747
Neurologic disorders, 726–745
    age-related changes in, 67–68, 766
    altered consciousness in, 726t, 726–730, 727t
    as surgical risk factor, 122
    brain death in, 745
    degenerative, 775–795
    diagnosis of, 748–757
        carotid Doppler studies in, 749–750, *751*
        cerebral angiography in, 750–752, *751*
        cisternal puncture in, 754
        computed tomography in, 749
        electroencephalography in, 754–755
        electromyography in, 757
        evoked potentials in, 757
        lumbar puncture in, 753–754, 755c–756c, *757*
        magnetic resonance imaging in, 749, *750*
        myelography in, *752*, 752–753
        nerve conduction studies in, 757
        positron emission tomography in, 749
        skull x-rays in, 748
        spinal x-rays in, 748–749
    functional, 795–800
    in elderly, 765–766, 832
    in hyperkalemia, 89, 90
    in hypokalemia, 86, 88
    in hyponatremia, 91
    in pernicious anemia, 477, 478
    increased intracranial pressure in, 730–738
    infectious and inflammatory, 767–775
    management of, 757–765
        intracranial surgery in, 757–761
        settings and providers for, 765
        spinal surgery in, 761–765, 763d
    mental status in, 726–730
    motor system dysfunction in, 739–742
    neoplastic, 828–832, 831t
    resources for, 2039–2040
    sensory system dysfunction in, 742–744
    speech and language dysfunction in, 738–739
    traumatic, 816–822
Neurologic function, in acute renal failure, 1395c–1396c
    in chronic renal failure, 1399t
    in heart disease, 183–184
    in HIV infection, 1466
Neuroma, acoustic, 828–832, 831t
    plantar digital, 910–911
Neuromuscular blockers, anesthetic, 141t
Neuromuscular function, hypercalcemia and, 97, 98–99
Neuromuscular transmission, 713
Neuron(s), 711–712, *712*

Neuron(s) (*Continued*)
    afferent, 711, *712*
    age-related loss of, 765
    efferent, 711–712, *712*
    impulse transmission via, 712–713, *714*
    loss of, in Alzheimer's disease, 766
    lower motor, 722
    motor, 711, *712*
    sensory, 711, *712*
    upper motor, 722
Neuropathy, diabetic, 1252d, 1253–1254
Neurosurgery, ablative, 1555t
Neurosyphilis, 1916
    treatment of, 1912t
Neurotoxicity, of chemotherapy, 1532, 1536t
Neurotransmitters, 713
    pain and, 1551–1552
Neurovascular assessment, in cast therapy, 857
    in musculoskeletal disorders, 849
    in traction, 862
Neutropenia, 1437
    chemotherapy and, 1531, 1536t–1538t
    in agranulocytosis, 491–493
Neutrophils, 429, *429*, *430*, 1432, *1432*, 1433t, 1435
    band, 445t
    in phagocytosis, 1436
    segmented, 445t
Nevus, dysplastic, 1633t
    pigmented, 1633t
Nevus flammeus, 1571
Niacin deficiency, clinical manifestations of, 1077t
Nicardipine (Cardene), 213, 215d
Nickel dermatitis, 1609t, 1609–1611
Nifedipine (Procardia), 213, 215d, 378t
Night sweats, in HIV infection, 1465
Nikolsky's sign, 1620
Nipple, discharge from, in mammary duct ectasia, 1853
Nipple retraction, in breast cancer, 1858, *1859*
    vs. age-related, 1880
Nipride (nitroprusside), 213, 213d, 378t, 380t
    for cardiogenic shock, 413
Nissen fundoplication, for hiatus hernia, 1042, *1042*, 1043–1044
Nitrates, 212d, 212–213
    for angina, 286, 287–289
    for heart failure, 275
    for myocardial infarction, 297
Nitrofurantoin (Furadantin), for prostatitis, 1734
Nitrogen loss, in burns, 1678
Nitroglycerin, 212d, 212–213
    for angina, 286, 287–289
    for bleeding esophageal varices, 1183
    for cardiogenic shock, 413
    for myocardial infarction, 297
Nitroprusside (Nipride), 213, 213d, 378t, 380t
    for cardiogenic shock, 413
Nitrous oxide, 139, 139t
Nocturia, 1335
Nocturnal enuresis, 1335–1336
Nodular goiter, 1315
    in elderly, 1323
Nodule, *1571*, 1572
Nomogram, total body surface area, 1525, *1526*

Nonbacterial prostatitis, sequential bacteriologic localization cultures for, 1704–1705

Noncardiogenic pulmonary edema, 686–688

Noncompliance, in asymptomatic disorders, 375–376
  in diabetes, 1246c–1248c, 1260d
  in hypertension, 376, 382d, 383
  with glaucoma therapy, 1981–1982

Nongonococcal urethritis, 1924–1925

Non-Hodgkin's lymphoma, 507t, 507–508
  nursing care guide for, 509c–511c

Nonhospital care, increase in, 17–21
  practice roles in, 26–29
  practice settings for, 21–29

Non–insulin-dependent diabetes (type 2), 1227, 1228t. See also *Diabetes mellitus.*

Non-rebreathing mask, 555t

Nonseminomatous testicular tumors, 1748–1752. See also *Testicular cancer.*

Nonsteroidal anti-inflammatory drugs (NSAIDs), 893d, 1553, 1554t. See also *Aspirin.*
  for ocular disorders, 1947
  for osteoarthritis, 893d, 897
  for rheumatoid arthritis, 892, 893d

Nontropical sprue, *1078*, 1078–1079
  malabsorption in, 1077t, 1077–1078

Noradrenalin, 726

Norepinephrine (Levophed), 1206t, 1215–1216, 1216t
  as vasoconstrictor, 173
  blood flow and, 329, 329t
  cardiac effects of, 405t
  hypersecretion of, from pheochromocytoma, 1292
  urinary assays of, 1293t

Normodyne (labetalol), 378t

North American Nursing Diagnosis Association (NANDA), 8–9

Nose. See under *Nasal.*

Nosebleed, 610–611

Nosocomial pneumonia, 641
  case study of, 928d–929d
  prevention of, 642d

NPO status, 124

NSAIDS. See *Nonsteroidal anti-inflammatory drugs (NSAIDs).*

Nuchal rigidity, 768, *768*

Nuclear medicine. See *Radionuclide scanning.*

Nucleolus, 1503, *1504*

5'Nucleotidase, assessment of, 1161t, 1162

Nucleus, cell, 1503, *1504*

Nummular eczema, 1608t

Nummular psoriasis, 1616–1619, 1617t

Nurse. See also *Medical-surgical nurse.*
  ambulatory care, 26–27
  circulating, 135, 143
  discharge planner, 26
  first assistant, 135
  home health, 27
  hospice, 27
  occupational health, 28
  practical, qualifications and responsibilities of, 25t
  public health, 28
  registered, qualifications and responsibilities of, 24t, 29
  school, 28
  scrub, 135
  visiting, 27

Nurse anesthetist, 135

Nurse practitioner, 4–5, 27–28
  certification of, 5t, 5–6

Nurse supervisor, of unlicensed assistive personnel, 26

Nurse-managed centers, 22

Nursing. See also *Medical-surgical nursing.*
  cultural aspects of, 12–14
  geriatric, 49. See also *Elderly.*
  in nonhospital settings, 26–29
  oncologic, resources for, 2042
  perioperative, 116–123
  school, 25–26
  spiritual aspects of, 13–14

Nursing care, components of, 3
  cultural competence in, 1230d–1231d
  technologically mediated, 28–29

Nursing care guide, for acute renal failure, 1395c–1398c
  for Addison's disease, 1282c–1283c
  for adrenalectomy, 1290c–1291c
  for amputation, 939c–942c
  for ascites, 1155c
  for assessment of elderly, 70c–74c, 70d–74d
  for burns, 1650c–1655c
  for cardiac arrest, 265c–268c
  for cardiac catheterization, 203c–205c
  for chronic lymphocytic leukemia, 497c–502c
  for cirrhosis, 1190c–1193c
  for conservative laryngectomy, 621c–625c
  for cystoscopy, 1354c–1356c
  for decubitus ulcer prevention, 70c
  for diabetes, for ketoacidosis, 1246c–1248c
    for self-management, 1244c–1246c
  for diagnostic testing for peripheral vascular disease, 341c
  for drug therapy in elderly, 56c–57c, 56d–57d
  for esophageal varices, 1191c–1192c
  for fracture reduction surgery, 920c–923c
  for hepatic disorders, 1155c–1158c
  for HIV infection, 1474c–1482c
  for hypocalcemic tetany, 1319c
  for hypothyroidism, 1303c–1305c
  for lobectomy, 588d–596d
  for lumbar puncture, 755c–756c
  for lumpectomy, 1870c–1874c
  for lymphoma, 509c–511c
  for nasal surgery, 613c–616c
  for osteosarcoma surgery, 939c–942c
  for pneumonectomy in lung cancer, 696, 700c–707c
  for radical neck dissection, 634c–637c
  for Raynaud's disease, 358c–360c
  for sexually transmitted diseases, 1890c–1900c
  for subtotal gastrectomy, 1034c–1041c
  for supraglottic laryngectomy, 621c–625c
  for temporary colostomy, 1085c–1093c
  for total joint replacement, 869c–872c
  for transfusion reaction, 459c–461c
  for urinary calculi, 1381c–1382c
  for varicose veins, 391c–392c

Nursing diagnoses, 8–9, 10t–11t

Nursing education, 3–5

Nursing history, 8

Nursing interventions, in nursing process, 9

Nursing Interventions Classification (NIC), 9

Nursing process, 8–12
  assessment in, 8
  evaluation in, 11–12
  implementation in, 11
  nursing diagnoses in, 8–9, 10t–11t
  planning in, 9–11

Nursing research, absorbent products for female urinary incontinence, 1339d
  aspirin for thrombosis prevention, 432d
  cognitive screening in head injury, 817d
  condom use in divorced/separated women, 1924d
  education for prostate cancer awareness in African-Americans, 1756d
  endotracheal tube cuff care, 562d
  gastrointestinal bleeding in stroke, 966d
  gender differences in coping with surgery, 120d
  hepatitis B immunization in elderly, 1175d
  in electrolytes and blood pressure, 100d
  mechanical ventilation in chronic obstructive pulmonary disease, 672d
  nurses' attitudes toward AIDS patients, 1470d
  nurses' attitudes toward euthanasia, 42b
  outpatient ocular surgery, 1950d
  oximetry probe sheaths, 545d
  patient and partner support in breast biopsy, 1850d–1851d
  patient teaching for colposcopy, 1782d
  recovery from myocardial infarction, 301d
  self-care after myocardial infarction, 299d
  side effects of intracavitary radiation therapy, 1833d, 1834
  Unna's boot dressings for skin grafts, 1676d

Nutrients, hepatic storage of, 1139

Nutrition. See also *Diet; Food.*
  after ileostomy, 1012d
  after intestinal resection, 1002
  as surgical risk factor, 120–121
  enteral. See *Enteral nutrition.*
  in amyotrophic lateral sclerosis, 777
  in blood cell formation, 441d
  in burns, 1678–1680
  in cancer, 1558–1560, 1560d
  in chronic obstructive pulmonary disease, 668, 669, 678d
  in colostomy, 1009, 1009d, 1010
  in Crohn's disease, 1067, 1069, 1069d
  in elderly, 51–52, 53d
    gastrointestinal function and, 65–66
  in emphysema, 670
  in endotracheal intubation, 563d
  in heart disease, 183d–185d, 184–185
  in hematologic disorders, 440–441, 441d, 452
  in HIV infection, 1470, 1472–1473, 1473d, 1477c–1478c
  in Hodgkin's disease, 506–507
  in iron deficiency anemia, 476
  in leukemia, 498c–499c, 502, 504d
  in lung cancer, 699d
  in mechanical ventilation, 563d
  in Parkinson's disease, 788–790, 789d
  in peritoneal dialysis, 1404
  in pneumonia, 646d
  in stroke, 813

Nutrition (*Continued*)
in supraglottic laryngectomy, 623c
in total laryngectomy, 630
in tracheostomy, 563d
in unconscious client, 728
postoperative, 155
in gastrectomy, 998t, 1000
in intestinal resection, 1003
in intracranial surgery, 761
pressure ulcers and, 1625, 1628, *1629*
total parenteral. See *Total parenteral nutrition.*
Nutritional assessment, for elderly, 52
for pressure ulcers, 1628, *1629*
Nutritional deficiencies, in alcoholism, 1139t, 1153
in hepatic disorders, 1139t, 1153–1154, 1154t
Nutritionist, qualifications and responsibilities of, 24t
Nystagmus, 742, 1943
Nystatin, for thrush, 1019t

O

Obesity, as surgical risk factor, 120–121
diabetes and, 1227, 1228t, 1232d
heart disease and, 186, 210
in Cushing's syndrome, 1286
vascular disease and, 338t
Obliterative cardiomyopathy, 306
Obstructive cirrhosis, 1181, 1181t. See also *Cirrhosis.*
Obstructive jaundice, 1140
Obstructive megaureter, ureterovesical junction obstruction and, 1382
Obtundation, 726t
Occipital lobe, 719, *719*
Occlusive dressings, 1583
Occult blood test, for colorectal cancer, 1513
Occupational factors, in cancer, 1508–1509
in prostate cancer, 1754
Occupational health, 23–25
Occupational health nurse, 28
Occupational lung diseases, 688–690
Occupational therapist, qualifications and responsibilities of, 24t
Occupational therapy, 884
for rheumatoid arthritis, 892–894
Octreotide (Sandostatin), for bleeding esophageal varices, 1183
Ocular complications. See also *Eye disorders.*
in HIV infection, 1466–1467
in hypertension, 375, 376
in renal failure, 1400
Ocular compress, 1967t
Ocular disorders. See *Eye disorders.*
Ocular fundus, examination of, 1944, *1944*
Ocular muscles, 1936, *1936*
examination of, 1943
weakness of, in myasthenia gravis, 782, 784
Ocularist, 1960
Oculomotor nerve, 723t
Ocusert, 1949, *1949*
Odynophagia, drug-induced, 1047t
in achalasia, 1044, 1045
in esophagitis, 1020
Ofloxacin, for gonorrhea, 1909–1910, 1911t, 1914

Ointments, 1579, 1580t
ophthalmic, administration of, 1949, *1949*, 1949t
Olfaction, age-related changes in, 61
Olfactory nerve, 723t
Oligodendroglia, 712, *713*
Oligodendroglioma, 828–832, 831t
Oligomenorrhea, 1775–1776
Oliguria, 1343
definition of, 1388t
in acute renal failure, 1389, 1390, 1391
in shock, 406, 407t
Ommaya reservoir, 1527
Oncogene, 1510
Oncologic nursing, resources for, 2042
Onychomycosis, 1600t, 1600–1601
Oocyte, 1768
Oophorectomy, 1786t
for ovarian cancer, 1837–1838
with hysterectomy, 1793–1794, *1794*. See also *Hysterectomy.*
Open pneumothorax, 692–693, *693*, 694
Open thoracotomy, 580t
Open-angle glaucoma, 1979–1982
Opening snap, 180
Open-lung biopsy, 580t
Ophthalmic assistant, 1960
Ophthalmic disorders. See *Eye disorders.*
Ophthalmic ointments and drops, administration of, 1949, *1949*
Ophthalmic photographer, 1960
Ophthalmic technician, 1960
Ophthalmic technologist, 1960
Ophthalmic ultrasonographer, 1960
Ophthalmic ultrasonography, 1945–1946, 1960
Ophthalmologist, 1960
Ophthalmopathy, infiltrative, in hyperthyroidism, 1307, *1307*, 1308
treatment of, 1308–1309
Ophthalmoscopy, 1944, *1944*
Opioids. See *Narcotics.*
Opportunistic infections, immunosuppression and, 1409, 1458, 1459t
in bone marrow transplant, 1451, 1453, 1454d
in HIV infection, 1466, 1467, 1470, 1476c–1477c
prevention of, 1464, 1472d, 1476c–1477c
Opsonization, 1437, 1439
defects in, 1437
Optic disk, *1936*, 1937
examination of, 1944, *1944*
Optic nerve, 723t
Optic tracts, 1938, *1938*
Optical aid, 1958–1959
Optical-to-tactile converters, 1959
Optician, 1960
Optional surgery, 119
Optometrist, 1960
Oral antidiabetic agents, 1239, 1239t, 1240d
for elderly, 1261
Oral bile acids, for gallstones, 1110–1111
Oral cancer, 1049–1053
clinical manifestations of, 1049–1050, *1050*
diagnosis of, 1050
etiology of, 1049
Internet connections for, 1056d
management of, 1050
pathophysiology of, 1049
self-examination for, 1053d

Oral cancer (*Continued*)
surgery for, 1050–1053
postoperative care in, 1051–1053
preoperative care in, 1050–1051
Oral candidiasis, 1017–1019, 1019t, 1602
in HIV infection, 1465
Oral care, after oral surgery, 1052, 1052d
in chemotherapy, 1529–1530, 1541t
in dehydration, 79
in endotracheal intubation, 563
in gastrointestinal intubation, 979
in hematologic disorders, 430–438, 439, 439d
in HIV infection, 1465, 1473d, 1478c
in leukemia, 499c–500c, 503
in nasal surgery, 615c
in radiation therapy, 1521d, 1523d
in sinus surgery, 604
in unconscious client, 729
postoperative, in transsphenoidal microsurgery, 1269, 1271c–1272c
with intermaxillary fixation, 1048, 1049d
Oral cavity, examination of, 968
self-examination of, 1053d
structure and function of, 951
Oral cholecystogram, 971–972
Oral contraceptives, for dysmenorrhea, 1776
for endometriosis, 1813, 1814d
heart disease and, 187
hepatotoxicity of, 1178t
smoking and, 211
Oral dryness, chemotherapy and, 1530, 1541t
in radiation therapy, 1520
Oral glucose tolerance test, 1229
Oral infections, 1017–1019, 1018t
Oral lesions, chemotherapy and, 1529–1530, 1541t
in elderly, nutrition and, 65–66
in hematologic disorders, 437–438, 439, 439d
in HIV infection, 1465, 1473d, 1478c
in radiation therapy, 1520–1521, 1521d
Oral mucosa, examination of, 968
Oral surgery, for cancer, 1050–1053
Orbicularis oculi muscle, 1936
Orchiectomy, 1708t, 1749, 1750–1752
for prostate cancer, 1759
Orchiopexy, 1708t
for cryptorchidism, 1739–1740, 1740d
Orchitis, 1731–1732
Oretic (hydrochlorothiazide), 377t
Organ donation, 45–46
Organ donors, criteria for, 1408
Organ of Corti, 1997
Organic brain syndrome, 832
Orgasm, female, 1769
male, 1698
Orinase (tolbutamide), 1239, 1239t, 1240d
Orogastric intubation, 976–980. See also *Gastrointestinal intubation.*
Oropharyngeal airway, 559, *560*
Oropharynx, *524*, *525*, 951
Orotracheal tube, 559, *560*. See also *Endotracheal intubation.*
Orthopedic disorders. See *Musculoskeletal disorders.*
Orthopedic surgery, 863–878
amputation, 868–878
external fixation devices and, *863*, 863–865

Orthopedic surgery (Continued)
   internal fixation devices and, 865, 865–867
   total joint replacement, 867–868, 868, 869c–872c
Orthopnea, 174
   in heart failure, 270, 277
Orthoptist, 1960
Orthostatic hypotension, 178
   in elderly, 64–65, 71c
   injury prevention in, 71c
Orthotopic hepatic transplant, 1196–1198
Osler's nodes, 234
Osmitrol (mannitol), 732d
   for increased intracranial pressure, 732
Osmoglyn (glycerin), for glaucoma, 1980
Osmolality, 75–76
Osmolarity, 75–76
Osmotic agents, for increased intraocular pressure, 1947
Osmotic diuretics, 732d
   for increased intracranial pressure, 731–732
Osseous labyrinth, 1996
Ossicles, auricular, 1996, 1996, 1997
Ossification, 838–839
   in bone repair, 840
   pathologic, 935
Osteitis deformans, 908
Osteoarthritis, 897–898
   nonsteroidal anti-inflammatory drugs for, 893d
Osteoblast, 838, 838, 839
Osteochondroma, 935–938, 936t
Osteoclast, 838, 838, 839
Osteocyte, 838, 838
Osteoid osteoma, 935–938, 936t
Osteoma, 935–938, 936t
Osteomalacia, 902–904
Osteomyelitis, 887–890
   acute, 888
   chronic, 888
   fungal, 889
   posttraumatic, 934
   Salmonella, 889
   syphilis, 889
   tuberculous, 888–889
Osteon, 838
Osteonecrosis, avascular, 935
Osteopenia, 904
Osteophytes, in osteoarthritis, 897
Osteoporosis, 67, 904–908
   in multiple myeloma, 511
   prevention of, estrogen replacement therapy for, 1772
   safety measures for, 71c
Osteosarcoma, 935–938, 936t, 938, 939c–942c, 942–943
   in Paget's disease, 908
Osteotomy, for rheumatoid arthritis, 892
Ostomate, 1006, 1010
Ostomy. See also Colostomy; Ileostomy; Urostomy.
Ostomy care, in gastrostomy, 986
Otalgia, 1998
Otitis externa, 2011–2012, 2012d
Otitis media, 2012–2103, 2014, 2103t
   brain abscess and, 771
   myringotomy for, 2005–2006, 2006
Otomycosis, 2011–2012
Otorrhea, 1998
   assessment of, 2000
Otosclerosis, 2015–2016, 2016

Otoscopy, 2000–2001, 2001
Ototoxic drugs, 1997, 1997t
   neomycin as, 1151d
Outcomes, expected, in nursing process, 9
Outpatient surgery, 115–116, 156t, 156–158, 157t
   facilities for, 22
   ocular, 1950d
Oval window, 1995–1996, 1996, 1997
Ovarian cancer, 1837–1838
   in elderly, 1838
Ovarian cystectomy, 1786t
Ovarian cysts, 1824–1825
   chocolate, 1813
Ovarian tumors, benign, 1824–1825
Ovary, palpation of, 1781
   in cancer, 1837
   structure and function of, 1207t, 1767, 1767–1768, 1768
Ovulation, 1768
   ovarian cancer and, 1837
   pain of, 1777
Ovum, fertilization of, 1769
Oxaprozin (Daypro), 893d
Oxidizing agents, burns from, 1686t. See also Chemical burns.
Oximetry, pulse, 544–545, 546
   probe sheaths for, 652d
Oxygen, partial pressure of, 540, 540t
   in oxyhemoglobin dissociation curve, 541, 541–542
   normal values for, 540t, 541
   SaO_2 and, 541
Oxygen consumption, 405t, 405–406
Oxygen delivery, 405, 405t
Oxygen diffusion, 540, 540t
Oxygen extraction ratio, 405t, 406
Oxygen masks, 555t
Oxygen tension, 540
Oxygen therapy, 556–559
   administration methods in, 555t, 556
   flow rate in, 556
   for adult respiratory distress syndrome, 687
   for angina, 288
   for carbon monoxide poisoning, 1659
   for cardiogenic pulmonary edema, 280
   for chronic obstructive pulmonary disease, 672, 675
   for heart failure, 279
   for hematologic disorders, 452
   for myocardial infarction, 296, 302
   for pneumonia, 645
   safety measures for, 556t, 556–557
   toxicity of, 556t
   transtracheal, 557, 557–559, 558d
Oxygen transport, 405t, 405–406
Oxygenation failure, 531
Oxyhemoglobin, 427, 540, 540t
Oxytocin, 1205t
   production of, 1209
Ozena, 601

P

P wave, 193, 194, 195
Pacemaker, artificial. See Pacing.
   junctional, 171
Pacemaker syncope, 176
Pacing, epicardial, 258
   external, 259, 259
   internal, 256–259, 257, 258

Pacing (Continued)
   temporary, 258–259
   transvenous, 258
Packed red cell transfusion, 453. See also Transfusion(s).
Packing, anal, 1074
   nasal, 604, 614c
   vaginal, 1800
$PaCO_2$, 540, 540t, 542–543
   normal values for, 540t, 541
Pads, incontinence, 1339d
Paget's disease of bone, 908
   alendronate for, 906d
Pain, abdominal, 964, 964t, 965
   characteristics of, 965
   sources of, 965t
   bladder, 1341–1342
   bone, 839, 846–847
     in hematologic disorders, 438
   chest, after cardiac arrest, 266c–267c
     assessment of, 188
     in heart disease, 175, 175t, 188, 285–289. See also Angina pectoris.
     in infective endocarditis, 235–236
     in myocardial infarction, 294, 295, 296, 300
     in pericarditis, 238, 239
     in pleuritis, 658
     noncardiac, 175
   definition of, 1551
   ear, 1998
     assessment of, 1999–2000
   gate-control theory of, 1551
   headache, 800, 801
   in abdominal aortic aneurysm, 368, 368d
   in achalasia, 1044, 1045
   in acute gastritis, 1024
   in acute pancreatitis, 1118, 1122
   in amputation, 875d–876d, 877
   in ankylosing spondylitis, 898, 899
   in anorectal abscess, 1072
   in appendicitis, 1065, 1065
   in arterial thromboembolism, 357
   in atherosclerosis, 362
   in burns, 1651c–1652c, 1670–1671
   in cancer, 1551–1558. See also Cancer, pain in.
   in cholecystitis, 1109
   in chronic pancreatitis, 1122–1124
   in compartment syndrome, 933
   in Crohn's disease, 1067, 1069
   in disc herniation, 793, 794–795
   in diverticular disease, 1082, 1083
   in elderly, 1015
   in endometriosis, 1813, 1814
   in epididymitis, 1729, 1730–1731
   in esophagitis, 1020
   in fibrocystic breast disease, 1854, 1856d
   in fractures, 916
   in gangrene, 333–334
   in genital herpes, 1902
   in glaucoma, 1979, 1981
   in gout, 899, 900, 901
   in hematologic disorders, 438
   in HIV infection, 1475c–1476c
   in intermittent claudication, 332, 332, 333–334
   in ischemic neuropathy, 332, 333–334
   in keratitis, 1967
   in laryngitis, 610
   in leukemia, 496, 503, 504d
   in multiple myeloma, 508, 512
   in necrotizing fasciitis, 1599, 1600

Pain (*Continued*)
in ocular trauma, 1989
in osteoarthritis, 897, 898d
in osteomalacia, 903, 904
in osteoporosis, 905
in osteosarcoma, 938
in peptic ulcer disease, 1026–1027, 1027t, 1029, 1032
in peritonitis, 1062, 1063
in postherpetic neuralgia, 1606–1607
in prostate cancer, 1760–1761
in prostatitis, 1735
in prostatodynia, 1735
in radical neck dissection, 634c, 637c
in reproductive disorders, in males, 1699
in respiratory disorders, 529
assessment of, 531
in rheumatoid arthritis, 891, 892, 893d, 895
in rib fractures, 690
in sexually transmitted diseases, 1890c–1891c
in sickle-cell crisis, 485, 486, 486d
in temporomandibular joint syndrome, 1998
in thromboangiitis obliterans, 352–354
in total joint replacement, 870c, 871c
in traction, 862
in ulcerative colitis, 1070
in vascular disorders, 331–334, 362, 363
in venous insufficiency, 332, 333–334
in venous thrombosis, 384, 385, 387
intensity of, rating scale for, *1558*
intermenstrual, 1777
ischemic, 331–334, 362, 363
joint, 846–847
in hematologic disorders, 438
low back, 911–913
menstrual, 1776–1777
muscle, 846–847
musculoskeletal, 846–847
neurotransmitters and, 1551–1552
ocular, 1939
of arterial ulcerations, 333–334
of gangrene, 333–334
on urination, 1335
ovulatory, 1777
phantom, 872–873
rectal, 1104
physiology of, 1551–1552, *1552*
postoperative, in cholecystectomy, 1117
in hemorrhoidectomy, 1098
in hysterectomy, 1799
in intracranial surgery, 760–761
in lobectomy, 592c–593c
in lumpectomy, 1871d
in mastectomy, 1865
in oral surgery, 1052
in pneumonectomy, 586
in spinal surgery, 764
in Whipple's procedure, 1130–1131
renal, *1341*, 1341–1342
response to, cultural factors in, 1379
rest, 332, 333–334
self-assessment of, 1558, *1558, 1559*
shoulder, in stroke, 809
ureteral, 1341–1342
urinary calculi and, 1379, 1381c
urinary tract, 1341–1342
visceral, 965, 965t
Pain management, 1552–1556. See also *Analgesia; Analgesics.*
cognitive-behavioral therapies in, 1553–1555

Pain management (*Continued*)
drug therapy in, 1552–1553, *1553*
flow chart for, 1556, *1557*
for ischemic pain, 333, 343
in elderly, 54t
in musculoskeletal disorders, 846–847
in myocardial infarction, 296
in osteoarthritis, 893d, 897
in rheumatoid arthritis, 892, 893d, 895
invasive therapies in, 1556, *1556*
nonsteroidal anti-inflammatory drugs in, 892, 893d
patient-controlled analgesia in, 847, 1553
physical therapies in, 1555–1556, *1556*
postoperative, 152–153
in cardiac surgery, 227
thermal applications in, 892
transcutaneous nerve stimulation in, 892
Pain perception, alterations in, *743*, 743–744
assessment of, 748
Pallor, 334, 1570
in anemia, 468
in heart disease, 182
in hematologic disorders, 434
Palmar psoriasis, 1616–1619, 1617t
Palpation, abdominal, 969
of abdomen, 192
of breast, 1845, *1845*
of chest, *181*, 190–191, 534–535
of distal pulses, 335, *336*, 338–339
of liver, 192, 969, 1159, *1160*
of ovary, 1781
in cancer, 1837
of prostate, 1702, *1702*
of pulses, 189, *190*
Palpebrae, 1935, *1936*
Palpebral conjunctiva, 1935–1936, *1936*
examination of, 1942, *1942*
Palpitations, 176–177
Pancreas, structure and function of, 957–958, *958*
Pancreatic abscess, fistula formation and, 1124–1126, *1125*
Pancreatic amylase, 956, 957, 958t
Pancreatic cancer, 1126–1131
chemotherapy for, 1128
cholecystojejunostomy for, 1127, *1127*
clinical manifestations of, 1127
diagnosis of, 1127
etiology of, 1126
incidence of, 1126
Internet connections for, 1113d
management of, 1127–1131
settings and providers for, 1128
pathophysiology of, 1126
radiation therapy for, 1128
Whipple's procedure for, 1128
Pancreatic enzymes, 957–958, 958t
in acute pancreatitis, 1118
in chronic pancreatitis, 1122
supplemental, for chronic pancreatitis, 1123d, 1124
for elderly, 1131
Pancreatic fistula, 1124–1126, *1125*
Pancreatic fluid, 957
Pancreatic function, in heart disease, 184
Pancreatic hormones, 1206t–1207t
Pancreatic juice, 956, 957, 958t
Pancreatic lipase, 956, 957, 958t
Pancreatic transplantation, for diabetes, 1239–1240
Pancreatic ultrasonography, 976

Pancreatitis, acute, 1118–1122
case study of, 1119d–1121d
in elderly, 1131
pancreatic fistula and, 1124–1126, *1125*
chronic, 1122–1124
in elderly, 1131
Pancreatoduodenectomy, radical, *1127*, 1127–1131
complications of, 1128
patient preparation for, 1128
postoperative care in, 1129–1131
postoperative course in, 1128
preoperative care in, 1128–1129
Pancuronium bromide (Pavulon), 141t
Pancytopenia, 480
in bone marrow transplant, 1451
Pannus, in rheumatoid arthritis, 890
Pansinusitis, 602
PaO$_2$, 540, 540t
in oxyhemoglobin dissociation curve, *541*, 541–542
normal values for, 540t, 541
SaO$_2$ and, 541
Papanicolaou test, 1513, 1779d, 1781–1782, *1783*, 1831
Papillary thyroid cancer, 1316
Papilledema, 733
brain tumors and, 828–829
Papule, *1571*, 1572
Paracentesis, for portal hypertension, 1144, 1145t
Paraesophageal hernia, 1041, *1042*
Parafollicular (C) cells, 1211, 1212
Paraldehyde, for seizures, 796, 797d–798d
Paralysis, 739
facial nerve, 829t–830t
in amyotrophic lateral sclerosis, 775–777
in Guillain-Barré syndrome, 773
in peripheral nerve injury, 828
in spinal cord injury. See *Spinal cord injury.*
Paralytic ileus, 1075–1077
after hysterectomy, 1795
in appendicitis, 1063, 1064t
in burns, 1679
in peritonitis, 1062
postoperative, 148t, 155, 996
Paranasal sinuses, *601*
inflammation of, 601–604
palpation of, *602*
surgery of, 603–604
Paraparesis, 739
Paraphenylenediamine dermatitis, 1609t, 1609–1611
Paraphimosis, 1737–1739
Paraplegia, 739
Parasympathetic nervous system, 725t, 726
in vascular control, 173
Parathyroid glands, autografting of, 1316
disorders of, 1316–1322
in elderly, 1324
injury to, in thyroidectomy, 1314
structure and function of, 1206t, *1212*, 1212t, 1212–1213, *1213*
Parathyroid hormone, 1206t, 1212–1213, *1213*
calcium and, 95
hypersecretion of, 1318–1322
hyposecretion of, 1316–1318
Paresis, 739. See also *Paralysis.*
Paresthesia, disc herniation and, 793, 794t, 795

Paresthesia *(Continued)*
  in arterial insufficiency, 334t
  in multiple sclerosis, 780
Parietal cells, 952
Parietal lobe, 719, *719*
Parietal pleura, 524–525, *525*
Parkinson's disease, *787,* 787–790, 789d
Parlodel (bromocriptine), for somatotropin
    hypersecretion, 1273
Paronychia, 1598t
Parotid glands, 951
Parotitis, postoperative, 148t
Paroxysmal atrial tachycardia, *244,* 244–
    245
Paroxysmal cough, 529
Paroxysmal nocturnal dyspnea, 174, 270
Partial rebreathing mask, 555t
Partial seizures, 796t
Partial thromboplastin time, 443t, 448
  in heart disease, 208–209
Partner notification, in gonorrhea, 1913–
    1914
  in syphilis, 1917, 1920
Passive motion device, 868, 914
Past-pointing test, 2001–2002
Patch tests, 1576–1577, *1577*
Pathologic fractures, in multiple myeloma,
    512
  in osteoporosis, 905, 906
Pathologic ossification, 935
Patient Self-Determination Act, 42–43
Patient teaching. See also *Internet connec-
    tions; Self-care.*
  discharge, 155, 156d
  for acute renal failure, 1398c
  for ambulatory surgery, 157–158
  for amputation, 875d–876d, 877–878
  for anaphylaxis prevention, 422d
  for anemia, 470, 470d
  for angina, 288
  for antacids, 1043
  for aplastic anemia, 482
  for appendectomy, 1066d
  for ascites, 1148–1149
  for asthma, 664–665
  for atherosclerosis, 362–363
  for bleeding disorders, 482d
  for blood glucose monitoring, 1242d,
      1244c–1245c
  for burns, 1683–1684, 1685d
  for cardiac catheterization, 201d, 203–
      204, 205d
  for cardiac disorders, 287d
  for cardiac valvular surgery, 315–316
  for cast therapy, 857d, 858
  for circumcision, 1737d
  for colostomy, 1006–1007, 1010–1011
  for coronary artery bypass graft, 291d,
      291–292
  for coronary artery disease, 284–285,
      285d, 289
  for diuretic therapy, 218d
  for diverticular disease, 1084d
  for drug therapy, 55, 55d–57d
  for dysrhythmias, 255–256
  for endocrine disorders, 1217–1218,
      1219d
  for genital herpes, 1906, 1906d, 1907d
  for heart failure, 273d, 279
  for hematologic disorders, 437, 442d
  for HIV infection, 1472, 1474c–1475c
  for hydrocelectomy, 1743d
  for hyperkalemia, 90
  for hypertension, 382d, 383d, 383–384

Patient teaching *(Continued)*
  for hypokalemia, 88–89
  for hyponatremia, 93
  for hypothyroidism, 1303c–1305c, 1306
  for hysterectomy, 1799–1800, 1800d
  for infection prevention, 440d
  for infective endocarditis, 235, 235d,
      236
  for insulin administration, 1236d–1237d
  for internal fixation devices, 866–867,
      867d
  for leukemia, 501c–502c, 503
  for lobectomy, 588c–589c
  for lung cancer, 698, 699d
  for mastectomy, postoperative, 1867,
      1867d
    preoperative, 1863
  for myocardial infarction, 301d, 302–303,
      303d
  for nasal surgery, 613c
  for orchiopexy, 1739
  for osteoarthritis, 898d
  for penile implant, 1724d
  for pneumonectomy, 585d, 706d
  for pneumonia, 646d
  for premenstrual syndrome, 1812d
  for prostatectomy, 1720d
  for radical neck dissection, 637c
  for Raynaud's disease, 356d, 360
  for rheumatoid arthritis, 896
  for sexually transmitted diseases, 1897c–
      1898c, 1901d
  for stoma care, in colostomy, 1006–1007,
      1010–1011, 1092c–1093c
    in tracheostomy, 566–567, 630, 631d,
        1092c
  for tonsillectomy, 607–608, 608d
  for total joint replacement, 869c–870c,
      872c
  for total laryngectomy, 630, 631d, 637
  for T-tube drainage, 1117d
  for tuberculosis, for drug therapy, 655,
      657
    for prevention, 656
  for venous stasis ulcers, 393
  for venous thrombosis, 388, 388d
  for vulvovaginal hygiene, 1805d, 1807d
  information sources for, 2037–2045
  postoperative, 129d, 131–133, 155, 156d
  preoperative, 129d, 129–133
Patient-controlled analgesia, 152, *152,*
    847
Pavulon (pancuronium bromide), 141t
Peak flow meter, 663, *663,* 667
Peau d'orange skin, in breast cancer, 1858,
    1859
Peck, Robert, 32
Pectus carinatum, 534, *534*
Pectus excavatum, 534, *534*
Pedicle flaps, 1587
Pediculosis pubis, 1928–1929
PEEP (positive-end-expiratory pressure),
    569. See also *Mechanical ventilation.*
Pelvic abscess, appendicitis and, 1064t
Pelvic examination, female, 1778–1781,
    1780
  in elderly, 1800
  patient preparation for, 1778–1779
  procedure for, 1779–1781, *1780*
  male, 1700–1703, *1702*
Pelvic exenteration, 1786t
  for cervical cancer, 1831–1832
Pelvic floor exercises, 1365, 1365d, 1779d,
    1817, 1817d

Pelvic fractures, bladder injury in, 1413–
    1414
  urethral injury in, 1415
Pelvic inflammatory disease (PID), antibi-
    otics for, 1912t
  chlamydial, 1920, 1921, 1923–1924. See
      also Chlamydia trachomatis *infec-
      tion.*
  in gonorrhea, 1909
Pelvic lymphadenectomy, in radical vul-
    vectomy, 1826–1830, 1829d
Pelvic radiation, sexual dysfunction and,
    1522
Pelvic supports, weakened, 1815–1819,
    1816
  in elderly, 1838
Pemphigus vulgaris, 1619–1620, *1620*
Penectomy, 1708t, *1746,* 1746–1748
Penicillin, for acute gingivitis, 1018t
  for necrotizing fasciitis, 1599
  for streptococcal pharyngitis, 237
  for syphilis, 1912t, 1917
  prophylactic, in sickle-cell anemia, 485
Penile cancer, 1744–1748, 1745t
  in elderly, 1761
Penile chancre, in syphilis, 1915, *1915*
Penile discharge, in chlamydia, 1921, 1922
  in gonorrhea, 1908, *1908*
Penile erection. See under *Erectile; Erec-
    tion.*
Penile implants, 1720–1724, *1721,* 1721t,
    1724d
Penile warts, 1063–1065, 1064t, *1926,*
    1926–1928
Penis, age-related changes in, 1725
  biopsy of, 1706
  examination of, 1700–1701
  hygiene for, 1702, 1728, 1729d
  structure and function of, 1695, *1696*
Pentothal (thiopental), for anesthesia,
    141t
  for increased intracranial pressure, 732
Pepsin, 952, 954, 958t
Peptic ulcers, assessment in, 1032
  bleeding in, 1029, *1029,* 1030d–1031d
  case study of, 1030d–1031d, 1030d–
      1301d
  clinical manifestations of, 1026–1027,
      1027t
  complications of, 1029
  diagnosis of, 1027
  diet in, 1027
  drug therapy for, 1027–1028
  etiology of, 1026
  hemorrhage in, 1029, *1029*
  in elderly, 1059–1060
  incidence of, 1026, 1027t
  Internet connections for, 1056d
  management of, 1027–1029
  nursing diagnoses and planning in,
      1032
  nursing interventions in, 1032–1033
  obstruction in, 1029
  pain in, 1026–1027, 1027t, 1032
  pathophysiology of, 1026, 1027t
  perforation in, 1029
  stress, 1033, 1679
    bleeding from, 966d
    in burns, 1679
    postoperative, 148t
  surgery for, 1028–1029, 1034c–1041c
Peptidase, 958t
Pepto-Bismol (bismuth subsalicylate), for
    H. pylori infection, 1028

Percussion, of abdomen, 192, 968–969
  of chest, 192
    diagnostic, 192, *535*, 535–536, *536*
    therapeutic, 553–555
  of liver, 1159, *1160*
Percutaneous cryosurgery, for prostate cancer, 1759
Percutaneous endoscopic gastrostomy, *982*, 982–983
  in esophageal cancer, 1055
  ostomy care in, 986
Percutaneous transhepatic cholangiography, 972
Percutaneous transluminal angioplasty, 343–344
Percutaneous transluminal coronary angioplasty (PTCA), for coronary artery disease, *292*, 292–293
  for myocardial infarction, 295
Perfusion scans, 548
Perianal area, examination of, 969
Pericardial effusion, 239d, 239–240
Pericardial fenestration, 240
Pericardial fluid, 164–165
Pericardial friction rub, 181, 236
Pericardial space, 164–165
Pericardiectomy, 240
Pericardiocentesis, 240
Pericardiostomy, 240
Pericarditis, 175, 238–239
  rheumatic, 236–237
Pericardium, 163–164, *164*
Perilymphatic fluid, 1996, 1997
Perimenopause, 1769
Perinatal transmission, of HIV, 1464
Perineal care, in abdominal perineal resection, 1104–1105
  in diarrhea, 964
  in prostatectomy, 1719
  in radical vulvectomy, 1828, 1829
  with body cast, 858
Perineal prostatectomy, 1710, *1710*, 1711, 1714t–1715t. See also *Prostatectomy.*
Perineal resection, abdominal. See *Abdominal perineal resection.*
Perinephric abscess, 1375
Perineum, female, 1766, *1766*
Perioperative nursing. See also *Surgery.*
  activities in, 116, 117t
  definition of, 116
  phases of, 116–123, 117t
  standards for, 116, 117t
Periorbital edema, in hypothyroidism, 1308, *1308*
Periosteum, 839
Peripheral angioplasty, 343–344
Peripheral arterial aneurysms, 371. See also *Aneurysm(s).*
Peripheral circulation, control of, 405
Peripheral iridectomy, for glaucoma, 1980
Peripheral nerves, injury of, 827–828
  regeneration of, 712, 827, *827*
Peripheral nervous system, anatomy and physiology of, 722–725, *724*
Peripheral neuropathy, diabetic, 1252d, 1254
  in acute renal failure, 1395c
  in burns, 1664–1665
Peripheral neurovascular dysfunction, in burns, 1664–1665
Peripheral vascular complications, of anesthesia, 140–141
  of casts, 856, 858
Peripheral vascular disease, 331–348

Peripheral vascular disease (*Continued*)
  angioplasty for, 343–344
  assessment in, 337–339
  bypass grafts for, 344–348, 345d
  clinical manifestations of, 331–337
  diagnosis in, 339t, 339–340, 340t, 341c, 342t
  drug therapy for, 343, 343d, 344d, 345t
  health history in, 337
  hypertension and, 373, 375
  in elderly, 348, 397–398
  lifestyle factors in, 338d, 338t
  management of, 342–348
    nonsurgical, 342–344
    setting and providers for, 348
    surgical, 344–348
  pain in, 331–334
  risk factors in, 337, 338t
    reduction of, 338d, 342–343
  skin changes in, 334t, 334–337
  stasis dermatitis in, 1611–1612, *1612*
  thromboangiitis obliterans and, 351–354
  varicose veins and, 386, 389–390, 391c–392c
  venous stasis ulcers and, 332, 333–334, 335, 386, 390–395
Peripheral vascular resistance, 328
Peripherally inserted central catheter, in total parenteral nutrition, 987
Peristalsis, 950
  duodenal, 956
  esophageal, 951
  gastric, 953–954, *954*
Peristaltic waves, 968
Peritoneal cavity, 951
Peritoneal dialysis, 1401–1404
  advantages and disadvantages of, 1401, 1401t
  assessment in, 1403
  care settings and providers for, 1407–1408
  catheters for, 1401–1402, *1402*
    care of, 1404d
    obstruction of, 1404
  complications of, 1403
  continuous ambulatory, 1402–1403
  continuous-cycle, 1403
  goals of, 1401
  intermittent, 1402
  nursing diagnoses and planning in, 1403
  nursing interventions in, 1403–1404, 1404d
  principles of, 1400
  procedure for, 1401–1403, *1402*
  uses of, 1400–1401, 1403
Peritoneoscopy, in hepatic disorders, 1163t
Peritoneum, parietal, 951
  structure and function of, 951
  visceral, 950, 951
Peritonitis, 1061–1063
  abdominal rigidity in, 969
  appendicitis and, 1063, 1064t
  perforated ulcer and, 1029
Peritonsillar abscess, 607–608
Periurethral blocking agents, for urinary incontinence, 1758
Pernicious anemia, 476–479
  in chronic gastritis, 1025, *1025*
  Schilling test for, 443t, 451, 478
  vs. folic acid deficiency, 479
PERRLA, 1942
Persistent generalized lymphadenopathy, 1465
Persistent vegetative state, 41

Personal care, in unconscious client, 729
Personality traits, cancer and, 1510–1511
  heart disease and, 187, 210, 303
Perthes' test, 340t
Pes planus, 910–911
Pessary, for uterine retrodisplacement, 1820
Petechiae, 1571
Pets, for elderly, 50
Pew Health Professions Commission report, 29
Peyer's patches, 1432
Pfannenstiel incision, 995t
pH, *102*, 102–104
  arterial blood, 540, 540t, 543, 544t
    oxygen transport and, 542
    $PaCO_2$ and, 542–543
    SaO_2 and, 542
  blood, 428
  buffer system and, 103, 104t
  in metabolic acidosis, 104
  in metabolic alkalosis, 106
  in respiratory acidosis, 108
  in respiratory alkalosis, 111
  normal values for, 102
  renal regulation of, *103*, 103–104, 104t, 1333
  respiratory control of, 103, *103*, 104t
  vaginal, maintenance of, 1884
Phacoemulsification, for cataract extraction, 1976
Phagocytes, *1432*, 1433, 1433t, 1436
Phagocytosis, 1433, 1435–1437, *1436*, *1437*
  defects in, 1437–1438
Phagosome, 1436, *1437*
Phantom limb sensation, 872–873
Phantom pain, rectal, 1104
Pharmacokinetics, age-related changes in, 52–58, 53d, 54t, 55d–57d
Pharmacology. See *Drug therapy.*
Pharyngitis, streptococcal, rheumatic fever and, 236, 237
Pharynx, *524*, 525
  examination of, 968
  structure and function of, 951
Phenobarbital (Luminal), for seizures, 796, 797d–798d
  hepatotoxicity of, 1178t, 1179
Phenothiazines, for chemotherapy-related nausea and vomiting, 1529
Phenytoin (Dilantin), for increased intracranial pressure, 732
  for seizures, 796, 797d–798d
Pheochromocytoma, 1292–1295
Phimosis, 1735–1737, *1736*
  penile cancer and, 1744
pHisoHex (hexachlorophene), 1581
Phlebitis, 384
  chronic venous insufficiency and, 388–394
Phlebothrombosis, 384
Phlebotomy, for polycythemia vera, 489–490
Phosphate, fluid distribution of, *85*
  parathyroid hormone and, 1213, *1213*
Phosphate buffer system, 103
Phosphate deficiency, clinical manifestations of, 1077t
Phosphodiesterase inhibitors, for heart failure, 274
Phospholine Iodide (echothiophate iodide), for glaucoma, 1979–1980
Phosphorus, calcium and, 95, 1213
  dietary sources of, 1318

Photocoagulation, for retinal tears, 1983
  laser, for diabetic retinopathy, 1253
Photophobia, 1939
Photopsia, 1039
  in retinal detachment, 1982
Photoreactive keratectomy, 1973, 1974
Photosensitivity, chemotherapy and, 1530, 1540t
Phthirus pubis, *1928*, 1928–1929
Physical therapy, for burns, 1682, 1684t
  in rheumatoid arthritis, 894
Physician, qualifications and responsibilities of, 24t
Physiologic cup, *1936*, 1937
  assessment of, 1944, *1944*
Physiologic pacemakers, 256
Pia mater, 714, *716*
Pigeon breast, 534, *534*
Pigmentation changes, age-related, 58, *58*
  chemotherapy and, 1530, 1539t–1540t
  generalized, 1570
  in Addison's disease, 1278, *1278*
  in Cushing's syndrome, 1286
  of lesions, 1570–1571
Pigmented lesions, 1631–1634
Pigmented nevi, 1633t
Pilocarpine, administration of, 1949
  for glaucoma, 1979
Pilonidal cyst, 1073t
Pindolol (Visken), 377t
Pineal gland, 1204–1208, 1207t
Pink eye, 1963–1964, *1964*, 1965d
Pinna, 1995, *1996*
Pins, in internal fixation, 865–867
  in traction, 860, *861*
    skin care for, 863t, 865
  Steinmann, 860, *861*
Pin-site care, 863t, 865
Piroxicam (Feldene), 893d
Pitressin (vasopressin), for bleeding esophageal varices, 1183
  for diabetes insipidus, 1275, 1276d
Pitting edema, 80, 80–81, 177
  in third-space shift, 82
Pituitary, anterior, *1208*, 1209
  disorders of, 1265–1274
  hypothalamus and, *1208*, 1208–1209, 1210
  posterior, *1208*, 1209
    disorders of, 1274–1277
  structure and function of, 1205t, *1208*, 1209–1210, *1210*, 1210t
Pituitary adenoma, 828–832, 831t, 1265–1269
  Cushing's syndrome and, 1285, 1287
  hyperthyroidism and, 1307
  somatotropin hypersecretion and, 1269–1274
  surgery for, 1266–1269, *1267*, 1270c–1272c
  in Cushing's disease, 1287
Pituitary disorders, 1265–1277
  etiology of, 1210
  hypothalamic dysfunction and, 1210
  hypothyroidism in, 1297, 1298–1301, 1301t
  in elderly, 1322–1323
  Internet connections for, 1295d
  of anterior lobe, 1265–1274
  of posterior lobe, 1274–1277
Pituitary hormones, 1206t, 1209–1210, 1210t
  hypersecretion of, acromegaly and, 1269–1274, *1273*

Pituitary hormones (*Continued*)
  gigantism and, 1272–1274
  in syndrome of inappropriate antidiuretic hormone, 1277
  pituitary adenoma and, 1265
  hyposecretion of, 1274
  in diabetes insipidus, 1274–1276, 1277d
  in hypopituitarism, 1274
Pityrosporum orbiculare, tinea versicolor and, 1603
Planning, in nursing process, 9–11
Plant alkaloids, in chemotherapy, 1524t, 1525
Plant dermatitis, 1609t, 1609–1611, *1610*
Plantar digital neuroma, 910–911
Plantar warts, 1603–1605, *1604*, 1604t
Plaque, *1571*, 1572
  atherosclerotic, *282*, 283
  in myocardial infarction, 293
Plaque psoriasis, 1616–1619, *1617*, 1617t
Plasma, 428–429
  fresh frozen, 455–456
  reference values for, 2024–2025
  substitutes for, 456d
  vs. serum, 429
Plasma cells, 1432, *1432*, 1433, 1433t, 1434
Plasma proteins, 428–429
Plasma volume, renal regulation of, 1333
Plasmapheresis, for myasthenia gravis, 783–784
  in Guillain-Barré syndrome, 773
Plastic surgery, 1590–1591, 1591t, 1592d
  for burns, 1682
  of breast, 1875–1880
    augmentation, 1879
    dermal mastopexy, 1880
    reconstructive, 1875–1879, *1876–1877*, 1879d
    reduction, 1879–1880
Platelet(s), 429, *429*, 430
  in inflammation, 1432
Platelet aggregation test, 443t, 447
Platelet antiaggregation therapy, for stroke, 807–808
Platelet count, 443t, 446–447
  normal values for, 1532t
  preoperative, 125t
Platelet transfusion, 453–455. See also *Transfusion(s)*.
Plates, orthopedic, 865–867
Plegia, 739
Plethysmography, 340t
Pleura, 524–525, *525*
Pleural effusion, empyema and, 657–658
  in pleuritis, 658
Pleural fluid, aspiration of, 550–552, *551*
Pleural friction rub, 537
Pleural needle biopsy, in tuberculosis, 652
Pleural space, 525
Pleuritis, 658–659
Plicae circulares, 955, *955*
Pneumatic antishock garment, 411
Pneumatic dilatation, esophageal, for achalasia, *1044*, 1045
Pneumatoscopy, 2001
Pneumococcal vaccine, 1447
Pneumoconiosis, coal workers', 688–691
Pneumocystis carinii pneumonia, in HIV infection, 1466, *1467*
Pneumonectomy, 580t, 581–586
  complications of, 581, 584, 703c
  discharge instructions for, 585d, 706c
  for lung cancer, 700d–707d

Pneumonectomy (*Continued*)
  incisions in, 580
  nursing care guide for, 700c–707c
  nursing interventions in, 582–586
  patient preparation for, 580–581, 700c–701c
  postoperative care in, 584–586, 701c–707c
  postoperative course in, 581–582
  preoperative care in, 582–583, 700c–701c
  procedure for, 581
  radical, 580t
  uses of, 581
Pneumonia, 641–647
  aspiration, 647
  assessment in, 644–645
  atypical, 641
  bacterial, 641
  causative organisms in, 641, 643t
  clinical manifestations of, 642–643
  clinical pathway for, 644d
  community-acquired, 641
  complications of, 645
  diagnosis of, 643
  etiology of, 641, 643t
  H. influenzae, 641
  hospital-acquired, 641
    case study of, 928d–929d
    prevention of, 642d
  immunization for, 646, 1447
  in chronic obstructive pulmonary disease, 671d, 678d
  prevention of, 671d
  in elderly, 707
  influenza and, 649
  Legionella, 641
  lung abscess and, 647–648
  management of, 643
  nursing diagnoses and planning in, 645
  nursing interventions in, 645–647, 646d
  opportunistic, 641
  P. carinii, in HIV infection, 1466, *1467*
  pathophysiology of, 641–642
  postoperative, 146t
  risk factors for, 642, 642d
  sputum color in, 644d
  viral, 641
Pneumonitis, hypersensitivity, 1488t, 1488–1489
Pneumothorax, 692–693, *693*, 694
  in chest tube drainage, 577, 578, 579
  in total parenteral nutrition, 987, 988
  pleuritis and, 658
Podophyllin, for anogenital warts, 1027, 1604
Poison ivy/oak/sumac, 1609t, 1609–1611, *1610*
Poisoning, chemical burns in, 1687
  toxins in, reference values for, 2029–2030
Polarization, membrane, 712–713, *714*
Pollen allergy, 601
Polycyclic lesions, 1573, *1574*
Polycythemia, in chronic obstructive pulmonary disease, 668
Polycythemia vera, 489–491
Polydipsia, in diabetes insipidus, 1275
  in diabetes mellitus, 1228, 1229
Polymenorrhea, 1775–1776
Polymeric enteral formulas, 981
Polymorphonuclear leukocytes, *429*, 1432, *1432*
Polyneuritis, postinfectious, 773
Polypectomy, nasal, 611, *611*

Polyphagia, in diabetes, 1228, 1229
Polyps, cervical, 1822–1823
  colonic, 1098–1100, *1099*
  endometrial, 1823
  nasal, 611, *611*
Polythiazide (Renese), 377t
Polyuria, 1343
  in acute renal failure, 1390
  in diabetes insipidus, 1275
  in diabetes mellitus, 1228, 1229
Pons, 720–721
Popliteal aneurysm, *371*, 371–372. See also
  Aneurysm(s).
Popliteal artery occlusion, 363–365
Porcine valves, 313, *313*
Portal circulation, 1135, *1136*
Portal cirrhosis, 1180–1193, 1181t. See also
  Cirrhosis.
Portal hypertension, 1139t, 1141–1149
  ascites in, 1142
    diuretics for, 1144d
    LeVeen shunt for, 1144–1145, *1146*
    management of, 1143d, 1144d, 1144–
      1145, 1145t, *1146*
    paracentesis for, 1144, 1145t
    sodium-restricted diet for, 1143d, 1144
  assessment in, 1145–1146
  clinical manifestations of, 1143
  definition of, 1141
  esophageal varices in, 1183–1193
    management of, 1183–1189
    nursing care guide for, 1191c–1192c
    nursing process for, 1189–1193
    in postnecrotic cirrhosis, 1181, *1182*
    management of, 1143d, 1144d, 1144–
      1145, 1145t, *1146*
  nursing diagnoses and planning in,
    1146–1147
  nursing interventions in, 1147–1149
  pathophysiology of, 1141–1143
Portal vein, 1135, *1136*
Portocaval shunt, for esophageal varices,
  1188, 1189
Portosystemic shunt, for esophageal varices, *1188*, 1189
Ports, chemotherapy, 1527, *1527, 1528*
Port-wine stain, 1571
Positional dyspnea, 174
Positioning, for aspiration prevention, 647
  for pressure ulcer prevention, 1630
  in heart failure, 278
  in increased intracranial pressure, 736
  in ischemic pain, 333
  in mechanical ventilation, 571
  in retinal detachment surgery, 1985
  in shock, 411, 421
  in vascular disorders, 333, 335–336
  of burn patients, 1683, 1684t
  of unconscious patient, 729
  postoperative, 131, 149
    in pneumonectomy, 702c
    in spinal surgery, 763d, 764
  surgical, 135, *136*, 143
Positive end-expiratory pressure (PEEP),
  569. See also *Mechanical ventilation*.
Positive-pressure ventilation, for chronic
  obstructive pulmonary disease
  (COPD), 672d
Positron emission tomography (PET), in
  heart disease, 198
  in neurologic disorders, 749
Postanesthesia care, assessment in, 143–
  144, 144t. See also *Postoperative period*.
  in ambulatory surgery, 157

Postanesthesia care *(Continued)*
  nursing interventions in, 144–149
  nursing process in, 144–149
Postanesthesia care unit (PACU), 131, 132–
  133, 143–149
  discharge from, 143–144, 144t, 150
  transfer from, 150
Posterior cerebral artery, 716, *717*
  stenosis of, 807t
Posterior chamber, 1937, *1937*
Posterior colporrhaphy, 1818–1819, 1819d
Posterior columns, 722
Posterior pelvic exenteration, 1786t
Posterior spinal artery, 716
Posterolateral thoracotomy incision, 580
Postgonococcal urethritis, 1925
Postherpetic neuralgia, 1606–1607
Posthitis, 1727–1728, 1729d
Postinfectious polyneuritis, 773
Postnasal drip, 529
Postnecrotic cirrhosis, 1181t, 1181–1193.
  See also *Cirrhosis*.
Postobstructive diuresis, 1378
Postoperative period, 143–156. See also
  Surgery.
  activity in, 153–154
  airway management in, 145, 146t, 151
  assessment in, 150
  body image and, 155
  breathing exercises in, 130, *130*, 151
  cardiac monitoring in, 145–149
  complications in, 146t–149t, 150–155
  coughing exercises in, 130, *131*, 151
  fluid management in, 145–149, 151
  gastrointestinal function in, 155
  in ambulatory surgery, 157
  in elderly, 159
  incentive spirometry in, 130–131, *131*,
    151
  leg exercises in, 131, *132*, 151
  nursing diagnoses and planning in, 144–
    145, 150–151
  nursing interventions in, 117t, 143–155
  nutrition in, 155
  patient teaching in, 129d, 131–133, 155,
    156d
  postanesthesia care in, 143–149, 144t
  shock in, 145–149
  thrombophlebitis prophylaxis in, 131,
    132, 151
  voiding in, 154–155
  wound care in, 147t, 153
Postprandial hypoglycemia, postgastrectomy, 998t
Post-streptococcal arthritis, 237
Post-transfusion hepatitis, 1171, 1171t. See
  also *Hepatitis, viral*.
Postural drainage, 553, *554*
  percussion in, 553–555
  vibration in, 555–556
Postural hypotension, 178
  in elderly, 64–65, 71c
  injury prevention in, 71c
Postural therapy, for uterine retrodisplacement, 1820, *1821*
Potassium, daily requirement for, 84
  deficiency of, 84–89. See also *Hypokale-
    mia*.
  dietary sources of, 183d
  excess of, 84–91, 89–91. See also *Hyper-
    kalemia*.
  fluid distribution of, 84, *85*
  functions of, 84
  normal values for, 84

Potassium *(Continued)*
  sources of, 84, 90
  supplemental, 86, 87d, 88d, 88–89
    for hypertension, 100d
Potassium chloride, for diabetic ketoacido-
  sis, 1249
Potassium iodide (SSKI), for hyperthyroid-
  ism, 1310, 1314
Potassium sparing diuretics, 377t. See also
  Diuretics.
Pouch, colostomy, *1008*, 1008–1009
  ileostomy, 1012, *1012, 1013*
  Kock, 1012, *1013*
Poverty, health care access and, 18
Povidone-iodine (Betadine), 1581
Power of attorney for health care, 42–43,
  44
Powerlessness, in cancer, 1545, 1549–1550
  in limb-girdle dystrophy, 786
  penectomy and, 1748
PPD test, for tuberculosis, 652, 1489
PQRST format, 188
PR interval, *194*, 195
Practical nurse, qualifications and respon-
  sibilities of, 24t
Prazosin (Minipress), 213, 213d, 378t
  for benign prostatic hyperplasia, 1753
Precapillaries, 324
Precapillary sphincter, 324, *328*
Prednisone, for canker sores, 1018t
Preferred provider organizations, 20–21
Pregnancy, burns in, 1690
  chlamydia in, 1920, 1921
  diabetes in, 1228
    diagnostic criteria for, 1229t
    starvation ketosis in, 1243
    urinary ketones in, 1243
  ectopic, chlamydial salpingitis and,
    1921
  genital herpes in, 1902–1903
  HIV transmission in, 1464
  surgery in, 123
  syphilis in, 1918
  vaginal candidiasis in, 1885
Preload, 403
  cardiac output and, 172
Premature atrial contractions, *243*, 243–244
Premature ejaculation, 1698–1699, 1699t
Premature junctional contractions, 247
Premature menopause, 1769
Premature ventricular contractions, *248*,
  248–249
Premenstrual syndrome, 1807–1810, 1809d,
  1809t
Preoperative period. See also *Surgery*.
  anxiety in, 130
  assessment in, 128–134
  coughing exercises in, 130, *131*
  deep-breathing exercises in, 130, *130*
  diagnostic procedures in, 123–124, 125t–
    127t, 130
  elimination in, 124, 133
  fluid restrictions in, 124, 133
  for anesthesia, 127t
  goals of, 129
  in ambulatory surgery, 156–157
  in elderly, 158–159
  incentive spirometry in, 130–131, *131*
  medications in, 127–128, 133
  nursing interventions in, 117t, 129–133
  nursing process in, 128–134
  patient teaching in, 129d, 129–133
  preoperative checklist in, 133, *134*
  skin preparation in, 124, 133

Prepuce, 1695
  inflammation of, 1727–1728
Presbycusis, 60–61, 766, 1997, 2019–2020
Presbyesophagus, 1059
Presbyopia, 60, 1961, 1970–1974
Presshear, 1623
Pressure garments, for burns, 1682, *1683*, 1684, 1685d
Pressure support ventilation, 569. See also *Mechanical ventilation*.
Pressure ulcers, 1622–1631
  antibiotics for, 1625–1626
  assessment in, 1626
  cleaning of, 1630–1631
  clinical manifestations of, 1623–1624
  Clinical Practice Guidelines for, 1623
  débridement of, 1625, 1625t
  diagnosis of, 1624
  dressings for, 1631
  etiology of, 1623, 1624t
  incidence of, 1622–1623
  management of, 1624–1626
  nursing diagnoses and planning in, 1626–1629
  nursing interventions in, 1629–1631
  nutrition and, 1624–1625, 1628, *1629*
  pathophysiology of, 1623
  prevention of, 70c, 279–280, 845, 1629–1630
    in unconscious client, 728
  reactive hyperemia and, 1623–1624, 1628
  re-epithelialization of, 1631, *1631*
  risk assessment for, 1626t–1627t, 1628
  risk factors for, 1623, 1624t, 1626t–1627t
  staging of, 1624, *1625*
Pretibial myxedema, in hyperthyroidism, *1307*
Preventive care, 14–15, 15t
Priapism, 1740–1741
  in autonomic dysreflexia, 823
Prick tests, 1446, *1446*, 1447
Primacor (milrinone), for heart failure, 274
Primary aldosteronism, 1289–1292
Primary biliary cirrhosis, 1181t, 1181–1193. See also *Cirrhosis*.
Primidone (Mysoline), for seizures, 796, 797d–798d
Prinivil (lisinopril), 213, 214d
Prinzmetal's angina, 286
Priority setting, in nursing process, 9
Prisms, 1958
Probenecid (Benemid), for gout, 900, 900d
Procainamide (Pronestyl), for dysrhythmias, 215, 216d
  for ventricular tachycardia, 25049
Procardia (nifedipine), 213, 215d, 378t
Procrit (epoetin alfa), 469, 470d
Progesterone, 1207t, 1814d
  for endometriosis, 1813, 1814d
  for fibrocystic breast disease, 1855
  in female hormonal cycle, 1768, 1769
Progestogens, 1814d
  for endometriosis, 1813
Progressive stroke, 806t
Progressive systemic sclerosis, 1494–1495
Projectile vomiting, 960
Prolactin, 1205t
Prolactin–inhibiting hormone, 1209t
Prolactin–releasing hormone, 1209t
Prone position, 135, *136*
Properidin pathway, 1440
Propofol, for anesthesia, 141t
Propranolol (Inderal), 214, 377t
  diabetic hypoglycemia and, 1250

Propranolol (Inderal) *(Continued)*
  for bleeding esophageal varices, 1183–1184
  for hyperthyroidism, 1308
Proprioception, alterations in, 743–744
Propylthiouracil, for hyperthyroidism, 1309, 1309t, 1314
Proscar (finasteride), for benign prostatic hyperplasia, 1753
Prostaglandin inhibitors, for dysmenorrhea, 1776
Prostaglandins, in blood pressure regulation, 1333
Prostate, age-related changes in, 1725
  biopsy of, 1705–1706, *1706*, 1707t
  enlarged. See *Benign prostatic hyperplasia*.
  palpation of, 1702, *1702*
  structure and function of, *1696*, 1697
  transurethral incision of, 1710
  transurethral resection of, *1710*, 1710–1711, 1714t–1715t
    clinical pathway for, 1755d
    for benign hyperplasia, 1753
Prostate cancer, 1754–1761
  alkaline phosphatase in, 1704
  chemotherapy for, 1759
  clinical manifestations of, 1511t, 1756
  cryosurgery for, 1759
  diagnosis of, 1756–1757
  etiology of, 1754
  hormone therapy for, 1759
  in elderly, 1761
  incidence of, 1754
  nursing care in, 1760d, 1760–1761
  pain in, 1760–1761
  pathophysiology of, 1754–1755
  patient teaching in, 1756d
  prostatectomy for. See *Prostatectomy*.
  prostate-specific antigen in, 1704
  psychosexual issues in, 1761
  radiation therapy for, 1758–1759
  risk factors for, 1511t
  screening for, 1704, 1756–1757, 1757t
  staging of, 1757, 1757t
  tumor markers in, 1757
Prostate disorders, Internet connections for, 1752d
Prostatectomy, 1708t, 1709–1720, 1757–1758
  case study of, 1716d–1717d
  complications of, 1712–1713, 1715t, 1758, 1760–1761
  contraindications to, 1711
  discharge instructions for, 1720d
  for benign hyperplasia, 1753, 1754
  impotence after, 1709t, 1713, 1715t, 1719–1720, 1761
  indications for, 1714t
  laser, 1754
  nursing care for, 1760–1761
  patient preparation for, 1711
  perineal, 1710, *1710*, 1711, 1714t–1715t
  postoperative care in, 1713–1720
  postoperative course in, 1711–1712
  preoperative care in, 1713
  radical, 1710, 1711, 1714t–1715t, 1757–1758
  retropubic, 1710, *1710*, 1711, 1714t–1715t
  simple, 1710, 1714t–1715t
  suprapubic (transvesical), 1710, *1710*, 1711, 1714t–1715t
  surgical approaches in, *1710*, 1710–1711, 1714t

Prostatectomy *(Continued)*
  transurethral, *1710*, 1710–1711, 1714t–1715t
    clinical pathway for, 1755d
    for benign hyperplasia, 1753
  urinary drainage in, 1712, 1714t
  urinary incontinence after, 1709t, 1712, 1715t, 1758, 1760, 1760d
  Walsh technique for, 1758
Prostate-specific antigen, 1704
  in screening, 1757, 1757t
  in staging and management, 1757
Prostatic acid phosphatase, 1704
Prostatic fluid, 1697
  sequential bacteriologic localization cultures of, 1704–1705
Prostatic stents, for benign prostatic hyperplasia, 1754
Prostatitis, 1733t, 1733–1735
  sequential bacteriologic localization cultures for, 1704–1705
Prostatodynia, 1733, 1733t, 1734
  sequential bacteriologic localization cultures for, 1704–1705
Prosthesis, after stapedectomy, 2015–2016, *2016*
  breast, 1866
  cardiac valve, 312–313, *312–314*
  cochlear, 2007–2008, *2008*
  joint (internal), 867–868, *868*, 869c–872c
  limb, lower extremity, 882–883, *883*
    temporary, 883–884
    upper extremity, 882, *882*, 883
  ocular, 1955–1956, 1956d, *1957*
  penile, 1720–1724, *1721*, 1721t, 1724d
Prosthetic intubation, for esophageal cancer, 1055, 1058
Prostigmin (neostigmine), for myasthenia gravis, 783, 783d
Prostigmin test, for myasthenia gravis, 783
Protective isolation, in hematologic disorders, 452
Protein, dietary sources of, 472d
Protein buffer system, 103
Protein deficiency, clinical manifestations of, 1077t
Protein loss, in burns, 1678
Protein metabolism, hepatic, 1137, 1137t
  in diabetics vs. nondiabetics, *1225*
  in hepatic disorders, 1161t, 1163–1164
  insulin in, 1223–1224
Protein studies, in hepatic disorders, 1163–1164
Protein-restricted diet, 1151d
  in hepatic encephalopathy, 1150, 1151d
  in renal failure, 1391d, 1400
Proteinuria, in diabetes, 1254
Prothrombin, *431*, 432, 433t, 447
Prothrombin complex, transfusion of, 456. See also *Transfusion(s)*.
Prothrombin time, 443t, 447–448
  in heart disease, 208–209
  in hepatic disorders, 1162t, 1164
Proton pump inhibitors, 1022d
  for peptic ulcers, 1028
Protoplasmic poisons, burns from, 1686t. See also *Chemical burns*.
Proximal convoluted tubules, 1331, *1331*
  in urine formation, 1332, *1332*
Pruritus, 1570
  antihistamines for, 1582
  cool-water bath for, 1583
  in eczema, 1608, 1609

Pruritus *(Continued)*
  in hematologic disorders, 440
  in jaundice, 1140–1141, 1141d
  in psoriasis, 1619d
  in renal failure, 1396c, 1399, 1400
    PUVA therapy for, 1583
  in sexually transmitted diseases, 1890c–
    1891c
  in vaginitis, 1805, 1885
  in vulvar cancer, 1826
  in vulvitis, 1803
  lice and, 1928, 1929
  management of, 1619d
  scabies and, 1929, 1930
Pseudoephedrine (Allerid), for retrograde
    ejaculation, 1699
Pseudohypoparathyroidism, 1316
Psoralen plus ultraviolet light (PUVA)
    therapy, 1582, 1584, 1618, 1619
Psoriasis, 1616–1619, *1617*, 1617t
  Internet connections for, 1639d
  PUVA therapy for, 1582, 1584, 1618,
    1619
Psoriatic arthritis, 1617
Psychosexual issues, in prostate cancer,
    1761
Psychosocial issues, in burn injury, 1680–
    1681
  in chronic obstructive pulmonary dis-
    ease, 678
  in male climacteric syndrome, 1725
  in menopause, 1771
PTCA. See *Percutaneous transluminal coro-
    nary angioplasty (PTCA).*
PTFE injection, for urinary incontinence,
    1758
Ptosis, in myasthenia gravis, 782, 784
Pubic lice, *1928*, 1928–1929
Public health departments, 23
Public health nurse, 28
Pull sheet, 794
Pulmonary angiography, 548
Pulmonary artery pressure, reference val-
    ues for, 685
Pulmonary artery pressure monitoring,
    200, 202–206, *206, 207*
  for cardiac output, 207
Pulmonary artery wedge pressure, 403,
    404
Pulmonary capacities, 538, *538*, 539t
Pulmonary circulation, *324*
Pulmonary complications, in radiation
    therapy, 1521
Pulmonary contusion, 695
Pulmonary disease, as surgical risk factor,
    121–122
Pulmonary edema, after pneumonectomy,
    584
  cardiogenic, 270, 280, 281d–282d
  diuretics for, 216, 217d, 218d
  noncardiogenic, 686–688
Pulmonary embolism, 386, 681–685
  case study of, 684d–685d
  clinical manifestations of, 681
  diagnosis of, 681–682
  etiology of, 681
  fat, 933
  management of, *682*, 682–683
  nursing process in, 683–684
  pathophysiology of, 681
  pleuritis and, 658
  postoperative, 146t
  prevention of, 682
  pulmonary hypertension in, 685–686

Pulmonary fibrosis, chemotherapy and,
    1532, 1535t
Pulmonary function studies, 537–539, *538,*
    539t
  in chronic bronchitis, 669, 674
  in emphysema, 671, 674
Pulmonary hygiene, 552–556, 587
  after lobectomy, 589c
  after pneumonectomy, 582–583, 585–586
  breathing exercises in, 130, 552–553
  in chronic obstructive pulmonary dis-
    ease, 672, 675–676
  in mechanical ventilation, 571
  in unconscious client, 728
  percussion in, 553–555
  postoperative, in cardiac surgery, 224–
    225, 227
    incentive spirometry in, 130–131, *131*
    incision splinting in, 130, *131*
  postural drainage in, 553, *554*
  vibration in, 555–556
Pulmonary hypertension, 685–686
  in chronic obstructive pulmonary dis-
    ease, 668
Pulmonary infarct, abscess and, 647
Pulmonary infections, in HIV infection,
    1466, *1467*
Pulmonary pain, vs. cardiac pain, 175
Pulmonary rehabilitation, for chronic ob-
    structive pulmonary disease, 673, *674*
Pulmonary toxicity, of chemotherapy,
    1532, 1535t
Pulmonary vascular resistance, 402t, 404
Pulmonary wedge pressure, 200, 202–206,
    206, 207
  for cardiac output monitoring, 207
Pulmonic valve, *164, 167, 167, 168, 171*
Pulse(s), *178–179*
  abnormal, 178–179, *179*
  amplitude of, 178, 338
  bigeminal, 179, *179*
  bounding, 178–179, *179*
  carotid, 178
    palpation of, 178
  distal, Doppler recording of, 335, *337,*
    339
    palpation of, 335, *336*, 338–339
  monitoring of, in hyperthyroidism, 1313
    in hypothyroidism, 1306
  normal values for, 178
  palpation of, 189, *190*
  radial, in hyperthyroidism, 1313
    in hypothyroidism, 1306
    self-monitoring of, 1306, 1313
  weak, 178, *179*
Pulse oximetry, 544–545, 545d, *546*
  probe sheaths for, 545d
Pulsus alternans, 179, *179*
Pulsus paradoxus, 179, *179*, 239
Punch biopsy, 1577–1578, *1578*, 1579d
  cervical, 1783
Pupil(s), age-related changes in, 1961
  examination of, 1942
  in increased intracranial pressure, 733
  in shock, 406, 407t
Pupillary accommodation, assessment of,
    1942
Pupillary light response, assessment of,
    1942
Purified protein derivative (PPD) test, 652,
    1489
Purine, dietary sources of, 901d
Purpura(s), 513–515, 1571
  thrombocytopenic, 513–515

Pursed-lip breathing, 130, 553
  in chronic obstructive pulmonary dis-
    ease, 676
Pustule, *1571*, 1572
PUVA therapy, 1582, 1584, 1618, 1619
Pyelography, antegrade, 1348t
  intravenous, 1346, 1347t, 1351
  retrograde, 1348t
Pyelonephritis, 1374–1375
Pyloric sphincter, 952, *952*
Pyloroplasty, for peptic ulcers, 1028–1209
Pylorus, 952, *952*
Pyogenic liver abscess, 1179
Pyramidal tract, 722
Pyrazinamide, for tuberculosis, 653, 653t,
    654t
Pyridostigmine (Mestinon), for myasthenia
    gravis, 783, 783d, 785
Pyridoxine deficiency, clinical manifesta-
    tions of, 1077t
Pyrosis, in esophagitis, 1020
  in hiatus hernia, 1041, 1043
Pyuria, in urethritis, 1373

Q

Q wave, 193, *194*, 195
QRS complex, 193, *194*, 195, *195*
Quadrantectomy, for breast cancer, *1861*
Quadriparesis, 739
Quadriplegia, 739
Quadruple rhythm, 180
Questran (cholestyramine), 343d
  for jaundice-related pruritus, 1141d
Quinethazone, 377t
Quinsy, 607–608

R

R wave, 193, *194*
Racial/ethnic groups, asthma in, 659
  cancer in, 1506–1507, 1506–1508, 1508,
    1509
  classification of, 373t
  cyanosis in, 182
  diabetes in, 1226, 1227
  glucose-6-phosphatase deficiency in, 488,
    488d
  hypertension in, 373
  immune response in, 1441
  lactase deficiency in, 1079–1081
  pallor in, 182
  prostate cancer in, patient teaching for,
    1756d
  risk factors for, 373t
  sickle-cell anemia in, *484,* 484–487, 485d,
    486t, 487d
Rad, 1517
Radial keratotomy, 1973, 1974
Radial pulse, in hyperthyroidism, 1313
  in hypothyroidism, 1306
  self-monitoring of, 1306, 1313
Radiation, cancer and, 1510
  for immunosuppression, 1449
Radiation recall, 1530
Radiation therapy, 1517–1523
  assessment in, 1522
  brachytherapy in, 1518–1519, *1519*
  cell damage in, 1517
  dosage in, 1518
  dose fractionation in, 1518
  external-beam, 1518, *1518*
  for basal cell epithelioma, 1637
  for bladder cancer, 1420, 1421

Radiation therapy (Continued)
  for brain tumors, 830
  for breast cancer, 1519, 1875
  for cervical cancer, 1832–1836
  for esophageal cancer, 1054–1055
  for hematologic disorders, 464
  for Hodgkin's disease, 505
  for lung cancer, 696, 1521
  for multiple myeloma, 511
  for oral cancer, 1050
  for pancreatic cancer, 1128
  for prostate cancer, 1758–1759
  for skin cancer, 1583–1584
  for testicular cancer, 1749
  for uterine cancer, 1836
  internal, 1518–1519, 1519, 1519c
    for breast cancer, 1519, 1875
  intracavitary, for cervical cancer, 1832–
      1836
    side effects of, 1833d
  megavoltage, 1518
  modes of, 1518–1519
  nursing interventions in, 1522–1523
  principles of, 1517
  radiosensitivity and, 1517
  safety precautions for, 1519, 1519t, 1520
  self-care in, 1523, 1523d
  side effects of, 1520–1523
  therapeutic uses of, 1517–1518
Radical cystectomy, for bladder cancer,
    1420–1421, 1421
Radical hysterectomy, 1793, 1794. See also
    Hysterectomy.
Radical mastoidectomy, 2006–2008, 2008
Radical neck dissection, 631–637
  neck exercises for, 632, 633, 637c
  nursing care guide for, 634c–637c
Radical nephrectomy, 1415–1418, 1418d
Radical pancreatoduodenectomy, 1127,
    1127–1131
  complications of, 1128
  patient preparation for, 1128
  postoperative care in, 1129–1131
  postoperative course in, 1128
  preoperative care in, 1128–1129
Radical pneumonectomy, 580t
Radical prostatectomy, 1710, 1711, 1757–
    1758. See also Prostatectomy.
Radical vulvectomy, 1826–1830
Radioactive iodine, for hyperthyroidism,
    1309–1310, 1313
Radioactive iodine uptake, 1300t
Radioallergosorbent testing, 1447
Radiographic contrast media, allergy to,
    201, 1346–1351
Radiography, in musculoskeletal disorders,
    850t
  KUB, 1347t
  of chest, in cardiac assessment, 192–193
    in respiratory disorders, 547, 547–548
    in tuberculosis, 652
    preoperative, 126t
  of skull, 748
    in fractures, 818
  of spine, 748–749
    preoperative, 125t–126t
Radioimmunoassays, 1445
  for cancer, 1513
Radioisotope scanning. See Radionuclide
    scanning.
Radiology, in musculoskeletal disorders,
    850t
  in urinary tract disorders, 1346–1351,
    1347t–1350t

Radiology (Continued)
  preoperative, 125t–126t
Radionuclide scanning, cardiac, 197–198
  hepatic, 1163t
  in cancer diagnosis, 1514
  in hematologic disorders, 452
  of urinary tract, 1350t
  preoperative, 127t
  thyroid, 1300t
  urinary tract, 1350t
  ventilation-perfusion, 548
Radionuclide venography, in venous insuf-
    ficiency, 340t
Radon, lung cancer and, 695
Rales, 537
Range-of-motion exercises, 741
  in rheumatoid arthritis, 895
  in unconscious client, 729
  postmastectomy, 1865–1866, 1867d, 1868
  shoulder, in stroke, 809
    postoperative, 583, 593c, 701c, 705c
Ranitidine (Zantac), 1022d
Rapid plasma reagin test, 1916–1917
Rash, chemotherapy and, 1530
  in drug eruptions, 1612, 1612–1613,
      1613t
  in Lyme disease, 901
  in syphilis, 1915, 1916
  in systemic lupus erythematosus, 1491,
      1491, 1492t
  in toxic shock syndrome, 1807
  scabies and, 1930
Raynaud's disease, 355–357, 356d
  nursing care guide for, 358c–360c
Raynaud's phenomenon, 356
  in scleroderma, 1494, 1495
Reactive hyperemia, 1623–1624, 1628
Receptive aphasia, 738–739, 814
Reconstructive surgery, 1590–1591, 1591t,
    1592d
  for burns, 1682
  of breast, 1867, 1875–1879, 1876–1877
Rectal. See also under Colorectal.
Rectal abscess, 1071–1074, 1072
Rectal examination, 969
  digital, prostate palpation in, 1702, 1702,
      1756–1757
Rectal opioids, 1554t
Rectocele, 1815–1819, 1816
  posterior colporrhaphy for, 1818–1819
Rectovaginal examination, 1781
Rectovaginal fistula, 1821–1822, 1822
Rectum, structure and function of, 956–
    957
  x-ray studies of, 971
Red blood cell(s), 429, 429, 430. See also
    under Erythrocyte(s).
  abnormalities of, 447t
  disorders of, 467–491
  in inflammation, 1432
  phagocytosis of, 1138
  production of, kidneys in, 1333
  sickled, test for, 443t, 448–449
  staining of, 446
  transfusion of, 453. See also Transfu-
      sion(s).
Red blood cell count, 443t, 444
Red blood cell indices, 443t, 446, 446t
Red reflex, 1944
Reduced hemoglobin, 427
Reducing agents, burns from, 1686t. See
    also Chemical burns.
Reduction mammoplasty, 1879–1880
Reed-Sternberg cell, 503

Reflex(es), assessment of, 748
  defecation, 957
  gastrocolic, 957
  gastroduodenal, 957
  light, tympanic membrane, 2001, 2001
  red, 1944
Reflex incontinence, 1336, 1340t, 1340–1341
Reflex sympathetic dystrophy, 935
Reflux, gastroesophageal, 1019–1023
  hiatus hernia and, 1041, 1043
  with tube prosthesis, 1055
Reflux esophagitis, 1019–1023
  hiatus hernia and, 1041, 1043
Refractive errors, 1970–1974
  assessment for, 1941–1942
  blurred vision and, 1938
  contact lenses for, 1971–1972, 1972d–
      1973d, 1974
  photoreactive keratectomy for, 1973,
      1974
  radial keratotomy for, 1973, 1974
Refractory period, in male sexual response,
    1698
Reframing, in pain management, 1555
Regional anesthesia, 137, 138t. See also An-
    esthesia.
Regional enteritis. See Crohn's disease.
Regional neurolytic blocks, 1555t
Registered nurse, qualifications and re-
    sponsibilities of, 24t
  future trends for, 29
Registered nurse first assistant, 135
Rehabilitation, after cochlear implant, 2008,
    2009
  cardiac, 229–230, 289
  for low back pain, 912
  in amputation, 878
  in fractures, 918–919
  in head injury, 820–821
  in long-term care facilities, 23
  in musculoskeletal disorders, 884
  in neurologic disorders, 765
  in spinal cord injury, 824
  in stroke, 808
  occupational therapy in, 884
  pulmonary, for chronic obstructive pul-
      monary disease, 673, 674
  vestibular, 2003
Rejection, in transplantation, 1409, 1409t
  of liver, 1197t, 1197–1198
Relaxation exercises, in vascular disease,
    354d
Relaxation therapy, in pain management,
    1555
Religious beliefs and practices, 13–14,
    1230d
  in death and dying, 34, 35t, 36, 40–41
REM sleep, 63–64
Renal. See also Kidney(s).
Renal artery, 1331, 1331
Renal biopsy, 1357–1358
Renal calculi. See Urinary calculi.
Renal calyx, 1330, 1330
Renal cancer, 1416–1418
  biopsy for, 1357–1358
Renal capsule, 1329–1330
Renal colic, urinary calculi and, 1379,
    1381c–1382c
Renal cortex, 1330, 1330, 1331
Renal disease, end-stage, 1399
  in diabetes, 1252d, 1254–1255
  malignant hypertension in, 375
  pain in, 1341, 1341–1342
  prevention of, 1418d

Renal failure, acute, 1388–1394
  activity intolerance in, 1397c
  assessment in, 1391–1392
  clinical manifestations of, 1389–1390
  clinical pathway for, 1392d
  cognitive impairment in, 1396c–1397c
  definition of, 1388t
  diagnosis of, 1390, 1392d
  dialysis in, 1391
  diet in, 1391, 1391d, 1392d
  diuretic phase of, 1390
  drug therapy for, 1390–1391, 1392d
  electrolyte imbalances in, 1389, 1390t
  etiology of, 1388
  fluid management in, 1391d, 1395c
  management of, 1390–1391, 1393d
  nursing diagnoses and planning in, 1394
  nursing interventions in, 1393d, 1394
  oliguric phase of, 1390
  onset phase of, 1389–1390
  pathophysiology of, 1388–1389
  patient teaching in, 1398c
  phases of, 1389–1390
  postrenal, 1388, 1389
  prerenal, 1388, 1389
  pruritus in, 1396c
    PUVA therapy for, 1584
  recovery phase of, 1390
  renal, 1388, 1389
  restless leg syndrome in, 1395c–1396c
  chronic, 1394–1400
    clinical manifestations of, 1399, 1399t
    definition of, 1388t
    diagnosis of, 1399
    dialysis in, 1400–1408
    diet in, 1366d, 1366–1367, 1391d
    end-stage renal disease in, 1399
    etiology of, 1394
    fluid management in, 1391d
    management of, 1399–1400
    pathophysiology of, 1394–1399
    pruritus in, 1396, 1400
      PUVA therapy for, 1583
    renal insufficiency in, 1399
    renal transplant in, 1408–1411
  hypercalcemia in, 97, 98
  hypertension and, 374, 375
  pyelonephritis and, 1374
  terminology for, 1388t
Renal function, acid-base balance and, 103, 103–104, 104t, 543
  age-related changes in, 66
  as cardiac risk factor, 122
  in electrical injury, 1688–1689
  in heart disease, 182–184, 183d
  in hypertension, 374, 375
  in shock, 406, 407t, 408
  in surgical patient, 122
Renal insufficiency, 1399
Renal medulla, 1330, 1330
Renal pain, 1341, 1341–1342
Renal parenchyma, 1330, 1330
Renal pelvis, 1330, 1330–1331
  cancer of, 1418–1419
Renal threshold, for glucose, 1227
Renal toxicity, of chemotherapy, 1532, 1543t
Renal transplant, 1408–1411
  complications of, 1409
  donors for, 1408
  immunosuppression for, 1409–1410
  nursing process in, 1410–1411

Renal transplant (Continued)
  procedure for, 1408, 1408–1409
  rejection in, 1409, 1409t
  self-care in, 1410d
  uses of, 1409
Renal trauma, 1411–1412, 1415–1416
Renal tumors. See also Renal cancer.
  varicocele and, 1744
Renese (polythiazide), 377t
Renin-angiotensin system, hypertension and, 373, 373
  in blood pressure regulation, 1333
  in heart failure, 270
  in shock, 406
Reperfusion rhythms, 297
Repolarization, 169, 170, 171
  membrane, 712, 714
Reproductive disorders, female. See also under Gynecologic.
  assessment in, 1777–1785
  diagnosis of, 1781–1785
    cervical biopsy in, 1783–1784, 1784
    colposcopy in, 1782d, 1782–1783
    endometrial biopsy in, 1785
    endometrial cytology in, 1784
    hysterosalpingography in, 1785
    hysteroscopy in, 1785
    Pap test in, 1513, 1779d, 1781–1782, 1783
    pelvic examination in, 1778–1781, 1780
    Schiller test in, 1782
    ultrasonography in, 1785
  drug therapy for, 1786
  functional, 1808–1815
  history in, 1778
  in elderly, 1800, 1838
  in HIV infection, 1467
  infectious and inflammatory, 1803–1808
  management of, 1786–1800
  neoplastic, 1822–1838
  risk reduction for, 1779d
  structural, 1815–1822
  surgery for, 1786–1800. See also Gynecologic surgery.
  male, assessment in, 1699t, 1700–1703
    clinical manifestations of, 1698–1699, 1699t
    diagnosis of, 1703–1706
      biopsies in, 1705–1706, 1706, 1707t
      blood tests in, 1704
      laboratory studies in, 1704
      semen analysis in, 1703–1704
      sequential bacteriologic localization cultures in, 1704–1705
      ultrasonography in, 1704–1705
      urethrocystoscopy in, 1704–1705
    history in, 1700, 1701
    in elderly, 1724–1725, 1761–1762
    infectious and inflammatory, 1727–1735
    Internet connections for, 1752d
    management of, 1707–1724
      settings and providers for, 1724
    neoplastic, 1744–1761
    pelvic examination in, 1700–1703, 1702
    risk reduction for, 1702d, 1703d
    structural, 1735–1744
    surgery for, 1707–1708, 1708t, 1709t
      complications of, 1708, 1709t
      patient preparation for, 1707–1708

Reproductive disorders (Continued)
    types of, 1708t
    resources for, 2043–2044
Reproductive history, 1887t
Reproductive system, female, age-related changes in, 68, 1771, 1800
  assessment of, 1777–1785
  health promotion for, 1779d
  structure and function of, 1765–1768, 1766–1768
  male, age-related changes in, 68, 1724–1725
    assessment of, 1699t, 1700–1703
    structure and function of, 1695–1698, 1696
Required surgery, 118
Research. See Nursing research.
Reserpine (Serpasil), 378t, 380t
Residual volume, 537, 538, 539t
Resistance vessels, 328
Resonance, on percussion, 536
Respiration. See also Breathing.
  accessory muscle of, 534
  artificial, in cardiopulmonary resuscitation, 262, 264t
  Biot's, 532, 533
  Cheyne-Stokes, 532, 533, 730
  definition of, 527
  depth of, 532, 533
  expiration in, 527, 528
  external, 527
  gas exchange in, 528
  gas transport in, 528
  in acid-base balance, 103, 103, 104t, 543
  inspiration in, 527, 527–528
  internal, 527
  Kussmaul's, 532, 533
    in diabetes, 1227, 1243
    in metabolic acidosis, 104, 105
  mechanics of, 528
  work of breathing in, 528
Respiratory acidosis, 108t, 108–111, 543
  hypercarbia and, 530
  in acute renal failure, 1390t
Respiratory alkalosis, 111t, 111–112, 543
  hypocarbia and, 530
Respiratory centers, 528
Respiratory disorder(s), 552–556
  artificial airways in, 559–567
  assessment in, 531–537, 532t
    auscultation in, 536, 536–537
    inspection in, 531–534
    palpation in, 534–535
    percussion in, 535, 535–536, 536
  chest tube in, 577–580
  diagnosis of, arterial blood gas analysis in, 540t, 540–545, 541, 544t
    blood studies in, 539–545, 540t, 541
    chest films in, 547, 547–548
    endoscopy in, 548–550
    lung biopsy in, 552
    pulmonary function studies in, 537–539, 538, 539t
    pulse oximetry in, 544–545, 545d, 546
    sputum studies in, 545–547
    thoracentesis in, 550–552
  drug therapy in, 574–575, 574d–576d
  in elderly, 587
  in HIV infection, 1466, 1467
  in immune disorders, 1443
  lower tract, 639–707
    asthma as, 659–668
    atelectasis as, 678–681

Respiratory disorder(s) (Continued)
  bronchiectasis as, 678
  chronic obstructive pulmonary disease as, 668–678
  circulatory, 681–688
  in elderly, 698–707
  infectious/inflammatory, 639–659
  Internet connections for, 665d
  neoplastic, 695–706
  occupational, 531, 688–690
  traumatic, 690–695
  management of, nonsurgical, 552–580
    settings and providers for, 596
    surgical, 580–587, 588–596c
  mechanical ventilation in, 567–574. See also Mechanical ventilation.
  occupational, 531, 688–690
  oxygen therapy in, 556–559. See also Oxygen therapy.
  patient history in, 531
  physical examination in, 531–537
  prevention of, 532d
  resources for, 2039
  respiratory therapy in, 552–556, 587. See also Respiratory therapy.
  traumatic, 690–695
  upper tract, 599–637
    in elderly, 637
    infectious and inflammatory, 599–610
    neoplastic, 616–637
    structural, 610–612
    traumatic, 612–616
Respiratory distress, in hypocalcemic tetany, 1317, 1318, 1319c
  in status asthmaticus, 660
  in transfusion reaction, 458, 462, 462d
  signs of, 532
Respiratory dysfunction, clinical manifestations of, 528–531
  in burns, 1655–1660, 1657t
    assessment of, 1658–1659, 1664
    management of, 1659–1660, 1664–1665
  in thoracic aortic aneurysm, 370
Respiratory failure, 530–531
  in adult respiratory distress syndrome, 686–688
Respiratory function, after cardiac arrest, 267c–268c
  age-related changes in, 65
  as surgical risk factor, 121–122
  in amyotrophic lateral sclerosis, 777
  in anesthesia, 140
  in ascites, 1147
  in elderly, 587
  in heart failure, 174–175, 270–271, 277, 278
  in metabolic acidosis, 104, 105, 106
  in metabolic alkalosis, 107, 108
  in myasthenia gravis, 782, 784, 785
  in respiratory acidosis, 108, 109, 110
  in respiratory alkalosis, 111, 112
  in shock, 406, 407, 407t
  in spinal cord injury, 826
  in surgical patient, 121–122
  postoperative, exercises for, 130, 130–131, 131, 151
    interventions for, 145, 146t, 151
    monitoring of, 145, 151
Respiratory infections. See also Pneumonia.
  in chronic obstructive pulmonary disease, 671d, 678d
    prevention of, 671d

Respiratory mucosa, 526
Respiratory rate, assessment of, 532
Respiratory rhythm, 532
Respiratory system, assessment of, 531–537, 532t. See also Respiratory disorder(s), assessment in.
  burns of, 1657t, 1658
  divisions of, 523
  health promotion for, 532d
  inspection of, 531–532
  lower, 523, 525, 526
  structure and function of, 523–528, 524–526
  upper, 523, 524
Respiratory therapists, 596
Respiratory therapy, 552–556, 596
  after lobectomy, 589c
  after pneumonectomy, 582–583, 585–586
  breathing exercises in, 130, 552–553
  in chronic obstructive pulmonary disease, 672, 675–676
  in mechanical ventilation, 571
  in unconscious client, 728
  percussion in, 553–555
  postural drainage in, 553, 554
  vibration in, 555–556
Respiratory zone, 526, 526–527
Rest. See also Bed rest.
  in chronic obstructive pulmonary disease, 676–677, 677, 678d
  in heart failure, 275, 279
  in hematologic disorders, 436, 452
  in hepatitis, 1173, 1177
  in myocardial infarction, 295–296, 302
Rest pain, 332, 333–334
Restless leg syndrome, in acute renal failure, 1395c–1396c
Restlessness, postoperative, 150
Restraints, postoperative, 150
Restrictive cardiomyopathy, 304, 306
Restrictive lung disease, burns and, 1658, 1664–1665
Resuscitation, cardiopulmonary. See Cardiopulmonary resuscitation (CPR).
  fluid. See also Fluid management.
    in burns, 1662
Retching, 960
Rete ridges, 1568, 1568
Reticular activating system, 720
  ascending, 720
Reticular formation, 720
Reticular lesions, 1573
Reticulocyte count, 443t, 444, 449
Reticulohistiocytes, 1568
Retina, 1936, 1937
  examination of, 1944, 1944
  function of, 1938
Retin-A (tretinoin), 1581–1582, 1615t
Retinal detachment, 1982–1985, 1983
Retinal holes, 1982–1985
Retinal tears, 1982–1985
Retinal vessels, examination of, 1944, 1944
Retinoids, 1581–1582
Retinopathy, diabetic, 1252d, 1253
  hypertensive, 375, 376
Retirement, 32
Retrograde ejaculation, 1699, 1699t
  after prostatectomy, 1709t, 1713, 1715t, 1719–1720
  after retroperitoneal lymphadenectomy, 1752
Retrograde pyelography, 1348t

Retroperitoneal lymphadenectomy, 1708t
  in testicular cancer, 1749–1750, 1752
Retropubic prostatectomy, 1710, 1710, 1711, 1714t–1715t. See also Prostatectomy.
Reverse Trendelenburg position, 135, 136
Reversible ischemic neurologic deficit, 806t
Rh blood group, 433
Rheumatic fever, 236, 237
Rheumatic heart disease, 236–237. See also Cardiac valvular disease.
  antibiotic prophylaxis in, 234–235, 237
  aortic stenosis in, 307–308
  infective endocarditis and, 233–236
  mitral regurgitation in, 309
  mitral stenosis in, 308–309
  pericarditis in, 238–239
Rheumatoid arthritis, 890–897
  arthrodesis for, 892
  assessment in, 894
  clinical manifestations of, 890–892, 891
  diagnosis of, 892
  drug therapy for, 892, 893d
  etiology of, 890
  Internet connections for, 896d
  management of, 892–894, 893d, 895
  nursing diagnoses and planning in, 894–895
  nursing interventions in, 895–896
  osteotomy for, 892
  pathophysiology of, 890
  support groups for, 896d
  synovectomy for, 892
  thermal applications for, 892
  total joint replacement for, 867–868, 868, 869c–872c
Rheumatoid factor, 892
Rheumatoid nodules, 892
Rhinitis, 599–601
  acute viral, 600, 600d
  allergic, 601, 1483–1486
    nasal polyps and, 611, 611
  atrophic, 601
  chronic, 601
    turbinate hypertrophy and, 611
  vasomotor, 601
Rhinoplasty, for deviated septum, 611–612
Rhinorrhea, 529, 531
  in rhinitis, 600–601
  in sinusitis, 601–602
RhoGAM, 1448
Rhonchi, 537
Rhus dermatitis, 1609t, 1609–1611, 1610
Rhytidectomy, 1591t, 1592d
Rhytidoplasty, 1591t, 1592d
Riboflavin deficiency, clinical manifestations of, 1077t
Ribs, 523, 525
  fractures of, 690–691
    flail chest and, 691, 691–692
  inspection of, 534
Rickets, 902–904
Rifampin, for tuberculosis, 653, 653t, 654t
Right bundle branch, 171
Right coronary artery, 164, 168, 168
Right ventricular afterload, 172
Rilutek (Riluzole), in amyotrophic lateral sclerosis, 775–776
Ringer's lactate, for hypovolemic shock, 411
  in fluid resuscitation, for burns, 1662
Ringworm, 1600t, 1600–1601, 1601
Rinne test, 2001

Risk for altered health maintenance. See *Patient teaching.*
Risk nursing diagnosis, 8
Risk reduction, 14t, 14–15
Rods, orthopedic, 865–867
    retinal, 1937
        electroretinography of, 1946
Role expectations, heart disease and, 187
Romberg test, 2001–2002
R-on-T phenomenon, 248, 249
Round ligaments, 1767, *1767*
Round window, 1995–1996, *1996,* 1997
Rubber band ligation, for hemorrhoids, 1097
Rubber dermatitis, 1609t, 1609–1611
Rubor, in vascular disorders, 334–335
Rugae, scrotal, 1696
Rule of nines, *1644,* 1645
Rupture, bladder, 1413–1414
Rural areas, health care access in, 1462d

S

S phase, of cell cycle, 1503, 1504, *1504*
S wave, 193, *194,* 195
S_1 heart sound, 179, *180*
    auscultation of, 191
S_2 heart sound, 179, *180*
    auscultation of, 191
S_3 heart sound, 179–180, *180*
    auscultation of, 191
S_4 heart sound, 180, *180*
    auscultation of, 191
Saccular aneurysm, 366, *366,* 367
Saccule, 1996
Sacrum, *715*
Saddle block, 137, 138t. See also *Anesthesia.*
Safe sex practices, for women, 1779d
Safety measures, after cataract surgery, 1977
    for ambulatory aids, 944
    for chemotherapy, 1528, 1528t
    for elderly, 944
    for eye patching, 1977
    for intracavitary radiation, 1835
    for pacemakers, 258, 259
    for radiation therapy, 1519, 1519t, *1520*
    for seizures, 772, 799, 799d
    for surgery, 143
    in Alzheimer's disease, 792
    in glaucoma, 1981
    in hypocalcemia, 97
    in mechanical ventilation, 570, 571
    in oxygen therapy, 556t, 556–557
    in Parkinson's disease, 789d
    in sensory disturbances, 744
    in stroke, 813
    postoperative, 149, 153
Salem sump pump, 977, *977*
Salicylates, 893d. See also *Aspirin.*
Salicylic acid, for warts, 1604
Saline breast implants, in augmentation mammoplasty, 1879
    in reconstructive surgery, *1876–1877,* 1876–1879, 1879d
Saline infusion. See also *Intravenous infusion.*
    for hyponatremia, 92–93
Saline inhalation method, for sputum collection, 546
Saliva, 951, 958t
Salivary amylase, 951, 958t
Salivary glands, 951

Salmonella osteomyelitis, 889–890
Salpingectomy, 1786t
Salpingitis, chlamydial, 1920, 1921
Salpingo-oophorectomy, for ovarian cancer, 1837–1838
    with hysterectomy, 1793, *1794.* See also *Hysterectomy.*
Salt. See *Sodium, dietary.*
Saluron (hydroflumethiazide), 377t
Sandostatin (octreotide), for bleeding esophageal varices, 1183
SaO_2, 540, 540t
    in oxyhemoglobin dissociation curve, *541,* 541–542
    measurement of, 544–545, *546*
    normal values for, 540t, 541
    PaO_2 and, 541
Saphenous vein, stripping of, 390, 392c
Sarcoma, 1505
    Ewing's, 942–943
    Kaposi's, in HIV infection, 1466, *1466*
    osteogenic, 936t, 938, 939c–942c, 942–943
Sarcomere, 840
Sarcoptes scabiei, 1929–1930
Scabies, 1929–1930
Scale, *1571,* 1572
    débridement of, 1583
Scalp, fungal infection of, 1600t, 1600–1601
    seborrheic dermatitis of, *1611,* 1611–1612
Scalp disorders, topical treatments for, 1583
Scalp hypothermia, in chemotherapy, 1530
Scalp injuries, 816–817
    management of, 817
        settings and providers for, 821
    nursing process in, 821–822
Scars, 1573
    burn, body image and, 1680, 1681
    hypertrophy of, 1682–1684
    keloid, 1632t–1633t
Schiller test, 1782
Schilling test, 443t, 451, 478
Schiøtz tonometer, 1945
School nurse, 28
School-based settings, 25–26
Sclera, *1936,* 1937, *1937*
    examination of, 1942, *1942*
Scleral buckle, for retinal detachment, 1983–1985, *1984*
Scleroderma, 1494–1495, *1495*
Sclerotherapy, for esophageal varices, 1186
    for hemorrhoids, 1097
    for varicose veins, 390, 392c
Scoliosis, 534, *534*
    assessment for, 848
SCOOP system, in transtracheal oxygen administration, *557,* 557–558, 558d
Scotomata, 742, 1939
Scratch tests, 1446, *1446,* 1447
Screening, cancer, 1511–1512, 1512d
    for chlamydia, 1921
    for colorectal cancer, 1100d
    for heart disease, 230
    for prostate cancer, 1704, 1756–1757, 1757t
    for sickle cell disease/trait, 485d
Screws, orthopedic, 865–867
Scrotum, age-related changes in, 1724–1725
    examination of, 1700–1701
    structure and function of, 1696, *1696*
    transillumination of, 1701

Scrub assistant, 135
Sebaceous cyst, 1572
Sebaceous glands, *1568, 1569,* 1569t
    in nonspecific immune response, 1435
Seborrheic dermatitis, 1611, *1611*
Seborrheic keratoses, 1632t
Secretin, 952, 953t
Secretory cells, gastric, 952
Sectral (acebutolol), 377t
Sedentary lifestyle, heart disease and, 187
Segmentation, 956
Segmented neutrophils, 445t
Seizure(s), focal (partial), 795, 796t
    generalized, 795, 796t
    in encephalitis, 772
    in meningitis, 772
    safety measures for, 772
Seizure disorders, assessment in, 798
    clinical manifestations of, 795, 796t
    diagnosis of, 795–796
    drug therapy for, 796, 797d–798d
    etiology of, 795
    Internet connections for, 779d
    management of, 796–797, 797d–798d
    nursing diagnoses and planning in, 798–799
    nursing interventions in, 799d, 799–800
    pathophysiology of, 795
    status epilepticus in, 795, 800
    surgery for, 796
Selective IgA deficiency, 1458
Selenium sulfide shampoo, for tinea versicolor, 1603
Self–blood glucose monitoring, in diabetes, 1241–1242, *1242,* 1242d, 1244c–1245c
Self-care. See also *Patient teaching.*
    after breast reconstruction, 1879d
    after corneal transplant, 1955d
    after cryosurgery, 1585c
    after dermatologic laser surgery, 1586, 1586d
    after intracavitary radiation, 1835d
    after myocardial infarction, 299d, 302–303
    after ocular surgery, 1953d
    after oral surgery, 1052, 1052d
    after plastic surgery, 1592d
    after skin biopsy, 1579d
    for homeless persons, 394–395
    for urinary tract infection prevention, 1372d
    in Addison's disease, 1282c–1283c, 1284d
    in Alzheimer's disease, 791d, 792
    in bleeding disorders, 482d
    in bone marrow transplantation, 1454d, 1454–1455
    in burns, 1683–1684, 1685d
    in chronic obstructive pulmonary disease, 673, *674,* 678
    in colostomy, 1006–1007, 1009–1011, 1010–1011, 1092c–1093c
    in diabetes, 1230–1243, 1244c–1246c, 1258–1259
        for long-term complications, 1252d
        in elderly, 1261–1262
    in diuretic therapy, 1144d
    in endocrine disorders, 1217–1218, 1219d
    in fibrocystic breast disease, 1856, 1856d
    in genital herpes, 1906d, 1906–1907
    in Guillain-Barré syndrome, 775
    in HIV infection, 1472, 1474d–1475d

Self-care *(Continued)*
  in hypothyroidism, 1303c–1305c, 1306
  in ileostomy, 1014d
  in immobility, 845–846
  in leukemia, 503, 504d
  in lung cancer, 698, 699d
  in menopause, 1774d, 1775
  in radiation therapy, 1523, 1523d
  in renal transplantation, 1410d
  in rheumatoid arthritis, 896
  in seizures, 799, 799d
  in sensory disturbances, 744
  in stroke, 812–813
  in urinary catheterization, 1362, 1364t
  in urinary tract disorders, 1365d, 1365–
      1366, 1366d
  information sources for, 2037–2045
  postoperative, for appendectomy, 1066d
      for hemorrhoidectomy, 1098d
      for herniorrhaphy, 1096d
  self-help devices for, 884
  with casts, 858, 922c–923c, 923–924
  with external fixation device, 864–865
Self-concept disturbance, in cancer, 1545,
    1549
Self-esteem, in elderly, 58
  in seizure disorders, 799–800
Self-examination, breast, *1846–1847*, 1846–
    1848
  for orofacial cancer, 1053d
  for skin cancer, 16
  for thyroid cancer, 1316
  testicular, *1703*, 1703d
  vulvar, 1779d
Self-help devices, 884
Semen, 1698
  analysis of, 1703–1704
  collection of, 1703–1704
  cryopreservation of, 1750
  ejaculation of, 1698
  reference values for, 2031
Semicircular canals, *1996*, 1996–1997
Semicomatose state, 726t
Semilunar valves, *164*, 167, *167*, *168*, 171
Seminal vesicles, structure and function of,
    1696, 1697
Seminiferous tubules, 1696
Seminoma, testicular, 1748–1752. See also
    Testicular cancer.
Sengstaken-Blakemore tube, *977*
  for esophageal varices, 1186–1188, *1187*,
      1191c–1192c, 1193
Senile dementia, 832
Senile hemangioma, 1632t
Senile keratosis, 1633t
Senile lentigo, 58, *58*
Senile miosis, 1961
Sensorineural hearing loss, 743, 1997–1998.
    See also *Hearing loss.*
  cochlear implant for, 2007–2008, *2008*
  in labyrinthitis, 2013–2014
  tinnitus and, 1998
Sensory aphasia, 738–739, 814
Sensory cortex, 719, *720*
Sensory function, age-related changes in,
    766
Sensory impairment, in stroke, 808, 813
Sensory neuron, 711, *712*
Sensory system assessment, 747–748
Sensory system dysfunction, 742–744, *743*
Sepsis, causative microorganisms in, 415t
  in burns, 1672
Septic shock, 413–416, 415t, 420. See also
    Shock.

Septic shock *(Continued)*
  in necrotizing fasciitis, 1599
  oxygen consumption in, 405–406
Sequential bacteriologic localization cul-
    tures, 1704–1705
Serial 7 test, 746
Seroma, postoperative, 147t
Serosa, gastrointestinal, 950
Serotonin, gastric secretion of, 952, 953t
  vasoconstriction and, 329t
Serous otitis media, 2012–2013, 2013t
Serpalan (reserpine), 378t, 380t
Serpasil (reserpine), 378t, 380t
Serpiginous lesions, 1573, *1574*
Serum, reference values for, 2024–2025
  vs. plasma, 429
Serum albumin, in hepatic disorders,
    1161t, 1163–1164
Serum creatinine, drugs affecting, 1346t
  in heart disease, 208
  in urinary tract disorders, 1345–1346,
      1346t
Serum electrolytes, preoperative, 125t
Serum folic acid, 443t, 450
Serum follicle-stimulating hormone, in
    males, 1704
Serum globulin, in hepatic disorders,
    1161t, 1163–1164
Serum glucose, in hepatic disorders, 1162t
Serum iron, 443t, 449–450
Serum lipids, in heart disease, 209
Serum luteinizing hormone, in males,
    1704
Serum osmolality, 75–76
Serum prostatic acid phosphatase, 1757
Serum protein electrophoresis, in hepatic
    disorders, 1161t, 1163–1164
Serum sickness, 1487–1488
Serum test profile (SMA 12), preoperative,
    125t
Serum thyroxine, assays of, 1299t, 1301t
Serum triiodothyronine, assays of, 1299t,
    1301t
Severe combined immunodeficiency
    (SCID), 1458
Sexual activity, HIV transmission and,
    1461–1463
Sexual dysfunction, after gynecologic sur-
    gery, 1787
  after mastectomy, 1867
  after prostatectomy, 1709t, 1713, 1715t,
      1719–1720, 1761
  after radical vulvectomy, 1829
  chemotherapy and, 1538t–1539t
  genital prolapse and, 1817
  in cancer, 1545, 1549
  in diabetes, 1254
  in elderly, 1761
  in menopause, 1771
  in radiation therapy, 1522
  in sexually transmitted diseases, 1899c–
      1900c
  male, clinical manifestations of, 1698–
      1699, 1699t
Sexual function, after hysterectomy, 1799,
    1800d
  age-related changes in, 68
    in females, 1838
    in males, 1725
  colostomy and, 1010, 1091c–1092c, 1106
  in spinal cord injury, 826–827
Sexual history, female, 1778
Sexual response, female, 1769
  age-related changes in, 1838

Sexual response *(Continued)*
  male, 1698
    age-related changes in, 1725
Sexually transmitted disease(s) (STDs),
    1883–1930
  anxiety in, 1898c–1899c
  assessment in, 1887t–1888t
  clinics for, 1883
  epididymitis in, 1728–1730
  history in, 1887t
  HIV infection as, 1461–1463
  incidence of, 1883
  Internet connections for, 1922d
  nursing care guide in, 1890c–1900c
  pain in, 1890c–1891c
  partner notification in, 1913–1914, 1917,
      1920
  patient teaching for, 1897c–1898c, 1901d
  physical examination in, 1888t
  prevention of, 1920
      condom use and, 1924d
  psychosocial assessment in, 1887t
  reporting of, 1883
  secondary infection in, prevention of,
      1891c–1893c
  sexual dysfunction in, 1899c–1900c
  sociocultural aspects of, 1919
  treatment compliance in, 1893c–1897c
  vaginitis in, 1804–1806, 1805t, 1883–
      1889
Shampoos, for seborrheic dermatitis, 1611
Sharps, safety precautions for, 1464, 1472d
Shattered kidney, 1411–1412
Shave biopsy, 1578, 1579d
Shaving, preoperative, 124
Shear, pressure ulcers and, 1623, 1630
Shift to the left, in white cell count, 1372
Shingles, 1606–1607
Shock, anaphylactic, 401, 417t, 417–418,
    420
    contrast media and, 1346
    insect stings and, 1621–1622, 1622d
    prevention of, 422d
    transfusion-related, 462
  assessment in, 418–419
  burn, 1660–1664, *1661*
  cardiogenic, 401, *411*, 411–413, 412t,
      419–420
  clinical manifestations of, 406, 407t
  compensatory stage of, 406–407, 407t
  distributive, 401, 420
  hemodynamic monitoring in, 402
  hemodynamics and, 402–405
  hemorrhagic, 409, 410t
  hypovolemic, 401, 408t, 408–411, *409*,
      419
  in elderly, 422
  in musculoskeletal disorders, 932
  nursing diagnoses and planning in, 420–
      421
  nursing interventions in, 421–422
  overview of, 401
  oxygen consumption in, 405t, 405–406
  oxygen delivery in, 405, 405t
  postoperative, 145–149, 146t
  progressive stage of, 407t, 407–408
  refractory stage of, 407t, 408
  septic, 401, 413–416, 415t, 420
  spinal (neurogenic), 401, 416–417, 420,
      823–824
  types of, 408–422
Shock position, 411
Shock-like symptoms, in fluid volume de-
    ficit, 77, 78

Short bones, 839
Short leg cast, 854t. See also *Cast(s)*.
Short-stay surgery, 115–116
Shoulder, bursitis of, 902
  tenosynovitis of, 902
Shoulder exercises, in stroke, 809
  postoperative, after mastectomy, 1865–
    1866, 1867d, *1868*, 1868t
    after thoracic surgery, 583, 586, 593c,
      701c, 705c
Shoulder pain, in stroke, 809
Shoulder prosthesis, 882, *883*
Shoulder spica cast, 855t. See also *Cast(s)*.
Shunt(s), 528
  arteriovenous, for hemodialysis, 1405,
    1405, 1406
  Denver, for ascites, 1145
  distal splenorenal, for esophageal vari-
    ces, *1188*, 1189
  intraocular, for glaucoma, 1980
  LeVeen, for portal hypertension, 1144–
    1145, *1146*
  surgical, for esophageal varices, *1188*,
    1189
  ventricular, for hydrocephalus, 802–804,
    803
SIADH. See *Syndrome of inappropriate anti-
  diuretic hormone (SIADH)*.
Sickle-cell anemia, *484*, 484–487, 485d,
    486t, 487d
  leg ulcers in, 437, 484, 487, 487d
Sickle-cell crisis, 484, 485
Sickle-cell test, 443t, 448–449
Sickledex, 443t, 448–449
Sighs, in mechanical ventilation, 570
Silent (painless) thyroiditis, 1296
Silicone breast implants, in augmentation
    mammoplasty, 1879
  in reconstructive surgery, *1876–1877*,
    1876–1879, 1879d
  mammography of, 1848–1849
Silicosis, 688, 689–691
Silver nitrate, for burns, 1674t
Silver sulfadiazine, for burns, 1674t
Simontons, 1544
Simple nontoxic goiter, 1314–1315, *1315*
Simple partial seizures, 796t
Simvastatin (Zocor), 216–217, 218d
Singultus, postoperative, 149t
Sinoatrial node, 169, *170*, 171
Sinus(es), paranasal, *601*
    inflammation of, 601–604
    palpation of, *602*
    surgery of, 603–604
Sinus arrhythmia, 242, *243*
Sinus bradycardia, 240–241, *241*
Sinus dysrhythmias, 178, 240–242, *241–
    243*
Sinus rhythm, 195, 196t
  normal, *241*
Sinus tachycardia, 241–242, *242*
Sinusitis, 601–604
  acute, 602–603
  brain abscess and, 771
  chronic, 603–604
Sitting position, 135, *136*
Sitz bath, for hemorrhoids, 1096, 1098,
    1098d
Skeletal muscle. See also *Muscle*.
  structure and function of, 840–842
Skeletal traction, 824, 826, 860, *861*. See
  also *Traction*.
  on, appendicular, 837
    37

Skeleton *(Continued)*
  structure and function of, 837–840, *838,
    840, 841*
Skene's glands, 1766
Skin, age-related changes in, 10–11, *58*,
    1591–1592
  atrophy of, 1573
  bacterial infections of, 1595–1600, *1596*,
    1597t–1598t, 1599d
  benign neoplasms of, 1632t–1633t, 1634–
    1636
  biopsy of, 1577–1578, *1578*, 1579d
    for melanoma, 1638
  culture of, 1576
  dermatophyte infections of, 1600t, 1600–
    1601, *1601*
  dry, 1608t
    in elderly, 58–59
  fungal infections of, 1600t, 1600–1603,
    1601, 1601d, *1602*
    in elderly, 1630
  hydration of, 1583
  in immune disorders, 1442
  in vascular insufficiency, 334t, 334–337,
    338, 362
  pigmented lesions of, 1631–1634
  structure and function of, 1567–1569,
    1568, 1569t
  sunreactive classification of, 1583t
  temperature of, in vascular disorders,
    334t, 335
  trophic changes in, 334
  viral infections of, 1603–1607
  yeast infections of, 1601–1603, *1602*
Skin cancer, 1636–1639
  basal cell, 1636–1637, *1637*
  clinical manifestations of, 1511t
  curettage and desiccation for, 1584–
    1585, 1637
  Internet connections for, 1639d
  melanoma as, *1638*, 1638–1639
  Mohs' micrographic surgery for, 1585,
    1637
  nursing care for, 1638–1639
  prevention of, 1636d
  radiation therapy for, 1583–1584
  risk factors for, 1511t
  self-examination for, 1053d, *1634–1635*,
    1635–1636
  squamous cell, 1637, *1637*
  vulvar, 1826–1830
  warning signs of, 1635–1636
Skin care, 1575d
  in acne, 1614
  in amputation, 875d–876d, 877, 878d,
    879
  in bed rest, 279–280
  in bone marrow transplant, 1453, 1453d
  in cast therapy, 858
  in chronic venous insufficiency, 393–395
  in colostomy, 1009–1010, 1086c–1087c,
    1092c–1093c
  in diarrhea, 964
  in enteral feeding, 986
  in fluid volume excess, 81
  in gastrointestinal intubation, 979–980
  in healed burns, 1683–1684, 1685d
  in hematologic disorders, 440
  in hypothyroidism, 1304c, 1306
  in immobility, 845
  in increased intracranial pressure, 737
  in jaundice, 1140–1141, 1156c–1157c
  in pancreatic fistula, 1125, 1126
  in portal hypertension, 1147–1148

Skin care *(Continued)*
  in radiation therapy, 1523d
  in stasis dermatitis, 393–395
  in unconscious client, 728
  in vascular disorders, 336–337, 355,
    355d
  in venous thrombosis, 387
  pin-site, 863t, 865
Skin color. See also *Pigmentation changes*.
  assessment of, 192
  changes in, 1570, 1575
    in anemia, 468
    in dark-skinned clients, 532, 1575
    in vascular disorders, 334t, 334–335
    inspection for, 532, 1575
Skin disorders, 1595–1640
  bullous, 1619–1621
  clinical manifestations of, 1570–1573
  color alterations in, 1570, 1575. See also
    Skin color.
  cryosurgery for, 1585, 1585d
  curettage and desiccation for, 1584–1585
  diagnosis of, 1575–1578, 1576t
  drug therapy for, 1579–1582
    topical, 1579–1581
  history in, 1574–1575
  in elderly, 1591–1592, 1630
  infectious, 1595–1607
  inflammatory, 1607–1619
  Internet connections for, 1639d
  lesions in, 1570–1573, *1571*
  management of, 1579–1591
    nonsurgical, 1579–1584
    settings and providers for, 1591
    surgical, 1584–1591
  neoplastic, 1631–1640
  occlusive dressings for, 1583
  of scalp, topical treatments for, 1583
  physical examination in, 1575
  radiation therapy for, 1583–1584
  resources for, 2043
  sensation alterations in, 1570
  temperature alterations in, 1570
  therapeutic baths for, 1583
  turgor alterations in, 1570
  wet dressings for, 1583
Skin flaps, 1587, *1587*
Skin grafts, 1587–1590, *1588, 1589*
  allograft, 1588–1590, 1675t
  assessment of, 1675–1676
  autograft, 1588–1590
    for burns, 1673–1678, *1675*, 1675t
  donor sites for, 1673, *1675*, 1678, 1678t
  dressings for, 1673, 1676d
  epidermal skin equivalent for, 1675
    for burns, 1673–1678
  heterograft, 1588–1590, 1673–1678, *1675*,
    1675t
    for burns, 1673–1678, *1675*, 1675t
  homograft, 1588–1590
    for burns, 1673–1678, *1675*, 1675t
  infection of, prevention of, 1677
  mesh, 1673, *1675*
  nursing diagnoses and planning for,
    1676–1677
  nursing interventions for, 1677–1678
  pain management for, 1678
  splints for, 1677
  Unna's boot for, 1676d
  xenograft, 1588–1590
Skin lesions, annular, 1573
  arciform, 1573
  arrangement of, 1573, *1574*
  bull's-eye, 1573

Skin lesions *(Continued)*
  chemotherapy and, 1530–1531, 1539t–
    1540t
  circinate, 1573
  confluent, 1573, *1574*
  depigmented, 1570–1571
  discrete, 1573, *1574*
  distribution of, 1573
  evolution of, 1573
  grouped, *1574*
  hyperpigmented, 1570–1571
  hypopigmented, 1570
  in HIV infection, 1466, *1466*
  in radiation therapy, 1520
  in scleroderma, 1494–1495, *1495*
  in syphilis, 1915, *1916, 1917*
  in systemic lupus erythematosus, 1491,
    1491
  iris, 1573
  linear, 1573*1574*
  polycyclic, 1573, *1574*
  precancerous, 1633t
  primary, 1573
  reticular, 1573
  satellite, 1602, *1602*
  secondary, 1573
  serpiginous, 1573
  shape of, 1573
  target, 1573
  types of, 1570–1573, *1571*
Skin preparation, for prostatectomy, 1711
  intraoperative, 135–136
  preoperative, 124
Skin sensation, alterations in, 1570
Skin tags, 58, 1632t
Skin temperature, alterations in, 1570
Skin tests, for hypersensitivity, 1489
Skin traction, 859–860, *860*. See also *Traction.*
Skin turgor, 1570
  in dehydration, 78
Skin wounds. See *Wound* entries.
Skinning vulvectomy, 1826
Skull, in Paget's disease, 908
  structure and function of, 713, *715*
  surgical decompression of, in increased
    intracranial pressure, 733
  x-ray films of, 748, 818
Skull fractures, 817–818, *818*. See also *Head
  injury.*
  depressed, *818, 917*
  management of, 818
    settings and providers for, 821
    nursing process in, 821–822
Sleep, age-related changes in, 63–64, 766
  in Parkinson's disease, 789d
Sleep disturbances, in keratitis therapy,
    1966–1967
  in menopause, 1771
Slit-lamp examination, 1945
Slobid. See *Theophylline (Slobid, Theodur).*
SMA 12, preoperative, 125t
Small intestinal resection, 1000–1015
  ileostomy in, 1011–1015. See also *Ileos-
    tomy.*
  patient preparation for, 1000
  postoperative care in, 1002–1003
  postoperative course in, 1001–1002
  preoperative care in, 1002
  procedure for, 1001
  uses of, 1000
Small intestine, ischemia of, in elderly,
    1106
  structure and function of, *955,* 955–956

Smegma, 1695
Smell, age-related changes in, 61
Smoke inhalation, 1657t, 1658
Smoker's face, 1592
Smoking, as surgical risk factor, 123
  by elderly, 65
  cancer and, 1509
  cessation of, for cardiac surgery, 219–
    220
  chronic bronchitis and, 669
  emphysema and, 670
  heart disease and, 186–187, 210, 211,
    285
  in atherosclerosis, 362
  in peptic ulcer disease, 1028
  in thromboangiitis obliterans, 352, 353
  lung cancer and, 695
  oral cancer and, 1049
  oral contraceptives and, 211
  premature atrial contractions and, 243–
    244, *244*
  second-hand smoke and, 1509
  skin changes from, 1592
  vascular disease and, 338t, 362
Smoking history, 531
Snellen chart, 1940–1941
Social isolation, hearing loss and, 2020
  in cancer, 1545–1546, 1550
  in HIV infection, 1472, 1479c–1480c
Social services, for rheumatoid arthritis patients, 896
Social worker, qualifications and responsibilities of, 25t
Sociocultural factors, in cancer, 1506–1508
  in communication, 666d–667d
  in health care access, 1462d–1463d
  in self-care for homeless persons, 394–
    395
  in sexually transmitted diseases, 1919d
Socioeconomic factors, in cancer, 1506–
    1508
  in health care access, 18, 1462d–1463d
Sodium, cardiac function and, 208
  cellular distribution of, 84, *85*
  deficiency of, 91–93. See also *Hypernatre-
    mia; Hyponatremia.*
  dietary, daily requirement for, 91
    in Addison's disease, 1284
    in heart failure, 275, 276d, 279
    restriction of, 382d, 1143d
      in fluid volume excess, 80, 81
      in heart failure, 275, 276d, 279
      in hypernatremia, 94
      in hypertension, 382d
      in portal hypertension, 1143d, 1144
    sources of, 184d
  excess of, 93–94. See also *Hypernatremia.*
  extracellular fluid volume deficit and,
    75–79, 77t
  function of, 91
  normal values for, 91
  regulation of, 91
  sources of, 93
Sodium bicarbonate. See *Bicarbonate.*
Sodium nitroprusside (Nipride), 213, 213d,
    378t, 380t
  for cardiogenic shock, 413
Sodium pentothal (Nembutal), for increased intracranial pressure, 732
Sodium polystyrene, for hyperkalemia, 89
Soft tissue abscess, 1595–1599, 1598t,
    1599d
Solar keratosis, 1633t
Solar lentigines, 58, *58*

Solutions, total parenteral nutrition, 986–
    987
Somatosensory evoked potentials, 757
Somatostatin, 1207t, 1209t
  gastric secretion of, 952, 953t
  in glucose metabolism, 1224
Somatotrope adenoma, somatotropin hypersecretion and, 1269–1274
Somatotropin, 1205t
  hypersecretion of, 1269
  in glucose metabolism, 1224
  reference values for, 1272
Somogyi phenomenon, 1250–1251
Sore throat, in peritonsillar abscess, 607–
    608
  in pharyngitis, 604–606, *605,* 606d
  in tonsillitis, 606, *606,* 606d
  postoperative, 149t
Sotalol (Betapace), for dysrhythmias, 215,
    216d
Spasms, bladder, after prostatectomy,
    1712, 1715t, 1718, 1719
  in hypocalcemia, 96
Spasticity, 840
  in multiple sclerosis, 780
Specimens, blood, arterial, 428, 543
    venous, 428, 545
  sputum, 546–547
Speculum examination, of cervix, 1780,
    1780
Speech. See also *Communication.*
  after total laryngectomy, 620–626, *626–
    628*
  esophageal, 618, *626*
Speech assessment, 738–739, 746–747
Speech center, of brain, 719
Speech pathologist, qualifications and re-
  sponsibilities of, 25t
Speech problems, 738–739
  in Parkinson's disease, 790
  in stroke, 814
Sperm, 1696
  transport of, 1697
Sperm banking, 1750
Spermatic cords, structure and function of,
    1696, 1697–1698
Spermatocelectomy, 1708t
Spermatogenesis, 1696
Sphenoid sinusitis, 602–604
Spherocytosis, hereditary, 482–484
Sphincter of Oddi, 957, *958*
Spica casts, 855t. See also *Cast(s).*
Spinal anesthesia, 137, 138t. See also *Anesthesia.*
Spinal arteries, 716
Spinal circulation, 716
Spinal cord, blood supply to, 716
  imaging of, *752,* 752–753
  lesions of, sensory alteration in, *743,*
    743–744
  major motor pathways of, 722
  structure and function of, *721,* 721–722,
    722
Spinal cord injury, 822–827
  autonomic dysreflexia in, 823, 825, 826
  clinical manifestations of, 823–824
  compression, 823, *823, 917*
  diagnosis of, 824
  etiology of, 822
  hyperextension, 822–823, *823*
  hyperflexion, 822, *822*
  management of, 824
  pathophysiology of, 822–823, *823*
  spinal cord syndromes in, 823, 824t

Spinal cord injury (Continued)
  spinal shock in, 823–824, 826
  subluxation, 823
Spinal cord syndromes, 823, 824t
Spinal fusion, 762–765, 763d
Spinal headache, epidural anesthesia and, 137
  lumbar puncture and, 754
Spinal nerves, 722–723, 724
  compression of, 793t
Spinal (neurogenic) shock, 416–417, 823–824
Spinal surgery, 761–765
  clinical pathway for, 763d
  complications of, 762
  nursing process in, 762–765
  postoperative care in, 762–765, 763d
  postprocedure course in, 762
  preoperative care in, 762, 763d
  procedure for, 761–762
  uses of, 761
Spinal tap, 753–754, 755c–756c, 757
  in subarachnoid hemorrhage, 815
Spinal traction, 824, 826, 861, 861. See also
    Traction.
Spine, disc herniation in, 792–795, 793,
      793t, 794d
  surgery for, 673d, 761–767
  immobilization of, 824, 825, 826
  magnetic resonance imaging of, 749
  myelography of, 752, 752, 753
  structure and function of, 713–714, 715
  x-ray films of, 748–749
Spiritual needs, in death and dying, 34,
      40–41
  in AIDS, 1482c
Spiritual nursing care, 13–14
Spirometry, 538–539
Spironolactone (Aldactone), 377t
  for heart disease, 216, 217d, 218d
  for portal hypertension, 1144, 1144d
  for primary aldosteronism, 1291
Spleen, hematologic functions of, 433, 435
  immunologic functions of, 1431–1432
  structure of, 433, 435
Splenectomy, 462–464
  defective opsonization and, 1437
  for aplastic anemia, 480
  for hereditary spherocytosis, 482
  for purpura, 514
  immunosuppression and, 1449
Splenomegaly, in hematologic disorders,
      441
  in infectious mononucleosis, 513
  in portal hypertension, 1142
  splenorenal for, 463–464
Splenorenal shunt, for esophageal varices,
      1188, 1189
Splinting, incision, 130, 131
  after thoracotomy, 582, 583, 585, 586
Splints, 881
  air, 883–884
  for fractures, 918
  for skin grafts, 1677
  in skeletal traction, 860
Spouse abuse, 19
Sprains, 913–914
Sprue, celiac, 1078–1079, 1079
  malabsorption in, 1077t, 1077–1078
Sputum, color of, in pneumonia, 644d
  examination of, 545–547
  expectoration of, 529
  from rupture abscess, 647
  in bronchiectasis, 679

Sputum (Continued)
  in chronic obstructive pulmonary dis-
      ease, 669t
Sputum culture, in tuberculosis, 652, 657
Sputum cytology, in lung cancer, 1513
Sputum specimen, collection of, 546–547
  in tuberculosis, 657
Squamous cell carcinoma, cervical, 1830–
    1836. See also Cervical cancer.
  of lung, 695–696
  of skin, 1637, 1637, 1638–1639
  of vulva, 1826–1830
ST segment, 193, 194, 195
Stab wounds, of brain, 819
  of heart, 316–317
  of kidney, 1411–1412
  of liver, 1194
  of spinal cord, 823
  of ureter, 1412–1413
Staging, cancer, surgery for, 1516
Stained red cell examination, 446
Standard precautions, 439t, 1464
  for hepatitis, 1176, 1177
  for HIV infection, 1464, 1472d
Standards of Clinical Nursing Practice,
    6–7, 7t
Stapedectomy, in otosclerosis, 2015–2016,
    2016, 2017d
Stapes, 1996, 1996, 1997
Staphylococcal infection, in toxic shock
      syndrome, 1807–1808
  infective endocarditis and, 234
  of breast, 1852–1853
Staphylococcal infections, of skin, 1595–
    1599, 1596, 1597t, 1599d
Starch bath, 1583
Starling law, 403, 403
Starvation ketosis, 1243
Stasis dermatitis, 1611–1612, 1612
Stasis ulcers, 332, 333–334, 334t, 335, 390–
    395
  in homeless persons, 394–395
  pain in, 332, 333–334
  venous thrombosis and, 386
Status asthmaticus, 660
  management of, 663
Status epilepticus, 795, 800
Steatorrhea, in chronic pancreatitis, 1123,
    1124
  in gluten-induced enteropathy, 1078
  in liver disease, 1138, 1153
  in malabsorption, 1077
Steinmann pins, 860, 861
Stem cells, 429, 430, 1430, 1431
  deficiency of, 1457–1458
  in thymus, 1430
Stents, coronary, 292–293, 293
  prostatic, for benign prostatic hyperpla-
      sia, 1754
  urethral, for benign prostatic hyperpla-
      sia, 1754
Stereotaxic surgery, for brain tumors,
    830
Sterility, after retroperitoneal lymphade-
      nectomy, 1752
  cryptorchidism and, 1739
  orchitis and, 1731
  varicocele and, 1743
Sterilization, female, 1793
  male, 1708t, 1708–1709, 1710, 1710d
Steroids. See Corticosteroids.
Stethoscope, 191
Stiff neck, in disc herniation, 793
  in meningitis, 768, 768

Stiffness, joint, in arthritis, 891, 892, 897–
      898
  posttraumatic, 933–934
Stings, insect, hypersensitivity to, 1483t,
    1621–1622, 1622d
Stirrup, 1996, 1996, 1997
Stockings, elastic compression, application
      of, 389d
  for varicose veins, 390
  for venous thrombosis, 388
Stokes-Adams syndrome, 176
Stoma, colostomy, 1009–1010, 1086c–1087c
  care of, 1009–1010, 1092c–1093c
  mucocutaneous separation in, 1005
  necrosis of, 1005
  patient teaching for, 1006–1007, 1010–
      1011, 1092c–1093c
  prolapse of, 1005, 1005
  retraction of, 1005, 1005
  stenosis of, 1005
  ileostomy, 1012, 1013, 1014d
  tracheostomy, 566–567, 630, 631d
  ureterostomy, 1423, 1424
Stomach. See also under Gastric; Gastroin-
    testinal.
  structure and function of, 952, 952–953,
    953
Stomatitis, chemotherapy and, 1529, 1541t
  in radiation therapy, 1520
Stones, kidney. See Urinary calculi.
Stool, fatty, in chronic pancreatitis, 1123,
    1124
  in gluten-induced enteropathy, 1078
  in liver disease, 1138, 1153
  in malabsorption, 1077
  in constipation, 961
Straight leg raise, 747, 912
Strains, 913
Strangulated hernia, 194, 1094
Stratum corneum, 1567, 1568, 1568, 1569t
  nails and, 1569
Stratum granulosum, 1568, 1568
Stratum lucidum, 1567, 1568
Strawberry hemangioma, 1571
Strength, assessment of, 747, 747t, 848
Streptococcal infection, arthritis and, 237
Streptococcal pharyngitis, 604–606, 605
  rheumatic fever and, 236, 237
Streptococcal tonsillitis, 606, 606
Streptokinase (Streptase), 217, 218
  for myocardial infarction, 295, 296d
  for pulmonary embolism, 682
Streptomycin, for tuberculosis, 653, 653t,
    654t
Stress, asthma and, 665
  cancer and, 1510–1511
  family, in cancer, 1546
  heart disease and, 187, 210, 285
  hypertension and, 373
  of surgery, 119
  premature junctional contractions and,
      247
  premenstrual syndrome and, 1807, 1810
  tension headache and, 800
  vascular disease and, 338t
Stress echocardiography, 199
Stress incontinence, 1338, 1340t, 1340–1341
  cystocele/urethrocele and, 1817
  Kegel exercises for, 1365, 1365d, 1779d,
      1817, 1817d
Stress response, in elderly, 1218
Stress testing, 195–197, 286
  in myocardial infarction, 298
  submaximal, 298

Stress ulcers, 1033, 1679
　bleeding from, 966d
　in burns, 1679
　postoperative, 148t
Striae, 1573
Striated muscle, 840–842. See also *Muscle.*
Stroke. See *Cerebrovascular accident (CVA).*
Stroke volume, 402, 402t
　cardiac output and, 172
Struvite calculi. See *Urinary calculi.*
Stump care, in amputation, 875d–876d, 877, 878d, *879*
Stupor, 726t
Stye (hordeolum), 1968t
Subacute bacterial endocarditis, 234
Subacute granulomatous thyroiditis, 1296
Subaortic stenosis, effort syncope in, 176
Subarachnoid hemorrhage, 814–816, *815*
　cerebrovascular accident and, 804, *805.* See also *Cerebrovascular accident (CVA).*
Subarachnoid screw, in intracranial pressure monitoring, 731, *731*
Subarachnoid space, 714, 814
Subclavian vein catheter, for hemodialysis, 1405, 1406
Subconjunctival hemorrhage, 1987–1989
Subcostal incision, 995t
Subcutaneous emphysema, 695
Subcutaneous fat, 1568–1569, 1569t
　age-related changes in, 51
　liposuction of, 1591t, 1592d
Subcutaneous opioids, 1554t
Subdural hematoma, 819–820, *820*
　in elderly, 832
　management of, settings and providers for, 821
　nursing process in, 821–822
Subdural space, 714
Sublimaze (fentanyl), for anesthesia, 141t
　transdermal, 1554t
Sublingual glands, 951
Subluxations, 915–916
Submandibular glands, 951
Submucosa, gastrointestinal, 950
Subphrenic abscess, appendicitis and, 1064t
Substance abuse, as surgical risk factor, 122–123
　HIV transmission and, 1463–1464
　infective endocarditis and, 234
Subtotal parathyroidectomy, for hyperparathyroidism, 1321
Subtotal thyroidectomy, 1310
　case study of, 1311d–1312d
　postoperative care in, 1314
Succinylcholine (Anectine), 141t
Sucralfate (Carafate), 1022d
　for peptic ulcers, 1028
Sucrase, 958
Suctioning, in endotracheal intubation, in unconscious client, 728
　in esophageal balloon tamponade, 1187, 1191c–1192c, 1193
　of tracheostomy tube, 566–567, 629–630
Suicide, assisted, 41, 42b
　bereavement in, 37–38
Sulcus, 718
Sulfamylon (mafenide acetate), for burns, 1674t
Sulfinpyrazone (Anturane), for gout, 900, 900d
Sulfonylureas, for diabetes, 1239, 1239t, 1240d

Sulfonylureas *(Continued)*
　in elderly, 1261, 1323
Sun exposure, avoidance of, in systemic lupus erythematosus, 1494c
　benign skin changes from, 1592
　minimization of, 1636d
　skin cancer and, 1636, 1637, 1638
　skin reaction to, 1583t
　sunscreen for, 1582, 1636d
Sun sensitizers, 1582
Sunburn, tendency for, 1583t
Sunreactive skin types, classification of, 1583t
Sunscreens, 1582, 1636d
Supine position, 135, *136*
Support groups, 2037–2045. See also *Internet connections.*
　for amputees, 878
　for ostomy clients, 1006, 1010, 1011
Suppressor T cells, 1433–1434, 1434t, 1439
Supraclavicular lymph nodes, *435.* See also *Lymph nodes.*
Supraglottic laryngectomy, 617–622. See also *Laryngectomy.*
　nursing care guide for, 619c–623c
　radical neck dissection in, *631,* 631–637
Suprane (desflurane), 139, 139t
Suprapubic catheters, 1362–1363
Suprapubic prostatectomy, 1710, *1710, 1711,* 1714t–1715t. See also *Prostatectomy.*
Supratentorial surgery, 757, 759t. See also *Intracranial surgery.*
Supraventricular tachycardia, paroxysmal, *244,* 244–245
Surgeon, 135
　assistant to, 135
Surgery, 115–159. See also specific sites and types.
　abdominal, paralytic ileus after, 1075–1077
　ambulatory, 115–116, 156t, 156–158, 157t
　　facilities for, 22
　anesthesia for, 136–142. See also *Anesthesia.*
　　preoperative management for, 127–128
　approach in, 119
　cancer, 1516–1517
　cardiac, 217–229
　　in heart failure, 275–276
　　valve-replacement, 234
　cardiovascular status and, 121
　consent for, 117–118
　definition of, 115
　diagnostic procedures for, 123–124
　　in elderly, 158
　draping for, 136
　economic factors in, 119–120
　elective, 118–119
　emergency, 118
　endocrine status and, 122
　extent of, 118
　fiberoptic/endoscopic, 119
　fluid and electrolyte balance and, 121
　for fracture reduction, 920c–923c
　for rheumatoid arthritis, 892
　gastrointestinal, 993–1015. See also *Gastrointestinal surgery.*
　hematologic status and, 122
　hepatic status and, 122
　immune status and, 121
　in diabetes, 1241

Surgery *(Continued)*
　in elderly, 158–159
　in pregnancy, 123
　infection prevention for, 143
　intracranial, 757–761
　intraoperative management in, 134–143. See also *Intraoperative period.*
　laser. See *Laser surgery.*
　legal issues in, 117–118
　limb reattachment, 930–932
　major, 118
　minor, 118
　Mohs' micrographic, 1585
　neurologic status and, 122
　nursing standards for, 116, 117t
　nutritional status and, 120–121
　optional, 119
　orthopedic, 863–878
　personnel in, 135
　plastic, 1590–1591, 1591t, 1592d
　　for burns, 1682
　positioning in, 135, *136,* 143
　postoperative management in, 143–156. See also *Postoperative period.*
　preoperative management in, 123–134. See also *Preoperative period.*
　psychosocial status and, 119, 120d
　renal status and, 122
　required, 118
　respiratory status and, 121–122
　risk factors in, 119–123
　routine drug therapy and, 122
　settings for, 115–116
　short-stay, 115–116
　sinus, 603–604
　skin preparation for, 124, 135–136
　substance abuse and, 122–123
　thoracic, 580–587, 588d–596d
　urgency of, 118–119
　urgent, 118
　vascular, 344–346
　　postoperative care in, 347–348
　　preoperative care in, 346–347
Surgical asepsis, 143
Surgical team, 135
Surgicenters, 22
Suturing, of skin wounds, 1586–1587, *1587*
Swallowing, 951
　difficult. See *Dysphagia.*
　painful. See *Odynophagia.*
　with prosthetic tube, 1055, 1058
Sweat glands, *1568,* 1569, 1569t
Swelling. See also *Edema.*
　of casted parts, 853
Sympathectomy, in thromboangiitis obliterans, 352
Sympathetic nervous system, 725t, 726
　in vascular control, 173
Synapse, 713
Synarthrodial joints, *841,* 842, 842t
Synchronized intermittent mandatory ventilation, 569. See also *Mechanical ventilation.*
　in weaning, 574
Syncope, in heart disease, 176
Syndrome of inappropriate antidiuretic hormone (SIADH), 83, 83t, 1277
　hyponatremia and, 91, 92
　in elderly, 1323
　in lung cancer, 696, 697, 698, 699d
Synovectomy, for rheumatoid arthritis, 892
Synovial fluid, 842
Synthroid (levothyroxine), for hypothyroidism, 1298, 1303c–1304c, 1305t

Syphilis, 1914–1920
  clinical manifestations of, 1914–1915, *1915, 1916*
  etiology of, 1914
  HIV infection and, 1917
  in pregnancy, 1918
  incidence of, 1914
  latent, 1914–1916
  pathophysiology of, 1914–1915
  primary, 1914, 1915
  secondary, 1914, 1915, *1916*
  stages of, 1914
  tertiary, 1914, 1915, 1916
Syphilis osteomyelitis, 889–890
Systemic lupus erythematosus, 1490–1494
  assessment in, 1492
  clinical manifestations of, 1491, *1491,* 1492t
  diagnosis of, 1491, 1492t
  etiology of, 1490
  management of, 1491–1492
  nursing diagnoses and planning in, 1492–1493
  nursing interventions in, 1493d, 1493–1494
  pathophysiology of, 1490–1491
Systemic sclerosis, 1494–1495
Systemic vascular resistance, 402t, 404
Systole, atrial, 165, *166,* 171, 191
  ventricular, 165, *166,* 171, 191
Systolic blood pressure, 177
Systolic hypertension, 372. See also *Hypertension.*
Systolic murmurs, 181

T

T cell(s), *429, 430,* 445t, *1432,* 1433t, 1433–1434
  CD4+. See *CD4+ cells.*
  cellular immunity and, 1433–1434, 1434t
  cytotoxic (killer), 1434, 1434t, 1439
  formation of, 1430, *1431*
  functions of, 1433–1434, 1434t
  helper, 1433, 1434t, 1439
  interaction of with B cells, 1434
  memory, 1434, 1434t
  suppressor, 1433–1434, 1434t, 1439
  types of, 1433–1434, 1434t
T wave, 193, *194*
T_3 (triiodothyronine). See *Triiodothyronine* (T_3).
T_3 resin uptake (T_3RU), 1299t, 1301t
T_4. See *Thyroxine* (T_4).
Tachycardia, 178
  in dehydration, 77, 78
  in elderly, 230
  paroxysmal atrial, *244,* 244–245
  sinus, 241–242, *242*
  ventricular, 248, *249,* 249–251
    in cardiac arrest, 261
Tachypnea, 532, *533*
Tactile fremitus, 535
Tactile sensation, age-related changes in, 61–63, 766
  alterations in, 743–744
  assessment of, 748
Tagamet (cimetidine), 1022d
  for peptic ulcers, 1024, 1028
Talk test, 284–285
Tamponade, balloon, for esophageal varices, 1186–1188, *1187,* 1191c–1192c, 1193

Tamponade *(Continued)*
  cardiac, 317
    in pericardial effusion, 239, 240
Tampons, toxic shock syndrome and, 1807–1808, 1808d
Tapazole (methimazole), for hyperthyroidism, 1309, 1309t
Tar preparations, 1579, 1583
  for psoriasis, 1579, 1618, 1619
Target lesion, 1573
Tarsal plate, 1935
Taste alterations, age-related, 61
  chemotherapy and, 1530
  in radiation therapy, 1521
T-bar, oxygen delivery via, 555t
Tea baths, for vaginitis, 1805–1806
Teaching. See *Patient teaching.*
Tears, 1935–1936
Technetium phosphate scanning, cardiac, 198
Teeth, care of. See *Oral care.*
  examination of, 968
Teflon injection, for urinary incontinence, 1367
Tegison (etretinate), 1581
Telangiectasia, 1571
Telemetry, 197
Telenursing services, 28–29
Telepaque tablets, for oral cholecystogram, 972
Telescopes, 1958
Temperature, skin, 1570
Temperature perception, alterations in, 743–744
Temporal lobe, 719, *719*
Temporomandibular joint syndrome, pain in, 1998
Tenckhoff catheter, for peritoneal dialysis, *1402*
Tendons, 842
Tenesmus, 1372
Tennis elbow, 902
Tenormin (atenolol), 214, 377t
Tenosynovitis, 902
TENS (transcutaneous electrical nerve stimulation), for rheumatoid arthritis, 892
Tensilon IV (edrophonium), in myasthenic vs. cholinergic crisis, 783
Tension headaches, 800. See also *Headache.*
Tension pneumothorax, 692–693, *693,* 694
Tentorium cerebelli, 714
Terazosin, for benign prostatic hyperplasia, 1753
Terbutaline, for asthma, 661, 662t
Terconazole, for vaginal candidiasis, 1884t, 1885
Terminal hair, 1569
Terminal illness. See *Death and dying.*
Testicular cancer, 1748–1752
  chemotherapy for, 1749
  classification of, 1749t
  clinical manifestations of, 1748
  cryptorchidism and, 1739
  diagnosis of, 1748–1749
  etiology of, 1748
  human chorionic gonadotropin in, 1704
  management of, 1749–1752
  orchiectomy for, 1708t, 1749, 1750–1752
  pathophysiology of, 1748
  radiation therapy for, 1749
  retroperitoneal lymph node dissection for, 1708t, 1749–1750, 1752
  staging of, 1749, 1749t
Testicular self-examination, *1703,* 1703d

Testicular torsion, 1739
Testis, age-related changes in, 1724
  inflammation of, 1731–1732
  structure and function of, 1207t, *1696,* 1696–1697
  undescended, 1696, 1739–1740
    orchiopexy for, 1739–1740, 1740d
Testosterone, 1207t
  endogenous, hair growth and, 1569
    measurement of, 1704
    secretion of, 1696–1697
  exogenous, for male climacteric syndrome, 1725
Tetanus immunization, 1447
  for burns, 1673
Tetany, after thyroidectomy, 1314
  hypocalcemic, 95–96, *96*
    after thyroidectomy, 1314
    in hypoparathyroidism, 1316
    nursing care guide for, 1319c
    nursing interventions for, 1318
    treatment of, 1317
  in metabolic alkalosis, 111, 1291
  in primary aldosteronism, 1291
  in respiratory alkalosis, 111
Tetracycline, for canker sores, 1018t
Tetrahydrocannabinol (THC), for chemotherapy-related nausea and vomiting, 1529
Thalamic lesion, hemianalgesia and, *743,* 743–744
Thalamus, 720
Thalassemia, 487–488
Thallium scanning, cardiac, 198
Theobromine, fibrocystic breast disease and, 1854
Theophylline (Slobid, Theodur), fibrocystic breast disease and, 1854
  for asthma, 661, 662t–663t
  for chronic obstructive pulmonary disease, 671, 673t
Thermal application, in musculoskeletal disorders, 850–853
  in rheumatoid arthritis, 892
Thermal injury. See also *Burns.*
  peripheral nerve, 828
Thermography, 852t
  breast, 1849
Thermotherapy, for benign prostatic hyperplasia, 1754
Thiamine deficiency, clinical manifestations of, 1077t
Thiazide diuretics, 377t. See also *Diuretics.*
  hepatic encephalopathy and, 1150
  hypercalcemia and, 97, 98
Thioamides, for hyperthyroidism, 1309, 1309t
Thiopental (Pentothal), for anesthesia, 141t
  for increased intracranial pressure, 732
Third-space fluid shift, 81t, 81–82
Thirst, in fluid volume deficit, 77
  increased, in diabetes insipidus, 1275
  in diabetes mellitus, 1228, 1229
Thoracentesis, 550–552, *551*
  diagnostic, 550–552
Thoracic aortic aneurysm, *367,* 370–371. See also *Aneurysm(s).*
Thoracic spine, *715.* See also under *Spinal; Spine.*
Thoracic surgery, 580–596
  complications of, 581
  incisions in, 580
  lobectomy, 587–588, 589c–596d

Thoracic surgery (Continued)
  nursing care guide for, 588d–596d,
    700c–707c
  patient preparation for, 580–581
  pneumonectomy as, 581–586, 700c–707c
  video-assisted, 587–596
Thoracic trauma, 690–695
  flail chest in, 691, 691–692
  hemothorax in, 694
  pneumothorax in, 692–693, 693, 694
  pulmonary contusion in, 695
  rib fractures in, 690–691
  subcutaneous emphysema in, 695
Thoracoscopic surgery, 587–596
Thoracostomy, incisions in, splinting of,
    582, 583
Thoracotomy, closed, 580t
  open, 580t
Thorax. See also Chest.
  lines of, 533
  structure and function of, 523–524, 525
Thorazine (chlorpromazine), hepatotoxicity
    of, 1178t, 1179
Three-point gait, 880–881
Throat, inflammation of, 604–606, 605
  sore, in peritonsillar abscess, 607–608
    in pharyngitis, 604–606, 605, 606d
    in tonsillitis, 606, 606, 606d
    postoperative, 149t
Throat culture, 604, 605, 605, 606
Thrombectomy, femoral vein, 386
Thrombin, 431, 432
  for coagulation disorders, 516d
Thromboangiitis obliterans, 351–354, 353d
  Raynaud's phenomenon and, 356
Thrombocytes. See Platelet(s).
Thrombocythemia, 446
Thrombocytopenia, 446–447
  in bone marrow transplant, 1450–1451
Thrombocytopenic purpura, 513–515
Thromboembolism. See also Thrombosis.
  arterial, 357–361
    in peripheral arterial aneurysm, 371,
      372
  embolectomy for, 346
  in gynecologic surgery, 1787
  postoperative, in hysterectomy, 1797,
    1799
  prevention of, in immobility, 845
Thromboendarterectomy, 365
Thrombolytic agents, 217, 218
  for myocardial infarction, 295, 296d, 297
  for pulmonary embolism, 682
  for venous thrombosis, 386
Thrombophlebitis. See Thrombosis.
Thromboplastin, 431, 432, 448
Thrombosis, 384–388. See also Thromboem-
    bolism.
  after prostatectomy, 1709t, 1712–1713
  assessment in, 386
  clinical manifestations of, 384
  deep, 384
  definition of, 357
  etiology of, 384
  in disseminated intravascular coagula-
    tion (DIC), 517–518
  in myocardial infarction, 293
  in peripheral arterial aneurysm, 371, 372
  management of, 385t, 385–386, 386t
  mesenteric, intestinal ischemia and, in
    elderly, 1106
  nursing diagnoses and planning in, 386–
    387
  nursing interventions in, 387–388, 388d

Thrombosis (Continued)
  pathophysiology of, 384
  postoperative, 131, 132, 146t, 151, 153–
    154
  prevention of, aspirin for, 432d
    postoperative, 131, 132, 151, 153–154
  risk factors for, 384, 384t
  superficial, 385
  venous, prevention of, 682
    pulmonary embolism and, 681
Thrombotic stroke, 804, 805. See also Cere-
    brovascular accident (CVA).
  case study of, 810d–812d
Thrombus, arterial, 357–361
  definition of, 357
  formation of, 384
  venous, 384–388
Thrush, 1017–1019, 1019t, 1602
  in HIV infection, 1465
Thymectomy, for myasthenia gravis, 784
  immunosuppression and, 1449
Thymic tumors, 698
Thymopoietin, 1207t
Thymus, structure and function of, 1204,
    1207t, 1430, 1430–1431
Thyroid, structure and function of, 1206t,
    1210–1212, 1211, 1212t
Thyroid adenoma, 1315
Thyroid cancer, 1315–1316
Thyroid crisis, 1308
Thyroid cysts, 1315
Thyroid disorders, 1295–1316. See also Hy-
    perthyroidism; Hypothyroidism.
  functional, 1296
  in elderly, 1323–1324
  infectious and inflammatory, 1295–1296
  Internet connections for, 1295d
Thyroid function, age-related changes in,
    68, 1323
Thyroid function tests, 1299t–1301t
  in hyperthyroidism, 1301t, 1308
  in hypothyroidism, 1298, 1301t
Thyroid hormone resistance, 1314
Thyroid hormones, 1206t, 1211, 1211–1212,
    1212t
  in hyperthyroidism, 1301t
  replacement, 1305t
    for elderly, 1323
    for hypothyroidism, 1298, 1305t
    patient teaching for, 1303c–1304c
Thyroid scan, 1300t
Thyroid storm, 1308
  postoperative, 1310
Thyroidectomy, parathyroid injury in,
    1314, 1316
  subtotal, case study of, 1311d
    postoperative care in, 1314
Thyroiditis, 1295–1296
  acute, 1296
  chronic (Hashimoto's), 1296
    hypothyroidism and, 1296, 1297
  De Quervain's, 1296
  silent (painless), 1296
  subacute granulomatous, 1296
Thyroid-stimulating hormone (TSH), 1209–
    1210, 1211, 1211–1212
  assays of, 1299t, 1301t
  in hyperthyroidism, 1301t
  in hypothyroidism, 1298, 1301t
Thyroid-stimulating immunoglobulins,
    1307
Thyrolar (liotrix), for hypothyroidism,
    1298, 1305t
Thyrotoxicosis, 1308

Thyrotropin, 1205t, 1209–1210, 1211, 1211–
    1212
Thyrotropin-releasing hormone (TRH),
    1205t, 1209t, 1211, 1211–1212
Thyrotropin-releasing hormone stimulation
    test, 1299t, 1301t
Thyroxine (T$_4$), 1206t, 1211, 1211–1212,
    1212t
  in hyperthyroidism, 1301t, 1306, 1307,
    1308
  in hypothyroidism, 1297, 1301t
  serum, 1299t, 1301t
Thyroxine-binding globulin, 1299t, 1301t
Tic douloureux, 829t–830t
Tick bites, encephalitis and, 769
  Lyme disease and, 901
Tidal volume, 537, 538, 539t
Tilting-disc valve, 312, 312
Timolol, 377t
  for glaucoma, 1979
Tinea, griseofulvin for, 1581
Tinea capitis, 1600t, 1600–1601
Tinea corporis, 1600t, 1600–1601
Tinea cruris, 1600t, 1600–1601, 1601
Tinea manuum, 1600t, 1600–1601
Tinea pedis, 1600t, 1600–1601, 1601
Tinea unguium, 1600t, 1600–1601
Tinea versicolor, 1603
Tinel's sign, 828
Tinnitus, 743, 1998
  assessment of, 2000
  in Meniere's disease, 2017–2019
Tissue expander, in breast reconstruction,
    1876
Tissue extravasation, in chemotherapy,
    1531
Tissue perfusion, in diabetes, 1259
Tissue plasminogen activator (TPA), 217,
    218
  for myocardial infarction, 295, 296d, 297
  for pulmonary embolism, 682
TNM staging system, 1513
Tobacco. See also Smoking.
  as carcinogen, 1509
  smokeless, oral cancer and, 1049
Tocainide (Tonocard), for dysrhythmias,
    215, 216d
Toenail. See Nail(s).
Tofranil (imipramine), for retrograde ejac-
    ulation, 1699
Tolazamide (Tolinase), 1239, 1239t, 1240d
Tolbutamide (Orinase), 1239, 1239t, 1240d
Tomography. See also Computed tomogra-
    phy.
  chest, 548
  in cancer diagnosis, 1514
Tongs, cervical, 824, 861, 861
Tongue, cancer of, 1049–1053. See also
    Oral cancer.
  examination of, 968
  in pernicious anemia, 1025, 1025
Tonocard (tocainide), for dysrhythmias,
    215, 216d
Tonometry, 1944–1945, 1945, 1979
Tonsil(s), examination of, 968
  immunologic functions of, 1432
Tonsillectomy, 607–608, 608d
Tonsillitis, 606, 606, 606d
  tonsillectomy for, 607–608
Tophi, 899, 899
Topical anesthesia, 137, 138t. See also An-
    esthesia.
Topical drugs, 1579–1581
  active ingredients in, 1579–1581

Topical drugs (Continued)
  occlusive dressings for, 1583
  vehicles for, 1579, 1580t
Topiramate (Topimax), for seizures, 796,
  797d–798d
Toradol (ketorolac), 893d
Toric lenses, 1970
Torticollis, 740
Total body surface area nomogram, 1525,
  1526
Total cholesterol, in hepatic disorders,
  1162t, 1164
Total eye rest, 1984
Total incontinence, 1336, 1340t, 1340–1341
Total iron-binding capacity, 443t, 450
Total joint replacement, 867–868, 868,
  869c–872c
Total laryngectomy. See Laryngectomy, total.
Total lung capacity, 539t
Total parenteral nutrition (TPN). See also
  Nutrition.
  assessment in, 988
  at home, 990, 990–993, 991d–993d
  catheter care in, 989, 990
  catheter infection in, 987
    prevention of, 989
  catheter insertion in, complications of,
    987
    technique for, 987
  complications of, 987–988
  dressing care in, 989
  hyperosmolar nonketotic syndrome in,
    992d–993d
  in unconscious client, 729
  infusion rate in, 989
  lipid administration in, 990
  nursing diagnoses and planning in, 988
  nursing interventions in, 988–989
  patient preparation for, 988–989
  procedure for, 987
  solutions for, 986–987
Total pelvic exenteration, 1786t
Total serum bilirubin, 1161t, 1163
Total serum protein, in hepatic disorders,
  1161t, 1163–1164
Total transfrontal hypophysectomy, for pituitary adenoma, 1267
Total transsphenoidal hypophysectomy,
  for pituitary adenoma, 1266, 1266–
  1269
  in Cushing's disease, 1287
Touch, age-related changes in, 61–63, 766
  alterations in, 743–744
  assessment of, 748
Toxic cirrhosis, 1181, 1181t. See also Cir-
  rhosis.
Toxic epidermal necrolysis, 1612
Toxic hepatitis, 1177t, 1177–1179, 1178t
  in elderly, 1198
Toxic nodular goiter, 1315
  in elderly, 1323
Toxic shock syndrome, 1807–1808, 1808d
Toxins, cancer and, 1508–1509
  reference values for, 2029–2030
T-piece, in ventilator weaning, 569
Trabeculoplasty, argon laser, for glaucoma,
  1980
Trachea, 525, 525
Tracheobronchial tree, 525, 526
Tracheoesophageal puncture, 618–626, 628
Tracheostomy, 564, 564–567, 565
  airway management in, 566–567, 624d–
  625d. See also Airway management.

Tracheostomy (Continued)
  airway obstruction in, 624d–625d, 629–
    630
  aspiration in, 618d–619d, 629–630
    pneumonia and, 647
  communication and, 567
  complications of, 565, 565
    in supraglottic laryngectomy, 620c–622c
  incision in, 564
  nursing process in, 566–567
  nutrition in, 563d
  permanent, 618, 618
    speech and, 620–626, 626–628
  procedure for, 565
  suctioning in, 566–567, 629–630
  tube in. See Tracheostomy tube.
  uses of, 564
  wound care in, 567
Tracheostomy care, 566–567, 629–630
  patient teaching for, 630, 631d
Tracheostomy collar, oxygen delivery via,
  555t
Tracheostomy tube, 564, 564–565
  changing of, 567
  removal of, 567
  suctioning of, 566–567, 629–630
Trachoma, 1920
Traction, 858–863
  application of, 861–862
  assessment in, 862
  in elderly, 885
    for hip fractures, 924–925
  manual, 859
  nursing diagnoses and planning in, 862
  nursing interventions in, 862–863
  principles of, 859
  purposes of, 858–859
  skeletal, 824, 826, 860–861, 861
  skin, 859–860, 860
  spinal, 824, 826, 861, 861
  straight, 859
  types of, 859t, 859–860, 860, 861
  vectored, 859
TRAM flap, in breast reconstruction, 1876–
  1879, 1877, 1879d
Trandate (labetalol), 378t
Transcultural issues, in communication,
  1231d
  in diet, 1230d
Transcultural nursing. See Cultural issues;
  Racial/ethnic groups.
Transcutaneous electrical nerve stimulation
  (TENS), 1556, 1556
  for rheumatoid arthritis, 892
Transdermal opioids, 1554t
Transesophageal echocardiography, 198
Transfrontal hypophysectomy, for pituitary adenoma, 1267
  in Cushing's disease, 1287
Transfusion(s), 452–463
  administration of, 458
  albumin, 456
  autologous, 453
    in hemolytic shock, 410
    nursing care guide for, 454c–455c
  blood sources for, 453
  clotting factor, 456–457
  cryoprecipitate, 456–457
  donors for, 453
  fresh frozen plasma, 455–456
  frozen red cell, 453
  granulocyte, 456
  HIV transmission via, 1464
  hyperkalemia and, 89, 90

Transfusion(s) (Continued)
  immune serum globulin, 457
  in aplastic anemia, 480
  in hemorrhagic anemia, 471
  in hereditary spherocytosis, 482
  in hypovolemic shock, 410
  in thalassemia, 487
  nursing care in, intratransfusion, 458
    posttransfusion, 458–462
    pretransfusion, 457–458
  packed red cell, 453
  plasma substitutes for, 456d
  platelet, 453–455
  prothrombin complex, 456
  whole blood, 453
Transfusion reaction, 458, 459c–461c, 461–
  462, 483, 488–489, 1486
  acute hemolytic, 461, 488–489
    case study of, 483
  anaphylactic, 462
  cytotoxic hypersensitivity in, 1486
  delayed, 462, 462d
  febrile nonhemolytic, 462
  management of, 462
  mild, 462
  nursing interventions in, 459c–461c, 462
  septic, 462
  types of, 462
Transient ischemic attack (TIA), 806t
  Alzheimer's disease and, 790, 791d, 792
Transillumination, of scrotum, 1701
Transitional cell carcinoma, of bladder,
  1419–1424. See also Bladder, cancer of.
  of renal pelvis and ureter, 1418–1419
Transjugular intrahepatic portosystemic
  shunt, for esophageal varices, 1188,
  1189
Translators, 666d–667d
Transperineal core needle biopsy, of prostate, 1705–1706, 1706, 1707t
Transplantation, bone marrow, 464, 1449–
  1455. See also Bone marrow transplantation.
  for aplastic anemia, 480
  cardiac, 227–229, 228
  corneal, 1954–1955, 1955d
  donors for, 1408
  graft rejection in, 1489
  hepatic, 1196–1198
  immunosuppression in, 1409–1410
    cyclosporine for, 1197d
  organ donation for, 46
  pancreatic, for diabetes, 1239–1240
  rejection in, 1409, 1409t
  renal, 1408, 1408–1411, 1409t, 1410d
Transrectal core needle biopsy, of prostate,
  1705–1706, 1706, 1707t
Transrectal fine-needle aspiration biopsy,
  of prostate, 1705–1706, 1706, 1707t
Transsphenoidal hypophysectomy, for pituitary adenoma, in Cushing's disease,
  1287
Transsphenoidal microsurgery, for pituitary adenoma, 1266, 1266–1269,
  1270c–1272c
  in Cushing's disease, 1287
Transtracheal oxygen therapy, 557, 557–
  559, 558d
Transurethral incision of prostate, 1710
Transurethral resection, for bladder cancer,
  1420
Transurethral resection of prostate, 1710,
  1710–1711, 1714t–1715t. See also Prostatectomy.

Transurethral resection of prostate
   (*Continued*)
   clinical pathway for, 1755d
   for benign hyperplasia, 1753
Transurethral resection syndrome, 1713
Transurethral Teflon injection, for urinary
   incontinence, 1367
Transvenous embolectomy, for pulmonary
   embolism, 682–683
Transverse rectus abdominis muscle flap,
   in breast reconstruction, 1876–1879,
   1877, 1879d
Transvesical prostatectomy, 1710, *1710*,
   1711, 1714t–1715t. See also *Prostatectomy.*
Trauma, bladder, 1413–1414, 1415–1416
   cardiac, 316–317
   laryngeal, 612–616
   renal, 1411–1412, 1415–1416
   thoracic, 690–695
   ureteral, 1412–1413, 1415–1416
   urethral, 1414–1416
   urinary tract, 1411–1416
Traumatic amputation, 930–932
Treadmill test, 195–197
   Doppler, in arterial insufficiency, 339t
Treatment, noncompliance in, in asymptomatic disorders, 375–376
   withdrawal/witholding of, 41, 42b
      advance directives for, 42–43, *43*, *44*
      Do Not Resuscitate (DNR) orders and,
      43–46, *45*
Treatment decisions, family involvement
   in, 1919d
Tremors, 740
   hepatic, 1150
   in Parkinson's disease, 787, *787*
Trench mouth, 1017–1019, 1018t
Trendelenburg position, 135, *136*
Treponema pallidum, 1914
Tretinoin (Retin-A), 1581–1582, 1615t
Triamcinolone, for eczema, 1608
Triamterene (Dyrenium), 377t
Trichlormethiazide (Metahydrin), 377t
Trichloroacetic acid, for genital warts, 1027
Trichomoniasis, 1804–1806, 1805t, 1884t,
   1885–1886, *1886*
   nursing care in, 1886–1889
   patient teaching in, 1901d
Tricuspid valve, *164*, 167, *167*, *168*, 171
Trigeminal nerve, 723t
Trigeminal neuralgia, 829t–830t
Trigger voiding, 1366
Triiodothyronine (T$_3$), 1206t, *1211*, 1211–
   1212, 1212t
   in hyperthyroidism, 1301t, 1306, 1307,
      1308
   in hypothyroidism, 1297, 1301t
   serum, assays of, 1299t, 1301t
Trimethadione, for seizures, 796, 797d–
   798d
Trimethaphan (Arfonad), 380t
Trochlear nerve, 723t
Troponin, in myocardial infarction, 294
Trousseau's sign, in hypocalcemia, 96, *96*
   in metabolic alkalosis, 111
   in respiratory alkalosis, 111
Truss, 1094
Trypsin, 956, 957, 958t
   in acute pancreatitis, 1118
T-tube drainage, in cholecystectomy, 1114,
   1114, 1116, 1117
   discharge instructions for, 1117d
   in liver transplant, 1197

Tubal ligation, 1793
Tube(s). See also *Intubation.*
   chest. See *Chest tube drainage.*
   endotracheal, 559–560, *560, 561, 564.* See
      also *Endotracheal intubation.*
   feeding, 981–984, *983*
   gastrointestinal, 976–978, *977.* See also
      Gastrointestinal intubation.
   typanostomy, 2005–2006, *2006*
Tube feeding, 980–986. See also *Enteral nutrition.*
Tube prosthesis, in esophageal cancer,
   1055, 1058
Tuberculin skin test, 652
Tuberculosis, 650–657
   assessment in, 655
   cavitation in, 650, *650*
   chest film in, 652
   clinical manifestations of, 651–652
   diagnosis of, 652
   drug therapy for, 653t–655t, 653–655
      compliance with, 656d, 657
   etiology of, 650–651
   Ghon's complex in, 650
   in elderly, 707
   incidence of, 650
   Internet connections for, 665d
   isolation in, 652
   latent, 650
      chemoprophylaxis for, 654–655, 655t
   management of, 652–655, 654t–655t
      settings and providers for, 655
   Mantoux test for, 652
   miliary, 650
   multi-drug–resistant, 650
   nursing diagnoses and planning in, 655–
      656
   nursing interventions in, 656–657
   of bone, 889–890
   pathophysiology of, 650–651
   pleural needle biopsy in, 652
   PPD test for, 1489
   prevention of, 653–655, 655t, 657d
      in health care providers, 652–653
      in home-care setting, 656d
   primary, 651
   risk factors for, 650, 650t
   secondary, 651
   sputum culture in, 652
      specimen collection for, 657
   tests for, 652
Tuberculosis Stat Test, 652
Tuberculous osteomyelitis, 889–890
Tubocurarine (Tubarine), 141t
Tumor(s), *1571, 1572.* See also *Cancer* and
   specific sites and types.
   ACTH-secreting, Cushing's syndrome
      and, 1285, 1286, 1287
   benign, 1505, *1505*
   bone, benign, 935–938, 936t
      malignant, 936t, 938–943
   brain, 828–832, 831t
   cardiac, 318
   malignant, 1505, *1505.* See also *Cancer.*
   ocular, 1991
   pituitary, 1265–1269, *1266, 1267*
Tumor debulking surgery, 1516
Tumor doubling time in, 1505–1506
Tumor markers, 1513
   in prostate cancer, 1757
Tunica adventitia, 323, *325*
Tunica intima, 323, *325*
Tunica media, 323, *325*
Tuning fork tests, 2001

Turgor, in dehydration, 78
   skin, 1570
Turner's sign, in acute pancreatitis, 1118
Turning, postoperative, 131
Twenty-four-hour urine collection, 1345,
   1345t
Two-point gait, 880
Tylectomy, *1861,* 1868–1874, 1869d–1874d
Tylenol (acetaminophen), 893d, 1553, 1554t
   hepatotoxicity of, 1178t
Tympanic cavity, 1995–1996, *1996*
Tympanic membrane, 1995, *1996,* 1997
   examination of, 2000–2001, *2001*
   in serous otitis media, *265, 266, 2014*
   perforation of, 2014–2015, *2015*
Tympanoplasty, 2003–2005, *2004*
Tympany, abdominal, 968
   on percussion, 536
Tyndall phenomenon, 1571
Typanostomy tubes, 2005–2006, *2006*
Type A personality, heart disease and, 187,
   188, 303

U

U wave, 193, *194*
Ulcer(s), *1571, 1573*
   aphthous, 1017–1019, 1018t
   arterial, 334t, 335
      pain in, 333–334
   corneal, 1965–1967
      fluorescein staining of, 1945
   Curling's, 1033, 1679
      bleeding from, 966d
      in burns, 1679
      postoperative, 148t
   Cushing's, 1033
   esophageal, drug-induced, 1047t
   gastric. See *Peptic ulcers; Ulcer(s), stress.*
   genital, in syphilis, 1915, *1915*
   in hematologic disorders, 437
   leg, in sickle-cell anemia, 437, 484, 487,
      487d
   oral, chemotherapy and, 1529, 1541t
   peptic, 1025–1033. See also *Peptic ulcers.*
   pressure, 1622–1631. See also *Pressure
      ulcers.*
   stress, 1033
      bleeding from, 966d
      postoperative, 148t
   venous stasis, 332, 333–334, 334t, 335,
      390–395
      in homeless persons, 394–395
      pain in, 332, 333–334
      venous thrombosis and, 386
Ulcerative colitis, *1066,* 1069–1071, *1070*
   ileostomy for, 1011–1015, 1071, *1071.* See
      also *Ileostomy.*
   in elderly, 1106
   Internet connections for, 1068d
   vs. Crohn's disease, 1072t
Ultrafast computed tomography, cardiac,
   199–200
Ultrasonography, breast, 1849
   Doppler, carotid, 749–750, *751*
      in arterial insufficiency, 339t
      in distal pulse recording, 335, *337,* 339
      in venous insufficiency, 340t
   gastrointestinal, 975–976
   hepatic, 1163t
   in cancer diagnosis, 1514
   in hematologic disorders, 451–452
   in male reproductive disorders, 1705
   ocular, 1945–1946, 1960
   pelvic, 1785

Ultrasonography (Continued)
in women, 1785
preoperative, 126t
urinary tract, 1349t
vaginal, 1785
Ultraviolet light plus psoralen (PUVA therapy), 1582, 1584, 1618, 1619
Ultraviolet radiation, for skin disorders, 1582, 1584
Umbilical hernia, 1093–1096, 1094
Unconsciousness, 726t, 726–730, 727t. See also Coma.
assessment in, 727, 727t
clinical characteristics of, 726t, 726–727
diagnosis of, 727
etiology of, 726
Glasgow Coma Scale for, 727, 727t
in heart disease, 184
management of, 727
nursing diagnoses and planning in, 727–728
nursing interventions in, 728–730
pathophysiology of, 726–727
terminology for, 726t, 726–727
Unconventional therapies, for cancer, 1544–1545
Unified Parkinson Disease Rating Scale, 787
Unilateral neglect, 813
United Ostomy Association, 1010, 1011
Universal pacemaker code, 256
Unlicensed assistive personnel, supervisor of, 26
Unna's boot, 390–392
for skin grafts, 1676d
Upper extremity prostheses, 882, 882, 883
Upper gastrointestinal endoscopy, 973, 973–974, 974, 975d
Upper gastrointestinal series, 970, 970–971
Upper midline incision, 994t
Upper motor neuron disease, 739, 740t
Upper motor neurons, 722
Upper paramedian (rectus) incision, 994t
Upper respiratory tract, structure and function of, 523, 524
Upper respiratory tract disorders, 599–637. See also Respiratory disorder(s).
in elderly, 637
infectious and inflammatory, 599–610
neoplastic, 616–637
structural, 610–612
traumatic, 612–616
Upper transverse incision, 995t
Urban areas, health care access in, 1462d
Urea, production of, 1137
Ureaplasma urealyticum, nongonococcal urethritis and, 1924–1925
Uremia, 1389
definition of, 1388t
in diabetes, 1254–1255
Ureter, cancer of, 1418–1419
dilation of, in urinary obstruction, 1377–1378, 1378
structure and function of, 1330, 1333–1334
traumatic injuries of, 1412–1413, 1415–1416
Ureteral calculi. See Urinary calculi.
Ureteral catheterization. See Urinary catheterization.
Ureteral dilatation, in benign prostatic hyperplasia, 1752–1753
Ureteral pain, 1341–1342
Ureteral stricture, 1383–1384
Uretero-ovarian ligaments, 1768
Ureteropelvic junction obstruction, 1380

Ureterosacral ligaments, 1767, 1767
Ureterosigmoidoscopy, 1421, 1421
Ureterostomy, 1421, 1421, 1423–1424
cutaneous, 1421, 1421
Ureterovaginal fistula, 1821, 1821–1822
Ureterovesical junction obstruction, 1380–1382
Urethra, balloon dilatation of, for benign prostatic hyperplasia, 1753
cancer of, 1424–1425
dilation of, 1386
structure and function of, 1334, 1335, 1696, 1697
traumatic injuries of, 1414–1416
Urethral catheterization. See Urinary catheterization.
Urethral discharge, in chlamydial infection, 1921, 1922
in gonorrhea, 1908, 1908
in nongonococcal urethritis, 1925
sequential bacteriologic localization cultures of, 1704–1705
Urethral obstruction, in benign prostatic hyperplasia, 1752–1753
Urethral pressure profile (UPP), 1360t
Urethral prolapse, 1815–1819, 1816
in elderly, 1368
Urethral sounds, 1386
Urethral stenosis, distal, 1386–1388
Urethral stents, for benign prostatic hyperplasia, 1754
Urethral stricture, 1385–1388
Urethritis, 1373–1374
gonococcal, 1908, 1908–1909. See also Gonorrhea.
nongonococcal, 1924–1925
chlamydial, 1920, 1921, 1924–1925. See also Chlamydia trachomatis infection.
postgonococcal, 1925
Urethrocele, 1815–1819, 1816
Urethrocystoscopy, 1705
Urethroplasty, 1386
nursing care in, 1387–1388
Urethrotomy, internal, 1386
nursing care in, 1387–1388
Urethrovaginal fistula, 1821, 1821–1822
Urge incontinence, 1338, 1340t, 1340–1341
Urgent care centers, 20
Urgent care settings, 21–22
Urgent surgery, 118
Uric acid calculi. See Urinary calculi.
Uric acid crystals, in gout, 899, 899
Uricosuric drugs, 900d
Urinalysis, 1344, 1344t
in musculoskeletal disorders, 851t
preoperative, 125t
Urinary calculi, 1378–1380
diet and, 1366–1367, 1367d, 1383d
hematuria and, 1342–1343
in hyperparathyroidism, 1320, 1321, 1322
nursing care guide for, 1381c–1382c
Urinary catecholamines, assays of, 1292, 1293t
Urinary catheterization, 1361–1363
after hysterectomy, 1795
catheters for, 1361
for meatal stenosis, 1386
indwelling catheter in, 1361–1362, 1362t, 1363
intermittent self-catheterization in, 1363, 1364t
postoperative, 154–155
in hysterectomy, 1795, 1798

Urinary catheretization (Continued)
in prostatectomy, 1712, 1714t, 1718, 1719
preoperative, 124
suprapubic catheter in, 1362–1363
Urinary diversion, in radical cystectomy, 1421, 1421
Urinary drain bags, 1362, 1363
Urinary flow rate, assessment of, 1359t
Urinary frequency, 1335
night-time, 1335
Urinary function, age-related changes in, 66
assessment of, in elderly, 66
Urinary hesitancy, 1336
Urinary incontinence, 1336–1341
absorbent products for, 1339d
after prostatectomy, 1709t, 1712, 1715t, 1758, 1760, 1760d
artificial urinary sphincter for, 1367, 1367, 1758, 1758
assessment in, 1340
catheterization for, 1361–1363, 1362d
Cunningham clamp for, 1760, 1760d
functional, 1339, 1340t
health history in, 1343
in elderly, 66, 1368, 1425
in menopause, 1771
in multiple sclerosis, 780, 781
in unconscious client, 729
Kegel exercises for, 1779d
nursing diagnoses and planning in, 1340
nursing interventions in, 1340–1341
periurethral blocking agents for, 1758
reflex, 1336, 1340t
stress, 1339, 1340t
cystocele/urethrocele and, 1817
total, 1336, 1340t
transurethral Teflon injection for, 1367
urge, 1338, 1340t
Urinary retention, 1336, 1337d–1338d
catheterization for, 1361–1363, 1362d
in autonomic dysreflexia, 823, 825, 826
in benign prostatic hyperplasia, 1753, 1754
in elderly, 1368
in males, 1699–1700
postoperative, 148t, 154–155, 996
in hysterectomy, 1795
in prostatectomy, 1718
in radical vulvectomy, 1829
in spinal surgery, 764
with penile implant, 1723–1724
Urinary sphincter, artificial, 1367, 1367, 1758, 1758
Urinary system, function of, 1331
Urinary tract disorders, assessment in, 1343–1344
catheterization in, 1361–1363, 1362d
clinical manifestations of, 1335–1343
diagnosis of, 1344–1361
bladder biopsy in, 1354–1357
blood studies in, 1345–1346, 1346t
cystoscopy in, 1352–1353, 1354c–1356c
radiologic studies in, 1346–1351, 1347t–1350t
renal biopsy in, 1357–1358
urine studies in, 1344t, 1344–1345, 1345t
urodynamic testing in, 1358–1361, 1359t–1360t
diet in, 1366d, 1366–1367, 1367d
drug therapy for, 1363–1365

Urinary tract disorders *(Continued)*
dysfunctional voiding in, 1335–1336
health history in, 1343–1344
hematuria in, 1342–1343
in elderly, 1368, 1425
incontinence in, 1336–1341
infectious and inflammatory, 1371–1377.
See also *Urinary tract infection (UTI).*
management of, nonsurgical, 1361–1367
settings and providers for, 1367–1368
surgical, 1367
neoplastic, 1416–1425
obstructive. See *Urinary tract obstruction.*
pain in, 1341–1342
physical examination in, 1344
resources for, 2041
risk reduction for, 1343d
self-care in, 1365–1366
traumatic, 1411–1416
urine color in, 1342, 1342t
urine odor in, 1342, 1342t
urine volume change in, 1343
Urinary tract infection (UTI), after prostatectomy, 1709t, 1712
catheterization and, 1362
cystitis in, 1371–1373
hematuria in, 1342–1343
in unconscious client, 729
postoperative, 148t
prevention of, 1372d, 1373
pyelonephritis in, 1374–1375
urethritis in, 1373–1374
urine culture in, 1344–1345
Urinary tract obstruction, 1377–1388,
1380–1385
at ureteropelvic junction, 1380
at ureterovesical junction, 1380–1382
causes of, 1377
hydronephrosis and, 1378, *1378*
hydroureter and, 1378, *1378*
lower tract, 1385–1388
care settings and providers for, 1386–
1387
meatal stenosis and, 1386–1388
postoperative care in, 1387–1388
preoperative care in, 1387
urethral strictures and, 1385–1388
management of, settings and providers
for, 1384
pathophysiology of, 1377–1378
postobstructive diuresis in, 1378
upper tract
care settings and providers for, 1384
postoperative care in, 1384–1385
preoperative care in, 1384
ureteral stricture and, 1383–1384
Urinary urgency, 1335
Urinary urobilinogen, 451
Urination. See *Voiding.*
Urine, blood in, 1342–1343. See also *Hema-*
turia
color of, changes in, 1342, 1342t
drain bags for, 1362, 1363
formation of, 1331–1332, *1332*
odor of, 1342, 1342t
reference values for, 2028–2029
storage of, 1334
Urine bilirubin, 1161t, 1163
Urine culture, 1344–1345
in cystitis, 1372
sequential bacteriologic localization,
1704–1705
Urine cytology, 1345
Urine magnesium tolerance test, 100

Urine output, in burns, 1669–1670
in dehydration, 78
in shock, 406, 407t
Urine sample, for urinalysis, 1344
for urine cytology, 1345
midstream, 1344
24-hour, 1345, 1345t
Urine tests, for glucose, in diabetes, 1242–
1243
for ketones, in diabetes, 1243, 1245c
Urine urobilinogen, 1161t, 1164
Urine volume, change in, 1343
Urobilinogen, 1138, *1138*
fecal, 1161t, 1164
urine, 1161t, 1164
Urobilinogen test, 443t, 451
Urodynamic testing, 1358–1361, 1359t–
1360t
Urogenital diaphragm, 1415
Urokinase, for myocardial infarction, 295,
296d
for pulmonary embolism, 682
Urolithiasis. See *Urinary calculi.*
Urologic disorders. See *Urinary tract disor-*
ders.
Urostomy, 1421, *1421*, 1423–1424
Urticaria, drug-related, 1612
Uterine bleeding, abnormal, 1775–1776
history in, 1778
in cervical cancer, 1830
in uterine cancer, 1836
Uterine cancer, 1836–1837
in elderly, 1838
Uterine fibromas, 1823–1824, *1824*
Uterine ligaments, 1766–1767, *1767*
Uterine myomas, 1823–1824, *1824*
Uterine prolapse, 1815–1819, *1816*
in elderly, 1368
vaginal packing for, 1800
Uterus, anteflexion of, 1819, *1820*
retrodisplacement of, 1819–1821, *1820,*
1821
structure and function of, *1766,* 1766–
1767, *1767*
Utricle, 1996
Uveal tract, *1936, 1937*

V

Vaccines, 1447. See also *Immunization.*
Vagina, structure and function of, *1766,*
1766, 1767
Vaginal atrophy, 1838
Vaginal bleeding, postoperative, in hysterectomy, 1795
Vaginal candidiasis. See *Vaginitis, candidal.*
Vaginal discharge, 1776
in atrophic vaginitis, 1806
in cervical cancer, 1830
in chlamydia, 1921, 1922
in gonorrhea, 1909
in trichomoniasis, 1885, *1886*
in vaginal candidiasis, 1885
in vaginitis, 1776, 1804–1805, 1805t
Vaginal dryness, in menopause, 1771
Vaginal fluid, constituents of, 1883–1884
organisms in, 1883–1884
Vaginal hygiene, patient teaching for,
1807d
Vaginal packing, 1800
Vaginal pH, maintenance of, 1884
Vaginal prolapse, 1815–1819, *1816*
in elderly, 1368
Vaginal ultrasonography, 1785

Vaginal warts, 1063–1065, 1064t, *1926,*
1926–1928
Vaginal-intestinal fistula, 1821–1822, *1822*
Vaginal-urinary fistula, *1821,* 1821–1822
Vaginectomy, 1786t
Vaginitis, 1804–1806, 1807d
atrophic, 1806–1807
candidal, 1804–1806, 1805t, 1884t, 1884–
1885
in HIV infection, 1467
nursing care in, 1886–1889
patient teaching in, 1901d
discharge in, 1776
Gardnerella vaginalis, 1884t, 1886–1889,
1901d
nonspecific, 1886
nursing care in, 1886–1889
sexually transmitted, 1883–1889
nursing care in, 1886–1889
patient teaching in, 1901d
trichomonad, 1884t, 1885–1889, *1886,*
1901d
Vagotomy, for peptic ulcers, 1028, *1028*
Vagus nerve, 723t
Valium (diazepam), hepatotoxicity of,
1178t
Valsalva maneuver, for paroxysmal atrial
tachycardia, 245
for serous otitis media, 2014d
in heart failure, 278
Valsalva voiding, 1365
Valve(s), cardiac, prosthetic, 312–313, *312–*
314
venous, in chronic venous insufficiency,
389, *389*
Valve replacement surgery, 234, 311–317.
See also *Cardiac valvular disease, sur-*
gery in.
Valvular disease. See *Cardiac valvular dis-*
ease.
Valvuloplasty, *310,* 310–311. See also *Car-*
diac valvular disease, surgery in.
Vanillylmandelic acid, hypersecretion of,
from pheochromocytoma, 1292
urinary assays of, 1293t
Varicella-zoster virus, 1606
herpes zoster and, 1606–1607
Varices, esophageal. See *Esophageal varices.*
Varicocele, *1743,* 1743–1744
Varicocelectomy, 1744
Varicose veins, 386, 389–390, 391c–392c
esophageal. See *Esophageal varices.*
venous thrombosis and, 386, 389
Vas deferens, ligation of, 1708t, 1708–1709,
1710, 1710d
structure and function of, *1696,* 1697
Vascular access, in hemodialysis, 1405,
1405, 1406
Vascular complications, in diabetes mellitus, 1252d, 1252–1255
Vascular disorder(s). See also *Peripheral*
vascular disease; Venous insufficiency.
aneurysms as, 365–372
arterial, 351–372
arterial thromboembolism as, 357–361
assessment in, 337–339
atherosclerosis as, 361–364
chronic arterial occlusive disease as,
363–365
clinical manifestations of, 331–337
diagnosis in, 339t, 339–340, 340t, 341c,
342t
drug therapy for, 343, 343d, 344d
foot care in, 355, 355d

Vascular disorder(s) *(Continued)*
  health history in, 337
  hypertensive, 372–384, 373–374, *374.* See also *Hypertension.*
  in elderly, 397–398
  Internet connections for, 361d
  lymphatic, 395–398
  management of, 342–348
    nonsurgical, 342–344
    surgical, 344–348
  obstructive, 354–365
  pain in, 331–334
  physical examination in, 337–338, 338t
  Raynaud's disease as, 355–357
  relaxation exercises in, 354d
  risk factors in, 337, 338t
    reduction of, 338d, 342–343
  skin care in, 355
  skin changes in, 334t, 334–337
  thromboangiitis obliterans as, 351–354
  venous, 384–395
Vascular headaches, 800–802
Vascular purpuras, 513–515
Vascular surgery, arterial bypass grafts in, 344–346, 364–365, *365, 366*
    postoperative care in, 347–348
    preoperative care in, 346–347
Vascular system, anatomy of, 323–328, *324–328*
Vasectomy, 1708t, 1708–1709, *1710,* 1710d
Vasoconstriction, in heart failure, 270
Vasoconstrictors, endogenous, 329, 329t
Vasodilators, 212d, 212–213
  endogenous, 329, 329t
  exogenous, for cardiogenic shock, 413
    for heart failure, 275
    for peripheral vascular disease, 345t
    intracavernosal injection of, priapism and, 1740–1741
Vasomotor rhinitis, 601
Vasopressin, endogenous. See *Antidiuretic hormone (ADH).*
Vasopressin (Pitressin), for bleeding esophageal varices, 1183
  for diabetes insipidus, 1275, 1276d
Vasopressin stimulation test, for diabetes insipidus, 1275
Vasospastic disorders, 355–357, 356d
Vasotec (enalapril), 213, 214d
VDRL test, 1916–1917
Vegetarian diet, vitamin B$_{12}$ deficiency and, 478
Vegetations, 234
Veins, 325–328, *327, 328*
  diameter of, blood flow and, 328
  elastic recoil of, blood flow and, 328
  structure and function of, 324, *324, 327*
  valves of, 328, *328*
  varicose, 386, 389–390, 391c–392c
    venous thrombosis and, 386, 389
Vellus hair, 1569
Vena cava filter, 386
  for pulmonary embolism, 683
Venereal disease. See *Sexually transmitted disease(s) (STDs).*
Venereal Disease Research Laboratory (VDRL) test, 1916–1917
Venereal warts, 1063–1065, 1064t, 1603–1605, 1604t, *1926,* 1926–1928
Venipuncture, 442
Venography, in venous insufficiency, 340t
  nursing care in, 342t
  radionuclide, in venous insufficiency, 340t

Venous blood specimen, 442, 545
Venous disorder(s), 384–395. See also *Peripheral vascular disease.*
  assessment in, 337–339
  chronic, 388–394
    venous thrombosis and, 386
  chronic venous insufficiency, 389–395
  diagnosis in, 339–340, 340t, 341c, 342t
  in thromboangiitis obliterans, 351–354
  management of, nonsurgical, 342–344
    surgical, 344–348
  pain in, 332–334
  skin changes in, 334t, 334–337
  thrombophlebitis as, 384–388
  varicose veins as, 386, 389–390, 391c–392c
  venous stasis ulcers as, 332, 333–334, 334t, 335, 386, 390–395
Venous insufficiency, 332. See also *Peripheral vascular disease.*
  chronic, 388–394
    varicose veins and, 386, 389–390, 391c–392c
    venous stasis ulcers and, 332, 333–334, 335, 390–395
Venous sinuses, cerebral, 716
Venous stasis ulcers, 332, 333–334, 335, 390–395
  in homeless persons, 394–395
  pain in, 332, 333–334
  venous thrombosis and, 386
Venous thrombosis, assessment in, 386
  chronic venous insufficiency and, 388–394
  clinical manifestations of, 384–385
  deep, 384
  etiology of, 384
  management of, 384–386, 385t, 386t
  nursing diagnoses and planning in, 386–387
  nursing interventions in, 387–388, 388d
  pathophysiology of, 384
  prevention of, 682
  pulmonary embolism and, 681
  risk factors for, 384, 384t
  superficial, 385
Venous valves, 328, *328*
Venous vascular disease, in elderly, 397–398
Ventilation, control of, 528
  mechanical. See *Mechanical ventilation.*
  mechanics of, *527,* 527–528
Ventilation/perfusion matching, 528
Ventilation-perfusion mismatch, in pulmonary embolism, 681
Ventilation-perfusion scan, 548
  in pulmonary embolism, 682
Ventilatory failure, 530–531
Ventral spinothalamic tract, 722
Ventricles, 165–167, *166*
Ventricular assist device, 229
Ventricular bigeminy, 248
Ventricular catheter, in intracranial pressure monitoring, 731, *731*
Ventricular conduction, 171
Ventricular couplets, 248
Ventricular diastole, 165, *166,* 171, 191
Ventricular diastolic gallop, 179
Ventricular dilatation, in heart failure, 269–270
Ventricular dysrhythmias, 248–251
  in myocardial infarction, 297
Ventricular fibrillation, *250,* 250–251
  in cardiac arrest, 261

Ventricular hypertrophy, in heart failure, 269
Ventricular shunt, for hydrocephalus, 802–804, *803*
Ventricular tachycardia, 248, *249,* 249–251
  in cardiac arrest, 261
Ventricular trigeminy, 248
Ventricular triplets, 248
Venturi mask, 555t
Venules, 325–328, *327*
Verapamil (Calan), 378t
  for dysrhythmias, 215, 216d
  for heart disease, 213, 215d
  for hypertrophic cardiomyopathy, 306
Verrucae. See *Warts.*
Vertebrae, 713–714, *715.* See also under *Spinal; Spine.*
Vertebral basilar artery, stenosis of, 807t
Vertebral compression fracture, 823, *823, 917*
Vertigo, 1996–1997, 1998–1999, *1999,* 1999t
  diagnosis of, 2001–2002
  in Meniere's disease, 2017–2019
  labyrinthitis and, 2013–2014
Very low-density lipoproteins (VLDL), heart disease and, 186, 209
Vesicants, burns from, 1686t. See also *Chemical burns.*
Vesicle, *1571,* 1572
Vesicouterine fistula, *1821,* 1821–1822
Vesicovaginal fistula, *1821,* 1821–1822
Vesicular breath sounds, 536–537
Vestibular dysfunction, rehabilitation in, 2003
  vertigo and, 1996–1997, 1998–1999, *1999,* 1999t
Vestibular function, assessment of, 2001–2002
Vestibular nerve, 723t
Vestibule, vaginal, 1765–1766, *1766*
  of inner ear, 1996
Vibration sense, 555–556
  assessment of, 748
Video-assisted thoracic surgery, 587–596
Videourodynamic study, 1360t
Villi, intestinal, *955,* 956
Vincent's disease, 1017–1019, 1018t
Vinegar douche, for atrophic vaginitis, 1806
Violence, domestic, 19
Violent deaths, bereavement in, 37–38
Viral encephalitis, 769–770
  nursing process in, 771–773
Viral hepatitis, 1169–1177. See also *Hepatitis, viral.*
Viral infections, of skin, 1603–1607
Viral keratitis, 1965–1967
Viral meningitis, 769
  nursing process in, 771–773
Visceral pain, 965, 965t
Visceral peritoneum, 950
Visceral pleura, 524–525, *525*
Vision, age-related changes in, 60, 766, 1961
  blurred, 1938
  color, 1937
    assessment of, 1943
    in elderly, 1992
  double, 1938
  physiology of, 1938, *1938*
Vision impairment, 742, *742,* 743–744, 1939, 1940t. See also *Eye disorders.*
  age-related, 60
  safety measures for, 71c

Vision impairment *(Continued)*
  gradual, 1939
  in atherosclerosis, 361
  in diabetes, 1252d, 1253
  in glaucoma, 1978, 1979, *1979*
  in hypertension, 375, 376
  in macular degeneration, 1985–1987, *1986*
  in multiple sclerosis, 779, 781
  in retinal detachment, 1982, *1983*
  in sickle-cell anemia, 485, 486
  in stroke, 807t, 808, 813
  nonoptical aids in, 1959, *1959*
  nursing process in, 743–744
  optical aids in, 1958–1959, *1959*, 1960d
  pituitary adenoma and, 1265, *1265*
  resources for, 2044
  sudden, 1939
  supportive treatment in, 1958–1959, *1959*, 1960d
Visiting nurse, 27
Visitors, family vs. nonfamily, 1919d
Visken (pindolol), 377t
Visual accommodation, assessment of, 1942
Visual acuity, assessment of, 1940–1942
Visual cortex, 719, *720*
Visual evoked potentials, 757, 1946
Visual field defects, 742, *742*, 744, 1940t
Visual fields, examination of, 1943
Visual pathways, 1938, *1938*
Vital capacity, 537–538, *538*, 539t
Vitamin(s), dietary sources of, 472d
  hepatic storage of, 1139
  supplemental, for hepatic disease, 1153–1154
Vitamin A, deficiency of, clinical manifestations of, 1077t
  dietary sources of, 472d
Vitamin B complex, dietary sources of, 472d
Vitamin B$_{12}$, deficiency of, clinical manifestations of, 1077t
  in chronic gastritis, 1025, *1025*
  pernicious anemia and, 451, 476–479
  postgastrectomy, 998t
  vegetarian diet and, 478
  parenteral, for pernicious anemia, 478
Vitamin C, dietary sources of, 472d
Vitamin D, calcium and, 1213
  deficiency of, clinical manifestations of, 1077t
  osteomalacia and, 902–904
  dietary sources of, 472d
  renal activation of, 1333
  supplemental, for hypoparathyroidism, 1317, 1318
  for osteoporosis, 905
  toxicity of, 1318
Vitamin K, deficiency of, acquired hypoprothrombinemia and, 517
  clinical manifestations of, 1077t
  for hepatic disorders, 1149
  hepatic storage of, 1139
Vitiligo, in Addison's disease, 1278, *1278*
  PUVA therapy for, 1582, 1584
Vitreous hemorrhage, in diabetes, 1253
Vitreous humor, 1937, *1937*
Vocal cords, *609*
  inflammation of, 608–610
Vocal fremitus, 535
Vocational nurse. See *Practical nurse.*
Voice, loss of, in laryngitis, 608–610

Voice sounds, 537
Voiding, Credé, 1365
  double, 1385
  dysfunctional, 1335–1336
    after hysterectomy, 1795
    after prostatectomy, 1712, 1715t, 1718
    catheterization in. See *Urinary catheterization.*
    cystocele and, 1817
    in benign prostatic hyperplasia, 1752–1753
    in cystitis, 1372, 1373
    in elderly, 1425
    in urethral trauma, 1415
    in urethritis, 1373
    in urinary obstruction, 1377–1378, 1382c
    meatal stenosis and, 1386
    resources for, 2041
    urethral stricture and, 1385
    urethrocele and, 1817
    urinary calculi and, 1377–1378, 1382c
  in elderly, 65–66, 1425
  in spinal cord injury, 823, 825, 826
  in stroke, 813–814
  painful/difficult, 1335
    in cystitis, 1372, 1373
    in urethritis, 1373
  physiology of, 1334–1335
  postoperative, 154–155
  trigger, 1366
  Valsalva, 1365
Voiding cystourethrogram, 1349t
Voiding diary, 1425
Volkmann's canals, 838, *838*
Voltaren (diclofenac), 893d
Voluntary muscle, 840–842. See also *Muscle(s).*
Volvulus, intestinal, 1074, *1074*
Vomiting, 959–961
  brain tumors and, 828
  chemotherapy and, 1529, 1530, 1540t
  complications of, 960
  in acute gastritis, 1024
  in intestinal obstruction, 1074, 1075
  in paralytic ileus, 1076
  in renal colic, 1379, 1381c
  nursing interventions in, 960–961
  pathophysiology of, 959–960
  projectile, 960
  with intermaxillary fixation, 1048
Vomiting center, 960
Vomitus, blood in, 960, 966
  assessment for, 1184d–1186d
    from esophageal varices, 1183, 1184d–1186d
  color of, 960
  contents of, 960
Von Willebrand's disease, *515*, 515–517
  cryoprecipitate for, 456–457
  Factor VIII concentrate for, 456–457
Von Zumbusch's psoriasis, 1616–1619, 1617t
Vulvar cancer, 1825–1830
  in elderly, 1838
  in situ, 1825–1826
  invasive, 1826–1830
Vulvar self-examination, 1779d
Vulvectomy, 1786t
  partial, 1826
  radical, 1826–1830
  skinning, 1826
  total, 1826
Vulvitis, 1803–1804, 1805d

Vulvovaginal hygiene, patient teaching for, 1805d, 1807d
Vulvovaginal warts, 1063–1065, 1064t6, *1926*, 1926–1928
Vulvovaginitis. See *Vaginitis.*

W

Walkers, 880, *880*
Walking, after stroke, 809, 812
  assistive devices for, 878–881, *880*
  intermittent claudication and, 332, 333–334
  postoperative, in hysterectomy, 1799
  with casts, 858
Walsh technique, for prostatectomy, 1758
Warfarin (Coumadin), 385t
  acquired hypoprothrombinemia and, 517
  after cardiac valvular surgery, 316
  for stroke, 807
  for venous thrombosis, 682
  therapeutic monitoring for, 208–209
Warm antibodies, in autoimmune hemolytic anemia, 1496
Warts, 1603–1605, *1604*, 1604t
  anogenital, 1603–1605, *1604*, 1604t, *1926*, 1926–1928
  common, 1603–1605, *1604*, 1604t
  filiform, 1603–1605, *1604*, 1604t
  flat, 1603–1605, *1604*, 1604t
  plantar, 1603–1605, *1604*, 1604t
Wasp stings, 1621–1622, 1622d
Water. See also under *Fluid.*
  body, 75–76, *76*
  topical application of, for skin disorders, 1582–1583
Water deprivation test, for diabetes insipidus, 1275
Water intoxication, 82–84, *83*, 83t
  in elderly, 112–113
Weak pulse, 178, *179*
Weakness, hyperkalemia and, 89, 90
  hypokalemia and, 86, 87–88
  hyponatremia and, 91, 92, 93
  in amyotrophic lateral sclerosis, 775–776, 777
  in hematologic disorders, 434, 436
  in limb-girdle dystrophy, 785–786
  in myasthenia gravis, 782, 785
Weaning, ventilator, 571–574
Weber's test, 2001
Wedge resection, 580t
Weight, age-related changes in, 51
  fluid component of, *76*
Weight loss, fluid loss and, 78
  in burns, 1679
  in chronic pancreatitis, 1122–1123
  in Crohn's disease, 1067
  in diabetes, 1228, 1229, 1232d
  in fluid volume deficit, 77
  in pancreatic cancer, 1127
Wellness, strategies for, 14t, 14–15
Wellness nursing diagnosis, 8
Wenckebach block, 251–252, *252*
Wernicke's aphasia, 738–739, 814
Wernicke's area, 719, *738*
Wertheim's operation, 1786t
Wet dressings, 1583
Wheal, *1571*, 1572
Wheelchair patients, pressure ulcer prevention for, 1630
Wheezes, 537
  in asthma, 660
Whiplash, 823

Whipple's procedure, *1127*, 1127–1131
  complications of, 1128
  patient preparation for, 1128
  postoperative care in, 1129–1131
  postoperative course in, 1128
  preoperative care in, 1128–1129
Whispered pectoriloquy, 537
White blood cell(s), 429, *429, 430*
  disorders of, 491–513
  polymorphonuclear, 1432, *1432*
  types of, *1432*, 1432–1433, 1433t
White blood cell count, 442–444, 443t
  differential, 443t, 444, 445t
    normal values for, 1532t
  normal values for, 1532t
  shift to the left in, 1372
White matter, 712
Winter itch, 1608t
Wires, in internal fixation, 865–867
  Kirschner, 860
Withdrawal, in alcoholism, in surgery, 122–123
Wolff's law, 840
Work. See also under *Occupational.*
Work of breathing, 528
Work preoccupation, 32
Wound, closure of, 1586–1587
Wound care, for pressure ulcers, 1630–1631
  in abdominal perineal resection, 1104–1105
  in amputation, 875d–876d, 877, 878d, *879*
  in burns, 1671–1678, 1685d. See also under *Burns.*
  in cardiac valvular surgery, 315
  in chemical burns, 1687
  in electrical injury, 1689, 1690
  in pancreatic fistula, 1125, 1126
  in tracheostomy, 567
  patient teaching for, 155, 156d
  postoperative, in oral cancer, 1052d

Wound contractures, in burns, 1682–1684, 1684t
Wound dehiscence/evisceration, abdominal, 996
  postoperative, 147t, 153
  in hysterectomy, 1788d–1789d, 1797
Wound healing, 153, *154*
  by granulation, 1587
  delayed, postoperative, 147t
  in burns, 1675–1676, *1677*
  in graft donor sites, 1678
Wound infection, postoperative, 147t
  in gastrointestinal surgery, 996
  prevention of, 153
Wrist, disorders of, 909–910
  fractures of, 927–930
Wytensin (guanabenz), 378t

X

Xanthelasma, 1961
Xanthoma, 1632t
Xenograft, cardiac valve, 313, *313*
  skin, 1588–1590
Xeromammography, 1849
Xerophthalmia, ectropion and, 1974
Xerosis, in elderly, 1630
Xerostomia, chemotherapy and, 1530, 1541t
  in radiation therapy, 1520
Xerotic eczema, 1608t
X-ray studies, chest, for lung cancer, 1514
  in cardiac assessment, 192–193
  in emphysema, 671
  in respiratory disorders, *547*, 547–548
  in tuberculosis, 652
  portable, 193
  preoperative, 126t
  in cancer diagnosis, 1514
  in musculoskeletal disorders, 850t

X-ray studies *(Continued)*
  preoperative, 125t–126t
  skull, 748
    in fractures, 818
  spinal, 748–749
  upper gastrointestinal, *970*, 970–971
Xylocaine (lidocaine). See *Lidocaine (Xylocaine).*

Y

Yeast infections, cutaneous, 1601–1603, *1602*
  vaginal, 1804–1806, 1805t, 1884t, 1884–1885
Yellow jacket stings, 1621–1622, 1622d
Yuppie flu, 1496–1497

Z

Zafirlukast, for asthma, 661, 662t
Zantac (ranitidine), for peptic ulcers, 1024, 1028
Zarontin (ethosuximide), for seizures, 796, 797d–798d
Zaroxolyn (metolazone), 377t
Zileuton, for asthma, 661, 662t
Zinc deficiency, clinical manifestations of, 1077t
Zocor (simvastatin), 216–217, 218d
Zoladex (goserelin acetate), for prostate cancer, 1759
Zona fasciculata, 1214, *1214*
Zona glomerulosa, 1213–1214, *1214*
  adenoma of, primary aldosteronism and, 1289–1292
Zona reticularis, 1214, *1214*
Zovirax (acyclovir), for genital herpes, 1903, 1904t
  for herpes simplex virus infection, 1581
Zyloprim (allopurinol), for gout, 900, 900d